# 三十年撷英

## 分子生药学发展

主审 · 黄璐琦

主编 · 袁媛 郑汉

上海科学技术出版社

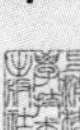

**图书在版编目（CIP）数据**

分子生药学发展三十年撷英 / 袁媛，郑汉主编.
上海 ： 上海科学技术出版社，2025. 8. -- ISBN 978-7
-5478-7280-2

Ⅰ. R93-53

中国国家版本馆CIP数据核字第2025SL3736号

**分子生药学发展三十年撷英**

主 审 黄璐琦
主 编 袁 媛 郑 汉

上海世纪出版(集团)有限公司
上 海 科 学 技 术 出 版 社 出版、发行
(上海市闵行区号景路159弄A座9F-10F)
邮政编码 201101 www.sstp.cn
上海颛辉印刷厂有限公司 印刷
开本 889×1194 1/16 印张 79.5
字数：3000千字
2025年8月第1版 2025年8月第1次印刷
ISBN 978-7-5478-7280-2/R·3328
定价：598.00元

# 内容提要

1995年，黄璐琦在《中国中药杂志》上发表《展望分子生物技术在生药学中的应用》一文，首次提出了“分子生药学”(Molecular Pharmacognosy)的概念。分子生药学至今已有近三十年的发展历程，这一学科的理论和技术已经成为解决中药领域中一些关键问题的重要工具，并逐渐成为中医药行业的热点。

本书选取三十年间分子生药学领域极具代表性的文章150篇，按主题分为学科发展、生药分子鉴定、道地药材遗传成因及中药活性成分合成生物学四个部分，以集中呈现分子生药学诞生三十年间的发展脉络、理论及技术创新、实际应用等方面内容，这些内容对相关科研及生产等领域的发展具有重要的指导价值。

本书可供中药学、药学、生物学相关专业技术人员参考阅读。

# 编　委　会

## 主　审

黄璐琦　中国中医科学院

## 主　编

袁　媛　中国中医科学院

郑　汉　中国中医科学院

## 编　委

（按姓名汉语拼音排序）

晁　志　南方医科大学

陈　同　中国中医科学院

陈瑞兵　海军军医大学

陈万生　上海中医药大学

陈晓亚　中国科学院植物生理研究所

陈宇航　成都医学院

程琪庆　湖北科技学院

崔光红　中国中医科学院

付　饶　四川大学

付雪晴　上海交通大学

高　杰　首都医科大学

高　伟　首都医科大学

高文远　天津大学

郭　娟　中国中医科学院

郭兰萍　中国中医科学院

胡添源　杭州师范大学

胡雅婷　首都医科大学

胡志敏　海军军医大学

华中一　中国中医科学院

黄　伟　湖北中医药大学

蒋　超　中国中医科学院

蒋周倩　首都医科大学

焦红红　陕西中医药大学

金效华　中国中医科学院

靳保龙　中国中医科学院

开国银　浙江中医药大学

黎　凌　上海交通大学

李旻辉　内蒙古科技大学包头医学院

梁宗锁　浙江理工大学

廖志华　西南大学

刘　娟　中国中医科学院

刘潺潺　南京中医药大学

刘春生　北京中医药大学
刘大会　湖北中医药大学
陆　续　中国药科大学
骆云峰　首都医科大学
麻鹏达　西北农林科技大学
马　莹　中国中医科学院
马春霞　山东省分析测试中心
马小军　中国医学科学院
毛柳英　北京中医药大学
彭丽华　浙江大学
申　业　中国中医科学院
沈思雨　首都医科大学
苏　平　中国中医科学院
唐克轩　崖州湾国家实验室
田晓轩　天津中医药大学
童宇茹　首都医科大学
屠李婵　浙大城市学院
王　健　中国中医科学院
王　娟　天津大学
王　升　中国中医科学院
王瑞杉　中国中医科学院
王学勇　北京中医药大学
王雅南　中国中医科学院
王真慧　吉林农业大学
王正鹏　中国中医科学院
吴啟南　南京中医药大学
肖　莹　上海中医药大学
薛哲勇　东北林业大学
杨　蕾　上海辰山植物园
杨东风　浙江理工大学
杨生超　云南农业大学
尹小建　中国科学院东北地理与农业生态研究所
虞慕瑶　北京中医药大学
袁　媛　中国中医科学院
张　磊　海军军医大学
张　阳　四川大学
张芳源　西南大学
张广辉　云南农业大学
张顺仓　扬州大学
张亚中　安徽省食品药品检验研究院
张逸风　首都医科大学
张重义　福建农林大学
赵瑜君　中国中医科学院
赵玉成　中国药科大学
郑　汉　中国中医科学院
周家伟　首都医科大学
周雍进　中国科学院大连化学物理研究所

# 序　言

分子生药学是在分子水平上研究生药的鉴定、质量形成、资源保护与生产的一门学科。其以生药分子鉴定为基础，以道地药材遗传成因研究为特色，以中药活性成分合成生物学生产为前沿，充分运用现代科技手段和前沿科技成果，立足于解决中药在生产、研究及应用方面的一系列问题。自 1995 年《中国中药杂志》刊登《展望分子生物技术在生药学中的应用》一文，首次提出了“分子生药学”（Molecular Pharmacognosy）概念，到 2000 年第一部《分子生药学》专著出版，学科成型，至今已经走过了三十个年头，分子生药学学科建设已取得了长足的发展。2006 年出版的《分子生药学(第二版)》，获得中华中医药学会著作一等奖；2015 年出版的《分子生药学(第三版)》，获第四届中国出版政府奖。2012 年由斯普林格(Springer)出版社出版了 *Molecular Pharmacognosy*，该书为第一本分子生药学外文专著，为学科发展提供了一个国际开放的交流平台。2020 年由斯普林格出版社出版了 *Molecular Pharmacognosy*（*Second Edition*）。

分子生药学作为一门交叉学科，已走过萌芽期、形成期、快速发展期，正逐渐步入成熟期，已形成了覆盖全国的分子生药学科研机构和学术队伍，建成了由全国重点实验室、重点学科、国家标准、学术期刊、国家奖项支撑的多元化学科平台，建立了面向本科生、硕士、博士研究生以及在职人员的多层次教学体系。2003 年，国家中医药管理局“生药分子鉴定”三级实验室建立。2008 年适合高等院校本科生使用的《分子生药学》教材首次出版，至今已有 5 版“十三五”“十四五”相关规划教材，在 40 余所高等院校开设了相关的本科生和研究生课程。2009 年，国家中医药管理局“道地药材生态遗传重点研究室”认定。2010 年，蕲蛇、乌梢蛇聚合酶链式反应法被《中华人民共和国药典》(2010 年版)收载，成为首个被《中华人民共和国药典》收载的中药分子鉴定方法，并获得当年中国专利优秀奖。2017 年，《中国中药杂志》设置分子生药学专栏；中国中西医结合学会分子生药学专业委员会成立。2018 年，中药领域首个国家自然科学基金重大项目“中药道地性研究”获得资助。2020 年，聚合酶链式反应法首次作为通用技术方法被《中华人民共和国药典》(2020 年版)收载，成为被《中华人民共和国药典》收载的首个分子生物学检查方法。2023 年，分子生药学被国务院学位委员会第八届中药学学科评议组列为中药学的二级学科，并入选国家中医药管理局高水平中医药重点学科；道地药材品质保障与资源持续利用全国重点实验获批成立，标志着分子生药学研究平台已达到国内领先水平。截至 2024 年，相关研究已获国家科技进步奖二等奖 6 项。此外，于 2012 年始，由中国中医科学院主办、各兄弟院校承办的分子生药学暑期班，已顺利举办 12 届，线下参会人员已累计 3 500 余人次，为广大从事分子生药学科研和教学工作的同仁提供了一个交流和学习的平台。

到目前为止，已有千余篇分子生药学相关的中英文论文先后发表在 *Nature Chemistry*、*Nature Communications*、*Molecular Plant*、*PNAS*、*Angewandte Chemie*、*Journal of the American Chemical Society*、*Trends in Plant Science*、*Science Bulletin*、*Plant Biotechnology Journal* 以及 *New Phytologist* 等国内外知名学术期刊上。本书精选了其中一部分具有代表性的论文及其他相关文献，意在回溯分子生药学三十载的发展历程，特别聚焦于中药分子鉴定、道地药材遗传成因、中药活性成分合成生物学生产这三大核心研究领域。本书编纂出版是分子生药学研究成果的一次系统总结，是一项重要的文献研究成果。

在学科不断深化与拓展的征途上，我深感荣幸，能与致力于分子生药学发展的同仁一道，共同为这一学科的发展贡献绵薄之力。

黄璐琦

2025 年 1 月

# 前　言

“分子生药学”(Molecular Pharmacognosy)是在分子水平上研究生药的鉴定、质量形成、资源保护及生产的一门学科。其以生药分子鉴定为基础，道地药材遗传成因研究为特色，中药活性成分合成生物学生产为前沿，充分运用现代科技手段和前沿科技成果，立足解决中药在生产、科研及应用方面的一系列问题。

分子生药学由黄璐琦院士 1995 年首次提出并得到快速发展，2000 年、2006 年及 2015 年分别出版《分子生药学》第一版、第二版及第三版，2008 年适合高等院校本科生使用的《分子生药学》教材出版，至今已有 5 版“十三五”“十四五”规划教材陆续出版，40 余所高等院校开设本科生和研究生课程。*Molecular Pharmacognosy* 分别于 2012 年与 2020 年由斯普林格(Springer)出版社相继出版两版。这些专著、教材的出版，向国内外同行介绍了分子生药学的新视角和新见解，讨论了分子生药学领域的热点和重点，并展望了新的研究方向。

历经三十年的建设和发展，分子生药学已走过萌芽期、形成期、快速发展期，逐渐步入成熟期，已被国务院学位委员会第八届学科评议组列为中药学二级学科。学科已形成了覆盖全国的科研学术队伍，建成由全国重点实验室、重点学科、国家标准、学术期刊、国家奖项支撑的多元化学科平台，建立面向本科、硕士、博士研究生以及在职人员的纵向多层次教学体系。在领域内专家、学者的共同努力下，分子生药学研究已达到全国领先水平。

本书按照时间顺序精选了 1995 年至 2024 年分子生药学发展三十年来具有代表性的中、英文论述及实验研究类文章 150 篇，涉及 36 家高校及科研院所，汇集院士、国家杰出青年基金项目获得者、教育部长江学者、中组部“万人计划领军人才”、中科院“百人计划”、国家优秀青年基金项目获得者、海外高层次人才引进计划、科协青年人才托举计划等高层次人才研究成果，聚焦生药分子鉴定、道地药材遗传成因、中药活性成分合成生物学三大核心研究领域。其中，属于科技部重点研发计划资助论文 68 篇，占比 45.3%；国家自然科学基金重大项目资助 20 篇，占比 13.3%；其他国家自然科学基金项目资助 101 篇，占比 67.3%。本书是分子生药学发展三十年成果的集中体现，也是本领域同仁共同努力的精彩见证。

分子生药学的研究内容极其丰富，涉及的研究机构、研究人员也非常广泛，本书所选文章仅是其中的一部分代表，可能难以十分完整、准确地反映分子生药学三十年发展的历程和成就。因此，对于未被本书收录的文章，其对分子生药学学科的发展贡献毋庸置疑，在此，对这些文章的作者也表示我们深深的敬意。

在编撰过程中，由于收录文章形式多样，内容各异，我们在整理过程中对文章做了适当的精简和整理工作，如读者在使用过程中需要更进一步了解相关文章内容，可检索原文阅读参考。由于本书篇幅较大，同时也限于我们的水平和编撰时间，书中可能存在一些不足之处，敬请广大读者在使用中给予批评指正。

编著者

2025 年 1 月

# 目　　录

## 第一篇　学科发展

001



## 第二篇　生药分子鉴定

025

## 第三篇 道地药材遗传成因

## 第四篇 中药活性成分合成生物学

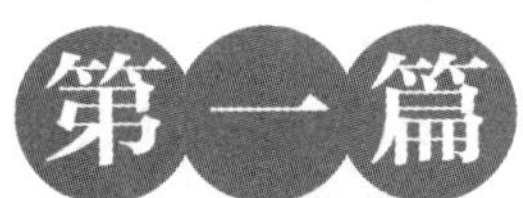

# 第一篇 学科发展

# 展望分子生物技术在生药学中的应用

生药学是研究生药(药材)的一门科学,是研究生药的名称、来源、形态、性状、组织、成分、效用及生产、采制、贮藏等的学科;是一门边缘学科,也是一门应用性学科,它是随着其他学科的发展而发展的。当今,分子生物技术是生命学科中最重要也是最先进的技术,且已广泛地运用于生命学科的各个领域,那么它是否也能在生药学科中得到应用呢?回答是肯定的。生药学的研究对象生药,一般认为是得自生物的药材,兼有生货原药之意,也就是说是由遗传物质DNA编码形成的生物,因此它与分子生物学有着结合的物质基础,这种物质基础为分子生物技术在生药学中的运用提供了理论上的依据。本文对分子生物技术在生药学中的应用进行了展望。

## 1 在鉴定方面的应用

我国药材种类繁多,资源丰富,然而来源复杂,品种混淆厉害。目前一直运用经典形态分类来研究药材来源,即鉴定生物物种。这种用形态分类学来划分物种是建立在个体性状描述和宏观观测水平上,得到的结论往往不完善,易引起争论,这就使生药的正本清源产生了困难。随着分子生物学和分子克隆技术的发展,现在可以根据遗传物质DNA在不同生物个体的差异来鉴别生物物种。如可利用限制性内切酶酶切片段长度多态性(RFLP)来研究品种间、属间的DNA的变异情况,从而揭示不同品种间的亲缘关系,为鉴别药材品种提供依据。同时这种方法也能为寻找新的药用资源提供线索。如天花粉蛋白是从栝楼 *Trichosanthes kirilowii* Maxim.根中提取,因其具有抗癌、中期引产和抑制艾滋病病毒等作用而引起世人的关注,很多学者正在寻找新的具有天花粉蛋白活性的蛋白。如香港中文大学的杨显荣等对葫芦科植物王瓜、木鳖、苦瓜等做了许多研究,发现有类似天花粉蛋白的引产活性,而木鳖、苦瓜等都不是栝楼属植物。根据亲缘关系相近的植物类群有相似的化学成分的理论,我们认为应该在同属植物中寻找,并且在国内的调查中发现作为天花粉入药的栝楼属植物有19种之多。因此,为寻找新的活性蛋白,首先就要搞清这19种植物间的亲缘关系,只有这样才能做到有的放矢,减少盲目性。以上是在鉴定药材来源方面的运用。

在药材鉴定上,虽然药材(不含矿物药)多不是新鲜的,DNA会有很大的降解,这似乎给DNA的分析带来了困难,但Mullis等人在1985年和1987年发展了1种聚合酶链式反应(PCR),能将原来痕迹量的DNA扩增到足以供实验人员方便进行检测与分析的数量,而且产物专一性强,不需进行特殊纯化,这种高速、高效、优质和全部自动化的优点使得PCR技术在短短几年中在分子生物学各个领域得到广泛应用。如20世纪90年代在PCR技术基础上发展起来的随机扩增的DNA多态性分析(RAPD),就可用于药材的鉴定,特别是贵重药材的鉴定。通过RAPD技术分析真伪药材的DNA多态性,找出真品特定的DNA片段,对此进行测序,进而制备DNA探针,来检测相应的药材,为生药学提供一个新的、便捷、准确的鉴定方法,相信这种方法尤其能运用于动物药的鉴定。

这种分子生物技术来鉴别药材,可称为"分子标记鉴别"。

## 2 在生产方面的应用

生药中绝大部分是植物药。为了扩大药源,保障质量,生产出更多更好的药材,药用植物中很大一部分都已引种栽培。如何有效地防治病虫害是栽培过程中所遇到的难题,目前防治病虫害的主要措施是施撒农药,这种方法不但危害人畜,而且污染环境。现在通过分子生物技术能使植物自身获得抗病虫害的能力,从而避免了上述问题。

在抗病毒方面,主要运用向植物转移病毒的外壳蛋白基因、利用植物病毒的卫星DNA基因及利用反义RNA等3种方法。如向植物转移病毒的外壳蛋白基因防治病毒工作做得最多的是对烟草花叶病毒(TMV)的防治:把烟草花叶病毒$U_1$株系的RNA中编码外壳蛋白(CP)的部分反转录成cDNA,把cDNA插入到带CaMV35S启动子的中间载体中,然后把这一中间载体引入根癌农杆菌,再把这种根癌农杆菌采用叶圆盘法转化烟草;再生的烟草(转基因烟草)高水平地表达了TMV的CP基因,对TMV表现出明显的抗性。这种转基因烟草已用于大田栽培。在继烟草花叶病毒外壳蛋白基因工程成功之后,现已有黄瓜花叶病毒(CMV)、马铃薯X病毒(PVX)的外壳蛋白基因分别在烟草、番茄和马铃薯中表达。在药用植物方面还未见报道。然而上述这些病毒对药用植物亦造成危害,据不完全统计,感染烟草花叶病毒的有白花曼陀罗、黄花败酱、八角莲;感染黄瓜花叶病毒的有太子参、丝瓜、白术、桔梗、毛当归、百合、车前草、牛蒡、蒲公英、青葙、马齿苋、虎杖等。因此,用分子生物技术使药用植物获得抗病毒能力,将有很大的市场,能产生很高的经济效益。

在抗虫害方面,1987年比利时学者把金云杆菌的δ毒素基因通过根癌农杆菌的Ti质粒转移到烟草中并得到表达。这种δ内毒素能杀死鳞翅目害虫,如烟草角虫在这种烟草上1天即停食,3天内死亡,并且δ内毒素基因在转基因烟草中能稳定表达和遗传。用这种方法已获得了抗虫的番茄和马铃薯等。而药用植物花果所受虫害主要来源于鳞翅目害虫,如豆荚螟危害白扁豆、黄芪等豆科植物;梨小食心虫危害木瓜、贴梗海棠等;棉铃虫危害白扁豆、穿心莲、丹参、牛蒡、颠茄等;白术术籽虫危害白术等。因此,这种方法的运用对保护以花果入药的药用植物有着重要意义。

另外,在抗虫等方面,英国曾把豇豆编码胰蛋酶抑制基因引入烟草。烟草具备制造胰蛋白酶抑制剂的能力,在昆虫吃了转化烟草后,虫体消化道内的胰蛋白酶活性得到抑制,蛋白在消化道内不能降解,害虫因得不到必需的营养而死去。这种方法可以防治各种害虫对植物的侵害。

总之,目前用分子生物学技术使植物自身获得抗病虫害的能力，主要应用在农作物上，把其运用到药用植物上，相信也能取得同样可喜的成果。

另外在药材生产上，自古就存在着药材道地性问题。如何看待这个问题？笔者认为药材的道地性是由同一种植物不同居群之间的差异形成的，其物质基础是化学成分或含量的不同，然而化学成分可能是由遗传因子产生的，也可能是地理-生态因子形成的。如水菖蒲 *Acorus calamus* L.根茎含油量和油中成分与染色体数有关，二倍体者芳香油中无β-细辛醚，三倍体者含20%～30%β-细辛醚，四倍体中β-细辛醚比三倍体高2倍，说明根茎含油量是由遗传因子控制的。又如生长在东北三省和苏、鄂的一叶楸含有左旋一叶楸碱，生长在北京近郊县的则多为右旋一叶楸碱，而一叶楸碱的旋光性和植物形态没有必然联系，其旋光性的差异可能是由于地理-生态因子的关系形成的。因此，通过分子生物技术如RFLP、RAPD比较不同居群之间在遗传物质DNA上的变化，可为揭示道地药材的“地道”之本质提供线索，并为药材的培育选种产生指导作用。

## 3 在获取有效成分方面应用

生药学的一个重大任务就是生药有效成分的提取和测定，对某一药材经过一系列繁琐而艰辛的分离提取及测定后得知其所含的有效成分，然而有效成分往往是微量的，如长春花碱、美登木碱等。如何获得更多有效成分一直是生药学的一个研究目标。20世纪80年代以来，分子生物技术的发展，为这一研究提供了新的方法，如转基因器官培养技术和反义技术等。转基因器官培养技术现主要是毛状根的培养，就是用发根农杆菌 *Agrobacterium rhizogenes* 转化植物，产生生长迅速、生产效能高而稳定的毛状根培养物，从而产生有效的次生物质。因为发根农杆菌含有Ri质粒，在感染植物细胞过程中可通过Vir区(致病区)片段的作用，将质粒上的T-DNA整合到植物细胞的DNA中，T-DNA在被感染的植物细胞中表达的表现型是从被感染的部位长出毛状根，将毛状根分离作为培养系统就能产生与自然根一样甚至更多的次生物质。如绞股蓝是1种含有80多种皂苷、具有人参样生理活性的药用植物，费厚满等为开发利用绞股蓝皂苷，用发根农杆菌的 $R_{1600}$ 菌株感染绞股蓝叶外植体，使外植株切口处出现毛状根，毛状根经Southern分析后，证明确已转化，在无激素的MS培养基中悬浮培养20天，致使毛状根中总皂苷含量约为自然根的2倍，并且在悬浮培养过程中，培养物向培养基中分出一定量的皂苷。这种方法已经在很多药用植物中得到运用。如在赛莨菪毛状根中分别得到了0.1%的东莨菪碱和0.3%的莨菪碱，含量均高于野生植株；在甘草毛状根培养物中检测到高于正常培养物含量的黄酮类化合物等；另外在颠茄和紫草等也得到运用。

反义技术是根据碱基互补原理，用反义DNA或RNA片段导入植物细胞，控制某一代谢途径上的关键酶活性，使之受到抑制或增强，而使活性成分含量提高。如木质素和黄酮类化合物都是苯内氨酸代谢产物。用反义技术调节亚麻属植物 *Linum flavum* L.毛状根中肉桂醇脱氢酶活性，抑制木质素的合成，使主要抗癌活性成分5-甲基鬼臼素含量提高。

总之，分子生物技术在生药学中的运用，在分子水平上研究生药的鉴定、生产和成分等，正如其在其他生命学科中运用一样，将使生药等的发展进入到一个崭新的发展阶段，并由此产生一门新的学科——分子生药学(Molecular Pharmcognosy)。

[黄璐琦.中国中药杂志，1995，20(11)：643-646.]

# 《分子生药学》评介

由黄璐琦博士任主编，多位博士、硕士参与编写的《分子生药学》由北京医科大学出版社于2000年6月正式出版。这是我国生药学界的一件大事。因为生药学这个学科的建立已经有近200年的历史，其间虽然也在不断地发展，然而对生药材鉴定技术而言，最初只是药材性状鉴别，也就是说对药材的外部形态特征、色泽、断面、质地、气味等进行药材真伪鉴别；其后则逐步发展为药材内部的细胞组织形态特征为依据，进行光学显微鉴别。随着科学的进步，观察超微结构的扫描电镜也在生药材鉴别当中应用了，其间还在真伪鉴别和质量研究中将理化方法引入，特别是以成分分析为依据，将各种光谱分析法应用得淋漓尽致，使生药学发展到一个新的高峰。黄璐琦同志于1995年还在攻读博士研究生阶段，就瞄上分子生药学这个尖端技术，因而潜心研究，很快发表了《展望分子生物技术在生药学中的应用》一文，并首次提出“分子生药学(Molecular Pharmacognosy)”这一概念。此文的发表引起了生药学界的强烈共鸣，一些志同道合者纷纷以各种方式提出自己的看法、商榷，鼓励其作进一步的探讨，使之更加系统化。正是这种共鸣和激励，经过数年的勤奋钻研，这部具有开拓性质的《分子生药学》终于正式出版了。它使原有的生药学跨入了一个新的时代，即分子生物学时代，从而也使生药学发展出一个新的分支学科“分子生药学”。我衷心祝贺这个新的分支学科的诞生和建立。使我特别高兴的是我干了几十年的中药鉴定科研工作，感到十分困惑的是环境因素常常给药材鉴定带来诸多干扰，尤其对药材近缘品种难以确定，而分子生药学技术是建立在遗传基因型基础之上的技术，它不受环境因素对药材原植物的一切影响，也不受检品性状(原药材、饮片或粉末)的影响，因而对药材近缘品种的检测有其独特的优越性。但是分子生物学在某些技术方面，也不是说就是十全十美的了。例如稳定性与重现性都还不够理想。DNA序列分析虽然好，既稳定又准确，用于种下一级分类亲缘关系研究最适宜，又能反映物种进化的历程，但仪器设备价格昂贵，一时较难普及等等。总之，《分子生药学》的出版，是新思想、新方法、新技术在中药和生药领域里的扩大应用，使我国生药学上了一个新台阶，这不仅能解决中药真伪鉴别上的一些难题，而且还可应用于药用植物分类学特别是近缘品种的认定、道地药材的品质评价、出土中药标本的鉴定以及对中药高产、优质、多抗性品种的培育、濒危紧缺中药资源的保护和持续利用等。这确实是一部好书，一部将分子生物学与中药研究相结合的好书。当今处于中药现代化之时，就是要把基因研究、转基因技术、克隆技术、RAPD方法以及利用基因芯片等技术鉴定药材品种等加以发展，应用于中医药这个在我国自然科学领域最有优势、最有特色的学科里，是最富生命力和广阔应用前景的。所以有人说“中药现代化就是将传统中医药的优势和特色与现代科学技术相结合，把中药推向国际”。我想“分子生药学”就是一个很好的例证。正是由于这部书作为第一次正式出版，其意义十分重大，且涉及分子生药学这个分支学科创立的大问题，因而它将作为我国药学特别是生药学发展史上的一件重大创举而载入我国药学史册。这里必需要说明的是分子生药学和传统生药学、现代生药学的关系问题，我认为它们永远是一种互补关系，而不是什么替代关系，因为它们使用的手段有所不同，解决的关键问题和取得的效果也不尽相同。在今后，要解决生药领域里的复杂疑难问题，看来是缺一不可，把这些手段统统加在一起联用或从中选择几种手段配合使用，才是更全面和更有效的办法。

该书为16开本，分3篇11章，约62万字。第一篇为概论，主要介绍分子生药学科产生的背景、理论基础和研究内容以及分子生药学与相关学科的关系等。第二篇为分子生药学研究方法及其基本技术，这是本书的核心内容，包括植物DNA和RNA方法与技术、分子杂交、遗传转化技术以及与分子生药学相关的因特网应用等。第三篇主要谈分子生药学的研究领域，如药用植物的分子系统学研究，药用植物种质资源的分子生物学研究，生药鉴定的分子标记研究，药用植物有效成分基因调控研究，药用植物转基因器官和细胞培养生产天然活性化合物等。书后有附录“名词解释”是对涉及分子生药学的一些名词如基因、标记基因、基因库、基因型、扩增、毛细管PCR、同工酶等70条左右有关专业名词作了恰当的解释，这对学习和从事分子生药学的人员来说更是给予了很大的方便。

当然《分子生药学》也还有不够尽善尽美之处，希望今后不断在理论上提高，在实践中总结补充而再版，使分子生药学这个新生事物更加成熟与完善。

该书可作为生药学研究生的专用教材和药科大学中医药大学本科生的生药学补充教材或选修教材，以及一般药学、中药学、生物学和农学等有关学科的研究参考用书。

［谢宗万.中国中药杂志，2001，26(3)：216.］

# Pharmacognosy in the 21st century

## 1 INTRODUCTION

The term pharmacognosy was first used between 1 811 and 1 815, and originally referred to “materia medica”, the knowledge of drug materials or pharmacology. It is derived from two Greek words, *pharmakon* (a drug) and *gignosko* (to acquire knowledge). Later on, pharmacognosy became restricted to that branch of pharmacy investigating “medicinal substances from the plant, animal and mineral kingdoms in their natural, crude, or unprepared state, or in the form of such primary derivatives as oils, waxes, gums, and resins”. Although this latter definition may have been appropriate for the descriptive and microscopical applications of pharmacognosy which were developed from the 19th century until the middle of the 20th century, it became necessary for the subject to be redefined as it subsequently broadened in scope to deal with the chemical components of crude drugs. For example, pharmacognosy was stated to be “an applied science that deals with the biologic, biochemical, and economic features of natural drugs and their constituents”. In a further attempt to update the scope of this field in a manner consistent with scientific activities ongoing at the beginning of the 21st century, pharmacognosy has recently been defined as “a molecular science that explores naturally occurring structure-activity relationships with a drug potential”.

The transition of pharmacognosy from a descriptive botanical discipline to one having more of a chemical focus was spearheaded in the US in the 1960s and 1970s by Arthur E. Schwarting, while he was at the University of Connecticut. Other early pharmacognosist pioneers of this trend in the US have included Egil Ramstad of Purdue University, Varro E. (Tip) Tyler of the University of Washington and Purdue University, Jack L. Beal of Ohio State University, and Norman R. Farnsworth of the University of Pittsburgh and the University of Illinois at Chicago, to name but a few. Some of the early pharmacognosists in the UK with a chemical focus in their work were James W. Fairbairn and Edward J. Shellard, both of the University of London, and Francis Fish, of the University of Strathclyde. There have been a great many other distinguished chemically-oriented pharmacognosists who have made equivalent scientific contributions in the last 40 or 50 years to those mentioned above, particularly in continental Europe and East Asia. Prominent among this illustrious group are René R. Paris of the University of Paris V in France, Egon Stahl, from the University of Saarbrücken in Germany, Ludwig Hörhammer and his successor, Hildebert Wagner, of the University of Munich, Otto Sticher of the Swiss Federal Institute of Technology, Zurich, Switzerland, and Japanese academics such as Shoji Shibata, of the University of Tokyo, and Tsunematsu Takemoto, of Tohoku University and later Tokushima Bunri University. All of those mentioned above, some of whom are still active in the field, built up academic groups that provided training to many younger pharmacognosists and natural product scientists. Examples of the work of some of these younger colleagues are included in the References of this review. Without the impetus such distinguished scientists provided, pharmacognosy as a discipline and speciality branch of academic pharmacy would not be anywhere near so well developed as it is at the onset of this new millennium.

Today, at the beginning of the 21st century, pharmacognosy teaching and research is pursued enthusiastically by its disciples in academic departments of pharmacy all over the world. Although the name pharmacognosy may be substituted in certain countries by terms such as phytochemistry or pharmaceutical biology, the areas of research embraced by natural products may include aspects of analytical chemistry, bioactive compound discovery, bioassay method development, biocatalysis, biosynthesis, biotechnology, cell biology, chemotaxonomy, clinical studies, cultivation of medicinal plants, ethnobotany, genetics, marine chemistry, microbial biotransformation, molecular biology, organic synthesis, pharmacology, phytochemistry, phytotherapy, the standardization of traditional medicines, taxonomy, tissue culture, and zoo-pharmacognosy (the study of self-medication of medicinal plants by primates and other animals). As elaborated on in an earlier review, research in pharmacognosy and natural products has undergone a great renewal of interest in recent years. Several specialist peer-reviewed international scientific journals on various aspects of pharmacognosy and natural products research have their main editorial offices in departments of pharmacy or pharmacognosy or else are edited by a trained pharmacognosist, including *Biochemical Systematics & Ecology*, the *Journal of Ethnopharmacology*, the *Journal of Natural Products* (formerly *Lloydia*), *Natural Medicines* (formerly *Shoyakugaku Zasshi*), *Pharmaceutical Biology* (formerly the *International Journal of Pharmacognosy*), *Phytomedicine*, *Phytotherapy Research*, *Planta Medica* (the *Journal of Medicinal Plant Research*), and the book series *The Alkaloids: Chemistry and Biology* (Academic Press, San Diego). Mention should also be made of a second extensive book series, *Medicinal and Aromatic Plants: Industrial Profiles* (Harwood Academic Publishers, Reading), to which many pharmacognosists have edited volumes or contributed chapters. World-wide, pharmacognosy-based scientific societies are flourishing, including the American Society of Pharmacognosy, Association Française pour l'Enseignement et la Recherche en Pharmacognosie (France), Gesellschaft für Arzneipflanzenforschung (Europe), the Korean Society of Pharmacognosy, and the Japanese Society of Pharmacognosy. These societies typically organize an annual meeting for members, award travel and research grants, and promote the publication of scientific journals and newsletters. The American Society of Pharmacognosy is most likely typical in welcoming into its membership ranks many talented natural products scientists who did not train in pharmacy as an under-graduate degree.

For about 50 years, the proportion of the under-graduate or professional pharmacy curriculum devoted to pharmacognosy has been in decline in certain countries, as noted by others. Moreover, fewer departments or schools of pharmacy have retained pharmacognosy as a discrete subject in the curriculum as other basic pharmaceutical and biomedical science and clinical aspects have become more prominent, particularly in the UK and the US. However, the situation is not all gloom and doom for the subject, since a recent analysis of faculty positions in pharmacognosy shows strong representations in pharmacy departments in countries such as France, Germany, Japan and Turkey. At this point in time, pharmacognosy is perhaps most strongly represented in Japan, where natural products has long been one of the strongest areas of chemistry, in large part because of the traditional use of natural remedies there. However, even in the UK and the US, the recent substantial increase in the use of herbal remedies in pharmacy practice has rekindled interest in pharmacognosy and natural products in general among pharmacists and pharmacy students alike. This increased interest in herbal products by the pharmaceutical profession has been paralleled by an increased awareness in this topic and other forms of alternative medicine by physicians.

The chemical aspects of pharmacognosy have benefited enormously from the widespread availability of powerful spectroscopic techniques, particularly mass spectrometry and nuclear magnetic resonance, coupled with effective chromatographic methods for the purification of organic molecules from crude solvent extracts. Some of the early phytochemical work in pharmacy departments tended to focus on looking for new sources of prescription drugs, for example, chemotaxonomic studies on bisindole alkaloids from the genus *Catharanthus* and indole alkaloids from *Rauwolfia* alkaloids. It was quickly realized in the more research-oriented pharmacy academic institutions, however, that it was necessary to incorporate an element of biological testing with phytochemical work. Incorporation of a bioassay into the process of chromatographic purification has permitted the purification of one or more bioactive substances from the crude extracts prepared from organisms by bioactivity-guided fractionation. Of particular mention here is the logistically simple brine shrimp lethality "bench top" bioassay developed by the pharmacognosist Professor Jerry L. McLaughlin and co-workers at Purdue University, which has been shown to be appropriate to direct the screening of cytotoxic and anti-tumour compounds from plants. This inexpensive in-vivo technique has become widely used in natural products chemistry and even synthetic organic chemistry laboratories around the world. Many primary and secondary bioassays appropriate for the screening of natural product crude extracts, purified chromatographic fractions, and pure isolates have been developed, and can be varied accordingly depending on whether the desired outcome of the research is a pharmaceutically or agrochemically relevant target compound.

In this review, two major facets of current research being conducted by pharmacognosy groups will be covered, namely, natural product drug discovery and the scientific investigation of herbal remedies (phytomedicines). Given the broad range of such activities that are taking place around the world, it is not possible to cover all of these in this review. However, the reader can be referred to recent literature for descriptions of aspects of biosynthesis, biotechnology, marine chemistry, pharmaceutical botany, and phytochemistry, compiled or being performed by pharmacognosy and pharmaceutical biology groups.

## 2 DRUG DISCOVERY FROM NATURAL PRODUCTS

The importance of drugs from animal, microbial, and higher plants is well established, with such natural products also serving as lead compounds for semisynthetic manipulation and as templates for total synthetic modification. It has been estimated that up to 50% of the prescriptions presently dispensed in the US may contain one or more natural product drugs, with this term broadly defined so as to include various types of molecular modification. While there was a trend in the middle of the 20$^{th}$ century to remove many old botanical drugs from official compendia, as many new synthetic and microbially-derived drugs appeared, several new small-molecule natural product-derived drugs have been introduced into therapy in western countries in recent years, including acarbose, artemether, capsaicin, docetaxel, dronabinol (the synthetic form of $\Delta^{9-}$ tetrahydrocannabinol), galanthamine, irinotecan, paclitaxel, tacrolimus (FK-506), and topotecan. This trend is likely to continue in the future, at least for the treatment of certain disease states, such as cancer and infectious diseases, based on the high proportion of compounds entering clinical trials that are either natural products per se, or semi-synthetic compounds based on natural product template molecules.

Accordingly, there remains considerable interest in the screening of organisms in drug discovery programmes, since structurally-novel chemotypes with potent and selective biological activity may be obtained, and considerable biodiversity exists. These organisms may be fungi, marine fauna and flora, microorganisms such as actinomycetes and bacteria, and plants. In a recent statistical survey, it was pointed out that when compared with libraries of synthetic substances, natural products offer the prospects of discovering a greater number of compounds with sterically more complex structures. The same authors determined that the origin of 30 000 bioactive natural products could be divided between animals (13%), bacteria (33%), fungi (26%) and plants (27%). The potential diversity of bacteria and fungi is particularly large, with some 5 000 out of >40 000 bacteria, and only 70 000 out of as many as 1.5 million fungi, having even been identified, let alone investigated in the laboratory. In the next few paragraphs, higher plants will be considered specifically, since this group of organisms has been studied the most by pharmacognosy groups around the world.

Only a relatively small percentage (5%～15%) of the approximately 250 000 higher plants has been systematically investigated for the presence of bioactive compounds. As many as 155 000 seed plants occur in the tropics, with some 120 000 in the tropical moist forests alone, attesting to their great biotic richness. Tropical rain forest plants occupy only 7% ～ 8% of the land surface on earth, but offer a disproportionate opportunity for the discovery of stucturally-novel, biologically-active substances. This has been attributed to the high humidity, elevated temperature, and species density, along with a continuous growing season, which have led tropical rain forest plants to produce specialized secondary metabolites as pollination attractants and as defensive substances against predators and parasites. However, there is a pressing need for the conservation of the biodiversity of the tropical rain forests as a consequence of the alarming degree of erosion due to increasing encroachment by human populations.

Plants offer the scientist searching for novel bioactive compounds the added advantage of ethnobotanical observations, since many species are used in systems of traditional medicine, mainly in developing countries. It has been estimated that nearly 75% of about 120 biologically active plant-derived substances used in the world were discovered by following up on leads from traditional medicine. However, great concern has been expressed about the prospects of indigenous knowledge of ethnomedicine lasting far into this new millennium. The ethnobotanist Mark Plotkin has reflected on the problem of the imminent loss of shamans in the world's tropical rain forests very adroitly, as follows: "In a conservation context, we stand at the end of a precipice. We are scrambling to find ways to save the rain forest, yet thousands of years of accumulated human wisdom — the knowledge to use the forest, without destroying it, to benefit human-kind — is going to vanish over that precipice within the next generation. Throughout the tropics the species are disappearing, but the knowledge to use those species is disappearing at an even faster rate. Each time one of these medicine men (or women) dies, it is as if a whole library has gone up in smoke".

Depending on the selection of the in-vitro and in-vivo bioassays used to monitor the crude extracts, chromatographic fractions, and pure isolates of a plant or other organism, natural products research can be focussed on a particular type of disease. Thus, the following paragraphs will summarize some of the progress made recently on the discovery of potential plant-derived anti-cancer agents and naturally occurring cancer chemopreventives in two separate multidisciplinary collaborative research projects at the University of Illinois at Chicago. Other groups in pharmacy academic institutions have described natural product research directed toward other disease targets, such as anti-fungal agents, anti-mycobacterial agents, anti-malarial agents, anti-viral agents, and hypoglycemic agents.

In the US, each day approximately 1 500 people die of cancer, with about double this number diagnosed with invasive cancer. On a world-wide basis, the incidence of cancer is superseding the increase in the population. Among the many advances in cancer therapy, cancer chemotherapeutic agents based on plant secondary metabolites have played a part, and there are now 11 such compounds based on four structural classes (bisindole alkaloids, camptothecin derivatives, epipodophyllotoxins, and the taxanes) used clinically in the US. The taxane diterpenoid, paclitaxel (Taxol; Figure 1, 1), is worthy of special mention, since this was the first chemically-unmodified plant constituent for over 25 years to have been approved by the Food and Drug Administration (FDA) in the US, when it came onto the market as an anti-cancer agent in the early 1990s. This compound, isolated initially with the trivial name taxol from the bark of the Pacific yew (*Taxus brevifolia* Nutt.; Taxaceae), is now produced semi-synthetically from 10-deacetylbaccatin Ⅲ (Figure 1, 2) extracted from ornamental yew species, and has become the biggest selling anticancer agent ever in the US, with sales of over $1 billion per year. Paclitaxel was listed as eighteenth in the 1999 list of top-selling medicines, and is now being used to treat an expanding range of cancer types. Needless to say, the clinical and commercial success of paclitaxel has played an extremely important role in stimulating further exploratory research to discover additional novel compounds from plants. In addition, several additional potential plant-derived anti-cancer agents are presently undergoing preclinical or clinical trials. Accordingly, there is an enduring interest in investigating the plant kingdom further, with the aim of discovering additional new classes of compounds with anti-cancer activity.

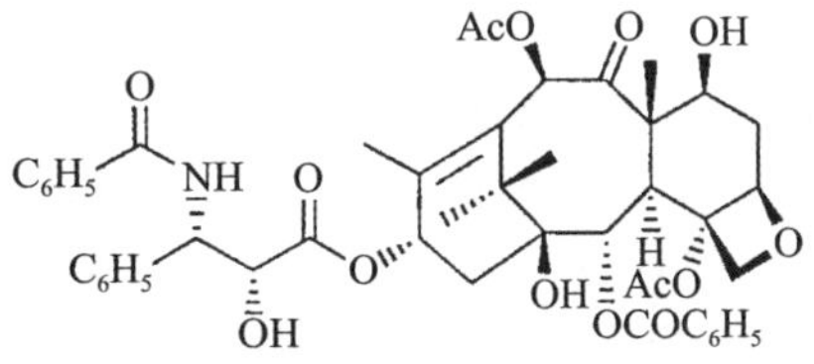

**1** paclitaxel (Taxol) 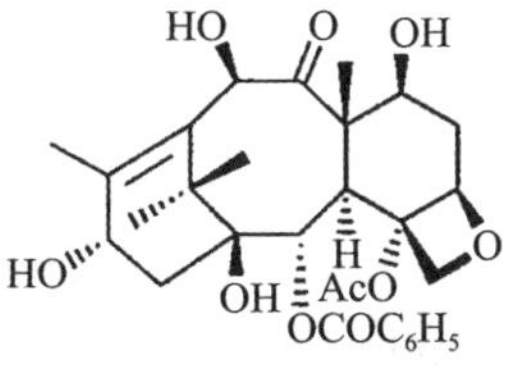 **2** 10-deacetylbaccatin Ⅲ

**Figure 1 Structures of paclitaxel (Taxol) and 10-deacetylbaccatin Ⅲ**

In an effort to discover novel anti-cancer agents of plant origin, our team at the University of Illinois at Chicago (UIC) is performing collaborative work with groups from a private research institute (Research Triangle Institute (RTI), Research Triangle Park, North Carolina) and a major pharmaceutical company (Bristol-Myers Squibb, Princeton, New Jersey). This project is funded by the US National Cancer Institute, under their National Cooperative Natural Products Drug Discovery Groups programme. This project is now in its third five-year phase, with Glaxo Wellcome Medicine Research Centre, Stevenage, UK having been the industrial partner with UIC and RTI during the period 1990 - 1995. Each year, 400 - 500 primary plant samples are collected, mainly from tropical regions, but also from the southern US. The species are identified by collaborating botanists in each host country, and priority is afforded to species that are endemic in the particular country concerned. Although as a policy decision, plants are not collected in this programme on an ethnomedical basis, for about 70% of the species collected there is no previous phytochemical or biological testing information available in the literature. Plants are collected only after formal signed agreements with host countries are in hand, with changes in the legal expectations, due primarily to international treaties (particularly the United Nations Convention on Biological Diversity convened in Rio de Janeiro in 1992) national legislation, and professional self-regulation, having made it much more difficult to collect samples for so-called biodiversity prospecting than was formerly the case. Our group has developed a standard extraction scheme suitable for the screening of dried plant samples, in which the chloroform-soluble extracts are subjected to a detannification step by washing with sodium chloride solution to remove vegetable tannins, which tend to interfere with protein-based bioassays. The organic-solvent crude extract of each plant acquisition is screened in a panel of about 25 cell-based and enzyme-inhibitory and receptor-binding mechanism-based in-vitro bioassays housed at the three primary sites in the consortial group, including high-throughput screening procedures at our partner pharmaceutical company. Before performing activity-guided fractionation of a promising lead, a dereplication step is taken, in an attempt to detect active compounds of previously known structure present in the crude extract. This involves subjecting the active extract in a standard HPLC system, passage through a UV detector at 280 nm, and splitting the stream into two. The smaller portion is treated and then passes into a mass spectrometer, while the larger portion is fractionated into a 96-well plate, with each well then evaluated in the bioassay in which the initial activity was found. In this manner, it is possible to obtain the masses of the active compounds in the wells and then to compare these data with information in the NAPRALERT and other data-bases. Several hundred biologically active compounds have been obtained in this collaborative project thus far, representative of a wide range of plant secondary metabolites. Examples of active compounds which have come from this programme to date are betulinic acid (Figure 2, 3) from *Ziziphus mauritiana* Lam. (Rhamnaceae), 15-oxozoapatlin (Figure 2, 4) from *Parinari curatellifolia* Benth. (Chrysobalanaceae), and the novel compound 4′-demethoxy-3′, 4′-methylenedioxy-methyl rocaglate (Figure 2, 5), from *Aglaia elliptica* Bl. (Meliaceae). Betulinic acid was shown to be selectively active for a human melanoma cancer cell line, and to exhibit in-vivo activity in a mouse xenograft model bearing human melanoma. Both 15-oxozoapatlin and 4′-demethoxy-3′, 4′-methylenedioxy-methyl rocaglate have been selected for in-vivo xenograft testing at the National Cancer Institute, following successful evaluation in a number of preliminary tests.

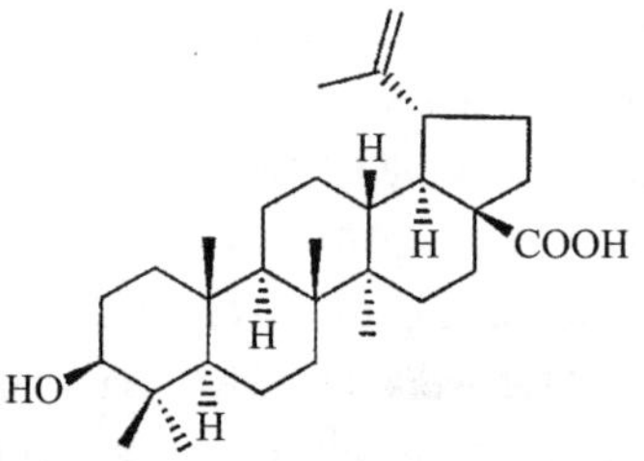

**3** betulinic acid

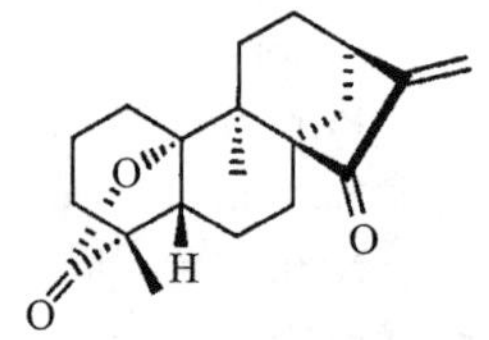

**4** 15-oxozoapatlin

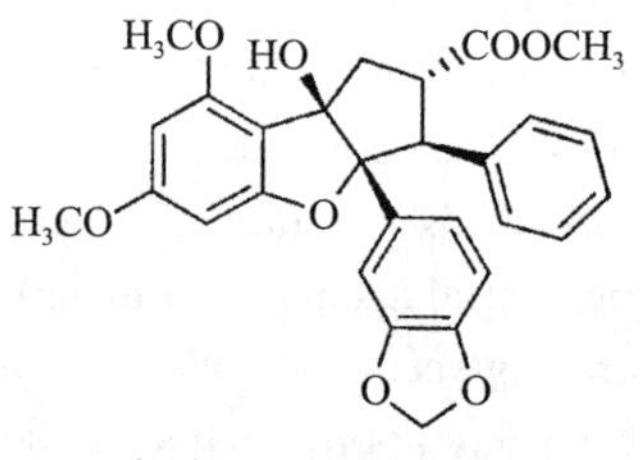

**5** 4′-demethoxy-3′,4′-methylenedioxy-methyl rocaglate

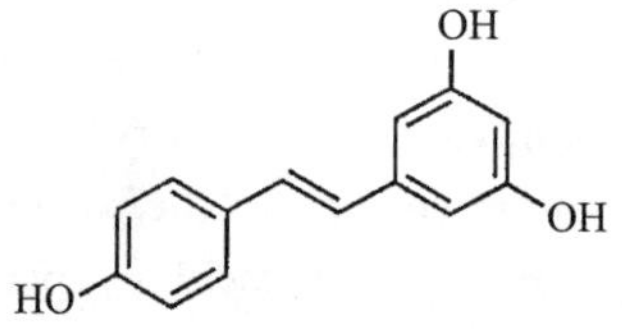

**6** *trans*-resveratrol

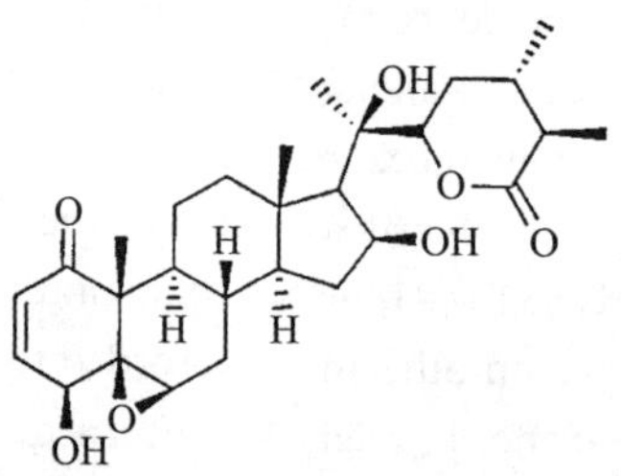

**7** withaphysacarpin

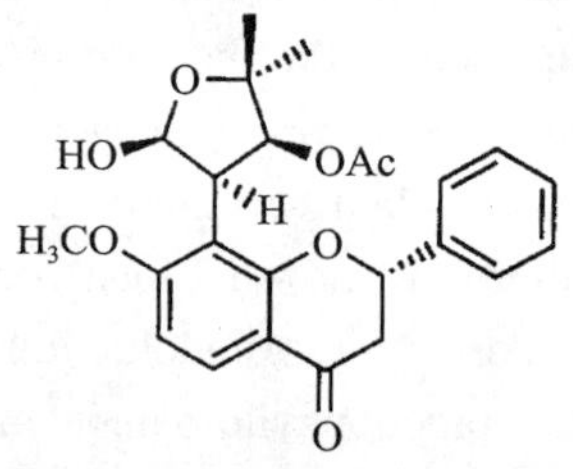

**8** tephrorin A

**Figure 2 Structures of promising bioactive natural products obtained from two drug discovery projects**

An alternative approach to combating cancer by intervention with natural products involves their use as potential cancer chemopreventive agents. Cancer chemoprevention has been defined as "a prevention or delay process of carcinogenesis in humans by the ingestion of dietary or pharmaceutical agents". There has been a considerable amount of work on the cancer chemopreventive effects of extracts and purified constituents of culinary herbs, fruits, spices, teas, and vegetables, which have been shown to inhibit the development of carcinogenesis in long-term animal models. However, at this point, there are no natural product-derived cancer chemopreventive drugs on the market, although a number of plant secondary metabolites are of interest for future clinical trials, including curcumin, ellagic acid, and phenethyl isothiocyanate.

In our collaborative project on cancer chemopreventive agents, which has been ongoing since 1991, novel compounds are also isolated from crude plant extracts by activity-guided fractionation, with a different panel of bioassays used than in the project described above on anti-cancer agents. The project is again funded by the US National Cancer Institute, with all of the laboratory work carried out at the University of Illinois at Chicago, and there being several different scientific components (plant acquisition, phytochemistry, in-vitro and in-vivo biology, synthetic chemistry, and technical core support). A primary focus of the overall project is on the collection of edible plants from around the world. Preliminary biological evaluation of an organic-soluble extract from each acquisition occurs in about ten in-vitro assays germane to each of the initiation, promotion, and progression stages of carcinogenesis. Biological follow-up testing is conducted using a mouse mammary organ culture assay, and, in a very few selected cases, in-vivo evaluation in a two-stage mouse skin and/or a rat mammary carcinogenesis model. As in the previously mentioned project, more than one hundred compounds have been isolated with activity in one or more bioassays, representative of a wide array of secondary metabolite structural types. Examples include resveratrol (Figure 2, 6) from *Cassia quinquangulata* Rich. (Leguminosae), with aphysacarpin (Figure 2, 7) from *Physalis philadelphica* Lam. (Solanaceae), and the new flavonoid, tephrorin A (Figure 2, 8), from *Tephrosia purpurea* Pers. (Leguminosae), which is a flavanone containing an unusual tetrahydrofuran moiety. Resveratrol, which also occurs in grapes and red wine, was found to be active as an inhibitor of cyclooxygenase 1, and then to show significant activity in the mouse mammary organ culture assay and in a full-term mouse skin carcinogenesis study. Both withaphysacarpin and tephrorin A are inducers of the phase Ⅱ drug metabolizing enzyme NAD(P)H: quinone reductase as evaluated in cultured Hepa 1c1c7 cells. Withaphysacarpin is of particular interest, since the fruits of its plant of origin (commonly known as the tomatillo) are used in the Latin American diet to produce green salsa, and in-vivo biological testing of this compound is currently taking place.

From the examples provided above from these two natural product projects related to cancer, it can be seen that interesting new biological observations may be made in a multidisciplinary setting for even very common compounds such as betulinic acid and resveratrol. Moreover, by strict adherence to activity-guided fractionation techniques, it is still possible to obtain new active compounds of considerable structural interest, even from comparatively well-investigated species such as *Tephrosia purpurea*. It can be expected that future natural product drug discovery projects will involve the need to go literally to the ends of the earth, to obtain previously unstudied organisms which may be logistically quite hard to obtain. In addition to the intended discovery of new drugs, such programmes can afford useful information concerning the protein and other cellular targets of small-molecule natural products. It is worth pointing out that natural product drug discovery projects, similar to the two described above, will increasingly require that participating pharmacognosists collaborate with scientists in other disciplines, such as analytical chemists, biochemists, biostatisticians, medicinal chemists, molecular biologists, organic chemists, pharmacologists, structural biologists, taxonomists, and toxicologists. Moreover, it is necessary for academic institutions to make a considerable investment in infrastructure in support of such research work. In addition to the need for properly equipped phytochemical and biological testing laboratories, it is also necessary to have access to facilities to process plants or other organisms (maintaining an inventory, taxonomic authentication, milling, small- and large-scale extraction, and storage), as well as having the appropriate means of cultivating selected species. A large amount of information is generated on the collection details of organisms, and on the biological data of extracts, chromatographic fractions and pure compounds, so it is necessary to process this information electronically. Central administrative support from the institution is also needed, as for example, the involvement of legal and international offices to help formulate agreements with authorities in the source countries of plants or other organisms of interest.

## 3 STUDIES ON HERBAL MEDICINES

In many developing countries of the world, there is still a major reliance on crude preparations of plants used in traditional medicines for their primary health care. In countries such as India and the People's Republic of China, the systems of traditional medicine are particularly well developed, and both of these have provided interesting new drug leads for potential development in western medicine. Moreover, a number of clinical evaluations of herbal medicinal preparations have already been conducted in certain western countries. As alluded to earlier, a major change has occurred in the interest of health professionals in western countries concerning the use of herbal remedies over the last decade, which in large part mirrors the increasing interest held by the public in terms of self-medication with botanical products. For pharmacognosists employed in institutions of pharmacy education, this new awareness of natural products has come as a major "shot in the arm", and a number of useful texts on the analysis, uses and/or potential toxicities of herbal remedies have appeared recently, which not only assist with teaching in pharmacy professional or undergraduate curricula but also serve as useful guides in pharmacy practice.

Not only has the "herbal remedy revolution" created new opportunities for the teaching of pharmacognosy, but also this phenomenon has served to stimulate research in a new field of direct relevance to human health care. There may be some who might well demur at what they see as the unchallenging prospect of working on phytomedicines, since much is already known about many of these. However, the eminent organic chemist, Professor Koji Nakanishi, of Columbia University in New York, has thrown down the gauntlet in terms of the types of research hurdles that will need to be overcome in future work on herbal remedies and related medicinal plants, as follows: "That natural medicines are attracting renewed attention is encouraging from both practical and scientific viewpoints; their efficacy has been proven over the centuries. However, to understand the mode of action of folk herbs and related products from nature is even more complex than mechanistic clarification of a single bioactive factor. This is because unfractionated or partly fractionated extracts are used, often containing mixtures of materials, and in many cases synergism is most likely playing an important role. Clarification of the active constituents and their modes of action will be difficult. This is nevertheless a worthwhile subject for serious investigators."

Many phytochemical and biological groups have already begun to perform laboratory work in a meaningful way on herbal remedies. For example, recent papers have appeared for common herbal remedies in terms of the development of analytical methodology; isolation procedures for reference compounds; the characterization of new chemical constituents; the identification, structure elucidation, biosynthesis and chemical reactivity of bioactive principles of phytomedicines; active compound mechanism of action determination; and the toxicological evaluation of phytomedicine components. A potentially far-reaching observation in terms of the safety of consuming certain herbal teas was made recently, when it was realized that two hepatotoxic otosenine-type pyrrolizidine alkaloid macroester constituents of the Chinese traditional medicine, *Ligularia hodgsonii* Hook. (Compositae), which is used as an antitussive, are soluble in both organic solvents and water. Although pyrrolizidine alkaloids based on otosenine are not particularly common, whenever they do occur in herbal teas they will thus be water-soluble when in the hydrophilic ionized form, and hence potentially toxic.

The concept of several active principles acting in a synergistic manner in herbal remedies may be somewhat unusual to pharmaceutical scientists who are more used to activity in a medicinal preparation being due to a single therapeutic agent. However, a recent example may be given of this phenomenon, with reference to constituents of the plant *Berberis freemontii* Torrey (Berberidaceae), a plant once used in Native American traditional medicine. It has been found that the anti-bacterial activity of berberine (Figure 3, 9) from *B. freemontii* against a resistant strain of *Staphylococcus aureus* was potentiated by the addition of two further constituents of the plant, the flavonolignan, 5′-methoxyhydrocarpin D (Figure 3, 10), and the porphyrin, pheophorbide *a* (Figure 3, 11). Although either compound 10 or 11 potentiated the effects of a subthreshold concentration of the alkaloid, neither possessed antibiotic activity when tested alone. Berberine is also present in high concentration levels in the widely used herbal remedy Goldenseal (the rhizomes of *Hydrastis canadensis* L.; Ranunculaceae), so it is possible that synergistic biological effects occur between this protoberberine alkaloid and other known or as-yet unidentified constituents of this phytomedicine.

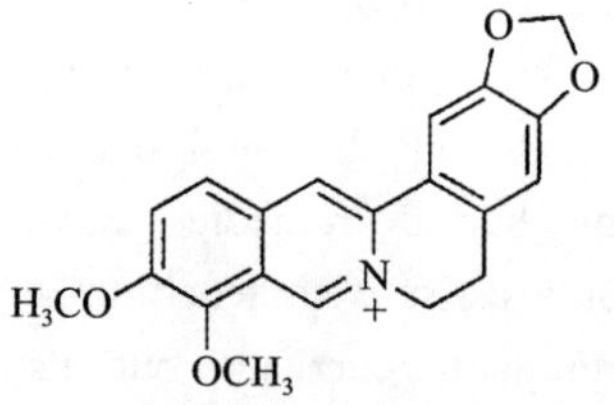

**9** berberine 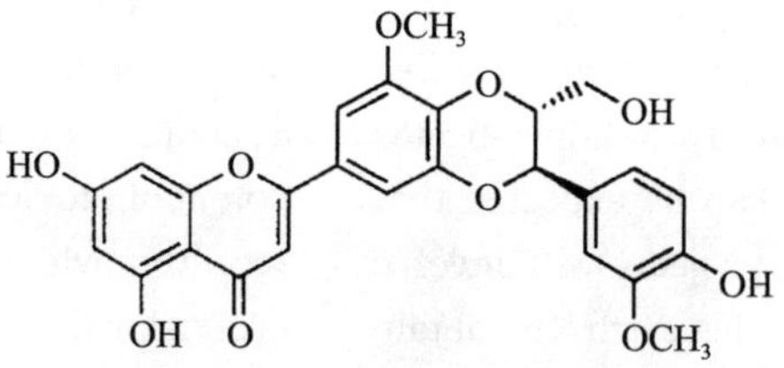 **10** 5′-methoxyhydnocarpin D 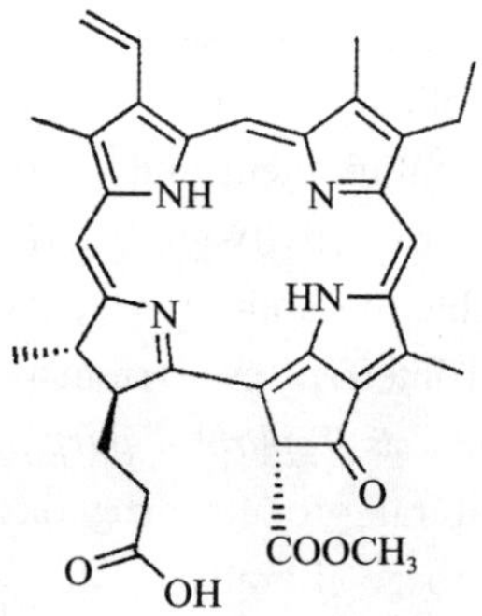 **11** pheophorbide *a*

**Figure 3 Structures of compounds showing synergistic antibacterial activity**

In a recent review article, Tyler has outlined some of the scientific challenges that ensuring the safe and effective use of herbal remedies will present the manufacturers of these products, in terms of bioavailability, phytoequivalence, standardization and other quality control, and the performance of properly designed clinical trials leading to the introduction of new phytomedicines. In the US, the passage of the Dietary Supplement Health and Education Act in 1994 led to the categorization of herbal medicines as "dietary supplements" for "health maintenance", and has resulted in the influx of hundreds of new plant products onto the shelves of pharmacies and health food stores. Many of these products have not been studied comprehensively, and are often of incompletely known chemical composition and/or pharmacodynamic activity, and there are sometimes concerns about their quality or potential interactions when co-administered with prescription drugs. This is in sharp contrast to the thoroughness in which single-agent synthetic or natural product therapeutic drugs must be evaluated before receiving approval by the US FDA. Perhaps the present state of affairs with regard to these new botanical dietary supplements is more in keeping with the situation which might have been expected at the turn of the 20th century than at the present time. Hence, there are numerous opportunities for those in academic and other institutions to perform highly socially relevant research on these products, not only in the field of pharmacognosy, but in the pharmaceutical sciences as a whole. The outlook for those wishing to perform such research in the US is particularly auspicious due to the recent inauguration of a new funding agency at the National Institutes of Health, namely, the National Center for Complementary and Alternative Medicine.

## 4 CONCLUSIONS

As we enter the 21st century and the new millennium, it may be argued that interest in pharmacognosy as a discipline and natural products in general is at an alltime high. The last decade has seen a greater use of botanical products among members of the general public through self-selection than ever before. This phenomenon has been mirrored by an increasing attention to herbal remedies (phytomedicines) as a form of alternative therapy by the health professions inclusive of pharmacy and medicine. The major new addition of herbal remedies to pharmacy practice has greatly increased the relevance of pharmacognosy as a didactic subject, and has augmented interest in this topic among pharmacy students. While pharmacognosy has always remained as a strong core discipline in the professional pharmacy curriculum in certain countries, it is not unreasonable to suggest that every school or department of pharmacy in future should have at least one faculty member who is thoroughly knowledgeable in the subject of herbal remedies. The various topics and scientific approaches to research in pharmacognosy and natural products continue to expand. As interest in the scientific components of natural drugs and foods increases in both the scientific community and the general public, there will be increased funding opportunities, but there will also be increased competition from those in disciplines outside of academic pharmacy institutions to perform this sort of research. Though pharmacognosists have valuable knowledge that can be extremely useful in natural products drug discovery efforts, these sorts of projects can be envisaged as becoming much more complex in the future, with an increasing number of scientific disciplines represented. It is to be hoped that as research in pharmacognosy becomes ever more specialized, the present strong and unified representation at international and national pharmacognosy meetings does not become fragmented. Young pharmacists and graduates with degrees in other science disciplines who are interested in entering a research career in pharmacognosy or natural products work should aim to have as broad a background as possible, and should gain an understanding of new developments that come to the fore, such as combinatorial biosynthesis, genomics, and proteomics. More flexibility will be required of new researchers of natural products than ever before, but because of the new tools available, the rewards in terms of inherent interest and the contribution to society will be correspondingly greater than they have ever been previously. There seems little question that pharmacognosy as a discipline will have a role to play for many more years, and that pharmacognosists can look to the future with a great deal of anticipation.

[A. Douglas Kinghorn. Journal of Pharmacy and Pharmacology, 2001, 53: 135-148.]

# From ethnobotany to molecular pharmacognosy: a transdisciplinary approach

## 1 SUMMARY

The following doctoral thesis consists of 3 major parts, which could be treated independently but are nonetheless closely related. In a first phase, 10 months of ethnobotanical fieldwork among the Yanomamï Amerindians in southern Venezuela was carried out. Fieldwork was based on an International Contract between the Swiss Federal Institute of Technology (ETH) Zurich and the Ministry of Environment (MARNR) of Venezuela, the elaboration of which was an integral part of the research process. The ethnobotanical study in 5 distant communities led to the collection of approximately 300 plant specimens and data about more than 650 plant species. It could be shown that the Yanomamï in Venezuela have a minor knowledge about medicinal plants than their relatives in Brazil. But the ethnobotanical study in many respects revealed the special importance of food plants, poisonous and magic plants, as well as the overall significance of plants in their culture. The role of palms in general and the medicinal species *Phyllanthus piscatorum* in particular, are discussed in detail. Bulk plant material of 10 culturally important species was collected for biological and phytochemical analysis. A preliminary screening of the raw extracts (*n*-hexane, DCM, MeOH) revealed several significant antibacterial, cytotoxic, and antifungal extracts. *Clathrotropis galucophylla* Cowan, a curare adjuvant, *Cupania scrobiculata* L. C. Rich., the bark of which is used in the preparation of a snuff drug, and *Phyllanthus piscatorum* H. B. K., a fish poison and medicinal plant were chosen for phytochemical analysis. The latter was subjected to bioactivity-guided fractionation. The phytochemical analysis of *C. scrobiculata* led to the isolation of 9 compounds belonging to 5 distinct chemical classes. 4 compounds were new to the literature. *P. piscatorum* yielded the highly bioactive arylnaphtalide lignan justicidin B and one new derivative which was called piscatorin. For the first time, justicidin B and piscatorin are shown to be the piscicidal principles of *P. piscatorum*, and to possess significant antifungal and antiprotozoal potential.

Due to an urgent need for novel bioassays in pharmacognosy, a reverse transcription — real time — PCR assay was developed to investigate inflammatory and cytotoxic events in human lymphocytes, such as the transcriptional activation of the NF-κB complex, the mRNA levels of pro-inflammatory and related genes, as well as genes involved in cell regulation and apoptosis. This functional transcriptomics assay allowed a differential analysis of the pharmacological potential of natural products. For the evaluation of the test system, several known substances were employed, such as curcumin, sesquiterpene lactones, hypericin, rotenone, and cyclosporin A. Other pharmacological experiments were carried out that led to new insights into the molecular mechanism of action of sesquiterpene lactones and other natural products. This transdisciplinary work resulted in 10 scientific publications (in 3 distinct areas).

## 2 ZUSAMMENFASSUNG

Die vorliegende Doktorarbeit besteht aus 3 Hauptteilen, die zwar unabhängig voneinander behandelt werden können, jedoch eng miteinander verknüpft sind. In der ersten Phase der Arbeit wurde während 10 Monaten eine ethnobotanische Untersuchung bei den Yanomamï Indianern in Südvenezuela durchgeführt. Diese Feldarbeit basierte auf einem internationalen Vertrag zwischen der Eidgenössischen Technischen Hochschule (ETH) Zürich und dem Umweltministerium (MARNR) Venezuelas. Der Vertrag stellte ein wichtiger Bestandteil des Forschungsprozesses dar. Die ethnobotanischen Untersuchungen in 5 verschiedenen Dörfern führte zu ca. 300 gesammelten Herbarbelegen und Daten über mehr als 650 Pflanzenarten. Es konnte gezeigt werden, dass die Yanomamï in Venezuela eine geringere Kenntnis über Medizinalpflanzen verfügen als ihre brasilianischen Nachbarn. Ferner wurde gezeigt, dass wilde Nahrungspflanzen, Gift- und magische Pflanzen von grosser Bedeutung sind. Die Stellung der Palmen im allgemeinen und die Bedeutung von *Phyllanthus piscatorum* im speziellen werden genauer diskutiert. Es wurden grössere Mengen Material von 10 kulturell wichtigen Pflanzen für biologische und phytochemische Analysen gesammelt. Ein erstes Screening der Rohextrakte (*n*-Hexan, DCM, MeOH) zeigte signifikante bakterizide, zytotoxische und fungizide Aktivitäten. Die Curarepflanze *Clathrotropis glaucophylla* Cowan, *Cupania scrobiculata* L. C. Rich., dessen Rinde als Zusatz für eine Schnupfdroge gebraucht wird, sowie das Fischgift und Medizinalpflanze *Phyllanthus piscatorum* H. B. K. wurden für phytochemische Studien ausgewählt, wobei *P. piscatorum* einer bioaktivitätsgeleiteten Fraktionierung unterworfen wurde. Die phytochemische Untersuchung von *C. scrobiculata* führte zur Isolierung von 9 Substanzen aus 5 verschiedenen chemischen Rassen. 4 Verbindungen wurden zum ersten Mal beschrieben. Die Untersuchung von *P. piscatorum* führte zur Isolierung des hochaktiven Lignans Justicidin B und einer neuen Verbindung, die als Piscatorin benannt wurde. Zum ersten Mal wird gezeigt, dass Justicidin B und Piscatorin die ichthyotoxischen Prinzipien von *P. piscatorum* darstellen und dass sie fungizide und antiprotozoale Eigenschaften aufweisen.

Basierend auf einem dringenden Bedarf an neuen und innovativen biologischen Testsystemen in der Pharmakognosie wurde ein reverse transcription — real time — PCR Biotest entwickelt, um entzündliche und zytotoxische Prozesse in humanen Lymphozyten zu untersuchen. Dabei wurde die transkriptionelle Aktivierung des NF-κB Komplexes, die mRNA Mengen der entzündlichen und anverwandten Gene, sowie Gene aus der Zellregulation und Apoptose analysiert. Dieses funktionelle Transcriptomics Testsystem erlaubte so eine differenzierte Analyse des pharmakologischen Wirkspektrums von bioaktiven Naturstoffen. Es wurden verschiende bekannte Verbindungen getestet, wie z. B. Curcumin, Sesquiterpen Laktone, Hypericin, Rotenon und Cyclosporin A. Weitere pharmakologische Untersuchungen erbrachten neue Erkenntnisse über die molekularen Wirkmechanismen von Curcumin und Sesquiterpen Lactonen. Diese transdisziplinäre Arbeit führte zu 10 wissenschaftliche Arbeiten in 3 verschiedenen Gebieten.

[Gertsch Jürg. Zürich: ETH Life, 2002.]

# 分子生药学:一门新兴的边缘学科

分子生药学(Molecular Pharmacognosy)是在分子水平上研究生药的分类与鉴定、栽培与保护及有效成分生产的一门科学,是生药学(Pharmacognosy)的一个极富前瞻性的分支。1995年,黄璐琦在《展望分子生物技术在生药学中的应用》一文中提出"分子生药学"这一概念。2000年6月,北京医科大学出版社出版了《分子生药学》一书,该书于2006年发行了第二版。同年,《分子生药学》进入本科生教材系列。迄今为止,全国已有不少中医院校或医学院校开设分子生药学课程。本文着重介绍了分子生药学产生的背景和意义、学科定位、10余年来取得的进展及其未来的发展方向。

## 1 分子生药学产生的背景

1.1 *生药及生药学的概念* 生药是指来源于植物、动物和矿物的新鲜品或经过简单的加工,直接用于医疗保健或作为医药用原料的天然药材。药用植物和动物是生药学的主体,占生药总量的99%以上。"生药"一词兼有生货原药之意,最早出现于明代太医院中规定"凡天下解纳药材,俱贮本院生药库","凡太医院所用药饵,均由……各地解来生药制造"。生药学(Pharmakognosie, Pharmacognosy)是应用本草学、植物学、动物学、化学(包括植物化学、药物分析化学、生物化学等)、药理学、中医学、临床医学和分子生物学(Molecular Biology)等学科的理论和知识,运用现代科学技术来研究生药的基源、鉴定、有效成分、生产、采制、品质评价及资源可持续性开发利用等的一门学科。这一词首见于1880年日本学者大井玄洞的译著《生药学》。通观生药学的研究内容,我国古代生药的研究内容主要包含在本草学中。现阶段,生药学与中药资源学和中药鉴定学学科的内涵和外延存在一定的交叉。

1.2 *生药学研究和发展的成就* 几十年来,生药学研究与实践在资源调查与整理、常用中药材品种整理与质量研究、资源的扩大与保护、资源的开发利用等方面取得了巨大的成就。通过3次全国范围的中药资源普查,已基本摸清了我国中药资源种类、分布、生态环境、蕴藏量、历史、生产利用情况以及传统使用经验等基本情况;对220种常用中药材开展了以品种整理为重点的系统研究;对71种常用中药材进行质量标准规范化研究;对400余种中药材进行了较深入的化学成分研究,填补了一大批中草药化学成分空白;筛选出800余种生物活性成分。从亲缘相近的同种属植物中成功地在我国找到国产安息香(*Styrax macrothyrsus*, *S. subniveus*, *S. hypoglaucus*)等进口药的国产资源。牛黄、麝香、虎骨、犀牛角、冬虫夏草等名贵中药人工制品或代用品研究均获成功。探索了药用部位的综合利用,如钩藤(*Uncaria rhynchophylla*)的药用部位由钩扩大到茎。中药人工繁殖及种植养殖迅速发展,国家从1999年开始推行中药材规范化种植,这些均大大缓解了野生资源的压力。这些年来,整理出版了一些具有代表性的大型著作,如《全国中草药汇编》《中药大辞典》《新华本草纲要》《中国中药资源》《中国中药区划》等。

1.3 *生药学面临的问题和局限* 作为一门不断成长分化的学科,生药学有其自身在研究领域、技术方法等方面的局限。比如,作为品种整理、资源调查、保护、开发利用的基础,生药鉴定是生药学的核心内容。生药材鉴定技术最初只是依据药材的外部形态特征、色泽、断面、质地、气味等进行药材真伪鉴别,其后逐步发展为对药材内部的细胞组织形态特征进行光学显微鉴别,对超微结构的扫描电子显微镜,以及对依据药材的理化性质开展的理化鉴别等,特别是各种光谱分析技术的应用,使生药学鉴定发展到一个新的高峰。但至今为止,生药鉴定仍存在很多无法解决的难题。例如,动物类药材由于药效成分不明确,特征不够鲜明而无法实现有效鉴别;又如,由于缺少有效的快速鉴别的技术,一些珍贵稀有的药材市场伪品严重。特别值得一提的是,多来源药材(一种中药来源于多种原植物)一直是影响中药材质量稳定性和均一性的关键问题之一。如黄芪原植物为豆科蒙古黄芪(*Astragalus membranaceus* Fisch. Bge. var. *mongholicus* Bge. Hsiao)或膜荚黄芪(*A. membranaceus* Fisch. Bge.);甘草原植物为豆科甘草(*Glycyrrhiza uralensis* Fisch.)、胀果甘草(*G. inflata* Bat.)或光果甘草(*G. glabra* L.)等。从生物学上来讲,每个物种都有其独特的遗传特性和表型特征,以及特定的对环境的适应方式,因此,将不同来源的药材视为一种中药显然是不合理的。为此,2005版《中华人民共和国药典》试图将多来源物种,按其来源不同拆分或合并,最终形成生物学上的物种与中药的种一一对应的关系。但由于很多多来源药材在进化中的分类地位存在争议,其系统关系不确定,基于遗传上的证据不足而无法确定其药材来源,导致无法对该多来源药材进行合并或拆分,这一计划并未很好实现,目前多来源问题仍是未来《中国药典》亟需解决的问题。例如,茅苍术[*Atractylodes lancea* (Thunb.) DC.]和北苍术[*A. chinensis* (DC.) Koidz.];多个来源的山银花,包括灰毡毛忍冬(*Lonicera macranthoides* Hand.-Mazz.)、红腺忍冬(*L. hypoglauca* Miq.)、华南忍冬(*L. confusa* DC.)等。可见,学科的发展对生药学提出了理论、方法及技术更新的要求。

1.4 *分子水平的研究成为生药学发展的必然要求* 20世纪末期,科学技术尤其是现代生物学及相关学科的飞速发展,极大地促进了生药学的发展,其他学科及相关知识的渗入使得生药学的研究内容不断扩大,技术方法不断更新,生药学科的内涵和外延也不断延伸,并产生了许多新的热点和难点问题。例如,如何认识生药的质量变异?其物质基础是什么?生药优质药材(特别是道地药材)是如何形成的,其形成的分子遗传与环境机理是什么?生药药效成分积累的生物学机理是什么?受什么因素影响?如何提高药效成分的含量?生药的种质资源具有怎样的特性，其与作物种质资源的研究有无不同等。这一个时期，人们开始意识到种质资源评价、珍稀濒危机制研究、次生代谢产物的调控等不少科学问题，已不仅仅是在有机体、组织、器官甚至细胞水平就可以揭示和解决，生药学的发展迫切要求在基因、蛋白质、酶等生物分子水平来阐释生药学的诸多生物学问题。生药来源于生物，但人们对其许多生物学的现象、规律及机理的研究和掌握却明显不足，而这些现象和规律的分子机理研究更是鲜有报道。可见，生产实践的需求，理所当然地将生药学的研究推进到分子水平。

1.5 *分子生药学是生药学与分子生物学学科交叉的必然产物* 自从1953年Watson和Crick对DNA结构的发现后，分子生物学迅速成为20世纪里发展最快，对人类影响最大的学科之一。分子生物学的飞速发展，极大地改变了人类对世界的认知，提高了人类改造自身和其他生物的能力，使与生物学有关的所有领域的分支学科，都发展到了分子水平。作为现代生命科学的"共同语言"，分子生物学的研究与发展一方面不断深化和提升本学科的理论和技术，使表现型和基因型的关系得到客观准确的阐释；另一方面不断地与其他学科进行广泛而深入的横向联系和交叉融合，以此开拓新的前沿领域和新的增长点，使得一大批交叉科学、边缘学科和前沿学科应运而生，例如分子遗传学、植物分子遗传学、分子系统学、分子生态学、蛋白组学、基因组学、代谢组学、微生物分子生态学、生物信息学等。分子生物学在生物医学各个领域渗透应用并飞速发展，由此产生了分子药理学、分子肿瘤学、分子病毒学、分子细胞生物学、分子生药学等相关学科。其中，作为分子生物学与生药学学科交叉的产物，分子生药学的形成和发展受到分子遗传学、分子系统学、分子生态学、保护生物学、药用植物育种学等诸多学科的启发，主要在核酸、蛋白等分子水平研究生药学的相关问题。分子生药学的产生，是生药学向微观深入研究发展的必然趋势之一。

## 2 分子生药学与生药学的关系及其产生的意义

2.1 *分子生药学与生药学的关系* 分子生药学不仅继承了传统生药学的内容和使命，更将赋予生药学新的任务和挑战。谢宗万分析了分子生药学和传统生药学、现代生药学的关系问题，认为"它们永远是一种互补关系，而不是什么替代关系，因为它们使用的手段有所不同，解决的关键问题和取得的效果也不尽相同"，并进一步指出"在今后，要解决生药领域里的复杂疑难问题，看来是缺一不可，把这些手段统统加在一起联用或从中选择几种手段配合使用，才是更全面和更有效的办法"。本文就生药学与分子生药学进行了系统的比较分析，足以看出分子生药学与生药学可以相互促进，但绝不可能相互替代(表1)。

**表1 生药学与分子生药学的区别及联系**

| | 生药学 | 分子生药学 |
|---|---|---|
| 概念 | 生药学是研究生药的基源、鉴定、有效成分、生产、采制、品质评价及资源可持续性开发利用等的一门科学 | 分子生药学是在分子水平上研究生药的分类与鉴定、栽培与保护及有效成分生产的一门科学，是生药学的一个极富前瞻性和前景性的分支 |
| 学科定位 | 面向应用，主要在个体和种群等较宏观水平开展生药真伪优劣的鉴别和质量评价，为生药资源生产及可持续利用提供依据 | 面向机理和应用，主要在分子水平研究生药的遗传背景、开展生药的分子鉴别、揭示次生代谢产物积累的分子机理、探索次生代谢产物的分子调控及生物合成，为生药的优质生产和保护提供依据 |
| 核心研究内容 | 识别鉴定生药基源<br>调查考证生药资源<br>制定生药的质量标准，并对其进行品质评价<br>为中药材规范化生产服务<br>资源开发 | 药用动植物的系统进化<br>药用动植物种质资源评价及保存<br>药用动植物濒危机制及保护<br>药用植物活性成分的生物合成及调控<br>药用动植物的道地性及分子机理<br>生药分子鉴定 |
| 主要研究方法 | 基源鉴定、性状鉴定、显微鉴定、理化鉴定、化学成分分析等 | DNA分析技术(分子杂交、分子标记技术、基因芯片、基因工程技术)、蛋白质分析技术(酶技术)、生物转化技术，以及生药学的常规分析方法(包括基源鉴定、显微鉴定、理化鉴定、化学成分分析)等 |
| 密切相关学科 | 本草学、中药资源学、中药鉴定学、中药化学、分析化学等 | 生药学、分子生物学、分子遗传学、分子生态学、植物生理学、生物学、遗传学 |

2.2 *分子生药学产生的意义* 生药学的主要任务为：在个体和种群等较宏观水平开展生药真伪优劣的鉴别和质量评价，为生药资源生产及可持续利用提供依据。相关研究涉及细胞(cell)、组织(tissue)、器官(organ)、有机体(organism)、种群(population)等层次，并在这些层次上形成了比较成熟和独立的理论和方法，如生药组织学、生药形态学等。分子生药学的主要任务为：在分子水平研究生药的遗传背景、开展生药的分子鉴别，揭示次生代谢产物积累的分子机理、探索次生代谢产物的分子调控及生物合成，为生药的优质生产和保护提供依据。分子生药学的产生，一方面将生药的研究层次向微观推进到基因(genes)水平，极大地丰富了以往对生药生命现象的认识；另一方面，由于不同基因或DNA片段的进化速度不同，其在进化中的特殊地位不同，所反映的遗传变异的尺度和水平也不同，这一点强化了人们对生药细胞、组织、器官、有机体、种群等层次的重新认识和思考。人们意识到生药作为一个生命体在不同研究水平所观察到的现象及规律的意义和局限，并试图通过对这些层次的全面分析和整合，得到一个生药的全貌。这样的努力提升了生药学研究的深度和广度，使生药学更多地摆脱唯象学，成为一门系统的现代科学。可以说，研究层次的改变导致了独特的视角，由此产生了独特的科学问题和解决思路、方法和理论，并最终导致了分子生药学学科的出现。我国生药学界前辈谢宗万先生认为2000年《分子生药学》"第一次正式出版，其意义十分重大，且涉及分子生药学

这个分支学科创立的大问题”。

## 3 分子生药学的研究内容、学科特色及技术方法

3.1 研究内容

3.1.1 生药分子鉴定 生药分子鉴定是分子生药学科的首要任务。作为可检测的遗传标记,DNA 标记具备准确性高、重现性好等特点,相对于传统鉴定方法(包括基原鉴定、性状鉴定、显微鉴定和理化鉴定),分子鉴定具有不受环境因素影响,也不受药材加工炮制后外观性状改变影响的优势。比在形态、组织和化学水平上的检测更能代表生药的变异类型。生药的分子鉴定最常用的技术有基于 PCR 与电泳技术相结合的 RAPD、SSR、AR-PCR、MARMS、APAPD 和 PCR-RFLP 等技术;基于 DNA 测序的 SNP 技术和 DNA 条形码技术。近年来,从国家科技期刊数据库中检索到生药分子鉴定的文献有百余篇,涉及天花粉、人参、当归、大黄、柴胡等诸多生药。

3.1.2 药用动植物的系统进化 药用动植物系统关系的确定,不但是其分类鉴别的基础,也是拓展近缘种,寻找替代品及开发新药源的基础。与传统的表型特征相比较,分子生物学方法受到环境的影响较少,因而更能反映出生物体在演变进化过程中的本质,其研究结果也更可靠。因此,利用 DNA 分子遗传标记、基因组序列分析、蛋白质分析及染色体计数等技术,从居群、个体乃至基因水平上,准确刻画药用动植物遗传背景差异和亲缘关系,进而构建基于叶绿体基因组基因和核基因组基因序列分析的重要药用动植物系统发育树,确定药用动植物系统关系及其在进化中的地位是分子生药学基础研究的重心。目前常用于分子系统学研究的主要基因种类有 *rbc* L、*mat* K、rps4、18s rRNA、ITS 等,其中前三者为叶绿体基因组基因,后二者为核基因组基因。相关研究已有不少报道,如白芷、瓜蒌、党参、苍术、芍药、厚朴、蛇等。

3.1.3 药用动植物种质资源评价及保存 种质资源(germplasm resources)也称遗传资源(genetic resources),是指选育新品种的基础材料,包括各种植物的栽培种、野生种的繁殖材料以及利用上述繁殖材料人工创造的各种植物的遗传材料。药用植物种质是影响中药质量和产量的重要因素,更是生药品种选育及资源可持续利用的物质基础。种质资源的收集、整理、保存及评价是药用动植物种质资源研究的主要内容。早些年,人们在品种选育的时候,就注意到红豆杉、人参、枸杞、地黄等很多中药种质资源在表型上的多样性。近年来,人们利用分子技术对石斛、厚朴、菊花、芍药、黄芩、白芷、苍术等种质资源的多样性、遗传结构、种质纯度、表型与遗传的相关性等进行了研究,为药用动植物种质资源的保护提供了丰富的遗传学资料。

3.1.4 药用动植物濒危机制及保护 遗传多样性对种群是否能适应环境变化、是否能长期存活都是非常重要的,如果没有遗传多样性,就没有能力应付变化的环境、进化的竞争。导致药用动植物濒危的内外因很多,其中,药用动植物种群遗传多样性低导致对环境的适合度降低是物种濒危的重要内在原因之一。因此,保护濒危物种的遗传多样性是濒危物种保护的基本目标。以 DNA 多态性分析为基础的分子标记和以基因组序列分析为基础的分子系统学,能直接测定 DNA 变异式样和确定保护的重点单元,并因种内群体的分衍和发展在本质上与物种的系统进化有相似的过程,可根据药用动植物的分子系统研究推测群体的发展状态和濒危程度,从而为生物多样性的测度与珍稀药用动植物资源保护对策的制定提供新的具有强操作性的手段。例如濒危药用植物荒漠肉苁蓉、杜仲、三七等。特别是目前用分子谱系地理学(molecular phylogeography)研究居群遗传变异方面取得的突破,为生药居群遗传变异研究提供了新的理论和研究方法。

3.1.5 药用植物活性成分的生物合成及调控 生药有效成分绝大多数来源于次生代谢产物,次生代谢产物的有无和多少决定着生药的品质。因此,研究药用植物次生代谢产物的形成机理,开展次生代谢产物的调控和生物合成,或进行次生代谢产物的基因工程,以此提高生药有效成分的含量,是分子生药学研究的新热点。例如,利用微生物转化体系对延胡索中镇痛成分延胡索乙素进行转化,得到了 2 个活性明显高于延胡索乙素的转化产物;利用转基因何首乌毛状根培养体系和转基因西洋参冠瘿组织培养体系转化外源性化合物香豆素类,大部分转化产物为糖基化产物。部分通过生物转化得到的新化合物,其活性超过了母体化合物。例如,利用小克银汉霉 AS3.970 转化雷公藤中雷公藤内酯,获得了 4 个新化合物且都具有对人肿瘤细胞株的细胞毒效应。目前,已建立毛状根培养系统的药用植物有紫草、长春花、人参、丹参、青蒿、甘草等数十种;进行有效成分基因调控研究的药用植物有罂粟、青蒿、丹参、红豆杉、喜树等数十种;利用根癌农杆菌感染石刁柏产生冠瘿瘤使其产生大量的喹啉生物碱,感染鬼针草产生大量的多炔类,感染长春花产生大量的生物碱,感染毛地黄产生大量的强心甾;利用转基因技术提高抗病虫害、抗旱抗盐等抗逆能力,或提高有效成分含量的药用植物有丹参毛状根、天仙子毛状根等。

3.1.6 药用动植物的道地性及分子机理 道地药材是古人对产于特定产地的优质中药材的称谓,其形成是特定的基因型,在特定的生境下受到复杂的调控,导致某些代谢过程的关键酶基因的表达产生了时空差异的产物。道地性研究一直是分子生药学研究的特色领域。生药道地性及其分子机理的研究,就是要在分子水平揭示道地药材居群水平的遗传变异,明确道地药材基因型特征,以及环境对道地药材基因表达的影响,从而揭示遗传因素对道地药材形成的贡献率。近年来,有学者指出道地性的遗传本质在居群水平通常是个量变的过程,它与种内其他非道地药材的区别主要表现为居群内基因型频率的改变;在个体水平表现为微效多基因控制的数量遗传,或是微效多基因和主基因联合控制的数量性状。目前药用植物次生代谢生物合成酶基因的克隆,相关转录控制因子的研究,及细胞在接受外界刺激时的信号传导研究等方面取得的成果均为从遗传、环境及信号传导等多方面来研究优质药材的形成机理提供了基础。目前,道地分子机理研究较多的生药有芍药、苍术、广藿香、厚朴、栀子等。

3.2 学科特色 分子生药学的学科特色既表现为这一学科研究和发展的困惑和困难,也是学科形成和发展的动力。学科特色主要体现在以下几个方面。

3.2.1 研究领域广泛,学科综合性很强 生药学本身就

是一门多学科综合的应用基础学科，分子生物学又是建立在生药学及其他诸多现代科学基础之上的边缘学科和综合学科，这一学科外延广泛且内涵丰富。研究中涉及生药学、分子生物学、分子遗传学、分子生态学、植物生理学、生物学、遗传学、中药化学、分析化学、生物化学等诸多学科的知识和技术，学科综合性很强，研究者个人知识背景及学科交叉的能力和素质对分子生药的研究及学科发展的影响很大。可见，复合型人才的培养，学科队伍的建设是分子生药学长期和艰巨的任务。

3.2.2 次生代谢产物积累的研究贯穿分子生药学 药用动植物与普通动植物相比，最大的区别是前者具有药用价值。由此造成了生药特殊的质量特性，即除了性状、气味、口感等外部特征外，次生代谢产物的积累及其种类和配比关系也是其质量标准的核心。纵观分子生药学的研究内容，不论是药用植物活性成分的生物合成及调控，还是分子鉴定(真伪优劣)、药用动植物的道地性(涉及药材的优质性)，或是药用动植物种质资源评价(包括品质评价)、药用动植物濒危机制及保护(优质药材更易濒危)，相关研究都与次生代谢产物的积累有直接或间接的关系。所以说次生代谢产物的积累贯穿分子生药学研究。分子水平观察和调控次生代谢产物的形成和积累是分子生药学重要内容，这一点与普通动植物，包括作物和林木等显著不同。

3.2.3 研究对象丰富多样，模式植物构建困难较大 分子生药学的研究对象为上万种药用动植物，其中常用药用动植物有数百种，与农作物、林木等研究对象相比(后者的常用种数目通常为几十种)，分子生药学的研究对象丰富多样。同时，作为贯穿分子生药学研究的主线，次生代谢产物形成机理复杂多样，其中公认的最核心的生物合成途径就有 5 条，各个途径彼此相差很大，且各途径内外部形成的复杂的代谢网络，造成以次生代谢产物的形成和积累为核心的分子生药学研究很难寻找到一个通用的理想的模式植物。

3.3 技术方法 分子生药学的常用技术方法主要包括：DNA 分析技术(分子杂交、分子标记技术、基因芯片、基因工程技术)、蛋白质分析技术(酶技术)、生物转化技术，以及生药学的常规分析方法(包括基源鉴定、显微鉴定、理化鉴定、化学成分分析)等。部分技术介绍如下。

3.3.1 DNA 分析技术 DNA 分析技术主要包括分子杂交、分子标记技术、基因芯片、基因工程技术等。

3.3.1.1 分子杂交 分子杂交(molecular hybridization)是确定单链核酸碱基序列的技术，主要用于核酸片段碱基序列的检测、鉴定及目标基因的定位等研究。主要包括固相杂交和液相杂交，其中固相膜核酸分子杂交技术又可分为菌落原位杂交(colony in situ hybridization)、斑点杂交(dot blotting)、Southern 印迹杂交(Southern blotting)、Northern 印迹杂交(Northern blotting)、组织原位杂交(tissue in situ hybridization)。

3.3.1.2 分子标记 是指以 DNA 多态性为基础的遗传标记技术。通过直接分析 DNA 的多态性，快速准确地测定 DNA 的差异性，可用于生药的鉴定、新药源的寻找开发等。

DNA 分子标记技术分以下几类。

(i) 以分子杂交为基础的分子标记技术 RFLP (restriction fragment length polymorphism)限制性内切酶片段长度多态性标记；VNTRs(variable number of tandem repeats)可变数量串联重复；DGGE－RFLP (denaturing gradient gel electrophoresis-RFLP)变性梯度凝胶电泳－RFLP。

(ii) 以 PCR 为基础的分子标记技术 RAPD(randomly amplified polymorphic DNA)随机扩增多态性 DNA；AP－PCR(arbitary primer-PCR)随机引物 PCR；DAF(DNA amplification fingerprinting)DNA 扩增产物指纹分析；SSCP (single strand conformation polymophism-RFLP)单链构象多态性；SCAR(sequence characterized amplified region)特征性片段扩增区域；CAPS(cleaved amplified polymorphism sequences)酶切扩增多态性序列，又称 PCR－RFLP；AFLP (amplified fragment length polymorphism)扩增片段长度多态性；AS－PCR(allele-specific PCR)等位基因特异 PCR；SPAR(single primer amplification reaction)单引物扩增的反应；SSR(simple sequence repeat)简单重复序列，又称微卫星 DNA(Microsatellite DNA)或 STR (short tandem repeat)短串联重复；ISSR(inter simple sequence repeat)inter－简单重复序列。

(iii) 以 PCR 和 RFLP 相结合的分子标记技术 AFLP (amplified fragment length polymorphism)扩增片段长度多态性。

(iv) 以逆转录 PCR 为基础的分子标记技术 RT－PCR (revert transcription PCR)逆转录 PCR；DD(differential display)差异显示；RDA(representative difference analysis)特征性差异分析；FQ－PCR(fluorescence quantitative polymerase chain reaction)荧光定量 PCR。

(v) 以测序为基础的分子标记技术(sequencing) SNP (single nucleotide polymorphisms)单核苷酸多态性；DNA barcoding 生物条形编码。

(vi) 基因芯片技术(DNA Chips) cDNA microarray cDNA 芯片；Oligo microarray 寡核苷酸芯片。

3.3.1.3 基因芯片 基因芯片技术系指将大量(通常每平方厘米点阵密度高于 400)探针分子固定于支持物上后与标记的样品分子进行杂交，通过检测每个探针分子的杂交信号强度进而获取样品分子的数量和序列信息的新型杂交和测序技术。这一技术由于可以一次性对样品大量序列进行高效、快速检测和分析，从而解决了传统核酸印迹杂交技术操作繁杂、自动化程度低、操作序列数量少、检测效率低等不足。可应用于基因表达谱测定、多态性分析、基因组文库作图及杂交测序等。在分子生药学中，目前主要应用于监测环境因素对道地药材基因表达的影响、主要有效成分调控基因的分析等研究。

3.3.1.4 DNA 重组技术 也称基因克隆或分子克隆，是基因工程操作的基础。它包括了一系列的实验技术，最终目的是把一个生物体中的遗传信息(DNA)转入另一个生物体。随着同源 DNA 重组技术的产生，基因工程将变得更为简易、快速和准确。该技术具有以下优点：无需使用限制性内切酶和连接酶；不改变 DNA 重组试验步骤；操作简单。目前，市售克隆载体很多。这一技术主要用于生药遗传改造及次生代谢产物的生物合成载体的构建等。

3.3.2 蛋白质分析 这一技术主要用于生药蛋白质水平变异的分析，包括蛋白质分离纯化的前处理、蛋白质的鉴定、蛋白质的盐析与透析及蛋白质的电泳技术(electrophoresis)、染色方法。其中，电泳技术包括：醋酸纤维素薄膜电泳(cellulose acetate membrane electrophoresis)；琼脂和琼脂糖凝胶电泳(agarose gel electrophoresis)；聚丙烯酰胺凝胶电泳(polyacrylamide gel electrophoresis, PAGE)；SDS-PAGE；印迹转移电泳(electrophoretic blot transfer)；聚丙烯酰胺凝胶等电聚焦(isoelectric focusing, IEF)；双向聚丙烯酰胺凝胶电泳(two-dimensional polyacrylamide gel electrophoresis)；免疫电泳(immunoelectrophoresis)。

3.3.3 生物转化技术 这一技术主要用于生药次生代谢产物积累的生物合成和生产研究，包括：(微生物、悬浮培养细胞或转基因器官)转化体系的构建和筛选；冠瘿瘤及毛状根获得及培养；添加底物诱导；生物转化产物的提取分离和鉴定等。

## 4 分子生药学的展望

4.1 生药资源永续利用的需求及技术发展导致特色领域成为热点 生药资源永续利用的需求与分子技术的优势相结合，最终决定着分子生药学研究的方向和热点。未来一段时间，分子生药学在药用动植物的系统进化、药用动植物濒危机制及保护、药用动植物道地性等原有的研究领域持续稳定发展，并将在以下领域形成热点。

4.1.1 分子鉴定稳步发展，biocoding 成为分子鉴定的重要方向 根据国家科技期刊数据库中检索结果，近年来，生药分子鉴定的文献处于快速增长阶段。随着分子生药学相关仪器及分子试剂成本的不断降低，分子生药学知识和技术将不断普及。作为分子生药学研究的核心和基础内容，分子鉴定将持续成为分子生药学的热点领域。与此同时，人们对分子鉴别的速度及方便程度提出新的要求和目标。因 DNA 条形码技术在物种鉴定方面拥有巨大的潜力，有望实现生药的快速和标准化鉴别，因而会在一段时间内成为分子生药鉴定的新热点。

4.1.2 次生代谢产物相关的功能基因组研究异军突起 基因组学(genomics)研究主要包括以全基因组测序为目标的结构基因组学(structural genomics)和以基因功能鉴定为目标的功能基因组学(functional genomics)，又被称为后基因组(postgenome)研究或后基因组学(postgenomics)。随着越来越多全基因序列的获得，人们在将基因组静态的碱基序列弄清楚之后，逐步转入对基因组动态的生物学功能学研究。次生代谢及其调控的分子机理是分子生药学的特色领域，促进和调控次生代谢产物合成是分子生药研究的重要目标之一。近年来，次生代谢途径的基础研究越来越受到重视，次生代谢产物的关键酶基因的研究取得积极进展。随着生药基因工程、组织培养、生物转化技术水平的整体提高，次生代谢产物相关的功能基因组研究异军突起，并将成为分子生药学研究中最富挑战和前景的方向之一。

4.1.3 基因组学、蛋白组学、代谢组学研究结果的整合和分析成为新热点 基因组学(genomics)、蛋白质组学(proteomics)、代谢组学(metabonomics/metabolomics)虽然均是在分子水平开展生药相关研究，但三者各有其优势和独特性，基因组学主要研究功能基因等基因层面的内容，蛋白质组学主要研究差异蛋白等蛋白质层面的内容，代谢组学主要研究次生代谢物，三者的分工不同。次生代谢产物是典型的多基因性状，其积累很大程度上受到环境尤其是环境胁迫的影响，主要在基因表达和蛋白水平发生变异。随着代谢组学、蛋白组学在分子生药研究中的不断拓展，将基因组、蛋白质组和代谢组三个不同层次的研究结果进行整合分析，从而获得超越三个组学各自领域的知识和信息将成为一种新的趋势。

4.1.4 核心种质构建形成新思路和新方法 核心种质(core collection)是种质资源的一个核心子集，以最少数量的遗传资源最大限度地保存整个资源群体的遗传多样性，同时代表了整个群体的地理分布。核心种质是生药种质资源群体研究和利用的切入点，可提高整个种质库的管理和利用水平。生药资源核心种质的构建模式主要参考农作物，后者通常是在已有种质资源库或已有大量种质资源的基础上，按照科学的取样方法与技术，从中选出约 10%样品，在一定程度上，代表了某一种及其近缘野生种的形态特征、地理分布、基因与基因型的最大范围的遗传多样性。与农作物种质资源研究形成明显区别的是，多数生药资源本身不具备种质资源库，而且不少野生、甚至珍稀濒危物种很难收集到大量种质。这一方面是由于生药资源研究基础较薄弱，另一方面，也与生药资源种类繁多，而且多数种质数量有限，种质资源库构建难度很大有关。显然，生药核心种质的构建模式无法也不该照搬农作物核心种质模式。在未来一段时间，如何发挥分子生药技术和方法在遗传多样性检测方面的优势，充分利用有限的材料，在分析药用动植物基因型上的差异，以及不同基因型对环境反应上的差异，特别是遗传结构的基础上，配合混合线性模型等统计分析，无偏预测生药性状的基因型值，用预测出的基因型值计算遗传材料间的遗传距离，准确评价不同材料间在遗传上的相似性，通过设计合理的抽样策略，构建生药核心种质库，并建立生药学核心种质构建的特有模式势在必行。

4.2 理论体系进一步完善 分子生药学从概念的提出到第一本《分子生药学》著作的出版历经 6 年时间，又经过了 8 年时间进入全国高等院校创新教材系列。在这短短十几年的时间里，越来越多的人参与到这一领域的研究中来，学科取得了突飞猛进的发展。随着研究的不断深入，许多分子层面的研究结果给人以新的启迪，人们对生药的认识不断深入。例如，生药多样性及种内变异的研究，使人们开始重新思考生药的标准化问题及解决策略；对次生代谢产物形成微效多基因及其与环境的互作，以及基因网络化和程序表达的认识，引发了人们对生药基因调控、品种选育的思考。又如，次生代谢产物的生物合成本身是个极复杂的系统工程，它有相对独立的一套理论、方法和技术，研究的深化要求人们对其在分子生药学学科中的地位进行思考。相应的思考会导致分子生药学理论体系的不断完善。

4.3 应用实践进一步加强 生药学是一门来源于实践的应用学科。虽然，有关分子层面机理的研究增加了分子生药学学科的理论成分，但分子生药学依然继承了生药学面向应用的这一属性，解决生药在生产实践和保护利用中的具体问题依然是学科发展的航标。分子生药学研究成果在实践中的应用是学科存在的意义所在，也是衡量学科健康发展的重要标志。目前，利用分子生药学技术对栝楼属的系统分类的结果同时被 *Flora of China*（第 19 卷）及 2000 年《中国药典》采纳是分子生药研究结果应用的典范。相信在不远的未来，这一领域的应用实践会进一步得到加强。

［黄璐琦，等. 中国科学，2009，39(12)：1101－1110.］

# 分子生药学栏目编者按

分子生药学是在分子水平上研究生药的鉴定、生产和成分的一门科学。1995 年，黄璐琦在《展望分子生物技术在生药学中的应用》一文中首次提出了“分子生药学”（Molecular Pharmacognosy）的概念。经过 20 余年的发展，分子生药学逐步建立了较为完善的理论体系、研究内容和技术方法。

2012 年，分子生药学成为国家中医药管理局重点学科（培育）。作为一门新兴的交叉学科，分子生药学学科已走过萌芽期、形成期、快速发展期，正在进入成熟期，已形成了覆盖全国的分子生药学科研机构和学术队伍，逐步建立了面向本科-硕士-博士研究生以及在职人员的纵向多层次学科教学体系，建成了由实验室-重点学科-学术期刊支撑的多元化的学科平台，在理论体系、研究平台、技术方法、学科队伍等方面均取得了显著的成绩。

## 1　理论体系建设

分子生药学理论体系不断发展完善，先后提出了道地药材形成的生物学本质及其 3 个模式假说、中药分子鉴定的使用原则、珍稀濒危常用中药资源 5 种保护模式、基于一个系统的“功能基因挖掘-合成途径解析-生物合成生产”的中药活性成分合成生物学研究模式等。2000 年，分子生药学第一本专著正式出版；2006 年，《分子生药学》第 2 版出版。2010 年《分子生药学》获得中华中医药学会著作奖一等奖。2012 年《分子生药学》（英文版）由 Springer 出版社发行，标志分子生药学获得了国际的认可。2015 年，出版了《分子生药学》第 3 版，其在对前 2 版进行补充和完善的基础上，增加了最新的研究方法和研究领域成果，丰富了分子生药学的内涵与外延。

## 2　研究平台建设

随着分子生药学在中药科研工作中的作用日益加强，目前国内大多数中医药院校均建有分子生药学实验室。2003 年，国家中医药管理局“生药分子鉴定”三级实验室建立。2006 年，沈阳药科大学与韩国东亚大学联合建立了“中韩分子生药学实验室”。2009 年，“国家中医药管理局道地药材生态遗传重点研究室”认定。2016 年，道地药材国家重点实验室培育基地的验收通过，成为行业内第一个局部共建的国家级重点实验室，标志着分子生药学研究平台达到国家领先水平。同时，蒙药分子生药学实验室、贵州特色分子生药学实验室、湖北道地药材分子生药学实验室等相继成立。

## 3　技术方法体系创建

将分子生物学与生药学相结合，发展具有中药特色的分子生药学技术方法是分子生药学学科建设的重要任务之一。其中蛇类饮片分子鉴定方法被《中国药典》（2010 年版）采纳，成为首个收载于《中国药典》的中药分子鉴定方法，标志着分子鉴定从实验室阶段进入应用阶段。2013 年提出了中药分子鉴别现场运用策略，开启了分子鉴定技术产品化和产业化进程。2014 年，“十二五”国家重点图书出版规划项目《中药分子鉴定操作指南》出版；2016 年，《中药资源转录组分析操作指南》出版，标志着具有中药特色的分子生药学技术体系正在建成。

## 4　学科队伍建设

2001 年，北京中医药大学和沈阳药科大学分别开展了分子生药学本科和研究生教学。2008 年，新世纪全国高等中医药院校创新教材《分子生药学》由中国中医药出版社出版。2015 年《分子生药学》入选国家卫生和计划生育委员会“十三五”研究生教材、2016 年《分子生药学》入选中医药行业“十三五”规划教材，标志着分子生药学独立完整教育体系的形成，目前国内 30 余所高等院校针对本科或研究生开设了分子生药学课程。自 2012 年起，在国家中医药管理局分子生药学继续教育重点项目的支持下，中国中医科学院中药资源中心联合中医药院校举办分子生药学暑期学术交流活动，先后有 530 余名研究生和青年教师代表参加，促进了分子生药学教学和科研水平提升，推动了分子生药学学科的发展。

在 2016 年江苏镇江举办的第五届分子生药学暑期研讨会上，与会专家认为分子生药学学科始终保持着快速发展的势头，且随着生命科学以及生物技术的发展，其内涵和外延都发生了很大的变化。分子生药学已形成了以“基础研究为重点，以创新研究为核心，以应用研究为目标”的学科建设思路，更加注重将理论与实践紧密结合，突出中医药特色，解决生药学的实际问题。分子生药学学科现阶段发展的主要任务“中药分子鉴定是基础、道地药材形成的分子机制是特色、应用合成生物学生产活性成分是前沿”，分子生药学研究领域的热点和重点正引领着中药资源、中药鉴定、中药品质形成与质量评价等研究的方向。

为响应与会专家建议，体现新形势下分子生药学学科蓬勃发展态势，鼓励多学科交叉融合与创新，《中国中药杂志》率先设立开放和包容的分子生药学专栏，稿件内容将涵盖分子生药学领域科研与教学的最新成果，将进一步推进各科研院所、高等院校分子生药学科研教学事业的发展，同时也对相关中药产业起到促进带动作用。

[黄璐琦.中国中药杂志，2017，42(2)：203－204.]

# 附

## 《分子生药学》(第一版)王永炎序

众所周知，中医治病有针灸、推拿、气功、中药等各种各样的方法。因此，古人早就有专门从事中药研究的学者，记载这种学问的书籍当时称为"本草"。汉代成书的《神农本草经》冠以三皇之一的神农氏为作者，这同《黄帝内经》托名黄帝的意义是一致的。当今人们则普遍认同，中华民族的兴衰从祖先起就与中医药防治疾病的卓越疗效联结在一起。

中药现在作为整个中医药研究领域的重要学科，与如今人们对疾病和健康的认识有关。只有当社会安定、人民丰衣足食时人们才有可能关心健康需要，这是一个进步，社会的需要是推动科学发展的动力。近年来中药的发展已不仅仅在于经验方的搜集、传统剂型的改革、新药的开发等，有些学者已开始注意从新思路、新方法、新技术方面去扩展新的研究领域，这种勇于探索的精神正是科学的精神。青年科学工作者黄璐琦博士主编的《分子生药学》正是这种勇于探索的代表著作。

科学发展进入20世纪末，有几个显著的特点：一是高度综合与高度分化的矛盾，科学越发展，学科分科也就越细越多，而任何一个实际问题的解决，都往往不是一个学科的事情，科学技术是一个有机的整体，既要注意其整体性，又要注意不断发展出来的新学科；二是继承与发展的矛盾，任何学科都是在继承与发展相结合的过程中，继承是源头、是基础，发展是目的、是归宿，在量变与质变的过程中不断发展；三是国际化的趋势，"科学是无国界的"在当今越来越被证实，如今世界上任何一个角落发生的重大科学技术发明与进步，都在迅速影响其他国家和地区。

分子生物学是在物理学与化学对生物学的交融和渗透下，逐渐由观察生命活动的现象深入到认识生命活动的本质，从而形成的一门学科。分子生物学不断发展，从20世纪后半期就对整个科学领域产生巨大影响。生药学本身也是在不断发展，翻开短短不到100年的教科书，对于生药学的认识就已大相径庭了。把分子生物学的方法引入到生药学的研究领域中，提出分子生药学研究领域，是一个进步。它从原来简单的方法带入，到系统接受，消化融合，达到一个新学科的产生。

分子生药学有很好的应用前景，主要表现在中药高产、优质、多抗性品种的培育，濒危紧缺中药资源的保护和持续利用以及中药新的、便捷、准确的分子标识鉴定方法的研究三方面，使生药学的研究对象不仅在组织、器官、有机体、居群等层次，而且使其扩展到基因层次，为过去不能很好解决的问题如道地药材的研究、药材品质的定向调控等提供新的方法和思路。

当然，这本《分子生药学》才刚刚起步，难免有疏漏，我们希望黄璐琦和他的同道们共同努力，在实践中不断摸索经验，学习国内外的新技术新方法，在理论上不断提高，使分子生药学更为成熟。

在《分子生药学》成书之际，庆贺黄璐琦博士等所取得的成就，爰为之序。

## 《分子生药学》(第一版)肖培根序

生药学(Pharmacognosy)是一门研究生药材的学科，已经有近200年的历史。随着历史的发展，其研究内容从组织形态，化学成分到化学分类，组织培养等，不断在发展和更新。现在大家对生药学的认识，普遍认为它是一门应用现代多学科的方法手段来解决生药材中各种技术和理论问题的专门学科。

到了20世纪中叶，随着DNA双螺旋结构的发现和确定，带来了分子生物学的迅猛发展。乃至科学界都认为：21世纪分子生物学将得到进一步发展并占有统治地位，而且将深刻影响到生命科学的各个领域。有鉴于此，美国生药学权威泰勒(Tyler)教授和他的同事在1996年出版的生药学新版本中，加强了生物技术方面的内容，取名为《生药学和药学生物技术》(Robbers JE. Speedie MK & VE Tyler：*Pharmacognosy and Pharmacobiotechnology*，Williams and Wilkins，Baltimors)。

无独有偶，以黄璐琦教授为代表的我国年轻一代的生药学科技工作者，以他们的敏锐洞察力预见到将先进的分子生物学的原理和方法引入到传统生药学科的重要性和必要性，并倡导提出它可以成为生药学学科中的一个分支学科——分子生药学（Molecular Pharmacognosy）的观点。他们身体力行，群策群力，结合他们各自的工作和本领域的新动向，编撰出版了这部《分子生药学》专著。应该说，他们这种勇于实践，敢于创新的精神是十分值得鼓励和赞扬的。

当然，要解决生药材在生产和研究中的各种具体问题，还需要从分子、细胞组织、器官、整体乃至群体的水平，从多个层次，多个角度应用各种方法手段才能获得满意的结果。但无疑从分子水平来研究生药材有利于从更加深入的层次和水平来阐明它们内在的各种客观规律，从而带动生药学的进一步发展。

从上述的各种意义，我不但乐于为这部著作作序，而且更要鞭策自己参加到这个行列中去，为我国生药学的蓬勃发展贡献自己的一份力量。

# 《分子生药学》（第二版）桑国卫序

2000年《分子生药学》的出版，为生药学科引入了新的理论方法和技术，使我国生药学上了一个新台阶，从而使生药学发展出一个新的分支学科“分子生药学”。自《分子生药学》第1版以来已经有五年的时间了，在这5年里，分子生药学作为一门学科取得了突飞猛进的发展，无论对生药学这一领域本身的建设，还是对研究生的教育都产生了深远的影响。目前，此书已被北京大学、复旦大学、华西医科大学等院校作为研究生的教材。

作为分子生药学的编著者，他们这5年来继续努力，不断完善分子生药学的理论和方法，在分子生药学的不同研究领域承担了多项国家级课题，先后获得中华中医药学会科学技术奖、中国中西医结合学会科学技术奖、中华医学会科学技术奖、北京市科技进步奖等，其中“栝楼属植物的系统演化及其药材的分子标识研究”获国家科学技术进步奖二等奖。与此同时，建立了国家中医药管理局的生药分子鉴定三级实验室，培养了多名从事分子生药学研究的硕士和博士，形成了一支蓬勃向上的科研队伍，这支年轻的队伍紧抓生药学科发展前沿，不断创新和拓展分子生药学的新领域，编著完成了第二版《分子生药学》。

第二版除对第一版内容进行修改完善外，还新增了道地药材形成的分子机理研究、珍稀濒危中药资源的遗传多样性分析和保护策略研究、药用植物的抗性基因工程研究、药用化学成分的生物转化及分子机理研究等章节。这些章节不仅是对最新工作进展的总结和提炼，更是对分子生药学研究领域的新的探索，这无疑会带来更大的挑战。我相信有这一群执着追求的年轻人，分子生药学这一学科的发展会越来越好。鉴于此，欣然为之序。

# 《分子生药学》（第三版）刘昌孝序

“分子生物学”（Molecular Biology）一词最早是1945年William Astbury在*Harvey Lecture*上应用。1953年Watson和Crick发现DNA双螺旋结构后，分子生物学迅速成为20世纪发展最快、对人类影响最大的学科之一。分子生物学的研究与发展不断深化和提升本学科的理论和技术，而且，分子生物学不断地与其他学科进行广泛而深入的交叉融合，以此开拓新的前沿领域和新的增长点，使得一大批交叉科学、边缘学科和前沿学科应运而生，如分子遗传学、植物分子遗传学、分子系统学、分子生态学、蛋白组学、基因组学等。

1995年，黄璐琦在《中国中药杂志》上发表《展望分子生物技术在生药学中的应用》一文，首次提出了“分子生药学”（Molecular Pharmacognosy）的概念。到现在为止，分子生药学已有近20年的发展历程。特别是在2000年，黄璐琦主编的《分子生药学》第一版在北京医科大学出版社出版，标志着一门崭新的生药学分支学科——分子生药学在国内诞生。此后，此书成为复旦大学、北京大学和华西医科大学等高校的研究生教材。2006年《分子生药学》第二版出版，2008年适合高等院校本科生使用的《分子生药学》教材出版。迄今，全国已有20余所高等院校开设本科生和研究生课程。2012年，黄璐琦主编的《分子生药学》（英文版）由Springer出版社发行，该书的出版，标志分子生药学获得了国际的认可。同年，分子生药学成为国家中医药管理局重点学科（培育）。经过近20年的建设和发展，分子生药学研究硕果累累。如建立高特异性聚合酶链反应技术鉴别中药材乌梢蛇真伪方法，被2010年版《中华人民共和国药典》收载，这是分子鉴别方法首次收载于国家药典；发现了一条丹参酮特有的二萜生物合成新途径等。与此同时，相继建立了国家中医药管理局生药分子鉴定三级实验室、国家中医药管理局道地药材生态遗传重点研究室、道地药材国家重点实验室培育基地，以及蒙药分子生药学实验室和贵州特色分子生药学实验室等研究平台。

作为分子生药学的开拓者和编著者，他们不断开展了一些创新的研究工作，以丰富和完善本学科的理论和方法，使分子生药学成了理论思想创新、研究方向稳定、技术水平领先、学术影响广泛、人才队伍不断壮大的一门日益成熟的交叉学科，成为生药学的一个极富前瞻性和生命力的分支。

第三版在前两版的基础上，紧跟科学前沿和最新发展动态，更加注重解决生药学的实际问题，特别是道地药材形成分子机制、分子育种、药用成分的生物合成等方面的工作。这是对分子生药学研究领域新的探索，无疑会带来更大的挑战。本人愿意与这群执着追求的年轻人一起，为分子生药学的发展贡献一份力量。鉴于此，欣然为之作序。

# Molecular Pharmacognosy(第一版)序

With its development over almost 200 years, pharmacognosy has existed as one applied science with comparably impeccable theory and technology. With the passage of time, it also faces various problems which cannot be solved by current technology and methodology, e.g., the exact identification of the "species" level of medicinal plants without flowers and fruits, sustainable uses of rarc and endangered medicinal resources, and directional control of the qualities of medical materials. All of these greatly need to be settled by introducing new technology and methodology.

Ever since the discovery of DNA's double helix structure and its semiconservative replication, the molecular biology technology has almost permeated into all the fields of life science, thus generating quite a number of interdisciplinary subjects. It can be clearly anticipated that molecular biology will still lead the development in life science in the twenty-first century. Without keeping out of the affair, pharmacognosy will combine with molecular biology and bring about new areas in its studies.

During the collision between pharmacognosy and molecular biology, how can we grasp and choose the binding point of the two? What is the theoretical basis for their binding? This is the problem I often pondered upon during my graduate studies. After continuous studies and thoughts as well as discussions with my teachers and classmates, I put forward the concept of "molecular pharmacognosy" in the article *Anticipation on the Application of Molecular Biological Technology in Pharmacognosy* published in 1995. I had never thought that its publication would arouse such strong resonance among so many scholars. They raised their own ideas, which encouraged me to do further researches. Along with 5-year research quest and practice, the rudiment of a new science, "molecular pharmacognosy", came into being with its own theory and technology.

In the past 15 years, owing to my research work and other researchers at home and abroad, the technology of molecular biology has been widely applied and practiced in relevant fields of pharmacognosy. Molecular pharmacognosy has been further developed theoretically and systematically. Up to now, the Chinese edition of molecular pharmacognosy has been copied twice with new research contents added in each edition, thus making the system of molecular pharmacognosy more abundant and more complete gradually. Besides, the course of molecular pharmacognosy has been opened up in Beijing University of Chinese Medicine, West China University of Medical Sciences, Fudan University, Huazhong University of Science and Technology, and other institutions of high learning. The innovative teaching material of molecular pharmacognosy was published in 2008. All of these sped up the advancement of the cultivation of research talents in molecular pharmacognosy and the subject's development.

Along with deeper researches of molecular pharmacognosy and more perfection of the subject's theoretical system, there are more researches in the field worldwide. Internationalization of molecular pharmacognosy, a new subject, is on schedule. Under this circumstance, we compiled this internationalized edition of molecular pharmacognosy in cooperation with experts and scholars in this field from Mainland China, Hong Kong, Taiwan. South Korea, and Japan in the hope for furthering the internationalized development of molecular pharmacognosy.

Initialized in the middle of 2010, this book is divided into nine chapters. The first chapter, "Emerging molecular pharmacognosy", mainly introduces the historical background, concepts, and research contents of molecular pharmacognosy as well as its relations with other subjects. "Methodology", being the second chapter, from the perspective of molecular pharmacognosy, introduces some common methods of molecular pharmacognosy researches and part of the new research thinking and methods, e.g., "Ingredient difference phenotypic cloning". Furthermore, some practical problems solved by molecular pharmacognosy have been discussed from the aspect of methodological application. The third chapter is "Molecular Identification of traditional medicinal materials". It mainly discusses the common methods to identify the Chinese medical molecules, and then, there is some exploration of molecular identification of the family, genus, inter-species, and under-species of original Chinese medical plants. The fourth chapter is "The mechanism of formation of Dao-di Herbs", with the specialty of Chinese herb Dao-di and theoretical hypothesis that have been formed as the main contents. The fifth chapter is "Seeking for new members of origin materials (a new usage of plant species) for CMM", centered on the introduction of the theory and methodology of pharmaphylogeny. The sixth chapter is "Gene modification of pharmic plants germplasm resources", with the main contents of the concept, classification, collection, and identification of pharmic plants' germplasm resources. The eighth chapter is "Regulation of the 'active constituents' production of medicinal plants". It mainly talks about the regulation of the active constituents' production of medicinal plants in biotransformation, generic engineering, and other methods. The ninth chapter is "Molecular mechanism and regulation on biosynthesis of active ingredients of medicinal plants", with the main contents of research overview, significance, as well as the basic strategies and ways of the biosynthesis of active ingredients of medicinal plants.

The publication of this book is intended to explicate the concept, theory, and methodology of molecular pharmacognosy and encourage more people in the same pursuit to solve more new problems of pharmacognosy with fully utilizing the developing technology and methodology of biology within the framework of molecular pharmacognosy.

It should be noted that compilation of this book is the fruit of all the international experts in the field of pharmacognosy. Considering the molecular pharmacognosy is a new inter-discipline to be further improved, we sincerely hope that more professionals will raise more advice and support to improve the maturity and development of molecular pharmacognosy.

# *Molecular Pharmacognosy*(第二版)序

With almost 200 years of development, pharmacognosy exists as an applied science with comparably impeccable theory and technology. As times advance, it faces various problems that cannot be solved by current technology and methodology, for example, the exact identification of the "species" level of medicinal plants, sustainable use of rare and endangered medicinal resources, and directional control of medical material quality. All of these issues greatly need to be settled by introducing new technologies and methodologies.

Ever since the discovery of DNA's double-helix structure and semi-conservative replication, molecular biology technology has permeated into almost all fields of life science, thus generating quite a number of interdisciplinary subjects. It can be clearly anticipated that molecular biology will lead the development of life science through-out the twenty-first century. Pharmacognosy will combine with molecular biology and bring about new areas of study.

During this collision between pharmacognosy and molecular biology, how can we grasp and choose the binding point of the two? What is the theoretical basis for their binding? This is the problem I often pondered upon during my graduate studies. After continuous study and thought, as well as discussions with my teachers and classmates, I put forward the concept of "molecular pharmacognosy" in an article titled "Anticipation on the Application of Molecular Biological Technology in Pharmacognosy", published in 1995. I had never thought that its publication would arouse such strong resonance among so many scholars. They raised their own ideas which encouraged me to do further research. Along with a 5-year research quest and practice, the rudiments of a new field, "molecular pharmacognosy", came into being with its own theories and technologies.

In the past 15 years, owing to the research work of the author and other researchers at home and abroad, the technology of molecular biology has been widely applied and practised in the relevant fields of pharmacognosy. Molecular pharmacognosy has been further developed theoretically and systematically. Up to now, the Chinese edition of *Molecular Pharmacognosy* has been copied three times, with new research contents added to each edition, thus making the system of molecular pharmacognosy more abundant and gradually more complete. Besides, the course of molecular pharmacognosy has been opened up at China Academy of Chinese Medical Sciences, Beijing University of Chinese Medicine, China Pharmaceutical University, Shenyang Pharmaceutical University, Tongji Medical College of Huazhong University of Science & Technology, Shanghai University of Traditional Chinese Medicine and other institutions of higher education. The innovative teaching material of molecular pharmacognosy was published in 2008. All of these have sped up the advancement of the cultivation of research talents in molecular pharmacognosy, as well as the subject's development as a whole.

Along with deeper studies of molecular pharmacognosy

and further perfection of the subject's theoretical system, there are an increasing number of studies in the field worldwide. The internationalization of molecular pharmacognosy, a new subject, is scheduled. Under this circumstance, this internationalized edition of *Molecular Pharmacognosy* was first published in 2013. This time, we have cooperated with experts and scholars in this field from multiple countries in the hope of furthering the internationalized development of molecular pharmacognosy and gradually making the field of molecular pharmacognosy more abundant and complete.

This second edition is divided into ten chapters. The first chapter, "Emerging Molecular Pharmacognosy", mainly introduces the historical background, concepts, and research contents of molecular pharmacognosy, as well as its relations to other subjects. The second chapter is "Molecular Identification of Traditional Medicinal Materials". It mainly discusses the common methods to identify Chinese medical materials and also explores the molecular identification of families, genera, species, and varieties of original Chinese medical plants and animals. The third chapter, "Seeking New Resource Materials for TCM", is centred on the introduction of the development of plant systematics, research methods of plant systematics, theoretical bases of the molecular systematics of medicinal plants, and some case studies on medicinal plant resources. The fourth chapter, "Phylogeography of Medicinal Plants", mainly introduces the background, basic theories, methods, application of molecular phylogeography in biological evolution, application of phylogeography in the evolution of medicinal plants, and a case studies on medicinal plant. The fifth chapter, "Salvation of Rare and Endangered Medicinal Plants", mainly discusses the theory, concept, method, and practice of protecting traditional Chinese medicine resources, and introduces reasons for the destruction of Chinese medicine resources, classification of endangered medicinal plants and animals, and specific examples of Chinese medicine resource protection. The sixth chapter, "Gene Modification of Medical Plant Germplasm Resources", mainly describes the concept, investigation, collection, and evaluation of medical plant germplasm resources. The seventh chapter, "Functional Genome of Medicinal Plants", introduces genomics, transcriptomics, proteomics, metabolomics, epigenomics, etc. The eighth chapter, "Molecular Mechanisms and Gene Regulation for Biosynthesis of Medicinal Plant Active Ingredients", mainly talks about the biosynthetic pathway, related functional genes, and regulation for the biosynthesis of active ingredients in medicinal plants. The ninth chapter, "Synthetic Biology of Active Compounds", contains an overview of synthetic biology in traditional Chinese medicine (TCM). The chapter describes the biological basis of synthesizing active ingredients of TCM, analyses key links in the study of synthetic biology in TCM, and discusses the application of synthetic biology for the sustainable utilization of TCM resources. The tenth chapter, "The Mechanisms of Dao-di Herb Formation", mainly focuses on China's special Dao-di herbs and the theoretical hypotheses of their formation mechanisms.

The publication of this book is intended to explicate the concepts, theories, and methodologies of molecular pharmacognosy and encourage more people in similar fields to solve more new problems of pharmacognosy by fully utilizing the developing technologies and methodologies of biology within the framework of molecular pharmacognosy.

Considering that molecular pharmacognosy is a new interdisciplinary field that needs to be further improved, we sincerely hope that more professionals will raise more attention and give more support to increasing the development of this emerging discipline.

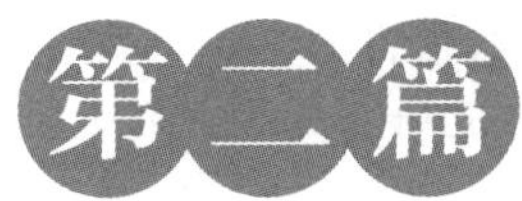

# 第二篇 生药分子鉴定

# 用随机扩增多态DNA(RAPD)技术鉴别中药材天花粉及其类似品

天花粉是很有价值的一味中药。从中提出的天花粉蛋白(trichosanthin)已广泛应用于早期和中期妊娠引产,治疗宫外孕、葡萄胎等疾病,近年又用于艾滋病的治疗。然而,全国各地所用天花粉的来源很多。据调查,不同植物来源的天花粉,其疗效也不完全一致,某些混淆品,如湖北栝楼根与木鳖子根,还有一定的副作用(表1)。为保证用药安全有效,我们已对这些天花粉商品作了药材性状和显微鉴定等方面的研究。为了探索药材鉴别上的新方法,根据随机扩增多态DNA(random amplified polymorphic DNA, RAPD)技术已成功地应用于遗传多样性的检测和品系鉴定,本文拟采用这一方法对不同来源的真伪天花粉商品进行鉴定,并对这一方法应用在中药材鉴定方面的问题进行初步探讨。

## 1 仪器和材料

1.1 仪器 1169型电脑全自动基因扩增仪(北京市新技术应用研究所);Micro-MB 3616型高速离心机(IEC公司,美国);UV-Ⅰ型多功能紫外透射仪(北京市新技术应用研究所)。

1.2 材料 取自中国中医研究院中药研究所标本室,为室温干燥后放入标本瓶中保存,材料经黄璐琦研究员鉴定(表1)。

**表1 商品天花粉的来源、贮存时间及使用概况**

| 类别 | 编号 | 名称 | 学名 | 产地 | 贮存时间 | 使用概况 |
|---|---|---|---|---|---|---|
| 大宗商品 | 1 | 栝楼 | *Trichosanthes kirilowii* Maxim. | 河南郑州 | 16年 | 粉多色白质佳,销全国 |
| | 2 | 栝楼 | *T. kirilowii* Maxim. | 湖北鄂州 | 1年 | |
| | 3 | 栝楼 | *T. kirilowii* Maxim. | 湖北蒲圻 | 1年 | |
| | 4 | 双边栝楼 | *T. rosthornii* Harms | 四川南川 | 20年以上 | 筋多,质量一般,习称川花粉 |
| | 5 | 双边栝楼 | *T. rosthornii* Harms | 四川南川 | 1年 | |
| 小宗商品 | 6 | 多卷须栝楼 | *T. rosthornii* Harms var. *multicirrata* S. K. Chen | 贵州罗甸 | 16年 | 广西习称"老品种",因产量少挖取不便,现已少用。 |
| | 7 | 黄山栝楼 | *T. rosthornii* Harms var. *huangshanensis* S. K. Chen | 产地不详 | 20年以上 | 湖北、江西多用此种 |
| | 8 | 黄山栝楼 | *T. rosthornii* Harms var. *huangshanensis* S. K. Chen | 江西婺源 | 当年 | |
| | 9 | 尖果栝楼 | *T. rosthornii* Harms var. *stylopodifera* L. Q. Huang | 贵州雷山 | 16年 | 筋多粉少,质量较差 |
| | 10 | 尖果栝楼 | *T. rosthornii* Harms var. *stylopodifera* L. Q. Huang | 贵州锦屏 | 16年 | |
| 混淆品或地区习惯用药 | 11 | 井冈山栝楼 | *T. jinggangshanica* Yueh | 江西井冈山 | 1年 | 江西西南部多用此种,质量与双边栝楼近似 |
| | 12 | 井冈山栝楼 | *T. jinggangshanica* Yueh | 江西井冈山 | 1年 | |
| | 13 | 湖北栝楼 | *T. hupehensis* C. Y. Cheng et C. H. Yueh | 四川南川 | 1年 | 味极苦,服后有不良反应 |
| | 14 | 湖北栝楼 | *T. hupehensis* C. Y. Cheng et C. H. Yueh | 四川南川 | 1年 | |
| | 15 | 长萼栝楼 | *T. laceribractea* Hayata | 四川南川 | 1年 | 两广使用较多,并调省外 |
| | 16 | 长萼栝楼 | *T. laceribractea* Hayata | 四川南川 | 1年 | |
| | 17 | 红花栝楼 | *T. rubriflos* Thorel et Cayla | 云南思茅 | 15年 | 质量极差 |
| | 18 | 糙点栝楼 | *T. dunniana* Levl. | 云南大理 | 15年 | 质量较差,不宜作天花粉用 |
| | 19 | 糙点栝楼 | *T. dunniana* Levl. | 云南德宏 | 15年 | |
| | 20 | 马干铃栝楼 | *T. lepiniana* (Naud.) Cogn. | 云南勐海 | 16年 | |
| | 21 | 趾叶栝楼 | *T. pedata* Merr. et Chun | 云南勐腊 | 15年 | 广西用治疮疖,偶有混用 |

（续表）

| 类别 | 编号 | 名称 | 学名 | 产地 | 贮存时间 | 使用概况 |
|---|---|---|---|---|---|---|
| | 22 | 王瓜 | *T. cucumeroides* (Ser.) Maxim. | 江西婺源 | 当年 | 有时混入 |
| | 23 | 木鳖 | *Momordica cochinchinensis* (Lour.) Spreng. | 产地不详 | 20年以上 | 四川、贵州、广西、湖北等地均曾误用，服后有不良反应 |
| | 24 | 三开瓢 | *Adenia cardiophylla* (Mast.) Engl. | 云南瑞丽 | 15年 | |
| | 25 | 异叶马瓞儿 | *Melothria heterophylla* (Lour.) Cogn. | 产地不详 | 20年以上 | 云南使用较多 |

注：①大宗商品：分布广，产量大，质量较佳。②小宗商品：分布较窄，产地自用，质量一般。③混淆品：质量极差或服后有不良反应。④地区习惯用药：产地使用有年，服后未见不良反应。

## 2 引物和试剂

2.1 引物 所用引物序列见表2，由华美生物工程公司合成。

**表2 本实验所用引物序列**

| 引物号 | 序列 5′→3′ |
|---|---|
| 1 | CAAACGTCGG |
| 2 | AGGGGTCTTG |
| 3 | GTGACGTAGG |
| 4 | AATCGGGCTG |
| 5 | GGGTAACGCC |
| 6 | CAGGCCCTTC |
| 7 | CAGCACCCAC |
| 8 | AGTCAGCCAC |

注：A为脱氧腺嘌呤核苷酸，C为脱氧胞嘧啶核苷酸，G为脱氧鸟嘌呤核苷酸，T为脱氧胸腺嘧啶核苷酸。

2.2 试剂 *Taq* DNA聚合酶（*Taq* DNA polymerase；U-P Biotech, Inc. USA）；琼脂糖（Agarose；Promega公司）；游离脱氧核苷三磷酸（deoxynucleoside triphosphate, dNTPs；Promega公司）；十六烷基三乙基溴化铵（cetyltriethylammonmium bromide, CTAB；Sigma公司）；溴化乙锭（Fluka公司）；水为高压灭菌后的去离子水；其余试剂为北京化工厂产的分析纯。

2.3 试剂的配制

2.3.1 所需贮存液的配制

2.3.1.1 0.5 mol/L EDTA溶液（pH 8.0） 在800 mL水中加入186.1 g二水乙二胺四乙酸二钠（EDTA-Na·$2H_2O$），在磁力搅拌器上剧烈搅拌，用氢氧化钠调节溶液的pH至8.0（约需氢氧化钠颗粒20 g），然后定容至1 L，分装后高压灭菌备用。

2.3.1.2 5 mol/L氯化钠溶液 在800 mL水中溶解292.2 g氯化钠，加水定容至1 L，分装后高压灭菌。

2.3.1.3 1 mol/L Tris-HCl溶液（pH 8.0） 在800 mL水中溶解121.1 g三羟甲基氨基甲烷[tris (hydroxymethyl) aminomethane, Tris]，加入浓盐酸42 mL调节pH至所需值。应使溶液冷至室温后方可最后调定pH，加水定容至1 L，分装后高压灭菌。

2.3.1.4 50×TAE电泳缓冲液的浓贮存液 Tris碱242 g，冰乙酸57.1 mL，0.5 mol/L EDTA（pH 8.0）100 mL，加蒸馏水配成1 L溶液。

2.3.2 所需缓冲液的组成

2.3.2.1 提取缓冲液 2%（*W/V*）CTAB，100 m mol/L Tris-HCl（pH 8.0），20 mmol/L EDTA，1.4 mol/L氯化钠，2%巯基乙醇。

2.3.2.2 沉淀缓冲液 1%（*W/V*）CTAB，50 mmol/L Tris-HCl（pH 8.0），10 mmol/L EDTA，1%巯基乙醇。

2.3.2.3 TE（pH 8.0） 10 mmol/L Tris-HCl（pH 8.0），1 mmol/L EDTA（pH 8.0）。

2.3.2.4 1×TAE电泳缓冲液 组成为0.04 mol/L Tris-乙酸，0.001 mol/L EDTA。由50×TAE稀释50倍而成。

## 3 方法

3.1 DNA模板的提取和浓度测定 取药材坚实部分粉碎，过中国药典4号筛，取少许置1.5 mL微型离心管中，立即加入保温60℃的提取缓冲液500 μL及巯基乙醇20 μL混匀，60℃保温40 min；加入等体积的氯仿-异丙醇（24∶1）抽提，轻轻颠倒混匀，10 000 r/min离心10 min，吸取上清液，加入1/10体积的10% CTAB溶液，再加入等体积氯仿-异丙醇（24∶1）重复抽提1次，吸取上清液加入等体积的沉淀缓冲液，室温下放置30 min以上，10 000 r/min离心10 min，小心弃上清液，分别用70%乙醇和无水乙醇各洗涤1次，弃掉洗液，挥干，以TE溶液40 μL溶解，用分光光度计测定DNA浓度，以确定模板用量。

3.2 聚合酶链式反应扩增（polymerase chain reaction, PCR） 反应体系总体积50 μL，其中引物为1 mmol/L，模板DNA约150 ng，*Taq*酶3U，dNTPs各0.05 mmol/L。扩增程序为预变性5 min，94℃ 40 s、72℃ 45 s、37℃ 45 s 40个循环，后延伸72℃ 5 min。取扩增产物10 μL于1.0%琼脂糖凝胶上用1×TAE电泳缓冲液电泳，紫外检测拍照。

## 4 结果与讨论

4.1 天花粉及其类似品的RAPD鉴别结果 本文选择了来源于13个种3个变种的天花粉及其类似品共26份样品，用8个扩增多态性好的引物（表2）分别进行RAPD扩增，得到清晰、稳定的条带共计 83 条(图 1)。将迁移率相同的带均作为同源位点处理,得到 1/0 数据(有计为 1,无计为 0)矩阵,按刘晓民等方法计算任意 2 个样品间的相似系数($s$)并得相似关系矩阵。将该矩阵取不同的 $\lambda$ 值($\lambda \in [0, 1]$)作不同的$\lambda$-截矩阵,采用编网法聚类,得树系图(见图 2)。结果表明,全部样品可被分成三大类,第一类是大宗商品和小宗商品(1～ 12 号),第二类是天花粉药材商品中最易混淆的湖北栝楼根(13, 14 号)和红花栝楼根(17 号),第三类全部是混淆品和地区习惯用药(15～16, 18～25 号)。这表明 RAPD 对不同植物来源的天花粉,尤其对来自不同组及组上水平的天花粉能够很好区分开来。其结果与物种间的亲缘关系基本一致。如湖北栝楼虽属大苞组,但因其根与正品天花粉极其相似,而显示出比其他大苞组植物与正品天花粉有更近的亲缘关系,本实验结果也恰好表明这一点(第一类正品天花粉与第二类湖北栝楼的关系比第三类更密切)。由此可见该方法具有一定的可靠性和实用价值。

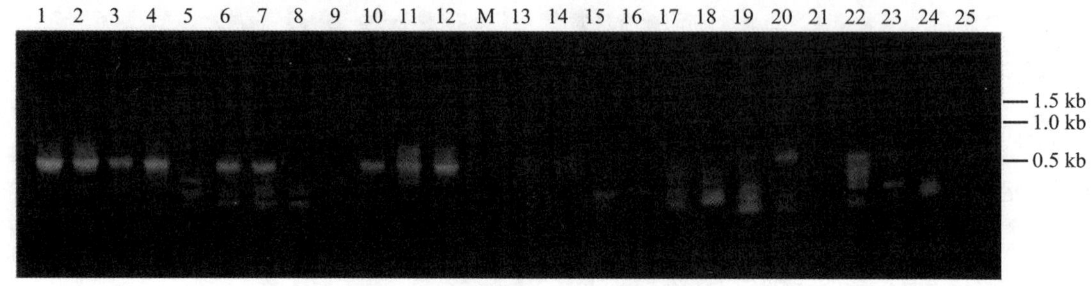


**图 1 5 号引物对 1～25 号样品 RAPD 扩增产物的琼脂糖凝胶电泳图谱(样品号码详见表 1)**

M:100 bp DNA ladder 分子标记物(Prmega 公司)。

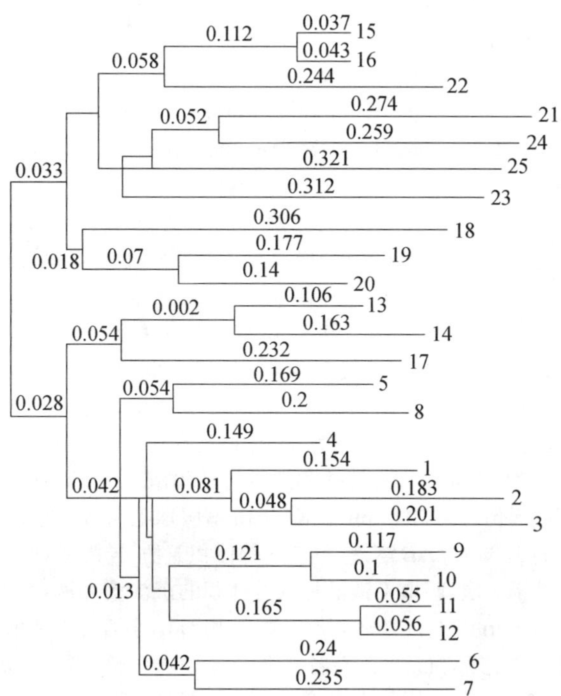


**图 2 RAPD 结果树系图(样品号码见表 1)**

4.2 RAPD 鉴别结果的影响因素分析

4.2.1 重复和污染问题 重复上述实验,结果稳定;空白对照表明本实验条件无明显污染。

4.2.2 样品的贮存时间与产地对 RAPD 结果的影响 在相同的贮存条件下,样品贮存时间的不同往往意味着 DNA 模板降解程度的不一致(图 3);而药材产地不同是指药材来自不同的地方居群(local population),居群间常存在比较大的遗传变异。因此,除了物种这一决定因素之外,样品的贮存时间与产地也可能直接影响 RAPD 结果,从而影响其对药材的鉴别结果。为此,本实验还对主要的天花粉及其类似品的不同(相同)贮存时间及产地的个体进行对照分析。树系图表明,贮存时间相同或非常相近的同一物种是最先聚类的(如 2 号和 3 号,9 号和 10 号,11 号和 12 号,13 号和 14 号,15 号和 16 号);而贮存时间相差很远的不能优先聚类(如 4 号和 5 号,7 号和 8 号,18 和 19 号)。为便于进一步分析,我们将贮存时间与产地作为可变条件对所对应的遗传距离作表(表 3),结果表明,贮存时间及产地相同所表现出的同一物种不同个体药材间的遗传距离显著小于二者或二者之一有变化所表现出的遗传距离,说明贮存时间及产地二者对 RAPD 结果都是有影响的。

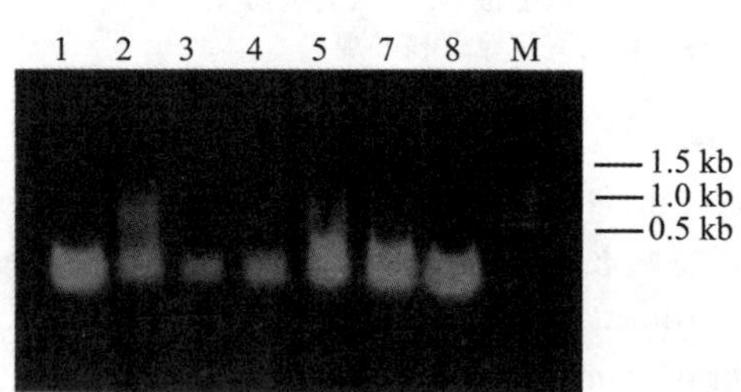


**图 3 不同贮存时间的样品 DNA 模板降解程度(样品号码详见表 1)**

M:100 bp DNA ladder 分子标识物(Promega 公司)。

**表 3 贮存时间及产地对同一物种不同个体间的遗传距离的影响**

| 条件 | | 样品编号 | 遗传距离 | 平均遗传距离 |
|---|---|---|---|---|
| 产地 | 贮存时间 | | | |
| 相同 | 相同 | 11、12<br>13、14<br>15、16 | 0.1111<br>0.2683<br>0.0811 | 0.1535 |
| 不同 | 相同 | 2、3<br>9、10<br>18、19 | 0.3846<br>0.2174<br>0.4286 | 0.3435 |

(续表)

| 条件 | | 样品编号 | 遗传距离 | 平均遗传距离 |
|---|---|---|---|---|
| 产地 | 贮存时间 | | | |
| 相同 | 不同 | 4、5 | 0.3191 | 0.3191 |
| 不同 | 不同 | 1、2<br>1、3<br>7、8 | 0.3750<br>0.4146<br>0.4444 | 0.4113 |

4.3 RAPD鉴别药材的可行性 在解决重复和污染问题后，在实际应用中虽然还有贮存时间和产地等因素将会对RAPD产生影响，但是，在待测样品与对照品对上述因素基本一致的情况下，由PCR产生的DNA指纹图谱基本不变，如人参与西洋参的鉴别；而在待测样品贮存时间和条件未知的情况下，本实验结果表明，采用多设对照品，取大量数据进行聚类分析，也能够使RAPD很好地应用于药材鉴别。这将为药材的鉴别提供新的方法。

[黄璐琦，等．药物分析杂志，1999，19(4)：233－238.]

# 栝楼属(*Trichosanthes* L.)的系统学研究

栝楼属(*Trichosanthes* L.)是葫芦科(Cucurbitaceae)中一个比较大的属，共有80多种，大多为雌雄异株，其分布地区为东亚及澳大利亚北部，其中我国有一半的种类。本属有多种药用植物，药用价值很高。《中华人民共和国药典》收载了本属植物3种，《中药志》收载了13种，具有止孕和抗艾滋病活性的天花粉蛋白(trichosanthin)就是从本属植物栝楼(*T. kirilowii* Maxim.)的块根中提取的。然而，作为本属的研究基础——分类学的研究，虽有很多学者做了大量的工作，但未达成共识；特别是栝楼这一复合种的研究，被称为"The most intractable taxonomic problem in eastern Asia Cucurbitaceae center"。这些问题严重影响了天花粉药材的使用。据我们对29省、市、区的调查，天花粉商品药材多达28种，其中来源同属近缘植物有19种，有些还具有很高的毒性，因此，急需理清本属的分类。为此，我们从世界范围栝楼属植物入手，采用经典的形态分类学为主，辅以细胞学、孢粉学和组织学等方法，期望能初步理清世界范围栝楼属植物中的种类及属下类群分划问题，解决一些误定和疑难种。同时，我们还采用了分子生物学的方法对栝楼植物，进行了初步的分析。

## 1 分类学研究

栝楼属是林奈于1753年依据蛇瓜 *T. anguina* L.建立，当时对该属植物仅记载了4种；到目前为止，已确认的栝楼属植物有80余种。本属植物通过长期演化，在花序、小苞片、果实及种子上常有差异而形成不同的近缘类群，因此，很多分类学家曾把本属分为各组或划分成不同的属。

我们在对国内进行广泛调查采集的基础上，从美国、英国、澳大利亚、泰国、马来西亚及日本等国的各大标本馆借来标本，系统研究整理了分布于世界各地本属植物的种类，确认有84种8变种，我国有37种6变种，是栝楼属植物的主要分布中心。

在初步理清种类的基础上，对栝楼属的属下划分依据形态学(如花序、小苞片及种子等)细胞学及孢粉学等特征，提出如下安排。

栝楼亚属 Subgen 1. *Trichosanthes*

小苞组 Sect. 1. *Trichosanthes*

叶苞组 Sect. 2. *Foliobracteola* C. Y. Cheng et C. H. Yueh

叶苞亚组 Subsect. 1. *Foliobracteola*

叶苞系 Ser. 1. *Foliobracteola*

全叶系 Ser. 2. *Ovifolia* C. H. Yueh et L. Q. Huang ser. nov.

Folia coriacea ovata integra vel raro tri-lobata.

Type：*T. smilacifolia* C. Y. Wu ex C. Y. Cheng et C. H. Yueh

柔毛亚组 Subsect. 2. *Villosae* C. H. Yueh et L. Q. Huang sect. nov.

Folia coriacea vel crasse chartacea, inflorescentia villosa floribus in brevi racemos vel paniculas dispositi raro sditanis.

Type：*T. subvelutina* F. Muell.

大苞组 Sect. 3. *Involucraria* (Ser.) Wight et Arn.

大苞亚组 Subscet. 3. *Bracteatae* C. Jeffrey ex S. K. Chen

复叶亚组 Subsect. 4. *Pedatae* (C. Y. Cheng et C. H. Yueh) C. Jeffrey

王瓜亚属 Subsgen. 2. *Cucumeroides* (Gaertn.) C. Y. Cheng et C. H. Yueh

王瓜组 Sect. 4. *Cucumeroides*

方子组 Sect. 5. *Tetragonosperma* C. Y. Cheng et C. H. Yueh

## 2 细胞学研究

栝楼属植物的细胞学研究报道较少。Darlington(1955)指出本属植物染色体基数为X=11。我们对16种本属植物进行了细胞学研究(表1)：方法是取用种子萌发的根尖为材料，经对二氯苯饱和水溶液处理，卡宝品红(carmine)染色和压片；每种植物观察细胞大约100个分裂相，按李懋学等的方法进行核型分析，核型对称性按Stebbins所确定的分类标准

**表 1 栝楼属植物染色体情况一览**

| 组别 | 种名 | 染色体数目(2n) | 倍性 | 最长染色体/最短染色体 | 绝对长度变异范围(μm) | 相对长度变异范围 | 核型公式 | 相对长度组成 | 核型对称型 |
|---|---|---|---|---|---|---|---|---|---|
| 王瓜组 | *T. chingiana* | 22 | 2 | 1.48 | 2.00～2.95 | 3.85～5.68 | 2n=2X=18m+4sm | 2n=22=10M2+12M1 | 2A |
| 小苞组 | *T. cucumerina* | 22 | 2 | 1.59 | 1.45～2.15 | 3.89～6.10 | 72n=2X=14m+8sm | 2n=22=2L+4M2+16M1 | 2A |
| 叶苞组 | *T. multicirrata* | 88 | 8 | 2.27 | 1.06～2.42 | 0.82～1.86 | | | B |
| | *T. kirilowii* | 88 | 8 | 1.86 | 0.69～1.45 | 0.85～3.89 | | | B |
| | *T. stylopodifera* | 88 | 8 | 3.27 | 0.71～2.32 | 0.65～2.12 | | | B |
| | *T. mianyangensis* | 88 | 8 | 40.8 | 7.00～3.48 | 0.62～2.48 | | | B |
| | *T. wuyuanensis* | 66 | 6 | 2.37 | 0.95～2.26 | 1.01～2.40 | | | B |
| | *T. truncata* | 22 | 2 | 2.08 | 1.44～2.98 | 3.63～7.55 | 2n=2X=16m(2SAT)+6sm | 2n=22=2L+6M2+14M1 | 2B |
| | *T. rosthornii* | 22 | 2 | 2.77 | 0.91～2.52 | 2.78～7.69 | | | B |
| | *T. scabrella* | 44 | 4 | 2.28 | 0.30～0.68 | 0.43～0.98 | | | B |
| 大苞组 | *T. laceribractea*(♀) | 22 | 2 | 2.15 | 2.11～4.53 | 2.99～6.43 | 2n=2X=2M(2SAT)+12m+8sm(2SAT) | 2n=22=4L+4M2+2M1+2S | 2B |
| | *T. laceribractea*(♂) | 22 | 2 | 2.38 | 1.33～3.17 | 2.69～6.41 | 2n=2X=17m(2SAT)+5sm | 2n=22=3L+8M2+10M1+1S | 2B |
| | *T. rubriflos*(♀) | 22 | 2 | 2.11 | 1.23～2.60 | 3.18～6.72 | 2n=2X=20m(2SAT)+2sm | 2n=22=2L+8M2+10M1+2S | 1B |
| | *T. rubriflos*(♂) | 22 | 2 | 2.68 | 1.05～2.81 | 2.65～7.13 | 2n=2X=19m(2SAT)+3sm | 2n=22=4L+7M2+8M1+3S | 2B |
| | *T. lepiniana* | 44 | 4 | 1.99 | 1.01～2.02 | 1.64～3.26 | | | A |
| | *T. hupehensis* | 22 | 2 | 2.05 | 1.17～2.40 | 3.48～7.13 | 2n=2X=18m(2SAT)+4sm | 2n=22=2L+8M2+12M1 | 2B |
| | *T. schizostroma* | 22 | 2 | 2.21 | 2.08～4.60 | 3.41～7.52 | 2n=2X=18m(2SAT)+4sm | 2n=22=2L+8M2+10M1+2S | 2B |
| | *T. pedata* | 22 | 2 | 1.75 | 1.68～2.94 | 3.76～6.58 | 2n=2X=18m+4sn(2SAT) | 2n=22=2L+4M2+16M1 | 2A |

划分，核型不对称性系数按 Arano 标准确定，染色体相对长度系数和相对长度公式按 Kuo et al. 方法。

实验结果显示本属染色体具有如下特点：①本属染色体的变化主要是数目的变化，即形成基数为 11 的整倍性的多倍体系列为演化趋势，而核型结构变异小，没有明显演化趋势。②多倍体与器官特化及地理分布规律性的相关不明显。③本实验所得到的染色体核型类型为 A、B 型，按 Stebbins 的分类原则，都属于较对称类型。同时，对在分类上有争议的 4 个种进行了分类的探讨，例如湖北栝楼（*T. hupehensis* C. Y. Cheng et Yueh）与花叶栝楼（*T. schizostroma* Hayata），在外部形态上没有稳定的区别，在染色体上核型都为 2n＝2X＝18m(2SAT)＋4sm，因此，两者应予合并。

## 3 孢粉学研究

我们观察了产于国外的本属 31 种及 1 变种的花粉在光学显微镜及扫描式电子显微镜下的形态特征。花粉材料均取自腊叶标本，光学显微镜的样品制备采用 Erdtman 醋酸酐分解法，扫描电镜样品的制备直接撒在粘于铜托上的双面胶带上，经真空镀膜直接观察。花粉描述采用 Erdtman 术语。

本属植物花粉的研究为属下划分提供了依据，具体特点如下：①复叶亚组在花粉上的特征为花粉体积较大，具粗网状纹饰，这与大苞组相近，从而支持将其并入大苞组作为一亚组。②柔毛亚组花粉为细网状或光滑，与大苞组不同，而近于叶苞组，同时因没有叶苞亚组所具有的明显的沟，支持在叶苞组中成一自然类群。③叶苞组中全叶系不仅在外部形态上，而且因其花粉光滑、不呈细网状，与叶苞系不同，支持全叶系的划分。④从花粉特征上支持一些植物的成立，如石垣栝楼 *T. ishigakiensis* E. Walk. 与中华栝楼 *T. rosthornii* Harms 的关系，两者不仅在外部形态上区别很大，如 *T. ishigakiensis* 为木质藤本，雄花为 2～6 条总状花序并生，*T. rosthornii* 为草质藤本，雄花或单生，或为一总状花序或两者并生，而且在花粉上两者也有区别，前者为粗网状，后者为细网状，因此，把两者合并是不妥的。

## 4 组织学研究

种子表皮的形态学研究在栝楼属植物的分类学研究中占有重要地位，为此，我们对本属 31 个种和 3 变种植物的种皮的组织构造进行了扫描电子显微镜的观察和比较（表 2）。所观察材料为成熟种子，用双面胶带固定于电子显微镜样品台上，经真空镀膜，在扫描电镜下直接观察其种脐、中部（王瓜亚属为侧臂中部）及合点 3 个部位。

**表 2 栝楼属植物种皮特征一览**

| 组名 | | | 种名 | 类型 |
|---|---|---|---|---|
| 小苞组 | | | 澳洲栝楼 *T. jonesii* sp. nov. | A, B |
| | | | 大方油栝楼 *T. dafangensis* N. G. Ye et S.J. Li | A |
| | | | 蛇瓜栝楼 *T. anguina* L. | C, D |
| 叶苞组 | 叶苞亚组 | 叶苞系 | 栝楼 *T. kirilowii* Maxim. | A, D |
| | | | 中华栝楼 *T. rosthornii* Harms | A, B |
| | | | 多卷须栝楼 *T. rosthornii* var. *multicirrata* | A |
| | | | 糙籽栝楼 *T. rosthornii* var. *scabrella* | A(B) |

（续表）

| 组名 | 种名 | 类型 |
|---|---|---|
| 全叶系 | 尖果栝楼 *T. rosthornii* var. *stylopodifera* | A, B, A |
| | 湘桂栝楼 *T. hylonoma* Hand.-Mazz. | A |
| | 绵阳栝楼 *T. mianyangensis* Yueh et R.G. Liao | A, B |
| | 大子栝楼 *T. truncata* C.B. Clarke | A |
| | 冲绳栝楼 *T. miyagii* Hayata | A, C |
| | 双序栝楼 *T. dieniensis* Merrill | A, C |
| | 菝葜叶栝楼 *T. smilacifolia* C.Y. Wu | D, A, B |
| | 沙捞越栝楼 *T. sarawakensis* sp. nov. | A |
| | 多籽栝楼 *T. pulleana* Cogn. | A, C |
| 柔毛亚组 | 绒毛栝楼 *T. subvelutina* F. Muell. | C |
| | 长果栝楼 *T. kerrii* Craib | B, D |
| | 密毛栝楼 *T. villosa* Bl. | D |
| 大苞组 大苞亚组 | 马干铃栝楼 *T. lepiniana* (Naud.) Cogn. | A, B, C |
| | 长萼栝楼 *T. laceribracteata* Hayata | A, B |
| | 湖北栝楼 *T. hupehensis* C. Y. Cheng et Yueh | A, B |
| | 糙点栝楼 *T. dunniana* Levl. | A(B) |
| | 红花栝楼 *T. rubriflos* Thorel ex Cayla | A, B |
| | 皱籽栝楼 *T. rugatisemina* C. Y. Cheng et Yueh | A, B |
| | 长方子栝楼 *T. fissibracteata* C. Y. Wu | A |
| | 单卷须栝楼 *T. unicirrata* sp. nov. | B |
| | 木梗栝楼 *T. grandiflora* Bl. | A, B |
| 复叶亚组 | 木基栝楼 *T. quinquefolia* C. Y. Wu | B, C |
| 王瓜组 | 喜马山栝楼 *T. ovigera* Bl. | A, D |
| | 王瓜 *T. cucumeroides* (Ser.) Maxim. | B(C) |
| | 喙果栝楼 *T. rostrata* Kitamura | C, D |
| | 短序栝楼 *T. baviensis* Gagnep. | C, D |
| 方子组 | 南洋栝楼 *T. beccariana* Cogn. | A |

实验结果表明本属种皮特征为 4 种类型——长方网型(A 型)、波浪型(B 型)、蜂窝型(C 型)、不规则型 (D 型),从种皮特征上很好地支持了对本属属下划分进行修改的合理性。如方子组种子表面特征为 A 型,有别于王瓜组中的 C 型为主,因此,支持王瓜组与方子组应是 2 个不同的自然类群。大苞组与叶苞组都以 A 型为主,兼顾其他 3 种类型,与别的组有明显不同,显示出在种皮表面特征上的相近性,但大苞组的 A 型条纹细,叶苞组的 A 型条纹粗,因此,种皮表面特征很好地表现出 2 组之间相近而又不同的关系。

## 5 分子系统生物学研究

如前所述,栝楼块根为重要中药材天花粉的来源,但其商品药材的来源很混乱,并且传统上只把雄株的根用作天花粉,因此急需引入新方法对其进行遗传变异分析并寻找快速有效的鉴定方法。

分子生物学实验方法已被越来越多地应用于植物系统发育研究中。用得较多的是核糖体 DNA(rDNA)和叶绿体 DNA,rDNA 转录了核糖体 RNA(rRNA),在染色体上以中等重复、连续的形式排列,每一个重复单位都有负责转录及转译 18S rRNA、5.8S rRNA 和 28S rRNA 的片段,其中 18S 和 28S 十分保守,在这 3 段 DNA 之间,有 2 个非编码转录片段,它们是中度保守区域;还有一个介于 28S rRNA 和下一个重复单位之间的非转录区 IGS,这是一段最不保守的区域。我们试图从 rDNA 的序列分析中寻找可用来进行遗传变异分析或类群鉴定的分子标记。

5.1 rDNA 的 RFLP 分析　RFLP(限制性片段长度多型性)分析是研究 DNA 多型性有效手段,对 rDNA 的 RFLP 分析已被成功用于多种生物的种间亲缘关系等方面的研究,但对于栝楼属植物的相关研究未见报道。因此,我们对栝楼居群内雌雄株共 9 个个体 rDNA 进行了 RFLP 分析。

植物材料及方法:在北京医科大学校园内的一个栝楼族群中随机选取了 4 个雌株和 5 个雄株。

总 DNA 提取方法按略加修改的 CTBA 法进行。所用探针是大豆的 rDNA 重复单位克隆。所用内切酶为 BamHⅠ、EcoRⅤ、HindⅢ、HinfⅠ、KpNⅠ、XbaⅠ、SmaⅠ、XhoⅠ(Pronega 公司)。

结果及讨论:限制性内切酶水解后的 rDNA 片段长度分析表明,栝楼雌雄株 rDNA 的拷贝长度为 14.0 kb,比葫芦科中近缘的南瓜属(*Cucurbita*)的 10 kb 和 11.5 kb 要大,是目前葫芦科报道中最长的 rDNA 拷贝。

RFLP 所能检测的 DNA 多态性主要是酶切位点的碱基突破,片段插入或缺失、片段倒位或易位等,因此其分辨能力与 DNA 中这些变异的多少有关。在本研究所检测的雌雄株 9 个个体中,雄株不同个体之间表现了较为丰富的多态性,而雌株较为均一;HindⅢ、XbaⅠ、HinfⅠ、XhoⅠ、BamHⅠ等酶在雌雄株 rDNA 上的酶切位点一致,而 EcoRⅠ、SmaⅠ、EcoRⅤ是在雌雄株 rDNA 上有着不同位点,但在雌雄株的不同个体之间却相一致,表明雌雄株在共同进化过程中所表现出的超异性。

在本研究中 EcoRⅠ、EcoRⅤ、SmaⅠ等是能较好地反映出栝楼 rDNA 多态性的限制性内切酶;BamHⅠ、HinfⅠ 2 种则能对栝楼 rDNA 酶解产生较多片段,这 5 种酶配合使用,就能基本上把栝楼 rDNA 的主要 RFLP 模式显示出来。但从目前的研究结果看,rDNA 的 RFLP 变化式样在栝楼居群变化较大,较难用于此复合种的遗传多样性分析。

5.2 rDNA 的 ITS 序列分析　rDNA 的 ITS1 及 ITS2 在被子植物中长度很保守,均 200～300 bp,易于进行 PCR 扩增及测序分析,同时它属于中度保守的序列,这些特点使短小的 ITS 区可提供足够多的信息作种或种以下系统分类研究及遗传变异分析,对本属的研究国内外还未见报道。在此我们报道栝楼植物 rDNA ITS 的序列。

植物材料与方法:栝楼叶子采自北京医科大学校园。DNA 提取方法同上,PCR 扩增方法参照瞿礼嘉等。DNA 测序在 ABI 373A DNA 自动测序仪上进行。

结果与讨论:测得的 ITS1 及 ITS2 的序列如下。

ITS1 序列—198 bp

TCGATTGCCTGAACATCAAACGACCCGCGAA
CGCTTTACAAACCTTCCGTGCAGGGGGGGAA
GCATCTTCCTTGCTTGCTCCCTCCCGGTGCCTA
AACCAAACCCCGGCGCAGGTCGGCAAGGAAC
TCAAACGAATTTGCCCGCCCCTTGCCCCGTGC
ACGGCTGGCGGGGGGCGTCTCATTCTTGTCG
TATTATTCA

ITS2 序列—215 bp

ATCGCTGCCCCCCCCACGCAACCCCCACTCAG
GTTCATTGCCAGACAAGGGCACACACTGGTC
TCCGATGCGCACCGTCGCGTGGATGGCTTAA
ATTCGAGTCCTTGGTGGTGTGATCAACTCGT
ACTGCTGTGACTCAGCCCGAGCACGTCCTCC
CAGTGAGCGAGGCTCCTATGCCGCCCTATGA
ATGTCGTGGGGAAAAACGATGCTCTCGA

栝楼的 ITS 区域与葫芦科中现已知的 ITS 区域相似性很高。在具体操作过程中，我们遇到了真菌的干扰，很多样品都有真菌的污染，使得这项测序工作很费时、费力，而且不能直接用 PCR 产物测序。因为我们的目的之一是想寻找一种能快速鉴定花粉正品的分子标记，所以我们现在正在试用无菌苗的随机扩增 DNA 多态性(RAPD)的方法及叶绿体 DNA 的片段分析方法。

[黄璐琦，等.江西中医学院学报，1999,11(2):75-78.]

# 中药白芷种质资源的 RAPD 分析

白芷为常用中药。按国内用药历史和习惯，现代所用商品药材均为栽培品，分为祁(禹)白芷和杭(川)白芷两大类。由于对其原野生植物来源尚未真正搞清，白芷类药材种名鉴定至今尚无统一的定论。据有关文献报道，祁(禹)白芷与分布于东北的兴安白芷(大活)为同种植物，定名为白芷 *Angelica dahurica* (Fisch.) Benth. et Hook.，而杭(川)白芷则分别作为独立种或共同作为白芷的变种，定名为 *A. dahurica* (Fisch.) Benth. et Hook. var *formosana* (Boiss.) Yen。因此，我们对上述兴安白芷、祁白芷、杭白芷三者进行了 RAPD 分析，探索相互间分子遗传关系和分类地位，为正确划分白芷的种类提供依据。

## 1 仪器、试剂和材料

1.1 仪器 PROGENE THERMAL CYCLER(Techne 公司，英国)；Micro-MB 3616 型高速离心机(IEC公司，美国)；UV-Ⅰ型多功能紫外透射仪(北京市新技术应用研究所)。

1.2 试剂 *Taq* 酶(U-P Biotech, Inc USA)；琼脂糖(Promega 公司)；dNTPs(Promega 公司)；CTAB(Sigma 公司)；溴化乙锭(Fluka 公司)；其余试剂为北京化工厂产的分析纯。

1.3 材料 取各种材料的新鲜叶子，见表 1。

**表 1 实验材料来源及多态位点百分率的比较**

| 编号 | 名称 | 个体数 | 来源 | 位点总数 | 多态位点数(%) |
|---|---|---|---|---|---|
| 1 | 杭白芷 | 8 | 浙江杭州药用植物园 | 40 | 20(50) |
| 2 | 杭白芷 | 4 | 江苏南京植物研究所 | 40 | 23(57.5) |
| 3 | 祁白芷 | 5 | 河北安国 | 40 | 18(45) |
| 4 | 兴安白芷 | 12 | 沈阳药科大学 | 40 | 9(22.5) |

注：引物数均 12。

## 2 实验方法

2.1 DNA 模板的提取和浓度测定 取新鲜叶片少许，置 1.5 ml Ep 管中，加入液氮用镊子研碎，立即加入 500 μL 保温 60℃的 2×CTAB 提取液[CTAB 2%，Tris-HCl(pH 8.0) 100 mmol/L，EDTA 20 mmol/L，NaCl 1.4 mol/L，巯基乙醇 2%]及 20 μL 巯基乙醇混匀，60℃保温 40 min；加入等体积的氯仿-异丙醇(24∶1)抽提，轻轻颠倒混匀，10 000 r/min 离心 10 min，吸取上清液，加入 1/10 体积的 10% CTAB 溶液，再加入等体积氯仿-异丙醇(24∶1)重复抽提 1 次，吸取上清液加入等体积的沉淀缓冲液[CTAB 1%，Tris-HCl(pH 8.0) 50 mmol/L，EDTA 10 mmol/L，巯基乙醇 1%]，室温下放置 30 min 以上，10 000 r/min 离心 10 min，小心去上清液，分别用 70%乙醇和无水乙醇各洗涤 1 次，弃掉洗液挥干。用分光光度计测定 DNA 浓度后进行 PCR 扩增。所用引物编号及其序列见表 2。

2.2 RAPD 扩增 反应体系总体积 50 μL，其中引物为 1 mmol/L，总 DNA 约 150 ng，*Taq* 酶 2 U，dNTPs 各 0.05 mmol/L。扩增程度为预变性 5 min，94 ℃ 40 s、38 ℃ 45 s、72℃ 45 s 40 个循环，后延伸 72℃ 5 min。取 10 μL 扩增产物于 1.0%琼脂糖凝胶上用 1×TAE 电泳缓冲液电泳，紫外检测拍照(图 1)。

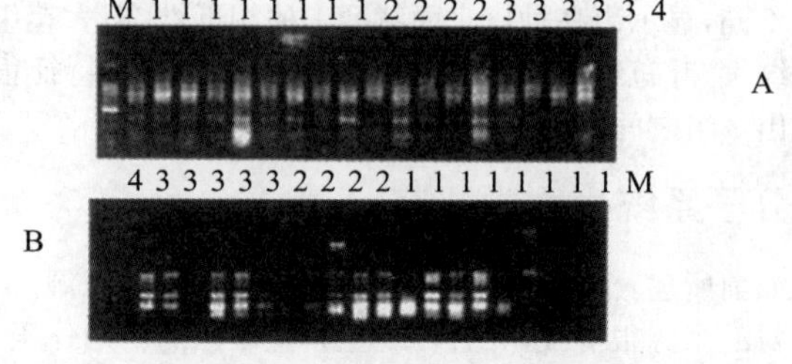


**图 1 样品不同个体以不同引物 RAPD 扩增产物的琼脂糖凝胶电泳图谱**

A. 3 号引物；B. 10 号引物。

表 2 RAPD 所用引物编号及其序列

| 编号 | 序列(5′→3′) |
|---|---|
| 1 | TCGGCGATAG |
| 2 | CAAACGTCGG |
| 3 | AGGGGTCTTG |
| 4 | GTGACGTAGG |
| 5 | AATCGGGCTG |
| 6 | GGGTAACGCC |
| 7 | CAGGCCCTTC |
| 8 | CAGCACCCAC |
| 9 | ACTCAGCCAC |
| 10 | TGCCGAGCTG<br>ATGATGAGATTCTTAG |
| 11 | TCCTCTCTTTGCTA<br>TCATGCCATATTGTTT |
| 12 | CGATTCAGCAGCAA |

2.3 *数据分析* 电泳图谱中的每一条带(DNA 片段)均为一个分子标记(Marker),并代表 1 个引物结合点。根据各分子标记的有无及其迁移率统计得到所有位点的二元数据,无带(隐性)计为 0,有带(显性)计为 1(强带和弱带的赋值均为 1)。对于多态位点,仅在重复实验中能稳定出现的差异带用于数据分析。用 RAPD 分析软件 RAPDistance Package-Version 1.04 中 Dice 的方法计算任意两个样品间的遗传距离,得到单株间和居群间的遗传距离,见表 3。

## 3 结果与讨论

3.1 琼脂糖电泳分析表明,在 RAPD 分析中 12 个 mer 随机引物在不同样品中共检测出 40 个位点,其中多态位点 26 个,占 65%;祁、杭白芷的多态位点的百分率分别是 45%、50%和 57.5%(表 1),近似于 Mosseler 等用 11 个引物在 *Picea glauca* 和 *Picea mariana* 各 3 个个体的研究中所得结果,显示出低水平的遗传变异,这可能与栽培过程中群体内和群体间的遗传多样性明显下降有关。

表 3 白芷单株间和居群间的平均遗传距离

| 操作分类单位 OTUs[1)] | 材料来源编号 | 1 | 2 | 3 | 4 |
|---|---|---|---|---|---|
| 1 | 1 | 0.113[2)] | | | |
| 2 | 2 | 0.179 | 0.166[2)] | | |
| 3 | 3 | 0.160 | 0.176 | 0.166[2)] | |
| 4 | 4 | 0.239 | 0.251 | 0.206 | 0[2)] |

注:[1)] Operational Taxonomic Unit 1-8 2-4 3-5 4-n; [2)] 居群内单株间的平均遗传距离。

3.2 RAPD 所得的遗传距离表明祁白芷与杭白芷中杭州居群的遗传距离(0.160)小于祁白芷居群内单株间的遗传距离(0.166),也小于杭白芷不同居群间的遗传距离(0.179);并且它们都低于与野生白芷的遗传距离,这证实了潘泽惠等的细胞学研究认为祁白芷不能与兴安白芷等同及祁、杭白芷关系密切等;并就此进一步得出祁、杭白芷应属同一类群,支持《中国植物志》把祁、杭白芷作为同种处理;但它们是否经兴安白芷栽培而来,有待在本实验的基础上研究它们与 *A. dahurica* 的近缘种类,如分布于河北、河南的 *A. porphyrocaulis* 和分布于台湾的 *A. formosana* 等进行比较研究,才能最终解决白芷类药材野生种质来源这一至今尚未解决的问题。

3.3 RAPD 分析显示出祁白芷与兴安白芷的遗传距离(0.206)相对杭白芷与兴安白芷的遗传距离(0.239 和 0.251)要小些,这与祁白芷在地理分布上更近于兴安白芷相符合,但其中是否有必然的联系有待进一步的研究。

[黄璐琦,等.中国中药杂志,1999,24(8):457-459.]

# 栝楼农家品种苗期的分子标识鉴别

栝楼(*Trichosanthes kirilowii* Maxim.)是常用中药瓜蒌、天花粉的来源植物。由于它是异花授粉植物,加上长期的栽培、选择,产区出现了很多植物类型,使栝楼质量变化较大。然而,这些栝楼变异类型只有等到果实成熟后才有明显区别,需用一种新技术能在营养期尤其是出苗期鉴别作用。为此,我们选择了 RAPD 这一分子标识法对山东长清等主产区的 3 个主流农家品种进行研究,以期使该方法能在药用植物的良种选育方面得到推广。

## 1 材料与仪器

1.1 *材料* 选用栝楼的幼叶见表 1,用硅胶快速干燥保存。所用引物序列见表 2,由华美生物工程公司合成。*Taq* 酶(U-P Biotech, Inc. USA);琼脂糖(Promega 公司);dNTPs(Promega 公司);CTAB(Sigma 公司);溴化乙锭(Fluka 公司);其余试剂均为分析纯。

表 1 材料来源、产量和质量

| 名称 | 产地 | 亩产(kg) | 质量 |
|---|---|---|---|
| 仁栝楼 | 山东长清伏牛镇 | 250～300 | 优 |
| 糖栝楼 | 山东长清伏牛镇 | 250～300 | 中 |
| 地栝楼 | 山东宁阳伏山镇 | 150～200 | 劣 |

表 2 本实验所用引物序列及其扩增结果

| 引物号 | 序列 5′→3′ | 特征条带大小(kb)[1] | | |
|---|---|---|---|---|
| | | 仁栝楼 | 糖栝楼 | 地栝楼 |
| 1 | TCGGCGATAG | | 0.5 | 0.7 |
| 2 | CAAACGTCGG | 0.9<br>0.2～0.3 | 0.7<br>0.2 | 0.8<br>0.2～0.3 |
| 3 | GGGTAACGCC | | 0.3<br>0.1～0.2 | 0.3<br>0.1～0.2 |
| 4 | CAGGCCCTTC | 0.9～1.0<br>0.6～0.7 | | |
| 5 | CAGCACCCAC | | 0.2～0.3<br>0.2 | 0.5<br>0.2～0.3<br>0.2 |
| 6 | ACTCAGCCAC | 0.3～0.4 | 0.3 | 0.3 |
| 7 | TGCCGAGCTG | | 0.1～0.2 | |

注：1) 该数值为目测估值。

1.2 仪器 1169 型电脑全自动基因扩增仪、UV-Ⅰ型多功能紫外透射仪(均为北京市新技术应用研究所产品)。Micro-MB 3616 型高速离心机(美国 IEC 公司)。

## 2 方法与结果

2.1 DNA 模板的提取 取材料少许置 1.5 mL Ep 管中，加入液氮用镊子研碎，立即加入 500 μL 保温 60℃的 2×CTAB 提取液[CTAB 2%，Tris-HCl (pH 8.0) 100 mmol/L，EDTA 20 mmol/L，NaCl 1.4 mol/L，巯基乙醇 2%]及 20 μL 巯基乙醇混匀，60℃保温 40 min；加入等体积的氯仿-异丙醇(24∶1)抽提，轻轻颠倒混匀，10 000 r/min 离心 10 min，吸取上清液，加入 1/10 体积的 10% CTAB 溶液，再加入等体积氯仿-异丙醇(24∶1)重复抽提 1 次，吸取上清液加入等体积的沉淀缓冲液[CTAB 1%，Tris-HCl (pH 8.0) 50 mmol/L，EDTA 10 mmol/L，巯基乙醇 1%]，室温下放置 30 min 以上，10 000 r/min 离心 10 min，小心去上清，分别用体积分数为 70%的乙醇和无水乙醇各洗涤 1 次，弃掉洗液，挥干。以 40 μL TE 溶液后进行 PCR 扩增。

2.2 PCR 反应 反应体系总体积 50 μL，其中引物为 1 mmol/L，核 DNA 约 150 ng，*Taq* 酶 3 U，dNTPs 各 0.05 mmol/L。扩增程序为预变性 5 min，94℃ 40 s，72℃ 45 s，37℃ 45 s 40 个循环，后延伸 72℃ 5 min。取 10 μL 扩增产物于 1.0%琼脂糖凝胶上用 1×TAE 电泳缓冲液电泳，紫外检测拍照。见表 2。

## 3 讨论

3.1 本实验所用材料为硅胶快速干燥的干叶，经检查 DNA 模板无降解现象，这为解决野外采样以及保存和运输上的困难提供了很大的方便。重复上述实验，结果稳定，空白对照表明本实验条件无明显污染。

3.2 在本研究中，7 个引物的扩增结果都呈现出多态性，其中 1、2、5 号引物能把三者明显地加以区别，是栝楼农家品种早期分子标识鉴别的首选引物；3、4、6、7 号引物的结果能将仁栝楼区别，而在糖栝楼和地栝楼之间则不能表现出区别条带，这是否能证明糖栝楼与地栝楼之间的亲缘关系较之与仁栝楼要近，还有待进一步研究。

3.3 RAPD 方法具有快速、有效、微量、方便的优点，Graham 等在葡萄栽品种的选育上已做了大量的工作，本实验对栝楼农家品种的早期鉴定也证实了这一点，因此其在药用植物育种方面也有广阔的应用前景。

[黄璐琦，等.中国药学杂志，1999，34(9)：642.]

# 蕲蛇及其混淆品高特异性 PCR 鉴别

蕲蛇为《中国药典》(2005 年版)一部收载的一种常用中药，来源于蝰科动物五步蛇 *Agkistrodon acutus* Güenther 的干燥体。有祛风、通络、止痉之功效。用于风湿顽痹，麻木拘挛，半身不遂，抽搐痉挛，破伤风，麻风疥癣。

蕲蛇作为贵重动物药材，临床功效确切，但商品来源复杂、药材形态鉴别困难，我们在收集实验材料的同时对市场上蕲蛇药材的流通情况进行了调查。流通商品中多以中介蝮蛇、山烙铁头、蝰蛇等经过加工后混作正品蕲蛇销售。这些品种与蕲蛇同科不同属，因其来源相近，故鉴定困难。此外，药材在加工处理时剖去内脏后，要进行干燥处理，皮上的花纹特征、颜色变得模糊，使得辨认困难，如百花锦蛇、玉斑锦蛇、滑鼠蛇、眼镜蛇等其大小、形态特征有与蕲蛇相近之处，这也是造成鉴定困难的另一重要原因。为了获取暴利，造假的手段越来越高明，一些造假者将蕲蛇蛇皮黏合其他动物的肉以增加份量。因此就要求鉴别者具备丰富的鉴别经验，如仅根据形态特征来进行鉴别已不能满足市场的需求。为深入研究蕲蛇药材分子遗传标记鉴别，寻找更为经济实用、准确便捷、稳定性高的鉴别方法，本文用高特异性 PCR 对蕲蛇药材及其混淆品进行了鉴别。

## 1 仪器、试剂及样品

1.1 仪器 ABI 9700 型全自动基因扩增仪(PE 公司);DYY－12 型电泳仪(北京六一仪器厂);Eppendorf 台式高速冷冻离心机(北京基因公司);SYNGENE 型紫外凝胶成像分析仪(北京基因公司)。

1.2 试剂 SDS、琼脂糖、蛋白酶 K、Tris 饱和酚均由 Promega 公司生产;溴化乙锭,Fluka 公司生产;dNTP、*Taq* DNA 聚合酶试剂盒由上海 Sangon 公司生产;其余试剂均为国产分析纯。

1.3 样品 用于高特异性 PCR 鉴别方法学研究的样品见表 1。所有样品均经中国药品生物制品检定所中药标本馆专家张继鉴定。

**表 1 样品原动物的来源及数量**

| 物种 | 编码 | 来源 | 数量 |
|---|---|---|---|
| 蕲蛇 *Agkistrodon acutus* Güenther | 1 | 江西樟树 | 2 |
| | 2 | 河北安国 | 2 |
| 百花锦蛇 *Elaphe moellendorffi* Boettger | 3 | 江西昌北 | 1 |
| | 4 | 河北安国 | 1 |
| 玉斑锦蛇 *Elaphe mandarinus* Cantor | 5 | 河北安国 | 1 |
| | 6 | 中国药品生物制品检定所 | 1 |
| 眼镜蛇 *Naja naja* Linnueus | 7 | 江西樟树 | 1 |
| | 8 | 中国药品生物制品检定所 | 1 |
| 滑鼠蛇 *Ptyas mucosus* Linnaeus | 9 | 河北安国 | 1 |
| | 10 | 中国药品生物制品检定所 | 1 |
| 蝮蛇 *Agkistrodon halys* Pallas | 11 | 河北安国 | 1 |
| | 12 | 中国药品生物制品检定所 | 2 |
| 山烙铁头 *Trimeresurus monticola* Güenther | 13 | 江西樟树 | 2 |
| | 14 | 中国药品生物制品检定所 | 1 |
| 蝰蛇 *Vipera russelli* Shaw | 15 | 江西樟树 | 2 |
| | 16 | 中国药品生物制品检定所 | 1 |

## 2 试验方法

2.1 蕲蛇 PCR 特异性鉴别引物的设计 将蕲蛇及其混淆品通用引物 Cyt *b* 的 PCR 扩增产物在上海生工生物公司进行测序,测序结果经 DNAMAN 软件对位排列后,分析正品、混淆品间序列差异,发现正链在 59～76 bp,互补链在 275～290 bp 为蕲蛇特异性位点。根据其设计高特异性的鉴别引物 HQSL－1 和 HQSH－1。扩增目的片段长度为 220 bp。

ORIGIN(部分序列如下所示)

| | | |
|---|---|---|
| 蕲蛇 1 | *GGAACCGTAATAAAGTCC*NCGTGCNATGTGGATGTAGATACAAATGAAAAANATTGAGGCGCCA－ATTGCGTGGATGTTTT | 138 |
| 蕲蛇 2 | GGAACCGTAATAAAGTCCNCGTGCNATGTGGATGTAGATACAAATGAAAAANATTGAGGCGCC－AATTGCGTGGATGTTTT | 138 |
| 山烙铁头 | GatnCanatccAtAcgngaCGTGCccTaTGGATGaAtcatacAAaacttcAtgcaatcngcgCAtcantGTtctTt-aTc. | 156 |
| 玉斑锦蛇 | cGtACacatcacAcGagatgtccCatatgGatgaatcATACAAAaccttcAtgcaatcGgcgCAtca. atgtttTtcaTc | 159 |
| 蝮蛇 | GatcCanatcnAtAcgagaCGT. CccTaTGGATGaAncatacAAaacttcAtgcaattGgcgCAtcantaTtctTtaTcT | 159 |
| 蝰蛇 | GattCacatcctAcGagatgtgcCtAacgGatgaatcAT-tCAAAacctccAtgcaatcGgcgCAtcT. atgtttTtcaTc | 159 |
| 滑鼠蛇 | GatcCanattatAcGngacgtncCctatgGatgaa-ccATACAAAatAttcAtgcaattagcgCAtcnaCtattcTt-TaTT | 160 |
| 眼镜蛇 | GattCacatcacgcGggacgtgcCttacg-GGtgaatcATACAAAaccttcAcgcaatcagcgCctcc. CtattcTtcaTc | 159 |
| 百花锦蛇 | GntcCacatnanAcGagacgtacCctgngGatgaatcATACAAAatcttcAtgcaattGgngCntcna. tattcTtcaTc | 159 |
| 蕲蛇 1 | GTGNATTGCTAGGAAAAATCCGGTNATTGTTTGTAATATTA...AGCANGTTAGTAATATN*GAT-CCAAAGTTTCATC*ATG | 291 |

| | | |
|---|---|---|
| 蕲蛇 2 | GTGNATTGCTAGGAAAAATCCGGTNATTGTTTGTAATATTA...<br>AGCANGTTAGTAATATNGATCCAAAGTTTCATCATG | 291 |
| 山烙铁头 | ....ATTatcAGG. gAccgCtctattaTtacccn. AatagcaacAGC. . tTcttTggctaN. gTCCtnc....CATgAgG | 284 |
| 玉斑锦蛇 | ....ATcagg....gActatattattaatTaTcctAatagcgacAG. catTcttTggatac. gTCCtgc....CATgA. G | 289 |
| 蝮蛇 | ....ATTatcAGG. AAccgCtctntnaTtacccTcAatagcaacAGCcttTcttTggctaNGgTCCtnc....CATgAaG | 294 |
| 蝰蛇 | ....ATcagg....AAccaCCctactaatTaTactcatagctacAt. cttTcttctgntat. gTannAc....CATgggG | 290 |
| 滑鼠蛇 | ....ATTatcAGGAAAccgCtctattaatTaccctAatagcaacAG. cttTcttTggctac. gTCCttc....CATg. aG | 291 |
| 眼镜蛇 | ....ATcagg....AAcAgCCctcctggtTaTccttatagcaacAG. cctTcttcggatac. gTCCtcc....CATgA. G | 289 |
| 百花锦蛇 | ....AnTatcAGGAAccgc. . ctattaatgantcttatagcaacAG. cctTcttTggctaN. gTCtgn.....CATg. aG | 288 |

2.2 模板DNA的提取 取蕲蛇及混淆品原动物的干燥肌肉组织约1g,参照王义权等的方法提取DNA模板。

2.3 特异性PCR鉴别 PCR反应体系25 μL,其中10 mmol/L Tris - HCl(pH 8.3),50 mmol/L 氯化钾,$Mg^{2+}$ 1.5 mmol/L,dNTP each 0.15 μmol/L,*Taq* 1 U(Takara Ex *Taq*),鉴别引物各0.15 μmol/L,模板DNA 50 ng。循环参数:95℃预变性4 min;95℃变性40 s,50℃退火1 min,72℃延伸30 s,25个循环;72℃延伸5 min。PCR反应选用不同的复性温度以寻找合适的反应参数。实验中设置无DNA模板的阴性对照。取5 μL反应液经1.8%琼脂糖凝胶电泳,EB染色,紫外凝胶分析检测,成像。

同时用扩增约308 bp的Cyt *b*基因片段的通用引物(L14841 5′AAAAAGCTTCCATC - CAACATCTCAG - CAT GATGAAA3′和H15149 5′ AAACTGCAGCCCCTCAGAAT GATATTTGTCCTCA3′)在55℃的复性温度下对上述用于PCR鉴别的模板DNA作阳性扩增对照。

## 3 结果

3.1 模板质量 蕲蛇药材及混淆品原动物提取的DNA模板用通用引物L14841和H15149扩增,得到约308 bp扩增带(图1A);表明样品中模板DNA质量符合PCR反应的要求。

3.2 序列测定 使用Cyt *b*通用引物对蕲蛇及混淆品进行PCR扩增后进行正反向测序,序列经Clustal X 1.8软件对位排列分析正、混品间DNA序列差异,设计出一对高特异性鉴别引物HQSL - 1和HQSH - 1(上海生工生物公司合成)。

3.3 高特异性PCR鉴别 用蕲蛇高特异性鉴别引物HQSL - 1和HQSH - 1对其原动物及混淆品DNA模板进行扩增。当复性温度为60℃和55℃时,蕲蛇正品及混淆品都没有扩增出特异性的条带(图1B);当复性温度降至50℃时,其反应具有高度特异性,仅正品蕲蛇有良好的单一扩增带,其余样品均无扩增带出现(图1C)。故特异性PCR循环参数确定为:95℃预变性4 min;95℃变性40 s,50℃复性1 min,72℃延伸30 s,25个循环;72℃延伸5 min。因此,依据鉴别引物扩增模板DNA有无扩增条带即可确定受试样品是否为正品。

3.4 PCR方法重现性考察 为了考察PCR方法的稳定性选取了Invitrogen公司、Promega公司、生工公司、华美公司、天为时代公司、博大生物公司 *Taq* DNA聚合酶及天为时代公司一管便捷式 *Taq* 酶试剂盒,使用相同的PCR仪(ABI - 9700)进行PCR高特异性鉴别。结果显示不同公司 *Taq* DNA聚合酶都得到了相同的鉴别结果。

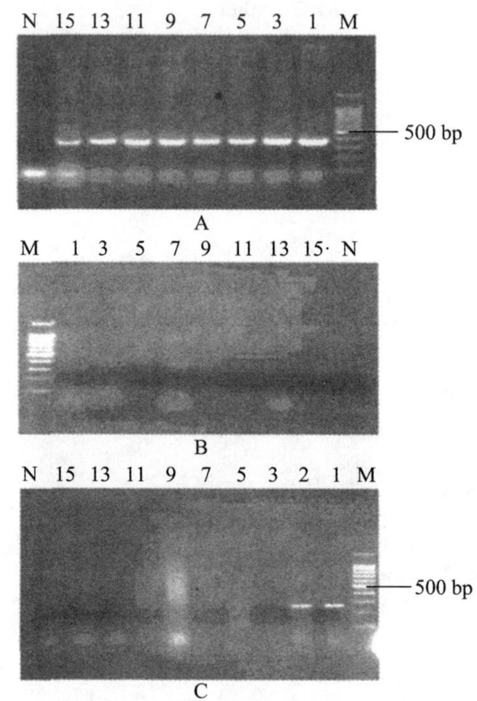


**图1 蕲蛇及其混淆品Cyt *b*片段扩增(A)、蕲蛇及其混淆品高特异性PCR鉴别(60℃或55℃,B)、蕲蛇及其混淆品高特异性真伪鉴别(50℃,C)**

1、2. 蕲蛇(*Agkistrodon acutus* Güenther);3. 百花锦蛇(*Elaphe moellendorffi* Boettger);5. 玉斑锦蛇(*Elaphe mandarinus* Cantor);7. 滑鼠蛇(*Ptyas mucosus* Linnaeus);9. 眼镜蛇(*Naja naja* Linnueus);11. 腹蛇(*Agkistrodon halys* Pallas);13. 山烙铁头(*Trimeresurus monticola* Güenther);15. 蝰蛇(*Vipera russelli* Shaw);N. 阴性对照;M. DNA markers (100 bp)。

## 4 讨论

4.1 市场调查 文献报道蕲蛇混淆品达一二十种,不同文献报道所涉及种类也存在较大差异。本次研究未能包括所有提及的混淆品,且实际调查中发现,有些混淆品在商品流通中出现的频率极低;另一些则由于在外观形态、大小上与蕲蛇相差很远,通过性状鉴别容易区分开来。所以寻找市场上充伪频率最高、来源相近、外观形态上与蕲蛇相近的品种,进行PCR鉴别才具有重要意义。当蕲蛇药材保持完整时,可通过外观形态的典型特征进行鉴定;但是当药材已经切成段进行销售时，性状鉴别就显得力不从心，这时从 DNA 分子水平进行检测就显出极大的优势。

4.2 引物设计 考虑到动物类药材由于贮藏方式不当或贮存过久，经常有虫蛀、发霉变质现象发生，加工炮制后其 DNA 均会存在不同程度的降解。所扩增的目的片段越长，扩增效率将会越低。因此实验中设计的特异性鉴别引物所扩增的目的片段长度为 220 bp，将不会受到药材 DNA 降解的影响。

4.3 PCR 方法的重现性考察 实验中使用进口及国产 *Taq* DNA 聚合酶进行验证。不同的 *Taq* 酶均得到相同的电泳结果，表明虽然不同的酶活力不同，但只要按各自的 PCR 反应体系加入相应的酶量则不会影响到鉴定结果。

［唐晓晶，黄璐琦，等．药物分析杂志，2006，26(2)：152－155.］

# 金钱白花蛇及其混淆品高特异性 PCR 的鉴别

金钱白花蛇为《中国药典》2005 年版一部收载的一种常用中药，来源于眼镜蛇科动物金钱白花蛇 *Bungarus multicinctus* Blyth 的干燥体，有祛风、通络、止痉之功效。金钱白花蛇作为动物药材临床功效确切，但商品来源复杂、药材形态鉴别困难，而且仅根据形态特征很难进行准确的鉴别。王义权等使用 PCR 高特异性鉴别引物已鉴定出金钱白花蛇的真伪，但所报道的混淆品数量少，有些通过形态特征即可排除，尚不能满足目前市场上混伪品的鉴定。为了深入研究金钱白花蛇类药材分子遗传标记鉴别，寻找到更为经济实用、准确便捷、稳定性高的鉴别方法，本研究用高特异性 PCR 对金钱白花蛇药材及其混淆品进行鉴别。

## 1 材料和方法

1.1 材料 用于高特异性 PCR 鉴别方法学研究的实验材料见表 1。用于验证实验的金钱白花蛇药材购自北京同仁堂、北京金象大药房、北京京隆堂、北京阳光同仁药房。所有实验材料均经中国药品生物制品检定所张继研究员鉴定。

**表 1 金钱白花蛇及其混淆品来源及数量**

| 编号 | 材料名称 | 拉丁学名 | 数量 |
|---|---|---|---|
| 1 | 金钱白花蛇[1] | *Bungarus multicinctus* | 2 |
| 2 | 金钱白花蛇[1] | *B. multicincutus* | 2 |
| 3 | 金钱白花蛇[1] | *B. multicincutus* | 2 |
| 4 | 金钱白花蛇[1] | *B. multicincutus* | 2 |
| 5 | 赤链蛇[2] | *Dinodon rufozonatum* | 2 |
| 6 | 赤链蛇[2] | *D. rufozonatum* | 2 |
| 7 | 赤链华游蛇[2] | *Sinonatrix annularis* | 2 |
| 8 | 赤链华游蛇[2] | *S. annularis* | 1 |
| 9 | 金环蛇[2] | *B. fasciatus* | 1 |
| 10 | 金环蛇[2] | *B. fasciatus* | 2 |
| 11 | 中国水蛇[2] | *Enhydris chinensis* | 1 |
| 12 | 中国水蛇[2] | *E. chinensis* | 1 |
| 13 | 双全白环蛇[2] | *Lycodon fasciatus* | 2 |
| 14 | 双全白环蛇[2] | *L. fasciatus* | 1 |
| 15 | 铅色水蛇[2] | *E. plumbea* | 2 |
| 16 | 铅色水蛇[2] | *E. plumbea* | 1 |

注：[1] 正品；[2] 混淆品；1、5、7、13、16 号样品购自江西樟树药材市场；2、6、8、10 号样品购自河北安国药材市场；3、12 号样品购自江西昌北药材市场；4、9、11、14、15 号样品购自中国药品生物制品检定所。

1.2 金钱白花蛇高特异性 PCR 鉴别引物的设计 对金钱白花蛇及其混淆品的 Cyt *b* 基因片段使用通用引物 L14841 5′AAAAAGCTTCCATCCAACATCTCAGCATGATGAAA 3′和 H15149 5′AAACTGCAGCCCCTCAGAATGATATTTGTCCTCA3′进行 PCR 扩增，对 PCR 产物测定其序列约 325 bp，经 DNAMAN 软件对位排列分析正、混品间 DNA 序列差异，设计出一对能特异性扩增金钱白花蛇 Cyt *b* 基因片段的鉴别引物 HJL－1 5′GACTTAGCTTTCTCATCTGTGATCCATATTA3′和 HJH－15′GCCTGCAGCCCCTCAGAATGATATTTGTCCTCA3′（上海生工生物公司合成）。序列见图 1。

1.3 模板 DNA 的提取 取金钱白花蛇及混淆品原动物干燥肌肉组织约 1 g，参照王义权等方法提取 DNA 模板。

1.4 特异性 PCR 鉴别方法 PCR 反应体系 30 μL，含 10 mmol/L Tris－HCl，pH 8.0，50 mmol/L KCl，0.1% Triton X－100，1.5 mmol/L $MgCl_2$，1.5 mmol/L dNTPs，高特异性鉴别引物 HJL－1 和 HJH－1 各 10 pmol/L，3 U *Taq* 酶和 DNA 模板约 150 ng。循环参数：95 ℃预变性 4 min；95 ℃变性 40 s，67 ℃退火 1 min，72 ℃延伸 30 s，25 个循环；72 ℃延伸 5 min。PCR 反应选用不同的复性温度以寻找合适的 PCR 鉴别反应参数。实验中设置无 DNA 模板的阴性对照。取 5 μL

```
ORIGIN
金钱白花蛇 TAACNTGCTTAATATTACAAACAATNACCGGATTTTCCTAGCAATNCACTATACAGGACTTAGCTTTCT     70
赤链蛇     ----c---c--nn-c------nt--a--a--n-----n-----n--c--------------n---n----    70
赤链华游蛇 ----c--t-c-gccc------tt--a--a--c--c--t--------c-----------a-----t-----    70
金环蛇     --g-c---c-----c------tt--a--------c-----------t-----c-----------t-----    70
中国水蛇   ----c---c-nt--c------tt--a--a--t--------------c-----------n--t--tg--n-    70
双全白环蛇 -t--c---c--n--c------tn--a--a--t--------------c-----n-----n-----tn--n-    70
铅色水蛇   ----c---c--gc-c--------tca--a--c--------------t-----c-----------cn-t--    70

金钱白花蛇 CATCTGTGATCCATATTACCACAT.CACACGGGATGTCCCCACGGGTGAANCATACAAAACATCCACGC    139
赤链蛇     a--g---------g-g--------.n-----a--c--a---tg---a----t---------tc-t--t--    139
赤链华游蛇 a-----t--------cg-a-----.------a--------at-t--a----t----------c-t--t--    139
金环蛇     a------------g-g--t-----.---g-----c--g--tt----------t----------c-t---n-    139
中国水蛇   a--t--------tg-g--------.t-t---n--c--n---t-t--a----c---------t--t--t--    139
双全白环蛇 a--t--------tg-g-------—c--t---a--c--g---t-t--a----c----------c-t--t--    140
铅色水蛇   a--a--t------g-g--t-----.-ct---a-----g--ta----a----t---t------c----t--    139

金钱白花蛇 AATTGGCGCCTCAATNTTTTCATTTGTATCTACATCCACATNGCACGNGGACTTTATTACGGTTCCTAN    209
赤链蛇     ------n--------a--c-----c--c-----t--t-----t-----a-----a-n---n--a-----c    209
赤链华游蛇 ---c-----a-----g--------c--c--------t--tg-c-----a-----a--c-----a-----c    209
金环蛇     ---c--------cc-a--c-----c----------c---t--c-----a-----c--c--t----ta--c    209
中国水蛇   ----a----a---c-a--c--t-----c--t--t-----t--t-----a-----a--c--t--c-.tata    208
双全白环蛇 ---------a-----a--c--t--c--c--t-----------t-----a-----a--c--t------ata    210
铅色水蛇   ---c-----a--t--g--------c--c--t----c------t-----a--g-----c-----c-----t    209

金钱白花蛇 CTAAACAAANAAGTNTGACTATCAGGAATCACCCTNTTAATTATCNTAATAGCCACANCCTTCTTNGGCT    279
赤链蛇     -----t-.-a-gaag—tga--atcaggaac-g-.c-attaatga--ct--tagca-cagcct-ctttgg    277
赤链华游蛇 -----t---a-t--a-----------g-ct-tat-a---------c-------g---g-a-----t--a-    279
金环蛇     -----t---g----t------------cag----cc-gg-----c-t-----a---g-------c--a-    279
中国水蛇   -ctc-a.t-a-gaag-ctgat-atcaggaac-g--c-attaat-acccta-tagca-cag.ct--ctctg    276
双全白环蛇 -ctc-act-a-gaag-ctgat-atcaggaac-g--c--tna.t-accctc-tagca-cagcct--ctttg    279
铅色水蛇   t--------ggg--g-------------c------ac-------ac-c-----t---t-t-----ct-g-    279

金钱白花蛇 ACGTACTACCATGAGGACAAATATCATTCTGAGGGGCTGCAGGCTTTAA                         326
赤链蛇     ctangtctg--.c-t--gg-ca-at--ca-tct-a-gg--t-cagttta                         324
赤链华游蛇 ----c--g-----------------------------------------                         325
金环蛇     ----c--c-----------------------------------------                         325
中国水蛇   g-tacg-c-ttcc-t--gg-ca-at--ca-tct-a-gg--t-cagttta                         325
双全白环蛇 g-tang-c-tncc-t--gg-ca-at--ca-tct-a-gg--t-cagttta                         328
铅色水蛇   -t---nn------------------------------------------                         325
```

**图 1　金钱白花蛇及其混淆品的 Cyt *b* 序列**

斜体序列为金钱白花蛇特异性鉴别引物。

反应液经 1.8% 琼脂糖凝胶电泳，EB 染色，紫外凝胶分析检测，成像。

同时用扩增约 320 bp 的 Cyt *b* 基因片段的通用引物，在 55 ℃的复性温度下对上述用于 PCR 鉴别的模板 DNA 作阳性扩增对照。

## 2　结果

2.1　*模板质量的研究*　金钱白花蛇药材及混淆品原动物提取的 DNA 模板用通用引物 L14841 和 H15149 扩增，得到约 320 bp 扩增带(图 2)；表明样品中模板 DNA 质量符合 PCR 反应的要求。

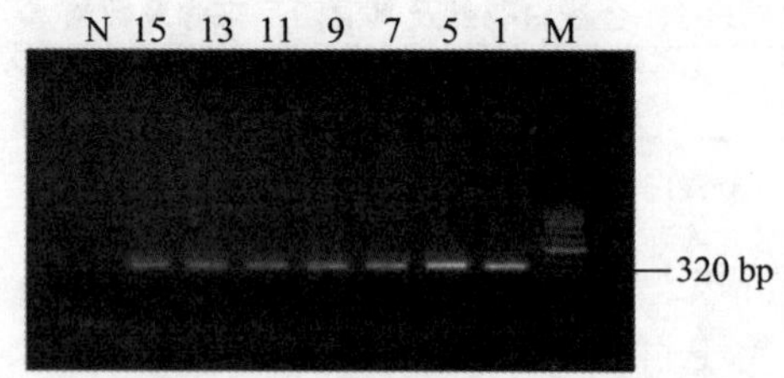


**图 2　通用引物 L14841 和 H15149 扩增(阳性对照)**

样品编号同表 1；N. 阴性对照；M. DNA marker(图 3～5 同)。

2.2　*高特异性 PCR 鉴别*　用鉴别引物 PCR 扩增金钱白花蛇原动物样品的 DNA。当复性温度为 60 ℃时，金钱白花蛇、金环蛇、中国水蛇、双全白环蛇在 230 bp 处扩增出条带(图 3)；当复性温度为 65 ℃时，金钱白花蛇、中国水蛇同时扩增出 1 条弱带(图 4)；当复性温度升至 67 ℃时，其反应具有高度特异性，仅正品金钱白花蛇有良好的单一扩增带，其余样品均无扩增带出现(图 5)；当退火和延伸温度合并为 67 ℃时，正品也未见扩增带出现；当复性温度升至 70 ℃时，所有样品均无扩增带出现。故特异性 PCR 循环参数确定为：95 ℃预变性 4 min；95 ℃变性 40 s，67 ℃复性 1 min，72 ℃延伸 30 s，25 个循环；72 ℃延伸 5 min。因此，依据鉴别引物扩增模板 DNA 有无扩增条带即可确定受试样品是否为正品。

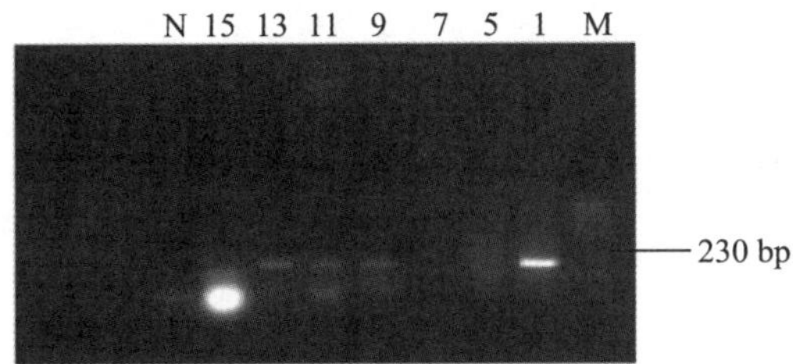


图 3 鉴别引物高特异性 PCR 鉴别(60 ℃退火)

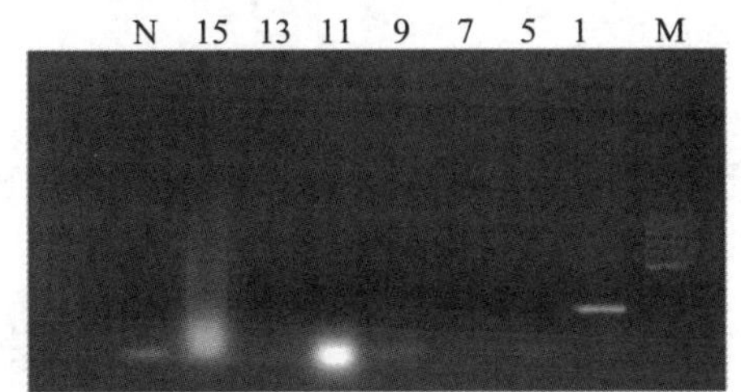


图 4 鉴别引物高特异性 PCR 鉴别(65 ℃退火)

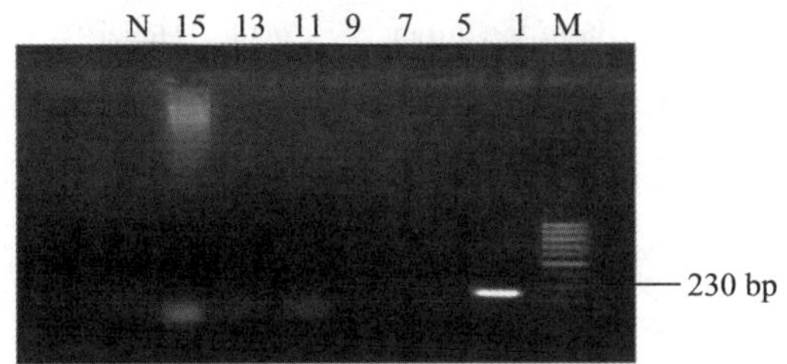


图 5 鉴别引物高特异性 PCR 鉴别(67 ℃退火)

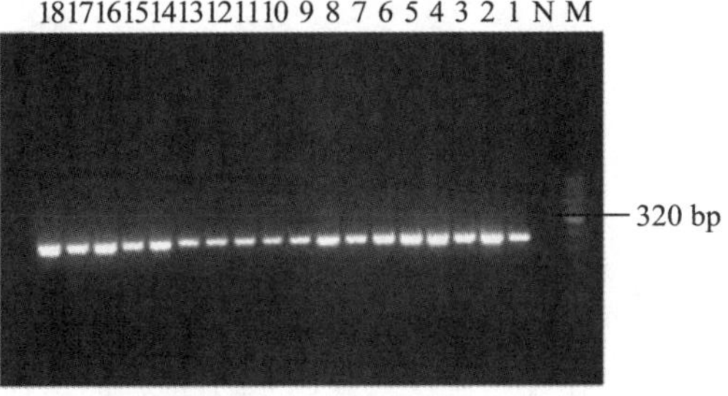


图 6 通用引物 L14841 和 H15149 扩增(阳性对照)

对购买的金钱白花蛇药材样品编号(编号与表 1 不同):1～5. 北京同仁堂药店;6～10. 北京金象大药房;11～14. 北京永安堂药房;15～18. 北京京隆堂药房(图 7 同)。

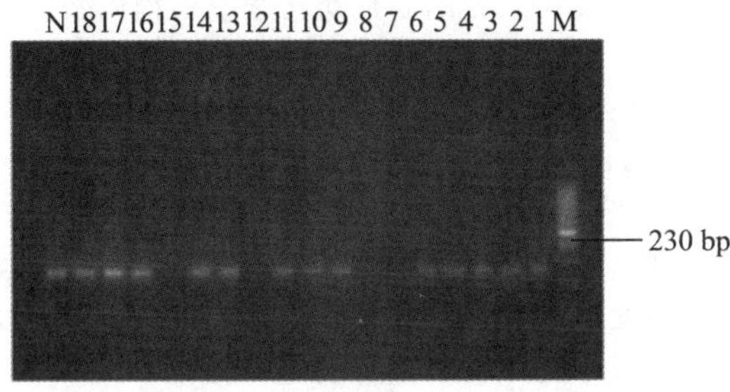


图 7 鉴别引物高特异性 PCR 鉴别(67 ℃退火)

2.3 *个体差异的研究* 因物种种内存在变异,本次实验针对动物类药材不同产地间物种的变异是否会影响 PCR 特异性鉴别结果进行了验证。将所有收集到的金钱白花蛇正品及混淆品原动物的 DNA 模板进行 PCR 鉴别,结果显示不同来源的正品金钱白花蛇在 230 bp 处出现扩增带,而混淆品均未见扩增带。表明金钱白花蛇及其混淆品同一物种的种内差异不会影响高特异性 PCR 鉴别的结果。

2.4 *市售金钱白花蛇药材特异性鉴别* 用金钱白花蛇鉴别引物,对北京同仁堂药店、北京金象大药房、北京阳光同仁药房、北京京隆堂随机购买的金钱白花蛇药材进行 PCR 鉴别,同时通用引物扩增作为阳性对照(图 6)。结果显示样品 1～5、8～10、12、15～18 在约 230 bp 处出现一条明亮的扩增带,表明为正品金钱白花蛇;而样品 6、7、11、14 均无扩增带出现,表明是金钱白花蛇的混淆品(图 7)。本结果与根据药材外观性状、显微鉴别的鉴定结果完全一致。

2.5 *PCR 方法稳定性考察* 为了考察 PCR 方法的稳定性选取了 Invitrogen 公司、Promega 公司、生工公司、华美公司、天为时代公司、博大生物公司 *Taq* DNA 聚合酶,使用相同的 PCR 仪(ABI-9700)进行 PCR 高特异性鉴别。结果显示不同公司 *Taq* DNA 聚合酶都得到了相同的鉴别结果。

## 3 讨论

3.1 *不同文献报道的金钱白花蛇混淆品种类存在较大差异* 实际调查中发现,有些混淆品在商品流通中出现的频率极低,一些则由于在外观上其形态、大小与金钱白花蛇相差甚远,通过性状特征容易区别。所以寻找充伪频率最高,来源相近,外观形态与金钱白花蛇相近的品种,进行 PCR 鉴别才具有重要意义。

3.2 *细胞色素 b(Cyt b)是动物体内编码蛋白质的基因,具有高度保守性* 而金钱白花蛇与其混淆品的 Cyt *b* 基因序列相近,所以提高退火温度并减少循环数来增加特异性就显得十分重要。使用鉴别引物在低温退火时会产生很多非特异性条带,通过摸索提高到 67 ℃时特异性最高。由于退火温度已经足够高,实验中还尝试将退火延伸合二为一完成整个扩增循环,既省时又提高特异性,但未得到期望的结果。

3.3 *动物类药材与植物药不同的是它不会固定生长* 金钱白花蛇产地遍及南方多省市,是否不同省市物种的种内差异会影响 PCR 鉴别的结果。取样时分别从不同地方收集到同一种的不同个体,有效避免了每个物种只有一个样品的弊端,从而消除了出现假阳性的可能。

3.4 *PCR 方法的稳定性一直以来倍受关注* 关于 PCR 鉴别方法稳定性的报道并不多见,但实际只有重复性好、稳定的方法才有可能得到广泛应用。实验中使用进口及国产 *Taq* DNA 聚合酶进行验证。不同的 *Taq* 酶均得到相同的结果,表明虽然不同的酶活力不同,但只要按各自的 PCR 反应体系加入相应的酶量,则不会影响到鉴定结果。

[冯成强,黄璐琦,等.中国中药杂志,2006,31(13):1050-1053.]

# 高特异性 PCR 方法鉴别乌梢蛇及其混淆品

乌梢蛇为《中国药典》(2005 版)一部收载的一种常用中药,来源于游蛇科动物乌梢蛇 *Zaocys dhumnades* Cantor 的干燥体。有祛风、通络、止痉之功效。用于风湿顽痹、麻木拘挛、半身不遂、抽搐痉挛、瘰疬恶疮。

鉴于乌梢蛇作为中药的临床功效确切,但商品来源复杂、药材性状鉴别困难的现状,我们对市场上乌梢蛇药材流通情况进行了调查。商品流通中多以红点锦蛇 *Elaphe rufodorsata* Cantor、黑眉锦蛇 *Elaphe taeniura* Cope、玉斑锦蛇 *Elaphe mandarinus* Cantor、王锦蛇 *Elaphe carinata* Guenther、灰鼠蛇 *Ptyas korros* Schlegel 等来混作正品药材进行销售,这些品种多数与乌梢蛇同科不同属;因其来源相近,造成鉴定困难。此外,药材在加工处理时剖去内脏后,要进行干燥熏黑处理,皮上的花纹特征、颜色几近消失,难以辨认,而且其大小、形态特征与乌梢蛇相近,这是造成其性状鉴别困难的另一重要原因。随着分子生物技术的发展,利用DNA分子遗传标记技术鉴别中药材的真伪已成为可能。王义权等通过对乌梢蛇及其混淆品线粒体 Cyt b 基因进行测序,通过对测序结果的比对分析来鉴别乌梢蛇的真伪,但因对 DNA 进行测序成本较高,操作有难度,不同人的测序结果会存在偏差,所以在实际应用中适用性不强。为了深入乌梢蛇类药材分子遗传标记鉴别研究,满足目前市场常见混伪品的鉴别要求,寻找更为经济实用、准确便捷、稳定性高的方法,本实验用高特异性 PCR 方法对乌梢蛇药材及其混淆品的原动物和炮制品进行鉴别。

## 1 材料与方法

### 1.1 材料

用于高特异性 PCR 鉴别方法学研究的实验材料见表 1。乌梢蛇炮制品购自北京同仁堂、北京京隆堂、北京阳光同仁药房、北京金象大药房。

表 1 实验材料的种类、来源和数量

| 编码 | 物种 | 来源 | 数量 |
|---|---|---|---|
| 1、2 | *Zaocys dhumnades* Cantor | Zhangshu, Jiangxi | 2 |
| 3 | *Zaocys dhumnades* Cantor | Anguo, Hebei | 1 |
| 4 | *Zaocys dhumnades* Cantor | Changbei, Jiangxi | 1 |
| 5 | *Elaphe rufodorsata* Cantor | Zhangshu, Jiangxi | 2 |
| 6 | *Elaphe rufodorsata* Cantor | Anguo, Hebei | 1 |
| 7 | *Elaphe mandarinus* Cantor | Anguo, Hebei | 1 |
| 8 | *Elaphe mandarinus* Cantor | Zhangshu, Jiangxi | 1 |
| 9 | *Elaphe radiata* Schlegel | Anguo, Hebei | 1 |
| 10 | *Elaphe radiata* Schlegel | NICPBP[1)] | 1 |
| 11 | *Ptyas korros* Schlegel | Zhangshu, Jiangxi | 1 |
| 12 | *Ptyas korros* Schlegel | NICPBP[1)] | 1 |
| 13 | *Elaphe taeniura* Cope | Zhangshu, Jiangxi | 2 |
| 14 | *Elaphe taeniura* Cope | Changbei, Jiangxi | 2 |
| 15 | *Elaphe carinata* Guenther | Zhangshu, Jiangxi | 3 |
| 16 | *Elaphe carinata* Guenther | Anguo, Hebei | 2 |
| 17 | *Dinodon rufozonatum* Cantor | Zhangshu, Jiangxi | 2 |
| 18 | *Dinodon rufozonatum* Cantor | Anguo, Hebei | 2 |
| 19 | *Natrix annularis* Hallowell | Zhangshu, Jiangxi | 2 |
| 20 | *Natrix annularis* Hallowell | Anguo, Hebei | 1 |
| 21 | *Naja naja* Linnueus | Zhangshu, Jiangxi | 1 |
| 22 | *Naja naja* Linnueus | NICPBP[1)] | 2 |
| 23 | *Ptyasmucosus* Linnaeus | Anguo, Hebei | 1 |
| 24 | *Ptyasmucosus* Linnaeus | Zhangshu, Jiangxi | 1 |

注:[1)] 中国药品生物制品检定所。

1.2 乌梢蛇高特异性 PCR 鉴别引物的设计 从 GenBank 下载正品原动物乌梢蛇及混伪品黑眉锦蛇、红点锦蛇、灰鼠蛇、眼镜蛇、赤链蛇、玉斑锦蛇、赤链华游蛇、王锦蛇、滑鼠蛇的原动物线粒体 12S rRNA 基因序列(GenBank 登录号依次为:AF236676、AF233940、AF236675、AF236680、AF236683、AF233939、AF236670、AF236677、AF236674、AY122828),经 DNAMAN 软件对位排列分析正、混品间 DNA 序列差异,设计出一对能特异性扩增乌梢蛇 12S rRNA 基因片段的特异性鉴别引物 HWL-1 和 HWH-1(上海生工生物公司合成)。乌梢蛇及其混淆品 12S rRNA 序列(约 800 bp)的部分序列,见表 2。

1.3 模板 DNA 的提取 取乌梢蛇及混淆品原动物和炮制品(醋炙乌梢蛇段)的干燥肌肉组织约 1 g,参照王义权等方法提取 DNA 模板。

1.4 特异性 PCR 鉴别方法 PCR 反应体系 25 μL,其中 10 mmol/L Tris-HCl (pH 8.3), 50 mmol/L 氯化钾, $Mg^{2+}$ 1.5 mmol/L, dNTP 各 0.15 μmol/L, *Taq* 1 U (Takara Ex *Taq*),引物各 0.15 μmol/L,模板 DNA 50 ng。循环参数:95 ℃预变性 4 min;95 ℃变性 40 s, 55～65 ℃复性 1 min, 72 ℃

**表 2　乌梢蛇及其混淆品 125 rRNA 序列(约 800 bp)的部分序列**

| 编码 | 物种 | 序　列 | |
|---|---|---|---|
| 1 | *Zaocys dhumnades* - 1 | GCCAGCAGCAGTAGTTAATATTAGGCCATAA*GCG*..*AAAGCTCGACCTAGCAAGGGGAC*.....*CACA*GGGCCGGTTAA | 219 |
| 1 | *Zaocys dhumnades* - 2 | ----------------------------------..-----------------------.....--------------- | 219 |
| 2 | *Elaphe taeniura* | --t--a----------a-----------------..-------t---------------...ca..-t----------- | 225 |
| 3 | *Elaphe rufodorsata* | ---------------a------------------..c------t-------------a...ctac-ta---------- | 223 |
| 4 | *Ptyas korros* | -------------------------t----a--..-----t-t-------------.--......t-t--------- | 214 |
| 5 | *Naja naja* | ---------------a------------------..c------t----------------...gcgtata.---------- | 224 |
| 6 | *Natrix annularis* | --------------tc----------------acc-------t------------a--gt.ta..at----------- | 220 |
| 7 | *Elaphe mandarinus* | --t-ca---------a---c-----------a--..c------t--------t---a----cttta-c-----t----- | 220 |
| 8 | *Dinodon rufozonatum* | ----c--------------------------..-------t-----------a--a-ttca..-c----------- | 222 |
| 9 | *Elaphe carinata* | -----------------a---------t-------c------t------------a--ac--tt....---------- | 223 |
| 10 | *Ptyas mucosus* | ...................................................................... | 0 |
| 1 | *Zaocys dhumnades* 1 | AATTTAAAA.GACTTGAC*GGTACCCCATAACAACCTAGAGGAGCCTG*TCTAATAACCGATACCCCACGATTAA.CCCAAC | 561 |
| 1 | *Zaocys dhumnades* 2 | ---------.---------------------------------------------------------------.------ | 561 |
| 2 | *Elaphe taeniura* | ---------.-----------g--t--a-c----------------------------------------a--.---g-- | 569 |
| 3 | *Elaphe rufodorsata* | ---------.--------------t--a-------------------------------------------c--.------ | 566 |
| 4 | *Ptyas korros* | ---------.--------------t--c------------------------------------------------a------ | 561 |
| 5 | *Naja naja* | ---------.-----------g--t--a----------------------------------------------.------ | 570 |
| 6 | *Natrix annularis* | --c------.-------------tt--c-c--c-----------------------------t----------.------ | 566 |
| 7 | *Elaphe mandarinus* | ---------a-------------t-t--c--------------------c---------------------c--.------ | 560 |
| 8 | *Dinodon rufozonatum* | --------.------------------c-------------------tc-g-----------t-----------.t----- | 567 |
| 9 | *Elaphe carinata* | --------.--------------g--t--a----------------------g----------t---------a-c--a-c- | 574 |
| 10 | *Ptyas mucosus* | --------.-----------------t--c---------------------c.------------tat------.---- | 313 |

注：斜体加粗部分为设计的特异性引物。

延伸 30 s，25 个循环；72 ℃延伸 5 min。PCR 反应选用不同的复性温度以寻找合适的 PCR 鉴别反应参数。实验中设置无 DNA 模板的阴性对照。取 5 μL 反应液经 1.8%琼脂糖凝胶电泳，EB 染色，紫外凝胶分析检测，成像。

同时用扩增约 400 bp 的 12S rRNA 基因片段的通用引物(L1091 5′ AAACTGGGATTAGATACCCCACTAT3′ 和 H1478 5′ TGACTGCAGAGGGTGACGGGCGGTGTGT3′)在 55 ℃的复性温度下对上述用于 PCR 鉴别的模板 DNA 作阳性扩增对照。

## 2　结果

2.1　模板质量研究　乌梢蛇药材及混淆品原动物和炮制品(醋炙乌梢蛇段)提取的 DNA 模板用通用引物 L1091 和 H1478 扩增，得到约 400 bp 扩增带(图 1)，表明样品中模板 DNA 质量符合 PCR 反应的要求。

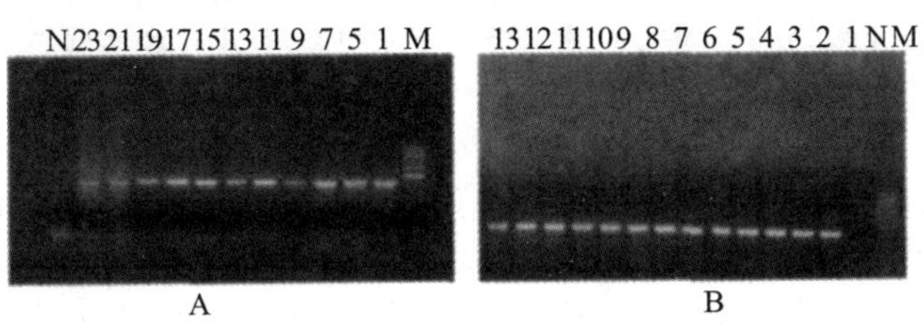


**图 1　12S rRNA 基因通用引物 L1091(A)和 H1478(B)扩增模板 DNA(阳性对照)**

2.2　高特异性 PCR 鉴别的研究　用鉴别引物 PCR 扩增乌梢蛇原动物样品的 DNA，当复性温度为 55 ℃时，乌梢蛇的正品有 2 条带，玉斑锦蛇、红点锦蛇、三索锦蛇有 1 条很弱的带(图 2A)；当复性温度为 60 ℃，乌梢蛇、赤链蛇同时扩增出 1 条带(图 2B)；当复性温度升至 65 ℃，25 个循环时，其反应具有高度特异性，仅正品乌梢蛇有良好的单一扩增带，其余样品皆无扩增带出现。当退火和延伸温度合并为 68 ℃时，正品也未见扩增带出现。故特异性 PCR 循环参数确定为：95 ℃预变性 4 min；95 ℃变性 40 s，65 ℃复性 1 min，72 ℃延伸 30 s，25 个循环；72 ℃延伸 5 min。因此，依据鉴别引物扩增模板 DNA 有无扩增条带即可确定受试样品是否为正品(图 3)。

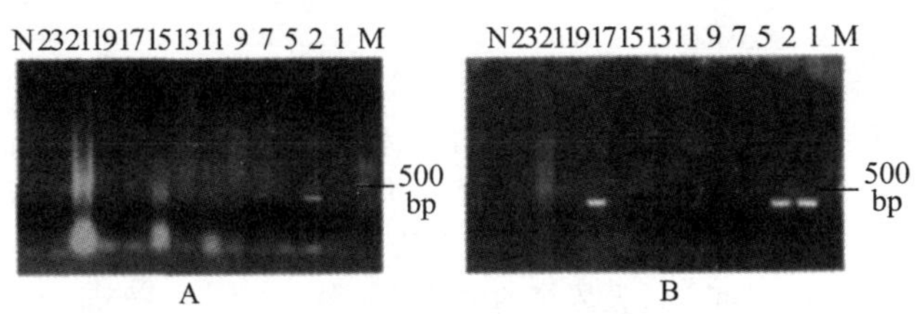


**图 2　退火温度 55 ℃(A)和 60 ℃(B)乌梢蛇鉴别引物 PCR 扩增**

2.3　个体差异的研究　因物种种内存在变异，本次实验针对动物类药材不同产地间物种的变异是否会影响 PCR 特异性鉴别结果进行了验证。将所有收集到的乌梢蛇正品及混淆品原动物的 DNA 模板进行 PCR 鉴别,结果显示不同来源的 4 个正品乌梢蛇在 320 bp 处出现扩增带,而混淆品均未见扩增带(图 3B)。表明乌梢蛇及其混淆品同一物种的种内差异不会影响高特异性 PCR 鉴别的结果。

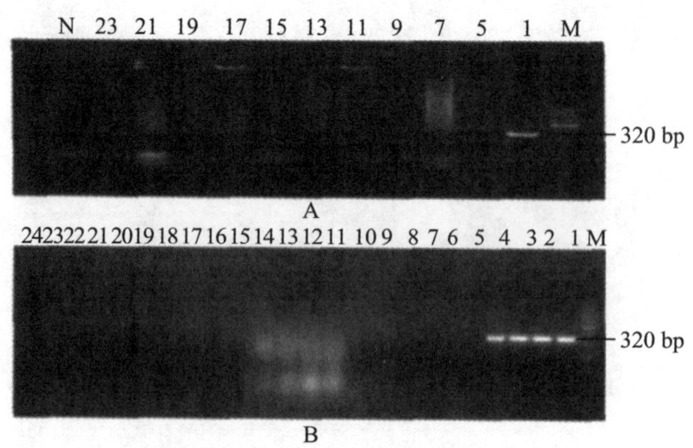


**图 3 退火温度 65 ℃乌梢蛇鉴别引物 PCR 扩增**

2.4 炮制品特异性鉴别的研究 用乌梢蛇鉴别引物,对北京同仁堂、京隆堂、阳光同仁药房、金象大药房随机购买的乌梢蛇药材炮制品进行 PCR 鉴别,结果显示,样品 1、2、3、4、6、8、11、12、13 在约 320 bp 处出现一条明亮的扩增带,表明为正品乌梢蛇;而样品 5、7、9、10 均无扩增带出现,表明是乌梢蛇的混淆品(图 4)。本结果与根据药材外观性状、显微鉴别的鉴定结果完全一致。

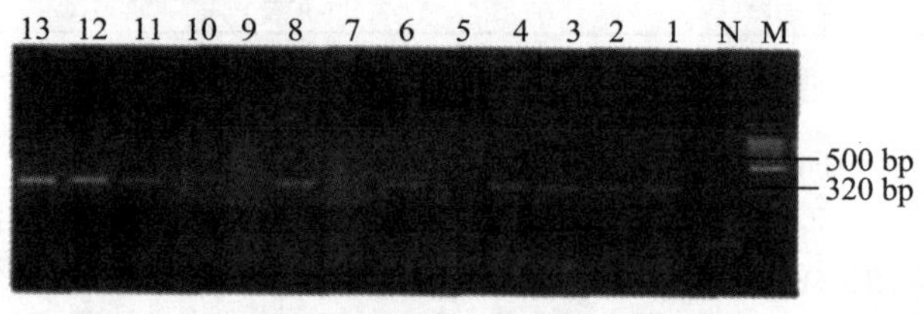


**图 4 65 ℃时乌梢蛇炮制品 PCR 鉴别反应**

N. 阴性对照;M. DNA marker;1～4. 北京同仁堂;5～7. 北京京隆堂;8～10. 北京阳光同仁大药房;11～13. 北京金象药房。

## 3 讨论

3.1 市场调查 文献报道的乌梢蛇混淆品达二三十种,不同文献报道的种类也存在较大差异,本次研究未能包括所有文献报道的混淆品。实际调查中发现,有些混淆品在商品流通中出现的频率极低,另一些则由于来源于非游蛇科,在外观上其形态、大小与乌梢蛇相差很远,通过性状特征容易区别开。所以本课题组寻找市场上充伪频率高、来源相近、外观形态上与乌梢蛇相近的品种,进行了 PCR 鉴别研究,这才具有重要意义。

3.2 药材炮制品的特异性鉴别 市售的乌梢蛇药材部分是经过醋炙的乌梢蛇段,失去个体的完整性,更利于不法商贩进行制假、掺假,以大量的混淆品来充当正品乌梢蛇。由于药材在醋炙过程中外观形态、皮和骨骼等会发生不同程度的改变,所以给乌梢蛇药材性状鉴别带来了更大的困难。而本研究显示,用 DNA 分子标记鉴别则能够更好地克服这个弊端,对乌梢蛇类药材的炮制品在 DNA 水平上进行准确鉴定。如将这对特异性引物加入 *Taq* 试剂盒配成鉴别试剂盒,PCR 时只需加入模板和引物,反应完成后即可直接电泳,使鉴别反应更加简化、便捷;供各级药检所用来鉴定药材及其炮制品,具有很大的应用价值。真正体现出了药材分子鉴别快速、准确可靠、易于操作的优点。

3.3 个体差异的研究 动物类药材由于其自身的特殊性,与植物药不同的是它不会固定生长。蛇类药材的产地遍布于全国,是否不同产地、人工繁殖或野生乌梢蛇种内差异会影响到 PCR 鉴别的结果,为此在收集样品时,分别从不同地方收集到同一种的不同个体,正品乌梢蛇药材达到 4 条,炮制品购自不同药店 13 件,有效避免了每个物种只有一个样品的弊端,从而消除了出现假阳性的可能。

[唐晓晶,黄璐琦,等.中国药学杂志,2007,42(5):333-336.]

# 动物药材分子鉴定研究策略

动物药材是祖国医药重要组成部分,临床上被广泛用于治疗疑难杂症、急重病证等。由于动物药材特别是多来源品种较为混乱,如虻虫、斑蝥等,而且大部分为贵重紧缺药材,通常多以粉末、中成药等形式入药,给动物药材的准确鉴定带来了极大的困难。过去传统的中药鉴定技术,主要是经验性的性状鉴别,这些方法虽然简便、快速,但对多来源药材、破碎药材、粉末药材以及中成药的鉴定有一定的局限性。随着现代科学技术的发展,显微鉴定、红外光谱、紫外吸收光谱、薄层色谱、凝胶电泳等方法也在动物药材的鉴定中起到了重要作用。近年来,分子生物学技术和方法不断更新,其理论和实验技术不断渗透到中药鉴定领域,中药鉴定涌现了一批中药材 DNA 分子鉴定技术,如 RFLP(restriction fragment length polymorphism,限制性片段长度多态性)、RAPD(random amplified polymorphic DNA,随机扩增多态性 DNA 标记)以及基因芯片技术等。DNA 分子鉴定技术不仅能对有形的动物药材整体及破碎部分器官组织进行准确的鉴定,而且还可以对以动物粉末、体液、分泌物和排泄物入药的生药及制剂进行有效的真伪鉴定、纯度检查与质量评价，为动物药材的鉴定带来了蓬勃生机，呈现出良好的发展前景。

## 1 动物药材分子鉴定研究现状

1.1 *基于线粒体 12S rRNA 基因序列的鉴别研究* 由于线粒体 12S rRNA 基因的进化速率较快，不同物种间序列差异大，有利于设计针对目标物种的高特异性引物，加上扩增该基因的稳定性和可重复性好，可以用来作为生物物种种属的鉴定，并在动物药材的分子鉴定中得到应用。利用该基因序列对蛇类药材进行鉴定的报道较多，主要集中在乌梢蛇、金钱白花蛇、蕲蛇及其混淆品的鉴定。如根据乌梢蛇及 10 种常见混淆品线粒体 12S rRNA 基因序列，设计一对专用于乌梢蛇的鉴别引物，从而建立一种简便、准确的乌梢蛇药材分子标记鉴别方法；结果表明，所设计的鉴别引物对正品乌梢蛇有高度的特异性。运用分子标记技术分别从药材蛇胆的胆衣和胆汁、原动物棕黑锦蛇的肌肉和胆汁中提取 DNA，经 PCR 扩增得到约 400 bp 的 12S rRNA 基因片段，并对该基因片段进行测序研究；结果表明，DNA 分子标记技术可用于中药材蛇胆和胆汁的鉴定，提示该技术也可用于其他动物分泌物类型药材的鉴别。有学者从乌龟 *Chinemys reevesii* 和其他 20 种产地为中国或东南亚国家的龟类组织材料中提取 DNA，扩增约 110 bp 的线粒体 12S rRNA 基因片段并进行序列分析，构建了 21 种龟类的 12S rRNA 基因片段序列数据库。序列比较的结果表明乌龟与其他 20 种龟类的这段序列均有差别，序列差异在 3.7%～15.7%。基于此，设计 1 对专用于鉴定中药材龟甲原动物乌龟的鉴别引物，对龟甲药材进行了分子鉴定。从 5 种海马药材中提取 DNA，用 PCR 技术扩增约 450 bp 的 12S rRNA 基因片段和约 490 bp 的细胞色素 b 基因片段；结果表明，用 DNA 序列分析方法得到的分子遗传标记可以鉴别所有 5 种海马。

1.2 *基于线粒体 Cyt b 基因序列的鉴别研究* Cyt *b* 基因是动物线粒体上一个编码蛋白质的基因，有一定的保守性。根据蛇类药材 Cyt *b* 基因片段序列的分析，表明这种在种内个体间的序列差异很小，而种间的序列差异却较大的 DNA 片段，正是物种鉴别的理想标记。因此，Cyt *b* 基因片段的 DNA 序列是鉴别蛇类药材原动物种类的一种良好分子标记。设计金钱白花蛇 PCR 鉴别的一对高度特异性引物，可以对金钱白花蛇及其伪品的 Cyt *b* 基因片段序列分析和 PCR 鉴别研究；结果表明，该对引物在对金钱白花蛇的 PCR 鉴别中，可以 100% 检出金钱白花蛇，并能在混合的药材粉末中检测出被检样品中是否含有金钱白花蛇组分。以同样的原理，利用 Cyt *b* 基因对蕲蛇药材及其市场收集样品进行了序列测定和分析；结果表明，Cyt *b* 基因序列是一种鉴别蕲蛇药材与其混淆品较好的分子遗传标记。类似的研究还有鸡内金及其伪品的分子鉴别研究，所设计的引物只扩增家鸡 DNA，而不扩增其他动物 DNA。利用 Cyt *b* 基因对鹿类中药材进行分子鉴定研究已见诸多报道。在对鹿类中药材的正品原动物梅花鹿、马鹿及其混伪品原动物的 Cyt *b* 基因全序列分析的基础上，设计一对专用于鉴定正品鹿类药材的位点特异性鉴别引物，建立鹿类中药材鹿茸、鹿鞭、鹿筋、鹿胎的 DNA 分子标记鉴定方法。建立的位点特异性 PCR 方法，能将正品鹿茸与其他近源种鹿茸药材鉴别开来，具有较高的特异性、重复性，可广泛应用于鹿类药材的鉴别。

## 2 动物药材分子鉴定研究存在的问题

2.1 *研究品种局限* 近几年，国内动物药材的 DNA 分子鉴定报道较多，但研究的品种比较局限，主要研究的品种集中在蛇类中药材、鹿类中药材、鸡内金、海马、龟甲等少数品种，而对于其他常用的品种研究不多，如中药材虻虫、斑蝥、蝉蜕、土鳖虫、水蛭、地龙、全蝎、蜈蚣等，急需在以后的研究工作中得到加强。

2.2 *参与单位较少* 文献报道显示，从事动物药材分子鉴定的研究机构主要是中国药科大学、沈阳药科大学、南京师范大学、北华大学、中国科学院昆明动物所、安徽大学、北京中医药大学、中国中医科学院中药研究所等少数院校和科研院所，加之从事动物药材鉴定和分类学的研究队伍不断缩减，使得全面而系统地开展动物药材分子鉴定面临巨大的挑战，急需呼吁各具有分子生物学技术的相关单位和从业人员联合研究，扩大规模。

2.3 *数据共享不足* 由于各自研究比较分散，品种局限，在分子鉴定的操作中，没有形成统一和规范的操作标准和规程，如药用动物遗传物质材料采集规范、动物药材 DNA 提取操作规范等，难以形成共享的分子鉴定数据信息系统，从而限制了相应技术和方法的推广应用。因此，急需制定实验技术使用规范流程，建立中国药用动物分子鉴定共享信息平台。

2.4 *实际应用不够* 有关动物药材的分子鉴定重点在基础研究，虽然在很多的报道中，均提示建立的方法具有简单、准确、快速、灵敏度高、重复性好等特点，但在实际操作中得到推广应用的很少。当然，基础研究到实际应用需要一定的积累，随着蕲蛇、乌梢蛇饮片 PCR 鉴别方法被 2010 年版《中国药典》收载，分子鉴别动物药材技术与方法，将逐步走向应用，有广阔的发展潜力及应用价值。

## 3 动物药材分子鉴定研究策略

3.1 *研究品种应逐步扩大* 根据 1985—1989 年开展的全国中药资源普查，我国中药资源共有 12 772 种，其中药用动物有 414 科、879 属、1 574 种；《中国中药资源志要》(1994 年)收载药用动物 1 590 种(414 科，879 属)；《中国动物药志》(1996 年)收载动物药 975 种，药用动物 1 546 种；《中华本草》(1999 年)收载动物药(药用动物)1 047 种；《动物本草》(2001 年)收载药用动物 1 567 种；目前，由中国中医科学院中药研究所牵头修订再版的《中国药用动物志》将收载药用动物约 1 800 种。可以看出，我国动物药材(药用动物)品种丰富。为此，应在进行临床常用的动物药材分子鉴定研究的基础上，逐步完成 2010 年版《中国药典》记载的动物药材品种的分子鉴定研究，并从药用动物科属的角度，进一步扩大样品，从而逐步拓宽研究品种和对象，开展全面深入研究。

3.2 *组织形式应联合攻关* 开展动物药材的分子鉴定，最为关键的是获得准确和足够的样品。由于动物药材的获得不同于一般的植物药材，尤其是珍稀濒危的野生动物，其样品的获得更是困难。为开展大规模的动物药材的分子鉴定研究，应以《中国药用动物志》修订再版工作为基础，抓住即将开展的全国中药资源普查的契机，进行全国范围药用动物的采样调查，在药材鉴定和动物分类学鉴定的基础上，采用适宜的分子鉴定技术进行鉴定研究。由于品种较多，分布复杂，采样工作艰苦，仅靠一个单位或一部分科研工作者难以完成，需要与动物药材相关的各大中专院校、科研机构、药监部门、林业部门等联合攻关，协调进行，从而建立动物药材分子鉴定的技术平台。

3.3 *加快分子鉴定试剂盒的开发与应用* 近几年来，针对某一类药材的鉴定，位点特异性鉴别 PCR 方法应用较为广泛。通过对正品药材及其伪、混品的某些 DNA 片段序列（如 12S rRNA，Cyt *b*）的研究，找出正品药材的特异性位点，从而设计高度特异性的鉴别引物；PCR 反应后，经过电泳检测便可准确鉴别样品的真伪。这种方法简便，可操作性强，容易推广应用。并且，这种方法在反复实验验证后，进一步优化各种条件，可以制成分子鉴定的试剂盒，从而可以在实际操作中推广应用。已经有学者根据对不同产地梅花鹿、马鹿、白唇鹿、水鹿线粒体 DNA 进行 PCR 扩增和序列测定，并与常见伪充药材来源动物线粒体 DNA 同位置序列比较，找到该 4 个鹿种的特征片段，建立中药材鹿鞭的分子分类学鉴定试剂盒；结果表明，该引物与相关试剂组成试剂盒后，可用于中药材鹿鞭与常见伪充药材牛鞭、驴鞭等的鉴别。因此，动物药材分子鉴定试剂盒的研制，应当大力提倡和推广，逐步将基础研究走向应用研究。

3.4 *全面启动中国动物药材 DNA 条形码研究计划* 与上述分子生物学技术相比，DNA 条形码（DNA barcoding）是利用一段标准 DNA 序列作为标记来实现快速、准确和自动化的物种鉴定，是分类学中辅助物种鉴定的新技术。这种新兴分类学技术引起了越来越多的生物学家关注，成为物种鉴定和分类学研究的新方向和研究热点。目前，作为国际生命条形码计划 4 个中心节点（加拿大、美国、欧盟和中国）之一，中国在世界生物 DNA 系统分类及条形码技术中占据相当重要的地位。植物（包括药用植物）DNA 条形码研究已经全面启动，动物条形码研究正在逐步开展。为此，对常用的动物药材也进行了有益尝试，制定了相应的操作规范，包括药用动物遗传物质材料采集规范、动物药材 DNA 提取操作规范等；下一步将联合国内各有关科研院所、大中专院校，全面启动中国动物药材 DNA 条形码研究计划，按照标准的操作规范，进一步扩大样品数量，完善标本的采集，利用分子生物学技术获得动物药材标准序列，构建动物药材 DNA 条形码分子鉴定的标准平台。

3.5 *建立中国动物药材分子鉴定标准数据库* 对《中国药用动物志》（修订版）收载药用动物种质资源（包括活体、标本、精子等）进行标准化整理、整合和数字化表达，建立“中国药用动物种质资源共享平台”；在此基础上，联合全国有关科研院校，制定、完善药用动物种质资源的描述标准、技术规程，逐步建立“中国动物药材分子鉴定数据库系统”，包括“中国动物药材 DNA 条形码数据库”“中国动物药材分子标识数据库”“中国动物药材分子鉴定基因序列数据库”等，实现信息数据共享。这不仅为动物药材的鉴定提供依据，而且为药用动物的分类及其遗传多样性研究奠定基础。

［黄璐琦，等. 中国中药杂志，2011，36(3)：234－236.］

# 中药材二维分子标记法及其构建

中药材的“真伪”“优劣”是保障药材质量最关键的 2 个要素。人们往往更重视中药“真伪”方面的鉴定。诚然，中药的“真伪”鉴定在药材资源长期依赖野生资源的匮乏时期，或者对于濒危药材以及贵重药材品种的鉴定等方面，确实保证了药材来源的准确性。然而，随着中药栽培技术的发展，栽培药材的比重越来越大，对于大宗普通药材品种来说，掺伪的可能性已大大降低，因而药材“优劣鉴定”将逐步成为中药鉴定研究的重点。

目前，包括基于分子鉴定方法在内的中药鉴定研究，大多存在“真伪”鉴定有余、“优劣”鉴定不足局面。究其原因，这与中药“真伪”鉴定远比“优劣”鉴别从方法学上容易实现有关。中药材真伪鉴定方法除基于中药材基原、性状、显微及理化等传统四大鉴定方法外，还运用基于 DNA 的诸多分子标记方法等，进行广泛而深入的研究。相对而言，中药材“优劣”方面的鉴定或评价，主要采用分析化学的方法，即通过鉴定和评价药材有效成分的“含量”，或有效成分指纹图分析各成分之间的比例等，对药材品质进行评价。这种化学分析方法对于“成品”药材的品质评价和鉴定发挥了不可替代的作用，然而对于药材的早期的“种子”“幼苗”及非采收期的药材的评价则无能为力。因此，需要建立新的方法，实现对中药材各个时期优劣的“动态”鉴定。这方面，采用功能基因的分子鉴定方法将有助于解决和填补这一中药鉴定领域“空白”。

综上，开展中药“真伪”和“优劣”2 个重要“维度”方面的鉴定研究，具有重要的意义。而如何建立中药“真伪、优劣”的二维鉴定的综合方法则是目前中药鉴定需要解决但面临巨大困难的瓶颈问题。近年来，随着分子标记技术及药材基原植物功能基因的研究的迅猛发展，不同药用植物居群间包括功能基因在内的基因序列普遍存在变异现象，为中药“真伪、优劣”评价的二维鉴定带来了新的契机，并奠定了良好理论基础。基于此，本文提出了中药“真伪、优劣”二维分子标记法及其策略构想，以期在分子水平同时解决中药“真伪、优劣”评价的 2 个核心问题。

## 1 中药材分子标记研究的现状

目前，一般的分子标记方法常用于不同药用植物种间或同一种、不同居群间的药用植物遗传多态性分析，缺乏针对药材品质的分子标记。以丹参为例:已有文献报道采用 RAPD、AFLP、ITS、ISSR 等标记方法对丹参进行了广泛研究,结果大多得出了不同产地丹参居群间遗传多态性比较丰富,居群间遗传变异明显,且某些居群内存在遗传均一性等的结论,并推断这些居群间的差异反映了丹参品种繁多、药材质量不稳定的内在遗传原因,但未见有效针对药材品质标记的研究报道。

随着后基因组时代的来临,功能基因成为引领时代的研究热点,药用植物次生代谢功能基因的研究也日益受到重视。越来越多的研究证据表明功能基因的遗传变异可对药材品质形成产生重要影响,这为新的分子标记策略提供了证据支持。

## 2 中药材二维分子标记法的方法

2.1 二维分子标记方法 二维分子标记法(2 - dimensional molecular marking method, 2DM)是基于分子标记技术以及功能基因分析方法,在分子水平同时研究中药材基原植物的种类、药材品种和品质的一种分子标记方法。该方法主要针对普通分子标记方法存在单一解决中药材"真伪"鉴定,忽略了"优劣"品质鉴定的不足,而提出的一种更为全面、综合鉴定中药材"真伪、优劣"的新策略和新方法。具体思路是在"真伪"鉴定方面:中药材 DNA—分子标记技术(包括 DNA 条形码技术)—中药材及其基原植物的真伪鉴定;在"优劣"鉴定方面:中药材 DNA 或 RNA—功能基因(包括功能基因编码区、非编码区)的序列变异及特征(核苷酸水平、氨基酸水平),表达水平、酶活性差异等—有效成分"有无""含量高低"的药材基因型的鉴定。简而言之,即"中药材物种相关的分子标记+中药材有效成分相关功能基因=中药材二维分子标记法",用公式表示为 2DM=marker1 (marker2 ……)+functional gene1 (gene2……)。

2.2 二维分子标记的原理与方法 中药材"真伪、优劣"的科学内涵归根结底与 DNA 的差异有关。这种差异主要体现在 2 个方面:种及以上水平上的差异,这种差异往往用于解决中药的"真伪"问题以及中药的多来源问题。种以下的水平,包括不同居群间、株系之间的差异,这方面常常用于解决药材品质的"优劣"问题。正是由于中药基原植物无论在"种"以上水平,还是在"种"以下水平均存在 DNA 信息间的差异,这些 DNA 信息差异可以表征在叶绿体 DNA、核 DNA、线粒体 DNA 以及功能基因 DNA 等碱基排列顺序的差异方面。因而可根据这一特点,设计包括基于 PCR 技术、分子杂交技术、测序技术等的检测方法,将这些 DNA 差异位点或碱基检测出来,结合统计学方法,系统分析由 DNA 差异所表达出来的"表型"包括如药材性状差异、品质差异等,在此基础上为各差异药材贴上 DNA"分子标签",这就是中药"真伪、优劣"二维分子标记方法的基本原理。

在"种"及以上水平的中药"真伪"鉴定方面,由于 DNA 序列信息差异较大,这种差异可通过叶绿体 DNA、核 DNA、甚至是动植物的线粒体 DNA 序列信息差异所表达出来。因此,在鉴定过程中,有多种技术手段可运用,如常见的基于 PCR 的分子标记技术 RAPD、ISSR、SSR、AFLP,黄璐琦等构建的 APAPD 方法等;测序技术如核 DNA 的 ITS、18S、5.8S、26S 等,叶绿体 DNA 的 16S、*rbc*L、*mat*K、*ndh*F、*rpo*C1、*rpo*B、*trn*H - *psb*A、*atp*F - *atp*H 等,以及线粒体的 *CO* Ⅰ、Cyt *b* 等,常用于"物种"DNA 条形码的分析鉴定。

在种以下水平,虽然种内 DNA 差异较种间的差异小,但越来越多的证据表明,不同产地、不同居群甚至不同株系的中药基原植物存在次生代谢功能基因变异,这种变异极有可能是产生中药材品质"优劣"的直接关联的分子基础。因此在"种"以下水平中药材的"优劣"鉴定方面,更应着重关注与有效成分生物合成(也称植物次生代谢)相关的功能基因的序列差异。因此可采用测序技术,SNP 分析技术、EST - SSR 技术等,分析和寻找特定药材"品质"相关的某一基因型作为中药材"品质"的分子标记。在此基础上,进一步分析该功能基因突变类型对次生代谢作用的影响,从而科学揭示中药材"优劣"品质形成的基因机制。

目前在中药材的定性标记方面,研究报道较多,在此不做赘述。在"定质"标记方面,其实植物领域已有许多研究报道。例如有报道对 35 个小麦品种的淀粉合成功能基因(*Wx - Bl* 基因)的研究结果发现,*Wx - Bl* 基因的多态性与直链淀粉含量密切相关,仅 *Wx - Bl* 基因第 4 内含子发生 2 个碱基的变异,就可导致直链淀粉含量超过 20%,而正常情况直链淀粉含量低于 20%。同样,在莱茵衣藻类胡萝卜素生物合成过程中,关键酶基因——*PDS* 基因发生突变,会导致有色类胡萝卜素生物合成明显升高。英国《自然遗传学》杂志重点报道了控制玉米产油量的功能基因。研究也显示,不同 $\beta$-香树脂醇合成酶基因变异类型会影响甘草酸的积累效率。上述文献报道提示,功能基因的微小变异可能导致目标产物的积累量产生显著差异,进而影响药用植物有效成分的积累,从而影响药材的品质,这为二维分子标记法关于"优劣"鉴定提供了文献证据支持。

## 3 二维分子标记优势与应用

3.1 具备对中药材"定性与定质"的双重标记优势 定性也即是指对药材"真伪"鉴定,"定质"即指对中药材的"优劣"鉴定。二维分子标记法(2DM)可实现同时对试验材料(中药材样本)实施种以上水平的"真伪"鉴定和种以下类群如不同品种、居群、株系等进行"优劣"鉴定和评价,这是二维分子标记法突出优势之一。

3.2 具有"真伪优劣"鉴定非时限性的特点 二维分子标记法的另一个突出优势是对中药材的鉴定不受采收时间和采收季节的限制,可对药材种子和幼苗进行筛选和评价,保障种植药材品种的均一性、药材品质的优良性,具有重要的科学意义和应用价值。

目前中药材的鉴定及评价往往是对采收药材的一种"既定事实的被动鉴定"。如果成品药材被鉴定为伪品或不合格"商品"的话,从劳力成本及资源成本来看,无疑是一种劳动力和资源的巨大浪费。因此若将这种"被动"鉴定转变为"主动"的动态鉴定,将鉴定时限大大提前,可避免重大资源浪费和经济损失。中药材二维分子标记法所具备的非时限性特点,正好可以实现对中药材药材种子和幼苗的"真伪优劣"鉴定,从而保障种植药材品种的均一性、药材品质的优良性,有利于从源头上控制药材的质量。目前本课题组正在开展丹参的这方面研究,已取得相应的初步成果。

3.3 具备发现中药材“优良”性状的隐性品种的优势 目前中药材来源混杂，遗传背景复杂，生物多样性明显。从药材质量控制方面来讲，这是中药材质量参差不齐的首要原因之一，是药材品质保障的一大“缺陷”。然而，从另一个角度来讲，其丰富的遗传多样性特点，必然出现药材品质的多样性或多元化特征，对寻找优良性状的分子标记而言，反而变成了一大“优势”。因此，如果从DNA信息分析角度，采用二维分子标记法，对某种具备“优良”特性或变异类型药材进行真伪和优劣进行定位和标记，极有可能从纷乱复杂的药材品种中发现某些虽然形态性状与普通品种一致，但却具有特定遗传信息和变异特征的隐性优良品种。这不仅对于中药材种质筛选产生重大影响，也将有可能对分子杂交育种提供重要的技术和材料支持。

3.4 应用实例 以中药材丹参 *Salvia miltiorrhiza* 为例：有报道采用DNA测序方法，对丹参及其近缘种的ITS序列进行分析，结果表明ITS1和ITS2两段序列在丹参种内保守，在属间有较大的差异，与外类群的差异最大，可作为中药丹参分子鉴定的标记，用于丹参及其近缘种的鉴别及系统学研究。王学勇等在前期研究工作基础上，建立了丹参EST-SSR标记方法，并通过已建立的实时荧光定量PCR方法，检测了不同产地丹参居群3个功能基因 *SmAACT*、*SmCMK*、*SmIPPI* 的表达水平，同时结合HPLC方法对丹参酮类成分含量检测结果，利用SAS 9.1软件对二者进行了相关性分析；结果表明，除 *SmIPPI* 表达水平与隐丹参酮呈低度正相关外，*SmAACT*、*SmCMK* 表达水平均与隐丹参酮含量呈中度正相关。鉴于 *SmAACT*、*SmCMK* 基因在丹参酮类合成途径上的关键作用，*SmAACT* 和 *SmCMK* 基因可作为丹参药材品质“优劣”鉴定的分子标记分析候选基因(图1)。目前正在对这2个功能基因的地理变异特征进行分析，以寻找能够对药材“优劣”进行标记的特异位点，从而实现丹参药材“优劣”的分子标记。因此，丹参的二维分子标记可用公式表示为：Sm2DM＝SmIT1(SmIT2)＋SmAACT(SmCMK)。其中SmIT1(SmIT2)为丹参的真伪标记，SmAACT(SmCMK)为丹参的优劣标记；将二者结合起来，实现丹参药材“真伪优劣”的二维分子标记。

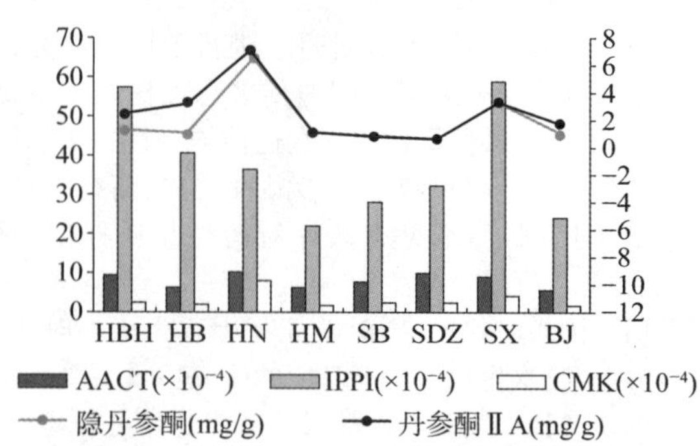


**图1 不同产地丹参功能基因表达量与有效成分含量的关系**

## 4 结语

中药鉴定学的科学内涵和本质是解决中药“真伪优劣”问题。建立新的研究策略和方法，在解决中药材真伪问题的同时，解决目前存在中药材“优劣”的动态(中药材基原植物发育的各个阶段)鉴定的瓶颈性难题，具有重要的科学意义和应用价值。

二维分子标记法既利用了一般分子标记对中药真伪鉴定的功能，又结合了功能基因在药材品质形成过程中的关键作用特点；既发挥了一般分子标记方法在“种”以上水平的鉴定优势，又强调了功能基因在种以下水平的不同居群间甚至是株系间药材品质“优劣”表征过程中的独特作用，达到了对中药材及其基原植物“真伪”和“优劣”的二维系统鉴定和评价的目的。二维分子标记法的提出和应用尝试，除了要求对中药材真伪及多来源的标准化鉴定外，再一次强调了中药材品质早鉴定、早评价、早知道的重要性。因此，充分利用中药材二维分子鉴定法的非时限性特点、具备发现阴性优良品种的能力，发挥其“定性、定质”优势，将在“主动”鉴定中药材药材种子和幼苗的品质，保障所种植药材品种的均一性和质量，避免造成劳力成本及资源的巨大浪费等方面发挥重要作用。

[黄璐琦，等. 中国中药杂志，2012，37(8)：1093-1095.]

# 基于双向位点特异性PCR的金银花真伪鉴别方法研究

金银花为忍冬科植物忍冬 *Lonicera japonica* Thunb. 的干燥花蕾或带初开的花，主要活性成分为绿原酸、木樨草苷等黄酮类物质。金银花临床应用非常广泛，《中国药典》成方和制剂中药中就有61个方剂以金银花作为主要的组成成分，现代药理实验证明其具有抑菌、抗炎、抗病毒、抗氧化、解热、镇痛、调节免疫、保肝、中枢兴奋和神经保护、抗心肌缺血等作用。

尽管在2005年版《中国药典》中已明确将忍冬作为金银花唯一植物来源，但之前各版《中国药典》根据临床疗效、地区用药习惯等，曾先后选定忍冬、红腺忍冬 *L. hypoglauca*、华南忍冬 *L. confusa*、水忍冬 *L. dasystyla* 等为金银花的基原植物。且2005年版《中国药典》同时规定红腺忍冬、华南忍冬、灰毡毛忍冬 *L. macranthoides* 和黄褐毛忍冬 *L. fulvotomentosa* 列为山银花药材基原植物。此外，由于不同地区均有金银花习用品，致使市场上流通的金银花一直非常混乱。

为保证用药安全，人们使用过多种方法对金银花进行真实性鉴定。然而金银花及其伪品的形态和化学成分高度相似，且传统形态学和化学鉴别常受到人为或环境因素的影响。与之相比，分子标记因具有稳定、不受器官和环境因素影响的特点，被用于金银花的分子鉴别。但目前已报道的金银花分子鉴别方法往往表现为重现性差（如ISSR）、样品用量大（如RFLP）、周期长（如DNA barcoding）、操作复杂（如SSR）等缺陷，不能满足实际需要，因此急需建立稳定、简便、通用性好的分子鉴别方法。

双向位点特异性PCR（bidirectional PCR amplification of specific alleles，Bi-PASA），可用于检测单个位点的核苷酸变异，具有共显性的特点。通过单个PCR反应即可鉴别真伪品，已成功用于人参、陈皮、藁本等中药材的真伪鉴别。本文通过使用双向位点特异性PCR技术，利用单个SNP位点在同一PCR反应中对金银花及其9个伪品进行鉴定，并尝试对真伪混杂品鉴别进行探索，为金银花真实性鉴别提供了简单快捷的方法。

## 1 材料与方法

1.1 植物 选取84份材料，包括来自10个产地的77份植物样品，其中忍冬29个、红腺忍冬8个、华南忍冬4个、灰毡毛忍冬6个、黄褐毛忍冬6个、水忍冬8个、金银忍冬 *L. maackii* 4个、郁香忍冬 *L. fragrantissima* 4个、新疆忍冬 *L. tatarica* 4个、繁果忍冬 *L. tatarica* cv. ‘Fanguo’ 4个，以及7批购自市场上经过炮制处理的药材进行双向位点特异性PCR。植物样品主要采自广西、河南、山东、江苏、湖南、北京、安徽地区，凭证标本保存于中国中医科学院中药研究所和广西药用植物园，见表1。

**表1 试验材料**

| 序号 | 编号 | 物种 | 产地 | 个数 | 鉴定人 |
|---|---|---|---|---|---|
| 1 | LJ2011_FQ | *Lonicera japonica* | 河南封丘 | 4 | 刘红彦 |
| 2 | LJ2011_LY | *L. japonica* | 山东临沂 | 6 | 李圣波 |
| 3 | LJ2011_MX | *L. japonica* | 河南新密 | 4 | 刘红彦 |
| 4 | LJ2011_NN | *L. japonica* | 广西南宁 | 4 | 吴庆华 |
| 5 | LJ2011_LYG | *L. japonica* | 江苏连云港 | 4 | 张燕 |
| 6 | LJ2012_YZ | *L. japonica* | 湖南永州 | 4 | 彭华胜 |
| 7 | LJ2011_HF | *L. japonica* | 安徽合肥 | 1 | 彭华胜 |
| 8 | LJ2011_GL | *L. japonica* | 广西桂林 | 2 | 余丽莹 |
| 9 | LH2011_NN | *L. hypoglauca* | 广西崇左 | 4 | 吴庆华 |
| 10 | LH2011_NN | *L. hypoglauca* | 广西桂林 | 4 | 吴庆华 |
| 11 | LC2011_GL | *L. confusa* | 广西桂林 | 3 | 吴庆华 |
| 12 | LC2011_LY | *L. confusa* | 山东临沂 | 1 | 李圣波 |
| 13 | LM2011_GL | *L. macranthoides* | 广西桂林 | 2 | 余丽莹 |
| 14 | LM2011_NN | *L. macranthoides* | 广西南宁 | 4 | 吴庆华 |
| 15 | LF2011_GL | *L. fulvotomentosa* | 广西桂林 | 6 | 余丽莹 |
| 16 | LD2011_GL | *L. dasystyla* | 广西桂林 | 4 | 余丽莹 |
| 17 | LD2011_CZ | *L. dasystyla* | 广西崇左 | 4 | 吴庆华 |
| 18 | LMa2012_BJ | *L. maackii* | 北京 | 3 | 彭华胜 |
| 19 | LMa2011_HF | *L. maackii* | 安徽合肥 | 1 | 彭华胜 |
| 20 | LFr2011_BJ | *L. fragrantissima* | 北京 | 4 | 郝近大 |
| 21 | LT2012_BJ | *L. tatarica* | 北京 | 4 | 郝近大 |
| 22 | LTc2012_BJ | *L. tatarica* cv. ‘Fanguo’ | 北京 | 4 | 郝近大 |
| 23 | LJ2011_NJ | *L. japonica* | 江苏南京（药材） | 2 | 郝近大 |
| 24 | LJ2011_BJ | *L. japonica* | 北京（药材） | 5 | 郝近大 |

1.2 SNP位点的筛选和引物设计 利用GenBank数据库中忍冬属植物的叶绿体 *trn*F-*trn*L 序列，通过ClastulW软件进行序列比对，分析结果表明忍冬的 *trn*F-*trn*L 序列625位为G，其他物种均为A。基于此SNP位点设计双向位点特异性PCR引物，引物序列见表2。

表2 引物及PCR反应条件

| 引物 | 序列(5′-3′) | PCR程序 |
|---|---|---|
| Lj-1F | GTTGACTGTCCTGTGTTGGT | 94℃ 5 min,35个循环(94℃ 30 s,61℃ 30 s,72℃ 45 s),72℃ 7 min |
| Lj-1R | GGATGAGAAATATAACGAATTTAG | |
| lj-2F | TTTATCCTTTTTTTGTTAGCGGTTGA | |
| lj-2R | CTATCCCGACCATTCCC | |
| *trn*L | GG TTCAAGTCCCTCTATCC | 94℃ 5 min,30个循环(94℃ 30 s,54℃ 30 s,72℃ 45 s),72℃ 7 min |
| *trn*F | ATTTGAACTGGTGACACGAG | |

注:A、G为增加特异性人为引入的错配。

1.3 基因组总DNA的提取、PCR扩增条件的确定 取100 mg干燥材料,使用CTAB法提取总DNA。取不同样品DNA,终浓度大约为10 mg/L,使用通用引物*trn*L和*trn*F进行PCR反应以检测模板DNA质量。PCR反应体系为2.5 μL 10×Ex *Taq* buffer, 2 μL 10 mmol/L dNTPs,引物各0.2 pmol, 0.5 U Ex *Taq*酶,约10 ng DNA模板。反应在Eppendorf公司的Mastercycler型PCR扩增仪上进行,反应程序见表2。反应结束后在PCR反应体系内加入5 μL 6×loading buffer,混匀后于EB染色的1%琼脂糖凝胶电泳检测,SYNGENE凝胶成像系统(GENE公司)观察、成像。

利用忍冬SNP鉴别引物Lj-1F和Lj-1R进行位点特异性PCR反应,并分别考察退火温度、PCR循环数、DNA模板用量、引物浓度、dNTP用量、*Taq*酶种类[r*Taq* DNA聚合酶(Takara大连生物有限公司)、Ex *Taq* DNA聚合酶(Takara大连生物有限公司)、*Taq* plus DNA聚合酶(生工生物(上海)有限公司)、*Taq* DNA聚合酶(Fermentas有限公司)]、*Taq*酶用量、不同PCR仪[9700型PCR仪(ABI公司)、PTC-100型PCR仪(MJ Research集团)、Mastercycler型PCR仪(Eppendorf公司)、TC-512型PCR仪(TECHNE公司)]对PCR反应稳定性的影响。依据最佳退火温度设计混淆品的基因型鉴别引物lj-2F和lj-2R,见表2。

1.4 双向位点特异性PCR鉴别 取不同样品DNA进行双向等位基因特异性PCR, PCR反应体系为2.5 μL 10×Ex *Taq* buffer, 2 μL 10 mmol/L dNTPs,引物Lj-1F、lj-2R各0.08 pmol,引物Lj-1R、lj-2F各0.2 pmol, 0.5 U Ex *Taq*酶,约10 ng DNA模板。反应在Eppendorf公司的Mastercycler型PCR扩增仪上进行。反应程序见表2。反应结束后在PCR反应体系内加入5 μL 6×loading buffer,混匀后于EB染色的1%浓度琼脂糖凝胶电泳检测,SYNGENE凝胶成像系统观察、成像。

在忍冬DNA提取液内加入混淆品的DNA,充分混合使得混淆品DNA依次占总DNA含量的1%、5%、10%、20%、50%、90%、100%。PCR反应体系及反应程序同上。

## 2 结果及讨论

2.1 双向位点特异性PCR引物设计 在Genbank数据库中共获得忍冬属植物叶绿体和ITS序列1 002条,分属于16个片段,利用生物信息学分析共筛选出4个忍冬特有SNP位点。利用位点特异性PCR方法对4个SNP位点进行验证,结果表明只有*trn*L-*trn*F 625位C/A位点被确认为忍冬SNP鉴别位点,用于设计引物进行双向位点特异性PCR。

双向位点特异性PCR又称四引物扩增受阻突变体系PCR,其主要是由于*Taq* DNA聚合酶缺少3′-5′外切酶校正活性,当引物3′端错配时造成PCR延伸效率降低、扩增受阻,因此可通过设计特异性引物对SNP位点的2个等位基因进行PCR扩增,具体策略见图1。多重位点特异性PCR通常需要2个以上位点来区分2种基因型,与其相比,双向位点特异性PCR只需要一个位点,且在一次PCR反应中即可区分2种基因型,在中药鉴定中具有更好的前景。

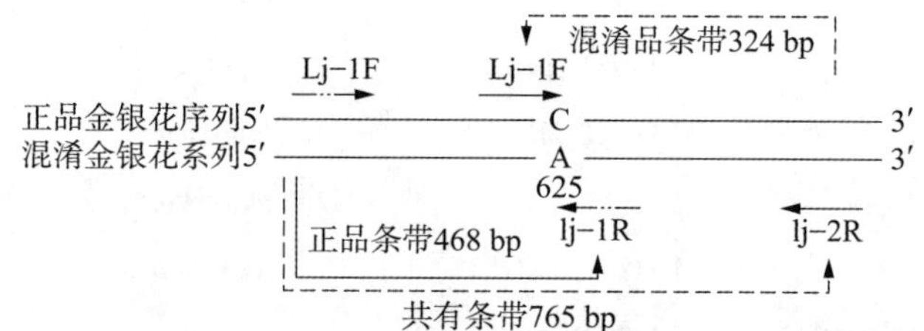


图1 Bi-PASA金银花真伪鉴别方法

2.2 PCR反应条件的确定 为获得最优的PCR反应条件,本文首先建立了单侧位点特异性PCR(amplification refractory mutation system, ARMS)方法,并对其反应条件进行优化,结果见表3。在此基础上设计另一侧引物,并对反应循环数及内外侧引物浓度比进行优化,以确定Bi-PASA的反应条件。实验结果表明,退火温度、*Taq*酶种类及用量对ARMS分型影响较大,且金银花ARMS及Bi-PASA分型的PCR条件中模板、引物、*Taq*酶的使用量均不宜太高,这与前人报道相符。由于Bi-PASA使用巢式引物,可能会造成正常PCR扩增受抑制的情况,王珂等优化Bi-PASA时认为1∶1或2∶1的内外侧引物浓度比结果较优;本文分析结果表明内外引物的浓度比为3∶1时,金银花Bi-PASA结果较好。

2.3 双向位点特异性PCR鉴别金银花及其伪品 利用设计的通用引物和双向特异性引物对29个忍冬个体、48个伪品个体及7批不同药店采购的金银花药材DNA进行PCR扩增,结果见图2。使用*trn*L-*trn*F通用引物均可扩增出1 050 bp的片段;使用金银花位点特异性PCR引物,只有金银花样品能扩增出468 bp的片段,而使用金银花伪品位点特异性PCR引物,伪品均可扩增出324 bp的片段,而正品不会扩增出任何条带。正反向引物所组成的双向位点特异性PCR

**表 3 不同 PCR 反应条件对金银花 ARMS 的影响**

| 因素 | 条件 | LJ | LH | LMac | LC | LFu | LD | LMaa | LFr | LT | LTc |
|---|---|---|---|---|---|---|---|---|---|---|---|
| 循环次数 | 30 | △ | — | — | — | — | — | — | — | — | — |
| | 32 | △ | — | — | — | — | — | — | — | — | — |
| | 33 | + | — | — | — | — | — | — | — | — | — |
| | 34 | + | △ | — | — | — | — | △ | — | △ | △ |
| $T_m$(℃) | 60 | + | + | △ | — | — | — | — | — | — | △ |
| | 61 | + | — | — | — | — | — | — | — | — | — |
| | 62 | △ | — | — | — | — | — | — | — | — | △ |
| *Taq* 酶量(U) | 0.25 | + | — | — | — | — | — | — | — | — | — |
| | 0.50 | + | — | — | — | — | — | — | — | — | — |
| | 1.00 | + | △ | △ | — | — | — | △ | △ | △ | △ |
| | 1.5 | + | + | + | △ | — | — | △ | △ | — | — |
| 引物浓度(pmol) | 0.125 | △ | — | — | — | — | — | — | — | — | — |
| | 0.25 | + | — | — | — | — | — | — | — | — | — |
| | 0.5 | + | + | + | — | — | — | — | — | — | — |
| DNA(ng) | 1 | △ | — | — | — | — | — | — | — | — | — |
| | 3 | △ | — | — | — | — | — | — | — | — | — |
| | 10 | + | — | — | — | — | — | — | — | — | — |
| | 30 | + | — | — | — | — | — | — | — | — | △ |
| | 90 | — | — | — | — | — | — | △ | — | — | △ |
| dNTP(nmol) | 5 | — | — | — | — | — | — | — | — | — | — |
| | 10 | △ | — | — | — | — | — | — | — | — | — |
| | 30 | + | + | △ | — | — | — | — | — | — | — |
| *Taq* 酶种类 | *Taq* plus | — | — | — | — | — | — | — | — | — | — |
| | *Taq* | — | — | — | — | — | — | — | — | — | — |
| | Ex *Taq* | + | — | — | — | — | — | — | — | — | — |
| | r*Taq* | + | — | — | — | — | — | — | — | — | — |
| 仪器 | Mastercycler | + | — | — | — | — | — | — | — | — | — |
| | TC-512 | — | — | — | — | — | — | — | — | — | △ |
| | 9700 | △ | — | — | — | — | — | — | — | — | — |
| | PTC-100 | + | + | — | — | — | — | — | — | — | — |

注：LJ. 忍冬；LH. 红腺忍冬；LMac. 灰毡毛忍冬；LC. 华南忍冬；LFu. 黄褐毛忍冬；LD. 水忍冬；LMaa. 金银忍冬；LFr. 郁香忍冬；LT. 新疆忍冬；LTc. 繁果忍冬；+. 亮条带；△. 暗条带；—. 无条带。

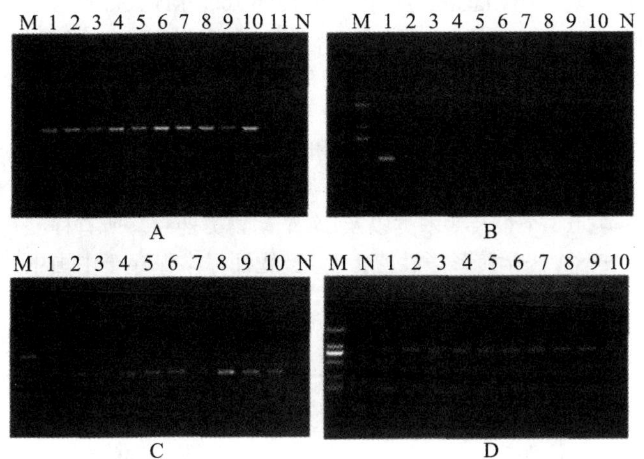


**图 2 双向位点特异性 PCR 鉴别忍冬及其伪品凝胶电泳**

A. 通用引物；B. 忍冬鉴别引物；C. 伪品鉴别引物；D. 双向位点特异性 PCR 引物；M. DL 2 000 marker；1. 忍冬；2. 红腺忍冬；3. 灰毡毛忍冬；4. 华南忍冬；5. 黄褐毛忍冬；6. 水忍冬；7. 金银忍冬；8. 郁香忍冬；9. 新疆忍冬；10. 繁果忍冬；N. 阴性对照。

引物，可在同一 PCR 反应中鉴别正品和伪品。

2.4 双向位点特异性 PCR 鉴别金银花 由于双向位点特异性 PCR 共显性的特点，对于金银花及其掺伪品，可通过双向位点特异性 PCR 条带进行区别。在忍冬中掺入 5%以上伪品时即可清晰的检测到伪品条带，见图 3。

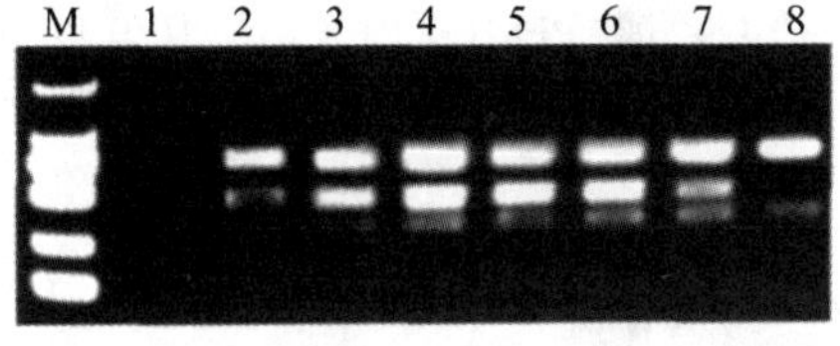


**图 3 不同比例忍冬-华南忍冬双向位点特异性 PCR**

M. DL 2 000 marker；1. 阴性对照；2～7. 分别为忍冬中掺杂了 1%、5%、10%、20%、50%、90% 的华南忍冬；8. 华南忍冬。

## 3 小结

单核苷酸多态性(SNP)在基因组水平上广泛存在,因其分布广泛、数量众多,双等位特性易于检测,常用来研究物种的起源与进化,进行物种的鉴定,在药材近缘种鉴别研究中具有重要意义。在基于SNP基因分型的鉴别研究中,双向等位基因特异性PCR仅通过单个SNP位点即可区分2种基因型,具有共显性、易于检测的特点,在药材真伪品快速检测方面具有独特的优势。本研究建立了双向等位位点特异性PCR方法,可用于鉴别金银花来源植物忍冬及其华南忍冬、灰毡毛忍冬等9种常用伪品,且通过单次PCR即可鉴别掺伪超过5%的混杂品,对于金银花"正本清源"和产业的可持续发展具有重要意义。

[蒋超,袁媛,等. 中国中药杂志,2012,37(24):3752-3757.]

# 使用碱裂解法快速提取药材DNA方法的研究

2010年版《中国药典》首次引入了中药材蕲蛇、乌梢蛇的聚合酶链式反应(PCR)鉴别方法。该方法通过消化液、裂解液、蛋白酶K裂解动物细胞,而后通过硅胶柱色谱纯化DNA获得模板DNA,所得DNA可成功用于蕲蛇、乌梢蛇的分子鉴定。然而该方法使用了商品试剂盒、蛋白酶K及硅胶纯化色谱柱,操作步骤多,费时较长,一般需要2～3 h才能得到模板DNA,不利于中药材的快速检测。而植物DNA提取的标准方法CTAB(十六烷基三甲基溴化铵)法或SDS(十二烷基硫酸钠)法需要使用经过酚/三氯甲烷抽提蛋白质、异丙醇沉淀DNA、乙醇洗涤等步骤。步骤烦琐、操作复杂,一般需要5 h以上才能获得药材DNA,无法满足DNA分子鉴定面临的样本量不断增大、检测强度增加的要求。

长期以来DNA的提取一直是DNA分析技术实验中最耗时、烦琐的步骤,严重制约分子鉴定方法的使用和推广。为达到快速提取DNA的目的,研究者先后提出了ROSE法、磁珠吸附法、Tris-ED-TA提取法等用于植物DNA的提取。尽管这些方法缩短了DNA提取的时间,但由于其仍然使用了加热、酚/三氯甲烷抽提、高速离心、沉淀等步骤,依然无法实现快速简便提取DNA的目的。DNA碱裂解法被认为是一种有效的DNA快速提取方法,已广泛用于小麦、玉米、花生、水稻等,在分子辅助育种、转基因植物鉴定、SSR鉴定等中起到了重要作用。DNA碱裂解法通过0.2 mol/L的氢氧化钠或氢氧化钾处理植物材料,裂解细胞并获得DNA,具有方法简单、操作步骤少、不需要使用酚等有毒试剂的特点。但由于植物材料差异巨大,难以找到通用的碱裂解试剂配方。NP-40、β-巯基乙醇、PEG(聚丙二醇)、甘氨酸、Tween 20、PVP(聚乙烯吡咯烷酮)都曾作为添加剂用于碱裂解试剂中,不同的碱浓度和中和试剂种类均影响了碱裂解提取的效率。

目前还未见使用碱裂解法提取中药材的报道。本研究尝试通过研究DNA提取过程中不同添加试剂对碱裂解法DNA提取的影响,筛选适合快速提取药材DNA的中和试剂,并将Triton X-100作为新的添加剂类型适用于碱裂解法提取中药材,建立一种具有广谱性、快速的药材DNA提取方法,为《中国药典》收载药材分子鉴定方法提供技术依据。

## 1 仪器与材料

1.1 仪器 PCR仪(ABI公司,型号:7500);电泳系统(北京市六一仪器厂);离心机(Eppendorf公司,型号:5810R);漩涡振荡器(Scientific Industrial公司);紫外凝胶成像分析仪(Syngene公司);核酸定量仪(Gene有限公司)。

1.2 试剂 氢氧化钠(北京化工厂);Tween 20(吐温20,Bio Basic公司);Triton X-100(曲拉通100,Bio Basic公司);PVP 40(聚乙烯吡咯烷酮40,北京江晨生物科技有限公司);PEG 4000(聚乙二醇4000,Merck公司);PVPP(聚乙烯聚吡咯烷酮,Sigma公司);甘氨酸(上海生工生物有限公司);r*Taq* DNA聚合酶(Takara公司,大连);DL2000 Marker(Takara公司,大连);琼脂糖(Invitrogen公司);Tris(三羟甲基氨基甲烷,Takara公司,大连);NaAc(醋酸钠,北京化工厂)。

1.3 药材 144个药材分别收集于北京市同仁堂药店、北京市永安堂大药房、安徽亳州康美中药城及中国中医科学院化学室,包括13个果实种子类、4个叶类、4个全草类、5个花类、101个根及茎木类以及17个动物类药材。所有样品均由安徽中医学院彭华胜博士鉴定,凭证标本保存于中国中医科学院中药研究所。实验材料详见表1。

**表1 实验样品详情**

| 编号 | 中药名 | 类别 | 炮制 | 来源 |
|---|---|---|---|---|
| 1 | 菟丝子(Semen Cuscutae) | 种子 | — | 同仁堂 |
| 2 | 五味子(Fructus Schisandrae Chinensis) | 果实 | — | 同仁堂 |
| 3 | 车前(Semen Plantaginis) | 种子 | — | 永安堂 |
| 4 | 葶苈子(Semen Descurainiae) | 种子 | — | 永安堂 |

（续表）

| 编号 | 中药名 | 类别 | 炮制 | 来源 |
|---|---|---|---|---|
| 5 | 决明子(Semen Cassiae) | 种子 | 炒制 | 中药所 |
| 6 | 牛蒡子(Fructus Arctii) | 果实 | — | 康美 |
| 7 | 紫苏(Folium Perillae) | 叶 | — | 同仁堂 |
| 8 | 藿香(Herba Pogostemonis) | 全草 | — | 同仁堂 |
| 9 | 石楠叶(Folium Photiniae) | 叶 | — | 永安堂 |
| 10 | 竹叶(Folium Bamboo) | 叶 | — | 中药所 |
| 11 | 荷叶(Folium Nelumbinis) | 叶 | — | 中药所 |
| 12 | 青蒿(Herba Artemisiae Annuae) | 全草 | — | 同仁堂 |
| 13 | 鸭趾草(Herba Commeli) | 全草 | — | 中药所 |
| 14 | 首乌藤(Caulis Polygoni Multiflori) | 茎 | — | 同仁堂 |
| 15 | 关木通(Caulis Aristolochiae Manshuriensis) | 茎 | — | 永安堂 |
| 16 | 合欢皮(Cortex Albiziae) | 皮 | — | 永安堂 |
| 17 | 厚朴(Cortex Magnoliae Officinalis) | 皮 | 蒸制 | 中药所 |
| 18 | 大血藤(Caulis Sargentodoxae) | 茎 | — | 中药所 |
| 19 | 厚朴(Cortex Magnoliae Officinalis) | 皮 | 姜制 | 中药所 |
| 20 | 杭白菊(Flos Chrysanthemi) | 花 | 蒸制 | 同仁堂 |
| 21 | 辛夷(Flos Magnoliae) | 花 | — | 同仁堂 |
| 22 | 红花(Flos Carthami) | 花 | — | 永安堂 |
| 23 | 金银花(Flos Lonicerae) | 花 | — | 永安堂 |
| 24 | 槐花(Flos Sophorae) | 花 | — | 中药所 |
| 25 | 夏枯草(Spica Prunellae) | 果穗 | — | 中药所 |
| 26 | 苍耳(Fructus Xanthii) | 果实 | — | 永安堂 |
| 27 | 枸杞子(Fructus Lycii) | 果实 | — | 永安堂 |
| 28 | 预知子(Fructus Akebiae) | 果实 | — | 中药所 |
| 29 | 吴茱萸(Fructus Evodiae) | 果实 | 甘草制 | 中药所 |
| 30 | 草豆蔻(Semen Alpiniae Katsumadai) | 种子 | — | 中药所 |
| 31 | 大枣(Fructus Jujubae) | 果实 | — | 中药所 |
| 32 | 山药(Rhizoma Dioscoreae) | 根茎 | — | 同仁堂 |
| 33 | 丹参(Radix Salviae Miltiorrhizae) | 根 | — | 同仁堂 |
| 34 | 人参(Radix Ginseng) | 根 | — | 永安堂 |
| 35 | 黄芪(Radix Astragali seu Hedysari) | 根 | — | 永安堂 |
| 36 | 山药(Rhizoma Dioscoreae) | 根茎 | 麸炒 | 永安堂 |
| 37 | 党参(Radix Codonopsis) | 根 | — | 永安堂 |
| 38 | 草乌(Radix Aconiti Kusnezoffii) | 根 | 煮 | 永安堂 |
| 39 | 川乌(Radix Aconiti) | 根 | 煮 | 永安堂 |
| 40 | 当归(Radix Angelicae Sinensis) | 根 | — | 中药所 |

（续表）

| 编号 | 中药名 | 类别 | 炮制 | 来源 |
|---|---|---|---|---|
| 41 | 大黄(Radix et Rhizoma Rhei) | 根 | 酒制 | 中药所 |
| 42 | 葛根(Radix Puerariae) | 根 | — | 中药所 |
| 43 | 桔梗(Radix Platycodonis) | 根 | — | 中药所 |
| 44 | 干姜(Rhizoma Zingiberis) | 根茎 | — | 中药所 |
| 45 | 三七(Radix Notoginseng) | 根 | — | 中药所 |
| 46 | 龙胆(Radix Gentianae) | 根 | — | 中药所 |
| 47 | 白术(Rhizoma Atractylodis) | 根茎 | — | 中药所 |
| 48 | 温郁金(Radix Curcumae) | 根 | — | 中药所 |
| 49 | 甘草(Radix Glycyrrhizae) | 根 | 蜜炙 | 中药所 |
| 50 | 黄连(Rhizoma Coptidis) | 根茎 | — | 中药所 |
| 51 | 姜黄(Rhizoma Curcumae) | 根茎 | — | 中药所 |
| 52 | 白芍(Radix Paeoniae Alba) | 根 | — | 中药所 |
| 53 | 黄芪(Radix Astragali seu Hedysari) | 根 | — | 中药所 |
| 54 | 川续断(Radix Dipsaci) | 根 | — | 中药所 |
| 55 | 黄芩(Radix Scutellariae) | 根 | — | 中药所 |
| 56 | 白土苓(Rhizoma Smilacis Glabrae) | 根茎 | — | 中药所 |
| 57 | 苦参(Radix Sophorae Flavescentis) | 根 | — | 中药所 |
| 58 | 何首乌(Radix Polygoni Multiflori) | 根 | 蒸制 | 中药所 |
| 59 | 附子(Radix Aconiti Lateralis Preparata) | 根 | — | 中药所 |
| 60 | 生川乌(Radix Aconiti) | 根 | — | 中药所 |
| 61 | 鸢尾(Radix Iris) | 根 | — | 中药所 |
| 62 | 玉竹(Rhizoma Polygonati Odorati) | 根茎 | 蒸制 | 康美 |
| 63 | 泽泻(Rhizoma Alismatis) | 块茎 | — | 康美 |
| 64 | 太子参(Radix Pseudostellariae) | 根 | — | 康美 |
| 65 | 石菖蒲(Rhizoma Acori Tatarinowii) | 根茎 | — | 康美 |
| 66 | 乌药(Radix Linderae) | 根 | — | 康美 |
| 67 | 藕节(Nodus Nelumbinis Rhizomatis) | 根茎节 | — | 康美 |
| 68 | 丹皮(Cortex Moutan Radicis) | 皮 | — | 康美 |
| 69 | 大黄(Radix et Rhizoma Rhei) | 根 | — | 康美 |
| 70 | 百合(Bulbus Lilii) | 鳞茎 | — | 康美 |
| 71 | 白薇(Radix Cynanchi Atrati) | 根 | — | 康美 |
| 72 | 羌活 (Rhizoma et Radix Notopterygii) | 根茎 | — | 康美 |
| 73 | 板蓝根(Radix Isatidis) | 根 | — | 康美 |
| 74 | 赤芍(Radix Paeoniae Rubra) | 根 | — | 康美 |
| 75 | 九节菖蒲(Radix Anemone) | 根 | — | 康美 |
| 76 | 巴戟天(Radix Morindae Officinalis) | 根 | — | 康美 |

（续表）

| 编号 | 中药名 | 类别 | 炮制 | 来源 |
|---|---|---|---|---|
| 77 | 延胡索(Rhizoma Corydalis) | 块茎 | — | 康美 |
| 78 | 升麻(Rhizoma Cimicifugae) | 根茎 | — | 康美 |
| 79 | 前胡(Radix Peucedani) | 根 | — | 康美 |
| 80 | 木香(Radix Aucklandiae) | 根 | — | 康美 |
| 81 | 漏芦(Radix Rhapontici) | 根 | — | 康美 |
| 82 | 天花粉(Radix Trichosanthis) | 根 | — | 康美 |
| 83 | 山豆根(Radix Sophorae Tonkinensis) | 根 | — | 康美 |
| 84 | 白芷(Radix Angelicae Dahuricae) | 根 | — | 康美 |
| 85 | 防风(Radix Saposhnikoviae) | 根 | — | 康美 |
| 86 | 防己(Radix Stephaniae Tetrandrae) | 根 | — | 康美 |
| 87 | 川芎(Rhizoma Ligustici Chuanxiong) | 根茎 | — | 康美 |
| 88 | 重楼(Rhizoma Paridis) | 根茎 | — | 康美 |
| 89 | 天门冬(Radix Asparagi) | 根 | — | 康美 |
| 90 | 苍术(Rhizoma Atractylodis) | 根茎 | — | 康美 |
| 91 | 穿山龙(Rhizoma Dioscoreae) | 根茎 | — | 康美 |
| 92 | 百部(Radix Stemonae) | 根 | — | 康美 |
| 93 | 莪术(Rhizoma Curcumae) | 根及根茎 | — | 康美 |
| 94 | 射干(Rhizoma Belamcandae) | 根及根茎 | — | 康美 |
| 95 | 秦艽(Radix Gentianae Macrophyllae) | 根 | — | 康美 |
| 96 | 苦参(Radix Sophorae Flavescentis) | 根 | — | 康美 |
| 97 | 香附(Rhizoma Cyperi) | 根茎 | — | 康美 |
| 98 | 山慈菇(Pseudobulbus Cremastrae) | 假鳞茎 | — | 康美 |
| 99 | 牛膝(Radix Achyranthis Bidentatae) | 根 | — | 康美 |
| 100 | 平贝母(Bulbus Fritillaria) | 鳞茎 | — | 康美 |
| 101 | 胡黄连(Rhizoma Picrorhizae) | 根茎 | — | 康美 |
| 102 | 千年健(Rhizoma Homalomenae) | 根茎 | — | 康美 |
| 103 | 半夏(Rhizoma Pinelliae) | 根茎 | — | 康美 |
| 104 | 茜草(Radix Rubiae) | 根 | — | 康美 |
| 105 | 葛根(Radix Puerariae) | 根 | — | 康美 |
| 106 | 甘草(Radix Glycyrrhizae) | 根 | — | 康美 |
| 107 | 高良姜(Rhizoma Alpiniae Officinarum) | 根及根茎 | — | 康美 |
| 108 | 三棱(Rhizoma Sparganii) | 根茎 | — | 康美 |
| 109 | 地榆(Radix Sanguisorbae) | 根 | — | 康美 |
| 110 | 郁金(Radix Curcumae) | 根 | — | 康美 |
| 111 | 藁本(Rhizoma Ligustici) | 根及根茎 | — | 康美 |
| 112 | 浙贝母(Bulbus Fritillariae Thunbergii) | 鳞茎 | — | 康美 |

（续表）

| 编号 | 中药名 | 类别 | 炮制 | 来源 |
| --- | --- | --- | --- | --- |
| 113 | 天麻（Rhizoma Gastrodiae） | 根茎 | — | 康美 |
| 114 | 天南星（Rhizoma Arisaematis） | 根茎 | — | 康美 |
| 115 | 独活（Radix Angelicae Pubescentis） | 根 | — | 康美 |
| 116 | 白及（Rhizoma Bletillae） | 根茎 | — | 康美 |
| 117 | 麦冬（Radix Ophiopogonis） | 根 | — | 康美 |
| 118 | 续断（Radix Dipsaci） | 根 | — | 康美 |
| 119 | 南沙参（Radix Adenophorae） | 根 | — | 康美 |
| 120 | 川牛膝（Radix Cyathulae） | 根 | — | 康美 |
| 121 | 贯众（Rhizoma Dryopteris） | 根茎 | — | 康美 |
| 122 | 柴胡（Radix Bupleuri） | 根 | — | 康美 |
| 123 | 红景天（Herba Rhodiolae） | 全草 | — | 康美 |
| 124 | 狗脊（Rhizoma Cibotii） | 根茎 | — | 康美 |
| 125 | 夏天无（Rhizoma Corydalis） | 根及根茎 | — | 康美 |
| 126 | 薤白（Bulbus Allii Macrostemonis） | 鳞茎 | — | 康美 |
| 127 | 玄参（Radix Scrophulariae） | 根 | 蒸制 | 康美 |
| 128 | 僵蚕（Bombyx Batryticatus） | 动物药 | 麸炒 | 中药所 |
| 129 | 土鳖虫（Eupolyphaga Seu Steleophaga） | 动物药 | — | 中药所 |
| 130 | 全蝎（Scorpio） | 动物药 | — | 中药所 |
| 131 | 地龙（Lumbricus） | 动物药 | — | 中药所 |
| 132 | 蟾皮（Cutis Bufonis） | 动物药 | — | 中药所 |
| 133 | 蛇蜕（Periostracum Serpentis） | 动物药 | — | 中药所 |
| 134 | 乌梢蛇（Zaocys） | 动物药 | — | 中药所 |
| 135 | 金钱白花蛇（Bungarus Parvus） | 动物药 | — | 中药所 |
| 136 | 王锦蛇（*Elaphe carinata*） | 动物药 | — | 中药所 |
| 137 | 黑眉锦蛇（*Elaphe taeniura*） | 动物药 | — | 中药所 |
| 138 | 山烙铁头（*Ovophis monticola*） | 动物药 | — | 中药所 |
| 139 | 赤链华游蛇（*Sinonatrix annularis*） | 动物药 | — | 中药所 |
| 140 | 中国水蛇（*Enhydris chinensis*） | 动物药 | — | 中药所 |
| 141 | 灰鼠蛇（*Ptyas korros*） | 动物药 | — | 中药所 |
| 142 | 玉斑锦蛇（*Elaphe mandarinus*） | 动物药 | — | 中药所 |
| 143 | 水赤链蛇（*Dinodon rufozonatum*） | 动物药 | — | 中药所 |
| 144 | 赤链蛇（*Dinodon rufozonatum*） | 动物药 | — | 中药所 |

注：同仁堂.北京同仁堂药店；永安堂.北京永安堂药店；康美.亳州康美中药城；中药所.中国中医科学院中药研究所。

## 2 DNA 提取

配制提取缓冲液 PA1－PA64，配方如表 2 所示。以人参、藿香、紫苏、金银花、车前子和金钱白花蛇作为根及茎木类、全草、叶、花、果实种子类、动物类中药材的代表，中药材 DNA 提取分别采用 2 种方法进行。

2.1 Tris 中和法 每种药材各取 64 份样品，每个样品粉末 1 mg，分别加入 96 孔微孔板中；1～64 份样品分别加入提取缓冲液 PA1－64 20 μL，使用漩涡振荡器振荡 10～15 s 混匀；煮沸 10～15 s，取出；每一孔内加入 0.1 mol/L Tris－HCl（pH=8.0）80 μL，轻微漩涡混匀；300×*g* 下离心 5 min；取上清用于 PCR 反应。

**表 2 碱裂解缓冲液配方**

| 缓冲液 | N | Tw | P | Pp | Tr | PEG | G | 缓冲液 | N | Tw | P | Pp | Tr | PEG | G |
|---|---|---|---|---|---|---|---|---|---|---|---|---|---|---|---|
| PA1 | + | | | | | | | PA33 | + | | + | + | + | | |
| PA2 | + | + | | | | | | PA34 | + | | + | + | | + | |
| PA3 | + | | + | | | | | PA35 | + | | + | + | | | + |
| PA4 | + | | | + | | | | PA36 | + | | + | | + | + | |
| PA5 | + | | | | + | | | PA37 | + | | + | | + | | + |
| PA6 | + | | | | | + | | PA38 | + | | + | | | + | + |
| PA7 | + | | | | | | + | PA39 | + | | | + | + | + | |
| PA8 | + | + | + | | | | | PA40 | + | | | + | + | | + |
| PA9 | + | + | | + | | | | PA41 | + | | | + | | + | + |
| PA10 | + | + | | | + | | | PA42 | + | | + | | + | + | + |
| PA11 | + | + | | | | + | | PA43 | + | | | + | + | + | + |
| PA12 | + | + | | | | | + | PA44 | + | + | + | + | + | | |
| PA13 | + | | + | + | | | | PA45 | + | + | + | + | | + | |
| PA14 | + | | + | | + | | | PA46 | + | + | + | + | | | + |
| PA15 | + | | + | | | + | | PA47 | + | + | + | | + | + | |
| PA16 | + | | + | | | | + | PA48 | + | + | + | | + | | + |
| PA17 | + | | | + | + | | | PA49 | + | + | + | | | + | + |
| PA18 | + | | | + | | + | | PA50 | + | + | | + | + | + | |
| PA19 | + | | | + | | | + | PA51 | + | + | | + | + | | + |
| PA20 | + | | | | + | + | | PA52 | + | + | | + | | + | + |
| PA21 | + | | | | + | | + | PA53 | + | + | | | + | + | + |
| PA22 | + | | | | | + | + | PA54 | + | | + | + | + | + | |
| PA23 | + | + | + | + | | | | PA55 | + | | + | + | + | | + |
| PA24 | + | + | + | | + | | | PA56 | + | | + | + | | + | + |
| PA25 | + | + | + | | | + | | PA57 | + | | | + | + | + | + |
| PA26 | + | + | + | | | | + | PA58 | + | + | + | + | + | + | |
| PA27 | + | + | | + | + | | | PA59 | + | + | + | + | + | | + |
| PA28 | + | + | | + | | + | | PA60 | + | + | + | + | | + | + |
| PA29 | + | + | | + | | | + | PA61 | + | + | + | | + | + | + |
| PA30 | + | + | | | + | + | | PA62 | + | + | | + | + | + | + |
| PA31 | + | + | | | + | | + | PA63 | + | | + | + | + | + | + |
| PA32 | + | + | | | | + | + | PA64 | + | + | + | + | + | + | + |

注：N. 0.5 mol/L 氢氧化钠；Tw. 2%吐温 20；P. 1%聚乙烯吡咯烷酮 40；Pp. 1%聚乙烯聚吡咯烷酮；PEG. 40%聚乙二醇 4000；Tr. 1%曲拉通 100； G. 1 mol/L 甘氨酸。

2.2 NaAc 中和法 每种药材各取 64 份样品，每个样品粉末 1 mg，分别加入 96 孔微孔板中；1～64 份样品分别加入提取缓冲液 PA1 - 64 20 μL，使用漩涡振荡器振荡 10～15 s 混匀；煮沸 10～15 s，取出；每一孔内加入 3 mol/L NaAc（pH=5.2）13.3 μL，轻微漩涡混匀，加入去离子水 66.7 μL；300×*g* 下离心 5 min；取上清用于 PCR 反应。

利用优化的 DNA 提取缓冲液 PA 和中和方法，对 144 个中药材样本进行提取。

## 3 PCR 扩增及电泳

分别将碱裂解法方法 1 和方法 2 所提取的 128 个人参、藿香、紫苏、金银花、车前子和金钱白花蛇基因组 DNA，调整 DNA 浓度为 100、20、4、0.4 ng/μL 后用于 PCR 反应。植物类药材使用 *psb*A - *trn*H 通用引物（上游引物：5′-GTTATGCATGAACGTAATGCTC - 3′；下游引物：5′-CGCGCATGGTGGATTCACAATCC - 3′）；动物类药材使用 *CO* Ⅰ通用引物（上游引物：5′- GGTCAACAAATCATAAAGATATTGG - 3′；下游引物：5′- TAAACTTCAGGGTGACCAAAAAATCA - 3′）。PCR 反应体系（25 μL）：2.5 μL 10×PCR buffer，2 μL 2.5 mmol/L dNTPs，10 μmol/L 引物各 1 μL，1 U r*Taq* 酶，1% PVP，0.2% BSA，1 μL DNA 模板。反应在 ABI 公司的 9700 型 PCR 扩增仪上进行。*psb*A - *trn*H 片段反应程序为：94 ℃ 预变性 10 min；94 ℃ 变性 30 s，56 ℃ 复性 45 s，72 ℃ 延伸 30 s，38 个循环；72 ℃ 延伸 10 min。*CO* Ⅰ片段反应程序为：94 ℃ 预变性 10 min；94 ℃ 变性 30 s，53～59 ℃ 复性 45 s，72 ℃ 延伸 30 s，38 个循环；72 ℃ 延伸 10 min。用于鉴

别乌梢蛇的引物及 PCR 条件参照唐晓晶等研究结果进行。用于鉴别金钱白花蛇的引物及 PCR 反应条件参照冯成强等的研究结果进行。反应结束后取 5 μL 反应液经 EB 染色的 1.5%琼脂糖凝胶电泳。

## 4 DNA 纯度、浓度分析及 PCR 扩增效率分析

使用核酸定量仪测定碱裂解法所提取 DNA 的 $A_{260}$、$A_{230}$ 及 $A_{280}$ 波长吸收，使用 SPSS 17.0 对 $A_{260}/A_{230}$ 及 $A_{260}/A_{280}$ 的数据进行分析，方法为 ANOVA 分析和单因素方差分析。对 100、20、4、0.4 ng/μL DNA 的 PCR 扩增结果进行统计，有条带记 1 分，无条带记 0 分。

## 5 结果与讨论

5.1 DNA 纯度与浓度分析 为筛选适合快速提取药材 DNA 的碱裂解试剂，本文研究了不同提取缓冲液配方的提取效果。结果表明，使用不同 DNA 提取缓冲液 PA 所得 DNA 纯度和浓度存在显著差异（表 3），其中缓冲液 PA14（含有 0.5 mol/L NaOH、1% Triton X－100、1% PVP）具有最佳的

**表 3 使用不同碱裂解缓冲液提取 DNA 的浓度、纯度及 PCR 成功率**

| 缓冲液 | DNA(ng/μL) | $A_{260}/A_{280}$ | $PCR_{SI}$ | 缓冲液 | DNA(ng/μL) | $A_{260}/A_{280}$ | $PCR_{SI}$ |
|---|---|---|---|---|---|---|---|
| PA1 | 302.46±98.40 | 1.35±0.19 | 32 | PA33 | 229.28±108.54 | 0.92±0.42 | 24 |
| PA2 | 368.37±227.22 | 1.26±0.10 | 34 | PA34 | 196.79±81.26 | 1.11±0.55 | 15 |
| PA3 | 374.09±147.07 | 1.14±0.14 | 25 | PA35 | 121.08±65.34 | 1.21±0.11 | 17 |
| PA4 | 489.10±243.34 | 1.33±0.14 | 28 | PA36 | 175.31±73.49 | 1.36±1.01 | 21 |
| PA5 | 185.20±128.27 | 0.51±0.22 | 22 | PA37 | 183.42±56.46 | 0.84±0.32 | 20 |
| PA6 | 412.63±218.42 | 1.24±0.16 | 35 | PA38 | 128.00±77.30 | 1.23±0.41 | 31 |
| PA7 | 402.90±212.07 | 1.25±0.15 | 30 | PA39 | 176.35±77.37 | 1.29±0.38 | 22 |
| PA8 | 264.01±45.05 | 1.19±0.43 | 33 | PA40 | 152.96±85.56 | 1.16±0.33 | 20 |
| PA9 | 361.07±107.07 | 1.00±0.72 | 23 | PA41 | 151.69±62.67 | 0.84±0.27 | 16 |
| PA10 | 272.14±129.27 | 1.29±0.29 | 27 | PA42 | 145.60±85.82 | 0.95±0.41 | 19 |
| PA11 | 245.93±113.24 | 1.26±0.64 | 36 | PA43 | 185.21±61.38 | 1.23±0.41 | 21 |
| PA12 | 230.69±110.17 | 1.13±0.52 | 31 | PA44 | 89.17±41.38 | 1.05±0.27 | 13 |
| PA13 | 163.27±83.57 | 1.25±0.18 | 27 | PA45 | 207.22±101.40 | 0.98±0.32 | 17 |
| PA14 | 284.62±116.24 | 1.52±0.23 | 43 | PA46 | 124.32±46.28 | 1.12±0.51 | 16 |
| PA15 | 238.53±106.66 | 1.48±0.29 | 40 | PA47 | 76.35±31.06 | 1.17±0.32 | 14 |
| PA16 | 149.42±57.53 | 1.16±0.26 | 25 | PA48 | 175.36±39.53 | 1.29±0.42 | 20 |
| PA17 | 177.45±94.53 | 1.26±0.14 | 29 | PA49 | 290.97±89.41 | 1.36±0.10 | 9 |
| PA18 | 175.04±59.72 | 1.25±0.17 | 38 | PA50 | 227.41±118.2 | 1.06±0.28 | 13 |
| PA19 | 128.04±77.30 | 1.14±0.63 | 31 | PA51 | 213.03±125.86 | 1.14±0.58 | 16 |
| PA20 | 193.18±50.79 | 0.84±0.32 | 33 | PA52 | 224.05±62.9 | 0.86±0.77 | 8 |
| PA21 | 177.89±76.31 | 0.84±0.27 | 21 | PA53 | 284.07±194.78 | 0.81±0.29 | 12 |
| PA22 | 176.35±77.37 | 1.19±0.53 | 24 | PA54 | 301.3±193.45 | 0.63±0.5 | 15 |
| PA23 | 149.40±82.59 | 1.07±0.24 | 22 | PA55 | 158.12±40.96 | 1.4±0.67 | 11 |
| PA24 | 354.87±149.96 | 1.22±0.30 | 19 | PA56 | 237.38±199.77 | 0.73±0.51 | 10 |
| PA25 | 265.86±154.38 | 0.94±0.33 | 29 | PA57 | 216.36±54.95 | 0.79±0.68 | 17 |
| PA26 | 199.57±104.68 | 1.07±0.22 | 26 | PA58 | 89.85±75.39 | 0.72±0.33 | 12 |
| PA27 | 240.95±114.37 | 1.35±0.42 | 22 | PA59 | 155.50±127.52 | 0.87±0.53 | 17 |
| PA28 | 206.40±85.93 | 1.23±0.42 | 21 | PA60 | 183.34±160.14 | 1.43±0.61 | 10 |
| PA29 | 238.53±163.27 | 1.14±0.35 | 18 | PA61 | 139.78±86.45 | 0.91±0.36 | 13 |
| PA30 | 235.28±114.58 | 1.19±0.14 | 27 | PA62 | 119.42±64.52 | 0.83±0.29 | 15 |
| PA31 | 244.89±98.18 | 1.24±0.2 | 26 | PA63 | 178.09±73.25 | 0.92±0.29 | 12 |
| PA32 | 197.59±70.72 | 1.19±0.53 | 15 | PA64 | 172.71±77.12 | 0.94±0.29 | 17 |

注：$PCR_{SI}$. PCR 扩增效率。

提取效果，使用该组合对6种代表中药材进行提取，其 $A_{260}/A_{280}$ 为1.52±0.23，总DNA浓度为284.62±116.24 ng/μL，PCR扩增成功率为100%。虽然使用缓冲液PA1-PA5，药材DNA浓度可达300 ng/μL以上，但其 $A_{260}/A_{280}$ 均低于PA14，表明DNA中可能具有较多的蛋白成分。

由于DNA中存在的杂质成分可能干扰了PCR的扩增效率，本研究将碱裂解法提取的DNA稀释为4个不同浓度，并考察了其对PCR扩增效率的影响。结果表明使用缓冲液PA14作为碱裂解液处理药材粉末时，金银花、人参、金钱白花蛇DNA浓度为100、20、4、0.4 ng/μL时均能扩出明显条带，且紫苏、车前子、藿香在20、4 ng/μL时也可扩出明显条带，而使用缓冲液PA34、PA44、PA47、PA52、PA56等时，PCR反应对DNA浓度具有非常严格的要求。

Tween 20、Triton X-100、PVP、PVPP、PEG、甘氨酸在DNA提取中具有不同的作用。本研究结果表明，使用加入Triton X-100的提取液，其药材DNA的PCR成功率最高，其次为Tween 20。Tween 20、Triton X-100均为表面活性剂，在DNA提取过程中有助于细胞膜的破裂，Xin和Shi等的研究均表明使用碱裂解法时加入Tween 20可获得更高的DNA浓度，这与本研究相符。

PVP、PVPP、PEG可去除植物多酚，同时PEG可提高碱裂解法中的 $OH^-$ 浓度。然而PEG和PVPP会降低DNA浓度，这与本研究结果相符，即使用含有PEG、PVPP的DNA提取缓冲液，其获得的药材DNA浓度较低。但另一方面，PVP和Triton X-100可以提高PCR稳定性从而增加PCR扩增成功率。本研究通过调整NaOH、PVP、Triton X-100在提取缓冲液中的浓度，提高了 $A_{260}/A_{280}$ 及PCR扩增效率，这可能是与去除PCR抑制剂有关。

然而，本实验结果还表明，随着添加物种类的增加，碱裂解法提取DNA的浓度有明显下降的趋势，且PCR扩增效率也随之降低。添加Tween 20、Triton X-100、PVP、PVPP、PEG、甘氨酸等试剂的其中1种或2种，药材DNA浓度降低不明显，且PCR扩增效率可保持在一个较高的水平；而在NaOH溶液内添加3种或3种以上试剂，DNA浓度显著减少，PCR扩增效率也显著降低。研究结果表明，在使用碱裂解法提取药材DNA时，适宜在缓冲液中添加1或2种试剂。

对Tris中和法和NaAc中和法提取DNA的纯度和浓度进行配对 $T$ 检验，结果表明使用2种中和方法提取的药材DNA浓度具有显著差异。使用Tris中和法提取药材DNA浓度显著高于NaAc中和法（$P<0.01$），但使用2种方法所得DNA纯度没有显著差异。

5.2 碱裂解法对样品的选择性　对于不同的样品，碱裂解法提取效果不同。64种不同的DNA提取缓冲液均对金银花具有最高的提取能力，DNA浓度平均为402.96±212.07 ng/μL。从药材类别看，碱裂解法提取DNA的浓度为：花＞种子＞茎＞动物药＞根＞叶。DNA纯度为：动物药＞花＞种子＞叶＞茎＞根。PCR扩增效率为：动物药＞花＞种子＞根＞茎＞叶。其中单纯的NaOH溶液提取动物药DNA即可扩增出PCR条带。且与植物药相比，动物药具有更高的 $A_{260}/A_{230}$ 值，为1.35±0.41。这可能是由于植物类药材具有细胞壁和多糖类成分，且药用成分多为次级代谢产物，而植物多糖、多酚及部分次级代谢产物均具有抑制PCR反应的效果；动物细胞不含植物多糖和细胞壁，成分较为单一，因此对PCR反应抑制效果不明显。

5.3 碱裂解法对中国药典收载DNA分子鉴别品种的适用性分析　2010年版《中国药典》收载了乌梢蛇、蕲蛇的高特异性PCR鉴别研究，然而该法操作时间长，花费比较高昂。为考察碱裂解法对中国药典收载品种DNA分子鉴别的适用性，本研究使用筛选的碱裂解缓冲液提取蛇类药材及伪品基因组DNA。分别使用COⅠ通用引物、乌梢蛇鉴别引物及金钱白花蛇鉴别引物对11个DNA样品进行PCR扩增，结果如图1所示。结果表明，使用乌梢蛇、金钱白花蛇、赤链华游蛇等11个DNA样品中均可扩出约650 bp的条带；使用乌梢蛇鉴别引物仅在乌梢蛇DNA中可扩出约330 bp条带，使用金钱白花蛇鉴别引物仅在金钱白花蛇DNA中扩出约240 bp条带，其余蛇类均无任何条带扩出。本研究结果表明，利用碱裂解法可在10 min内提取出蛇类样品的DNA，并可保障中国药典收载乌梢蛇鉴别方法的实施。

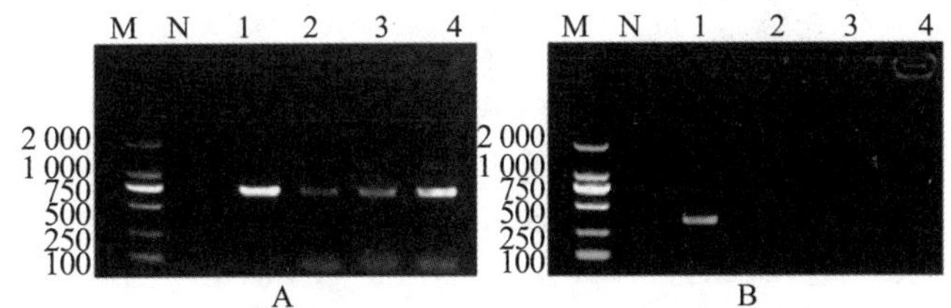


**图1　使用碱裂解法提取DNA用于乌梢蛇的鉴别**

A. *CO*Ⅰ通用引物；B. 乌梢蛇鉴别引物；M. DL 2000 marker；N. 阴性对照。1. 乌梢蛇（Zaocys）；2. 金钱白花蛇（Bungarus Parvus）；3. 王锦蛇（*Elaphe carinata*）；4. 赤链华游蛇（*Sinonatrix annularis*）。

5.4 碱裂解法提取中药材DNA有效性分析　为进一步研究碱裂解法DNA提取在中药材品种的适用范围，使用优化的DNA提取缓冲液PA14对144个不同类别的中药材DNA进行提取，结果如图2所示。所提取药材DNA浓度为354.87±154.96 ng/μL，$A_{260}/A_{230}$ 值为1.17±0.24。由于*psb*A-*trn*H引物对不同药材的PCR反应条件存在差异，本实验分别选择退火温度为53、56、59 ℃进行PCR扩增，并对扩增结果进行统计分析。结果表明，123个药材（85.4%）DNA获得了PCR扩增产物，其中花类、果实种子类及动物类药材DNA获得了100%的PCR成功率。炮制过的药材PCR成功率明显降低，其中制何首乌、玄参及发汗处理的厚朴均无法扩出任何条带。这可能与炮制过程尤其是蒸和煮处理导致DNA极度降解有关。同时部分未炮制药材如藁本、温郁金、泽泻等也未得到PCR扩增产物，可能存在的原因包括：采收、加工过程中的DNA降解；药材干燥后细胞壁结构致密，氢氧化钠裂解不充分；中药材产生的次级代谢产物对PCR的抑制作用；*psb*A-*trn*H引物并不适合用于这些药材的PCR扩增。

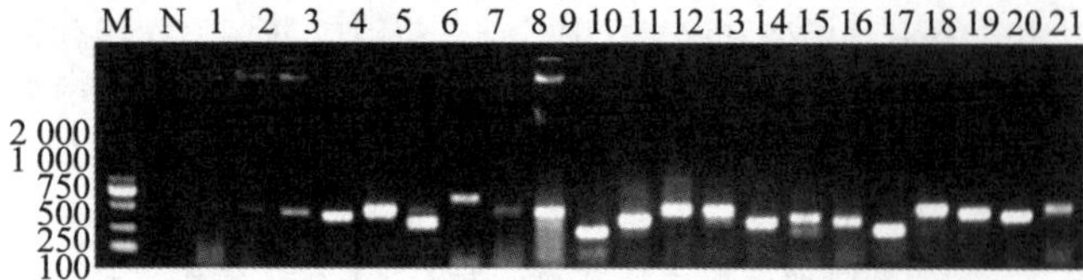


**图 2 DNA 提取缓冲液 PA14 提取中药材 DNA 作为模板的 *psbA* - *trnH* 引物 PCR 扩增结果**

M. DL 2000 marker；N. 阴性对照（negative control）；1. 郁金（Radix Curcumae）；2. 合欢皮（Cortex Albiziae）；3. 当归（Radix Angelicae Sinensis）；4. 金银花（Flos Lonicerae）；5. 人参（Radix Ginseng）；6. 车前子（Semen Plantaginis）；7. 防风（Radix Saposhnikoviae）；8. 广藿香（Herba Pogostemonis）；9. 红花（Flos Carthami）；10. 苦参（Radix Sophorae Flavescentis）；11. 辛夷（Flos Magnoliae）；12. 预知子（Fructus Akebiae）；13. 丹参（Radix Salviae Miltiorrhizae）；14. 延胡索（Rhizoma Corydalis）；15. 桔梗（Radix Platycodonis）；16. 浙贝母（Bulbus Fritillariae Thunbergii）；17. 白芍（Radix Paeoniae Alba）；18. 鸭跖草（Herba Commeli）；19. 首乌藤（Caulis Polygoni Multiflori）；20. 山药（Rhizoma Dioscoreae）；21. 党参（Radix Codonopsis）。

## 6 讨论

6.1 *碱裂解法的优点* 相对传统的 CTAB 和 SDS 法以及广泛用于各种试剂盒的硅胶柱吸附法，碱裂解法具有操作步骤少，提取速度快，价格低廉，不需要大型仪器，可大规模高通量提取的优点，非常适合用于药材 DNA 的快速检测与鉴定。同时，DNA 经由碱裂解之后，由于 Taq DNA 聚合酶更易于接近目的片段，对于 GC 富集区 DNA 扩增具有明显增强效果。Bourke 等的研究表明，氢氧化钠处理能抑制高度降解材料中 PCR 抑制剂对 PCR 扩增效率的影响。与新鲜植物不同，药材的采收、加工、运输、炮制等过程中均会造成 DNA 不同程度的降解，碱裂解法对降解 DNA 的提取有一定的优势。

6.2 *碱裂解法在中药材DNA提取中的不足* 由于碱裂解法使用强碱处理样本，在裂解细胞、变性蛋白质、降解 RNA 的同时也打断了 DNA 链。研究表明，碱裂解法处理之后的样本 DNA 一般降解到 1 kb 以下，对于 1 kb 以上的片段甚至 600 bp 的片段，PCR 扩增效率有所降低。尽管 Rogers 和 Collard 等研究均表明在各种 DNA 快速提取方法中，碱裂解法的成功率和实用性均具有明显的优势，但其 DNA 提取成功率依然小于 CTAB 法，在本研究中利用碱裂解法可有效地提取 85.4%的药材 DNA。由于碱裂解法没有使用纯化 DNA 的步骤，其 DNA 的 $A_{260}/A_{280}$ 一般小于 1.6，$A_{260}/A_{230}$ 小于 1.0 无法用于 DNA 杂交等实验。

6.3 *小结* 综上所述，DNA 快速提取一直是制约中药材分子鉴定的关键步骤。碱裂解法具有操作简单、提取速度快、通量大的特点，已被广泛用于动物、植物、微生物、法医研究的各个领域。本文通过研究药材碱裂解法 DNA 提取的条件，筛选获得含有 0.5 mol/L 氢氧化钠、1% PVP、1% Triton X - 100 的缓冲液可用于中药材生品和炮制材料 DNA 的提取，对于动物和植物药材均具有良好的效果，仅在 10 min 内即可提取出中药材 DNA，并可用于 PCR 反应，对于中药材分子标记及快速 DNA 检测研究具有重要意义。

［蒋超，袁媛，等. 药物分析杂志，2013，33（7）：1081 - 1090.］

# 中药材分子鉴别现场运用的策略与实践

中药材基原真伪鉴别是中药学研究领域中的重要研究方向和首要问题，中药材是否“正本清源”直接影响到用药安全。由于中药材基原具有多样性、复杂性的特点，易受到物种延续性、变异性、地域性和复杂性等因素的影响。因此，对中药材基原鉴别可以从源头上控制中药的质量，对保障中药生产和中药产业的健康发展起到举足轻重的作用。利用分子生物学技术依据遗传物质 DNA 在不同生物个体的差异鉴别生物物种，可为中药材品种鉴别提供依据。近 20 年间，以 PCR 技术为基础的中药分子鉴别技术因其不受外界环境的影响、具有较好的客观性，逐渐被业内认可。其中乌梢蛇、蕲蛇分子鉴别方法被《中国药典》（2010 年版）收载。笔者认为，对中药鉴定技术的需求不仅仅局限于实验室应用，未来将更主要应用于广泛的实际生产与贸易交流环节。随着分子鉴别技术的发展，构建中药材分子鉴别现场运用模块系统有望实现在产地、药市、药房等进行药材现场分子鉴别，将对中药鉴定学科和中药产业的可持续发展将起到推动作用。

## 1 中药材分子鉴别现场运用的意义和需求

1.1 *分子鉴别现场运用是常规检测手段的延伸* 对中药材真伪品的检测通常采用眼看、手摸、嘴尝、鼻闻等方法，正确辨别药材真伪品需要较高的专业技能和长时间经验积累。目前能够熟练掌握这一技能的人才缺乏，且面对种类繁多的中药材，鉴定人员存在主观判断力差异，也影响鉴定的结果。分子鉴别现场运用可以在短时间内实现对药材真伪品的检测，且不受药材外观形态、个体大小和完整性的影响，有利于提高中药材质量监管的科学性和管理效力。

1.2 *高通量检测是分子鉴别现场运用的重要优势* 在药材抽检的过程中，按照中药材或中药饮片抽验工作程序，样品数量巨大。发展高通量检测技术是缩短检测时间、减少工作量、节约检测成本的重要途径。

1.3 *仪器设备简单、成本低廉将有利于分子鉴别现场运用的推广* 近年来，许多学者利用分子生物学技术对中药鉴定方法进行了广泛的研究，并取得了丰富的成果。如杨俊宝等筛选获得2个RAPD引物，可以用于鉴别半夏和掌叶半夏。蒋超等利用EST-SSR技术对金银花、山银花进行了鉴别方法的研究。DNA条形码技术也被认为是中药鉴别的重要方法之一。荆志伟等用基因芯片技术对中药石斛的不同种属进行了鉴别研究，将16个不同种属石斛的ITS序列固定在玻片上制作了基因芯片，用于其中5种石斛的鉴定。然而这些方法目前仅止于实验室阶段，由于其操作繁琐、检测需要大型仪器、耗时长、成本高，难以实现在产地、药市、药房等进行现场鉴别，极大地限制了分子鉴别技术的使用范围和推广程度。

在日常监督工作中对于廉价药材的检测或者对技术较复杂、操作过程繁琐的检测指标进行大批量样品筛检时，往往面临时间和经费的双重困难。利用分子鉴别现场运用系统有望有效解决这一难题。

1.4　*在有毒中药、珍稀濒危药材、贵重药材鉴别方面具有广阔的发展潜力*　分子鉴别现场运用系统，对药材需求量少，仅需0.1g药材就可以进行鉴别反应。因此，对于一些价格昂贵或珍稀濒危的药材，该系统具有更广阔的发展潜力。

1.5　*中药材快速检测工作模式的探讨*　将快速检测车及现场快速检测仪器作为主要工作平台，依托快检实验室开展工作。形成涵盖现场快速检测的药材分子快速检测模式。现场采集的样本可以通过快速检测仪器获得结果，如需实验室检测或需进一步确证，则将样品送回快检实验室获得检测结果。

## 2　中药材分子鉴别现场运用存在的困难及解决方案

2.1　*中药材DNA快速提取*　CTAB法、SDS法等是中药材DNA提取的常用方法，在这些方法中常使用65℃水浴使细胞裂解、蛋白质变性，从而使DNA被释放出来，水浴时间一般为30 min至2 h，这很难满足中药材分子鉴别现场运用的需求。本课题组开发了一种基于碱裂解法的中药材DNA快速提取方法，并申请发明专利，在此基础上研制了中药材DNA快速提取试剂盒。试剂盒中主要包括溶液A和B。简要操作过程：将药材粉末加入溶液A后震荡1 min，再加入溶液B震荡1 min，静置后取上清待用。笔者利用这种方法对市售的180余种药材包括果实类、种子类、花类、全草类、皮类、根类药材及炮制品进行了DNA提取，并选择叶绿体*psb*A-*trn*H序列通用引物进行PCR反应及琼脂糖凝胶电泳检测，结果表明85%药材DNA获得了PCR扩增条带，其中花类、果实种子类及动物类药材DNA获得了100%的PCR成功率，但炮制过的药材PCR成功率明显降低。

2.2　*药材真伪鉴别DNA标记的开发及其快速检测*　获取药材正品及其市场常见混淆品的核酸信息，并利用生物信息学分析软件对相关序列进行分析，筛选药材真伪鉴别DNA标记，收集不同产地、不同批次的药材正品及其混淆品样品，对真伪鉴别DNA标记进行验证。RAPD、RFLP、ISSR、DNA条形码等DNA标记已被用于中药材的真伪鉴别，但这些鉴别DNA标记检测的方法大多以PCR技术为基础，荧光定量法、测序法、限制性内切酶酶切法、质谱法、基因芯片等方法也被用于鉴别标记的检测。但这些方法大多操作复杂、价格昂贵、检测时间长，而且需要大型的仪器设备，因此并不适合于现场鉴别。

单核苷酸多态性SNP(single nucleotide polymorphisms)作为新一代的分子标记，具有数量多、覆盖密度大、遗传稳定性强、多态性丰富的优势，且由于SNPs一般只有2个等位基因，在检测时只需要通过一个简单的"+/-"方式即可进行基因分型，使得其检测易于实现自动化。基于SNP标记，在病原微生物检测、疾病诊断等研究中陆续开发了一些可用于现场快速鉴别的技术，简化了对仪器和实验室条件的要求、缩短了检测时间，具有很好的发展前景。如等温扩增技术，包括Q复制酶反应(QBRA)、链置换扩增技术(SDA)、切口酶恒温扩增技术(NEMA)、转录依赖的扩增技术(TAST-MA，3SR，NASBA)、解旋酶扩增技术(HAD)、滚环扩增技术(RCA)、环介导等温扩增技术(LAMP)、单引物等温扩增技术(SPIA)等，为中药材现场鉴别中的鉴别DNA标记快速检测试剂盒开发提供了思路。

## 3　研究实例

3.1　*中药材分子鉴别现场运用的整体方案*　从实际出发，基于药材真伪鉴别DNA标记，设计了一套用于中药材分子现场鉴别的模块系统(图1)，包括药材DNA快速提取模块、药材鉴别DNA标记检测模块和保障模块。

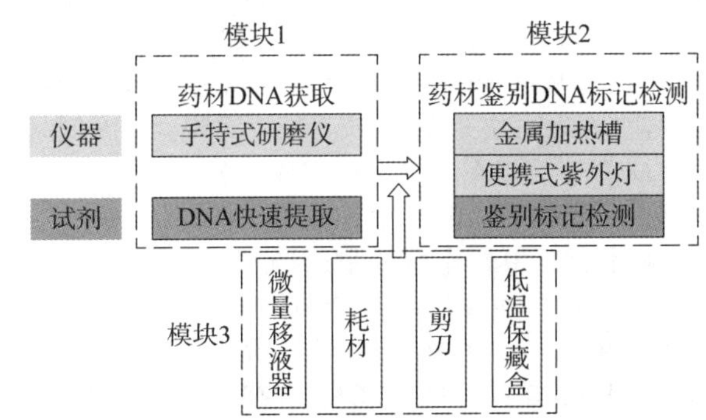


**图1　中药材分子鉴别现场运用模块系统组成**

3.1.1　*药材DNA快速提取模块*　①手持式研磨仪。配置锂电池，适合野外使用。②中药材DNA快速提取试剂盒，包括溶液A和B，常温保存。

3.1.2　*药材鉴别DNA标记检测模块*　①微型金属加热槽。配置锂电池或车载电源，可用于65±5℃ DNA扩增反应。②便携式紫外灯。配置锂电池，适合野外使用，用于荧光检测，配备小型暗箱。③鉴别DNA标记的快速检测试剂盒。

3.1.3　*保障模块*　①微量移液器。②微量离心管。③吸头、吸头盒。④锋利的剪刀。⑤低温保藏盒，用于储存DNA聚合酶，配置冰袋。

现场鉴别模块系统拥有完善和简单的操作流程，操作时间控制在40～60 min，仪器装置简单、成本低，操作人员无需掌握较好的专业知识，经过简单训练即可进行中药材快速鉴别。

3.2 金银花分子鉴别现场运用研究

3.2.1 金银花真伪鉴别DNA标记的开发 通过对GenBank收录的忍冬属植物叶绿体*trn*L - *trn*F序列进行对比分析，获得金银花真伪鉴别SNP位点，并依据该SNP位点设计特异性引物，对84份金银花基原植物及其市售饮片、混淆品进行双向位点特异性PCR扩增，根据真伪品的特异性条带进行金银花药材鉴别，确定了金银花真伪鉴别SNP。

3.2.2 鉴别DNA标记的快速检测技术 利用已获得的金银花真伪鉴别SNP，开发了一种改良LAMP技术，通过设计特异性引物，于65℃在DNA聚合酶的作用下进行扩增反应。反应产物加入适量的SYBR Green染料，在紫外灯下进行检测，正品样本即可检测产生荧光，混淆品样品则不产生荧光。在此基础上开发了金银花鉴别DNA标记快速检测试剂盒。包括：溶液C. 缓冲液(常温保存)；溶液D1 - 4. 特异性引物(常温保存)；溶液E. DNA聚合酶(低温保存)；溶液F. SYBR Green染料(常温保存)；溶液G. 正对照；溶液H. 负对照。

3.2.3 金银花分子鉴别现场运用操作规程 ①用剪刀剪碎药材，取少量样品用手持式研磨仪磨成粉末。②取少量粉末放置于2 mL离心管中，使用中药材DNA快速提取试剂盒进行DNA提取。③使用鉴别DNA标记快速检测试剂盒进行药材的真伪检测。依次在0.2 mL离心管中加入溶液C、溶液D、2 μL DNA提取液、溶液E，放置于微型金属加热槽中，在65℃条件下进行DNA扩增反应。反应30 min后，冷却至室温。加入溶液F，混匀后在紫外灯下进行检测。实验设置正、负对照。④判定标准：产生荧光即为正品样本，不产生荧光则为混淆品样品。

[袁媛，黄璐琦. 中国中药杂志，2013，38(16)：2553 - 2555.]

# 快速PCR方法在金银花真伪鉴别中的应用

自Millus等1985年发明PCR技术以来，PCR已成为分子生物学研究中的最基本和普遍手段之一。由于PCR的重要性，为了提高实验效率、节约成本，对该技术的改良从未停止过。早在1991年，Yap等通过更改PCR条件以缩短PCR反应时间。而Wittwer等通过使用毛细管进行PCR反应，即利用热空气注入法快速控温，从而减少升降温的时间，使得30个PCR循环可以在30 min内完成。在此基础上，提出了快速PCR(rapid PCR)的概念。

准确、快速是中药分子鉴别的核心需要。目前已报道的中药分子鉴别方法，如RAPD、SSR、SCAR、PCR - RFLP、AS - PCR、AFLP及DNA条形码等均依赖于PCR技术。快速PCR与其相结合，将缩短PCR反应时间、提高效率，有利于中药分子鉴别技术的现场运用和推广。

本文基于已建立的金银花位点特异性PCR真伪鉴别方法，对PCR的反应程序进行了优化，并引入了荧光染料法对真伪鉴别结果进行检测，结合药材DNA快速提取技术，可将金银花真伪分子鉴别时间控制在30 min左右，为实现药材分子鉴别的现场运用提供技术支撑。

## 1 材料

1.1 药材 选取来自不同产地的8个忍冬正品及9种16个忍冬属伪品材料进行快速位点特异性PCR研究。植物样品采自广西、河南、山东、北京、安徽地区，凭证标本保存于中国中医科学院中药资源中心和广西药用植物园，见表1。

**表1 试验材料**

| 序号 | 物种 | 拉丁名 | 产地 | 个数 | 鉴定人 |
|---|---|---|---|---|---|
| 1 | 忍冬 | *Lonicera japonica* | 河南封丘 | 4 | 刘红彦 |
| 2 | 忍冬 | *L. japonica* | 山东临沂 | 4 | 李圣波 |
| 3 | 红腺忍冬 | *L. hypoglauca* | 广西崇左 | 2 | 吴庆华 |
| 4 | 华南忍冬 | *L. confusa* | 山东临沂 | 1 | 李圣波 |
| 5 | 灰毡毛忍冬 | *L. macranthoides* | 广西南宁 | 2 | 吴庆华 |
| 6 | 黄褐毛忍冬 | *L. fulvotomentosa* | 广西桂林 | 2 | 余丽莹 |
| 7 | 水忍冬 | *L. dasystyla* | 广西桂林 | 2 | 余丽莹 |
| 8 | 金银忍冬 | *L. maackii* | 安徽合肥 | 1 | 彭华胜 |
| 9 | 郁香忍冬 | *L. fragrantissima* | 北京 | 2 | 郝近大 |
| 10 | 新疆忍冬 | *L. tatarica* | 北京 | 2 | 郝近大 |
| 11 | 繁果忍冬 | *L. tatarica* cv. 'Fanguo' | 北京 | 2 | 郝近大 |

1.2 仪器 GeneAmp 9700 型 PCR 扩增仪(Applied Biosystem 公司);5810 R 型高速冷冻离心机(Eppendorf 公司);VORTEX-2 GENIE 漩涡震荡仪(Scientific Industries 公司);DYY-12 型电脑三恒多用电泳仪(北京六一仪器厂);HE99X-15-1.5 型电泳槽(Hoefer 公司);SYNGENE 凝胶成像系统(Gene 公司);ZF-7A 型手持式紫外灯(上海谷村电子光学仪器厂)。

1.3 试剂 琼脂糖购自 Promega 公司;溴化乙啶购自 Fluka 公司;r*Taq* DNA 聚合酶、Ex *Taq* 聚合酶、SpeedStar HS *Taq* DNA 聚合酶、2 000 bp DNA Marker 购自 TaKaRa 公司;Apta*Taq* fast DNA 聚合酶 Mix 购自 Roche 有限公司、Transfast *Taq* DNA 聚合酶购自 Transgen 有限公司;10 000× SYBR 购自 Invitrogen 公司;其他试剂均为国产分析纯。

## 2 方法

2.1 快速位点特异性 PCR 引物设计 此前,本课题组已验证金银花 *trn*L-*trn*F 序列 625 位 G/T 变异可以准确鉴别金银花及其同属伪品,本文据此位点设计快速 PCR 鉴别引物。通过 Premier Primer 5.0 (http://www.premierbiosoft.com/primerdesign/)设计快速位点特异性 PCR 引物,调整参数使上游引物为 3′末端与 625 位 G/T 的 SNP 位点互补,$T_m$ 值为 65~70 ℃,在引物 3′末端倒数第二位引入人为错配,PCR 产物长度为 60~100 bp。引物命名为 LJ-RAPID-1F 和 LJ-RAPID-1R,由上海生工生物科技有限公司合成。

2.2 基因组总 DNA 的提取 取 20 mg 干燥材料,使用碱裂解法提取总 DNA,所提取 DNA 稀释 50 倍用于 PCR 反应。通用引物对 *trn*L F/*trn*L R 用于 PCR 反应以检测 DNA 质量,PCR 反应体系包含 2 μL 10×r*Taq* buffer, 1 μL 10 mmol/L dNTPs, 0.25 μmol/L 上游及下游引物、0.5 U 快速 *Taq* 酶、1 μL 20% PVP 40 溶液、0.5 μL 10 g/L BSA 溶液、1 μL(约 10 ng)DNA 模板,反应程序见表 2。

**表 2 引物及 PCR 反应条件**

| 引物名 | 序列(5′-3′) | 反应条件 |
|---|---|---|
| LJ-RAPID-1F | TTATCCTTTTTTTGTTAGCGGTTTC | 94 ℃ 1 min;95 ℃ 30 s,68 ℃ 30 s,30 个循环;94 ℃ 5 min |
| LJ-RAPID-1R | CTCAGATCTATTTGTAAAGAAGTAAGGTGG | |
| *trn*L F | CGAAATCGGTAGACGCTACG | 94 ℃ 30 s,56 ℃ 30 s,72 ℃ 45 s,35 个循环;72 ℃ 7 min |
| *trn*F R | ATTTGAACTGGTGACACGAG | |

2.3 PCR 扩增条件的确定 取不同样品 DNA 用于确定快速位点特异性 PCR 反应条件。20 μL PCR 反应体系包含 2 μL 10×r*Taq* buffer,1 μL 10 mmol/L dNTPs,0.25 μL 10 μmol/L 上游及下游引物,0.5 U 快速 *Taq* 酶,1 μL 20% PVP 40 溶液,0.5 μL 10 g/L BSA 溶液,1 μL(约 10 ng)DNA 模板。PCR 反应在 9700 型 PCR 扩增仪上进行。由于 Yap 等报道 94 ℃预变性 1 min 即可实现全基因组解链,而本课题组前期证实 94 ℃预变性 1 min 可实现 PCR 产物的有效扩增,依此设定初始反应程序见表 2,在此基础上开展 PCR 反应条件的优化。

反应结束后在 PCR 反应体系内加入 2 μL 100×SYBR Green I(Invitrogen 公司),混匀后于 365 nm 紫外波长肉眼下检测荧光。另取 PCR 反应产物,加入 5 μL 6×Loading buffer (Takara 公司)混匀后于 EB 染色的 1%琼脂糖凝胶电泳检测,SYN-GENE 凝胶成像系统观察、成像。

利用忍冬 SNP 鉴别引物 LJ-RAPID-1F 和 LJ-RAPID-1R 进行快速位点特异性 PCR 反应,并分别考察退火温度(66、68、70、72 ℃)、PCR 循环数(27、30、33 个循环)、变性温度(95、91、89、87、85、83 ℃)、变性和退火时间(10、5、3、1 s)、*Taq* 种类(r*Taq* DNA 聚合酶,SpeedStar HS *Taq* DNA 聚合酶,Apta *Taq* fast DNA 聚合酶 Mix, Transfast *Taq* DNA 聚合酶)、不同 PCR 仪[9700 型 PCR 仪(ABI 公司),PTC-100 型 PCR 仪(MJ Research 集团),Mastercycler 型 PCR 仪(Eppendorf 公司),TC-512 型 PCR 仪(Techne 公司)]对 PCR 反应稳定性的影响。

2.4 PCR 产物检测 在 PCR 扩增产物中加入 2 μL 100×SYBR Green I 于 365 nm 紫外波长下检测荧光,出现强烈绿色荧光则表明有扩增。

## 3 结果与分析

3.1 碱裂解法提取金银花类材料 DNA 由于碱裂解法提取的 DNA 无法通过凝胶电泳检测,故本文使用通用引物进行扩增,以检测 DNA 提取效果。1%琼脂糖凝胶电泳检测结果表明,利用 *trn*L F/*trn*F R 引物,忍冬及其 9 个同属混淆品均获得约 1 050 bp 大小的扩增产物,与 *trn*L-*trn*F 片段大小一致见图 1,说明碱裂解法提取的 DNA 可以满足 PCR 反应的要求。

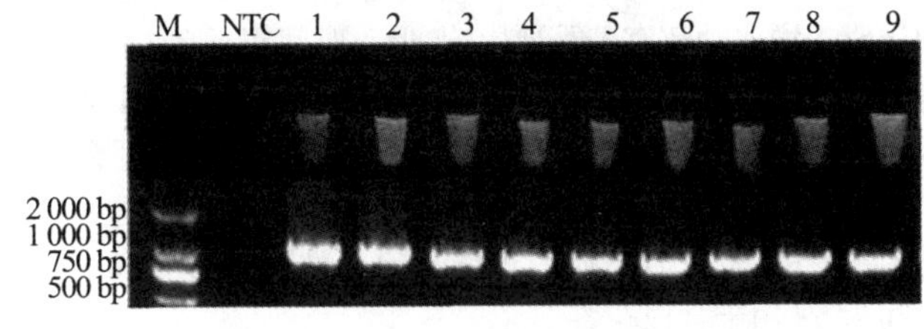


**图 1 *trn*L F/*trn*F R 通用引物扩增**

M. DL 2 000 marker;1. 忍冬;2. 红腺忍冬;3. 灰毡毛忍冬;4. 华南忍冬;5. 黄褐毛忍冬;6. 水忍冬;7. 金银忍冬;8. 郁香忍冬;9. 新疆忍冬;NTC. 无模板对照。

3.2 PCR 反应条件的确定 与 AS-PCR 一样,快速位点特异性 PCR 要求严格的退火温度、循环数,循环数过高或退火温度过低均会导致假阳性的分型结果。为获得最适反应条件,本文依次分析了退火温度、循环数、变性温度、变性和退火时间、*Taq* 酶种类及不同的 PCR 仪对 PCR 反应稳定性的影响。结果表明,使用快速 AS-PCR 鉴别引物扩增时,如当退火温度为 66℃时,伪品也有荧光。当退火温度为 70、72℃时,均无荧光。当退火温度为 68℃时,仅正品有荧光,所以本文金银花快速 AS-PCR 鉴别的最佳退火温度选择 68℃,见图 2A。

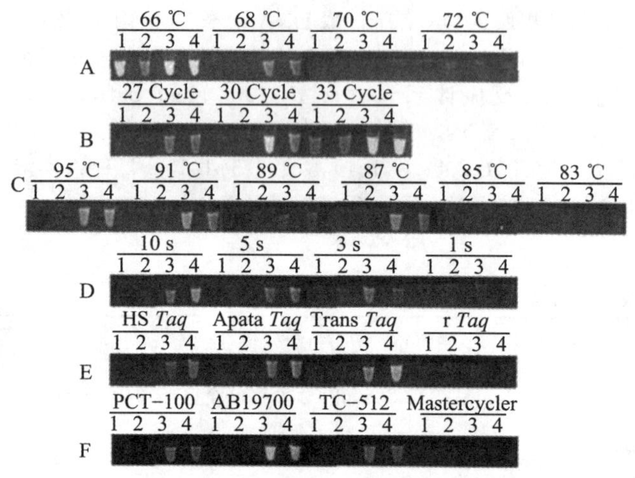

**图 2 不同因素对快速位点特异性 PCR 的影响**

A. 退火温度;B. 循环数;C. 变性温度;D. 变性时间,其中退火时间与变性时间一致;E. *Taq* 酶种类的影响,其中 HS *Taq* 为 SpeedStar HS *Taq* DNA 聚合酶,Apta *Taq* 为 Apta *Taq* fast DNA 聚合酶 Mix,Trans *Taq* 为 Transfast *Taq* DNA 聚合酶,r*Taq* 为 TaKaRa r *Taq* DNA 聚合酶;F. 不同 PCR 仪的影响,其中 PCT-100 完成 PCR 时间为 30 min;ABI 9700 为 26 min;TC-512 为 28 min;Mastercycler 为 18 min;1. 灰毡毛忍冬;2. 红腺忍冬;3. 忍冬(河南);4. 忍冬(山东)。

减少 PCR 反应时间,在退火温度为 68℃,逐渐减少循环数。当循环数为 27 个循环,PCR 产物出现弱荧光,见图 2B。然而,当选用 27 个循环时,变性-退火/延伸的时间低于 20 s 时即无法扩增出条带,故最终选择循环数为 30。

在此基础上,变性温度高于 85℃(图 2C),变性及退火时间大于 3 s(图 2D)才能有效鉴别金银花真伪品。随着变性温度的降低,PCR 成功率降低,当变性温度低于 85℃时无法获得 PCR 产物,该结果与 Yap 等的报道一致。变性及退火时间同样对扩增成功率有着重要影响,退火时间超过 3 s 才能获得有效的扩增,这可能与 PCR 起始过程中 DNA 聚合酶结合模板-引物复合物需要时间有关。由于不同 PCR 仪温度会有所差异,升降温时变温所需时间有所差别,为增加快速 PCR 鉴别金银花的适用性,本研究最终选定变性温度为 87℃,退火时间为 5 s 用于金银花鉴别。

在所选择的 4 种 DNA 聚合酶中,3 种快速 DNA 聚合酶 SpeedStar HS *Taq* DNA 聚合酶、Apta *Taq* fast DNA 聚合酶 Mix、Transfast *Taq* DNA 聚合酶均能实现金银花真伪鉴别(图 2D)。对金银花快速 PCR 不同 PCR 仪扩增时的稳定性进行考察,结果表明,PCT-100、ABI 9700、TC-512 型 PCR 仪均可用于金银花快速 PCR 鉴别(图 2F)。而 Mastercycler 型 PCR 仪未获得扩增,可能是由于其完成 PCR 所用时间太短(18 min),升降温速度太快,反应不完全引起的。

3.3 快速位点特异性 PCR 鉴别金银花 使用快速 AS-PCR 对金银花及其 9 种同属伪品进行扩增,PCR 扩增条件为 87℃预变性 1 min;87℃变性 5 s,68℃延伸 5 s,30 个循环。反应结束后在扩增产物中加入 2 μL 100×SYBR Green Ⅰ 于 365 nm 紫外波长下检测荧光。金银花正品显示出明亮绿色荧光,而伪品不发出荧光,取 5 μL 进行凝胶电泳,仅金银花扩出约 100 bp 大小的条带,伪品无条带,见图 3。

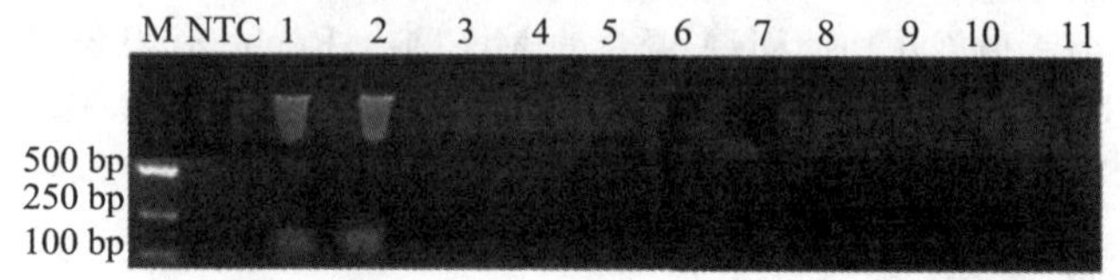

**图 3 快速位点特异性 PCR 鉴别金银花类中药材荧光检测**

M. DL 2000 marker;NTC. 空白对照;1. 金银花(山东);2. 金银花(河南);3. 红腺忍冬;4. 灰毡毛忍冬;5. 华南忍冬;6. 黄褐毛忍冬;7. 水忍冬;8. 金银忍冬;9. 郁香忍冬;10. 新疆忍冬;11. 繁果忍冬。

## 4 讨论

4.1 金银花快速 PCR 反应的实现 经典的 DNA 分子鉴定过程一般包括 DNA 提取、目标核酸或目标信号的扩增和产物检测 3 个方面。为达到快速鉴定的目的,须尽量缩短这 3 步的时间。DNA 提取是制约 DNA 分子鉴定用时的首要因素,传统的 CTAB 法或 SDS 法一般需 4 h 以上才能获得 DNA,试剂盒常用的硅胶柱法一般需要 1~2 h 才能获得 DNA,并且需要进行反复离心,操作繁琐,难以满足快速鉴别的要求。故本研究采用了碱裂解法进行 DNA 提取,由于碱裂解法只有裂解和中和 2 步,DNA 提取用时大约 5 min。研究结果表明,碱裂解法适用于金银花及其伪品 DNA 提取,所得 DNA 满足分子鉴定要求。

制约 DNA 分子鉴定的第 2 个因素是 PCR 扩增过程,常规 PCR 扩增一般需时 2~3 h,主要是进行 30~40 个循环的变性-退火-延伸需时较长。由于 *Taq* DNA 聚合酶延伸速度一般为 1~6 kb/min,用于鉴定的 PCR 片段一般 300~1 000 bp,故传统上常选择 0.5~2 min 的延伸时间,造成扩增反应用时很长。为达到快速扩增的目的,PCR 产物长度应尽可能短,故本文进行金银花鉴别引物设计时,设定引物距 SNP 鉴别位点上下游 1~30 bp,所得 PCR 产物≤100 bp。另一方面,减少 PCR 循环过程中升降温的温差,采取两步法进行 PCR 扩增,也可以缩短 PCR 的反应时间。为减少升降温用时,本文设计的引物 $T_m$ 与延伸温度基本一致。Yap 等的研究表明,PCR 产物变性远较全基因组变性容易,极端情况时 92℃下 1 s 即可实现短产物变性,所以本文首先尝试降低变性温度以减少升降温温差,最终发现 87℃时达到金银花 PCR 产物变性的临界点,选择该温度用于金银花分子鉴定。在此基础上,逐步缩短变性-退火/延伸的时间,最终达到了快速扩增的目的。

经典的 PCR 产物检测方法为凝胶电泳方式,需要经过制胶、胶凝、电泳和成像 4 步,需用时 1 h 以上。当使用 SYBR

Green Ⅰ荧光染料时，产物检测过程为染色、成像2步，用时约2 min，极大缩短了检测时间。

本文通过利用常规PCR仪，建立了金银花真伪快速PCR鉴别技术，并结合药材DNA快速提取技术和荧光检测技术，有望在短时间内完成药材分子鉴别过程，且仅需PCR仪、操作简单，为中药材分子鉴别技术的推广和应用提供技术保障。

4.2 快速PCR在中药分子鉴定应用的展望 随着PCR技术的快速发展，研究者对检测时间有了越来越高的要求，希望在保证PCR反应灵敏度和特异性的条件下尽可能缩短PCR时间、提高检测效率，快速PCR技术应运而生。快速PCR技术在临床检验和司法检测中已有广泛应用，然而目前尚未见到快速PCR用于中药鉴定的报道。

建立准确、快速、高通量、低成本的鉴别方法一直是中药鉴定的追求。相对传统性状和理化鉴别来说，基于PCR的分子鉴别操作相对复杂、耗时相对较长，制约了中药分子鉴别的应用和推广。与经典PCR相比，快速PCR的程序更为简单，检测速度明显提高，基本能满足中药快速、准确鉴别的要求，在中药分子鉴别中具有良好的应用前景。

建立快速PCR检测方法主要包括以下几种策略：改变PCR程序，即缩短变性-退火-延伸的时间。提高酶与模板的亲和力，即缩短PCR启动时间、提高*Taq*酶延伸速度。改进PCR仪的升降温速度，即增加热传导率。改变PCR进行方式，即在硅基芯片上实现微池静态PCR或平流PCR。由于目前商品化的快速*Taq*酶已经很成熟，而常规PCR仪在今后较长一段时间内仍会是主流仪器，因此通过优化PCR程序，在常规PCR仪上进行快速PCR将成为中药快速PCR鉴别的一个研究方向。而便携式PCR仪的问世及其商业化，将促进在野外、药市或药房进行PCR分子鉴定，此时PCR反应和产物检测时间可能会成为制约DNA分子鉴定的瓶颈。快速PCR的实现，能提高单位时间检测通量，促进现场检测技术的发展和应用。

[蒋超，袁媛. 中国中药杂志，2014，39(19)：3668－3672.]

# 中药分子鉴定发展中的若干问题探讨

近20年间，国内外学者一起致力于运用生物技术对中药进行研究，尤其是分子标记技术在中药鉴定中的应用是目前最令人鼓舞的进展之一。蛇类药材的分子鉴别方法成为《中国药典》(2010年版)收载的第一个中药分子鉴别方法，标志着这一技术已从实验室研究进入广泛应用阶段。与传统中药鉴别方法相比，中药分子鉴别具有准确性高、重现性好等特点，且不受样品形态的限制，原药材、饮片、粉末乃至含有生药原型的中成药(丸剂、散剂等)均可应用。由于其所需检样量少，对珍稀药材及化石标本的鉴定更具应用价值。但随着中药分子鉴别快速发展的同时，也存在一些误区和问题，值得探讨。

## 1 中药分子鉴定使用原则

随着分子生物技术的高速发展，大量药用动、植物的基因序列已见发表，动植物DNA条形码的开发已成为科研热点之一。这些公共基因资源为各科研领域的发展提供了宝贵的基础，也加速了中药分子鉴定技术的开发与应用。但由于生物进化机制的复杂性，如多倍化现象(如大黄属植物)、基因水平转移(如菟丝子属)、杂交(如独活属、白珠属)、基因渗入、辐射物种形成(如石斛属、龙胆属)和物种谱系分选不完全等，经常造成物种树与基因树不一致，导致DNA条形码序列在一些物种间没有鉴别力。因此，即使药材真伪品来源于不同物种，其DNA条形码序列也可能完全一致，以致会导致错误的鉴别结论。中药分子鉴定的本质是物种的界定，物种的概念有生物学的种和分类学的种，生物学种的界限是生殖隔离，分类学种的界定是根据分类学特征(如形态特征、DNA序列特征等)的差异，在植物中，很多种间没有明显的生殖隔离，出现大量的过渡类型，导致分类学种界定的困难。如何界定某种中药的物种界限和种内变异幅度，是中药分子鉴定的瓶颈问题，分子系统学是解决这一瓶颈问题的有力工具，缺乏分子系统学分析的中药分子鉴定，就好比"盲人摸象"，难免盲目性和片面性，必然是不可靠的。为此提出中药分子鉴定的二步法：首先建立被鉴定中药所在属完全物种取样(包括药用和非药用的种)的分子系统数据库，然后将被鉴定中药在该数据库中进行比对判断其归属。数据库涵盖物种的全面与否决定了该鉴定系统的可靠程度。

另一方面，中药材种类繁多，使用历史悠久，来源复杂；有些药材来自野生，有些药材来自栽培，它们的进化历史不尽相同。加上异地引种和商业贸易的发展，人为改变了居群间、种间的基因流，使药用植物间发生杂交或基因渐渗程度进一步增强，在栽培药用植物中出现了明显的种质混杂情况。因此，某味药材分子鉴别方法的建立不能证明其他药材品种也具备建立分子鉴定方法的条件，需要采取个案分析原则，即针对具体的药材品种进行个案评估，逐步进行推进，在了解和把握品种具体情况前，不应作出中药分子鉴别使用的结论和决定，更不能简单地予以全盘通过或者全盘否定。

在明确药材物种树与基因树一致的前提下，可以选择合适的基因片段进行中药分子鉴别。由于物种的生活型(木本与草本)、物种形成方式(渐进式分化与适应性辐射)等存在极大的多样性，物种间基因的进化速率存在很大的差异。这使得基因标记在某一类群可能分辨率很高而在另一类群却很低，甚至没有分辨度。到目前为止，还没有一个理想基因标记可以分辨所有的植物类群，因此一味地去寻找高分辨率的“万能标记”可能是中药分子鉴定的误区。在中药DNA条形码的选择上一个可行的办法是“分阶层的鉴定体系”，即先在整个植物界确定一个进化速率适中的基因片段作为核心条形码，然后再在科或属级水平寻找高进化速率的基因作为辅助条形码。当前对于陆生植物核心条形码已经达成共识（*mat*K+*rbc*L或ITS），而在特定类群基于药用植物基因组筛选辅助条形码并建立标准可能是未来中药分子鉴定的发展方向之一。

总之，中药分子鉴别技术应建立在科学、客观的基础上，遵循在一定系统学研究背景，采取个案分析原则建立分阶层的鉴定体系，为中药分子鉴定使用提供依据。

## 2 中药分子鉴定研究领域中的热点问题

“真伪优劣”是中药鉴定领域的核心问题。就中药分子鉴别而言，其研究的重点应侧重于解决传统鉴别中的难点和热点问题，如多来源药材鉴别、产地鉴别、年限鉴别、成药鉴别等。

2.1 *多来源药材鉴别* 受到历史、地理和人为因素的影响及研究手段的限制，长期以来我国中药材存在多来源的现象。2010年版《中国药典》中收载140余种多来源的药材。按一药一名一标准的原则，科学、客观地逐步解决中药材长期存在的同品名来源问题是未来重要的研究方向，也是《中国药典》要求和规定的理想目标。

药材多来源的生物学内涵即亲缘关系相近的近缘种或相近的分类单位。原动植物的分类地位的确定对多来源药材的鉴别有显著作用。现今多来源药材的研究主要集中于同种药材不同来源的主要化学成分及显微鉴别，如淫羊藿研究，分子水平的鉴别研究尚处于起步阶段。解决多来源药材的问题，在结合形态学考察的前提下，针对特定的问题选择合适的分子片段开展多来源药材的分子鉴定。通常使用核基因组ITS序列、叶绿体基因的非编码区序列或线粒体 *CO* Ⅰ基因对植物较低分类阶元及动物物种进行鉴定分类。遵循中医临床用药经验，对常用的多来源药材进行深入研究，基于系统学的鉴定方法与体系，从居群水平搞清楚中药原动植物的分类地位。按照中药分子鉴定使用原则，在分子系统学研究基础上开展多来源药材的分子鉴定，以期对我国常用多来源中药材进行进一步的系统研究与鉴定分类。

2.2 *产地鉴别* 药材的质量因其产地不同而存在差异，已成为业界公论。从总体上来看，近现代药材被划分为川药、广药、云药、贵药、怀药、浙药、关药、北药、西药、南药十大类别。从单一品种来看，按照产地命名的药材种类繁多，如当归可分为岷归、云归、川归、窑归等；菊花可分为亳菊、滁菊、贡菊和杭菊等。随着对“道地药材认证”“地理标识产品认证”等工作的重视，对产地鉴别标记的开发已成为迫切需要解决的关键技术问题。

除提取传统区域性状鉴别特征外，分子鉴定有望成为产地鉴别的有力工具，主要体现在以下3种手段：①利用分子谱系地理学基本理论，分析不同产地药材单倍型，构建网状进化树，并结合单倍型和进化树筛选可进行产地鉴别的分子标记。②利用遗传学理论，筛选与药材活性成分积累相关的功能基因，通过比较其在不同产地药材功能基因的变异程度差异，筛选可用于进行产地鉴别的分子标记。③利用代谢组学等技术筛选获得产地特征成分标记物（群），利用免疫检测技术制备成分相关抗体（群），并建立免疫检测芯片、试剂盒或检测试纸条。

2.3 *年限鉴别* 大多数中药材均为多年生，其有效成分积累随时间变化呈现一定的规律性。药材的质量因生长年限不同而存在差异，其功效也有区别。如生长4年以上的黄芩宿根称“枯芩”，善清上焦肺火，主治肺热咳嗽痰黄；生长2～3年的黄芩称“子芩”，善泻大肠湿热，主治湿热泻痢腹痛。传统认为人参、黄连等部分根及根茎类药材须生长5年以上才能采收，厚朴等须生长15年以上才能采收使用。目前年限鉴别的主要方法是传统性状鉴别，如人参通过芦头形状和芦碗数目来判断年限，依赖于药工的经验，难以实现鉴定方法的定量化、标准化。

分子鉴定有望成为中药材年限鉴定的有力工具。梁加贝等利用端粒酶活性和端粒长度随生长年限变化的规律，建立了不同年限人参的端粒长度鉴别方法，并建立了对应的数学模型。程春松等利用端粒酶切长度分析（TRFs）对不同年限石柱人参及赤芍端粒长度进行了进一步研究，发现石柱人参及赤芍端粒均随生长年限延长而变短，表明平均端粒长度的缩短可作为年限鉴别的依据。解决多年生中药材年限鉴别问题，将理论研究转化为实际应用工具还需要更多深入的工作。

2.4 *成药鉴别* 中成药的定性鉴别通常是利用其原料药的形态、组织学特征、化学成分的物理和化学性质等进行鉴别，常用的方法包括性状鉴别、显微鉴别、色谱法、化学定性法、物理常数测定法、升华法、光谱法等。但由于中成药剂型种类繁多，给其原料鉴定工作带来了许多困难。薄层色谱法是目前中成药鉴别的常用方法之一，《中国药典》收录的一些中成药大部分都采用该方法进行定性鉴别，如复方丹参滴丸、复方鱼腥草片等。然而薄层色谱法根据特征性化学成分有无对中成药中原料药材生药基原进行鉴别不够客观、准确，如对含有金银花中成药的鉴别，一般只检测成药中是否含有绿原酸，然而金银花及其混淆品中均含有绿原酸，因此无法判断在中成药中投放的原料药材是金银花还是山银花。另外，显微技术也是中成药鉴别的主要方法之一，但超微粉碎技术的出现使药粉直径常常不足10 μm，导致无法使用光学显微技术对中成药进行鉴定。

分子鉴定技术应用于中成药鉴别，不受化学成分的影响，即使没有性状或显微鉴别经验的人员也能够进行中成药鉴别。蒋超等建立了基于位点特异性PCR技术的中成药金银花原料分子鉴别方法，利用该方法可有效检测成药中投放的原料药材是金银花还是其混淆品。崔占虎等利用序列分析技术尝试对中成药中的复杂原料进行鉴定，采用梯度扩增、克隆测序结合生物信息学分析等手段，从市售连翘败毒丸的19种原料中鉴定出其中的10种，为中成药鉴别研究提供的新思路。

## 3 中药分子鉴别的技术创新

随着中药分子鉴别的快速发展，对其的要求也越来越高。作为传统鉴别技术的有益补充，中药分子鉴别不仅要在实验室中使用，而且被要求进一步运用于野外、药市、药房和生产企业等各个环节。针对这种情况，袁媛等提出了中药分子鉴别现场运用的策略，按照中药分子鉴别的基本步骤，即DNA提取技术、扩增反应、检测和真伪判定，通过开发新方法，并结合已有技术，进行有效的选择、优化、整合，形成“积木式”的模块化技术体系，即针对具体检测对象的实际情况，在各个环节上选择最优技术，从而搭建最适技术体系，用于中药快速、现场鉴别。

中药分子鉴别的发展除了依赖于人们对生命活动认识的逐步加深，还取决于先进仪器和技术在该领域的应用。以核酸扩增为例，核酸扩增可分为目标扩增（靶扩增）、探针扩增和信号扩增3种方法。其中目标扩增包括PCR、反转录PCR、巢式PCR、多重PCR、随机引物PCR、实时荧光定量PCR、依赖核酸序列的扩增（NASBA）、环介导等温扩增（LAMP）、转录介导扩增（TMA）、链置换扩增（SDA）等；探针扩增包括连接酶链反应（LCR）和多重链接依赖探针扩增（MLPA）；信号扩增包括滚环扩增（RCA）、分支DNA（bDNA）和杂交捕获扩增（HCR）等。目前在中药分子鉴定中常用的是PCR技术，但NASBA、LAMP、TMA、SDA等核酸等温扩增技术，由于其检测的灵敏度和特异性都得到很大提高，因而在炮制品、中成药等分子鉴定中将发挥更强的作用。随着分子生物学、化学等技术的不断发展，中药分子鉴定将向着快速、简便和高度自动化的方向发展。未来基因测序、基因芯片技术、免疫检测技术、荧光标记技术等检测方法将在中药鉴定领域中得到广泛的发展与应用。

中药分子鉴别是一个应用性很强的领域，尽管考虑的只是药材的“真伪优劣”，容易只关注药用的物种，然而这些物种的准确界定离不开其所在属完全物种取样的分子系统学研究。因此，从中药鉴别的实际出发，基于分子系统学理论，建立尽可能全面涵盖所有物种（包括药用和非药用物种）的系统数据库和药用物种的居群数据库，才能确保鉴定的正确性和可靠性。在此基础上研发满足实际需要的分子鉴定技术，以达到快速、现场、高通量、低成本的中药鉴定目的，将实验室成果进一步转化，服务于中药产业。

［黄璐琦，等．中国中药杂志，2014，39(19)：3663－3666.］

# 基于熔解曲线分析技术的鹿茸药材分子鉴别

鹿茸始载于《神农本草经》，具有壮肾阳、益精血、强筋骨、调冲任、托疮毒的功效，能够提高机体工作能力、减轻疲劳，改善睡眠、饮食及蛋白质代谢障碍，增加肾脏利尿功能。鹿茸正品为鹿科动物梅花鹿 *Cervus nippon* Temminck 或马鹿 *C. elaphus* Linnaeus 的雄鹿未骨化密生茸毛的幼角。作为名贵中药材品种，鹿茸在市场上供不应求且价格昂贵，导致市售饮片常出现各种混伪品，如驯鹿、白唇鹿、水鹿等常见动物的幼角饮片。赵磊等对梅花鹿茸、马鹿茸、花马杂交鹿茸、麋鹿茸及驯鹿茸等5种鹿茸的常规成分、无机元素和氨基酸含量进行了测定，结果表明梅花鹿茸、麋鹿茸与其他3种鹿茸无机元素存在差异。因此，鹿茸真伪鉴别方法的开发对于保证药材品质具有重要的作用。

现代化学分析技术是一种常用的鹿茸品种鉴定和质量评价方法。王树春等建立了中药材鹿茸（花鹿茸）的X衍射Fourier谱分析，张丽等通过应用粉末X射线衍射Fourier指纹图谱鉴定法对3支马鹿茸和1支花鹿茸中药材进行分析鉴定，并获得了马鹿茸的对照X射线衍射Fourier指纹图谱及特征标记峰值。但化学成分积累往往受到多种因素的影响，导致鉴别图谱稳定性不高、背景较复杂。

分子标记技术由于具有微量、快速、特异性强、准确可靠、对样本要求较低等特点，已广泛用于中药鉴定领域。张蓉等利用鹿茸动物线粒体细胞色素C氧化酶亚基Ⅰ（*CO*Ⅰ）基因设计了一对鹿科动物DNA条形码通用引物，通过PCR扩增、序列分析、构建系统进化树等步骤建立了鹿茸饮片DNA条形码鉴别方法，但该方法操作比较复杂、耗时长。王学勇等根据鹿科鹿属种动物Cyt *b* 序列建立鹿茸药材位点特异性PCR鉴别方法，但其主要基于已知真伪品的DNA变异设计鉴别标记、建立鉴别方法，但对于未知伪品仍难以实现有效的鉴别。

高分辨率熔解曲线（high resolution melting，HRM）是结合饱和荧光染料、未标记探针和实时荧光定量PCR的一种新的检测基因突变与基因分型的分子诊断技术。早在20世纪70年代HRM的概念就已经提出并应用于相关的研究实验，后经由Ririe等进一步发展，有高通量、低成本、简单快捷、结果准确、灵敏度和特异性高和真正闭管操作等优点，在疾病诊断、种质资源鉴定等方面广泛应用。本文基于动物DNA条形码 *CO*Ⅰ序列，采用高分辨率熔解曲线分析，建立鹿茸药材正品熔解曲线，并通过比对鹿茸药材DNA扩增熔解曲线的峰形和 $T_m$ 位置来鉴别鹿茸药材真伪。

## 1 材料

LightCycler480型实时荧光定量PCR仪（Roche公司），5810R型低温冷冻离心（Eppendorf公司），ND－100型核酸蛋白分析仪（Gene公司），DDZ－11型电池式电动骨钻（上海医疗器械集团）。

TIANDZ柱式骨骼DNAout购自北京天恩泽公司；LightCycler480 High Resolution Melting Master购自Roche公司；三氯甲烷购自北京化工厂，均为国产分析纯。

鹿茸药材包括马鹿、梅花鹿及其混伪品，共计25个样品，分别购自湖南、重庆、昆明、成都、玉林、亳州、新疆鹿场，样品由金世元教授鉴定，药材标本保存于中国中医科学院中药资源中心，见表1。

表 1 材料来源

| 序号 | 物种 | 药材 | 数量 | 来源 |
|---|---|---|---|---|
| 1 | 梅花鹿 *Cervus nippon* | 鹿茸 | 1 | 新疆鹿场 |
| 2 | 梅花鹿 *C. nippon* | 鹿茸 | 1 | 新疆 |
| 3 | 梅花鹿 *C. nippon* | 鹿茸 | 1 | 蕲春 |
| 4 | 梅花鹿 *C. nippon* | 鹿茸 | 2 | 亳州药材市场 |
| 5 | 梅花鹿 *C. nippon* | 鹿茸片 | 1 | 湖南药材市场 |
| 6 | 梅花鹿 *C. nippon* | 鹿茸片 | 1 | 重庆药材市场 |
| 7 | 马鹿 *C. elaphus* | 鹿茸 | 2 | 新疆鹿场 |
| 8 | 马鹿 *C. elaphus* | 鹿茸 | 3 | 亳州药材市场 |
| 9 | 马鹿 *C. elaphus* | 鹿茸片 | 2 | 昆明药材市场 |
| 10 | 马鹿 *C. elaphus* | 鹿茸片 | 1 | 成都药材市场 |
| 11 | 马鹿 *C. elaphus* | 鹿茸片 | 1 | 玉林药材市场 |
| 12 | 驯鹿 *Rangifer tarandus* | 鹿茸 | 3 | 新疆鹿场 |
| 13 | 驯鹿 *R. tarandus* | 鹿茸 | 2 | 亳州 |
| 14 | 白唇鹿 *Gervus albirostris* | 鹿茸 | 2 | 亳州 |
| 15 | 白唇鹿 *G. albirostris* | 鹿茸 | 2 | 亳州 |

## 2 方法

2.1 DNA 提取 取药材样品，经过 75%乙醇表面消毒后，利用骨钻钻取 20 mg 样品粉末，采用 TIANDZ 柱式骨骼 DNAout 提取鹿茸总 DNA，作为模板用于熔解曲线分析。

2.2 PCR 扩增与熔解曲线分析 分别以不同来源的鹿茸药材 DNA 为模板，调整 DNA 质量浓度为 10～100 mg/L，在 Light Cycler 480 型实时荧光定量 PCR 仪上进行 PCR 扩增及熔解曲线分析。PCR 反应体系 20 μL，包括 2× High Resolution Melting Master Mix 10 μL，$MgCl_2$（25 μmol/L）1.6 μL，引物（10 μmol/L）各 0.4 μL，模板 DNA 1 μL，dd$H_2O$ 6.6 μL。PCR 反应及熔解曲线程序：95 ℃ 预热 10 min；PCR 扩增 95 ℃ 30 s，60 ℃ 30 s，72 ℃ 45 s，45 个循环；熔解曲线分析 95 ℃ 1 min，40 ℃ 1 min，66 ℃ 1 s；40 ℃冷却，10 s。*CO* Ⅰ引物序列为：RonM-tl 5′-TGTAAAAGGAGGGC-CAGTGGMGCMCCMGATATRGCATTCCC-3′；VRL-tl 5′-CAGGAAACAGCTATGACTAGACTTCTGGGTGGCCAAAGAATCA-3′。

2.3 熔解曲线模型的建立 随机选取不同来源的 4 支梅花鹿鹿茸和 7 支马鹿鹿茸，以 *CO* Ⅰ序列为引物，采用高分辨率熔解曲线分析，建立鹿茸药材正品熔解曲线模型，并对其精密度、重复性进行考察。

2.4 PCR 反应体系适用性分析 考察 DNA 模板浓度、引物浓度、$Mg^{2+}$ 浓度对鹿茸药材熔解曲线峰形和 $T_m$ 的影响，从而确定可依据峰形和 $T_m$ 鉴别鹿茸药材真伪品的适合条件。

## 3 结果与分析

3.1 熔解曲线模型的建立 随机选择不同来源的梅花鹿 4 支、马鹿鹿茸 7 支，分别提取其 DNA，并进行熔解曲线分析，结果表明梅花鹿熔解曲线为双峰，其 $T_m$ 分别为（81.96±0.07）、（84.51±0.03）℃；马鹿熔解曲线为双峰，其 $T_m$ 为（82.58±0.13）、（85.95±0.05）℃，见图 1。

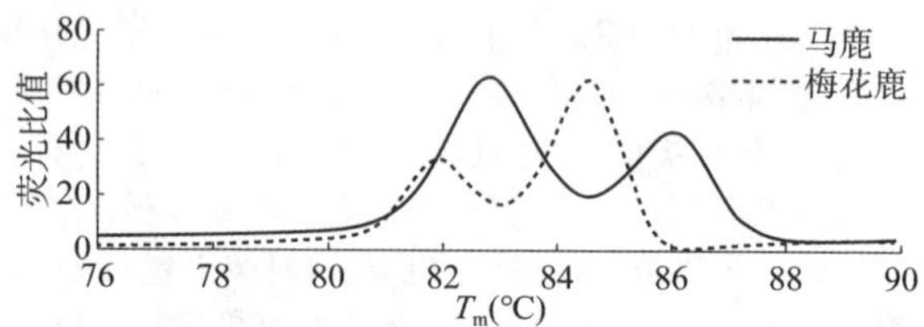


图 1 鹿茸药材熔解曲线模型

对同一支梅花鹿茸 DNA 样品，进行熔解曲线分析，重复 3 次，其熔解曲线峰形一致，$T_m$ 的 RSD 为 0.04%～0.16%、0.01%～0.07%。对同一支马鹿茸 DNA 样品，进行熔解曲线分析，重复 3 次，其熔解曲线峰形也一致，$T_m$ 的 RSD 分别为 0.01%～0.06%、0.01%～0.05%。

3.2 PCR 反应体系适用性分析

3.2.1 DNA 模板浓度 选取质量浓度分别为 785.4、157.3、31.4、6.1 mg/L 梅花鹿模板 DNA 和质量浓度分别为 524.5、104.8、20.5、4.1 mg/L 马鹿模板 DNA，以 *CO* Ⅰ序列作为引物进行扩增，获得熔解曲线，并分析不同浓度模板 DNA 对鹿茸熔解曲线峰形和 $T_m$ 的影响，见图 2。结果表明，模板 DNA 在 10～100 mg/L 均可获得稳定、均一的熔解曲线，可用于鹿茸药材分子鉴别。

3.2.2 引物浓度 参考 LightCycler480 High Resolution Melting Master 说明书，在反应体系中选取引物浓度梯度为 0.1、0.2、0.3、0.4 μmol/L。以 50 mg/L 梅花鹿 DNA 作为模板，获得其熔解曲线，并分析不同引物浓度对鹿茸熔解曲线峰形和 $T_m$ 的影响（图 2）。结果表明，引物为 0.2 μmol/L 时鹿茸模板 DNA 均获得稳定、均一的熔解曲线，可用于鹿茸药材分子鉴别。

3.2.3 $Mg^{2+}$ 浓度 参考 LightCycler480 High Resolution Melting Master 说明书，在反应体系中选取 $Mg^{2+}$ 浓度梯度为 1.5、2.0、2.5、3.0 mmol/L。以 50 mg/L 梅花鹿 DNA 作为模板，获得其熔解曲线，并分析不同 $Mg^{2+}$ 浓度对鹿茸熔解曲线峰形和 $T_m$ 的影响（图 2）。结果表明，$Mg^{2+}$ 浓度为 2.0 mmol/L 时鹿茸模板 DNA 均获得稳定、均一的熔解曲线，可用于鹿茸药材分子鉴别。

3.3 鹿茸真伪品鉴别 从市场上随机选取鹿茸药材 5 支，在模板 DNA 质量浓度为 10～100 mg/L、引物浓度为 0.2 μmol/L，$Mg^{2+}$ 浓度为 2.0 mmol/L 的条件下进行熔解曲线分析，其获得的熔解曲线峰形和 $T_m$ 与正品鹿茸药材熔解曲线模型一致。

随机选取 3 支驯鹿样品和 3 支白唇鹿样品，在上述相同的条件下进行熔解曲线分析，并与正品鹿茸药材熔解曲线模型进行比较，其峰形存在明显差别，见图 3。

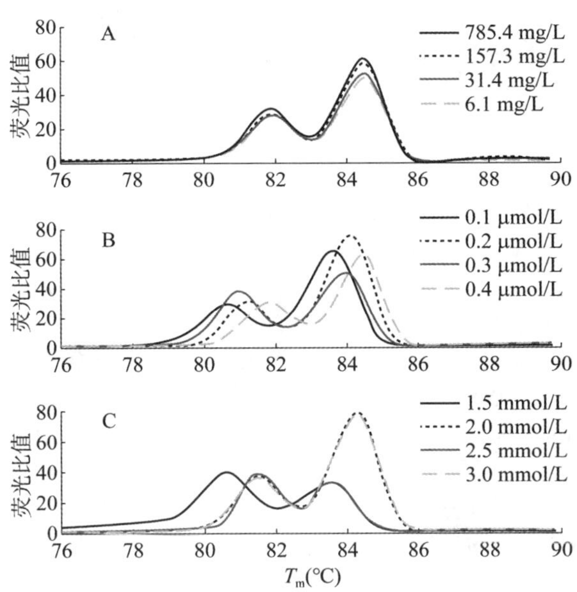


**图 2 熔解曲线模型的优化**

A. DNA 模板浓度;B. 引物浓度;C. $Mg^{2+}$ 离子浓度条件。

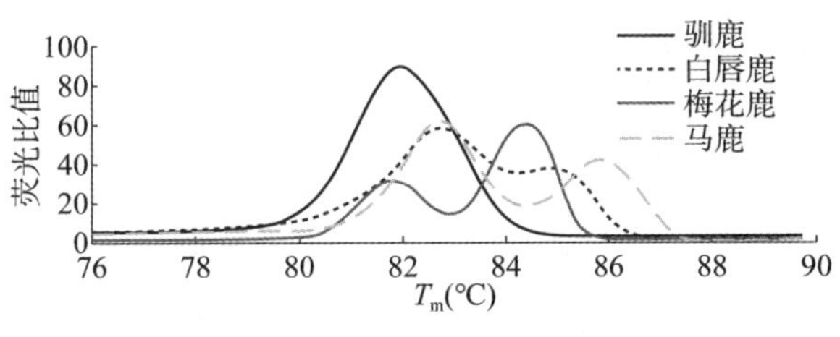


**图 3 鹿茸真伪品鉴别**

驯鹿熔解曲线为单峰,其 $T_m$ 为 82.14±0.07℃;白唇鹿熔解曲线为双峰,两峰未明显分开,其主峰 $T_m$ 为 83.39±0.05℃。

## 4 讨论

4.1 *高分辨熔解曲线技术在鹿茸药材鉴定的实现* 随着分子鉴定技术的不断发展,利用 DNA 熔解曲线技术鉴定中药材的方法不断出现,如蒋超等利用酶切-熔解曲线分析建立了一种新的 SNP 分型方法并在金银花、苍术药材鉴定中应用等。与前期研究者相比,本实验中采用了饱和荧光染料和更加精密的定量 PCR 仪。由于饱和染料与非饱和染料在与 DNA 结合位置上的差异,导致以 SYBR Green 为代表的非饱和染料,存在染料再分布容易造成误差大、特异性弱的问题。与 DNA 结合如要达到饱和,必须高浓度加入,但过高浓度会抑制 PCR 反应。而以 LC Green 为代表的饱和染料,在不抑制 PCR 反应的浓度下即可占据双链 DNA 碱基对。此外,当双链 DNA 局部解链时,游离下来的染料亦不会重新结合到 DNA 分子上去。所以荧光强度的降低可精准地反映出 DNA 分子的解链情况。

本实验首先对不同来源的梅花鹿、马鹿样品建立了鹿茸正品熔解曲线标准模型,然后对样品 DNA 浓度、引物浓度、$Mg^{2+}$ 浓度等影响因素进行条件优化。由图 2 进行分析,样品 DNA 浓度、$Mg^{2+}$ 浓度对熔解曲线峰形和位置影响较小;引物浓度对熔解曲线峰形影响较小,位置影响较大。而优化后,鹿茸模板 DNA 均获得稳定、均一的熔解曲线,具有较高的稳定性和重复性。

本研究建立了基于熔解曲线分析技术鉴别鹿茸药材方法,选择 *CO* Ⅰ 序列作为鉴别引物,在 DNA 模板 10~100 mg/L,引物浓度为 0.2 μmol/L,$Mg^{2+}$ 浓度为 2.0 mmol/L,退火温度为 60℃,45 个循环条件下鹿茸药材 DNA 均可获得稳定、均一的熔解曲线。鹿茸药材熔解曲线模型特征是:梅花鹿熔解曲线为双峰,其 $T_m$ 分别为(81.96±0.07)、(84.51±0.03)℃;马鹿熔解曲线为双峰,其 $T_m$ 分别为(82.58±0.13)、(85.95±0.05)℃。利用该模型,通过比对熔解曲线峰形和 $T_m$,即可在未获得伪品信息的情况下进行鹿茸药材真伪鉴别,对于鹿茸药材的质量控制具有重要意义。

4.2 *高分辨熔解曲线技术在中药分子鉴定中的展望* 核苷酸双链的热稳定性由其碱基组成、长度和 GC 含量决定,序列改变会引起升温过程中双链核苷酸解链行为的改变。结合实时荧光 PCR 技术,通过在线监测核苷酸双链熔解过程中荧光信号积累的变化,可以直观地看到双链熔解曲线随温度变化而变化,从而实现对 PCR 产物差异进行分析,即实时 PCR 熔解曲线分析。在使用高精密度仪器的基础上,配合饱和染料出现了 HRM 分析技术。

本实验是在分子鉴定方面将 DNA 条形码技术(DNA barcoding)与高分辨熔解曲线技术(high resolution melting, HRM)相结合,不仅发挥 DNA 条形码技术在动物药材鉴定方面的优势,而且又发挥了高分辨熔解曲线技术准确、高通量、快速、可视化的特点。与 X 衍射 Fourier 谱分析相比,熔解曲线分析图谱稳定性较强,背景单一;与 DNA 条形码、位点特异性 PCR 等鉴别方法相比,熔解曲线分析无需凝胶电泳、操作简单,整个实验可在 2 h 内完成,而且更加精确。以白唇鹿与马鹿熔解曲线比较为例,两者扩增产物进行序列比对,只存在 10 bp 左右的碱基差异,凝胶电泳无法完全区分,而在熔解曲线图谱上却存在明显差异(图 3)。本实验未对 PCR 程序中循环次数进行筛选、优化,以目前结果推测,PCR 程序中循环次数完全可以从 45 个循环降低到 30 个循环,即可进一步缩短时间。同时 HRM 技术也可以用于药材掺假品快速检测方面的应用。HRM 技术由于较为精准,有比较苛刻的实验条件和操作要求,但无需任何特殊的荧光探针和荧光标记物,成本不高。

HRM 技术给分子鉴定带来了简便的检测方法。随着 HRM 设备和染料的改进,这项技术还会继续迅速发展,可以减少大量的测序工量。由于 HRM 对 PCR 产物没有破坏性,所以在通过 HRM 初筛后的 PCR 产物,还可以再进行测序,这使得其非常适合于中药材真伪品的高通量分子检测。

HRM 技术与 DNA 条形码技术的结合,通过比对药材 DNA 扩增熔解曲线的峰形和 $T_m$ 位置来鉴别药材真伪。该方法具有快速、高通量、低成本等优点,为中药鉴定提供新的技术支持。

[陈康,袁媛,等.中国中药杂志,2015,40(4):619-623.]

# 双分子标记法的构建及在中药研究中的应用

笔者2012年提出了中药"真伪""优劣"二维分子标记法及其策略构想，以期在分子水平同时解决中药"真伪、优劣"评价的2个核心问题。经过近3年的研究实践，发现"优劣"鉴定方面的功能基因研究难度较大，导致该方法研究进展缓慢。而随着代谢标识物研究快速发展，为上述策略构想的实施提供新的方向和支撑。为此本文提出了双分子标记法及其构想，以期促进二维分子标记法构建，从分子水平对中药的真伪优劣进行鉴定及评价研究的进一步发展。

## 1 双分子标记法的构建

1.1 *双分子标记法的提出* 目前，中药鉴定与评价的分子标识主要侧重于单一DNA分子标记对中药不同种属间的鉴别(黄芪、川贝母、洋金花等)及对不同居群间的遗传多样性的分析，或根据单指标化学成分评价同一中药不同来源、不同产地、不同发育阶段的质量差异。但由于中药的原植物生物进化机制复杂，杂交、基因转移、多倍化现象、栽培种质混杂等会导致DNA序列信息在一些物种间没有鉴别力或产生错误的鉴定结论。中药是多成分的复杂体系，通过单一或部分指标性成分来评价其质量优劣，无法体现其整体效应，存在一定局限性。

双分子标记法(bimolecular marking methods，简称BIMM)是基于DNA分子标记和代谢标识物相结合的分析方法，在分子水平同时研究中药的种类、区别和质量差异的一种分子标记方法。DNA分子标记用于中药物种的遗传信息分析，代谢标识物的定性及定量分析完成对中药物质基础的评价。

1.2 *双分子标记法的原理与方法* DNA分子标记是指能反映中药物种个体或种群间基因组中某种差异的特异性DNA片段，主要来源有核糖体基因ITS、18S，叶绿体基因如*mat*K、*rbc*L、*psb*A-*trn*H、*trn*L-*trn*F等，动物中线粒体*CO* Ⅰ基因的DNA序列信息。目前获得DNA分子标记的主要技术方法包括RFLP、AFLP、RAPD、ISSR、SRAP、SSR，基于DNA序列分析的SNP及测序等。

中药的代谢产物是治疗疾病的物质基础，是人类药物的重要来源。代谢产物的研究及其质量优劣关系到用药的有效性、安全性及稳定性。中药植物药中有效成分多为其次生代谢产物，动物药中多为初生代谢产物。中药代谢产物成分复杂，能够评价中药质量的代谢产物是代谢标识物。目前多以单指标代谢标识物评价中药质量，该方法操作性强、相对有效，但也存在不足：个别或部分代谢标识物难以体现其整体效应。随着代谢组学高通量、高灵敏度和高精准度的各种谱学分析技术的发展，这种无选择性的接近全景代谢物的分析使得不同来源、不同产地、不同年限、不同部位等中药的代谢标识物-主要活性化合物或者代谢中间产物的发现成为可能。

根据不同的研究对象，筛选合适的DNA分子标记，通过对其多态性的分析，获取不同研究对象的特征DNA序列。应用LC-MS、GC-MS、Tof-MS和QTof-MS等分析仪器对中药进行全景代谢谱测定，通过应用多种统计分析手段(如主成分分析、聚类分析等)分析来自不同类别的中药的数据，寻找可以有效区分其类别的标识性化合物。综合比较DNA分子标记与代谢标识物分析的关系，建立与药材品质紧密连锁的双分子标记技术平台，双分子标记法结合基因组和代谢组2个方面进行研究，将中药的遗传信息多态性与其表型性状化学成分的定性与定量分析相结合，不仅从DNA序列信息上找出差异，亦结合其代谢物的有无和含量差异，进行中药的鉴定与质量评价，双分子标记法技术流程见图1。

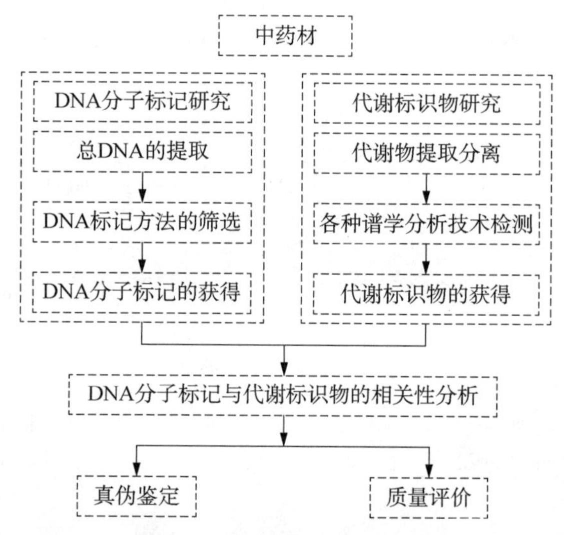


**图1 双分子标记法技术流程**

## 2 双分子标记法在中药研究中的应用

2.1 *多来源药材的鉴别研究* 2010年版《中国药典》中收载140多种多来源的药材，如何科学客观地逐步解决中药材长期存在的同品名多来源问题是中药鉴别研究的重点和难点问题。对于多基原的鉴别研究，本质是解决其生物学的近缘种或相近的分类单位的鉴别问题。如贝母属植物鳞茎多做贝母用，产于浙江的浙贝母长于清肺化痰，产于四川、西藏、云南等地的川贝母长于润肺止咳，其来源复杂，鉴定难度大。

在形态学考察的前提下，可以针对特定的物种选择合适的分子标记开展多来源药材的鉴定研究。双分子标记法中的DNA分子标记能够部分完成从种及种上水平的分类和鉴别，即真伪鉴别。根据药用植物亲缘学理论，亲缘关系相近的物种不仅在形态上相似，其所含的次生代谢产物往往也比较相似。但单一或某几个化学成分往往无法完成对近缘物种的鉴别。通过代谢组学技术进行全景式扫描，可以获得用于近源物种鉴定的特异性代谢标识物或标识物组合。这些代谢标识物的确定不仅是对DNA分子标记的补充，亦避免了由于近缘物种的种质交流、谱系分选不彻底等问题导致的DNA分子标记研究中的阴性或假阳性结果。综上所述，同时运用DNA分子标记及代谢标识物双标记可以有效进行不同基原药材的鉴别研究。

2.2 年限鉴别的研究 中药中根、根茎类、皮类药材，如人参、三七、赤芍、龙胆、延胡索、黄芪、黄芩、黄连、苍术、厚朴、杜仲等多是多年生。其临床疗效的物质基础多为次生代谢产物，这些代谢产物的积累随时间变化呈现出一定的规律性，故药材的疗效和质量与其生长年限有着紧密的联系。

中药不同年限鉴别的本质是解决其生物学不同发育阶段的鉴别问题。目前关于年限的鉴别主要通过宏观层面的传统的器官层次的性状鉴别，如通过芦头形状和芦碗数判断人参年限等。梁加贝等通过端粒酶的长度和端粒酶活性随生长年限的变化规律建立了不同年限人参的鉴别方法。程春松等发现石柱人参及赤芍端粒均随着生长年限延长而变短，为中药年限的DNA分子鉴别研究做出了有益的尝试与探索。中药次生代谢产物的积累随时间变化呈现一定规律性，因此可以通过代谢组学技术对同一药材不同生长年限或发育阶段的代谢物成分进行分析，尝试找出合适的代谢标识物及变化规律。通过双分子标记法可以在DNA分子标记完成真伪鉴别的基础上，通过代谢标识物完成对年限的鉴定。

2.3 产地的鉴别研究 中药次生代谢产物的积累因环境因素不同发生变化。药材的质量因产地不同存在差异。临床用药上，历代医家习用道地药材。道地药材是指在特定自然条件、生态环境的地域所产的药材，因生产较为集中、栽培技术与采收加工有一定讲究，较同种药材其他地区所产者品质佳、疗效好。药名前标有“川”“云”“广”等字样，说明药材的质量与地理分布有着密切的关系。同种异地产出的药材在质量上有明显差异，导致其药效差异很大。

对于中药不同产地的鉴定研究其本质是解决其种下不同居群水平的鉴别问题。不同产地药材的鉴别中，除去传统区域性状鉴别特征外，可以利用分子谱系地理学的理论，运用DNA分子标记寻找用于产地鉴别的分子标记。但不同产地间中药的基因交流较为频繁，存在种质混杂严重现象，在一些物种中，无法寻找出能鉴别出所有产地的DNA分子标记。因此可通过代谢组学技术对不同产地药材进行分析，寻找具有产地特征的代谢标识物并研究其变化规律，结合DNA分子标记的信息与代谢产物的化学信息进行综合分析，从而达成产地鉴定的目的。

2.4 优良种质研究 中药中很大一部分都已引种栽培，但引种多存在盲目性，品种混乱。自留种、各地农家栽培类型构成家种中药的主要品种来源，往往造成中药产量低、质量差现象。在中药的品种改良中不仅需考虑其产量，还需考虑其有效成分的含量高低。目前中药的育种研究工作较为薄弱，仅少数几个中药有品系的系统研究，如人参（大马牙，二马牙）、地黄（北京1号，北京2号，金状元，85－5等）、杭菊花（大洋菊，早小洋菊，红心菊）、柴胡（中柴1号，中柴2号，中柴3号）等。双分子标记法以中药主要次生代谢产物指标性成分的组成和含量为优良种质标准，寻找与药材品质相关的DNA分子标记，筛选构建优质的中药分子标记图谱；通过代谢组学分析技术对其化学成分指标进行分析，分析中药资源的遗传差异与药材品质的相关性。从整体上评价中药不同种质间的化学差异，筛选出一批有效成分含量高的优良种质资源，为中药优良种质的鉴定、筛选及品质改良等提供科学依据和技术支持。

2.5 寻找和开发新的药物资源 近年来，随着回归自然理念的畅行，中医药产业兴起，对中药资源的需求愈发加大。为此应不断探索新药源，提供新药物和新产品。系统进化关系和植物化学成分分类学揭示亲缘关系越亲近的物种，其体内所含的有效化学成分越近似。通过DNA分子标记的研究可以掌握中药类群间亲缘关系，探讨其系统演化关系，完成其分子系统进化关系的研究。从而依据肖培根院士提出的药用植物亲缘学理论，再结合对中药的整体物质组成的化学表征和活性成分的测试，通过统计学的相关性分析代谢标识物的研究，寻找和扩大新药源，为开发新药提供思路。

2.6 为中药的植物新品种权保护提供技术支持 我国自1999年4月加入国际植物新品种保护联盟（UPOV）以后便开始受理国内外植物新品种权申请。随着我国对知识产权保护力度的不断加大和人们对于植物新品种权的日益重视，我国的植物新品种保护名录持续扩大，新品种权申请量逐年递增。然而目前我国对于中药新品种的保护力度较小，表现在列入保护名录的中药种类和申请量均很少。植物新品种权授予时考察的主要技术指标是该申请品种的特异性（distinctness）、一致性（uniformity）和稳定性（stability）（简称DUS测试）。进行DUS测试的基础是植物的性状，主要从形态学上进行考察。然而中药与其他植物相比具有自身特性：一方面，中药的不同品种不仅从形态性状上进行区分，而且更加注重其活性成分有无和含量的高低，仅用DUS测试的形态性状难以全面反映中药新品种的所有特征；另一方面，中药某些代谢产物的种类或含量具有较好的特异性，不仅能成为区别不同来源的中药，而且可以成为区别同一来源不同品种的重要指标。目前DNA分子标记技术已经成功应用于植物新品种保护中DUS测试近似品种辅助筛选和植物真实性鉴定，因此通过对中药双分子标记的研究，能弥补中药DUS测试的不足，作为DUS测试的重要补充，为中药的植物新品种权保护提供技术支持。

## 3 小结

目前，国内外已有开始用DNA分子标记和代谢标识物来研究中药的真伪优劣，如笔者所在研究团队利用DNA分子标记成功对黄芪原植物进行了鉴别研究，以及使用AFLP技术联合GC－TOF－MS的代谢组学研究对黄芪药材的研究等。但尚未系统地提出其相关理论基础和运用方向。本文的撰写就是希望更多的研究者能开展相关工作，使双分子标记法在中药研究中发挥更大作用。

[黄璐琦，等.中国中药杂志，2015，40(2)：165－168.]

# 动物药材分子鉴别现状与策略

动物药材在中医药行业中具有重要地位，《中华人民共和国药典》2010版（以下简称《中国药典》）收载了蕲蛇、乌梢蛇的特异性PCR鉴别方法，成为中外药典收载的第一个中药分子鉴定方法，标示着DNA鉴定手段已从实验室进入了广泛应用阶段。2011年作者曾对动物药材分子鉴定研究的现状及问题进行了总结和分析，并提出扩大研究品种、加快动物药材分子鉴定试剂盒的研制和推广，全面启动动物药材DNA条形码研究计划，建立动物药材分子鉴定标准数据库等研究策略等。在过去的5年里，随着分子生物学技术的发展和分子鉴定理论不断完善，中药分子鉴定原则的提出，中国动物药材DNA条形码的发展与分子鉴定数据库的建立，相继研制推出了蕲蛇、乌梢蛇、冬虫夏草等动物药材分子鉴定试剂盒，表明2011年提出的动物药分子鉴定的策略与目标已初步完成。目前已通过DNA分子标记鉴定的动物药材包括土鳖虫、地龙、蜈蚣、水蛭等虫类；蛤壳、珍珠母等介类；金钱白花蛇、乌梢蛇、蛤蚧等蛇蜥类；龟甲、穿山甲、鹿茸、鹿角、羚羊角、鳖甲等角甲类；阿胶等胶霜类；麝香、蛇胆等囊胆类；桑螵蛸等外分泌物类药材以及海龙、海马等海洋药物（详见表1）。动物药材DNA分子鉴定技术开始呈现多样性，鉴定范围从属、种鉴别扩大到居群、品种与产地，检测材料也从原动物、药材、饮片扩大到中成药，鉴定需求正在逐步从定性检测向定量检测方向发展。

## 1 动物药材分子鉴定关键问题

1.1 *动物分类学基础及分子鉴定标准化* 动物药材的分子鉴定，首先依赖于对其原动物进行准确的分类学鉴定。然而不同种类动物的分类学研究进展存在严重的不平衡，如相对于鸟类、兽类等大型动物，昆虫等无脊椎动物的分类研究进展缓慢，导致其物种的区分、鉴定和命名工作远未完成。加之世界范围传统分类学研究人员的缺乏，且如不具备相关形态学经验，仅依靠检索表难以完成动物的准确分类鉴定，也造成部分动物药材的原动物分类基础薄弱。

另一方面，在获取标准动物药材之后，还需采取标准化手段建立动物药材分子鉴定方法。以动物通用条形码标记*CO* Ⅰ为例，根据国际生命条形码数据标准，每个DNA条形码都要有完整的凭证标本信息、采集信息和测序峰图的原始文件，且应及时上传生命条形码数据系统（BOLD，http://boldsystems.org/）和/或GenBank（http://www.ncbi.nlm.nih.gov/genbank/）数据库。而事实上，早期分类学研究团队发表的数据常不能严格执行以上要求，导致后续以此类研究为基础的动物药材分子鉴定工作，存在假阳性或假阴性可能。

目前在已完成《中国药用动物志》的基础上，中国动物药材DNA条形码研究计划制定了统一的"药用动物DNA条形码试验样品采（收）集规范"，以及实验研究基本路径和实施方案；通过各协作组专家、同仁的齐心努力，已顺利完成了蛇类、蛤蚧类、哈蟆油类、龟甲类、水蛭类、海马类、鱼类、虻虫类、桑螵蛸、斑蝥、鹿茸类、羚羊角类等十二大类正品及其伪混品之分子系统学及*CO* Ⅰ和/或Cyt *b* DNA条形码鉴定研究，以期为动物药材准确、快速鉴定奠定理论与技术基础。

1.2 *种下水平鉴定问题* 与植物药类似，在动物药（如阿胶）中同样存在道地药材鉴别、野生与家养品鉴别等难题。而目前最为通用的动物DNA条形码技术是物种水平鉴定的工具，其分子标记的选择可有效区分同属近缘物种。而针对种下水平（如不同地理居群、品种与产地），随着高通量测序技术普及，可依赖基因组（包括线粒体基因组）、转录组数据，设计开发新的分子标记。且细胞器基因组本身，也有望作为"超级条形码"，解决快速分化的近缘物种鉴定问题。

**表1 部分代表性动物药材DNA分子鉴定汇总**

| 药材品种 | 技术 | 备注 | 内容简述 |
|---|---|---|---|
| 阿胶 | 特异性PCR | 药材 | 基于驴、马、猪、牛的SINE序列差异开发了一对驴特异性PCR引物，仅驴皮胶能产生约80 bp条带 |
| 鳖甲 | 特异性PCR | 原动物 | 比较山瑞鳖、缘板鳖、斑鼋、中华鳖12S序列，设计特异性引物，55℃退火下仅正品有扩出320 bp条带 |
| 鳖甲 | DNA条形码 | 原动物 | 比较了GenBank上中华鳖、山瑞鳖、缘板鳖等的*CO* Ⅰ序列，各物种可形成相对独立的分支 |
| 鳖 | PCR-RFLP | 种系 | 太湖、黄河、台湾、日本品系中华鳖NADH4、COXI和NADH5-NADH6扩增产物酶切图谱均不相同 |
| 龟甲 | 特异性PCR | 药材 | 通过比较龟甲原动物乌龟及其18种混伪品12S序列，设计了一对龟甲特异性PCR引物扩增乌龟及其他18种龟的DNA模板，正品乌龟均可获得180 bp特异性条带，混伪品无条带 |
| 龟甲 | DNA条形码 | 原动物 | 以*CO* Ⅰ为条形码构建系统发育树，龟甲基原动物形成独立一支与其他8种常见伪品相互区分 |

（续表）

| 药材品种 | 技术 | 备注 | 内容简述 |
|---|---|---|---|
| 冬虫夏草 | 定量 PCR | 药材 | 比较正品及古尼虫草等 ITS 序列，设计冬虫夏草特异性反应的实时荧光 PCR 引物和探针，检测限低至 0.1 pg |
| 冬虫夏草 | LAMP | 药材 | 针对冬虫夏草的 CS2 基因设计环介导等温扩增（LAMP）引物组，65 ℃时恒温反应 1 h，可特异性鉴别冬虫夏草及其 6 种常见混伪品，其检测限达 6 pg/mL |
| 冬虫夏草 | PCR－RFLP | 药材 | 利用 ITS 基源的一个 SNP 位点，设计引物并进行 PCR－RFLP 分析，冬虫夏草可被 Sac Ⅱ酶切形成 488 bp 和 128 bp 的两个条带，伪品古尼虫草无法酶切 |
| 冬虫夏草 | SCAR | 药材 | 从随机引物 CAGCGACAAG 转化出一个 SCAR 标记用于鉴别冬虫夏草、古尼虫草、亚香棒虫草和细虫草 |
| 冬虫夏草 | DNA 条形码 | 药材 | 以 ITS 为条形码构建系统发育树，冬虫夏草形成独立支可与其他 12 种伪品相区分，亦可通过 BLAST 鉴定 |
| 冬虫夏草 | 侧流试纸条 | 原动物 | 从 EF－1α 分别设计冬虫夏草、古尼虫草和北虫草带标记的特异性引物，扩增产物经侧流试纸条可肉眼鉴定 |
| 蛇类药材 | DNA 条形码 | 原动物 | 对 3 种药典品种及 20 种常见蛇类 *CO* Ⅰ 产物测序，各物种在系统发育树形成独立的支，可相互鉴定 |
| 蛇类药材 | 快速 PCR | 药材 | 设计蕲蛇、乌梢蛇、金钱白花蛇特异性引物，对 3 种蛇类正品及 18 种伪品进行快速 PCR 扩增，产物加入荧光染料 SYBR Green Ⅰ直接显色，仅正品出现绿色荧光，伪品无荧光 |
| 蛇类药材 | 多重 PCR | 原动物 | 从随机引物 OPF－14 中分别转化出蕲蛇、乌梢蛇、金钱白花蛇的 SCAR 引物，50℃退火进行多重 PCR 分别扩出 459 bp、499 bp 和 254 bp 的条带，伪品滑鼠蛇、眼镜蛇等 6 种蛇类无条带 |
| 乌梢蛇 | DNA 条形码 | 原动物 | 使用 *CO* Ⅰ 为条形码，乌梢蛇与其他滑鼠蛇等 17 种蛇类可相互区分，各物种支持度达 100% |
| 乌梢蛇 | 特异性 PCR | 市售药材 | 设计的特异性引物可鉴别乌梢蛇及市场常见伪品，65 ℃退火下仅正品扩出 320 bp 条带 |
| 蕲蛇 | 特异性 PCR | 市售药材 | 设计基于 Cyt *b* 的特异性引物鉴别蕲蛇与 9 种混伪品，50 ℃退火下仅正品蕲蛇产生约 220 bp 的扩增带 |
| 金钱白花蛇 | 特异性 PCR | 市售药材 | 设计的特异性引物可鉴别金钱白花蛇及市场常见的 20 种伪品，仅正品有 565 bp 条带 |
| 金钱白花蛇 | PCR－RFLP | 原动物 | 利用 *CO* Ⅰ 序列上的 SNP 位点差异鉴别金钱白花蛇及 11 种常见混伪品，金钱白花蛇可被 SpeI 和 BstEII 双酶切 |
| 蛇蜕 | DNA 条形码 | 原动物 | 使用 *CO* Ⅰ 为条形码对 23 种蛇蜕进行扩增构建系统发育树，各物种可按科属相互区分 |
| 蛇胆 | DNA 测序 | 药材 | 提取蛇胆和原动物 DNA，从 12S 上设计引物扩增，产物测序后经 BLAST 比对鉴别蛇胆、鸭胆并发现伪品 |
| 蛤蚧 | 特异性 PCR | 药材 | 从 12S 序列上设计的特异性引物鉴别蛤蚧及 15 种伪品，仅正品 55 ℃退火下扩出 400 bp 条带 |
| 蛤蚧 | DNA 条形码 | 原动物 | 使用 *CO* Ⅰ 来源的 150 bp 微型条形码（Mini-Bar）鉴别蛤蚧及其伪品，种内多态性为 4%，种间为 33.5% |
| 蛤蚧 | RAPD | 产地 | 使用 21 对 RAPD 引物对 6 个不同地域（河池、南宁、桂林、百色、越南、泰国）的蛤蚧进行扩增，与系统发育分析，发现国内蛤蚧聚为一支，再与越南蛤蚧聚为一支，最后与泰国蛤蚧聚为一支，与地理分布一致 |
| 海龙 | RAPD | 药材 | 使用引物 LJ09、LJ192 进行 RAPD 扩增可鉴别拟海龙、刁海龙、尖海龙、粗吻海龙、海蠋鱼、宝珈海龙 |
| 海龙 | DNA 测序 | 原动物 | 结合 12S、16S 和 Cyt *b* 序列对海龙科动物建立系统发育树，尖海龙和刁海龙可形成独立支与其他物种鉴定 |
| 海马 | SSR | 原动物 | 利用 35 对 SSR 引物扩增，依其条带有无形成特征指纹图谱可准确鉴别包括 4 种药用海马在内的 10 种海马 |
| 海马 | PCR－RFLP | 杂交鉴定 | 扩增 S7 基因和 Tmo－4c4 基因片段，分别使用 Ms1I 及 BsrBI 酶切鉴定灰海马、吻海马及其杂交种 |
| 海马 | DNA 条形码 | 原动物 | 使用 Cyt *b* 序列对包含 4 种海马基原动物的 22 个物种进行了系统进化分析，表明线纹海马、三斑海马、刺海马可与其他海马相互区分 |

（续表）

| 药材品种 | 技术 | 备注 | 内容简述 |
|---|---|---|---|
| 海马 | DNA条形码 | 药材 | 使用 *CO* Ⅰ作为条形码对海马属21个物种进行了系统进化分析，表明海马5种基原动物线纹海马、三斑海马、刺海马、小海马可与其他海马相互区分 |
| 鹿茸 | LNA-MCA | 产地 | 对俄罗斯、中国、加拿大、新西兰等4国家的马鹿茸ATPase 8基因进行扩增，使用荧光标记的锁核酸（LNA）作为探针进行熔解曲线分析，发现其熔解曲线类型和位置均不相同，可用于这4个国家的鹿茸产地鉴别 |
| 鹿茸 | HRM | 药材 | 使用高分辨率熔解曲线分析梅花鹿、马鹿、驯鹿的 *CO* Ⅰ扩增产物，熔解曲线峰型位置均不相同 |
| 鹿茸 | RAPD | 药材 | 提取线粒体DNA，使用随机引物GAGCGTCGAA扩增，梅花鹿、马鹿、驯鹿条带位置不同 |
| 鹿茸 | AS-PCR | 原动物 | 鹿茸特异性PCR引物可鉴别梅花鹿、马鹿茸及9种鹿科鹿属其他鹿科动物的茸，仅正品有323 bp条带 |
| 鹿茸 | DNA条形码 | 原动物 | 以 *CO* Ⅰ为条形码，对包括鹿茸正品基源动物梅花鹿、马鹿在内的3种鹿科动物及GenBank上6种混伪品序列构建系统发育树，发现马鹿分为两个独立分支，但各物种可相互区分 |
| 鹿鞭 | PCR-SSCP | 药材 | 从Cyt *b* 序列设计特异性引物扩增鹿鞭及其伪品，产物经由10%变性聚丙烯凝胶电泳进行单链构象多态性（SSCP）分析，梅花鹿、马鹿、驯鹿鞭分别为AA型、AB型和ABC型，牛鞭无扩增 |
| 鹿类药材 | 多重PCR | 药材 | 从16S和D-loop上分别设计特异性引物进行多重PCR，不同鹿产生不同带型：梅花鹿（307 bp）、塔河马鹿（272 bp）、马鹿（230 bp）、加拿大鹿（307和246 bp）、驯鹿（141 bp）；并用于鹿茸、鞭、血等鉴定 |
| 鹿肉 | TaqMan PCR | 原动物 | 从ERF基因序列设计的特异性引物鉴别鹿肉，使用TaqMan荧光定量法，对梅花鹿混伪检测限达0.1% |
| 虎骨 | AS-PCR | 药材 | 从Cyt *b* 序列设计的特异性引物鉴别虎骨，使用荧光定量PCR扩增，混伪检测限达0.5% |
| 水蛭 | 序列分析 | 原动物 | 对水蛭基原物种日本医蛭、宽体金线蛭、尖细金线蛭和相近物种菲牛蛭、光润金线蛭及八目石蛭的 *CO* Ⅰ、12S和16S基因进行测序并构建分子系统树，发现每种水蛭均形成独立分支，可用于6种水蛭的分类鉴别 |
| 貂心 | 特异性PCR | 原动物 | 从Cyt *b* 序列设计的特异性引物鉴别貂心与其伪品鸡、鸭、鹅、兔等的心，仅貂心扩出310 bp条带 |
| 蛤蟆油 | 特异性PCR | 药材 | 从Cyt *b* 序列上设计引物鉴别蛤蟆油基原动物中国林蛙及其8种伪品，仅中国林蛙扩出240 bp特异性条带 |
| 穿山甲 | DNA条形码 | 药材 | 使用 *CO* Ⅰ作为条形可鉴别亚洲穿山甲和非洲穿山甲物种，并可区分马来穿山甲和中华穿山甲药材 |
| 角类药材 | DNA条形码 | 药材 | 以 *CO* Ⅰ为条形码，羚羊角、鹿茸等可与对应伪品山羊角、水牛、原羚或红鹿等10个物种相互区分 |
| 羚羊角 | DNA条形码 | 原动物 | 使用 *CO* Ⅰ为条形码，对羚羊角基原动物赛加羚羊及其混伪品鹅喉羚、普氏原羚、藏羚羊、蒙古瞪羚、藏原羚、山羊及绵羊进行 *CO* Ⅰ片段测序并构建系统发育树，除普氏原羚与蒙古瞪羚外均可相互区分鉴定 |
| 广地龙 | 特异性PCR | 市售药材 | 从12S序列上设计的特异性引物鉴别广地龙及其9种伪品，66℃退火仅正品扩出360 bp条带 |
| 桑螵蛸 | DNA条形码 | 市售药材 | 提取桑螵蛸药材DNA，使用 *CO* Ⅰ构建系统发育树，证实大刀螳螂和巨斧螳螂分别为团螵蛸和黑螵蛸的基原动物，小刀螂和薄翅螳螂为长螵蛸基原动物 |
| 鸡内金 | 特异性PCR | 原动物 | 从Cyt *b* 上设计特异性PCR引物鉴别家鸡、3种伪品内金源动物（鸭、鹅、鸽）和4种其他动物，61℃退火下仅正品扩出约500 bp条带 |
| 蜈蚣 | DNA条形码 | 药材 | 以 *CO* Ⅰ为条形码对正品少棘及伪品多棘等5种蜈蚣构建系统进化树、各物种除少棘和赤蜈蚣外可相互区分 |

（续表）

| 药材品种 | 技术 | 备注 | 内容简述 |
|---|---|---|---|
| 麝香 | DNA条形码 | 原动物 | 比较麝香3种原动物及伪品麝鼠等4种伪品GenBank中*CO* Ⅰ序列，系统发育树各物种形成相对独立的支 |
| 蛤壳 | DNA条形码 | 原动物 | 比较了蛤壳基原动物文蛤、青蛤和8种伪品GenBank中*CO* Ⅰ序列，系统发育树正伪品可相互分开 |
| 珍珠母 | DNA条形码 | 原动物 | 比较蚌科18个物种ITS序列发现褶纹冠蚌为单系群可与其他物种区分，三角帆蚌分支地位不稳定 |
| 羚羊清肺散 | DNA条形码 | 中成药 | 使用引物对LCO1490/HCO2198扩增羚羊角粉、羚羊清肺散等7种中成药，测序后与对照药材建树鉴别 |
| 牙疼一粒丸等 | 二代测序 | 中成药 | 中成药DNA提取，*trn*L内含子和16S rRNA片段扩增，PCR产物使用454焦磷酸测序法进行高通量序列测定，测序结果与NCBI网站Nt/Nr数据库进行比对确定物种归属的办法，对牙痛一粒丸等15种中成药中的原料药材进行了分子鉴定，首次引入了中药成方制剂直接测序分析的方法 |
| 羚羊清肺丸 | 特异性PCR | 中成药 | 从12S，16S，Cyt *b* 和*CO* Ⅰ序列上设计了多对赛加羚羊和山羊特异性引物用于鉴别羚羊清肺丸中的羚羊角 |
| 大黄䗪虫丸 | 克隆测序 | 中成药 | 16S、*CO* Ⅰ-MiniBar引物对大黄䗪虫丸进行扩增，产物克隆测序，经BLASTn比对可鉴别出蛴螬、虻虫等 |
| 蛇类药材 | CCP-FRET | 中成药 | 设计蕲蛇、乌梢蛇、金钱白花蛇特异性引物，对3种蛇类正品及23种伪品进行荧光扩增，加入阳离子聚合物PFP产生荧光共振能量转移，正品发出绿色荧光，伪品为蓝色荧光，并对含蛇类中成药进行了鉴定 |
| 活血止痛胶囊 | 16S测序 | 中成药 | 使用蜚蠊目通用引物扩增活血止痛胶囊16S可获得475 bp片段，测序结果与土鳖虫相一致 |

## 2 动物药材分子鉴定研究现状

目前中药分子鉴定技术，较为公认的方式有3类：①DNA扩增指纹，如AFLP（amplified fragment length polymorphism，扩增长多多态性）、RAPD（randomly amplified polymorphic DNA，随机扩增多态性DNA）、ISSR（inter-simple sequence repeat，简单重复序列间区多态性）以及由之派生出的SCAR（sequence-characterized amplified region，序列特异性扩增区）等。②分子杂交信号，如Southern杂交及DNA芯片技术等。③核酸序列分析，如DNA测序、DNA barcoding技术（DNA条形码技术）、AS-PCR（allele-specific PCR，位点特异性PCR技术）、HRM分析（high resolution melting，高分辨率熔解曲线分析）以及派生出的依据序列差异进行区分的各种新型扩增与检测方法等。这些方法多已应用于动物药材分子鉴定。

2.1 *DNA扩增指纹技术* 系指使用通用引物对基因组进行扩增，通过扩增条带差异进行检测（RAPD、AFLP、DAMD、SSR等）或对扩增条带进行后续处理（RAPD-SCAR等）以鉴定中药的技术，如通过RAPD技术依其条带差异鉴别中药材海龙以及从RAPD中转化出虫草特异性的SCAR鉴别冬虫夏草等。DNA扩增指纹技术只要筛选通用引物即可鉴定，不需要待测物种的基因组信息，能在短时间内筛选大量位点信息，尤其适合于物种及以下分类阶元的鉴定；鉴定过程可无需DNA测序，成本较低。主要缺陷包括引物较短（9～10 bp），DNA聚合酶、扩增体系、反应条件等变化都可能影响实验重复性，最终影响鉴定结果。同时由于扩增指纹是一种随机扩增技术，不区分目标序列与外源污染物，而微生物易滋生的特点致使其在动物药鉴定中应用困难。近年来随着DNA序列的积累和基于特异性序列鉴别技术的发展，DNA扩增指纹技术在动物药鉴定日渐减少，但对种下遗传多样性分析和居群鉴定方面仍有一定优势，亦有选择重现性好的特异性条带进行测序转化为SCAR标记进行动物药鉴定的研究。

2.2 *分子杂交信号技术* 系指将待测单链核酸与已知序列的单链核酸序列通过碱基配对形成可以检测的双螺旋片段，通过靶序列凝胶电泳图谱差异（Southern杂交）或固定在固相基质上不同位置的探针分子杂交信号（DNA芯片杂交）进行鉴定的一种技术，其中DNA芯片杂交因其探针密度大、检测方便等优势广泛用于物种鉴定。如Geoffrey等根据常见肉类16S rRNA序列差异设计特异性探针点制于芯片上，通过PCR扩增含探针序列的16S区域后在芯片上进行杂交，可同时鉴别牛、羊、猪、马等32种肉类，混伪检出限可达1%。DNA杂交技术最大的优势是中到高通量的信息位点集成，能同时检测混合生物样本中的多个组分，利于掺杂检测，结合探针短，可用于部分降解的材料，并且根据不同探针标记类型可鉴定未知遗传背景（如SSH杂交，suppression subtraction hybridization）和已知遗传背景的物种，适合的分类元可从种上到种下（如DArT芯片，diversity arrays technology）；但与基于PCR的方法相比，DNA分子杂交技术耗时长，且较松弛的杂交条件可能产生交叉杂交而导致假阳性，同时探针筛选和条件确定工作量大，由于目标DNA只与特定的探针结合，对于中高通量芯片来说物料消耗大，成本高。目前DNA分子杂交技术在植物药和食品鉴定中研究较多,还未见有动物药DNA分子杂交技术的研究报道。近年来DNA条形码研究积累了大量物种序列信息,针对条形码上序列变异信息设计特异性探针点制芯片,通过样品条形码片段扩增后进行芯片杂交和荧光信号分析从而进行物种鉴定,从而依据科属制作全物种鉴定芯片表现出一定优势。

2.3 核酸序列分析技术 核酸序列是遗传信息的直接载体,能直接反映物种的遗传变异从而实现中药的分子鉴别。随着DNA测序技术的发展,测序通量不断增加同时价格大幅下降,利用DNA测序可以获得大量信息标记,进而开发出简单、特异的分子鉴定方法。目前已有多种基于核酸序列分析的鉴定方法。

2.3.1 DNA测序鉴定 指扩增目的基因后对序列进行测序,通过生物信息学分析判断物种归属的方法。目前DNA测序鉴定中最引人瞩目的方法是DNA条形码技术,该方法通过选择一对通用引物,扩增一段物种间有足够变异、易于扩增、相对较短(~700 bp)的DNA片段,测序后通过特定的生物信息学方法与构建的DNA条形码数据库进行比对从而鉴定物种。与其他的鉴定方法相比,DNA条形码最大的特点是通用性,并且易于实现数据共享构建全球统一的数据库进行鉴定,在动物物种鉴定中尤为成功。《中国药典》2015版收载的中药DNA条形码鉴别指导原则即为本法。

自Paul Hebert等对包括脊椎动物和无脊椎动物11门13 320个物种的线粒体细胞色素C氧化酶亚基1(cytochrome coxdase Ⅰ, *CO* Ⅰ)基因序列比较分析提出DNA条形码概念以来,*CO* Ⅰ作为动物通用DNA条形码已获得公认。我国全面启动动物药DNA条形码计划时间较晚,研究尚处于初级阶段,许多动物药并未测定DNA条形码数据;对药典中45个动物药材的51基原物种的*CO* Ⅰ序列进行了分析,表明除节肢动物门外,其在物种水平和属水平上均能达到准确鉴定。但在部分节肢动物类群中,*CO* Ⅰ序列在容易产生混伪品的同属近缘物种间,分辨率时而不够理想。除*CO* Ⅰ外,Cyt *b*、Nad、12S rRNA与16S rRNA序列也有望作为候选条形码或条形码组合进行动物药鉴定。另一方面,对于遗传关系复杂、分类学基础薄弱的物种,依据DNA条形码序列重建的系统发育关系常与已有分类学认知存在不一致,其所揭示的隐存物种多样性,物种间关系争议,需要谨慎细致的个案分析。

2.3.2 特异性扩增鉴定 系指在正伪品差异序列上设计特异性引物进行扩增,利用引物与正品DNA序列完全匹配可进行扩增产生特定长度条带,伪品因引物与序列不匹配发生阻滞无法产生条带从而进行鉴定的一种方法。依据正伪品序列差异大小与引物位置,基于PCR的方法可分为特异性PCR和位点特异性PCR(AS-PCR, allele-specific PCR)。基于扩增阻滞的原理,改变扩增方法,可实现特异性LAMP(loop-mediated isothermal amplification,环介导等温扩增技术)、特异性HDA(helicase dependent amplification,解旋酶依赖扩增)等其他特异性扩增鉴定方式;改变检测方法,可实现特异性荧光定量PCR鉴定,快速PCR鉴定,荧光共振能量转移(FRET, forster resonance energy transfer)鉴定,微流控芯片鉴定及DNA试纸条鉴定等;改变扩增体系,特异性PCR亦可组合成多重特异性PCR鉴定,如对蛇类药材、鹿类药材的鉴定。

主要的特异性扩增鉴定方法中,特异性PCR利用正伪品间序列变异大的区域或正品特有序列区域设计引物,因DNA序列差异大,正伪品间遗传间断明显,特异性和稳健性均较好,在动物药鉴定中应用广泛,如阿胶、龟甲、蛤蚧、鸡内金等的鉴定,2010年起《中国药典》收载的蕲蛇和乌梢蛇聚合酶链式反应鉴别即为本法;位点特异性PCR则根据单个SNP变异位点,利用Taq DNA聚合酶缺少3′—5′外切酶校正活性,当引物3′端与混伪品错配时造成扩增阻滞无法产生条带从而区分正伪品,已用于冬虫夏草、鹿茸等动物药鉴定。特异性扩增鉴定技术对于任意具有序列差异的物种均可鉴定,高效、快速,操作简便、仪器依赖性低、易于制成试剂盒推广,目前已有蕲蛇、乌梢蛇、龟甲等的鉴定试剂盒面世;该方法的主要缺点是不同中药鉴定引物需单独设计,不利于建立数据库共享,对于一些含有PCR阻抑物的动物药,可能产生假阴性结果,特异性鉴定引物设计时需要大量测序及条件优化工作。

2.3.3 PCR-RFLP鉴定 系指在正伪品差异区域两侧序列设计共有引物进行PCR扩增,对扩增产物使用合适的内切酶进行酶切,根据酶切条带谱图差异鉴别的一种方法。如对冬虫夏草、金钱白花蛇等药材的鉴定,2012年起《中国药典》收载的川贝母的聚合酶链式反应-限制性内切酶酶切图谱多态性鉴别即为本法。该方法具有良好的重现性和准确性,适合于较低阶分类元尤其是多基源的近缘物种的中药鉴定,与基于测序的方法相比操作简单、仪器依赖性低、易于制成试剂盒推广;PCR-RFLP不足之处主要是要求正伪品差异序列/差异SNP位点位于限制性内切酶的识别位点上,并且其序列差异正好导致酶切能力改变,对于一些具有内切酶阻抑物的动物药,导致酶切不完全,PCR-RFLP引物设计时需要考虑酶切前后片段分离度并且扩增序列内不含有额外的限制性内切酶识别位点。

2.3.4 高通量测序技术 高通量测序技术(high throughput sequencing)是测序技术发展的一个里程碑,通过把整个基因组序列片段化后,通过不同手段把DNA片段分散从而使各个片段分离并测序,可以对数百万个DNA分子进行同时测序。目前所说的高通量测序技术主要是指454焦磷酸测序、Illumina及Ion torrent二代测序以及单分子测序技术。高通量测序技术在鉴定上的突出优点是能同时对大量序列进行并行测序,通过生信分析可对基因组、转录组及甲基化组等组学数据进行分析获得大量分子标记,能对未知混合生物样本进行物种解析。如Coghlan ML等对牙痛一粒丸等15种中成药*trn L*内含子和16S rRNA片段的PCR扩增产物进行高通量测序,测序结果进行高通量BLAST比对解析中成药中物种基源,发现标称含有羚羊角的中药存在山羊角序列。

## 3 动物药材分子鉴别研究发展方向

3.1 鉴定标记和DNA提取方法开发多元化 不同动物药材的来源、炮制、存储、市场销售情况千差万别,不能奢求一种方法满足所有的鉴定需求。例如,由于动物药材含有大量营养成分,在存储、运输、加工过程中易滋生细菌、真菌、寄生虫和仓储害虫。虽然进行DNA提取前处理时常须对动物药材表面进行乙醇擦拭和紫外杀菌处理，但药材内部仍可能藏有细菌、真菌和仓储害虫等，难以避免DNA污染。且对于水蛭、虻虫等吸血性动物来说，其体内可能含有其他物种血液，在使用 *CO*Ⅰ、Cyt *b* 等DNA条形码鉴别方法时，会同时扩增药材及其污染物种基因片段，影响鉴别的准确性。因此，选择专属性高的分子标记是保证动物药材鉴定准确的重要发展方向。

另一方面，由于一些动物类药材如胶类、贝壳类、分泌物、皮膜药材，DNA降解严重或含量较低，造成DNA提取困难、PCR扩增难度也很大；骨骼药材DNA提取时因须进行脱钙处理，用时较长。这些困难也阻碍了分子鉴定技术的推广。针对此类样品，摸索固定最适宜的DNA提取条件，开发短片段分子标记是较合理的解决策略。

3.2 加强标准研究和制定 《中国药典》2015版共收载动物药材50种，其中仅31种载有鉴定方法，而冬虫夏草、海龙、海马、蛇蜕、金钱白花蛇、鹿角、蜂蜜等常用动物药项下无任何鉴定方法(表2)。具有鉴定项的动物药则多以显微和薄层鉴定为主，专属性和特异性不强，仅蕲蛇、乌梢蛇鉴别项下收载PCR鉴定方法。除了《中国药典》以外，有关动物药材及饮片分子鉴定标准重点应加强行业标准、团体标准和企业标准的制定工作，推进技术方法广泛应用。

**表2 《中国药典》2015版中收载的动物药鉴定方法**

| 编号 | 药材名 | 鉴定项数 | 检查项 | 含量项 | 编号 | 药材名 | 鉴定项数 | 检查项 | 含量项 |
|---|---|---|---|---|---|---|---|---|---|
| 1 | 九香虫 | 薄层1 | 1 | 0 | 26 | 海龙 | 0 | 0 | 0 |
| 2 | 土鳖虫 | 显微1+薄层1 | 4 | 0 | 27 | 海螵蛸 | 显微1+理化1 | 1 | 1 |
| 3 | 瓦楞子 | 0 | 0 | 0 | 28 | 桑螵蛸 | 显微1 | 3 | 0 |
| 4 | 牛黄 | 性状2+薄层2 | 3 | 2 | 29 | 蛇蜕 | 0 | 1 | 0 |
| 5 | 乌梢蛇 | 性状1+PCR 1 | 0 | 0 | 30 | 猪胆粉 | 薄层1 | 4 | 1 |
| 6 | 水牛角 | 显微1 | 0 | 0 | 31 | 鹿角 | 0 | 0 | 0 |
| 7 | 水蛭 | 薄层1 | 6 | 1 | 32 | 鹿角胶 | 质谱1 | 6 | 1 |
| 8 | 石决明 | 0 | 0 | 1 | 33 | 鹿角霜 | 0 | 1 | 0 |
| 9 | 冬虫夏草 | 0 | 0 | 1 | 34 | 鹿茸 | 理化1+薄层1 | 0 | 0 |
| 10 | 地龙 | 显微1+薄层2 | 6 | 0 | 35 | 羚羊角 | 显微1 | 0 | 0 |
| 11 | 虫白蜡 | 0 | 3 | 0 | 36 | 斑蝥 | 薄层1 | 0 | 1 |
| 12 | 血余炭 | 0 | 1 | 0 | 37 | 蛤壳 | 显微1+薄层1 | 2 | 1 |
| 13 | 全蝎 | 显微1 | 1 | 0 | 38 | 蛤蚧 | 显微1+薄层1 | 0 | 0 |
| 14 | 牡蛎 | 显微1+薄层1 | 2 | 1 | 39 | 蜈蚣 | 0 | 3 | 0 |
| 15 | 体外培育牛黄 | 性状1+理化*3+薄层1 | 2 | 2 | 40 | 蜂房 | 0 | 3 | 0 |
| 16 | 龟甲 | 薄层1 | 0 | 0 | 41 | 蜂胶 | 性状1+薄层1 | 5 | 1 |
| 17 | 龟甲胶 | 理化1+质谱1 | 5 | 1 | 42 | 蜂蜡 | 0 | 0 | 0 |
| 18 | 阿胶 | 质谱1 | 4 | 1 | 43 | 蜂蜜 | 0 | 6 | 1 |
| 19 | 鸡内金 | 0 | 2 | 0 | 44 | 蝉蜕 | 0 | 0 | 0 |
| 20 | 金钱白花蛇 | 0 | 0 | 0 | 45 | 蕲蛇 | PCR 1 | 0 | 0 |
| 21 | 珍珠 | 显微1+理化2 | 2 | 0 | 46 | 僵蚕 | 显微1 | 5 | 0 |
| 22 | 珍珠母 | 显微1+理化2 | 2 | 0 | 47 | 蟾酥 | 性状1+理化2+薄层1 | 3 | 1 |
| 23 | 哈蟆油 | 液相1 | 0 | 0 | 48 | 鳖甲 | 0 | 0 | 0 |
| 24 | 穿山甲 | 显微1+薄层1 | 2 | 0 | 49 | 麝香 | 性状3+显微1+液相1 | 2 | 1 |
| 25 | 海马 | 0 | 3 | 0 | 50 | 水牛角浓缩粉 | 0 | 3 | 1 |

注：* 理化鉴定指通过简单试剂颜色或状态变化检测的方法。

3.3 扩大技术推广范围 目前仅在经济较发达地区科研院所、部分省级药检部门、极少数大型医药企业建有动物药材分子鉴定实验室，大部分机构和医药企业不具备动物药材分子检验能力，严重制约了分子鉴定技术的推广应用。随着动物药材分子鉴定技术改良、PCR鉴定试剂盒的商业化生产，逐步解决基础条件薄弱问题，重点加强科研和检验人员队伍建设，增加检验品种数量，扩大技术培训范围，将有力地促进动物药材分子鉴定技术的应用。

## 4 展望

DNA分子标记作为遗传信息的直接载体，不受外在形态、发育阶段、取样部位和生境差异的影响，在缺乏特征成分的动物药鉴定中体现出明显的优势。DNA序列仅由A、T、C、G四种碱基组成，易于搭建数据库实现数据共享。相对于小分子标记物，DNA标记选取可以应对属、种乃至种下的不同层级，具有特异性高、灵敏度好的特点，且其检测方法可以多向拓展，因而近年来在动物药材鉴定领域得以快速发展。未来动物药材分子鉴定应进一步加强动物分类学基础研究、扩大研究品种，完善基础数据库建设，针对复杂多来源药材和关键技术难点开发更为有效、快速的检测方法（如单碱基延伸及其他信号扩增技术等），促进标准制定或修订和产业化发展。

［黄璐琦，等．中国现代中药，2017，19(1)：1－8.］

# 金银花配方颗粒的位点特异性PCR鉴别研究

中药配方颗粒是由单味中药饮片经水提、浓缩、干燥、制粒而成，在中医临床配方后，供患者冲服使用的粉状或颗粒状产品。配方颗粒具有携带方便、服用简单、易于调制、适合工业化生产的特点，同时实现了中药同批内产品物质基础的均质性要求，解决了中药长期以来质量不均的问题。自2001年7月，国家食品药品监督管理总局制定了《中药配方颗粒管理暂行规定》规定配方颗粒纳入中药饮片管理范畴以来，中药配方颗粒快速发展，经过10余年的试点，中药配方颗粒已超过600多品种，并广泛应用于600多家医院中。

然而，由于中药配方颗粒已完全失去了传统中药饮片的鉴别特征，其鉴别与监管已成为制约配方颗粒产业的瓶颈问题之一。由于生产、控制工艺的不同，中药配方颗粒一直处于“试点”阶段，尚缺乏统一可控的质量标准，在生产、流通、使用环节上技术监管难度较大，导致中药配方颗粒存在出现以伪充真、以次充好现象的风险，影响配方颗粒的临床功效。

作为质量控制的上游环节，配方颗粒的基原鉴定直接决定了其质量与疗效。由于配方颗粒系经提取加工形成的颗粒状制剂，已失去所有形态学辨识特征，无法通过性状和显微检测的方式进行鉴别；而在理化鉴别方面目前配方颗粒一般只通过薄层色谱和高效液相色谱进行鉴别，但使用个别指标成分进行定性分析对于近似种，尤其是同属近缘物种的鉴定具有很大困难；且对一些配方颗粒品种，因尚无专属性指标性成分而难以建立化学鉴定方法。因此，目前急需建立准确性高、稳定性好的方法用于配方颗粒原料物种的鉴定。

DNA分子鉴定是指通过比较药材、饮片的DNA差异来鉴别药材、饮片的方法。分子鉴定具有稳定、准确、特异性好、不受生物发展阶段与储藏加工影响等特点，受到了国内外研究者广泛关注，已建立多种中药材及中药饮片的分子鉴定方法，甚至也有对中成药乃至其汤剂进行分子鉴定的报道。其中蕲蛇、乌梢蛇饮片分子鉴别方法已经作为国家标准率先收录于2010年版《中国药典》中。2016年8月国家药典委员会发布的《中药配方颗粒质量控制与标准制定技术要求（征求意见稿）》也明确提出“对于来源复杂的原料药材，必要时采用DNA分子鉴别技术进行物种真伪鉴别”。

选择合适的分子标记，建立特异性DNA分子鉴定手段，可解决配方颗粒物种基原鉴别的难题，有助于建立统一可控的配方颗粒质量标准，规范其生产、流通、用药过程的监管，为产品追溯及仲裁提供依据。金银花配方颗粒（Jinyinhua formula granule）由金银花药材水提后加工而成，是临床最为常用的配方颗粒之一。本研究以金银花配方颗粒为例，运用位点特异性PCR技术对金银花的基原植物及配方颗粒进行鉴定，分析DNA分子鉴定技术对配方颗粒基原鉴定的适用性，以期为中药配方颗粒质量控制与标准制定研究提供依据，为配方颗粒生产、流通、用药安全提供保障。

## 1 材料

1.1 植物材料 依托第四次全国中药资源普查标本库，收集金银花配方颗粒正品基原植物忍冬 *Lonicera japonica* Thunb.及其同属混伪品短柄忍冬、红腺忍冬、华南忍冬、黄褐毛忍冬、灰毡毛忍冬、金银忍冬、盘叶忍冬、华南忍冬、西南忍冬、细毡毛忍冬、新疆忍冬原植物材料，使用硅胶干燥，凭证标本保存于中国中医科学院中药资源中心，见表1。

**表1 植物材料**

| 序号 | 物种 | 拉丁名 | 标本号 | 产地 |
|---|---|---|---|---|
| 1 | 忍冬 | *Lonicera japonica* | 511129120721034 | 四川乐山沐川 |
| 2 | 忍冬 | *L. japonica* | LJ0410 | 河南郑州新密 |
| 3 | 忍冬 | *L. japonica* | LJ0411 | 河南郑州新密 |
| 4 | 忍冬 | *L. japonica* | LJ0412 | 河南郑州新密 |

（续表）

| 序号 | 物种 | 拉丁名 | 标本号 | 产地 |
| --- | --- | --- | --- | --- |
| 5 | 忍冬 | *L. japonica* | LJ0413 | 河南郑州新密 |
| 6 | 忍冬 | *L. japonica* | LJ0401 | 河南郑州新密 |
| 7 | 忍冬 | *L. japonica* | LJ0402 | 河南郑州新密 |
| 8 | 忍冬 | *L. japonica* | LJ0403 | 河南郑州新密 |
| 9 | 忍冬 | *L. japonica* | LJ0404 | 河南郑州新密 |
| 10 | 忍冬 | *L. japonica* | LJ0405 | 河南郑州新密 |
| 11 | 忍冬 | *L. japonica* | LJ0406 | 河南郑州新密 |
| 12 | 忍冬 | *L. japonica* | LJ0407 | 河南郑州新密 |
| 13 | 忍冬 | *L. japonica* | LJ0408 | 河南郑州新密 |
| 14 | 忍冬 | *L. japonica* | LJ0409 | 河南郑州新密 |
| 15 | 忍冬 | *L. japonica* | SDYT2 | 山东临沂莒南 |
| 16 | 忍冬 | *L. japonica* | SDYT3 | 山东临沂莒南 |
| 17 | 忍冬 | *L. japonica* | SDYT20 | 山东临沂莒南 |
| 18 | 忍冬 | *L. japonica* | SDYT21 | 山东临沂莒南 |
| 19 | 忍冬 | *L. japonica* | YNKM13 | 云南昆明 |
| 20 | 忍冬 | *L. japonica* | YNKM14 | 云南昆明 |
| 21 | 忍冬 | *L. japonica* | YNKM15 | 云南昆明 |
| 22 | 忍冬 | *L. japonica* | YNKM16 | 云南昆明 |
| 23 | 忍冬 | *L. japonica* | 259 | 湖南永州 |
| 24 | 忍冬 | *L. japonica* | 260 | 湖南永州 |
| 25 | 忍冬 | *L. japonica* | 261 | 湖南永州 |
| 26 | 忍冬 | *L. japonica* | 262 | 湖南永州 |
| 27 | 忍冬 | *L. japonica* | 292 | 湖南永州 |
| 28 | 忍冬 | *L. japonica* | ZB4 | 安徽合肥 |
| 29 | 忍冬 | *L. japonica* | WD3 | 湖北十堰武当山 |
| 30 | 忍冬 | *L. japonica* | WD4 | 湖北十堰武当山 |
| 31 | 忍冬 | *L. japonica* | WD5 | 湖北十堰武当山 |
| 32 | 忍冬 | *L. japonica* | BJ1 | 北京房山窦店镇 |
| 33 | 忍冬 | *L. japonica* | BJ2 | 北京房山窦店镇 |
| 34 | 忍冬 | *L. japonica* | BJ3 | 北京房山窦店镇 |
| 35 | 忍冬 | *L. japonica* | BJ4 | 北京房山窦店镇 |
| 36 | 忍冬 | *L. japonica* | 5328220302 | 云南西双版纳勐海 |
| 37 | 忍冬 | *L. japonica* | 4308210089YC | 湖南张家界慈利 |
| 38 | 短柄忍冬 | *L. pampaninii* | LDB090101 | 广西南宁 |
| 39 | 短柄忍冬 | *L. pampaninii* | LDB090102 | 广西南宁 |
| 40 | 红腺忍冬 | *L. hypoglauca* | LSV090103 | 广西南宁 |
| 41 | 红腺忍冬 | *L. hypoglauca* | LS090101 | 广西南宁 |
| 42 | 红腺忍冬 | *L. hypoglauca* | LS090102 | 广西南宁 |

（续表）

| 序号 | 物种 | 拉丁名 | 标本号 | 产地 |
|---|---|---|---|---|
| 43 | 红腺忍冬 | *L. hypoglauca* | LSV090103 | 广西南宁 |
| 44 | 红腺忍冬 | *L. hypoglauca* | LS090101 | 广西南宁 |
| 45 | 红腺忍冬 | *L. hypoglauca* | LS090102 | 广西南宁 |
| 46 | 红腺忍冬 | *L. hypoglauca* | LSP090101 | 广西南宁 |
| 47 | 华南忍冬 | *L. confusa* | YC511529201406150241 | 不详 |
| 48 | 华南忍冬 | *L. confusa* | LTF010401 | 中国科学院植物园 |
| 49 | 华南忍冬 | *L. confusa* | LTF010403 | 中国科学院植物园 |
| 50 | 华南忍冬 | *L. confusa* | LTF010405 | 中国科学院植物园 |
| 51 | 华南忍冬 | *L. confusa* | LTF010402 | 中国科学院植物园 |
| 52 | 华南忍冬 | *L. confusa* | LY090101 | 广西南宁 |
| 53 | 黄褐毛忍冬 | *L. fulvotomentosa* | LF090101 | 中国科学院植物园 |
| 54 | 灰毡毛忍冬 | *L. macrathoides* | 433125D00110812020 | 湖南保靖普戎镇 |
| 55 | 灰毡毛忍冬 | *L. macrathoides* | LM010405 | 中国科学院植物园 |
| 56 | 金银忍冬 | *L. maackii* | DJY20120629001 | 四川成都都江堰 |
| 57 | 金银忍冬 | *L. maackii* | LMA020101 | 天津大学 |
| 58 | 金银忍冬 | *L. maackii* | LMA020102 | 天津大学 |
| 59 | 金银忍冬 | *L. maackii* | LMA020103 | 天津大学 |
| 60 | 金银忍冬 | *L. maackii* | LMA020104 | 天津大学 |
| 61 | 金银忍冬 | *L. maackii* | LMA020105 | 天津大学 |
| 62 | 金银忍冬 | *L. maackii* | LMA020106 | 天津大学 |
| 63 | 金银忍冬 | *L. maackii* | LMA020107 | 天津大学 |
| 64 | 金银忍冬 | *L. maackii* | LMA020108 | 天津大学 |
| 65 | 金银忍冬 | *L. maackii* | LMA020109 | 天津大学 |
| 66 | 金银忍冬 | *L. maackii* | LMA020110 | 天津大学 |
| 67 | 金银忍冬 | *L. maackii* | LMA010401 | 中国科学院植物园 |
| 68 | 金银忍冬 | *L. maackii* | LMA010402 | 中国科学院植物园 |
| 69 | 金银忍冬 | *L. maackii* | LMA010403 | 中国科学院植物园 |
| 70 | 金银忍冬 | *L. maackii* | LMA010404 | 中国科学院植物园 |
| 71 | 盘叶忍冬 | *L. tragophylla* | LX010401 | 中国科学院植物园 |
| 72 | 华南忍冬 | *L. confusa* | 4305211205160010 | 邵阳邵东水东江乡 |
| 73 | 华南忍冬 | *L. confusa* | LHY120610017 | 不详 |
| 74 | 西南忍冬 | *L. bournei* | 5328010489 | 云南西双版纳景洪 |
| 75 | 细毡毛忍冬 | *L. similis* | 511781120604058LY | 四川达州万源丝罗乡 |
| 76 | 细毡毛忍冬 | *L. similis* | LSV090102 | 中国科学院植物园 |
| 77 | 新疆忍冬 | *L. tatarica* | LT0104011 | 中国科学院植物园 |
| 78 | 新疆忍冬 | *L. tatarica* | LT010402 | 中国科学院植物园 |
| 79 | 新疆忍冬 | *L. tatarica* | LT010403 | 中国科学院植物园 |
| 80 | 新疆忍冬 | *L. tatarica* | LT010404 | 中国科学院植物园 |

1.2 配方颗粒 从华润三九医药股份有限公司、北京中医药大学附属东直门医院、中国中医科学院附属西苑医院购买金银花配方颗粒样品，共计 17 批，见表 2。

表 2 金银花配方颗粒样品

| 序号 | 品牌 | 批号 | DNA (mg/L) | $A_{260}$/$A_{280}$ |
|---|---|---|---|---|
| 1 | 华润三九医药 | 1502001W | 76.7 | 1.43 |
| 2 | 华润三九医药 | 1502001S | 58.3 | 1.42 |
| 3 | 华润三九医药 | 1501001W | 49.5 | 1.43 |
| 4 | 北京康仁堂医药 | 2016040249 | 25.8 | 1.51 |
| 5 | 江阴天江药业 | 1511105 | 43.6 | 1.52 |
| 6 | 江阴天江药业 | 1510213 | 33.7 | 1.56 |
| 7 | 江阴天江药业 | 1601072 | 54.9 | 1.61 |
| 8 | 北京康仁堂医药 | 2016042831 | 53.7 | 1.65 |
| 9 | 北京康仁堂医药 | 2016042832 | 37.0 | 1.67 |
| 10 | 北京康仁堂医药 | 2016042833 | 79.3 | 1.58 |
| 11 | 北京康仁堂医药 | 2016042834 | 27.2 | 1.81 |
| 12 | 北京康仁堂医药 | 2016042835 | 35.5 | 1.68 |
| 13 | 北京康仁堂医药 | 2016042836 | 58.8 | 1.66 |
| 14 | 北京康仁堂医药 | 2016042837 | 23.6 | 1.67 |
| 15 | 北京康仁堂医药 | 2016042838 | 19.1 | 1.74 |
| 16 | 北京康仁堂医药 | 2016042839 | 23.4 | 1.75 |
| 17 | 北京康仁堂医药 | 2016042840 | 18.8 | 1.82 |

1.3 仪器 Veriti™ 96 孔梯度 PCR 仪(Applied Biosystems 公司);5810R 型高速冷冻离心机(Eppendorf 公司);DYY-12 型电脑三恒多用电泳仪(北京六一仪器厂);SYNGENE 凝胶成像系统(Gene 公司)。

1.4 试剂 SpeedSTAR HS *Taq* DNA 聚合酶、MightyAmp DNA 聚合酶和 DL2000 DNA Marker 均购自 Takara 公司。

## 2 方法

2.1 DNA 提取

2.1.1 植物 DNA 提取 使用改良 CTAB 法提取金银花及其混伪品基原植物 DNA,使用 200 μL dd $H_2O$ 溶解,-20℃保存。

2.1.2 配方颗粒 DNA 提取 使用改进的硅胶吸附柱法进行提取,取 20 mg 配方颗粒置于 2.0 mL 微量离心管中,加入 1 000 μL 提取缓冲液,充分漩涡混匀至配方颗粒全部溶解,56℃水浴 15 min;取出,冷却至室温,5 000×*g* 离心 5 min;取 750 μL 上清,加入至 G2 硅胶吸附柱,12 000×*g* 离心 1 min;弃穿透液,加入 700 μL 漂洗缓冲液,12 000×*g* 离心 1 min;取出离心柱转移至一新的 2.0 mL 微量离心管中,使用 50 μL 洗脱液洗脱。

2.2 鉴别引物设计 基于金银花基原植物忍冬及其同属混伪品间 SNP 鉴别位点(*trn*L-*trn*F 序列 625G/A),设计金银花配方颗粒特异性鉴别引物 Jinyinhua-1. F/R 和 Jinyinhua-2. F/R。使用 Primer Premier 5.0 设计引物,参数为:引物长 18~25 nt,GC 为 40%~60%,$T_m$ 位于 50~60℃,扩增产物大小为 100~200 bp,引物由生工生物工程(上海)股份有限公司合成,见表 3。

表 3 特异性 PCR 鉴别引物及其反应条件

| 引物 | 序列(5′-3′) | 产物(bp) | PCR 反应程序 |
|---|---|---|---|
| Jinyinhua-1. F | AGTCCCTCTATCCCCAAA | 106 | 95℃ 5 min,45 个循环(95℃ 20 s,63℃ 20 s,72℃ 20 s),72℃ 5 min |
| Jinyinhua-1. R | TGGATGAGAAATATAACGAATTAG | | |
| Jinyinhua-2. F | CCTTTTTTTGTTAGCGGTTAC | 237 | 95℃ 5 min,45 个循环(95℃ 20 s,55℃ 20 s,72℃ 20 s),72℃ 5 min |
| Jinyinhua-2. R | GGTCCTGGAATTTCTTGGAT | | |
| LJ-1. F | GTTGACTGTCCTGTGTTGGT | 468 | 94℃ 5 min,45 个循环(94℃ 30 s,61℃ 30 s,72℃ 45 s),72℃ 7 min |
| LJ-1. R | GGATGAGAAATATAACGAATTTAG | | |

2.3 金银花真伪鉴别方法的建立 取金银花及其混伪品 DNA,使用设计的鉴别引物进行扩增,用于确定位点特异性 PCR 反应条件。25 μL PCR 反应体系包含 2×MightyAmp Buffer Ver. 2 预混液 12.5 μL,MightyAmp DNA Polymerase (1.25 U/μL) 0.6 μL、10 μmol/L 上游及下游引物各 0.25 μL,20%聚乙烯吡咯烷酮-40(PVP-40)溶液 1 μL,10 g/L 牛血清蛋白(BSA)溶液 0.5 μL,DNA 模板 1 μL(约 10 ng)。PCR 反应在 Veriti™ 型 96 孔梯度 PCR 扩增仪上进行。初始反应程序见表 3。取 PCR 反应产物,加入 5 μL 6×Loading buffer (Takara 公司)混匀后于溴化乙锭(EB)染色的 2.0%琼脂糖凝胶电泳检测,SYNGENE 凝胶成像系统观察、成像。根据蒋超等的方法对 PCR 反应条件进行考察,确定可鉴别金银花及其混伪品的位点特异性 PCR 退火温度、循环数和 DNA 浓度范围。

2.4 金银花配方颗粒真伪方法的建立 根据"2.3"项的结果,筛选出特异性鉴别引物 Jinyinhua-1. F/Jinyinhua-1. R,取金银花基原植物、混伪品及配方颗粒 DNA,考察退火温度(57、59、61、63、65℃)、PCR 循环数(35、40、45、50 个循环)、*Taq* 种类(SpeedSTAR HS *Taq* DNA 聚合酶、Mighty-Amp DNA Polymerase)、不同 *Taq* 酶量(0.25、0.75、1.25 U)对 PCR 鉴别结果稳定性的影响。筛选出最适鉴别条件,对金银花配方颗粒进行位点特异性 PCR 鉴别。

2.5 序列测定及分析 金银花配方颗粒特异性 PCR 扩增阳性产物,使用 Sanger 法进行测序,由北京睿博兴科科技有限公司完成。对获得的序列,使用 BLASTn 程序在 NCBI

核酸数据库中进行比对，以判断鉴别结果的准确性。

2.6 检出限 调整金银花、混伪品及配方颗粒的总DNA至50 mg/L，并进行逐级稀释依次获得浓度分别为50、10、2、0.4 mg/L的DNA。以所稀释的DNA为模板进行位点特异性PCR，以扩出条带的最低浓度确定检测限。

## 3 结果与分析

3.1 金银花位点特异性PCR鉴别结果 凝胶电泳结果表明，所有样品仅金银花特异性鉴别引物Jinyinhua－1. F/R在退火温度>53℃扩出条带，当退火温度为59、61、63℃时仅金银花出现特异性鉴别条带，混伪品无条带。大于30个循环时，金银花样品均出现明显条带，30～45个循环时，金银花出现特异性鉴别条带。DNA浓度在0.5～100 mg/L时均可获得扩增。因此，本文最终确定的金银花特异性PCR的反应参数为95℃预变性5 min后，(95℃ 20 s，63℃ 20 s，72℃ 20 s)共40个循环，并使用该条件对金银花及其同属混伪品进行扩增，结果金银花均出现条带，混伪品无条带，见图1。

3.2 金银花配方颗粒的位点特异性PCR鉴别 根据"3.1"项获得的金银花位点特异性PCR鉴别体系，对金银花配方颗粒PCR鉴别反应参数进行筛选和优化，见表4。使用优化后的PCR反应条件对不同来源金银花配方颗粒或基原植物进行扩增，均可获得约100 bp的特异性条带，配方颗粒扩增条带亮度较基原植物条带弱；配方颗粒特异性PCR产物测序峰图与基原植物峰图一致，且与金银花*trn*L－*trn*F序列完全相同，见图2。

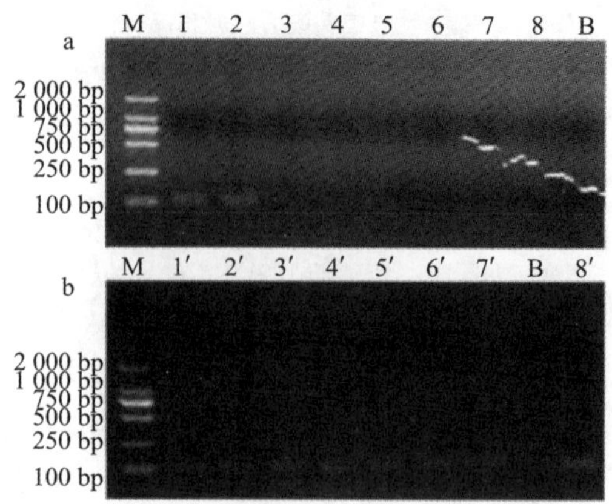


**图1 金银花位点特异性PCR鉴别**

a. 金银花及其混伪品鉴别结果；b. 不同产地金银花鉴别结果；1. 金银花(山东)；2. 金银花(河南)；3. 短柄忍冬；4. 红腺忍冬；5. 灰毡毛忍冬；6. 华南忍冬；7. 金银忍冬；8. 黄褐毛忍冬；1′. 河南；2′. 山东；3′. 云南；4′. 湖南；5′. 湖北；6′. 四川；7′. 北京；8′. 安徽；M. DL 2000 marker；B. 空白对照(dd $H_2O$)。

**表4 金银花配方颗粒位点特异性PCR鉴别条件优化**

| 实验因素 | 适宜条件 | 最佳条件 |
|---|---|---|
| 退火温度(℃) | 61～65 | 63 |
| *Taq* 酶 | MightyAmp DNA Polymerase | MightyAmp DNA Polymerase |
| PCR循环数 | 40～45 | 45 |
| DNA聚合酶浓度(U) | 0.75～1.25 | 0.75 |

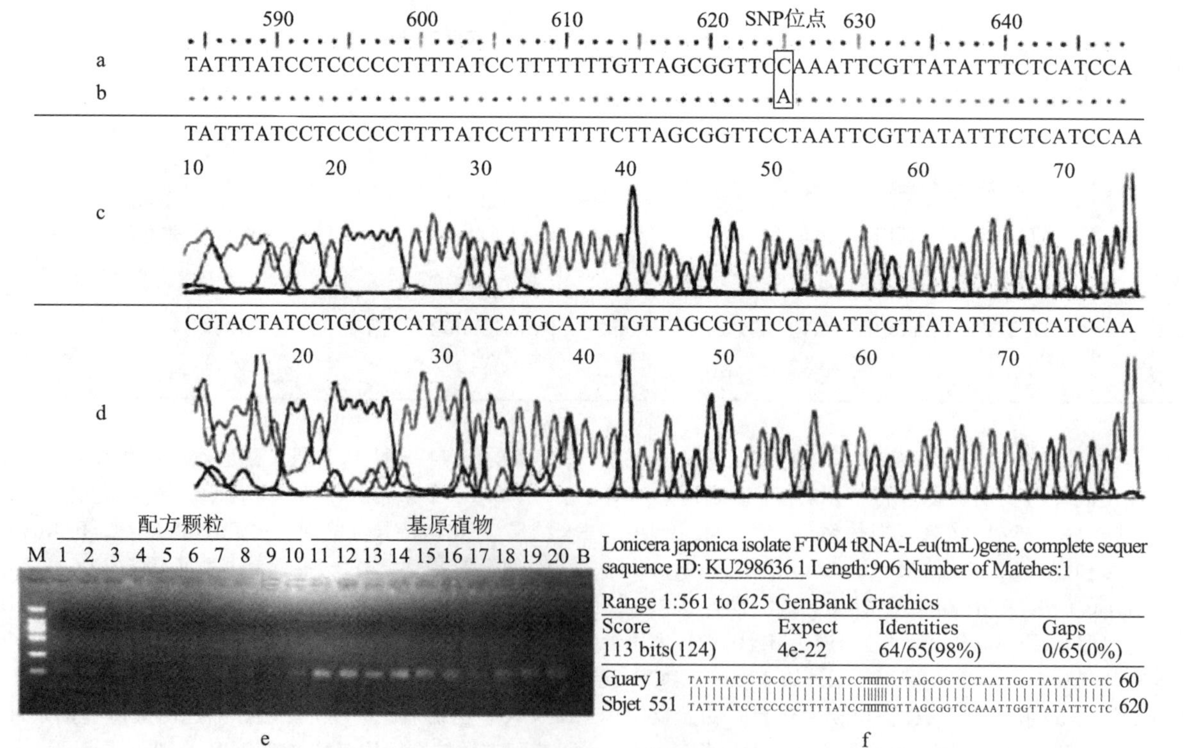


**图2 金银花配方颗粒鉴别**

a. 金银花序列；b. 混伪品序列；c. 金银花配方颗粒测序峰图；d. 金银花基原植物测序峰图；e. 金银花配方颗粒位点特异性PCR；f. 金银花配方颗粒BLAST比对；M. DL 2000 DNA marker。1～10. 不同厂家金银花配方颗粒：1～2. 华润三九；3～4. 江阴天江；5～10. 康仁堂。11～20. 不同产地金银花基原植物：11～12. 河南；13～14. 山东；15～16. 云南；17～18. 湖南；19～20. 湖北。B. 空白对照(dd $H_2O$)。

BLAST 结果表明，配方颗粒特异性扩增产物序列与 GenBank 数据库中相似性最高的是金银花 *trn*L－*trn*F (KU298636.1)，一致性为 98%，仅有 1 个 T/A 变异，经核对引物序列表明，该 SNP 位点位于引物倒数第二位，是为了增加特异性而人为引入的错配。

3.3 检出限 使用优化后的 PCR 反应条件，对不同浓度的金银花配方颗粒 DNA 模板进行位点特异性 PCR 扩增。DNA 模板浓度在 50～10 mg/L 时，金银花配方颗粒均能扩增出约 110 bp 的特异性鉴别条带；降低至 2 mg/L 后，部分厂商配方颗粒无法扩增，见图 3。

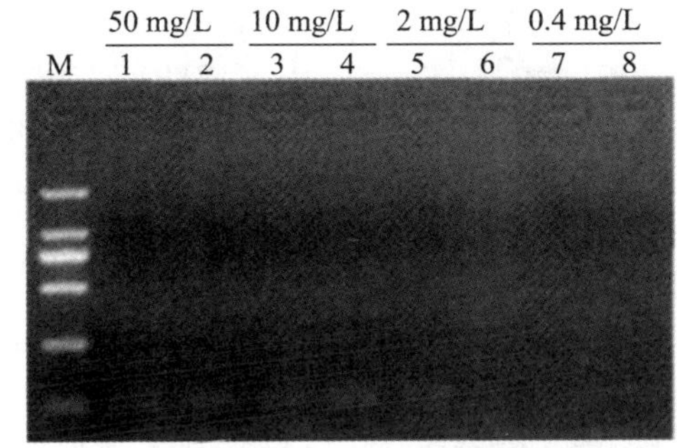


**图 3 金银花配方颗粒位点特异性 PCR 鉴别的检出测试**

M. DL 2000 marker；1、3、5、7. 厂商 1；2、4、6、8. 厂商 2。

## 4 讨论与展望

中药配方颗粒是一种经水煮沸提取 1 h 以上并加入辅料制成的颗粒状饮片，已完全失去了原药材的性状与显微鉴别特征，难以用传统鉴定方法对其真实性进行有效鉴定，无法满足《中药配方颗粒质量控制与标准定技术要求（征求意见稿）》提出的“对栽培、养殖或野生采集的药用动植物，应准确鉴定其种，不同种的中药材不可相互混用”的要求。本研究运用位点特异性 PCR 技术，对金银花配方颗粒及其基原植物进行鉴别。经过优化 DNA 提取方法后，药材与配方颗粒均成功提取到 DNA，采用凝胶电泳或测序比对均能成功鉴定到物种。动植物 DNA 经长时间煮沸提取后会发生严重降解，DNA 降解程度类似古 DNA 样品，难以存留超过 200 bp 的 DNA 片段。本研究使用了 3 对不同扩增长度的鉴别引物进行 PCR 反应，仅 Jinyinhua－1. F/R 引物在金银花配方颗粒中获得扩增产物，长度约 100 bp，其结果与崔占虎等在水提液中获得的片段长度类似。

本研究结果证明，即使在长时间煮沸提取的中药配方颗粒中，也有短片段 DNA 存留，可以使用特异性 PCR 的方式对其物种基原进行鉴定。由于不同中药品种具有不同性质，其配方颗粒加热提取时间、加水用量、辅料用量、干燥方法均有不同，应根据配方颗粒的性质和制备工艺，考察并选择合适的 DNA 提取方法，寻找高稳定性 DNA 片段，遵循中药分子鉴定使用原则，使用短片段扩增与鉴定的方式建立配方颗粒 DNA 分子鉴别方法，并测试方法对原料药的适用性，从而建立覆盖原料、中间体、成品的配方颗粒真实性鉴别及溯源体系。由于配方颗粒 DNA 片段短，辅料干扰性大，基于 SNP 或短序列扩增的特异性鉴别技术，如位点特异性 PCR、快速 PCR、实时荧光定量 PCR、环介导等温核酸扩增技术及高分辨率熔解曲线鉴别技术等在中药配方颗粒产业的原料收购、加工及市场流通、产品追溯与仲裁等方面将起到更好的控制和监管的作用，发挥更大的经济效益和社会效益。

［蒋超，袁媛. 中国中药杂志，2017，42(13)：2484－2490.］

# 基于 *COI* 与 *SRY* 序列建立梅花鹿、马鹿及其杂交鹿茸的分子鉴别方法

鹿茸是我国传统名药之一，始载于《神农本草经》，具有促进生长发育、强壮身体、抗炎、免疫调节、抗衰老、促进创伤愈合等功能。《中国药典》规定鹿茸基原为鹿科动物梅花鹿 *Cervus nippon* Temminck 或马鹿 *C. elaphus* Linnaeus 的雄鹿未骨化密生茸毛的幼角。作为名贵中药材品种，鹿茸在市场上供不应求且价格昂贵。

杂交有利于提高畜牧产量，我国的茸鹿种间和亚种间的杂种优势利用一直处于国际领先水平。早在 1958 年吉林省吉林市龙潭山鹿场即用本交的方法开展家养马鹿(♀)与梅花鹿(♂)杂交（简称马・花杂交）试验研究，随后茸鹿的杂交育种技术得到推广与应用。其中，马・花杂交被认为经济性状最佳杂交组合之一。导致中药市场中除了出现驯鹿、白唇鹿、水鹿等常见动物的茸片等混伪品，还常出现马・花杂交鹿茸或花・马杂交鹿茸。而这些鹿茸品质特征并不一致，如赵磊等对梅花鹿茸、马鹿茸、花马杂交鹿茸等 5 种鹿茸的常规成分、无机元素和氨基酸含量进行了测定，结果表明梅花鹿茸与花马杂交鹿茸无机元素等营养成分存在差异。另一方面，也缺乏准确可靠的杂交鹿茸鉴别方法，依据外部形态、显微特征、理化性状的传统鉴定方法对马鹿与梅花鹿的杂交鹿茸鉴定存在很大困难。因此，对鹿茸药材进行正本清源，特别是对杂交鹿茸的鉴别，对保障药材质量具有重要的意义。

分子标记方法具有灵敏性高、准确性好、客观性较强等优势，目前在鹿茸等贵重药材及其原动物的分子鉴定方面有不少文献报道，比如基于 *CO* Ⅰ 或 Cyt *b* 片段的鹿茸类药材分子鉴定的相关文献报道。而以 *CO* Ⅰ 基因是线粒体 DNA，属于细胞质遗传，只能作为鉴别其母本的证据，因此，为了建立对

杂交鹿的分子鉴别，还需要Y染色体的上基因作为父本的鉴别标记，其中，Y染色体上的 *SRY* 基因作为哺乳动物的性别决定基因，在不同物种间 *SRY* 基因的位置、大小、结构等均不相同。因此，*SRY* 基因在分子进化领域得到了广泛应用。本实验拟利用 *CO* Ⅰ和 *SRY* 基因建立梅花鹿、马鹿及其杂交鹿的鹿茸样本的分子鉴别方法。

## 1　材料

1.1　仪器　微量分光光度计(Nanodrop 2000，Thermo Scientific公司)；Veriti PCR仪(Applied Biosystems)，5810R型低温冷冻离心(Eppendorf公司)，ND－100型核酸蛋白分析仪(Gene公司)，DDZ－11型电池式电动骨钻(上海医疗器械集团)。

1.2　试剂及样品　TIANDZ柱式骨髓DNAout购自北京天恩泽公司；DL 2000 plus DNA Marker购自Takara公司；多重PCR 5×Master Mix购自NEB公司，Fast*Taq* DNA聚合酶购自TransGen公司。三氯甲烷购自北京化工厂，均为国产分析纯。鹿茸药材包括马鹿、梅花鹿及其混伪品，共计48个样品，分别购自新疆、吉林、安徽、湖南、重庆、广西、云南、北京、广州等地，样品由金艳鉴定，药材标本保存于中国中医科学院中药资源中心，见表1。

表1　材料信息

| 序号 | 材料 | 名称 | 杂交鉴定情况(拉丁名) | 来源 | 数量 |
|---|---|---|---|---|---|
| 1 | 鹿角 | 梅花鹿 | *Cervus nippon* | 新疆乌鲁木齐 | 4 |
| 2 | 鹿角 | 杂交鹿 | 马・花杂交 | 新疆乌鲁木齐 | 2 |
| 3 | 鹿角 | 马鹿 | *C. elaphus* | 新疆乌鲁木齐 | 3 |
| 4 | 鹿角 | 杂交鹿 | 马・花杂交 | 吉林双阳 | 3 |
| 5 | 鹿角 | 梅花鹿 | *C. nippon* | 吉林双阳 | 4 |
| 6 | 鹿角 | 马鹿 | *C. elaphus* | 吉林双阳 | 4 |
| 7 | 鹿茸 | 驯鹿 | *Rangifer tarandus* | 北京 | 2 |
| 8 | 鹿茸 | 水鹿 | *Rusa unicolor* | 北京 | 2 |
| 9 | 鹿茸饮片 | 梅花鹿 | 待检药材 | 安徽亳州 | 3 |
| 10 | 鹿茸饮片 | 马鹿 | 待检药材 | 安徽亳州 | 5 |
| 11 | 鹿茸饮片 | 梅花鹿 | 待检药材 | 北京 | 3 |
| 12 | 鹿茸饮片 | 马鹿 | 待检药材 | 北京 | 5 |
| 13 | 鹿茸饮片 | 梅花鹿 | 待检药材 | 广东广州 | 1 |
| 14 | 鹿茸饮片 | 马鹿 | 待检药材 | 湖南长沙 | 1 |
| 15 | 鹿茸饮片 | 马鹿 | 待检药材 | 广西玉林 | 1 |
| 16 | 鹿茸 | 梅花鹿 | 待检药材 | 新疆乌鲁木齐 | 1 |
| 17 | 鹿茸饮片 | 马鹿 | 待检药材 | 新疆乌鲁木齐 | 1 |
| 18 | 鹿茸饮片 | 马鹿 | 待检药材 | 重庆 | 1 |
| 19 | 鹿茸饮片 | 马鹿 | 待检药材 | 辽宁沈阳 | 1 |
| 20 | 鹿茸饮片 | 马鹿 | 待检药材 | 云南昆明 | 1 |

## 2　方法

2.1　基因组DNA的提取和纯化　取药材样品，经过75%乙醇表面消毒后，利用骨钻钻取20 mg样品粉末，饮片则直接粉碎，采用TIANDZ柱式骨髓DNAout提取鹿茸总DNA，作为模板用于鹿茸DNA鉴别研究。

2.2　通用引物扩增 *CO* Ⅰ与 *SRY* 基因序列　应用通用引物 *CO－F* 与 *CO－R* 扩增 *CO* Ⅰ基因序列。PCR反应程序为：95℃ 5 min；95℃ 30 s，45℃ 1.5 min，72℃ 1.5 min，5个循环；95℃ 1 min，50℃ 1.5 min，72℃ 1 min，35个循环；72℃ 7 min。获得PCR产物通过1.2%琼脂糖凝胶电泳，并用EB染色观察，由生工(上海)有限公司测序。

应用通用引物 *SR－F* 与 *SR－R* 扩增 *SRY* 基因序列，PCR反应程序为：95℃预变性23 min；95℃变性30 s，58℃退火30 s，72℃延伸2 min，35个循环；72℃延伸7 min。获得PCR产物通过1.2%琼脂糖凝胶电泳，并用EB染色观察，由生工(上海)有限公司测序。

2.3　鉴别标记获得与引物设计　根据测序所获得的受试样品的 *CO* Ⅰ，*SRY* 基因序列，并从NCBI数据库中下载梅花鹿、马鹿、驯鹿、水鹿等物种的 *CO* Ⅰ、*SRY* 基因序列，利用ClustulX 2.1软件进行同源对齐，校对后分析其特异性SNP位点，并从特异性SNP位点中筛选合适的鉴别位点，使用Primer Premier 5.0设计出梅花鹿、马鹿的特异性鉴别引物。以梅花鹿 *CO* Ⅰ序列JF700150.1为参照，选择 *CO* Ⅰ序列第391位的梅花鹿特异性SNP位点C作为鉴别位点，设计特异识别梅花鹿的引物 *CCnF*；而以第106位的马鹿特异性SNP位点C作为鉴别位点，设计特异识别马鹿的引物 *CCeF*；并设计共同的反向引物 *CCR*。梅花鹿 *SRY* 序列AB915321.1为参照，选择 *SRY* 序列第69位的梅花鹿特异性SNP位点C作为鉴别位点，设计特异识别梅花鹿的引物 *SCnF*；而以第446位的马鹿特异性SNP位点G作为鉴别位点，设计特异识别马鹿的引物 *SCeF*；并设计共同的反向引物 *SCR*。设计的特异性鉴别引物序列见表2，由生工(上海)有限公司合成。

表2　所用引物

| 名称 | 序列(5′—3′) |
|---|---|
| *SR－F* | AGCTTAGCAGTTACTTCCCATGC |
| *SR－R* | CGGCTGGACTGTAAACATCG |
| *CO－F* | GGTCAACAAATCATAAAGATATTGG |
| *CO－R* | TAAACTTTCAGGGTGACCAAAAAATCA |
| *CCeF* | TACTCTGCTTGGAGACCAC |
| *CCnF* | GCTTCAGTAGACCTGTCC |
| *CCR* | TTGTATTTAGGTTTCGGTCTGTT |
| *SCnF* | GGACTCCATGTGAATGTAATCTTTCAGAAC |
| *SCeF* | GCATTGCTTAAATCATGTTTTATTTTAAG |
| *SCR* | TAACAGATGATCAAAAACTAAACAAAACTAAA |

2.4　双位点特异PCR扩增及电泳　分别基于 *CO* Ⅰ与

*SRY* 基因序列，利用梅花鹿及马鹿的特异鉴别引物与通用反向引物分别构建1个双位点特异PCR体系：总体积20 μL，其中包括 *Taq* DNA聚合酶1 U，5×Master Mix 4 μL，2 μmol/L特异鉴别引物各1 μL，2 μmol/L共同反向引物2 μL，灭菌蒸馏水补足20 μL。通过设置退火温度梯度(52、54、56、58、60 ℃)考察不同退火温度对双位点特异PCR扩增稳定性的影响。利用所构建的双位点特异PCR体系，选择最合适退火温度对候选样品进行双位点特异PCR扩增检测，循环数设置35个循环。待PCR扩增反应结束后，向反应体系加6 μL 6×Loading buffer，混匀，取混合产物8 μL点样于1.5%的琼脂糖凝胶上，于200 V电压的条件下电泳8～10 min，经EB显色，最后于凝胶成像仪观察记录结果。

## 3 结果分析

3.1 引物设计 根据测序结果及从NCBI数据库中下载梅花鹿、马鹿、驯鹿、水鹿等物种的 *CO* Ⅰ、*SRY* 基因序列，分析梅花鹿、马鹿的特异性SNP位点，并从特异性SNP位点中筛选合适的鉴别位点。以梅花鹿 *CO* Ⅰ序列JF700150.1为参照，选择 *CO* Ⅰ序列第391位的梅花鹿特异性SNP位点C作为鉴别位点。为提高鉴别能力，把第389位点的碱基由A替换为T，设计特异识别梅花鹿的引物 *CCnF*；而以第106位的马鹿特异性SNP位点C作为鉴别位点，并把第104位点的碱基由G替换为C，设计特异识别马鹿的引物 *CCeF*；并设计共同的反向引物 *CCR*，则可通过PCR扩增获得232 bp的梅花鹿特异片段，而产生518 bp的马鹿特异片段。以梅花鹿 *SRY* 序列AB915321.1为参照，选择 *SRY* 序列第69位的梅花鹿特异性SNP位点C作为鉴别位点，而把第67位点的碱基由T替换为A，设计特异识别梅花鹿的引物 *SCnF*；而以第446位的马鹿特异性SNP位点G作为鉴别位点，而把第444位点的碱基由T替换为A，设计特异识别马鹿的引物 *SCeF*；并设计共同的反向引物 *SCR*。通过PCR扩增可获得803 bp的梅花鹿特异片段，产生425 bp的马鹿特异片段，见图1和表2。

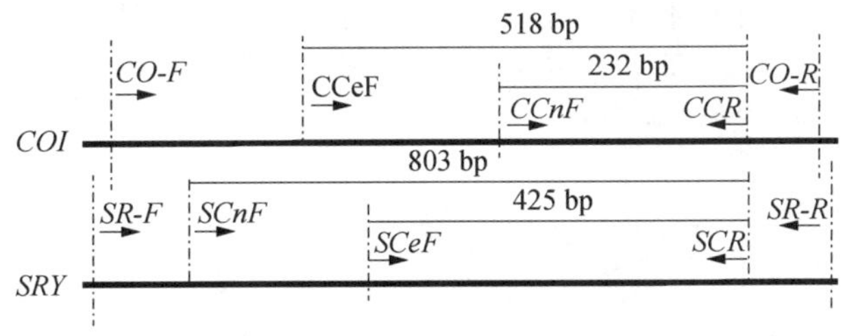


**图1 梅花鹿与马鹿鉴别引物设计**

3.2 建立双位点特异PCR鉴别受试梅花鹿、马鹿与其杂交鹿样品 基于基因序列，利用梅花鹿特异鉴别引物 *CCnF* 及马鹿特异鉴别引物 *CCeF* 与通用反向引物 *CCR* 构建1个双位点特异PCR体系。另外，基于 *SRY* 基因序列，利用梅花鹿特异鉴别引物 *SCnF* 及马鹿特异鉴别引物 *SCeF* 与通用反向引物 *SCR* 构建另一个双位点特异PCR体系。通过退火温度梯度实验，分析退火温度对PCR反应效率的影响；结果显示，这2个反应体系在退火温度52～60 ℃条件下均能扩增出梅花鹿与马鹿相应的特异鉴别条带。

选择退火温度56 ℃，使用以上建立的反应体系，分别对不同来源的梅花鹿、马鹿与其杂交鹿的鹿角样品进行鉴别，受试8个梅花鹿鹿角样品，7个马鹿鹿角样品及5个马·花杂交的鹿角样品分别检测到相应的阳性特异性条带，而驯鹿与水鹿等阴性样品则扩增不到条带。表明该体系具有特异性，可以直接鉴别梅花鹿、马鹿与其杂交鹿的鹿茸样，见图2。

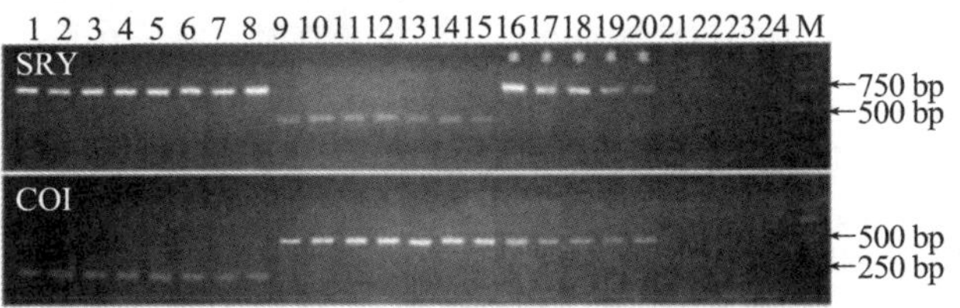


**图2 特异性PCR鉴别梅花鹿、马鹿及其杂交鹿样品凝胶电泳**

1～8. 梅花鹿样品；9～15. 马鹿样品；16～20. 杂交鹿；21～22. 驯鹿；23～24. 水鹿；M. marker。

3.3 对市场流通的待测鹿茸样品进行鉴别分析 利用以上建立的双位点特异PCR体系，对重流通市场中收集的8批待测的梅花鹿鹿茸样品、16批待测的马鹿鹿茸样品进行鉴别，结果显示受试8个待测的梅花鹿鹿茸样品的 *CO* Ⅰ、*SRY* 基因序列均属于梅花鹿，表明其父母本均为梅花鹿。而16个待测的马鹿鹿茸样品的 *CO* Ⅰ基因序列均属于马鹿，而其中有3个样品的 *SRY* 基因序列并不属于马鹿，而属于梅花鹿，表明其父本为梅花鹿，即为马·花杂交的鹿茸样品(见星号标注)，见图3。

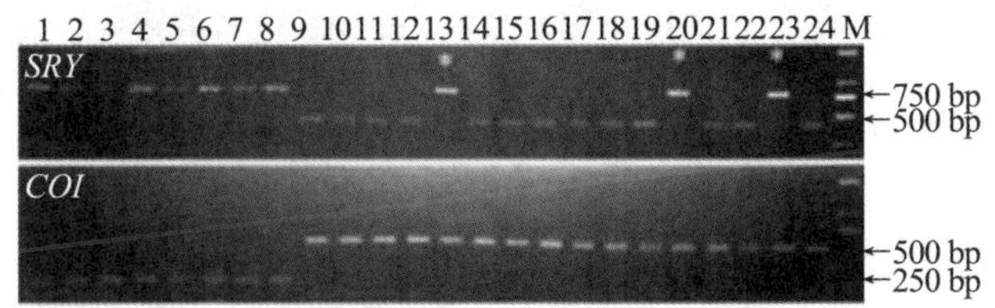


**图3 特异性PCR鉴别梅花鹿、马鹿及其杂交鹿样品凝胶电泳**

1～8. 梅花鹿待测品；9～24. 马鹿待测品；M. marker。

## 4 讨论

杂交育种是选育新品种主要途径，是育种工作最重要的方法。农林杂交育种主要以经济效益为导向，育种目标包括提高抗逆、产量、品质等。对于药用动植物，育种目标既要提高入药部位的生物产量，更要提高药用成分的相对含量。其中，对于鹿茸的生产，我国早在1958年就把杂交育种技术应用于鹿茸的生产，并经1987—1992年大规模推广应用，大幅度提高养鹿业生产力和经济效益。而对于中药，杂交育种还要考虑对中药药性的影响。因此，如何鉴别杂交基原的中药材是中药分子鉴定领域重要关注点。目前，对杂交鹿茸药性药效是否与亲本一致仍无完善评价方法，且缺乏准确区分杂交与非杂交品的方法。本研究对市场流通的鹿茸样品随机选样进行鉴别分析，在24个马鹿鹿茸的待测样品就发现有3个是马·花杂交鹿茸，可见市场流通的杂交鹿茸比例较高。据报道，马·花杂交F1生长速度显著高于花·马杂交F1，呈母本显性遗传，成年时体重和体型与母本鹿（马鹿）的相近，且茸生长快，其生长天数短，而茸质嫩，再生茸大、嫩又成型。而其茸型和肉质又多能呈父本显性遗传，不仅是最佳的茸肉兼用型鹿，还是茸血兼用鹿，具有较高的经济效益，这可能是市场流通中的具有较高比例的马·花杂交鹿茸的原因。而马·花杂交鹿茸的药用价值还有待进一步研究分析。

目前以线粒体序列建立的鹿茸分子鉴别方法，只能作为鉴别其母本的证据，对杂交鹿无法进行直接鉴别。为了建立杂交鹿茸的分子鉴别方法，本研究利用Y染色体的*SRY*基因作为父本的鉴别标记。目前，*SRY*基因在分子进化领域得到了广泛应用：如蔡欣等利用*SRY*基因多态性对牦牛与其他家牛属动物及其父系进化关系分析；周盼伊等利用*SRY*基因进行家养梅花鹿品种Y染色体遗传多样性和父系遗传结构分析；苏莹等利用Y染色体*SRY*基因对马鹿的遗传多样性进行研究。以上研究均表明*SRY*基因多态性可进行哺乳动物父本的溯源分析。因此，本研究选择*SRY*作为杂交鹿的父本鉴定标记，结合母本标记基因*CO*Ⅰ，可有效进行杂交鹿的父母本鉴定。

本研究分别基于*CO*Ⅰ与*SRY*基因序列建立了2个双位点特异PCR体系，用于鉴别鹿茸样品的父母本来源，初步建立了杂交鹿茸的鉴定方法。本研究过程中，试图把2个双位点特异PCR体系优化成1个多重PCR体系，发现在同一PCR系统中，基于*SRY*基因的鉴别引物扩增效率很低，且不稳定，推测是同一样品中基因组DNA拷贝数远远低于线粒体DNA的拷贝数，导致PCR扩增时扩增效率显著低于基于*CO*Ⅰ的鉴别引物。后续可通过降落PCR方法等进一步优化，构建有效稳定单一的多重PCR鉴别方法，可更简便进行杂交鹿茸的分子鉴定。本研究结果对杂交鹿茸鉴别也具有实际应用价值，也为后续进行杂交鹿茸的品质评价时提供有效的鉴别方法。

[魏艺聪，袁媛. 中国中药杂志，2017，42(23)：4588-4592.]

# 金银花种质资源DNA身份证构建及遗传相似性分析

中药材品质与其种质和产地密切相关。其中种质是指生物体亲代传递给子代的遗传物质，它往往存在于特定品种或品系中；在长期自然与人工选择过程中，形成了中药材诸多农家品种或品系，在遗传物质上会发生变化，导致植株形态、药材产量与质量均呈现出不同程度的差异。如金银花为忍冬科植物忍冬 *Lonicera japonica* Thunb. 的干燥花蕾或带初开的花，随着金银花市场需求量的逐年增加，新产区不断得到发展，盲目引种的现象比较普遍，致使种质混乱，药材产量与质量差异显著。目前报道的有关金银花的种质农艺性状分类研究、显微性状的研究，只能将金银花分为毛花系与鸡爪花系两大类，并不能将不同种质的金银花准确区分。

另一方面，在中药材质量控制体系中首先需要考虑建立中药材物种、变种、品种、品系等遗传稳定性评价方法，但目前大多数研究仅局限于物种一致性。DNA指纹图谱(DNA fingerprint)是以DNA标记为基础，可将品种之间彼此区分开的电泳图谱，目前已被应用于中药材种质分型、种源追溯等。本研究以金银花为例，在利用SSR分子标记技术建立58个农家种DNA身份证的基础上，通过计算不同农家种间遗传相似系数，依据其遗传一致性对农家种间关系进行分类，为金银花种质资源鉴定、新品种选育、完善中药材质量控制方法提供依据。

## 1 材料

1.1 植物 本研究收集了来自中国20个产地的58个金银花农家种，其中亚特红为红白忍冬（忍冬变种，非金银花），共计1025份样本；硅胶干燥，凭证标本保存于中国中医科学院中药资源中心。实验材料见表1。

**表1 58份金银花植物材料**

| 序号 | 品种名 | 采样地 | 采样量 | 采样日期 |
|---|---|---|---|---|
| 1 | 河北红银花 | 河北巨鹿堤村乡 | 15 | 2013-05-31 |
| 2 | 河北九丰一号 | 河北巨鹿堤村乡 | 18 | 2013-05-31 |
| 3 | 河北小鸡爪花 | 河北巨鹿堤村乡 | 14 | 2013-05-31 |
| 4 | 河北小线花 | 河北巨鹿堤村乡 | 13 | 2013-05-31 |
| 5 | 河北叶里齐 | 河北巨鹿堤村乡 | 21 | 2013-05-31 |
| 6 | 河北山花子 | 河北巨鹿堤村乡 | 25 | 2013-05-31 |
| 7 | 河北一线红 | 河北巨鹿堤村乡 | 10 | 2013-05-31 |
| 8 | 河北大麻花 | 河北巨鹿堤村乡 | 28 | 2013-05-31 |
| 9 | 河北大毛花 | 河北巨鹿堤村乡 | 11 | 2013-05-31 |
| 10 | 河北四季花 | 河北巨鹿堤村乡 | 15 | 2013-05-31 |

（续表）

| 序号 | 品种名 | 采样地 | 采样量 | 采样日期 |
|---|---|---|---|---|
| 11 | 河北大站花 | 河北巨鹿堤村乡 | 16 | 2013 - 05 - 31 |
| 12 | 河北大线花 | 河北巨鹿堤村乡 | 10 | 2013 - 05 - 31 |
| 13 | 河北大鸡爪花 | 河北巨鹿堤村乡 | 20 | 2013 - 05 - 31 |
| 14 | 河北金丰一号 | 河北巨鹿堤村乡 | 10 | 2013 - 05 - 31 |
| 15 | 河北巨花一号 | 河北巨鹿堤村乡 | 30 | 2013 - 05 - 31 |
| 16 | 河南野生 1 | 河南新密尖山乡 | 8 | 2013 - 05 - 28 |
| 17 | 河南大毛花 | 河南新密尖山乡 | 54 | 2013 - 05 - 28 |
| 18 | 河南野生大毛花 | 河南新密尖山乡 | 5 | 2013 - 05 - 28 |
| 19 | 河南野生 2 | 河南新密尖山乡 | 2 | 2013 - 05 - 28 |
| 20 | 河南小毛花 | 河南新密尖山乡 | 5 | 2013 - 05 - 28 |
| 21 | 河南线花 | 河南新密尖山乡 | 33 | 2013 - 05 - 28 |
| 22 | 江苏亚特 | 江苏连云港 | 20 | 2013 - 05 - 25 |
| 23 | 江苏大毛花 | 江苏连云港 | 30 | 2013 - 05 - 25 |
| 24 | 江苏九丰一号 | 江苏连云港 | 20 | 2013 - 05 - 25 |
| 25 | 江苏鸡爪花 | 江苏连云港 | 30 | 2013 - 05 - 25 |
| 26 | 江苏-河南引种 | 江苏连云港 | 20 | 2013 - 05 - 25 |
| 27 | 江苏红 | 江苏连云港 | 10 | 2013 - 05 - 25 |
| 28 | 江苏巨花一号 | 江苏连云港 | 20 | 2013 - 05 - 25 |
| 29 | 江苏四季花 | 江苏连云港 | 20 | 2013 - 05 - 25 |
| 30 | 山东大毛花 | 山东临沂农科院 | 13 | 2013 - 05 - 21 |
| 31 | 山东四季花 | 山东临沂农科院 | 9 | 2013 - 05 - 21 |
| 32 | 山东鸡爪花 | 山东临沂农科院 | 13 | 2013 - 05 - 21 |
| 33 | 山东红金 | 山东临沂农科院 | 13 | 2013 - 05 - 21 |
| 34 | 山东中花一号 | 山东临沂农科院 | 17 | 2013 - 05 - 21 |
| 35 | 山东野生 3 | 山东临沂莒南 | 5 | 2013 - 05 - 22 |
| 36 | 山东亚特红蕾 | 山东临沂莒南 | 30 | 2013 - 05 - 22 |
| 37 | 山东亚特立本 | 山东临沂莒南 | 30 | 2013 - 05 - 22 |
| 38 | 山东亚特青蕾 | 山东临沂莒南 | 30 | 2013 - 05 - 22 |
| 39 | 山东亚特良种 | 山东临沂莒南 | 30 | 2013 - 05 - 22 |
| 40 | 山东-美国引种 | 山东临沂莒南 | 10 | 2013 - 05 - 22 |
| 41 | 山东-意大利引种 | 山东临沂莒南 | 10 | 2013 - 05 - 22 |
| 42 | 广西-山东引种 | 广西乐业甘田镇园艺场 | 20 | 2014 - 05 - 17 |
| 43 | 云南亚特红 | 云南昆明官渡 | 20 | 2014 - 04 - 13 |
| 44 | 云南亚特 | 云南昆明 | 20 | 2014 - 04 - 13 |
| 45 | 湖南九丰一号 | 湖南攸县石羊塘镇田星村 | 20 | 2014 - 05 - 04 |
| 46 | 重庆-山东引种 | 重庆江北余盛镇华山村 | 20 | 2014 - 05 - 18 |
| 47 | 重庆-陕西引种 | 重庆垫江 | 4 | 2014 - 05 - 18 |
| 48 | 重庆垫江金银花 | 重庆垫江 | 20 | 2014 - 05 - 18 |

(续表)

| 序号 | 品种名 | 采样地 | 采样量 | 采样日期 |
|---|---|---|---|---|
| 49 | 湖北野生 | 湖北黄冈罗田骆驼坳镇 | 10 | 2014-05-05 |
| 50 | 湖北-河北引种 | 湖北黄冈罗田大崎乡 | 12 | 2014-05-06 |
| 51 | 安徽-山西引种 | 安徽宣城广德邱村镇赵村 | 21 | 2014-05-08 |
| 52 | 陕西金花三号 | 陕西咸阳杨陵崔家沟 | 20 | 2014-05-22 |
| 53 | 河南尖山大毛花 | 河南新密尖山乡山居 | 5 | 2014-05-16 |
| 54 | 河南封丘大毛花 | 河南封丘鲁岗乡 | 20 | 2014-05-16 |
| 55 | 宁夏-山东引种 | 宁夏固原官厅乡城儿山村 | 10 | 2014-06-18 |
| 56 | 甘肃亚特 | 甘肃武威凉州清水乡 | 20 | 2014-06-16 |
| 57 | 北京亚特红 | 北京房山窦店镇芦山村 | 20 | 2014-05-27 |
| 58 | 北京亚特立本 | 北京房山窦店镇芦山村 | 20 | 2014-05-27 |

1.2 *仪器* PCR仪(ABI公司),电泳系统(北京六一仪器厂),高速冷冻离心机(德国Eppendorf),SYNGENE凝胶成像系统(Gene公司),混合型球磨仪(德国Retsch),Bio-rad电泳仪(美国),HH-2数显恒温水浴锅(国华电器有限公司),MDF-192低温冰箱(日本Sanyo公司)。

1.3 *试剂* 2×CTAB提取液,10%过硫酸铵(APS),10×TBE buffer (pH 8.3),10%硝酸银溶液,3% NaOH溶液,DNA *Taq* 聚合酶(Takara公司),50 bp DNA Marker (Takara公司),TEMED。

## 2 方法

2.1 *总DNA提取* 样品采集后硅胶干燥,取20～100 mg,使用2步CTAB法提取样品总DNA,并进行DNA浓度和纯度测定,调整终浓度为50～100 mg/L用于进一步研究。

2.2 *混合样本池的构建* 先以单株样本基因组DNA为模板分别进行PCR扩增,然后将每个PCR产物等浓度混合构建混合池。

2.3 *SSR标记来源* 通过ssr.pl程序(http://www.gramene.org/db/markers/ssrtool)搜索大毛花和鸡爪花基因组序列(本课题组保存),识别标准为:二、三、四、五、六核苷酸重复基序的重复次数分别为10、9、8、7、6、5、4、3次。然后以大毛花基因组序列作为数据库,使用Blastn(http://blast.ncbi.nlm.nih.gov/Blast.cgi)寻找大毛花对鸡爪花的同源序列;以鸡爪花基因组序列作为数据库,使用Blastn寻找鸡爪花对大毛花的同源序列。2次比对识别标准均为 $e \leqslant 1\times10^{-30}$、score≥100、匹配数 $b=1$。

2.4 *SSR引物设计和PCR扩增* 应用引物设计软件Primer Premier 5.0和Primer 3.0设计引物。引物设计的序列来源于大毛花和鸡爪花的共同同源序列,二者彼此为模板相互同源,遵循设计的基本原则设计引物,引物由北京生工生物工程(上海)股份有限公司合成。PCR反应体系(25 μL)为:2.5 μL 10×PCR buffer,1 μL 2.5 mmol/L dNTPs,10 μmol/L引物各0.25 μL,2.5 U r*Taq* 酶,0.2 μL,1 μL DNA模板。反应程序为:94 ℃预变性5 min;94 ℃变性30 s,46～51 ℃复性30 s,72 ℃延伸30 s,35个循环;72 ℃延伸7 min。产物用2%琼脂糖凝胶电泳后,经8%非变性聚丙烯酰胺凝胶电泳,银染检测多态性条带。

2.5 *数据处理* 染色体上等位基因多态性是通过同一个位点上PCR扩增、电泳的条带的大小、有无及数量而确定的。经聚丙烯酰胺凝胶电泳得到的图谱上的每一条带记为一个位点,同一片段大小位点处有带记为"1",无带记为"0",用Excel软件统计整理。采用PopGene32 (version 1.32)软件计算SSR位点的有效等位基因数(Effective number of alleles, $N_e$)、Shannon-weaver多样性指数(Shannon's information index, $H$)和各农家种间的Nei's遗传相似系数($G_s$);每个SSR位点的多态性信息含量(polymorphic information content,PIC)按公式 $PIC=1-\Sigma f_{i2}$ 计算,$f_i$ 表示i位点的基因频率;并利用NTSYS pc version 2.10e软件根据Nei's遗传相似系数采用UPGMA方法进行聚类分析。

## 3 结果与分析

3.1 *SSR引物设计及筛选* 通过Blastn筛选大毛花和鸡爪花的基因组序列,共获得13 083对同源序列对,其中1 697对SSR存在差异,从中筛选出分布平均的22对引物用于PCR扩增和聚丙烯酰胺凝胶电泳,SSR引物信息见表2。

利用上述22对SSR引物在58个金银花农家种上进行PCR扩增,均可得到有效的PCR产物,从中筛选出多态性较强、扩增带型稳定、重复性较好的7对引物,占所用引物的29.2%,共检测到68个等位基因,扩增出的片段大小在100～700 bp。

每对引物可以检测到6～11条数目不等的多态性条带,平均可检测到8条。每对引物扩增的有效等位基因数为1.483～1.778,平均每对引物为1.632。Shannon-Weaver多样性指数($H$)变化范围为0.292～0.428,平均值为0.366,有4对引物高于均值。58份金银花农家种材料的多态性信息含量(PIC)平均值为0.833,变化范围为0.736～0.885,其中引物SSR9412929的PIC值最高,见表3。根据Bostsein的研

表 2　22 对引物信息

| 引物名称 | 引物序列(5′-3′) | |
|---|---|---|
| | 正向 | 反向 |
| SSR9168125 | TAAACGCTTGGCTAAAAATAC | TGATGGTGGTGTAAATAGGTG |
| SSR9231057 | TAACCTTTCATACGCCCTC | ATAATGACACCTCTATCCCTAAC |
| SSR9239135 | CCAAGCAACAAAGAGAACAT | TCTCCATTGCCTACATTTTC |
| SSR9240957 | TTTTTTCTCAATAATCCAAGTAAG | TGTTGTCAATGGCGTTAGG |
| SSR9282941 | TTCACAGCAGAAAGGGAG | TGACTGATTCAACAACCTACC |
| SSR9397534 | ACGCCTCTGTGGAATCTC | CGTAGCTCTTTGGGTGC |
| SSR9508438 | TGTCACACATTCTCCCTAACC | TGAGTATATTTTTAGAAGGCTGG |
| SSR9545025 | TAAGGTGGCGTTGAAGGAG | TTCTGTCATATTCTTCTGCTCATC |
| SSR9565972 | CACCCCGAGCACAGAGG | ACATTTTTGAGCCACACTTTTC |
| SSR8504433 | GGACGTACAAATGGAACAATG | AGGAAATACAAATAACTAAGAGCG |
| SSR8883380 | ATGAAGCTGCAATACAGAATCC | CCACAATGGGCACAACACT |
| SSR9008219 | CGTGGGGAACATTTAATCAT | CAAAAAGCCGTAGAAGAACC |
| SSR9118060 | TGGACAACAAGGCAAGG | AAAAGAAACCAAAAGAATAAGAG |
| SSR9122370 | TGGGAGAAGGAGATGAGC | ATAGTTTGATTATATTCGGGC |
| SSR9130459 | CAAAATATAAACAAGGAAACAAC | TATTGCTTATGTATGCTCTCG |
| SSR9131651 | CTAATGATGCTCACTTGACTTTTG | AAGTGAACTAAGAGCGTCATTTG |
| SSR9308616 | GAACATCCATCGTTGCGTG | TTGCGGTGATTCGAGAGC |
| SSR9412929 | TTAGCGGGTTGGGTCTC | ATGAGCCAAATGACCAGG |
| SSR9417243 | CGTTTTTGTTTTGATTCATCTCTG | ACCACCTAAAAGAAAGTGCGTC |
| SSR9547421 | CTTATTTTGAGGGGTATTTTGG | GGCAAAGATAGTAAGGACGG |
| SSR9553121 | TCGTCCAAGTCCCATCC | CGTTAAGAGCTGCACCAT |
| SSR9562432 | CCTTTCAATCCCATTCATCTG | GCAATCACTATCCACCACCTG |

表 3　SSR 多态性引物的特征

| 引物 | 等位位点数 | 有效等位基因数 $N_e$ | 多样性指数 $H$ | 多态性信息含量 PIC |
|---|---|---|---|---|
| SSR9008219 | 8 | 1.657 | 0.376 | 0.831 |
| SSR9118060 | 11 | 1.563 | 0.334 | 0.865 |
| SSR9122370 | 7 | 1.778 | 0.428 | 0.826 |
| SSR9308616 | 6 | 1.483 | 0.292 | 0.735 |
| SSR9412929 | 11 | 1.620 | 0.366 | 0.885 |
| SSR9553121 | 9 | 1.596 | 0.359 | 0.848 |
| SSR9562432 | 8 | 1.730 | 0.407 | 0.841 |

究，PIC 值是衡量等位信息含量和变异程度高低的理想指标，当 PIC>0.5 时该位点为高度多态位点，0.25<PIC<0.5 时为中度多态位点，PIC<0.25 时为低度多态位点。本研究筛选的 7 个 SSR 引物标记位点均为高度多态性位点，表明这些 SSR 位点可从分子水平解释其基因型差异，具有丰富的遗传差异性，可作为有效的标记来构建 58 份金银花农家种的 DNA 身份证。

3.2　*金银花农家种 DNA 身份证的构建*　采用 7 对 SSR 核心引物构建 58 个金银花农家种 DNA 身份证，见表 4，部分引物聚丙烯酰胺凝胶电泳图谱见图 1。其中引物 SSR9118060 可以区分 27 个不同农家种，引物 SSR9008219 可以区分 19 个不同农家种，引物 SSR9122370 可以区分 20 个不同农家种，引物 SSR9308616 可以区分 10 个不同农家种，引物 SSR9412929 可以区分 23 个不同农家种，引物 SSR9553121 可以区分 18 个不同农家种，引物 SSR9562432 可以区分 26 个不同农家种。然后随机选择 20 株对所建立的 DNA 身份证进行验证，结果表明利用上述 7 对核心引物组合可以将 58 个金银花农家种准确区分。

3.3　*遗传相似系数分析*　根据 7 对 SSR 引物所检测出的 68 个多态性位点，采用 PopGene32(vesion1.32)软件计算各农家种间的 Nei's 遗传相似系数($G_s$)，并利用 NTSYS pc version 2.10e 软件根据 Nei's 遗传相似系数采用 UPGMA 方法进行聚类，遗传相似系数变异范围为 0.3667～0.9167，见图 2。

表 4 部分农家种的 DNA 身份证

| 序号 | SSR9008219 | | | | | | | | SSR9118060 | | | | | | | | | | | SSR9122370 | | | | | | | SSR9308616 | | | | | |
|---|---|---|---|---|---|---|---|---|---|---|---|---|---|---|---|---|---|---|---|---|---|---|---|---|---|---|---|---|---|---|---|---|
| | a | b | c | d | e | f | g | h | i | g | k | l | m | n | o | p | q | r | s | t | u | v | w | x | y | z | aa | ab | ac | ad | ae | af |
| 1 | 0 | 1 | 1 | 1 | 0 | 1 | 1 | 1 | 0 | 0 | 1 | 1 | 0 | 1 | 1 | 0 | 1 | 1 | 0 | 0 | 1 | 1 | 1 | 0 | 0 | 1 | 0 | 0 | 0 | 0 | 0 | 0 |
| 2 | 0 | 0 | 0 | 1 | 0 | 0 | 0 | 0 | 0 | 0 | 0 | 0 | 0 | 1 | 1 | 0 | 1 | 1 | 1 | 0 | 0 | 0 | 1 | 0 | 1 | 0 | 0 | 0 | 0 | 0 | 1 | 1 |
| 3 | 0 | 0 | 1 | 1 | 1 | 1 | 1 | 0 | 0 | 0 | 0 | 0 | 0 | 1 | 0 | 0 | 1 | 1 | 0 | 0 | 0 | 1 | 1 | 1 | 1 | 0 | 0 | 0 | 0 | 0 | 1 | 1 |
| 4 | 0 | 0 | 1 | 1 | 0 | 0 | 0 | 0 | 0 | 1 | 0 | 0 | 0 | 1 | 1 | 0 | 1 | 1 | 0 | 0 | 0 | 0 | 1 | 1 | 1 | 0 | 0 | 0 | 0 | 0 | 1 | 1 |
| 5 | 0 | 0 | 1 | 0 | 0 | 0 | 0 | 0 | 0 | 0 | 0 | 0 | 0 | 1 | 1 | 0 | 1 | 1 | 0 | 0 | 0 | 0 | 1 | 0 | 1 | 0 | 0 | 0 | 0 | 0 | 1 | 1 |
| 6 | 0 | 1 | 1 | 0 | 0 | 0 | 0 | 0 | 0 | 1 | 1 | 0 | 1 | 1 | 0 | 0 | 0 | 1 | 1 | 0 | 0 | 0 | 1 | 0 | 1 | 0 | 0 | 1 | 0 | 0 | 1 | 1 |
| 7 | 0 | 1 | 1 | 1 | 1 | 0 | 1 | 0 | 0 | 1 | 1 | 0 | 1 | 1 | 1 | 0 | 1 | 1 | 1 | 0 | 1 | 0 | 0 | 0 | 1 | 1 | 0 | 0 | 0 | 1 | 0 | 1 |
| 8 | 0 | 1 | 1 | 1 | 1 | 0 | 1 | 0 | 0 | 1 | 0 | 0 | 1 | 0 | 0 | 0 | 0 | 0 | 0 | 0 | 1 | 1 | 0 | 0 | 1 | 1 | 0 | 1 | 0 | 0 | 1 | 1 |

| 序号 | SSR9412929 | | | | | | | | | | | SSR9553121 | | | | | | | | | SSR9562432 | | | | | | | |
|---|---|---|---|---|---|---|---|---|---|---|---|---|---|---|---|---|---|---|---|---|---|---|---|---|---|---|---|---|
| | ag | ah | ai | aj | ak | al | am | an | ao | ap | aq | ar | as | at | au | av | aw | ax | ay | az | ba | bb | bc | bd | be | bf | bg | bh |
| 1 | 1 | 0 | 1 | 0 | 0 | 0 | 0 | 1 | 0 | 1 | 0 | 0 | 0 | 0 | 0 | 1 | 0 | 1 | 1 | 1 | 0 | 0 | 1 | 1 | 0 | 1 | 1 | 1 |
| 2 | 1 | 1 | 0 | 0 | 1 | 1 | 0 | 0 | 1 | 1 | 0 | 0 | 0 | 1 | 0 | 1 | 0 | 0 | 1 | 0 | 0 | 0 | 1 | 1 | 1 | 1 | 0 | 1 |
| 3 | 1 | 0 | 0 | 0 | 1 | 0 | 0 | 1 | 1 | 1 | 0 | 0 | 0 | 1 | 0 | 1 | 0 | 0 | 0 | 0 | 0 | 0 | 1 | 0 | 1 | 0 | 0 | 1 |
| 4 | 1 | 0 | 0 | 0 | 0 | 1 | 0 | 1 | 1 | 1 | 0 | 0 | 0 | 1 | 0 | 1 | 0 | 0 | 1 | 1 | 1 | 1 | 0 | 1 | 1 | 1 | 1 | 0 |
| 5 | 1 | 0 | 0 | 0 | 0 | 1 | 0 | 0 | 1 | 1 | 0 | 0 | 0 | 1 | 1 | 0 | 0 | 0 | 1 | 1 | 1 | 0 | 0 | 1 | 1 | 1 | 0 | 0 |
| 6 | 1 | 0 | 0 | 0 | 1 | 1 | 0 | 1 | 1 | 1 | 0 | 0 | 0 | 0 | 0 | 1 | 0 | 1 | 0 | 0 | 0 | 0 | 0 | 1 | 1 | 0 | 0 | 1 |
| 7 | 1 | 0 | 0 | 0 | 0 | 1 | 0 | 0 | 1 | 1 | 0 | 0 | 0 | 1 | 1 | 0 | 0 | 0 | 0 | 1 | 0 | 0 | 0 | 1 | 0 | 0 | 0 | 1 |
| 8 | 1 | 0 | 0 | 0 | 1 | 1 | 1 | 1 | 1 | 1 | 0 | 0 | 0 | 0 | 1 | 1 | 0 | 1 | 0 | 1 | 1 | 0 | 0 | 1 | 1 | 0 | 0 | 1 |

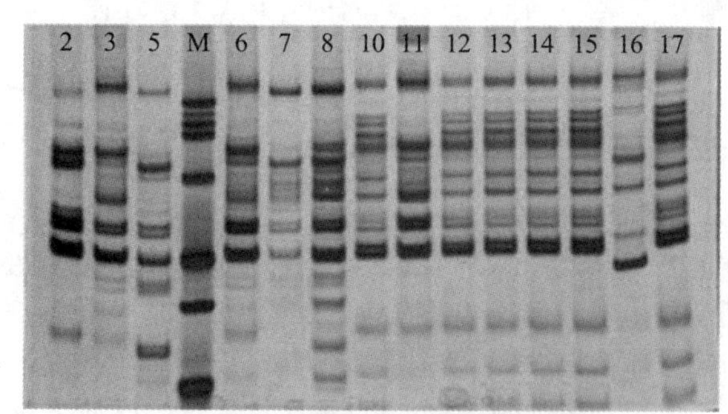


**图 1 引物 SSR9412929 的聚丙烯酰胺凝胶电泳图谱**

M. marker；数字为金银花农家种编号。

基于农家种间遗传相似系数可将金银花农家种遗传一致性分成 A、B、C、D 4 个等级，见表 5。A 等级如 38 号山东亚特青蕾与 39 号山东亚特良种，其同属一个育种体系且产区一致，二者遗传相似系数为 0.9167，表明其遗传背景高度一致。B 等级如河北省巨鹿县堤村乡采集的农家种 12 号河北大线花、15 号河北巨花一号、13 号河北大鸡爪花、14 号河北金丰一号遗传相似系数为 0.8167～0.8833，推测其具有相似的遗传背景。C 等级如河南密县采集的 18 号河南野生大毛花、21 号河南线花、20 号河南小毛花，遗传相似系数为 0.6667～0.7833；22 号江苏亚特、44 号云南亚特、56 号甘肃亚特均引种于山东亚特(37 号)，其遗传相似系数为 0.5833～0.7667。该类样本间遗传一致性降低，可能与种质差异或引种后种质混乱导致遗传变异有关。D 等级如不同产区、不同种质的 5 号河北叶里齐和 20 号河南小毛花的遗传相似系数为 0.4333，说明其遗传背景存在明显差异。

## 4 讨论

4.1 *DNA 身份证的构建* 传统药材品种鉴定方法一般采用形态学方法，对一些亲缘关系较近、性状差异较小的品种以及一些因跨地区引种而产生表型差异的品种很难鉴定。采用 SSR 分子标记技术建立中药材 DNA 指纹图谱并构建其身份证，因不受引种栽培等外界环境的影响，可以有效区分表型特征相似的近缘物种、种质资源以及农家种。本研究采用的 58 份金银花农家种产地几乎涵盖了全国金银花主产地区，所构建的 58 个金银花农家种 DNA 身份证可为金银花种质数据库的建设奠定基础；随着金银花新品种的不断出现，需要不断更新品种信息和对核心引物进行完善。

4.2 *遗传一致性分析* 遗传相似系数可以反映种质间的亲缘关系，从基于遗传相似系数进行的聚类分析结果可以发现，多数产地相近的金银花农家种表现出较为密切的亲缘关系，这与丝瓜等园艺作物种质资源评价结果相似。

种质资源是中药材生产和育种的源头，通过药用植物种质资源研究提高中药材质量是目前迫切需要解决的问题。作为优质药材代名词的道地药材也可以被看作为特殊的“种

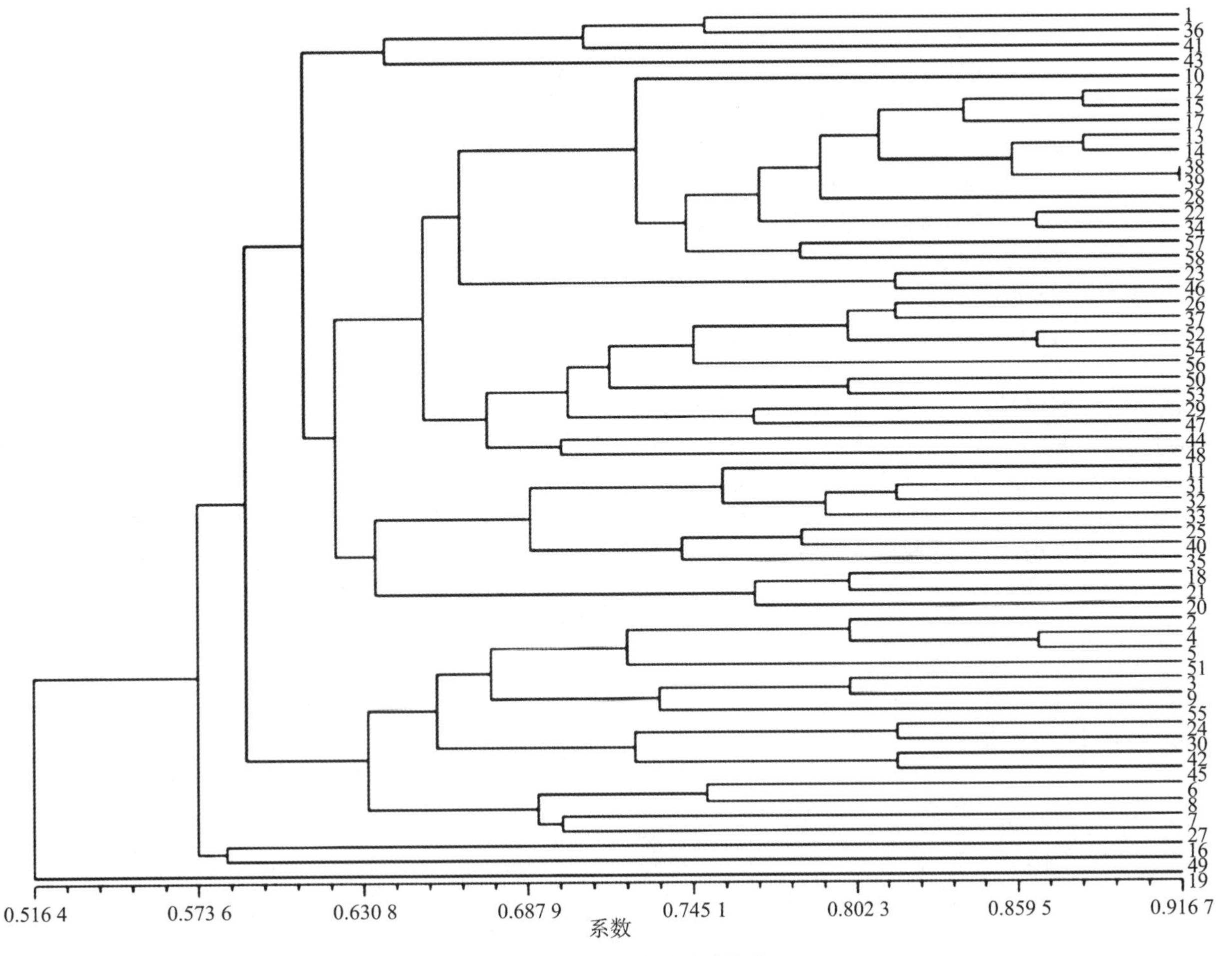

图2 58个金银花农家种的聚类

表5 遗传一致性评价

| 遗传相似系数 | 置信区间(95%) | 一致性分级 |
|---|---|---|
| $G_s \geq 0.9$ | [0.9985,1.0000] | A |
| $0.8 \leq G_s < 0.9$ | [0.8192,0.8350] | B |
| $0.55 \leq G_s < 0.8$ | [0.6369,0.6434] | C |
| $G_s < 0.55$ | [0.4924,0.5007] | D |

质”。袁媛在建立道地药材评价体系中提出首先要建立对照道地药材,在此基础上开展药材一致性评价研究,以期为道地药材特征辨识提供支撑。随着中药材栽培产区不断扩大,出现种植混乱、盲目引种等问题,使得同种异地产出的药材在质量与药效上存在差异。因此,建立中药材物种、变种、品种、品系等遗传一致性评价方法,是建立完整道地药材评价与中药材质量控制体系中不可缺少的一部分,是对种质资源保护与利用的基础。本研究以金银花为例,分析58个金银花农家种间亲缘关系,并根据遗传相似系数将58个农家种遗传一致性分为4类,为金银花引种栽培溯源、新品种培育、道地药材评价研究提供依据。

[朱凤洁,袁媛.中国中药杂志,2018,43(9):1825-1831.]

# 红天麻、乌天麻及其杂交天麻的PCR鉴别

天麻作为我国名贵中药材,具有良好的药用价值。据2015年版《中国药典》规定,天麻来自兰科植物天麻 *Gastrodia elata* Bl.的干燥块茎,具有息风止痉、平抑肝阳、祛风通络的功效。《中国植物志》记载周铉在广泛野外调查观察的基础上,结合人工栽培经验,将我国天麻分为如下5个变型:红天麻(原变型)*G. elata* f. *elata*、乌天麻 *G. elata* f. *glauca*、绿天麻 *G. elata* f. *viridis*、黄天麻 *G. elata* f. *flavid* 和松天麻 *G. elata* f. *alba*。其中红天麻产自黄河流域与长江流域诸省,其种子发芽率和产量高,适应性和耐旱性强;乌天麻产自贵州西部、云南东北部至西北部,其块茎含水量低、干品品质好;二者的天麻素和多糖含量均较高,被作为栽培的优良品系。

杂交技术是一种根据杂种优势原理培育具有父母本优良性状新品种的方法，目前在水稻、棉花、高粱等作物上已广泛使用。为了提高天麻产量与质量，湖北等地培育出红乌杂交天麻，其天麻素含量远高于亲本，但随之也加剧了天麻种质混乱、质量和产量不稳定等问题。在生产中，天麻种质鉴定基本采用传统性状鉴定方法，如观察茎秆颜色、块茎形状、环纹数量等；该方法具有一定的局限性，即鉴别特征易受到环境等外因的影响。因此建立一种快速、准确、稳定的红天麻、乌天麻及其杂交天麻鉴别方法，对保证药材质量与天麻的栽培育种具有重要意义。

聚合酶链式反应(polymerase chain reaction，PCR)是一种模拟自然DNA复制过程的体外酶促合成特异性核酸片段技术，具有操作简单、快速、灵敏度高、特异性强的特点，在品系、杂交品鉴别上已有成功应用。本研究拟在已获得天麻全基因组序列的基础上，利用重测序获得红天麻和乌天麻鉴别位点，并运用特异性PCR方法建立红天麻、乌天麻及其杂交天麻鉴别方法。

## 1 材料

1.1 植物样品 红天麻、乌天麻及其杂交天麻分别采自贵州大方、云南昭通、陕西宁陕、湖北英山和湖北宜昌，由金艳副研究员鉴定，标本保存于中国中医科学院中药资源中心，见表1。

**表1 试验材料**

| No. | 材料名称 | 拉丁名 | 来源 | 数量 |
|---|---|---|---|---|
| 1 | 红天麻 | *Gastrodia elata* f. *elata* | 陕西宁陕 | 4 |
| 2 | 红天麻 | *G. elata* f. *elata* | 湖北英山 | 8 |
| 3 | 红天麻 | *G. elata* f. *elata* | 湖北宜昌 | 6 |
| 4 | 乌天麻 | *G. elata* f. *glauca* | 贵州大方 | 4 |
| 5 | 乌天麻 | *G. elata* f. *glauca* | 云南昭通 | 14 |
| 6 | 乌天麻 | *G. elata* f. *glauca* | 湖北宜昌 | 4 |
| 7 | 红乌杂交天麻 | — | 贵州大方 | 3 |

1.2 仪器 Veriti™型PCR仪，GeneAmp 9700型PCR仪(美国Applied Biosystem公司)；PTC-100型PCR仪，SYNGENE SYNGENE型凝胶成像系统(Gene公司)；TC-512型PCR仪(上海Techne公司)。

1.3 试剂 Ex *Taq* DNA聚合酶(批号RR001B)，SpeedSTAR HS *Taq* DNA聚合酶(批号RR070 A)，r*Taq* DNA聚合酶(批号R001B)，Mighty Amp DNA聚合酶(批号R071 A)，均购自大连TaKaRa公司；FastPfu Fly DNA聚合酶(批号M10527)购自北京NEB公司；2×T5 Super PCR Mix(colony，批号TSE005)购自北京擎科新业生物技术有限公司；*Taq* DNA聚合酶267S(批号M0267)，*Taq* DNA聚合酶273S(批号M0273)，均购自北京NEB公司；6×Loading buffer(批号9156)，购自大连TaKaRa公司；Trans2K DNA Marker(批号BM101)，Trans2K Plus DNA Marker(批号BM111)，均购自北京全式金生物技术有限公司。

## 2 方法

2.1 DNA提取 用70%乙醇擦拭刀片，刮取适量天麻样品，放入液氮中，用高通量组织研磨仪打成粉末，取10～30 mg粉末至2.0 mL离心管中，使用经典CTAB法提取DNA：加入900 μL 65℃预热的CTAB提取缓冲液、10 μL β-巯基乙醇和少许PVP，混匀，65℃水浴30 min，其间不时轻摇混匀；冷却至45℃以下，加等体积氯仿-异戊醇混合液，温和摇动，12 000 r/min离心10 min；吸取约700 μL上清液至2.0 mL离心管，加入700 μL氯仿-异戊醇混合液，混匀，12 000 r/min离心5 min；吸取500 μL上清液至1.5 mL离心管，加入330 μL异丙醇，混匀，−20℃放置30 min；4℃下12 000 r/min离心，弃上清；加入500 μL 70%乙醇，悬浮DNA，12 000 r/min离心5 min；弃上清，加入500 μL无水乙醇，悬浮DNA，12 000 r/min离心5 min；弃上清，挥干乙醇，加入75 μL灭菌水，待DNA溶解，4℃保存。

2.2 引物设计 根据天麻重测序的结果，筛选红天麻与乌天麻的SNP位点，选取变异位点两端保守序列，使用软件Primer Premier 5.0设计特异性引物，由生工生物工程(上海)股份有限公司合成，见表2。

**表2 本实验所用引物**

| 名称 | 序列(5′-3′) |
|---|---|
| W291-F | CAATCCAGGCTTATGATGC |
| W291-R | TATTTTCATTTATGTCAATTAACG |
| H255-F | CCTTATTACTTCCATGTGTGTC |
| H255-R | TTTCTTCATAATTGCCGG |

2.3 PCR扩增条件的确定 分别使用上述2对鉴别引物对红天麻、乌天麻及其杂交天麻总DNA模板进行扩增，初始PCR反应体系：反应总体积为25 μL，包含10×PCR缓冲液2.5 μL，dNTPs(10 mmol/L) 1.5 μL，上、下游引物各0.5 μL，r*Taq* DNA聚合酶1.5 U，DNA模板1 μL，用无菌双蒸水补足剩余体积。初始反应程序：95℃预变性5 min，35循环(95℃ 30 s，56℃ 20 s，72℃ 30 s)，72℃终延伸10 min，15℃保温。PCR反应结束后，取反应产物5 μL，加入2 μL 6×Loading buffer，混匀后点样于溴化乙锭(EB)染色的2.0%琼脂糖凝胶上，200 V电压条件下电泳8～10 min，置SYNGENE凝胶成像系统观察。

分别考察：退火温度、PCR循环数、DNA模板量、*Taq*酶种类、*Taq*酶用量，确定最佳反应体系和反应参数，并使用最佳条件对天麻样品进行PCR鉴别，验证该体系是否能稳定、准确地鉴别红天麻、乌天麻及其杂交天麻。

## 3 结果与分析

3.1 红天麻特异性PCR鉴别条件的考察 使用引物H255-F/H255-R对天麻DNA进行PCR扩增，考察退火温度、PCR循环数、DNA模板量、*Taq*酶种类、*Taq*酶用量、PCR仪型号等因素影响，结果见表3。当退火温度为48℃，PCR循环数为48，使用1.75 U r*Taq* DNA聚合酶，且DNA模板量为300 ng时，红天麻及红乌杂交天麻在255 bp时可获得最优条带，见图1。

3.2 乌天麻特异性PCR鉴别条件的考察 使用引物W291-F/W291-R进行PCR扩增，考察退火温度、PCR循环数、DNA 模板量、*Taq* 酶种类、*Taq* 酶用量、PCR 仪型号等因素影响，结果见表 4。当退火温度为 48 ℃，PCR 循环数为 48，使用 1.75 U r*Taq* DNA 聚合酶，且 DNA 模板量为 300 ng 时，乌天麻及红乌杂交天麻在 291 bp 时可获得最优条带，见图 2。

3.3 红乌杂交天麻特异性 PCR 鉴别 分别使用引物 W291－F/W291－R 和 H255－F/H255－R 进行 PCR 扩增，反应条件见"3.1"与"3.2"，红乌杂交天麻分别在 255、291 bp 处出现单一明亮的特异性鉴别条带，见图 1、2。

**表 3 红天麻特异性 PCR 条件考察**

| 参数 | 考察条件 | 适宜范围 | 最优条件 |
|---|---|---|---|
| 退火温度(℃) | 46,47,48,49 | 46～49 | 48 |
| PCR 循环数 | 31,33,35,37 | 31～37 | 33 |
| *Taq* 酶种类 | r*Taq* DNA 聚合酶，Ex *Taq*DNA 聚合酶，Speed Star HS *Taq*DNA 聚合酶，Mighty Amp DNA 聚合酶，FastPfu Fly DNA 聚合酶，2×T5 Super PCR Mix，*Taq* DNA 聚合酶 267S，*Taq* DNA 聚合酶 273S | r*Taq* DNA 聚合酶，*Taq* DNA 聚合 267S，*Taq* DNA 聚合酶 273S | r*Taq* DNA 聚合酶 |
| *Taq* 酶用量(U) | 1.25，1.50，1.75，2.00 | 1.25～2.00 | 1.75 |
| DNA 模板量(ng) | 100，300，1 000，3 000 | 100～3 000 | 300 |

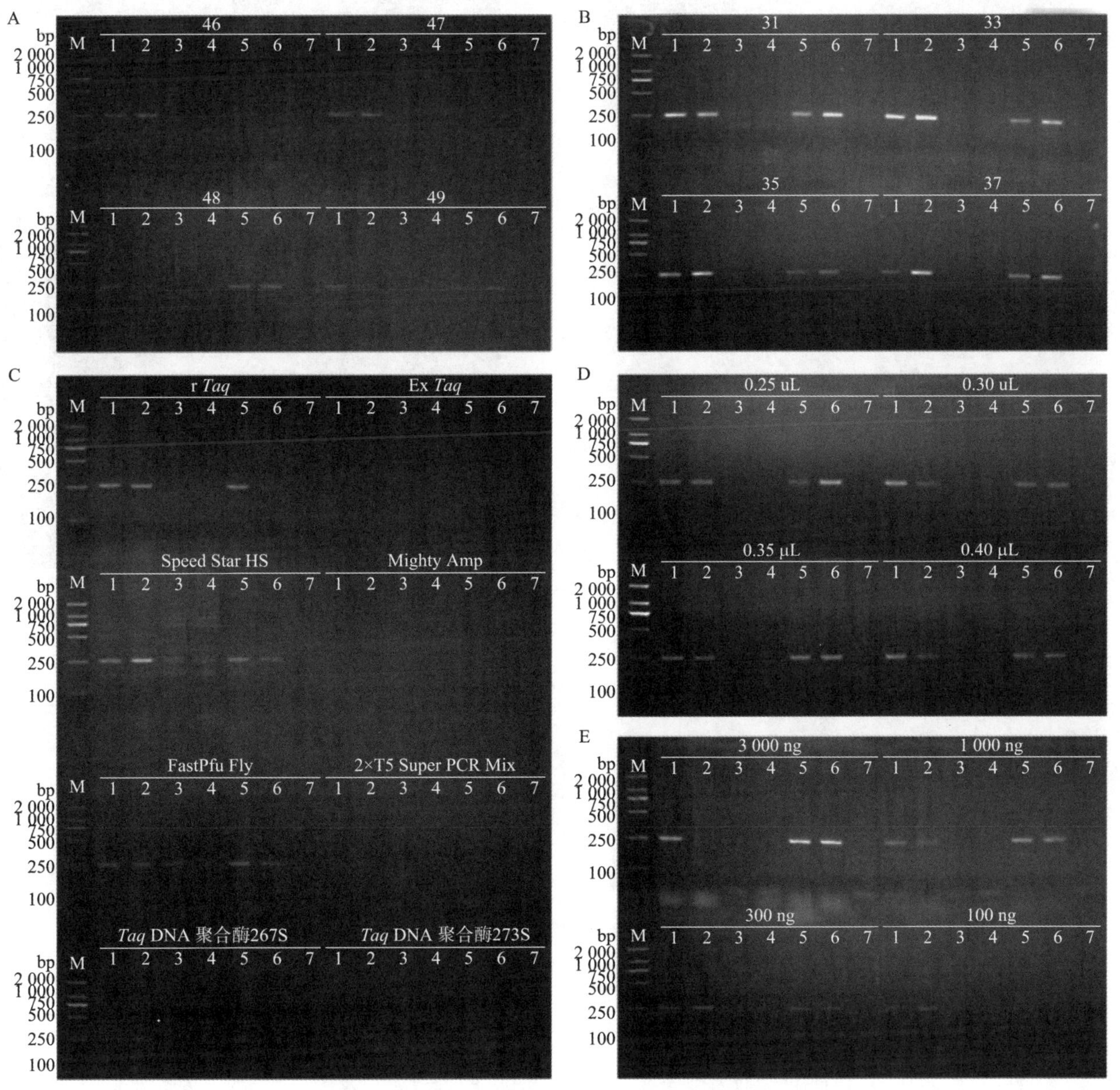


**图 1 不同条件对红天麻、红乌杂交天麻特异性 PCR 鉴别结果的影响**

A. 退火温度；B. 循环数；C. 酶种类；D. *Taq* 酶用量；E. DNA 模板量。1、2. 红天麻；3、4. 乌天麻；5、6. 红乌杂交天麻；7. 空白对照，以 $ddH_2O$ 为模板(图 2、3 同)；M. DL 2 000 marker。

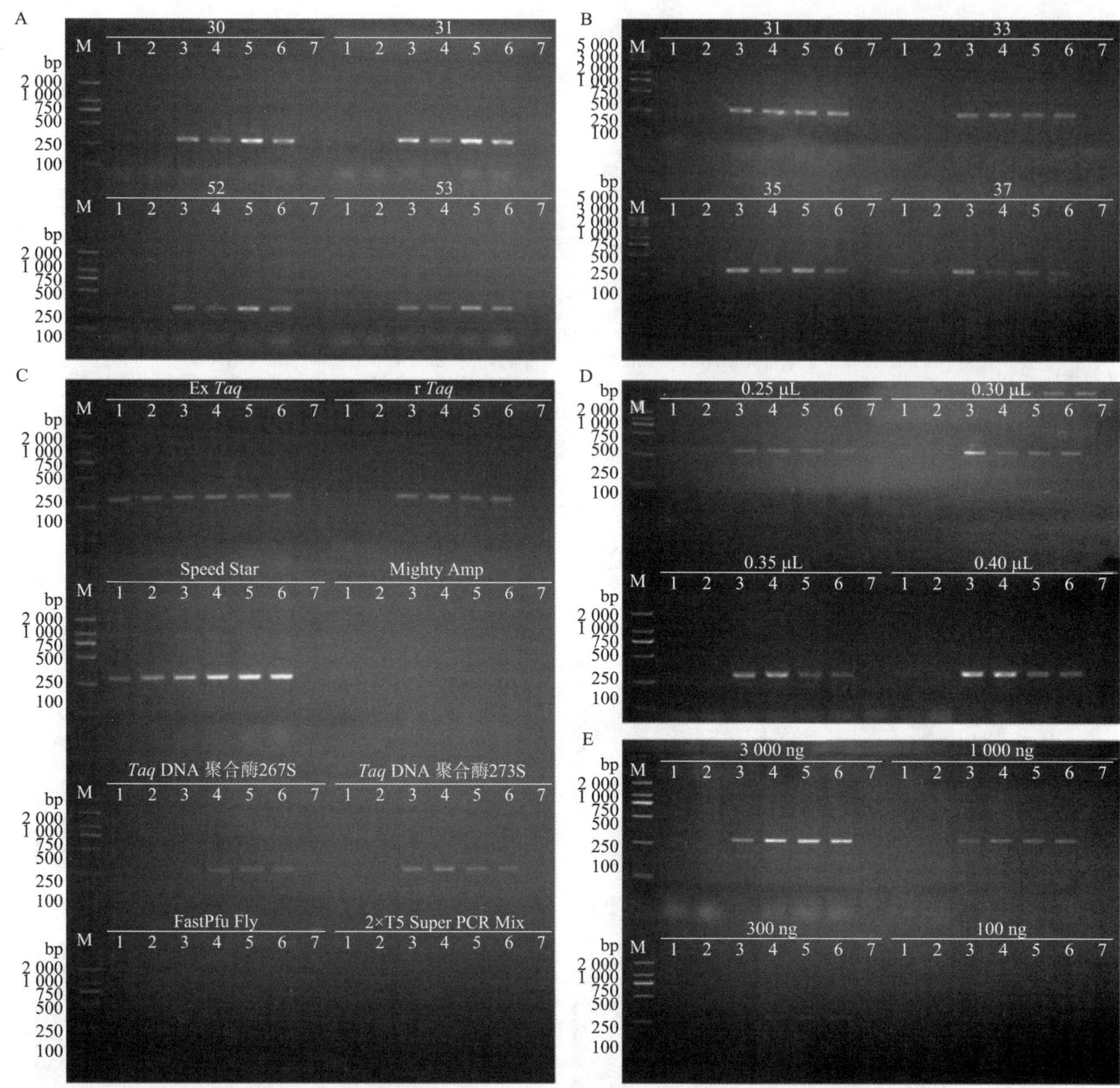


**图 2 不同条件对乌天麻、红乌杂交天麻特异性 PCR 鉴别结果的影响**

M. DL 2000 marker；DL 2000 plus marker。

**表 4 乌天麻特异性 PCR 条件考察**

| 参数 | 考察条件 | 适宜范围 | 最优条件 |
|---|---|---|---|
| 退火温度(℃) | 50,51,52,53 | 50～53 | 51 |
| PCR 循环数 | 31,33,35,37 | 31～37 | 31 |
| *Taq* 酶种类 | r*Taq* DNA 聚合酶，Ex *Taq*DNA 聚合酶，Speed Star HS *Taq*DNA 聚合酶，Mighty Amp DNA 聚合酶，FastPfu Fly DNA 聚合酶，2×T5 Super PCR Mix，*Taq* DNA 聚合酶 267S，*Taq* DNA 聚合酶 273S | r*Taq* DNA 聚合酶，*Taq* DNA 聚合 267S，*Taq* DNA 聚合酶 273S | r*Taq* DNA 聚合酶 |
| *Taq* 酶用量(U) | 1.25,1.50,1.75,2.00 | 1.25～2.00 | 1.75 |
| DNA 模板量(ng) | 100,300,1 000,3 000 | 100～3 000 | 300 |

3.4 耐受性考察 为测试不同 PCR 仪对红天麻、乌天麻及其杂交天麻鉴别结果的影响，分别使用 Veriti、ABI 9700、PTC-100 以及 TC-512 型基因扩增仪进行 PCR 扩增，均可获得正确的鉴别结果，见图 3。

3.5 适用性考察 根据“3.1”和“3.2”项下确定的最优PCR鉴别体系和条件（红天麻：95 ℃预变性5 min；95 ℃变性30 s，48 ℃退火30 s，72 ℃延伸30 s，33个循环；72 ℃再延伸5 min。乌天麻：95 ℃预变性5 min；95 ℃变性30 s，51 ℃退火30 s，72 ℃延伸30 s，31个循环；72 ℃再延伸5 min），对采集的天麻样品进行PCR扩增，产物经2%琼脂糖凝胶电泳检测。结果显示，样品1～18号红天麻与41～43号红乌杂交天麻在255 bp处均出现单一明亮条带；样品19～40乌天麻与41～43号红乌杂交天麻在291 bp处均出现单一明亮条带，表明该体系能稳定准确鉴别红天麻、乌天麻及其杂交天麻，见图4。

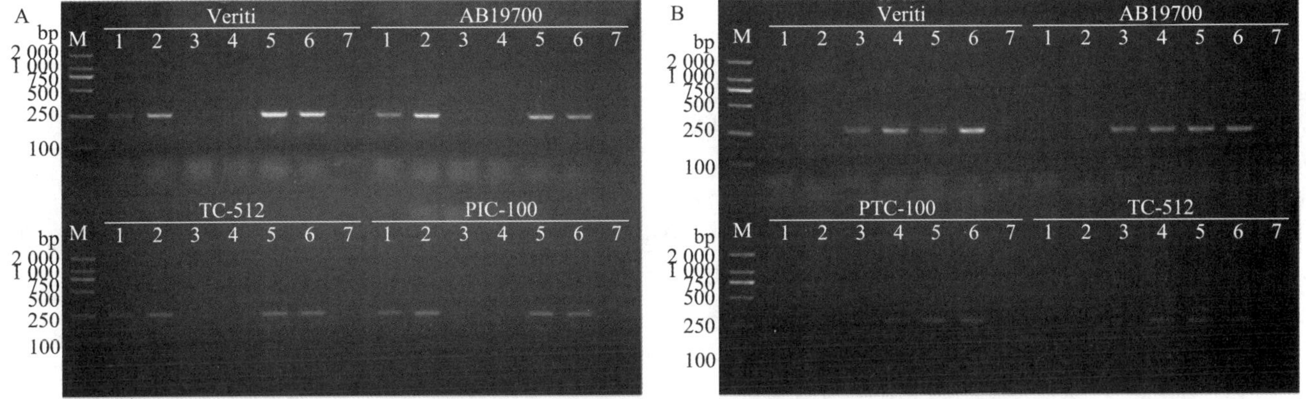


**图3 不同仪器对红天麻、乌天麻、红乌杂交天麻特异性PCR鉴别结果的影响**

M. DL 2000 marker；A. 引物H255－F/H255－R；B. 引物W291－F/W291－R（图4同）。

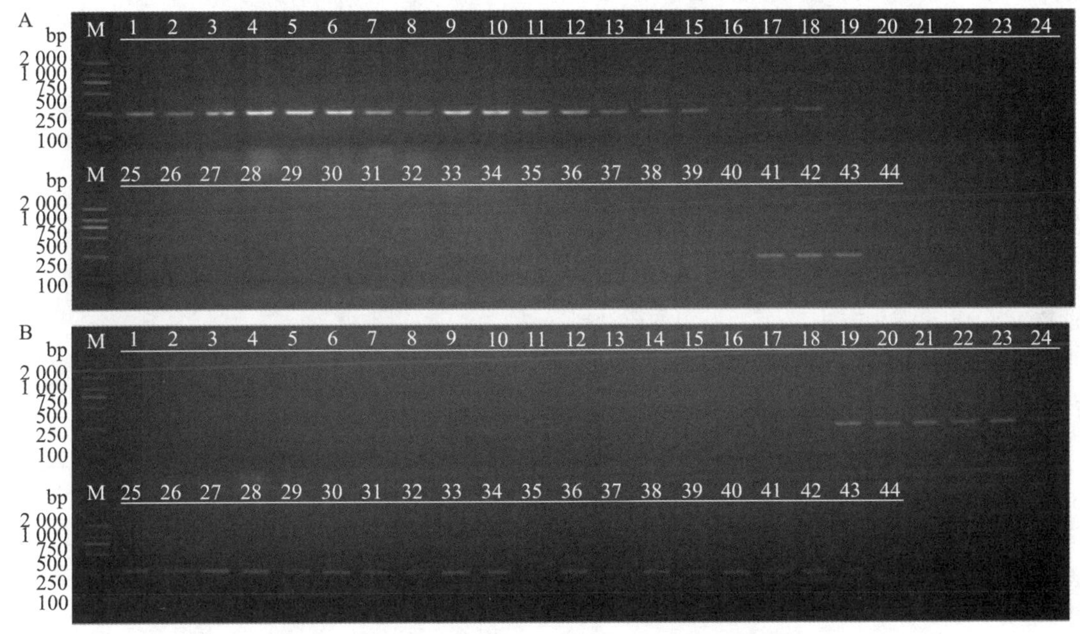


**图4 特异性PCR鉴别红天麻、乌天麻及红乌交天麻样品凝胶电泳**

1～18. 红天麻样品；19～40. 乌天麻样品；41～43. 红乌杂交天麻样品；44. 空白对照（以$ddH_2O$为模板）。

## 4 小结

杂交育种是选育中药材优良新品种的主要途径之一。云南、陕西、湖北等地先后进行了天麻杂交育种的研究，提高了天麻的产量。但由于异地盲目引种导致中药材种质混乱，且缺乏对杂交天麻及其父本、母本品种权保护等，引起天麻质量和产量不稳定等问题。

品种鉴别一直是中药鉴定中的难点。传统上对乌天麻、红天麻及其杂交天麻的鉴别主要基于茎的颜色、花的形态与颜色等特征，仅在开花期可以进行观察，且鉴别结果主观性强、依赖个人经验。特异性PCR技术已被证实是中药材真实性客观鉴别的一种常用技术，本研究根据红天麻、乌天麻重测序筛选SNP位点设计鉴别引物，并分别对影响特异性鉴别的PCR反应条件和反应程序中的关键因素进行了考察，确定了最优PCR鉴别条件，建立红天麻、乌天麻及其杂交天麻特异性PCR鉴别方法。该方法效率高、成本低、稳定且特异性强，可为天麻新品种选育、种质资源保护等提供技术支持，为中药材品种鉴别提供一种新的途径。

［李慧，袁媛，黄璐琦，等. 中国中药杂志，2020，45（15）：3666－3671.］

# 霍山石斛的 PCR - RFLP 鉴别研究

霍山石斛来源于石斛属植物霍山石斛 *Dendrobiumhuoshanense* C.Z. Tang et S.J. Cheng 的新鲜或干燥茎，分布于安徽霍山及邻近地区，具有益精强阴、生津止渴、养胃清热之功效，长于润喉清音。霍山石斛因物种名贵、价格较高、有利可图，许多商家把铁皮石斛、铜皮石斛等宣传成霍山石斛进行销售；部分不良商家仿冒霍山石斛“枫斗”加工方法，把小的铁皮石斛、紫皮石斛、河南石斛等加工成霍山石斛独有的龙头凤尾形状，即使业内人士也很难辨认，其伪品产量日益增大，市场混乱。

由于霍山石斛资源匮乏，霍山石斛的物质基础研究薄弱，无法建立专属的薄层色谱和高效液相色谱等理化鉴别方法。目前人们主要通过传统的性状鉴别和显微鉴别方法来区分霍山石斛及其混伪品，但石斛的种类繁多，在实际工作中，很难通过外观性状和显微鉴别霍山石斛和其近源种石斛，迫切需要建立快捷而简便的真伪品鉴定方法。近年来，学者们对聚合酶链反应-限制性内切酶酶切长度多态性（polymerase chain reaction-restriction fragment length polymorphism, PCR - RFLP）的研究突飞猛进，并广泛应用于中药的真伪鉴定与质量评价等相关研究。PCR - RFLP 鉴别法即在 PCR 的基础上，对特异片段进行切割，如果酶切位点发生了突变，便不能被切割，可以通过琼脂糖凝胶电泳法检测。本研究建立了霍山石斛的 PCR - RFLP 鉴别方法，为霍山石斛的质量控制提供了一种新的分析方法。

## 1 材料与方法

1.1 *仪器* GeneAmp 9700、Veriti 和 PTC - 100PCR 仪（Applied Biosystem 公司和 Gene 公司），Gel Doc XR＋凝胶成像系统（Bio-Rad 公司），PowerPac 电泳仪（Bio-Rad 公司），ML204 万分之一电子分析天平（Mettler 公司），Milli-Q 纯水仪（Millipore 公司），Vortex-Genie 2 旋涡振荡仪（Scientific industries 公司），Centrifuge 5418 离心机（Eppendrof 公司）。

1.2 *试剂* TSpeedStar HS Taq（Takara 公司）；10000× Genegreen 核酸染料（TianGen 公司）；DL2000 DNA Marker（Takara 公司）；*Alu* I 限制性内切酶（NEB 公司）；聚乙烯吡咯烷酮（Diamond）；牛血清蛋白（绿叶生物公司）；十六烷基三甲基溴化铵（国药集团）；β-巯基乙醇（国药集团）；其他试剂均为国产分析纯。

1.3 *材料* 选取 40 批次霍山石斛药材和 21 种其他石斛药材共 110 批进行 PCR - RFLP 鉴别研究，见表 1。

表 1 试验材料详表

| 编号 | 材料名称 | 批次 |
|---|---|---|
| 1 | 霍山石斛 *D. huoshanense* | 40 |
| 2 | 铁皮石斛 *D. officinale* | 15 |
| 3 | 细茎石斛 *D. moniliforme* | 15 |
| 4 | 河南石斛 *D. hennanense* | 2 |
| 5 | 鼓槌石斛 *D. chrysotoxum* | 5 |
| 6 | 齿瓣石斛 *D. devonianum* | 5 |
| 7 | 金草石斛 *D. clavatum* | 1 |
| 8 | 金耳石斛 *D. hookerianum* | 1 |
| 9 | 罗河石斛 *D. lohohense* | 1 |
| 10 | 美花石斛 *D. loddigesii* | 1 |
| 11 | 疏花石斛 *D. henryi* | 1 |
| 12 | 杯鞘石斛 *D. gratiosissimum* | 1 |
| 13 | 金钗石斛 *D. nobile* | 5 |
| 14 | 流苏石斛 *D. fimbriatum* | 5 |
| 15 | 兜唇石斛 *D. aphyllum* | 1 |
| 16 | 球花石斛 *D. thyrsiflorum* | 2 |
| 17 | 束花石斛 *D. chrysanthum* | 2 |
| 18 | 晶帽石斛 *D. crystallinum* | 2 |
| 19 | 长苏石斛 *D. brymerianum* | 2 |
| 20 | 尖刀唇石斛 *D. heterocarpum* | 1 |
| 21 | 报春石斛 *D. polyanthum* | 1 |
| 22 | 肿节石斛 *D. pendulum* | 1 |

## 2 实验方法

2.1 *差异限制性酶切位点的获得和 PCR 引物设计* 通过 RAD（restriction site associated DNA）测序技术对包含细茎石斛复合体所有物种在内的 22 种石斛样品进行测序分析，利用 BioEdit 软件进行同源对齐，手动矫正后分别分析霍山石斛和近源种石斛的 SNP 位点。使用 Primer Premier 5.0 软件设计霍山石斛特异性鉴别引物。

2.2 *基因组总 DNA 提取* 使用改良 CTAB 法进行石斛药材基因组总 DNA 的提取，方法如下：取石斛药材 1 g，置于粉碎机中研磨粉碎，过 40 目筛；称取 0.05 g 粉末转移至 2.0 mL 的微量离心管中，加入已高压灭菌的 CTAB（十六烷基三甲基溴化铵）沉淀液 1000 μL、PVP 40 粉末 0.02 g、β-巯基乙醇 10 μL，混匀，65 ℃ 水浴保温 20 min，离心（转速为 12000 r/min）10 min，弃上层清液。沉淀加入已高压灭菌的 CTAB 沉淀液 1000 μL，混匀，再 65 ℃ 水浴保温 5 min，离心（12000 r/min）5 min，弃上层清液，重复此步骤 2～4 次。沉淀加入已灭菌的 CTAB 提取液 1000 μL、PVP 40 粉末 0.02 g、β-巯基乙醇 10 μL，混匀，65 ℃ 水浴保温 30 min，加入氯仿-异戊醇(24∶1)900 μL,充分振荡混匀,离心(12 000 r/min)10 min。转移 750 μL 上层清液至另一新的 2.0 mL 微量离心管中,加入氯仿-异戊醇(24∶1)750 μL,充分振荡混匀,离心(12 000 r/min)10 min。转移 500 μL 上层清液至另一新的 2.0 mL 微量离心管中,加入异丙醇溶液 330 μL,置 −20 ℃放置 0.5 h。取出,离心(转速为 12 000 r/min)10 min,弃上层清液,沉淀用 70%(体积分数)乙醇洗涤 2 次,37 ℃挥干乙醇,用灭菌水 100 μL 溶解,即得基因组总 DNA,−20 ℃密闭保存待用。

2.3 PCR - RFLP 分析

2.3.1 PCR 扩增 本试验采用 25 μL PCR 扩增反应体系,包括 10×PCR 缓冲液 2.5 μL,dNTP(2.5 mmol/L)1 μL,*Taq* DNA 聚合酶(5 U/L)0.3 μL 和模板 2 μL,上下游鉴别引物各 0.2 μL,10 mg/mL 牛血清蛋白 0.5 μL,25%聚乙烯吡咯烷酮 0.2 μL,无菌超纯水 18.1 μL。反应程序见表 2。取反应产物 5 μL,加入 6×Loading buffer 2 μL,混匀后于 Genegreen 染色的 1.5%琼脂糖凝胶电泳检测,SYNGENE 凝胶成像系统成像。

**表 2 引物及 PCR 反应条件**

| 引物名 | 序列(5′-3′) | 反应条件 |
|---|---|---|
| HuoShan - F | ATTCTTCATCAAGTTTAGTGCATTC | 95 ℃预变性 5 min;95 ℃变性 10 s,56 ℃退火 10 s,72 ℃延伸 20 s,45 个循环;72 ℃延伸 5 min |
| HuoShan - R | AGAGCTGATGGGCCTTTGA | |

2.3.2 RFLP 分析 另取石斛及其混伪品 PCR 产物进行 RFLP 分析,反应总体系为 20 μL,反应体系包括 10×酶切缓冲液 2.0 μL,PCR 反应液 17.5 μL,*Alu* I(10 U/μL)0.5 μL。酶切反应在 37 ℃水浴反应 0.5 h。取反应产物 5 μL,加入 6×Loading buffer 2 μL,混匀后于 Genegreen 染色的 1.5%琼脂糖凝胶电泳检测,SYNGENE 凝胶成像系统成像。

2.4 条件考察 在确定单对引物对相应石斛药材的特异性 PCR 条件后,对可能影响 PCR 鉴别准确性和稳定性的主要条件进行考察,包括循环数、退火温度、不同仪器、DNA 模板量、酶切时间、冻融稳定性、适用性。

## 3 结果

3.1 差异限制性酶切位点的获得和 PCR 引物设计 通过对霍山石斛和近缘种石斛的序列比对分析,发现霍山石斛与其混伪品在 Tag C12722046 的序列上存在一个 T/G 的 SNP 位点,其中霍山石斛为 T,混伪品均为 G,此位点位于 *Alu* I 限制性内切酶识别序列(5′…AG^CT…3′)上,通过特异性酶切可以使得混伪品可被切开,霍山石斛无法切开。设计霍山石斛鉴别引物 5′- ATTCTTCATCAAGTTTAGTGCATTC - 3′和 5′- AGAGCTGATGGGCCTTTGA - 3′,依次命名为 HuoShan. F 和 HuoShan. R。该引物可使酶切前后片段长度差异相对较大,大小在 100~250 bp 之间,便于对凝胶电泳条带进行区分。见图 1。

3.2 条件考察结果 考察结果见表 3。

3.2.1 循环数 取霍山石斛及其近伪品,使用霍山石斛鉴别引物进行 PCR 扩增。设定不同的循环数进行扩增,结果在 35 循环时条带黯淡不可见,40 循环时可见微弱条带,45 循环时所有样品均扩增获得较明亮条带,最终确定循环数 45 进行鉴别反应。见图 2。

3.2.2 退火温度 取霍山石斛及其近伪品,使用霍山石斛鉴别引物进行 PCR 扩增。分别设定退火温度为 52~58 ℃进行 PCR 反应,结果 52~58 ℃时均能扩增获得明亮条带,各温度下条带无明显区别。最终确定 56 ℃作为 PCR 退火温度。见图 3。

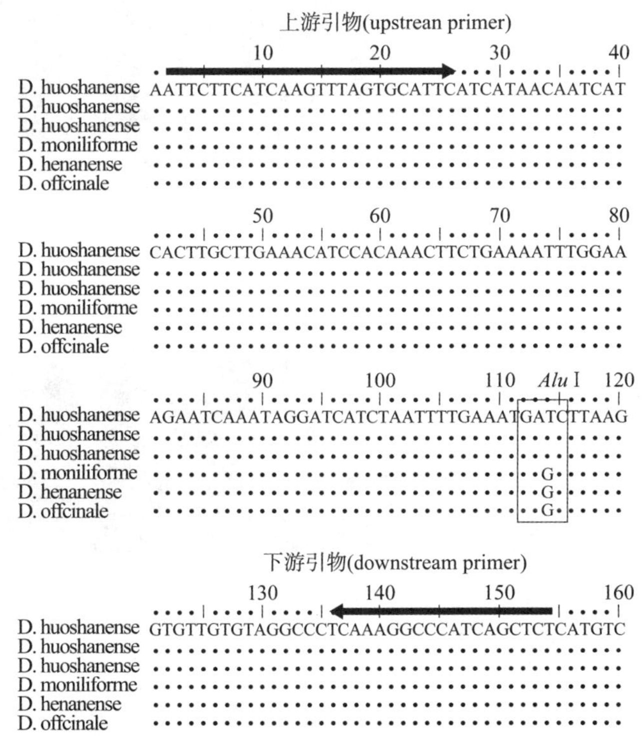


**图 1 霍山石斛 PCR - RFLP 引物设计结果**

**表 3 霍山石斛 PCR - RFLP 条件考察结果**

| 参数 | 参数值 | 最优条件 |
|---|---|---|
| 循环数 | 35、40、45 | 45 |
| 退火温度(℃) | 52、54、56、58 | 56 |
| PCR 仪 | ABI 9700、Veriti、PTC - 100 | 均可使用 |
| DNA 模板量(ng) | 1、5、10、25 | 25 |
| 酶切时间(min) | 15、30、120、240 | 30 |

3.2.3 PCR 仪器选择 霍山石斛及其近伪品,使用霍山石斛鉴别引物进行 PCR 扩增。分别用 ABI 9700、Veriti 以及 PTC - 100 型基因扩增仪进行 PCR 扩增,结果表明霍山石斛及其伪品均能扩增得到 153 bp 的亮带。见图 4。

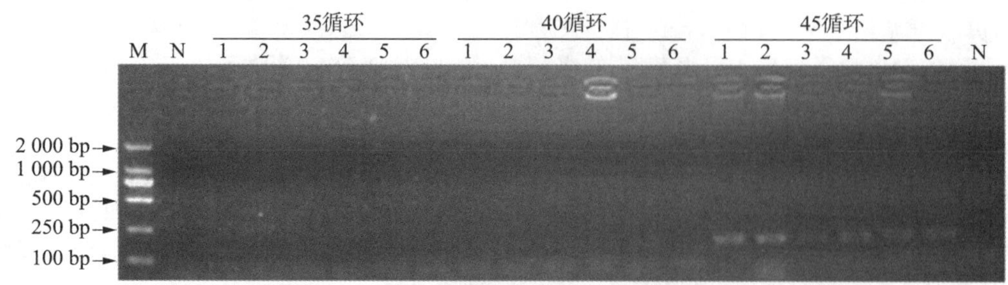


**图 2 不同循环数对霍山石斛 PCR 鉴别结果的影响**

M. marker；1、2. 霍山石斛(*D. huoshanense*)；3、4. 铁皮石斛(*D. officinale*)；5、6. 细茎石斛(*D. moniliforme*)。

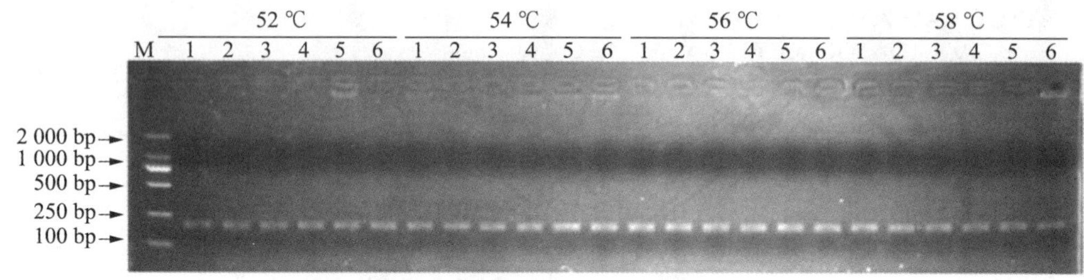


**图 3 不同退火温度对霍山石斛 PCR 鉴别结果的影响**

M .marker；1、2. 霍山石斛(*D. huoshanense*)；3、4. 铁皮石斛(*D. officinale*)；5、6. 细茎石斛(*D. moniliforme*)。

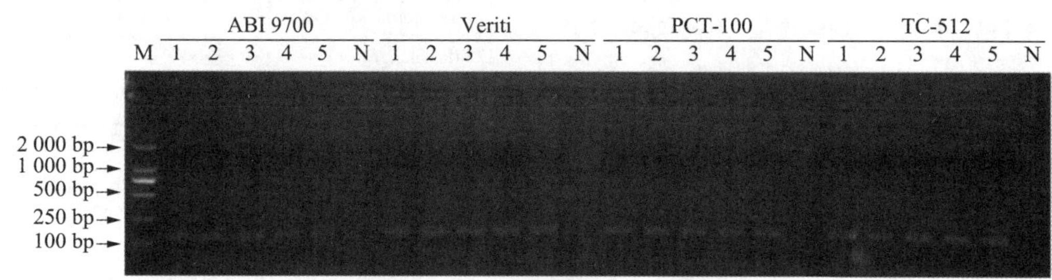


**图 4 不同仪器对霍山石斛 PCR 鉴别结果的影响**

M. marker；1、2. 霍山石斛(*D. huoshanense*)；3、4. 铁皮石斛(*D. officinale*)；5. 细茎石斛(*D. moniliforme*)；N. 空白对照。

3.2.4 DNA 模板量 取霍山石斛及其近伪品提取的 DNA，稀释成不同浓度。使用霍山石斛鉴别引物进行 PCR 扩增，设定 PCR 循环数为 45，退火温度为 56℃进行 PCR 扩增，结果 1～5 ng 时，PCR 扩增量小，条带不清晰；每个 PCR 体系中 DNA 模板量在 10 ng 以上时，能扩出较明亮条带；DNA 在 25 ng 模板量时获得明亮条带。见图 5。

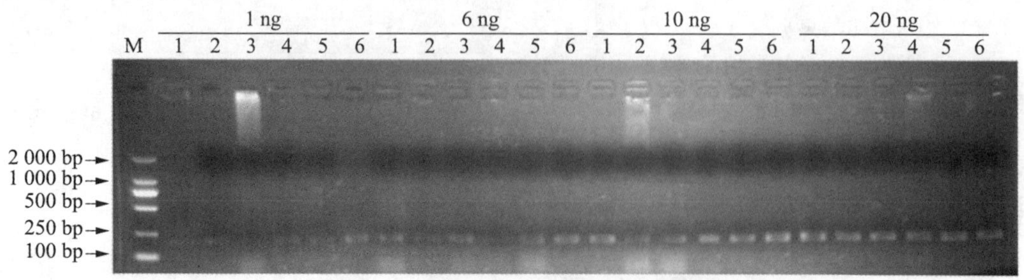


**图 5 不同 DNA 浓度对霍山石斛 PCR 鉴别结果的影响**

M. marker；1～2. 霍山石斛(*D. huoshanense*)；3、4. 铁皮石斛(*D. officinale*)；5、6. 细茎石斛(*D. moniliforme*)。

在确定 PCR 条件的同时，对酶切条件进行了考察。取霍山石斛和铁皮石斛各 2 个进行 PCR 扩增，并取扩增产物进行酶切反应；取 *Alu* I 限制性内切酶进行酶切，设定酶切时间为 10～240 min。结果不同酶切时间下霍山石斛均不能酶切，为约 150 bp 的单一条带；而铁皮石斛均被酶切为 2 条带（其中 1 条大小约 40 bp，凝胶电泳不可见），未出现星活性现象。为达到最佳酶切效果，取中间的 30 min 作为酶切时间。见图 6。

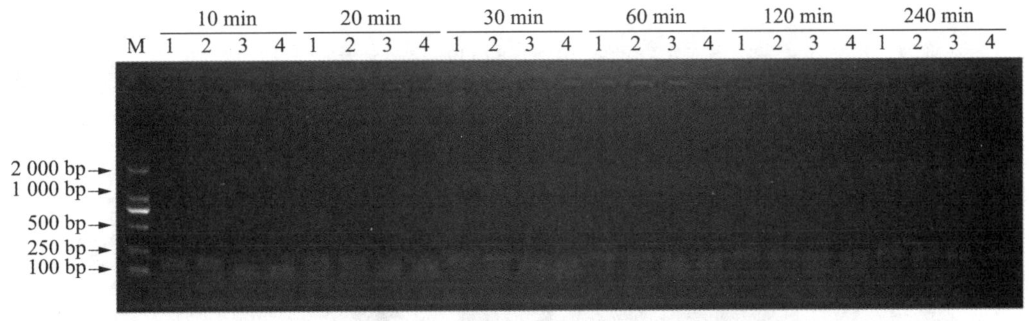


**图 6　不同酶切时间对霍山石斛 PCR 鉴别结果的影响**

M. marker；1、2. 霍山石斛（*D. huoshanense*）；3、4. 铁皮石斛（*D. officinale*）。

3.2.5　重复性考察　取 3 批霍山石斛样品，提取 DNA，配制 PCR 扩增体系，进行 PCR 鉴别测试。结果，对于 PCR 体系的重复性考察电泳结果而言，经 10 次 PCR 扩增试验重复，电泳结果皆一致，说明此方法重复性好。见图 7。

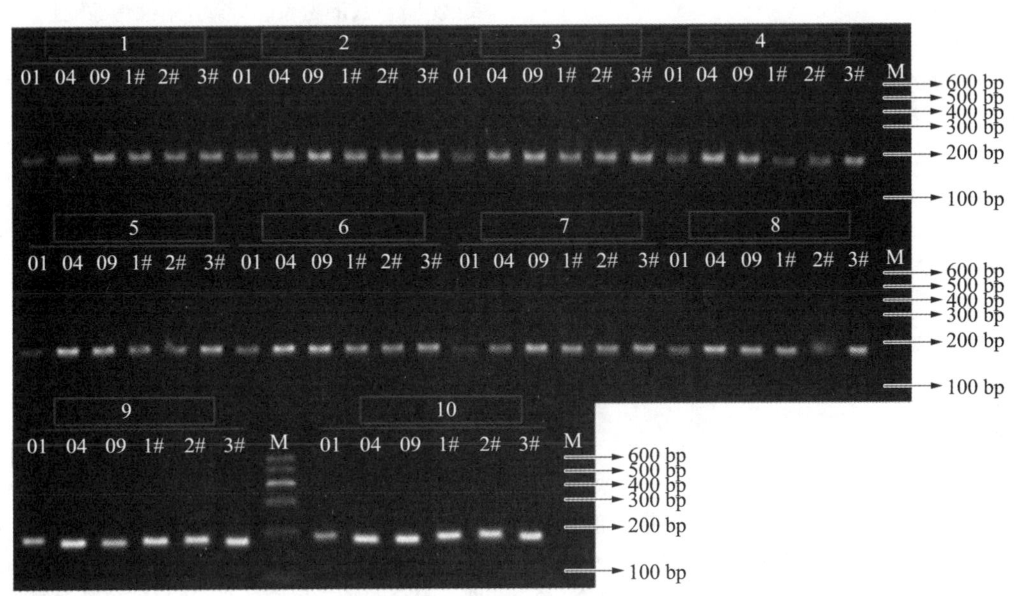


**图 7　重复性考察电泳结果**

3.2.6　冻融稳定性考察　取 3 批霍山石斛样品，提取 DNA，配制 PCR 扩增体系，反复冻融 1、2、3、4、5、6、7、8 次后进行 PCR 鉴别测试。结果对于霍山石斛 3 份正伪品 DNA 的 PCR 扩增，PCR 体系在反复冻融 8 次时仍能与冻融一次的结果一致，皆扩增出条带亮度一致的目的条带，目的条带大小为 153 bp，说明此 PCR 扩增体系反复冻融性好。见图 8。

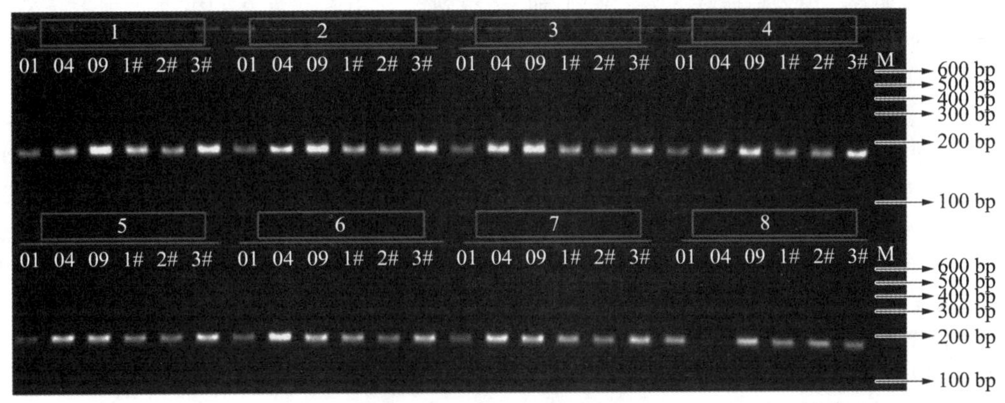


**图 8　冻融稳定性考察电泳结果**

3.3 方法适用性考察 采用上述确定的优化体系，对收集的霍山石斛和近伪品样品进行扩增，不同种类、来源石斛均可产生约 153 bp 条带，经 *Alu* Ⅰ酶切后，近伪品均产生大小约为 113 bp 和 40 bp 的 2 条条带，而正品霍山石斛均无法酶切；表明该体系能稳定、准确地鉴别霍山石斛。典型图谱见图 9。

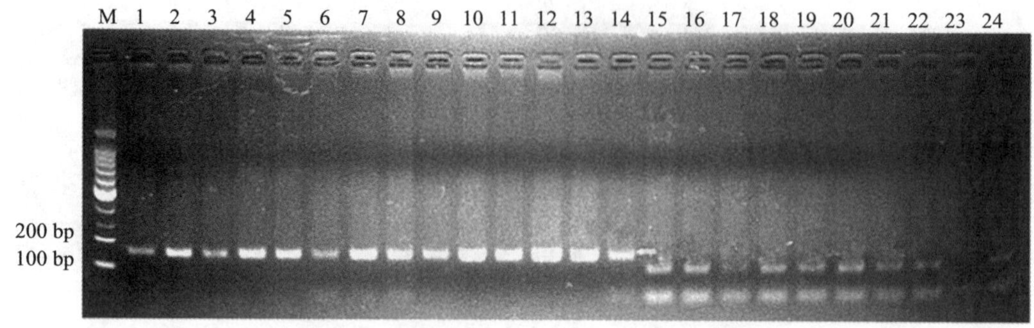


**图 9 霍山石斛及其近伪品典型鉴别图谱**

M. marker；1～14. 霍山石斛（*D. huoshanense*）；15～24. 霍山石斛的近伪品（near-forgery of *D. huoshanense*）。

## 4 讨论

DNA 提取一直是石斛类药材分子鉴定的难点。石斛中含有大量的多糖，在 DNA 提取过程中很难与 DNA 分离。本实验采用改良 CTAB 法提取石斛类样品的 DNA，首先将多糖类成分去除，可以提取纯度较高的 DNA 模板。

本试验共收集霍山石斛及其近伪品 110 批作为研究样本，通过简易基因组测序、引物的设计、DNA 提取方法的改良、实验参数的考察、系统适用性考察，建立了霍山石斛的分子鉴别方法。结果表明，本实验建立的 PCR - RFLP 方法可以有效鉴别霍山石斛的真伪。

［胡冲，张亚中，等. 药物分析杂志，2020，40(12)：2109 - 2115.］

# 《中国药典》聚合酶链式反应法的建立

聚合酶链式反应（polymerase chain reaction，PCR）是一种用于扩增 DNA 片段的分子生物学技术，可以指数形式扩增极其微量的 DNA，对检测样品要求低、操作简便，具有高特异性、高灵敏度、高效率和高忠实度，目前已广泛用于动物、植物、微生物鉴别以及重组制品特性评价和质量控制，并在法医、生物医学、食品科学、农业科学、检验检疫、动植物分类与鉴别等领域快速发展。

目前使用 PCR 技术鉴别生物基原、动植物品种、种质纯度、微生物检验检疫等的国家标准、行业标准及地方标准已超过 470 项，其中多项标准涉及药用物种种属来源的鉴别，如“GB/T 21106 动物源性饲料中鹿源性成分定性检测方法 PCR 方法”“HS/T 13 牛、羊、鹿源性成分鉴别方法 实时荧光 PCR 方法”“SN/T 3033 燕窝的分子生物学鉴别方法 实时荧光 PCR 法和双向电泳法”“SN/T 3957 冬虫夏草真伪鉴别 实时荧光 PCR 方法”“SN/T 4452 出口虎、豹、狮源性成分定性检测方法 PCR - RFLP 方法”等。除各物种鉴别标准外，国家标准化管理委员会也发布了食品、农业、微生物检验检疫等领域 PCR 相关总则或规程。

2010 年蕲蛇、乌梢蛇 PCR 鉴别方法被收载于《中国药典》一部，川贝母 PCR - RFLP 方法被收载于 2010 年版《中国药典》增补本，金钱白花蛇 PCR 鉴别方法被收载于 2015 年版《中国药典》增补本，霍山石斛 PCR - RFLP 方法被收载于 2020 年版《中国药典》。随着 PCR 相关技术研究的深入与普及，国家药典委员会讨论通过在 2020 年版《中国药典》四部中列入聚合酶链式反应法，该通则是在对大量中药、生化药原料药鉴别研究的实验基础上，参照现行《中国药典》标准及国家、行业、团体标准及其他国外药典标准部分研究成果拟定形成。涉及的工作包括如下 4 项。

第一，《中国药典》一部收载的蕲蛇 PCR 鉴别法、乌梢蛇 PCR 鉴别法、金钱白花蛇 PCR 鉴别法、川贝母 PCR - RFLP 鉴别法、霍山石斛 PCR - RFLP 鉴别法。

第二，《中国药典》三部收载的生物制品生产检定用动物细胞基质制备及检定规程、皮内注射用卡介苗多重 PCR 鉴别试验、乙型脑炎减毒活疫苗转录酶活性检查法、注射用重组人白细胞介素 - 11（酵母）基因稳定性检查、重组乙型肝炎疫苗（汉逊酵母）种子批菌种、重组人表皮生长因子凝胶（酵母）、重组人表皮生长因子滴眼液（酵母）菌种来源的检定。

第三，《中国药典》四部收载的通则 3304 SV40 核酸序列检查法、通则 3306 血液制品生产用人血浆病毒核酸检测技术要求、指导原则 9107 中药材 DNA 条形码分子鉴定法指导原则。

第四，其他标准包括国家标准“GB/T 34408 - 2017 天然皮革牛、羊、猪源性成分定性 PCR 检测方法”“GB/T 25165－2010 明胶中牛、羊、猪源性成分的定性检测方法 实时荧光 PCR 法”“CB/T 21101－2007 动物源性饲料中猪源性成分定性检测方法 PCR 方法”等；《美国药典》（USP 40 指导原则 1125－1127）、《欧洲药典》（EP 9.0 通则 2.6.21）、《英国药典附录ⅩⅣ》《日本药典》（JP 17 基本信息）；行业标准“SN/T 1119－2002 进口动物源性饲料中牛、羊源性成分检测方法 PCR 方法”；中华中医药学会团体标准“中药分子鉴定通则”“金银花快速 PCR 鉴定”“金钱白花蛇快速 PCR 鉴定”等。

本文介绍了 2020 年版《中国药典》聚合酶链式反应法（通则 1001）起草说明，并对该通则在中药、生化药等应用前景进行展望，为中药材、生化药准确、可靠鉴别及其他药品检定提供基本规范。

## 1 聚合酶链式反应法定义及原理

PCR 是指 DNA 片段的特异性体外扩增过程，其特异性依赖于与目的 DNA 片段两端互补的寡核苷酸引物。PCR 基本原理为双链 DNA 在高温下发生变性解链成为单链 DNA，当温度降低后又可以复性成双链，通过温度变化控制 DNA 的变性和复性，加入引物、DNA 聚合酶、脱氧核糖核苷三磷酸（dNTP）及相应缓冲液，完成特定 DNA 片段的体外复制。

PCR 法按原理和用途可分为常规 PCR 法、实时定量 PCR 法（quantitative real-time PCR，qPCR）等。常规 PCR 法系利用供试品中一段特征 DNA 片段设计引物进行 PCR 扩增，并通过比较供试品组和对照组 PCR 产物片段大小或数量进行结果判定的核酸检测方法，也可结合限制性内切酶酶切多态性技术（restriction fragment length polymorphism，RFLP）、片段分析或核酸测序技术对扩增产物进行测定，主要用于动、植物源性中药材和饮片，原材料，中间体，原料药与辅料等种属鉴别，也可用于其他药品质量控制中特征 DNA 片段的检定。

## 2 PCR 法通则起草说明

2.1 *仪器一般要求的依据* 所用仪器包括电子天平、离心机、冰箱、恒温仪、紫外分光光度仪、可对温度进行连续控制并实现核酸指数级扩增的 PCR 仪、具有稳压直流电源和平板电泳槽电泳仪、紫外凝胶成像仪（或紫外透射仪）等。仪器应定期进行校准。

使用 PCR 法进行测定的一般步骤包括样品前处理和 DNA 提取、PCR 反应、凝胶电泳与凝胶成像等。电子天平用于样品前处理时的取样称量，离心机主要用于 DNA 提取过程中的固液分离和柱纯化分离，冰箱用于 DNA、酶的保存，恒温仪用于 DNA 提取时的孵育，紫外分光光度计用于 DNA 浓度和质量的测定，PCR 仪用于 PCR 扩增，具有稳压直流电源和平板电泳槽电泳仪用于凝胶电泳，紫外凝胶成像仪（或紫外透射仪）用于凝胶成像，上述仪器均为进行 PCR 必不可少的仪器。

2.2 *样品前处理依据* 药品种类众多、形态多样，来源于动物、植物、微生物的不同部位，具有异质性；且垂体后叶素、肝素钠等动物源性生化药原材料、中间体、原料药与辅料的形态、性质也不同，取样方法存在差异。

由于 PCR 样品用量小，首先应通过一定手段对样品进行均质处理。由于不同中药、动物源性生化药原辅料、中间体性质不一，取样部位和取样量应根据样本进行分别规定，中药材需按药材和饮片取样法（通则 0211）取样。由于药材表面往往具有细菌、霉菌、其他药材附着、污染物等情况，且可能存在样品间交叉污染，应先去除外源污染和附着物，依次使用 75%乙醇和无菌双蒸水擦拭表面后晾干，以确保供试品准确性。动物源性生化药品原辅料、中间体可根据样本来源和样本类型适当处理后取样，如骨骼、全蝎等可参照药材和饮片取样法取样，血清等液体样品在取样前应充分混匀。

供试品通常使用液氮研磨和组织研磨仪进行粉碎，液氮研磨可使样品保持低温状态，防止 DNA 降解，而组织研磨仪可同时粉碎多份样品，可有效避免样品间的交叉污染，粉碎粒度小，均质性强。由于 PCR 鉴别具有很高的灵敏度，供试品前处理应严格与其他区域隔离并严格防止交叉污染。进行 PCR 法的实验室应满足实验室分区要求，实验室要求可参考国家标准“GB/T 27403－2008 实验室质量控制规范 食品分子生物学检测”。

2.3 *模板 DNA 制备方法选择依据* 获得高质量 DNA 是 PCR 法成功的前提，提取的 DNA 应符合 PCR 反应及其产物检测的要求，即 DNA 含量、完整性、纯度应满足扩增、酶切和电泳检查等步骤的要求。常用的药品 DNA 提取方法包括十六烷基三甲基溴化铵（cetyltriethyl-ammnonium bromide，CTAB）法、十二烷基硫酸钠（sodium dodecyl sulfate，SDS）法、DNA 碱裂解法等。其中 CTAB 法可通过调整提取缓冲液中盐浓度去除 DNA 中的多糖、蛋白质、色素及多酚类杂质，且可通过增加聚乙烯吡咯烷酮（PVP）及 β-巯基乙醇的含量来防止植物细胞中多酚类物质的氧化。SDS 法可通过调整 SDS 浓度和蛋白酶 K 含量对骨类、角甲类、壳类药品进行 DNA 提取。与 CTAB 和 SDS 法相比，DNA 碱裂解法的试剂组成简单、操作步骤少，且不需要使用酚等有毒试剂，被认为是一种具有良好前景的药品快速 DNA 提取方法。在 DNA 提取过程中，也可以采用基于上述或其他原理的等效 DNA 提取试剂盒，目前常用试剂盒多采用硅胶膜离心柱法。

2.3.1 *中药材和饮片* 由于中药材所含成分复杂，且在标准研制过程中发现不同供试品需要选择合适的 DNA 提取方法才能达到最佳 DNA 提取效果，如川贝母 PCR－RFLP 鉴别使用了新型植物基因组提取试剂盒，蕲蛇和乌梢蛇一般使用动物基因组 DNA 提取试剂盒进行 DNA 提取。为确保通则的通用性和规范性，对 DNA 提取方法仅给予原则性的规定，即要求模板 DNA 的质量和浓度应满足核酸扩增的基本要求，原则上模板 DNA 质量浓度宜不低于 10 ng/μL，$A_{260}/A_{280}$ 宜在 1.8～2.0。

2.3.2 *动物源性生化药品* 目前多种商品化试剂盒可用于动物源性生化药品 DNA 的提取纯化，应根据样品类型（如固体或液体样品，细胞或非细胞样品等）选择适用的提取方法与试剂盒。对于部分 DNA 含量极低或含有大量 PCR 反应抑制成分（如蛋白质等）的原材料或辅料，可根据样品特点进行合适前处理后，采用商品化试剂盒提取基因组 DNA。原则上动物源性生化药品模板 DNA 质量浓度宜不低于 10 ng/μL，$A_{260}/A_{280}$ 宜在 1.8～2.0，但对于小牛血清、糜蛋白酶原等DNA含量极低的样品，在不影响后续PCR反应的前提下，可不要求准确测定 $A_{260}$ 及 $A_{280}$。若DNA提取液的浓度过低，需相应地加大取样量或减少最终DNA产物的溶解体积。

2.4 引物选择的依据

2.4.1 中药材和饮片 特异性PCR反应鉴别法是《中国药典》收载中药材和饮片PCR检测的主要方法，其原理是根据正伪品药材间碱基存在差异的一段特定区域DNA序列，设计特异性的正品鉴别引物，建立PCR反应及其产物检测方法，根据凝胶电泳条带的大小及有无区分正品和伪品，从而实现中药材及饮片的鉴别。

《中国药典》蕲蛇、乌梢蛇饮片、金钱白花蛇项下收载的PCR鉴别法，其原理属特异性PCR反应鉴别法。除此之外，该方法还已广泛应用于龟甲、鹿茸、蜈蚣、蛤蚧、鸡内金等动物药材及饮片；人参、西洋参、太子参、三七、前胡、半夏、大黄、白及、黄芪、贝母、何首乌、泽泻等根和根茎类，西红花、金银花等花类，木通、杜仲、紫苏、石斛等茎类，莱菔子、紫苏子、菟丝子、白术种子等种子类，麻黄、淫羊藿、薄荷等全草类药材和饮片的鉴别。

由于中药材和饮片PCR法中每种正品或正品的每个基原均需根据其基原物种特征设计特异性引物，具体引物序列不做统一规定，需依照品种项下要求。《中国药典》已收载中药PCR鉴别品种及其引物序列见表1。

**表1 《中国药典》收载中药PCR鉴别引物**

| 品种 | 方法名称 | 收载时间 | 上游引物序列（5′-3′） | 下游引物序列（5′-3′） | 产物大小（bp） |
|---|---|---|---|---|---|
| 蕲蛇 | PCR | 2010年版 | GGCAATTCACTACACAGCCAACATCAACT | CCATAGTCAGGTGGTTAGTGATAC | 342 |
| 乌梢蛇 | PCR | 2010年版 | GCGAAAGCTCGACCTAGCAAGGGGACCACA | CAGGCTCCTCTAGGTTGTTATGGGGTACCG | 351 |
| 川贝母 | PCR-RFLP | 2010年版第一增补本 | CGTAACAAGGTTTCCGTAGGTGAA | GCTACGTTCTTCATCGAT | 306～308 |
| 金钱白花蛇 | PCR | 2015年版第一增补本 | GAAATTTCGGCTCTATGCTTATAACCTGTCTTT | GGAATCTTATCGATATCTGAATTAGTA | 565 |
| 霍山石斛 | PCR-RFLP | 2020年版 | ATTCTTCATCAAGTTTAGTGCATTC | AGAGCTGATGGGCCTTTGA | 153 |

2.4.2 动物源性生化药品 参考"GB/T 21101-2007 动物源性饲料中猪源性成分定性检测方法 PCR方法""SN/T 1119-2002 进口动物源性饲料中牛、羊源性成分检测方法 PCR方法"以及GenBank公共核酸数据库等资料，确定猪、牛、羊源性成分鉴别引物，序列见表2。

**表2 动物源性生化药品猪、牛、羊源性成分鉴别引物**

| 用途 | 引物名称 | 靶物种 | 上游引物序列（5′-3′） | 下游引物序列（5′-3′） | 产物大小(bp) |
|---|---|---|---|---|---|
| 猪源性成分鉴别引物 | PidF/PidR | *Sus scrofa domestica* | GCCTAAATCTCCCCTCAATGGTA | GCCTAAATCTCCCCTCAATGGTA | 212 |
| 牛源性成分鉴别引物 | BidF/BidR | *Bos taurus domesticus* | GCCATATACTCTCCTTGGTGACA | GTAGGCTTGGGAATAGTACGA | 271 |
| 羊源性成分鉴别引物 | SidF/SidR | *Ovis aries* | TATTAGGCCTCCCCCTTGTT | CCCTGCTCATAAGGGAATAGCC | 293 |

2.5 核酸扩增方法确定的依据 除另有规定外，核酸扩增可采用PCR反应或PCR-RFLP反应进行。

2.5.1 PCR反应 PCR反应体系和PCR反应条件需要依据各药品特征制定。

一般来说，PCR反应体系应由脱氧核糖核苷三磷酸（dNTPs，含脱氧核糖核苷三磷酸dATP、dCTP、dGTP、dTTP各2.5 mmol/L）、引物溶液（10～30 μmol/L）、耐热 *Taq* DNA聚合酶（具有5′-3′聚合酶活性）1～2.5 U及其缓冲液（含镁离子）、模板和无菌水组成，总体积为25或30 μL。

扩增程序应包括变性、退火、延伸3个基本步骤，还可包括预变性、终延伸。预变性时间一般为94 ℃保温3～5 min，对于鸟嘌呤和胞嘧啶所占比例较高的品种，可适当延长预变性时间至10 min或升高预变性温度至98 ℃。PCR循环可以为3步或2步PCR循环，反应循环次数一般在30～40次，退火温度一般在45～65 ℃。当PCR反应产物长度小于500 bp时，退火延伸时间一般在20～45 s。终延伸温度一般为72 ℃或68 ℃，可根据使用的 *Taq* DNA聚合酶特性决定。特异性PCR对反应条件要求严格，其退火温度、酶量、引物量、循环数、模板浓度、*Taq* 酶种类均可影响鉴别结果。

PCR反应条件的关键参数包括温度、时间和循环次数，基于PCR原理3步骤而设置变性-退火-延伸3个温度点。关键参数与引物序列特征密切相关，特异性PCR引物序列严格依赖于正伪品间碱基存在差异的一段特定区域及其上下游DNA序列特征。反应体系和反应条件需要依据各药材和饮片品种特征制定，《中国药典》已收载中药PCR鉴别引物及其反应条件，见表3。琼脂糖凝胶电泳图谱显示，蕲蛇、乌梢蛇在300～400 bp有1条条带，金钱白花蛇在500～750 bp有1条条带，混伪品无条带，见图1。

**表3 《中国药典》收载中药PCR鉴别法PCR扩增条件**

| 品种 | PCR反应体系 | PCR反应参数 |
|---|---|---|
| 蕲蛇 | 10×PCR缓冲液2.5 μL，dNTP(2.5 mmol/L)2 μL，鉴别引物(10 μmol/L)各0.5 μL，高保真DNA聚合酶(5 U/μL)0.2 μL，模板DNA 0.5 μL，无菌双蒸水18.8 μL | 95℃预变性5 min，循环反应30次(95℃ 30 s，65℃ 45 s)，延伸(72℃)5 min |
| 乌梢蛇 | 10×PCR缓冲液2.5 μL，dNTP(2.5 mmol/L)2 μL，鉴别引物(10 μmol/L)各0.5 μL，高保真DNA聚合酶(5 U/μL)0.2 μL，模板DNA 0.5 μL，无菌双蒸水18.8 μL | 95℃预变性5 min，循环反应30次(95℃ 30 s，65℃ 45 s)，延伸(72℃)5 min |
| 川贝母 | 10×PCR缓冲液3 μL，二氯化镁(25 mmol/L)2.4 μL，dNTP(30 mmol/L)0.6 μL，鉴别引物(30 μmol/L)各0.5 μL，高保真 *Taq* DNA聚合酶(5 U/μL)0.2 μL，模板DNA 1 μL，无菌超纯水21.8 μL | 95℃预变性4 min，循环反应30次(95℃ 30 s，55～58℃ 30 s，72℃ 30 s)，72℃延伸5 min |
| 金钱白花蛇 | 10×PCR缓冲液2.5 μL，dNTP(10 mmol/L)1 μL，鉴别引物(10 μmol/L)各0.2 μL，*Taq* DNA聚合酶(5 U/μL)0.2 μL，模板DNA 1 μL，25%聚乙烯吡咯烷酮1 μL，10 g/L牛血清蛋白0.5 μL，无菌双蒸水18.4 μL | 95℃预变性5 min，循环反应30次(95℃ 30 s，60℃ 45 s)，延伸(72℃)5 min |
| 霍山石斛 | 10×PCR缓冲液2.5 μL，dNTP(10 mmol/L)1 μL，鉴别引物(10 μmol/L)各0.2 μL，*Taq* DNA聚合酶(5 U/μL)0.2 μL，10 g/L牛血清蛋白1 μL，25%聚乙烯吡咯烷酮1 μL，模板1 μL，无菌超纯水18.4 μL | 95℃预变性5 min，循环反应40次(95℃ 10 s，56℃ 20 s，72℃ 20 s)，72℃延伸5 min |

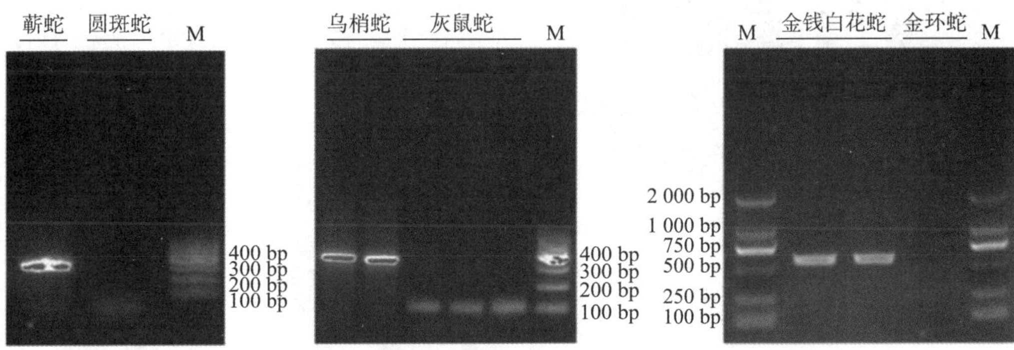


**图1 蕲蛇、乌梢蛇、金钱白花蛇PCR鉴别**

M. DNA相对分子质量标准(图2～4同)。

动物源性生化药品猪、牛、羊源性成分鉴别PCR反应体系和反应参数为：①PCR反应体系，2×PCR预混液12.5 μL，引物(2.5 mmol/L，鉴别引物(10 μmol/L)各0.5 mL，模板DNA 10 μL，灭菌水1.5 μL。②PCR反应参数，95℃预变性5 min，循环反应35次(95℃ 30 s，57℃ 30 s，72℃ 30 s)，72℃延伸5 min。使用该条件对小牛脾匀浆、小牛血清、垂体后叶粉、糜蛋白酶原、玻璃酸酶、肝素钠等样品的种属来源进行PCR测定，结果与经过测序验证的猪、牛、羊对照品结果相一致，在进行牛源性成分种属鉴别时，含有牛源性成分样本在200～300 bp有1条DNA条带，猪、羊样本均无DNA条带；在进行猪源性成分种属鉴别时，含有猪源性成分样本在200～300 bp(近200 bp处)有1条DNA条带，牛、羊样本均无DNA条带；在进行羊源性成分种属鉴别时，含有羊源性成分样本分别在200～300 bp(近300 bp处)有1条DNA条带，牛、猪样本均无DNA条带，见图2。通过对多批次实际样品进行检测，结果均具有良好的特异性、重现性和重复性。

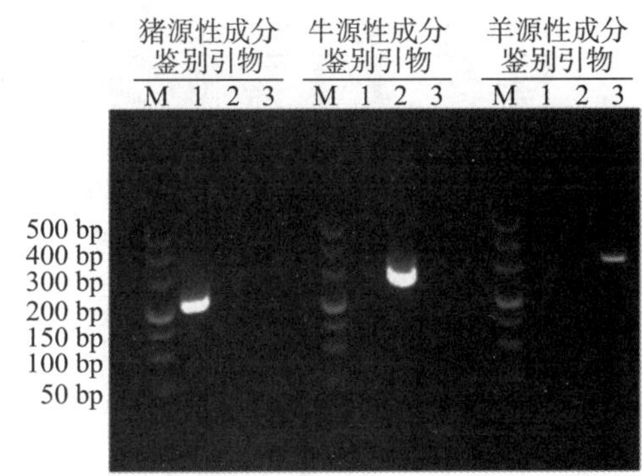


**图2 脾脏匀浆样品猪、牛及羊源性成分PCR鉴别**

1. 牛脾匀浆样品；2. 猪脾匀浆样品；3. 羊脾匀浆样品(图4同)。

2.5.2 PCR-RFLP反应 PCR-RFLP是一种利用

PCR扩增目的DNA片段，再使用特定的核酸内切酶消化扩增产物，通过分析酶切条带大小及多态性，从而检测酶切位点处是否发生突变的一种技术。一般来说，酶切体系由10×酶切缓冲液、限制性内切酶、扩增产物、无菌双蒸水组成，总体积为20～30 μL。由于PCR－RFLP严格依赖于限制性内切酶的种类，即要求鉴别位点位于限制性内切酶的识别序列上，从而导致识别位点的改变。因此需要根据正伪品差异序列特征，选择对应的限制性内切酶种类，以及酶切温度和时间。常规限制性内切酶的酶切反应时间为2～6 h，快速限制性内切酶的酶切反应时间不超过30 min，时间过长容易产生星活性，导致鉴别结果错误。

《中国药典》川贝母、霍山石斛项下收载的聚合酶链式反应-限制性内切酶长度多态性方法，其原理属PCR－RFLP反应鉴别法。此外，该方法还已广泛应用于人参、半夏、何首乌、大黄、石斛、木通、泽泻、绞股蓝、金银花、紫草等中药材鉴别。其步骤主要包括PCR反应和酶切反应，其中PCR反应同特异性PCR反应鉴别法。反应体系和反应条件需要依据各药材和饮片品种特征制定。《中国药典》已收载中药PCR鉴别品种及其酶切反应条件见表4，使用对应限制性内切酶对PCR产物进行酶切，川贝母在100～200 bp有2条条带，霍山石斛在100～200 bp有1条条带，且PCR产物与酶切产物条带位置一致，见图3。

**表4 《中国药典》收载中药PCR鉴别法酶切条件**

| 品种 | 内切酶 | 酶切反应体系 | 酶切反应参数 | 产物大小(bp) |
|---|---|---|---|---|
| 川贝母 | *Sma* Ⅰ | 10×酶切缓冲液2 μL，PCR反应液6 μL，*Sma* Ⅰ内切酶(10 U/μL)0.5 μL，无菌超纯水11.5 μL | 32℃水浴保温2 h | 125＋183 |
| 霍山石斛 | *Alu* Ⅰ | 10×酶切缓冲液2 μL，PCR反应液17.5 μL，*Alu* Ⅰ内切酶(10 U/μL) 0.5 μL | 37℃水浴保温30 min | 113＋40 |

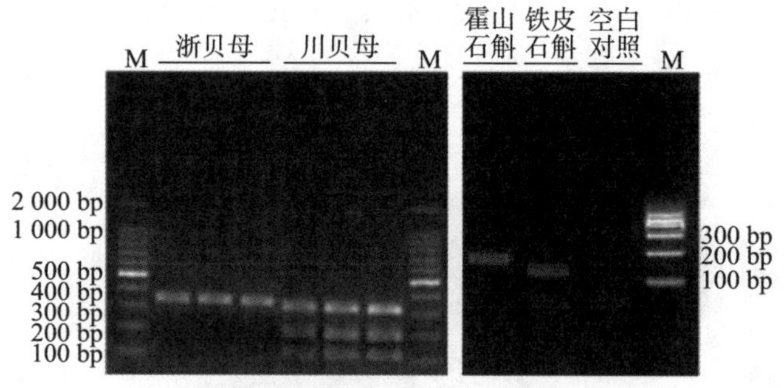


**图3 川贝母、霍山石斛PCR－RFLP鉴别法琼脂糖凝胶电泳图谱**

动物源性生化药品PCR测定时采用PCR－RFLP，其反应条件和酶切条件均通过多批次的实验研究结果确定，见表5。牛、猪、羊源性成分种属鉴别时分别使用BidF/BidR，PidF/PidR，SidF/SidR引物对进行PCR扩增，扩增后取产物，分别使用限制性内切酶*Dpn* Ⅱ，*Mnl* Ⅰ，*Sau*3AI进行酶切，含牛源性成分样本分别在200～300 bp，及50～100 bp(近100 bp)各有1条DNA条带；含猪源性成分样本在150～200 bp有1条DNA条带，含羊源性成分样本在200～300 bp，及50～100 bp各有1条DNA条带，见图4。通过对小牛脾匀浆、小牛血清、垂体后叶粉、糜蛋白酶原、玻璃酸酶、肝素钠等不同批次样品进行检测，其扩增方法和酶切方法均具有良好的重现性和重复性。

**表5 动物源性生化药品猪、牛、羊源性成分鉴别酶切条件**

| 品种 | 内切酶 | 酶切反应体系 | 产物大小/bp |
|---|---|---|---|
| 猪 | *Mnl* Ⅰ | 10×酶切缓冲液2 μL，PCR反应液6 μL，*Mnl* Ⅰ内切酶(10 U/μL) 1 μL，无菌双蒸水11 μL | 198＋16 |
| 牛 | *Dpn* Ⅱ | 10×酶切缓冲液2 μL，PCR反应液10 μL，*Dpn* Ⅱ内切酶(10 U/μL) 1 μL，无菌双蒸水7 μL | 214＋57 |
| 羊 | *Sau*3AI | 10×酶切缓冲液3 μL，PCR反应液17.5 μL，*Sau*3AI内切酶(10 U/μL) 1 μL，无菌双蒸水9.5 μL | 202＋91 |

注：酶切反应参数均为37℃水浴保温1 h。

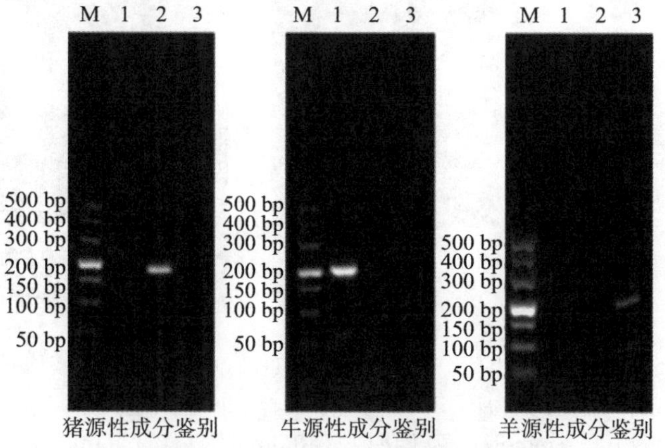


**图4 脾脏匀浆样品猪、牛及羊源性成分鉴别酶切**

2.6 *反应产物检测依据* DNA片段可通过琼脂糖凝胶电泳法进行反应产物检测。大量实验数据证明，琼脂糖凝胶电泳已成为成熟PCR或酶切产物检测技术，PCR反应产物检测采用供试品与对照品/对照药材DNA扩增/酶切产物凝胶电泳结果进行对比的方式进行。由于不同检测批次凝胶电泳迁移速度、迁移时间不同，需要对照DNA相对分子质量标准判断产物片段凝胶电泳迁移位置，DNA相对分子质量标准应含有用于结果判定的相对分子质量条带。琼脂糖凝胶电泳法适合分离片段大小差异为50～1 000 bp的反应产物，根据产物片段大小选择合适浓度的琼脂糖凝胶；对于片段小于1 000 bp的产物，制备的琼脂糖凝胶质量分数应在1%～3%，见表 6。

**表 6 琼脂糖浓度与线性 DNA 片段大小参考表**

| 琼脂糖凝胶质量分数(%) | 分离线性 DNA 的有效范围(bp) |
|---|---|
| 0.7 | 800～12 000 |
| 1 | 500～10 000 |
| 1.2 | 300～7 000 |
| 1.5 | 200～3 000 |
| 2.0 | 50～2 000 |

由于 PCR 鉴别具有很高的灵敏度,为避免在实验过程中由于操作不当引入的外源污染或样品交叉污染,需同时进行对照试验,阳性对照使用对照品或对照药材,阴性对照使用无菌双蒸水,保证实验的可靠性。

2.7 *质量控制要求的依据* 质量控制是检测结果质量保证体系中最重要、最关键的环节之一。由于 PCR 具有极高的灵敏度,能将微量 DNA 模板放大,微量的试剂、器具、耗材、气溶胶或样品交叉污染可能造成假阳性结果;而检测人员的错误操作或试剂、耗材的失效则易造成假阴性结果。

在进行 PCR 检测时应根据《中国药典》通则 3306 要求建立涵盖检测人员、检测实验室、仪器设备、结果质量控制和管理体系的质量控制系统。除酶等具有生物活性的试剂外,或另有规定不能灭菌的试剂外,进行 PCR 检测的试剂与耗材均应根据灭菌法(《中国药典》通则 1421)进行灭菌。实验室生物安全和污染废弃物可根据《实验室生物安全通用要求》(GB 19489)进行处理。在此基础上,还可参考国家标准"GB/T 27403 实验室质量控制规范 食品分子生物学检测"的相关要求。

## 3 方法适用性要求的确定依据

PCR 检测结果受 DNA 聚合酶性质、PCR 仪控温能力、升降温速度及其他条件的影响。在进行 PCR 检测时,应首先进行方法适用性试验,以确认所采用方法适合于该供试品的测定。进行方法适用性确认时,可选择已知含有待测物种成分的样品作为阳性样品,已知不含待测物种成分的样品作为阴性样品,按建立的方法进行操作,阳性样品应在预期位置出现DNA 条带,阴性样品应无 DNA 条带或 DNA 条带数量与位置与预期不一致,空白对照应无条带。若测定条件以及供试品来源、部位、加工、制备工艺、干扰物质、储藏等因素可能影响测定结果时,应重新对所用方法的专属性等进行确认。

方法适用性确认可采用中国合格评定国家认可委员会(China National Accreditation Service for Conformity Assessment, CNAS)、中国计量认证(China Metrology Accreditation, CMA)通常采取的实验室能力验证的方式进行。能力验证通常采用 2 种方式进行:①实验室间比对。②上级实验室样品检测。其核心为上级实验室发布的样本,按照规定的方法学进行检测,看结果偏差是否在可接受的范围。

3.1 *中药材和饮片* PCR 测定的方法适用性确认可选择已知正品和同属(或近缘属)常见混伪品,在不同时间进行 3 次(及以上)试验,正品样本用待确认的方法检测结果应为阳性,混伪品样本检测结果应为阴性,可视为符合方法适用性的要求。

3.2 *动物源性生化药品* 动物源性原材料最主要的物种来源为猪、牛、羊,进行猪源性成分 PCR 测定适用性确认时已知猪源性样本使用待确认的方法检测应为阳性,已知的牛或羊源性样本使用待确认的方法检测应为阴性,牛、羊猪源性成分 PCR 测定方法适用性确认方式同猪源性鉴别。

## 4 展望

PCR 已成为 DNA、RNA 检定方法的基础。PCR 法纳入《中国药典》将进一步规范中药、生化药及生产加工过程中涉及核酸的生物制品、重组产品的种属鉴别和质量控制,在药品的真伪检定、原料药监控、微生物污染管控、进出口管理及检验检疫发挥重要作用。目前 PCR 法多通过凝胶电泳进行定性检测,相信随着 PCR 技术进一步深入和普及,实时荧光定量 PCR 等定量检测技术也有望逐步纳入《中国药典》,形成更加完善的生物核酸检测标准体系。环介导等温扩增技术(loop-mediated isothermal amplification, LAMP)、重组酶辅助扩增技术(recombinase polymerase amplification, RPA)等新型 DNA 扩增技术不断发展,有助于解决 PCR 技术对仪器的依赖问题,应用于中药、生化药品的快速检测。

[袁媛,等. 中国中药杂志,2020,45(19):4537-4543.]

# Analysis of the age of *Panax ginseng* based on telomere length and telomerase activity

Ginseng, which is the root of *Panax ginseng* C. A. Meyer (Araliaceae), has been used in Chinese medicine for thousands of years as a stimulant and dietary supplement. In European and American countries, ginseng phytomedicines have been used to increase physical and mental performance, provide resistance to stress and disease, and prevent exhaustion for decades. Ginseng plants begin flowering in their fourth year, and the roots can live for hundreds of years after maturing at 4 - 6 years of age. The older the root, the higher its medicinal value because of the higher concentration of ginsenosides, which are the active chemical compounds in ginseng. However, chemical analyses often require gram quantities of dried ginseng material, and it is difficult to extract such quantities while leaving the ginseng intact; thus, chemical analysis greatly decreases the ginseng's value. Therefore, effective methods for identifying the age of ginseng roots are urgently needed to improve quality control and protect the interests of ginseng consumers.

Telomeres, which are specialized structures at the physical ends of eukaryotic chromosomes that consist of highly conserved, repeated DNA sequences, shorten with each round of DNA replication because DNA polymerases cannot completely replicate linear DNA molecules. In gymnosperms, telomere length can be used to predict the future replicative capacity of cells. Highly significant correlations between telomere length and age have been observed in humans, Australian sea lions, martins and dunlins and different stages of barley. Therefore, telomere shortening can be used as a marker of cell replication and aging. Telomerase activity has been detected in plants using a polymerase chain reaction (PCR)-based telomerase repeat amplification protocol (TRAP) assay. Telomerase appears to be developmentally regulated in plants, which is similar to what occurs in humans. These reports indicate biological correlations between telomere length and age. However, plant telomeres are maintained by telomerase. Telomere lengths remain stable in tomato leaves, whereas they change cyclically, lengthening and shortening with age, in the needles of *Pinus longaeva*. After the first plant telomere sequence was cloned from *Arabidopsis*, nearly all plant telomeres were found to consist of the heptanucleotide repeat (TTTAGGG) n. *Arabidopsis*-type repeats have also been found in *P. ginseng*. However, researchers have not yet ascertained whether *Arabidopsis*-type repeats are located in telomeres or their relationship with age.

In this study, we combined traditional identification methods and measurements of telomere length in ginseng plants of known age. Preliminary investigations indicated that telomere length was slightly positively correlated with the age of the ginseng plant. Analysis of telomerase activity in different parts of the plant further revealed that the main root was the most active meristematic region. Therefore, we used this tissue to evaluate telomere length. Determination of telomere terminal restriction fragment (TRF) lengths in *P. ginseng* specimens of different ages demonstrated that the telomeres in the main roots showed a significant increase in TRF length with plant age that could be used for age estimation for 2 - 8 years.

## 1 RESULTS

Fluorescence *in situ* hybridization to determine telomere sequences The telomeres of most higher plant species are composed of the repeated sequence (TTTAGGG) n. To investigate *P. ginseng* telomeres comprising the same repeat, we using the complementary end digoxigenin-labeled, telomere-specific oligonucleotide $(CCCTAAA)_3$ as a probe to perform *in situ* hybridization. Hybridization signals visualized as green fluorescence demonstrated that *Arabidopsis*-type telomeric sequence repeats, $(TTTAGGG)_n$, were located in the chromosomes of *P. ginseng* (Fig. 1).

**Figure 1 *In Situ* Localization of TTTAGGG Telomeric Motifs on *P. ginseng* Chromosomes**

The the digoxigenin-dUTP nick tag sequence $(CCCTAAA)_5$ telomeric probe was hybridized with adventitious root of *P. ginseng* metaphase chromosomes and counterstained with propidium iodide.

Growth rings in the roots of *P. ginseng* from Ji'an The paraffin sections of *P. ginseng* rhizomes of different ages collected from Ji'an revealed distinct growth rings in the xylem of secondary roots, and the number of growth rings in the main root was consistent with an age of 1 - 6 years (Fig. 2).

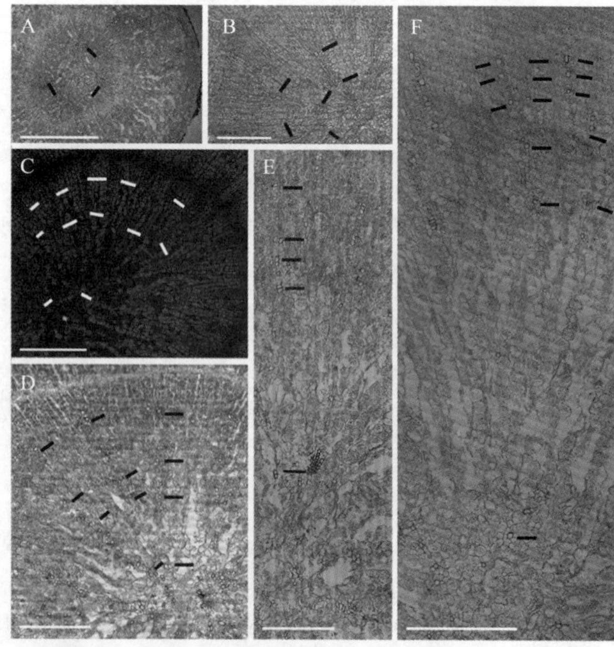


**Figure 2 The growth rings in the ginseng root of 1~6 years**

(A), (B), (C): 1 year ginseng root, 2 year ginseng root, 3 year ginseng root, Bar=1 000 μm; (D), (E), (F): 4 year ginseng root, 5 year ginseng root, 6 year ginseng root, Bar=500 μm.

However, microscopy analysis showed that the growth rings of the ginseng specimens did not precisely reflect age after 6 years.

Telomeric activity of different ginseng tissues A representative TRAP analysis image that was used to quantify telomerase activity is shown in Fig. 3. Average telomerase activities in various tissues and different stages of plant development were assayed using TRAP, and the results indicated that the main root showed the highest average telomerase activities of all of the examined tissues. Because telomerase can lengthen telomeres, and the activity of telomerase may be correlated with age, the main roots were used for further analyses.

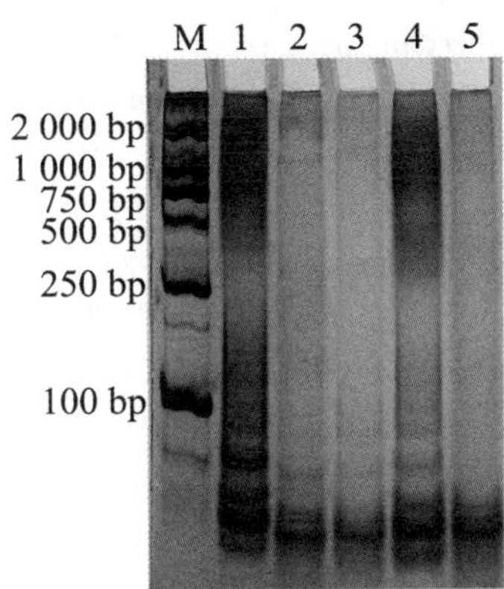


**Figure 3 Developmental Regulation of Telomerase Expression in 5 years *P. ginseng***

Telomerase activities in various tissues and different stages of plant development were assayed by TRAP, using 47F as the forward primer and PTelC3 as reverse primers. Lane1: tap root; Lane2: leaves; Lane3: stems; Lane4: root tips; Lane5: seeds.

Tangential cryo-sectioning of 400 μm sections of samples from 5-year-old *P. ginseng* tissues, followed by densitometric quantitation of telomerase activity (in relative units), revealed the highest telomerase activity in the cambium and adjacent zones of differentiating secondary xylem (Fig. 4).

Analysis of TRF lengths in ginseng of different ages DNA fragments were analyzed through DNA gel blot hybridization using the $(CCCTAAA)_3$ oligonucleotide as a probe. A representative Southern blot image that was used to quantify TRFs is shown in Fig. 5a, b, where the hybridization signals represent telomeric regions. The autoradiograph was scanned and imported as a TIFF-format image to measure TRF length. The location of the peak intensity could not be accurately determined by eye. Therefore, an easy-to-use system that was able to determine the distributions of telomeric regions based on copy number and calculate statistics was employed. The unbiased TRF measure software Telotool was used to measure the TRF lengths of ginseng roots. A plot of the relative telomere copy number versus molecular weight was created, which

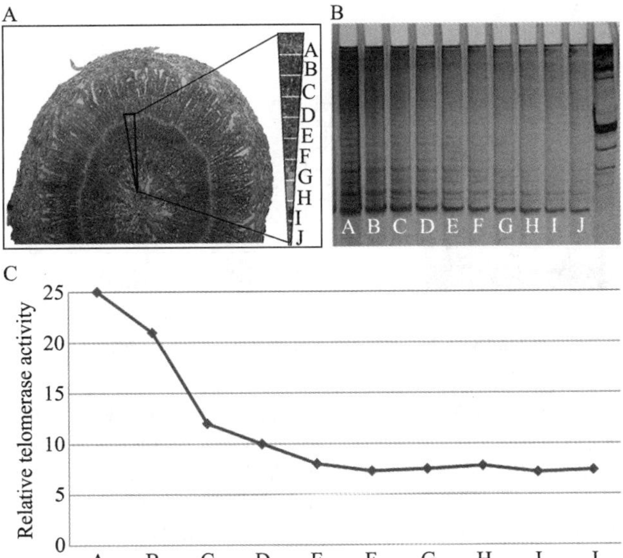


**Figure 4 Anatomical observation of 5 years *P. ginseng* by tangential cryosectioning**

Aseries of 400-um-thick tangential cryosections (A)～(J) was taken for each sample: tissues at different stages were isolated by tangential cryosectioning; (B) Telomerase activities in various tissues and different stages of plant development were assayed by TRAP, using 47F as the forward primer and PTelC3 as reverse primers; (C) Densitometric quantization revealed higher relative telomerase activity (relative units) in cambiums.

provided the user with a realistic picture of the actual distribution of telomeric lengths. The measurements of TRF length for each sample using Southern hybridization was repeated three times.

We investigated the correlation between TRF length and plant age using *P. ginseng* samples of known age from Ji'an and Fusong. First, DNA fragments were analyzed through Southern hybridization using the $(CCCTAAA)_3$ oligonucleotide as a probe for telomeric DNA (Fig. 5a). Although observations made by eye are not precisely accurate, this easy-to-use method is convenient and allowed rapid analysis of the telomeres of ginseng roots by determining copy number. A general model for age-related TRF length in ginseng was introduced. Eleven models were simulated using SPSS 20.0 software, and the most suitable linear fitting curve was determined. The obtained results satisfied the 83% confidence limits ($R^2 = 0.832$, $F = 79.029$, $Sig. = 0.000$), and it was found that TRF length was significantly positively correlated with age after 3 years (Fig. 5b), which indicated that TRF length could be maintained via telomerase activity as tissues developed. Based on these results, we propose a mathematical model through which telomere length can be used to predict *P. ginseng* age:

$$y = 0.827x + 8.231$$

where, $x$ is age, and $y$ is TRF length.

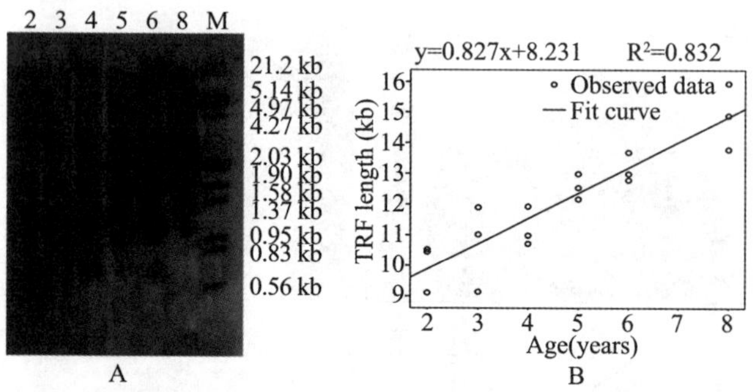


**Figure 5 Southern hybridization images used for measurement and quantization of TRF length**

(A) Lane M: DNA Molecular Weight Marker Ⅲ, Digoxigenin-labeled (Roche). Numbers 2, 3, 4, 5, 6, 8 means different years of *P. gensing* samples collected from the city of Ji'an, Jilin province, China. (B) Data fitting results and the trend of variation of TRF length with different ages. Overall, average TRF length increased with ages in main root (The following 1 cm of "ginseng lutou").

## 2 DISCUSSION

Scientific identification of the potency of traditional Chinese medicines is crucial to ensure their authenticity and effectiveness. Authenticity can be assured based on several factors: the geographic origin or cultivation source of the species; proper harvesting and processing methods; and growth stage. These factors are all important for the quality of Chinese herbal medicines. Because bioactive secondary compounds accumulate as medicinal plants such as *P. ginseng*, *Salvia miltiorrhiza* and *Coptis chinensis* age, older plants usually serve as better medicinal herbs. However, in the pursuit of economic efficiency, a number of inappropriate strategies, including the use of growth hormones and swelling agents as well as continual transplantation, have been employed to simulate age. Therefore, the quality of Chinese herbal medicines is difficult to determine. This study aimed to establish a reliable and effective method for identifying the age of ginseng that complements traditional methods of age determination.

Gymnosperms and dicotyledonous angiosperms generally undergo primary and secondary growth, whereas monocots usually lack secondary growth. The retention of stem-cell-like meristematic cells plays a critical role in perennial longevity. Stem-cell-like meristematic cells are located in the cambium. Accordingly, when environmental conditions change periodically, associated with different growing seasons, the cambium cell cycle is activated, and the tissue layers form rings (termed growth rings) during each individual period of growth. Arx, Schweingruber and Dietz indicated that growth rings could be an effective biomarker for estimating age in the roots of dicotyledonous perennial herbs. In the present study, growth-ring characteristics were clearly present in 1- to 6-year-old ginseng top roots. However, when the ginseng specimens were older than 6 years, dry, decayed channels emerged within the cambium rings, making the growth rings difficult to distinguish and influence age estimation. Therefore, this method can only be applied over a minimum age range, and a new marker was required for estimation of the age of older ginseng samples.

Telomere length and telomerase activity are useful biomarkers for age prediction in animals and plants due to their close association with cell proliferation. However, it was unclear whether telomerase activity is related to the mechanisms maintaining stem cells in meristems. Our analyses of several *P. ginseng* tissues showed that telomerase activity was highest in the cambium. Telomerase expression in plants is very similar to that in humans. In plants, telomerase activity is highest in the meristem and reproductive organs, whereas there is little or no activity in the endosperm, leaves and stems. In *Ginkgo biloba*, tissues with a high percentage of dividing cells also exhibit high levels of telomerase activity, which is consistent with our results. We found that the sampled tissue had a substantial impact on the age estimation in *P. ginseng*. The main root samples contained most of the organized cambium and annual growth rings. We found that telomere length in the main roots was positively correlated with plant age. However, due to sampling limitations, ginseng plants of older ages were difficult to sample. Therefore, our mathematical model is only suitable for a certain range of ginseng ages.

A Study that examined TRF branch length in detail suggested that telomere branch lengths increase with age to some extent in *G. biloba*, in accord with the results of the present study. Our analyses indicate that ginseng telomere length increases significantly with age; however, in contrast to the progressive shortening of TRFs observed in somatic cells as animals aging, telomere length and telomerase activity change in different patterns during plant development. Telomere lengths have been observed to be stable in tomato leaves in four-week-old to six-month-old plants, and they do not significantly change during plant ontogenesis or leaf senescence in *Melandrium album* and *Arabidopsis thaliana* or during cyclical changes of lengthening and shortening in size associated with age in *Pinus longaeva*. Furthermore, telomeres do not shorten during increased tissue differentiation from embryonic to adult stages in *Hordeum vulgare* and *Pinus sylvestris*, whereas they show decreased lengths during *Betula pendula* tissue culture, while increased lengths are observed with age in *G. biloba*. These results suggest that the relationship between telomere length and plant development is complex and may be affected by the species and lines involved as well as environmental stress and telomerase and stem cell activities. The present study indicates that telomere length in the top roots of *P. ginseng* increases with age, as observed in the leaves and calli of *G. biloba*. Interestingly, many studies show that ginsenoside Rgl, which is one of the main biologically active components of ginseng, can decrease telomere shortening and reinforce telomerase activity in delayed hematopoietic stem cells and reduce senescence in human somatic cells. Similar results were found for a *G. biloba* extract, which significantly augmented endothelial progenitor cell telomerase activity to prevent the cells from entering senescence. These results imply that the increase in telomere length with age observed in ginseng and ginkgo may be related to the bioactive components of these plants, which may maintain telomere length by the telomerase mechanism or/and the ALT mechanism. The correlation between telomere length and telomerase activity in *P. ginseng* that was demonstrated here suggests that telomere length and telomerase activity might play essential roles in directly or indirectly regulating the life span of *P. ginseng*.

**Table 1 The Ginseng samples collected from two different districts**

| Age (year) | 2 | 3 | 4 | 5 | 6 | 8 |
|---|---|---|---|---|---|---|
| Fusong | √ | √ | √ | √ | √ | |
| Ji'an | √ | √ | √ | √ | √ | √ |

Ginseng samples of known age were collected from the Ji'an and Fusong districts of Jilin Province, China, in mid-August, 2010 and 2013. The samples were taxonomically identified by Prof. Shiquan Xu, Institute of special animal and plant science, Chinese Academy of Agricultural Sciences. All samples consist of 3 individuals every year.

[梁加贝，蒋超，黄璐琦，等. Scientific Reports, 2015, DOI: 10.1038/srepo7985.]

# Commercialized non-*Camellia* tea: traditional function and molecular identification

## 1 INTRODUCTION

Tea (the leaves from *Camellia* plants) has been one of the most widely consumed non-alcoholic beverages in the world for thousands of years. It plays important roles in commerce, health, and culture. However, many other kinds of plants have been widely used as tea as well. These are not from *Camellia* (Theaceae), and are called non-*Camellia* tea, such as kuding tea, huangqin tea, laoying tea. More than 20 kinds of non-*Camellia* tea are reportedly used within the Chinese culture. Modern pharmacology studies have reported that non-*Camellia* tea may prevent and/or treat chronic metabolic diseases, by producing hypolipidemic, hypoglycemic, or hypotensive actions. Moreover, most kinds of non-*Camellia* tea have also been used as medicine for disease prevention and treatment in folklore.

In recent years, with the increasing international demand for herbal medicines, non-*Camellia* tea has attracted increasing attention. However, original plants of non-*Camellia* tea are confused, and some adulterants have begun to appear in the market. Furthermore, fatalities and serious illnesses have occurred after drinking non-*Camellia* teas, caused by overdose, mislabeled products, or allergic reactions. For instance, kuding tea is suitable for high blood pressure, body fat or hot body, but not for the person whose body 'slants cold' in traditional Chinese medicine theory. According to this theory, a person whose body 'slants cold' will receive no improvement from ingestion of kuding tea and symptoms may appear or worsen, including abdominal pain, severe diarrhea and other symptoms. The significant differences in chemical components among different kinds of the original plants could account for such variations in responses. Finally, undefined compounds in some of these teas may be dangerous to health.

Identification of non-*Camellia* tea is difficult, partly due to a lack of unified standards. Traditionally, morphological features remain as the main basis of taxonomy. However, many of these commercial products are dried and processed, rendering the authentication by morphological methods very difficult. When morphological characteristics are absent, a DNA barcoding technique can identify and detect species utilizing one or a few DNA fragments. DNA barcoding technique is a supplement to traditional authentication method which has been able to solve some identification problems. In this study, we randomly collected non-*Camellia* tea from the medicinal material market in China. Using DNA barcoding technique, the original plants from which the teas were derived were identified to (1) explore which DNA regions are better for the authentication of non-*Camellia* tea traditionally used by Chinese people and (2) evaluate their safety.

## 2 MATERIALS AND METHODS

2.1 Plant materials We collected 37 commercialized tea samples, including 33 kinds of non-*Camellia* tea and 4 kinds of *Camellia* tea from 16 provinces (Yunnan, Sichuan, Guangxi, etc.) in China during 2012, and recorded the detailed information of these medicinal non-*Camellia* tea samples, including the local tea name, collecting location and time, and therapeutic effects (Table 1). All the samples were pressed and deposited at the Herbarium of the Institute of Medicinal Plant Development (IMPLAD).

**Table 1 Summary of sample collecting location and time, original plants and traditional function of non-*Camellia* tea**

| Local commodity name | Collecting location and time | Original plant | Use part | Traditional function |
|---|---|---|---|---|
| **Non-*Camellia* tea** | | | | |
| Baixue tea | Yunnan Province May 2012 | *Thamnolia vermicularis* (Ach.) Asahina<br>*T. subuliforms* (Ehrh.) W. Culb. | Leaves | Clearing away heat and remove toxic material, relieving cough, reducing sputum, anti-inflammatory |
| Big leaf kuding old tea | Guangxi Province June 2012 | *Ilex latifolia* Thunb.<br>*I. kaushue* S. Y. Hu | Leaves | Quenching thirst, improving eyesight, relieving restlessness, refreshing oneself, dissolving phlegm, increasing secretion of urine, relieving sore throat |
| Big leaf kuding tender tea | Guangxi Province June 2012 | *Ilex latifolia* Thunb.<br>*I. kaushue* S. Y. Hu | Leaves | Quenching thirst, improving eyesight, relieving restlessness, refreshing oneself, dissolving phlegm, increasing secretion of urine, relieving sore throat |
| Duosuike sweet tea | Sichuan Province May 2012 | *Lithocarpus litseifolius* (Hance) Chun | Leaves | Reducing fever and causing diuresis, nourishing the liver and kidney, regulating the stomach to descend stomach-qi, moistening the lung to arrest cough |
| Fengwei tea | Wenshan, Yunnan Province May 2012 | *Elsholtzia bodinieri* Vant.<br>*E. heterophylla* Diels | Leaves | Relieving exterior syndrome by dispersion, regulating flow of qi, harmonizing the stomach |
| Gongju tea | Huangshan city, An'hui Province July 2012 | *Chrysanthemum morifolium* Ramat. | Flowers | Expelling wind and clearing away heat, clearing liver-fire to treat eye disease, and eliminating toxic substances |
| Guangxi sweet tea | Guangxi Province June 2012 | *Rubus suavissimus* S. Lee | Leaves, and branch | Clearing away heat and removing toxic material, promoting the secretion of saliva or body fluid, moistening the lung, relieving a cough, relieving sore throat |
| Hongxue tea | Yunnan Province May 2012 | *Lethariella cashmeriana* Korw.<br>*L. cladonioides* (Nyl.) Krog<br>*L. sernanderi* (Motyka) Obermayer<br>*L. zahlbruckneria* (Dr.) Krog | Leaves | Clearing heart-fire to regain consciousness, relieving pain, hyperlipidemia, anti-fatigue, anti-inflammatory |
| Huangqin tea | Inner Mongolia Autonomous Region September 2012 | *Scutellaria baicalensis* Georgi<br>*S. scordifolia* Fisch. ex Schrank<br>*S. amoena* C. H. Wright<br>*S. viscidula* Bunge | Herbs | Heat-clearing and damp-drying drug, purging fire for removing toxin, anti-inflammatory, promoting digestion |
| Jiaogulan tea | Hunan Province July 2012 | *Gynostemma pentaphyllum* (Thunb.) Makino | Leaves | Anti-fatigue, anti-hypoxia, enhancing immunity, hyperglycemic and hypolipidemic |
| Kuqiao tea | Liangzhou, Sichuan Province May 2012 | *Fagopyrum tataricum* (L.) Gaertn. | Seeds | Hyperglycemic, hypolipidemic, enhancing immunity, et al |
| Laoying tea | Guangyuan, Sichuan Province May 2012 | *Litsea coreana* Levl. var. *lanuginosa*<br>*Actinodaphne cupularis* (Hemsl.) Gemble | Leaves | Diabetes, expelling dampness, anti-diarrhea, stop burping, promoting digestion, et al |

(Continued)

| Local commodity name | Collecting location and time | Original plant | Use part | Traditional function |
|---|---|---|---|---|
| Liangwang tea | Yunnan Province May 2012 | *Nothopanax delavayi* (Franch.) Harms ex Diels | Leaves, and flowers | Clearing away heat and removing toxic material, relaxing muscles and bones, promoting digestion, et al |
| Luobuhongma tea | Xinjiang Uygur Autonomous Region July 2012 | *Apocynum venetum* L. | Leaves, and flower | Hypotensive, anti-radiation, anti-aging, preventing bronchitis and cold |
| Luobubaima tea | Xinjiang Uygur Autonomous Region July 2012 | *Apocynum hendersonii* Hook. | Leaves, and flowers | Reducing fever and causing diuresis, flat liver resting to restore energy, hypotensive, hypolipidemic, anti-inflammatory, anti-anaphylaxis |
| Luohan tea | Guangxi Province June 2012 | *Engelhardtia roxburghiana*. Wall. | Leaves | Clearing away heat and removing toxic material, engendering liquid and allaying thirst, relieving summer-heat, removing dampness |
| Lvluohua tea | Tibet Autonomous Region July 2012 | *Epipremnum aureum* (Linden & André) G. S. Bunting | Flowers | Hypoglycemic, anti-bacterial, anti-inflammatory, hypotensive |
| Mabiancao tea | Shanxi Province June 2012 | *Verbena officinalis* L. | Herbs | Clearing away heat and removing toxic material, promoting blood circulation to induce menstrual, diuretic swelling, preventing attack of malaria |
| Niubaiteng sweet tea | Guangxi Province June 2012 | *Hedyotis hedyotidea* (DC.) Merr. | Stems, leaves | Clearing away heat, dispelling wind, eliminating dampness, detumescence detoxification, et al |
| Paraguay tea | Bei Jing August 2012 | *Ilex paraguariensis* St. Hilaire. | Leaves | Curing dyspepsia, antiobesity effect |
| Qingqianliu tea | Jiangxi Province August 2012 | *Cyclocarya paliurus* (Batal.) Iljinsk. | Leaves | Engendering liquid and allaying thirst, clearing away heat and removing toxic material, enhancing physical strength, prolonging life |
| Sishi tea | Wuyuan, Jiangxi Province August 2012 | *Scoparia dulcis* L. | Herbs | Dispelling wind and relieving cough, clearing away heat, removing dampness by dieresis |
| Shen tea | Yunnan Province May 2012 | *Clerodendranthus spicatus* (Thunb.) C. Y. Wu ex H. W. Li | Leaves | Clearing heat and expelling damp, removal of stone and increasing secretion of urine |
| Shiliang tea | Guangxi Province June 2012 | *Chimonanthus salicifolius* S. Y. Hu<br>*C. Zhejiangensis* M.C. Liu<br>*C. nitens* Oliv. | Leaves | Dispelling wind to relieve exogenous syndrome, regulating qi-flowing for strengthening spleen, anti-diarrhea |
| Shiya tea | Guangxi Province June 2012 | *Adinandra nitida* Merr. ex Li | Leaves | Engendering liquid and allaying thirst, anti-inflammatory, clearing away heat and removing toxic material |
| Small leaf kuding tea | Sichuan Province. May 2012 | *Ligustrum robustum* (Roxb.) Blume | Leaves | Cooling and refreshing antipyretic, dieresis |
| Tianyeju tea | Yunnan Province May 2012 | *Stevia rebaudiana* Bertoni | Leaves | Helping to produce saliva and slake thirst, hypotensive, hypoglycemic |
| Vine tea | Zhangjiajie, Hunan Province June 2012 | *Ampelopsis grossedentata* (Hand. -Mazz.) W. T. Wang | Stems, leaves | Clearing away heat and removing toxic material, diminishing inflammation and relieving sore throat, hypotensive and hypolipidemic |
| Xiangsiteng tea | Guangxi Province June 2012 | *Abrus precatorius* Linn. | Stems, leaves | Helping to produce saliva, moistening lung, clearing heat, induce diuresis diuresis |
| Xiangfeng tea | Hebei Province July 2012 | *Chimonanthus salicifolius* S. Y. Hu | Leaves | Promoting digestion, treating liver-stomach disharmony, et al |
| Yaowang tea | Xi'an, Shangxi Province July 2012 | *Potentilla fruticosa* L.<br>*P. glabra* Lodd. var. *mandshurica* | Leaves, flowers | Clearing away heat, invigorating the stomach, regulating the menstrual function |

(Continued)

| Local commodity name | Collecting location and time | Original plant | Use part | Traditional function |
|---|---|---|---|---|
| Yeju tea | Zhejiang Province August 2012 | *Chrysanthemum indicum* L. | Flowers | Clearing away heat and removing toxic material, dispersing wind and heat, dispersing blood stasis, improving eyesight, hypotensive, et al |
| Zhegu tea | Wanning, Hainan Province. August 2012 | *Mallotus oblongifolius* (Miq.) Muell. Arg. | Leaves | Neutralizing the greasy, promoting digestion, eliminating summer-heat, prevention and treatment of common cold |
| **Traditional tea** | | | | |
| Black tea | Fujian Province March 2012 | *Camellia sinensis* | Leaves | Strengthening tendons and bones, anti-fatigue, preventing cold |
| Green tea | Chongqing Province June 2012 | *Camellia sinensis* | Leaves | Refreshing oneself, resolving phlegm, promoting digestion, inducing diuresis, detoxify |
| Tieguanyin tea | Fujian Province March 2012 | *Camellia sinensis* | Leaves | Exciting the brain, inducing diuresis strong heart, antiaging, anticancer and detoxification |
| Xihulongjing tea | Hangzhou, Zhejiang Province August 2012 | *Camellia sinensis* | Leaves | Refreshing oneself, resolving phlegm, promoting digestion, inducing diuresis, detoxify |

2.2 DNA barcoding Four candidate barcodes (*rbc*L, *mat*K, *psb*A-*trn*H and ITS2) were selected based on previous barcoding studies. We isolated the total genomic DNA from approximately 100 mg of dried powder from each sample using the cetyl trimethylammonium bromide method. Extracted DNA was stored in sterile microcentrifuge tubes at −20℃.

The selected regions were amplified by polymerase chain reaction (PCR) on a PCR system 9 700 thermocycler (Gene Co., USA). DNA was amplified in 20 μL of reaction mixtures containing 1 U Ex *Taq* polymerase with 10×Ex *Taq* buffer (100 mmol/L pH 8.3 Tris-HCl, 500 mmol/L of KCl) (Takara, China), 1.25 mmol/L of deoxyribonucleotide triphosphate, 0.05 mmol/L of each primer, and 20 ng of template DNA. Primers and reaction conditions used in the present study were listed in Table 2. The amplified products were sequenced in forward directions with the primers used for amplification in the Beijing Genomics Institute (China). Sequences were assembled and aligned using Bioedit Sequence Alignment editor version 7.0.9.

**Table 2 Primers and reaction conditions used in the present study**

| Gene name | Name of primer and primer sequence 5′-3′ | PCR reaction condition |
|---|---|---|
| *rbc*L | 724R: TCGCATGTACCTGCAGTAGC<br>1F: ATGTCACCACAAACAGAAAC | 95℃ 5 min<br>94℃ 30 s, 56℃ 30 s, 72℃ 100 s, 35 cycles<br>72℃ 7 min |
| *mat*K | 3F: CGTACAGTACTTTTGTGTTTACGAG<br>1R: ACCCAGTCCATCTGGAAATCTTGGTTC | 95℃ 5 min<br>94℃ 30 s, 52℃ 30 s, 72℃ 100 s, 32 cycles<br>72℃ 7 min |
| *psb*A-*trn*H | *trn*H: CGCGCATGGTGGATTCACAATCC<br>*psb*A: GTTATGCATGAACGTAATGCTC | 94℃ 4 min<br>94℃ 30 s, 58℃ 45 s, 72℃ 100 s, 32 cycles<br>72℃ 7 min |
| ITS2 | ITS2F: ATGCGATACTTGGTGTGAAT<br>ITS2R: GACGCTTCTCCAGACTACAAT | 95℃ 5 min<br>95℃ 30 s, 56℃ 30 s, 72℃ 100 s, 35 cycles<br>72℃ 7 min |

2.3 BLASTN and phylogenetic analysis BLASTN and the nearest distance method were used to identify obtained relative accurate identification of species. First, the measured DNA sequences from non-*Camellia* tea were determined using BLASTN against the NCBI databases to identify the original plants of non-*Camellia* tea with similarity over 95%. To optimize correct identifications, DNA sequences of four candidate regions (*rbc*L, *mat*K, ITS2, *psb*A-*trn*H) from non-*Camellia* tea were determined from the best reciprocal hits. In most cases this corresponded to the sequence with the highest BLAST score. Second, in order to find a suitable reference sequence, all of *rbc*L, *mat*K, *psb*A-*trn*H, and ITS2 were extracted from the National Center for Biotechnology Information (NCBI) database according to the names of origin plant of the non-*Camellia* tea. After cluster and phylogenetic analysis, individual sequences were eliminated because of their ambiguous nucleotides shorter than 100 bp. Finally, the download sequences including 29 *rbc*L, 26 *mat*K. 22 *psb*A-*trn*H, and 29 ITS2 (Table 3) combining with the sequences of commercial non-*Camellia* tea were used to construct phylogenetic trees by Mega 5.0 and Clustal X with a bootstrap value of 1000 replicates, respectively. Preliminary trees were reconciled by setting the bootstrap value greater than 50%, yielding a more credible consensus tree.

## 3 RESULTS

3.1 Traditional uses According to the literature (Table 1), original plants of 33 kinds of non-*Camellia* tea are distributed across 29 genera in 22 families. The most widely used plant portions are leaves (26), followed by flowers (7), herbs (3), stems (3), and the least used plant portions are seeds (1) and branches (1). The investigated non-*Camellia* teas have a variety of therapeutic applications (Table 1). The non-*Camellia* teas have been mainly used for three therapeutic effects: ① heat-clearing tea (20), such as vine tea, qingqiangliu tea, yeju tea. ② digestant tea (8), such as laoying tea, zhegu tea, liangwang tea. ③ health tea (9), such as jiaogulan tea, kuqiao tea, lvluohua tea.

3.2 DNA extraction, PCR, and sequencing success All samples were extracted through CTAB method successfully. At the same time, the PCR success rates of *rbc*L, *mat*K, *psb*A-*trn*H and ITS2 were 91.9% (34/37), 75.8% (28/37), 78.4% (29/37) and 100% (37/37), respectively. All the PCR products were sequenced successfully. In all sequences, *rbc*L sequence lengths ranged from 625 bp to 692 bp; *mat*K sequence lengths ranged from 780 bp to 860 bp. *psb*A-*trn*H sequence lengths were from 196 bp to 587 bp, and ITS2 sequence lengths were from 426 bp to 506 bp.

3.3 Species identification based on BLASTN The *rbc*L, *mat*K, *psb*A-*trn*H, and ITS2 sequences of the non-*Camellia* teas were also blasted against the NCBI database with maximum identity that are greater than 95% using an *e*-value below 0.0 to determine the difference between the original plants. The closest match in the database was recorded and DNA sequences of non-*Camellia* tea were determined from the reciprocal best hits.

Taking into account the uncertainties arising from incomplete databases, shared barcodes, ambiguous common names and sequencing without success, BLASTN analysis of the *rbc*L data showed 32 commercialized samples were assigned to species, one sample to genus, and one sample was not recorded in the GenBank (Table 3). But because *rbc*L identification ability is limited, only 11 commercialized samples matched with the original plants, including 7 kinds of non-*Camellia* teas and 4 kinds of traditional tea (Table 4).

**Table 3 The sequence information in GenBank**

| Species | Genbank no. | | | |
|---|---|---|---|---|
| | *rbc*L | *mat*K | *psb*A-*trn*H | ITS2 |
| *Abrus precatorius* (1-2) | JN407285; JF738654 | JN407125 | JN406972 | AF467015 |
| *Actinodaphne cupularis* | — | — | — | HQ697213 |
| *Apocynum venetum* | — | — | — | DQ449485 |
| *Ampelopsis grossedentata* | JQ182479 | JF953244 | JF437070 | — |
| *Camellia sinensis* (1-2) | JN654337 | AJ429305; JN654321 | GQ487359 | FJ004887 |
| *Chimonanthus nitens* | — | — | — | AY786094 |
| *Chimonanthus zhejiangensis* | — | AY525341 | — | AY786106 |
| *Chimonanthus salicifolius* | HQ427177 | HQ427325 | HQ427018 | AY786102 |
| *Chrysanthemum × morifolium* | — | EU334382; HM989758 | EF091621 | EF091597 |
| *Chrysanthemum indicum* | JF949971 | — | JF949971 | EF577298;JN315940 |
| *Clerodendranthus spicatus* | GQ464985 | FJ513161 | FJ513103; GQ464982 | HM595465 |
| *Cyclocarya paliurus* (1-2) | AY263942; AY147094 | AY147098 | — | AF179583 |

(Continued)

| Species | Genbank no. | | | |
|---|---|---|---|---|
| | *rbc*L | *mat*K | *psb*A-*trn*H | ITS2 |
| *Dasiphora fruticosa* | — | AB458578 | JN044379 | — |
| *Engelhardia roxburghiana* | — | — | — | AF303801 |
| *Epipremnum aureum* (1-2) | JQ734504; JN090003 | JN090088 | — | — |
| *Fagopyrum tataricum* | JN187117 | JF829984 | JQ807577 | AB000339 |
| *Gynostemma pentaphyllum* | AY968523 | AY968451 | EF621687 | FJ980303 |
| *Hedyotis hedyotidea* | HM752999 | HM753079 | HM640314; HM640334 | HQ148756 |
| *Ilex aquifolium* | — | JN896160 | — | — |
| *Ilex kaushue* | JF942007 | JF954101 | JN044945 | — |
| *Ilex latifolia* | JF942011 | HQ427289 | JN044949 | AF200592;AY140215 |
| *Ilex paraguariensis* | FJ394634 | GQ248141 | GQ248322 | FJ394705 |
| *Lethariella cashmeriana* | — | — | — | AF297743;DQ980014 |
| *Lethariella sernanderi* | — | — | — | AF297744 |
| *Ligustrum robustum* | JF942292 | JF954385 | JN045240 | — |
| *Litsea coreana* | — | — | — | AF272286 |
| *Lithocarpus litseifolius* | — | EF057121 | — | EF057112 |
| *Mallotus oblongifolius* | JF738963 | — | — | — |
| *Poacynum pictum* | — | — | — | DQ451830 |
| *Potentilla fruticosa* | PFU06818 | — | AM114863 | AF163478 |
| *Scutellaria amoena* | HQ676585 | JX981408 | HQ680371 | — |
| *Scutellaria baicalensis* | GQ374130 | JX981417; HQ676586; FJ513169 | HQ680366 | JF421544; FJ609732 |
| *Scutellaria scordifolia* | HM590110 | HQ839713 | FJ513143 | FJ546875 |
| *Scutellaria viscidula* | HQ676583 | HQ676587 | HQ680369 | — |
| *Scoparia dulcis* | JQ593281 | JQ588687; JQ588683 | — | AY963776 |
| *Stevia rebaudiana* | AY215182 | AY215865 | AY215611 | AB457301 |
| *Thamnolia vermicularis* | — | — | — | JQ409350 |
| *Verbena officinalis* (1-3) | HM850444; JF950020; JN893754 | HM850974 | GQ435188; HE966861 | GQ434586 |

— Species without the gene sequence in NCBI.

The *mat*K analysis data showed 24 commercialized samples were assigned to species, 4 to family. As one common primer of DNA barcoding, *mat*K is suitable for genera identification. In this report, only 13 commercialized samples matched the designation of the original plants: 11 kinds of non-*Camellia* teas and 2 kinds of traditional teas (Table 4).

BLASTN analysis of the *psb*A-*trn*H data indicated 26 samples were assigned to species, 1 to family, and 2 were not recorded in GenBank. Only 13 commercialized samples matched the designation of the original plants: 12 kinds of non-*Camellia* teas and 1 kind of traditional tea (Table 4).

The ITS2 BLASTN result indicated 30 commercialized samples were assigned to species, 4 to genera, 3 to family. Of these, 23 commercialized samples matched the designation of the original plants: 21 kinds of non-*Camellia* teas and 2 kinds of traditional teas (Table 4).

In summary, using one or more DNA data by BLASTN analysis, 23 non-*Camellia* teas were assigned to their original plants successfully.

3.4 Species identification based on phylogenetic tree

Some original plants of the non-*Camellia* tea listed on labels lacked GenBank records. So the reference databases only

**Table 4 BLASTN identification result of non-*Camellia* tea**

| No. | Commodity tea name | *rbc*L | *mat*K | *psb*A-*trn*H | ITS2 |
| --- | --- | --- | --- | --- | --- |
| BYC-1 | Paraguay tea | *Ilex* sp. | *Ilex aquifolium* | *Ilex paraguariensis* # | *Ilex paraguariensis* # |
| BYC-2 | Baixue tea | *Ampelopsis brevipedunculata* | *Ampelopsis grossedentata* | *Ampelopsis grossedentata* | Caprifoliaceae |
| BYC-3 | Blank tea | *Camellia sinensis* # | *Camellia sinensis* # | *Camellia cuspidata* | *Camellia sinensis* # |
| BYC-4 | Big leaf Kuding tender tea | *Ilex kaushue* # | *Ilex aquifolium* | *Ilex pentagona* | *Ilex latifolia* # |
| BYC-5 | Big leaf Kuding old tea | N | N | N | *Ilex latifolia* # |
| BYC-6 | Duosuike sweet tea | *Quercus nigra* | Fagaceae | *Quercus phillyraeoides* | *Lithocarpus* sp. |
| BYC-7 | Fengwei tea | *Elsholtzia stauntonii* | *Mosla chinensis* | *Mosla chinensis* | Lamiaceae |
| BYC-8 | Gongju tea | *Chrysanthemum mutellinum* # | *Chrysanthemum* × *morifolium* # | *Chrysanthemum indicum* | *Chrysanthemum morifolium* # |
| BYC-9 | Green tea | *Camellia sinensis* # | Compositae | *Camellia cuspidata* | *Camellia* sp. |
| BYC-10 | Guangxi sweet tea | N | N | N | *Rubus crataegifolius* |
| BYC-11 | Hongxue tea | *Panax ginseng* | N | N | *Scutellaria baicalensis* |
| BYC-12 | Huangqin tea | *Scutellaria rehderiana* | *Scutellaria baicalensis* # | *Scutellaria baicalensis* # | *Scutellaria baicalensis* # |
| BYC-13 | Jiaogulan tea | *Gynostemma pentaphyllum* # | *Gynostemma pentaphyllum* # | *Gynostemma pentaphyllum* # | *Gynostemma pentaphyllum* # |
| BYC-14 | Kuqiao tea | *Panax ginseng* | N | N | *Stevia rebaudiana* |
| BYC-15 | Laoying tea | *Litsea japonica* | *Cinnamomum brenesi* | N | *Litsea coreana* # |
| BYC-16 | Liangwang tea | *Macropanax dispermus* | *Schefflera heptaphylla* | *Metapanax delavayi* # | *Metapanax delavayi* # |
| BYC-17 | Luobuhongma tea | *Apocynum cannabinum* | *Apocynum cannabinum* | *Apocynum cannabinum* | *Apocynum venetum* # |
| BYC-18 | Luobubaima tea | *Apocynum cannabinum* | *Apocynum cannabinum* | *Apocynum cannabinum* | *Poacynum hendersonii* # |
| BYC-19 | Luohan tea | *Engelhardtia fenzelii* | *Alfaropsis roxburghiana* # | Unknown | *Engelhardtia roxburghiana* # |
| BYC-20 | Lvluohua tea | *Edgeworthia chrysantha* | Thymelaeaceae | Thymelaeaceae | *Edgeworthia chrysantha* |
| BYC-21 | Mabiancao tea | *Verbena bracteata* | *Verbena rigida* | *Verbena stricta* | *Verbena officinalis* # |
| BYC-22 | Niubaiteng sweet tea | *Hedythyrsus* sp. | *Hedyotis hedyotidea* # | *Hedyotis hedyotidea* # | *Hedyotis hedyotidea* # |
| BYC-23 | Qingqianliu tea | Unknown | *Cyclocarya paliurus* # | Unknown | *Cylocarya paliurus* # |
| BYC-24 | Sishi tea | *Bacopa* sp. | N | *Gratiola neglecta* | *Callicarpa poilanei* |

(Continued)

| No. | Commodity tea name | *rbc*L | *mat*K | *psb*A-*trn*H | ITS2 |
|---|---|---|---|---|---|
| BYC-25 | Shen tea | *Clerodendranthus spicatus* # | N | N | *Orthosiphon aristatus* # |
| BYC-26 | Shiliang tea | N | *Chimonanthus salicifolius* S. Y. Hu# | *Chimonanthus salicifolius* # | *Chimonanthus salicifolius* S. Y. Hu# |
| BYC-27 | Shiya tea | *Panax ginseng* | N | N | *Adinandra elegans* |
| BYC-28 | Tianyeju tea | *Stevia rebaudiana* # | *Stevia rebaudiana* # | *Stevia rebaudiana* # | *Stevia rebaudiana* # |
| BYC-29 | Tieguanyin tea | *Camellia sinensis* # | Compositae | *Camellia chekiangoleosa* | *Camellia* sp. |
| BYC-30 | Vine tea | *Ampelopsis brevipedunculata* | *Ampelopsis grossedentata* # | *Ampelopsis grossedentata* # | Compositae |
| BYC-31 | Xihulongjing tea | *Camellia sinensis* # | *Camellia sinensis* # | *Camellia sinensis* # | *Camellia sinensis* # |
| BYC-32 | Xiangsiteng tea | *Abrus precatorius* # | *Abrus precatorius* # | *Abrus precatorius* # | *Abrus precatorius* # |
| BYC-33 | Xiangfeng tea | *Panax ginseng* | *Chimonanthus salicifolius* # | *Chimonanthus salicifolius* # | *Chimonanthus zhejiangensis* # |
| BYC-34 | Small leaf Kuding tea | *Panax ginseng* | N | *Ligustrum robustum* # | *Ligustrum robustum* # |
| BYC-35 | Yaowang tea | *Potentilla fruticosa* # | *Draba lanceolata* | N | *Dasiphora phyllocalyx* |
| BYC-36 | Yeju tea | *Chrysanthemum mutellinum* | *Chrysanthemum* × *morifolium* | *Chrysanthemum indicum* # | *Chrysanthemum indicum* # |
| BYC-37 | Zhegu tea | *Mallotus* sp. | N | *Mallotus apelta* | *Mallotus* sp. |

N, Sequencing without success; Unknown, not identification using DNA barcoding. # Identification results are correct.

comprised 29 *rbc*L, 26 *mat*K, 22 *psb*A-*trn*H and 29 ITS2 sequences obtained by downloading all the sequences that yielded an *e*-value of 0.0 in the initial BLAST searches, and the measured DNA sequences comprised of 34 *rbc*L, 28 *mat*K, 32 *psb*A-*trn*H and 37 ITS2. All the sequences were also used to construct phylogenetic trees using Mega 5.0 and Clustal X, with a bootstrap value of 1000 replicates, respectively. Moreover, we reconciled preliminary trees by setting the bootstrap value greater than 50% to yield a more credible consensus tree.

In the *rbc*L, *mat*K, *psb*A-*trn*H and ITS2 tree, 13 (39%), 10 (30%), 8(30%) and 12(36%) commercialized samples of identification result accord with the original plants of non-*Camellia* tea, respectively (Fig. 1).

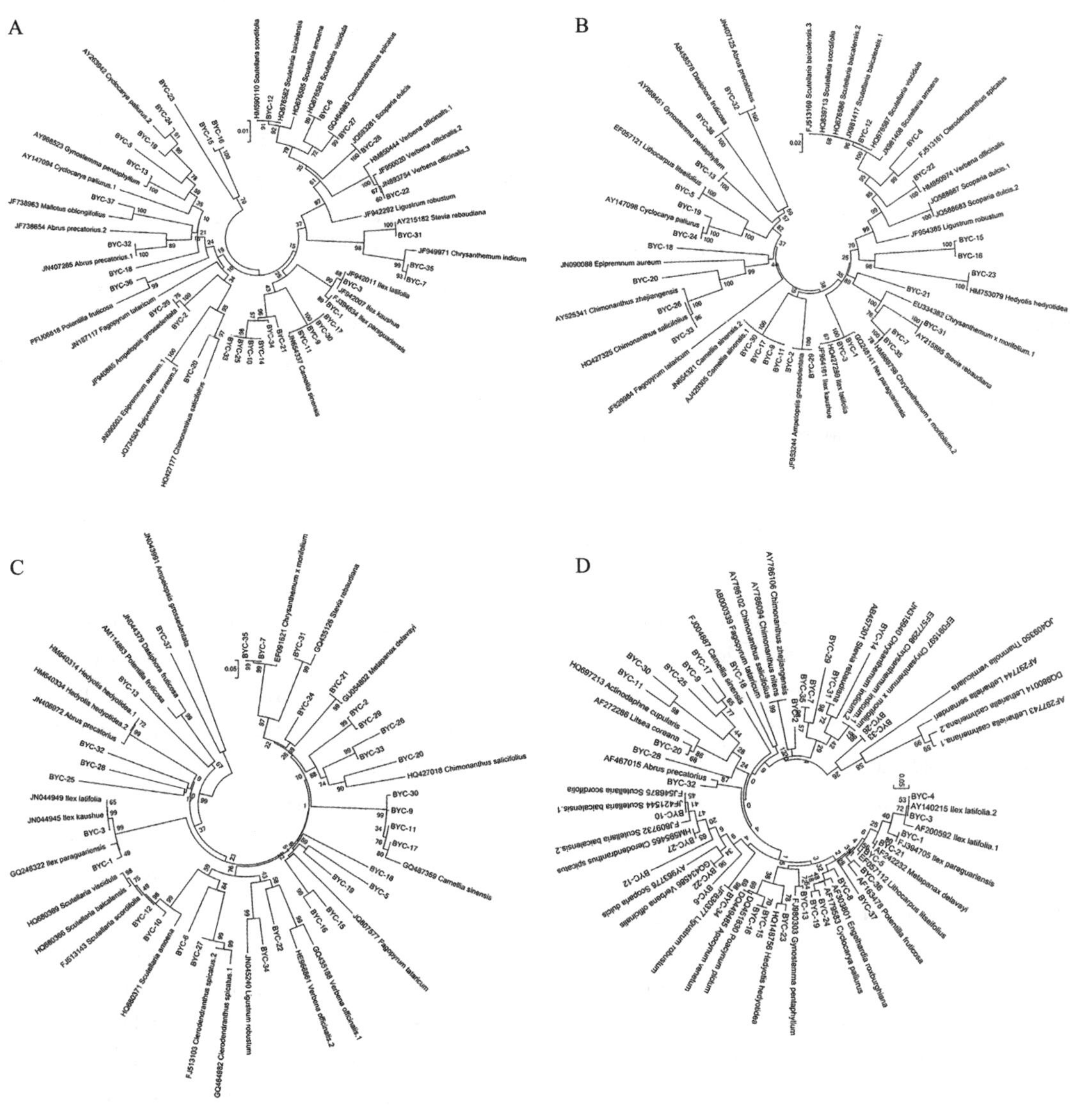


**Figure 1 Phylogenetic trees constructed by DNA barcoding sequences**

(A) *rbc*L; (B) *mat*K; (C) *psb*A-*trn*H; (D) ITS2.

## 4 DISCUSSION

4.1 Non-Camellia tea of misidentification and potential risk Non-*Camellia* tea has been widely used in China for centuries. However, correct identification of some of these teas has remained a problem. According to our investigation, some non-*Camellia* teas from several original plants are used wildly in different regions. For instance, Huangqin tea comes from at least four original plants of the *Scutellaria* genus, including *Scutellaria baicalensis*, *S. scordifolia*, *S. amoena*, *S. viscidula*, etc. They were distributed in more than ten provinces in China. However, it is not easy to distinguish differing species of the same genus. Based on experience, the villagers generally seek to collect the herb that has the similar morphological species. Even some people collected other genus species to use as Huangqin tea, such as *Dracocephalum rupestre*. Therefore, it is of great importance to establish an unequivocal identification system for quality control of non-*Camellia* tea for safety and optimum therapeutic use.

4.2 Accuracy of authentication based on BLASTN and phylogenetic tree In our BLASTN results, 11, 11, 12 and 21 non-*Camellia* teas were identified by *rbc*L, *mat*K, *psb*A-*trn*H and ITS2, respectively. That means the ITS2 have more different loci than chloroplast regions. Of course, the plant species lacking GenBank records should not be ignored.

In all phylogenetic trees, yeju tea, gongju tea and all down-loaded species from *Chrysanthemum* were grouped in a clade with strong support, but both samples did not match with their original plants. It means that yeju tea, gongju tea can be identified at genera level by a signal DNA barcoding marker. At the same time, the possibility of mixed-use between yeju tea and gongju tea also should be considered. The identification of genera also existed in *Ilex* (paraguay tea and big leaf kuding tea) in *rbc*L and ITS2 trees. However, additional data are needed for further authentication. *Chimonanthus* (shiliang tea and xiangfeng tea) became more interesting and different because of the diverse plant materials of shiliang tea. Further research with broader sampling of these species will advance the identification work.

Laoying tea is from *Litsea coreana* var. *lanuginose* (Lauraceae) and *Actinodaphne cupularis* (Hemsl.) Gemble (Lauraceae), and the major original plant is the former. In the ITS2 tree, all downloaded sequences of species from Lauraceae were in the same clade with the BYC-20 as sister group, and the commercial sample has much closer relationship with *L. coreana*. This means that laoying tea can be most accurately identified by ITS2.

Finally, some non-*Camellia* teas, such as hongxue tea, baixue tea, lvluohua tea and kuqiao tea, were not accurately matched to their original plants in all trees, indicating significant errors associated with the accuracy of DNA barcording among these species. The limited data in all trees among these species probably contribute to these errors. These results show that commercial non-*Camellia* teas should be identified with more accurate DNA barcoding sequences and broader sampling techniques.

4.3 Safety evaluation based on BLASTN and phylogenetic tree Consumers have become more interested in the beneficial effects of tea to improve health. However, non-*Camellia* tea is not easily identified by morphological characteristics in the market. Adulteration and misidentification are common in the non-*Camelliaea* teas market, which might be malgenic or lethal. Several kinds of non-*Camelliaea* tea (*e.g.*, *Verbena officinalis* L.) are considered abortifacients, and, if unknowingly consumed by a pregnant woman, could cause miscarriage. Luobuma tea from *Apocynum* (Apocynaceae) also is difficult to morphologically distinguish from some toxic plants in Apocynaceae. In our study, *V. officinalis* L. was accurately identified by DNA barcoding. Luobuhongma tea and luobubaima tea were identified at the genera level by BLASTN and both samples were grouped in a branch separated with other kinds of non-*Camelliaea* tea. However, we did note that DNA barcoding technology can't identify some of non-*Camellia* teas, such as fengwei tea, vine tea and sishi tea. This is because there are only a limited number of these sequences from original plants in GenBank. As a consequence, it is not easy to evaluate the safety of non-*Camelliaea* teas. More original plant sequences need to be submitted to GenBank in order to improve the safety of non-*Camellia* teas.

## 5 CONCLUSIONS

Non-*Camellia* tea has been ingested for centuries for cultural and health purposes. These teas have been used to protect health and prevent diseases, such as cancer, hyperlipidemia, hypertension and hyperglycemia. In recent years, with the development and utilization of non-*Camellia* tea, only few non-*Camellia* teas have been developed into beverages, such as jiaogulan tea and kuding tea. But published data concerning the toxicity of some kinds of non-*Camellia* tea are very limited; the pharmacological activity and mechanisms of action for most kinds of non-*Camellia* tea have not been systematically studied. Additional research on all of these aspects of non-*Camellia* tea is needed.

In this study, molecular results revealed that DNA barcoding technology is a viable and effective method to identify non-*Camelliaea* tea. DNA barcoding technology can offer an effective method to help provide more accurate ingredient labels to consumers, thereby helping improve the safety of food and botanicals. This is particularly pertinent in an increasingly global economy where longer and more complex market chains increase distances between suppliers and consumers, and where regulatory agencies are becoming more stringent with food and botanicals.

[龙平，李旻辉，肖培根，等. Acta Pharmaceutica Sinica B, 2014, 4(3):227-237.]

# Entire industrial chain botanical origin authenticity control of ginseng formula granule products using simple PCR-based identification

## 1 INTRODUCTION

Chinese herbal medicines (CHMs) are derived from botanical, animal, or mineral sources. They play a vital role in healthcare in Asia countries, and their use is increasing in Western countries. According to China's National Bureau of Statistics, the global herbal industrial output of CHMs was estimated to be USD $107 billion in 2017, and with an annual growth rate of 37.9% from 2011. Botanical medicines are the most important CHMs in China. They account for more than 90% of all CHM types and exhibit significant biological activity in phytochemicals and pharmaceuticals.

Accurate identification of botanical medicine at the species level is extremely difficult for some materials, especially during downstream material processing in the industrial chain. To protect the vital interests of patients, guaranteeing the safety of CHMs is a fundamental need that requires distinguishing botanical medicines from their inferior substitutes, adulterants, or counterfeits. For instance, inaccurate identification of herbal materials has caused several serious safety issues that have attracted global attention. As highlighted in recent reports, misidentification of *Aristolochia* and related plants that contain aristolochic acids caused kidney failure, as well as cancers of the liver and urinary tract. Products that substituted American ginseng (*Panax quinquefolius*) for Korean ginseng (*P. ginseng*) have also been reported. The nature of the pharmacological effects in those CHMs are different, because Korean ginseng is "warm" and usually used to treat a "yang deficient" conditions, whereas American ginseng is "cool" and is usually used to treat a "yin-deficient" conditions. Substituting one for the other can place a patient at risk. In addition, products with adulterants are often morphologically and chemically similar to the authentic product.

Derived from the root of *P. ginseng*, ginseng formula granule is one of the most important Chinese herbal industrial products. To convert botanical materials into formula granule, an industrial chain begins with the crude ginseng drug and undergoes a series of herbal preparation procedures — processing, heat reflux extraction, vacuum concentration, spray drying, and granulation. During these processes, the morphological appearance, microscopic characteristics, and phytochemical profiles vary greatly because of extract manipulation, formulation process, and storage conditions. In addition, morphological appearances and some microscopic characteristics are destroyed during extraction and granulation; thus, traditional identification methods fail at these stages. Consequently, it is hard to establish a uniform authenticity control method in the formula granule industrial process.

In recent years, DNA-based molecular approaches have become a popular species identification tool for their high specificity, robustness, and reliability from the original plant to the commercial products. Several DNA-based methods have been applied to identify the authenticity of ginseng in different industrial stages, including the original plant, powder, decoction, extract, and numerous commercial ginseng preparations. Ginseng formula granule is the final product in the industrial chain. At this stage, identification with DNA-based molecular tools is relatively difficult — hot temperature extraction and drying procedures fragment the DNA, but species identification requires an excessively long amplification region. Fortunately, in several recent studies, DNA fragments shorter than 200 bp were amplifiable from highly processed materials, including decoctions and formula granules, using a series of DNA extraction and purification procedures. Therefore, a PCR-based method could serve as a uniform botanical origin authenticity control for the entire ginseng formula granule industrial chain.

In this study, a rapid and reliable allele-specific PCR identification method was developed as a uniform tool for botanical origin authenticity control of ginseng drugs, extract, and formula granule in the entire industrial chain. *P. ginseng*-specific primers and non-*P. ginseng* ginseng-specific primers were employed to identify authentic species and adulterants in the same sample. The method was proven capable of distinguishing *P. ginseng* from related species and detecting adulterants in ginseng products.

## 2 MATERIALS AND METHODS

2.1 Samples Information identifying plant samples and crude drug materials that were tested in this study are shown in Table S1 (273 sample batches). The crude drugs (authentic *P. ginseng* and the closely related species) were obtained from different herbal markets in China and were identified morphologically by experts according to methods described in Chinese Pharmacopoeia 2015. These were used as reference materials to establish molecular identification methods. Samples were stored at −20℃ until use to prevent degradation of the DNA. To remove potential contamination, all samples were washed with 75% alcohol and sterilized water prior to DNA extraction. Herbal extracts and formula granules were collected from six different granule companies (Table 1, Fig. 1). All tested samples were deposited in the National Resource Centre for Chinese Materia Medica, China Academy of Chinese Medical Sciences, Beijing, China.

**Table 1 Herbal extracts and formula granules used in this study**

| NO. | Samples | Origin | Voucher |
|---|---|---|---|
| 1 | Ginseng granules | CR | 1507001S, 1408001S, 1509001S, 1507001S, 1504001S, 1401001W, 1501001S, 1509002S, 1706002S, 1601001W, 1701001S, 1704001S, 1702001S |
| 2 | Ginseng granules | BTC | 1700631, 17013592 |
| 3 | Ginseng granules | JTP | 1706038, 1706083, 20171106001, 1701120, 2017110685, 2017110691 |
| 4 | Ginseng granules | Yifang | 7060701, 7032361 |
| 5 | Ginseng granules | Neo | 1604055 |
| 6 | Ginseng granules | Spring | 161017 |
| 7 | American ginseng granules | CR | 1602001S, 1606001S, 1405001S, 1702001S, 1509001W, 1703001S, 1704005S |
| 8 | American ginseng granules | JTP | 1611803, 1704806, 1508803 |
| 9 | American ginseng granules | Yifang | 6095031, 7071421, 6086892, 7026202, 5060721, 412383T |
| 10 | American ginseng granules | BTC | 17003152, 16008833 |
| 11 | American ginseng granules | Spring | 160209 |
| 12 | Notoginseng granules | CR | 1504001W, 1502001S, 1504001S, 1307001S, 1504001S, 1406002S, 1706002S, 1708001W, 1501001S |
| 13 | Notoginseng granules | BTC | 1619122 |
| 14 | Notoginseng granules | JTP | 1704117, 1707187, 1708093 |
| 15 | Notoginseng granules | Yifang | 7062881 |
| 16 | Notoginseng granules | Spring | 170711 |
| 17 | Ginseng extraction | CR | 170102C, 7170801C, 7171001C, 7170802C |
| 18 | American ginseng extracts | CR | 161201C, 161202C, 160601C |
| 19 | Notoginseng extracts | CR | 5171101C, 5171102C, 5171103C |

CR: China Resources Co., Ltd. BTC: Beijing Tcmages Pharmaceutical Co. Ltd. JTP: Jiangyin Tianjiang Pharmaceutical Co., Ltd. Yifang: Guangdong Yifang Pharmaceutical Co., Ltd. Neo: Sichuan Neo-Green Pharmaceutical Technology Development Co., Ltd. Spring: Spring 9 Department of modern traditional Chinese Medicine Co., Ltd.

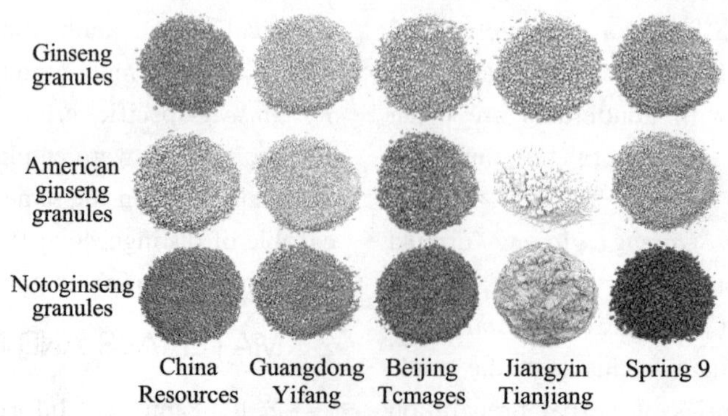


**Fig. 1 Morphology of ginseng, American ginseng, and Notoginseng formula granules from five major formula granule manufacturers**

2.2 Genomic DNA extraction Plant and crude drug materials were frozen in liquid nitrogen and ground to a fine powder with a MM 400 Mixer Mill (Retsch Technology GmbH, Haan, Germany). Genomic DNA was extracted from approximately 30 mg of drug powder using a DNeasy Plant Mini Kit (QIAGEN, CA, USA) according to the manufacturer's protocol.

In total, 50 mg of formula granule samples was dissolved in 1 500 μL of DNA Binding Buffer (Thermo Scientific, Waltham, USA) by vortex and incubated at 56℃ for 20 min. Undissolved debris was removed by centrifugation at 5 000× g for 2 min. 1 000 μL of supernatant was added twice to G2 Purification Columns (GeneJET Gel Extraction Kit, Thermo Scientific, Waltham, USA) and centrifuged at 12 000 × g for 1 min. Then the manufacturer's instructions were followed to obtain 50 μL genomic DNA, and kept at −20℃ before use. The concentration of the isolated DNA and the ratios of the absorbances at 260 nm - 280 nm ($OD_{260}/OD_{280}$ ratio) and 260 nm - 230 nm ($OD_{260}/OD_{230}$) were measured with a NanoDrop ND-1000 spectrophotometer (Gene, Hong Kong, China).

2.3 Oligonucleotide primers DNA sequences of 18S rDNA and chloroplast *trn* L-F region of *Panax* L. were retrieved from the GenBank database (https://www.ncbi.nlm.nih.gov/genbank/). Haplotype sequences were aligned using the multiple sequence alignment program ClustalW in BioEdit 7.2.5 and analyzed with DnaSP version 5.10. Specific identification primers were designed using Primer Premier 5.0 software (PREMIER Biosoft International, USA) for the indicated genes. To detect the presence of PCR-amplifiable fragments in formula granule, primers were designed to generate different length amplicons. All primers were synthesized by Sangon Biotech (Shanghai, China). The nucleotide sequences are shown in Fig. 2 and Table 2.

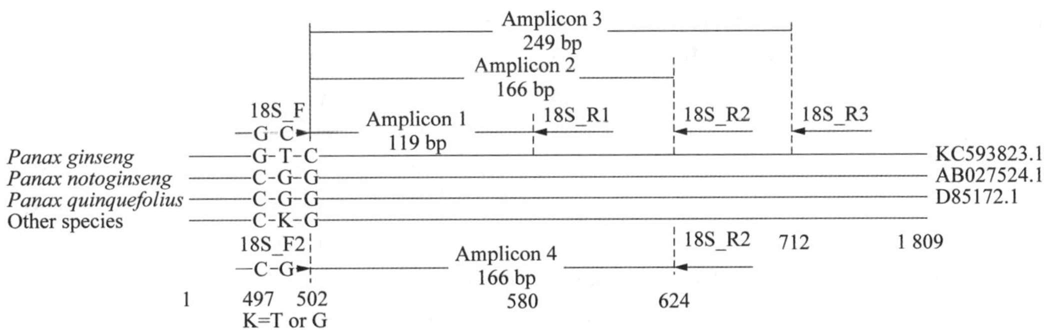


**Fig. 2 *P. ginseng*-specific primers and adulterant specific primers. SNPs are shown in red or green sequence**

For interpretation of the references to colour in this figure legend, the reader is referred to the web version of this article.

**Table 2 Primer sets for amplification and sequencing**

| Primer Name | Primer sequences (5'→3') | Amplicons Size (bp) | Annealing Tm (℃) |
|---|---|---|---|
| 18S_F | ATAACAATACCGGGCTGATAC | — | — |
| 18S_F2 | ATAACAATACCGGGCTCAAAG | — | — |
| 18S_R1 | TATTGGAGCTGGAATTACCGC | 119 | 60 |
| 18S_R2 | CAAAGTCCAACTACGAGCTTTTT | 166 | 60 |
| 18S_R3 | GCCAGTTAAGGACAGGAG | 249 | 60 |
| trnL_F1 | ACGGGGAGGTAGTGACAAT | 83 | 56 |
| trnL_R1 | CGTTAAGGGATTTAGATTGTACTC | | |
| trnL_F2 | TTTTATATGAAAACGGAAGAATTG | 204 | 56 |
| trnL_R2 | CGACGGATTTTCCTCTTACTAA | | |

The underline letter represents of artificial mismatch base.

2.4 PCR amplification and sequencing PCR was performed in a total volume of 25 μL containing 12.5 μL of 2×MightyAmp Buffer Ver. 2 ($Mg^{2+}$, dNTP plus) (Takara, China), 0.6 μL of MightyAmp DNA Polymerase Ver. 2 (1.25 U/μL, Takara), 0.4 μL each of the forward and reverse primers (10 μmol/L, Sangon), and 3 μL (approximately 30 ng) of genomic DNA. Amplification was performed in a Veriti™ thermal cycler (Applied Biosystems, Foster City, CA, USA) with the following cycling conditions: an initial denaturation at 94℃ for 5 min; 40 cycles of 94℃ for 20 s, indicated annealing temperatures for 20 s, and 72 ℃ for 1 min; and a final extension at 72 ℃ for 2 min. After the reaction, products were held at 4 ℃. The PCR products were analyzed by running 5 μL on 2.5% agarose gels (Invitrogen, California, USA) with ethidium bromide (10 mg/mL) in 1× Tris-Acetate-EDTA solution buffer for 25 min at 180 V. The agarose gel was visualized under UV light and images were taken on a GBOX gel documentation system (Syngene, UK). Negative control reactions (using $ddH_2O$ instead of genomic DNA) were simultaneously performed in every DNA extraction and PCR amplification to ensure that the authentication did not result from DNA contamination in the reagents.

PCR products were purified by a Purification Kit (Spin-column) (TransGen, Beijing, China) and bidirectionally sequenced using PCR-derived primers. The dideoxy chain termination method was performed by Ruiboxinke bioTech Co. Ltd., Beijing, China. The sequences were submitted to sequence similarity analysis against the NCBI nucleotide database (https://www.ncbi.nlm.nih.gov/nuccore), and query sequences were identified to species level with best similarity.

## 3 RESULTS

3.1 Ginseng-specific SNPs identified from Genbank/EMBL database Chloroplast DNA sequences of *mat*K, *rbc*L, *trn* L-F, and *psb*A-*trn*H; mitochondrial DNA genes sequences of 12S, NAD, and COXI; and nuclear DNA sequences of 18S rDNA and internal transcribed spacer (ITS) from all available *Panax* species were retrieved from the Genbank/EMBL database to eliminate intraspecific variation. Sequences were aligned with multiple sequence alignment software BioEdit for *in silico* analysis of ginseng-specific SNPs. Four SNPs were discovered, of which two SNPs were located at 18S rDNA (KC593832.1, 497 G>C, 502 C>G), one was located at *trn* L-F (KT161169.1, 508 T>A) and one was located at *rbc*L (KT161190.1, 67 T>C).

3.2 Small amplicons for DNA identification of ginseng formula granules To determine the amplifiable content of ginseng crude drugs and formula granules, a series of primers generating different amplicon sizes were designed and used for specific PCR reactions (Fig. 2). Five primers targeting 18S rDNA or the chloroplast *trn* L-F region of *Panax* L. were tested in ginseng crude drugs and formula granules. PCR amplifications yielded single size amplicons in all crude drug reaction systems except trnL_F1/trnL_R1 primer pairs. This indicated that despite being dried or processed, relatively long amplifiable DNA fragments still existed in the crude drugs. However, as shown in Fig. 3, only small amplicons shorter than 200 bp could be amplified successfully from ginseng formula granules. The highest intensity PCR bands were 166 bp, obtained from the 18S_F/18S_R2 primer pair. This set was selected to establish a ginseng medicine authentication system. A new primer pair 18S_F2/18S_R2 was also designed and used to detect adulterants in ginseng formula granules (Fig. 2, amplicon 4).

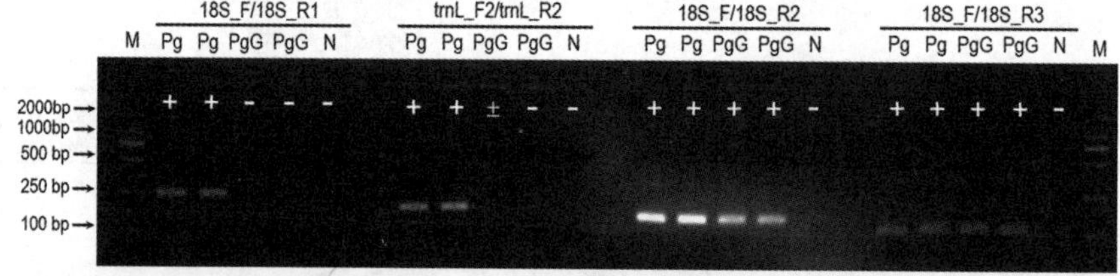


**Fig. 3 PCR amplification of ginseng crude drugs and formula granules using primers targeted to 18S rDNA or the chloroplast *trn* L-F region**

Pg: Korean ginseng crude drug; PgG: ginseng formula granules; M: DL 2000 DNA marker; N: Negative control ($ddH_2O$ as template). Symbols +, − and ± in electrophoresis lane represent brilliant, absent, and weak band, respectively.

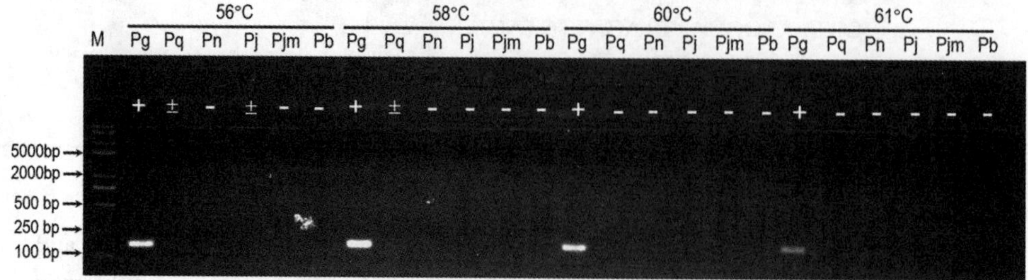


**Fig. 4 Influence of annealing temperature on ginseng identification**

Pg: Korean ginseng; Pq: American ginseng; Pn: Notoginseng; Pj: *P. japonicus*; Pjm: *P. japonicus* var. *major*; Pb: *P. japonicus* var. *bipinnatifidus*; M: DL 2000 plus DNA marker; N: Negative control ($ddH_2O$ as template). Symbols +, − and ± in electrophoresis lane represent brilliant, absent, and weak band, respectively.

To determine the 166 bp amplicon of ginseng formula granules, PCR products were sequenced and submitted to BLAST against the NCBI nucleotide database to obtain a 100% identical match with *P. ginseng* 18S ribosomal RNA gene (KM036295.1).

3.3 Optimizing PCR amplification conditions for authentication of *P. ginseng* products Primer specificity was the critical consideration for accurate PCR results. Several factors, including the annealing temperature, temperature cycles, and properties of thermophilic DNA polymerase contribute to the specificity of discrimination. Six major *Panax* species, namely *P. ginseng* (Korean ginseng), *P. quinquefolius* (American ginseng), *P. notoginseng* (Notoginseng), *P. japonicus*, *P. japonicus* var. *major*, and *P. japonicus* var. *bipinnatifidus*, are widely used in Asian medicine. They are vulnerable to adulteration or misidentification. To establish an accurate and robust approach for identifying *P. ginseng* products, *P. ginseng* and its primary adulterants were tested, and a PCR amplification condition was optimized.

Gradient PCR was carried out on an Applied Biosystems Veriti™ thermal cycler to determine the best annealing temperature (56 - 61 ℃) for *P. ginseng*-specific primers. Strong reaction products were observed from 56 ℃ to 61 ℃. However, when the annealing temperature was 56 ℃ or 58 ℃, weak bands were detected in American ginseng PCR products (Fig. 4). Therefore, to avoid false positive results, 61 ℃ was selected as the optimal annealing temperature for PCR amplification. Various kinds of thermophilic DNA polymerase were selected to test the specificity of the reaction. 166 bp PCR amplicons were generated from all crude drugs. However only MightyAmp Ver 2.0 polymerase (Takara Co., Ltd., Kyoto, Japan) and T5 Super PCR Mix (Tsingke, Beijing, China) could successfully amplify this amplicon from ginseng formula granules (Fig. 5 and S1). The number of thermocycles was also optimized by varying from 31 to 40. All cycle conditions showed excellent capacity to discriminate between ginseng and its adulterants (Fig. S2). Considering the severe DNA degradation in ginseng extract and formula granules, 40 was selected as the optimal cycle number for the identification of ginseng and its adulterants.

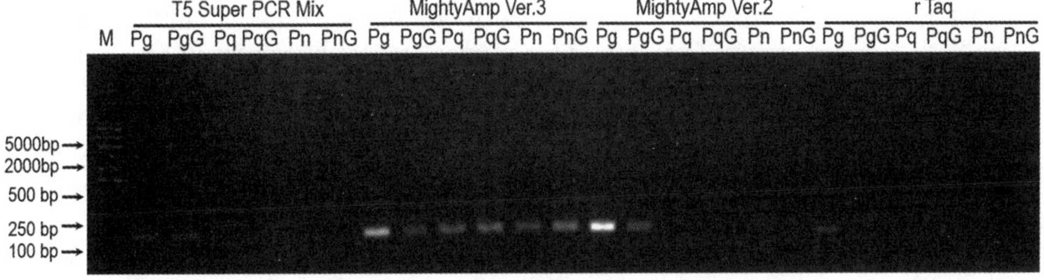


**Fig. 5 Influence of different thermophilic DNA polymerases on ginseng identification**

Pg: Korean ginseng crude drug; PgG: ginseng formula granules; Pq: American ginseng crude drug; PqG: American ginseng formula granules; Pn: Notoginseng crude drug; PnG: Notoginseng formula granules; M: DL 2000 plus DNA marker; N: Negative control ($ddH_2O$ as template).

In the same manner, the annealing temperature and thermal cycles were optimized in the range of 56 - 62 ℃ and 31 - 40 cycles with the adulterant specific primer set 18S_F2/18S_R2 to obtain the optimum conditions of 60 ℃ and 40 cycles (Figs. S3 and S4).

3.4 Establishing species-specific PCR for origin authenticity control of ginseng formula granule products To confirm the accuracy of *P. ginseng*-specific SNPs in Korean ginseng samples, more than 250 batches of ginseng samples were collected from prevalent production areas (Table S1) for testing with *P. ginseng*-specific primers. All *P. ginseng* samples yielded a 166 bp fragment after agarose electrophoresis, and no cross-reactivity was found with adulterants.

Genomic DNA of ginseng products, including crude drugs, herbal extracts, and formula granules, were extracted and subjected to specific PCR using *P. ginseng*-specific primer set 18S_F/18S_R2 and adulterant-specific primer set 18S_F2/18S_R2, with their respective optimized thermocycling programs. As shown in Fig. 6A, by using the *P. ginseng*-specific primers, a 166 bp fragment was amplified from the 18S region in all Korean ginseng crude drugs, herbal extracts, and formula granules from different manufacturers. No amplification was observed from American ginseng or Notoginseng DNA. When using the adulterant specific primers, a 166 bp fragment was amplified in all American ginseng and Notoginseng PCR products, whereas no amplification was observed from Korean ginseng DNA (Fig. 6b). This indicated that the primers were effective in distinguishing authentic *P. ginseng* from adulterant species after the complete formula granule industrial chain. To evaluate detection limit of the allele-specific identification method, DNA samples were serially diluted to 30, 6, 1 and 0.2 ng, respectively. PCR products of crude drugs, herbal extracts, and formula granules were observed for the 1 ng DNA templates by using the *P. ginseng*-specific and adulterant specific primers both, and there was no significant difference between 30 and 6 ng (Figs. S5 and S6). Therefore, by utilizing optimized PCR cycling parameter with specific primers 18S_F/18S_R2 to examine ginseng derived materials and 18S_F2/18S_R2 to examine non-*P. ginseng* derived materials, sample authenticity could be determined for the entire formula granule industrial chain.

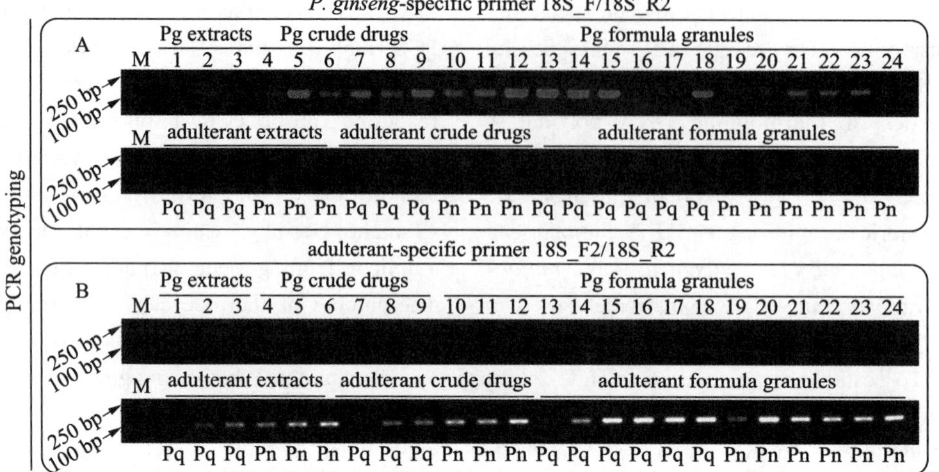


**Fig. 6 Allele specific PCR for identification of ginseng crude drugs, herbal extracts and formula granules. DNA was amplified using *P. ginseng*-specific primer 18S_F/18S_R2 and adulterant specific primers 18S_F2/18S_R2 within the 18S region.**

M: DL 2000 plus DNA marker; Pg: Korean ginseng; Pq: American ginseng; Pn: Notoginseng; lane 1 - 24 represent samples from different production areas or manufacturers, 1 - 3: China Resources Co., Ltd., 4 - 9: samples from prevalent production areas; 11 - 13, 14 - 16, 17 - 19, 18 - 21, 22 - 24 represent samples from the five formula granule manufacturers of China Resources, Beijing Tcmages, Jiangyin Tianjiang, Guangdong Yifang and Spring 9, respectively.

## 4 DISCUSSION

4.1 DNA extraction method and amplification fragment selection in ginseng products Accurate species identification is critical for the efficacy and safety control of herbal products. A reliable method is required to validate the authenticity of herbal products for production quality, particularly for herbal market consumers. However, compared to the extensive traditional identification methods developed in the upstream production of the herbal industrial chain, the quality control of intermediate and terminal products is not well established, particularly for the heavily processed formula granules. Two critical steps were the major constraints to establish a reliable method for authentication: 1) retrieval of fragmented DNA and removal of PCR inhibitors from heavily processed materials, and 2) amplification of a specific target sequence using well-designed specific primers. As indicated in previous studies, intact DNA fragments decrease exponentially with increasing fragment size according to the random degradation model. In addition, ubiquitous PCR inhibitors like polyphenols, polysaccharides, tannic acid, and other secondary metabolites in herbal products could co-precipitate with nucleic acid and chelate metal ions to inhibit PCR amplification. The presence of PCR inhibitors would also inhibit large-sized DNA fragment amplification. Therefore, only small amplicons could be retrieved from highly degraded materials. As indicated in previous studies, fragments shorter than 200 bp are amplifiable in animal formula granules of Hirudo and Zaocys, and botanical formula granules of Lonicerae Japonicae Flos and Radix Achyranthis Bidentatae.

Because ginseng products undergo a series of preparative procedures, genomic DNA degrades at an accelerated rate. Ginseng plant materials can be amplified with lengths greater than 1 000 bp, while crude drugs only yield ≤ 500 bp amplicons. Only short PCR products of ≤ 121 bp were observed after 120 min of boiling to generate ginseng decoction. In this study, only small amplicons of shorter than 200 bp could be amplified successfully in ginseng extract or formula granule.

Furthermore, retrieval of amplifiable DNA fragments is also highly affected by the presence of PCR inhibitors. Numerous classical DNA extraction methods including cetyltrimethylammonium bromide (CTAB), sodium dodecyl sulfate (SDS), and several column-based methods were performed to extract DNA from ginseng extracts and ginseng granules. However, these methods failed to yield PCR products (data not shown). In this study, it was found that G2 Purification Columns (Thermo Scientific) could remove the contaminants present in ginseng extract and ginseng granule as well as in plant material and crude drugs.

Amplification fragment selection was the other critical step to reliably identify ginseng products. 18S rDNA was chosen for amplification since ribosomal polymorphisms are highly suited for distinguishing species. Because ribosomal DNA occurs at a high copy number (approximately 30 000 copies per genome) in most species, some of it may survive DNA damage and degradation. The copy number of ribosomal DNA is even higher than that of mitochondrial (mtDNA) or chloroplast DNA (cpDNA) in plants. Several cpDNA-derived primers were used to amplify small amplicons (87 - 204 bp) from *P. ginseng* products, but none of them could amplify PCR products from ginseng formula granule. This result is consistent with several previous studies of ginseng decoction and Radix Achyranthis Bidentatae formula granule.

4.2 Specific PCR identification methods have potential for authenticity control in the whole herbal industrial chain

Specific PCR is an accurate method to identify biological origin with species-specific primers. When artificial nucleotide mismatches were introduced to the end of the identifying primer, specific PCR possessed the capacity to differentiate single SNPs in closely-related species. As each species could have its own highly specific primers to present a single band on gel electrophoresis, simplex or multiplex PCR could be developed to assess the authenticity of herbal products. Many PCR-based methods have been applied for quality control at several stages of the herbal industrial chain. However, the different properties of the intermediate products led to difficulty in developing a uniform quality control method for DNA extraction and primer selection.

In this study, a uniform specific PCR identification approach was established to authenticate all critical materials in the entire ginseng industrial chain. As illustrated in Fig. 7, *P. ginseng*-specific and non-*P. ginseng* primers were designed and tested on all critical materials of the ginseng granule industrial chain. By using the uniform DNA extraction method, identification primers, PCR amplification system, and gel electrophoresis, PCR products of *P. ginseng* crude drugs, herbal extracts, and formula granules were observed. 166 bp fragments were generated with *P. ginseng*-specific primers, whereas non-*P. ginseng*-specific primers generated the same fragment sizes from adulterant species. Therefore, this approach may be explored for botanical origin authenticity control in the entire herbal industrial chain. If coupled to quantitative PCR, the ratio of authentic to adulterant herbs can be determined. This method is applicable to other crop industrial chains with appropriate primer selections.

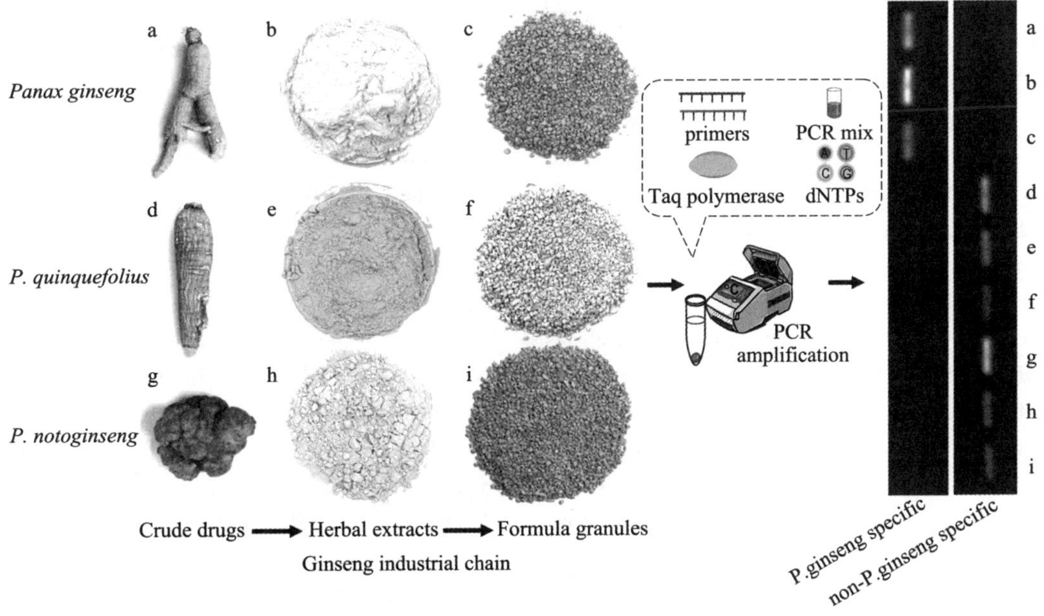


**Fig. 7 18S rDNA-based allele-specific PCR as a uniform method for the botanical origin authenticity control of the ginseng granule industrial chain**

## 5 CONCLUSION

Small fragments shorter than 200 bp were amplifiable during the manufacturing process including processing, pulverization, water extraction, desiccation, and granulation. Allele-specific PCR was sensitive enough to be used as a tool for the identification of botanical origin in highly processed plant materials. Moreover, coupled with adulterant-specific primers, the method can be applied as a uniform and effective high-throughput technique for authenticity analyses of ginseng products in the entire ginseng granule industrial chain.

[蒋超,袁媛,等. Industrial Crops & Products, 2018, 123 (2018): 556 - 562.]

# Towards comprehensive integration and curation of chloroplast genomes

Dear Editor,

Chloroplasts are semi-autonomous genetic organelles that contain their own DNA. Since the first chloroplast genome was sequenced in 1986, chloroplast genomes have been extensively utilized as fundamental tools in plant phylogenetics and genetically modified to produce protein drugs, especially in the fight against COVID-19. More chloroplast genome sequences could not only help us learn more about plant diversity and evolution, but they could also help chloroplast biotechnological applications by codon optimization and identifying non-conserved intergenic spacer regions and regulatory sequences that are needed for genetic engineering. Consequently, the chloroplast genomes of numerous plant species, particularly economically significant crops, have been continuously sequenced. Powered by high-throughput sequencing, over 7 000 plant chloroplast genomes have been deposited in the National Center for Biotechnology Information (NCBI) organelle genome database, of which over 50% have been sequenced in the last 3 years (1 082, 1 175, and 1 539 were sequenced in 2019, 2020, and 2021, respectively). With the accumulation of data, inaccurate taxonomic information, disunity of genomic terms, and other attendant problems have emerged, provoking significant challenges in employing chloroplast genomes. Many efforts have been made, but current databases still suffer from a lack of comprehensiveness and data curation, as well as incomplete data collection. Most existing curated databases are taxon-specific (e. g., cpGDB for spermatophytes and OGDA for algae) or limited to certain data types (e. g., ChloroMitoSSRDB for simple sequence repeats [SSRs]), which could be further improved by incorporating more comprehensive data. Additionally, each published organelle genome database covers only a fraction of chloroplasts, and thousands of chloroplast genomes are still dispersed in different nucleotide databases. Therefore, there is an urgent need to establish an integrated portal with a comprehensive collection and curation of chloroplast genomes.

Here, we developed the Chloroplast Genome Information Resource (CGIR), an integrated platform (https://ngdc.cncb.ac.cn/cgir) comprising 19 388 chloroplast genome assemblies and their corresponding meta-information (Figure 1a). The CGIR comprises five modules: (1) genomes, (2) genes, (3) SSRs, (4) barcodes, and (5) DNA signature sequences (DSSs; Figure 1b). The 'Genomes' module displayed 19 388 chloroplast assemblies from 11 946 different species (Figure 1c). Noticeably, among all assemblies, we sequenced 1 170 assemblies from 718 species, of which the chloroplast genomes from 307 species were reported for the first time, including one family (Juncaginaceae) and 53 genera. In addition to boosting the number of sequenced species, newly added assemblies allow a group of species to have chloroplasts from many individuals. Compared to the NCBI Organelle Genome Database and CpGDB, with only one component for each species, multiple assemblies with explicit taxonomic information can provide more information for plant phylogeny. The taxonomic information of assemblies was curated in accordance with *The Catalogue of Life Checklist 2021* to eliminate disunity across different databases and contributors (Figure 1d). Functional information on plant species was integrated into the CGIR according to the *World Checklist of Useful Plant Species*. The 'Genes' module contains information on genes as well as their associated coding DNA sequence (CDS) and protein sequence (Figure 1e). To ensure a high-quality dataset, we first unified gene names by curating incorrect capitalization, spelling mistakes, extra characters in gene names, and synonymous gene names (Figure 1f). More importantly, not only was uniformity achieved, but corrections were also made. For example, the gene NADH-ubiquinone oxidoreductase chain 6 (*nad6*) should be encoded in the mitochondrial genome. However, this gene was observed in some chloroplast genome annotations, such as *Bulbophyllum reptans* (GenBank accession: NC_058531.1). By manual curation, we confirmed that *nad6* in NC_058531.1 was *ndhG* (Figure 1f).

To better utilize these chloroplast genomes, the remaining three modules contained three commonly used DNA markers developed based on chloroplast genomes. The 'Barcodes'

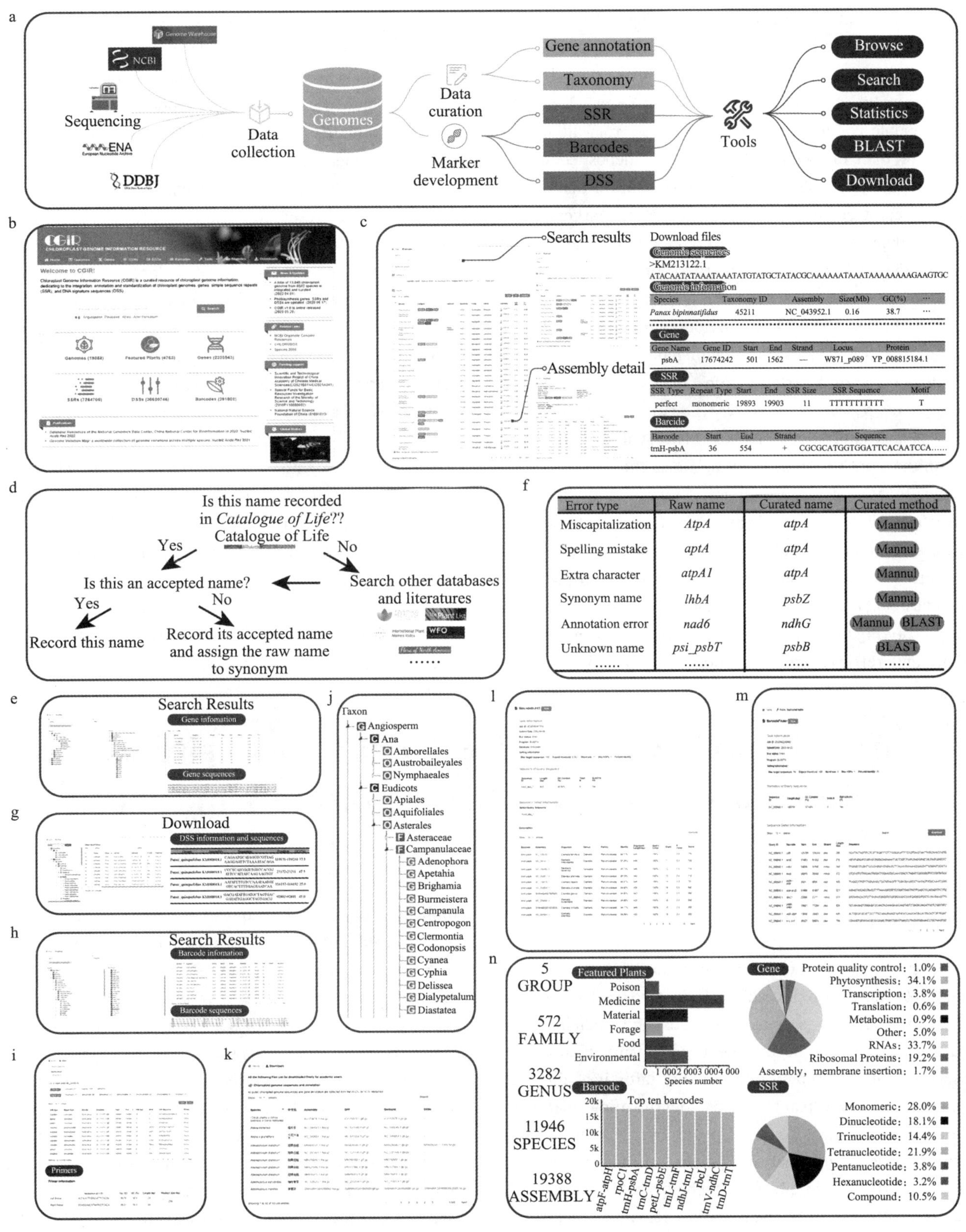


**Figure 1 Architecture of the CGIR**

(a) Design and construction of the CGIR, (b) the CGIR homepage, (c) the Genome module, (d) the curation model of taxonomic information, (e) the Gene module, (f) the curation model of gene annotation, (g) the Barcode module, (h) the DSS module, (i) the SSR module, (j) the Taxonomy tree view, (k) the Download module, (l) BarcodeBlast, (m) BarcodeFinder, and (n) the statistics of CGIR.

module contains DNA barcodes extracted from 29 different loci using the electronic PCR approach (Figure 1g), making the CGIR an excellent complement to traditional DNA barcode databases (e. g., Barcode of Life Data System [BOLD]), which are mainly from *rbc*L and *mat*K loci. The 'DSS' module contains the candidate DSSs from all species with more than one chloroplast assembly deposited in the CGIR (Figure 1 h). DSS is a species-level marker that can be used as a complement to conventional DNA markers. The 'SSR' module comprises 7 284 705 SSRs and their associated primers (Figure 1i), far exceeding that of any other plastid SSR database.

In addition, the CGIR provides various methods for viewing, searching, and downloading data. To help users find the genome of a certain taxon, the 'Genomes' module allows users to search by species name, as well as class, order, genus, and family names. The synonyms are also listed in the search results, enabling researchers to determine whether to use these assemblies (Figure 1c). Because chloroplast data are always used in inter-species comparisons, the CGIR also provides a taxonomy tree view for users who are concerned with specific aspects of chloroplast data (e. g., *rbc*L gene, CDS sequences) in higher taxa (Figure 1j). Using this view, users can browse, search, and retrieve gene, barcode, and DSS data at any taxonomic level. A separate download module is also provided for easy data downloads (Figure 1k). Additionally, the 'BarcodeBLAST' tool allows users to search their barcode sequences against those deposited in the CGIR using BLAST (Figure 1l), and the 'BarcodeFinder' tool can help users to identify barcode regions in their uploaded chloroplast sequences (Figure 1m).

In general, the integration of high-throughput sequencing, public genomic resources, and careful manual curation guaranteed both the quantity and quality of chloroplast data in the CGIR, making it the largest comprehensive chloroplast repository available (Figure 1n). The CGIR will be a valuable resource for researchers working on phylogenetics and chloroplast genetic engineering. The curated taxonomy information and molecular markers are of tremendous value to plant phylogenetics; the labelled featured plants and corrected gene information will assist researchers in identifying suitable research objects and locating intergenic spacer regions, both of which are necessary for designing chloroplast engineering vectors. In future, the CGIR will be continuously updated to incorporate more types of data.

[华中一,章张,袁媛,等. Plant Biotechnology Journal, 2022, 20: 2239-2241.]

# Accurate identification of taxon-specific molecular markers in plants based on DNA signature sequence

## 1 INTRODUCTION

Vascular plants include more than 300, 000 known species, playing an irreplaceable role in terrestrial ecosystems and offering benefits, such as food, fuel, and medicine. The need for sustainable development and plant biodiversity conservation has prompted international initiatives aimed at developing accurate plant species identification methods. Several methods have been proposed over the past years based on genetic information, pollen, chemistry profiles, and using artificial intelligence techniques. However, the accurate identification of plant species remains a significant challenge because of the tremendous diversity of plants.

Among the existing methods, DNA-based methods have become increasingly popular, and various molecular markers have been developed. Generally, these DNA markers can be classified into two types: taxon-specific and DNA barcode markers. Taxon-specific markers, such as derived cleaved amplified polymorphic sequences (dCAPS) and sequence characterized amplified regions (SCAR), were applied based on the presence-absence variance (PAV) of the marker. In contrast to taxon-specific markers, DNA barcodes use universal primers instead of taxon-specific primers to amplify fragments and identify species based on nucleotide dissimilarity. Since the launch of the Barcode of Life Data System (BOLD), DNA barcoding has become a globally accepted method for taxonomists, ecologists, and conservation biologists. Two chloroplast DNA barcodes (*rbc*L + *mat*K) have been recommended as core plant barcodes and the internal transcribed spacer (ITS) and ITS2 with higher discriminatory power have subsequently been proposed as complementary markers. The universal primers of DNA barcodes also enable the combination of DNA barcoding and high-throughput sequencing (HTS), which can identify species from mixtures containing multiple taxa. Nonetheless, introgression induced by gene flow, incomplete lineage sorting due to retention of ancestral polymorphisms, adaptive radiation triggered by natural selection, and numerous other ongoing processes are common in plant evolution, consequently making DNA barcoding incapable of clustering conspecifics with clear discontinuities from other species, and therefore, unable to provide well-defined species boundaries such as taxon-specific markers.

Taxon-specific $k$-mers, also referred to as DNA signature sequences (DSS), are nucleotide sequences with constant length for identifying species by PAV and are promising for plant species identification. Originally, DSSs were used for microbial identification and have become emerging molecular markers for plant identification because of the overwhelming accumulation of chloroplast genomes. Nevertheless, whether DSS markers can be used over a wide taxonomic range, that is, its universality, remains poorly explored. HTS technologies make it feasible and desirable to identify DSS markers from several publicly available chloroplast genomes. The purpose of this study was to conduct large-scale data analysis to identify DSS markers from chloroplasts, confirm their universality and discriminatory power, and compare them with existing methods.

## 2 MATERIALS AND METHODS

2.1 Collection of plant chloroplast genomes A total of 4 356 chloroplast assemblies covering 3 899 species (216 families, 1 512 genera) were used in this study. Of these, 3 623 assemblies covering 3 535 species were obtained from NCBI Organelle Genome Resources (https://www.ncbi.nlm.nih.gov/genome/organ elle/), 16 assemblies covering 16 species were downloaded from the Genome Warehouse (GWH) at the National Genomics Data Center, and 717 assemblies covering 434 species were sequenced and assembled in our study and then deposited in GWH. All data from the public databases were accessed on 30 June 2020. To minimize potential errors caused by plant name synonyms, the species name of each assembly collected from the public database was curated in accordance with The Catalogue of Life Checklist 2021. The full list of accession numbers for the plastid genome sequences analysed in this study is summarized in Table S1.

2.2 An in silico pipeline for DSS candidate identification We have developed an in silico pipeline called IdenDSS for DSS candidate identification (https://github.com/Hua-CM/IdenDSS). IdenDSS requires two categories of species as input: the target species whose DSSs need to be identified and the background species from which the target species should be distinguished. In brief, four steps were followed for identifying DSS candidates. The first step was to generate all possible $k$-mers from one of the target species' chloroplast assemblies using the sliding window method by setting a fixed-length (default 40 bp) sliding window with a 1-bp step. Second, after deredundancy, the nonredundant $k$-mers were blasted against other assemblies of the target species to identify $k$-mers conserved in the target species. These conserved non-redundant $k$-mers were then blasted against the chloroplast assemblies of the background species. Lastly, $k$-mers present in the background species assemblies were removed, and the rest were considered as DSS candidates.

2.3 Validating DSS using HTS data sets The DSSs were validated according to a previously published procedure with minor modifications. For a specific species, HTS data sets used for DSS validation were categorized into two types: conspecific data sets, containing whole-genome sequencing (WGS) reads from conspecific samples, and background data sets, containing WGS reads from other species. The background data set is further divided into two types: the common data set: an HTS data set containing WGS reads from 12 common fruits, vegetables, and crops; and the congeneric data set: an HTS data set containing WGS reads from congeneric species. The common data set was downloaded from the SRA (detailed in Table S2), whereas other data sets were generated in this study according to the methods described in Library Construction and high-throughout sequencing and deposited in the GSA at the NGDC under the accession number CRAOO4065 (detailed in Table S3). Only DSS candidates of 165 species were validated because the tested species must have a conspecific data set and a congeneric data set, but most of the 3 899 species did not have the corresponding WGS data set. FastK software was used to determine whether DSS candidates appeared in the HTS data sets. To exclude questionable or incorrect DSS due to sequencing errors, a "detectable" $k$-mer was identified if it could be detected at least twice. If a DSS candidate could only be detected in a conspecific data set but not in the background data set, the DSS candidate was considered as a DSS. For each species, the precision of the DSS candidate was calculated using the following equation:

$$\text{Precision}=\frac{\text{No. of DSSs}}{\text{No. of DSS candidates}}$$

We created random subsets with different numbers of sequenced nucleotides ($10^6$, $10^7$, $10^8$, $10^9$, and $5\times10^9$) from the original FASTQ files and validated the DSS using each subset.

2.4 Evaluating the sampling number of DSS candidates for achieving a DSS DSS candidates and DSSs validated in 165 species were used to evaluate the sampling number of DSS candidates required to achieve a DSS. Specifically, a set of species (i.e., 10, 20, 30, 40, 50, 60, 70, 80, and 90) were sampled from the 165 species. For each species, different numbers of DSS candidates (i.e., 1, 2, 3, 4, 5, 10, 20, 30, 40, 50, 60, 70, 80, 90, and 100) from different combined DSS candidates were sampled. The proportion of species that possessed at least one DSS among the sampled species was recorded. We performed a bootstrap internal validation procedure with 1 000 bootstrap resamples.

2.5 Validating DSS using PCR amplification and sanger sequencing Two case studies were conducted to investigate the applicability of validating DSS using polymerase chain reaction (PCR) amplification and Sanger sequencing. The first case study was conducted on *Panax ginseng* and *P. quinquefolius* as these were the predominant and valuable *Panax* species. The global ginseng market is worth more than US$ 2 billion. Although multiple DNA markers for *Panax* have been reported, identification methods using multilocus DNA barcode markers or super DNA barcodes based on complete chloroplast genomes are neither convenient nor economical. The second case study involved *Atractylodes japonica*, *A. macrocephala*, and *A. lancea*. *A. lancea* has a long history of use as an important herb in eastern Asia. However, several congeneric species, such as *A. japonica* and *A. macrocephala*, are frequently found as adulterants in *A. lancea* rhizomes, either deliberately or unintentionally. Currently, there is no established molecular marker for the identification of *A. lancea*.

Plant DNA was extracted using the DNeasy Plant Mini Kit (Qiagen Co. Ltd.). The selected DSSs and corresponding primer details used in the case studies are presented in Table S4. All primers were designed using Primer 3. Briefly, the 25 μL PCR system contained 12.5 μL 2× *Taq* Master Mix, 1.0 μL PCR forward primer (10 μmol/L), 1.0 μL PCR reverse primer (10 μmol/L), 1.0 μL cDNA, and 9.5 μL $dH_2O$. PCR amplification was conducted on a Veriti 96 PCR system (Applied Biosystems) under the following conditions: initial denaturation at 95 ℃ for 10 min; 35 cycles of amplification at 94 ℃ for 15 s, 55 ℃ for 10 s, and 72 ℃ for 30 s; and a final extension at 72 ℃ for 5 min. PCR products were evaluated using 1.5% agarose gel electrophoresis. Positive PCR products were purified using a PCR Products Purification Kit (Spin-column) (TransGen) and bidirectionally sequenced using PCR-derived primers. The dideoxy chain termination method was performed at the Beijing Genomics Institute, China.

2.6 Library construction and high-throughput sequencing DNA was extracted as described in the previous section. In all HTS experiments performed in our study, sequencing libraries were generated using the NEB Next Ultra DNA Library Prep Kit for Illumina (NEB) following the manufacturer's recommendations, and library quality was assessed on the Agilent Bioanalyser 2 100 system (Agilent Technologies). The 150-bp paired-end reads were generated on an Illumina Hiseq 4 000 platform (Illumina Inc.).

2.7 Identification of DNA barcode sequences The barcode regions and corresponding primers used in this study are listed in Table S5. To identify the target barcodes for each assembly, BLAST (version 2.9.0+) was applied with the following parameters: -task blastn-short-evalue 10. The sequences between the primer target sequences in the assembly were considered as barcode sequences.

2.8 Evaluation of DNA barcodes' universality and discriminating power First, all available angiosperm sequences of the barcodes (as of 11 November 2020) were downloaded from the NCBI nucleotide data-base using query expressions detailed in Table S6. For example, the following query expression was used for *rbcL*: "((rbcL [Title]) AND Magnoliopsida [Organism]) AND 200: 4 000 [Sequence Length]". Second, the obtained records were filtered to remove sequences whose origin plants were not in the chloroplast data set. Third, the filtered sequences were used as query sequences, and the BLAST+ program (version 2.9.0+) was applied to query the reference data-base for each sequence with an E-value of less than $1\times 10^{-5}$. The evaluation was only carried out in the barcode region, with records from more than 100 species. Identification was considered successful if the query sequence had the closest match with a conspecific individual in the reference database. The bootstrap method was applied to calculate bias-corrected 95% confidence intervals with 1 000 *bootstrap* replicates.

## 3 RESULTS

3.1 Identification of DSS candidates in 3 899 angiosperms The process of identifying DSSs is divided into two parts: identifying DSS candidates and validating the DSSs from these candidates (Figure 1). We do this because, while the bioinformatic pipeline for identifying DSS candidates in silico could be standardized, researchers may weigh and consider a variety of factors when selecting appropriate techniques for validating DSSs, such as economics and technical difficulty. Nonetheless, an important prerequisite to obtaining the DSSs of a specific species is obtaining an adequate number of DSS candidates.

We first introduced a pipeline called IdenDSS for identifying DSS candidates, which overcomes two major issues in the previous method. ① Every time the target or background species are altered, the database must be recreated, requiring the creation of 3 899 databases to identify DSS candidates for 3 899 species. ② the maximum length of *k*-mer was restricted to 32 bp in the previous method.

Using the IdenDSS pipeline, we assessed and optimized four factors that may affect the identification of DSS candidates (DSS length, assembly numbers, background

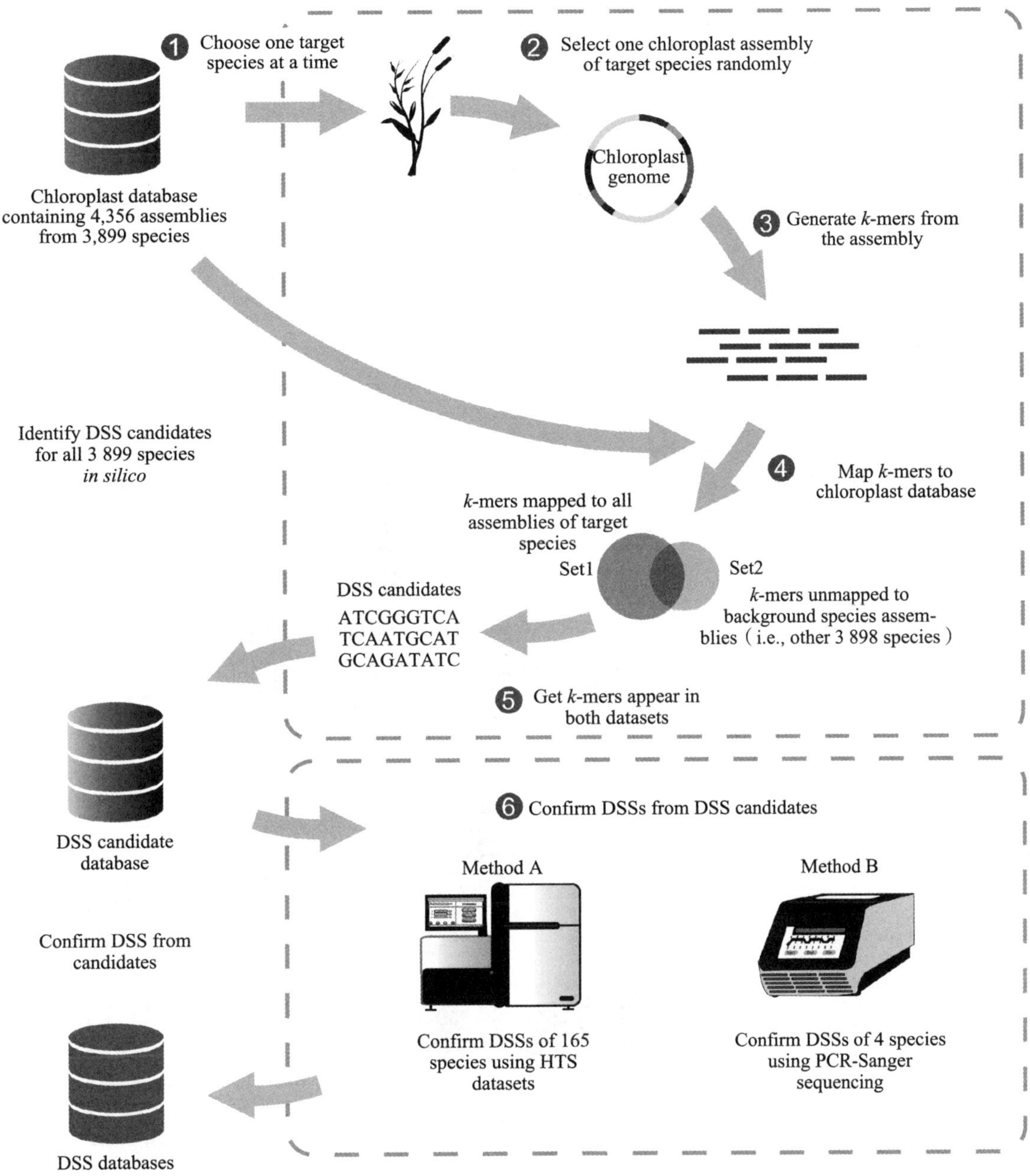


**Figure 1 Workflow for identifying DNA signature sequence (DSS) in the present study**

First, the chloroplast database containing 4 356 assemblies from 3 899 species is established. Next, an in silico pipeline is applied to identify the DSS candidates of each species. For each species, all possible *k*-mers from one of target species chloroplast assemblies were generated at a fixed *k*-mer length. Then, the nonredundant *k*-mers were blasted against other assemblies in the chloroplast database. The *k*-mers mapped to all assemblies of target species were recorded as Set1. The *k*-mers unmapped to background species (i.e., the other 3 898 species in the present study) were recorded as Set2. The *k*-mers appearing in both Set1 and Set2 are considered as DSS candidates. After identifying DSS candidates of all 3 899 species, a DSS candidate database is created using all achieved DSS candidates. Then, polymerase chain reaction (PCR)-sanger sequencing and HTS are used to validate the DSSs of four species and 165 species, respectively, using 40 bp DSS candidates in the constructed database.

species number, and related species). At 20, 30, 40, 50, and 60 bp *k*-mer length, the numbers of species without DSS candidates were 130, 106, 91, 89, and 95, respectively (Figure 2a, Table S7). Based on the above results, a shorter *k*-mer length tends to yield more species without DSSs. We noticed that there were 83 species with no DSS candidates for all five *k*-mer lengths (Table S7). Of the 83, 62 had multiple assemblies. The proportion of species with multiple assemblies was greater than the proportion of species with multiple assemblies in the entire data set (Fisher's test, $P<0.01$). We also found that for all five testing lengths, species with only one assembly presented more DSS candidates than species with multiple assemblies (Figure 2b, Table S8). This result suggests that assembly number has a substantial impact on the identification of DSS candidates. For 369 species with multiple assemblies, our results showed that when the $k$-mer length was 40 bp, the number of species with DSS candidates was the highest, and the proportion of species with DSS candidates was 82.38% (Figure 2c). We also used these 369 species to investigate whether the number of DSS candidates decreased with increasing numbers of background species. Our results showed that the number of DSS candidates remained stable when the number of background species was >1 000 (Table S9). As molecular markers for closely related species are known to be limited, we further used congeneric species to evaluate their effect on the identification of DSS candidates. Aside from the species that had no sequenced congeneric species, the number of congeneric species had no significant influence on the distribution of species without DSS candidates ($P > 0.05$, Kolmogorov-Smirnov test, Figure 2d). However, this result has limitations because the species with sequenced congeneric

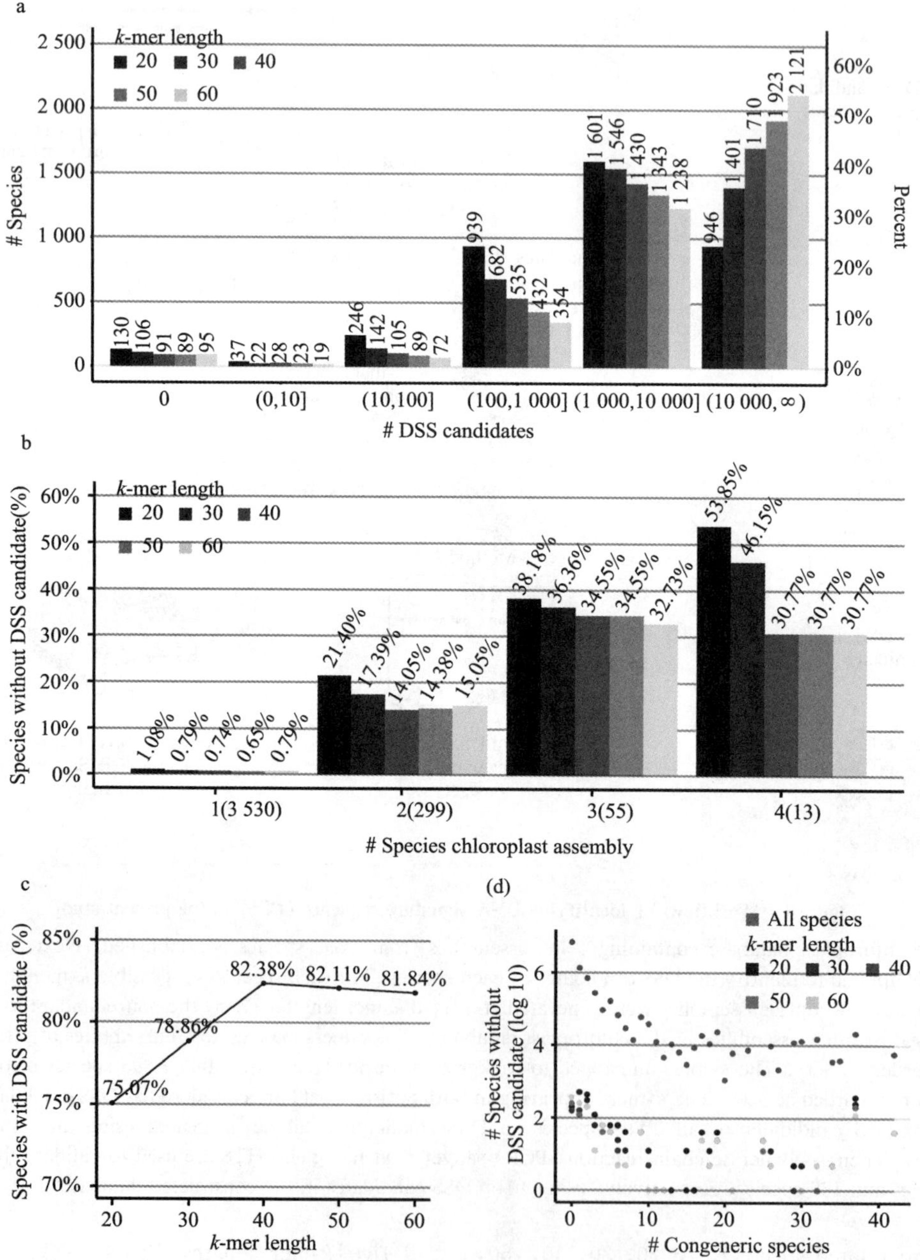


**Figure 2 The DNA signature sequence (DSS) candidates in angiosperms**

(a) Number of species by considering different number of DSS candidates. (b) Proportion of species without DSS candidates by considering different number of species chloroplast assemblies. Numbers in parentheses indicate the number of species with corresponding number of assemblies in 3 899 species. Two species possessing five assemblies not shown. (c) Proportion of species with DSS candidate under different $k$-mer lengths in 369 species with multiple assemblies. (d) Number of species without DSS candidate by considering different number of congeneric species.

species used in our study represent only a small fraction of plants, and even among these, closely related species cannot be fully portrayed by congeneric species because the degree of species differentiation varies across genera. We will further investigate the influence of closely related species in future case studies. Based on the aforementioned results, we propose two principles for the identification of DSS candidates in plants: ① Species to identify DSS should have at least two chloroplast assemblies; the more assemblies, the better the results. ② the optimal *k*-mer length is 40 bp.

In addition, we found that DSS candidates could appear successively. For example, when the *k*-mer length is set to 40 bp, supposing that there are three DSS candidates identified from positions 1 - 40, 2 - 41, and 3 - 42, these three DSS candidates form a "combined DSS candidate". Thus, we investigated the combined DSSs in the collected genomes (Figure S1 - S2) and found that the number of combined DSS candidates was positively correlated with the number of DSS candidates.

3.2 DSS validation using PCR and sanger sequencing

3.2.1 Case study 1 Because our data set comprised only one *P. ginseng* assembly and one *P. quinquefolius* assembly, we added an extra *P. ginseng* assembly (accession number: KM067390.1) and a *P. quinquefolius* assembly (accession number: KT028714) in this case study based on the principles proposed above for identifying DSS candidates. A total of 1 681 and 2041 DSS candidates (from 64 and 69 combined DSS candidates, respectively) were identified in *P. ginseng* and *P. quinquefolius*, respectively. Taking efficiency and cost into account, five *P. ginseng* and five *P. quinquefolius* DSSs were randomly selected and tested. We found that all five *P. ginseng* DSS candidates and four of the five *P. quinquefolius* DSS candidates were successfully distinguished from *each other* (Figure 3a), indicating that these DSS candidates were DSSs.

3.2.2 Case study 2 Five *A. lancea* DSS candidates and five *A. macrocephala* DSS candidates were randomly selected from the 646 and 1 327 DSS candidates identified in this study (from 30 and 53 combined DSS candidates, respectively). The results (Figure 3b) showed that two of the five *A. macrocephala* DSS candidates could distinguish *A. macrocephala* from the other two species. In contrast to *A. macrocephala*, none of the five *A. lancea* DSS candidates could distinguish *A. lancea* from *A. japonica*. These results indicate that two *A. macrocephala* DSS candidates, but none of the *A. lancea* DSS candidates, were DSSs.

We hypothesize that none of the selected *A. lancea* DSS candidates could separate *A. lancea* from *A. japonica* due to a bias induced by the lack of background species because *A. japonica* chloroplasts were not included in our 3899-species data set. To validate this hypothesis, one sample of *A. japonica* was collected and sequenced, and its chloroplast sequence (accession no. GWHAZVW01000000) was added to the background data set, based on which *A. lancea* DSS candidates were reidentified. Only one DSS candidate was identified (Figure 3c) and further validated as a DSS.

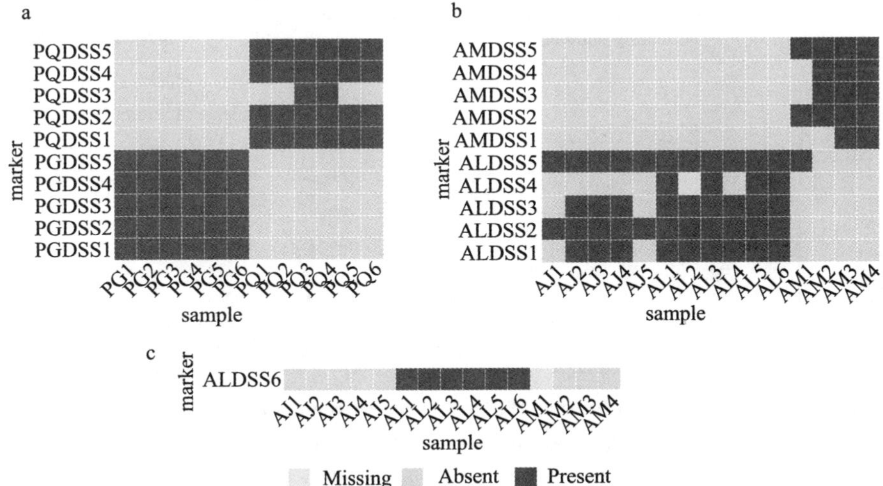


**Figure 3 The validation of DNA signature sequences (DSSs) using polymerase chain reaction (PCR) and sanger sequencing**

(a) the PAV of *P. ginseng* and *P. quinquefolius* DSS candidates in *panax* samples. PG1 - PG6 are six *P. ginseng* samples, PQ1 - PQ6 are six *P. quinquefolius* samples. PGDSS1 - PGDSS5 are five *P. ginseng* DSS candidates, PQDSS1 - PQDSS5 are five *P. quinquefolius* DSS candidates. (b) the PAV of *A. lancea* and *A. macrocephala* DSS candidates in *Atractylodes* samples. AJ1 - AJ4, AL1 - AL5, and AM1 - AM5 are four *A. japonica*, five *A. lancea*, and five *A. macrocephala* samples, respectively. ALDSS1 - ALDSS5 are five *A. lancea* DSS candidates, AMDSS1 - AMDSS5 are five *A. macrocephala* DSS candidates. (c) the PAV of the *A. lancea* DSS candidates after adding *A. japonica* into background species. Missing, the failure of PCR amplification; absent, the DNA sequence in the amplification product was not identical to the DSS candidate; present, the DNA sequence in the amplification product was identical to the DSS candidate.

3.3 HTS-based DSS validation Large-scale validation of DSS candidates was performed using WGS data generated from HTS. According to the principles mentioned above, we set the $k$-mer length at 40 bp to identify DSS candidates, and a DSS candidate was regarded as such if it could be detected exclusively in the conspecific data set but not in the background data set. In total, WGS was performed on 165 species and their DSSs were validated using the HTS method (Tables S3 and S8).

Because the library size influences the detection of $k$-mer in HTS, we compared the proportion of DSS validated from DSS candidates, that is, the precision of DSS candidates, under five different library sizes to obtain a suitable library size. The higher the precision of the DSS candidates, the more reliable they are. Except for six species that do not exhibit any DSS at any sequencing depth, the highest precision of DSS candidates was achieved in 132 of the 159 species when the library size was 1 Gb or 100 Mb (Figure 4a, Table S10).

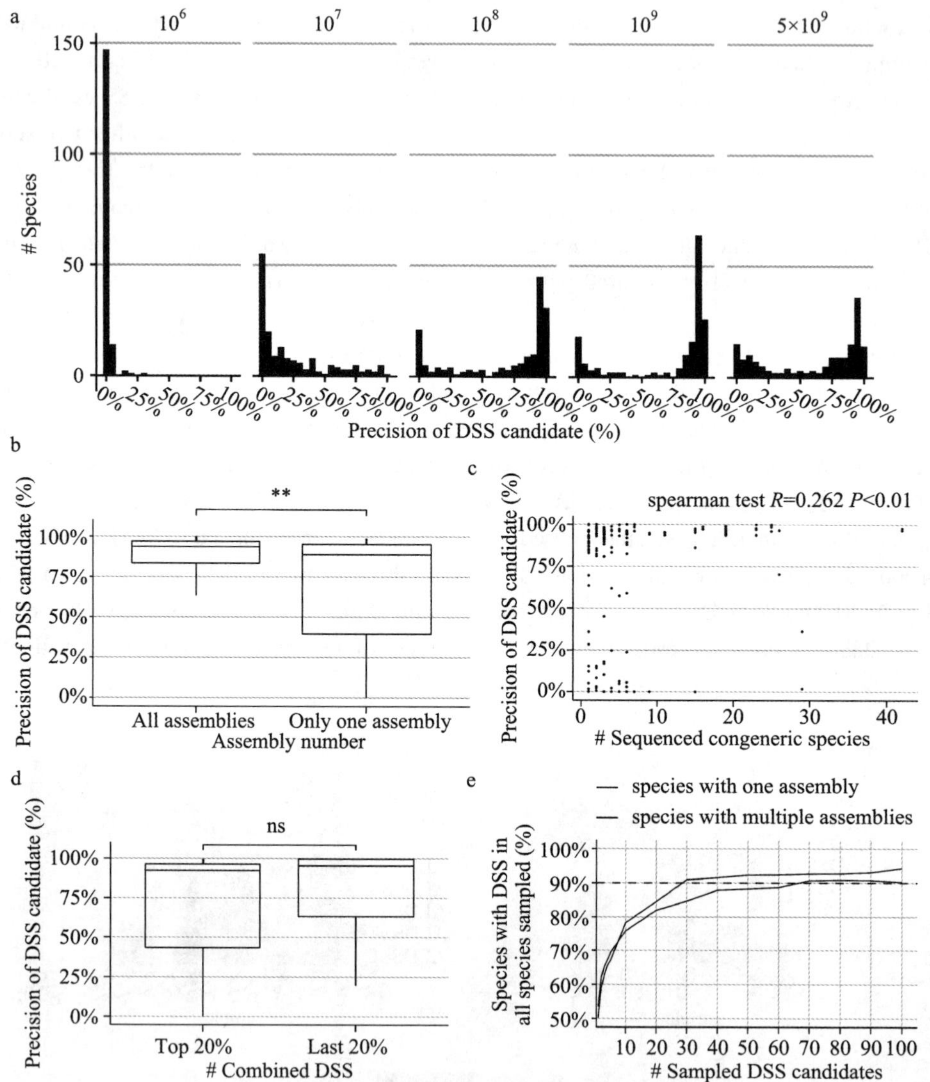


**Figure 4 The validation of DSSs using HTS and factors affecting the precision of DSS candidates**

(a) Histogram of the number of species over different precision of DSS candidates. The DSSs were validated on data sets of five different library size ($10^6$, $10^7$, $10^8$, $10^9$, and $5\times10^9$ bp sequenced nucleotides). (b) the precision of DSS candidates using different number of assemblies. (c) Correlation between the precision of DSS candidates and the number of sequenced congeneric species. (d) Precision of DSS candidates in species with different numbers of DSSs. (e) the probability that one DSS is present under different sampling number of DSS candidates when the number of sampling species is 40.

** $P<0.01$; ns, not significant.

We then investigated the influence of three factors on the precision of DSS candidates using their precision under $10^9$ sequenced nucleotides. First, regarding the number of assemblies, we compared the precision of DSS candidates identified from all assemblies (Table S10) with those identified from individual assemblies (Table S11) using 94 species with multiple assemblies in 165 species. The results demonstrated that the precision of the DSS candidates based on all assemblies was relatively high (Figure 4b). Second, we found that the precision of DSS candidates and congeneric species numbers was weakly correlated ($r = 0.262$, $P < 0.01$; Spearman's test, Figure 4c). For the third factor, the influence of the number of DSSs was assessed. Biologically, DSSs from the same combined DSS are the same markers. Thus, the precision of DSS candidates in the top and last 20% of species ranked by the number of combined DSS candidates, rather than the number of DSSs, were compared. The precision of the DSS candidates in the last 20% was not lower than that in the top 20% (Figure 4d). Our results suggest that for a given species, the number of DSS candidates and closely related species has no effect on the precision of DSS candidates, but the presence of multiple assemblies did. To increase the precision of the DSS candidates, we suggest using multiple assemblies to identify DSS candidates for each species.

Moreover, benefitting from the DSSs of 165 species validated by the HTS method, we investigated another question: How many DSS candidates need to be tested to achieve a DSS? Is testing five DSS candidates sufficient for most species to achieve at least one DSS, such as *P. ginseng*? This question is critical if DSSs must be validated using a low-throughput PCR-based method. To this end, we evaluated the probability of at least one DSS being present under different sampling numbers of DSS candidates. Because the precision of DSS candidates is related to the chloroplast assembly number, we separately evaluated the sampling number of DSS candidates in 71 species with one assembly and 94 species with multiple assemblies to eliminate bias. In addition, to remove sampling bias, we sampled different numbers of species (ranging from 10 to 40), and similar results proved that there was no species bias (Figure 4e, Figure S2). For 94 species with multiple assemblies, more than 90% of the species achieved at least one DSS when the number of DSS candidates sampled was over 40 (Figure 4e, Table S12), whereas for species with one assembly, more than 70 sampling DSS candidates were needed to achieve the same effect (Figure 4e, Table S12).

### 3.4 Comparison of DSS-based methods and DNA barcoding

To compare the discriminatory power and universality of DSSs with DNA barcoding, we collected 29 DNA barcoding regions from the chloroplast data set (see Methods), resulting in 103,307 barcode sequences (Table 1). Consistent with previous studies, the discriminatory power of most chloroplast barcodes at the species level was approximately 66%, with a descending order with the top five barcodes being *atpF-atpH* (66.67%), *rps*16 (66.66%), *trnL-trnF* (66.50%), *matK* (62.50%), and *trnH-psbA* (60.00%) (Table 1). It is not surprising that DSS, a species-specific marker, has a lower universality than most DNA barcode markers (Figure 5) (the universality of four primary barcodes were: *trnL-trnF* [98.23%], *trnH-psbA* [98.08%], *rbcL* [85.66%], *matK* [87.46%]).

**Table 1 The discriminatory power and universality of DNA barcodes**

| Barcode | Number of sequences | Number of species (without prior records) | Family discrimination success (95% confidence interval) | Genus discrimination success (95% confidence interval) | Species discrimination success (95% confidence interval) |
|---|---|---|---|---|---|
| *accD* | 3679 | 3254(2962) | 47.96%-48.00% | 31.00%-31.31% | 19.00%-19.19% |
| *atpB* | 1317 | 1186(950) | 87.88%-88.00% | 81.82%-82.00% | 63.00%-63.64% |
| *atpF-atpH* | 4327 | 3825(3557) | 99.00%-100.00% | 93.94%-93.94% | 66.67%-66.67% |
| *atpI-atpH* | 4412 | 3797(3769) | — | — | — |
| *matK* | 3408 | 3022(908) | 96.00%-96.97% | 91.00%-91.00% | 62.00%-63.00% |
| *ndhF-rpl32* | 1302 | 1160(1133) | — | — | — |
| *ndhJ* | 2388 | 2075(1997) | — | — | — |
| *ndhJ-trnL* | 4193 | 3741(3740) | — | — | — |
| *petL-psbE* | 4298 | 3832(3820) | — | — | — |
| *psaI-accD* | 3526 | 3121(3092) | — | — | — |
| *psbB-psbH* | 2367 | 2091(2025) | — | — | — |
| *psbD-trnT* | 3645 | 3211(3192) | — | — | — |
| *psbJ-petA* | 3937 | 3546(3496) | — | — | — |
| *psbK-psbI* | 4199 | 3743(3671) | — | — | — |

(Continued)

| Barcode | Number of sequences | Number of species (without prior records) | Family discrimination success (95% confidence interval) | Genus discrimination success (95% confidence interval) | Species discrimination success (95% confidence interval) |
|---|---|---|---|---|---|
| *rbcL* | 3 752 | 3 340(1 093) | 95.00%-95.88% | 84.85%-85.00% | 56.00%-56.57% |
| *rpl14-rpl36* | 4 142 | 3 664(3 648) | — | — | — |
| *rpl32-trnL* | 3 765 | 3 341(3 274) | — | — | — |
| *rpoB* | 4 210 | 3 765(3 271) | 67.78%-68.54% | 57.83%-58.33% | 34.12%-34.88% |
| *rpoC1* | 4 318 | 3 847(3 078) | 88.78%-89.47% | 77.55%-78.00% | 45.83%-46.39% |
| *rps12-rpl20* | 2 464 | 2 217(2 197) | — | — | — |
| *rps16* | 3 749 | 3 364(2 374) | 96.97%-96.97% | 90.72%-90.91% | 65.31%-66.00% |
| *rps16-trnK* | 3 772 | 3 321(3 293) | — | — | — |
| *trnC-trnD* | 4 110 | 3 670(3 652) | — | — | — |
| *trnD-trnT* | 3 865 | 3 468(3 446) | — | — | — |
| *trnH-psbA* | 4 314 | 3 824(2 787) | 98.00%-98.99% | 92.00%-93.00% | 60.00%-60.00% |
| *trnL-trnF* | 4 290 | 3 830(2 693) | 100.00%-100.00% | 93.00%-93.00% | 66.00%-67.00% |
| *trnV-ndhC* | 4 266 | 3 671(3 647) | — | — | — |
| *ycf1* | 2 486 | 2 068(1 851) | 97.40%-97.44% | 90.54%-90.79% | 60.76%-61.33% |

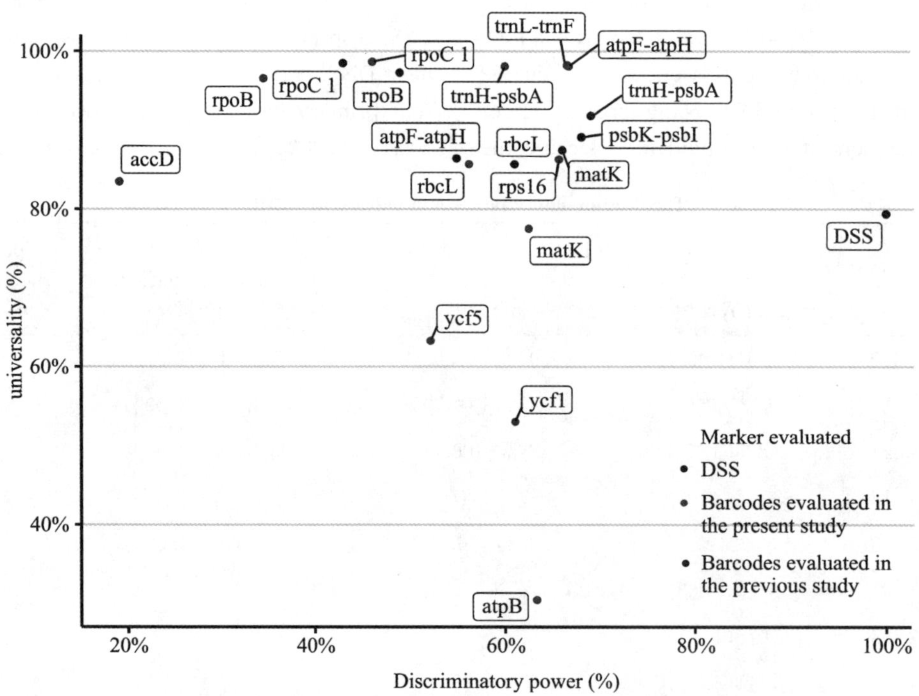


**Figure 5 The universality and discriminatory power of different markers**

The data of barcodes evaluated in a previous study was obtained from CBOL working group (2009).

Furthermore, DNA barcodes for multiple regions of many species have been reported for the first time. For example, 3 752 *rbcL* sequences were obtained from 3 340 species in our study, of which 1 093 had no prior *rbcL* records in GenBank. This was also observed in regions of less concern such as *atpI-atpH*, *ndhJ-trnL*, and *petL-psbE*. These results also indicated that our identified DNA barcodes from the existing plastid data set could be a supplementary source of DNA barcodes.

## 4 DISCUSSION

4.1 The best practice for identifying DSS We split the process of identifying DSSs into two: identifying DSS candidates and validating DSSs from these candidates. First, for identifying DSS candidates, we noticed that DSS candidates of species with multiple assemblies had higher precision (Figure 4b). We speculate that this is because some false-positive interspecies variations can be eliminated by intraspecies variations reflected in multiple assemblies. This also explains why species with multiple assemblies are more likely to possess no DSS candidates than those with only one assembly (Figure 2b). Furthermore, there should be an optimal *k*-mer length for identifying DSS candidates using multiple assemblies because both intraspecies and interspecies variations increase with *k*-mer length simultaneously. According to subsequent analysis, the optimal length was 40 bp (Figure 2c).

Although multiple assemblies can improve the precision of DSS candidates, there may still be false-positive DSS candidates due to sequencing errors, random mutations, etc.; thus, validating DSS is necessary. A potential barrier preventing researchers from using PCR-based methods is the possibility that too many candidates must be tested to achieve a DSS. Our results showed that 90% of the species acquired DSS after testing 40 DSS candidates (Figure 4e, Table S12). In addition, the number of DSS candidates is not linearly correlated with the probability of DSS presence, implying that most species do not have to go through a test of 40 DSS candidates to acquire a DSS. For species with multiple assemblies, five DSS candidates achieved a 67% probability of finding at least one DSS and 10 DSS candidates, corresponding to 78% (Figure 4e).

The HTS method can rapidly screen the DSSs from DSS candidates. *Based on the HTS-based validation of 165 species, we found that* the optimal sequencing amount for DSS validation was 1 Gb. One possible explanation for the 1 Gb overwhelming the 5 Gb data set is that the probability of reads containing DSS sequences generated from the nuclear genome rather than the chloroplast genome increases with sequencing depth. Therefore, 100 Mb - 1 Gb sequencing data should be optimal for validation of DSS candidates in most plants based on the trade-off between reducing bias from the background species nuclear genome and increasing the likelihood of detecting DSS candidates from target species.

Apart from the factors discussed above, background species are another critical, yet challenging issue. In this case study, we obtained 30 combined DSS candidates from a background species data set that did not include *A. lancea*. However, only one of these has been proven to be a DSS marker that can distinguish *A. lancea* from *A. japonica*. In contrast, *A. macrocephala* DSS candidates identified using the same data set did not exhibit this deficiency. Although it is difficult to estimate how frequently this problem is likely to occur, increasing the background species may address this issue to some extent because the number of DSS candidates remains stable when the number of background species is over 1 000. Nonetheless, it is preferable for researchers to sequence the chloroplast genome of closely related species that need to be distinguished from the target species but are not available in public databases. In the case of genus *Atractylodes*, we speculate that the capability of DSS to distinguish species not included in the background data set may be affected by affinity because *A. japonica* is more closely related to *A. lancea* than *A. macrocephala*.

Based on our results, we propose five principles for identifying DSS candidates: ① species to identify DSS should have at least two chloroplast assemblies, and the more assemblies, the better the results. ② the optimal *k*-mer length for DSS is 40 bp. ③ closely related species that need to be distinguished should be included in background species. ④ when using the HTS method to validate DSS, the optimal sequencing amount is 1 Gb. ⑤ when using low-throughput methods to validate DSS, testing 40 DSS candidates should be sufficient.

4.2 Do all species possess DSSs? To evaluate a molecular marker, two touchstones used in DNA barcoding can be consulted: ① Universality: which loci can be routinely amplified and sequenced across land plants? ② Discrimination: Which loci enable most species to be distinguished? DSSs are constant-length nucleotide sequences that can detect the presence of a taxon and distinguish it from background species; thus, the discriminatory power of DSS was 100%. Therefore, the most critical question for DSS application is the universality of DSS (i.e., do all species possess DSSs?). Because we split the process of identifying DSSs into two processes, the universality of DSS can be calculated by the following formula:

$$\text{The universality of DSS} = \frac{\text{Species with DSS candidates}}{\text{All species}} \times \frac{\text{Species with DSS}}{\text{Species with DSS candidates}} \times 100\%$$

To identify DSS candidates for a specific target species, a key issue is defining what the "background species" in the DSS definition is. Theoretically, in terms of plant identification, the background species comprise all other plant species, except for the target species. However, in practical applications, it is neither possible nor necessary to include all other plants because only a few of them have been sequenced. In this study, we use other 3 898 species as background species when the DSS of each species was identified. In compliance with the principles proposed above, we used the results of species with multiple assemblies and HTS-based validation results using 1 Gb sequencing data to evaluate the universality of DSS. As a result, 304 of 369 species (82.38%) with multiple assemblies were DSS candidates, and the HTS-based validation showed that DSSs could be found in 159 of 165 species (96.36%) with DSS candidates. Therefore, the universality of the DSSs was 79.38% (82.38%×96.36%). A potential concern may be that for a specific species, the number of DSSs may decrease with an increase in background species, especially for closely related species. Our results demonstrated that when the number of background species was over 1000, the number of DSS candidates did not decrease significantly with increasing numbers of background species. Our results also indicated that the number of closely related species did not influence the occurrence of DSS candidates (Figure 2d) or the precision of DSS candidates (Figure 4c).

4.3 Future prospects for DSS Efficient plant species identification methods are the basis of plant biodiversity conservation; however, there is still a long way to go. DSS markers can be used as powerful supplements to address the issue that DNA barcoding does not perform well in certain taxa to some extent. *Gentiana* spp. are derived from multiple lineages and undergo radiative speciation. A previous study reported that the discriminatory power of single-locus DNA barcodes ranged from 60% to 74.42% in *Gentiana* and the discriminatory power of multi-locus barcodes ranged from 71.43% to 88.24%. In our study, the DSSs of four *Gentiana* spp. were validated, showing high precision of DSS candidates at 99.8%, 93.6%, 96.3%, and 94.3% for *G. rigescens*, *G. scabra*, *G. trifloral*, and *G. manshurica*, respectively (Table S2).

Another valuable aspect of DSS is that it is PCR-free. The detection of plant components unidentifiable by morphology from mixtures (e.g., food, herbal products, and environmental samples) can portray the biodiversity of environmental samples and improve the oversight of trade in endangered species. Metabarcoding is a powerful tool for detecting plant components in mixtures, but it is hampered by low amplification efficiency because DNA in complex mixtures always degrades due to heating, pH changes, and other factors. In contrast, DSS is PCR-free when combined with HTS because it is simple to obtain reads longer than 100 bp using HTS. This strength makes DSS a promising tool for detecting components of plant origin in complex mixtures.

[华中一，黄璐琦，袁媛，等. Molecular Ecology Resources，2023，23：106－117.]

# Phylogenomic analysis of *Bupleurum* in Western Sichuan, China, including an overlooked new species

## 1 INTRODUCTION

*Bupleurum* L., comprising about 210 species accepted nowadays, is one of the largest genera of the family Apiaceae. It has long been recognized as a natural group distinctively characterized by its members having simple leaves, mostly parallel veins, and conspicuous bracts/bracteoles. Infrageneric classification and phylogeny of the genus was of interest to plant taxonomists from the early days. The first use of section names in *Bupleurum* can be dated back to 1 848. Wolff published a comprehensive revision of the genus that classified it into 5 sections, and his classification is the most widely used for about a century. Shu et al. carried out a numerical taxonomic study in 1998 and divided the Chinese *Bupleurum* species into subgenus *Longifolia* and subgenus *Eubupleura* (including section *Ranunculoidea* and section *Falcata*). Neves & Watson suggested dividing *Bupleurum* into two subgenera (subg. *Penninervia*, subg. *Bupleurum*) based on phylogenetic analyses of nuclear ribosomal internal transcribed spacer (nrITS) sequences of 35 taxa. Although the previous researches have deepened our understanding of the genus, it is still hard to say being sufficient.

China harbors abundant diversity of *Bupleurum*. In *Flora of China* published in 2005, 42 species, 16 varieties and 6 forms were recorded. After revisions of He et al. and Pimenov, etc. in recent years, it was acknowledged there are 47 species, 1 subspecies, 6 varieties and 5 forms of *Bupleurum* in China, most of which have reputed medicinal values in treating fever and liver ails, as observed in many wild species of Apiaceae.

In the western part of Sichuan Province in Southwestern China, i.e., some areas of Aba Zang and Qiang Autonomous Prefecture near Chengdu, including Wenchuan, Mao County, Songpan, and so on, the steep mountains and plateaus lead to the differentiation and formation of

*Bupleurum* species. Closely related species discovered and reported in this region include *B. wenchuanense* R.H. Shan & Y. Li, *B. chaishoui* R. H. Shan & M. L. Sheh, *B. malconense* R.H. Shan & Y. Li, *B. sichuanense* S.L. Pan & P.S. Hsu, *B. microcephalum* Diels, etc. Most of them are quite morphologically similar and the differences between each other are subtle, thus their identification is notoriously difficult. And also, their genetic relationship remains unclear.

Phylogenomics, especially that based on the whole chloroplast (cp) genome sequences, has been proved highly efficient in resolving complicated phylogenetic problems of taxonomically complexed plant groups, and in differentiating and identifying closely related species. We've made some efforts in elucidating phylogeny of Chinese *Bupleurum* through phylogenomic means. We sequenced cp genomes of two woody *Bupleurum* species (*B. gibraltaricum* Lam. and *B. fruticosum* L.) endemic to Mediterranean and made comparative analysis with some Chinese species, confirming the division of 2 subgenera (subg. *Penninervia*, subg. *Bupleurum*) and revealing their divergence time; we also analyzed the sequences of whole cp genomes of 4 Southwest China endemic alpine *Bupleurum* species and suggested phylogenetic affinity in the genus might be closely related to geographical distribution; and we proposed the phylogenetic position of *B. sikangense* C.B. Wang, X.G. Ma & X.J. He as well. As a continuation of the work, we made a phylogenomic analysis of the above-mentioned species distributed in western Sichuan, based on both cp genome and 45 s nuclear ribosomal DNA (nrDNA, including 16 s rRNA-ITS1-5.8 s rRNA-ITS2-26 s rRNA), in order to untangle the complicated relationship among them, and to seek suitable molecular markers for species identification.

Additionally, in the ongoing study on *Bupleurum* investigation, the authors encountered a population in which the individuals obviously belonged to this genus in Wenchuan county years ago. For all the time, the authors had been regarding the plants in this population as *B. chaishoui*. Until recently, the authors obtained some specimens of *B. chaishoui* in its type locality and had a deeper understanding of the species. The authors realized that the plants met before is unique in its leathery dimorphic leaves and represent an overlooked new species, and then named it as *B. pseudochaishoui*. It was thus described here.

## 2 MATERIALS AND METHODS

Plant materials In this study, 65 plant samples, representing 29 *Bupleurum* species were collected in the summer of the years of 2014 through 2020, from North, Northeastern, Northwestern and Southwestern China, including 20 samples of the six above-mentioned species in Western Sichuan (Table 1). The voucher specimens were deposited in the herbarium of the University (Southern Medical University herbarium, SMU, to be listen in the Index Herbarium).

**Table 1 Sources of material and GenBank accession numbers**

| Taxa | Locality | Voucher | Accession number | | |
|---|---|---|---|---|---|
| | | | cp genome | nrDNA | ITS |
| *Bupleurum pseudochaishoui* Z. Chao sp. nov. | Wenchuan. Sichuan | Chao Z 1682502 | **OQ460239** | **OQ627439** | **OQ506349** |
| | Wenchuan. Sichuan | Chao Z 2020080849 | **OQ460238** | **OQ627450** | **OQ651273** |
| | Wenchuan. Sichuan | Liuli 0908102 | | | JF757223 |
| *B. chaishoui* R.H. Shan & M.L. Sheh | Songpan, Sichuan | Chao Z 1682703 | **OQ460228** | **OQ627440** | **OP433488** |
| | Maoxian, Sichuan | Chao Z 1683102 | **OQ460233** | **OQ627442** | **OP433487** |
| | Maoxian, Sichuan | Chao Z 1773003 | **OQ460227** | **OQ627445** | **OP433486** |
| | Heishui, Sichuan | Zhang DJ et al., s.n. | | | **OP433484★** |
| | Maoxian, Sichuan | Yuan CQ & Wang NH 92043 | | | **OP433489★** |
| *B. malconense* R. H. Shan & Y. Li | Danba, Sichuan | Chao Z 1780601 | | | **OP433483★** |
| | Deqin, Yunnan | Chao Z 1782001 | | | **OP433482★** |
| | Jinchuan, Sichuan | Chao Z & Huang R 2020080421 | **OQ460229** | **OQ627451** | **OP433478** |
| | Jinchuan, Sichuan | Chao Z & Huang R 2020080422 | **OQ460230** | **OQ627452** | **OP433481** |
| | Rangtang, Sichuan | Ma XG 10091401 | | | HQ687945 |
| | Ma'erkang, Sichuan | Ma XG 09092103 | | | GU269879 |
| *B. microcephalum* Diels | Ma'erkang, Sichuan | Chao Z 1683101 | **OQ460232** | **OQ627441** | **OP433476** |
| | Xiaojin, Sichuan | Chao Z 1780302 | | | **OP433474★** |
| | Songpan, Sichuan | Chao Z 1773104 | **OQ460231** | **OQ627446** | **OP433473** |
| | Lixian, Sichuan | Ma XG 090801403 | | | GU269882 |

(Continued)

| Taxa | Locality | Voucher | Accession number | | |
|---|---|---|---|---|---|
| | | | cp genome | nrDNA | ITS |
| *B. sichuanense* S.L. Pan & P.S. Hsu | Wenchuan. Sichuan | Chao Z 1682501 | **OQ460234** | **OQ627438** | **OP433472** |
| | Maoxian, Sichuan | Chao Z 1682601 | | | **OP433471**★ |
| | Maoxian, Sichuan | Chao Z 1773001 | **OQ460235** | **OQ627444** | **OP433470** |
| | Wenchuan. Sichuan | Chao Z & Zhang DG 0308052 | | | DQ285447 |
| | Maoxian, Sichuan | Yuan CQ & Wang NH 92044 | | | **OP433477**★ |
| *B. wenchuanense* R.H. Shan & Y. Li | Wenchuan. Sichuan | Chao Z 1683103 | **OQ460237** | **OQ627443** | **OP433468** |
| | Maoxian, Sichuan | Chao Z, Zhang DG 0308051 | | | DQ285461 |
| | Maoxian, Sichuan | Chao Z & Huang R 2020080639 | **OQ460236** | **OQ627449** | |
| | Wenchuan. Sichuan | Ma XG 090831 | | | HQ687964 |
| *B. angustissimum* (Franch.) Kitag. | China | Wang H 00031289 | MT534600 | | |
| | Wuqi, Shaanxi | Chao Z 1981601 | | **OR493965** | **OR502915** |
| | Jingbian, Shaanxi | Chao Z 1681802 | | **OR493964** | **OR502914** |
| | Shuozhou, Shanxi | Wang CB 09010 | | | HQ824721 |
| | Tongxin, Ningxia | Wang CB 09091 | | | GU570631 |
| *B. bicaule* Helm | China | Wang H 00031282 | MT534603 | | |
| | Zalainuo'er, Neimenggu | Chao Z 2082302 | | **OR493966** | **OR502916** |
| | Chenba'erhu, Neimeng | Chao Z 2082401 | | **OR493967** | **OR502917** |
| | Neimenggu, China | Wang ZX 20100912 | | | HQ824722 |
| | Manzhouli, Neimenggu | Wang CB 09066 | | | HQ824723 |
| *B. boissieuanum* H. Wolff | China | zhc20111019 - 15 - 2 | OQ621980 | | |
| | Taibai, Shaanxi | Chao Z 1680902 | **OR508810** | **OR493968** | |
| | Chengkou, Chongqing | Chao Z 1882603 | **OR508811** | **OR493969** | |
| | Kongtongshan, Gansu | Wang CB 09078 - 4 | | | GU570624 |
| | Taibaishan, Shaanxi | Wang CB 09132 | | | HQ687905 |
| *B. candollei* Wall. ex DC. | China | / | MT261183 | | |
| | Dali, Yunnan | Chao Z 1782501 | | **OR493970** | **OR502917** |
| | China | Xie H 040517002 | | | DQ285471 |
| | Kunming, Yunnan | Wang CB 20081105 | | | GU269873 |
| *B. chinense* DC. | Zhashui, Shaanxi | Zhang F 611026LY0126 | MN337347 | | |
| | Feixi, Anhui | Chao Z 2171901 | **OR508812** | | |
| | Shexian, Heibei | Chao Z 2020081983 | **OR508815** | **OR493973** | **OR502921** |
| | Shijiazhuang, Heibei | Chao Z 2020081458 | **OR508813** | **OR493971** | **OR502919** |
| | Wuling, Beijing | Feng CQ 200508 | | | EU001334 |
| | Dabieshan, Anhui | Wang CB 09017 | | | GU570615 |
| *B. commelynoideum* H. Boissieu | Kangding, Sichuan | Chao Z 1682303 | **OR508818** | **OR493976** | **OR502924** |
| | Kangding, Sichuan | Chao Z 1682201 | **OR508816** | **OR493974** | **OR502922** |
| | Kangding, Sichuan | Chao Z 1682203 | **OR508817** | **OR493975** | **OR502923** |
| | Kangding, Sichuan | Chao Z 1780605 | | **OR493977** | **OR502925** |
| | Kangding, Sichuan | Chao Z 2020080217 | | **OR493978** | **OR502926** |
| | Daocheng, Sichuan | Wang CB 09141 | | | HQ687920 |
| | Daofu, Sichuan | Ma XG 182 | | | HQ687926 |
| *B. densiflorum* Rupr. | China | / | MT261184 | | |
| | Tianshan, Xinjiang | Wang CB 09165 | | | GU570611 |
| *B. dracaenoides* Huan C. Wang, Z.R. He & H. Sun | China | / | MT387201 | | |
| | China | Wang HC 20110148 | | | JQ365173 |

(Continued)

| Taxa | Locality | Voucher | Accession number | | |
|---|---|---|---|---|---|
| | | | cp genome | nrDNA | ITS |
| *B. euphorbioides* Nakai | Kangwon-do, Korea | Anonymous TKMII-33-2 | MT821948 | | |
| | Changbaishan, Jilin | Wang CB 09038-5 | | | GU570619 |
| *B. falcatum* L. | Suihua, Heilongjiang | Zhang GX & Wang H 23000503 | MT075716 | | |
| | South Korea | / | NC027834 | | |
| | Japan | Wei XQ 86 | | | GU570605 |
| | Lixian, Sichun | Ma XG 09092201 | | | GU570639 |
| | Hanyuan, Sichuan | Chao Z 2020072901 | **OR508820** | **OR493980** | **OR502928** |
| | Xiangfen, Shanxi | Chao Z 2020081878 | **OR508821** | **OR493981** | **OR502929** |
| | Toyama, Janpan | Chao Z 2009100601 | **OR508819** | **OR493979** | **OR502927** |
| *B. fruticosum* L. | Cultivated, London | Chao Z 1871201 | MW497417 | **OQ627447** | **OP433467** |
| | Estremadura, Portugal | Neves 33 | | | AF479297 |
| *B. gibraltaricum* Lam. | Cultivated, London | Chao Z 1871202 | MW497418 | **OQ627448** | **OP433466** |
| | Sevilla, Spain | Neves 35 | | | AF479851 |
| | Sevilla, Spain | Neves & Watson 51 | | | AF479852 |
| *B. hamiltonii* N.P. Balakr. | Bijie, Guizhou | Anonymous HPCH0003 | MW262986 | | |
| | China | Wang QZ & Pu FD 348618 | | | EU001338 |
| | Kunming, Yunnan | Wang CB 20081101 | | | GU205475 |
| | Huize, Yunnan | Chao Z 1782703 | | **OR493982** | **OR502930** |
| *B. kaoi* Liu, C.Y. Chao & Chuang | Miaoli, Taiwan | TAIE: 47911 | OK050523 | | |
| | Taiwan, China | / | | | AM711598 |
| *B. kweichowense* R.H. Shan | Jiangkou, Guizhou | Chao Z 1882001 | MW135454 | **OR493983** | **OR502931** |
| *B. latissimum* Nakai | South Korea | / | MT821949 | | |
| | Korea | / | NC 033346 | | |
| | South Korea | / | | | AY551292 |
| *B. longiradiatum* Turcz. | Ningan, Heilongjiang | Chao Z 1481902 | **OR508823** | **OR493985** | **OR502933** |
| | Tieli, Heilongjiang | Chao Z 1481601 | **OR508822** | **OR493984** | **OR502932** |
| | Jiamusi, Heilongjiang | Wang CB 09034-1 | | | GU570618 |
| *B. marginatum* Wall. ex DC. | China | / | MT261187 | | |
| | Weishan, Yunnan | Wang ZX 2010091101 | | | HQ687955 |
| | Ranwu, Xizang | Chao Z 1781102 | **OR508826** | **OR493988** | **OR502936** |
| *B. marginatum* var. *stenophyllum* (H. Wolff) R.H. Shan et Y. Li | Lintao, Gansu | Zhang GX 62000301 | MT075712 | | |
| | Nielamu, Xizang | Yu Y 00107 | | | HQ687952 |
| | Huize, Yunnan | Chao Z 1782702 | **OR508825** | **OR493987** | **OR502935** |
| | Jianshui, Yunnan | Chao Z 1782601 | **OR508824** | **OR493986** | **OR502934** |
| *B. pusillum* Krylov | China | / | MT261188 | | |
| | Qinghai Lake, Qinghai | Ma XG 09151 | | | HQ824728 |
| *B. rockii* H. Wolff | Lijiang, Yunnan | Chao Z 1782301 | MW135455 | **OR493989** | **OR502937** |
| | Lijiang, Yunnan | TEW008 | MW135456 | **OR493990** | **OR502938** |
| *B. scorzonerifolium* Willd. | Lindian, Heilongjiang | Zhang GX & Wang H 23000403 | MT075715 | | |
| | Zhangbei, Hebei | Anonymous, 130722LY0211 | MT239475 | | GU570604 |
| | Zibo, Shandong | Pang YL 2007007 | | | GU570604 |
| | Chuzhou, Anhui | Wang ZX 2010071102 | | | HQ687960 |
| | E'erguna, Inner Mongolia | Chao Z 2082403 | | **OR493991** | **OR502939** |

(Continued)

| Taxa | Locality | Voucher | Accession number | | |
|---|---|---|---|---|---|
| | | | cp genome | nrDNA | ITS |
| *B. shanianum* X.G. Ma & X.J. He | Baima Snow Mountain, Deqin, Yunnan | Chao Z 1782002 | MW135452 | **OR493992** | **OR502940** |
| *B. sibiricum* Vest ex Roem. & Schult. | China | / | MT261190 | | |
| | Daqingshan, Neimeng | Pan SL 0519 | | | DQ285457 |
| | Chifeng, Neimeng | Chao Z 1980701 | | **OR493993** | **OR502941** |
| *B. sikangense* X.J. He & C.B. Wang | Mangkang, Xizang | Chao Z 1780701 | MW263066 | **OR493994** | **OR502942** |
| | Mangkang, Xizang | Chao Z 1781901 | MW263067 | **OR493995** | **OR502943** |
| *B. smithii* H. Wolff | Guyuan, Ningxia | Chao Z 1582502 | MN854381 | **OR493996** | **OR502944** |
| | Wuzhong, Ningxia | Chao Z 1582702 | MN854382 | **OR493997** | **OR502945** |
| | Tianzhu, Gansu | Chao Z 2180101 | **OR508827** | **OR493998** | **OR502946** |
| | China | Xie H 040727001 | | | DQ285455 |
| | Minhe, Qinghai | Ma XG 09080410 | | | GU570637 |
| *B. thianschanicum* Freyn | China | / | MT261192 | | |
| | China | Wang F 04-0111 | | | EU220927 |
| | Zhaosu, Xinjiang | Tuozi 780580 | | | GU570608 |
| *B. triradiatum* Adams ex Hoffm. | China | / | MT261193 | | |
| | Tianshan, Xinjiang | Chao Z 1573001 | | **OR494000** | **OR502948** |
| | Hami, Xinjiang | Anonymous 039 | | | GU570635 |
| *B. yinchowense* R.H. Shan & Y. Li | China | / | MT261194 | | |
| | Suide, Shanxi | Wang CB 09101 | | | GU570629 |
| | Jixian, Shaanxi | Wang CB 09008 | | | HQ687966 |
| | Yulin, Shaanxi | Chao Z 1681701 | **OR508829** | **OR494001** | **OR502949** |
| | Zichang, Shaanxi | Chao Z 2280101 | **OR508830** | **OR494002** | **OR502950** |
| | Jingbian, Shannxi | Chao Z 2280105 | **OR508831** | **OR494003** | **OR502951** |
| *B. yunnanense* Franch. | Kangding, Sichuan | Chao Z 1682301 | MW135450 | | |
| | Lijiang, Yunnan | Chao Z 1782303 | MW135453 | **OR494004** | **OR502952** |
| | Kunming, Yunnan | Wang QZ & Pu FD 374574 | | | EU001349 |
| | Shangri-la, Yunnan | Ma XG 10090302 | | | HQ687969 |
| *Apium graveolens* L. | Guangzhou, Guangdong | Chao Z 2019042602 | **OR508809** | **OR501374** | **OR502913** |
| *Centella asiatica* (L.) Urb. | China | Chao Z 2019042601 | MN854377 | **OR501373** | **OR502953** |
| *Cryptotaenia japonica* Hassk. | Guangzhou, Guangdong | Chao Z 2019042603 | **OR508832** | **OR501376** | **OR502954** |
| *Foeniculum vulgare* Mill. | Guangzhou, Guangdong | Chao Z 2019042604 | **OR508833** | **OR501377** | **OR502955** |

Sequences with accession number in bold face were obtained in this study; those marked with "★" were acquired through PCR amplification and Sanger sequencing. "/" means voucher specimen information unavailable.

Specimens of other Chinese *Bupleurum* species, especially those distributed in Western Sichuan, which were deposited in the major herbaria of China including China National Herbarium (PE), Herbarium of Department of Biology, Sichuan University (SZ), Herbarium of Chengdu Institute of Biology, Chinese Academy of Sciences (CDBI), Kunming Institute of Botany Herbarium (KUN) and Herbarium of College of Life Sciences, Northwest Agriculture & Forestry University (WUK), were also consulted and inspected on site or through Chinese Virtual Herbarium (CVH) website.

Morphological inspection  The morphological characters of taxonomic significance in *Bupleurum*, i.e., the number, shape and size of bracteoles, comparison of bracteoles length and umbellule size, the number and length of rays, the number and size of florets, the shape, size and texture of leaves, of *B. pseudochaishoui* were inspected, and were compared with the related species, *B. wenchuanense*, *B.*

*chaishoui*, *B. malconense*, *B. sichuanense*, and *B. microcephalum*. The data were acquired from at least 10 individuals of living materials or herbarium specimens, and were also checked in accordance with the descriptions in *Flora of China*. For measurements of some quantitative traits, such as plant height, leaf size, the number of small flowers, etc., 50 pieces of data were collected for each item, then the variation ranges were summarized and recorded.

DNA extraction Genomic DNA was isolated from the silica gel dried leaves of each sample using DNAsecure Plant Kit (TIANGEN Biotech Co, Ltd., Beijing, China). After purification, concentration of the extracted DNAs was determined on a NanoDrop 2000C spectrophotometry (Thermo Fisher, US).

ITS region amplification and sequencing ITS region of some samples (those with ITS accession number marked by "★" in Table 1) were amplified and sequenced. The universal primers ITS-p4 and ITS-p5 were used. PCR amplification was performed in a 15 μL reaction system containing 6 μL of 2× *Taq* Plus PCR MasterMix (Tiangen Biotech Co, Ltd., Beijing, China), 2 μL of DNA template, 0.5 μL of each primer (10 mM), and 6 μL of $ddH_2O$. The PCR products were purified and sequenced bidirectionally by Ruibo Biotech Co. Ltd. (Guangzhou, China). The sequences have been deposited in GenBank, and the accession numbers were listed in Table 1. We also downloaded several ITS sequences of the related species from GenBank (Table 1).

Skimmed genome sequencing The purified genomic DNAs were subjected to genome skimming performed on an BGISEQ-500 sequencer by BGI Genomics (Shenzhen, China). For each sample, a total of 3.0 Gb sequence data was obtained.

Whole cp genome and nrDNA assembly and annotation Whole cp genomes of the samples were assembled using GetOrganelle v1.7.4 software (Jin et al., 2020). The published cp genome of *B. chinense* DC. (GenBank accession number: MN337347) was used as the reference genome. Bowtie 2 was first called to filter out plastid-like reads, and then SPAdes was called for assembly. The cp genome was annotated using GeSeq and Plastid Genome Annotator (PGA) software, and the tRNAs in the genome were identified by tRNAscan-SE v2.0.7 and ARAGORN v1.2.38. The annotated genomes, together with the reference genome, were input into Geneious v22.2.2 for comparison to determine start and stop codons, as well as to manually correct the possible errors. Finally, the cp genome was physically mapped into a loop using the online software OGDRAW. The assembled and annotated cp genome sequences were deposited in GenBank (http://www.ncbi.nlm.nih.gov/) under accession numbers OQ460227 - OQ460239 (Table 1).

nrDNAs were also assembled using GerOrganelle v.1.7.3 software, and the output contigs were compared and annotated with the reference genome in Geneious v22.2.2.

Genome structure and comparative analysis The cp genome characteristics of the six species of *Bupleurum* were described, including the overall genome structure, the size of each part of the genome, and the GC content of the genes, which was acquired using Geneious v22.2.2. Multiple genome alignments of 13 sequences were done using the Mauve v2.4.0 plugin in Geneious v22.2.2, with default parameters.

To determine the expansion/contraction of IR, genes distributed within and next to the boundaries of LSC, SSC and IR regions were compared and manually mapped to visualize them.

To investigate the highly variable regions (divergence hotspots), 13 complete chloroplast sequences of six *Bupleurum* species, were compared using MAFFTv. 1.3.7. Subsequently, the cp genomes of *Bupleurum* species were paired and visualized using the Shuffle LAGAN mode in mVISTA, with the cp genome of *B. chinense* (GenBank access number: MN337347) as a reference. Using DnaSP v6.0, the nucleotide diversity (pi) in the cp genome sequence was calculated through sliding window analysis, with a window size of 600 bp and a step size of 200 bp.

Some other parameters, such as simple sequence repeats (SSRs), short dispersed repeats (SDRs), nonsynonymous (Ka) and synonymous (Ks) substitution rates, were also investigated. (Supplementary File S1, Figures S1, 2).

Molecular phylogenetic analysis In order to get insight into the phylogenetic relationship among the *Bupleurum* species, maximum likelihood (ML) analyses and Bayesian inference (BI) analyses based on the whole cp genome, the coding sequences (CDS), the highly variable regions, the nrDNA, and the ITS region were performed respectively. Besides the sequences obtained in this study, the previously reported cp genome and ITS sequences of Chinese *Bupleurum* species were also downloaded from Genbank and incorporated into phylogenetic analysis (Table 1).

The best model was obtained under AIC criteria using ModelFinder for molecular modeling of the dataset (Table 2). For ML analyses, IQ-tree 1.6.12 was used, and the reliability of each branch was assessed using bootstrap values (number of replicates set to 1 000). As for BI analyses, MrBayes 3.2.7a was used, and Markov chain Monte Carlo (MCMC) analysis was run for a total of 20 million generations, with samples taken every 1 000 generations. In the phylogenetic tree construction, *Centella asiatica* were used as outgroup species, and the resulting tree files were visualized and embellished using iTOL v. 6. 1. 2 software.

**Table 2 Best models for ML and BI analyses**

| dataset | whole chloroplast genome | the coding sequences (CDS) | nrDNA | ITS |
|---|---|---|---|---|
| ML | TVM+R10+F | GTR+F+R3 | GTR+F+R5 | GTR+F+G4 |
| BI | GTR+F+I+G4 | GTR+F+I+G4 | GTR+F+G4 | GRT+F+G4 |

## 3 RESULTS

Chloroplast genome and nrDNA features A total of 13 cp genomes from the six *Bupleurum* species were obtained. Size of these cp genomes ranges from 155 012 bp (*B. pseudochaishoui*) to 155 715 bp (*B. wenchuanense*). All of them exhibit a typical quadripartite structure, consisting of a small single copy (SSC) region (17 368 - 17 524 bp), a pair of inverted repeat (IR) regions (52 250 - 54 902 bp) and a large single copy (LSC) region (83 282 - 85 491 bp) (Table 3, Figure 1). The overall GC contents are highly similar (37.7%- 37.8%) (Table 3).

Genes and its arrangement in the cp genomes of the six *Bupleurum* species are almost the same. Each cp genome encodes 114 genes, including 80 protein-coding genes (PCG), 4 rRNA genes, and 30 tRNA genes. There're 60 PCGs and 22 tRNA genes in the LSC region, 12 PCGs and 1 tRNA gene in the SSC region. In the IR region, for 12 of the 13 cp genomes, there're 20 gene repeats, including 8 PCGs, 7 tRNA genes and 4 rRNA genes, except for one *B. wenchuanense* sample (voucher 2020080639), which has 2 extra PCGs (*rpl*22 and *rps*3) and thus a total of 22 genes in the IR region. Among these 114 genes, eighteen genes are found with introns, 15 of which containing one intron, while the other three (*clp*P, *ycf*3, and *rps*12) containing two introns. Incomplete copies of *ycf*1 and *rps*19 in the IR region are considered as pseudogenes. (Table 3, Table 4, Figure 1).

The nrDNA sequences of the six *Bupleurum* species are 5 821 - 5 824 bp in length. The nrDNA is composed of five segments, i.e., the small-subunit rRNA gene (18s rDNA), internal transcribed spacer 1 (ITS1), the 5.8S rRNA gene, internal transcribed spacer 2 (ITS2), and the large-subunit rRNA gene (26s rDNA). The length of each segment is 1 809 bp, 214 - 217 bp, 163 - 164 bp, 227 - 228 bp, and 3 406 - 3 407 bp respectively. The overall nrDNA GC content is 54.4%; among the five segments, ITS regions have higher GC content (with a value of 57.9%~58.7%). (Table 5).

Comparative analysis of chloroplast genome and nrDNA structure Results of Mauve pairwise analysis indicate that no rearrangement has occurred in coding and noncoding regions of the cp genomes of the six *Bupleurum* species (Figure 2), implying that the cp genomes are conservative.

The genes *rpl*22 and *rpl*2 are located on the left and right sides of the LSC/IRb junction respectively, while the gene *rps*19 crosses the JLB line (70 bp occurring in the IR region). The *ndh*F gene is at the right side of the IRb/SSC junction and 14 - 26 bp away from the boundary. Traversing the SSC and IRa region is the gene *ycf*1; a fragment of 1 877 - 1 902 bp in length of the gene is located in the IR region. The gene *trn*H lies 4-bp away from the JLA line (IRa/LSC boundary) to the right (Figure 3).

There's an obvious expansion in the IR region of a *B. wenchuanense* sample (voucher 2020080639). In this sample, as mentioned above, genes *rpl*22 and *rps*3 are found in the IR region. Generally, these two genes were located in the LSC region. The *rps*3 gene is crossing the junction of LSC/IRb (JLB) and LSC/IRa (JLA). (Figure 3).

**Table 3 Summary on chloroplast features of six *Bupleurum* species**

| | *B. chaishoui* | *B. microcephalum* | *B. sichuanense* | *B. malconense* | *B. wenchuanense* | *B. pseudochaishoui* |
|---|---|---|---|---|---|---|
| Total length (bp) | 155 272 - 155 592 | 155 048 - 155 080 | 155 533 - 155 544 | 155 441 - 155 562 | 155 080 - 155 715 | 155 012 |
| Total GC content (%) | 37.7 | 37.8 | 37.7 | 37.7 | 37.8 | 37.8 |
| IRa length (bp) | 26 295 - 26 322 | 26 125 - 26 133 | 26 295 - 26 311 | 26 309 - 26 311 | 26 129 - 27 451 | 26 134 |
| IRb length (bp) | 26 295 - 26 322 | 26 125 - 26 133 | 26 295 - 26 311 | 26 309 - 26 311 | 26 129 - 27 451 | 26 134 |
| SSC length (bp) | 17 368 - 17 456 | 17 511 - 17 524 | 17 493 - 17 494 | 17 468 - 17 494 | 17 521 - 17 531 | 17 530 |
| LSC length (bp) | 85 314 - 85 492 | 85 258 - 85 319 | 85 428 - 85 450 | 85 325 - 85 476 | 83 282 - 85 301 | 85 214 |
| Number unique genes | 114 | 114 | 114 | 114 | 114 | 114 |
| Protein coding | 80 | 80 | 80 | 80 | 80 | 80 |
| tRNA genes | 30 | 30 | 30 | 30 | 30 | 30 |
| rRNA genes | 4 | 4 | 4 | 4 | 4 | 4 |

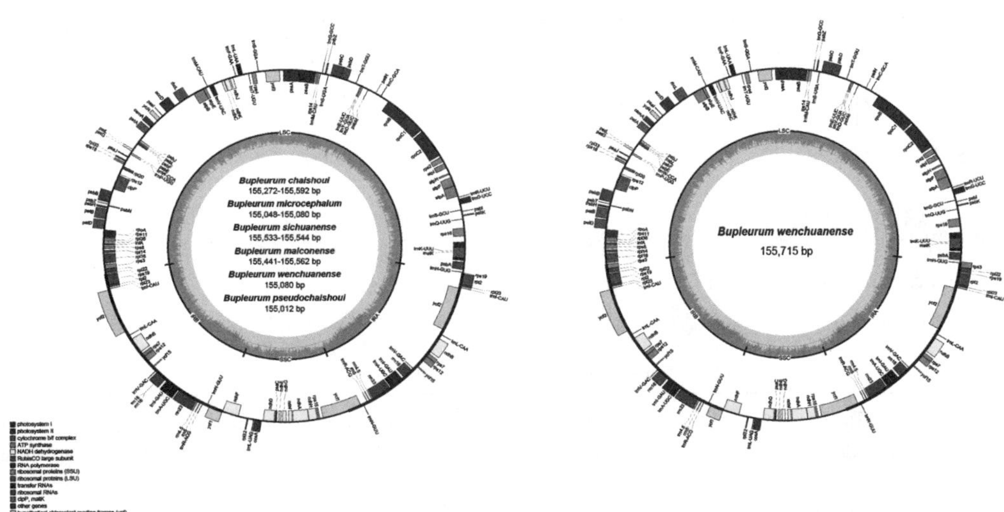


**Figure 1 cp genome map of the six *Bupleurum* species Genes shown outside of the larger circle are transcribed clockwise, while genes shown inside are transcribed counterclockwise. Thick lines of the smaller circle indicate IRs and the inner circle represents the GC variation across the genic regions**

Highly variable regions & nucleotide polymorphism in the chloroplast genomes and nrDNA We compared and mapped whole chloroplast gene alignments among 13 sequences of six *Bupleurum* species using mVISTA, using the published cp genome of *B. chinense* (No. MN337347) as the reference. The results showed that the divergence in the noncoding regions was greater than that in the coding regions, and a high degree of divergence in the 13 cp genomes appeared at intergenic spacers, including *trn*K-*rps*16, *atp*F-*atp*H, *atp*H-*atp*I, *trn*C-*pet*N, *pet*N-*pet*M, *ndh*C-*trn*V, *pet*A-*psb*J, *acc*D-*psa*I, *rps*15-*ycf*1, *rpl*32-*trn*L, and *trn*V-*rps*7. The coding regions were more conserved, and *trn*L, *rpo*C, *pet*D, *ycf*2, *ndh*A and *ycf*1 were the more divergent coding regions of these species. (Figure 4).

**Table 4 List of genes encoded in six *Bupleurum* plastomes**

| Gene Category | Genes | Number |
| --- | --- | --- |
| Ribosomal RNAs | *rrn*4.5$^{(\times2)}$; *rrn*5$^{(\times2)}$; *rrn*16$^{(\times2)}$; *rrn*23$^{(\times2)}$ | 8 |
| Transfer RNAs | *trn*A-UGC$^{(\times2)a}$; *trn*C-GCA; *trn*D-GUC; *trn*E-UUC; *trn*F-GAA; *trn*fM-CAU; *trn*G-GCC; *trn*G-UCC$^{a}$; *trn*H-GUG; *trn*I-CAU$^{(\times2)}$; *trn*I-GAU$^{(\times2)a}$; *trn*K-UUU$^{a}$; *trn*L-CAA$^{(\times2)}$; *trn*L-UAA$^{a}$; *trn*L-UAG; *trn*M-CAU; *trn*N-GUU$^{(\times2)}$; *trn*P-UGG; *trn*Q-UUG; *trn*R-ACG$^{(\times2)}$; *trn*R-UCU; *trn*S-GCU; *trn*S-GGA; *trn*S-UGA; *trn*T-GGU; *trn*T-UGU; *trn*V-GAC$^{(\times2)}$; *trn*V-UAC$^{a}$; *trn*W-CCA; *trn*Y-GUA | 37 |
| Subunits of photosystem Ⅰ | *psa*A; *psa*B; *psa*C; *psa*I; *psa*J; *ycf*3$^{b}$; *ycf*4 | 7 |
| Subunits of photosystem Ⅱ | *psb*A; *psb*B; *psb*C; *psb*D; *psb*E; *psb*F; *psb*H; *psb*I; *psb*J; *psb*K; *psb*L; *psb*M; *psb*N; *psb*T; *psb*Z | 15 |
| ATP-dependent protease subunit P | *clp*P$^{b}$ | 1 |
| Large subunit of rubisco | *rbc*L | 1 |
| NADH dehydrogenase | *ndh*A; *ndh*B$^{(\times2)a}$; *ndh*C; *ndh*D; *ndh*E; *ndh*F; *ndh*G; *ndh*H; *ndh*I; *ndh*J; *ndh*K | 12 |
| Ribosomal protein (large subunit) | *rpl*2$^{(\times2)a}$; *rpl*14; *rpl*16$^{a}$; *rpl*20; *rpl*22; *rpl*23$^{(\times2)}$; *rpl*33; *rpl*32; *rpl*36 | 11 |
| Small subunit of ribosomal proteins | *rps*2; *rps*3; *rps*4; *rps*7$^{(\times2)}$; *rps*8; *rps*11; *rps*12$^{(\times2)b}$; *rps*14; *rps*15; *rps*16$^{a}$; *rps*18; *rps*19 | 14 |
| DNA-dependent RNA polymerase | *rpo*A; *rpo*B; *rpo*C1; *rpo*C2 | 4 |
| Subunits of ATP synthase | *atp*A; *atp*B; *atp*E; *atp*F$^{a}$; *atp*H; *atp*I | 6 |
| C-type cytochrome synthesis gene | *ccs*A | 1 |

(Continued)

| Gene Category | Genes | Number |
|---|---|---|
| Subunits of cytochrome b/f complex | *pet*N; *pet*A; *pet*L; *pet*G; *pet*B[a]; *pet*D[a] | 6 |
| Envelop membrane protein | *cem*A | 1 |
| Maturase | *mat*K | 1 |
| Hypothetical chloroplast reading frames | *ycf*1; *ycf*2(×2) | 3 |
| Subunits of Acetyl-CoA-carboxylase | *acc*D | 1 |
| Pseudogenes | *inf*A; *rps*19★; *ycf*1★; *ycf*15(×2) | 5 |
| Total | 114 single-copy genes, 134 in total. | |

(×2): Two gene copies in the IRs; a: Gene containing one intron; b: Gene containing two introns; ★ means the incomplete copy located in the IR of the gene stradding the IR and LSC/SSC regions. Gene rps3(×2) and rpl22(×2) are in one of the Bupleurum wenchuanense sequences.

In order to assess the sequence divergence level of these *Bupleurum* species, the nucleotide diversity (Pi) of the cp genomes and nrDNAs were calculated.

The Pi values of the whole cp genome of the six species range from 0.00 – 0.06, and the two IR regions were significantly less divergent than the LSC and SSC regions. The spacer regions between genes were found with higher Pi values than the coding regions. Totally there're 7 spacer regions with Pi values greater than 0.01; the spacer with the highest Pi value was *rpl*32-*trn*L ($P>0.06$), followed by *pet*A-*psb*J ($P>0.02$), and consecutively, *trn*K-*rps*16, *atp*F-*atp*H, *atp*H-*atp*I, *ndh*C-*trn*V and *rps*15-*ycf*1 ($P>0.01$). Only two coding regions (*trn*L-UAA and *ycf*1) had Pi values higher than 0.01, and the *ycf*1 gene has higher value. (Figure 5A).

The concatenated nrDNA sequences of the six *Bupleurum* species have 65 variation sites and 54 parsimony-informative sites, accounting for 1.12% and 0.93% of the total sequences, respectively. The Pi value of the whole sequence was 0 – 0.044, and the variant regions were mainly concentrated in the transcribed spacer region (ITS), with a mean value of 0.029 (range 0 – 0.044) for ITS1, 0.007 (range 0 – 0.036) for 5.8S rRNA and 0.023 (range 0 – 0.044) for ITS2. 18S rRNA and 26S rRNA were more conserved, with a mean value of 0.001 (range 0 – 0.025) for 18S rRNA and 0.002 (range 0 – 0.036) for 26S rRNA. (Figure 5B).

Phylogenetic analysis Figures 6A – D shows the results of maximum likelihood (ML) analysis and Bayesian inference (BI) analysis of chloroplast whole genomes, protein-coding genes, the nrDNA and ITS region respectively, for the studied *Bupleurum* species. The phylogenetic trees estimated by ML and BI analyses showed similar topologies with high bootstrap support values and strong posterior probabilities for most nodes. The trees constructed based on the cp genome, protein-coding genes, and nrDNA were essentially alike. *Bupleurum* species formed a monophyletic clade which was sister to the other three species of Apioideae and could be divided into two main subclades, one consisting of *B. fruticosum* and *B. gibraltaricum* from the Mediterranean region (clade A), and the other consisting of all the remaining Chinese species (clade B).

**Table 5 Summary on nrDNA (18S-ITS1-5.8S-ITS2-28S) features of six *Bupleurum* species**

| | *B. chaishoui* | *B. microcephalum* | *B. sichuanense* | *B. malconense* | *B. wenchuanense* | *B. pseudochaishoui* |
|---|---|---|---|---|---|---|
| Total length (bp) | 5822 | 5823 | 5821 | 5821 | 5824 | 5824 |
| 18S rRNA length (bp) | 1809 | 1809 | 1809 | 1809 | 1809 | 1809 |
| ITS1 length (bp) | 216 | 216 – 217 | 213 – 214 | 214 – 215 | 216 | 216 |
| 5.8S rRNA length (bp) | 163 | 163 – 164 | 163 – 164 | 163 – 164 | 164 | 164 |
| ITS2 length (bp) | 227 – 228 | 227 | 228 | 227 | 228 | 228 |
| 26S rRNA length (bp) | 3406 – 3407 | 3407 | 3407 | 3407 | 3407 | 3407 |
| Total GC content (%) | 54.4 | 54.4 | 54.4 | 54.4 | 54.4 | 54.4 |
| ITS GC content (%) | 58.3 | 58.0 – 58.2 | 58.7 | 58.8 | 57.9 – 58.4 | 58.4 |

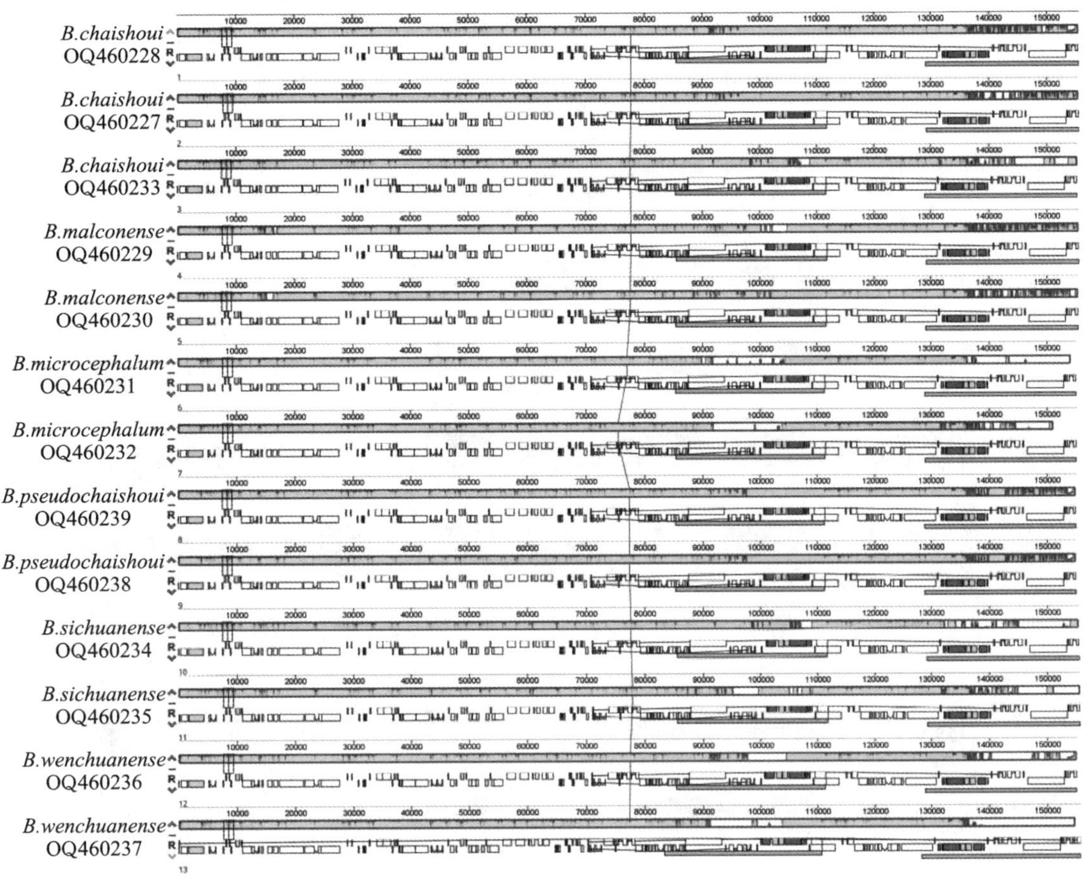


**Figure 2 MAUVE alignment of the six *Bupleurum* species Locally collinear blocks are represented by continuously colored regions**

The clade of Chinese species in subgenus *Bupleurum* can be further divided into clades C and D. In all trees, the constituent species of these two clades are consistent. A small one (clade C) was composed of *B. hamiltonii* N. P. Balakr., *B. candollei* Wall. ex DC., *B. yunnanense* Franch., *B. marginatum* Wall. ex DC. and its variety *B. marginatum* var. *stenophyllum* (H. Wolff) R. H. Shan & Y. Li. A large one (clade D) included more than 20 species; the six species produced in western Sichuan are all in this large clade.

Topology of clade D in the chloroplast-based trees and nuclear gene-based trees showed difference to some extent. The number of branches, the composing species of each branch, and the position of the branches, were quite different; for example, the position of *B. chaishoui*, the relationship between *B. microcephalum* and *B. wenchuanense* (See below, Discussion section, and Figure 6). Nevertheless, all four phylogenetic trees showed that the new species *B. pseudochaishoui* were closely related to *B. wenchuanense* and *B. microcephalum*; they were either forming/mixing in a separating branch (CP, CDS and nrDNA trees) or locating in adjacent branches (ITS tree). Similarly, *B. malconense* and *B. sichuanense* are closely related species of *B. chinense* and *B. yinchowense* R. H. Shan & Y. Li (Figures 6A-D).

The position of *B. chaishoui* varied in different trees. In the CP tree, it's close to *B. malconense*-*B. sichuanense*-*B. chinense*-*B. yinchowense* group, and then merged with *B. kweichowense* R. H. Shan and *B. sikangense*. In the CDS tree, it joined with *B. kweichowense* first, then *B. malconense*-*B. sichuanense*-*B. chinense*-*B. yinchowense* group and *B. sikangense*. In the NR tree, it's adjacent to the branch of *B. sikangense* and *B. commelynoideum* H. Boissieu, and then aggregated with *B. rockii* H. Wolff and *B. triradiatum* Adams ex Hoffm. successively. It's noticeable that in the ITS tree, *B. chaishoui* formed an independent branch sister to other species, neighboring to *B. sikangense* and *B. commelynoideum* branch.

The nrDNA phylogenetic tree has the highest resolution in differentiating the six *Bupleurum* species, in which each species formed a monophyletic branch.

## 4 DISCUSSION

Differences in gene and structure of chloroplast genomes among *Bupleurum* species We described for the first time the cp genomes of six species of *Bupleurum* from western Sichuan Province, China, providing important insights into the cp genome characteristics of members of this genus. Our

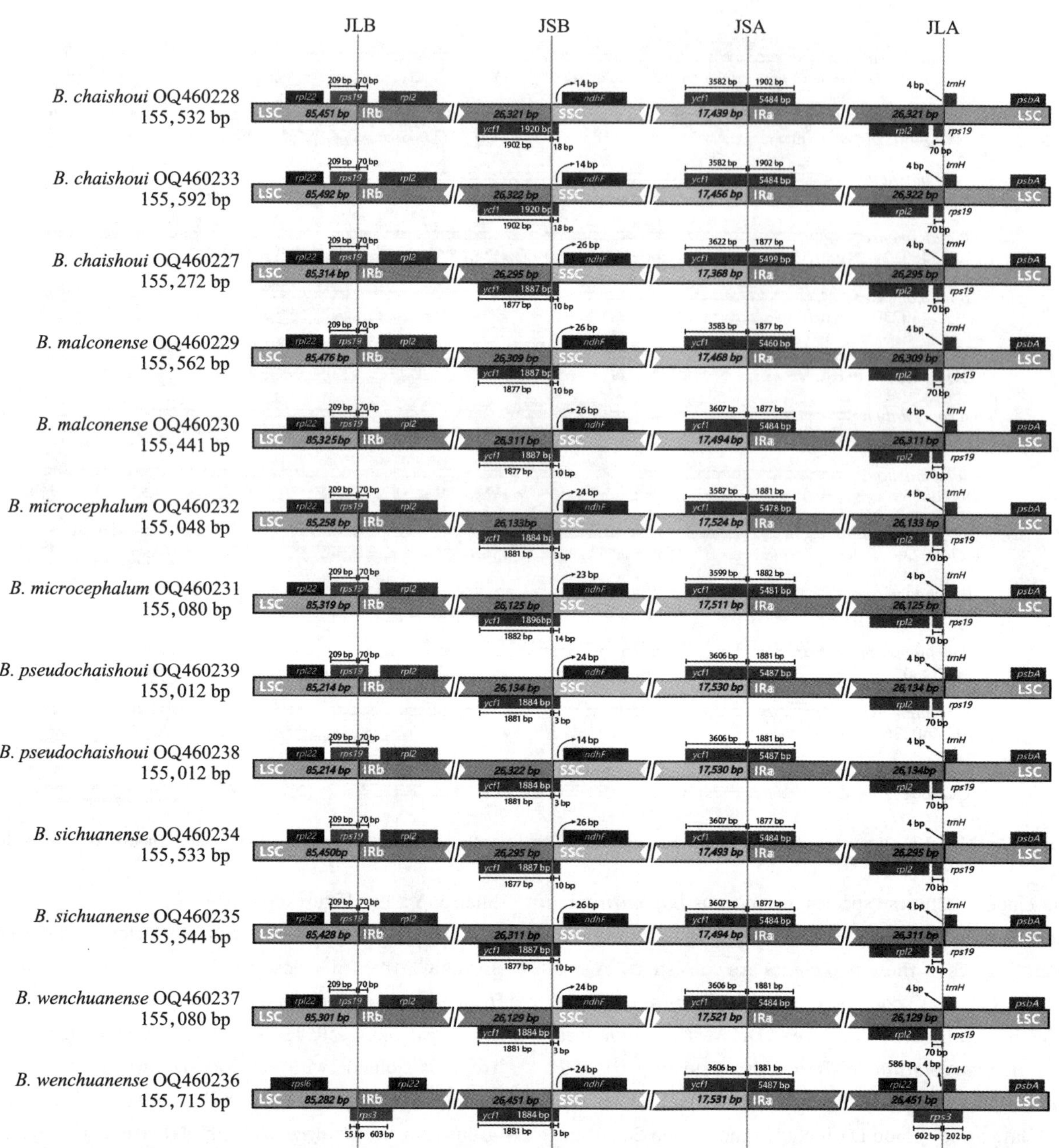


**Figure 3 Comparison of the LSC, SSC and IR junction among the six *Bupleurum* species**

JLB, junction line between LSC and IRb; JSB, junction line between SSC and IRb; JSA, junction line between SSC and Ira; JLA, junction line between LSC and IRa.

results show that the cp genomes of *Bupleurum* species are extremely similar, indicating that they are highly homogeneous in terms of cp genome structure, gene content and tendency of SDRs and SSRs. The cp genomes of the six *Bupleurum* species differ in size by only a few hundred bp (155 012 - 155 712 bp), consistent with the description that the cp genomes of *Bupleurum* species show only minor differences in size (~1 kb) (Huang et al., 2021a). Many mutational events occurring in the cp genome, including substitutions, insertions and deletions (InDels), inversions, genomic rearrangements and translocations (Abdullah et al., 2021), did not occur in any of the six *Bupleurum* species.

It has been reported that IR region contraction and expansion is a common phenomenon in cp genomes, and that changes in the size of the cp genome are usually the result of IR region expansion and that these variants can be observed in both closely and distantly related plant species and may lead to pseudogene production, gene duplication and deletion of individual copies of genes. Comparative analysis of IR boundaries showed the same distribution of genes at the LSC/IR junction in the cp genomes of the six *Bupleurum* species, with minor differences in gene length (*ycf*1 and *rps*19) at the SSC/IR junction. The *ycf*1 sequence located at the IRa and SSC boundaries was identified as a pseudogene

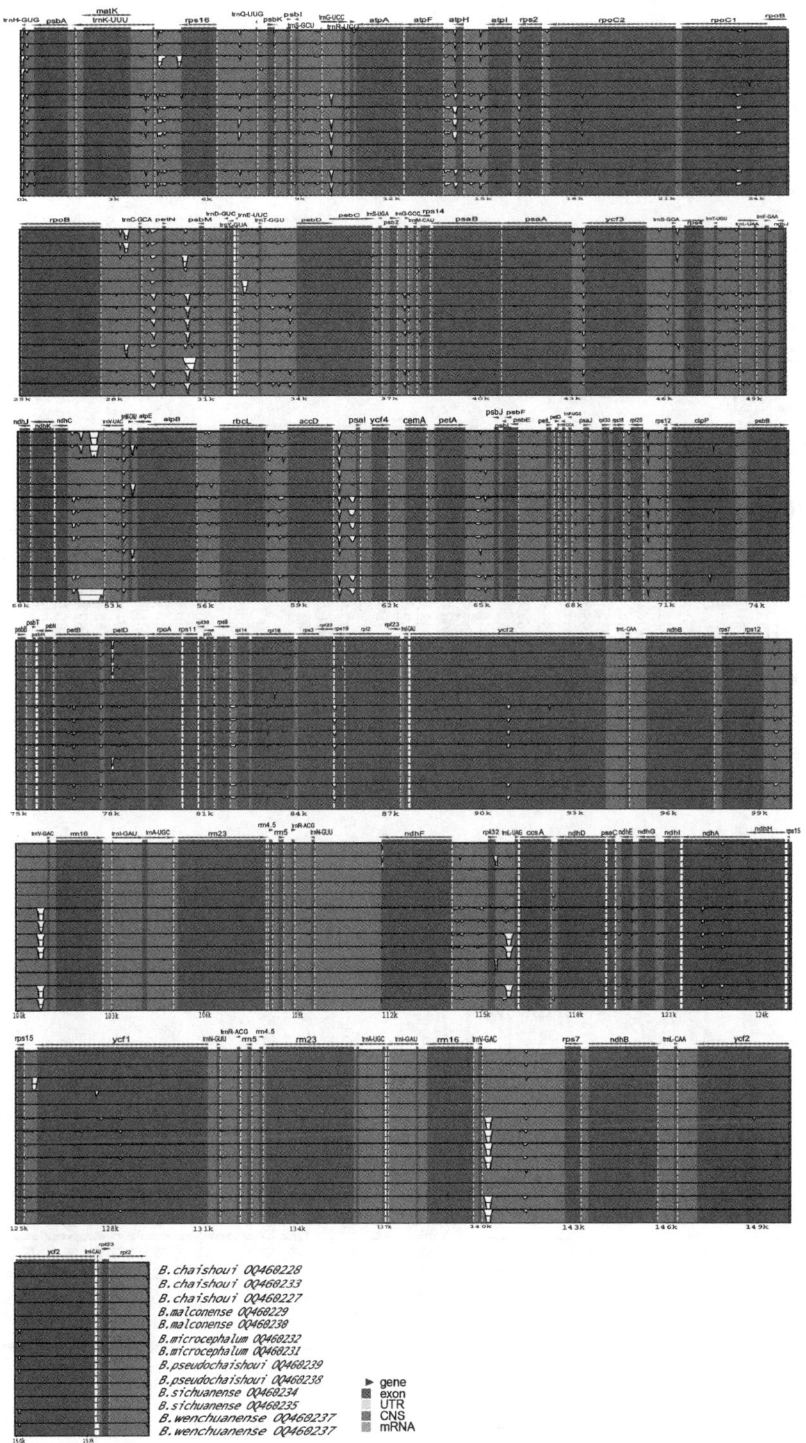


**Figure 4 Comparison of the six *Bupleurum* species cp genomes using the mVISTA alignment program, with *B. chinense* as a reference**

because it was truncated and was an incomplete duplicate of a normal copy. In the cp genome of a sample (*B. wenchuanense* voucher 2020080639), expansion of the IR region was found occurred, resulting in inconsistency between LSC/IR and SSC/IR border genes to other *Bupleurum*. The expansion was due to duplication of genes in IR (*rpl*22 and *rps*3). Variation in the number of duplicated genes in angiosperm cp genomes is common and different numbers of duplicated genes can be observed in different species, but IR expansion within species is somewhat uncommon. This phenomenon was once observed in the cp genome of *Sinopodophyllum hexandrum*. We performed read mapping analysis and confirmed such an expansion in the very sample of *B. wenchuanense* (Figure S4). However, the overall gene number and order remains consistent and reflects the significant conserved nature of chloroplasts in this species.

Highly variable regions in cp genome presumed as potential molecular markers Inspired by Dong's research

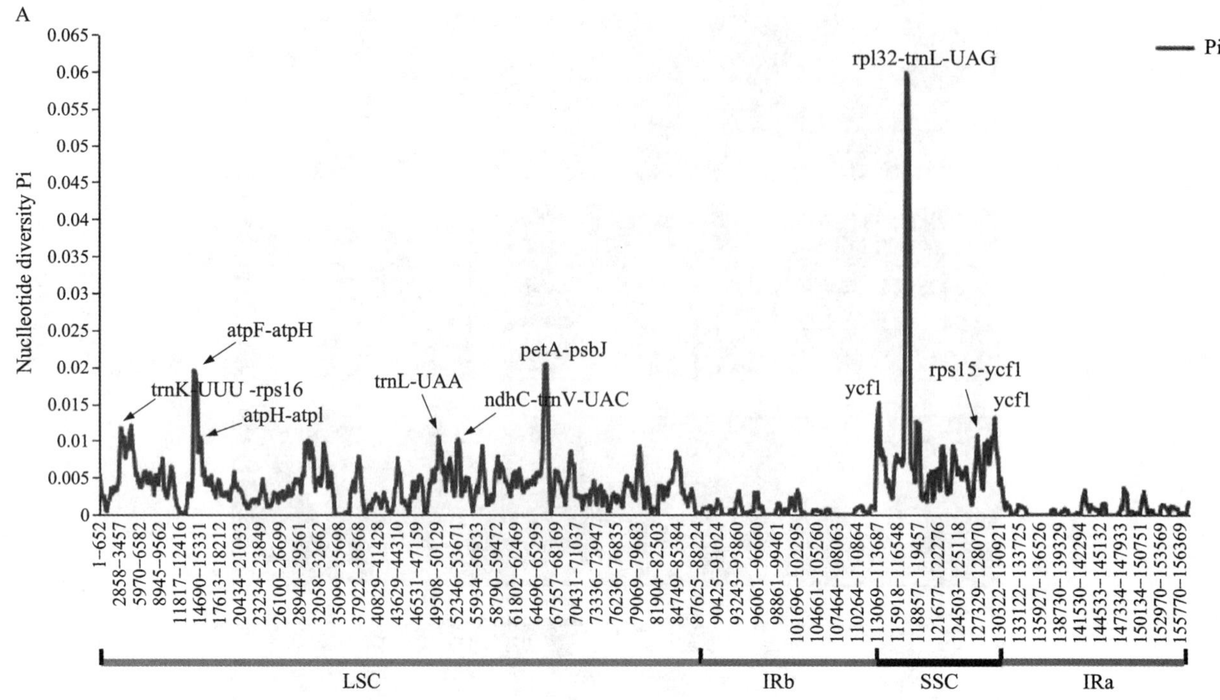


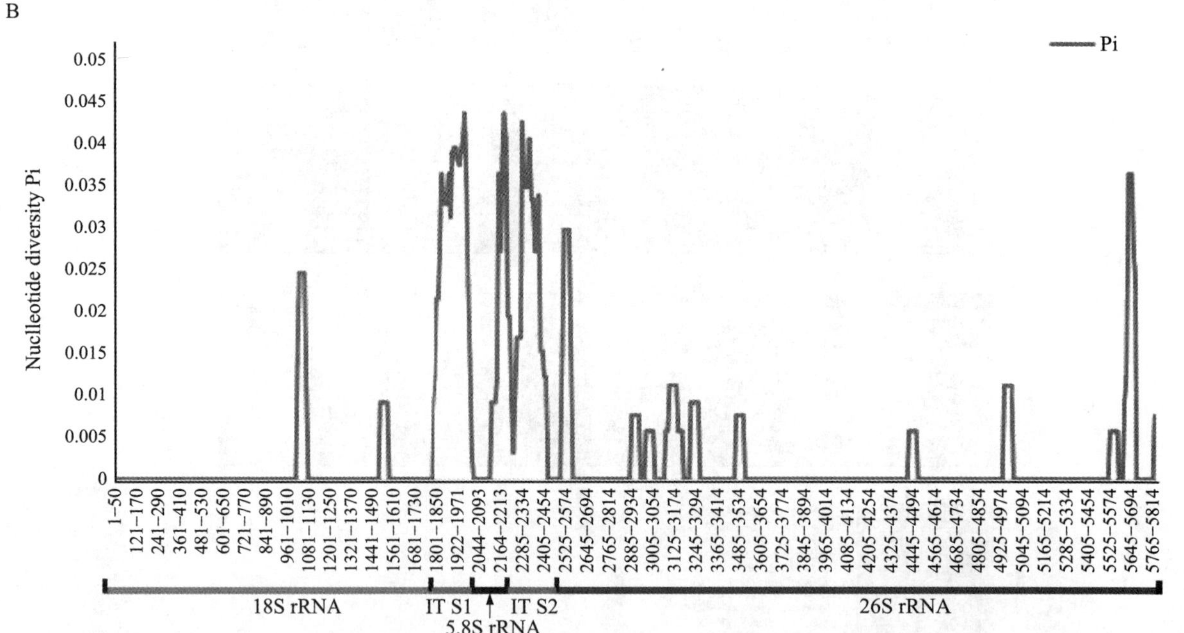


**Figure 5 Comparative analysis of the nucleotide diversity (Pi) value among the six *Bupleurum* species**

(A) cp genome; (B) nrDNA. X-axis: nucleotide position, Y-axis: nucleotide diversity value.

work, highly variable regions in cp genome have been generally thought to be potential molecular markers for phylogeny and identification of plant species. In some cases, the highly variable regions worked well in resolving phylogeny and identifying species, but in some other cases they were not so effective; more often, their effectiveness has not been evaluated. In order to assess whether the they can work in *Bupleurum* phylogenetic analysis and species identification; we checked the highly variable regions in cp genomes of the six *Bupleurum* species.

We found that the non-coding intergenic spacer regions have considerable diversity over the protein-coding regions, which was consistent with most previous studies. Seven spacer regions (*rpl*32-*trn*L, *pet*A-*psb*J, *atp*F-*atp*H, *trn*K-*rps*16, *atp*H-*atp*I, *ndh*C-*trn*V, and *rps*15-*ycf*1), and two coding regions (*trn*L-UAA and *ycf*1) were found to be highly variable ($P>0.01$). However, the discovered highly variable regions were not all the same as the previously reported ones in *Bupleurum*. The spacer regions *pet*A-*psb*J, *trn*K-*rps*16 and the gene *ycf*1 are the highly variable regions found in common in these studies on *Bupleurum* cp genomes. There is evidence supporting the *ycf*1 gene as one of the core plastid DNA barcodes in land plants. The *rpl*32-*trn*L, *pet*A-*psb*J gene have also been reported to show very high nucleotide per site diversity in several genera, and indeed the Pi values of the *rpl*32-*trn*L spacer regions of these six *Bupleurum* species were also much higher than the other regions in the present study, so *rpl*32-*trn*L together with *pet*A-*psb*J, *trn*K-*rps*16, and *ycf*1 were considered as having potential to be used as high-resolution DNA barcodes to identify species of *Bupleurum*.

We constructed phylogenetic trees of the six *Bupleurum* species using the four screened potential molecular markers independently and in combination, and found the trees were in similar topology to the whole cp genome and CDS trees, i. e., the six species were divided into two clades. But in each tree, there's species group that cannot be clearly separated (Figures S3A - F). The "potential" disappears in reality. Therefore, we propose that in similar studies in the future such presumed molecular markers should be verified.

Phylogenetic relationship inferred from cpDNA and nrDNA  The backbone of phylogenetic trees constructed based on the complete cp genomes, protein-coding sequences, nrDNA of the six *Bupleurum* species were highly silimar; and they were consistent with those acquired in the previous studies. The results confirmed *Bupleurum* is a monophyletic group and supported the treatment of its independent tribe status in subfamily Apioideae. The two main subclades represented the two subgenera in the genus, subgenus *Penninervia* and subgenus *Bupleurum*, respectively. The two clades (clade C and clade D in Figure 6) of Chinese *Bupleurum*, as well as the species included in each one, were also in concordance with the earlier researches.

*B. microcephalum*  In the six *Bupleurum* species in Western Sichuan, *B. microcephalum* and *B. malconense* were considered to be the most closely related species. The leaves of *B. microcephalum* are linear, extremely long, soft and thin, while the leaves of *B. malconense* are more than half shorter than that of *B. microcephalum*, and the texture is hard. But in all phylogenetic trees, *B. microcephalum* forms a clade with *B. wenchuanense*, and *B. pseudochaishoui*; in the tree based on nrDNA and ITS, it forms a sister branch to the latter two species. This is not consistent with the previous concepts that it's close to *B. malconense*. The three species in this clade all have solitary stem, which is different from species that have caespitose rootstock and numerous stems in the other clade.

*B. sichuanense* and *B. malconense*  *B. sichuanense* was established in 1992 by Pan and Hsu. In the original species description, it was pointed out *B. sichuanense* was closely related to *B. malconense*, and was differ from the latter in its short and tender cauline leaves, more umbel rays (6～7), and bracteoles not longer than the pedicel (<2 mm). In *Flora of China*, it was synonymized with *B. malconense*. Our molecular phylogenetic analysis proved their intimate relationships. In the phylogenetic trees constructed with the whole cp genomes, the CDS regions and the high variable regions, neither of the two formed a separate clade. In the nrDNA ITS tree, more than 10 sequences derived from these two species tangled together; but in the tree based on the nrDNA, *B. sichuanense* and *B. malconense* were clearly separated, implying they were two independent species. We checked the specimens of *B. malconense* and *B. sichuanense* deposited in Chinese Virtual Herbarium and those we collected and were of the opinion that the nrDNA correctly reflects the relationship between the two species. The results also implied the nrDNA might serve as a more suitable molecular marker for *Bupleurum* phylogenetic analysis and species identification.

The close relationship of *B. sichuanense* and *B. malconense* to *B. chinense* and *B. yinchowense* was disclosed almost 15 years ago. Their intimate relationship has once again been proven in this study. *B. chinense* is the officially recognized origin species of the crude drug of Chaihu. There is a need for molecular marker to distinguish *B. chinense* from the other three closely related species. It seems nrDNA and ITS perform better than cpDNA does for such a purpose.

*B. chaishoui* and the nucleocytoplasmic conflict  Phylogenetic trees constructed from cp genome and nrDNA show different topologies, indicating the existence of nuclear cytoplasmic conflicts. The position of *B. chaishoui* is an obvious example. Phylogenetic trees constructed from both nrDNA and ITS sequences support that *B. chaishoui* is closely related to *B. sikangense* and *B. commelynoideum*, while in the phylogenetic trees constructed from the whole cp genome sequence and CDS sequence, *B. chaishoui* is closely related to *B. malconense*; the latter is consistent with the opinion in FRPS that stated *B. chaishoui* and *B. malconense* are similar in morphology; The two species, together with the third species in the same clade, *B. sichuanense*, share a common morphological feature, i. e., the caespitose rootstock.

The inconsistencies in the topology of the gene trees acquired from the two different set of chloroplast and nuclear genomic data is a widespread phenomenon caused by a variety of reasons, including gene duplication and loss, horizontal gene transfer, incomplete lineage sorting, and hybridization introgression, etc. The most common reason for this phenomenon was believed to be chloroplast capture caused by hybridization. It was also reported cp genome-

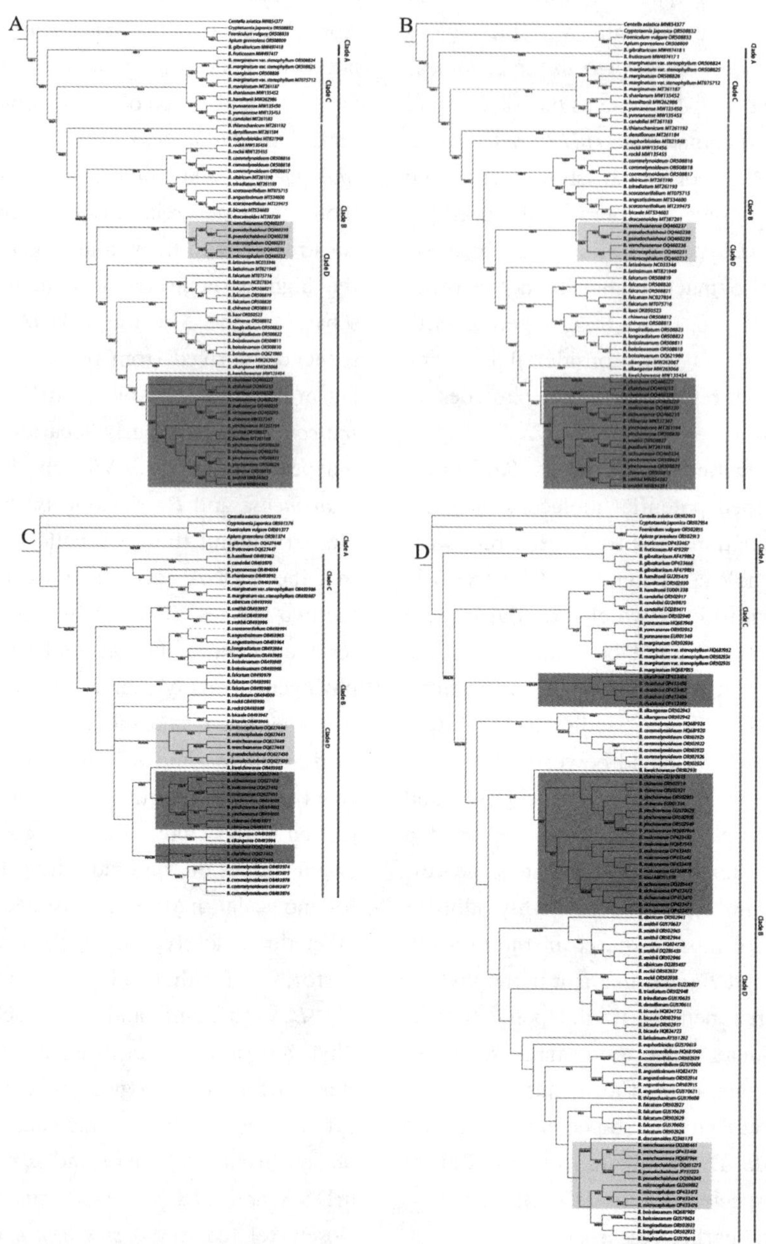

**Figure 6 Phylogenetic trees showing the relationship between *Bupleurum* species (BS>70, PP>0.95 obtained by ML/BI methods are shown above the branches)**

(A) Phylogenetic tree based on the whole cp genome; (B) Phylogenetic tree based on protein-coding genes; (C) Phylogenetic tree based on the nrDNA; (D) Phylogenetic tree based on the ITS region.

based phylogenetic relationships were often found to be related to geography rather than morphology. The Hengduan Mountains-Western Sichuan area is one of the diversity centers of *Bupleurum* species, and more than half of the species in China can be found in this region. The complex terrain and landforms, and diverse climate of ancient and modern times in the region have created opportunities for natural interspecific hybridization, and the results of phylogenetic trees suggest the possibility of ancient chloroplast capture events. Moreover, the widespread presence of hybridization in biological taxa has gained increasing recognition. However, compared to its complex biodiversity, there are still very few clearly described hybridization events in the genus *Bupleurum*. In-depth researches in this aspect are expected in the future to reveal the important value of hybridization for the formation and maintenance of biodiversity of *Bupleurum*.

The overlooked new species The materials collected from Weizhou Town and Shuixi Town of Wenchuan (voucher Chao Zhi 1682502 and Chao Zhi & Huang Rong 2020080849) had been overlooked and mistakenly acknowledged as *B. chaishoui* for years, recently we realized it represents a new species and named it *B. pseudochaishoui*. These two samples formed distinct clade in all phylogenetic trees, supporting its status as an independent species.

*B. pseudochaishoui* shows distinguishable morphological character to its allies. Its leaves are coriaceous and some shiny. The basal leaves are long petiolated and the blades are quite large, blade broadly ovate-elliptic to lanceolate elliptic; the middle and upper cauline leaves are much smaller, long lanceolate, with no petiole (Figure 7). In Chinese *Bupleurum*, only *B. longiradiatum* Turcz. (Northeastern, Northern and Northwestern China) and *B. aureum* Fisch. ex Hoffm. (Xinjiang) have basal leaves with blades of such a similar shape and size to *B. pseudochaishoui*.

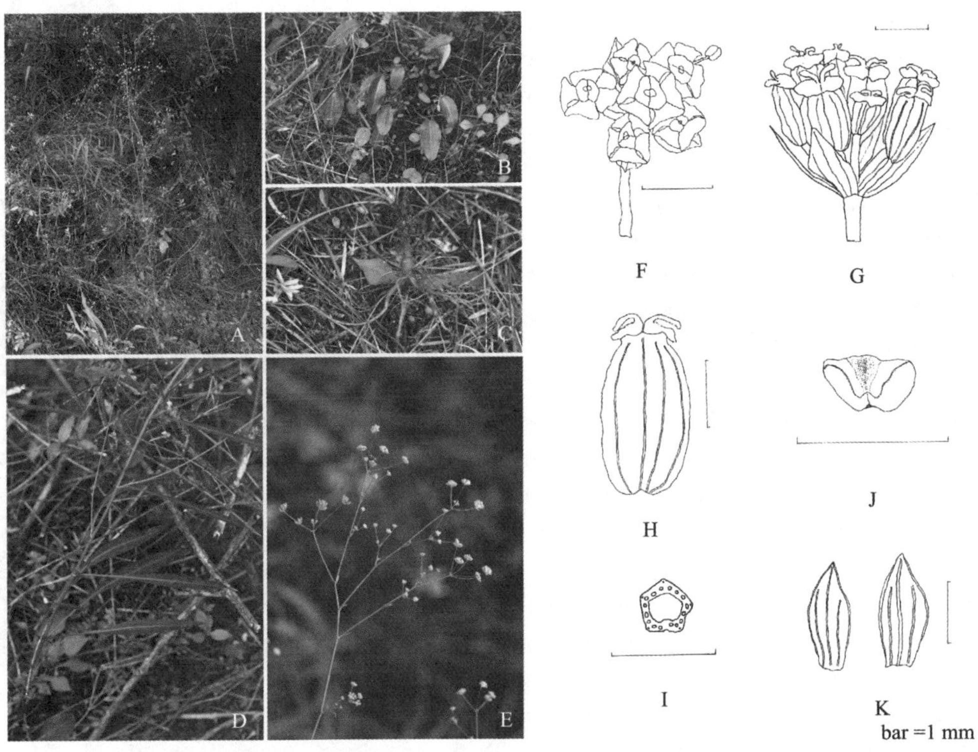


**Figure 7 *Bupleurum pseudochaishoui* Z. Chao sp. nov.**

(A) habitat and individual plant; (B) basal leaves; (C) root; (D) middle cauline leaves; (E) Compound umbels; (F) umbellule; (G) infructescence; (H) cremocarp; (J) petal; (K) bracteole; (I) schizocarp transverse section.

Molecular data indicated that *B. wenchuanense* is the most intimately related species to *B. pseudochaishoui*, but it differs from the new species in its numerous, rosette-caespitose oblanceolate basal leaves and subulate to squamose middle and upper leaves, and the (1-)2-3 very unequally rayed umbels, 1-4-flowered umbellules.

*B. chaishoui*, the species which we previously misrecognized as *B. pseudochaishoui*, has caespitose numerous stems, and lanceolate to elliptic cauline leaves; the shape and size of cauline leaves vary greatly, especially those born on the same node or adjacent nodes are very unequal; the upper ones often grow in a reflexed way (Figure 8). On the contrary, *B. pseudochaishoui* has solitary stem, and its cauline leaves often are not reflexed.

In the areas neighbor to Southwestern China, there are another two *Bupleurum* species having basal leaves with broadly oval lamina, namely *B. lanceolatum* Wall. ex DC. in Himalayas in India and Western Pakistan and *B. gilesii* H. Wolff in Western Pakistan and Afghanistan. The upper cauline leaves are of similar shape to the basal and lower leaves in *B. lanceolatum*, and short condensed main stem and numerous branches from the base in *B. gilesii*, make them easily to be distinguished from *B. pseudochaishoui*.

## 5 CONCLUSION

Comparative analysis of the cp genomes and nrDNA sequences of six *Bupleurum* species from western Sichuan Province, China revealed their conserved structure. Phylogenetic analysis based on nrDNA proved the monophyly of each species. Incongruence between nuclear and plastome gene trees was observed, which may be attributed to chloroplast capture. For overall consideration, *B. sichuanense* was thought to be an independent species different from *B. malconense*; *B. chaishoui* was supposed to be close relative to these two species, and they all shared the characteristic of having caespitose numerous stems. The other three species with solitary stem, *B. microcephalum*, *B. wenchuanense* and *B. pseudochaishoui*, were close in consanguinity. The new species, *B. pseudochaishoui*, was described and illustrated.

Taxonomy *Bupleurum pseudochaishoui* Z. Chao, sp. nov. (Figure 7).

Diagnosis: —This new species is easily distinguishable in the genus by its leathery dimorphic leaves, i.e., basal leaves with relatively large ovate-lanceolate blade and extremely long petiole, and lanceolate middle leaves. Molecular data implied it is closely related to *B. wenchuanense*, but the latter differs in its numerous, rosette-caespitose oblanceolate basal leaves and subulate to squamose middle and upper leaves, and the (1-)2-3 very unequally rayed umbels, 1-4-flowered umbellules.

Type: —CHINA. Sichuan Province: Wenchuan county, Buwa Village, growing on mountain slopes, 31°29′42.24″N, 103°35′43.01″E, elevation 2 000 m, 25 August 2016 (fl. & fr.), *Chao Zhi 1682502* (holotype, Southern Medical University herbarium, SMU)!.

Description: — Perennial herb. Taproot 10-15 cm long and 5-8 mm in diameter, stout, brownish, the head often inflated and annulated, lower part always branched and longitudinally finewrinkled, with sparse small horizontal protuberance. Rhizome present at the top of the root, lignified, 3-10 cm long. Stem solitary, solid and rigid, surface obviously striped, 80-120 cm high; base woody, sometimes tinged purple; middle and upper part slightly tortuous, much branched, branches 10-30 cm long. Leaves leathery, bright green, abaxial surface light green, margin narrowly white-cartilaginous; basal and the lower leaves large, blade broadly ovate-elliptic to lanceolate elliptic, 5-13 cm×2.5-4.5 cm, 5-7 nerved, apex rounded-obtuse or acute, base cuneate or broadly cuneate, tapering into long petiole up to 17 cm, slightly expanded into a sheath at the base, clasping; middle-part leaves long lanceolate, 10 cm×1 cm, nerves 5-7, often white-colored on both sides of the midvein, apex acute or acuminate, base tapering and clasping; upper leaves gradually smaller. Inflorescence much-branched, umbels numerous, 1.5-3 cm across; bracts 1-5, ovate or squamose, unequal, 1-3 mm×0.2-1 mm, 1-3 veined; rays 3-5, slender, unequal, 0.5-2.5 cm long; bracteoles 5, slightly membranous, ovate or lanceolate, 1.5-2 mm×0.8-1 mm, longer than pedicels, slightly shorter than umbellules, apex acuminate, 3-veined; umbellules 2-4 mm across, (5) 8-10 (12)-flowered; florets about 1 mm in diameter. Petals pale yellow, slight brown convex at the top of the inflex, ligule slightly ladder-shaped, apex obviously 2-lobed, lobes obtuse; pedicels 1-1.5 mm long; stylopodium yellow, thick discoid, wider than ovary. Fruit oblong, 2 mm×1 mm, brownish brown to dark brown, ribs not very obvious, vittae 3 in each furrow, 4 on commissure; fruit stalk about 2 mm long. Fl. Jul-Sep, fr. Aug-Oct.

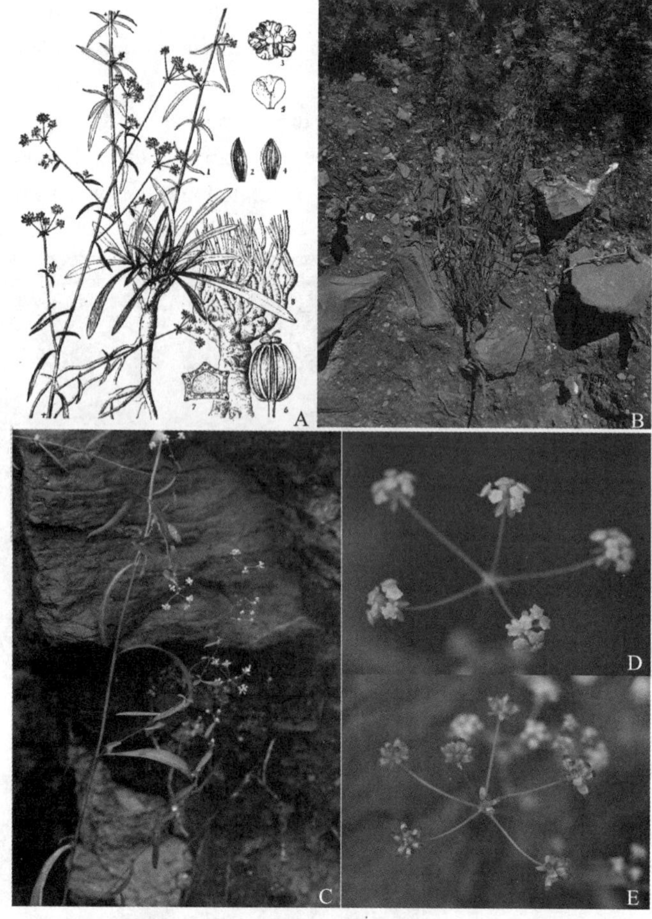

**Figure 8** ***Bupleurum chaishoui* R. H. Shan et M. L. Sheh**
(A) Illustration in FRPS; (B) individual plant; (C) middle cauline leaves; (D) Compound umbels; (E) infructescence.

Habitat and distribution: —The new species was found only in its type locality. It inhabits shrubs on mountain slopes, at an elevation about 2 000 m. Fl. and fr. July-Sept.

Etymology: —The epithet refers to it has been previously mistaken as *B. chaishoui*.

A key to the six most closely related species of *Bupleurum* in the region of Western Sichuan is given as follows:

1. Stem usually numerous, caespitose.

2. Cauline leaves lanceolate to elliptic, very unequal at the same node, 1.2-9 cm×0.3-1.2 cm, upper leaves usually reflexed ······································· *B. chaishoui* R.H. Shan & M.L. Sheh

2. Cauline leaves linear, similar in size, upper leaves not reflexed.

3. Involucel bracts less than 2 mm long, shorter than the pedicel; leaves tender, at most 8 cm long; rays of umbel usually 6-7 ······································· *B. sichuanense* S.L. Pan & P.S. Hsu

3. Involucel bracts more than 2 mm long, exceeding the pedicel; leaves firm, up to 15 cm long; rays of umbel usually less than 5 ·······································

………………… *B. malconense* R.H. Shan & Y. Li

1. Stem single, not caespitose.

4. Rays of umbel (1)2－3, very unequal; upper leaves small, subulate or squamose, few; stem much-branched … *B. wenchuanense* R.H. Shan & Y. Li

4. Rays of umbel more than 4; leaves conspicuous and numerous.

5. Basal and cauline leaves uniform, linear, very long and narrow, herbaceous, soft, abaxially slightly glaucous ………………… *B. microcephalum* Diels.

5. Leaves coriaceous; the basal and lower ones large, blade broadly ovate-elliptic to lanceolate elliptic, petiole quite long; the middle and upper ones long lanceolate ……………………………………………… ………… *B. pseudochaishoui* Z. Chao sp. nov.

［晁志，等. Frontiers in Plant Science, 2023, 14, DOI: 10. 3389.］

# A novel biological sources consistency evaluation method reveals high level of biodiversity within wild natural medicine: a case study of *Amynthas* earthworms as "Guang Dilong"

## 1 INTRODUCTION

The evaluation of batch similarity/consistency is a fundamental issue in traditional Chinese medicine (TCM) quality control. Due to a lack of effective trait discovery and bioactivity assessment methods, biological sources evaluation has become an indispensable means in evaluating TCM within and between batches, particularly in animal-based traditional medicines. Specifically, approximately 80% of all Chinese herb sources are wild, and assessments of the inter-/intra-species level biodiversity of wild medicinal resources are constantly insufficient. Following the exploitation of wild resources, unanticipated biodiversity may exist in natural medical materials as species with similar morphological characteristics and sympatric distribution, resulting in high heterogeneity when processed to TCM and Chinese patent medicine. Establishing proper and efficient approach to evaluate the biological composition consistency of medicinal resources, at both of inter-/intra-species level, has become one of the key priorities in the internationalization and modernization of TCM.

Over the past decade, molecular methods such as DNA barcoding have provided an accurate and efficient strategy for identifying species and distinguishing the authentic ones from the adulterants in various types of traditional medicines. Furthermore, DNA barcoding can also speed up the identification of distinct lineages, and accelerate the discovery of the cryptic/undescribed inter-/intra-species level biodiversity. However, as traditional DNA barcoding identifies single specimens based on individual DNA sequencing reactions, it is often unsuitable for bulk commercial materials. The ongoing development of DNA metabarcoding which combines next-generation sequencing (NGS) with DNA barcoding has enabled the identification of a large number of samples with high throughput and low cost. Aside from detecting species level diversity, recent studies have demonstrated its ability to distinguish intraspecific genetic variation from environmental samples. Moreover, as cytochrome c oxidase I (COI) has a natural high intraspecies variability for metazoan, the mini-barcode (100－250 bp) designed within the COI region, combined with DNA metabarcoding, would simultaneously characterize the intra- and inter-species genetics of bulk animal-based medicinal materials, even in samples with degraded DNA.

The dried bodies of earthworms such as "Dilong" are widely used to treat inflammation, thrombus, asthma, and pyretic. According to the *Chinese Pharmacopoeia*, species *Amynthas aspergillum* (Perrier, 1872) (synonym *Pheretima aspergillum*), *Metaphire vulgaris* (Chen, 1930) (synonym *P. vulgaris*), *M. guillelmi* (Michaelsen, 1895) (synonym *P. guillelmi*) and *A. pectieniferus* (Michaelsen, 1931) (synonym *P. pectinifera*) were official recorded as the original medicinal materials of "Dilong". The first one is known as "Guang Dilong", and mainly distributed in Guangdong province, Hainan province and Guangxi Zhuang Autonomous Region (Guangxi) in China. According to the authors' investigation, residents tend to collect this medical species in the wild at harvest time more than they breed them due to their relatively low price compared to human cost. In addition to *A. aspergillum*, there are a large number of sympatrically distributed Megascolecidae species that resemble each other in morphological characters, where new species are continually discovered. Moreover, the rapid growth in price in recent years led to the emergence of intended adulterations and substitutions in medicinal markets, making the actual biological composition of "Guang Dilong" more confusing. The biological composition stability of medical materials should benefit from the fixation of producing areas. Nevertheless, while the alpha taxonomic classification of Megascolecidae in south China is still ongoing, information on the sympatric distribution of multiple cryptic species and relative taxa abundance is still too limited to inform the selection of suitable collection or breeding sites. On the other hand, although multiple methods were developed for the authentication of *Amynthas* species, so far there is no reasonable biological composition assessment approach suitable for batch consistency evaluation of "Guang Dilong".

In this study, taking "Guang Dilong" as an example, a novel strategy based on DNA metabarcoding combined with minibarcode was proposed for batch-to-batch biological sources consistency evaluation of TCM. High levels of interspecific and intraspecific genetic diversity were discovered in medical materials from various production regions and Chinese patent medicines. Notably, even the two subgroups of *A. aspergillum* that were revealed here differed significantly in chemical compositions and biological activities. Fortunately, the subsequent analysis of locally acquired "decoction pieces" samples confirmed the geographic areas with constant *Amynthas* species composition. The inter-/intra-biodiversity display in our approach could be taken as an innovative indicator of batch consistency evaluation, and our strategy should be conducive to the fixation of the producing area and the establishment of entire industrial chain origin quality consistency control and quality traceability systems.

## 2 MATERIALS AND METHODS

2.1 Local cytochrome c oxidase I dataset preparation and evaluation of molecular markers Previous reports have validated 658 bp Folmer region of COI gene amplified by LCO1490/HCO2198 as the "standard" marker for the DNA barcoding of earthworms. To set up a local reference database, 1 575 *Amynthas* and *Metaphire* COI sequences were first collected from BARCODE OF LIFE DATA (BOLD; http://boldsystems.org) and GenBank. After trimming with primers LCO1490 (5′-GGTCAACAAATCATAAAGATATTGG-3′) and HCO2198 (5′-TAAACTTCAGGGTGACCAAAAAATCA-3′), the sequences without species level taxonomic information, containing transcription terminators, or below 500 bp in length, were removed. Finally, 689 sequences from 99 species were preserved in our local dataset.

The LCO1490 and HCO1777 (5′-ACTTATATTGTTTATACGAGGGAA-3′) primer pair, which has been successfully used to identify degraded earthworm components in reptile feces samples, was selected as the marker, owing to the relative small size of the PCR product (281 bp). To further assess the universality of primer HCO1777 for *Amynthas* and *Metaphire* species, the nucleotide diversity (Pi) value of each locus in our database was calculated and screened using DnaSP to determine whether the primer binding sites among different species were conserved. To evaluate the taxonomic resolution of the LCO1490/HCO1777 marker, the amplicon regions were extracted in silico from our reference dataset, and after selecting the optimal fitting model determined by the ModelFinder implemented in IQ-TREE v1.6.12, the ML phylogenetic tree was constructed using IQ-TREE with 1 000 bootstrap replicates.

2.2 Sample collection and pretreatment To investigate the biodiversity within "Guang Dilong", 5 075 earthworm (Table 1) samples regarded as "Guang Dilong" were collected in the wild from 18 locations of Guangxi from September 2017 to June 2019, and made into dried decoction pieces by local farmers under the authors' supervision. Although the morphological characteristics of earthworms were lost in processed samples, this acquisition method ensured convenient sample collection, transportation, and storage, and maximized the numbers of samples. We assumed that this operable method could be adopted by other rapid biodiversity assessment practice on herbal medicine. In addition, 301 processed samples were bought from Baise Market of Traditional Chinese Medicine, Guangxi. To test the results of our species distribution pattern, three batches of 2 796 dried earthworms (Table 1) collected from assigned sites were obtained from Youbo Pharmaceutical Co., Ltd. in April 2018. Finally, to uncover the cryptic biodiversity within the TCM product, three kinds of Chinese patent medicine containing "Dilong" (earthworm) were incorporated into the experiment in June 2019 as GX (batch number: 17 083 634), NX1 - NX23 (batch numbers 130 524, 141 127, 1 501 116, 141 016, 150 534, 140 817, 140 968, 141 042, 1 411 145, 150 211, 150 533, 1 407 137, 150 535, 150 543, 150 544, 150 545, 150 546, 150 547, 150 848, 150 556, 150 557, 150 558 and 1 501 122), and SH (batch number 17 013 914).

As metabarcoding allows for the pooling of hundreds of samples and their sequencing in a single sequencing run, for each collection site or product batch, 0.02 g of muscle was cut off individually from the abdomen and packed into a single tube. One point five percent (*W*/*V*) sodium dodecyl sulfate (SDS) lysate was used to pre-process samples after powdering. The mixture was incubated at 65 ℃ for 20 min and centrifuged at 3 000 revolutions per minute (r/min) for 5 min. Approximately 200 μL of supernatant was stored for further DNA extraction.

2.3 DNA extraction and amplification Total genomic DNA from each group sample was extracted using TIANamp

**Table 1 Sample information**

| Sample name | Sampling place/source | Coordinate | Sampling time | Number of individuals |
|---|---|---|---|---|
| BB | Bobai county | 22°06′N, 109°87′E | 2017.11 | 213 |
| BL | Dayantang village, Beiliu city | 22°43′27″N, 110°18′20″E | 2018.11 | 428 |
| BS | Bought from Baise drug market | 23°54′18.21″N, 106°36′53.87″E | 2018.11 | 301 |
| CL | Changle town | 21°49′21.67″N, 109°24′26.52″E | 2017.11 | 340 |
| CT | Caotang village, Changle town | 21°88′N, 109°39′46″E | 2017.11 | 398 |
| DJ | Dujiao village, Changle town | 21°49′21.67″N, 109°24′26.52″E | 2018.11 | 230 |
| DQ | Daqiao town, Luchuan county | 22°15′1.67″N, 110°12′58.36″E | 2018.11 | 260 |
| DX | Dongxing town, Dongxing county | 21°32′20.25″N, 107°58′6.08″E | 2018.11 | 260 |
| DY | Dayantang village, Beiliu city | 22°43′27″N, 110°18′20″E | 2018.11 | 210 |
| HX | Huoxing village, Changle town | 21°87′16″N, 109°44′52″E | 2017.11 | 307 |
| LC | Luchuan county | 22°19′26″N, 110°15′35″E | 2017.11 | 410 |
| MP | Mapo town, Luchuan county | 22°29′36.74″N, 110°13′3.80″E | 2018.11 | 240 |
| PS | Poshan village, Changle town | 21°49′21.67″N, 109°24′26.52″E | 2018.11 | 220 |
| SC | Songshuyuan village, Shikang town | 21°80′04″N, 109°34′51″E | 2017.11 | 307 |
| ST | Santang town, Bobai county | 22°11′2.83″N, 110°01′370.3″E | 2018.11 | 170 |
| TD | Tiandong county | 23°35′58.99″N, 107°07′19.10″E | 2017.11 | 260 |
| WL | Pubei county | 22°27″N, 109°55′E | 2018.11 | 240 |
| XWC | Xuwu village, Changle town | 21°76′7″N, 109°42′58″E | 2017.11 | 302 |
| ZH | Zhanghuang town, Pubei county | 22°0′37.79″N, 109°27′20.93″E | 2018.11 | 280 |
| dlA[a] | Hepu county, batch number: 170506 | N/A | 2018.04 | 1001 |
| dlB[a] | Beiliu county, batch number: 170510 | N/A | 2018.04 | 902 |
| dlC[a] | Bobai county, batch number: 170509 | N/A | 2018.04 | 893 |

[a] Samples purchased from assigned sites and provided by pharmaceutical company.

Genomic DNA Kit (Tiangen Biotech Co., Ltd., China). The quality and concentration of the extracted DNA were determined using NanoDrop 2000. A 281 bp long segment of the 5′ terminus of the COI gene was amplified using primers LCO1490 and HCO1777. The amplification products were then pooled to construct the final libraries. To distinguish amplicons originating from different samples, tag oligonucleotides were ligated to each side of the primers, as shown in Supporting Information Table S1. As "tag jumps" between different indexed samples during library preparation and sequencing could lead to false assignment of sequences and artificially inflate diversity, each PCR amplification was carried out with matching tags to minimize tag jumps. PCR reactions were carried out at a final volume of 25 μL containing 12.5 μL 2×Gflex buffer (containing 1 mmol/L of $Mg^{2+}$ and 200 μmol/L of each dNTP), 0.5 μL Tks Gflex DNA Polymerase (1.25 U/μL) (Takara Dalian, China), 1 μL DNA template, 0.5 μL forward, and 0.5 μL reverse primers. The reaction condition that followed was predenaturation at 94 ℃ for 1 min; 40 cycles of denaturation at 98 ℃ for 10 s, annealing at 48 ℃ for 15 s, extension at 68 ℃ for 30 s; and final extension at 68 ℃ for 5 min. Extraction blanks and PCR blanks were included for each batch of DNA extraction to ensure no carryover contamination occurred. The PCR products were isolated on 1.5% agarose gel electrophoresis and purified using the Agarose Gel DNA Purification Kit Version 2.0 (Takara Dalian, China).

2.4 Amplicon sequencing data processing The amplification products were sequenced using 2 × 250 bp paired-end protocol on the Illumina Hiseq 2500 platform. Pair-end reads were demultiplexed using fastq-multx and assigned to each sample according to the unique tags. Then the primer sequences were trimmed using bbduk. The amplicon sequence variants (ASVs) were identified after quality control, joining of paired ends, removal of chimeras, removal of non-target-length sequences, and denoising using the DADA2 method. In contrast with traditional Molecular Operational Taxonomic Units (MOTUs), which cluster multiple sequences to represent taxons at species level, ASVs generally stand for unique haplotypes. Rarefaction curves were inferred to define the rarefaction value for normalizing the ASVs table using the Vegan R Package. Subsequently, the alpha-diversity indexes (Shannon) and betadiversity were measured using R package phyloseq. To analyze the phylogenetic relationship between ASV sequences, Bayesian inference (BI) and maximum-likelihood (ML) methods were performed using MrBayes and IQ-TREE and based on GTR+G and GTR+F+I+G4 model, respectively.

2.5 Taxonomy assignment of amplicon sequence variants and molecular operational taxonomic units Two species delimitation methods were utilized to identify the MOTUs from the representative ASV sequences. The automatic barcoding gap discovery (ABGD) method was used to identify the genetic distance at which a "barcoding gap" occurs and then sort the ASVs into putative species, with the default settings being $P_{min}=0.001$, $P_{max}=0.1$, Steps=10, $X$ (relative gap width)=1.5, and Nb bins=20; and with K2P distances. The Bayesian version of Poisson Tree Processes (bPTP) analysis was also run for delimiting species on a rooted MrBayes consensus tree. The Bayesian tree was uploaded to https://species.h-its.org/ptp/and the number of MCMC generations was set as 500000.

The taxonomic information of each ASV/MOTU was determined using two methods based on sequence similarity and phylogenetic placement, separately. The first strategy was BLAST-MEGAN. BLAST search against the local database was conducted as -outfmt 5, -evalue 10, -max_target_seqs 5, -gapopen 5, -gapextend 2, and -num_threads 16. Subsequently, the BLAST results were visualized using MEGAN community edition version 6.10.8 and parsed to assign the optimal hits to appropriate taxa in the NCBI taxonomy. MEGAN parameters were set as: minimum score=50, maximum expected=0.01, top percent=10, minimum support percent=0.01, minimum support=1, and weighted LCA algorithm. The minimum identity to query would be set as 97% for species level identification, or 93% to obtain taxonomic information at a relatively high level for queries that could not be identified as exact species. The phylogenetic-based taxonomic assignment was performed as our second strategy. The ASVs queries were aligned with our local COI reference dataset and placed on the COI reference ML tree using pplacer followed by taxonomic classification with the pplacer guppy tool.

For that MOTUs failed to be identified at the species level, our cooperators in Shanghai Jiao Tong University were entrusted with the use of a professional database for identification. To verify the authenticity of MOTUs, whose Linnaean species name cannot be specified finally, 7 earthworms were randomly selected from the dried products purchased from the Baise Market of Traditional Chinese Medicine. After DNA extraction, PCR amplification and Sanger sequencing, the 658 bp Folmer regions of COI gene were obtained. Two individuals with 100% similarity to Megascolecidae sp2 were screened out. Whole-genome shotgun sequencing of 2 samples was carried out on the Illumina Hiseq X Ten platform (PE150; insert size, 350 bp).

Quality assessment of raw reads was performed using Trimmomatic version 0.36 by removing low-quality and adaptercontaminated reads. Subsequently, remaining high-quality reads were assembled into contigs using NOVOPlasty version 3.1. The parameters were set as: insert size=350, read length=150, type=mito, gene range=10000-20000, $k$-mer=39. The preliminary mitochondrial genome annotations were conducted in MITOS web server, under default settings and the invertebrate genetic code for mitochondria, followed by manual corrections of the start and stop codons in Geneious based on the previously published mitochondrial genome of *Metaphire californica*.

To verify the phylogenetic status of the presumed species, protein-coding sequence (CDS) on mitochondrial genome of 2 Megascolecidae sp2 individuals and 18 other pheretimoid species were extracted and concatenated by PhyloSuite with default parameters, then the phylogenetic tree was constructed using ML algorithms with TIM2+F+R8 model in IQ-TREE v1.6.12 and visualized using iTOL (https://itol.embl.de/).

2.6 Analysis of intraspecies subgroups within "Guang Dilong" samples that identified as A. aspergillum When inspecting the intraspecies biodiversity within *A. aspergillum*, two subgroups were discovered and the "barcoding gap" between them based on genetic distance was depicted by MEGA (10.1.8) and R package ggplot2 (v3.3.5). Subsequently, a haplotype network was constructed to illustrate the relationships among haplotypes using Population Analysis of Reticulated Trees (PopART) version 1.7.

To verify the authenticity of these two subgroups, one individual from each subgroup was selected for whole-genome sequencing. To compare the overall similarities of mitochondrial genomes, pairwise alignments were performed in the mVISTA program (http://genome.lbl.gov/vista/mvista/submit.shtml), under LAGAN mode using the annotation of *A. aspergillum* (GenBank accession number: NC_025292, BINs ID: ACH7381) as reference.

To determine whether two subgroups of *A. aspergillum* have the same chemical composition and pharmacodynamic action, 19 samples (11 of subgroup 1 and 8 of subgroup 2) were selected randomly from our samples.

The UHPLC-Q-TOF/MS system used to describe the

chemical profile was composed of Agilent 1 290 UHPLC instrument (Agilent Technologies, Waldbronn, Germany) and Agilent 6546 Q-TOF mass spectrometer (Agilent Corporation, Santa Clara, CA, USA). The MS data were acquired in positive dual Agilent Jet Steam Electron Spray Ionization (AJS ESI) mode. Chromatographic separation was performed on a Waters ACQUITY BEH Amide column (2.1 mm×100 mm, 1.7 μm) at 35 ℃, and at a flow rate of 0.4 mL/min. The mobile phase comprised (A) 0.15% aqueous formic acid (contained 5 mmol/L ammonium formate and 5 mmol/L ammonium acetate) and (B) 0.15% acetonitrile formic acid (contained 1 mmol/L ammonium formate and 1 mmol/L ammonium acetate) using gradient elutions of 10% A at 0 - 3 min, 13%- 25% A at 10 - 15 min, 50% A at 21 - 23 min, and 10% A at 24 min; the re-equilibration time of gradient elution was 4 min. The related Q-TOF/MS parameters were as follows: gas temp 350 ℃, drying gas 10 L/min, nebulizer 50 psi, sheath gas temp 350 ℃, sheath gas flow 10 L/min, vcap 4 500 V, skimmer 65 V, and fragmentor 175 V. The acquisition rate was 1 spectra/s and the mass range was set as 100 - 1 700 *m/z*. The collision energy was set as 10 V to obtain MS/MS information. Nineteen sample solutions were mixed at a certain volume to prepare for the QC sample for precision evaluation. To investigate the natural grouping situation and obtain the difference variable, the mass and retention time lists were used for principal component analysis (PCA) and orthogonal partial least-squares discriminant analysis (OPLS-DA) using SIMCA-P software (Version 14.1).

Considering the medicinal properties of "Guang Dilong", the anti-coagulation activity of two subgroups was assessed using thrombin-fibrinogen assay. Furthermore, 0.2 g of the sample was weighed and extracted with 1 mL water in an ultrasonic water bath at 40 ℃ for 40 min. Afterwards, the solution was centrifuged at 14,000 r/min for 5 min. The supernatant was filtered using a 0.22 μm nylon membrane. Aliquot (100 μL) of the filtrate solution was transferred to a 2 mL centrifuge tube that contained 200 μL fibrinogen (5 mg/mL, PBS). Then, the mixture was incubated for 5 min in a 37 ℃ water bath, after which 2 μL thrombin (10 U/mL, normal saline) was added to the mixture every 4 min until a fibrous precipitate was observed. For the blanks (negative controls), the earthworm solution was replaced with distilled water and a procedure similar to the one above was carried out. The consumed thrombin solution was used to calculate the anticoagulation activity of earthworms based on the following Eq. (1):

$$U = \frac{C_1 V_1}{C_2 V_2} \tag{1}$$

where $U$ represented anti-coagulation potency per gram; $C_1$ represented the concentration of thrombin solution; $V_1$ represented the consumption volume of thrombin solution; $C_2$ represented the concentration of earthworm solution; and $V_2$ represented the volume of earthworm solution. If the consumption volume of thrombin was less than that of the negative control, the earthworm sample was regarded as lacking anti-coagulation activity. To verify whether the difference in efficacy between the two subgroups is stable, in addition to above samples, 12 subgroup 1 and 8 subgroup 2 *A. aspergillum* individuals were subsequently included.

2.7 Biodiversity analysis of earthworm samples Prior to the biodiversity analyses at haplotype level, ASV total abundances in each sample were rarefied (resampled with replacement) to the minimum number of reads found (58 905 read counts). The relative read abundance (*i.e.*, the value of each taxon divided by the total reads per sample) of MOTUs were calculated and plotted using the R package ampvis2. Samples from the same collection site were grouped in the heat-map. The alpha- and beta-diversity of samples based on ASVs and MOTUs were analyzed. The Shannon index as a measure of entropy, indicated the richness and evenness of the taxa present. With respect to beta diversity, 18 batches of samples collected in the wild were included, and Principal co-ordinates analysis (PCoA) was performed using Bray-Curtis distance analysis.

To observe the influence of geographic distribution on the species level (MOTUs) biodiversity, the capture locations (geographical coordinates) were entered into the GenGIS (v2.5.1) software to generate the distribution map.

For 3 batches of the samples of earthworm decoction pieces supplied by pharmaceutical companies and 25 batches of Chinese patent medicine, the relative abundance of taxa was analyzed as previously mentioned.

## 3 RESULTS

3.1 Evaluation of LCO1490/HCO1777 marker for Amynthas and Metaphire species discrimination Compared to the standard COI 5′ region, the amplicon of LCO1490/HCO1777 with a length of 281 bp was more suitable for degraded samples, such as processed natural medicine products. While the universality of LCO1490 for metazoan had been validated by numerous studies, the conservation of the HCO1777 primer binding region was further assessed in our *Amynthas* and *Metaphire* local dataset (Supporting Information Appendix A). As shown in Fig. 1, HCO1777 was located in a region with low variability compared with its neighboring areas. Furthermore, the LCO1490/HCO1777 amplicon sequences of *A. aspergillum* clustered into one branch stably on the ML phylogenetic tree, and the species level discrimination ability of this short marker was acceptable for *Amynthas* and *Metaphire* species (Supporting

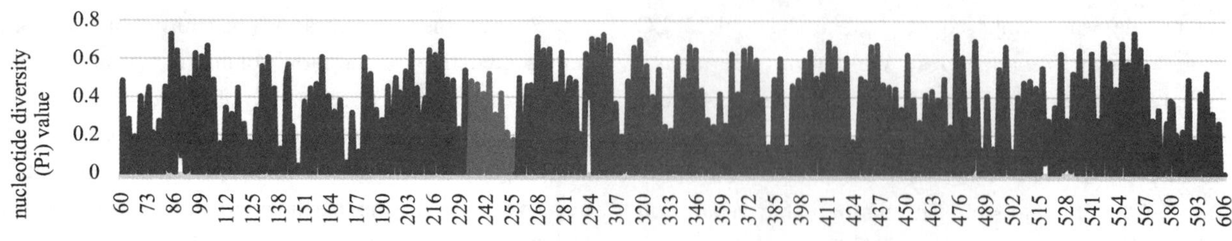


**Figure 1 Nucleotide diversity (Pi) value of HCO1777 primer region across local COI barcode dataset comprising 689 sequences from 99 *Amynthas* and *Metaphire* species**

The value on the horizontal axis represented the base position starting next to the 3′ end of LCO1490, and the orange section represented the location of primer HCO1777.

Information Fig. S1). At the same time, after sanger sequencing of 15 individuals, it was found that the identification results of the two markers were consistent (Supporting Information Table S2). The 658 bp "classic" COI regions and the 232 bp regions of these samples were presented as Supporting Information Appendix B.

3.2 Sequencing data filtering and clustering for "Guang Dilong" samples collected in the wild A total of 34 107 981 raw pair-end reads were generated, and 31 065 432 clean reads were obtained after trimming the adapter and removing low-quality sequences. The number of clean reads for each sample was presented in Supporting Information Table S3. First, 512 ASVs were detected using the DADA2 algorithm. After filtering out ASVs whose read count coverage was <100 and checking for stop codons, a total of 358 ASVs associated with particular COI haplotypes remained, while 302 of them were identified as earthworms (Supporting Information Table S4).

3.3 Species level taxon identification for "Guang Dilong" samples Rarefaction analysis (ASVs counts based) showed that the sequencing effort covered the haplotypes present in the samples, as curves approached saturation (Supporting Information Fig. S2). To infer the taxonomic assignment of 302 "Guang Dilong" ASVs, both similarity-based and phylogeny-based identification procedures were performed. Not surprisingly, 233 ASVs were identified as *A. aspergillum* using both methods, *i.e.*, the certified "Guang Dilong" described in *China Pharmacopoeia*. Using the BLAST-MEGAN approach, only ASV_180 and ASV_189 were identified as *Amynthas* sp. and ASV_131 and ASV_170 as Megascolecidae sp. Among the rest, and the taxonomic status of other 65 ASVs could not be assigned. Furthermore, the phylogenetic placement strategy additionally identified 38 ASVs as *A. aspergillum* and provided additional taxonomic information for the 31 ASVs remaining (18 ASVs as *Amynthas* sp. and 13 as Megascolecidae sp.), as shown by Supporting Information Table S5.

For all haplotypes with exact or ambiguous taxon names revealed from "Guang Dilong" samples, species delimitation methods were applied to identify species level biodiversity. The ABGD method clustered 31 ambiguous ASVs into 7 molecular operational taxonomic units (MOTUs), and 271 *A. aspergillum* ASVs into the final one (Supporting Information Table S6). Meanwhile, the bPTP analysis of the

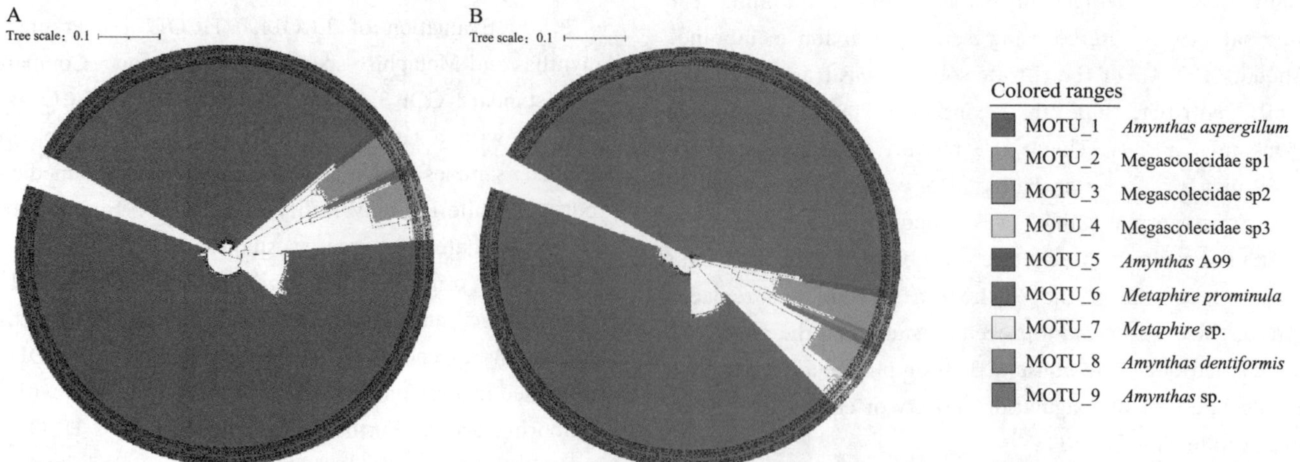


**Figure 2 Species delimitation of "Guang Dilong" COI ASVs based on the bPTP method**

(A) Bayesian tree; (B) ML tree. The light blue circular ball in the figure represents the node support rate of each branch, and the larger the sphere, the greater the node support rate. The ABGD result was similar to that of bPTP, except that MOTU_4 and MOTU_7 were clustered into a single MOTU by ABGD.

**Table 2 Taxonomic identification information of nine MOTUs**

| MOTU ID | Contained ASVs ID (No. of ASVs) | BLAST against public dataset | Phylogenetic replacement using public dataset (support percent) | BLAST against professional dataset constructed by taxonomists on pheretimoid earthworms (ASVs as queries) | Final identification result |
|---|---|---|---|---|---|
| MOTU_1 | ASV_1, ASV_2, ASV_3, ASV_4 ..., ASV_360, ASV_361, ASV_363, ASV_365, ASV_366, ASV_368 (271) | 233 ASVs identified as *Amynthas aspergillum*, while the other 38 ASVs could just be identified as *Amynthas* sp. | *A. aspergillum* (100) | *A. aspergillum* (ASV_5 ASV_6 ASV_13 ASV_21 ASV_79 ASV_90) | *A. aspergillum* |
| MOTU_2 | ASV_8, ASV_41, ASV_133, ASV_156, ASV_168, ASV_181, ASV_207, ASV_267, ASV_327(9) | Not assigned | *Amynthas* sp. (71.06 - 77.95) | Not assigned (ASV_8, ASV_41) | Megascolecidae sp1 |
| MOTU_3 | ASV_10, ASV_20, ASV_80, ASV_194, ASV_268, ASV_276, ASV_280, ASV_296, ASV_347(9) | Not assigned | Megascolecidae sp. (91.22 - 99.99) | Not assigned (ASV_10, ASV_20, ASV_80) | Megascolecidae sp2 |
| MOTU_4 | ASV_25, ASV_34, ASV_92, ASV_304, ASV_323, ASV_332(6) | Not assigned | *Amynthas* sp. (67.38 - 74.67) | Not assigned (ASV_25, ASV_34, ASV_92) | Megascolecidae sp3 |
| MOTU_5 | ASV_112, ASV_119(2) | Not assigned | *Amynthas* sp. (63.22, 65.51) | *Amynthas* A99 (ASV112, ASV119) | *Amynthas* A99 |
| MOTU_6 | ASV_131, ASV_170(2) | Megascolecidae sp. | Megascolecidae sp. (84.09, 75.61) | *Metaphire prominula* Qiu & Jiang (ASV_131, ASV_170) | *M. prominula* Qiu & Jiang |
| MOTU_7 | ASV_160(1) | Not assigned | Megascolecidae sp. (58.57) | *Metaphire* sp. (ASV_160) | *Metaphire* sp. |
| MOTU_8 | ASV_180(1) | *Amynthas* sp. | Megascolecidae sp. (72.79) | *Amynthas dentiformis* Sun & Jiang (ASV_180) | *A. dentiformis* Sun & Jiang |
| MOTU_9 | ASV_189(1) | *Amynthas* sp. | *Amynthas* sp. (99.99) | *Amynthas* sp. (ASV_189) | *Amynthas* sp. |

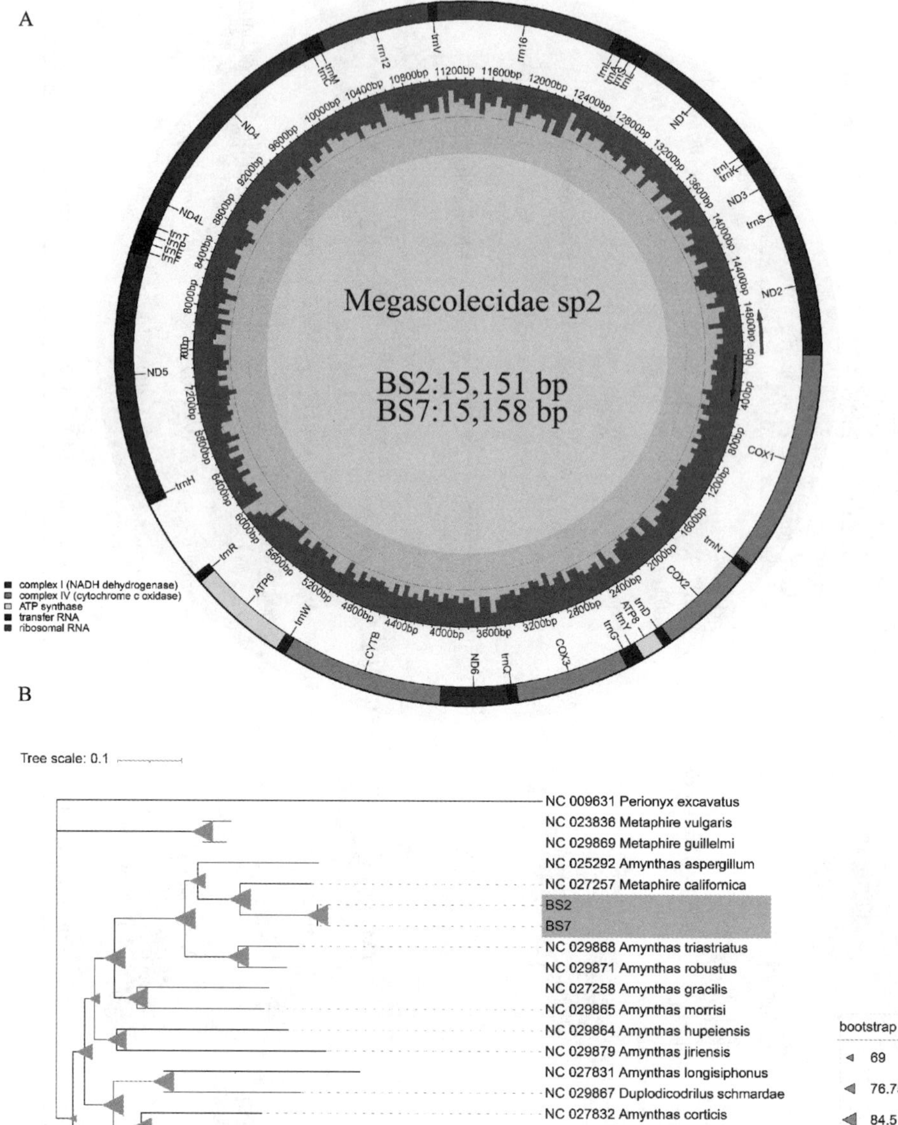


**Figure 3 Mitochondrial genomes of two individuals within Megascolecidae sp2**

(A) Physical map of the mitochondrial genome. The gray part in the inner ring indicates the percentage of GC content; (B) Phylogenetic analysis of Megascolecidae sp2 and 18 other pheretimoid species based on the mitochondrial genome.

COI gene data based on the ML tree identified 9 MOTUs as shown in Fig. 2. Conversely, given the ABGD result, the ASV_160 grouped with 6 other ASVs by ABGD was further classified as an independent MOTU (MOTU_7) by bPTP.

With the aid of collaborators in Shanghai Jiaotong University, typical ASVs of each MOTU were selected and used to search against a professional COI barcoding dataset constructed by taxonomists on pheretimoid earthworms. Finally, taxonomic identification results of 9 MOTUs containing 302 ASVs were presented in Table 2. In addition to MOTU_1 as *A. aspergillum*, MOTU_6, MOTU_7, MOTU_8 and MOTU_9 were identified as *Metaphire prominula* (Qiu & Jiang), *Metaphire* sp., *Amynthas dentiformis* (Sun & Jiang), and *Amynthas* sp., respectively. Notably, ASV112 and ASV119 within MOTU_5 matched with the COI region of a specimen called HN201702-01 and collected from Longtang Town, Haikou City, Hainan Province, China. Their respective identity percentages were 100% and 99.6%. According to the taxonomic description, this specimen should belong to the *Amynthas corticis*-group and be listed as a new species temporarily named as *Amynthas* A99, owing to its unique morphological characters of four pairs of spermathecal pores in 5/6-8/9, special male pore zone, cecum, and spermatheca caecus. The morphological description is presented in Supporting Information Fig. S3. Formal description of the new species will be published in another paper.

For the MOTUs that could not be assigned to the professional dataset, further validation on genome level was conducted. For MOTU_3 (Megascolecidae sp2), two corresponding individuals were determined, and the entire mitochondrial genome was constructed. The mitochondrial genomes of two individuals were 15 151 and 15 158 bp in length, respectively. These two genomes had a high degree of similarity (99.9%), and the same genetic composition and structure. Each of them encoded 37 unique genes, including 13 coding sequences, 22 tRNA, and 2 rRNA genes (Fig. 3A, Supporting Information Table S7). The "classic" 658 bp-COI region was extracted from mitogenome and then searched against BOLD and GenBank nt databases. Both the ML phylogenetic analysis (Fig. 3B) and the BLAST identification results confirmed that, the nucleotide data of this putative species, at least, had never been recorded in the public database.

3.4 Intraspecies subgroups hidden in "Guang Dilong" samples that identified as A. aspergillum As shown in Fig. 4A, as the haplotype network, two major groups were uncovered within *A. aspergillum* ASVs, comprising 38 ASVs, which was not classified as *A. aspergillum* by BLAST-based method, and the 233 other ASVs. Moreover, the ambiguous "barcoding gap" (c, minimum interspecific distance exceeded the maximum intraspecific distance) was observed in Fig. 4B. Both the maximum intra-group and minimum inter-group genetic distance (Kimura 2-parameter model) were 5.40%, and the average intra- and inter-group genetic distances were 2.04% and 7.46%, respectively. Considering the sympatric distribution pattern and the species delimitation results described above, these two groups were regarded as subgroups within species *A. aspergillum*, rather than two distinct species, although the genetic distance between them was neither in the intraspecies nor interspecies range for earthworm species. It is worth nothing that, multiple genetic distance distribution peaks were observed in the "barcoding gap" plot, and three ASV clusters within subgroup 1 in the haplotype network directly corresponded with BOLD BINs ACH7381, ACB6697, and AAK1097 within *A. aspergillum*, whereas the subgroup 2 was consistent with BOLD BINs ACB6847.

Furthermore, 11 subgroup 1 samples (5 from BINs ACH 7381 and 6 from BINs ACB 6697) and 8 subgroup 2 samples were selected to assess the influence of these intraspecific diversities within *A. aspergillum* on the quality of "Guang Dilong". The 658 bp "classic" COI regions of these samples were presented as Supporting Information Appendix C. The maximum intra-group and minimum inter-group genetic distances (Kimura 2-parameter model) were 2.65% and 9.50%, respectively, and the average intra- and inter-group genetic distances were 1.32% and 1.02%, respectively. The comparison of mitochondrial genomes in two *A. aspergillum* subgroups was revealed using mVISTA, and we observed approximately identical gene order and organization among them (Fig. 4C). Notably, not only the COI gene, but also the other genes of mitochondrial genome of subgroup2 (BINs ID ACB6847) differed from the reference sequence (BINs ID ACH7381, subgroup1) much than subgroup1 (BINs ID ACB6697), especially for the noncoding regions.

However, we failed to identify sufficiently distinguishable morphological characters between the two subgroups with distinct genetic variation (Supporting Information Fig. S4).

Subsequently, the untargeted metabolomics strategy based on UHPLC-Q-TOF/MS was applied to compare chemical components, as shown in Fig. 4D. The QC samples as the data normalization tool were mainly distributed at the origin of the coordinates of the PCA plot, thereby indicating acceptable analytical precision. Significantly, samples of subgroup 1 were distributed in the second and third quadrants, and subgroup 2 samples mainly existed in the first and fourth quadrants. The OPLS-DA plot (Supporting Information Fig. S5A) displayed the obvious separation between two types of samples. To validate the accuracy of OPLS-DA, a 200-step permutation experiment was performed. As shown in Fig. S5B, the rightmost points of $R^2$ and $Q^2$ both exceeded those of the other points. Cumulative $R^2(Y)$ and $Q^2(Y)$ values ($R^2=0.98$, $Q^2=0.75$) close to 1 indicated a reliable model. Considering variable importance in projection (VIP)>1 as the criteria, 161 variables (chemical compounds) (Supporting Information Table S8) were screened out, and within them, 18 compounds were unambiguously identified. Then, all variables were qualitatively analyzed using Agilent MassHunter Qualitative Analysis (version B.07.00). As illustrated in Fig. 4E, stachydrine, Lyso-PAF C-16, nicotinic acid, adenosine, and 3′-AMP/AMP had relatively high content in subgroup 2, while the 13 other ingredients such as L-pipecolic acid, Arg-Ala, Val-Arg, phenylalanine, Leu-Arg/Ile-Arg, alanine betaine, Ile-Val/Leu-Val, Pro-Arg, His-Gln, His-Val, His-Ala, Leu-Pro/Ile-Pro, and *O*-acetyl-L-serine exhibited relatively high content in subgroup 1. Although most of these compounds were regarded as primary metabolites of earthworms, certain ingredients such as Stachydrine, Lyso-PAF C-16, and nicotinic acid have been reported to display bioactivities as anti-inflammatory, cardioprotective, or lipid metabolism regulation. Among 18 previously identified differential compounds, lyso-platelet-activating factor (lyso-PAF), the platelet-activating factor (PAF) precursor, could promote platelet aggregation by induction of free $Ca^{2+}$

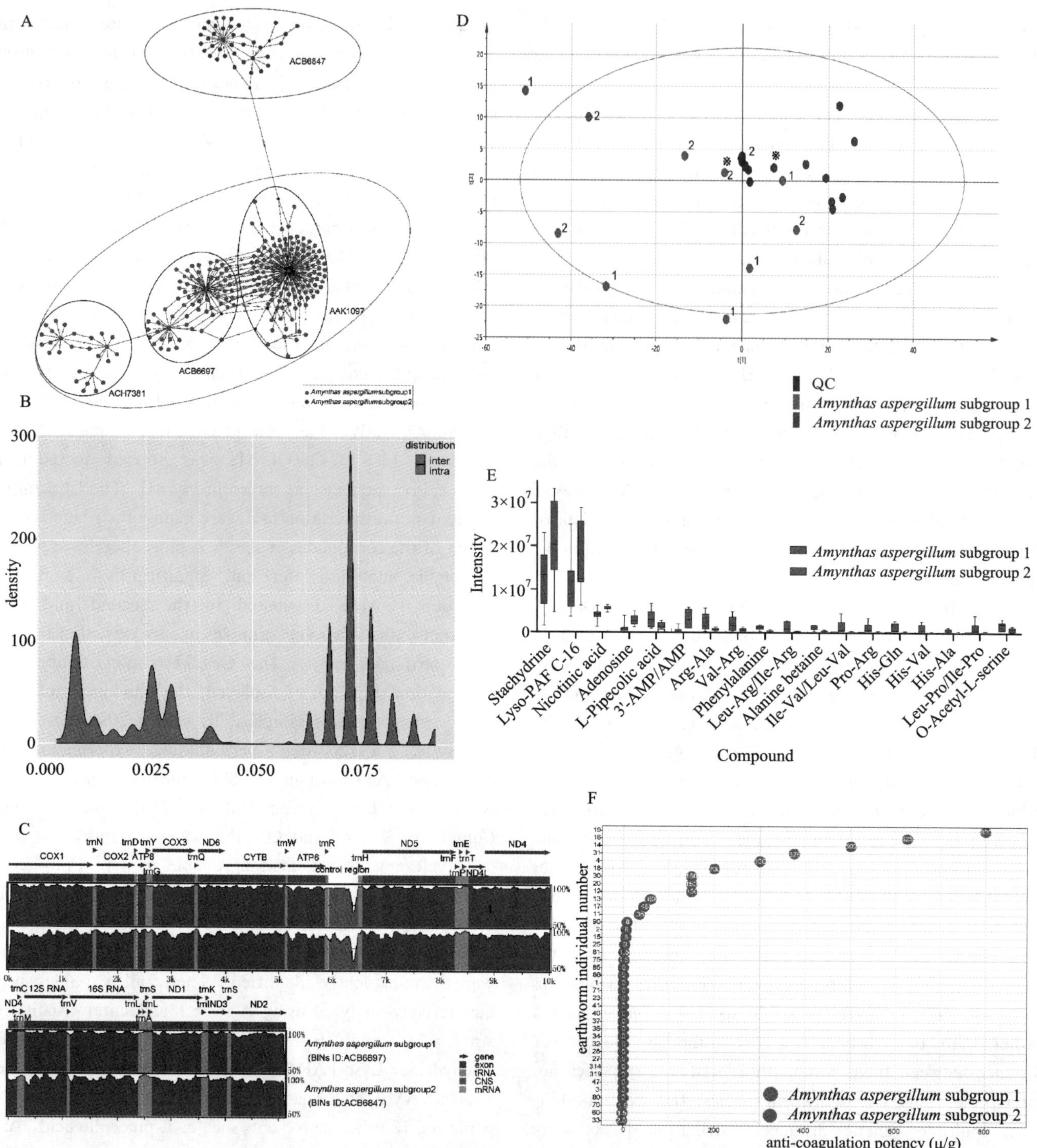


**Figure 4 Intraspecies level biodiversity within *Amynthas aspergillum* samples**

(A) Haplotype network of 302 ASVs within MOTU_1 (*Amynthas aspergillum*), and the corresponding BOLD BINs number was indicated; (B) Barcoding gap analysis between two subgroups; (C) Comparison of the mitochondrial genome sequences of two subgroups of *Amynthas aspergillum* using mVISTA alignment program, using the annotations of *A. aspergillum* (GenBank accession number: NC_025292, BINs ID: ACH7381) as reference. The vertical scale indicates the percentage of identity, ranging from 50% to 100%; (D) The PCA results between two subgroups: subgroup 1 samples with BINs ID: ACH 7381 (indicated as 1) and ACB 6697 (indicated as 2), and subgroup 2 samples with BINs ID: ACB6847. The QC samples were mainly distributed at the origin of the coordinates the PCA plot, which indicated acceptable analytical precision; (E) 18 differential chemical compositions were identified in two subgroups; (F) anti-coagulation potency of *Amynthas aspergillum* subgroup 1 and subgroup 2 samples. Two subgroups of individuals used for whole-genome skimming sequencing.

increase and coagulation factor-Ⅲ secretion. It is worth noting that, as the non-targeted metabolomics emphasized on the comprehensive analysis of detectable small molecules, the anticoagulant ingredients such as potential bioactive peptides may not be fully represented. The exact active substances of this kind of earthworm responsible for anticoagulant effects would require further research to be elucidated. With respect to anti-coagulation activity, the non-parmetric Mann—Whitney U-Test ($P$=0.0001) showed significant bioactivity difference between two subgroups, and the average potency of subgroup 1 significantly exceeded that of subgroup 2 (Fig. 4F).

3.5 Overall biodiversity of the earthworm collected in the wild As illustrated in Fig. 5A and B, except sample BS used as control and purchased at the local market, among the other 18 samples collected in the wild, the relative read abundance of *A. aspergillum* accounted for more than 80%. Fig. 5C showing the PCoA plot using Bray-Curtis distance and Supporting Information Fig. S6 showing the geographic distribution map present three samples: SC, CT, and XWC that were geographically adjacent in Hepu County and had similar earthworm species composition. While DQ in Luchuan had a relative severe unintentionally substitution by Megascolecidae sp1, the proportions of *A. aspergillum* in the other 14 sampling sites exceeded 98% and were grouped together in the beta-diversity analysis. Generally, our results indicated that the locations we selected, as part of the traditional producing areas for "Guang Dilong", had a relatively stable species composition.

Furthermore, considering the impact of genetic variation on pharmaceutical effect, the intraspecies level biodiversity was observed in these samples. Within the 18 samples, only 5 samples were occupied by single the *A. aspergillum* subgroup (subgroup 1), and 9 samples whose >10% of read abundance levels were occupied by the minor subgroup type. Samples that were subgroup 1-predominant, subgroup 2-predominant, or with middle type were clustered into different groups in Fig. 5D.

As illustrated in Fig. 5B, the distribution of the Shannon entropy index based on the MOTUs, subgroups, or ASVs were irrelevant to each other, which indicated the complication of intraspecific biodiversity, especially for the ASVs level. Six samples: BL, DY, BB, HX, PS, and LC, had an ASVs Shannon value that exceeded 1. Interestingly, sample PS comprising only *A. aspergillum* subgroup 1 had a relatively high alpha-diversity level based on ASVs, which implied the richness of germlines on this collection site. According to the composition of 302 earthworm ASVs, the 14 samples where *A. aspergillum* was absolutely predominant (>98%) were divided into 3 groups, as shown in Fig. 5E.

3.6 Testing traditional Chinese medicinal product samples containing earthworms To further test our hypothesis that the source control of medical material "Guang Dilong" could benefit from the biodiversity pattern uncovered, three batches of 2 796 dried earthworms collected from assigned sites were provided by a related pharmaceutical company for taxon identification. For these samples, a total of 5,753,904 paired-end reads of COI amplicon were generated. As a result, 105 ASVs were obtained, and rarefaction curve (Supporting Information Fig. S7) analysis indicated that the sequencing depths were sufficient for reliable results. The identification information of these ASVs was listed as Supporting Information Table S9. As shown in Fig. 6, while *A. aspergillum* subgroup 1 accounted for most of the proportion, *A. aspergillum* subgroup 2 and a few proportions of *A. dentiformis*, as unintentional substitution, were observed. This result was consistent with the species distribution we reported above.

For 25 Chinese patent medicine samples containing "Dilong" (earthworm), 10 593 960 paired-end reads and 304 ASVs were obtained, 37 ASVs of which were assigned to earthworms. As shown in the right section of Fig. 6, the sources of the earthworm components of GX and SH were subgroup 1 and subgroup 2 of *A. aspergillum*, individually. While the main component for NX was identified as *M. vulgaris*, one kind of source of "Dilong" included in *Chinese Pharmacopoeia*, *Metaphire tschiliensis* (Michaelsen, 1928) as common adulterant of "Dilong" recorded in the previous survey was also detected (percent ranging from 0 to 17.3%). Due to the limitation of resources yield, Chinese patent medicine companies prefer purchasing medical materials from different but relative stable geographic locations, and this may be one of the main causes of the species level diversity among different Chinese patent medicine samples.

## 4 DISCUSSION

4.1 The advantage of DNA metabarcoding combined with minibarcode in the discovery of biodiversity within batches of medical materials As demonstrated in previous research studies, a large amount of cryptic biodiversity concealed amidst natural medical materials has not been discovered yet. DNA barcoding provided an effective tool for the discovery of cryptic species in the field of ecology and taxonomy. However, because DNA degradation occurs during TCM manufacturing processing, the DNA fragments in extraction are frequently too short to be the template for "standard" DNA barcoding amplification, whose amplicon usually exceeds 500 bp. DNA mini-barcode with short DNA segments ranging from 100 to 250 bp and sufficient variable sites could address the difficulties associated with "standard" DNA barcoding. As indicated by Lo et al., DNA fragments of approximately 300 bp could be successfully amplified in herbs that have been boiled for 60 min, and PCR products of ≤120 bp were even observed for 120 min of the boiled sample. So far, several studies have explicitly highlighted

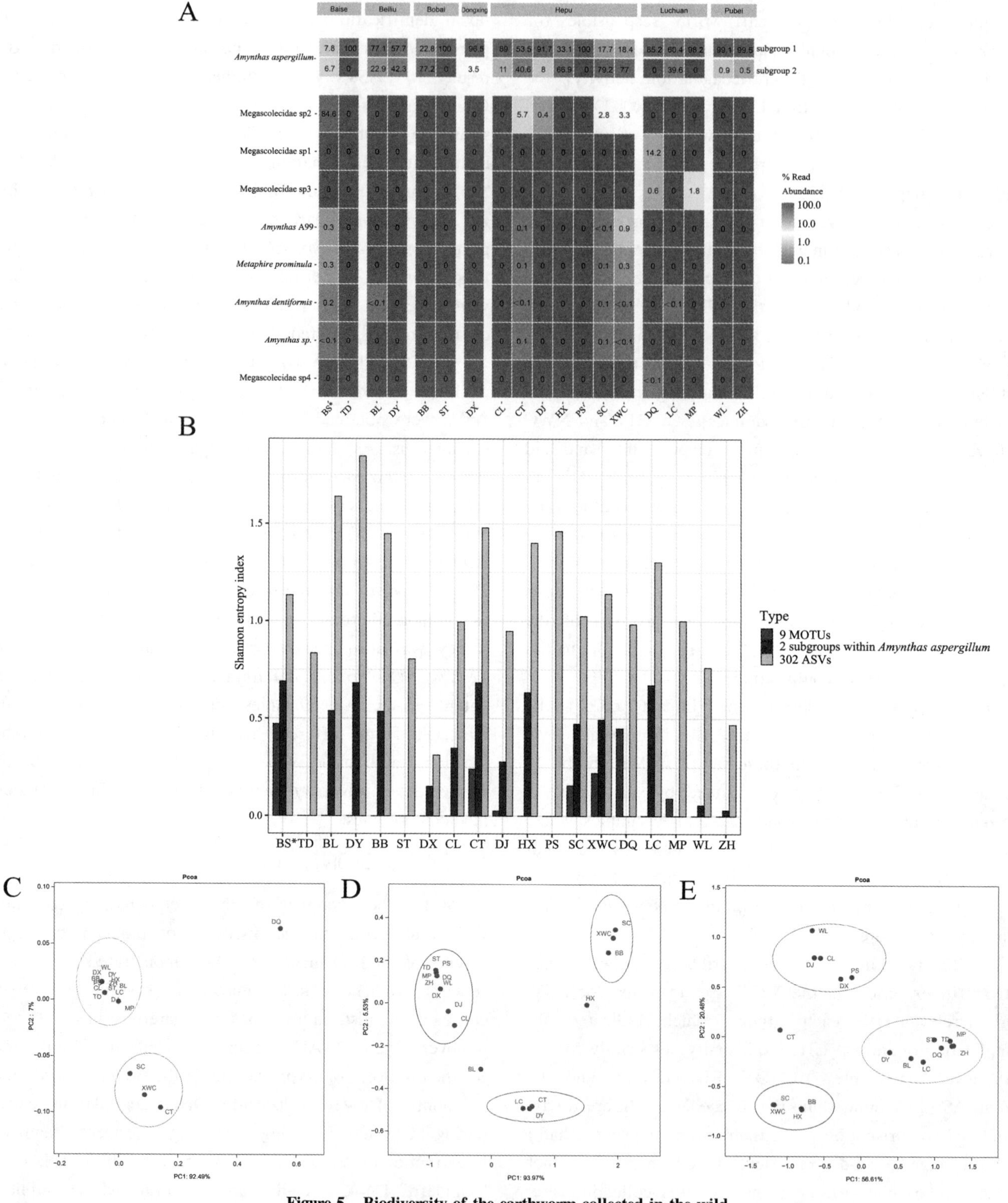

**Figure 5 Biodiversity of the earthworm collected in the wild**

(A) Heat map reflecting the species composition on 19 different collection sites; (B) Shannon index reflecting the alpha diversity within each sample; (C-E) Bray-Curtis PCoA (beta diversity) used to qualitatively examine differences in biological composition on MOTUs, *A. aspergillum* subgroups and ASVs level, separately. * Bought from Baise local market.

that the DNA mini-barcode expands the DNA barcoding method for assessing the quality of processed TCM materials.

For animals, 658 bp region in the gene encoding mitochondrial COI is one of the most important standard barcoding genes. The key advantage of COI as a marker for DNA metabarcoding is that reference databases have been well established and are actively developed and extended. If the goal is to identify the species present in the sample, COI

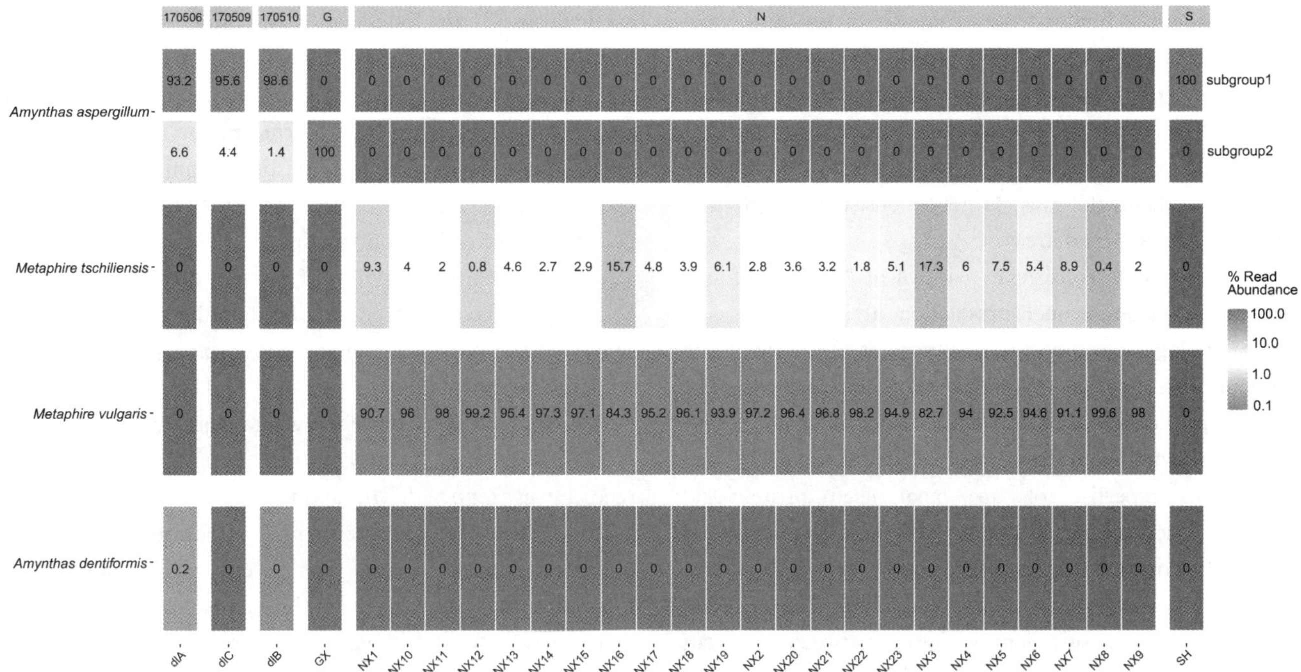


**Figure 6 Heat map reflecting the species composition of 3 batches of decoction pieces and 25 Chinese patent medicines**

is the best choice due to the availability of extensive public reference databases. Besides, the COI locus differs from many other metabarcoding loci (*e.g.*, 18S, 16S, 12S, ITS) in that it is a protein coding gene, imparting strict expectations of amplicon sequence read properties that can be exploited in metabarcoding bioinformatics. In this study, to avoid the difficulty caused by DNA degradation, we selected a pair of primers that amplified the 281 bp fragment in COI 5′ region, which has been confirmed to be able to successfully identify earthworm components in feces.

A common concern for the mini-barcode is whether it can provide enough molecular polymorphism to differentiate species. However, Yeo et al. recently observed that there was no significant difference between species-level identification performance of the full-length COI Folmer barcode and mini-barcode exceeding 200 bp across a large range of metazoan taxa, based on species delimitation algorithms. In our study, the 232 bp marker we selected had a variation ratio that was consistent with that of the 658 bp "standard" COI sequence for *Amynthas* and *Metaphire* species, as shown in Fig. 1. Moreover, the mini-barcode ASVs identified as the same species based on the reference dataset, were clustered into single MOTU through species delimitation methods, indicating the reliable accuracy of the mini-barcode on species inference. In addition, 15 individuals were randomly selected to amplify a 658 bp Folmer region of the COI gene using LCO1490/HCO2198, and a 232 bp segment of the 5′ end of the COI gene with primers LCO1490/HCO1777, respectively, and the results of Sanger Sequencing showed that the identification results of the two markers were consistent (Table S2). In short, the 232 bp mini-barcode on COI genes was suitable for the biodiversity discovery of earthworms.

Another factor that limited the biodiversity survey on batched natural medicinal materials was the relatively high human resource and experimental costs of the regular individual identification method, such as DNA barcoding. DNA metabarcoding, simultaneous DNA barcoding of all specimens in a bulk sample using NGS platforms, allows for time- and cost-effective assessments of uncovered diversity. To our knowledge, this study was the first application of metabarcoding on batched commercial TCM materials. In addition to species level (MOTUs) assignment, haplotype level (ASVs) information was obtained. Although unavoidably affected by PCR and sequencing error, metabarcoding bioinformatic pipeline as DADA2 could generate an error model based on the quality of sequencing run and use this model to distinguish between the predicted "true" biological variation (ASVs) and that was likely generated by systematic error. Ideally, these single-nucleotide level variations represent oligotypes within pool samples, which allow for description of intraspecific diversity. Particularly for the COI barcode region, sequences that cannot be properly translated were excluded to further eliminate non-authentic ASVs, as nuclear mitochondrial pseudogenes (numts) and erroneous sequences.

Although the exact quantitative ability of metabarcoding has always been tested towing to primer bias, the relative abundances of MOTUs or ASVs were still comparable between samples under the same experimental and bioinformatic processes. Diversity monitoring would benefit from this kind of read abundance comparison, even without a reference database and taxonomy assignment. In this study, the species composition revealed from samples collected in the wild was largely consistent with that purchased from assigned areas.

4.2 The batch consistency control of "Guang Dilong" would benefit from proper production area selection and effective biological composition assessment approach The taxonomic identification of earthworm mainly relies on the morphological characteristics such as spermathecal pores, female pores and male pores, genital papillae, etc., and requires the expertise of an experienced professional taxonomist. More importantly, most of these characteristics would be destroyed during the preparing process of medicinal materials. Significantly, DNA barcoding uses DNA fragments exhibiting sufficient variation between different species to identify species. Except for the identification of unknown specimens, DNA barcoding can speed up the designation of distinct lineages, and accelerate the discovery of the cryptic/undescribed earthworm species. However, as traditional DNA barcoding identifies single specimens based on individual DNA sequencing reactions, it is often unsuitable for bulk commercial materials.

In this study, through mini-barcode and DNA metabarcoding, thousands of *Amynthas* earthworm individuals used as medicinal materials were treated in batches, and high interspecies and intraspecies diversity was demonstrated. Besides the intentional and unintentional adulteration, even the subgroups within *A. aspergillum* revealed here differed in chemical compositions and biological activity, indicating the need for origin control for this kind of wild source medicine.

Fortunately, this study identified the producing areas where *A. aspergillum* as the genuine source in the Pharmacopoeia taking overwhelming majority of the local earthworm community. As the discrimination result of subsequent commercial samples implied, it was feasible to stabilize the species origin of wild TCM by controlling their geographical origin. This study also provided an identification tool for earthworm medical materials, such as mini-barcode primers pair and reasonable species genetic distance threshold. Combined with the power of DNA metabarcoding, it could support the large-scale sampling needed for time- and costefficient assessment of commercial materials.

Recently, the rising demand for TCM products in treating cardiovascular and cerebrovascular diseases has led to additional consumption of earthworm medicinal materials. Driven by growing market demand, over-harvesting may lead to a decline or loss of the biodiversity among earthworms. In the long term, more attention should be paid to the domestication and breeding of earthworms. The producing areas selected by this study could be regarded as artificial breeding bases. Furthermore, the intraspecies level diversity obtained elucidates existing germplasm resources, offers guidelines for *in-situ* conservation, and the core germplasm collection construction.

From a biology point of view, the Megascolecidae MOTUs that could not be identified at the species level also suggested the presence of numerous cryptic species or species without standard barcodes yet. For MOTU_5, identified as new species *Amynthas* A99, which was first collected in Hainan Province, China, a new geographic distribution record was reported. In addition, two subgroups whose genetic distance was neither in the intraspecies nor interspecies range were discovered within species *A. aspergillum*. Based on high-throughput method as DNA metabarcoding, the biodiversity assessment on abundant commercial TCM materials collected in the wild may elucidate studies on taxonomy and ecology.

4.3 Data availability statement The datasets presented in this study are accessible from online repositories. The names of the repository/repositories and accession number (s) are accessible here: https://www.ncbi.nlm.nih.gov/genbank/, (NCBI accession number: ON553959), https://www.ncbi.nlm.nih.gov/genbank/, (NCBI accession number: ON553960). Illumina data sets have been deposited in the NCBI Sequence Read Archive (SRA) under accession numbers: SRR19586215, SRR19446212 and SRR19855328.

## 5 CONCLUSIONS

To our knowledge, this was the first biological sources consistency evaluation of batched natural medicinal materials based on the well-evaluated mini-barcode and DNA metabarcoding. The earthworms as "Guang Dilong" were distinguished at haplotype level, from both commercially available medical materials and Chinese patent medicine. Although there were significant differences between two subgroups within *A. aspergillum* in terms of chemical compositions and biological activity, the hypothesis that the stability of biological composition would benefit from producing areas fixation was proved when the biodiversity pattern was uncovered at relatively fine geographical levels (*e.g.*, village or town). We believe that, due to the advancement of handheld highthroughput sequencing technology and the declining sequencing cost, the origin control strategy described in this study should be introduced to improve the batch consistency of TCM, and to obtain the species community diversity information of medical materials depending on wild resources, particularly for taxa for which basic taxonomic and biodiversity works are woefully insufficient. In addition to stabilizing the biological source, the intraspecific biodiversity revealed by this method also offers guidelines for *in-situ* conservation and breeding bases construction.

[邢志美,黄璐琦,田晓轩,等. Acta Pharmaceutica Sinica B, 2023, 13(4):1755-1770.]

# Cationic conjugated polymer fluorescence resonance energy transfer for DNA methylation assessment to discriminate the geographical origins of Lonicerae Japonicae Flos

## 1 INTRODUCTION

The geographical origins of crops and foods have received increasing attention in recent decades, and discrimination of the geographical origin has become a major problem for consumers, merchants, farmers, and food authorities. Geographical origins frequently have a tight association with food quality and flavor, and clear geographical origins of food usually assist manufacturers in obtaining customer acceptance and premium prices. Moreover, fraud and incorrect labeling of geographical origin are detrimental to consumers and damage the reputations of legitimate producers.

*Lonicerae japonicae flos* (LJF) is widely used to manufacture teas and health products in China, and LJF cosmetics have gained popularity in recent years owing to antioxidant and antiallergic effects. A previous survey suggested that overall LJF consumption will surpass 13 500 tons in 2021, with around 50% of LJF being used to make scented tea and soft drinks. Chinese legislators have introduced the National Geographical Indication Product (NGIP) designation for food with special geographical characteristics, and LJF cultivated in Mixian in Henan and Pingyi in Shandong have had NGIP labels since 2012 and 2010, respectively. In addition to Henan and Shandong provinces, additional emerging production regions for LJF include the Beijing, Guangxi, Yunnan, Ningxia, Hubei, Shaanxi, Gansu, Anhui, Chongqing, Hebei, and Jiangsu provinces of China. A previous study revealed that biologically active components, such as chlorogenic acid and galuteolin, are present at high and stable levels in LJF from regions with NGIP labels, and these may contribute to a better flavor and quality of LJF. LJF with verified origins and a NGIP label delivers a premium price, while geographical origin fraud influences the reputation and price of NGIP-labeled LJF. Therefore, it is of importance to achieve geographical origin control for LJF.

Several mass spectrometric, spectroscopic, and DNA fingerprinting methods have been used to discriminate the geographical origin of foods. Using isotope ratio mass spectrometry (IRMS) and inductively coupled plasma mass spectrometry (ICP-MS), trace elements and isotopes coupled with chemometrics have been assessed for geographical origin discrimination. δD, Mn, and Fe were selected out of 37 elements and 2 water isotopes to discriminate U.S. Washington State wines from other wines, while $\delta^{34}$S, Mn, and Mg made a greater contribution to the geographical authentication of Asian rice than 3 other stable isotopes and 23 elements. Ultraperformance liquid chromatography (UPLC), gas chromatography, near-infrared spectroscopy (NIRS), and Fourier transform infrared spectroscopy (FTIR) are also widely employed for food geographical authentication. On the basis of differences in chemical composition, UPLC was used to distinguish German white asparagus from asparagus cultivated in other regions, and NIRS combined with multivariate analysis was developed to protect green coffee and walnuts from geographical origin mislabeling. Molecular biological methods for geographical origin determination have surged in recent decades, and DNA fingerprinting, such as simple sequence repeat (SSR) and single nucleotide polymorphism (SNP), has been shown to be feasible for geographical origin discrimination for sesame oil and olive oil.

DNA methylation involves the addition of a methyl group to cytosine without a change in the DNA sequence. An abundant presence of 5′-cytosine-phosphate-guanosine-3′ (CpG) in the 5′-untranslated region (5′-UTR) of the gene is termed as the CpG island. Increasing attention has been focused on the role of DNA methylation in responses to environmental stress. Previous studies have revealed that variation in DNA methylation among geographically distinct subpopulations influences the transcription of related genes and further affects phenotypes when plants adapt to environmental change. Although DNA methylation holds the potential for geographical origin discrimination as a result of a close relationship with environmental differences, direct use of DNA methylation as a molecular marker for geographical origin discrimination has been rare to date.

Methods for detecting the DNA methylation status of a specific CpG island surged in clinical detection depending upon biosensors based on fluorescence, electrochemistry, colorimetry, mass spectrometry, surface plasmon resonance, etc. Digoxigenin and biotin were used as amplification tags for accurate analysis of methylated DNA in clinical plasma, showing high sensitivity of electrochemical biosensors. Using the ligase chain reaction-based colorimetric assay, DNA methylation can be visualized by color changes of gold nanoparticles, which indicates the merit of direct observation and simple instrumentation of the colorimetric method. Mass spectrometry and surface plasmon resonance possess high sensitivity and accuracy in DNA methylation detection through measuring changes of the molecular weight or refractive index, while the expensive instruments limit their wider application. Fluorescence resonance energy transfer (FRET) became the most popular analytical technique in DNA methylation detection as a result of advantages of high sensitivity, easy operation, and field portability. The cationic conjugated polymer (CCP)- FRET method has been developed to detect DNA methylation for screening and differential diagnosis of colon cancer, and the quantum-dot-based FRET method contributed to detect DNA methylation levels of three tumor suppressor genes for cancer diagnosis. FRET refers to a non-radiative energy transfer process from a light-sensitive donor to an acceptor. In comparison to other FRET donors, CCPs have merits of efficient light harvesting, good optical amplification properties, and the ability to form complexes with negatively charged DNA through electrostatic interaction.

The aim of this study is to distinguish the geographical origins of LJF by the DNA methylation level of epigenetic markers. Through metabolomic and bioinformatic analysis, 13 CpG islands in the chlorogenic acid and iridoid biosynthetic pathways were discovered with a putative association with LJF geographical origin. Then, the CCP-FRET method was used to determine the DNA methylation levels of LJF from diverse geographical origins. A total of 10 reliable epigenetic markers were screened and validated using orthogonal partial least squares discriminant analysis (OPLS-DA), and effective models were constructed for geographical origin discrimination of LJF. The study showed that DNA methylation difference has the potential to be a powerful tool for LJF geographical authentication.

## 2 MATERIALS AND METHODS

2.1 Chemicals and Reagents High-performance liquid chromatography (HPLC)-grade methanol, acetonitrile, and formic acid were obtained from Thermo Fisher Scientific (Waltham, MA, U. S. A.). Distilled water was obtained from Watson's Water Company (Guangzhou, China).

MspJI methylation-sensitive restriction endonuclease (5 000 U/mL), 10× CutSmart buffer, 15 μmol/L enzyme activator, and bovine serum albumin (BSA) were purchased from New England Biolabs (Ipswich, MA, U. S. A.). The 2× SYBR Premix Ex *Taq*II, 50× ROXII, 10× Fast Buffer I, dNTP mixture (2.5 mmol/L each), 5 U/μL SpeedSTAR HS Taq DNA polymerase, 10× SAP buffer, and 1 U/μL shrimp alkaline phosphatase (SAP) were obtained from TakaRa Bio, Inc. (Shiga, Japan). Fluorescein-labeled 2′-deoxyuridine-5′-triphosphate (Fl-dUTP, 25 μmol/L) was purchased from PerkinElmer (Waltham, MA, U. S. A.). Primers used in this study were synthesized by Sangon Biotech (Shanghai, China).

2.2 LJF Samples Fresh LJF was collected from 14 geographical regions for metabolomic analysis. The geographical origins and coordinates of each LJF are listed in Table S1 of the Supporting Information. Freeze-dried fine LJF powder (0.1 g) was added to 1.5 mL of 80% methanol and treated ultrasonically at 100 Hz for 30 min. The extracted solution was centrifuged at 4 000 r/min for 10 min at 4 ℃, and the supernatant was subjected to UPLC with quantitative time-of-flight tandem mass spectrometry (Q-TOF-MS/MS).

LJF from 39 Chinese geographical regions was collected to determine DNA methylation levels. The LJF samples were collected from the field in the LJF plantation located in different geographical regions. *Lonicera japonica* Thunb. with verified germplasm was cultivated in corresponding plots. Each plot was sampled by a five point sampling method. The germplasm, geographical origin, latitude, and longitude of each sample were recorded and are listed in Table S2 of the Supporting Information.

2.3 UPLC-Q-TOF-MS/MS Analysis was performed using an ACQUITY UPLC H-Class system (Waters, Milford, MA, U. S. A.) equipped with a quaternary pump, vacuum degasser, autosampler, and thermostatically controlled column compartment coupled to micrO-TOF-Q MS with an Apollo II ESI source (Bruker, Billerica, MA, U. S. A.). Samples were separated on an ACQUITY UPLC BEH C18 column (2.1×50 mm, 1.7 μm, Waters, Milford, MA, U. S. A.) at 30 ℃ using 0.1% (*V*/*V*) formic acid in water (A) and 0.1% (*V*/*V*) formic acid in acetonitrile (B). The elution gradient was 5% B at 0-1 min, 5%-13% B at 1-4 min, 13% B at 4-6 min, 13%-40% B at 6-11 min, and 40%-80% B at 11-18 min. The flow rate was maintained at 0.4 mL/min. Electrospray ionization (ESI) source conditions were as follows: capillary voltage, 5 500 V; drying gas ($N_2$)

flow rate, 6 L/min; and temperature, 220 ℃. MS and MS/MS data were obtained in negative mode with the mass range set to 50 - 1 500 Da.

2.4 Bioinformatic Analysis Chlorogenic acid biosynthesis genes in LJF have been previously reported. The iridoid biosynthesis pathway (map00902) was visualized using the Kyoto Encyclopedia of Genes and Genomes (KEGG) database (https://www.kegg.jp/). Iridoid biosynthesis genes in LJF were identified from the National Center for Biotechnology Information (NCBI) database (www.ncbi.nlm.nih.gov) using BLAST ($E < 10^{-5}$). The coding sequences of the chlorogenic acid and iridoid biosynthesis genes in LJF were obtained from the NCBI database (www.ncbi.nlm.nih.gov) and are included in the Supporting Information. The 5′-UTR sequences of chlorogenic acid and iridoid biosynthesis genes were obtained from the *L. japonica* genome (assembly ASM2146441v1 in NCBI) and are shown in the Supporting Information. CpG islands were predicted using MethPrimer (http://www.urogene.org/methprimer2/), with the following parameters: methylation window width, 100 bp; obs/exp, 0.6; and GC content, > 40%. Following the prediction results in Tables S6 and S7 of the Supporting Information, the sequence of CpG islands was obtained from the 5′-UTR sequence and is given in the Supporting Information.

2.5 DNA Methylation Determination by CCP - FRET A modified cetyltrimethylammonium bromide method was used to extract genomic DNA from LJF. Genomic DNA was divided into two parallel samples: one was digested with MspJI restriction endonuclease, and the other was treated with inactivated MspJI. Briefly, 2 μL of 10 × CutSmart buffer, 0.6 μL of enzyme activator (15 μmol/L), 1 μL of MspJI (5 000 U/mL) or inactivated MspJI, 1 μL of 100 × BSA, and 100 ng of DNA template were mixed in a 20 μL digestion reaction. To obtain inactivated MspJI, MspJI was incubated at 65 ℃ for 15 min. MSPJI digestion was carried out at 37 ℃ for 2 h, followed by inactivation at 65 ℃ for 15 min, and samples were then held at 4 ℃.

The digested and mock digested DNA were amplified to incorporate the fluorescein label. Briefly, 2 μL of 10× Fast Buffer I, 1.5 μL of dNTP mixture (2.5 mmol/L each), 0.2 μL of SpeedSTAR HS Taq DNA polymerase (5 U/μL), 0.2 μL of paired primers (10 μmol/L each), 2 μL of Fl - dUTP (25 μmol/L), and 2 μL of MspJI-digested DNA or inactivated-MspJI-treated DNA were mixed in a 20 μL polymerase chain reaction (PCR) reaction. PCR was performed using a Veriti PCR system (Applied Biosystems, Waltham, MA, U.S.A.) with initial denaturation at 94 ℃ for 2 min, 30 cycles of denaturation at 94 ℃ for 20 s, annealing and extension at $T_m$ (Table S3 of the Supporting Information) for 20 s, and then incubation at 72 ℃ for 2 min, followed by holding at 4 ℃. The primers used in PCR are shown in Table S3 of the Supporting Information.

Prior to the fluorescence measurement, 3 μL of 10× SAP buffer and 2 μL of shrimp alkaline phosphatase (1 U/μL) were added to the PCR products, followed by incubation at 37 ℃ for 20 min and inactivation at 80 ℃ for 15 min to degrade the remaining Fl - dNTPs. Following this, the mixture was held at 4 ℃. For fluorescence detection using FRET, 80 μL of 25 mmol/L 4-(2-hydroxyethyl)-1-piperazineethanesulfonic acid (HEPES), 25 μL of 15 mmol/L poly {9, 9-bis [(6′-*N*, *N*, *N*-trimethylammonium) hexyl] fluorenylene phenylene dibromide} (PFP), and 20 μL of purified PCR products were added to a 96-well microtiter plate. The mixture was shaken vigorously for 15 s, and the fluorescence intensities at 425 and 530 nm were measured using a Varioskan Flash Spectral Scanning Reader (Thermo Fisher Scientific). CpG methylation levels were calculated as $RC_{FRET} = I_{530}/I_{425}$ and $E = 1 - RC_{FRET}/RC_{FRET0}$.

2.6 DNA Methylation Determination by Methylation-Dependent Quantitative Polymerase Chain Reaction (MD-qPCR) The procedure for genomic DNA isolation and MSPJI digestion was the same as that of section 2.5. Briefly, 2 μL of MspJI-digested DNA or inactivated MspJI-treated DNA, 10 μL of 2 × SYBR Premix Ex *Taq*II, 0.2 μL of paired primers (10 μmol/L), and 0.4 μL of 50 × ROX II were mixed in a 20 μL quantitative polymerase chain reaction (qPCR) reaction. Mixtures were prepared in 96-well qPCR plates on ice and transferred to a 7 500 Real-Time PCR System (Roche, Basel, Switzerland). Reactions were performed by incubation at 50 ℃ for 2 min, initial denaturation at 95 ℃ for 5 min, 45 cycles of denaturation at 95 ℃ for 5 s, and annealing at $T_m$ (Table S3 of the Supporting Information) for 30 s and extension at 72 ℃ for 45 s. The primers used in qPCR are shown in Table S3 of the Supporting Information. The CpG methylation level was calculated using the following equation: $E = 1 - 2^{C_t\,\text{MspJI digestion}} / 2^{C_t\,\text{inactivated MspJI digestion}}$.

2.7 Data Analysis Principal component analysis (PCA) and OPLS-DA were performed using SIMCA-P 14.1 (http://umetrics.com/products/simca). Cluster analysis was performed using SPSS (version 20.0, IBM, Armonk, NY, U.S.A.). An elevation map of China was obtained using ArcGIS10.5 (http://www.arcgis.com/features/).

## 3 RESULTS AND DISCUSSION

3.1 UPLC - Q-TOF-MS Metabolomic Analysis of LJF of Different Geographical Origins To acquire a comprehensive metabolic profile of LJF, large-scale untargeted UPLC - Q-TOF-MS was carried out. The metabolome of LJF from 14 geographical regions, including Guangxi, Yunnan, Ningxia,

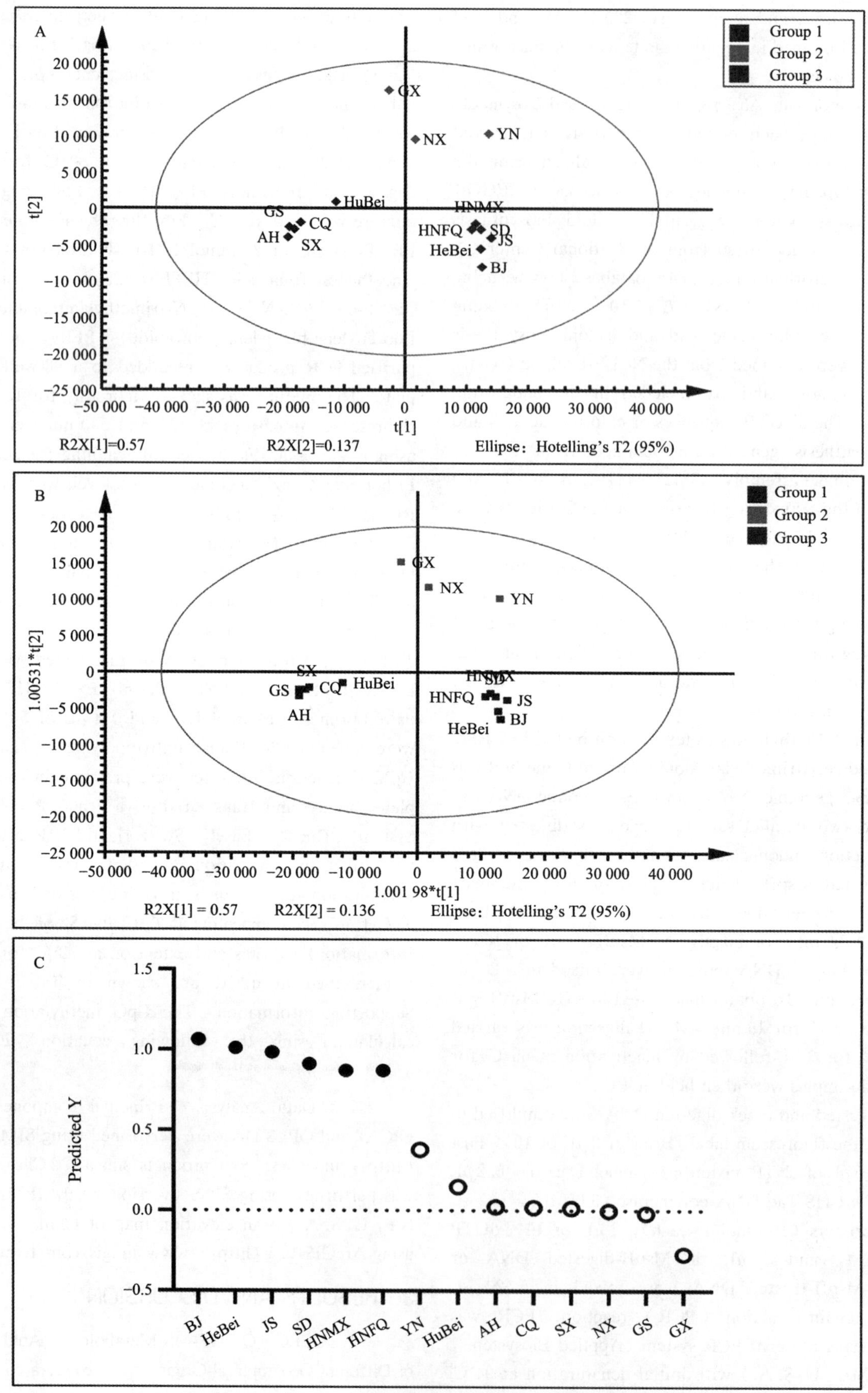


**Figure 1 Chemometrics based on LJF metabolomics**

(A) PCA of metabolomics ($R^2X$=0.707 and $Q^2_{(cum)}$=0.551). (B) OPLS-DA based on LJF metabolomics ($R^2X$=0.705, $R^2Y$=0.944, and $Q^2_{(cum)}$=0.85). (C) Predicted $Y$ plot of OPLS-DA. The solid circles represent geographical origins marked red in panels A and B.

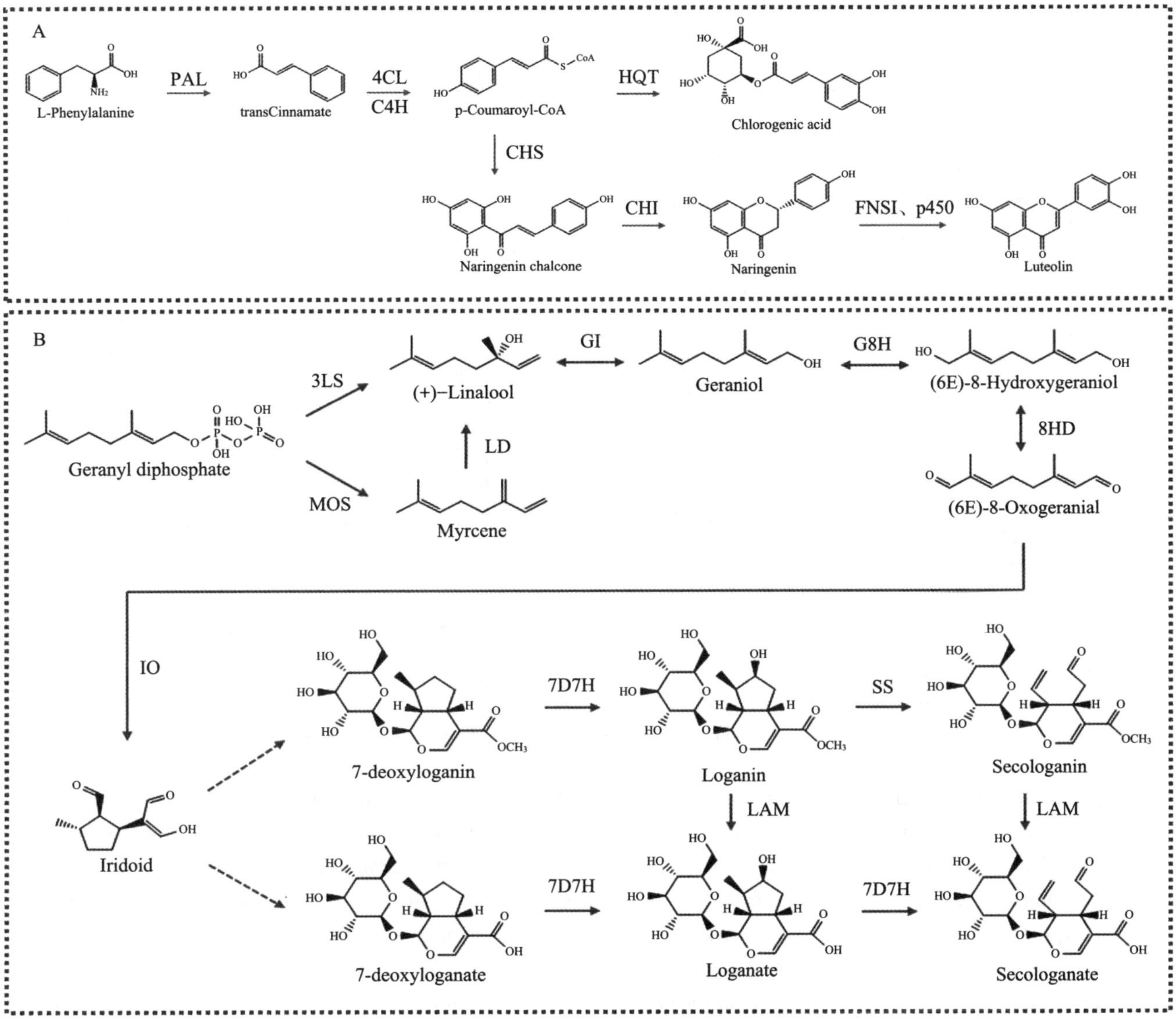

**Figure 2 Biosynthetic pathways for (A) chlorogenic acids and (B) iridoids in LJF**

PAL, phenylalanine ammonia lyase; 4CL, 4-coumarate coenzyme A ligase; C4H, cinnamate 4-hydroxylase; CHS, chalcone synthase; CHI, chalcone isomerase; FNSI, flavone synthase; HQT, hydroxycinnamoyl-coenzyme A quinate hydroxycinnamoyl transferase; 3LS, (3*S*)-linalool/(*E*)-nerolidol synthase; 7D7H, 7-deoxyloganic acid 7-hydroxylase; 8HD, 8-hydroxygeraniol dehydrogenase; G8H, geraniol 10-hydroxylase; IO, iridoid oxidase; LAM, loganic acid methyltransferase; MOS, (*E*)-*β*-ocimene/myrcene synthase; SS, secologanin synthase.

Shaanxi, Hubei, Gansu, Anhui, Chongqing, Mixian in Henan, Fengqiu in Henan, Hebei, Shandong, Jiangsu, and Beijing, was constructed. Chemometrics was performed to assess the geographical classification potential of the metabolic fingerprints obtained.

Unsupervised PCA with unit variance scaling was conducted to visualize the effects of geographical origins on metabolites in LJF, with the model parameters ($R^2X=0.707$ and $Q^2_{(cum)}=0.551$) indicating that 70.7 and 55.1% of the total variation could be explained and predicted, respectively (Figure 1A). As shown in the PCA plot, a tight cluster of LJF from Henan, Hebei, Shandong, Jiangsu, and Beijing demonstrated that LJF of these geographical origins had similar chemical compositions (Figure 1A). Previous research has shown that LJF from Henan and Shandong have high and stable levels of active compounds, and these regions are in close geographical proximity. Thus, LJF from Henan, Hebei, Shandong, Jiangsu, and Beijing were classified into the same group and are marked in red in Figure 1A.

OPLS-DA was used to further analyze which chemicals contributed to geographical discrimination based on PCA classification. In the OPLS-DA score plots, LJF from Henan, Hebei, Shandong, Jiangsu, and Beijing were clearly distinguished from LJF from other regions (Figure 1B). According to the MS data of the available reference standards, 22 compounds were identified in LJF, and

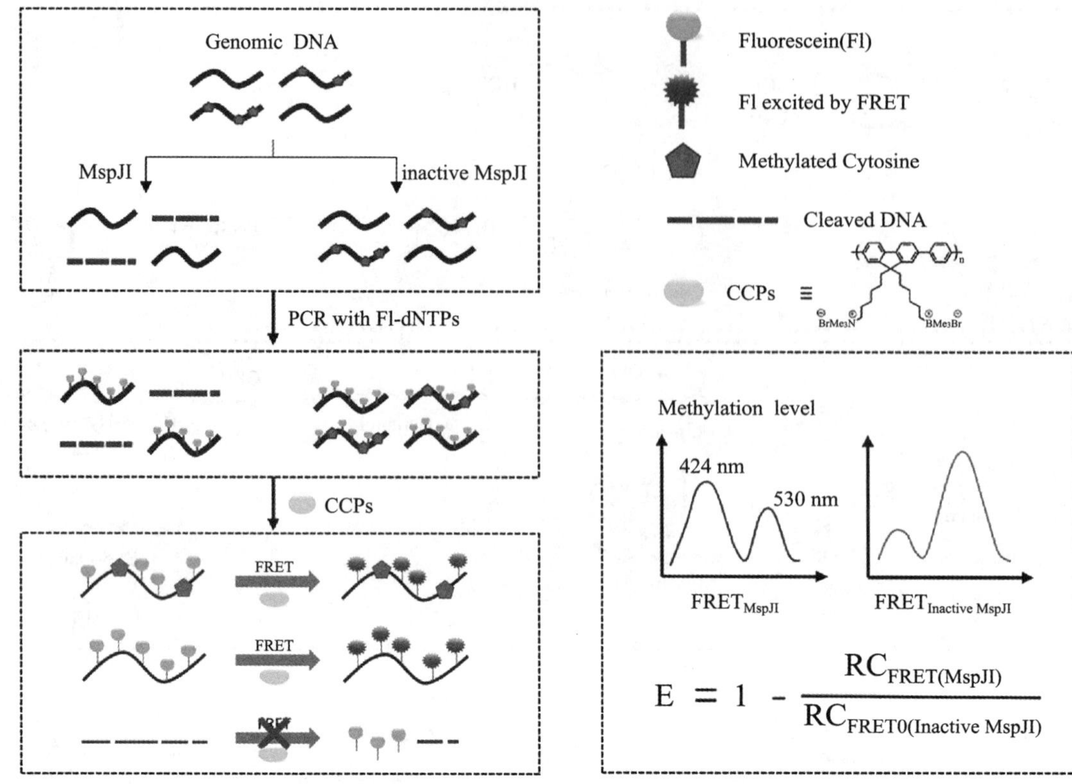


**Figure 3 Schematic of the CCP - FRET method for determining DNA methylation**

detailed information on these chemical constituents was listed in Table S4 of the Supporting Information. As shown in Figure 1C and Table S5 of the Supporting Information, LJF cultivated in these six regions were characterized by higher levels of cryptochlorogenic acid, isochlorogenic acid C, loganic acid, and secoxyloganin. High variable importance in projection (VIP>2.0) for the four variables in the OPLS-DA model revealed contributions to group separation. The results imply that chlorogenic acids and iridoids have the potential to discriminate the geographical origins of LJF, consistent with previous research. Therefore, the chlorogenic acid and iridoid biosynthesis pathways were used to identify epigenetic markers for discrimination of the LJF geographical origin.

3.2 Geographically Related Epigenetic Marker Screening Figure 2A depicts the biosynthetic pathway for chlorogenic acids in LJF. The 5′-UTR sequences of chlorogenic acid biosynthetic genes, including phenylalanine ammonia lyase (*PAL*), 4-coumarate coenzyme A ligase (*4CL*), cinnamate 4-hydroxylase (*C4H*), chalcone synthase (*CHS*), chalcone isomerase (*CHI*), hydroxycinnamoyl-coenzyme A quinate hydroxycinnamoyl transferase (*HQT*), and flavone synthase (*FNS*) are presented in Table S6 of the Supporting Information. DNA methylation prediction result showed that CpG islands were present in the 5′-UTR of *PAL3*, *4CL1*, *4CL2*, *CHS2*, *CHI2*, and *C4H1* (Table S6 of the Supporting Information).

The biosynthetic pathway of iridoids in LJF is shown in Figure 2B. By reference to the monoterpene synthesis pathway (map00902) in the KEGG database, (*E*)-*β*-ocimene/myrcene synthase (*MOS*), loganic acid methyltransferase (*LAM*), (*3S*)-linalool/(*E*)-nerolidol synthase (*3LS*), 8-hydroxygeraniol dehydrogenase (*8HD*), geraniol 10-hydroxylase (*G8H*), secologanin synthase (*SS*), 7-deoxyloganic acid 7-hydroxylase (*7D7H*), loganic acid methyltransferase (*LAM*), and iridoid oxidase (*IO*) were identified as critical genes in the LJF iridoid biosynthetic pathway. The coding and 5′-UTR sequences of the above genes were obtained from the NCBI database and the *L. japonica* genome (assembly ASM2146441v1) and are given in the Supporting Information. CpG islands were screened, and the results indicated that seven genes, including *3LS*, *MOS1*, *MOS2*, *8HD1*, *IO1*, *SS7*, and *7D7H2*, contained CpG islands in the 5′-UTR regions (Table S7 of the Supporting Information).

Several studies have shown that DNA methylation regulates gene expression, which, in turn, affects the content of metabolites. The above bioinformatics results showed abundant CpG islands present in the LJF chlorogenic acid and iridoid biosynthesis pathways, implying a probable link between these CpG islands and metabolic differences in chlorogenic acid and iridoid contents. Given that chlorogenic

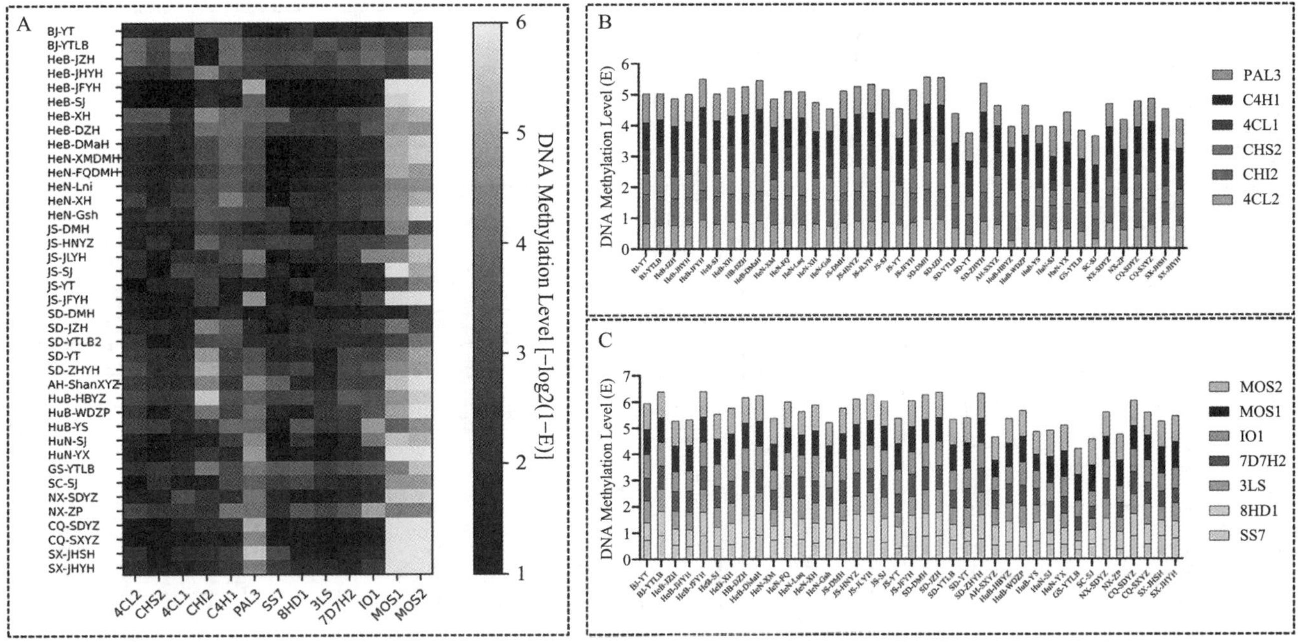

**Figure 4 DNA methylation level of LJF of different geographical origins**

(A) Heatmap for DNA methylation levels of LJF samples as determined by the CCP－FRET method. Stacked bar charts showing the DNA methylation level of (B) chlorogenic acid biosynthesis genes and (C) iridoid biosynthesis genes in LJF samples as determined by the MD-qPCR method.

acids and iridoids contributed significantly to LJF geographical discrimination, the above 13 CpG islands screened in this study may have the potential to classify LJF geographical origins.

3.3 Principle of CCP－FRET The CCP－FRET method has been widely applied in DNA methylation detection for diagnosis of cancers and tumors in the clinic. The schematic of the CCP－FRET approach for determining DNA methylation levels of CpG islands is shown in Figure 3. Genomic DNA of LJF was divided into two parallel samples. One sample was digested using MspJI methylation endonuclease with $5'$-$^{m}$CNNR(N)$_9$-$3'$ as the recognition sequence, and then the fluorescein label was incorporated using PCR to represent the amount of unmethylated DNA fragments. A second sample was conducted for a parallel operation but treated with inactivated MspJI to represent the total amount of DNA fragments. When PFP was added, negatively charged amplicons bound to positively charged PFP as a result of strong electrostatic interactions, and Fl fluorescence was detected via FRET, with fluorescence intensity linearly correlated with the amount of Fl. As residual Fl was removed using shrimp alkaline phosphatase, the Fl signal reflects Fl－dNTPs incorporated into amplicons, which directly represents the amount of undigested fragments in the initial genomic DNA. Here, parameter $E$ was defined for measuring the DNA methylation level of CpG islands, and background was subtracted on the basis of mock digestion with inactivated MspJI. The relevant equation is shown in Figure 3, where $RC_{FRET(MspJI)}$ refers to the FRET ratio for the MspJI-treated sample and $RC_{FRET0(inactive\ MspJI)}$ gives the FRET ratio for sample treated with inactivated MspJI. Because the CCP－FRET method detected DNA methylation levels based on the proportion of methylated fragments in genomic DNA, the result was independent of the initial amount of DNA in the sample.

3.4 DNA Methylation in LJF of Different Geographical Origins To differentiate LJF of 39 geographical origins, the DNA methylation levels in 13 CpG islands, including PAL3, 4CL1, 4CL2, CHS2, CHI2, C4H1, 3LS, MOS1, MOS2, 8HD1, IO1, SS7, and 7D7H2, were determined using the CCP－FRET method. As shown in Figure 4A, the heatmap revealed a potential relationship between CpG methylation levels and LJF geographical origins. In comparison to other samples, LJF from Gansu, Sichuan, Ningxia, Chongqing, and Shaanxi revealed low CpG methylation levels on CHS2, 8HD1, 3LS, and 7D7H2 but high levels on MOS1 and MOS2 (Figure 4A). Because Gansu, Sichuan, Ningxia, Chongqing, and Shaanxi are all located in Western China, the results imply that geographical proximity may lead to similar methylation patterns. In contrast, the CpG methylation levels on PAL3, MOS1, and MOS2 were lower in LJF from Hunan, Hubei, and Anhui, also implying that LJF from adjacent provinces had similar CpG methylation levels (Figure 4A). LJF from Beijing had clearly different methylation performances on 4CL2, CHS2,

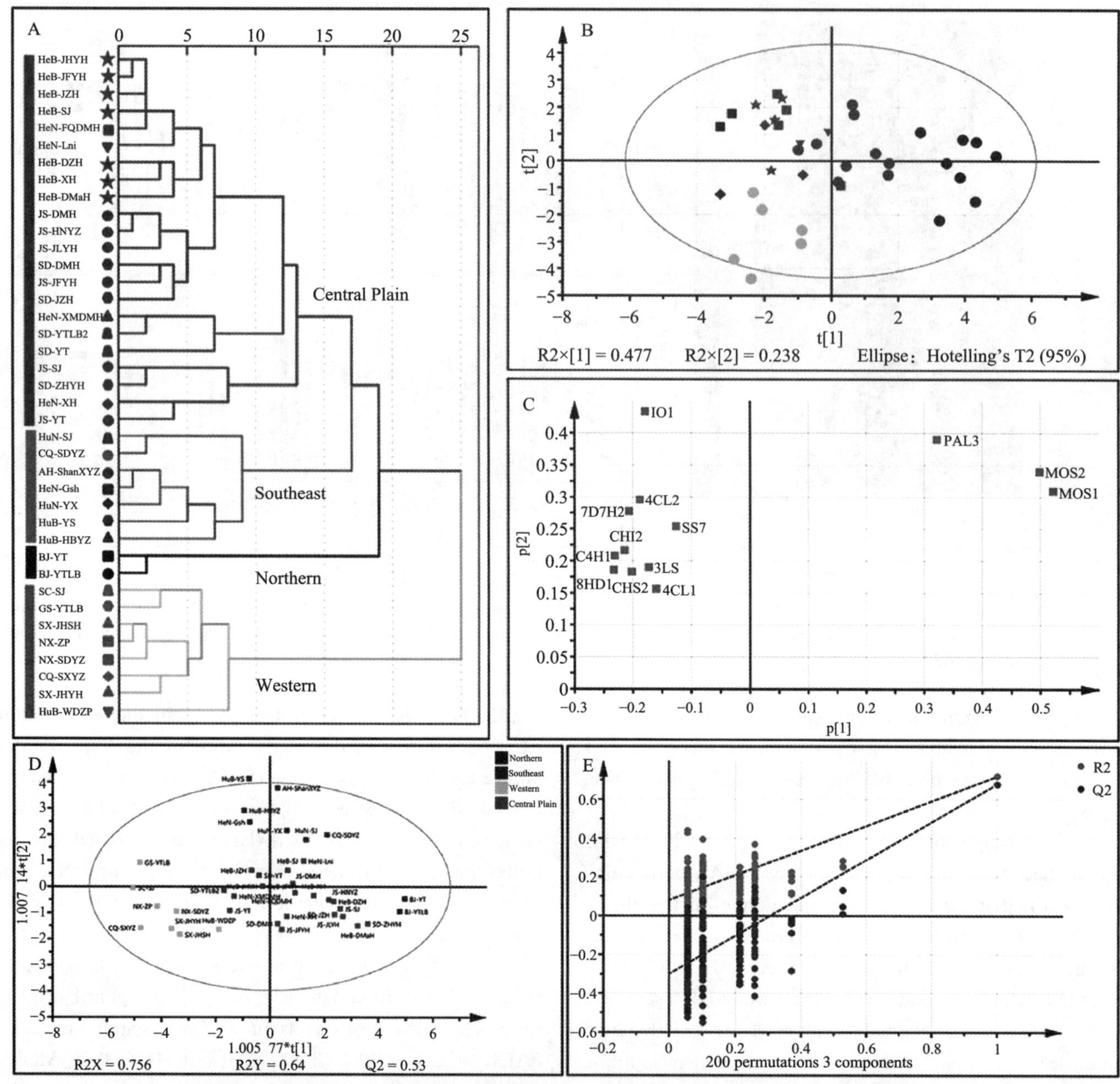


**Figure 5　Discrimination of geographical origin for LJF based on the DNA methylation difference**

(A) Cluster analysis of LJF samples based on CpG methylation levels. The different shapes represent different geographical origins in each group. (B) PCA score plot for LJF samples. The different shapes of dots represent different LJF germplasms: square, Da-mao-hua; solid inverted triangle, Ji-zhua-hua; hollow inverted triangle, Xian-hua; circle, Xiao-mao-hua; and star, wild or undetermined strain. (C) Loading scatter plot of PCA. (D) OPLS-DA score plot for LJF samples. (E) Two hundred times permutation test plot for the OPLS-DA model.

4CL1, CHI2, SS7, 8HD1, and 3LS and can be distinguished from LJF of other geographical origins (Figure 4A). The above results demonstrated a close relationship between CpG methylation levels and LJF geographical origins.

MD-qPCR is another sensitive method for CpG methylation detection and has had wide application in clinical investigations. To validate the reliability of the CCP-FRET method for DNA methylation analysis, MD-qPCR was simultaneously conducted to determine CpG methylation in LJF (panels B and C of Figure 4). Pearson's correlation coefficient between the CpG methylation level determined by CCP-FRET and that determined by MD-qPCR was 0.84 ($P<0.01$; $n=494$), showing high consistency between the two methods. The above result confirms that the CCP-FRET method has good reliability for DNA methylation determination in LJF.

The CCP-FRET method had high sensitivity, with only nanogram amounts of DNA template required for DNA methylation detection. In comparison to the commonly used methylation-sensitive restriction enzyme *Hpa*II, MspJI used in this study was able to improve the accuracy of DNA methylation determination owing to a broader recognition site. Moreover, the CCP - FRET method for CpG methylation determination has the merits of simple operation and use of commonly available instruments. In conclusion, the CCP - FRET method may be more pervasive for determining the DNA methylation status of LJF in the future.

3.5 Discrimination of LJF Geographical Origins On the basis of the CpG methylation levels of LJF plants of different geographical origins, cluster analysis was conducted to classify the geographical origins of LJF. As shown in Figure 5A, LJF of different geographical origins clustered into four branches, representing LJF plants from the Central Plain of China, Southeast China, Northern China, and Western China.

PCA was used to visualize the relationship between geographical origins and CpG methylation levels in LJF, with the model parameters ($R^2X = 0.715$ and $Q^2_{(cum)} = 0.484$) indicating that 71.5 and 48.4% of the total variation could be explained and predicted, respectively. Consistent with the classification of cluster analysis, LJF of 39 different geographical origins were clearly classified into four groups, which suggests that DNA methylation differences in 13 CpG islands, including PAL3, 4CL1, 4CL2, CHS2, CHI2, C4H1, 3LS, MOS1, MOS2, 8HD1, IO1, SS7, and 7D7H2, can be used for discrimination of geographical origin in the LJF (Figure 5B). The loading plot for the principal components indicated that CpG methylation levels in 4CL1, 3LS, and SS7 contribute less to LJF geographical origin discrimination (Figure 5C).

Finally, 10 CpG islands on PAL3, 4CL2, CHS2, CHI2, C4H1, MOS1, MOS2, 8HD1, IO1, and 7D7H2 were used as epigenetic markers for discriminating geographical origin in LJF. As shown in Figure 5D, OPLS-DA was able to validate that CpG methylation levels in these 10 CpG islands could successfully distinguish geographical origins of LJF. Consistent with cluster analysis and PCA classification, LJF of different geographical origins were well-differentiated into four groups representing the Central Plain of China, Southeast China, Northern China, and Western China (Figure 5D). The OPLS-DA model had good fitting and prediction abilities, as reflected in the evaluation parameters: $R^2X_{cum} = 0.756$, $R^2Y_{cum} = 0.64$, and $Q^2_{cum} = 0.53$. In addition, a 200 times permutation test was performed to determine whether the OPLS-DA model was overfitting. As shown in Figure 5E, all permuted $R^2$ and $Q^2$ values to the left are lower than the original points to the right, indicating that the OPLS-DA model is valid.

Extensive introduction and domestication in past decades have led to a complex germplasm distribution for LJF, as revealed in previous research and shown in Table S2 of the Supporting Information. Molecular markers based on DNA sequences have been greatly affected by extensive introduction and, thus, have limitations for geographical authentication, while DNA methylation differences are primarily related to environmental stress and are less influenced by introduction and domestication. As shown in Figure 5A, the classification result indicates that the geographical difference obviously has more contribution than different genotypes in cluster analysis. In Figure 5B, different shapes indicate different germplasms of LJF, and LJF from the Central Plain of China incorporates several germplasms but was successfully separated from the other groups. These results indicate that the different genotypes have a limited influence on geographical origin discrimination of LJF. The attempt to distinguish geographical origins of LJF based on DNA methylation status may provide a new approach for geographical discrimination.

LJF cultivated in Henan and Shandong has been registered as a NGIP based on geographically related characteristics, including consistent quality and unique flavor. In this study, LJF from Henan, Shandong, Hebei, and Jiangsu had similar metabolic profiles and DNA methylation levels and were classified into the Central Plain of China (Figure 1 and panels A and B of Figure 5). Notably, this discrimination of LJF origins is supported by previous geographical classifications based on numerical taxonomy of agronomic traits, restriction fragment length polymorphism, and differences in the content of chlorogenic acids. As shown in the elevation map (Figure 5F), Henan, Shandong, Hebei, and Jiangsu (marked red) have a close geographical distance and similar altitude and latitude and share a similar climate. The results here indicate that LJF from Hebei and Jiangsu have similar characteristics to LJF from Henan and Shandong and have potential for NGIP labeling. In this study, LJF from Henan, Shandong, Hebei, and Jiangsu were successfully distinguished from LJF of other origins, which provides a reference for improving the traceability and authenticity of LJF geographical origins.

To further explore the contribution of geographical characteristics, multivariate analysis of variance was conducted upon the data combining metabolomics data, DNA methylation data, germplasm, elevation, latitude, and longitude of LJF samples. As shown in Table S8 of the Supporting Information, the $p$ values of Pillai's trace, Wilk's lambda and Roy's largest root were less than 0.05 when elevation and latitude were used as fixed variables. This result indicated that elevation and latitude have significant influence on DNA methylation status and metabolite content of LJF samples. The test of between subject effects showed that elevation and latitude both have significant correlation on the DNA methylation level of IO1, 4CL2, MOS1, PAL3, 4CL1, C4H1, CHS2, MOS2, 3LS, 7D7H2, and contents of loganic acid, loganin, secoxyloganin, cryptochlorogenic acid, isochlorogenic acid B, and isochlorogenic acid C (Table S9 of the Supporting Information). The above results contributed to elucidate the modulation of the DNA methylation status and metabolites under different geographical characteristics.

Different from geographical classification based on metabolomics, LJF samples from Beijing were further divided into an independent group according to DNA methylation differences (Figures 1A and 5A). This classification based on DNA methylation status combined with cluster analysis was partially supported by a previous study of LJF and corresponds to the characteristic environment of Beijing. Furthermore, the geographical classification result by DNA methylation levels was based on more LJF samples compared to metabolomic analysis, which can improve the reliability of analysis. When a plant is subjected to environmental stress, response at the epigenetic level will be antecedent to that at the metabolic level, which may explain why geographical classification results based on the DNA methylation difference were more reliable than classification based on metabolomics. It is worth noting that LJF samples from Northern China are insufficient according to the *L. japonica* Thunb. less distributes in Northern China. Considering that this may compromise the reliability of the OPLS-DA model, more LJF samples from Northern China will be collected in the future to improve our study.

In conclusion, differences in DNA methylation were determined to address the critical problem of discriminating the LJF geographical origin. A total of 10 CpG islands, including PAL3, 4CL2, CHS2, CHI2, C4H1, MOS1, MOS2, 8HD1, IO1, and 7D7H2, were selected as epigenetic markers for discriminating the geographical origin of LJF. On the basis of DNA methylation levels determined by the CCP-FRET method, LJF of 39 geographical origins were successfully classified into four groups using PCA and OPLS-DA models. Furthermore, LJF from Henan, Shandong, Hebei, and Jiangsu showed similar geographical characteristics and were successfully distinguished from LJF of other origins. This study indicated that DNA methylation differences have great potential to discriminate among the geographical origins of food. Epigenetic markers identified in this study may provide a reference for the geographical traceability of LJF products.

[王正鹏，黄璐琦，袁媛. Journal of Agricultural and Food Chemistry, 2023, 71: 12346-12356.]

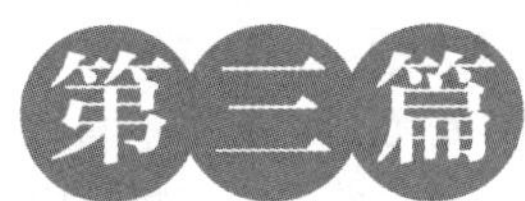

# 第三篇 道地药材遗传成因

# “道地药材”的生物学探讨

道地药材是一个约定俗成的概念，是一个古代药物标准化的概念。它以固定产地生产、加工或销售来控制药材质量，保证了药材的货真质优，得到医者与患者的普遍认可。它的产生是以实践经验为依据，经得起临床的考验，有着丰富的科学内涵，已引起诸多学者的关注，并进行了有关的研究。这些研究无论是采用传统的方法或是现代科学手段，也无论是引种栽培、成分分析或提高临床疗效诸方面，都取得了很大的成绩，积累了丰富的经验。应该说，在几千种中药当中，道地药材是研究得比较深入的部分，但距离阐明药材道地性的科学内涵还相差甚远，还没有对中药学术的振兴产生重大影响，究其原因就是没有从药材(除矿物药)来源于生物这一本质出发进行阐述。作者现仅从理论上谈谈个人的认识。在本文的讨论中，仅以生物药道地药材为内容(以下简称“道”)，不涉及矿物药和合成药及生物药的加工、销售对其道地性的影响。

## 1 道地药材的生物学内涵

药材(除矿物药)来源于生物，都有着生物的内涵。生物是由基因(gene)、细胞(cell)、器官(organ)、有机体(organism)、居群(population)、群落(community)等6个主要的生物层组成的，这一多层次结构模式被称为“生物学谱”(biological spectrum)。每一层次都有其自身的科学问题，有相应的研究方法，如细胞生物学和分子生物学及其方法，人们在认识生物时都是从其所处的层次逐渐向宏观和微观两个方面发展，药材研究也不例外，如在药材的鉴定上，就有细胞层次的鉴定——显微鉴定，器官层次的鉴定——性状鉴定及有机体层次的鉴定——基原鉴定。

如果进一步向宏观方向发展到居群层次研究药材，那就涉及道地药材的研究。历代本草对“道地药材”的论述主要体现以下几个方面：①中医理论指导。②工艺技术的体现。③同种异地。④异种异质。在这些方面中涉及生物学范畴的为后2种，并以同种异地为“道地药材”的基础，而异种异质指物种不同。在南北朝及其以前，这是道地药材形成的主要原因，唐宋以后，这种现象逐渐减少，发展至今它早不作道地药材来看待，而是作为就地取材，扩大资源来考虑。因此，“道地药材”的生物内涵是同种异地.即同一物种因其具有一定的空间结构，能在不同的地点上形成大大小小的群体单元，其中如果某一群体产生质优效佳的药材，即为道地药材，而这一地点则被称为药材的“道地产地”。这个同一物种在不同地点上形成的群体单元，在生物学上就称为“居群”。因此，“道”在生物学上就是指某一物种的特定居群，这里的“特定”不是由研究者根据研究目的方便划定的，而是由一定的土壤、光热及阴湿等环境所决定的，有着比较稳定的边界，是一个比较稳定的“地方居群”(local population)，是在特定的空间和时间里生活着的自然的或人为的同种个体群。

## 2 道地药材形成中的生物学原理

道地药材的形成有其历史条件、地理条件和生长的环境因子(土壤、气候)及人为因子等，其形成模式有生境主导型、种质主导型、技术主导型、传媒主导型以及各种多因子关联决定型，但与生物这一本质相关的模式只有前2种，其形成原理可解释为“道”所具有的有效成分含量高，临床疗效好等特征，是不同产地同一药材的不同表现。这种表现的差异正同进化生物学中的“变异”，是由自身的遗传本质——基因型所决定的，受一定的环境条件影响。从生物学上说，“道”的形成应是基因型与环境之间相互作用的产物，可用公式表示：

表型＝基因型＋环境饰变

所谓表型，指“道”可被观察到的结构和功能特性的总和，包括药材性状、组织结构、有效成分含量及疗效等。这里的环境饰变(environmental modification)，是指由生境引起的表型的任何不同遗传的变化。基因有产生某一特定表型的潜力，但不是决定着这一表型的必然实现，而是决定着一系列的可能性，究竟其中哪一个可能性得到实现，要看环境而定。因为，器官的生长和性状的表现，都必须依靠来源于周围生境的物质，在合适的生境中产生“道”所具有的特别表型特征。反之，在其他生境中该基因的这种调控则可能发生“弥散”(penetrant)，出现一种不确立性，比如生长在东北三省、苏、皖、浙、鄂的一叶楸[*Securinega suffruticosa*(Pall.) Rehd.]含有左旋一叶楸碱(*l*-securinine)，生长在北京近郊县多为右旋(*d*-securinine)，承德附近6个县一叶楸碱具有左、右两种旋光性。生物类药材的同一基因在不同的外界环境条件下，有着不同的表型，称为表型可塑性(phenotyic plasticity)。表型可塑性，说明为什么不同产地的同一种药材质量和疗效有着差别。与可塑性相关的另一个概念是耐受性，即是指生物对极端环境的耐受能力，或者指生物所生存的环境因素范围。“道地产区”常被认为是这一环境范围内最适宜植物生长的地方，即该物种的某居群在某生境下表现出最大的适应性。但应该清楚地认识到，决定药材疗效的物质基础是有效成分，有些有效成分在正常条件下没有或很少，只有当受到外界刺激(如干旱、严寒、伤害)时才会产生，这类物质属异常二次成分，被称为保护素(phytoalexin)，而这种对生物残酷的环境是处于这一生物的分布区的边缘，可见“道地产区”不仅在药材分布区的密度中心，也有可能在边缘，如甘草、大黄、枸杞、防风等药材的道地产区，这在实际应用上的意义就在于提示了建立道地药材生产基地时不能仅考虑适合药材生长的区域。

当一个药材种具有较广的分布区时，它的各个不同地区的居群往往具有不同的基因型，或称地方性特化基因型(local specialized genotype)，而这些基因型是由于不同的生态或地理的条件长期选择作用塑造而成，是产生"道"的遗传本质。可以说，"道"是对一特殊的界限明确的一套环境条件的基因型反应的产物，属"药材"的"生态型"。相同的环境条件，可产生同样的和基本相似的生态型，因而生态型可以是多地起源，这也是为什么药材也可以有多个"道地产区"的原因所在。

## 3 道地药材研究的生物学问题和方法

居群的特征可分为数量特征、空间特征、遗传特征 3 个方面，而"道"这一特殊居群除上述 3 个特征外，还有"药效特征"，它属于药材学范畴，这里不作讨论。

3.1 数量特征 主要指"道"在"道地产区"的密度，对其研究常常是"道"管理、采挖和质量评价的基础。影响密度的 4 个参数是出生率、死亡率、迁入率和迁出率。①出生率(natality)是泛指任何生物个体或居群产生新个体的能力，可分为最大出生率(maximum natality)和实际出生率(realized natality)。最大出生率是指在理想条件下(既无任何生态因子限制，仅受生理因子限制)的出生率，实际出生率是指在具体的生境中最终实现的出生率。②死亡率(mortality)是指居群内个体死亡的百分率，同样也分为最低死亡率(minimum mortality)和生态死亡率(ecological mortality)，比较出生率与死亡率可指明"道"未来产量的变化趋势，比较最大和实际的出生率、死亡率就能知道道地产区生境的变化趋势，在研究一个"道"时，只有通过连续多年的观察和记录，特别是详细记录出生率和死亡率，并通过分析和模拟，才能找出影响"道"的主要生态因子，避免单从土壤或其他单一因素考虑。③迁入(immigation)是指其他居群内个体通过扩散进入到该研究居群的过程。在"道"生产上这种迁入常常是伴随着人为的栽培引种而发生，引种药材质量的好坏，不仅影响当年每亩药材的产量和质量，而且因这种迁入能打破"道"与非"道"之间的隔离，导致居群间基因的流动，改变整个"道"的遗传组成，给整个产区以后的生产带来影响。如在茅苍术生产栽培中，其致命弱点在于常异花授粉性产生的实生后代普遍存在有效成分变异，它使后代难以保持亲代的优良品质，所以目前 60% 以上的植物性道地药材在人工栽培时是采用无性繁殖方式。但是，长期的无性繁殖，后代始终是前代营养体的继续，植株得不到复壮机会，得不到新的基因，致使品种生活力下降。因此，防止"道"的品种退化，加强人工选择，施行科学留种应引起高度重视。④迁出(emigration)是指居群内个体移出的过程，它往往造成居群内个体数量的减少，同时会使该居群向外扩张，占领新的领地。这种现象的发生会导致道地产区扩大和迁移，影响因素是多方面的，有气候、土壤、温度以及人为因素。一般而言，在研究迁入和迁出时的困难是居群边界的不易确定，而"道"这一特殊居群中却有着比较固定的边界，使得这一研究相对比较容易。

3.2 空间特征 是指居群内个体在空间分布及其动态，居群大体上有 3 种分布类型：随机分布、均匀分布和群集分布。"道"在产区内的自然状态常常属于群集(cluped)这一分布型，即是个体成群或成团分布，这就使得"道"有着不同的密度分布，可称"道地药材密度"，就是单位面积或体积内的个体数目。这一分布密度是对生境差异产生的结果，同时也受气候、环境的变化及季节变化的影响。有人指出，气候因素决定植物的分布范围，土壤因素决定植物分布范围内的密度。研究"道"与生境的相互作用，要从"道地药材密度"入手，不仅是比较道地产区与非道地产区之间的生境变化，而且更要揭示造成这一密度分布的原因所在。如盛产白术的江西安福县的 3 个乡，相距最多 40 公里，海拔及地理位置也极相近，但 3 个乡的白术生产质量有所差异，究其原因主要为土壤质地不同。可以说，"道地药材密度"是道地产区内同种药材的质量参差不齐的生物学表现。

上述这些数量特征和空间特征都受生态因子左右，各个生态因子的影响总是相互联系作用的，每个生态因子对于同一种药材的影响是不同的，这一点决定于它与其他因子的配合。另外，必须区别出生态环境各个因子之间的直接关系和间接关系。水分状况、热量状况、土壤溶液的成分都是属于直接影响因素；地形、成土等都是通过直接因子起作用的，属间接因子。过去的研究着重在直接生态因子方面，但间接因子的重要意义并不小于直接因子，对此，已引起不少学者的关注，如 GBS 的制约效应。总之，他们的研究属居群生态学的研究范围。

3.3 "道"的另一个重要特征就是"遗传特征" 由于"道"在"产区"多是以人为方式进行无性繁殖而不单单是通过有性繁殖来进行基因交换，形成一个在个体组成、数量以及遗传结构上有一定界限的地方繁育居群(或称孟德尔式群体)，因此，"道"应看成一个具有共同基因库的由交配和亲缘关系联系起来的同一物种的个体。研究其遗传特征就是要针对其特点，即要揭示在"道"之内及与非"道"之间的遗传变异大小、变化规律及其影响因素。"道"与非"道"之间和"道"之内存在大量的遗传变异这一事实，早已为人们所观察和意识到，比如伊克昭盟甘草，就可分为河地草、梁地草及淮地草等 3 种，它们在外部形态、组织构造和化学成分上都有明显区别，但它们在遗传上的变异程度却没有进一步研究。可见过去的研究多为形态标记研究，即为个体特征描述和宏观观测，这样得到的结论往往是不完善的，易引起争论。

近年来，人们通过分子生物学方法比较不同生物在基因表达产物(蛋白质)乃至遗传物质(核酸)本身的异同性来研究遗传变异。这些方法目前主要指同工酶，RFLP、RAPD、AP-PCR 等技术。其中后 3 种方法研究对象是遗传物质本身，不像形态学标记和同工酶标记是研究基因转录翻译后加工的产物，甚至是多基因型的表现型，因此不受显隐性关系、环境条件和发育阶段的影响，成为研究居群遗传变异的重要方法，越来越被重视和采用。

造成遗传变异因素是主要为繁育系统、分布范围和种子传播机制。繁育系统在居群遗传结构的形成过程中起着十分关键的作用，如自交种的遗传变异的 51% 存在于居群之间，相当于异交风媒植物的 5 倍，动物授粉的物种介于这两个极端之间。

分布区的大小对遗传变异有显著影响，由于居群范围小，使近亲繁殖的机会增加，使遗传多样性造成损失，遗传变异相应减少。

种子散播机制也明显影响遗传变异的分布，靠重力、附着和果实破裂而散播种子的遗传变异大，其后代向外扩展的能力有限，从而加强居群间的分化。因此，以这种方式传播后代，就会使“道”与非“道”之间的遗传变异比靠风力来传播种子的要大得多，“道地性”会更加明显。

总之，“道”包含的遗传变异越多，产生外部形态、组织结构及化学组成差异的基础越厚，会使居群间的分化进一步加深，这种分化又会随着居群地理分布范围的加大；表现为“地理宗”的分化，当“地理宗”间出现进一步趋异时就可能导致新种的形成，目前已有学者认为白芷、牡丹、牛膝、花椒、艾叶等“道”的变异大于或等于种间的差异。因此，研究“道”是研究生物进化的很好材料，这也是“道”的生物学意义之一。

以上方面是居群遗传学的研究主题。居群生态学和居群遗传学组成了居群生物学，也提出了“道”的生物学问题和研究方法。

## 4 小结

“道”是指生物学上的“居群”，是一个具有共同基因库的由交配和亲缘关系联系起来的同一物种的个体群。它的形成，是由基因型与环境饰变共同作用的结果，具有数量特征、空间特征、遗传特征和药效特征。对其的生物学研究是用居群生态学和居群遗传学的方法研究上述特征及其影响因素，突破过去研究只是找出“道”或“道地产区”的旧框框和旧模式，使研究是从药材来源于生物这一本质问题开始，产生的结果将更具“道地性”，并为研究生物进化提供素材。

[黄璐琦，等.中国药学杂志，1997，32(9)：563-566.]

# 珍稀濒危中药资源保护的相关问题探讨

我国幅员辽阔，纵跨热带、温带和寒温带，地质、地貌格局复杂多变，物种多样，极其丰富，植物种类约占世界总数的11%。据全国大规模中药资源普查表明，我国中药资源已达12 772种，其中药用植物11 118种，药用动物1 547种。随着国民经济的发展和社会日趋进步，人们对健康状况的关注程度提高，医疗、保健等用药需求量猛增；与此同时，在世界范围内，新药开发投入经费的不断增加，研究难度的逐渐加大，使从野生药用动植物中发现和寻找新化合物、新结构已成为一种趋势。这些在不同程度上加大了中药资源的压力。加之，长期以来，对合理开发利用中药资源的认识不足，一些地区不同程度上对中药资源进行了掠夺式的过度采收(捕猎)，目前，很多中药资源蕴含量下降，甚至耗竭，一些种类濒临灭绝，因此，对珍稀濒危中药资源进行保护已迫在眉睫。为了更好地开展此项工作，本文试从珍稀濒危中药资源的现状和保护入手，结合国际保护公约和协议的介绍，探讨我国珍稀濒危中药资源保护所存在的问题及相关的对策。

## 1 珍稀濒危中药资源的现状和保护

上述种种原因使得一些药用种类出现衰退甚至濒临灭绝，有些种类的优良种质正面临消失和解体。药用动物如黑熊、马鹿、林麝、大(小)灵猫、中国林蛙、蛤蚧、玳瑁等40个种类的资源显著减少，已影响了近30种动物药材的市场供应；药用植物如甘草、光果甘草、羌活、单叶蔓荆、黄皮树、银柴胡、肉苁蓉、三叶半夏、新疆阿魏和紫草等100多种资源量普遍下降，影响60多个药材品种的医疗用药。黑长臂猿、原麝、海南坡鹿等近20种动物和见血封喉、峨嵋野连、八角莲、凹叶厚朴、杜仲、小勾儿茶、野山参、黑节草等30多种植物，因野生资源稀少，以致无法提供商品或只能提供少量商品；高鼻羚羊(又称赛加羚羊)、印度犀、野马和厦门文昌鱼等4种野生动物资源几近绝迹。为此，我国自20世纪80年代以来，在保护濒危野生药用植物方面做了大量的工作，制定了一系列的法令法规。1984年我国公布了第一批珍稀濒危保护植物名录，1987年国务院发布了“国家重点保护野生药材物种名单”，1988年国家环境保护局主持编写《中国珍稀濒危植物》一书于1989年在国内出版(现以《中国植物红皮书》正式在国际上发行)，共收保护物种388种，药用物种约102种，其中属于常用中药约33种。黑龙江、内蒙古和新疆还制定了地方性中药资源保护法规。在“八五”“九五”期间，“濒危动物药资源保护与开发研究”被列为国家科技攻关项目。通过积极开展科学研究，研制和寻找出不少代用品，如人工麝香、人工牛黄，人工犀角(正在攻关)，山羊角代替羚羊角，水牛角代替犀角等，研究牛骨、猪骨、狗骨代替虎骨等；在药用植物保护方面，建立自然保护区，实施就地保护，截至1993年全国有自然保护区700多个，占国土面积的6.8%。这些自然保护区保护了大量药用植物物种，如长白山自然保护区受到保护的药用植物有900多种，峨眉山自然保护区保护的药用植物有1 655种。各地还建立了一些药用生物保护区，如黑龙江先后建立了五味子、防风、龙胆、桔梗、黄柏、黄芩、马兜铃等药材的36个保护区；广西的龙虎山、猫儿山保护区；云南的药山、海子坪保护区等，为保护各地的特产及野生药材做出贡献。同时，积极开展野生变家种的研究。目前，我国家种的大宗药用植物就有150多种，种植面积达440多万亩，据初步统计，由野生变为家种的药用植物不下60种，主要有防风、龙胆、柴胡、甘草、辽细辛、五味子、半夏、山茱萸、何首乌、天麻等，引种国外药用植物约30余种，主要有颠茄、丁香、毛花洋地黄、安息香、大风子等。总之，通过积极创造条件，多方面努力发展我国珍稀濒危中药资源的保护事业，为我国传统中医药的持续发展打下了坚实的物质基础。

## 2 珍稀濒危中药资源保护的相关国际公约及协议

目前有关动植物保护的国际公约或协议不少，世界各国也有相关法令，并且有的行之有效，为保护生物物种多样性做出了贡献。现简要介绍一些对我国珍稀濒危中药资源保护有影响的公约和协议。

2.1 国际动物保护公约及协议

2.1.1 濒危野生动物国际贸易公约(The Convention on International Trade in Endangered Species of Wild Fauna and Flora, CITES) 1973年在美国华盛顿签署,又称华盛顿公约,我国于1980年正式加入。CITES设立目的主要在于建立野生物种输入、输出国之间合作管理,以确实防止公约指定名录内物种的非法国际贸易行为。公约条文共25条,对于全世界濒绝、渐危物种贸易管制的原则,各会员国应采取的措施,会员国大会、国内立法的配合,公约的签署、修订、入会、争端解决等都有详细规定。

2.1.2 国际重要湿地公约(Convention on Wetlands of International Importance, Especially as Waterfowl Habitat,又称 Ramsar Convention) 1971年于伊朗拉姆萨尔签约,故又称拉姆萨尔公约。公约重点是重视特殊水鸟,加强湿地的保育及适当利用。该公约共有12条条文,对于重要湿地名单的制定、管理计划的研究与执行、湿地自然保护区的设定、国际合作、会员大会的召开、会议代表的组成等均有明文规定。

2.1.3 世界文化及自然遗产保护公约(Convention for the Protection of the World Culture and Natural Heritage) 1972年在联合国教科文组织(UNESCO)支持下于法国巴黎签署,该公约共38条,主要目的在于保护世界主要遗产名册内的自然及文化地区。凡人类文化遗产、特殊生物群系、濒危动植物的栖息地都有资格被列入名册保护。

2.1.4 生物多样性公约(Convention on Biological Diversity) 1992年于巴西正式缔约。公约共有42条,对生物多样性的保护和永续使用、监测、域内保育、域外保育、遗产资格的取得、生物技术的处理及其受益分配、缔约国会议、争端解决、签署、加入、退出等均有详细规定。

2.2 区域性公约

2.2.1 欧共体自然栖地及野生动植物保育公约(Directive on the Conservation of Natural Habitats and of the Wild Fauna and Flora) 1992年5月21日由欧洲共同体(The Council of the European Communities)于比利时布鲁塞尔(Brussels)完成研订。规定欧洲共同体各成员国应保育其辖内之濒临绝种的动植物及天然栖地,以维持生物多样性。在详细的附表中,他们已列出必须特别保育的自然栖地类型168个,必须特别保育之动植物632种,并规定各会员国应该设立特别保育区(special areas of conservation)。

2.2.2 欧洲野生物及自然栖地保育公约(Convention of the Conservation of European Wildlife and Natural Habitats) 1979年签约于伯恩(Bern)。

2.2.3 西半球自然及野生物保育公约(Convention on Nature Protection and Wildlife Preservation in the Western Hemisphere) 1940年签约于华盛顿。

2.2.4 非洲自然及自然资源保育公约(African Convention on the Conservation of Nature and Natural Resources) 1968年签约于阿尔及尔。

2.2.5 东南亚国协自然及自然资源保育协议(ASEAN Agreement on the Conservation of Nature and Natural Resources) 1985年签约于吉隆坡。

2.2.6 东南亚及太平洋地区植物保护协议(Plant Protection Agreement for the South-East Asia and Pacific Region) 1956年签约于意大利罗马。

2.2.7 东非保护区及野生动植物协议(Protocol Concerning Protected Areas and Wild Fauna and Flora in the Eastern African Region) 1985年签约于内罗毕。

2.2.8 加勒比海地区保护区及野生物协议(Protocol Concerning Specially Protected Areas and Wildlife in the Wider Caribbean Region) 1990年签约于金斯敦(Kingston)。

2.2.9 南太平洋地区自然资源及环境保护公约(Convention for the Protection of the Natural Resources and Environment of the South Pacific Region) 1986年签署于努美阿(Noumea)。

## 3 珍稀濒危中药资源保护所面临的问题及相应的对策

3.1 正确对待国际社会的意见和批评 我国中医药记载和曾经使用过被视为野生动植物保护的旗舰物种如犀牛角和虎骨等,招致了不同层次、不同来源的各种批评,乃至抨击。诚然,在这众多的批评中,有不少是由于缺乏对我国传统医药的正确理解,缺乏基本知识以及错误翻译所致;然而,对国际社会的批评也不能一概而论地认为是恶意中伤。原因是中医药界与野生动植物保护组织,特别是野生动植物保护主管部门之间缺乏沟通,未能有效地宣传自己;为此,在1997年召开的CITES成员国第10次会议上首次讨论传统医药问题时,我国政府介绍了中医药文化在保护药用动植物和代用品研究方面所做的努力和取得的成就,使得本次会议通过了传统药的决议,对传统药特别是中国的传统医药文化和价值给予积极的肯定,并增加了肯定人工培植和人工繁殖作用的内容,体现了只有相互沟通才能理解。因此,对于中医药与野生动植物保护的关系,我们的态度是:我们加入和遵守CITES公约,我们现有的12 000多种中草药中,有80%以上系以植物原产为基础制作而成,并且常用的种类均有栽培品种,仅有一小部分中成药含有动物药成分。在利用及保护之间寻求一种平衡已成为我国传统医药事业发展的动力之一,野生动植物的保护已经成为中医药发展不可缺少的重要组成部分。

3.2 客观评价珍稀濒危中药材的疗效 由于古代科学技术发展水平的局限以及目前条件的限制,部分珍稀濒危中药材缺乏必要的科学研究,对前人记载的功效不能进行客观评价。因此,我们应通过科学研究正确区分哪些是传统中医药中的精华,哪些是确有疗效,应当加以坚持开发;哪些因受眼前利益驱动,或悖谬误传,将会对未来的用药基础构成威胁。只有搞清这些问题,才能切实遵循"保护为先,利用为后"或"保护与利用并重"的原则,才能为濒危物种替代物的研究提供客观标准。

3.3 加强科研,为保护立法和强化管理打下坚实的基础 为了加强珍稀濒危中药资源的保护立法,健全相关的法制法规,加大执法力度,急待开展以下的科研工作。

3.3.1 本底资料的调查工作 在全国范围内有针对性地调查濒危中药材的种类、数量,分析种群区系的分布特点(包括广布种与濒危种),绘制地理分布图,了解当前保护现状等,这是一项巨大而重要的工程,是基础研究,是濒危程度评价的前提。

3.3.2 珍稀濒危程度的量化标准 中药材珍稀濒危程度应该有一个全面的、科学的而且必须是实用性强的评价标准,目前国内对此研究尚少,是一个亟待解决的标准化问题。评价标准除充分考虑动植物分类学特点外,还应考虑药用价值对物种、族群的影响,应从分布特点、野生资源量、栽培状况、保护现状、开发利用、药典收载等方面细化量化标准。评价时需特别注意影响因素间的权重系数、交互作用。据此标准划分濒危程度,确定保护等级,制定具体的保护措施及奖惩办法等。

3.3.3 中药材致濒原因的研究 要对濒危物种及其遗传多样性进行有效保护,必须查明中药材致濒因子,这有赖于基础研究的加强。如查明濒危物种的种群动态、繁育系统、极端环境压力下的抗逆性、人为干扰对物种的影响等,从而可以揭示濒危中药材生活史薄弱环节,区分致濒的内在机制和外部原因,为物种保育、人工栽培或驯养提供科学依据。研究表明:银杉遗传变异水平低,族群间又强烈分化,势必造成族群内严重近交,产生近交衰退等一系列后果,最终导致银杉的进一步濒危。因此对银杉保护应采取特殊策略,即应该保护较多族群,对于特定等位基因的单株和亚族也应予以保护。而鹅掌楸族群遗传多样性并不比广布品种的低,其濒危过程是一个时间和空间的渐变过程,是内部和外部不良环境条件综合作用的结果。总之造成中药材濒危原因十分复杂,有内因、外因,也有内、外因综合作用,不能一概而论,更不能以偏概全。对保护物种需找出致濒因子,才能实施有效的保护。

[黄璐琦,等.世界科学技术,2001,3(6):46-49.]

# 中药材道地性研究的现代生物学基础及模式假说

道地药材是中医临床长期、反复实践中产生的、公认的优质中药材,它的形成与我国特有的生态地理、文化背景及中医药理论有关。由于道地药材独特的优良品质,其经济价值往往不同一般。近年来,对道地药材的掠夺性开发加之生态环境的人为破坏,致使许多道地药材濒于灭绝。因此,开展道地药材的研究不仅能体现中医药特色,而且是保证中医药持续发展的需要。应该说,在几千种中药当中,道地药材是研究得比较深入的部分。尤其是近些年来,运用多学科的理论和方法对道地药材进行研究,使道地药材的研究更加全面和系统,并取得了很大的成绩,但距离阐明药材道地性的科学内涵,从理论上有所创新来振兴中药学术还相差很远。为此,作者在回顾道地药材研究现状,找出问题的基础上,着重分析其研究所遵循的途径及相互关系,提出应结合现代生物学的研究方法,为今后道地药材的研究提供参考。

## 1 道地药材研究现状及问题

道地药材研究主要是从本草考证、药材性状、有效成分、药效、生态环境、遗传基因、栽培和采收加工技术等方面进行研究。

1.1 本草考证方面的研究 主要是对主流本草,二十六史各道、州、府、郡进贡药材史料,历代地理志,方志,清宫医案等有关道地药材的资料进行分析整理,通过这些研究明确许多道地药材的来源和产地。如对地黄、当归等药材的本草考证,发现这些药材的道地产区分别为河南怀庆、甘肃的岷县。但是这方面的研究,目前主要集中在主流本草和药材史料的研究,相比之下对于历代地理志,方志方面的考证较少。

1.2 药材性状、有效成分及药效方面的研究 道地药材性状的研究,主要集中在药材的外观形态、色泽等,并借助其他学科的技术来研究道地药材的性状,客观地评价药材的道地性。如肖小河等在研究附子的道地性时,借助计算机对药材进行三维重建与显示。

对于道地药材的有效成分方面的研究,主要利用色谱法和光谱法对道地药材和非道地药材中有效成分或指标性成分进行研究,比较异同。如:张重义等采用紫外分光光度法对怀山药道地产区与非道地产区药材质量进行分析,发现不同产地怀山药中的淀粉、蛋白质、浸出物、多糖含量不同,但道地产区怀山药中淀粉、多糖含量较高。近来越来越多的学者采用化学指纹图谱和模式识别等对道地药材加以识别鉴定。王荣等、陈闽军等、王雁等、马英丽等分别采用化学指纹图谱和模式识别的方法对大黄、川芎、三七、黄芪等药材的道地性进行了分析。道地药材药效的研究,目前文献报道较少。有研究报道甘肃礼县所产掌叶大黄的止血有效率高于陕西的非道地药材,而对正常人的副作用也低于非道地大黄。

1.3 生态环境方面的研究 主要研究太阳辐射的强度、水分、温度、土壤等生态因子以及地质背景方面对道地药材形成的影响,其中研究较多的为土壤的性质。范俊安等在测定四川道地药材味连、雅连、川芎、贝母、天麻、郁金、枳壳、麦冬、川乌、白芷、党参中所含微量元素铁、铜、锌、锰、锶、氟、碘、钴、锂、铍、铅、汞的量都高于非道地药材。张重义等比较了5个不同产区同一种质金银花的地质背景,分析土壤理化状况,发现道地金银花产区土壤受其成土母质影响,道地金银花最适合的土壤类型是中性或稍偏碱性的砂质土壤,且要求土壤的交换性能较高。范俊安等研究表明生态系统中GBS(地质背景系统)制约效应对川产道地药材产生影响。

1.4 遗传基因方面的研究 道地药材的形成从生物学

角度来看应是基因型和环境之间相互作用的产物。近年来,国内外从DNA分子水平上来研究中药材道地性取得了许多进展。如高文远等采用了RAPD的方法对当归药材的道地性进行分析,说明不同产地当归居群的遗传背景具有丰富的多样性,为当归药材道地性提供了基因水平上的参考信息;郭宝林等采用RAPD方法研究丹参主要居群的遗传关系及药材的道地性问题,研究表明山东和河南产的丹参也可认为是丹参的道地药材。

1.5 栽培和采收加工技术方面的研究 道地药材除少数野生品外,已多数属于栽培品。千百年来对药材不断精心培育和采取特殊的栽培技术与管理措施,是形成道地药材重要成因之一。这部分研究较少,而且也不系统,大部分道地药材的独特的采收加工及栽培技术的机理没有得到阐明,只知其然,不知其所以然。

1.6 道地药材研究存在的问题 通过对道地药材研究现状进行分析可见,道地药材的研究存在以下几个问题:①没有从道地药材是一个涉及遗传、环境以及人文这一复杂系统出发,树立起系统复杂性科学的思想观念,即使有多学科的联合研究,但相互之间没有进行有机的联系。对研究所取得的成果只是进行孤立地分析,没有遵循科学的规律,围绕相应的假说和理论,进行阐述和验证。②忽视了"自然等级理论"和"尺度效应",如对气候、气象条件的研究尺度过粗,只考虑年温差、年降水等气象因子,忽视微生态气象因子在植物生长阶段的时间变化规律。③观察分析没有把数学作为基本工具,对研究样本的代表性、全面性及结果等没有进行统计数学详尽的量化分析及处理。

## 2 道地药材的研究途径及相互关系的分析

道地药材研究所存在的问题概括起来主要是方法学的问题。从学科角度上看以现代生物学为基础并结合数理化等多学科的方法联合攻关是研究道地药材的必然趋势,在此过程中,将不断引进新的方法和理论,使道地药材的研究从不同层次和角度开展起来,对此,很难加以综合概括,但从主要途径上来分析,可概括为理论研究、实验研究和观察分析这3条途径。理论研究着重在中医药理论指导下,对道地药材的生物学本质,物质基础及形成机理等方面进行探讨,提出相应的假说;实验研究除目前进行的遗传及化学成分、药理药效分析外,还着重进行生态学的实验研究,即:实验室实验、野外实验和自然实验;观察分析主要应用数学作为基本工具。"任何一门科学,只有在成功地应用了数学,才算真正达到了完善的地步。"这句19世纪的名言,为运用数学研究道地药材指明了方向。

如何理解理论研究、实验研究和观察分析以及这三者的关系?这需要模式的介入。模式(pattern)意味着可重复的一致性(repeated consistency)。道地药材是控制药材质量的模式,它是怎样出现的?它又怎样在时间和空间上发生改变?识别模式是极为重要的,但不能仅停留在对模式的描述上,需要理解这些模式是怎样产生的,或者是说,是哪些机理(过程)导致了所观察到的模式,它们的相互关系如图1所示。

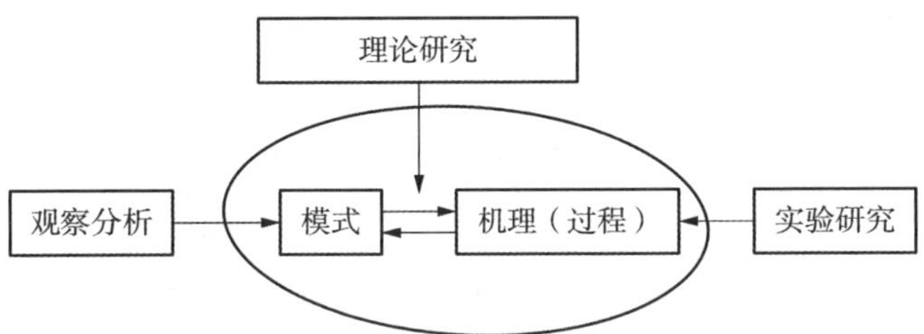


**图1 理论研究、实验研究及观察分析三者之间的相互关系**

科学研究通常的次序是先观察,识别模式,后进行理论化解释。而且一旦理论解释已经建立,它就可以引导人们进行有目的的观察或实验。或者说根据一定前提条件,经理论化逻辑推导,能促使人们发现一些以前没有注意到的现象;而发现这些现象又反过来说明了理论解释的正确性。所以,理论研究不仅在于解释已有的模式,而且还可以引导人们得到新的发现,同时对这些新观察到的模式也给出了相应的机理解释。对于任意一组模式,可能的过程往往有许多。鉴别这些过程中的哪一个(或哪一些)在自然界中是真正起作用的机理往往需要采用受控实验的研究途径。对于任何一门科学,实验都是极端重要的,这一点毋庸置疑。但是对实验途径的过度强调也可能会带来另外一种风险。许多生物学家被灌输了只相信实验科学的传统教育。我们知道,许多科学进步是从一种学说起步的,而且许多假说的验证并不完全依靠实验方法,例如天文学、地质学。此时,对模式的验证是通过解释已获得的资料和预测尚未记录在卷的新发现而实现的。这种研究方法在生物学、进化生物学、分类系统学、生物地理学、古生物学等宏观生物学领域内恐怕都是常见的,并且也确实取得了成功。

以上概略地说明了道地药材研究的3个主要途径及相互关系。很明显,没有哪个途径是最重要的或者是最不重要的,3个途径互相重叠,互相补充,缺一不可。理论的价值体现在解释观察到的模式和做出进一步能够检测的预测,观察的价值在于产生假说和检验理论预测;而实验的价值就是检验假说和理论预测。确立那些内在过程可以导致观察到的模式(假说形成)是摆在道地药材研究面前的首要任务。

## 3 道地药材所具有的模式及分析

中药系统演进的基本规律用现代生物学的观点来看,即是用进废退,去伪存真,优胜劣汰,择优而立,道地自成。道地药材的演变是一个与生态环境、遗传变异和人文密切相关的复杂系统的自适应过程。在这一过程中定要显现出特征和规律,产生相应的模式或假说。Tilman提出,应该首先研究哪些具有广泛一般性的模式,它不仅仅是由于这样的模式最明显,重复性最好,而且还由于它们提供了一个框架,使得相对特殊一些的模式能够在这个框架内得到更有效的研究。每种道地药材都有其自身所特有的性质,一般性的模式往往意味存在着一个一般性起因。目前,通过分析和总结前人的研究成果,认为道地药材有如下的模式假说。

3.1 道地药材的道地性越明显,其基因特化越明显 道地药材的生物内涵是同种异地,即同一物种因其具有一定的空间结构，能在不同的地点上形成大大小小的群体单元，其中如果某一群体产生质优效佳的药材，即为道地药材。这个同一物种在不同地点上形成的群体单元，在生物学上就称为“居群”。因此，“道地药材”在生物学上就是指某一物种的特定居群，这里的“特定”不是由研究者根据研究目的方便划定的，而是由一定的土壤、光照及阴湿等环境所决定的，有着比较稳定的边界，是一个比较稳定的“地方居群”，是在特定的空间和时间里生活着的自然的或人为的同种个体群。从生物学上说“道地药材”的形成应是基因型与环境之间相互作用的产物，可用公式表示：表型＝基因型＋环境饰变。所谓表型，指“道地药材”可观察到的结构和功能特性的总和，包括药材性状、组织结构、有效成分含量及疗效等。这里的环境饰变是指由生境引起的表型的任何不同遗传的变化。基因有产生某一特定表型的潜力，但不是决定着这一表型的必然实现，而是决定着一系列的可能性，究竟其中哪一个可能性得到实现，要看环境而定。因为，器官的生长和性状的表现，都必须依靠来源于周围生境的物质，在适合的生境中产生“道地药材”所具有的特别表现型特征。反之，在其他生境中该基因的这种则可能发生“弥散”，出现一种不确定性。当1个药材种具有较广泛的分布区时，它的各个不同地区居群往往具有不同的基因型或称地方性特化基因型（local specialized genotype），而这些基因型是由于不同的生态或地理的条件长期选择作用塑造而成，是产生“道地药材”的本质。因此，药材种越是广布种，越需要择地而生，其道地性越明显，其基因特化越明显。如高文远等对当归道地药材的RAPD分析，显示地理分布距离越小，当归的遗传差异越小，反之，越大。郭宝林等对厚朴道地性的遗传学证据分析，代表厚朴各道地产区的不同种之间的遗传差异明显。

3.2 “边缘效应”能促进道地药材的形成 边缘是事物的边界状态，度的概念的具体赋值。边缘效应的存在具有普遍性，“边缘效应”能促进道地药材的形成，主要在以下3个方面：①“边缘效应”能促进生物多样性的形成，并成为道地药材产生和确定的基础。中药道地药材发现和确立的过程，实质上就是对生物多样性的选择性应用，既有在物种之间进行的优选，也有对物种内多样性的选择。其中前者的优选在南北朝及其以前，是道地形成的主要原因；唐宋以后，这种现象逐渐减少，发展至今它早不作道地药材看待，而是作为就地取材，扩大资源来考虑。因此，生物多样性是道地药材产生和确立的基础。边缘效应长期以来被认为对生物多样具有重要影响，对于生物多样性的研究和保护具有特定的价值，在特定的生境中有望产生较高的生物多样性。其原因是：在边缘地带会有新的微观环境，导致有高的生物多样性；边缘地带会为生物提供更多的栖息场所和食物来源，允许有特殊需求的物种散布和定居，从而有利于异质种群的生存，并增强了居群个体觅食和躲避自然灾害的能力，允许有较高的生物多样性。因此，边缘效应所产生的结果能成为道地药材形态和遗传变化的基础。②“边缘效应”是促进道地药材化学变异的因素之一。决定药材疗效的物质基础是有效成分，有些有效成分在正常条件下没有或很少，只有当受到外界刺激（如各种生态因子）才会产生。这类物质属异常二次成分，被称为保护素（phytoalexin），边缘效应常常促使这些保护素产生或得到进一步加强。究其原因是因为在边缘地带各种生态因子并不仅仅是简单的加成关系，还有一种非加成性关系。任何物种对同一种生态因子的利用强度与其他生态因子的现有水平有关。对特定的物种来说，它们一旦与边界异质环境处于合适的生态位相“谐振”，各因子之间就会产生强烈的协同效应。③“边缘效应”是道地药材形成中人文在生态系统空间分布上的体现。作为中药系统演进的三大动力：遗传变异、环境饰变和人文作用（含生产技术、临床选择、文化传播、市场交通、社会政治等）对道地药材形成的贡献大小虽不一致，但都是促进了道地药材的形成。其中人文作用在道地药材形成的生态系统空间分布表现出了“边缘效应”。由于边缘气候和边缘景观的影响，集中分布了暖湿、温湿、温干及冷干型的植物区系成分和多种植被类型，包括森林、森林草原、灌木丛及草原等，这些生态系统也是多种类型动物的集中分布区，而其边缘带往往是动物的南北迁徙、高原和平原之间迁徙的必经之地。这就使得人更有效地介入各生态系统的食物链中取得食物。山地森林生态系统为其提供了丰富的猎物和木材；高原半干旱地带又是牧畜的好场所；河谷平原则是农耕的发源地；而平原上众多的河流湖泊提供了丰富的渔业资源；林缘、水边又是多种果树、谷类和小动物的集中分布区，因而是最佳的采集场所。所以，这种边缘地带是人居住最多和最早的地区。据文献记载和考古发掘的结果，河南省的中部和北部、山西省南部、陕西省的关中盆地、河北省的西南部和山东省的西部属，是人类较早居住、生产力较为发达的地区。目前，这些地区也是道地药材的集中分布区。

3.3 道地药材的化学组成有其独特的自适应特征 道地药材是中医临床长期、反复实践中产生的公认的优质中药材，其良好的临床疗效的物质基础是其化学组成的独特特征。如作者对茅苍术道地药材的挥发油组成特征分析显示，茅苍术挥发油主要组分的含量明显不同于非道地南苍术，茅苍术总挥发油含量显著低（$P<0.01$），其归一化百分率含量大于1%的组分数目显著高（$P<0.01$），苍术酮加苍术素的含量极其显著高，而茅术醇加β-桉叶醇的含量极其显著低（$P<0.01$），苍术酮、茅术醇、β-桉叶醇及苍术素呈现出一种特定配比关系（0.70～2.0）：（0.04～0.35）：（0.09～0.40）：1。

总之，道地药材是一个复杂系统，它的每一个元素之间的相互作用不可能都被研究，必须有所取舍，选择哪些并忽略哪些就代表在头脑中对模式起因已形成了假说。上述3条模式的提出就是基于这一思路，从道地药材发展的动力学因素考虑提出“边缘效应”，从道地药材的生物学本质提出“特化基因型”，从道地药材的药物属性提出“独特的化学特征”。这将促使理论研究、实验研究及观察分析能围绕一中心进行有机的联系，并有目的克服“自然等级理论”和“尺度效应”所带来的困难。可以说对这些模式特征和规律的分析探讨，不仅是继承了传统道地药材的理论，而且是对系统复杂性科学研究的剖析。

[黄璐琦，等.中国中药杂志，2004，29(6)：494-496，610.]

# 中药白芷种质资源的系统研究

白芷是常用中药。现用商品白芷药材为栽培品，分为川(杭)白芷和祁(禹)白芷两大类。由于对其原野生植物来源未能真正搞清楚，因此中药白芷的种名鉴定曾有过多次变化，一直没有统一的定论。如对北方栽培的祁(禹)白芷，《中国药典》2000年版定名为 *Angelica dahurica* (Fisch. ex Hoffm.) Benth. et Hook. f.，而《中国植物志》则将其定名为上述植物的栽培变种 *A. dahurica* cv. Qibaizhi Yuan et Shan。实际上 *A. dahurica* 是一类东亚野生种类，在我国主要分布于东北地区，又称为兴安白芷、大活，当地另作药用，其药材外形和药效与历来本草所载的白芷有相当的差异。对于南方栽培的川(杭)白芷的命名，则是各不相同，分别有 *A. taiwaniana* de Boiss.、*A. dahurica* var. *formosana* Yen、*A. dahurica* cv. Hangbaizhi Yuan et Shan、*A. anomala* Ave-Lall. 等。因此，由于名称的不统一，在有关的研究报道中造成一定程度的混乱，严重影响了临床用药的安全和有效。

从上述情况可以看出，中药白芷的野生种质来源应当是伞形科当归属植物 *A. dahurica* 的近缘种类，包括原变种兴安白芷 *A. dahurica* Benth. et Hook. f. ex Franch. et Sav. 和变种台湾白芷 *A. dahurica* var. *formasana* (de Boiss.) Yen(《中国植物志》称台湾独活)。另外，根据我们对标本、文献资料的调查，认为还有一种植物雾灵当归(或称紫茎独活)应当纳入研究对象之中。兴安白芷与雾灵当归的分布情况为：兴安白芷分布于我国的东北地区以及俄罗斯的远东地区、朝鲜半岛和日本；雾灵当归主要分布于我国的华北和中原地区(山西、河北、河南等省)，以及邻近的西北、东北的省区(陕西、宁夏、辽宁、内蒙古)。另外，这2种野生植物的根，在东北的有些地区被称为"大活"或"独活"入药，能发表、祛风除湿，用于治疗伤风头痛、风湿性关节痛及腰腿酸痛等症，与中药白芷的效用不尽相同。

对此，本文从形态解剖、染色体、化学成分、分子系统学等各个层面上，主要以4类栽培白芷及其3种近缘野生植物兴安白芷、台湾白芷和雾灵当归为研究样本，对中药白芷的原植物来源进行分析研究。

## 1 形态解剖研究

对川白芷(四川遂宁)、杭白芷(浙江杭州、江苏射阳)、祁白芷(河北安国)、禹白芷(河南禹县)4种栽培白芷及其3种近缘植物兴安白芷 *A. dahurica* Benth. et Hook.(黑龙江桃山，吉林延边)、台湾白芷 *A. dahurica* var. *formasana* Yen(台湾台中)和雾灵当归 *A. porphyrocaulis* Nakai et Kitagawa(河北兴隆雾灵山)的野生形态和果实解剖特征进行研究，结果将上述7个样本分为以下3个组。

1.1 川、杭、祁、禹4类白芷和台湾白芷　其主要特征是：花瓣淡黄绿色，分果背棱隆起呈峰状，有延伸的短翅。

1.2 兴安白芷　其主要特征7为：花瓣白色，分果背棱呈平台状或圆丘状隆起，无翅。茎紫色，有光泽；叶开张宽阔，末回裂片多为长圆形，卵形。

1.3 雾灵当归　其主要特征为：花瓣白色，分果背棱呈平台状或圆丘状隆起，无翅。茎紫色但常带有绿色条纹；叶较窄，末回裂片多为披针形至长圆形。

因此，从形态、解剖特征来看，川、杭、祁、禹4类栽培白芷之间没有明显的区别，并且与近缘野生植物台湾白芷甚为相似；而它们与另2种近缘野生植物兴安白芷、雾灵当归之间则存在着明显的区别。

## 2 染色体核型和花粉形态研究

对同样的上述7个样本进行染色体核型和花粉形态的研究。研究结果表明：在染色体的核型上，7个样本均为二倍体植物；核型基本一致，几乎对称至稍不对称；各对染色体相对长度较为一致；第3或第4对具中部着丝点染色体上有小的随体。总之，7个样本的核型较为近似，同时在当归属中又较为独特。但其中，雾灵当归与其他几个样本有较明显的差异。在核型公式上，比其他几个样本少一对中部着丝点染色体而多一对近端部着丝点染色体；随体位于第3对染色体而不是第4对上。此外，兴安白芷、台湾白芷的核型与4个栽培样本的核型公式一致；但又都与栽培样本有一定程度的差异。而4个栽培样本的染色体核型极为相似，不存在细胞分类学上的差别。

在花粉形态上，杭白芷、祁白芷与3个野生近缘种之间存在着相当的一致性，如花粉极面观均为近圆形，赤道面观均为类圆形，萌发孔均为边萌发孔，外壁纹饰均为网状纹，体积大小指数均在19～24等，这些都说明它们的亲缘关系相当近。同时，彼此之间在萌发孔沟、外壁纹饰等方面也存在着一些细微的区别，从这些区别来看，栽培白芷与台湾白芷更为接近。

## 3 香豆素类化学成分的研究

植物体内所含化学成分的类型、种类，取决于植物的种类。在伞形科植物中，香豆素类成分具有较高的分类学意义；同时，作为中药使用的白芷类植物，香豆素类成分是目前已知的主要活性成分。因此，对中药白芷及其野生近缘植物进行香豆素类成分的比较，有着化学分类的理论意义和药材鉴别的实用价值。因此本研究运用高效液相及与标准品对照的方法对川、杭、祁、禹白芷4种栽培类型和他们的近缘野生植物兴安白芷、台湾白芷和雾灵当归进行了香豆素类成分的比较分析。为了利于对结果的考察比较，还增加了同属2种野生植物黑水当归 *A. amurensis* Schischk. 与芷叶白芷 *A. baizhioides* (Mss.)作为外类群。前者分布于我国东北地区，当地部分地区有将其根与兴安白芷的根部当作"大活"作为地方用药使用的历史；后者分布于我国云南省丽江玉龙雪山，形态与白芷相近。

从所得液相图谱的总体类型来看，4 类中药白芷和 3 种野生近缘植物兴安白芷、台湾白芷和雾灵当归的峰形基本一致，故可归为一个大类型；而这一类型和芷叶白芷、黑水当归三者之间进行比较，则峰型的差别十分明显，说明所含以香豆素类为主的化学成分无论在化合物种类还是在含量方面都存在着很大的差异。

进一步观察比较可以发现，在 4 类栽培白芷和台湾白芷的图谱中，可以清晰见到 suberosin 峰，而在其他样本中则看不到，而且，就主要的峰而言，看不出有明显的差别。各种香豆素类成分的含量和互相之间的比例上虽然有一定的差别，但这种程度的差别即使在同一场所采得的同一种植物的不同个体之间也会存在，在化学分类上可以忽略不计。而在其余的 2 个样本中，兴安白芷与雾灵当归峰 1 与峰 2 的比例截然不同。

综上所述，从香豆素类成分的角度来看，可以认为，4 类栽培白芷与 *A. dahurica* 的 3 个野生变种兴安白芷、台湾白芷和雾灵当归确为近缘植物，而与另外 2 种当归属野生植物亲缘关系相对比较远；而在 *A. dahurica* 的 3 个野生变种中，台湾白芷又与栽培白芷最为接近。至于 4 类栽培白芷之间，则看不出有意义的区别。

## 4　分子遗传学研究

为提供分子遗传依据以澄清中药白芷的原植物问题，我们采用 RAPD 和 ITS 序列分析的方法，在分子水平上对上述 4 类栽培白芷和 3 个野生近缘种兴安白芷、台湾白芷和雾灵当归之间的关系进行研究（表 1）。此外，由于黑水当归 *A. amurensis* Schischk 与兴安白芷近缘，都分布于我国东北地区，部分地区有将其根与兴安白芷的根都当作“大活”作为地方用药使用的历史。因此，我们选择了黑水当归作为外缘类群。

表 1　样品来源及编号

| 编号 | 名称 | 植物学名 | 来源 |
|---|---|---|---|
| 1 | 台湾白芷 | *Angelica formosana* de Bioss. | 台湾台中 |
| 2 | 川白芷 | *A.* spp. | 四川遂宁 |
| 3 | 兴安白芷 | *A. dahurica* (Fisch. ex. Hoffm.) Benth. et Hook. f. ex. Franch. et. Sav. | 黑龙江佳木斯 |
| 4 | 黑水当归 | *A. amurensis* Schischk. | 黑龙江佳木斯 |
| 5 | 祁白芷 | *A.* spp. | 河北安国 |
| 6 | 雾灵白芷 | *A. porphyrocaulis* Nakai et Kitagawa | 河北兴隆雾灵山 |
| 7 | 杭白芷 | *A.* spp. | 浙江杭州 |
| 8 | 禹白芷 | *A.* spp. | 河南禹县 |

从 40 个 RAPD 引物中筛选出 29 个效果较好的引物，共得到 206 条带，其中多态性条带为 182 条，占 88.3%。图 1 所示为引物 W19 和 W20 的扩增结果。树系图（图 2）表明 4 种商品白芷之间具有密切的关系；并与台湾白芷关系密切。

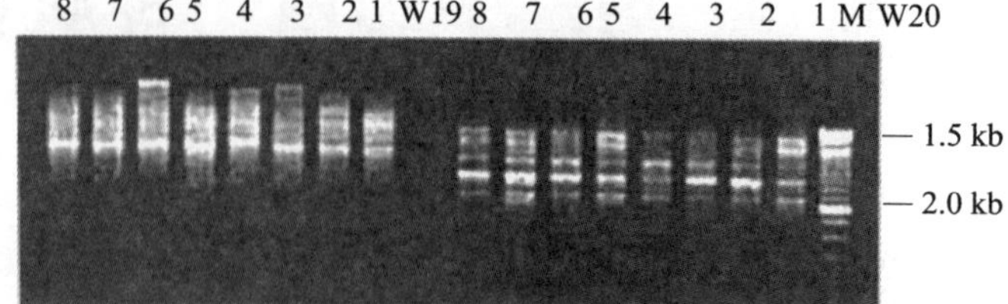


**图 1　各样品以引物 W19 和 W20 所得的 RAPD 结果**

各样品的编号同表 1；Lane M：100 bp DNA ladder。

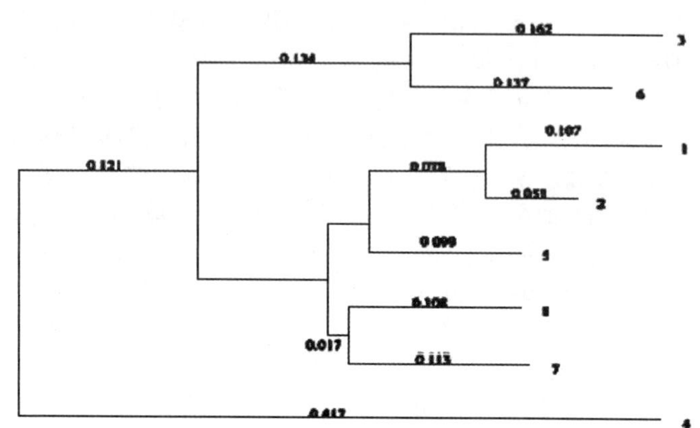


**图 2　RAPD 分析所得的树系图**

各样品的编号同表 1。

各样品扩增所得 ITS 1 序列为 439 bp，ITS 2 序列为 410 bp。进行排序和同源性比较，4 种商品白芷的序列与台湾白芷是完全相同的。对台湾白芷、兴安白芷、雾灵当归和黑水当归的 ITS 1、ITS 2 与 ITS 1+ITS 2 分别进行最大简约树（图 3，P1、P2、P3）和邻接树（图 3，N1、N2、N3）的计算，6 组数据得到 2 种树型。ITS 序列分析结果表明 4 种商品白芷与台湾白芷所测序列是完全相同的，应归属于同一类群。

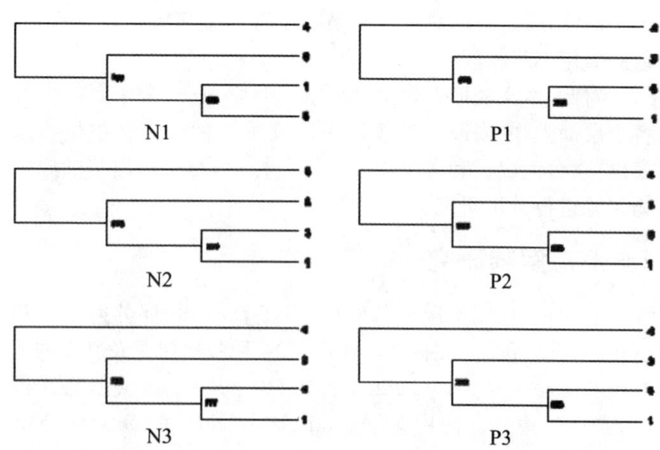


**图 3　根据 PHYLIP 3.57c 中 DNAPARS 建立的最大简约树（P1，P2，P3）和用 neighbor-joining 程序构建的分支树（N1，N2，N3）**

每个分支旁标注的数字为 bootstrap 值（1 000 次重复抽样）；N1 和 P1 由 ITS 1 计算而得，N2 和 P2 由 ITS 2 计算而得，N3 和 P3 由 ITS 1+ITS 2 计算而得；各样品的编号同表 1。

关于台湾白芷、兴安白芷、雾灵当归3者之间的关系，对于三者及其外缘类群黑水当归的ITS 1和ITS 2序列以及ITS 1+ITS 2分别进行最大简约法和邻接法的分支分析得到2种树型，其中5组数据(图3，N1、N3、P1、P2、P3)得到的树型Ⅰ为台湾白芷与雾灵当归构成1个单系类群，二者又与兴安白芷构成1个单系类群；另有1组数据(图3，N2)得到的树型Ⅱ为台湾白芷与兴安白芷构成1个单系类群，二者又与雾灵当归构成1个单系类群。在2种树型中，台湾白芷，兴安白芷，雾灵当归3者都并为1个单系类群，且都得到较高的靴带支持率(69.0%～99.9%)。有关三者之间的关系，支持台湾白芷与雾灵当归关系更密切的树型Ⅰ获得了5组数据的支持，而支持台湾白芷与兴安白芷更为密切的树型Ⅱ仅得到1组数据的支持。但是从bootstrap值来看，在3个简约树中(P1，P2，P3)，台湾白芷与雾灵当归单系类群的分支支持率仅有33.3%，在3个邻接树中(N1，N2，N3)，N1、N3的台湾白芷与雾灵当归单系类群的分支支持率分别为83.3%和77.7%，N2的台湾白芷与兴安白芷单系类群的支持率为69.0%，相差不大。因此，综合本研究结果，台湾白芷、兴安白芷、雾灵当归三者具有密切的亲缘关系，具有共同祖先；而在此单系类群内部，三者并未形成明显的归属关系。因此本研究结果倾向于将三者视为互相独立的种。此结论也得到了形态和解剖学及地理分布的支持。

## 5 结论

综合上述全部研究结果，并结合本草和各野生种的分布情况，已可确认当代使用的中药白芷(包括川白芷、杭白芷、祁白芷和禹白芷)的野生种质来源为目前仅分布于我国东南地区(以台湾省为主)的台湾白芷。这对于中药白芷的生产标准化和使用规范化都具有相当重要的意义，同时也为中药白芷的野生种质资源保护提出了明确的对象。同时，在植物分类学方面，对白芷的近缘植物兴安白芷、雾灵当归、台湾白芷之间的分类学关系也做出理由比较充分的推断。

[黄璐琦.江西中医学院学报，2004，16(6)：5-7.]

# 药用植物种质资源研究的发展——核心种质的构建

药用植物种质资源是中药生产的源头，是进行中药材品种改良、新品种培育及遗传工程的物质基础，尤其是野生近缘植物和古老的地方种是长期自然选择和人工选择的产物，具有独特的优良性状和抵御自然灾害的特性。如人参、地黄、浙贝母在长期的人工种植过程中，由于自然选择及长期的生态适应形成了一些地方品种、农家品种，是极其宝贵的自然财富。种质资源越丰富，研究越深入，在中药材品种改良、新品种培育越有针对性和预见性。因此，所掌握的种质资源数量和对其性状表现及遗传规律的研究是十分重要的。

为了人类的生存和持续发展，世界上的有识之士早就开始注意并从事生物资源的抢救和保存活动，特别是对农业、林业物种资源。目前，国家已经开始重视药用植物资源的保护与保存工作，例如，国家科技基础条件平台"药用植物种质资源标准化整理、整合及共享试点"项目的实施。通过对药用植物种质资源平台建设，能提供种质的保护及保存、栽培育种、生物技术研究、中药基础理论研究、中医临床研究等方面的信息，也为我国中医药事业的创新能力做出贡献。随着对药材种质资源的调查研究及优良种质的评价与利用研究的深入，如何利用现有的条件有效的保存种质资源成为下步开展种质资源研究的关键和基础。为此，借鉴农作物成功的经验，对药用植物核心种质及其构建进行探讨，提出对核心种质的研究是药用植物种质资源发展的必然趋势。

## 1 核心种质的内涵和药用植物核心种质的特性

种质资源的征集保存对药用植物新品种的选育、特异种质材料的利用以及种质创新具有重要意义，世界各国相继建立了不同植物的种质资源库，以保存地方品种及其野生近缘种。随着种质资源的不断征集和积累，种质资源库变得越来越大，极大地提高了种质资源的管理费用，增加了特异种质材料筛选、挖掘的难度。Frankel和Brown于1984年最早提出核心种质(core collection)的概念。认为核心种质是保存的种质资源的一个核心子集，以最少数量的遗传资源最大限度地保存整个资源群体的遗传多样性，同时代表了整个群体的地理分布。因此核心种质可以作为种质资源群体研究和利用的切入点，从而提高整个种质库的管理和利用水平。一般来讲，核心种质是从现有的种质中按照科学的取样方法与技术，选出约10%样品组成，在一定程度上，代表了某一种及其近缘野生种的形态特征、地理分布、基因与基因型的最大范围的遗传多样性。对于促进种质交流、利用以及基因库管理具有重要的学术和实用意义。核心种质的材料必须具有最大的遗传差异，这些差异主要表现为不同材料在基因型上的差异，以及不同基因型对环境反应上的差异，因此如何准确地评价不同材料间在遗传上的相似性则是合理构建核心种质的前提。

根据核心种质的定义，从药用植物的特点出发，认为药用植物核心种质应具有如下特性：①核心种质组成应包括和体现当前药用植物的主要变异类型。②核心种质彼此间要有异质性，最大限度地避免遗传上的重复。③核心种质存在动态交流和调整，而不是一成不变。④包含生产实践所需要的优异农艺性状或基因。⑤包含临床疗效所需要的有效成分及其调控基因。

## 2 药用植物核心种质的内容和研究的理论依据

2.1 药用植物核心种质的内容　药用植物核心种质的

研究内容主要包括 4 个方面:①数据的收集整理。这些数据包括药用植物种质资源现有的基本数据、评价鉴定数据和特征数据;基本数据是指有关材料收集地、起源地的生态地理状况或分类体系等有关信息;评价鉴定数据包括质量、产量及抗性等信息;特征数据是指包括形态、生化、分子标记在内的表征某材料特征数据。数据的收集要求尽可能全面,以满足研究的需要。②数据分析。将具有相似特点的种质材料分组,例如可以根据分类学、地理起源、生态类型、遗传标记、农艺性状等数据来分组。③样品的选择。按照分组的材料,以合理的取样方法和比例选取核心种质。④核心种质的管理。核心种质建立后,要制定科学的管理制度和利用体系,并根据需要不断调整、充实、完善核心种质,以保证核心种质的有效利用。为了便于种质资源的保存与研究利用,应构建种质资源的四级结构:保留种质、初级核心种质、核心种质和核心应用种质。应该指出,核心种质建立后并非一劳永逸,而要随着研究的深入、对资源认识和进一步收集以及应用的新需求,及时对其内容和结构进行调整和充实。

2.2 药用植物核心种质研究的理论依据

2.2.1 药用植物遗传多样性研究的深入 近年来,随着计算机技术和分子生物技术的发展,特别是以 PCR 为基础的分子标记技术如雨后春笋般地涌现出来,给生物遗传多样性的研究带来了极大的便利,同时这一技术也深入到药用植物遗传多样性这一研究领域,尤其是珍稀濒危的药用植物资源。例如,杜仲、肉苁蓉、人参等。对遗传多样性的研究可以揭示物种或居群的进化历史,也能为进一步分析其进化潜力和未来的命运提供重要资料,尤其有助于物种稀有或濒危原因及过程的探讨。我国药用植物的种类多,开发应用历史悠久,在医疗界的作用很大,这在全世界是无与伦比的。对药用植物遗传多样性的深入研究,为药用植物核心种质的构建提供了有力的保障。

2.2.2 道地药材的优质性 药用植物在长期的生存竞争及与自然界双向选择的过程中,与产地的生态环境建立了密切的联系。中药材有特定的分布区,不同产地的同一药材质量迥异,成为中药材的道地性。道地药材是优质中药材,是药用植物中用量大,范围广的品种,因此当前应备受重视、并予以重点研究和保护的类型。道地药材由于长期适应特定自然地理环境条件,原物种在长期的变异和分化过程中形成了具遗传稳定性的生态型或变异宗,且品质各异,差异很大。优良的种质资源是道地药材品质形成的内因。优良的种质资源的获得有赖于加强道地药材种质资源的保存和系统研究,有赖于关键性种质资源的发现和利用。因此,对道地药材从形态和遗传特性上进行研究,探讨其优质性,可以为药用植物核心种质的构建打下坚实的理论基础。

## 3 药用植物核心种质研究的特色和方法

3.1 药用植物核心种质研究的特色

3.1.1 建立药用植物核心种质库是一项系统工程,需要进行大量而深入的研究 药用植物种质资源的保护有别于一般植物,在我国占有特殊的地位。药用植物种质资源大多数散布在深远山区,野生性状较强,调查收集任务繁重,保护难度大。药用植物也不同于大田作物,大田作物的产量、品质等经济性较药用植物易于控制,且适应性广。其品质如淀粉、蛋白质、蔗糖、脂肪酸等在植物体内的含量高。药用植物作为中药材,要考虑到有效成分含量,其有效成分一般为植物的次生代谢产物,含量极微。同时药用植物种质资源带有明显的地域性,药用植物的品种比农作物更强调地域性;多年生种类多,栽培种类繁多。由于上述的特点,加之未受到应有的重视,因此,药用植物种质资源库的构建工作难度大,进展缓慢。

我国在药用植物的调查、收集和整理方面居于世界领先水平。但对种内的变异资源,尤其是本地品种资源,缺乏科学的系统整理和研究。对中药材种质资源进行收集整理,一方面摸清家底掌握我国药用植物资源的基本情况,从根本上解决目前中药材生产上的品种混杂现象,利于进一步合理保护和研究。另一方面通过调查和整理,系统评价后从中发现一些优良品质,选育出相对稳定的中药材优良品种。因此,建立药用植物核心种质,是一项系统工程,需要进行大量而深入的研究。然而,核心种质一旦构建,就可以将有限的人力物力集中于数量较少的资源研究上,从而方便药用植物优异种质的发掘和利用。

3.1.2 药用植物核心种质的构建是种质资源保存的必然趋势,已有一些先进技术可以借鉴 建立药用植物种质资源库的工作量大,建立核心种质库是必然趋势。目前,建立药用植物核心种质的工作只是一种设想,但在农业等领域有很多技术经验可以借鉴。

对于药用植物来说,建立核心种质是全新的探索,尚需要进行大量的研究工作,如取样方法的选择、取样比例的确定、对所建立的核心种质检验方法的确定、保存方法的确定等。前人的经验将为药用植物的核心种质的构建提供技术方法和理论依据。

3.1.3 构建药用植物核心种质应加强道地药材的研究 就像中药资源的任何研究都离不开道地性研究一样,核心种质的研究也是如此,而且应该更加深入。因为道地药材是最优质的中药材,因此研究道地药材的优良性状和品质,对建立核心种质是十分重要的一个环节。

近年来,由于掠夺式的开发自然资源,生态环境恶化,不少的名贵道地药材种类处于濒危状态,如天麻、人参、虫草、贝母、砂仁等。栽培药材品种退化,质量下降,最终导致道地性丧失。为了保证道地药材的质量稳定和增产增收,必须加强道地药材的种质资源的收集、保存和研究,改良和稳定道地药材物种居群形状,培育优质高产、抗逆性强的品种。这就为药用植物核心种质的研究提出了新的要求。

3.1.4 构建药用植物核心种质不仅要考虑遗传多样性还要考虑有效成分的多样性 药用植物的品质包括内在质量和外观性状两部分。内在质量主要指有效成分的含量。因此构建核心种质时,药材的有效成分是重要的考核指标。同时,药用植物种质的优良与稳定性也是构建核心种质的关键所在。

进行药用植物的核心种质的构建,要从源头上把关,即首先要鉴定出优良的种质。因此对进入核心种质的药用植物的基源必须进行鉴定,明确到种、变种、生态型、化学型、居群或栽培品种。如苍术在中国境内广泛分布,研究表明,其主要药效成分挥发油在种内存在很大变异,表现出不同的化学型,苍术道地药材的挥发油组成特征明显不同于其他产地苍术，苍术道地药材良好的临床疗效的物质基础是其独特的化学组成。这些研究结果对药用植物核心种质的构建意义重大。

3.2 药用植物核心种质研究的方法 进行种质资源研究，特别是种质遗传多样性的研究，在核心种质构建中具有重要意义。药用植物核心种质的研究除准确的度量不同遗传材料间的遗传相似度以及合理高效的抽样方法外，还应包括化学成分变化的多样性和稳定性。

3.2.1 遗传多样性的研究方法

3.2.1.1 分子标记技术 分子标记技术在遗传学的建立和发展过程中有着举足轻重的作用，是检测种质资源遗传多样性，构建核心种质的有效工具。利用分子标记对种质资源的分类、遗传多样性、优异基因的定位及核心种质的构建等研究具有重大的理论和实践意义。目前，用于作物种质资源鉴定及育种的分子标记主要有限制性片断长度多态性(restriction fragment length polymorphism，简称 RFLP)、随机扩增多态性DNA(random amplified polymorphic DNA，简称 RAPD)、扩增片断长度多态性(amplified fragment length polymorphism，简称 AFLP)、微卫星 DNA(microsatellite DNA)又称简单重复序列(simple sequence repeat，简称 SSR)以及原位杂交(in situ hybridization)等。有人提出在种质资源保存研究过程中，对于核心种质构建、基因性状鉴定、品种指纹图谱建库时，用 SSR 技术进行分子标记为最佳，该方法优点是多态性高，易于观察比较。

3.2.1.2 DNA序列分析 由于遗传信息储存在染色体和细胞器基因组的 DNA 序列中，故染色体水平和 DNA 水平的遗传多样性就显得格外引人注目。DNA 测序是检测遗传多样性最彻底的方法，早期都用放射性标记。近来，PCR 应用于测序提高了灵敏度。各种新的基因克隆方法的发明，使生物 DNA 全序列分析成为可能，对中草药有效成分进行 DNA 测序，提供了细胞学和分子生物学的新证据，利用现代生物技术建立中草药种质资源基因库，对世界范围的植物分类也是很有意义的。

3.2.1.3 凝胶电泳 凝胶电泳技术是分子生物学技术中一种十分重要的实验手段，应用于核苷酸序列分析、分子标记、分子杂交等各个方面。张琼光等人对优良种源区域内厚朴的两种类型植株的种质资源进行电泳分析，以探索优质种子的鉴别方法，凝胶电泳技术为优质种质资源的选择和质量控制，提供了一条新的途径。

3.2.1.4 近亲交配成自交 自交(即近亲交配，inbreed)是最常被使用的育种方法，以这种方法得到的子代以 Fn 来表示，F 的原文意义为“子代的世代数”(Filial generation)，其用意在于：由少数的亲本即可展开育种；近亲交配可将基因纯化，以选拔带有大型生长基因的个体或带有优美个体基因的个体。但是，自交(累代)数目增加会产生一些问题，包括畸形的产生及个体小型化等，所以自交次数建议不要大于 6。遗传育种工作十分强调自交或近亲交配，因为只有在自交或近亲交配的前提下才能使供试材料具有纯合的遗传组成，从而才能确切地分析和比较亲本及杂种后代的遗传差异，研究性状遗传规律，更有效地开展育种工作。

随着生物技术的不断运用与发展，人们将不仅能更加充分的利用现有种质资源，还可以通过基因重组创造新的种质类型，极大地丰富药用植物的种质资源，实现中药资源的长期可持续发展战略。因此，只有利用先进的分子生物技术对种质资源进行研究，扩大繁殖，促进其更新，才能保证资源的永续利用。种质资源是药用植物育种的物质基础，没有优异的种质资源很难培育出优良的新品种，进一步寻找和创造出更多具有特殊价值的种质资源将是今后生物技术运用的一项重要内容。

3.2.2 化学成分多样性的研究方法 中药指纹图谱(finger printing)借用 DNA 指纹图谱发展而来。最先发展起来的是中药化学成分色谱指纹图谱，特别是高效液相色谱(HPLC)指纹图谱。HPLC 具有很高的分离度，可把复杂的化学成分进行分离而形成高低不同的峰组成一张色谱图，这些色谱峰的高度和峰面积分别代表了各种不同化学成分和其含量。整个色谱图表征了该样品所含化学成分的多少和量的大小。目前，中药指纹图谱的研究已如火如荼地展开，是中药研究的热点之一，可以在药用植物核心种质的构建中得到有效的利用。

3.2.3 抽样方法 构建遗传资源核心种质的另一个重要环节是核心材料的抽样，不同的抽样方法直接影响核心材料的抽取。目前构建核心种质的方法是先对样品进行遗传分类，根据分类结果采用一定的抽样比率和抽样策略抽取核心材料。构建核心种质采用的抽样方法主要有随机抽样(R)、按常数抽样(C)、按比率抽样(P)、按对数抽样(L)和按遗传变异度抽样(G)。

确定合理的取样比率是构建作物核心种质的重要环节，各种核心种质构建中往往根据原始群体的大小调整抽样比率。对于大容量的资源群体一般采用较低的抽样比率，如 10%；而较小的群体则采用较高的抽样比率，如 20%或 25%等。随着核心种质容量的变小，保存的遗传变异及结构对其容量的大小将非常敏感。可以利用不同的方法对种质进行分类(计算机聚类关联规则等)在方法上可以进行改进。

评价核心样品对整个种质资源多样性的代表性是核心种质研究中的又一重点和难点。根据核心种质的概念，构建核心种质时要选择有代表性、异质性和多样性、类型齐全的样本作为核心种质。因此，可以选择了多样性指数、表型方差、变异系数、表现型分布频率方差、表型保留比例、最大值离差及最小值离差等参数作为初选指标。农业上有人利用无偏预测的基因型值进行核心种质构建方法的研究；同时采用多种系统聚类和核心种质的抽样方法构建水稻核心种质，探讨构建水稻核心种质的最佳方法和途径。

3.2.4 其他 核心种质的保存也是研究的重点。目前世界种质资源日益枯竭，大量有用基因损失，特别是那些不产籽植物或种子寿命短的植物更为严重，因此寻找合适的方法保存种质资源显得非常重要。贮存种质资源是一个涉及人力、财力和科学技术的复杂问题。为此全世界都在广泛深入地进行研究，并采取了综合贮存的策略，即田间基因圃、种子库、原位保存、设备保存、DNA 保存、花粉贮藏、离体保存基因库等。近年来运用超低温保存技术已日益成为一种较为理想的保存种质资源的新方法。药用植物应根据本身的特殊性，保存方式方法上也有待于进行更深入的研究。

## 4 结语

由于核心种质最大程度地去除了种质资源中的遗传重复，以极少的种质数量即囊括了原资源群体中的全部或大多数变异类型，这无疑为解决当前巨大的资源收集量与资源深入评价及有效利用之间所存在的突出矛盾提供了一个十分有利的契机，从而极大地推动和促进种质资源研究的进一步发展。首先，核心种质的构建有助于了解现有种质资源遗传多样性的组成特点和分布状况，以及其潜在的利用价值，进而对于今后种质资源的引种、收集工作，包括引种方向、引种类型、材料等的确定具有重要的指导作用。其次，核心种质的构建可以有效地加强和实现我们对重点材料的重点保护和管理，防止和避免遗传多样性，特别是优异种质和基因的丢失。第三，核心种质实际上提供了一套规模急剧减少而遗传多样性又十分丰富且具有代表性的样品集，这使得在现阶段即能够采用一系列先进手段和方法有目的、有重点地进行重要性状遗传规律的研究，以及优异种质、基因的筛选与克隆，避免工作中的盲目性，从而尽快提高种质资源的研究水平和利用效率。

在中药现代化系统工程中，药用植物种质资源是根本，对药用植物核心种质的研究不仅可以为保护中药种质和遗传资源，加强优选优育和中药种源研究，防止品种退化，解决品种源头混乱的问题提供一条出路。同时，收集中药品种、产地、药效等相关的数据，对加强中药材野生变家种家养研究，植保技术研究，发展绿色药材，加强中药材新品种培育，开展珍稀濒危中药资源的替代品研究都有很好地推动作用。

综上所述，核心种质的研究为加强和实现种质资源的有效管理及开发利用提供了一个十分便利的条件和途径。目前，我国药用植物核心种质的研究还处于初级阶段，还有巨大的发展空间。除技术问题外，药用植物核心种质的构建还涉及其他综合因素，需要人们提高认识。核心种质在药用植物种质资源的建设中刚刚兴起，有待于引起社会的重视，并加以大力支持。在世界范围内，核心种质研究的规模普遍较小，而且缺乏统一的技术模式或技术体系。药用植物核心种质的研究可以为世界范围内的核心种质的构建提供研究实例和方法。

[黄璐琦，等. 中国中药杂志，2005，30(20)：1565－1568，1586.]

# 药用植物受威胁及优先保护的综合评价方法

随着经济和医疗保健事业的飞速发展，中药资源的需求出现了空前的增长，从中药中提取有效成分应用于化妆品、食品及工业原料的研究也越来越深入，这些原因在不同程度上加大了中药资源的压力。加之长期以来，对开发利用中药资源的认识不足，一些地区不同程度上对中药资源进行了掠夺式的过度采收(捕猎)，致使很多中药资源蕴含量下降，甚至耗竭，一些种类濒临灭绝，因此，对珍稀濒危中药资源进行保护已迫在眉睫。然而，提到中药资源的保护，首先必须确定其保护对象，由于中药资源的绝大部分来源于药用植物，其保护的重点是药用植物的保护。为此，制定评价药用植物受威胁及优先保护的量化体系尤为重要。

对药用植物受威胁及优先保护的评价，应该制定一个较全面的、科学的、系统的、实用性强、操作性强和可量化的评价体系。目前，此类研究报道较少，王年鹤等提出过初步定量化评价标准的研讨，从药用价值、分类学意义、分布及生境要求、野生资源量等 8 个方面进行评价，其评价标准已经提出了初步的定量方法，受到了普遍的赞同，并且被《中药资源学》《野生植物资源学》等引用。笔者认为评价时还应该从其他方面进行细化和量化，而且影响因素之间侧重点有所不同，其权重系数也存在差别。例如：药用植物的价值方面，随着科学技术的发展，药用植物已不仅仅作为药用，还可应用于工业、食品加工业等领域，除此之外，有的应用价值目前还没有确定，但是已经在做这方面的研究，如一旦确定，此种药用植物的应用将大大增加，势必造成潜在的需求危机；再如，药用植物不仅具有药物的特征，而且还具有植物的一般特征，包括它的遗传特征、生长特征、分布特征等。这些因素都与药用植物资源的利用、保护有密切关系。因此，考虑到上述种种因素，在前人的基础上，对药用植物受威胁及优先保护综合评价方法作了进一步的探讨。

## 1 药用植物受威胁及优先保护综合评价方法的制定原则及其体系

1.1 制定原则 影响药用植物受威胁及优先保护的因素很多，而且某些因素之间会相互作用。通过对药用植物资源的全面考察和综合分析，将各因素进行细化和量化，按药用植物面临的现状给予一定的分值，然后将其综合评定。本着实用性和可操作性的原则，现将评定标准划分为价值系数(coefficience of value，Cv)、分布系数(coefficience of distribution，Cd)、生物学系数(coefficience of biology，Cb)、资源现状系数(coefficience of present situation，Cs)等 4 个大项，其中每一大项又包括若干小项，即价值系数包括药用价值、经济价值、学术价值、潜在价值；分布系数包括药用植物地域性特征、特有种情况、药材道地性特征；生物学系数包括种型分类学特征、可再生能力特征、生长周期特征；资源现状系数包括野生资源量、栽培现状、药材来源现状(分原植物来源和药材商品来源)、保护现状。

1.2 综合评价体系 将上述 15 个小项分别按不同程度给予一定的分值，初步制定了药用植物受威胁及优先保护综合评价体系(表 1)。

表 1 药用植物受威胁及优先保护综合评价项目表

| 系数项 | | 具体评分标准项 | 分值 |
|---|---|---|---|
| 价值系数(Cv) | 药用价值 | 常用种类,被《中国药典》收载 | 3 |
| | | 较常用种类,被《中国药典》收载 | 2 |
| | | 不常用种类,被《中国药典》收载,或被地方标准收载,已形成商品 | 1 |
| | | 一般民间药,未被《中国药典》收载,未形成商品 | 0 |
| | 经济价值 | 除药用外,用于化妆品,食品和工业原料 | 3 |
| | | 除药用外,用于化妆品,食品或工业原料三者之二 | 2 |
| | | 除药用外,用于化妆品,食品或工业原料三者之一 | 1 |
| | | 仅供药用 | 0 |
| | 学术价值 | 孑遗植物或在研究系统发育等方面有重要价值 | 1 |
| | | 无明显学术价值 | 0 |
| | 潜在价值 | 已通过研究,有价值,待开发 | 2 |
| | | 正在进行研究,价值待明确 | 1 |
| | | 目前尚未进行研究,或已经研究过,未发现其价值 | 0 |
| 分布系数(Cd) | 药用植物地域性特征 | 分布于 1 个或相邻的 2 个省某山地局部区域内,生境特殊 | 3 |
| | | 分布于 3～6 个省或某一大区域内 | 2 |
| | | 6 个以上省内有分布,但不超过全国省份的一半 | 1 |
| | | 全国广泛分布,分布省份超过全国省份的一半 | 0 |
| | 药用植物特有种情况 | 某省特有 | 3 |
| | | 区域特有 | 2 |
| | | 中国特有 | 1 |
| | | 非中国特有 | 0 |
| | 药材道地性特征 | 道地产区仅为 1 个区域 | 3 |
| | | 道地产区为 2 个区域 | 2 |
| | | 道地产区为 2 个以上区域 | 1 |
| | | 无道地性 | 0 |
| 生物学系数(Cb) | 种型分类学特征 | 单种科型,科内仅 1 属 1 种植物 | 4 |
| | | 单种属型,属类仅 1 种植物 | 3 |
| | | 少种科型,科内仅 2～3 种植物 | 2 |
| | | 少种属型,属内仅 2～3 种植物 | 1 |
| | | 多种属型,属内种数多,一般 4 种以上 | 0 |
| | 可再生能力特征 | 主要依靠有性繁殖的木本或寄生植物 | 3 |
| | | 主要依靠有性繁殖的草本 | 2 |
| | | 主要依靠无性繁殖 | 1 |
| | | 有性繁殖和无性繁殖均可 | 0 |
| | 生长周期特征 | 生长 3 年以上才可供利用 | 2 |
| | | 生长 2～3 年可供利用 | 1 |
| | | 生长 1 年内可供利用 | 0 |
| 资源现状系数(Cs) | 野生资源量 | 极少 | 3 |
| | | 少 | 2 |
| | | 尚多 | 1 |
| | | 多 | 0 |
| | 栽培现状 | 栽培种不能替代野生种或现无栽培技术 | 3 |
| | | 栽培技术不稳定,没有推广应用 | 2 |
| | | 栽培技术成熟,但只有 1 省为栽培基地 | 1 |
| | | 栽培技术成熟, 2 省或以上设有栽培基地 | 0 |
| | 药材来源现状:原植物来源 | 1 种来源 | 3 |
| | | 2 种来源 | 2 |

（续表）

| 系数项 | 具体评分标准项 | 分值 |
|---|---|---|
| 药材来源现状：药材商品来源 | 3 种来源 | 1 |
| | 3 种以上来源 | 0 |
| | 药材商品主要来源于野生 | 2 |
| | 药材商品来源于野生和栽培 | 1 |
| | 药材商品主要来源于栽培 | 0 |
| 保护现状 | 目前未受到保护 | 2 |
| | 自然保护区内有分布 | 1 |
| | 有专题保护区已作重点保护 | 0 |

根据表 1 中 4 大系数项的相对重要程度，综合分析药用植物资源的特点，并征求有关专家的意见，反复研究讨论，对权重比例进行了分配。相比较而言，药用植物资源的价值和现状对其受威胁及优先保护的评定更加重要，其权重比例也应稍大，因此，将 4 大系数权重比例确定为：价值系数 0.30；分布系数 0.20；生物学系数 0.20；资源现状系数 0.30。

将表 1 中 4 大系数项的各项指标进行评分，再将 4 个系数分别按比例计算后相加，可以对各种药用植物受威胁及优先保护程度进行评价，从而确定受威胁级别，同时为各种药用植物保护的迫切性和重要性提供依据。分值越高，受威胁程度越严重，需要保护的迫切性也越强。为了便于比较，将 4 个系数相加后的值定为级别系数（coefficience of grade，Cg）来计算评价结果。公式为 Cg＝Cv×0.30＋Cd×0.20＋Cb×0.20＋Cs×0.30，其中 4 个系数（即 Cv，Cd，Cb，Cs）的计算公式统一为：C＝该系数各指标所得分之和/该系数各指标总分之和。

按计算结果，受威胁级别及保护等级作如下划分：①Cg＝0.70～1.00；受威胁级别：一级；保护等级：Ⅰ级，亟待加以保护。②Cg＝0.55～0.69；受威胁级别：二级；保护等级：Ⅱ级，应积极加以保护。③Cg＝0.40～0.54；受威胁级别：三级；保护等级：Ⅲ级，需注意保护。④Cg 值在 0.40 以下，定为安全种。

1.3 评价体系中的几点说明 ①价值系数中常用种类、较常用种类和不常用种类的划分主要依据《新编中药志》。②分布系数中药用植物地域性特征的评定主要参见《中国中药区划》，药用植物特有种情况主要参见《中国植物红皮书——珍稀濒危植物》。③资源现状系数中野生资源量的评定主要参考《中国常用中药材》和《中国中药区划》。④资源现状系数中药材来源现状包括原植物的来源和药材商品的来源两种情况，其中原植物来源主要参见《中国药典》的收载，如黄芪为豆科植物蒙古黄芪或膜荚黄芪的干燥根，其评分时定为 2 种来源，记 2 分。药材商品来源主要参见《中国常用中药材》。

## 2 综合评价方法应用举例

应用此评价体系，以临床常用的中药材人参、黄芪、大黄、贝母、细辛为例（表 2），进行了综合评价，其结果与《中国植物红皮书——珍稀濒危植物》《中国珍稀濒危保护植物名录》中收载的受威胁级别及优先保护的等级基本相近。因此，作者认为此药用植物受威胁及优先保护评价方法具有一定的可行性。

**表 2 5 味中药材综合评价结果**

| 系数项 | | 人参 | 黄芪 | 大黄 | 贝母 | 细辛 |
|---|---|---|---|---|---|---|
| 价值系数 | 药用价值 | 3 | 3 | 3 | 3 | 3 |
| | 经济价值 | 3 | 3 | 2 | 1 | 2 |
| | 学术价值 | 1 | 0 | 0 | 0 | 0 |
| | 潜在价值 | 2 | 1 | 1 | 1 | 1 |
| | Cv | 1.00 | 0.78 | 0.67 | 0.56 | 0.67 |
| 分布系数 | 地域性特征 | 2 | 1 | 1 | 2 | 0 |
| | 特有种情况 | 2 | 0 | 0 | 0 | 0 |
| | 药材道地性特征 | 3 | 2 | 1 | 3 | 3 |
| | Cd | 0.78 | 0.33 | 0.22 | 0.56 | 0.33 |
| 生物学系数 | 种型分类学特征 | 0 | 0 | 0 | 0 | 0 |
| | 可再生能力特征 | 2 | 2 | 2 | 0 | 2 |
| | 生长周期特征 | 2 | 2 | 2 | 1 | 2 |
| | Cb | 0.44 | 0.44 | 0.44 | 0.11 | 0.44 |

（续表）

| 系数项 | | 人参 | 黄芪 | 大黄 | 贝母 | 细辛 |
|---|---|---|---|---|---|---|
| 资源现状系数 | 野生资源量 | 3 | 2 | 0 | 1 | 0 |
| | 栽培现状 | 3 | 0 | 0 | 2 | 0 |
| | 原植物来源 | 3 | 2 | 1 | 0 | 1 |
| | 商品来源 | 2 | 1 | 1 | 2 | 1 |
| | 保护现状 | 0 | 0 | 2 | 0 | 0 |
| | Cs | 0.85 | 0.38 | 0.31 | 0.38 | 0.15 |
| 级别系数 Cg | | 0.80 | 0.50 | 0.43 | 0.42 | 0.40 |
| 受威胁级别 | | 一级 | 三级 | 三级 | 三级 | 三级 |
| 保护等级 | | Ⅰ级 | Ⅲ级 | Ⅲ级 | Ⅲ级 | Ⅲ级 |

## 3 讨论

要实现药用植物资源的可持续利用，就必须处理好开发利用与保护管理之间的密切关系，加强保护是为了更好地利用。确立保护对象需要一个客观的、可操作的、定量的标准去综合评价一种药用植物受威胁的程度。作者是从药用植物资源的角度出发，根据其自身的特点，用价值系数、分布系数、生物学系数、资源现状系数等 4 个大的方面去评定一种药用植物的受威胁程度，最后用级别系数表示其评定结果，从而确立受威胁级别及保护等级。这种综合评价的方法实用性强，具有可操作性，并且其结果能较客观地反映药用植物资源的整体状况。

在药用植物受威胁及优先保护评价标准制定过程中，不仅较全面地、系统地考虑到药用植物作为资源的可利用方面，而且对药用植物具有植物的特性加以了强调。综合评价方法的某些问题还有待进一步探讨，例如在评价的过程中，植物的野生资源量有的记载不详，尤其对于有着悠久栽培历史的中药材，如地黄、牛膝、白芍、附子、枸杞等，因栽培产量丰富，其野生资源状况无统计资料，但要评定一种药用植物的受威胁程度，野生资源量又是一个不可缺少的重要方面。

［黄璐琦，等. 中国中药杂志，2006，31(23)：1929－1932.］

# 道地药材的属性及研究对策

道地药材的理念根植于传统中医药理论，来源于生产实践，它是一项古人评价中药材质量的独特标准。谢氏指出："道地药材就是指在特定自然条件、生态环境的地域内所产的药材，且生产较为集中，栽培技术、采收加工也都有一定的讲究，以致较同种药材在其他地区所产者品质佳、疗效好、为世所公认而久负盛名者称之。"近年来，不少学者就道地性的表现形式及科学内涵、道地药材的形成机理、道地药材的质量评价及鉴别等问题展开研究和讨论，并已取得卓有成效的研究结果。

作为中医药的精髓，药材的道地性既有来源于历史和文化的属性，又涉及遗传、环境及生产实践等方方面面。笔者从药材道地性所蕴含的科学内涵和文化属性相结合的角度，对其研究对策进行探讨。

## 1 道地药材是自然与人文结合的典范

作为一个约定俗成的概念，道地药材的优良品质，除了中医临床疗效外，还包括药材的外观性状、采收加工和贮藏运输方式，甚至可能也可以包括它的传播方式、市场口碑等能让道地药材增值的任何因素。为此，肖氏根据中药系统演进的三大动力——遗传变异、环境饰变和人文作用（含生产技术、临床选择、文化传播、市场交通、社会政治等），及其对道地药材形成的贡献大小不一致这一事实，将道地药材形成模式分为生境主导型、种质主导型、技术主导型、传媒主导型以及各种多因子关联决定型。可见，道地药材不是个纯粹的自然科学概念，它除了具有自然科学的属性，还同时具有它的文化属性和经济属性。有学者将自然科学与人文科学比做人类的一双眼睛，指出它们是认识世界的两大工具。承认道地药材具有人文科学的成分，就不能完全套用自然科学的思路和方法研究道地药材。只有尊重道地药材这个客观事实，分清道地药材这一概念所涵盖的自然科学问题和人文科学的问题，并采用相应的手段去研究这些问题和解决这些问题，才能真正认清道地药材的科学本质。

因此，必须要承认道地药材是个已经存在的客观事实，不论其化学组成的特征是什么，目前药理药效学能否证明其良好疗效，也不论其遗传上的特异性是否被揭示，环境对道地药材的影响是什么，它作为一个被广泛称誉的地理产品，其经济价值、市场信誉及产品的号召力都已使它成为一个货真价实的"优质"产品，既道地药材的身份无须怀疑。一个道地药材的产生可能起源于特点产地、特定加工、特定遗传背景、特定文化背景、特定传播方式等诸多原因中的一个或多个原因的共同作用，甚至不排除来源于历史上的一个非常偶然的原因。它成为道地药材的原因可能会被最终揭示，也可能会永远遗失在历史的长河里，但它作为道地药材的属性却实实在在地留了下来，这个特定的属性就是它产于某个特定的地方，并被广泛承认具有优良的品质，而且可以创造巨大的经济价值。

为此，道地药材的科学研究中最重要的就是要尊重科学研究规律，不论是使用自然科学还是人文科学手段，都应尊重学科本身的要求和规范，最主要的就是不能用自然科学的结果去揭示和怀疑道地药材的人文科学内涵。总之，只有将自然科学和人文科学进行完美结合，才能更科学更客观地揭示道地药材的本质。

## 2 与地理标志的接轨有利于揭示道地药材的文化属性

地理标志（geographical indications）和原产地命名制度在国外已经有100多年的历史。法国一开始主要利用该制度对其国内生产的香槟酒和其他一些酒类进行保护。WTO成立后，《与贸易有关的知识产权协议》（TRIPs协议）明确将地理标志纳入了知识产权的保护范围，地理标志成了当今世界普遍关注的一项知识产权。我国自1999年实施地理标志产品保护制度以来，已对500多个地理标志产品实施保护。2005年7月，国家质检总局新颁布的《地理标志产品保护规定》正式施行。

TRIPs第22条第1款将地理标志明确定义为"地理标志系指标示某商品来源于某成员领域内，或来源于该领域中的某一地区或地方，而该商品的特定质量、信誉或其他特征主要与该地理标志来源相关联的标志"。简单地说，地理标志具有如下特点：①在汉语地理标志通常的结构是"地理名称＋商品名称"，如绍兴黄酒、镇江香醋、（河南）道口烧鸡、（辽宁）盘锦大米等。②结构中的地理名称具有真实性，能够说明所标示商品或服务的真实原产地。③地理标志所表示的商品或服务具有独特的品质、声誉或其他特征。④地理标志与其所标示商品、服务的质量、声誉或其他特征之间存在密切联系。这是地理标志的最本质特征。一个普通的地理产品名称之所以能够发展为地理标志，关键是因为商品的质量、声誉或其他特征与该原产地内的特殊的自然环境以及人为因素有密切关系。这里的自然因素是指该地域所具有的特殊的地理环境、气候、土壤、水质、物种等；这里的人为因素通常是指独特的传统生产工艺、配方、秘诀等。如新疆葡萄、西湖龙井茶等，都是当地独有的地貌、气候、土壤、植物等自然生态环境，加上千百年来独具特色的采制工艺，形成其独特的品质特征。

分析地理标志的特征，有助于我们认识道地药材与地理标志的关系。从形式上看，不少道地药材在药名前多冠以地名，以示其道地产区。如西宁大黄、宁夏枸杞、川贝母、川芎、秦艽、辽五味、关防风、怀地黄、密银花、亳菊花、宣木瓜、杭白芷、浙玄参、江枳壳、苏薄荷、茅苍术、建泽泻、广陈皮、泰和乌鸡、阿胶、代赭石等，这一点与地理标志有异曲同工之妙。更重要的是，地理标志协议强调产品原产于某一地域，且其主要品质、声誉或其他特征与该地理原产地密切相关，这一点与道地药材完全一致。中药道地药材从选种、育苗、栽培、收获到加工成品，无不是当地人民数百年来辛勤的充满智慧的劳动与自然环境的完美结合，因此，其药材优良品质在很大程度上可以说就是"天、药、人合一的作品"，即道地药材是自然的恩赐与特定地域人民聪慧大脑完美结合的产物。由此可见，道地药材的内涵里包括地理标志所要求的所有本质特征，即道地药材是一类典型的地理标志产品。

地理标志作为知识产权的一种，是一种无形的财产权，其具有的巨大的经济价值，体现为促成该商品具有某种独特的品质、声誉或其他特征的人的智力成果。与一般产品相比，地理标志产品是具有高质量、高知名度、高附加值的产品。同时，地理标志与其标示的商品或服务的质量密切相关，它具有区别于其他同类产品的功能。可见，将道地药材的概念与被世界广泛理解并接受的地理标志和地理标志产品的概念接轨，不但有利于提醒人们重视道地药材的文化属性，还可以借鉴国际上地理标志产品研究的理论体系及思路方法，来研究和阐述道地药材的科学内涵。同时，利用地理标志产品保护制度，通过地理标志产品命名及其控制手段，确定道地药材生产条件和生产标准，保证药材的质量和特色，不仅有利于保护中药道地药材的文化精髓，促进道地药材研究和发展，也是道地药材走向国际化的必由之路。近年来，已有不少中药申请了地理标志，长白山人参、长白山的"中国林蛙"油、云南的"文山三七"等，为中药道地药材地理标志的推行积累了经验。

## 3 连续变异的理念是揭示道地药材科学属性的钥匙

越来越多有关种内变异的研究表明，种内变异对中药材表型性状、遗传变异及质量变异有巨大影响。如中药中所含化学成分是道地性的物质基础，但不同产地同种中药材中的同一个化学成分或有或无，或多或少，甚至存在数量级的差别，如甘草、龙胆、乌头、黄芪、大黄、麻黄等；有时种内化学成分变异会远远超过种间的变异，如苍术、关苍术。对此，黄氏等指出，道地药材包含的遗传变异越多，产生外部形态、组织结构及化学组成差异的基础越厚，其居群间的分化越深，这种分化又会随着居群地理分布范围的加大，表现为"地理宗"的分化，当"地理宗"间出现进一步趋异时就可能导致新种的形成。而道地药材在生物学上就是指某一物种的特定居群，是由一定的土壤、光热及阴湿等生境所决定的，有着比较稳定的边界，是一个比较稳定的"地方居群"（local population），是在特定的空间和时间里生活着的自然的或人为的同种个体群，即道地药材的生物内涵是同种异地。

而作为一个种下的特定居群，道地药材与非道地药材居群之间存在着一系列的过渡性和模糊性。肖氏等指出，中药的优劣是源于种内居群的连续变异，道地药材与非道地药材间既连续又间断，是量变、渐变。道地药材本身的模糊性与质量评价工作的明晰性、品质变异的复杂多样性与品质评价等级的阶层正是道地药材质量评价产生困惑的根本原因。黄氏进一步分析了道地药材的分子机理和遗传本质，指出"道地性"所表现出来的连续性，如性状特征、次生代谢产物等的连续性是多基因控制的结果，即“道地性”是多基因性状，表现为连续变异。并指出道地药材性状变异、化学成分变异所呈现出连续变异的特点，是其长期进化过程中适应地理环境的连续变异的结果。

针对多基因的表达容易受环境影响，以及环境连续变异的特点，道地药材研究中应高度重视尺度效应（包括遗传学尺度、生态学的尺度及由此引起的药材质量变异的尺度）对研究结果的影响。同时，只有借鉴数量统计学的理论和方法，利用频率、均数、方差等统计学指标，同时，配合适当的多变量分析手段或模糊综合评判手段，对道地药材质量进行综合评价，并在居群水平上研究遗传与环境的交互作用，才能充分认识道地药材居群内和居群间（组内和组间）的连续变异，并最终揭示道地药材的品质特征和生物学本质。郭氏等针对苍术种内的连续变异，利用单株取样大量的方法，结合均数分析、方差分析、主成分分析、聚类分析等统计方法，揭示了苍术道地药材挥发油组分的特征，即总挥发油含量显著低，其归一化百分含量大于1%的组分数目显著高，苍术酮加苍术素的含量极其显著高，而茅术醇加β-桉叶醇的含量极其显著低，苍术道地性在挥发油组分中的表现主要为苍术酮、茅术醇、β-桉叶醇及苍术素呈现出的一种特定配比关系。作者同时采用居群遗传结构的分析，通过随机扩增多态性（RAPD）方法，证实茅山苍术在长期适应环境的过程中，已经发生遗传分化。类似研究，为道地药材的居群生物学研究探索了方法。

总之，道地药材的优质性具有连续性、相对性和模糊性，它只是个量的概念，表现为适度的含量，特定的配比等，而非质的差别。连续变异作为遗传与环境交互作用的表现形式和必然结果，在某个特定的域值表现为药材的“道地性”，因此，连续变异的研究必将成为揭示道地药材生物学本质的一把金钥匙。

［黄璐琦，等．中国中医药信息杂志，2007，14(2)：44－46.］

# 环境胁迫下次生代谢产物的积累及道地药材的形成

植物的生存环境并不总是适宜的，植物生长发育的过程中经常受到各种环境胁迫（environmental stress，也称逆境）。20世纪80年代以来，植物对逆境的反应及机制研究引起人们的高度重视，植物抗逆性研究在代谢机理、基因定位和遗传研究等方面取得重要进展。当前，植物整体抗逆性概念的出现和整体抗逆性研究的开展，使植物抗逆性研究进入一个崭新的阶段。

次生代谢产物（secondary metabolites）通常是中药的主要药效成分。次生代谢产物在植物药体内的分布和代谢，及次生代谢产物的分类、化学、药理药效等已进行了大量研究，但对环境影响中药次生代谢产物形成和积累的研究较少，尤其是环境胁迫对中药次生代谢产物积累的影响刚刚起步。近年来，不少学者就环境对道地药材形成的影响进行了研究。郭兰萍等研究发现，道地药材苍术的形成中受到缺钾及高温胁迫；黄璐琦等指出了道地药材形成的逆境效应理论。本研究旨在将中医药理论与现代生物学及生态学理论结合起来，借鉴植物次生代谢产物的研究成果，探讨逆境对中药次生代谢产物积累及道地药材形成的影响。

## 1 环境胁迫与植物生长的关系

植物的环境胁迫因素分为物理、化学和生物3大类。其中物理类包括干旱、水涝、热害、冻害、辐射、电损伤、风害等；化学类包括营养缺乏、元素过剩、毒素、重金属毒害、pH过高或过低、盐碱、农药污染、空气污染等；生物类有竞争、抑制、化感作用、病虫害、有害微生物等。植物对逆境的抗性叫抗逆性。它通常是植物在长期适应环境中获得，或通过人工选育获得。植物抗逆性可体现在群体、个体、组织器官、细胞、生理代谢、分子、基因等不同水平。

植物本身是否能有效地运用自身的防御机制去抵制环境胁迫是决定其生存繁育的关键。多种因素决定植物如何适应环境胁迫，如植物的基因型和发育环境，胁迫的严重程度和持续时间，植株适应胁迫和任何多重胁迫的协同效应的时间长短，等等。通常，植物通过多种反应机制抵抗胁迫，无法补偿均衡的严重胁迫将导致植株死亡。

植物体可以与受到和识别的环境信号组成应激性反应。进行环境胁迫识别后信号被传输到细胞内和植物体全部。典型的环境信号传导导致细胞水平基因的表达，反过来又可以影响植物体的发育和代谢。植物体通常是以细胞和整个生物有机体抵抗环境胁迫。逆境下，植物会在形态结构、组织细胞及分子水平不同层次做出反应，如植物形态结构、生理生化、渗透调节、植物激素水平、膜保护物质及活性氧平衡、逆境蛋白形成等诸多环节发生变化，涉及植物水分、光合、呼吸、物质代谢等过程。

总体上讲，植物可以通过避逆和耐逆2种方式来抵抗逆境。前者指植物通过对生育周期的调整来避开逆境干扰，在相对适应的环境中完成生活史；后者指植物处于不利环境时，通过代谢反应来阻止、降低或修复由逆境造成的损伤，使植物仍保持正常的生理活动。

## 2 环境胁迫对植物次生代谢产物积累的影响

近年来，环境胁迫对植物次生代谢的影响引起国内外逆境生理学研究的重视。人们认识到，植物在受到生物或非生物因子侵染时，能通过体内抗性基因的表达，合成并积累一系列具有抗病作用的低相对分子质量化合物，来抵抗病原菌的侵害，这类物质通称为植保素（phytolexin）。植保素通常是些次生代谢产物，它是植物体在次生代谢过程中产生的一大类小分子化合物。次生代谢产物是相对于初生代谢产物（primary metobolities）而言的，后者是植物维持生命活动所必需的，而次生代谢产物并非是维持细胞正常生命活动和植物正常生长发育所必需的。常见的次生代谢产物包括生物碱、黄酮、萜类、蒽醌、香豆素、木质素等。

次生代谢产物是植物长期进化中适应环境的产物，其公认的生态学功能主要是抗病、抗虫、抗环境胁迫等。迄今为止，已发现有几百种次生代谢产物有参与植物抗真菌、细菌、病毒甚至线虫的作用，而且感染病虫害会使植物次生代谢产物增加。如感染茎点毒（一种真菌病原体），可以导致苜蓿叶中异黄酮成分芒柄花素苷和苜蓿素的积累。许多研究表明，植物在受虫害损伤后，在次生代谢方面一个最明显的变化是酚类化合物含量的增加。此外，虫害诱导植物产生的挥发物中，萜烯类物质是其中最主要的组成部分。同时，越来越多的研究表明，多种物理、化学胁迫会引起植物体内次生代谢产物积累的增多。Tang 等发现，万寿菊 *Tagetes erecta* 在水分胁迫条件下（干旱），所含酚类物质的含量明显高于其在水分充足时的含量。Josep 等发现 $CO_2$ 浓度增高使迷迭香体内单萜含量增加。还有不少学者报道在养分缺乏等环境胁迫条件下，植物产生的用于防御的次生代谢物质的数量增加。何丙辉等发现干旱胁迫对槲皮素含量的提高有一定的促进作用，遮荫处理对提高银杏幼树叶片中药用成分含量有显著的促进作用。Hall 等研究发现，随着营养胁迫程度的增强，向日葵 *Helianthus annuus* 产生的酚类物质含量相应增加。Bettina 等研究发现紫外光胁迫后，转 MtIFS1 基因的苜蓿和对照组株系的 HPLC 色谱图中，出现了一系列峰，与异黄酮的生物合成一致。

近年来，不少学者对逆境下植物的基因表达进行了研究，在基因水平揭示了逆境对植物次生代谢的影响。郎印海等综述了高等植物在厌氧、热激、盐分胁迫、养分胁迫、紫外辐射等各种逆境条件下，基因表达更替的系列过程，提出基因表达变化对作物适应逆境条件的意义。王少峡等研究发现 DREB 转录因子由逆环境胁迫诱导产生后，可激活其他多达 12 个依赖 DRE 顺式作用元件的抗逆功能基因，引起脯氨酸及蔗糖含量提高，从而增强植株对多种逆境（旱、冻及盐）的抵抗性。张玉秀等对编码一种菜豆 DnaJ-like 蛋白的 PvSR6（phaseolus vulgaris stress related）基因进行 Northem 杂交表明，PvSR6 基因在未处理的菜豆叶片中表达较少，重金属（$Hg^{2+}$ 和 $Cd^{2+}$）、机械损伤、紫外辐射、高温和水杨酸等环境胁迫能强烈地促进其基因的转录，推测 DnaJ-like 蛋白在保护细胞膜和酶蛋白的结构和功能及提高植物的抗逆性方面有重要作用。这些研究对揭示逆境影响植物次生代谢基因表达有重要意义。

## 3 环境胁迫影响次生代谢产物的假说

植物在长期生长中，已经适应了自然环境，当自然环境发生剧烈改变，特别是在环境胁迫的情况下，植物将发生一系列变化来适应环境，提高生存竞争力。其中，产生对植物具有保护作用的次生代谢产物具有重要意义。

当前，在次生代谢产物随环境变化的机理方面，根据次生代谢产物的产生是否需要成本，及次生代谢产物的产生是个主动的过程还是被动的过程，形成了不同的假说。

3.1 生长/分化平衡（growth/differentiation balance，GDB）假说 GDB 假说认为，在资源充足时，植物以生长为主，而在资源匮乏时，植物以分化为主，任何对植物生长影响超过对植物光合作用影响的环境因子（如营养匮乏、$CO_2$ 浓度升高，低温等）都会导致次生代谢产物的增多。这一假说的理论基础是植物的生长发育在细胞水平可分为生长和分化 2 个过程，前者主要指细胞的分裂和增大，后者主要包括细胞的特化和成熟。次生代谢产物是细胞特化和成熟过程中生理活动的产物，因此，随植物生长年龄的增大和老化含量增大，如人参、三七、黄连等不少中药材都必须种够一定的年限，药效成分含量才能达到用药要求。

3.2 碳素/营养平衡（carbon/nutrient balance，CNB）假说 CNB 假说认为，植物体内以碳（C）为基础的次生代谢产物（如酚类、萜烯类等）与植物体内的 C/N（碳素/营养）比呈正相关，而以氮（N）为基础的次生代谢物质（如生物碱等含 N 化合物）与植物体内的 C/N 比呈负相关。这一假说在一定程度解释了不同植物次生代谢产物累积量与碳素/营养平衡的关系，并成功地预测了许多有关植物营养及光照对其次生代谢产物的影响。CNB 假说的理论基础是植物营养对其自身生长的影响大于其对光合作用的影响。在营养胁迫时，植物生长的速度大为减慢，而光合作用的变化不大，植物会积累较多的碳、氢元素，体内 C/N 比增大。因此，以 C 为基础的酚类、萜烯类物质增多；反之，在遮荫条件下，光合作用降低，体内 C/N 比降低，酚类、萜烯类物质减少。研究发现，益母草生物碱含量由北向南减少，相反，青蒿、苍术等药材的挥发油（萜类）含量由北向南增多，与我国光温条件由北向南的变化趋势有一定相关性。这一现象，似乎可以用 CNB 假说来解释。

3.3 最佳防御（optimum defense，OD）假说 OD 假说认为，植物只有在其产生的次生代谢产物所获得的防御收益大于其生长所获得的收益时，才产生次生代谢产物。该假说的理论基础是，植物次生代谢产物的产生是以减少植物生长的机会成本为代价的。环境胁迫条件下，植物生长减慢，此时，产生次生代谢产物的成本较低。同时，植物受损的补偿能力较差，次生代谢产物的防御收益增加。因此，环境胁迫条件下，植物会产生较多的次生代谢产物。

3.4 资源获得（resource availability，RA）假说 RA 假说认为，由于自然选择的结果，在环境恶劣的自然条件下生长的植物，具有生长慢而次生代谢产物多的特点，而在良好的自然条件下生长的植物，具有生长较快且次生代谢产物少的特点。即植物潜在的生长速度降低时，植物产生的用于防御的次生代谢产物的数量就会增加。这一假说的理论依据是，环境胁迫条件下，植物生长的潜在速度较慢，受到损害时，其损失的相对成本较高。

以上 4 个假说，前两者将植物次生代谢产物的形成和积累视为由于外界环境变化引起植物体内物质积累的一个被动过程，而后两者认为植物次生代谢产物的产生是根据其产生成本的变化而变化的主动过程。忽视由于视角不同造成的差异，这几个假说从不同的角度提出了一个共同的结论，即环境胁迫条件下，植物次生代谢产物的数量会增加。

## 4 环境胁迫与道地药材的关系

4.1 环境对道地药材形成的影响 道地药材是中医药的精髓，它在传统中医药中是优质药材的代名词。道地药材的形成与中药的优良种质和特定自然环境密不可分。为此，不少道地药材在药名前多冠以地名，以示其道地产区。如西宁大黄、宁夏枸杞、川贝母、川芎、秦艽、辽五味、关防风、怀地黄、密银花、亳菊花、宣木瓜、杭白芷、浙玄参、江枳壳、苏薄荷、茅苍术、建泽泻、广陈皮、泰和乌鸡、阿胶、代赭石等。古人对环境影响道地药材的记述很多，如“诸药所生，皆有境界”“一方土地出一方药也”“离其本土，其质同而效异”等。如果说“天人合一”是中医学的基本思想，则“天药合一”就是古人认识道地药材的基本思路，《内经》指出“岁物者，天地之专精也”，说的即是这个意思。

现代生物学认为道地药材的生物学本质为表型变异＝遗传变异＋环境饰变，可见，道地药材的表型可塑性与自然环境关系密切。近年来，自然环境对中药道地性形成的影响受到空前的重视，不少学者开展了相关研究，积累了大量的本底资料和有益的研究结果。但总体看来，研究结果零散，有待进一步系统整理突破。

通常，经过长期对环境的适应，药用植物已经选择了较为适宜的自然环境，当自然环境的突然改变或在环境胁迫条件下，植物通过物理手段与其他植物竞争有限资源的能力大为降低，此时化学的方法就会上升为其竞争的重要手段。次生代谢产物是植物保护素，环境胁迫下，植物通过向外界环境释放次生代谢产物(释放到环境中的次生代谢产物又被称为化感物质)来抑制其他植物的生长，以提高自身的竞争能力。由于环境胁迫(如干旱、严寒、伤害、高温、重金属等)能刺激植物次生代谢产物的积累和释放。在这个意义上讲，逆境可能更利于中药道地性的形成。如郭兰萍等研究发现，苍术道地药材茅山苍术在生长发育过程中土壤酸化严重，养分状况不理想，并受到严重的缺钾胁迫。同时发现，高温是苍术生长发育的限制因子，而茅山地区几个与温度有关的气候因子均为其整个分布区的最高值，其道地产区处于苍术整个分布区的东南边缘。作者认为植物积累次生代谢产物所需的适宜生境与其生长发育的适宜生境可能并不一致，甚至相反，即药用动植物生态适宜性概念与普通生物的生态适宜概念并不完全相同。黄璐琦等明确提出逆境能促进道地药材的形成，并进一步指出道地药材的这种“逆境效应”，可能导致其道地产区在物理空间上位于其整个分布区的边缘，并由此产生“边缘效应”。

4.2 环境胁迫影响药材道地性的研究 植物整体抗逆性指的是植物在整个生命活动过程中(包括生长发育和果实种子收获贮藏休眠期)，具有由基因控制的、能够抵抗各种外来环境胁迫的能力，使生长发育、产量、生活力受到有限危害水平，它可以反映在分子、细胞、组织器官、个体植株、群体甚至整个生态系统的不同水平上。作为中药适应特定自然环境的最佳表型，临床疗效好、药效成分含量高是道地药材最重要的优良品质。此外，中药的道地性还包括外观性状好、高产、易贮藏、抗虫、抗病性强等诸多优良性状的全部或部分。由于道地性是个综合指标，其环境适应的机制涉及道地药材生长发育的多方面，与植物的整体抗逆性有关。因此，借鉴植物整体抗逆性理念，可以为环境胁迫下药材道地性的研究提供很好的思路和方法。

如首先，根据整体抗逆性的内涵，如抗性的多重性、抗性表现形式的多样性、抗性表现的阶段性、抗性效应的整体性等，观察和认识道地药材的抗逆性；然后，根据将抗性分类，如抗寒、抗旱、抗高温、抗盐碱、抗病虫、抗辐射、抗缺素、抗药等，分析植物是单抗、多抗、兼抗、综合抗性及整体抗性；最后，以道地药材表型与生境及基因型的相互关系为切入点，采用对比试验，从分子、细胞和个体的不同水平上，深入研究道地药材对干旱、盐胁迫和养分亏缺等逆境信息的感受、传递和信号转导机制，研究道地药材抗逆基因的功能、表达的调控机制，及其适应逆境的生理及分子机制，从而最大限度地挖掘道地药材自身的生物学潜力，为利用基因工程方法培育道地药材抗逆优质品种，改进抗逆高效的栽培措施，大幅度提高道地药材产量并保证道地药材的质量提供新思路。

近来，人们已经认识到，环境影响道地性的研究应是在能够人工控制的实验地进行，因为在这样的地方可以模拟一种或一种以上的影响道地药材存活及品质的关键环境因子，可以设置一系列的梯度用于研究道地药材在这些环境条件下的表型变异趋势。而且，实验应是以对比实验的方式进行，既要考察不同处理间的变化，也要考察时间序列上道地药材表型的变异。同样，环境胁迫对道地药材影响的研究也主要以受控试验的方式进行。

同时，随着植物抗逆性研究的广泛开展，人们日益认识到环境胁迫之前所处的条件(预先条件)对决定植物能否克服这种胁迫有重要影响。不少研究表明，在预先条件中经历适度的胁迫，会提高植物抗下一次胁迫的能力。道地药材是长期适应逆境的产物，道地性可能是在经历了无数次环境胁迫中获得。为此，在研究逆境影响道地药材的试验中，设置预先胁迫可能会有更有意义的发现。

[黄璐琦，等.中国中药杂志，2007，32(4)：277－280.]

# 道地药材形成的分子机制及其遗传基础

近年来，道地药材研究一直是中药研究的热点问题之一，不少学者就道地性的科学内涵，道地药材形成的机制，道地药材的质量评价及鉴别等问题展开研究和讨论。人们认识到，道地药材是遗传变异和自然选择的结果，属“药材”的“生态型”或“化学型”，次生代谢产物既是道地药材的物质基础也是其最重要的表型特征之一。换言之，道地药材的形成是特定的基因型，在特定的生境下受到复杂的调控，导致某些代谢过程的关键酶基因的表达产生了时空差异的产物。

作者在分析道地性内涵及生物学特征及其分子机制研究的基础上，探讨道地性的遗传学本质，并提出道地药材分子机制研究中应注意的问题。

## 1 道地性的内涵及特征

道地性可以看作是道地药材特有属性的简称，主要通过道地药材的质量性状(外观、所含次生代谢产物等)、遗传性状、生境特征等特性来体现。人们从自身利用的角度出发，通常将道地药材的特征归纳为以下几点：地域性(与特定的产地分不开)、优质性(中医临床公认的优质药材)、具有文化内涵(品质与生产和加工有关)、具有较高经济价值(较同种药材的单价较高)。

从生物学角度出发，“道地性”与道地药材的表型、遗传背景及环境三者有关，它是遗传、环境及药材表型三者在长期协同进化过程中，在某个特定时空上的一个反映。由于环境因素包含时间和空间2种信息，道地性可以被视为时间和空间交互作用，及其在药材自身遗传背景、形态特征及次生代谢产物等所有方面表现出来的一种综合特征。换言之，道地性与药材的遗传特征、表型特征及特定的时间和空间有关，在药材的生物学上主要概况为以下几个方面的特征。

1.1 特异性 道地药材通常在居群水平会呈现出某种共同的特定性，如皮薄、个大、高产、肉厚、油多等。这种特异性是特定空间、特定时间、特定表性、特定遗传背景的综合。作者曾指出“道地药材的化学组成有其独特的自适应特征”。郭兰萍及欧阳臻等发现苍术道地药材茅山苍术呈现出一种特定比例；刘玉萍发现藿香道地药材石牌藿香与其他非道地产区的藿香为不同化学型。而这种特异性表现在其药用价值上，就成为优质性。道地药材是公认的优质中药材，它的优质性是个综合指标。就药材本身而言，它可能包括临床疗效好、药效成分含量高、外观性状好、高产、易贮藏、抗虫、抗病性强等诸多优良性状的全部或部分。其中，临床疗效好、药效成分含量高是道地药材最重要的优良品质。

1.2 地域性 作为特定地理环境的产物，道地性被认为是特定种质长期适应环境的结果。我国历代医家对此早有深刻认识，所谓“诸药所生，皆有其界”，又云“凡用药必须择土地所宜者，则药力具用之有据”，再如“离其本土，则效异”中的“本土”即包括土壤、水、光、温度、地形等环境因子。现代生物学认为道地药材是同种异质，是道地药材原物种在其分布产地的种系与区系的发生发展过程中，长期受孕育该物种的历史环境条件影响而形成的某一特殊的居群，这个居群可以是生态宗、地理宗、地方宗、化学宗、生理宗或者是栽培变种、变型、品系、农家品种等。作者曾认为道地药材作为一类典型的地理标志产品，特定的地理环境是其形成的必要条件。为此，不少道地药材在药材前冠以地名，如阳春砂、宣木瓜、茅苍术、岷当归、关黄柏、江油附子、石柱黄连、东阿阿胶，以及四大川药、四大怀药、浙八味等。由此可见，道地药材这一概念形成和发展的全过程都离不开特定产地，其本质是同一药材在不同产地中质量最佳者，特点地域(即道地产区)是道地药材生产的必要条件，离开了道地产区也就不存在道地药材的概念。

1.3 连续性和迁延性 从一个较大的范围来看，环境条件中的大多数空间变异是梯度的，而不是间断的或陡峭的。因此，如果居群或种适应于环境的话，那它们的变异也是梯度的、连续的，按照环境梯度形成一个形态特征逐渐过渡的倾群。目前不少学者都把具有广泛分布区的种内大部分变异，包括生态型及化学型，看成是由数量性状上有变化的遗传级差，亦即梯度变异所构成。作为一个开放的复杂系统，道地药材的形成是长期适应环境的结果，属于种内变异。既然环境因素是道地药材形成的根本动力，则时间和空间的连续性造就药材遗传与表型的连续性。比如不少连续分布的物种，其化学成分的变异通常也会呈现出连续变异的特点，如薄荷、菊花、苍术、甘草、麻黄等等，其道地药材与非道地药材的化学成分通常只是量变而非质变。与此同时，道地药材是进化的产物，也依然处于进化的过程中，因此，其道地性的内涵不是永恒不变的。其中，道地产区的变迁是其道地性内涵改变的最直接的证据。历史上，不少道地药材的道地产区都发生过变迁，如人参、芍药等。道地产区的改变可能是由于人类对道地药材认识的深入，也可能是环境改变的结果。就生物学而言，既然道地性是遗传、环境及药材表型三者协调进化的结果，环境的改变也必然带来遗传与表型的改变，由此造成道地药材的迁延性。这种迁延在生物学上多是长期进化的结果，而非突发事件。

## 2 道地药材分子机制研究

道地药材的分子机制的研究，就是要在分子水平揭示道地药材居群水平的遗传变异，明确道地药材基因型特征，以及环境对道地药材基因表达的影响，从而揭示遗传因素对道地药材形成的贡献率。根据研究目的，将相关研究归纳为以下几个方面。

2.1 道地药材遗传多样性研究及分子鉴别 居群水平的遗传多样性(遗传变异)一直是道地药材分子研究的基础和热点。不少学者就道地药材的遗传多样性展开研究。随机扩增多态性(RAPD)、扩增酶切片段多态性(AFLP)及简单重复序列区间(ISSR)等多种分子标记技术被用于乌头、人参、枳壳、芍药、苍术、半夏、厚朴、石斛等道地药材的遗传多样性的评价。研究发现，不同药材的遗传多样性水平差异极大。在观察遗传多样性的同时，不少学者希望找到道地药材特有的分子标记，从而可以在分子水平实现道地药材的鉴别。有学者比较了用于中药材鉴定的分子标记技术，主要有SCAR、RFLP、RAPD、PCR-RFLP、DNA测序和位点特异性鉴别PCR等，指出位点特异性鉴别PCR技术以其简单、快速、准确、重现性好、成本低、抗污染等优点，应用前景广阔。陈毓亨等应用RAPD技术，在供试的12个地区24个样品中，发现所研究的21个引物中，有9个引物仅见于2个地区间高含量紫杉烷样品的共同的特征条带，认为这些条带可能与紫杉烷的形成有一定关系，为道地药材分子鉴别标记的寻找提供了线索。

2.2 道地药材遗传分化及进化遗传学研究 居群水平的遗传分化是道地药材形成的遗传学基础。遗传分化越明显,道地药材与同种其他居群药材的差异越明显。ISSR,RAPD等分子技术被用于明党参、苍术、芍药、厚朴等道地药材遗传分化的测定。作为物种进化的重要环节,通过遗传分化分析,可以推测道地药材在进化树中的位置,及其与其他居群及近缘种的关系。左云娟等采用ISSR技术分析来自江西省樟树市昌傅镇和黄岗镇的江枳壳品种臭橙、柚子橙、鸡子橙、勒橙和香橙共27个样品的遗传关系。杜娟等采用AFLP方法研究了全国10个主要产地的野生或栽培半夏不同种源之间遗传关系,发现遗传关系的远近与其总生物碱含量差异趋势一致。

2.3 道地药材地理变异及环境适应性研究 作为特定地理环境的产物,地理变异及其环境适应性研究是道地药材研究的关键和特色。张君毅等运用PCR扩增后直接测序,认为半夏rDNA变异与其地理分布相关。张英等研究认为广藿香的地理分布和其IIS1、IIS2基因型具有良好的相关性。韩建萍等运用AFLP研究发现地理位置相近的栀子种群聚为一类。陈大霞等ISSR分析发现来源于同一地区的部分黄连种质聚在一起,呈现出一定的地域性分布规律。赵桂仿等应用RAPD技术研究发现阿尔卑斯山黄花茅遗传分化沿海拔梯度发生,而且亚居群间的遗传分化和它们的海拔高度(地理距离)呈有意义的正相关。刘玉萍等利用PCR直接测序,发现广藿香基因序列分化与其产地所含挥发油变异类型呈良好相关性。郭水良RAPD研究表明,8个车前种群的遗传分化与地理位置、海拔高度有联系。道地药材的地理变异反映了道地药材的环境适应性。针对道地药材的形成可能是适应环境胁迫的结果,有学者提出了道地药材形成的逆境效应。周洁等开展了环境胁迫下道地药材苍术在分子水平的适应性反应,发现缺钾、干旱胁迫下苍术挥发油积累及保护酶系统发生系列改变。但环境胁迫下道地药材基因表达有待进一步深入。

2.4 道地药材种质资源评价及品种选育 特定的遗传背景是道地药材形成的遗传学基础。作者曾指出,道地性越明显,其基因特化越显著。为此,不少学者就道地药材种质资源展开研究,试图为道地药材的形成提供遗传学上的证据。当前,丹参、桔梗、人参、银杏等道地药材的种质资源的遗传多样性得到研究,为道地药材的分子育种提供了依据。

2.5 道地药材功能基因表达及调控研究 道地性归根结底是道地药材所拥有的基因型受到特定生境(道地产区)中环境因子诱导后表达的产物。因此,基因表达是道地药材研究的重要环节,而功能基因表达的调控是道地药材研究的目标之一。揭示道地药材和非道地药材在基因表达方面的差异是道地药材功能基因研究的重要内容。但由于环境中生态因子众多,加上生态因子作用的综合性,致使影响道地药材形成的生态主导因子无法确定,或者即使确定了,主导因子也通常是多个生态因子综合组成。加上基因表达对研究所用RNA材料的要求较高,且通常需要通过对比实验来完成,造成道地药材基因表达及调控实验目前主要集中在实验室中。同时,由于细胞培养和组织培养周期较短,材料均匀性较好,相关研究多是在细胞和组织水平,抑或在转基因获得的毛状根植物中开展。如黄新等利用mRNA差异显示技术研究茉莉酸甲酯对红豆杉细胞mRNA表达的差异。李娟等考察了碳源、氮源、有机成分对HBsAg转基因人参细胞生长和HBsAg表达量的影响。毛莹等研究发现$Cu^{2+}$、$Zn^{2+}$能显著诱导丹参金属硫蛋白基因的表达。刘峻等研究了真菌诱导子影响人参毛状根总苷的合成量。以上研究,虽然距离真正地实现道地药材功能基因的表达和调控尚有一段距离,但为道地药材功能基因表达和调控研究积累了思路和方法。

2.6 道地药材转基因及生物安全性评价 近年来,转基因工程研究在中药材研究中取得较快进展,转基因工程的生物安全性评价也日益引起人们的重视。韩立敏等用农杆菌EHA105介导的叶盘转化法,获得了7个丹参转基因株系。冯丽玲等克隆并通过叶盘共培养法已获得一批表现卡那霉素抗性的转基因青蒿植株。宋永波等用高压纸层析电泳证实了根癌农杆菌C58对西洋参茎的转化成功。但真正意义上的道地药材转基因工程的进展,有赖于道地药材分子机制研究总体水平的提高,特别是道地药材功能基因研究取得的实质性进展,首先必须找到与道地性直接相关的功能基因,才有望真正实现道地药材的转基因工程。

## 3 道地性的遗传本质及其研究对策

3.1 道地性的遗传本质 通过上述关于道地性的内涵和生物学特征,以及道地药材分子机制研究的现状的综述,可以初步得到以下的印象:道地药材在生物学上,既表现出某种确定性(特异性、地域性),也有其不确定性(连续性和迁延性);道地药材的分子机制取得了极大的进展,但其分子机制的研究成果主要是集中在一些分子现象的积累上,如道地药材遗传多样性及遗传分化程度的高低、道地药材地理变异的相关性大小、道地药材种质资源的多样性及其与品质的关联性、道地药材功能基因表达及调控研究相关研究的初步探索等,至今未见到有关道地药材遗传学本质的研究报道和学术探讨。

那么,道地药材生物学特性的不确定性产生的遗传学基础是什么?道地药材分子现象的遗传学本质是什么?基因特化的表现是什么?为什么众多的研究至今未找到道地药材特有的基因?有没有一个道地药材特有的"道地基因"?作者根据进化遗传学及数量遗传学的理论,在居群和个体2个水平就道地药材形成的遗传本质进行探讨,以期从根本上梳理道地药材的分子机制。

3.1.1 在居群水平表现为基因频率的改变 现代群体遗传学将进化定义为基因频率的改变。并用下面的公式表示:进化 =遗传变异+变异的不均等传递+物种形成。其中遗传变异主要指个体水平的基因突变、重组及基因流;变异的不均等传递主要指居群水平的自然选择和遗传漂变,即生物适应环境过程中产生的居群水平的遗传分化;而物种的形成则是指物种水平的生殖隔离。中性理论进一步阐明进化的实质是中性突变,适者生存,即遗传上的突变是随机的,中性的,但只有适应环境的突变才被保存下来。可见进化是针对居群及其以上水平而言,其中遗传变异是进化的源泉,环境是进化的动力。如果说物种的更替是进化的最终表现形式或结果,则新物种形成前的居群水平的遗传分化则可以被视为进化过程中的表现形式。

在生物学上,道地药材通常是指种内的不同居群,尚未达到生殖隔离，即未达到新物种的形成。换言之，道地药材可被视为物种进化中的一个阶段或状态，其与同种内其他居群个体尚未达到生殖隔离，基因交流仍在发生。由此可知，道地药材的遗传变异在居群水平通常是个量变的过程，它与种内其他非道地药材区别主要表现为居群内基因型频率的改变。可见，道地药材的基因特化，主要表现为道地居群内某种基因型频率的增高或降低。这就是道地药材遗传多样性或高或低，其与同种其他居群的遗传分化或大或小，但不论在性状上，还是遗传上都很难找到道地药材独有的表型特征或分子标记的根本原因。但可以设想，如果在群体水平寻找多数道地药材所共有的某种特征或分子标记，还是有望实现的。

3.1.2 在个体水平的表现为微效多基因控制的数量遗传 遗传学上将遗传变异根据其表现形式分为决定质量性状(qualitative)的变异和决定数量性状(quantitative)的变异2种。质量性状表现为不连续变异，由少数主基因(major gene)决定，符合孟德尔定律；数量性状表现为连续变异。经典数量遗传学理论认为，数量性状由微效多基因(multiple gene)控制，数量性状基因型值是控制该性状的所有基因加性效应的总和。近年的研究表明，在许多数量性状的遗传变异中，既有众多微效基因的作用，也有主基因的作用，即这些性状应属于微效多基因和主基因联合控制的混合性状，且这些基因往往具有多效性，即不只对一个特征产生影响，对其他特征也有程度不同的影响。

决定数量性状的遗传变异很容易受环境影响，并与环境发生交互作用。即数量性状由遗传变异，环境变异及基因与环境的交互作用三部分组成。多基因虽然按孟德尔方式遗传，但其控制的表型变异相对于非遗传变异，或至少是相对于总变异其效应较小，因此在表型分布中不能分辨出非连续性。于是，非连续的、定量的基因型变异就可能产生光滑的、连续的表型变异。即环境的修饰作用可能掩饰基因型的非连续变异，从而使表型上呈现连续变异，从而使性状变异变的平滑、不可检测。

根据上面介绍，道地药材在生物学上具有特异性、地域性、连续性、迁延性等特点，这些特点在生物学上都是适应环境变异的结果，特异性是适应环境异质性的结果，连续性是适应环境因子连续变异的结果，迁延性是适应历史上环境因子变迁的结果。作者曾撰文指出，“连续变异的理念是揭示道地药材科学属性的钥匙”，可见，道地性在生物学表现为易受环境影响的呈现连续变异的数量性状。这既是道地药材的鉴别至今未得到有效解决的原因，也是道地药材无法通过品种选育，及异地移栽等手段移栽到其他产地，并令其优良品质不发生改变的原因。可见，道地性在个体水平表现为微效多基因控制的数量遗传，或是微效多基因和主基因联合控制的数量性状。诸多的现代研究早已证实了这一点，比如次生代谢产物是中药道地性最直接最重要的指标之一，其代谢的步骤繁多而复杂，代谢的每个步骤都有至少1个基因在起作用，因此，次生代谢产物是典型的多基因性状。当前已初步了解的各类次生代谢产物，如萜类、烯类、生物碱、黄酮、蒽醌、香豆素等一系列物质的生物合成，不论通过的是哪种次生代谢途径，都要经过相当多的代谢步骤，并涉及大量的关键酶基因。例如，黄曲霉素(aflatoxin)B1合成途径中的各个步骤，已知至少包括22种酵素基因，超过20个酵素步骤参与黄曲霉素B1生合成。同样，植物的株高、分蘖数、生物量等生物学性状也都是众所周知的多基因性状。

控制数量性状的数量性状基因座位(quantitative trait loci，QTL)是数量性状研究的重要武器。QTL作为一特定染色体片段，控制同一性状的1组微效多基因的集合或基因簇(gene cluster)。研究表明，1个数量性状的QTL并不很多，一般为4～8个。每个QTL为1个孟德尔因子，它可能是1个基因，也可能是由2个或2个以上的基因组成的基因群。可见，如果有1类基因与药材的道地性有明显关联，且可被称之为“道地基因”，则该道地基因更像是由控制数量性状的数量性状基因座位构成。因此，借鉴QTL检测方法，如候选基因分析(candidate gene approach)，或标记-QTL连锁分析(mark-QTL linkage analysis)，可能为道地基因的寻找提供线索。

3.2 道地性遗传本质研究中应注意的问题

3.2.1 高度重视道地药材研究的尺度 道地药材是生物进化过程中的产物，道地性归根结底地理变异的一种表现形式，其遗传本质在居群水平为基因频率的改变。换言之，道地药材在基因水平表现为一种概率，该概率只有在居群水平才有显著意义，就个体水平而言，道地药材与非道地药材间既连续又间断，是量变、渐变。

尺度效应认为，当观测、试验、分析或模拟的时空尺度发生变化时，系统特征也随之发生变化。为此，道地药材研究应高度重视尺度效应，相关观察研究必须在居群水平展开，而且该居群必须以道地药材的实际分布区为依据，而非人为划定的居群。可见，居群水平的遗传变异、遗传分化、分子鉴别、地理变异式样及居群水平的分子适应机制等，既是道地药材关注的热点，也是揭示道地性的必由之路。

此处尺度效应不只包括生态学上的尺度，也包括遗传学尺度。也就是说，居群水平开展道地药材分子机制研究，不只是说将研究范围确定在居群这一等级上，更重要的是，在选择道地药材研究的相关基因时，要高度关注所分析基因进化速率，可参照各种基因在系统进化分析中的地位，选择用于种下群体间变异的基因进行研究。同样，各种分子技术，也分别适应于具有不同变异速率的分子检测，应根据研究目的慎重选择。

3.2.2 充分利用数量遗传学的理论和方法 前面指出，道地药材在居群水平表现为基因频率的改变，在个体水平的表现为微效多基因控制的数量遗传，这使得道地药材无论在基因水平还是表型上都呈现出数量特征。正是这种数量特征及其表现出来的连续性，为道地药材鉴别、质量评价及分子机制研究带来了困惑。

在研究形态数量变异过程中，很难确定具体是哪一个基因在起作用，而只能从数量遗传的角度加以研究。数量遗传学或生统遗传学是遗传学方法和生物统计学结合的产物，主要研究连续变异的理论及研究方法。道地药材的数量遗传特征，使得数量遗传学方法技术可能成为未来道地药材分子机制研究的重要的手段。利用数量遗传学的概念和实验方法，研究道地药材遗传的物质基础、性状的连续变异，尺度问题，均值分量和变异分量、互作和连锁、基因和有效因子、选择进展等问题，将成为揭示道地药材分子机制的重要手段。特别值得一提的是，对QTL的研究构成了正在形成的分子数量遗传学的主体，也成为人们研究数量性状遗传的最有力的武器，道地基因的研究应对QTL给予高度重视。

3.2.3 重点关注基因与环境的交互作用 根据数量遗传理论，形态数量特征的最终表现形式，是各方面因素综合作用的结果。形态数量特征的发育受多方面的影响，包括直接的加性或非加性遗传效应、母性效应、基因型与环境的相互作用，以及环境的随机影响等。其中，基因与环境间的互用是多基因遗传的重要特点，其互作有许多形式，最主要的有：一是环境通过施加于某一群体的选择压而影响该群体的遗传结构；二是基因型和环境可能借助于它们在发育中的相互作用所产生的非遗传效应，而在决定直接观察的个体和居群间的差异上表现为互作。这两种互作对道地药材的形成都有重要作用。

遗传变异和生态环境的交互作用，大大丰富了中药材原物种种质的多样性和种质资源，为道地药材品质形成提供了生态生物学基础。因此，对遗传与环境的交互作用的研究是揭示道地药材分子机制研究的关键，也必将成为道地药材研究的热点和难点。

［黄璐琦，等.中国中药杂志，2008，33(20)：2303－2308.］

# 药用植物功能基因克隆新方法——成分差异表型克隆法

在后基因组时代，功能基因成为关注和研究热点。这些功能基因的研究往往是建立在基因序列比较清楚的情况下进行的。药用植物功能基因与农作物相比，其分子遗传研究背景往往比较薄弱，这给药用植物有效成分生物合成相关基因的克隆研究带来了较大困难。目前药用植物常用的基因克隆方法是基于PCR为基础的同源克隆法，该方法虽然具有简便经济等优点，但是其前提要求所克隆的目的基因信息清楚，至少需要从其他物种获取含有该基因序列信息。这在药用植物有效成分代谢途径不明确，有效成分次生代谢关键酶的编码基因未知的情况下，基于PCR同源克隆方法显得无能为力。为此，如何在药用植物遗传背景比较薄弱的情况下克隆药用植物有效成分的生物合成的功能基因，从基因水平上调控药用植物有效成分的生产等问题，已经成为严重制约药用植物次生代谢基因工程研究的技术瓶颈。经典的功能基因克隆方法，是基于同位素示踪法获悉具体次生代谢途径内的基础上普遍采用的同源克隆方法。由于该方法操作起来有一定难度，再加上同位素发射性污染等因素，一定程度上限制了其广泛应用。笔者介绍了一种药用植物有效成分生物合成途径(或次生代谢途径)及其功能基因克隆研究的新思路与方法，即“成分差异表型克隆法”。该方法不需要清楚有效成分具体代谢途径和目的功能基因同源序列信息，具有克隆速度快、高通量等优点。这无疑为解决药用植物次生代谢的基因调控和相关基因工程研究的瓶颈问题提供了新的研究思路和有效的手段。结合药用植物功能基因研究现状，就本方法的概念、原理和方法、优势与应用并以丹参功能基因克隆为研究实例进行介绍。

## 1 药用植物功能基因研究的现状

药用植物功能基因研究，特别是次生代谢相关功能基因的研究存在的最大困难是遗传信息背景即基因信息基础较薄弱。与农作物不同，绝大多数药用植物遗传背景信息非常少。王伟等对2300种药用植物的基因组、蛋白质及表达序列标签(EST)的注册统计表明，66%的药用植物没有核酸序列报道，77%的药用植物没有蛋白质序列注册。据报道，药用植物功能基因克隆主要集中于长春花、青蒿、甘草、红豆杉、天麻、银杏、雪莲、毛地黄、葛等32属42种药用植物，其中黄酮类(酚类)合成基因、细胞色素P450基因克隆最多。药用植物功能基因研究日本最多，美国次之，德国第3，中国第4。美国对长春花、红豆杉有关的基因克隆走在世界前沿。德国在生物碱合成，包括长春花和萝芙木中的生物碱主要合成酶基因的克隆研究较多。日本药用植物基因克隆主要包括了黄连、杜仲、甘草、紫草、黄芪、人参以及天仙子等。

笔者在检索NCBI 的公共数据库(http://www.ncbi.nih.gov/，Revised：September 15，2008.)中发现，目前在GenBank注册的序列中，丹参 *Salvia miltiorrhiza* 核酸序列10423条(包含EST)，蛋白氨基酸序列51条；人参 *Panax ginseng* 的核酸序列10449条，蛋白氨基酸序列424条；银杏 *Ginkgo biloba* 核酸序列20096条，蛋白氨基酸序列405条；藏红花 *Crocus sativus* 核酸序列6812条，蛋白氨基酸序列62条；薄荷 *Mentha haplocalyx* 核酸序列8条，蛋白氨基酸序列8条；东北红豆杉 *Taxus cuspidata* 核酸序列199条，蛋白氨基酸序列44条。然而，在诸多基因核苷酸序列或氨基酸序列当中，功能基因特别是与有效成分次生代谢相关的功能基因的研究报道极少。以丹参为例，在Genbank注册的10399条核苷酸序列中，与丹参酮类成分次生代谢相关的功能基因，目前只报道如下几条HMGR(AAU87798)，DXR(ABJ80680)，以及笔者注册的CMK(ABP96842)，它们分别位于萜类化合物次生代谢的上游途径，甲羟戊酸(MVA)途径和1-去氧木糖-5-磷酸(DXP)途径。因此，在药用植物有效成分次生代谢途径及其相关功能基因克隆研究时，首先遇到的困难就是药用植物遗传背景基础薄弱。

药用植物有效成分次生代谢途径不清楚是药用植物有效成分功能基因克隆研究的又一难点之一。有效成分次生代谢的基因调控研究重点和难点往往是次生代途径中下游的功能基因的克隆。虽然药用植物有效成分化学结构明确，但其在植物体内的次生代谢途径不清楚，给功能基因的克隆研究和后续的次生代谢基因工程研究等带来了巨大困难。目前水稻和拟南芥基因组测序工作均已完成。正如人基因组测序工作完成以后进入后基因组时代即功能基因研究时代一样，植物的后基因组时代也聚焦于功能基因的研究。此间，参照拟南芥基因信息，许多重要的植物功能基因将被发现。然而，药用植物有效成分与拟南芥次生代谢产物结构往往相差很远，代谢途径差异较大，很难根据拟南芥提供的基因组信息，基于基因的保守结构域，设计合成寡核苷酸简并引物，克隆获得次生代谢相关的功能基因。由于大多数药用植物有效成分次生代谢途径不清楚，按相似序列同源克隆的方法克隆药用植物有效成分相关功能基因极为困难。所以说新的克隆思路和策略将是解决问题的关键所在。

## 2 药用植物功能基因研究新方法的提出

鉴于药用植物研究的特殊性，采用相似基因同源克隆的方法往往难以获得新的功能基因，更不用说次生代谢途径的研究。因此，迫切需要一种理想的药用植物功能基因克隆方法，以推动整个药用植物功能基因研究的快速发展。在这里，笔者首次提出并成功实践了“有效成分差异→功能基因表达差异→功能基因克隆→次生代谢途径”的研究思路和方法。

2.1 *成分差异表型克隆法的概念* 成分差异表型克隆法(ingredient difference phonetypical cloning)，是基于植物次生代谢产物的差异(包括某类成分含量差异和某些成分的有无)为表型特征，运用差异表达基因相关克隆技术来获取次生代谢相关未知基因的一种克隆思路和方法，属于表型克隆的范畴。该方法具有高通量、快速，克隆效率高等特点，适用于未知次生代谢途径中未知功能基因的克隆以及次生代谢途径研究，是该方法的最突出优势。

2.2 *成分差异表型克隆法的原理与方法* 植物细胞在外界环境变化如各种胁迫、诱导子刺激等异常状态下，常有些与次生代谢有关的基因特异性表达或表达异常地增高，导致次生代谢产物特异性生产或积累急剧增加，与正常条件培养的对照组比较，人为造成药用植物有效成分差异和基因表达差异，通过各种差异表达基因克隆技术如差异显示 PCR、抑制性消减杂交和 cDNA 微阵列(cDNA microarray)等技术克隆所需要的次生代谢相关的目的功能基因。

因此，在进行成分差异表型克隆法实验设计时，首先考虑在人为可控条件下，如何促使有效成分差异最大。比如人为地加入诱导子，重金属等促使植物细胞受到异常状态刺激，次生代谢活动增强，迅速特异的产生或快速积累次生代谢产物(有效成分)。其次，经测定并比较对照组与刺激组有效成分的含量差异，选择有效成分差异最大(有效成分有无或含量高低)的 2 组样本做基因表达差异研究。最后，筛选出表达差异大的基因克隆，测序、分析和验证后，进行全长序列的克隆、功能验证等工作。成分差异表型克隆实验流程见图 1。

在这里，有效成分含量测定一般采用高效液相色谱方法，若关注挥发油类成分可采用气相色谱方法，若导致未知成分的差异可选用液-质联用技术测定并分析化学成分结构特点，以获得药用植物最明显的成分差异性状。成分差异表型克隆法可引入目前所有的差异表达克隆研究技术。目前差异表达

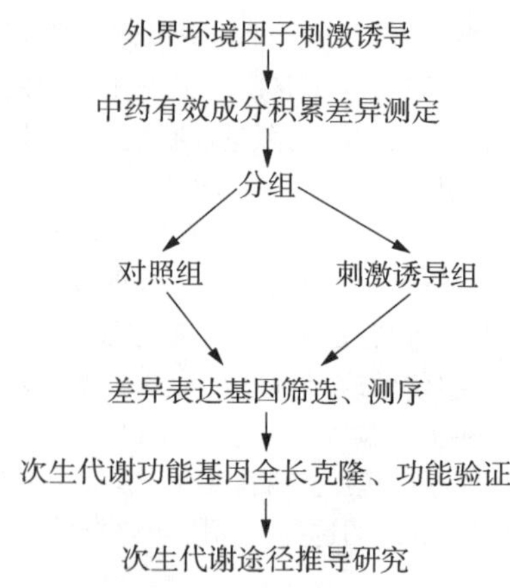


**图 1 成分差异表型克隆法实验流程**

的基因克隆技术主要有消减杂交(subtractive hybridization, SH)，mRNA 差异显示技术(mRNA differential display reverse transcription PCR, DDRT-PCR)、抑制消减杂交(suppression subtractive hybridization, SSH)和 cDNA 微阵列技术(cDNA microarray)等。

2.3 *成分差异表型克隆法的优势与应用*

2.3.1 *优势* 成分差异表型克隆方法最突出的优点是高通量，效率高，一次能同时克隆次生代谢途径上的多个功能基因。如果把功能基因克隆视为钓鱼的话，基于相似基因的同源克隆 1 次只能钓取 1 条鱼，而差异基因表型克隆法可以 1 次网罗数条鱼，速度快、效率高。

以诱导子作为外界环境刺激因子，依托丹参基因芯片的技术平台，采用成分差异表型克隆方法克隆得到了丹参有效成分次生代谢相关的 6 个功能基因见表 1。在这些基因中，1 个基因参与了丹参水溶性成分酚酸类成分的代谢(Sm4CL)，5 个基因参与了丹参酮类化合物次生代谢(SmAACT, SmCMK, SmIPP, SmFPPS, SmKS)，并在 GenBank 上注册了 5 个与丹参酮成分代谢相关的功能基因。

**表 1 丹参次生代谢途径关键基因编码的酶、催化前体物质及产物**

| GenBank 注册号 | 编码的酶 | 催化前体物质 | 催化产物 |
|---|---|---|---|
| — | 4-香豆酸-CoA 连接酶(Sm4CL) | 4-香豆酸 | 4-香豆酸 CoA |
| F635969 | 乙酰 CoA 酰基转运酶(SmAACT) | 乙酰 CoA | 乙酰乙酰 CoA |
| EF534309 | 4-(5′-焦磷酸胞苷)-2-C-甲基-*D*-赤藓醇激酶(SmCMK) | 4-(5-焦磷酸胞苷)-2-C-甲基-*D*-赤藓醇 | 4-(5-焦磷酸胞苷)-2-C-甲基-*D*-赤藓醇-2-磷酸 |
| EF635967 | 异戊烯基焦 δ 异构酶(SmIPP) | 羟甲基丁烯基-4-磷酸 | 异戊烯基焦磷酸 |
| EF635968 | 法呢基焦磷酸合成酶(SmFPPS) | 牻牛儿基焦磷酸(GPP) | 法呢基焦磷酸(FPP) |
| EF635966 | 内根-贝壳杉烯合酶(SmKS) | 古巴焦磷酸 | 内根-贝壳杉烯 |

2.3.2 应用 系统揭示次生代谢与外界环境刺激因子之间的生物网络关系，有利于阐明次生代谢功能基因表达调控机制。以诱导子作为外界环境刺激因子为例：诱导子与细胞膜上受体的结合，这一过程会引起膜成分的变化以致引起膜的通透性、膜内离子分布的变化。诱导子作为外界信号作用胞质膜而引起膜上发生变化，到引起胞内基因启动、酶活性改变的过程应该是一个级联过程，这中间需要有物质充当胞内信使，也即第二信使。目前人们由实验推出的主要第二信使包括 $Ca^{2+}$、cAMP、磷酸肌醇、G2 蛋白、水杨酸、茉莉酮酸及其甲氧基酯以及植物细胞壁组成成分等。诱导子信号被传递到细胞内以后，通过控制次生代谢途径中关键酶的合成来调节次生代谢产物的合成。

采用成分差异表型克隆法克隆得到了丹参信号转导相关的蛋白，应激原蛋白，水通道及金属相关蛋白酶基因等与次生代谢调控相联系的一些基因，为进一步阐述有效成分功能基因表达的调控机制奠定了基础(表 2)。

**表 2 成分差异表型克隆法克隆得到丹参次生代谢功能基因的相关调控基因**

| 克隆号 | 获得的差异表达基因 | 诱导组与对照组表达差异倍数 |
|---|---|---|
| chip44d06 | 水通道(PIP2;8/PIP3B) | 1.610 |
| chip39b01 | CBL-交互作用蛋白激酶 | 2.025 |
| chip31h02 | DNA 结合/转录因子 | 0.465 |
| chip36h12 | 变应原 Cora 1 | 3.455 |
| chip41b06 | 硫酸根载体蛋白 | 2.515 |
| chip45h02 | 胁迫与致病响应蛋白 | 2.765 |
| chip19g08 | 致病响应蛋白-10 | 2.345 |
| chip29h02 | 金属硫蛋白-1(MT-1) | 0.285 |

## 3 讨论

药用植物有效成分克隆方法和策略的局限是限制药用植物功能基因克隆的瓶颈之一。目前药用植物功能基因的克隆普遍采用同源性为基础的 PCR 克隆策略。此法虽然简单，经济，但它只能克隆相关物种上已克隆出的相似基因，使简并引物扩增效率不高，在 PCR 扩增时有一定的偶然性和随机性，不具备高通量克隆功能基因的能力。此法克隆药用植物有效成分生物合成上游途径相关酶基因具有一定可行性，但对于下游未知途径、未知或同源性较低的已知基因序列的新基因的克隆几乎不可能。基因差异表达在植物领域研究比较广泛，但主要集中在植物胚胎发育、形态发生、信号传导、植物抗逆、抗病、抗虫等基因的鉴定与克隆的研究方面。例如 Wilkinson 等克隆了番茄成熟基因，Nemoto 等从小麦中克隆到几个新的盐反应早期响应基因等，主要是通过比较同一类细胞在不同生理状态下或在不同生长发育阶段基因表达的差异。药用植物与一般植物研究的侧重点不同，它主要关注有效成分次生代谢及其含量，目前，根据成分变化应用基因差异表达克隆的研究报道还比较少。

成分差异表型克隆法的提出，将研究者视线再一次聚焦到药用植物有效成分这一重要而特殊的研究对象上来。跟农作物性状与遗传信息的关系一样，药用植物有效成分(次生代谢产物)跟遗传信息(基因)紧密联系。成分差异表型克隆研究为了最大限度地消除外界不可控因素的影响，其理想状态是对药用植物采用统一可控制的培养条件，外加人为的刺激(外因)比如加入诱导子等，促使药用植物细胞产生成分最大差异性状，通过基因差异表达克隆技术获取相应的目的功能基因。

此外，植物的次生代谢往往受外界环境因子的影响。因此，成分差异表型克隆方法可广泛用于道地药材形成机制的研究中，研究道地药材有效成分的次生代谢、基因与环境互作之间的交互网络关系。可以预见，随着药用植物资源研究的不断深入、药用植物道地药材形成机制研究的逐步展开，功能基因组研究的日益白热化，成分差异表型克隆法的应用将迅速促进功能基因组与药用植物研究紧密结合，推动药用植物现代化的快速发展。

[王学勇，黄璐琦，等. 中国中药杂志，2009，34(1)：14-17.]

# 探讨道地药材研究的模式生物及模型

道地药材(geoherbs)是中医临床长期、反复实践中产生和公认的优质中药材，它的形成与我国特有的生态地理、文化背景及中医药理论等有关。面对这样一复杂的，特别是包含有人文科学的系统，选择适合的研究思路与方法极其重要。道地药材在临床上的确切疗效是其科学价值的核心，物质成分是产生疗效的基础，因此研究道地药材物质基础的生物学成因十分关键。道地药材物质基础的表现形式(表型)包括药材性状、组织结构、有效成分的组成和含量及其疗效等，其取决于道地药材原植物的基因型及其所处的环境，即“表型＝基因型＋环境饰变”。这是道地药材物质基础生物学成因的核心理论假说，为使这一假说得到证实，作者在唇形科药用植物丹参 *Salvia miltiorrhiza* Bunge 的研究基础上，设计了相关的实验模型，同时探讨以丹参为模式生物来研究道地药材的前景。

## 1 道地药材研究的问题探讨

前人对道地药材的研究主要是从本草考证、药材性状、有效成分、药效、生态环境、遗传基因、栽培和采收加工技术等多方面进行。通过对道地药材研究现状进行分析，道地药材的研究存在以下几个问题：①没有从道地药材是一个涉及遗传、环境以及人文这一复杂系统出发，树立起系统复杂性科学的思想观念，即使有多学科的联合研究，但相互之间没有进行有机的联系。②对研究所取得的成果只是进行孤立地分析，没有遵循科学的规律，围绕相应的假说和理论，进行阐述和验证。③观察分析没有把数学作为基本工具，对研究样本的代表性、全面性及结果等没有统计学的量化分析及处理。为更有效率的解决道地药材研究中的问题，首先应该剖析出道地药材这一复杂系统的核心部分，在此基础上，根据相关的假说来设计研究模型，进行受控实验，运用系统生物学的思路和方法进行研究。

道地药材的物质基础主要包括其种源(遗传物质基础)和化学物质基础等。由于中药材复杂的化学组成及其多靶点、多途径的作用机制，现在的研究水平很难得到全面的解析和控制，然而这些物质基础产生的内因之一取决于生物体本身的遗传物质，因此种源对每一种道地药材来说是相对固定的。一般认为道地药材的生物内涵是同种异地，即同一物种因其具有一定的空间结构，能在不同的地点上形成大大小小的群体单元，其中如果某一群体产生质优效佳的药材，即为“道地药材”。对于道地药材化学物质基础来说，主要包括初生代谢物：多糖、脂肪、蛋白和核酸等；次生代谢物：生物碱、酚类、黄酮、蒽醌、木质素、香豆素、萜类、甾类、皂苷、多炔类、有机酸等；金属和非金属元素等等。它们可能都是道地药材良好药效的物质基础，但一般认为次生代谢物是药理活性中最为重要的部分。

植物次生代谢是植物在长期进化中对生态环境适应的结果。许多植物在受到病原微生物侵染后，产生并积累用以增强自身抵抗力的小分子抗生物质，如很多具有药用价值的萜类、生物碱和异黄酮等。某些次生代谢物与植物寄生物宿主专一性及寄生物与宿主间的相互作用有关，如植物的黄酮类成分与根瘤菌共生固氮、酚类物质与根癌农杆菌 T-DNA 转移，都有密切联系。还有些次生代谢物与植物异株相克、种子传播、吸引昆虫授粉以及防御捕食有关。甚至在正常条件变化以及不良环境对次生代谢物质的积累也会造成影响，如树荫对黄酮类的积累就会造成影响。这表明植物次生代谢物的产生和积累主要是由特定的遗传基础与其所处的环境中的各种因子相互作用所决定。因此探明有效成分、基因型和环境三者的关系是研究道地药材物质基础的生物学成因核心的内容。

## 2 道地药材研究的模式生物及模型

模式生物通常指人们研究生命现象过程中长期、反复作为实验材料的物种，并且从模式生物的研究中得出的生命规律往往代表了许多物种的共同规律。人们在对模式物种的形态、解剖、生理、生化、细胞及遗传进行全面分析和归纳的基础上，把它们作为典范，将研究得出的规律，推演到相关的生物物种中，从而加快其他生物物种的研究。一般每种模式生物只能在一两个研究领域中拥有自己的优势，如果蝇在生物遗传学研究中的地位是不可动摇的；粗糙脉孢菌是生物化学研究中的重要模式生物；高等植物中的玉米是遗传分析的典型材料，生物界著名的 Barbara MoClintock 有关转座因子的理论就是以玉米作为研究材料，从而成了分子遗传学发展史上的重要里程碑；其他还有大肠杆菌、啤酒酵母、小鼠，线虫和拟南芥等生物都在自己的领域中扮演重要的角色。整体说来模式生物应该有以下特征：取材方便、生物周期短、遗传背景较清晰、实验方法通用、具有遗传改造和表型分析手段、有利于同行的交流等。

对道地药材这一复杂系统来说，如果能够借鉴模式生物的方法学，选择具有代表性的道地药材，针对相关关键问题进行系统深入的研究，揭示共性问题，树立研究典范，将有很大的现实意义。作者根据道地药材物质基础生物学成因研究的特征，初步认为其模式生物必须具备以下条件：生物材料来源广；遗传背景较清楚；药效成分研究较清楚，并且分析技术成熟；具备相关生物学研究手段和技术；具有建立实验模型的潜力；分布区域广且生态环境多样等。结合以上特征，基于本课题组对丹参 *S. miltiorrhiza* 所进行的系统研究，现提出丹参作为道地药材研究的模式生物具有一定的基础和优势。

2.1 丹参为模式生物的基础

2.1.1 丹参分布区广，道地性明确 丹参 *S. miltiorrhiza* 为唇形科 Labiatae 鼠尾草属 *Salvia* 植物。其分布区广，南起江西、湖南，北达辽宁，西至四川、陕西、甘肃等省；分布环境多样，野生丹参常见于海拔 120～1 300 m 的山地丘陵中的山坡、草丛、林下、溪谷旁；对环境干扰较敏感，喜光、温和湿润的环境，耐寒、怕旱、怕涝等。丹参药材各产地药效成分的质和量存在显著的差异，道地性显著。在针对丹参的遗传、环境和化学成分等三方面的关系研究中，初步认为，同产地不同丹参品种(系)之间其有效成分的含量存在显著性差异，并且同一丹参品种(系)在不同产地种植其有效成分的含量也存在显著性差异；同时，丹参有效成分的积累与土壤因子之间的关系存在基因型差异，脂溶性成分与水溶性成分积累与土壤因子的关系有明显的不同。这些进一步说明，丹参有效成分的积累与遗传和环境密切相关，为研究丹参道地药材物质基础生物学成因提供了良好基础。

2.1.2 丹参药效及其物质基础清晰 丹参药材中主要含有以脂溶性的二萜醌类和水溶性的酚酸类化合物组成的多组分物质，其发挥药效的物质基础取决于所含的多种化学成分的综合作用。目前在丹参植物中已经分离得到多种具有抗菌、调节内分泌等作用的脂溶性化合物，主要包括丹参酮Ⅰ、丹参酮$Ⅱ_A$等。丹参水溶性成分主要为丹参素、丹酚酸 A 和丹酚酸 B，还有迷迭香酸、紫草酸等，这些成分主要有抗氧化、内皮细胞的保护、心脏和血管作用等。近来对丹参作用机制有了进一步的研究又发现其具有抗肿瘤等作用。丹参药材化学物质的分析检测水平也较成熟，建立了一批如 HPLC-$MS^n$，HPLC-DAD-ESI-$MS^n$ 等特异性强和灵敏度高的方法。

2.1.3 丹参次生代谢成分的生物合成途径已有较好的研究基础 丹参为遗传多样性较丰富的物种；染色体数目为 2n=2x=14，基因组较小；并且丹参次生代谢产物种类多，主要包含萜类和苯丙烷类两大代谢途径来源的次生代谢成分，是研究药用植物次生代谢途径及其调控的较好模式物种。丹参脂溶性的成分主要是丹参酮等二萜醌类化合物。目前,由于国际上对生物合成植物激素赤霉素和裸子植物红豆杉中二萜类次生代谢产物紫杉醇的关键基因的克隆和功能研究,相关生物合成途径已逐渐明晰,这为丹参中二萜类化合物的生物合成方面的研究提供了较好基础。

近来针对丹参酮类成分生物合成途径的研究取得巨大的进展。本研究组以丹参毛状根为材料,运用基因芯片分析技术得到了多个参与丹参酮类生物合成途径的关键酶基因以及相关调控基因的信息,并经过多种克隆技术得到了以下酶的全长 cDNA:来源于 MVA 途径的乙酰 CoA C 酰基转运酶(acetyl-CoA: acetyl-CoA C-acetyltransferase, AACT),3 羟基-3-甲基戊二酰 CoA 还原酶(3-hydroxy-3-methylglutaryl-CoA reductase, HMGR)基因;来源于 DXP 途径的 5′-焦磷酸胞苷-2-C 甲基-D 赤藓醇激酶[4-(cytidine 5-diPhospho)-2-C-methylerythritol kinase, CMK], DXP 还原异构酶(1-deoxy-D-xylulose 5-Phosphate reductoisom erase, DXR)基因;在中游途径中包括异戊烯基焦磷酸异构酶(IPP isomerase, IPI)、法呢基焦磷酸合成酶(famesyl pyrophosphate synthetase, FPS)、牻牛儿基牻牛儿基二磷酸合酶(geranylgeranyl diphosphate synthase, GGPS)等关键酶基因;下游途径中克隆到了重要的类贝壳杉烯合酶(entkaurene synthase like, KSL)和柯巴基焦磷酸合酶(copalyl diphosphate synthase, CPS)以及相关 P450 酶基因;并且得到相关转录因子和 microRNA 的生物信息;相关基因的功能鉴定和转基因等工作正在进行。

丹参水溶性酚酸类化合物,除丹参素和咖啡酸等几种单苯环物质可由氨基酸直接氧化脱氨生成外,其余均可视为由咖啡酸与丹参素酯化缩合产生。根据 Yamamoto 等的工作,将迷迭香酸生物合成途径加以概括。苯丙氨酸解氨酶(PAL)是苯丙氨酸进入此代谢途径的限速酶,4-香豆酸辅酶 A 连接酶(4CL)催化产生活化形式的 4-香豆酰 CoA 是后续分支途径的前体分子之一。4-香豆酰 CoA 和由酪氨酸经酪氨酸 α 酮戊二酸转氨酶(TAT)的氧化脱氨和羟基苯丙酮酸还原酶(HPR)的还原作用产生的 4 羟基苯乳酸,在迷迭香酸合成酶(RS)作用下首先生成 2 氧-(4 香豆酰)-3-(4-羟基苯)乳酸(迷迭香酸生物合成途径中一个重要的中间产物),最后由细胞色素 $P_{450}$ 蛋白-CYP98A6 的催化生成迷迭香酸。对丹参的研究 Zhao Shujuan 等克隆和分析了参与丹参水溶性酚酸类生物合成中的关键酶基因 4-香豆酸辅酶 A 连接酶(4CL)基因 Sm4CL1 和 Sm4CL2,并初步证明 Sm4CL2 比 Sm4CL1 在此途径中扮演更重要的角色。

2.1.4 丹参有丰富的研究材料 丹参的生物工程方面的研究有相当基础,有丹参组培苗,多倍体材料,水培苗,不定根,愈伤组织,毛状根,细胞培养系等各种组织器官水平的实验材料,并且有获得以上实验材料的成熟技术。基于次生代谢积累的功能基因组学的研究中,丹参的萜类和酚酸类的生物合成途径中的功能基因研究已经逐步深入,相关技术如 DNA 和 RNA 提取分析技术;基因克隆和基因芯片技术;原核和真核验证体系;转基因技术(过表达和 RNA 等)和代谢组学分析等高精度的分析技术已基本成熟。

2.2 “丹参毛状根”研究模型及其他相关研究模型的建立 针对道地药材物质基础生物学成因的模式假说:表型=基因型+环境饰变,以丹参为生物载体建立了相关的模型,用受控实验来验证这一假说。本研究组建立了“丹参毛状根”研究模型,并针对模型的特性进行研究:①再现性,作为研究道地药材的模型要考察毛状根和其原型(即原药材)之间的相似性,包括化学成分,毒性以及药效等,来阐明毛状根是否具有再现原药材的特性。②稳定性,毛状根的核 DNA 的稳定性、rol 基因遗传稳定性、化学成分稳定性等。③实用性,在证明毛状根模型具有稳定性和再现性的基础上,对其作为模型的实用性进行了研究,主要包括:模拟环境因子,即通过改变毛状根培养条件,如温度、光照、矿物营养水平、pH、激素诱导等研究其生长量和有效成分含量的变化,确定不同环境条件下的表型变异;模拟遗传因子,即通过改变毛状根的遗传物质,如转基因、化学诱变,或利用不同基因型丹参的毛状根研究其生长状况和有效成分含量的变化,确定表型变异的遗传机制;并考察毛状根是否便于取材和作为模型是否易于建立和使用等多方面进行了系统评价。表明该模型具备相似性、可重复性、开放性、易用性、定量和定性相结合等特征,可以在以下几方面进行道地丹参成因的研究:①道地丹参生物学特征的环境影响因子。②基因型对道地丹参生物学特征的影响。③道地丹参形成中功能基因的作用。④道地丹参形成中环境与遗传因子的相互作用等。

其他以组培丹参或转基因丹参苗为材料的研究模型正在研究和评价,主要内容包括:①分析遗传因子对同一环境下丹参的影响。②研究较大环境因子(如人工气候室)对同一遗传背景的丹参的影响。③用于“丹参毛状根”研究模型的放大验证。这些将能对道地药材物质基础生物学成因的研究有重大的突破。

## 3 展望

建立可控的研究模型及树立模式生物来集中研究道地药材的生物学成因,在研究方法的可控性及相关指标和因子的可数据化;研究的系统性和全面性;各类资源的优化配置等方面拥有很多优点,这有望在道地药材研究中取得突破进展。丹参作为各“模型”的载体生物,以其在化学物质基础、药理、细胞和分子生物学等方面深入研究的基础,认为丹参可以作为模式生物来研究道地药材生物学成因。

[黄璐琦,等.中国中药杂志,2009,34(9):1063-1066.]

# 基于同源基因功能分化的药用植物活性成分变异机制研究

搞清药用植物活性成分变异的机制一直是中药资源和中药鉴定研究领域的热点问题，其对于药材质量控制具有重要的意义。中药材来源复杂，表现为同属多来源药材均可作为一种药材入药，如膜荚黄芪和蒙古黄芪均为药材黄芪的基原植物；同一药材不同部位也可作为不同药材使用，如葫芦科植物栝楼或双边栝楼的干燥成熟果皮可作为瓜蒌皮使用，干燥成熟种子可作为瓜蒌子使用，干燥根可作为天花粉使用；不同产地的药材，其化学成分也因所生长环境的不同而不同。

尽管入药物种或部位具有相似性，但在药效上仍然存在一定的差异。药效上的相似与差异主要由活性成分的异同来决定，而目前中药活性成分评价主要集中在化学和药理学领域，但由于植物中存在数以万计的化合物，利用化学分析手段始终不能满足对中药材所有成分进行分析，因此存在着一定的缺陷。利用药理学手段进行评价则需要选择合适、可靠的药理研究模型，工作量较大。从植物本身来看，活性成分的形成和积累与其体内基因及基因调控网络密切相关，即活性成分的异同是由基因的变异决定的。随着高通量测序技术的发展和成本的降低，已经有大量的药用植物通过 RNA-seq 进行了转录组研究，获得了基因序列。然而，完成转录组测序仅是功能基因组研究的第一步，更大的挑战在于搞清基因序列的遗传信息与其所执行的生物学功能。本文详细介绍了同源基因、基因重复的概念和分类，并重点展望了重复基因功能分化在药用植物活性成分变异分子机制研究中的作用，旨在为药材质量控制基础研究提供新的思路。

## 1 同源基因的正确注释是研究药用植物活性成分变异的重要前提

研究基因序列的遗传信息与其所执行的生物学功能，首先取决于对基因序列的正确注释。目前基因注释的方法主要依赖于生物信息学分析，同源性在基因注释中是一个极其重要的概念，同源基因一般不会有完全一致的核苷酸序列，因为同源基因在出现后会独立的发生随机突变，但它们的序列组成相似，大部分未突变的核苷酸位置相同。因此，一个新的基因序列被确认后，根据同源性可从数据库中找到已知序列的同源基因，并依据进化的相关性可从已知同源基因推测新基因的功能。同源基因分为直向同源基因（orthologous gene）和共生同源基因（paralogous gene）两类。

1.1 直向同源基因与种间变异 直向同源基因指 2 种或 2 种以上不同物种之间的同源基因，它们来自物种分隔之前同一祖先的同源序列。直系同源的序列通常具有相似的结构和生物学功能，即功能高度保守甚至近乎相同，且其在近缘物种间可以相互替换，一般是编码生命活动必需的关键性调控蛋白、酶或辅酶的基因。基因组学、功能基因组学、分子系统学、进化生物学等生命科学领域多个学科的研究均依赖于直系同源基因的识别，如物种新发现基因的功能预测、系统发生关系的构建及重现基因的进化历史等。许多直系同源基因均具有序列变化速度与进化距离相当、调控途径相似且能够重现物种进化历史等特征。由于系统发育树的构建需要不同群体间的直系同源基因，因此完整、正确的直系同源基因识别是重现基因进化过程重要的前提。

目前发现的功能千变万化的基因最初都是由少量祖先基因通过基因加倍、变异和功能域重组产生的。因此，通过基因序列的比较，可从同一物种或不同物种中找到同源的基因成员。随着药用植物转录组数据的增加，鉴定和区分这些具有相同或者不同功能的同源基因以及对控制元件进行识别，已成为药用植物功能基因组研究的重要内容之一。同时，识别直系同源基因可以帮助重建进化历史，了解垂直遗传关系和谱系特有的基因丢失以及基因水平转移，对于解析药用植物种及品种间活性成分变异将具有重要的意义。

1.2 共生同源基因与药用植物器官间活性成分变异 共生同源基因（paralogous gene），指同一物种内部的同源基因，其常为多基因家族的不同成员，其共同的祖先基因可能存在于物种形成之后，也可能存在于物种形成之前。祖先基因的复制及其突变形成了基因家族，这是增加基因组复杂性的一个重要途径。多基因家族是真核生物基因组的共同特征，即因基因加倍和趋异产生了许多在 DNA 序列组成上基本一致而略有不同的成员。同一家族的基因成员在序列组成上相似，且担负类似的生物学功能，如苯丙氨酸解旋酶（PAL）在金银花中存在 3 个成员，在黄芩中存在 4 个成员，这些基因成员具有相似的功能，但它们在个体发育的不同阶段表达。比较基因家族中各个成员间的序列差异，可追踪基因的进化轨迹，研究基因复制及功能分化对于解析药用植物器官间活性成分变异将具有重要的意义。

## 2 重复基因的功能分化是形成药用植物活性成分变异的基础

2.1 基因重复 基因重复现象是生物界广泛存在的，遍布原核和真核生物，特别是高等被子植物在进化过程中由于经历了多次多倍化过程，产生了大量的重复基因。由于重复基因的进化可以诱导基因表达模式的分化从而满足物种发育的需求，因此基因重复是推动植物进化最重要的驱动力，也是产生新功能基因的重要来源。

研究重复基因对于揭示重复基因结构变异及其功能分化具有重要意义。根据重复区域的大小，基因重复可分为：小规模基因重复，即单个基因重复；大规模基因重复，包括部分基因组重复以及整个基因组重复（多倍体化）。单个基因和部分基因组重复主要通过不等交换产生，而全基因组重复是由有丝分裂或减数分裂过程中的错误引发决定的。单个基因重复可以导致同一个基因组内存在2个或2个以上拷贝(copy)的同源基因序列,从而可能造成功能上的冗余(redundant),并受到剂量效应的调节。

2.2 重复基因的亚功能化与新功能化 由于通过基因重复拷贝不同的表达分化以及选择作用可以促使植物加快应对胁迫环境生理反应机制的进化,从而产生适应特殊环境条件的多样性形态特征,所以基因重复在植物环境适应性及进化过程中起着重要作用。重复基因的保留机制一直是人们关注的热点问题之一。经过自然选择的作用,保留下来的重复基因,除了因其中1个拷贝发生突变导致非功能化(nonfunctionalization)而形成为假基因(pseudogene)外,大致面临以下2种不同的命运:新功能化(neofunctionalization),即其中1个拷贝保留了原始的功能,另1个拷贝获得了新的功能。重复基因间的表达分化是重复基因产生新功能非常重要的一步,其可以提高基因的功能和表达的复杂性,有助于促进植物形成特异性的防御机制。由于选择压力的松弛,基因重复产生的冗余基因得以在加速碱基替换速率的同时,各自积累不同的遗传变异,使基因的结构和功能发生改变,分化产生适用于新的生存环境相应的功能或表达调节机制。所以环境胁迫相关联的重复基因,包括大量作为植保素的次生代谢产物相关重复基因,更倾向发生基因表达分化。亚功能化(subfunctionalization),即2个拷贝发生了亚功能化,分担了原基因的功能,而它们合起来的功能则涵盖了祖先基因功能。基因亚功能化同样也主要是由于自然选择压力松弛,导致重复基因不同拷贝的表达具有时空性,即在表达时间和组织特异性方面产生明显分化,且各自分担了祖先基因的部分功能而被选择作用所保留,且突变积累主要发生在基因表达或转录调控区。

随着基因组研究的深入,重复基因保留进化模式也被不断地更新和完善,在一定范围内阐释重复基因不同水平的进化方式。其中DDC(duplication degeneration complementation)模型,即重复基因亚功能化拷贝可被随机遗传漂变保留固定,拷贝间功能互补,共同完成原祖先基因的功能;SNF(subneofunctionalization)模型认为,在长期进化过程中,发生亚功能化的基因可能各自形成了新的功能。

## 3 药用植物基因功能分化决定其活性成分的变异

3.1 活性成分部位差异的分子机制 药材赤芍和白芍均来源于植物芍药 *Paeonia lactiflora* 的干燥根,长久以来关于它们的分类标准始终存在争论,如花色、产地、加工方式等。目前市场上出售的白芍一般为去皮干燥根,而赤芍为干燥根,本课题组首先利用芍药转录组数据获得芍药苷(paeoniflorin)和没食子酸(gallic acid)生物合成途径关键酶基因家族成员序列,并分别选择具有相同成分的牡丹转录组和不具有芍药苷、具有没食子酸的石榴 *Punica granatum*、刺果毒漆藤 *Rhus radicans*、马桑 *Coriariane palensis* 转录组中的直向同源基因作为对照,构建系统进化树。在此基础上,对14个活性成分相关同源基因功能多样性进行预测。结果表明,芍药没食子酸生物合成途径中的PLaroDE共生同源基因可能具有相同的功能,而它们的直向同源基因在石榴、刺果毒漆藤、马桑中也存在。结合基因表达分析结果,预测aroDE同源基因在芍药的不同组织中具有相似的表达谱,且与芳香族氨基酸含量有关。芍药苷生物合成途径上的PLDXPS共生同源基因可能具有不同的功能,且在芍药不同组织中的表达谱不一致,暗示其功能分化可能影响化学成分的分化。通过比较芍药根与根皮基因表达谱,还发现芍药苷及其芳香族氨基酸衍生物生物合成相关基因 *PLaroDEs*、*PLMVK*、*PLPMK*、*PLMVD*1在根皮中的转录水平显著高于去皮根,与根皮中该类成分含量高一致,支持了依据根皮的有无作为药材白芍、赤芍分类的标准。

3.2 活性成分物种差异的分子机制 2010年版《中国药典》中收载的金银花类药材包括两类,即金银花(忍冬)、山银花(红腺忍冬、华南忍冬、红腺忍冬、黄褐毛忍冬)。绿原酸和木樨草苷是金银花的主要活性成分,本课题组对金银花转录组进行分析,共获得14.9 GB数据,对获得的数据进行分析,共获得4万余个UniGene。以金银花化学成分为切入点,围绕酚酸类、萜类、脂肪酸生物合成途径,初步构建了金银花活性成分基因调控网络,筛选获得用于评价金银花化学质量的关键酶。在此基础上,重点比较了忍冬与红腺忍冬、灰毡毛忍冬、华南忍冬中绿原酸和木樨草素生物合成途径关键酶同源基因的结构及其在花蕾和叶中表达模式的变异,其与活性成分变异具有一致性。以上分析结果为进一步理解金银花类药材不同部位间活性成分变异以及药用物种的利用提供了依据。

3.3 展望 药用植物活性成分相关基因家族成员功能分化是研究基因变异决定活性成分变异机制的重要内容之一。依赖药用植物转录组数据,克隆获得活性成分相关直向同源基因和共生同源基因,建立药用植物基因数据库。在基因进化理论和方法的指导下,对药用植物重复基因功能分化进行分析,并与活性成分种类和数量变化相结合,从分子生药学角度揭示药用植物物种、部位、产地间活性成分差异的机制,从而为指导药材质量控制提供理论依据。

[袁媛,黄璐琦,等.中国中药杂志,2015,40(6):1023-1026.]

# 表观遗传与药材道地性研究探讨

近年来对药材道地性研究已经有很多论述,黄璐琦等从生物学角度出发,认为药材道地性与其表型、遗传背景及环境有着密切的关系,且道地药材具有特异性、地域性、连续性和迁延性特征。道地药材通常在居群水平存在某些特异性表型特征，如茅山苍术断面可见明显的棕红色油腺，俗称“朱砂点”；铜陵凤丹皮的主要特点是肉厚、木心细、香味浓等，这些独特的表型特征均与药用植物的生长发育有着密切的关系。

除经典遗传之外，表观遗传现象如DNA甲基化、组蛋白修饰、非编码RNA等在植物的生长发育中也发挥重要作用。伴随着表观遗传学研究的不断深入，将药材道地性与表观遗传相联系是未来研究的重点方向之一。本文主要从植物生长发育表观调控和道地药材特征研究入手，探讨基于表观遗传的药材道地性形成机制研究前景，为道地药材质量评价和鉴别提供依据。

## 1 表观遗传的范畴

表观遗传学(epigenetics)又称“表遗传学”“外遗传学”以及“后遗传学”，在生物学和特定的遗传学领域，其研究的是在不改变DNA序列的前提下，通过某些机制引起可遗传的基因表达或细胞表现型的变化。“表观遗传”的概念由发育生物学家Conrad Waddington在20世纪40年代提出，最初用来描述基因之间以及基因与环境间的相互作用，后来被进一步定义为在不改变基因的编码序列或上游启动子区域的情况下，生物表型、形态或分子层级的改变。

表观遗传学作为阐明基因组功能及基因表达的关键研究领域之一，已成为生命科学研究热点。DNA编码的遗传信息为生命活动提供遗传物质基础，而表观遗传调控则提供了何时、何地、以何种方式去应用遗传指令，它与经典遗传学共同组成了完整的基因调控网络。表观遗传学的研究内容主要包括DNA甲基化、染色质重塑和基因组印迹等方面，其中因染色质重塑、组蛋白修饰及组蛋白H3的特殊甲基化均通过调节DNA甲基化信号改变表型性状的遗传特征，目前对DNA甲基化的研究最为活跃。

## 2 DNA甲基化与基因表达调控

甲基化是基因组DNA的一种主要表观遗传修饰形式，是调节基因功能的重要手段。DNA甲基化(DNA methylation)是指在DNA甲基转移酶(DNA-methyltransferases, DN-MTs)的催化下，CpG二核苷酸中的胞嘧啶被选择性地添加甲基，形成5-甲基胞嘧啶。DNA甲基转移酶可分为2种：一种是维持甲基化酶(DNMT1)，它能使半甲基化的DNA双链分子上与甲基胞嘧啶相对应的胞嘧啶甲基化，可参与DNA复制双链中新合成链的甲基化；另一种是重新甲基化酶，如Dnmt3a和Dnmt3b等，它们使去甲基化的CpG位点重新甲基化。DNA甲基化一般与基因的沉默相关，而DNA去甲基化则与基因的活化相关。

DNA甲基化在植物基因组防御、调控基因表达以及控制植物的生长和发育中起重要作用，对植物本身有着积极的意义。DNA甲基化可调控特定的内源基因表达，即抑制rRNA基因的表达、控制重复基因家族全部基因的表达、植物启动子区的DNA甲基化通常抑制转录，但基因编码区的甲基化一般不会影响基因表达。

## 3 表观遗传与特异性表型

表型特征的形成过程是十分复杂的，不同产地、不同种质、不同发育阶段均会对药用植物表型产生影响。与药材道地性特异性表型相关的功能基因在内外环境下选择性的表达难以用经典遗传学的理论和方法来诠释。越来越多的证据表明，表观遗传修饰与物种间和物种内的表型变异有关，甚至从宏观上会影响物种的进化。目前已有一些表观遗传对植物表型差异影响的报道，如郑小国等论述了表观遗传学对植物株高、生育期、花型、果实着色以及应对环境胁迫等方面的影响。汪媛媛和王子成研究了DNA甲基化抑制剂5-氮杂胞嘧啶核苷(5-azaC)对菊花的影响，发现5-azaC处理能够影响丛生芽的分化、株高和根长等表型性状，且低浓度5-azaC处理可以使菊花提前开花。

同时表观遗传也会影响药用植物次生代谢产物的积累，本项目组发现尽管金银花、红金银花活性成分生物合成关键酶基因的表达存在显著差异，但其序列基本不变。倪竹君等利用5-azaC处理石斛组培苗，分析石斛苗生长变化、生物活性物质含量及其相关基因表达变化，发现多糖含量和生物碱含量明显上升，编码生物碱合成酶的基因相对表达量均显著上调，说明5-azaC去甲基化修饰处理可能激活了这些生物碱合成相关基因表达，从而证实了DNA去甲基化修饰对石斛次生代谢产物的生物合成具有重要的调控作用。

作为表观遗传修饰的重要调控方式，DNA甲基化或组蛋白修饰可以直接干扰转录因子与其识别位点的结合，进而影响基因转录的正常进行。因此，分析药材功能基因在内外环境下选择性表达遗传信息的分子机制，并结合表型分析结果开展药材道地性特征形成的表观遗传学机制研究，将为道地药材特征辨识提供理论支撑。

## 4 表观遗传与道地药材地域性

环境因子在道地药材形成中的作用毋庸置疑，但环境因子究竟是如何通过修饰道地药材的基因型而发生作用的，生态因子与道地药材次生代谢产物积累又有着怎样的关系，至今缺少直接的和系统地实验研究的揭示和证明。针对这些问题，表观遗传学研究将可以给予解答。

近年来的研究对环境因素影响植物表观遗传变化进行了一些探讨，温度、水分、高盐、重金属等非生物胁迫能够通过诱导DNA甲基化的动态变化调控逆境应答基因的表达，从而提高植物对环境的适应能力。如铝、百草枯、盐、冷等胁迫诱导了烟草中*NtGPDL*(glycerophosphodiester-ase-like protein)基因编码序列的去甲基化，从而促进该基因的表达。植物对环境胁迫诱导的应答或抗性可以是短暂时，也可以是长期的，这种获得抗性也可以是跨代遗传的，后者称为植物胁迫记忆或印记。植物胁迫记忆与逆境诱导的DNA甲基化变异能够遗传有着密切的联系，蒲公英*Taraxacum officinale*无性系DNA甲基化的研究揭示胁迫处理组中甲基化位点改变的比例比对照组的高，而且发现DNA甲基化的改变能够延续到它们的后代。经历胁迫的植物后代即使在没有胁迫条件下，也显示出基因组整体的超甲基化状态。这种超甲基化可能是植物采取的一种胁迫环境下维持基因组稳定性的防御机制。经历非生物胁迫的拟南芥后代对胁迫的抗性得到增强，如以根长度为指标，重金属离子处理的植物后代对相同的离子胁迫也有较强的耐性。经历胁迫的植物后代也增强了对其他胁迫的交叉抗性，如盐胁迫增强了植物后代对其他胁迫的交叉抗性。

由此可见，不同生态胁迫对同一品种的长期影响可能会形成独特的药材表观遗传模式，从而产生药材道地性表型特征。而不同产地间药材表观遗传的变异可以来自随机的表观突变，但更主要还是来源于由环境变化产生的压力。从表观遗传的角度来看，变异的诱因一方面是药材环境适应性变化的选择者，另一方面在环境压力的选择下，表观突变速率往往远高于基因突变，体现了环境因素是道地药材形成的根本动力，而时间和空间的连续性造就药材遗传与表型的连续性。

新的表观遗传修饰可以是一个种群中多个个体同时发生。尽管这样突变可以通过表观遗传复位的方式被损耗，但只要环境压力保持足够长的时间，在种群中总的表观突变频率可以在十几代内迅速达到一个稳定的频率。针对个体来说，对比发生率极低的基因突变率，多个表观突变可以在同一个体中同时发生，因此针对环境波动有更好的适应性。因此，与 DNA 序列信息相比，表观突变作为道地药材地域性形成的主要驱动力更具有说服力。

## 5 DNA 甲基化、组蛋白修饰的技术手段已经较为成熟

目前表观遗传学差异研究主要集中在 DNA 甲基化、组蛋白共价修饰和 miRNA 表达等方面，其研究手段和技术方法已日趋成熟，具体可划分为基因组 DNA 甲基化检测技术，如甲基化敏感扩增多态性(methylation sensitive amplification polymorphism, MSAP)法、亚硫酸盐测序(bisulfite sequencing PCR, BSP)法、甲基化 DNA 免疫共沉淀(methylated DNA immunoprecipitation, MeDIP or mDIP)法、高分辨率溶解曲线(high-resolution melting, HRM)法等。组蛋白共价修饰检测技术，目前最常用的为染色质免疫共沉淀技术，在实际应用中可以将 ChIP 与生物芯片或测序技术相结合，在全基因组或基因组较大区域上高通量分析 DNA 结合位点或组蛋白修饰的方法。miRNA 检测技术，如 Northern blot、实时荧光定量 PCR 和 DNA 芯片法等。这些方法体系的建立已为道地药材表观遗传研究提供了良好的技术平台。

## 6 展望

从学科角度上看，以现代生物学为基础并结合数理化等多学科的方法联合攻关被认为是研究道地药材的必然趋势。随着对生命认识程度的加深，在后基因组时代，表观遗传学已成为阐明功能基因表达模式变异的关键研究领域之一。越来越多的情况表明，在遗传背景基本一致的前提下，道地药材表型差异是对环境及适应性的结果，而表观遗传对药材道地性形成的影响更大。因此，体现道地药材生物学本质的特化基因型研究，应将经典遗传与表观遗传相结合，科学、客观地反映各个地区不同的生态或地理条件长期选择而形成的道地药材的遗传本质。

不同产地环境因子变异也是促进道地药材表型及化学变异的因素之一，表观遗传改变作为中等时间或空间尺度内的行为，可以对不同种类的外部或内部刺激做出快速反应，且药用植物也可以在环境变化和应激状态下改变表观遗传状态，从而产生新的表型以适应环境，并可将其传递给下一代，这对于诠释“道地药材发展的动力学因素——边缘(逆境)效应”“道地药材的药物属性——独特的化学特征”有着重要的理论意义。

[袁媛，黄璐琦，等. 中国中药杂志，2015，40(13)：2079－2083.]

# 中药微生态与中药道地性

道地性(geoherbalism)是中医关于药材品质的重要理论，是在中医哲学理论体系下对药材疗效与环境关系的综合认知和评价。道地药材(Dao-di herbs)是指经过中医临床长期应用优选出来的，产在特定地域，与其他地区所产同种中药材相比，品质和疗效更好，且质量稳定，具有较高知名度的中药材。道地药材是传统公认品质优良、疗效确切且产生于某一特定生态地理环境的一类中药材。在长期医疗实践过程中，“道地药材”成为优质中药材的代名词，成为评价中药材品质的综合性标准。培育和发展道地药材，是历代祖国医药学者孜孜不倦的追求。开展中药道地性研究是保障中药材质量和中医药临床疗效的关键。

自 20 世纪 70 年代开始，我国许多学者以中医药理论为指导，运用先进科学技术和现代化研究手段，采用多学科综合分析模式，对道地药材的形成规律和实质展开了全面而系统的研究。胡世林等将古人对道地药材认识归纳为天药相应、地造灵药，提出“多因协同”的药材品质观；肖小河等将地道药材划分为：生境主导型、种质主导型、技术主导型、传媒主导型和多因子关联决定型等形成模式；王永炎等将古代对道地药材“环境”的认识分为道地的“朴素生境观”、道地的“小环境观”和道地的“整体观”3 个阶段。黄璐琦等指出“道地性形成＝遗传机制＋环境机制”；万德光等提出药材品质形成的多层次理论。

近年来，研究者逐渐认识到药用植物内生菌、根际微生物等中药微生态的因素以各种不同的方式直接或间接地影响着药材生长、性状、代谢、化学成分等，进而造就道地药材与非道地药材品质及效用的差异，并将微生态纳入中药道地性形成机制的核心研究中。现今，逐步形成一门新兴交叉学科——中药微生态学(traditional Chinese medical microecology, TCMM)。揭示中药微生态结构的形成及其变化规律与药材品质效用之间的关系，是中药微生态学研究的主要任务之一。

本文系统论述了中药微生态分布的地域性特征以及在此基础上对道地药材种质建成、产量与发育、活性成分积累、毒性、采收与炮制与加工、贮存等各环节的影响，提出道地性形成的中药微生态观，以期为中药道地性的科学内涵和评价体系提供新的研究思路，为道地药材资源可持续生产提供指导，同时推动中药微生态理论的进一步发展。

## 1 中药微生态与道地药材地域性的关系

道地药材同时具有2个重要的特定属性：一是具有特定的产地属性，二是具有优良的品质。

“道”是我国古代的一种行政区划。唐代贞观十三年(639年)，唐太宗为了加强控制地方，依据地理形势划全国为十道。后唐玄宗将十道再加细分为十五道，下设州、县。至后世几经变更，曾有“领道”“道尹”等类似称谓。因而“道地药材”可以理解为由某个或某几个行政区划所出产的优质药材。

道地药材产生于特定的生态地理环境，长期受独特的生长环境作用而形成。特定产区是药材道地性的内在成因和外在标签。我国历代医药家无一不重视中药材的产地属性。自《神农本草经》就有“土地所出，真伪陈新，并各有法”的经典论述；陶弘景《本草经集注》认为“诸药所生，皆有境界”。《新修本草》指出“离其本土，则质同而效异”。唐代孙思邈强调“古之医者，用药必依土地，所以治十得九”。宋代《本草衍义》言“用药必择州土所宜者，则药力具，用之有据”。并将产地用于药物命名中，如《神农本草经》记载的巴豆、蜀椒、秦椒、秦皮、阿胶等，以及后来的川芎、川贝母、田七，闻名遐迩的四大怀药、浙八味等。

道地性之“地”即特定的生态环境，包括气候因子、土壤因子、地形地貌、栽培条件等各种生态因子。不同地域中的生态因子组合形成各不相同的药材生长外生环境，同时也导致了不同的土壤微生物群落结构。土壤微生物通过改善土壤养分和理化状态影响药用植物的营养，有的长期与药用植物相互作用，成为后者根际、叶围中紧密关联的伴生菌群，甚至成为药用植物生命体内部不可分割的一部分，即内生菌群，并随着宿主的繁殖而垂直传播。各地特定的伴生、内生菌群和宿主共同构成特定的“中药微生态系统”，产生特定的中药微生态效应，导致在不同产地形成有差异的药材品质。因此，厘清和利用土壤微生物、内共生微生物的地理分异规律、成因，对理解中药的道地性，培育道地药材意义重大。

1.1 *土壤微生物的地理分异规律* 土壤是药用植物生存的根本，大量的土壤微生物与药用植物之间发生着极其复杂的相互作用。特定环境条件形成特定的土壤微生态系统，进而对中药品质的形成特定的影响。

首先，在大的空间尺度下，受气候和地理因素的影响，土壤微生物群落结构及其多样性呈现出一定的分布格局，即土壤微生物呈纬度多样性梯度(latitudinal diversity gradient)变化规律——高纬度土壤微生物多样性低，低纬度土壤微生物多样性高。例如，一些 *Roseivivax* 出现在纬度较高的地区，而在低纬度地区并没有出现。但是，土壤微生物的纬度地带性不同于高等植物，前者更加容易受到微区环境因子如土壤pH、降水、温度、成土母质、土壤营养状况、伴生植物类群等多个方面的干扰。

在区域距离的尺度(1～260 km)下，群落间的差异不随地理距离的增加而增加，决定群落结构的主要因素是物理化学环境，最显著的有年降水量和土壤中钠、铵的水平等。据Liu J等的测定，在引起土壤细菌群落变异的相关因子中，地理距离的贡献率为14.75%，而土壤pH和土壤碳含量等环境因子的贡献率高达37.52%。

在局域距离的尺度(25～1 000 m)下，土壤微生物结构变异程度存在距离衰减关系，即2个地点相距越远，它们之间的微生物群落差异越大。地理距离比土壤类型更能影响土壤微生物群落组成：地区相同但土壤类型不同，其土壤微生物组成虽然明显不同，但彼此间的差异性却远不及那些土壤类型相同而地区不同的土壤。

此外，药用植物本身对土壤微生物的组成有积极的作用，植物功能类群组成影响土壤微生物群落组成。同一田块中，在药用植物根系分泌物的作用下，根际及根表面的微生物种群密度、种类及活性均要明显高于非根际土，形成比耕作土层更加复杂和高丰度的根际微生态系统，产生强烈的根际效应，影响根际能力，提高药材对环境的适应性，促进养分的吸收等。

土壤微生物的地理分异规律对中药的道地性形成具有重要的意义。研究者对道地产区和非道地产区药用植物土壤微生物组成进行了比较研究，人参、滇重楼、仙鹤草、牡丹、天麻等多种药材土壤菌群结构均显示出产地差异性。且道地产区的土壤微生物往往更加丰富，存在更多的地域专属性的菌株。袁小凤等研究发现土壤细菌多样性与芍药苷的累积呈显著正相关，道地产区磐安杭白芍的芍药苷含量相当高，其道地性与磐安土壤微生态环境关系密切。仇有文等对中药白术 *Tractylodes macrocephala* Koidz 土壤菌群做了深入调查，发现高产土壤中细菌、放线菌、真菌等微生物区系均极显著高于白术产量一般的土壤和低产土壤，说明土壤中丰富的微生物益于药材品质与生产，是药材道地性形成过程中不容忽视的因素和重要的生物资源。

1.2 *药用植物内生菌的地域性* 在土壤微生物的时空分异背景下，因离散度和距离等隔离因素限制，同一地区的植物受到明显的局域性菌群的感染，这些本地菌在大的分类学水平上(如门、纲、目、科的水平)可能与其他地方相似，但在小的分类学水平上(如属、种的水平)却有所不同。与来自其他地区的植物相比，同一地区的植物内部有更多相似的微生物群落，经过长期的积累逐渐形成鲜明的微生态地域特征。李淑彬等采用终端限制片段长度多态性(terminal restriction fragment length polymorphism，T-RFLP)技术分析著名南药高良姜的内生细菌菌群，发现道地产区的高良姜以海洋螺菌、红杆菌、交替假单胞菌等海洋细菌及热带根瘤菌、沼泽考克菌相对丰度较高。可见，宿主药用植物生长的海岸环境是影响其内生菌种群组成的重要因素。

不同产地，药用植物内生菌群结构、分布和数量等存在必然差别。印度尼西亚产和日本产出的金鸡纳中的内生菌在属水平上表现出物种组成上的差异。刘学周等比较了不同产地西洋参内生菌群结构，发现吉林珲春、长白、抚松、靖宇、集安5个产地中，高海拔的产地(吉林长白山)西洋参内生菌优势种群向芽孢杆菌属 *Bacillus* 集中，有群落单一化趋势，奇异度较高；低海拔的产地（吉林省珲春）西洋参内生菌种群丰富度较高，分布较均匀，奇异度较低，呈现出类似于土壤微生物分布的地带性规律。

牡丹、杜仲、川芎、丹参、银杏等近100种药用植物被陆续报道具有内生菌地域分布差异性，尤其以道地产区与非道地产区之间的差别最为显著。一方面，道地产区所产药材内生菌的生物多样性通常最为丰富；另一方面，道地产区药材通常携带更多的特有内生菌。Yang G等从3种类型的牡丹中共检出26个真菌属，其中仅8个真菌属为共有类群，10个真菌属仅见于道地药“凤丹”*Paeonia ostii* ‘Feng Dan’，4个真菌属仅见于“洛阳凤丹”*P. ostii* ‘Luoyang Feng Dan’，另4个真菌属仅见于“洛阳红”*P. suffruticosa* ‘Luoyang Hong’。

1.3 中药内生菌群结构地域性形成的主要因素　造成中药内生菌群结构地域性差异的原因大致有二。一是外环境综合因素。Yang G等对3种牡丹的研究结果显示，同一生长环境下的不同品种之间内生真菌群落结构相似性高于不同产地环境的同一品种，说明与牡丹品种相比，地理环境即外环境综合因素对牡丹内生真菌多样性的影响更为重要。

二是宿主选择。内生菌的自然分布具有明显的宿主限制性。环境中的某些微生物可能通过随机定植的方式侵染宿主植物，但更多的菌是否能够成功定植却受宿主的遗传特性决定。内生菌定植过程中，少数微生物类群充当“中心”菌群，宿主基因型及非生物因子对“中心”菌群起着决定性的作用；“中心”菌群再通过与其他微生物之间的互作，间接影响后者的定植，最终形成特定的微生物群落结构。尤其是在小的分布范围内，生态环境差异不大，微生态结构更多地受到宿主选择性的影响而形成各自特定的特异性菌群组合。邓毅等比较研究了同为甘肃所产的乌拉尔甘草野生品与栽培品的内生菌群，发现丝核菌属仅见于野生品、木霉属仅见于栽培品；且二者的内生真菌和内生细菌优势菌种均有不同。2个品种的药材活性成分及药理作用呈现差异，很可能与宿主对“中心”菌群的决定作用以及由此形成的特定内生菌群结构有关。

综上可见，中药微生态结构是宿主祖代生活轨迹与当代生存环境状态之间综合作用的结果，携带着重要的环境信息，特定的内生菌群式样是对药材生产地小环境的表征，可以成为道地药材的地域性标签，在分子标记和化学成分指纹图谱之外提供一种道地药材产地溯源的新思路。采用生态学统计方法综合分析道地产地微生物地理分异规律，对在中药微生态学的层次上阐释药材道地性的形成机制具有重要的学术价值，在发展道地药材生产、区划制定和产地溯源，保护道地药材的声誉和中药特色等方面具有重要现实和战略意义。

## 2　中药微生态促进道地药材优质种质

种质指遗传物质相对一致的同种生物的个体群。优良的中药材种质是道地药材形成的基本保证。中药微生态系统中的许多菌群能增强或赋予宿主药用植物抗病、抗旱、抗寒、抗盐碱等特性，从而优化药材种质，促进中药的道地性形成。

2.1 中药微生态增强道地药材的抗病虫能力　药用植物在生长过程中，面临多种致病菌侵袭的风险，优良的道地药材往往具有较好的抗病能力。研究表明，病害的严重程度与拮抗性内生菌的数量成负相关，即内生菌数越少，病害越重。丰富的内生菌及其根际土壤中的多种微生物通过各种机制帮助宿主植物与病原菌进行“免疫抗衡”：①内生菌及根际微生物合成抗生素类物质，在药用植物体内转运，利于发挥防病作用。研究证明，接入了抗生素高产菌株的宿主，比野生型植株具有更强的抗病能力。②内生菌及根际微生物合成细菌素、细胞壁降解酶类等，能水解病原菌的细胞壁、细胞膜，使原生质外流。③部分内生菌及根际微生物与病原菌具有相似的生态位，相互形成营养竞争关系，通过竞争和定殖优势抑制病原菌的繁殖发展，达到抗衡制约的效果。④还有部分内生菌及根际微生物能诱导宿主产生抗性，例如通过合成并积累水杨酸等物质等，激活宿主复杂的防御信号通路，促进药用植物抗病基因表达。⑤内生菌构成细胞外屏障，帮助药用植物隔离病原菌侵袭。Soliman S S M等研究发现木腐真菌将杀菌剂紫杉醇隔离在胞内疏水体中，再通过胞吐分泌释放到胞外。之后，疏水小体合并形成一道显著的细胞外屏障。这一过程中，内生菌类似于动物免疫细胞，充当一种自主的、抗病原体的哨兵，监测维管系统，增强宿主的免疫力。⑥某些内生菌及根际微生物能产生噬铁素，造成病原菌铁缺乏而无法正常生长繁殖。⑦内生菌可以产生多种对食草动物和昆虫具有毒性的生物碱。值得注意的是，微生态菌群需要达到一定的种群密度才能起到有效的抗病效果。因此，因菌群结构差异导致的药用植物的抗病能力的大小只是程度上的差别。

2.2 中药微生态增强道地药材的抗旱能力　菌根真菌（arbuscular mycorrhiza fungi，AMF）是公认的能提高植物抗旱性的微生物，帮助宿主药用植物从环境中吸收利用更多的水分，改善水分代谢循环功能。①某些AM菌能降低根部或根细胞的水势，促进根部的吸水能力，保持了根内水分，增强了宿主的御旱、耐旱和抗旱性。甘草是我国的保护中药，也是一种典型的沙生耐旱植物，AM如*Glomus moseae*、*G. etumicatum*通过增加甘草根部可溶性糖和脯氨酸含量，降低根部水势。石斛是气生兰科药用植物，具有较好的耐旱性能。陈连庆等研究发现越是干旱，铁皮石斛*Dendrobium candidum* Wall. ex Lindl.菌根感染率越高，菌根繁殖力越强，细胞内菌根真菌菌丝团结构生长发育越强烈，并伴有针状结晶体出现。龚记熠从野生金钗石斛内分离到的内生真菌株能增加宿主根部脯氨酸和可溶性糖含量，大大提高了石斛气生菌根细胞的渗透压。②AM菌提高宿主体内抗氧化系统（SOD，CAT，POD）的活性，降低脂质过氧化水平，从而帮助宿主在干旱胁迫条件下生长、提高其抗旱能力。③部分AM菌上调根系水孔蛋白基因的表达，增加根系对水的吸收能力。著名的道地药材宁夏枸杞*Lycium barbarum* L.具有较强的耐旱性，胡文涛等发现夏枸杞根系通过招募AM真菌中的内球囊霉*Rhizophagus irregularis*上调根系上水孔蛋白基因*LbPIP*2-1、*LbTIP*3-7以及根内球囊霉水孔蛋白基因*RirAQP*2的表达。④AM真菌还能增加叶片的气孔导度和蒸腾速率、叶片相对水分含量，降低叶片温度，从而保障宿主在轻、重度水胁迫条件下的仍然能进行正常的光化学反应。

2.3 中药微生态增强道地药材的耐盐能力　盐胁迫会造成植物水分状况的变化，导致植物生理性干旱，影响其生理功能的正常进行。研究表明，盐胁迫与正常环境下相比，药用植物微生态结构差异显著。例如在正常情况下*Medicago* *truncatula* 内生菌群以 *Brucella inopinata*、*Sphingobium xenophagum*、*Shinella granuli* 丰度较高，而在高盐胁迫下内生菌群却以 *Enterobacter kobei*、*Halomonas lutea*、*Thalassospira povalilytica*、*Pseudomonas stutzeri* 居多。Yaish MW 等发现枣椰树 *Phoenix dactylifera* L. 中的一些内生菌曾报道从盐水和海洋环境中分离获得，这些内生菌很有可能有利于 *Phoenix dactylifera* L. 的耐盐性。中华补血草是一种典型的盐生药用植物，生长于沿海潮湿盐土，主要分布于我国南北沿海地区及台湾等地。冯维维等从江苏沿海滩涂所产的中华补血草中分离筛选获得菌株的 NaCl 盐耐受范围多数为 0～13%，呈现了突出的盐胁迫耐受性。在盐胁迫条件下，内生菌与菌根真菌自身菌丝可能通过直接吸收作用，及改善药用植物菊花的矿质营养状况和内源激素平衡状况的间接作用，增加菊花根、叶中的含水量，缓解因盐过量而导致的植物生理干旱，增强宿主在盐环境中的忍耐力。Lubna 从 *Chenopodium album* 根部分离获得的内生真菌 *Aspergillus flavus* CSH1 则通过调节植物内源激素及抗氧化系统，显著提高 *Glycine max* L. 高盐胁迫耐受能力。

2.4 中药微生态增强道地药材的抗寒能力 植物在受冷害刺激时，叶片细胞膜受到低温伤害，电解质渗出，且温度越低，渗出越快。贾炜等从南极苔藓中分离到一株木霉菌株 NTYM－0112 能有效减少低温胁迫对植物膜结构造成的破坏，减少叶片可溶性糖的外渗，对植物的抗寒性具有积极的促进作用。木麻黄类原产于热带和亚热带地区，耐寒性能差。但接种不同菌根菌可以使短枝木麻黄的主要保护酶 SOD、POD、CAT 活性在低温胁迫条件下显著提高，并在 0～4℃达到最高值，同时使 MDA 含量和细胞膜透性显著降低，从而提高宿主植物抗寒能力。当然，各菌株处理的升降幅度存在显著差异，其中，内生菌根菌苏格兰球囊霉 *Glomus caledonium* Nicoison & Ceelemann 和外生菌根菌多根硬皮马勃 *Scleroderma polyrhizum* Pers. 对短枝木麻黄耐寒性的促进效果最佳。可见，微生态资源极具增加宿主药用植物抗寒的潜力。

综上说明，在各种胁迫生境中，植物会形成特定的内生菌群结构，而这些内生菌群对宿主植物适应特殊的生境提供极大的帮助，赋予道地药材较好的抗逆性品质。同时，一定胁迫压力，更能诱导药用植物合成特定的次生代谢产物。因此，抗性品系的药用植物往往同时也产生更加丰富和含量较高的活性成分。

## 3 中药微生态促进道地药材产量

3.1 中药微生态对道地药材的促生作用 产量高是药材道地性重要的组成部分。微生态对药用植物的促生促产作用已得到广泛证实。一方面，内生菌或根际微生物可以合成植物生长调节剂，如 IAA、吲哚乙腈、乙烯、生长素、细胞激动素、赤霉素、脱落酸、玉米素、玉米素核苷等，间接调节植物内源激素的含量水平，对宿主植物的生长起促进作用。Arora P 等从喜马拉雅山脉西北部的 4 个不同地点所产甘草的 1 019 个组织片段中分离到 266 株内生真菌，这些内生菌全都能产生浓度不等的 IAA。张集慧等对不同种类的兰科药用植物所获得的内生真菌不仅能够不同程度地产生 IAA，还能产生赤霉素($GA_3$)，吲哚乙酸、脱落酸(ABA)、玉米素(z)，玉米素核苷(ZR)。药用植物中华补血草中分离筛选出的内生与根际细菌中有 7 属 18 株都具有 1－氨基环丙烷－1－羧酸 ACC 脱氨酶活性，可以催化乙烯的前体 ACC，从而影响植物生长时的乙烯水平，其中有 13 个株菌的 ACC 脱氨酶含量较高，9 株菌能产生 IAA。因此，感染内生菌的植物一般都表现出比未感染植株生长快速的特点。例如，将丹参内生真菌球毛壳菌 *Chaetomium globosum* D38 活菌回施于丹参幼苗，丹参的生长明显受到促进。

另一方面，内生菌、菌根真菌发达的菌丝帮助宿主植物吸收矿物营养物质磷、钙、锌等。郭兰萍等研究发现接种 VA 菌根真菌可以促进药用植物苍术根系对土壤养分的吸收，影响苍术根际区有机质组成，提高苍术根际土壤微生物的功能多样性及代谢活性，从而显著促进苍术的营养生长，同时不会造成苍术挥发油质量的变异。中华补血草中分离出的内生菌中能够解磷。赵杨景等将从兰科植物分离出的内生真菌接种于大花蕙兰，其中 GC945 菌使幼苗吸收 N 和 K 的量比增施矿质营养但不接种真菌的处理(CK2)分别提高了 175.7%、97.5%；GC943 菌使植株对 P 的吸收量比 CK2 处理提高了 7 倍；幼苗茎叶干重比 CK2 处理提高了 173.2%～250.1%。

再者，多种根际微生物及内生菌具有固氮作用，提高宿主药用植物的 N 素营养。甘肃道地药材党参、黄芪和当归种植地的根际土壤中固氮微生物资源十分丰富，杜文静等从中共分离得到根瘤菌属 *Rhizobium*、中华根瘤菌属 *Sinorhizobium*、芽孢菌属 *Bacillus*、短波单孢菌属 *Brevundimonas*、无色杆菌属 *Achromobacter*、农杆菌属 *Agrobacterium* 等 28 株具有固氮酶活性的菌株。冯维维等从中华补血草中分离出内生菌中 11 株可以固氮。

中药微生态的促生作用通常并不是单一的，而是多管齐下。Kumar A 等从姜黄根状茎中分离筛选了 6 株内生菌，即分别来自厚壁菌门、γ-变形菌门、拟杆菌门的 *Bacillus cereus*、*B. thuringiensis*、*Bacillus* sp.、*B. pumilis*、*Pseudomonas putida* 以及 *Clavibacter michiganensis* 表现出对姜黄根状茎生长的多方面的促进作用，包括合成重氮化、磷酸盐和钾的增溶，生长素合成以及水解酶的产生等。

3.2 中药微生态促进道地药材药用部位的发育 道地药材良好的生长发育形成典型的性状特征，通常也成了性状鉴别的重要依据。某些药材离开本土，移栽他地之后，性状也随之改变。研究发现，在药用植物的生长发育过程中，某些土壤微生物或内生菌感染还会引起宿主器官发育的变化。例如，土壤真菌拟康氏木霉(*Trichoderma pseudokoningii* SMF2)能合成一类 peptaibols 抗菌肽康宁霉素(trichokonis, TKs)，其主要生物活性成分为康宁霉素 Ⅵ(TK Ⅵ)。适当浓度的 TK Ⅵ能促进植物主根伸长，同时能促进可见侧根数量明显增加；而高浓度的 TK Ⅵ却显著抑制植株生长。部分菌群通过分泌生长调节剂途径(如 3.1 所述)影响宿主发育，也有部分菌群通过相关基因调控通路干预植物的器官发育。Song Y 等研究表明，名贵中药三叶青 *Tetrastigma hemsleyanum* Diels & Gilg ex Diels 葫芦状块根中的数个内生真菌菌株可以调控宿主膨胀素基因 *Th-exp* 的表达。其中，镰刀菌属 *Fusarium* 菌株 TH15、TH26 可以上调根茎叶各部

*Th-exp* 基因的表达；*Plectosphaerella* 属菌株 TH12 及刺盘孢属 *Colletotrichum* 菌株 TH09 则可以下调根茎叶各部 *Th-exp* 基因的表达；菌株 TH14 在茎、叶部位能上调该基因表达，在根部则发挥相反的效用。由此可见，伴生或共生微生物的分布和丰度可能影响药材的发育及器官形态建成，这种影响具有植物部位效应及菌群综合效应。有产地特性的中药微生态结构则可能造成药材产量及性状上的差别，进而形成具特定形态的道地药材。

## 4 中药微生态参与道地药材有效成分的形成

内生菌感染会导致超过三分之一的宿主基因表达发生显著变化，引发宿主代谢的重新编程，以初级代谢为代价促进次级代谢。各类药用植物中均存在某些内生菌种类能干预宿主药用植物合成活性成分，促进宿主体内次生代谢产物的形成和累积（表 1）。来自不同药用植物的不同内生菌群，可能促进同一类活性成分的合成。

**表 1 近年来中药微生态参与道地药材有效成分合成的研究案例**

| 内生菌 | 药用植物 | 次生代谢产物类型 |
|---|---|---|
| 深绿木霉 *Trichoderma atroviride* D16 | 丹参 *Salvia miltiorrhiza* | 丹参酮 tanshinone |
| 球毛壳菌 *Chaetomium globosum* D38 | 丹参 *S. miltiorrhiza* | 丹参酮 tanshinone<br>二氢丹参酮Ⅰ dihydrotanshinone Ⅰ<br>隐丹参酮 cryptotanshinone<br>丹参酮$Ⅱ_A$ tanshinone $Ⅱ_A$<br>丹酚酸 salvianolic acid |
| 茎点霉 *Phoma glomerata* D14 | 丹参 *S. miltiorrhiza* | 丹酚酸 C salvianolic acid C |
| 拟茎点霉属 *Phomopsis* | 黄连 *Coptis chinensis* | 小檗碱 berberine |
| 链格孢属 *Alternaria* sp. | 喜树 *Camptotheca acuminate* | 喜树碱 camptothecin (CPT) |
| 拟茎点霉属 *Phomopsis* sp. | | 10-羟基喜树碱 10-hydroxycamptothecin |
| 镰孢属 *Fusarium* sp. | | |
| 刺盘孢属 *Colletotrichum* sp. | | |
| 腐皮镰刀菌 *F. solani* | 喜树 *C. acuminata* | 喜树碱 camptothecin (CPT)<br>甲氧基喜树碱 9-methoxycamptothecin<br>羟基喜树碱 10-hydroxycamptothecin |
| 曲霉属 *Aspergillus* | 银杏 *Ginkgo biloba* | 银杏内酯 C 及结构类似物 ginkgolide C and similar structure compounds |
| 盘长孢属 *Gtoeosporium* | | |
| 色串孢属 *Tolura* | | |
| 丝菌属 *Phacodium* | | |
| 枝霉属 *Rhinocladiella* sp. | 雷公藤 *Tripterygium wilfordii* | 细胞松弛素类 cytochalasins |
| 无孢菌群(暂定) | 海南粗榧 *Cephalotaxus hainanensis* | 细胞松弛素类 cytochalasins |
| 拟茎点霉 *Phomopsis theicola* BCRC 09F0213 | 小梗木姜子 *Litsea hypophaea* | 细胞松弛素类 cytochalasins |
| 曲霉属 *Aspergillus* sp. | 半夏 *Pinellia ternata* | 细胞松弛素类 cytochalasins |
| 木霉菌 *Trichoderma gamsii* | 三七 *Panax notoginseng* | 木霉酮 trichoderpyrone |
| 尖孢镰刀菌 *F. oxysporum* | 长春花 *Catharanthus roseus* | 长春碱 vincristine |

内生菌对宿主代谢的干预机制主要包括诱导及转化。前者是在内生菌所携带的某些组分，作为信号转导途径中的信号分子，诱导宿主植物特定基因的表达，从而激活植物的特定次生代谢途径，导致活性成分显著积累。例如，来自内生真菌深绿木霉 *Trichoderma atroviride* D16 的诱导子能显著促进丹参酮成分的生物合成。内生真菌球毛壳菌 *Chaetomium globosum* D38 提取物能增强丹参酮生物合成途径中 5 个关键基因的转录活性，且比活真菌所起到的促进作用要强得多。由此说明，内生菌的代谢产物对宿主基因表达产生了调控作用。能引起宿主产生一系列生理生化过程的、高度专一性的生化信号物质，被称为“诱导子”或“诱导物”。真菌产生的诱导物多是细胞壁降解物和葡聚糖、糖蛋白、壳聚糖（chitosan）、几丁质（chitin）、环糊精（cyclodextrin）、寡糖（oligosaccharide）、小肽、脱乙酰几丁质、不饱和脂肪酸（polyunsaturated fatty acids）等。目前，利用内生菌诱导子调控药用植物次生代谢产物合成已经成为中药活性成分生物合成的重要手段。

此外，内生菌合成的某些关键酶，能将植物体内活性成分的结构类似物前体转化成为有效的活性成分。著名的抗疟药青蒿素是一类具有过氧桥结构的倍半萜内酯类化合物。青蒿素的生物活性与过氧键密不可分，但是催化青蒿酸形成青蒿素的环内过氧键合酶却一直没有找到。Yan W 等最终研究发现催化这类反应的环内过氧键合酶元件来源于黄花蒿的共生真菌，由此解开了过氧桥合成的世界难题。喜树内生真菌腐皮镰刀菌 *Fusarium solani*、拟茎点霉属 *Phomopsis* sp.、链格孢属 *Alternaria* sp.、镰孢属 *Fusarium* sp. 及刺盘孢属 *Colletotrichum* sp. 等能合喜树缺乏的关键酶，进而将喜树产生的某种前体物质转化成喜树碱及其类似物，这也就是无菌条件下导致喜树碱大量减少的主要原因。郭从亮等从人参中筛选到一株活性菌株，可特异性地转化三七总皂中的人参皂苷 $Rb_1$，获得人参皂苷 Rd 和稀有人参皂苷 C-K，且发酵 12 d 后人参皂苷 C-K 的转化率高达 11.62%。植物内生菌的生物转化产物，多是萜类、生物碱、皂苷、黄酮、酚类和多烃类等能产生疗效的有效化合物。

不同产地的中药材，由于所处生态环境的差异、药材本身所产生的遗传变异，以及由此所导致的内生菌群结构的区别，必然影响宿主植物的代谢网络以及有效成分的积累。例如印度尼西亚产和日本产出的金鸡纳中的内生菌组成在属水平上存在差异，虽然其部分内生菌也具有产金鸡纳生物碱的能力，但与印尼金鸡纳内生菌相比，日本金鸡纳内生菌的产量非常小，特别是奎宁的总含量远小于印度尼西亚。川西高原地区 7 个产地的野生药用植物桃儿七根茎和根中鬼臼毒素含量存在极明显差异，松潘牟尼沟产地的含量最高，质量分数达 2.65%；红原打西坝含量最低，质量分数仅为 1.68%。该研究表明，即使是同在川西高原区域，气候、温度等相差不远的前提下，不同产地间仍然有如此明显的差异。

综上所述，结构及功能多样的微生态系统以各自不同的方式影响着药材性状、生长、发育、抗性、次生代谢过程等，最终导致道地药材与非道地药材品质的差异。内生菌的生物转化作用为道地中药活性成分的生产及新活性成分的开发等方面提供了广阔的前景。值得注意的是，微生物与药用植物药效成分含量之间可能存在"量-效"关系。例如，丛枝菌根真菌 *Glomus mosseae* 对名贵中药三七有效成分积累具有促进作用，但随着丛枝菌根侵染强度的增加，三七皂苷 $R_1$、人参皂苷 $Rg_1$、人参皂苷 $Rb_1$、人参皂苷 Rd 以及这 4 种皂苷的总产量均出现明显的先增加后下降的趋势。即丛枝菌根具有低侵染增加皂苷积累，高侵染转而降低皂苷积累的现象。只有当丛枝菌根适度侵染时，三七才具有最大的生物量和最高的皂苷含量及皂苷产量。

## 5 中药微生态时空波动与道地药材采收时节的关系

中药采收有很强的季节性。元代李杲谓："根、叶、花、实，采之有时……失其时，则气味不全。"又有"三月茵陈四月蒿，五月采回当柴烧"的农谚。恰当的种植年限与采收时节是中药质量的保障，而药用植物代谢产物的累积与其生长发育过程及中药微生态的动态波动不无关系。滇重楼根茎的药用品质具有典型的生境依赖性，种植年限增加会引起重楼药用品质下降明显。该药用植物根际土壤微生物资源丰富，分布规律为细菌数量＞放线菌数量＞真菌数量；随着种植年限的增加，真菌与解钾细菌数量呈逐年增加趋势，而细菌、放线菌、解无机磷细菌与解有机磷细菌数量则呈逐年减小的变化趋势。二年生苍术根际区土壤中细菌、放线菌、真菌普遍低于一年生样品，三者分别下降 46.14%、31.93%、49.15%，土壤细菌、放线菌及真菌三者的比例改变。同样的规律见于怀地黄道地产区河南省焦作、地黄主产区山西省临汾、牡丹道地产区南陵，其根际细菌和放线菌数量随着药用植物生长年限的增加均呈下降趋势；但根际真菌数量呈先降后升的趋势。总体上，药用植物根际微生物随种植年龄的增加有从高肥的"细菌主导型"向低肥的"真菌主导型"趋势发展。

药用植株发育阶段的不同，其体内的生理生化代谢存在差异，也会引起内生菌组成发生波动。孙剑秋考察了杜仲、连翘、秦岭连翘、卵叶连翘、细叶小檗、青麸杨 6 种药用植物的枝条内生菌群年际变化规律，结果显示一年生枝条的内生真菌定植率和分离率为11.4%～75%和 0.15～1.03，二年生枝条为 66.7% ～97.5% 和 0.97 ～1.58，三年生枝条为 87.5%～100%和 1.23～1.85。可见，药用植物枝条内生菌群呈均逐年增多的规律。

中药微生态结构波动的原因一方面与气候的季节性波动有关，在适宜的温湿度下，菌群生长和繁殖繁盛；另一方面则与共生和伴生的药用植物的代谢活动密切相关。研究表明，土壤微生物数量与植株生长发育旺盛程度呈正相关。宿主植物生长周期中新陈代谢最旺盛的时期，是土壤释放易吸收可利用养分最多的时期，又是植物吸收养分、根系分泌最多的时期，因此该时期土壤微生物数量最多。当然，除了微生物数量以外，在植物生长的各阶段，根际菌群优势种在科、属和 OTU 水平上也在发生着明显的变化。一方面，种植年限增加会引起土壤微生态区系的变化、根际区土壤养分缺乏、土壤化感物质增加，降低药用植物对营养物质的吸收利用；另一方面，随着种植年限的增加，根际有益真菌迅速减少而土传病害病原菌开始富集，导致病虫害的发生增多，进而造成药材药用品质下降。轮作或休作的措施常被用来解决连作后的药材品质下降或栽培障碍的问题，林贵兵等证实该过程实际上为土壤微生物群落结构调整及种群数量自然恢复并重新建立土壤生态系统平衡的过程。

药材采收的时节应当在药材本身的次生代谢产物及活性物质的积累最为丰富的时候，这个时候是其微生态结构的动态变化最适宜于药材品质最终形成的时节。否则，微生态系统的进一步演替波动也可能造成药材药效和品质的下降。对药材采收时间与中药微生态规律的深入研究对维持或调节药材高效生产具有深远的科学意义。

## 6 中药微生态与道地药材加工及炮制

中药微生态与道地药材加工炮制的关系主要体现在两个方面。第一，植物药材本身带有一定微生物，生产、加工和贮存过程也会引入微生物，尤其是中药发酵制剂最易受到微生物污染。有害微生物生长繁殖影响药材质量，分泌真菌毒素通过口服进入人体后给患者健康和生命带来安全隐患。常见的中药有害真菌包括曲霉属、青霉属、镰刀属中的部分真菌，分泌的真菌毒素有黄曲霉毒素（aflatoxin，AFT）、赭曲霉毒素（oehrotoxins）、伏马菌素（fumonisins）、T－2 毒素（T－2 toxin)、玉米赤霉烯酮(zerolaenone)等。其中,毒性最强的黄曲霉毒素(aflatoxins, AF)主要为黄曲霉 *Aspergillus flavus* Link 和寄生曲霉 *A. parasiticus* Speare 产生的一类次级代谢产物,具有致畸、致癌、致突变性。药材的加工和炮制过程可以有效杀灭和控制大多数微生物,减少或避免有害微生物生长繁殖带来的危害。此外,药用植物合成的某些成分也可以反过来抑制有害微生物的生长繁殖。例如,姜黄、丁香、肉桂等多种药用植物的挥发油能有效抑制黄曲霉毒素合成作用,且安全性较好,耐药性小。研究者把姜黄挥发油制备成脂质体,可完全抑制霉菌生长和黄曲霉毒素的产生,具有极大开发前景。

第二,发酵炮制是中药炮制的主要方法,通过微生物生长代谢和生命活动炮制中药可以大幅度改变其药性,还能降低毒副作用,提高有效成分提取率,促进有效成分的吸收和利用。例如半夏的中的某些毒性成分对各种黏膜有刺激性,使人出现咽喉肿痛、呕吐等症状。利用微生物中所含的酶类可以将半夏中某些有毒物质进行分解和转化,使其毒性降低。此外,大黄、喜树碱、三七、马钱子、何首乌、雷公藤等多种毒性中药均可通过微生物转化作用降低其毒副作用。值得注意的是,某些微生物的存在对药材活性的保持具有积极的作用,但炮制过程对中药微生态菌群结构产生强烈的影响。部分中药经加工后药效比生品降低,其中是否与中药微生态的变化有关尚未可知。目前,对炮制加工过程中中药微生态结构的变化规律还知之甚少。通过现代生物技术分析药材炮制、加工及贮藏过程中的微生态结构变化及其与饮片药效之间的联动关系是中药微生态学的重要任务。

## 7 中药微生态与中药毒性

部分中药中自身含有毒性物质,例如乌头属植物川乌、草乌、附子、雪上一枝篙等所含的生物碱具有程度不等的毒性。中药毒性在一定程度上制约了某些种类中药的临床应用。厘清中药毒性的来源,减低或消除中药毒性是中药国际化发展道路上不可忽视的环节。

研究表明,植物内生菌也能合成有毒性的化合物。例如,苦马豆素(swainsonine, SW)是豆科黄芪属 *Astragalus* 和棘豆属 *Oxytropis* 中有毒植物的主要毒性成分,是导致动物中毒的根本原因。此外,旋花科番薯属 *Ipomoea* 和 *Turbina*,锦葵科黄花稔属 *Sida* 等 6 个属约 60 多种植物也含有 SW。近年来,已证实内生真菌弯曲牙管蠕孢菌 *Undifilum* spp. 是 SW 产生的主要因素。另一种内生真菌香柱菌 *Epichloë* 则通过生产二萜生物碱和吲哚二萜生物碱及其衍生物使得宿主对摄食动物产生毒性效应。某些药用植物毒性成分的合成也离不开内生菌的参与或介导:乌头内生真菌枝孢菌 *Cladosporium cladosporioides* 可合成与标准品的化学结构相一致的乌头碱成分;雷公藤内生真菌镰刀菌属 *Fusarium* sp. NS-1 能合成雷公藤甲素;从马兜铃内生真菌 *Colletotrichum* sp. 的发酵产物中分离得到 7-hydroxy-10-oxodehydrodihydrobotrydial、格链孢酚、5-甲氧基格链孢酚、链格孢毒素1、腾毒素和二氢腾毒素共计 6 个化合物,其中前 4 个化合物对肺癌细胞和乳腺癌细胞有细胞毒活性。这些毒性物质往往是也有效成分,合理使用能带来显著的治疗效果,但过强的毒副作用也限制了中药的使用。

内生菌的代谢转化作用可以降低或消除宿主的有毒次生代谢产物。例如,内生真菌中的拟青霉属 *Paecilomyces* sp.、木霉菌属 *Trichoderma* sp.、枝孢菌属 *Cladosporium* sp. 能对麻疯树仁中含有毒性特性的佛波酯(phorbol esters, PEs)产生解毒效应。此外,土壤中有毒物质的积累对植物的生长造成很大的影响,甚至对植物造成严重的毒害。根际微生物中的某些无致病假单胞菌具有很强的分解烃类化合物的能力,对除草剂、农药、原油、甲醇等多种有害物质及污染物具有转化和分解效用,减少了污染物的吸收。这些菌群资源在解决中药的重金属富集和农残等问题上具有广阔的应用前景。

综上,中药的安全性是临床用药的基本要求。中药毒性可能源于微生态也有望消除于微生态。利用中药微生态对中药毒性物质进行转化修饰,在稳定或增强药效的基础上,降低甚至消除毒副作用,应当成为中药效用研究的重要内容。

## 8 菌物药的道地性

在中药的大家族中还有一类重要成员——微生物类中药,通常称菌物药,主要是大型真菌。中国药用真菌物种丰富,被记述的药用菌达 450 余种。中国菌物药的使用历史已逾 2 500 年,自《神农本草经》起记载菌物药 13 种——冬虫夏草、灵芝、茯苓、猴头菌、木耳、香菇等,至《中华本草》收载菌物药已达 134 种;2015 年版《中国药典》中收载的菌物药有灵芝、茯苓、雷丸、马勃、猪苓、冬虫夏草等 11 种。其中,著名菌物药茯苓 *Poria cocos* (Schw.) Wolf 自古"以云南产者……最正地道",为广大用药者所认同和推崇,其质优品佳在国内乃至国际上都享有极高的信誉。马芳等比较分析了大别山与云南两大茯苓产区 7 个产地的茯苓皮成分及含量,结果表明不同产地茯苓皮的红外光谱具有明显的地域性差异;大别山产区的茯苓皮中草酸钙含量较高,而云南省的茯苓皮中硅酸盐含量较高;产地地域跨度小则茯苓皮成分含量相似,产地地域跨度大则茯苓皮成分差异大。灵芝,多孔菌科真菌赤芝 *Ganoderma lucidum* (Leyss. ex Fr.) Karst. 或紫芝 *G. sinense* Zhao, Xu et Zhang 的干燥子实体,在我国已有 2 000 多年的应用史。赖长江生和 Chen Y 先后利用近红外(near infrared, NIR)技术比较研究不同地理来源灵芝的质量,结果均表明不同产地的灵芝样品之间确实存在差异,且类群差异明显。松茸 *Tricholoma matsutake* (S. Ito et Imai) Sing. 是珍贵的外生菌根菌,具有较高的食药用价值。李强等研究发现,四川各地区松茸可分为 2 个品质群,凉山州的木里县、盐源县、冕宁县、会东县松茸品质群富含蛋白质、脂肪、氨基酸与维生素;而小金、雅江、盐边松茸品质群富含纤维素与矿质元素含量高。环境、气候与土壤生态等因素综合作用造成了四川松茸独特的品质和产地差异性。上述研究可证,药用菌物同药用植物一样,其品质具有显著的地域特性,地理环境和生态因子是其道地品质形成的重要原因。

## 9 中药微生态与道地药材引种

道地药材虽质优效佳,但由于野生资源不断减少,药材需求量日益增加,土地利用规划改变,拉动地方经济等各种原因,需要对某些中药进行异地引种栽培。

在引种过程中发现，引种的产地、产区不同，药材的产量、化学成分，甚至性状等皆不同。如质量较佳的山东平邑、临朐的丹参引种至四川中江引种后，质量变为较次；山东沂南、河北行唐的丹参由引种前的质量较次变为引种后质量较佳。原产地为山东平邑的金银花引种至宁夏贺兰后，大白期绿原酸含量及各个花期总黄酮含量明显低于原产地。甘肃陇西等9个柴胡引种地之间相互比较，所产有效成分含量存在较大差异。原产于南美洲秘鲁的濒危珍稀药材资源玛咖于2003年玛咖在中国云南引耕成功，比较研究云南丽江、会泽、香格里拉以及秘鲁4个产的玛咖质量，发现其主要功效成分并不相同，其中丽江玛咖中主要含有脯氨酸和二糖，会泽玛咖中主要含有脯氨酸和苄基-芥子油苷，香格里拉玛咖中主要含有咪唑类生物碱B和二糖，而秘鲁玛咖中主要含有脯氨酸和二糖，其他共有成分如精氨酸、脯氨酸等的含量在4个产地也不一致。

有效成分的改变是引种中药适应新生境必然表现，造成该现象的原因极有可能与其微生态结构的重组有关。中药柱冠粗榧自然分布区在日本，中国江西庐山等地虽有引种，但生长不良。Langenfeld A等对比研究了日本原产和法国引种的柱冠粗榧的内生菌群，发现日本内生菌群的丰度高于法国，内生菌群的分类学组成明显不同。*Pestalotiopsis cocculi* BG35在法国较为丰富，在日本较为罕见；而对 *Nigrospora oryzae*、*Phomopsis* sp.（BG3）、*Diaporthe eres*、*Coniochaeta velutina* 来说，情况正好相反。在54个类群中，只有6个类群为两国共有菌种，并且为在全球广布种。引种法国后，柱冠粗榧捕获了当地存有的世界广布性的部分菌群；而在原产地，大多数内生菌群为日本当地或亚洲区域分布的分离株。

综上所述，药用植物在异地引种后，功效成分均要发生不同程度的变化，主要原因应在于环境的改变。在适应新生境的过程中，药材建构新的微生态结构，必然影响原有的植物次生代谢网络，从而导致活性成分积累的变化。具有悠久传统栽培模式的药材、单道地种和狭域野生种类长期适应原产地独特的生长环境和特有的栽培方式，轻易异地引种可能导致微生态结构的不平衡，增加土传病害风险，影响药材原有的优良品质。

## 10 小结和展望

为了适应不同产地环境，中药微生态系统协助甚至诱导宿主建立抗性、调整性状和药材产量、积累次生代谢产物，形成药材鲜明的“地域性”差异。这些差异在长期的人为选择过程中可能发展为某地中药材的重要优势，最终形成中药材的道地性。微生态是自然界中始终存在的一种生态关系，但因其所涉及的微生物群具有极高的多样性、宿主差异性、时空波动性、菌群之间互作的复杂性、菌株变异性以及定植随机性，加上绝大多数菌种难以纯化培养，导致对中药微生态的认识很晚，重视不足。

几十年来，对中药微生态的探究大致历经了中药微生态资源的广泛挖掘阶段、功能菌株的筛选及初步利用阶段、功能基因及关键酶基因的克隆阶段、利用功能菌对中药活性成分加以转化和诱导合成的阶段。尽管当前中药微生态研究已经发展到分子代谢层次，但多数研究关注少数菌株的个别功能在特定药材上的作用效果，换一种药材或条件就难再重现，因此研究结果的代表性、普遍性比较欠缺，对中药微生态的利用更是十分局限。当然，这与中药微生态结构本身的地域性、宿主选择性、生态关系的复杂性等有关。

随着以组学为代表的现代分子生物技术、信息科学技术、AI技术、各种观测技术等新兴技术的不断涌现，中药微生态这一复杂的生态关系将会由模糊走向清晰，并渗透到中药品质与道地性理论研究及应用性研究的方方面面，尤其是以下方向将会成为未来的研究热点。①基于中药微生态介导的道地性化学成分的生源途径挖掘，例如内生菌介导青蒿素过氧桥形成的这一重要代谢途径的挖掘，可以极大增加药效成分体外合成的种类和成功率。②基于微生态量效关系的中药代谢合成生物反应器的研究和开发。中药微生态系统在诱导或介导宿主活性成分合成与积累过程中存在复杂的量效关系。因此，在利用宿主活细胞制备中药活性成分生物反应器，必须将微生态与宿主之间的量效关系纳入考察范围。③基于中药微生态结构重构的道地药材仿生种植研究。道地中药具有特定的中药微生态结构，在人工控制的条件下进行中药“道地微生态结构”的重构，将会使药材的品质、抗性等逐渐接近于原生道地药材。④基于中药微生态的产地鉴别条码溯源技术研究。特定产地的中药材携带特定的菌群结构，该特定结构即为相应产地的“天然标识”，可以作为不同产地来源的同类甚至同种药材鉴别及产地溯源的“身份标签”。⑤基于微生态的中药减毒增效技术及道地药材加工工艺的研究。某些微生物直接合成或诱导合成了中药中的毒性物质，另一些微生物则能转化并降低这些物质的毒性。对中药微生态系统中大量微生物资源的筛查和利用，有望在中药栽培源头或药材加工过程中实现对药材的增效减毒。

[何冬梅，黄璐琦，等.中国中药杂志，2020，45(2)：290-302.]

# 道地药材分子生药学研究进展和发展趋势

随着分子生物学成为现代生命科学的共同语言，其理论与技术不断与中药学交叉融合、广泛联系，以此开拓出新的研究领域和增长点。1995年在《展望分子生物技术在生药学中的应用》中首次提出了“分子生药”。分子生药学是在分子水平上研究中药的鉴定、质量的形成及活性成分生产的一门学科，目前它已形成14个研究方向，包括中药资源分子系统学、中药资源功能基因组、中药分子鉴定、中药资源活性成分的生物合成和代谢调控、珍稀濒危中药资源保护、中药资源活性成分的生物技术生产、中药资源分子标记辅助育种等。

2000年《分子生药学》的出版，标志着分子生药学学科的建立并进入快速发展期。在这一时期DNA分子标记技术广泛应用于中药资源研究，一系列中药资源遗传多样性、分子系统学研究成果呈现强劲的增长趋势，为中药材品种整理和质量标准化研究、中药资源保护与可持续利用提供了新的策略。自2009年利用454测序技术进行青蒿转录组研究起，目前已发表了200余种中药资源转录组、基因组，以基因的结构、表达、调控为核心的分子生药学研究日新月异，为中药理论创新、中药质量有效控制和中药材新品种定向选育奠定基础。2012年分子生药学成为国家中医药管理局重点培育学科，并于2017年、2019年分别出版了"十三五"中医药行业规划教材、国家卫生健康委员会规划教材、国家卫计委研究生规划教材，已在30余家高等院校开设本科生或研究生课程。

道地药材是中药质量评价的原创综合性指标。道地药材及其形成机制研究是一项复杂的工作，是中药资源研究成果的集中体现，也是分子生药学重要的研究内容。1997年在《"道地药材"的生物学探讨》中首次提出了"道"是生物学上的"居群"，它的形成是由基因型和环境饰变共同作用的结果。道地药材的表型包括药材性状、组织结构、活性成分组成及药效，特定基因的存在是其产生特定表型的基础，而适宜的生境则是产生特定表型的推动力。2004年在《中药材道地性研究的现代生物学基础及模式假说》中又提出理论研究、实验研究和观察分析是道地药材研究的主要途径，以及道地药材研究的三个模式假说，即道地药材应具有特定化学成分组成、独特基因型和"边缘效应"。随着道地药材研究的深入，越来越多的实验证据表明道地药材化学成分组成等表型是由其内在基因及其基因调控网络决定的，并受到生长环境、采收阶段、产地加工方式等外因的影响。

## 1 道地药材"优形、优质"特征

根据"辨证论治"是中医理论结合实际治病原则的精髓，谢宗万提出了中药品种经验鉴别的精髓在于"辨状论质"的观点，这是对药材质量系统性和整体性传统经验认识的一种体现。辨状的内容包括辨药材的形状、大小、色泽、表面特征、质地、断面、气味等；论质则有两方面的结论：一是药材的真伪，二是优劣评判，也就是有效性。

随着科学技术的发展，以计算机视觉和人工智能为核心的现代多层次表型采集技术的出现使得对生物的表型研究已经发展到精确的表型鉴定。在国家自然科学基金重大项目"中药道地性研究"中提出了道地性表型可表现为药材的"优形"和"优质"，并体现为药材使用上的"优效"。在狭义上，"优形"指道地药材具有公认的性状特征，"优质"指其具有独特的化学成分组成，"优效"指其在临床功效上优于非道地药材；在广义上，"优质"泛指道地药材的优良品质，包含"优形"和"优效"。本文论述的道地药材"优形、优质"属狭义上的特征。

道地药材"优形、优质"特征的提出，拓宽了传统药材辩状的范畴，其核心思想是通过获取高质量、可重复的性状数据，进而量化分析基因型和环境互作效应及其对中药质量的影响，为中药材现代化质量控制体系建立奠定基础。通常认为，化学成分是中药发挥临床疗效的物质基础，也是药材质量评价的主要指标，但目前有关中药药效物质及其作用机制尚存在争论。而从生物学本质上来看，药材的"优形"和"优质"特征是统一的。

大量的现代科学研究结果表明，药材性状特征和化学成分均受到相同基因或基因调控网络控制。目前研究比较清楚的是颜色相关成分和基因，如柑橘不同品种其果皮因类胡萝卜素组成和含量的多态性呈现出不同的色泽，利用红橘（红色果皮）×枳（黄色果皮）的双假测交遗传群体和自然群体关联分析锁定到类胡萝卜素裂解酶编码基因CCD4b的顺式调控元件是红色果皮性状形成的主效遗传位点。在传统鉴别中存在着许多有关"以色论质"的药材，如《增订伪药条辨》记载丹参"皮色红，肉紫有纹……为最佳"。现代研究表明色红主要是由于丹参根周皮中含有红色的丹参酮类成分所致，且该类成分含量越高、红色越深。目前已初步解析了丹参酮类成分的生物合成途径，相继发现了2个萜类合酶、3个CYP76家族成员可催化生成丹参酮基本碳骨架次丹参酮二烯、铁锈醇、柳杉酚、四氢丹参新酮等多种化合物，这些基因的克隆和功能研究将为进一步解析丹参根皮红色变异机制奠定基础。同时，成分的组成和比例也可以影响颜色的形成，如4-香豆酸辅酶A连接酶基因被认为与玫瑰粉红色的形成有关，而二氢黄酮醇4-还原酶基因的低水平表达可能与白色形成有关；通过比较银杏金黄色叶片与绿叶在细胞学、生理学和转录组学方面的差异，发现金黄色叶片中叶绿素和类黄酮含量较低、类胡萝卜素含量较高，与叶绿素生物合成相关基因表达下调、类胡萝卜素生物合成相关基因表达上调相一致，说明类胡萝卜素与叶绿素比例的变化是导致叶色变黄的主要因素。

另一方面，药材性状特征和化学成分均受到生物"生长与防御权衡"机制的影响。当植物在面临不良环境胁迫时，往往会以抑制正常生长为代价，消耗更多的代谢资源用于激活防御系统，以抵抗胁迫对自身的伤害，而这些代谢资源往往在药材中作为活性成分存在，是"优质"的重要物质基础。如木瓜为蔷薇科植物贴梗海棠的干燥近成熟果实，夏、秋二季果实绿黄时采收，有机酸、总黄酮含量在近成熟果实中累积到较高水平，且随着果实的成熟逐渐下降；有机酸、总黄酮均为植物防御物质，其积累与果实大小呈负相关。化学成分在性状表型特征的形成过程中发挥了重要作用，如激素是控制"生长与防御权衡"的主要因素之一，茉莉酸可以帮助植物进行能量物质的分配，使其适应复杂的生长环境；水杨酸可以通过基础亮氨酸拉链家族转录因子AaTGA6调节青蒿素的生物合成；油菜素内酯和脱落酸被认为是金荞麦种子大小的重要调节因子，油菜素内酯也可以通过调节细胞数量和大小控制莲子的大小。在植物体内存在某些具有激素样作用的化合物，如三萜类成分在植物体内也可能发挥类激素作用，从而调控植物的生长发育。研究表明，燕麦中的三萜类成分β-amyrin会阻塞根表皮细胞发育，导致"superhairy"根表型的形成。

## 2 道地药材特定的基因组结构及其特征

药材"优形、优质"特征实质上属于生物的复杂性状，其形成是由基因组结构及其特征决定的。药材“优形、优质”特征可分为质量性状和数量性状，质量性状为表现不连续变异的性状，如花的颜色；大多数性状为数量性状，受多基因控制。随着基因组大数据时代的到来，挖掘“优形、优质”特征重要功能基因、解析药材性状演化的遗传基础、揭示药材质量的生物内涵已成为分子生药学的主要研究内容之一。如通过比较基因组研究发现青蒿中的萜类合酶基因家族显著扩张，且是目前已测植物物种中萜类合酶基因最多的物种之一。倍半萜青蒿素是一种从青蒿中分离得到的有效抗疟药物，其生物合成途径已经基本解析清楚，而腺毛特异性转录因子 AaORA 可以正向调节青蒿素和青蒿酸的合成。AaHD1 是茉莉酸调控分泌型腺毛发育的重要因子之一，且以 AaTCP14－AaORA 转录激活复合体为核心，参与茉莉酸响应的多个转录因子组成了青蒿素生物合成的多层次调控网络，揭示了青蒿“以腺毛特征论青蒿素成分”的机制。同时在全基因组水平上可比较物种间、品种间基因组结构及其特征的差异，利用基因序列差异可建立道地药材 DNA 指纹图谱，结合性状、化学特征形成道地药材特征辨识体系，用于保证其基原可靠。

## 3 道地药材的表型可塑性

当生物体的结构、形态和功能还未达到成熟和稳定水平时，容易受环境因素的影响而产生变异，这种表型可塑性是相同基因型在不同环境下产生不同表型的能力，而药材“优形、优质”特征的形成也是其对所处生长环境适应的一种表现。表型可塑性被认为受遗传控制，包括基因和表观遗传调控。基因表达水平的变化受到环境的影响，不同等位基因对环境的敏感性也存在很大差异。来自外部环境的信号被生物体识别，召集不同的转录因子，激活不同结构基因的转录，产生不同的表型，从而形成生物体对不同环境信号的响应。另一方面，表观遗传是指在基因组 DNA 序列没有改变的情况下，基因的表达调控和性状发生了可遗传的变化，主要包括 DNA 甲基化、组蛋白修饰、非编码 RNA 等。其中 DNA 甲基化是调节基因功能的重要手段之一，启动子区的 DNA 甲基化通常会抑制基因的转录，从而影响生物的表型。如 NO 处理下石斛的 DNA 甲基化水平发生改变、DNA 甲基化水平变异会影响菊花的生长和花的发育，DNA 甲基化通路在果实发育与成熟、生物和非生物胁迫、根瘤发育和根瘤固氮中也具有重要作用。非编码 RNA 也可参与生物表型、环境应激反应、代谢的调控，如茉莉酸甲酯处理下商陆 miRNA 可靶向茉莉酸生物合成酶基因的转录；通过整合 mRNA 和 miRNA 分析，揭示山药块茎发育的基因调控模式，发现 miRNA160、miRNA396、miRNA535 和 miRNA5021 可能参与了山药细胞分裂和分化的调控；并参与调控萜类、萜内酯类、黄酮类、皂苷类成分的生物合成。

道地药材“优形、优质”特征的形成与其性状表型相关基因在内外环境下的选择性表达密切相关，其基原物种在特定生长区域内呈现出一定的形态结构、生理机制、遗传特性等特征。由于这种生物对环境的适应是相对的，使得道地药材对环境因子的适应性具有一定的界限范围，其上限和下限之间的生态区域即为道地药材的分布区。道地药材特征的可塑性不仅表现为多种环境因素的综合影响，还是其基原物种通过自身调控机制缓冲、平衡、抵抗或促进环境影响的整合性结果。当道地药材被引种到界限范围以外的产区，其表型可能发生改变而影响药材的道地性。

## 4 道地药材分子生药学研究和未来发展建议

道地药材是一个复杂的生物系统，具“优形、优质”特征、特定的基因组结构和基因特征以及表型可塑性。道地药材形成的分子生药学研究涉及多领域、多层面、多技术，通过认识“优形、优质”相关基因或蛋白质的物理与化学特性，进一步解析基因和蛋白质构成的相互作用网络，是诠释道地药材形成的基础和关键。种群进化、复杂性状形成、防御、植物全能性将成为道地药材分子生药学研究领域最受关注的科学问题。

4.1 道地药材形成机制研究的新方法 目前道地药材形成机制研究方法大体可分为两个层次：一是以基因组、转录组、代谢组等为核心技术，二是以 DNA 分子标记、基因克隆、基因表达、基因体内或体外功能验证为核心技术，用于解析“优形、优质”相关基因及其基因调控网络。随着生命科学的发展，一些新的技术和方法被用于生物表型特征的研究，也将有助于推动道地药材形成机制的深入解析。

4.1.1 表型组分析 植物表型组是指由基因型和环境互作产生的植物全部表型，包括植物物理、生理和生化特征和性状，可以系统反映植物的结构和生长发育过程。基于数量分类的表型精准度量已成为深入认识生命现象形成规律的基础，是系统解析生命复杂系统的突破口。目前植物表型组研究方法主要包括以下几个方面。

4.1.1.1 高通量、高分辨率的表型组研究平台 随着遥感技术、机器人技术、计算机视觉和人工智能的发展，越来越多的现代多层次表型采集技术被应用于植物表型组研究。通过配备自动、半自动或手动的成像系统和传感器，可对植物进行连续监测，并获取高通量的实时动态数据。按照观测尺度大体可分为两类平台：①受控实验研究：利用多参数、高通量植物表型测量设备和图形一体化采集分析软件，对植物或组织进行自动、无损的特征数据采集，用于表征植物生长发育、响应环境胁迫等特征及其变化规律。针对根系在土壤中的特殊性，还可利用高分辨率扫描仪对根系图像进行采集，或利用 X 射线进行电子计算机断层扫描对根系实施原位成像分析。②田间实验研究：利用装置于固定监测塔、移动监测设备、大型田间作物扫描平台、小型飞行器的光谱检测设备，通过对植物地上部分光谱信号的收集，用于表征植物的性状、水分、叶绿素、营养成分、病害等特征。

成像和信号的采集主要依赖于不同类型的传感器，如可见光成像主要被用于植物的颜色、大小、叶片形态、植株骨架结构等分析，叶绿素荧光成像主要用于光合作用的研究，近红外成像主要用于植物中水分、氮含量和无机盐等的无损检测，高光谱成像可通过对特征光谱检测进而表征与其关联的生理特征，3D 激光扫描可通过 360 度的云点扫描构建植株的立体成像。基于机器学习的方法是进行表型检测和计数最有前景的方法，利用该方法可实现表型特征的识别、分类、量化和预测。

4.1.1.2 高分辨率质谱成像研究平台 质谱成像技术是基于质谱发展起来的一种分子成像技术，其可以通过直接扫描生物样本，同时获得多种化合物的分子结构信息和空间分布特征，弥补了传统光学显微镜的不足，已成为生物学、化学等研究领域的关键技术之一。利用高分辨率质谱成像系统可对植物的种子、根、茎、叶片以及穗轴等进行可被化检测，研究植物生长发育过程中的空间分布特征。如在对贯叶连翘蒽醌类化合物定位的研究中，利用高分辨率质谱成像系统可确定蒽醌类化合物位于根部的外皮层和内皮层，对控制水分运输、防止病虫害具有重要意义。

4.1.2　单细胞测序　生命体基本上为多细胞生物，其均从单个细胞发育而来，细胞与细胞之间是存在差异的，其基因组与转录组等遗传信息也是存在差异的。传统的测序方法是在多细胞水平上进行的，难以获得细胞间异质性的信息，而单细胞测序技术是一种单细胞水平上的测序，其可以从混杂的样品中筛选出异质性信息。利用单细胞测序可以以精确的方式跟踪和构建生命体所需的各种组织、器官、系统发育轨迹，揭示每个细胞分裂和分化、与相邻细胞协调功能等变化，并获得全新的细胞类型。

目前植物单细胞 RNA 测序技术已比较成熟，利用该技术对拟南芥根组织进行细胞水平基因表达谱分析，解析了根生毛细胞的发育路径；比较了根组织热激响应转录调控的细胞异质性，发现新的细胞类型特异表达基因、细胞状态特异的发育调控因子等。在进行植物单细胞 RNA 测序时，易受到细胞壁等因素的限制，需要根据研究的物种和组织类型，对解离酶的选择、解离酶的处理时间等条件进行优化。此外，单细胞 CHIP-seq、单细胞 Hi-C、单细胞全基因甲基化组等测序技术也将会应用于植物的单细胞研究，从基因、转录、表观水平等多维度观测单一细胞，从整体了解单一细胞内不同事件是如何发生以及如何与其他事件相互联系的。在单细胞水平上，揭示道地药材基原物种的组织、器官发育过程，将为阐明道地药材“优形”特征的形成奠定基础，是未来重要的研究方向之一。

4.1.3　基因编辑技术　基因编辑技术主要是利用序列特异性核酸酶在特定基因位点产生 DNA 双链断裂，借助编辑受体自身的 DNA 修复系统在非同源末端连接过程中产生的随机 Indels 或在同源重组修复过程中插入或替换相应的基因片段，最终实现基因组序列的突变。

基因功能鉴定和新品种选育离不开突变体的获得，但目前对道地药材基原物种突变体重视不足；传统上突变体的获得主要依靠自然突变、物理或化学诱变以及 T-DNA 随机插入等手段，但对于中药材基原物种来说，上述方法存在突变效率低、突变位点随机、实验周期长等缺陷。将纳米材料生物大分子传递系统应用于道地药材基原物种的基因编辑研究中，在功能基因组研究的基础上，在特定位点上引入核苷酸变异，实现基因的定点编辑能高效地获得目标突变体，从而加快道地药材“优形、优质”特征形成机制研究及其定向育种的进程。

4.2　道地药材“优形、优质”特征表征及其形成研究的核心任务

4.2.1　量化“优形、优质”特征　在传统鉴别经验的基础上，利用图像识别、人工智能等技术对道地药材“优形”特征进行量化，利用质谱分析、化学计量学等技术对道地药材“优质”特征进行量化，结合表型组、质谱成像等技术对道地药材“优形、优质”特征进行关联和统一，为实现道地药材特征辨识、进一步进行道地药材基因型与环境互作机制研究奠定基础。

4.2.2　阐释“外在优形”与“内在优质”的相关性　以道地药材“形、色、质、味”鉴别特征为核心，在基因组、转录组、代谢组、表型组、表观组研究的基础上，结合颜色数字化、高分辨质谱成像技术、激光切割技术、电镜技术、共聚焦显微镜联合组织化学技术等，进行“优形、优质”基因挖掘及功能鉴定，探究药材“外在优形”与“内在优质”的相关性，为阐明道地药材形成机制奠定基础，为指导药材种植生产、品种选育提供依据。

4.3　道地药材“优形、优质”特征的定向诱导和新品种选育的新方案　以道地药材“优形、优质”特征为目标，筛选相关表型标记、遗传标记和化学标记，并建立道地药材评价体系，指导中药材“安全、有序”生产。利用基因编辑、人工诱变等技术构建药材基原物种突变体，并结合分子标记辅助育种进行中药材新品种选育。

4.3.1　系统选育法结合多组学技术　在种质资源收集和整理的基础上，建立种质资源圃；应用系统选育法，基于表型组、代谢组、DNA 分子标记、活性评价分析等方法，经多代自交纯化，逐步淘汰不良品种，综合筛选获得“优形、优质”候选品系及新品种。

4.3.2　基于功能基因标记的分子设计育种　在获得全基因组序列的基础上，利用遗传群体初定位和精细定位“优形、优质”关键基因，结合表型组、代谢组分析结果，筛选关键基因特异表达株系作为候选品系进行新品种选育。

4.3.3　基于人工诱变技术的新品种选育　基于物理、化学等定向诱导手段或基因编辑技术获得突变材料，并通过表型观测、成分分析、活性评价等方法，筛选获得“优形、优质”特征明显、变异性状稳定的新品系或新品种。

## 5　结语

伴随着中医药的起源和发展，道地药材的产生和形成同样经历了漫长的经验认知过程。所谓万变不离其宗，利用分子生药学理论和技术开展道地药材研究仍需尊重传统法则、守正创新，从“辨状论质”到“优形、优质”的特征化、标准化，实现从经验判断到规律研究的转化和提升。道地药材的现代研究需要集合表型组、代谢物定性定量分析、细胞生物学、分子生物学、植物生理学等多种技术手段，对药材“优形、优质”特征进行定量表征，利用和吸收生命科学发展最新成果，揭示道地药材形成机制。并积极探索应用转化途径，进行“优形、优质”特征定向诱导和新品种选育，将有助于道地药材良种繁育、建立生产技术标准体系和等级评价制度，推动中药质量提升和产业高质量发展。

[袁媛，黄璐琦. 科学通报，2020，65(12)：1093－1102.]

# 论基于基因组学的中药材定向培育策略与展望

近年来，我国中药材种植面积持续增加，2021 年已达 9 000 万亩，中药材产量达到 495.2 万吨。目前中药材品种选育以常规育种为主，选育及推广的优良中药材品种数量还相对较少，且多为药用植物的引种驯化，即对野生药用植物进行人工培育，使野生变为家种，在种质纯化、杂交育种、生物育种等研究领域基础薄弱。对优质、抗病、抗逆、耐贮藏等新品种选育的研究起步较晚、水平较低，难以满足规模化、现代化中药农业发展的需求。为了推动和加快中药材品种选育和种业发展，亟需重视和加强中药种质创新的研究和实践，形成具有中药特色的种质创新途径。

获得具有优良性状的亲本是新品种选育的首要步骤，育种核心种质的选择与合理组配首先是对地方品种、外来品种或野生近缘种进行表型与性状鉴定，将优良目标性状转到中间材料，创制具有有利性状及其等位基因的新种质，进而利用这些新种质培育新品种。地方品种又称农家品种、传统品种、地区性品种，是在当地自然或栽培条件下，经长期自然或人为选择形成的品种，对当地自然或栽培环境具有较好的适应性；外来品种是相对于地方品种而言，一般指从国外原产地引入到新地区并定植的生物种，也可以泛指非本土原产的各种外域物种；野生种质包括野生近缘种，具有很强的广适性与抗性，具有较高的利用价值。育种核心种质的选择与合理组配应更侧重于识别特定的性状来源和实现新的性状组合，以及在早期子代中进行选择，以提供具有良好特征的种质资源，作为新亲本用于育种中。

中药材种质创新的过程主要包括种质资源的收集与保存、种质资源鉴定、种质资源评价等，研究周期较长，一般为 5～10 年。随着高通量测序等技术的发展，基因组学的理论与方法广泛应用于种质资源研究，种质资源的创新与利用在研究思路与技术上得到了全新变革。基因组学不仅为中药材种质资源的收集与利用提供了理论指导，提高了优良基因发掘和种质创新效率，也为加快中药材新品种选育提供了理论方法。本文根据目前中药材品种选育面临的瓶颈问题，系统论述中药材种质创新的主要内容、关键技术、基础平台等，为基于基因组学的中药材品种选育研究提供思路和方法，以期进一步推动中药材种业的高质量发展。

## 1 中药材品种选育现状

中药材良种直接影响药材的质量和临床疗效，中药材品种选育多参考传统农作物品种选育方式，较重视产量、活性成分含量、抗性等选育指标，目前采用的选育方法包括选择育种、诱变育种、倍性育种、杂交育种、分子育种等(表 1)。

**表 1 中药材品种选育的主要方法**

| 方法 | 定 义 | 优 点 | 缺 点 |
| --- | --- | --- | --- |
| 选择育种 | 对现有品种群体中出现的自然变异进行性状鉴定、选择并通过品系比较试验、区域试验和生产试验培育新品种 | 获得的品种稳定，变异频率小 | 育种周期长，效率低，预见性差 |
| 诱变育种 | 利用物理、化学和生物因素诱发植物发生可遗传的变异，然后根据育种目标进行选择，从而育成新品种 | 变异范围广，变异率高，育种周期短，稳定性强，大幅度改良某些性状，可获得稀有突变 | 有利变异少，需大量处理材料，诱变方向和性质不能控制，改良数量形状效果差，有盲目性 |
| 倍性育种 | 根据育种目标要求，采用染色体加倍(或减半)的方法选育植物新品种。包括单倍体育种和多倍体育种 | 培育出的植物产量高，或次生代谢产物含量高 | 结实率低，发育迟 |
| 杂交育种 | 通过人工杂交将两个或两个以上亲本的优良性状综合到一个个体中，继而在分离的后代群体中，通过人工选择和比较鉴定，获得新品种 | 使生物体不良性状集中同一个体，具有预见性 | 育种年限长，需连续自交才能育出优良性状 |
| 分子育种 | 在分子水平上进行育种，分为基因工程育种和分子标记辅助育种 | 可实现基因的直接选择和聚合，育种周期短 | 基因工程育种成本高，育种体系不完善，基因功能平台较弱 |

中药材新品种的培育源于对药用植物的人工培育或者野生药用植物的开发，目前中药材品种选育模式存在以下挑战：①中药材种类繁多，大部分药材的育种研究基础薄弱，栽培驯化程度相对较低。②引种是植物在其遗传性适应范围内的迁移，这种适应范围受到基因型的严格制约，同一植物种类的不同品种间在适应性上存在差异，其对环境变异的自体调节能力与品种基因型的杂合性程度有关，但目前在中药材野生变家种的过程中，极少关注基因型对引种驯化程度的影响。③种质基因杂合度普遍较高，品种选育多以选择育种为主，人工杂交等方法的应用相对滞后。④选育目标多与产量、抗性、指标性成分含量相关，是否对药材品质产生影响或存在临床安全用药风险尚存在争论。⑤目前仅少数中药材进行了全基

因组测序，且大部分中药材没有开展DNA身份证等相关研究，导致目前中药材新品种确权难。

针对上述情况，应根据对中药材质量的实际需求，通过对控制“优形优质”性状关键基因的驯化，加强中药材种质创新研究，在较短时间内将自然界中的野生植物物种转变为家养品种。为了减少对外界环境的依赖性，植物可采取形态、生理和行为等多种机制保持其“内稳态”，但内稳态机制不能完全摆脱环境的限制，植物仅在一定范围内具有生态适应性。因此，应优先考虑以基因型鉴定为核心，选育具有基因型、外观形状、化学成分“内稳态”特征的中药材种质，以保证中药材质量的稳定可控。

## 2 中药材种质创新的主要内容

中药材种质创新的本质是为了提高种质资源的可利用性，获得可用于育种的材料，其基本内容包括种质扩增、改良与创新。

2.1 收集和引进　系统进行中药材种质资源的收集，建立种质资源圃。

2.2 鉴定和评价　对种质进行系统鉴定，包括物种鉴定、基因型鉴定、产量性状和药用性状鉴定、生物和非生物逆境抗性鉴定，遴选优异种质。筛选适用于作为育种亲本的高纯合度种质，研究杂种优势群，明确改良途径。

2.3 改良和创新　通过自交或其他手段选育纯系；以道地药材“优形优质”特征为育种目标，配制循环选系的基础群体，创制育种新材料。

2.4 群体构建　供体群体：针对育种目标要求和限制因素，构建供体群体（如产量性状、药用性状、生物和非生物逆境抗性性状等），用作育种的基因供体。育种群体：针对育种目标要求，创建具有不同种质基础和性状特征的循环改良群体。群体改良：采用轮回选择方法改良群体遗传结构，提高优良等位基因频率，获得新一轮改良群体，并创制优良育种新材料。

2.5 数据采集与信息管理系统　数据采集：构建适宜的育种管理软件，建立系统的田间性状数据采集系统。收集育种新材料的性状信息，以及分子数据。数据库建设：建立公共数据库，实现数据分类、存储、处理、共享及维护等。

## 3 基于基因组的中药材种质创新关键技术

3.1 遗传多样性分析　遗传多样性一般指种内的遗传多样性或称遗传变异，包括居群水平、个体水平、组织和细胞水平以及分子水平。遗传多样性不仅包括遗传变异高低，也包括遗传变异分布格局即居群的遗传结构。检测遗传多样性的方法从形态学水平、细胞学（染色体）水平、生理生化水平，逐渐发展到分子水平。例如，通过使用21对SRAP（sequence-related amplified polymorphism）引物对100份紫苏种质资源进行遗传多样性分析，结果显示，紫苏种质遗传多样性较为丰富，各群体之间遗传差异性大，组内差异不显著，组内群体遗传纯合度高。利用12个EST-SSR标记对14个厚朴自然居群的遗传多样性和遗传结构进行分析，结果表明，14个厚朴自然居群可以按分布区域划分为3个类群，其中西部类群的遗传多样性高于中部和东部居群，不同居群间的历史迁移率较低且不对称。药用植物遗传多样性研究为中药种质资源的评价、保护、核心种质的构建奠定基础。

3.2 种质纯合度分析　遗传背景混杂是目前中药材育种亟需突破的关键瓶颈，快速筛选高纯合度种质，获得遗传稳定育种材料，对药用植物纯系育种研究具有重要意义。中药材种质资源遗传多样性较丰富，可从自然群体或栽培群体中筛选纯合度高的种质进行纯系育种，进而获得纯系品种作为育种材料。

建立高效、便捷的高纯合度种质材料筛选方法，有利于加速中药材纯系育种的进程。传统上，种质纯度的检验主要通过田间实验完成，费时且受环境影响较大。目前，利用高通量测序数据和分子标记法实现了对种质纯合度的快速评估，如利用PCR-RFLP法从15份天麻种质材料中筛选获得10份高纯合度种质材料（纯合度≥95%）。在实际应用中，将分子标记技术与基因组重测序结合，用低成本的分子标记分析，从大量样品中初步筛选高纯合度的种质材料，再对初筛获得的种质材料进一步重测序并精确评估，最终获得可用于纯系育种的材料。

3.3 多倍体鉴定　多倍体在生物界广泛存在，是新物种形成的驱动力之一，在物种进化、环境适应中发挥重要作用。多倍化是物种形成及植物育种的重要途径，多倍体药用植物在茎粗、叶大、花大、果实大、代谢产物含量高等特性中表现出一定优势，可用于克服远缘杂交种不育性、创制不亲和材料中间亲本等。但由于某些药用植物存在成熟期长、体型巨大、个体分散、多倍体发生率低等生物学特点，建立快速筛选天然多倍体种质的方法具有重要意义。

目前多倍体鉴定方法包括形态学鉴定、染色体计数鉴定、流式细胞术法鉴定及分子标记技术鉴定。由于分子标记多态性不仅表现为不同个体的某一基因位点存在多态性，也表现为同一个体的同源染色体之间存在多态性，利用分子标记技术可进行多倍体种质的筛选，基本解决了单纯利用细胞学手段鉴定多倍体对实验材料高限制条件的问题。例如，利用5个ISSR分子标记分析菘蓝四倍体株系遗传稳定性，结果表明，其株系8～36代之间均未产生变异条带。

3.4 DNA分子身份证鉴定　传统的形态、生理和生化指标难以对数量种类繁多的品种资源进行准确鉴定，利用分子标记构建DNA分子身份证在种质资源鉴定与评价中已成为发展趋势。分子身份证是指基于DNA指纹图谱信息，利用基因分型技术选取若干个固定的基因位点或特异性序列进行种质鉴定，选出具有唯一性的基因位点和序列标记组合，将电泳结果数字化，以条形码或二维码的形式表示。DNA分子身份证可以通过计算机自动识别实现对种质的快速比对。目前已建立滇皖产区铁皮石斛、枸杞、当归等中药材的SSR分子身份证，利用一段极短的物种特异性DNA序列（20～50 bp）构建的DNA分子身份证也已应用在西洋参、冬虫夏草、银杏等药材中。

3.5 稀有等位基因鉴定　稀有等位基因通常是根据它们的相对频率来定义的，即等位基因频率小于某个指定值的等位基因可以称为稀有等位基因。稀有等位基因是非常宝贵的遗传改良资源，如粉果人参可能蕴藏着稀有基因型，是优质、高产、多抗等品种遗传改良的潜在基因来源。在野生资源驯化的过程中,稀有基因可能会出现丢失的情况,如野生甜瓜种质的平均 Shannon's index (I) 值和 polymorphism information content (PIC)值比栽培种质高,说明野生种质的多样性更为丰富,包含更多的稀有基因。目前大部分中药种质资源还处于驯化早期阶段,因此需要加强对其稀有基因的保护。

在育种过程中,人工选择涉及数千个位点,包括编码和非编码区域,常导致核苷酸多样性的减少和稀有等位基因比例增加。通过稀有等位变异分析和基于 PCA、K-means 聚类的遗传关系分析也可以对种质资源中的非杂交后代进行鉴定。

3.6 *关键性状相关基因挖掘* 全基因组关联分析(genome-wide association study, GWAS)是一种针对全基因组范围内的遗传变异进行基因分型,寻找某一群体内性状与分子标记或候选基因间关系的分析方法。GWAS 对于连锁标记开发、目的基因挖掘和复杂性状的遗传研究具有重要作用。利用 GWAS 挖掘和研究调控道地药材"优形优质"性状基因及其分子标记,有助于加快中药材优异种质的鉴定和优良品种的培育。

随着 100 余种药用植物全基因组测序的完成,利用高通量数据对中药种质资源复杂性状开展 GWAS 研究越来越便利。与数量性状座位(quantitative trait locus, QTL)方法相比,GWAS 具有不需要构建作图群体和一次性可同时检测多个等位基因位点的优势。用全基因组重测序和 GWAS 分析获得 1 个三七根腐病抗性相关位点,为三七抗病品种选育奠定基础。利用 GWAS 挖掘出 24 个与菊花耐寒性显著关联的 SNP 位点,其中 5 个与脚芽期相关,11 个与现蕾期相关,5 个与盛花期相关,3 个与盛花期舌状花相关;5 个 SNP 位点的表型效应值均小于−4℃,为优异等位变异位点;在此基础上,鉴定 5 个菊花耐寒性候选基因。基于全基因组测序结果,对检测到的变异进行注释,最终筛选出 30 个 SNPs 标记用于紫苏高产新品种的鉴定与筛选,并选育丰产新品种。

## 4 中药材新品种培育的基础平台建设

4.1 *核心种质构建* 核心种质是指收集保存种质资源的一个核心子集,该子集以最少数量的遗传资源最大限度地保存整个种质资源群体的遗传多样性,同时代表整个群体地理分布的多样性。中药材种质资源丰富,遗传基础广泛。不同于一般农作物,药用植物种质资源通常分布于深远山区,且多为多年生植物,为种质的收集和调查,遗传资源的保存、研究和利用带来了困难,因此构建药用植物核心种质是保护其遗传资源变异的重要途径。基于药用植物的特点,黄璐琦等人总结了其核心种质的特性,认为药用植物核心种质组成应包含并体现该物种的主要变异类型。不同种质间应存在异质性,才能最大限度地避免遗传上的重复。核心种质不可一成不变,而应当存在动态调整,还需包含生产实践所需要的优良农艺性状、临床疗效所需要的活性成分及相应的调控基因。

核心种质的构建需要收集的数据主要包括:①有关材料原生境的生态地理状况、育种体系和分类体系等基本信息。②包括形态、生化、分子标记等在内的表征某材料特征的特征数据。③包括质量、产量及抗性等信息的评价鉴定数据。

分子标记具有不受环境和生长时期影响、操作简便、快速稳定的优势,随着分子生物学技术的发展,在核心种质构建的特征数据收集中广泛应用。例如,利用 ISSR 标记对 11 个省(市)的 129 份山茱萸样品的遗传多样性进行分析,基于随机、位点取样策略和 SM、Jaccard、Nei & Li 遗传距离相结合的方法,最终确定 34 份资源可作为山茱萸核心种质。这些核心种质保留了原种质 26.36% 的样品,遗传多样性指数的保留率为 100.0%。结合 13 个表型性状的分析,进一步证明了基于 ISSR 标记构建的山茱萸核心种质能够代表原种质的遗传多样性。

对药用植物种质资源进行鉴定与评价时,除了产量等经济性状,还需要对活性成分含量进行评估。例如,采用 SRAP 分子标记对全国 44 个居群的 327 份何首乌样品进行研究,基于比例取样和聚类取样策略,结合化学成分研究结果,最终确定何首乌核心种质由 37 份样品组成,包括 3 份何首乌成分含量较为优异的样品,为何首乌优良种质的筛选提供材料基础。

4.2 *种质基因库构建* 种质改良的主要目标是对基因型的改良,以提高目标基因的频率。对于单一药材基原植物,通过收集保存其种质资源,建立种子繁殖或无性繁殖的种群,并利用保存的种质资源建立基因库,为种质改良提供重要的参考基因型。

目前药用植物遗传资源基因库的建设、管理和利用面临着诸多挑战。在基因库中,对新品种选育具有直接贡献的遗传资源仅占一小部分。相对于水稻、大豆、芝麻等作物,对药用植物基因组学和功能基因组学的研究还比较薄弱,尤其是对于复杂性状形成规律的研究还很不充分。

对基因库中的资源进行种质鉴定和遗传多样性分析,可指导种质资源的保存与管理工作。缩小基因库和品种选育之间的距离,对提高中药种质资源的利用效率具有重要的意义。针对药用植物种质资源的特点,需要构建符合实际育种需求的种质基因库。种质基因库应包含 3 个模块:①种质材料。收集、鉴定并保存药用植物种质资源,特别是核心种质中具有任何实用或潜在遗传功能价值的生物材料,包括种子、离体器官、组织、细胞和 DNA 等。②遗传信息资源。包括基因组信息(基因编号、基因座位置、不同数据库的基因功能注释、重要农艺性状的候选基因等数据)、变异信息(SNP 位点、SSR 等)、分子标记(物种鉴定标记、品种鉴定标记和表型性状关联标记)。③信息共享平台。整合药用植物种质鉴定与评价数据,建立基因数据共享平台,实现种质资源数据信息的远程查询、分析、下载,以及材料资源线上预订服务,促进育种信息交流、共享与利用。

4.3 *管理系统平台建设* 目前,我国中药材育种还处于起步阶段,缺乏标准化、规范化的育种管理体系。对育种过程中种质资源的收集调查、相关育种材料的选取、选育试验方案的选择、育种各阶段性状数据的调查记录、管理与分析等均缺乏数字化、信息化及有效存储方案的支持,导致整体育种效率低下。构建有效的管理系统平台可系统集成育种过程中种质的表型、基因型、杂交策略和谱系数据,并对其进行数据统计分析和可视化管理,辅助育种工作者进行育种决策,提升育种效率,实现中药材品种选育的全流程追溯。

由中国中医科学院中药资源中心自主研发的中药种质资源管理系统是连接种质资源与育种研究之间的桥梁,可用于亲本及其品种的定向培育，总体上根据育种需求分为 4 个功能模块。

4.3.1 数据库后台 建立基础种质资源库，对种质资源档案数据进行记录管理，包括对种质护照信息、表型信息、基因信息等数据的新增、编辑、删除、导出。①种质护照信息：种质编号、名称、物种学名、来源地、亲本子代等基础信息。②表型信息：为支持不同的药材品种的性状采集，由用户自定义重要的表型数据字段，确定填写的数据类型，如数字、日期、选项、文本等，并可按植物学特征性状、农艺学特征性状、经济学性状、抗逆性状等类型分类。③基因信息：关联种质相关的基因数据。

4.3.2 数据库前端 针对开放数据提供种质资源和品种数据检索查询、比对，为育种材料筛选提供便利工具。①通过输入种质资源编号、名称查询护照信息、表型信息、基因信息等详细数据。②选择多项性状特征进行筛选匹配，并根据特征匹配数按序显示筛选出的种质资源。③在筛选匹配出来的种质资源或品种中，选择多个种质或品种进行各项性状对比。

4.3.3 选育管理与分析 ①育种材料选择：根据育种目标在种质资源库中选取相关育种供体材料和基础品种，并添加为育种对象。②田间试验信息管理：支持对田间试验的基本信息记录管理，包含试验编号、试验地概况、气象资料记载、各阶段性状信息采集任务管理等，功能包括新增、编辑、删除等。③选育试验信息管理：针对选育试验进行种质资源和新品种的系谱管理，记录试验类型，并根据记录的亲本子代信息以树状图可视化种质的系谱情况，每种种质均可向上或向下对亲本或子代进行追溯。④新品种库管理：对育种性状数据进行审定，对种质资源进行新品种评估、申请，通过审定的新品种则纳入新品种库。

4.3.4 种质采集程序 于 PC 端建立资源采集任务，使用手机端程序实现采集种质的基本信息、采集地信息、鉴定信息、采集信息、表型信息等的现场数据记录。功能包括新增、编辑、删除及种质资源库纳入申请等。

## 5 展望

5.1 中药材种质资源收集鉴定是一项公益性的基础工作 公益性、基础性是中药材种质资源收集鉴定的基本特征，是尽快提升中药材种业科技创新能力的前提。重视和加强中药材种质资源的发掘和创制、重要基因发掘利用、育种理论与技术的突破，建立中药材亲本及其品种定向培育研究共享平台(图 1)，将为提升中药材种业科技创新能力提供有效支撑。

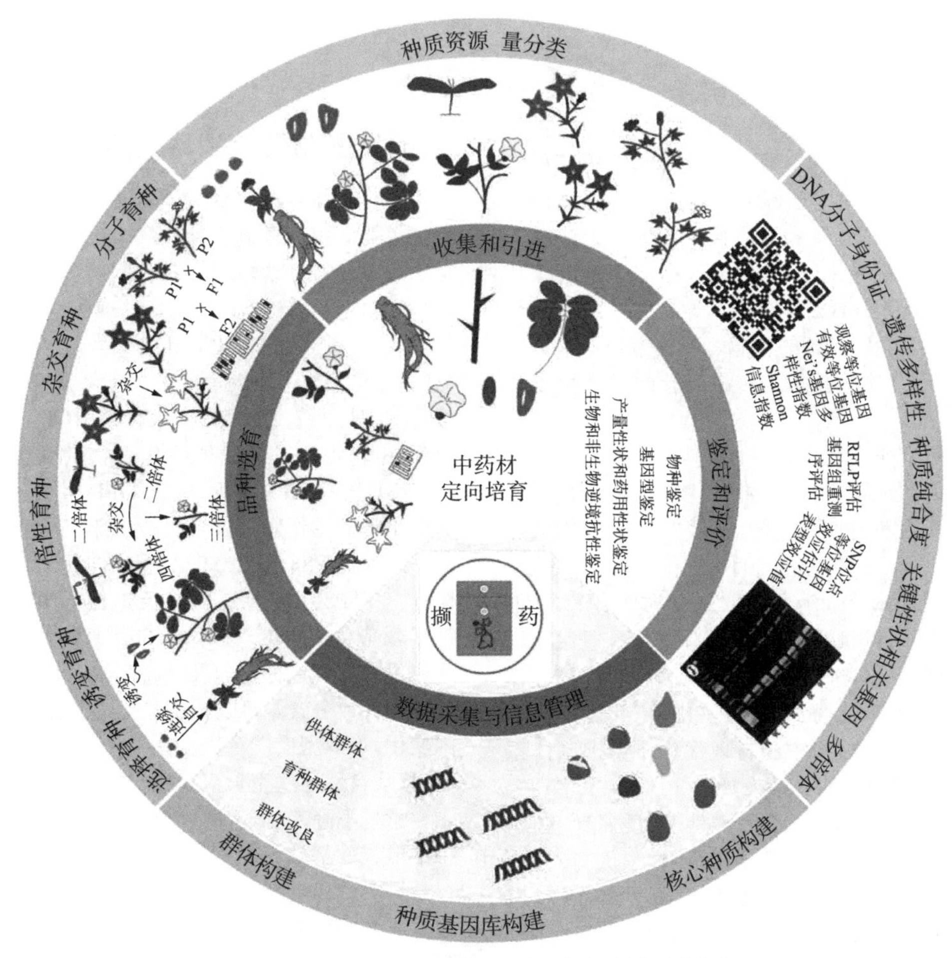


**图 1 现阶段中药材种质资源研究与创新的基本框架**

5.2 基于中药材种质资源杂合度高的特点有序进行中药材育种核心种质及其品种定向培育研究 中药材种质资源的杂合度普遍较高，是中药材育种核心种质及其品种定向培育研究的“双刃剑”：一方面，高杂合度导致遗传多样性丰富，为中药材种质创新和优良品种选育提供了坚实的物质基础和巨大的潜力；另一方面，高杂合度也是导致种质混乱这一长期困扰中药材产业高质量发展难题的关键因素，必须重视纯系育种的研究。可依据杂合度评估结果，选择合适的繁育方式，如杂合度较低，可采用杂交育种等；如杂合度较高，可采用无性繁殖等。

5.3 具“内稳态”特征的中药材种质创新和新品种选育是现阶段主要任务之一 保障和提高中药材质量是中医药振兴发展的主要任务之一。中药材种质创新和新品种选育是从源头保障中药材质量的关键，中药材新品种选育目标应兼顾产量和质量。从理论上，植物的生长和次生代谢产物的积累往往遵循“生长-防御”平衡的理论，即植物次生代谢产物含量与其器官大小呈负相关，这对兼顾产量和质量的中药材品种选育需求来说是一个挑战，需要选择符合中药特色的选育目标。对以工业原料供应为需求的中药材，可以选择明确功能成分或指标性成分作为选育目标；但面对以保障高质量饮片供应的传统种植需求，由于中药材通过多成分、多靶点、多信号通路发挥治疗疾病的作用，具有“天然组合化学库”之称，因此其选育目标不能仅局限于单一成分，而应着重于“内稳态”特征，即具有稳态的外观形状和代谢谱。

5.4 利用基因组学技术助力中药材品种选育研究 相对于一般农作物，中药材生长周期较长，且遗传背景复杂，常规选育需要耗费较多的时间和精力，具有清晰遗传背景的中药材育种材料匮乏。分子标记辅助育种在一定程度上加快了育种的进程，但目前中药材新品种选育研究的相关基础仍相对薄弱。基因组学技术可为种质资源分类鉴定、遗传多样性评估、核心种质筛选、复杂性状相关基因挖掘提供新工具，用于解析中药材品质特征遗传机制，筛选获得“优形优质”相关的基因或分子标记，加快中药材种质资源的创新与利用，提升中药材品种选育效率。

[袁媛，黄璐琦．科学通报，2024，69(4－5)：499－509.]

# 再论道地药材“优形、优质、优效”特征成因及研究模式

传统上，道地药材被认为是优质中药材的代名词，是古代辨别优质中药材质量的综合标准。而“辨状论质”是中药材传统经验的总结，即通过“形、色、气、味、质”等外在特征进行归纳分类，判断中药品质的真伪优劣。尽管化学分析方法在药材质量检测中得到了广泛应用，但它们被认为逐渐偏离了传统的质量控制模式。运用现代分子生物学原理和技术深入解析中药传统经验鉴别“辨状论质”的科学内涵成为弥补这一鸿沟的必要途径，有助于为现代技术与传统经验的融合提供有力的支持。

依据现代生命科学研究成果及发展趋势，笔者提出道地药材可表现为“优形”(公认药材性状)和“优质”(独特化学成分组成)特点，并体现为药材使用上的“优效”(优于非道地药材的临床功效)。道地药材“优形、优质、优效”(excellent shape, high quality, superior effect, EHS，简称“三优”)特征的提出，拓宽了传统药材辨状的范畴，其核心思想是通过获取高质量、可重复的性状数据，进而量化分析基因型和环境互作效应及其对中药质量的影响，为加快推进中医药和现代数字技术相互融合和相互促进、建立中药材现代化质量控制体系奠定基础，推动中医药事业的可持续发展。

近年来，随着对中药道地性的自然属性、物质属性、药物属性研究的逐步深入，丰富和完善了道地药材“三优”特征的科学内涵。将本草文献、产区调查与数量分类学结合，对道地药材“优形”“优质”特征进行诠释和量化，并依据其独特的表型、生理、成分特征提出道地药材研究的模式生物及模型。

## 1 道地药材“三优”特征的科学内涵

1.1 “独特化学型”是“优质”特征形成的基础 “优质”特征主要体现为道地药材具有优势活性成分(群)及独特的生物合成及调控体系，其与药用植物活性成分的积累与其生长特性和生态学特性有关，主要表现为品种、产区生态因子、采收等人工栽培措施导致活性成分含量、成分比例的变化，形成“独特化学型”。如樟通常被分为龙脑型、樟脑型、芳樟醇型、桉叶油型和橙花叔醇型 5 种化学型，萜类合酶(terpene synthase, TPS)是形成这些化合物的关键酶，研究结果显示 CcTPS1 和 CcTPS9 均可催化 GPP 生成冰片基焦磷酸，并在磷酸水解酶的作用下得到(+)-龙脑，产物占比分别为 0.4%、89.3%；CcTPS3 和 CcTPS6 均可催化 GPP 生成单一产物芳樟醇，CcTPS6 还可与 FPP 反应生成橙花叔醇；CcTPS8 与 GPP 反应生成 1,8-桉叶油(30.71%)，表明其基因多样性是形成优势活性成分(群)及独特生物合成体系的决定因素。

活性成分含量、成分比例可随生长时间延长在一定范围内变化，如醇型广藿香无菌苗的百秋李醇含量均低于广藿香酮，移栽自然环境生长后，百秋李醇含量呈上升趋势，广藿香酮含量呈下降趋势，但醇型仍为其“独特化学型”，是其“优质”特征形成的基础。

1.2 “优质”特征是联系“优形”和“优效”的纽带 优势活性成分(群)具有双重作用，其可作为“优效”的物质基础，“优效”特征体现为道地药材临床应用的有效性和安全性，即表现为“质优效佳”；也可参与调控“优形”的形成，是其在长期进化过程中逐渐形成环境适应性特征，即道地药材具有独特

的药用植物器官形态特征和药材感官鉴别特征，表现为“形质合一”。

“形神合一”是中医学对于生命整体性的重要认识。与“形神合一”相似，道地药材“形质合一”反映了植物体内各部分之间保持着密切的相互协调关系，且与外界环境密切联系。从生物学本质上来看，药材的“形质合一”的具体表现为：①药材性状特征和化学成分均受到相同基因或基因调控网络控制。②药材性状特征和活性成分均受到生物“生长与防御的权衡”机制的影响。③活性成分在植物体内参与调控药用植物的生长发育。如西洋参原产北美，我国于20世纪70年代引种成功。引种驯化导致西洋参的“优形优质”特征显著改变。与野生西洋参相比，国产栽培西洋参的侧根数减少，人参皂苷 $Rg_1$ 含量降低。利用选择清除分析在栽培群体中筛选到397个受选择基因，结合根、叶比较转录组分析发现其中21个基因在西洋参根中显著高表达，并注释到包括Expansin-like细胞膨胀蛋白基因和β-半乳糖苷酶基因等与植物细胞壁发育相关的受选择基因；体内外实验进一步证明，PqEXLA1和PqEXLB1作为影响细胞生长和 $Rg_1$ 积累的枢纽基因，在西洋参引种驯化过程中发挥调节植物生长和防御平衡的关键功能。

## 2 道地药材“三优”特征形成的主导型模式

道地药材“三优”特征受到品种基因型和产区生态因子交互作用的影响，可体现为气候主导型、生产措施主导型、种质主导型。

2.1 气候主导型 以人参为例，由于人参吉林、云南等产区存在温度等生态因子差异，导致二醇型人参皂苷（如人参皂苷 $Rb_1$、Rd等）、齐墩果酸型人参皂苷（如人参皂苷Ro等）含量的变化，不定根（习称为“艼”）和侧根（习称为“腿”）数量、主根长度和周长等根形特征（习称为“体”）变化，以及对DOX引起心肌细胞毒性的保护作用、对阿霉素诱导心衰的保护作用等变化。人参皂苷 $Rb_1$ 可保护血管内皮、抗动脉粥样硬化作用，可通过恢复钙稳态、抑制细胞凋亡和炎症坏死来减轻心脏毒性，与人参“艼”等根形特征的形成相关联，其具体机制是：人参皂苷 $Rb_1$ 可通过调控 *WOX*11 等基因的表达，从而影响不定根等根形特征形成和人参皂苷生物合成。

适当的冷胁迫可促进细胞中人参皂苷的积累以及3-hydroxy -3-methylglutaryl-CoA reductase（HMGR2），squalene epoxidase（SE1），squalene synthase（SS），dammarenediol synthase（DS-Ⅱ），and β-alanine C-28 hydroxylase（CYP716A52v2）等基因表达水平。而持续冷冻（5℃ 12 h）会诱导PPT型人参皂苷，间歇冷冻（25℃ 12 h和5℃ 12 h）会刺激PPD型人参皂苷的积累。短期冷胁迫也明显降低了人参的根鲜重和干重，增加丙二醛、脯氨酸、可溶性糖和可溶性蛋白质的浓度，超氧化物歧化酶、过氧化物酶和过氧化氢酶的活性也明显增加，直根（韧皮部和木质部）和须根中的原人参三醇型人参皂苷浓度以及叶片中的原人参二醇型人参皂苷浓度显著增加；但随着冷胁迫时间的延长，所有抗氧化酶的活性都有所下降。在人参皂苷 $Rg_1$ 和Re积累之前，冷胁迫会引发ABA的积累。用去甲二氢愈创木脂酸（NDGA）抑制冷胁迫人参不定根中ABA的生物合成，可降低 *DDS* 和 *PPTS* 基因的表达水平，抑制人参皂苷 $Rg_1$ 和Re的积累；而在NDGA处理的人参不定根中外源添加ABA，可分别恢复 *DDS* 和 *PPTS* 基因的表达水平，以及人参皂苷 $Rg_1$ 和Re的积累。这些结果表明，ABA参与了人参不定根在冷胁迫下人参皂苷 $Rg_1$ 和Re的合成。冷胁迫通过影响膜脂过氧化激活抗氧化酶系统以减轻氧化损伤，进而调控根型和人参皂苷含量的变化，这可能是导致人参道地产区分布和药材“优形优质”差异的重要因素。

2.2 生产措施主导型 以三七为例。通过对故宫博物院馆藏的清代贡品三七和市售不同规格三七进行形态学观察和比较，发现清代贡品与为市售120头规格三七相当。在此基础上对近代三七药材特征及其栽培模式变迁进行文献考证，发现120头规格可代表清代最大药材质量，且随着时代变迁，三七药材质量呈逐渐增加的趋势，现今以20头代表最大药材质量。与清代相比，三七当代栽培模式呈现低温、低降水量及高施肥量的趋势，推测栽培模式的改变对三七外观性状和内在化学成分产生影响。

三七是一种耐阴和对氮敏感的物种，常见的栽培措施包括使用架棚遮阴、施肥等。氮（N）是限制叶片光合作用的主要因素，施用低浓度氮肥可通过减慢卡尔文循环和光反应速度抑制光合能力，而高浓度氮肥则由于其促进失活的Rubisco形式增加导致光合能力抑制，随着施用有机肥增加，根干产量和三七皂苷含量呈先增后减的趋势。光照强度可影响三七总皂苷含量以及达玛烯二醇-Ⅱ合酶（DS）和CYP716A47的表达水平。适当的种植密度可通过平衡淀粉和蔗糖等初级代谢和IAA、人参皂苷等次级代谢，有利于三七的生长和人参皂苷的积累。但在高种植密度下，强烈的种内竞争导致了植物激素水杨酸（SA）和茉莉酸（JA）、抗氧化剂龙胆二糖、草酸、脱氢抗坏血酸和其他抗胁迫相关代谢物的积累；而在低密度、种内竞争小的情况下，通过上调半乳糖代谢扰乱了正常的碳水化合物代谢，使得干生物量和人参皂苷含量明显较低。

收集120头和20头规格三七原植物根组织，对二者的外观性状、显微结构、转录组分析、细胞壁成分及活性成分含量进行比较。比较转录组分析结果表明，在20头三七中PnGAP和PnEXPA4基因显著高表达，其被报道与植物细胞壁形成有关，且表达水平受环境温度、湿度、磷含量等影响。显微结构分析结果表明，20头三七具有更厚的韧皮部、木质部细胞壁和导管壁，并具有更高含量的木质素、纤维素及胼胝质。化学成分分析结果表明，20头三七中人参皂苷 $Rb_1$ 含量显著增高，120头三七中三七素含量显著增高。实时荧光定量PCR测定结果表明，与活性成分人参皂苷生物合成相关的 *FPS*、*CYP716A47*、*CYP716A53v2* 基因转录水平在20头三七中显著增高，与植物生长调节物质赤霉素生物合成相关的 *GGPPS* 基因表达水平在20头三七中也显著增高。酵母单杂交及凝胶阻滞实验显示，在120头三七中高表达的 *PnPHL8* 低磷响应转录因子，可体外特异性结合 *PnGAP*、*PnGGPPS3* 及 *PnCYP716A47* 启动子。因此推测 *PnPHL8* 可能参与协同负调控三七细胞壁结构、根的生长与人参皂苷生物合成，进而影响三七“优形优质”。由于三七皂苷具有降低血瘀大鼠的全血黏度、纤维蛋白原含量等血液流变学指标的作用，因此清代以来三七栽培模式的改变，是否进一步影响三七临床应用还有待于进一步研究。

2.3 种质主导型

2.3.1 种间水平 以人参属为例。同属于五加科的人参和三七均含有人参皂苷等生物活性成分，对神经系统和免疫系统疾病具有多种药理作用。然而，根据传统中医理论，人参补气而三七活血，两者的应用明显不同。研究表明，人参含有较多的多糖和氨基酸，对心血管疾病、神经疾病、癌症和糖尿病有较好的保护作用；而三七则含有较多的皂苷、挥发油和多炔类化合物。在药理作用方面，对脑血管疾病有较好的保护作用。基于单拷贝基因的系统发生树表明，三七和人参的分化在6.0～17.1百万年前，二者存在显著的遗传分化，与三七相比，参与调控细胞壁组成和结构的基因家族在人参和西洋参中显著扩张，表明其在人参属药用植物根系形态建成中发挥重要作用。目前已从人参属中分离并鉴定出约300种人参皂苷，其中人参皂苷二醇型（如人参皂苷 $Rb_1$ 等）、三醇型（如人参皂苷Re等）和齐墩果酸型（如人参皂苷Ro等）均对人参不定根生长具有低浓度促进、高浓度抑制的作用。与三七相比，SOC1-like和FUL-like亚类转录因子仅在人参和西洋参基因组中存在，且SOC1-like亚类转录因子PgMADS41和PgMADS44通过调控细胞壁膨胀蛋白基因表达参与根系的生长，同时通过调控人参皂苷关键酶基因表达影响Ro的生物合成，而人参皂苷Ro也参与调控SOCl-like基因的表达。

2.3.2 种下水平 以天麻为例。目前市场上流通的天麻商品多为红天麻、乌天麻或杂交天麻，根据天麻基因组重测序结果，筛选获得特异性单核苷酸多态性变异位点，可用于鉴定不同品系乌天麻、红天麻。《本草纲目》记载“天麻目黑头旋，风虚内作，非此不能除，为治风神药，名定风草”，热板致痛和醋酸致痛实验结果表明，与空白对照组比较，红天麻可显著提高小鼠的痛阈值，红天麻和乌天麻均具有一定的镇痛作用。红天麻和乌天麻的差异成分琥珀酸、L-焦谷氨酸可显著提高小鼠的痛阈值，丁香酸、天麻素、琥珀酸、L-焦谷氨酸均具有一定的镇痛作用，其中琥珀酸、L-焦谷氨酸的镇痛作用更佳。

与大多数种子植物相比，天麻线粒体基因组扩张至1 339 kb，推测其对异养植物的生长发育具有关键作用。琥珀酸是柠檬酸循环的中间产物之一，其可被琥珀酸脱氢酶重新氧化，通过线粒体复合体Ⅰ的反向电子传递产生大量活性氧ROS。琥珀酸含量的变化导致天麻多糖、氨基酸等能量代谢物质和细胞氧化应激反应的变化，从而影响块茎的发育。如线粒体二羧酸-三羧酸载体蛋白（dicarboxylate-tricarboxylate carrier，DTC）负责二羧酸、三羧酸的转运，参与甘油酸酯的产生、氮的同化、ATP合成等。而线粒体分裂蛋白DRP1被认为通过依赖蛋白的内吞作用在细胞质分裂、细胞扩张、细胞生长和细胞壁/质膜生物合成中发挥重要作用。通过农杆菌介导转化法分别获得天麻GeDTC和GeDRP1E基因的拟南芥互补突变体、马铃薯过表达株系，结果发现，与拟南芥突变体相比，GeDTC和GeDRP1E基因互补突变体株高、结实率表型得以恢复；与野生型马铃薯相比，GeDTC基因过表达株系微型薯体积变小、质量更轻、有机酸含量降低，但淀粉含量没有显著变化，而GeDRP1E基因过表达株系微型薯体积、质量显著增大，淀粉含量显著增高，推测GeDTC和GeDRP1E通过参与调节线粒体的形态影响拟南芥植株、马铃薯微型薯的生长发育。

## 3 道地药材研究模式生物及方法体系

模式生物（model organisms）通常指人们研究生命现象过程中长期、反复作为实验材料的物种，并且从模式生物的研究中得出的生命规律往往代表了许多物种的共同规律。模式生物是现代生命科学研究领域的重要组成部分，人们在对模式物种的形态、解剖、生理、生化、细胞及遗传进行全面分析和归纳的基础上，把它们作为典范将研究得出的规律推演到相关的生物物种中，从而加快其他生物物种的研究。一般来讲，模式生物具有取材方便、生物周期短、遗传背景较清晰、实验方法通用、具有遗传改造和表型分析手段、有利于同行的交流等特征。

针对道地药材这一复杂系统，黄璐琦等提出如果能够借鉴模式生物的方法学，选择具有代表性的道地药材，对相关关键问题进行系统深入的研究，揭示共性问题，树立研究典范，将有很大的现实意义。并以丹参为例，基于其具有分布区广和道地性明确、药效及其物质基础清晰、次生代谢成分的生物合成途径已有较好的研究基础、研究材料丰富、已建有“丹参毛状根”“组培丹参”“转基因丹参”研究模型等条件，认为丹参可以作为模式生物来研究道地药材的生物学成因。

随着科学研究技术的不断发展，以丹参作为药用模式植物而开展的化学成分分离、药理学研究、生物合成研究、组学研究和代谢工程研究更加深入。多个研究团队发表了丹参不同品种、组织部位的转录组和基因组信息，并利用单分子实时测序（SMRT）技术解析药用器官根组织的发育规律，为活性化合物生物合成和调控的分子机制提供了重要依据。丹参酮类成分生物合成及其调控机制研究已取得突破性进展，GGPP在二萜合酶或环化酶以及多个CYP450的作用下经过多步酶促反应生成丹参酮类化合物的最终产物。丹参中酚酸类成分大多是丹参素和迷迭香酸的衍生物，近年来丹酚酸途径中的解析主要集中于可催化迷迭香酸生成的CYP98A亚家族，以及催化迷迭香酸与多个小分子通过特殊反应生成丹酚酸类化合物的漆酶（lactase，LAC）基因的鉴定。

丹参高效遗传转化体系和基因编辑系统已建立并运用，利用三靶点CRISPR/Cas9系统对SmCYP76AK2和SmCYP76AK3基因进行编辑，形成的突变体中5种主要丹参酮类物质的含量均显著降低。在丹参RNAi转基因毛状根体系中，抑制SmCYP71D375基因表达导致隐丹参酮、丹参酮 $Ⅱ_A$ 等含量显著降低。通过建立了一个丹参原生质体-植株再生系统，可用于无转基因CRISPR/Cas9介导的基因编辑，成功靶向编辑了7个调控丹参中水溶性和脂溶性活性成分生物合成的转录因子基因（MYB28、MYB36、MYB39、MYB100、bZIP1、bZIP2和MYB98），通过单次转染实现了这些基因的高效敲除，一些关键转录因子基因如MYB98的敲除可显著降低根中活性成分的含量；而bZIP1和bZIP2的敲除可提高根中脂溶性成分的含量。

在上述工作的基础上，利用丹参模式生物可建立用于道地药材“三优”特征研究的方法体系。

3.1 道地药材“性效关系”表征方法体系 在整体、细胞、分子水平上，表征丹参“活血祛瘀、通经止痛、清心除烦、凉血消痈”等核心功效，进而探究其“性-效”关系的分子靶点。如通过网络药理学分析，发现迷迭香酸、丹酚酸B和丹参素可通过40多个靶点和16条途径发挥抗动脉粥样硬化的作用。通过构建“功效-药理药效-靶点-成分”的多维网络，预测丹参活血化瘀的潜在功效标志物包括丹酚酸B、丹酚酸A、丹参酮ⅡA、丹参酮Ⅰ等成分，其中丹酚酸B、丹参酮ⅡA等成分在不同产地之间存在较大差异，可作为“优效”评价的指标成分。

3.2 基于“优质”特征的道地药材质量评价体系 鉴于“优质”特征是联系“优形”和“优效”的纽带，因此可选择代表“优形”“优效”的“优质”特征建立道地药材质量评价体系。丹参酮和丹酚酸是丹参的主要活性成分，即“优质”特征成分。如利用HPLC测定丹参根系不同年龄、不同直径和不同组织中8种脂溶性及水溶性成分的含量，可为评估多年栽培丹参根龄提供依据。通过UPLC和GC-MS技术检测定丹参酮类成分，并结合其基因表达水平，证实生源途径上游基因、中游中间体化合物与下游丹参酮类化合物含量之间的统一关系，可建立丹参质量“以点带面”评价方法。

质谱成像技术也被应用于丹参的质量评价中，利用非靶向代谢组学与DESI-MSI技术，绘制了丹参发育过程中代谢物分布图谱。利用MALDI-MSI技术实现了正常生长丹参与连作丹参中丹参酮类、丹酚酸类、寡糖类、脂肪酸类、胆碱类、小分子有机酸类、多胺类等多类代谢物分子的可视化分析。通过不断更新迭代的质量检测技术在模式丹参中的应用，逐渐揭开“色紫红者为佳”与高丹参酮含量丹参之间的“形质合一”特征，丰富了道地药材质量评价体系。

3.3 基于“优形优质”特征的道地药材稳态综合控制体系 丹参为常异花授粉植物，生态适应强，种质资源丰富，其品种基因型、产区生态因子、生产措施等复杂因素对道地药材“优形优质”形成具有综合效应。HPLC分析结果表明，‘陕黄’等4个丹参品系的丹参酮Ⅰ、隐丹参酮、丹参酮ⅡA、原儿茶酸、迷迭香酸、丹酚酸B含量存在差异。白花丹参 *Salvia miltiorrhiza* f. *alba* C. Y. Wu et H. W. Li 是常见的一种变型，在山东等地已广泛种植，其叶中总黄酮、总酚酸含量与紫花丹参显著不同。在产地调查中，还发现了一种根皮呈现砖红色的丹参种质，采用高分辨液质联用技术发现其丹参酮ⅡA与丹参酮Ⅰ几乎检测不到，但其二氢丹参酮Ⅰ和隐丹参酮含量与正常丹参种质相比变化不大，丹参二醇B与丹参二醇C含量显著低于正常种质。

采用超高效液相色谱(UPLC)及超高效液相色谱-三重四极杆质谱联用技术(UPLC-QQQ-MS)同时测定来自山东、河南、陕西、四川、安徽共408份丹参中23种化学成分的含量，并对数据进行多元统计分析，发现17种酚酸类及6种丹参酮类成分在不同产地丹参中均存在显著差异，其中山东的丹参样品中丹参酮类成分含量最高，四川的样品中丹酚酸B含量最高，安徽丹参的紫草酸、丹酚酸Y、丹酚酸A、丹酚酸D和丹酚酸E等的含量最高。产区生态因子也是影响丹参药效组分变化的重要因素，如不同产区土壤中的无机元素与丹参酮类成分存在强相关性，其中土壤钾(K)、钠(Na)、钛(Ti)、全氮为影响丹参药材中丹参酮类成分的主要土壤因子，其与土壤Ti呈正相关，与Na、K、全氮呈负相关。环境因子可以通过激素信号介导转录因子调控表型(活性成分)的形成，如丛枝菌根真菌参与促进了丹参生物量的增加及活性成分的积累，并且能够抵御致病菌如尖孢镰刀菌的侵害，而茉莉酸信号能够促进丛枝菌根真菌与植物的相互作用。此外，在栽培方式、采收、加工及贮藏等多个环节中，也同样会显著影响丹参药材品质。

利用丹参模式生物可以不断优化道地药材形成机制的模式研究方法，利用基因组及重测序技术阐明品种基因型对丹参“优形优质”的影响，并通过比较不同产地相关环境因子包括气候条件、土壤微生物、栽培措施等对丹参“优形优质”特征形成的影响，建立道地药材稳态综合控制体系，即在一定温度、降水、土壤微生物群落组成等生态因子条件下，按照固定的中药材生产规范进行操作，通过改变环境因素，间接干预内在机制，定向获得具有明显“优形优质”表型、丹参酮及酚酸含量稳定的丹参药材。

## 4 展望

4.1 建立药用模式植物综合研究平台 据统计，在 *Cell*、*Nature*、*Science* 等期刊上发表的有关生命过程和机制的研究，80%以上都是借助模式生物材料完成，在成熟的模式体系中完成机制的创新更被科研界所认可。目前对道地药材品质及其形成机制的研究多局限在活性成分形成机制上，而对“优形”研究鲜有报道，“形质合一”的形成机制仍不清楚。为了全面、系统阐释道地药材形成的生物学本质，须要进一步整合道地药材生物学研究数据和方法，建立药用模式植物综合研究平台。

该平台应在原有的基础上，包括组学数据、自然群体或杂交群体等种质资源、外观形状等表型谱定量工具、“优形优质”关联基因挖掘技术、稳定的基因编辑体系和基因功能验证技术、多类型受控实验体系和生态效应研究技术等。目前由本团队自主研发的中药种质资源管理系统，包括基础种质资源库、种质采集程序、选育管理与分析等模块，可对种质护照信息、表型信息、基因信息等档案数据进行记录管理，可针对开放数据提供种质资源和品种数据检索查询、比对，支持对育种过程涉及的材料选择、田间试验信息管理、选育试验信息管理、新品种库管理等，并可于PC端建立资源采集任务，使用手机端程序实现采集种质的基本信息、采集地信息、鉴定信息、采集信息、表型信息等的现场数据记录，可用于自然群体或杂交群体等种质资源收集与鉴定、外观形状等表型谱定量数据查询、比对、分析等工作。同时本团队开发了中药多维度核酸数据资源平台(IMP，https://www.bic.ac.cn/IMP)，目前已收录了480个高质量的药用植物基因组，整理了28 327 656个基因，以及2 547个转录组测序样本，涵盖了多个器官、组织、发育阶段和胁迫刺激，为中药核酸数据资源的利用提供了一个标准化的信息平台。

正向遗传学研究是解析植物个体或群体间表型差异所对应的分子遗传基础的通用手段，在建立理想的研究群体基础上，利用全基因组选择等技术有针对性的挖掘与“优形优质”特征相关的基因，进一步揭示其形成机制是未来重要的研究方向之一。

4.2 建立药用模式植物突变体库 突变体库是一种人工构建的大量可变突变形式的基因库，它包含的基因序列形态多样，包括自然发生或人工诱导的突变体。在道地药材研究过程中，应加强对自然发生或人工诱导的药用植物突变体的研究，特别是开展针对具有“优形优质”性状的突变体筛选和创制工作，有助于深化道地药材形成机制研究。

突变体库的建立是进行功能基因组学研究的必要组成部分。拟南芥、水稻等模式植物突变体库被广泛应用，为发现控制生物体内多种形态的生物功能分子奠定了基础，目前尚未有关药用植物突变体库建立的报道。与拟南芥相比，药用植物如丹参具有独特的表型、生理、成分特征，利用拟南芥突变体库进行丹参功能基因的相关研究，存在一定的局限性，不能完全反映功能基因在丹参体内的生物学功能，也可能丢失一些新知识。因此，建立丹参突变体库对于完善其作为道地药材模式生物是十分必要的，可利用诱变及基因编辑等技术逐步建立突变体库，选育双单倍体及优质纯合系群体，丰富丹参种质资源，为深入研究基因型与环境因子互作对道地药材形成影响的机制奠定基础。

4.3 建立可用于其他药用植物功能基因研究的模式生物 模式生物是指可作为实验模型以研究特定生物学现象的生物，研究模式生物得到的结论，通常可适用于其他生物。由于药用植物种类众多，道地药材形成机制复杂，一方面可利用丹参等药用植物较为成熟的基因资源和研究体系，根据多类型“优形优质”特征，建立适宜的研究模型，推动其他药用植物的研究进程。另一方面，模式生物也可多元化，不同模式物种的优势不同，如丹参适合作为二萜类和酚酸类活性成分以及“辨色论质”研究的模式生物，青蒿适合作为倍萜类活性成分以及“腺毛发育与成分”研究的模式生物，甘草适合作为黄酮类活性成分以及“断面特征与成分”研究的模式生物，等等。第三，目前药用模式生物的生长周期较长，选择或通过合成生物学手段创制生长周期更短的种质，优化药用模式植物及其道地药材研究模型，是未来重要的研究方向之一。

4.4 道地药材“优形优质”特征研究热点 道地药材“三优”特征研究目前仍处于起步阶段，需要开展更为深入和广泛的基础性工作，以揭示其遗传基础、生物学特性、生态适应性等方面的机制，为优化药用植物定向育种、规范化栽培、药材质量提升提供科学依据，进一步推动道地药材的可持续利用和发展。

未来的研究热点方向包括：①揭示药材特化“优形”性状的形成机制及其生物适应性规律，鉴定与传统公认“优形”特征关联的化学成分，深入解析“优质”物质对药材生长的调控机制。②解析药材“三优”特征共生功能体的调控机制，重点关注种质纯化、细胞壁可塑性、微生物群落等对药特征为基础的道地药材稳态综合控制体系。在此基础上，形成基于核心功效基因型的中药材定向育种体系，以及基于精准调控“三化”特征共生功能体组成的中药材现代化高效栽培技术体系。

[袁媛，黄璐琦，等. 中国中药杂志，2024，DOI：10.19540.]

# The jasmonate-responsive AP2/ERF transcription factors AaERF1 and AaERF2 positively regulate artemisinin biosynthesis in *Artemisia annua* L.

## 1 INTRODUCTION

Artemisinin (*Qinghaosu* in Chinese), a sesquiterpene lactone with an endoperoxide bridge, was first isolated from *Artemisia annua* over 30 years ago. Artemisinin and its semi-synthetic derivatives are extensively used in the treatment of malaria, mostly in artemisinin-based combination therapies (ACTs) so as to reduce resistance. *A. annua* is the only natural source of artemisinin; however, its content in plants is relatively low (0.1%～0.8% by dry weight). Engineering metabolic pathways of *A. annua* plants holds a great potential for increasing artemisinin production, but the success relies highly on deep understanding of the artemisinin biosynthesis pathway and the regulation of the enzyme genes.

Plants of *A. annua* produce a rich amount of monoterpenes and sesquiterpenes. Because of the great medical value of artemisinin, many investigations have been devoted to clarifying its biosynthetic pathway (Figure 1). The first committed step—cyclization of farnesyl diphosphate (FDP) into the sesquiterpene intermediate—is catalyzed by the sesquiterpene synthase, amorpha-4, 11-diene synthase (ADS). CYP71AV1, a cytochrome P450 monooxygenase, catalyzes the oxidation of amorpha-4, 11-diene to artemisinic acid, via artemisinic alcohol and artemisinic aldehyde intermediates. Recent reports show that a double bond reductase, DBR2, catalyzes the reduction of the Δ11(13) double bond of artemisinic aldehyde, and an aldehyde dehydrogenase, ALDH1, catalyzes the oxidation of both artemisinic and dihydroartemisinic aldehydes. Most of these enzymes are localized in the two apical cells of glandular trichomes, indicating that at least the initial steps of artemisinin biosynthesis occur in these cells.

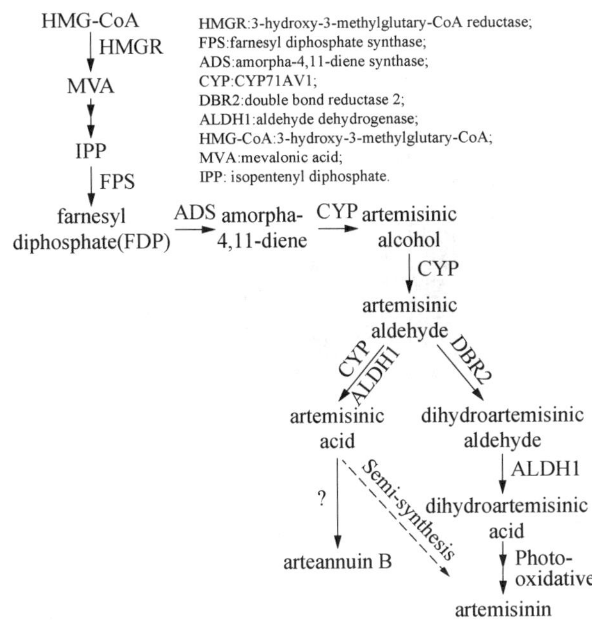


**Figure 1 The artemisinin and arteannuin B biosynthetic pathway**

In comparison with the great progress made in cloning enzymes of the artemisinin pathway and engineering the pathways in microorganisms, much less is known about the regulatory mechanisms of artemisinin biosynthesis in plants. A WRKY transcription factor, *AaWRKY1*, was reported to positively regulate the transcription of *ADS* by binding to the W-box in its promoter. In addition, we found that overexpression of *AtCRY1*, a blue light receptor of *Arabidopsis*, led to increased accumulation of artemisinin, implying a correlation between light signaling and artemisinin biosynthesis.

Plants have developed structurally diverse and tightly regulated secondary metabolites to battle against herbivores and pathogens, and accumulation of these metabolites in plants is often regulated directly or indirectly by phytohormones. It is well known that the phytohormones of jasmonate (JA), salicylic acid (SA), and abscisic acid (ABA) aid plants in survival from the biotic and abiotic stresses by triggering a *de novo* synthesis of protective metabolites and proteins. Of these, JA has been shown to regulate secondary metabolism in many plant species. It up-regulates alkaloid biosynthesis in tobacco, terpenoid indole alkaloid biosynthesis in *Catharanthus roseus*, and it also stimulates the *de novo* biosynthesis of vitamin C in plant cell suspensions. Recent reports showed that JA treatment of *A. annua* plants resulted in enhanced artemisinin production, possibly by stimulating both the glandular trichome formation and the sesquiterpene accumulation in glandular trichome. However, transcription factors involved in JA regulation of artemisinin biosynthesis have not been reported.

Transcription factors of the APETALA2/ethylene response factor (AP2/ERF) family are characterized by the presence of DNA binding AP2 domain, which consists of ~60 conserved amino acid residues. Based on the number of AP2 domains and the existence of other domains, such as B3 DNA binding domain, this family can be divided into five subfamilies: AP2, DREB, ERF, RAV, and the fifth (comprising members not assigned to other four groups), of which the ERF subfamily constitutes the largest group. Members of the AP2/ERF family function as key regulators in both plant development and stress responses. For example, in *Arabidopsis*, the AP2 subfamily members targeted by miR172 are important in phase transition, the DREB members are predominantly involved in the regulation of abiotic stress response, and most ERF factors participate in biotic stress response and hormone (ethylene, JA, and SA) signaling. There have been reports that AP2/ERF family transcriptional factors play an important role in plant secondary metabolism. For example, overexpression of the JA-inducible AP2/ERF-domain transcription factor *ORCA3* of *C. roseus* led to increased expression of several metabolic biosynthetic genes and consequently increased accumulation of terpenoid indole alkanoids in suspension cells. Further investigation revealed that ORCA3 activated *strictosidine synthase* (*Str*) expression by directly interacting with a JA- and elicitor-responsive element (JERE) in its promoter regions.

Considering the important role of AP2/ERF factors in JA signaling and plant secondary metabolism, as well as the positive role of JA on artemisinin biosynthesis, it is interesting to ask whether these transcription factors are involved in the regulation of artemisinin biosynthesis. By characterization the genes of two JA-responsive AP2/ERF subfamily transcriptional factors (*AaERF1* and *AaERF2*) isolated from an *A. annua* glandular trichome cDNA library, we show that both of them are able to bind to the *cis*-elements of *ADS* and *CYP71AV1* promoters and activate their expression; overexpression of the two AP2/ERF genes results in increased accumulation of artemisinin and artemisinic acid in transgenic *A. annua* plants.

## 2 RESULTS

Induction of *ADS* and *CYP71AV1* Expression by MeJA To investigate the effects of JA on artemisinin biosynthesis, genes encoding the general mevalonate (MVA) pathway enzymes of 3-hydroxy-3-methylglutaryl coenzyme A reductase (HMGR) and farnesyl diphosphate synthase (FPS), as well as the artemisinin pathway enzymes of ADS and CYP71AV1 were analyzed for their spatial patterns of expression and responses to methyl jasmonate (MeJA). Quantitative RT-PCR (qRT - PCR) showed that the transcript levels of *ADS* and *CYP71AV1* were high in inflorescences, moderate in young leaves, and low in mature leaves and stems (Figure 2A)—a pattern that was consistent with the report that artemisinin content was 4-11-fold higher in inflorescences than in leaves of *A. annua* L. When young plants were treated with MeJA, expression level of *ADS* was increased rapidly and peaked within 1 h post treatment, followed by a quick decline (Figure 2B). The response of *CYP71AV1* to MeJA treatment was relatively slow but lasted longer, with the maximum transcript level occurring at 9 h post treatment (Figure 2B). The expression of *HMGR* and *FPS* genes was, however, neither expressed highly in inflorescences nor responded to MeJA treatment (Figure 2A and Supplemental Figure 1). These results indicate that JA promotes expression of key enzyme genes of the artemisinin biosynthesis pathway.

To find out *cis*-elements responsible for the MeJA induction of *ADS* and *CYP71AV1* expression, promoter regions of the two genes were scanned with PLACE software (www. dna. affrc. go. jp/htdocs/PLACE/signalscan. html) for putative transcription factor binding sites. We found that both promoters contained CRTDREHVCBF2 (CBF2) and RAV1AAT (RAA) motifs, which were reported to be the binding sites of AP2/ERF transcription factors, implying that transcription factors of this family might participate in transcriptional regulation of *ADS* and *CYP71AV1*.

Isolation and Characterization of AaERF1 and AaERF2 To isolate the candidate AP2/ERF family transcription factors, we searched expressed sequence tags (ESTs) from a glandular trichome cDNA library of *A. annua* for conserved AP2 domain sequences, which retrieved seven cDNA fragments. Subsequent qRT-PCR analyses showed that two of them were highly expressed in inflorescence (Figure 2A) and responsive to MeJA treatment (Figure 2C).

By 5′-rapid amplification of cDNA ends (5′-RACE), full-length cDNAs of the two genes were isolated and named *AaERF1* and *AaERF2*, respectively. *AaERF1* contains an open reading frame (ORF) encoding a protein of 253 amino acids, whereas the protein encoded by *AaERF2* contains 204 amino acids. Both AaERF1 and AaERF2 contain only one conserved DNA-binding domain (AP2/ERF domain), which shows a high sequence identity (79.7%) between each other. In the AP2/ERF domain, the 14 th alanine and the 19th aspartic acid along with a WLG motif are highly conserved (Supplemental Figure 2A). AaERF1 and AaERF2 share a very low sequence identity (~10.6%) except for the conserved AP2/ERF domain. Based on the sequence information and domain structure, AaERF1 and AaERF2 both belong to the ERF subfamily. Members of this subfamily have been reported to function as either activators or suppressors of defense genes, and play important roles in cross-talk of ethylene and JA signaling pathways. The ERF subfamily can be further divided into six groups (B1-B6) according to the conserved amino acid residues and the existence of other motifs. B1 group members share a conserved EAR repression domain and act as transcription

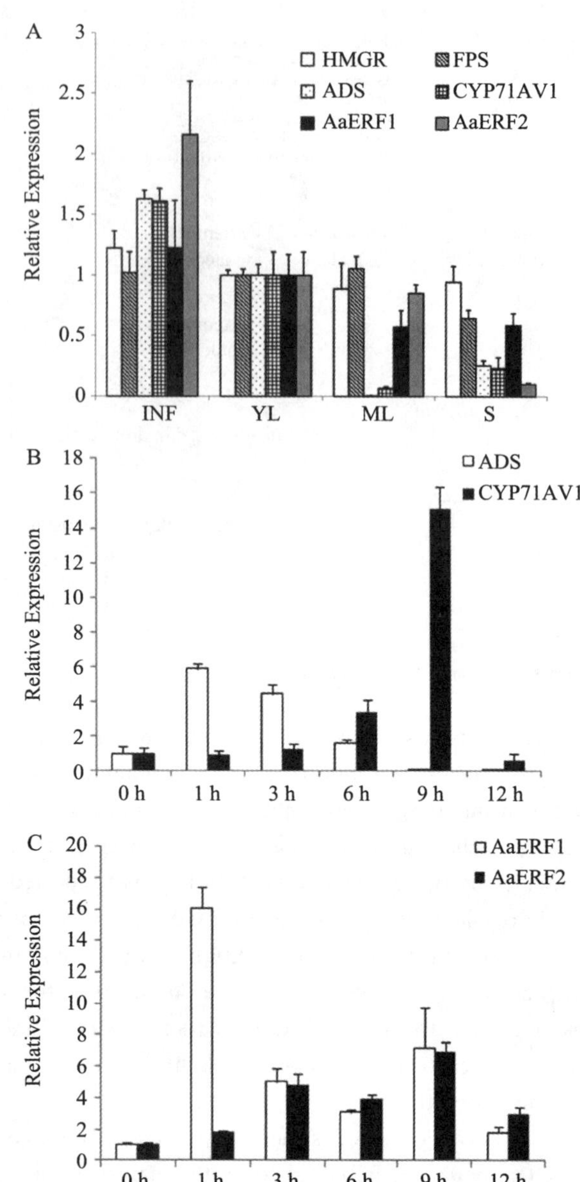


**Figure 2 Expressions of *ADS*, *CYP71AV1*, *AaERF1*, and *AaERF2* in plants of *A. annua* and their response to mejA elicitation**

(A) Expression levels of *HMGR*, *FPS*, *ADS*, *CYP71AV1*, *AaERF1*, and *AaERF2* in inflorescence (INF), young leaves (YL, from the 1/3 upper stem), mature leaves (ML, from the 1/3 lower stem), and stem (S). *ACTIN* was used as the internal standard. (B) *ADS* and *CYP71AV1* expression in response to MeJA treatment. The 4-week-old plants were dipped in DMSO or MeJA solution (50 μmol/L). Young rosette leaves were collected at 0, 1, 3, 6, 9, and 12 h of the treatment for qRT-PCR analysis. (C) *AaERF1* and *AaERF2* expression in response to MeJA treatment. Plant materials used were the same as described in (B). *ACTIN* was used as an internal control. Error bars indicate SD of three technical replicates, and the results were consistent in three biological replicates.

repressors, whereas B3 group is consisted of transcription activators, such as AtERF1, AtERF2, AtERF5, of which AtERF2 functions positively in plant defense and JA-dependent responses. Sequence comparison and phylogenetic analysis place both AaERF1 and AaERF2 in the B3 group (Supplemental Figure 2B). Moreover, AaERF1 shows 63% protein sequence identity to tomato LeERF1 Whereas AaERF2 is 51% identical to *Nicotiana sylvestris* NsERF4; both LeERF1 and NsERF4 are involved in ethylene-mediated wounding responses.

Expression and Induction Patterns of *AaERF1* and *AaERF2* The expression patterns of both *AaERFs* in *A. annua* plants were then compared to those of the artemisinin pathway genes. According to qRT-PCR, both *AaERF1* and *AaERF2* exhibited a spatial expression pattern similar to that of *ADS* and *CYP71AV1*, with the highest level of transcripts in inflorescence, and a moderate level in young leaves (Figure 2A).

It has been reported that artemisinin accumulation in plants and cultured cells was increased after treatment with MeJA. We then treated the 4-week-old *A. annua* plants with various phytohormones, including MeJA, SA, auxin (3-indole acetic acid, IAA), gibberellic acid ($GA_3$), 1-aminocyclopropane-1-carboxylate (ACC, a precursor of ethylene). We found that, among the five hormones tested, MeJA was most effective in inducing *ADS* and *CYP71AV1* expressions (Supplemental Figure 1). Importantly, expression of both *AaERFs* also responded to MeJA treatment. The transcript level of *AaERF1* was increased rapidly and peaked within 1 h after MeJA treatment, followed by a quick decline (Figure 2C), whereas the *AaERF2* response to MeJA treatment was relatively slow but lasted longer, with the highly elevated transcript level occurring between 3 and 9 h post treatment (Figure 2C). Together, the expression patterns and sequence information suggested that both AaERF1 and AaERF2 may serve as transcription factors in mediating the MeJA regulation of artemisinin pathway genes.

Activation of *ADS* and *CYP71AV1* Promoters by AaERF1 and AaERF2 To determine the subcellular localization of AaERF1 and AaERF2, the ORFs of *AaERF1* and *AaERF2* wcrc in-frame fused to the yellow fluorescent protein (YFP) derivative VENUS, respectively. After transferring the constructs into onion epidermal cells, the florescence was observed exclusively in nuclei; by contrast, cells transformed with 35S: VENUS showed florescence throughout the cell (Figure 3). These data indicate that both AaERF1 and AaERF2 proteins are nuclear-localized, consistently with their putative role as transcription factors.

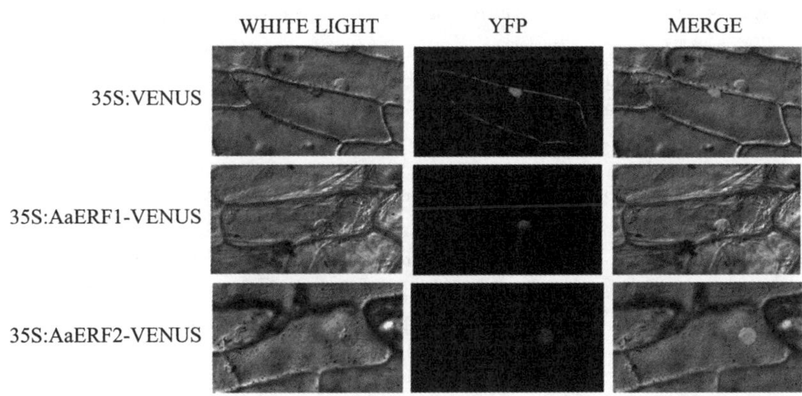


**Figure 3 Nuclear localization of AaERF1 and AaERF2 proteins in onion epidermal cells**

Onion epidermal cells were transiently transformed with constructs harboring AaERF1-VENUS, AaERF2-VENUS, or a control VENUS, respectively, under the control of 35S promoter. Bright-field (left), fluorescence (middle), and the corresponding overlay (right) images of cells were shown.

To test whether AaERF1 and AaERF2 could bind to promoters of *ADS* and *CYP71AV1*, yeast one-hybrid assays were performed. Triple repeated RAA and CBF2 motifs were integrated into the genome of yeast cells, respectively. After introducing *AaERF1* and *AaERF2* into the yeast strains, we found that the two ERF factors indeed were able to bind to both the CBF2 and the RAA motifs, respectively, and AaERF2 appeared to have a higher affinity than AaERF1 to these two DNA motifs (Figure 4A).

To further examine the binding activities of AaERF1 and AaERF2 to the *ADS* and *CYP71AV1* promoters, an electrophoretic mobility shift assay (EMSA) was performed. The recombinant protein of HIS-AaERF1 showed binding activities to both the 3×RAA and the 3×CBF2 fragments (Figure 4B and 4C). The DNA-binding specificity was then confirmed in a competition experiment with excess amounts of the unlabeled probes of 3 × RAA and 3 × CBF2, respectively (Figure 4B and 4C). Similarly, the recombinant

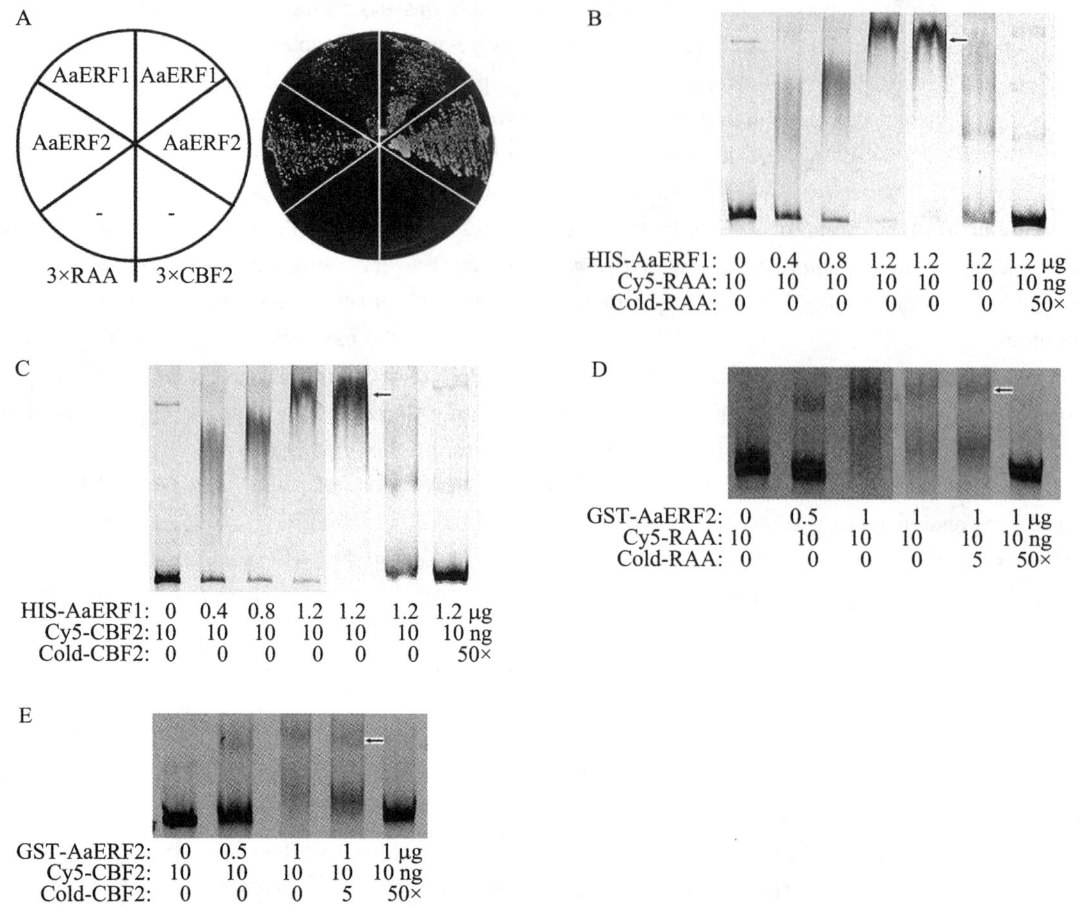


**Figure 4 Binding assay of AaERF1 and AaERF2 to RAA and CBF2 *cis*-elements**

(A) Diagram and the result of yeast one-hybrid assay for the interaction between each AaERF protein with DNA motifs. Triple RAV1 - AAT (RAA) motif and CRTDREHVCBF2 (CBF2) motif were used as bait, respectively. Yeast cells carrying pGAD424, pGAD - AaERF1, or pGAD - AaERF2 were grown for 3 d at 30 ℃ on SD/-His/-Leu base with 10 mM 3-amino-1, 2, 4-triazole (3-AT). (B, C) EMSA analysis of binding of AaERF1 protein to the RAA and CBF2 *cis*-elements. Ten micrograms of Cy5-labeled RAA (B) or CBF2 (C) were incubated with different concentrations HIS - AaERF1 fusion protein (0, 0.4, 0.8, and 1.2 μg) at 25 ℃ for 30 min to compete with cold probes (0, 5, 50×) and then analyzed by electrophoresis. (D, E) EMSA analysis of binding of AaERF2 protein to the RAA and CBF2 *cis*-elements. Ten micrograms of Cy5-labeled RAA (D) or CBF2 (E) were incubated with different concentrations of the GST - AaERF2 fusion protein (0, 0.5, and 1 μg) at 25 ℃ for 30 min to compete with cold probes (0, 5, 50×) and then analyzed by electrophoresis. The bands were clarified with a solid black arrow.

protein of GST - AaERF2 with improved solubility also interacted with the 3×RAA and 3×CBF2 DNA fragments (Figure 4D and 4E). Thus, data gained from both yeast one-hybrid assay and *in vitro* EMSA support that AaERF1 and AaERF2 recognize and interact with the RAA and CBF2 palindromes present in *ADS* and *CYP71AV1* promoters.

To provide more evidence that *AaERFs* regulate *ADS* and *CYP71AV1* transcription, an *Agrobacterium*-mediated transient expression assay was performed. The promoter fragments of *ADS* (~2 kb) and *CYP71AV1* (~1.3 kb) were used to drive the *GUS* reporter gene, respectively, and the ORF of either *AaERFs* was overexpressed under the control of the 355 promoter (Figure 5A). Each promoter - *GUS* construct was then co-transferred with either 35S: *AaERF1* or 35S: *AaERF2*, respectively, into tobacco (*Nicotiana benthamiana*) leaves. We found that both AaERF1 and AaERF2 increased the *GUS* reporter gene expression. Based on *GUS* transcript abundance, up to threefold increase in the *ADS* promoter activity was achieved by AaERF2, and that of *CYP71AV1* promoter was increased about sixfold by AaERF1 (Figure 5B).

AaERF1 and AaERF2 Promote Artemisinin Biosynthesis

Since AaERF1 and AaERF2 could bind to the *ADS* and *CYP71AV1* promoters and enhance gene transcription, it was then interesting to further analyze the role of the two transcription factors in regulating artemisinin biosynthesis in plants of *A. annua*. Both *AaERF1* and *AaERF2* were overexpressed in *A. annua* under the control of the 35S

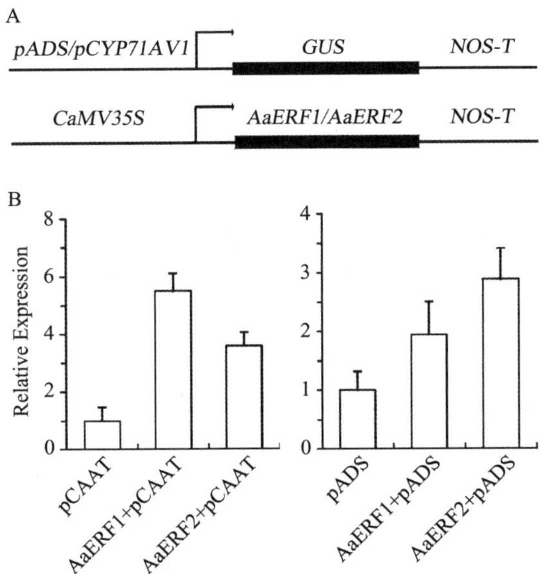


**Figure 5 Enhancing *ADS* and *CAAT* (*CYP71AV1*) promoter activities by AaERF1 and AaERF2.**

(A) Schematic diagram of the reporter (pADS/pCAAT: GUS) and effector (35S: *AaERF1/AaERF2*) constructs used in the co-expression experiment. The constructs were co-transformed into leaves of 1-month-old tobacco (*N. benthamiana*). After growing in a greenhouse for 3 d, leaves were harvested for qRT-PCR analysis.
(B) qRT-PCR analysis of the *GUS* gene expression in transiently transformed *N. benthamiana* leaves. AaERF1 and AaERF2-activated *GUS* gene expression in pCAAT: *GUS* (left) and pADS: *GUS* (right) reporters, respectively. *NbACTIN1* (*ACTIN1* of *N. benthamiana*) was used as the internal standard. Error bars indicate SD of three technical replicates, and the results were consistent in three biological replicates.

promoter, respectively. The transgenic plants were first confirmed by semi-qRT-PCR and genomic DNA-based PCR on kanamycin-resistant gene (Supplemental Figure 3), and then three transgenic lines for each gene were chosen for further analysis.

In the overexpression (ox) plants examined, transcripts of *AaERF1* and *AaERF2* were increased by about twofold, respectively (Figure 6A and 6B). Consequently, expression levels of *ADS* and *CYP71AV1* were also elevated drastically, ranging from 2- to 8- and 1.2- to 5-fold, respectively (Figure 6A and 6B). The expression of *DBR2* was also moderately increased, whereas the expression leaves of the upstream MVA pathway enzyme genes of *HMGR* and *FPS* were barely or only slightly changed (Supplemental Figure 4). The artemisinin and artemisinic acid contents in mature leaves of the 3-month-old *A. annua* plants were analyzed by high-performance liquid chromatography (HPLC). Comparedto the wild-typecontrol, artemisinin and artemisinic acid levels were increased by 19%~67% and 11%~76% in *AaERF1-ox* transgenic plants, and by 24%~51% and 17%~121% in *AaERF2-ox* plants, respectively (Figure 6C and 6D).

To further prove the function of *AaERF1* and *AaERF2* in regulation of artemisinin biosynthesis *in planta*, we down-regulated their expression by an RNA interference (RNAi) approach. In the dsRNA transgenic lines, the expression of *AaERF1* and *AaERF2* was suppressed to 27%~62% and 19%~55% of the wild-type level, respectively. Consequently, *ADS* and *CYP71AV1* transcript levels were reduced to 35%~13% and 38%~7% of the wild-type level in *AaERF1-ds* plants, and to 9%~4% and 12%~3% in *AaERF2-ds* plants, respectively (Figure 7A and 7B). As a result of reduced *ADS* and *CYP71AV1* gene expression, the contents of artemisinin and artemisinic acid were decreased to 76%~58% and 55%~30% of the wildtype level in *AaERF1-ds* plants. In *AaERF2-ds* plants the reduction was 70%~51% for artemisinin and 69%~37% for artemisinic acid, respectively (Figure 7C and 7D). We did not observe any morphological difference between AaERF overexpression or RNAi transgenic lines and the wild-typc plants (QT). These data demonstrate clearly that *AaERFs* are positive regulators of *ADS* and *CYP71AV1* and contribute to the production of artemisinin and artemisinic acid in plants.

## 3 DISCUSSION

The phytohormone JA plays an important role in many aspects of plant life, including flower development, root growth, leaf senescence, and particularly plant response to biotic and abiotic stresses that are party achieved by enhancing biosynthesis of secondary metabolites, including terpenoids. For example, our previous investigation showed that, in rice, JA induced the expression of *OsTPS3*, a sesquiterpene synthase gene, leading to increased release of (E)-β-caryophyllene. In suspension-cultured cells of cotton (*Gossypium arboreum*), accumulation of the sesquiterpene aldehyde gossypol and expression of the sesquiterpene synthase [(+)-δ-cadinene synthase] gene were strongly induced by treatments of JA and a fungal elicitor. In *C. roseus*, regulation of biosynthesis of terpenoid indole alkaloids biosynthesis was mediated by *ORCA3*, an AP2/ERF subfamily transcriptional factor. In this investigation, we found that stimulation of artemisinin biosynthesis in *A. annua* by JA was also mediated by the AP2/ERF subfamily members AaERF1 and AaERF2, which directly bound to promoter regions of *ADS* and *CYP71AV1*. These suggest that, despite diverse chemical structures and biological functions of plant terpenoids, similar regulatory mechanisms exist in plants of different taxa. Considering the signaling functions of JA and defense functions of plant secondary metabolites, how such regulatory mechanism is established and maintained during evolution is an interesting subject of further investigation.

The basic helix-loop-helix transcription factors play important roles in plant organ development, light signaling,

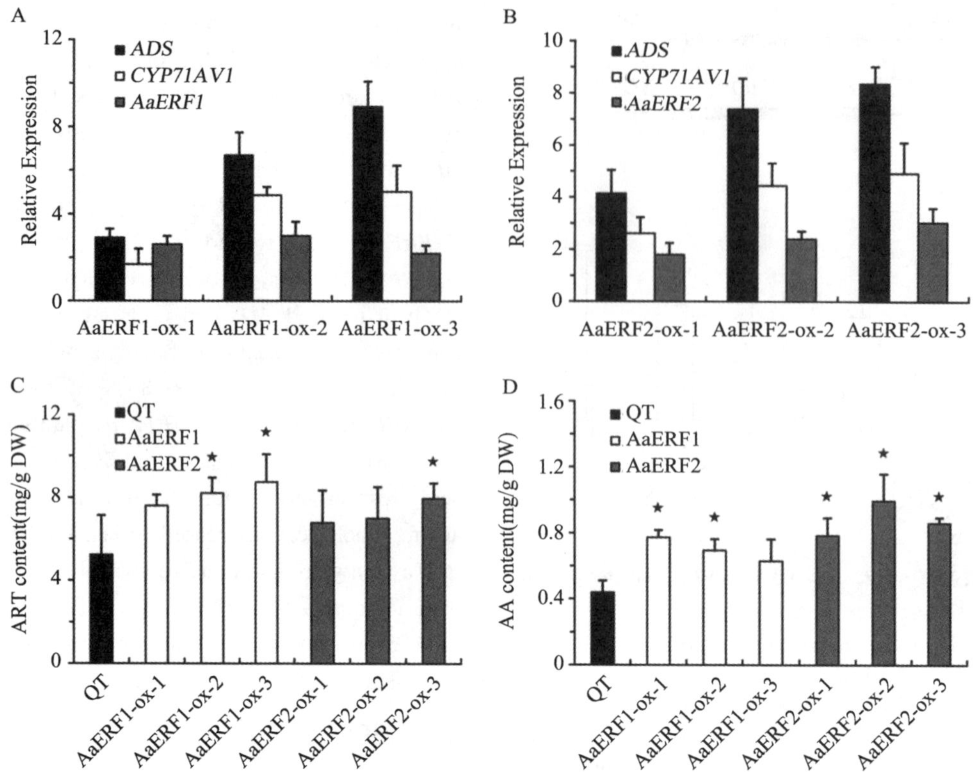


**Figure 6 Elevated expression of *ADS* and *CYP71AV1*, and artemisinin (ART) and artemisinic acid (AA) contents in *A. annua* overexpressing *AaERF1* or *AaERF2*. Untransformed plants of *A. annua* cv. QiuTe (QT) were used as control**

(A) Expression of *AaERF1*, *ADS*, and *CYP71AV1* in leaves of the 3-month-old plants transformed with 35S: *AaERF1* (AaERF1-ox). *ACTIN* was used as the internal standard; for each gene, the expression level relative to *ACTIN* in the control plant (QT) was taken as 1. Error bars indicate SD of three technical replicates, and the results were consistent in three biological replicates. (B) Expression of *AaERF2*, *ADS*, and *CYP71AV1* in leaves of the 3-month-old plants transformed with 35S: *AaERF2* (AaERF2-ox). (C) Contents of artemisinin (ART) in leaves of AaERF1-ox and AaERF2-ox transgenic plants, determined by HPLC. The content of ART was compared to dry weight of sample. Error bars indicate SD of three biological replicates. Asterisks denote Student's $t$-test significance compared with QT (* $P<0.05$). (D) Contents of artemisinic acid (AA) in leaves of AaERF1-ox and AaERF2-ox transgenic plants, determined by HPLC. The content of AA was compared to dry weight of sample.

stress response, and plant secondary metabolism. The *Arabidopsis* bHLH transcription factor AtMYC2 has long been considered a central regulator of JA signaling pathway, mediating both developmental and stress responses. Recently, AtMYC3 and AtMYC4 were reported to act additively with AtMYC2 to regulate different subsets of JA responses. It was also reported that the homologous protein in *C. roseus*, CrMYC2, mediated the JA signaling and terpenoid indole alkaloid biosynthesis by binding to the promoter region of the AP2/ERF transcription factor gene *ORCA3*. Coincidentally, in tobacco, NtMYC2 positively regulated nicotine biosynthesis not only by binding to the G-box in the biosynthetic genes' promoters, but also via activating *NIC2*-locus *ERF* genes that functioned redundantly with NtMYC2 in up-regulating nicotine biosynthesis. It should be interesting to investigate whether both types of transcription factors are also involved in artemisinin biosynthesis in *A. annua*. Isolation and characterization of *cis*-elements in promoter regions of *AaERFs* will facilitate our understanding of the signaling network in regulating sesquiterpene biosynthesis in *A. annua*.

Artemisinin is an effective ingredient for malaria treatment; however, its utilization has been limited due to low yield in plants of *A. annua*. Despite the great potential of engineering microbes to produce artemisinin, until now, only artemisinic acid has been produced in large quantities. In tobacco, heterologous expression of *ADS* and *CYP71AV1* led to the production of amorpha-4, 11-diene and artemisinic alcohol, and additional expression of *DBR2* and *ALDH1* led to the accumulation of dihydroartemisinic alcohol. However, no artemisinin was detected, largely due to unclarified remaining steps in the artemisinin biosynthesis pathway. Therefore, further elucidation of the artemisinin biosynthetic pathway and the regulatory mechanism is of great importance.

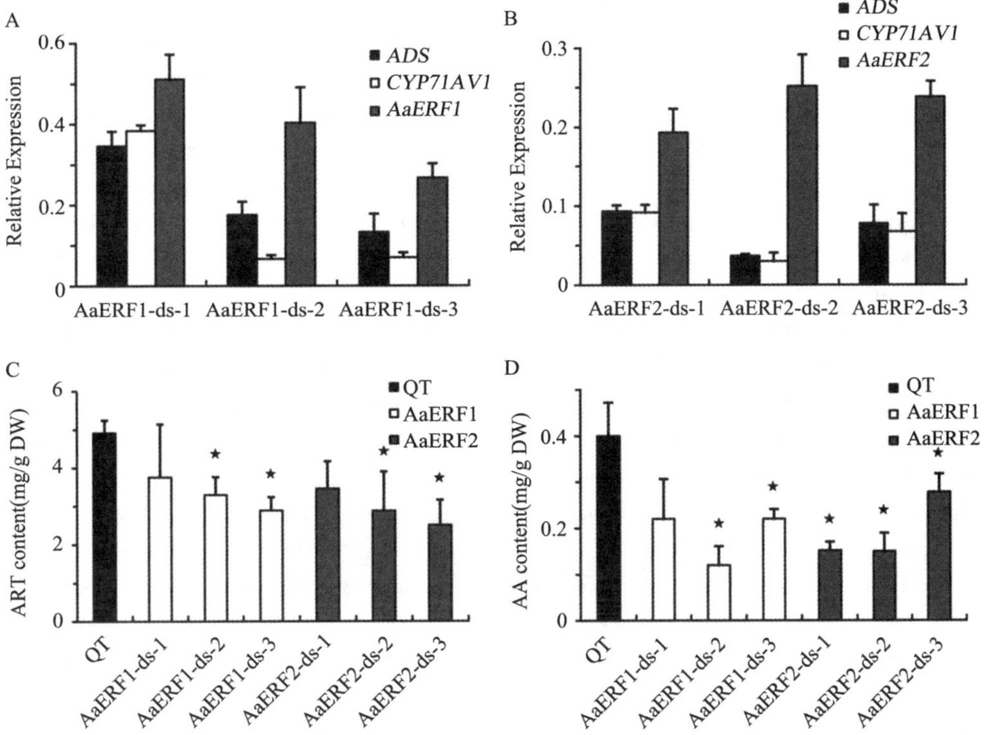


**Figure 7 Reduced expression of *ADS* and *CYP71AV1*, and ART and AA contents in *A. annua* expressing the dsRNA targeting *AaERF1* or *AaERF2*. Untransformed plants of *A. annua* cv. QiuTe (QT) were used as control**

(A) Expression of *AaERF1*, *ADS*, and *CYP71AV1* in the leaves of the 3-month-old AaERF1-ds plants. *ACTIN* was used as the internal standard; for each gene, the expression level relative to *ACTIN* in the control plant (QT) was taken as 1. Error bars indicate SD of three technical replicates, and the results were consistent in three biological replicates. (B) Expression of *AaERF2*, *ADS*, and *CYP71AV1* in leaves of the 3-month-old AaERF2-ds plants. (C) Contents of artemisinin (ART) in leaves of AaERF1-ds and AaERF2-ds transgenic plants, determined by HPLC. The content of ART was compared to that of the sample. Error bars indicate SD of three biological replicates. Asterisks denote Student's *t*-test significance compared with QT (* $P<0.05$). (D) Contents of artemisinic acid (AA) in leaves of AaERF1-ds and AaERF2-ds transgenic plants, determined by HPLC. The content of AA was compared to that of the sample.

Biosynthesis of plant secondary metabolites usually involves multiple enzymes, increasing the target metabolite production in the host plant by overexpressing one or two enzymes, or engineering one organism to produce specialized secondary metabolites of another organism by heterologous expression of enzymes, and is often inefficient. Regulatory components often target the key steps or even the whole biosynthetic pathway. We have shown that overexpression of the two AP2/ERF-type transcription factors, AaERF1 and AaERF2, resulted in increased artemisinin accumulation in transgenic *A. annua* plants. Therefore, engineering the regulatory mechanism, especially transcription factors, is of great potential in engineering plant secondary metabolism. In addition, blocking other competing pathways, such as sterol and β-caryophyllene biosynthesis, could enrich precursors for artemisinin formation. Combining these two strategies will shed new light on increasing artemisinin production. As artemisinin content increases obviously in the full-flower stage and correlates closely to trichome changes, the control of *A. annua* phase transition and trichome density is worthy of further investigation.

## 4 METHODS

Plant Materials and Phytohormone Treatments *A. annua* L. cv. QT was used in this investigation, and the seeds were obtained from Sichuan Province, China. Plants of *A. annua* L. and *Nicotiana benthamiana* were grown in a greenhouse with 14/10-h light/dark photoperiod at 26 ℃. For MeJA treatment, plants of *A. annua* were dipped in MeJA solution (50 μmol/L) for 1, 3, 6, 9, and 12 h, as indicated, and the DMSO solution was used as mock. For other phytohormone (MeJA, SA, IAA, $GA_3$, ACC), the leaves of 4-week-old *A. annua* plants were collected at 4-h post treatments. For tissue expression pattern analysis, the 2-month-old plants were transferred to 12/12-h photoperiod for flowering. After another month, different parts were collected; leaves on the 1/3 upper stem were defined as young leaves and those on the 1/3 lower stem as mature leaves.

Isolation of cDNAs Based on expressed sequence tags (ESTs), full-length cDNAs of *AaERF1* and *AaERF2* were obtained by 5′-rapid amplification of cDNA ends (5′-PACE), using the GeneRacer Kit (CLONTECH Laboratories, Inc.). An adaptor primer (forward) and two gene-specific primers (reverse) were used for isolation. All the primers used in this investigation are listen in Supplemental Table 1.

Transgenic Plants Confirmation and Expression Analysis The genomic DNA of kan-resistant and control plants was isolated as follows: 1-month-old plant material of 0.2 g was ground to powder and 0.6 mL buffer (100 mmol/L Tris, 50 mmol/L EDTA, 0.5 mol/L Nacl, 10 mmol/L β-mercaptoethanol) added, and it was boiled for 10 min before centrifugation at 13 000 rpm for 10 min. The supernatant was mixed with isopropanol and placed at −20 ℃ for 30 min, centrifuged at 13 000 rpm under 4 ℃, and the precipitate was dissolved as templates for PCR analysis.

Total RNAs were prepared with Trizol reagent (Invitrogen). One microgram total RNA was used as a template for reverse transcription with oligo (dT) as primer in a 20-μL reaction system, using the RNA PCR (AMV) kit (Promege). Quantitative real-time RT-PCR (qRT-PCR) was performed with the SYBR-Green PCR Mastermix kit (Takara) on a Mastercycler ep RealPlex2 (Eppendorf) monitor. The relative expression level of each gene was determined as described previously and the transcript level of *A. annua ACTIN* (EU531837) was used as a control.

Plant Transformation The full-length coding regions of *AaERF1* and *AaERF2* were amplified by PCR with stick *Pst*I and *BamH*I ends, and inserted into the binary vector pCAMBIA2300 under the control of the CaMV 355 promoter. Each construct was introduced into *Agrobacterium tumefaciens* strain EHA105 for plant transformation, which was performed as previously described. The defined ORF fragments of *AaERF1* (183 - 517 bp downstream of ATG codon) and *AaERF2* (39 - 359 bp downstream of ATG codon) were PCR-amplified for RNAi constructs (for primers, see Supplemental Table 1), followed by inserting into the modified pCAMBIA2300 under the control of the 355 promoter. Plants of the wild-type *A. annua* L. cv. QT were used for transformation. The rest of the plants that were not transformed were used as control for both gene expression and HPLC analysis. At least three independent control lines (QT) were tested in these experiments and the mean value was shown as the control.

Protein Subcellular Localization The full-length coding regions of *AaERF1* and *AaERF2* were in-frame fused to the N-terminus of the *VENUS* gene with a glycine linker under the control of the 355 promoter. The AaERF1-linker-VENUS and AaERF2-linker-VENUS fusions as well as the VENUS control vectors were bombarded into onion epidermal cells by particle bombardment (Bio-Rad). Transformed cells were cultured on MS medium for 24 h in dark and images were obtained with an LSM510 laser scanning confocal microscope (Zeiss), with argon laser excitation at 488 nm and a 505 - 550-nm emission filter set.

Yeast One-Hybrid Assay The binding assay utilizing MATCHMAKER yeast one-hybrid system (Clontech) was performed according to the manual. The triple tandem copies of the CRTDREHVCBF2 motif (5′-AGGTCGACCG ATAGGTCGACCGATAG GTCGACCGAT-3′) and the RAV1AAT motif (5′-CTCAACATTGTCTCAACATT GTCTCAACATTGT-3′) were inserted into pHISi-1 between *Sacl* and *Xbal* as baits, respectively. These two bait constructs were linearized and integrated into the genome of yeast strain *YM4271*. The preys were the ORFs of *AaERF1* and *AaERF2* in-frame fused with the GAL4 activation domain in pGAD424 between *BamH*I and *Pst*I. The preys were then introduced into yeast cells previously transformed with baits, with balnk pGAD424 plasmid as control. The positively transformed clones were analyzed on SD/-His/-Leu medium with different concentrations of 3-amino-1, 2, 4-triazole (3-AT).

Electrophoretic Mobility Shift Assay The ORF of *AaERF1* was inserted into the expression vector pET32a (Novagen) between the *Sac*I and *Sal*I sites, and the ORF of *AaERF2* was inserted into the expression vector pGEX-4T-1 (Amersham Pharmacia Biotech) between the *Bam*HI and *Sal*I sites so as to increase protein solubility. The recombinant AaERF1 and AaERF2 proteins were purified according to the instruction manual. The probe sequences were the same as those used in yeast one-hybrid assay except for labeled with Cy5 on both ends. The DNA fragment and purified proteins were incubated at 25 ℃ for 30 min and then separated with native polyacrylamide gel electrophoresis (PAGE). The fluorescence was detected with a FUJIFILM FLA-9000 image scanner.

Transient Expression Assay With an *Xba*I stick end (5′) and a *Sma*I blunt end (3′), the 2 037-bp fragment of *ADS* promoter (DQ448297) and a 1 274-bp fragment of *CYP71AV1* promoter (CN 200910045041) were fused with β-glucuronidase (*GUS*) reporter gene and cloned into the binary vector pBI101, respectively. The ORFs of *AaERF1* and *AaERF2* were inserted into the binary vector pCAMBIA1300 between *BamH*I and *Sal*I sites under the control of 355 promoter. These constructs (including modified pCAMBIA1300 as a control) were then introduced into *A. tumefaciens* strain GV3101, respectively. For transient transformation, the *Agrobacterium* clones were inoculated in 2 mL LB culture (containing appropriate selection antibiotics) and grew overnight at 28 ℃ with rotation at 200 rpm, followed by transferring into 50 mL LB containing 20 μmol/L acetosyringone and 10 mmol/L MES (pH 5.7) for additional culture for 16 - 20 h. Cells were collect by centrifugation at 5 000 rpm for 5 min at 4 ℃, re-suspended in a transformation solution (10 mmol/L $MgCl_2$, 10 mmol/L MES, pH 5.7, 150 μmol/L acetosyringone) and kept for at least 3 h at room temperature. The *Agrobacterium* suspensions of reporter and effecter were mixed and infiltrated into tobacco leaves using a syringe. The infiltrated plants were grown in a greenhouse for an additional 3 d and total RNAs in the infiltrated leaves were used for qRT - PCR. Quantitative analysis was performed at least three times throughout this investigation.

Chemical Analysis　Contents of artemisinin and artemisinic acid were determined by high-performance liquid chromatography (HPLC) as described, with slight modification. Leaves of ~1 g from the 3-month-old *A. annua* plants were collected and dried overnight at 50 ℃. The material was pestled into fine powder and extracted with 60 ml petroleum ether (boiling range 30 - 60 ℃) for 3 h at 55 ℃ and then evaporated till dryness. The residue was dissolved in 1 mL ethanol with supersonic for 2 min. The suspension was centrifuged at 12 000 rpm for 5 min and the supernatant was mixed with 640 μL 0.2% (*W/V*) NaOH and incubated at 50℃ for 30 min. The solution was cooled to room temperature before 800 μL of 0.05 mol/L acetic acid and 200 μL of an internal standard (ethyl-4-hydroxybenzate) were added. After filtering with a nitrocellulose filter (0.45 μm), the samples were used for HPLC (Agilent, Eclipse plus C18 analytical column 4.6× 150 mm, 5 μm) analysis with a mobile phase of 0.01 mol/L sodium phosphate buffer (pH 7.0): methanol (50 : 50) at a flow rate of 1 mL/min, and artemisinin was detected at 260 nm.

For artemisinic acid analysis, plant material was extracted in 50 mL methanol for 2 h, centrifuged at 12 000 r/min for 5 min, and the supernatant was evaporated until dry. The residue was dissolved in 6 mL of ethyl ether and 10 mL water, and the aqueous layer was re-extracted with 20 mL ethyl ether. The extracts were washed with 15 mL 5% sodium hydroxide solution, centrifuged at 12 000 r/min for 5 min, and the under layer was adjusted with 12 mol/L HCl to pH 1.0. After stirring the mixture at room temperature for 30 min and extraction three times with 5 ml ethyl ether, the extracts were evaporated to dryness and dissolved with 1 mL methanol for HPLC analysis. The artemisinic acid was detected at 210 nm with a mobile phase of acetonitrile: 0.5% acetic acid (55 : 45, *V/V*) at a flow rate of 1 mL/min.

[于宗霞,陈晓亚,等. Molecular Plart, 2012, 5(2): 353 - 365.]

# Analysis of integrated multiple 'omics' datasets reveals the mechanisms of initiation and determination in the formation of tuberous roots in *Rehmannia glutinosa*

## 1 INTRODUCTION

*Rehmannia glutinosa* Libosch, commonly known as Chinese foxglove or Sheng Di Huang, is a perennial herbaceous medicinal plant of the Scrophulariaceae family. This species has a cultivation history in China of more than 1 000 years and is traditionally used as a medicine for nourishing *Yin* to restore the bodily balance of *Yin* and *Yang* and supplementing 'blood elements' according to Chinese medicine. Modern pharmacological studies have demonstrated that *R. glutinosa* can strengthen immunity, exhibits anti-inflammatory and anti-tumour effects, and ameliorates diabetes and liver disorders. *R. glutinosa* produces over 70 active pharmaceutical compounds that include a variety of polysaccharides, aminoacids, and iridoid compounds. These compounds are synthesized in the tuberous roots of *R. glutinosa*, which are usually processed into three medicinal forms, i.e. fresh, dry, and steamed. Although the tuberous root is the primary medicinal composition of *R. glutinosa*, studies of its formation have been scarce.

The reproductive properties of the tuberous roots of *R. glutinosa* are similar to those of *Ipomoea batatas* (sweet potato) and *Manihot esculenta* (cassava). The tuberous roots are derived from the swelling of fibrous roots (FRs), which are developed from adventitious roots (ARs). In contrast, the tubers of *Solanum tuberosum* (potato), corms of *Allium cepa* (onion), and rhizomes of *Nelumbo nucifera* (lotus) originate from the expansion of an underground stem. The formation of this underground storage organ involves three common processes: induction, initiation, and formation. The formation of storage organs is induced by similar environmental and endogenous factors, such as photoperiod, high sucrose, and hormone changes. However, distinct storage organs may require different level of specific factors, such as the length and intensity of light, and the concentration and composition of hormones. The appearance of the cambium cells in FRs signals the initiation of tuberous root formation. The formation of *R. glutinosa* tuberous root is anatomically and physiologically similar to that of sweet potato; the vascular cambium first develops within the protoxylem in FRs, followed by the appearance of an anomalous cambium. Subsequent continuous division and expansion in the cambium cells lead to a rapid increase in FR diameter. The mechanisms of storage organ formation have been studied extensively in sweet potato and potato, and many key regulatory proteins have been identified using molecular biology methods. The developmental process of *R. glutinosa* tuberous roots is less well characterized, particularly at the molecular level.

The transition from FRs to tuberous roots is a complex biological process involving many specific genes and proteins. Transcriptome and proteome techniques can efficiently detect these gene and protein changes. RNA-Seq (RNA sequencing) technology is a cost-effective quantification approach that exhibits high reproducibility and accuracy and produces broad real-time dynamic transcriptional profiles at low cost. Isobaric tag for relative and absolute quantification (iTRAQ) enables qucik identification of protein profiles and the exact quantification of differentially expressed proteins (DEPs). Integration of proteomics and transcriptomics is a favoured approach for the detection of differentially expressed genes (DEGs) and proteins with complementary strengths. In this study, transcriptomic and proteomic approaches were combined to identify key genes and proteins associated with the initiation of tuberous root formation.

Tuberous roots are derived from FRs, but not all FRs are destined to become tuberous roots, and the control mechanism for this transition is unknown for all the plants with tuberous roots. Many studies have indicated that miRNAs play important roles in cell fate determination in root development. A study on the root development process of the model plant *Arabidopsis* indicated that miR165/6 determine the fate of root cells. In potato, miR172/miR156 act as long-distance signalling molecules to regulate tuber formation. sRNA transcriptome (sRNAome) sequencing has become the conventional method for detecting specific miRNAs. To identify the specific miRNAs that are closely involved in the transition process, a mutant FR incapable of forming tuberous roots is needed. However, such a mutation is rare in *R. glutinosa*. A minority of FRs stopped tuberous roots development at mature stage of *R. glutinosa*. These FRs, designed as unexpanded fibrous roots (UFRs), provide an alternative approach to explore the transition mechanisms in the absence of an FR mutation.

Morphological analysis, biomass statistics analysis, and an anatomical survey of tuberous roots at different development stages were performed to elucidate the characteristics of the anatomical and physiological states. Based on these analyses, representative tuberous root development stages were defined. Initiated fibrous roots (IFRs) at seedling stages and UFRs at mature stage were also collected. The following two analyses were then conducted: ① tuberous roots (initiated tuberous root, ITRs) at key developmental stages was compared with IFRs using RNA-Seq and iTRAQ to identify the crucial genes and proteins that are closely related to the initiation of FRs. ② the differentially expressed miRNAs in ITRs compared with UFRs as well as their targets were identified through sRNA and degradome sequencing to determine the miRNAs involved in the fate of FRs. By integrating various datasets, the aim was to elucidate the molecular mechanisms underlying the determinant processes of FR transition, which may enable improved economic production of *R. glutinosa*.

## 2 MATERIALS AND METHODS

The full methods can be found in the Supplementary Methods at *JXB* online.

Plant material preparation *R. glutinosa* 'Wen 85-5' was planted at Wen Agricultural Institute, Jiaozuo City, Henan Province, China. Sample collection started when seedlings sprouted 2 cm above ground approximately 20 days after planting (DAP). Additional samples were collected at 60, 80, 100, and 120 DAP. Two types of FRs (fibrous roots at seeding stages and mature stages) were simultaneously collected at 40 DAP and 120 DAP. These roots were used for anatomical and other analyses to understand the key stages of tuberous root development. The tuberous roots at key developmental stages and the two types of FRs were then used for the construction of various libraries, as shown in Fig. 1. In addition, parts of *R. glutinosa* were shaded using a sunshade net with 60% and 90% light transmittance at 40 DAP to investigate the role of light in tuberous root initiation.

RNA sequencing and data analysis After isolation, purification, and digestion of total RNA, sequencing was performed using an Illumina HiSeq 2000 (Beijing Genomics Institute). The reads passing quality control from RNA-Seq were then aligned to an RNA-Seq reference sequence. The number of aligned reads for each gene was used to calculate gene expression level through RSEM software. The NOISeq software was used to identify DEGs among the samples. Thresholds of fold change $\geqslant 2$ or $\leqslant -2$ and diverge probability $\geqslant 0.8$ were applied to assess the significance of the differences in transcription.

Protein sequencing and data processing Proteins from different samples were labelled with the iTRAQ reagent,

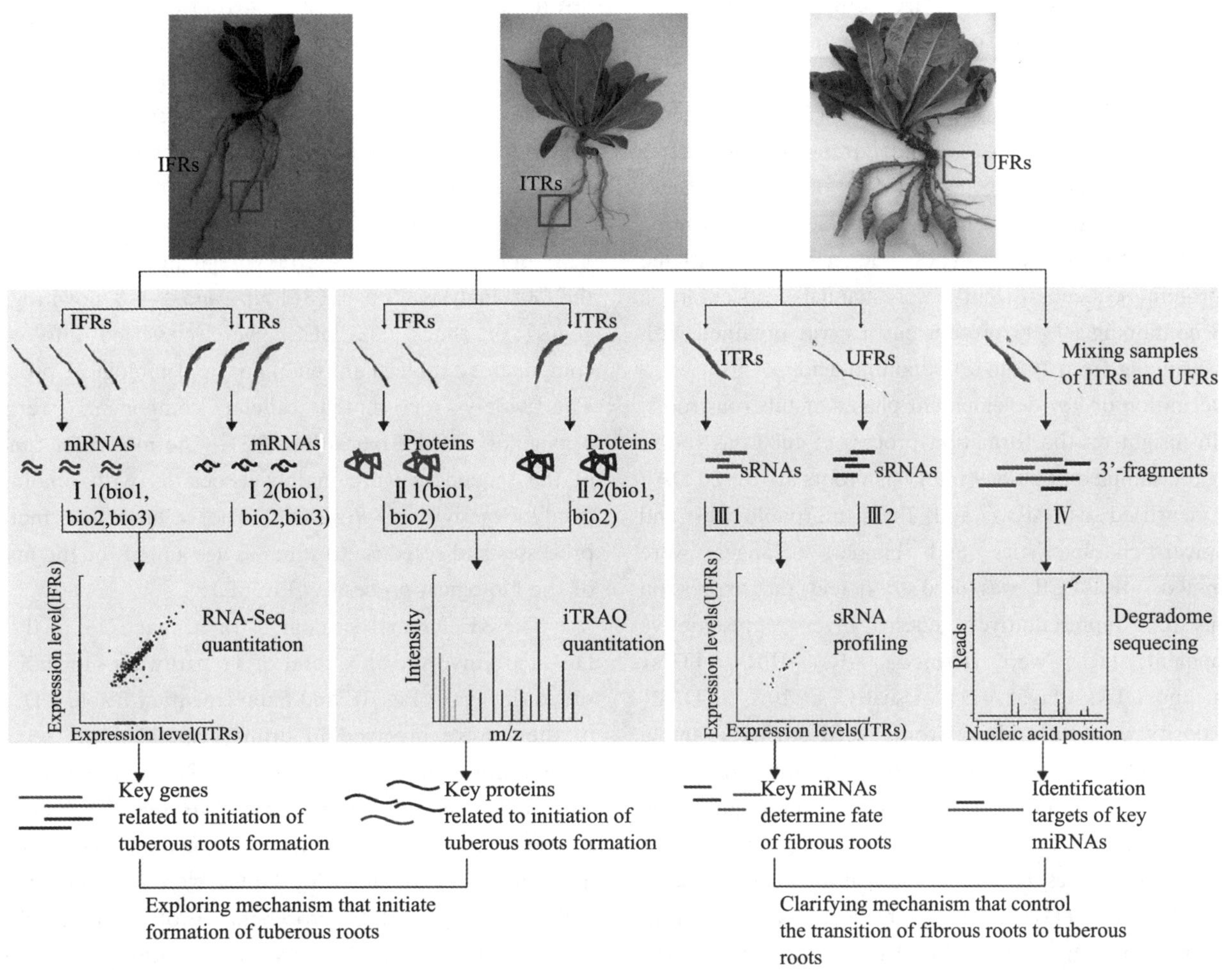


**Fig. 1 Overview of the experimental procedure and the material composition for the construction of each library**

and were then subjected to strong cation exchange fractionation. The fractions were separated using combined nanoflow HPLC, followed by analysis of mass spectral using Q-Exactive. The peptides were analysed using a protein database that was translated from the *R. glutinosa* transcriptome using Mascot 2.2 using the parameters of peptide false discovery rate (FDR) $\leqslant 0.01$ and protein FDR $\leqslant 0.01$. The threshold value adopted for significant differential expression among the samples was 0.77-fold for downregulated proteins and 1.30-fold for upregulated proteins, with $P<0.05$.

sRNA sequencing and data processing Total RNA was separated by 15% denaturing PAGE to recover sRNAs with a length of 18 – 30 nt. The sRNAs were then purified and used for cDNA synthesis, which was then sequenced on an Illumina HiSeq 2000. The known miRNAs were identified by BLASTN searches against the miR Base 20.0 database with default parameters. Candidate precursor miRNAs were predicted using MIREAP, and confirmed by quantitative (q) RT-PCR (forward primers can be found in Supplementary Table S1).

Degradome sequencing and data analysis RNA fragments with a poly(A) tail were isolated from the total RNA of each example. A series of steps, including ligation of 5′ RNA adaptors, digestion, ligation of double-stranded DNA adaptor, purification, and amplification were conducted and sequencing was done on an Illumina HiSeq 2000. The raw sequencing reads were processed by Illumina's Pipeline v1.5 to obtain clean reads, which were them used to identify potentially cleaved targets.

qRT-PCR analysis Differential mRNAs and miRNAs were validated by qRT-PCR (miRNA forward primers are given in Supplementary Table S2, mRNA primers in Supplementary Table S3). The expression pattern of the key genes (primers are provided in Supplementary Tables S4 and S5), and key miRNAs (primers provided in Supplementary Table S6) and their targets was analysed by qRT-PCR.

## 3 RESULTS

Construction of the R. glutinosa transcriptome and proteome reference library A root and leaf transcriptome library for *R. glutinosa* has been previously constructed. The root library was deposited at NCBI with the accession number SRX269425 and yielded 99 708 unigenes with a mean length of 348 bp using the software SOAPdenovo (http://soap.genomics.org.cn/). To improve the quality and length of the sequences, 94 544 leaf unigenes assembled from the leaf library (SRX269426) were combined with root unigenes to form a more complete *R. glutinosa* transcriptome. After removing the overlapping sequences, a set of 87 665 unigenes with a mean length of 554 bp was obtained, representing 41.82 Mbp of total sequence. These unigenes were translated into protein sequences, and after manual inspection, a library containing 50 796 protein entries was obtained with lengths ranging from 100 to 3 000 amino acids.

Definition of key development phases of tuberous roots To gain insight on the formation process of tuberous roots, roots were sampled at 20-day intervals (roots at 10 - 20 DAP were identified as ARs) and their morphological and anatomical characteristics and biomass changes were determined. qRT-PCR was used to detect the expression patterns of representative genes. Five representative development stages were defined: ARs, IFRs, ITRs, MTRs, and LTRs (Fig. 2A-D). Usually, at 10 - 20 DAP, the majority of ARs erupted from 'seed stocks', and a fraction rapidly developed into IFRs. In the process of tuberous root formation, IFRs represent a key point in the transition from FRs to tuberous roots in which the vascular cambium, which cues FRs to develop into tuberous roots, appears (Fig. 2B). ITRs represent a critical point in tuberous root formation in which the vascular cambium and anomalous cambium that characterize the development of FRs into tuberous roots are initiated (Fig. 2B). Therefore, the periods in which IFRs develop into ITRs are the most critical times for the initiation of the swelling of FRs.

Furthermore, expansion of FRs in a single plant was not a synchronous process; FRs may be initiated early, late, or not at all (Fig. 2A). Therefore, the root systems after the ITRs consist of two types of roots: tuberous roots at different development states and FRs in an unexpanded state. The FRs coexisted with LTRs (named as UFRs) that could not transform into tuberous roots and are very similar to mutants that lack the ability to trigger the expansion process. These UFRs are different from FRs at the seeding stage, which can develop into tuberous roots in the next stage (Fig. 2A), or ARs, a proportion of which are induced into IFRs. The fate of ARs and IFRs in subsequent stages in uncertain; it is difficult to study the determinant of FR fate using ARs and IFRs, and thus UFRs were an optimal control material.

Identification of DEGs in ITRs compared with IFRs To identify the genes that are involved in IFR expansion, ITR and IFR libraries were constructed from three biological replicates each using RNA-Seq technology (Supplementary Results). Differential transcription between the two RNA-Seq libraries was identified by a fold change ≥2 or ≤−2 with a divergence probability ≥0.8, resulting in a set of 1 827 up- and 4 205 downregulated transcripts in ITRs compared with IFRs (Fig. 3A and Supplementary Table S7). To determine the roles of these DEGs detailed NR, GO, and KEGG analyses were performed. The NR analysis revealed that 4 155 of 6 032 DEGs were well annotated, including 1 244 upregulated and 2 911 downregulated genes in ITRs. In the GO analysis, 3 049 (871 up- and 2 178 downregulated genes) of the 6 032 DEGs were classified into cellular components, molecular functions, and biological processes. The widely represented cellular components were cell organelles and cell parts (Fig. 3C). The molecular functions of the sequences were mainly associated with binding and catalytic activities (Fig. 3D). The cellular and metabolic processes and response to stimulus accounted for the majority of the biological processes (Fig. 3E).

The KEGG analysis demonstrated that 2 902 of the 6 032 DEGs are involved in a total of 12 pathways (including 116 sub pathways) (Fig. 3F and Supplementary Table S8). Most of these were involved in primary metabolism, secondary metabolism, and compound metabolism; these metabolic pathways may be closely related to the development of tuberous roots and bioactive compound synthesis. In addition, large numbers of DEGs were also annotated as DNA processing, RNA processing, protein biogenesis, and protein modification. Notably, the 232 significantly induced genes are involved in plant hormone metabolism and signal transduction, and 27 are involved in cell cycle regulation.

Verification of DEPs between ITRs and IFRs To further elucidate the molecular mechanisms underlying the formation of tuberous roots at the protein level, iTRAQ was used to identify DEPs between ITRs and IFRs in two biological replicates each. A. total of 9 897 high-quality peptides were obtained using the *R. glutinosa* protein database translated from RNA-Seq. After merging the two replicates, 4 636 non-redundant proteins were identified and qualified. Significantly different proteins potentially involved in response to initiation of tuberous root formation were selected based on a 95% interval level and cut-off values of 1.30-fold for upregulated proteins and 0.77-fold for downregulated proteins. Finally, 450 proteins were identified as DEPs in ITRs compared with IFRs, of which 172 were increased and 278 were decreased in the ITR library (Fig. 3A and Supplementary Table S9).

The DEPs were also analysed using the GO and KEGG databases to explore the possible roles of these proteins in expanding IFRs. Among the 450 DEPs, 227 were subcategorized into 32 hierarchically structured GO classes, including 18 biological processes, 7 cellular components, and 7 molecular functions. Cell part and cellular organelles were the most

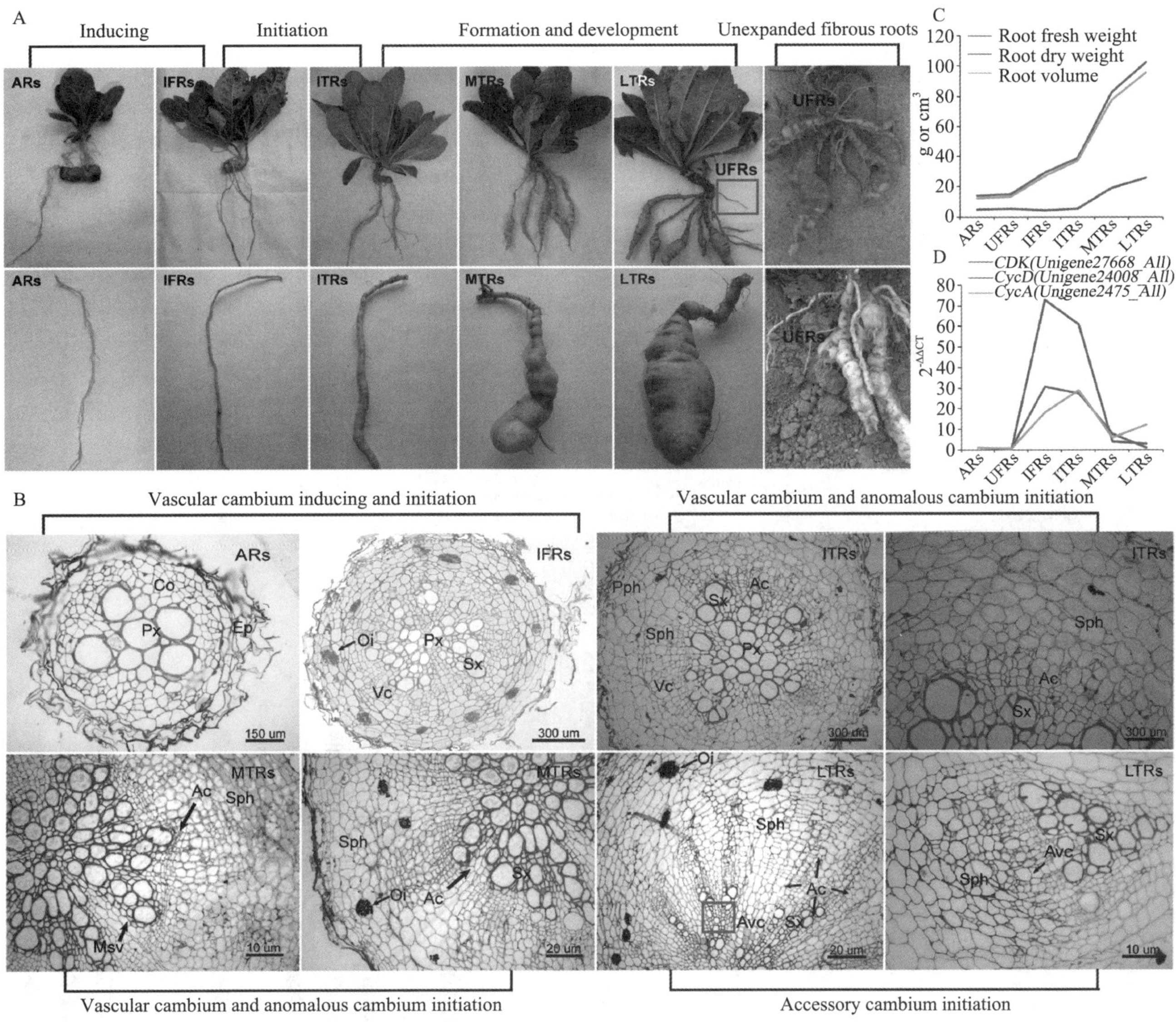


**Fig. 2 The definitions of critical developmental stages.**

(A) The phenotype of whole plants and their tuberous roots, and (B) anatomical characteristics of tuberous roots at different developmental stages, in which ARs are sprouted from 'seed stock', and its histological characteristics consist of epidermis, cortex, and microtubule (at ARs). Some ARs elongate vertically, and the vascular cambium fragment begins to appear toward the pericycle (at IFRs). The central parts of FRs begin swelling, the vascular cambium ring has started to divide, and the anomalous cambium also forms (at ITRs). Some accessory cambium appears in the secondary phloem, and the continuous division of these cambium cells leads to rapid swelling of FRs (at MTRs and LTRs). (C) Changes in the root weight and root volume and (D) changes in the expression of genes related to cell cycle throughout tuberous root formation. C and D indicate that the root biomass increases gradually and peaks sharply at ITRs, whereas the expression of cell division-related genes peak at IFRs. Ac, anomalous cambium; Avc, accessory cambium; Co, cortex; Ep, epidermis; Msv, meristems around the vessel; Oi, oleoplast; Pph, primary phloem; Px, protoxylem; Sph, secondary phloem; Sx, secondary xylem; Vc, vascular cambium.

frequently involved subcategories in the cellular component (Fig. 3C), whereas catalytic activity, binding, and transporter activity were the most frequent categories in molecular function (Fig. 3D). In the biological process, the most frequent categories were metabolic processes, cellular processes, and response to stimulus (Fig. 3E). To determine which biological pathways were active when IFRs was initiated, classification of the 450 DEPs into 104 KEGG pathways revealed that these proteins mainly participated in metabolism, protein synthesis, and signal transduction (Fig. 3F, Table S5 and Supplementary Table S10). Within the metabolism category, most of the proteins related to amino acid metabolism, glucose metabolism, and fatty acid metabolism were significantly enhanced in tuberous roots, and the proteins that were involved in calcium and the MAPK signalling pathways were also enhanced. In addition, the KEGG pathway analysis also revealed that the most active pathways in tuberous roots involved transcription, cell cycle,

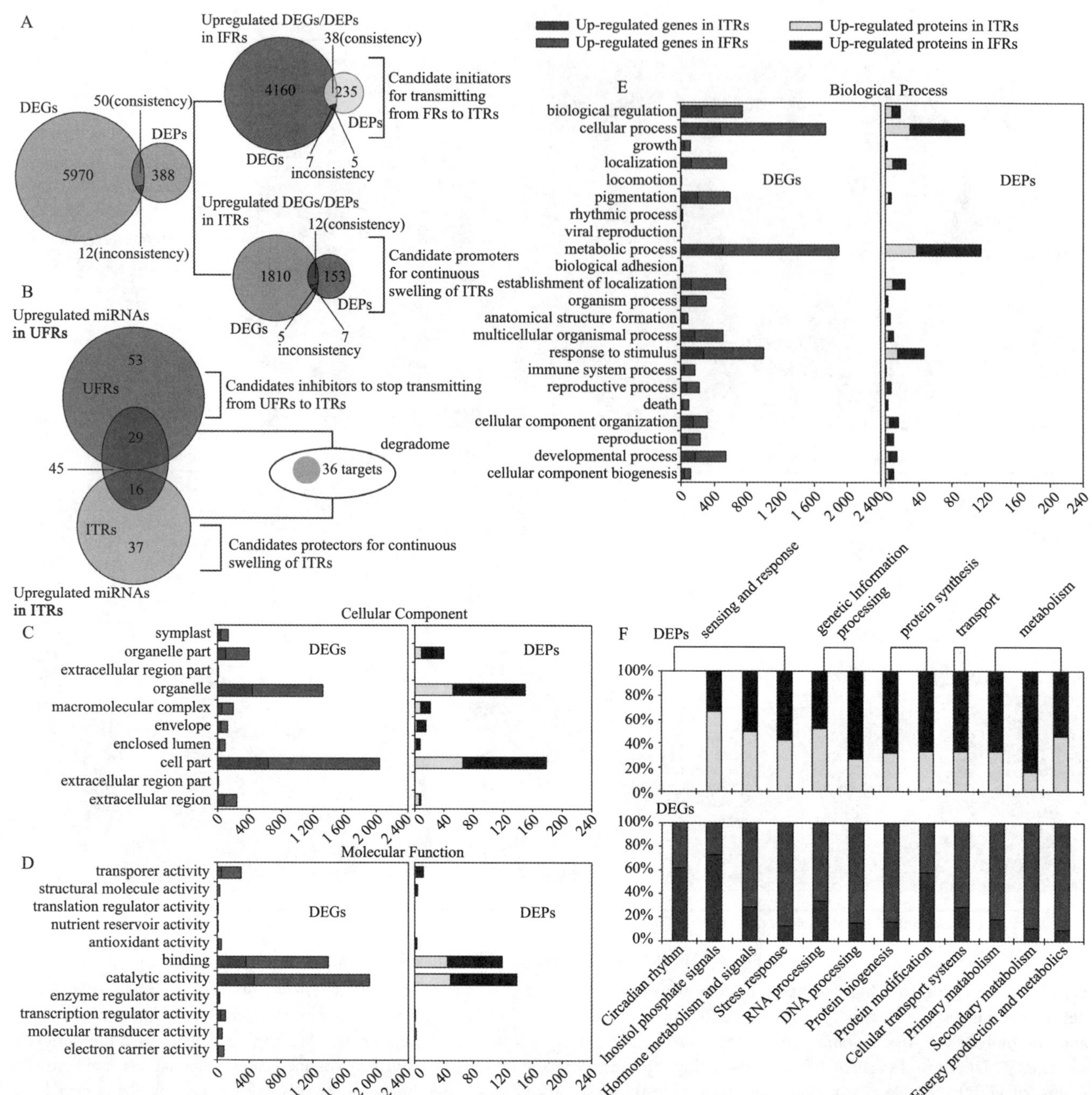


**Fig. 3 Numbers/functional categories of DEGs and DEPs in ITRs compared with IFRs and differential miRNAs in ITRs compared with UFRs**

(A) Numbers of DEGs and DEPs upregulated in either ITRs or IFRs and numbers of overlapping genes/proteins. (B) Numbers of upregulated miRNAs in either ITRs or UFRs, numbers of overlapping miRNAs in both ITRs and UFRs, and numbers of miRNA targets in the degradome. (C-E) GO and (F) KEGG categories for DEGs and DEPs.

and cellular transporters.

Comprehensive analysis of DEGs and DEPs in ITRs compared with IFRs This study revealed large numbers of DEGs and DEPs in ITRs compared with IFRs using RNA-Seq and iTRAQ experiments. There was remarkably little overlap between the DEGs and DEPs; of the 6 032 DEGs, only 62 were present in the list of 450 DEPs (Fig. 3A and Supplementary Table S11). Nevertheless, up-or downregulation trends of the functional categories in which the DEGs and DEPs were involved were very similar (Fig. 3C-F). To clarify the mechanism of tuberous root formation in terms of DEGs and DEPs, they were grouped by the functional categories they are involved in based on NR, GO, and KEGG annotations. For simplicity, when the DEGs or DEPs participated in more than one biological process, only the more prevalent role was considered. As a result, 6 032 DEGs and 450 DEPs were placed into 16 manually curated functional categories, which included light signalling, hormone metabolism and signalling, signal transduction, and transcription, etc. (Fig. 4A). The complete list is provided in Supplementary Tables S7 and S9.

qRT-PCR was used to define the temporal patterns of key DEGs and DEPs involved in light signalling, hormone metabolism, signal transduction, cell division, and cell enlargement to further determine the mechanisms of these genes. Seven genes (*BEL29*, *BEL1*, *CONSTANS*, *Photoperiod-respone protein*, *GATA transcription factor*, and two *Phototropins*) responded to light and exhibited varying degrees of increased expression from IFRs to MTRs compared with ARs, except for LTRs (Fig. S1A, B). The expression of two genes related to auxin (IAA) signalling, *ARF* and *PCNT115*, increased at five stages and to higher levels in IFRs and ITRs, reaching their highest expression in IFRs (Supplementary Fig. S1C). The expression of two genes (*ARR* and *UGT76C1*)

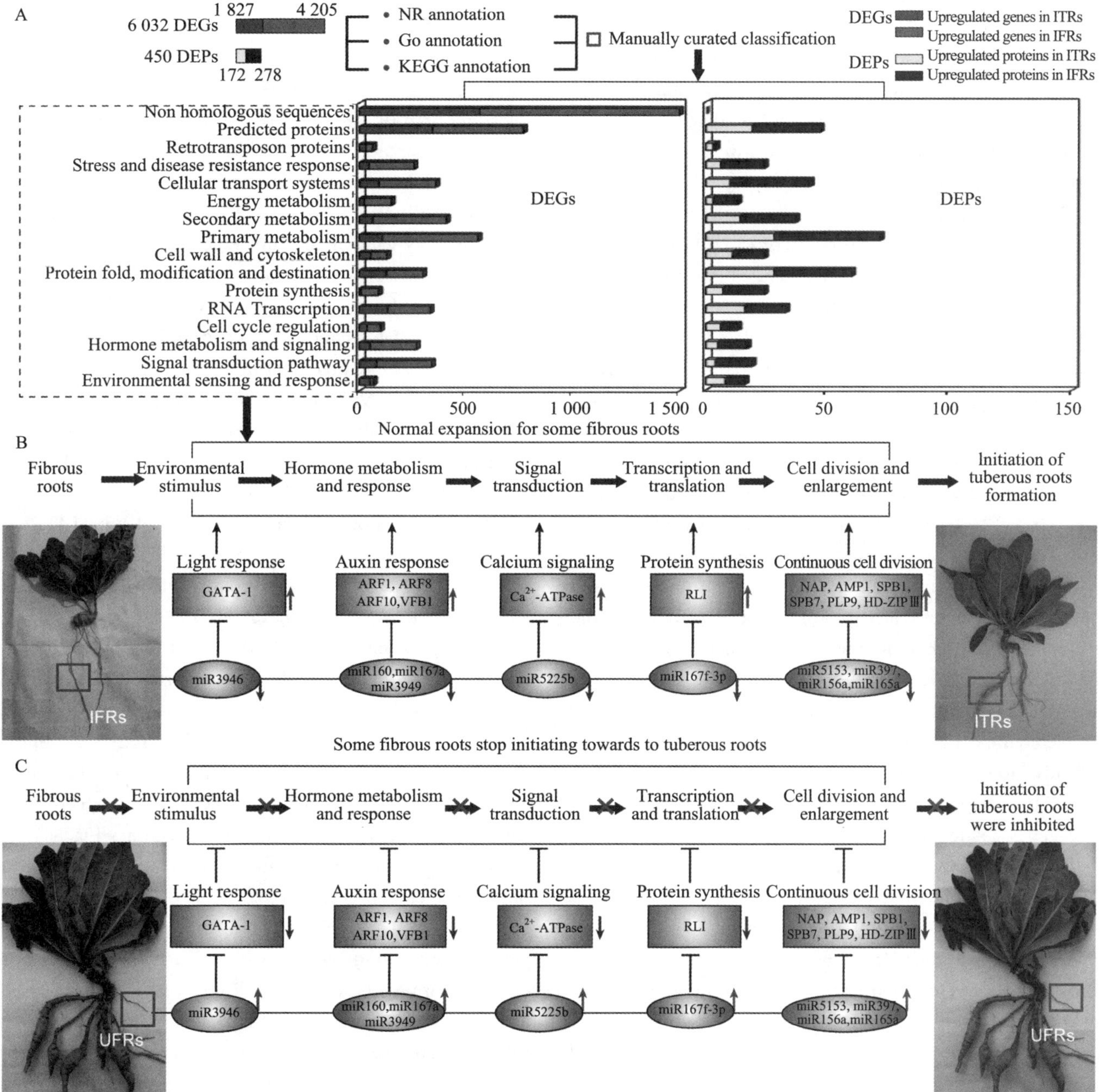


**Fig. 4** (A) The manually curated functional categories of DEGs and DEPs as determined by integrating NR, KEGG, and GO annotation information. (B) The transition process from IFRs to tuberous root is initiated through some essential processes, in which the key genes were kept highly expressed through downregulating the miRNAs that target them in ITRs. The green arrow and ellipse indicate specific miRNAs that were downregulated in IFRs as confirmed by sequencing data. The red arrows and box represent the corresponding target genes upregulated in IFRs as confirmed by qRT-PCR. (C) The transition process from UFRs to tuberous root is terminated by degrading the key genes involved in the essential processes for expansion, which is caused by upregulating related miRNAs in the UFRs. The red arrow and ellipse indicate specific miRNAs that were upregulated in UFRs as confirmed by sequencing data. The green arrow and box represent the corresponding targets being downregulated in UFRs as confirmed by qRT-PCR.

involved in cytokinin (CK) metabolism and signalling was largely enhanced in IFRs and ITRs, particularly IFRs (Supplementary Fig. S1D). A lipoxygenase related to jasmonic acid (JA) synthesis was more highly expressed from IFRs to LTRs compared with ARs, whereas the expression of a gene (*BAK*) related to brassinosteroid (BRs) signalling peaked in IFRs (Supplementary Fig. S1E). Three genes (*ACS*, *ERF*, and *AP2/ERF*) related to ethylene metabolism and signalling had the highest expression in all stages (Supplementary Fig. S1F). Two genes that are associated with abscisic acid (ABA), *ABA-8-oxidase* and *PYL8*, were most highly expressed in IFRs, ITRs, and MTRs (Supplementary Fig. S1G). Two genes that are closely related to gibberellin (GA) synthesis were expressed at relatively low levels from IFRs to MTRs (Supplementary Fig. S1H). Quantitative analysis demonstrated that the genes related to the biosynthesis and response to IAA, CK, ABA, ethylene, JA, and BRs were upregulated in IFRs. Genes related to GA synthesis and response were downregulated. The expression of most of the genes (related to IAA, CK, BRs, and JA) was maximal during the initiation stages (IFRs and ITRs), and some (related to ABA and ethylene) had relatively higher expression in the elongation and pre-expanding stages (MTRs and LTRs). These results indicate that IFRs are key stages for the swelling of FRs in which IAA, CK, BRs, and JA may promote division of the meristem cell, whereas ABA and ethylene antagonize GA.

Genes related to signal transduction, cell division, and transcription were selected for profiling during the development of tuberous roots. The expression of two *CDPK*s, two *CaMbindings*, two *CBLs*, and a *CBP* peaked in IFRs and ITRs (Fig. 5A), and two *MAPKs* peaked in IFRs (Supplementary Fig. S1J). The expression of two *PIP4K* gradually increased from IFRs to MTRs and peaked in ITRs and MTRs (Supplementary Fig. S1K). The expression of three genes related to the cell cycle, including the *CDK*, *Cyclin*, and *FtsZ* genes, peaked in IFRs and ITRs (Supplementary Fig. S1L). The majority of essential genes that are related to transcription, such as *Myb*, *MADS*, *WRKY*, *bHLH*, *and MYC*, were more highly expressed from IFRs to MTRs, and some genes (*NAP* and *GRAS*) were only highly expressed in IFRs (Supplementary Fig. S1M, N). The other genes related to cell extension and expansion, including *tubulin* (*β/α-tubulin*), *Extension*, and *XET*, were highly expressed at stages from IFRs to LTRs (Supplementary Fig. S1O, P). These results indicate that cell divisions mainly occur in IFRs and ITRs accompanied by cell enlargement, whereas cell enlargement continuously occurs from IFRs and LTRs. In conclusion, the expression pattern of these genes reflected a series of developmental events that are closely regulated (Supplementary Fig. S2).

**Capturing the differential expression of miRNAs in ITRs compared with UFRs** To screen for the miRNAs that control the expansion of FRs, sRNA libraries were sequenced from ITRs and UFRs (Supplementary Results). The sRNAs detected by sequencing were processed using a series of rigorous steps. Finally, 196 and 207 known miRNAs were identified in the sRNA libraries of ITRs and UFRs, respectively (Supplementary Table S12). Based on the application of a set of strict identification criteria, 23 unique sequences of 18 pre-miRNAs across the two libraries could be considered candidate novel miRNAs that were not registered in miR Base, and five of these contained miRNA* sequences (Supplementary Fig. S3 and Supplementary Table S13). The presence of 20 of the 23 candidate miRNAs was verified by RT-PCR, and 20 miRNAs were finally amplified from the cDNA template (Supplementary Fig. S4).

A comparison of the miRNA abundance between the ITR and UFR libraries revealed significantly different levels of 14 novel miRNAs and 121 known miRNAs. A total of 82 miRNAs were more abundant in UFRs than in ITRs, and the remaining miRNAs exhibited the opposite trend (Fig. 3B; Supplementary Tables S12 and S13). Of these miRNAs, 37 miRNAs were specifically expressed in ITRs, and 53 were only observed in the UFR library (Fig. 3B).

**Construction of a degradome library of mixed ITRs and UFRs and identification of target genes of differentially expressed miRNAs in ITRs compared with UFRs** To identify the roles of the above differentially expressed miRNAs, a mixed degradome library of ITRs and UFRs was constructed and ~17.9 million raw reads of 3′ cleavage fragments obtained (Supplementary Fig. S5). These reads were filtered to exclude any structural RNAs and ~14.4million clean reads were kept for further analysis. In these reads, 374380 (38.22%) unique reads could be mapped to the transcriptome of *R. glutinosa* (Supplementary Fig. S6). The software CleaveLand was used to identify the degraded targets for each of the miRNAs that differed in expression between ITRs and UFRs. The abundance of each sequence was plotted along with each unigene target, and the degradation targets were divided into five categories (0-4) according to their relative abundance. A total of 36 target mRNAs were identified in the degradome library, of which sixteen targets were classified in category 0, eight in category 1, and twelve in categories 2, 3, and 4 (Supplementary Fig. S7 and Supplementary Table S14). These target genes belonged to 27 miRNAs (10 up- and 17 downregulated in the ITR sRNA library); 28 of the target genes were functionally annotated, and eight had unknown function (Supplementary Table S14). An analysis of the targets revealed that several key genes involved in the formation of tuberous roots were

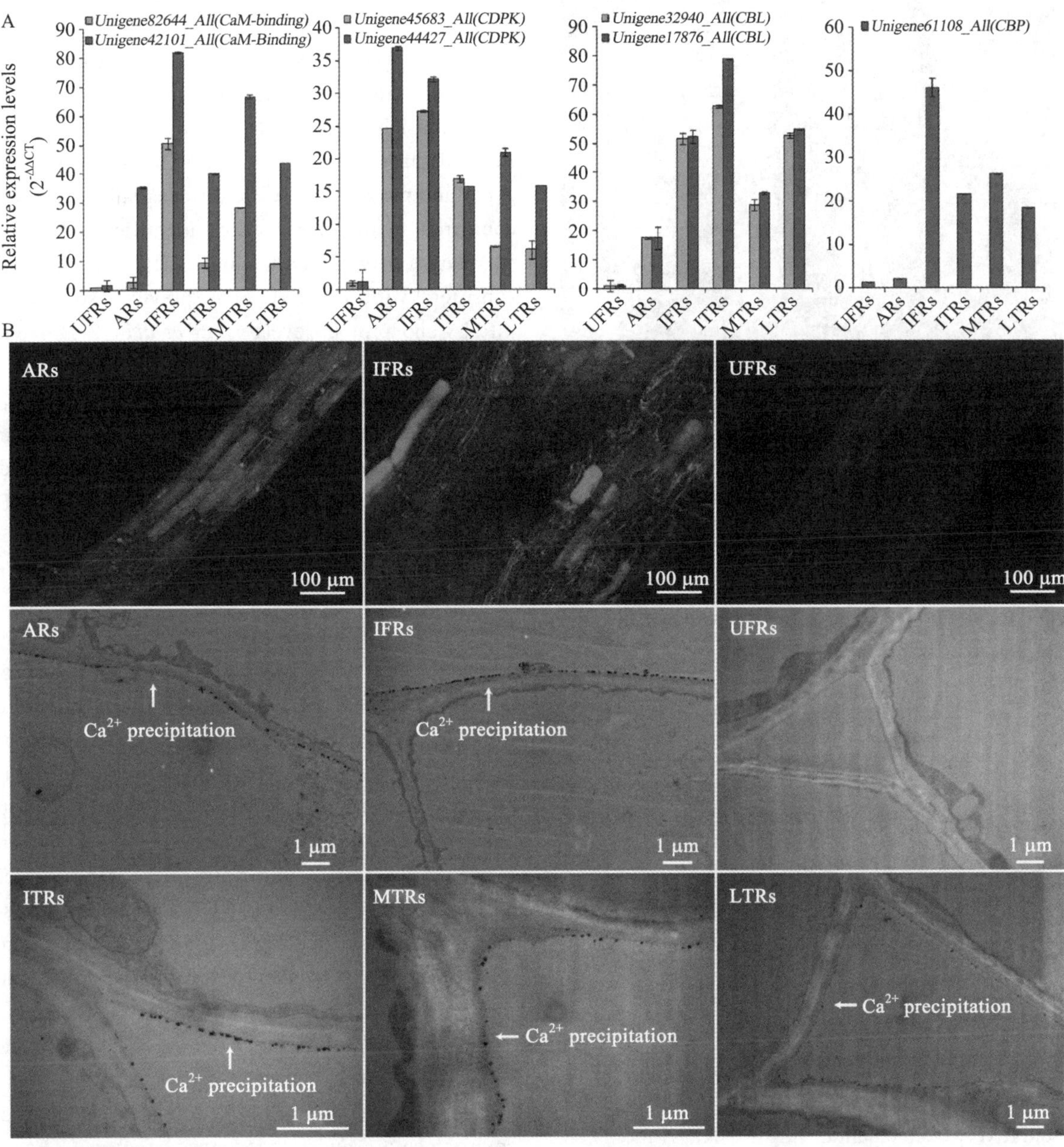


**Fig. 5** (A) Expression patterns of calcium signalling-related genes at different developmental stages of tuberous root. (B) $Ca^{2+}$ concentrations at different developmental stages of tuberous root formation as determined by staining with a fluorescent dye and potassium pyroantimonate precipitation. Fluorescent signals and calcium precipitation were barely observed in UFRs, whereas the other stages displayed obvious calcium signal traces. These results indicate that calcium signalling plays an important role during tuberous root formation.

completely regulated by miRNAs; these miRNAs were thus considered key candidate regulators of the expansion of FRs.

**Expression pattern analysis of differential miRNAs in ITRs compared with UFRs and their corresponding targets during tuberous root formation** To understand the roles of these miRNAs during the formation of tuberous roots, the 16 differentially expressed miRNAs and their targets identified in the degradome were quantified by qRT-PCR. UFRs were used as controls, and the normal formation process of tuberous roots (ARs, IFRs, ITRs, MTRs, and LTRs) was used as the treatment. The abundance of each of the 12 upregulated miRNAs in the UFRs in the sequencing data, including miR167a, miR160a, miR156a, miR165a, miR5153, miR5225b, miR6150, miR5340, miR3946, miR167f-3p, miR397, and miR3949, gradually decreased with the development of tuberous roots compared with that in UFRs, except for LTRs (Fig. 7A). Notably, the targets of these miRNAs exhibited opposite trends, i.e. the higher the expression of each miRNA, the lower the transcript levels of the corresponding target (Fig. 7A). However, among the four miRNAs that were upregulated in the ITRs based on sequencing data, miR171-3p had the highest

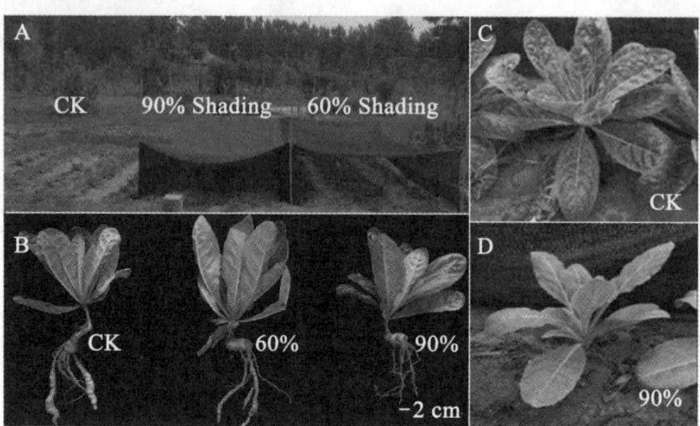


**Fig. 6 Effects of light on transformation of FRs towards ITRs**

(A) The shading experiments were conducted in three plots. In one plot, the plants were grown under natural light; in other plots, the plants were shaded by a sunshade net with 90% and 60% light transmittance, respectively. (B, C, D) Appearance of the plants grown under normal light and shaded light.

expression at the IFR, ITR, and MTR stages, and its target exhibited a corresponding decrease in expression. novel _ miRl _ 3p appeared to be more abundant only in ITRs, MTRs, and LTRs, and its target exhibited little change and maintained a level of few transcripts. miR535 and miR5054 were strongly induced during the early stages of tuberous root development, and the expression of their targets significantly decreased throughout tuberous root formation (Fig. 7B).

## 4 DISCUSSION

The transition from fibrous roots to tuberous roots is a complex, successive process in which initiation is the most critical step and involves the activation of the cambium cells. A root exhibiting specific developmental stages with characteristics of cambium differentiation is therefore necessary to uncover the mechanisms of tuberous root formation. In this study, the representative developmental stages AR, IFR, ITR, MTR, and LTR were clearly defined based on their specific characteristics (Fig. 2A-D). Based on the analysis of anatomical characteristics and the expression patterns of key genes in different stages of tuberous roots (Fig. 2B, D), the stages described above can be roughly divided into three periods: induction (AR to IFR), initiation (IFR to ITR), and formation (MTR to LTR); however, there are no obvious boundaries between the successive stages (Fig. 2A, B). This lack of distinct boundaries indicates that the induction and initiation of tuberous root formation are inseparable processes; induction still occurs when tuberous roots have been initiated.

At the IFR stage, the vascular cambium has already appeared. Typically, IFRs have begun the process of transforming into tuberous roots. In the ITR stage, the circular vascular cambium and anomalous cambium is already well formed (Fig. 2B), which implies that IFRs have completed the initiation process. In this study, RNA-Seq and iTRAQ technology were used to explore the differences between ITRs and IFRs at the transcription and protein levels to provide insight into which 'events' occur from the start to the end during fibrous roots initiation. Large numbers of genes and proteins that were differentially expressed in ITRs compared with IFRs were identified. However, the correlation between DEGs and DEPs was poor (Fig. 3A), consistent with the results of previous studies comparing mRNA and protein levels (Lan *et al.*, 2012; Wu *et al.*, 2014). Despite this lack of overlap, the DEGs and DEPs are involved in similar molecular processes(Fig. 3C F), and the identical functional roles revealed by the DEGs and DEPs point to the same biological regulatory events during the initiation of IFRs. Therefore, the DEGs and DEPs were integrated into identical function categories to provide a clear and comprehensive picture of the IFR initiation process (Fig. 4A).

The transition from ARs to LTRs is a dynamic process involving successive and uninterrupted regulations. For example, hormone response, cell division, and cell expansion were involved continuously during tuberous roots formation. Thus, among genes/proteins with the same function, a subset of them is highly expressed in IFRs, whereas others are expressed in ITRs (Supplementary Tables S7 and S9). However, overall, significantly more genes/proteins were upregulated in IFRs than in ITRs, particularly those related to hormone and calcium sig-nalling. This upregulation reflects the large number of proteins that play important roles in the initiation of FRs towards ITRs.

Light signalling triggers the onset of tuberous root initiation A series of studies in potato and sweet potato have revealed that the onset of storage organ formation is induced by both environmental and endogenous factors. For potato, photoperiodic control is very important for tuber initiation, particularly under short-day conditions, and an appropriate photoperiod is also required for lotus and onion. To verify the role of light during the initiation of tuberous root formation, *R. glutinosa* IFRs were shaded using a sunshade net, which completely blocked the transformation of IFRs towards ITRs (Fig. 6A-D). This result clearly demonstrated that adequate light, particularly high-intensity light, is essential for the swelling of IFRs. Some genes, such as *Photoperiod response protein*, *Lateral organ boundaries protein*, and *GATA transcription factor*, which have been identified as important members in photoperiodic regulation, were significantly induced in IFRs (Supplementary Table S7). Genes related to light signalling transduction, including *Phototropin*, *CONSTANS*, *light sensitive hypocotyls*, and *COP-interactive proteins*, were predominantly expressed in

ITRs (Supplementary Tables S7 and S9). Furthermore, the abundance of these genes was gradually enhanced during the initiation and formation of tuberous roots (Supplementary Fig. S1A, B). However, their peaks and expression patterns were obviously different, suggesting that light regulation is very critical throughout tuberous root formation and that some genes, including *Photoperiod response protein*, *GATA transcription factor*, and *CONSTANTS*, might be more beneficial during induction and initiation, whereas others are more important for the continuous development of tuberous roots (Supplementary Fig. S2). Although these genes have not been identified as key factors in the induction of storage organ initiation, important processes, such as light response, clock rhyme, and morphogenesis, are modulated by these genes. Light-response proteins may have distinct biological effects in different organs. For example, in *Arabidopsis*, lateral roots are regulated by root-localized phyB, whereas root-localized phytochrome is required for the regulation of root elongation.

Moreover, genes detected in the roots may also be transcribed in the leaves and then transported to the root. For potato, *stBEL5* mRNA is transmitted to stolon tips through the phloem, followed by translation into protein to regulate the initiation of storage organ formation. Ten *BELs* genes with sequences similar to *stBEL5* that were upregulated in ITRs were continuously expressed throughout initiation of tuberous root formation, suggesting a function similar to that of potato *stBEL5* (Supplementary Fig, S1A and Supplementary Table S7), Although potato tubers and *R. glutinosa* tuberous roots are derived from different organs, a similar regulation system might exist. Therefore, these genes/proteins might participate in the light-signal-regulated initiation of tuberous root formation via different mechanisms.

Phytohormones are critical factors for regulating tuberous root formation A study of *R. glutinosa* demonstrated that tuberous roots can be generated by application of exogenous hormones. Hormones are known to be critical inducing factors in the regulation of the onset and formation of storage organs in sweet potatoes and potatoes. IAA maintains the meristematic state in cambial cells, increasing the number of xylem elements and promoting cell expansion. CK stimulates cell division by regulating the transition from Gl to S phase and is involved in the activation of the vascular cambium in sweet potato. JA induces tuberous root formation by stimulating the enlargement of meristematic cells in sweet potato and potato. BRs control root meristem size and xylem differentiation. Recently, several studies have reported that BRs promote root nodule formation by altering polyamine content and that polyamines increase the tuber number in potato. A few studies in potato demonstrated ethylene-inhibited elongation of the stem and ethylene-stimulated tip swelling, with a more in-depth analysis demonstrating that ethylene promotes tuber formation by inhibiting GA biosynthesis. ABA is mainly associated with cell differentiation in the vascular cambium and is involved in storage root thickening by activating the cell division of the secondary meristem in the xylem. ABA has also been proposed to be an antagonist of GA. In contrast to the hormones described above, GA is commonly considered as an inhibitor of potato tuber formation, and a high GA content inhibits tuber formation in potato.

In this study, dramatic changes were detected in the expression of genes/proteins related to IAA, CK, ethylene, ABA, and JA at the IFR stage. These genes are involved in hormone metabolism and signal transduction pathway, the majority of which were upregulated in IFRs (Supplementary Fig. S1C-G, Supplementary Tables S7 and S9). Genes/proteins associated with GA were inhibited throughout tuberous root formation (Supplementary Fig. S1H and Supplementary Table S7), suggesting an important role of hormonal regulation during tuberous roots initiation. The typical anatomical characteristics of IFRs indicate that the primary cambium has undergone cell division (Fig. 2B). The analysis of gene and protein expression in the present study suggests that IAA, CK, and BRs induce and maintain the cell division of cambium cells.

Multiple signalling pathways are activated to regulate the initiation of tuberous root formation Cellular processes are usually triggered by specific stimuli and by hormones involving a series of signalling pathways. In this study, the expression of phospholipid signalling-related genes/proteins was increased in ITRs (Supplementary Tables S7 and S9). Phospholipid signalling plays important roles in root growth, pollen development, and vascular formation, and participates in cell cycle progression, cell division, and hormone regulation. These roles suggest that phospholipid signalling is important for continuous tuberous root formation. Notably, phospholipid — calcium signalling systems regulate potato tuberization. Calcium signalling is thought to be involved in nearly every aspect of plant growth and development, including control of cell division, cell differentiation, and stress responses. In the $Ca^{2+}$ signalling system, the $Ca^{2+}$-binding proteins CDPK, CaM, and CBL recognize and transmit $Ca^{2+}$ signals and activate downstream genes. Many studies have demonstrated that the mRNA abundances of CaM and CDPK peak at the point of tuber initiation in potato and that the inhibition of these proteins with specific inhibitors halts tuberization. The $Ca^{2+}$ signals are a possible mediator of the response to tuberization stimuli. Several studies have reported the involvement of a CaM-binding kinesin protein (KCBP) in cell division in the swelling of potato tubers. In this study, there was an increase in IFRs in the expression of calcium signalling-related genes, including 11 *CDPKs*, six *CBLs*, seven *CBPs*, and 21 *CaMs*, and of calcium signalling-related proteins, including a CDPK, a CaM, and three CBPs (Supplementary Tables S7 and S9). This provides further evidence that calcium signalling is involved in the initiation of tuberous root formation. Furthermore, to demonstrate the role of $Ca^{2+}$ during tuberous root formation, $Ca^{2+}$ distribution in root cells at different developmental stages was analysed using Fluo-3/AM and pyroantimonic acid staining. These results indicate that the $Ca^{2+}$ concentration and calcium signalling-related genes were significantly increased throughout tuberous root formation and confirm that calcium signalling participates in tuberous root formation (Fig. 5A, B). In addition, several MAPK signalling-related genes and proteins were upregulated in IFRs, indicating that MAPK signalling participates in the initiation of tuberous root formation (Supplementary Tables S7 and S9). MAPK signalling is not known to be involved in tuberous root formation, but, similar to calcium signalling, it is an important regulator of cell cycle control, and hormone and stress responses. In particular, MAPKs are required for cell cycle re-entry from both G1 and G2 phases.

A set of transcription factors participate in the initiation of tuberous root formation  Previous studies of sweet potato have identified many important families of transcription factors that participate in the initiation of tuberous root formation, including Myb, MADS-box, GRAS, and Nck-associated protein (NAP). MADS-box family transcription factors are involved in cell proliferation during storage root formation in sweet potato. In some plants, MYB and AP2/ERF transcription factors are important cellular regulators involved in root radial patterning, xylem/phloem differentiation, meristem maintenance, asymmetric cell division, cell wall synthesis, and secondary metabolism. WRKY family transcription factors play important roles in hormone responses, calcium signalling, and MAPK signalling. NAP transcription factors are associated with cell division and growth. The basic helix-loop-helix (bHLH) family of transcription factors are key regulators in a variety of developmental processes.

In this study, a set of transcription factor-related genes were found differently expressed in ITRs compared with IFRs at the transcript level, including three *SCL*, six *MADS-box*, 45 *MYB*,13 *MYC*, 24 *WRKY*, 11 *GRAS*, 15 *NAP*, 23 *HD-Zip*, 18 *bHLH*, and 93 other candidate transcription factors (Supplementary Table S7). In addition, several transcription factors, including one NAP and four other candidate transcription factors, were found differentially regulated in ITRs compared with IFRs at the protein level (Supplementary Table S9). In summary, numerous transcription factors have been identified that were differentially expressed in ITRs compared with IFRs. Some were upregulated in IFRs, whereas others were upregulated in ITRs at the transcript or protein levels (Table S1, S2 in Dataset S5). This differential expression indicates that these transcription factors may have specific roles in different developmental stages (the transcription factors expressed at each stage are summarized in detail in Supplementary Fig. S2). Among these transcription factors, MYC2, NAP, GRAS, and WRKY may play a greater role in the induction and initiation of tuberous root formation. The active expression of these proteins indicates multiple essential roles during tuberous roots formation, including cell proliferation activation, cell cycle regulation, and cell division maintenance. They are also valuable candidates for further studies to clarify the control mechanisms of tuberous root formation.

miRNAs determine the transition of FRs to tuberous roots Specific environmental and endogenous factors induce FRs to form tuberous roots. However, only some of the FRs are designated to form tuberous roots, whereas others remain in their original form. miRNAs play important roles in determining the fate of the root cell and regulating tuber formation. In this study, differential expression sRNA profiling of ITRs and UFRs was performed. These UFRs lose the ability to develop into tuberous roots and were used to screen key miRNAs in the control of FR expansion. Thirty-six reliable targets of differentially expressed miRNAs were identified (Supplementary Fig. S7 and Table S14). Analysis of these targets revealed that differential miRNAs regulate key processes for initiating expansion of FRs in tuberous root development by regulating the DEGs and DEPs (Fig. 4). More importantly, the expression of the targets were also confirmed in the RNA-Seq and qRT-PCR results (Fig. 7 and Supplementary Table S15). These results strongly suggest that miRNAs control the transition of FRs to tuberous roots.

miR3946 was highly expressed in UFRs; its target is a GATA-1 zinc finger protein that participates in light-mediated and circadian-regulated gene expression. The high expression of miR3946 in UFRs results in degradation of the GATA-1 transcript, blocking the light signalling, which is the key factor in the formation of tuberous roots. The miR167a targets two *ARF* genes (*ARF1* and *ARF8*), and miR160 targets three *ARF* genes (an *ARF22* and two *ARF18*). These analyses demonstrate that IAA is involved in the initiation of FRs; however, the higher abundance of miR160 and miR167a in UFRs may terminate the IAA response by interfering with ARF production. The target of miR3949 is Vier F-box protein 1 (VFB1). This study demonstrated that the decreased expression of VFB1-4 reduces

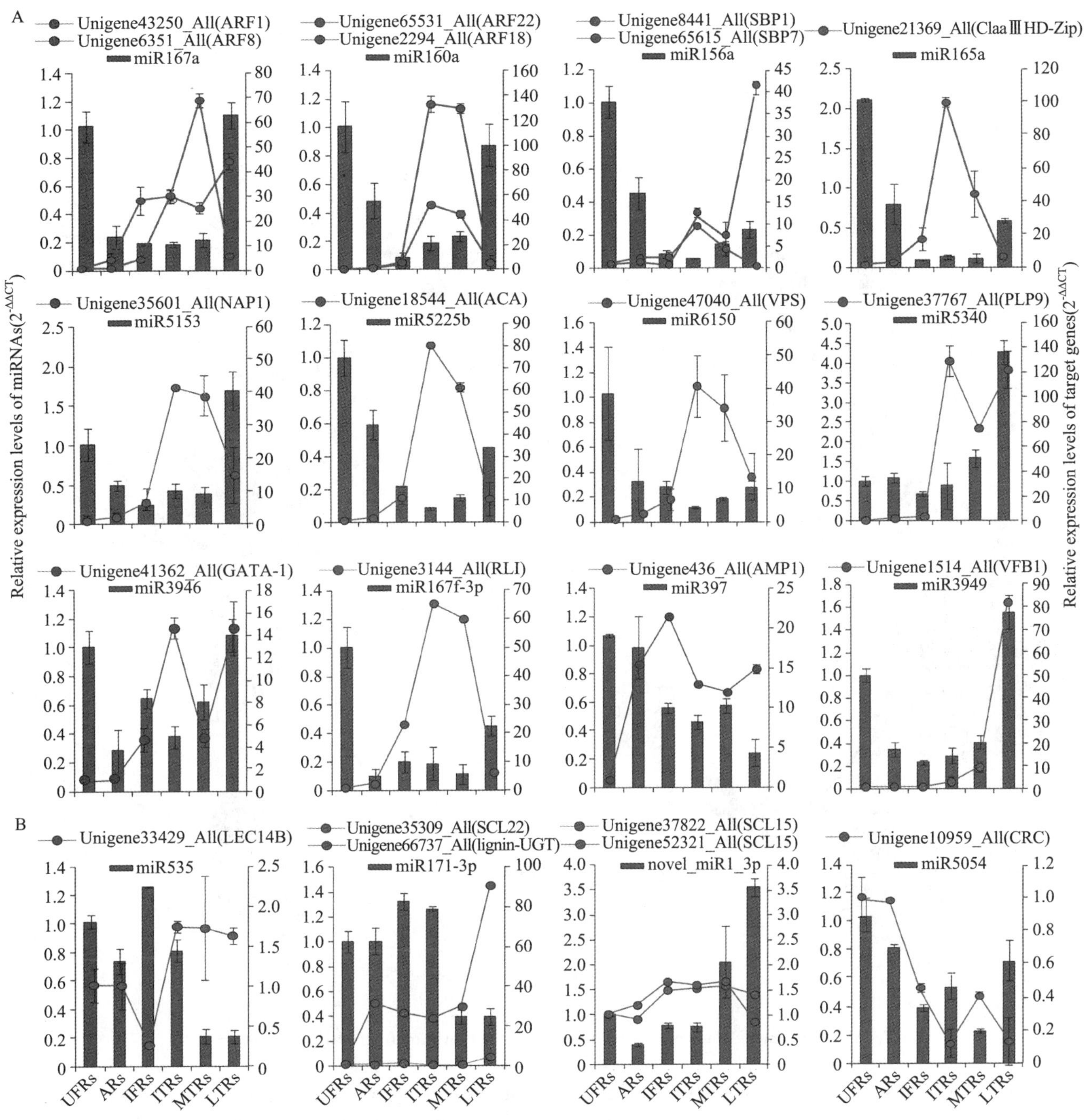

**Fig. 7 Temporal expression of differential miRNAs in UFRs compared with ITRs and their targets at different developmental stages of tuberous root formation**

the IAA response, suggesting that VFB1 plays a role in the IAA response but was stopped in UFRs by the high expression of miR3949. The target of miR5225b is ACA, whose products participate in calcium signalling. The upregulation of miR5225b in UFRs might affect calcium signalling of UFRs. NAP is a target of miR5153. In yeast, NAPl and CDK maintain cell division, and a mutant of NAPl leads to cell cycle arrest in G1. In lotus, a NAP1 mutation resulted in large numbers of hairy roots. In *Arabidopsis*, root elongation growth is blocked when the *NRP1* genes are simultaneously knocked out. Therefore, NAPl plays critical roles in promoting cell division and cell enlargement. Its production is degraded by miR5153 in UFRs, suggesting that the cell cycle may terminate earlier in UFRs.

The higher expression of miR397 in UFRs targets the aminopeptidase M1 protein gene (*AMP1*), a critical protein in plant root development. In plants, MI metalloproteases are also required for meiosis, mitosis, and hormonal or nutrient homeostasis. As an Ml metalloprotease, AMP1 is closely related to cell mitosis. However, its mRNA might be degraded in UFRs by miR397, suggesting that cell mitosis is

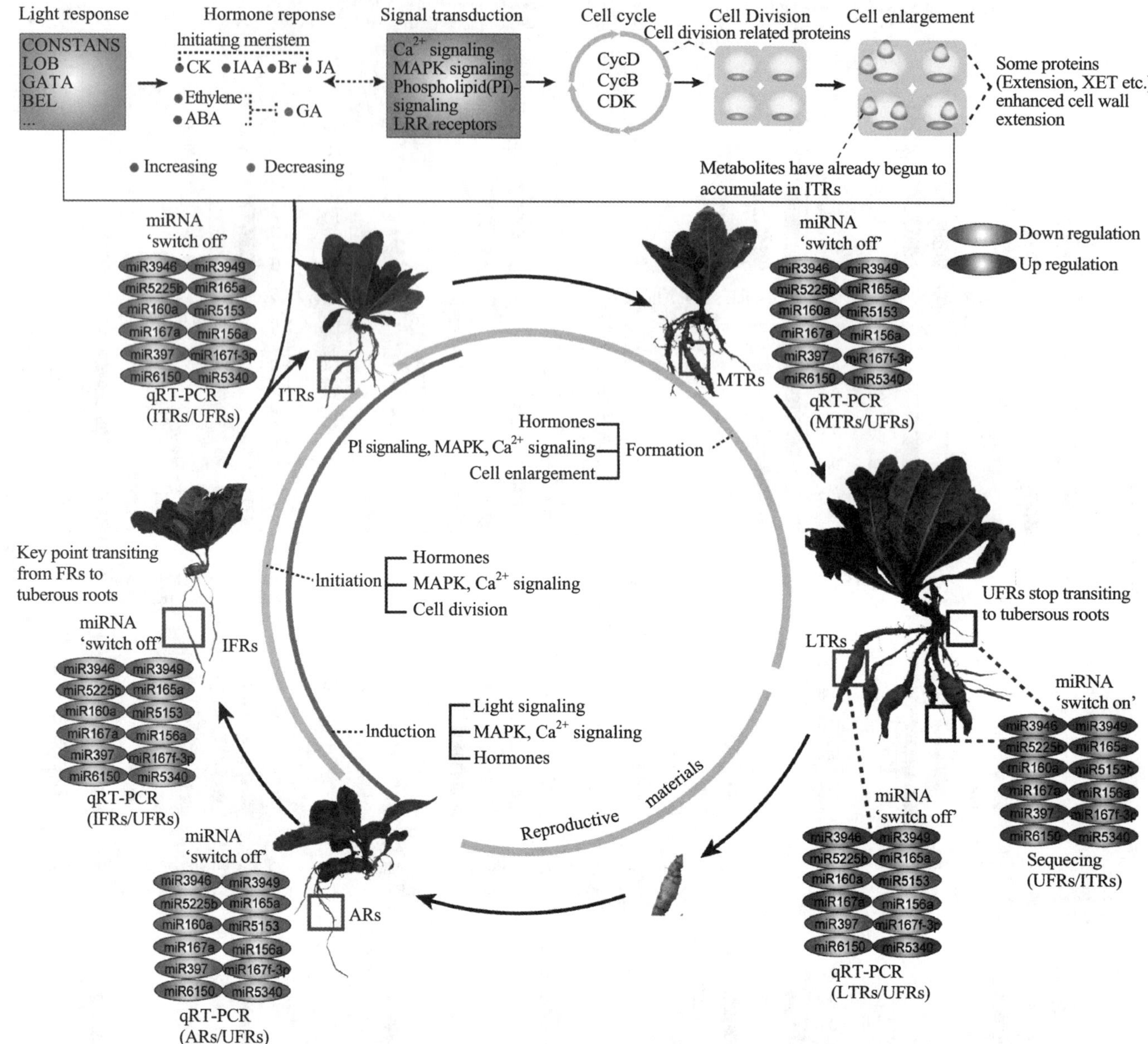


**Fig. 8 Initiation and determinant mechanisms for the transition from FRs to tuberous roots**

also arrested in UFRs. The target of miRNA165a and miRNA165-3p is a class Ⅲ HD-Zip protein, which promotes the initiation of cambium and the differentiation of vascular cambium. In *Arabidopsis*, miR165/6 determines the xylem patterning by regulating class Ⅲ HD-Zip. The greater abundance of miR165a in UFRs thus disturbs cambium cell initiation and xylem differentiation. miR156a targets four squamosa promoter binding-like (*SPB*) genes, whose products are required for vegetative growth, fruit development, and plant morphogenesis. An excess of miR156a in UFRs interferes with the further development of UFRs. miR5340 targets two patatin-like protein 9 (*PLP9*) genes with nutrient reservoir activity that therefore regulate growth of plant meristem. The high level of miR5340 expression in UFRs hinders this nutrient storage activity. Because miR167f-3p and miR167a, respectively, target an RNase L inhibitor (RLI) and a ribosomal protein S1 (rpsA), they play an extremely important role in translation and ribosome biogenesis in eukaryotes. The high expression of miR167f-3p and miR167a in UFRs thus hinders their protein synthesis.

In contrast, with the greater abundance of miRNA171-3p, novel _miR1_3p in ITRs targets scarecrow-like protein (SCL), the products of which are mainly involved in the positive regulation of GA signalling and in the promotion of AR generation. The upregulation of miRNA171-3p and novel _miR1_3p reduced the effects of GA and lateral root production in ITRs. In addition, miRNA171-3p also targets a lignin glucosyltransferase that is related to lignin synthesis; however, lignin is a critical inhibitor of the initiation of cambium cells in fibrous roots of sweet potato. The high expression of miRNA171-3p in ITRs eliminated the adverse effects of lignin for the initiation of tuberous root formation.

In conclusion, the UFR-specific miRNAs might terminate the transformation of UFRs into tuberous roots by preventing processes that are essential for the initial expansion of IFRs, as demonstrated by the analysis of DEG and DEP data. These processes include light signalling, calcium signalling, protein synthesis, control of cell cycle, and cell division (Fig. 4B, C and Supplementary Fig. S2). One possible scenario for the mechanism of control of FR expansion by miRNAs is outlined in Fig. 8, although the details remain to be elucidated. Interestingly, 12 upregulated miRNAs in UFRs were maintained at very low levels in ARs, IFRs, ITRs, and MTRs as determined by qRT-PCR (Fig. 7), suggesting that specific miRNAs in UFRs must be repressed during the normal formation of tuberous roots. Consequently, these miRNAs can be considered as 'switches' whose 'on' or 'off' position significantly affects the development of tuberous roots (Fig. 8).

[李明杰，陈新建，张重义. Journal of Experimental Botany, 2015, 66(19): 5837-5851.]

# The *Gastrodia elata* genome provides insights into plant adaptation to heterotrophy

Symbiotic associations between plants and fungi (mycorrhizae) began about 450 million years ago. Most mycorrhizal associations are mutualistic, such that the host plant and mycorrhizal fungi exchange nutrients with each other. However, mycoheterotrophs have evolved a special type of plant-fungi symbiosis in which a plant gets fixed carbon and other nutrients from fungal partners, rather than from photosynthesis. One of the most interesting characteristics of orchids is the reliance on fungi for seed germination and nutrient absorption, for example, through formation of mycorrhiza with fungi. Over 99% of orchids show partial mycoheterotrophy in which young plants obtain carbon (C) nutrients from fungi prior to the development of green leaves, while adult plants are autotrophic. The extreme type of mycoheterotrophy in orchids is obligate mycoheterotrophy, in which plants are achlorophyllous (lack chlorophyll) throughout their life cycle and therefore fully dependent on fungi for nutrition.

*Gastrodia elata* (Orchidaceae) is an orchid popularly used in traditional Chinese medicine that has a fully mycoheterotrophic lifestyle with highly reduced leaves and bracts in scape, although field guides and systematists often refer to the plants as leafless. During its life cycle, in associates with at least two types of fungi: *Mycena* for seed germination and *Armillaria mellea* for plant growth. To obtain nutrition, it forms an association with *A. mellea* and more than 80% of its ~36-month lifespan is spent underground as a tuber (Fig. 1a). These features of the plant are putative adaptions to its obligate mycoheterotrophic lifestyle. *G. elata* thus offers the possibility of obtaining a valuable insight into the genetic basis of mycoheterotrophy. Here we present a high-quality reference genome assembly of *G. elata* (Orchidaceae), and use it to investigate the molecular basis of its full mycoheterotrophic life cycle. The observations presented here will be of value for functional ecological studies seeking to understand the mechanisms and evolutionary basis of plant-fungal associations.

## 1 RESULTS

Sequencing and annotation  The genome of a *G. elata* individual was sequenced using a whole-genome shotgun (WGS) approach (Supplementary Table 1). Through K-mer distribution analysis, the genome size was estimated to be 1.18 Gb (Supplementary Fig. 1). The assembly consisted of 3 779 scaffolds, with a scaffold N50 of 4.9 Mb (total length= 1 061.09 Mb) and contig N50 of 68.9 kb (total length = 1 025.5 Mb) (Supplementary Table 2). Overall, 98.51% of the raw sequence reads could be mapped to the assembly, suggesting that our assembly results contained comprehensive genomic information (Supplementary Table 3). Gene region completeness was evaluated by RNA-Seq data (Supplementary Table 4): of the 80,646 transcripts assembled by Trinity, 98.66% could be mapped to our genome assembly, and 94.41% were considered as complete (more than 90% of the transcript could be aligned to one continuous scaffold). The completeness of gene regions was further assessed using CEGMA (conserved core eukaryotic gene mapping approach): 239 of 248 (96.37%) conserved core eukaryotic genes from CEGMA were captured in our assembly, and 217 (87.5%) of these were complete (Supplementary Table 5).

Much of the *G. elata* genome (66.18%) was occupied by transposable elements (TEs). Class Ⅰ (retrotransposons) and Class Ⅱ (DNA transposons) TEs accounted for 55.94%

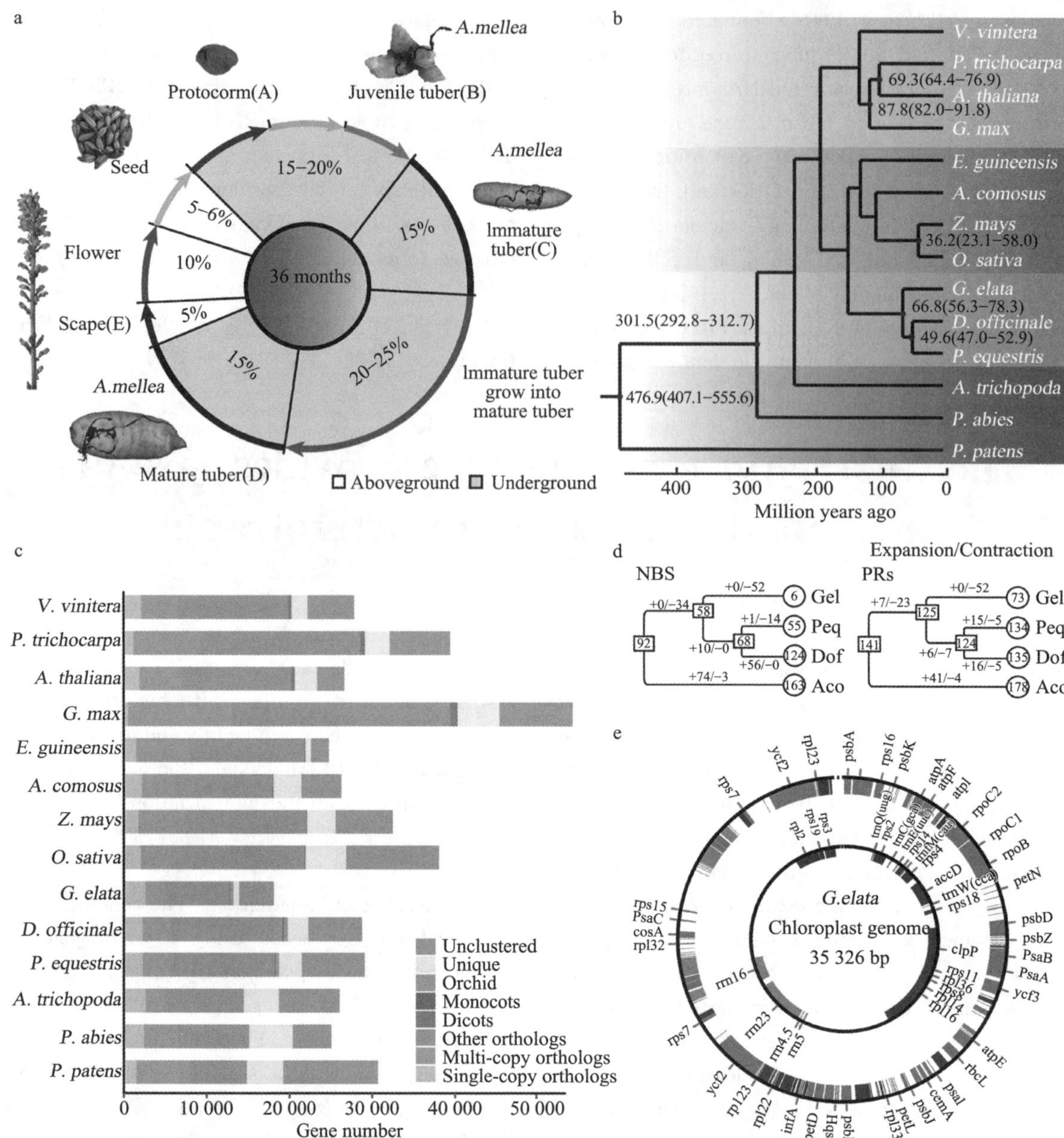


**Fig. 1 *Gastrodia elata* life cycle and gene-family contraction**

**a.** The main developmental stages of *G. elata*. Seeds develop into a protocorm stage without requiring *A. mellea* (A). The protocorm then differentiates into a corm stage after commencing its association with *A. mellea*; note that lateral buds develop into juvenile tubers (B). Young and immature tubers (C). Mature tuber with an emergent young scape (D). Scape (stem and inflorescence) of mature plants (E). **b.** Phylogenetic tree of 14 plant species including *G. elata*. The red dot represents a calibration point determined from the timetree website. **c.** Bar graph of the number of protein-coding genes in each of the species. Single-copy orthologs include common orthologs with one copy in specific species. Multi-copy orthologs include common orthologs with multiple copy numbers in specific species. Other orthologs include genes from families shared in 2–13 species. 'Eudicot' clusters with eudicots. 'Monocots' clusters with monocotyledonous plants. 'Orichd' clusters with *G. elata*, *P. equestris*, and *D. officinale*. 'Unclustered' include genes that cannot be clustered into gene families. **d.** Analysis of gene numbers in the genomes of four species for the nucleotide-binding site gene family (NBS), the pathogenesis-related protein (PR) family (Gel *G. elata*, Peq *P. equestris*, Dof *D. officinale*, Aco *A. comosus*). Numbers in circles represent the number of family members in each genome, and numbers with plus or minus signs indicate, respectively, the number of duplicated or deleted genes. **e.** The plastid genomes of *P. equestris* (outer circle) and *G. elata* (inner circle). Red, protein; orange, rRNA; green, tRNA; gray, genes lost from the plastid genome of *G. elata*.

and 4.38% of the genome, respectively (Supplementary Table 6). Long terminal repeats (LTRs) formed the most abundant category of TE, with LTR/Gypsy and LTR/Copia occupying 45.04% and 7.10% of the genome, respectively (Supplementary Table 7). Global activity of LTRs was similar between *G. elata* and *Phalaenopsis equestris*, while *Dendrobium officinale* presented a recent burst of LTR activities (Supplementary Fig. 2a). Compared to *P. equestris*, all LTR families in *G. elata* had fewer members, except a substantive expansion of del family (Supplementary Table 8 and Supplementary Fig. 2b). Through a combination of ab initio prediction, homology search, and RNA sequence-aided prediction, 18,969 protein-coding genes were predicted in the *G. elata* genome. Of these genes, 81.6% were functionally annotated (Supplementary Table 9) and 88.69% had detectable transcripts in an RNA-seq analysis of protocorms, tubers (juvenile, immature, and mature tubers), and scapes (Supplementary Table 10). Our transcriptomics analysis revealed that there were 10,548 differentially expressed genes among the five growth stages; these differentially expressed genes clustered into five distinct groups that were representative of the particular stages of growth of *G. elata* (Supplementary Fig. 3, Supplementary Table 11 and Supplementary Note).

Phylogeny and whole-genome duplication Comparison of the sequenced genomes of the orchid species *G. elata*, *P. equestris*, and *D. officinale* in-dicated that they diverged approximately 67 million years ago(Fig. 1b and Supplementary Fig. 4). Two ancient whole-genome duplication (WGD) events are evident in the *G. elata* genome; these events can also be discerned in the genomes of *P. equestris* and *D. officinale* suggesting they occurred prior to the divergence of the three orchid species (Supplementary Fig. 5). The older WGD event might represent the heWGD event shared by most monocots, while the younger WGD event were likely shared by all extant orchids and might contribute to the divergence of orchid, as suggested in *Apostasia shenzhenica* genome.

Extensive gene lost in *G. elata* genome Compared to *P. equestris* (29,431 protein-coding genes) and *D. officinale* (28,910 protein-coding genes), *G. elata* has a relative small proteome size(18,969 protein-coding genes). The estimated proteome size of *G. elata* is the smallest theoretical proteome so far identified among angiosperm genomes (Supplementary Table 12). Comparison of *G. elata*, *P. equestris*, and *D. officinale* genes that have functional annotation information revealed global gene set reduction in the *G. elata* genome. For example, almost all second level gene ontology (GO) categories had fewer genes in *G. elata* than in the other two species, and 9 of these categories (16.7%) were significantly reduced (Fisher's Exact test, $P<0.05$, Supplementary Fig. 6 and Supplementary Table 13). We also found that several Pfam domain families were significantly reduced in the *G. elata* genome (Supplementary Table 14). Among the 14 angiosperm used in the phylogenetic analysis, *G. elata* had the lowest number of gene families; moreover, *G. elata* had on average the lowest number of genes in each gene family (Fig. 1c, and Supplementary Table 15). This consistently low number of genes and gene families suggests that many gene families have been eliminated from the *G. elata* genome, and further suggests that many of the remaining gene families have contracted. Gene family expansion and contraction analysis based on maximum likelihood modeling of gene gain and loss confirmed that 3 586 gene families had undergone contraction in *G. elata*, much more compared to the other two orchid genomes (Supplementary Fig. 7 and Supple-mentary Table 16). A Benchmarking Universal Single-Copy Orthologs (BUSCO) analysis, which assessed 956 orthologous groups with genes present as single-copy in at least 90% of plant genomes, revealed that 195 (20.4%) highly-conserved genes were missing from the *G. elata* genome. This rate of absence is much higher than in the genomes of the 13 land species that were included in this analysis (Supplementary Table 17). All of these analyses indicate that *G. elata* has undergone extensive gene losses, even for genes that were conserved in other plant species that have also undergone extensive lost events.

The absence of these genes is unlikely to be due to genome assembly problems because 98.66% of the transcripts assembled from transcriptome data could be mapped to the assembly. Another possibility is that several genes were missed due to gene prediction problems. By mapping RNA reads onto the annotated genome, we found that the majority of RNA reads (>86%) from all *G. elata* tissues could be mapped to annotated exon regions (Supplementary Table 18). This rate of mapping was comparable to that achieved in the well-annotated rice genome and higher than in the *P. equestris* genome (Supplementary Table 18). Through analysis of gene synteny among *G. elata* and *P. equestris* and *D. officinale*, we detected 2 961 gene deletion events in *G. elata* versus *P. equestris*, and 3 120 gene deletion events in *G. elata* versus *D. officinale* (Supplementary Table 19). Further TBLASTN searches of these deleted genes recovered less than 3% of them. Of these genes, fewer than 15% were supported by RNA-seq data (Supplementary Table 19). Both the RNA mapping results and the synteny deletion analysis confirmed that our gene prediction was comprehensive; thus, the possibility of missing gene annotations was low. Finally, PCR amplification of 18 lost genes (*atp*D, *atp*G, *Ihc*A, *Ihc*B, *psa*D, *psa*F, *psa*L, *psa*N, *psb*O, *psb*R, *psb*Y, *psb*27, *psb*28, *pet*C, *pet*E, *ICS*, *DHAR*, and *TRX*) confirmed that all were absent from the *G. elata* genome (Supplementary Figs. 8, 9 and Supplementary Table 20). Thus, the global gene losses in *G. elata* represent evolutionary events, and might be the result of adaption to an obligate mycoheterotrophic lifestyle.

Both pseudogenizations and genome rearrangements contributed to the gene lost process of *G. elata*. We found 876 and 1 080 pseudogenes in *G. elata* using *P. equestris* and

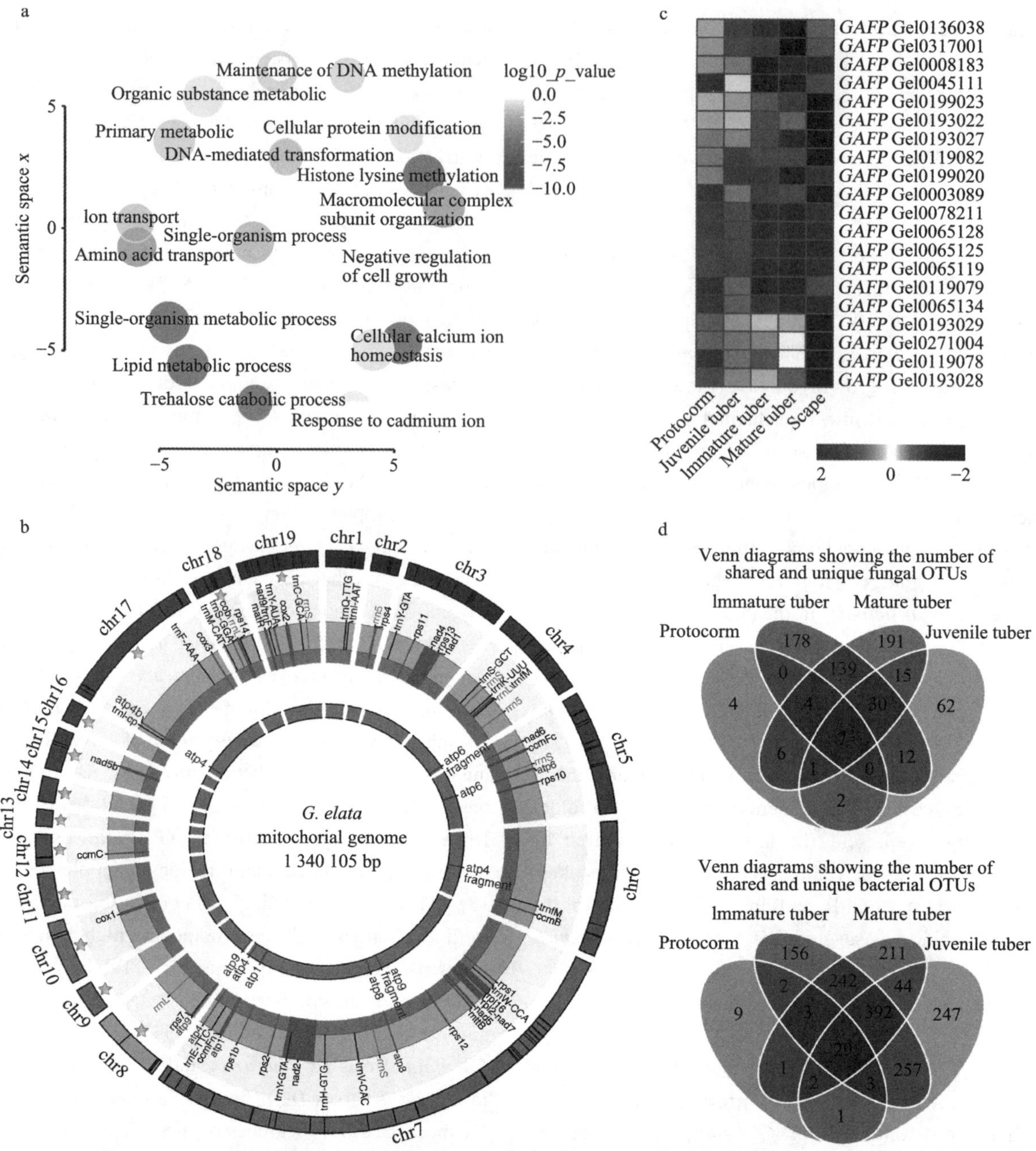


**Fig. 2 Gene expansion in *G. elata* and microbial community analysis**

**a.** REViGO semantic similarity scatter plot of Biology Process Gene Ontology terms for expanded genes in *G. elata*. In semantic spaces, the proximity between circles represents relatedness(similarity) of the GO terms. Similar GO terms are close together in the plot. The axes in the plot have no intrinsic meaning, but were used to measure pairwise similarities between GO terms. Color indicates degree of enrichment for each process presented as the *P*-value from the hyper-geometric test. **b.** The draft mitochondrial genome of *G. elata*. Nineteen contigs are manually displayed as a circle, including 12 circular contigs in orange(ornamented with stars) and 7 linear contigs(in blue). The genes are indicated in the middle circle, and are color coded as follows: *trn* (blue), *rrn* (light blue), *atp*(red), and other protein-coding genes (black). The duplicated *atp* genes and their fragments are detailed in the inner circle. The duplicated genes are suffixed with 'b', and the gene fragments are suffixed with 'fragment'. **c.** Gene expression heat map of the normalized RNA-Seq data for genes encoding the monocot mannose-binding lectin antifungal proteins (GAFP) in *G. elata*. The units indicate the expression levels of different gene members of *GAFP* in the protocorm, juvenile tuber, immature tuber, mature tuber, and scape of *G. elata*(only shown where the gene expression level RPKM$>1$, $n=3$). **d.** Venn diagrams showing the number of shared and unique fungal and bacterial operational taxonomic units (OTUs) based on the ITS and 16S sequence analyses in protocorms, juvenile tubers, immature tubers, and mature tubers of *G. elata*. OTUs showed the composition and abundance of the microbe species, which were defined at 3% dissimilarity.

*D. officinale* genes as seeds, respectively (Supplementary Tables 21 - 24). Through a whole-genome alignment between *G. elata* and *P. equestris*, we found 487 genes were lost due to local rearrangements (SV genes, Supplementary Tables 25 and 26). Functional genes in *G. elata* were located closer to transposable elements than to pseudogenes and SV genes, suggesting that transposable element did not play significant role during the gene lost processes in *G. elata* (Supplementary Fig. 10). Thus the gene lost processes in *G. elata* might be dominated by random mutations as we found many pseudogenes in *G. elata*. Notably, compared with the genomes of *P. equestris*, *D. officinale*, *A. comosus* (pineapple, used in this study as an outgroup) and *Arabidopsis thaliana* (used in this study as an outgroup), the *G. elata* genome has a reduced number of genes related to plant resistance to pathogens, such as the NBS (the nucleotide-binding site) gene family, PR (pathogenesis-related) gene family, and genes of antioxidant proteins (Fig. 1d, Supplementary Fig. 11 and Supplementary Table 27). For example, the *ICS* gene, which is known to function as a primary modulator of salicylic acid-based plant defense responses, is absent from the *G. elata* genome, illustrating the loss of a key gene for systemic acquired resistance (Supplementary Figs. 8, 9 and Supplementary Table 27).

Degeneration of photosynthesis system  As *G. elata* does not perform photosynthesis, it was unsurprising that genes enriched for 'chloroplast' and 'plastid' annotations were strongly represented among the missing genes (Supplementary Table 28). To further investigate the putative functions of missing genes, we examined genes related to the photosynthetic apparatus, namely Photosystem I, Photosystem II, Cytochrome $b_6f$, Cytochrome $C_6$, ATP synthase, and Rubisco. Of the 35 nuclear genes coding for photosynthetic apparatus proteins (NEP), only 12 were present in the *G. elata* genome; this is significantly fewer than in *A. thaliana*, *A. comosus*, *P. equestris*, and *D. officinale* (Supplementary Tables 28, 29). We assume that these genes were non-functional because their full complements of subunits were not present.

We also sequenced and assembled the plastid genome of *G. elata*. We found that the plastid genome of *G. elata* (35, 326 bp) was dramatically restructured and reduced in size, in a similar manner to the reduction in gene number observed for the nuclear genome (Fig. 1e), compared to the plastid genomes of *P. equestris* (148, 958 bp) and *D. officinale* (152,221 bp), the two other orchid species with sequenced genomes. The plastid genomes of these two species comprise two single-copy regions (a large and a small single-copy region) and the two identical large inverted repeats (IRs) encode 75 and 76 genes, respectively, that are most associated with photosynthesis. The *G. elata* plastid genome has lost one IR and encodes only 19 protein-coding genes (Fig. 1e), suggesting that *G. elata* is an ancient mycoheterotroph and that its plastid genome is in the last stage of a degradation ratchet, i. e., retention and loss of the five core nonbioenergetic genes. Excluding the possibility that these genes were missed by our genome assembly, the transcriptome sequencing analysis indicated that none of the deleted plastid or nuclear encoded genes were expressed in *G. elata*, while the five core nonbioenergetic genes, *trnE*, *aacD*, *clpP*, *ycf1*, and *ycf2*, were moderately to highly expressed in all five stages in *G. elata* (Supplementary Tables 30, 31). These results clearly show that both the plastid and nuclear genomes of *G. elata* have lost most of the genes required for photosynthesis, although the highly degraded plastome is still essential for this full mycoheterotroph.

Expansion of mitochondrial genome  Although the *G. elata* genome has clearly undergone extensive gene loss, we found that 430 gene families (19 by a significant margin), containing 1 532 genes(184 by a significant margin), showed expansion in *G. elata* compared to *P. equestris*, *D. officinale*, and *A. comosus* (Supplementary Fig. 7 and Supplementary Tables 32, 33). These genes are enriched for GO terms related to several metabolic proccsses (Fig. 2a, Supplementary Table 32). We speculate that these expanded genes are related in some way to the functional requirements of the obligate mycoheterotrophic lifestyle of *G. elata*. We first sequenced and assembled the mitochondrial genome to explore this idea, and the mitochondrial genome *G. elata* is markedly expanded in size (1 339 kb, Fig. 2b) compared to the mitochondrial genomes of most other seed plants. Thirty-seven protein-coding genes were annotated, and one subunit of mitochondrial ATP synthase, atp4, had two copies in the mitochondrial genome of *G. elata* and was highly expressed in the cortex layer (Supplementary Table 34). In addition, 36 of the genes had detectable expression in mature tubers (epidermis, cortex, and parenchymal cell) using a tissue-specific qPCR-based analysis (Supplementary Table 34).

Management of symbiotic microbials  We next explored how gene expansion in *G. elata* may have contributed to its association and interactions with fungal microbiota. The monocot mannosebinding lectin antifungal protein family (GAFP) of *G. elata* contains 20 genes, compared to only 3 in *A. comosus* and 0 in *A. thaliana* (Supplementary Table 27). GAFP proteins have been documented to inhibit the growth of both ascomycete and basidiomycete fungal plant pathogens in vitro. More than 80% of the *GAFP* genes were highly expressed in protocorms and juvenile tubers, the growth stages that occur before *G. elata* establishes a stable symbiotic association with *A. mellea* (Fig. 2c). 4-Hydroxybenzyl alcohol ($p-$PA), the precursor of the phytoalexin gastrodin is a major phenolic compound of *G. elata*. The expression of $p-$PA biosynthesis genes (e. g., cinnamate 4-hydroxylase, *C4H*, alcohol dehydrogenase, *ADH*, hydroxybenzaldehyde synthase, *HBS*) was relatively high in protocorms and juvenile tubers. Ultra performance liquid chromatography coupled with quadrupole time-of-flight mass spectrometry

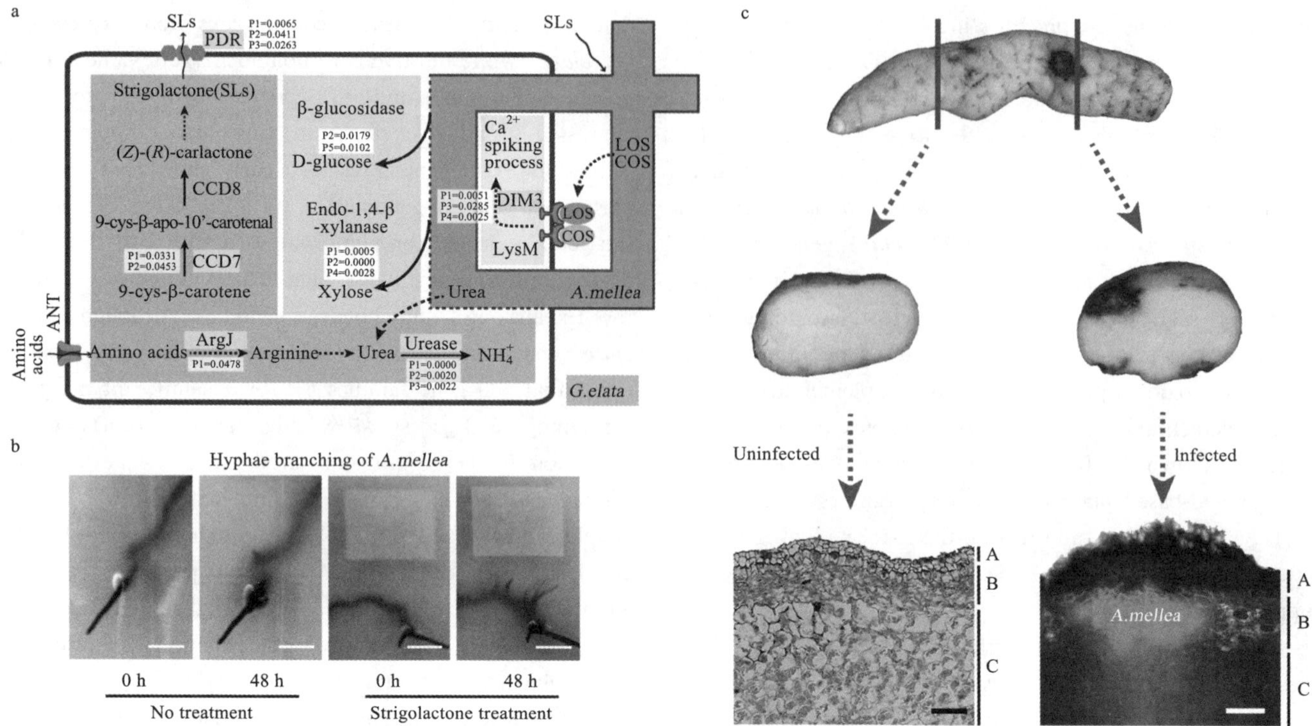


**Fig. 3 Strigolactone as a putative signal compound in *G. elata* in its mycoheterotrophic symbiotic relationship with *A. mellea***

**a.** Overview of proposed signaling and nutrition transfer in *G. elata*. The red-labeled genes are expanded in the *G. elata* genome and *P*-value of Fisher's exact test of gene number $<0.05$(Supplementary Tables 38, 40,41). ANT, ANT1-like aromatic and neutral amino acid transporters; ArgJ, glutamate N-acetyltransferase; CCD, carotenoid cleavage dioxygenases; COS, chitooligosaccharides; DMI3, does-not-make-infections 3 subfamily; LOS, lipochitooligosaccharides; LysM, LysM-receptor-like kinases; PDR, ABC transporter. P1, *P*-value of Fisher's exact test of gene number in *G. elata* genome compared to *P. equestris*, *D. officinale*, *A. comosus*, and *A. thaliana*; P2, *P*-value of Fisher's exact test of gene number in *G. elata* genome compared to *A. thaliana*; P3, *p*-value of Fisher's exact test of gene number in *G. elata* genome compared to *A. comosus*; P5, *P*-value of Fisher's exact test of gene number in *G. elata*, *P. equestris*, and *D. officinale* genome compared to *A. comosus* and *A. thaliana*. **b.** Branching of *A. mellea* hyphae was significantly promoted after strigolactone treatment(Supplementary Fig. 13). Scale bar was 5 mm. **c.** Cross sections and micrographs of immature *G. elata* tubers in association with *A. mellea* (A, epidermis; B, cortex; C, inner parenchyma cells, Supplementary Fig. 14). The black scale bar on the left was 100 μm and the white one on the right was 20 μm.

(UPLC-ESI-Q-TOF-MS) metabolite analysis revealed that *p*-HA is present in *G. elata* tubers but not in *A. mellea* hyphae(sampled from tuber, wood, and PDA medium). *S*-(*p*-HA)-glutathione was detected in both *G. elata* tubers and in *A. mellea* hyphae sampled from tubers (Supplementary Fig. 12, Supplementary Table 35), which putatively suggests that *G. elata* may transport this phytoalexin to *A. mellea* and prevent the excessive growth of *A. mellea*. To investigate the effect of *A. mellea* on microbial management in *G. elata*, we performed a 16S ribosomal (rRNA) and rDNA ITS sequencing analysis and found that the diversity of bacterial and microbial species was significantly lower during the protocorm stage than at other growth stages ($P<0.05$), which was consistent with the pattern of gene expression of *GAFP* (Fig. 2c, d, Supplementary Tables 36, 37). This increased diversity of bacteria and fungi during the juvenile tuber to mature tuber periods implies that a compatible mycorrhizal fungus (*A. mellea*) can affect the structure of the microbial community associated with its host and greatly reduce the antifungal and antibacterial activities as a symbiotic association with *A. mellea* is established.

Signaling and nutrition transfer in *G. elata* Without the ability to perform photosynthesis, *G. elata* depends completely on its symbiotic fungus for nutrition. It is thus obvious that the signaling pathways related to the establishment of this symbiotic relationship are crucial for *G. elata*. Some of the mechanisms underlying the symbiotic interaction between *G. elata* and *A. mellea* are similar to those for interactions between other plants and arbuscular mycorrhizal (AM) fungi. The *G. elata* genome contains many of the genes known to participate in AM associations (Fig. 3a, Supplementary Table 38). Key genes for biosynthesis and secretion of strigolactone were expanded in *G. elata* (e.g., carotenoid cleavage dioxygenases, CCDs, for biosynthesis and ABC transporters, PDRs, for secretion) (Supplementary Table 38). It is known that strigolactone can stimulate hyphal branching and development of arbuscular mycorrhizal fungi, which increases the chances of an encounter with a host plant. We conducted growth assays and confirmed that strigolactone had similar branch-inducing effects in *A. mellea* (Fig. 3b, Supplemental Fig. 13). The expanded number of genes encoding CCDs and PDRs suggests that *G. elata* has enhanced its ability to interact with *A. mellea* to increase the efficiency of the establishment of the symbiotic relationship essential for its nutrition and metabolism. Calmodulin-dependent protein kinase genes of the *does-not-make-infections 3* subfamily (*DMI3*) were also doubled or tripled in *G. elata* (10 genes) compared to *P. equestris* (3 genes), *D. officinale* (5 genes), and *A. comosus* (4 genes); these genes participate in the $Ca^{2+}$ spiking process that has been shown to regulate the colonization of plants by fungi.

After *A. mellea* colonizes *G. elata*, fungal growth is restricted to its cortex layer (Fig. 3c, Supplemental Fig. 14). We performed a tissue-specific qPCR-based analysis of 10 genes in *G. elata* tubers and found that PDR transcripts, which mediate secretion of strigolactone to the extracellular space, were highly abundant in the cortex layer (Supplementary Fig. 15). This finding suggests that *G. elata* may preferentially guide *A. mellea* to colonize its cortex layer. Similarly to ATP synthases, we found that some glycoside hydrolases from gene families that have expanded in the *G. elata* genome were also highly expressed in the cortex layer, supporting the idea that *A. mellea* hyphal walls are digested in the cortex layer of *G. elata* tubers (Supplementary Table 39). The expanded endo-β-1, 4-D-xylanase and β-glucosidase may have become neofunctionalized to cleave fungal glycan substrates during the digestion of hyphal walls of *A. mellea* (Fig. 3a, Supplementary Table 40).

Given that the ANT1-like aromatic and neutral amino acid transporters (ANT) are known to translocate arginine (Arg), which is a key component in nitrogen translocation in arbuscular mycorrhizal fungi, it seems likely that Arg in *G. elata* is related to mycoheterotrophic symbiosis (Fig. 3a, Supplementary Table 41). It is known that arginases can hydrolyze Arg into urea in mycelia, which is further hydrolyzed to ammonium and carbonic acid by ureases. Although *P. equestris*, *D. officinale*, *A. comosus* and *A. thaliana* have only one copy of glutamate Nacetyltransferase (ArgJ), an enzyme of the arginine biosynthesis pathway, *G. elata* has three copies (Supplementary Fig. 11 and Supplementary Table 41). The number of genes encoding ureases is drastically expanded in *G. elata* (9 genes) compared with *P. equestris* (2 genes), *D. officinale* (2 genes), *A. comosus* (1 gene), and *A. thaliana* (1 gene) (Supplementary Table 41). This suggests that urea metabolism might be an important source of nitrogen for *G. elata* (Fig. 3a).

Conclusion The extensive deletion and expansion of genes, especially the global reduction of gene complements in almost all functional categories in the *G. elata* genome, provides a powerful example of how a plant with a fully heterotrophic life cycle has made use of genome plasticity to achieve extensive neo-functionalization and gene loss. Our results establish a unique opportunity for researchers to understand how plants that have abandoned photosynthesis continue to persist and thrive.

## 2 METHODS

Plant materials and DNA preparation The experimental materials of *Gastrodia elata* were harvested from Xiaocaoba in Yunnan Province (latitude 27.79°N longitude 104.24°E) located in the southwestern China. Genome sequencing and assembly was done on the scape of beige-scape *G. elata*. Five transcriptomes were sequenced from five different *G. elata* tissues (protocorm, juvenile tuber, immature tuber, mature tuber, scape). Four different *G. elata* tissues (protocorm, juvenile tuber, immature tuber, mature tuber) were collected to investigate the diversity of microbial communities. High-quality genomic DNA was extracted using the Qiagen DNeasy Plant Mini Kit.

Genome sequencing and assembly Multiple paired-end and mate-pair libraries were constructed with a spanning size that ranged from 180 bp to 20 kb. Sequencing was conducted on an Illumina HiSeq 2 500 platform. In total, 179.1 Gb raw sequencing reads were produced (Supplementary Table 1). Raw sequencing reads were subjected to filtering to remove: ① low quality reads with low quality bases (>50% bases with *Q*-value ≤8). ② reads with Ns>10% of the read length. ③ reads with adapter contamination. ④ duplicated reads caused by PCR during library construction. Filtered data were assembled using ALLpaths-LG (version 44 080), where overlapping paired-end reads with an insert size of 230 nucleotides were used as fragment libraries, and all other libraries (>230 nucleotide insert size) were used as jumping libraries. The Allpaths-LG assembly was run with default settings, then a gap filling step was carried out using GapCloser based on the paired-end information of the paired-end reads that had one end mapped to the unique contig and the others located in the gap region (http://sourceforge.net/projects/soapdenovo2/files/GapCloser).

Genome-quality evaluation To evaluate the completeness of the assembly and the uniformity of the sequencing, all the paired-end reads were mapped to the assembly using BWA. The mapping rate was 98.51% and the genome coverage was 99.84%. This result suggested that our assembly results contained almost all the information in the reads (Supplementary Table 3). Gene region completeness was evaluated from the scape tissue, of 80, 646 transcripts assembled by Trinity, 98.66% could be mapped to our genome assembly, and 94.41% were considered as complete (more than 90% of the transcript could be aligned to one continuous scaffold). CEGMA (Core Eukaryotic Genes Mapping Approach) defined a set of conserved protein families that occur in a wide range of eukaryotes, and identified their exon-intron structures in a novel genomic sequence. Through mapping to the 248 core eukaryotic genes, a total of 239 genes with a ratio of 96.37% were found in *G. elata* (Supplementary Tables 5). Genome completeness was also assessed using BUSCO gene set analysis version 2.0 which includes a set of 956 single-copy orthologous genes specific to Plantae.

Repetitive elements identification  A combined strategy based on homology alignment and de novo search was used to identify repeat elements in the *G. elata* genome. For de novo prediction of transposable elements (TEs), we used RepeatModeler (http://www.repeatmasker.org/RepeatModeler.html), RepeatScout, and LTR-Finder with default parameters. For alignment of homologous sequences to identify repeats in the assembled genome, we used RepeatProteinMask and RepeatMasker (http://www.repeatmasker.org) with the rebase library. Transposable elements overlapping with the same type of repeats were integrated, while those with low scores were removed if they overlapped more than 80 percent of their lengths and belonged to different types (Supplementary Table 7).

Dynamics of long terminal-repeat retrotransposons  Intact Long terminalrepeat retrotransposons (LTR) were identified by searching the genomes of *G. elata*, *D. officinale* and *P. equestris* with LTRharvest from Genome Tools v1.5.1. The candidate sequences were filtered by two-step procedure to reduce false positives. First, LTRdigest was used to identify the primer binding site (PBS) motif based on the predicted tRNA sequences from tRNAscan-SE, and only elements contained PBS were retained; then protein domains (pol, gag and env) in candidate LTR retrotransposons were identified by searching against HMM profiles collected by Gypsy Databas (GyDB). Elements contained gag domain, protease domain, reverse transcriptase (RT) domain and integrase domain, which were considered as intact. Second, families of these intact LTR retrotransposons were clustered using the previously described method. Finally, LTRs that did not contain protein domains or that belonged to families with less than 5 members were discarded. The EMBOSS program distmat was used to estimate LTR divergence rates between the 5′- and 3′- LTR sequences of the intact LTRs (Supplementary Fig. 2).

Gene prediction  Gene prediction was conducted through a combination of homology-based prediction, ab initio prediction and transcriptome-based prediction methods. Protein repertoires of plants including *A. comosus*, *Amborella trichopoda*, *Arabidopsis thaliana* (phytozomev10), *Brachypodium distachyon* (phytozomev10), *D. officinale*, *O. sativa* (phytozomev10), *P. equestris*, *Vitus vinifera* (phytozomev10), *Sorghum bicolor* (phytozomev10) and *Zea mays* (phytozomev10) were downloaded and mapped to the *G. elata* genome using TBLASTN ($E$-value $\leqslant 1e^{-5}$). The BLAST hits were conjoined by Solar software. GeneWise (version 2.4.1) was used to predict the exact gene structure of the corresponding genomic region on each BLAST hit. Homology predictions were denoted as "Homology-set". RNA-seq data derived from protocorm, juvenile tuber, immature tuber, mature tuber, and scape(Fig. 1a) were assembled by Trinity (version 2.0). The Trinity assembly included 183,515 contigs with an average length of 592 bp. These assembled sequences were aligned against the *G. elata* genome by PASA (Program to Assemble Spliced Alignment). Valid transcript alignments were clustered based on genome mapping location and assembled into gene structures. Gene models created by PASA were denoted as PASA-T-set (PASA Trinity set). Besides, RNA-seq reads were directly mapped to the genome using Tophat (version 2.0.8) to identify putative exon regions and splice junctions; Cufflinks (version 2.1.1) was then used to assemble the mapped reads into gene models (Cufflinks-set). Augustus (version 2.5.5), GeneID (version), GeneScan (version 1.0), GlimmerHMM (version 3.0.1), and SNAP (version) were also used to predict coding regions in the repeat-masked genome. Of these, Augustus, SNAP and GlimmerHMM were trained by PASA-H-set gene models. Gene models generated from all the methods were integrated by EvidenceModeler (EVM). Weights for each type of evidence were set as follows: PASA-T-set > Homology-set > Cufflinks-set > Augustus > GeneID = SNAP = GlimmerHMM = GeneScan. The gene models were further updated by PASA2 to generate UTRs, alternative splicing variation information, which generated 26,872 gene models. Gene models only supported by ab initio evidence were filtered out. To reduce the possibility of missing and poorly annotated genes, we invested additional effort in annotating some gene families that could be missed by automated genome annotation, such as NBS-encoding genes. In total, 1943 protein sequences containing an NB-ARC domain were searched against the *G. elata* genome using TBLASN with a threshold of $1e^{-5}$. All BLAST hits in the genome, together with 5 000 bp flanking regions on both sides, were annotated by the GeneWise program. The resulting predictions were surveyed to verify whether they encoded NBS or LRR motifs using Pfam. We also focused on other genes, such as those related to photosynthesis, and transporter, and these were manually annotated through a combination of BLAST search and motif verification. Ultimately, a comprehensive non-redundant reference gene set was produced that contained 18 969 protein-coding gene models. Functional annotation of the protein-coding genes was carried out using BLASTP ($E$-value cut-off $1e-05$) against two integrated protein sequencing databases, SwissProt and TrEMBL. Protein domains were annotated by searching against InterPro (Version 5.16) and Pfam (Version 3.0) database, using InterProScan (version 4.8) and HMMER (version 3.1b1) (http://hmmer.janelia.org), respectively. The GO terms for genes were obtained from the corresponding InterPro or Pfam entry. The pathways in which the genes might be involved were assigned by BLAST against the KEGG databases (release 20150831) with the $E$-value cut-off of $1e^{-5}$.

Identification of pseudogenes Pseudogenes in the *G. elata* genome were identified by searching against *G. elata* intergenic regions using *D. officinale* or *P. equestris* protein sequences as the seed sequences (TBLASTN, $E$-value cut-off $1e^{-5}$). Before the BLAST search, regions of the 18,969 true genes were masked. The BLAST hits were conjoined by Solar software. GeneWise was used to predict the pseudogene structures with the '-pseudo' parameter. Pseudogenes were then classified by PseudoPipe. The PseudoPipe program applies a set of sequence identity and completeness cut-off to report a final set of good-quality pseudogene sequences. We used the following cutoffs: amino acid (AA) sequence identity >30% and match length >50 AA to filter out false positives. GeneWise results that fulfilled the cut-off criteria were denoted as high-confidence pseudogenes. High-confidence pseudogenes were then assigned to three categories. ① Processed/retrotransposed pseudogenes (PSSDs), which formed through retrotransposition. Retro-transposition occurred by reintegration of a cDNA, a reverse transcribed mRNA transcript, into the genome at a new location. ② Duplicated pseudogenes (DUPs), which formed through gene duplication, following by decay of genes, include frameshifts or premature stop codons. ③ Pseudogenic fragments (FRAGs), which were fragments that have high-sequence similarity to known proteins, but were too decayed to be reliably assessed as processed or duplicated. We used the following criteria to classify PSSDs, DUPs, and FRAGs: ① PSSDs, exon number=1, $0.7<$align ratio$\leq 0.95$, $0.3\leq$identity$\leq 0.95$. ② DUPs, exon number>1, $0.3\leq$identity$\leq 0.95$, and existing insertion, deletion, termination, or frameshift. ③ FRAGs, exon number=1, align ratio$<0.7$, $0.3\leq$identity$\leq 0.95$.

Gene family construction Whole protein-coding gene repertoires from 14 plant genomes including *G. elata*, *A. comosus*, *A. trichopoda*, *O. sativa* (phytozome v10), *Z. mays* (phytozomev10), *D. officinale*, *P. equestris*, *Elaeis oleifera*, *A. thaliana* (phytozomev10), *V. vinifera* (phytozomev10), *Populus trichocarpa* (JGI), *Glycine max* (phytozomev10), *Picea abies*, *Physcomitrella patens* (ASM242v1) were used to construct a global gene family classification. To remove redundancy caused by alternative splicing variations, we retained only gene models at each gene locus that encoded the longest protein sequence. To exclude putative fragmented genes, genes encoding protein sequences shorter than 50 amino acids were filtered out. All-against-all BLASTp was employed to identity the similarities between filtered protein sequences in these species with an $E$-value cut-off of $1e^{-7}$. The OrthoMCL method was used to cluster genes from these different species into gene families with the parameter of "-inflation 1.5".

Phylogenetic tree reconstruction Protein sequences from 74 single-copy gene families were used for phylogenetic tree reconstruction. MUSCLE was used to generate multiple sequence alignment for protein sequences in each single-copy family with default parameters. Then, the alignments of each family were concatenated to a super alignment matrix. The super alignment matrix was used for phylogenetic tree reconstruction through maximum likelihood (ML) methods. Before ML reconstruction, we used ProtTest to select the best substitution models. The JTT+I+G+F model was selected as the best-fit model, and RAxML was used to reconstruct the phylogenetic tree.

Species divergence time estimation Divergence time between 14 species was estimated using McMctree in PAML with the options 'correlated molecular clock' and 'JC69' model. A Markov Chain Monte Carlo analysis was run for 20 000 generations, using a burn-in of 1 000 iterations. Five calibration points were applied in the Present study (Fig. 1): *P. equestris* and *D. officinale* divergence time (47～52.9 million years ago), *O. sativa* and *Z. mays* divergence time (24 - 84 million years ago), *A. thaliana* and *P. trichocarpa* divergence time (65 - 89 million years ago), *P. trichocarpa* and *G. max* divergence time (56 - 89 million years ago), and root of land plants (407 - 557 million years ago).

Gene family expansion and contraction Expansion and contractions of orthologous gene families were determined using CAFÉ 2.2 (Computational Analysis of gene Family Evolution). The program uses a birth and death process to model gene gain and loss over a phylogeny. Large changes in gene family size in a phylogeny were tested by calculating $p$-values on each branch using the Viterbi method with a randomly generated likelihood distribution. This method calculates exact $p$-values for transitions between the parent and child family sizes for all branches of the phylogenetic tree. Enrichment of Gene Ontology terms for *G. elata* expanded gene families were summarized and visualized using REVIGO (small list, similarity (0.5), SimRel similarity measure).

The expanded and contracted families focused on in this

study were confirmed using Fisher's exact test. For each gene family, we compared the gene count of the tested family in *G. elata* (copy number of the tested family as numerator, total number of genes of the whole genome as denominator) versus the frequency in *D. officinale*, *P. equestris*, *A. comosus*, and *Arabidopsis thaliana* (phytozomev10). In addition, phylogenetic trees were constructed for each family to confirm gene gain or loss events. The extreme case of gene lost was that one gene was absent in the *G. elata* genome. To avoid false positive gene absence events caused by missing gene annotations, a TBLASTN search against the *G. elata* genome was carried out using protein sequences derived from other plant genomes.

PCR verification of lost genes Total genomic DNAs were extracted by hexadecyl trimethyl ammonium bromide (CTAB) method from *G. elata*, *A. thaliana*, *A. comosus*, and *D. officinale*. PCR was carried out using SpeedSTAR™ HS DNA Polymerase (TaKaRa, Japan) and specific gene primers (Supplementary Table 20). PCR products were verified by agarose gel electrophoresis (Supplementary Figs. 8 and 9).

Whole-genome duplication analysis A homolog search within the *G. elata* genome was performed using BLASTP ($E$-value $< 1e^{-7}$), and MCscanX was used to identify syntenic blocks within the genome. For each gene pair in a syntenic block, the 4DTv (transversion substitutions at fourfold degenerate sites) distance was calculated, and values of all gene pairs were plotted to identify putative whole-genome duplication events in *G. elata*.

Inferring syntenic gene deletions in *G. elata* Proteins of *G. elata*, *P. equestris* and *D. officinale* were aligned using the BLASTp algorithm ($E$-value $<1e^{-7}$). Alignments with matches of at least 30% identity and coverage higher than 30% were retained for comparison. The best reciprocal BLAST pairs between different genomes were extracted as putative orthologous gene pairs. Then, using gene location information in each species, we identified micro-synteny gene blocks between *G. elata* and the other two orchids. Putative gene loss events were traced from the synteny table using the flanking gene method. Given three genes A, B, and C in order, if gene A and C were presented as collinear orthologs in two genomes, but B was missed in one of the genome(for example, *G. elata*), then gene B was denoted as a possible lost gene in *G. elata*. To avoid false positives due to the failure of gene annotation, the *G. elata* intergenic genomic sequence between A and C was extracted, and a GeneWise prediction in this intergenic region was carried out using the B protein sequence from *P. equestris* as seed. If the predicted protein could be aligned to the seed protein with coverage >70%, and did not contain frameshift or premature stop codon mutations, this gene loss event was defined as a false positive and filtered out (Supplementary Table 19).

Plastid genome Total genomic DNA was extracted using a modified CTAB from silica-dried tissues of *G. elata* (Supplementary Table 42). The DNA was sheared to 500 bp, and sequencing libraries were generated using the NEBNext Ultra DNA Library Prep Kit (according to the manufacturer's protocol) for sequencing on an Illumina Hiseq 2 500 at the State Key Laboratory of Systematics and Evolutionary Botany, Chinese Academy of Sciences. The raw reads were filtered using NGSQCTOOLKIT v 2.3.3. The cleaned reads were mapped to *Calanthe triplicata* in GENEIOUS 9.0 (Biomatters, Inc., Auckland, New Zealand; http://www.geneious.com). Used reads were exported and assembled using SOAPDENOVO2. The plastid sequences were extracted from the total contigs using BLASTN 2.2.29+ and the *C. triplicata* plastome(GenBank ID: NC_024544) as subject sequence. The finished plastome scaffolds were reoriented according to the *C. triplicata* reference plastome. The boundaries of IRs were determined by BLAST, and finished manually. The plastomes of *G. elata* were determined using DOGMA with an *e*-value of 5, a 60% cut-off for protein-coding genes and 80% cut-off for tRNAs; the GENEIOUS annotation tool was used to determine the plastomes of *C. triplicata* and *Oncidium* Gower Ramsey (GenBank ID: NC_014056.1) as references. Linear plastome maps were drawn using OGDRAW.

Mitochondrial genome Mitochondria were isolated from all *G. elata* tissues except the rhizome using previously described centrifugation methods. A modified CTAB method was used to extract mt-DNAs. The purified mt-DNAs were sequenced on an Illumina Hiseq 2 500 to generate 100 bp paired-end reads at the State Key Lab of Systematic and Evolutionary Botany, Chinese Academy of Sciences (Beijing).

Eleven million raw reads were generated from sequencing and trimmed using Trimmomatic v0.35 to produce low quality reads. All sequenced plant mitochondrial genomes were downloaded from NCBI and used as a local blast database. To minimize the possibility of contaminated reads from plastid or nuclear genomes, filtered reads were first mapped to the local database and mapped reads were subsequently imported into Geneious v10.1.3 (Biomatters, Inc., Auckland, New Zealand; http://www.geneious.com) for initial assembly. The contigs generated by the initial assembly were used as seeds for further iterative mapping and extension processes. Velvet and Geneious were alternatively used during assembly with multiple combinations of k-mer lengths.

In most cases, the extension process of the assembly worked well. In particular, when the head and tail of a contig had an overlapping region and could not be further extended, this contig could be reasonably connected into a circle. Although several circles were produced during assembly, some problems did arise in the extension process. For example, some contigs were displayed as single lines because their boundaries were too difficult to determine due to poly structures or repeats in the mitogenome. The final assembled results were verified by remapping and some ambiguous regions with low coverage were further checked by PCR. Overall, 19 contigs with a total length of 1 340 105 bp were assembled including 12 circles (ranging from 13.5 to 120.6 kb) and 7 single lines (837 015 bp).

The assembled contigs were firstly annotated by NCBI-BlastN based on the local database with an *e*-value $<1e^{-6}$. Then, the boundaries of each gene were confirmed by Mitofy and exported as Sequin formatted files. tRNA genes were further predicted by tRNAscan (http://lowelab.ucsc.edu/tRNAscan-SE/) (Supplementary Table 43).

Transcriptome library and gene expression analysis The paired-end reads for protocorm, juvenile tuber, immature tuber, mature tuber, scape samples were mapped to the *G. elata* genome using TopHat. The total numbers of aligned reads were normalized by gene length and sequencing depth for an accurate estimation of expression level. We used these normalized read counts (RPKM) as the expression level for each gene. Then, DESeq was used to identify differentially expressed genes (Supplementary Tables 44 - 58). A repeated bisection method and a top-down hierarchical clustering algorithm in gCLUTO (http://glaros.dtc.umn.edu/gkhome/cluto/gcluto/overview) were used to generate the expression profiles of all differently expressed genes.

RNA extraction and quantitative PCR Four different *G. elata* tissues (epidermis, cortex, parenchymal cell A and B) were collected from three mature tuber samples. Total RNAs were extracted using TRIzol® Reagent (Thermo Fisher Scientific, USA) according to the manufacturer's instructions. The concentrations and purities of the total RNAs were assessed by a spectrophotometric analysis at 260 and 280 nm. One μg of total RNA was reverse transcribed at 42 ℃ using TransScript® Reverse Transcriptase (TransBionovo Co, China) and Oligo$(dT)_{18}$ according to the manufacturer's recommendations. Prior to use in qPCR, cDNA was diluted 1 : 5 with $H_2O$.

The qPCR reactions were performed in duplicate for each condition using the KAPA SYBR® FAST qPCR Master Mix (KapaBiosystems, USA) and LightCycler® 480 Real-Time PCR System (Roche, Switzerland). Each reaction consisted of 20 μL containing 1 μL of cDNA and 200 nmol/L of each primer (Supplementary Tables 59 and 60). The cycling conditions were: denaturation at 95 ℃ for 3 min; followed by 45 two-segment cycles of amplification at 95 ℃ for 10s, and 60 ℃ for 30s in which fluorescence was automatically measured, and one three-segment cycle of 95 ℃ for 5s, 65 ℃ for 1min, and 95 ℃ for 30s. The baseline adjustment method of the LightCycler® 480 software was used to determine the Ct in each reaction. β-actin was selected as the internal control and the expression levels of tested genes were determined using the comparative Ct ($2^{-\Delta\Delta Ct}$) method.

Diversity of microbial communities Four different *G. elata* tissues (protocorm, juvenile tuber, immature tuber, mature tuber) were collected and total genomic DNAs were extracted using hexadecyl trimethyl ammonium bromide (CTAB). The 16S V4 and ITS1 genes in all sample were amplified using the universal primers 515F-806R and ITS5-1737F with a barcode as a marker for distinguishing samples. The PCR was performed with Phusion® High-Fidelity PCR Master Mix (New England Biolabs, Ipswich, MA, UK). PCR products were mixed in equidensity ratios. Then, the mixed PCR products were purified with Qiagen Gel Extraction Kit (Qiagen, Germany). Sequencing libraries were generated using a TruSeq® DNA PCR-Free Sample Preparation Kit (Illumina, USA) following the manufacturer's recommendations and index codes were added. The library quality was assessed on a Qubit® 2.0 Fluorometer (Thermo Scientific) and Agilent Bioanalyzer 2100 system. The library was sequenced on an Illumina HiSeq 2 500 platform and 250 bp paired-end reads were generated.

High-quality sequences were clustered into OTUs defined at 97% similarity. These OTUs were applied for diversity, richness and rarefaction curve analyses using MOTHUR. Taxonomic assignments of OTUs that reached the 97% similarity level were made using the QIIME (quantitative insights into microbial ecology) software package through comparison with the SILVA, Greengene, and RDP databases. Venn diagrams were generated to identify the mutual and specific taxons between groups using R software (http://www.r-project.org/).

Microscopy For identification and analysis of *G. elata* infected by *A. mellea*, hand sections were cut through the infection point of an immature tuber, and the sections were then embedded in agar plates. Images were captured using a Zeiss AX10 fluorescence microscope with × 10 water immersion lenses. Owing to the spontaneous blue fluorescence, both visible and DAPI filters were used to observe the hyphae of A. *mellea* with fluorescent microscopy (Zeiss AX10).

To analyze tissue and cell structures of *G. elata* uninfected by *A. mellea*, paraffin sections (10 μm thickness) were obtained using a Thermo Scientific MicRoM HM 325 sliding microtome. For light microscopic observations of the highly lignified hyphae of A. *mellea*, sections were stained with Fast Green stain reagent to investigate the infected cells of *G. elata*. After staining, sections were washed by PBS three times, dehydrated through an alcohol (50%, 80%, 90%, 95%, 100%), cleared in xylene, sealed with neutral gum, and observed using a fluorescence microscope (Zeiss AX10).

Quantification of *p*-HA and *S*-(*p*-HA)-glutathione About 0.35 g of frozen fresh *G. elata* were homogenized and ultrasonically extracted for 30 min in four volumes (g/mL) water. After centrifugation (13 000 r/min, 10 min), 100 μL aliquots of supernatant were mixed with 10 μL of rutin (101.0 μg/mL) for quantification of *p*-HA (λ 270 nm, Rt 6.8 min) and S-(*p*-HA)-glutathione (*m/z* 412.12, Rt 8.9 min) using an UPLC-PDA-ESI-Q-TOF-MSE method. The injection volume was 1 μL. The contents were determined by the peak intensity ratios of the analyte to rutin (*m/z* 609.14, 15.5 min).

Hyphal-branching assay Hyphal branching in *A. mellea* fungi was evaluated in vitro by the paper disk diffusion method. Primary hyphae were cultured in PDA medium containing 20 g/L glucose, 4 g/L potato powder and 14 g/L agar. The dishes were cultured in the dark for 5-7 days at 23 ℃. Secondary hyphae emerge from primary hyphae and grow upward in a negative geotropic manner in the gel; the growth of secondary hyphae was used for the assay. Test samples were first dissolved in acetone then diluted with 70% ethanol in water. The concentration of test sample solutions of natural 5-deoxy-strigol was adjusted with reference to the calibration of synthetic (±)-5-deoxy-strigol in an HPLC analysis. Paper disks (1 cm in length, 8 mm in width) loaded with 15 μL of test sample solution were placed in front of the tips of the secondary hyphae. The control was on the opposite direction of the paper without 5-deoxy-strigol. Hyphal branch patterns were analyzed at 24 h and 48 h after treatment. The sample was scored as positive for hyphal branching if new hyphal branches formed from the treated secondary hyphae. The assay was repeated at least twice, using between three and five dishes for each concentration.

Data availability Genome data were deposited in GenBank under accession number PVEL00000000 and transcriptome sequence reads were deposited in the Sequence Read Archive (SRA) under accession number SRX2879747. The standard flowgram format(SFF) files related with bacterial and fungal communities were also deposited in the SRA under study accession SRX2875242 and SRX2876148. Plastid genome data were deposited in GenBank under accession number MF163256. Mitochondrial genome data were deposited in GenBank under accession numbers MF070084-MF070102.

[袁媛，金效华，黄璐琦，等. Nature Communications, 2018, DOI: 10, 1038.]

# Jasmonate promotes artemisinin biosynthesis by activating the TCP14-ORA complex in *Artemisia annua*

## 1 INTRODUCTION

Artemisinin, a sesquiterpene lactone, and its semisynthetic derivatives (artemether and artesunate) are famous for their use in the treatment of malaria. To decrease the high risk of drug resistance when using a single drug, such as chloroquine, mefloquine, and sulfadoxine-pyrimethamine, to treat malaria, the use of artemisinin-based combination therapies has been proposed by the World Health Organization. In plants, *Artemisia annua* is the only natural source of artemisinin, and the artemisinin content in this plant is very low (0.01 to 1.0% by dry weight). The low artemisinin content and unstable supply of plant-derived artemisinin have motivated the semisynthetic production of artemisinin in yeast. However, the limited production in engineered yeast cannot meet the high demand for artemisinin production, and *A. annua* plants are still the major suppliers of this compound.

So far, available evidence indicates that the glandular secretory trichomes (GSTs) of *A. annua* are biofactories for artemisinin biosynthesis and accumulation, and the artemisinin biosynthetic pathway has been well elucidated (fig. S1A). Briefly, farnesyl diphosphate synthase (FPS) catalyzes the production of farnesyl diphosphate (FPP) from isopentenyl diphosphate and isomer dimethylallyl diphosphate, which are produced from both the cytosolic mevalonic acid pathway and the plastidial methylerythritol diphosphate pathway. The first committed step of artemisinin biosynthesis is the cyclization of FPP to amorpha-4,11-diene by amorpha-4, 11-diene synthase (ADS). Amorpha-4, 11-diene is then successively oxidized to yield artemisinic alcohol, artemisinic aldehyde, and artemisinic acid (AA) by cytochrome P450-dependent hydroxylase (CYP71AV1) along with the reduced form of nicotinamide adenine dinucleotide phosphate: cytochrome P450 oxidoreductase or alcohol dehydrogenase 1. In addition, artemisinic aldehyde is converted to dihydroartemisinic aldehyde by double bond reductase 2 (DBR2). Then, aldehyde dehydrogenase 1 (ALDH1) catalyzes the formation of dihydroartemisinic acid (DHAA) from dihydroartemisinic aldehyde. Last, AA and DHAA may be transported to the trichome subcuticular space and then converted to arteannuin B (AB) and artemisinin by an enzyme-independent reaction. It is noteworthy that artemisinic aldehyde is the last common intermediate of the two pathways leading to AB and artemisinin. Consequently, to produce high levels of artemisinin, efficient reduction of artemisinic aldehyde to dihydroartemisinic aldehyde by DBR2 is necessary.

Although the artemisinin biosynthetic pathway has been elucidated, the transcriptional regulation of this pathway remains largely unknown. Several lines of evidence suggest that transcription factors play pivotal roles in plant specialized metabolism, including in artemisinin biosynthesis. An *A. annua* WRKY transcription factor, AaWRKY1, was reported to be a positive regulator of *ADS* and *CYP71AV1* expression. The jasmonate (JA)-responsive *A. annua* GST-specific WRKY1 (AaGSW1) was found to promote artemisinin biosynthesis by directly binding to and activating the *CYP71AV1* promoter. Artemisinin biosynthesis is positively regulated by the basic helix-loop-helix (bHLH) transcription factor AaMYC2, which promotes the expression of *CYP71AV1* and *DBR2*, and the basic leucine zipper transcription factor AabZIP1 (basic leucinezipper 1), which promotes the expression of *ADS* and *CYP71AV1*. In addition, several APETALA2/ETHYLENE-RESPONSIVE FACTOR (AP2/ERF) proteins, including AaERF1, AaERF2, and AaTAR1, have also been shown to positively regulate artemisinin biosynthesis by up-regulating *ADS* and *CYP71AV1* expression. Moreover, *A. annua* octadecanoid-responsive AP2/ERF (*AaORA*) has been shown to be a trichome-specific AP2/ERF transcription factor that activates artemisinin biosynthesis by up-regulating *ADS*, *CYP71AV1*, and *DBR2* expression. Furthermore, it was recently reported that *AaORA* is a direct target of AaGSW1 and that *AaORA* expression is also up-regulated after JA treatment, suggesting that an AaORA-related regulatory module is important for JA responses. It is worth mentioning that AaORA is a close homolog of CrORCAs in *C. roseus* and *NIC2*-locus ERFs in *Nicotiana tabacum*, and members of these families play vital roles in the synthesis of terpenoid indole alkaloids (TIAs) and nicotine. Likewise, both CrORCA2 and CrORCA3 are downstream components of JA signaling pathways and are regulated by CrMYC2. Thus, the results from these previous studies indicate that AP2/ERF proteins are crucial regulators of plant specialized metabolism and hormone signaling. However, except for these few examples, very little is known about AP2/ERF regulatory networks, especially the candidate partners, and the mechanism by which AaORA regulates artemisinin biosynthesis in *A. annua* is completely unknown.

Other transcription factors in addition to those mentioned above might also play important roles in specialized metabolism, such as the members of the TEOSINTE BRANCHED 1/CYCLOIDEA/PROLIFERATING CELL FACTOR (TCP) family. Members of this family, which was discovered in 1999, contain a noncanonical bHLH and are divided into two groups on the basis of the bHLH motif: class Ⅰ [PCF (proliferating cell nuclear antigen factor) or TCP-P] and class Ⅱ (TCP-C). In *Arabidopsis thaliana*, class Ⅰ TCP proteins specifically recognize the sequences GGNCCCAC, GGNCC, or GCCCR (R = A or G), and class Ⅱ TCP proteins specifically recognize the sequence G (T/C) GGNCCC. In plants, TCP proteins function as key regulators of plant developmental processes, hormonal pathways, the circadian clock, and immunity, and several members of this family play key roles in plant metabolism. However, the role of TCP proteins in artemisinin biosynthesis is unknown and needs to be further investigated.

Apart from transcription factors, the plant hormone JA plays a key role in artemisinin biosynthesis. Spraying *A. annua* with methyl JAs (MeJAs) increased artemisinin content by up-regulating the transcription of artemisinin biosynthetic genes and promoting GST formation. Overexpression of allene oxide cyclase, a key enzyme in JA biosynthesis, increased JA content and promoted artemisinin biosynthesis by up-regulating the expression of *FPS*, *CYP71AV1*, and *DBR2*. It is worth mentioning that these genes are also up-regulated by overexpression of the JA-responsive transcription factor, *AaORA*, suggesting that JA signaling may activate artemisinin biosynthesis by modulating AaORA activity.

JA signaling has been well studied in the model plant *A. thaliana*. Several JASMONATE ZIM-DOMAIN (JAZ) proteins, which are key regulators of JA signaling, act as repressors by recruiting members of the TOPLESS family of transcriptional corepressors through the adaptor protein, Novel Interactor of JAZ. The JAZ repressors interact with transcriptional activators, such as MYC2, to inhibit their transcriptional activation activity. The activity of the JAZ repressors is regulated, in turn, by the JA receptor, CORONATINE INSENSITIVE 1 (COI1), which is an F-box protein that plays a role in E3 ubiquitin ligase Skp/Cullin/F-box complex ($SCF^{COI1}$)-mediated proteasomal degradation. Following the conjugation of JA to isoleucine to form the active hormone JA-isoleucine (JA-Ile), JA-Ile binds to COI1 to facilitate the formation of COI1-JAZ complexes, leading to the ubiquitination and subsequent degradation of the JAZ proteins, which liberates transcriptional activators involved in diverse JA-mediated responses. In *A. annua*, it was reported that AaJAZ8 repressed the transcriptional activation activity of HOMEODOMAIN PROTEIN 1 (AaHD1), which regulates JA-mediated trichome development and artemisinin content. Nevertheless, further study is needed to determine whether AaJAZ8 affects the activation of other transcriptional regulators of artemisinin biosynthesis.

In this study, we identified AaTCP14 as a novel interactor of AaORA and demonstrated that AaORA and AaTCP14 form a complex that modulates artemisinin biosynthesis by directly activating the expression of *DBR2* and *ALDH1*. The repressor AaJAZ8 interacts with both AaORA and AaTCP14, which reduces the interaction between AaORA and AaTCP14. Moreover, AaJAZ8 attenuates the activation of *DBR2* by repressing the AaTCP14-AaORA complex. MeJA treatment induces the degradation of AaJAZ8 and liberates the AaTCP14-AaORA complex, leading to activation of the *DBR2* promoter, which subsequently promotes JA-induced artemisinin accumulation. Thus, our research reveals a novel mechanism underlying JA-mediated control of artemisinin biosynthesis.

## 2 RESULTS

Identification of AaTCP14 as an AaORA-interacting protein  AaORA significantly activated the promoters of four key genes involved in artemisinin biosynthesis, *ADS*, *CYP71AV1*, *DBR2*, and *ALDH1*, in dual-luciferase (LUC) assays (Fig. S1B), which is consistent with the positive role of AaORA in artemisinin biosynthesis. However, interactions between AaORA and the promoters of these genes were not detected in yeast one-hybrid (Y1H) assays (Fig. S1C), implying that AaORA might fulfill its positive regulatory function, in part, by interacting with other DNA-binding transcription factors.

To identify putative AaORA-interacting transcription factors and to elucidate the molecular basis for AaORA control of artemisinin biosynthesis, a Y2H screen for AaORA-interacting proteins was performed using an *A. annua* complementary DNA (cDNA) library constructed from the youngest leaves and meristem. Deletion analysis revealed that full-length AaORA had autonomous transcriptional activation activity (Fig. S2); therefore, a truncated version of the AaORA protein, AaORAΔN1 (C terminus of AaORA), lacking autonomous transcriptional activation activity was used as the bait. An initial screen identified AaTCP14, a TCP transcription factor with high similarity to TCP14 proteins from *A. thaliana* and *Gossypium raimondii* (Fig. S3 and S4), as the dominant interactor of AaORA (9 of 23 positive clones). The physical interaction between AaORA and AaTCP14 was further confirmed by both Y2H (Fig. 1A) and in vitro GST pulldown assays with proteins purified from *Escherichia coli* (Fig. 1B).

BiFC assays were performed to verify the AaORA-AaTCP14 interaction in plant cells. When AaORA-cYFP (the C-terminal fragment of YFP) was transiently coexpressed with AaTCP14-nYFP (the Nterminal fragment of YFP) in *Nicotiana benthamiana* leaf cells, reconstituted YFP fluorescence was observed in the nucleus. By contrast, no YFP fluorescence signals were observed when AaORA-cYFP and nYFP or cYFP and AaTCP14-nYFP were coexpressed (Fig. 1C). These results suggest that AaORA interacts with AaTCP14 in planta. Coimmunoprecipitation (Co-IP) assays further demonstrated that AaORA associates with AaTCP14 in *N. benthamiana* leaf cells (Fig. 1D). Together, these results demonstrate that AaORA directly interacts with AaTCP14 in vitro and in vivo.

*AaTCP14* and *AaORA* have similar expression patterns and AaTCP14 is a nuclear-localized protein  To investigate the spatial and temporal expression pattern of *AaTCP14*, we analyzed the expression levels of *AaTCP14* in leaves at different positions and in different tissues using quantitative real-time polymerase chain reaction (qRT-PCR). *AaTCP14* expression was high in young leaves (leaf 1 and leaf2) and then gradually decreased during leaf development (Fig. 2, A and B). This expression pattern is similar to that of artemisinin biosynthetic genes and *AaORA* (Fig. 2, A and B). In addition, *AaTCP14* transcripts were also detected in other organs. *AaTCP14* was most highly expressed in trichomes; moderately expressed in leaves, shoots, flowers, and buds; lowly expressed in the stems; and very lowly expressed in the roots (Fig. 2C).

To more precisely determine the expression patterns of *AaTCP14*, we transformed wild-type (WT) *A. annua* with *1391Z-proTCP14-GUS* (β-glucuronidase), where expression of the GUS reporter is driven by the 1828-base pair (bp) promoter sequence of *AaTCP14*. Histochemical GUS staining of *1391Z-proTCP14-GUS* transgenic lines revealed GUS activity in young leaves and stems, especially in the two types of trichomes, T-shaped non-GSTs (TSTs) and GSTs (Fig. 2D). No GUS activity was observed in *A. annua* plants transformed with the empty vector (Fig. 2D). The expression pattern of the GUS reporter correlated well with the expression patterns determined using qRT-PCR (Fig. 2C).

There is accumulating evidence that the phytohormone MeJA plays a positive role in artemisinin biosynthesis. *AaORA* expression was gradually induced by MeJA and peaked at 9 hours after MeJA treatment (Fig. 2E). Thus, we wanted to know whether *AaTCP14* had the same expression pattern as *AaORA* under MeJA treatment. On the basis of qRT-PCR analysis, *AaTCP14* expression was robustly induced at 3 hours and also peaked at 9 hours after MeJA treatment

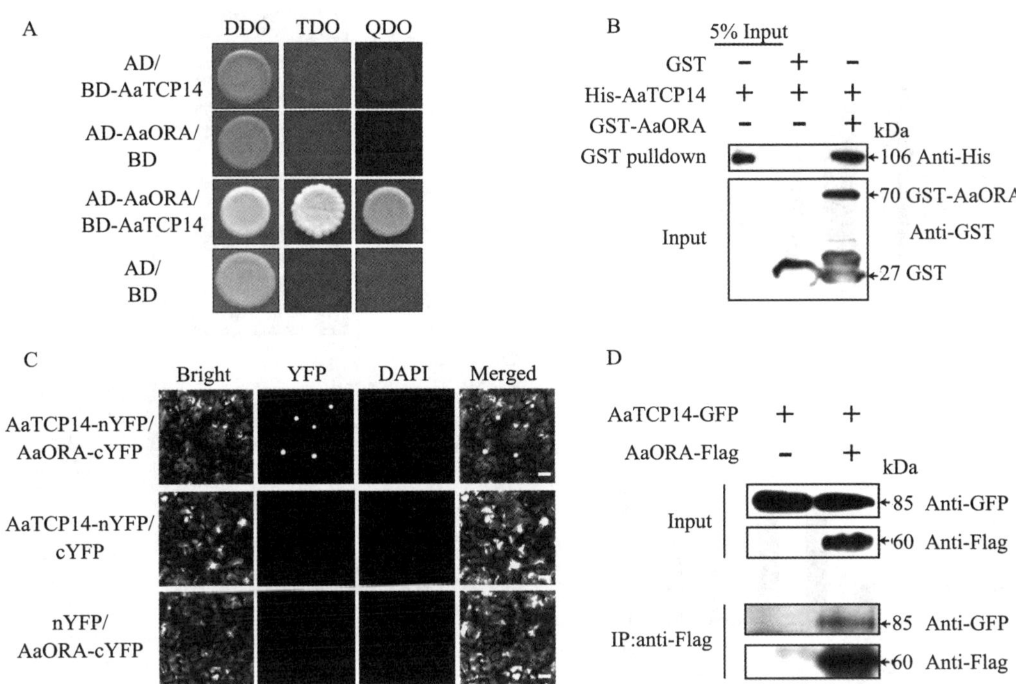


**Fig. 1 AaTCP14 protein interacts with AaORA**

(**A**) Y2H analysis of AaTCP14 interaction with AaORA. Yeast cells transformed with different combinations of constructs containing AaTCP14 fused with the DNA binding domain (BD-AaTCP14), AaORA fused with the activation domain (AD-AaORA), the BD alone, and the AD alone were grown on two different selective media, SD/-Trp/-Leu/-His (TDO) and SD/-Trp/-Leu/-His/-Ade (QDO), and the control medium SD/-Trp/-Leu (DDO). Pictures were taken after 4 days of incubation at 30 ℃. Y2H assays were repeated three times, and representative results are shown. (**B**) In vitro pulldown assays of AaTCP14 and AaORA recombinant proteins. His-AaTCP14 proteins were pulled down with GST-AaORA and further detected on Western blots probed with anti-His antibody. Experiments were carried out three times, and representative results are shown. (**C**) Bimolecular fluorescence complementation (BiFC) analysis of the interaction between AaTCP14 and AaORA in *N. benthamiana* cells. AaTCP14 was fused to the N-terminal fragment of yellow fluorescent protein (AaTCP14-nYFP), and AaORA was fused to the C-terminal fragment of YFP (AaORA-cYFP). Colocalization of reconstituted YFP and nuclei was determined by 4′, 6-diamidino-2-phenylindole (DAPI) staining. Three independent transfection experiments were performed. Scale bars, 20 μm. (**D**) Co-IP studies of AaTCP14 and AaORA complex formation in *N. benthamiana* leaves. Total protein extracts from *N. benthamiana* leaves infiltrated with constructs harboring AaTCP14-GFP and AaORA-Flag were immunoprecipitated with anti-Flag antibody. The coimmunopre-cipitated proteins were detected by anti-GFP antibody. Experiments were repeated three times and similar results were obtained.

(Fig. 2E). Thus, these results suggest that *AaTCP14* and *AaORA* have similar expression patterns in response to MeJA treatment, which also induces artemisinin biosynthesis.

To determine where the AaTCP14 protein functions within the cell, we next determined the subcellular localization of an AaTCP14-YFP fusion protein. In contrast to YFP, which was distributed throughout the cell, the AaTCP14-YFP fusion protein was observed exclusively in nuclei (Fig. 2F) in *N. benthamiana* leaf cells, suggesting that AaTCP14 is a nuclear-localized protein, consistent with its potential function as a transcriptional regulator.

Overexpression of *AaTCP14* increases artemisinin content, and attenuated expression of *AaTCP14* reduces artemisinin production in *A. annua* To investigate the physiological role of AaTCP14, *AaTCP14* was overexpressed in *A. annua* plants. Three independent *AaTCP14* overexpression lines, named AaTCP14-5, AaTCP14-28, and AaTCP14-31, were selected for subsequent analysis. The transcript levels of *AaTCP14* in these lines were significantly higher than those in WT plants (Fig. 3A). The expression levels of *ADS*, *CYP71AV1*, *DBR2*, and *ALDH1* were also dramatically increased in *AaTCP14* overexpression plants compared with WT (Fig. 3B). This suggests that AaTCP14 may activate the transcription of artemisinin biosynthetic genes. Furthermore, the expression levels of *AaWRKY1*, *AaMYC2*, *AaGSW1*, and *AaORA*, which are involved in different pathways positively regulating artemisinin biosynthesis, were significantly up-regulated in the *AaTCP14* overexpression lines (Fig. S5, A to D). Up-regulation of these genes may, in turn, activate *ADS*, *CYP71AV1*, and *DBR2* expression. In addition, the expression levels of some well-known JA biosynthetic genes, including *AaAOC* and *AaOPR3*, were higher in *AaTCP14* overexpression lines than in WT, but the expression levels of *AaAOS* and *AaOPCL1* were not (Fig. S5, E to H). Up-regulation of *AaAOC* could enhance the JA content, which, in turn, would activate artemisinin

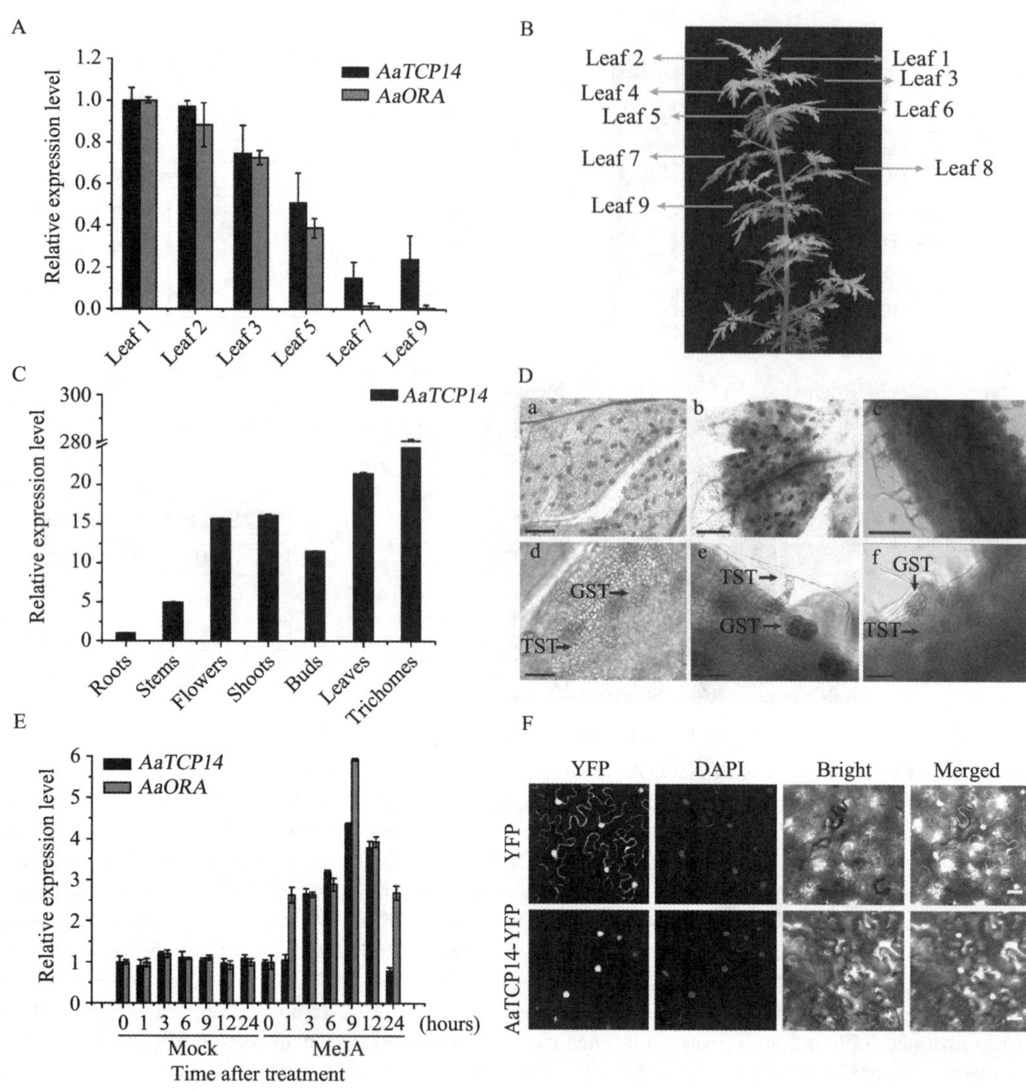


**Fig. 2 Expression pattern and subcellular localization of AaTCP14**

(**A**) Relative expression levels of *AaTCP14* and *AaORA* in leaves at different positions. The expression levels of *AaTCP14* and *AaORA* in leaf 1 were set as 1. *Actin* was used as an internal control. The data represent the means±SD of three replicates from three independent *A. annua* plants. (**B**) Animage of a 3-month-old *A. annua* plant labeled with the leaves numbered as in (A). (**C**) Relative expression levels of *AaTCP14* in roots, stems, flowers, shoots, buds, leaves, and trichomes were measured by qRT-PCR. The expression level of *AaTCP14* in roots was set as 1. *Actin* was used as an internal control. The data represent the means±SD of three replicates from three independent *A. annua* plants. (**D**) GUS expression (blue staining) in *A. annua* plants transformed with the *1391Z-GUS* empty vector (control plants) and *1391Z-proTCP14-GUS*. (**a** and **d**) Leaves of control plants. (**b** and **e**) Leaves of *1391Z-proTCP14-GUS* plants. (**c** and **f**) Stems of *1391Z-proTCP14-GUS* plants. Scale bars, 200 μm (a to c) and 50 μm (d to f). (**E**) Relative expression levels of *AaTCP14* and *AaORA* in plants treated with MeJA (100 μmol/L) over 24 hours. *Actin* was used as an internal control. The data represent the means±SD of three replicates from three independent experiments. (**F**) Subcellular localization of AaTCP14. Colocalization of AaTCP14-YFP and nuclei was determined by DAPI staining. YFP was used as a negative control. Three independent transfection experiments were performed. Scale bars, 20 μm.

biosynthesis. Together, these results indicate that AaTCP14 has the potential to enhance artemisinin yield. Consistent with the up-regulation of genes involved in artemisinin biosynthesis, high-performance liquid chromatography (HPLC) analysis showed that the artemisinin and DHAA contents in *AaTCP14* overexpression lines increased by 80% to 120% and 10% to 120%, respectively, compared with WT (Fig. 3C and Fig. S6A), whereas the AA content decreased by 45% to 69% in *AaTCP14* overexpression plants (Fig. S6B). These results indicate that AaTCP14 positively promotes artemisinin biosynthesis.

To further verify the biological role of *AaTCP14* in controlling artemisinin biosynthesis, we silenced *AaTCP14* expression by transforming *A. annua* with the antisense vector *pHB-ANTCP14*. Three candidate *AaTCP14* antisense transgenic plants, named ANTCP14-43, ANTCP14-53, and ANTCP14-60, were chosen for subsequent analysis. The expression level of *AaTCP14* in these antisense lines was

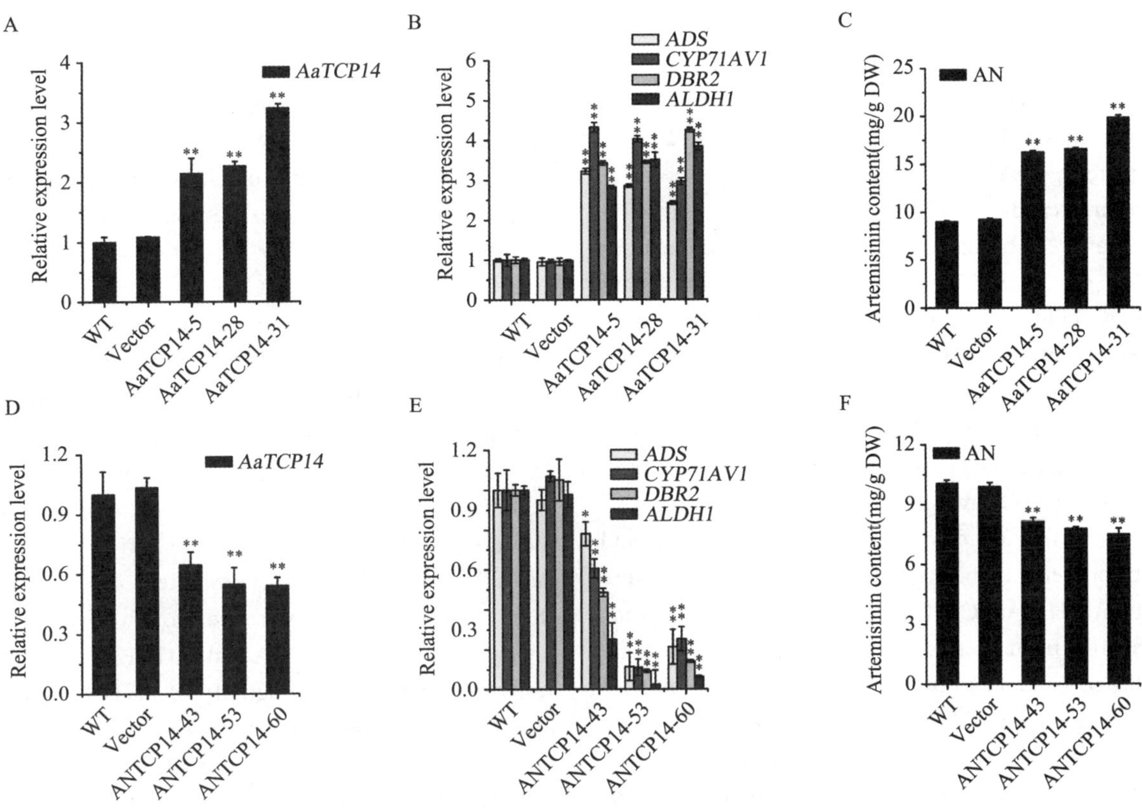

**Fig. 3 Analysis of *AaTCP14* transgenic plants.**

(**A** and **D**) Expression levels of *AaTCP14* in different *A. annua AaTCP14* overexpression (A) and antisense lines (D), plants transformed with the empty vector, and WT plants. *Actin* was used as the internal standard. (**B** and **E**) Expression levels of *ADS*, *CYP71AV1*, *DBR2*, and *ALDH1* in different *A. annua AaTCP14* overexpression (B) and antisense lines (E), plants transformed with the empty vector, and WT. *Actin* was used as the internal control. (**C** and **F**) HPLC analysis of artemisinin (AN) in the leaves of different *A. annua AaTCP14* overexpression (C) and antisense lines (F), plants transformed with the empty vector, and WT. All data represent the means±SD of three replicates from three cutting propagations. * $P<0.05$, ** $P<0.01$, Student's *t* test.

significantly reduced compared with WT (Fig. 3D), and the expression levels of *ADS*, *CYP71AV1*, *DBR2*, and *ALDH1* were significantly down-regulated compared with WT (Fig. 3E). The expression levels of *AaWRKY1*, *AaMYC2*, *AaGSW1*, and *AaORA* were also down-regulated in the *AaTCP14* antisense plants (Fig. S5, I to L), which probably contributed to decreased *ADS*, *CYP71AV1*, and *DBR2* expression. Moreover, the expression levels of *AaAOC* and *AaOPR3* decreased in *AaTCP14* antisense plants, but the expression levels of *AaAOS* and *AaOPCL1* did not (Fig. S5, M to P). This is consistent with the gene expression changes observed in the *AaTCP14* overexpression plants and suggests that AaTCP14 regulates JA biosynthesis through *AaAOC* and *AaOPR3*. Together, these results indicate that AaTCP14 plays a positive role in controlling artemisinin biosynthesis. Consistent with this, the contents of artemisinin, DHAA, and AA in *AaTCP14* antisense plants were reduced by 19 to 25%, 20 to 72%, and 11 to 37%, respectively (Fig. 3F and Fig. S6, D and E). No obvious morphological differences were observed in either the *AaTCP14* overexpression or antisense transgenic plants compared with the *A. annua* plants transformed with the empty vector (control plants, labeled as vector) (Fig. S6, C and F). Together, these results indicate that AaTCP14 is a positive regulator of artemisinin biosynthesis and may be a good target in efforts to increase artemisinin production through genetic engineering of A. *annua*.

AaTCP14 enhances the transcription of both *DBR2* and *ALDH1* by binding to their promoters To further investigate whether AaTCP14 directly affects *ADS*, *CYP71AV1*, *DBR2*, and *ALDH1* expression, we used dual-LUC assays. When AaTCP14-GFP (green fluorescent protein) was expressed in *N. benthamiana* leaf cells harboring the $DBR2_{pro}$: LUC or $ALDH1_{pro}$: LUC plasmids, the promoter activities of *DBR2* and *ALDH1*, respectively, significantly increased compared with the GFP control (Fig. 4, A and B). However, the activities of the *ADS* and *CYP71AV1* promoters were not obviously altered (Fig. 4B).

Together, these results suggest that AaTCP14 is a positive regulator of *DBR2* and *ALDH1*.

Previous studies suggested that TCP family proteins directly bind to the TCP binding site (TBS) in the promoter sequence of target genes in *A. thaliana*. Promoter analysis revealed two similar TBS motifs (*D1* and *D2*; 1 721 and 1 461 bp upstream of ATG, respectively) in the promoter of *DBR2* and three candidate TBS motifs (*A1*, *A2*, and *A3*; 1 285, 827, and 219 bp upstream of ATG, respectively) in the *ALDH1* promoter (Fig. 4, C and D). Y1H assays showed that binding of the pB42AD-AaTCP14 fusion protein, but not pB42AD alone, to three tandem repeats of the *D2* motif or the *A1* motif strongly activated the expression of the *LacZ* reporter gene (Fig. 4, E and F), indicating that AaTCP14 binds to the *D2* and *A1* motifs in the *DBR2* and *ALDH1* promoters, respectively.

Next, to further confirm AaTCP14 binding to *D2* and *A1*, electrophoretic mobility shift assays (EMSAs) were conducted with His-AaTCP14 and His-TF (trigger factor) proteins purified from *E. coli*. As shown in Fig. 4 (I and J), a single shifted band was observed in the presence of both His-AaTCP14 and a labeled DNA probe containing the *D2* or *A1* motif (D2q or A1q, shown in Fig. 4, G and H). The intensity of this band decreased with increasing concentrations of a cold competitor, and no band was observed when His-TF was added in place of His-AaTCP14 (Fig. 4, I and J). Moreover, mutations in the *D2* or *A1* motifs markedly attenuated the band intensity (Fig. 4, G to J), indicating that AaTCP14 specifically bound to the *D2q* and *A1q* motifs. Together, these results demonstrate that AaTCP14 positively regulates *DBR2* and *ALDH1* expression by directly binding to their promoters.

AaTCP14 and AaORA synergistically promote artemisinin biosynthesis, and the function of AaORA is partly dependent on AaTCP14  We have shown that the AaTCP14 and AaORA proteins interact (Fig. 1), that the genes encoding these proteins share similar expression patterns (i.e., in leaves sampled from different positions and in response to MeJA treatment) (Fig. 2, A and E), and that both proteins activate the *DBR2* and *ALDH1* promoters (Fig. 4 and Fig. S1B). These results prompted us to examine whether AaORA affects the AaTCP14-mediated transactivation of *DBR2* and *ALDH1* under MeJA treatment. To test this, we used dual-LUC assays to evaluate the promoter activity of *DBR2* and *ALDH1* with the effectors AaTCP14 and AaORA delivered individually or in combination in the presence or absence of MeJA in *N. benthamiana* leaf cells. AaTCP14 and AaORA alone were able to significantly activate the *DBR2* and *ALDH1* promoters, and this induction was significantly enhanced by coexpressing AaORA and AaTCP14 (Fig. 5, A to C). These results suggest that AaORA elevates the transcriptional activation activity of AaTCP14 through direct protein interactions (Fig. 1). It should be noted that MeJA treatment strengthened the activation of the *DBR2* and *ALDH1* promoters by AaTCP14, AaORA, and AaTCP14-AaORA (Fig. 5, B and C), suggesting that AaTCP14 and AaORA may act as downstream components of JA signaling pathway and cooperatively activate the expression of *DBR2* and *ALDH1*.

Next, to check whether the AaORA-AaTCP14 interaction affects the ability of AaTCP14 to bind to the *DBR2* and *ALDH1* promoters, we performed EMSAs using DNA fragments D2q and A1q (labeled in Fig. 4, G and H), respectively, as probes. The addition of an increasing amount of His-AaORA fusion protein, which was purified from *E. coli*, had a negligible effect on the ability of His-AaTCP14 to bind to *DBR2* and *ALDH1* (Fig. S7, A and B), indicating that AaORA does not affect the ability of AaTCP14 to bind to these promoters in vitro. Together, these observations support the notion that the physical interaction between AaORA and AaTCP14 may promote the transcriptional activation activity of AaTCP14 but does not affect its DNA binding ability.

To evaluate the importance of the AaTCP14-AaORA complex in artemisinin biosynthesis, we generated transgenic *A. annua* plants simultaneously overexpressing *AaTCP14* and *AaORA*. Three candidate *AaTCP14-AaORA* co-overexpression lines, named AaTCP14-AaORA-6, AaTCP14-AaORA-15, and AaTCP14-AaORA-16, were chosen for further analysis. The expression levels of *AaTCP14* and *AaORA* in these lines were significantly higher (2.5- to 4.0-fold and 12- to 31-fold, respectively) than those in WT (Fig. 5D). The expression levels of *DBR2* and *ALDH1* dramatically increased in *AaTCP14-AaORA* coexpression plants compared with both WT and plants overexpressing only *AaTCP14* (Fig. 5E), indicating that AaTCP14 and AaORA cooperatively activate the transcription of *DBR2* and *ALDH1*. This finding is consistent with the enhancement of *DBR2* and *ALDH1* promoter activation by coexpressing *AaTCP14* and *AaORA* in *N. benthamiana* leaf cells (Fig. 5, A to C). Furthermore, HPLC analysis showed that the levels of artemisinin, DHAA, and AA were significantly increased in *AaTCP14-AaORA* co-overexpression plants compared with WT and plants overexpressing only *AaTCP14* (Fig. 5F and Fig. S6, G and H). No obvious morphological differences were observed between *AaTCP14-AaORA* coexpression plants and *A. annua* plants transformed with the empty vector (Fig. S6I). Together, these results indicate that AaTCP14 and AaORA synergistically regulate artemisinin biosynthesis and may form a protein complex that enhances artemisinin production.

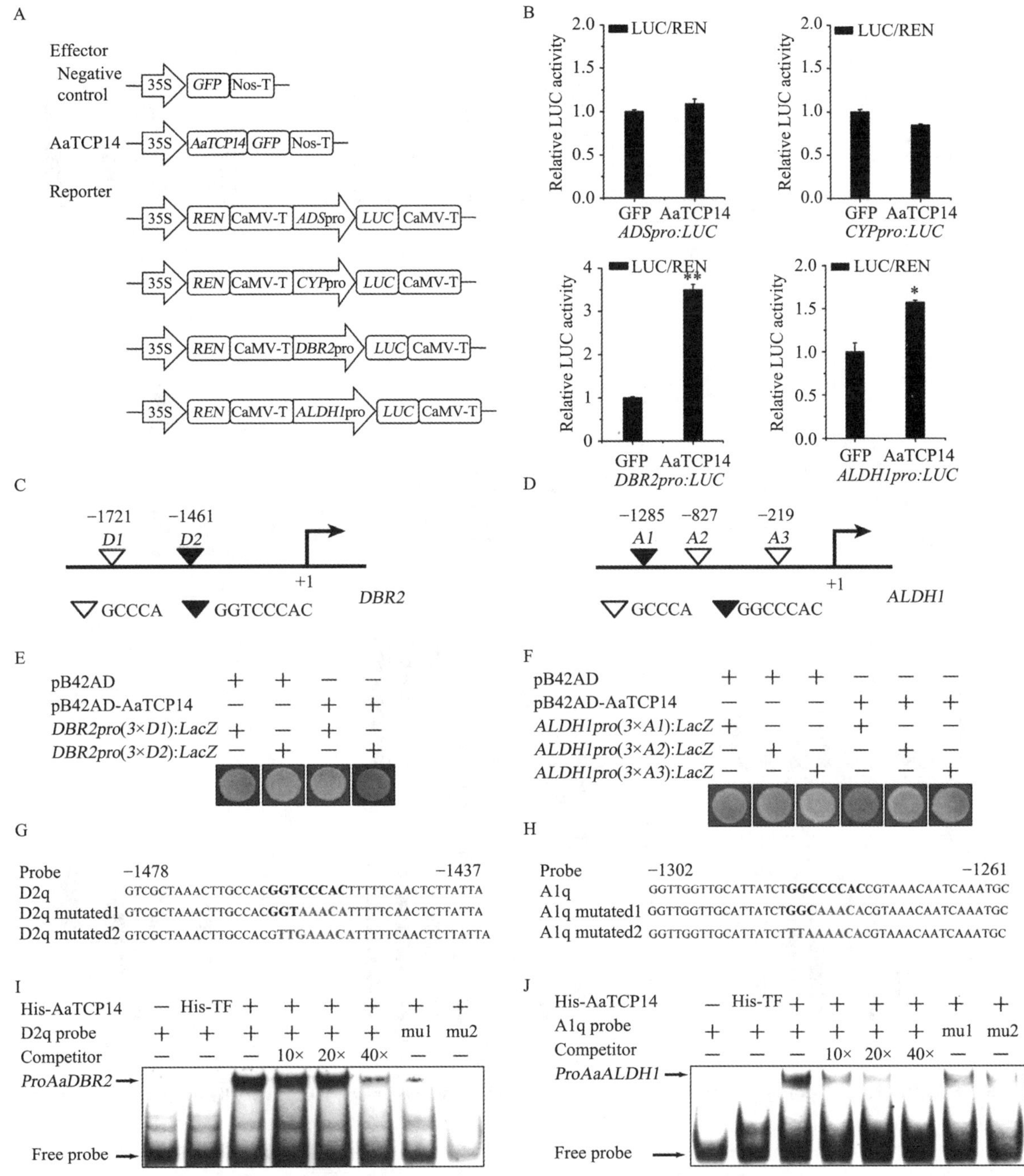


**Fig. 4 AaTCP14 is a transcriptional activator of *DBR2* and *ALDH1***

(**A**) Schematic diagrams of the effector (pCambia1300-AaTCP14-GFP) and reporter (35S: REN-ADS/CYP/DBR2/ALDH1$_{pro}$: LUC) plasmids used in dual-LUC assays. CYP, CYP71AV1; REN, *Renilla* luciferase; LUC, firefly luciferase. (**B**) Dual-LUC assay in *N. benthamiana* cells using the constructs shown in (A). The GFP effector was used as a negative control, and the LUC/REN ratios of GFP were set as 1. Three independent transfection experiments were performed. The data represent the means ± SD of three replicates from three independent experiments. $^{*}P < 0.05$, $^{**}P < 0.01$, Student's *t* test. (**C** and **D**) Schematic diagrams of the *DBR2* and *ALDH1* promoters. The positions of potential TBS DNA binding sites (*D1* and *D2* and *A1*, *A2*, and *A3*) are shown as black and white triangles and are numbered on the basis of their distance from the translational start site (ATG), which is set as +1. (**E** and **F**) Y1H assays showing that AaTCP14 binds to the TBS motifs of *DBR2* and *ALDH1*. Three tandem repeats of each motif were used as baits. Yeast cells coexpressing pB42AD, pB42AD-AaTCP14, and the DNA motifs from the *DBR2* and *ALDH1* promoters were grown on selective medium, SD/-Trp/-Ura, containing X-gal (20 mg/liter), and pictures were taken after 4 days of incubation at 30 ℃. Blue plaques indicate protein-DNA interactions. The Y1H assays were repeated three times, and representative results are shown. (**G** and **H**) The sequences of WT and mutated probes used for EMSAs. Class I TCP binding motifs are shown in bold, and the mutated nucleotides are indicated in red. (**I** and **J**) EMSAs showing that AaTCP14 binds to the *D2q* motif from *DBR2* and the *A1q* motif from *ALDH1*. Unlabeled D2q and A1q were used as cold competitors, and two labeled mutated D2q and A1q probes were tested as negative controls. 10×, 20×, and 40× indicate the fold excess of cold competitors relative to that of the labeled probe. His-TF protein was used as a negative control.

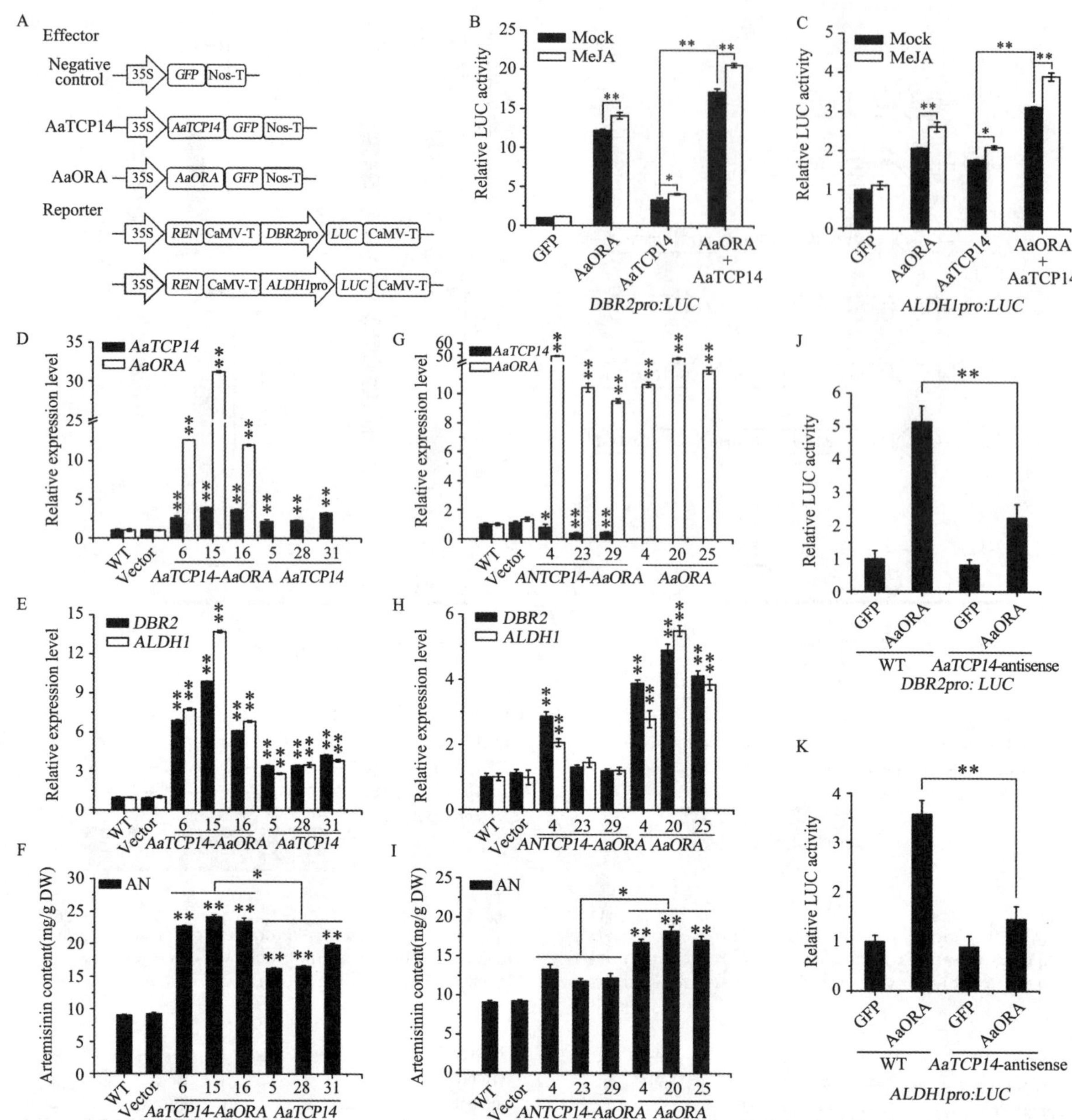

**Fig. 5 AaTCP14 and AaORA synergistically promote artemisinin biosynthesis, and AaORA is partly dependent on AaTCP14**

(**A**) A schematic representation of the constructs used in dual-LUC assays. (**B and C**) Activation of the *DBR2* (B) and *ALDH1* (C) promoters by AaORA and AaTCP14 proteins in the presence or absence of MeJA in *N*. *benthamiana* leaves. The GFP effector in the mock treatment served as a negative control, and the LUC/REN ratios of GFP were set as 1. Three independent transfection experiments were performed. The reporter strain harboring *DBR2pro*: *LUC* or *ALDH1pro*: *LUC* was mixed with the effector strains harboring *35Spro*: *AaTCP14* and *35Spro*: *AaORA* at a ratio of 1∶1∶1. The data represent the means±SD of three replicates from three independent experiments. * $P<0.05$, ** $P<0.01$, Student's *t* test. (**D and E**) Expression levels of *AaTCP14* and *AaORA* (D) and *DBR2* and *ALDH1* (E) in different *A*. *annua* plants including *AaTCP14*-*AaORA* co-overexpression (*AaTCP14*-*AaORA*), *AaTCP14* overexpression lines, and plants transformed with the empty vector. *Actin* was used as the internal standard. WT plants served as controls. The data represent the means ±SD of three replicates from three cutting propagations. ** $P<0.01$, Student's *t* test. (**F**) HPLC analysis of artemisinin (AN) in the leaves of different *A*. *annua* plants including *AaTCP14*-*AaORA* and *AaTCP14* overexpression lines, plants transformed with the empty vector, and the WT control. The data represent the means±SD of three replicates from three cutting propagations. * $P<0.05$, ** $P<0.01$, Student's *t* test. (**G and H**) Expression levels of *AaTCP14* and *AaORA* (G) and *DBR2* and *ALDH1* (H) in different *A*. *annua* plants including the *AaTCP14* antisense-*AaORA* overexpression (*ANTCP14*-*AaORA*), *AaORA* overexpression lines, and plants transformed with the empty vector. *Actin* was used as the internal standard. WT plants served as controls. The data represent the means±SD from three replicates from three cutting propagations. * $P<0.05$, ** $P<0.01$, Student's *t* test. (**I**) HPLC analysis of artemisinin (AN) in the leaves of different *A*. *annua* plants including the *ANTCP14*-*AaORA*, *AaORA* overex-pression lines, plants transformed with the empty vector, and the WT control. The data represent the means±SD of three replicates from three cutting propagations. * $P<0.05$, ** $P<0.01$, Student's *t* test. (**J and K**) Dual-LUC experiments showing the activation of the *DBR2* (J) and *ALDH1* (K) promoters by AaORA in *A*. *annua* protoplasts from WT and *AaTCP14* antisense (*ANTCP14*) lines. GFP was used as a negative control, and the LUC/REN ratios of GFP in WT *A*. *annua* were set as 1. Three independent transfection experiments were performed. The data represent the means±SD of three independent experiments. Student's *t* test, ** $P<0.01$.

To determine whether the function of AaORA is dependent on AaTCP14, we generated transgenic *A. annua* plants only overexpressing *AaORA* and plants simultaneously overexpressing *AaORA* and silenced *AaTCP14*. Three candidate *AaORA* overexpression lines, AaORA-4, AaORA-20, and AaORA-25, and three *AaTCP14* antisense-*AaORA* overexpression lines, ANTCP14-AaORA-4, ANTCP14-AaORA-23, and ANTCP14-AaORA-29, were chosen for further analysis. The expression levels of *AaORA* in the *AaORA* overexpression and *AaTCP14* antisense-*AaORA* overexpression plants were notably higher than those in WT (Fig. 5G). The expression levels of *AaTCP14* in the *AaTCP14* antisense-*AaORA* overexpression plants were markedly lower than those in WT (Fig. 5G). The expression levels of *DBR2* and *ALDH1* in the *AaTCP14* antisense-*AaORA* overexpression plants were higher than those in WT but lower than those in *AaORA* overexpression plants (Fig. 5H). Consistently, the artemisinin content in the *AaTCP14* antisense-*AaORA* overexpression plants were higher than those in WT but lower than those in *AaORA* overexpression plants (Fig. 5I). Dual-LUC assays were also performed to evaluate the regulation of the *DBR2* and *ALDH1* promoters by AaORA in protoplasts from WT and *ANTCP14 A. annua* lines. The transactivation of the *DBR2* and *ALDH1* promoters by AaORA was much lower in cells with less *AaTCP14* expression than in WT cells (Fig. 5, J and K). Collectively, these results demonstrate that the enhancement of artemisinin production by AaORA is partly dependent on AaTCP14.

AaJAZ8 negatively regulates artemisinin biosynthesis and interacts with both AaTCP14 and AaORA  It has been reported that JA induces artemisinin accumulation by activating artemisinin biosynthetic genes or JA-responsive transcription factors. In contrast, JAZ proteins function as negative regulators that repress diverse JA responses by suppressing various positive transcriptional regulators. In *A. annua*, the JAZ protein encoded by *AaJAZ8* was previously found to repress the transcriptional activation activity of AaHD1, which is involved in trichome development and artemisinin content. In our study, we found that *AaJAZ8* is broadly expressed and is most highly expressed in trichomes (Fig. S8A). Moreover, *AaJAZ8* expression is induced by MeJA treatment, and the level of AaJAZ8 protein is regulated by MeJA through the 26S proteasome (Fig. S8, B and C), suggesting the potential role of AaJAZ8 in controlling JA-mediated artemisinin accumulation. To functionally characterize AaJAZ8 and determine its role in artemisinin biosynthesis, we generated transgenic plants overexpressing *AaJAZ8*. The expression levels of *ADS*, *CYP71AV1*, *DBR2*, and *ALDH1*, determined by qRT-PCR analysis, were lower in *AaJAZ8* overexpression lines than in WT plants (Fig. S8D), and the artemisinin content was concomitantly decreased (Fig. S8E). Because the jas domain of JAZ proteins is essential for JA-mediated protein degradation, we also overexpressed a dominant form of *AaJAZ8* (*AaJAZ8*Δ*jas*) that lacks the jas domain to disrupt JA-mediated AaJAZ8 protein degradation. The expression levels of *ADS*, *CYP71AV1*, *DBR2*, and *ALDH1* were lower in *AaJAZ8*Δ*jas* overexpression lines than in WT plants (Fig. S8F). Together, these results suggest that AaJAZ8 attenuates JA-induced artemisinin biosynthesis in *A. annua*.

Considering that *AaTCP14*, *AaORA*, and *AaJAZ8* are all induced by MeJA (Fig. 2E and Fig. S8B) and that AaORA is a putative downstream regulator of JA signaling, there may be a possible connection between *AaTCP14*, *AaORA*, and *AaJAZ8*. Hence, we examined whether AaJAZ8 could physically interact with AaTCP14 or AaORA. Y2H assays revealed that both AaTCP14 and AaORA interact with AaJAZ8 (Fig. 6A). Intriguingly, among all the AaJAZ proteins (AaJAZ1 to AaJAZ9), only AaJAZ8 interacted with AaTCP14, and apart from AaJAZ7, all AaJAZ proteins (AaJAZ1 to AaJAZ6, AaJAZ8, and AaJAZ9) interacted with AaORA (Fig. S9A), indicating that AaTCP14 and AaORA are common targets of AaJAZ8. MYC2 is a key regulator of JA signaling and is also a general target of JAZ proteins in *Arabidopsis*. AaMYC2 and AaJAZ1 to AaJAZ4, which were previously reported to interact, were used as positive controls, and parallel experiments showed clear interactions of AaMYC2 with all other AaJAZ proteins (AaJAZ5, AaJAZ6, AaJAZ8, and AaJAZ9) except AaJAZ7 (Fig. S9A). Next, the pairwise interactions of AaJAZ8 with AaTCP14 and AaORA were validated by performing BiFC assays. As expected, when the AaJAZ8-cYFP construct was transiently coexpressed with AaTCP14-nYFP or AaORA-nYFP in *N. benthamiana* leaf cells, strong YFP fluorescence signals were observed in the nucleus (Fig. 6B), indicating that AaJAZ8 interacts with AaTCP14 and AaORA in plant cells.

To further substantiate this result, we performed transient colocalization assays, expressing YFP-AaJAZ8, cyan fluorescent protein (CFP)-AaTCP14, and CFP-AaORA, either individually or together, in *N. benthamiana* leaf cells. As anticipated, AaJAZ8 colocalized with AaTCP14 and with AaORA in the same nuclear bodies (NBs) (Fig. 6C). AaJAZ8-AaTCP14 and AaJAZ8-AaORA interactions in *N. benthamiana* leaf cells were also confirmed by LUC complementation assays (Fig. 6D). Together, these results suggest that AaJAZ8 specifically interacts with AaTCP14 and AaORA in plant cells. Next, Y2H assays were carried out to map which domain of AaJAZ8 is responsible for its interaction with AaTCP14 and AaORA. AaJAZ8Δjas, which contains only the ZIM domain, was capable of interacting with AaTCP14

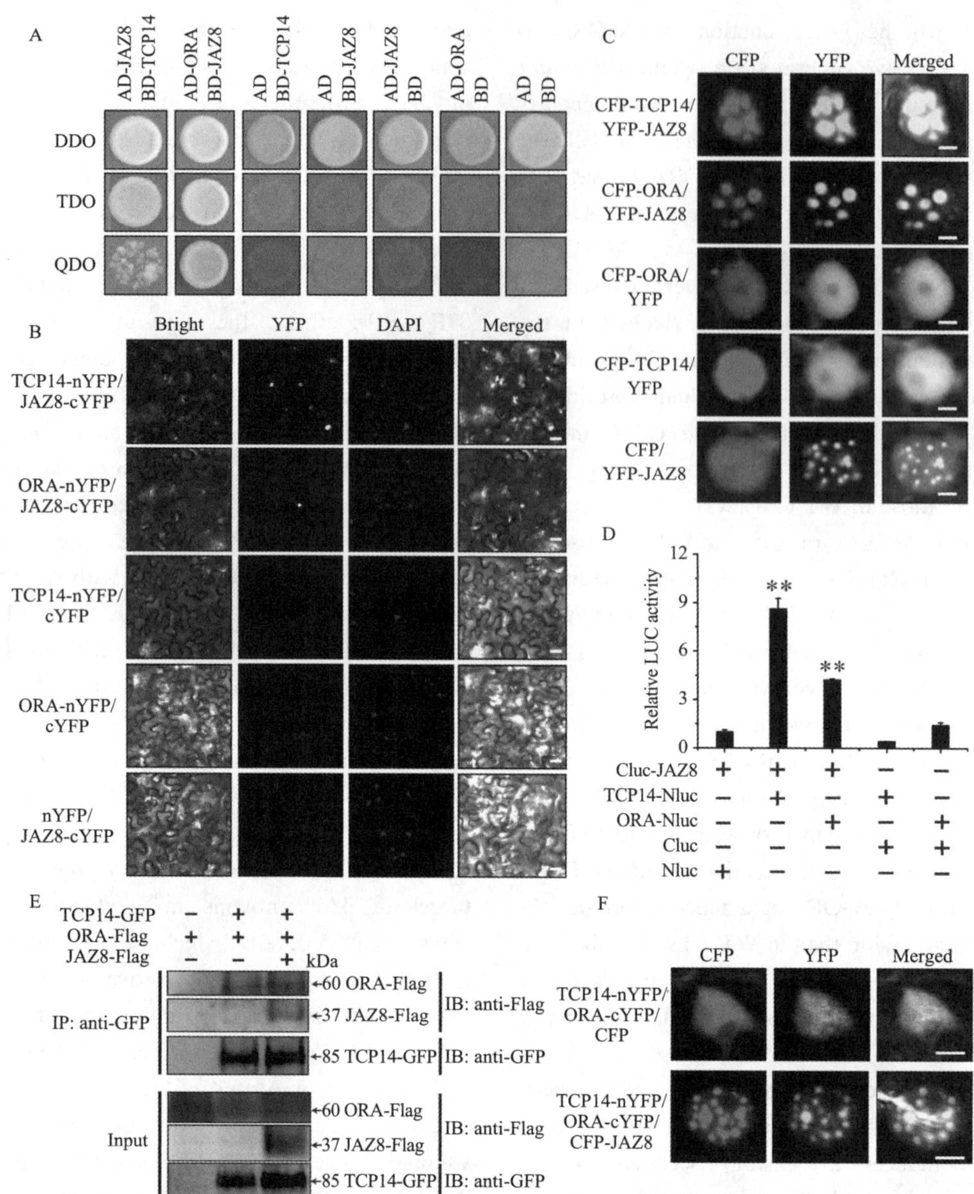


**Fig. 6 AaJAZ8 interacts with both AaTCP14 and AaORA**

(**A**) Y2H assays to detect the pairwise interactions between AaJAZ8, AaTCP14, and AaORA. AaORA and AaJAZ8 were fused with the activation domain (AD), and AaTCP14 and AaJAZ8 were fused with the binding domain (BD). Yeast cells harboring bait and prey plasmids were grown on two types of selective media, QDO and TDO, and the control medium, DDO. Pictures were taken after 4 days of incubation at 30℃. The Y2H assays were repeated three times, and representative results are shown. (**B**) BiFC analysis to detect the pairwise interactions between AaTCP14, AaORA, and AaJAZ8. AaTCP14 and AaORA were fused to the N-terminal fragment of YFP (TCP14-nYFP and ORA-nYFP), and AaJAZ8 was fused to the C-terminal fragment of YFP (JAZ8-cYFP). Colocalization of reconstituted YFP and nuclei was determined by DAPI staining. Three independent transfection experiments were performed. Scale bars, 20 μm. (**C**) Colocalization of AaTCP14 and AaJAZ8 and of AaORA and AaJAZ8 to the same NBs in *N. benthamiana* cells. *N. benthamiana* leaves were infiltrated with *A. tumefaciens* strains harboring different combinations of CFP-TCP14, CFP-ORA, and YFP-JAZ8 fusion protein constructs, and CFP-TCP14 and YFP, CFP-ORA and YFP, and CFP and YFP-JAZ8 were cotransformed as negative controls. Pictures were taken after 60 to 72 hours of incubation at 23℃. Three independent transfection experiments were performed. Scale bars, 5 μm. (**D**) LUC complementation assay to detect the pairwise interactions between AaTCP14, AaORA, and AaJAZ8. AaJAZ8 was fused to the C-terminal fragment of LUC (Cluc-JAZ8), and AaTCP14 and AaORA were fused to the N-terminal fragment of LUC (TCP14-Nluc and ORA-Nluc). LUC activity of Cluc-JAZ8 and Nluc was set to 1. Three independent transfection experiments were performed. The data represent the means±SD of three independent experiments. ** $P<0.01$, Student's *t* test. (**E**) Co-IP analysis of TCP14-GFP, ORA-Flag, and JAZ8-Flag in *N. benthamiana* leaves. Total protein extracts from *N. benthamiana* leaves infiltrated with *A. tumefaciens* harboring TCP14-GFP, ORA-Flag, and JAZ8-Flag fusion protein constructs were immunoprecipitated with anti-GFP antibody. The coimmunoprecipitated proteins were detected by anti-Flag antibody. Similar results were obtained in three independent experiments. (**F**) Colocalization of TCP14-nYFP, ORA-cYFP, and CFP-JAZ8 in the same NBs in *N. benthamiana* leaves. Colocalization of TCP14-nYFP, ORA-cYFP, and CFP was used as the negative control. After *A. tumefaciens* infiltration, pictures were taken after 60 to 72 hours of incubation at 23℃. Three independent transfection experiments were performed. Scale bars, 5 μm. IB, immunoblotting.

and AaORA, but truncated versions of AaJAZ8 (AaJAZ8ΔZIM) that lacked the ZIM domain could not (Fig. S9B).

Subsequently, Co-IP assays were performed to examine the interactions between all three proteins. When AaORA-Flag and AaJAZ8-Flag were coexpressed with AaTCP14-GFP in *N. benthamiana* leaf cells, both AaORA and AaJAZ8 were coimmunoprecipitated with AaTCP14 (Fig. 6E). To further explore the interaction between AaJAZ8 and the AaTCP14-AaORA complex, we transiently coexpressed AaTCP14-nYFP and AaORA-cYFP with CFP, and strong YFP fluorescent signals corresponding to reconstituted YFP were observed uniformly throughout the nucleus (Fig. 6F). However, when AaTCP14-nYFP and AaORA-cYFP were coexpressed with AaJAZ8-CFP, we found that the reconstituted YFP colocalized with AaJAZ8 in the same NBs (Fig. 6F) in *N. benthamiana* leaf cells, suggesting that AaJAZ8 brings the AaTCP14-AaORA complex to the NBs.

To gain more insight into the interactions between AaTCP14, AaJAZ8, and AaORA, we mapped the domains of AaORA that interact with AaTCP14 and AaJAZ8. We found that AaORAΔN1, which contains only the C terminus of AaORA, was capable of interacting with AaTCP14, but truncated versions of AaORA (AaORAΔC1, AaORAΔC2, and AaORAMC) that lacked the C-terminal domain could not (Fig. S9C). However, the N-terminal or C-terminal domain of AaORA alone was sufficient for interacting with full-length AaJAZ8 (Fig. S9C). These results suggest that AaORA uses different domains for the AaTCP14-AaORA and AaJAZ8-AaORA interactions.

AaJAZ8 attenuates the binding between AaTCP14 and AaORA  To investigate whether AaJAZ8 regulates the interaction between AaTCP14 and AaORA, we performed Y3H assays. When all three proteins were coexpressed in yeast cells, there was a significant reduction in growth density on selective medium (SD/-T/-L/-H/-A/-M) compared with yeast cells coexpressing only AaTCP14 and AaORA (Fig. 7A). β-Galactosidase (β-gal) activity assays further demonstrated that AaJAZ8 substantially repressed AaTCP14-AaORA interaction (Fig. 7B). These results were independently verified by a competitive LUC complementation assay, where the AaJAZ8-Flag fusion protein was coexpressed with split LUC-tagged AaTCP14 and AaORA proteins in *N. benthamiana* leaf cells. Compared with the Cluc-Flag (Cluc: C-terminal fragment of LUC) negative control, AaJAZ8-Flag significantly reduced the relative LUC activity generated by the interaction between AaTCP14-Nluc and Cluc-AaORA in living cells (Fig. 7C), indicating that AaJAZ8 inhibited the AaTCP14-AaORA interaction.

Next, deletion analysis was performed to map the domain of AaTCP14 that is responsible for the interaction with AaORA and AaJAZ8. Y2H assays showed that truncated versions of AaTCP14 that include the C terminus, TCP14ΔN1 and TCP14ΔN2, interacted with AaORA and AaJAZ8 (Fig. 7D). In contrast, truncated proteins that lacked the C terminus, TCP14ΔC1, TCP14ΔC2, and TCP14MC, were unable to interact with AaORA or AaJAZ8 (Fig. 7D), indicating that the C-terminal domain of AaTCP14 is necessary and sufficient for interaction with AaORA and AaJAZ8. Collectively, these results suggest that AaJAZ8 serves as a competitor of AaORA binding to the C terminus of AaTCP14 and thereby prevents the interaction of AaTCP14 and AaORA.

AaJAZ8 represses the transcriptional activation activity of the AaTCP14-AaORA complex  It is well known that JAZ repressors have a negative effect on the transcriptional function of their targets, and both AaTCP14 and AaORA are targets of AaJAZ8 (Fig. 6). To test whether AaJAZ8 affects the transcriptional activation activity of the AaTCP14-AaORA complex, we performed dual-LUC assays in the presence or absence of MeJA in *N. benthamiana* leaf cells (Fig. 7E). In the absence of MeJA, we found that AaTCP14, AaORA, and AaTCP14-AaORA increased the promoter activity of *DBR2*. However, coexpression with AaJAZ8 significantly decreased the promoter activity of *DBR2* in the presence of all tested combinations of AaTCP14, AaORA, and AaTCP14-AaORA, demonstrating that AaJAZ8 represses the transcriptional activation activity of AaTCP14 and AaORA. Because AaJAZ8 attenuates the interaction between AaTCP14 and AaORA (Fig. 7, A to C), these results support the notion that AaJAZ8 represses the transcriptional activation activity of the AaTCP14-AaORA complex at least in part through inhibiting the interaction between AaTCP14 and AaORA.

In the presence of MeJA, the activation of the *DBR2* promoter by AaTCP14, AaORA, and the AaTCP14-AaORA complex increased. Application of MeJA suppressed the inhibitory effect of AaJAZ8 by triggering its degradation through the 26S proteasome (Fig. 7E and Fig. S8C), suggesting that JA can reverse the AaJAZ8-mediated interference with the transcriptional function of AaTCP14 and AaORA. In accordance with these results, the *AaTCP14* overexpression lines had higher levels of JA-induced artemisinin accumulation compared with *A. annua* plants transformed with the empty vector (Fig. S10A), while the *AaTCP14* antisense lines had lower levels of JA-induced artemisinin accumulation compared with *A. annua* plants transformed with the empty vector (Fig. S10B). These results indicate that the transcriptional function of the AaTCP14-AaORA complex is negatively regulated by AaJAZ8 through its disruption of AaORA and AaTCP14 interaction and also demonstrate that JA mediates artemisinin biosynthesis via the AaORA-AaTCP14 complex.

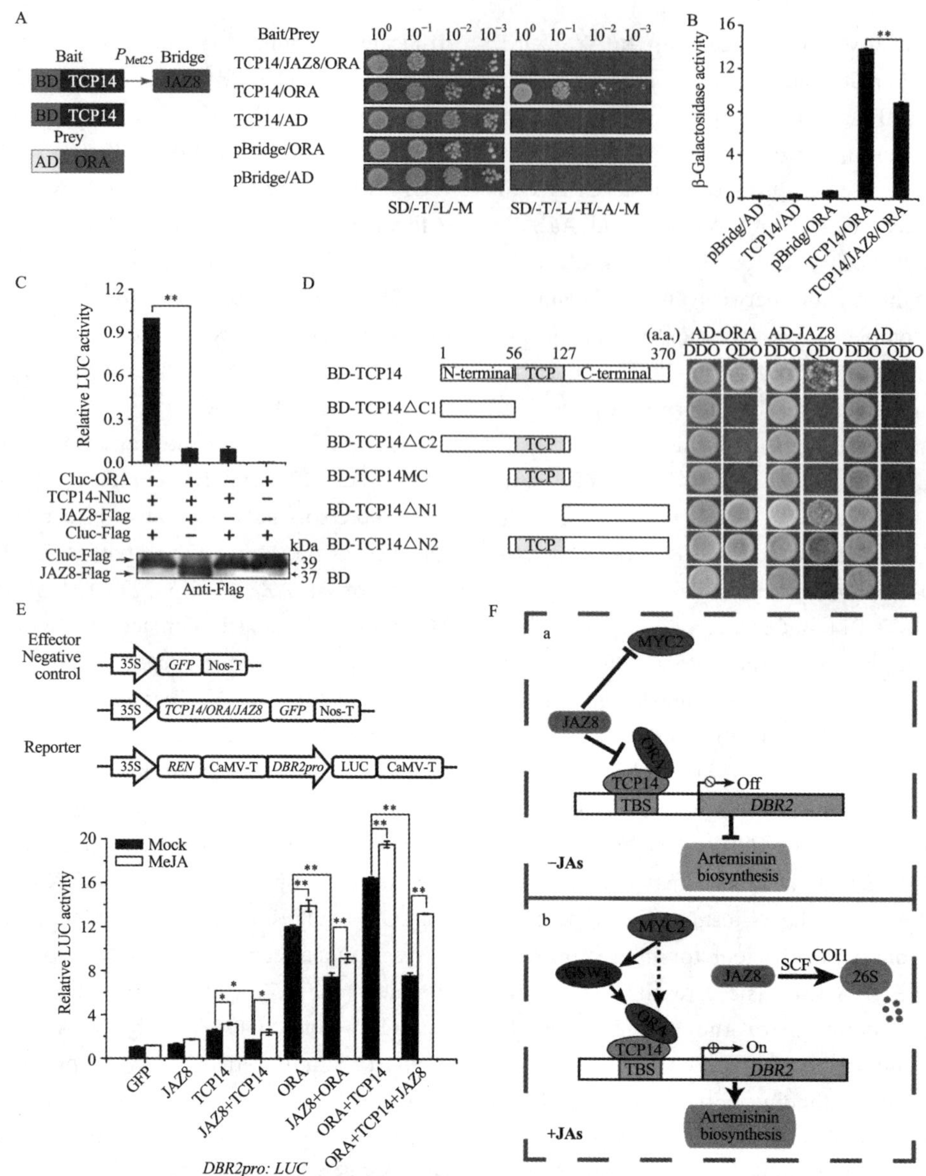

**Fig. 7 AaJAZ8 interferes with the interaction between AaORA and AaTCP14 and attenuates the transcriptional activation activity of AaTCP14 and AaORA**

(**A**) Y3H assays of the influence of JAZ8 on TCP14-ORA interaction. Left, schematic representation of the bait and prey constructs used in Y3H assays. ORA was fused with the activation domain (AD), and TCP14 was fused with the binding domain (BD). $P_{Met25}$ is an inducible promoter that drives the expression of the bridge protein, JAZ8. Right, yeast cells harboring bait and prey plasmids were grown on two types of selective media, SD/-Trp/-Leu/-Met (SD/-T/-L/-M) and SD/-Trp/-Leu/-His/-Ade/-Met (SD/-T/-L/-H/-A/-M), and pictures were taken after 4 days of incubation at 30℃. The different dilutions, $10^0$, $10^{-1}$, $10^{-2}$, and $10^{-3}$, are shown at the top of the figure. The Y3H assays were repeated three times, and representative results are shown. (**B**) β-Gal activities of yeast in (A) were measured in the presence or absence of JAZ8. The promoter driving *JAZ8* expression was suppressed by methionine. The data represent the means±SD of three replicates from three independent experiments. Student's *t* test, $^{**}P<0.01$. The β-gal activity assays were repeated three times, and similar results were obtained. (**C**) LUC complementation assay showing that JAZ8 inhibits TCP14-ORA interaction. The LUC activities of Cluc-ORA, TCP14-Nluc, and Cluc-Flag were set to 1. The data represent the means±SD of three replicates from three independent experiments. $^{**}P<0.01$, Student's *t* test. The bottom panel shows a Western blot of proteins isolated from *N. benthamiana* cells. JAZ8-Flag and Cluc-Flag fusion proteins were detected using anti-Flag antibody. Three independent transfection experiments were performed. (**D**) Y2H analysis showing the interactions between ORA, JAZ8, and full-length and truncated versions of TCP14. Left, schematic representations of the truncated TCP14 proteins used in this experiment. Numbers indicate the amino acid (a.a.) positions of the truncated TCP14 variants. The location of the TCP domain is indicated by a yellow box. Right, transformed yeast cells were grown on the selective medium, QDO, and the control medium, DDO, and pictures were taken after 4 days of incubation at 30℃. (**E**) Dual-LUC experiment showing that MeJA treatment partially recovers the activation of the *DBR2* promoter by AaTCP14 and AaORA in the presence of AaJAZ8. The LUC/REN ratio of GFP in the mock treatment was set as 1. Three independent transfection experiments were performed. The data represent the means±SD of three replicates from three independent experiments. $^{*}P<0.05$, $^{**}P<0.01$, Student's *t* test. (**F**) A working model depicting how JA signaling regulates the *DBR2* promoter via interactions between TCP14-ORA and JAZ8. (**a**) In the absence of JA, JAZ8 interacts with both TCP14 and ORA and disrupts the TCP14-ORA complex. This attenuates the transcriptional activation activity of the TCP14-ORA complex at the *DBR2* promoter, decreasing artemisinin biosynthesis. In addition, JAZ8 interacts with MYC2 and may suppress MYC2-mediated artemisinin biosynthesis. (**b**) In the presence of JA, JAZ8 is recognized by COI1 (the JA receptor) and degraded by the 26S proteasome. In the absence of JAZ8, the ORA and TCP14 proteins form a TCP14-ORA complex and synergistically activate the *DBR2* promoter, enhancing artemisinin biosynthesis. In addition, the degradation of JAZ8 releases MYC2, and MYC2 directly or indirectly activates the expression of its target gene *GSW1* and the downstream gene *ORA* to enhance JA-regulated artemisinin biosynthesis. Solid arrow, direct regulation. Broken line arrow, hypothetical direct links. T-bars, negative interactions. 26S, 26S proteasome.

## 3 DISCUSSION

Malaria is a global health problem, with 216 million new cases and 445,000 deaths observed worldwide in 2016. Artemisinin and its derivatives can rapidly kill *Plasmodium* parasites, thereby treating malaria efficiently. However, current artemisinin production is not sufficient to meet global needs. The artemisinin biosynthetic pathways have been well elucidated and involve four key enzymes, ADS, CYP71AV1, DBR2, and ALDH1. JA enhances artemisinin content by both elevating the expression levels of these key enzymes and increasing the number of GSTs. Although JA-responsive transcription factors regulate the activities of *ADS*, *CYP71AV1*, and *DBR2*, the exact mechanism of how these genes interact with the JA pathway is far from being completely understood. Therefore, identification and characterization of JA-responsive protein complexes and transcriptional networks that regulate the expression of these four key enzymes are important for understanding how artemisinin metabolism is regulated. In a previous report, the trichome-specific AP2/ERF transcription factor AaORA was found to be a positive regulator of the *ADS*, *CYP71AV1*, and *DBR2* genes. However, the mechanism by which AaORA regulates JA-mediated artemisinin biosynthesis has remained unclear. In this study, we identified a novel interactor of AaORA that functions in the regulation of artemisinin biosynthesis. AaTCP14 and AaORA interact in vitro and in vivo. Moreover, AaTCP14 directly binds to and activates the *DBR2* and *ALDH1* promoters. AaTCP14 and AaORA synergistically interact to control the expression of these two genes, and the regulation of *DBR2* and *ALDH1* expression by AaORA is at least partially dependent on AaTCP14. Moreover, the repressor AaJAZ8 interacts with both AaTCP14 and AaORA and disrupts the AaTCP14-AaORA complex, which results in decreased *DBR2* promoter activity. JA induces AaJAZ8 degradation and derepresses the AaTCP14-AaORA complex to promote artemisinin biosynthesis. Thus, we propose that plants have evolved an intricate mechanism for regulation of specialized metabolism through the JA signaling pathway.

AaTCP14 belongs to the class I TCP gene family, members of which are involved in a myriad of plant developmental processes, hormone signaling, and plant metabolism. Here, we found that AaTCP14 is JA responsive and directly activates the *DBR2* and *ALDH1* promoters in vivo and in vitro (Figs. 2E and 4). Furthermore, the overexpression and down-regulation of *AaTCP14* activated and repressed, respectively, the expression of artemisinin biosynthetic genes (Fig. 3, B and E), transcription factors in positively regulating artemisinin biosynthesis, and JA biosynthetic genes (Fig. S5). The expression levels of these genes may ultimately contribute to the increase and decrease of the artemisinin content in *AaTCP14* overexpression and antisense transgenic plants, respectively (Fig. 3, C and F), indicating that AaTCP14 could be used for engineering artemisinin biosynthesis in *A. annua*.

Notably, AaTCP14 directly binds to the GGTCCCAC or GGCCCCAC sites in the *DBR2* and *ALDH1* promoters, respectively (Fig. 4). Both of these sites are consensus binding sites (GGNCCCAC) of class Ⅰ TCP family transcription factors, suggesting that other members of the class Ⅰ TCP family may also have the potential to regulate artemisinin biosynthesis by interacting with similar binding sites. Thus, further investigation is needed to determine whether other members of the TCP family are also involved in regulating artemisinin biosynthesis. In addition, we also found a putative class Ⅱ TBS in the *AaGSW1* promoter (GTGGTCCC, −2 098 bp upstream of ATG), which partially overlaps with a putative class Ⅰ TBS (GGTCC, −2 096 bp upstream of ATG), indicating that artemisinin biosynthesis may be coregulated by both class Ⅰ and class Ⅱ TCP proteins. In *Arabidopsis*, class Ⅰ and class Ⅱ TCPs are known to coregulate SOC1-dependent flowering at multiple levels. However, the precise mechanism by which class Ⅰ and class Ⅱ TCP proteins coregulate artemisinin biosynthesis awaits further investigation.

In plants, numerous cellular functions are often highly coordinated through protein-protein interactions. TCP family members are known to synergistically or antagonistically interact with a variety of proteins to regulate a wide spectrum of biological processes. For example, the ubiquitin receptors DA1, DAR1, and DAR2 modulate AtTCP14/15 stability to regulate endoreduplication in *Arabidopsis*. AtTCP3 interacts with R2R3-MYB (myeloblastosis) proteins and enhances their transcriptional activation activity, leading to the promotion of flavonoid biosynthesis in *Arabidopsis*. AtTCP14 and DELLA regulate plant height by regulating GA (gibberellin) signaling in florescence shoot apex in *Arabidopsis*. In this case, DELLA binds to the DNA binding domain of AtTCP14 and blocks its ability to bind DNA. Intriguingly, we found that AaORA is an important interaction partner of AaTCP14 based on several lines of evidence. First, AaTCP14 and AaORA interact in vitro and in vivo (Fig. 1). In addition, AaTCP14 and AaORA share similar expression patterns (Fig. 2, A and E). Moreover, AaTCP14 and AaORA synergistically regulate the activity of the *DBR2* and *ALDH1* promoters (Fig. 5, A to C) and promote their expression (Fig. 5E). As a result, artemisinin content is higher in *AaTCP14-AaORA* co-overexpression lines compared to *AaTCP14* overexpression lines (Fig. 5F). The regulation of *DBR2* and *ALDH1* by AaORA at least partially depends on AaTCP14 (Fig. 5, G to K). Biochemical analysis suggests that AaTCP14 provides the DNA binding ability, while AaORA has strong transcriptional activation activity (Fig. 4 and Fig. S1B). Thus, these paired transcription factors act together to increase the artemisinin content in *A. annua* plants.

AaORA has an AP2 DNA binding domain, and its close homolog ORCA3 in *C. roseus* can specifically bind and activate the promoter of the TIA biosynthetic gene *STR* (*strictosidine synthase*). In our study, in addition to *DBR2* and *ALDH1*, AaORA also activated the promoters of *ADS* and *CYP71AV1* (Fig. S1B). However, AaTCP14 failed to activate the *ADS* or *CYP71AV1* promoters (Fig. 4B). This indicates that AaORA may also regulate artemisinin biosynthesis independently of AaTCP14. Consistent with this notion, we found that additional positive regulators of artemisinin biosynthesis also interact with AaORA in a Y2H screen, suggesting that AaORA might promote artemisinin biosynthesis in *A. annua* through interactions with other proteins. The precise mechanism by which AaORA controls artemisinin biosynthesis will require further investigation.

JA has been found to activate artemisinin production. Both *AaTCP14* and *AaORA* are JA responsive. Work in *C. roseus* has revealed that CrMYC2 directly activates the promoter of *CrORCA3*, a homolog of *AaORA*, to regulate alkaloid biosynthesis. Similarly, AaMYC2, a central transcription factor acting downstream of the JA signaling pathway, directly activates the expression of the JA-responsive gene *AaGSW1*, and AaGSW1 activates the expression of *AaORA* and promotes JA-mediated artemisinin biosynthesis (Fig. 7F). Thus, it is possible that AaMYC2 positively regulates *AaORA* expression in both a direct and an indirect manner. The expression levels of *AaMYC2* were up-regulated and down-regulated in *AaTCP14* overexpression and antisense transgenic plants, respectively (Fig. S5, B and J), indicating that *AaMYC2* expression is regulated by AaTCP14. This may be a consequence of the regulation of JA biosynthesis by AaTCP14, as AaTCP14 activates the expression of the JA biosynthetic genes *AaAOC* and *AaOPR3* (Fig. S5, F and G). Thus, a positive feedback loop between JA signaling and AaTCP14 may allow rapid response to JA for biological processes controlled by AaTCP14, such as artemisinin biosynthesis. Given that most of the abovementioned JA biosynthetic and JA-responsive genes have been reported to promote artemisinin biosynthesis, AaTCP14 might positively regulate artemisinin biosynthesis by directly or indirectly influencing the JA biosynthesis and signaling pathways.

We uncovered another connection between the AaTCP14-AaORA complex and the JA signaling pathway by identifying AaJAZ8 as an interacting partner for both AaTCP14 and AaORA. JAZ proteins were identified as targets of the $SCF^{COI1}$ complex and repress diverse JA-regulated plant responses by interacting with and attenuating the activity of their downstream transcription factors. JAZ1 affects the interactions between bHLHs [GL3 (Glabra 3), EGL3 (Enhancer of GL3), and TT8 (Transparent Testa 8)] and MYBs [MYB75 and GL1 (Glabra 1)] proteins by directly interacting with these proteins and thus regulates JA-mediated anthocyanin accumulation and trichome initiation in *Arabidopsis*. A recent study demonstrated that AtJAZ3 and AtTCP14 do not directly interact, but the *Pseudomonas syringae* type III effector HopBB1 bonds with both AtJAZ3 and AtTCP14 to bring the complex to the proteasome for protein degradation. This process releases the subset of JA responsive genes regulated by AtTCP14 to modulate pathogen virulence in *Arabidopsis*. Unlike AtJAZ3-HopBB1-AtTCP14, we uncovered direct interactions between AaJAZ8, AaTCP14, and AaORA. AaJAZ8 directly interacts with the AaTCP14-AaORA complex, and this modulates the transcriptional activation of key genes that encode artemisinin biosynthesis enzymes by AaTCP14-AaORA in a JA-responsive manner (Figs. 6 and 7). In JA-elicited cells, AaJAZ8 is degraded, which allows the formation of the AaTCP14-AaORA complex to activate *DBR2* expression (Fig. S8C and Fig. 7E). The interference of the AaTCP14-AaORA complex by AaJAZ8 may be due to the competition of binding between AaORA and AaJAZ8 to the C terminus of AaTCP14 (Fig. 7, A to D). Although we found that only AaJAZ8 (out of nine AaJAZ proteins tested) could interact with AaTCP14, we cannot rule out the possibility that these AaJAZ proteins interact with other AaTCP proteins. The JA-responsive regulation of artemisinin biosynthesis reveals a delicate balance wherein plants were involved to cope with the changing environment. Specialized metabolites, such as artemisinin, are already known to affect plant growth when they overaccumulate; thus, plants need to fine-tune the production of these metabolites, generating the appropriate amount to deal with the biotic stresses with less penalty of growth.

In recent years, it has been found that some JAZ proteins fulfill their functions by forming specific tripartite complexes. In *Arabidopsis*, AtJAZs repress the transcriptional activation activity of the AtMYC-AtMYB complex by competing with AtMYBs (MYB28, MYB29, MYB76, MYB34, MYB51, and MYB122) for interaction with AtMYCs (MYC2, MYC3, and MYC4) to regulate glucosinolate biosynthesis. AtJAZs also interact with and repress the AtbHLH-AtMYB complex to control stamen and pollen development. The AtJAZ-AtMYC-AtMYB and AtJAZ-AtbHLH-AtMYB complexes are similar to the AaJAZ8-AaTCP14-AaORA complex in that JAZs repress the transcriptional activation activities of these complexes to regulate downstream target genes, suggesting that the use of

JA signaling to regulate processes, such as specialized metabolism, is a common strategy. Recent work showed that injury induces $Ca^{2+}$/calmodulin-dependent phosphorylation of AtJAV1, which disintegrates the AtJAV1-AtJAZ8-AtWRKY51 complex and de-represses JA biosynthesis in *Arabidopsis*. This complex is distinct from the AtJAZ-AtMYC-AtMYB, AtJAZ-AtbHLH-AtMYB, and AaJAZ8-AaTCP14-AaORA complexes. In the AtJAV1-AtJAZ8-AtWRKY51 complex, AtJAZ8 enhances the repression of the *AOS* promoter by both AtJAV1 and AtWRKY51, but in the case of AtJAZ-AtMYC-AtMYB, AtJAZ-AtbHLH-AtMYB, and AaJAZ8-AaTCP14-AaORA, JAZ represses the transcriptional activation activity of AtMYC-AtMYB, AtbHLH-AtMYB, and AaTCP14-AaORA, suggesting the common usage of JAZ for different transcriptional regulation purposes.

Do JAZs change the DNA binding ability of their downstream genes? In *Arabidopsis*, DELLAs interact with the AtTCP14 DNA recognition domain and block AtTCP14 activity by keeping it from binding to its targets (*32*). By contrast, AaJAZ8 interacts with the C-terminal region of AaTCP14, and not the DNA recognition domain; hence, it is unlikely that AaJAZ8 alters the DNA binding ability of AaTCP14 (Fig. S7C).

On the basis of our current findings, we propose a working model for JA regulation of artemisinin biosynthesis. Briefly, in the absence of JA, AaJAZ8 interacts with both AaTCP14 and AaORA and disrupts the AaTCP14-AaORA complex. This attenuates the transcriptional activation function of AaTCP14-AaORA and decreases activation of the *DBR2* promoter (Fig. 7F), thus impeding artemisinin biosynthesis. By contrast, in the presence of JA, AaJAZ8 is recognized by COI (the JA receptor) and degraded by the 26S proteasome. The released AaTCP14 and AaORA proteins and the AaTCP14-AaORA complex synergistically activate the *DBR2* promoter to enhance artemisinin biosynthesis (Fig. 7F). Given that AaMYC2 positively regulates artemisinin biosynthesis, potentially by activating *AaORA* expression in a direct and indirect manner (*17*, *18*, *25*), and that JAZ repressors, including AaJAZ8, interact with AaMYC2 (Fig. S9A), it is possible that AaJAZ8 may function at different transcriptional regulatory layers to fine-tune artemisinin biosynthesis in response to JA signaling. This model provides a foundation for deepening our understanding of the molecular mechanisms of JA regulation of specialized metabolism in plants.

Together, our data indicate that JA enhances artemisinin biosynthesis in *A. annua* through three mechanisms: ① increasing the transcriptional activation of the *DBR2* promoter by AaTCP14, AaORA, and the AaTCP14-AaORA complex. ② degrading the repressor protein AaJAZ8, thereby freeing AaTCP14, AaORA, and the AaTCP14-AaORA complex to activate the transcription of *DBR2*. ③ facilitating the formation of AaTCP14-AaORA, which, in turn, enhances *DBR2* promoter activity (Fig. 7F).

## 4 MATERIALS AND METHODS

Plant materials and hormone treatments  The high-artemisinin cultivar of *A. annua* L., named "Huhao 1," which originated in Chongqing and was further subjected to several years of selection in Shanghai, was used for all *A. annua*-related assays. For in vitro culture, seeds of *A. annua* were first surface sterilized in 70% ethanol for 3 min and washed three times with sterile water. This was followed by sterilization in 20% sodium hypochlorite solution for 10 min and then five washes with sterile water. These seeds were sown on Murashige and Skoog medium (Sigma-Aldrich, USA) with 3% sucrose and 0.6% agar (pH 5.7). *A. annua* and *N. benthamiana* plants were grown in pots at 23±2 ℃ under a 16-hour light/8-hour dark photoperiod.

For MeJA treatment, 10-day-old *A. annua* seedlings were sprayed with 100 μmol/L MeJA (Sigma-Aldrich, USA). For the mock treatment, seedlings were sprayed with 0.1% ethanol. Seedling samples were collected at 0, 1, 3, 6, 9, 12, and 24 hours after treatment. To analyze artemisinin content in *AaTCP14* transgenic plants after MeJA treatment, the 2-month-old cutting propagations of *AaTCP14* overexpression, antisense, and control plants (*A. annua* plants transformed with the empty vector) were sprayed with 100 μmol/L MeJA or 0.1% ethanol (mock treatment) and sampled at 48 hours for artemisinin extraction.

RNA extraction and qRT-PCR  Leaves of 3-month-old *A. annua* at different positions (labeled in Fig. 2B) and different tissues of 4-month-old *A. annua*, including roots, stems, flowers, shoots, buds, leaves, and trichomes, were harvested. To analyze the expression of *TCP14*, *ADS*, *CYP71AV1*, *DBR2*, *ALDH1*, *WRKY1*, *MYC2*, *GSW1*, *ORA*, *AOS*, *AOC*, *OPR3*, and *OPCL1* in *AaTCP14* overexpression lines and *AaTCP14* antisense lines; the expression of *TCP14*, *ORA*, *DBR2*, and *ALDH1* in *AaTCP14*-*AaORA* co-overexpression lines and *AaTCP14* antisense-*AaORA* overexpression lines; the expression of *ORA*, *DBR2*, and *ALDH1* in *AaORA* overexpression lines; and the expression of *JAZ8*, *ADS*, *CYP71AV1*, *DBR2*, and *ALDH1* in *AaJAZ8* overexpression lines, the leaves of 3-month-old transgenic plants were collected. *A. annua* plants transformed with empty vector (control plants, labeled as vector) and WT plants were used as controls. RNA was extracted using the total plant RNA Extraction Kit (Tiangen Biotech, China) according to the manufacturer's instructions. cDNA was synthesized from 1.0 μg of total RNA using the PrimeScript 1 st Strand cDNA Synthesis Kit

(Takara, Japan) according to the manufacturer's instructions. The expression levels of genes were normalized to the expression of *A. annua Actin*. qRT-PCR analysis was performed as previously described (*22*). All primers used for qRT-PCR are listed in table S1.

Co-IP assays and degradation of the AaJAZ8 protein For Co-IP assays with two and three proteins, the full-length coding sequences of *AaTCP14*, *AaORA*, and *AaJAZ8* were cloned from the *A. annua* meristem cDNA library and inserted into the pCambia 1300-GFP or pCambia1300-Flag vectors to yield the following constructs: 1300-AaTCP14-GFP, 1300-AaORA-Flag, and 1300-AaJAZ8-Flag with GFP or Flag tag, respectively (primer information is provided in table S1). Five-week-old *N. benthamiana* leaves were transformed by injection of *Agrobacterium* strain GV3101 cells harboring the indicated combinations of 1300-AaORA-Flag, 1300-AaTCP14-GFP, and/or 1300-AaJAZ8-Flag. After incubation at 23 ℃ for 72 hours, the leaves were ground to a fine powder in liquid nitrogen and resuspended in extraction buffer[50 mmol/L tris-HCl(pH 7.5), 150 mmol/L NaCl, 1 mmol/L EDTA (pH 8.0), 0.2% Triton X-100, and protease inhibitors including 100 μmol/L Pefabloc (Sigma-Aldrich, USA), 100 μmol/L cocktail(Roche, Switzerland), and 50 μmol/L MG132 (Calbiochem, USA)]. After incubation on ice for 20 min, the protein suspensions were centrifuged at 14,000 r/min for 10 min. For two-protein Co-IP, the supernatant was incubated with 2 μL of anti-Flag antibody (Sigma-Aldrich, USA) for 1 hour at 4 ℃. For three-protein Co-IP, the supernatant was incubated with 15 μL of anti-GFP antibody (GenScript, Nanjing, China) for 1 hour at 4℃. Next, 20 μL of prewashed Protein G Sepharose (GE Healthcare, Amersham, UK) was added, and the mix-ture was incubated for 2 hours at 4 ℃. Then, the immunoprecipitates were washed four times with extraction buffer and resuspended with 2×SDS sample buffer [500 mmol/L tris-HCl, 12.5% SDS, 25% glycerol, bromophenol blue (0.33 mg/mL), and 10% 2-mercaptoethanol]. Subsequently, the samples were boiled at 100℃ for 10 min and centrifuged for 10 s before they were separated by 12% SDS-PAGE (polyacrylamide gel electrophoresis). Proteins were transferred to polyvinylidene fluoride (PVDF) membranes and detected using anti-GFP (Abmart, China) or anti-Flag antibody (Sigma-Aldrich, USA).

To evaluate the degradation of AaJAZ8, 5-week-old *N. benthamiana* leaves were transformed by injection of *Agrobacterium* strain GV3101 cells harboring 1300-AaJAZ8-Flag. After incubation at 23℃ for 48 hours, the leaves were pretreated with or without 100 μmol/L MG132 (Calbiochem, USA) for 1 hour and then treated with 50 μmol/L MeJA for 0, 0.5, 1, 2, and 4 hours. The JAZ8-Flag proteins were extracted and detected using anti-Flag antibody (Sigma-Aldrich, USA).

Dual-LUC assays For the transient transcriptional activity assays in *N. benthamiana* leaves, the full-length coding sequences of *AaORA*, *AaTCP14*, and *AaJAZ8* were inserted into the pCambia1300-GFP vector (effectors), and the promoter regions upstream of the start codons of *UBQ* (a homolog of *AtUBQ10*) (~1.7 kb), *ADS* (~ 2.9 kb), *CYP71AV1* (~1.2 kb), *DBR2* (~2.3 kb), and *ALDH1* (~2.3 kb) were ligated into the pGREENII0800-LUC vector (reporters). Infiltration and detection were performed as described previously with a few modifications. The *Renilla* LUC (REN) gene in pGREENII0800-LUC was used as an internal control. Empty pCambia1300-GFP was used as the negative control for the effector. GV3101 strains harboring indicated combinations of effectors and reporters were cotransformed into 5-week-old *N. benthamiana* leaves. Plants were incubated for 72 hours at 23 ℃ to allow expression of the transgenes. For hormone treatment in dual-LUC assays, *N. benthamiana* leaves were treated with 50 μmol/L MeJA or 0.05% ethanol (mock treatment) for another 4 hours before the sample was collected. For the transient transcriptional activity assays in *A. annua* protoplasts, protoplasts from 14-day-old WT and *AaTCP14* antisense *A. annua* mesophyll cells were prepared and transfected, as previously described. The reporters and effectors were cotransformed into the WT and *AaTCP14* antisense protoplasts in the indicated combinations, and after transformation, the transformants were cultured in the light for 8 hours. The reporters (*DBR2* and *ALDH1* promoters) were used at 6 μg per transfection, and effectors (GFP and GFP-AaORA) were used at 10 μg per transfection. All experiments were repeated at least three times for each plasmid combination. Firefly LUC and REN activities were analyzed using commercial dual-LUC reaction reagents (Promega, USA) according to the manufacturer's instructions. The LUC activity was normalized to REN activity, and the relative LUC/REN ratios were used to represent the activity of the promoter. For each combination, LUC/REN ratios from at least three independent transformations were determined. All primers used for these constructs are listed in table S1.

Y1H assays For Y1H experiments, the full-length coding sequences of *AaORA*, *AabZIP1*, and *AaTCP14* were amplified using the primers in table S1 and ligated into the pB42AD vector. The promoter sequences of *ADS*, *CYP71AV1*, *DBR2*, and *ALDH1*; three tandem copies of the *E1* motif from *ADS* promoter; the *D1* and *D2* motifs from the *DBR2* promoter; and the *A1*, *A2*, and *A3* motifs from the *ALDH1* promoter were ligated into the pLacZ vector. Various combinations of pB42AD-AabZIP1, pB42AD-AaORA, and pB42AD-AaTCP14 and different promoters and

DNA motifs were cotransformed into the yeast strain EGY48. Combinations of pB42AD and different promoters and DNA motifs were also cotransformed into the yeast strain EGY48 as negative controls. The transformants were cultivated on SD/-Trp/-Ura plates, and positive clones were transferred to and grown on SD/-Trp/-Ura plates with X-gal for blue color development. All primers used to amplify promoters and DNA motifs are listed in table S1.

Y2H assays The *A. annua* cDNA library for Y2H experiments was constructed by OE BioTech (Shanghai, China) by cloning cDNA synthesized from the mRNAs of the youngest leaves and meristem of *A. annua* into the prey vector pGADT7 (Takara, Japan). The fulll-ength coding sequence of *AaORA* and truncated sequences including *AaORAΔC1*, *AaORAΔC2*, *AaORAMC*, *AaORAΔN1*, and *AaORAΔN2* were amplified by PCR using the indicated primers (table S1) and inserted into the bait vector pGKBT7 (Takara, Japan). These recombinant constructs were introduced into the yeast strain AH109 and tested for autoactivation and toxicity. Because of the strong autoactivation of full-length *AaORA*, we used *AaORAΔN1* (C terminus of AaORA) for Y2H screening assays, which were performed according to the Matchmaker Gold Y2H system's user manual (*Yeast Protocols Handbook*; Takara, Japan).

For additional Y2H experiments to test for specific interactions and to map the protein domain of AaTCP14, AaJAZ8, or AaORA involved in paired interactions, the full-length coding sequences of *AaORA*, *AaMYC2*, and *AaTCP14* and truncated sequences including *AaTCP14ΔC1*, *AaTCP14ΔC2*, *AaTCP14MC*, *AaTCP14ΔN1*, and *AaTCP14ΔN2* were amplified using the listed primers (table S1). In addition, the full-length coding sequences of the *JAZ* genes (*AaJAZ1*, *AaJAZ2*, *AaJAZ3*, *AaJAZ4*, *AaJAZ5*, *AaJAZ6*, *AaJAZ7*, and *AaJAZ9*), AaJAZ8, and the truncated variants *AaJAZ8ΔZIM* and *AaJAZ8Δjas* were amplified using the listed primers (table S1). All the aforementioned amplicons were cloned into the pGADT7 or pGKBT7 vectors. Various combinations of plasmids were cotransformed into the yeast strain AH109 according to the manufacturer's instructions (Takara, Japan), and bait-only or prey-only controls were tested with empty pGADT7 or pGBKT7. The transformants were cultivated on DDO plates, and positive clones were transferred to and grown on TDO and/or QDO plates. Yeast cells were photographed after 4 days of growth at 30 ℃ to record growth. All experiments were repeated three times with similar results.

Y3H assays For Y3H assays, the full-length coding sequences of *AaTCP14* and *AaJAZ8* were cloned into the pBridge vector (Takara, Japan) to create DNA binding domain fusion proteins. *AaJAZ8* was inserted into the same pBridge vector driven by the *MET25* promoter to provide Met repression. The full-length coding sequence of *AaORA* was cloned into the pGADT7 vector. Y3H assays were based on the Matchmaker GAL4 three-hybrid systems (Takara, Japan). The combinations pBridge-AaTCP14-AaJAZ8 and pGADT7-AaORA, and pBridge-AaTCP14 and pGADT7-AaORA were cotransformed into the yeast strain AH109. The recombinant vectors were transformed with empty pGADT7 or pBridge as controls. The transformants were cultivated in liquid SD/-Trp/-Leu media to $OD_{600}$ (optical density at 600 nm) = 0.6 and then diluted to different concentrations. Six-microliter dilutions of suspended yeast were plated on solid medium containing SD/-T/-L/-M and SD/-T/-L/-H/-A/-M. Yeast growth was observed after incubation for 4 days at 30 ℃. β-Gal assays were performed to quantify protein interaction according to the manufacturer's instructions (Takara, Japan), using chlorophenol red β-D-galactopyranoside (Roche, Switzerland) as the substrate. The experiments were repeated three times, and the primers used are listed in table S1.

Electrophoretic mobility shift assays For protein expression and purification, the full-length coding sequences of *AaORA*, *AaTCP14*, and *AaJAZ8* were cloned into the pCold-TF vector (Takara) to produce His-tagged fusion proteins. The pCold-AaORA, pCold-AaTCP14, and pCold-AaJAZ8 constructs were transferred into *E. coli* strain Rosetta (DE3) (TransGen Biotech, China). The empty pCold-TF vector was introduced into *E. coli* strain Rosetta (DE3) and was used as the negative control. Expression of His fusion proteins in Rosetta cells was induced by adding 0.2 mmol/L isopropyl β-D-1-thiogalactopyranoside (IPTG) to the culture medium and incubating the cells for 14 hours at 16 ℃. The fusion proteins were purified using Ni-NTA (nitrilotriacetic acid) agarose (Invitrogen, USA) according to the manufacturer's instructions.

EMSAs were performed as previously described with minor modifications using the DIG Gel Shift Kit, 2nd Generation (Roche) according to the manufacturer's instructions. For these assays, 0.5 μg of recombinant His-TF, 0.5 μg of recombinant His-AaTCP14, and 0.5, 1, 2, and 4 μg of recombinant His-AaORA and His-AaJAZ8 were used. The D2q, D2q-mutated1, D2q-mutated2, A1q, A1q-mutated1, and A1q-mutated2DNA probes from the *DBR2* and *ALDH1* promoters were synthesized by Sangon (Shanghai, China). The mutated probes were designed as previously described. The primers and probes used in the EMSAs are listed in table S1.

BiFC assays The BiFC assays were performed as previously described. For the generation of the BiFC vectors, the full-length cDNAs of *AaORA*, *AaTCP14*, and *AaJAZ8* were cloned into pEarleyGate 201-YN (N terminus of YFP) and pEarleyGate 202-YC (C terminus of YFP) to obtain AaORA-cYFP, AaORA-nYFP, AaTCP14-nYFP, and AaJAZ8-cYFP and then transformed into *Agrobacterium* strains GV3101. The indicated vector combinations were cotransformed into 5-week-old *N. benthamiana* leaves. After incubation at 23 ℃ for 60 to 72 hours, YFP signals were observed by confocal laser microscopy (Leica TCS SP5-II). Nuclei were stained with DAPI (Sigma-Aldrich, USA). Three biological repeats were conducted for all experiments. The primers are listed in table S1.

Subcellular localization and colocalization assays For subcellular localization experiments, the GV3101 strains harboring pHB-AaTCP14-YFP or pHB-YFP were transformed into 5-week-old *N. benthamiana* leaves. YFP signals were analyzed 60 to 72 hours after infiltration by confocal laser microscopy (Leica TCS SP5-II). Nuclei were stained with DAPI (Sigma-Aldrich, USA). Three biological repeats were performed to verify these results.

For two- and three-protein colocalization assays, the full-length cDNAs of *AaORA*, *AaTCP14*, and *AaJAZ8* were ligated into the pHB-CFP and pHB-YFP vectors to obtain AaORA-CFP, AaTCP14-CFP, AaJAZ8-CFP, and AaJAZ8-YFP. GV3101 strains harboring AaTCP14-CFP and AaJAZ8-YFP, AaORA-CFP and AaJAZ8-YFP, or AaTCP14-nYFP, AaORA-cYFP, and AaJAZ8-CFP were cotransformed into 5-week-old *N. benthamiana* leaves. Meanwhile, GV3101 strains harboring AaORA-CFP and YFP, AaTCP14-CFP and YFP, CFP and AaJAZ8-YFP, or AaTCP14-nYFP, AaORA-cYFP, and CFP were also transformed into 5-week-old *N. benthamiana* leaves as negative controls. After incubation at 23 ℃ for 60 to 72 hours, YFP and CFP signals were observed by confocal laser microscopy (Leica TCS SP5-II). Three biological repeats were performed to verify these results. The primers are listed in table S1.

In vitro pulldown assays For protein expression and purification, the full-length coding sequences of *AaORA* and *AaTCP14* were cloned into the pGEX4T-1 (GE Healthcare) and pCold-TF (Takara, Japan) vectors to produce GST-tagged fusion protein and His-tagged fusion protein, respectively. The pGEX4T-1-AaORA and pCold-AaTCP14 constructs were then transferred into *E. coli* strain Rosetta (DE3). Expression of GST and His fusion proteins in Rosetta cells was induced by adding 0.2 mmol/L IPTG to the culture medium and incubating the cells for 14 hours at 16 ℃. The GST-AaORA and His-AaTCP14 fusion proteins were purified according to the manufacturers' instructions using glutathione-agarose 4B (GE Healthcare) beads and Ni-NTA agarose (Invitrogen), respectively.

For the pulldown assay, equal amounts (100 μL) of purified GST or GST-AaORA and His-AaTCP14 were mixed and incubated with glutathione-agarose 4B beads for 10 hours at 4 ℃ in 250 μL of pulldown buffer [40 mmol/L Hepes-KOH (pH 7.5), 10 mmol/L KCl, 3 mmol/L $MgCl_2$, 0.4 mol/L sucrose, 1 mmol/L EDTA, 1 mmol/L dithiothreitol, 0.2% Triton X-100, and protease inhibitors] with agitation. The beads were then centrifuged at 2 000*g* for 1 min at 4 ℃ and washed five times with 1× PBS buffer [137 mmol/L NaCl, 8.1 mmol/L $Na_2HPO_4 \cdot 12H_2O$, 2.68 mmol/L KCl, 1.47 mmol/L $KH_2PO_4$, and 1 mmol/L phenylmethylsulfonyl fluoride (pH 7.4)]. Bound proteins were eluted by boiling with 5 × sample buffer, and the released proteins were separated by 12% SDS-PAGE. Proteins were transferred to PVDF membranes and detected using anti-His (Abmart, China) or anti-GST (Abmart, China) antibody.

Plant transformation and phenotype analysis The overexpression constructs pHB-AaTCP14-Flag, 1305-AaORA-GFP, pHB-AaJAZ8, and 1300-AaJAZ8Δjas (a jas-domain deletion version of *AaJAZ8* cDNA); the antisense construct pHB-ANTCP14; the co-overexpression construct 1305-AaTCP14-Myc-AaORA-GFP; and the 1305-AaTCP14 antisense-AaORA overexpression construct were transferred into *Agrobacterium tumefaciens* strain EHA105 and then used to transform *A. annua*, as previously described. The phenotype of *A. annua* plants transformed with the empty vector (control plants) and *AaTCP14* overexpression, *AaTCP14* antisense, and *AaTCP14-AaORA* co-overexpression lines were observed at the indicated times under normal conditions.

LUC complementation assay For the LUC complementation assays, the full-length coding sequences of *AaORA* and *AaTCP14* were ligated into pCAMBIA-Nluc and pCAMBIA-Cluc, respectively, and the full-length *AaJAZ8* coding sequence was ligated into pCAMBIA-Cluc. The TCP14-Nluc, ORA-Nluc, Cluc-ORA, and Cluc-JAZ8 constructs were introduced into *A. tumefaciens* strain GV3101. GV3101 strains harboring the indicated constructs were co-infiltrated into *N. benthamiana* leaves, as previously described.

For the competition LUC complementation assay, GV3101 strains harboring JAZ8-Flag, Cluc-ORA, and TCP14-Nluc were co-infiltrated into *N. benthamiana* leaves. A GV3101 strain harboring Cluc-Flag instead of JAZ8-Flag was co-infiltrated as a control. Leaf discs were taken 3 days later and ground to powder in liquid nitrogen. Then, the relative LUC activities were measured with a LUC kit (Promega, USA) according to the manufacturer's instructions (Promega, USA). The primers are listed in table S1.

GUS expression in *1391Z-proTCP14-GUS* transgenic *A. annua plants* To construct *1391Z-proTCP14-GUS*, the 1 828-bp promoter region upstream of the start codon of *AaTCP14* was amplified with specific primers (table S1) from the *A. annua* genomic DNA library and inserted into the pCambia1391Z vector. Then, the plasmids *1391Z-proTCP14-*

*GUS* and *1391Z-GUS* were introduced into *A. annua* plants using *Agrobacterium*-mediated genetic transformation, as described previously. Histochemical staining for GUS activity in transgenic plants was conducted as previously described with minor modifications. Leaves and stems were stained in a GUS staining solution [1 mmol/L 5-bromo-4-chloro-3-indolyl-β-D-glucuronic acid, 100 mmol/L $Na_2HPO_4$, 50 mmol/L $KH_2PO_4$, 10 mmol/L $Na_2EDTA$, 0.5 mmol/L $K_3Fe(CN)_6$, 0.5 mmol/L $K_4Fe(CN)_6$, and 0.1% (V/V) Triton X-100] and incubated at 37℃ for 12 to 24 hours in the dark. After GUS staining, 70% ethanol was used to remove chlorophyll. *A. annua* plants transformed with the empty vector were processed in parallel as negative controls.

Measurement of artemisinin, DHAA, and AA content Leaves collected from 3-month-old *AaTCP14* transgenic *A. annua* plants; *AaTCP14-AaORA* co-overexpression, *AaTCP14* antisense-*AaORA* overexpression, *AaORA* overexpression, and *AaJAZ8* overexpression *A. annua* plants; *A. annua* plants transformed with the empty vector; and WT plants grown in the greenhouse were dried at 50℃ overnight and then ground to powder. Dried leaf powder (0.1 g) was extracted twice with 2 ml of methanol under ultrasound for 30 min. Then, the samples were centrifuged for 5 min at 12 000 r/min, and the supernatant was filtered through a nitrocellulose filter (0.22 μmol/L). The concentrations of artemisinin, DHAA, and AA in the final samples were measured by HPLC, as described previously.

**SUPPLEMENTARY MATERIALS**

Supplementary material for this article is available at http://advances.sciencemag.org/cgi/content/full/4/11/eaas9357/DC1.

Fig. S1. A schematic diagram of the artemisinin biosynthetic pathway and its regulation in *A. annua*, and AaORA activates the *ADS*, *CYP71AV1*, *DBR2*, and *ALDH1* promoters.

Fig. S2. Y2H assay showing the regions of AaORA with autoactivation activity.

Fig. S3. Alignment of the protein sequences of AaTCP14 and 29 related proteins.

Fig. S4. Phylogenetic analysis of TCP14 proteins from *A. annua* and other plants.

Fig. S5. Relative expression levels of transcription factors positively regulating artemisinin biosynthesis and JA biosynthetic genes in *AaTCP14* transgenic plants.

Fig. S6. Characterization of *A. annua* transgenic plants.

Fig. S7. Neither AaORA nor AaJAZ8 affects the ability of AaTCP14 to bind DNA.

Fig. S8. The expression patterns of *AaJAZ8*, MeJA-induced AaJAZ8 degradation, and analysis of artemisinin biosynthesis in *A. annua* plants overexpressing *AaJAZ8* or *AaJAZ8Δjas*.

Fig. S9. AaTCP14 and AaORA interact with AaJAZ proteins and mapping of the domains involved in the interaction between AaJAZ8, AaORA, and AaTCP14 using Y2H assays.

Fig. S10. Artemisinin content in *AaTCP14* transgenic plants under MeJA treatment.

Table S1. List of primers used in this study.

[马亚男,唐克轩. Science Advances, 2018, 4: eaas9357.]

# The genome of *Artemisia annua* provides insight into the evolution of Asteraceae family and artemisinin biosynthesis

## 1 INTRODUCTION

Malaria is a global health problem: in 2016 alone, there were an estimated 216 million new cases of malaria, 445,000 deaths, and nearly 1 one billion people living in areas with a high risk of the disease. Artemisinin, an edroperoxide sequiterpene lactone, is an effective antrimalarial compound that is synthesized in the glandular trichomes of the Chinese mddicinal plant *Artemisia annua*. Due to her discovery of the anti-malaria function of artemisinin, which has saved millions of lives, the Chinese scientist Youyou Tu received a Nobel Prize in Physiology or Medicine in 2015. Artemisininbased combination therapies (ACTs) are recommended by the WHO for treatment of uncomplicated malaria caused by the *Plasmodium falciparum* parasite.

Currently, the supply of ACTs is reliant on the agricultural production of artemisinin. However, plant-based production sometimes cannot meet the global demand due to the low amount of artemisinin produced in *A. annua* leaves (0.1%–1.0% of dry weight). Alternatively, a semi-synthetic system can be used for the production of artemisinin, in which yeast are engineered to synthesize its precursor, artemisinic acid. However, the semi-synthetic production of artemisinin is expensive and thus cannot replace its agricultural production at present. The use of the whole *Artemisia* plant as a malaria therapy was found to be more effective than a comparable dose of pure artemisinin, and was shown to be able to overcome resistance to pure artemisinin in a rodent malaria model and human clinical trial. Moreover, parasite resistance to artemisinin has recently been confirmed by the WHO in the Greater Mekong subregion. Besides its anti-malarial activity, many other therapeutic effects of artemisinin on diseases such as cancer, tuberculosis, and diabetes have been reported. Hence, artemisinin is a potential multi-functional compound and is of high medicinal value. There is a considerable interest in increasing the artemisinin content of *A. annua* and an urgent need to identify other potential anti-malarial compounds.

Artemisinin is synthesized from isopentenyl pyrophosphate via farnesyl pyrophosphate, which is converted to amorpha-4,11-diene by the action of amorpha-4,11-diene synthase (ADS). The next reaction is the three-step oxidation of amorpha-4, 11-diene to artemisinic acid, via artemisinic alcohol and artemisinic aldehyde, through the action of a cytochrome P450 monooxygenase (CYP71AV1). Artemisinic aldehyde is converted by artemisinic aldehyde Ä11 (13) reductase (a double-bond reductase, DBR2) into dihydroartemisinic aldehyde. ALDH1 (aldehyde dehydrogenase 1) then catalyzes the oxidation of artemisinic aldehyde and dihydroartemisinic aldehyde to produce artemisinic acid and dihydroartemisinic acid, respectively (Supplemental Figure 1). The conversion of dihydroartemisinic acid to artemisinin occurs via a light-induced non-enzymatic photochemical oxidation process.

In the last two decades, metabolic engineering has been demonstrated to be a useful approach to increase artemisinin content in *A. annua*. Previous studies employed several metabolic engineering strategies to enhance artemisinin production, including overexpression of artemisinin biosynthetic pathway genes, overexpression of transcription factors (TFs) that can enhance the expression of artemisinin biosynthetic genes, and overexpression of the ADP-FPS fusion gene to stimulate substrate channeling. However, in these reports either *A. annua* cultivars producing low levels of artemisinin (0.02% - 0.4% of dry weight) were used as transgenic recipients, or the improvement of artemisinin content was not as efficient when high-artemisinin-producing cultivars (0.8% - 1.0% of dry weight) were used as transgenic reciplents. Moreover, most of previous studies focused only on modifying the upstream or downstream parts of the artemisinin biosynthetic pathway, and thus were unable to effectively boost the entire metabolic flux toward artemisinin biosynthesis. This may be one of the reasons for the failure to obtain transgenic *A. annua* lines with high artemisinin content. Recently, a synthetic biology strategy for artemisinin biosynthesis, in which the complete biosynthetic pathway of artemisinic acid, the precursor of artemisinin, is introduced into tobacco plants, has also been reported. However, whether this strategy allows efficient artemisinin production in other plant species needs to be further studied.

*A. annua* is a member of the Asteraceae, the largest family of flowering plants, which comprises more than 23 000 species, including many with considerable medicinal, ornamental, and economic importance. A major impediment to the exploitation of these resources in basic and breeding sciences has been the absence of reference genome sequences; to date, only the sunflower genome has been released, although some transcriptome and metabolomics datasets are available. Here, we report a high-quality draft genome sequence of *A. annua* obtained by an integrative approach combining short-read sequencing (Illumina and Roche 454) and long-read sequencing (PacBio RSII), which is highly effective in assembling complex genomes such as that of *A. annua*. We also performed transcriptomic analyses, and identified some novel genes involved in the biosynthesis of artemisinin or other terpenoids based on the genomic and transcriptomic data. We demonstrate that the availability of a reference genome sequence coupled with RNA sequencing (RNA-seq) is helpful for metabolic engineering of important secondary metabolites, leading to improvement in artemisinin production.

## 2 RESULTS

Genome Sequencing, Assembly, and Annotation We generated a high-quality draft genome sequence of a high-artemisinin-producing *A. annua* cultivar, Huhao 1, a highly heterozygous diploid ($2n = 2x = 18$ chromosomes). According to standard 17-mer curves, the heterozygosity of the *A. annua* genome is 1.0%-1.5% (Supplemental Figure 2). The DNA sequencing reads were obtained using Illumina, Roche 454, and PacBio sequencing technologies. A total of 442 gigabases (Gb) of high-quality Illumina reads, 3.1 Gb of Roche 454 reads, and 22 Gb of PacBio long reads (Supplemental Tables 1 - 3) were generated, resulting in ~260× coverage of the *A. annua* genome. The total genome assembly amounted to 1.74 Gb, consisting of 39 579 scaffolds, with a scaffold N50 of 104.86 kb and a contig N50 of 18.95 kb (Table 1). The completeness of the genome assembly was evaluated by using the Core Eukaryotic Genes Mapping Approach (CEGMA) and Benchmarking Universal Single-Copy Orthologs (BUSCO). CEGMA results indicated that 98.0% of core eukaryotic genes were contained in our assembly (243 out of 248 core eukaryotic genes) (Supplemental Table 4). Based on BUSCO analysis 89.2% of plant sets were identified as complete (1 284 out of 1 440 BUSCOs) (Supplemental Figure 3). Completeness of the assembled

**Table 1 *A. annua* genome assembly and annotation statistics**

| | |
|---|---|
| Chromosome number (2*n*) | 18 |
| Estimate of genome size | 1.74 Gb |
| Number of scaffolds | 39 579 |
| N50 of scaffolds | 104 858 bp |
| Number of contigs | 197 282 |
| N50 of contigs | 18 950 bp |
| GC content | 31.5% |
| Number of protein-coding genes | 63 230 |
| Average gene density (per 100 kb) | 4.78 |
| Mean gene length | 3 803 |
| Mean coding sequence length | 994 |
| Total size of coding regions | 85.29 Mb |
| Fraction of coding regions | 4.76% |
| Fraction of protein-coding genes | 18.19% |
| Repetitive elements share in genome | 61.57% |

genome sequence was also estimated by mapping a multiple-sourced eval dataset, including 166 full-length genes and 86 708 unigenes from the NCBI database, 19 168 transcripts from Roche 454 sequencing, and 79 190 Trinity-assembled transcripts, to the assembled genome. All of the 166 full-length gene sequences completely mapped to the assembly. Of 19 168 Roche 454 transcripts, 91.8% and 94.7% were successfully mapped to the genome with the "hard" and "soft" criteria, respectively. Of the 12 616 (66 574) Trinity-assembled transcripts, 85.1% (78.9%) were successfully mapped to the genome with >90% coverage and 89.2% (84.8%) mapped with >70% coverage, while 75.8% and 86.6% of the unigenes were mapped with the "hard" and "soft" criteria, respectively (Supplemental Table 5). We identified mitochondrial and chloroplast contigs from the sequenced genome data by performing a BLAST search against plant mitochondrial and chloroplast genome sequences from the NCBI Organelle Genome Resources using alignment length ≥10 kb as a threshold. We found nine and ten contigs putatively associated with the mitochondrial and chloroplast genomes, respectively (Supplemental Tables 6 and 7).

By combining homology-based and *de novo* approaches, we found that 61.57% of the assembled *A. annua* genome consists of repetitive elements; 60.10% of the genome was predicted to consist of interspersed repeats and transposable elements, while 1.47% was predicted to be tandem repeats (Supplemental Table 8). Of the repetitive elements, 32.66% could not be classified into any known gene family, and the most abundant characterized elements were LTRs (long terminal repeats), which accounted for 22.69% of the genome. Next, proteincoding gene models were constructed using a pipeline combining *de novo*, homology-based, and EST-aided prediction, resulting in 63 226 protein-coding gene models. The predicted gene structures were further refined using a transcriptome sequencing dataset. Prediction of alternatively spliced forms of these protein-coding genes identified 6 758 splice variants for 3 064 genes. Of the predicted gene models, 54 317 (85.9%) were supported by transcriptome data from at least one of nine organs/tissues (young leaf, old leaf, bud, flower, stem, seed, root, epidermis, and mixed trichome cells), indicating the high accuracy of the gene predictions (Supplemental Figure 4). Among 41 518 genes supported by transcriptome data with transcripts per kilobase per million (TPM) >1, more than 28 870 were expressed in buds, whereas only about 20 000 expressed genes were detected in trichomes (Supplemental Figure 5). A total of 41 884 genes (66.2%) were assigned to gene ontology (GO) categories, of which 26 752 fell within the "metabolic processes" category (Figure 1A).

The *A. annua* genome we report here is one of a few sequenced Asteraceae genomes. Orthologous clustering of the predicted *A. annua* proteins with those of 16 other representative green plants revealed that 7 522 *A. annua* genes distributed among 2 899 families are common to these species. A total of 36 435 *A. annua* genes clustered with those from at least one of the 16 genomes. Another 2 496 genes, from 871 families, grouped only with genes from *Helianthus annuus*. These genes are referred to as Asteraceae-specific genes. Further comparison of *A. annua*, *H. annuus*, *A. thaliana*, and *S. lycopersicum* proteins revealed 8 401 clusters of genes distributed among all four eudicot genomes and 3 739 gene families that were unique to *A. annua* (Figure 1B). These *A. annua* specific gene families were enriched in genes involved in the GO-defined biological processes such as SCF-dependent proteasomal ubiquitin-dependent protein catabolism, shade avoidance, stomatal movement, and nitrate metabolism, as well as those associated with the transferase activity and kinase activity (Supplemental Table 9).

Evolution and Gene Family Expansion Analysis A phylogenetic tree was constructed based on a concatenated sequence alignment of the 67 single-copy genes shared by the *Artemisia* genus and 16 other green plant species (Figure 1C). In this phylogenetic tree, *A. annua*, as expected, clustered with *H. annuus*, another Asteraceae species, and these two species were most closely related to the Solanaceae family. Although the 67 single-copy genes already provided phylogenetic signals that allowed for phylogeny construction of the 16 green plant species, accurate dating of the divergence

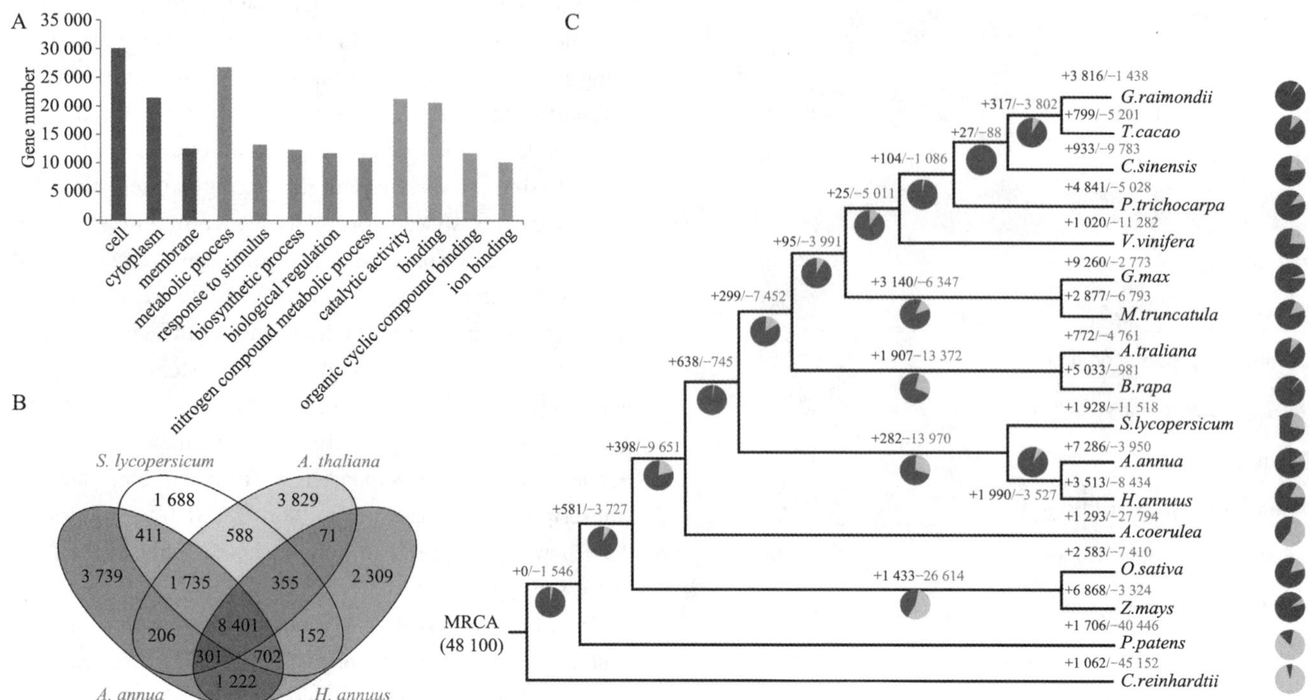


**Figure 1 Characterization of *A. annua* genome evolution and gene family expansion**

(**A**) Gene Ontology (GO) functional classification. (**B**) Protein clusters shared between *A. annua* and other more phylogenetically distant plant species. *A. annua* is a representative of the *Artemisia* genus, *Helianthus annuus* is a representative of the *Helianthus* genus, *Solanum lycopersicum* is a representative of the *Solanum* genus, and *Arabidopsis thaliana* is a representative of the *Arabidopsis* genus. (**C**) The phylogenetic tree was constructed from a concatenated alignment of 67 single-copy genes from 17 plant species. Gene family expansion is indicated in red, and gene family contraction is indicated in green; the corresponding proportions among total changes are shown using the same colors as in the pie charts. MRCA, most recent common ancestor.

times between Asteraceae and other families still requires a larger gene set. We identified the gene families that have expanded or contracted in the *Artemisia* lineage. In total, 7 286 gene families were expanded in *A. annua*, whereas 3 950 gene families were contracted (Figure 1C). Gene family expansion in *A. annua* has resulted in a notably large number of genes, making *A. annua* to be one of the genome-sequenced plant species with the largest number of genes compared with the other 50 plant species with sequenced genomes listed by Michael and Jackson. Notably, 2 717 TFs were identified in *A. annua* (Supplemental Table 10), which is substantially more than the number in most sequenced plant genomes, and three TF families, C3H, FAR1 and Nin-like, were particularly larger than their counterparts in the other plant species.

The diverse array of secondary metabolites that are synthesized by *A. annua* provides protection against pests, pathogens, and herbivores across its natural range of habitats. An important class of these defense compounds is terpenoids, including artemisinin, which are synthesized and stored in glandular trichomes. In this regard, a striking feature of the *A. annua* genome is the existence of unusually large gene families related to terpene biosynthesis and the expansion of several prenyltransferase families (Figure 2A). The terpene synthase (TPS) family genes are generally divided into seven clades, whereas in most plants the majority of TPS genes fall into one or two clades, indicating lineage-specific expansion. We found 122 putative TPS genes in the *A. annua* genome, most of which belonged to the TPS-a and TPS-b subfamilies. Phylogenetic analysis of putative full-length TPSs from 11 sequenced plant genomes revealed that *A. annua* and *H. annuus* TPSs were clustered together in each subclade. The presence of Asteraceae-specific members of the TPS-a and TPS-b subfamilies indicates lineage-specific expansion of the TPS family (Figure 2B). The positions of TPS genes from the model flowering plant *A. thaliana* on the branches of the TPS-a and TPS-b clades indicate that almost all of the Asteraceae TPS genes arose by gene duplications that occurred after the divergence of the Asteraceae lineage from the *Solanum lycopersicum* and *A. thaliana* lineages.

Genomic and Transcriptomic Analyses of the Artemisinin Biosynthetic Pathway and Its Regulation  Although the artemisinin biosynthetic pathway has been extensively studied

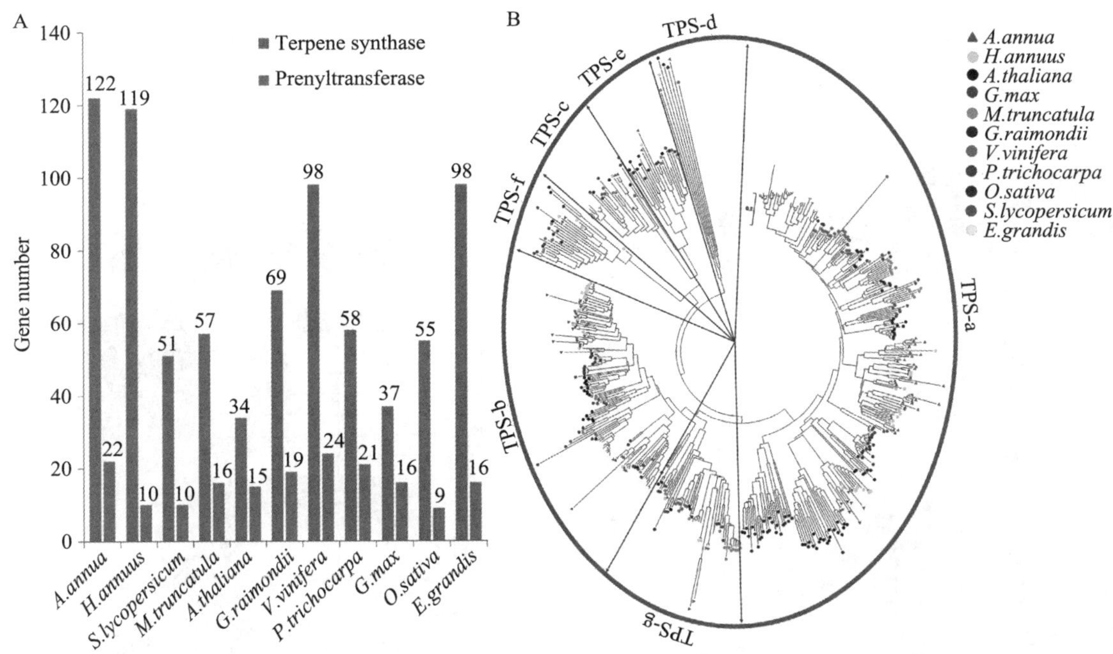


**Figure 2 Interspecific phylogenetic analysis and classification of terpene synthase genes from *A. annua* and 10 other sequenced plant genomes**

(**A**) Comparison of terpene synthase and prenyltransferase genes in *A. annua* and 10 other sequenced plant genomes. BLAST analysis of the genomes was performed using the terpene synthase and prenyltransferase conserved domain by HMM.

(**B**) Phylogenetic tree of terpene synthases (TPS). Putative full-length TPS proteins (>400 amino acids in length) identified in 11 sequenced plant genomes, including 88 from *A. annua*, 51 from *H. annuus*, 30 from *S. lycopersicum*, 40 from *M. truncatula*, 33 from *A. thaliana*, 54 from *G. raimondii*, 43 from *V. vinifera*, 44 from *P. trichocarpa*, 24 from *G. max*, 41 from *O. sativa*, and 69 from *E. grandis*, were subjected to phylogenetic analysis. The scale bar (0.2) shows the number of amino acid substitutions per site.

and some key components and enzyme-catalytic steps for artemisinin biosynthesis have been well characterized, by combining genomic and transcriptomic analyses we obtained some new insights about this biosynthetic pathway and their transcriptional regulation in *A. annua*. Analysis of the *A. annua* genome revealed that the copy numbers of *DXR*, *FPS*, *ADS*, and *ALDH1* were in line with both previous transcriptomic sequencing reports (Figure 3A). However, as for gene *HMGR* (3-hydroxy-3-methylglutaryl coenzyme A reductase), two genes (AA201470 and AA271980) in the *A. annua* genome were annotated as *HMGR* and showed 97% nucleotide sequence identity to the previously reported *A. annua HMGR1* (GenBank: AF142473.1) and *Chrysanthemum* × *morifolium HMGR2* (GenBank: KT809341.1) genes, respectively, whereas Graham et al. and Ma et al. reported four contigs and three contigs for *HMGR*, respectively. Moreover, through genomic sequence alignment we showed that these two *HMGR* genes shared less than 50% nucleotide sequence identity. Therefore, we consider them to be two different genes rather than two alleles. Similarly, two copies of *CYP71AV1* and *DBR2* were found in the *A. annua* genome (Figure 3A). The two *CYP71AV1* paralogs have 97% nucleotide sequence identity (Supplemental Figure 6); one paralog (AA566140) was located on scaffold QH_S14321(37.6 kb) and based on RNA-seq analysis was highly expressed in trichomes, and in buds and young leaves that have a large number of trichomes, while the other paralog (AA502080) was located on scaffold QH_S10223 (58.7 kb) and showed basal expression in all the organs/tissues examined (Figure 3A). PCR analysis using genomic DNA further confirmed that there are two copies of *CYP71AV1* in *A. annua*. The two *DBR2* (AA049700 and AA049710) paralogs also have extremely high nucleotide sequence identity, but unlike *CYP71AV1*, the two *DBR2* paralogs were tandem repeated on scaffold QH_S00290 (316.65 kb) and showed a similar expression profile. The two *DBR2* paralogs were both highly expressed in trichomes, and in buds and young leaves (Figure 3A).

The biosynthesis of plant secondary metabolites is usually species, organ, or tissue specifi, as exemplified by artemisinin, which is only synthesized and stored in the glandular trichomes on plant surfaces. The expression of biosynthetic pathway genes is known to be regulated by a number of TFs, and most of the known artemisinin metabolism-related genes were found to be expressed at higher levels in young leaves and buds, or in bud trichomes (Figure 3A). Several TFs in *A.*

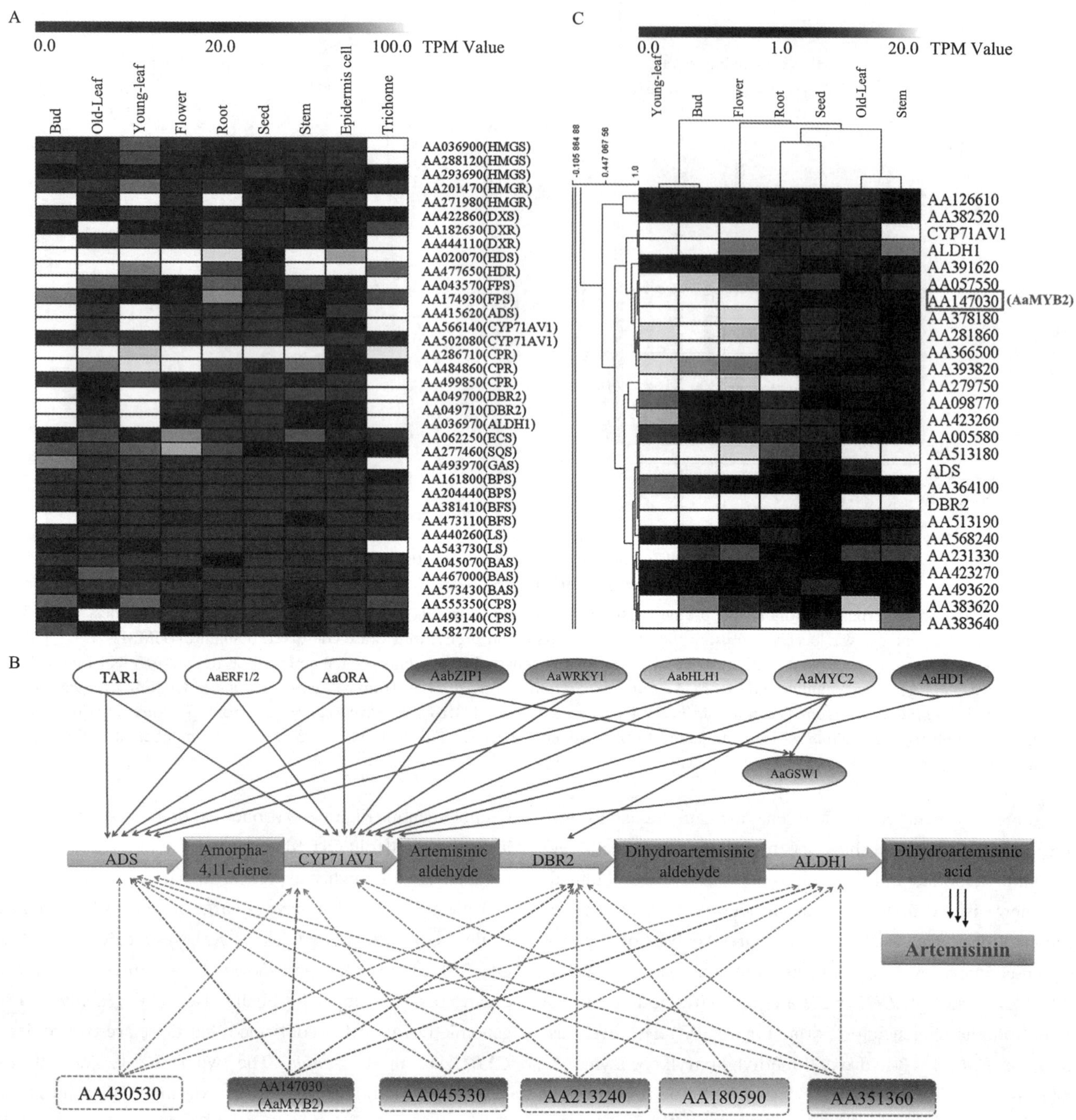


**Figure 3 Artemisinin-related gene expression in selected tissues and the artemisinin biosynthesis transcriptional regulatory network**

(**A**) Copy number and expression levels of genes functioning in the artemisinin biosynthetic pathway and its competitive pathway. (**B**) Hierarchical clustering heatmap analysis coupled with Pearson correlation analysis of the MYB transcription factor family (part of the MYB family in *A. annua*) and artemisinin biosynthetic pathway genes (*ADS*, *CYP71AV1*, *DBR2*, and *ALDH1*) using MeV4.9 software. AaMYB2 is marked by a red box. (**C**) Transcription factors bind the promoters of artemisinin biosynthetic pathway genes such as *ADS*, *CYP71AV1*, *DBR2*, and *ALDH1*. The activation of gene expression results in an increase in artemisinin content in *A. annua*. ADS, amorpha-4,11-diene synthase; CYP71AV1, cytochrome P450 monooxygenase; CPR, cytochrome P450 reductase; DBR2, artemisinic aldehyde Ä11 (13) reductase; ALDH1, aldehyde dehydrogenase 1. Red solid arrows represent transcription factors reported previously and demonstrated to bind to the promoters of pathway genes (TAR1, AaERF1/2, AaORA, AabZIP1, AaWRKY1, AabHLH1, AaMYC2, AaHD1, AaGSW1). Red dotted arrows represent the induction of pathway gene expression by the predicted AaMYB2 transcription factor. Blue dotted arrows represent putative transcription factors identified by hierarchical clustering heatmap analysis coupled with Pearson correlation analysis that may regulate artemisinin biosynthetic pathway genes. Different colors indicate different transcription factor families.

*annua* such as the basic helix-loop-helix family gene *AaMYC2*, the WRKY family gene *AaGSW1*, and the HD-ZIP family gene *AaHD1* have already been demonstrated to regulate artemisinin biosynthesis. To investigate the transcriptional regulatory network underlying artemisinin biosynthesis, we performed hierarchical clustering (HCL) heatmap analysis coupled with Pearson correlation analysis using MultiExperiment Viewer (MeV4.9.0) software as previously described. We identified several groups of TFs with expression patterns that were significantly correlated with those of *ADS*, *CYP71AV1*, *DBR2*, and *ALDH1*, and as such might be involved in regulating artemisinin biosynthesis (Figure 3B), including some TFs that have already been shown to be involved in artemisinin biosynthesis, such as AaORA, a member of the AP2/ERF family (Supplemental Figures 10-14). In addition, we identified an MYB family TF, AaMYB2 (AA147030), a member of the R2R3-MYB clade, which closely clustered with artemisinin biosynthesis-specific genes based on expression pattern, similar to AaORA (Figure 3C). MYB TFs participate in a range of plant developmental processes and the biosynthesis of secondary metabolites. However, little is known about whether this TF family is associated with artemisinin biosynthesis.

Metabolic Engineering of Artemisinin Biosynthesis

The information obtained by genome sequencing and RNA-seq has potential value in enhancing artemisinin content through metabolic engineering. Overexpressing a single artemisinin biosynthetic pathway gene (such as *FPS* and *HMGR*) has been partially successful, but has not resulted in substantial increases in artemisinin accumulation. HMGR is responsible for the conversion of HMG-coenzyme A into mevalonic acid, the precursor of isopentenyl diphosphate, and its expression level was low in trichomes when compared with that of *ADS*, *CYP71AV1*, and so forth. FPS, the enzyme responsible for generating farnesyl pyrophosphate, the immediate substrate for the biosynthesis of sesquiterpenes including artemisinin, is a key enzyme located at a branching point of artemisinin biosynthesis. DBR2, the enzyme responsible for converting artemisinic aldehyde to dihydroartemisinic aldehyde, is another crucial enzyme in the formation of artemisinin, sitting in the downstream position in artemisinin biosynthesis. To increase artemisinin

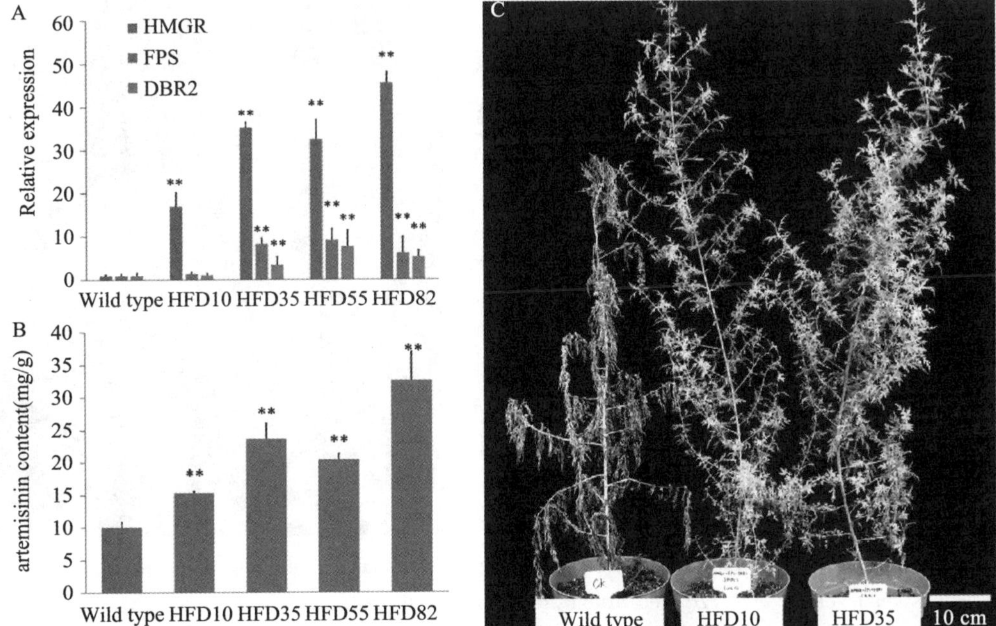


**Figure 4 Genome and RNA-Seq guided plant metabolic engineering to increase artemisinin content in A. *annua***

(**A**) Relative expression levels of *HMGR*, *FPS*, and *DBR2* in wild-type and four independent transgenic *A. annua* overexpression lines determined by qPCR. (**B**) HPLC analysis of artemisinin content in wild-type and four independent *HMGR*, *FPS*, and *DBR2*-overexpressing transgenic *A. annua* lines. (**C**) Three-month-old transgenic *A. annua* lines overexpressing *HMGR*, *FPS*, and *DBR2* (middle and right) and wild-type (left) after 3 g/l glyphosate ammonium treatment. Data represent the means ± SE from three replicates. The *â-actin* gene (GenBank: EU531837.1) was used as the control for gene expression normalization. Statistical significance was determined by two-independent-samples *Æ* test (** $P<0.01$). Asterisks indicate the differences between wild-type and transgenic lines.

content, we generated transgenic *A. annua* lines simultaneously overexpressing *HMGR* (AA201470), *FPS*, and *DBR2* (Figure 4A and Supplemental Figure 7). We found that many transgenic lines showed high artemisinin content in the leaves, among which line HFD82 had the highest artemisinin content (3.2%, dry weight) as determined by high-performance liquid chromatography (HPLC) analysis (Figure 4B and Supplemental Figure 8). The artemisinin contents of these lines were further confirmed by liquid chromatography-mass spectrometry analysis (Supplemental Figure 9). In addition to having high artemisinin content, because the *EPSPS* gene encoding 5-enolpyruvylshikimate-3-phosphate synthase that confers resistance to glyphosate was used as a selection marker during plant transformation, the transgenic lines overexpressing *HMGR*, *FPS*, and *DBR2* exhibited resistance to the herbicide glyphosate (Figure 4C and Supplemental Figure 7) and thus can potentially be used for large-scale cultivation.

We also produced transgenic *A. annua* lines with constitutive overexpression of *AaMYB2*, in which the transcript levels of *AaMYB2* showed a 1.2- to 7.4-fold increase compared with those in the wild-type plants. As expected, the transcript levels of genes in the artemisinin biosynthetic pathway, including *ADS*, *CYP71AV1*, *DBR2*, and *ALDH1*, showed substantial increases in *AaMYB2*-overexpressing lines (Figure 5A). Compared with the wild-type plants, the artemisinin and dihydroartemisinic acid contents were 51% - 103% and 83% - 144% higher, respectively, in the *AaMYB2*-overexpressing lines (Figure 5B), which showed no morphological or developmental abnormalities (Figure 5C). These results indicate that AaMYB2 is a positive regulator of artemisinin biosynthesis.

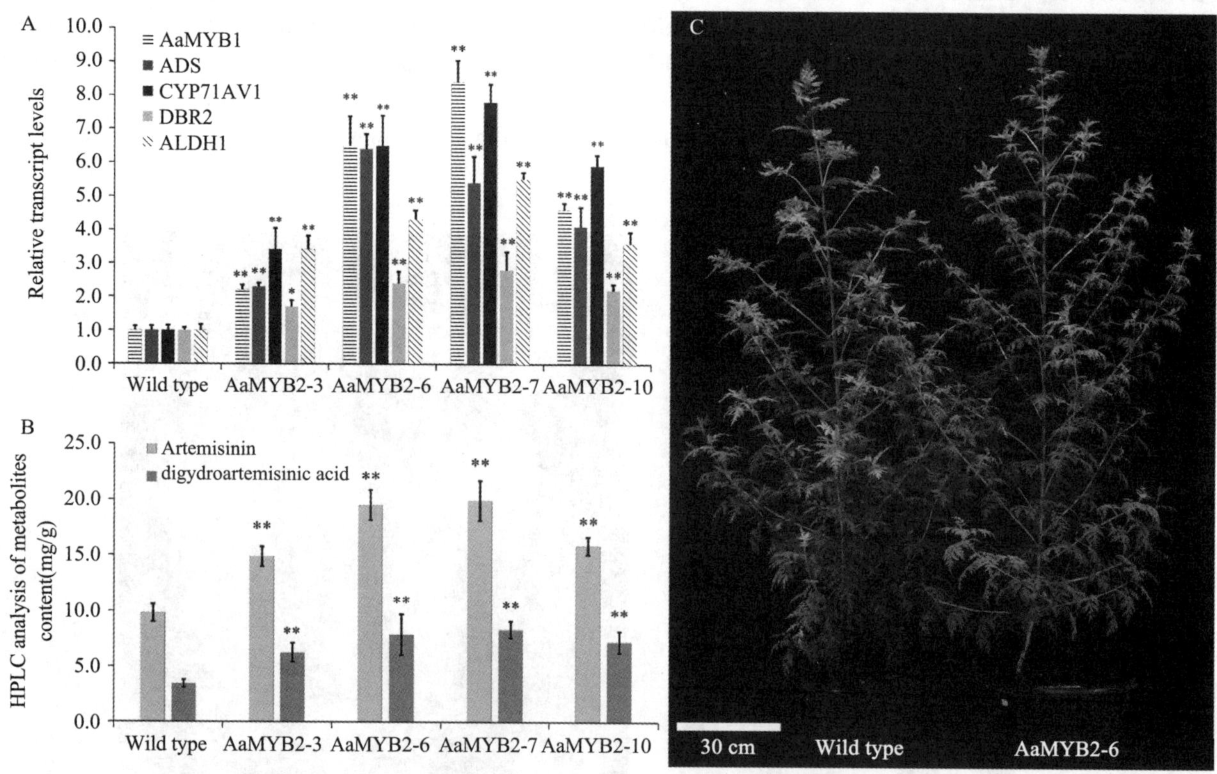


**Figure 5 The AaMYB2 transcription factor positively regulates artemisinin biosynthesis in *A. annua***

(**A**) Relative expression levels of *AaMYB2* and artemisinin biosynthetic pathway genes (*ADS*, *CYP71AV1*, *DBR2*, and *ALDH1*) in wild-type and four independent *AaMYB2*-overexpressing transgenic *A. annua* lines determined by qPCR. (**B**) HPLC analysis of artemisinin and dihydroartemisinic acid contents in wild-type and four independent *AaMYB2*-overexpressing transgenic *A. annua* lines. Data represent the means±SE from three replicates. The *â-actin* gene was used as the control for normalization. (**C**) No morphological difference is observed between wild-type and an *AaMYB2*-overexpressing transgenic *A. annua* line.

Statistical significance was determined by two-independent-samples Æ test (* $P<0.05$; ** $P<0.01$). Asterisks indicate the differences between wild-type and *AaMYB2*-overexpessing lines.

## 3 DISCUSSION

The *de novo* assembly of large genomes with a high degree of heterozygosity remains a particular challenge. For example, self-incompatibility is the most common mode of outcrossing in the Asteraceae (Hiscock, 2000), which might result in high heterozygosity. It is both technically challenging and time-consuming to generate haploid, pure lines with low heterozygosity. The *A. annua* genome is highly heterozygous (heterozygosity is 1.0% - 1.5%, shown in Supplemental Figure 2), with a high density of LTRs and low GC content. Such characteristics are barriers to the assembly of diploid genome sequences generated using only short-read sequencing (Roche 454 or Illumina), whereas the PacBio RSII sequencing platform generates long reads, thereby faciliting the sequence assembly and enhancing the assembly quality. The integrated PacBio strategy used here was highly effective in assembling the complex *A. annua* genome.

Analysis of the *A. annua* genome revealed that 871 gene families might be unique to the Asteraceae family. Due to its morphological complexity and the large number of species, systematic analysis of this family has been challenging for taxonomists. Our phylogenetic analysis, based on sequence alignment of 67 single-copy genes, supports the traditional phylogeny. For example, of the species tested, *A. annua* and *H. annuus* showed the closest evolutionary relationship to *S. lycopersicum* (*Solanum* family), which is consistent with a previous tomato genome sequence report, indicating the usefulness of the *A. annua* genome in phylogenetic studies.

The *A. annua* genomic and associated transcriptomic datasets provide not only new insights into the artemisinin biosynthetic pathway and its regulation but also valuable tools for artemisinin metabolic engineering. Previous studies manipulating artemisinin biosynthesis in *A. annua* mainly focused on either upstream or downstream of the artemisinin biosynthetic pathway, resulting in increased but still limited artemisinin accumulation in transgenic *A. annua* lines. Multiple enzymatic steps are involved in artemisinin biosynthesis, implying that there may be more than one enzymatic step limiting the metabolic flux into artemisinin biosynthesis. In this study, by simultaneously overexpressing multiple genes functioning in the upstream (*HMGR*), midstream (*FPS*), and downstream (*DBR2*) of the artemisinin biosynthetic pathway, which may effectively boost the entire pathway, we obtained transgenic *A. annua* lines with significantly increased artemisinin content. Thus, an efficient strategy to increase the production of plant secondary metabolites might be to simultaneously enhance the expression of genes encoding enzymes functioning in different steps in a biosynthetic pathway or to overexpress the TFs such as AaMYB2 that regulate the expression of multiple genes in a biosynthetic pathway. *AaMYB2* closely clustered with artemisinin biosynthesis-specific genes based on expression pattern, and we found that overexpression of this gene could significantly enhance artemisinin and dihydroartemisinic acid content in transgenic *A. annua* lines. This also implies that the other TF genes that clustered with the artemisinin biosynthetic pathway genes may have similar functions, and as such represent candidate genes for metabolically engineered enhancement of artemisinin levels.

In short, our study adds abundant valuable information to the limited genomic resources of Asteraceae, one of the biggest plant families with diverse specialized metabolites. The *A. annua* genome and transcriptome data we provide here should be valuable for both fundamental biological research and applied breeding programs. The transgenic *A. annua* lines with high artemisinin content generated in this study should be a useful aid in enhancing the global supply of artemisinin from plant sources.

## 4 METHODS

Sample Preparation, DNA Extraction, and RNA Extraction The *A. annua* cultivar used for sequencing, “Huhao 1” is a high artemisinin producer variety originating from Youyang, the major and traditional *A. annua* growing area, and was developed at Shanghai Jiao Tong University after several years of selection. *A. annua* plants were grown in the university greenhouse and fresh young leaves were collected from 4-month-old plants. External contaminants were removed by washing with Milli-Q water three times, then leaves were frozen in liquid nitrogen and stored at −80 ℃ until DNA extraction. Genomic DNA (gDNA) was extracted using the CTAB method with phenol - chloroform followed by RNase A and proteinase K treatments to remove RNA and protein contamination.

Total RNA was extracted from seven organs/tissues (young leaf, old leaf, bud, flower, stem, seed, and root) collected from five independent plants, using the Column Plant RNAout kit (TIANDZ, China). The trichome cells and epidermal cells were collected by laser capture microdissection (LCM) as described previously. The mRNA from seven tissues was enriched using an Illumina TruSeq RNA Library Prep Kit, which involves poly (A) pull-down using oligo-dT attached magnetic beads, following the manufacturer's standard protocol. Total RNA from LCM samples was extracted using the RNeasy Micro Kit (Qiagen, Germany), and mRNA was amplified in a two-round amplification using the TargetAmp kit (Epicenter Biotechnologies, USA) following the manufacturer's instructions. The DNA and RNA quantity and size distribution were verified using a Bioanalyzer (Agilent Technologies, USA).

Library Construction and DNA Sequencing A shotgun library with an insert size of 300- to 800-bp was prepared from 1 ìg of gDNA using the Roche GS DNA Library Preparation Kit following the manufacturer's standard protocol (Roche, Switzerland), and 3-Gb sequence data were produced by a Roche 454 GS FLX. The paired-end (PE) libraries with different inserts (170 300, and 800 bp) were prepared using a standard protocol (Illumina, USA). The three PE libraries were sequenced (2× 150- bp reads) on a HiSeq 2 500 (Illumina), generating 169 Gb of sequence data. The 500-bp library was sequenced (2×300- bp reads) on a MiSeq (Ilumina) and 56 Gb of sequence data were generated. Mate-pair-end (MP) libraries with varied insert sizes (3, 5,8, 10, and 20 kb) were constructed using the Cre-Loxp Inverse PCR Paired-End (CLIP-PE) method and sequenced in the 2 × 150-bp format on a HiSeq 2 500 (Illumina), generating 217 Gb of sequence data. Four flowcells were used on the HiSeq 2 500 and another four on MiSeq. Samples were not multiplexed with those from other species.

For the PacBio sequencing library construction and sequencing, 5 ìg of gDNA, extracted from the fresh young leaves of five plants, was sheared using a Covaris g-TUBE (Covaris, USA) followed by purification via binding to pre-washed AMPure XP beads (Beckman Coulter, USA). Sheared gDNA was end-repaired using the PacBio DNA Template Prep Kit 2.0 (Pacific Biosciences, USA) and then ligated with blunt adapters, followed by exonuclease incubation to remove all unligated adapters and DNA. The final "SMRT bells" were annealed with primers and bound to the proprietary polymerase using the PacBio DNA/Polymerase Binding Kit P4 (Pacific Biosciences) to form the "Binding Complex". After dilution, the library was loaded onto the PacBio *RS*II sequencer with DNA Sequencing Kit 2.0 (Pacific Biosciences) and an SMRT Cell 8 Pac V3 for sequencing. A primary filtering analysis was performed on the sequencer, and the secondary analysis was performed using the SMRT analysis pipeline version 2.1.0 (Pacific Biosciences).

Genome Assembly and Evaluation The 1.5% heterozygosity along with the high repetitive content (62%) of the *A. annua* genome poses a challenge for assembly with next-generation sequencing short reads. Extremely fragmental contigs with N50 lengths of 100-200 bp were obtained when we used the Illumina PE and MP sequencing method and assembly recipe. To alleviate the effects of the complex genome and short reads, we sequenced a 2× 300 MiSeq pair-end library with an insert size of 500 bp and merged read pairs to obtain long reads using FLASH. Although the volume of the Roche 454 data is small compared with Illumina data, the Roche 454 data were fed to Newbler (v2.9, Roche) at an early stage of the assembly process to construct the core contigs. *A. annua* Roche 454 data were solely sequenced with 12 flowcells, resulting in a total of 3.1 Gb with a mean read length of 585 bp. The samples were not multiplexed with those of other species. Newbler (v2.9, Roche) was run with default parameters except that "large Genome" and "heterozygote Mode" were set to true.

Considering the complexity of the *A. annua* genome, we sequenced five different mate-pair libraries with insert sizes of 3, 5, 8, 10, and 20 kb. All mate-pair reads were processed by Trimmomatic to remove the adapters and low-quality sequences before genome assembly. After evaluation, cleaning, and some quality trimming, these mate-pair reads were mapped to core contigs to extract contig pairing information. SSPACE (v3.0) was used to collect, calculate, and summarize the information and generate the genome scaffolds.

To obtain the final genome assembly with better assembly continuity, we used a 2-step gap-closing process to close sequence gaps within the scaffolds. First, GapCloser was used to close small-sized gaps with Illumina pair-end reads. Second, for the remaining larger-sized gaps, PacBio long reads, which have longer single sequence lengths, were used to cross and fill some of these gaps. PBJelly2 was applied in this process to ensure the quality of the consensus sequence from local assembly around the gaps. The assembled genome sequences were searched again for vector and *Escherichia coli* genome sequences to remove contaminant sequences.

We mapped all contigs onto each other using Lastz and, when two contigs were more than 95% identical over more than 90% of the shorter contig, we discarded the shorter sequence to filter out homologous contigs. Based on this criterion, 173 highly homologous contigs were removed. Since the 1.5% heterozygosity of the *A. annua* genome was not high enough to require the assembly of two separate genome sets, we did not screen out secondary haploid scaffolds from the assembly and retained this information for subsequent analysis.

The completeness of the final genome assembly was evaluated by using CEGMA and BUSCO. We performed a BUSCO testing run for sequenced plant genomes using version 3 run _BUSCO. py software with the embryophyta protein set (run _BUSCO. py -i plant _ species. fa -o plant _ species -l embryophyta _ odb9/-m proteins). We also collected a multiple-sourced eval dataset and mapped these sequences to the assembled genome to evaluate the completeness.

Estimation of the Genome Size The genome size (G) of *A. annua* was estimated based on the occurrence distribution from 17-mer resampling of sequencing reads, calculated with the equation $G=N_{17mer}/D_{17mer}$, where $N_{17mer}$ is the number of total 17-mers and $D_{17mer}$ is average sequence depth. For $N_{17mer}$, low-frequency 17-mers, which possibly resulted from sequencing errors (depth <3), were excluded from the calculation to alleviate the deviation from sequencing error. The total genome assembly was 1.74 Gb. The total K-mer (K = 18) number was 154 863 960 403, and the volume peak was 88. The genome size can be estimated as (total K-mer number) / (volume peak), which is 1 759 817 732 bp.

RNA-Seq Two micrograms of *A. annua* mRNA were enriched using the Illumina TruSeq RNA Library Prep Kit (Illumina), which uses oligo (dT)-attached magnetic beads to pull down poly (A) RNA. The *A. annua* mRNA was then used to synthesize cDNA using a non-strand-specific SuperScript Double-Stranded cDNA Synthesis Kit (Invitrogen, USA), and the library was constructed using the Roche shotgun-library-preparation method. In total, 625 Mb of transcriptome sequence was generated using a Roche 454 GS FLX instrument. The mRNA from nine organs/tissues (young leaf, old leaf, bud, flower, stem, seed, root, epidermal cells, and trichome cells) of *A. annua* were converted into RNA-seq libraries and sequenced using an Illumina HiSec2 500, and 237 577 070 pairs of 100-bp roads were generated.

Low-quality raw read sequences were removed using Trimmomatic (version 0.30). Cleaned reads were then mapped to the genome of *A. auuna* using TopHat2 software. Reads courts were calculated with HTsep using BAM results from TopHat2, and TPM values were then calculated for every gene in the tissues analyzed.

Gene Prediction The repeat-masked *A. annua* genome sequence was used for gene predictions. Three predictors, Fgenesh, GeneMark, and Augustus, were used for *ab into* gere prediction with default parameters, and for Fgenesh and Augustus, *A. thaliana* was selected as the species template. For each locus, predicted genes from Fgenesh, GeneMark, and Augustus were annotated based on BLAST searches against the NCBI nr, UniProt, and KEGG protein databases. The predicted gene with the highest score from BLAST was considered the best prediction and selected as the gene model of the locus. All steps were performed using in-house peri scripts. The selected gene predictions were improved using PASA with two cycles of annotation comparison. Sequence improvement included adding untranslated regions, exon boundary adjustments, merging genes, and adding alternative transcripts.

In total 205 982 transcripts were constructed from about ~237 million pairs of PE llumina (Hiseq2 500) RNA-seq reads from nine organ/tissue libraries. In total 19 168 transcript assemblies were constructed from ~0.8 million Roche 454 RNA-seq sequences using Trinity with default parameters: Trinity release 2014-07-17, Trinity. pl -seqType fq - JM 500G-full _ cleanup - output Artemisia _ output -left All _ paired _1 fq-right All _ paired _2 fq - single All _ unpaired. fq - CPU 24. An additional 86 708 *A. annua* unigenes were downloaded from the NCBI public database.

We evaluated the possibility that the high number of gene models in our assembly were false positives by using *A. annua* predicted proteins as queries in searches against the NCBI hr protein databases. Among the 63 226 predicted *A. annua* proteins, 59 190 proteins were similar to the nr proteins (E-value$<1e^{-5}$), and 54 586 proteins were similar to the nr proteins (E-value $<1e^{-10}$). Furthermore, the predicted *A. annua* genes were validated by BLASTN (2.2.26 version) searches against the sunflower genes (https://sunflowergenome.org/), the *A. annua* transcripts assembled from RNA-seq sequences, and the downloaded *A. annua* unigenes. Of the 63 226 predicted genes, 55 198 genes (87.3%) were similar to sunflower genes (E-value$<1e^{-10}$), and 55091 genes (87.1%) were supported by the unigenes or transcripts (E-value$<1e^{-50}$, overall length coverage>50% of the predicted gene).

The 63 226 predicted genes encode 66 920 transcripts. The lengths of the transcripts (mRNA) range from 153 to 16465 bp, and the average length is 1 324 bp. For the predicted genes, the average number of exans per gene is 5.2, the average exon length is 219 bp, and the average intron length is 655 bp.

Gene Family Analysis OrthoMCL was used to define gene families across 17 plant genomes. Besides the predicted proteins from *A. annua*, we used the following sources to obtain proteins from 16 other species: *Aquilegia coerulea*, *Brassica rapa*, *Chlamydomonas reinhardti*, *Citrus sinansis*, *Glycine max*, *Gossypium raimondii*, *Helianthus annuus*, *Physcomitrella patens*, *Populus trichocarpa*, *Theobroma cacao*, *Vitis vinifera*, *and Zea mays* (version 10.1, http://genome.jgi.doe.gov/pages/dynamicOrganism Download.jsf?organism = Phytozome V10.1); *Arabidopsis thaliana* (version 10, https://www.arabidopsis.org/); *Medicago truncatula* (version 4.0, http://medicago.jcvi.org/medicago/display.php? pageName = General§ion = Download); *Solanum lycopersicum* (version 2.4, http://solgenomics.net/organism/solanum_lycopersicum/genome); and *Oryza sativa* (version 7.0, http://rice.plantbiology.msu.edu/). All protein sets were filtered for a minimum protein length of 50 amino acid residues. An all-against-all comparison was performed using BLASTP with the thrashold E-value$<1e^{-5}$. For defining gene families, the Markov cluster algorithm was used to cluster the BLASTP results into groups of homologous proteins at an inflation factor of 1.5.

The output of OrthoMCL was parsed to identify gene families. A concatenated alignment of single-copy genes was performed using ClustalW with default settings. The phylogenetic tree was constructed using maximum parsimony with the MEGA program (version 6.0) with 1 000 bootstrap replicates. Computational analysis of changes in gane family size in 17 plant genomes was done using CAFE.

Identification of Transcription Factors We refined the TF prediction pipeline by updating the hidden Markov model (HMM) profiles used to identify TFs. The HMM profiles were downloaded from Pfam (version 27.0) for most signature domains. The predicted *A. annua* proteome and eight other sequenced plant proteomes were scanned using HMMER suite (http://hmmer.janelia.org/) based on pfam profiles to identify TFs, after which TFs were assigned to different families according to assignment rules.

ldentification of Terpene Synthase Genes The protein sequences were scanned using pfamscan based on the HMMER suite. The TPSs were identified by screening with the HMM profiles of the PFAM motifs PF01397 (N-terminal TPS domain) and PF03936 (TPS, metal binding domain). The require ment for the presence of both domains was strict.

Phylogeny Reconstruction of TPS Proteins Putative full-length TPSs (>400 amino acids in length) identified in 11 sequenced plant genomes, including 88 from *A. annua*, 51 from *H. annuus*, 30 from *S. lycopersicum*, 40 from *M. truncatula*, 33 from *A. thaliana*, 54 from *G. raimondii*, 43 from *V. vinifera*, 44 from *P. trichocarpa*, 24 from *G. max*, 41 from *O. sativa*, and 69 from *E. grandis*, were subjected to phylogenetic analysis. To perform phylogeny reconstruction, we performed multiple protein sequence alignments of the TPS homologs using Clus-talW with the default settings. The neighbor-joining trees were constructed using the MEGA program (version 6.0) with 1000 bootstrap replicates.

Hierarchical Clustering Analysis Using RNA-Seq Data Hierarchical clustering analysis based on RNA-seq data was performed using MultiExperiment Viewer (MeV4.9.0) software to predict potential TFs involved in the biosynthesis of artemisinin. Sample clustering was carried out using the HCL method, and the evolutionary distances were computed with Poisson correction and average linkage clustering.

Construction of Transforming Vectors and Transformation of *A. annua* The full-length open reading frames (ORFs) of *HMGR* (AA201470), *FPS*, and *DBR2* from *A. annua* were cloned from young leaf cDNA using gene-specific primers and then ligated into the modified pCAMBIA1305.1 vector with a glyphosate selection marker gene, and with expression driven by the CaMV35S promoter (Supplemental Figure 7, Supplemental Table 11). The full-length ORF of *AaMYB2* was cloned from *A. annua* young leaf cDNA using AaMYB2-F and AaMYB2-R primers (Supplemental Table 11) and then ligated into the $pHB^+$ vector under the control of the CaMV35S promoter.

The resulting constructs were introduced into *Agrobacterium tumefaciens* strain EHA105, and *A. annua* transgenic plants were generated as described previously.

Gene Expression and HPLC Analyses The relative transcript levels of all *A. annua* genes tested were measured by qPCR. The relative transcript levels were normalized to the transcript abundance of *A. annua â-actin* (GenBank: EU531837.1). For qPCR analysis, mRNA was extracted using the RNAprep pure Plant Kit (Tiangen, China) and reverse transcribed into cDNA using the PrimeScript RT Master Mix (TaKaRa, China). PCR amplification was performed in a Roche LightCycler96 (Roche) using the SYBR Green qPCR Master Mix (Tiangen) according to the manufacturer's instructions. The thermal profile for SYBR Green qPCR was 95℃ for 2 min, followed by 40 cycles of 95℃ for 20s, 54℃ for 20 s, and 72℃ for 20 s. Samples for HPLC analysis were prepared as described previously. Artemisinin standard was purchased from Sigma and dihydroartemisinic acid standard was obtained from Guangzhou Honsea Sunshine Bio Science and Technology (Sunshine Bio, China).

［沈乾，张立达，唐克轩，等. Molecular Plant, 2018, 11: 776-788.］

# The *Coix* genome provides insights into Panicoideae evolution and papery hull domestication

## 1 INTRODUCTION

*Coix lacryma-jobi* L., commonly known as adlay or Job's tears, is a widely cultivated crop in East and Southeast Asia. In China, people have used *Coix* seeds for food and brewing beer since ~8000 years ago. *Coix* seeds have higher protein content than most of the common cereals, and are a nutritionally balanced food. In addition, Coix is a key ingredient in traditional Chinese herbal medicine. The Kanglaite drug extracted from *Coix* seeds has been widely used to cure cancer and reduce the side effects of other treatments. With the re-recognition of *Coix*'s nutrition and medical function, *Coix* demand is increasing rapidly, and it has now been introduced to almost all tropical and subtropical zones of the world.

In traditional taxonomy, *Coix*, *Sorghum*, *Zea*, and *Setaria* are all Panicoideae. Based on characteristic inflorescence, *Sorghum* and *Setaria* are classified into

Andropogoneae and Paniceae, respectively. *Coix* and *Zea* belong to Maydeae. *Coix* is the only genus in Asia ever considered as a possible progenitor of maize. However, analysis of repetitive sequences indicated that *Coix* was closer to *Sorghum* than to *Zea*. In addition, *Zea mays* has a recent whole-genome duplication (WGD) event, which is associated with ancient tetraploids and ongoing gene loss. Whether it is also this case in *Coix* needs to be investigated. Even now, the evolutionary relationship of these genera in Panicoideae is still controversial, owing to lack of a sequenced *Coix* genome.

Wild *Coix* grain is encapsulated in a stony hull and the cultivated *Coix* in a papery one. The stony hull is thick and difficult to dehull, whereas the papery one is thin and easily removed. Papery hull is considered to be a key domestication trait in *Coix*. A stony hull in the wild species contributes to their fitness in adverse environments. However, stony hulls impede seed germination, production and processing in agriculture. During domestication of seed crops, the stony hull of the wild progenitors would be one of the most notable obstacles faced by ancient humans. Hence, selection of papery hulls and even exposed kernels is a key step in domestication of many important seed crops including barley, maize, and wheat. This trait is usually controlled by a small number of key genes as revealed in maize, legume, barley, and oil palm. However, whether this is also applied to the hull domestication of *Coix* still needs to be investigated.

Despite the importance of *Coix*, the related genomic and genetic research is very limited. Here, we report a chromosomal-scale genome assembly of *Coix aquatica*, a wild relative of the cultivated *Coix chinensis*, as well as a genetic map and seed hull transcriptome. Comparative genomic analysis showed that *Coix* is more closely related to sorghum than maize. Using this-omics information, we successfully revealed the physiology, transcriptome, and QTLs behind the key step in *Coix* domestication: from stony hull to papery hull.

## 2 RESULTS

Genome Sequencing, Assembly, and Annotation The genome of *C. aquatica* Daheishan (DHS, $2n = 2x = 20$), which was selected from wild *Coix* and used as a perennial grass for herbivores (Supplemental Figure 1), was *de novo* sequenced and assembled using integrated technologies of Illumina and SMRT. We obtained 82 Gb of data, which contained 8 783 914 clean reads with an average length of 9 kb, N50 of 14 kb, and N90 of 6 kb (Supplemental Figure 2A). K-mer analysis showed that the C. *aquatica* genome size was about 1.66 Gb (Supplemental Figure 2B), which is almost identical to the estimated 1.68 Gb using flow cytometry. The assembled genome is 1.62 Gb, containing 4 519 contigs with an N50 of 751 kb (Table 1). The assembled sequences cover 99.84% of 807 129 741 Illumina short reads, 97.82% of 458 core eukaryotic genes, and 95.76% of 1 440 core land-plant genes, respectively (Supplemental Figure 3A). Using Hi-C technology, the contig N50 was further improved to 2.24 Mb, and 1 595-Mb contig sequences were anchored onto ten pseudo-chromosomes with a maximum and minimum length of 184 Mb and 136 Mb, respectively (Supplemental Table 1). Among them, the order and direction of 1 500-Mb contig sequences were determined (Table 1). The Hi-C assembly accuracy was also confirmed by normalized contact matrix (Supplemental Figure 3B).

In total, 39 629 protein-coding genes were predicted by integrated approaches (Table 1), including *ab initio*, homologous, and prediction based on RNA sequencing (RNA-seq) (Supplemental Figure 4A). Among them, 37 336 genes were annotated at least by one of gene ontology (GO), KEGG, KOG, TrEMBL, and Nr databases (Supplemental Figure 4B). In *C. aquatica* genome, total exon length, mean total exon length per gene, and mean exon length were 56.6 Mb, 1 428 bp, and 310 bp, respectively (Figure 1A), which were closer to that of *Sorghum bicolor* and *Z. mays* rather than *Setaria italica* and *Oryza sativa* (Figure 1A).

**Table 1 Summary of *C. aquatica* genome assembly and annotation**

| Category | Number | N50 (kb) | Size (Mb) | Percentage of assembly |
|---|---|---|---|---|
| Contigs | 4 519 | 751 | 1 619 | NA |
| Correction | 3 005 | 2 241 | 1 615 | 99.8 |
| Anchored | 2 385 | NA | 1 595 | 98.8 |
| Oriented | 1 000 | NA | 1 500 | 92.9 |
| Predicted coding genes | 39 629 | NA | 56.6 | 3.5 |
| Repeat sequences | 527 996 | NA | 1 218 | 75.4 |

NA, not applicable.

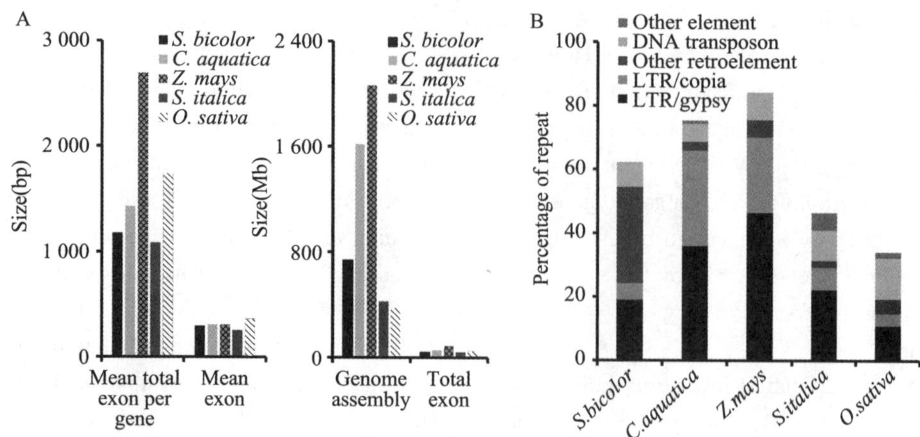


**Figure 1　Comparative analysis of the genome structure of *C. aquatica*, *S. bicolor*, *Z. mays*, *S. italica*, *O. sativa*, *H. vulgare*, and *A. thaliana***

(**A**) Comparison of the protein-coding gene structure. (**B**) Comparison of the repetitive element structure.

The *C. aquatica* genome has a total repetitive element content of 75.39%, comprising 68.64% retroelemerits, 5.72% DNA transposons, and 1.03% other elements (Table 1 and Figure 1B). Most of the retroelements are long terminal repeat (LTR), including 36.07% *gypsy* and 29.83% *copia* (Figure 1B). The repetitive element content in *C. aquatica* (75.39%) was between that of *S. bicolor* (62%) and *Z. mays* (84%), but far from *S. italica* (46%) and *O. sative* (34%) (Figure 1B). However, the ratio of *gypsy/copia* in *C. aquatica* was the lowest in the five compared species, suggesting that *copia* amplification had higher contribution to genome evolution in *C. aquatica* than in the other species.

Evolutionary Analysis of *Coix*　Predicted genes in *C. aquatica*, *S. bicolor*, *Z. mays*, *S. italica*, *O. sativa*, *Hordeum vulgare*, and *Arabidopsis thaliana* were clustered into 19 589 gene families, which covered 34 169 genes of *C. aquatica*. These genes were classified into 5 881 single-copy, 7 558 multiple-copy, 2 755 unique, and 17 975 other genes (Figure 2A). Among them, 2 755 unique genes were clustered into 655 gene families mainly involved in photosynthesis, ribosome biogenesis, oxidative phosphorylation, and protein processing in endopiasmic reticulum (Supplemental Table 2). These genes may explain the high biomass and protein content of *C. aquatica* (Supplemental Figure 1A and 1D). A phylogenetic tree was constructed based on 2 882 shared single-copy genes (Figure 2A). The results showed that Panicoideae was split ~49.6 million years ago (Mya), *S. italica* was spilt ~23.9 Mya, and *Z. mays* was split ~13.1 Mya (Figure 2A), which are close to the reported ~48, ~27, and ~13 Mya, respectively. *C. aquatica* and *S. bicolor* were located in the same branch and diverged ~10.0 Mye, which was very close to the divergent time of *Z. mays* (Figure 2A). In addition, *C. aquatica* and *S. bicolor* shared the largest number of gene families, followed by *C. aquatica* and *Z. mays*, *C. aquatica* and *S. italica*, and *C. aquatica* and *O. sativa* (Figure 2B). Furthermore, the synteny between *C. aquatica* and *S. bicolor* was higher than that between *C. aquatica* and *Z. mays* (Figure 2C). Together, these results suggest that *C. aquatica* is more closely related to *S. bicolor* than to *Z. mays* on the whole-genome level. We detected a recent WGD event in *Z. mays*, which was not found in *S. bicolor* (Figure 2D), in agreement with previous reports. Interestingly, *C. aquatica* has a recent segmental genome duplication event that is independent from the one in *Z. mays* (Figure 2D). However, we cannot determine the exact order of genome duplication and divergent times among *Z. mays*, *C. aquatica*, and *S. bicolor* because they are very close to each other (Figure 2A and 2D), and the molecular clock may run at different rates in different lineages or over different time spans.

We found 1 647 gene families expanded and 603 gene families contracted in *C. aquatica* (Figure 2A). The expanded gene families were mainly involved in photosynthesis, ABC transporters, oxidative phosphorylation, ribosome, Isoquinoline alkaloid biosynthesis, plant - pathogen interaction, and other pathways (Supplemental Table 3), which may contribute to high biomass and biotic resistance of *C. aquatica*. Among them, there were 41 NB-ARC domain gene families, and the total number of genes in *C. aquatica* is more than other compared species excluding *H. vulgare* (Supplemental Figure 5A). Moreover, another family, GF_58, involved in benzoxazinoid (BX) biosynthesis, was also expanded (Supplemental Figure 5B). It has been documented that BXs play important roles in plant resistance

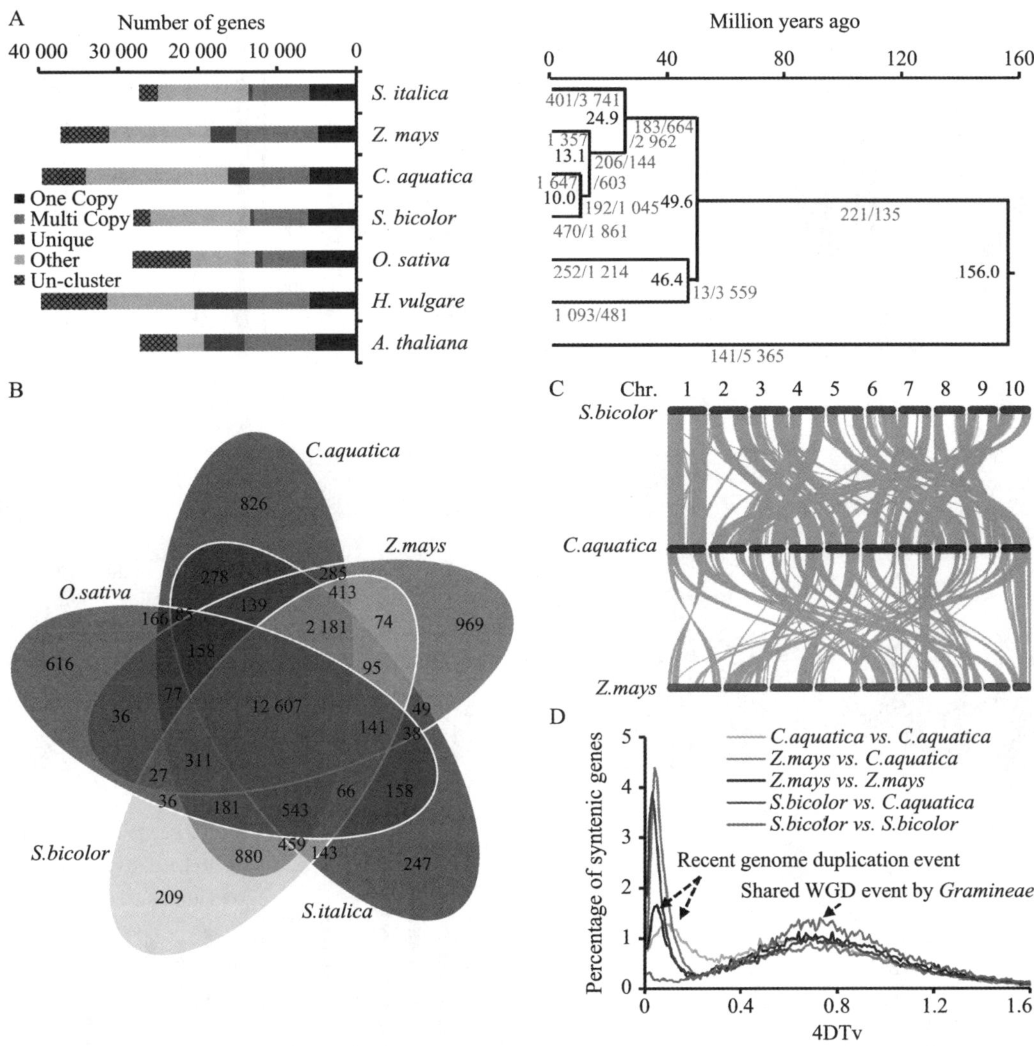


**Figure 2 Evolutionary analysis of the *C. aquatica* genome**

(**A**) Left: family clustering of predicted genes. Right: phylogenetic tree based on shared single-copy gene families. Divergent times are indicated above the tree, and the number of expanded and contracted gene families are shown in red and blue numbers on the branches, respectively. (**B**) Number of shared and unique gene families. (**C**) Syntenic blocks between *C. aquatica*, *S. bicolor*, and *Z. mays*. (**D**) Distribution of four-fold degenerate sites of the third codons (4DTv) for percentage of syntenic genes from *C. aquatica*, *S. bicolor*, and *Z. mays*. Two whole-genome duplication (WGD) events were indicated by the peaks (4DTv=0.08 and 0.68).

to pests and diseases.

Characterization and Transcriptome of *Coix* Seed Hull

The selection of papery hull was a milestone in *Coix* domestication. Thus, we characterized the differences between two contrasting hull types in wild DHS (stony hull) and cultivated Xiaobaike (XBK, papery hull) (Figure 3A and Supplemental Figure 6B). We found that the hull of XBK (~171 μm) was significantly thinner than that of DHS (~460 μm) (Figure 3B). We also measured seed hull pressure resistance (SHPR), the minimum strength required to break the hull of a mature seed in dehulling. The SHPH of XBK was only one-fiftieth that of DHS (Figure 3C). This makes seeds of cultivated *Coix* much easier to dehull by human beings, especially in ancient times when there were few effective processing tools available. Furthermore, the germination rate of hulled seeds was 91.3% in XBK but only 25.7% in DHS, while the corresponding values for denulled seeds were about the same (90%) (Supplemental Figure 8A and 8B). Hindering of dehulling and seedling establishment by the stony hull may ascribe to its thickness.

To further investigate the structurai differences between papery hull and stony hull, we compared cross-sections of seed hulls (Figure 3D). XBK hull has fewer vascular bundles than DHS hull, and sclerenchyma cells around the vascular bundles in XBK hull were significantly smaller than in DHS. In addition, these differences were also found between other

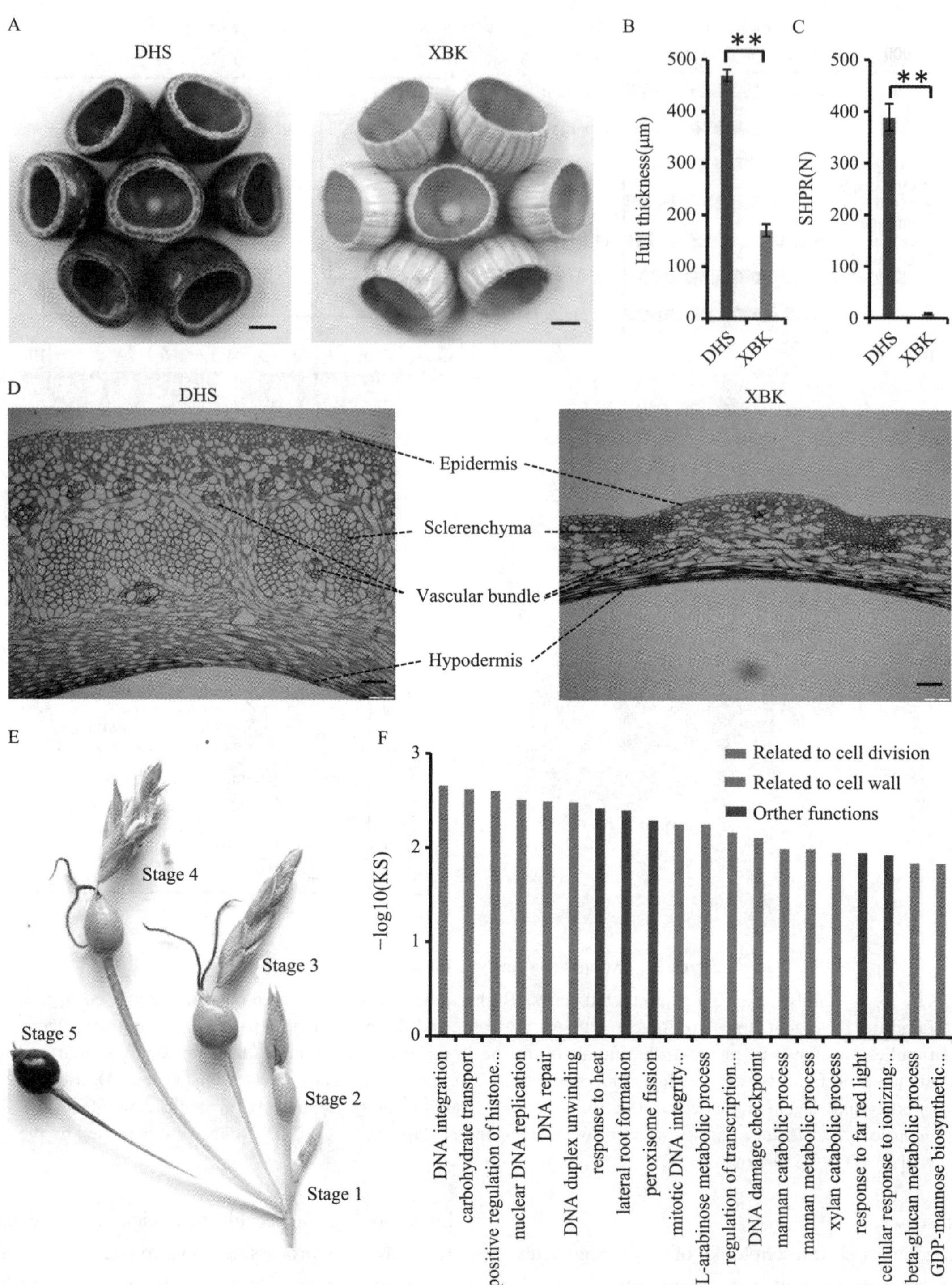


**Figure 3 Comparison of seed hull of Daheishan (Stony Hull) and Xiaobaike (Papery Hull)**

(**A**) Hull cross section of Daheishan (DHS) and Xiaobaike (XBK). Scale bar represents 2 mm. (**B**) Hull thickness of DHS and XBK (mean±SD; two-sided *t*-test ($n=30$), ** $P \leqslant 0.01$). (**C**) SHPR of DHS and XBK (mean±SD; two-sided *t*-test ($n=51$), ** $P \leqslant 0.01$). (**D**) Hull structure of DHS and XBK. Scale bar represents 50 μm. (**E**) Hulls at different developmental stages co-exist in a typical *Coix* inflorescence. Stage 1, emerging; stage 2, fast-enlarging; stage 3, late-enlarging; stage 4, early-maturing; stage 5, late-maturing. (**F**) The 20 most enriched biological process GO terms among DEGs in stage-2 hull.

wild and cultivated *Coix* accessions (Supplemental Figure 7 and Supplemental Table 4). To track the developmental process of the hull, we divided *Coix* hull development into five stages according to the shape and growing speed of the hull (Figure 3E). At stage 2 (Supplemental Figure 8C), hull thickness of DHS and XBK was still comparable but XBK hull started to have fewer vascular bundles than DHS hull. The sclerenchyma cells around the vascular bundles in XBK hull were slightly smaller than in DHS. At stage 3 (Supplemental Figure 8C), the XBK hull became significantly thinner than the DHS hull. The sclerenchyma cells in XBK hull were less developed while they were well enlarged in DHS. These differences were maintained to the maturing stages (stage 4 and stage 5) (Supplemental Figure 8C). These results showed that the number of vascular bundles and size of sclerenchyma cells determined the difference in hull thickness between wild and cultivated *Coix*.

At stage 4, *Coix* hull stops enlarging and has the shape and thickness of a mature hull (Supplemental Figure 8C). Thus, transcriptomes of hulls at stages 1 - 3 (Supplemental Figure 9A) were analyzed to find differentially expressed genes (DEGs) associated with hull formation between DHS and XBK. The number of DEGs at stage 2 was greater than that at stage 1 and stage 3 in cell division, carbohydrate transport and metabalism, and cell wall biogenesis (Supplemental Figure 9B). GO enrichment showed that these DEGs at stage 2 were mainly involved in DNA integration, carbohydrate transport, positive regulation of histone acetylation, nuclear DNA replication, mitotic DNA integrity checkpoint, L-arabinose metabolic, and xylan catabolic (Figure 3F and Supplemental Figure 10). By clustering these DEGs into 20 subclusters (Supplemental Figure 11A), we found that subcluster 18 was the most significantly downregulated in XBK. These genes were enriched in glutathione metabolic, L-arabinose metabolic, regulation of transcription from RNA polymerase II promoter, and DNA strand elongation involved in mitotic DNA replication (Supplemental Figure 11B). These results and the morphology differences suggested that inhibition of cell division and wall biogenesis contributed to the thinner hull in XBK.

Mapping of QTLs Contributing to SHPR A genetic map was constructed with an "immortalized $F_2$" population derived from a cross between DHS and XBK. The map contains 230 Indel markers and covers 1 570.12 cM with an average interval of 6.83 cM (Supplemental Figure 12 and Supplemental Table 5). Ninety percent of the markers are consistent with the physical map (Supplemental Table 5). Using the genetic map and $F_2$ population, QTL mapping of SHPR, heading date, plant height, and number of tillers was conducted (Supplemental Figure 12 and Supplemental Table 6). In the $F_2$ population, besides the parental phenotypes (thick black hull and thin white hull, hereafter termed TKB hull and TNW hull), two recombinant phenotypes (thick white hull and thin black hull, hereafter TKW hull and TNB hull) were also observed (Figure 4A and 4B; Supplemental Table 7). The average SHPR of the four hull types was significantly different, with the highest to the lowest being TKB, TKW, TNB, and TNW hull, respectively (Figure 4B), revealing that thick/thin is more associated with SHPR than black/white. To resolve the puzzle of the association between hull color and SHPR, we measured the contents of mineral elements in different hull types. We found that the contents of multiple mineral elements, including Ca, Cu, K, Mg, Si, P, Zn, and S, were higher in the white hulls than in the black ones (Supplemental Figure 13).

We consistently detected two QTLs for SHPR. One was *Ccph1* (*Coix chinensis papery hull 1*) flanked by markers yyIndel0226 and yyindel0732 in Chr. 8, and the other was *Ccph2* (*Coix chinensis papery hull 2*) neighboring marker yylndel0715 in Chr. 6 (Supplemental Figure 12). *Ccph1* explained 61%, 69%, and 74% of phenotypic variance in three independent experiments, and the corresponding values for *Ccph2* were 8%, 6%, and 5%, respectively (Supplemental Table 6). Furthermore, we constructed a $BC_{4(DHS)}$ population by backcrossing an $F_1$ plant to the double-recessive parent XBK (*ph1ph1ph2ph2*) four times. The substituted chromosome segments containing QTLs of SHPR in the population were confirmed by the 230 Indel markers of the genetic map (Supplemental Figure 14 and Supplemental Table 8). We found that *Ccph1* and *Ccph2* segments were both heterozygous in all the tested TKB hull plants (*PH1ph1PH2ph2*). *Ccph1* segments were heterozygous and *Ccph2* segments homozygous in TKW hull plants (*PH1ph1ph2ph2*), and this was reversed in TNB plants (*ph1ph1PH2ph2*). Together, these results convincingly demonstrated that *Ccph1* and *Ccph2* coordinately regulate SHPR, and *Ccph1* specifically governs hull thickness while *Ccph2* solely regulates hull color.

Fine Mapping of *Ccph1* and *Ccph2* To narrow down the region of *Ccph1*, we genotyped an additional 1 276 $F_2$ individuals with markers yyIndel0226 and yyIndel0732. On the basis of the *Coix* genome, three new Indel markers (yylndel0893, yylndel0894, and yylndel0903) were developed (Supplemental Table 9), and *Ccph1* was mapped within yyIndel0903 and yyIndel0894. With two additional singlenucleotide polymorphism (SNP) markers (ZN1 and PK1), we fine mapped *Ccph1* to an interval of 250 kb between ZN1 and PK1, using 14 286 $F_2$ plants (Figure 4C). The region contains *EVM0025867* encoding an uncharacterized protein, *EVM0018786*, related to DNA recombination and a gap (Supplemental Table 10). To find clues as to what genes may be in the gap, we checked the synteny sequence in *S. bicolor* genome corresponding to *Ccph1* region (Supplemental Figure 15). The *S. bicolor* segment contains only two putative protein-coding genes. One is *LOC110435847*, encoding an uncharacterized protein, and the other is *LOC8070685*, encoding a putative Harbinger Transposase

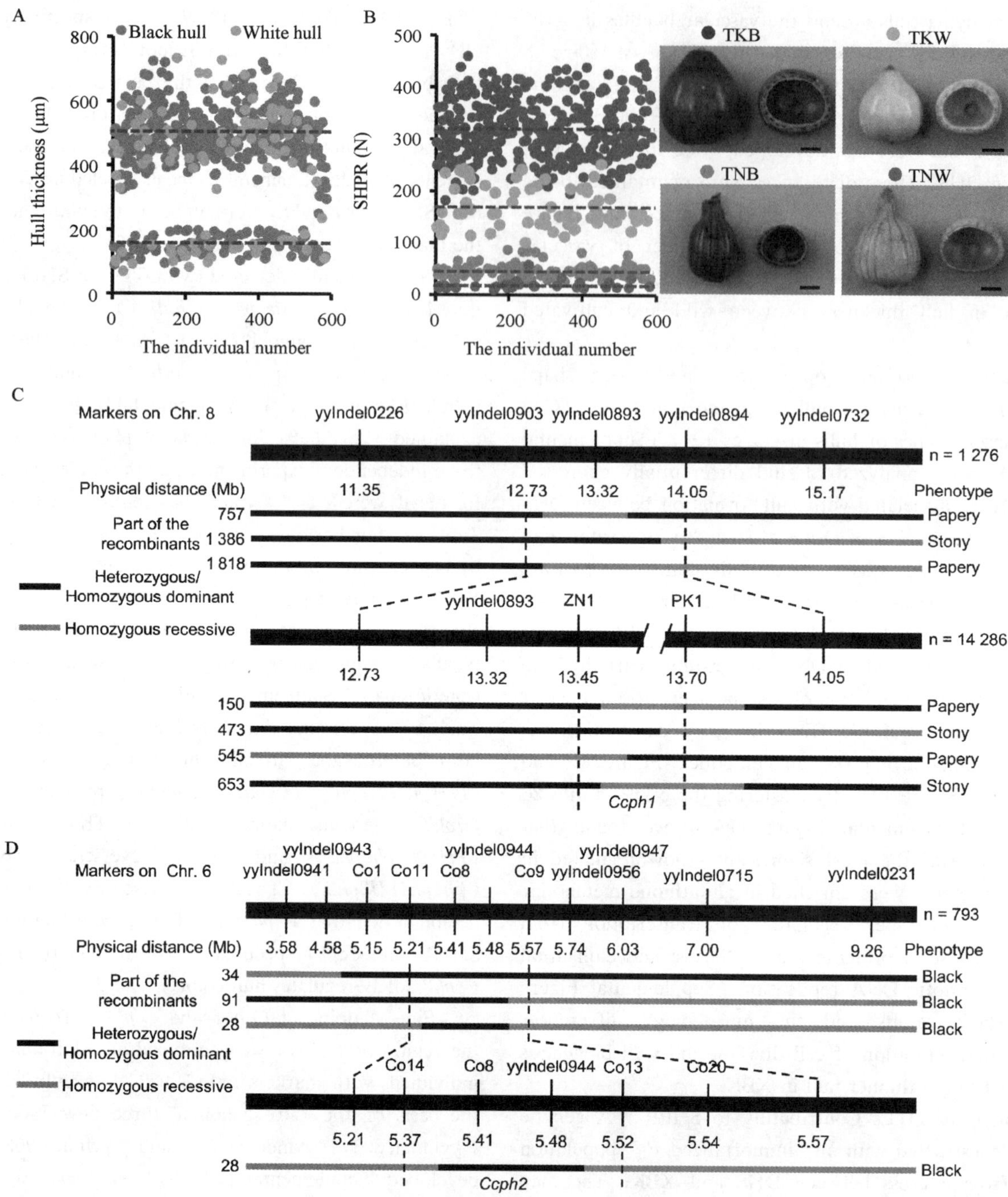


**Figure 4 Fine mapping of *Ccphl* and *Ccph2***

(**A**) Distribution of hull thickness. Hull thickness was clearly clustered into two groups (mean. $n = 5$). (**B**) Distribution of SHPR. Four types of hulls are clearly distinguished. TKB, thick black hull; TKW, thick white hull; TNB, thin black hull; TNW, thin white hull (mean, $n=5$). Scale bar represents 2 mm. For (**A**) and (**B**), 551 $F_2$ individuals in the "immortalized $F_2$" population were used, and the dotted red lines represent the average thickness and SHPR in different hull types. (**C**) Fine mapping of *Ccphl*. (**D**) Fine mapping of *Ccph2*.

Derived 1 (HARBI1). Similarly, *Ccph2* was fine mapped to a 146-kb region between two SNP markers, Co14 and Co13 (Figure 4D). The genome sequence of this region carries 10 predicted protein-coding genes (Supplemental Table 10), among which *EVM0013000* encodes a putative β subunit of adaptor protein (AP) complex 3.

## 3 DISCUSSION

The comprehensive information of the wild *C. aquatica* genome would provide an excellent resource for genetic improvements for this crop and its close relatives including sorghum and maize. Many valuable traits of wild *Coix* have been identified, such as higher medicinal components and protein level, long duration of staying green, and waterlogging resistance. Discovery and utilization of the functional genes for these traits would help to breed new elite *Coix* cultivars. Furthermore, as a helophyte, *Coix* has excellent disease resistance, especially against pathogens that tend to burst under a humid environment. This is probably due to the expanded gene families with NB-ARC domain and gene families involved in biosynthesis of defensive metabolites, such as GF_58 (Supplemental Figure 5A and 5B). These advantages of *Coix* may benefit resistance breeding of maize and sorghum, which suffer greatly from humid-induced diseases.

The mutation of *tga1* (*teosinte glume architecture 1*) in teosinte, the progenitor of maize, causes glume thinning, which leads to the exposed and readily utilized kernels in maize. In *Coix*, we showed that a similar trait was controlled by a major QTL, *Ccph1*. Anatomic and transcriptome analysis suggested that recessive *Ccph1* in cultivated *Coix* leads to inhibition of cell division and wall biogenesis (Figure 3F; Supplemental Figures 9B and 11). We fine mapped *Ccph1* to a region of 250kb (Figure 4C), which contains a gene with unknown function, a gene involved in DNA recombination, and possibly a gene of unknown function and a *HARBI1* in the gap revealed by the synteny between *Coix* and *Sorghum* genome (Supplemental Figure 15). However, which gene is the real *CcPH1* and how it regulates hull thickness still need further investigation. Interestingly, *Ccph2*, another major QTL of SHPR, is also associated with hull color. In the fine-mapped region of *Ccph2* (Supplemental Table 10), a gene *EVM0013000* encoding AP3-β was annotated. AP complexes display a conserved function of selection and packaging of cargo proteins in the eukaryotic cell. Furthermore, mutation of AP3-β caused defective pigment biogenesis in fruit fly, mouse, and human. Based on the plant-specific role of AP3-β in vacuolar biogenesis and function, it is likely that AP3-β also regulates pigment accumulation in *Coix* hull. Besides, this gene could negatively affect the transportation and accumulation of mineral elements in the hull (Supplemental Figure 13). The higher accumulation of mineral elements in the white hulls might make them more fragile, thus leading to a lower SHPR.

The *C. aquatica* genome together with the mapping population, genetic map, and transcriptome data set have offered a powerful platform for evolutionary study and functional genomics, and will facilitate the molecular breeding of this important crop. Using these toolboxes, we demonstrated that papery hull in cultivated *Coix* might be caused by both abnormal cell division and development. We further found this trait to be controlled by two major QTLs, which are separately associated with hull thickness and color. These findings greatly enhanced our understanding of the domestication of this crop. As the first sequenced species in *Coix* genus of Gramineae, *C. aquatica* genome bridges the sequenced sorghum and maize, and will help in studies of the evolution of grass crops.

## 4 METHODS

4.1 Plant Materials Daheishan (DHS, $2n = 2x = 20$), possessing a stony hull (thick and black), was selfed for seven generations from a wild *C. aquatica* plant collected from Jinghong, China. DHS is bred as a perennial grass (Supplemental Figures 1 and 6). In this study, it was used for whole-genome sequencing and as one parental line of the "immortalized $F_2$" population. Xiaobaike (XBK, $2n = 2x = 20$) was the most widely cultivated *Coix* in China and has a papery hull (thin and white). Besides hull feature, the two varieties have significant differences in many important agronomic traits, including plant height, number of tillers, and heading date (Supplemental Figure 6). In addition, a mini-core collection of 10 wild and 10 cultivated *Coix* accessions were used for anatomic analysis (Supplemental Figure 7 and Supplemental Table 4).

4.2 Preparation of Samples Genomic DNA of DHS, XBK, 551 $F_2$ individuals, and 84 $BC_{4(DHS)}$ individuals were isolated from 7-day-old leaves using a conventional CTAB (cetyl trimethylammonium bromide) method. Total RNA of DHS and XBK were isolated from 2-month-old mixed tissues (root, stem, and leaf) for RNA-seq to predict encoding genes and develop markers. Total RNA of DHS and XBK were isolated from hulls at stage 1 - 3 for RNA-seq to analyze DEGs with three replicates. All samples were collected and flash-frozen in liquid nitrogen. Total RNAs were isolated using the E. Z. N. A. Plant RNA Kit (Omega Bio-Tek) according to the manufacturer's standard protocol. The quality of RNAs was then checked using an Agilent 2 100 Bioanalyzer.

4.3 Genome Sequencing and Assembly Genome sequencing of DHS was performed using SMRT sequencing on a PacBio RS II sequencer (Pacific Biosciences) following the manufacturer's standard protocol. We acquired about 50× clean reads using Pacific Biosciences SMART analysis software v1.2.

With the aid of module of Canu v1.5, clean reads longer than 500 bp were selected with the settings 'genomeSize = 3 500 000 000' and 'corOutCoverage = 80'. Reads overlapping were detected through a highly sensitive overlapper MHAP v2.12 ('corMhapSensitivity = low/normal/high'), and errors were corrected using falcon _ sense method ('correctedErrorRate = 0.025'). The corrected reads were assembled into contigs using Canu v1.5. The iterative polishing of assembly was achieved by aligning Illumina paired-end reads (~72× PE150 reads) into contigs using Pilon v1.22. Furthermore, the assembly was evaluated by mapping Illumina reads, recoveries of core eukaryotic genes from CEGMA v2.5, and core landplant genes from BUSCO v2. According to the previous Hi-C assembly procedure, the contigs were broken into fragments with a length of 500 kb and then were clustered by LACHESIS software using Hi-C data. The number of the Hi-C read pairs between any two bins (500 kb each bin) was computed as the signal of contact intensity. The frequent contacts between adjacent DNA regions within contigs were confirmed by an invariable, strong and broad diagonal in the contact matrix after some manual adjustments. Finally, the contigs were clustered, ordered, and oriented into pseudo-chromosomes by Hi-C data. The gaps of pseudo-chromosomes were filled, and Illumina reads were used to correct base-calling again. Finally, the interaction of adjacent Hi-C sequences was checked for assessing the assembly.

4.4 Genome Annotation Using LTR FINDER v1.05, MITE-Hunter, RepeatScout v1.0.5, and PILER-DF v2.4, transposable element (TE) was predicted by homolog-based and *de novo* strategies. These repeats were then merged together using Repbase to form a *C. aquatica* repetitive sequence database. Finally, the database was used to identify and annotate TEs by RepeatMasker v4.0.6. *De novo*, homolog-based, and transcriptome-based strategies were combined to predict the gene model. Genscan, Augustus v2.4, GlimmerHMM v3.0.4, GeneID v1.4, and SNAP v2006-07-28 were used in the *de novo* prediction. GeMoMa v1.3.1 was used for homolog-based prediction. In the transcriptome-based prediction, unigenes were first parametrically and non-parametrically assembled, respectively, then were predicted by TransDecoder v2.0, GeneMarkS-T v5.1, and PASA v2.0.2, respectively. All the predicted gene structures were integrated into a consensus set with EVM v1.1.1. The predicted genes were annotated according to alignments against databases including GO, KEGG, KOG, TrEMBL and Nr using BLAST v2.2.31 (*E* value $\leqslant 1\times10^{-5}$). In addition, noncoding RNA, including microRNA, rRNA, and tRNA, were predicted by Infenal v1.1 and tRNAscan-SE v1.3.1 according to the Rfam and miRbase databases. Pseudogenes were predicted by GenBlastA v1.0.4 alignment and GeneWise v2.4.1.

4.5 Comparative Genomic Analysis OrthoMCL was used to cluster the gene families. The sequences of shared single-copy gene families in *C. aquatica*, *S. bicolor*, *Z. mays*, *S. italica*, *O. sativa*, *H. vulgare*, and *A. thaliana* were used to construct phylogenetic trees using PhyML, and divergent time, including fossil time points of *O. sativa* versus *H. vulgare*, *A. thaliana* versus *S. bicolor*, *O. sativa* versus *S. italica*, and *S. italica* versus *Z. mays*, were estimated with Macmctree. Based on results of phylogenetic trees and gene family clustering, analysis of expanded and contracted gene family was performed with CAFÉ and annotated using Pfam. Syntenic block analysis was performed by MCScanX. The 4DTV method was adapted to identify genome duplication events in the *S. bicolor*, *Z. maize*, and *C. aquatica* genomes.

4.6 RNA Sequencing, Marker Development, and DEG Analysis RNA-seq libraries of mixed tissues (root, stem, and leaf) and hull tissues of stage 1 - 3 were prepared and sequenced on a HiSeq 2 500 system with a PE150 strategy following the manufacturer's instructions (Illumina, USA). All low-quality reads were filtered using in-house perl script as follows: ① reads with ≥10% unidentified nucleotides (N). ② reads with >10 nucleotides aligned to the adapter, allowing ≤10% mismatches. ③ reads with >50% bases having Phred quality <5. About 6 Gb of clean reads were aligned to genome using HISAT2 v2.0.4 with the default parameters, then were assembled by String Tie v1.3.0 with parameters "- max-intronlen 20 000 - min-intronlen 20 -p 10."

Based on the RNA-seq data of mixed tissues (root, stem, and leaf), the SNP and Indel were identified by GATK4 and SAMtools with default parameters. Intersection of the two methods was used as the candidate marker set for genetic map construction and fine mapping.

In DEG analysis, FPKM was used as measurement of the expression level to calculate gene expression by String Tie v1.3.0 with the default parameters. Pearson's correlation coefficient was used to measure the correlation between biological replicates. DEseq was then used to analyze DEGs at fold change ≥2 and false discovery rate (FDR) <0.01. Finally, these DEGs were performed functional enrichment using Blast2GO. The *P* value was calculated using two-sided Fisher's exact test and was further corrected with the Benjamini-Hochberg procedure.

4.7 Construction of Population Using an $F_1$ plant derived from the cross between DHS and XBK, an $F_2$ population and a $BC_{4(DHS)}$ population were developed. The $F_2$ population contains 551 individuals. As *Coix* is perennial under controlled conditions and can be propagated through cutting at the stage of flowering time, the initial $F_1$ plant and all the $F_2$ individuals are permanently maintained. Thus, the $F_2$ population is an "immortalized $F_2$" population. The $BC_{4(DHS)}$ population was created by backcrossing the $F_1$ plant to the double-recessive parent XBK four times.

4.8 Phenotyping The "immortalized $F_2$" population was grown in Jinghong, China in 2017 - 2018 and Chengdu, China in 2018. Heading date, plant height, and number of tillers at heading stage were recorded. Five mature seeds were randomly selected from each $F_2$ individual to measure SHPR and hull thickness, and color recorded. SHPR was recorded as the minimum pressure to break the hull of a mature seed by putting the seed laterally on a pressure detector (YYD-1 type, Zhejiang Top Instrument). To measure hull thickness, we sliced the hull crosswise at the middle position, then measured it under an anatomical microscope. The hull was classified as thick if thicker than 230 μm, or thin if thinner than 200 μm. Hull color was recorded as white or black.

*Coix* has an indefinite inflorescence, and hulls at different developmental stages co-exist in a typical *Coix* inflorescence (Figure 3E). Based on shape and growing speed, *Coix* hull development can be divided into five stages, namely emerging, fast-enlarging, late-enlarging, early-maturing, and late-maturing. Stage 2 is the vital and fastest growing stage. For anatomical observation, hulls at stages 2－5 were sliced crosswise as used to measure thickness and used for making paraffin sections. After staining with safranin O-fast green, the sections were observed under a microscope.

For the germination assay, hulled and dehulled seeds of DHS and XBK were cultivated in an incubator (28 ℃, relative humidity 80%, light/dark 16 h/8 h), and the germination rate was recorded every 2 days until the 20th day.

For measurement of mineral element contents of hull, 2-g hulls from each of 10 random individuals for each hull type (TKB, TKW, TNB, and TNW) in the "immortalized $F_2$" population were harvested and then mixed together. In total, four mixing pools, together with DHS and XBK, were tested using reported methods.

A two-sided *t*-test and least significant difference test were performed for corresponding phenotypic measures in IBM SPSS.

4.9 Construction of Genetic Map and QTL Mapping

Previously identified Indels from DHS and XBK were used to design primers with Primer 3, and 891 Indel markers were selected from the marker set to verify polymorphism between the parents. Finally, 230 reliable markers were used to genotype the 551 individuals in the "immortalized $F_2$" population. Linkage analysis and QTL mapping were carried out using QTL IciMapping. Markers were grouped at LOD= 3.0, and QTLs were mapped by the ICIM-ADD method with LOD ⩾ 2.5. Phenotypic data from multiple environments together with genotypic data were used for QTL analysis. The QTLs that were found in at least two environments were considered candidates. To confirm the chromosome segments containing QTLs of SHPR, we subjected $BC_{4(DHS)}$ individuals to genotyping analysis using 230 markers covering the whole genome of DHS as illustrated in Supplemental Figure 14.

To fine map *Ccph1* and *Ccph2*, we developed and verified more Indel and SNP markers within flanking markers from a previous marker set of RNA-seq. At the same time, we used an additional $F_2$ population of 15 562 individuals to identify more recombinants in a linkage block. Primers of these markers are listed in the Supplemental Table 9.

## 5 ACCESSION NUMBERS

The *C. aquatica* genome assembly has been deposited in the National Center for Biotechnology Information under BioProject accession code PRJNA509097. Other sequence release data will be deposited under the same BioProject and will be available upon acceptance of the manuscript.

[郭超，王雅南，周树峰，等. Molecular Plant, 2019, 13: 309－320.]

# *Ii*WRKY34 positively regulates yield, lignan biosynthesis and stress tolerance in *Isatis indigotia*

## 1 INTRODUCTION

Polyploids often present novel phenotypes that are not found in their diploid progenitors, including enhanced organ size, biomass and stress tolerance, etc. These traits often have some adaptive significance, allowing polyploids to increase their chances of being selected by nature, which we called "polyploidy vigor". The appearance of polyploidy vigor is demonstrated under complex genetic control, involving changes in gene expression through increased variation in dosage-regulated gene expression, epigenetic regulation and regulatory interactions. Therefore, study on the gene expression related to the altered phenotype is crucial to clarify the underlying molecular mechanisms of polyploidy vigor, and will prompt the discovery of rational intervention strategies towards desired phenotypes.

*Isatis indigotica* Fort., belonging to the family Cruciferae, is a prevalent Chinese medicinal herb. The root of *I. indigotica* (Radix Isatidis), with Chinese name "Ban Lan Gen", is frequently used for the treatment of hepatitis, influenza and various kinds of inflammation. Lignans, mainly including lariciresinol and its derivatives, have been identified as effective antiviral components of *I. indigotica*. In our previous study, the tetraploid *I. indigotica* ($2n=28$) with greater yield, higher lignans accumulation and enhanced stress resistance was obtained from its natural diploid progenitor ($2n=14$). An *Arabidopsis thaliana* whole genome Affymetrix gene chip (ATH1) was used to survey the variation of gene expression between tetraploid and diploid *I. indigotica*, and results revealed a coordinated induction and suppression of 715 and 251 ploidy-responsive genes in tetraploid *I. indigotica*, involving in various developmental, signal transduction, transcriptional regulation and metabolic pathways. Some of them, such as a stomatal developmental gene *IiSDD1*, two signal transduction genes *IiCPK1* and *IiCPK2*, and a lignan biosynthetic pathway gene *IiPAL*, have been characterized to explore their contribution to the favorable physiological consequences after polyploidization. More recently, transcriptomic analysis of diploid and tetraploid *I. indigotica* indicated that the differentially expressed genes (DEGs) were mainly involved in cell growth, cell wall organization, secondary metabolite biosynthesis, stress response and photosynthetic pathways. Nevertheless, further studies are required to explore the mechanisms of the autotetraploidy vigor of *I. indigotica*.

Transcription factors (TFs) play essential roles in plants by controlling the expression of genes involved in various cellular processes, and are recognized to be particularly important in the process of crop domestication and are targets of molecular breeding of crops. The comprehensive survey of global gene expression performed by ATH1 revealed eight TFs tend to be significantly higher in tetraploid than in diploid *I. indigotica*, and among them there are 4 *WRKY* genes. Since the physiological role of WRKY TFs are widely related to diverse developmental processes, stress responses, and specialized metabolism, we reason that their expression variation in diploid and tetraploid *I. indigotica* might associate with altered phenotypes.

In the present study, a total of 64 *IiWRKY* genes (*IiWRKY1* - *64*) were first identified in *I. indigotica* transcriptome. In particular, *IiWRKY34* expression, significantly higher in tetraploids than in diploids, positively correlated with lariciresinol accumulation. Over-expression and RNAi analysis indicated that *IiWRKY*34 is able to regulate lariciresinol biosynthesis, meanwhile, its upregulation improves root development, and enhances salt and drought stress tolerance. This study provides new insights into the genetic bases underlying the superiority of tetraploid *I. indigotica* compared to its diploid progenitor, as well as a potential target for genetic improvement of *I. indigotica* herb.

## 2 MATERIALS AND METHODS

2.1 Identification and characterization of IiWRKY genes The homologous of *WRKYs* from the assembly of diploid *I. indigotica* transcriptome sequences were searched using the BLASTx algorithm from *A. thaliana* WRKYs (*At*WRKYs) and Chinese cabbage WRKYs (*Bra*WRKYs) respectively retrieved from The *Arabidopsis* Information Resource (http://www.arabidopsis.org/) and *Brassica* Database (BRAD, http://brassicadb.org/brad/). The Pfam database (pfam, http://pfam.janelia.org/) and the Simple Modular Architecture Research Tool (SMART, http://smart.embl-heidelberg.de/) were used to identify the putative WRKY proteins. The ProtParam tool (http://web.expasy.org/protparam) was further used to analyze the chemical and physical characteristics of these *Ii*WRKY proteins.

2.2 Bioinformatics analysis of IiWRKYs The amino acid sequence alignments of *Ii*WRKYs alone, or along with *At*WRKYs were performed using CLUSTALX version 2.0.12. Phylogenetic relationships were analyzed using the Neighbor-Joining method with pairwise deletion option in MEGA 5.05. The putative polyploidy-responsive *Ii*WRKYs were identified through comparative analysis of orthologous genes between *I. indigotica* and *Arabidopsis*. According to the multiple sequence alignment and the previously reported classification of *At*WR-KYs, the *Ii*WRKYs were assigned to different groups and subgroups. The possible conserved motifs were further detected by MEME. *Ii*WRKY protein interactions were constructed by using STRING software (http://string-db.org/).

2.3 Integrated analysis of IiWRKYs expression and lariciresinol accumulation Tetraploid *I. indigotica* was generated followed the methods as described by Qiao using *I. indigotica* ($2n=14$) as the diploid donor. The supposed diploid and tetraploid plants were sampled to analyze ploidy levels using Quanta SC Flow Cytometer (Beckman Coulter, Brea, CA, USA). The hairy root culture was derived after infection of diploid and tetraploid *I. indigotica* plantlets with a Ri T-DNA bearing *Agrobacterium rhizogenes* bacterium (C58C1). Methyl jasmonate (MeJA, 0.5 μmol/L) treatment was performed on the day 18 post-inoculation, and the hairy roots were harvested at various time points (0, 1, 3, 6, 12 and 24 h). The harvested hairy roots, along with roots of diploid and autotetraploid *I. indigotica*, were used for RNA isolation and lariciresinol content determination.

Total RNAs were extracted using TRIzol Reagent (Thermo, Waltham, MA, USA), and the mRNAs were reversely transcribed by oligo dT to generate cDNA as a template. Real-time quantitative PCR (RT-qPCR) was used to analyze the transcripts of *IiWRKY33*, *IiWRKY34*, *IiWRKY48*, *IiWRKY49* and *IiWRKY50*. Gene-specific DNA primers for these *IiWRKYs* and the *I. indigotica* actin gene reported by Li et al. were listed in Supporting Information Table S1. The RT-qPCR was performed according to manufacturer's instruction (Takara, Beijing, China). Quantification of the gene expression was done with comparative CT method. Three independent biological samples were analyzed. Experiments were performed in triplicate, and the results were represented by their mean ± standard deviation (SD).

Lariciresinol content was determined by triple-quadrupole mass spectrometer (Agilent 6410, Agilent, Santa Clara, CA, USA) following our previously published methods. Multiple reaction monitoring mode was used for lariciresinol quantification with a selected transition of *m/z* 359 → 329. Lariciresinol standard was purchased from Sigma—Aldrich (St. Louis, MO, USA).

Correlations between *IiWRKYs* expression and lariciresinol accumulation were calculated by the Pearson correlation coefficient using *R* according to the co-occurrence principle between mRNA and metabolite levels.

2.4 Plasmid vector construction and transgenic hairy roots generation The coding sequence of *IiWRKY34* was amplified by PCR using gene-specific primers *IiWRKY34*-F and *IiWRKY34*-R (Table S1). The PCR products were digested with *Bcl* I and *Spe* I, and ligated into plasmid PHB-flag to generate PHB-*IiWRKY34*-flag. For construction of the RNAi vector, an appropriate 351 bp fragment of *IiWRKY34* was amplified by PCR using primers *IiWRKY34*-s*Nco*I-a*Sal*I and *IiWRKY34*-s*Kpn*I-a*Xba*I (Table S1). The PCR products were then subcloned in opposite orientations on either side of the Pdk intron of the pCAMBIA1300-pHANNIBAL vector to generate plasmids pCAMBIA1300-*IiWRKY34*. After sequencing confirmation, the above two plasmids, together with PHB-flag and pCAMBIA1300-pHANNIBAL as vector controls (control check, CK), were introduced separately into leaf explants of diploid *I. indigotica* by using *Agrobacterium tumefaciens* C58C1 strain and the generated hairy roots were screened using hygromycin. Hairy root lines generated through transformation with the blank C58Cl strain were used as wild-type (WT) control.

The hairy roots were cultured as described by Chen et al. The fresh weight (determined as the difference between the whole flask with and without the harvested root tissues) was recorded at Day 9, 18, 27, 36, and 45 post-inoculation. The hairy roots harvested at the Day 45 were used for DNA extraction, RNA extraction, metabolite determination, microscopic analysis and phloroglucinol-HCl staining.

Genomic DNA was subjected for PCR analysis to detect exogenous *IiWRKY34* transformations using primers *IiWRKY34*-ovx-F and *IiWRKY34*-ovx-R (designed specifically to cover the gene sequence and the vector sequence, Table S1). For RNAi transgenic hairy roots, primers JDPDK-1F and JDPDKR (Table S1) were used to detect the inserted *IiWRKY34* fragment. The transformed status of hairy roots was also verified for the presence of genes *hpt* and *rolb* or *rolc*. PCR-positive hairy roots were analyzed for *IiWRKY34* expression by using RT-qPCR analysis as described above.

The content of lignans was determined by LC—MS as described above. The selected transitions of *m/z* were 179→146 for conifer alcohol, 357→151 for pinoresinol, 359→329 for lariciresinol, 361→164 for secoisolariciresinol, 519→357 for pinorcsinol 4-*O*-glucopuranoside, and 685 → 523 for secoisolariciresinol diglucoside, respectively. All the standards were purchased from Sigma—Aldrich.

Microscopic analysis of hairy roots was done essentially as described by De & Aronne. Phloroglucinol-HCl staining was conducted to detect lignans, lignins, or wall-bound phenolics and derivatives, based on our previously published protocols.

2.5 Expression profile of IiWRKY34 in different tissues and under various treatments Leaves of 2-month-old diploid *I. indigotica* seedlings were sprayed with salicylic acid (SA, 100 μmol/L), MeJA (100 μmol/L) or NaCl (200 mmol/L) and sampled at 0, 1, 3, 6, and 12 h after treatment. For drought treatment, the seedlings were subjected to 2.5% polyethylene glycol (PEG) for the indicated times. For UV-B treatment, the seedlings were exposed to 1 500 J/$m^2$ UV-B light for 30 min, and then sampled at 0, 20, 40, 60 and 80 min during treatment, and at 30, 60, and 120 min post-treatment. The expression level of *IiWRKY34* in different tissues (roots, stems, leaves and flowers) and under various treatments was examined using RT-qPCR analysis as described above.

2.6 Determination of ROS level, proline content and total antioxidant capacity of transgenic hairy roots under stress treatments The *IiWRKY34* overexpression and depression, along WT type hairy roots (20 g) were respectively subjected to salt and drought treatments by adding NaCl (75 mmol/L) and PEG (2.5%) into the liquid culture medium. After treatment for 5 days, reactive oxygen species (ROS) level was detected using the red fluorescence probe dihydroethidium (Vigorous, http://www.vigorousbiol.com/) following the methods as described by Wang et al. Free proline content was determined as described by Bates et al. Total antioxidant activities were evaluated for trolox equivalent antioxidant capacity (TEAC) using the methods as described by Zhang et al.

2.7 Trasscript profiling The Illumina HiSeg2000 platform (San Diego, CA, USA) was used to investigate gene expression profile of thet ransgenic and WT harity roots (3 groups × 5 biological replicates) harvested at the day 45 after inoculation. The raw reads were first generated using Solexa GA pipeline 1.6. After the removal of low-quality reads, the retained high-quality reads were mapped to previous annotation of *I. indigotica* transcriptome. Tags were assigned to have significantly differential expression if they had a *P*-value of $<0.05$, a false discovery rate (FDR) of $<0.05$, and an estimated absolute fold-change $>2$ in sequence counts across libraries. These DEGs were further applied for Gene Ontology (GO) enrichment analysis and Kyoto Encyclopedia of Genes and Genomes (KEGG) pathway enrichment analysis to find out their biological implications or the involved pathway.

2.8 Untargeted metabolite profiling Metabolites from 15 different samples (100 mg of fresh weight, 3 groups ×5 biological replicates) were extracted according to Lisec et al. and determined by GC - TOF/MS (Agilent 7890, Agilent). The programs of temperature-rise was set as followed: 70℃ for 2 min, 10℃/min rate up to 140℃, 4℃/min rate up to 240℃, 10℃/min rate up to 300℃ and staying at 300℃ for 8 min. Full-scan method with range from 50 to 600 ($m/z$) was used. The total mass of signal integration area was normalized for each sample, and the normalized data were imported into Simca-P software (version 11.5, http://www.umetrics.com/simca), employing PLS-DA model using the first principal component of VIP (variable importance in the projection) values (VIP>1) combined with Student's *t* test (*t*-test, $P<0.05$) to find differentially expressed metabolites. The volcano plot was used to reveal significantly altered metabolite features *via* delineating a log transformation plot of the fold-change difference ($\log_2$ fold change value as *x*-axis) and the level of statistical significance ($-\log_{10} P$ value as the *y*-axis) of each metabolite. Metabolite alterations between *IiWRKY34*-OVX and *IiWRKY34*-RNAi lines were depicted in a map drawn according to KEGG pathway database.

2.9 Data mining The assembly of transcriptome sequences was searched for *IiWRKYs* and the lariciresinol biosynthetic genes using our previously published protocols, and these gene expression patterns in different *IiWRKY34* transgemic lines (15 samples) were visualized with a heat map using the $\log_2$-transformed data in Multi-Experiment Viewer (version 4.9.0). Genes with different expression patterns were grouped through hierarchical clustering. Accordingly, a heat map showing lignans accumulation in different *IiWRKY34* transgenic lines was also constructed.

Correlation among *IiWRKY34*, lariciresinol biosynthetic genes and lignans were constructed using the Pearson correlation coefficient according to the co-occurrence principle. The correlation network was generated using Cytoscape (version 3.6.0).

2.10 EMSA The *IiWRKY34* coding sequence was amplified using primers *IiWRKY34*-pET-F and *IiWRKY34*-pET-R (Table S1), and inserted into pET32a vector (Novagen, Darmstadt, Germany) between the sites NcoI and SacI to generate pET-*IiWRKY34* plasmid. This plasmid was then transformed into the *Escherichia coli* BL21 strain, and the recombinant protein was purified by using a His Spin Trap column (GE Healthcare, Buckinghamshire, UK). EMSA was performed using biotin-labelled probes and a Light-Shift chemiluminescent EMSA kit (Thermo, Chicago, IL, USA). To design biotin-labelled probes, a 1 500-bp upstream region of *Ii4CL3* was amplified following the instructions of the Genome Walker Kit (Clontech, Mountain View, CA, USA), and analysed for the presence of W-boxes (C/T) TGAC (T/C). The biotinlabelled probes (Table S1) were synthesized by Sangon Biotech Company (Shanghai, China).

2.11 Dual luciferase assay The coding sequence of *IiWRKY34* was subcloned into the PHB vector (Biovector, Beijing, China) to generate the effector, and the promoter of *Ii4CL3* was fused into the vector pGreenII 0800 (Biovector) to generate a reporter. The reporter and effector constructs were then separately transformed into *A. tumefaciens* strain GV3101. The bacterial cells were resuspended in MS medium with 10 mmol/L methylester sulfonate and 150 μmol/L acetosyringone to $OD_{600}=0.6$ and then incubated at room temperature for 3 h. The bacteria-harboring constructs were infiltrated into tobacco leaves according to Zhang et al. The leaves were collected after 48 h for dual-LUC assays using a Dual-Luciferase Reporter Assay System according to the manufacturer's instructions (Promega, Madison, WI, USA). Three independent biological replicates were measured for each sample.

2.12 Statistics Experiments were performed in triplicate, and statistical analysis was performed using SPSS 22.0 software. Paired, two-tailed Student's *t*-test was used to compare group differences. *P*-values$<0.05$ were regarded as statistically significant.

2.13 Data availability The nucleotides and amino acid sequences of *IiWRKYs* (*IiWRKY1* to *IiWRKY64*) are deposited in the GenBank databases under the accession numbers (MN480587 to MN480650). The raw RNA-seq read data are accessible through accession number PRJNA491805 (http://www.ncbi.nlm.nih.gov/sra/).

## 3 RESULTS

3.1 Identification and characterization of WRKY genes in *I. indigotica* A total of 64 putative *IiWRKY* genes

(*IiWRKY1* to *IiWRKY64*) were identified (Supporting Information Table S2). The ORFs were extracted from the putative *IiWRKY* sequences, and then converted into amino acid sequences (Supporting Information Table S3). Detailed information about each *IiWRKY* is given in Table 1.

**Table 1 Identification of *WRKY* genes in *I. indigotica***

| Group | Subgroup | Gene ID | Gene locus ID | CDS (bp) | ORF (aa) | Mass (kDa) | pI | Atortholog | | |
|---|---|---|---|---|---|---|---|---|---|---|
| | | | | | | | | *At*Gene ID | *At*Locus | Identity (%) |
| Ⅰ | | *IiWRKY3* | comp12944_c0_seq1 | 1 443 | 480 | 52.36 | 5.47 | *AtWRKY32* | AT4G30935.1 | 74.07 |
| Ⅰ | | *IiWRKY5* | comp14011_c0_seq1 | 594 | 197 | 22.08 | 8.86 | *AtWRKY20* | AT4G26640.1 | 90.86 |
| Ⅰ | | *IiWRKY14* | comp22052_c1_seq1 | 717 | 238 | 26.16 | 9.30 | *AtWRKY44* | AT2G37260.1 | 84.45 |
| Ⅰ | | *IiWRKY17* | comp22961_c0_seq1 | 1 392 | 463 | 50.46 | 8.73 | *AtWRKY58* | AT3G01080.1 | 76.33 |
| Ⅰ | | ***IiWRKY33*** | **comp27067_c0_seq1** | **1 548** | **515** | **56.76** | **8.37** | ***AtWRKY33*** | **AT2G38470.1** | **84.95** |
| Ⅰ | | *IiWRKY36* | comp27813_c0_seq2 | 972 | 323 | 36.24 | 9.45 | *AtWRKY26* | AT5G07100.1 | 74.53 |
| Ⅰ | | *IiWRKY37* | comp27813_c0_seq4 | 375 | 124 | 14.46 | 9.56 | *AtWRKY26* | AT5G07100.1 | 77.65 |
| Ⅰ | | ***IiWRKY48*** | **comp32055_c0_seq1** | **1 065** | **354** | **39.73** | **7.70** | ***AtWRKY25*** | **AT2G30250.1** | **71.00** |
| Ⅰ | | ***IiWRKY49*** | **comp32055_c0_seq2** | **1 224** | **407** | **45.56** | **7.19** | ***AtWRKY25*** | **AT2G30250.1** | **84.54** |
| Ⅰ | | *IiWRKY53* | comp32270_c3_seq7 | 1 521 | 506 | 54.83 | 8.67 | *AtWRKY4* | AT1G13960.1 | 89.17 |
| Ⅰ | | *IiWRKY54* | comp32270_c3_seq8 | 1 548 | 515 | 56.23 | 6.98 | *AtWRKY3* | AT2G03340.1 | 83.43 |
| Ⅰ | | *IiWRKY60* | comp34055_c0_seq1 | 1 431 | 476 | 52.80 | 8.70 | *AtWRKY1* | AT2G04880.2 | 76.72 |
| Ⅱ | **a** | ***IiWRKY34*** | **comp27256_c0_seq2_1** | **909** | **302** | **33.43** | **7.55** | ***AtWRKY40*** | **AT1G80840.1** | **88.12** |
| Ⅱ | a | *IiWRKY51* | comp32255_c0_seq1_1 | 762 | 253 | 28.16 | 8.80 | *AtWRKY60* | AT2G25000.1 | 72.14 |
| Ⅱ | a | *IiWRKY52* | comp32255_c0_seq2_2 | 729 | 242 | 26.81 | 8.61 | *AtWRKY60* | AT2G25000.1 | 74.00 |
| Ⅱ | b | *IiWRKY11* | comp19028_c0_seq1 | 1 587 | 528 | 58.63 | 6.39 | *AtWRKY61* | AT1G18860.1 | 77.91 |
| Ⅱ | b | *IiWRKY13* | comp20394_c0_seq1 | 1 368 | 455 | 50.41 | 6.79 | *AtWRKY47* | AT4G01720.1 | 82.81 |
| Ⅱ | b | *IiWRKY21* | comp26285_c0_seq1 | 1 539 | 512 | 56.04 | 5.94 | *AtWRKY42* | AT4G04450.1 | 80.63 |
| Ⅱ | b | *IiWRKY31* | comp26827_c0_seq1 | 885 | 294 | 33.43 | 8.12 | *AtWRKY9* | AT1G68150.1 | 73.73 |
| Ⅱ | b | *IiWRKY39* | comp28388_c0_seq1 | 1 173 | 390 | 43.18 | 6.17 | *AtWRKY36* | AT1G69810.1 | 67.65 |
| Ⅱ | b | *IiWRKY55* | comp32451_c1_seq1 | 1 617 | 538 | 58.46 | 5.48 | *AtWRKY31* | AT4G22070.1 | 88.27 |
| Ⅱ | b | *IiWRKY61* | comp36248_c0_seq1 | 1 728 | 575 | 62.32 | 8.81 | *AtWRKY72* | AT5G15130.1 | 85.23 |
| Ⅱ | c | *IiWRKY2* | comp12464_c0_seq1 | 972 | 323 | 36.56 | 5.94 | *AtWRKY49* | AT5G43290.1 | 70.37 |
| Ⅱ | c | *IiWRKY6* | comp14046_c0_seq1 | 1 236 | 411 | 46.24 | 6.37 | *AtWRKY48* | AT5G49520.1 | 81.88 |
| Ⅱ | c | *IiWRKY10* | comp17362_c0_seq1 | 585 | 194 | 22.38 | 6.30 | *AtWRKY59* | AT2G21900.1 | 78.71 |
| Ⅱ | c | *IiWRKY15* | comp22285_c0_seq2 | 465 | 154 | 18.02 | 8.48 | *AtWRKY8* | AT5G46350.1 | 83.77 |
| Ⅱ | c | *IiWRKY19* | comp24875_c0_seq2 | 192 | 63 | 7.39 | 9.39 | *AtWRKY50* | AT5G26170.1 | 93.65 |
| Ⅱ | c | *IiWRKY22* | comp26365_c0_seq1 | 618 | 205 | 23.2 | 5.88 | *AtWRKY51* | AT5G64810.1 | 85.50 |
| Ⅱ | c | *IiWRKY23* | comp26532_c0_seq1 | 939 | 312 | 34.85 | 6.62 | *AtWRKY28* | AT4G18170.1 | 83.85 |
| Ⅱ | c | *IiWRKY24* | comp26532_c0_seq2 | 930 | 309 | 34.63 | 8.24 | *AtWRKY28* | AT4G18170.1 | 66.87 |
| Ⅱ | c | *IiWRKY25* | comp26532_c0_seq3 | 852 | 283 | 31.95 | 7.74 | *AtWRKY71* | AT1G29860.1 | 79.79 |
| Ⅱ | c | *IiWRKY26* | comp26532_c0_seq4 | 861 | 286 | 32.16 | 6.46 | *AtWRKY71* | AT1G29860.1 | 64.86 |
| Ⅱ | c | *IiWRKY28* | comp26776_c0_seq1 | 528 | 175 | 20.20 | 9.51 | *AtWRKY57* | AT1G69310.1 | 90.12 |
| Ⅱ | c | *IiWRKY29* | comp26776_c0_seq5 | 999 | 332 | 36.95 | 6.98 | *AtWRKY57* | AT1G69310.1 | 78.98 |
| Ⅱ | c | *IiWRKY30* | comp26776_c0_seq9 | 540 | 179 | 20.73 | 9.63 | *AtWRKY57* | AT1G69310.1 | 90.00 |
| Ⅱ | c | *IiWRKY32* | comp26972_c0_seq2 | 441 | 146 | 16.77 | 9.37 | *AtWRKY75* | AT5G13080.1 | 85.81 |
| Ⅱ | c | *IiWRKY35* | comp27574_c0_seq1 | 1 113 | 370 | 41.52 | 7.32 | *AtWRKY23* | AT2G47260.1 | 80.86 |
| Ⅱ | c | *IiWRKY38* | comp27813_c0_seq7 | 576 | 191 | 21.52 | 7.00 | *AtWRKY56* | AT1G64000.1 | 82.50 |
| Ⅱ | c | *IiWRKY40* | comp28803_c0_seq1_1 | 519 | 172 | 19.82 | 8.97 | *AtWRKY12* | AT2G44745.1 | 89.40 |
| Ⅱ | c | *IiWRKY41* | comp28803_c0_seq2_2 | 399 | 132 | 15.51 | 9.30 | *AtWRKY12* | AT2G44745.1 | 94.70 |

(Continued)

| Group | Subgroup | Gene ID | Gene locus ID | CDS (bp) | ORF (aa) | Mass (kDa) | pI | Atortholog | | |
|---|---|---|---|---|---|---|---|---|---|---|
| | | | | | | | | *At*Gene ID | *At*Locus | Identity (%) |
| | c | *IiWRKY56* | comp32704_c0_seq5 | 432 | 143 | 16.51 | 9.01 | *AtWRKY45* | AT3G01970.1 | 75.84 |
| | d | *IiWRKY8* | comp16130_c0_seq1 | 1 038 | 345 | 37.72 | 9.62 | *AtWRKY11* | AT4G31550.2 | 82.61 |
| | d | *IiWRKY45* | comp31187_c4_seq1 | 1 041 | 346 | 38.24 | 9.75 | *AtWRKY74* | AT5G28650.1 | 85.26 |
| | d | *IiWRKY46* | comp31187_c4_seq3 | 996 | 331 | 36.74 | 9.51 | *AtWRKY39* | AT3G04670.1 | 89.46 |
| | d | *IiWRKY47* | comp31456_c3_seq4 | 588 | 195 | 21.83 | 9.44 | *AtWRKY15* | AT2G23320.1 | 90.97 |
| | **d** | ***IiWRKY50*** | **comp32075_c0_seq1** | **687** | **228** | **25.35** | **9.64** | ***AtWRKY21*** | **AT2G30590.1** | **84.65** |
| | d | *IiWRKY62* | comp37405_c0_seq1 | 1 038 | 345 | 37.81 | 9.77 | *AtWRKY7* | AT4G24240.1 | 77.93 |
| | e | *IiWRKY7* | comp15334_c0_seq1 | 1 269 | 422 | 45.77 | 5.17 | *AtWRKY14* | AT1G30650.1 | 82.45 |
| | e | *IiWRKY9* | comp17232_c0_seq1 | 900 | 299 | 32.35 | 6.39 | *AtWRKY22* | AT4G01250.1 | 91.33 |
| | e | *IiWRKY12* | comp19645_c0_seq1 | 870 | 289 | 31.64 | 5.60 | *AtWRKY35* | AT2G34830.1 | 82.33 |
| | e | *IiWRKY16* | comp22855_c0_seq1 | 828 | 275 | 30.59 | 5.09 | *AtWRKY69* | AT3G58710.2 | 87.73 |
| | e | *IiWRKY18* | comp24498_c0_seq1 | 777 | 258 | 28.91 | 5.52 | *AtWRKY65* | AT1G29280.1 | 91.98 |
| | e | *IiWRKY43* | comp30090_c0_seq1 | 552 | 183 | 20.37 | 4.57 | *AtWRKY27* | AT5G52830.1 | 74.16 |
| | e | *IiWRKY44* | comp30090_c0_seq3 | 1 047 | 348 | 38.68 | 4.93 | *AtWRKY27* | AT5G52830.1 | 73.86 |
| | e | *IiWRKY64* | comp46853_c0_seq1 | 921 | 306 | 34.08 | 6.27 | *AtWRKY29* | AT4G23550.1 | 86.18 |
| Ⅲ | | *IiWRKY1* | comp7344_c0_seq2 | 786 | 261 | 29.77 | 5.66 | *AtWRKY67* | AT1G66550.1 | 53.64 |
| | | *IiWRKY4* | comp13639_c0_seq2 | 894 | 297 | 33.32 | 6.01 | *AtWRKY70* | AT3G56400.1 | 71.59 |
| | | *IiWRKY20* | comp25578_c2_seq1 | 870 | 289 | 32.90 | 5.71 | *AtWRKY46* | AT2G46400.1 | 75.67 |
| | | *IiWRKY27* | comp26620_c0_seq1 | 1 020 | 339 | 37.96 | 5.63 | *AtWRKY54* | AT2G40750.1 | 74.65 |
| | | *IiWRKY42* | comp29870_c0_seq1 | 999 | 332 | 36.76 | 6.46 | *AtWRKY41* | AT4G11070.1 | 69.37 |
| | | *IiWRKY57* | comp33243_c1_seq1 | 423 | 140 | 15.71 | 8.44 | *AtWRKY55* | AT2G40740.1 | 65.44 |
| | | *IiWRKY58* | comp33243_c1_seq4 | 804 | 267 | 29.92 | 6.91 | *AtWRKY55* | AT2G40740.1 | 52.28 |
| | | *IiWRKY59* | comp334956_c0_seq1 | 933 | 310 | 34.83 | 6.06 | *AtWRKY30* | AT5G24110.1 | 75.56 |
| | | *IiWRKY63* | comp39251_c0_seq1 | 774 | 257 | 29.73 | 6.10 | *AtWRKY62* | AT5G01900.1 | 80.15 |

Words in 'bold font' indicate the polyploidy-responsive *I. indigotica WRKY* genes and their corresponding information. CDS, coding sequence; ORF, open reading frame; bp, base pair; aa, amino acids; pI, isoelectric point.

Sequence alignment of the unique DNA-binding domain, spanning approximately 60 amino acids of all 64 *Ii*WRKYs revealed that all *Ii*WRKYs contain the highly conserved DNA binding domain composed of the conserved WRKYGQK sequence followed by a $C_2H_2$- or $C_2HC$-type zinc finger motif (Supporting Information Fig. S1), which is the most prominent structural feature of WRKY protein. These IiWRKYs were classified into 3 large groups including groups Ⅰ (12), Ⅱ (43) and Ⅲ (9) according to the structures of their WRKY domains, and the 43 group-Ⅱ *Ii*WRKYs were further classified into 5 distinct subgroups (Ⅱa-e) according to different conserved motif distributions (Table 1). Phylogenetic and structural analysis of *Ii*WRKYs were shown in Supporting Information Fig. S2. Moreover, a phylogenetic tree including 64 *Ii*WRKYs and 72 *At*WRKYs was shown in Supporting Information Fig. S3. Results indicated that *Ii*WRKYs evolved from group Ⅰ to group Ⅱ and finally to group Ⅲ, paralleled with a WRKY evolutionary process observed in several other plant species.

3.2 Identification of putative polyploidy-responsive IiWRKYs Generally speaking, proteins from the same taxonomic group probably have the same origin and exhibit relatively conserved function. Since *I. indigotica* and *Arabidopsis* belong to the same family (Cruciferae), we use *Arabidopsis* database to predict *Ii*WRKYs functions in the present study. Orthologous WRKYs between *I. indigotica* and *Arabidopsis* were summarized in Table 1.

In our previous survey of the gene expression difference between tetraploid and diploid *I. indigotica via* ATH1 by using 22,810 probe sets, the *WRKY* genes, corresponding to *Arabidopsis* probe sets *AtWRKY33* (At2g38470), *AtWRKY25* (At2g30250), *AtWRKY40* (Atlg80840) and *AtWRKY21* (At2g30590), tend to be significantly higher in the tetraploids than in the diploids. Here, the orthologous gene comparative analysis between *I. indigotica* and *Arabidopsis*, clearly pinpointed the *IiWRKYs* with high homology to these *Arabidopesis* probe sets (Table 1), revealing in fact *IiWRKY33* (orthologous to *AtWRKY33*), *IiWRKY34* (orhologous to

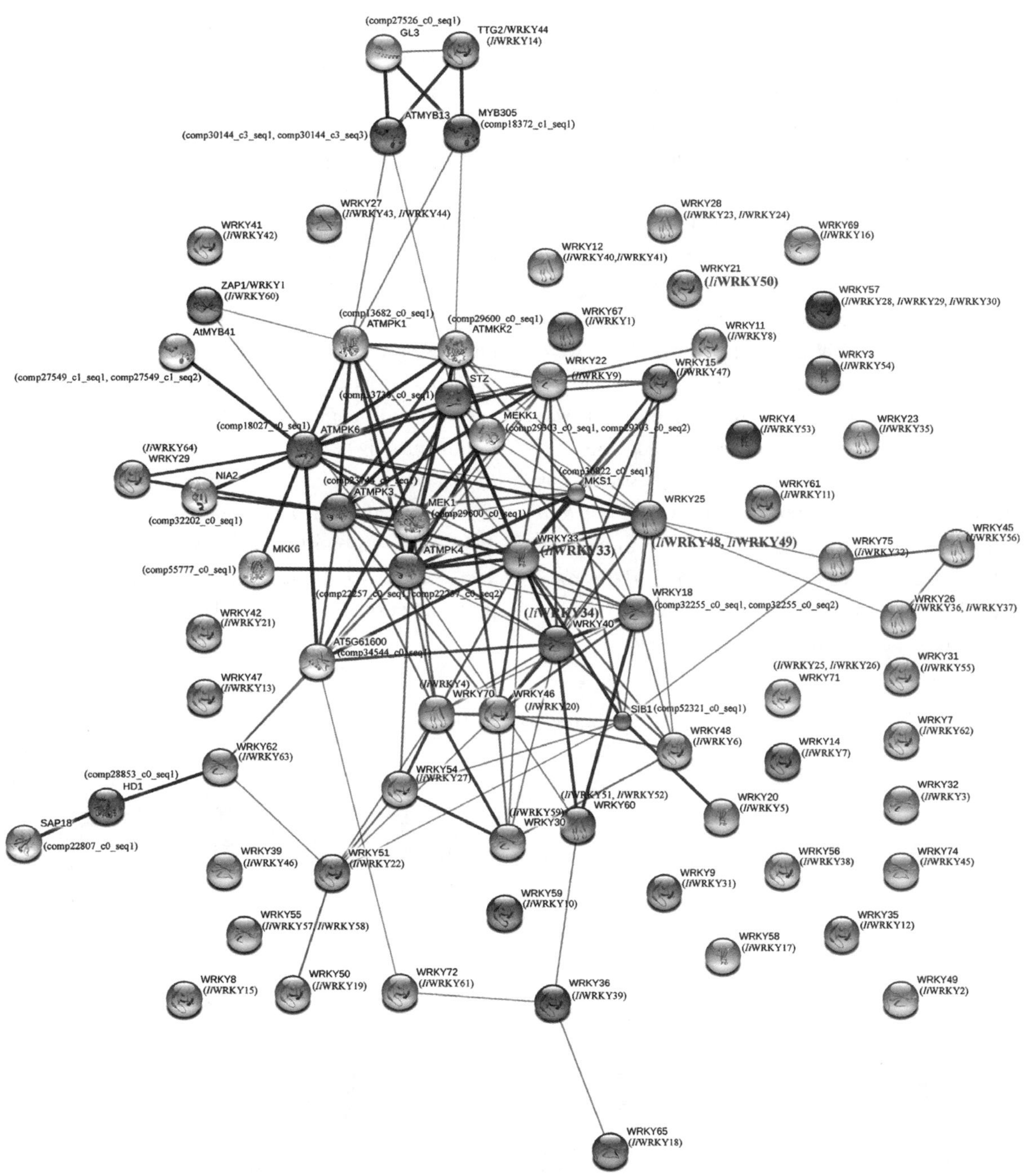


**Figure 1 The interaction network of 64 *Ii*WRKY proteins identified in *I. indigotica* and related proteins in *Arabidopsis***

Stronger associations are represented by thicker lines. The polyploidy-responsive *Ii*WRKYs are denoted with red color.

*AtWRKY40*), *IiWRKY48* (orthologous to *AtWRKY25*), *IiWRKY49* (orthologous to *AtWRKY25*) and *IiWRKY50* (orhologous to *AtWRKY21*) were precisely those polyploidy-responsive ones. *IiWRKY48* and *IiWRKY49* are paralogous genes, with 71% and 84.54% of identity to *AtWRKY25*, respectively.

An interaction network was constructed associated with WRKY *Arabidopsis* orthologs using *Ii*WRKYs. As shown in Fig. 1, many *Ii*WRKYs are involved in an interaction network that largely participate in plant defence regulatory pathways, as most factors affect plant stress responses, including STZ (salt tolerance zinc finger), HD1 (involved in jasmonic acid and ethylene-dependent pathogen resistance) and SIB1 (involved in responses to pathogen infection, jasmonic acid and SA stimulus), etc. Interestingly, *Ii*WRKY33 (orthologous to *At*WRKY33), *Ii*WRKY34 (orthologous to *At*WRKY40), *Ii*WRKY48 (orthologous to *At*WRKY25) and *Ii*WRKY49 (orthologous to *At*WRKY25), which were predicted polyploidy-responsive, respresent central nodes in the interaction networks that become activated by numerous elicitors and may integrate signaling from various stresses. However, *Ii*WRKY50, another polyploidyinduced member, was not integrated in the network.

3.3 Integrated analysis of polyploidy-responsive IiWRKYs and lariciresinol The ploidy levels of diploid and tetraploid *I. indigotica* were confirmed *via* flow cytometric analysis as shown in Supporting Information Fig. S4. RT-qPCR analysis indicated that the transcript levels of *IiWRKY33*, *IiWRKY34*, *IiWRKY48*, *IiWRKY49* and *IiWRKY50* in roots of tetraploid *I. indigotica* were significantly higher than that of diploid ones ($P<0.05$), and the fold changes were comparable with our microarray findings. *IiWRKY33*, *IiWRKY34*, *IiWRKY48*, *IiWRKY49* and *IiWRKY50* were responsive to MeJA treatment in both diploid and tetraploid *I. indigotica* hairy roots, but with different patterns. It was obvious to note that *IiWRKY34* was more responsive to MeJA than other members, and its expression was dramatically up-regulated at 1 h post-treatment then lasted to the end of the experiment in both samples. It was interesting to note that the expression pattern of *IiWRKY33*, *IiWRKY34*, *IiWRKY48*, *IiWRKY49* and *IiWRKY50* in the induced hairy roots of tetraploid *I. indigotica* greatly differed from that in its original roots, suggesting the expression of these *IiWRKY* genes is under strict developmental and tissue-specific control. LC-MS analysis showed roots of tetraploid *I. indigotica* accumulated more lariciresinol than diploid progenitor ($P<0.05$), consistent with our earlier finding that tetraploid *I. indigotica* exhibited higher antiviral effect compared with its diploid counterpart. In addition, MeJA treatment greatly triggered lariciresinol production in both diploid and tetraploid *I. indigotica* hairy roots, but with different patterns that in diploids lariciresinol accumulation increased gradually and peaked at 12 h, whereas in tetraploids it decreased gradually until 3 h and then continuously increased from 3 to 24 h post treatment (Fig. 2A).

A correlation analysis between the above *IiWRKYs* and lariciresinol presented as a heat map (Fig. 2B) indicated that *IiWRKY34* was most highly correlated with lariciresinol with a correlation coefficient of 0.812, suggesting *IiWRKY34* probably positively regulated lariciresinol production.

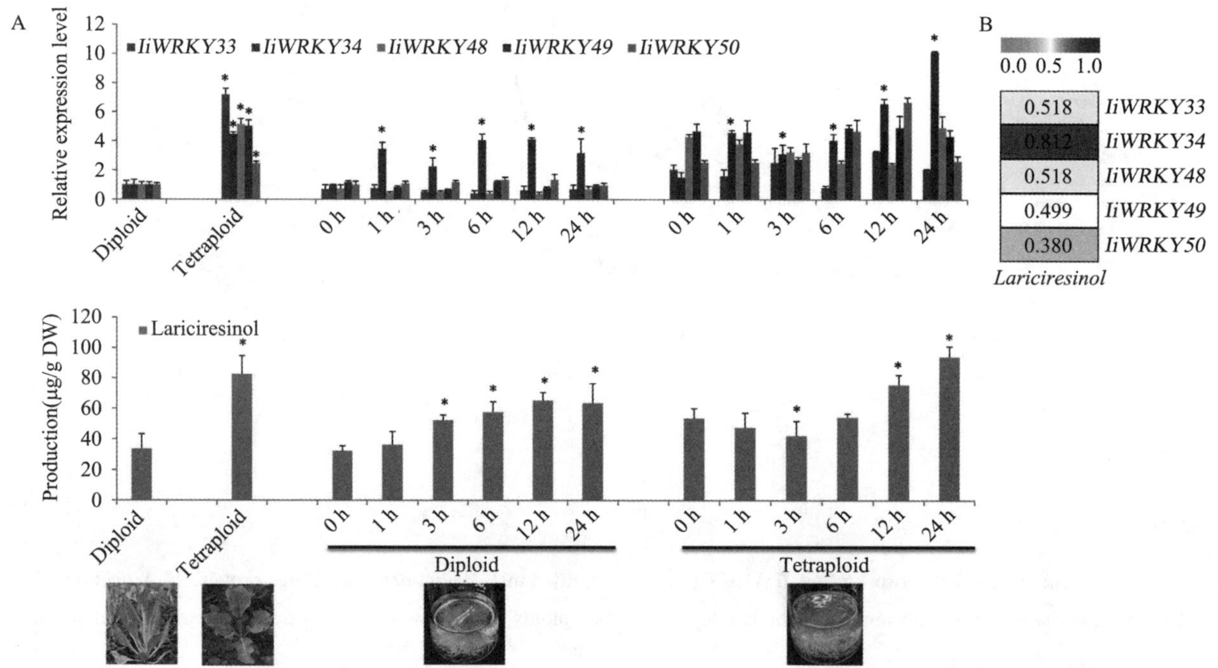


**Figure 2 Integrated analysis of *IiWRKYs* expression and lariciresinol production**

(A) *IiWRKY33*, *IiWRKY34*, *IiWRKY48*, *IiWRKY49* and *IiWRKY50* expression and lariciresinol production in response to autopolyploidy as well as MeJA treatment. Quantitative PCR analysis showing *IiWRKY33*, *IiWRKY34*, *IiWRKY48*, *IiWRKY49* and *IiWRKY50* expression relative to the control lines (diploid *I. indigotica*) set at 1. Data were expressed as means±SD ($n=3$). Asterisks represent significant difference at 0.05 level by Student's *t*-test. (B) Heat map showing *IiWRKY* — lignan correlation coefficients.

3.4 IiWRKY34 positively regulates lignan biosynthesis in *I. indigotica* hairy roots The role of *Ii*WRKY34 in lignan biosynthesis was investigated using a transgenic hairy root assay (Fig. 3). Two constructs (PHB-*IiWRKY34*-flag and pCAMBIA1300-*IiWRKY34*, Supporting Information Fig. S5) were generated for over-expression and RNA interference analysis (*IiWRKY34*-OVX and *IiWRKY34*-RNAi), respectively. The transformants were identified by PCR analysis: all the hairy roots contained the *rolb* or *rolc* gene, which indicated successful transformation of pRiA4.

The hygromycin resistance gene *hpt* was detected in both transgenic and CK lines. In addition, transgenic lines also contained *IiWRKY34*-specific fragments (Supporting Information Fig. S6).

RT-qPCR analysis indicated that *IiWRKY34* expression level was successfully regulated through genetic manipulation that transgenic roots overexpressing *IiWRKY34* showed a dramatic increase in *IiWRKY34* expression, whereas *IiWRKY34*-RNAi roots showed a significant reduction compared with WT and CK ($P<0.05$, Fig. 3G). It was interesting to note *IiWRKY34*-OVX roots grew fast and vigorously with thick branches whereas *IiWRKY34*-RNAi roots grew slowly with slender branches (Fig. 3A). At the Day 45 after inoculation, the biomass of *IiWRKY34*-OVX and *IiWRKY34*-RNAi roots were approximately 3.7- and 0.3-fold of WT respectively, and no significant difference was detected between WT and CK (PHB, P1300) lines during the whole hairy root culture period (Fig. 3F). The morphology of different transgenic roots at the Day 45 was shown in Fig. 3B, and these roots were used to microscopic analysis and phloroglucinol-HCl staining. Microscopic analysis showed that when compared with WT and CK controls, the interfascicular fibers and xylem cells of *IiWRKY34*-OVX roots were relatively compacted with a higher lignification level, on the contrary those of *IiWRKY34*-RNAi counterparts were dispersed and had a lower lignification level (Fig. 3C). Phloroglucinol-HCl staining showed *IiWRKY34*-OVX roots presented a violet-red colour, whereas *IiWRKY34*-RNAi counterparts presented a weaker browning compared with WT and CK (Fig. 3D). Similar color was also found in their corresponding eluents (Fig. 3E). These results indicate that *IiWRKY34* positively improves the accumulation of lignans, lignins, and/or wall-bound phenolics and derivatives.

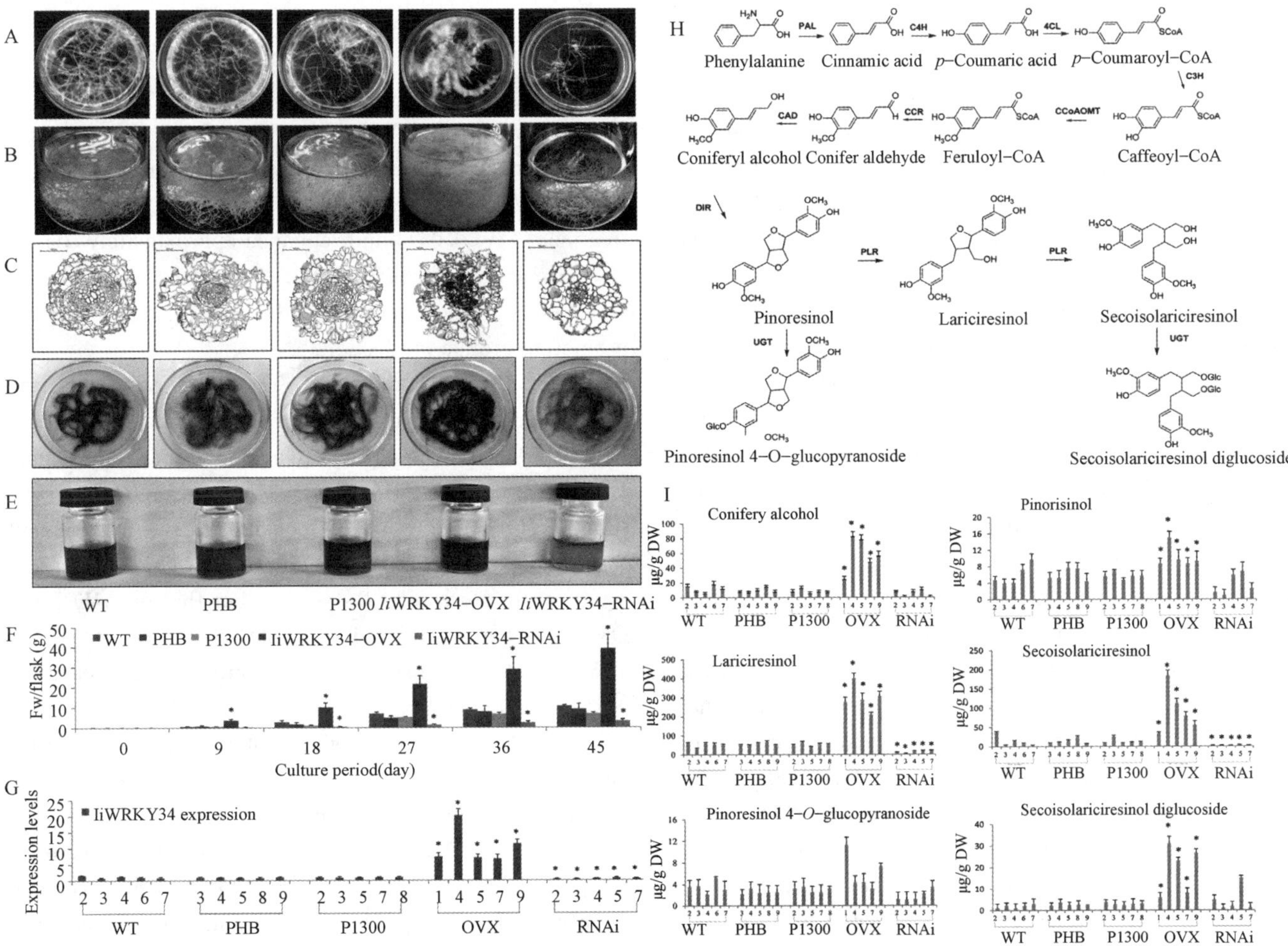


**Figure 3 Phenotype analysis of *IiWRKY34* transgenic hairy roots**

Phenotype of developed root lines on solid medium for 20 days (A), and their corresponding root culture in liquid medium for 45 days (B). (C) Cross sections of hairy roots stained with safranin O/fast green FCF. Bar=100 μm. Phenotype (D) and eluents (E) of hairy roots after phloroglucinol-HCl staining. (F) Biomass accumulation during the culture period. *IiWRKY34* transcript expression (G) and lignan content (I) in different lines. Quantitative PCR analysis showing *IiWRKY34* expression relative to the wild-type lines (WT-2) set at 1. (H) lignan biosynthetic pathway. Data were expressed as means±SD ($n=3$). Asterisks represent significant difference at 0.05 level by Student's $t$-test.

To test whether *Ii*WRKY34 positively improves the pharmaceutically important lignans, 6 compounds involved in lariciresinol biosynthetic pathway (Fig. 3H) were determined by LC-MS. Results showed that overexpression of *IiWRKY34* dramatically enhanced the production of the 6 lignans, and line OVX-4, with the highest *IiWRKY34* expression (20-fold of WT, Fig. 3G), produced the most abundant conifer alcohol (82.8 μg/g DW), pinoresinol (14.9 μg/g DW), lariciresinol (400.4 μg/g DW), secoisolariciresinol (184.5 μg/g DW), and secoisolariciresinol diglucoside (31.1 μg/g DW), which were ~6.7-, 2.5-, 7.6-, 14.1-and 16.4-fold more than in WT, respectively. In contrast, RNAi suppression of *IiWRKY34* decreased the production of conifer alcohol, lariciresinol, secoisolariciresinol, and pinoresinol 4-*O*-glucopuranoside with different degrees. There was no significant difference in lignan content between CK and WT lines (Fig. 3I).

3.5 IiWRKY34 positively improves salt and drought stress tolerance in *I. indigotica* hairy roots Expression of *IiWRKY34* was examined in various organs of 2-month-old *I. indigotica* seedlings, result showed that it was abundantly expressed in roots, stems and leaves, but only slightly expressed in flowers. *IiWRKY34* responded to drought, salt, SA, MeJA and UV-B treatments, but with different patterns of variation. After drought and salt treatment, the expression level of *IiWRKY34* increased gradually and reached a maximum at 6 h after treatment, which was approximately 7.3- and 24.2-foid, respectively, higher than that before treatment. When *I. indigotica* was treated with SA, *IiWRKY34* expression increased sharply at 1 h and peaked at 6 h (29.1-fold of that before treatment). Paralleled with MeJA-treated *I. indigotica* hairy roots (Fig. 2A), *IiWRKY34* expression in *I. indigotica* seedlings was induced by MeJA at 1 h (28.0-fold of that before treatment) post-treatment but decreased at 3 h, and then gradually increased afterward. For UV-B treatment, *IiWRKY34* expression gradually increased until 60 min and decreased at 80 min under UV-B, but its expression then increased after UV-B was turned off, and the expression level at 120 min achieved approximate 31.6-fold of that before treatment (Supporting Information Fig. S7). These results indicate that *IiWRKY34* can be significantly induced when subjected to environment stresses, which is in agreement with that *IiWRKY34* is involved in plant defence regulatory pathways as indicated in Fig. 1.

Both bioinformatics analysis (Fig. 1) and stress induction (Fig. S7) suggested a role of *IiWRKY34* in stress response. Thus, its capacity for stress tolerance was further investigated using transgenic hairy roots. Results showed *IiWRKY34* expression indeed could positively improve salt and drought stress tolerance. As shown in Fig. 4A, after 5 days of salt or drought treatment, both WT and *IiWRKY34*-OVX roots grew well as normal, but *IiWRKY34*-RNAi counterparts showed an early senescence phenotype with severe growth retardation compared with that without treatment (CK).

The intracellular ROS level in the WT and transgenic hairy roots was tested by fluorescence staining. Under normal conditions (CK), *IiWRKY34*-OVX root tips displayed a lower level of ROS whereas *IiWRKY34*-RNAi displayed a relatively higher level compared to WT. After salt or drought treatment, ROS accumulation enhanced in both WT and RNAi roots (especially in RNAi ones), while its accumulation in *IiWRKY34*-OVX roots still stayed at a low level as that in CK (Fig. 4B). These results imply that *Ii*WRKY34 may reduce the ROS level to confer salinity and drought stress tolerance.

Since proline accumulation is widely recognized as a sign of stress tolerance in plants, we examined whether the proline content in transgenic hairy roots was altered. Under salt or drought stress condition, both WT and *IiWRKY34*-OVX lines accumulated more proline than CK, and the proline content of *IiWRKY34*-OVX lines was much higher than that of WT. In contrast, the proline accumulation in *IiWRKY34*-RNAi lines was significantly decreased after salt treatment ($P<0.05$), and remained approximately constant after drought condition (Fig. 4C). These results indicate that *Ii*WRKY34 may enhance salt and drought stress tolerance by promoting proline production.

Moreover, we measured TEAC to investigate the physiological effects of transgenic hairy roots. Compared with WT, *IiWRKY34*-OVX lines showed an approximate 1.5-fold increase in TEAC level, whereas *IiWRKY34*-RNAi showed a reduction by 1-s. After salt and drought treatment, the TEAC level of both WT and *IiWRKY34*-RNAi lines significantly decreased ($P<0.05$), but that of *IiWRKY34*-OVX was barely changed (Fig. 4D). This result indicates *Ii*WRKY*34* may maintain total antioxidant capacity to confer stress tolerance.

3.6 Gene expression profiles of transgenic *I. indigotica* hairy roots Totally, 144,731 isogenes were identified by assembly. Differences in gene expression of the 3 groups (*IiWRKY34*-OVX, *IiWRKY34*-RNAi and WT hairy roots, 5 lines in each group) were shown in Fig. 5. Gene expression from individual groups showed a distinct sample separation (Fig. 5A), and a larger variation was found between *IiWRKY34*-OVX and *IiWRKY34*-RNAi lines compared with other pairwise samples that a total of 15,178 unigenes showed differential expression containing up-regulated and down-regulated ones (Fig. 5B). GO amotations indicated that these DEGs distributed in biological process, cellular component and molecular function categories with distinct

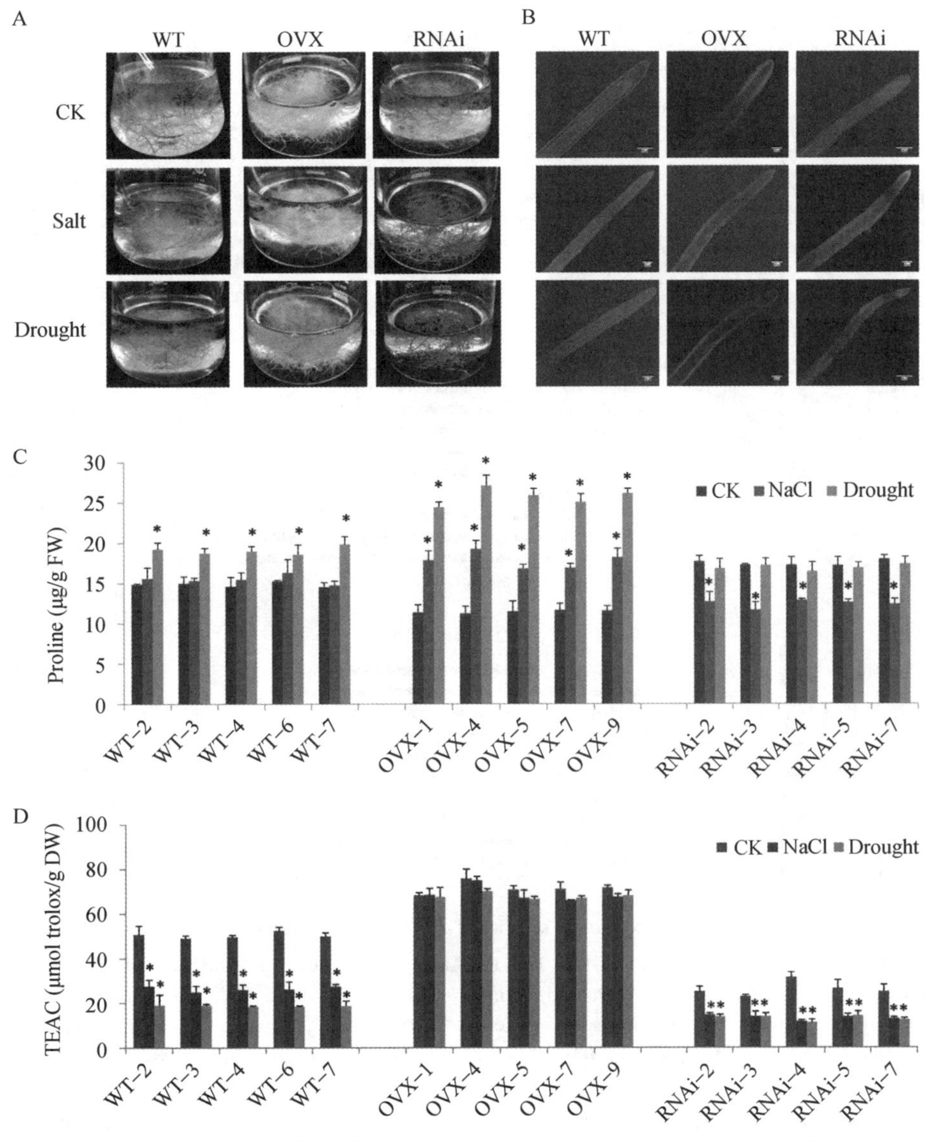


**Figure 4 Performance of *IiWRKY34* transgenic hairy roots under salt and drought stresses**

(A) Growth of transgenic hairy roots in 75 mmol/L NaCl, 2.5% PEG or liquid culture medium only for 5 days. ROS level (B), proline content (C) and trolox equivalent antioxidant activities (D) in different lines. The untreated wild-type hairy roots were designated as the control. Data were expressed as means±SD ($n=3$). Asterisks represent significant difference at 0.05 level by Student's $t$-test.

patterns (Supporting Information Fig. S8). KEGG pathway enrichment analysis indicated that these DEGs were involved in biosynthesis of amino acids, carbon metabolism and phenylpropanoid, etc. The top 10 enriched pathways *via* pairwise contrasts presented in Fig. 5C distinguished a prominent variation between *IiWRKY34*-OVX and *IiWRKY34*-RNAi samples, and there were a total of 60 DEGs (17%) involved in phenylpropanoid biosynthesis.

The transcript levels of 64 *IiWRKY* in WT, *IiWRKY34*-OVX and *IiWRKY34*-RNAi hairy roots were presented as a heat map in Fig. 5D. As expected, *IiWRKY34* expression in *IiWRKY34*-OVX lines was higher than WT, whereas lower in *IiWRKY34*-RNAi counterparts, and the fold changes were paralleled well with that examined by RT-qPCR (Fig. 3G), indicating that the RNA-Seq expression profile is robust and gene expression level obtained from this database is reliable. It was interesting to note that *IiWRKY33*, *IiWRKY48* and *IiWRKY49*, which were found highly responsive to autopolyploidy (Fig. 2A), displayed a similar expression pattern with *IiWRKY34* and they grouped together, indicating they may associate with each other in some manners.

3.7 Metabolite profiling of transgenic *I. indigotica* hairy roots To assess the impact of *Ii*WRKY34 on the metabolic shifts, nontargeted metabolic profiling was performed using GC—TOF/MS. Totally, 662 independent analytes were obtained from 15 samples. Differentially expressed metabolites (VIP>1, $P<0.05$) in the 3 groups

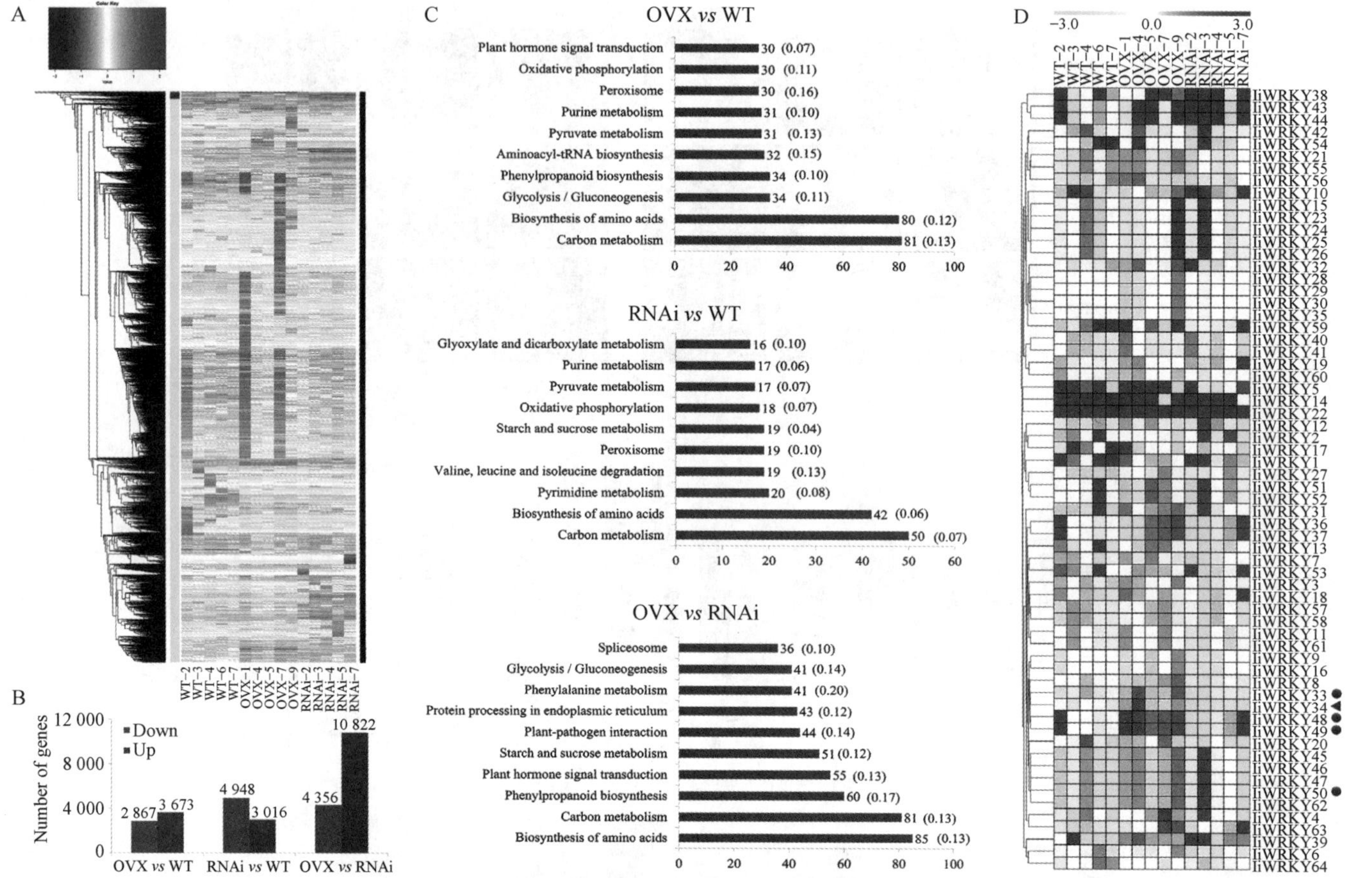


**Figure 5 Gene expression profiles of *IiWRKY34* transgenic hairy roots**

(A) Heat map showing DEGs in *IiWRKY34*-OVX, *IiWRKY34*-RNAi and WT lines. (B) Number of DEGs *via* pairwise contrasts of *IiWRKY34*-OVX, *IiWRKY34*-RNAi and WT roots with fold-change $>2$ and FDR $<0.05$. (C) Numbers of DEGs in the top ten enriched pathways. In parentheses: percentage of the total number of genes in the respective pathway. (D) Expression profiles of 64 *IiWRKY*s in different lines. *IiWRKY33*, *IiWRKY34*, *IiWRKY48*, *IiWRKY48* and *IiWRKY50* are highlighted with red markers.

(*IiWRKY34*-OVX, *IiWRKY34*-RNAi and WT hairy roots, 5 lines in each group) were shown in Fig. 6. Similar with gene expression profiles (Fig. 5A), metabolite accumulation from individual groups also showed a distinct sample separation (Fig. 6A). Variation between *IiWRKY34*-OVX and *IiWRKY34*-RNAi lines was more significant than that between other pairwise samples, there were 113 and 52 metabolites found decreased and enhanced in abundances for *IiWRKY34*-OVX *versus* *IiWRKY34*-RNAi samples, respectively (Fig. 6B and Supporting Information Table S4). Generation of volcano plots further visualized the significantly altered metabolite features in *IiWRKY34*-OVX, *IiWRKY34*-RNAi and WT hairy roots (Fig. 6C).

To integrate both primary and secondary metabolism that had been modified by *IiWRKY34* expression, we used a pathway scheme to summarize the metabolic changes (VIP$>$1, $P<0.05$) in *IiWRKY34*-OVX compared with *IiWRKY34*-RNAi roots. As shown in Fig. 6D, there were significantly higher amounts of phenylpropanoids such as flavonoids and lignans, whereas the basic sugar and the products of the TCA cycle, were reduced significantly, indicating that *Ii*WRKY34 appeared to reprogram primary metabolism, driving carbon flux towards specific secondary metabolism.

3.8 Regulatory network of IiWRKY34 for lignan biosynthesis Metabolic analysis revealed that *IiWRKY34* positively regulated lignans production. To have a systematic view on the variation of lignan biosynthesis pathway, we examined abundances of 37 transcripts coding 9 catalytic genes (Supporting Information Tables S5) and 6 metabolites involved in lariciresinol biosynthesis in WT, *IiWRKY34*-OVX and *IiWRKY34*-RNAi hairy roots (5 lines in each group). The RNA-Seq expression profile indicated that lariciresinol biosynthetic genes responded to *IiWRKY34* transgene with various patterns (Fig. 7A). The accumulation levels of six lignans (Fig. 3I) were normalized and presented as a heat map in Fig. 7B. Correlation coefficient cut-off values were applied to construct *IiWRKY34*-pathway genes—lignans correlation networks. Fig. 7C presents one example with a cut-off $R>0.5$: a total of 11 pathway genes are correlated with *IiWRKY34* and at least one lignan,

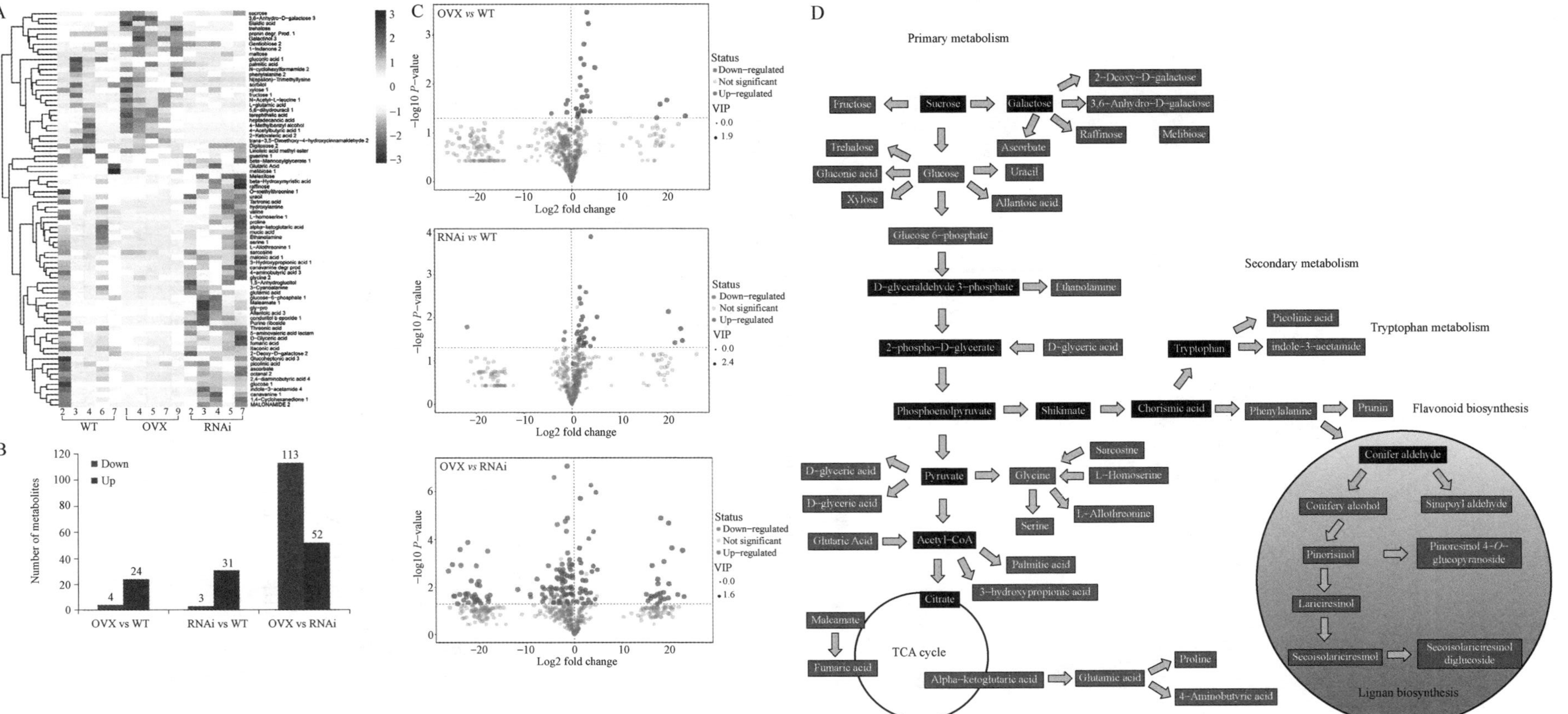


**Figure 6 Metabolite profiling of *IiWRKY34* transgenic hairy roots**

(A) Heat map showing differentially expressed metabolites of *IiWRKY34*-OVX, *IiWRKY34*-RNAi and WT lines. (B) Number of metabolites with significant changes in concentration (VIP>1, $P<0.05$) *via* pairwise contrasts. (C) Volcano plot of differentially expressed metabolites *via* pairwise contrasts. (D) Pathway scheme summarizing the metabolic changes in *IiWRKY34*-OVX compared with *IiWRKY34*-RNAi transgenic roots. Metabolites which changed significantly (VIP>1, $P<0.05$) are highlighted in red (for increased) and blue (for decreased), metabolites without significant changes are highlighted in black.

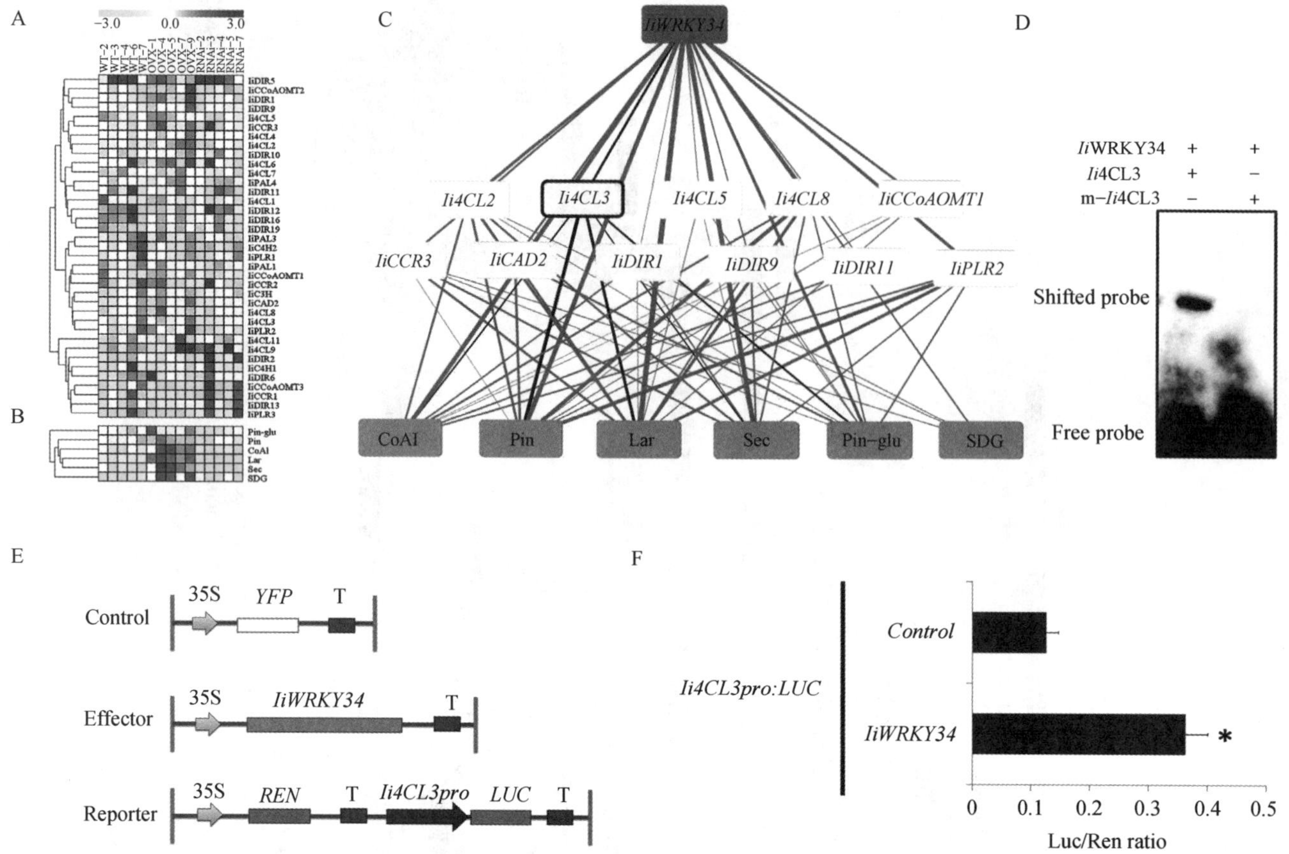


**Figure 7 Regulatory network of *IiWRKY34* for lignan biosynthesis**

Heat maps showing expression profiles of lignan biosynthetic genes (A) and lignan accumulations (B) in *IiWRKY34*-OVX, *IiWRKY34*-RNAi and WT lines. (C) *IiWRKY34*-lignan pathway genes-lignans correlation network with a cut-off $R > 0.5$. *IiWRKY34*, pathway genes and lignans are drawn in red, yellow and green, respectively. The thickness of lines represents the level of correlation. *IiWRKY34*-*Ii4CL3*-lignans correlation was highlighted by black lines. (D) *IiWRKY34* specifically binds to the promoter of *Ii4CL3*. (E) Schematic diagram of the reporter and effector constructs used in the transient dual luciferase assay. (F) Transient dual luciferase analysis showing *IiWRKY34* activation of the transcription of *Ii4CL3* in *N. benthamiana* leaves. LUC/REN represents the luciferase/renilla ratio of $n = 3$ independent experiments; Data were expressed as means ± SD. Asterisk represents significant difference at 0.05 level by Student's *t*-test.

indicating *Ii*WRKY34 may improve lignan biosynthesis by modulating these lignan biosynthetic genes. Among these genes, one *Ii4CL* family member *Ii4CL3* has been demonstrated as a key rate-limiting enzyme of lariciresinol production, severing as a hub gene of lignan regulatory network in our earlier study. In order to test whether *Ii*WRKY34 regulate lignan by direct interacting with *Ii*4CL3, EMSA was performed using *Ii*WRKY34 recombinant protein and the promoter of *Ii4CL3*. Result showed *Ii*WRKY34 indeed specifically bound to the W-box in the promoter region of *Ii4CL3*. There are two W-boxes in the 1 500-bp *Ii4CL3* promoter region (Supporting Information Fig. S9), and the biotin-modified probe representing the two TGAC core elements formed a DNA — protein complex with *Ii*WRKY34. Mutation of the two elements disrupted protein binding, and no retarded band representing complex formation was observed in the binding assay (Fig. 7D). Dual luciferase assay was further used to investigate how *Ii*WRKY34 regulate *Ii4CL3* by direct binding to its promoter sequence (Fig. 7E). Result showed *Ii*WRKY34 activated the promoter of *Ii4CL3 in vivo*, as evidenced by a higher value of LUC/REN than the control (Fig. 7F), supporting the hypothesis that *Ii*WRKY34 interacts with the promoter of *Ii4CL3* and thus activates its transcription.

## 4 DISCUSSION

Yield potential, medicinal compounds concentration and stress tolerance capacity are 3 classes of traits determining the quality of herbs. Tetraploid *I. indigotica* has been appealing to people because of its greater yield, higher bioactive compounds accumulation and enhanced stress tolerance compared to its diploid counterpart. Elucidation of the underlying molecular basis of the significantly qualitative difference is of great importance for the improvement of *I. indigotica*.

In the present study, *IiWRKY33*, *IiWRKY34*, *IiWRKY48*, *IiWRKY49* and *IiWRKY50*, which express especially higher in tetraploid *I. indigotica* than diploids, were proposed to be particularly important in the trait development seen in the tetraploids. An interaction network constructed using *Arabidopsis* database revealed *Ii*WRKY33, *Ii*WRKY34, *Ii*WRKY48 and *Ii*WRKY49 located as hub genes and associated with various defence regulatory pathways (Fig. 1), suggesting they might have contributed to the higher stress resistance of tetraploid *I. indigotica*. Previous reports of their *Arabidopsis* homologues *At*WRKY33 (orthologous to *Ii*WRKY33), *At*WRKY40 (orthologous to *Ii*WRKY34) and *At*WRKY25 (orthologous to *Ii*WRKY48 and *Ii*WRKY49) confirmed the reliability of this functional protein association network. For instance, overexpression of *At*WRKY25 and *At*WRKY33 increased salt tolerance and ABA sensitivity, *At*WRKY40 was induced in response to microbial pathogen infection as well as MeJA treatment, *At*WRKY25 was involved in plant defense against *Pseudomonas syringae*, and also acted as a cold resistance gene. Another polyploidy-responsive member *Ii*WRKY50, not found integrated in the network, was designated as a calmodulin binding protein according to the protein annotation of its *Arabidopsis* ortholog *At*WRKY21. Since calcium serves as an important second messenger in plants, and changes in calcium concentration are closely related to plant responses to various stimuli, the expression of calcium-related proteins such as *Ii*WRKY50 might indirectly influence plant performance. To sum up, it can be conceived that, during plant development, the up-regulation of *WRKY* caused by the environmental stresses (*e. g.*, pathogen, salinity, coldness, drought, etc.) would result in higher stress tolerance, thus prompting higher growth performance (*e. g.*, higher yield and enhanced metabolites biosynthetic efficiency). Therefore, we can expect that the up-regulation of *WRKY* TFs (*IiWRKY33*, *IiWRKY34*, *IiWRKY48*, *IiWRKY49* and *IiWRKY50*) induced by autopolyploidy suggested tetraploid *I. indigotica* had a much stronger adaptation capacity than diploid progenitor. Paralleled with our previous report of *IiSDD1*, a gene specialized in stomatal density and distribution, this work implies a key advantage of "fast-evolution" by artificial breeding. Why did the polyploid become more adaptable than the diploid one? A possible mechanism is: the changed expression of critical genes, such as transcription factor *IiWRKYs* and functional gene *IiSDD1*, prompts the regulatory effect more significantly. This study proposes that WRKY not only participates in the defense/stress responses, but also associates with polyploidy vigor. The molecular mechanism of how tetraploidization leads to the expression changes of these critical genes is worth investigating in the future.

For medicinal plants, the concentration of pharmaceutical compounds is the most important factor affecting the practice of medicine. Compared with diploid *I. indigotica*, the tetraploids accumulate more lignans including lariciresinol and its derivatives, which present effective antiviral ingredients of *I. indigotica*. The potency of plant-specific signaling molecules jasmonates, such as MeJA, to elicit secondary metabolism in cell cultures has made them powerful tools to cause the genetic diversity and help to unravel the complex cellular process. Here, MeJA-elicited diploid and tetraploid *I. indigotica* hairy roots harvested at different time points, along with the original roots of diploid and tetraploid *I. indigotica*, were employed as a resource of genetic variation to explore the potential correlation between polyploidy-responsive *IiWRKYs* (*IiWRKY33*, *IiWRKY34*, *IiWRKY48*, *IiWRKY49* and *IiWRKY50*) and lariciresinol. Result showed *IiWRKY34* was positively correlated with lariciresinol with a high correlation coefficient value ($R = 0.812$), suggesting *Ii*WRKY34 probably participated in lariciresinol biosynthesis. Further evidence for a role of *IiWRKY34* in the regulation of secondary metabolites has been found in its orthologs from other plants. For instance, *Ga*WRKY1, also an ortholog of *At*WRKY40, regulates the production of gossypol in cotton; *Cr*WRKY13, another ortholog of *At*WRKY40, is involved in biosynthesis of terpenoidindole alkaloids in *Catharanthus*. Therefore, we further investigated the effect of *IiWRKY34* expression in lariciresinol biosynthesis using transgenic hairy root assays. Overexpression and RNAi analysis demonstrate that *Ii*WRKY34 is an activator of lignans including lariciresinol, and it also plays a positive role in biomass accumulation (Fig. 3), as well as salt and drought tolerance as indicated by the changes of ROS level, proline content and total antioxidant capacity of transgenic hairy roots under stress conditions (Fig. 4).

Since large alterations were observed in the developmental phenotype for *IiWRKY34*-transgenic hairy roots, their molecular phenotype was characterized by changes to both transcript and metabolism. Generally speaking, both transcriptome and metabolome profiling from individual groups (*IiWRKY34*-OVX, *IiWRKY34*-RNAi and WT hairy roots, 5 lines in each group) showed a distinct sample separation (Figs. 5A and 6A), indicating *IiWRKY34* expression made a marked effect on reshaping molecular phenotype of *I. indigotica*. Pathway classification of the DEGs revealed that *Ii*WRKY34 appeared to affect both primary and secondary metabolism, including carbon metabolism, starch and sucrose metabolism, amino acids biosynthesis and phenylpropanoid biosynthesis, etc (Fig. 5C). Measurement of metabolic shifts supported this conclusion, and *IiWRKY34* expression can drive carbon flux to specific overaccumulations of phenyl-propanoids including flavonoids and lignans (Fig. 6). However, the content of the downstream compounds in the biosynthetic pathway of macrocyclopropanediol did not change significantly, suggesting *Ii*WRKY34 modulated the flux not through genetic regulation of the enzymatic steps involved in this pathway. Therefore, *Ii*WRKY34 modifications on lignan accumulations are the combined outcome of a much more complex interplay of various metabolic pathways, not merely due to the activated phenylpropanoid biosynthetic steps.

To get insight into the specific molecular mechanism of *Ii*WRKY34 for lignan biosynthesis, a *IiWRKY34*—lignan pathway genes—lignans network (Fig. 7C) was constructed based on transcript—metabolite correlation. *Ii4CL3*, which has been demonstrated as a hub gene for lignan biosynthesis, was found to be a potential target gene of *Ii*WRKY34. EMSA and dual luciferase assays demonstrated that *Ii*WRKY34 indeed activated the transcription of *Ii4CL3* by binding to the promoter (Fig. 7D and F). These results indicate that *Ii*WRKY34 modulates lignan biosynthesis, at least in part, due to regulate *Ii*4CL3, revealing the regulatory network of *Ii*WRKY34 for lignan biosynthesis is robust and the identified target genes are worthy to be intensively investigated.

## 5. CONCLUSIONS

Numerous genes that individually control plant growth, secondary metabolism and stress response have been identified. Compared with these genes, *Ii*WRKY34 has large pleiotropic effects on an array of traits, including yield, lignan biosynthesis and stress tolerance, which are inferred to has contributed significantly to the high level of polyploidy vigor of *I. indigotica*. Strong expression of *IiWRKY34* in tetraploid *I. indigotica* corresponded well with greater yield, higher lignan accumulation and enhanced stress tolerance of the tetraploids. The major effects of *Ii*WRKY34 will prompt the possibility of this gene based molecular marker-assisted selection and transformation for the improvement of herbs instead of individually manipulating the component traits using multiple genes of small effects.

[肖莹，陈万生，张磊，等. Acta Pharmaceutica Sinica B, 2020, 10(12): 2417-2432.]

# The ERF-Ⅶ transcription factor SmERF73 coordinately regulates tanshinone biosynthesis in response to stress elicitors in *Salvia miltiorrhiza*

## 1 INTRODUCTION

Tanshinones are a group of abietane diterpenoid natural products synthesized in the root of *Salvia miltiorrhiza*, commonly called Danshen, a well-known traditional Chinese medicine. To date, over 40 tanshinones and structurally related compounds have been identified in Danshen, such as cryptotanshinone (CPT), tanshinone ⅡA (Tan ⅡA), dihydrotanshinone (DHT), and tanshinone Ⅰ (Tan Ⅰ), which reportedly provide clinical benefits for treating cardiovascular diseases. Tanshinone biosynthesis is initiated by cyclization of (E, E, E)-geranylgeranyl diphosphate (GGPP) into copalyl diphosphate (CPP) by CPP synthase (CPS1), and further cyclization and rearrangement into miltiradiene by kaurene synthase-like (KSL1). CPS1 was identified to be involved in tanshinone biosynthesis in the root, while it has been postulated that CPS2 is involved in tanshinone biosynthesis in aerial tissues of Danshen. CYP76AH1 catalyzes a unique four-electron oxidation cascade on miltiradiene to produce ferruginol. CYP76AH3 oxidizes ferruginol at two different carbon centers to obtain 11-hydroxy ferruginol and 11-hydroxy sugiol. CYP76AK1 hydroxylates the C-20 of two of the resulting intermediates into 11, 20-dihydroxy ferruginol and 11, 20-dihydroxy sugiol. Notably, *CPS1*, *CPS2*, *KSL1*, *CYP76AH1* and *CYP76AH3* are located in a major tanshinone biosynthetic gene cluster in Danshen, which raises questions about how the expression of these disparate genes are co-regulated during tanshinone metabolite biosynthesis.

Tanshinones accumulate in the stems, leaves, flowers, and most notably the roots of *S. miltiorrhiza*. The synergistic effect of a combination of biotic elicitor yeast and abiotic elicitor $Ag^+$ can induce tanshinone accumulation in hairy roots of *S. miltiorrbiza* more effectively than a single elicitor. The plant hormone methyl jasmonate (MeJA) can also induce the accumulation of tanshinones in hairy roots of *S. miltiorrbiza*. However, the induction of tanshinone biosynthesis using only yeast or silver ions in Danshen cell culture, or the combined elicitor of yeast and silver ions in the Danshen hairy roots, has been shown to be stronger than that of MeJA alone. The transcriptome and metabolome of Danshen hairy roots induced by a combination elicitor ($YE+Ag^{+}$) suggest that biotic and abiotic stress elicitors induce transcription factors through the jasmonic acid signal pathway, which in turn induces the biosynthesis of tanshinones. In addition to MeJA, plant hormones such as gibberellin, salicylic acid and abscisic acid (ABA) can also induce the accumulation of tanshinones in hairy roots. However, the mechanism by which signaling pathway networks regulate tanshinone biosynthesis is still largely unknown.

With the completion of the Danshen draft genome, and now that elicitor-responsive transcriptomic data are available many transcription factors have been found to be implicated in the regulation of tanshinone biosynthesis. However, analyses have mostly concentrated on the genes encoding enzymes in the terpenoid precursor and the carbon skeleton formation stages. For examplc, SmERF1L, SmMYB9b, and SmWRKY1 up-regulate *DXR1*, the second key enzyme in the methylerythritol 4-phosphate (MEP) pathway, and SmMYB9b also up-regulates the isopentenyl transferase *GGPPS*. Furthermore, SmbHLH10, SmERF6, SmERF128, and SmWRKY2 up-regulate the diterpene synthase *CPS1*, and SmERF6 and SmERF128 positively regulate the diterpene synthase *KSL*. There are still few studies on the transcriptional regulation of genes involved in the post-modification stage of the diterpene tanshinone skeletons. At present, only SmERF128 has been found to regulate *CYP76AH1* in the miltirone branch pathway.

The ERF family in Arabidopsis is classified into 12 subgroups based on the sequence homology and the presence of conserved functional domains. Generally, ERFs involved in the biosynthesis of secondary metabolites belong to group Ⅸ, while group Ⅶ ERFs are known for their roles in stress-inducible responses to excessive water, such as flooding and hypoxia. Group Ⅶ ERFs contain a characteristic MCGGAII/L N-terminal conserved motif, and members of this group also bind the canonical GCC-box element through the AP2 domain. Overexpressing group Ⅶ member HRE1 in Arabidopsis can increase pyruvate decarboxylase (PDC) and alcohol dehydrogenase (ADH) activity in the fermentation pathway under hypoxic stress, leading to increased ethanol production. However, there are few reports linking group Ⅶ ERFs to the regulation of secondary metabolites.

In this study, we report the regulatory function of a group Ⅶ ERF transcription factor previously unknown in *S. miltiorrhiza*, SmERF73, which participates in the regulation of tanshinone biosynthesis in response to elicitors of biotic and abiotic stress. Overexpression of *SmERF73* in *S. miltiorrhiza* led to the up-regulation of seven tanshinone pathway genes as well as the upstream MEP pathway, consequently enhancing the accumulation of tanshinones in roots. Consistent with this finding, RNA interference (RNAi) -mediated knockdown of SmERF73 in *S. miltiorrhiza* plants resulted in down-regulation of the expression of these seven genes and decreased tanshinone accumulation. Furthermore, SmERF73 can directly and specifically bind to GCC cis-elements *in vitro* and *in vivo*, thereby activating the transcription of at least four genes (*DXR1*, *CPS1*, *KSL1* and *CYP76AH3*) essential for tanshinone biosynthesis. Moreover, yeast two-hybrid (Y2H) and split-luciferase complementation assays showed that SmERF73 interacts with the SmJAZ3 repressor. Taken together, our results revealed that SmERF73 coordinately regulates the expression of several genes necessary for tanshinone biosynthesis in response to stress elicitors through GCC-box binding, and the transcriptional regulation of tanshinone biosynthesis in *S. miltiorrhiza* also exhibits a limited response to the jasmonic acid (JA) signaling pathway.

## 2 MATERIALS AND METHODS

Plant material, growth conditions, and stress treatment The *Salvia miltiorrhiza* Bunge (Danshen) plants used in this study were *S. miltiorrhiza* var. *miltiorrhiza* with purple flowers. Flowers, leaves, stems, and roots were collected from 2-yr-old plants. Tissue-cultured seedlings of Danshen were grown on Murashige and Skoog (MS) medium (PhytoTechnology Laboratory, Shawnee Mission, KS, USA) with 3% sucrose and 0.5% agar at pH 5.6. Hairy roots of Danshen were derived from plantlets infected with *Agrobacterium rhizogenes* strain C58C1. Danshen plants and *Nicotiana benthamiana* seedlings were grown in a glasshouse.

Yeast extract (YE) and $Ag^{+}$ elicitors were used in the combined treatment and prepared as described previously. Combined elicitors of YE and $Ag^{+}$ were added to the Danshen hairy root medium at respective final concentrations of 100 μg/mL and 30 μmol/L, and hairy roots were harvested at 0, 1, 2, 4, 8, 12, 24 and 36 h post-induction. Methyl jasmonate was dissolved in ethanol and added at a final concentration of 100 μmol/L into the hairy root medium, and hairy roots were harvested at the aforementioned time intervals. All treatments were replicated with at least three independent biological experiments.

RNA extraction and gene expression analysis Total RNA was isolated with Plant RNA Purification Reagent (Invitrogen) according to the manufacturer's instructions. Reverse transcription and real-time polymerase chain reaction (PCR) were performed. Primers are listed in Supporting Information Table S1.

Multiple sequence alignments and phylogenetic analysis Multiple sequence alignments were constructed using BioEdit v. 7.0. A phylogenetic analysis was conducted in Mega v. 8.0

using the neighbor-joining method with 1 000 bootstrap replicates. For sequence logo generation, the results of the previous multiple sequence alignments in BioEdit were submitted to WebLogo v. 3.

Protein subcellular localization  To determine subcellular localization, the full-length cDNA of *SmERF73* was cloned into the transient expression vector pE3025 in-frame with the green fluorescent protein (GFP) gene. For each construct, 1 μg of plasmid was used to coat 0.5 mg of 1.6 μm-diameter gold microcarriers and bombarded into living onion epidermal cells using the Helios Gene Gun System (Bio-Rad). Transformed cells were cultured on MS medium in darkness for 24 h and observed under an Axio Imager A2 fluorescence microscope (Zeiss, Jena, Germany) with an excitation wavelength of 488 nm and an emission wavelength of 515 - 530 nm.

Generation of transgenic plants  To produce the *SmERF73* overexpression and knockdown constructs, the full-length cDNA and a 456 bp fragment of *SmERF73* were cloned into the binary vectors pK7WG2D and pK7GWIWG2D (Ⅱ), respectively, using Gateway technology. The constructs were introduced into *Agrobacterium tumefaciens* strain EHA105 via a freeze-thaw transformation method. Transgenic plants were obtained via *Agrobacterium* mediation using a leaf disc. Ten independent lines were screened by quantitative polymerase chain reaction (qPCR), and three lines were used in these experiments for gene expression and metabolite analyses.

Chemical analysis  Roots were collected from 2-yr-old Danshen plants and lyophilized overnight using an FDU-1110 freezer dryer (Eyela, Tokyo, Japan). The samples were accurately weighed and sonicated in methanol at a ratio of 1 : 30 (*W/V*) for 30 min using an SB-800 DTD sonicator (Ningbo Xinzhi, China; power, 100 W; frequency, 40 kHz). The resulting supernatant was filtered through a 0.22 μm filter (Pall, Ann Arbor, MI, USA) for subsequent ultra-performance liquid chromatography coupled withtriple-quadrupole tandem mass spectrometry (UPLC-TQ-MS) analysis.

Liquid chromatography analysis was performed on an Acquity UPLC I-Class system (Waters, Milford, MA, USA) equipped with an online vacuum degasser, a binary pump, an autosampler, and a thermostat column compartment. An Acquity UPLC BEH C18 column (100 mm×2.1 mm internal diameter, 1.8 μm) was used for separation. The binary gradient of water containing 0.1% formic acid (A) and acetonitrile (B) at a constant flow rate of 0.5 mL/min was applied with an injection volume of 1.0 μL. The column oven temperature was held at 40℃. The linear gradient conditions were optimized as follows: 0 min, 60% B; 3.5 min, 70% B.

An AB Sciex API 6500 triple quadrupole mass spectrometer with an electrospray ion source (Applied Biosystems, Foster City, CA, USA) was used. The MS spectra were acquired in positive ion mode, which was carried out by optimization of the production obtained from the fragment of the isolated precursor ion for each analyte. The ion spray potential was 5 500 V, and the source temperature was set at 550 ℃. Once the productions were chosen, the multiple reaction monitoring MRM conditions for each standard were further optimized to achieve maximum sensitivity (Table 1).

Experiments included three biological replicates with three technical replicates each, and the statistical significance was evaluated using a Student's *t*-test in Spss v. 16.0.

**Table 1  Mass spectra properties of tanshinones**

| Analyte | $t_R$ (min) | Quantitative ion pairs $m/z$ | Declustering potentials (DP/V) | Collision energy (CE/V) | Cell exit potential (CXP/V) |
|---|---|---|---|---|---|
| Cryptotanshinone | 1.99 | 297.1/254.1 | 222 | 39 | 11 |
| Tanshinone ⅡA | 2.93 | 295.1/249.1 | 205 | 32 | 22 |
| Tanshinone Ⅰ | 1.94 | 277.1/178.2 | 191 | 52 | 22 |
| Dihydrotanshinone | 1.37 | 279.1/205.0 | 209 | 39 | 8 |

Electrophoretic mobility shift assay (EMSA)  The full-length cDNA of *SmERF73* was cloned into pMAL-c2X. Recombinant proteins were purified using Amylose Resin High Flow (NEB, Ipswich, MA, USA). Electrophoretic mobility shift assays were performed using the Light Shift Chemiluminescent EMSA kit (Thermo Fisher Scientific, Waltham, MA, USA) according to the manufacturer's instructions. The binding reactions were performed using 1 μg of MBP-SmERF73 incubated with a 125 fmol probe in binding buffer (1% NP-40, 5 mmol/L $MgCl_2$, 50 ng Poly (dI: dC) and 2.5% glycerol) for 30 min at room temperature. The reaction mixtures were separated in 6% native polyacrylamide gel electrophoresis (PAGE) gel. Biotin activity was detected according to the manufacturer's instructions.

Yeast one-hybrid assay  A Matchmaker Gold yeast one-hybrid system (Clontech, Mountain View, CA, USA) was used according to the manual. The tandem copies of the *GCC*-box, *proDXR1*$^{866}$, *proCPS1*$^{1042}$, *proKSL1-L*$^{857}$, *proKSL1-S*$^{289}$ and *proCYP76AH3*$^{630}$ were inserted into the pAbAi vector as bait. These bait constructs were integrated separately into the genome of the Y1HGold to generate six bait reporter strains. The minimal inhibitory concentrations of Aureobasidin A (AbA) were determined for bait using SD/− Uracil (Ura) agar plates containing 100 - 800 ng/mL AbA. *SmERF73* was inserted into the pGADT7 vector as prey. The pGADT7-*SmERF73* construct was introduced into the bait reporter strains, with a blank pGADT7 plasmid serving as a negative control. Positive transformants were selected on SD/−Leucine (Leu) with an appropriate concentration of AbA medium. Yeast cells were grown for 3d at 30 ℃.

Chromatin immunoprecipitation − quantitative polymerase chain reaction (ChIP-qPCR) assay Chromatin immunoprecipitation assays were performed as previously described, with minor modifications. Mouse polyclonal SmERF73 antibody was generated against a synthesized peptide (CYDGQSQSPPPPSNPPPDTV) of SmERF73. A total of 4 g of 45-d-old roots were cross-linked with 1% (*V/V*) formaldehyde under vacuum for 10 min and then sonicated. The SmERF73/DNA complexes were immunoprecipitated by ERF73 antibody and GammaBind G Sepharose (GE Healthcare, Pittsburgh, PA, USA) together for at least 4 h at 4 ℃. The precipitated DNA was purified using a DNA purification kit (Qiagen, Amtsgericht Düsseldorf, Germany) and the enriched DNA fragments were determined by qPCR using the specific primers listed in Table S1. Chromatin precipitated without antibody was used as a negative control, while the isolated chromatin before precipitation was used as an input control. All ChIP assays had three biological replicates.

Transient expression in *N. benthamiana* Transient expression assays were performed in *N. benthamiana* leaves as previously described. The *DXR1*, *CPS1*, *KSL1*, and *CYP76AH3* promoters were cloned into the binary vector pGWB35 to generate the reporter constructs $DXR1_{pro}$ : *LUC*, $CPS1_{pro}$ : *LUC*, $KSL1_{pro}$ : *LUC*, and $CYP76AH3_{pro}$ : *LUC*, and with the binary vector pGWB17 to generate the effector construct *35Spro* : *SmERF73*. A low-light cooled CCD imaging apparatus (Lumazone 1300B; Roper Scientific, Trenton, NJ, USA) was used to capture the LUC image and to quantify luminescence intensity. The leaves were sprayed with 1 mmol/L luciferin and were placed in darkness for 3 min before luminescence detection. Relative LUC activity $cm^{-2}$ infiltrated leaf area was calculated using WINVIEW32 software. Each data column contained at least 12 replicates, and three independent experiments were performed.

Yeast two-hybrid assays Full-length cDNA of *SmERF73* and *SmJAZ3* were cloned inframe in pGADT7 and pGBKT7 vectors (Clontech), respectively. The pGADT7 and pGBKT7 constructs were cotransformed into yeast strain AH109 and selected on SD/− Leu/− Trp medium. The resultant co-transformed cells were then streaked on triple dropout medium (SD/− His/− Leu/− Trp) followed by incubation at 30 ℃ for 48 h.

Split-luciferase complementation assays in *N. benthamiana* The split-luciferase complementation assays were performed in *N. benthamiana* leaves as described previously. The SmJAZ3 and SmERF73 coding regions were cloned into the pCM1307-NLuc and pCM1307-CLuc vectors, respectively. The LUC activity was measured using a cooled CCD imaging camera (IVIS Spectrum, PerkinElmer, Waltham, MA, USA). The calculation of relative LUC activity was as described in the 'Transient Expression in *N. benthamiana*' section.

RNA-seq and data analysis The root tissues of three independent RNAi transgenic lines (*Ri-2*, *Ri-3*, and *Ri-7*) and one empty vector (EV) transgenic line (material from three plants pooled per line) were collected, and total RNAs were extracted as described earlier. RNA-seq library preparation and paired-end sequencing were both performed using an Illumina HiSeq 6 000 platform (Novogene, Beijing, China). Differentially expressed genes (DEGs) with a $\log_2$ foldchange ($|\log_2 FC|$) $\geq 1$ and an adjusted $q$-value $\leq 0.005$ were identified using the $DEG_{SEQ}$ R package. The Gene Ontology (GO) and KEGG enrichment analysis of the DEGs was implemented using the $GO_{SEQ}$ R package and KOBAS software, respectively. The RNA-seq data have been deposited in the National Center for Biotechnology Information (NCBI) archive under accession no. PRJNA670263.

## 3 RESULTS

The ERF-VII transcription factor SmERF73 in *S. mitiorrhiza* was identified in the stress elicitor-induced transcriptome Previous work in Danshen hairy root has shown that the expression of tanshinone biosynthetic genes, and the tanshinone content in tissues, could be induced using combined biotic (YE) and abiotic ($Ag^+$) elicitors. To identify ERFs associated with tanshinone biosynthesis, we used co-expression analysis to mine the Danshen transcriptome generated under YE+$Ag^+$ treatment (NCBI SRA under accession no. SRX317052), and found that five of the nine considerably upregulated *ERFs* had peak expression at 12 h (Fig. 1a). We then compared the expression of these genes in root and leaf transcriptomes and found that the expression of *isotig10181* was highest in roots (Fig. S1), which is consistent the fact that roots are the accumulation organ for tanshinones. Based on the above analysis, we choose *isotig10181* for further research.

Isotig10181 contains a 780 bp open reading frame (ORF) encoding a protein of 259 amino acids. To further predict the function of isotig10181, we reconstructed a phylogenetic tree using 122 AtERFs from Arabidopsis and 20 other previously described ERFs for their involvement in plant secondary metabolism. Consistent with the findings of a previous report, these ERFs were classified into 12 groups (Ⅰ to Ⅹ, Ⅵ-L, and Ⅹb-L), and isotig10181 was clustered with five ERF-VII proteins from Arabidopsis (Figs 1b, S2; Table S2). Alignment of isotig10181 with the Arabidopsis ERF-Ⅶ group (AtERF71-75) further showed a highly conserved N-terminal MC motif (MCGGAⅡ/L motif), a putative NLS (nuclear localization signal), a conserved DNA-binding domain (AP2/ERF domain), a CMVⅡ-3 motif (E/A/GxxxxR/KxxK/S) in the 5′-flanking region of the AP2/ERF domain, and a CMVⅡ-5 motif (LWS (I/L/Y)) in the C-terminal regions of this group (Fig. 1c, Fig. S3). Based on the conservation of the CMVⅡ-1, CMVⅡ-3, and CMVⅡ-5 motifs, isotig10181 distinctly belonged to the ERF-Ⅶ group and was thus designated as SmERF73 (Fig. 1b).

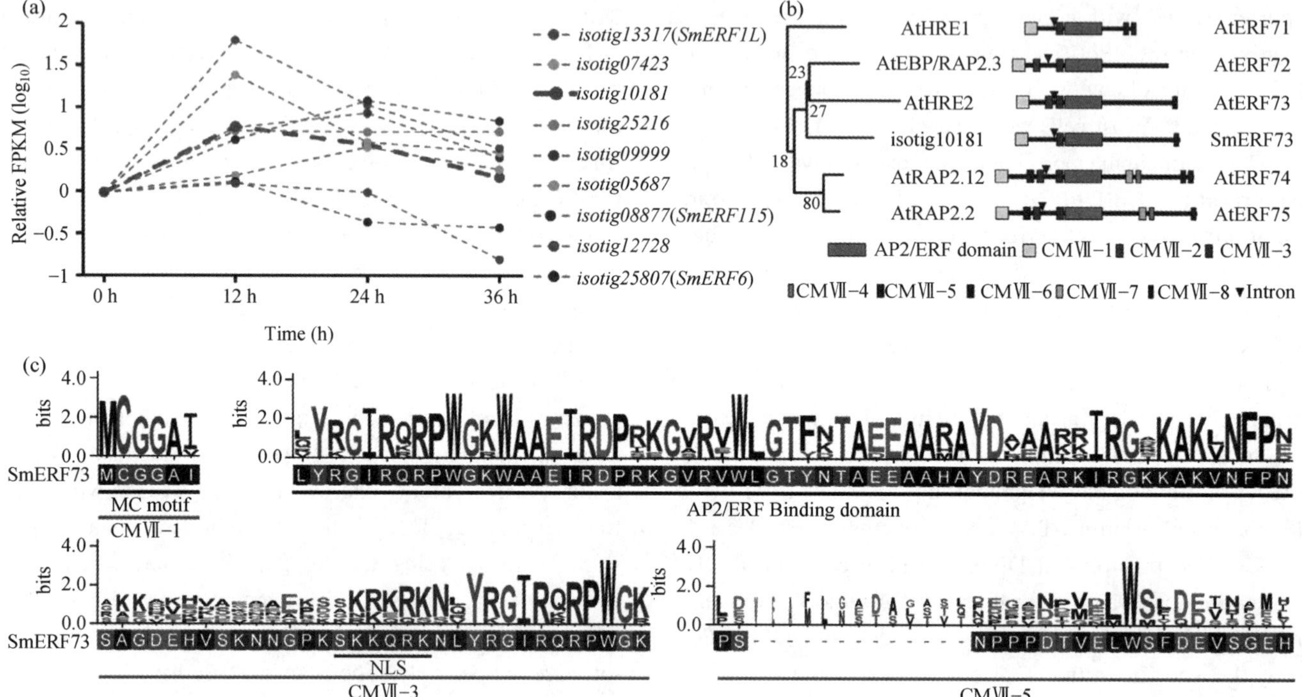


**Fig. 1 Transcriptome profile during the stress response in Danshen hairy root revealed isotig10181 —an ERF-Vll group transcription factor**

(a) The transcriptomic expression profiles during YE+$Ag^+$-mediated stress induction revealed significant differential up-regulation of several putative *ERFs* (dashed lines) including the previously unreported *isotig10181* (red dashed line). The $x$-axis represents the duration of YE+$Ag^+$ exposure in h; the $y$-axis represents the fragments per kilobase of transcript per million mapped reads (FPKM) expression value ($\log_{10}$). Hairy root treatment for 0 h was set to 1. (b) Phylogenetic reconstruction of isotig10181, designated SmERF73, with Arabidopsis ERFs showed clustering with group ERF-VII. The arrowheads represent introns, the grey boxes represent the AP2/ERF domain, and the colored boxes represent conserved motifs. Bootstrap values from 1 000 replicates were used to assess the robustness of the Jones-Taylor-Thornton (JTT) neighbor-joining tree. (c) Multiple sequence alignment and logo plots of group VII ERFs illustrate the conservation of the N-terminal MC motif (MCGGAII/L motif), the putative nuclear localization signal (NLS), and a conserved DNA-binding domain (AP2/ERF domain). The group VII conserved motifs (CMVII-1, 3, 5) are indicated by a horizontal red line.

*SmERF73* silencing decreased tanshinone metabolite accumulation, while its overexpression enhanced tanshinone biosynthesis in Danshen To determine whether SmERF73 functions as a regulator for tanshinone biosynthesis, we generated *SmERF73* RNA interference lines of Danshen (*Ri-SmERF73*). Ten independent transgenic lines were identified by qPCR analysis of *SmERF73* transcription (Fig. S4c), and three *SmERF73-RNAi* lines (*Ri-2*, *Ri-3* and *Ri-7*) with substantially reduced expression were selected for further analysis. Seven tanshinone biosynthesis genes, including two MEP pathway genes (*DXS2*, *DXR1*), two diterpene synthases (*CPS1*, *KSL1*), and three genes encoding P450 enzymes reported to participate in the miltirone branch pathway (*CYP76AH1*, *CYP76AH3*, and *CYP76AK1*), were selected to identify the effects of *SmERF73* knockdown on the expression patterns of tanshinone biosynthesis genes in the transgenic lines.

In the RNAi transgenic lines, *SmERF73* transcription was suppressed to 0.16- to 0.26-fold that of the empty vector (EV) control. Expression of the upstream MEP genes *DXS2* and *DXR1* was reduced to 0.16- to 0.36- and 0.19- to 0.60-fold of that of the control group, respectively; expression levels of the diterpene skeleton biosynthetic genes *CPS1* and *KSL1* were reduced to 0.06- to 0.57- and 0.09- to 0.32-fold, respectively; and expression of the miltirone branch pathway genes *CYP76AH1*, *CYP76AH3*, and *CYP76AK1* was reduced to 0.05- to 0.36-, 0.06- to 0.14-, and 0.09- to 0.13-fold, respectively (Fig. 2).

To determine the metabolic effects of *SmERF73* suppression, we measured the tanshinone content in mature roots of 2-yr-old plants from three independent *SmERF73-RNAi* lines using UPLC-TQ-MS. Compared to the EV control lines, cryptotanshinone Ⅰ (CPT), tanshinone ⅡA (Tan ⅡA), dihydrotanshinone Ⅰ (DHT), and tanshinone Ⅰ (Tan Ⅰ) accumulations were reduced to 38%~58%, 55%~71%, 55%~57% and 76%~85% of control levels, respectively, in the *SmERF73-Ri* transgenic plants (Fig. 2). These results indicated that suppression of *SmERF73* by RNAi led to a reduction in biosynthetic pathway gene expression, as well as a reduction in tanshinone accumulation.

To determine how tanshinone biosynthesis may lead to other transcriptional or physiological alterations in Danshen, we also generated *SmERF73* overexpression (OE) lines in *S. miltiorrhiza* (*OE-1*, *OE-6* and *OE-10*), which were confirmed by qPCR (Fig. S4d). The transcript levels of *SmERF73* in OE lines were increased 2.62- to 4.15-fold relative to EV control lines. Furthermore, the expression of upstream MEP pathway genes *DXS2* and *DXR1* increased 1.91- to 2.08-fold and 1.17- to 1.53-fold, respectively, relative to controls; the expression of diterpene skeleton biosynthetic genes *CPS1* and *KSL1* increased 1.09- to 3.92-fold and 1.71- to 1.96-fold, respectively, relative to control lines; and expression levels of miltrone branch pathway genes *CYP76AH1*, *CYP76AH3* and *CYP76AK1* were 1.03- to 1.55-, 1.96- to 4.46- and 1.08- to 2.64-fold higher than those of the control group (Fig. 2).

To determine the metabolic content of *SmERF73-OE* lines, we measured tanshinone content in mature roots of the 2-yr-old plants of three independent lines using UPLC-TQ-MS. We found that in *SmERF73-OE* transgenic plants cryptotanshinone Ⅰ (CPT), tanshinone ⅡA (Tan ⅡA), dihydrotanshinone Ⅰ (DHT), and tanshinone Ⅰ (Tan Ⅰ) accumulated to 93%~168%, 97%~162%, 109%~224%, and 143% ~ 237% of the contents in the EV controls, respectively (Fig. 2). These results showed that overexpression of *SmERF73* induced the expression of tanshinone biosynthetic genes, and generally stimulated the accumulation of tanshinones in transgenic Danshen, thus suggesting that SmERF73 is likely a positive regulator of tanshinone biosynthesis.

Transcriptomic analysis reveals a positive role of SmERF73 in tanshinone biosynthesis  To fully reveal the transcriptional regulatory function of SmERF73 in *S. miltiorrhiza*, we performed RNA-seq experiments using *SmERF73*-RNAi lines (*Ri-2*, *Ri-3* and *Ri-7*) and the EV control line. We identified a total of 5 489 differentially expressed genes (DEGs), including 3 105 that were down-regulated and 2 384 that were up-regulated in *Ri-3* vs EV lines (Fig. S5a).

To better understand the involvement of SmERF73 in the regulation of secondary metabolism, and all down- and up-regulated DEGs in *Ri-3* vs EV lines were assigned to 104 KEGG pathways. KEGG analysis revealed that these down-regulated DEGs were enriched in the ribosome, plant-pathogen interaction, plant hormone signal transduction, and multiple secondary metabolic pathways in the *Ri-3* vs EV group, which included terpenoid backbone biosynthesis and diterpenoid biosynthesis (Fig. S5d), while triterpenoid biosynthesis genes were in the up-regulated group (Fig. S5e).

To elucidate the molecular mechanism of SmERF73-mediated tanshinone biosynthesis, the expression of tanshinone biosynthetic genes was investigated. We investigated 42 unigenes that encoded 22 enzymes involved in tanshinone biosynthetic pathways (Fig. 3 and Table S3). The expression of genes in the mevalonate (MVA) pathway, such as *HMGR1-3*, exhibited a significant decrease in Ri-7 Danshen lines, while the expression of the genes in the MEP pathway, such as *DXS1*, *DXS2* and *DXR1* showed a significant decrease. Isoprenyl diphosphate synthase genes, such as *SSU II.1*, *LSU*, *FPPS* and *GGPPS1*, and diterpene synthases (*CPS1*, *KSL1*) were significantly down-regulated in RNAi lines. In addition to the three P450 enzymes involved in the miltirone branch pathway (*CYP76AH1*, *CYP76AH3* and *CYP76AK1*), 53 P450s were also found to be down-regulated, while 14 P450s were up-regulated (Table S4). This indicates that SmERF73 may potentially regulate the down-stream tanshinone biosynthetic pathways.

Also, the expression levels of monoterpene synthase (*Sabinene Synthase*) and sesquiterpene synthase (*Sesquiterpene Synthase1*, *Sesquiterpene Synthase12*, and *gamma-cadinene synthase*) genes were significantly down-regulated in RNAi lines (Fig. 3; Table S5), while the expression level of a triterpene synthase gene (*Squalene Monooxygenase*) was slightly increased (Fig. 3; Table S6).

SmERF73 localized to nuclei and was up-regulated by stress elicitors and methyl jasmonate  A nuclear localization signal, SKKQRK, was identified in SmERF73 via multiple sequence alignment (Fig. S3). To determine the subcellular localization of SmERF73, the ORF of *SmERF73* was fused in-frame to GFP. The *35Spro::SmERF73-GFP* fusion construct and *35Spro::GFP* empty vector control were transformed into onion epidermal cells by bombardment. The SmERF73-GFP fusion protein was observed exclusively

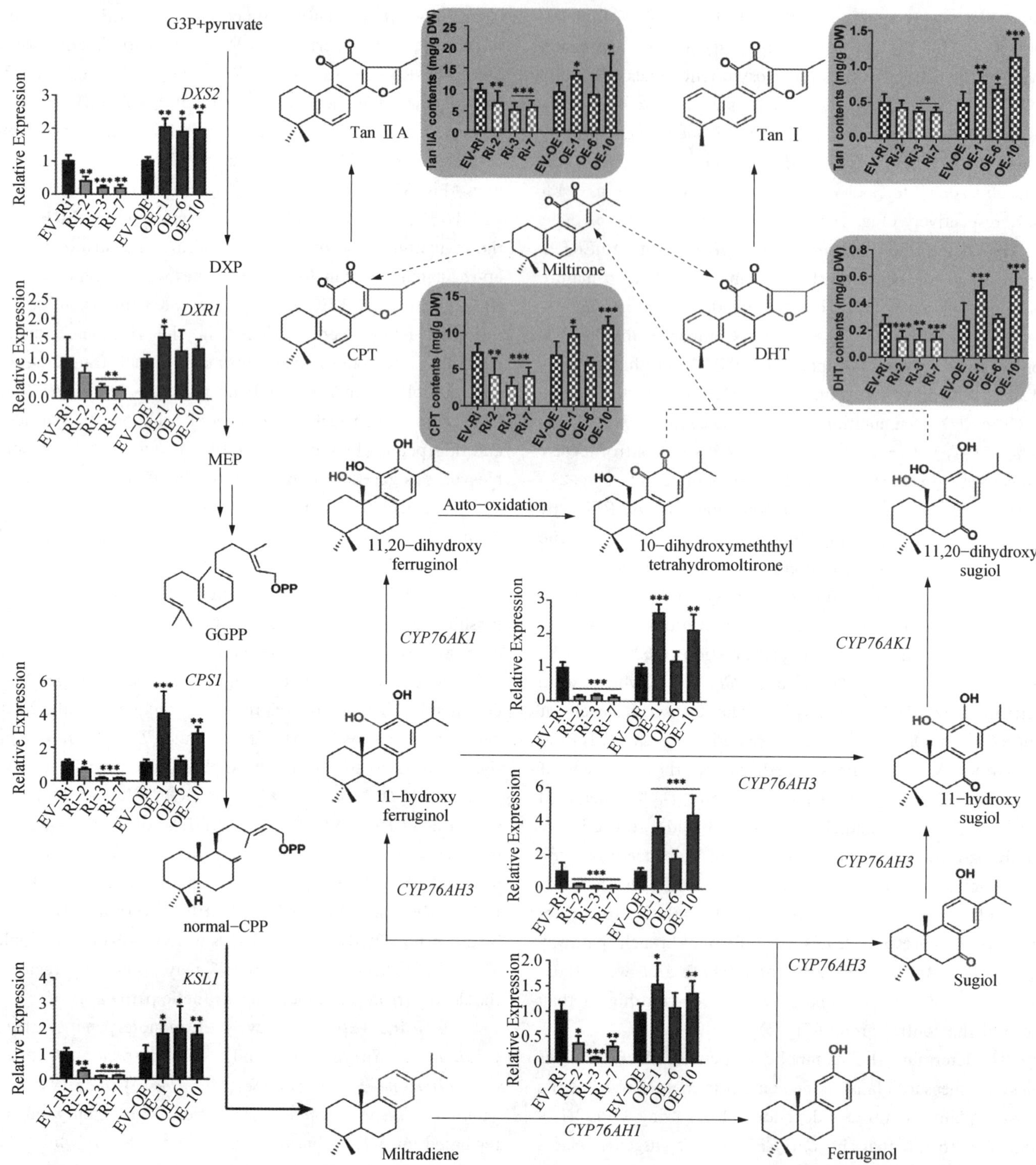


**Fig. 2** ***SmERF73*-silenced lines show reduced tanshinone biosynthetic gene expression and metabolite accumulation, while *SmERF73*-overexpression lines exhibit the inverse response**

A diagram of the tanshinone biosynthesis pathway in *Salvia miltiorrhiza* with corresponding relative expression levels of individual genes in 2-yr-old *SmERF73* RNAi (Ri), overexpression (OE) and control (EV) lines, indicating positive regulatory effects. Root contents (upper right) of cryptotanshinone Ⅰ (CPT), tanshinone ⅡA (Tan ⅡA), dihydrotanshinone (DHT), and tanshinone Ⅰ (Tan Ⅰ) were determined byultra-performance liquid chromatography coupled withtriple-quadrupole tandem mass spectrometry (UPLC-TQ-MS). Solid arrows represent single enzymatic steps; dashed arrows represent multiple enzymatic steps. CPS, copalyl diphosphate synthase; DXS, 1-deoxy-D-xylulose-5-phosphate synthase; DXP, 1-deoxy-D-xylulose 5-phosphate; DXR, 1-deoxy-D-xylulose-5-phosphate reductoisomerase; G3P, Glyceraldehyde 3-phosphate; GGPP, Geranylgeranyldiphosphate; KSL, kaurene synthase; MEP, 2C-methy-D-erythritol-4-phosphate; normal-CPP, *normal*-Copalyl diphosphate. *ACTIN* was used as the internal standard; for each gene, the expression level relative to *ACTIN* in the control plant (i.e. empty vector, EV) was set as 1. Data are shown as the mean ± SD ($n = 3$). Statistical significance was determined by Student's $t$-test: *, $P < 0.05$; **, $P < 0.01$; ***, $P < 0.001$.

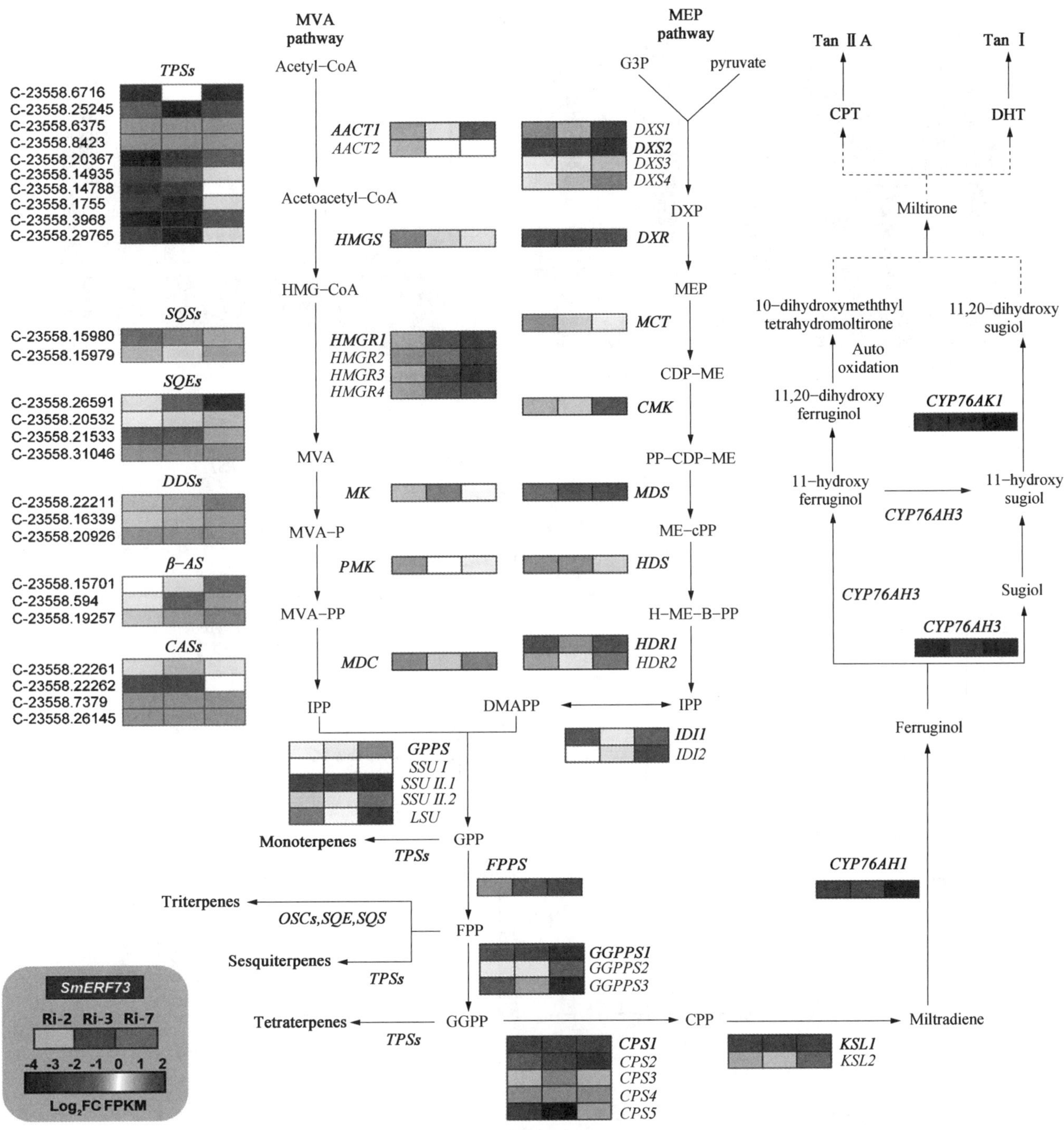


**Fig. 3 SmERF73 not only affects tanshinone blosynthesis, but also some terpene synthases**

Heat map showing expression fold changes ($\log_2$ FC) of terpene-related genes in *Ri-2*, *Ri-3* and *Ri-7* compared with the empty vector (EV) lines. The fragments per kilobase of transcript per million mapped reads (FPKM) value and adjusted *P*-value (q-value) of each gene are shown in Supporting Information Tables S3 - 56. $q$-value $<0.005$ and $|\log_2(\text{folchange})|>1$ was set as the threshold for significant differential expression.

in nuclei; by contrast, cells transformed with 35S-GFP showed fluorescence in the cytoplasm (Fig. 4a). The data showed that SmERF73-GFP localized to the nucleus, which is consistent with its putative role as a transcription factor in the nucleus.

Although tanshinones primarily accumulate in roots, trace amounts have also been detected in aerial organs. We collected four tissues (flowers, leaves, stems and roots) and quantified the relative expression levels of *SmERF73* and four tanshinone biosynthetic genes. The expression of *SmERF73* was significantly higher in roots and stems than in flowers and leaves. For *DXR1*, *CPS1*, *KSL1* and *CYP76AH3*, the expression levels of two diterpene synthase genes (*CPS1* and *KSL1*) were expressed 50-fold higher in roots than in flowers (Fig. 4b).

Based on our previous results, we selected a combined set of seven genes for analysis of YE + $Ag^+$-induced co-

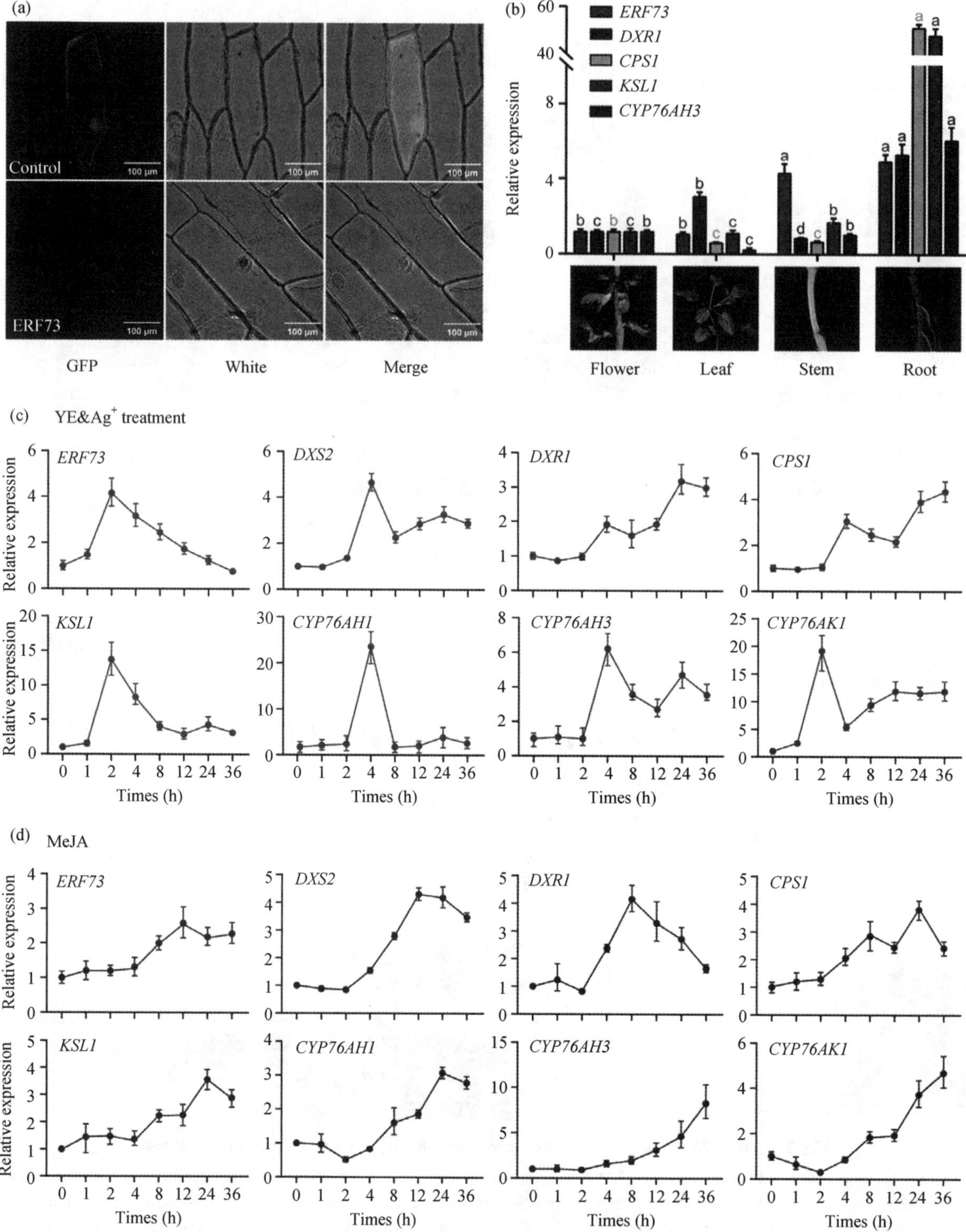


**Fig. 4 *SmERF73* localizes to nuclei with the highest target gene expression in roots**

(a) Transient expression of SmERF73-GFP fusion proteins shows localization to the nucleus in onion epidermal cells. Green fluorescent protein (GFP) fluorescence (left); bright-field (middle); merged images (right). (b) Relative expression levels of *SmERF73* and its putative targets *DXR1*, *CPS1*, *KSL1* and *CYP76AH3* in flower, leaf, stem, and root tissues of 2-yr-old plants at the flowering stage. The expression levels for five genes in flowers were set to 1, with *ACTIN* used as the internal control. Data are shown as the mean±SD ($n=3$), and the different letters indicate values that vary significantly at $P<0.05$ (one-way ANOVA). (c, d) Relative expression analysis by reverse transcription-quantitative polymerase chain reaction (RT-qPCR) of *SmERF73* and seven tanshinone biosynthesis genes (*DXS2*, *DXR1*, *CPS1*, *KSL1* *CYP76AH1*, *CYP76AH3* and *CYP76AK1*) in 21-d-old hairy roots treated with a combined yeast extract (YE) and $Ag^+$ elicitor treatment or 100 μmol/L methyl jasmonate (MeJA), respectively. *ACTIN* was used as an internal control; for each gene, the expression level relative to *ACTIN* in the control was set at 1. Data are shown as the mean±SD ($n=3$).

expression, including *DXS2*, *DXR1*, *CPS1*, *KSL1*, *CYP76AH1*, *CYP76AH3* and *CYP76AK1*. The transcriptional responses by *KSL1*, *CYP76AH1*, and *CYP76AK1* were significantly higher than that of controls, with *KSL1* and *CYP76AK1* exhibiting peak expression at 2 h and *DXS2*, *CYP76AH1*, and *CYP76AH3* peaking at 4 h post-treatment. *DXR1* and *CPS1* expression continued to increase over 24 h post-treatment. Furthermore, we examined the expression pattern of *SmERF73* induced by YE+$Ag^+$, and our results showed that *SmERF73* expression increased rapidly and peaked within 2 h post-treatment, followed by a slow decline (Fig. 4c). This trend suggested that *SmERF73* responds rapidly to YE+$Ag^+$ exposure. These results together show that YE+$Ag^+$ induces expression of *SmERF73* and other genes encoding tanshinone biosynthetic enzymes.

Previous reports have indicated that MeJA induces the expression of tanshinone pathway genes, as well as the accumulation of tanshinones. When Danshen hairy roots were treated for 36 h with 100 μmol/L MeJA, *SmERF73* expression slowly increased (Fig. 4d), while *DXR1* expression peaked at 8 h, *DXS2* at 12 h, and *CPS1*, *KSL1* and *CYP76AH1* at 24 h. By contrast, *CYP76AH3* and *CYP76AK1* expression continued to increase over 36 h (Fig. 4d). Taken together, these results show that MeJA induces the expression of *SmERF73*, as well as that of other tanshinone biosynthetic genes.

SmERF73 specifically binds to GCC cis-elements of *DXR1*, *CPS1*, *KSL1*, and *CYP76AH3 in vitro* The previous results showed that the expression levels of *DXS2*, *DXR1*, *CPS1*, *KSL1*, *CYP76AH1*, *CYP76AH3* and *CYP76AK1* genes declined in *SmERF73-RNAi* lines, while the expression of these genes was elevated in *SmERF73-OE* lines. To better understand the relationship between SmERF73 and these putative target genes, we further investigated whether SmERF73 directly binds to their respective promoter regions *in vitro*. First, we analyzed the promoter sequences of these genes and found that four of the seven promoters (*DXR1*, *CPS1*, *KSL1* and *CYP76AH3*) contained either a predicted ERF binding element (GCCGCC) or a GCC-like element (GCCGCCGCCGCC).

We then performed yeast one-hybrid assays to examine whether SmERF73 was able to bind the GCC motif. After introducing pGADT7-*SmERF73* into yeast strains that contained either 3×GCC or 2×GCC-like elements, we found that SmERF73 factors indeed interacted with the tandem repeated GCC motifs. (Fig. 5a). To further test whether SmERF73 bound these motifs within the native promoter regions of *DXR1*, *CPS1*, *KSL1*, and *CYP76AH3*, we then integrated the *proDXR1*$^{866}$, *proCPS1*$^{1042}$, *proKSL1-L*$^{857}$, *proKSL1-S*$^{289}$ and *proCYP76AH3*$^{630}$ individually into the genomes of yeast cells. After introducing pGADT7-*SmERF73* into each of the respective yeast strains, we found that all five strains carrying the target promoters were able to grow on selective media (Fig. 5a), thus indicating that SmERF73 also binds to the full GCC-containing promoter fragments for each of the putative targets.

To further demonstrate that SmERF73 binds directly to the GCC elements, we performed an EMSA using SmERF73-MBP (malE) fusion protein expressed in *Eicherichia coli*. When the 3×GCC and 2×GCC-like elements were used as labeled probes (Fig. 5b), a DNA-SmERF73 protein complex was strongly detected (lane 3) (Fig. 5c). However, binding activity was abolished by a G>T mutation of the 5′GCC base, resulting in a TCCTCC motif (lane 5; Fig. 5c). Furthermore, the cold competing probes (100-fold concentration of unlabeled 3×GCC and 2×GCC-like elements) attenuated the binding of SmERF73 to the labeled probes (lane 4) (Fig. 5c). Then, to further confirm the binding ability of ERF73 to the above four GCC motifcontaining promoter regions, we synthesized 30–34 bp DNA fragments of the *DXR1*, *CPS1*, *KSL*, and *CYP76AH3* GCC-box regions as specific probes for EMSA (Fig. 5b). We found that SmERF73-MBP (malE) was able to bind the promoter fragments of each of these tanshinone biosynthesis genes (lane 3) (Fig. 5d), but failed to bind DNA probes containing a TCCTCC mutant variant (lane 5). Similarly, a high concentration of unlabeled DNA probes competitively inhibited the binding of SmEFR73 to the GCC probes (lane 4). These results provide strong evidence confirming that SmERF73 binds to both the GCC-box as well as the native promoters of at least four tanshinone biosynthectic genes.

SmERF73 directly binds the promoters of tanshinone biosynthetic genes *in vivo* to activate their expression To confirm that SmERF73 targets the promoters of tanshinone biosynthetic genes *in vivo*, we performed ChIP-qPCR assays using the root tissue of wild-type plants and an anti-SmERF73 antibody. Chromatin without SmERF73 antibody was used as a negative control. We first analyzed the full genomic DNA sequences of *DXR1*, *CPS1*, *KSL1* and *CYP76AH3* and located the GCC-box (box), 5′ untranslated region (5′UTR), and 3′ untranslated region (3′UTR) (Fig. 6a–d). According to their positions, we designated five fragments (P1, P2, box, 5′UTR and 3′UTR) within these genes, where only the box fragment contains the GCC-motif.

The ChIP-qPCR results showed that SmERF73 binds the *DXR1*, *CPS1*, *KSL1* and *CYP76AH3* promoters *in vivo*, and specifically that SmERF73 binds more tightly to the GCC-box-containing fragment than to other fragments. These results together suggest that SmERF73 binds to the GCC-box of the tanshinone biosynthetic genes and in turn regulates their transcription (Fig. 6e–h).

Then, to further verify whether ERF73 positively

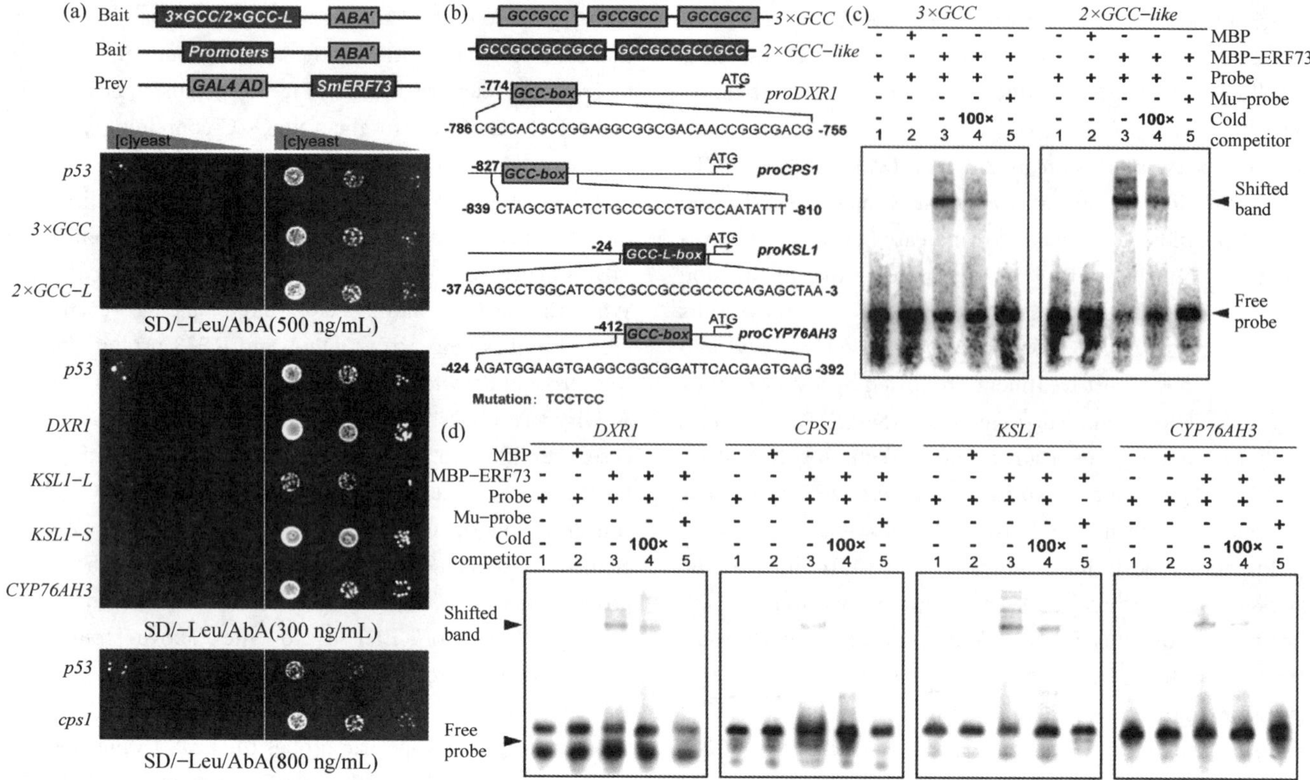


**Fig. 5 SmERF73 binds to the GCC-box in the *DXR1*, *CPS1*, *KSL1*, and *CYP76AH3* promoter *in vitro***

(a) Plasmid structure of pABAi-promoters and pGADT7-SmERF73 (top). SmERF73 protein binds to triple (3×) or double (2×) tandem repeats of GCC or GCC-like motifs, respectively, as bait. Using the promoter fragments *proDXR1*$^{866}$, *proKSL1-L*$^{857}$, *proKSL1-S*$^{289}$, *proCYP76AH3*$^{630}$, and *proCPS1* as bait, SmERF73 was shown to bind *DXR1*, *KSL1-L* (long), *KSL1-S* (short), *CYP76AH3*, and *CPS1*. Grey triangles represent the dilution ratio of the yeast suspension. The numbers in the construct name indicate the distance from the start codon. (b) Schematics of *cis*-elements in electrophoretic mobility shift assay (EMSA) probes. Yellow boxes represent GGC motif promoters; green boxes represent GCC-like promoters. Numbers indicate fragment positions in their respective promoter regions. G(C)>T(A) mutated residues are indicated in red. (c) Electrophoretic mobility shift assays showing that SmERF73 specifically binds to the GCC-motif. (d) Electrophoretic mobility shift assays showing that SmERF73 specifically binds to promoter fragments of tanshinone biosynthesis genes. In (c) and (d), an excess of the cold, unlabeled probe was used as a competitor (lane 4), and those with a mutated binding motif as mu-probe (lane 5); free and bound DNA bands, black arrow.

regulates the tanshinone biosynthetic genes, we performed transient expression assays in *N. benthamiana* leaves. The *proDXR1*$^{866}$, *proCPS1*$^{1042}$, *proKSL1-L*$^{857}$ and *proCYP76AH3*$^{630}$ promoter regions were used to drive the luciferase gene (LUC) as fusion reporters, with ERF73 overexpressed under the control of the 35S promoter as an effector (Fig. 6i). Detection of LUC luminescence indicated that co-expression with the SmERF73 transcription factor increased the expression of the *DXR1pro::LUC*, *CPS1pro::LUC*, *KSL1pro::LUC*, and *CYP76AH3pro::LUC* reporters compared to controls lacking the *35Spro::SmERF73* (Fig. 6j－m). These results indicated that SmERF73 can thus transcriptionally up-regulate these four tanshinone biosynthetic genes.

SmERF73 closely interacts with the transcriptional repressor SmJAZ3　Previous experiments found that *SmERF73* was induced by MeJA (Fig. 4d), leading us to hypothesize that SmERF73 is potentially involved in the JA signaling pathway. To investigate this hypothesis, we performed yeast two-hybrid assays to test for possible interactions between 11 jasmonate-ZIM domain (JAZ) repressor proteins and SmERF73 in Danshen. We found that only SmJAZ3 interacted with SmERF73 in yeast, whereas the other 10 JAZ proteins did not (Figs 7a, S6).

We then used split-luciferase complementation assays to confirm the interaction between SmERF73 and SmJAZ3 *in planta*. SmERF73 fused to the C-terminal fragment of LUC (CLuc-SmERF73) and SmJAZ3 fused with the N-terminal fragment of LUC (SmJAZ3-NLuc) were transiently co-expressed in *N. benthamiana* leaves via *Agrobacterium*-mediated infiltration. The results showed that co-expression of SmJAZ3-NLuc with CLuc-SmERF73 generated a significantly stronger luminescence signal than the control pairs in *N. benthamiana* leaves (Fig. 7b, c), thus verifying that SmERF73 physically interacts with SmJAZ3.

## 4 DISCUSSION

In this study, we identified an ERF-VII group transcription factor, SmERF73, which is essential for elicitor-inducible

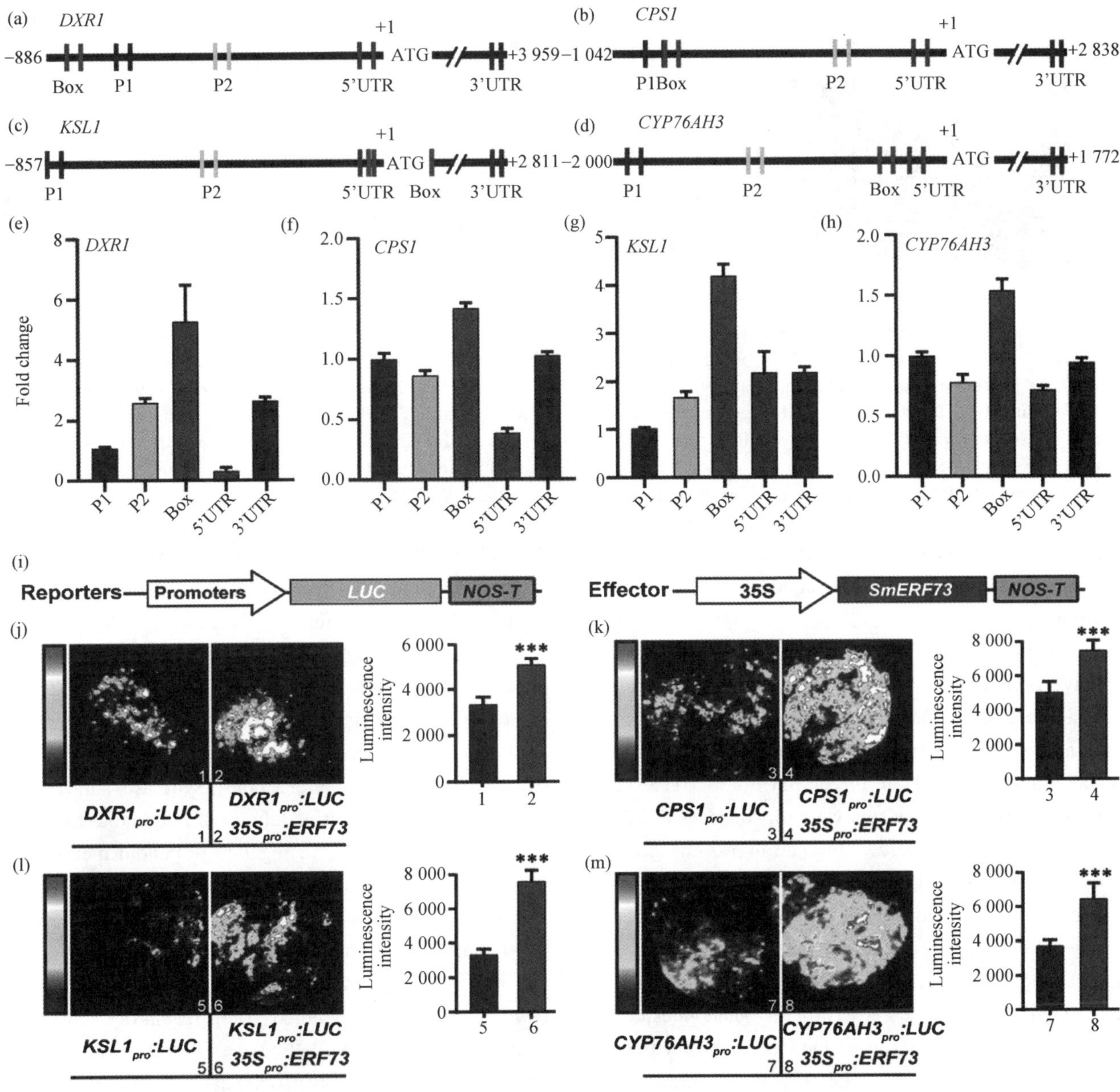

**Fig. 6 SmERF73 is specifically recruited to the GCC and GCC-like boxes *in vivo* and activates transcription of *DXR1*, *CPS1*, *KSL1*, and *CYP76AH3* in tobacco**

(a - d) Schematics of tanshinone pathway gene promoter regions. The horizontal black line represents the full promoter region used for chromatin immunoprecipitation—quantitative polymerase chain reaction (ChIP-qPCR); the red lines represents the GCC-box, the green lines represents the 5′untranslated region (5′UTR), the purple lines represent the 3′ untranslated region (3′UTR), the blue lines represent P1, and the yellow lines represent P2. The numbers indicate the nucleotide positions relative to translational start site (ATG, +1). Error bars represent SDs of three independent replicates. (e - h) The results of the ChIP-qPCR analyses show that SmERF73 interacts with tanshinone biosynthetic gene promoter motifs *in vivo*. Protein/DNA complexes were immunoprecipitated from 45-d-old wild-type seedlings with or without the anti-SmERF73 antibodies. Chromatin without SmERF73 antibody was used as a negative control. For each promoter, five DNA fragments (P1, P2, box, 5′UTR and 3′UTR) were used to determine the enrichment of the DNA fragment containing the GCC-box. The fold enrichment represents the binding efficiency ratio of antibody: no antibody. Data are normalized against input DNA and shown as a relative enrichment of DNA immunoprecipitated with anti-SmERF73 (control). Data are shown as the mean ± SD ($n=3$). (i) Schematics of luciferase reporter and effector constructs. The *proDXR1*$^{866}$, *proCPS1*$^{1042}$, *proKSL1-L*$^{857}$ and *proCYP76AH3*$^{630}$ constructs were each used to drive the LUC reporter; *35S::SmERF73* was used as an effector. (j - m) Transient expression assays of SmERF73 transcriptional activation of tanshinone pathway genes. Luminescence imaging of *N. benthamiana* leaves at 72 h after infiltration. Higher luminescence intensity was observed in co-expression of SmERF73 with *DXR1pro:LUC*(j), *CPS1pro:LUC*(k), *KSL1pro:LUC*(l), or *CYP76AH3pro:LUC* (m). Quantitative analysis of luminescence intensity was determined. These experiments were repeated three times with similar results. Values are means±SD of 12 independent measurements. Error bars indicate SD. Asterisks denote significant difference according to Student's *t*-test: *, $P<0.05$; **, $P<0.01$; ***, $P<0.001$.

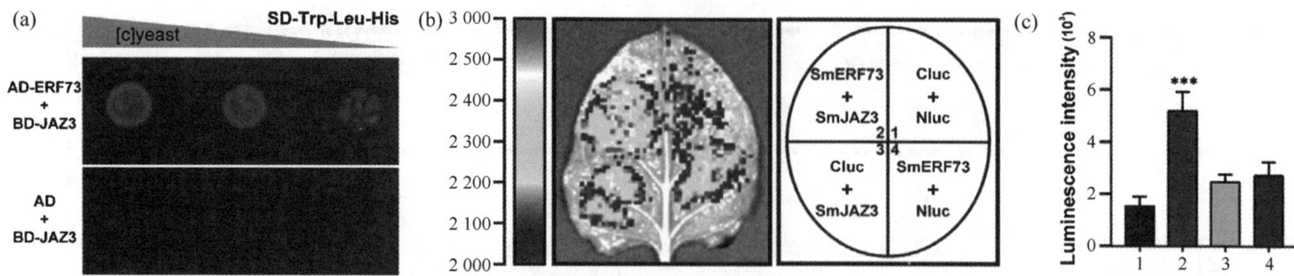


**Fig. 7 SmERF73 closely interacts with SmJAZ3 protein**

(a) Interactions between SmERF73 and SmJAZ3 in yeast two-hybrid assays. AD-SmERF73, SmERF73 fused to activation domain; BD-SmJAZ3, SmJAZ3 fused to GAL4 DNA binding domain. The empty AD/BD-SmJAZ3 combination served as a negative control. (b, c) Split-luciferase complementation assays show that SmERF73 interacts with SmJAZ3 in *Nicotiana benthamiana*. CLuc-SmERF73, SmERF73 fused to C-terminal fragment of LUC (CLuc); SmJAZ3-NLuc, SmJAZ3 fused to N-terminal fragment of LUC (NLuc). *Nicotiana benthamiana* leaves were infiltrated with *Agrobacterium* strains containing the indicated construct pairs, and LUC signals were collected 50 h post infiltration. Values are means ± SD of three independent measurements. Error bars indicate SD. Asterisks denote significant difference according to Student's *t*-text: *, $P<0.05$; **, $P<0.01$; ***, $P<0.001$.

production of tanshinones, and coordinately regulates the expression of seven genes in the tanshinone biosynthesis and upstream MEP pathways.

The gene clusters for specialized metabolic pathways in plants have been found in diverse monocot and dicot plant species, and are required for the synthesis of different kinds of secondary metabolites (terpenes, alkaloids, and cyanogenic glycosides). Four terpene synthase (TPS) and cytochrome P450 (CYP) clusters were all found in the draft genome of *S. miltiorrhiza*. In an improved genome assembly of Danshen, the five genes encoding enzymes identified as being involved in tanshinone biosynthesis, including three diterpene synthases, *SmCPS1*, *SmCPS2* and *SmKSL1*, and two CYPs, *CYP76AH1* and *CYP76AH3*, were located in a large biosynthetic gene cluster in chromosome 6. SmERF73 can influence the production of tanshinones by coordinately regulating the transcriptional expression of seven key enzyme-encoding genes, including two diterpene tanshinone skeletons, *CPS1* and *KSL*, diterpene tanshinone skeleton postmodification genes, *CYP76AH1*, *CYP76AH3* and *CYP76AK1*, and the upstream MEP pathway genes *DXR1*, *DXS2* (Fig. 2). However, based on *in vivo* and *in vitro* experimental analysis, SmERF73 can only selectively bind to GCC-box promoter elements of four tanshinone biosynthetic genes (*DXR1*, *CPS1*, *KSL1*, and *CYP76AH3*) (Figs 5, 6). In this way, SmERF73 can directly bind to cis-elements of three of the five genes in the tanshinone biosynthetic gene cluster, thereby regulating the biosynthesis of tanshinone. These enzymes may control the flow of isoprenoid metabolism in tanshinone biosynthesis. CPS1 and KSL1 are involved in the formation of the abietane-type diterpene quinone skeleton of tanshinones, and they are fused with other related synthases to significantly increase the miltiradiene production in yeast. SmCYP76AH3 oxidizes ferruginol at two different carbon centers to obtain 11-hydroxy ferruginol and 11-hydroxy sugiol, thereby forming a branch in the tanshinone biosynthetic pathway. SmERF73 directly or indirectly acts on the key enzyme-encoding genes in the biosynthesis of tanshinone, transcriptionally regulates genes in the plastid MEP isoprenoid precursor pathway, and increases the expression of the diterpenoid synthase and skeletal modification genes. Ultimately, it is reasonable to speculate that SmERF73 is likely to regulate terpenoid metabolic flux to increase the accumulation of tanshinone products.

With the mining of large-scale genome data, several in-depth studies have emerged describing the structure, origin, and function of plant biosynthetic gene clusters. However, few studies have detailed the regulatory mechanisms controlling plant biosynthetic gene clusters, especially at the transcriptional level. In particular, OsTGAP1 (a bZIP transcription factor) in rice, Bl (a bHLH transcription factor) in cucumber and GAME9 (an AP2/ERF transcription factor) in potato and tomato were all shown to coordinately regulate biosynthetic gene clusters in their respective species. Metabolic gene clusters are commonly described as co-regulated, co-expressed, or coordinately regulated. Plant biosynthetic gene clusters can be co-expressed under the induction of biotic and abiotic elicitors and exogenous plant hormones. For example, eight of the nine genes involved in cucurbitacin C synthesis were induced by drought stress and exogenous ABA treatment. Similarly, we found that a suite of tanshinone biosynthesis genes regulated by SmERF73 are co-expressed following exposure to both biotic and abiotic stress elicitors, as well as exogenous MeJA (Fig. 4c, d). Furthermore, this co-regulated cluster of secondary metabolite biosynthetic genes regulated by transcription factors also shows coordinated

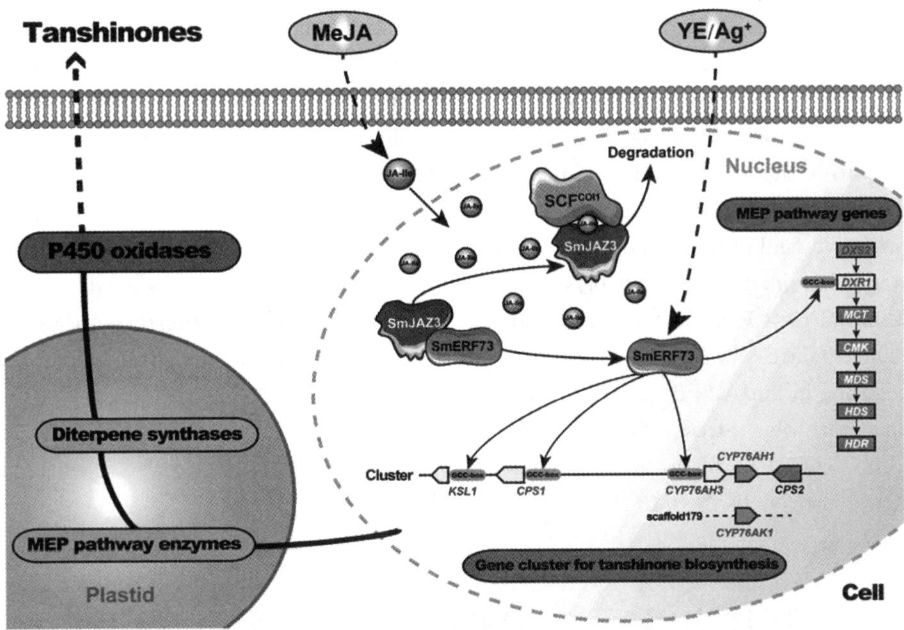


**Fig. 8 Model for coordinated regulation of tanshinone biosynthesis by SmERF73**

Exogenous methyl jasmonate (MeJA) induces endogenous JA-Ile biosynthesis, subsequently stimulating interaction between the SmJAZ3 repressor and $SCF^{COI1}$ ubiquitin ligase, leading to SmJAZ3 degradation via the 26S proteasome. Derepression of SmJAZ3 allows the SmERF73 transcription factor to activate the expression of tanshinone biosynthetic genes through binding to the GCC-box promoter motifs. SmERF73 thus co-regulates the transcription of tanshinone biosynthesis genes as well as upstream methylerythritol 4-phosphate (MEP) pathway genes, thereby stimulating the accumulation of tanshinone pathway metabolites.

patterns of expression in both SmERF73-overexpression and -interference lines in Danshen (Fig. 2), similar to that observed for Bl in cucumber and GAME9 in potato and tomato. While transcription factors typically appear to co-regulate gene clusters through binding to specific DNA motifs, other unknown factors may also indirectly mediate regulation of these clusters, such as CAME9 binding to cis elements in the promoter of some genes in the gene cluster cooperatively with an MYC transcription factor. SmERF73 can directly bind to the promoter of four of the seven tanshinone biosynthesis genes that it was shown to regulate, and the regulation mechanisms of the other three genes require further elucidation. Interestingly, SmERF73 in Danshen can also activate the expression of upstream MEP pathway genes in addition to the tanshinone gene cluster, similar to OsTGAP1 in rice.

The majority of ERFs shown to participate in secondary metabolite biosynthesis are members of group IX, such as *CrORCA4* in *Catharanthus roseus*, and *AaERF1/2* and *AaORA* in *Artemisia annua*. For example, overexpression of *CrORCA4* led to a dramatic increase of terpenoid indole alkaloid (TIA) accumulation in *C. roseus* hairy roots, and overexpression of either *AaERF1/2* or *AaORA* in *A. annua* plants increased transcript levels of both amorpha-4, 11-diene synthase gene (*ADS*) and *CYP71AV1*, leading to increased production of artemisinin. The group VII ERFs have been previously reported to perform essential roles in the regulation of abiotic and biotic stress responses (particularly the response to low-oxygen stress. However, SmERF73 in Danshen increases tanshinone accumulation through the transcriptional activation of diterpene biosynthetic genes. Thus, involvement of the ERF- VII group in lowoxygen stress implies a potential role for SmERF73-mediated tanshinone production in the stress response, which can be further explored in future studies.

In our previous work, transcriptomic changes in Danshen hairy roots induced by the combined elicitor ($YE+Ag^+$) led us to speculate that biotic and abiotic stress may promote the accumulation of tanshinones by inducing transcription factors through the jasmonic acid signal pathway. Overexpression of *SmJAZ3/8/9* in Danshen hairy roots led to reduced contents of tanshinones, whereas silencing of *SmJAZ3/8/9* resulted in the accumulation of these compounds. We used Y2H to investigate possible interactions between SmERF73 and eleven *S. miltiorrhiza* JAZ proteins. Only SmJAZ3 was found to closely interact or bind with SmERF73, suggesting that SmJAZ3 may block SmERF73 transcriptional activation of tanshinone biosynthetic genes during the JA response. However, the expression patterns of SmERF73 and diterpene tanshinone biosynthetic genes induced by MeJA are inconsistent with those induced by $YE+Ag^+$ (Fig. 4d). Studies have confirmed that the elicitor YE has a greater impact on terpene biosynthesis-related genes, while MeJA has significant effects on phenylpropane metabolic pathwayrelated genes. The expression of SmERF73 is likely to be controlled not only by the JA signal pathway but also by multiple signal pathways. Further research will clarify the mechanism of SmERF73 regulation of the expression of tanshinone pathway genes.

Based on our cumulative findings, we propose a model for the JA-dependent regulation of tanshinone biosynthetic gene expression by SmERF73 (Fig. 8). In this model, exogenous MeJA could induce limited biosynthesis of endogenous JA-Ile, resulting in SmJAZ3 degradation via the $SCF^{COI1}$-26S proteasome pathway. Stress elicitors ($YE + Ag^{+}$) could also induce SmERF73 by as-of-yet unknown pathways. Free SmERF73 then binds the GCC-box elements to coordinately activate the near-simultaneous transcription of tanshinone biosynthetic genes *DXR1*, *CPS1*, *KSL1* and *CYP76AH3*, leading to increased accumulations of tanshinone compounds. This coordination of transcription by SmERF73 could potentially modulate the biosynthesis of select tanshinone intermediates, thereby providing a useful tool for engineering the production of individual compounds. Furthermore, this mechanism provides insight into how tanshinone biosynthesis is mediated by JA or biotic and abiotic stress in *S. miltiorrhiza*, thus laying a foundation for further study of the biological roles of tanshinone metabolites in plants.

[郑汉，黄璐琦，申业，等. New Phytologist, 2021, 231: 1940-1955.]

# AaWRKY9 contributes to light- and jasmonate-mediated to regulate the biosynthesis of artemisinin in *Artemisia annua*

## 1 INTRODUCTION

Malaria is an extremely serious health problem and caused *c*. 405 000 deaths globally in 2018 according to the World Malaria Report 2019. Artemisinin Combination Therapies are currently recommended by the World Health Organization as the preferred drug to fight the malaria. Artemisinin, a sesquiterpene lactone, isolated from *A. annua*, is extensively used to treat malaria. Considerable efforts have been expended to determine the artemisinin biosynthetic pathway (Supporting Information Fig. S1). The genes encoding enzymes in artemisinin biosynthetic pathway have been isolated. Amorpha-4, 11-diene synthase (ADS), cytochrome P450 monooxygenase (CYP71AV1), cytochrome P450 reductase (CPR), artemisinic aldehyde Δ11 (13)-double bond reductase (DBR2), an aldehyde dehydrogenase (ALDH1), an alcohol dehydrogenase (ADH1) and cytochrome $b_5$ monooxygenase (CYB5) were involved in the biosynthesis of artemisinic acid (AA) and dihydroartemisinic acid (DHAA). The conversions of DHAA to artemisinin and AA to arteannuin B are regarded as nonenzymatic photo-oxidation reactions. In *A. annua*, artemisinin is synthesised in the glandular trichomes, which contain two stalk cells, two basal cells and three pairs of secretory cells.

Although the biosynthetic pathway of artemisinin has been clearly elucidated, the mechanism underlying the transcriptional regulation of the genes in this pathway remains largely unknown. Several transcription factors (TFs) involved in artemisinin biosynthesis have been identified in *A. annua*. For example, APETALA 2/ ETHYLENE RESPONSIVE FACTOR (ERF) proteins, namely AaERF1, AaERF2, AaORA and AaTAR1, have been shown to positively regulate artemisinin biosynthesis by activating the expression of *AaADS*, *AaCYP71AV1* and *AaDBR2*. AaWRKY1 was also found to increase artemisinin content by activating the expression of *AaADS*, *AaCYP71AV1* and *AaDBR2* in *AaWRKY1*-overexpression lines. There is evidence that plant hormones such as jasmonate (JA) also play important roles in artemisinin biosynthesis regulation. For instance, the glandular trichome-specific WRKY TF AaGSW1 directly binds to W-boxes in the promoters of *AaCYP71AV1* and *AaORA*, and positively regulates their expression, in response to JA. Similarly, the JA-responsive basic helix—loop—helix TF AaMYC2 was found to promote artemisinin biosynthesis through direct binding to the G-box of the *AaDBR2* promoter, activating the expression of *AaCYP71AV1* and *AaDBR2*. In addition, AaJAZ8, a repressor in the JA signalling pathway, suppresses the transcriptional activation activity of the AaTCP14-AaORA complex, which directly binds to and activates the *AaDBR2* and *AaALDH1* promoters; after AaJAZ8 is degraded by JA treatment, the AaTCP14—AaORA complex is released, resulting in the enhancement of artemisinin biosynthesis. Therefore, the results from the previous studies showed that JA signalling is crucial for regulating artemisinin accumulation in *A. annua*.

Energy from the sun is not only essential for photosynthesis and plant longevity, but also plays significant roles in various development and growth processes. Plants have evolved complex transcriptional networks involved in the response to light and perceive light signals via phytochromes, cryptochromes, phototropins and UVR8. In *A. annua*, overexpression of the blue-light receptor cryptochromel gene *AtCRY1* from Arabidopsis was found to enhance artemisinin production by activating the expression of *FPS*, *ADS* and *CYP71AV1*. In addition, Zhang *et al*. found that both red-light and blue-light signals have the potential to increase artemisinin accumulation by promoting the transcription of artemisinin biosynthetic genes; they found that the artemisinin content was observably higher under red-light and blue-light conditions than under the white light, infrared light and darkness. Previously, we have reported that the expression of artemisinin biosynthesis genes significantly decreased under darkness in comparison with light conditions. Transcriptome analysis of *A. annua* leaves treated with methyl jasmonate (MeJA) under light or dark conditions showed that light-dependent JA signalling can significantly promote artemisinin biosynthesis. Recently the bZIP TF ELONGATED HYPOCOTYL 5 (HY5), which is involved in light signalling was found to activate artemisinin biosynthesis by directly binding to the promoter of *AaGSW1*. However, the mechanism underlying the interaction of light and JA signalling in relation to artemisinin biosynthesis regulation is still unresolved in *A. annua*.

Here, we demonstrate that AaWRKY9 plays an important role in regulating artemisinin biosynthesis through the light-dependent JA signalling pathway. We found that AaWRKY9 positively regulated artemisinin accumulation by binding to the promoters of *AaDBR2* and *AaGSW1*. A key TF in the light signalling pathway, AaHY5, activated the expression of *AaWRKY9* and bound to its promoter. In addition, the repressor AaJAZ9 in the JA signalling pathway interacted with AaWRKY9 and suppressed its transcriptional activation activity. Our results indicated that AaWRKY9 contributes to light and JA signalling to regulate the biosynthesis of artemisinin in *A. annua*.

## 2 MATERIALS AND METHODS

Plant materials *Artemisia annua* L. (Huhaol) seeds were harvested from Chongqing, China and bred selectively in Shanghai for several years. *A. annua* and *Nicotiana benthamiana* plantlets were placed in a glasshouse with a 16 h:8 h, light:dark photoperiod at 24 ℃.

Light treatments were carried out in an E-30 LED growth chamber (Percival, Boone, IA, USA) with a blue and red-light-emitting diode at 22 ℃. Mean photon flux densities [μmol/($m^2$ · s)] were measured by an Li250 quantum photometer (Li-Cor, Lincoln, NE, USA). Four-wk-old *A. annua* seedlings were transferred into the dark, then sampled at 0, 0.5, 3, 6, 9, 12 and 24 h. *A. annua* seedlings pretreated in darkness for 24 h were exposed to blue or red light with 5, 10 and 40 μmol/($m^2$ · s) PPFD. The leaves were collected after 0, 0.5, 3, 6, 9, 12 and 24 h under blue-light (470 nm) or red-light (680 nm) conditions [5, 10, 20 and 40 μmol/($m^2$ · s) PPFD]. The leaves were sampled at 0, 0.5, 3, 6, 9, 12 and 24 h under blue-light or red-light conditions. For hormone treatments, 2-wk-old *A. annua* seedlings were treated with 100 μmol/L MeJA and water with 0.1% of ethanol was used as a mock treatment. The leaves were collected at 0, 0.5, 1.5, 3, 6, 9, 12 and 24 h after treatment. All samples were separately collected from five seedlings, frozen in liquid nitrogen and stored at −80 ℃. The cutting seedlings of overexpression and antisense transgenic plants, the control plants transformed with the empty vector and wild-type *A. annua* plants were cultivated in continuous white light for 2 wk. Then half of them were transferred to the dark conditions for 24 h. After the independent pretreatment, the cutting seedlings were sprayed with 100 μmol/L MeJA and 0.1% ethanol (as mock) under the light and dark conditions. The leaves were sampled at 24 and 48 h for artemisinin analysis. Three biological replicates were performed for each treatment.

RNA extraction, transcriptome sequencing and qRT-PCR Total RNA was extracted from different tissues (young leaves, old leaves, buds, roots, stems, flowers and trichomes) and from leaves at various developmental stages of 5-month-old plants *A. annua* using the RNAprep Pure Plant Kit (Tiangen, Beijing, China) as described previously. First-strand cDNA for qRT-PCR was synthesised from the total RNA using the PrimeScript™ RT Master Mix (TaKaRa, Shiga, Japan). cDNA libraries for RNA-sequencing (RNA-seq) were constructed from the total RNA of plants treated with blue or red light [40 μmol/($m^2$ · s) PPFD] for 0, 6 and 24 h using the Illumina TruSeq™ RNA Sample Prep Kit (Illumina, San Diego, CA, USA). Subsequently, the cDNA libraries were sequenced at Shanghai Majorbio Biopharm Biotechnology Co. Ltd (Shanghai, China). The raw data were filtered before *de novo* transcriptome assembly. To obtain high-quality clean reads, the adapter sequences, low-quality or empty reads were removed using TRIMMOMATIC (v. 0.30). The remaining high-quality clean reads were used for *de novo* transcriptome assembly using Trinity software (http://trinityrnaseq.sourceforge.net/) helped by *A. annua* reference genome. All the TF genes and the transcript levels of putative genes in different tissues (seed, root, leaf, bud and trichome) were identified according to the *A. annua* reference genome. Hierarchical clustering analysis based on RNA-seq data was performed using MultiExperiment Viewer software to predict potential TFs involved in the biosynthesis of artemisinin.

The first leaves of 3-month-old transgenic plants were collected to analyse the expression of *ADS*, *CYP71AV1*, *DBR2*, *ALDH1*, *AaWRKY9*, *AaJAZ9*, *AaORA*, *AaGSW1*, *AaTCP14* and *AaMYC2*. Real-time qPCR was carried out using the SuperReal PreMix Plus (SYBR Green) Kit (Tiangen, Beijing, China) using *β-ACTIN* of *A. annua* as the reference gene. qRT-PCR assays were performed as previously described. Three biological repeats were measured for each sample. All the primers used in this study are listed in Table S1.

Dual-LUC assays The effector genes *AaWRKY9*, *AaJAZ9* and *AaHY5* were inserted into pHB vector. The promoters of *ADS*, *CYP71AV1*, *DBR2*, *ALDH1*, *AaWRKY9* and *AaGSW1* were cloned into the pGREEN0800-LUC vector as reporters. The empty pHB vector was used as the effector control. The recombinant reporter vectors were transformed separately into *Agrobacterium tumefaciens* strain GV3101 with the plasmid pSoup19, and the recombinant effector vectors were transformed into GV3101. The strains harbouring the recombinant vectors were injected into *N. benthamiana* leaves. After incubation for 48 h, the leaves were treated with 50 μmol/L MeJA for 4 h and water with 0.05% ethanol was used as the control. Equally sized leaves were collected for dual-LUC assays according to the manufacturer's instructions (Promega). All experiments for each combination were repeated in triplicate. All the primers used in this study are listed in Table S1.

Subcellular localisation To determine the subcellular localisation of the AaWRKY9 protein, the yellow fluorescent protein (YFP) was fused to the Nterminal domain of AaWRKY9 under the control of the CaMV35S promoter. The recombinant plasmid (pHB—YFP—AaWRKY9) and the empty vector control were transferred into GV3101, then separately co-transformed into *N. benthamiana* leaves with a strain containing the p19 plasmid. YFP signals were observed by confocal laser microscopy (Leica TCS SP5-II) after 48 h of incubation.

Molecular cloning of promoters and promoter-GUS fusions for expression in *A. annua* The promoter sequences of *AaWRKY9 and AaJAZ9* were predicted using the *A. annua* reference genome. The predicted promoter regions of *AaWRKY9* (1 177 bp) and *AaJAZ9* (1 799 bp) were amplified using specific primers and inserted into the *BamH*I and *Nco*I sites of pCAMBIA1391. The recombinant plasmids were transformed into *A. tumefaciens* strain EHA105 for *A. annua* plant transformation. GUS staining was performed as previously described.

Construction and transformation of *A. annua* The full-length coding regions of *AaWRKY9* and *AaJAZ9* were cloned into separate pHB—Flag vectors. To construct the antisense lines, a 500-bp nonconserved domain in the coding region of *AaWRKY9* was cloned into the pHB vector. The constructs (pHB—Flag—*AaWRKY9*, pHB—anti-*AaWRKY9* and pHB—*AaJAZ9*—Flag) and the pHB vector were transferred into strain EHA105 for *A. annua* plant transformation.

Measurement of artemisinin, DHAA and AA content Fresh leaves from overexpression, antisense, transgenic lines transformed with the empty vector and wild-type plants were collected, dried at 50 ℃ for 48 h and ground to powder. Each sample (0.1 g) was extracted twice with 1 ml methanol. After centrifuging at 13 586*g* for 10 min, the supernatant was collected to measure artemisinin, DHAA and AA content, as described previously. All assays were repeated three times.

Yeast-one-hybrid and electrophoretic mobility shift assays The open reading frames of *AaWRKY9* and *AaHY5* were amplified and inserted into the pB42AD vector. Three tandem copies of the W-box motifs in the promoter of *CYP71AV1* (C1—C3), *DBR2* (D1—D7), *ALDH1* (A) and *AaGSW1* (G1—G4) were cloned into separate pLacZ vectors. Three tandem copies of the G-box motifs in the promoter of *AaWRKY9* were also ligated into the pLacZ vector. The recombinant pB42AD plasmids and pLacZ vectors with the motifs were transferred into the yeast strain EGY48A. The empty vector pB42AD and the motifs were used as the negative controls. The clones were transferred to SD/—Trp/—Ura medium containing X-gal and cultivated at 30 ℃ for 2 d after selection on the SD/—Trp/—Ura plates.

The full-length coding sequences of *AaWRKY9* and *AaHY5* were cloned into the pCold-TF vector (TaKaRa, Japan). The recombinant vectors and empty vector were transferred into *E. coli* strain Rosetta (DE3) (TransGen Biotech, Beijing, China). His fusion protein expression was induced by adding 200 μmol/L isopropyl-D-1-thiogalactopyranoside (IPTG) and incubating at 16 ℃ for 14 h and purified using nitrilotriacetic acid (Ni-NTA) agarose (Invitrogen Life Technologies). Electrophoretic mobility shift assays (EMSA) assays were performed using the LightShift® Chemiluminescent EMSA Kit according to the manufacturer's instructions (Thermo Fisher Scientific, Waltham, MA, USA). The biotin-labelled W5, W5-mutant, W4, W4-mutant, G and G-mutant probes were synthesised by Sangon (Shanghai, China). All primers are listed in Table S1.

Yeast-two-hybrid and pull-down assays Construction of a cDNA library of *A. annua* for yeast-two-hybrid (Y2H) experiments was carried out by OE BioTech (Shanghai, China) using mRNAs from the youngest leaves and meristem. The open reading frame of *AaWRKY9* was cloned into the pGBKT7 vector. Y2H screening assays were performed using the Matchmaker Gold Y2H system's user manual (TaKaRa, Japan) as previously described. For Y2H assays, *AaJAZ9* was inserted into the pGADT7 vector. The combinations of recombinant plasmids were transferred into yeast stain AH109. The positive clones cultivated on SD/−Leu/−Trp agar medium plates were transferred to SD/−Leu/−Trp/−His and SD/−Leu/−Trp/−His/−Ade medium plates. The results were observed after 3 d.

For pull-down assays, the full-length coding sequence of *AaJAZ9* was cloned into the pGEX4T-1 vector (GE Healthcare), then transformed into *E. coli* strain Rosetta (DE3) to synthesise the GST-AaJAZ9 protein. His-AaWRKY9 protein was produced in *E. coli* strain Rosetta (DE3) harbouring the pCold-*AaWRKY9* plasmid. The pull-down assay was carried out as previously described. All the experiments were repeated three times.

Bimolecular fluorescence and co-immunoprecipitation assays  For bimolecular fluorescence complementation (BiFC) assays, the open reading frame of *AaJAZ9* was cloned into the pxy104 vector and the full-length coding region of *AaWRKY9* was inserted into the pxy106 vector. The recombinant plasmids (pxy104−*AaJAZ9* and pxy106−*AaWRKY9*) and the empty vectors were transferred into GV3101. Subsequently, combinations of the plasmids were co-transformed into *N. benthamiana* leaves. Confocal laser microscopy (Leica TCS SP5-II) was used to observe the YFP signals.

For co-immunoprecipitation (CoIP) assays, the open reading frame of *AaJAZ9* was inserted into the pHB−YFP vector. The recombinant plasmids (pHB−Flag−*AaWRKY9* and pHB−*AaJAZ9*−YFP) and the empty vectors were transformed to GV3101. *N. benthamiana* leaves were injected with the combinations of the stains harbouring the plasmids. After incubation for 48 h, the leaves were collected and ground to powder using liquid nitrogen. CoIP assays were carried out as previously described. For each sample, 15 μl of Protein G Sepharose (GE Healthcare, Bucks, UK) and 10 μl of the rabbit anti-GFP antibody (GenScript, Nanjing, China) were incubated for 2 h at 4 ℃. The total proteins from tobacco were added into the Protein G Sepharose, then incubated for 2 h at 4 ℃. The proteins were detected using anti-GFP (AbMart, Shanghai, China) and anti-Flag antibody (Sigma-Aldrich).

Accession numbers  Sequence data in this article were deposited in the GenBank databases under the following accession numbers: AaORA (JQ 797708), AaWRKY9 (PWA78774.1), AaWRKY1 (FJ390842.1), AaGSW1 (KX465128.1), AaWRKY75b (KX465129.1), HaWR KY9 (XP_021988131.1), LsWRKY9 (XP_023730594.1), CcW RKY9 (XP_024980454.1), AcWRKY9 (PSS02849.1), GhW RKY9 (XP_016719407.1), AtWRKY9 (NP_176982.1), AtWRK Y45 (NP_186846.1) AtWRKY1 (NP_178565.1), *proADS* (DQ448294), *proCYP71AV1* (FJ870128), *proDBR2* (KC118523.1) and *proALDH1* (KC118525.1).

Raw RNA-seq data are available from the NCBI Sequence Read Archive (SRA; accession no. PRJNA669960).

## 3 RESULTS

Blue and red light induce the expression of artemisinin biosynthesis genes  *Artemisia annua* seedlings cultivated in the light for 2 wk were transferred to dark conditions for 24 h. qRT-PCR results showed that the expression levels of the artemisinin biosynthetic genes *AaADS*, *AaCYP71AV1*, *AaDBR2* and *AaALDH1* were significantly reduced after the dark treatment (Fig. S2a, b), indicating that light plays a critical role in artemisinin biosynthesis in *A. annua*. As demonstrated before, *A. annua* seedlings grown under red and blue light had higher levels of artemisinin and AA accumulation in comparison with those grown under white and infrared light. Therefore, in this study, red and blue light were used to treat *A. annua* seedlings. The seedlings cultivated in light and pretreated darkness for 24 h, were transferred to blue light at 5, 10, 20, or 40 μmol/($m^2$ · s) PPFD for 24 h. qRT-PCR analysis revealed that only the expression of *AaDBR2* was significantly higher compared with the 0 h under 5 μmol/($m^2$ · s) PPFD (Fig. S3a) and the expression of both *AaCYP71AV1* and *AaDBR2* was significantly increased under 10 μmol/($m^2$ · s) PPFD (Fig. S3b). Enhancing the intensity of blue light [20 and 40 μmol/($m^2$ · s) PPFD] observably increased the transcriptional levels of *AaADS*, *AaCYP71AV1*, *AaDBR2* and *AaALDH1* (Fig. S3c, d). Similarly, the expression of *AaADS*, *AaCYP71AV1*, *AaDBR2* and *AaALDH1* was significantly higher under 10, 20 and 40 μmol/($m^2$ · s) PPFD red-light conditions (Fig. S3f-h), but the transcript levels of these genes did not change when *A. annua* seedlings were exposed to lower intensity red light [5 μmol/($m^2$ · s) PPFD] (Fig. S3e). Overall, these results indicated that blue and red light induced the expression of artemisinin biosynthesis genes in *A. annua*.

Identification of blue- and red-light-induced TF genes involved in artemisinin biosynthesis by RNA-seq  To identify light-induced TFs regulating the artemisinin biosynthesis, samples treated with blue-light and red-light [40 μmol/($m^2$ · s) PPFD] treatment for 0, 6, 24 h were used for transcriptome sequencing. The sequencing reads were mapped against the reference genome. We found that the expression levels of *AaADS*, *AaCYP71AV1*, *AaDBR2* and *AaALDH1* were significantly higher after seedlings pretreated in the dark for 24 h were exposed to blue and red light for 6 and 24 h (Fig. S4a, b). In total, 172 TF genes from the blue-light RNA-seq data and 111 TF genes from the red-light RNA-seq data exhibited expression patterns similar to those of the artemisinin biosynthetic genes.

To obtain the candidate light-regulated TFs regulating artemisinin biosynthesis, hierarchical clustering analysis with the artemisinin biosynthetic genes was performed using the RNA-seq data from different *A. annua* tissues. Thirteen TF genes from the blue-light RNA-seq data and nine TF genes from the red-light RNA-seq data were identified (Fig. S5a, b). Four TF genes (AA532500, AA213240, AA046070 and AA041930) were induced by both blue-light and red-light treatments, one of which (AA532500) encoded the AaORA protein, which positively regulates artemisinin biosynthesis by activating the expression of *AaADS*, *AaCYP71AV1* and *AaDBR2*. qRT-PCR analysis confirmed the RNA-seq results, indicating that the expression patterns of 15 candidate genes were consistent with the RNA-seq data (Fig. 1). The transcript levels of the 15 candidate genes in different tissues were further analysed by qRT-PCR, revealing that 13 genes showed an expression pattern similar to that of *AaORA* (Fig. S6). Subsequently, the dual-LUC system was used to identify the function of the candidate TFs related to artemisinin biosynthesis, revealing that an unknown WRKY protein (AA213240) could observably activate the expression of *CYP71AV1*, *DBR2* and *ALDH1* (Fig. 2). Therefore, AA213240, assigned the name *AaWRKY9*, was chosen for further study. AaWRKY9 clustered with HaWRKY9, CcWRKY9 and LsWRKY9 in a phylogenetic tree (Fig. S7a), and alignment of the AaWRKY9 protein with several WRKYs showed that AaWRKY9 contained the conserved WRKY domain (Fig. S7b).

AaWRKY9 is a glandular trichome-specific TF in *A. annua* To investigate the expression pattern of *AaWRKY9*, the expression levels of *AaWRKY9* in different tissues and leaves at different developmental stages were analysed by qRT-PCR. *AaWRKY9* was highly expressed in two types of trichomes and expressed at low levels in stems and roots (Fig. 3a). *AaWRKY9* expression was high in the youngest leaf (leaf 0) and then rapidly decreased with leaf ageing (Fig. 3b), which was similar to the expression pattern observed for the four artemisinin biosynthetic genes.

To further analyse the expression pattern of *AaWRKY9* in *A. annua*, the promoter of *AaWRKY9* was cloned and inserted into pCAMBIA1391Z carrying a GUS reporter gene. Transgenic plants expressing pCAMBIA1391Z — *proAaWRKY9* — GUS were generated. Histochemical GUS staining was only active in glandular trichomes of young leaves (Fig. 3c). GUS activity was not observed in the old leaves from the transgenic plants, nor in the young leaves of wild-type *A. annua*.

To determine the subcellular localisation of AaWRKY9 protein, the yellow fluorescent protein (YFP) was fused to the N-terminal domain of the AaWRKY9 under control of the CaMV35S promoter. The YFP — AaWRKY9 fusion protein was exclusively localised in nuclei (Fig. 3d), implying that AaWRKY9 regulates transcription as a TF in nuclei. These results indicated that AaWRKY9 is a glandular trichome-specific TF in *A. annua*.

The expression of *AaWRKY9* responds to both light and JA signals AaWRKY9 was identified from the RNA-seq data of blue-light-and red-light-treated plants, so we further confirmed the expression pattern of *AaWRKY9* in the dark and in response to blue-light and red-light treatments by qRT-PCR. These results showed that the expression level of *AaWRKY9* was observably reduced after the dark treatment (Fig. 3e) and significantly increased after the blue-light and red-light treatments [40 μmol/($m^2$ · s) PPFD] of plants pretreated with dark conditions for 24 h (Fig. 3f, g), which have similar expression patterns as those of the artemisinin biosynthetic genes (Fig. S3d, h); these expression patterns are similar to those of the artemisinin biosynthetic genes (Fig. S3d, h), suggesting that the expression of *AaWRKY9* is induced by light.

Previous research has indicated that artemisinin production is enhanced by treatment with the phytohormone MeJA (Maes *et al.*, 2011). We performed qRT-PCR analysis to check the expression of *AaWRKY9* after MeJA treatment. The results indicated that the transcript level of *AaWRKY9* was significantly induced by MeJA (Fig. 3 h). The expression of *AaWRKY9* increased by 1.5 h after MeJA treatment, peaked at 3 h and then decreased (Fig. 3h). Taken together, our results revealed that the expression of *AaWRKY9* increased in response to both light and JA signals.

Overexpressing *AaWRKY9* increases artemisinin content and knock-down of *AaWRKY9* reduces artemisinin accumulation in *A. annua* To explore the function of *AaWRKY9*, *35S*::*AaWRKY9* transgenic *A. annua* lines were generated. Three independent lines (OE-*AaWRKY9*-2, OE-*AaWRKY9*-20 and OE-*AaWRKY9*-28) were chosen for further analysis. The transcript levels of *AaWRKY9* were markedly increased by 2.4 - 3.5-fold compared with that of wild-type (Fig. 4a). The expression levels of *AaADS*, *AaCYP71AV1*, *AaDBR2* and *AaALDH1* were also significant higher in the *AaWRKY9* overexpression lines (Fig. 4b). HPLC analysis indicated that *AaWRKY9* overexpression transgenic lines produced 1.6 - 2.2-fold more artemisinin compared with the control (Fig. 4c). In addition, both the DHAA and AA contents were significantly increased in overexpressed transgenic lines (Fig. 4c). In addition, when we analysed the expression of *AaORA* and *AaGSW1*, which encodes TFs regulating artemisinin biosynthesis, in the overexpression lines, we found that *AaGSW1* expression was markedly upregulated (Fig. 4b).

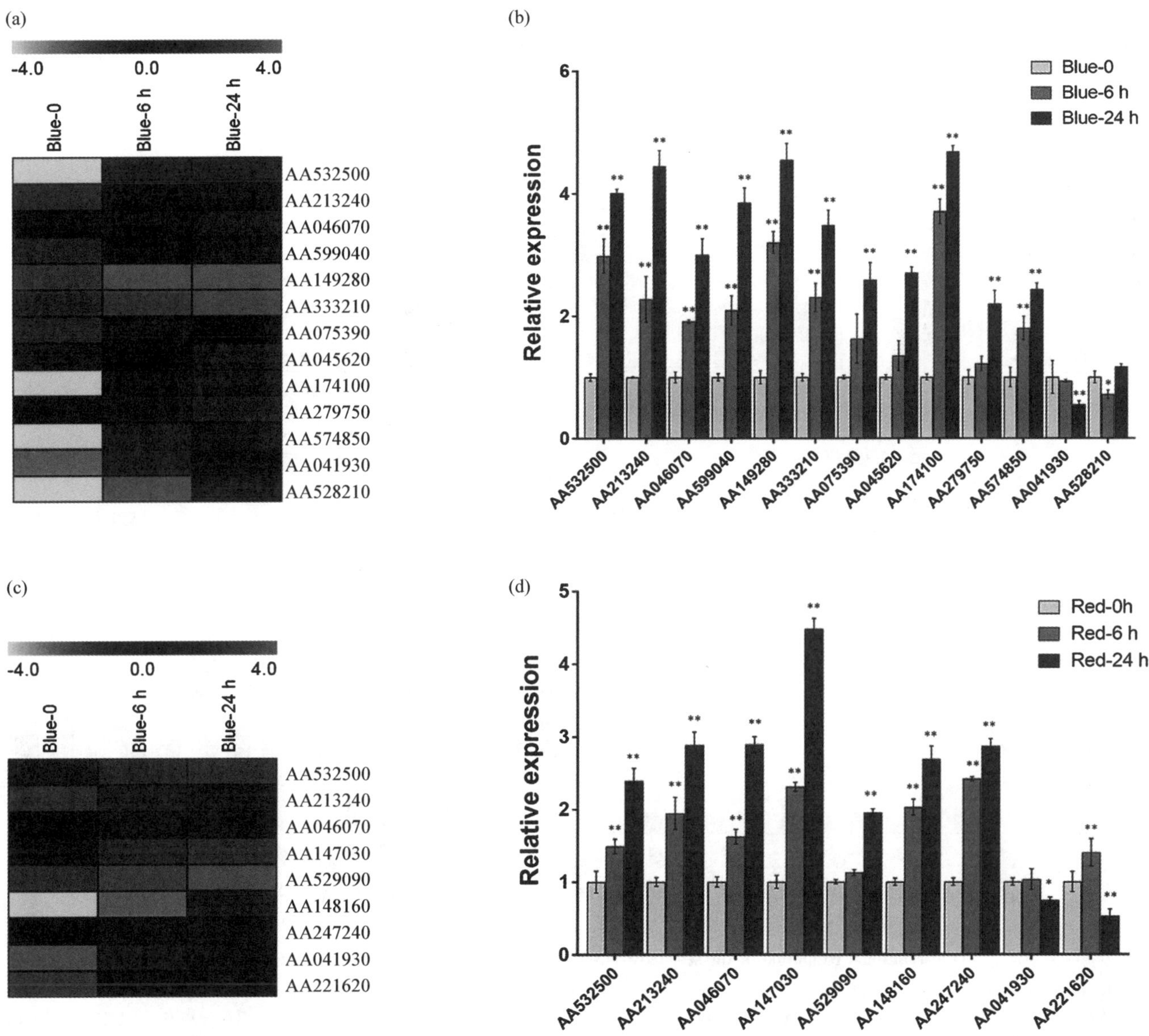


**Fig. 1 Heatmaps of the expression levels of candidate genes determined by RNA-sequencing and qRT-PCR analysis**

(a, c) Heatmap showing the expression levels of selected transcription factor genes from (a) the blue-light RNA-seq data and (c) the red-light RNA-seq data. Colour saturation represents the value of $\log_2$ RPKM (reads per kilobase per million) for the selected genes. (b, d) qRT-PCR analysis of the selected transcription factor genes from (b) the blue-light RNA-seq data and (d) the red-light RNA-seq data. *ACTIN* was used as an internal control. The expression level of genes at 6 and 24 h are comparisons relative to the expression level of genes at 0 h. Data represent the means±SD from three technical replicates. Asterisks denote a significant difference of light treatments relative to the 0 h control as determined by Student's *t*-test: **, $P<0.01$; *, $P<0.05$.

To further identify the function of AaWRKY9 in regulating artemisinin production, we downregulated *AaWRKY9* expression in *A. annua* using the antisense vector pCYP71AV1 - anti*AaWRKY9* under the control of the glandular trichomespecific promoter *AaCYP71AV1*. We selected three independent lines (anti*AaWRKY9*-8, anti*AaWRKY9*-15 and anti*AaWRKY9*-29) for further analysis. Compared with wild-type, the expression of *AaWRKY9* in antisense lines was significantly lower (Fig. 4d). qRT-PCR analysis showed that suppressing the expression of *AaWRKY9* resulted in a decrease in the transcript levels of *AaADS*, *AaCYP71AV1*, *AaDBR2* and *AaALDH1* (Fig. 4e). Consistent with the downregulation of artemisinin biosynthetic genes, the contents of artemisinin, DHAA and AA in the *AaWRKY9* antisense lines were decreased by 35%～45%, 21%～30% and 40%～63%, respectively (Fig. 4f). Moreover, the transcript level of *AaGSW1* was downregulated in *AaWRKY9* antisense lines, compared with wild-type plants (Fig. 4e). We also analysed the density of glandular trichomes in the transgenic plants. The results showed that there was no significant difference in glandular trichomes between the transgenic plants and wild-type plants (Figs S8, S9). These results indicated that

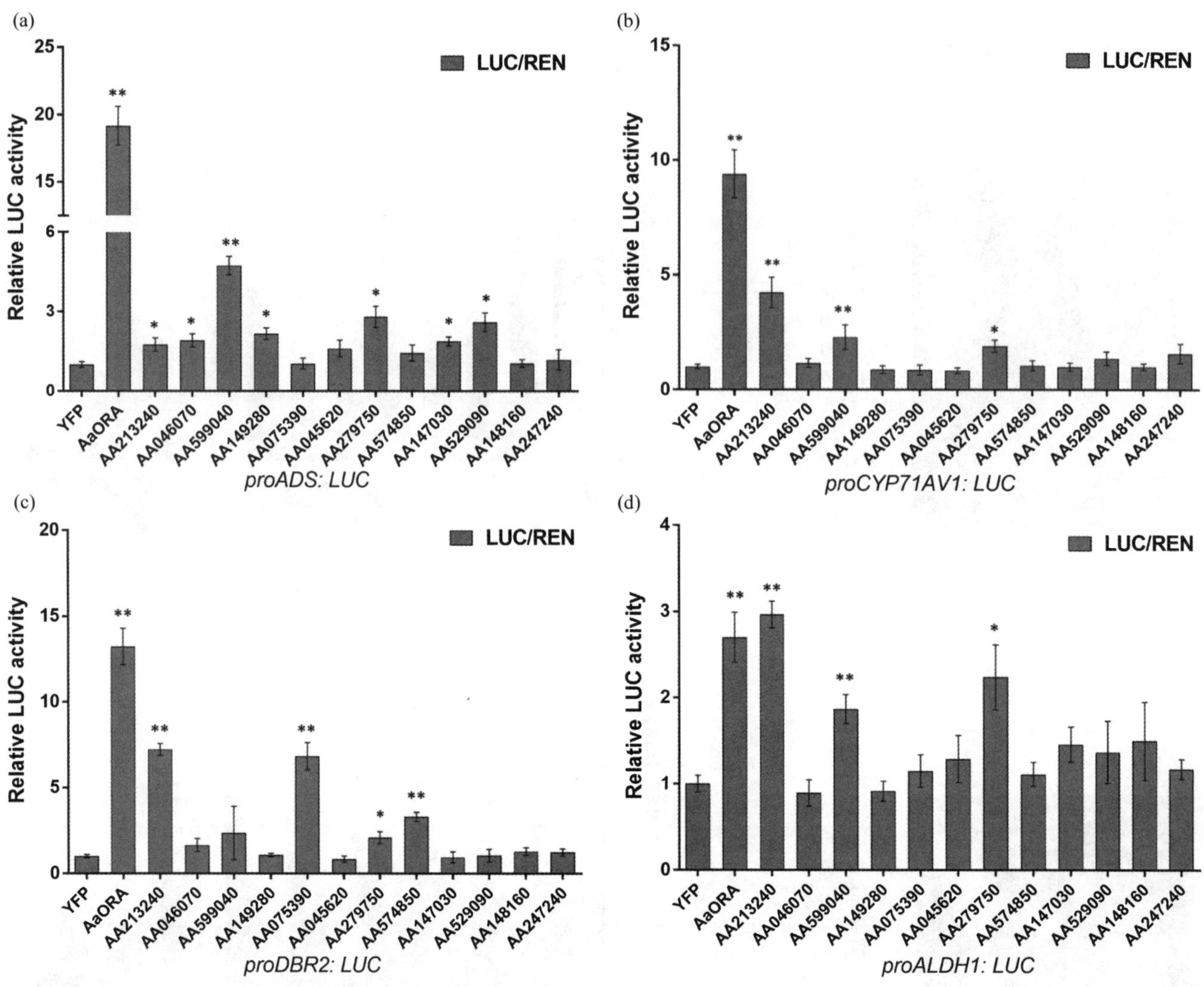


**Fig. 2 Transcriptional regulation of the selected transcription factors (TFs) involved in artemisinin biosynthesis**

Dual-LUC assay showing the effects of the selected transcription factors on the promoter activation of (a) *AaADS*, (b) *AaCYP71AV1*, (c) *AaDBR2* and (d) *AaALDH1*. The empty vector pHB—YFP was used as the control. The relative LUC activity of the selected TFs are comparisons relative to the LUC/REN ratio of pHB—YFP. Data represent the means±SD from three biological replicates. Asterisks denote a significant difference of the selected TFs relative to pHB—YFP as determined by Student's *t*-test: **, $P<0.01$; *, $P<0.05$.

AaWRKY9 is a positive TF controlling artemisinin biosynthesis.

AaWRKY9 activates the transcription of *AaDBR2* and *AaGSW1* by binding to their promoters Using dual-LUC assays, we found that AaWRKY9 could observably activate the promoters of *AaCYP71AV1*, *AaDBR2* and *AaALDH1* (Fig. 2). Previous experiments demonstrated that WRKY proteins could specifically bind to the W-box (T) TGAC(C/T) in the promoters of genes. Prediction of W-boxes in the promoters of *AaCYP71AV1*, *AaDBR2* and *AaALDH1* revealed three W-box fragments (W1, W2 and W3; 1 146, 616 and 235 bp upstream of ATG, respectively) in the promoter of *AaCYP71AV1* (Fig. S10a), seven W-box fragments (W1, W2, W3, W4, W5, W6 and W7; 1 411, 976, 490, 479, 176, 117 and 20 bp upstream of ATG, respectively) in the promoter of *AaDBR2* (Fig. 5a) and one W-box fragment (W1; 872 bp upstream of ATG) in the promoter of *AaALDH1* (Fig. S10b). To better understand the mechanisms of AaWRKY9 regulation of the artemisinin accumulation, Y1H assay was carried out. The results indicated that AaWRKY9 only bound to one of the W-box fragments (W5) in the promoter of *AaDBR2* (Fig. 5b). To further confirm this result, EMSA was performed using the His-AaWRKY9 protein. This assay demonstrated that His-AaWRKY9 could bind to the W-box (W5) in the promoter of *AaDBR2* (Fig. 5c). When the His-AaWRKY9 protein was replaced by His-TF expressed using the pCold empty vector, we could not detect the signal (Fig. 5c). In addition, the band intensity was significantly lower when the mutation was introduced into the W-box (W5) in the *AaDBR2* promoter (Fig. 5c).

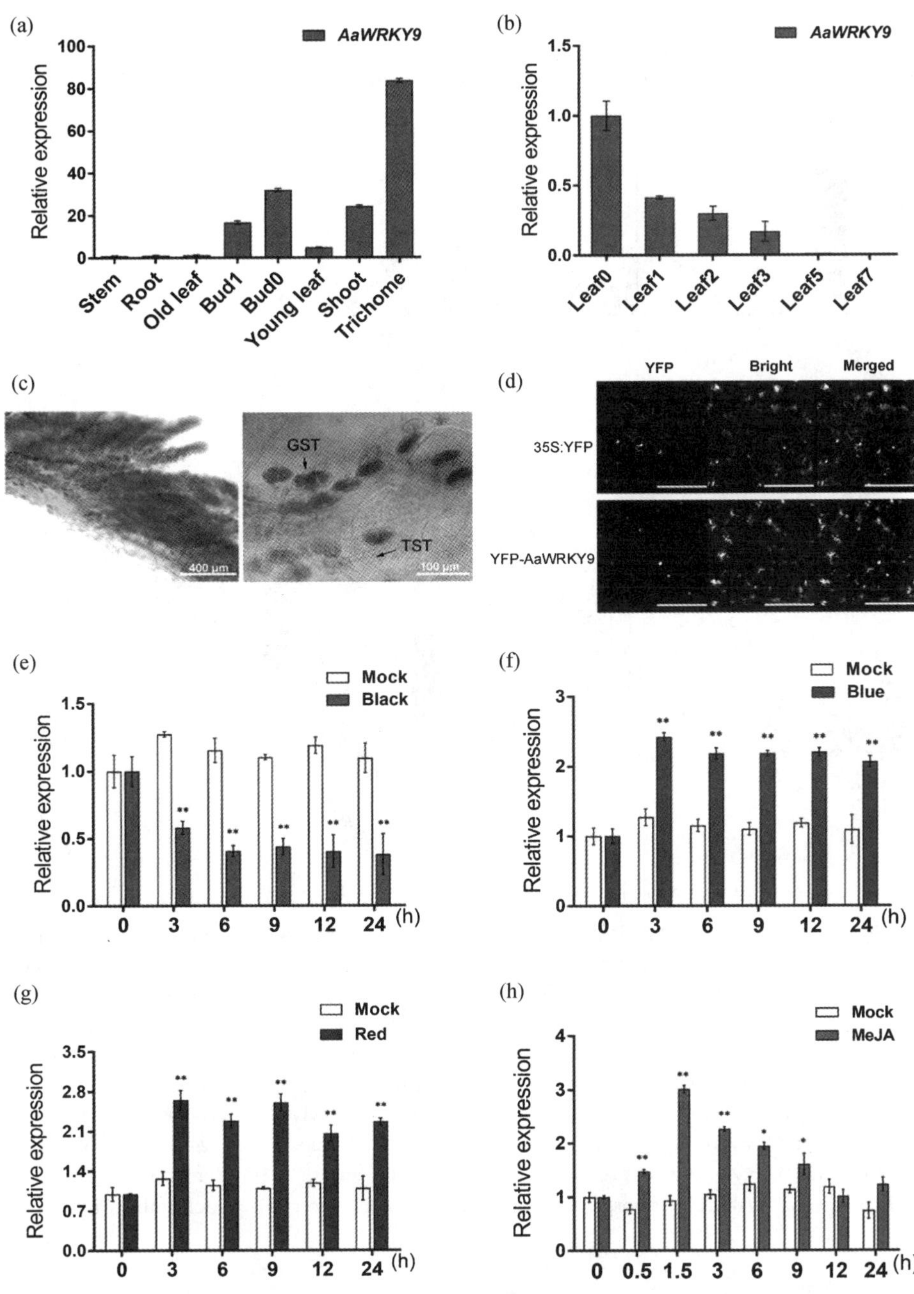


**Fig. 3 Expression pattern and subcellular localisation of AaWRKY9**

(a) Expression levels of *AaWRKY9* in stem, root, old leaf, bud1, bud0, young leaf, shoot and trichome of *Artemisia annua*. Bud0 and bud1 were gathered 5 and 12 d after budding. Expression levels of *AaWRKY9* in root, old leaf, bud1, bud0, young leaf, shoot and trichome are comparisons relative to the expression level in stem. (b) Expression levels of *AaWRKY9* in different developmental ages of *A. annua*. Leaf0 (meristem), Leaf1 (first leaf below meristem), Leaf2, Leaf3, Leaf5 and Leaf7 were collected from the main stem of 5-month-old *A. annua* plants. Expression levels of *AaWRKY9* in Leaf1, Leaf2, Leaf3, Leaf5 and Leaf7 are comparisons relative to the expression level in leaf0. *ACTIN* was used as an internal control. Data represent the means ± SD from three biological replicates. (c) GUS staining of *proAaWRKY9-GUS* transgenic *A. annua*. GST, glandular trichome; TST, T-shaped trichome. (d) Subcellular localistation of AaWRKY9. YFP signal was used as the control. Bars, 20 μm. (e) Relative expression of *AaWRKY9* in the dark. (f, g) Expression levels of *AaWRKY9* in the leaves of *A. annua* exposed to (f) blue light with 40 μmol/($m^2$ · s) PPFD and (g) red light with 40 μmol/($m^2$ · s) PPFD after pretreatment in darkness for 24 h. White light was used as a mock treatment. (h) Expression level of *AaWRKY9* in the leaf of *A. annua* treated with 100 μmol/L methyl jasmonate (MeJA); 0.1% ethanol was used as a mock treatment. Relative expression levels of *AaWRKY9* at different treatment times are comparisons relative to the expression level at 0 h. *ACTIN* was used as an internal control. Data represent the means ± SD from three biological replicates. Asterisks denote a significant difference of MeJA treatments relative to the 0 h control as determined by Student's *t*-test: **, $P < 0.01$; *, $P < 0.05$.

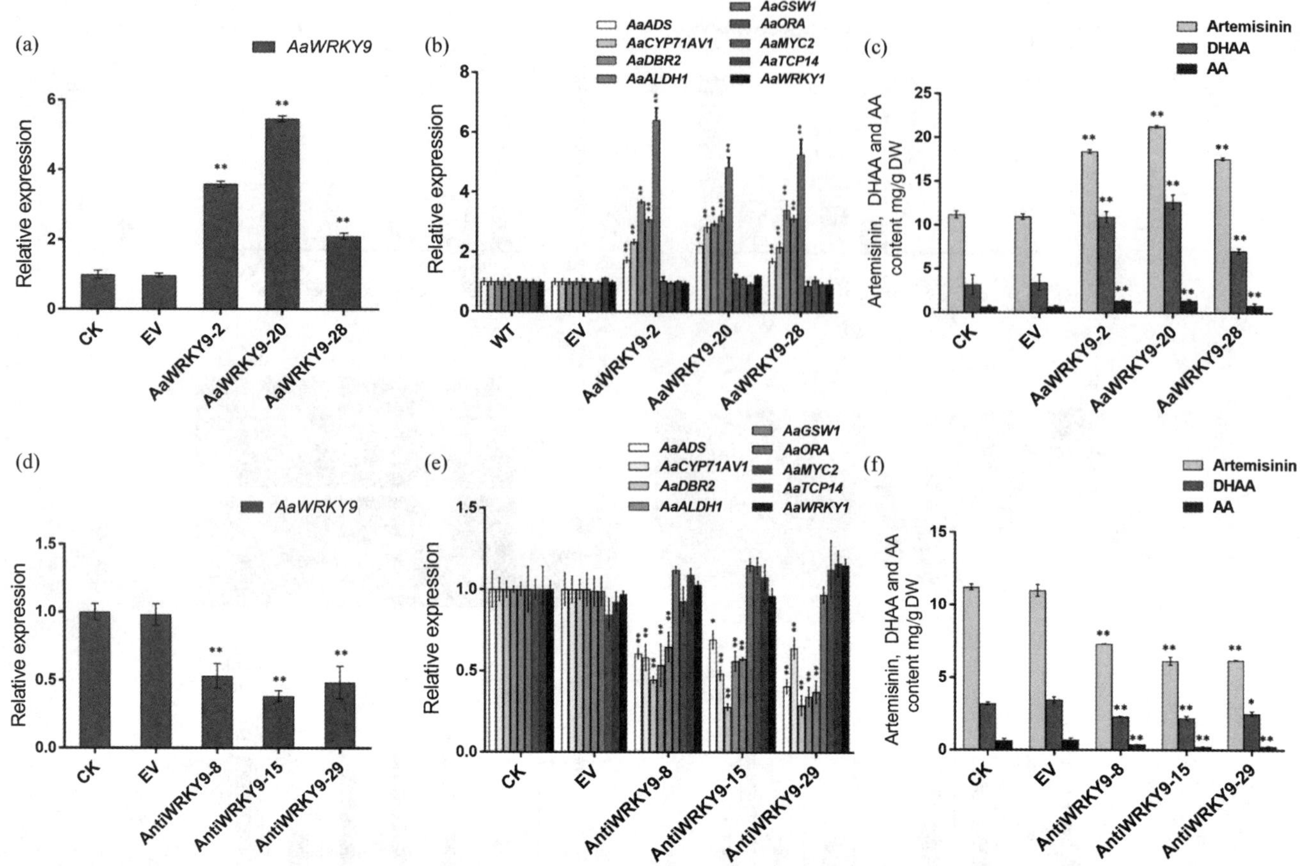


**Fig. 4 AaWRKY9 positively regulates artemisinin biosynthesis in *Artemisia annua***

(a, d) Expression levels of *AaWRKY9* in *AaWRKY9* overexpression (a), *AaWRKY9* antisense (d), and empty vector (EV) transgenic *A. annua* plants and wild-type *A. annua* plants (CK). Expression levels of *AaWRKY9* in transgenic *A. annua* plants are comparisons relative to the expression level of *AaWRKY9* in wild-type plant. (b, e) Expression levels of *AaADS*, *AaCYP71AV1*, *AaDBR2*, *AaALDH1*, *AaGSW1* and *AaORA* in *AaWRKY9* overexpression (b), *AaWRKY9* antisense (e), empty vector (EV) transgenic *A. annua* and wild-type *A. annua* plants. Expression levels of these genes in transgenic *A. annua* plants are comparisons relative to the expression level of these genes in wild-type plant. *ACTIN* was used as an internal control. (c, f) The contents of artemisinin, dihydroartemisinic acid (DHAA) and artemisinic acid (AA) in the leaves of *AaWRKY9* overexpression (c), *AaWRKY9* antisense (f), and empty vector (EV) transgenic *A. annua* plants and wild-type *A. annua* plants. All contents are comparisons relative to the contents of wild-type *A. annua* plants. Data represent the means ± SD from three biological replicates. Asterisks denote a significant difference of *AaWRKY9* transgenic lines relative to wild-type plant as determined by Student's *t*-test: **, $P < 0.01$; *, $P < 0.05$.

We found that overexpressing *AaWRKY9* increased the expression level of *AaGSW1*, while downregulating the expression of *AaWRKY9* resulted in a decrease of the transcript level of *AaGSW1* (Fig. 4b, e). To further demonstrate if AaWRKY9 could bind to the promoter of *AaGSW1*, the promoter sequence of *AaGSW1* was analysed and four W-box fragments (W1, W2, W3 and W4; 1 373, 1 327, 1181 and 325 bp upstream of ATG, respectively) were identified (Fig. 5d). A Y1H assay indicated that AaWRKY9 only bound to the W-box (W4) in the promoter of *AaGSW1* (Fig. 5e) and EMSA confirmed that His-AaWRKY9 directly bound to this W-box (Fig. 5f). In conclusion, our data suggested that the AaWRKY9 protein positively regulates artemisinin biosynthesis by directly binding to the W-boxes in the promoters of *DBR2* and *AaGSW1* and activating their expression.

AaHY5 enhances the transcription of *AaWRKY9* by directly binding to its promoter HY5 plays an important role in mediating light control of gene expression. In Arabidopsis, HY5 interacts with the ubiquitin E3 ligase CONSTITUTIVE PHOTOMORPHOGENIC1 (COP1), and is degraded by COP1 via the 26S proteasome pathway in the dark. However, under light conditions a decrease in the level of COP1 protein in the nucleus allows for accumulation of HY5. Similarly, AaHY5 interacts with AaCOP1 and is also degraded by AaCOP1 in darkness in *A. annua*. It was reported that AaHY5 positively regulates artemisinin biosynthesis by activating the expression of *AaGSW1*. That *AaWRKY9* was identified in the blue-light and red-light treatment RNA-seq data, and our finding that its expression

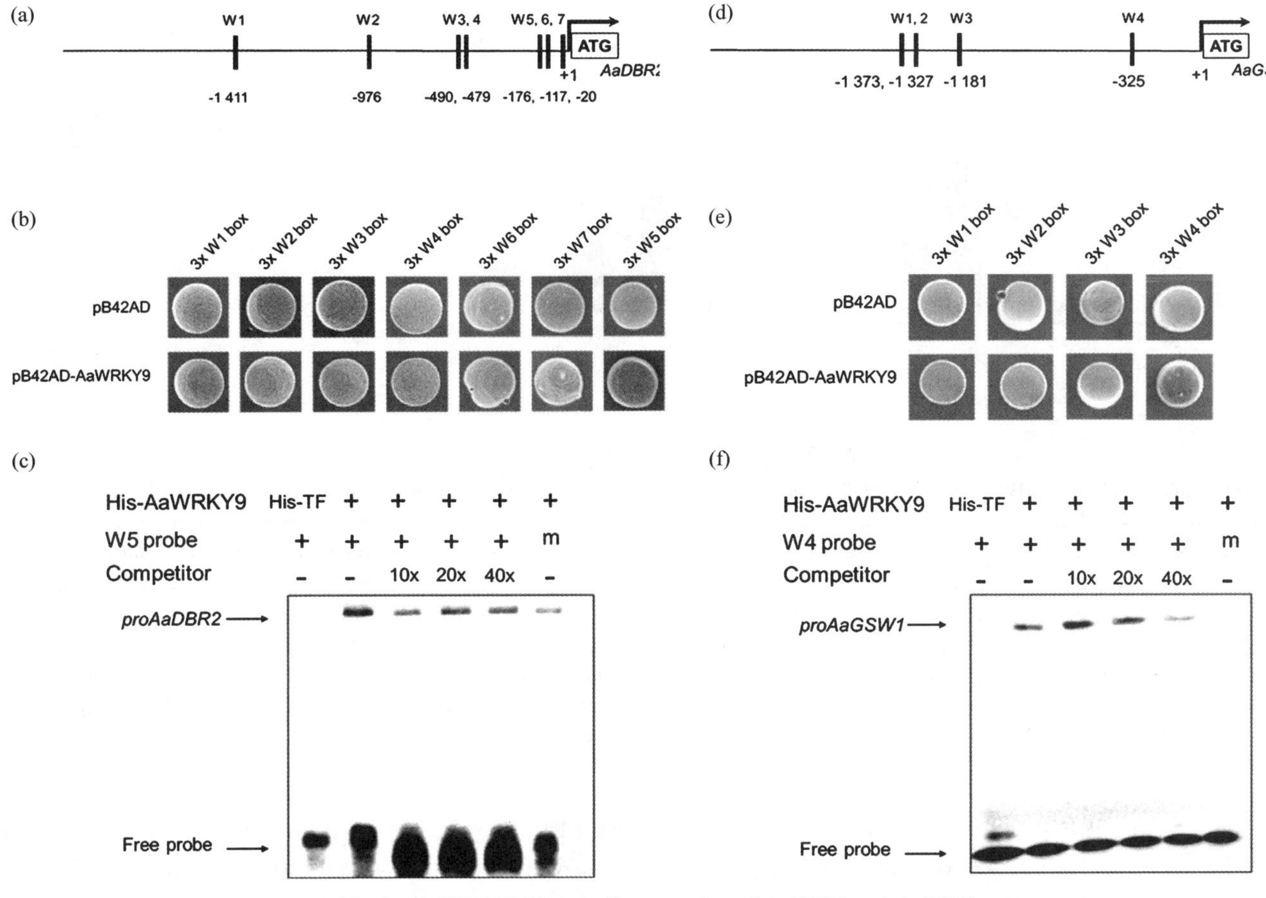


**Fig. 5 AaWRKY9 binds to the promoters of *AaDBR2* and *AaGSW1***

(a and d) Schematic diagrams of the *AaDBR2* and *AaGSW1* promoters. The black lines represent the positions of the potential W-box (W1 - 7) in the *AaDBR2* promoter (a) and the potential W-box (W1 - 4) in the *AaGSW1* promoter (d). The numbers indicate the distance from the translational start site (ATG). (b, e) AaWRKY9 binds to W-boxes in the promoters of *AaDBR2* and *AaGSW1*. EGY48A yeast expressing pB42AD or pB42AD-*AaWKY9* and W-box fragments were grown on SD/—Ura/—Trp medium (20 mg/L X-gal). The blue plaques show protein—DNA interactions. (c, f) EMSA showing AaWRKY9 binds to W-boxes in the promoters of *AaDBR2* and *AaGSW1*. The His—AaWRKY9 fusion protein and the labelled probe were used. Unlabelled probe was used as a cold competitor. 10×, 20× and 40× represent 10-fold, 20-fold and 40-fold molar excess of unlabelled probe, respectively. His-TF protein was included as a negative control. m, mutated probe.

was induced by light after the pretreatment in the dark for 24 h (Fig. 3), indicate that AaWRKY9 mediates light signals to positively regulate artemisinin biosynthesis. We determined the transcript levels of *AaWRKY9* in *AaHY5* overexpression and RNAi transgenic lines. The results showed that the expression of *AaWRKY9* was observably increased in *AaHY5* overexpression lines and significantly decreased in *AaHY5* RNAi lines (Fig. 6a). We found there were two G-box motifs in the promoter of *AaWRKY9*. To determine whether AaHY5 controls the expression of *AaWRKY9*, dual-LUC and Y1H assays were performed. The dual-LUC assay demonstrated that AaHY5 activated the promoter of *AaWRKY9* (Fig. 6b). The EMSA assay indicated that AaHY5 directly bound to the G-box (CACGTT) in the promoter of *AaWRKY9 in vitro* (Fig. 6c). Therefore, our data indicated that AaHY5 binds to the promoter of *AaWRKY9* and activates its transcription.

### The repressor protein AaJAZ9 interacts with AaWRKY9

A previous study showed that JA promotes artemisinin production by activating artemisinin biosynthetic genes. Here, we observed that *AaWRKY9* was induced by MeJA (Fig. 3h). To further explore the function of AaWRKY9 in artemisinin biosynthesis, we performed a Y2H screen using an *A. annua* cDNA library to identify AaWRKY9 interacting partners. The jasmonate ZIM-domain (JAZ) protein AaJAZ9 was identified as an interacting protein and the AaJAZ9—AaWRKY9 interaction was further confirmed by a Y2H assay (Fig. 7a). BiFC and CoIP assays were used to detect the interaction between AaWRKY9 and AaJAZ9 *in vivo*. When AaJAZ9-nYFP and cYFP-AaWRKY9 were co-expressed in the leaves of *N. benthamiana*, YFP fluorescence was detected in the nucleus (Fig. 7b). No signal was observed when AaJAZ9—nYFP and cYFP or nYFP and cYFP—AaWRKY9 were transiently co-expressed (Fig. 7b).

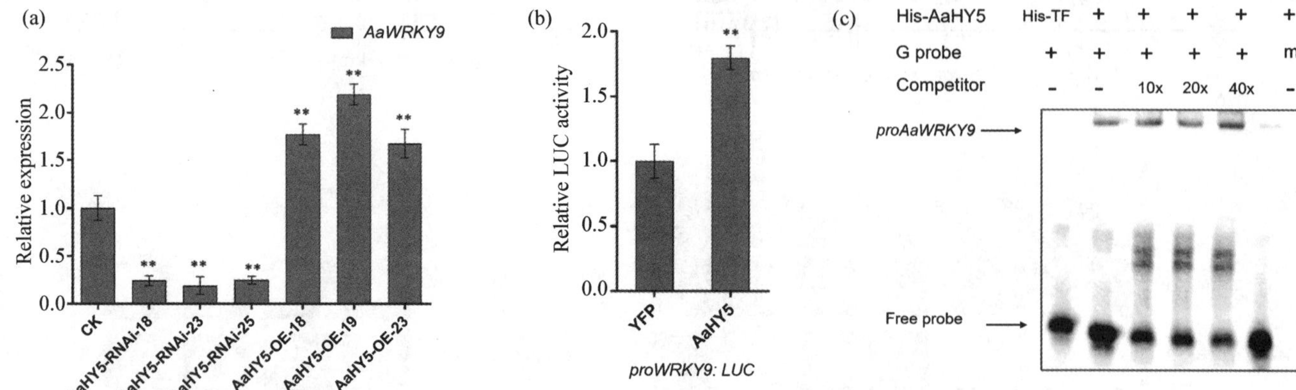


**Fig. 6 AaHY5 is a transcriptional activator of *AaWRKY9***

(a) Expression levels of *AaWRKY9* in *AaHY5* overexpression and, *AaHY5* RNAi transgenic *Artemisia annua* and wild-type *A. annua* plants (CK). Expression levels of *AaWRKY9* are comparisons relative to the expression level in wild-type plant. Values represent the means ± SD from three biological replicates. Asterisks denote a significant difference of *AaWRKY9* transgenic lines relative to wildtype plant as determined by Student's *t*-test: **, $P<0.01$; *, $P<0.05$. (b) Dual-LUC assay showing that AaHY5 activates the expression of *AaWRKY9*. The empty vector pHB—YFP was used as the control. The relative LUC activity of AaHY5 are comparisons relative to that of pHB—YFP. Asterisks denote a significant difference of AaHY5 relative to pHB—YFP as determined by Student's *t*-test: **, $P<0.01$; *, $P<0.05$. (c) EMSA showing AaHY5 binds to G-boxes in the promoters of *AaWRKY9*. The His—AaHY5 fusion protein and the labelled probe were used. Unlabelled probe was used as a cold competitor. 10×, 20× and 40× represent 10-fold, 20-fold and 40-fold molar excess of unlabelled probe, respectively. His-TF protein was included as a negative control.

Consistently with this, a CoIP assay indicated that AaWRKY9 interacted with AaJAZ9 *in vivo* (Fig. 7c). Moreover, a pull-down assay further proved that AaWRKY9 interacted with AaJAZ9 (Fig. 7d). Taken together, these results demonstrated that AaWRKY9 interacted with the repressor protein AaJAZ9.

AaJAZ9 represses the transcriptional activation function of AaWRKY9 JAZs are negative regulators of JA-mediated plant responses. In *A. annua*, AaJAZ proteins (AaJAZ1-6, AaJAZ8 and AaJAZ9) were shown to interact with AaMYC2. AaJAZ8 negatively regulates artemisinin biosynthesis by repressing the activity of the AaTCP14—AaORA complex and also interacts with AaHD1 to control the development of the glandular trichomes. qRT-PCR analysis indicated that the expression of *AaJAZ9* was highest in trichomes and lowest in shoots (Fig. S11a). In leaves, expression was lowest in the youngest leaf (leaf 0) and slowly increased as the leaves aged (Fig. S11b). In *pAaJAZ9-GUS* transgenic plants, GUS staining was observed in the entire leaf and strong staining was also observed in the glandular trichomes (Fig. S11c). In addition, the expression of *AaJAZ9* was induced by MeJA treatment (Fig. S11d).

To investigate whether AaJAZ9 repressed the function of AaWRKY9 in enhancing artemisinin accumulation, dual-LUC assays were performed. When AaJAZ9 was co-expressed with AaWRKY9 in tobacco, AaJAZ9 reduced the activation of the *AaCYP71AV1*, *AaDBR2*, *AaALDH1* and *AaGSW1* promoters by AaWRKY9 (Fig. 8). We also used dual-LUC assays to test the transcriptional activation activity of AaWRKY9 in the presence and absence of MeJA. The promoters of *AaCYP71AV1*, *AaDBR2*, *AaALDH1* and *AaGSW1* were observably activated by AaWRKY9 in the presence of MeJA (Fig. 8). The results also suggested that AaJAZ9 repressed the transcriptional activation function of AaWRKY9 in the absence of MeJA. The transcriptional activation activity of AaWRKY9 was significantly enhanced, when AaJAZ9 was degraded by the MeJA treatment. To analyse the role for AaWRKY9 in the interaction of light and JA signalling, the cutting propagations of *AaWRKY9* overexpression, antisense, the empty vector transgenic plants and wild-type *A. annua* plants were cultivated in continuous white light for 2 wk. Then half of these plants were transferred to the dark conditions for 24 h. After the independent pretreatment, the cutting seedlings were sprayed with 100 μmol/L MeJA and 0.1% ethanol (as mock) under the light and dark conditions, respectively. The leaves were sampled at 24 and 48 h for artemisinin analysis. The results showed that the *AaWRKY9*-2 overexpression cutting seedlings accumulated more artemisinin after JA-induced compared with the mock treatment in light (Fig. 9a); by contrast, the artemisinin content in *antiWRKY9*-15 antisense cutting seedlings after JA-induced showed no obvious change (Fig. 9b). In darkness, we found that artemisinin contents in transformants with empty vector and wild-type *A. annua* plants were not obviously increased after spraying with MeJA at 24 and 48 h (Fig. 9c, d). The artemisinin content was also

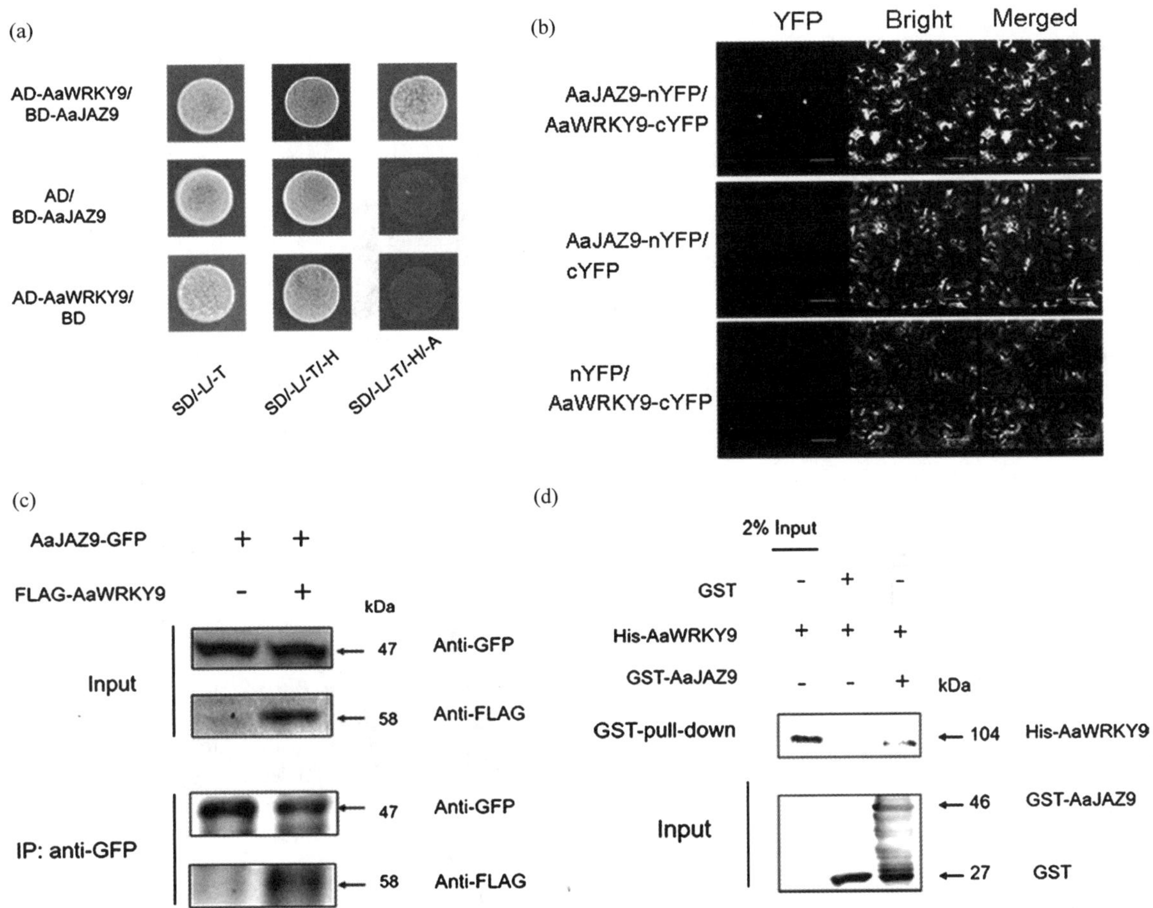


**Fig. 7 AaWRKY9 interacts with AaJAZ9 *invitro* and *invivo***

(a) Yeast two-hybrid (Y2H) analysis of AaWRKY9 interaction with AaJAZ9. Transformed yeast cells were grown on control medium (SD/—Trp/—Leu), and selective media (SD/—Trp/—Leu/—His and SD/—Trp/—Leu/—His/—Ade). Pictures were taken after 4 d of incubation at 30℃. Y2H assays were repeated three times, and representative results are shown. (b) Bimolecular fluorescence complementation (BiFC) analysis of the interaction between AaWRKY9 and AaJAZ9 in *Nicotiana benthamiana* cells. The N-terminal fragment of YFP was fused to the N-terminus of AaWRKY9 (nYFP-AaWRKY9), and AaJAZ9 was fused to the C-terminal fragment of YFP (AaJAZ9-cYFP). Three independent transfection experiments were performed. Bars, 20 μm. (c) Co-immunoprecipitation studies of AaWRKY9 and AaJAZ9 complex formation in *N. benthamiana* leaves. Total protein extracts from *N. benthamiana* leaves infiltrated with constructs harbouring FLAG-AaWRKY9 andAaJAZ9-YFP were immunoprecipitated with anti-GFP antibody. The co-immunoprecipitated proteins were detected by anti-FLAG antibody. Experiments were repeated three times and similar results were obtained. (d) *Invitro* pull-down assays of AaWRKY9 and AaJAZ9 recombinant proteins. His-AaWRKY9 proteins were pulled down with GST-AaJAZ9, and detected on western blots probed with anti-His antibody. Experiments were carried out three times and representative results are shown.

not obviously promoted in both *AaWRKY9-2* overexpression and *antiWRKY9*-15 antisense cutting seedlings at 24 and 48 h in the absence of MeJA compared with the mock treatment (Fig. 9c, d).

## 4 DISCUSSION

Artemisinin, a sesquiterpene lactone with an endoperoxide bridge that was isolated from the traditional herbal medicinal plant *A. annua*, is an effective drug for malaria, and artemisinin-based combination therapy is worldwide the first-line treatment for falciparum malaria. The phytohormone JA, which plays crucial roles in regulating plant development responses to biotic and abiotic stresses, and secondary metabolism, has also been shown to improve artemisinin content by increasing the expression levels of artemisinin biosynthetic enzyme genes and JA-responsive TF genes. For example, the contents of artemisinin, DHAA, and AA increased 49%, 28% and 80%, respectively, upon MeJA treatment, which increased the density of glandular trichomes and activated the expression of artemisinin biosynthetic genes. Light plays an important role in artemisinin biosynthesis. AaHY5, a light-dependent member of the bZIP transcription factors, was isolated from *A. annua*. The analysis of *AaHY5* transgenic plants and yeast-one-hybrid assays demonstrated that AaHY5 positively regulated artemisinin biosynthesis by binding to the promotor of *AaGSW1*. Furthermore, it was reported that JA increased the artemisinin biosynthesis in a light-dependent manner.

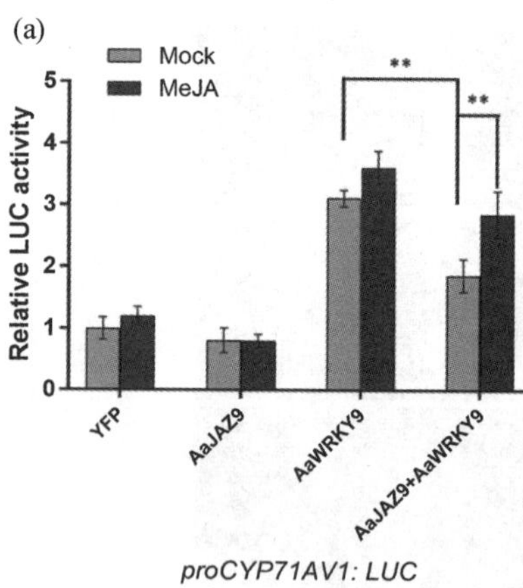


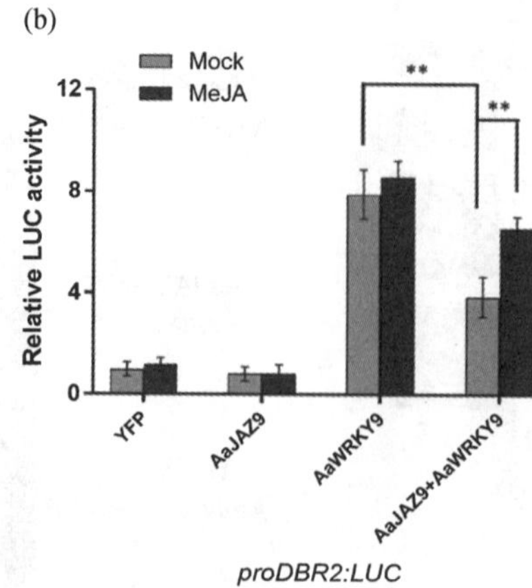


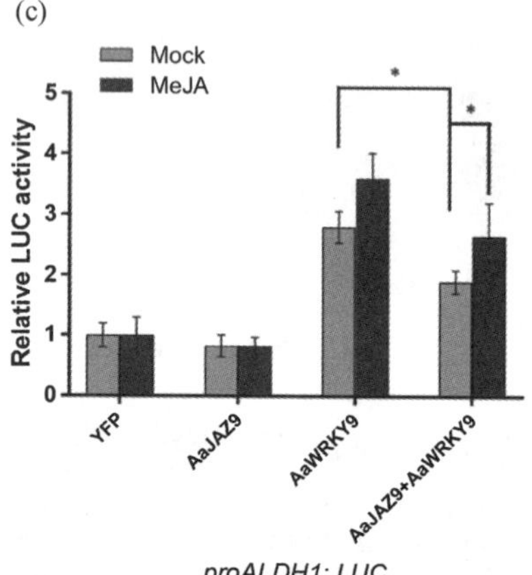


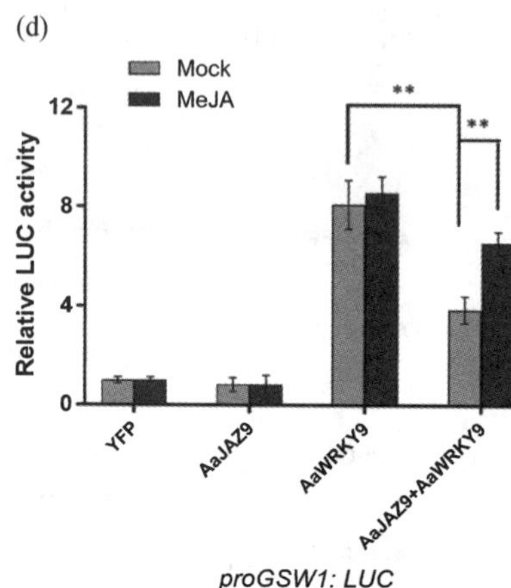


**Fig. 8 AaJAZ9 protein represses the transcriptional activation function of AaWRKY9**

(a–d) Activation of the *AaCYP71AV1* (a), *AaDBR2* (b), *AaALDH1* (c), and *AaGSW1* (d) promoters by the AaJAZ9 and AaWRKY9 proteins in the presence and absence of methyl jasmonate (MeJA) in *Nicotiana benthamiana* leaves. The YFP effector in the mock treatment served as a negative control, and the relative LUC activity of AaJAZ9 and AaWRKY9 proteins are comparisons relative to the YFP controls. The relative LUC activity of AaJAZ9 and AaWRKY9 proteins in the presence of MeJA are comparisons relative to mock treatment. Three independent transfection experiments were performed. Data represent the means ± SD from three biological replicates. Student's *t*-test: **, $P < 0.01$; *, $P < 0.05$.

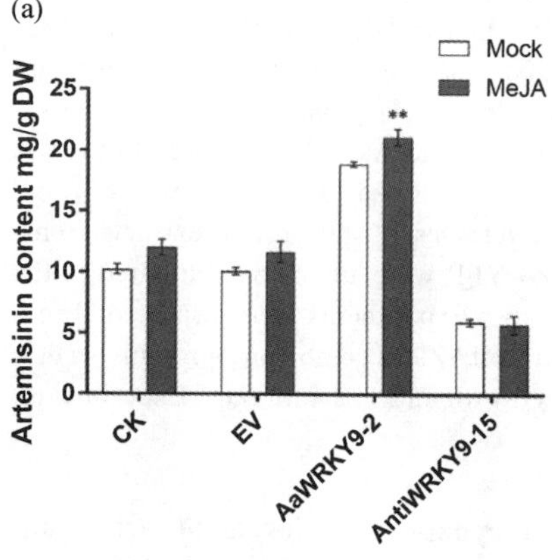


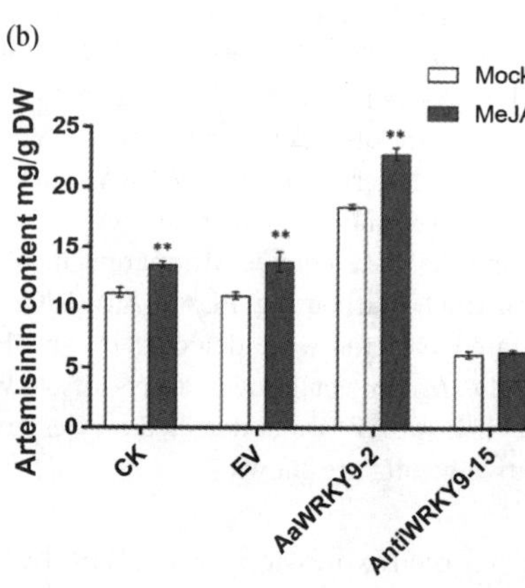


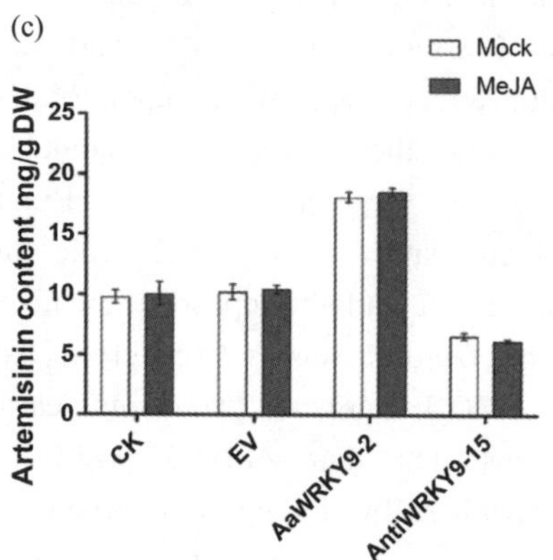


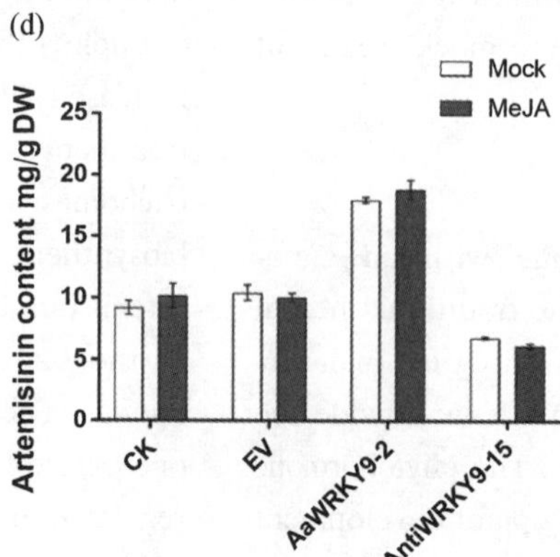


**Fig. 9 Artemisinin content in *AaWRKY9* transgenic plants with methyl jasmonate (MeJA) treatment in light and darkness**

The cutting seedlings of *AaWRKY9* overexpression, antisense, the empty vector transgenic plants, and wild-type *Artemisia annua* plants were sprayed with 100 μmol/L MeJA and 0.1% ethanol (as mock) in light and darkness. The leaves were sampled for artemisinin analysis at (a) 24 h and (b) 48 h in light after MeJA treatment, (c) 24 h, and (d) 48 h in darkness after MeJA treatment. The error bars represent the means ± SD (standard deviation) from three biological replicates. Asterisks denote a significant difference of MeJA treatment relative to the 0 h control as determined by Student's *t*-test: **, $P < 0.01$; *, $P < 0.05$.

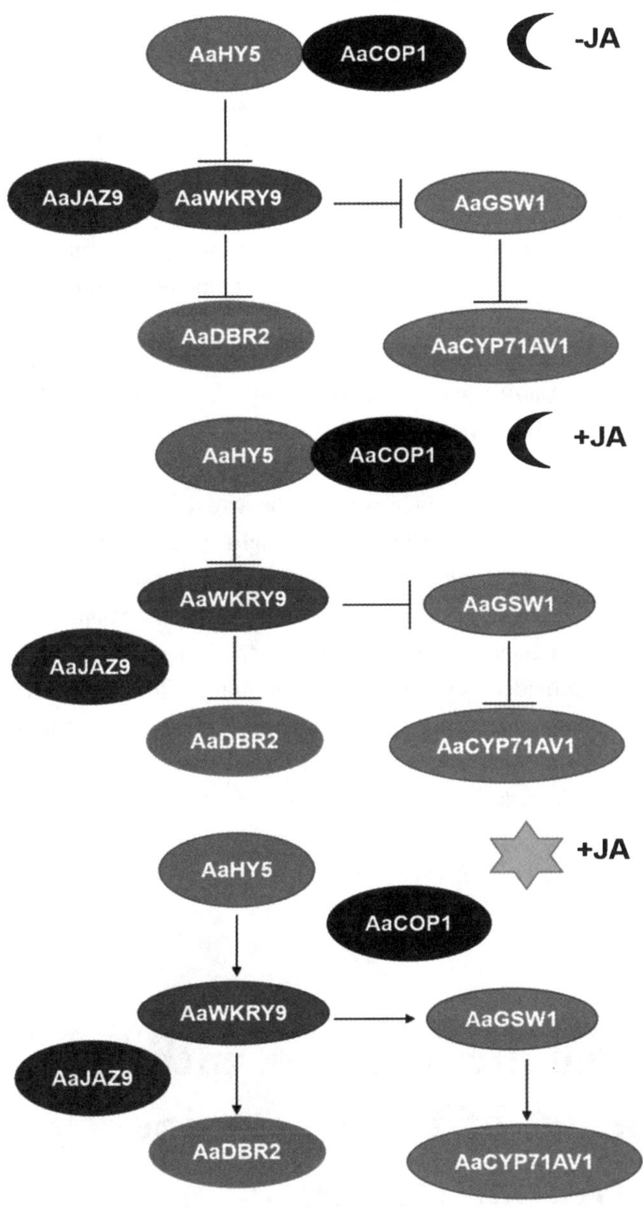


**Fig. 10 A working model showing that AaWRKY9 contributes to light and jasmonate (JA) signalling to regulate the biosynthesis of artemisinin**

(a) AaHY5 is degraded by the ubiquitin E3 ligase AaCOP1 to repress the transcription of *AaWRKY9* in dark, and AaJAZ9 interacts with AaWRKY9 in the absence of JA. (b) In the darkness, AaJAZ9 is degraded in the presence of JA. But the interaction between AaHY5 and AaCOP1 also inhibits the transcription of *AaWRKY9*. (c) AaHY5 increases the transcription of *AaWRKY9* in the light, and AaJAZ9 is degraded by the JA signal, resulting in promotion of artemisinin biosynthesis by AaWRKY9.

The fact that light and JA play important roles in artemisinin biosynthesis and that the increase in artemisinin by JA is light dependent, suggested that these pathways interact. In Arabidopsis, COP1 interacts with MYB75 to reduce the production of anthocyanin, implying there were the interaction of light and JA signals to regulate anthocyanin biosynthesis. Li *et al*. reported that MeJA promoted anthocyanin biosynthesis through increasing the expression levels of DFR, UF3GT and LDOX under far-red light, indicating that MeJA promoted anthocyanin accumulation dependent on the phyA signalling pathway.

In this study, we found that a trichome-specific transcription factor, AaWRKY9, positively regulates artemisinin biosynthesis by directly binding to the promoters of the artemisinin biosynthesis genes *AaDBR2* and *AaGSW1* (Figs 4,5). The contents of artemisinin, DHAA and AA were observably higher in transgenic *A. annua* lines overexpressing *AaWRKY9* compared with the wild-type due to the activation of the expression of *AaADS*, *AaCYPAV1*, *AaDBR2* and *AaALDH1* (Fig. 4a — c). In addition, the contents of artemisinin, DHAA and AA were 35%～45%, 21%～30% and 40%～63% lower, respectively, in *AaWRKY9* antisense lines compared with wild-type (Fig. 4d, f). We found that *AaWRKY9* was induced by MeJA (Fig. 3h) and that AaWRKY9 interacted directly with a JA repressor, AaJAZ9, in Y2H, BiFC, CoIP and pull-down assays (Fig. 7). When AaWRKY9 and AaJAZ9 were co-expressed, AaJAZ9 repressed the transcriptional activation activity of AaWRKY9 (Fig. 8). In the presence of MeJA, the transcriptional activity of AaWRKY9 was observably increased even when it was co-expressed with AaJAZ9 (Fig. 8). In addition, qRT-PCR analysis showed that the expression of *AaWRKY9* was observably reduced in the dark (Fig. 3e). In addition, the transcript level of *AaWRKY9* showed a significant increase with blue-light and red-light treatment after pretreatment under dark conditions for 24 h (Fig. 3f, g). Dual-LUC and EMSA assays indicated that AaHY5 activated the transcription of *AaWRKY9* by binding to the G-box motif of the *AaWRKY9* promoter (Fig. 6). In conclusion, our findings indicated that that AaWRKY9 contributes to light and JA signalling to regulate the biosynthesis of artemisinin in *A. annua* through the following mechanisms:

4.1 In the dark AaHY5 is degraded by the ubiquitin E3 ligase AaCOP1, leading to decreased transcription of *AaWRKY9*, and in the absence of JA the interaction between AaJAZ9 and AaWRKY9 decreases the activation of the *AaDBR2* and *AaGSW1* promoters (Fig. 10a).

4.2 In the presence of JA in the dark AaJAZ9 is degraded, but the interaction between AaHY5 and AaCOP1 also inhibits the transcription of *AaWRKY9* (Fig. 10b).

4.3 In the light AaHY5 increases the transcription of *AaWRKY9* and AaJAZ9 is degraded by the JA signalling pathway, resulting in AaWRKY9 promotion of artemisinin biosynthesis (Fig. 10c).

As mentioned, our results further demonstrate that AaWRKY9 also contributes to light and JA signalling to regulate artemisinin biosynthesis in *A. annua* and provides a novel molecular mechanism for the interaction of light and

JA signals to regulate secondary metabolism in plants.

In *A. annua*, several WRKY TFs have been reported to regulate artemisinin biosynthesis, the first of which was AaWRKY1. Analysis of *AaWRKY1* transgenic plants suggested that AaWRKY1 promoted artemisinin accumulation by activating the expression of *ADS* and *CYP71AV1*. Subsequently, the WRKY family gene *AaGSW1* was cloned from *A. annua*. AaGSW1 clusters with AtWRKY75 from Arabidopsis and positively regulates artemisinin biosynthesis by binding to the *AaCYP71AV1* promoter. Both *AaWRKY1* and *AaGSW1* are induced by MeJA. However, little information is known about the mechanism connecting WRKY TFs with the JA signalling pathway. We suggest that AaWRKY9 and the JA signalling pathway are connected through the repressor AaJAZ9. Together, our findings indicated that WRKY TFs interacted with JAZs to respond to JA signalling.

Several candidate TFs identified from the RNA-seq data could activate artemisinin biosynthesis (Fig. 2). AaORA forms a positive regulator complex with AaTCP14 and promotes artemisinin biosynthesis via the JA signalling pathway. In this study, the transcription of *AaORA* was also induced by light (Fig. 1). Hao *et al*. found that the expression of AaORA was upregulated in *AaHY5*-overexpression lines and significantly decreased in *AaHY5*-RNAi lines. However, they did not find a binding site of AaHY5 in the promoter of *AaORA*, demonstrating that *AaORA* might not be activated by AaHY5. In addition, we found that the candidate gene *AA599040* was also induced by MeJA (Fig. S12). These results indicated that AaORA and AA599040 might integrate light and JA signalling to trigger artemisinin biosynthesis through another regulatory network, indicating that artemisinin biosynthesis is regulated by a complex regulatory network. Based on our findings, we also identified some TFs, such as AaORA and AA599040, induced by both light and JA signals. As we mentioned above, AaORA and AA599040 might have other mechanisms of regulation artemisinin biosynthesis, and the relation between AaORA or AA599040 and COP1 could be explored in further studies. Interestingly, the artemisinin content was higher following bluelight and red-light treatment than after treatment with white light. In agriculture, the strategy of blue-light or red-light combined with MeJA treatment might further enhance artemisinin production. Taken together, our study provided new insights into the interaction of different signalling pathways in the regulation of terpene biosynthesis in plants, and also revealed a novel candidate gene for metabolic engineering and enhancement of artemisinin production.

[付雪晴,唐克轩,等. New Phytologist, 2021, 231: 1858-1874.]

# SmKFB5 protein regulates phenolic acid biosynthesis by controlling the degradation of phenylalanine ammonia-lyase in *Salvia miltiorrhiza*

## 1 INTRODUCTION

*Salvia miltiorrhiza* Bunge is a well-known medicinal plant in the Lamiaceae family that exhibits great efficacy for the clinical treatment of cardiovascular and cerebrovascular diseases in China and, to a lesser degree, in Japan, the USA, and some European countries. With its short life cycle, undemanding growth requirements, significant medicinal value, mature genetic transformation technique, and relatively small genome size, *S. miltiorrhiza* has become a model medicinal plant.

Phenolic acids, including caffeic acid, rosmarinic acid, and salvianolic acid B, are the major group of bioactive constituents and secondary metabolites of *S. miltiorrhiza*, which possess anti-oxidant, anti-cancer, and anti-inflammatory bioactivities, and enhance memory function. Among the phenolic acids, salvianolic acid B is referred to in the Chinese Pharmacopoeia as one of the marker constituents for evaluating the quality of *S. miltiorrhiza*. Phenolic acids are mainly synthesized through phenylpropanoid- and tyrosine-derived branch pathways, and most genes encoding biosynthetic enzymes including phenylalanine ammonia-lyase (PAL), cinnamate-4-hydroxylase (C4H), 4-coumarate-CoA ligase (4CL), tyrosine aminotransferase (TAT), hydroxyphenyl pyruvate reductase (HPPR), rosmarinic acid (RAS), and CYP98A14 have been cloned and characterized. In addition, several of the genes encoding enzymes in the phenolic acid biosynthetic pathways are present as small gene families in *S. miltiorrhiza*. For example, the *PAL* gene family has three members in the *S. miltiorrhiza* genome.

Because of the wide interest in phenolic acids, considerable efforts have focused on understanding the regulatory mechanisms of the different branches of their biosynthetic pathway. It is generally believed that transcription factors regulate the expression of structural genes of the biosynthetic pathway at the transcriptional level, which greatly affects the accumulation of phenolic acids. For example, an array of transcription factors, primarily belonging to the bHLHs, bZIPs, MYBs, WRKYs, and ERFs, act as positive or negative regulators either singly or together and constitute a complex, hierarchically organized network, modulating the transcription of the phenolic acid biosynthetic enzymes. Substantial research has examined the transcriptional regulation of phenolic acid biosynthesis, but little is known about the multifaced regulatory mechanisms controlling phenolic acid biosynthesis beyond the transcriptional level. Protein ubiquitination is one of the most widespread post-translational modifications that regulate protein function in response to developmental and environmental stimuli in prokaryotes and eukaryotes. In recent years, increasing numbers of studies have indicated that protein ubiquitination plays an important role in regulating secondary metabolite biosynthesis.

Protein ubiquitination involves sequential reactions catalyzed by three enzymes, namely ubiquitin-activating enzyme (E1), ubiquitin-conjugating enzyme (E2), and ubiquitin protein ligase enzyme (E3). E3 ligase plays critical roles in recognizing and binding specifically to the substrate in a temporally and spatially regulated manner. In most cases, the target protein conjugating with ubiquitin is recognized and degraded by the 26S proteasome, and the released ubiquitin is recycled. In the E3 ligase family, the SCF (SKP1-CUL1-F-box protein) ubiquitin ligases play fundamental roles in a range of diverse cellular processes. F-box proteins, in addition to the loosely conserved F-box motif that binds to SKP1, usually carry one of a variety of typical protein-protein interaction domains that confer substrate specificity to the SCF complexes. As one of the protein superfamilies, F-box proteins are widely distributed in yeasts, plants, and mammals. The *Arabidopsis thaliana* and *Medicago sativa* genomes contain nearly 700 and 1 000 F-box protein encoding genes, respectively, which are categorized into different subfamilies according to the presence of additional protein—protein interaction domains near the C-terminus. One subfamily of the F-box family, the Kelch motif-containing F-box (KFB) proteins, was initially identified in *Drosophila melanogaster*. To date, 103, 46, 36, and 31 KFBs have been identified in *A. thaliana*, *Oryza sativa*, *Vitis vinifera*, and *S. miltiorrhiza*, respectively. Several KFBs have been characterized and shown to have functions in the circadian clock, photoperiodic flowering, growth, and development. In addition, in recent years KFB proteins have been shown to be involved in the regulation of the phenylpropanoid pathway. The phenylpropanoid pathway is also one of the up-stream pathways of phenolic acid biosynthesis in *S. miltiorrhiza*. However, it remains unclear how SmKFB protein regulates phenolic acid biosynthesis in *S. miltiorrhiza*.

In a previous study, we identified 31 SmKFBs from *S. miltiorrhiza* and predicted that SmKFB5 may be a regu-lator that is involved in phenolic acid biosynthesis. In this study, to gain insights into the molecular basis of the role of SmKFB5 in phenolic acid biosynthesis, we systematically explored the potential protein—protein interactions of the phenolic acid biosynthetic enzymes by yeast two-hybrid (Y2H) assays. Here, we show that SmKFB5 protein physically interacts with and mediates the proteolytic turnover of three SmPAL isozymes, and that disturbing *SmKFB5* expression consequently affects the biosynthesis of phenolic acids.

## 2 MATERIALS AND METHODS

Molecular cloning and bioinformatics analysis of SmKFB5 The full-length ORFs of *SmKFB5*, *SmPAL1*, *SmPAL2*, and *SmPAL3* were amplified by PCR with gene-specific primers (Supplementary Table S1) and then inserted into the Gateway entry vector pGP-B2E. The conserved domain of SmKFB5 was predicated by Conserved Domains database on the NCBI website (https://www.ncbi.nlm.nih.gov/cdd/).

Yeast two-hybrid assays The full-length cDNAs of *S. miltiorrhiza* phenolic acid biosynthetic genes and *SmKFB5* were isolated by PCR using the primers described in Supplementary Table S1. The ORFs of these genes were cloned into pGADT7 and pGBKT7 using the Infusion® cloning method. The Y2H screen and the pairwise verification were performed according to the manufacturer's instructions (Clontech, Beijing, China).

Bimolecular fluorescence complementation assay and subcellular localization To generate the subcellular localization and bimolecular fluorescence complementation (BiFC) construct, we subcloned the full-length *SmPAL1-3* genes and the full-length or truncated *SmKFB5* gene into the 063075-DEST, 063076-DEST, and pGWB506 vectors from their entry vector pGP-B2E to generate $YFP^C$-SmKFB5, $YFP^C$-F^SmKFB5 (in which the F-box domain was removed), $YFP^N$-SmPALs, GFP-SmKFB5, GFP-F ^ SmKFB5, and GFP-SmPALs. *Agrobacterium* strain GV3101 carrying these vectors ($OD_{600}=0.6$) was infiltrated alone or jointly into tobacco (*Nicotiana benthamiana*) leaves according to the experimental purpose. The fluorescence of the expressed fusion protein was detected 3 days after infiltration. Fluorescence images were captured with a Leica TCS SP5 laser scan confocal microscope (Leica, Wetzlar, Germany).

Assay for the transient expression of SmPAL in tobacco leaves and PAL activity The ORFs of *SmPAL* genes were cloned by PCR using the primers described in Supplementary Table S1. The PCR fragments were recombined into pCAMBIA1300-3 × FLAG using the Infusion® cloning method to generate SmPAL1-FLAG, SmPAL2-FLAG, and SmPAL3-FLAG. *Agrobacterium* strain GV3101 carrying the SmPAL expression vector was mixed with an equal volume of an *Agrobacterium* strain ($OD_{600}$ = 0.6) carrying GFP-SmKFB5 or the empty pGWB506 vector and was infiltrated into tobacco leaves. At 3 days after infiltration, the total soluble proteins were extracted with lysis buffer containing 25 mmol/L Tris—HCl (pH 7.5), 150 mmol/L NaCl, 1 mmol/L EDTA, 10% glycerol, 0.2% Nonidet P-40, 10 mmol/L DTT, and 1× protease inhibitor cocktail. The ratio of leaf fresh weight to extraction buffer was 1 g/mL. The concentration of total protein was measured by using a Bradford protein assay kit (TaKaRa, Dalian, China). The proteins were examined by immunoblotting with anti-FLAG monoclonal antibody (Sigma-Aldrich, Burlington, MA, USA). Actin was used as the reference protein and was detected by immunoblotting with anti-plant actin mouse monoclonal antibody (3T3) (Abbkine, Wuhan, China). The PAL enzymatic assays were performed following the protocol described by Song and Wang.

Protein degradation assays in vivo For the protein degradation assay in rice, we isolated rice protoplasts from 7- to 9-day-old seedlings of *O. sativa* cv. Nipponbare. Protoplast preparation and transfection were carried out according to the procedures described previously. After transfection with 8 μg SmPALs-FLAG and 8 μg GFP-SmKFB5 or GFP-F ˆ SmKFB5 plasmids by using the polyethylene glycol-mediated transfection approach and incubation for 4 h, the proteasome inhibitor *MG132* (Sigma-Aldrich, Burlington, MA, USA) was added to the protoplasts to a final concentration of ~50 μmol/L. The protoplasts were sampled at 12 h after treatment and extracted with lysis buffer as described above. For the protein degradation assay in tobacco, tobacco leaves were first infiltrated with *Agrobacterium* strain GV3101 carrying the SmPAL expression vector ($OD_{600}$=0.5) mixed with an equal volume of an *Agrobacterium* strain carrying GFP-SmKFB5 or the empty pGWB506 vector ($OD_{600}$=0.15). One day after the first infiltration, each half leaf was reinfiltrated with infiltration buffer with 50 μmol/L MG132 or DMSO and left for 1 day before harvesting. Leaves were ground in liquid nitrogen and extracted with lysis buffer as described above. The concentration of total protein was measured by using a Bradford protein assay kit (TaKaRa, Dalian, China).

Co-immunoprecipitation assay Tobacco leaves transiently expressing SmPALs-FLAG fusion proteins and the Myc-F ˆ SmKFB5 fusion protein either individually or in co-expression were sampled 3d after infiltration. We extracted the total soluble proteins from homogenized tobacco leaves with a buffer consisting of 25 mmol/L Tris—HCl (pH 7.4), 150 mmol/L NaCl, 1 mmol/L EDTA, 1% NP-40, 5% glycerol, and 1× protease inhibitor cocktail. For binding the FLAG fusion protein, we mixed 20 μL of anti-FLAG antibody-conjugated magnetic agarose beads (GenScript, Nanjing, China) with the crude protein extracts and gently agitated them for 1 - 2 h at 4 ℃. The magnetic beads were collected using a magnetic separator and washed five times with 1 mL of PBS buffer (pH 7.4). The FLAG proteins were eluted from the magnetic beads with 160 μL 2× SDS-PAGE sample buffer and incubated at 100 ℃ for 10 min. Immunoprecipitated samples (35 μL) were separated by SDS-PAGE. The proteins were examined by immunoblotting with anti-FLAG monoclonal antibody and anti-Myc monoclonal antibody (Abmart, Shanghai, China).

Generation of SmKFB5 transgenic plants To construct the plant overexpression vector, full-length *SmKFB5* was subcloned into the binary vector pK7WG2R from the entry vector pGP-B2E. To construct the plant gene editing vector, the DNA sequence of *SmKFB5* was submitted to the Cas-Designer website to design sgRNA. A pair of complementary oligos was synthesized by Personalbio (Shanghai, China) and annealed to generate sgRNA. The sgRNA was then cloned into the CRISPR/Cas9 vector pICSL002218A via restriction enzyme digestion and recombination. The vectors were transferred into *S. miltiorrhiza* by *Agrobacterium rhizogenes* ATCC15834 to generate transgenic hairy roots.

Protein extraction from hairy roots and western blot To examine the protein levels of endogenous SmPAL, we extracted the total soluble proteins from homogenized transgenic hairy roots with 100 mmol/L Tris-HCl buffer, pH 8.0, containing 25 mmol/L EDTA, 500 mmol/L NaCl, 50 mmol/L DTT, 3% PVPP, 2% β-mercaptoethanol, 1% SDS, and 1× complete protease inhibitor cocktail. The total protein was separated on 12% SDS-PAGE gel and transferred on to a polyvinylidene fluoride membrane using the western blot transfer system (Tanon, Shanghai, China). We synthesized peptides C-HVQSAEQHNQDVNSL and used them to generate the anti-PAL polyclonal antibody (HUABIO, Hangzhou, China) that we then employed in the hybridization assay. The verification of the specificity of the anti-PAL antibody is shown in Supplementary Fig. S1. Anti-PAL was used as primary antibody at a dilution of 1 : 5000 in 5% (*W/V*) skim milk with Tris-buffered saline (TBS)-Tween buffer. Horseradish peroxidase-conjugated goat anti-rabbit IgG (BBI, Shanghai, China) was used as secondary antibody at a dilution of 1 : 10000 in 5% (w/v) skim milk with TBS-Tween buffer. The signal was developed using SuperSignal™ West Pico PLUS Chemiluminescent Substrate (Thermo, Shanghai, China) and detected using a Chemiluminescent Analyzer (Tanon, Shanghai, China).

Plant materials and growth conditions The hairy-root culture system of *S. miltiorrhiza* described by Xing *et al.* was used. Samples of fresh hairy roots of *S. miltiorrhiza* weighing 0.2 g were inoculated into 100 mL triangular flasks containing 50 mL of hormone-free 1/2 Murashige and Skoog liquid medium. The flasks were then placed on an orbital shaker at 110 rpm and incubated at 25℃ in the dark. Methyl jasmonate (MeJA; Sigma-Aldrich) was dissolved in ethanol to a concentration of ~100 mmol/L and then sterilized by filtering through 0.22 μm filters. MeJA treatment of the root cultures was performed on the 18th day after inoculation; MeJA was added to the growth medium to a final concentration of ~100 μmol/L. Hairy roots treated with pure ethanol were used as the control. Hairy roots were sampled at 0, 12, and 24 h after treatment. The samples were immediately frozen in liquid nitrogen and stored at −80℃ for RNA and protein extraction.

Transcriptional analysis by real-time quantitative PCR Total RNA was extracted from liquid stored hairy roots of *S. miltiorrhiza* using the RNAprep pure Plant Kit (Tiangen, Beijing) and then reverse transcribed with a PrimeScript™ RT reagent Kit (TaKaRa, Dalian, China) according to the manufacturer's instructions. RNA integrity was analyzed on a 1.0% agarose gel. RNA quantity was determined using a NanoDrop 2000 Spectrophotometer (Thermo Scientific, USA). The obtained cDNA was used as the template for real-time quantitative PCR (RT−qPCR) analysis using QuantStudio™ Flex6 System (Applied Biosystems, Foster City, CA, USA) with SYBR Green reagents (TaKaRa, Dalian, China). The primers used are listed in Supplementary Table S1. *SmActin* and *SmUBQ10* were used as an internal control. RT−qPCR was performed with the following conditions: 30 s pre-denaturation at 95 ℃, followed by 40 cycles of 5s at 95 ℃ and 30s at 58 ℃. Quantification of gene expression was done with the $2^{-\Delta\Delta Ct}$ method. Experiments were performed in triplicate for each biological replicate, and the results are represented are means ±SD.

Phenolic acid extraction and HPLC analysis Phenolic acids were extracted from 1-month-old hairy roots and analyzed by HPLC according to the methods described in Yu *et al.*, with minor modifications. The hairy roots were dried at 45℃ in a drying oven. The dried hairy roots were ground to a powder with a homogenizer (ALLSHENG, Hangzhou, China). A 20 mg sample of the powder was soaked in 2 ml of 70% methanol overnight and then sonicated for 1 h. The supernatant obtained by centrifugation (12 000 g, 20℃, for 10 min) was used for HPLC analysis in a Waters HPLC system (Milford, MA, USA) consisting of a 1 525 binary pump, an automatic sample injector, and a Waters 2 998 photodiode array detector (PDA). HPLC separation was performed with a SunFire C18 column (4.6 mm×250 mm, 5 μm particle size) at 30℃. Empower 3 software (Milford, MA, USA) was used for data acquisition and analysis. The sample injection volume was 20 μL and the PDA detection wavelength for the water-soluble phenolic acids was 280 nm. Separation was achieved by elution using a linear gradient with solvent A (acetonitrile) and solvent B (0.026% phosphoric acid solution); the HPLC gradient program is shown in Supplementary Table S2. The standard curves of caffeic acid, rosmarinic acid, and salvianolic acid B are shown in Supplementary Fig. S2.

Luciferase assays The *SmKFB5* promoter fragment was cloned into the pGreenII 0800-LUC vector to generate a reporter construct. The effector construct was generated by cloning the *SmMYC2a* gene into the pGreenII 62-SK vector. The recombinant vectors were transformed into *Agrobacterium* GV3101. Tobacco leaves were infected with the mixed *Agrobacterium* strains. Fluorescence was detected using a Chemiluminescent Analyzer (Tanon, Shanghai, China).

## 3 RESULTS

Isolation and characterization of *SmKFB5* The full-length cDNA sequence of *SmKFB5* contained an ORF of 1 029 bp in length and encodes a putative 343-amino acid protein. Sequence analysis by the Conserved Domains website indicated that SmKFB5 protein contained an N-terminal F-box domain that may interact with SKP1 protein to form an SCF-type E3 complex. In addition, SmKFB5 also contains three Kelch repeat domains near the C-terminus, which is responsible for interacting selectively with the target proteins, therefore conferring specificity on this complex (Fig. 1).

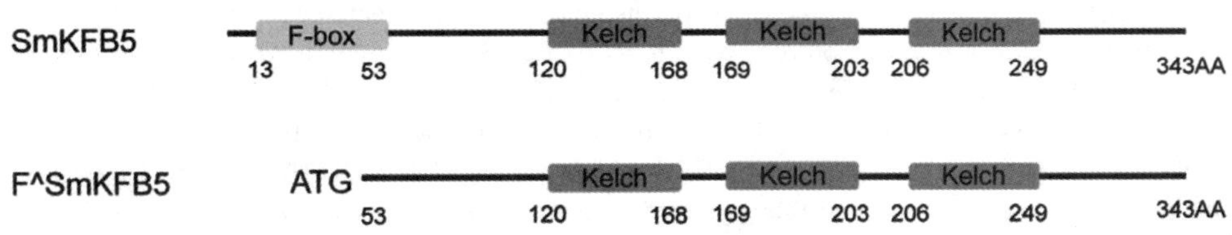


**Fig. 1 Schematic diagram showing the predicted F-box and Kelch repeat domains of SmKFB5 and F^SmKFB5**

SmKFB5 interacts physically with PAL isozymes Previously, based on the results of phylogenetic and gene expression analyses, we speculated that SmKFB5 was potentially related to phenolic acid biosynthesis. In order to verify this, we first examined whether SmKFB5 interacted physically with *S. miltiorrhiza* phenolic acid biosynthetic enzymes via a Y2H assay. The results showed that the yeast transformants harboring the expressed SmKFB5 and SmPAL isozymes effectively activated the expression of four independent reporter genes (*lacZ*, *HIS3*, *ADE2*, and *MEL1*), resulting in a substantial rescue of growth of blue yeast colonies on SD/-Ade/-His/-Leu/-Trp medium containing X-α-Gal (Fig. 2A). By contrast, SmKFB5 showed a nearly indiscernible interaction with other phenolic acid enzymes in Y2H assays under the same conditions (Supplementary Fig. S3). These *in vitro* data suggested that SmKFB5 had a strong interaction with all three SmPAL isozymes.

To further examine whether the SmKFB5 and SmPAL isozymes interacted *in planta*, we conducted a BiFC assay by transiently co-expressing the N-terminus of SmKFB5 fused with the C-terminal half of yellow fluorescent protein ($YFP^C$) and the N-terminus of the SmPAL isozymes fused with the N-terminal half of yellow fluorescent protein ($YFP^N$) in tobacco leaf cells. Unexpectedly, we failed to detect any complementary chimeric fluorescence signals when $YFP^C$-SmKFB5 was co-expressed with any of the $YFP^N$-SmPALs in the leaves of tobacco (Fig. 2B). Based on the literature, we knew that, as a part of SCF-type E3 ligase, F-box protein specifies the protein substrates for degradation via the ubiquitin-26S proteasome. We speculated that the interaction of SmKFB5 with SmPAL might attenuate the stability of SmPAL, leading to its rapid degradation. The N-terminal F-box motif of the KFB proteins is required to mediate the interaction of the KFB proteins with SKP1 to form a functional SCF-type E3 ligase. Therefore, we constructed a truncated F^SmKFB5, in which we removed

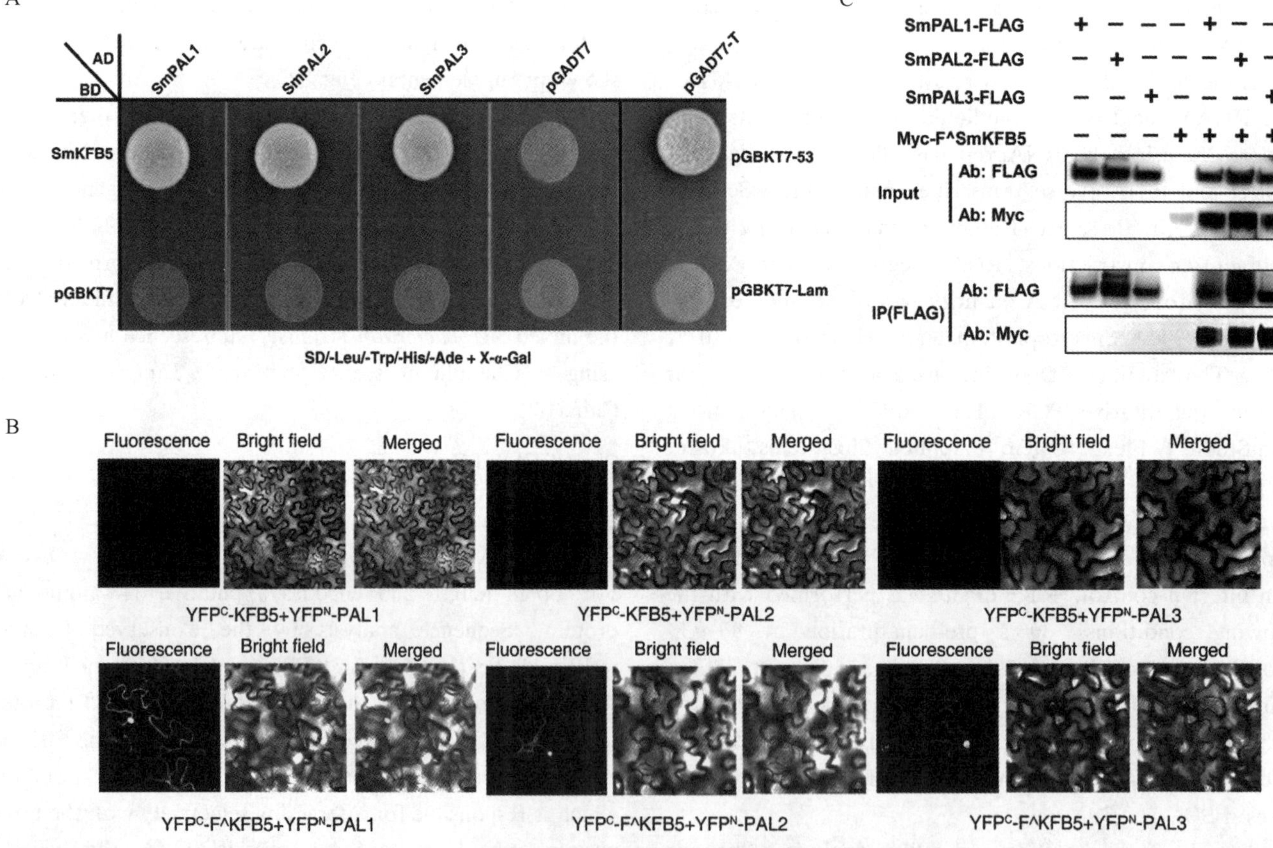


**Fig. 2 Interaction of SmKFB5 with SmPAL isozymes**

(A) Yeasts carrying activation domain (AD) (pGADT7-SmPAL1-3) and binding domain (BD) (pGBKT7-SmKFB5) vectors were grown on quadruple dropout (-Leu/Trp/His/Ade) synthetic defined medium supplemented with X-α-Gal. Yeast harboring pGBKT7-53 and pGADT7-T vectors served as a positive control; yeast harboring pGBKT7-Lam and pGADT7-T vectors served as a negative control. (B) BiFC assay for SmKFB5 or truncated SmKFB5 (F^SmKFB5) fused with $YFP^N$ at their N-termini and SmPAL1-3 fused with $YFP^C$ at their N-termini. The SmKFB5 and F^SmKFB5 fusion constructs were co-infiltrated with SmPAL1-3 constructs into tobacco leaves. (C) Co-IP of SmPALs-FLAG fusion proteins with Myc-tagged F^SmKFB5 protein. Crude lysates (Input) were immunoprecipitated with anti-FLAG antibody and then detected with anti-FLAG antibody for the SmPAL-FLAG fusion protein and anti-Myc antibody for the truncated SmKFB5 (F^SmKFB5) tagged with Myc.

the predicted F-box domain of SmKFB5 (Fig. 1), and then produced a YFP$^C$-F^SmKFB5 construct and co-expressed it with YFP$^N$-SmPALs. Co-expression of these fusion proteins produced strong yellow fluorescence signals (Fig. 2B). This suggested that the BiFC signals obtained with the co-expression of YFP$^C$-F^SmKFB5 and YFP$^N$-SmPALs reflected the specific interaction of SmKFB5 and SmPAL isozymes.

To further examine whether the SmPALs and SmKFB5 protein form protein complexes *in planta*, we conducted coimmunoprecipitation (Co-IP) assays by transiently co-expressing SmPALs-FLAG and the truncated Myc-SmKFB5 (F^SmKFB5) fusion protein in tobacco leaf cells. Crude proteins were immunoprecipitated using anti-FLAG antibody-conjugated magnetic agarose beads. Although the F^SmKFB5 fused with the Myc tag was present at only a low level in the crude cell lysates (Fig. 2C, Input), it was coimmunoprecipitated by the anti-FLAG antibody when it was co-expressed with SmPALs-FLAG. Thus, these results indicated that the SmPALs and truncated SmKFB5 fusion proteins could bind together in living cells. To confirm that the Co-IP of the FLAG- or Myctagged fusion proteins was not a consequence of the spontaneous binding of the tagged fragments, we used a Myc-GFP fusion protein as a negative control. We co-expressed the control GFP-Myc fusion protein with SmPALs-FLAG fusion proteins and found that Co-IP with anti-FLAG antibody-conjugated magnetic agarose beads produced no signal, whereas Myc-GFP was detected with anti-Myc antibody (Supplementary Fig. S4). These data confirmed the specific interactions of the SmPALs and SmKFB5 protein *in vivo*.

To examine whether the F-box motif we removed from SmKFB5 influenced the subcellular location of SmKFB5 protein, the N-terminal of either SmKFB5 or F^SmKFB5 fused with green fluorescent protein (GFP) was transiently expressed in tobacco leaves. The fusion proteins showed a similar cytosolic and nuclear distribution, suggested that removing the F-box motif did not influence the subcellular location of SmKFB5 (Fig. 3). In addition, we also transiently expressed GFP-SmPALs fusion proteins in tobacco leaves. The GFP-SmPALs localized primarily to the cytosol and showed a less extensive network-like strand distribution and nuclear periphery localization (Fig. 3). Previous studies have found that PALs were localized mostly in the cytosol and some isozymes also partially localized on the surface of the endoplasmic reticulum, findings that were consistent with those of our study. In addition, the common cytosolic localization of SmKFB5 and the SmPAL proteins also supports their interactions *in vivo*.

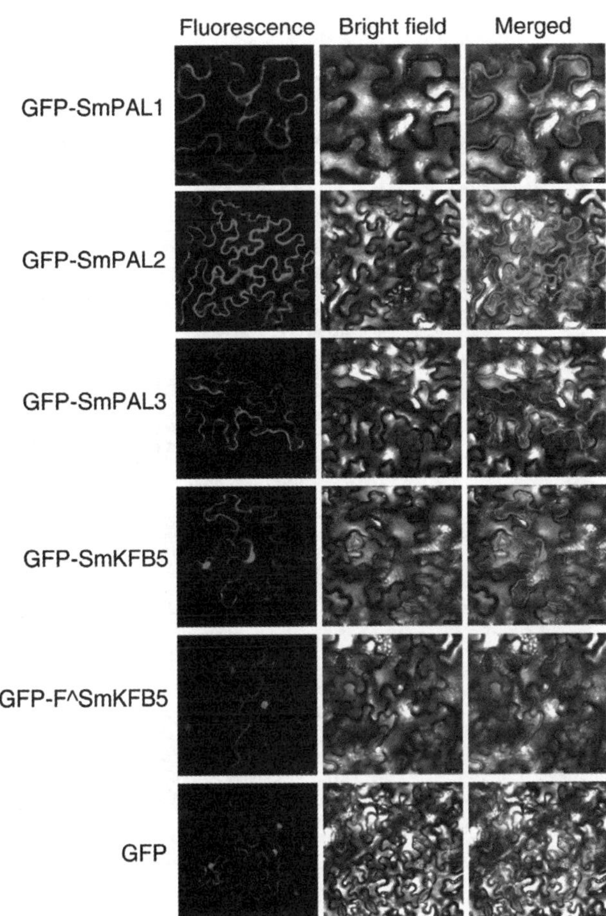


**Fig. 3 Subcellular localization of GFP-SmKFB5, truncated GFP-F^SmKFB5, and SmPAL1-3 fusion proteins transiently expressed in tobacco leaves**

SmKFB5 attenuates the stability of SmPAL isozymes

To evaluate the hypothesis that SmKFB5 mediates the turnover of the SmPALs, we first examined whether the interaction of SmKFB5 protein with the SmPAL isozymes affected SmPAL activity. We expressed a 35S: SmPALs-FLAG expressing cassette in combination with a 35S: GFP-SmKFB5 or 35S: GFP expressing cassette in 1-month-old tobacco leaves. 35S: SmPALs-FLAG co-expressed with 35S: GFP was regarded as the control. Leaves expressing SmPALs with GFP, SmKFB5, and F^SmKFB5 were collected and homogenized. The crude protein extracts from the infiltrated leaves were used for measuring the activity of the SmPAL enzymes in converting L-phenylalanine to *trans*-cinnamic acid. Co-expression of the SmPAL-FLAG fusion proteins with GFP-SmKFB5 decreased SmPAL activity by 70%-90% compared with the control (Fig. 4A).

To verify whether the reduction of activity of SmPAL isozymes resulted from the degradation of SmPAL protein, we examined the stability of the SmPALs-FLAG fusions by western blotting with an anti-FLAG antibody. The signal for SmPALs-FLAG fusions was absent in extracts from leaves co-expressing SmPAL with full-length SmKFB5 protein. In contrast, the signal of SmPALs was essentially unchanged when they were co-expressed with either free GFP or GFP-F^SmKFB5 (Fig. 4B). To explore whether degradation of

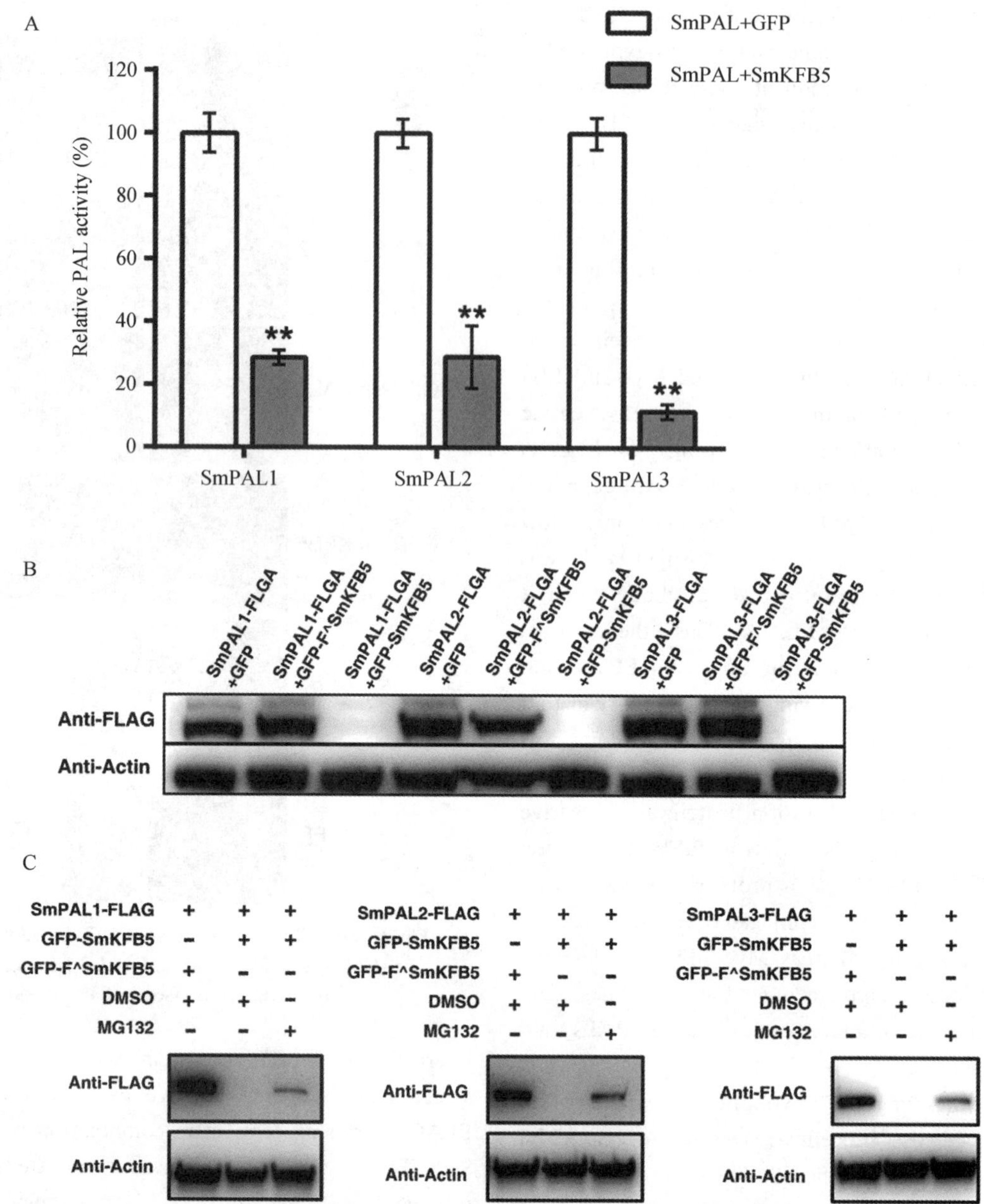


**Fig. 4 SmkFB5 proteins attenuate the stability of SmPALs**

(A) Relative activity of SmPAL isozymes in crude extracts from tobacco leaves co-expressing SmPALs with GFP or GFP-SmKFB5. Data are the mean ±SD from three biological replicates. Asterisks indicate significant differences (** $P<0.01$; *t*-test). (B) Immunoblot detection of the stability of the SmPAL-FLAG fusion proteins using anti-FLAG antibody in tobacco leaves co-infiltrated with GFP, GFP-SmKFB5, or GFP-F^SmKFB5 constructs. Anti-β-actin was used as a protein loading control. (C) Degradation of SmPALs via the plant 26S-proteasome pathway. SmPALs-FLAG and GFP-SmKFB5 or GFP-F^SmKFB5 were co-expressed in rice protoplasts. After 4 h, the protoplasts were treated with DMSO or MG132 and cultured for an additional 12 h, and protoplast proteins were extracted for western blot analysis.

SmPAL proteins occurs via the ubiquitin-26S proteasome pathway, we carried out protein degradation assays using rice protoplasts. We used the proteasome inhibitor MG132 to treat rice protoplasts transiently co-expressing SmPALs-FLAG and GFP-SmKFB5 fusion proteins. As shown in Fig. 4C, the intensity of the SmPALs-FLAG bands was stronger in the presence of MG132 than in the presence of DMSO. In addition, we also carried out protein degradation assays in tobacco leaves in which SmPALs-FLAG and GFP-SmKFB5 fusion proteins were co-expressed following *Agrobacterium* infiltration. After 24 h, half of the transformed leaves were infiltrated with 50 μmol/L MG132 or an equal volume of DMSO and cultivated for an additional 24 h, and leaves were then harvested for western blot analysis. As shown in Supplementary Fig. S5, when the leaves were infil-trated with 50 μmol/L MG132, the degradation of SmPALs was substantially inhibited. These results indicated that the degradation of SmPALs occurred via the 26S proteasome. Taken together, the changes in SmPAL activity and stability in the co-expression experiments indicated that SmKFB5 mediated the degradation of the SmPAL isozymes via the ubiquitin-26S proteasome pathway.

Up-regulation of *SmKFB5* in *S. miltiorrhiza* impairs the synthesis of phenolic acids To further explore the potential role of *SmKFB5* in the regulation of phenolic acid biosynthesis *in vivo*, we stably overexpressed *SmKFB5* driven by a constitutive 35S promoter in *S. miltiorrhiza* hairy roots. Data on the SmKFB5-overexpressing transgenic lines are shown in Supplementary Fig. S6.

The expression level of *SmKFB5* was higher in the generated transgenic lines than in the wild type, albeit with large variation among the independent transgenic events (Fig. 5A). Overexpression of *SmKFB5* in *S. miltiorrhiza* did not significantly change the expression of the endogenous *SmPAL* genes in some lines (Supplementary Fig. S7), whereas the level of SmPAL protein, detected with an anti-SmPAL peptide antibody, was reduced substantially in the transgenic lines highly expressing *SmKFB5* (Fig. 5B).

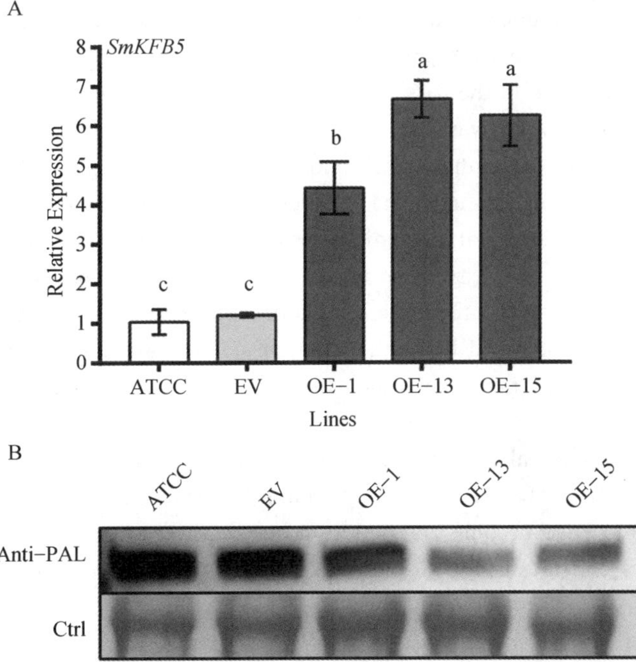


**Fig. 5 Molecular analysis of SmKFB5-overexpressing hairy roots**

(A) Relative expression of *SmKFB5* in the overexpressing lines (OE-1, OE-13, and OE-15) and controls (ATCC, EV). The ATCC and EV hairy roots were developed using *A. rhizogenes* ATCC15834 without vector and ATCC15834 with empty vector, respectively. Data are the mean ± SD from three biological replicates. Different letters indicate significant differences ($P<0.05$; Tukey's multiple comparison test). (B) Western blot analysis of the protein levels of SmPAL isozymes in the transgenic overexpressing lines using polyclonal antibody against SmPAL.

Salvianolic acid B, rosmarinic acid, and caffeic acid have usually been regarded as the representative compounds of the phenolic acids in *S. miltiorrhiza*. As shown in Fig. 6, the transgenic *SmKFB5*-overexpressing lines showed a substantial decrease in the amounts of caffeic acid, rosmarinic acid, and salvianolic acid B, coincident with the alteration in the stability of SmPAL in these lines. Specifically, the concentration of caffeic acid, rosmarinic acid, and salvianolic acid B in hairy root declined by ~15%-40%, ~29%-63%, and ~50%-60%, respectively, in the transgenic lines; this decrease was evident particularly in the OE-13 line, in which the expression of *SmKFB5* was higher than the other transgenic lines. These data indicated that the overexpression of *SmKFB5* promoted the turnover of endogenous SmPAL enzymes, thus disturbing phenolic acid biosynthesis.

Knockout of *SmKFB5* in *S. miltiorrhiza* enhances the synthesis of phenolic acids To further examine the effect of SmKFB5 on the stability of SmPAL, we used CRISPR-Cas9 gene editing technology to generate mutant lines. Data on the *smkfb5* mutants are shown in Supplementary Fig. S8. We used anti-SmPAL peptide antibody to detect the abundance of endogenous SmPAL in the three biallelic mutant lines. As shown in Fig. 7, stronger PAL signals were observed in the three knockout *smkfb5* mutants compared with the controls. These data further suggested that SmKFB5 was responsible for the turnover of PAL proteins *in vivo*.

Quantification of the concentration of accumulated phenolic acids in *smkfb5* hairy roots revealed increases of ~14% - 22% for caffeic acid, ~ 28% - 46% for rosmarinic acid, and ~17% - 38% for salvianolic acid B relative to the controls (Fig. 8). These data indicate that SmKFB5 indeed negatively affects phenolic acid biosynthesis. The results also indicate that it is likely that additional control factors exist for regulating PAL activity.

Expression of *SmKFB5* is suppressed by MeJA MeJA as an elicitor can up-regulate the expression of key genes in the phenolic acid biosynthetic pathway, including *SmPALs*, and the consequent accumulation of a set of phenolic acid metabolites, including caffeic acid, rosmarinic acid, and salvianolic acid B. To evaluate whether SmKFB5 is involved in jasmonate (JA) signaling, which, in turn, can regulate SmPALs and phenolic acid biosynthesis, we quantified the transcriptional changes of *SmKFB5* and the *SmPAL* genes in hairy roots treated with MeJA. As expected, the expression of *SmPAL1* and *SmPAL3* was sharply up-regulated by 5-fold and 11-fold, respectively, after 12 h of exposure. By contrast, the expression levels of *SmPAL2* and *SmKFB5* were suppressed, with their levels of expression decreased by ~2-fold compared with that in the control hairy roots (Fig. 9A). In addition, the total protein abundance of SmPALs was increased with the extension of MeJA treatment time to 24 h (Fig. 9B).

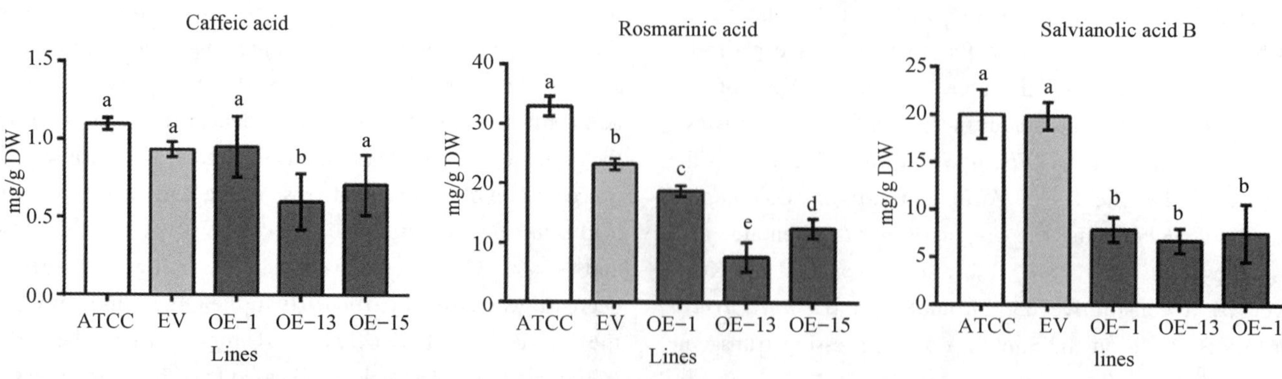


**Fig. 6 HPLC analysis of the accumulation of phenolic acids in *SmKFB5*-overexpressing hairy roots**

Data are the mean±SD from three biological replicates. Different letters indicate significant differences ($P<0.05$; Tukey's multiple comparison test).

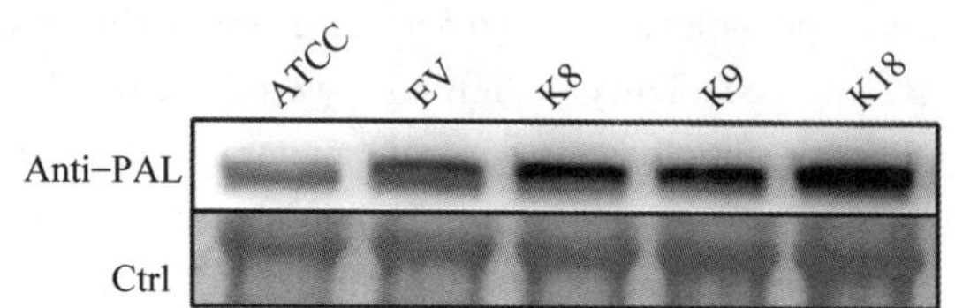


**Fig. 7 Protein levels of SmPAL isozymes in *SmKFB5*-knockout hairy roots**

Western blot analysis of the protein levels of SmPAL isozymes in three *SmKFB5*-knockout lines (K8, K9, and K18) and controls (ATCC, EV). The ATCC and EV hairy roots were developed using *A. rhizogenes* ATCC15834 without vector and ATCC15834 with empty vector, respectively.

We found a G-box motif in the promoter of *SmKFB5* (Supplementary Fig. S9A). *MYC2* is a JA-responsive gene and can bind to the G-box *cis*-element. Therefore, we explored whether MYC2 can regulate the gene expression of *SmKFB5*. As shown in Supplementary Fig. S9B, SmMYC2a could significantly inhibit the expression of *SmKFB5* in a luciferase reporter assay. These data implied that during the process of MeJA promoting the biosynthesis of phenolic acids, both transcriptional and post-translational controls are implemented in *S. miltiorrhiza*—that is, by up-regulating the transcription of the key biosynthetic genes, *SmPALs*, and reducing the level of *SmKFB5*, thus modulating the stability of SmPAL proteins, to maximize the synthesis of phenolic acids as a plant defense mechanism.

## 4 DISCUSSION

Plant secondary metabolites have been considered as a treasure because they represent an important source of pharmaceuticals. In excess of 30% of medicinal products are sourced directly from plants, and over 60% of the drugs introduced in the past 20 years are based on plant extracts or their close derivatives.

The biosynthesis of secondary metabolites is regulated at multiple levels, including product inhibition, transcriptional and translational regulation, post-translational inactivation and proteolysis, enzyme organization/subcellular compartmentation, and metabolite feedback regulation. However, with regard to phenolic acid biosynthesis, most studies have focused on transcriptional regulation. In our study, we found that SmKFB5 regulates the activity of SmPALs at the post-translational level to regulate the accumulation of phenolic acids. PALs are encoded by a family of genes in most plants and have become one of the most extensively studied types of enzymes in higher plants because of their key role in the

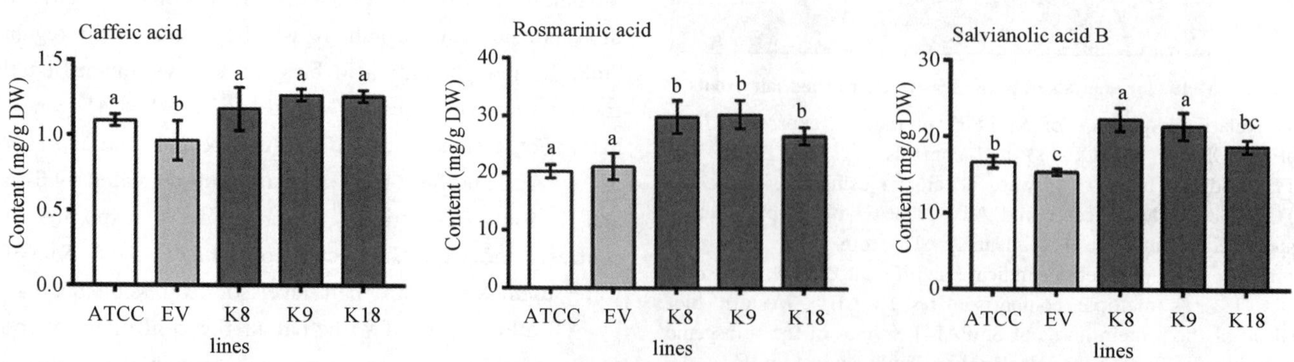


**Fig. 8 HPLC analysis of the accumulation of phenolic acids in *SmKFB5*-knockout hairy roots**

Data are the mean ±SD from three biological replicates. Different letters indicate significant differences ($P<0.05$; Tukey's multiple comparison test).

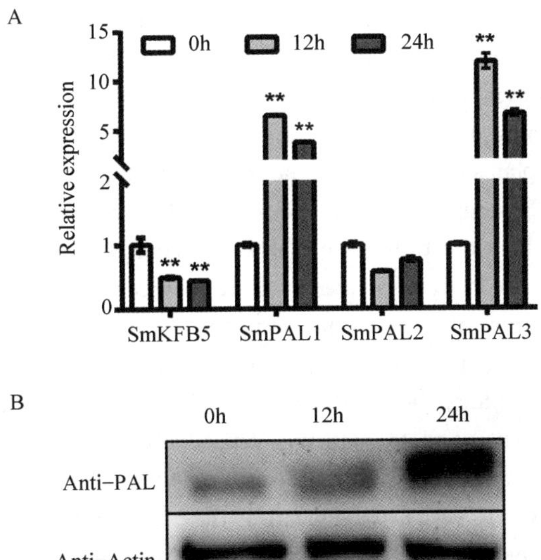


**Fig. 9 The gene and protein expression pattern in hairy roots of *S. miltiorrhiza* treated with MeJA.**

(A) Relative gene expression levels of *SmKFB5* and *SmPAL*s in hairy roots of *S. miltiorrhiza* treated with MeJA. Eighteen-day-old hairy roots were grown on 6, 7-V medium supplemented with 100 μmol/L MeJA for 12 h and 24 h. The expression level in untreated samples (0 h) was set at 1. Data are the mean ±SD from three biological repeats. Asterisks indicate significant differences (** $P<0.01$; $t$-test). (B) Western blot analysis of the protein levels of SmPAL isozymes in hairy roots of *S. miltiorrhiza* treated with MeJA. Anti-β-actin was used as a protein loading control.

biosynthesis of a large variety of plant-specific phenylpropanoid derivatives. In *S. miltiorrhiza*, three *SmPAL* genes have been isolated through searching the *S. miltiorrhiza* genome. Of these genes, *SmPAL1* and *SmPAL3* were highly expressed in roots and leaves of *S. miltiorrhiza*, whereas *SmPAL2* was predominantly expressed in stems and flowers. A previous study indicated that in *SmPAL1*-RNAi lines the total content of phenolic acids was decreased by 20%~70% compared with untransformed plantlets and a vectorcontrol line, and this decrease was accompanied by lower PAL activity. Some researchers proposed an inactivation mechanism that reversibly converts PAL to its inactive form. Protein modification by phosphorylation is a way to turn the activity of some biosynthetic enzymes on and off. However, the catalytic activity of PAL was unaffected by phosphorylation in French bean and popular. Earlier studies also revealed that environmental factors can transiently increase the cellular level of PAL; after the initial increase, PAL often rapidly declines to basal or near-basal levels, suggesting that the decline in PAL might be due to its proteolytic turnover. These data imply the complex regulation of PAL activity at post-translational levels. In our study, evidence from *in vitro* and *in planta* experiments suggested that SmKFB5 functions as a negative regulator specifically controlling phenolic acid biosynthesis via mediating the degradation of SmPALs through the ubiquitin-26S proteasome pathway.

The ubiquitin-26S proteasome pathway is a rapid and precise regulatory mechanism for selective protein degradation in plants and is also an integral part of plant physiological processes such as growth, development, and response to environmental stresses. There is increasing evidence that the ubiquitin-26S proteasome pathway plays a crucial role in plant secondary metabolism regulation. A group of *A. thaliana* KFB proteins (AtKFB01, AtKFB20, AtKFB39, and AtKFB50) have previously been found to interact with AtPALs, which mediate PAL ubiquitination and subsequent degradation and negatively regulate plant phenylpropanoid biosynthesis. SmKFB5 is phylogenetically related to AtKFB1, AtKFB20, AtKFB39, and AtKFB50, suggesting that SmKFB5 could have a similar function in phenylpropanoid biosynthesis in *S. miltiorrhiza*. In this study, we tested SmKFB5 pairwise with 11 phenolic acid biosynthetic enzymes in a Y2H assay. The results showed that SmKFB5 interacted only with SmPAL1-3 among the 11 enzymes that were tested (Supplementary Fig. S3), further supporting that SmKFB5, like its homolog AtKFBs, is involved in mediating PAL proteolysis. However, unlike AtKFB1, AtKFB20, AtKFB39, and AtKFB50, which showed different interaction preferences for PALs, SmKFB5 showed a strong and similar interaction with all three SmPALs in a Y2H assay under the same conditions (Fig. 2A). In the BiFC assay, when we co-expressed full-length *SmKFB5* and *SmPALs* in the leaves of tobacco, we failed to detect any complementary chimeric yellow fluorescence signals (Fig. 2B). F-box proteins are widely distributed in plants; nearly 700 F-box protein genes but only 21 *SKP1* genes have been isolated from the *A. thaliana* genome, suggesting that any given SKP1 protein may interact with many F-box proteins and, conversely, the same F-box protein may bind to multiple SKP1 proteins. In addition, most F-box proteins tested also interacted with other plant or non-plant (yeast) SKP1 proteins. Therefore, the F-box protein SmKFB5 might interact with tobacco SKP1 to form a functional SCF-type E3 ligase, which promoted the ubiquitination and degradation of SmPALs, resulting in the failure to observe fluorescent signals. The F-box protein binds to the SKP1 protein through the F-box domain to form a functional SCF-type E3 ligase. Subsequently, we removed the predicted F-box domains of SmKFB5 and then co-expressed fusions of the truncated proteins ($YFP^{C}$-F^-SmKBF5) with $YFP^{N}$-SmPALs. Co-expression of these fusion proteins produced strong chimeric fluorescence signals (Fig. 2B). This result argues for an interaction of SmKFB5 with SmPALs, and preliminarily suggests that SmKFB5 mediates SmPALs degradation via the ubiquitin-26S proteasome system. Furthermore, the co-expression of a GFP-SmKFB5 fusion protein and the individual SmPAL-FLAG fusion proteins substantially decreased the PAL activity by ~71%—88% compared with the co-expression of GFP and individual SmPAL isozymes (Fig. 4A). This biochemical property is consistent with the co-expression of individual AtKFB1, AtKFB20, AtKFB39, or AtKFB50 with SmPALs leading to reduced PAL activity. We used anti-FLAG antibody to verify whether the reduction of PAL activity resulted from the degradation of PAL protein. The signals for PAL-FLAG fusions were absent in extracts from leaves co-expressing full-length SmKFB5 protein with the individual SmPALs (Fig. 4B). In contrast, we observed no protein degradation when free GFP or truncated KFB was co-expressed with each SmPAL protein (Fig. 4B), suggesting that SmKFB5 specifically targets SmPAL isozymes and mediates their selective degradation. This also confirmed that the failure to detect complementary chimeric fluorescence signals when full-length $YFP^C$-SmKFB5 and individual $YFP^N$-SmPALs were co-expressed was likely due to proteolysis of SmPALs as a result of SmKFB5 mediating the ubiquitin-26S proteasome system. This effect of SmKFB5 on the stability of SmPALs was evidenced further by manipulating *SmKFB5* expression *in planta*; knockout or overexpression of *SmKFB5* in hairy root resulted in a reciprocal change in the endogenous level of the SmPAL proteins and the content of phenolic acids (Figs 5 - 8), suggesting that SmKFB5 control SmPALs stability in living cells.

PAL, as the first rate-limiting enzyme in the phenylpropanoid pathway, controls the partitioning of primary metabolic flux into a variety of desirable phenolic acids; therefore, it is an ideal target for enhancing phenolic acid biosynthesis. Generally, up-regulating the transcription of *SmPAL* genes is a way to increase the biosynthesis of phenolic acids. However, it is difficult to boost the activity of PAL by genetically manipulating the level of *PAL* gene expression in plants. For example, when a bean *PAL* gene, driven by the 35S promoter, was expressed in tobacco, the transgenic plants exhibited a series of unusual phenotypes, including fluorescent lesions, altered leaf shape and texture, reduced lignification in xylem, stunted growth, and altered flower morphology and pigmentation. Genetic analysis of a transformant with severe symptoms showed that symptom development was the result of PAL activity and a reduction in the content of soluble phenylpropanoid products. Furthermore, the expression of the endogenous tobacco *PAL* gene was also suppressed. The brown planthopper (BPH) is the most destructive pest of rice and causes losses of billions of dollars annually. BPH feeding induced the expression of *OsPAL* genes, leading to increased biosynthesis and accumulation of salicylic acid and lignin. As a result, the plants gained increased resistance to BPH. *OsPAL6* was overexpressed in the susceptible rice variety 02428 to confirm the role of OsPAL6 in BPH resistance. Unexpectedly, the transgenic lines showed greater susceptibility to BPH than the parental 02408 plants. RT—qPCR analysis showed that the reduction of BPH resistance could be caused by co-suppression of *OsPAL6* in the transgenic plants. Of course, there are also events that increase the activity of PAL through overexpression. In addition, PALs are usually encoded by a multigene family in most plants. For example, four, five, and eight *PALs* have been identified in the genome of *A. thaliana*, *Populus trichocarpa*, and *O. sativa*, respectively. It is difficult to overexpress multiple *PAL* genes at the same time, and boosting *PAL* gene expression usually causes abnormal phenotypes. In our study, we found that knocking out *SmKFB5* significantly enhanced PAL stability and thus its cellular concentration and activity, consequently leading to an increase in the production of phenolic acids (Fig. 8). This feature offers a unique opportunity to overcome the obstacles in directly manipulating PAL to produce the desired phenolic acids.

Jasmonic acid and its cyclic precursors and derivatives, collectively referred to as JAs, constitute a family of oxylipins that have been found to induce the biosynthesis of many secondary metabolites, including phenolic acids, in *S. miltiorrhiza*. The JA-ZIM domain (JAZ) proteins, which are substrates of the $SCF^{COI1}$ complex, function as negative regulators to repress diverse JA responses, probably by directly inhibiting various transcriptional regulators. Upon perception of a JA signal, $SCF^{COI1}$ mediated JAZ protein degradation to release the related transcription factors, which consequently resulted in the activation of target genes.

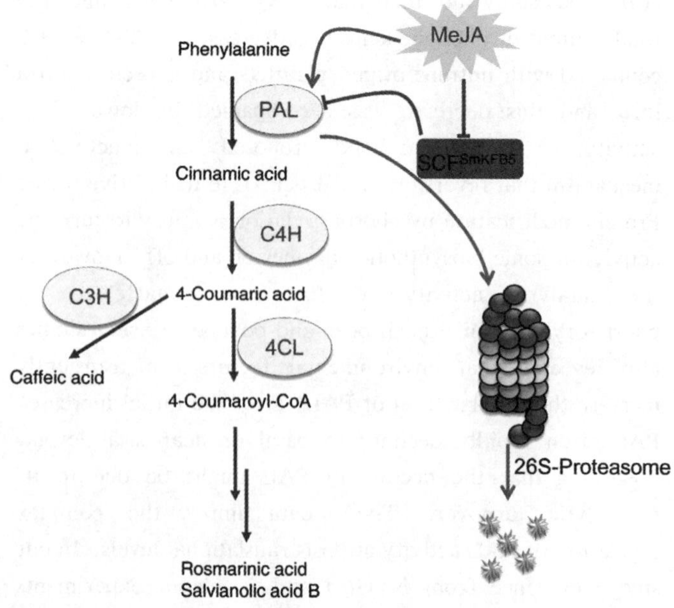


**Fig. 10 Model for the role of SmKFB5 in MeJA/JA signal responses and phenolic acid accumulation**

In *S. miltiorrhiza*, a series of JA-responsive transcription factors, including bHLH, AP2/ERF (APETALA2/ethylene-response factors), and MYB, have been characterized. These transcription factors specifically bind to *cis*-acting elements in the promoter of biosynthetic genes and regulate their expression to control the accumulation of phenolic acids. In our study, we found that *SmKFB5*, which codes for an F-box protein, confers specificity on the SCF complex, and its gene expression was suppressed by MeJA. Based on these results and previous studies, we propose a model to describe the role of SmKFB5 in the modulation of MeJA (or JA) to enhance phenolic acid biosynthesis (Fig. 10). MeJA treatment repressed the expression of *SmKFB5* and thus inhibited SmKFB5-mediated degradation of the SmPAL proteins. Furthermore, MeJA also up-regulated the transcript level of *smPALs*. The increased abundance of SmPAL protein enhanced the biosynthesis of phenolic acids. In the absence of JA, SmKFB5 mediates SmPAL degradation via the ubiquitin-26S proteasome pathway to maintain the level of SmPAL at basal or near-basal levels and retard or stop the biosynthesis of phenolic acids. Taken together, our results extend our understanding of how JA is involved in enhancing the biosynthesis of phenolic acids and provide a valuable target for the genetic improvement of phenolic acid accumulation in *S. miltiorrhiza*.

[于海征，韩蕊莲，梁宗锁，等. Journal of Experimental Botany, 2021, 72(13): 4915-4929.]

# High-throughput screening and spatial profiling of low-mass pesticides using a novel $Ti_3C_2$ MXene nanowire (TMN) as MALDI MS matrix

## 1 INTRODUCTION

Pesticides with various groups have been widely used over the past few decades, but extensive and incorrect use of these toxic compounds may seriously contaminate the environment and pose risks to human health. Thus, there is an urgent demand for a fast, sensitive, and reliable screening method to monitor pesticide residuals quantitatively and efficiently. Mass spectrometry (MS) is an irreplaceable analytical technique for detecting pesticides because it has significant instrumental flexibility and analytical capability within a wide range of metrologic criteria. Nowadays, the determination of pesticide residues is usually performed by liquid chromatography/gas chromatography-mass spectrometry (LC/GC-MS) as well as hybrid methods of high-performance liquid chromatography (HPLC), ultra-performance liquid chromatography (UPLC), and tandem mass spectrometry.

Most of the MS techniques mentioned are efficient; nonetheless, these methods require complicated sample preparation procedures prior to the determination of pesticides, have difficulties in the separation process, and they are laborious and time-consuming, which has led to conventional pesticide analysis of foodstuffs being minimized. In addition, these methods cannot detect different kinds of pesticides simultaneously using a small sample volume and, therefore, are unable to screen large numbers of samples. Therefore, a more sensitive and high-throughput MS method for detecting toxic pesticides is strongly desired.

Matrix laser desorption/ionization mass spectrometry (MALDI MS) has been proposed as an alternative analytical tool for pesticide analysis. It has the advantages of fast analysis speed, accurate quality measurement, and simple sample processing to detect pesticides. Furthermore, MALDI MS not only allows the rapid detection of analytes in liquid samples but can also directly visualize the distribution of molecules in tissue using the mass spectrometry imaging (MSI) technique. These advantages show the tremendous potential of MALDI MS in tracking molecular trajectories, which can unambiguously reveal the translocation mechanism of agrochemicals in real samples. However, this technique encounters challenges for the detection of pesticides in the small molecule range with a mass-to-charge ratio ($m/z$) $<$ 500 Da because of the traditional organic compound matrices, such as α-cya-no-4-hydroxycinnamic acid (CHCA) and 2,5-dihydroxybenzoic acid (DHB) which can produce serious background interference at $<$ 500 Da, and easily form non-uniform co-crystallization between matrices and small-molecule analytes. To circumvent the problem of background signal interference, inorganic materials such as porous silicon, carbon nanomaterials, and gold nanoparticles (NPs) have been proposed as background-free alternatives to traditional organic matrices. However, their low solubility, inhomogeneous nature, and cluster production often hinder the use of these materials as matrices. It remains a great challenge to detect low-mass pesticides (<500 Da) using the above inorganic materials.

The main driving force for MALDI MS analysis of nanomaterials is the photo-thermal conversion process. Thus, MXene, as a new series of two-dimensional (2D) materials, is one of the most promising materials for MALDI MS analysis because of its extremely high photothermal conversion ability originating from the electron-phonon coupling effect. MXenes share a common stoichiometry of $M_{n+1}X_nT_x$ (n = 1, 2, or 3) to the chemical formula, where M represents an early transition metal (such as Ta, Ti, Mo, and Cr), X denotes carbon and/or nitrogen, and Tx refers to surface functional groups (such as —O, —OH, —F, and —Cl). Among the MXene materials, $Ti_3C_2$ (also denoted as $Ti_3C_2T_x$) has emerged as one of the most attractive 2D metal carbides. The existence of numerous highly active surface groups (—O, —F, and —OH) on exfoliated $Ti_3C_2$ may provide additional opportunities to interact with pesticides by hydrogen-bonding interactions and to support metal ion ($Na^+/K^+$) enrichment and transfer, which could enhance the ionization efficiency of pesticides. Two studies investigated the effect of typical sheet-like $Ti_3C_2$ as a matrix for MALDI MS, demonstrating that sheet-like $Ti_3C_2$ has a comparatively higher MALDI MS efficiency than conventional nanomaterials such as graphene oxide (GO), multi-walled carbon nanotubes (MWCNTs), single-walled carbon nanotubes (SWCNTs), $MoS_2$ nanoflakes, and $TiO_2$ nanoparticles. Nevertheless, its low photoluminescence and large diameter (500 nm) may reduce the optical absorption of typical sheet-like $Ti_3C_2$ and the reproducibility of MALDI analysis results, which has a large impact on quantitative analysis and MALDI MSI resolution. The properties of $Ti_3C_2$ still need to be improved as a matrix in MALDI MS analysis and imaging of low-mass pesticides in different samples.

Previous studies reported that nanowires (NWs) of $SnO_2$, $TiO_2$, and ZnO, and carbon nanotubes, performed much higher MALDI MS efficiency compared to these metal nanoparticles because of their higher optical absorptivity, lower heat capacity, improved thermal confinement effect, and smaller diameter below 200 nm. The NWs not only improve the dispersion of nanomaterials and the homogeneity of sample spots, but also significantly increase the laser energy absorption capacity in MALDI MS. Furthermore, recent studies reported that $TiO_2$ and $SiO_2$ nanowire films, which were prepared on a polished semiconductor surface, could be utilized for MALDI MSI of complex biological samples. The properties of the nanowires were found to be suitable for MALDI MS analysis. Notably, the electrical conductivity of MXene is highly dependent on the flake size. Investigations of $Ti_3C_2$ MXene nanowires (TMN) have not been reported, and the potential of TMN as a functional matrix as well as the measurement of pesticides in complex samples have never been explored. To the best of our knowledge, the TMN matrix has never been used for MALDI MSI.

In this work, we aim to prepare a novel $Ti_3C_2$ MXene nanowire (TMN) by a facile synthesis method and study the efficiency of TMN as a matrix for MALDI MS analysis of different kinds of pesticides in positive ion mode. The synthesis route for TMN is fast and green. The results showed that the TMN matrix possessed significant advantages, including high sensitivity, good dispersibility, low background noise, good salt tolerance, and good reproducibility for MALDI MS analysis of pesticides. The as-prepared TMN matrix was also successfully employed for the analysis of residual pesticides from traditional Chinese herb extracts. More importantly, the TMN film was synthesized through a simple hydrothermal self-assembly process by dropping an amount of TMN on an indium tin oxide (ITO) slide and drying at 60 ℃ without any chemical addition or modification. The TMN matrix is useful for MALDI-MSI to study the tissue-specific distribution of residual pesticides and various secondary metabolites in the intact root of the medicinal plant *P. quinquefolium* at a high resolution.

## 2 MATERIALS AND METHODS

2.1 Chemicals and materials CHCA, DHB, and trifluoroacetic acid (TFA) with a purity of >99% were purchased from Sigma-Aldrich (St. Louis, MO, USA). HPLC-grade ethanol was provided by Shanghai Aladdin Biochemical Technology Co., Ltd. (Shanghai, China). Methamidophos, isoprocarb, carbofuran, imidacloprid, diniconazole, and indoxacarb were purchased from Sigma Aldrich (St. Louis, MO, USA). HPLC-grade acetonitrile (ACN) and methanol (MeOH) were obtained from Merck (Darmstadt, Germany). Ultrapure water (18.2 MΩ cm, TYP-10 S, Taiping-M) was used in this study.

2.2 Synthesis of the materials Monolayer $Ti_3C_2$ was obtained from Beike 2D Materials Co., Ltd. (Jiangsu, China). TMN was prepared through a modified facile hydrothermal process, and the TMN film was synthesized by a self-assembly process. The detailed synthesis methods and measurements of material characterization are described in the Supplementary Information.

2.3 Sample preparation for MALDI MS analysis The TMN solution was prepared at a concentration of 1.0 mg/mL in water. DHB and CHCA were dissolved in 0.1% TFA buffer (ACN/water, 70 : 30, *V/V*) and 0.1% TFA buffer (ACN/MeOH/water, 70 : 25 : 5, *V/V*) at a concentration of 20 mg/mL, respectively. The graphene oxide (GO) solution was prepared at a concentration of 1.0 mg/mL in water. Three types of samples were prepared for MALDI MS analysis in this study. The first type included the standards of imidacloprid (100 mmol/L), carbofuran (100 mmol/L), methamidophos (100 mmol/L), diniconazole (100 mmol/L), indoxacarb (100 mmol/L), and isoprocarb (100 mmol/L) and their mixture. The second type was a mixture of standard methamidophos (100 mmol/L) and salts (NaCl 0 - 100 mmol/L) or proteins (BSA, 5 mg/mL). The third was a mixture of the six pesticide standards and the extracts of *Panax ginseng* (*P. ginseng*) roots or *Ginkgo biloba* leaves. The detailed method of sample preparation is described in Supplementary Information.

2.4 MALDI MSI of intact P. Quinquefolium root Intact *P. quinquefolium* roots were collected from Weihai Garden, China. After digging it out of the soil, the root of *P. quinquefolium* was spiked with diniconazole (10 mmol/L) and then flash-frozen in liquid nitrogen for 20 s and transferred to a −80℃ refrigerator. The frozen ginseng root was sectioned to a thickness of 10 μm on a cryo-cut microtome (Thermo CryoStar NX50 NOVPD, Bremen, Germany) at −20℃ and mounted onto the surface of TMN film-coated ITO glass slides. Then, all root sections were transferred to a closed container and vacuum dried for 10 min.

2.5 MALDI MS and MSI instrumentation All measurements were performed on a Rapiflex MALDI Tissuetyper™ TOF/TOF MS (Bruker Daltonics, Billerica, MA, USA) in positive mode. The MS instrument was equipped with a nitrogen laser and operated using a 355 nm Smartbeam II laser. The laser was fired at a frequency of 5 000 Hz, and raw mass spectra data were collected in the $m/z$ range of 100 - 700. MS calibration was performed using DHB and CHCA matrix ions (Bruker Daltonics, USA). For the detection of liquid samples, a 1 μL nanomaterial matrix solution was pipetted onto the stainless-steel ground sample plate and then completely air-dried, followed by the addition of 1 μL of analyte solution being dropped on top of the matrix and dried again. Meanwhile, the DHB and CHCA matrices were treated to the opposite order of matrix and sample addition following the principle of "sample-first and matrix-second" before MALDI MS tests were done. The dried plates were then detected by MALDI MS. The spatial resolution of MALDI MSI was set at 100 μm for *P. quinquefolium* root imaging.

2.6 Data analysis Data analysis was performed using FlexAnalysis Version 4.0 (Bruker Daltonik GmbH) and FlexImaging 5.0 (Bruker Daltonics, USA). MSI was analyzed and viewed using SCiLS Lab 2018b software (GmbH, Bremen, Germany). Database searching for metabolite identification was performed using the Human Metabolome Database, Metlin, Massbank, National Institute of Standards and Technology (NIST), and Lipidmaps, as previously described.

## 3 RESULTS AND DISCUSSION

3.1 Characterization of the TMN materials The TMN was prepared by a fast and green route, which is described in Section 2.2, and Supplementary Information. Ultraviolet—visible (UV—Vis) absorption was investigated to examine the optical characteristics of TMN (Fig. 1(a)). In comparison with $Ti_3C_2$ MXene, TMN exhibited a stronger absorption peak from 310 to 365 nm, which was attributed to the formation of $TiO_2$ nanoparticles and the $n-\pi^*$ transition of the C=O bond. The strong UV absorption of TMN at 355 nm is well matched with the typical wave-length of the laser (355 nm) available in MALDI MS, facilitating laser energy absorption and transfer, and qualifying TMN as a MALDI matrix. Fourier transform infrared (FT-IR) measurements were performed to characterize the functional groups associated with the surface of TMN (Fig. 1(b)). The FT-IR spectrum of TMN showed identical vibrations, including −OH at 3 254 $cm^{-1}$, C=O at 1 636 $cm^{-1}$, O—H at around 1 330 $cm^{-1}$, and C − F at 1 120 $cm^{-1}$. The vibration at 3 120 $cm^{-1}$ was ascribed to the − NH groups of TMN, revealing that the surfaces of the TMNs were passivated by −NH groups. Transmission electron microscopy (TEM) images showed that spindle-like TMNs were successfully prepared with an average size of 80 nm (Fig. 1(c)). The lattice of TMN is clearly displayed in the high-resolution TEM (HRTEM) image, exhibiting good crystallinity and a lattice space of 0.458 nm, assigned to the (004) plane of $Ti_3C_2$ (Fig. 1(c)). The HRTEM results indicated that TMN had the pristine structure of MXene owing to its relatively low synthesis temperature and the protection of surface-NH groups under a reducing environment created by ammonia. Elemental mapping showed homo-geneous distributions of Ti, C, O, and N, confirming that the spindle-like TMNs originated from $Ti_3C_2$ and the introduction of N and O during the TMN preparation process (Fig. 1(e)). Fig. 1(c) shows that TMN has a clear reduction in particle size compared with MXene, which may improve the electrical conductivity, and thus assist it as a useful matrix in MALDI MS.

The X-ray powder diffraction (XRD) pattern of TMN is shown in Fig. 1(d). A previous study reported that the XRD pattern of $Ti_3C_2$ presented typical peaks at 9.12° and 18.12° corresponding to the (002) and (004) peaks, respectively. As shown in Fig. 1(d), the (002) and (004) peaks of TMN shift to lower angles when compared with the untreated MXene, as previously reported, indicating the successful formation of TMN by interrupting the MXene flakes. The clear peak at around 25.5° (2θ) suggests the

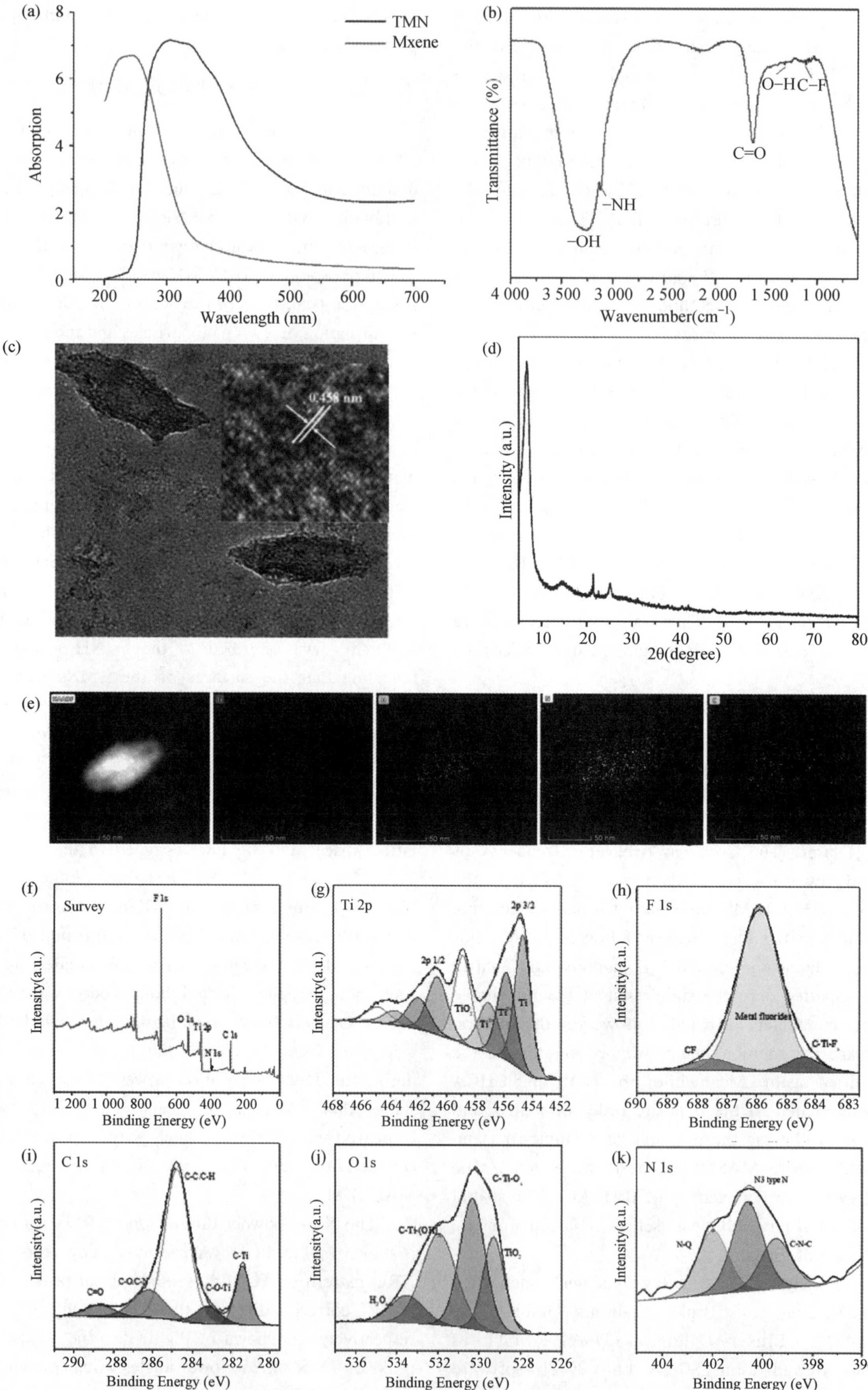


**Fig. 1** (a) UV—visible absorption spectra of the Mxene and TMN; (b) FT-IR spectrum of the TMN; (c) TEM and HRTEM (inset) images of the TMN; (d) XRD pattern of the TMN; (e) HRTEM image in dark field, and Ti, O, N, C element mapping image of TMN; (f) Survey XPS spectrum, and (g－k) high-resolution XPS spectra of (g) Ti 2p (h) F 1s, (i) C 1s, (g) O 1s and (k) N 1s for TMN.

formation of $TiO_2$ on the surface of TMN. The disappearance of the peaks at around 60° (2θ) indicates full delamination of MXene and no crystallographic stacking of the MXene sheets. X-ray photoelectron spectroscopy (XPS) was performed to investigate the chemical composition and bonding configuration of TMN (Fig. 1 (f)). The results confirmed the presence of C, Ti, O, F, and N Fig. 1(g-k). In the $Ti_{2p}$ spectrum displayed in Fig. 1(g), the predominant species found at 455.1 eV and 461.3 eV were Ti atoms including Ti, $Ti^{2+}$, $Ti^{3+}$ and $TiO_2$, which bonded to the surface terminations of O and F species (-Ox and -Fx). Fig. 1 (h) shows the $F_{1s}$ spectra of the TMN, revealing the C—F band (687.5 eV) in TMN. As showed in Fig. 1 (i), the $C_{1s}$ peaks at 288.6 eV, 286.1 eV, 284.8 eV, 283.4 eV, and 281.4 eV corresponded to C=O, C—O/C—N, C—C, C—O—Ti, and C—Ti band, respectively. Fig. 1(j) shows the $O_{1s}$ spectrum of TMN. According to the peak positions, $H_2O_{ads}$, C—Ti- $(OH)_x$, C—Ti-$O_x$, and $TiO_2$ are presumed to exist in this material. Fig. 1 (k) indicates the $N_{1s}$ XPS spectrum of the TMN, and reveals three peaks that may represent the N-Q (quaternary N), pyridinic C—N—C, and N3 type N. These results confirm the formation of polyaromatic structures containing C—N and C=N in the prepared TMN.

Taken together, the characterization results show that TMN was successfully prepared with an exfoliated and oxidized structure compared to $Ti_3C_2$. Abundant, highly active surface sites (-O, —NH, and —OH) were introduced into the TMN. In MALDI MS, the interaction between the matrix and analyte could affect the laser desorption ionization process. Multiple aromatic chromophores, —OH groups, and —NH groups not only modify the solubility and stability of the TMN but also make it a proton and electron donor or acceptor, thereby assisting it as a useful matrix in MALDI MS analysis.

3.2 Use of TMN as matrix for MALDI MS analysis of pesticides The performance of TMN as a matrix for MALDI MS analysis of the pesticide mixture was evaluated. Different types of typical pesticides with molecular weights <700 Da were selected as model analytes, including an organophosphorus pesticide (methamidophos), an organochlorine pesticide (isoprocarb), a carbamate pesticide (carbofuran), a neonicotinoid pesticide (imidacloprid), a triazole pesticide (diniconazole), and an oxadiazine pesticide (indoxacarb) (Table S1). The performance of different matrices (including TMN, GO, and two conventional organic matrices, DHB and CHCA, in the detection of the above typical pesticides were compared. Notably, GO, a two-dimensional carbon nanomaterial, was recently identified as a valuable matrix for MALDI; thus, it was also compared in this study.

The results are shown in Fig. 2, and the $m/z$ values of the feature peaks for the pesticides are listed in Table S1. From Fig. 2, TMN clearly displayed the best performance among the four tested matrices. With TMN as a MALDI MS matrix (Fig. 2 (a)), all six pesticides could be detected with the strongest peak intensities without background interference as cation adducts with sodium and/or potassium such as $[M+Na]^+$ and $[M+K]^+$ of methamidophos at $m/z$ 164.1 and 180.2, isoprocarb at $m/z$ 216.2 and 232.3, carbofuran at $m/z$ 244.2 and 260.3, imidacloprid at $m/z$ 278.7 and 294.8, diniconazole at $m/z$ 349.2 and 365.3, indoxacarb at $m/z$ 550.8 and 566.9, respectively. With TMN as a matrix, the $[M+H]^+$ signals were relatively suppressed compared to the $[M+Na]^+$ and $[M+K]^+$ signals, which is consistent with a previous study using $Ti_3C_2$ as a matrix. In the case of GO as a matrix (Fig. 2 (b)), peaks of $[M+Na]^+$ and $[M+K]^+$ of methamidophos at $m/z$ 164.1 and 180.2, $[M+K]^+$ of carbofuran at $m/z$ 260.3, $[M+Na]^+$ of imidacloprid and indoxacarb at $m/z$ 278.6 and 550.9 were observed, but no peaks corresponding to isoprocarb and diniconazole could be observed. As in a previous study, the GO matrix may suffer from aggregation, which largely limits its performance in MALDI MS analysis. Using the conventional organic matrix DHB, only the characteristic $[M+Na]^+$ and $[M+K]^+$ ions of carbofuran and indoxacarb at $m/z$ 244.2, 260.3, 550.8, and 566.9, respectively, and $[M+Na]^+$ ion of imidacloprid at $m/z$ 278.7 (Fig. 2 (c)) were observed. This could be because many background peaks made spectrum interpretation complicated and difficult. Finally, when using CHCA as a matrix (Fig. 2 (d)), only a weak peak of $[M+H]^+$ of imidacloprid at $m/z$ 256.7, and a peak of $[M+Na]^+$ of diniconazole at $m/z$ 365.3 were observed, while peaks for other compounds were absent, again indicating that the conventional organic matrix was not suitable for small molecule analysis.

Fig. S1 shows the MALDI MS spectra of TMN as a matrix without any analyte. From the MS spectra, it can be observed that no matrix peak existed in the low mass range in the positive ion mode when directly ionizing TMN, indicating that it is very suitable for the analysis of low mass pesticides. The distinct MALDI MS efficiency of TMN is mainly ascribed to its specific structure. The introduction of C—N and C=N bonds significantly enhanced the laser absorption and energy transfer ability of TMN. Meanwhile, the $N_{1s}$ XPS spectrum showed that TMN possessed N-Q (quaternary N), pyridinic C—N—C, and N3 type N. The pyridinic nitrogen atoms can act as Lewis bases and benefit from accepting protons. Furthermore, because $TiO_2$ is also known as a matrix for MALDI MS analysis, its existence in TMN could facilitate synergistic effects for MALDI MS detection of small compounds. In addition, the highly oxidized

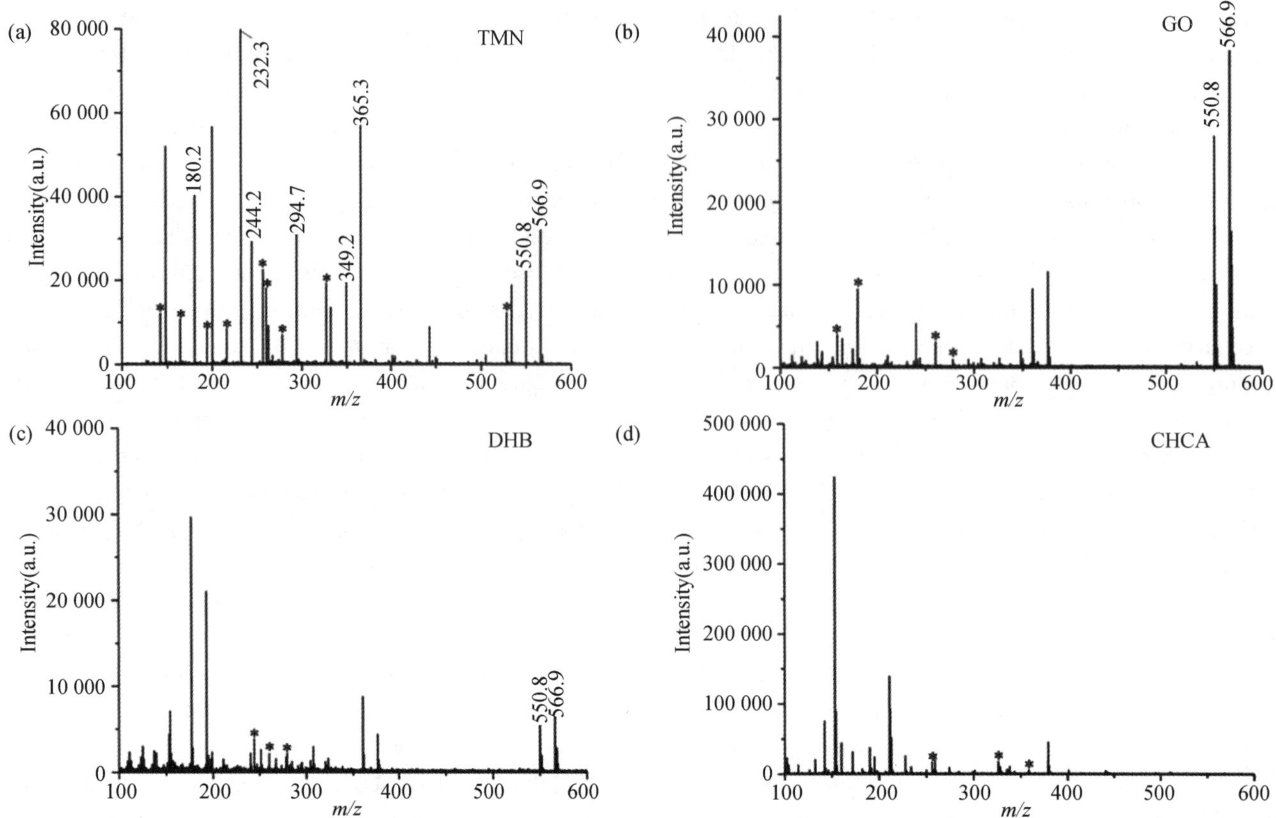


**Fig. 2 Comparison of different matrix for MALDI MS analysis of pesticides**

(a) using TMN, (b) using GO, (c) using DHB, and (d) using CHCA.

structure of TMN improves the band gap energy, dispersity, and laser energy absorption capacity. As a result, compared with GO, the signal response of the pesticide molecule based on the TMN matrix was higher. This indicates that TMN is a promising platform for MALDI MS analysis of diverse pesticides.

3.3 Analytical performance of TMN matrix Assay validation of TMN as a matrix for MALDI MS was performed with the selected analytes in the positive ion mode. The concentrations of pesticides loaded onto the TMN matrix decreased until their S/N ratios were below 3. Table S1 displays the limits of detection (LODs; signal-to-noise ratio (S/N) = 3) for typical pesticides. The LODs for all pesticides were at part per trillion (ppt) or even sub-ppt levels (0.1 - 500 pg/mL), which are much lower than the maximum residue limits (MRLs) reported in the European Union pesticides database. Such a high sensitivity makes screening possible with a very small amount of liquid sample, that is, even a single drop of liquid sample.

The reproducibility was investigated using diniconazole as a model analyte and GO and TMN as the matrix separately. When using GO as the matrix, the analysis of pesticides obtained shot-to-shot relative standard deviations (RSDs; $n=18$) of 28.5% - 38.5% and sample-to-sample RSDs ($n=15$) of 29.8%- 33.8% (Table S1). For the TMN situation, the analysis had a better reproducibility with the shot-to-shot RSDs ($n=18$) of 5.6%- 10.5% and sample-to-sample RSDs ($n = 15$) of 4.5% - 9.5% (Table S1). Reproducibility is a topic in MALDI MS analysis, because the co-crystallization process of analytes with a conventional organic matrix could result in "hot spots." Here, the result showed that with TMN as a matrix, the problem of "hot spots" could be avoided.

Biological samples usually contain high concentrations of salt, which leads to decreased ionization efficiency and analyte signal inhibition in MALDI MS analysis. The salt tolerance of TMN in positive ion mode was tested using methamidophos ($m/z$ 180.2, $[M+K]^+$) as a model analyte, which was diluted with a 0 - 100 mmol/L NaCl solution for further analysis. As shown in Fig. 3a, as the concentration of NaCl increased, the signal intensity of the methamidophos decreased slightly. When the concentration of the NaCl solution was increased to 100 mmol/L, a high S/N ratio of methamidophos ($m/z$ 180.2, $[M+K]^+$) could still be detected. Protein endurance is also crucial for MALDI MS analysis of complex biological samples. When 5 mg/mL BSA was added, the peak intensity of methamidophos did not change significantly (Fig. 3b).

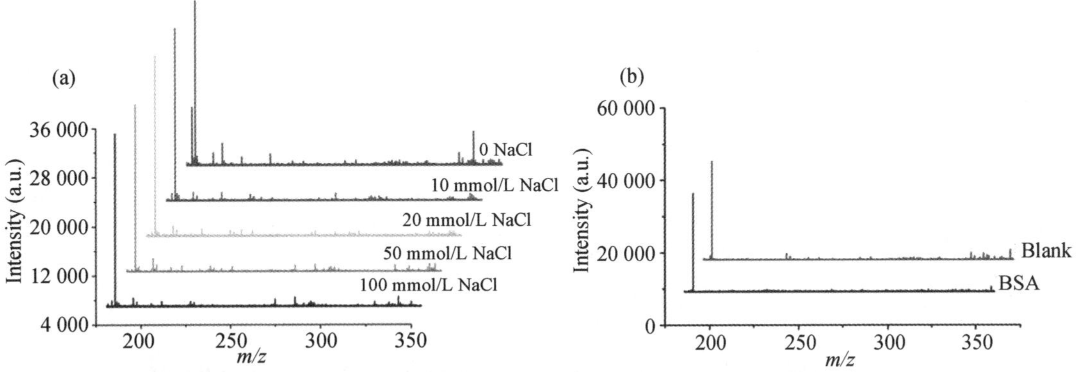


**Fig. 3 MALDI MS spectra of methamidophos ($m/z$ 180.2, $[M+K]^+$) analyzed using TMN as the matrix in positive ion mode with (a) no additional salt and 10, 20, 50, and 100 mmol/L NaCl, and (b) no additional protein and 5 mg/mL BSA**

The suitability of TMN as a matrix was further tested for the identification and screening of toxic pesticides in two traditional Chinese medicines (*P. ginseng* and *G. biloba*). A mixture of six pesticides (100 mmol/L) was spiked into the prepared extracts of *P. ginseng* and *G. biloba*, and analyzed. As shown in Fig. 4a - b, the signal peaks of the six pesticides were detected and marked with asterisks, and the detailed MS peaks according to $[M+Na]^+$ or $[M+K]^+$ are shown in Table S2. To accurately quantify the pesticide, 10 ng/mL D-fenthion (Isotopic) was added to a 0 - 50 ng/mL diniconazole solution, and a calibration curve was plotted using the ion intensity ratio of D-fenthion ($[M+K]^+$, $m/z$ 318.2) to diniconazole ($[M+K]^+$, $m/z$ 365.3). As shown in Fig. 4c, the regression equation was $y = 0.1367x + 0.8135$ with good linearity ($R^2 > 0.99$), which could meet the analytical requirements of pesticides in biological samples.

Therefore, TMN could be utilized as a matrix for MALDI MS analysis to detect pesticides in a small amount of liquid sample with high salinity and protein endurance without additional pretreatment. Overall, these results demonstrate that TNM is an efficient matrix for MALDI MS analysis of low-mass pesticides.

3.4 Visualization of spatial distribution of pesticides and secondary metabolites in P. Quinquefolium root

Insights into the distribution of pesticide residues in plants are of utmost importance for understanding the fate of pesticides. A visualization strategy for the tracking of pesticides is needed. However, the applications of traditional organic matrices (such as DHB and CHCA) in MALDI MSI to image small-molecule pesticides are limited owing to the issue of enormous noise interference. In addition, the various sizes of conventional organic matrix crystals and the homogeneity of matrix spraying across the specimen by organic matrices will largely affect the spatial resolution of MALDI MSI.

Recently, the capability of nanomaterial matrix-assisted MALDI MSI for the visualization of the spatial distribution of small molecule metabolites in tissues has attracted attention owing to its matrix-free application and highly reduced background noise in the low $m/z$ range. Since TMN exhibited superior ability for MALDI MS analysis of various pesticides in liquid samples, the performance of the TMN self-assembly film as a matrix of MALDI MSI was evaluated. The root of *P. quinquefolium* with diniconazole residual was employed as a model to detect the feasibility of TMN assembly film as a MALDI MSI matrix because it is a popular herbal product containing various small bioactive compounds and is vulnerable to pesticide contamination. Without the matrix spraying procedure, the homogeneous TMN film addresses the challenge of traditional organic matrices with outstanding advantages. The results demonstrated high-resolution mapping of small secondary metabolites and pesticides simultaneously in the roots of *P. quinquefolium* by TMN-film-assisted MALDI MSI.

Fig. 5 shows the distinct tissue-specific distributions of the relative abundance of various endogenous compounds (e.g., amino acids, sugars, and fatty acids) and xenobiotic compounds (pesticides) in *P. quinquefolium* roots obtained by TMN film-assisted MALDI MSI in positive ion mode. For amino acids, alanine ($[M+Na]^+$, $m/z$ 112.1) with the highest intensity was relatively homogenously distributed across the root, whereas serine ($[M+Na]^+$, $m/z$ 128.1) was mainly accumulated in the phloem and medulla of the root (Fig. 5b - c). The spatial distributions of aspartic acid ($[M+K]^+$, $m/z$ 172.1) and glutamate acid ($[M+K]^+$, $m/z$ 186.1) were similar and mainly accumulated in the phloem of the root (Fig. 5d and Fig. 5f). In the case of arginine ($m/z$ 175.2), it was mainly distributed in the xylem (Fig. 5e). The plant growth hormone salicylic acid ($[M+K]^+$, $m/z$ 177.1) and citric acid ($[M+K]^+$, $m/z$ 193.1) were visualized in *P. quinquefolium* root, with the former mainly distributed in the cambium and phloem, and the latter in the medulla and xylem (Fig. 5g-h). Choline ($[M+H]^+$, $m/z$ 105.1), an important precursor of

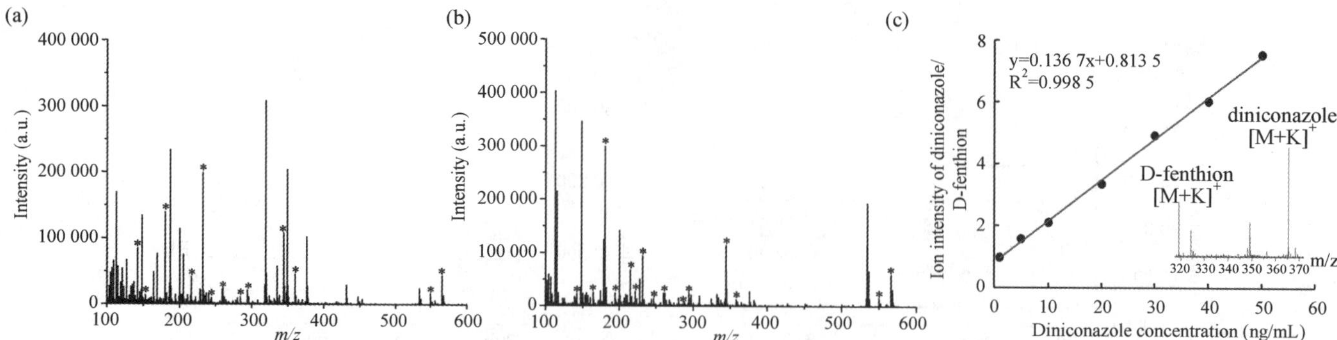


**Fig. 4 MALDI MS spectrum of six pesticides in (a) an extraction of *P. ginseng* sample and (b) an extraction of *G. biloba* sample using TMN as the matrix. (c) Calibration curves used for the quantitative determination of diniconazole was obtained by plotting the ion intensity ratio of D-fenthion ([M+K]$^+$, *m/z* 318.2) to diniconazole ([M+K]$^+$, *m/z* 365.3)**

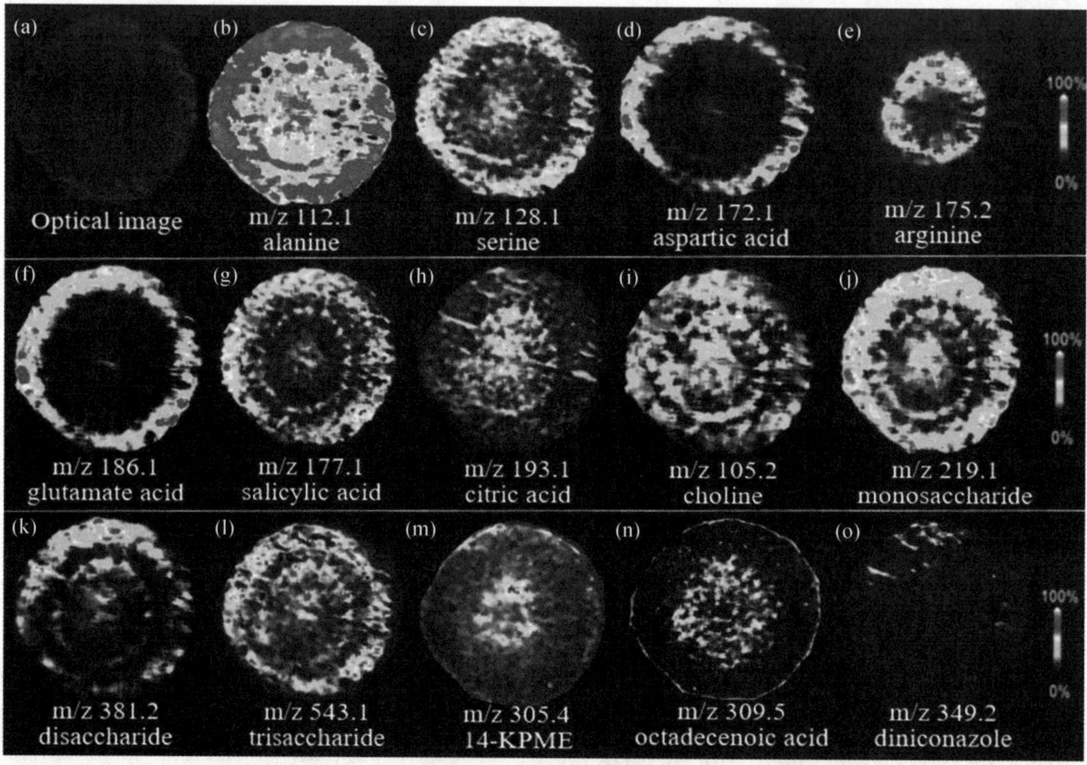


**Fig. 5 Spatial distributions of pesticide and endogenous metabolites observed in *P. quinquefolium* root in positive ion mode using TMN self-assembly film as matrix. The step size is 100 μm. The colored bars represent the relative signal intensity**

The above *m/z* images were obtained from the same *P. quinquefolium* root. (a) Optical scan image of *P. quinquefolium* root slice; (b) *m/z* 112.1 as alanine; (c) *m/z* 128.1 as serine; (d) *m/z* 172.1 as aspartic acid; (e) *m/z* 175.2 as arginine; (f) *m/z* 186.1 as glutamate acid; (g) *m/z* 177.1 as salicylic acid; (h) *m/z* 193.1 as citric acid; (i) *m/z* 105.2 as choline; (j) *m/z* 219.1 as monosaccharide; (k) *m/z* 381.2 as disaccharide; (l) *m/z* 543.1 as trisaccharide; (m) *m/z* 305.4 as 14-keto pentadecanoic methyl ester(14-KPME); (n) *m/z* 309.5 as octadecenoic acid; (o) *m/z* 349.2 as diniconazole.

glycerophosphatidylcholine (lecithin) synthesis, was observed throughout the root (Fig. 5i). Highly abundant ions of monosaccharide ([M+K]$^+$, *m/z* 219.1), disaccharide ([M+K]$^+$, *m/z* 381.2), and trisaccharide([M+K]$^+$, *m/z*543.1) were mainly observed in the medulla, cambium, and phloem (Fig. 5j-l). Additionally, disaccharide ([M+K]$^+$, *m/z* 381.2) was co-localized with trisaccharide ([M+K]$^+$, *m/z*543.1). In the case of fatty acids, 14-keto pentadecanoic methyl ester (14-KPME) ([M+K]$^+$, *m/z* 305.4) and octadecenoic acid ([M+Na]$^+$, *m/z*309.5) with relatively low intensity were observed in the medulla and xylem, respectively (Fig. 5m - n). One MS image of diniconazole ([M+Na]$^+$, *m/z* 349.3) was clearly acquired (Fig. 5o), indicating that the distribution of low-mass pesticides can be visualized by TMN film-assisted MALDI MSI.

Various analytical methods have been developed for the

detection of metabolites in plant tissues, such as a combination of laser microdissection and HPLC MS analysis, which usually involve complex processes. However, TMN film-assisted MALDI MSI detection provided a much more convenient analysis method for plant tissue-specific metabolite analysis. The localization of endogenous compounds was related to the chemical information of the plant, contributing to the understanding of particular biological functions and the biosynthetic pathway of secondary metabolites in plant tissue. The high concentration of various bioactive small molecules (e. g., amino acids) in phloem supports the hypothesis that some secondary metabolites are mainly in the most vulnerable parts of the plant to defend against insects. The localization maps of endogenous compounds were also useful for optimizing the component-specific extraction of *P. quinquefolium*.

Some pesticides have been identified to interact with endogenous metabolites in plants, which could regulate the activity and expression of endogenous metabolites. It is vital to simultaneously understand the distribution of pesticides and the distribution of endogenous metabolites to regulate their uptake and distribution by structural design, facilitating fewer negative effects on ecosystem pollution. From these observations, TMN-film-assisted MALDI MSI can be considered a powerful tool for visualizing tissue specific distributions of secondary metabolites and pesticides in complex biological samples owing to its high sensitivity and broad molecular coverage. In view of the potential of TMN film-assisted MALDI MSI for a *P. quinquefolium* root, this approach will open new paths for deeper insights into the interactions between endogenous metabolites and pesticides. Compared with the available methods, this simple method is available for most laboratories without matrix spray or tedious nanomaterial preparation processes, which may contribute to the wider application of this strategy.

## 4 CONCLUSION

In summary, a novel TMN was successfully prepared as an effective MALDI matrix for pesticide analysis and in situ imaging of biological samples. The TMN matrix demonstrated good performance in pesticide analysis, including simplicity, high throughput, good repeatability, high selectivity, and sensitivity. The LOD for each selected pesticide by this method was much lower than the MRLs, as required in the European Union pesticides database. More importantly, the results demonstrate the practical application of this method by quantitatively detecting pesticides in traditional Chinese herbal products. Furthermore, the application of TMN assembly film can avoid inhomogeneous matrix deposition and provide high MS signal sensitivity and stability for MALDI MS imaging of secondary metabolites in plant tissues. Successful MALDI MS imaging of intact *P. quinquefolium* roots in positive ion modes revealed tissue-specific distributions of various endogenous metabolites (e. g., amino acids and saccharides, fatty acids, alkaloids, and plant hormones) and xenobiotic pesticides. This method may provide guidelines for the precise use of agrochemicals to avoid uncontrolled spread and off-target applications. The TMN-assisted MALDI-MS method has potential applications in the field of pesticide residue detection.

[马春霞,黄璐琦,等. Chemosphere, 2022, 286(2022): 131826.]

# Genome sequencing reveals chromosome fusion and extensive expansion of genes related to secondary metabolism in *Artemisia argyi*

## 1 INTRODUCTION

*Artemisia* is a large plant genus in the Asteraceae family that comprises approximately 500 species and subspecies. These species are mainly distributed in the temperate northern hemisphere regions and most are widely used in various fields such as herb, food, cosmetics, spices, forage and ornamentals. In 2015, the discovery of artemisinin, an antimalarial ingredient isolated from *Artemisia annua*, won the Nobel Prize in Physiology or Medicine, drawing global attention to study other species of the genus *Artemisia*.

Previous cytogenetic studies have contributed to the knowledge of the systematic and evolutionary relationship within the *Artemisia* species. Three basic chromosome numbers were reported in the genus based on numerous chromosome counts from approximately 373 taxa; $x=9$ is the most common (85.6%), and $x = 8$ is less frequent (9.7%). Both basic chromosome numbers exhibited polyploid series, with known levels up to 16x for $x=9$ and hexaploid for $x=8$. In addition, a chromosome number of $2n=34$ occurs in a few species, such as *Artemisia vulgaris*, *Artemisia rubipes* and *Artemisia argyi*, suggesting that a third base number $x = 17$ may exist. The diversity of chromosome number and polyploidy level results in a 7.4-fold variation in *Artemisia* genome size, from 4.11 Gb of *A. dolosa* ($2n=2x=18$) to 30.45 Gb of *A. medioxima* ($2n=16$ $x=144$). The chromosome numbers observed in *Artemisia* species suggest that, in addition to polyploidization, variation in basic chromosome numbers may also play an important role in the evolution of the genus. Chromosomal fusion and fission are considered the predominant causes for the evolution of basic chromosome numbers in animal and plant kingdoms. For example, the origin of human chromosome 2 was derived from head-to-head fusion of two ancestral ape chromosomes. Chromosome fusion affects genetic diversity and environmental adaptation of *Heliconius*. Large-scale chromosomal fission/fusion events promote the speciation of the wild *Morus notabilis* ($x = 6$) and the cultivated *Morus alba* ($x=14$). There are far more examples of chromosome fusion that could be discussed. In *Artemisia*, fluorechrome-banded karyotypes of *A. vulgaris* provide some evidence that a centric (Robertsonian) chromosome fusion may also occur and cause the reduction of its basic chromosome number from $x=9$ to $x=8$. However, despite a wide knowledge of cytological studies on *Artemisia*, the role of chromosome fusion in basic chromosome numbers variation of *Artemisia* has not been fully verified and highly valued.

Among the *Artemisia* genus, *A. argyi* (also called 'Chinese mugwort') is one of the well-known species and is widely distributed in Asian countries, such as China, Korea and Japan. The dried leaves of *A. argyi*, known in Chinese as 'Aiye', have been used as TCM (traditional Chinese medicine) for about 3 000 years. *A. argyi* was first recorded in 'Shi Jing' (a famous China classical literature) near 1 100 BC and was first recognized as medicine in 'Wu Shi Er Bing Fang' in the Han Dynasty (A. D. 220). In addition, the medical applications of *A. argyi* were also listed in many other classic clinical and medical literature such as 'Huang Di Nei Jing', 'Ming Yi Bie Lu', 'Jin Gui Yao Lve' and 'Ben Cao Gang Mu'. In the long-term practice of traditional Chinese medicine, *A. argyi* is believed to have the properties of bitterness, warmth and pungency and has the effects of dispelling cold and dampness, warming menstruation, haemostasis, and preventing abortion. Recent pharmacological studies have demonstrated that *A. argyi* also exhibits anti-inflammatory, anti-allergic, antimicrobial, antioxidant and anticancer activities. Clearly, *A. argyi* has a long history of application and is still widely used in clinical practice. In 2020, the annual value of the *A. argyi* market was over 40 billion RMB, making it the largest herbal medicine industry chain in China. In addition, acupuncture and moxibustion (world-renowned medicinal products derived from *A. argyi*) were recognized as the World Intangible Cultural Heritage in 2010, and traditional Chinese medicine/therapy (including moxibustion) has been recommended by WHO (World Health Organization) in 2019. Therefore, acupuncture and moxibustion have successfully spread worldwide as a reliable alternative therapy for multiple diseases. As the major source of moxibustion, *A. argyi* is also becoming increasingly popular worldwide.

These amazing economic and medicinal values of *A. argyi* are due to the large number of secondary metabolites in its leaves, which include volatile oils, flavonoids, terpenoids, phenolic acids and other compounds. More than 100 nature metabolites have been identified in *A. argyi* volatile oil, primarily comprising monoterpenes, sesquiterpenes and their derivatives. These metabolites contribute to the aromatic odours of *A. argyi* and pharmacological activities against asthma, eczema and cough. *A. argyi* leaves are also rich in flavonoids, including flavonoids, flavonols, flavonols and chalcone. Among them, eupatilin, jaceosidin, apigenin, luteolin, quercetin, and naringin are representative components and have been proven to have biological activities for preventing oxidative damage, inflammation, allergies and tumours. Remarkably, eupatilin has been confirmed as the pharmacodynamic component of Stillen® (DA-9601) which has been approved as a phytomedicine for gastritis in Korea. Thereby, it is necessary to investigate the biosynthesis pathways of these active secondary metabolites in *A. argyi*.

However, despite the huge economic and medical value, *A. argyi*'s evolution and the molecular basis of the biosynthesis of the abundant active ingredients are rarely reported due to the lack of a high-quality reference genome. Here, we constructed a chromosome-level genome of *A. argyi* through an integrative approach combining PacBio sequencing (SMRT sequencing high fidelity, HiFi) and high-throughput chromatin conformation capture (Hi-C) technology. In addition, whole-genome duplication (WGD) events and expansion and contraction of gene families in the *A. argyi* genome were also investigated through phylogenetic and comparative genomic analysis. Furthermore, pivotal candidate genes involved in the biosynthesis of terpenoids and flavonoids were also identified based on genomic and transcriptomic analyses. Briefly, as the first chromosome-level genome in *Artemisia*, this reference genome will provide valuable resources for exploring the genetic and evolutionary biology of *A. argyi* and other *Artemisia* species.

## 2 RESULTS

*Artemisia argyi* genome sequencing, assembly and annotation

Qichun (Hubei Province) is the authentic production area of *A. argyi* in China. Based on preliminary resource evaluation, a highly volatile oil- and flavonoid-producing *A. argyi* cultivar, 'Xiang Ai' from Qichun, was selected for *de novo* genome sequencing and assembly (Figure 1a). The somatic cells of *A. argyi* contained 34 chromosomes by the cytological observation method (Figure 1b) and the genome size was approximately 7.44 Gb by flow cytometry estimation (Figure S1). A 21-mer analysis of genome survey sequencing shows that *A. argyi* is a tetraploid, with a monoploid genome size of ~1.96 Gb and a whole-genome size of ~7.84 Gb (Figure S2). Compared to 12 other genome-sequenced species in Asteraceae (*Erigeron breviscapus*, *Helianthus annuus*, *Lactuca sativa*, *Artemisia annua*, *Cynara cardunculus*, *Conyza canadensis*, *Chrysanthemum nankingense*, *Chrysanthemum seticuspe*, *Carthamus tinctorius*, *Mikania micrantha*, *Tanacetum cinerariifolium*, *Taraxacum kok-saghyz* Rodin), *A. argyi* features the largest and most complex genome. It was also estimated that the genome of *A. argyi* had a relatively high heterozygosity (2.36%) and a large proportion of repetitive sequences (75.86%) (Figure S2, Table S1), which increased the challenge of *de novo* assembly of this genome.

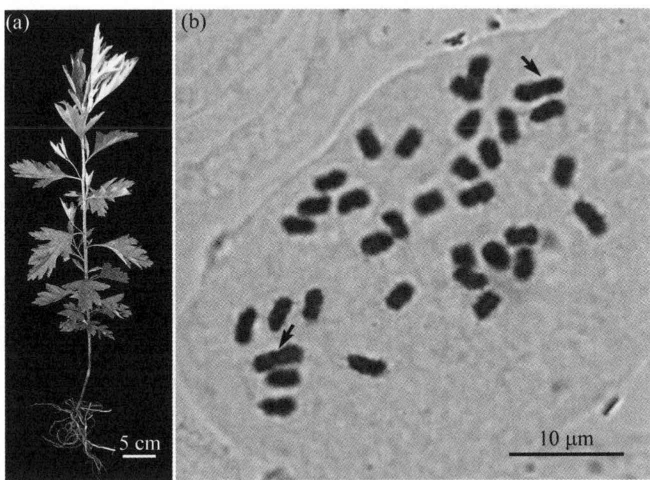


**Figure 1 Plant morphology and somatic chromosome number of *A. argyi***

(a) A plant of *A. argyi* cultivar 'Xiang Ai'. (b) The karyotype of *A. argyi*.

To overcome the assembly challenging of the *A. argyi* genome caused by polyploidy, high heterozygosity and repetitive sequences, an integrated strategy was adopted by combining Illumina short paired-end reads, PacBio long high-fidelity (HiFi) reads, and Hi-C sequencing (Figure S3). A total of 161.3 Gb of PacBio circular consensus sequencing (CCS) reads with an average length of 15 154 bp and 19-fold whole-genome coverage was obtained from 7 flow cells of the PacBio Sequel II platform (Table S2). These CCS reads were assembled into an initial genome with a total length of approximately 8.03 Gb, containing 10 274 contigs, with an N50 of 8.32 Mb and a longest contig of 43.52 Mb (Table S3) by Hifiasm assembly. Subsequently, a total of 407 Gb clean Hi-C paired-end reads were used for scaffold extension and chromosome mounting (Table S4). With the assistance of Hi-C sequence data, the assembled contigs were anchored to 34 super-scaffolds, which covered 91.4% (7.34 Gb) of the size of the assembled genome (Tables S5 and S4). In summary, the chromosome-level *A. argyi* genome assembly has a total size of approximately 8.03 Gb, containing 12 449 scaffolds, with a scaffold N50 size of 206.40 Mb and a contig N50 of 6.25 Mb (Table 1 and Figure 2a).

**Table 1 Major features of the *Artemisia argyi* genome assembly**

| Assembly feature | Size/Number | |
|---|---|---|
| | Hifi assembled | Hi-C Anchored |
| Assembly size (Mb) | 8 029.08 | 8 030.38 |
| GC (%) | 35.46 | 35.46 |
| Repeat (%) | 73.59 | 73.59 |
| Number of scaffolds | — | 12 449 |
| Scaffold N50 size (Mb) | — | 206.40 |
| Scaffold N90 size (Mb) | — | 180.30 |
| Longest scaffolds (Mb) | — | 342.73 |
| Number of contigs | 10 274 | 15 063 |
| Contig N50 size (Mb) | 8.32 | 6.25 |
| Contig N90 size (Mb) | 1.46 | 0.64 |
| Longest contig (Mb) | 43.52 | 40.67 |

To assess the completeness of the assembly of *A. argyi* genome, the Illumina short reads and PacBio isoform sequencing (Iso-Seq) data were aligned to the assembled genome, resulting in high mapping rates of 99.89% and 99.70%, respectively (Table S6). Furthermore, benchmarking universal single-copy orthologue (BUSCO) analysis was also employed to assess the quality of the assembly. The obtained results showed that 95.5% (2 221 out of 2 236 BUSCOs) of the BUSCOs were completely present in the *A. argyi* genome (2 192 of the 2 236 BUSCO genes were complete) (Table S7). In short, these results demonstrated that the assembled *A. argyi* genome had high completeness.

We further applied a combination of ab initio and homologybased approaches to identify the repetitive sequences. A total of 73.59% of the assembly was identified as repetitive sequences, including 1.37% DNA transposons, 1.29% interspersed nuclear elements (LINEs) and 39.08% long terminal repeats (LTRs) (Table S8). In addition, higher ratio of *Gypsy* than *Copia* elements was observed, each accounting for 24.47% and 13.80% of the genome, respectively, which is similar to the genomic characteristics of other Asteraceae species such as sunflower, stevia, and lettuce. Next, combined with RNA-seq and full-length transcriptome data generated from seven different tissues and organs (root, rhizome, stem and leaf A-D) (Data S1), a total of 279 294 high-quality protein-coding genes were annotated for this tetraploid-resolved genome. We attempted to separate the subgenomes by using *K*-mers to examine the potential bias in genome characteristics. However, we failed to distinguish homologous chromosome pairs into distinct A and B subgenomes using the enrichment pattern of *K*-mers. Therefore, we selected the longest chromosome from each pair of homologous chromosomes as one set of chromosomes of *A. argyi*, except for chromosome 10, because it was fused from chromosomes 8 and 9 (We address this further below). This monoploid genome contained 64 354 genes. We also counted the genes in contigs that were not anchored into chromosomes and 29 534 genes were obtained. The gene number ranks *A. argyi* as the most gene-enriched species among the sequenced Asteraceae plants, and this gene number is about 2.5 times the average number of genes (36 795) reported for plant genomes. The average lengths of gene and coding DNA sequence (CDS) were 3 416 and 1 256 bp, respectively, with an average of 5 exons and 4 introns per gene (Table S9). A total of 93.87% and 93.98% of these genes were functionally annotated in the Nr and TrEMBL databases, and 72.30% of the genes were classified by Gene Ontology (GO) terms, and 31.13% of the genes were annotated to Kyoto Encyclopedia of Genes and Genomes (KEGG) pathways (Table S10). In addition, 1033 miRNAs, 19784 tRNAs, 310 rRNAs and 3 606 SnRNAs were identified in the *A. argyi* genome (Table S11).

Comparative genomic analysis of *A. argyi* To gain insights into the evolution of the *A. argyi* genome, a comparative genomic analysis was performed using *Arabidopsis thaliana*, *Vitis vinifera* and six other Asteraceae species (*A. annua*, *C. nankingense*, *E. breviscapus*, *H. annus*, *L. sativa* and *C. tinctorius*). According to the sequence homology among these nine species, 93 888 protein-coding genes (including 64 354 genes in the monoploid genome of *A. argyi* and 29 534 genes in scattered contigs) comprised 3 384 single-copy orthologues, 14 817 multiple-copy orthologues, 18 902 unique paralogues, 36 066 other paralogues and 20 719 unclustered genes (Figure 2b and Table S12). These genes were clustered into 27 915 gene families; among them, 5 321 (19.06%) gene families contained 18 902 unique genes in *A. argyi* (Table S13). GO enrichment analysis showed that the biological functions of these specific gene families were enriched in RNA-directed DNA polymerase activity (GO: 0003964), DNA polymerase activity (GO: 0034061), nucleotidyltransferase activity (GO: 0016779) and zinc ion binding (GO: 0008270) (Figure S5 and Data S2). Meanwhile, KEGG enrichment results showed that these genes were mainly enriched in pathways involved in phagosome (ko04145), protein processing in endoplasmic reticulum (ko04141), mismatch repair (ko03430) and terpenoid backbone biosynthesis (ko00900) (Figure S6 and Data S3). Furthermore, gene family evolution analysis showed that 40.04% (11 177/27 915) of the gene families were expanded and 14.15% (3 951/27 915) of the gene families were contracted in the *A. argyi* genome (Figure 2b). Compared to the other six species in the Asteraceae family, whose contracted genes were larger than the expanded genes, the number of expanded gene families in *A. argyi* was approximately three times that of the contracted gene families. GO enrichment analysis indicated that the functions of the expanded genes were significantly related in terms of binding, catalytic activity, photosynthetic electron transport in photosystem II and oxidoreductase activity (Figure S7 and Data S4). KEGG analysis revealed that expanded genes were enriched in photosynthesis, DNA replication, homologous recombination and several secondary metabolic pathways (Figure S8 and Data S5). In particular, several markedly expanded genes were identified including *PsbA* genes (encoded photosystem II P680 reaction center protein D1) in PSII, replication factor A1 (*RPA1*) participating in homologous recombination and DNA replication, and heat shock protein genes (*HSPs*, *HSP40*, *HSP70*, *HSP73*) and terpene synthase genes (*TPSs*) (Table S14). It is well known that these genes are related to plant growth and stress responses. Given the ability of *A. argyi* to adapt to a wide variety of habitat conditions, these largely expanded genes may contribute to its successful expansion across the landscape and rapid growth.

Subsequently, we constructed a time-calibrated phylogenetic tree by using a concatenated sequence alignment of 944 singlecopy orthologues shared by these nine species. These results verified the close evolutionary relationship between *A. argyi* and *A. annua*, and the divergence time of *A. argyi* and *A. annua* was approximately 7.4 million years ago (Mya). The most recent common ancestor (MRCA) of *A. argyi* and *A. annua* diverged from the MRCA of *C. nankingense* ~9.3 Mya, which together diverged from the MRCA of *E. breviscapus* ~41.3 Mya and further from the MRCA of *L. sativa* ~52.2 Mya (Figure 2b).

Whole-genome duplication (WGD) is considered the

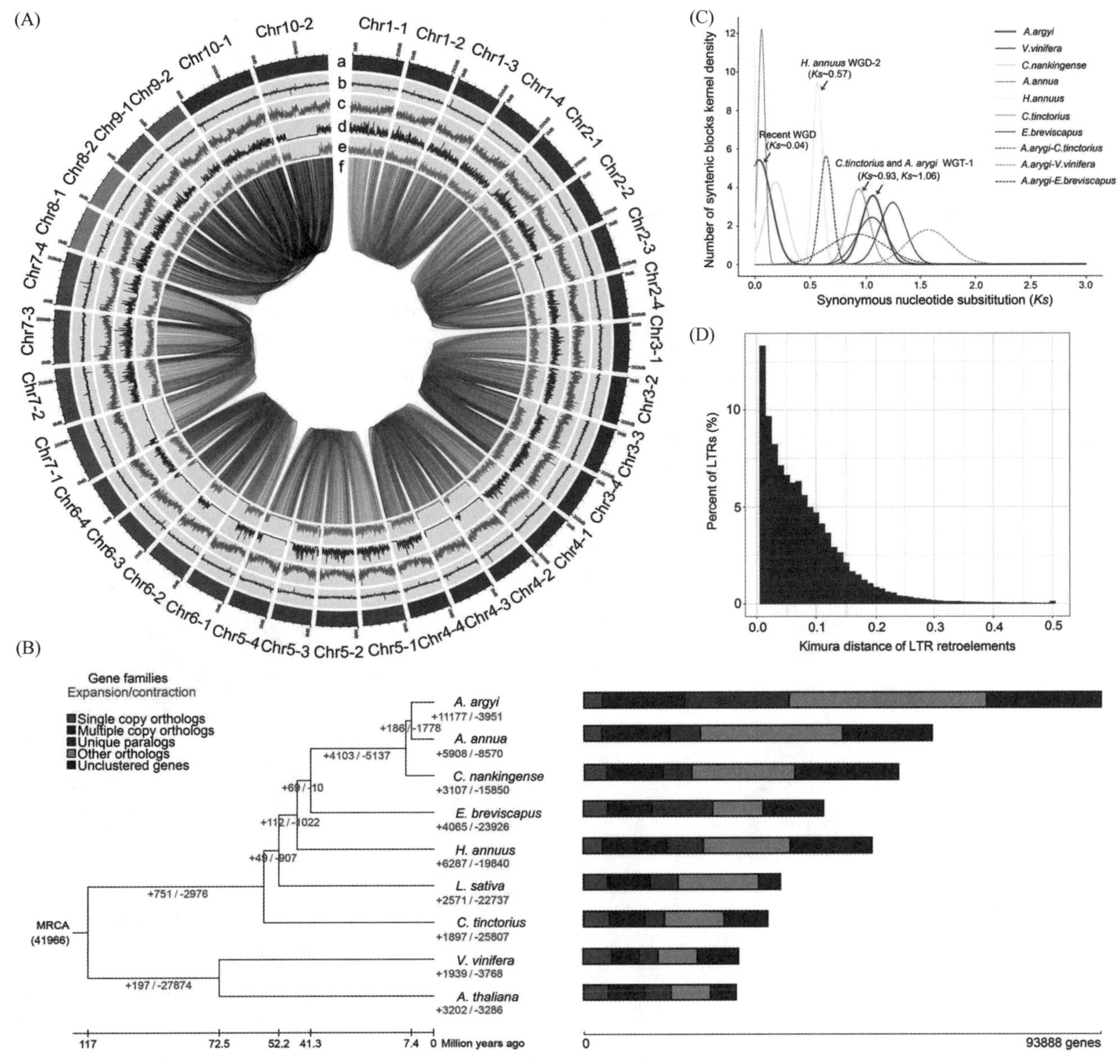


**Figure 2 Assembly and genomic features of the *A. argyi* genome**

(A) The circos diagram of *A. argyi* draft. (a) the genomic landscape of the 34 *A. argyi* pseudochromosomes. (b) the density of gene. (c) repeat coverage. (d) the density of SNP. (e) the density of Indel. f. synteny relationship between pseudochromosomes. (B) Phylogenetic tree of seven species from the Asteraceae based on the information of single copy genes. And Arabidopsis and *V. vinifera* were used as the outgroup. The expanded gene families were marked with green and the contracted gene families were marked with red. (C) The *Ks* distributions of paralogous genes in *A. argyi*, *A. annua*, *C. nankingense*, *H. annuus*, *E. breviscapus* and *C. tinctorius* of the Asteraceae, and the eudicot species *V. vinifera*. (D) Kimula distance of LTR retroelements.

main factor driving genome evolution and expansion. In *A. argyi*, the WGD events were examined by distributions of synonymous substitutions (*Ks*) within genes in syntenic blocks compared with six other species (*A. annua*, *C. nankingense*, *H. annuus*, *E. breviscapus*, *C. tinctorius* and *V. vinifera*). The distribution of *Ks* for the paralogous genes of the *A. argyi* genome showed two prominent peaks at ~0.04 and ~1.06, indicating that *A. argyi* has experienced two rounds of WGD (recent WGD and WGT-1) events. We further estimated that the most recent WGD event of *A. argyi* occurred at ~2.2 Mya, which was a species-specific duplication event and did not occur in the genomes of *E. breviscapus*, *H. annuus* and *C. tinctorius*, but occurred in *A. annua* and *C. nankingense*. The WGT-1 event in *A. argyi* was a conserved whole-genome triplication event shared with *E. breviscapus*, *C. tinctorius* and other Asterid-II plants, occurring at approximately 62.9 Mya. Moreover, the *Ks* dot plot of retained paralogues in *A. argyi* genome also supported the occurrence of the WGD events (Figure 3a). Based on the *Ks* value (~0.6) of orthologous peaks for *A. argyi* and *E. breviscapus*, we predicted that their divergence time was ~38.2 Mya, which was close to the phylogenetic results. The relative age (Kimura distance) computed for LTR retroelements also indicates a recent increasing transposon activity (Figure 2d). The most recent WGD event and the recent outbreak of LTRs in *A. argyi* may be one of the most important reasons for its large genome size.

Chromosome fusion in the *A. argyi* genome Synteny analysis showed that the 34 pseudochromosomes of *A. argyi* comprised 10 homologous groups, of which seven groups each had four sets of monoploid chromosomes, and three groups had two chromosomes in each (Figure S9). Moreover, each of the four chromosomes in the 1 - 7 chromosome groups can be divided into two subgroups according to the gene synteny analysis, which indicates that *A. argyi* is an allotetraploid (Figure S10), and this result was also consistent with that of survey analysis. Importantly, the length of chromosome 10 was almost the sum of the lengths of chromosomes 8 and 9 (Figure 3a and Table S5), and intragenome synteny analysis showed that chromosomes 8 and 9 shared close syntenic regions with chromosome 10 (Figure 3b). In addition, 11 780 (92.05%, total 12 797) genes on chromosome 10 were homologous with the genes on chromosomes 8 and 9 based on the BLAST results. Together, these data allow us to postulate that the ancestral 8 and 9-like chromosomes were fused into the chromosome 10 in *A. argyi*, and chromosome 10 appears as the end-to-end fusion of ancestral 8 and 9-like chromosomes, accompanied by at least one inversion and two intrachromosomal translocation events (Figure 3b).

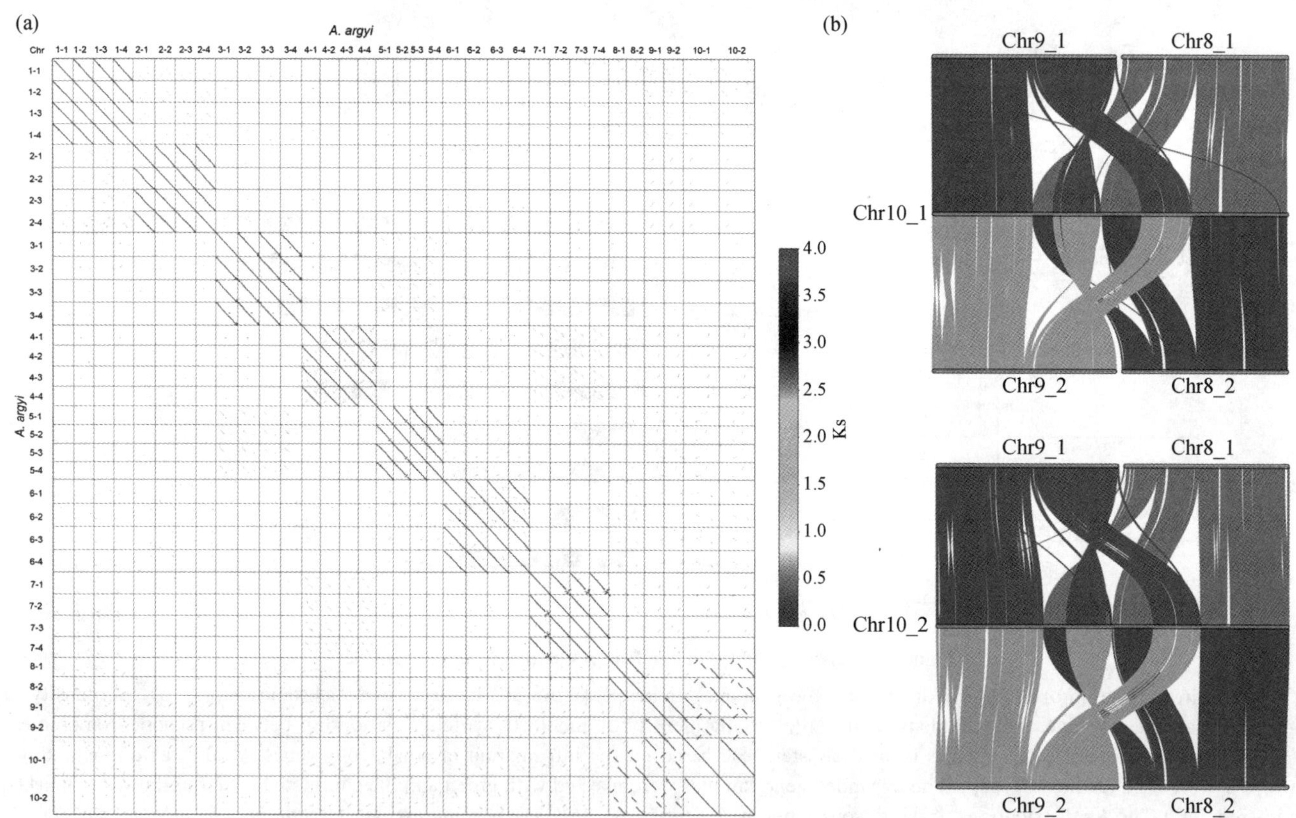


**Figure 3 Chromosomal collinearity patterns and chromatin structures between chromosome 10 and chromosomes 8 and 9**

(a) Syntenic dot plot between all chromosomes of *A. argyi*. (b) Syntenic blocks between chromosomes 8, 9 and 10.

By comparing the number of homologous genes on chromosome 10 with those on chromosomes 8 and 9, we found that 1129 genes were missing and that 1017 genes were newly formed on chromosome 10. These genes were mainly concentrated in the biological process category, including heme transport, iron coordination entity transport (lost genes), snRNA binding and oxidative phosphorylation (novel genes) (Data S6). In addition, by comparing the expression levels of homologous genes on chromosome 10 with those on chromosomes 8 and 9, we found that 411 genes were upregulated and 404 genes were downregulated on chromosome 10. GO enrichment analysis showed that the biological functions of these upregulated genes were significantly enriched in response to external biotic stimulus and cellular response to salicylic acid stimulus, and the downregulated genes were enriched in the methylerythritol 4-phosphate pathway (Data S7).

Genes involved in flavonoid biosynthesis Eupatilin, jaceosidin, hispidulin, schaftoside, isoschaftoside and vitexicarpin are representative bioactive flavonoids in *A.*

*argyi* that contribute to versatile pharmacological effects such as anti-inflammatory, antioxidation and anti-tumor effects. Ultra-performance liquid chromatography (HPLC) was used to quantify these flavonoids in seven different tissues (roots, rhizome, stem, and four different developmental stages of leaves A - D) of 'Xiang Ai'. The obtained results showed that these bioactive flavonoids were more abundant in leaves than in other tissues. Among them, the content of eupatilin was the highest, and it increased with the growth stage of leaves (Figure S11). However, the genes that participated in the biosynthesis of these flavonoids such as hispidulin, jaceosidin and eupatilin in *A. argyi* remain largely unknown. Based on extensive investigations of the flavonoid biosynthesis pathway in other plants, we proposed the possible biosynthesis routes of these compounds in *A. argyi* (Figure 4a, c).

In total, 44 candidate genes encoding 12 key enzymes in flavonoid biosynthesis pathway were identified by homologue searching and functional annotation. Of note, nearly half of the candidates especially were expanded genes and the number of phenylalanine ammonia-lyase (*PAL*), 4-hydroxylase (*C4H*), hydrox-ycinnamoyl transferase (*HCT*), chalcone synthase (*CHS*), flavanone hydroxylase (*F3'H*, *F3H*) homologues in *A. argyi* was dramatically increased relative to that in Arabidopsis (Table S15). We mapped these genes to *A. argyi* genome and found that the *PAL* exhibited tandem repeats on chromosomes 5 (Data S8). Subsequently, a transcriptomic analysis was performed using samples from roots and leaf organs (Figure S12) to identify differentially expressed genes (DEGs) between different tissues and different developmental stages of leaves. Based on their expression patterns, almost all candidate genes were expressed in seven selected tissues, but the expression levels of the first four genes in this pathway, especially the expression levels of *HCT* genes in root samples, were higher than those in leaf samples, while the expression levels of the downstream genes, especially the *CHS* genes, were higher in leaves than in roots (Figure 4b). HCT is a key enzyme in lignin synthesis, while CHS is the first rate-limiting enzyme in plant flavonoid synthesis. Therefore, the expression patterns of the *HCT* and *CHS* genes were crucial for the regulation of lignin and flavonoid synthesis in *A. argyi*,

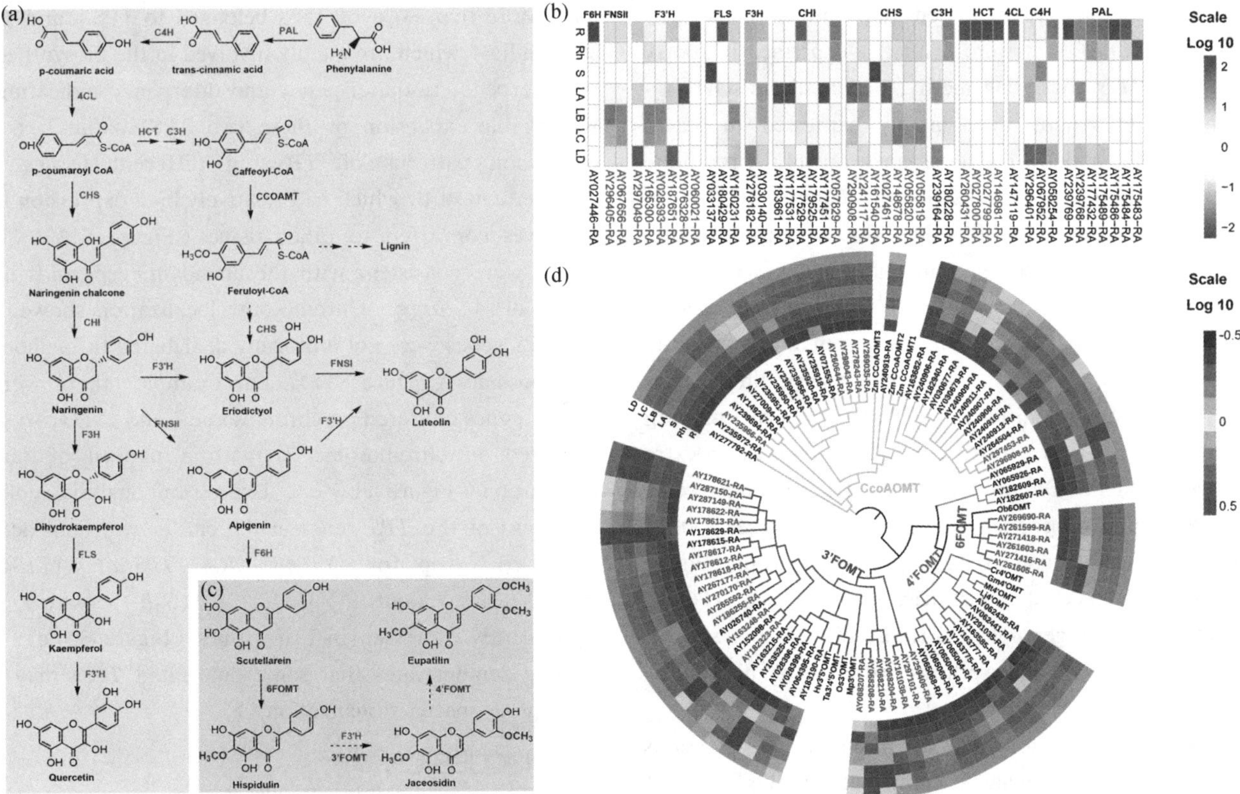


**Figure 4 The identification and expression profiles of genes related to the biosynthesis of flavonoids in *A. argyi***

(a) The proposed flavonoid biosynthesis pathway in *A. argyi*. Red fonts represented the abbreviations of enzymes participating in the catalytic steps. And the full names of relative enzymes were shown in Data S9. (b) The expression patterns of candidate genes involved in flavonoids biosynthesis pathway in different tissues. The expanded genes were marked in red. R, root; Rh, rhizome; S, stem; LA, leaf buds, 0 day; LB, young leaves 15 days; LC, mature leaves 30 days; LD, old leaves 45 days. (c) Proposed biosynthesis pathways for hispidulin, jaceosidin and eupatilin. (d) Expression profile and phylogenetic tree of all members of the flavonoid *O*-methyltransferase (*FOMT*) gene family in *A. argyi*. The genes in red were expanded genes.

which probably facilitates its rapid adaptation to heterogeneous environments. Furthermore, most of the DEGs involved in flavonoid biosynthesis were upregulated in the leaf tissues, and this correlates well with the fact that flavonoids, for example, hispidulin, jaceosidin and eupatilin, are mainly enriched in *A. argyi* leaves.

Flavonoid O-methyltransferase (FOMT) is a key enzyme for the postmodification of flavonoid compounds. Studies have confirmed that *O*-methylated flavonoids have stronger antioxidant, anti-inflammatory, and anti-cancer functions. In consideration of the active ingredients, including hispidulin, jaceosidin, eupatilin and vitexicarp, in *A. argyi* that were all *O*-methylated flavonoids, we further investigated the whole-genome *FOMT* genes in *A. argyi* using the conserved domain and the reported *FOMT* genes as queries. A total of 83 FOMT were identified. Phylogenetic analysis showed that these FOMTs were clustered into five main subclades based on their catalytic sites including 31 3′ FOMT, six 6FOMT, 10 4′ FOMT, 32 caffeoyl-CoA *O*-methyltransferase (CCoAOMT) and four unclassified FOMTs (Figure 4d). We found that almost all types of *FOMTs* were significantly expanded in the *A. argyi* genome and exhibited a pattern of tandem duplication (Data S9). Most of the *CCoAOMTs* were primarily expressed in roots, while the *FOMTs* catalysing methylation at the 3′-OH, 4′-OH and 6-OH groups were mainly expressed in leaves (Figure 4d). Hispidulin has a methoxy on its C6 position, indicating that its enzymatic synthesis requires 6FOMT to mediate C6-methoxylation. Based on the chemical structure and a previous study, scutellarein may be a precursor for hispidulin biosynthesis. Jaceosidin is a di-methoxyflavone with one methyl group on the C6 position of the A ring and another on the C3′position of the B ring, suggesting that its synthesis requires an additional 3′FOMT by comparison with hispidulin. Eupatilin is a trimethoxyflavone that has an extra methyl group at the C4′ position of the B ring compared to jaceosidin, suggesting that there may be a 4′ FOMT catalysing the conversion of jaceosidin to eupatilin (Figure 4c). In summary, the identification of these *FOMT* candidates based on genomic and transcriptome analyses will accelerate the enzymatic synthesis pathway of hispidulin, jaceosidin, and eupatilin.

Genes involved in terpenoid biosynthesis  Volatile oil is a significant pharmacodynamic component in the leaves of *A. argyi* due to a rich content of terpenoids. The volatile oil from *A. argyi* leaves contains abundant monoterpenoids and sesquiterpenoids(Figure 5a). Although terpenoids are diverse and have various structures, they all come from the common precursors isopentenyl pyrophosphate (IPP) and dimethylallyl pyrophosphate (DMAPP). IPP and DMAPP are mainly produced through the mevalonate pathway (MVA) pathway in the cytoplasm and the methylerythritol phosphate(MEP) pathway in the plastid. Candidate genes participating in MVA and MEP pathways were screened by using the methods of homoloy searching and functional annotation. The obtained results indicated that a total of 66 genes encoding 14 gene families were involved in these two pathways in *A. argyi* (Figure 5b). These genes were widely distributed on *A. argyi* chromosomes, especially on chromosomes 7 (Data S10). The key genes identified in the MEP pathway were greatly expanded compared with the genes identified in the MVA pathway. RNA-seq analysis demonstrated that genes related to the MEP pathway were more specifically expressed in leaves than those in the MVA pathway (Figure 5c), indicating that the terpenoids in *A. argyi* leaves mainly come from the MEP pathway.

Terpene synthase (*TPS*) family genes are responsible for the biosynthesis and structural diversity of terpenoids. We found that *TPS* genes were extremely expanded in the *A. argyi* genome. In total, we identified 135 *TPS* genes in the *A. argyi* genome (Data S11). According to phylogenetic analyses, these TPSs were grouped into five subfamilies, including TPS-a, TPS-b, TPS-c, TPS-d and TPS-e/f (Figure 6a). More than 80% of TPSs belonged to TPS-a and TPS-b subfamilies, which are mainly involved in the biosynthesis of monoterpene, sesquiter-pene, and diterpene, indicating the remarkable expansion of these two TPS subfamilies. The expression patterns of *TPSs* in different tissues were analysed, most of which had relatively high expression levels in leaves compared to other tissues (Figure S13). These results were consistent with the abundant terpenoids in the leaves of *A. argyi*. Chromosome localization showed that the *TPS* genes were not uniformly distributed throughout the chromosomes (Figure S14). For example, there were 12 *TPS-a* genes clustered on chromosome 6 and 13 *TPS-b* genes clustered on chromosome 3, with a pattern of tandem duplication (Figure 6b, c). Expression analysis indicated that most of the *TPS* genes in the cluster were not actively expressed, except for *AY184877-RA* (*TPS-a*), *AY184880-RA* (*TPS-a*) and *AY075453* (*TPS-b*), which were significantly expressed in leaf tissues (Figure 6b, c). This finding demonstrates that some duplicated *TPSs* may have undergone neofunctionalization.

## 3 DISCUSSION

The high-quality *A. argyi* genome sequence in this study represents the first species in the genus *Artemisia* for which chromosome-level assembly has been constructed. This well-annotated genome will be the foundation for evolutionary and molecular biological studies of this economically and medicinally important plant. However, the high heterozygosity (2.36%), large proportion of repetitive sequences (75.86%)

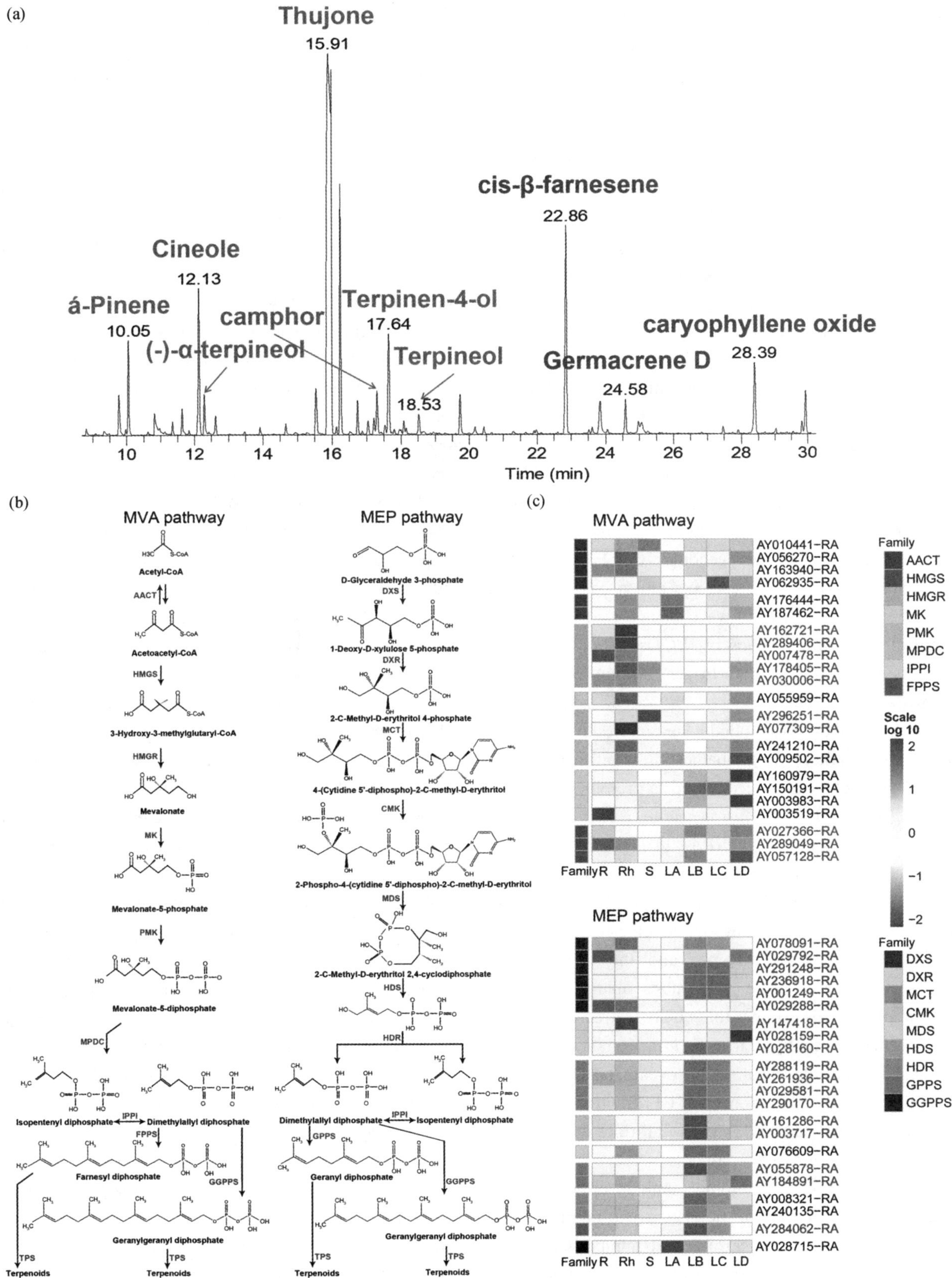


**Figure 5 Volatiles compounds in *A. argyi* leaves and their biosynthesis pathways**

(a) Gas chromatogram of volatile oils from *A. argyi* leaves. Monoterpenes and sesquiterpenes were marked green and red, respectively. (b) The proposed MVA and MEP pathways in *A. argyi*. Red fonts indicated the abbreviations of enzymes participating in these two pathways. And the full names of these enzymes were listed in Data S10. (c) The expression patterns of candidate genes involved in MVA and MEP pathways in different tissues. The expanded genes were marked in red. R, root; Rh, rhizome; S, stem; LA, leaf buds, 0 day; LB, young leaves 15 days; LC, mature leaves 30 days; LD, old leaves 45 days.

and polyploidy (allotetraploid) present significant challenges for the genome assembly of *A. argyi*. In this study, an integrated strategy combing PacBio long HiFi reads, Hi-C sequencing and Illumina short reads greatly facilitated the assembly of the complex polyploidy *A. argyi* genome. Compared with the other 14 species in Asteraceae whose genomes have been released, *A. argyi* features the largest genome with a size of 8.03 Gb. The scaffold N50 (206.4 Mb) of the *A. argyi* genome was the longest among them, and the contig N50 (6.25 Mb) is only shorter than that of safflower. In brief, the *A. argyi* genome is the fifth chromosomal-level genome in Asteraceae, and the first chromosome-level genome in *Artemisia*.

WGD events and TE amplification are the main causes of large genomes. Here, the analysis of *Ks* distribution indicated that two rounds of WGD events occurred in the *A. argyi* genome (Figure 2c). The most recent WGD (~2.2 Mya) is an *A. argyi* and its closely related species (*A. annua* and *C. nankingense*) specific event, which is distinct from the WGD-2 event in the sunflower genome. Combined with a WGT-γ event occurring in all eudicots and a basal WGT-1 event occurring in Asteraceae, we conclude that *A. argyi* underwent at least three rounds of WGDs. The additional WGD events may also contribute to gene family expansion. In comparison with other sequenced Asteraceae species, we found that the number of expanded gene families in *A. argyi* was approximately three times that of the contracted gene families (Figure 2b), which accounts for a prominently large number of genes in the *A. argyi* genome. In particular, *PsbA* genes in photosystem II, *RPA1* in DNA replication, *HSPs* and *TPS* were markedly expanded, all of which participate in plant growth and development and stress responses. Moreover, the transposable elements occupied 73.59% of the *A. argyi* genome, and the LTR/Gypsy subfamilies (24.47%) were the most abundant. The distribution of *Ks* also hints that LTR retrotransposons explosion occurred recently in the *A. argyi* genome (Figure 2d). Together, the additional WGD event and the recent proliferation of LTRs in *A. argyi* may be responsible for the expansion of the genome and may play vital roles in *A. argyi* adaptations to challenging environments.

Variation in basic chromosome numbers is not a rare phenomenon in some genera in the Asteraceae family, such as *Melampodium* whose basic chromosome numbers are $x=11$, 9 and 14. *Artemisia* is reported to have at least two basic chromosome numbers, with $x=9$ being the common chromosome number and $x=8$ being less frequent. The somatic chromosome numbers of *A. argyi* also exhibited considerable variation, including $2n=18$, 34 and 36, through chromosome count and karyotype analysis. The number of basic chromosomes of *A. argyi* is nominally $x=9$. Chromosomal fusion/fission and polyploidy are the main causes of chromosome number evolution. Our chromosomal-scale genome of *A. argyi* provides reliable evidence for the chromosome number variation of this species. Synteny analysis showed that the 34 chromosomes of *A. argyi* comprise 10 homologous groups, of which seven groups each have four sets of monoploid chromosomes, and three groups have two chromosomes in each, and chromosomes 8 and 9 shared closely syntenic regions and high rates of homologous genes with chromosome 10 (Figure 3a, b). We proposed that the ancestral 8- and 9-like chromosomes were fused into chromosome 10 in *A. argyi*. This single fusion explains the odd base chromosome number of *A. argyi*. More-over, the existence of $x=8$ base chromosomes suggests that the fusion may occur before allohybridization. Polyploidy and variation in basic chromosome numbers in *Artemisia* may facilitate the species differentiation and survival in extremely arid habitats.

Flavonoids and terpenoids are the main medicinal active ingredients in *A. argyi*. Based on the high-quality genome, we proposed backbone biosynthetic pathways of flavonoids and terpenoids and identified the key gene families in both pathways. In plants, the biosynthesis of flavone *O*-methyl derivatives is catalysed by FOMTs, which transfer the methyl group of S-adenosyl-L-methionine (SAM) to the hydroxyl group of flavonoids. Thus, FOMTs play significant roles in the biosynthesis of *O*-methylated flavones in *A. argyi*. In this study, a relatively complete biosynthetic pathway for the three *O*-methylated flavones, hispidulin, jaceosidin, and eupatilin, was conjected based on synergistic analysis of genome sequencing, transcriptomics and metabolomics. A large number of *FOMT* genes were identified in the *A. argyi* genome, and the *FOMTs* catalysing methylation at the 3′-OH, 4′-OH and 6-OH groups are important candidates for the synthesis of hispidulin, jaceosidin and eupatilin (Figure 4). For terpenoid synthesis, The high and special expression of genes in the MEP pathway in *A. argyi* genome demonstrates that this pathway is a main source of terpenoid precursors. *A. argyi* leaves contain more than 100 kinds of terpenoids (mainly rich in monoterpenes and sesquiterpenes), and the diversity of terpenoids is mainly determined by *TPS* family genes. Whole-genome-wide identification of *TPS* family genes shows that the extensive expansion of *TPS-a* and *TPS-b* subfamily genes (Figure 6) in the *A. argyi* genome may be one explanation for the accumulation of diverse monoterpenes and sesquiterpenes. We also found remarkable tandem duplications in the *FOMT* and *TPS* family genes, which may contribute to the high contents of flavonoids and volatile oil in *A. argyi*.

In conclusion, our study of a high-quality *A. argyi* genome provides valuable information for the finite genomic resources of complicated polyploids in *Artemisia* and offers a

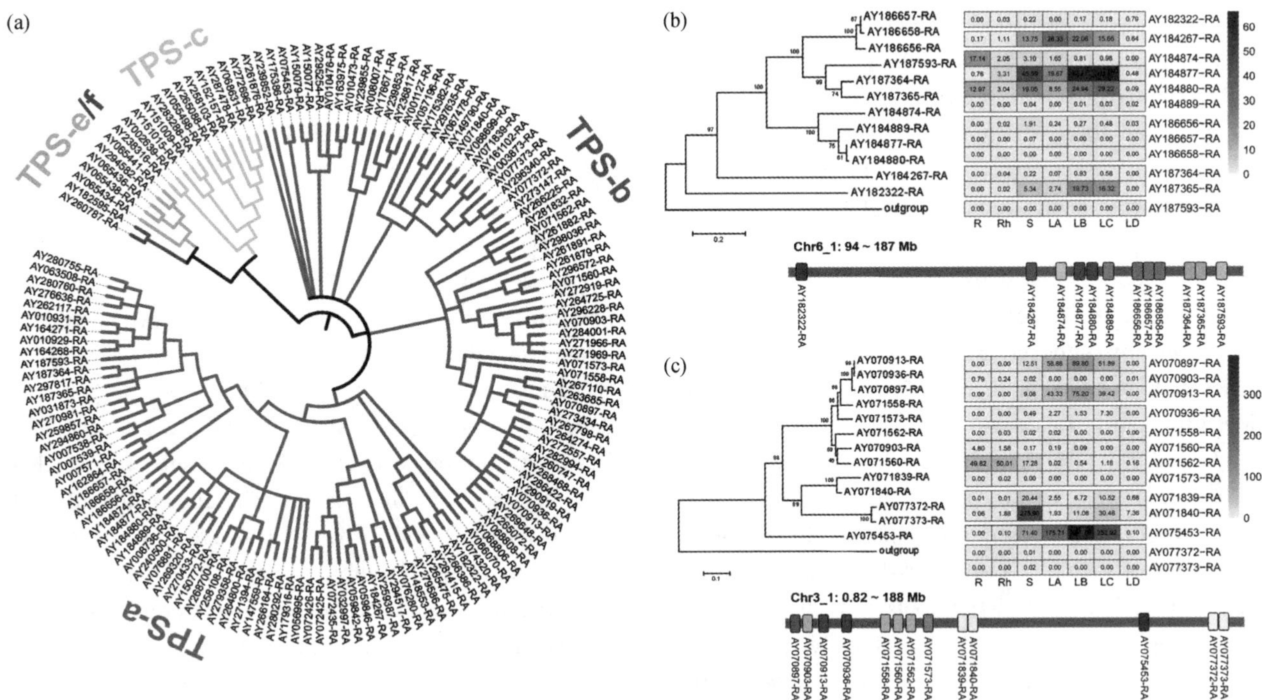


**Figure 6 Expansion of terpene synthase-encoding genes and their gene clusters on chromosomes in the *Artemisia argyi* genome**

(a) Phylogeny of TPSs identified in *A. argyi* genome. (b) Phylogeny, expression profiles and chromosomal position of *TPS-a* clade gene cluster on Chr6_1. The outgroup gene of the phylogenetic tree was *TPS-e* subfamily gene with gene ID *AY065441-RA*. (c) Phylogeny, expression profiles and chromosomal position of *TPS-b* clade gene cluster on Chr3_1. The outgroup gene of the phylogenetic tree was *TPS-e* subfamily gene with gene ID *AY294582-RA*.

comprehensive insights into the mechanism of economically and medicinally important traits and environmental adaptation.

## 4 METHODS

Plant materials The cultivated mugwort 'Xiang Ai' was used for the construction of the reference genome. The young leaves of 90-day-old 'Xiang Ai' plants were sampled to extract high-quality genomic DNA for genome sequencing and Hi-C analysis. Roots®, rhizomes (Rh), stems (S), leaf buds (0 day, LA), young leaves (15 days, LB), mature leaves (30 days, LC) and old leaves (45 days, LD) of 'Xiang Ai' were collected for RNA-seq analysis.

Flow cytometry The nuclear DNA content of 'Xiang Ai' was measured by flow cytometry according to the method described previously. Briefly, leaves from 'Xiang Ai' and *Chrysanthemum nankingense* plants were finely chopped with a razor blade in 2 mL Galbra'th's buffer, respectively. After the suspension was filtered through a 48 μm nylon membrane, 200 μL of PI (50 μg/mL) and 100 μg/mL RnaseA were added immediately. Following 30 min of incubation on ice, the samples were detected by flow cytometry (BD FACSCalibur, BD Biosciences, Wuhan, China).

Estimation of genome size Illumina-seq generated approximately 215 Gb of clean reads, which were subjected to *K*-mer analysis to estimate the genome size of 'Xiang Ai'. The 21-mer frequency distribution was shown in Figure S2.

Whole-genome sequencing For PacBio SMRT sequencing, high-quality DNA from 'Xiang Ai' was first sheared and concentrated to construct 15-Kb DNA sequencing libraries and subsequently run on a PacBio Sequel II platform according to the manufacturer's instruction with seven cells.

For genome survey sequencing, 5 150-bp paired-end (PE) libraries were constructed for sequencing on an Illumina NovaSeq 6 000 platform and ~ 215 Gb of raw sequencing data were obtained.

For Hi-C sequencing, two Hi-C libraries digested with *Mbo*I restriction enzyme were sequenced on BGI MGISEQ-2000 to generate ~422 Gb of valid data from 150 PE reads.

Genome assembly and evaluation Briefly, we performed *de novo* assembly using HiCanu v 2. 2 and Hifiasm (version 0. 13-r308) and the result showed that the Hifiasm assembly (N50 = 8. 32 Mb with 10 274 contigs) was better than the HiCanu assembly (4. 69 Mb with 48 227 contigs). Then, the draft genome from the Hifiasm assembly was further assembled into scaffolds with Hi-C data using the 3D-DNA pipeline (version 180 922). These scaffolds were roughly split by Juicebox (version 1. 11. 08) and another round of scaffolding by 3D-DNA. Genome assembly completeness was assessed by BUSCOs and transcriptome data.

Genome annotation Transposable elements of *A.*

*argyi* assembly were identified by homology- and *de novo*-based methods. Repbase (version 2017-01-27) was used to build the homology repeat library. Then, RepeatModeler v2.0.1 was used to construct the *de novo* repeat library. Finally, RepeatMasker v4.1.0 was used to annotate the repetitive elements in the Repbase and the *de novo* repeat library.

Protein coding genes of *A. argyi* genome were annotated by MAKER according to three complementary methods: *de novo* prediction, homology-based prediction and transcriptome-based prediction. First of all, Isoseq3 was employed to identify full-length high-quality transcripts from PacBio Sequel II. HISAT2 (version 2.1.0) and Cufflinks (version 2.2.1) were used to predict the genes by using the RNA-seq data and the assembled genome. In the second round, Augustus v 3.2.1, GeneMark-ES Suite v 4.61_ lic and SNAP (version 2013-02-16) tools were used for gene model training for *de novo* prediction. Finally, precise gene annotation was performed by using non-redundant proteins from *Artemisia annua* and *Helianthus annuus* based on the homology-based approach. Complete BUSCO hits were used to evaluate the gene annotation results of *A. argyi* genome. Following the gene annotation, BLAST analyses against several functional databases (NR, EggNOG, SwissProt and TrEMBL) were performed on the predicted protein-coding genes to identify homologous proteins in other species using diamond (version v 2.0.4.142). In addition, possible GO terms were obtained using the SwissProt database and Trembl database ID mapping. Gene pathways were accomplished with KEGG analysis by using KOBAS v 3.0.

tRNAs were annotated by tRNAscan-SE (version 1.3.1), rRNAs were annotated by BLASTN (version 2.10.1). miRNAs and snRNAs were annotated by searching the Rfam database (version 14.5) using BLASTN and INFERNAL (version 1.1.2).

Sequence alignment and variation analysis  Burrows-Wheeler Aligner (BWA, version 0.7.17) software was used to map all clean reads to the assembled genome with the methods described by He *et al*. In brief, SAMtools (version 1.9) were employed to convert the mapping results into the BAM format. Picard package (Version 1.96) was used for the filtration of duplicated reads. Genome Analysis Toolkit (GATK, version 3.8-0-ge9d806836) was used to realign reads around Indels. Variations were detected with both SAMtools mpileup and GATK HaplotypeCaller packages, and only concordance results were retained. Raw variations were filtered by GATK VariantFiltration packages with the following parameters '-- filter-name FilterQual -- filter-expression "QUAL <60.0" -- filter-name FilterQD -- filter-expression "QD <20.0" -- filter-name FilterFS -- filter-expression "FS> 13.0" -- filter-name FilterMQ -- filter-expression "MQ<30.0" -- filter-name FilterMQRankSum -- filter-expression "MQRankSum<−1.65" -- filter-name FilterReadPosRankSum -- filter-expression "ReadPosRankSum <−1.65"-- cluster-window-size 10 -- cluster-size 2'. SNPs within 10 bp with an indel were removed. Finally, SnpEff software was used to annotate the identified SNPs and Indels.

Gene family, phylogenomic analysis and WGD identification  Gene families of *A. argyi* genome and *Arabidopsis thaliana*, *Vitis vinifera* and six other Asteraceae species were identified by OrthoMCL (version 2.0.9) with default parameters. RaxML (version 8.2.12) were used to construct the phylogenetic tree by using the single-copy orthologues of the nine species. The divergence times of *A. thaliana* and *A. argyi* from TimeTree (http://timetree.org/) were used for calibration and the divergence times of phylogenetic tree were estimated by r8s (version 1.81). The expanded and contracted gene families were calculated by CAFE (version 4.2) in each lineage. WGD events in the *A. argyi* genome were searched according to the WGDi pipeline.

RNA sequencing  Total RNA of different tissues was extracted using TRIzol reagent. An mRNA sequencing library of seven different tissues was constructed on an Illumina Novaseq 6 000 platform by 150 bp PE sequencing. For full-length transcriptome sequencing, a mixed RNA library from different tissues was prepared according to the PacBio ISO-Seq experimental workflow and subsequently run on a PacBio Sequel II platform. For RNA-seq analysis, 2 μg RNA from each sample was sequenced on the Illumina platform. Three replications were performed for each sample.

Gene identification in flavonoid and terpenoid biosynthesis pathways  The protein sequences of the enzymes (PAL, C4H, 4CL, HCT, C3H, CHS, CHI, F3H, and FLS) in flavonoid biosynthesis pathways of *A. thaliana* were obtained from the TAIR database, and those for F3′H and FNSII in fleabanes, FNSI in parsley and celery, and F6H in soybean were obtained from previous studies and the NCBI database. These sequences were blasted against the *A. argyi* protein sequences using BLASTP (*E*-value $< 1e^{-5}$).

Functional proteins involved in the MEP and MVA pathways of terpenoid backbone biosynthesis in *A. thaliana* were obtained from the TAIR database. Homologues of these proteins in the genome of *A. argyi* were investigated by BLASTP with an *E*-value cutoff of $1e^{-5}$. Fragments per kb of exon model per million mapped fragments (FPKM) not <10 were selected for heatmap analysis.

Identification of terpene synthase genes (*TPSs*) and flavonoid *O*-methytransferase (*FOMTs*)  The protein sequences of TPSs were identified by screening with functional motifs PF01397 and PF03936. A total of 146 *TPS* genes were predicted in the 'Xiang Ai' genome. There are 11 genes were removed manually, since it was not possible to calculate genetic distance by MEGA6.

We searched the candidate *FOMT* genes by the combination of conserved domain (PF01596) and homologue-based BLAST, and repetitive sequences were removed. A total of 83 *FOMT* genes were predicted in the *A. argyi* genome. 11 selected FOMT proteins downloaded from NCBI based on high gene homology and genome annotation were subjected to phylogenetic analysis.

Phylogenetic reconstruction of TPSs and FOMTs The neighbour-joining trees were constructed using the MEGA6 software. Heatmap analysis based on RNA-seq data was performed by the pheatmap package in R language (version 1.0.12).

HPLC analysis of flavonoids Agilent 1 260 Infinity HPLC system (Agilent Technologies) was used for HPLC analyses. The flavonoids were separated by ZORBAXRRHD Eclipse Plus 95A C18 column (2.1 × 100 mm, 1.8 μm, Agilent) and detected at 330 nm by UV. The mobile phases were acetonitrile (A) and 0.1% phosphoric acid (B) with the flow rate of 0.4 mL/min. The separation gradient conditions were as follows: 0 - 0.5 min, 2%～5% A; 0.5 - 7 min, 5% ～ 25% A; 7 - 11 min, 25% ～ 330% A; 11 - 14 min, 30%～33% A; 14 - 19.5 min, 33%～45% A; 19.5 - 20.5 min, 45%～85% A; 20.5 - 27 min, 85%～98% A; 27 - 28 min, 98%～2% A.

## 5 ACKNOWLEDGEMENTS

We appreciate the funding support from the key project at the central government level: The ability establishment of sustainable use for valuable Chinese medicine resources (2060302), National key research and development program (No: 2017YFC1700704), the young qihuang scholars of the national administration of TCM, the special fund for the construction of modern agricultural industrial technology system (CARS-21, CRAS-23), Hubei Province outstanding young and middle-aged scientific and technological innovation team -Traditional Chinese medicine ecological agriculture (T2021008), innovation team and talents cultivation programme of national administration of traditional Chinese medicine. (No: ZYYCXTD-D-202005), and the Nature Science Foundation of Hubei Province (2021CFB225). We appreciate the support for computational work from BioSmartSeek company.

[苗玉焕，刘大会，黄璐琦，等. Plant Biotechnology Journal, 2022, 20: 1902 - 1915.]

# Comparative physiological responses and transcriptome analysis revealing the metabolic regulatory mechanism of *Prunella vulgaris* L. induced by exogenous application of hydrogen peroxide

## 1 INTRODUCTION

*Prunella vulgaris* L., belonging to the family Lamiaceae, is an important medicinal plant that is widely used for the treatment of mastitis, thyroid gland malfunctions, infectious hepatitis, hypertension, pulmonary tuberculosis, sore throat infections, nephritis and oedema in Northeast Asia, the Middle East, and Europe. In southeastern cities of China, *P. vulgaris* is usually used as an ornamental plant, and the material composing the functional herbal tea, as well as *P. vulgaris* seedling fresh leaves, have been eaten as a vegetable since the Ming Dynasty. In recent years, *P. vulgaris* has been widely planted in South China to conserve wild populations and increase the supply of medicinal material. Approximately 60 million kilograms of *P. vulgaris* are processed into Chinese patented medicine and functional herbal tea every year. However, the long-term "Chemical Agriculture" planting mode of *P. vulgaris* leads directly to a decline in the quality of its medicinal materials, which seriously reduces the safety and effectiveness of clinical medication. Therefore, understanding the formation mechanism of the active components is essential to improve the quality of *P. vulgaris* medicinal materials.

Polyphenolic and triterpene acids are two of the major bioactive components of *P. vulgaris* and possess antioxidant, anti-inflammatory, and antitumour functions. We typically believe that polyphenolic (e.g., rosmarinic acid) and triterpene (e.g., ursolic acid and oleanolic acid) contents are important criteria for evaluating the quality of *P. vulgaris*. Our previous studies have shown that the accumulation of polyphenolic and triterpene acids occurs in *P. vulgaris* plants suffering from abiotic stress, UV-B radiation, UV-B/A removal, drought stress, and soil nutrient element deficiency and is mediated by key signal molecules ($H_2O_2$). Therefore, studying the $H_2O_2$ signal transduction mechanisms of *P. vulgaris* polyphenolic and triterpene acids will provide new ideas for complex secondary metabolite biosynthesis to improve medicinal material quality and clinical efficacy.

$H_2O_2$ is an important reactive oxygen species (ROS) in medicinal plants and plays a central role in the regulation of many biological processes, e. g., growth, development and response to abiotic stresses. In response to abiotic stress, $H_2O_2$ is also a signalling molecule that activates the formation of secondary metabolites. Similar studies have confirmed that $H_2O_2$ can induce polyphenolic synthesis in *Scrophularia striata*, phenolic and flavonoid accumulation in *Mentha pulegium* L. and triterpene saponin synthesis in *Aralia elata* (Miq.) Seem. In addition to $H_2O_2$, salicylic acid (SA) and jasmonic acid (JA), two key signalling molecules, are also considered to regulate the defence response of medicinal plants to various biotic and abiotic stresses. Our recent study showed that exogenous MeJA treatments upregulated the expression of phenylpropanoid biosynthesis-related genes, consequently leading to increased phenolic and flavonoid contents in *P. vulgaris*. However, the underlying $H_2O_2$ and endogenous phytohormone crosstalk mechanisms modulating *P. vulgaris* secondary metabolite biosynthesis remain unknown.

Recently, transcriptome sequencing technology has been used to analyse the response of *P. vulgaris* to growth, development, and abiotic stress and to explore its molecular biosynthesis mechanism. For example, performed transcriptome sequencing of *P. vulgaris* roots, stems, leaves, and flowers from the seedling, bud, and flowering stages. Transcriptome sequencing was reported to be significantly enriched in the phenylpropanoid biosynthesis, flavonoid biosynthesis and isoquinoline alkaloid biosynthetic pathways of KEGG. RNA-seq technology was used to analyse the flowering (leaves and spicas) and nonflowering (leaves) parts of *P. vulgaris* plants under field conditions, and it was found that the flowering process involves plant hormone signal transduction and sugar metabolism, among other processes. By comparing spica (Prunellae Spica) of *P. vulgaris* under low, medium, and high NaCl stress transcriptome sequencing results, we found that the KEGG pathways were primarily concentrated in translation, signal transduction, carbohydrate metabolism, energy metabolism, lipid metabolism and amino acid metabolism. However, the molecular mechanisms modulating the *P. vulgaris* response to exogenous $H_2O_2$ stress remain unknown.

This study reports the physiological and transcriptomic mechanisms that occur during exogenous $H_2O_2$ treatment of *P. vulgaris*. Quantitative changes in the photosynthetic index, antioxidant enzyme system, nonenzymatic antioxidant system, osmotic regulating substance, endogenous hormone, secondary metabolites, and gene expression associated with bioactive ingredients and hormone synthesis in *P. vulgaris* were investigated under different exogenous $H_2O_2$ treatments. Important metabolic regulatory substances were filtered out, and upstream regulatory genes and their participating pathways were determined. This study could provide a basis for exploring the metabolic regulatory mechanisms in response to $H_2O_2$ stress in *P. vulgaris* and other related medicinal plants of the Lamiaceae family.

## 2 MATERIALS AND METHODS

2.1 Plant materials and growth conditions  The *P. vulgaris* seeds used in the experiment were purchased in Queshan County, Henan Province, P.R. China in June 2020 and identified as *P. vulgaris* (family Lamiaceae) mature seeds by Professor Yuhang Chen from the College of Pharmaceutical Sciences of Chengdu Medical College. The mature seeds were air-dried, sterilized with 2% $H_2O_2$ solution for 2 min, and rinsed in distilled water several times. The seeds (mixed with sand at a 1 : 1 ratio) were sown in a medicinal garden (latitude: 30° 49′ 32.41″ N, longitude: 104° 12′ 7.3″ E, altitude: 471 m) at Chengdu Medical College (Chengdu city, Sichuan Province, P. R. China) on June 30, 2020. Under normal conditions, the seeds were germinated on moist filter soil surfaces at 20 - 25 ℃ for 7 - 10 days. *P. vulgaris* seedlings were grown naturally (26 ℃/15 ℃, 16/8 h day/night) under the same fertilizer and water conditions. Uniform seedlings of *P. vulgaris* (six-leaf stage) were transplanted into plastic pots (top-down diameter 17×8 cm, height 12 cm) and transferred to an experimental greenhouse on 20 April 2021. The soil characteristics of *P. vulgaris* in the experimental fields and transplanting pots were measured according to. The results are shown in Supplementary Table S1. The pots were filled with 800 g of nutrient soil (3 : 1 ratio of sandy loam soil: vermiculite), pH: 7.05, soil organic matter: 24.57 g/kg, hydrolysable-N: 85.89 mg/kg, available-P: 15.28 mg/kg, available-$K_2O$: 150.27 mg/kg, and each pot contained 3 seedlings. The *P. vulgaris* seedlings were grown in an experimental greenhouse with a temperature regimen of 26 ℃/15 ℃ (day/night), photoperiod of 16 h/8 h (day/night), relative humidity of 55 - 65%, and photosynthetically active radiation (PAR) of 1 200 μmol/($m^2$ · s).

2.2 Application of exogenous $H_2O_2$ treatments  The experiment was conducted in the medicinal garden of Chengdu Medical College under natural conditions. On 15 May 2021 (three weeks after transplanting into pots), the pots of *P. vulgaris* plants (florescence stage) were individually divided into five groups, with ten replicates, and each replicate contained 10 *P. vulgaris* plants. *P. vulgaris* was treated with two treatments: control (distilled water)

(CK group) and 2.0 mmol/L $H_2O_2$ ($H_2O_2$ group) (Chengdu Kelong Reagent Chemical Factory, Chengdu, China). The treatment solutions were applied to the plants in the form of an exogenous spray. Approximately 100 mL of treatment solution was sprayed on each pot. Fresh leaves of *P. vulgaris* from each treatment were stochastically collected, harvested after 24 h, immersed in liquid nitrogen, and transferred to a −80 ℃ refrigerator for subsequent analysis. Moreover, these groups of *P. vulgaris* leaf samples were collected and dried in a dryer at 60 ℃ to a constant weight. The samples were ground into powder and passed through a 60-mesh sieve for later use.

2.3 Physiological analysis

2.3.1 Leaf photosynthetic attributes The photosynthetic parameters including net photosynthesis rate (Pn), intercellular $CO_2$ concentration (Ci), stomatal conductance (Gs), transpiration rate (Tr) and instantaneous water-use efficiency (WUEi) were determined by a hand-held photosynthesis analysis system (SY - 1020, Shiyakeji, Shijiazhuang, China) during morning hours from 9:00 am to 11:30 am on sunny days. Three fully mature *P. vulgaris* leaves were measured in each treatment. Light intensity, carbon dioxide concentration, air temperature, and relative humidity remained at approximately 1 200 μmol/($m^2$ · s) PAR, 500 ± 10 μmol/L, 23 ± 2 ℃, and 70% ± 1%, respectively. Chlorophyll contents were measured for each treatment using a SPAD - 502 (Konica Minolta, Tokyo, Japan) portable chlorophyll metre. The SPAD value is an indicator of chlorophyll content.

2.3.2 $H_2O_2$ content, enzyme activities and osmotic regulating substances Leaf enzymatic activity was measured with some modifications in accordance with the method of. First, fresh leaf samples (0.5 g) of *P. vulgaris* from the control and $H_2O_2$ stress treatments after 24 h were extracted with 4.5 mL of 0.1 mol/L phosphate buffer (pH 7.28). After centrifugation at 10,000 *g* and 4 ℃ for 10 min, the supernatants were used as the crude enzyme extract for the following assays. Each treatment was performed for three biological repeats.

Leaf superoxide dismutase (SOD, EC 1.15.1.1), catalase (CAT, EC 1.11.1.6), peroxidase (POD, EC 1.11.1.7), ascorbate peroxidase (APX, EC 1.11.1.11), phenylalanine ammonia-lyase (PAL, EC 4.3.1.5), and polyphenol oxidase (PPO, EC 1.14.18.1) activities and soluble protein, soluble sugar, free proline (Pro), malondialdehyde (MDA), $H_2O_2$ and glutathione (GSH) contents were determined using commercial test kits (Nanjing Jiancheng Bioengineering Institute, Nanjing, China) · $H_2O_2$, soluble protein, soluble sugar, Pro, MDA, and GSH contents and POD, SOD, CAT, APX, PPO, and PAL activities were measured at wavelengths of 405 nm, 595 nm, 630 nm, 520 nm, 532 nm, 420 nm, 420 nm, 470 nm, 550 nm, 405 nm, 290 nm, 420 nm, and 290 nm, respectively, using a 752 UV/Vis spectrophotometer (Shanghai Jinghua Technological Instrument, Shanghai, China), and each experiment included three biological replicates. The results were calculated according to the formula shown in the commercial test kits. The units of soluble protein are expressed in gprot/L; soluble sugar and Pro in μg/g proteins; $H_2O_2$ in mmol/g proteins; POD, SOD, CAT, PPO, APX, and PAL in U/mg proteins; GSH in mg/g proteins; and MDA in nmol/mg proteins.

2.3.3 Phenolic acids, flavonoids, and triterpenoic acids The contents of phenolic acids (e.g., rosmarinic acid, salviaflaslde, and caffeic acid), flavonoids (e.g., hyperoside), and triterpenoic acids (e.g., oleanolic acid and ursolic acid) were measured by high-performance liquid chromatography (HPLC) in accordance with the modified method of Chen et al. Into a conical flask was weighed 0.5 g of dried *P. vulgaris* powder and 10 mL of 80% methanol solution, followed by sonication at 40 ℃ for 60 min. After centrifugation, the supernatants were filtered with a 0.22 - μm organic filter membrane, and the filtrate was used as the test solution. The test solution (10 μL) was injected onto an Agilent C18 column (150 mm × 4.6 mm, 5 μm) (Agilent Technologies Inc., Santa Clara, California, USA) for analysis on a high-performance liquid chromatograph (Prominence-I, LC - 2030 C 3D Plus, Shimadzu Co., Tokyo, Japan). The mobile phase consisted of chromatographic acetonitrile (solvent A) and 0.1% phosphoric acid solution (solvent B), the flow rate was 0.8 mL/min, the column temperature reached 30 ℃ (with a run time of 45 min), and detection wavelengths were monitored at 325 nm (caffeic acid, salviaflaside, and rosmarinic acid) and 360 nm (hyperoside). The mobile phase consisted of chromatographic methanol (90%) and 0.2% acetic acid solution (10%), the flow rate was 0.8 mL/min, the column temperature was 18 ℃ (with a run time of 30 min), and the detection wavelength was 210 nm (ursolic acid and oleanolic acid).

Total flavonoids and total phenolics were determined by UV spectrophotometry (UV - 752, Shanghai Jinghua Technological Instrument, Shanghai, China). The dried *P. vulgaris* leaf powder (0.5 g) was added to 50% ethanol at a ratio of 1 : 40 for ultrasonic extraction for 30 min. After filtration, 2 mL of the filtrate was placed into a 10-mL volumetric flask, and the total flavonoid content was determined at 510 nm. The dried *P. vulgaris* powder (0.25 g) was weighed into a 50 - mL corked conical flask with 25 mL 70% ethanol for 60 min of ultrasonic extraction. After filtration, 0.1 mL filtrate was placed into a 10 - mL volumetric flask, and the total phenolic content was measured at 760 nm.

2.3.4 Phytohormone contents The plant endogenous hormones jasmonic acid (JA), salicylic acid (SA), abscisic acid (ABA), and indole-3-acetic acid (IAA) in fresh leaves of *P. vulgaris* were determined using liquid chromatography-mass spectrometry (LC-MS/MS) (API QTRAP 5 500, AB Sciex, Palo Alto, California, USA).

Approximately *P. vulgaris* leaves (1.0 g) were ground in liquid nitrogen, added to a precooled (4℃) solution of 80% isopropanol —19% distilled water —1% hydrochloric acid, mixed and extracted by maceration at 4℃ for 16 h, shaking 2-3 times. The sample was centrifuged at 4℃ for 5 min at 15,000 g. The supernatant was aspirated, and the extraction solution was added to the residue and repeated once, combining the supernatant extracts. The extract was concentrated and redissolved in 50% methanol/water to 1 mL, filtered with a 0.22-μm PTFE membrane and placed in a sample bottle, and the sample was aspirated and flowed into an XB-C18 100 A column (2.1×100 mm, 2.6 μm) (Agilent Technologies Inc., Santa Clara, California, USA) for LC-MS analysis.

2.4 Transcriptome analysis of *P. vulgaris*

2.4.1 RNA extraction, cDNA library construction and sequencing *P. vulgaris* mixed sample RNA was extracted using the GeneMark Plant Total RNA Purification Kit (GeneMarkBio, Taiwan, China) and analysed by agarose gel electrophoresis for RNA degradation and contamination. The RNA purity, concentration and integrity were tested with a Nanodrop, Qubit, and Agilent 2 100 Bioanalyzer (Agilent Technologies Inc.), respectively. After oligo(dT) enrichment of poly (A)-containing mRNA, mRNA was reverse transcribed into cDNA using the SMARTer PCR cDNA synthesis Kit (Clontech, Mountain View, California, USA). Polymerase chain reaction (PCR) amplification of the synthesized cDNA and large-scale PCR using magnetic beads were used to screen fragments to obtain sufficient cDNA. The full-length cDNA was fragmented, end-repaired and joined with SMRT dumbbell connectors to construct a full-length transcriptome library. Bluepippin was used to screen full-length cDNA fragments with different lengths and construct the Iso-Seq library, which was then subjected to SMRT sequencing on the Pac-Bio Sequel platform.

2.4.2 Full-length transcript analysis, transcript correction and deredundancy After the sequencing was completed, the original downstream data were dejunctioned, and low-quality reads were removed. SMRTlink V8.0 software was used to process the output data. Self-correction was performed to obtain a circular consensus sequence (CCS). CCS was divided into two types of sequences, full-length nonchimeric (FLNC) and nonfull-length (nFL), by testing whether they included primer and poly (A) sequences. The hierarchical n* log(n) algorithm was used to cluster FLNC sequences. Finally, the full-length sequence was polished to obtain the consistent sequence after polishing for subsequent analyses. The second-generation data were corrected by LoRDEC software for polished consensus sequences to further improve the sequencing accuracy. CD-HIT software was used to remove redundant and similar sequences from *P. vulgaris* transcripts.

2.4.3 Gene function annotation and quantification of gene expression levels To obtain comprehensive information on gene function, sequences were annotated for gene function after redundancy using CD-HIT soft-ware using the following databases: NCBI nonredundant protein sequences (NR), NCBI nonredundant nucleotide sequences (NT), protein families (Pfam), clusters of orthologous groups of proteins (KOG/COG), a manually annotated and reviewed protein sequence database (Swiss-Prot), Kyoto Encyclopaedia of Genes and Genomes (KEGG), and Gene Ontology (GO).

Quantification of gene expression levels: The RNA of *P. vulgaris* leaves in the CK and $H_2O_2$ groups was extracted, and three biological repeats of the two treatments were sequenced using the Illumina HiSeq 2 500 platform (Illumina Inc., California, USA). The obtained sequences were mapped to *P. vulgaris* full-length transcriptome sequences, the readings mapped to each gene were calculated, and the relative gene expression level was standardized by FPKM (number of fragments per thousand base transcripts per million mapping reads).

2.4.4 Differential expression analysis The differential expression of FPKM in the CK and $H_2O_2$ groups was analysed using the DESeq R package (1.18.0). The *P* value was adjusted using the method of Benjamini and Hochberg to control the error detection rate. DESeq discovered that genes with an adjusted $|\log_2(\text{fold change})|>1$ and $P$ value $<0.05$ were considered to be differentially expressed genes (DEGs). We used the GOseq R package and KOBAS software to perform GO and KEGG enrichment statistics for DEGs.

2.5 Quantitative real-time PCR (RT-qPCR) analysis RNA from *P. vulgaris* samples in the CK and $H_2O_2$ groups was extracted using a plant RNA extraction kit (MiniBEST, Takara, Dalian, China). The sequences of 30 metabolism-related genes and transcription factor-related genes, with β-actin as the internal reference gene, were selected and synthesized with Primer 5 designed primers (Premier Biosoft International, Palo Alto, California, USA) and Shanghai Biotechnology Services Co., Ltd. (Shanghai, China), as shown in Supplementary Table S2. cDNA was synthesized using the PrimeScript™ RT reagent Kit with the gDNA Eraser (Perfect Real Time) kit (TaKaRa). cDNA was diluted 5-fold, and according to the procedure outlined in the

TB Green ® Premix Ex Taq™ II (Tli RNaseH Plus) kit (TaKaRa), 1 μL of cDNA, 6.25 μL of 2×TB Green Premix Ex Taq (Tli RNaseH Plus), 0.5 μL of upstream and downstream primers, and 4.25 μL of $ddH_2O$ were mixed and finally detected using a CFX96 Real-Time PCR instrument (Bio-Rad Laboratories, Hercules, California, USA). The RT-qPCR procedure was as follows: predenaturation at 95℃ for 30 s, denaturation at 95℃ for 5 s and annealing at 60℃ for 30 s for 40 cycles. The results were compared with the Ct method ($2^{-\Delta\Delta Ct}$) to calculate the relevant gene expression.

2.6 Statistical analysis IBM SPSS Statistics for Windows software (version 21.0, IBM Corp., Armonk, New York, USA) was used for single factor analyses of variance. GraphPad Prism 8.0 (GraphPad Software Inc., San Diego, California, USA) and Origin 2019 (OriginLab, Hampton, Massachusetts, USA) software were used for plotting. The significant difference test was based on Fisher's least significant difference (LSD) method, and $P<0.05$ indicated a significant difference. All experiments were performed using three biological replicates. The data are expressed as means±SDs.

## 3 RESULTS

3.1 Physiological analysis

3.1.1 Photosynthetic attributes The photosynthetic index and pigments in *P. vulgaris* leaves were determined (Table 1). Under $H_2O_2$ stress conditions, Pn significantly increased 2.5-fold after the 24-h treatment period compared with nontreated plants. Tr was significantly higher (increases of 1.9-fold) in $H_2O_2$-pretreated plants during the 24-h period than in unstressed control plants. After 24 h, the Ci and WUEi values were significantly higher (1.2-fold and 4.3-fold) in $H_2O_2$-pretreated plants than in untreated control plants, respectively. In contrast, Gs declined by 9% after 24 h in the $H_2O_2$-treated groups. Additionally, the chlorophyll content (SPAD value) significantly increased by 17% in $H_2O_2$-pretreated plants compared with untreated control plants.

**Table 1 Variations in Pn, Tr, Ci, WUEi, Gs, and SPAD of *P. vulgaris* leaves under exogenous $H_2O_2$ application**

| photosynthetic attributes | CK | $H_2O_2$ |
|---|---|---|
| Pn {$CO_2$[μmol/(m² · s)]} | 16.07±0.32 b | 39.75±0.62 a |
| Tr {$H_2O$ [μmol/(m² · s)]} | 3.53±0.23 b | 6.68±0.17 a |
| Ci (μL/L) | 410.10±3.96 b | 491.50±8.33 a |
| WUEi (mmol/mol) | 2.61±0.13 b | 11.34±0.17 a |
| Gs {$H_2O$ [μmol/(m² · s)]} | 0.35±0.02 a | 0.32±0.01 a |
| SPAD (mg/g) | 47.40±0.81 b | 55.60±0.40 a |

Results are the mean±SD of three replicates. ANOVA and LSD analyses were performed. Different letters in lines indicate a significant difference at $P<0.05$. Pn: net photosynthesis rate; Ci: intercellular $CO_2$ concentration; Gs: stomatal conductance; Tr: transpiration rate and WUEi: instantaneous water-use efficiency; SPAD: chlorophyll content.

3.1.2 Osmotic adjustment substances To explore $H_2O_2$-pretreated *P. vulgaris* plant responses to osmotic damage, the contents of soluble protein, soluble sugar, MDA, and Pro were determined (Table 2). The MDA and Pro contents in *P. vulgaris* leaves increased significantly after 24 h of $H_2O_2$ pretreatment, by 1.8-fold and 1.2-fold, respectively, compared with those in unstressed control plants. The *P. vulgaris* leaf soluble sugar content was markedly elevated by 14% after 24 h of $H_2O_2$ pretreatment. In contrast, compared with control conditions, there was no significant change in soluble protein content after 24 h of $H_2O_2$ pretreatment.

**Table 2 Effects of exogenous $H_2O_2$ application on osmotic adjustment substances in *P. vulgaris* leaves**

| Osmotic adjustment substances | CK | $H_2O_2$ |
|---|---|---|
| MDA (nmol/mg prot) | 1.41±0.15 b | 2.51±0.07 a |
| Pro (μg/g) | 85.53±4.30 b | 102.39±2.06 a |
| Soluble sugar (μg/g prot) | 8.55±0.07 b | 9.74±0.07 a |
| Soluble protein (gprot/L) | 2.63±0.14 a | 2.64±0.18 a |

Results are the mean±SD of three replicates. ANOVA and LSD analyses were performed. Different letters in lines indicate a significant difference at $P<0.05$. MDA: malondialdehyde; Pro: free proline.

3.1.3 $H_2O_2$ content and antioxidant systems The content of $H_2O_2$, antioxidant enzyme activities, and nonenzymatic antioxidants in *P. vulgaris* leaf samples pretreated with distilled water and 2.0 mmol/L $H_2O_2$ were measured after 24 h of exogenous $H_2O_2$ stress (Fig. 1). At 24 h, the $H_2O_2$ content increased and was 18% higher than that in the control (Fig. 1A). The POD activity in pretreated plants increased by 12% compared with that in nontreated plants (Fig. 1B). However, $H_2O_2$ caused a decrease in SOD, CAT, and APX activities values that were 13%, 21%, and 38% lower, respectively, compared with normal conditions (Fig. 1C - E). In addition, the GSH content increased significantly to values that were 74% higher in $H_2O_2$-treated plants than in unstressed control plants (Fig. 1F). A lower level of AsA content (decreased of 12%) was also found in *P. vulgaris* leaves that were treated with $H_2O_2$ than in nontreated plants (Fig. 1G). Furthermore, GO analysis showed that the most abundant GO terms in the "molecular function" category were related to antioxidant activity, implying that *P. vulgaris* improved antioxidant capacity when subjected to $H_2O_2$ stress (Supplementary Fig. S1C). Finally, the expression of genes encoding SOD, CAT, and APX (Fig. 1H) was lower and POD was greater in *P. vulgaris* leaves that were treated with $H_2O_2$ compared with unstressed control plants (Fig. 1H).

3.1.4 Phytohormones and their metabolism-related genes

The contents of JA, SA, ABA, and IAA in *P. vulgaris* leaf samples pretreated with distilled water and 2.0 mmol/L $H_2O_2$ were measured after 24 h of exogenous $H_2O_2$ stress

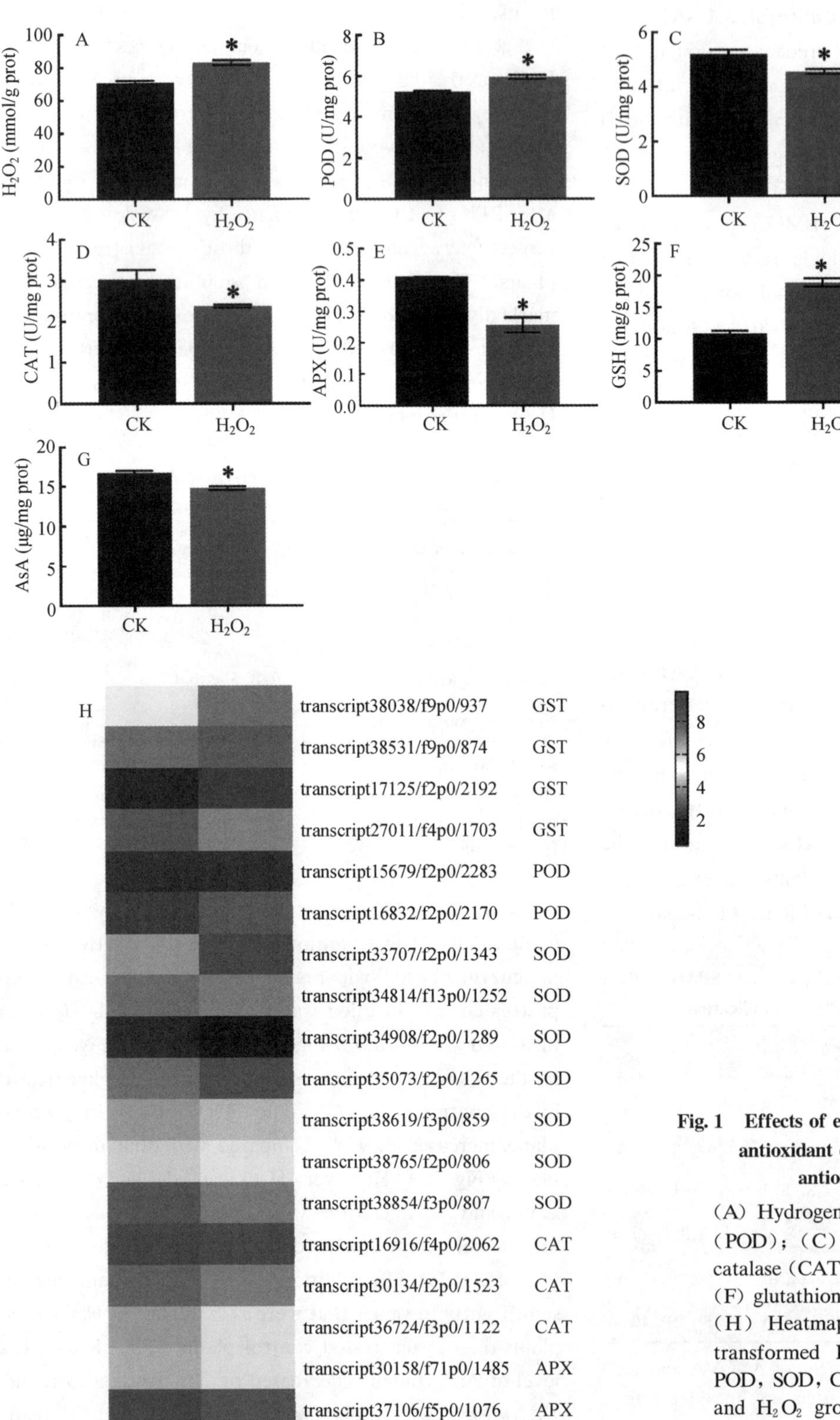


**Fig. 1 Effects of exogenous $H_2O_2$ treatment on $H_2O_2$ content, antioxidant enzyme activities, and nonenzymatic antioxidants in *P. vulgaris* leaves**

(A) Hydrogen peroxide ($H_2O_2$); (B) peroxi-dase (POD); (C) superoxide dismutase (SOD); (D) catalase (CAT); (E) ascor-bate peroxidase (APX); (F) glutathione (GSH); (G) ascorbic acid (AsA). (H) Heatmaps were constructed based on $log_2$-transformed FPKM expression values of GST, POD, SOD, CAT, and APX DEGs between the CK and $H_2O_2$ groups. Results are the mean ± SD of three replicates. * indicates significant differences among the treatments at $P < 0.05$ according to ANOVA and LSD analyses.

(Fig. 2). In *P. vulgaris*, exogenous $H_2O_2$ application significantly increased the contents of JA and SA compared with control plants (increases of 1.5- and 11-fold, respectively) (Fig. 2A–B), which showed that $H_2O_2$ could enhance the contents of JA and SA to upregulate the related synthase expression levels of phytohormones in $H_2O_2$-stressed

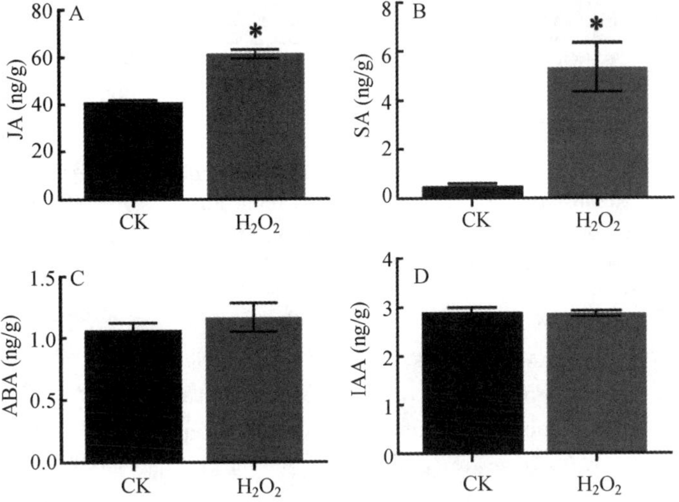


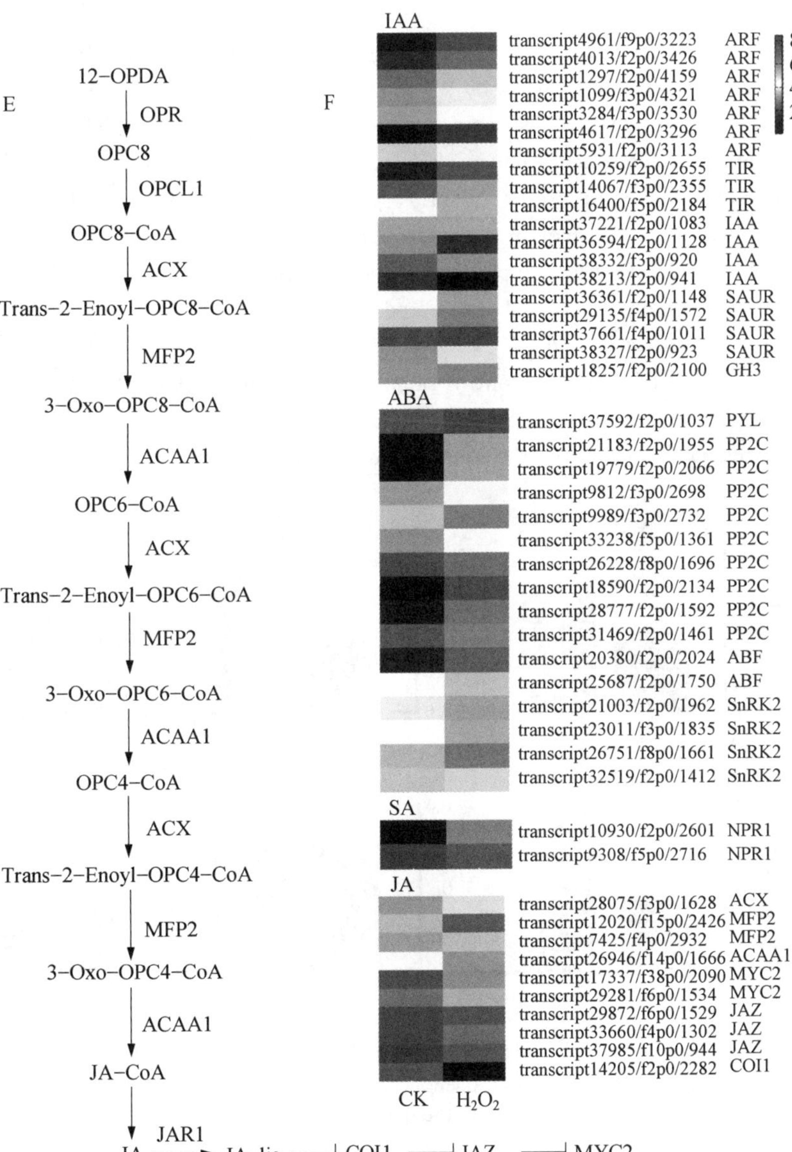


**Fig. 2 Effects of exogenous $H_2O_2$ treatment on plant endogenous hormone contents in *P. vulgaris* leaves**

(A) jasmonic acid (JA), (B) salicylic acid (SA), (C) abscisic acid (ABA), and (D) indole-3-acetic acid (IAA). Results are the mean ± SD of three replicates. * indicates significant differences among the treatments at $P < 0.05$ according to ANOVA and LSD analyses. (E) Comparison of the transcriptional regulation by $H_2O_2$ of JA synthesis and transduction pathways be-tween the CK and $H_2O_2$ groups of *P. vulgaris*. Red indicates upregu-lated DEGs in response to $H_2O_2$ stress, and blue indicates downregulated DEGs. (F) Heatmaps were constructed based on $\log_2$-transformed FPKM expression values of plant hormone signalling pathway DEGs between the CK and $H_2O_2$ groups. $1_2$-OPDA: 12-oxo-phytodienoic acid; OPCL1: OPC-CoA ligase 1; OPR: 12-oxophytodie-noate reductase; OPC: (8-[(1 R, 2 R)-3-Oxo-2-{(Z)-prent-2-enyl} cyclopentyl] octanoate); ACX: acyl-coenzyme A oxidase; ACAA1: acetyl-CoA acyltransferase 1; MFP: glyoxysomal fatty acid beta-oxidation multifunctional protein MFP; JA: jasmonic acid; JAR1: jas-monic acid-amido synthetase JAR1; MYC2: transcription factor MYC2; JAZ: jasmonate ZIM domain protein; COI1: coronatine-insensitive protein 1; SA: salicylic acid; ABA: abscisic acid; IAA: indole acetic acid; ARF: auxin response factor; TIR: protein transport inhibitor response; SAUR: SAUR family protein; GH3: auxin responsive GH3 gene family; PYL: abscisic acid receptor PYL; PP2C: protein phosphatase 2 C; ABF: ABA responsive element binding factor; SnRK2: serine/threonine-protein kinase SRK2A; NPR1: BTB/POZ domain and ankyrin repeat-containing protein NPR1.

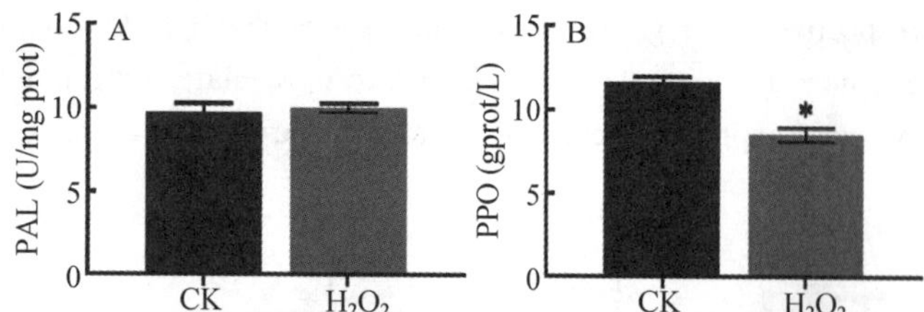


**Fig. 3 Effects of exogenous $H_2O_2$ treatment on PAL and PPO activities in *P. vulgaris* leaves**

(A) Phenylalanine ammonia lyase (PAL) and (B) polyphenol peroxidase (PPO). Results are the mean±SD of three replicates. * indicates significant differences among the treatments at $P<0.05$ according to ANOVA and LSD analyses.

*P. vulgaris*. Consistent with the JA content, *PvACAA1*, *PvMFP2*, and *PvACOX* expression levels were observably upregulated after $H_2O_2$ pretreatment in *P. vulgaris* leaves (Fig. 2E - F). Similar to the JA content, $H_2O_2$ accumulation in $H_2O_2$-stressed *P. vulgaris* activated *PvNPR1* gene (a key regulator of SA synthesis) expression to promote SA accumulation (Fig. 2F).

The ABA content was found to have no significant increased (a slightly increase by 9%) in *P. vulgaris* under $H_2O_2$ stress (Fig. 2C). The gene expression levels of ABA biosynthesis-related genes under $H_2O_2$ treatment, including abscisic acid receptor PYL (*PvPYL*), protein phosphatase 2C (*PvPP2C*), serine/threonine-protein kinase SRK2A (*PvSNRK2*), and ABA responsive element binding factor (*PvABF*), were increased compared with the control (Fig. 2F). In contrast, the *P. vulgaris* leaf IAA content was slightly lower than that in control samples. Consistent with the IAA content, elevated $H_2O_2$ generated a significantly downregulated effect on the relative expression levels of *PvAUX/IAA* and *PvGH3* (Fig. 2D - F).

3.1.5 Secondary metabolism-related enzyme activities The effects of exogenous $H_2O_2$ stresses on PAL and PPO activities are shown in Fig. 3. PAL activity in *P. vulgaris* leaves was enhanced by 3% after 24 h in the $H_2O_2$-stressed groups, but the values were not significantly changed compared with those in the control plants (Fig. 3A). Interestingly, the leaf PPO activity of $H_2O_2$-pretreated plants was significantly reduced by 27% compared with that of nontreated plants after a 24-h period (Fig. 3B).

3.1.6 Secondary metabolite contents and its metabolism-related gene expression The polyphenolic and triterpenoid contents of *P. vulgaris* leaf samples were studied after $H_2O_2$ pretreatment for 24 h (Fig. 4). Compared with the control group, the total phenolic, total flavonoid, rosmarinic acid, hyperoside, and salviaflaside contents were obviously increased (increases of 1.8 - fold, 1.7 - fold, 1.2 - fold, 2.0 - fold and 1.6 - fold, respectively), whereas the caffeic acid content decreased by 7%, but there was no significant difference during $H_2O_2$ pretreatment (Fig. 4A - F). Furthermore, the oleanolic acid content was significantly increased by 2.1 - fold in response to 24 h of $H_2O_2$ stress, and the ursolic acid was increased by 26% but was not significant in unstressed control plants (Fig. 4G - H).

The mechanism underlying $H_2O_2$-induced polyphenolic production in *P. vulgaris* was investigated, and it was found that transcriptional expression of *PvPAL*, *PvC4H*, *Pv4CL*, *PvTAT*, *PvHPPR*, *PvHPPD*, *PvCSE*, *PvRAS*, and *PvCYP98A* in the CK and $H_2O_2$ groups responded to the biosynthesis of *P. vulgaris* polyphenols (Fig. 5A). This result showed that the transcript expression levels of *Pv4CL*,

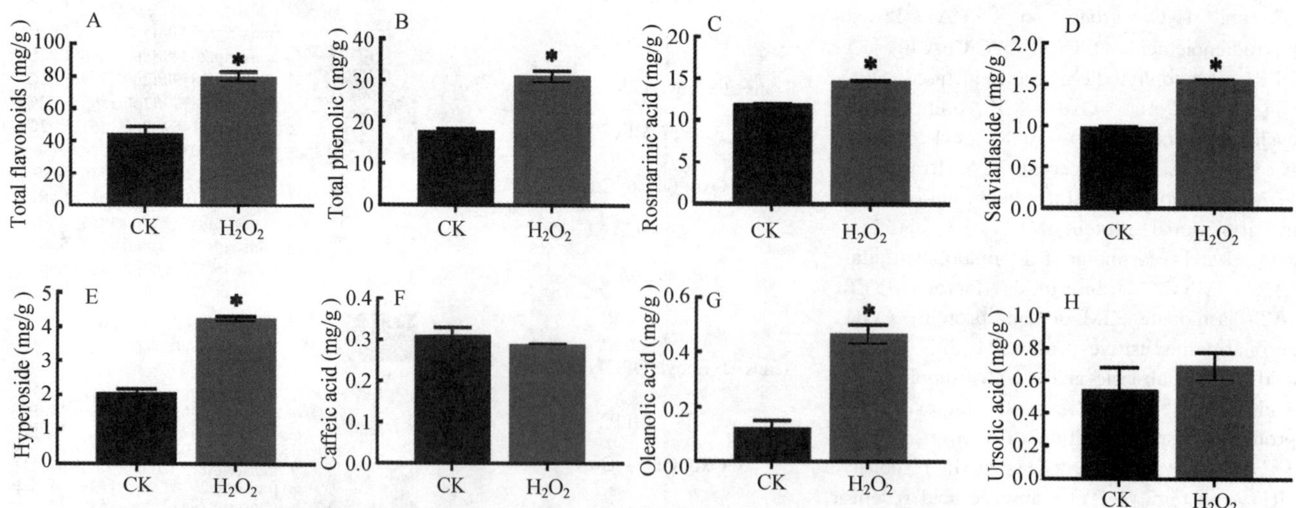


**Fig. 4 Effects of exogenous $H_2O_2$ treatment on phenolic acid, flavonoid, and triterpene acid contents in *P. vulgaris* leaves**

(A) Total flavonoids; (B) total phenolics; (C) rosmarinic acid; (D) caffeic acid; (E) salviaflaside; (F) hyperoside; (G) oleanolic acid; (H) ursolic acid. Results are the mean±SD of three replicates. * indicates significant differences among the treatments at $P<0.05$ according to ANOVA and LSD analyses.

*PvHPPR*, *PvHPPD*, *PvCSE* and *PvCYP98A* were upregulated significantly in response to 24 h of $H_2O_2$ stress compared with the control group. However, the transcript expression of *PvPAL* and *PvRAS* was not affected by $H_2O_2$ stress (Fig. 5B). Furthermore, administration of $H_2O_2$ was able to inhibit the transcript expression of *PvTAT* and *PvC4H*, which downregulated their relative expression levels (Fig. 5B).

Treatment of *P. vulgaris* leaves with distilled water and $H_2O_2$ to study the transcriptional expression levels of terpenoid biosynthesis-related genes, including the mevalonate

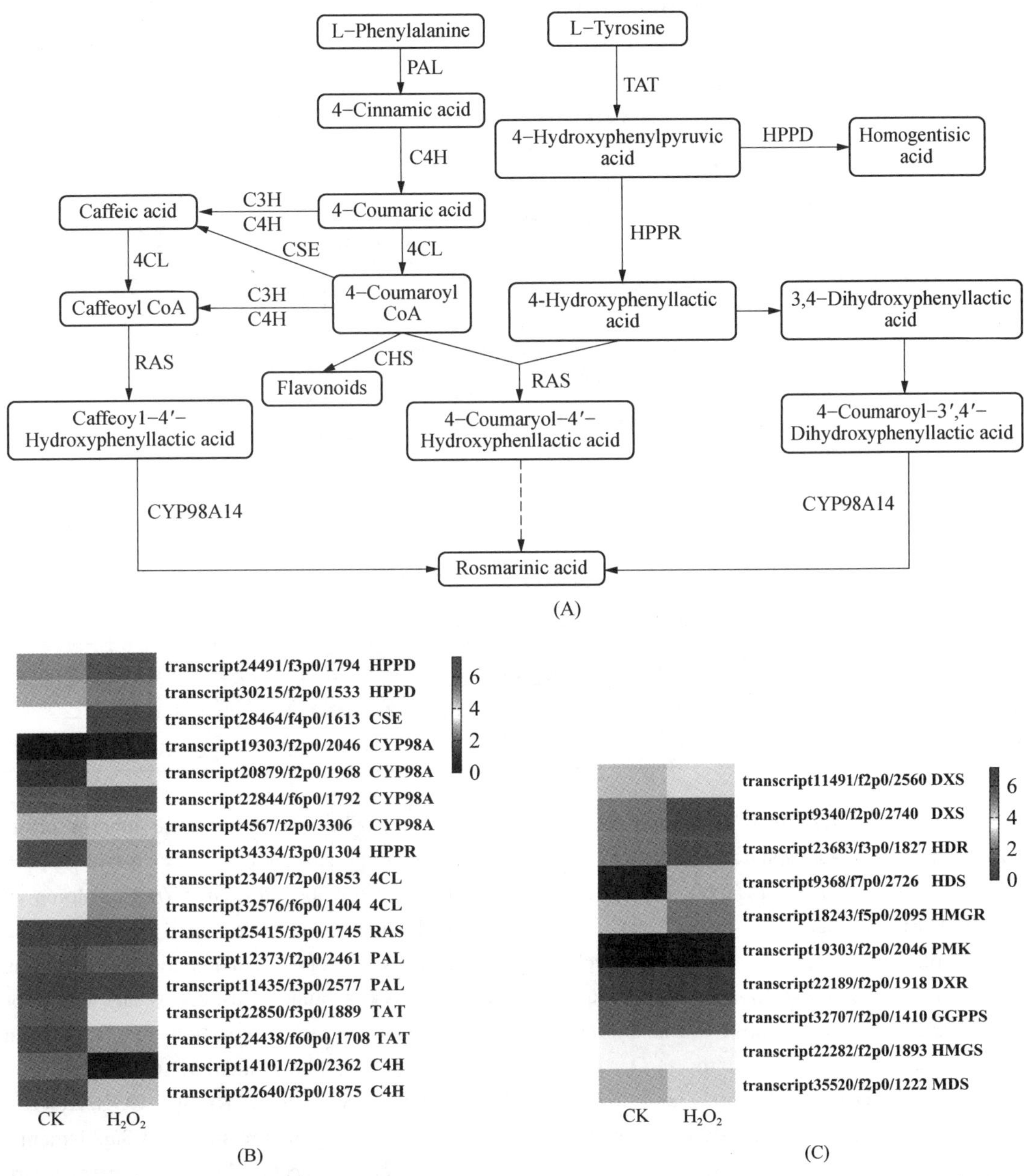


**Fig. 5** (A) DEGs involved in the phenylpropanoid biosynthesis pathway in the transcriptome profile of *P. vulgaris* in response to $H_2O_2$. Red indicates DEGs that were dramatically upregulated in response to $H_2O_2$ stress, blue indicates DEGs with significant downregulation. (B) Heatmaps were constructed based on $log_2$-transformed FPKM expression values of polyphenolic DEGs between the CK and $H_2O_2$ groups. (C) Heatmaps were constructed based on $log_2$-transformed FPKM expression values of triterpenoid pathway DEGs between the CK and $H_2O_2$ groups. (D) DEGs involved in the triterpenoid biosynthesis pathway in the transcriptome profile of *P. vulgaris* in response to $H_2O_2$ application. PAL: phenylalanine ammonia lyase; C4H: cinnamate 4-hydroxylase; C3H: p-coumarate 3-hydrolase; 4CL: 4-hydroxy cinnamoyl CoA ligase; HPPR: hydroxyphenylpyruvate reductase; HPPD: hydroxyphenylpyruvate dioxygenase; RAS: rosmarinic acid synthase; TAT: tyrosine aminotransferase; CSE: caffeoyl shikimate esterase; CHS: Chalcone synthase; CYP98A: cytochrome P450 CYP98A; MVK: mevalonate kinase; MVD: mevalonate 5-dinhophate decarboxylase; AACT: acetyl-CoA acyltransferase; HMGS: 3-hydroxy-3-methylglutaryl-CoA; HMGR: 3-hy-droxy-3-methylglutaryl-CoA reductase; PMK: phosphomevalonate kinase; DXS: 1-deoxy-D-xylulose 5-phosphate synthase; DXR: 1-deoxy-D-xylulose 5-phosphate reductoisomerase; MCT: MEP cytidyltransferase; MDS: 2-C-Methy-D-eryth-ritol2,4-cyclodiphosphate synthase; HDS: hydroxymethylbutenyl 4-dipho-sphatesynthase; HDR: 4-hydroxy-3-methylbut-2-enyldiphosphatereductase; IDI: iso-pentenyl diphosphate isomerase; GGPPS: geranylgeranyl diphosphate synthase; CMK: 4-(cytidine 5-diphospho)-2-C-methylerythritol kinase.

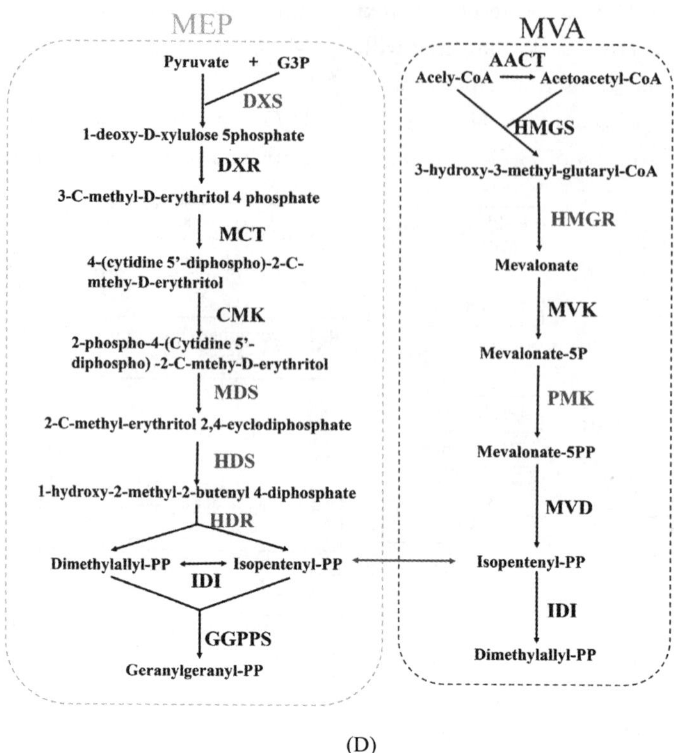


(D)

**Fig. 5** (continued)

**Table 3 Statistics for the polymerase reads**

| Sample | Polymerase read bases G | Polymerase reads | Polymerase read length mean | Polymerase read N50 |
|---|---|---|---|---|
| *P. vulgaris* leaves, stem, spicas | 23.5 Gb | 471,436 | 49,841 | 103,935 |

(MVA) pathway (e.g., *PvHMGS*, *PvHMGR*, and *PvPMK*) and 2-C-methyl-D-erythritol-4-phosphate (MEP) pathway (e.g., *PvDXS*, *PvDXR*, *PvMDS*, *PvHDS*, *PvHDR*, and *PvGGPPS*), were measured (Fig. 5D).

Based on the obtained results, the expression levels of *PvDXS*, *PvHDS*, *PvHDR*, and *PvHMGR* were upregulated after $H_2O_2$ treatment. However, the *PvMDS* expression level was downregulated in response to $H_2O_2$ stress. Additionally, *PvDXR*, *PvGGPPS*, *PvPMK*, and *PvHMGS* gene expression levels were not significantly different under $H_2O_2$ stress (Fig. 5 C).

3.2. Transcriptome analysis

3.2.1 Transcriptome sequencing, transcript analysis correction and gene function annotation To explore the effects of exogenous $H_2O_2$ on *P. vulgaris* leaves, we performed a transcriptome analysis of leaves treated with distilled water and $H_2O_2$ for 24 h. In total, 471,436 polymerase reads (23.5 Gb) were generated during PacBio Sequel sequencing (Table 3). To improve the accuracy of the data, the full-length transcriptome was calibrated and redundantly sequenced several times, and the length frequencies of the transcripts before and after redundancy and the distribution of sequence lengths after redundancy were counted (Table 4). Transcripts of 39,136 reads were available before the full-length transcriptome was calibrated and redundantly sequenced, and the number of genes after redundancy was 21,415. The majority of the transcripts were in the 1 - 3 kbp range, with an average length of 2 175 bp.

The functional annotation of 21,415 unigenes was normalized and the redundancy removed in seven databases, including Nr, Swiss-Prot, KEGG, COG/KOG, GO, Nt, and Pfam, and the results are shown in Supplementary Fig. S1A. The number of successfully annotated transcripts in at least one database was 20,406, the number of successfully annotated transcripts in all seven databases was 10,280, and the numbers of unigenes successfully annotated to the Nr, Swiss-Prot, KEGG, KOG, GO, Nt, and Pfam databases were 20,288, 17,984, 20,235, 13,617, 15,536, 17,901, and 15,536 entries, respectively.

In addition, to obtain the gene sequence similarity between *P. vulgaris* and related species, the total unigenes of *P. vulgaris* obtained from different treatments were annotated against the NR library, and the results showed that the *P. vulgaris* gene sequences had the highest homology

**Table 4 Length-frequency distribution statistics of transcripts before and after deredundancy**

| Sample | Transcripts length interval | <500 bp | 500 - 1 kbp | 1 - 2 kbp | 2 - 3 kbp | > 3 kbp | Total |
|---|---|---|---|---|---|---|---|
| Before deredundancy | Number of transcripts | 26 | 1 339 | 17 813 | 13 279 | 6 679 | 39 136 |
| After deredundancy | Number of Genes | 13 | 884 | 9 987 | 7 033 | 3 498 | 21 415 |
| Sequence length after deredundancy | | | | | | | |
| Sample | Total nucleotides | Total number | Mean length | Min length | Max length | N50 | N90 |
| After deredundancy | 46,577,397 | 21 415 | 2 175 | 377 | 8 401 | 2 357 | 1 412 |

with *Sesamum indicum*, followed by *Erythranthe guttata*, *Salvia miltiorrhiza*, and *Dorcoceras hygrometricum* (Supplementary Fig. S1B).

The GO functional classification statistics revealed 29,716 unigenes annotated to biological process, 153, 516 unigenes annotated to cellular component and 194, 736 unigenes annotated to molecular function. Biological process had the highest distribution in metabolic process and cellular process, with 7 502 and 6 856 unigenes, respectively. The cellular component had a relatively average and low gene abundance. The genes for binding and catalytic activity accounted for more than 90% of molecular function, with 9 808 and 7 562 genes, respectively (Supplementary Fig. S1C).

To further investigate its biochemical function, the genes were annotated into the KEGG database, and 20,235 genes were found to be annotated to 358 metabolic pathways of the 5 major KEGG pathways. The most annotated pathways were "carbon metabolism" (ko01200, 484), "biosynthesis of amino acids" (ko01230, 381), "plant hormone signal transduction" (ko04075, 283), and "starch and sucrose meta-bolism" (ko00500, 169). The pathways associated with secondary metabolism were "phenylpropanoid biosynthesis" (ko00940, 90), "flavonoid biosynthesis" (ko00941, 30), "flavone and flavonol biosynthesis" (ko00944, 2), "terpenoid backbone biosynthesis" (ko00900, 76), "diterpenoid biosynthesis" (ko00904, 12), and "sesquiterpenoid and triterpenoid biosynthesis" (ko00909,17) (Supplementary Fig. S1D).

3.2.2 Analysis of differentially expressed genes (DEGs) We sequenced the transcriptomes of two groups (control leaves (CK), $H_2O_2$-treated leaves ($H_2O_2$)) consisting of three replicates. In all 3 374 DEGs, 1 442 upregulated and 1932 downregulated genes were found between the CK and $H_2O_2$ groups of *P. vulgaris* leaves that matched the padj<0.05 and $|\log_2 \text{FoldChange}|>1$ (Fig. 6).

GO analysis between the CK and $H_2O_2$ groups showed that 1 436, 331, and 747 DEGs were annotated into "biological process", "cellular component" and "molecular function", respectively (Fig. 7). The biological process classification DEGs were mainly enriched in "metabolic

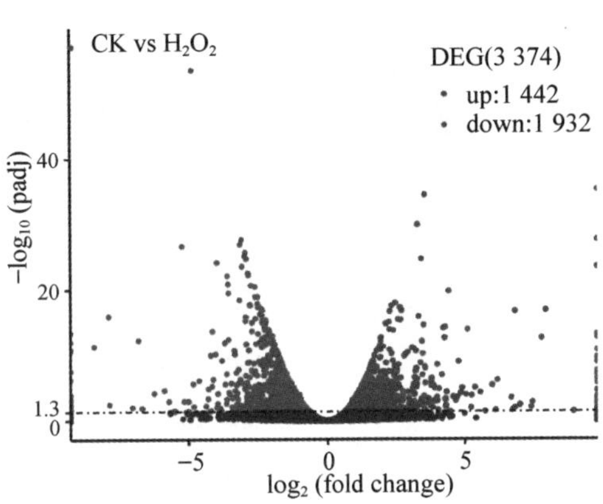


**Fig. 6 Differential gene volcano map in the CK vs · $H_2O_2$ group**

process", "single-organism metabolic process", and "oxidation-reduction process". The molecular function classification DEGs were enriched in "catalytic process activity" and "oxidoreductase activity". These results indicated the role of $H_2O_2$ in cell metabolism, biological regulation and the oxidative stress response.

To explore metabolic pathways and gene functions, we discovered 557 upregulated DEGs that were annotated into 95 KEGG pathways between the CK and $H_2O_2$ groups. Fig. 8 shows the first 20 enrichment pathways; among them, "plant hormone signal transduction", "starch and sucrose metabolism", "ubiquitin mediated proteolysis", "peroxisome", and "glycerolipid metabolism" had the most upregulated DEGs. Additionally, 5, 8, and 37 DEGs were obviously upregulated in polyphenol-, terpenoid- and plant hormone signal transduction-related pathways, respectively (Supplementary Table S3).

3.2.3 Transcription factor (TF) expression Transcription factors are important regulators of gene regulatory networks in abiotic stress. Between the CK and $H_2O_2$ groups, there were 240 differentially expressed TFs from 56 different TF families, of which 128 were upregulated and 112 were downregulated. The top 30 are shown in Fig. 9A. The results showed that $H_2O_2$ stress caused the differential expression of many TFs, most of which were from the bHLH, WRKY and MYB families. These

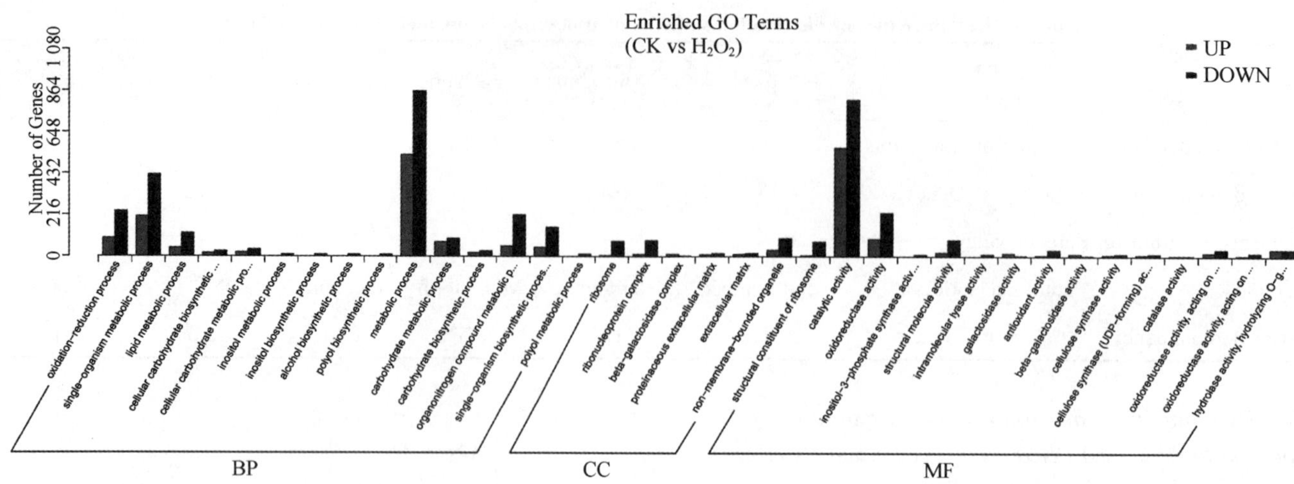


Fig. 7 GO classification of differentially expressed genes in the CK vs · $H_2O_2$ group

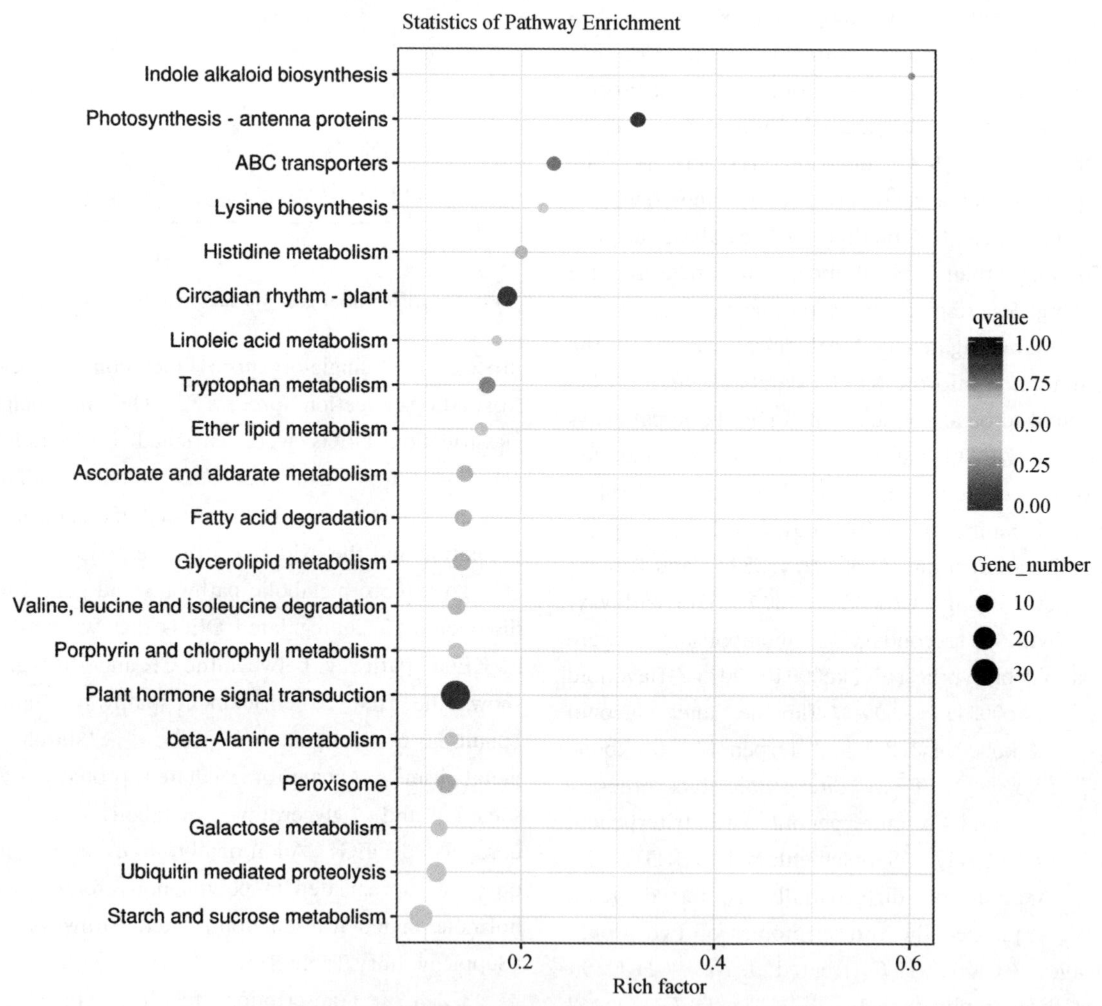


Fig. 8 The top 20 KEGG pathways enriched in DEGs between CK and $H_2O_2$

differentially expressed TFs were also considered to have the function of regulating antioxidant capacity. The cis elements in the promoter regions of genes related to secondary metabolites (phenolic acids, flavonids, and triterpenes acids) were analysed, and bHLH, WRKY and MYB had numerous binding sites (Fig. 9B - D) · $H_2O_2$ may modulate the expression of genes related to secondary metabolism by regulating the response of TFs to $H_2O_2$ stress.

3.2.4 RT-qPCR validation of the RNA-Seq results

To verify the transcriptome data, RT-qPCR was used to verify the expression of 29 DEG genes in *P. vulgaris* leaves after $H_2O_2$ treatment. As shown in Fig. 10, the expression

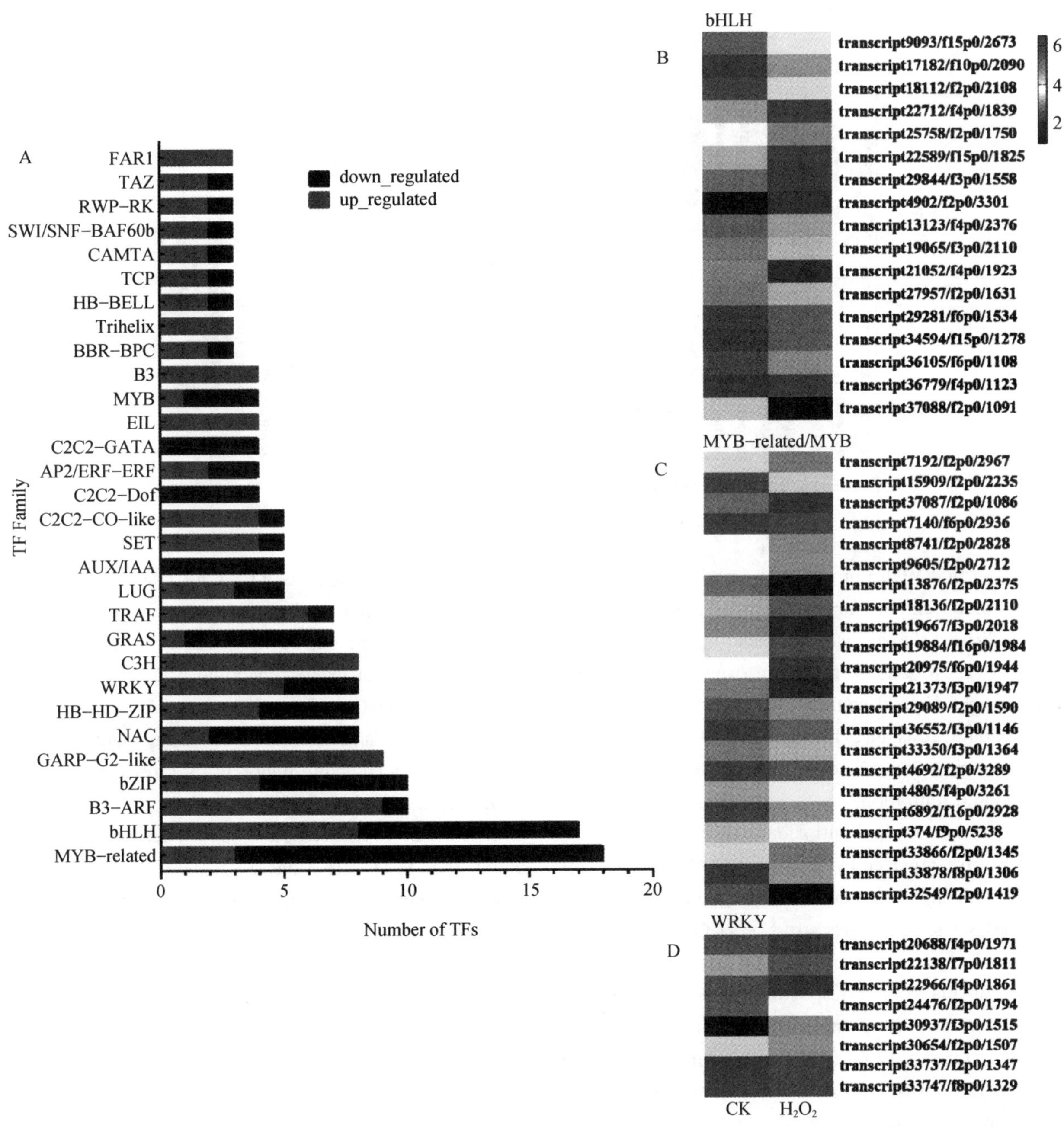


**Fig. 9** (A) The numbers of differentially expressed transcription factors between the CK and $H_2O_2$ groups. (B)-(D) Heatmaps were constructed based on $\log_2$-transformed FPKM expression values of bHLH, MYB-related/MYB, and WRKY TFs between the CK and $H_2O_2$ groups.

profiles of all validation genes were similar to those detected by sequencing. These findings showed the high reliability of the transcriptome data and their to reflect actual transcriptome changes.

# 4 DISCUSSION

4.1 Photosynthesis and chlorophyll analysis Plant photosynthesis can lead to the acquisition of carbon and energy, which are extremely sensitive to abiotic stress. Photosynthetic efficiency is closely related to chlorophyll content, and a suitable concentration of $H_2O_2$ can significantly improve the photosynthesis capability in many crops and medical plants. In the present study, spraying of exogenous $H_2O_2$ after 24 h significantly increased Pn due to the higher chlorophyll contents in *P. vulgaris* plants under oxidative stress. In addition, exogenous $H_2O_2$ decreased Gs in oxidatively stressed plants after 24 h. These studies indicated that *P. vulgaris* could clearly increase Pn by reducing the stomatal limitation following 24 h of $H_2O_2$ stress. In addition, WUEi is a crucial index of plant adaptation and defence to oxidative stress. The results of this study showed that WUEi increased in $H_2O_2$-free plants after

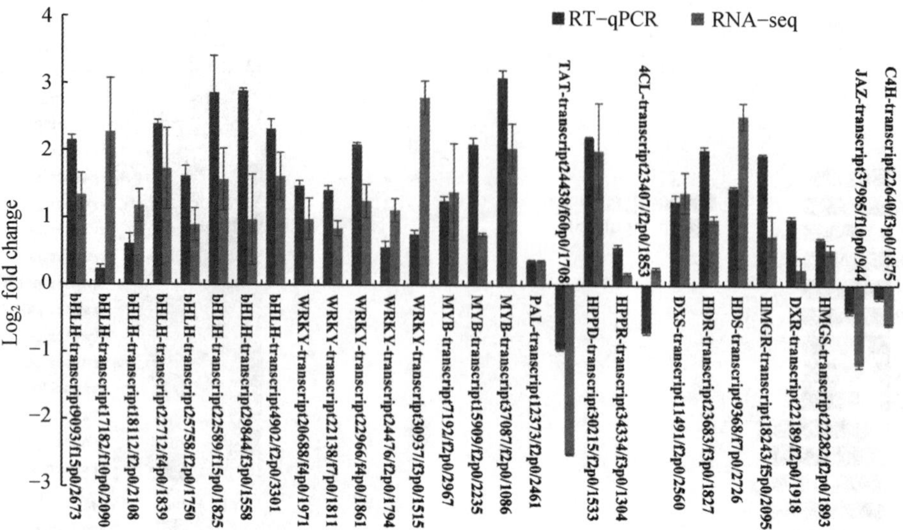


**Fig. 10 Validation of the RNA-Seq results by RT - qPCR**

Data are presented as the mean±SD of three replicates.

24 h, indicating that WUEi might be an important factor for *P. vulgaris* plant enhancement of antioxidant tolerance. This study indicated that *P. vulgaris* could help to retain the green colour of leaves and protect them from $H_2O_2$ injury by increasing the chlorophyll content. Therefore, *P. vulgaris* exerts antioxidant resistance by increasing the chlorophyll content, enhancing the photosynthetic capacity, and the reducing stomatal limitation.

4.2 $H_2O_2$ content and antioxidant systems When *P. vulgaris* plants are damaged by exogenous $H_2O_2$, antioxidant signalling is invoked, which in turn adjusts and controls the defence response to oxidative stress · $H_2O_2$ is a crucial signalling molecule, and it can regulate the growth and development of plants and respond to various biotic and abiotic stresses. The endogenous $H_2O_2$ content increased significantly after exogenous $H_2O_2$ spraying for 24 h (Fig. 3A), which was consistent with previous research results. These results demonstrated that exogenous $H_2O_2$ spraying resulted in the accumulation of endogenous $H_2O_2$ in *P. vulgaris*.

*P. vulgaris* prevents oxidative injury by activating the antioxidant defence system, including antioxidases of POD, CAT, SOD, and APX. As a crucial antioxidant enzyme, POD can catalyse the translation of $H_2O_2$ to $H_2O$ and $O_2$. In this research, the POD activity of *P. vulgaris* plants in the $H_2O_2$ group was significantly higher than that in the CK group, which may be due to the increased expression of POD genes under $H_2O_2$ in *P. vulgaris* leaves (Fig. 1B). The expression of genes encoding POD was upregulated under oxidative stress in rice. Therefore, we surmise that *P. vulgaris* scavenging $H_2O_2$ capacity may be connected with POD activity.

*P. vulgaris* leaf SOD, CAT, and APX activities significantly decreased under 24 h stress conditions (Fig. 1C-E), which may be due to the significant downregulation of the expression of genes encoding SOD, CAT, and APX under 24 h $H_2O_2$ pretreatment in *P. vulgaris* leaves. Moreover, the activities of these antioxidant enzymes also showed a larger decline under $H_2O_2$ stress, which may lead to higher levels of $H_2O_2$, MDA and Pro during 24 h of $H_2O_2$ pretreatment (Fig. 1A; Table 2). Therefore, these results imply that $H_2O_2$ stress has a greater effect on *P. vulgaris* leaves enzymatic antioxidant system. Similar results were reported in previous studies.

*P. vulgaris* leaves contain nonenzymatic antioxidants such as ascorbate (AsA) and glutathione (GSH), and the AsA-GSH cycle enzymes are well coordinated and can render better tolerance to oxidative stress. In this research, GSH levels were highly increased under $H_2O_2$ stress compared to the control, which is due to GSH playing a central role in antioxidant defence systems. More interestingly, the expression of glutathione S-transferase (GST) genes was greater in leaves subjected to the $H_2O_2$ treatment (Fig. 1H), which can catalyse GSH combination with peroxide products and reduce the content of $H_2O_2$ in cells. In addition, the AsA content decreased significantly under $H_2O_2$ stress, which might lead to more $H_2O_2$ and MDA accumulation under $H_2O_2$ conditions. Therefore, *P. vulgaris* can mitigate $H_2O_2$-induced ROS damage by enhancing POD activity and GSH accumulation.

4.3 Osmotic adjustment substances Plants undergo physiological changes under stress, and the ultimate objective is to maintain cell homeostasis to support normal growth and development. Previously, when plants were stressed by exogenous $H_2O_2$, soluble sugar, soluble protein, MDA and Pro played an important role in maintaining homeostasis, but different plant species have different osmoregulation functions. Studies have shown that there are differences in important osmotic regulators of *P. vulgaris* under exogenous $H_2O_2$ stress. First, as a membrane lipid peroxide, MDA content can directly reflect the extent of membrane peroxidation. Second, as a physiologically compatible solute, Pro can be added as needed to maintain the beneficial osmotic potential between cells and their surrounding environment. Under $H_2O_2$ stress, the increase in MDA and Pro in the 24 h period was higher (1.8-fold and 1.2-fold) than that in untreated plants, which showed that the damage to lipid peroxidation was unfavourable. This phenomenon might be connected to the observation that 24 h-treated *P. vulgaris* plants have a stronger antioxidant system, which can remove reactive oxygen species (ROS) damage caused by $H_2O_2$ stress.

As cell osmotic regulators, soluble proteins and soluble sugars can improve the antioxidant capacity of plants by the regulating cell osmotic potential, which is similar to our previous research. The soluble protein content in *P. vulgaris* leaves was not significantly changed by 24 h of $H_2O_2$ application, possibly because more free amino acids participate in phenylpropanoid metabolism, generating more secondary metabolites to defend against $H_2O_2$-induced stress. In addition, the soluble sugar content in *P. vulgaris* leaves was slightly enhanced after 24 h of $H_2O_2$ treatment, possibly due to the generation of sugars functioning as true ROS scavengers; additionally, sugars and phenolic compounds synergistically scavenge ROS in plants and enhance stress resistance. Moreover, sugars not only directly participate in biochemical compound synthesis and energy production but are also involved in maintaining membrane stability. Interestingly, the $H_2O_2$ group soluble sugar content did not change significantly compared with the CK group, which might be because the accumulation of $H_2O_2$ exceeded the soluble sugar content. Thus, this study indicated that *P. vulgaris* plants could adapt to adversity by adjusting the ROS concentration by synthesizing and accumulating more compatible solutes after damage caused by $H_2O_2$ stress, and osmotic regulatory substances play important roles in the $H_2O_2$ stress response.

4.4 Phytohormones and their metabolism-related genes

The phytohormones JA and SA can regulate the protective response to $H_2O_2$ stress through $H_2O_2$-induced signalling pathways. This study confirmed that the accumulation of $H_2O_2$ in *P. vulgaris* leaves was related to the upregulation of jasmonate synthesis and jasmonate-related synthase gene transcription.

We confirmed that $H_2O_2$ accumulation in *P. vulgaris* leaves was connected with the upregulation of JA biosynthesis-related synthase genes (e.g., *PvACAA1*, *PvMFP2*, and *PvACOX*). More interestingly, the transcription levels of JA downstream synthases, such as jasmonate ZIM-domain (JAZ), myelocytomatosis 2 (MYC2), COI1 protein, and MYC2-targeted BHLH1 (MTB1), were inhibited, resulting in the reduced decomposition of JA (Fig. 2E-F). These results are consistent with the $H_2O_2$-activated JA signalling mechanism in $H_2O_2$-stressed *Aquilaria sinensis*. In addition, exogenous $H_2O_2$ stress leads to an accumulation of JA and increases polyphenolic biosynthesis and transcript levels of phenylpropanoid synthases (e.g., *Pv4CL*, *PvHPPR*, and *PvCYP98A*) and terpenoid synthases (e.g., *PvDXS*, *PvHDS*, *PvHDR*, and *PvHMGR*). In conclusion, $H_2O_2$ can accelerate the accumulation of JA and subsequently promote polyphenolic (phenolic acids and flavonoids) and triterpene acid production.

SA is an absolute signalling molecule that participates in a variety of physiological processes. A large number of studies have confirmed that SA protects plants from oxidative damage by regulating the redox balance. Exogenous $H_2O_2$ induced an increase in SA content in *P. vulgaris* leaves (Fig. 2B). Correspondingly, the transcript level of the primary gene involved in SA biosynthesis (*PvNPR1*, a key regulator of SA synthesis) was upregulated in $H_2O_2$-pretreated *P. vulgaris* plants, which further upregulated phenolic acid, flavonoid, and triterpene acid biosynthesis, as well as the transcription of polyphenolics and terpenoid-related synthases by exogenous $H_2O_2$ application. These results confirmed that the accumulated $H_2O_2$ could activate SA and regulate the biosynthesis of polyphenols and triterpene acids. Nevertheless, the interaction between $H_2O_2$ and SA is complicated, and the mechanism underlying the interaction between $H_2O_2$ and SA during $H_2O_2$-induced phenolic acid, flavonoid, and triterpene acid formation requires further research.

As a crucial endogenous plant hormone, ABA plays a role in the plant response to different abiotic stress chemical signals. In this study, we discovered that the ABA content increased by 9% when *P. vulgaris* was subjected to $H_2O_2$ application (Fig. 2C). On the one hand, the increase in ABA promotes stomatal closure, enables *P. vulgaris* plants to confine water loss through transpiration, and improves the water condition of plants with the increase in root hydraulic conductivity. On the other hand, the increase in ABA can upregulate the phenolic biosynthesis pathway following exposure to oxidative stress. Additionally, the expression levels of genes related to ABA biosynthesis (e.g., *PvPYL*, *PvPP2C*, *PvSNRK2*, and *PvABF*) were upregulated in *P. vulgaris* leaves under $H_2O_2$ stress (Fig. 2F). These results indicated that the ABA increase might be linked with $H_2O_2$

tolerance as a signalling molecule for controlling stomatal closure and antioxidant defence.

Abiotic stress decreases the IAA content in leaves of plants. This study showed that with increasing $H_2O_2$ levels, the IAA content in *P. vulgaris* leaves was slightly lower than that in control samples (Fig. 2D). Additionally, $H_2O_2$ stress decreases the relative expression levels of *PvAUX/IAA* and *PvGH3* (two central auxin-related gene families). Moreover, plant phenolics, as chemical messengers or physiological regulators, limit IAA synthesis (monohydroxy B-ring flavonoids) or inhibit IAA catabolism (dihydroxy B-ring flavonoids). Additionally, a negative relationship was observed between IAA and total flavonoid content ($R=-0.39$). Taken together, these results show that $H_2O_2$ induces phenolic acid and flavonoid production to suppress IAA biosynthesis.

4.5 Secondary metabolism-related enzyme activities

During oxidative stress, *P. vulgaris* plants accumulate secondary metabolites for adaptation and defence. Phenylalanine ammonia-lyase (PAL) catalyses phenylalanine deamination from primary metabolism to necessary secondary phenylalanine/phenolic metabolism in *P. vulgaris* plants. In this research, PAL activity in *P. vulgaris* leaves increased in response to $H_2O_2$ stresses (Fig. 3A). The increase in PAL activity triggered the reaction of the phenylpropanoid pathway to produce specific phenylpropanoid derivatives, such as phenolic compounds and flavonoids. Phenolic and flavonoid compounds of *P. vulgaris* play a crucial role in reducing oxidative damage because they are involved in ROS elimination. Interestingly, PAL activity did not show a marked increase in *P. vulgaris* leaves, which suggests that suppression of PAL activity is induced by higher $H_2O_2$ and polyphenol contents. Additionally, our previous research indicated a positive linear relationship between PAL activity and both the total phenolic acid content and flavonoids of *P. vulgaris* ($R=0.949^{**}$ and $R=0.914^{**}$, respectively). Taken together, these results indicate that the increased PAL activity is related to the *P. vulgaris* plant tolerance response to $H_2O_2$ stresses.

In contrast, PPO activity was significantly lower in *P. vulgaris* plants under $H_2O_2$ stress (Fig. 3B). In general, the PPO activity and gene expression levels induced in plant leaf tissues can help plants reduce abiotic stress. Interestingly, a downregulation of PPO activity in leaves by high $H_2O_2$ stress suggests that the decrease in PPO activity could be developed by *P. vulgaris* to improve the antioxidative action of phenolic compounds. Previous studies have reported similar results.

4.6 Secondary metabolite contents and its metabolism-related gene expression Phenolic acids and flavonoids are two crucial secondary metabolites in *P. vulgaris*. Abiotic stress produces ROS such as $H_2O_2$, and $H_2O_2$ also induces a large amount of phenolic acid and flavonoid synthesis in *P. vulgaris* plants. Compared with the CK group, the application of $H_2O_2$ stress produced 1.8-fold and 1.7-fold increases in total phenolics and total flavonoids, respectively (Fig. 4A - B). These findings are similar to those in a previous study showing that when *P. vulgaris* suffered from adverse stress and destruction of the primary antioxidant defence system, polyphenolics (e.g., phenolic acids and flavonoids) acted as a secondary antioxidant system to scavenge ROS · $H_2O_2$ mainly acts on phenylalanine branch synthesis genes (e.g., PAL, C4H, and 4CL) in the synthesis of phenolic acids and flavonoids in *P. vulgaris* (Fig. 5A). Exogenous application of $H_2O_2$ produced higher *PvPAL* gene expression and significantly upregulated the gene expression of *Pv4CL* (Fig. 5B). Among them, 4CL serves as an important branch point of the branched pathways leading to the generation of phenolic acids and flavonoids. Moreover, enzymatic analysis indicated that the recombinant protein of *Sm4CL2* had a strong substrate affinity for *p*-coumaric acid. In addition, similar to our previous study, the increased $H_2O_2$ content could upregulate the expression level of the *PvPAL* gene, thus promoting the production of phenolic acids and flavonoids (Fig. 5B). Interestingly, treatment with $H_2O_2$ significantly downregulated the expression level of phenylalanine synthase genes (e.g., *PvC4H*), which indicated that the related gene expression did not show a trend consistent with the change in phenolic acid content. In addition, the phenylpropanoid metabolism-related synthase gene expression levels were in agreement with polyphenol content, suggesting that $H_2O_2$ accumulation in *P. vulgaris* leaves activated PAL activity and *PvPAL* and *Pv4CL* gene expression to promote phenolic acid and flavonoid accumulation.

Rosmarinic acid and salviaflaside are the main phenolic components and show high antioxidant activity in *P. vulgaris*. In *P. vulgaris*, the rosmarinic acid and salviaflaside contents were clearly increased (increases of 1.2-fold and 1.6-fold, respectively) compared with the results obtained with the control treatment (Fig. 4C - D). Previous research confirmed that the rosmarinic acid content of *P. vulgaris* plants significantly increased in response to abiotic stress (e.g., UV-B radiation, UV-B/A removal, drought stress, and soil nutrient element deficiency) and was mediated by a key signalling molecule ($H_2O_2$). This $H_2O_2$-induced stress generates a large amount of endogenous $H_2O_2$ production, which further activates and upregulates the expression levels of the four genes in the phenylalanine and tyrosine branches of the rosmarinic acid synthesis pathway (e.g., *PvPAL*, *Pv4CL*, *PvHPPR*, and *CYP98A14*), thereby providing sufficient substrates to maintain the metabolic pathway level required for rosmarinic acid synthesis. To date, the metabolic enzymes *PAL*, *4CL*,

*HPPR*, and *CYP98A14* in *Salvia miltiorrhiza* (as a Labiatae model herb) have been functionally analysed. Overexpression of *SmPAL*, *Sm4CL*, *SmHPPR*, and *SmCYP98A14* significantly increased the production of rosmarinic acid. Interestingly, salviaflaside enhanced *P. vulgaris* leaf performance, probably due to β-glucosidase activity, and its gene expression levels were dramatically activated by $H_2O_2$ stress, similar to previous studies. These results revealed that $H_2O_2$ played an important role in increasing *PvPAL*, *Pv4CL*, *PvHPPR*, and *CYP98A14* expression levels in the rosmarinic acid synthesis pathway and thus enhanced rosmarinic acid and salviaflaside production against ROS damage induced by $H_2O_2$ stress in *P. vulgaris* plants.

Caffeic acid is a crucial phenolic component in *P. vulgaris*. In this research, the caffeic acid content in *P. vulgaris* leaves that decreased by 7% under $H_2O_2$ pretreatment was not significantly different from that in nontreated plants (Fig. 4F). Transcriptome analysis indicated that $H_2O_2$ acted on the phenylalanine branch in the process of caffeic acid synthesis in *P. vulgaris* leaves and reduced the content of caffeic acid by downregulating the expression of related genes (e. g., cinnamate 4-hydroxylase (*PvC4H*) and coumarate 3-hydroxylase (*PvC3H*)). These results implied that $H_2O_2$ strongly inhibits the transcript levels of the *PvC4H* and *PvC3H* genes, resulting in a decrease in the 4-coumaric acid content in the caffeic acid biosynthesis pathway. Interestingly, a higher transcript level of *Pv4CL* accelerated the coenzyme A (CoA) connection and catalysed the process of 4-coumaric acid to 4-coumaroyl-CoA and caffeic acid to caffeoyl-CoA, with similar results found in a previous study. In addition, the caffeic acid content was not significantly reduced compared to that in the control samples, which was due to the higher transcript level of *PvCSE* accelerating the catalysis of 4-coumaroyl-CoA to caffeic acid. Taken together, these results showed that $H_2O_2$ stress strongly inhibits caffeic acid accumulation by suppressing the catalytic product (4-coumaric acid: a precursor of caffeic acid) or downregulating the expression of the *PvC4H* and *PvC3H* genes and accelerating the decomposition of 4-coumaric acid and caffeic acid, accompanied by activation of the *Pv4CL* gene transcript level.

Hyperoside is the major flavonol glycoside compound and is an effective ROS scavenger in *P. vulgaris*. In this study, $H_2O_2$ treatment significantly induced a 2.0-fold increase in the hyperoside content of *P. vulgaris* leaves compared with the control treatment (Fig. 4E). Moreover, we observed that the transcript levels of 2 hyperoside biosynthetic genes (e.g., *PvPAL* and *Pv4CL*) were induced in *P. vulgaris* leaves under $H_2O_2$-induced stress (Fig. 5B). PAL and 4CL encode two enzymes that act early in hyperoside biosynthesis, and 4CL is a key branch point of the branched pathways leading to the production of hyperoside. In addition, our previous study also indicated a significant positive correlation between the hyperoside content and both the $H_2O_2$ content and PAL activity of *P. vulgaris* ($R = 0.994^{**}$, $R = 0.972^{**}$, respectively). Therefore, we hypothesized that $H_2O_2$ could upregulate the activity of the *PvPAL* and *Pv4CL* genes in hyperoside biosynthesis and that hyperoside could be used as an antioxidative regulator to eliminate ROS and enhance $H_2O_2$ stress tolerance in *P. vulgaris*.

Ursolic acid and oleanolic acid are the most widespread components and demonstrate antioxidant activity in *P. vulgaris*. MVA and 2-C-methyl-D-erythritol-4-phosphate (MEP) are two pathways for terpenoid synthesis; among them, triterpenoids (e. g., ursolic acid and oleanolic acid) are mainly synthesized via the MVA pathway. In this study, we found that elevated $H_2O_2$ levels enhanced the production of triterpenoids in *P. vulgaris* leaves (Fig. 4G - H). Correspondingly, the gene transcript levels of two main synthase genes (*PvHMGR* and *PvPMK*) in the MVA pathway and the main synthase genes (two for *PvDXS*, one for *PvHDS*, and one for *PvHDR*) in the MEP pathway were upregulated by exogenous $H_2O_2$ application (Fig. 5C). Our previous study showed that UV solar exclusion significantly stimulated ursolic acid and oleanolic acid production in *P. vulgaris* plants. Gene expression analysis showed that abiotic stress (e.g., UV-B irradiation, phosphate (Pi) deficiency, and silver cation ($Ag^+$)) upregulated the expression of terpenoid (e. g., tanshinone, dihydrotanshinone I, and cryptotanshinone) biosynthesis-related genes in *S. miltiorrhiza*, such as *SmDXS*, *SmHMGR*, and *SmPMK*. Moreover, a tanshinone biosynthesis-related enzyme gene (*SmHDR*) of *S. miltiorrhiza* could be promoted by exogenous MeJA treatment. Furthermore, overexpression of *SmDXS1*, *SmDXS2*, *SmHMGR1*, and *SmHMGR2* could significantly enhance tanshinone synthesis in *S. miltiorrhiza*. Additionally, previous studies have confirmed that HMGR and PMK are two key metabolic enzymes that participate in triterpene biosynthesis. Based on this information, $H_2O_2$ is a key signalling molecule that induces triterpene acid synthase transcription to catalyse oleanolic acid and ursolic acid accumulation against oxidative damage induced by high $H_2O_2$ levels in *P. vulgaris* plants. Elucidating the mechanism of $H_2O_2$-induced triterpene acid formation in *P. vulgaris* requires further research.

4.7 Analyses of DEG expression profiles Stress induces damage to cellular components of plant cells, such as nucleic acids, proteins and membrane lipids, resulting in metabolic dysfunction. To better understand how $H_2O_2$ plays a role in *P. vulgaris* plants, we used transcriptome sequencing to study the effect of $H_2O_2$ on gene expression under exogenous $H_2O_2$ stress.

To better comprehend how $H_2O_2$ plays a role in *P. vulgaris*, we used transcriptome sequencing to study the impact of $H_2O_2$ on gene expression after exogenous $H_2O_2$ stress. We screened 3 374 DEGs in the CK and $H_2O_2$ groups: 1 442 upregulated and 1 932 downregulated DEGs. Most genes were enriched in cell metabolism, biological regulation and response to oxidative stress in the GO analysis. Our results indicated that $H_2O_2$ influenced phytohormone metabolism after $H_2O_2$ application. Phytohormone contents (e.g., JA, SA, and ABA) are crucial regulatory factors for polyphenolic and terpenoid metabolism in medicinal plants. According to the KEGG pathway annotation, "plant hormone signal transduction", "starch and sucrose metabolism" and "biosynthesis of amino acids" were three of the most abundant KEGG pathways in this study (Supplementary Fig. S1D). Phytohormones are crucial signalling molecules that participate in growth and development, and phytohormone metabolism (e.g., JA and SA) promotes polyphenolic and terpene production affected by $H_2O_2$ application. For example, the $H_2O_2$ supply improved the phytohormones (e.g., JA and SA) and sesquiterpene biosynthesis of *Aquilaria sinesis*. Moreover, our previous study also found that exogenous methyl jasmonate (MeJA) treatment induced the expression of *PvPAL*, *Pv4CL*, *PvC4H*, and *PvTAT*, resulting in a significant increase in total flavonoids, total phenolics, rosmarinic acid, and hyperoside. Moreover, *P. vulgaris* amino acid and soluble sugar accumulation can regulate the permeability of abiotic treatment. This research showed that $H_2O_2$ regulated endogenous hormone-, amino acid- and carbon metabolism-related gene expression in *P. vulgaris* plants after $H_2O_2$ application.

In addition, numerous DEGs were annotated into the "secondary metabolism" pathway, which is primarily involved in the $H_2O_2$ signalling pathway. Our previous studies have indicated that abiotic stress helps to improve the antioxidant tolerance of *P. vulgaris* by activating the $H_2O_2$ signalling pathway. Moreover, correlational research has indicated that osmotic stress induces an increase in $H_2O_2$ levels, which activate polyphenol and terpenoid synthase gene expression to cause further responses by polyphenol and terpenoid biosynthesis. In the present study, $H_2O_2$ upregulated the expression of phenylalanine and terpenoid synthase genes and increased phenolic acid, flavonoid, and triterpenoid acid production in *P. vulgaris* leaves (Fig. 4). Polyphenol and triterpenoid acid accumulation in *P. vulgaris* could be involved in ROS scavenging under abiotic stress, such as UV-B radiation, UV-B/A removal, drought, and N, P, and K deficiency. An increasing number of polyphenol and terpenoid biosynthesis-related genes have been identified and shown to be related to antioxidation and plant hormone synthesis. Moreover, a few TFs are closely related to phenol/terpenoids, including bHLHs (e.g., bHLH51 and bHLH148), MYBs (e.g., MYB1 and MYB98), and WRKYs (e.g., WRKY1 and WRKY2), which can induce the expression of key enzyme genes in the synthesis pathway of active components. Therefore, $H_2O_2$ may have enhanced *P. vulgaris* antioxidant tolerance by activating polyphenol and terpenoid biosynthesis-related gene expression.

4.8 Analyses of $H_2O_2$-responsive TFs TFs play a vital role in abiotic stresses through gene regulatory networks and are the main participants in oxidative stress signalling. Most TFs make up the main hub of the signalling transduction network, such as bHLH, WRKY, MYB, AP2/ERF, GRAS, bZIP, WD40, and NAC. In this research, 240 differentially expressed TF-encoding genes were found between the CK and $H_2O_2$ groups, principally from the bHLH, WRKY, and MYB families (Fig. 9).

In *P. vulgaris*, bHLH TF members were the most abundant. As one of the most vital transcriptional regulatory gene families, bHLHs play a crucial role in regulating the biosynthesis of phenolic acids, flavonoids, and terpenoids in medicinal plants. Compared with the CK group, eight secondary metabolism-related TFs were upregulated in the $H_2O_2$ group (Fig. 9B). Previous studies have shown that *SmbHLH51* and *SmbHLH148* participate in phenolic acid biosynthesis as well as flavonoids, and *SmbHLH148* participates in the JA signalling pathway of *S. miltiorrhiza*. For instance, overexpression of *SmbHLH51* and *SmbHLH148* significantly increased phenolic acid and rosmarinic acid production, accompanied by the upregulation of *SmPAL*, *SmTAT*, *SmHPPR*, *Sm4CL*, *SmRAS*, and *SmCYP98A14*. *SmbHLH51* overexpression significantly increased the production of flavonoids, accompanied by the upregulation of *SmDFR* and *SmANS*. *SmbHLH148* overexpression can activate terpenoid biosynthesis-related gene expression, such as *SmDXS*, *SmDXR*, and *SmHMGR*, and the expression of *SmJAZs* involved in JA signalling pathways. In addition, *SmMYB1* and *SmMYB98* promoted polyphenols (e.g., phenolic acid, flavonoids and rosmarinic acid) and terpene accumulation in *S. miltiorrhiza* by activating the expression of several key enzyme genes, such as *SmPAL*, *Sm4CL*, *SmHPPR*, *SmCYP98A14*, and *SmDXS*. Furthermore, *SmWRKY1* and *SmWRKY2* are two regulatory TFs in *S. miltiorrhiza* and have been demonstrated to significantly elevate the transcription of *SmDXS*, *SmDXR*, and *SmCPS* genes encoding enzymes, resulting in an increase in terpenoid production. Therefore, $H_2O_2$ affects *P. vulgaris* polyphenol and terpenoid acid biosynthesis under $H_2O_2$ pretreatment by regulating TF expression.

## 5 CONCLUSIONS

Overall, physiological analysis revealed that *P. vulgaris* plants can alleviate $H_2O_2$ stress through multiple mechanisms. First, *P. vulgaris* could enhance photosynthetic capacity by promoting photosynthetic pigment synthesis and the net photosynthetic rate; second, *P. vulgaris* enhanced oxidation tolerance by mediating antioxidant systems and osmotic regulatory substances; third, *P. vulgaris* had higher jasmonic acid (JA) and salicylic acid (SA) but lower indole-3-acetic acid (IAA) accumulation in leaves. In addition, there were 3 374 DEGs between the CK and $H_2O_2$ groups, and the GO analysis indicated that *P. vulgaris* could respond to exogenous $H_2O_2$ by regulating cellular metabolism and biological processes. KEGG pathway investigation further showed that $H_2O_2$ plays a crucial role in phytohormone signal transduction, carbon, amino acids, and secondary metabolites. In addition, $H_2O_2$ can trigger JA and SA accumulation to promote phenolic acids, flavonoids, and triterpene acids by activating the expression of phytohormones and secondary metabolite-related enzyme genes. Furthermore, $H_2O_2$ affects *P. vulgaris* secondary metabolite biosynthesis by regulating bHLH, WRKY, and MYB TF expression. This study provides important information on the metabolic regulatory mechanisms by which exogenous $H_2O_2$ influences secondary metabolite production in *P. vulgaris*.

[胡金玉，陈宇航，等. Industrial Crops & Products, 2023, 192:116065.]

# SmbHLH60 and SmMYC2 antagonistically regulate phenolic acids and anthocyanins biosynthesis in *Salvia miltiorrhiza*

## 1 INTRODUCTION

*Salvia miltiorrhiza*, *Lamiaceae* family, is a medicinal herb widely used in Chinese medicine for treatments of cardiovascular and cerebrovascular diseases. The composition and concentration of phenolic acids and liposoluble tanshinones are associated with their health-promoting properties. Caffeic acid (CA), salvianolic acid B (SAB), salvianolic acid A (SAA) and rosmarinic acid (RA) are the main bioactive phenolic acids identified and reported to have anti-oxidant, anti-inflammatory, anti-atherosclerosis, anti-tumor, and anti-diabetic activities. High economic value and increasing market demands for enhanced content of phenolic acids derive current researches focus on the regulation of phenolic acid biosynthesis pathways.

In plants, the phenolic acid biosynthesis pathway has been extensively studied and in *S. miltiorrhiza* two upstream pathways have been characterized: the phenylpropane metabolic pathway and the tyrosine-derived metabolic pathway (Fig. S1). In the phenylpropane metabolic pathway, L-phenylalanine is sequentially metabolized by phenylalanine ammonia-lyase (PAL), cinnamic acid 4-hydroxylase (C4H) and 4-coumarate: CoA ligase (4CL) to generate one of the precursors, 4-coumaroyl-CoA. In parallel, tyrosine conversion is catalyzed by tyrosine aminotransferase (TAT), 4-hydroxyphenylpyruvate reductase (HPPR) and additional uncharacterized enzymatic steps to form the other precursor, 3,4-dihydroxyphenyllactic acid. Subsequently, the two precursors will be used to generate rosmarinic acid catalyzed by rosmarinic acid synthase (RAS) and cytochrome P450-dependent monooxygenase (CYP98A14). The formation of additional phenolic acids by these two precursors may occur by yet unknown step(s).

4-coumaroyl-CoA is an important precursor in the phenylpropanoid pathway taking part in the production of numerous phenylpropanoids including anthocyanins. The latter is extremely important secondary metabolites, widely distributed among higher plants, serve as important natural pigments and have strong antioxidant activity, and are therefore beneficial for the human diet. So far, a major part of the anthocyanin biosynthesis pathway in *S. miltiorrhiza* has been characterized including chalcone synthase (SmCHS), chalcone isomerase (SmCHI), flavone synthase (SmFNS), flavanone 3-hydroxylase (SmF3H), flavonoid 3′-hydroxylase (SmF3′H), flavonoid 3′,5′-hydroxylase (SmF3′5′H), flavonol synthase (SmFLS), dihydroflavonol 4-reductase (SmDFR), and anthocyanidin synthase (SmANS). However, only a few works studied the regulation mechanism of anthocyanins in *S. miltiorrhiza*.

Many elicitors including gibberellins (GAs), methyl jasmonate (MeJA), abscisic acid (ABA), salicylic acid (SA), yeast extract (YE), $Ag^+$, nitric oxide (NO), and hydrogen peroxide ($H_2O_2$) have been proven to increase the phenolic acids accumulation. In addition, MeJA has been used to increase the content of anthocyanins. However, the mechanism in which MeJA-induced phenolic acid and anthocyanin regulation in *S. miltiorrhiza* is still largely unknown.

The basic helix-loop-helix (bHLH) TF family plays an extremely important role in secondary metabolism regulation. It was also shown that bHLHs can bind to specific promoter regions in their targeted genes, such as E-box (CANNTG) or G-box (CACGTG). Currently, 127 bHLH TFs were found in *S. miltiorrhiza* by genome mining, some of which were discovered to be involved in the regulation of secondary metabolism. For example, SmbHLH3 negatively regulates phenolic acid biosynthesis by modulating *SmTAT1* and *SmHPPR1*. RA, SAB and CA levels were increased by 2.87, 4.00 and 5.99 times, respectively, as compared to the control in SmbHLH148. SmbHLH10 increased the accumulation of tanshinone in the roots of *S. miltiorrhiza*. SmbHLH92 and SmbHLH37 have been confirmed to negatively regulate phenolic acids biosynthesis pathways while SmbHLH51 functions as a positive regulator. SAB biosynthesis, in *S. miltiorrhiza*, triggered by MeJA is also regulated by SmbHLH53 presumably with a dual-role. MYELOCYTOMATOSISs (MYCs), another type of bHLH TFs, were also shown to take a central role in secondary metabolites regulation. For example, AaMYC2, a jasmonate-responsive TF, positively regulates artemisinin biosynthesis in *Artemisia annua*. In *Catharanthus roseus*, CrMYC2 has been proved to be essential for the accumulation of alkaloids. In *S. miltiorrhiza*, SmMYC2 plays a role as a core transcription factor in the MeJA-mediated phenolic acid secondary metabolism signaling pathway by actively binding to *SmPAL1*, *SmTAT1* and *SmCYP98A14* promoters altering their expression, leading to the accumulation of phenolic acids. Still, in *S. miltiorrhiza*, the mechanism in which SmMYC2 regulates MeJA-mediated phenolic acid and anthocyanin biosynthesis is not fully understood. Our data suggest that by forming a heterodimer, SmbHLH60 and SmMYC2 antagonistically regulate anthocyanin and phenolic acid biosynthesis. Our new findings reveal the molecular regulation mechanism of SmbHLH60 and SmMYC2 and elucidate the MeJA-mediated regulation of secondary metabolites regulation in *S. miltiorrhiza*.

## 2 MATERIALS AND METHODS

Plant materials *S. miltiorrhiza* seedlings were grown in the greenhouse of Zhejiang Chinese Medical University. *S. miltiorrhiza* seedlings were cultured on Murashige and Skoog (MS) medium at 25 ℃, which were lighted for 16 h and dark for 8 h. *Nicotiana benthamiana* was cultivated in a greenhouse at 25 ℃, under the same conditions as *S. miltiorrhiza*. *S. miltiorrhiza* hairy roots were grown on 1/2 MS solid medium and cultured in the dark in a greenhouse at 25 ℃. For culture in a flask, the hairy roots were cultured in 100 mL 1/2 MS liquid medium at 120 rpm for 50 days in the dark.

Isolation and characterization of SmbHLH60 *SmbHLH60* was found to be one of the most significantly down-regulated bHLH genes in RNA-Seq data, and the full-length cDNA was amplified using specific primers (Table S1). ClustalX and MEGA 6.0 software were used for sequence alignment and phylogenetic tree analysis. The phylogenetic tree was constructed based on the amino acid sequence with the neighbor-joining method and then optimized with the iTOL tool. All protein sequences including SibHLH130 (XP_011087339.1), SibHLH130-like (XP_011093536.1), PjbHLH130 (GFQ08151.1), OebHLH130-like (XP_022896111.1) used in multiple sequence alignment were download from NCBI database.

Gene expression profile assay For RNA isolation, different tissues of one-year-old *S. miltiorrhiza* plants, including roots, lateral roots, stems, xylems, phloems, leaves and young leaves were collected and performed using the Tiangen Plant RNA Extraction Kit. Followed by reverse transcription and qRT-PCR for *SmbHLH60* gene detection, *SmActin* was used as an internal reference. Exogenous plant hormones including 100 μmol/L methyl jasmonate (MeJA) was used to spray one-month-old *S. miltiorrhiza* seedlings and sampled at 0, 1, 2, 4, 6, 8, 12, 24 h after treatment for RNA extraction, followed by reverse transcription and qRT-PCR to detect *SmbHLH60* gene expression. The relative quantitative analysis method ($2^{-\Delta\Delta CT}$) was used to calculate the relative gene expression, and *SmActin* was used as the internal reference gene and all experiments were repeated with more than three biological replicates.

Subcellular localization of SmbHLH60 To determine the subcellular localization of SmbHLH60, the open reading frame (ORF) of *SmbHLH60* was cloned and constructed into the pHB-YFP vector driven by the CaMV 35S promoter to form the SmbHLH60-YFP fusion protein (Fig. S2B). The negative control was performed by an empty pHB-YFP vector. The fusion vector was transformed into *Agrobacterium tumefaciens* GV3101 strain. Then the transformed GV3101 was injected into five-week-old *N. benthamiana* leaves while pHB-YFP was used as a negative control. To confirm the position of the nucleus, 10 mg/mL 4′, 6-diamidino-2-phenylindole dihydrochloride (DAPI) solution was injected into *N. benthamiana* leaves 4 h before observing the fluorescence signal. Then the fluorescence signal was observed by laser confocal microscope (Zeiss, Germany) under the excitation of 405 nm and 488 nm laser. All experiments were repeated with more than three biological replicates.

Generating S. miltiorrhiza hairy roots The complete ORF of *SmbHLH60* was cloned into the pCAMBIA2300$^{+}$

vector containing the CaMV 35S promoter to form the pCAMBIA2300$^+$ - *SmbHLH60* recombinant vector (Fig. S2A). For the knockout vector, sgRNA was designed according to the 5′- G - 19base - NGG - 3′ principle, which was constructed on the pCAMBIA2300$^+$ vector (Fig. S2A). *SmbHLH60* sgRNA was driven by the AtU6 promoter, and hSpCas9 was by the CaMV 35S promoter with pCAMBIA2300$^+$ serving as a control vector. The above vectors were transformed into C58C1 and then used to infect *S. miltiorrhiza* for hairy roots. The hairy root DNA was extracted by the CTAB method and the positive clones were identified with specific primers (Table S1). All experiments were repeated with three biological replicates.

Quantitative real-time PCR (qRT-PCR) Tissues including taproots, lateral roots, xylems, phloems, stems, leaves, and tender leaves of *S. miltiorrhiza* were collected and ground into a powder with liquid nitrogen to extract total RNA and follow the steps in the Tiangen plant total RNA extraction kit. The qRT - PCR experiments were used to detect the results with Thermo Fisher quantitative master mix and the Applied Biosystem Step One Real-Time PCR System (Applied Biosystems, USA) and the *SmActin* was used as an internal control. All experiments had three biological replicates.

Measuring the accumulation of phenolic acids and anthocyanins in hairy roots 0.1 g of dried hairy root powder was weighed for phenolic acid extraction with 80% ethanol solution (4 : 1, *V*/*V*), and ultrasonic extraction was performed for 30 min. The extract was dissolved in 2 mL of distilled water after vacuum rotary steaming. HPLC was used to detect each component in the phenolic acid extract, and the content was calculated by substituting it into the standard curve. In addition, 0.02 g of dried hairy root powder was weighed and mixed in 1 mL of 1% (v/v) hydrochloric acid methanol solution (hydrochloric acid: methanol=1 : 99), at 100 rpm, 20 ℃ overnight for total anthocyanin extraction. Then samples were centrifugated at 12, 000 rpm and the supernatant was taken for further analysis. Samples were mixed similar volume of chloroform and the absorbance of the extract at 530 nm and 657 nm wavelengths were detected by spectrophotometry. Anthocyanin content Q (antho-cyanin) = $(A530 - 0.25 \times A657) \times M^{-1}$, and M is the dry weight of plant tissue. All measurements were carried out in three biological replicates.

Yeast one-hybrid assay (Y1H) The complete *SmbHLH60* ORF sequence was constructed on the pB42AD vector to form a recombinant vector, and the E/G-box in the promoters of key genes of phenolic acid and anthocyanin biosynthesis were constructed on the pLacZ2u vector. The recombinant plasmid was co-transformed into yeast strain EGY48, followed cultured on SD/-Ura/-Trp medium for 48 h. Then the positive colony was picked and tested for growth of monoclonal strains on SD/-Ura/-Trp/Raf/Gal medium with X-gal for 48 h. Empty vectors pB42AD and pLacZ2u were used as negative controls. We performed the Y1H experiment more than three biological replicates.

Electrophoretic mobility shift assay (EMSA) The ORF of *SmbHLH60* was inserted into the vector pCold-His. Recombinant protein SmbHLH60-His was expressed in *E. coli* BL21 (DE3) and purified using a protein purification kit with a His-tag, which was purchased from Shanghai Sangon Co., Ltd. Probe fragments from the promoter of *SmTAT1* and *SmDFR* were synthesized by Shanghai Sangon Co., Ltd. The 5×EMSA binding buffer was purchased from Beyotime Biotechnology Co., Ltd. (Shanghai, China), and the chemiluminescence detection kit was purchased from Thermo Fisher Scientific (Shanghai, China), and the fluorescence was detected using a C300 image scanner (Azure Biosystems, USA). SmbHLH60 - His purified protein was combined with probes of *SmTAT1pro* and *SmDFRpro* by adding 5× binding buffer (Beyotime Biotechnology Co., Ltd.) at 25 ℃ for 25 min. Then follow the previously reported method. EMSA experiment was repeated with three biological replicates.

Dual-luciferase assay (dual-LUC) Promoters about 2 000 bp of all key enzyme genes involved in phenolic acid and anthocyanin biosynthesis were constructed to pGreen0800-LUC vector. The recombinant vector was then transferred to *A. tumefaciens* GV3101. The *N. benthamiana* was then transformed instantaneously by infiltrating the *Agrobacterium* mixture into the back of the leaves. After 48 h, samples were taken from the infected site, and the extract was detected using a dualluciferase reporter analysis system (Promega, Madison, USA), and the fluorescence values were detected. All dual-LUC experiments were repeated for more than three biological replicates.

Bimolecular fluorescent complementary assay (BiFC) To verify the interaction between SmbHLH60 and SmMYC2, the full-length ORF of *SmbHLH60* and *SmMYC2* were constructed on pXY106 - nYFP and pXY104 - cYFP, respectively, and then transformed into *A. tumefaciens* GV3101. The resuspended *Agrobacteria* were mixed and injected into *N. benthamiana* leaves for transient expression. Then *N. benthamiana* plants were placed in a greenhouse at 26 ℃ for 48 h, and the yellow fluorescence was observed by laser confocal microscope (Zeiss, Germany) under the excitation of 488 nm lasers previously described. This experiment was repeated with three replicates.

GST pull-down assay The complete ORFs of *SmbHLH60* and *SmMYC2* were respectively constructed on the pCold-His vector and pGEX - 4T - 1 vector, which were transformed into *E. coli* BL21 (DE3) for protein expression, using His-tag and GST-tag protein purification kit (Shanghai Sangon

Co., Ltd) for purification, respectively. SmMYC2 - GST was incubated with GST magnetic beads (Shanghai Sangon Co., Ltd) at 26℃ for 30 min to form a GST-target protein complex. Subsequently, SmbHLH60-His recombinant protein was added for the binding reaction at 4℃ overnight. After 3000 rpm centrifugation, the supernatant was aspirated and used for input detection by anti-GST and anti-His. Then, the magnetic beads were washed 3 times with wash buffer, the supernatant was discarded. Finally, the elution buffer was added to elute the protein, which was taken for electrophoresis and western blot detection by anti-His. This experiment had three biological replicates.

## 3 RESULTS

SmbHLH60 expression pattern analysis *SmbHLH60* was found to be one of the most significantly down-regulated bHLH genes in MeJA-mediated RNA-Seq data (Fig. 1A). To examine the involvement of *SmbHLH60* in the MeJA signaling pathway, exogenous MeJA was applied to the whole plant, and the expression of *SmbHLH60* was examined by qRT - PCR. *SmbHLH60* expression was significantly decreased in MeJA-treated samples as compared to control (0 h) from 1 h, reaching the lowest levels at 6 h (Fig. 1B). These results showed good accordance with our previous RNA-seq data. In addition, *SmbHLH60* showed an opposite expression pattern with *SmMYC2* and genes involved in phenolic acid biosynthesis such as *SmPAL1*, *SmC4H*, *SmTAT1*, *SmHPPR*, *SmRAS* and *SmCYP98A14* after MeJA treatment (Fig. 1A). Meanwhile, we analyzed the expression patterns of *SmbHLH60* and the previously characterized *SmbHLHs* under MeJA treatment. We found that the expression of *SmbHLH92*, a negative regulator in the biosynthesis of phenolic acid, decreased in MeJA-mediated RNA-seq data (Fig. S5), which showed a similar expression pattern to *SmbHLH60*. Therefore, we speculated that SmbHLH60 may participate in the negative regulation of phenolic acid. Total phenolic acid accumulation in the leaf of *S. miltiorrhiza* was the highest among the three tissues (root, leaf and stem) (Fig. S6). Tissue expression profile showed that *SmbHLH60* expressed the highest in leaf, especially in young leaf (Fig. 1C). Meanwhile, *SmMYC2* was found to have the highest expression in the leaf. These results support that SmbHLH60 might participate in the regulation of phenolic acids. Therefore, we focused on the research of *SmbHLH60*.

Isolation and characterization of SmbHLH60 *SmbHLH60* sequence contained an 1 185 bp of an open reading frame, encoding a 394 amino acids protein with a size prediction of 43.58 kDa. To explore the evolutionary relationship between SmbHLH60 and 167 bHLH TFs in *Arabidopsis thaliana*, the phylogenetic tree was constructed, which showed that SmbHLH60 was high homology with AtbHLH130 (Fig. S3). The latter is known as FLOWERING BHLH4 (FBH4) and it was reported to activate CONSTANS (CO) with FBH1, FBH2, and FBH3 redundantly as part of the flowering regulatory mechanism in *A. thaliana*. The result of BLAST-Protein (BLASTP) analysis showed that SmbHLH60 has the highest identity (60.58%) to *Sesamum indicum* bHLH130. All proteins, including SibHLH130-like, PjbHLH130, OebHLH130-like contained the basic helix-loop-helix conserved domain at the Cterminus (Fig. 2A). Subcellular localization assay was used to explore the location of SmbHLH60 in cells. SmbHLH60-YFP fluorescence was observed in the nucleus using a laser confocal microscope, while the YFP signal of pHB-YFP was distributed in the cell nucleus and cytoplasm, and DAPI appeared in the nucleus (Fig. 2B).

Generation of SmbHLH60-overexpression and SmbHLH60-CRISPR hairy roots To decipher the role of *SmbHLH60* in phenolic acid and anthocyanin accumulation, transgenic lines were generated. Recombinant vectors pCAMBIA2300$^{+}$ - *SmbHLH60* and pCAMBIA2300$^{+}$ - *SmbHLH60* - CRISPR/Cas9 were separately transfected into the modified *A. tumefaciens* C58C1 harboring *A. rhizogenes* A4 Ri plasmid. For infecting explants of *S. miltiorrhiza* to obtain genetically modified hairy roots. Fig. S4 showed the results that the positive *SmbHLH60* - OE lines were identified with primer in Table S1. EV means hairy roots which derive from infecting with *A. rhizogenes* C58C1 containing empty vector (pCAMBIA2300$^{+}$) plasmid, which was used as a negative control. The CRISPR/Cas9 knockout lines used target sequence-specific primers to amplify about 400 bp sequence for sequence determination. The sequencing results and sequencing diagrams were shown in Fig. 3C - D, and the TGG was the PAM sequence. Four *SmbHLH60* overexpression (*SmbHLH60* - OE) and four CRISPR/Cas9 knockout lines (*SmbHLH60* - CRISPR) were used for further analysis (Fig. 3A). In *SmbHLH60* - OE lines, the expression levels of *SmbHLH60* were significantly higher as compared to the control. Conversely, expression levels of *SmbHLH60* were much lower in the knockout lines as compared to the control (Fig. 3B).

SmbHLH60 reduces the phenolic acid accumulation Total polyphenol content was determined using Folin-Phenol reagent was the highest in the knockout lines, then in the control, and the lowest levels were detected in the *SmbHLH60* overexpression hairy root lines (Fig. 4A). HPLC analysis confirmed our results with total phenolic acids (TS) of 32.77 ± 1.75 mg/g in the knockout lines, significantly higher than the control line with 22.07 ± 2.55 mg/g, while the TS content in *SmbHLH60* overexpression hairy roots was 12.88 ± 3.21 mg/g significantly lower than the control line

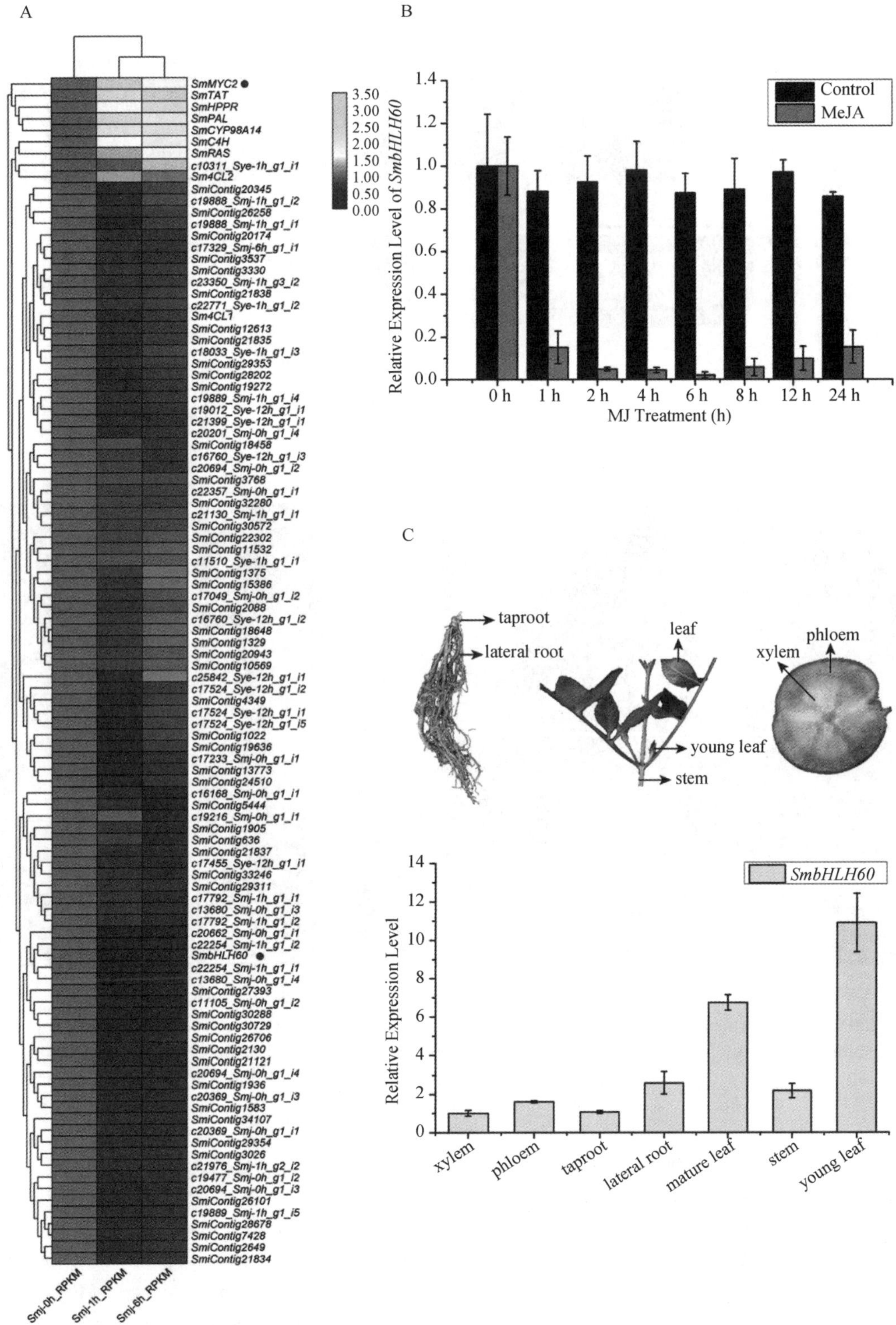


**Fig. 1 Expression profiles analysis of *SmbHLH60***

(A) The analysis of *SmbHLH60* expression pattern in MeJA-induced transcriptome library at 1 h and 6 h. The heat map was produced using TBtools. The yellow color indicated high expression levels, and the blue color indicated low expression levels. A total of 89 bHLH TFs showed decreased expression after MeJA treatment revealed in the transcriptome library. The expression of *SmbHLH60* decrease obviously after MeJA treatment at 1 h (B) The effect of exogenous MeJA on the expression of *SmbHLH60*. The expression of *SmbHLH60* was detected under MJ treatment for 0 h, 1 h, 2 h, 4 h, 6 h, 8 h, 12 h, 24 h. *SmbHLH60* was drastically decreased under the regulation of MeJA in the whole plant. (C) *SmbHLH60* gene expressions in different tissues of *S. miltiorrhiza*. The transcription level of *SmbHLH60* was detected in the xylem, phloem, taproot, lateral root, mature leaf, steam and young leaf respectively. All experiments were repeated three times, and the error bars represented the standard deviation of the three replicates. (For interpretation of the references to color in this figure legend, the reader is referred to the web version of this article.)

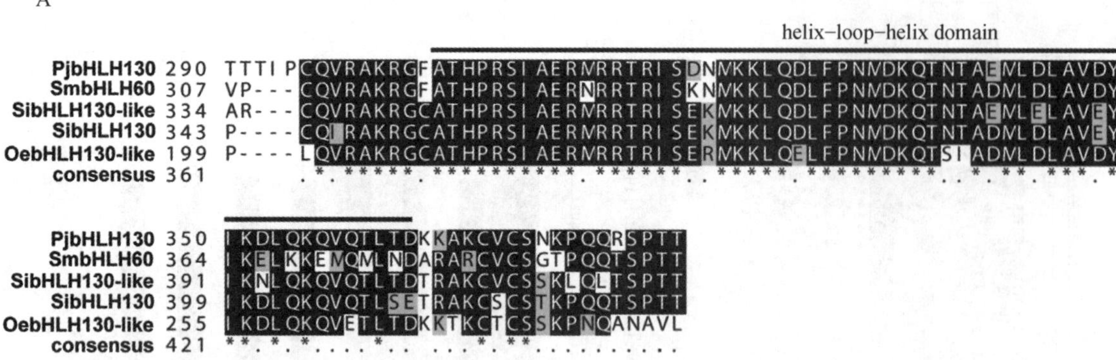


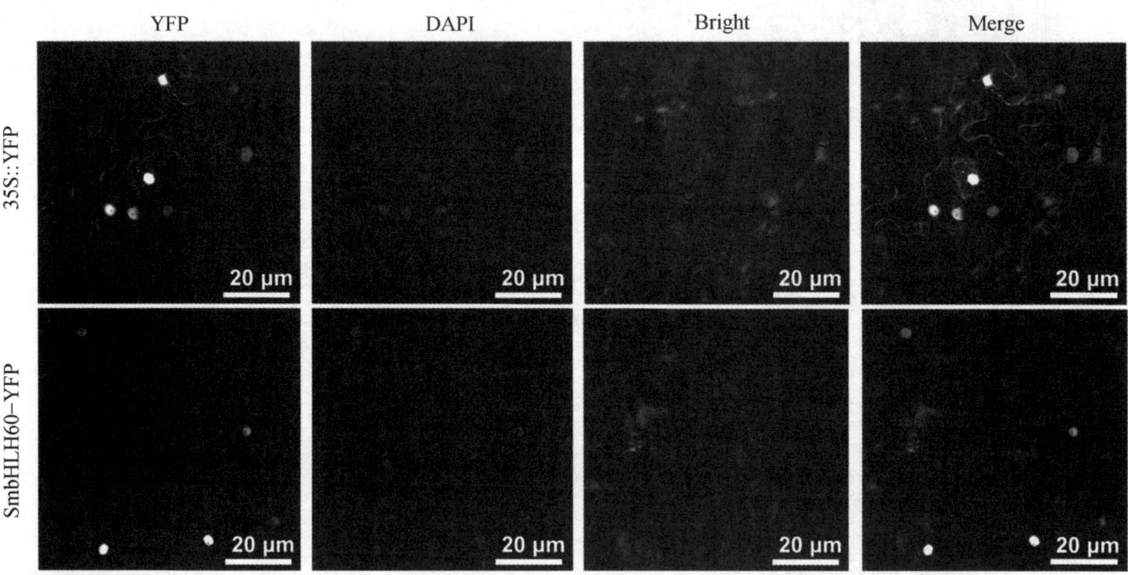


**Fig. 2 Characterization and subcellular localization of SmbHLH60**

(A) ClustalX was performed for multiple sequence alignment. Multiple amino acid sequence alignments of bHLH TFs including SibHLH130 (XP_011087339.1), PjbHLH130 (GFQ08151.1), OsbHLH130 - like (XP_022896111.1) and SibHLH130 - like (XP_011093536.1). (B) Subcellular localization of SmbHLH60 in *N. benthamiana* leaf epidermal cells. YFP fluorescence and DAPI signals were observed at 488 nm and 405 nm.

(Fig. 4B). In accordance with our chemical profiling, the expression level of genes involved in the biosynthesis of phenolic acid *SmPAL1*, *SmC4H1*, *Sm4CL2*, *SmTAT1*, *SmHPPR1*, *SmRAS1* and *SmCYP98A14* were significantly higher in the *SmbHLH60* - CRISPR lines as compared to the control. The expression levels in the *SmbHLH60* - OE lines were significantly lower as compared to the control line (Fig. 4C).

SmbHLH60 negatively regulates anthocyanin biosynthesis The initial steps of the phenylpropanoid pathway provide the precursors for the biosynthesis of phenolic acids and anthocyanins. Total anthocyanin extracts from hairy roots of different lines exhibited inconsistent colors (Fig. 5A). Therefore, we examined if the effect on color accumulation is directly or indirectly related to the anthocyanin biosynthetic pathway. In the *SmbHLH60* - CRISPR lines, the total anthocyanins were significantly increased, about twice the control. In the *SmbHLH60* - OE lines, the anthocyanin content was significantly reduced, which was about 42% lower than the control (Fig. 5B). Expression of genes involved in the biosynthesis of anthocyanins including *SmCHS*, *SmFLS*, *SmF3H*, *SmF3′H*, *SmF3′5′H*, *SmANS* and *SmDFR* was significantly higher in the *SmbHLH60* - CRISPR lines as compared to the control, while in the latter it was significantly higher as compared to the *SmbHLH60* - OE lines (Fig. 5C).

SmbHLH60 binds and transcriptionally inhibits the promoters of SmTAT1 and SmDFR SmbHLH60 caused a decrease in phenolic acid and anthocyanin, so we selected 11 genes (7 key enzyme genes of phenolic acid biosynthesis and

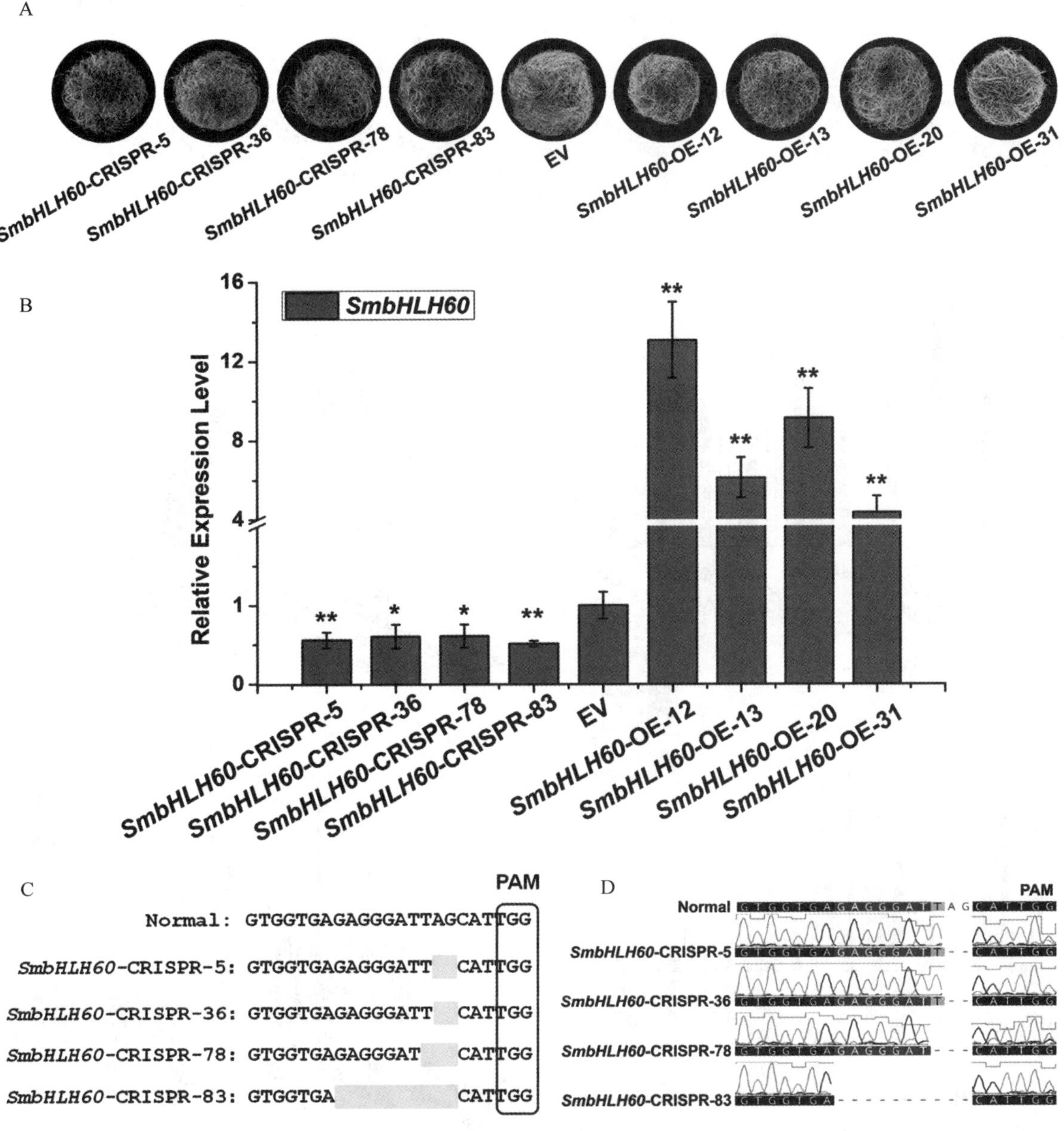


**Fig. 3 Generation of transgenic hairy roots**

(A) Hairy roots were cultured for 50 days in 1/2 MS. Four knockout lines and four overexpression lines were used for cultivation and subsequent experiments. (B) Transcript-level expression of *SmbHLH60* in *SmbHLH60* - CRISPR lines and *SmbHLH60* - OE lines were tested by qRT - PCR and error bars represented the standard deviation of three biological replicates (*, $P<0.05$; **, $P<0.01$). (C-D) CRISPR/Cas9 system knocks out hairy root. TGG was the PAM sequence. After being edited with CRISPR/Cas9 system, line 5 and line 36 lacked 2 bases, line 78 lacked 3 bases, and line 83 lacked 10 bases.

4 key enzyme genes of anthocyanin biosynthesis) whose transcription level decreased significantly in the *SmbHLH60* - OE lines and increased in the *SmbHLH60* - CRISPR lines for dual-LUC experiments. The results showed that *SmTAT1*, *SmPAL1*, *SmRAS1* (phenolic acid biosynthesis pathway) and *SmDFR* (anthocyanin biosynthesis pathway) were significantly transcriptionally repressed by *SmbHLH60* (Fig. 6A - B, S7). Further investigation showed that SmbHLH60 only bound to the G-box element in the promoter of *SmTAT1* and *SmDFR* as performed by Y1H (Fig. 6C - D). EMSA was performed to further verify whether SmbHLH60 is bound to the promoters of *SmTAT1* and *SmDFR*, and the pCold-His protein was used as a negative control. The band of the protein-probe complex was detected only in the presence of the SmbHLH60-His fusion protein, indicating that SmbHLH60 can bind to *SmTAT1* and *SmDFR* by the G-box in its promoter (Fig. 6E - F). These results revealed that *SmTAT1* and *SmDFR*, the target genes of SmbHLH60, were transcriptionally inhibited by SmbHLH60, which was consistent with the expression of

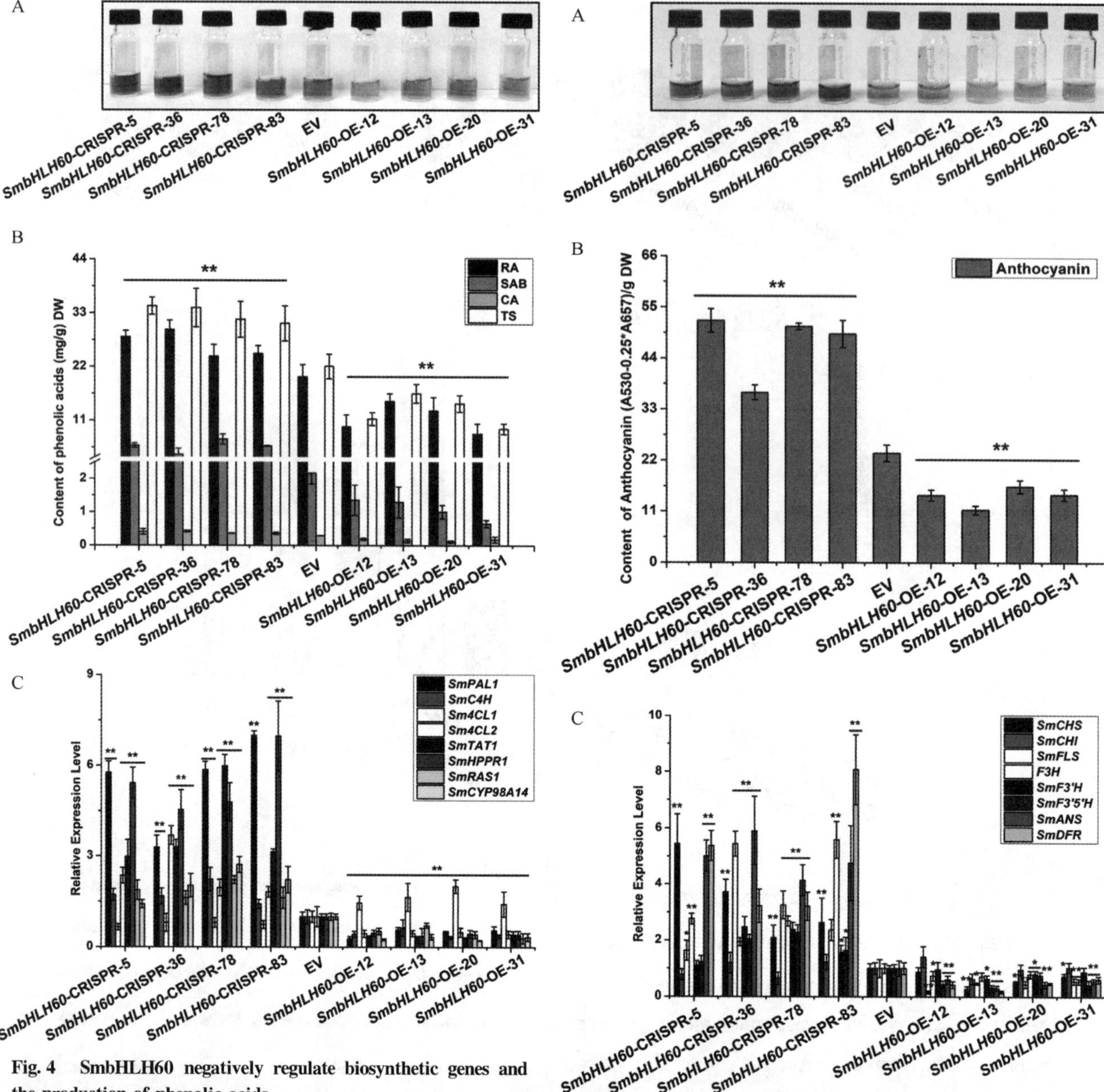


**Fig. 4 SmbHLH60 negatively regulate biosynthetic genes and the production of phenolic acids**

(A) Color of total phenolic acids (TS) extracts of transgenic hairy roots. Folin-Phenol was used for staining of total phenolic acid extract. The shade of color represented the total content of phenolic acid. (B) Determination of total phenolic acid and three main phenolic acids including rosmarinic acid (RA), salvianolic acid B (SAB), caffeic acid (CA) by HPLC. The content determination of each hairy root line was repeated three times, and error bars represented the standard deviation of three biological replicates (*, $P<0.05$; **, $P<0.01$) (C) qRT-PCR was used to detect gene expressions of key enzymes in phenolic acid biosynthesis. Transcription levels of genes involved in phenolic acid biosynthesis were detected in *SmbHLH60*-CRISPR lines and *SmbHLH60*-OE lines respectively. All experiments were repeated three times, and error bars represented the standard deviation of three biological replicates (*, $P<0.05$; **, $P<0.01$).

**Fig. 5 *SmbHLH60* transgenic lines negatively regulate biosynthetic genes and total anthocyanins**

(A) Color of anthocyanin extracts of transgenic hairy roots. The hydrochloric acid-methanol solution was used to extract total anthocyanins ($V:V=1:99$). The picture showed the product after the extraction of total anthocyanins. (B) Determination of total anthocyanins. The anthocyanin extract was mixed with an equal volume of chloroform and detected by a microplate reader (*, $P<0.05$; **, $P<0.01$). (C) qRT-PCR was used to detect gene expression of key enzymes in anthocyanin biosynthesis. All experiments were repeated three times, and error bars represented the standard deviation of three biological replicates (*, $P<0.05$; **, $P<0.01$).

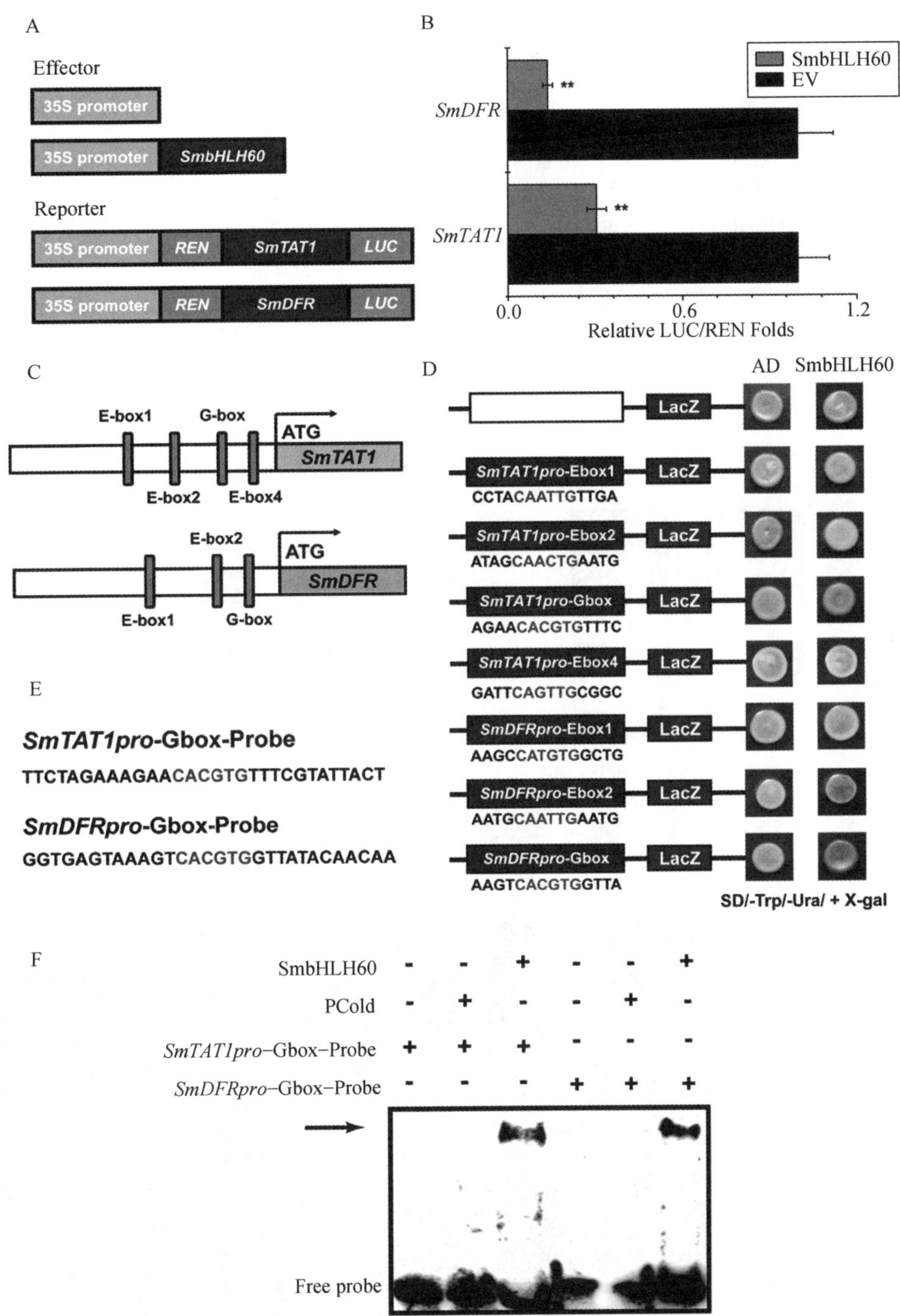


**Fig. 6 SmbHLH60 can bind to the G-Box motif in the promoter region of *SmTAT1* and *SmDFR***

(A) Schematic diagram of constructs used in assays of transient transcriptional activity. (B) SmbHLH60 repressed promoters of *SmTAT1* and *SmDFR*, and the relative LUC activity was normalized to the *Renilla* (REN) luciferase. pGreen0800 - *SmTAT1pro* - LUC and pGreen0800 - *SmDFRpro* - LUC were co-injected with pHB - *SmbHLH60* respectively into tobacco epidermal cells for promoter activity determination. All experiments were carried out in three biological replicates and error bars represented the standard deviation of three biological replicates (*, $P<0.05$; **, $P<0.01$). (C) The positions of E/G-box elements in *SmTAT1pro and SmDFRpro* for Y1H and EMSA analysis. (D) The Y1H assays showed that SmbHLH60 bound to the G-box in the promoters of *SmTAT1* and *SmDFR*. Two vectors including pB42AD - *SmbHLH60* and pLacZ2u-E/G-box were transferred into EGY48 yeast, which was placed on a medium containing X-gal for selection. (E) Probe sequences used in the EMSA experiment including CACGTG conserved sequence. (F) Specific binding of SmbHLH60 to G-box in the promoters of *SmTAT1* and *SmDFR*. The third lane of the DNA-protein complex was detected, indicating that SmbHLH60 was directly bound to the probe containing the G-box element.

*SmTAT1* and *SmDFR* in our qRT-PCR results.

SmbHLH60 interacts with SmMYC2 to form a heterodimer

Interestingly, the Y2H results showed that SmbHLH60 and SmMYC2 could interact directly (Fig. 7A). BiFC and

GST pull-down were performed to clarify the interaction between SmbHLH60 and SmMYC2. In BiFC assays, the peptides nYFP and cYFP were combined to excite fluorescence only when nYFP-SmbHLH60 and SmMYC2 - cYFP combined, otherwise there was no fluorescence excitation (Fig. 7B). In the GST pull-down assay, the SmbHLH60 - His fusion protein in the experimental group and input was detected through the His antibody, while GST protein and SmMYC2 - GST fusion protein were detected through the GST antibody. SmbHLH60 - His was incubated with SmMYC2 - GST and GST, respectively. The result of the western blot (WB) assay found that the luminescence signal was only detected in the group where SmbHLH60 - His and SmMYC2 - GST were incubated together, while no band was detected in the group incubated with SmbHLH60 - His and GST (Fig. 7C). These results indicated that an interaction existed between SmbHLH60 and SmMYC2.

SmbHLH60 attenuates the transcriptional activation effect of SmMYC2 on SmTAT1 and SmDFR The discovery that SmMYC2 and SmbHLH60 target the same genes provoked

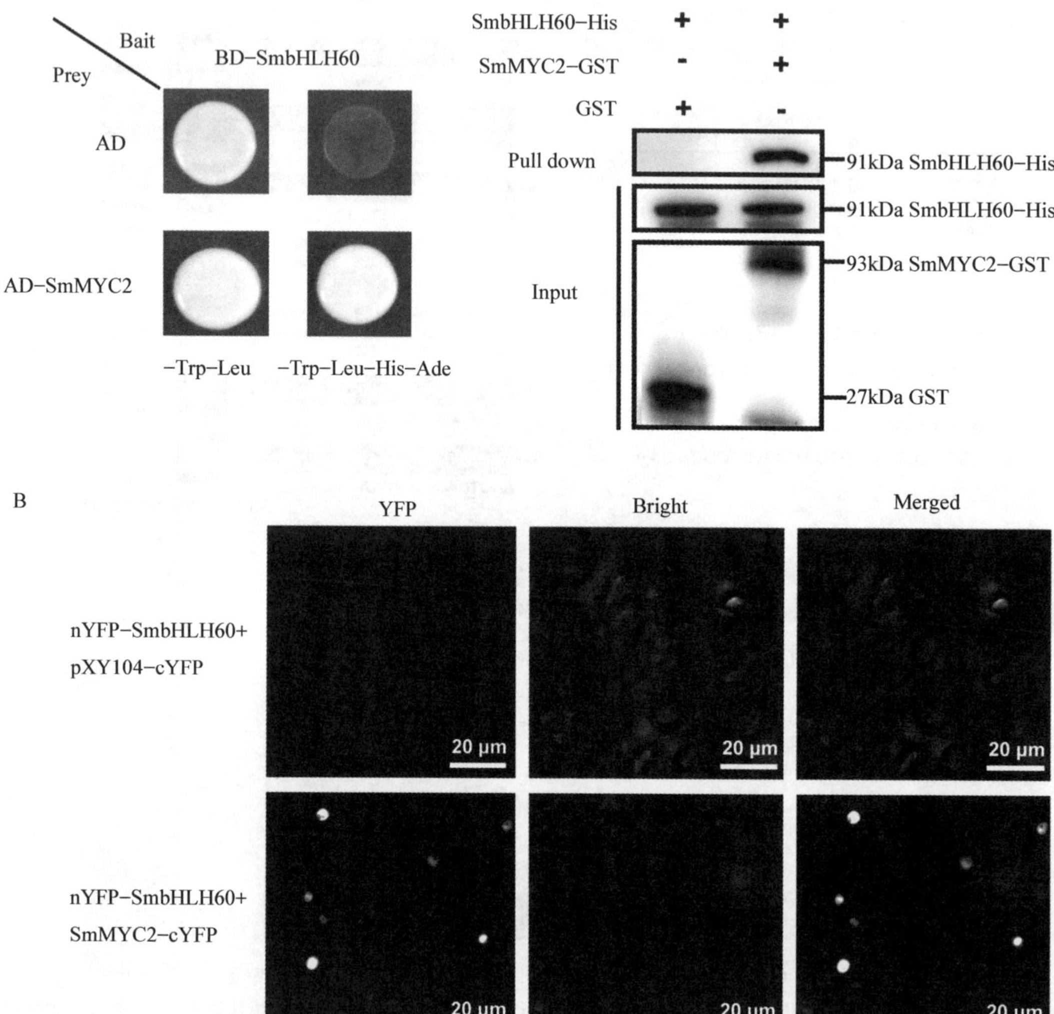


**Fig. 7 SmbHLH60 interacted with SmMYC2 *in vitro* and *in vivo***

(A) Yeast-two-hybrid assay showed SmbHLH60 can interact with SmMYC2. The ORF of *SmMYC2* and *SmbHLH60* were connected to pGADT7 and pGBKT7, respectively. After AD - MYC2 and BD - SmbHLH60 were co-transformed, the yeast could grow normally on the SD/-Trp/-Leu/-His/-Ade medium. (B) Bimolecular fluorescent complementary assays to detect the interaction between SmbHLH60 and SmMYC2. The ORFs of *SmbHLH60* and *SmMYC2* were constructed on the pXY - 106 - nYFP vector and pXY - 104 - cYFP vector, respectively. Fluorescence could only be detected when nYFP-SmbHLH60 was combined with SmMYC2 - cYFP, scale bar was 20 μm. (C) GST pull-down assay verified that SmbHLH60 could interact with SmMYC2. The fusion protein SmbHLH60 - His and SmMYC2 - GST were incubated together with magnetic beads. The final results were detected with the anti-His.

us to further investigate the molecular mechanism underlying this finding. Dual-LUC was performed to explore the effect of SmMYC2 and SmbHLH60 on *SmTAT1* and *SmDFR* transcription activation. Our results showed that SmMYC2 can activate *SmTAT1* and *SmDFR*, while SmbHLH60 can attenuate the expression of *SmTAT1* and *SmDFR* when SmMYC2 and SmbHLH60 existed alone. However, the transcriptional activation levels of *SmTAT1* and *SmDFR* were weakened when SmMYC2 and SmbHLH60 acted as the co-effector (Fig. 8A - B), suggesting that SmbHLH60 competed with SmMYC2 to bind to the promoters of *SmTAT 1* and *SmDFR*. Especially, the SmMYC2 - SmbHLH60 interaction did not affect the ability of SmbHLH60 to bind to the G-box probes of *SmTAT1pro* and *SmDFRpro* (Fig. 8C - D). To study the relationship between SmbHLH60 and SmMYC2, we detected the transcription level of SmMYC2 in SmbHLH60 transgenic plants. The transcription level of *SmMYC2* decreased in *SmbHLH60* -OE hairy roots, but

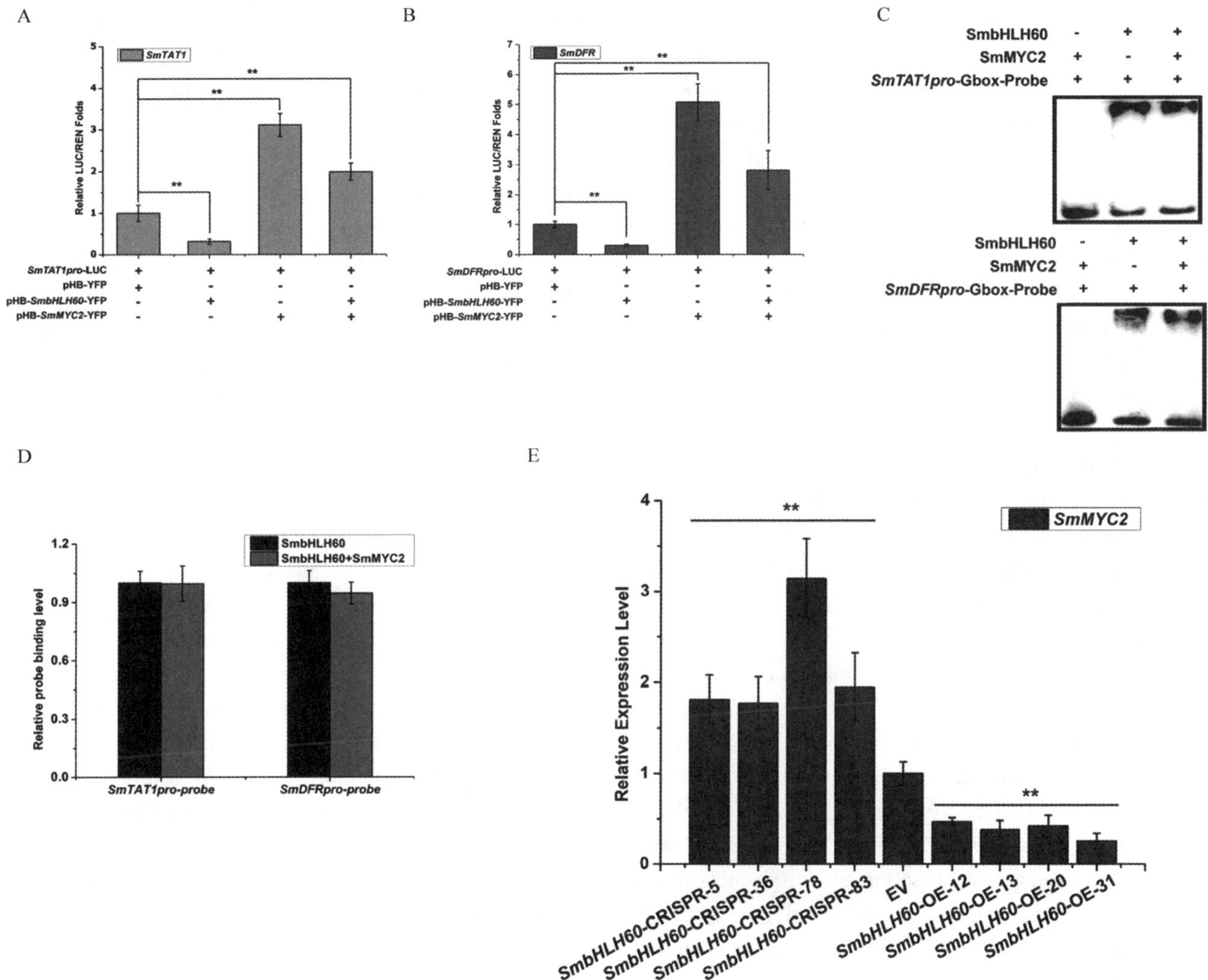


**Fig. 8 Competition between SmbHLH60 and SmMYC2 attenuates a promoter-dependent transcriptional activation of *SmTAT1* and *SmDFR***

(A) Effectors SmbHLH60 and SmMYC2 were co-transformed with reporters *SmTAT1pro* - LUC. We mixed pHB - SmbHLH60 with pHB - MYC2 and injected it with pGreen0800 - *SmTAT1* - LUC into tobacco epidermal cells and tested the results. (B) Effectors SmbHLH60 and SmMYC2 were co-transformed with reporters *SmDFRpro* - LUC. pHB - *SmbHLH60* and pHB - *MYC2* were mixed, which were injected with pGreen0800 - *SmDFR* - LUC into tobacco epidermal cells and detected the results. All data were means of three biological replicates with error bars indicating standard deviation (*, $P<0.05$; **, $P<0.01$). (C) EMSA was used to detect whether the SmbHLH60 - SmMYC2 interaction would affect the ability of SmbHLH60 to bind to the *SmTAT1* and *SmDFR* promoters by EMSA. SmMYC2 and SmbHLH60 were separately or mixed and then incubated with the biotin-labeled probes *SmTAT1pro* and *SmDFRpro* for EMSA. (D) The gray value of the bound probe was statistically used to detect whether the SmMYC2 - SmbHLH60 interaction would affect the binding of SmbHLH60 to the *SmTAT1pro* and *SmDFRpro*. All gray values were means of three biological replicates with error bars indicating standard deviation (*, $P<0.05$; **, $P<0.01$). (E) qRT - PCR was performed to detect the transcription level of *SmMYC2* in *SmbHLH60* transgenic plants. The relative quantitative analysis method ($2^{-\Delta\Delta CT}$) was used to calculate the relative gene expression, and *SmActin* was used as the internal reference gene. All experiments were repeated three times, and error bars represented the standard deviation of three biological replicates (*, $P<0.05$; **, $P<0.01$).

increased in *SmbHLH60* - CRISPR hairy roots (Fig. 8E). Meanwhile, the expression of *SmbHLH60* was also detected in *SmMYC2* - OE lines, which showed that *SmbHLH60* was decreased (Fig. S9). These results indicated that SmbHLH60 and SmMYC2 function as antagonistic regulators of phenolic acid and anthocyanin biosynthesis by direct regulation of *SmTAT1* and *SmDFR*.

## 4 DISCUSSION

MeJA has a central role in plant growth, development and adaptation to the environment. In *S. miltiorrhiza*, MeJA promotes anthocyanin, tanshinones and phenolic acids accumulation. Additionally, the effect of MeJA was also shown in the gene expression level. However, the molecular mechanism (s) underlying the regulation of secondary metabolites, and more specifically for phenolic acids in *S. miltiorrhiza*, is still unknown. Generally, MeJA regulates secondary metabolic pathways through a cascade of transcription factors to regulate downstream key enzyme genes, which ultimately leads to changes in the accumulation of metabolites. The molecular mechanism of how these key enzyme genes are regulated by the JA pathway is to be further analyzed.

The bHLH transcription factor, MYC2, was shown to act as a core regulator in the MeJA signaling pathway. In a previous report, it was found that SmMYC2, the core transcription factor for JA signaling, is a positive regulator of *SmPAL1*, *SmTAT1* and *SmCYP98A14* (37, 41). However, the mechanism by which SmMYC2 regulates JA-mediated phenolic acid biosynthesis remains unclear. In this study, a novel interactor of SmMYC2 that functions as a negative regulator in phenolic acid biosynthesis. Moreover, SmbHLH60 binds to and represses the promoters of *SmTAT1* and *SmDFR*. SmbHLH60 and SmMYC2 antagonistically interact to regulate *SmTAT1* and *SmDFR* expression. Therefore, we propose that plants regulate the biosynthesis of phenolic acid and anthocyanin mediated by the bHLH complex in *S. miltiorrhiza* through the JA signaling pathway.

SmbHLH60 may be involved in MeJA-mediated phenolic acid biosynthesis as a negative regulator MeJA has been proven to be an effective inducer that can cause the accumulation of phenolic acid. To explore the molecular mechanism of phenolic acid accumulation in *S. miltiorrhiza* which is regulated by MeJA, the MeJA-mediated transcriptome data in *S. miltiorrhiza* was analyzed. We identified 89 bHLH transcription factors that are down-regulated by MeJA, of which *SmbHLH60* was one of the most significantly down-regulated genes (Fig. 1A). SmbHLH92 have been characterized to negatively regulate phenolic acid biosynthesis. Interestingly, *SmbHLH92* showed reduced transcription levels in MeJA-mediated RNA-seq data while *SmMCY2* increased in RNA-seq data (Fig. S5). The expression pattern of *SmbHLH60* after MeJA treatment is consistent with *SmbHLH92*. These results suggest that SmbHLH60 may be a negative regulator.

In previous research, SmMYB1 has been proved to promote phenolic acid biosynthesis show a consistent expression pattern with the expression of genes in the biosynthetic pathway of phenolic acid increased significantly after MeJA treatment. However, *SmbHLH60* showed an expression pattern opposite to key enzyme genes including *SmPAL1*, *SmC4H*, *SmTAT*, *SmHPPR*, *SmRAS* and *SmCYP98A14*. These results indicated that SmbHLH60 may hold a negative regulatory role in the MeJA-mediated biosynthesis of phenolic acid. Therefore, we decided to focus on deciphering the role of this gene in regulating phenolic acid biosynthesis.

SmbHLH60 negatively regulates the biosynthesis of phenolic acid in S. Miltiorrhiza by repressing SmTAT1 It was found that total phenolic acids in hairy roots increased significantly after *SmbHLH60* was knocked out, which was 1.48 times that of the control line. Conversely, the content of phenolic acids decreased by 40% compared with the control in the *SmbHLH60* - OE lines (Fig. 4B). These results showed SmbHLH60 exhibited an opposite effect to SmMYC2. Several important genes of the phenolic acid biosynthesis pathway, including *SmPAL1*, *SmC4H*, *Sm4CL2*, *SmTAT 1*, *SmHPPR1*, *SmRAS1*, and *SmCYP98A14*, were suppressed in the presence of *SmbHLH60*. Meanwhile, the expression of these genes increased when *SmbHLH60* was knocked out (Fig. 4C). The reason for the detection of Sm4CL2 expression is that previous studies have shown that *Sm4CL2* may play a more important role in synthesizing phenolic acids. Among them, the expression of *SmPAL1*, *SmTAT1* and *SmHPPR1* increased significantly in the *SmbHLH60* - CRISPR lines. RA and SAB levels were significantly decreased in accordance with the downregulation of *SmPAL1* confirming the importance of *SmPAL1* in phenolic acid biosynthesis. Overexpression of *SmTAT1* led to a significant increase of the RA and SAB content than the wild type. Furthermore, the expression of *SmTAT1* and *SmHPPR1* was associated with the biosynthesis of RA and SAB after being treated with MeJA or other treatments, suggesting that the tyrosine conversion is a rate-limiting step in the biosynthesis of phenolic acids. These results support the hypothesis that SmbHLH60 acts as a negative regulator of the biosynthesis of phenolic acids.

We detected 7 possible candidate target genes in phenolic acid biosynthesis of SmbHLH60 by dual-LUC (Fig. 6B, S7). Our results showed that SmbHLH60 transcriptionally repressed *SmPAL1*, *SmTAT1* and *SmRAS1*, which indicated that

*SmPAL1*, *SmTAT1* and *SmRAS1* might be the target genes of SmbHLH60. Furthermore, Y1H and EMSA results showed that SmbHLH60 bound to the G-box of *SmTAT1pro* (Fig. 6D, F). Interestingly, SmbHLH60 did not bind to the E-box of *SmTAT1pro* (Fig. 6D). *SmTAT1* is the first committing enzymatic step in the tyrosine pathway. It is worth noting that our investigation demonstrated that SmbHLH60 regulates *SmTAT1* expression by direct binding to its G-box (CACGTG) promoter region. These results revealed that SmbHLH60 bound to the promoter of *SmTAT1* and suppress its expression to reduce phenolic acid biosynthesis in *S. miltiorrhiza*.

SmbHLH60 represses the expression of SmDFR to negatively regulate anthocyanin biosynthesis The total anthocyanins were extracted and it was found that the color of the *SmbHLH60* transgenic hairy root extract was significantly different from that of the control (Fig. 5A). Therefore, we are curious whether SmbHLH60 directly caused the difference in the color of anthocyanin extracts. As a result, total anthocyanin content in the knockout line reached twice that of the control line. Conversely, in hairy roots overexpressing *SmbHLH60*, the total anthocyanin content was only 59% of the control line (Fig. 5B). The expression of key genes in anthocyanin biosynthesis, including *SmCHS*, *SmFLS*, *SmF3H*, *SmF3′H*, *SmF3′5′H*, *SmANS* and *SmDFR* were decreased to varying degrees in the *SmbHLH60* - *OE* lines. Especially, *SmFLS*, *SmANS* and *SmDFR* are significantly suppressed. On the contrary, these genes showed an upward trend in *SmbHLH60* - CRISPR lines (Fig. 5C). The expressions of *SmCHI*, *SmANS* and *SmDFR* were significantly up-regulated in the *SmbHLH60* - CRISPR lines. These results indicated that SmbHLH60 negatively regulates biosynthesis not only phenolic acids but also anthocyanins.

Dual-LUC assays verified that SmbHLH60 can transcriptionally repress the expression of *SmDFR*, but it has no regulatory effect on other several anthocyanin genes (*SmF3H*, *SmCHS*, *SmANS*) (Fig. 8B, S7). Subsequently, we wonder whether SmbHLH60 binds to the G-box binding site in the *SmDFR* promoter. The dihydroflavonol reductase (DRF) is an important key enzyme in the pathway of anthocyanin biosynthesis. For example, the biosynthesis of anthocyanins in apples is regulated by DFR activity. DFR catalyzes a significant step in the biosynthesis of anthocyanins and proanthocyanidins by reducing dihydroflavonols to anthocyanins. Besides, *SmDFR* has been identified in *S. miltiorrhiza* and few reports that TFs directly regulate anthocyanin biosynthesis have been reported. Our results found that SmbHLH60 directly bound to the G-box but not E-box of the *SmDFR* promoter. As we predicted, SmbHLH60 directly regulated the expression of *SmDFR* and reduced total anthocyanins in hairy roots.

In addition to phenolic acid and anthocyanin, we also found that SmbHLH60 may also negatively affect the accumulation of tanshinones. However, the molecular mechanism requires further research in the future (Fig. S8).

SmbHLH60 and SmMYC2 antagonistic function in a bHLH heterodimer to regulate the biosynthesis of phenolic acids and anthocyanins bHLH-type TFs usually function as homodimer or heterodimer. Although SmbHLH53 has been reported to interact with SmMYC2, the mechanism by which they regulate phenolic acid biosynthesis remains unclear. Different types of transcription factors can also form complexes to regulate downstream target genes. For instance, SmMYB1 has been reported to form a complex with SmMYC2 to regulate *SmCYP98A14* and to induce phenolic acid accumulation. In this study, we identified that the SmbHLH60 interacted with SmMYC2 through the Y2H assays (Fig. 7A). BiFC and GST pull-down assays also verified the interaction between SmMYC2 and SmbHLH60 (Fig. 7B-C). These results revealed that SmbHLH60 directly interacted with SmMYC2 to form a heterodimer.

SmMYC2 has been reported to bind to *SmTAT1* and promote its transcriptional activation. Interestingly, we found that SmbHLH60 bound to and transcriptionally repressed *SmTAT1* expression (Fig. 6B - C). SmbHLH60 repressed the expression of *SmDFR* in contrast to the results that SmMYC2 promoted the transcriptional activation of *SmDFR* as was demonstrated by dual-LUC assay (Fig. 8A - B). Y1H results showed that SmMYC2 was bound to the *SmTAT1pro* and *SmDFRpro*, which indicated that *SmTAT1* and *SmDFR* were target genes for SmMYC2 (Fig. S10A). Thus, we postulate that SmbHLH60 and SmMYC2 antagonistically regulate *SmTAT1* and *SmDFR* by binding different elements of *SmTAT1* and *SmDFR*. In order to verify our hypothesis, we performed dual-LUC assays by co-injecting SmMYC2 and SmbHLH60 into *N. benthamiana* leaves with *SmTAT1* and *SmDFR*, respectively. The promotion effects of SmMYC2 on *SmTAT1* and *SmDRF* were impaired when SmbHLH60 was present (Fig. 8A - B). Interestingly, we found that the SmMYC2-SmbHLH60 interaction did not affect the ability of SmbHLH60 to bind to the *SmTAT1* and *SmDFR* promoters (Fig. 8C - D). Y1H results also showed that the binding sites of SmbHLH60 and SmMYC2 to *SmTAT1pro* and *SmDFRpro* were different (Fig. S10B). This result also implied that the binding sites of SmMYC2 and SmbHLH60 were not the same although both bound to the promoter of *SmTAT1*. Furthermore, we found that the expression of *SmMYC2* was decreased in *SmbHLH60* - OE hairy roots, but increased in *SmbHLH60* - CRISPR hairy roots (Fig. 8E). In the contrast, *SmbHLH60* was repressed in *SmMYC2* - OE lines (Fig. S9). These results indicate that SmbHLH60 and SmMYC2 antagonistically control phenolic acid and anthocyanin biosynthesis by competing with the promoters of *SmTAT1* and *SmDFR*. Furthermore, we found that SmbHLH60 interacted with SmJAZ-1like, SmJAZ8 and SmJAZ9 (Fig. S11A - B). Based on these results, we speculate that SmbHLH60 may form an inhibitory complex with JAZs to participate in phenolic acid biosynthesis. However, how the SmJAZs, SmbHLH60 and SmMYC2 work together to regulate phenolic acid and anthocyanin biosynthesis still needs more exploration in the future.

A new model-SmbHLH60 as a negative regulator for the production of phenolic acids and anthocyanins  We proposed a new hypothetical working model for the SmbHLH60 and SmMYC2 antagonistic regulation of phenolic acid and anthocyanin biosynthesis mediated by MeJA in *S. miltiorrhiza* (Fig. 9). In the absence of MeJA, *SmTAT1* and *SmDFR* are repressed by the SmbHLH60. Meanwhile,

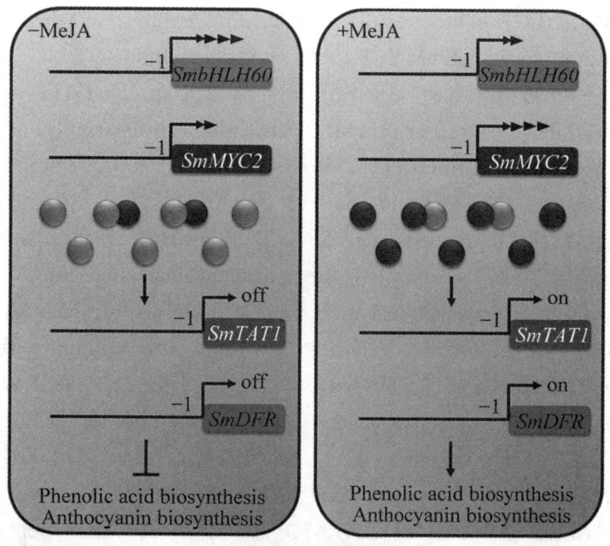


**Fig. 9  Proposed mechanism for the regulation of phenolic acids biosynthesis by SmbHLH60 in *S. miltiorrhiza***

SmbHLH60 and SmMYC2 antagonized the regulation of phenolic acid biosynthesis. Under the treatment of MeJA, *SmbHLH60* was suppressed and the expression of *SmMYC2* was increased, which led to the increase in the expressions of *SmTAT1* and *SmDFR*, resulting in the production of phenolic acid and anthocyanin increased ultimately.

SmbHLH60 and SmMYC2 form a heterodimer, which inhibited the transcriptional activation of SmMYC2 on *SmTAT1* and *SmDFR*. However, MeJA leads to a decrease in the expression of *SmbHLH60* while increasing the expression of *SmMYC2*. Furthermore, these changes in expression result in a reduction of the inhibitory effect of *SmTAT1* and *SmDFR* and enhancement of the transcriptional activation by SmMYC2. Finally, this complexed bHLH-JA dependent regulation results in increased production of phenolic acids and anthocyanins in *S. miltiorrhiza*. In summary, our discovery provides novel insights into the regulatory mechanism of bHLH-type TFs as heterodimers in the regulation of secondary metabolites which lays a foundation for further research of MeJA-mediated biosynthesis in plants.

## 5 CONCLUSIONS

In this study, a bHLH negatively regulated by MeJA was identified and characterized, named SmbHLH60. SmbHLH60 regulates phenolic acid and anthocyanin biosynthesis in *S. miltiorrhiza* roots. The expression of *SmbHLH60* was negatively correlated to the phenolic acid and anthocyanin concentrations as was shown in the OE and knockout lines. Key biosynthetic genes involved in the anthocyanin and phenolic acid production were up-regulated in the *SmbHLH60* - CRISPR lines and down-regulated in the *SmbHLH60* - OE lines. Furthermore, we have elucidated the molecular machinery in which SmbHLH60 regulates secondary metabolites. SmbHLH60 can directly bind *SmTAT1* and *SmDFR* and repress their expression through their promoters. A SmbHLH60-SmMYC2 dimer takes part in the regulation of phenolic acid and anthocyanin biosynthesis in *S. miltiorrhiza*. These results shed new light on the role of bHLH transcription factors in the biosynthesis of phenolic acids and anthocyanins through heterodimers in *S. miltiorrhiza*, and provide new insights for the analysis of the MeJA-mediated regulation network of secondary metabolites.

[刘书灿，郭新红，开国银，等. Journal of Advanced Research，2022,42:205 - 219.]

# OpNAC1 transcription factor regulates the biosynthesis of the anticancer drug camptothecin by targeting loganic acid *O*-methyltransferase in *Ophiorrhiza pumila*

## 1 INTRODUCTION

According to a recent World Health Organization (WHO) report, about one in six deaths is caused by cancer. Camptothecin (CPT) is a pentacyclic quinoline alkaloid initially isolated from the *Camptotheca acuminata*. It exhibits excellent antitumor activity by selectively binding and preventing the function of DNA topoisomerase I (TOP I) in humans. Such an inhibitory effect does not occur in cells of the CPT-producing plants due to the specific mutations within their TOP I. Two CPT-derivatives (Topotecan and Irinotecan) have been clinically approved for diverse cancer treatments, such as ovarian and non-small-cell lung cancers. Currently, the camptothecin production still relies on natural sources, such as the woody plants *C. acuminata* (Nyssaceae), *Nothapodytes foetida* (Icacinaceae). However, the plant-based camptothecin is far more cost effective in meeting demand. Therefore, looking for alternative plant sources of camptothecin is crucial.

The *Ophiorrhiza* genus with more than 300 species world-wide belonging to the Rubiaceae family, are mainly found in wet tropical forests of Southeast Asia and used as a common folk herbal medicine. In China, 68 species, including 47 endemics, are recorded and most of the *Ophiorrhiza* genus plants are distributed to the south of the Yangtze River. Among them, *Ophiorrhiza pumila* has been confirmed to produce camptothecin in all parts of the whole plant and often can be found in clusters in wet or shallow water silt. In addition, other *Ophiorrhiza* genus plants, such as *O. mungos*, *O. hirsutula*, and *O. pectinate*, produce camptothecin. The CPT-producing herbaceous plant *O. pumila* grows relatively fast, has complete reference genomes, accumulates high camptothecin content, and has reliable protocols for *Agrobacterium rhizogenes*-mediated hairy root transformation. All of the above attributes place it as a suitable model plant for studying camptothecin biosynthesis and regulation.

Camptothecin, a kind of monoterpene indole alkaloid (MIA), is synthesized using strictosidine as the precursor in *O. pumila* (Figure S1). Strictosidine is condensed from secologanin, providing the monoterpenoid moiety in the iridoid pathway, and tryptamine, providing the indole moiety in the shikimate pathway by strictosidine synthase (STR). In the post-strictosidine pathway, several intermediates have been identified to be involved in camptothecin production in *O. pumila*. However, the catalyzing enzymes have not been identified. Alternatively, strictosidinic acid, and not strictosidine, serves as the sole precursor for camptothecin biosynthesis in *C. acuminata*. In general, strictosidine is the precursor for camptothecin biosynthesis in *O. pumila*, whereas strictosidinic acid is used as the intermediate in *C. acuminata*, which confers metabolite diversity in these two CPT-producing plants from different families. Loganic acid *O*-methyltransferase (LAMT) catalyzes the conversion of loganic acid into loganin in strictosidine-producing plants such as *Catharanthus roseus* and *O. pumila*, and the conversion of loganic acid to secologanic acid is catalyzed by secologanic acid synthase (SLAS) in strictosidinic acid-producing *C. acuminata*. However, the involvement of OpLAMT synthase in camptothecin biosynthesis and its active sites, catalyzing the conversion of loganic acid to loganin, is still largely unknown.

Metabolic engineering using pathway-specific transcription factors (TFs) is an effective strategy to achieve increased camptothecin yields; some TFs, including ERF, MYB and WRKY, have been demonstrated to participate in the regulation of camptothecin production in *O. pumila*. Out of five ERF TF family genes (*OpERF1* - *OpERF5*), *OpERF2* has been shown to positively regulate the iridoid biosynthesis branch of camptothecin biosynthesis. Moreover, *O. pumila* hairy roots overexpressing *OpMYB1* showed reduced camptothecin accumulation. Four *O. pumila* WRKY TFs regulating camptothecin biosynthesis have been identified in our previous studies. Recent studies have found that NAC (NAM, ATAF and CUC) proteins can regulate plant metabolism; these include TaNAC019 in wheat, AaNAC1 in *Artemisia annua*, and SmNAC1 in *Salvia miltiorrhiza*. However, whether NAC protein(s) regulate camptothecin biosynthesis in *O. pumila* is still unknown.

Here, we showed that the high accumulation of camptothecin in the roots corresponds to the expression of its bio-synthetic genes. We identified two *OpLAMT* candidate genes, whereas only OpLAMT1 demonstrated a catalytic activity in converting loganic acid to loganin. Loganin or camptothecin was not identified in the *OpLAMT1* knock-out lines. Four key residues in the *OpLAMT1* were critical for the enzyme catalytic activity and were identified in the OpLAMT1 protein for the first time. The transcription factor OpNAC1 was also targeted as a candidate gene using co-expression network analysis. OpNAC1 was found to inhibit camptothecin biosynthesis by directly suppressing the expression of *OpLAMT1* in homodimer forms. Thus, two different camptothecin metabolic engineering strategies, including biosynthetic genes and transcription factors, are reported here and can serve as a foundation for further large-scale camptothecin production in CPT-producing plants.

## 2 RESULTS

Camptothecin biosynthesis was differentially activated in *O. pumila* tissues *Ophiorrhiza* genus plants comprise more than 300 species belonging to the Rubiaceae family, and *O. pumila* is representative among them and contains the anticancer drug camptothecin (Figure 1A). High-performance liquid chromatography (HPLC) was used to quantify the camptothecin content in different tissues of *O. pumila*. The results showed that camptothecin accumulation in the roots was higher compared with the stems and leaves (Figure 1B). In order to present global expression difference profiling in *O. pumila*, genomics and transcriptomics data were constructed. Before genome sequencing, the genome size of *O. pumila* was first determined using short Illumina PE150 sequencing, and was estimated to be ~459.96 Mb with the low heterozygosity of 0.06% and repetition (56.24%) (Figure S2; Table S1). Three different sequencing technologies, including PacBio Sequel II sequencing (~ 133-fold sequence coverage), Illumina NovaSeq 6 000 sequencing (~147-fold sequence coverage), and Hi-C genomic sequencing (~ 130-fold sequence coverage), were applied to obtain the whole-genome information for *O. pumila*. The final 456.90 Mb genome assembly contained 200 contigs, with contig N50 as 14.75 Mb and a maximum length of 40.19 Mb; 451.27 Mb (98.77%) was anchored onto 11 near chromosome-scale scaffolds, of which the N50 of the scaffold was 41.38 Mb, and the maximum chromosome length was 61.23 Mb (Dataset S1; Figures 1C, S3 - S5; Tables S2 - S4). The core gene statistics was assessed using BUSCO (Benchmarking Universal Single-Copy Orthologs) analysis to verify the sensitivity of gene prediction and the completeness of the genome assembly; the results showed that 95.3% of BUSCOs were tagged and 93.8% of BUSCOs were completed covered (Table S5). Thus, the reference genome of CPT-producing *O. pumila* was constructed and used for Rubiaceae evolution analysis, camptothecin biosynthesis, and transcriptional regulation explorations.

Then, *ab initio* prediction, homologue annotation, and cDNA-based annotation strategy were used to annotate the *O. pumila* genome. In total, 21,448 genes encoding proteins with an average gene length of 3,519 bp, an average coding sequence size of 1,333 bp, with a mean of 5.23 exons per gene were predicted (Figures S6 - S8; Table S6). Predictions of biological functions were assigned to 21,094 genes (98.35%), based on their homologies to reference organism in the TrEMBL, InterPro, Swiss-Prot, Kyoto Encyclopedia of Genes and Genomes [KEGG] and Gene Ontology [GO] databases (Figure S9; Table S7). Here, 64.73% of the *O. pumila* genome was comprised of transposable elements (TEs) that were identified using a combination of *ab initio* and homology-based repetitive sequences approaches. The two most abundant types of repetitive elements were long terminal repeat (LTR) retrotransposons and DNA transposons (49.35% and 8.91% of the nuclear genome, respectively) (Table S8). Several key genomic features of *O. pumila* are illustrated using a Circle plot (Figure 1C). Thus, the high-quality, near chromosome-level reference genome assembly and annotation of *O. pumila* could serve as the genome resource for the *Ophiorrhiza* genus and Rubiaceae family.

Gene clustering was performed for *O. pumila* with nine other plant species. In total, 19,810 *O. pumila* genes (92.36%) were clustered into 13,833 gene families, which included 7,434 (22.00%) gene families shared by all 10 species; 167 (2.20%) specific families in *O. pumila* were also identified (Figure S10; Table S9). GO and KEGG term enrichment analysis revealed that those genes unique to *O. pumila* were involved in strictosidine and indole alkaloid biosynthesis (Figure S11). In total, 489 common single-copy gene families among the 10 species were selected to construct a phylogenetic tree. The results showed that *O. pumila*, *Coffea canephora*, and *Gardenia jasminoides* lay on a branch and diverged from other euasterids at ~ 60.2 million years ago (Mya) (54.5 - 66.2 Mya), and that *O. pumila* and other Rubiaceae plants diverged at ~40.5 Mya (33.9 - 50.5 Mya) (Figure S12). The distribution of synonymous substitution rates per gene (Ks) between collinear paralogous genes of *O. pumila*, *Arabidopsis thaliana*, *Vitis vinifera*, *C. canephora*, and *G. jasminoides* genome were used to identify whole-genome duplication (WGD) events, and the results showed that three Rubiaceae plants did not show signs of any recent WGD (Figure S13). Also, synteny analyses comparing the genomes of *O. pumila* with *C. canephora* and *G. jasminoides* did not show evidence of a WGD event, and only one typically matching region in *O. pumila* with a similar level of divergence was found (Figure S14). These three Rubiaceae species generally had a closer genetic relationship, which was consistent with

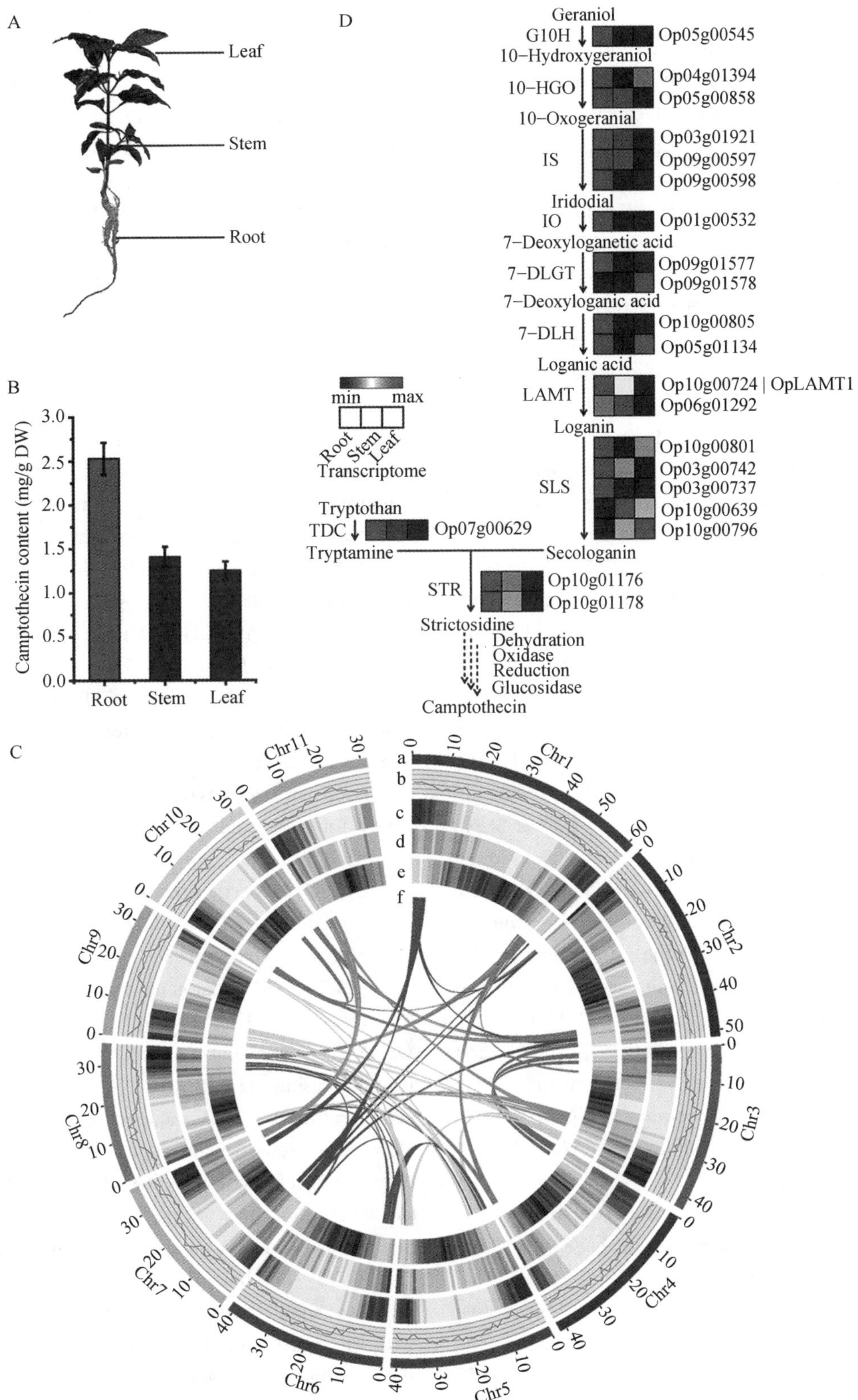


**Figure 1 The camptothecin accumulation and biosynthesis in different *Ophiorrhiza pumila* plant tissues**

(A) CPT-producing *O. pumila* plant. (B) The content of camptothecin in three different tissues (roots, stems and leaves) was detected by HPLC-DAD. Error bars represent the SD of three biological replicates. (C) Characteristics of the 11 chromosomes of *O. pumila*. From the outer to the inner ring are: a, chromosome length; b, GC content in 1 Mb windows; c, gene density in 1 Mb windows; d, density of long retrotransposon terminal repeats in 1 Mb windows; e, density of DNA transposable elements in 1 Mb windows; f, intragenomic synteny information. (D) The transcriptional levels of candidate camptothecin biosynthetic genes. HPLC, high-performance liquid chromatography.

their phylogenetic placement.

A high-quality genome sequence and an annotation dataset for *O. pumila* were used to identify candidate genes potentially involved in camptothecin biosynthesis and transcriptional regulation. In total, 64 candidate genes encoding 32 enzymes for the intermediate strictosidine in the camptothecin biosynthetic pathway were identified using the MIA-related biosynthetic genes from the genome databases of *C. acuminata*, *C. roseus*, and *G. jasminoides* (Figure 1D; Datasets S2 - S4; Table S10). To further analyze MIA biosynthesis at the transcriptional level in *O. pumila*, three different tissues (roots, stems and leaves) were selected for transcriptome sequencing. Then, the gene expression in *O. pumila* was annotated and analyzed using the new *O. pumila* genome assembly obtained in this study. We found a spatial correlation between candidate genes involved in intermediate strictosidine biosynthesis to the accumulation pattern of camptothecin in the tissues analyzed (Figure 1D). In total, 192 cytochrome P450 (CYP450) encoding genes were annotated in the *O. pumila* genome, which is likely to include enzymes involved in the biosynthesis of camptothecin (Figure S1; Dataset S4).

OpLAMT1, and not OpLAMT2, catalyzes the conversion of loganic acid to loganin in *O. pumila* LAMT catalyzes loganic acid to loganin in strictosidine-producing plants, such as *C. roseus* and *O. pumila*, whereas SLAS catalyzes loganic acid to secologanic acid in strictosidinic acid-producing *C. acuminata*. Thus, strictosidine is the only precursor for camptothecin biosyn-thesis in *O. pumila*, whereas strictosidinic acid is used as the intermediate in *C. acuminata*, which confers metabolite di-versity in these two CPT-producing plants. We identified two *OpLAMT* in *O. pumila* (Figures 2A, S15), and both *OpLAMT1* and *OpLAMT2* were expressed in all detected tissues. The expression level of *OpLAMT1* in roots was higher than in other tissues, whereas the expression level of *OpLAMT2* was higher in the stems (Figure 1D).

OpLAMT1 and OpLAMT2 were expressed in *Escherichia coli*, enzymatic assays showed that OpLAMT1, but not OpLAMT2, catalyzed loganic acid to loganin (Figures 2B, S16). In order to further map the active domains of LAMT protein from *O. pumila*, the recombinant OpLAMT1 with a His-tag was heterologously expressed and purified under optimized conditions (Figure S17). Kinetic analysis of OpLAMT1 indicated that the values for *Km* and *kcat* were 0.475 mmol/L and 0.003 57 $s^{-1}$, respectively (Figure 2C; Table S11). The effect of the temperature and pH on the catalytic reaction toward loganin was optimal at 40℃, pH 7.0, and metal ions did not affect the OpLAMT1 enzyme activity (Figure 2D - F). In addition, recombinant OpLAMT1 purified from *E. coli* cells could not catalyze secologanic acid (Figure S18).

Bioinformatics analysis revealed that OpLAMT1 was a member of the SABATH methyltransferase family, and the overall structure of OpLAMT1 consisted of a Rossmann-like domain for binding methyl donor *S*-adenosyl-homocysteine (SAH) and an α-helical domain for surrounding the methyl accepter substrate loganic acid (Figure S19). According to molecular docking results, the carboxylate group of loganic acid was engaged and oriented for methyl transfer by residue Thr-323, and the cavity of OpLAMT1 was occupied by several polar residues (Tyr - 169, His - 172, Trp - 173, His - 255, Gln - 283) that were within the hydrogen-bonding distance from the substrate loganic acid (Figure 2G). In addition, the volume of solvent-accessible surface for OpLAMT1 was calculated as ~2028 $Å^3$ by PROTEINS PLUS (Figure S19). To further investigate the role of key catalytic residues in the functioning of the active site pocket of OpLAMT1, six mutants (Y169A, H172A, W173A, H255A, Q283A, and T323A) were generated using site-directed mutagenesis (Figure 2G). The catalytic reaction indicated that the Y169A, H172A, W173A, and H255A displayed no catalytic activity for loganic acid. In contrast, the activity of mutant Q283A amounted to just 10% of that of the wild-type, and the mutant T323A showed slightly lower activities compared with wild-type protein (Figures 2G, H, S20). Thus, four essential catalytic residues of OpLAMT1 were identified.

*OpLAMT1* participates in the camptothecin biosynthesis in *O. pumila* To explore the role of *OpLAMT1* in camptothecin biosynthesis, *OpLAMT1* overexpression (*OpLAMT1 - OE*) transgenic hairy root lines was generated (Figures 3A - G, S21). In addition, three homozygous *OpLAMT1* knock-out (*OpLAMT1 - KO*) hairy root lines mediated using the CRISPR/Cas9 system were also obtained according to the DNA sequencing results (Figures 4A, B, S22, S23). No noticeable appearance changes and dry weight effects were observed in the *OpLAMT1 - KO* and *OpLAMT1 - OE* hairy root lines (Figures 3G, 4A, S24). Metabolic analysis showed that camptothecin and loganin contents in *OpLAMT1 - KO* hairy root lines were barely detected, but increased significantly in the *OpLAMT1 - OE* lines compared with the control lines (Figures 3H, I, 4C, D). Accordingly, the content of loganic acid, LAMT substrate, was significantly improved in the *OpLAMT1 - KO* hairy root lines (Figure 4E). The autofluorescence properties of camptothecin provided another straightforward method to investigate the relative concentrations of camptothecin in different trans-genic lines by comparing the fluorescence intensity. Comparing the fluorescence pattern in the hairy root between *OpLAMT1 - KO* lines and the control, low to no fluorescence was observed from the *OpLAMT1 - KO* lines

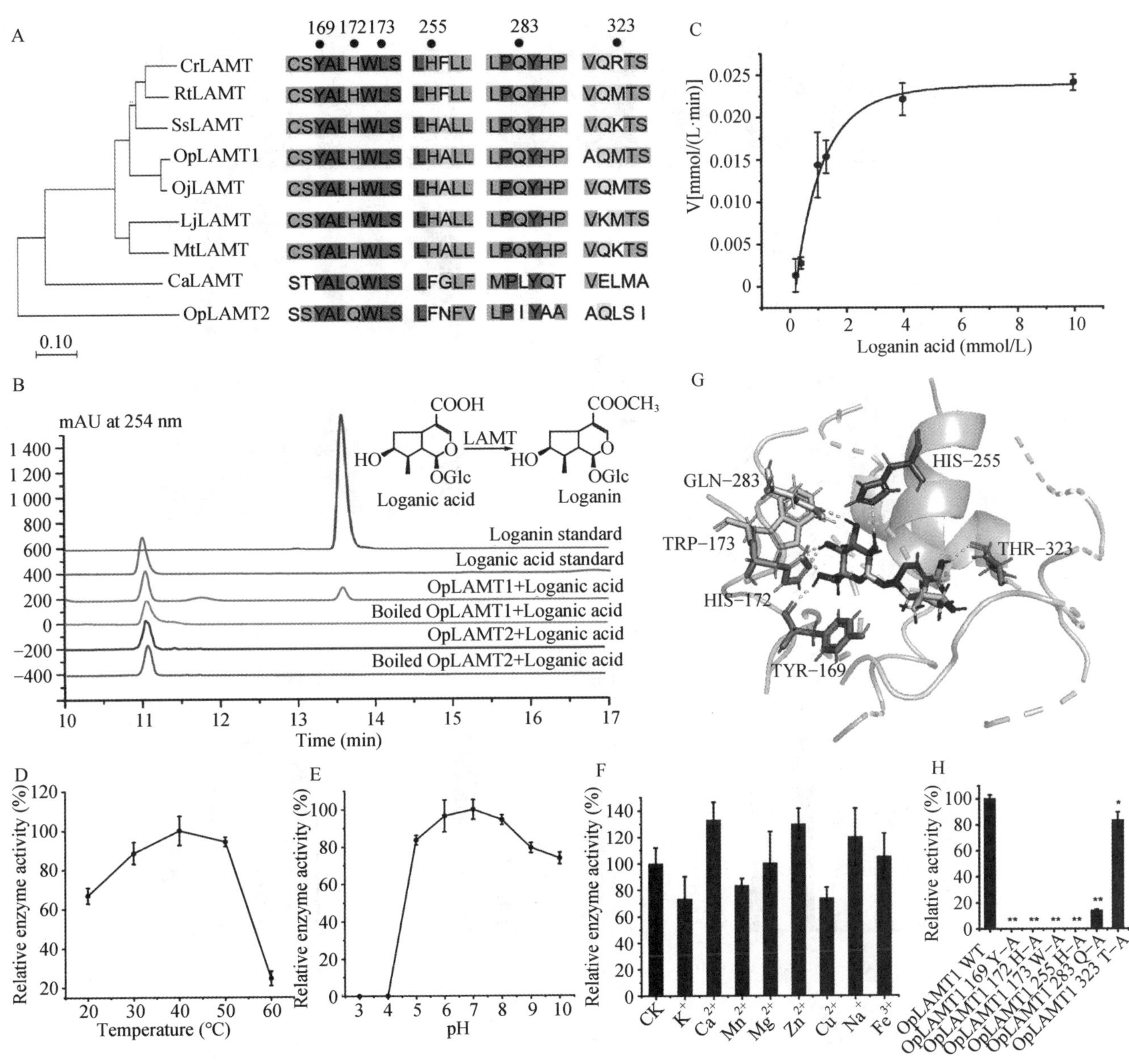


**Figure 2 Structural of OpLAMT1 and enzyme activity assay**

(A) Phylogenetic relationship and protein sequence alignment of OpLAMT1 and LAMT homologues from other species. (B) HPLC traces illustrate repre-sentative compound peaks for the target products of OpLAMT1. (C) Enzyme kinetics of OpLAMT1 calculated from the Michaelis－Menten equation. (D) The effect of the temperature (20－60 ℃) on the catalytic reaction was evaluated and the activity toward loganin was optimal at 40 ℃. (E) A variety of buffers from a pH range of 3.0 to 10.0 was used to examine the effect of pH on the activity of the purified recombinant OpLAMT1, and the activity toward loganin peaked at pH 7.0. When the pH was less than 4.0, OpLAMT1 had no activity. (F) The effect of metal ions on OpLAMT1 enzyme activity. Most metal ions did not affect the OpLAMT1 enzyme activity. Three biological repeats were conducted for all experiments. (G) Docking results for loganic acid of OpLAMT1. (H) Relative activities of OpLAMT1－WT and the mutated OpLAMT1.

(Figure 4F). Similarly, the fluorescence intensity of *OpLAMT1－KO* hairy root extracts was significantly lower than that of the control. Conversely, the fluorescence intensity in the *OpLAMT1－OE* lines was slightly higher than in the controls (Figure S25). These results suggested that *OpLAMT1* was indeed rate-limiting in loganin and camptothecin biosyn-thesis and genetic manipulation of *OpLAMT1* is effective in modulating camptothecin accumulation.

OpNAC1 negatively regulates camptothecin biosynthesis

To further study the transcriptional regulation of camptothecin biosynthesis in *O. pumila*, 1,189 TFs were identified in the genome and were divided into 57 families. The bHLH, MYB, ERF, C2H2, and NAC families were the five most dominant classes, each with more than 60 genes (Data S5; Figure S26). The construction of a co-expression network revealed a total of 672 candidate TFs that may be involved in the regulation of camptothecin biosynthesis,

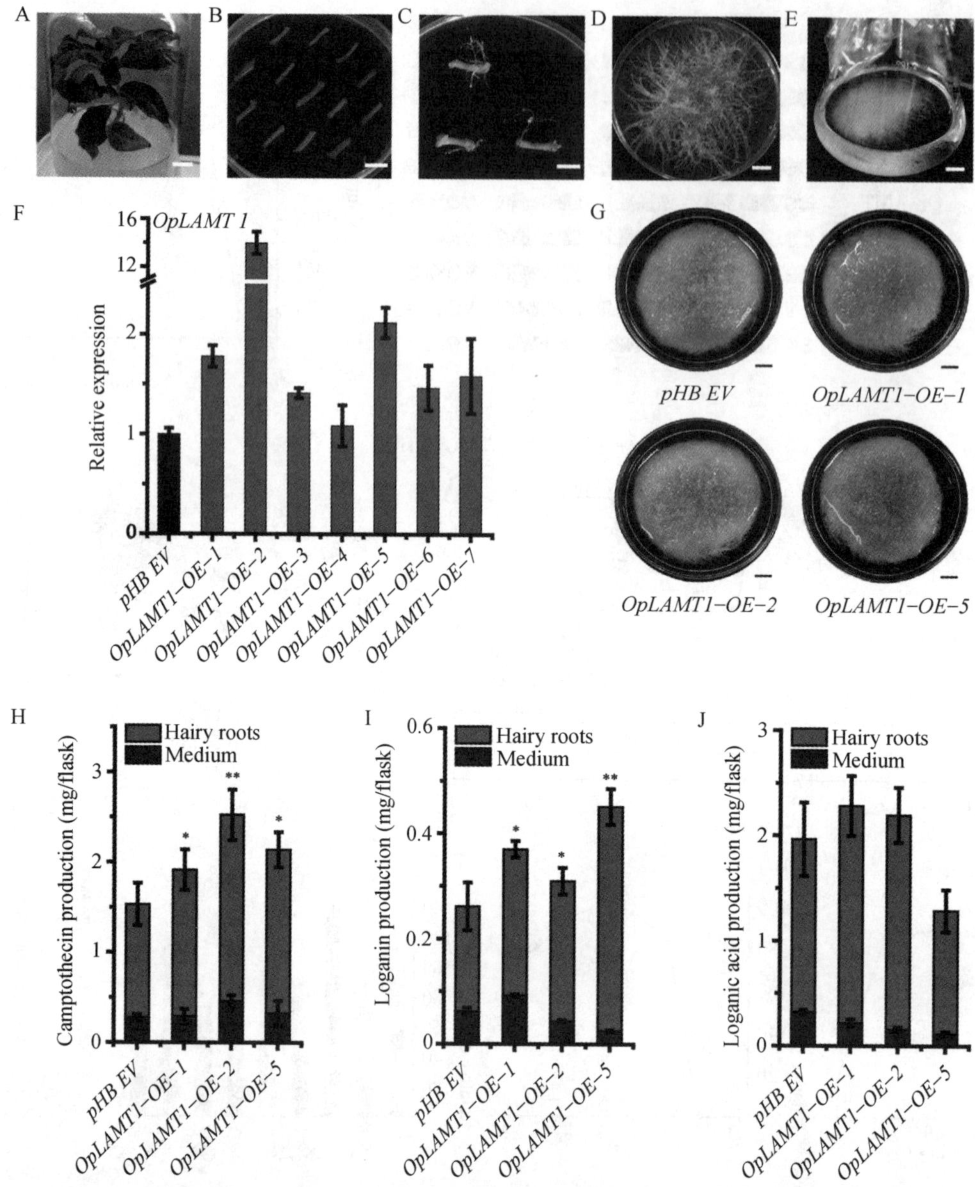


**Figure 3 Analysis of camptothecin biosynthesis in the *OpLAMT1* -*OE* transgenic hairy root lines**

(A-E) Generation of transgenic *Ophiorrhiza pumila* hairy root lines. (A) *O. pumila* explants on B5 medium. (B) *O. pumila* stems precultured on B5 medium. (C) Hairy roots differentiated from infected *O. pumila* explants. (D) Isolated monoclonal hairy roots. (E) Hairy root monoclones cultured in B5 liquid medium. Scale bars: 1 cm. (F) The relative transcript levels of *OpLAMT1* in the *OpLAMT1* - *OE* transgenic hairy root lines were detected by qRT-PCR. (G) The phenotype of the *OpLAMT1* -*OE* transgenic hairy root lines (scale bars: 1 cm). (H-J) The production of camptothecin, loganin, loganic acid in *OpLAMT1* -*OE* transgenic hairy root lines was detected by HPLC. Error bars represent the SD of three biological replicates. Student's *t*-test: ** $P<0.01$; * $P<0.05$. HPLC, high-performance liquid chromatography.

including MYB (67 genes), ERF (47 genes), bHLH (44 genes), NAC (43 genes), C2H2 (42 genes), bZIP (31 genes), WRKY (26 genes), and so on (Figure 5A). The expression of *OpNAC1* in *O. pumila* roots was significantly higher than in the stems and leaves, correlating with the camptothecin biosynthetic genes (Figures 5B, S27). To further investigate the potential regulatory function of OpNAC1 in the camptothecin biosynthetic pathway, the potential binding sites of NAC TFs (NACRS motif, C/TACG) in about 3,000 bp promoter regions of 10 camptothecin biosynthetic genes were analyzed. Yeast-one-hybrid (Y1H) assays were performed to corroborate the specific binding affinity of OpNAC1 to the NACRS element in the promoter of *OpLAMT1* (Figure S28). Thus, possible functions of *OpNAC1* in regulating camptothecin biosynthesis were furtherly determined. First, OpNAC1 owned the conserved domain: A, B, C, D, and E motifs, and the phylogenetic analysis placed OpNAC1 in the NAP subfamily. Transient

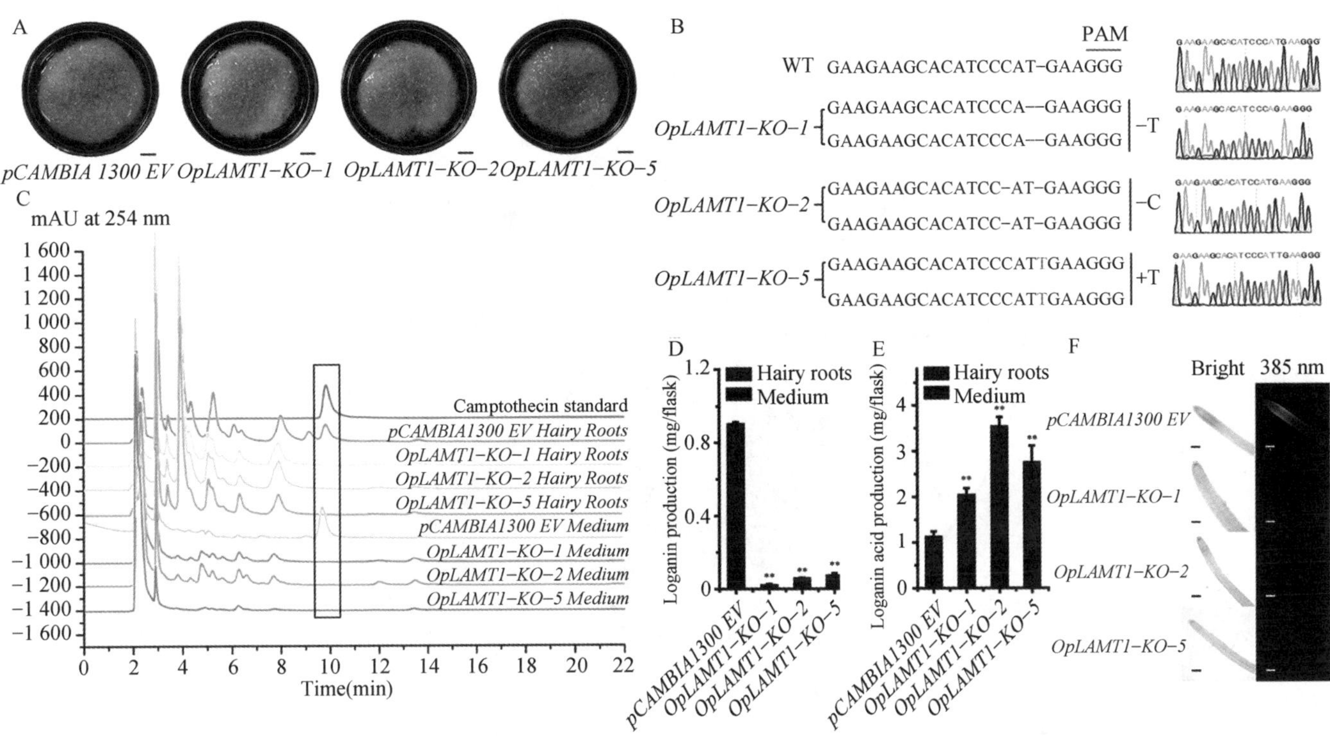


**Figure 4 Analysis of camptothecin biosynthesis in the *OpLAMT1*-*KO* transgenic hairy root lines**

(A) The phenotype of the *OpLAMT1*-*KO* transgenic hairy root lines (scale bars: 1 cm). (B) Genomic OpLAMT1 DNA sequences from different *OpLAMT1*-*KO* transgenic hairy root lines were detected by DNA sequencing. The original sequence of *OpLAMT1* is displayed at the top; the PAM (GGG) area is highlighted in the red line. Detailed DNA insertions and point mutations of the *OpLAMT1* sequence in different *OpLAMT1*-*KO* transgenic hairy root lines are presented on the right. (C) HPLC detection of camptothecin accumulation in *OpLAMT1*-*KO* transgenic hairy root lines. (D, E) The concentrations of loganin and loganic acid in *OpLAMT1*-*KO* transgenic hairy root lines. Error bars represent the SD of three biological replicates. (F) The camptothecin distribution in the *OpLAMT1*-*KO* transgenic hairy root lines (scale bars: 200 μm). HPLC, high-performance liquid chromatography.

transformation assays revealed that the OpNAC1 fluorescent signal was only detected in the nucleus of *Nicotiana benthamiana* leaves cells expressing OpNAC1-YFP (Figures S29-S31). *OpNAC1*-*OE* and *OpNAC1*-*KO* transgenic hairy root lines were generated (Figures 6A, B, S32, S33). Out of the 28 positive transgenic *OpNAC1*-*OE* hairy root lines, three *OpNAC1*-*OE* lines (*OpNAC1*-*OE*-*21*, *OpNAC1*-*OE*-*27*, *OpNAC1*-*OE*-*28*) with the highest expression levels were selected for further analysis (Figure 6C). Then, the *OpNAC1* gene was amplified for DNA sequencing in 25 positive CRISPR/Cas9 lines carrying *OpNAC1* sgRNA and three homozygous *OpNAC1*-*KO* hairy root lines (*OpNAC1*-*KO*-*1*, *OpNAC1*-*KO*-*12*, *OpNAC1*-*KO*-*25*) were obtained according to the DNA sequencing results (Figure 6D). In the *OpNAC1*-*KO* hairy root lines, the expression levels of *OpNAC1* were 0.31 to 0.73 times that of the control (Figure 6E).

Compared with the controls, no phenotypic changes or changes in the root dry weight were observed in the *OpNAC1*-*OE* and *OpNAC1*-*KO* hairy root lines (Figures 6A, B, S34). In the *OpNAC1*-*OE* lines, a 23%-45% reduction in camptothecin production was observed. Conversely, camptothecin production in the *OpNAC1*-*KO* lines was significantly higher than in the control lines (Figure 6F, H). Accordingly, the relative transcript levels of camptothecin biosynthetic genes, including *OpLAMT1*, *OpSLS1* and *OpSTR1*, were reduced significantly in the *OpNAC1*-*OE* hairy root lines compared with the control. An opposite trend was observed in the *OpNAC1*-*KO* lines (Figure 6G, I). Altogether, these results suggested a negative regulatory role played by OpNAC1 in camptothecin biosynthesis.

OpNAC1 binds to the promoter of *OpLAMT1* and suppresses its expression To further investigate the regulatory mechanism of OpNAC1 in camptothecin biosynthesis, Y1H assays were performed to corroborate the binding affinity of OpNAC1 to the NACRS element in the promoter of camptothecin biosynthetic genes. The results showed that OpNAC1-GAL4 activated the *LacZ* reporter of *pOpLAMT1*-*NACRS* (Figure 7A). To further confirm the role of OpNAC1 in the transcription of *OpLAMT1*, Dual-LUC assays were carried out using *N. benthamiana* leaves (Figures 7B, S35). Compared with the pHB-YFP control, the suppression ability on *pOpLAMT1* of OpNAC1-YFP driven by the 35S promoter was detected. The reporter gene

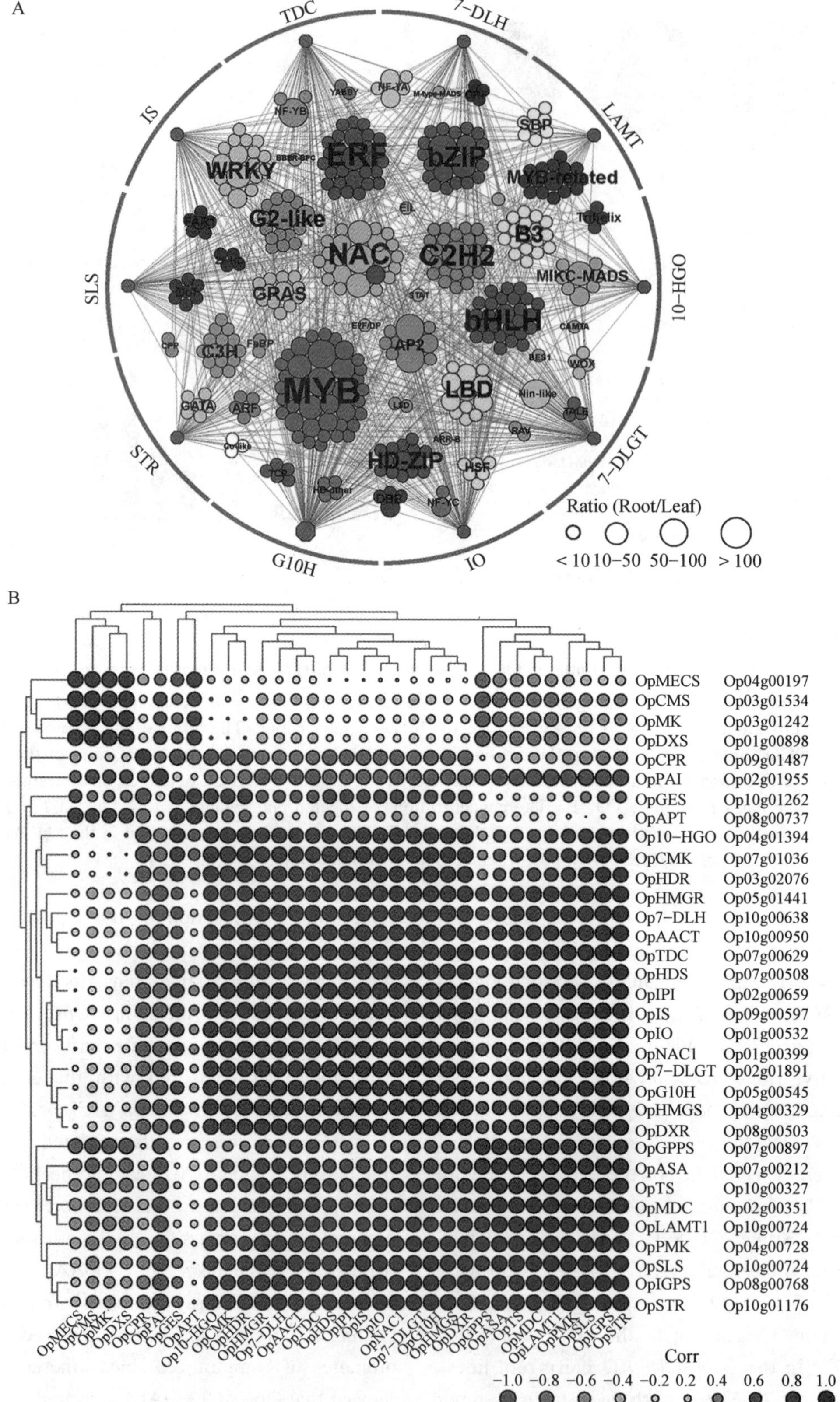


**Figure 5 Co-expression network of transcription factors and camptothecin biosynthetic genes**

(A) The hexagons represent camptothecin biosynthetic genes and the colored solid circles represent transcription factors. The larger circle means the higher expression levels of transcription factors in roots compared with leaves. The edges are drawn when the linear correlation coefficient is >0.95, with *e*-value <0.05. The red solid circle represented the *OpNAC1* gene and other OpNACs are shown in light red. (B) Cluster heatmap shows the expression correlations between *OpNAC1* transcription factor gene and 32 camptothecin biosynthetic genes.

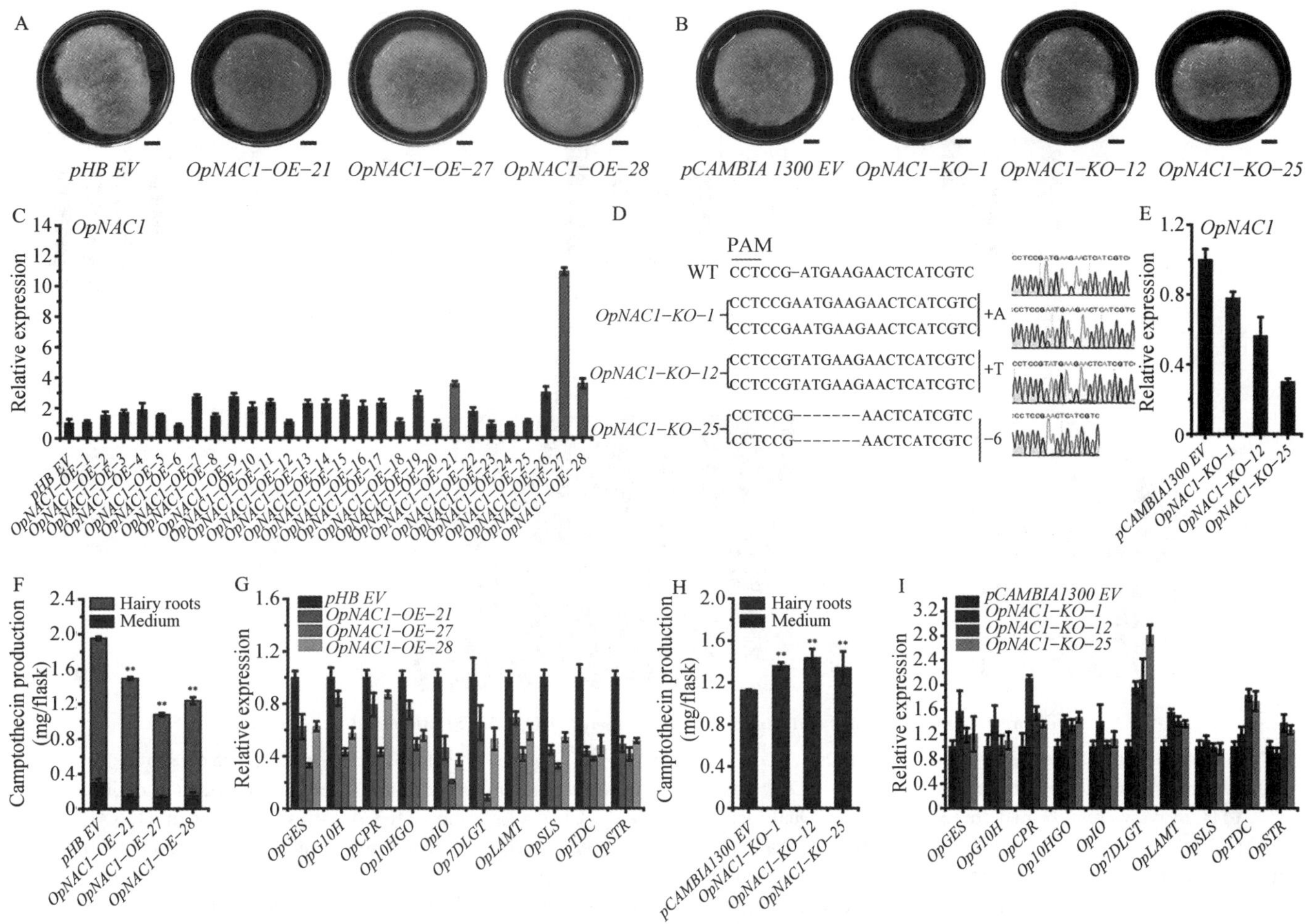


**Figure 6 Analysis of camptothecin biosynthesis in the *OpNAC1 - OE* and *OpNAC1 - KO* transgenic hairy root lines**

(A, B) The phenotype of the *OpNAC1 - OE* and *OpNAC1 - KO* transgenic hairy root lines (scale bars: 1 cm). (C, E) The relative transcript levels of *OpNAC1* in the *OpNAC1 - OE* and *OpNAC1 - KO* transgenic hairy root lines were detected by qRT - PCR. (D) Genomic OpNAC1 DNA sequences from different *OpNAC1 - KO* transgenic hairy root lines were detected by DNA sequencing. The original sequence of OpNAC1 is displayed at the top; the PAM (CCT) area is highlighted by the red line. Detailed DNA insertions and point mutations of the OpNAC1 sequence in different *OpNAC1 - KO* transgenic hairy root lines are presented on the right. (F, H) The concentration of camptothecin in *OpNAC1 - OE* and *OpNAC1 - KO* transgenic hairy root lines. Error bars represent the SD of three biological replicates. (G, I) The expression levels of camptothecin biosynthetic genes in the *OpNAC1 - OE* and *OpNAC1 - KO* transgenic hairy root lines. The average transcriptional expression level of each gene in the two control hairy root lines was set to 1. The *OpUBQ* gene was used as a housekeeping gene. Error bars represent the SD of three technical replicates.

was not activated in the constructs of the mutated promoter in the NACRS element (Figure 7B). Furthermore, the content of loganin, intermediate in the iridoid pathway of camptothecin biosynthesis, was significantly decreased in *OpNAC1 - OE* hairy root lines and slightly increased in *OpNAC1 - KO* lines, consistent with the camptothecin production (Figure 7C, D). These results confirmed that OpNAC1 inhibited camptothecin biosynthesis through the suppression of *OpLAMT1* expression.

NAC proteins have been reported to form homodimers in various plants. To investigate whether OpNAC1 forms homodimers, OpNAC1 was inserted into the plasmids pGADT7 - GAL4 and pGBKT7 - GAL4 and co-transformed into yeast in various combinations. The full-length version and deletion construct of OpNAC1 (N-terminal NAC domain region and C-terminal region) interacted with the full-length OpNAC1 protein in yeast-two-hybrid assays (Y2H) (Figure 7E). Similarly, the full length of nYFP-OpNAC1 could interact with the cYFP-OpNAC1, which indicated that the OpNAC1 protein could form homodimers shown by the bimolecular fluorescence complementation (BiFC) assays (Figure 7F). Thus, OpNAC1 negatively regulated camptothecin biosynthesis by directly binding and suppressing *OpLAMT1* in homodimer forms (Figure 7G).

## 3 DISCUSSION

High-throughput sequencing facilitates research in CPT-producing plants　Camptothecin is one of the most promising anticancer drugs with additional pharmacological properties including antiviral and antifungal activities. More

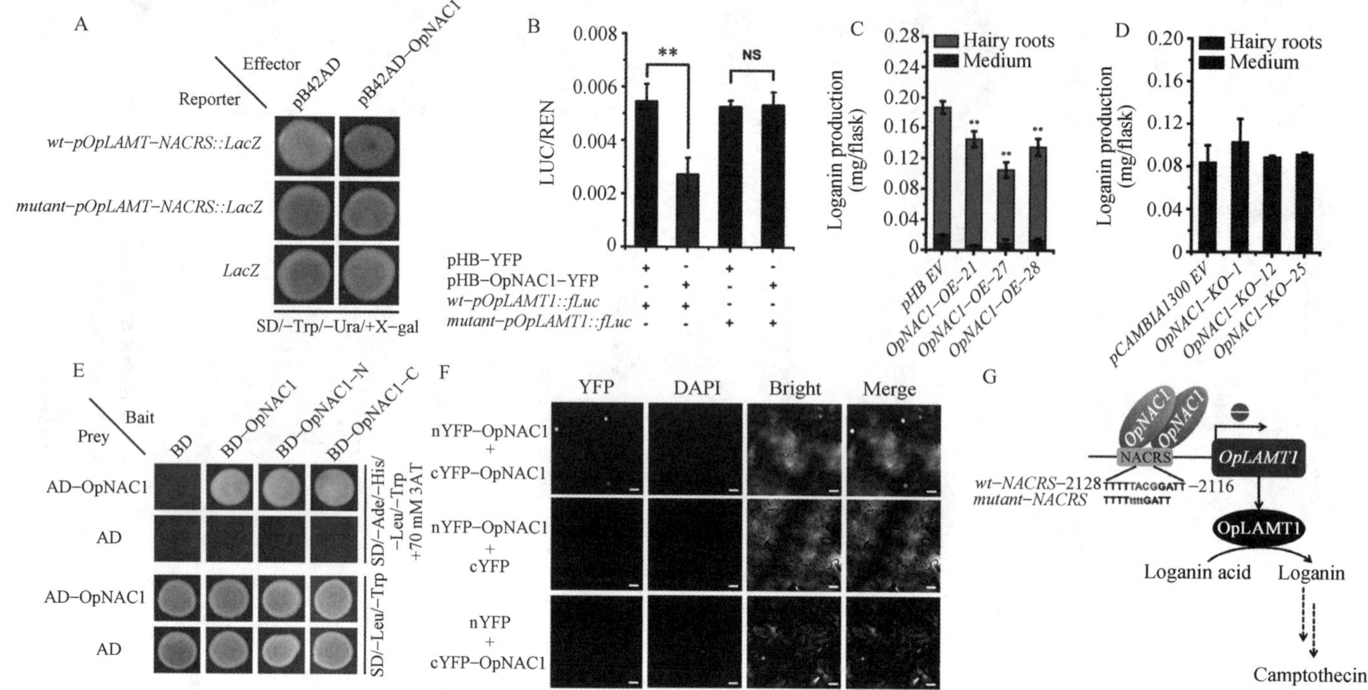


**Figure 7 OpNAC1 binds and suppresses the promoter of *OpLAMT1* in homodimer forms**

(A) Yeast-one-hybrid (Y1H) assay indicates that OpNAC1 binds to the NACRS in the *OpLAMT1* promoter. Yeast cells transformed with different combi-nations of constructs were grown on SD/−Ura/−Trp/+X-gal medium. Photographs were taken after 4 d of incubation at 30℃. Y1H assays were repeated three times. (B) Dual-luciferase (Dual-LUC) assays shows the suppression effect of OpNAC1 on the *OpLAMT1* promoter. The *OpLAMT1* promoter and *OpLAMT1* promoter containing a NACRS motif mutant were fused to the firefly luciferase reporter gene. A transient Dual-LUC assay determined the promoter activity in *Nicotiana benthamiana* leaves. The relative LUC activity was normalized to that of the reference *Renilla* (REN) luciferase. Error bars indicate SD ($n=3$). Student's $t$-test: ** $P<0.01$; NS, no significance. (C, D) The production of loganin in *OpNAC1-OE* and *OpNAC1-KO* transgenic hairy root lines was detected by HPLC. Error bars represent the SD of three biological replicates. Student's $t$-test: ** $P<0.01$. (E) The interaction of OpNAC1 was verified by yeast-two-hybrid assay. Yeast cells transformed with different combinations of constructs were grown on selective medium SD/−Trp/−Leu/−His/−Ade and the control medium SD/−Trp/−Leu. Photographs were taken after 4 d of incubation at 30℃. Y2H assays were repeated three times. (F) Interactions of OpNAC1 examined by bimolecular fluorescence complementation (BiFC) in *N. benthamiana* leaves. OpNAC1 was fused in the vectors pXY104-YC and pXY106-YN. Scale bar: 20 μm. (G) Regulatory model of camptothecin biosynthesis by OpNAC1. HPLC, high-performance liquid chromatography.

than 10 CPT-producing plant species have been discovered from different families, such as Nyssaceae, Icacinaceae, Apocynaceae, and Rubiaceae. In the *Ophiorrhiza* genus of the Rubiaceae family, CPT-producing *O. pumila* is a representative folk medical plant. To explore the chemodiversity of *O. pumila*, complete $^{13}$C-based metabolome labeling and $^{15}$N-based stable isotope labeling for *O. pumila* were performed. Metabolomics analysis showed that MIAs accumulated in a tissue-specific manner, with the highest levels in the root and hairy root, and lower levels in the leaf tissues. Consistent with the accumulation of MIAs in *O. pumila*, the expression of iridoid biosynthesis-related genes is also tissue specific, with high expression in the root and hairy root, and low expression in leaf and cell suspension culture. For mining camptothecin biosynthetic functional genes, detecting gene transcription levels is of great significance. Before whole-genome information was available, genetic studies on CPT-producing plants such as *C. acuminata*, *N. nimmoniana*, and *O. pumila* were mainly carried out at the transcriptional level. In this study, the transcriptomes of different tissues in CPT-producing *O. pumila* were established, which provided a valuable data resource for analyzing the expression of camptothecin biosynthetic genes. The expression of camp-tothecin biosynthetic genes was high in the roots of *O. pumila*, consistent with camptothecin accumulation.

Several genomes of CPT-producing plants, such as *C. acuminata* and *O. pumila* are currently available. The first published *C. acuminata* genome assembly was created in 2017, producing an assembly of 1,394 scaffolds spanning 403.2 Mb. To improve this short-reads-based assembly, the 414.95 Mb genome of *C. acuminata* was re-sequenced and anchored onto 21 pseudo-chromosomes. In addition, the 11 chromosome-level reference and phased genome assembly of *O. pumila* was reported, with 21 assembly gaps and a contig N50 of 18.49 Mb. In this study, the genome size of CPT-producing *O. pumila* was estimated to be ~459.96 Mb with a low heterozygosity of 0.06% and repetition (56.24%) by short Illumina PE150 sequencing (Figure S2; Table S1), which exhibited the simple genome characteristics. The background of sterile *O. pumila* material was relatively pure after reproducing for many generations using the tissue culture system in our group. In total, 11 near chromosome-scale genomes of *O. pumila* with low error and high mapping rates were generated. Our *O. pumila* genome assembly had fewer genes than the previously published genome, with 21,448 vs. 32,389 genes. However, we annotated longer genes on average (3,519.28 bp compared with 3,117.94 bp) and more exons per gene (5.23 compared with 4.47) (Table S6). BLAST alignment between our genes and those in the previously published Op_genome assembly showed 11,480 genes with significantly shorter gene lengths that were missing in our new *O. pumila* genome (*P*-value$<2.2e^{-16}$) (Dataset S1; Figure S7). MCScanX analysis of these two *O. pumila* genome assemblies revealed a total of 12,634 1∶1 orthologous genes with no significant difference in their lengths (Dataset S1; Figure S8). Furthermore, there were 2,731 and 452 genes in our new *O. pumila* genome, which had two and three matches in previously published Op_genome assembly according to MCScanX (Dataset S1). The three Rubiaceae plants *O. pumila*, *C. canephora*, and *G. jasminoides* had a close genetic relationship based on a whole-genome phylogenetic comparison, and the genomes did not show signs of any recent WGD (Figure S12), which was consistent with their previously assigned phylogenetic placement. Thus, a high-quality chromosome-scale genome assembly combined with the transcriptome of CPT-producing *O. pumila* was constructed in this study.

Metabolic engineering strategies for camptothecin production in CPT-producing plants  LAMT catalyzes the synthesis of loganin by adding methyl to loganic acid in strictosidine-producing plants, such as *C. roseus* and *O. pumila*. In contrast, loganic acid is directly converted to secologanic acid by SLAS in strictosidinic acid-producing *C. acuminata*. Thus, the camp-tothecin biosynthesis in *O. pumila* utilizes strictosidine as the exclusive intermediate, and strictosidinic acid is used as the intermediate in *C. acuminata*. Hence, at least two diverse metabolic pathways can lead to camptothecin production in CPT-producing plants. In our study, loganin and camptothecin were not detected in *OpLAMT1-KO* hairy root lines. Furthermore, we identified four critical residues of OpLAMT1 protein catalyzing the loganic acid to loganin, suggesting that OpLAMT1 plays pivotal roles in camptothecin biosynthesis. Therefore, OpLAMT1 is a strong candidate for the regulation of camptothecin metabolic engineering.

Genetic engineering of biosynthetic enzymes to study and improve camptothecin production in CPT-producing plants has been demonstrated. For example, suppression of tryptophan decarboxylase (TDC) or secologanin synthase (SLS) in *O. pumila* hairy roots by RNA interference led to a decrease in camptothecin content. Overexpression of *strictosidine synthase* (*STR*) and *geraniol 10-hydroxylase* (*G10H*) from *C. roseus* led to an increase in camptothecin levels. Camptothecin was significantly reduced in the *OpG10H* and *OpSLS* knock-out hairy root lines. The co-introduction of these two biosynthetic genes in *O. pumila* hairy roots resulted in higher camptothecin accumulation.

The use of hormones and transgenic technology to regulate TFs can often spontaneously regulate the transcription of biosynthetic enzymes, thereby efficiently changing metabolic pathways. To date, TFs such as WRKY, MYB, ERF and bZIP have been found to participate in the regulation of camptothecin biosynthesis in CPT-producing plants. In *O. pumila*, *OpERF2* has been reported to positively regulate the iridoid biosynthesis of camptothecin. *OpMYB1* can act on the indole synthesis branch of camptothecin biosynthesis, downregulating the expression level of *OpTDC* and inhibiting the biosynthesis of camptothecin. Additionally, four WRKY TFs are involved in camptothecin biosynthesis in *O. pumila*, *OpWRKY2* enhances camptothecin biosynthesis by regulating the expression of *OpTDC*, *OpWRKY6* negatively regulates camptothecin biosynthesis by directly downregulating gene expression in the iridoid and shikimate pathways, whereas *OpWRKY1* and *OpWRKY3* play a regulatory role by binding to the W-box on the *OpCPR* promoter. Alternatively, the NAC TFs are characterized by a conserved region known as the NAC domain at their N terminus, involved in DNA recognition, dimerization, and binding, whereas their C terminus is highly diverse. Recent studies have found that NAC TFs can regulate plant metabolism, and NAC proteins have been reported to form homodimers in various plants. In this study, the full-length 1 134 bp open reading frame (ORF) fragment of *OpNAC1* was cloned and encoded a 377 amino acid protein that belonged to the NAP subfamily and shared the conserved NAC domain-containing A, B, C, D, E motifs (Figures S29, S30). We have shown that OpNAC1 functions as a repressor and negatively regulates camptothecin biosynthesis by directly binding to *OpLAMT1* in homodimer forms. Therefore, this study provided an effective strategy for camptothecin production using metabolic engineering and a new perspective for improving the germplasm resources of *O. pumila*.

## 4 MATERIALS AND METHODS

Plant materials  *Ophiorrhiza pumila* used for expression analysis and genetic transformation was collected from

Fujian Province (Fujian, China) in 2006. It was cultured in growth chambers at Zhejiang Chinese Medical University (Zhejiang, China) at 24 ℃ under a 16 h light photoperiod. For the reference genome sequencing, *O. pumila* sterile plants were cultured on a solid B5 medium (pH 5.5), and the leaves of *O. pumila* were used to isolate the DNA for genome sequencing. Different tissues of *O. pumila* (roots, stems and leaves) were used for transcriptomic analyses. Explants of stems from 1-month-old *O. pumila* sterile plants were collected for *A. rhizogenes* infection to generate transgenic hairy roots. *N. benthamiana* plants were grown in pots in a growth chamber at 24 ℃ under a 16 h light photoperiod for subcellular localization experiments, Dual-LUC and BiFC assays.

Quantitative detection of metabolites by high-performance liquid chromatography  The quantitative detection of different metabolites in different tissues and transgenic hairy roots of *O. pumila* was determined by HPLC. Different tissues (roots, stems, and leaves) of 5-month-old *O. pumila* seedlings and different transgenic hairy root lines cultured in 100 mL B5 liquid medium for 45 d were collected and freeze dried to grind into powder. For the camptothecin measurement in different tissues and transgenic hairy roots of *O. pumila*, 1 mL methanol was added to 20 mg powder, followed by 30 min of ultrasonication, and determined as previously described. For loganic acid and loganin measurement in different transgenic hairy root lines, 100 mg dried hairy root powder was extracted with 10 mL ethanol: water (4 : 1, v/v) and sonicated for 30 min, and were determined as previously described. Three replicates for each tissue sample were used.

Transcriptome sequencing *O. pumila*  Total RNA was extracted from three different tissues (roots, stems, leaves) of *O. pumila* using the Omini Plant RNA Kit (DNaseI) (Kangwei Company, China). The quality assessment was conducted using an Agilent Bioanalyzer® 4200 TapeStation. A Qubit RNA BR Assay Kit (Thermo Fisher Scientific, USA) was used to determine the concentration of each total RNA sample. RNA-Seq libraries were prepared using the VAHTS Stranded mRNA-seq Library Prep Kit (Vazyme, China) and sequenced on an Illumina NovaSeq 6000 System (Illumina, USA) to generate RNA-Seq PE150 reads. We removed adapters and discarded reads with >10% N bases and reads having more than 20% low-quality bases (quality scores below 5) from these libraries using the NGS QC Toolkit v 2.3.344.

Recombinant protein expression and OpLAMT1 enzyme activity assay  Full-length cDNAs of *OpLAMT1* (1,146 bp) and *OpLAMT2* (1,083 bp) were separately cloned from the *O. pumila* cDNA library by PCR amplification and inserted into the pET30a-His expression vector with a His-tag using the ClonExpress II One Step Cloning Kit (Vazyme, China). *E. coli* strain Top10 was used as the cloning host for plasmid construction, and *E. coli* BL21 (DE3) was used as the host for recombinant protein production. Single colonies for each construct were inoculated into 10 mL Lysogeny broth (LB) medium, followed by culture at 37 ℃ for 12 h. Then the culture was transferred into 400 mL of fresh LB medium with kanamycin until the $OD_{600}$ reached 0.6. For protein expression, isopropyl-β-D-thiogalactoside (IPTG) was added to the cultures to induce protein production over 12 h at 25 ℃.

To optimize the conditions of OpLAMT1 protein expression, different concentrations of IPTG (2, 1, 0.5, 0.3, and 0.1 mmol/L) were added to the cultures to induce protein production over 12 h at different temperatures (37 ℃, 30 ℃, 25 ℃, 20 ℃, and 15 ℃). After collection by centrifugation, the cell pellets in 30 mL of lysis buffer (Sangon Biotech, B548117, consisting of 20 mmol/L potassium phosphate buffer, pH 7.5, 100 mmol/L NaCl and 5% glycerol) were suspended and lysed by sonication in an ice bath. After centrifugation at 5,000 r/min for 10 min, the supernatant was added onto a column loaded with $Ni^{2+}$ resin. Then, lysis buffers containing increasing concentrations of imidazole (25, 50, 100, 250, and 400 mmol/L) were used to wash the column. Each fraction was sampled using SDS-PAGE analysis. The target proteins on a PD - 10 column were concentrated and desalted, and the protein concentration were determined using the Bradford assay and bovine serum albumin (BSA) to generate a standard curve.

To optimize the conditions of the OpLAMT1 protein catalytic reaction, a typical enzymatic assay in 100 μL aliquots of a reaction mixture containing 20 mmol/L phosphate-buffered saline (PBS) buffer with eight different pH (pH 3 - 10), 1 mmol/L loganic acid, and 1 mmol/L *S*-adenosyl methionine (SAM) in the presence of loganic acid methyltransferase (LAMT) (1 mg/mL) was performed. The reaction mixtures at different temperatures (20 ℃, 30 ℃, 40 ℃, 50 ℃, and 60 ℃) were incubated for 2 h and the reactions were quenched with the addition of 100 μL of methanol and vortexing for 5 min. After centrifugation at 12,000 *g* for 5 min and filtration, a 10 μL sample was used for HPLC-diode array detection (HPLC - DAD) analysis. The column applied for analysis was an Agilent Eclipse Plus C18 column (4.6 × 150 mm, 3.5 μm) on an Agilent 1260 Infinity II system with the temperature set at 35 ℃. Mobile phases A ($H_2O$+0.1% formic acid) and B (methanol) were run in the following gradient program at 0.8 mL/min: 0 - 30 min 10%-100% B; 30 - 31 min 100%-10% B; 31 - 36 min 10% B. In total, 5 μL of sample was injected for analysis. OpLAMT1 assays were monitored at 254 nm by the extracted ion chromatogram of the products.

Homology modeling was performed with SWISS-MODEL using the closest template available. The results were inspected and rendered with PyMOL. Protein docking and binding energy calculation were done with SYBYL, using local search parameters and default docking parameters. The SYBYL software preprocessed the protein, including removing water molecules, hydrogenation and charges, and extracting the original ligands in the structure. To further investigate the role of key catalytic residues in the functioning of the active site pocket of OpLAMT1, six mutants (Y169A, H172A, W173A, H255A, Q284A, and T323A) were generated through site-directed mutagenesis.

Yeast-one-hybrid assay For Y1H assays, the full-length *OpNAC1* ORF fragment was amplified and cloned into the effector plasmid pB42AD. The triple tandem copy of the *pOpLAMT1* NACRS-containing region (TTTTTACGGATT) and its mutant (TTTTTtttGATT) were inserted into the reporter plasmid pLacZ between *Eco*RI and *Xho*I, respectively. Y1H assays were performed as previously described. Effector and reporter plasmids were co-transformed into yeast strain EGY48. Transformants were cultured on SD/−Ura/−Trp medium for 48 h and tested on SD/−Ura/−Trp medium with 5-bromo-4-chloro-3-indolyl-β-D-galactopyranoside (X-gal) for 24 h. Empty pB42AD and pLacZ plasmids were co-transformed into yeast and used as the negative controls. All primers used to amplify *OpNAC1*, and DNA motifs are listed in Dataset S6.

Dual-LUC assays To investigate the ability of OpNAC1 to transcriptionally activate the camptothecin biosynthetic genes, ~3,000 bp promoters of 10 camptothecin biosynthetic genes were analyzed and cloned into the pGreenII 0800-LUC vector. The reporter constructs were obtained by inserting the native promoter of 10 CPT-biosynthetic genes into the pGreenII 0800-LUC vector to drive the expression of the firefly luciferase gene. The *Renilla* luciferase gene driven by *CaMV 35S* promoter was used as an internal control. The assembled vectors were co-transformed with the helper plasmid pSoup19 into *A. tumefaciens* strain GV3101. The *A. tumefaciens* strain GV3101 containing pHB-*OpNAC1*-YFP was used as an effector, and pHB-YFP was used as a negative control. Infiltration and detection were performed as previously described, with minor modifications. The reporter strains were mixed with effector strains harboring either pHB-*OpNAC1*-YFP or pHB-YFP at a ratio of 1∶1. Leaves were collected after 48 h and Dual-LUC assays were performed using the Dual-Luciferase Reporter Assay System according to the manufacturer's instructions (Promega, Madison, WI, USA). Three biological replicates per treatment were measured. All primers used to amplify promoters are listed in Dataset S6.

Yeast two-hybrid assays For yeast-two-hybrid analysis, we inserted the ORF of *OpNAC1* into the pGBKT7 and pGADT7 vectors to create pGBKT7-*OpNAC1* and pGADT7-*OpNAC1*, respectively. The two constructs were co-transformed into yeast strain AH109. pGADT7-*OpNAC1* and pGBKT7, pGADT7 and pGBKT7-*OpNAC1*, pGBKT7 and pGADT7 were used as negative controls. The transformants were cultured on SD/−Leu/−Trp medium and tested on SD/−Ade/−His/−Leu/−Trp medium.

BiFC assays BiFC assays were performed as previously described. For the generation of the BiFC vectors, the full-length cDNA of *OpNAC1* was cloned into pXY104-YC (C terminus of YFP) and pXY106-YN (N terminus of YFP) to obtain OpNAC1-cYFP, OpNAC1-nYFP and then transformed into *Agrobacterium* strains GV3101, respectively. The indicated vector combinations were co-transformed into 5-week-old *N. benthamiana* leaves. After 60-72 h of incubation, YFP signals were observed using LSM880 confocal laser microscopy (Carl Zeiss, Germany). Nuclei were stained using DAPI (Sigma-Aldrich, USA). Three biological OpNAC1 negatively regulates camptothecin biosynthesis repeats were conducted for all experiments. The primers are listed in Dataset S6.

Statistical analyses All experiments in this study were conducted with at least three biological replicates. All data are presented as the mean±standard deviation (SD). Paired two-tailed Student's *t*-test was used with a significance threshold of $P<0.05$ to test the differences between control and treated samples/transgenic hairy root lines.

Data availability statement The data that support the findings of this study are openly available in China National GenBank Database (CNGB) Nucleotide Sequence Archive with project accession ID: CNP0002219. Accession number: PacBio sequencing reads (CNX0351651); Illumina HiSeq sequencing reads (CNX0351652); Hi-C sequencing reads (CNX0350500); transcriptome sequencing reads (CNX0372332, CNX0372333 and CNX0372334).

[郝小龙，开国银，等. Journal of Integrative Plant Biology, 2023.65(1):133-149.]

# Reshuffling of the ancestral core-eudicot genome shaped chromatin topology and epigenetic modification in *Panax*

Polyploidy or whole genome duplication (WGD) is a ubi-quitous phenomenon in angiosperms and all extant flowering plants likely evolved from a polyploid ancestor. Recurring polyploidization and (re) diploidization events in flowering plants led to highly dynamic plant genomes. However, it remains poorly characterized how these often-cyclical genome doubling/diploidization processes have contributed to angiosperm evolution and diversification.

It is evidenced that all extant core-eudicots share an ancient WGD, usually referred to as the γ-triplication event. The ancestral core-eudicot genome was restored to a diploid karyotype, and most of the extant core-eudicot species experienced additional paleo-polyploidization events during their independent diversification processes. Frequent genome doubling followed by independent diploidization and chromosomal rearrangement processes have provided extant core-eudicots with structural genomic and phenotypic diversity. An example of such genome structural evolution is cotton (*Gossypium*) where, following polyploidization, both large genomic fragment reorganization (i.e., chromosome fusion and fission) and individual gene repertoire evolution (i.e., biased genetic fractionation) have generated phenotypic novelty and species diversification. However, relatively little is understood about how reshuffling of the duplicated ancestral core-eudicot genome affected genome plasticity of extant core-eudicot plants and the underlying mechanisms responsible for the genetic and epigenetic partitioning of a duplicated genome. The genus *Panax* (Araliaceae) includes four diploids, three tetraploids and one species complex. It has been shown that this genus shares the core-eudicot γ triplication and has undergone two additional *Panax*-specific WGDs (Pg-β and Pg-α). In particular, as a medically important genus, all ginseng species contain a large number of secondary metabolites. These attributes make the ginseng genus an ideal system to elucidate how the reshuffling of the duplicated (or better triplicated) ancestral core-eudicot genome has affected genome structure, epigenetic regulation and secondary metabolites diversity of extant plant species after repeated polyploidization and (re)diploidization events.

In this study, we assemble chromosomal-level reference genomes of one diploid (experienced γ and Pg-β) and three closely related tetraploid (experienced γ, Pg-β and an additional, more recent, Pg-α duplication) *Panax* species. We infer the evolutionary history of the seven ancestral core-eudicot chromosomes (Eu1-Eu7) in the four *Panax* species. Based on this paleo-polyploidization framework of the genus *Panax*, our genome-wide comparisons of the three-dimensional (3D) genome architecture and cytosine methylation and gene expression dynamics (mRNA, lncRNA and small RNA) further reveal that reorganization of the ancestral genome structure is associated with the reconfirmation of chromatin topology and epigenetic regulation divergence in extant *Panax* genomes. Our study thus provides a genome-wide landscape view of how polyploidization and subsequent (re) diploidization contribute to genome structure plasticity and metabolomic diversity of extant *Panax* species.

## 1 RESULTS

Genome assembly, gene annotation and quality control Our chromosome analyses confirmed the diploid ($2n=2x=24$) and tetraploid ($2n=4x=48$) karyotypes of the four *Panax* species (Supplementary Fig. 1). Genome sizes of the four species were estimated by genome survey (Table 1 and Supplementary Fig. 2) and flow cytometry (Supplementary Fig. 3), respectively. To obtain reliable inference of the karyotype evolution, we employed three different strategies to de novo assemble the four *Panax* species (Supplementary Note 1-2). The resulting assemblies were 1.96 Gb and 2.02 Gb for *P. stipuleanatus* and *P. japonicus*, with a contig N50 of 2.88 Mb and 1.58 Mb for the two species, respectively (Table 1). Total lengths of the assembled genomes were relatively larger for *P. ginseng* (3.36 Gb) and *P. quinquefolius* (3.57 Gb), with a contig N50 of 19.75 Mb and 0.87 Mb for the two species, respectively. Genome annotation of the four *Panax* species identified 41,224-74,307 protein-coding genes (Table 1).

Assessments of the genome quality revealed high gene completeness (BUSCO = 93.00 — 95.14%) and genome contiguity (LAI=7.13—16.24) for all four species (Table 1). In particular, genome contiguity measures of *P. stipuleanatus* (LAI = 12.85) and *P. japonicus* (LAI = 16.24) were comparable to the model species *Arabidopsis thaliana* (LAI=15.62) and *Vitis vinifera* (LAI=14.58), although the two *Panax* species had much larger genome sizes. Genome collinearity analyses showed that, while the four species varied dramatically in genome size, they still maintained high collinearity across the 12 orthologous chromosomes (Supplementary Fig. 4). Based on the genome collinearity and sequence homoeology to diploid relatives, we further separated the 24 chromosomes of the three tetraploid species as two subgenomes (Supplementary Table 1). Phylogenetic inference based on orthologous genes revealed that subgenome B of the three tetraploid species clustered with the diploid *P. notoginseng* while subgenomes A formed a monophyletic clade (Supplementary Fig. 5). These genomic features together corroborated the quality of the genome assemblies of the four *Panax* species.

**Table 1 Statistics of genome features of the four *Panax* species**

| Genome information | P. stipuleanatus | P. japonicus | P. ginseng | P. quinquefolius |
|---|---|---|---|---|
| Genome size (Gb)[a] | 2.15 | 2.09 | 3.41 | 3.60 |
| Total length of contigs (Gb) | 1.96 | 2.02 | 3.36 | 3.56 |
| GC content (%) | 35.24 | 33.93 | 34.25 | 34.11 |
| N50 length (contig) (Mb) | 2.88 | 1.22 | 19.75 | 0.87 |
| Predicted genes | 41,224 | 74,307 | 65,913 | 64,247 |
| Average transcript length (bp) | 1280 | 1267 | 1389 | 1394 |
| Average CDS length (bp) | 1037 | 1061 | 1119 | 1149 |
| Average exon length (bp) | 273 | 265 | 270 | 264 |
| Average intron length (bp) | 925 | 916 | 835 | 891 |
| BUSCO (%) | 93.10 | 93.00 | 95.14 | 93.93 |
| LTR Assembly Index (LAI) | 12.85 | 16.24 | 7.13 | 7.99 |

[a]Genome size was estimated by genome survey.

**Reconstruction of the ancestral karyotype in the modern *Panax* genome** The polyploidization history of the four *Panax* species was estimated by calculating synonymous substitution rates (Ks) between homologous gene pairs. Our results confirmed that the genus *Panax* experienced the core-eudicot-shared γ triplication and two additional lineage-specific duplications (Pg - α and Pg - β) (Supplementary Fig. 6). Likewise, we also identified the other previously inferred paleo-polyploidizations (i.e., Dc - β) in *Daucus carota* (carrot) and *Lactuca sativa* (lettuce). Karyotype evolution of the ancestral core-eudicot genome in extant *Panax* species was inferred by analyzing genome collinearity between grape (putative post-γ core-eudicot genome) and the above selected six species (extant core-eudicot genomes). Our genome-wide comparisons identified more collinear orthologous genes (referred to as ancestral genes) in the four *Panax* species (16,010 - 31,729) than those of carrot (13,985) and lettuce (14,087) genomes (Supplementary Table 2). In particular, these ancestral genes tend to be retained in *Panax* genomes as large contiguous genomic blocks, i.e., on average about 17 - 20 (95% confidence interval (CI)) ancestral genes localized in each of these collinear genomic blocks (Supplementary Figs. 7 - 16 and Supplementary Table 2). In contrast, a smaller number of collinear ancestral genes have been retained in the carrot (95% CI: 12—13) and lettuce (95% CI: 11—12) genomes ($t$-test, $P$ value$<$0.01). Together, our results indicate that the ancestral core-eudicot genome has been well-preserved in modern *Panax* genomes, even after several rounds of polyploidization-diploidization.

Based on genome collinearity analyses, we identified 26 post-γ and four post-Pg-β chromosomal fusion events in the *Panax* genomes, 10 and 20 of the post-γ events were also characterized in lettuce and carrot genomes, respectively (Supplementary Figs. 8 - 16). Given the shared ancestral (γ) and lineage-specific (i.e., Pg-α and Pg - β) polyploidization/(re) diploidization histories of the six extant core-eudicot species, we propose an evolutionary framework wherein the 21 (after hexaploidy/triplication) post - γ ancestral core-eudicot chromosomes (A1 - A7, B1 - B7 and C1 - C7) were rearranged into eight pre-Pg-β ancestral chromosomes (Ar1 - Ar8) through the identified 26 post-γ chromosomal fusions (Fig. 1 and Supplementary Figs. 8 - 16). Thereafter, the post-Pg-β genome (Ar1a - Ar8a and Ar1b - Ar8b) was structured into the ancestral *Panax* genome (Pa1 - Pa12) via four post-Pg-β chromosomal fusion events (Fig. 1). Among the extant *Panax* genomes, we also identified three chromosomal rearrangements, including one fragmental inversion on *P. stipuleanatus* chromosome 4, one reciprocal translocation between *P. stipuleanatus* chromosomes 8 and 9, and one inversion on *P. notoginseng* chromosome 6 (Fig. 1 and Supplementary Figs. 17 and 18).

The above inferences have revealed the evolutionary transformation of the seven ancestral core-eudicot chromosomes

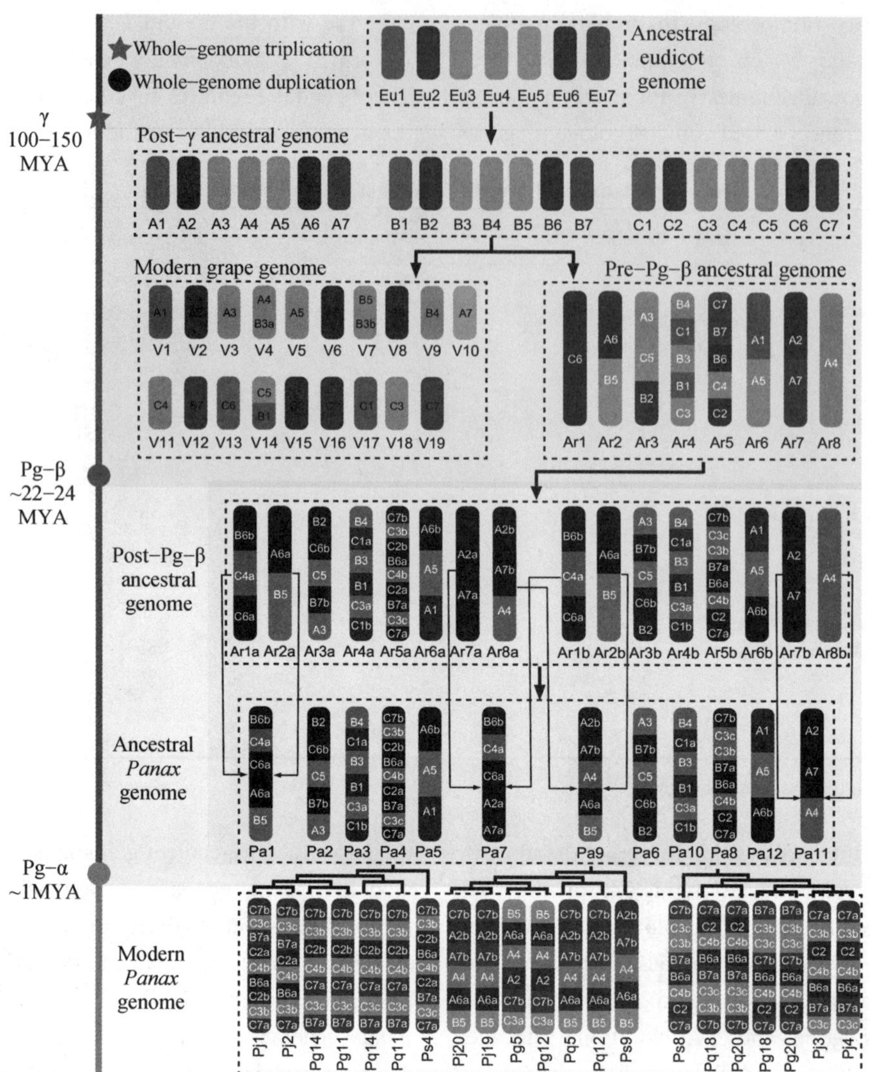


**Fig. 1 Evolutionary rearrangements of the ancestral core-eudicot genome to generate the genome of extant ginseng species**

The ancestral core-eudicot genome is hypothesized to contain seven chromosomes (Eu1 - Eu7) marked with seven different colors. The post-γ ancestral genome consists of three chromosomal compartments (A1 - A7, B1 - B7 and C1 - C7) which were reunited into the same nucleus some 100 - 150 million years ago (MYA). The extant grape genome (V1 - V19) has evolved from the post-γ karyotype through one chromosomal fission and two fusions. In parallel, the post-γ ancestral genome was structured into a pre-Pg-β karyotype with eight chromosomes (Ar1 - Ar8). The pre-Pg-β karyotype was doubled about 22 - 24 MYA (Ar1a - Ar8a and Ar1b - Ar8b) but further reorganized into the ancestral *Panax* genome with 12 chromosomes (Pa1 - Pa12). After the Pg-α duplication, one fragment conversion and two translocations occurred in the four extant *Panax* species (Ps, *Panax stipuleanatus*; Pj, *Panax japonicus*; Pg, *Panax ginseng*; Pq, *Panax quinquefolius*). Red star, green and orange circles present the γ triplication, Pg - β and Pg - α duplication, respectively.

(Eu1 - Eu7) into 42 homoeologous genomic regions (referred as to duplicated ancestral core-eudicot chromosome) in extant *Panax* genomes after the γ triplication (3×) and Pg-β duplication (2×) (Fig. 1). We then allocated all identified collinear genes to the 42 ancestral core-eudicot chromosomes (Fig. 2a and Supplementary Data 1). In the *P. stipuleanatus* genome, for example, biased genetic fractionation of the gene duplicates was a general phenomenon in all the 42 ancestral core-eudicot chromosomes, with only 993 (6.7% of total) of the ancestral genes retaining more than half (> 3) of the duplicate pairs (Supplementary Data 1). In addition, our comparisons also showed that genes duplicated by the more recent Pg-β duplication (6 484 gene pairs) were less fractionated compared to those derived from the more ancient γ triplication (4 143 gene pairs). Further genome-wide comparisons of the fractionation pattern confirmed that gene duplicates derived from the same ancestral gene showed different retention rates along the ancestral core-eudicot chromosomes (Supplementary Fig. 19). For example, even though the six homologous genomic regions (marked with

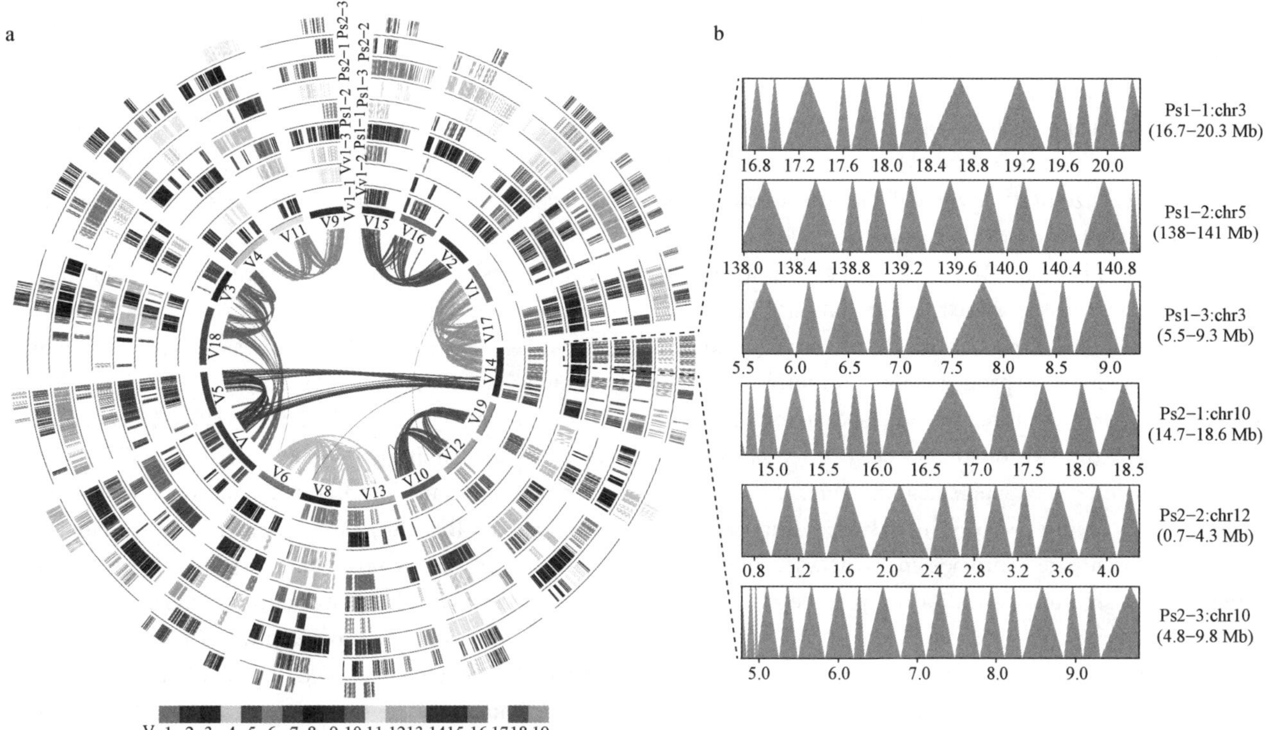


**Fig. 2 Global alignment of ginseng genomic regions to the grape genome and chromatin topology of the paleo-polyploidization-derived homologous regions in ginseng**

(a) Collinearity was determined by genes (referred to as ancestral core-eudicot gene) that were collinear between ginseng and grape genomes. The 19 extant grape chromosomes (V1 - V19) in the innermost circle are color-coded to different colors according to the color bar at the bottom. Curved lines within the inner circle connect homoeologous genes duplicated by the γ triplication. Colors of these curved lines correspond to the seven ancestral core-eudicot chromosomes (Eu1 - Eu7). A genomic region in grape has three and six homologous regions compared to itself and ginseng genomes, respectively. The three grape circles (Vv1 - 1, Vv1 - 2, and Vv1 - 3) are the result of the core-eudicot γ triplication. The middle three (Ps1 - 1, Ps1 - 2, and Ps1 - 3) and outside three (Ps2 - 1, Ps2 - 2, and Ps2 - 3) circles are also the result of the core-eudicot shared γ triplication plus the Pg-β duplication, respectively. The short lines within each genomic region of the nine circles represented the predicted ancestral core-eudicot genes. Grape genes have initials "Vv" or "V" and ginseng genes "Ps". Colors of these core-eudicot genes represent their physical locations on the 19 grape and 12 ginseng chromosomes, respectively. The six homologous genomic regions included in black dashed line were selected to compare chromatin topology. (b) From top to bottom are the topological association domain-like (TADs-like) structures of the six selected homologous genomic regions. Both the top three (extant *Panax* chromosome 3, 3, and 5) and bottom three (extant *Panax* chromosome 10, 10, and 12) regions resulted from the γ triplication, while the top and bottom three homologous genomic regions, in turn, resulted from the Pg-β duplication (giving rise to Ps1 and Ps2). The numbers on *x*-axis indicate physical positions on extant ginseng chromosomal segments. Triangle size represents the length of each TAD on the ginseng chromosome. Source data are provided as a Source Data file.

purple color in Fig. 1) in the extant *P. stipuleanatus* genome (chromosomes 2, 4, 6, 7, 8, and 11) were duplicated from the same ancestral core-eudicot chromosome Eu2, the numbers of retained ancestral genes differed dramatically along the γ-derived triplicates (i.e., among the Ps1 - 1/Ps1 - 2/Ps1 - 3 or Ps2 - 1/Ps2 - 2/Ps2 - 3) (Supplementary Fig. 19 and Supplementary Data 2). In contrast, Pg-β-derived gene duplicates (i.e., between Ps1 - 1 and Ps1 - 2, Ps1 - 2 and Ps2 - 2 or Ps1 - 3 and Ps2 - 3) showed similar gene fractionation rates along the ancestral core-eudicot chromosomes.

We next focused on how these ancestral genes duplicated in the different WGDs evolved in the diversification process of extant *Panax* species. Our pan-genomic analyses assigned these ancestral genes to 29, 499 orthogroups, only 1 836 (6.2% of the total) of which were specific to each of the seven extant *Panax* genomes (one diploid and six tetraploid genomes) (Supplementary Table 3). Further collinearity comparisons revealed that 6 874 (32.6%- 49.4%) of these ancestral genes have been retained in the seven extant *Panax* genomes as collinear orthologous genes (Supplementary Table 4 and Supplementary Data 3). Among the three tetraploid species, we identified 13,679 (52.1% of the total) and 14, 550 (57.6%) collinear orthologous genes in the subgenomes A and B, respectively (Supplementary Table 5 and Supplementary Data 4). It is notable that while the three tetraploid species showed high genome collinearity (see

Supplementary Fig. 4), *P. japonicus* possesses a substantially smaller genome (2.02 Gb) compared to *P. ginseng* (3.36 Gb) and *P. quinquefolius* (3.57 Gb) (see Table 1). This phenomenon can be explained, at least partially, by the different evolutionary history of long terminal repeats (LTRs). For example, compared to *P. ginseng*, the increased genome size of *P. quinquefolius* was likely due to the post-speciation (<1 MYA) burst of unknown LTRs (Supplementary Figs. 12 - 13). In contrast, while *P. japonicus* experienced the shared pre-speciation LTR burst, the majority of the *Copia*, *Gypsy* and other unknown retrotransposons have expanded more recently. Distinct expansion patterns of the three retrotransposon families were also observed for the two diploid species, *P. stipuleanatus* and *P. notoginseng* (Supplementary Figs. 20 - 21). Together, these features suggest that biased fractionation, together with broad-scale chromosomal rearrangements have resulted in extensive diversification of genome structure in extant *Panax* species.

Association between core-eudicot genome repatterning and chromatin topology The evolutionary rearrangement of chromosomes and genome content can profoundly affect chromatin topologies. Evidence from cotton and other plant species confirmed that polyploidization reshapes the chromatin topology of newly formed polyploid genomes. However, it is largely unknown how the reshuffling of the ancestral core-eudicot genome affected the remodeling of chromatin topology in extant eudicot genomes. Based on the above described paleo-genomic framework, we investigated whether the chromatin topology observed in the extant *P. stipuleanatus* genome was associated with the evolutionary history of the ancestral core-eudicot genome. We assume that, if all the duplicated ancestral core-eudicot chromosomes were fully preserved, the 42 homologous genomic regions in extant *Panax* genomes would have maintained similar chromatin topologies. However, our inference of the ancestral core-eudicot karyotype evolution revealed considerable DNA-based genomic structural variation in the extant *Panax* species. Therefore, we wondered whether the chromatin topologies of duplicated ancestral chromosomes were randomly reestablished in the extant *P. stipuleanatus* genome. To this end, we studied the 3D genome architecture of *P. stipuleanatus* at the chromosome level. Genome-wide comparisons of chromatin interactions at 100 Kb resolution identified 12 interaction blocks corresponding to the *Panax* chromosomes (Supple-mentary Fig. 22a). This observed higher level of intrachromosomal interactions compared to interchromosomal interactions (*t*-test, $P<0.01$) indicates remodeling of chromatin topology in the *Panax* genome during the polyploidization/(re)diploidization processes.

To further examine this phenomenon, we compared the chromatin topologies between the homologous genomic regions derived from γ and Pg-β based on the same interaction matrix. Our analyses revealed that the post-Pg-β chromosome pairs (Ar1a - Ar8a and Ar1b - Ar8b in Fig. 1) showed no significantly higher values of the chromosomal interaction (estimated by the log2-normalized frequencies of the valid read pairs among the different genomic regions) compared to the other duplicated chromosomes (*t*-test, $P=0.45$). For example, the overall chromatin interaction between the chromosomes Chr2 (Ar3a) and Chr6 (Ar3b) (from −7.083 to −8.808) was similar to the other inter-chromosomal comparisons (i.e., Chr2 vs. Chr3 (Ar4a) and Chr6 vs. Chr3) (from −7.236 to −9.051) (Supplementary Fig. 22b). Similarly, most of the eight post-Pg-β chromosome pairs also differ in the activated (A)/ inactivated (B) chromatin compartments (Supplementary Figs. 23 - 25 and Supplementary Data 5). This trend was more evident in the distribution pattern of submegabase topologically associating domain-like (TAD-like) structures, where the total number and length of TAD-like structures varied dramatically between the post-Pg-β chromosome pairs (Fig. 2b, Supplementary Figs. 26 - 28 and Supplementary Data 6). Nevertheless, the epigenetic modification patterns of TAD-like structures were broadly consistent with previous observations, with the TAD-like regions showing hyper-methylation at cytosine sites and lower levels of gene expression compared to the border regions (Supplementary Fig. 29). These features indicate that chromatin topology remodeling of the duplicated ancestral core-eudicot chromosomes has further increased the 3-D genome diversity of the extant *Panax* species.

It is notable that the degree of intrachromosomal interaction was broadly consistent with the reorganization patterns inferred from comparison to the ancestral core-eudicot chromosomes (Eu1 - Eu7) (Fig. 3a, b and Supplementary Figs. 23 - 25). A general pattern was that chromatin interactions between the homologous genomic regions derived from the same ancestral core-eudicot chromosome were stronger than those between genomic regions from different ancestral chromosomes. For example, both the extant *P. stipuleanatus* chromosomes 2 and 6 are homologous to the post-γ ancestral chromosomes B2 (purple frame) and C6b (blue frame) (Fig. 3b). Levels of the chromatin interaction within the two segments were significantly stronger compared to those between the two segments and the other genomic regions (*t*-test, $P<0.01$). In line with this, we also observed that the A/B compartment switching genomic regions broadly overlapped with ancestral chromosome fusion/fission sites (Fig. 3a, b and Supplementary Figs. 23 - 25). Nevertheless, we did not find a similar correlation between the TAD-like structure and the ancestral core-eudicot karyotype (Fig. 3c), possibly due to localized regional DNA sequence divergence. Together, these results suggest that while the chromatin topologies (compartment A/B and TAD-like) of duplicated ancestral core-eudicot chromosomes were reestablished in extant ginseng genome, their intrachromosomal interactions have been largely maintained during the polyploidization/(re) diploidization processes.

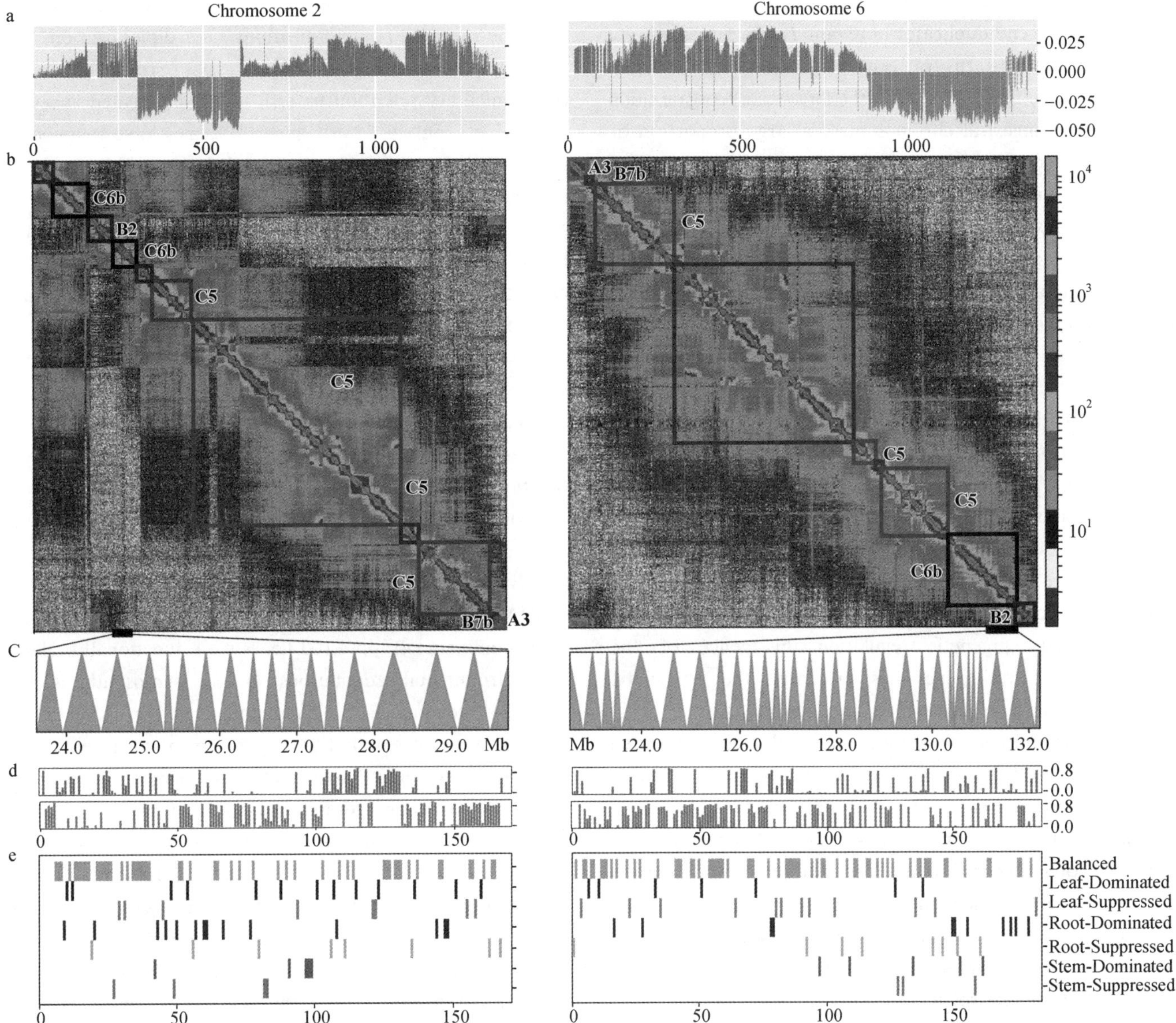


**Fig. 3 Three-dimensional (3-D) genome architecture, cytosine methylation and gene expression patterns in extant *Panax stipuleanatus* genome**

(a) Activated A (red) and inactivated B (blue) compartments at 100 Kb resolution on extant *Panax* chromosomes 2 and 6. The two chromosomes were duplicated through the Pg-β duplication event. *X*- and *Y*-axis are the numbers of 100 Kb sliding bins and PCA eigenvectors of A/B compartments, respectively. Coordinates from left to right on chromosome 2 mirrored those on chromosome 6. (b) Heatmap of the chromatin interaction map at 100 Kb resolution. The color scheme on the right indicates the levels of chromatin interaction between the 100 Kb sliding bins. Colored boxes within the heatmap represent the ancestral core-eudicot chromosomes. Colors and names of these ancestral core-eudicot chromosomes are the same as in Fig. 1. The gray color box represents the homologous genomic region that was lost in extant grape genome. (c) Distribution pattern of topological association domain-like (TAD-like) structures on the post-γ segment C6b. The C6b segment on extant chromosomes 2 and 6 were duplicated by Pg-β. The *x*-axis indicates the physical position on extant *P. stipuleanatus* chromosomes. Each triangular shape represents a TAD-like structure. (d) Cytosine methylation of the duplicated ancestral core-eudicot genes on the two homologous segments C6b derived from Pg-β. Red and blue lines are, respectively, singletons and retained duplicates in the two segments C6b. *X*- and *Y*-axis denote the number of ancestral genes and methylation level, respectively. e Expression patterns of the duplicated ancestral core-eudicot genes in the two segments C6b. *X*-axis is the number of ancestral core-eudicot genes. Colors of these expressed genes indicate the seven expression patterns. Source data are provided as a Source Data file.

**Epigenetic regulation divergence of the duplicated ancestral genes** Reorganization of the ancestral core-eudicot chromosomes resulted in a nested pattern of duplicated genes and genomic regions and an altered chromatin topology. We then examined whether this repatterning of the ancestral core-eudicot genome has also promoted epigenetic regulation divergence of gene duplicates in extant *Panax* genomes. By comparing the patterns of gene expression and cytosine methylation, we found that, after the large-scale reorganization of duplicated ancestral chromosomes, a large proportion of the retained gene duplicates showed tissue-biased expression (39.7% of the total) (Supplementary Data 7) and differential cytosine methylation (21.1%) (Supplementary Data 1). Taking the Pg-β duplicate segment C6b as an example, the above comparisons revealed remodeling of the chromatin topologies of the two homologous regions in the extant *Panax* genome (see Fig. 3a-c). Here, our biased fractionation analyses further confirmed that only 69 (24.7% of the total) Pg-β-derived genes retained both duplicate pairs (Supplementary Data 7). In contrast, 98 (35.1%) and 112 (40.1%) ancestral genes evolved back to singleton status (i.e., lost their duplicate again) on each of the two C6b duplicated segments. Both the singleton genes as well as the retained duplicates differed in patterns of gene expression and cytosine methylation (Fig. 3d, e), which indicates that epigenetic regulation divergence of the duplicated ancestral genes has promoted the epigenetic regulation divergence of extant *Panax* species.

We next addressed how these ancestral genes duplicated by distinct WGDs interact in the highly plastic *Panax* genome. Our analyses of the gene co-expression network revealed that the retained genes derived from the seven ancestral core-eudicot chromosomes exhibited similar degrees of functional connection in extant *Panax* genomes (Supplementary Fig. 30 and Supplementary Table 6). In the leaf tissue, for example, while the total numbers of genes identified in the leaf-related regulatory module varied among the seven ancestral core-eudicot chromosomes (from 217 to 388), functionally important genes showed nearly equal contributions to the leaf development processes ($t$-test, all $P$ values $> 0.01$), i.e., photosynthesis, kinase and synthase (Fig. 4a, Supplementary Fig. 30 and Supplementary Table 7). A similar phenomenon was also observed in the overall epigenetic regulation dynamics, where the duplicated ancestral core-eudicot chromosomes did not show dramatic changes in patterns of gene expression and cytosine methylation in extant *Panax* genomes (Fig. 4b, c and Supplementary Fig. 31).

The above observations indicate that while the genomic regions duplicated from the same ancestral core-eudicot chromosome (Eu1 - Eu7) showed dramatic biased genetic fractionation and divergence in epigenetic regulation, genes retained on each of the duplicated genomic regions had similar functional contributions to the tissue development of extant *Panax* species. We then examined whether the genes retained within these duplicated ancestral core-eudicot chromosomes were involved in similar molecular functions after the repeated polyploidizations/(re) diploidizations. As expected, biased fractionation has resulted in a complementary retention pattern of the duplicated ancestral genes, i.e., only 6.7% of ancestral genes have retained all copies of their duplicates (see in Supplementary Data 1). In particular, the retained genes on each of the duplicated ancestral core-eudicot chromosome are involved in similar KEGG pathways, i.e., 62.6 - 78.6% of the KEGG pathways shared in more than half (>3) of the duplicated ancestral chromosomes (Supplementary Fig. 32). Likewise, the majority of the balanced-expression genes also shared similar molecular functions among the duplicated ancestral core-eudicot chromosomes (Supplementary Fig. 33). In contrast, tissue-dominant orsuppressed genes showed functional divergence among the duplicated ancestral core-eudicot chromosomes. This phenomenon is associated with gene functions, where balanced-expression genes were mainly enriched in basic cellular activities (i.e., TCA cycle, mRNA surveillance and ubiquitin mediated proteolysis), but tissue-dominant orsuppressed genes were functionally related to environmental adaptations (i.e., photosynthesis and nitrogen metabolism) (Supplementary Fig. 34). These observations suggest that the complementary retention of gene duplicates may have - at least partly - dealt with functional redundancy in extant *Panax* species.

It is notable that the regulatory non-coding RNAs (lncRNAs and small RNAs) exhibited relatively higher expression divergence than protein-coding genes among the duplicated ancestral core-eudicot chromosomes (Fig. 4d and Supplementary Fig. 35). Non-coding RNAs are RNA molecules transcribed from the genome but not translated into proteins. Both the lncRNAs and small RNAs play crucial regulatory roles in a variety of biological processes by modulating gene expression at the transcriptional and post-transcriptional levels. Here, the observed high expression divergence of non-coding RNAs suggest that DNA-based structural reorganization may have impacted birth-death (expressed-silent) of these RNA molecules among the duplicated ancestral core-eudicot chromosomes. Together, our findings suggest that, while the evolutionary dynamics of individual ancestral genes varied dramatically at both genetic and epigenetic levels, overall patterns of the molecular function and epigenetic regulation remained relatively stable among the duplicated eudicot ancestral core-eudicot chromosomes in extant *Panax* species.

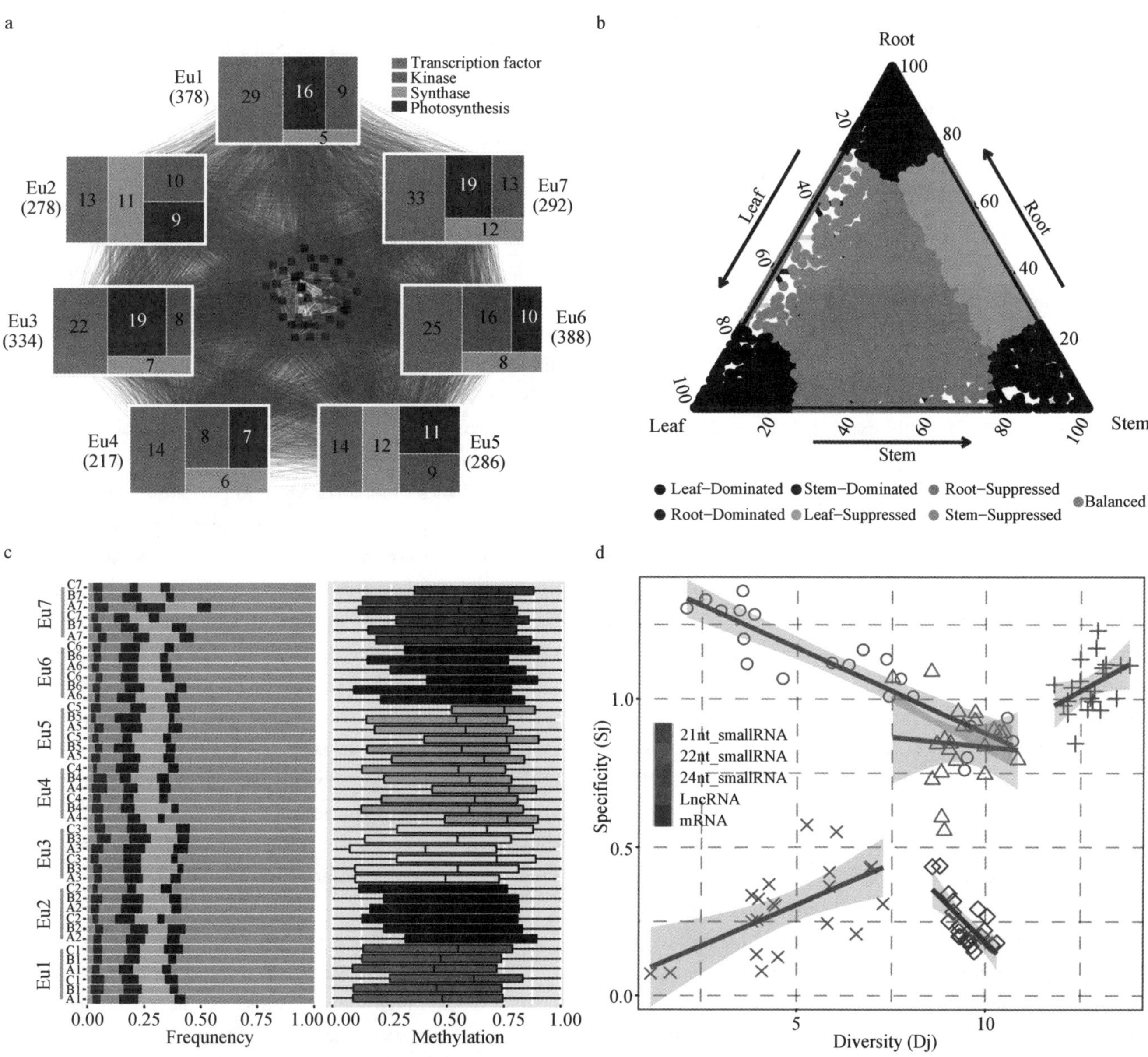


**Fig. 4 Evolutionary dynamics of the ancestral core-eudicot genes in extant *Panax stipuleanatus* genome**

(a) Co-expression network of the ancestral core-eudicot genes involved in the leaf development in extant *P. stipuleanatus* species. Eight gene clusters were defined according to their originations. Eul - Eu7 are the seven ancestral core-eudicot chromosomes. Numbers below each ancestral chromosome (Eul - Eu7) are the total identified ancestral genes. Gray dots in the middle are the ancestral genes that cannot be unassigned to the seven ancestral chromosomes. Gray lines indicate the ancestral gene interaction. Colors and numbers represented the functions and numbers of ancestral genes involved in the leaf development. (b) Ternary plot of expression patterns of ancestral genes in extant *P. stipuleanatus* genome. Each circle is a triad showing relative expression abundance in leaf, root and stem tissues for each ancestral gene. Triads in vertices correspond to the three tissue-dominant expression categories, whereas triads close to edges and between vertices correspond to three tissue-suppressed expression categories. Balanced triads are shown in gray. (c) Percentage of triads in each category of the ancestral genes (left) and boxplot of cytosine methylation for the ancestral genes (right). The 42 bars from top to bottom represent the duplicated ancestral core-eudicot chromosomes (Eul - Eu7). Each ancestral chromosome contains six homologous genomic regions in extant *P. stipuleanatus* genome. Colors of the seven types of genes and names of each ancestral chromosome are the same as in Fig. 1. All ancestral genes identified in the 42 genomic regions were used to the statistical analyses. In right panel, the lower and upper whiskers of each colored box are the lowest (0.00) and highest (1.00) cytosine methylation level, respectively. The black solid lines within each box are media values. Lengths of the boxes are the interquartile range. (d) Expression dynamics of the protein-coding genes and non-coding RNAs of the 42 duplicated ancestral chromosomes in the leaf, root, and stem tissues. *X*- and *Y*-axis are expression diversity (Dj) and specificity (Sj) of the ancestral genes. Each symbol represents an ancestral chromosome. Differences in Dj and Sj values indicate high expression diversity among the ancestral chromosomes and expression specificity among the three tissues. The edges of each shade area are the error bands. Source data are provided as a Source Data file.

Evolutionary contributions of the duplicated ancestral core-eudicot genes to metabolomic diversity The evolutionary role of paleo-polyploidization in genome evolution and phenotypic diversification of angiosperms has long been of interest. Our comparative analyses revealed that the repeated poly-ploidization/(re)diploidization processes have resulted in high dynamics of genome structure and epigenetic regulation of extant *Panax* species. Here, we further investigated whether this reshuffling of the ancestral core-eudicot genome has also promoted phenotypic diversification. Our results showed that, while the post-polyploidization genome contraction is observed at both the chromosomal and individual gene levels, gene families related to secondary metabolites were significantly expanded in the *Panax* genus and other selected eudicot species, especially those involved in the phenylpropanoid, sesquiterpenoid and triterpenoid biosynthesis pathways (Supplementary Figs. 36 - 38). Plant secondary metabolites are low molecular weight organic compounds, which not only function as signal molecules to regulate plant growth and development, but also mediate interactions with various biotic and abiotic stresses. In eudicots, the majority of secondary metabolites, such as terpenoids, steroids and cyanogenic glycoside, are catalyzed by the cytochrome P450 (CYP) superfamily. We explored the evolutionary roles of polyploidization-derived CYPs in the diversification of plant secondary metabolites.

As the largest family of enzymes in plant metabolism, all CYPs in angiosperms were derived from 11 ancestral genes with variable patterns of post-polyploidy retention and additional duplication. Here, we identified candidate genes of nine major *Arabidopsis* CYP clades in *Panax* and other representative eudicot species (Supplementary Fig. 39). As expected, these extant core-eudicot species possessed distinct copy numbers of the nine CYP clades (Supplementary Fig. 39). In the ginseng genus, for example, highly variable copy numbers of the CYPs among the WGD-derived genomic regions (i.e., post-Pg-β chr2 and chr6) are possibly due to the independent retention of duplicated CYPs during the polyploidization/(re)diploidization processes (Supplementary Fig. 40 and Supplementary Data 8). At the epigenetic regulation level, compared to the total number of genes that showed hypermethylation [mean: 57.1% (95% CI: 49.6%-50.1%)] and balanced expression (60.3%) (Supplementary Data 7), the CYPs were preferentially hypomethylated [mean: 24.0% (95% CI: 20.1%-27.9%)] and exhibited tissue-biased expression (79.3%) (Supplementary Data 9), which suggests that biased genetic fractionation and divergent epigenetic regulation of the duplicated CYPs may have promoted the diversification of secondary metabolites in extant *Panax* species.

We next focused specifically on the ginsenosides, which are the major triterpene saponin and found almost exclusively in *Panax* species. Triterpene saponins are one of the largest and most structurally diverse plant-specialized metabolites, which play important roles in, for example, plant antifungal and antibacterial activities. In eudicots, the subfamily CYP716 (belonging to CYP85 clade) is a major contributor to the diversification of triterpenoid biosynthesis. Through analyzing the paleo-polyploidization history of the CYP716 subfamily, our results showed that the ginseng genus contained five (A, D, E, S, and Y) CYP716 subgroups, with the A and Y subgroups preserving both ancestral duplicates (Fig. 5a and Supplementary Fig. 41). The five CYP716 subgroups not only neofunctionalized for oxidation and hydroxylation at different carbon positions (Fig. 5a), but also showed expression-level subfunctionalization in leaf and root tissues (Fig. 5b). More importantly, neofunctionalization and expression-level subfunctionalization of the lineage-specific protopanaxadiol synthase (Y-subgroup) and protopanaxatriol synthase (S-subgroup) genes, together with the eudicot-common oleanolic acid synthase gene (A-subgroup) and other key genes (i.e., UGTs) of the ginsenoside biosynthesis, have facilitated the evolution of the immense diversity in structure and function of ginsenosides in *Panax* genus. Our metabolic analyses further confirmed that both dammarane-type (synthesized by S and Y subgroups) and oleanane-type (synthesized by A subgroup) ginsenosides showed different concentrations in leaf and root tissues (Fig. 5c and Supplementary Figs. 42 and 43).

## 2 DISCUSSION

Polyploidy is a universal phenomenon in the evolutionary history of all angiosperm plants. Studies from across the entire phylogenetic spectrum of angiosperms have clearly illustrated the critical roles of polyploidization in genome evolution and species diversification. Genome collinearity analyses have also confirmed that reshuffling of ancestral genome blocks following polyploidy resulted in great diversity of genome architecture in extant plant species. In this study, focusing on the genus *Panax*, our comparative analyses revealed that while the ancestral core-eudicot genome has experienced three rounds of WGDs ($\gamma$, Pg-β and Pg-α), all these duplicated ancestral core-eudicot chromosomes (Eu1 - Eu7) are still preserved—at least to some extent—in extant *Panax* species. In particular, *Panax* species possess a relatively more conserved ancestral core-eudicot genome relative to some other extant eudicots, such as carrot and lettuce, although each of these extant species experienced additional paleo-polyploidization events after the $\gamma$ hexaploidy event.

Using this paleo-genomic framework, we further examined whether this reshuffling of the ancestral core-eudicot genome

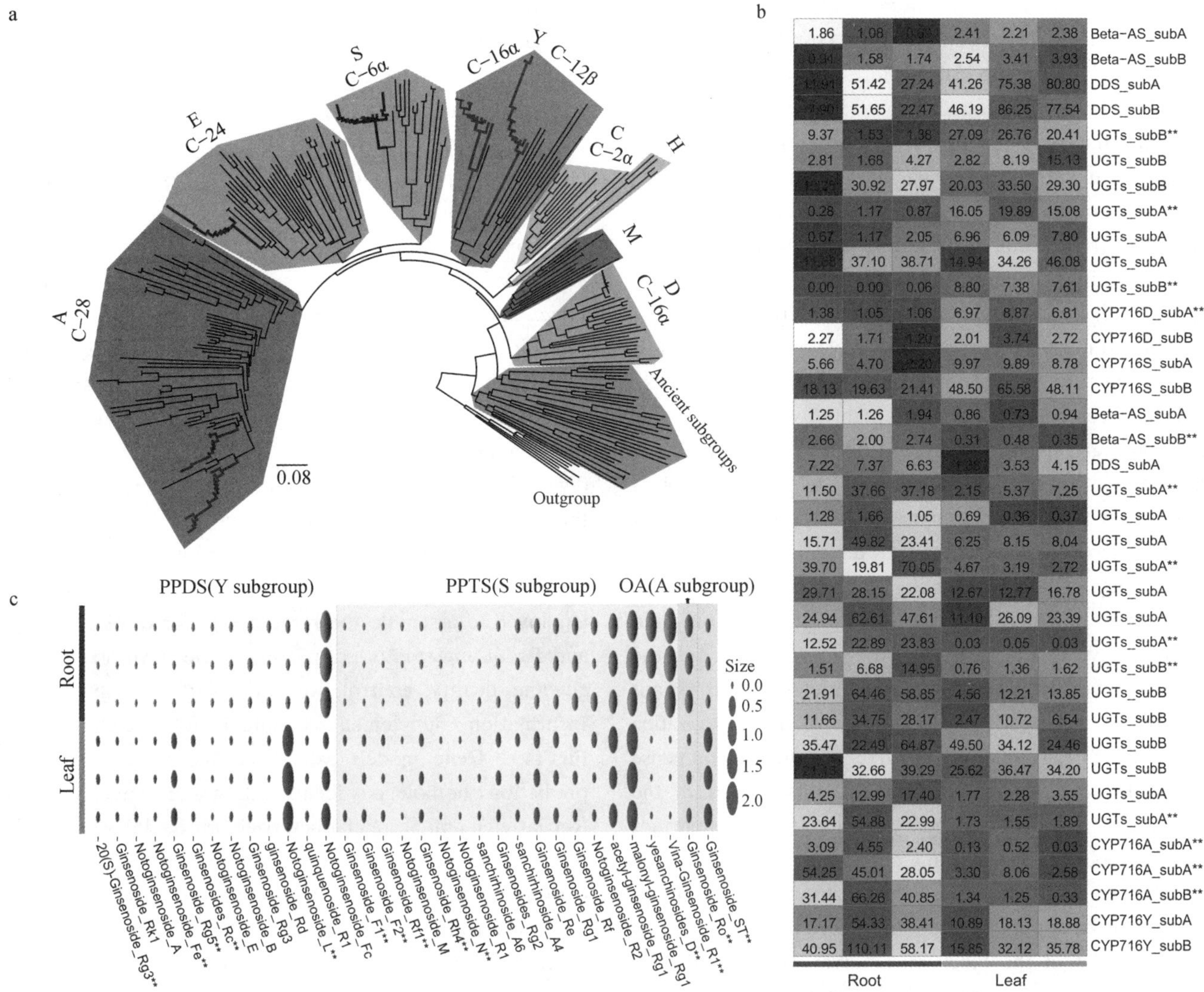


**Fig. 5 Functional diversification of the CYP716 subfamily and triterpenoid biosynthesis genes**

(a) Functional divergence of the subgroups in CYP716 subfamily. Each colored clade represents a subgroup that was derived from an ancestral CYP716 gene during polyploidization/diploidization processes. Branches marked with red color are *Panax* species. Oxidation and hydroxylation of the carbon positions are shown for each clade. (b) Expression divergence of the triterpenoid biosynthesis genes in root and leaf tissues. Numbers in the heatmap are the normalized gene expression levels based on transcriptome data. Name of each gene is shown on the right. The five subgroups of CYP716 were derived from paleo-polyploidizations. The "subA" and "subB" originated by Pg-α. The other major genes involved in triterpenoid biosynthesis in ginseng species are also shown in the heatmap. (c) Metabolic analyses of the triterpenoid biosynthesis in ginseng root and leaf tissues. Name of each ginsenoside is shown at the bottom. Red, green and purple colors indicate the two dammarane and one oleanane type ginsenosides, respectively. The ginsenoside ST marked with gray color is unknown. **, indicates significant difference (Wald test) between the root and leaf tissues. Exact *P* values of these comparisons are shown in the Source Data file.

has caused remodeling of chromatin topology in extant *Panax* genomes. Compared to neo-polyploid species, i.e., cotton and wheat, recent polyploidization has reshaped the chromatin topologies between the subgenomes at a smallscale level. Our comparisons showed that chromatin topologies (A/B compartment and TAD-like structure) of the duplicated ancestral core-eudicot chro-mosomes (Eu1 - Eu7) were extensively remodeled in extant *Panax* species. Of special significance, we show that while all seven ancestral core-eudicot chromosomes underwent substantial changes in DNA-based genome structure, chromatin interactions within the same ancestral chromosome have been largely maintained in extant ginseng genomes after the cyclic polyploidization-diploidization processes. These findings provide a paleo-polyploidization perspective of how reshuffling of the ancestral core-eudicot genome has defined the reestablishment of chromatin topology in derived extant eudicot species.

Genome contraction after polyploidization is a common phenomenon at both the chromosomal and individual gene level. Evidence from diverse neo-polyploid species and experimental aneuploid lines have illustrated that gene dosage balance and divergence in molecular function or gene expression have determined the post-polyploidization retention of the gene duplicates. Here, we show that biased genetic fractionation, together with divergent epigenetic regulation, likely played important roles in reshaping the duplicated ancestral core-eudicot chromosomes during polyploidization and (re)diploidizations. In particular, although the reshuffling of the ancestral core-eudicot genome has resulted in genome structure diversity and epigenetic regulation divergence, genomic regions derived from the seven ancestral chromosomes likely have similar functional contributions to tissue development of extant *Panax* species.

It has been proposed that the highly dynamic nature of the genome architecture has acted as a key factor in the diversification of polyploid species. We here showcase plant secondary metabolites as examples to illustrate the important roles of paleo-polyploidization/(re) diploidization processes in promoting metabolic diversity of extant eudicot plants. Our results revealed that preferential retention and regulation divergence of CYP genes have promoted the qualitative diversification of secondary metabolites in extant *Panax* species. Of significance, neo- and sub-functionalization within the CYP716 subfamily has likely resulted in immense diversity in structure and function of ginsenosides in the *Panax* genus. The plant secondary metabolites are important determinants in regulating plant development as well as the responding to various biotic and abiotic stresses. Our findings suggest that different evolutionary events have played important roles in the biochemical diversity of CYPs and consequently the ecological adaptation of *Panax* species.

## 3 METHODS

Plant materials, DNA and RNA extraction, and karyotype characterization To address the evolutionary reorganization of the ancestral core-eudicot genome in extant *Panax* species, we collected samples of one diploid (*P. stipuleanatus*, $2n = 2x = 24$) and three tetraploid (*P. ginseng*, *P. japonicus* and *P. quinquefolius*, $2n=4x=24$) species (Supplementary Note 1). Genomic DNAs was extracted from fresh mature leaves using the TianGen plant genomic DNA kit (Tianjin, China). Total RNA was extracted from leaf, stem and root tissues using the TianGen plant RNA kit. Genomic DNA and RNA for genome assembly and gene annotation were obtained from the same individual of each species. Total RNAs (mRNA, lncRNA and small RNA) for gene expression comparison were isolated from leaf, stem and root tissue of three individuals for each species using the TianGen plant RNA kit (Tianjin, China). The haploid genome size of the four species was estimated by flow cytometry with three technical replicates. Karyotypes of the four species were visualized using OLYMPUS BX53 (Olympus Corporation, Japan).

Genome sequencing, assembly and gene annotation Three de novo assembly strategies were employed to reconstruct the reference genomes of the four *Panax* species (Supplementary Note 1). Briefly, short insert libraries (350 bp) of *P. stipuleanatus* and *P. japonicus* were constructed by Illumina Novaseq (Tianjin, China) and sequenced using the Illumina Novaseq platform (Illumina, USA). Then, ~20 Kb SMRTbell libraries were generated for each of the two *Panax* species and sequenced on the PacBio RSII platform (PacBio, USA). In addition, DNA fragments longer than 50 kb were used to construct a 10× Gemcode library with a Chromium instrument (10× Genomics) and sequenced using the Illumina Novaseq platform (Illumina, USA). Finally, digested genomic DNA was used to construct Hi-C library for the two species and sequenced using the Illumina Novaseq platform (Illumina, USA). In contrast, two alternative strategies using the Nanopore platform (Nanopore, UK) was employed to assemble the reference genomes of *P. ginseng* and *P. quinquefolius*, respectively. De novo assembly and genome quality control were detailed in Supplementary Information (Supplementary Note 1 and 2; Supplementary Fig. 44). Gene models were predicted based on de novo prediction, homologous identification and Unigene clusters. Repeat elements were characterized using LTR-FINDER and RepeatScout and annotated using RepeatMasker with the parameter "-nolow-no_is-norna-engine wublast".

Ancestral karyotype inference and ancestral gene characterization The ancestral core-eudicot karyotype was constructed by identification of collinear genomic blocks among the *Vitis vinifera* (grape), *Daucus carota* (carrot), *Lactuca sativa* (lettuce) and the four *Panax* species using ColinearScan using a pipeline developed in previous studies. In brief, the grape is the most conserved genome among all extant core-eudicot plants and did not experience additional polyploidization events after its split from the common core-eudicot ancestor. Carrot and lettuce are the most closely related species with assembled reference genomes to *Panax*. Protein sequences and genome annotations of the three selected species were obtained from Phytozome (https://phytozome. jgi. doe. gov/pz/portal. html). Paleo-polyploidization histories of the selected species have been well-documented; all of which have experienced the core-eudicot shared $\gamma$ triplication and followed by additional species-specific duplications/triplications (i.e., Dc-$\alpha$ and Dc-$\beta$). In addition, we inferred the karyotype of the ancestral *Panax* genome by identification of collinear genomic blocks among the four extant *Panax* species. Orthologous genes among the four *Panax* species were determined using the BLAST with an *e* value cutoff of $10^{-5}$. Then, these homologous genes were used to identify collinear genes. The maximal gap length between neighboring genomic blocks was set to 50 genes. Large gene families with >30 members were excluded from the genome collinearity analysis. Putative ancestral core-eudicot genes were defined as those genes shared among at least two subgenomes of the four *Panax* species. Based on the polyploidization history of the four *Panax* species, we defined the top two homologous genes (duplicated by Pg-β) as in-paralogous and the other four homologous genes (duplicated by γ) as out-paralogous, respectively. The order of the ancestral core-eudicot genes on genomic region of *Panax* chromosomes was determined using ColinearScan. Based on the collinear genomic regions, overall genome collinearity was then visualized using WGDI (https://github.com/SunPengChuan/wgdi). In addition, we also calculated the synonymous mutation rate (Ks) between colinear homologous genes using the YN00 program in the PAML (v4.9 h) package with the Nei-Gojobori approach. The median Ks value of each collinear genomic region was applied to infer the polyploidization history. In brief, we used the kernel smoothing density function to generate $K_S$ distribution curve. Then, Gaussian multipeak fitting of the curve was further generated by using the gaussian approximation function in WGDI. Orthologous gene families of the four *Panax* species were identified using OrthoFinder. Then, gene family amplification and contraction analysis were performed using CAFE software with default parameters. Full-length LTR retrotransposons in the *Panax* species were characterized using LTR-harvest and LTR-finder. Insertion time of each LTR retrotransposon family was estimated using the formula: age=K/2r, where K is the Kimura 2-parameter distance and r is the mutation rate of $1.3\times10^{-8}$ for the these *Panax* species.

Chromatin topology and DNA methylation A total of 1,408,300,221,000 bp Hi-C data of the *P. stipuleanatus* (718.5× genome coverage) were obtained from the Illumina Novaseq platform (Illumina, USA). Clean short Illumina reads were mapped to the reference genome using bowtie2 (version 2.2.3). Only uniquely valid read pairs were retained for the subsequent interaction analyses. The Hi-C interaction matrix was constructed according to the pipeline developed by previous study. Briefly, we utilized the ICE method to remove potential Hi-C data bias caused by restriction fragment length, GC content and mapping of reads. Interaction matrices at various resolutions (genome partitioned into bins of different sizes) were constructed using HiC-Pro and visualized by HiC-Explorer. Genome-wide Hi-C resolutions were defined as 100 kb for compartment A/B and 20 kb for TAD-like structure, respectively, based on interaction maps. Identification of activated and inactivated compartment was performed at 100 kb resolution using the matrix2compartment module in Cworld software. In brief, the expected score within the matrix was calculated using lowess smoothed average over the intra-interactions. The eigenvalues of the principal component were plotted to ascribe the bins to two types of compartments. Positive and negative eigenvalues denoted the compartment A and B, respectively. Enrichments of respective genomic compositions and epigenetic markers in each 100 kb bin were summarized and compared in terms of their compartment origins (compartment A/B), and visualized by ggplot2. Topologically associated domain-like structures were identified by the insulation score method at a 20 kb resolution with default parameters. Exact TAD-like structure boundaries and interior regions were specifically framed out using Hidden Markov Model. Then, we converted the real TAD-like structure into a visualized format. Cytosine methylation (5mC) was calculated using Nanopolish. Expression patterns of protein-coding genes were estimated using DESeq2.

Expression patterns of protein-coding genes and small RNAs Clean non-coding RNA reads were mapped onto the reference genomes with HISAT2. In parallel, the short non-coding RNA reads were also assembled by StringTie. The program GffCompare (http://ccb.jhu.edu/software/stringtie/gffcompare.shtml) was used to compare the assembled transcripts to annotated protein-coding genes. Long non-coding RNAs (lncRNAs) were then identified as transcripts >200 nucleotides in length which lack protein-coding potential. Those lncRNAs that were expressed in only one replicate and with TPM<1 were excluded. For the small RNAs, the clean reads were aligned and analyzed with reference genomes using ShortStack (version 3.8.3) with default settings. The identified non-coding RNAs were extracted with customer Perl scripts. The number of total metabolites were estimated for the leaf and root tissues of the four species using non-targeted metabolomics. The overall quantity of the metabolites was estimated and normalized based on the total peak area in the sample. Variable importance in projection (VIP) produced by PLS-DA, ANOVA, and fold change (FC) were applied to discover the contributable variable for classification. Tissue-biased metabolites were defined according to the following parameters, including VIP>1, $P$ value<0.05, and FC≥2 or FC≤0.5.

Total RNAs of three *Panax* species (*P. stipuleanatus*, *P. ginseng*, and *P. quinquefolius*) was extracted from root, stem and leaf tissues using an RNA extraction kit (Tiangen, Beijing, China) based on the manufacturer's instructions. RNA libraries were constructed by Novoseq (Tianjin, China) and sequenced using Illumina Novoseq (Illumina, CA, USA). Clean reads were aligned to the reference genomes using HISAT with default parameters. Raw mapped read counts were calculated using the prepDE. py script provided by StringTie. Differences in transcription level of each gene were estimated using DESeq2. Differentially expressed genes (DEGs) were defined according to the 2-FC differences ($P < 0.05$) at the transcription level between different samples. Functional annotation of the genes was performed based on the KEGG and GO databases. Venn diagram were drawn with Venn Diagram. Expression patterns of the protein-coding genes were estimated according to a previous study. In brief, the relative expression level of a single gene was calculated based on the transcripts per million (TPM) for the three tissues within the triad as follows

$$\text{Expression(Leaf)} = \frac{TPM(Leaf)}{TPM(Leaf) + TPM(Root) + TPM(Stem)} \quad (1)$$

$$\text{Expression(Root)} = \frac{TPM(Root)}{TPM(Leaf) + TPM(Root) + TPM(Stem)} \quad (2)$$

$$\text{Expression(Stem)} = \frac{TPM(Stem)}{TPM(Leaf) + TPM(Root) + TPM(Stem)} \quad (3)$$

where TPM(Leaf), TPM(Root), and TPM(Stem) represent the expression level of each gene in leaf (Eq. 1), root (Eq. 2) and stem (Eq. 3) tissues, respectively. The normalized expression value was calculated for each one of the three tissues and for the average across all expressed tissues. The values of the relative contributions of each tissue per triad were used to plot the ternary diagrams using the R package ggtern.

Cytochrome P450 gene family member identification Orthologs of the CYP 450 superfamily in the ginseng genus and other selected species were identified using BLAST. We downloaded CYP450 members identified in *Arabidopsis* (con-taining 288 members, https://drnelson. uthsc. edu/cytochromeP450. html) and *P. ginseng* (containing 484 members) as references in this analysis. We aligned each species' genome to the references, using blastp (-outfmt 6,-e value $1e^{-5}$, -num_threads 20, -num_alignments 100 and identity $\geqslant 40\%$), and received many potential terms. In addition, we required that the identical amino acid sites accounted for $\geqslant 40\%$ (for Panax species) or $\geqslant 20\%$ (for other species) of the reference gene sequence in each potential term (which will be classified into retained terms), when the CYP450 data set from *P. ginseng* (KPG) was used as reference. Finally, we compared previous terms with potential terms when the CYP450 data set from Arabidopsis was used as reference, and only overlapped terms that met the following requirements (identical amino acid sites accounted for $\geqslant 40\%$ of its own gene sequence and $\geqslant 20\%$ of the Arabidopsis gene sequence in each term) were kept for further analyses.

Reporting summary Further information on research design is available in the Nature Research Reporting Summary linked to this article.

## 4 DATA AVAILABILITY

The raw total sequence reads and four genome assemblies have been deposited into the National Center for Biotechnology Information under the BioProject number PRJNA752920 with BioSample accessions SAMN20855168, SAMN20855173, SAMN20855195 and SAMN20855167. We also deposited the genome assemblies of the four *Panax* to Genome Warehouse in National Genomics Data Center, Chinese Academy of Sciences/China National Center for Bioinformation, under the project number PRJCA006678. Source data are provided with this paper.

[王真慧，刘宝，李霖锋，等. Nature Communications, 2022,13:1902.]

# Transcriptional regulatory network of high-value active ingredients in medicinal plants

High-value active ingredients in medicinal plants have attracted research attention because of their benefits for human health, such as the antimalarial artemisinin, anticardiovascular disease tanshinones, and anticancer Taxol and vinblastine. Here, we review how hormones and environmental factors promote the accumulation of active ingredients, thereby providing a strategy to produce high-value drugs at a low cost. Focusing on major hormone signaling events and environmental factors, we review the transcriptional regulatory network mediating biosynthesis of representative active ingredients. In this network, many transcription factors (TFs) simultaneously control multiple synthase genes; thus, understanding the molecular mechanisms affecting transcriptional regulation of active ingredients will be crucial to developing new breeding possibilities.

## 1 TRANSCRIPTIONAL REGULATORY NETWORKS

Many active ingredients have been isolated and identified from medicinal plants, including terpenoids, alkaloids, saponins, and phenolic acids, which have crucial roles in the development of drugs and promotion of human health (Figure 1). Many environmental responses and specific accumulation of active ingredients in medicinal plants depend on transcriptional regulatory networks of hormone signals. Here, we review the transcriptional regulation of artemisinin, tanshinone, salvianolic acid, Taxol, vinblastine, and ginsenoside biosyntheses, which mainly involve jasmonic acid (JA), abscisic acid (ABA), salicylic acid (SA), gibberellic acid (GA), ethylene (Eth), and indole acetic acid (IAA) signaling.

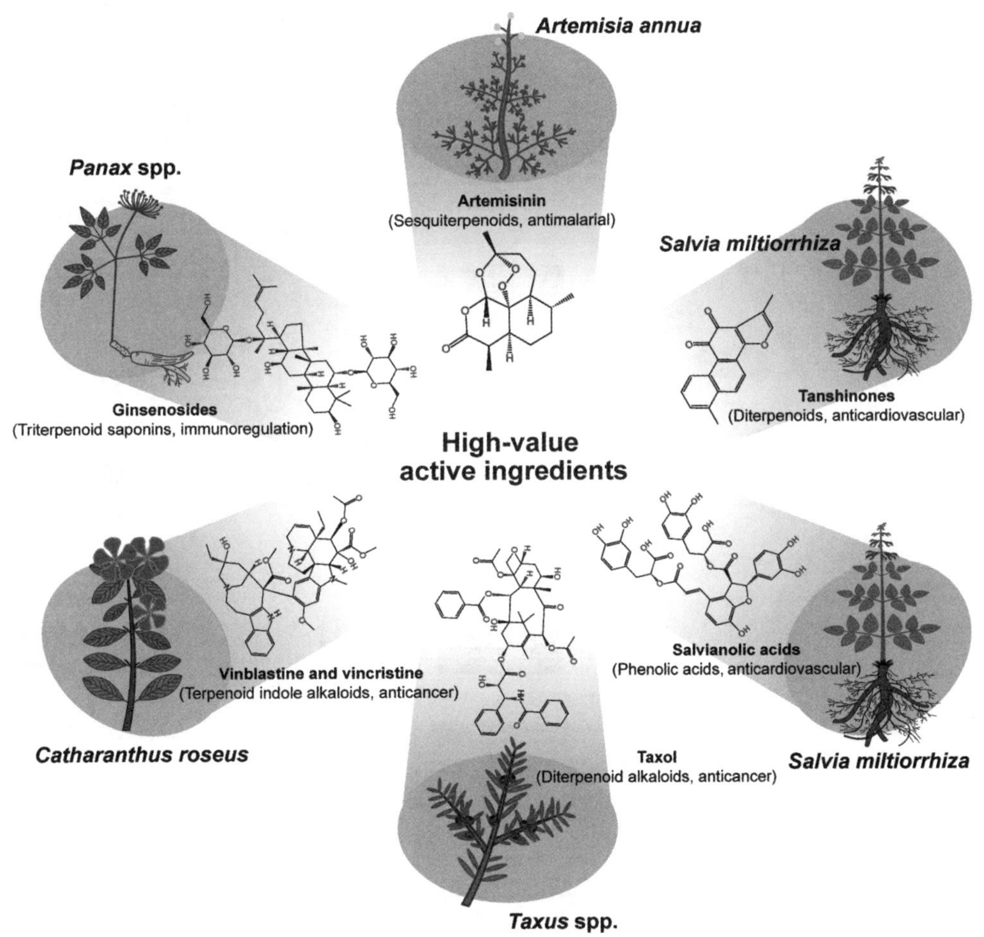


**Figure 1 Main medicinal plants and their active ingredients**

Sesquiterpenes, artemisinin in *Artemisia annua* L.; diterpenoid, tanshinones in *Salvia miltiorrhiza* Bge.; phenolic acid, salvianolic acid B in *S. miltiorrhiza*; diterpenoid alkaloid, Taxol in *Taxus* spp; terpenoid indole alkaloid, vinblastine and vincristine in *Catharanthus roseus* L.; and triterpenoid saponin, ginsenosides in *Panax* spp.

## 2 ANTIMALARIAL SESQUITERPENOID: ARTEMISININ

Artemisinin, a sesquiterpene endoperoxide lactone, is a highly effective antimalarial drug isolated from a traditional Chinese medicinal plant, *Artemisia annua*. However, the artemisinin content of *A. annua* is relatively low, representing 0.1% - 1% of the plant leaf dry weight. Therefore, there is an urgent need to develop a method to increase the artemisinin content in *A. annua* to promote a high-quality, stable, and swift supply of artemisinin.

Transcriptional regulatory network of artemisinin biosynthesis TFs that respond to various hormones and environmental signals have been shown to be regulators in artemisinin biosynthesis, demonstrating the involvement of a complex transcriptional regulatory network (Figure 2), as described below.

Jasmonate-induced artemisinin biosynthesis JA has an important role in the regulation of artemisinin biosynthesis. AaWRKY1, the frst identified methyl jasmonate (MeJA)-induced TF in *A. annua*, regulates artemisinin biosynthesis by binding to the W-box of the *ADS* promoter. JA-responsive AP2/ERF TFs, AaERF1 and AaERF2, bind directly to the CRTDREHVCBF2 (CBF2) and RAV1AAT (RAA) motifs of the *AaADS* and *AaCYP71AV1* promoters to positively regulate their expression. In addition, AaERF1

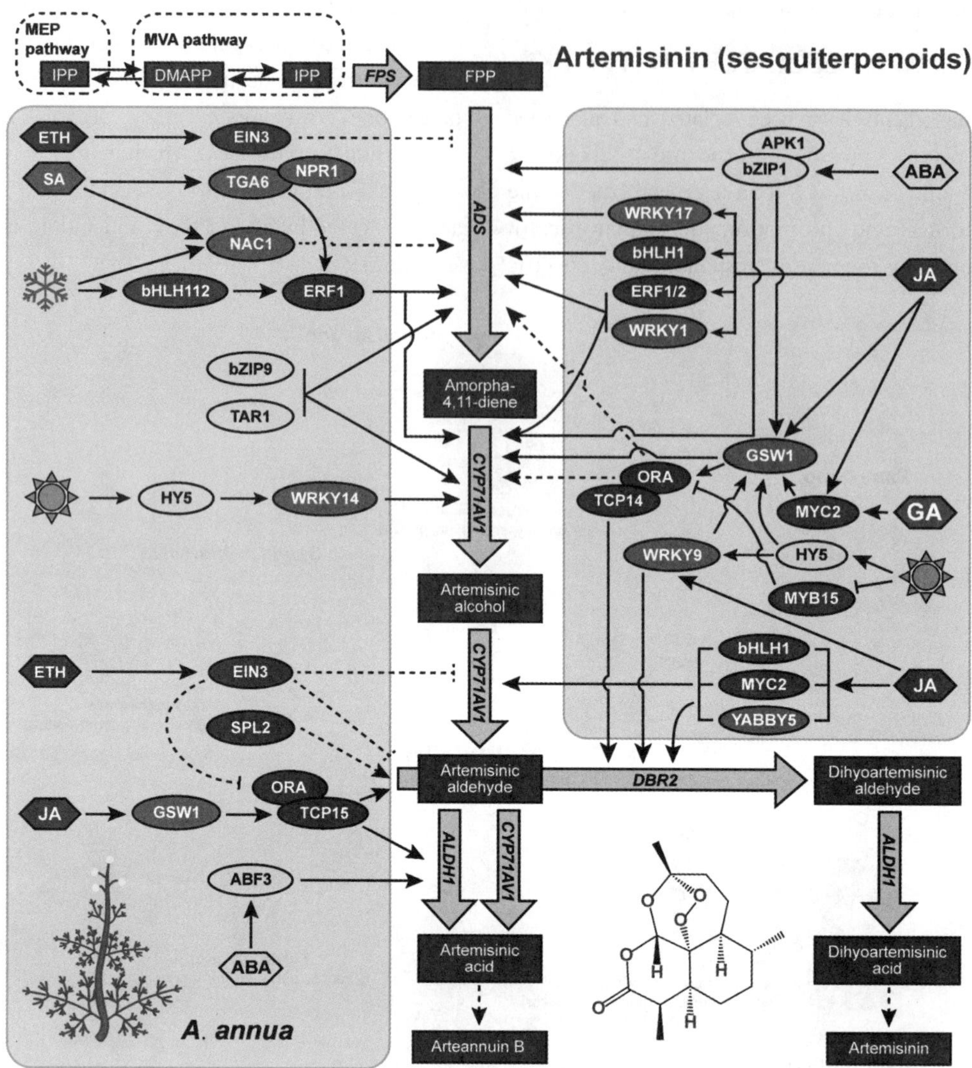


**Figure 2 Transcriptional regulatory network of artemisinin biosynthesis in *Artemisia annua***

The artemisinin-specific biosynthetic pathway starts with a cyclization reaction, in which amorpha-4, 11-diene synthase (ADS) converts FPP into amorpha-4, 11-diene. Cytochrome P450 monooxygenase (CYP71AV1) oxidizes amorpha-4, 11-diene to form artemisinic alcohol, which is further catalyzed into artemisinic aldehyde. This is then converted into dihydroartemisinic acid by artemisinic aldehyde D11 (13) reductase (DBR2), and aldehyde dehydrogenase (ALDH1). Alternatively, CYP71AV1 and ALDH1 catalyze the artemisinic aldehyde to form artemisinic acid. The conversion from dihydroartemisinic acid to artemisinin and artemisinic acid to arteannuin B are also regarded as nonenzymatic photooxidized reactions.

activates expression of defense marker genes, positively regulating resistance to *Botrytis cinerea* in *A. annua*. AaERF3 is also an AP2/ERF TF responding to MeJA. Subsequently, Lu *et al*. reported a trichome-specific TF AaORA as a positive regulator of both artemisinin biosynthesis and resistance to *B. cinerea*. AaTCP14 was identified by Y2H screening for AaORA-interacting proteins, and activates the transcription of both *AaDBR2* and *AaALDH1* by directly binding to the TCP-binding site of their promoters. In addition, AaJAZ8 represses the function of the AaTCP14 - AaORA complex. These findings demonstrate that the AaTCP14 - AaORA complex promotes JA-induced artemisinin biosynthesis. MYC2 TFs are also considered to be involved in JA signaling. In *A. annua*, AaMYC2 promotes artemisinin accumulation by activating the expression of *AaCYP71AV1* and *AaDBR2*. Studies of *A. annua* genomics and transcriptome have opened a new biological era, particularly for transcriptional regulation. For instance, a glandular trichome-specific WRKY protein AaGSW1, which positively regulates the transcript level of *AaCYP71AV1* and *AaORA* to increase artemisinin content, was identified using co-expression analysis. Additionally, AabHLH1, AaYABBY5, and AaWRKY17, induced by MeJA treatment, have been characterized as positive regulators of artemisinin biosynthesis.

These studies demonstrate the research focus on resolving the mechanisms of JA-induction of artemisinin biosynthesis. As a result, WRKY, bHLH, ERF, TCP, and

YABBY TFs were identified to promote artemisinin biosynthesis mediating JA signaling.

Abscisic acid-induced artemisinin biosynthesis ABA regulates many important plant physiological processes, such as seed germination, seedling establishment, and responses to drought, cold, and pathogen stresses. Endogenous ABA treatment increases artemisinin content in *A. annua* by activating artemisinin biosynthetic gene expression. Thus, understanding the mechanism by which ABA regulates artemisinin biosynthesis is important for improving artemisinin accumulation in *A. annua*. In a global expression analysis of bZIP genes, the ABA-responsive factor AabZIP1 was identified as a positive regulator of artemisinin biosynthesis by upregulating *AaADS* and *AaCYP71AV1* expression. Zhong *et al*. identified another ABA-responsive factor, AaABF3, which could activate *AaALDH1* expression through direct bind to the *AaALDH1* promoter, enhancing artemisinin accumulation. Artemisinin content and drought tolerance were markedly increased in transgenic plants overexpressing *AaPYL9*. The ABA-responsive kinase AaAPK1 inhibits phosphorylation of AabZIP1. However, only a few TFs involved in ABA-mediated regulation of artemisinin biosynthesis have been reported.

Light-induced artemisinin biosynthesis Many physiological processes throughout the plant life cycle are strongly influenced by light, including seed germination, hypocotyl growth, anthocyanin accumulation, gravitropism, phototropism, stomatal development, vegetative growth, root development, and flowering. Overexpression of the arabidopsis (*Arabidopsis thaliana*) blue light receptor cryptochrome1 (*AtCRY1*) in *A. annua* significantly increased the artemisinin content. Additional TFs involved in light signaling were identified in *A. annua* after completion of genome sequencing. AaHY5 interacts with AaCOP1 and positively regulates artemisinin biosynthesis by controlling the activity of *AaGSW1*. An R2R3 - MYB, AaMYB15, is induced by both dark conditions and JA. Furthermore, AaMYB15 inhibits artemisinin biosynthesis by directly binding to the *AaORA* promoter. In a recent study, AaWRKY14 was shown to activate *AaCYP71AV1* expression.

Signal crosstalk in regulating artemisinin biosynthesis Previous studies revealed the complexity of the transcriptional regulatory network of artemisinin biosynthesis in *A. annua*, *including* significant crosstalk, such as between light and JA and between JA and ABA. Completion of a high-quality draft of the *A. annua* genome allowed deeper exploration of the mechanisms underlying transcriptional regulation of artemisinin biosynthesis. It was found that JA promotion of artemisinin biosynthesis is light dependent, although the mechanism remained unclear. More recently, transcriptome analysis revealed the glandular trichome-specific AaWRKY9 as a positive regulator of artemisinin accumulation through binding to the W-box element in the *AaDBR2* and *AaGSW1* promoters. Yeast one-hybrid (Y1H) and electrophoretic mobility shift assay (EMSA) analyses showed that AaHY5 activated expression of *AaWRKY9*. AaWRKY9 also interacts with AaJAZ9, and AaJAZ9 suppresses transcriptional activation of AaWRKY9. These results indicate that AaWRKY9 mediates light- and JA-induced upregulation of artemisinin biosynthesis in *A. annua*. A recent study showed that a dual JA- and ABA-responsive TF, AaTCP15, interacts with the positive regulator AaORA and directly increases the expression of *AaDBR2* and *AaALDH1* by binding to their promoters. Overexpression of *AaTCP15* increased artemisinin production. Y1H and EMSA analyses indicated that the dual JA- and ABA-responsive protein AaGSW1 bound to the promoter and activated expression of *AaTCP15*. The interaction between these two signaling pathways indicates a complex and layered transcriptional regulatory network governing artemisinin biosynthesis, and a complex relationship between specialized metabolism and biotic/abiotic signaling.

TFs involved in other signaling pathways, such as SA, Eth, and cold stress, are also reported to regulate artemisinin biosynthesis. The SA-responsive TF AaNAC1 upregulates artemisinin biosynthesis and enhances tolerance to drought and *B. cinerea* in *A. annua*. The SA-induced TF AaTGA6 forms a complex with AaNPR1 and AaTGA3, binding to the *AaERF1* promoter to increase artemisinin biosynthesis. AabHLH112 activates *AaERF1* via promoter binding in response to cold stress. It was previously shown that Eth suppresses the expression of artemisinin synthase genes, and that a key TF in the Eth signaling pathway, AaEIN3, negatively regulates artemisinin biosynthesis by repressing expressions of *AaADS*, *AaCYP71AV1*, *AaDBR2*, and *AaORA*. AaSPL2 and AabZIP9 are also positive regulators of artemisinin biosynthesis. Taken together, these findings reveal the transcriptional regulatory network affecting artemisinin biosynthesis, although further studies are needed to fully understand the components and their relationships.

## 3 ANTICARDIOVASCULAR DISEASE DITERPENOIDS AND PHENOLIC ACIDS: TANSHINONES AND SALVIANOLIC ACIDS

Two main active ingredients are obtained from *Salvia miltiorrhiza*: lipophilic diterpenoid quinones (including tanshinone I, dihydrotanshinone I, cryptotanshinone, and tanshinone IIA) and hydrophilic phenolic acids (e.g., danshensu and salvianolic acid A/B). These two types of ingredient have a synergistic effect in treating cardiovascular disease through anticardiac fibrosis, antithrombotic, antiapoptosis, antioxidant, antiinflammation, platelet aggregation inhibitory, angiogenesis inhibi-tory, and vasoprotective effects.

Transcriptional regulation of tanshinone and salvianolic acid biosyntheses Importantly, TFs can regulate the accumulation of active ingredients by acting at multiple steps throughout biosynthetic pathways. Over the past few decades, TFs belonging to multiple families [e. g., MYB, bHLH, MYC, ERF, WRKY, NAC, bZIP, GRAS, and Squamosa promotor binding protein-like (SPL)] have been reported to mediate tanshinone and salvianolic acid biosynthesis regulation in response to hormone signaling (Figure 3).

JA-induced tanshinone and salvianolic acid biosyntheses

MYB TFs have critical roles in a variety of plant processes. MYB proteins are the most common TFs involved in tanshinone and salvianolic acid biosyntheses. SmMYB111, an R2R3-MYB TF, promotes salvianolic acid accumulation; SmMYB111 interacts with SmTTG1 and SmbHLH51 to form a complex. Expression of *SmMYB111* is significantly downregulated by MeJA, GA, or SA treatment. SmMYB97 mediates JA signaling to positively regulate tanshinone and phenolic acid biosyntheses through interactions with SmJAZ8. The results of Y1H and transient transcriptional activity assays indicated that SmMYB97 could bind to the promoters of *SmPAL1*, *SmTAT1*, *SmCPS1*, and *SmKSL1*. The MeJA-responsive SmMYB1 and SmMYB2 can bind to the promoter of *CYP98A14* and activate its expression.

MYC2 has a pivotal role in the JA signaling pathway. SmMYC2a and SmMYC2b interact with SmJAZ1 and SmJAZ2. Furthermore, they also positively regulate tanshinone and phenolic acid biosyntheses in hairy roots. SmMYC2 activates the expression of *SmTAT1*, *SmPAL1*, and *SmCYP98A14*, leading to an increase in Sal B content, while SmbHLH37 downregulates Sal B biosynthesis in transgenic *S. miltiorrhiza*.

JA-inducible ERF TFs involved in tanshinone and phenolic acid biosyntheses have also been studied. SmERF73 is induced by MeJA, yeast extract (YE), and $Ag^+$, positively regulating tanshinone biosynthesis by directly binding to promoters of *SmDXR1*, *SmCPS1*, *SmKSL1*, and *SmCYP76AH3*. Additionally, SmERF73 interacts synergistically with SmJAZ3 to mediate JA signaling. Furthermore, SmERF73 controls tanshinone biosynthesis in *S. miltiorrhiza*. Moreover, overexpressing *SmERF115* increases the phenolic acid content. Y1H and EMSA assays indicated that SmERF115 directly binds to the *SmRAS1* promoter. Likewise, SmERF1L1 positively regulates tanshinone and phenolic acid biosyntheses by activating the *SmDXR* promoter.

Two WRKY TFs (SmWRKY1 and SmWRKY2) have been identified as positive regulators of tanshinone biosynthesis. *SmWRKY1* expression is induced by MeJA, SA, and nitric oxide (NO), and directly activates the *SmDXR* promoter. *SmWRKY2*, responding only to MeJA, activates both *SmDXS2* and *SmCPS1*, but only binds to the W-box in the *SmCPS1* promoter.

Several negative TFs involved in JA signaling are reported to regulate tanshinone and phenolic acid biosyntheses. Lateral organ boundaries domain (LBD) proteins are TFs in the JA signaling pathway. Lu *et al*. identified SmLBD50 from genome databases of *S. miltiorrhiza*. Overexpressing *SmLBD50* significantly reduced the total phenolic acid and anthocyanin content. In addition, SmLBD50 interacts with SmJAZ1, SmMYB36/97, SmbHLH37, and SmMYC2a/b. Recently, the JA-induced TF SmNAC2 was reported to negatively regulate Tan I and Tan IIA accumulation in *S. miltiorrhiza*, but an increasing content of tanshinone was obtained in *SmNAC2*-RNAi transgenic roots.

ABA-induced tanshinone and salvianolic acid biosyntheses

ABA treatment significantly increases phenolic acid accumulation in *S. miltiorrhiza* hairy roots. The expression of *SmbZIP1* is elevated by ABA treatment. Overexpressing *SmbZIP1* increases the phenolic acid content by upregulating both *SmC4H1* and *SmHPPR* expressions through binding to the *SmC4H1* promotor only. Conversely, phenolic acid production was significantly decreased in *Crispr-SmbZIP1* hairy roots. SPLs have a significant role in plant growth and development. In *S. miltiorrhiza*, the expression of *SmSPL6* and *SmSPL7* is reduced after ABA, IAA, or MeJA treatments. Separately, SmSPL6 is a positive regulator of phenolic acid biosynthesis by directly binding to the promoters of *Sm4CL9* and *SmCYP98A14*, while SmSPL7 inhibits phenolic acid biosynthesis by binding to the *Sm4CL9* and *SmTAT1* promoters. Additionally, ABA-responsive SmSnRK2.6 interacts with SmAREB1 to increase the accumulation of rosmarinic acid (RA) and Sal B. Expression of *SmbHLH148* can be induced at high levels by ABA and moderately induced by MeJA and GA. Overexpressing *SmbHLH148* results in an increase in tanshinone and phenolic acid accumulation in hairy roots through the upregulation of *SmHMGR 1-3*, *SmDXS2*, *SmDXR*, *SmGGPPS*, *SmCPS1*, *SmKSL1*, *SmCYP76AH1*, *SmPAL1*, *SmC4H1*, *SmTAT*, *SmHPPR*, *SmRAS*, and *SmCYP98A14*.

GA-induced tanshinone and salvianolic acid biosyntheses

Exogenous GA promotes tanshinone accumulation in *S. miltiorrhiza* hairy roots. GRAS proteins are plant-specific TFs involved in GA signaling. Suppressing *SmGRAS1* and *SmGRAS2* expression results in decreased tanshinone accumulation and increased levels of GA and phenolic acids. Research has indicated that SmGRAS1 interacts with SmGRAS2 and directly binds the *SmKSL1* promoter. Similarly,

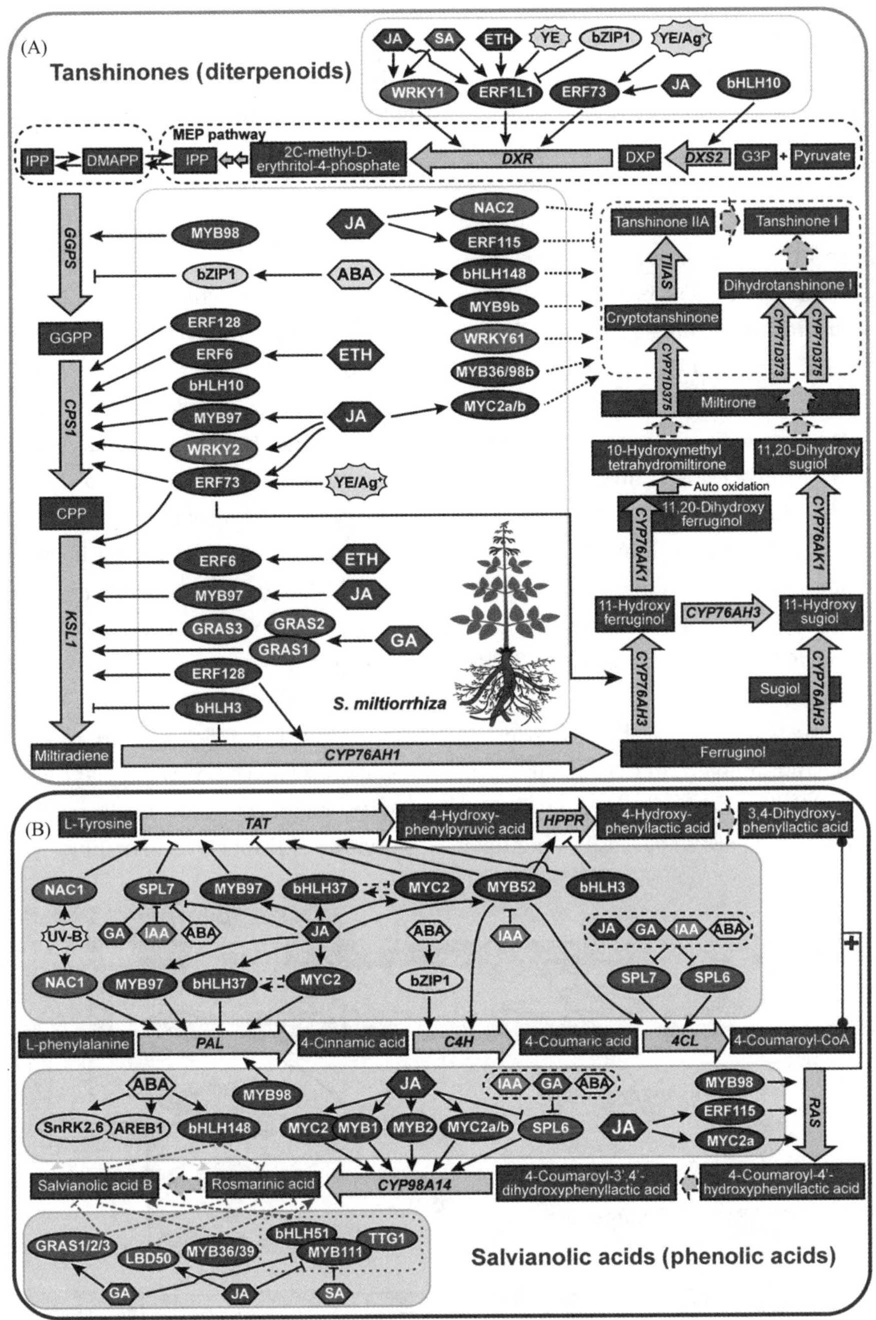


**Figure 3 Transcriptional regulation of tanshinones and phenolic acids biosynthesis in *Salvia miltiorrhiza***

(A) Transcriptional regulation of tanshinone biosynthesis. Tanshinone biosynthesis is initiated by cyclization of (E, E, E)-geranylgeranyl diphosphate (GGPP) into copalyl diphosphate (CPP) by CPP synthase (CPS1) and further cyclization and rearrangement to miltiradiene by kaurene synthase-like (KSL1). CYP76AH1 catalyzes a unique four-electron oxidation cascade on miltiradiene to produce ferruginol. CYP76AH3 oxidizes ferruginol at two different carbon centers to obtain 11-hydroxy ferruginol and 11-hydroxy sugiol. CYP76AK1 hydroxylates the C-20 of two of the resulting intermediates into 11,20-dihydroxy ferruginol and 11, 20-dihydroxy sugiol. CYP71D373 and CYP71D375 catalyze hydroxylation at carbon-16 (C16) and 14,16-ether (hetero)cyclization to form the D-ring. TIIAS acts as a dehydrogenase catalyzing furan ring aromatization and converts cryptotanshinone to tanshinone ⅡA. Notably, *CPS1*, *KSL1*, *CYP76AH1*, and *CYP76AH3* are located in one major tanshinone biosynthetic gene cluster in *S. miltiorrhiza*, which raises questions about how the expression of these disparate genes is coregulated during tanshinone metabolite biosynthesis. (B) Transcriptional regulation of phenolic acid biosynthesis. Phenolic acid biosynthesis is initiated by a tyrosine-derived and phenylpropanoid pathway in *S. miltiorrhiza*. L-Tyrosine is catalyzed by tyrosine aminotransferase (TAT) and 4-hydroxyphenylpyruvate reductase (HPPR) successively into 3, 4-dihydroxyphenyllactic acid. The phenylpropanoid pathway is initiated by the catalytic action of phenylalanine ammonia-lyase (PAL) on phenylalanine, which is then catalyzed by cinnamate 4-hydroxylase (C4H) and p-coumaroyl coenzyme A ligase (4CL) into 4-coumaroyl-CoA. 3, 4-dihydroxyphenyllactic acid and 4-Coumaroyl-CoA are precursors of phenolic acid biosynthesis. These are then catalyzed by rosmarinic acid synthase (RAS) to form 4-coumaroyl-4′-dihydroxyphenyllactic acid and 4-coumaroyl-3′,4′-dihydroxyphenyllactic acid, which are then converted into rosmarinic acid by SmCYP98A14. Finally, salvianolic acid B is formed by an as-yet unresolved multistep reaction.

SmGRAS3 was found to positively regulate tanshinone biosynthesis by activating the *SmKSL1* promoter in *S. miltiorrhiza* hairy roots.

Other factors inducing tanshinone and salvianolic acid biosynthesis In addition, the Eth-responsive TF SmERF6 binds to and activates the *SmKSL1* and *SmCPS1* promoters, and also regulates tanshinone biosynthesis. SmNAC1 mediates upregulation of salvianolic acid biosynthesis under UV-B irradiation through directly binding to the CATGTG and CATGTC motifs of the *SmPAL3* and *SmTAT3* promoters. Low phosphate ion (Pi) conditions induce SmMYB98b to promote tanshinone biosynthesis. SmMYB36, SmMYB9b, SmbHLH10, SmERF128, SmMYB98, and SmWRKY61 are also identified as positive regulators of tanshinone biosynthesis. SmMYB39 and SmbHLH3 inhibit phenolic acid and tanshinone biosyntheses, whereas SmMYB52 promotes Sal B biosynthesis by activating the expression of *SmTAT1*, *Sm4CL9*, *SmC4H1*, and *SmHPPR1* involved in Sal B biosynthetic pathways.

Significant efforts have been made to reveal the mechanisms of regulation controlling tanshinone and phenolic acid biosyntheses. Most of the TFs involved (e.g., *SmMYB111*, *SmbHLH148*, and *SmWRKY1*) are induced by multiple hormones, suggesting the existence of interactions among hormones in regulating secondary metabolism. However, the mechanisms underlying multihormone-mediated regulation of tanshinone and phenolic acid biosyntheses require further exploration.

## 4 ANTICANCER DITERPENOID ALKALOID: TAXOL

Taxol is a complex tetracyclic diterpenoid mainly produced in plants within the *Taxus* genus, including *Taxus chinensis*, *Taxus brevifolia*, *Taxus wallichiana*, *Taxus baccata*, *Taxus cuspidate*, and *Taxus media*. It is a well-known chemotherapy agent that is effective against a variety of cancers. Direct extraction from *Taxus* plants is the primary method of obtaining Taxol.

Transcriptional regulation impacting Taxol biosynthesis Several TFs, including members of the AP2/ERF, WRKY, MYC, and MYB families, have been found to regulate the expression of genes related to Taxol biosynthesis (Figure 4). Phytohormones, such as JA, GA, auxin, ABA, and Eth, are involved in the regulation of Taxol biosynthesis to maintain a balance between plant growth and defense. MYC family members may mediate the regulation of Taxol biosynthesis through JA signaling.

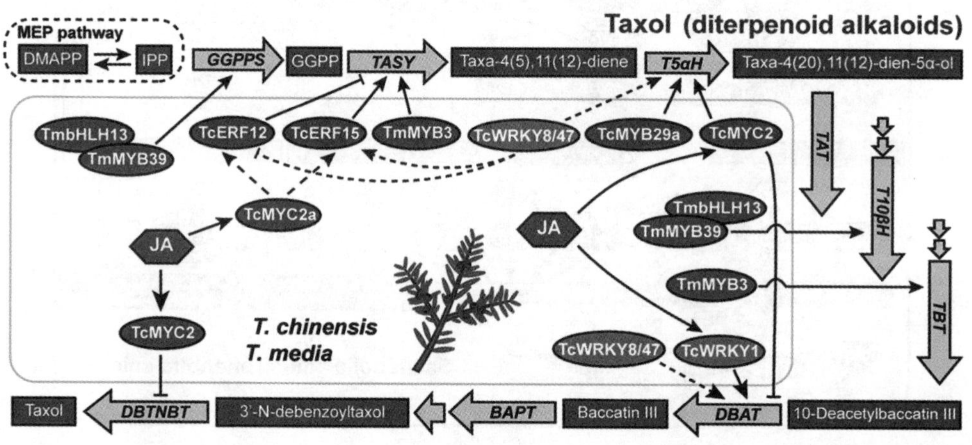


**Figure 4 Transcriptional regulation of taxol biosynthesis in *Taxus chinensis* and *Taxus media*.**

Taxol as a tetracyclic diterpene, featuring 11 chiral centers, is biosynthesized by a complex metabolic pathway. To date, over 20 enzymes have been identified in the Taxol biosynthetic pathway. Taxadiene synthase (TASY) catalyzes (E,E,E)-geranylgeranyl diphosphate (GGPP) to form 10-deacetylbaccatin III (10-DAB). Taxane 5α-hydroxylase (T5αH) catalyzes taxa-4(5),11(12)-diene into taxa-4(5),11(12)-diene-5α-ol. Taxadiene is decorated to baccatin III via catalysis by a series of enzymes, such as taxadienol 5α-*O*-acetyl transferase (TAT), taxane-2α-*O*-benzoyltransferase (TBT), and 10-deacetylbaccatin III-10-*O*-acetyltransferase (DBAT). DBAT catalyzes 30′-N-debenzoyl-20′-deoxytaxol synthesis. 3′-N-debenzoyl-2′-deoxytaxol-N-benzoyltransferase (DBTNBT) is involved in the formation of Taxol.

TcJAMYC1 negatively regulated the promoters of the last three late pathway genes (*TcDBBT*, *TcBAPT*, and *TcDBTNBT*) by the transient overexpression of TcJAMYC2 in *Taxus* cultured cells. TcJAMYC2 represses *TcBAPT* expression, while the promoters of *TcDBAT*, *TcDBBT*, *TcBAPT*, and *TcDBTNBT* are downregulated by TcJAMYC4. TcMYC2a also controls the expression of *TcTASY*, *TcTAT*, *TcDBTNBT*, *TcT13OH*, and *TcT5αH* via ERF regulators in *T. chinensis*. Two AP2/ERF TFs, TcERF12 and TcERF15, function as negative and positive factors, respectively, by binding to the GCC-box in the JA-response element of the *TcTASY* promoter in *T. chinensis*. JAZs can bind with MYCs to inhibit transcriptional activity. Interactions between JAZs and MYCs have also been detected in *T.*

*media*; these interactions inhibit MYC transcriptional activities. The expression levels of 27 AP2/ERF genes are tightly correlated with regulation of Taxol biosynthetic genes in *T. chinensis*. Further phylogenetic and structural analyses of AP2/ERF genes aided the functional characterization of the key AP2/ERF genes related to Taxol biosynthesis. A phytochemical analysis revealed that an R2R3-MYB factor, TmMYB3, increased Taxol biosynthesis by activating transcription of *TmTBT* and *TmTASY* in *T. media*. TcMYB29a, an ABA-responsive R2R3-MYB TF, upregulates Taxol biosynthesis in cell suspension culture of *T. chinensis* by upregulating the expression of *TcTASY*, *TcT5αH*, and *TcDBTNBT*. Subsequently, bimolecular fluorescence complementation (BiFC) and Y2H assays revealed an interaction between TmMYB39 and TmbHLH13, suggesting that TmMYB39 functions in transcriptional regulation of Taxol biosynthesis through a 'MYB - bHLH' module, *trans*-activating *TmGGPPS* and *TmT10OH* expression. The miRNA-mediated *TcMYB* post-transcriptional regulation revealed that 18 TcMYBs were targeted by miR858 miR159 and miR828, providing a basis for identifying key candidate TcMYBs involved in Taxol regulation in *T. chinensis*. A plant-specific WRKY TF, TcWRKY1, enhanced *TcDBAT* expression in *T. chinensis* suspension cells by targeting W-box *cis*-elements. Two other WRKY TFs, TcWRKY8 and TcWRKY47, significantly upregulate *TcDBAT*, *TcT5αH*, and *TcERF15* expression, but downregulate *TcERF12* expression. Interestingly, fermentation broth of the endophytic fungus KL27 - FB isolated from *T. chinensis* effectively enhanced Taxol production in needles by regulating the expression of genes related to the terpene and Taxol biosynthetic pathways. Differentially expressed genes included TFs and genes involved in hormone biosynthesis and signal transduction. Only a few TFs were considered to have important roles in regulating genes in the Taxol biosynthetic pathway. Other factors involved in hormone signaling positively regulate taxol biosynthesis, but the associated regulatory machinery remains unknown.

## 5 ANTICANCER TERPENOID INDOLE ALKALOIDS: VINBLASTINE AND VINCRISTINE

*Catharanthus roseus*, commonly known as one of the most valuable medicinal plants worldwide, produces more than 100 bioactive terpenoid indole alkaloids (TIAs). Vinblastine and vincristine isolated from *C. roseus* are widely used in the clinical treatment of cancers, including breast, liver, and ovarian cancers. Both compounds also have antibacterial, antidiabetic, and diuretic properties.

Transcriptional regulation of vinblastine and vincristine biosyntheses The vinblastine and vincristine biosynthetic pathways in *C. roseus* comprise more than 35 enzymatic steps and are transcriptionally regulated by an intricate system (Figure 5). Two JA-responsive plant-specific AP2/ERF TFs, ORCA2 and ORCA3, were characterized as critical regulators of TIA biosynthesis. Y1H screening showed that ORCA2 has a key role in JA- and elicitor-induced TIA biosynthesis and binds to the GCC-box-like element of the *CrSTR* promoter. Overexpressing *ORCA3* upregulated the expression of *CrDXS*, *CrTDC*, *CrSTR*, *CrCPR*, and *CrAS* in cell suspension cultures, but did not affect *CrG10H* or *CrDAT* expression. EMSA assays indicated that ORCA3 binds the promoters of *CrTDC*, *CrSTR*, and *CrCPR*. However, the transcript levels of TIA biosynthetic genes in cell suspension cultures differ from the results observed in hairy roots. ORCA3 also activates transcription of *CrAS*, *CrDXS*, and *CrSTR*, and inhibits *CrSGD* expression in hairy roots, but upregulating *ORCA3* had no effect on *CrTDC*, *CrG10H*, *CrCPR*, CrGBFs, or *ORCA2* expression. Overexpressing *ORCA2* not only significantly promoted the expression of structural genes (e.g., *CrAS*, *CrTDC*, *CrSTR*, *CrPRX*, *CrSGD*, and *CrDAT*), but also upregulated the expression of several TF genes (e.g., *ORCA3*, *CrZCTs*, and *CrMYC2*) in *C. roseus* hairy roots. Treating *C. roseus* with artemisinic acid or inoculating it with fungal endophytes upregulated *ORCA3* expression and increased vindoline accumulation. Co-expression analysis of ORCA genes showed that ORCA3, ORCA4, and ORCA5 engaged in intracluster regulation. ORCA6 activates the *STR* promoter in tobacco cells. These results demonstrate that ORCAs are crucial in vinblastine and vincristine biosynthesis. Overexpressing *CrERF5* by transient transformation in *C. roseus* strongly activated the expression of TIA biosynthetic genes and increased secologanin, catharanthine, and vinblastine accumulation. An MeJA-induced AP2/ERF CrCR1 was found to negatively regulate vindoline and serpentine biosyntheses. These results demonstrate that JA-induced AP2/ERF TFs are important regulators of TIA biosynthesis.

AtMYC2 binds to the JA-responsive element (JRE) of the ORCA3 promoter and activates its expression in arabidopsis. CrMYC2 also positively regulates *ORCA3* expression via binding to the JRE of the promoter, enhancing catharanthine and tabersonine accumulation. In a protoplast assay, CrMYC2 activated *ORCA6* expression. The bHLH TF BIS1 was also shown to activate the expression of several genes based on co-expression analysis of RNA-sequencing data, which was further proven in *C. roseus* cell culture. The JA-responsive protein BIS2 interacts with BIS1 to activate promoters of the iridoid biosynthesis genes. *BIS2* overexpression in *C. roseus* increased monoterpene indole alkaloid (MIA) production, whereas silencing *BIS2*

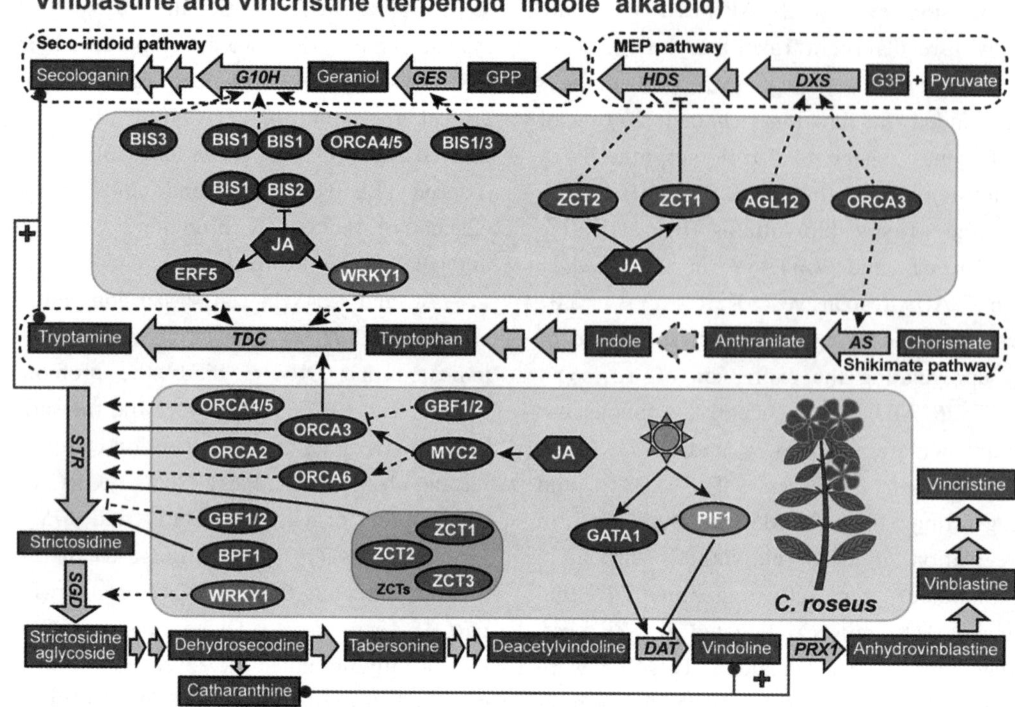


**Figure 5 Transcriptional regulation of terpenoid indole alkaloid (TIA) biosynthesis in *Catharanthus roseus***

The early stage of alkaloid biosynthesis involves the shikimate pathway. The synthesis of chorismate is catalyzed by anthranilate synthase (AS) and tryptophan decarboxylase (TDC). In the secoiridoid pathway, the common precursor secologanin is synthesized from geranyl diphosphate (GPP) through a series of catalytic reactions by geraniol synthase (GES), geraniol 10-hydroxylase (G10H), and so on. All TIAs in *C. roseus* derive from strictosidine, which is produced by the coupling of tryptamine from the indole pathway and secologanin from the iridoid pathway by strictosidine synthase (STR). Strictosidine is converted into strictosidine aglycoside by strictosidine β-glucosidase (SGD). Then, vindoline is synthesized via hydroxylation by tabersonine-16-hydroxylase (T16H) and deacetoxyvindoline4-hydroxylase (D4H), and by acetylation by deacetylvindoline acetyl CoA acetyltransferase (DAT). PRX1 catalyzes the coupling of vindoline and catharanthine to produce the direct precursor of vinblastine and vincristine, anhydrovinblastine. Finally, vinblastine and vincristine are derived from anhydrovinblastine.

decreased MIA accumulation. The JA-induced *BIS3* is clustered on the same genomic scaffold with *BIS1* and *BIS2*. *BIS3* promotes loganic acid biosynthesis by activating the transcription of all iridoid pathway genes and *BIS1* and *BIS2* in flower petals overexpressing *BIS3*.

The MYB-like protein CrBPF1 was identified in Y1H screening with the YE- and JA-responsive gene *CrSTR*. Overexpressing *CrBPF1* upregulated both transcriptional activator and repressor genes, suggesting that CrBPF1 acts as integrating signals to balance TIA biosynthesis in C. *roseus*. The JA-, GA-, and Eth-induced CrWRKY1 activates the expression of several synthase genes, such as *CrAS*, *CrSGD*, and especially *CrTDC*, but represses the expression of the transcriptional activator genes *ORCA2*, *ORCA3*, and *CrMYC2*. Two bZIP TFs, CrGBF1 and CrGBF2, form homo- and heterodimers, and CrGBF dimerization interacts with CrMYC2 to repress transcription of *CrMYC2* and key enzyme genes in the TIA pathway. Three C2H2-type zinc finger proteins (CrZCT1, CrZCT2, and CrZCT3) induced by YE and JA repress the expression of *CrSTR* and *CrTDC* by binding to their promoters, and also inhibit ORCA activities. CrZCT2 binds the *CrHDS* promoter, and CrZCT1 and CrZCT2 (but not CrZCT3) repress *CrHDS* promoter activity.

A Leu-Leu-Met domain GATA TF, CrGATA1, is involved in light signaling and regulates the expression of key vindoline pathway genes in *C. roseus* seedlings. Phytochrome interacting factor (CrPIF1) represses promoter activities of *CrGATA1* and *CrDAT* via binding to the promoter G/E-box region. A root-specific MADS-box TF, Agamous-like 12 (AGL12), selectively increases *CrDXS* and *CrG10H* expression in *C. roseus* suspension cells. Shen *et al*. selected JA-responsive miRNAs using small RNA-sequencing and genome-wide expression analysis, and predicted 519 potential cro-miRNAs targeting auxin response factors (ARFs) through *in silico* target prediction, and demonstrated that CrARF16 represses TIA biosynthesis by auxin-mediated binding and downregulation of key TIA pathway genes.

## 6 IMMUNOMODULATING TRITERPENOID SAPONINS: GINSENOSIDES

Ginsenosides are key active ingredients in *Panax* plants, which are used worldwide as medicinal and functional herbs and show multiple pharmacological effects on nervous system and immune diseases. Ginsenosides comprise both dammarane-type tetracyclic triterpenoid saponins and oleanane-type pentacyclic triterpenoid saponins.

Transcriptional regulation of ginsenoside biosynthesis Due to the diffculty of developing a mature genetic transformation system in *Panax*, few studies have addressed ginsenoside biosynthetic regulation. Such studies have mainly focused on JA-mediated regulatory mechanisms (Figure 6). PgMYB2, a MeJA-responsive TF, specifically binds the MBS II motif of *PgDS*, and may upregulate ginsenoside biosynthesis. *PgLOX6* overexpression upregulated the expression of *PgWRKY1*, *PgWRKY22*, *PgAP2*, *PgDELLA*, *PgERF3*, and

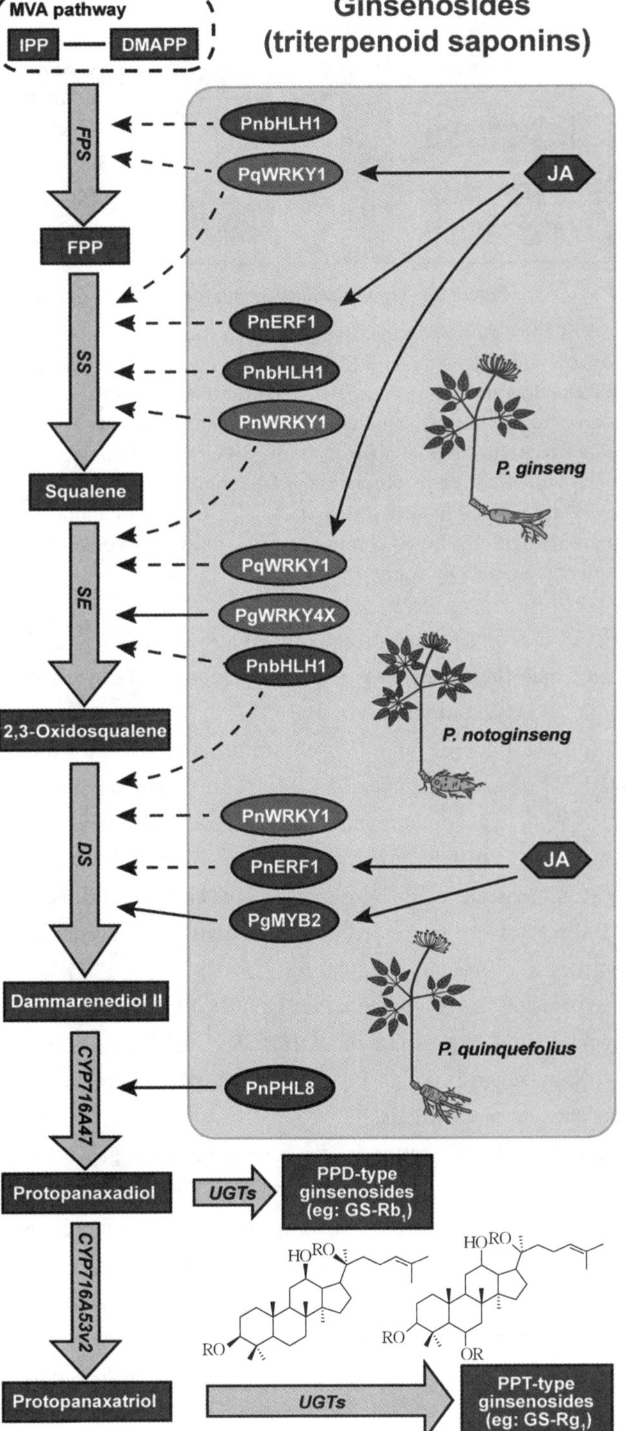


**Figure 6 Transcriptional regulation of ginsenoside biosynthesis**

Ginsenosides are main active ingredients in *Panax* spp, comprising both dammarane-type tetracyclic triterpenoid saponin and oleanane-type pentacyclic triterpenoid saponin. Consistent with most triterpenoids, upstream precursor of ginsenosides are biosynthesized mainly through the mevalonate (MVA) pathway, obtaining isopentenyl pyrophosphate (IPP) and dimethylallyl pyrophosphate (DMAPP), which are converted into 2,3-oxidosqualene by geranyl pyrophosphate synthase (GPS), farnesyl diphosphate synthase (FPS), squalene synthase (SS), and squalene epoxidase (SE), representing the mid-stage of ginsenoside biosynthesis. Oleanane-type ginsenosides represented by ginsenoside Ro are synthesized by β-amyrin synthase (β-AS) followed by CYP716A52v2. Dammarenediol-II synthase (DS) cyclizes 2,3-oxidosqualene into dammarenediol-II, which is then hydroxylated and oxidized by cytochrome P450 monooxygenase (CYP450). CYP716A47 oxidates the C-12 site of dammarenediol-II to produce protopanaxadiol (PPD), while CYP716A53v2 further oxidates the C-6 site of PPD to obtain protopanaxatriol (PPT). Glycosylation catalyzed by UDP-glucosyltransferase (UGT) contributes to the diversity and bioactivity formation of ginsenosides. UGT74AE2, UGT71A27, UGT94Q2, UGTPg29, UGTPg45, PnUGT5, and UGRdGT participate in the formation of PPD-type ginsenosides, represented by ginsenoside $Rb_1$ and ginsenoside Rd, while UGT71A27, UGTPg100, UGTPg101, and PnUGT3 have important roles in conversion into PPT-type ginsenosides, represented by ginsenoside $Rg_1$ and ginsenoside Re.

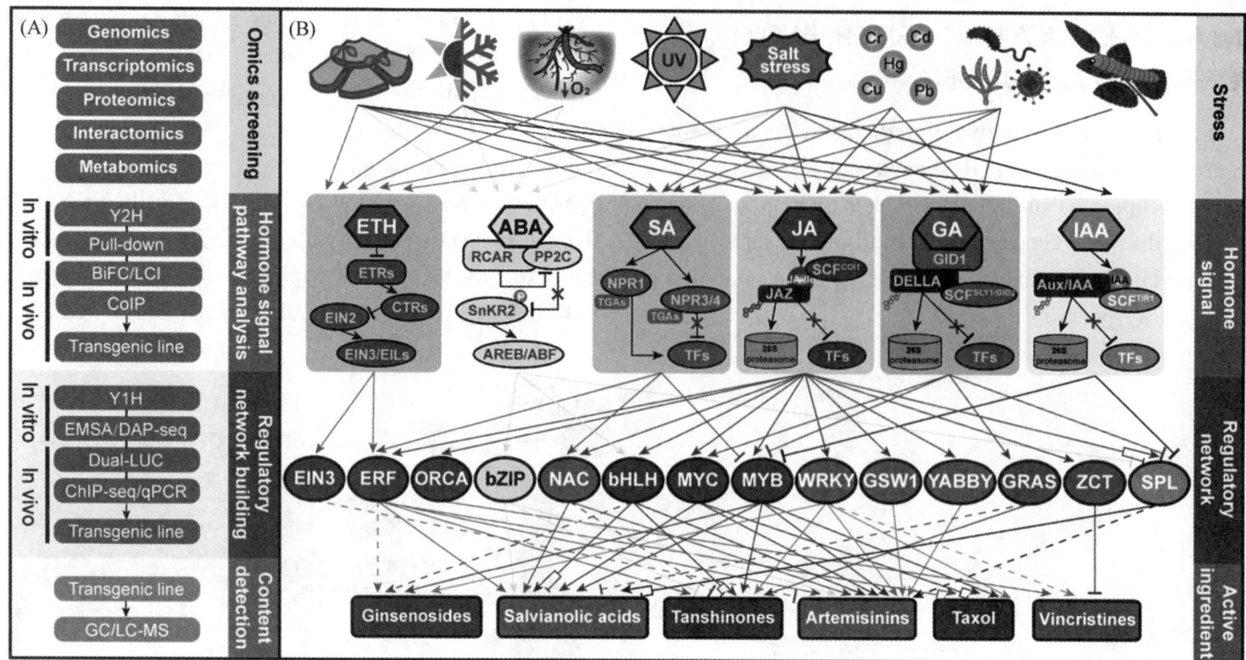


**Figure 7 Transcriptional regulatory network of active ingredients and multi-omics integration in medical plants**

(A) Omics data and molecular biology technology can be used to decipher the molecular mechanism of transcriptional regulation of active ingredients. (B) Transcriptional regulatory network of active ingredients is the most important tie between the production and environment in medical plants. Multi-omics integration can effectively identify transcription factors (TFs) involved in multiple families and the various signaling pathways that regulate active ingredient biosynthesis in medical plants. Abbreviations: ABA, abscisic acid; BiFC/LCI, bimolecular fluorescence complementation/firefly luciferase complementation imaging; ChIP-seq, chromatin immunoprecipitation sequencing; CoIP, co-immunoprecipitation; DAP-seq, DNA affinity purification and sequencing; EMSA, electrophoretic mobility shift assay; Eth, ethylene; GA, gibberellic acid; GC/LC-MS, gas chromatography/liquid chromatography-mass spectrometry; IAA, indole acetic acid; JA, jasmonic acid; LUC, luciferase; SA, salicylic acid; TF, transcription factor.

*PgMYC2*, leading to overproduction of ginsenosides, which indicates that these TFs may regulate ginsenoside biosynthesis through the JA pathway via PgLOX6. Members of the PgbHLH III (d+e) and IV subfamilies, PgWRKY8 and PgWRKY9, were upregulated by MeJA treatment, whereas PgWRKY1-7 was downregulated. In *Panax notoginseng*, MeJA-induced PnERF1 promotes the expression of *PnDS* and *PnSS* to increase levels of ginsenoside $Rg_1$ and Re. PnERF2 and PnERF3 were predicted to participate in ginsenoside biosynthesis through regulating *PnDS* and *PnSE*. Overexpression of the JA-inducible *PqWRKY1* in arabidopsis upregulated the expression of *AtHMGR*, *AtFPS2*, *AtSS1*, and *AtSE2*, suggesting that PqWRKY1 is a positive regulator of ginsenoside biosynthesis.

Ginsenoside biosynthesis is regulated through other means in addition to JA signaling. PgWRKY4X, induced by an effective fungal elicitor *Chaetomium globosum*, increases ginsenoside biosynthesis through binding to the TGAC motif of *PgSE*. *PgTIFY10A*, *PgTIFY10B*, and *PgMYB108* are activated by *Cylindrocarpon destructans* and affect ginsenoside accumulation. PgWRKYs are reportedly correlated with CYP716A53v2, and may modulate ginsenoside biosynthesis. PnbHLH1 activates the expression of *PnFPS*, *PnSS*, *PnSE*, and *PnDS*, while PnWRKY1 activates transcription of *PnSS*, *PnSE*, and *PnDS* to promote ginsenoside accumulation. PnPHL8, a MYB-CC TF related to the phosphate starvation response, was reported to specifically bind to the P1BS motif of *PnCYP716A47*, and may contribute to increased production of ginsenoside $Rb_1$.

## 7 CONCLUDING REMARKS AND FUTURE PERSPECTIVES

Numerous studies have demonstrated the complex and multilayered mechanisms affecting transcriptional regulation of active ingredient biosynthesis in medicinal plants, which is a current research hotspot in molecular pharmacognosy. Numerous TFs that belong to multiple families and are induced by various hormones have been shown to regulate the biosynthesis of active ingredients. Global screening methods using genomics, transcriptomics, proteomics, interactomics, and metabolomics have greatly advanced the process of characterizing active ingredients in medicinal plants. These methods have allowed researchers to discover active ingredients, decipher the associated biosynthetic pathways, and dissect the mechanisms of transcriptional regulation governing their biosyntheses (Figure 7A). A decade ago, homology-based cloning was the main method used to identify TFs related to both artemisinin and tanshinone biosyntheses. New data from medicinal plant genome and transcriptome databases have made research into transcriptional regulatory networks easier. However, current knowledge of transcriptional regulatory networks is far from sufficient. Further investigations are required to understand relevant protein-protein interactions and mechanisms related to miRNA and post-translational regulation. This will lead to better understanding of the transcriptional regulatory networks controlling active ingredient biosynthesis in medicinal plants. Epigenomics, phenomics, and advanced bioinformatics can also reveal the mechanisms involved in transcriptional regulation of active ingredient biosynthesis, providing a theoretical basis for breeding new plant varieties with high levels of desirable active ingredients.

Hormones are key signals required for plant resistance to abiotic and biotic stresses, such as drought, hypoxia, UV radiation, heavy metal, pathogens, and herbivores. The transcriptional regulation network acts as the bridge between environmental signals and production of active ingredients, explaining why adverse conditions promote accumulation of active ingredients in medicinal plants (Figure 7B). Future research should focus on a deeper understanding of the transcriptional regulation mediated by hormones, environmental factors, and their crosstalk. Understanding the molecular mechanisms affecting transcriptional regulation of active ingredients, such as how many TFs simultaneously control multiple synthase genes, has opened the door to exciting new breeding possibilities. For example, the highest artemisinin content in *AaTCP14*-overexpressing plants was an increase of 120%. Overexpressing *AaWRKY9* doubled the artemisinin content. The content of CPT, Tan ⅡA, DHT, and Tan I in overexpressing *SmERF73* lines increased to 93%-168%, 97%-162%, 109%-224%, and 143%-237% of the levels in control lines, respectively.

Of the medicinal plants discussed in this article, *S. miltiorrhiza* is a promising model for research into the molecular mechanisms underlying transcriptional regulation of diterpenoid biosynthesis. The tanshinone biosynthesis pathway occurs in *S. miltiorrhiza*, and we have sufficient knowledge of the transcriptional regulatory network, as well as a mature genetic transformation system for the homozygous genome of this species. We predict that, in the foreseeable future, precise genome-editing techniques can be used to increase the accumulation of desirable active ingredients in medicinal plants by specifically modifying transcriptional regulatory networks (also see Outstanding questions).

[郑汉，黄璐琦，唐克轩，等. Trends in Plant Science, 2023,28(4):429-445.]

# Evolution-guided multiomics provide insights into the strengthening of bioactive flavone biosynthesis in medicinal pummelo

## 1 INTRODUCTION

In the Citrus genus, pummelo (*Citrus maxima* or *Citrus grandis*) is a basic species derived from the near northeastern India, northern Myanmar and northwestern Yunnan and more recently originated compared with *Citrus*-related genera (such as *Atalantia*) and wild citrus species (such as *Citrus mangshanensis*). Pummelo is used not only for fresh eating but also used as a medicinal plant for some landraces. The dried immature pummelo fruit peel, including all of flavedo and a small amount of albedo, was processed into traditional Chinese medicines, named Huajuhong that were one of the important treatment medicines of the COVID-19 in China (Figure 1a). The medicines have efficient functions in reducing the risk of inflammatory diseases, oxidative stress, diabetes, dyslipidemia, endothelial dysfunction and atherosclerosis, due to the high abundance of flavanones, flavones and limonoids. Many studies have been shown that secondary metabolites were selected during the evolution and origin process of crops, such as carotenoids, sugar and cucurbitacin in watermelon, polyol/monosaccharide, cinnamyl alcohol and pectin in peach, and lignin and cellulose in coconut. Despite the detailed origin of pummelo, the changes in the metabolome in the origin process of pummelo are largely unknown.

With the development of metabolome detection technologies, over 200 000 metabolites have been detected in medicinal plants, crops and model plants. Subsequently, metabolome-transcriptome association analysis (MTA) and mGWAS were used to find the regulatory network of metabolites. The regulatory network of metabolites during the developmental stages of *Senna tora*, sweet orange and

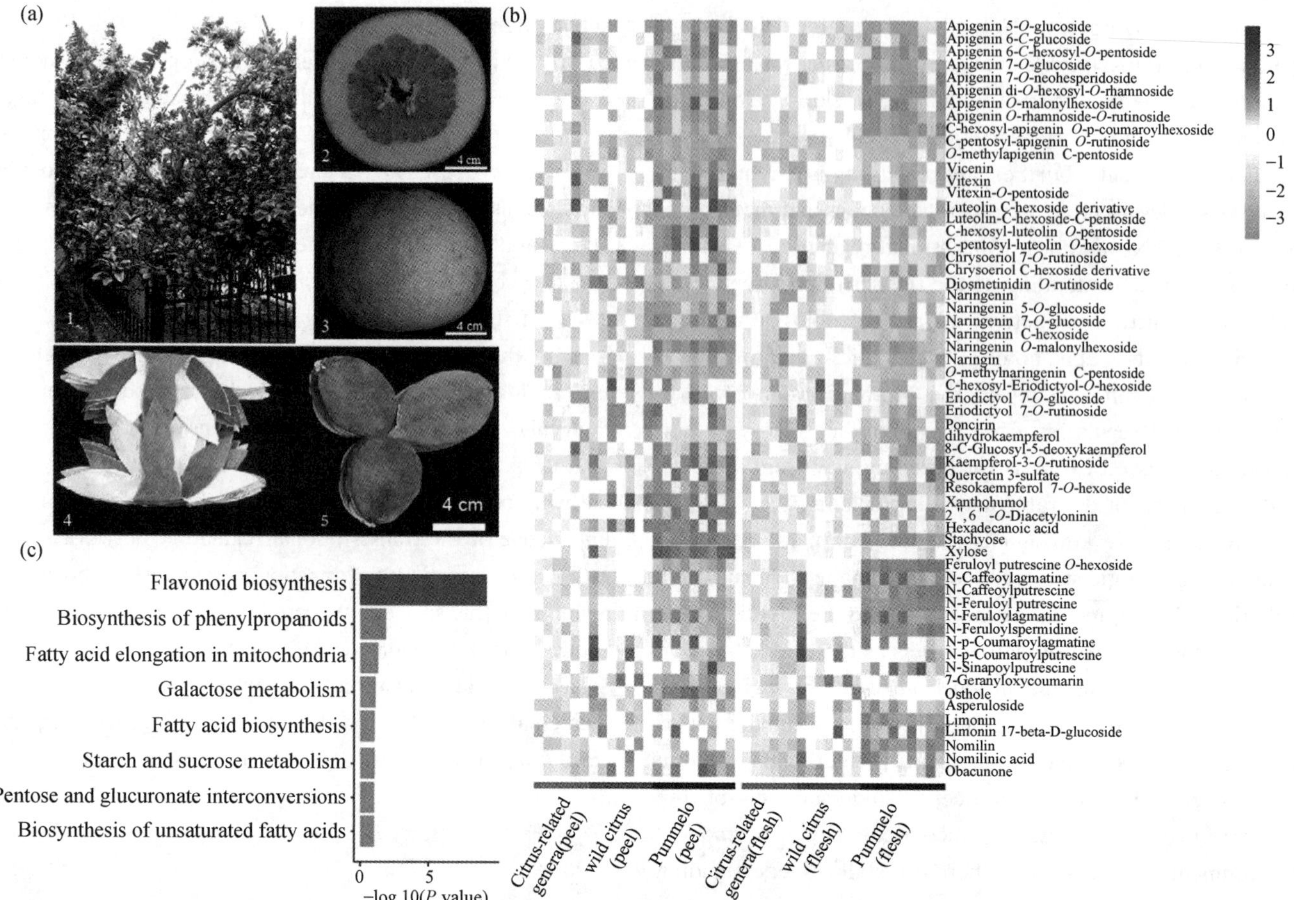


**Figure 1 Characteristics of pummelo medicines and metabolic changes during the origin process of pummelo**

(a) The 100-year-old HZY-T king tree (1), equatorial (2) and shape (3) of HZY-T mature fruit, seven claws (4) and three claws (5) Huajuhong medicines made from HZY-T immature fruit peel, scar bar=4 cm. (b) Heatmap of 59 metabolites that were higher levels in both flesh and peel of pummelo fruit compared with *Citrus*-related or wild citrus species ($P<0.05$, fold change>2). *Citrus*-related genera ($n=6$), wild citrus species ($n=7$), pummelo ($n=9$). Red represents high levels; sky blue represents low levels. (c) KEGG enrichment results of 59 metabolites with higher levels in pummelo.

kiwifruit have been described by MTA. Meanwhile, based on mGWAS, researchers have also identified many genes involved in the regulatory and synthesis of phenylpropanoids, flavonoids and terpenoids in Qingke, rice and tomato, respectively. Due to the limits of population numbers, the mGWAS has rarely been used to identify the regulatory network of bioactive metabolites in medicinal plants.

Bioactive metabolite synthetic pathways, such as the flavonoid pathway, phenylpropanoid pathway and terpenoid pathway, are usually regulated by MYBs, interacting with *chalcone synthase* (*CHS*), *chalcone isomerase* (*CHI*), *flavanone 3-hydroxylase* (*F3H*), *flavonol synthase* (*FLS*), *cinnamate 4-hydroxylase* (*C4H*), *squalene synthase* (*SQS*) and *oxidosqualene cyclases* (*OSCs*). Some structural variations (SVs) and single nucleotide polymorphisms (SNPs) were generated in the promoters and body of MYBs during the evolutions or domestications of apple, strawberry and chilli pepper, which changed the expression and activity of MYBs and affected the levels of malic acid, anthocyanins and apsaicinoid metabolites, respectively. However, the relationships between the changed genomic basis and bioactive metabolites accumulated in medicinal plants have been less studied.

In this study, we present a high-quality reference genome of HuazhouYou-tomentosa (HZY-T). Combining metabolome, genome and transcriptome analysis, we described the relationships between the genomic variation and metabolome changes during the origin process of pummelo, generated a bioactive metabolite regulatory network in HZYs fruit peel, and identified an important gene responsible for the high abundance flavonoids in pummelo fruit peel compared with *Citrus*-related genera and wild citrus species.

## 2 RESULTS

The metabolic profile of pummelo To investigate the contribution of metabolites to the formation of medicinal-purpose cultivars in pummelo and metabolic changes during the origin process of pummelo, we analysed metabolome of peel and flesh in six *Citrus*-related genera, seven wild citrus species and nine pummelo species (Table S1). A total of 403 metabolites were detected in 22 accessions (Table S2). Principal component analysis (PCA) of metabolites divided 22 accessions into three groups, including *Citrus*-related genera, wild citrus species and pummelo (Figure S1a, b). Compared with *Citrus*-related genera or wild citrus species, 59 kinds of metabolites were at higher levels in both peel and flesh of pummelo. These metabolites included 2 kinds of carbohydrates, 1 kind of chalcone, 2 kinds of coumarins, 1 kind of flavanol, 11 kinds of flavanones, 21 kinds of flavones, 4 kinds of flavonols, 5 kinds of limonoids, 2 kinds of lipids, 9 kinds of phenamines and 1 kind of terpenoid (Figure 1b, Table S2). KEGG enrichment analysis revealed that metabolites with higher levels in pummelo (MHLPs) were mainly enriched in flavonoid biosynthesis and biosynthesis of phenylpropanoids (Figure 1c).

Of these MHLPs, 21/59 metabolites have anti-inflammatory, anticancer and anti-oxidative function to varying degrees and others, which were identified as bioactive metabolites; 22/59 metabolites were bioactive metabolite derivatives (Table S2). Among the bioactive metabolites and their derivatives, there are 18 kinds of flavones, 11 kinds of flavanones, 5 kinds of limonoids, 4 kinds of flavonols, 2 kinds of coumarins, one kind of chalcone, one kind of flavanol and one kind of terpenoid, such as vitexin, apigenin 7-*O*-neohesperidoside, naringin, naringenin 7-*O*-glucoside, limonin, nomilin, 7-geranyloxycoumarin, obacunone and xanthohumol, which is consistent with the metabolic basis of Huajuhong medicines. Most bioactive metabolites and their derivatives were flavones and flavanones. Therefore, two flavones (vitexin and apigenin 7-*O*-neohesperidoside) and one flavanone (naringin) were analysed for their anti-inflammatory function. The results indicated that vitexin, naringin and apigenin 7-*O*-neohesperidoside inhibited the expression of the proinflammatory cytokines (*COX-2* and *IL-6*) induced by lipopolysaccharide (LPS) *in vitro* and exhibited anti-inflammatory activity (Figure S2a, b). Collectively, the formation of pummelo medicinal value was highly correlated with the origin of pummelo.

Genomic characterization of a medicinal pummelo accession HZY-T is one of the most important pummelo medicinal plants and is most widely processed in Hujuhong medicines. A 100-year-old HZY-T tree, also named king tree, was found in Huazhou, Guangdong Province (Figure 1a). We *de novo* assembled a high-quality genome of the tree king. The genome was sequenced using a combination of PacBio long reads from the PacBio Sequel platform, Illumina short reads and chromosome conformation capture (Hi-C) technology. The assembled genome of HZY-T is 349.07 Mb with a contig N50 of 1.74 Mb and nine chromosomes (Table S3, Figure 2a). To verify the quality of the assembly, we confirmed that 99.8% of the HZY-T Illumina sequences could be mapped to the assembled genome. Assembly completeness was 99.1% by BUSCO assessment. Meanwhile, we ordered the assembled contigs and oriented them into nine pseudochromosomes using Hi-C data (Figure S3). We annotated 26 924 genes for HZY-T, which were distributed with an increase in density toward the ends of the pseudomolecules (Figure 2a). Meanwhile, we used a fourfold degenerate site at each SNP of 22 pummelo accessions (Table S4), including HZY-T, HZY-S and 20 published accessions (Wang *et al.*, 2018), to perform the PCA analysis, which showed that pummelo accessions were divided into HZYs and other pummelo accessions (Figure 2b). The phylogenetic tree of pummelo based on the above SNPs also showed that the HZYs were grouped into one class (Figure S4).

HZY-T and ten high-quality genomes of Aurantioideae species from CPBD (http://citrus.hzau.edu.cn/), including *Clausena lansium*, *Murraya paniculate*, *Luvunga scandens*, *Aegle marmelos*, *Atalantia buxifolia*, *Poncirus trifoliata*, *Citrus mangshanensis*, *Citrus ichangensis*, *Citrus maxima* 'Wanbaiyou' and *Citrus maxima* 'Majiayou', were used to construct a phylogenetic tree and added to the time of fossil. The results reflected that these accessions diverged into three groups, *Citrus*-related genera, wild citrus species and pummelo, and the *Citrus*-related genera and wild citrus species had an earlier evolutionary origin than pummelo (Figure 2c), which is consistent with the conclusion previously reported. To investigate the genome changes during origin process of pummelo, we identified the 1 405 expanded gene families from *Citrus*-related genera/wild citrus species to pummelo (Table S5). These gene families were mainly enriched in flavonoids-, sterol- and phenylpropanoid biosynthetic process (Table S6, Figure 2d). We also identified 7 091 genes with SVs in pummelo compared with *Citrus*-related genera/wild citrus species (Figure 2a, Table S7).

Transcriptome analysis of genes correlated with flavonoids To investigate MHLPs transcriptional regulatory networks over the course of the HZYs fruit growth cycle, we collected two HZYs (HZY-T and HZY-S) flavedo and albedo of fruit peel in six developmental stages that were 45 DAF (days after flowering), 65 DAF, 85 DAF, 115 DAF, 145 DAF and 185 DAF, for a total of 24 samples (Figure 3a). Among these stages, the first three stages were usually considered the harvested and processed time of Huajuhong medicines. Analysis of 59 MHLPs in six different developmental stages of two HZYs fruit flavedo and albedo, showed that the accumulation of most bioactive metabolites and their derivatives were at higher levels in the pre-developmental

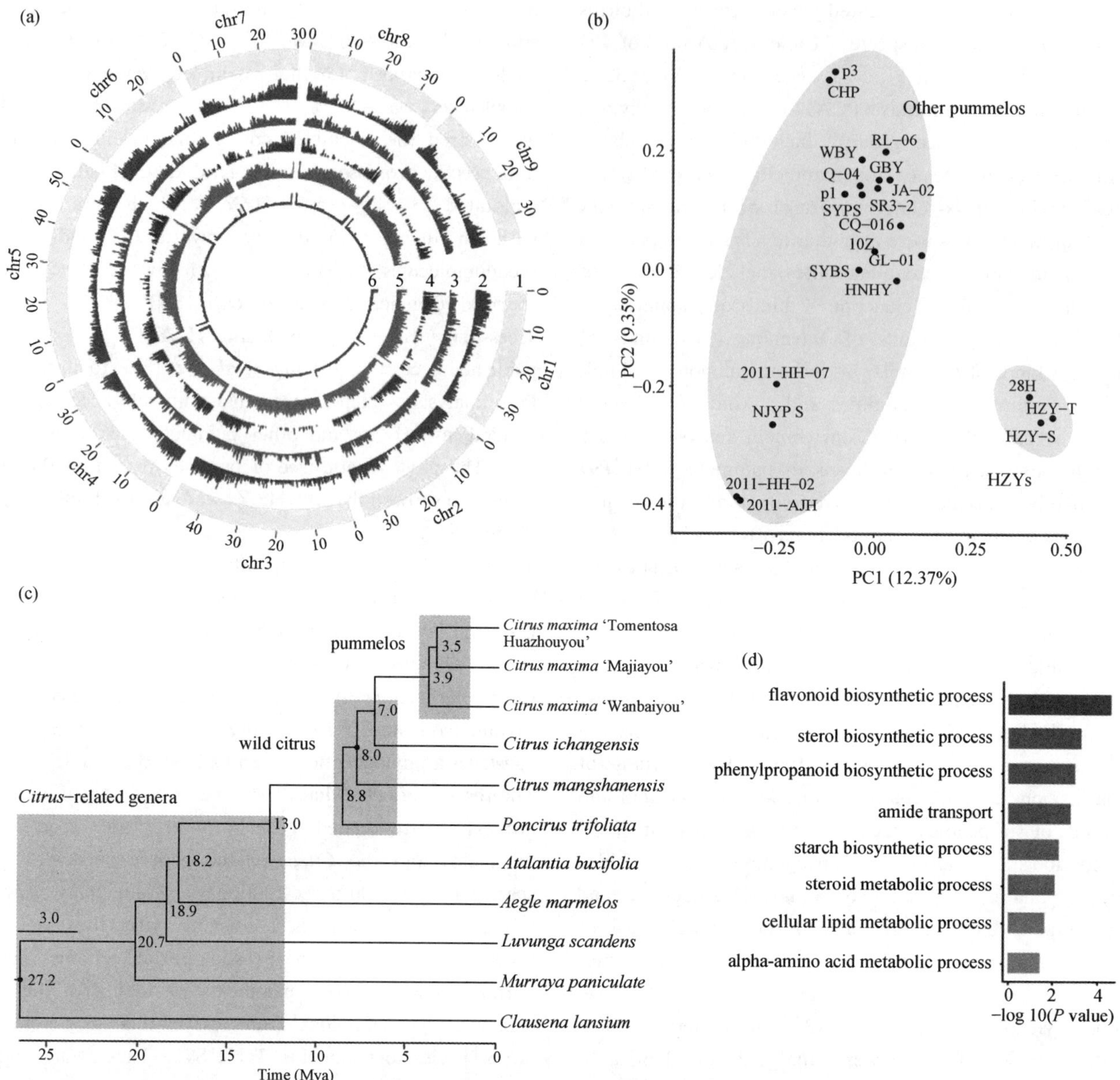


**Figure 2 Genome features of HZY-T pummelo**

(a) Overview of the HZY-T genome assembly. 1: Chromosomes, 2: Gene density, 3: SNP density, 4: density of SVs from 11 genomes, 5: TE density, 6: GC content. The SNPs and SVs were identified using the HZY-T reference genome. (b) PCA of 22 pummelo accessions based on fourfold degenerate site SNPs. (c) Phylogenetic tree of citrus subfamilies based on orthologous genes. Mya, million years ago. (d) Gene Ontology enrichment analysis of genes that were expanded in pummelo compared with *Citrus*-related genera or wild citrus species.

stages of fruit flavedo and albedo, which was a reason why the first three stages were harvested and processed in Huajuhong medicines (Figures S5 and S6). In addition, the PCA-based MHLPs displayed first three stages were closer in both two HZYs (Figure S7a).

Furthermore, we constructed the transcriptome profile in 24 samples and approximately 493.13 Gb of clean data were filtered (Table S8). Subsequently, the fragments per kilobase of exon model per million mapped fragments (FPKM) of 26 924 genes were calculated (Table S9). Similar to the metabolome results, the PCA of the transcriptome also showed that the first three stages were closer in both two HZYs (Figure S7b). We removed the genes with a standard deviation = 0 in six developmental stages of flavedo or albedo. A total of 22 596 and 22 403 genes were filtered in flavedo and albedo, respectively (Table S10). Subsequently, we used the gap statistic to determine the optimal number of clusters, and the numbers in flavedo and albedo were 7 and 8, respectively (Figure S8), which reflected that the two tissues have different regulatory network. Because flavedo was mainly source of Huajuhong medicines, we analysed the transcriptome regulatory

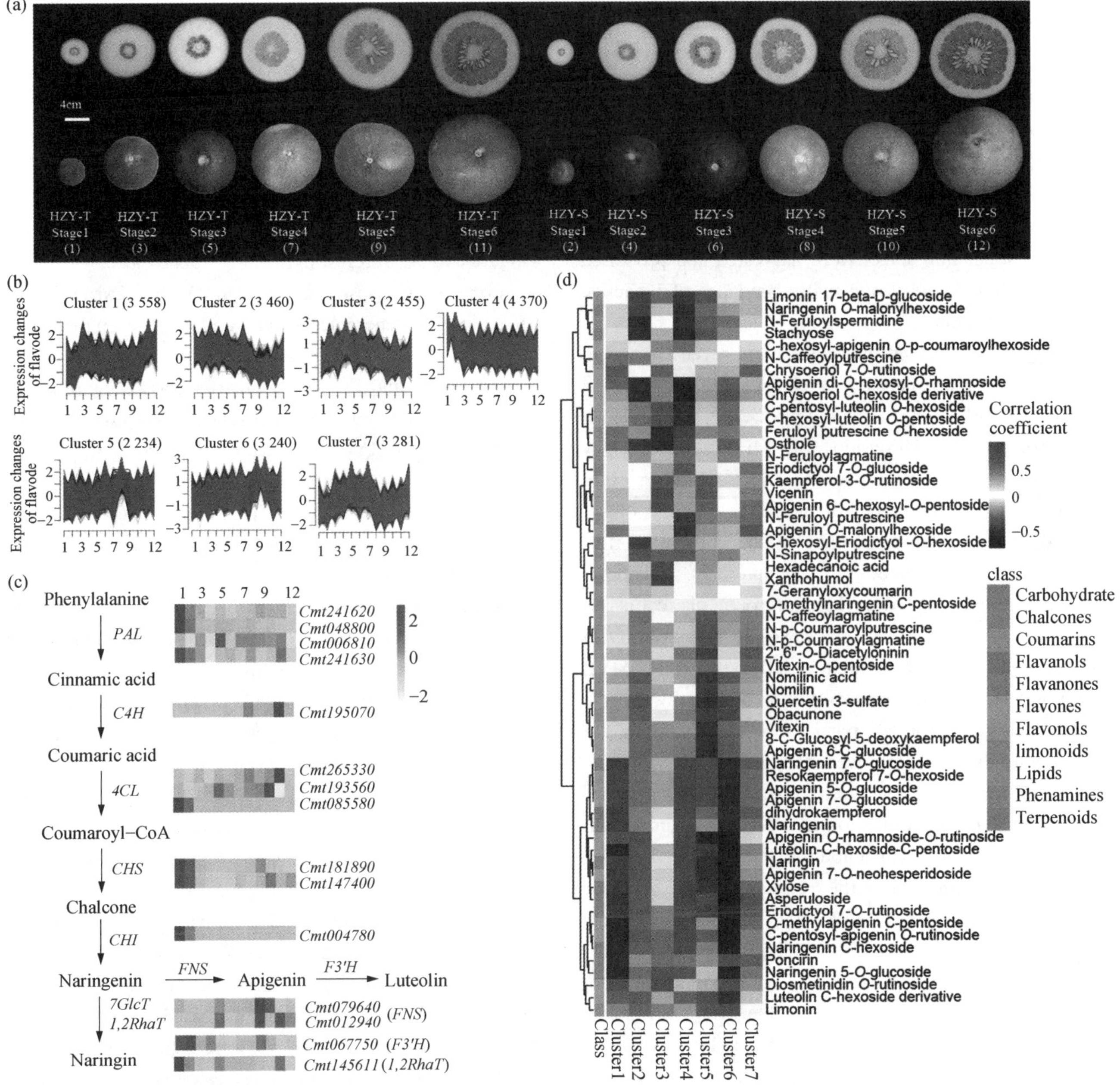


**Figure 3 Dynamics of MHLPs and gene expression in different developmental stages of HZYs fruit flavedo**

(a) Six developmental stages of HZY-T and HZY-S fruit. Bar, 4 cm. (b) Fuzzy c-means clustering identified seven distinct temporal patterns of gene expression in the flavedo. 1,3,5,7,9 and 11 represent stages 1-6 of HZY-T fruit, respectively. 2,4,6,8,10 and 12 represent stages 1-6 of HZY-S fruit, respectively. The *y*-axis represents log2-transformed, normalized intensity ratios in each stage. (c) The relative expression of flavone and flavanone pathway genes. Red represents high expression, and white represents low expression. (d) Heatmap showing the correlation coefficient values between gene clusters and MHLPs in flavedo. Red indicates positive correlation; blue indicates negative correlation.

network in flavedo and applied the fuzzy c-means algorithm to cluster gene expression profiles in six stages of flavedo, and the seven distinct clusters of temporal patterns displayed different gene expression in flavedo (Figure 3b).

Among these clusters, cluster 1 represented gene expression that is upregulated then downregulated then upregulated, and stage 6 were highest, cluster 2 represented gene expression that was downregulated then upregulated, and stage 5 was lowest. Cluster 3 represented gene expression that is upregulated then downregulated, cluster 4 represented gene expression that is downregulated, cluster 5 represented gene expression that are upregulated, cluster 6 represented gene expression that is upregulated then downregulated, and stage 5 was highest. Cluster 7 represented gene expression that is upregulated then downregulated then upregulated, which displayed a bimodal expression pattern. Because flavones and flavanones were more than half of MHLPs, we analysed the expression of genes involved in flavone and flavanones pathway, *PAL* (*phenylalanine ammonialyase*), *C4H*, *4CL* (4-coumarate — CoA ligase), CHS, CHI, FNS (flavone synthase), F*3′H* (*flavonoid 3′-monooxygenase*) and *1,2RhaT* (1,2-rhamnosyltransferase), which reflected that *PAL*, *CHS*, *CHI*, *F3′H* and *1*, *2RhaT* were downregulated, and *C4H*, *4CL* and *FNS* were upregulated then downregulated (Figure 3c), which further explained that pre-developmental stages were harvested and processed time of Huajuhong, due to the high abundance of bioactive flavones and flavanones.

Subsequently, we used the MHLPs and seven clusters to perform co-expression analysis, which reflected the potential regulatory networks of these metabolites (Figure 3d, Table S11). Among these relationships, 32 MHLPs were highly positively correlated with cluster 2, and 28 MHLPs were highly negatively correlated with cluster 5 ($|r| > 0.3$). Therefore, the potential genes that regulated these MHLPs existed in clusters 2 and 5. For example, the flavonols, including 8-C-glucosyl-5-deoxykaempferol, quercetin 3-sulphate and resokaempferol 7-*O*-hexoside were positively correlated with cluster 2, which included the R2R3-MYB transcription factor that regulates the flavonol pathway.

Identification of flavone regulatory genes Among the MHLPs, more than one-third were flavones, such as vitexin, apigenin 7-*O*-glucoside, apigenin di-*O*-hexosyl-*O*-rhamnoside and apigenin 7-*O*-neohesperidoside, which are important bioactive metabolites in Huajuhong medicines (Figure S2a, b). To provide insight into the regulatory mechanism of flavones, we performed mGWAS in 154 pummelo accessions. Flavones, including vitexin, apigenin 7-*O*-glucoside and apigenin di-*O*-hexosyl-*O*-rhamnoside were co-mapped to a significant SNP, located at Chr5: 27438929 (Figure 4a, Tables S12 - S14). The SNP is located 615 kb from *Cg5g022560* that is *Cmt069590* in HZY-T. Cmt069590, named CmtMYB108, was grouped into the MYB transcription factor family that usually regulates the flavonoids pathway. Meanwhile, we found that *Cmt069590* grouped cluster 5, upregulated during the developmental stage, which was highly negative correlated with flavones in the MTA of the HZYs fruit flavedo (Figure 3d). We also found that gene expression was highly negative correlated with flavone biosynthesis pathway genes, including *PAL* (*Cmt048800*), *CHS* (*Cmt181890*), *FNS* (*Cmt079640*) and *F3′H* (*Cmt067750*), which were downregulated during the developmental stage (Figure 4b). Collectively, CmtMYB108 was a potential regulator of flavone pathway.

Due to the higher levels of flavones in pummelo than in *Citrus*-related genera or wild citrus species, we analysed whether *CmtMYB108* was selected during the origin process of pummelo. The gene coding sequences in the citrus subfamilies were obviously divided into three groups, including *Citrus*-related genera, wild citrus species and pummelo (Figure 4c). Meanwhile, we randomly selected two *Citrus*-related genera accessions, two wild citrus accessions and three pummelo accessions to analyse the expression of *CmtMYB108*, which indicated that the expression of *CmtMYB108* was significantly lower in pummelo than in *Citrus*-related genera/wild citrus species (Figure 4d). Interestingly, we found a 0.6 - 0.9-kb deletion ~ 3-kb upstream of *CmtMYB108* existed in five *Citrus*-related genera accessions, and an ~30-bp insertion ~ 380-bp upstream of *CmtMYB108* existed in five *Citrus*-related genera and three wild citrus species (Figure S9). In addition, a miniature inverted-repeat transposable element (MITE) and an MYC motif were found in the 0.6 - 0.9-kb deletion of *Citrus*-related genera, and an unknown motif was found in the ~ 30-bp insertion (Figure S9). Collectively, the two SVs maybe explain the low expression of *CmtMYB108* in pummelo.

CmtMYB108 Negatively regulates the flavone pathway To further confirm the function of *CmtMYB108*, we transiently overexpressed it in *N. benthamiana* leaves, which suggested that the total content of flavonoids was significantly decreased in overexpressed *N. benthamiana* leaves (Figure 5a, b). Meanwhile, *CmtMYB108* was overexpressed in sweet orange by *Agrobacterium*-mediated transformation. Metabolome analysis revealed that 15 flavones and 3 flavanones were significantly decreased in transgenic sweet orange (Figure 5f). These decreased flavones and flavanones are also consistent with the bioactive metabolites and their derivatives of MHLPs. Compared with wild-type sweet orange leaves, the expression level of *CmtMYB108* was significantly increased, and the flavone pathway genes, *PAL* and *FNS* were significantly decreased in overexpressed sweet orange leaves (Figure 5c, Table S8). Interestingly, the expression levels of *PAL* and *FNS* were higher in pummelo compared with *Citrus*-related genera/wild citrus species (Figure 5d, e), which is consistent with the accumulation of flavones and the expression levels of *CmtMYB108*.

To verify whether *CmtMYB108* negatively regulates the flavone pathway, the promoters of *FNS* and *PAL* were cloned for interaction analysis. A dual luciferase (LUC) transcriptional activity assay was performed in tobacco leaves, which confirmed that CmtMYB108 binds to the promoters of two genes and represses their expression levels (Figure 5g, h, Figure S10). Yeast one-hybrid assays (Y1H) also revealed that CmtMYB108 interacted with the promoter of *FNS* (Figure 5i). Hence, these results revealed that CmtMYB108 is a negative regulator of flavone synthesis that

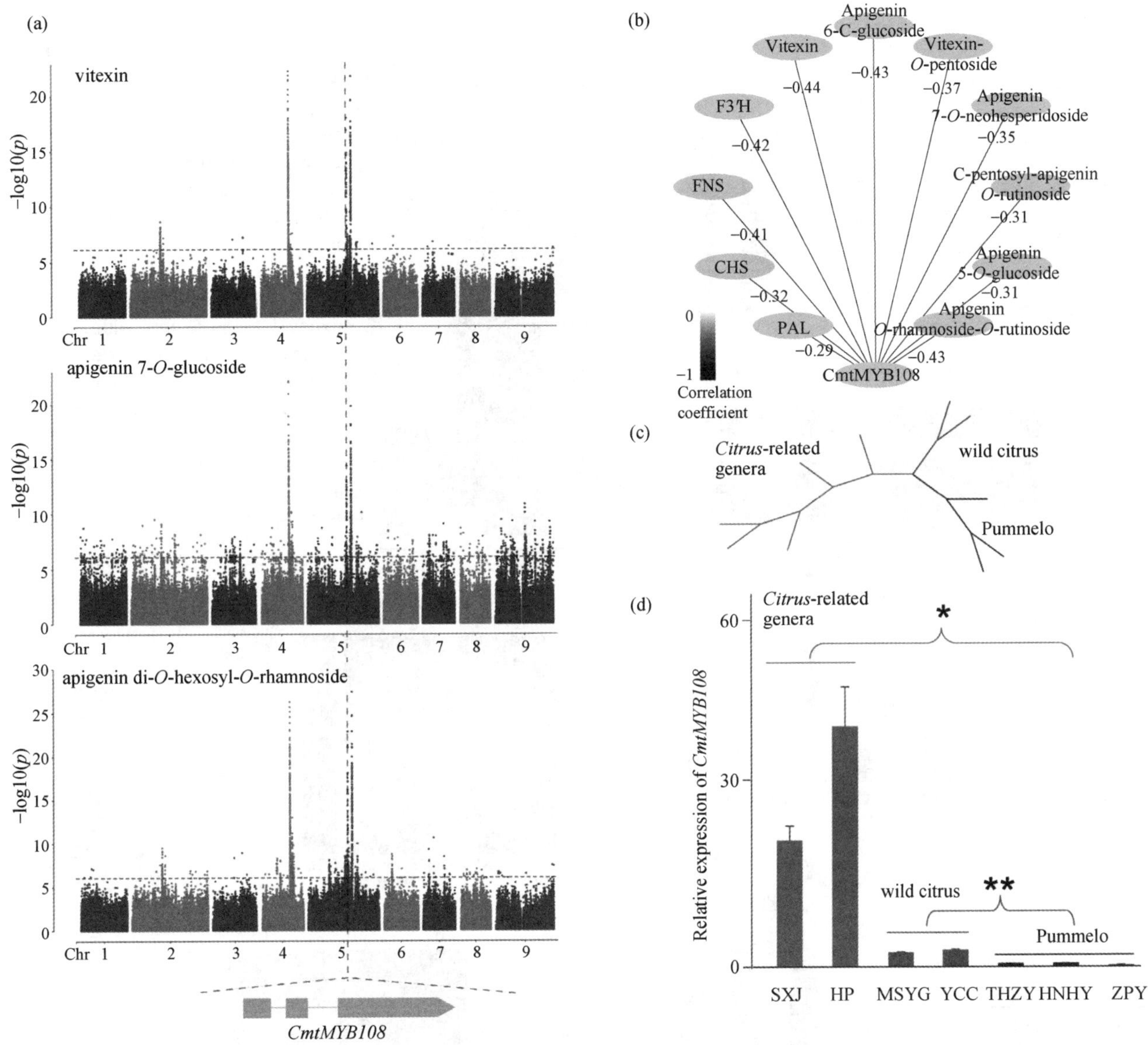


**Figure 4 The identification and variation of *CmtMYB108***

(a) Manhattan plots of vitexin, apigenin 7-*O*-glucoside, apigenin di-*O*-hexosyl-*O*-rhamnoside. (b) Networks were established from correlations among flavones levels, expression of *CmtMYB108* and flavone biosynthesis pathway genes. Pearson correlation coefficient values were calculated for each pair, different line colour represents different correlation coefficient value, and grey number represent each pair correlation coefficient values. (c) Neighbour-joining tree of *CmtMYB108* coding sequence of *Citrus*-related genera, wild citrus species and pummelo. (d) Relative expression of *CmtMYB108* in the fruit peel of *Citrus*-related genera (SXJ, *Glycosmis pentaphylla*. HP, *Clausena lansium*), wild citrus species (MSYG, *Citrus mangshanensis*. YCC, *Citrus ichangensis*) and pummelo (HZY-T, *Citrus maxima* 'Huazhouyou-Tomentosa'. HNHY, *Citrus maxima* 'Huanonghongyou'. ZPY, *Citrus maxima* 'Zipiyou').

functions by directly binding to the promoter of *FNS* and repressing its expression.

## 3 DISCUSSION

In this study, we profiled the changes in metabolite levels in the origin process of pummelo, which displayed that 59 metabolites (MHLPs) were significantly higher levels in pummelo. These MHLPs included 21 bioactive metabolites and 22 bioactive metabolite derivatives, accounting for 73% of the MHLPs number, and most bioactive metabolites and their derivatives were flavones, flavanones and limonoids, which is consistent with the metabolic basis of the medicinal value of Huajuhong medicines (Table S2). For example, vitexin and apigenin 7-*O*-neohesperidoside grouped flavones, and naringin grouped flavanones have anti-inflammatory function, similar to previous studies (Figure S2a,b), limonin and nomilin grouped limonoids were reported to have anti-inflammatory, anti-cancer, anti-obesity. Therefore, the metabolic basis of pummelo medicines is consistent with most MHLPs.

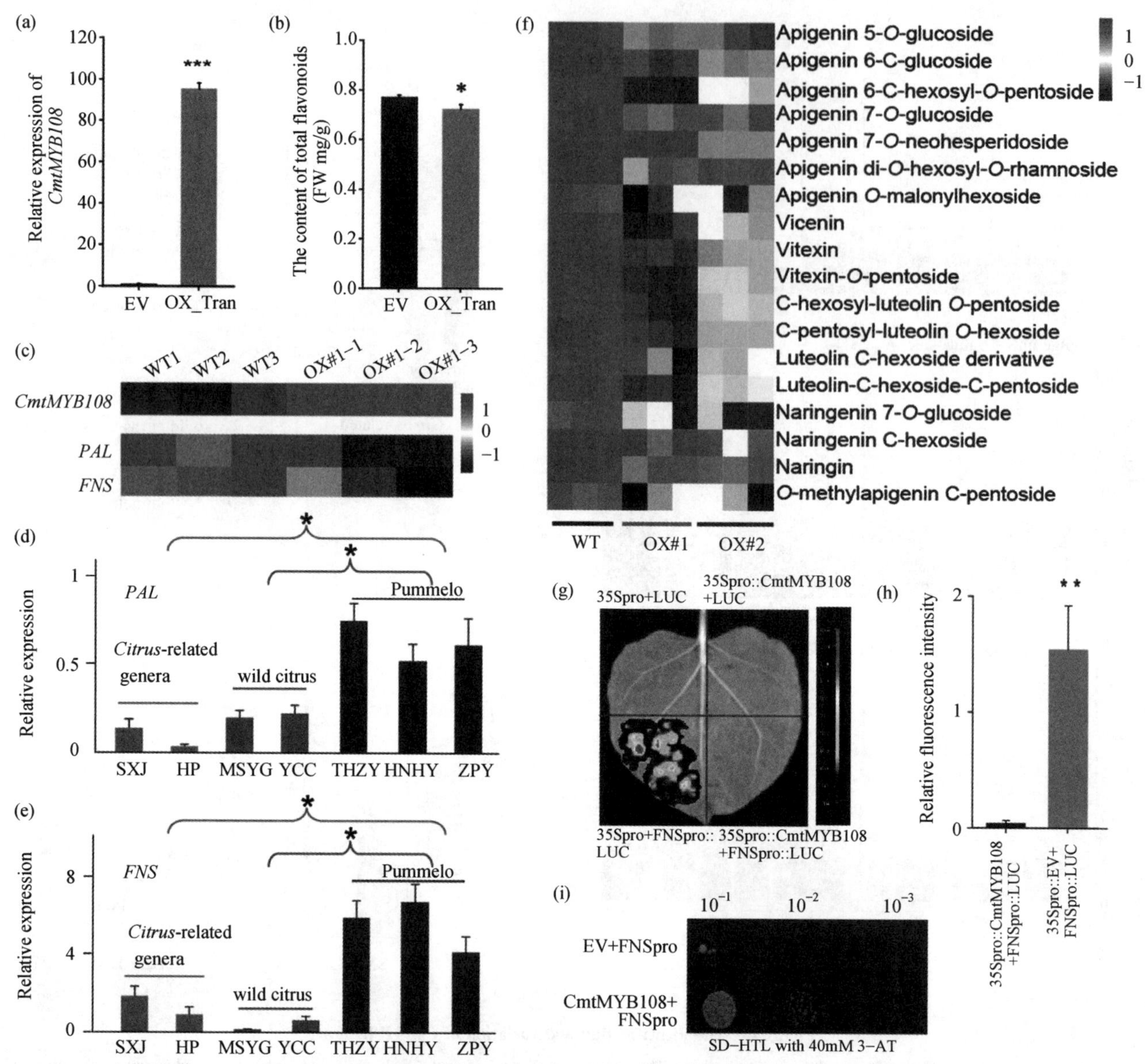


**Figure 5 Functional analysis of *CmtMYB108***

(a) The relative expression of *CmtMYB108* in *N. benthamiana* leaves. EV: empty vector; OX Tran: *CmtMYB108* transiently overexpressed in *N. benthamiana* leaves. (b) The total content of flavonoids in *N. benthamiana* leaves. (c) The expression of *CmtMYB108*, *PAL* and *FNS* in sweet orange leaves. WT: wild type sweet orange; OX#1: *CmtMYB108* overexpressed in sweet orange. (d-e) Relative expression of *CmtMYB108*, *PAL* and *FNS* in the fruit peel of *Citrus*-related genera, wild citrus species and pummelo. (f) Heatmap showing that the content of flavones and flavanones significantly decreased in *CmtMYB108* overexpression lines. WT: wild type; OX#1: overexpressed *CmtMYB108*, OX#2: grafting line and the scion come from OX#1. (g) Transient transactivation assays in *N. benthamiana* leaves with firefly luciferase (LUC) reporter genes. (h) The relative fluorescence intensity in 35Spro::CmtMYB108+FNSpro::LUC and 35Spro::EV+FNSpro::LUC *N. benthamiana* leaves. (i) *CmtMYB108* directly bound to the promoter of *FNS* in the Y1H assay.

HZYs were the most wide source of Huajuhong medicines. We assembled the HZY-T genome with chromosome levels and high completeness (99.1%), which is better than the previous genome with contig levels and low completeness (94.1%). Gene family analysis found that the expanded gene families in pummelo were enriched in the flavonoid biosynthetic process, phenylpropanoid biosynthetic process, response to oxidative stress and response to water deprivation. Pummelo was diverged approximately 7 Mya (Figure 2c) in the near northeastern India, northern Myanmar and northwestern Yunnan with high light, and gradually spread to southeast Asia and south of China. Due to the appearance of the quaternary glaciations, the climate has obviously become low temperature and drought after the time of pummelo divergence. In previous studies, many plants enhanced their adaptability against UV-B, low temperature and drought by increasing the levels of secondary metabolites, such as flavonoids and phenylpropanoid. Pummelo may also adapt to changing environments with high light, low temperature and drought by accumulating high content of flavones and flavanones. Therefore, the origin processes of pummelo may indirectly promote the medicinal value formation of pummelo by enhancing its adaptability to harsh environment.

We found an R2R3 MYB transcription factor CmtMYB108 that repressed the flavone pathway and decreased the levels of flavones and flavanones, such as apigenine 7-*O*-neohesperidoside, vitexin, luteolin-C-hexoside-C-pentoside and naringin. Previous studies have been identified many transcription factor functions by MAT or mGWAS, including glycerophospholipid metabolism regulators in Rice Metabolic Regulation Network results, steroidal glycoalkaloids in the MicroTom Metabolic Network of tomato results, and aromatic phenolamide biosynthesis regulators in the mGWAS results of Qingke. Although the MAT of sweet orange has been reported, this study mainly focused on the accumulation mechanism of sucrose and acid that affected the fruit taste. Utilizing the MAT of HZY-T and HZY-S fruit flavedo, we systematically showed the regulatory network of bioactive metabolites in pummelo medicinal plants (Figure 3d, Table S11). In addition to identifying the new regulator network, we also confirmed the previously reported regulators that MYB42 increased the limonoids levels in *Citrus*. Collectively, multiomics analysis played an important role in determining the regulatory mechanism of bioactive metabolites in medicinal plants.

Transcription factors that regulate flavone biosynthesis are less known in plants compared with flavonol, anthocyanin and flavanol biosynthesis. Previous studies have shown that *GtMYBP3* and *GtMYBP4* in gentian flowers positively regulate flavone biosynthesis, while *CmMYB012* inhibits flavone biosynthesis in response to high temperatures in chrysanthemum. In this study, multiomics analysis revealed that a novel R2R3 MYB transcription factor *CmtMYB108* potentially negatively regulated flavone biosynthesis. Overexpression of *CmtMYB108* in sweet orange significantly reduced the content of flavones in transgenic lines (Figure 5f). However, *CmtMYB108* overexpressed sweet orange showed growth defects with abnormal growth, dwarfing and minimal leaves. Only one transgenic seedling with medium expression level of *CmtMYB108* survived, which might be due to the inhibition of flavones, the essential metabolites for plant growth and development. In addition, previous studies reported that overexpression of *AtMYB62*, homologous gene of *CmtMYB108* in *Arabidopsis*, also led to abnormal development, dwarfing and growth retardation in *Arabidopsis*. Further detection found that the expression levels of the flavone pathway genes *PAL* and *FNS* were significantly upregulated in pummelo compared with *Citrus*-related genera and wild citrus species (Figure 5d, e). Through the LUC assay, we found that CmtMYB108 inhibited the promoter activities of *PAL* and *FNS*, and the Y1H experiment showed that only the *FNS* promoter could be bound by CmtMYB108 (Figure 5g-i, Figure S10). The above results indicated that CmtMYB108 could directly bind and inhibit the expression of *FNS*, thereby inhibiting the synthesis of flavones. MITEs are short non-autonomous DNA transposons, that are widely studied in plants and found to exist in promoters or other regulatory regions to play important roles in gene expression regulation. Here, two SVs, including MITE, MYC motif and unknown motif, were observed in the promoter region of *CmtMYB108* in *Citrus*-related genera and wild citrus species (Figure S9), which may decrease the expression of *CmtMYB108* in pummelo, indirectly increase expression of *PAL* and *FNS* and result in a higher content of flavones in pummelo.

In conclusion, our study elucidates the formation of bioactive flavones during the origin process of pummelo. HZY-T was regarded as a representative to explain the changes in the genome during origin process of pummelo. We also constructed MHLPs transcriptional regulation networks. Furthermore, a novel R2R3 MYB transcription factor, CmtMYB108, was identified by multiomics analysis to regulate the synthesis of flavones by directly inhibiting the promoter activity of *FNS*. In addition, the two SVs in the promoter region of *CmtMYB108* were identified, which maybe result in a decrease in the expression of *CmtMYB108* in pummelo, and promote the accumulation of flavones. This study provides a new reference for the improvement and breeding of medicinal citrus in the future.

## 4 METHODS

Plant materials The 72 samples (three biology replicates) of HZY-T and HZY-S were from Huazhou, Guangdong province from April to September 2021. Five to 10 fruit were randomly divided into three replicates. The fruits were washed with tap water, then the flavedo and albedo were separated and placed in liquid nitrogen followed by storage at −80℃. The 22 accessions fruit peel and flesh for metabolism analysis were collected from Yunnan province, Guangxi province and Hubei province in the years of 2019 and 2020 (Table S1, https://doi. org/10.6084/m9. figshare. 22261738). The fruit samples were ripe, a normal size and healthy. Nine to 15 fruit were randomly divided into three replicates. Each piece of fruit was washed with tap water. The flesh was separated and placed in liquid nitrogen followed by storage at −80℃ until further analysis.

Metabolite profiling All the chemicals were of analytical reagent grade. Gradient-grade methanol, acetonitrile and acetic acid were purchased from Merck Company, Germany. The water was doubly deionized with Milli-Q water purification system (Millipore, Bedford, MA). Standards were purchased from ANPEL, Shanghai, China, BioBioPha Co., Ltd. and Sigma-Aldrich, USA.

The freeze-dried fruits were crushed using a mixer mill (MM 400, Retsch) with zirconia beads for 1.8 min at 15 Hz. A 100 mg mass of powder was weighted and extracted overnight at 4 ℃ with 1.0 mL of 70% aqueous methanol. Following centrifugation at 10 000 g for 10 min, the extracts were filtered (SCAA - 104, 0.22 μm pore size; ANPEL, Shanghai, China) before LC-MS analysis. The sample extracts were analysed using an LC-ESI-MS/MS system (Shim-pack UFLC SHIMADZU CBM30A system, http://www.shimadzu.com.cn/; MS, SHIMADZU LCMS-8060, http://www.shimadzu.com.cn/). The analytical conditions were as follows, UPLC: column, Shim-pack GISS C18 (pore size 1.9 μm, dimensions 2.1 × 100 mm); solvent system, water (0.04% acetic acid): acetonitrile (0.04% acetic acid); gradient program, 95:5 *V/V* at 0 min, 5:95 *V/V* at 12.0 min, 5:95 *V/V* at 13.2 min, 95:5 *V/V* at 13.3 min, 95: 5 *V/V* at 15.0 min; flow rate, 0.4 mL/min; temperature, 40 ℃; and injection volume: 2 μL.

Population structure analyses by metabolomics principal component analysis plots were used to infer the structure of the *Citrus*-related genera, wild citrus species and pummelo. The data matrix was generated from *Citrus*-related genera, wild citrus species and pummelo with 403 metabolites which represented the contents of each metabolite in average of two biological repeats. PCA was performed with log2-transformed metabolite data. PCA was performed with FactoMineR and factoextra packages in R version 3.6.2. Significantly difference analysis was performed with wilcox. test in R version 3.6.2.

The anti-inflammation function identification of vitexin, apigenin 7-*O*-neohesperidoside and naringin RAW 264.7 macrophages were grown in Dulbecco's Modified Eagle's Medium (DMEM) with high glucose (4.5 g/L) (Hyclone, GE Healthcare, Little Chalfont, UK) containing 10% fetal bovine serum (FBS) supplemented with 1% penicillin and streptomycin at 37 ℃ and 5% CO2—95% air under humidified conditions. The concentrations of vitexin, apigenin 7-*O*-neohesperidoside and naringin were 3 μmol/L. In brief, the RAW 264.7 macrophages were routinely cultured in a 12-well for 24 h. Then, the cells were co-treated with flavones or flavanones (3 μmol/L) and LPS (1 μg/mL) for additional 18 h under cell culture conditions.

Library construction and sequencing HZY-T sample for genome assembly and HZY-S were re-sequenced were selected from Huazhou, Guangdong province. Extraction of genomic DNA from leaf tissue using TIANGEN BIOTECH (BEIJING) DNAquick Plant System from HZY-T and HZY-S, respectively. The 150-bp paired-end libraries of HZY-T and HZY-S were then constructed using the Illumina Genomic DNA Sample Preparation Kit, and sequencing was performed using Illumina NovaSeq 6 000 platforms. For PacBio long-read sequencing, we use the protocol then released by PacBio to construct the SMRTbell libraries (20 kb) of HZY-T, then use Pacbio Sequel platform II for sequencing. A total of 7 995 694 (~100×) Pacbio subreads were obtained. In addition, an Hi-C libraries were created from tender leaves of HZY-T by Novogene (Beijing, China), A total of 92.1 million (~100×) 150 bp paired-end reads were produced on the Illumina NovaSeq 6 000 platform.

Genome assembly The HZY-T genome size is first estimated using GCE (v1.0.2). Then use Canu (v2.0) to correct (parameter 'maxThreads = 20, minReadLength = 2 000, minOverlapLength = 500, corOutCoverage = 150, corMinCoverage= 2'), trim (parameter 'maxThreads= 20 minReadLength = 2 000, minOverlapLength = 500') and assemble (parameter' maxThreads = 25, genomeSize = 363 m, correctfedErrorRate=0.035′). The PacBio subreads to obtain a diploid HZY-T genome.

In order to obtain the HZY-T haploid genome, we first used Minimap2 to map the trimmed Pacbio subreads to the initial diploid genome. Then use purge_ dups to remove redundancy and get the main haploid assembly. Finally, the Nextpolish was used to polish the haploid assembly with a short read-long sequence and rimmed Pacbio subreads. After finishing these steps, a preliminary evaluation of the quality of contigs by assembled size, N50, longest sequence was undertaken. BUSCO was used to evaluate the completeness.

For HZY-T pseudochromosome construction, we first mapped the clean Hi-C reads to the polished assembly using BWA. Then, the contigs is anchored to scaffolds using ALLHiC (parameter '-e AAGCTT-k 10'). We finally aligned the ALLHiC assembly against the pummelo genome (Citrus grandis (L.) Osbeck. cv. 'Wanbaiyou' v1.0) using NUCmer in MUMMER4 with default parameters to determine the pseudochromosome order.

Genome mapping, variant calling and population analyses Raw Illumina reads was processed to remove adapter sequences and low-quality reads by Fastp. The cleaned reads were mapped to the reference genome using BWA-MEM. Then mapped reads were sorted and the duplicated reads were removed by Sortbam and MarkDuplicates tools in the GATK package. The UnifiedGenotyper of GATK was then used to call variants. The fourfold synonymous third-codon transversion (4DTV) file was extracted in VCF file by SnpEff. The PCA was performed by PLINK and GCTA using 4DTV file.

Gene family analysis and phylogenetic tree The longest

proteins of 11 genomes were filtered. The gene families were identified by OrthoFinder. The gene family's number of each genome was computed by CAFÉ. For Phylogenetic tree analysis, we used MUSCLE (v3.8.31) to multiple sequence alignment. The conserved sequences were extracted and merged by Gblocks_0.91b and SeqKit, respectively. Then we used RAxML to construct the ML tree.

Transposable elements and genes annotation for HZY-T The genome sequences were used to build a *de novo* TE library using the RepeatModeler software. The TE library was used to identify repeat sequences in particular genomes using RepeatMasker. Gene models were annotated based on ab initio gene predictions, homology searches and RNA-seq. For ab initio gene predictions, AUGUSTUS, GlimmerHMM and SNAP were employed using default parameters. The protein databases were constructed by integrating the amino acid sequences from the published genomic protein sequences of Citrus. Homology searching was then conducted using genome threader. In addition, RNA-seq reads were generated from a mixture of tissues. The Trinity software was utilized to perform genome-guided and de novo transcript assembly. The PASA software was used to update the protein-coding gene annotations by incorporating PASA alignment evidence, correcting exon boundaries, adding UTRs and modelling alternative splicing based on the PASA alignment assemblies. All of the gene structures predicted using the aforementioned methods were combined using the EVM software.

Structural variation analysis The longest 30× PacBio/Nanopore reads were mapped to the reference by NGLMR. The resulting alignments were sorted and indexed by Samtools. Initial SV callings were performed by Sniffles, SVs supported by at least five reads were left. We filtered low-quality SVs (flag: UNRESOLVED) and removed duplicate SV calls (SVs at the same position for multiple pairs of breakpoints). Next, we merged SVs from all individuals using SVRVIVOR with parameters "200 - 1 1 - 1 - 1 - 1 merged.vcf". The merged SVs were used as input to force call all the SVs across all samples using Sniffles with parameter-Ivcf enabled. Finally, we merged the called SVs again to obtain a fully genotyped multi-sample SVs. The merged SVs were added to the genome of *C. sinensis* to construct a graph-based genome with the vg pipeline.

Transcriptome analysis Raw Illumina reads were processed to remove adapter sequences and low-quality reads by Fastp. The cleaned reads were mapped to the reference genome using HISAT2. Then mapped reads were sorted by Samtools. FPKM values were calculated by Subreads in R software.

Determination of total flavonoid content The total flavonoid content of tobacco leaf was measured with an aluminium chloride method. Briefly, 0.5 g fresh leaf was powdered and extracted with 10 mL 80% methanol, shaking at room temperature for 2 h, and centrifuged at 1400 g to get the supernatant. Then prepare the reaction according to the following steps: 0.5 mL supernatant, 2.25 mL $ddH_2O$ and 0.15 mL 5% $NaNO_2$ were mixed and shaken for 6 min, then added 0.3 mL 10% $AlCl_3$ solution, shaken for 5 min, finally added 1 mL 1 mol/L NaOH solution and immediately measured the absorbance at 510 nm with a spectrophotometer. Rutin was used as the standard curve to calculate the content of total flavonoids.

Plasmid construction and stable transformation in citrus The coding sequence of CmtMYB108 was isolated from HZY-T pummelo by PCR and cloned into a pK7WG2D overexpression vector. The vector was then transformed into epicotyls of Anliu sweet orange by using A. tumefaciens strain EHA105 described previously. The explants were screened by GFP and then the expression levels of CmtMYB108 were identified by qPCR. The positive transgenic seed lines were potted in a controlled greenhouse for subsequent studies.

Dual luciferase transcriptional activity assay About 2 kb of DNA sequences upstream of the translational start codon of *FNS* (*Cmt079640*) and *PAL* (*Cmt241630*) were amplified by PCR from genomic DNA of 'Anliu' sweet orange. The fragments were subsequently inserted into a pGreenII 0800-LUC to generate reporter vectors, which were then transformed into *A. tumefaciens* GV3101 (with plasmid pSoup-p19) competent cells. The effector vector was a CmtMYB108 overexpression vector pK7WG2D described above, and an empty pK7WG2D vector was used as a control. Both vectors were also transformed into GV3101 (pSoup-p19) competent cells. The GV3101 cells containing effector and reporters were mixed to a proportion of 5 : 1 and then injected into leaves of *N. benthamiana*. 3 days after injection, the surface of the transfected leaves was treated with 0.2 mmol/L luciferin and kept for 5 min in darkness. LUC activity was measured using a NIGHTSHADE imaging apparatus (LC 985). The primers used for these experiments are listed in Table S15.

Yeast one-hybrid assay analysis The promoters of *CsFNS* and *CsPAL* were ligated into the pHIS2 vector (Clontech) which contains a HIS3 nutritional reporter gene. The bait plasmids were then integrated into a yeast strain Y187. 3 - AT (3-amino-1, 2, 4-triazole) was used for inhibiting the self-activation of the bait vectors. Full length of CmtMYB108 was ligated into the pGADT7 vector (Clontech) and then transferred into yeast cells containing bait vectors. pGADT7 empty vector used as negative control. The positive interactions could be detected by the growth of yeast cells on histidine-deficient media.

RNA extraction and gene expression analysis RNA extractions from all frozen samples were performed as described in a previous study. Then, 1.0 mg of the extract was digested with 4× gDNA wiper (Vazyme Biotech) to remove the genomic DNA, followed by the addition of 5× HiScriptII Q RT supermix to synthesize first-strand cDNA for further analysis. The relative expression of candidate genes, including *CmtMYB108* and its target genes (*PAL* and *FNS*), was quantified using quantitative RT-PCR with the SYBR FAST qPCR Kit (YEASEN) and the LC480 Fast Real Time System. qRT-PCR was performed using gene-specific primers (Table S15) and equal amounts of cDNA from three independent biological replicates with three technical replicates for each biological replicate. Relative expression levels were calculated using the $2^{-\Delta\Delta Ct}$ method.

[郑伟康，黄璐琦，马兆成，等. Plant Biotechnology Journal，2023，21：1577－1589.]

# Profiling of phytohormone-specific microRNAs and characterization of the miR160-ARF1 module involved in glandular trichome development and artemisinin biosynthesis in *Artemisia annua*

## 1 INTRODUCTION

Malaria is a global health problem with 241 million cases in 87 endemic countries in 2020. *Artemisia annua* L. has gained increasing attention for its widespread use in the extraction of a potent drug for malaria, artemisinin. Artemisinin is a sesquiterpenoid produced in glandular trichomes of *A. annua*. The oral delivery of artemisinin in the form of dried *A. annua* leaves has proven highly effective even against parasite strains resistant to artemisinin combination therapy and intravenous artesunate. In addition to antimalarial benefits, artemisinin has many other biological and pharmacological properties, including antiviral, anticancer, and antischistosomal effects. Therefore, artemisinin has been considered to be a promising multifunctional natural product. The relatively low content (0.1%-1.0% of dry weight) of artemisinin in *A. annua* is a serious limitation to the commercialization of the drug. Although semisynthesis of artemisinin via artemisinic acid can be obtained from genetically modified yeast, the semisynthetic production of artemisinin is expensive and thus cannot replace its agricultural production at present. Hence, regulating artemisinin biosynthesis in *A. annua* to increase its content remains the desirable approach to resolve the contradiction between supply and demand.

Concerted attempts have been made to elucidate the biosynthetic pathway of artemisinin and its regulatory mechanisms in *A. annua*. In the last three decades, three primary metabolic engineering strategies have been developed to optimize the production of artemisinin in *A. annua*: ① overexpressing artemisinin biosynthetic pathway genes (*ADS*, *CYP71AV1*, *DBR2*, and *ALDH1*). ② overexpressing transcription factors (TFs) involved in artemisinin biosynthesis and glandular trichome formation. ③ applying exogenous phytohormones. Methyl jasmonate (MeJA), salicylic acid (SA), abscisic acid (ABA), and gibberellins (GAs) are effective elicitors for enhancing artemisinin accumulation by inducing the expression of genes encoding TFs that regulate the artemisinin biosynthetic pathway genes or increase the glandular trichome density in *A. annua*. *Aa*MYC2, a JA-response bHLH TF, can bind to the G-box-like cis-elements present in both *CYP71AV1* and *DBR2* promoters and then strongly activate their expression. *Aa*TCP15, a JA and ABA dual-responsive teosinte branched1/cycloidea/proliferating (TCP) TF, is essential for JA- and ABA-induced artemisinin biosynthesis and functions by directly binding to and activating the promoters of *DBR2* and *ALDH1*, two genes encoding enzymes for artemisinin biosynthesis. Glandular trichome initiation occurs at the G1 to S and G2 to M stages, and MeJA may specifically delay the switch from G1 to S and prolong the G1 phase. Consequently, exogenous treatment with JA stimulates artemisinin production in *A. annua*, as well as the formation of glandular trichomes. Similarly, the external application of ABA can activate the TF *Aa*bZIP1, directly regulating the accumulation of artemisinin by stimulating the expression of *ADS*, *FPS*, and *CYP71AV1*. Some studies have revealed that SA applications are able to increase artemisinin content by 54% in two different ways: converting the dihydroartemisinic acid into artemisinin due to the burst of ROS and positively affecting the expression of artemisinin-related biosynthetic enzymes. In addition, the expression of some enzyme genes such as the β glucosidase gene, to increase glandular trichome density can improve artemisinin content.

In addition to the TF, increasing evidence suggests that the miRNA-TF module has emerged as a key regulator of phytohormone response pathways in planta by affecting their metabolism. For instance, the phytohormone-responsive miR156-SPL module is involved in phase changes, leaf trichome development, anthocyanin biosynthesis, and plant responses to salt stress in *Arabidopsis thaliana*. Similarly, the miR156 - SPL module has been proven to function in regulating developmental phase transition and flowering and in the spatiotemporal regulation of sesquiterpene biosynthesis. For instance, miR156 plays a role in regulating the formation of (*E*)-β-caryophyllene in the flowering stage by targeting SPL9, which is a positive regulator of *TPS21* in sesquiterpene biosynthesis. These studies implicate the possibility that miRNAs are involved in artemisinin synthesis. Thus, further systematic characterization of the miRNA is still needed to reveal their regulatory mechanisms in artemisinin biosynthesis.

Although computational predictions and high-throughput sequencing of miRNAs have been performed previously for *A. annua*, the miRNAs related to artemisinin synthesis cannot be accurately screened in the absence of reference genomes. Herein, in view of the diverse regulatory effects of phytohormones on artemisinin synthesis, a pipeline to identify candidate miRNAs under various hormone stress conditions was designed to decipher the regulatory roles of miRNAs in artemisinin biosyn-thesis in *A. annua* at the genome-wide level. Sequencing and bioinformatic methods were used for the first time to profile miRNAs in *A. annua* with ABA, MeJA, and SA treatment. Furthermore, the phytohormone-responsive miR160-ARF1 module was identified as a negative regulator in repressing glandular trichome development and artemisinin biosynthesis in *A. annua*. Collectively, these findings provide not only new insights into the important roles of the miRNA-TF module in the development of glandular trichomes and the regulation of artemisinin biosynthesis but also a new strategy to engineer plants for high and stable production of artemisinin in the future.

## 2 RESULTS

Profiling of miRNAs in *A. annua* To study the post-transcriptional regulation, regarding especially miRNAs involved in the molecular regulation of artemisinin biosynthesis, 10 small RNA (sRNA) libraries were constructed from aerial tissue of *A. annua* treated with DMSO and MeJA, SA and ABA at different time points. The numbers of raw reads and valid reads, which were obtained from one control and nine treatments, are summarized in Table S1. The size distributions of the unique valid sRNAs (Figure 1a) and total valid sRNAs (Figure 1b) in the 10 libraries showed strikingly similar patterns. The valid reads ranging from 20 to 24 nucleotides were approximately 89% and 90% in the total and unique sequences, respectively, with 21- and 24-nt reads being the most dominant sRNA species, consistent with evidence found in the dicotyledonous plants.

To identify the conserved miRNAs from 10 *A. annua* libraries, all valid reads were mapped onto the genome of *A. annua* and the sequences of known plant miRNAs, such as miRNA precursors and mature miRNAs registered in miRbase 21.0. The sequences mapped to miRBase were identified as conserved miRNA, and those mapped to the *A. annua* genome only were considered novel miRNAs. The criteria of the blast search required no more than two mismatches in the first 16 nt of the miRNA and three mismatches in total between the specific miRNAs and pre-miRNAs in miRBase. All detected miRNAs were categorized into Groups 1 - 4 (gp1 - 4), and members of gp4 were identified as novel miRNA candidates. Interestingly, the numbers of miRNAs varied among families. The miR156 family was the largest (42 members), followed by the miR169 family (25 members), and more than 1/3 of miRNA families had only one miRNA member (Figure 1c). Following the BLASTn search and further sequence analysis, 224 conserved miRNAs belonging to 33 families in the small RNA library were found to be orthologues of known miRNAs from other plant species, which were previously deposited in the miRBase database (Figure 1d). The distribution of the conserved miRNA family in *A. annua* was highly similar to those of *Artichoke*, *Jerusalem artichoke*, and other species belonging to Compositae, and was significantly different from those of other species. In total, 61 pre-miRNAs, corresponding to 52 mature miRNAs, were identified as novel miRNA candidates that were not registered in miRBase. The number of miRNAs was counted and normalized to the total reads of sRNAs. The expression levels of miRNA families of miR156, miR166, miR167, miR393, miR171, and miR160 were high in our pooled *A. annua* sample. Precursors forming hairpin structures for the novel miRNAs were predicted, with folding free energies ranging from −157.8 to −35.5 kcal/mol (Table S2). The lengths of precursors of the novel miRNAs ranged from 81 nt (PC-5p-1705_6778) to 252 nt (PC-5p-1284_9299).

Response patterns of miRNAs to phytohormones To systematically identify miRNAs in *A. annua* that respond to phytohormones and may be involved in the biosynthesis of artemisinin, the differential expression of miRNAs in 10 libraries was analysed and compared based on the normalized read counts generated from the high-throughput sequencing. Generally, the majority of miRNAs (77, 68.0% of the

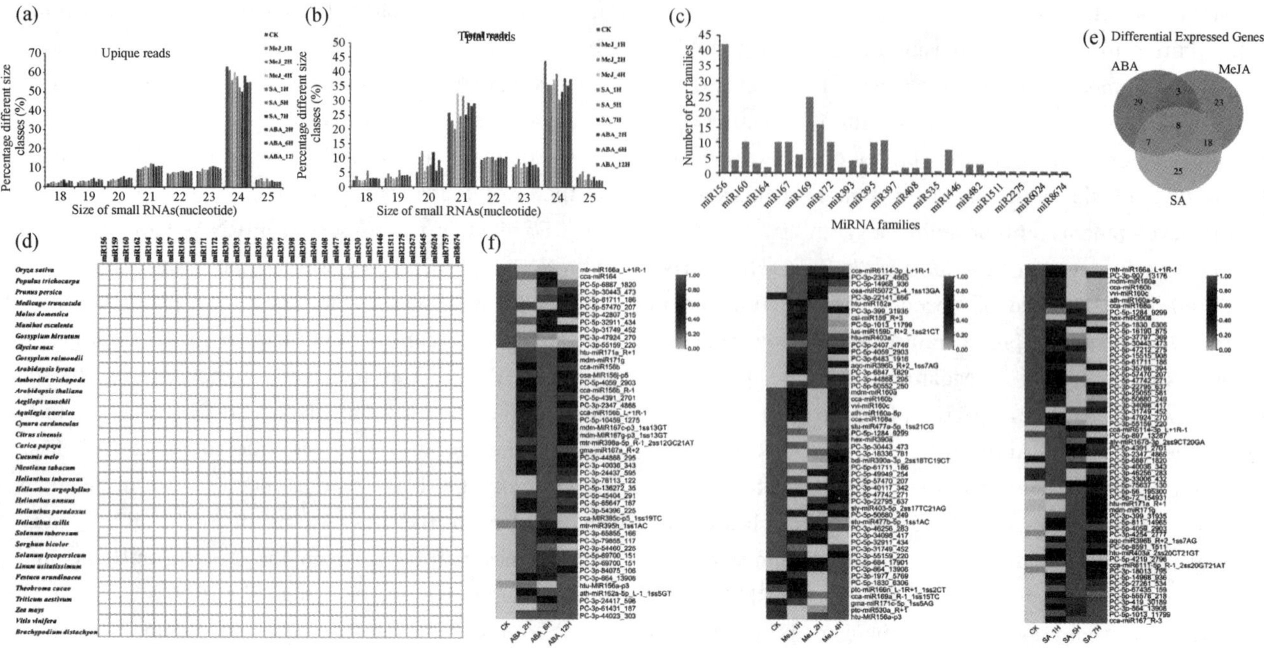

**Figure 1 miRNA features of *Artemisia annua***

(a) Length distribution of unique sRNAs in *A. annua* sequencing samples. (b) Length distribution of total sRNAs in *A. annua* sequencing samples. (c) Number of conserved miRNA families from *A. annua*. (d) Conserved miRNA families in *A. annua* and across species. (e) Venn diagram showing the overlap of significantly differentially expressed miRNAs between the control and ABA-, SA-, and MeJA-treated in *A. annua* groups. (f) Differentially expressed miRNA analysis. Heatmaps show the significantly differential expression of miRNAs ($P<0.05$) under ABA, MeJA, and SA treatment in *A. annua*. Red indicates higher levels of miRNA and green indicates lower levels. The absolute signal intensity ranges from 0 to +1.0, with corresponding colour changes from green to red.

differentially expressed miRNAs) were upregulated in hormone-treated samples compared with their levels in the control. There were 23 MeJA-specific miRNAs, of which 13 miRNAs were conserved and 10 miRNAs were novel. Four conserved miRNAs and 21 novel miRNAs were specific to SA treatment. Meanwhile, 12 conserved miRNAs and 17 novel miRNAs were specific to ABA treatment. Additionally, one conserved miRNA and 2 novel miRNAs were found in the ABA and MeJA treatments but not in the SA treatment. Similarly, 3 conserved miRNAs and 4 novel miRNAs were detected only in the ABA and SA treatments, whereas 8 conserved miRNAs and 10 novel miRNAs were detected only in the MeJA and SA treatments. In comparing the three treated groups with each other, only 8 novel miRNAs were all significantly differentially expressed, but the expression levels were low (Figure 1e). In total, 41 known miRNAs and 72 novel miRNAs were found to be differentially expressed in at least two pairwise comparisons when stricter criteria of total expression abundance $>10$ and $P$-value $\leqslant 0.05$ were used in hormone-treated groups compared with the mock treatment group. The heatmap of potential differentially expressed miRNAs is illustrated in Figure 1f.

qRT-PCR was used to investigate the miRNA expression profiles of the selected miRNAs. As shown in Figure 2, the sequencing and the qRT-PCR results showed that miR156 expression first increased and then decreased with ABA treatment. Conversely, the miR160 showed a trend of first decreasing and then increasing again with MeJA treatment, but miR160 showed a continuous decreasing trend after SA treatment. miR171 was significantly differentially expressed by ABA or SA induction, and miR159 was significantly differentially expressed by ABA or MeJA induction. In comparing results from qPCR and sequencing analyses, the expression levels of these miRNAs between qPCR and sequencing analyses were consistent (Figure 2). Therefore, three conserved miRNAs (miR159, miR160, and miR171), which respond to the induction of two hormones, were used as candidates for artemisinin biosynthesis.

Identification of miRNA target genes in *A. annua* by degradome sequencing Multiple studies have indicated that miRNAs may directly target TFs that affect plant development and various secondary metabolism processes. Degradome sequencing combines the advantages of high-throughput deep sequencing, computer analysis, and RACE to search for miRNA-guided cleaved sites in mRNAs and was used as an efficient strategy to globally identify small RNA targets in this study. Through degradome sequencing, among the 224 miRNAs of the 33 known miRNA families, 190 could be searched for their potential targets, yielding 254 genes (Table S3). Among the 345 novel miRNAs, there

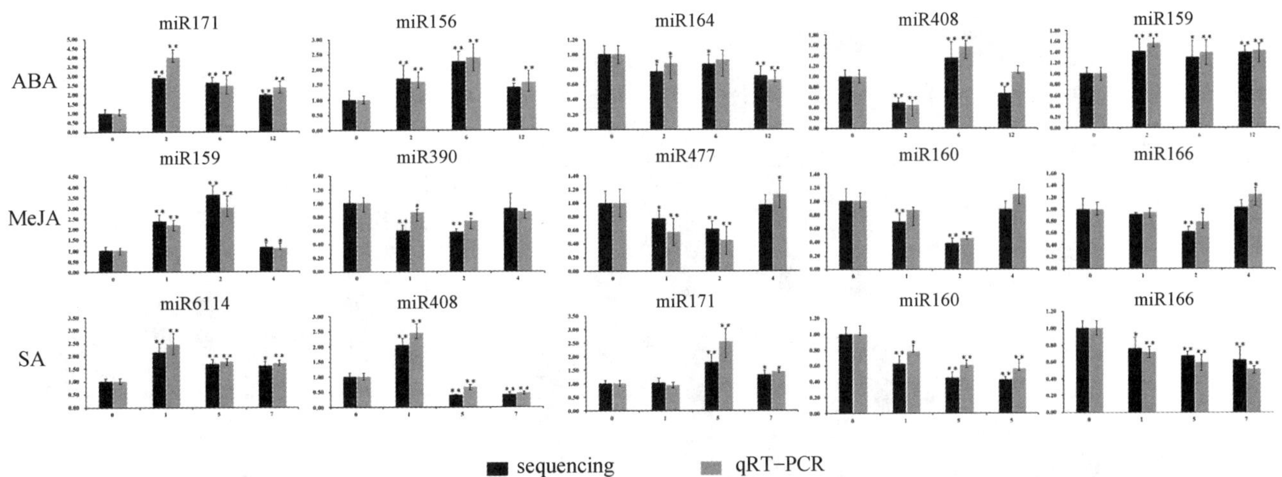


**Figure 2 Confirmation of the expression levels of selected miRNAs in *Artemisia annua* by qRT-PCR**

The horizontal axis represents the time after hormone treatments (hours), and the vertical axis represents the relative expression of miRNAs. The black bar represents the deep sequencing, and the grey bar represents the qRT-PCR. The expression levels of these miRNA were confirmed using stem-loop qRT-PCR. *Actin* was used as a loading control in qRT-PCR. The data are represented as the mean plus SD of $n=3$ biological replicates. * $P<0.05$, ** $P<0.01$, Student's $t$ test.

were 328 predicted targets (Table S3). The detailed annotation of each miRNA target is shown in Table S3. One-half of the conserved miRNA targets (131 of 258) were TFs, including SPL, GRAS, AP2, ARF, MYB, and NAC. Other conserved miRNA targets, such as CYP85A1, COMT1, and GA2OX1, are involved in secondary metabolism.

According to Gene Ontology (GO) annotation classification, the category containing the most target genes was 'biological process', which was subcategorized into the 25 biological processes displayed in Figure S1, and regulation of transcription process (GO: 0006355), oxidation-reduction process (GO: 0055114), and auxin-activated signalling pathway (GO: 0009734) were the most significantly enriched terms (Figure S1). Kyoto Encyclopedia of Genes and Genomes (KEGG) enrichment analysis of 72 miRNAs/miRNA families and 184 target genes revealed that plant hormone signal transduction (ko04075), monoterpenoid biosynthesis (ko00902), plant-pathogen interaction (ko04626), and purine metabolism (ko00230) pathways were the most important pathways (Figure S2). Therefore, the focus of the further study was on miRNAs in the plant hormone signal transduction category.

In the present study, we also found expression changes for several miRNAs involved in the regulation of transcription and auxin signalling. For instance, miR160 showed a 3.78-fold change in abundance under SA or MeJA treatment (Figures 1f, 2), highlighting it as a candidate for having a regulatory role in artemisinin synthesis. miR160 was predicted to target an Auxin_resp domain TF, which functions as a hormone-responsive TF. ARF TFs are also regulated by miR160 and function in plant growth and the response to stress in *A. thaliana*. Based on the above, an attempt was made to identify the function of miR160 in *A. annua*.

miR160 regulates artemisinin biosynthesis and glandular trichome development Since some of the predicted or validated ARFs targeted by miR160 are orthologous to the tomato ARFs involved in the formation of trichomes, we theorized that miR160 might also be involved in glandular trichome development in *A. annua*. To test this hypothesis, *MIR160* overexpression vectors were transformed into the *Agrobacterium strain* GV3101, which was then introduced into *A. thaliana* Col-0 by the *Agrobacterium*-mediated floral dip method. Three candidate *MIR160* overexpression lines (named *35S: miR160*), *35S: miR160*-5, 8, and 13, were chosen for further analysis. For each transgenic line, three 2-week-old third leaves were used to count the number of trichomes. For comparison, a significantly decreased trichome density was found on the first two rosette leaves in *35S: miR160* transgenic lines, with a 43%-77% decrease compared to wild-type (WT) plants (Figure 3a).

To further characterize the role of miR160 in *A. annua*, *MIR160* overexpression and suppression constructs were transferred into *Agrobacterium* EHA105 and genetically transformed into *A. annua*. In total, 13 independent *35S: miR160* lines and 15 independent *MIR160* knockdown lines (named STTM160) were obtained (Figure 4a, b). The transcript abundance of *MIR160* in selected transgenic *A. annua* plants was detected using qPCR. Reasonably, upon the comparison of the miRNA abundance with WT plants, the expression level of *MIR160* was found to be upregulated in the *35S:miR160* lines, while that of miR160 was reduced in the STTM160 lines (Figure 4c). The RNA-Seq data showed that the expression levels of *AaADS*, *AaCYP71A1*, *AaALDH1*, and *AaDBR2* were significantly reduced in the

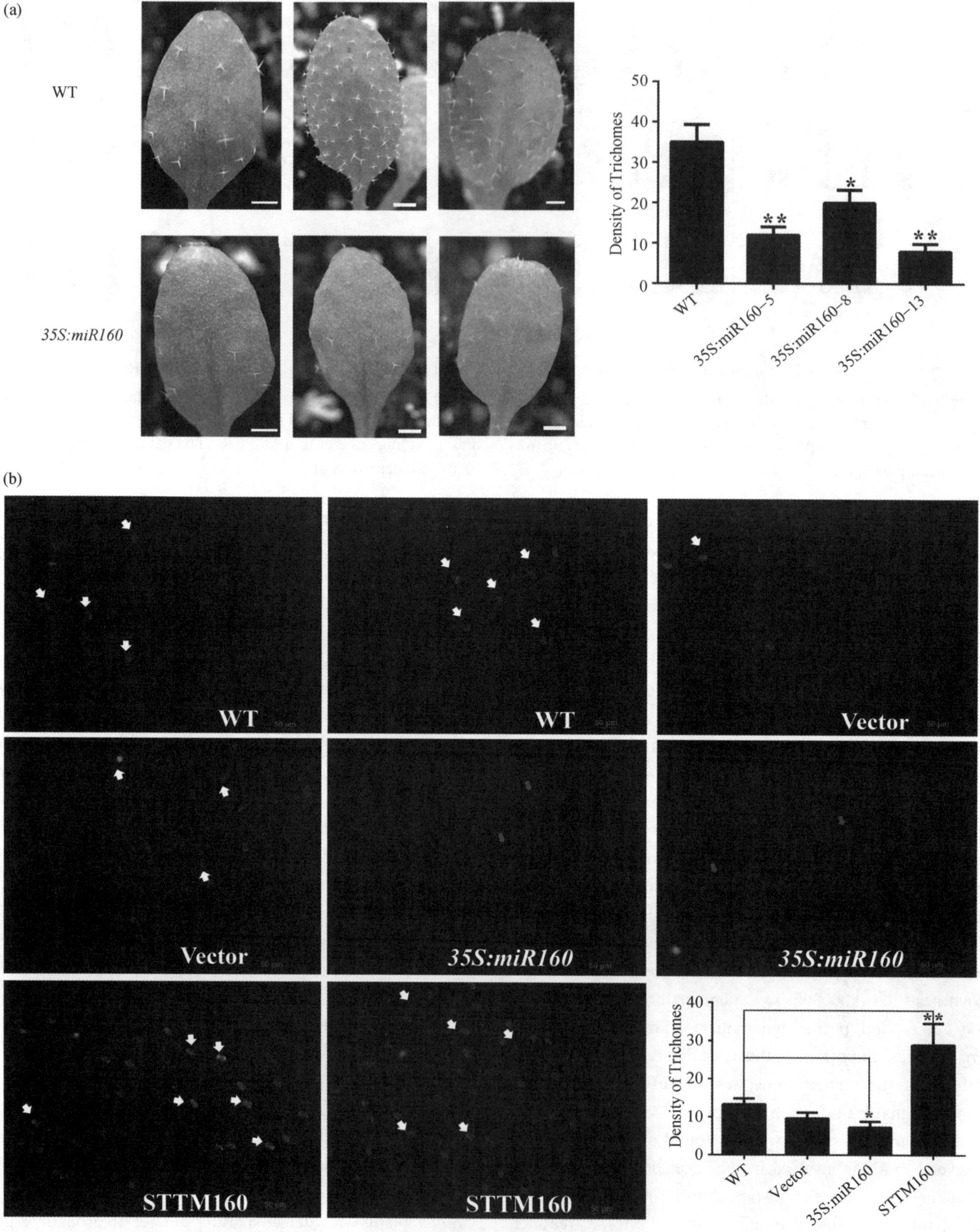


**Figure 3 Density of trichomes in leaves of transgenic *Arabidopsis thaliana* and *Artemisia annua* plants**

(a) Leaf surface and density of trichomes in leaves from WT plants and *35S*:*miR160* transgenic *A*. *thaliana* plants. The number of trichomes decreased significantly compared with WT. Bars represent 1 mm. * $P<0.05$, ** $P<0.01$, Student's *t* test. (b) The adaxial surface was observed using fluorescence microscopy of leaves and the density of glandular trichomes in leaves from *35S*:*miR160* and STTM160 transgenic *A*. *annua* lines, plants transformed with the empty vector, and WT plants. Bars represent 50 μm. * $P<0.05$, ** $P<0.01$, Student's *t* test.

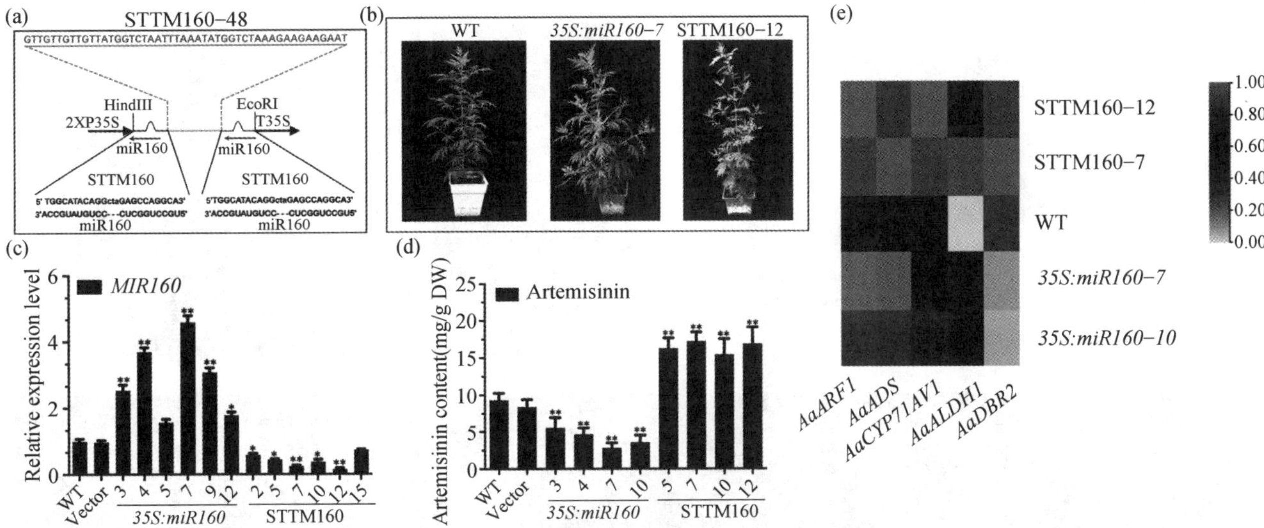


**Figure 4 Analysis of miR160 transgenic *Artemisia annua* plants**

(a) Schematic representation of STTM constructs used for silencing miR160 via *Agrobacterium tumefaciens*-mediated transient expression. Green indicates the spacer region and the spacer sequence. Purple indicates the bulge sequences in the miRNA-binding sites. (b) Different phenotypes among the *35S*: *miR160*, STTM160, and WT lines. (c) Expression levels of *MIR160* in the different *35S*: *miR160* and STTM160 lines, plants transformed with the empty vector, and WT plants. *Actin* was used as the internal standard. All data represent the means±SDs of three replicates from three cutting propagations. * $P<0.05$, ** $P<0.01$, Student's *t* test. (d) HPLC analysis of artemisinin in the leaves of different *35S*: *miR160* and STTM160 lines, plants transformed with the empty vector, and WT plants. All data represent the means±SDs of three replicates from three cutting propagations. * $P<0.05$, ** $P<0.01$, Student's *t* test. (e) Expression analyses of *AaARF1*, *AaADS*, *AaCYP71AV1*, *AaALDH1*, and *AaDBR2* in WT, suppressed lines, and overexpression lines. Heatmaps show the significantly differential expression of genes ($P<0.05$) in *A. annua*. Rows represent differentially expressed artemisinin biosynthesis genes, and columns represent group comparisons. Red indicates higher levels of gene expression and green indicates lower levels. The absolute signal intensity ranges from 0 to +1.0, with corresponding colour changes from green to red.

*35S*: *miR160* lines. Conversely, the expression levels of these four enzymes were greatly increased greatly in the miR160 repression lines compared with the control (Figure 4e). Moreover, overexpressing miR160 dramatically decreased glandular trichome density, and the autofluorescence of many glandular trichomes exhibited a strong reduction on the *35S*: *miR160* plant leaves (shown by red arrows), indicating defective glandular trichomes (Figure 3b). The most severe reduction in glandular trichome density correlated with the highest expression level of *35S*: *miR160-7*, while the glandular trichome density of STTM160 plants was increased significantly and showed strong green autofluorescence (shown by white arrows) compared with the controls. Consistent with the downregulation of genes involved in artemisinin biosynthesis, liquid chromatography-tandem mass spectrometry (LC-MS/MS) analysis showed that the artemisinin contents in *35S*: *miR160* lines decreased by 40%-70% compared with WT. In contrast, the artemisinin contents in STTM160 lines increased by 65%-81% compared with WT plants (Figure 4d). These results indicate that miR160 is a key regulator of glandular trichome formation and artemisinin biosynthesis.

ARF1 mRNA cleavage is directed by miR160 To investigate the underlying mechanisms by which miR160 regulates artemisinin biosynthesis, we tried to identify its target genes. Seven target genes (AA320180, AA003210, AA004030, AA122040, AA203930, AA487720, and AA072530) were found to have been cleaved at their miR160-specific cleavage sites according to the available *A. annua* degradome sequencing data, indicating that they could be the target genes of miR160 (Figure S3). All of the above seven target genes encode ARF family proteins with ARF motifs and are named ARF1 to ARF7. A phylogenetic analysis based on protein sequences showed that the predicted target genes are highly conserved and can be divided into two clades (Figure S4). Predicted miRNA targets were then validated using RNA ligase-mediated 5′ RACE PCR. The cleavage products of *ARF1* and *ARF6* mRNA fragments generated by miR160 processing were successfully detected (Figure 5a). Sequence analysis of the amplified products from 25 independent cDNA clones suggested that the cleavage sites were located in the middle of the miR160 complementary region. The cleavage site of the miR160/*ARF1* pair was between the 10th and 11th nucleotides of miR160, whereas *ARF6* was mapped to the paired miR160 at the 9th or 10th nucleotide from the 5′-end (Figure 5a). In conclusion, these results demonstrate that miR160 may regulate divergent aspects of artemisinin biosynthesis by targeting *ARF* genes.

To verify the preferential targeting of *ARF*s by miR160,

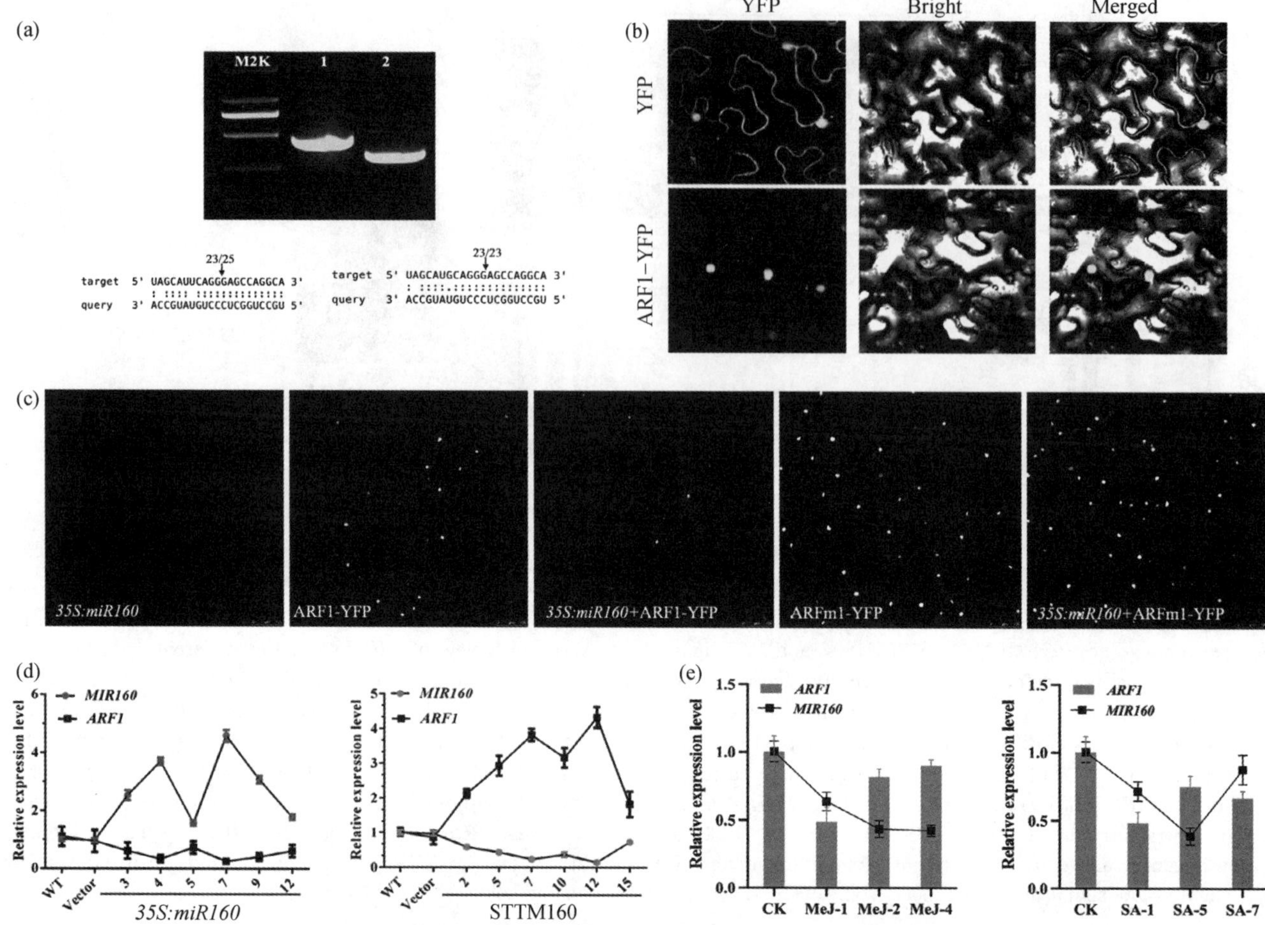


**Figure 5 Experimental validation of *ARF1* as a target gene of miR160**

(a) Nested PCR products of 5′ RACE. Vertical arrows indicate the 5′ termini of the miRNA-guided cleavage products, as identified by 5′ RACE, with the frequency of clones shown. (b) Subcellular localization of ARF1. YFP was used as a negative control. Three independent transfection experiments were performed. (c) miR160 targeting of ARF1 was verified in *Nicotiana benthamiana* leaves. The indicated constructs were transformed or cotransformed into *N. benthamiana* leaves, and the expression of ARF1 was imaged. Experiments were performed three times. (d) The expression profiles of *MIR160* and the target gene *ARF1* by qPCR in *35 S:miR160* and STTM160 transgenic *A. annua* lines. All data represent the means±SDs of three replicates from three cutting propagations. (e) The expression profiles of *miR160* and the target gene *ARF1* by deep sequencing in treated *A. annua*. The green bar represents the *ARF1*, and the black lines represent *miR160*. All data represent the means±SDs of three replicates from three cutting propagations. The data are represented as the mean plus SD of $n=3$ biological replicates. * $P<0.05$, ** $P<0.01$, Student's $t$ test.

we transiently performed a yellow fluorescent protein (YFP)-based reporter assay in *Nicotiana benthamiana* as described in a previous report. As a negative control, we used a primer to introduce six mismatched nucleotides in the miR160/ARF mRNA complementary region of the *ARF* mRNA sequence without changing the encoded amino acid sequences, and the mutant was designated ARFm (Figure S5). Constructs harbouring ARF or ARFm fused with YFP under the control of the CaMV35S promoter were transiently transformed (either individually or with *35S:miR160*) into *N. benthamiana* leaf cells by infiltration. The expression of ARF-YFP was evaluated by confocal microscopy. In contrast to YFP, which was distributed throughout the cell, a strong YFP signal was detected only in the nuclei of the transformed cells expressing ARF1 or ARFm1 (Figure 5c), sug-gesting that ARF1 has a putative role in the control of transcription (Figure 5b). As shown in Figure 5c, when ARF1 and miR160 were coexpressed in tobacco leaf epidermal cells, YFP signals were substantially reduced, showing that miR160 inhibits the expression of ARF1. In contrast, the YFP signals were not greatly affected in cells coexpressing ARF1m6-YFP and miR160. Oppositely, miR160 did not silence the potential target gene ARF6 (Figure S6). Notably, the level of the *MIR160* transcript was highest in the transgenic line *35S:miR160*-5, while the expression of *ARF*1 was most reduced. The expression of *ARF*1 was also increased significantly in the STTM lines (Figure 5d). The inverse expression pattern of *MIR160* and *ARF1* was also observed after phytohormone treatments (Figure 5e). In summary, these data suggest that miR160 may regulate artemisinin biosynthesis through its target gene *ARF1*.

ARF1 positively regulates artemisinin biosynthesis by activating *AaDBR2* expression The results of 5′ RACE and transient expression experiments prompted us to investigate the effect of ARF1 on artemisinin biosynthesis. Given that miR160 overexpression results in reduced artemisinin production (Figure 4d), RNA interference (RNAi) of ARF1 was performed to assess whether ARF1 knockdown would produce the same phenotype. As shown in Figure 6a, the abundances of *ARF1* transcripts were confirmed to be greatly reduced by 41%–87% in ARF1-RNAi plants, and four indepen-dent lines (ARF1-RNAi-3, ARF1-RNAi-4, ARF1-RNAi-7, and ARF1-RNAi-8) were chosen for further metabolism analysis. As expected, the contents of artemisinin in ARF1-RNAi plants were reduced by 18%–44% (Figure 6c).

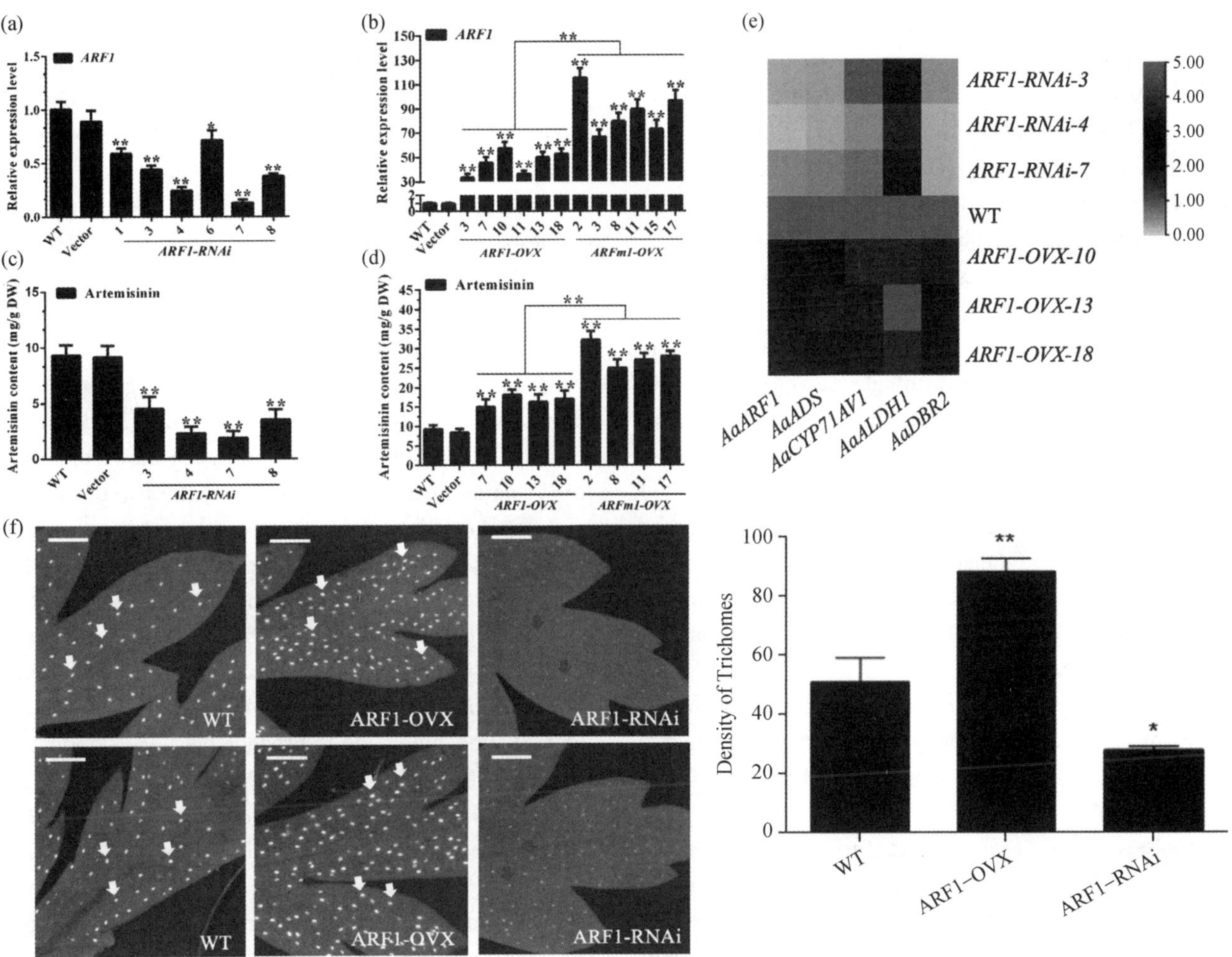


**Figure 6 Analysis of *ARF1* transgenic plants**

(a) Expression levels of *ARF1* in different *Artemisia annua* plants including *ARF1-RNAi* lines, and plants transformed with the empty vector. *Actin* was used as the internal standard. WT plants served as controls. All data represent the means±SDs of three replicates from three cutting propagations. * $P<0.05$, ** $P<0.01$, Student's *t* test. (b) Expression levels of *ARF*1 in different *A. annua* plants including *ARF1-OVX* lines, *ARFm1-OVX* lines, and plants transformed with the empty vector. *Actin* was used as the internal standard. WT plants served as controls. All data represent the means±SDs of three replicates from three cutting propagations. * $P<0.05$, ** $P<0.01$, Student's *t* test. (c) HPLC analysis of artemisinin in the leaves of different *A. annua* plants, including *ARF1-RNAi* lines, plants transformed with the empty vector, and WT plants. All data represent the means± SDs of three replicates from three cutting propagations. * $P<0.05$, ** $P<0.01$, Student's *t* test. (d) HPLC analysis of artemisinin in the leaves of different *A. annua* plants, including *ARF*1-*OVX* lines, *ARF*1-*OVX* lines, plants transformed with the empty vector, and WT plants. All data represent the means±SDs of three replicates from three cutting propagations. * $P<0.05$, ** $P<0.01$, Student's *t* test. (e) Expression analyses of *AaARF1*, *AaADS*, *AaCYP71AV1*, *AaALDH1*, and *AaDBR2* in the WT, suppressed, and overexpression lines. Heatmaps show the significantly differential expression of genes ($P<0.05$) in *A. annua*. Rows represent differentially expressed artemisinin biosynthesis genes, and columns represent group comparisons. Red indicates higher levels of gene expression and green indicates lower levels. The absolute signal intensity ranges from 0 to +5.0, with corresponding colour changes from green to red. (f) The adaxial surface was observed using fluorescence microscopy of leaves and the density of glandular trichomes in leaves from ARF1-OVX and ARF1-RNAi transgenic *A. annua* lines and WT plants. Bars represent 250 μm. * $P<0.05$, ** $P<0.01$, Student's *t* test.

To further investigate whether miR160 regulates artemisinin by negatively regulating *ARF1* expression, *ARF1* or its mutant sequence *ARFm1* with six mismatches to miR160 were overexpressed. *ARF1* mRNA levels increased <57.6-fold in ARF1 - OVX plants but were 66.7 - 115.5 times higher in ARFm1 - OVX plants than in empty vector controls (Figure 6b). In agreement with the *ARF1* transcript level, metabolism analysis showed that the ARFm1 - OVX lines accumulated higher artemisinin contents than the ARF1 - OVX lines. The artemisinin contents increased by 61% - 94.6% and 168.8% - 246.2% in the ARF1 - OVX and ARFm1 - OVX lines compared with WT lines, respectively (Figure 6d). Based on our RNA-Seq data, the expression levels of artemisinin pathway genes (*AaADS*, *AaCYP71A1*, *AaALDH1*, and *AaDBR2*) were significantly enhanced after *ARF1* overexpression. Meanwhile, compared with the WT, the expression levels of these four enzymes were greatly reduced in ARF1 - RNAi lines (Figure 6e). Furthermore, overexpressing *ARF1* also increased glandular trichome density and the autofluorescence of glandular trichomes on ARF1 - OVX plant leaves (shown by white arrows). However, compared with the WT lines, the glandular trichome density of ARF1 - RNAi plants was decreased significantly and showed weak green autofluorescence (shown by blue arrows) (Figure 6f). These results confirm that *ARF1* is the target of miR160 and is intimately involved in the regulation of glandular trichome formation and artemisinin biosynthesis.

To investigate the underlying mechanisms by which ARF1 regulates artemisinin biosynthesis, we performed a yeast one-hybrid assay (Y1H), an electrophoretic mobility shift assay (EMSA), and transient dual-luciferase (dual-LUC) analysis. ARF TFs are reported to commonly bind to the GAGACA box (AuxRE) of the promoter region and achieve subsequent promotion or repression of expression. To identify the potential binding sites of ARF1, the Plant CARE cis-regulatory element database (http://bioinformatics.psb.ugent.be/webtools/plantcare/html/) was used to analyse the promoters of artemisinin pathway genes (*AaADS*, *AaCYP71AV1*, *AaALDH1*, and *AaDBR2*), which showed that only *AaADS* and *AaDBR2* promoters contain a putative AuxRE. Y1H assays showed that the binding of the *p*B42AD - ARF1 fusion protein, but not *p*B42AD alone, to three tandem repeats of the D2 motif strongly activated the expression of the *LacZ* reporter gene (Figure 7a, b), indicating that ARF1 binds to the D2 motif of the *AaDBR2* promoter *in vivo*. However, interactions between ARF and the promoters of the *AaADS* gene were not detected in Y1H assays, implying that ARF might fulfil its positive regulatory function in part by interacting with *AaDBR2*.

Furthermore, EMSAs were performed (Figure 7c), and a single shifted band was observed only in the presence of both GST-ARF1 and the labelled DNA probe containing the D2 motif. The intensity of the shifted band decreased with increasing concentrations of a cold competitor, and no band was observed when the control protein GST-TF was added in place of GST-ARF1. The results of EMSAs indicated that ARF1 can bind to the D2 motif of the *AaDBR2* promoter *in vitro*. In dual-LUC assays, when ARF1 - YFP was transiently expressed in *N. benthamiana* leaf cells harbouring the DBR2pro: LUC plasmid, the promoter activities of *AaDBR2* significantly increased compared with the YFP control (Figure 7d, e). These results demonstrate that ARF1 positively regulates *AaDBR2* expression by directly binding to its promoters. In conclusion, this study illustrates that miR160 negatively regulates artemisinin synthesis by degrading the positive TF ARF1 of the artemisinin pathway gene *AaDBR2*.

## 3 DISCUSSION

Plant miRNAs play an important regulatory role in secondary metabolism by targeting mRNA degradation. Although miRNA-TF modules have been shown to be critical for regulating secondary metabolic synthesis, the regulatory mechanism of artemisinin synthesis has not been elucidated. Phytohormone treatments, including MeJA, ABA, and SA, have been reported to increase the artemisinin content in *A. annua* by both elevating the biosynthetic levels and the glandular trichome density. Thus, we systematically mapped phytohormone-responsive miRNA profiles in *A. annua* for the first time, intending to broaden our understanding of the biological functions of miRNAs in the biosynthesis of artemisinin. Many novel phytohormone-specific miRNAs, which have not been reported in previous works were successfully discovered. In total, we identified 47 conserved miRNA families in the 10 libraries, of which miR156 was the largest (Figure 1c). This finding is consistent with recent reports of salt stress-regulated miRNAs in *Medicago sativa* and drought-responsive miRNAs in *Camellia sinensis*. The lower abundance and fewer identified targets of novel miRNAs compared to conserved miRNAs suggest that the majority of them may not be functional, whereas the abundantly expressed conserved miRNAs may be the dominant small RNA regulators of artemisinin biosynthesis.

It is well known that miRNAs work by suppressing the expression of target genes. Genome-wide analysis of the degradome was performed, and numerous target transcripts of known and novel miRNAs were identified. To assess the miRNA-mediated regulation of artemisinin biosynthesis, we searched specifically for miRNA targets of identified miRNAs among annotated genes of the artemisinin biosynthesis pathway. However, no miRNA targets were found among

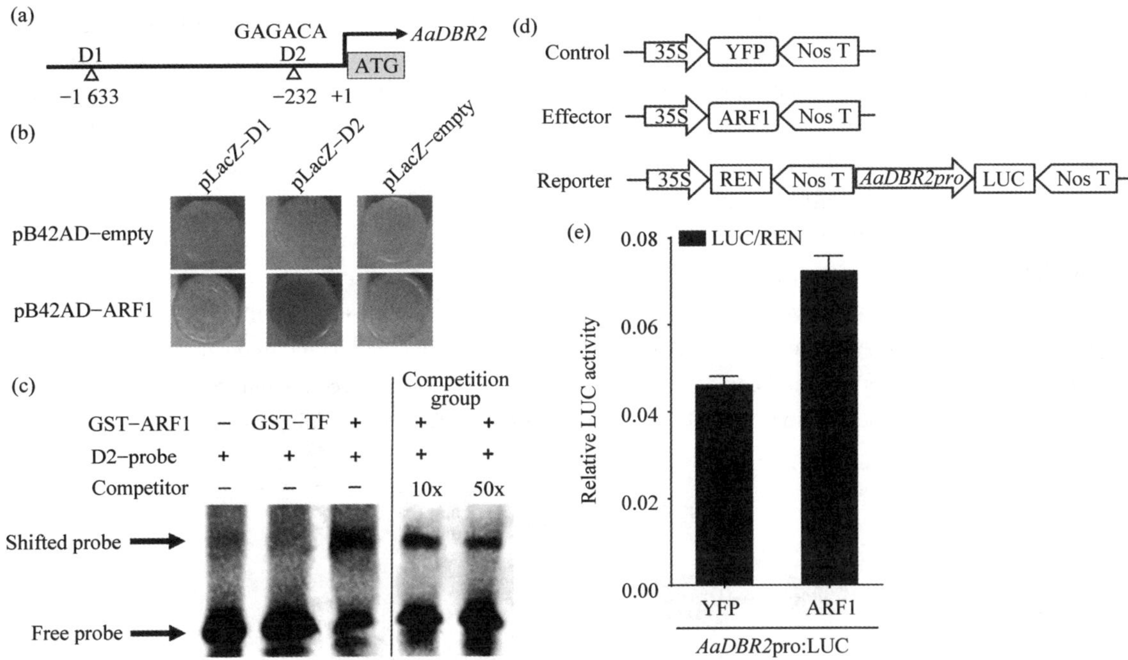


**Figure 7 ARF1 directly activates the expression of AaDBR2**

(a) Schematic diagrams of the *AaDBR2* promoters. The black triangles represent the positions of the 'GAGACA' cis-elements in the *AaDBR2* promoter. (b) Yeast one-hybrid assay of protein-DNA interactions. Empty vectors were used as a negative control. Representative results are shown. (c) EMSA showing ARF1 binding to the second GAGACA box of the *AaDBR2* promoter. An unlabeled D2 probe was used as a cold competitor, and GST-TF protein was used as a negative control. The fold excesses of cold competitors relative to that of the labelled probe are indicated as 10× and 50×. The EMSAs were also repeated three times, and representative results are shown. (d) Schematic representation of the control, effectors, and reporters used in the dual-LUC assays. (e) LUC reporter constructs harbouring *AaDBR2* promoters were used as reporters (*AaDBR2*pro:LUC). Effector constructs harbouring full-length ARF1 were driven by the CaMV35S promoter. The LUC activities were normalized to Renilla (REN) luciferase activities. The YFP driven by the 35S promoter was used as a negative control.

these pathway genes, which implied that the regulation of the artemisinin pathway by miRNA is not direct but may be achieved through the miRNA-TF module. We then predicted that some miRNAs might regulate artemisinin biosynthesis through phytohormone signal transduction during hormone stress. However, their exact functions remain to be verified in future investigations.

miR160 was the most abundant in our sequencing samples and was differentially expressed in response to MeJA and SA treatments (Figure 1f). Overexpression of miR160 resulted in decreased glandular trichome density and artemisinin content in *A. annua*, which reveals that miR160 mediates the regulation of glandular trichome development and artemisinin biosynthesis. Unexpectedly, miR160 also exhibits functions involved in tri-chome development in *A. thaliana*, although the regulatory patterns of glandular trichome and nonglandular trichome development are generally believed to be different.

The members of the miR160 family are reported to be able to regulate the auxin signal transduction pathway by targeting genes of the ARF family and play central roles in plant growth and development. In *A. thaliana* and tomato (*Solanum lycopersicum*), multiple ARF TFs are downregulated by miR160 through a translational mechanism. In *A. thaliana*, ARF10/16/17, which repress auxin activity, is important for the development of reproductive and vegetative tissues under the control of miR160. Additionally, miR160 targets ARF10/16/17 to regulate the auxin/cytokinin balance during nodule formation in soybean. Overexpression of *SlARF10* has been shown to alter leaf size resulting in leaflets with extremely narrow blades. Auxin-responsive ARF4 is highly expressed in type Ⅱ, Ⅴ, and Ⅵ trichomes and positively regulates trichome formation in tomato leaves, although it has not been shown to be regulated by miR160. Our RACE results demonstrated direct cleavage of target mRNAs by miR160 (Figure 5a), but we cannot exclude the possibility that miR160 may also regulate its target translational repression at the post-transcriptional level. In this study, we found that *ARF1* was a positive regulator of artemisinin biosynthesis and glandular trichome formation in *A. annua*. We found that ARF1 could affect artemisinin biosynthesis by directly regulating the expression of *DBR2* in the artemisinin pathway. However, the mechanism of its regulation of glandular trichome development remains to be further explored.

As in *A. thaliana* and tomato, ARFs always function in

the transcriptional regulation of secondary metabolism with miR160 building blocks. However, there is no evidence of a direct link between the module and the biosynthesis of artemisinin. In this study, we provide solid evidence that miR160 - ARF1 in *A. annua* regulates glandular trichome development and artemisinin biosynthesis in a module fashion (Figure 8). Our results provide novel insights into the miRNA-mediated regulation of gene expression and artemisinin biosynthesis in *A. annua*. However, the mechanism by which the miR160-ARF1 module responds to phytohormones and regulates glandular trichome development still needs to be further explored to fill the gap in knowledge of the phytohormone regulation network involved in artemisinin synthesis. Furthermore, in addition to the artemisinin pathway gene *DBR2*, whether there is a regulatory relationship between the miR160-ARF1 module and other well-defined artemisinin synthesis-related TFs (such as *AaHD1*, *AaHD8*, and *AaMIXTA1*) also deserves further exploration. In conclusion, this study clarified the biological functions of the miR160-ARF1 module in regulating artemisinin synthesis and glandular trichome development, supplemented the regulatory network of phytohormone-induced artemisinin synthesis, and provided a new idea for the breeding of high-quality *A. annua*.

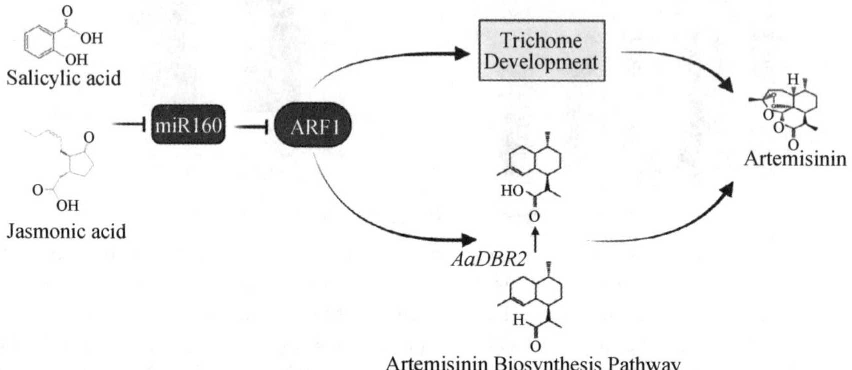


**Figure 8 Proposed model for the regulatory roles of the miR160-ARF1 module involved in artemisinin biosynthesis in *Artemisia annua***

## 4 METHODS

Plant materials The high-artemisinin cultivar of *A. annua* L., named 'Huhao 1', which originated from Chongqing was used for all *A. annua*-related assays. The seeds were first surface-sterilized with 70% ethanol for 1 min, followed by 10% sodium hypochlorite solution for 10 min, and then rinsed four times with sterile water. After that, the seeds were sown on Murashige and Skoog (MS) medium (Sigma-Aldrich) with 88 mmol/L sucrose and 0.7% agar (pH 5.8) and incubated with a photoperiod of 16/8 h light/dark with 7 500 lux at 26 ℃.

The *Arabidopsis* (*A. thaliana*) WT and transgenic plants used in this work were Col-0 ecotypes grown in pots in a growth chamber under a 24 ℃ and 16-h light/8-h dark photoperiod. For *in vitro* culture, seeds were surface-sterilized in 10% sodium hypochlorite solution and 0.01% Triton X - 100 for 5 min and washed three times in sterile distilled water. After conducted for 3 d at 4 ℃, the seeds were sown on plates containing MS solid medium composed of MS basal salts and 20% sucrose solidified with 0.6% agar at pH 5.7. The plates were sealed and incubated in a controlled-environment growth chamber.

Hormone treatments For hormone treatments, 30-day-old *A. annua* seedlings were sprayed with MeJA (100 μmol/L), ABA (100 μmol/L), or SA (100 mmol/L), whereas water with 1‰ concentration of DMSO was used as a mock treatment (CK). Seedling samples were collected at 1, 2, and 4 h after spraying with MeJA, 1, 5, and 7 h after spraying with SA, and 2, 6, and 12 h after spraying with ABA. These treated samples were denoted MeJ_1H, MeJ_2H, MeJ_4H, SA_1H, SA_5H, SA_7H, ABA_2H, ABA_6H, and ABA_12H. To reduce the differences between individuals, at least 50 seedlings were collected as samples at a single time point. For each group, three individual seedlings were used as biological repeats. Pooled seedling samples were collected and frozen in liquid nitrogen immediately and stored at −80 ℃ for further analysis.

Transcriptome sequencing and *de novo* assembly analysis Total RNA was extracted using the Total RNA Purification Kit, TRK1001 (LC Sciences, Houston, TX, USA). All RNA samples were treated with DNase I (TaKaRa, Dalian, China) to avoid genomic DNA contamination. RNA quality and purity were checked using denaturing 1.0% (p/v) agarose gel electrophoresis and a NanoDrop 2000 spectrophotometer (Thermo Fisher Scientific, Waltham, MA, USA) at 260/280 nm (ratio >2.0). The total RNA quantity and purity were analysed using an Agilent 2 100 Bioanalyzer and an RNA 1 000 Nano LabChip Kit (Agilent, CA, USA) with RIN >7.0. mRNAs with poly (A) tails were purified from the total RNA, using oligo (dT) magnetic beads, and then fragmented with an RNA fragmentation kit with two rounds of purification. Then, the cleaved RNA fragments were reverse-transcribed to create the final cDNA library following the protocol for the TruSeq Stranded mRNA Library Prep Kit (Illumina, San Diego, CA, USA), and the average insert size for the paired-end libraries was 300 bp (±50 bp). Paired-end sequencing was performed on an Illumina HiSeq2000 (LC Sciences) following the vendor's recommended protocol. *De novo* assembly of the transcriptome was performed with Trinity. Trinity groups transcripts into clusters based on shared sequence content. Such a transcript cluster is very loosely referred to as a 'gene'. The longest transcript in the cluster was chosen as the 'gene' sequence (aka Unigene).

Small RNA sequencing and miRNA identification Total RNA from the aerial tissue of *A. annua* of the control and treated samples was extracted using the EASYspin Plus Plant RNA Kit (Aidlab Bio, Beijing, China) according to the manufacturer's protocol. Ten small RNA libraries (CK, MeJ_1H, MeJ_2H, MeJ_4H, SA_1H, SA_5H, SA_7H, ABA_2H, ABA_6H, and ABA_12H) were constructed by Solexa/Illumina sequencing (LC Bio, Hangzhou, China). The raw RNA reads generated by next-generation sequencing (NGS) from the 10 sRNA libraries were processed to remove 5′ and 3′ adapters and contaminated and low-quality sequences, as well as those smaller than 18 nt, through Illumina's Genome Analyzer Pipeline V1.5. The filtered reads were subjected to a further filtration step to remove the common RNA families (rRNA, tRNA, and snRNA) with a proprietary pipeline script ACGT101 - miR v4.2 (LC Sciences). Then, the remaining clean and unique reads were aligned against the latest miRBase database, version 22.0 (http://www.mirbase.org/), using the BLAST algo-rithm to identify known miRNAs. The stem-loop hairpin structures were aligned to sequencing reads and mature miRNAs from miRBase using Bowtie. Ten groups of miRNAs were revealed through bioinformatics analysis of sRNA sequencing based on the classification method. The read distribution was checked to meet the principles for miRNA prediction and authentic miRNAs were regarded as described previously. The miRNA sequencing raw data are available at NCBI SRA (BioProject ID: PRJNA756118).

Degradome sequencing, target identification, and analysis Equal amounts of RNA samples treated with MeJA, ABA, or SA at different time points were mixed to generate 10 degradome libraries. The extracted sequencing reads with lengths of 20 and 21 nt were then used to identify potentially cleaved targets by the Cleveland pipeline. Then, the degradome reads were mapped to the *A. annua* genome data. The targets selected were categorized as 0, 1, 2, 3, and 4 as in a previous study. Based on the signatures (and abundances) along the hormone-treated *A. annua* transcriptome data, t-plots were built for high-efficiency analysis of the potential miRNA targets. Finally, all of the identified potential target genes were subjected to an NCBI search using the BLASTX algorithm and GO analysis. The degradome sequencing raw data are available at NCBI SRA (BioProject ID: PRJNA756886).

Differentially expressed target gene analysis To discover the expression profiles of the target genes, 10 independent libraries were constructed from each of the RNA samples from 10 different hormone treatment durations. For each library, all of the sequences were processed to filter out the adapter and low-quality sequences. Then, all of the clean tags were mapped to the assembled unigenes of *A. annua* for annotation. The reads per kb per million reads method was used to calculate the gene expression level. Then, a rigorous algorithm method was performed to identify the differentially expressed genes between the two samples. The false discovery rate method was used to determine the *P* value threshold in multiple tests and analyses. The significantly differentially expressed genes among all of the different samples were judged by the following thresholds: $P$ value $< 0.005$, false discovery rate $\leqslant 0.001$, and the absolute value of log2 ratio $\geqslant 1$. The heatmap of the differentially expressed miRNAs was constructed using the ggplot2 package in R (version 3.1.3).

RNA extraction and quantitative PCR analysis Total RNA was extracted from the young leaves of *A. annua* plants using the TransZol Up Plus RNA Kit (Transgene, Beijing, China) and total small RNAs were extracted from *A. annua* using the miRNA Isolation Kit (Invitrogen, Carlsbad, CA, USA). One microgram of RNA was used to prepare first-strand cDNA using TransScript First-Strand cDNA Synthesis SuperMix (Transgene). First-strand cDNA was also synthesized from the total small RNAs using a miRNA First Strand cDNA Synthesis Kit (Sangon, Shanghai, China). qRT-PCR was performed on a Dice Real-Time PCR machine (TaKaRa, Tokyo, Japan) using the TransStart Top Green qPCR SuperMix Kit (Transgene) according to the manufacturer's instructions. Stem-loop-specific reverse transcription for miRNAs was performed as described previously. The relative expression levels of genes were normalized to the expression of *A. annua* Actin. All gene expression data are from three biological replicates with three technical replicates for each biological sample. All primers used for stem-loop qRT-PCR are listed in Table S4.

Prediction of miRNA targets and 5′ RACE mapping of miRNA target cleavage sites A modified procedure for RNA ligase-mediated rapid amplification of 5′ cDNA ends (RLM - 5′ RACE) was conducted with the FirstChoice RLM-RACE kit (Invitrogen) to map the cleavage sites of target transcripts. Briefly, 250 μg of a mixture of total RNA from the aerial parts of *A. annua* were subjected to an Oligotex mRNA Mini Kit (Qiagen, Hilden, Germany) for poly(A) mRNA isolation. Poly (A) mRNA was directly ligated to the 5′ RACE RNA Oligo adapter (45 nucleotides) from the FirstChoice RLM-RACE Kit without alkaline phosphatase and tobacco acid pyrophos-phatase treatment. The oligo (dT) (15-mer) primer was used to synthesize cDNA with reverse transcriptase. The resulting cDNA samples were amplified by nested PCR according to the manufacturer's protocols. ARF outer and inner primers were designed for the lateral outer and inner PCRs (Table S5). Inner PCR products were cloned into the *Trans1-T1* vector (Transgene) and sequenced. For each target, 25 single clones were sequenced.

Plasmid construction For the miR160 overexpression construct, the sequence (153 bp) containing the *MIR160* foldback was amplified from *A. annua* genomic DNA and inserted into the plant expression vector PHB-flag under the control of the 35S promoter of cauliflower mosaic virus (CaMV) using *Spe*I and *Bam*HI. The resulting construct was verified by DNA sequencing and named *35S:miR160*. The STTM160 sequence was constructed to silence the activity of miR160, which contained two copies of imperfect miR160 binding sites with a 48 nt linker, and each copy had a cleavage-preventive bulge containing three additional nucleotides (CTA) that was made using the method according to the reference. The STTM160 module was inserted between the 35S promoter and the 35 S terminator in the PHB-flag vector, and the resulting construct was named STTM160.

To verify the direct target genes of miR160 and analyse the subcellular localization of the target genes, the open reading frames (ORF) of *ARF1* and *ARF6* were amplified and inserted into the expression vector PHB-YFP using *Hin*dIII and *Bam*HI under the CaMV35S promoter to generate PHB - ARF1 - YFP or PHB - ARF6 - YFP fusion protein.

For site-directed mutagenesis, six-point mutations of ARF1 and ARF6 in the nucleotide sequences of the miR160 complementary sites were designed according to the procedure of Chen using the Hieff Mut™ Multi Site-Directed Mutagenesis Kit with *ARF1* or *ARF6* mutagenesis forward and reverse primers (Table S6) (Yeasen, Shanghai, China). The resulting clones were designated PHB - ARFml - YFP and PHB - ARFm6 - YFP, respectively. Correct mutagenesis was verified by sequencing. For ARF1 - overexpression vector construction, the coding region of *ARF1* was amplified and inserted into the vector PHB-flag using the *Spe*I and *Bam*HI restriction sites to generate the ARF1 - PHB construct. To construct the *ARF1* RNAi vector, a less conserved region at the C-terminus of ARF1 (510 bp) was amplified by PCR from ARF1 cDNA. The fragment was placed in forward and reverse orientation on the two ends of the pyruvate orthophosphate dikinase intron to generate the ARF1 - RNAi construct. All primers used for plasmid construction are listed in Table S3.

*Agrobacterium tumefaciens* infiltration in *Nicotiana benthamiana* The plasmids PHB - ARF1 - YFP, PHB - ARF6 - YFP, PHB - ARFml - YFP, and PHB - ARFm6 - YFP were transformed into *A. tumefaciens* strain GV3101 and transiently infected into epidermal cells of *N. benthamiana*. Infiltration and detection were performed according to the protocols described previously with minor modifications. The transformed *A. tumefaciens* cells were resuspended in MS liquid medium buffer with 10 mmol/L methylester sulfonate and 150 μmol/L acetosyringone at $OD_{600}$ = 0.6 and incubated at room temperature for at least 3 h before being infiltrated into the abaxial air spaces of 5-week-old *N. benthamiana* plants. For the coinfiltration experiments, equal volumes of an *Agrobacterium* culture containing *35S:miR160* ($OD_{600}$ = 1.75) and PHB - ARF1 - YFP, PHB - ARF6 - YFP, PHB - ARFml - YFP, or PHB - ARFm6 - YFP ($OD_{600}$ = 0.25) were mixed before infiltration into *N. benthamiana* leaves. After incubation at 23℃ for 60 to 72 h, YFP signals were observed with a Leica TCS SP5 confocal laser scanning microscope (Leica Microsystems, Wetzlar, Germany). The PHB - YFP construct was used as the negative control. Three biological repeats were performed to verify these results.

Plant transformation and phenotype analysis The resulting plasmids *35S:miR160* and STTM160 were introduced into the *Agrobacterium strain* GV3101, and *A. thaliana* Col - 0 WT plants were transformed with these constructs using the *Agrobacterium*-mediated floral dip method. Progeny from self-fertilized primary transformants was grown in soil for observation of the glandular trichome phenotype.

The overexpression constructs *35S:miR160*, ARF1 - PHB, and STTM160; the construct version resistant to miR160 cleavage, ARFml - PHB; and the RNAi construct RNAi-ARF1 were transferred into *A. tumefaciens* strain EHA105 as described above. The transformation of *A. annua* was carried out according to a previous description. The phenotypes of *A. annua* plants transformed with the empty vector (control plants), *35S:miR160* overexpression and STTM160 silencing were observed at the indicated times under normal conditions. Fresh leaves were placed under a 488 nm excitation wavelength, and the glandular trichome fluorescent signal was imaged on an Olympus BX43 microscope. The total number of glandular trichomes was counted in a 1-mm2 leaf area to measure the glandular trichome density using the ImageJ software.

Measurement of artemisinin content using HPLC-MS/MS Leaves were collected from 3-month-old *35S:miR160*,

STTM160, ARF1-PHB, ARFm1-PHB, and RNAi-ARF1 transgenic *A. annua* plants; *A. annua* plants were transformed with the empty vector; and WT plants grown in the greenhouse were dried at 50 ℃ overnight and ground to powder. Dried leaf powder (0.1 g) was extracted twice with 2 mL of methanol under ultrasound for 30 min. After centrifugation at 16 000 × *g* for 5 min, the supernatant was filtered through a 0.22-μm microfiltration membrane. The concentrations of artemisinin in the final samples were measured by HPLC/MS-MS.

Yeast one-hybrid assay The Matchmaker Gold Yeast One-Hybrid System (Clontech, Suzhou, China) was constructed to investigate the DNA binding properties of the ARF1 protein. The auxin-responsive TGTCTC elements of the *DBR2* promoter were cloned into the *p*LacZ vector, and the ORFs of ARF1 were amplified and inserted separately into the yeast expression vector *p*B42AD. The empty *p*B42AD vector was used as a negative control. Different combinations were cotransformed into the yeast strain EGY48a. The cotransformed yeast cells were cultivated on the SD-Trp-Ura medium, and the SD-Trp-Ura medium with X-gal was used as a selection medium. All primers are listed in Table S6.

Electrophoretic mobility shift assay The ARF1 ORF was cloned into the pGEX-4T-1 vector to produce GST-tagged fusion proteins. The pGEX-4T-1-ARF1 construct and the negative control empty pGEX-4T-1 vector were transformed into the *Escherichia coli* strain *Transetta* DE3 (TransGen, Beijing, China). Then, 0.75 mmol/L isopropyl β-D-1-thiogalactopyranoside was added to induce the expression of the fusion protein for 16 h at 16 ℃ after the *Transetta* DE3 strains were cultured to $OD_{600}$ = 0.6. GST-tag Purification Resin (Beyotime Biotech, Shanghai, China) was used to purify the fusion proteins from the pGEX-4T-1-ARF1 and empty pGEX-4T-1 vectors.

The 50 bp biotin-labelled oligonucleotides for the D2 elements were synthesized (Genewiz, Suzhou, China) and equimolar pairs were annealed. EMSAs were performed using the Light-Shift Chemiluminescent EMSA Kit (Thermo) according to the manufacturer's instructions. Two micrograms of recombinant protein and 100 fmol biotin-labelled DNA with binding reaction buffer were incubated for 20 min at 25 ℃. An ultraviolet (UV) cross-linker was used to cross-link the DNA after blotting it on a positively charged nylon membrane. The biotin-labelled DNA was detected by chemiluminescence and exposed to X-ray film. The probes and primers used in the EMSA are listed in Table S6.

Dual-LUC assay For the dual-LUC assay, PHB-ARF1 was transformed into *A. tumefaciens* strain GV3101 as an effector. The promoter of *DBR2* was fused to the firefly luciferase gene on the plasmid *p*Green Ⅱ 0800-LUC into GV3101 to act as the reporter. Then, the incubated *Agrobacterium* cells were harvested by centrifugation and resuspended in MS medium (containing 10 mmol/L MES and 150 mmol/L acetosyringone) to an $OD_{600}$ of 0.6. The reporter construct AaDBR2pro: LUC was mixed with the effector strain GV3101 harbouring 35Spro: ARF1 in a 1 : 1 ratio and injected into tobacco leaves after 3 h of incubation at room temperature. After incubation for 48 h under low-light conditions, the leaf samples were collected for the dual-LUC assay. The dual-LUC assays were performed using the Promega Dual-Luciferase Reporter Assay system according to the manufacturer's instructions. The probes and primers used in the dual-LUC assay are listed in Table S6.

[郭志英，陈瑞兵，张磊，等. Plant Biotechnology Journal, 2023, 21: 591-605.]

# Genome-wide analysis of *Panax* MADS-box genes reveals role of *PgMADS41* and *PgMADS44* in modulation of root development and ginsenoside synthesis

## 1 INTRODUCTION

MADS-box transcription factors (TFs) are found in animals, fungi, and plants. Plant MADS-box TFs display more diverse functions, and can be largely divided into type I and II lineages based on their evolutionary origin. Type II MADS-box classes are divided into MIKC* and MIKCc subfamilies based on their structural characteristics; the latter contains 12 clades. Type II TFs are involved in numerous aspects of plant development and morphogenesis, but those participated in flower development and flowering transition are most studied.

In recent years, few studies have emphasized on the function of some MADS-box TFs in regulating root growth and development. In the lateral root cap and epidermis of *Arabidopsis thaliana*, the SOC1-like clade genes, *AGL19* is specifically expressed. *AGL20* plays an essential role in lateral root growth and is related to P and S nutritional regulation. *AGL42* expression is enriched in quiescent center cells of its root meristem. *XAL2/AGL14* regulates meristem homeostasis in root, and its mutants cause development of shorter primary roots. ANR-like clade genes (*AGL17*, *AGL21*, and *ANR1*) are specifically expressed in roots and *ANR1* overexpression has strongest effect on lateral and primary root growth. *AGL21* positively stimulates lateral root initiation. *XAL1* is mainly expressed in the phloem and atrichoblast cells of root vascular and epidermis. Involvement of some MADS-box TFs has also been identified in secondary metabolite regulation. In rubber plant, *HbMADS4* and *HblMADS24* regulate *HbSRPP* and *HbFPS1*, respectively, and are involved in natural rubber (cis-1, 4-polyisoprene) biosynthesis. In tomato, *TAGL11*, *TAGL12*, and *TAGL1* influence carotenoid accumulation during fruit ripening and autocatalytic ethylene synthesis regulation. In Cineraria, *ScAG* and *ScAGL11* participate in anthocyanin biosynthesis as inhibitory factors and influence the bicolor pattern appearance.

MADS-box TFs have been identified in many species, such as *Vitis vinifera*, *Phyllostachys edulis* and *Dimocarpus longan*, but not in *Panax*, which is a well-known medicinal and dietary plant that has been used for thousands of years. Approximately 20 species have been identified; however, the most common include *P. ginseng*, *P. quinquefolium*, and *P. notoginseng*. The active components of *Panax* are ginsenosides, which are divided into dammarane-, ocotillol-, oleanane-, and malonyl-type.

The ginsenoside content is generally believed to be related to aspects of root development, such as weight, main root length and diameter, branch root number and diameter, and fibrous root number and length. In this study, we performed a genome-wide investigation of MADS-box TFs in three common *Panax* plants, and found SVP, SOC1 and ANR1-like clade genes mainly expressed in root tissues. We used a ginseng adventitious root culture platform to demonstrate that the expression of two SOC1-like genes, *PgMADS41* and *PgMADS44* were induced by exogenous ginsenoside Ro in the process of adventitious root growth in *P. ginseng*, and they could regulate the expression of cell wall expansion and ginsenoside synthesis-related genes by binding to their promoters *in vitro*. On this basis, *PgMADS41* and *PgMDS41* also increased lateral and primary root growth in transgenic *A. thaliana*. Therefore, we speculated that SOC1-like clade genes *PgMADS41* and *PgMADS44* may be involved in root development and ginsenoside accumulation in *P. ginseng*. The research provides new insights into the coordinated regulation of morphology and active compounds of medicinal plants, for better understanding of root formation and genetic improvement in *Panax* plants.

## 2 MATERIALS AND METHODS

2.1 Panax samples and treatment Four-year-old *P. ginseng* collected in Ji'An City, Jilin Province, in September 2020, was divided into different tissues, including lateral root (FERT), periderm (PM), cortex (CX), and stele (SE) of the primary root, rhizome (RE), shoot (ST), stem (SM), leaf (LFBE), leaf peduncle (LFPE), fruit (FTFH), and fruit peduncle (FTPE) (Fig. S1) after the statistics of main root length and lateral root number were finished, a total of 20 independent biological replicates were obtained. Four-year-old *P. quinquefolius* collected in Weihai City, Shandong Province, in June 2021. The 14 independent biological replicates were collected, as well as the main root length and lateral root number were investigated. All samples were clearly marked, instantly frozen in liquid nitrogen and stored at −80 ℃ for ginsenoside content detection, RNA-seq, qRT-PCR and Pearson's correlation analysis. Samples and data of *P. notoginseng* came from our laboratory.

2.2 MADS-box gene family identification in three Panax genomes *P. ginseng*, *P. notoginseng*, and *P. quinquefolius* protein sequences were downloaded from http://ginsengdb.snu.ac.kr/index.php, http://www.plantkingdomgdb.com and our laboratory (unpublished data), respectively. *A. thaliana* MADS-box protein sequences were obtained from the TAIR website (http://www.arabidopsis.org/) (Text S1). Hidden Markov Model (HMM) profiles SRF-TF (PF00319) and K-box (PF01486) were obtained from Pfam (https://pfam.xfam.org/).

BLASTP and HMM searches were used to identify all possible MADS-box genes in the three *Panax* genomes. First, the known MADS-box proteins from *A. thaliana* were used as queries to search for the *Panax* MADS-box genes with BLASTP (e-value $< 1e^{-5}$), and the sequence identity and alignment ratio ≥50% as a candidate protein sequence. Next, PfamScan was used to determine whether the candidate protein sequence contained the corresponding domain of the reference gene. Finally, all candidate protein sequences were examined using the NCBI Batch Conserved Domains search (https://www.ncbi.nlm.nih.gov/Structure/bwrpsb/bwrpsb.cgi).

2.3 Subcellular localization, conserved motif, gene structure, and phylogenetic classification analysis of MADS-box gene family The subcellular locations of the *Panax*

MADS-box TFs were predicted by WoLF PSORT (https://wolfpsort.hgc.jp/). The conserved motifs were predicted using Multiple Em for Motif Elicitation (MEME Suite 5.4.1) website (https://meme-suite.org/meme/tools/meme) with maximum 10 motifs (between 10 and 100 optimum width and any number of repetitions), and annotated with the Pfam database. The gene structures were analyzed by the GSDS 2.0 online software (http://gsds.gao-lab.org/). MADS-box protein sequences were aligned by Clustal W. A phylogenetic tree was constructed with neighbor-joining method (1 000 bootstrap) in MEGA 7.0 software.

2.4 Identifying key enzyme genes in ginsenoside synthesis and cell wall expansion genes in P. ginseng The common precursor molecule for different types ginsenoside biosynthesis is 2, 3-oxidosqualene, which is then modified through various cytochrome P450 enzymes and glycosyltransferases to produce various types ginsenosides. The key enzymes involved in ginsenoside synthesis include *HMGR*, *MVD*, *FPS*, *SS*, *SE*, *DDS*, *β-AS*, *CYPs*, and *UGTs* genes. The amino acid sequence of acetyl-CoA *C*-acetyltransferase (*AACT*; KJ804173.1), 3-hydroxy-3-methylglutaryl-CoA synthase (*HMGS*; KJ804167.1), 3-hydroxy-3-methylglutaryl-CoA reductase (*HMGR*; KJ804166.1, KM386694.1, KM386695.1), mevalonate kinase (*MVK*; JQ957844.1), phosphomevalonate kinase (*PMVK*; KC439363.1), mevalonate diphosphate decarboxylase (*MVD*; GQ455989.2), farnesyl diphosphate synthase (*FPS*; DQ087959.1), squalene synthase (*SS*; GU183406.1), squalene epoxidase (*SE*; DQ386734.1), dammarenediol synthase (*DDS*; AB265170.1), β-amyrin synthase (*β-AS*; AB014057.1), *CYP716A52v2* (JX036032.1), *CYP716A47* (JN604536.1), *CYP716A53v2* (JX036031.1), and UDP-glycosyltransferase (KP795113.1, KP795114.1, KF377585.1, JX898529.1, JX898530.1, KM401911.1) were download from the NCBI (Text S2).

The 35 cell wall expansion protein sequences of *A. thaliana* were obtained from the TAIR website (Text S3). Using the same method as that described above to identify the key enzyme genes in ginsenoside synthesis, and cell wall expansion genes in the *P. ginseng* genome. The Pfam domain is shown in Table S1.

2.5 Related genes expression analysis in Panax RNA-seq of different *Panax* tissues was performed to detect the expression patterns of MADS-box TFs, cell wall expansion and ginsenoside synthesis related genes. Three biological replicate sequencing libraries were prepared from each tissue, and sequenced for paired-end reads using Illumina HiSeq PE150 by Novogene (Beijing, China). Gene expression levels were estimated in fragments per kilobase of transcript per million mapped reads (FPKM) using featureCounts v1.5.0-p3. The RNA-seq data of different tissues of *P. quinquefolius* from our laboratory (unpublished data) and of *P. notoginseng* (SRP151328) from the NCBI SRA database were obtained to generate a heatmap using the TBtools software.

2.6 P. ginseng adventitious roots culture, treatment, and growth conditions Adventitious root cultures of *P. ginseng* were preserved and subcultured as previous description. Ginsenoside Ro was dissolved in dimethyl sulfoxide (DMSO). The standard compound was prepared at a stock concentration of 10 mmol/L and added to Murashige and Skoog (MS) solid medium for subsequent adventitious root culture. The roots were placed on 90 mm disposable sterile petri dishes containing 0, 5, 10, and 50 μmol/L Ro in MS solid medium and cultured for 45 d to analyze root phenotypes, gene expression levels, and ginsenoside content. This experiment was performed in 40 biological replicates for each treatment.

2.7 Extraction and quantitative detection of ginsenosides The fresh ginseng samples were frozen in a mortar with liquid nitrogen, and then 0.1 g of each sample was accurately weighed and placed into a 5 mL centrifuge tube. After that, the extraction solvent of ethanol (2 mL, 70%) was added to each tube and ultrasonically extracted for 30 min at 25 ℃ and 25 KHz (SCIENT ultrasonic processor, Ningbo, China). After centrifuged at 13 000 rpm for 10 min, the sample supernatants were subsequently filtered through a 0.2 μm membrane filter prior to analysis. Four biological replicates were performed for each sample.

The standards of Ro (CAS: 34367-04-9, HPLC ≥98%), Rb1 (CAS: 41753-43-9, HPLC ≥98%), and Re (CAS: 51542-56-4, HPLC ≥98%) were purchased from Yuanye Bio-Technology Co., Ltd. (Shanghai, China), and the content of ginsenoside was determined by ultra-performance liquid chromatography coupled to a triple quadrupole mass spectrometry (UPLC-QQQ-MS). The mobile phase consisting of 0.05% formic acid in water (A) and 0.1% (v/v) formic acid in acetonitrile (B), and the linear elution gradients were: 20% B (0-0.5 min), 20-80% B (0.5-3 min), 80-98% B (3-3.1 min), 98% B (3.1-5 min), 98-20% B (5-5.1 min), 20% B (5.1-8 min). The flow rate was set at 0.5 mL/min. The ACQUITY UPLC BEH C18 column (2.1 mm×100 mm, 1.7 μm; Waters) was used with a temperature of 40 ℃, sample plate temperature of 4 ℃, a sample volume of 1 μL, and analysis time of 8 min. Electrospray ionization was used with 1 107.50/945.5 (*m/z*) (ESI-) for Rb1, 945.60/637.40 (m/z) (ESI-) for Re, and 955.60/793.40 (*m/z*) (ESI+) for Ro. The monitoring method was set for multiple reaction monitoring. The pressure of the curtain gas was 30 psi, the ionization voltage was 4 500 V, the spray gas pressure was 50 psi, the auxiliary heating gas pressure was 50 psi, and the ion source temperature was 550 ℃. MultiQuant software was used to process the data.

2.8 Subcellular localization of PgMADS41 and PgMADS44 *PgMADS41* and *PgMADS44* CDS (coding sequence), without the stop codon, were cloned into the pCAMBIA1300 vector under *AtUBQ10* promoter control to construct *AtUBQ10*::*PgMADS41* - *EGFP* and *AtUBQ10*::*PgMADS44* - *EGFP* recombinant plasmids. The fusion constructs and the *AtUBQ10*:: *EGFP* empty vector were individually transferred into *N. benthamiana* leaves by *Agrobacterium* mediated transfection method. The enhanced green fluorescent protein (EGFP) fluorescence was detected by confocal microscope (Zeiss, LSM 880, Germany) with excitation and emission wavelengths of 488 and 594 nm, respectively.

2.9 Genes promoters cloning and analysis Promoter sequences of *CYP716A52v2* - *4*, *β*-*AS* - *13*, *PgEXLB5*, *PgEXPA18*, *PgEXPA13*, and *SE* - *4* were isolated using a Genome Walking Kit (Takara Bio, Beijing, China) with the primers listed in Table S2 following the manufacturer's instructions. The putative CArG motif was identified using New PLACE.

2.10 Yeast one-hybrid (Y1H) assay The three tandem copy sequences of each CArG motif in *CYP716A52v2* - *4*, *β* - *AS* - *13*, *SE* - *4*, *PgEXLB5*, *PgEXPA13*, and *PgEXPA18* were individually cloned into the pAbAi vector at *Sac* I and *Xho* I sites. The CDS of *PgMADS41* and *PgMADS44* were separately cloned into the pGADT7 vector as prey at *EcoR* I and *Xho* I sites (AD - *PgMADS41*, AD - *PgMADS44*). The Y1H was performed with the Matchmaker Gold yeast one-hybrid. system (Clontech) following the manufacturer's manual. All primers used are summarized in Table S2.

2.11 Dual-luciferase reporter assay The promoters (genomic sequence before ATG) of *PgEXLB5* (1 363 bp), *PgEXPA18* (506 bp), *PgEXPA13* (913 bp), *CYP716A52v2* - *4* (1852 bp), *SE* - *4* (650 bp) and *β*-*AS* - *13* (1 500 bp) were cloned and fused to pGreenII 0800 - LUC to construct reporters ($PgEXPA18_{pro}$: *LUC*, $PgEX-PA13_{pro}$: *LUC*, $CYP716A52v2-4_{pro}$: *LUC*, $SE-4_{pro}$: *LUC* and $\beta-AS-13_{pro}$: *LUC*). With the CaMV 35S promoter, the CDS sequences of *PgMADS41* and *PgMADS44* were individually cloned into pGreen Ⅱ 62 - SK to generate the effector vectors *35S*::*PgMADS41* and *35S*::*PgMADS44*. The pGreen Ⅱ 0800-LUC empty vectors were co-expressed with the effector as a negative control (*35S*::*PgMADS41* + LUC and *35S*:: *PgMADS44* + LUC). *Agrobacterium tumefaciens* GV3101 (pSoup) was cultured overnight to obtain $OD_{600}$ values of approximately 1.0. The supernatant was discarded after centrifugation (4 000 r/min, 10 min), resuspended in infiltration medium (10 mmol/L MES, 10 mmol/L $MgCl_2$, and 10 μmol/L acetosyringone), and incubated for 3 h at 25 ℃ without shaking. The transformation method followed that of a previous study. There were eight biological replicates were contained for each transformation. The Dual-Luciferase® reporter assay system (Promega) was used to detect the firefly LUC (Luciferase) and REN (Renilla) luciferase activities, and the ratio of LUC/REN was calculated, which were normalized to 1 in the negative control group. All primers listed in Table S2.

2.12 A. thaliana growth and genetic transformation *A. thaliana* plants used in this research were maintained in Col-0 background. The T-DNA insertion line *soc1* (SALK_138131C) was purchased from AraShare (https://www.arashare.cn/index/), the homozygous mutant was identified by PCR, and the *soc1* gene expression level was detected by qRT-PCR (n=3). The CDS of *PgMADS41* and *PgMADS44* were cloned into pCAMBIA3301 vectors at the sites of *Bgl* II and *BstE* II for overexpression plasmid construction. Using the *Agro-bacterium*-mediated floral dip method, two recombinant plasmids were introduced into *soc1* and Col-0 *A. thaliana*, respectively. First-generation seeds of the *PgMADS41* and *PgMADS44* transgenic plants were directly sown in the soil and grown under greenhouse conditions for one week, and then sprayed with 1% (*V*/*V*) Basta (containing 20% glufosinate ammonium) to select positive transgenic plants. Positivity was further verified by PCR and qRT-PCR, and homozygotic lines were selected for three generations. Seeds of homozygous transgenic material, *soc1* mutant, and Col - 0 were sown in 1/2 MS medium vernalized at 4 ℃ for 2 d in the dark and cultured under 16 h light/8 h dark conditions at 22 ℃ for 8 d to calculate the number of lateral roots, and the length of primary roots, which was measured using Image J software. The total of biological replicates was 40 for each line. The plant samples were collected, instantly frozen in liquid nitrogen, and stored at −80 ℃ for PCR, qRT-PCR, and Pearson's correlation analysis.

2.13 PCR and qRT-PCR analysis The Hi-DNAsecure Plant Kit (TransGen Biotech, Beijing, China) was used to extract DNA from 20-day-old *soc1* mutants, transgenic *A. thaliana* seedlings, and the leaf of *P. ginseng*. The extracted DNA was used as a template to identify the homozygous *soc1* mutants, positive transgenic of *A. thaliana*, *PgMADS41* and *PgMADS44* genes cloning, as well as promoters cloning for cell wall expansion and ginsenoside synthesis-related genes in *P. ginseng* by PCR, respectively.

Frozen tissue samples (100 mg), including *A. thaliana* samples, different tissues of *Panax* plant, adventitious root cultures, were pulverized in liquid nitrogen and total RNA was extracted with the EASY-spin Plant RNA Kit (Aidlab Biotech, Beijing, China). The cDNA was synthesized using

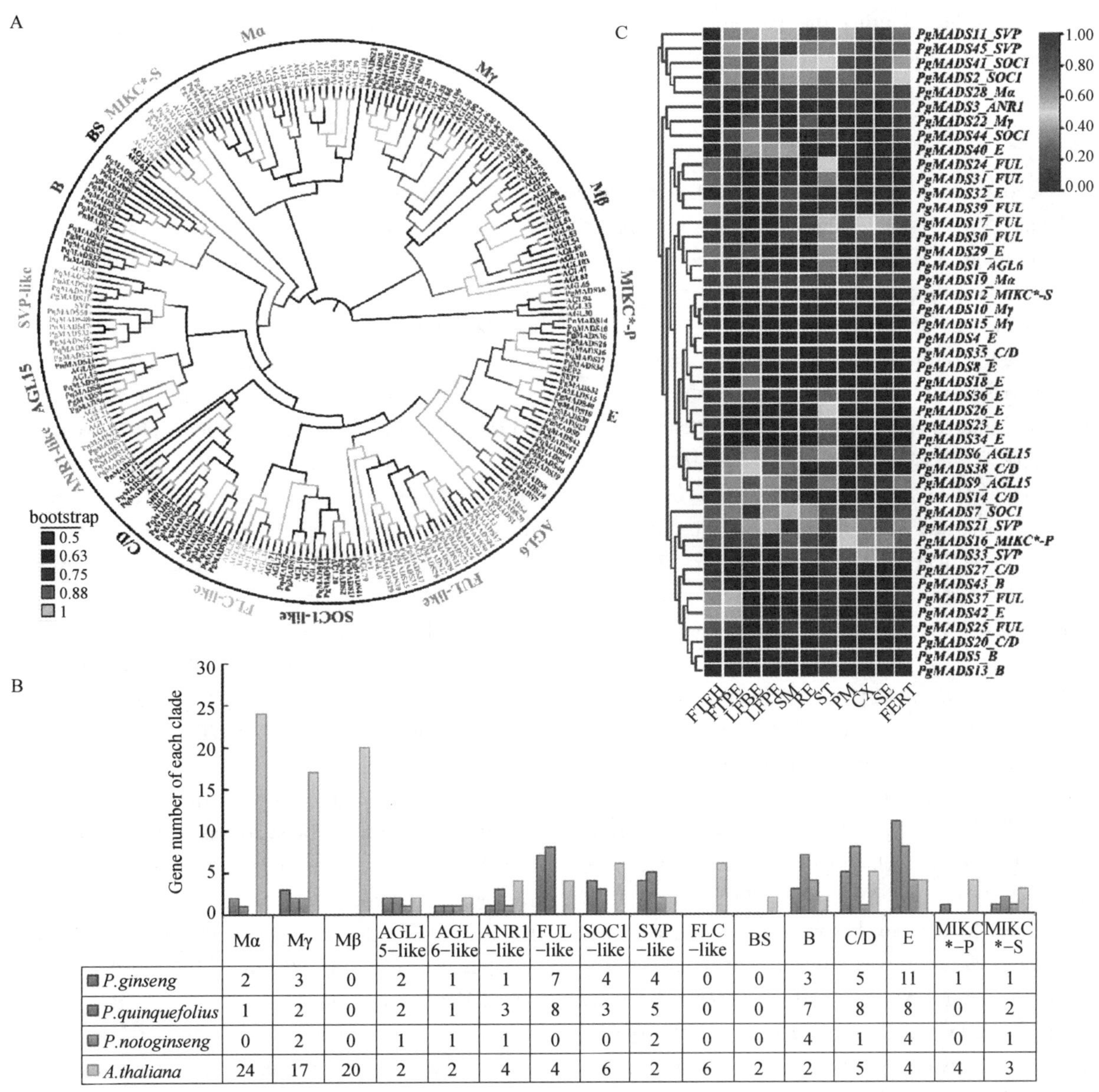


| | Mα | Mγ | Mβ | AGL15-like | AGL6-like | ANR1-like | FUL-like | SOC1-like | SVP-like | FLC-like | BS | B | C/D | E | MIKC*-P | MIKC*-S |
|---|---|---|---|---|---|---|---|---|---|---|---|---|---|---|---|---|
| *P.ginseng* | 2 | 3 | 0 | 2 | 1 | 1 | 7 | 4 | 4 | 0 | 0 | 3 | 5 | 11 | 1 | 1 |
| *P.quinquefolius* | 1 | 2 | 0 | 2 | 1 | 3 | 8 | 3 | 5 | 0 | 0 | 7 | 8 | 8 | 0 | 2 |
| *P.notoginseng* | 0 | 2 | 0 | 1 | 1 | 1 | 0 | 0 | 2 | 0 | 0 | 4 | 1 | 4 | 0 | 1 |
| *A.thaliana* | 24 | 17 | 20 | 2 | 2 | 4 | 4 | 6 | 2 | 6 | 2 | 2 | 5 | 4 | 4 | 3 |

**Fig. 1 Phylogenetic tree and expression profile of the MADS-box TFs in *Panax***

(A) Phylogenetic relationships and subfamily designations in MADS-box proteins based on the neighbor-joining method with MEGA 7.0. The reliability of the predicted tree was tested by bootstrapping with 1 000 replicates. Values higher than 50% are shown with different colours in the branch. These proteins were divided into 15 clades and are represented by different colours. (B) The number of each clade genes in *Panax* and *A. thaliana*. (C) Heatmap showing the expression profiles of MADS-box TFs in different tissues, including lateral root (FERT), primary tissues of periderm (PM), cortex (CX) and stele (SE), rhizome (RE), shoot (ST), stem (SM), leaf (LFBE), leaf peduncle (LFPE), fruit (FTFH), and fruit peduncle (FTPE) of four-years old *P. ginseng*. The colour gradient from red to blue indicates change inexpression values from high to low. (For interpretation of the references to colour in this figure legend, the reader is referred to the web version of this article.)

the TransScript II First-Strand cDNA Synthesis SuperMix Kit (TransGen Biotech, Beijing, China). TransStart® Tip Green qPCR SuperMix (TransGen Biotech, Beijing, China) was used for qRT-PCR to quantify the related genes expression. The *EF-1α*, *GAPDH*, and *26S-2* used as a reference gene for *P. ginseng*, *P. quinquefolius* and *P. notoginseng*, respectively. While in *A. thaliana*, *Atactin2* was used as a reference gene. Expression levels of the target genes were analyzed by relative quantification based on the comparative $2^{-\Delta\Delta Ct}$ method. All primers are summarized in Table S2.

2.14 Statistical analysis IBM SPSS version 21.0 (IBM Corp., Armonk, NY, United States) were used for all statistical analyses. Student's *t*-test at $P<0.05$ was used to analyze the significant difference between control and treatment. The data are presented as means±standard error of the mean (SEM). GraphPad Prism 9 (GraphPad Software, La Jolla, CA, United States) were used to construct the graphs. Relationships between root phenotype (root length and lateral root number) and relative gene expression were evaluated using the Pearson's correlation analysis. The data were tested for normality (Shapiro-Wilk normality test) before analysis of variance.

## 3 RESULTS

3.1 Genome-wide identification of MADS-box gene family in Panax To investigate whether MADS-box TFs are involved in root growth and ginsenoside biosynthesis in *Panax*, we identified them in three common *Panax* plants. The protein sequences of *P. ginseng* and *P. notoginseng* were downloaded from the public database, and of *P. quinquefolius* from our laboratory (unpublished data). Using BLASTP and domain searches, we identified 45 (*PgMADS1* - *PgMADS45*), 50 (*PqMADS1* - *PqMADS50*), and 17 genes (*PnMADS1* - *PnMADS17*) on the genomes of tetraploid *P. ginseng* and *P. quinquefolius*, and diploid *P. notoginseng*, respectively. Most MADS-box TFs are predicted to be located in the nucleus, with few in organelles such as chloroplasts, cytoplasm, and mitochondria (Table S3).

Based on *A. thaliana* MADS-box TFs classification, a phylogenetic tree was constructed, which revealed that the *Panax* MADS-box TFs were divided into type I (Mα, Mβ, and Mγ clades) and type II classes (MIKCc and MIKC* subfamilies) (Fig. 1A). Type II class genes were further classified into 11 clades, including B, C/D, E, BS, SVP-like, ANR1-like, SOC1-like, FUL-like, FLC-like, AGL15, and AGL6. *Panax* MADS-box TFs were unevenly distributed across all clades. Mα clade was only present in *P. ginseng* and *P. quinquefolius*, Mγ clade was present in three species, and Mβ clade was absent in *Panax*. In the type II class, there were seven clades in three *Panax* plants, including B, C/D, E, SVP-like, ANR1-like, AGL15, and AGL6. However, SOC1 and FUL-like clades were only found in *P. ginseng* and *P. quinquefolius*, whereas BS and FLC-like clades were absent in *Panax* (Fig. 1B). Most *Panax* MADS-box TFs within the same clade showed similar gene structures and highly conserved motifs (Figs. S2 and 3).

To further explore the possible function of MADS-box TFs in *Panax* root growth, we analyzed the expression patterns of MADS-box TFs based on RNA-Seq data. SOC1-like (*PgMADS2/7/41/44*), ANR1-like (*PgMADS3*), SVP-like (*PgMADS11/45*), and Mγ (*PgMADS22*) clade genes were widely expressed in the root tissues of *P. ginseng*, particularly in the periderm (PM), cortex (CX), stele (SE), and lateral root (FERT) (Fig. 1C, Table S4). In addition to SOC1-like (*PqMADS7/11/19*), SVP-like (*PqMADS47* - *50*), ANR1-like clade genes (*PqMADS12* - *14*), and Mγ (*PqMADS25*), the FUL-like clade genes (*PqMADS22* - *24*, *PqMADS29*) were also abundantly expressed in the root tissues of *P. quinquefolius* (Fig. S4, Table S4). A few MADS-box TFs were identified in diploid *P. notoginseng*, and only two SVP-like clade genes (*PnMADS16/17*) and one clade E gene (*PnMADS12*) were strongly expressed in roots and fibril (Fig. S4, Table S4). These findings suggest that MADS-box TFs from the SVP, SOC1, and ANR-like clades may play important roles in *Panax* root formation. Pearson's analysis furtherly showed the significantly positive correlations between these gene expressions with the main root length and lateral root number of *Panax* (Table S5).

3.2 Ginsenosides content and expression pattern of ginsenosides-biosynthesis related genes in P. ginseng roots Ginsenosides include protopanaxadiol (PPD) (e.g., Rb1), proto-panaxatriol (PPT) (e.g., Re) and oleanolic acid-type (e.g., Ro). To investigate the tissue distribution of different types of ginsenosides, UPLC - QQQ - MS was used to detect ginsenoside content in different tissues of *P. ginseng*. The results showed that Rb1 was enriched in the rhizome (RE), primary root (PYRT), and stem (SM), while Re was mainly enriched in PYRT, FERT, and fruit (FTFH), and oleanane-type ginsenoside Ro was found in subterranean tissues, including ST, RE, PYRT, and FERT (Fig. 2B).

It has been reported that the expression patterns of essential ginsenoside biosynthesis-related genes affect the distribution of ginsenosides in leaves, fruits, stems, rhizomes, and roots. According to the reported sequence, we identified 112 ginsenoside biosynthesis-related genes in *P. ginseng*, including *HMGR*, *MVD*, *FPS*, *SS*, *DDS*, *β - AS*, *CYPs*, and *UGTs* (Text S2). Using RNA-seq data, we found that the distribution of different types of ginsenosides was consistent with the gene expression profiles (Fig. 2A, Table S6). For instance, Rb1 downstream biosynthesis genes (*UGT71A27*, *UGT74AE2*, and *UGRdGT*) were present in almost all tissues, but the key Re biosynthesis genes (*CYP716A53v2* and *UGTpg100*) were mainly present in primary roots. *β - AS* and *CYP716A52v2* are the key genes involved in Ro, and were found to be strongly expressed in shoots (ST), followed by root tissues. Most of the terpenoid backbone genes, such as *MVD*, *FPS*, *SS*, and *SE*, had higher expression level in the underground than in the aboveground tissues, which is consistent with the finding that ginsenosides mainly accumulate in the root tissues.

MADS-box genes can regulate the synthesis of secondary metabolites by binding to specific DNA sequences known as CArG elements in downstream gene promoters. We scanned the 1 500 bp promoter region of 112 ginsenoside synthesis genes and found that the promoter regions of 98 genes contained at least one CArG motifs (Table S7), indicating possible involvement of MADS-box TFs in terpenoid biosynthesis in *P. ginseng*.

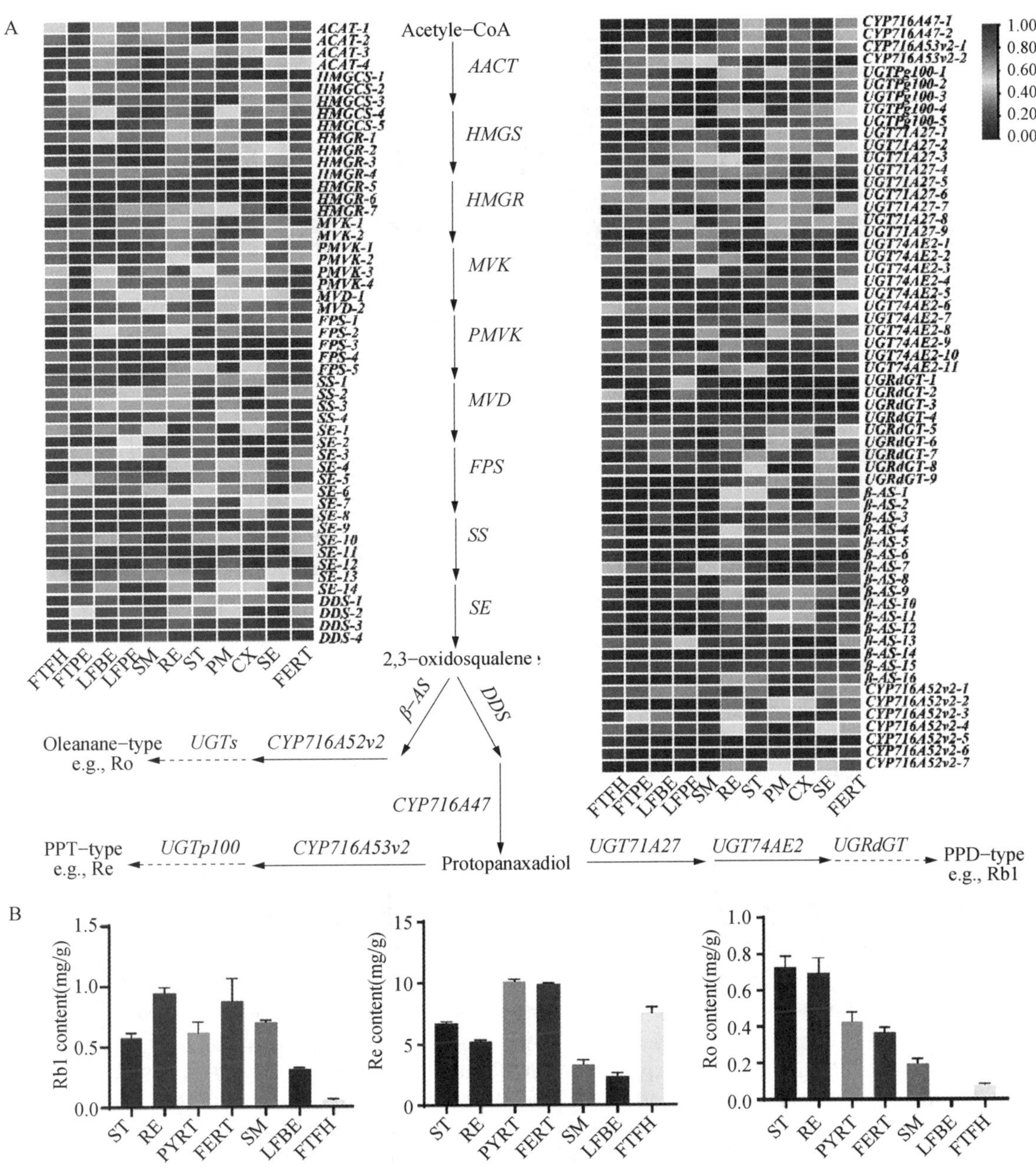


**Fig. 2 Gene expression patterns involved in ginsenoside biosynthesis**

(A) Ginsenoside biosynthetic pathway and gene expression patterns are shown. Heatmap showing the expression profiles of ginsenoside genes in different tissues, including FERT, PM, CX, SE, RE, ST, SM, LFBE, LFPE, FTFH, and FTPE. The colour gradient from red to blue indicates change in expression values from high to low. *AACT*, acetyl-CoA *C*-acetyltransferase; *HMGS*, 3-hydroxy-3-methylglutaryl-CoA synthase; *HMGR*, 3-hydroxy-3-methylglutaryl-CoA reductase; *MVK*, mevalonate kinase; *PMVK*, phosphomevalonate kinase; *MVD*, mevalonate diphosphate decarboxylase; *FPS*, farnesyl diphosphate synthase; *SS*, squalene synthase; *SE*, squalene epoxidase; *DDS*, dammarenediol synthase; β-*AS*, β-amyrin synthase; *CYP*, cytochrome P450; *UGTs*, UDP-glucuronosyltransferase. (B) Ginsenoside content in different *P. ginseng* tissues is shown. PYRT stands for primary root that consists of CX, SE and PM parts. For interpretation of the references to colour in this figure legend, the reader is referred to the web version of this article.

3.3 Exogenous ginsenoside Ro increased the expression levels of PgMAD41 and PgMAD44, and affected the number of adventitious root branches in P. ginseng Ginsenosides have been shown to affect the development of *Panax* plants. In *P. ginseng*, the dammarane-type ginsenosides Re and Rb1 can be involved in the growth and development of adventitious roots by regulating the expression level of *PgWOX11*. The distribution of oleanane-type Ro differs from these two ginsenosides in that it is mainly accumulated in the subterranean tissues (Fig. 2B), but whether it has similar or different functions is unclear. To explore the biological function of Ro, we treated adventitious root

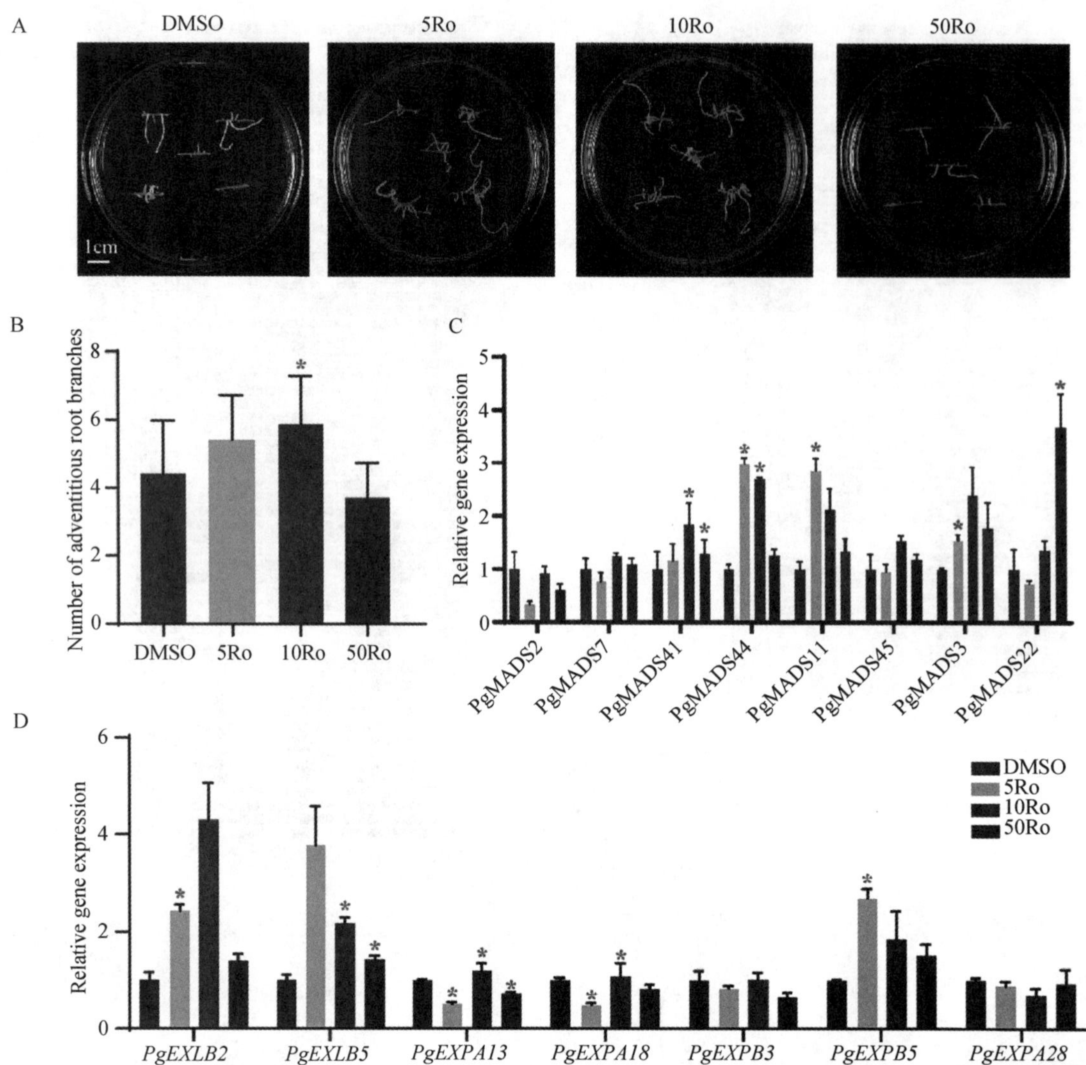


**Fig. 3 Characteristics of cultured adventitious roots of *P. ginseng* by ginsenoside treatment**

(A) Effects of treatment with different concentrations of Ro on root phenotype. Bar=1 cm. (B) Root branching pattern with different ginsenoside treatment (n=30). (C) Changes in the expression of SOC1-clade (*PgMADS2*, *PgMADS7*, *PgMADS41*, and *PgMADS44*), the SVP-like clade (*PgMADS11* and *PgMADS45*), ANR1-like clade gene (*PgMADS3*) and Mγ clade gene (*PgMADS22*) following treatment with Ro in cultured ginseng adventitious root after 45 d (n=3). (D) Changes in the expression of seven expansion genes (*PgEXLB2*, *PgEXLB5*, *PgEXPA13*, *PgEXPA18*, *PgEXPB3*, *PgEXPB5*, and *PgEXPA28*) following treatment with Ro in cultured ginseng adventitious root (n=3). * indicates significantly different values ($P<0.05$) by Student's *t*-test.

cultures of *P. ginseng* with different concentrations of Ro as the elicitor. Concentration of 10 μmol/L promoted adventitious root branching (Fig. 3A and B). We then investigated whether Ro treatment affected the expression of SOC1-like (*PgMADS2*, *PgMADS7*, *PgMADS41*, and *PgMADS44*), ANR1-like (*PgMADS3*), and SVP-like (*PgMADS11* and *PgMADS45*) clade genes, which were mainly expressed in roots (Fig. 1C). *PgMADS41* and *PgMADS44* expression levels were significantly upregulated when treated with 10 μmol/L Ro (Fig. 3C), suggesting that these two genes response to the Ro elicitor and maybe participate in growth and development of adventitious roots.

Expansion proteins are involved in cell wall extension and relaxation, which influence root system development. In *P. notoginseng*, increasing the expression of expansion gene *PnEXPA4* increased root size. Therefore, we investigated whether cell wall expansion genes also play significant roles in the development of *P. ginseng* roots. Fifty expansion genes of *P. ginseng* were identified in its genome (Fig. S5, Text S3), of which seven genes (*PgEXLB2*, *PgEXLB*5, *PgEXPA13*, *PgEXPA18*, *PgEXPB*3, *PgEXPB5*, and *PgEXPA28*) were specifically expressed in the lateral roots (Fig. S6, Table S8). We detected their expression levels in adventitious roots treated with 10 μmol/L Ro and discoverd that the expression levels of *PgEXLB5*, *PgEXPA13*, and P*gEXPA18* were significantly upregulated (Fig. 3D), and their expression patterns were similar to those of *PgMADS41* and *PgMADS44* TFs.

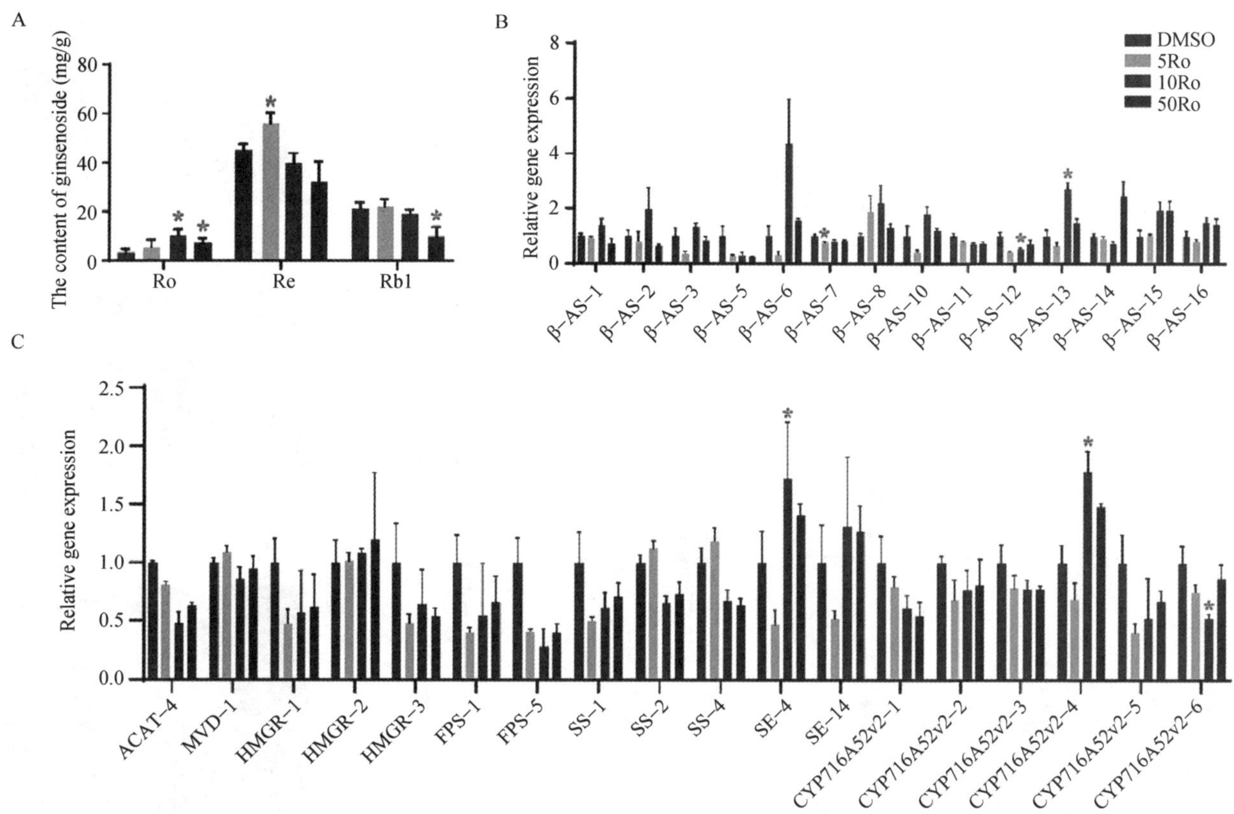


**Fig. 4 Changes of ginsenosides content and ginsenoside biosynthetic genes expression in cultured adventitious roots of *P. ginseng* by ginsenoside treatment**

(A) The content of ginsenoside Ro, Re and Rb1 in cultural ginseng adventitious roots. n=4. (B, C) Changes in the expression of 32 genes related to Ro biosynthesis (*β-AS*-1~3, *β-AS*-5~8, *β-AS*-10~16, *CYP716A52v2*-*1*~*6*, *ACAT*-4, *MVD*-1, *HMGR*-*1*, *HMGR*-2, *HMGR*-3, *FPS*-*1*, *FPS*-5, *SS*-1, *SS*-2, *SS*-4, *SE*-4, and *SE*-*14*) following treatment with Ro in cultured ginseng adventitious root (n=3). * indicates significantly different values ($P<0.05$) by Student's $t$-test.

3.4 Exogenous ginsenoside Ro improved ginsenoside Ro content and ginsenosides biosynthesis in adventitious roots of P. ginseng Using UPLC-QQQ-MS, we also found that the ginsenoside Ro content was significantly increased by treatment with 10 μmol/L Ro, whereas that of Rb1 and Re did not change significantly (Fig. 4A). *β-AS*, *CYP716A52v2*, and terpenoid skeleton-related genes are involved in oleanolic acid Ro biosynthesis. The expression levels of 32 Ro biosynthesis-related genes, including 14 *β-AS* and 6 *CYP716A52v2* genes, one *ACAT*, three *HMGRs*, one *MVD*, two *FPS*, three *SS*, and two *SE* that were greatly expressed (PKPM > 10) in root tissues (Fig. 2A), were examined in adventitious roots treated with 10 μmol/L Ro. The results revealed that the expression levels of *β-AS*-13, *CYP716A52v2*-*4*, and *SE*-*4* were significantly upregulated (Fig. 4B and C), similar to those of *PgMADS41* and *PgMADS44* (Fig. 3C). These findings suggest that *PgMADS41* and *PgMADS44* possibly regulate ginsenoside accumulation.

3.5 Expansion and ginsenoside synthesis-related genes were directly regulated by PgMADS41 and PgMADS44 In the promoter regions of *PgEXPA18*, *PgEXPA13*, *PgEXLB5*, *CYP716A52v2*-*4*, *β*-*AS*-*13* and *SE*-*4* genes, one (*PgEXPA18*), two (*PgEXPA13*), four (*PgEXLB5*), four (*CYP716A52v2*-*4*), five (*β*-*AS*-*13*) and one (*SE*-*4*) CArG motifs were identified, respectively (Fig. 5A), suggesting that *PgMADS41* and *PgMADS44* may play a regulatory role by binding to the promoters. To demonstrate this mechanism, Y1H assays were performed to verify the efficacy of specific binding sites of *PgMADS41* and *PgMADS44*. The results showed that they can interact with the CArG motif at cis3 and cis4 sites of *CYP716A52v2*-*4*, but not at cis1 and cis2 site motifs. In the genes of *β*-*AS*-*13*, they can only bind to the motifs of cis3 and cis4 rather than the other three sites (cis1, cis2, and cis5). The genes had different binding abilities to *PgEXLB5*; in addition to cis4 site motif, *PgMADS41* can also bind to the cis3 site. Simultaneously, they can interact with the CArG motif of *SE*-*4* and bind to the cis1 site of *PgEXPA13* (Fig. 5B).

Furthermore, the dual-luciferase reporter assay was performed to verify that *PgMADS41* and *PgMADS44* positively regulate the expansion and ginsenoside synthesis genes. The complete promoter regions of *CYP716A52v2*-*4*$_{pro}$, *β*-*AS*-*13*$_{pro}$, *SE*-*4*$_{pro}$, *PgEXLB5*$_{pro}$, and *PgEXPA13*$_{pro}$

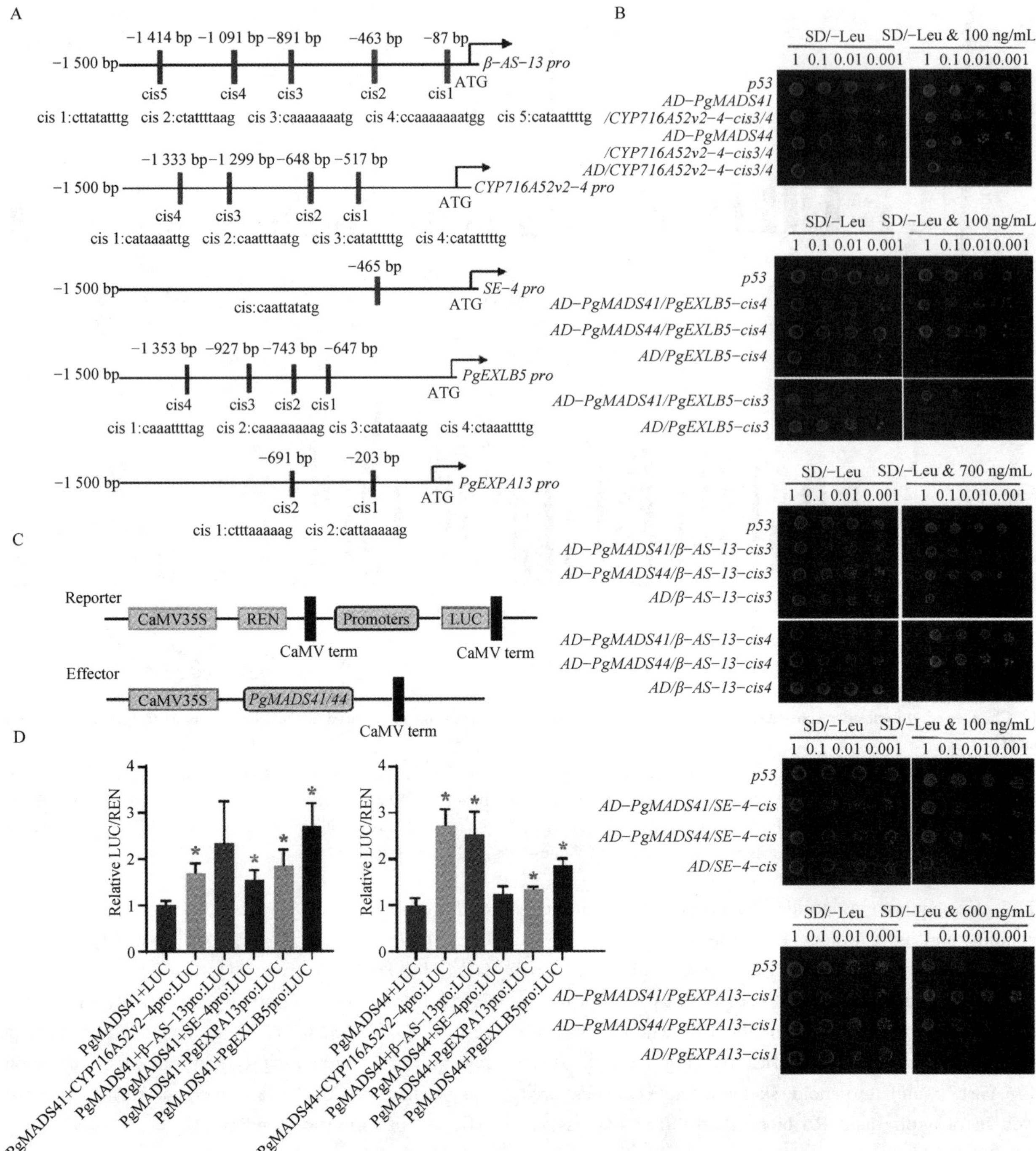


**Fig. 5 *PgMADS41* and *PgMADS44* promote expansion and ginsenoside synthesis genes expression**

(A) Diagram of the *CYP716A52v2-4*, *β-AS-13*, *SE-4*, *PgEXLB5*, and *PgEXPA13* genes promoter region containing the putative CArG motif. (B) Yeast-one-hybrid assay. The CDS of *PgMADS41* and *PgMADS44* were constructed into pGADT7 and the fragment containing the CArG motif of expansion, and ginsenoside synthesis genes promoter was cloned into PAbAi vector, respectively. Different yeast culture dilutions (1 : 1, 1 : 10, 1 : 100, and 1 : 1 000) were grown on SD/-Leu medium with or without AbA. (C) Effector and reporter constructs used in transient dual-luciferase assays. (D) Transient transactivation assays. Schematic illustration of the effector and reporters used in the transient transactivation assays. The *PgMADS41* and *PgMADS44* effector were under the control of the CaMV 35S promoter. The *CYP716A52v2-4*$_{pro}$, *β-AS-13*$_{pro}$, *SE-4*$_{pro}$ and *PgEXLB5*$_{pro}$, and *PgEXPA13*$_{pro}$ promoters were individually fused to the LUC gene as reporters. The firefly LUC and REN activities luciferase were detected by transient dual-luciferase reporter assays, and LUC:REN ratio was calculated. The REN activity was used as an internal control. Values are mean±SEM, n≥8. * indicates significantly different values ($P<0.05$) by Student's *t*-test.

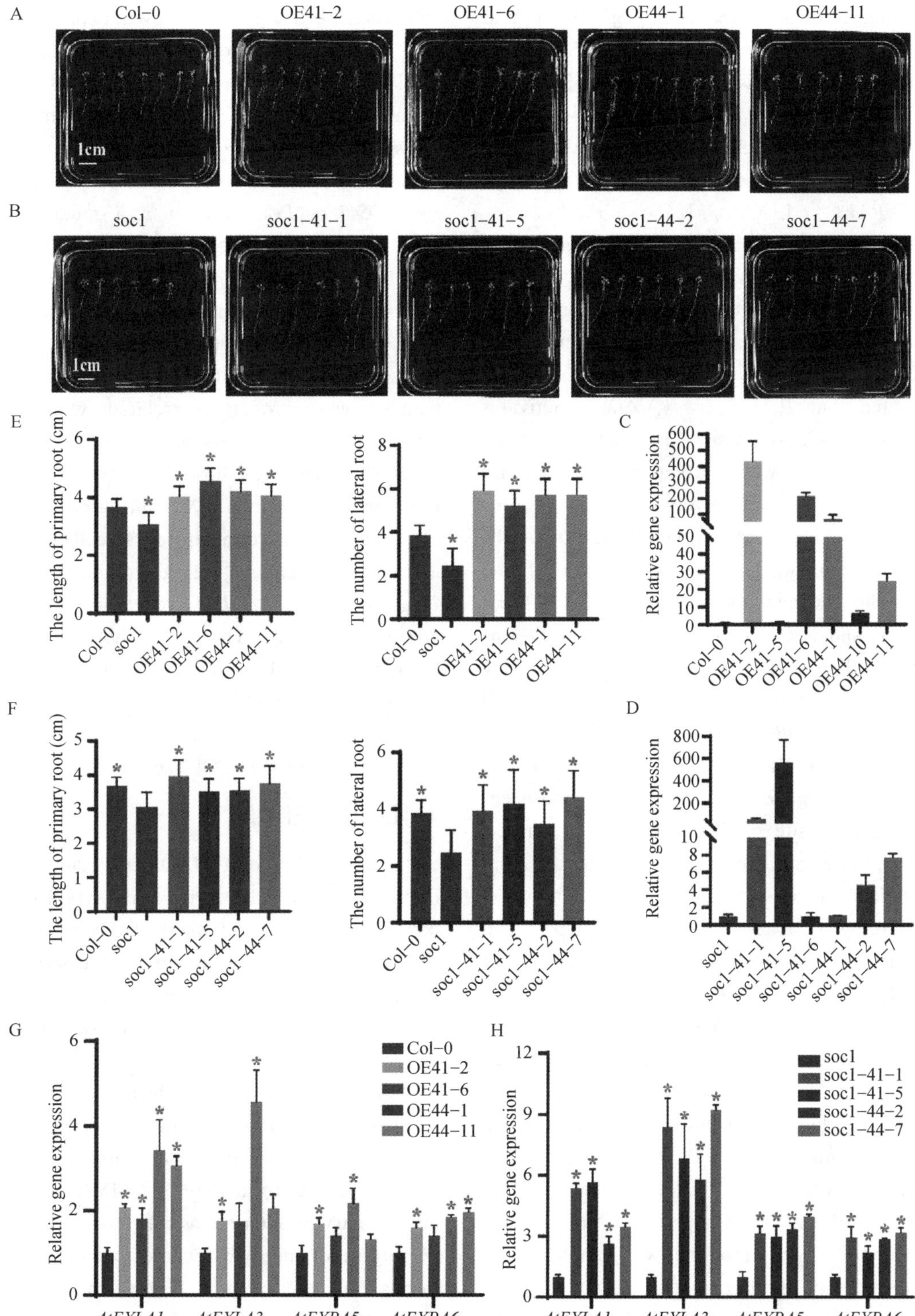


**Fig. 6 *PgMADS41* and *PgMADS44* promote primary root growth and increase the number of lateral roots**

(A, B) Morphology of ten-day-old seedlings for homozygous transgenic materials (bar=1 cm). (C, D) Expression level of *PgMADS41* in three independent lines of over-expression homozygous transgenic plants (*OE41-2*, *OE41-5*, and *OE41-6*), *PgMADS44* in *OE44-1*, *OE44-10* and *OE44-11*, *PgMADS41* in three independent lines of complementary homozygous transgenic plants (*socl-41-1*, *socl-41-5* and *socl-41-6*), *PgMADS44* in *socl-44-1*, *socl-44-2* and *socl-44-7* lines, respectively (n=3). (E, F) Primary root length and lateral root numbers in over-expression and complementary homozygous transgenic plants, respectively (n=32). The significance is compared with Col-0 in over-expression and with *socl* in complementary homozygous transgenic plants. (G, H) Changes in the expression of four expansion genes (*AtEXLA1*, *AtEXLA3*, *AtEXPA5*, and *AtEXPA6*) in the over-expression and complementary homozygous transgenic plants (n=3). * indicates significantly different values ($P<0.05$) by Student's *t*-test. Data are presented as means±SEM.

were fused to the LUC as a reporter; *PgMADS41* and *PgMADS44* were cloned into the pGreen - 62 - SK vector controlled by the 35S promoter as an effector (Fig. 5C). The LUC/REN ratio in *N. benthamiana* leaves cotransformed with *PgMADS41*/*CYP716A52v2* - $4_{pro}$: LUC, *PgMADS44*/*CYP716A52v2* - $4_{pro}$: LUC, *PgMADS41*/*PgEXPA13* $_{pro}$: LUC, *PgMADS44*/*PgEXPA13* $_{pro}$: LUC, *PgMADS41*/*PgEXLB5* $_{pro}$: LUC, and *PgMADS44*/ *PgEXLB5* $_{pro}$: LUC significantly increased, as compared to the co-expression of empty vector. In addition, *SE* - $4_{pro}$: LUC was also significantly upregulated by *PgMADS41*, and *β* - *AS* - $13_{pro}$: LUC was upregulated by *PgMADS44* (Fig. 5D). Y1H and dual-luciferase reporter assays demonstrated that *PgMADS41*/*PgMADS44* activates expansion and ginsenoside synthesis gene transcription by binding to their promoters, which affects root growth and ginsenoside accumulation in *P. ginseng*.

Finally, the subcellular localization of these two TFs was determined to confirm the cellular location of the protein action. The recombinant vectors of *AtUBQ10*:: *PgMADS41* - *EGFP* and *AtUBQ10*:: *PgMADS44* - *EGFP*, as well as empty *AtUBQ10*:: *EGFP* vector, were separately transformed into *N. benthamiana* leaves. The GFP fluorescence signals of *AtUBQ10*:: *PgMADS41* - *EGFP* and *AtUBQ10*:: *PgMADS44* - *EGFP* were clearly detected in the nuclei of leaves cells (Fig. S7). This result was consistent with the Wolf Psort website prediction (Table S3) and a previous study, indicating that the *PgMADS41* and *PgMADS44* TFs played a role in the nuclei.

3.6 Heterologous expression of PgAMDS41 and PgMADS44 genes promoted the lateral and primary root growth in A. thaliana *PgMADS41* and *PgMADS44* are homologous to *AtSOC1* (AT2G45660.1) in *A. thaliana*. These two SOC1-like genes also contain relatively conserved MADS and K domain, and a divergent C-terminal region (Fig. S8). Except for the lower number of lateral roots in homozygous *soc1* mutants (Fig. S9), the primary root length was shorter than that in Col - 0 *A. thaliana*. After defining the root phenotype of the *soc1* mutant, we transformed *PgMADS41* and *PgMADS44* into the *soc1* mutant and obtained complementary homozygous transgenic plants *soc1* - *41* - *1*, *soc1* - *41* - *5*, and *soc1* - *41* - *6* for *PgMADS41*, and *soc1* - *44* - *1*, *soc1* - *44* - *2*, and *soc1* - *44* - *7* for *PgMADS44*. We also generated overexpression homozygous transgenic plants in Col - 0 *A. thaliana*, named *OE41* - *2*, *OE41* - *5*, and *OE41* - *6* for *PgMADS41*, and *OE44* - *1*, *OE44* - *10*, and *OE44* - *11* for *PgMADS44*, respectively. Expression analysis revealed that the mRNA transcript levels of *PgAMDS41* and *PgMADS44* genes were detected in all transgenic plants, but found differences in their expression levels (Fig. 6C and D). The *OE41* - *5*, *OE44* - *10*, *soc1* - *41* - *6*, and *soc1* - *44* - *1* lines were not used for further verification because of their lower expression levels.

To determine whether *PgAMDS41* and *PgMADS44* had similar functions to *AtSOC1*, the seeds of Col - 0, *soc1* mutans, and complementary and overexpression homozygous transgenic plants were germinated on 1/2 MS medium. Phenotypic statistics results revealed that over-expression of *PgMADS41* or *PgMADS44* in *soc1* mutant partially rescued the fewer number of lateral roots and shorter primary root length phenotype (Fig. 6B and F). The over-expressing plants in the Col - 0 background can stimulate more lateral root growth and longer root lengths (Fig. 6A and E). Pearson's correlation analysis also reflected the lateral root number was strongly correlated with *PgMADS44* and *PgMADS41* genes expression level ($r>0.7$, $P<0.05$) (Table S9). These findings show that *PgMADS41* and *PgMADS44* function similarly to *AtSOC1* during root growth.

In addition, we quantified 35 cell wall expansion genes in each *A. thaliana* transgenic line to demonstrate that *PgMADS41* and *PgMADS44* regulation of expansion genes to affect root growth. The results showed increased expression levels of *AtEXLA1*, *AtEXLA3*, *AtEXPA5*, and *AtEXPA6* in transgenic lines (Fig. 6G and H; Figs. S10 and 11). These findings suggest that regulatory networks of root growth exist in plants between the SOC1-like clade TFs and expansion genes.

## 4 DISCUSSION

4.1 The type II MADS-box class genes play a more important biological functions than type I in Panax MADS-box TFs participate in many biological processes, such as root growth and development, and secondary metabolite biosynthesis. MADS-box gene families have been identified for >30 plant species so far, with varying gene numbers in different plants.

Phylogenomic analysis shows that *P. notoginseng* was the first diverged species and formed ~2.32 MYA, and tetraploids *P. ginseng* and *P. quinquefolius* were the last diverged species formed ~0.77 MYA and with much closer evolutionary relationship as compared to *P. notoginseng*. *P. ginseng* experienced two whole-genome duplication (WGD) events, and the recent 2.2 MYA of which contributed to duplicated genes, resulting in twice as many genes as that in diploid *P. notoginseng*. We also discovered that the number of MADS-box TFs in *P. ginseng* (45) was almost the same as that in *P. quinquefolius* (50), which was more than twice that in *P. notoginseng* (17) (Fig. 1B).

The numbers of MADS-box TFs in different species are variable because of the different birth- and-death rates of MADS-box TFs after gene duplication. *P. ginseng* has a larger genome size and has experienced two WGD events, but with much lower number of MADS-box TFs than *Arabidopsis* (107) owing to the severe contraction of type I genes. One explanation for this phenomenon may be related to the fact that type I genes have faster rates of gain and loss than type II genes. However, the number of type II subfamily genes in *P. ginseng* (40) and *P. quinquefolius* (47) was approximately equal to that in *A. thaliana* (46) (Fig. 1B), signifying the type II class genes are conserved in *Panax*. This is further supported by the results of gene structure analysis: type II genes in *Panax* have many introns, whereas type I genes lack them (Fig. S2). Genes with more introns are considered to be better conserved.

Similarly, type II class genes may have more significant biological functions than type I genes in plant development. For instance, *SVP* genes contribute to stem elongation in wheat, are associated with dormancy in grapes, and respond to water deficit and drought resistance in *A. thaliana*, the ANR1-like clade genes control lateral root growth and response to nitrate, and the SOC1 clade genes exhibit relatively high expression in roots. In *Panax*, the SVP, SOC1, and ANR1-like clade genes were mainly expressed in root tissues (Figs. 1C and S4), strongly correlated with the root length and lateral root number (Table S5). These results suggest that the retention duplication of SVP, SOC1, and ANR1-like clade genes may have important in the growth, development, and defense of *Panax* plants during evolution.

4.2 SOC1-like clade genes of PgMADS41 and PgMADS44 can regulate cell wall expansion genes expression to act as an important positive regulator of root growth The adventitious root culture platform of *Panax* is widely utilized as an essential research material to explore the morphology, gene expression, and metabolite profile metabolic variations in diverse root types because of its unique features of easy control and relative stability. Exogenous Re and Rb1, as non-phytohormone regulatory tools, can regulate the adventitious root branching through the *PgWOX11* TFs. Ro is mostly accumulated in underground tissues, such as rhizomes, dormant buds, and roots (Fig. 2B), has a special defensive role against insects, and is an endogenous signaling molecule of ginseng in response to abiotic stress. We also found that Ro has a comparable root development to that of Re; it can significantly increase the number of adventitious root branches (Fig. 3A). This molecular mechanism may be related to the increased expression levels of SOC1-like clade genes (Fig. 3C). In transgenic *A. thaliana*, overexpression of *PgMADS41* and *PgMADS44* in *soc1* mutant can rescue the fewer lateral roots and shorter primary root phenotype (Fig. 6B). Currently, most studies on the function of SOC1-like genes are related to flowering time, whereas the regulatory function of root development is poorly understood. Our results provide more scientific evidence for the function of SOC1-like genes in root development.

Expansion proteins are involved in the extension and relaxation of cell walls, ensuring flexibility and integrity of cells during fast-growing roots. Plant expansions contain α-expansin (EXPA), β-expansin (EXPB), expansin-like A (EXLA), and expansin-like B (EXLB) subfamilies. In *P. notoginseng*, cell wall architecture is involved in root size, which is enlarged with the increasing expression of the EXPA subfamily gene of *PnEXPA4*, whereas in *A. thaliana*, *AtEXPA5* is involved in the development of primary roots. In soybean, EXLB subfamily gene *GmEXLB1* overexpression increases the number of lateral roots. The EXLA subfamily gene *AtEXLA2* is mainly expressed in lateral roots. Expansion genes can be regulated by transcription factors such as *SOC1*. In this study, we found that the EXLB and EXPA subfamily genes of *PgEXLB5* and *PgEXPA13* were highly expressed in the lateral roots of *P. ginseng*, which can be directly regulated by SOC1-like clade *PgMADS41* and *PgMADS44* TFs during adventitious root development (Fig. 7). In addition, overexpression of *PgMADS41* and *PgMADS44* genes in *A. thaliana* can also increase *AtEXLA1*, *AtEXLA3*, *AtEXPA5*, and *AtEXPA6* expression levels (Fig. 6G and H). *PgEXPA13* is homologous to *AtEXPA6* and *AtEXPA5*, and the *AtEXLB* and *AtEXLA* genes are closely related (Fig. S5). Therefore, we speculated that *PgMADS41* and *PgMADS44* can influence root development by regulating the expression of EXPAs and expansion-like (EXLs) subfamily genes in *P. ginseng* (Fig. 7). We preliminarily demonstrated a regulatory relationship between SOC1 TFs (*PgMADS41* and *PgMADS44*) and cell wall expansion genes (*PgEXLB5* and *PgEXPA13*) in *P. ginseng*, which may affect the root growth of ginseng and provide gene resources for improving the productivity of ginseng in the future.

4.3 PgMAD41 and PgMADS44 act as important positive regulators in the Ro ginsenoside biosynthesis Ginseng has a thinner primary root, a longer rhizome, and more lateral roots that contain greater amounts of ginsenosides. Oleanolic acid-type Ro ginsenosides are abundant in wild *P. ginseng*, and mainly accumulate in underground tissues, which is related to the diversity of ginsenoside synthesis gene expression patterns (Fig. 2). However, few studies have focused on the molecular mechanisms underlying the coordinated relationship between morphological characteristics and active compound synthesis genes. In tea, MYB TFs can regulate shoot development and the accumulation of catechins, caffeine, theanine, and terpenoids. In *P. notoginseng*, diterpene and triterpenoid biosynthesis, as well as cell wall structure and root size, can be regulated in coordination by *PnPHL8* TF. *β-AS* and *CYP716A52v2* are the key genes involved in oleanolic acid Ro biosynthesis, and downregulation of *β-AS* gene expression can reduce oleanolic acid ginsenoside. *CYP716A52v2* overexpression distinctly enhanced the Ro content. *SE* is the key rate-limiting enzyme in the formation of (3*S*)-2, 3-oxidosqualene, which is common precursor molecule for various ginsenoside biosynthesis. In addition to the regulation of the *PgEXLB5* and *PgEXPA13* genes, which affect root growth, we also demonstrated that *PgMADS41* and *PgMADS44* can regulate the *β-AS-13*, *CYP716A52v2-4*, and *SE-4* expression to affect ginsenoside accumulation (Fig. 7). This study provides further evidence for the coordinated involvement of TFs in root development and secondary metabolite accumulation, and a new genetic strategy for ginseng breeding.

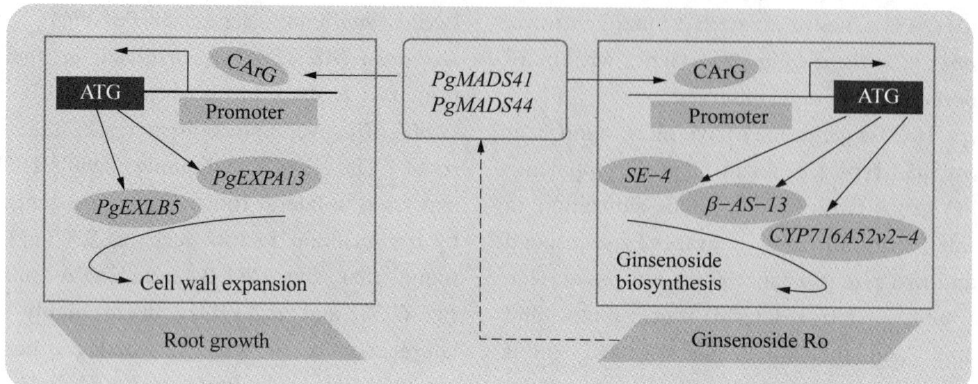


**Fig. 7 Proposed model describing the function of *PgMADS41* and *PgMADS44* in *P. ginseng***

## 5 CONCLUSION

This study is the first to comprehensively analyze the MADS-box gene family in three *Panax* plants. Compared with *Arabidopsis* homologous genes, the number of type I genes was reduced, while that of type II subfamily genes was similar in *Panax*. The type II subfamily genes, SVP, SOC1, and ANR1-like clade genes, are mainly expressed in the root tissues of *Panax*, which may play important regulatory roles in ginseng root development. Two MADS-box TFs genes, *PgMADS41* and *PgMADS44*, belonging to the SOC1-like clade, were identified, which improved the expression levels of cell wall expansion genes (*PgEXLB5* and *PgEXPA13*) and ginsenoside biosynthesis-related genes (*CYP716A52v2-4*, *β-AS-13*, and *SE-4*). *PgMADS41* and *PgMADS44* promoted primary root growth and increased the number of lateral roots in *A. thaliana* seedlings.

Supplementary data to this article can be found online at https://doi.org/10.1016/j.ijbiomac.2023.123648.

[焦红红，袁媛，黄璐琦，等. International Journal of Biological Macromoledes, 2023,233:123648.]

# DNA methylation regulates biosynthesis of tanshinones and phenolic acids during growth of *Salvia miltiorrhiza*

## 1 INTRODUCTION

Epigenetic regulation refers to the heritable changes in chromatin structure and biochemical properties without changing the DNA sequence. DNA methylation plays a crucial role in plant growth, development, biotic and abiotic stresses response, and biosynthesis of secondary metabolites. DNA methylation is a dynamic process in plants that involves multiple coordinated processes, including de novo methylation, maintenance methylation, and demethylation. In Arabidopsis (*Arabidopsis thaliana*), the RNA-directed DNA methylation (RdDM) pathway can establish DNA methylation in CG, CHG, and CHH (H=A, T, or C) contexts by recruiting structural DOMAINS REARRANGED METHYL TRANSFERASE 2 (DRM2). The DNA METHYLTRANSFERASE 1 (MET1) and CHROMOMET HYLASE3 (CMT3) are involved in maintaining the CG and CHG DNA methylation, respectively, while DNA demethylation is initiated by 5-mC DNA glycosylases-apurinic/apyrimidinic lyases, including REPRESSOR OF SILENCING 1 (ROS1), DEMETER (DME), and DEMETER-like (DMLs).

Secondary metabolites are intermediate products of cellular metabolism catalyzed by various enzymes that naturally occur within the plant cells, which are not only involved in plant growth and stress response processes but also serve as precursors of primary metabolites. Recent studies have shown that the dynamics of genome-wide DNA methylation levels regulate with the biosynthesis and accumulation of secondary metabolites in plants. For instance, in the case of strawberries (*Fragaria* × *ananassa*), a reduction in genome-wide DNA methylation levels during ripening has been linked to an increase in anthocyanin content. A series of upregulated genes involved in anthocyanin biosynthesis have been identified according to transcriptome and methylome analysis in strawberries. Both apple (*Malus domestica*) and peach (*Prunus persica*) treated with DNA methylation inhibitor (5-azacytidine, 5-azaC) exhibited a reduction in genome-wide methylation levels and upregulation of genes related to anthocyanin biosynthesis, ultimately promoting anthocyanin accumulation. Overexpression of *AtROS1* in tobacco (*Nicotiana tabacum*) could increase the promoter of demethylation of flavonoid biosynthesis-related genes and activate the gene expression; while silencing of *CaMET1-like1* in pepper (*Capsicum annuum*) fruit resulted in reduced DNA methylation and carotenoid accumulation. These results suggest that genome-wide DNA hypomethylation could promote the accumulation of secondary metabolites in some plants, but the opposite is also true. A substantial increase in carotenoid content during orange (*Citrus sinensis*) fruit ripening is accompanied by an increase in genome-wide methylation levels. In tomato (*Solanum lycopersicum*) fruit, the content of secondary metabolites such as lycopene, lutein, and β-carotene were substantially reduced when treated with 5-azaC. Thus, DNA methylation plays key roles in secondary metabolites regulation in plants.

*Salvia miltiorrhiza*, as a medicinal model plant, has been widely used in the treatment of metabolic disorders and cardiovascular diseases, and its therapeutic effects are highly associated with 2 types of secondary metabolites: fat-soluble tanshinones and water-soluble salvianolic acids. The tanshinones biosynthesis is initiated from the mevalonate (MVA) pathway in the cytoplasm or the 2-*C*-methyl-d-erythritol 4-phosphate (MEP) pathway in the plastid. Both pathways produce isopentenyl diphosphate or dimethylallyl diphosphate as intermediates, which can be catalyzed by geranyl diphosphate synthase (GPPS) or geranylgeranyl diphosphate synthase (GGPPS) to produce the diterpenoid precursor geranylgeranyl diphosphate via the MEP pathway. Subsequently, geranylgeranyl diphosphate is successively catalyzed by a series of enzymes including copalyldiphosphate synthase (CPS) and kaurene synthase-like (KSL) to produce miltiradiene; an important intermediate in the tanshinones branched pathway. The final production of tanshinones is catalyzed by cytochrome P450 terminal oxygenases (CYP450s) represented by CYP76A and CYP71D. The biosynthetic precursors of salvianolic acid are phenylalanine and tyrosine. The phenylalanine pathway produces 4-coumaroyl-CoA through a series of catalysis by phenylalanine ammonia-lyase (PAL), cinnamate 4-hydroxylase (C4H), and 4-Coumarate-CoA ligase (4CL). In the tyrosine-derived pathway, a series of enzymes: tyrosine aminotransferase (TAT), hydroxyphenylpyruvate reductase (HPPR), and an unknown cytochrome P450-related enzyme catalyze the production of 3, 4-dihydroxyphenyllactic acid. The products of both pathways are then catalyzed by rosmarinic acid synthase (RAS) and cytochrome P450 to produce rosmarinic acid (RA), which is further catalyzed to produce salvianolic acid.

Recent studies have demonstrated that treatment of *S. miltiorrhiza* hairy roots with 5-azaC led to a 1 to 1.5-fold increase in the content of tanshinone, and demethylation was observed in the promoter region of the *CPS* gene. Li et al. reported that DNA methylation levels in 2-yr-old *S. miltiorrhiza* roots were reduced in July compared to March. These findings suggest that the biosynthesis of tanshinone in *S. miltiorrhiza* may be regulated by DNA methylation. However, the impact of global DNA methylation on secondary metabolites biosynthesis in *S. miltiorrhiza* remains largely unknown. To investigate the regulatory role of DNA methylation in tanshinones and salvianolic acid biosynthesis in *S. miltiorrhiza*, we combined targeted metabolite assays, whole-genome bisulfite sequencing, and transcriptome sequencing across 3 growth stages. We found that tanshinones and phenolic acid content gradually increased during growth in *S. miltiorrhiza* roots. Remarkably, we observed a considerable surge in global DNA methylation levels during early root growth, coinciding with the upregulation of pivotal methylation enzyme genes. These changes corresponded with marked modifications in the expression of key genes that are responsible for tanshinones and salvianolic acid biosynthesis. Our results provide clues to unravel the dynamic nature of DNA methylation during *S. miltiorrhiza* root growth and elucidate its profound involvement in tanshinones and phenolic acid accumulation.

## 2 RESULTS

Dynamic changes of tanshinones and phenolic acid content in roots during *S. miltiorrhiza* growth To evaluate the dynamic changes in the content of tanshinones and phenolic acids during the root development, roots grown for 40 d, 60 d, and 90 d (referred to as r40, r60, and r90, respectively; Fig. 1A) were used for target metabolic analysis. A total of 5 tanshinones and 3 phenolic acids were detected (Fig. 1, B and C). Notably, the contents of most tanshinones (cryptotanshinone, tanshinone I, tanshinone IIA, and rosmariquinone) and phenolic acids (rosmarinic

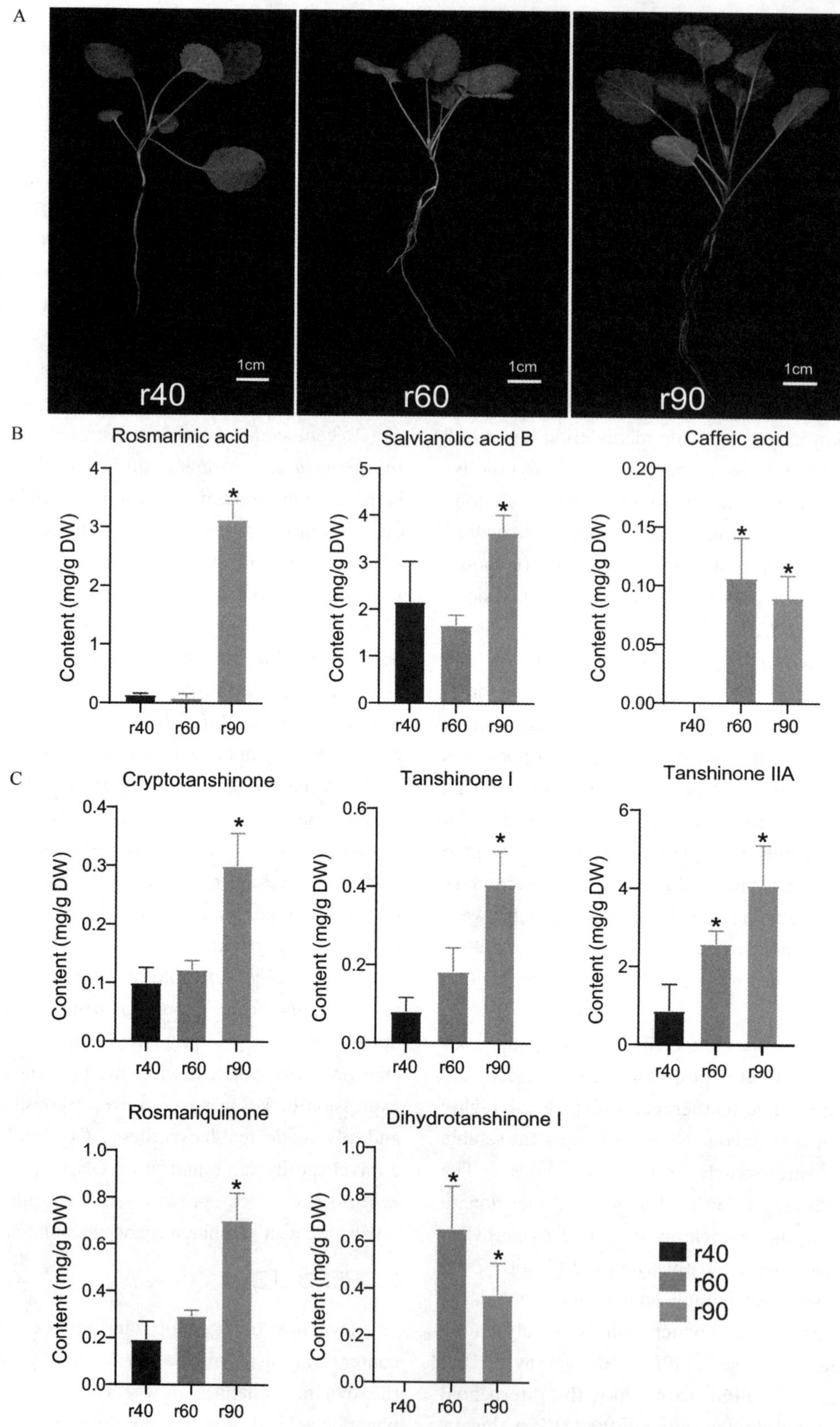


**Figure 1 Root growth and targeted metabolites accumulation of *Salvia miltiorrhiza***

(A) The roots of *Salvia miltiorrhiza* at different growth stages. r40, r60, and r90 indicate the root grown at 40, 60, and 90 d, respectively. (B) Changes in the content of phenolic acids. (C) Changes in the content of tanshinones. Each bar shows the mean ± SE of triplicate assays. * Indicates a statistically significant difference as relative to the value at r40 for each metabolite at $P < 0.05$, respectively. Student's *t* test. Scale bars.

acid and salvianolic acid B) showed a gradually increasing trend as the root growth. For example, the fold-changes of cryptotanshinone, tanshinone I, tanshinone IIA, rosmariquinone, rosmarinic acid, and salvianolic acid B were 3.0, 5.0, 4.7, 3.6, 22.3, and 1.7, respectively, in r90_VS_r40 group. In addition, caffeic acid and dihydrotanshinone I have the highest content at r60, and both of them could not be detected at r40. Compared to r40, the contents of all the metabolites at r90 significantly increased. These results indicated that the root growth was accompanied by the accumulation of tanshinones and phenolic acids in *S. miltiorrhiza*.

Characteristics of the *S. miltiorrhiza* DNA methylome In order to investigate whether the DNA methylation dynamics associate with tanshinones and phenolic acid accumulation during root growth in *S. miltiorrhiza*, we performed whole-genome bisulfite sequencing using r40, r60, and r90 and generated single-base resolution maps of DNA methylation. To ensure accuracy and reliability of the data, we prepared 3 biological replicates for each growth stage and evaluated the correlation between replicates. The result showed high correlation coefficients for all 3 samples (Supplemental Fig. S1). Over 123 million reads were sequenced per replicate, yielding more than 40 G raw data, and approximately 55% of the reads were mapped to the reference genome using Bismark, covering more than 81% of the genomic cytosines in each sample, with a Q30 score exceeding 90.18%, resulting in an average of > 13-fold coverage (Supplemental Table S1). The bisulfite conversion rate for all libraries was higher than 99.40% (Supplemental Table S1). The sequencing coverage and depth of our data are comparable to those of other plants, such as *Arabidopsis* and orange, indicating that the data are valid and reliable for further analysis.

From the global DNA methylation analysis, we observed that the DNA methylation levels in CHH context of r90 (59.53% in CG, 42.87% in CHG, 15.63% in CHH) were higher than r40 (59.56% in CG, 43.32% in CHG, 13.58% in CHH) and r60 (59.84% in CG, 43.63% in CHG, 13.53% in CHH), which was also consistent among the 3 biological replicates (Fig. 2A). We found that 911.46 million and 783.69 million cytosines were methylated at r40 and r60, respectively, including 206.72 million (22.68%) and 190.53 million (24.31%) in mCG; 173.97 million (19.09%) and 160.73 million (20.51%) in mCHG; and 530.77 million (58.23%) and 432.43 million (51.18%) in mCHH, respectively. However, the number of methylated cytosines was comparatively higher at r90 than r40 and r60, with 946.72 million methylated cytosines. Intriguingly, the mCHH site (561.86 million, 59.35%) was substantially increased in r90 compared to the mCG and mCHG contexts (Fig. 2B). This indicated that the methylation level and the number of methylated cytosines were higher at r90 than r40 and r60, especially in CHH context. As a result, both the rise in total mC quantity and the increase in the level of existing mC methylation may have contributed to the increase in DNA methylation from r40 to r90. The genome-wide average methylation levels of 8 chromosomes were shown in Fig. 2C. Our data showed that the DNA methylation level was higher in TE-rich regions in all 3 contexts, but lower in gene-rich regions, which is consistent with previous studies in *Arabidopsis* and rice, indicating a conserved methylation feature in the genome of *S. miltiorrhiza*.

DNA methylation patterns in genes and transposable element regions We examined the DNA methylation profiles in genes and transposable element (TE) regions and their flanking regions within 2 kb. As shown in Fig. 3, we found that different stages exhibited a highly consistent pattern of CG, CHG, and CHH methylation in both gene and TE regions. Additionally, the lowest DNA methylation levels were observed near the transcription start site of genes. As for TE regions, the DNA methylation levels in CG, CHG, and CHH contexts were substantially higher than that in the flanking regions, particularly in CG and CHG contexts. Although the DNA methylation patterns were similar among different stages, the DNA methylation levels increased in CHH context at r90 compared to r40 and r60, regardless to genes or TE regions (Fig. 3).

Given that approximately 62.12% of *S. miltiorrhiza* genome consists of TE sequences, we investigated the relationship between DNA methylation and TEs. Firstly, we profiled the DNA methylation patterns of different TEs in the *S. miltiorrhiza* genome (Supplemental Fig. S2) and found that LTR_Gypsy, DNA/Helitron, and DNA/DTT were more abundant (154 974 for LTR_Gypsy, 219 274 for DNA/Helitron, and 217 583 for DNA/DTT). We also observed that CG and CHG methylation levels were relatively stable and high across all TE types, although the methylation levels were low in CHH context, the DNA methylation levels were increased for all TE types at r90 compared to r40 and r60 (Fig. 4A, Supplemental Table S2). Specifically, we monitored a total of 374 295 TEs with increased levels of CHH methylation at different stages of *S. miltiorrhiza*, among which the main TE types were DNA/DTT (88 408, 23.62%), DNA/Helitron (74 260, 19.84%), and LTR/Gypsy (57 529, 15.37%) (Fig. 4, B and C).

Next, we investigated the relationship between DNA methylation and TE length. As shown in Fig. 4D, we roughly divided TEs into 6 groups according to their lengths (rank1: ≤100 bp, rank2: 101 to 200 bp, rank3: 201 to 500 bp, rank4: 501 to 1 000 bp, rank5: 1 001 to 5 000 bp, rank6: >5 000 bp), the DNA methylation levels of TEs with

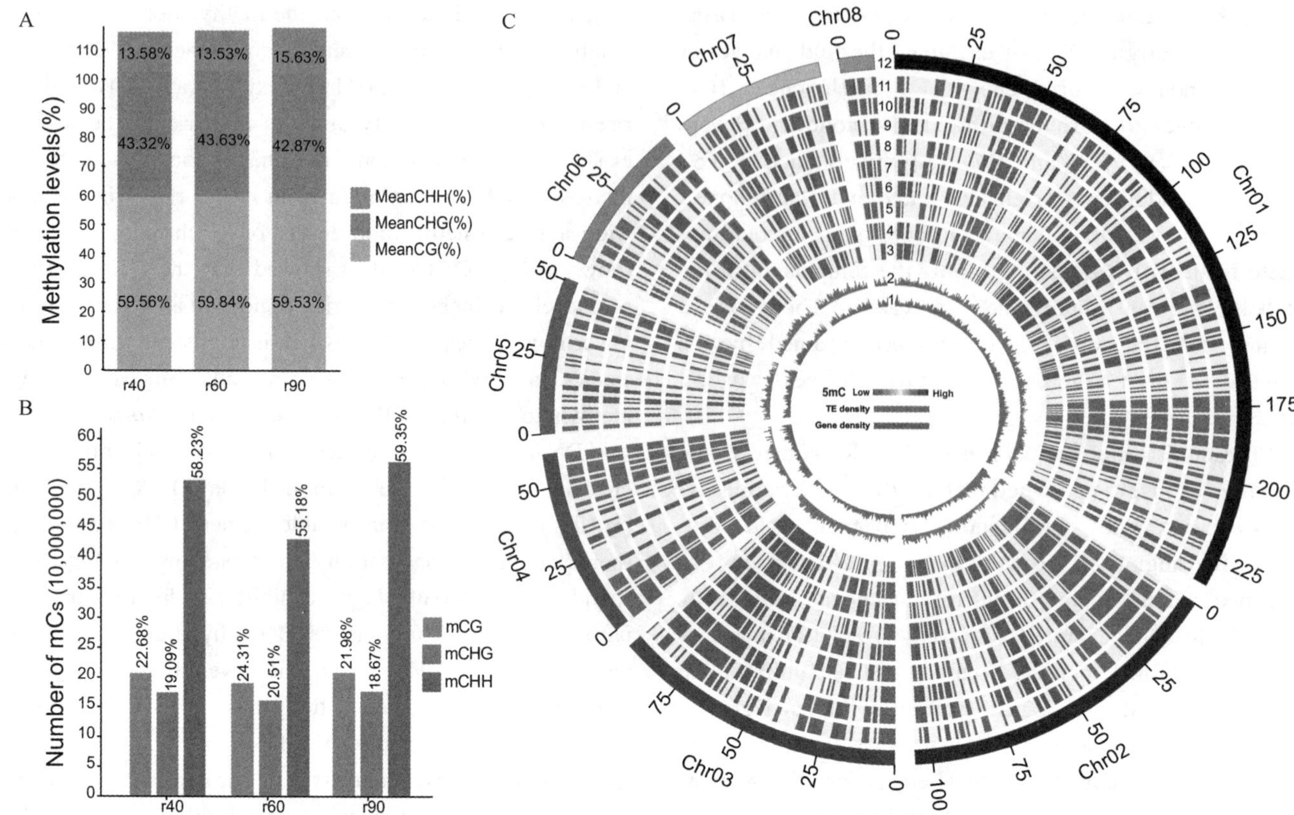


**Figure 2  DNA methylation landscape of *S. miltiorrhiza* root at different stages**

(A) Genome-wide average DNA methylation levels of r40, r60, and r90 in CG, CHG, and CHH contexts, respectively. (B) The relative proportion of methyl-cytosines in CG, CHG, and CHH contexts of r40, r60, and r90. (C) Circos plot showing the gene density, TE density, and DNA methylation levels of all 3 contexts at 3 stages. (1): gene density; (2): TE density; (3), (4), (5): DNA methylation levels in the CG, CHG, and CHH contexts at r40, respectively; (6), (7), (8): DNA methylation levels in the CG, CHG, and CHH contexts at r60, respectively; (9), (10), (11): DNA methylation levels in the CG, CHG, and CHH contexts at r90, respectively.

500 to 5 000 bp length were higher in CG and CHG, while the DNA methylation levels of TEs with < 500 bp were higher in CHH.

Characterization of differential methylation sites (DMCs) and differential methylation regions (DMRs) at different periods of *S. miltiorrhiza* growth  Differences in DNA methylation between different growth stages can be quantitatively characterized by differential methylation sites (DMCs) and differential methylation regions (DMRs). We used r40 as the control to identify the DMCs and DMRs for other growth stages. In total, we identified 642 019 DMCs in r60_VS_r40 group, of which 319 644 were hyper-methylated DMCs (49.79%) and 322 375 were hypo-methylated DMCs (50.21%), and 809 026 DMCs in r90_VS_r40 group, of which 455 937 (56.36%) were hyper-DMCs and 353 089 (43.64%) were hypo-DMCs. The number of DMCs in the r60_VS_r40 and r90_VS_r40 stages was comparable in CG and CHG methylation. However, in CHH, the number of DMCs in r60_VS_r40 was substantially lower than in r90_VS_r40. We found 185 872 significantly differentially methylated CHH sites in r90_VS_r40, of which hyper-DMCs accounted for 156 996 (84.46%) (Fig. 5A), indicating an increased DNA methylation occurred in the CHH context in r90_VS_r40.

In addition, the number of the mCHH-DMRs (31 310 and 84 720) in each comparison group (r60_VS_r40 and r90_VS_r40) was much larger than the number of mCG-DMRs (21 322 and 18 838) and mCHG-DMRs (24 594 and 19 660). In CHH context, we identified 19 025 and 78 599 hyper-DMRs in r60_VS_r40 and r90_VS_r40, respectively. The number of hyper-DMRs in r90_VS_r40 was considerably higher than that in r60_VS_r40 (Fig. 5B). Subsequently, we sought to investigate the distribution of DMRs overlapping gene features in the r90_VS_r40, including promoters, exons, introns, and intergenic regions. We found that DMRs were mostly enriched in the intergenic (63.86%), followed by the promoter (21.65%) and gene body (14.49%) (exon: 10.69%, intron: 3.80%), either for hyper-DMRs or hypo-DMRs (Fig. 5C). These results indicated that DMRs primarily occurred in intergenic regions. Additionally, we obtained 14 391 hyper-DMRs from promoter regions, suggesting that gene expression regulation may be influenced

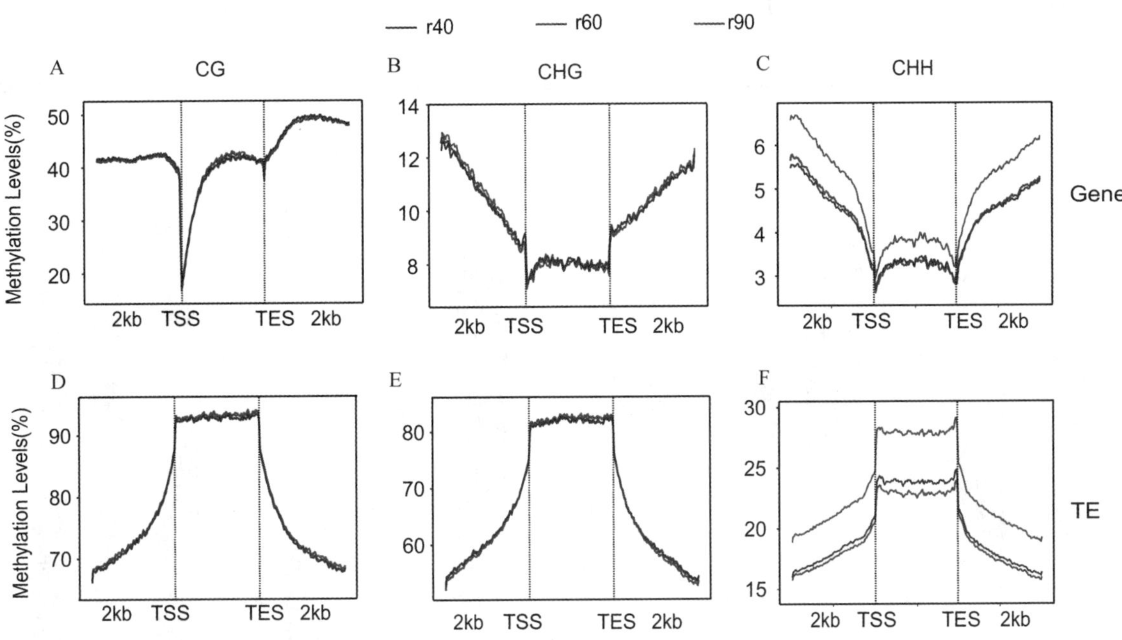


**Figure 3 DNA methylation patterns of gene and TE regions**

(A to C) Average DNA methylation levels across genes and their flanking regions within 2 kb. (D to F) Average DNA methylation levels across TEs and their flanking regions within 2 kb. The dashed line indicates the transcription start site (TSS) and transcription end site (TES).

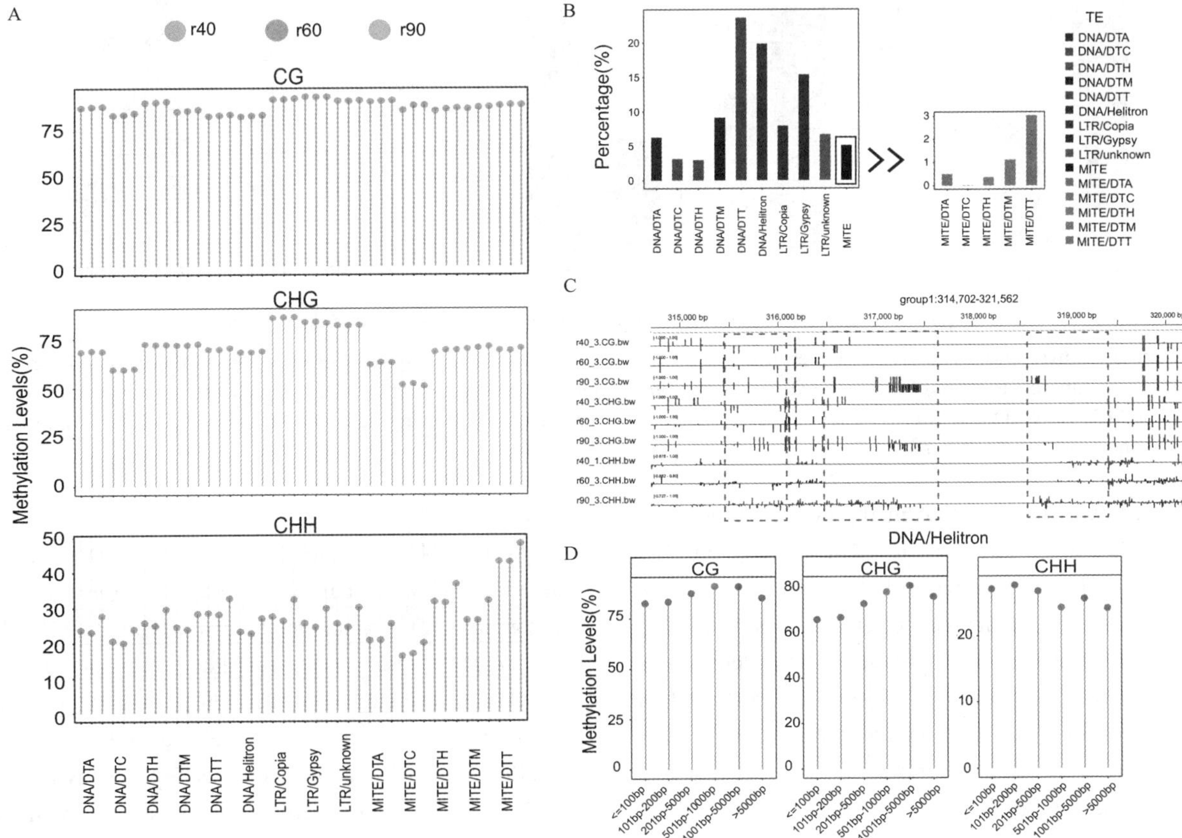


**Figure 4 Methylation profiles of different transposable elements (TEs) in *S. miltiorrhiza* genome**

(A) DNA methylation of different types of TEs in CG, CHG, and CHH contexts for 3 stages, blue: r40, red: r60, green: r90. (B) Percentage of different types of TE with increased CHH methylation at r90 compared to r40 and r60. (C) Representative TEs (DNA/Helitron) with increased CHH methylation at r90. (D) DNA methylation levels of TEs with different lengths in different contexts.

by promoter region methylation (Fig. 5, B and C). We examined the relationship of DMRs among the 3 contexts and analyzed the overlap between CG-, CHG-, and CHH-DMRs in r90_VS_r40. Only a small number of DMRs were present in all 3 contexts, indicating that various types of methylation underwent different methylation modifications (Fig. 5D).

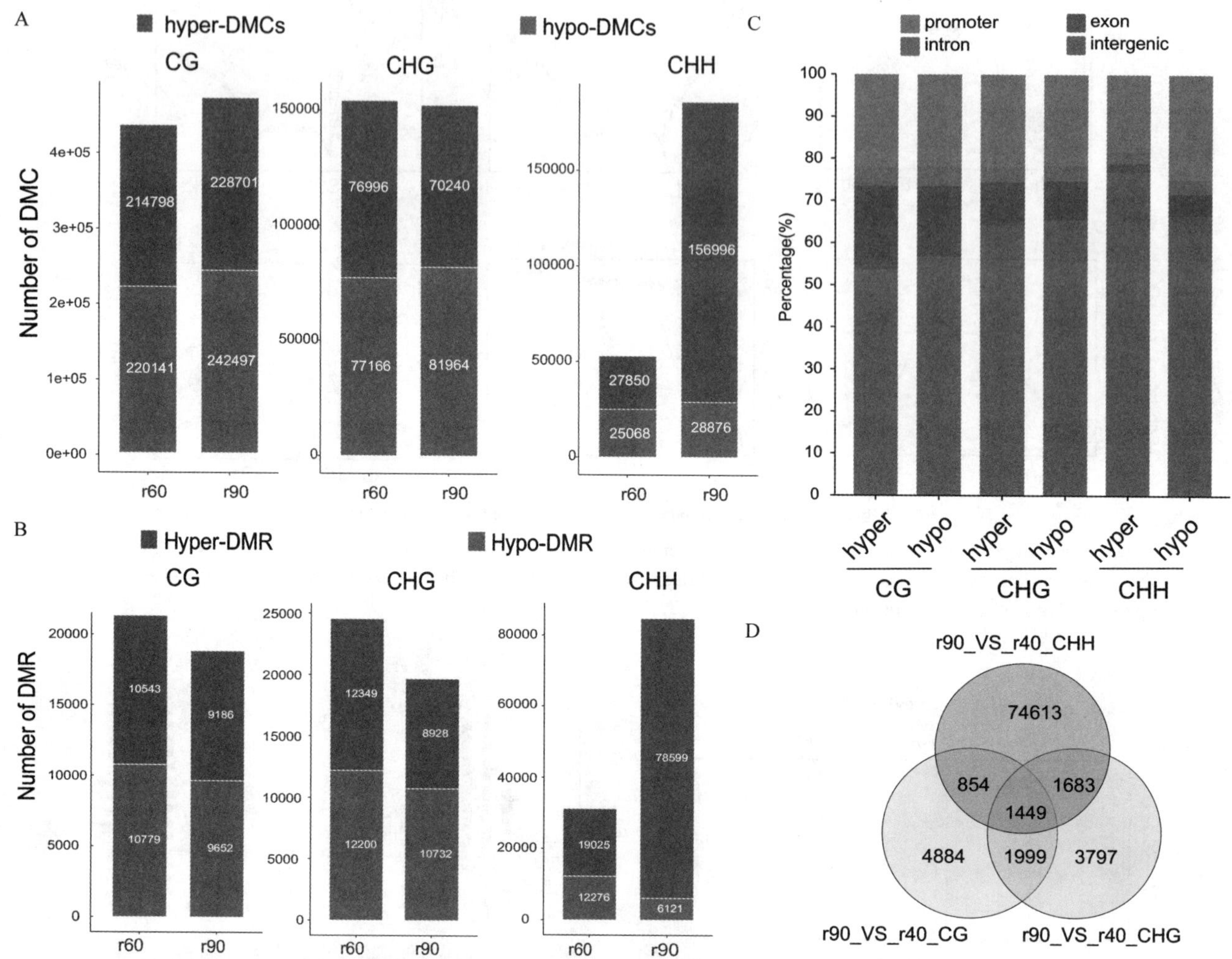


**Figure 5 Characterization of differential methylation regions during root growth**

(A) Number of differentially methylated sites at r60 and r90 compared to r40. (B) Number of differentially methylated regions at r60 and r90 compared to r40. (C) The relative proportion of genomic features over-lapping with DMRs in the group of r90_VS_r40. DMRs were divided into hypo- and hyper-DMRs. (D) Venn diagram showing the overlap among CG, CHG, and CHH-DMRs in the group of r90_VS_r40.

Increased expression of DNA methylesterase genes along with *S. miltiorrhiza* roots growth The increase in DNA methylation levels with growth of *S. miltiorrhiza* roots could potentially be attributed to either enhanced DNA methylesterase activity or reduced DNA demethylase activity. To investigate these possibilities, we examined the expression levels of DNA methylation-related genes at the 3 different growth stages of *S. miltiorrhiza*. We first annotated DNA methylation-related genes in the genome of *S. miltiorrhiza* from scratch and identified 8 genes, including 3 DNA demethylase homologs and 5 methylesterase homologs, then we constructed 2 phylogenetic trees for DNA demethylase protein sequences and DNA methylesterase protein sequences using the maximum likelihood method (Fig. 6, A and B).

As for DNA demethylase genes, *SmDME*, *SmDML*, and *SmROS1* were barely expressed in the roots of *S. miltiorrhiza* (Fragments Per Kilobale Million (FPKM)$<$5) (Fig. 6A). These results implied that increased DNA methylation through the 3 different growth stages could not be attributed to the decreased expression of DNA demethylase genes. As for the other 5 genes involved in the RdDM pathway and maintenance of DNA methylation, *SmAGO4-1* and *SmAGO4-2* were highly expressed at the 3 growth stages while the expression levels of *SmCMT2* and *SmDRM1* showed an upward trend. Although *SmDDM1* exhibited higher expression levels at r60 compared to r40 and r90, its expression levels still relatively higher than the

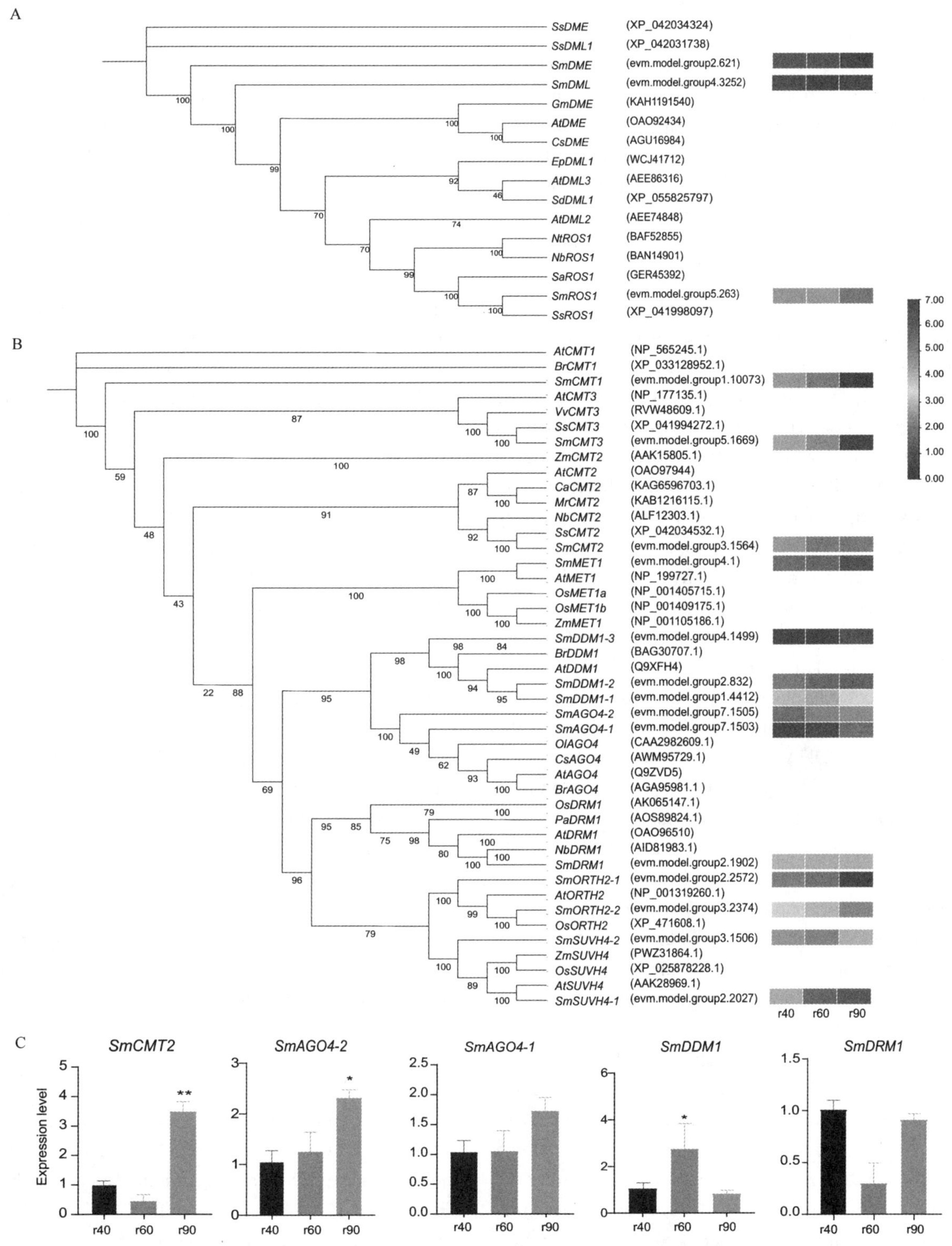


**Figure 6 Expression of genes involved in DNA methylation and demethylation**

(A) Phylogenetic tree of DNA demethylase genes in *Arabidopsis* (At), *Citrus sinensis* (Cs), *Nicotiana tabacum* (Nt), *Euphorbia peplus* (Ep), *Glycine max* (Gm), *Nicotiana benthamiana* (Nb), *Solanum dulcamara* (Sd), *Striga asiatica* (Sa), *Salvia splendens* (Ss), and *S. miltiorrhiza* (Sm), and heatmap showing expression levels of DNA demethylase genes at r40, r60, and r90. Bootstrap numbers shown at nodes are the percentage of 1000 replicates. (B) Phylogenetic tree of DNA methylesterase genes in *Arabidopsis* (At), *Brassica rapa* (Br), *Cucurbita argyrosperma* (Ca), *Castanea sativa* (Cs), *Nicotiana benthamiana* (Nb), *Morella rubra* (Mr), *Olea europaea* (Ol), *Oryza sativa* (Os), *Phalaenopsis aphrodite* (Pa), *Salvia splendens* (Ss), *Zea mays* (Zm), and *S. miltiorrhiza* (Sm), and heatmap showing expression levels of DNA methylesterase genes at r40, r60, and r90. Expression levels were shown as log2 (Fragments Per Kilobale Million (FPKM) + 1). Bootstrap numbers shown at nodes are the percentage of 1 000 replicates. (C) RT-qPCR results of DNA methylesterase genes. The normalized gene expression levels at r40 were arbitrarily set to 1. Each bar shows the mean±SE of triplicate assays. * or ** indicates a statistically significant difference as relative to the value at r40 for each gene at $P<0.05$ or 0.01, respectively. Student's *t* test. Scale bars.

control at r90 (Fig. 6B).

The expression levels of the above mentioned 5 methylesterase genes were further detected at the 3 different growth stages by reverse transcription quantitative polymerase chain reaction (RT-qPCR; Fig. 6C). The results showed that the expression of *SmAGO4-1* and *SmAGO4-2* showed an increasing trend as the growth of *S. miltiorrhiza*, in which the expression of *SmAGO4-2* was significantly higher in r90 than in r40. The expression of *SmDDM1* and *SmDRM1* was close to each other throughout r40 and r90, but in r60, *SmDDM1* displayed the highest expression while *SmDRM1* showed the lowest expression. The RT-qPCR results of *SmCMT2* and *SmDDM1* were consistent with the expression trends observed from the RNA-seq. Although there were slight differences in the expression trends of *SmAGO4-1*, *SmAGO4-2*, and *SmDRM1* between RT-qPCR and RNA-seq; these 3 genes still exhibited relatively high expression levels at r90 stage (Supplemental Table S3). Based on these observations, we hypothesize that the increase in DNA methylation in CHH during *S. miltiorrhiza* growth is mainly caused by the elevated expression of a series of DNA methylation-related genes.

Association between tanshinones and salvianolic acid biosynthesis and DNA methylation levels To identify the relationship between DNA methylation changes and gene expression, transcriptome sequencing was performed on r40, r60, and r90 roots using the same materials as those used for DNA methylome sequencing. We identified 24 102 differentially methylated genes (DMGs) and 2 412 differentially expressed genes (DEGs) in the group of r90_VS_r40. Specifically, among hyper DMGs, 27.53% DEGs were upregulated and 39.14% were downregulated, while among hypo DMGs, 9.77% DEGs were upregulated and 15.44% were downregulated (Fig. 7A).

To examine the biological function of DEGs regulated by DNA methylation during root growth, we performed Kyoto Encyclopedia of Genes and Genomes (KEGG) enrichment analysis. We observed a significant enrichment of the downregulated DEGs regulated by hyper-methylation in pathways ($P<0.05$) including metabolism, amino acid metabolism, and biosynthesis of other secondary metabolites (Supplemental Fig. S3A). The upregulated DEGs were primarily associated with pathways related to ribosome, plant hormone signal transduction, and transcription factors (Supplemental Fig. S3B). Additionally, we observed that upregulated DEGs regulated by hypomethylation were significantly enriched in the metabolism (Supplemental Fig. S3C) whereas downregulated DEGs were enriched in no KEGG pathways. Further analysis showed that for hyper-DMRs, both downregulated DEGs and upregulated DEGs, their hyper-methylation occurred mainly in the promoter region (downregulated DEGs: 70%; upregulated: 80%). Similarly, the upregulated DEGs regulated by hypomethylation also occurred mainly in the promoter region (66.67%).

To examine the expression of genes involved in the tanshinone and phenolic acid biosynthetic pathway at different growth stages in *S. miltiorrhiza*, we first searched the *S. miltiorrhiza* genome and identified the homologs of tanshinone and phenolic acid biosynthetic pathway genes. We found that most of these genes were differentially expressed at different growth stages (Fig. 7B). For example, *SmCPS5*, *SmCYP71D464*, *SmGGPPS1*, and *SmGPPS* are important enzymes involved in tanshinones biosynthesis, and *SmHPPR-1* is important enzymes involved in phenolic acid biosynthesis; we found that these genes were highly expressed during the r90 stage of root growth in *S. miltiorrhiza*. In addition, one member of the phenolic acid biosynthesis inhibitor (*SmHPPD*) was significantly downregulated in r90 compared to the r60 and r40. We also observed that these DEGs were associated with increased DNA methylation. Further investigation revealed that *SmHPPD* hyper-methylation occurred primarily in the promoter region, while *SmCPS5*, *SmCYP71D464*, *SmGGPPS1*, *SmGPPS*, and *SmHPPR-1* hyper-methylation occurred primarily in the gene body region. Figure 7, C to E visually showed the DNA methylation of 3 representative genes. We found that *SmCYP71D464* DNA hyper-methylation mainly occurred in the CHH sequence context, while *SmHPPR* and *SmHPPD* mainly occurred in the CG context at 3 stages. In summary, our results suggested that the upregulation of tanshinone and phenolic acid biosynthetic pathway genes and downregulation of phenolic acid synthesis inhibitors were accompanied by increase in gene body or promoter methylation, which probably promotes the accumulation of active components.

## 3 DISCUSSION

As an epigenetic modification, DNA methylation is involved in various biological processes in organisms, including transcriptional regulation, genome stability, and silencing of TEs. The application of DNA methylome and transcriptome co-analysis has become a prevalent approach in studying the intricate process of plant development in diverse species, such as *Lonicera japonica*, *S. lycopersicum*, *Fragaria × ananassa*, and *C. annuum*. In this study, we conducted analyses of DNA methylome, transcriptome, and targeted metabolites in different growth stages of *S. miltiorrhiza* to accurately describe the role of DNA methylation in the accumulation of tanshinones and phenolic acids in roots.

The DNA methylation sequencing data revealed that approximately 55% of the reads could be uniquely mapped to the *S. miltiorrhiza* reference genome, which is comparable to the mapping rates in *S. miltiorrhiza* (47% to 65%) and rice (*Oryza sativa*) (49% to 65%). Whole-genome bisulfite sequencing revealed that, similar to sweet orange (*C. sinensis*), the DNA methylation level of the entire *S. miltiorrhiza* genome increased during its growth process, with hyper-methylation observed in CHH context. The consequences of DNA methylation establishment in the context of CHH (H = A, C, or T) currently remain unknown. However, for plants such as maize (*Zea mays*) and rice, in which CHH methylation levels can be easily detected, there is clear evidence suggesting that CHH methylation may play a role in regulating the sexual reproduction and developmental processes of these species. The *S. miltiorrhiza* samples selected for this study had not yet undergone the flowering stage, and it is possible that methylation in the CHH context also plays a vital role in the developmental process of *S. miltiorrhiza*.

The proportion of repetitive sequences in plant genomes has a substantial contribution to the genome-wide methylation level. In the *S. miltiorrhiza* genome, repetitive sequences, primarily derived from TEs, account for approximately 60% of the genome, which is close to that of sugar beet (*Beta vulgaris*). Despite the difference in genome size between sugar beet and *S. miltiorrhiza*, it is noteworthy that both species exhibit higher levels of TE methylation compared to gene methylation in CG, CHG, and CHH contexts. This observation underscores the importance of TE as a key determinant of genome-wide methylation levels in these plants. During the growth process of *S. miltiorrhiza*, TEs also experience an increase in genome-wide DNA methylation levels in CHH context, which may reflect the role of asymmetric methylation in transposon silencing. Compared to the gene body regions, TE regions exhibit stable and high levels of DNA methylation in CG and CHG, suggesting that *S. miltiorrhiza* may share a similar genome-wide DNA methylation pattern shaped primarily by TEs, as observed in maize (*Z. mays*). Therefore, sustained and stable hyper-methylation of the root TE region contributes to genomic stability.

DNA methylation levels are dynamically regulated by DNA methyltransferases and demethylases. In the process of tomato (*S. lycopersicum*) ripening, DNA hypo-methylation is attributed to increased expression of *SlDML2*, while in oranges, DNA hyper-methylation during maturation is due to decreased expression of DNA demethylases (*CsDME*, *CsDML1*, *CsDML4*, and *CsDML3*). In our study, we observed higher expression of DNA methyltransferases, such as *SmCMT2*, *SmDDM1*, and *SmDRM1*, and key genes in the RdDM pathway, such as *SmAGO4*, in the growth process of *S. miltiorrhiza*, while the expression of DNA demethylase genes was relatively lower. These results suggest that the increased expression of a series of DNA methyltransferase-related genes contributes to the increase in DNA methylation during *S. miltiorrhiza* growth. Overall, the expression of DNA methyltransferase and demethylase genes plays an important role in plant growth, root development, and fruit maturation.

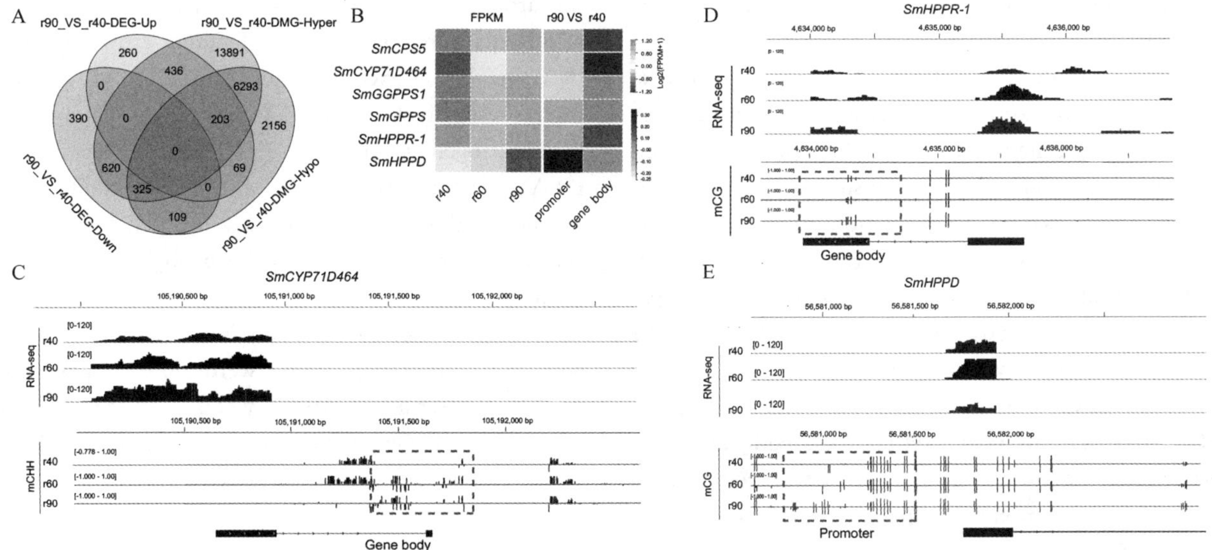


**Figure 7 Analysis of gene expression associated with changes in DNA methylation**

(A) Venn diagram of DMGs and DEGs in r90_VS_r40 group. DEG was determined using DESeq2 with $P<0.05$. (B) The gene expression levels and DNA methylation levels of genes involved in the biosynthesis pathways of tanshinones and salvianolic acid. (C to E) The Genome Browser shows the DNA methylation and expression of the representative tanshinone and salvianolic acid biosynthesis-related genes. The levels of DNA methylation are indicated by the height of the vertical bar on each track.

Gene expression is regulated by the level of DNA methylation, and the methylation of gene body and promoter regions has received extensive attention. During the growth of *S. miltiorrhiza* roots, the expression of 4 tanshinone (*SmCPS5*, *SmCYP71D464*, *SmGGPPS1*, *SmGPPS*) and 1 phenolic acid (*SmHPPR-1*) biosynthetic pathway genes was increased. Additionally, the methylation level of the gene body of these genes also showed a concomitant rise, suggesting that gene body methylation may have a positive regulatory effect on gene expression. Early studies have proposed that there are a large number of gene body methylation genes in angiosperm genomes, and gene body methylation is associated with transcription process to some extent. However, the potential mechanisms underlying gene body methylation dependent gene activation have not been definitively clarified. There is a substantial body of inconsistent or even contradictory research on gene body methylation. Consequently, the function and potential importance of gene body methylation remain subject to debate. It is worth noting that gene body methylation is associated with high levels of gene expression, and has positive effect on genes expression levels and stabilization. Gene body methylation is predominantly observed in angiosperms, and the majority of methylated genes are constitutively expressed. This suggests that gene body methylation may not lead to transcriptional repression. As for the regulation of promoter methylation on gene expression, it is generally believed that the hyper-methylation of promoter region will inhibit gene expression. In this study, the expression of the competitive inhibitor gene *SmHPPD* is negatively regulated by promoter methylation levels. This is consistent with the results of most previous studies.

In our forthcoming investigation, we will undertake knock-down and overexpression experiments targeting DNA methyltransferase-related genes in *S. miltiorrhiza* root, aiming to unravel the intricate mechanisms underlying DNA methylation's influence on the regulation of crucial enzyme genes involved in tanshinones and salvianolic acid biosynthesis. By meticulously monitoring alterations in the components of tanshinones and phenolic acids, alongside the dynamic shifts in the expression patterns of key enzyme genes, we anticipate gaining a more profound comprehension of the intricate interplay between DNA methylation and the biosynthetic pathways of these bioactive compounds. Crucially, this exploration holds great promise in augmenting the yield of bioactive constituents derived from *S. miltiorrhiza* root.

## 4 CONCLUSIONS

In conclusion, targeted detection of tanshinones and phenolic acids during different growth stages of *S. miltiorrhiza* roots revealed an increase in the content of 4 tanshinones (cryptotanshinone, tanshinone I, tanshinone IIA, and tosmariawinone) and 2 phenolic acids (rosmarinic acid and salvianolic acid B) as the roots grew. Whole-genome bisulfite sequencing and transcriptome sequencing analysis showed a gradual increase in genome-wide DNA methylation, primarily occurring in gene bodies, TEs, and their flanking regions in CHH context. These changes in DNA methylation were associated with high expression of a range of methylase genes, such as *SmCMT2*, *SmDDM1*, *SmAGO4*, and *SmDRM1*. In addition, the expression levels of many tanshinone biosynthesis genes (*SmCPS5*, *SmCYP71D464*, *SmGGPPS1*, and *SmGPPS*) and phenolic acid biosynthesis genes (*SmHPPR-1* and *SmHPPD*) have altered because of hyper-methylation. Hyper-methylation predominantly occurred in the promoter region of *SmHPPD*, while gene body hyper-methylation was observed in *SmCPS5*, *SmCYP71D464*, *SmGGPPS1*, *SmGPPS*, and *SmHPPR-1*. These methylation patterns potentially contribute to the accumulation of tanshinones and phenolic acids in *S. miltiorrhiza*. However, the underlying molecular mechanisms by which DNA methylation influences these changes in gene expression require further investigation.

## 5 MATERIALS AND METHODS

Plant materials Danshen (*S. miltiorrhiza*) was cultivated in the key laboratory of plant secondary metabolism at Zhejiang Sci-Tech University, under mild climatic conditions with sufficient light, moist air, and fertile soil. The temperature was approximately 18 ℃, and the air humidity was around 80% during the growth period.

Roots were collected at 3 different growth stages; r40, r60, and r90 referred as to 40-d-old, 60-d-old, and 90-d-old roots, respectively. The roots were immediately frozen in liquid nitrogen and stored at −80 ℃ for subsequent DNA and RNA extraction. Ten to 30 *S. miltiorrhiza* plants of uniform size and without visible defects were used for each growth stage. The experiment included 3 biological replicates and 2 technical replicates.

Targeted metabolites analysis The samples (40-d-old, 60-d-old, and 90-d-old roots) were thoroughly washed with deionized water and blotted dry. Subsequently, 0.5 g of the sample was weighed and dried in an oven at 45 ℃ for 48 h to ensure complete drying. Once dried, the sample was ground into a fine powder using a micro collision cell crusher. A quantity of 0.03 g of the root powder was then carefully added to a 2 mL centrifuge tube, and 1.0 mL of 70% v/v methanol was added to the tube. The mixture was allowed to stand for 12 h at 4 ℃ and was then subjected to ultrasonic extraction for 1 h using an ultrasonic extractor. During the extraction process, the tube was shaken up and down every

15 min. Following this, the treated samples were centrifuged at 12 000×*g* for 10 min to physically separate the supernatant from the solid residue. The supernatant was then carefully collected using a 2 mL syringe and passed through a 0.22 μm membrane to remove any impurities, before being collected in an injection vial. These samples were subsequently used for analysis. The target metabolites were identified by HPLC that was equipped with Waters 2 695 with a Waters 2 998 diode array detector, a Waters SunFire C18 column and data acquisition using Empower 2 software with a loading volume of 20 μL.

The mobile phase consists of 0.02% v/v phosphoric acid in water (solvent A) and acetonitrile (solvent B) with a gradient elution at a flow rate of 1 mL/min and a column temperature of 30 ℃. The peaks of the tanshinones were recorded at 270 nm, while the phenolic acids were detected at 288 nm. To determine the tanshinone and phenolic acid content, the external standard method of analyte peak area was employed. For all samples, 3 replicates were used to ensure the consistency and accuracy of the results obtained.

Whole-genome bisulfite sequencing data analysis DNA was extracted from *S. miltiorrhiza* roots using a plant genomic DNA kit (Tiangen Biochemical Technology Co., Ltd.) according to the manufacturer's instructions. The concentration and purity of DNA were measured using a nanodrop 2000 ultra-micro UV spectrophotometer (Thermo). For each stage, 3 biological replicates were designed, and 9 bisulfite sequencing libraries were constructed accordingly. The libraries were sequenced on the Illumina Novaseq platform, and paired-end 150 bp sequences were generated at Novogene Technologies Ltd (Beijing, China).

FastQC v0.11.9 was used to filter raw data reads to obtain clean reads. Bismark v0.23.1 with default parameters was used to align the bisulfite-treated clean data to the *S. miltiorrhiza* genome (https://ngdc.cncb.ac.cn/search/?dbId=gwh&q=PRJCA003150). Bowtie2 v2.4.5 was then used to construct the index. Accordingly, whole-genome bisulfite sequencing processed versions were obtained from sequence read segments, and these read segments were aligned to the reference genome in a directed manner. Finally, the cytosine methylation information of each site was extracted. DMR was identified by BatMeth2 and the methylKit package in R v4.0.5 (https://www.r-project.org), which detects DMRs with a dynamic fragment strategy of 500 bp as the window and 500 bp as the step size. *t* test was applied to filter significant DMRs by *q*-value of $<0.01$ and methylation difference threshold percentage (methdiff) > 25 as the standard for CG context, and methylation difference thresh-old percentage (methdiff)>20 as the standard for CHG context, while difference > 10 for CHH context. After that, DMGs were identified using bedtools v2.30.0. Methylation levels of different genomic regions (both gene and TE regions) were obtained using BatMeth2, and graphs were generated using the ggplot2 package in R v4.0.5. IGV_2.12.3 was used to display DNA methylation levels in gene and TE regions as well as in flanking regions. Sequence regions where the main body region (5′ to 3′ of the transcript start site) or promoter region (2 kb upstream of the transcript start site) of gene overlaps with the DMR are identified as DMG (Supplemental Table S3).

Transcriptome sequencing data analysis Transcriptome sequencing was performed using the same material as for DNA methylation sequencing, with 3 biological replicates at each stage. Total RNA was extracted using a polysaccharide polyphenol plant total RNA extraction kit (Tiangen Biochemical Technology Co., Ltd.) according to the instructions, and RNA integrity and purity were measured by a nanodrop. 2000 ultra-micro UV spectrophotometer (Thermo). One gram RNA was prepared for each sample to construct a transcriptome library, which was then sequenced by Novogene Technologies, Inc. The constructed libraries were then sequenced on the Illumina NovaSeq platform, and 150 bp paired-end reads were generated. Trimmomatic v0.39 was used to filter the raw reads and then generate clean data. These clean reads were mapped to the *S. miltiorrhiza* genome using HISAT2 v2.2.1. Gene expression was calculated by RSEM v1.3.1. DEGs were identified by DEseq2, with screened criteria as fold change≥2 and $P<0.05$. The correlation between replicates in diagrams was made by using the psych (https://personality-project.org/r/psych/) package in R v4.0.5.

RNA extraction and RT-qPCR analysis RNA samples were extracted from *S. miltiorrhiza* roots using an RNA Extraction Kit (Vazyme, Nanjing, China). Total RNA samples (500 ng) were transcribed into cDNA using a Reverse Transcription Kit (Accurate Biology, Hunan, China). SYBR Green Premix qPCR Kit (Accurate Biology, Hunan, China) and QuantStudio 6 Flex Real-Time PCR System (Thermo Fisher, USA) were used to analyze the expression of related genes as described in Fig. 6C. The experiments were performed using the following operating parameters: initial denaturation of the samples at 95 ℃ for 30 s, followed by 40 amplification cycles. Each cycle consisted of denaturation at 95 ℃ for 5 s and annealing at 60 ℃ for 30 s. The final stage of dissociation was 95 ℃ for 15 s, 65 ℃ for 1 min, and 95 ℃ for 15 s. The specific information regarding the primer sequences can be found in Supplemental Table S4. Each sample underwent 3 biological replicates and 3 technical replicates.

Identification of DNA methylation-related genes First, the protein sequences of DNA methylation-related genes in the *Arabidopsis* genome were obtained from NCBI, and then DNA methylesterase genes were searched in the *S. miltiorrhiza* genome using the Blastp v2.11.0 program. Finally, IQtree v2.2.0 was used for sequence alignment and phylogenetic tree construction based on maximum likelihood method (- m MFP - bb 1000 - T AUTO).

KEGG enrichment analysis KEGG enrichment analysis was performed using TBtools for upregulated DEGs and downregulated DEGs, and KEGG terms with *P*-values of $< 0.05$ were used for further analysis.

Statistical analysis All the statistical analyses were carried out using independent sample *t* tests by SPSS 25 software (IBM SPSS Statistics, Chicago, USA). Pairwise comparisons were determined using Student's *t* tests ($^{*}P<0.05$, $^{**}P<0.01$). Each reaction was performed on 3 biological replicates.

Accession numbers Sequence data from this article can be found in the GenBank/EMBL data libraries under accession numbers OR683668 - OR683685.

[何心雨,张顺仓,杨东风,等. Plant Physiology, 2024, 194(4):2086 - 2100.]

# The ERF transcription factor LTF1 activates DIR1 to control stereoselective synthesis of antiviral lignans and stress defense in *Isatis indigotica* roots

## 1 INTRODUCTION

The accumulation level of bioactive metabolites and the ability to resist stresses determine the quality of medicinal plants. Lignans are a large group of natural products derived from the oxidative coupling of two coniferyl alcohol molecules. Owing to the stress-resistant function and biological activities, lignans are important for plant growth and human health. Therefore, it is of great significance to elucidate the biosynthesis and regulation mechanism of lignans for the guidance of optimizing plants, whether to improve the stress resistance or the content of active lignans.

Plants are not motile and thus they must endure a variety of stresses, especially the root-based environmental stresses underground, such as high salinity and pathogen infection. Fortunately, plants have evolved powerful defense mechanisms in roots to withstand and adapt to their environments. When environmental stress signals are sensed, plants can directly resist stresses by regulating the accumulation of secondary metabolites with the guidance of multistage signal transduction. Plants produce a series of secondary metabolites to govern interactions with and adaptation to their biotic and abiotic environments. Lignans are ubiquitously present in all plants that contain lignin (most land plants) and have long been considered as potential metabolites that increased tolerance to stress. After the activity against in-sects of the lignans sesamin, asarin and pinoresinol was first proposed through *in vitro* tests in 1942, a series of stress-resistant lignans were discovered *in vitro*. Western red cedar (*Thuja plicata*) accumulates relatively large amounts of lignans, which are derived from plicatic acid in the heartwood, as part of a complex system that may increase pest and disease resistance. Pinoresinol, as one of the simplest lignans, is synthesized from two molecules of coniferyl alcohol through 8 - 8′ radical coupling reactions and has antihelminthic and antifungal activities *in vitro*. Our previous study found that the synthesis and accumulation of pinoresinol and its derivatives were regulated by methyl jasmonate (MeJA) in *Isatis indigotica*, suggesting its potential involvement in the response to stresses. However, the actual stress-resistant potential *in vivo* and the application potentiality to increase plant tolerance of lignans remains to be confirmed.

Lignans have also received wide attention as leading compounds of novel drugs for the treatment of tumor and virus infection, as well as healthy diets to reduce the risks of lifestyle-related non-communicable diseases. Sesamin and its metabolites exhibited anti-hypertensive, anticancer, immunomodulatory, and anti-inflammatory activities. It is worth noting that the activities of most lignans are closely related to the stereo configuration of lignans. The (−)-podophyllotoxin (isolated from *Podophyllum* plants) and its semi-synthetic derivatives, (−)-etoposide, (−)-teniposide, and (−)-etopophos, are clinically utilized to treat testicular and small-cell lung cancer. (−)-gossypol, instead of (+)-gossypol, is the bioactive form with anti-spermatogenic activity in mammals. These active lignans with specific stereo configurations are typically distributed in specific tissues at low content levels and are even accumulated only in some endangered plants, which hinders the efficient and stable production. Therefore, understanding and exploiting the mechanisms of lignan stereoselective synthesis and regulation will prompt the discovery of rational intervention strategies toward desired plant improvement for higher lignan content and stronger plant defense.

The biosynthetic pathways of lignans and flavonoids share the upstream of shikimate and phenylpropanoid pathways to produce phenolic acids that are further converted to the lignan precursor coniferyl alcohol (Supporting Information Fig. S1). In this process, chorismic acid is first converted to L-phenylalanine, which is used to synthesize cinnamic acid by phenylalanine ammonia-lyase (PAL). Cinnamic acid is then hydroxylated by a cytochrome P450 monooxygenase (CYP) cinnamate 4-hydroxylase (C4H) to form *p*-coumaric acid. Furthermore, the sequential reactions catalyzed by 4CL (4-(hydroxy) cinnamoyl CoA ligase), CCoAOMT (caffeoyl CoA *O*-methyltransferase), CCR (cinnamoyl CoA reductase), and CAD (cinnamyl alcohol dehydrogenase) achieve the biosynthesis of coniferyl alcohol. The pathway of all lignans in plants is started from a common first step, the electron coupling reaction of coniferyl alcohol to produce the key lignan molecule pinoresinol with stereo configuration, which is accomplished by Dirigent (DIR) protein, followed by the production of diverse lignan structures through specific downstream enzymes, such as pinoresinol-lariciresinol reductase (PLR), CYP, and UDP-glucotransferase (UGT), etc.. DIR as the first step of the lignan pathway mediates the regio- and stereoselectivity of bimolecular phenoxy radical coupling reactions for (−)-pinoresinol or (+)-pinoresinol biosynthesis, which preliminarily determines the stereo configuration of lignans in a plant. In addition, DIRs are also involved in the formation of Casparian strips in roots and the atroposelective synthesis of gossypol. Lignan synthesis is very sensitive to environmental changes. Although several stress- and phytohormone-responsive transcript factors have been identified to explain the susceptible perturbation of lignan biosynthesis, these affect all are indirectly mediated through up-stream genes of phenylpropanoid and aromatic alcohol pathway (phenylalanine ammonia-lyase, PAL; coumarate3-hydroxylase, C3H; 4-coumarate: CoA ligase, 4CL; cinnamoyl-CoA reductase, CCR) rather than the actual lignan pathway, which suggests that the effect of these transcription factors on lignan synthesis is probably a side effect, and the actual regulatory target is the stress-resistant flavonoids and lignin. Therefore, the transcription factor that directly regulates lignan synthesis has not been discovered so far, that is, the specific regulatory mechanism of lignan response and adaptation to environmental stress is still unclear.

The root of *I. indigotica* (Radix Isatidis), with the Chinese name "Ban Lan Gen", is frequently used for the treatment of influenza and hepatitis because of antiviral lariciresinol glucosides and indole alkaloids, as well as their derivatives. Therefore, this study aims to elucidate the stereoselective synthesis and the response mechanism to stresses of antiviral lariciresinol glucosides in *I. indigotica*, which can guide the improvement of the herbal quality of Radix isatidis. Here, we found that the (−)-lariciresinol glucosides are the primary antiviral components in *I. indigotica* roots, which are synthesized through continuous stereoselective reactions catalyzed by DIR1/2, PLR, and UGT71B2. Two of the 19 DIRs (DIR1 and DIR2) were identified in *I. indigotica* roots mediating the regio- and stereoselective synthesis of (−)-pinoresinol, which is further converted to (−)-lariciresinol and (+)-secoisolariciresinol by lariciresinol glucosides by UGT71B2, although UGT71B2 prefers to react with (+)-lariciresinol. Constitutive overexpression of DIR1 and DIR2 in hairy roots significantly increased lignan and lignin biosynthesis because of their regioselectivity; furthermore, overexpression enhanced the hairy root resistance to biotic and abiotic stresses, which suggested the definite stress-resistant function of lignans *in vivo*. Despite having redundant biochemical functions, the expression patterns of DIR1 and DIR2 are completely different. DIR1 is specifically localized in the cell periphery of vascular regions in mature roots and is regulated by a variety of phytohormones synergistically or antagonistically. Furthermore, we identified an ERF transcriptional regulator LTF1 that regulates lignan biosynthesis through DIR expression in response to abiotic and biotic stresses. LTF1 is the first transcription factor found to directly and specifically regulate the lignan pathway, and its regulatory target DIR is the first common step for the lignan synthesis in plants and the decisive step for lignan configuration. Lignans are ubiquitously present in all plants that contain lignin, and this study provides evidence of a novel mechanism by which the plant ERF-DIR module regulates lignan synthesis in response to stresses. In particular, the ERF-DIR module will be an ideal engineering target for enhancing plant stress resistance while increasing the content of valuable lignans, such as antiviral lignans in *I. indigotica*.

## 2 MATERIALS AND METHODS

2.1 Plant material and growth conditions Flowers, leaves, stems, petioles, and roots were collected from 8-month-old plants. To collect sterilized seedlings, seeds of *I. indigotica* were surface sterilized in 75% ethanol for 1 min and then in sodium hypochlorite solution with 1.7% active chlorine for 15 min. After rinsing thoroughly five times with sterile distilled water, the seeds were placed on Murashige and Skoog (MS) medium (PhytoTech, USA) with 3%

sucrose and 0.5% agar (pH 6.0).

2.2 sgRNA design and CRISPR/Cas9 vector construction LTF1 was selected as the target locus for editing, and the sgRNA was designed by an online web tool (http://crispr.mit.edu/). Two potential 20-bp sequences followed by PAM from the ORF of LTF1 (no introns of the LTF1 DNA sequence) were used for the CRISPR/Cas9-mediated efficient targeted mutagenesis of LTF1 according to published protocols.

2.3 Construction of plant overexpression vectors To create overexpression hairy roots, the coding sequences of DIR1, DIR2, and LTF1 were separately cloned into the *p*HB-X-myc vector with *Bam*H I and *Sac* I restriction sites. The empty vector *p*HB-X-myc was used as the control without exogenous gene insertion into the vector.

2.4 Plant transformation of hairy roots The transgenic hairy roots were cultured through the induction of *Agrobacterium rhizogenes* C58C1 harboring the proper plasmids as described by reference. The hairy roots were weighed each week and harvested after 9 weeks for DNA extraction, RNA extraction, metabolite determination, microscopic analysis, phloroglucinol-HCl staining, GUS staining, and induction assays according to corresponding protocols.

2.5 Bioinformatics analysis Phylogenetic analysis was performed using the neighbor-joining method with the pairwise deletion option in MEGA 5.05. The *cis*-elements of promoters were predicted using the PANTCARE tool (http://bioinformatics.psb.ugent.be/webtools/plantcare/html).

2.6 Protein heterologous expression The coding sequences of DIRs were separately constructed into *p*PICZ$\alpha$ for protein expression in *Pichia pastoris*. The expression process was performed according to the reference. The day after, the sample was subjected to a nickel-nitrilotriacetic acid (Ni-NTA) agarose affinity column for further purification.

The *p*ET28a vector was transformed into *Escherichia coli* BL21 (DE3) for the expression of LTF1, PLR, and UGT71B2. The expression was induced with 0.5 mmol/L IPTG followed by continued growth at 16℃ and 110 rpm for 16 h. The protein was extracted by sonication and purified by a Ni-NTA agarose affinity column for EMSAs.

2.7 Catalytic assays In a total reaction mixture volume of 250 μL, a final concentration of 400 mmol/L MES (pH 6.0), 0.5 U/mL laccase (Sigma, product number 40 452), and 1 mg/mL coniferyl alcohol was maintained along with purified DIR enzymes. The reaction mixture without DIRs served as a control. The reaction mixture was incubated at 30℃ and 500 rpm for 4 h and then quenched by adding 500 μL of ethyl acetate. Finally, the mixture was centrifuged to remove proteins and filtered through a 0.22 μm filter prior to analysis by high-performance liquid chromatography-tandem mass spectrometry (HPLC - MS - MS). The assays of enzyme activity for PLR and UGT71B2 were performed as previous methods.

2.8 Chemical extraction Lignans were extracted from 500 mg of powdered lyophilized tissues. The samples were extracted two times in 15 mL methanol and sonicated for 10 min. Combined extracts were then centrifuged for 30 min at 4 000 rpm, and the supernatant was evaporated and dissolved in 1 mL 50% (*V*/*V*) of methanol for further β-glucosidase (Sigma, product number 49 290) hydrolysis and determination.

Lignin extraction was performed from 10 g powdered lyophilized tissues by nitrobenzene oxidation. Lignin is oxidatively cleaved to form aromatic carbonyl compounds, *i.e.*, syringaldehyde and vanillin as the main products. Vanillin and syringaldehyde were used as markers for guaiacyl- and syringyl-type lignin, respectively. The samples were mixed in 27 mL methanol and centrifuged after 10 min. The precipitate was then washed twice with 60℃ deionized $H_2O$ and dried at 50℃ in an oven. The 0.2 g solid residues were mixed in 7 mL basic solution (2 mol/L NaOH and 0.5 mL nitrobenzene), loaded into a stainless-steel reactor and heated up to 170℃ for 2.5 h. In case of high-pressure conditions in this step, we paid close attention to safety. After cooling, the reactor was opened to collect the supernatant, which was then adjusted to pH 3.0 with 1 mol/L HCl and extracted twice with chloroform at room temperature. The combined organic phases were dried with nitrogen and dissolved in 500 μL methanol for further experiments.

2.9 Chemical analysis Lignan analysis was performed by high-performance liquid chromatography (HPLC) with detection by mass spectrometry (MS) on an Agilent Technologies 1 200 system coupled to an Agilent Technologies 6 410 quadrupole mass spectrometer (Santa Clara, CA). The enzymatic reaction products of DIRs were subjected to chromatography by a Superchiral R-OZ column (4.6 mm × 250 mm, 5 μm) for chiral analysis using the constructed methods (Supporting Information Table S2). The associated Agilent MassHunter and OpenLAB software packages were used for data collection and analysis. Lignan extracts from LTF1 - OVX hairy roots were subjected to chromatography by an Agilent ZORBAX SB - C18 (2.1 mm × 100 mm, 3.5 μm) column (Supporting Information Table S3). Lignin extractions were subjected to chromatography on an Agilent HPLC 1 260 equipped with a UV detector and an Agilent tc-C18 column (4.6 mm × 250 mm, 5 μm) (Supporting Information Table S4).

2.10 Stress treatment, qRT-PCR, and heatmap construction The hairy roots were treated with NaCl (200 mmol/L), $H_2O_2$ (200 μmol/L), flg22 (1 μmol/L), ABA (50 μmol/L), ethephon (50 μmol/L) and ABA + ethephon

(50 μmol/L) separately and then sampled at designated time points for gene expression analysis. Total RNA was extracted using the Plant RNA Extraction kit (Takara, Japan) and then reverse transcribed into complementary deoxyribonucleic acid (cDNA) using the PrimeScript TM kit (Takara, Japan). The PP2A4 gene of *I. indigotica* was selected as the internal reference gene. Primers and standard curves for qPCR analysis are listed (Supporting Information Dataset 1, Fig. S2). The heatmap was constructed with log2 transformed and normalized expression data by TBtools.

2.11 Bioinformatics analysis Phylogenetic analysis was performed using the neighbor-joining method with the pairwise deletion option in MEGA 5.05 (Supporting Information Datasets 2 and 3). The *cis*-elements of promoters (Supporting Information Dataset 4) were predicted using the PlantCARE tool (http://bioinformatics.psb.ugent.be/webtools/plantcare/html).

2.12 Subcellular localization The gene ORF was fused in a frame with a yellow fluorescent protein (YFP) and driven by the 35S cauliflower mosaic virus promoter. The constructs were introduced into the *A. tumefaciens* strain GV3101 for infiltration and transient expression in *Nicotiana benthamiana epidermal* cells. We collected and recorded the results after 2 days of transformation at an excitation wavelength of 511 nm and an emission wavelength in the range 520 - 548 nm. The YFP fluorescence signal was imaged using a Leica TCS SP5 laser confocal scanning microscope (Leica Microsystems, Germany).

2.13 β-Glucuronidase staining (GUS) analysis The gene promoter was collected from the genomic DNA through PCR and subcloned into the *p*CAMBIA1301 vector. The constructs were transformed into the *A. tumefaciens* strain C58C1, which was used for the transformation of hairy roots. Hairy roots were analyzed by histochemical GUS staining. The stained samples were visualized under an Olympus BX43 light microscope (Olympus, Japan).

2.14 Histochemical staining Histochemical staining was performed on sections cut from the maturation zone of hairy roots. The hairy roots were embedded in 7% agarose before being transversely sectioned at a thickness of 50 μm using a vibratome (Leica VT1000S, Germany). The phloroglucinol-HCl staining method was used to detect the deposition and composition of lignans, lignin, or wall-bound phenolics and derivatives. All sections were observed under an Olympus BX43 microscope (Japan).

2.15 Y1H assay In Y1H experiments, LTF1 was amplified and cloned into the *p*GADT7 - REC2 vector. The sequence containing the GCCGCC elements of the promoter of pathway genes was cloned into the *p*His2.1 vector. The combination of *p*GADT7 - REC2 - LTF1 and *p*His2.1 - GCC was transformed together into the yeast strain Y187 for cultivation on SD-Leu-Trp selection medium. The empty *p*GADT7 - REC2 vector and the mutated *p*His2.1 - TCC were used as negative controls. Different combinations were transformed into the yeast strain Y187 to verify the binding of LTF1 to the promoters.

2.16 Electrophoretic mobility shift assays The biotin-labeled oligonucleotides in this experiment were synthesized by the Genewiz company (Suzhou, China). EMSAs were performed using the EMSA/Gel-Shift Kit (Pierce, USA) according to the manufacturer's instructions. After blotting on a positively charged nylon membrane, a UV cross-linker was used to cross-link the DNA. The biotin-labeled DNA was detected by chemiluminescence and exposed to X-ray film.

2.17 Luciferase assay The coding sequence of LTF1 was subcloned into the *p*GreenII 62 - SK vector (Biovector, Beijing, China) to generate the effector, and the promoters of pathway genes were fused into the vector pGreenII 800-LUC (Biovector) to generate reporters. The empty vectors *p*GreenII 62 - SK and *p*GreenII 800-LUC were used as controls for the effector and reporter, respectively. The constructs were then separately transformed into *A. tumefaciens* strain GV3101. Then, the incubated cells were harvested by centrifugation and resuspended in an MSS medium with 10 mmol/L methylester sulfonate (MES) and 150 mmol/L acetosyringone. Cultures were then grown to an $OD_{600}$ of 0.6 and incubated at room temperature for 3 h. Effector- and receptor-containing cells were mixed at a ratio of 1 : 1 and dispensed into tobacco leaves. LUC activity was measured using a cooled CCD imaging system after 2 days (Lumazone 1300B; Roper Scientific, Trenton, NJ, USA). The leaves were sprayed with 1 mmol/L luciferin and placed in darkness for 3 min before luminescence detection. Three independent biological replicates were measured for each sample.

## 3 RESULTS

3.1 Stereochemical analysis of lignans in I. indigotica Stereochemical differences in the lignans of wild-type *I. indigotica* were investigated (Supporting Information Fig. S3). With the exception of flowers, (±)-lariciresinol is the major constituent of lignans in the vascular-rich organs of *I. indigotica*, including the root, stem, and leaf. Treatment with β-glucosidase significantly increased the lignan content, indicating that lignans were mainly present in the form of glucosides. To characterize the level of lignan synthesis more accurately, the content levels of all lignans in this study were determined based on the aglycone form, which occurs after glycoside hydrolysis. Lignans in roots and flowers have similar stereochemical characteristics, that is, (−)-pinoresinol, (−)-lariciresinol and (+)-secoisolariciresinol are predominant (Supporting Information Fig. S3d), implying the presence of potential (−)-pinoresinol-forming DIR (defined as (−)-DIR) protein which directs the selective synthesis of lignans.

3.2 Stereoselective synthesis of antiviral lignans in I. indigotica roots To completely characterize the whole stereoselective biosynthesis pathway of lignans, the stereochemical function of pathway enzymes DIR, PLR, and UGT was studied.

To predict functional members of the DIR family, an unrooted phylogenetic tree was created based on the amino acid sequences of 19 potential DIRs of *I. indigotica* and 16 known DIRs (Supporting Information Fig. S4, Dataset 2). Cluster I, consisting of four *I. indigotica* DIRs (DIR1, 2, 3, and 4) and four known (−)-DIRs from flax (*Linum usitatissimum*) and *Arabidopsis thaliana*, corresponds to the previously defined DIR-a subfamily. Of these, the high expression of DIR1 and DIR2 in roots suggests their potential involvement in root lignan biosynthesis (Fig. 1a). Recombinant proteins DIR1 and DIR2 were expressed in *pichia pastoris* and then tested for their biochemical function in *in vitro* reaction mixtures containing *Trametes versicolor* laccase for one-electron oxidation and coniferyl alcohol as a substrate. Reactions with both DIR1 and DIR2 had significant stereo-selectivity and produced (−)-pinoresinol in enantiomeric excess (ee), which identified DIR1 and DIR2 as (−)-DIR proteins (Fig. 1b). DIR1 and DIR2 produced (−)-pinoresinol in 45.8±2.3% and 71.0±1.8% ee with the addition of 6.4 μmol/L DIR protein, respectively.

To further study the physiological function of DIRs *in vivo*, DIR1- and DIR2-overexpressing hairy roots (DIR1-OVX and DIR2-OVX) of *I. indigotica* were constructed. Quantitative RT-PCR (qRT-PCR) analysis showed that the transcription of DIR1 and DIR2 was successfully increased in the corresponding over-expression hairy roots (Supporting Information Fig. S5). Analysis of stereochemical differences in lignan accumulation indicated that the content of all lignan stereoisomers in DIR-OVX was increased (Fig. 1c - e). Of these, the content of (−)-pinoresinol-derived lignans in DIR1-OVX and DIR2-OVX hairy roots increased to 1.55±0.09 folds (36.5±2.2 μg) and 2.52±0.25 folds (59.2±5.8 μg/g) of control (23.6 ± 1.3 μg/g), respectively (Fig. 1f). Similarly, the content of (+)-pinoresinol-derived lignans (total content of (+)-pinoresinol, (+)-lariciresinol and (−)-secoi-solariciresinol), compared to the control (1.0±0.1 μg/g), was increased by 3.05±0.49 folds (3.0±0.5 μg/g) and by 6.91 ± 1.12 folds (6.8 ± 1.1 μg/g) in DIR1-OVX and DIR2-OVX hairy roots, respectively. The increase in content may be a result of the DIR-mediated regioselectivity of the 8 - 8′ oxidative coupling of coniferyl alcohol. Surprisingly, coniferyl alcohol content was also significantly increased in both DIR1-OVX (7.0±1.1 μg/g) and DIR2-OVX (32.2 ± 13.4 μg/g) hairy roots, which presents an alternative reason for the overall increase in lignan content (Supporting Information Fig. S6a). Unexpectedly, the ee of (−)-pinoresinol-derived lignan in both DIR1 - OVX (84.8±2.5%) and DIR2-OVX (79.5±1.5%) hairy roots was slightly decreased compared to the control (92.0±0.9%), which may be due to excess substrate coniferyl alcohol and saturation of DIR function (Supporting Information Fig. S6b). *In vitro*, a gradual decrease in the ee of (−)-pinoresinol with increasing coniferyl alcohol concentration supports this hypothesis (Fig. S6c). In conclusion, DIR1 and DIR2 as highly expressed (−)-DIR determine (−)-pinoresinol derived lignans as dominant lignan configuration in *I. indigotica* roots (Fig. 1g).

In previous studies, we reported that PLR is the key enzyme that catalyzes the continuous synthesis of lariciresinol and secoisolariciresinol from pinoresinol. Here, we found that PLR also exhibits significant substrate selectivity, which contributes to the preferential accumulation of (−)-lariciresinol and (+)-secoisolariciresinol in roots (Supporting Information Fig. S7). *In vitro* catalytic assays showed that PLR was able to indiscriminately convert (+)-pinoresinol and (−)-pinoresinol to (+)-lariciresinol and (−)-lariciresinol, respectively; however, PLR only showed low activity in stereoselectively catalyzing (−)-lariciresinol to generate (+)-secoisolariciresinol. Thus DIR1/2 and PLR jointly determine that (−)-lariciresinol derived lignans are the dominant form in roots.

Glycosylation is important for the synthesis of many active natural products. UDP-glucoside transferase UGT71B2 was previously identified as a key enzyme catalyzing lariciresinol to antiviral lariciresinol glucosides. However, the activity to different stereo configurations of lariciresinol remains to be investigated. To validate the stereoselectivity of UGT71B2, recombinant UGT71B2 expressed in *E. coli* was reacted with totally racemic (±)-lariciresinol as the sugar-acceptor, producing two glucosides (peaks 8 and 9) and one diglucoside (peak 10) (Supporting Information Fig. S8a). Owing to the difficulty in the chiral separation of glucosides by chromatographic analysis, the remaining concentrations of substrates were used to analyze the stereoselectivity of UGT71B2 (Fig. S8b). The unequal amounts of remaining substrates (+)-lariciresinol and (−)-lariciresinol indicated that UGT71B2 was able to react with both configurations and also displayed stereoselectivity, favoring reaction with (+)-lariciresinol over (−)-lariciresinol (Fig. S7).

In conclusion, the stereo configuration of lignans in *I. indigotica* is determined by the first key enzyme DIR from the beginning, and PLR and UGT71B2 further refine it, ultimately achieving lignan accumulation with specific

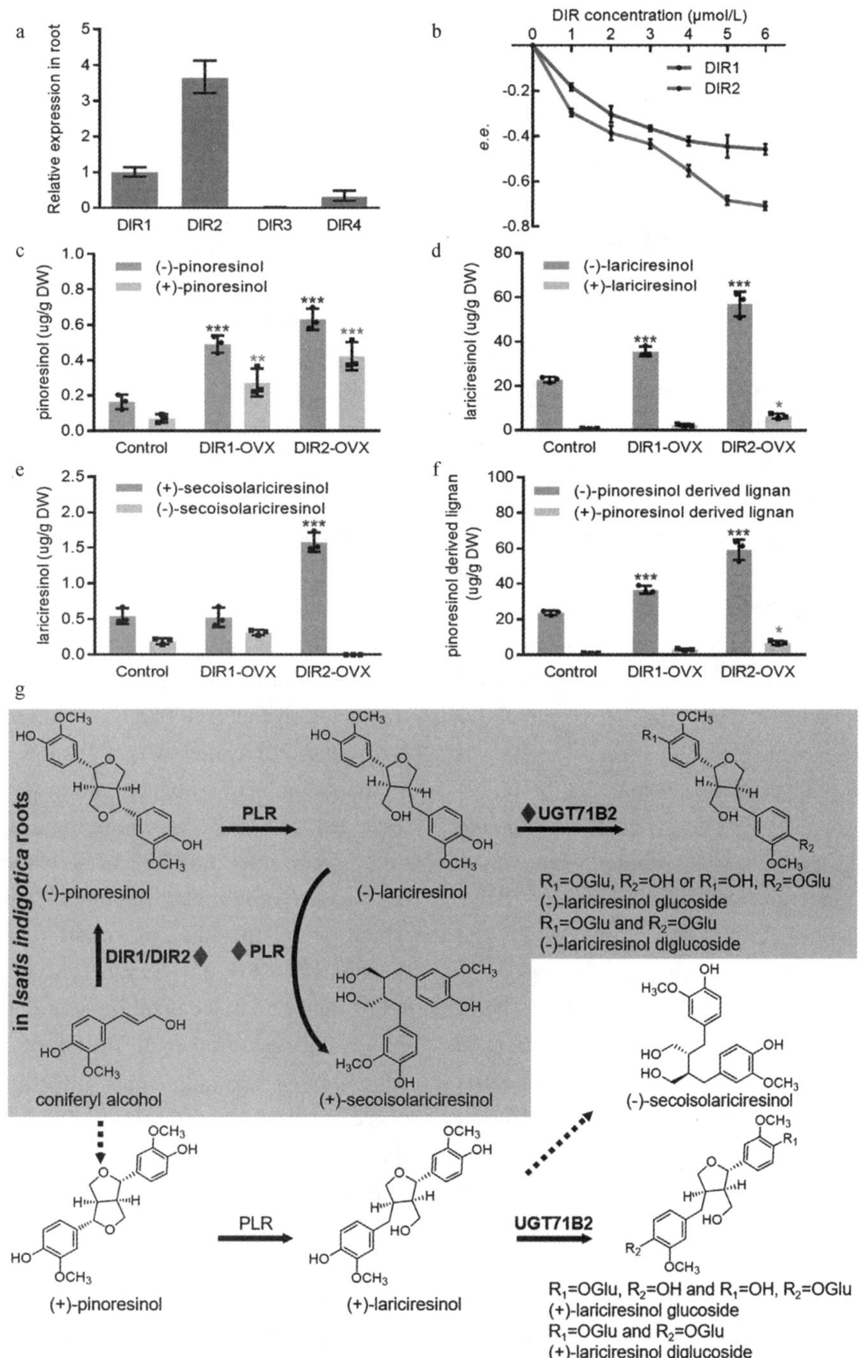


**Figure 1 Stereoselective synthesis of lignan glucosides in *I. indigotica* roots**

(a) Expression levels of the cluster I DIRs in *I. indigotica*. (b) Enantiomeric excess (ee) of (−)-pinoresinol with increasing amounts of recombinant DIR1 and DIR2. Chiral HPLC - MS/MS analysis of (−)-pinoresinol/(+)-pinoresinol (c), (−)-lariciresinol/(+)-lariciresinol (d), (−)-secoisolariciresinol/(+)-secoisolariciresinol (e) and total pinoresinol-derived lignan (f) contents in transgenic plants. The (−)-pinoresinol-derived lignan content is equivalent to the sum of (−)-pinoresinol, (−)-lariciresinol and (+)-secoisolariciresinol content, and the (+)-pinoresinol-derived lignan content means the sum of (+)-pinoresinol, (+)-lariciresinol and (−)-secoisolariciresinol content. Statistical analysis was performed tween control and over-expressing hairy roots by using Two-way ANOVA multiple comparisons ($^{*}P<0.05$, $^{**}P<0.01$, $^{**}P<0.001$). All data represent the mean of three biologically independent samples and error bars show standard deviation. (g) Stereoselective synthesis of lignan glucosides in *I. indigotica* roots. DIR1 and DIR2 mediates the stereoselective synthesis of (−)-pinoresinol; PLR is able to indiscriminately convert (+)-pinoresinol and (−)-pinoresinol to (+)-lariciresinol and (−)-lariciresinol, respectively, and only show low activity in stereoselectively catalyzing (−)-lariciresinol to generate (+)-secoisolariciresinol; UGT71B2 is able to react with both configurations of lariciresinol and also displayed stereoselectivity, favoring reaction with (+)-lariciresinol over (−)-lariciresinol. In conclusion, (−)-pinoresinol-derived ligans, including (−)-lariciresinol, (+)-secoisolariciresinol and (−)-lariciresinol glucosides, are the primary lignan component in *I. indigotica* roots. Green background represents stereoselective pathway of antiviral lignans in *I. indigotica* roots. Arrows represent the reactions *in vitro*. Dotted arrows represent reactions that do not happen in *I. indigotica* roots. The red squares represent the stereoselective steps in the root.

stereoconformation, which determines that the dominant antiviral lignan in *I. indigotica* roots is (−)-lariciresinol derived lignans including (−)-lariciresinol glucosides (Fig. 1g).

3.3 DIRs enhance stress resistance by mediating an increase in lignan and lignin content As the first key enzyme of the lignan pathway, 22 *At*DIRs in *A. thaliana* were shown to exhibit specific expression patterns in different tissues and in response to different hormones. In parallel, the expression of different *At*DIRs significantly varies following biotic and abiotic stress-related treatments. Each DIR in spruce, conifer, and sugarcane also shows its own unique expression patterns in different tissues and in response to different stress and hormone treatments. These results imply that DIR may be the key gene for plant lignans to respond to environmental stresses, but the transcriptional regulation mechanism has not been well explained.

To investigate whether the DIRs contribute to plant defense through lignan biosynthesis, we first tested their response to biotic and abiotic stresses. NaCl (300 mmol/L) and $H_2O_2$ (200 μmol/L) treatments were used to assess salt and oxidative tolerance, respectively; Flg22 (1 μmol/L) treatment was used to simulate biotic stress for triggering immunity (Fig. 2). Upon stress stimulation, there was a rapid and robust increase in the expression of DIRs, especially DIR1 (Fig. 2a). Compared with DIR2, the expression of DIR1 was more significantly increased by $55.12\pm25.45$ folds at 6 h following $H_2O_2$ treatment. NaCl and Flg22 increased the expression of DIR1 by $5.79\pm3.08$ and $31.32\pm7.04$ folds at 0.5 h, respectively. The expression of DIR2 was induced at 0.5, 6, and 0.5 h after the different stress treatments. These results suggest that DIR1 expression may play an important role in plant defense, especially in response to oxidative stress.

We next investigated the stress resistance of control and overexpression hairy roots (Fig. 2b). After 9-day cultivation, the growth rate and biomass of DIR1-OVX and DIR2-OVX hairy roots were significantly higher than those in the control following NaCl and $H_2O_2$ treatment, suggesting that DIR1 and DIR2 were involved in tolerance to abiotic stresses. Flg22 is often used to induce plant immune responses caused by microorganisms without causing actual damage to the plants. Although the hairy roots of the control and overexpression lines had similar growth rates (biomass of ~10 g), the inducible expression by Flg22 implied the involvement of the DIR proteins in response to biotic stresses (Fig. 2a). In addition to the increase of lignan levels in DIR overexpressing roots (Fig. 1c–e), we also found an increase in lignin content (both S- and G-type lignin) (Supporting Information Fig. S9), which is important for plant defense; further-more, S/G ratio values decreased from 1.64 to 1.17 and 1.45 in the DIR1-OVX and DIR2-OVX hairy roots, respectively (Fig. 2c and d), which could be caused by the increased content of coniferyl alcohol (Supporting Information Fig. S6). Furthermore, fluorescence localization of GFP indicated that both DIR1 and DIR2 specifically localize in the cell periphery, which allows them to perform biological functions extracellularly (Fig. 2e). These results suggest that DIRs, especially DIR1, participate in the regulation of stress resistance by mediating lignan and lignin biosynthesis in *I. indigotica* (Fig. 2c).

3.4 LTF1 positively regulates stress resistance through lignan biosynthesis Given that a typical ERF binding element (GCCGCC box) was found in the promoter of DIR1, the ERF transcription factor may regulate DIR1 expression and lignan synthesis (Supporting Information Fig. S10). ERF transcription factors play an important role in the response to biotic and abiotic stresses. Through "gene-metabolite" network analysis, we previously predicted that an ERF transcription factor, lignan biosynthesis-associated transcription factor 1 (LTF1), which is highly expressed in roots, was correlated with lignan biosynthesis. Comparison of the amino acid sequences along with phylogenetic analysis indicated that LTF1 was homolog to the unknown ERF1B of other Cruciferae (*Rs*ERF1 of *Raphanus sativus* and *Br*ERF1 of *Brassica rapa*) and seemingly clustered with *At*ERF1, which was thought in plant defense with unknown mechanisms (Fig. 3a, Supporting Information Dataset 3). LTF1 subcellular localization was determined by transiently expressing an N-terminal fusion of ERF1 to GFP in *N. benthamiana* leaves by agroinfiltration. The specific fluorescence localization of the LTF1-GFP fusion protein indicated that it functioned as a transcription factor in the nucleus (Fig. 3b). The transcriptional pattern showed that LTF1 was highly expressed in roots, which was similar to the accumulation characteristics of lignans (Fig. 3c and d).

Biosynthesis of antiviral lignans in *I. indigotica* is originated from phenylalanine and is accomplished by three cooperative pathways including the phenylpropanoid pathway, aromatic alcohol pathway, and lignan pathway (Fig. 3e). The gene transcript abundance detected by qPCR showed that the expression pattern of LTF1 was very similar to that of DIR1, as well as some other pathway genes (*e.g.*, PLR and CCR) (Fig. 3f). These results suggest that LTF1 is strongly associated with lignan biosynthesis in roots and is a strong candidate gene for mediating stress resistance. By the way, the low expression levels of DIR1 and DIR2 are consistent with the weak stereoselective synthesis of (−)-pinoresinol derived lignans in stems and leaves (Supporting Information Fig. S3e and f).

From the above screening, LTF1 was selected and further characterized. The expression of LTF1 was rapidly

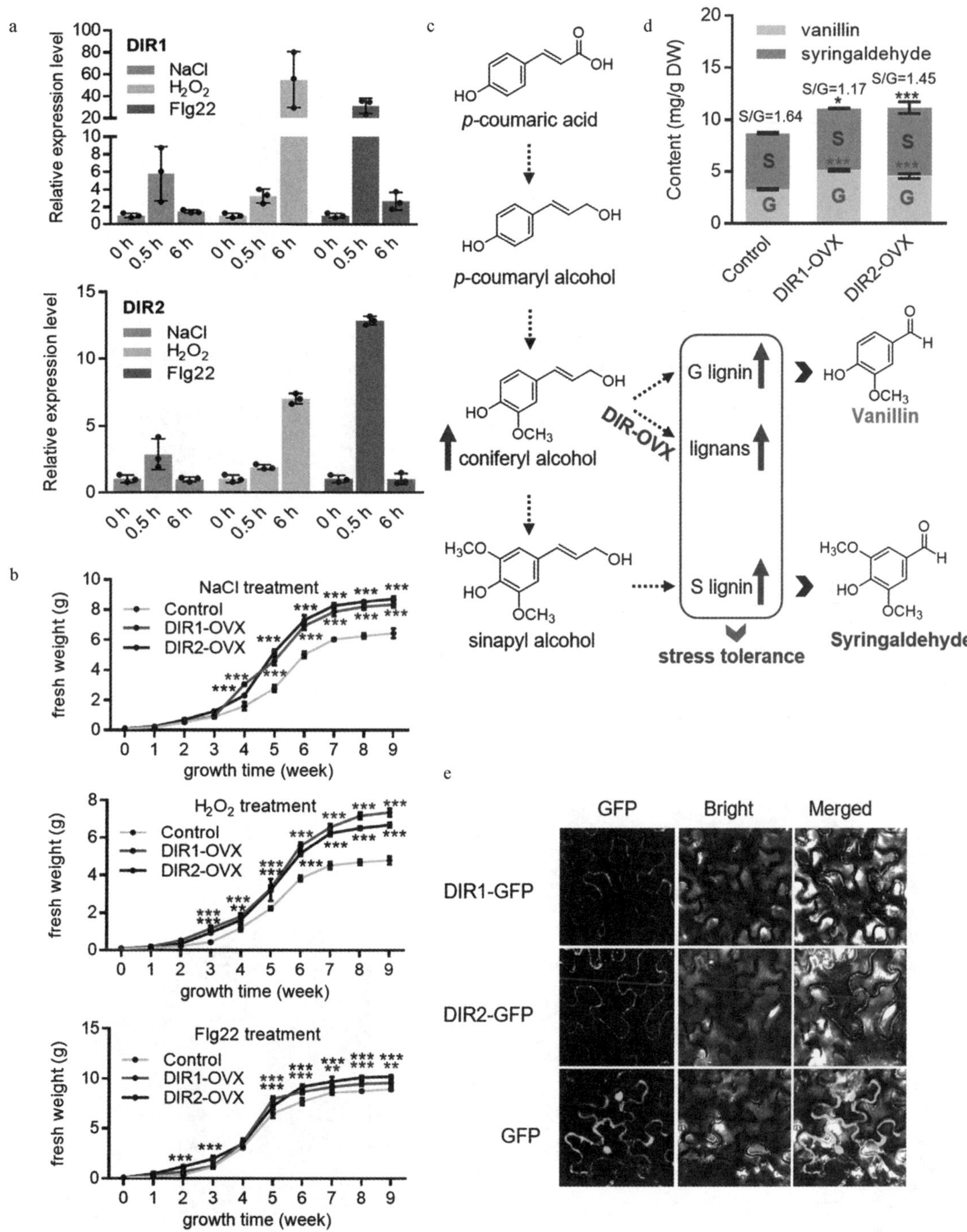


**Figure 2 Stress resistance by DIR1 and DIR2 in plants**

(a) qRT-PCR analysis of DIR1 and DIR2 induction by NaCl, $H_2O_2$ and Flg22 treatment. (b) Growth curves of control and overexpression hairy roots after NaCl, $H_2O_2$ and Flg22 treatment. (c) Metabolic mechanism by which DIR exerts stress resistance. (d) Lignin analysis in control and overexpression hairy roots. (e) Subcellular localization of DIR1 and DIR2 in *N. benthamiana* leaf epidermal cells. Statistical analysis was carried out by using Two-way ANOVA ($^{**}P<0.005$, $^{***}P<0.001$).

induced by salt, $H_2O_2$, and Flg22 over 6 h, and the expression peaked at 0.5, 6, and 0.5 h, respectively, for the different stress treatments (Supporting Information Fig. S11). The expression of defense- and stress-responsive genes in response to biotic and abiotic stresses are modulated by the antagonistic interactions between multiple components of the ABA and ethylene signaling pathways. Considering that phytohormones play an important role in the response to stresses, we asked whether ethephon (ET) and ABA affect the induction of LTF1 expression. The results of qRT-PCR indicated that ET significantly triggered LTF1 expression after 1 h of treatment, which was highly similar to the expression pattern of DIR1 and DIR2 (Fig. 4a). The response intensity of DIR1 and DIR2 to ET was significantly higher

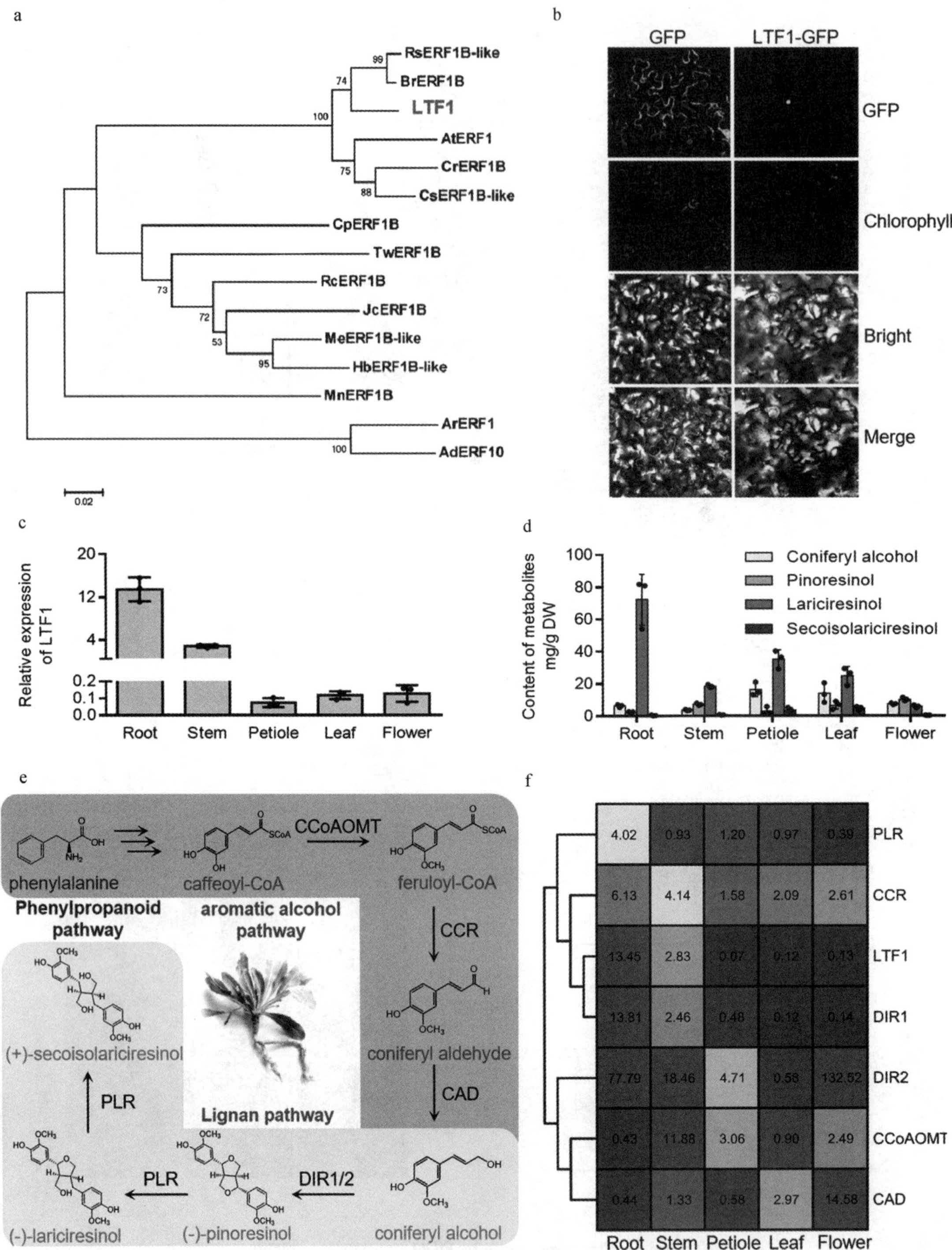


**Figure 3　Expression patterns of LTF1**

(a) Phylogenetic analysis of LTF1. (b) Transient expression of LTF1 - GFP fusion in *N. benthamiana* leaves. Image shows nuclear localization of LTF1 - GFP. LTF1 expression (c) and lignan contents (d) in different organs of *I. indigotica*. (e) Biosynthetic pathway of lignans. (f) Cluster analysis of gene expression patterns in different organs. Gene expression levels from low to high are represented by the transition from blue to red. Values represent relative expression levels.

than that of other pathway genes, implying that DIR may be a key step of the lignan pathway in response to environmental changes. Conversely, LTF1 was inhibited after 0.5 h of ABA treatment and gradually recovered at later time points (Fig. 4b). It should be noted that DIR1 and DIR2 had completely different responses to ABA, and only DIR1 maintained the same expression pattern as LTF1. Furthermore, LTF1 induction by ET treatment was suppressed by ABA, which was again consistent with DIR1 (Fig. 4c). These results imply that LTF1 may regulate lignan biosynthesis through DIR1, rather than DIR2, and mediate stress resistance. The GUS staining assays also showed that $P_{LTF1}$ : GUS and

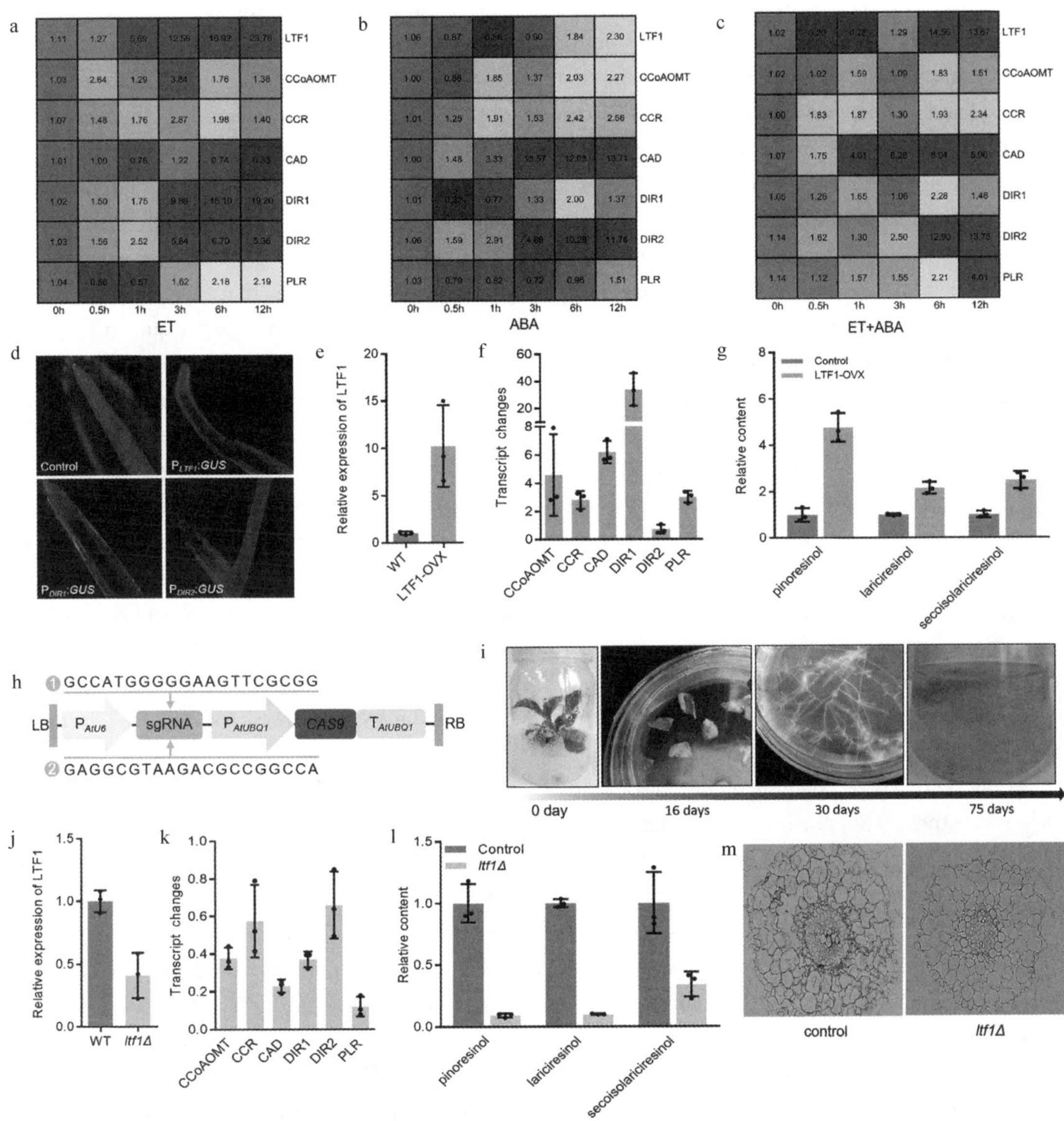


**Figure 4 LTF1 positively regulates lignan biosynthesis in the roots of *I. indigotica***

Heatmap of the expression patterns of lignan pathway genes in response to ET (a), ABA (b) and ET + ABA (c). (d) Analysis of GUS activity driven by the LTF1, DIR1 and DIR2 promoters in hairy roots. (e) Relative expression of LTF1 in LTF1-OVX hairy roots. (f) The changes in transcript expression of ligan pathway genes in LTF1-OVX hairy roots. (g) The relative level of lignans in LTF1-OVX hairy roots compared to the control. (h) The design of sgRNA for LTF1 editing. (i) The induction and cultivation *I. indigotica* hairy roots. (j) Relative expression of LTF1 in *ltf1Δ* hairy roots. (k) The changes in transcript expression of ligan pathway genes in *ltf1Δ* hairy roots. (l) The relative level of lignans in *ltf1Δ* hairy roots compared to the control. (m) Cross sections of hairy roots stained with phloroglucinol-HCl.

$P_{DIR1}$: GUS expression principally occurred in the vascular strand of mature root tissues, while $P_{DIR2}$: GUS was principally expressed in root tips, which further suggests a potential regulatory relationship between LTF1 and DIR1 (Fig. 4d).

To test this conjecture, we first overexpressed LTF1 in LTF1-OVX hairy roots, where the expression level of LTF1 was successfully increased $10.23 \pm 4.31$ folds compared to the control (Fig. 4e). As expected, DIR1 expression levels were dramatically increased by $33.80 \pm 12.00$ folds (Fig. 4f). Conversely, the expression level of DIR2 in the LTF1-OVX hairy root was only $0.72 \pm 0.33$ folds of that in the control. Clearly, these results indicated a significant positive regulation of DIR1 by LTF1. Metabolite analysis indicated a $4.76 \pm 0.61$ folds increase in pinoresinol content in the LTF1-OVX hairy root compared to the control (Fig. 4g). The increase of pinoresinol content was also transmitted to downstream, which increased the accumulation levels of lariciresinol and secoisolariciresinol by $2.15 \pm 0.26$ and $2.47 \pm 0.37$ folds, respectively. The results of qRT-PCR indicated that abiotic and biotic stresses also triggered the LTF1 expression, which was very similar to the response of DIR1 (Fig. S11). Growth curve analysis showed that overexpression of LTF1 made hairy roots grow better under the stress treatments (Supporting Information Fig. S12). Based on these results, we conclude that LTF1 can respond to environmental stresses through phytohormones, thereby positively regulating DIR1 expression and lignan biosynthesis to increase stress resistance.

To verify the necessity of LTF1 in stress resistance by lignans, we tried to mutate the LTF1 gene in hairy roots through the CRISPR/Cas9 system. Based on the previously constructed genome of *I. indigotica*, two potential high-scoring 20-bp sequences followed by the NGG (PAM sequence) from the open reading frame (ORF) of LTF1 were designed and cloned into a construct harboring a chimeric single guide RNA (sgRNA) driven by the *A. thaliana* U6-26 promoter ($P_{AtU6}$) (Fig. 4h). The constructs were transformed into *A. rhizogenes* to infect wounded young leaves for generating hairy roots (Fig. 4i). Heterozygous and biallelic mutations that produced superimposed sequence chromatograms of LTF1 were decoded using the Degenerate Sequence Decoding method. Sequencing data revealed that sgRNA1 and sgRNA2 generated 10 and 12 hairy root lines containing mutations with corresponding mutation rates of 52% and 47%, respectively (Supporting Information Table S1). Of these, seven mutations were homozygous, with mutations occurring in the same DNA locus in both alleles (Supporting Information Fig. S13). Others were non-homozygous mutations, including six heterozygous mutations (wild type/single mutation) and nine biallelic mutations (two distinct variations). Most mutations generated by sgRNA1 caused a single nucleotide insertion of A or T, whereas many mutations produced by sgRNA2 had multiple nucleotide deletions. Three hairy root lines (lines 1-5, 1-18, and 2-1) with significantly reduced expression of LTF1 were selected by qRT-PCR and used for further analysis (Fig. 4j). The qPCR results showed that the expression of lignan pathway genes was reduced to varying extents upon mutation of LTF1 (Fig. 4k). The expression of DIR1 and DIR2 in *ltf1Δ* hairy roots was 0.37±0.04 folds and 0.66±0.18 folds of that in control hairy roots. Combined with the results of tissue localization experiments, these results show that DIR1 expression is likely controlled by LTF1, while LTF1 does not regulate the expression of DIR2 (Fig. 4d). Unexpectedly, the expression of other pathway genes was also inhibited in *ltf1Δ* hairy roots, especially PLR, which was decreased most significantly to only 0.12 ± 0.05 folds of the control, suggesting that LTF1 is essential for the normal expression of PLR. Metabolite analysis revealed that the contents of pinoresinol, lariciresinol, and secoisolariciresinol were significantly reduced to 0.09±0.02, 0.10±0.01 and 0.34±0.10 folds of the control, respectively (Fig. 4l). Phloroglucinol-HCl staining of cross sections of hairy roots shows that the *ltf1Δ* hairy root had a weaker browning of vascular regions visually compared to the control, which reveals that LTF1 is necessary for the accumulation of lignans, lignin, and/or wall-bound phenolics and derivatives (Fig. 4k). Thus, it is reasonable that the growth of *ltf1Δ* hairy roots was worse than that of the control (Supporting Information Fig. S12). Based on these results, we preliminarily conclude that LTF1 plays a stress-resistant function by regulating the expression of the lignan pathway gene DIR1, and LTF1 is also critical for the expression of other genes in the pathway, especially PLR.

3.5 LTF1 directly upregulates DIR1 for stress defense

Previous results indicated that the expression of the stress resistance-related DIR1, instead of DIR2, was significantly elevated in the LTF1-OVX line and decreased in the *ltf1Δ* line. To investigate the underlying mechanisms by which LTF1 regulates DIR1 expression and lignan biosynthesis, we found a typical ERF binding element (GCCGCC box) in the DIR1 promoter (Supporting Information Fig. S9). Considering that the homolog of LTF1 in other plants, can directly regulate gene expression by binding to the GCC box, we speculate that DIR1 may also be directly regulated by LTF1. To test this hypothesis, the yeast one-hybrid assay (Y1H), electrophoretic mobility shift assay (EMSA), and transient luciferase analysis were performed.

We first performed Y1H assays to determine whether LTF1 was able to directly bind the DIR1 promoter sequence ($P_{DIR1}$) containing the GCC box. Y1H assays were carried out with the addition of 50 mmol/L 3-AT to inhibit the self-activating effect (false positive result) and the results showed that LTF1 was indeed able to bind the 3×GCC element in the DIR1 promoter to activate the expression of the reporter gene HIS3, which allowed yeast to grow on selection plates (-T/-L/-H/+50 mmol/L 3-AT) (Supporting Information Fig. S14, Fig. 5a). Conversely, all negative controls, including the use of the mutated 3×TCC element ($P_{mutDIR1}$), failed to grow clones on the selection plate.

Next, $P_{DIR1}$ was used as a labeled probe for EMSAs, and the results showed a distinct shift band of the DNA-LTF1 complex (column 2) (Fig. 5b). Binding activity was gradually diluted by the unlabeled probes (columns 3-6) and the labeled mutated probes with the TCCTCC box (columns 7-10). These results provide strong evidence that LTF1 binds to the native promoter of DIR1 through the GCCGCC *cis*-element.

To further verify whether LTF1 positively regulates the transcription of DIR1, we performed transient expression assays in *N. benthamiana* leaves (Fig. 5c). The DIR1 promoter region $P_{DIR1}$ was used to drive the luciferase gene (*LUC*) as the reporter, and LTF1 was overexpressed under

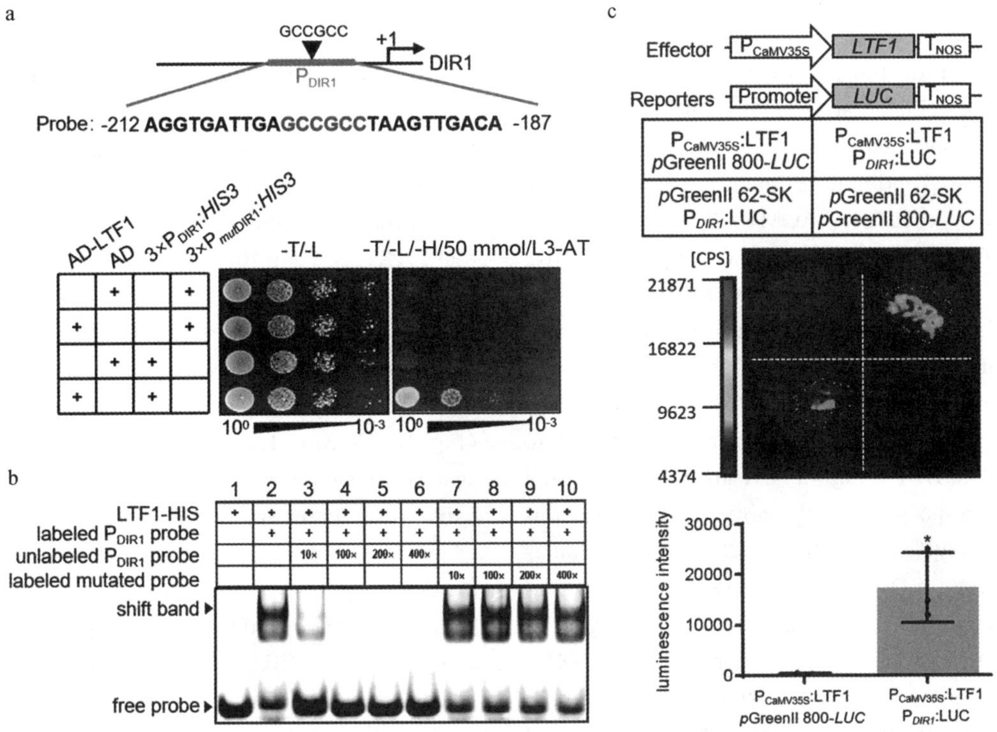


**Figure 5 LTF1 directly binds to the GCC box of the DIR1 promoter and activates its transcription**

(a) Promoter of DIR1. (b) Y1H assays showing that the LTF1 protein binds to triple (3×) tandem repeats in the $P_{DIR1}$ sequence of the DIR1 promoter. Black triangles represent the dilution ratio of the yeast suspension. (c) EMSAs showing that LTF1 specifically binds to the $P_{DIR1}$ sequence of the DIR1 promoter. An excess of the unlabeled probe (lines 3 - 6) and labeled mutated probe (lines 7 - 10) were used as competitors. The free and bound DNA bands are indicated by black arrows. (d) Transient luciferase analysis showing that higher luminescence intensity was observed following coexpression of *LTF1* and $P_{DIR1}$ : *LUC*. Quantitative analysis of luminescence intensity was performed. Statistical analysis was carried out by using Student's *t*-test (one-tailed, * $P<0.05$).

the control of the CaMV35S promoter ($P_{CaMV35S}$) as the effector. Detection of LUC luminescence indicated that overexpression of LTF1 ($P_{CaMV35S}$ : LTF1) significantly increased the LUC signal of the reporter ($P_{DIR1}$ : LUC) compared to controls lacking $P_{CaMV35S}$ : LTF1.

In conclusion, combined with the analysis of hairy roots, these results showed that LTF1 can transcriptionally upregulate lignan biosynthesis through the first key enzyme DIR1.

## 4 CONCLUSIONS AND DISCUSSIONS

In addition to the involvement in the process of plant defense, lignans have various activities to protect human health. Lignans are the main antiviral components in the *I. indigotica* root. However, the stereo configuration of lignans and their stereoselective biosynthetic pathway in *I. indigotica* are unclear, which may threaten the safety of medicine use and make it difficult for plant improvement. Although lignans have been considered key players in plant stress resistance, the long-sought-after mechanism of lignan biosynthesis in response to the environment has remained elusive.

In this study, we systematically identified the stereoselective biosynthesis of lignans in the *I. indigotica* root, which determined (−)-lariciresinol glucosides as antiviral lignans. First, we found that two of the 19 DIRs (DIR1 and DIR2) were highly expressed in the *I. indigotica* root, showed stereoselectivity *in vitro* by guiding the synthesis of (−)-pinoresinol, and showed significant regioselectivity *in vivo*, thereby promoting the accumulation of lignans in roots (Fig. 1). In the consequent step, PLR showed stereoselectivity for the substrate and catalyzed the formation of specific configurations of (−)-lariciresinol and (+)-secoisolariciresinol. The last step of antiviral (−)-lariciresinol glucoside biosynthesis involved the reaction of UGT71B2 with (−)-lariciresinol. The biochemical functions of DIR1, DIR2, PLR, and UGT71B2 explain the lignan composition in the roots of *I. indigotica* (Supporting Information Fig. S3).

In addition, we showed that overexpression of DIR1 and DIR2 increased biosynthesis of lignan and lignin, resulting in significantly enhanced stress tolerance of hairy roots to NaCl, $H_2O_2$, and Flg22 (Fig. 2). Additionally, we observed a high consistency between the expression patterns of DIR1 and LTF1 (tissue localization, phytohormone response, and stress induction). We found that LTF1 directly activates DIR1 to enhance plant defense ability through lignan biosynthesis, which sheds light on the potential application of lignan biosynthesis in improving plant stress tolerance (Figs. 4 and 5). As shown in Fig. 4, the expression levels of some other pathway genes were changed in LTF1 overexpressed and mutated plants. Among the gene promoters available to us (CCoAOMT, DIR2 and, PLR) (Supporting Information Dataset 4), only the DIR2 promoter contains many *cis*-elements related to stress response and binding sites of MYB transcription factors (Supporting Information Fig. S10), which imply the different regulatory mechanisms for DIR2 expression. The fact that DIR2 shows a completely different response to phytohormones than DIR1 (Fig. 4a-c), and CCoAOMT and PLR are also less responsive to phytohormones, support this hypothesis. Notably, although DIR2 has a similar biochemical function to DIR1, the response level to stresses of DIR2 is much weaker than that of DIR1 (Fig. 2a), indicating that DIR1 is more like a supplement for DIR2 under environmental stresses, making lignan synthesis more efficient. Given that methyl jasmonate (MeJA) is a vital plant cellular regulator that mediates defense responses against biotic and abiotic stresses, including drought, salinity, and pathogen infection, the MeJA induced transcript abundance of all identified genes of the lignan pathway and DIR family members were analyzed through the previously constructed transcriptome data (Supporting Information Fig. S15). As expected, all genes of the lignan pathway are highly expressed in the root. The transcript abundance of five members of the DIR family (DIR1, DIR2, DIR9, DIR11, and DIR17) is higher in the root. Interestingly, of the all identified lignan pathway genes, only DIR1 can significantly respond to MeJA treatment. Conversely, the expression of DIR2 is always at a relatively high level in the root. These results confirm our conclusion that DIR1 is vital for the environmental response of *I. indigotica* roots through regulating lignan biosynthesis.

We developed a CRISPR/Cas9-guided gene-editing system for *I. indigotica* to construct *ltf1Δ* hairy roots, which showed extreme lignan defects and stress susceptibility (Fig. 4). Conversely, the content of lignan and the defense against stresses were significantly increased in LTF1-OVX hairy roots. Based on this data, we propose a working model of the *I. indigotica* stress response in which LTF1 responds to environmental stresses through phytohormone-related signal transduction, directly binding to the DIR1 promoter and activating DIR1 expression in the cell periphery of vascular regions in mature roots and further triggering the accumulation of lignin and the stereoselective synthesis of lignans (Fig. 6). Furthermore, the increased content of lignan and lignin lead to higher stress resistance in *I. indigotica*.

Although transcription factors AP2/ERF049 of Soloist sub-family and WRKY34 in our previous studies have been proven to affect lignan synthesis through PAL and 4CL of phenylpropanoid pathway, and CCR of aromatic alcohol pathway, which all are not direct regulation of the lignan

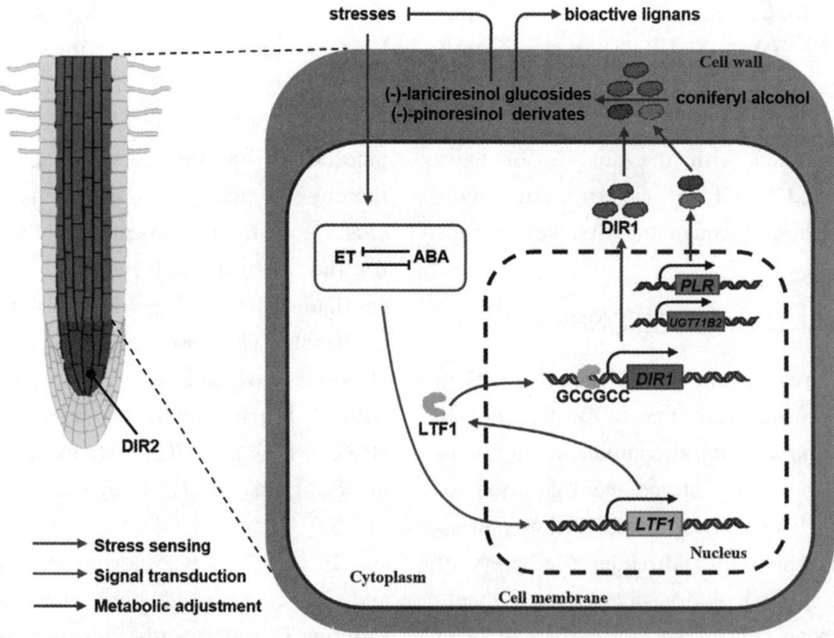


**Figure 6 Proposed working model depicting the roles of LTF1-DIR1 module in lignan biosynthesis and stress defense**

The stresses are sensed by diverse receptors and the perceived signals further trigger stress-specific signal transduction. The multilevel transduction ultimately activates LTF1, which further binds to the promoter of DIR1 to up-regulate the expression of DIR1. The DIR1 protein is specifically localized in the cell periphery of vascular regions in mature roots to direct the accumulation of lignin and the stereoselective synthesis of lignans and thus plays a role in stress defense.

pathway. The LTF1 of the ERF subfamily in this study is the first transcription factor directly activating lignan biosynthesis through DIR, the common key gene of all lignan biosynthesis in plants. As reported, DIR and homologs thereof are found in at least 104 studied terrestrial plants but not in aquatic organisms (such as algae), bacteria and mammals, indicating that the DIR family may originate from and be present in vascular plants to withstand the stresses on land. Most members of the DIR family in *A. thaliana* (15 of 22) and *I. indigotica* (9 of 19) are highly expressed in roots, further implying that vascular plants may have evolved the DIR family and their specific functions during the process of land colonization. As an increasing number of DIR proteins have been characterized, there is no doubt that some DIRs with regio- and stereoselectivity mediate the specific production of (+)- or (−)-pinoresinol. In addition to the identified pinoresinol-forming DIRs, there are at least 20, 35, and 17 DIRs with unknown functions in *A. thaliana*, *Picea spruce*, and *I. indigotica*, respectively. Considering that their expression levels all show temporal and spatial specificity, as well as inducibility, it is reasonable to speculate that they could have specific biological functions in response to stress. For example, a Dirigent domain-containing protein identified in *A. thaliana* mediates resistance to floods and droughts by regulating the formation of the Casparian strip in the root. Therefore, more efforts are needed to unravel the mystery of DIR functions in plant defense. This study verified that the root-specific DIRs (DIR1 and DIR2) of *I. indigotica* are involved in stress resistance (salt, oxidative and pathogen stress in this study) *in vivo* through overexpression experiments, and this finding suggests that the DIRs in other plants with the same biochemical function in mediating the selective biosynthesis of lignans should play a role in stress resistance. The inducibility of these genes by phytohormones and stresses further supports this hypothesis. In the signal transduction process, whether in response to biotic stress or abiotic stress, $H_2O_2$ is an important signaling molecule, and $H_2O_2$ is detrimental to biomolecules when its levels exceed the cellular capacity for detoxification. As polyphenolic compounds, lignans may achieve stress resistance by eliminating ROS, and this idea has been verified by pharmacological experiments. On the other hand, the free radical oxidative coupling reaction of coniferyl alcohol to generate pinoresinol can consume $H_2O_2$, and the increase in DIR expression can significantly enhance the number of reactions (Fig. 1 and Supporting Information Fig. S5). Thus, the expression of DIRs is significantly upregulated under stresses in *I. indigotica*, and this probably enhances the consumption of $H_2O_2$ by the free radical oxidation coupling reaction, which in turn increases resistance to stresses.

In addition to stress defense for plants, lignans with the specific stereo configuration often have important physiological functions in humans, such as the functions of (−)-podophyllotoxin as pharmaceuticals for cancer treatment. In particular, chemically-modified derivatives of (−)-podophyllotoxin, teniposide, etoposide, and etoposide are widely used in cancer chemotherapy. Although lignan glucosides are the main antiviral active component of *I. indigotica*, their stereo configurations are still unclear. This study indicated that 3 enzymes (DIR, PLR, and UGT) with stereoselectivity cooperate to synthesize (−)-pinoresinol derived lignans and antiviral (−)-lariciresinol glucosides in *I. indigotica* roots. The overexpression of DIR1 and DIR2 in hairy roots proved that DIR1 and DIR2 were involved in the *in vivo* synthesis of (−)-pinoresinol derived lignans, and also significantly increased the content of antiviral lignans and stress resistance. Therefore, we believe that DIR is an ideal target to engineer plants that accumulate valuable lignans, which will increase the content of lignans while also improving stress resistance.

[陈瑞兵,陈万生,张磊,等. Acta Pharmaceutica Sinica B, 2024,14(1):405-420.]

# ZnO-*S. cerevisiae*: an effective growth promoter of *Astragalus memeranaceus* and nano-antifungal agent against *Fusarium oxysporum*

## 1 INTRODUCTION

*Astragalus memeranaceus* has been used to treat diseases for thousands of years, which is the dried root of legume *A. membranaceus* (Fisch.) Bge. var. *mongholicus* (Bge.) Hsiao or *A. membranaceus* (Fisch.) Bunge. *A. memeranaceus* can resist viruses and preserve the myocardium, and exhibits other biological activities, including anti-aging, anti-infective, cytoprotective, anti-inflammatory, and antioxidant. The main bioactive components are triterpene glycosides, flavonoids, saponins, and alkaloids, among which astragaloside IV is an important triterpenoid. Astragaloside IV has effects of anti-inflammatory, antifibrotic, antioxidant stress, anti-asthma, anti-diabetes, and is a natural neuroprotective agent for neurological disorders.

Due to destructive exploitation, cultivation are main resource, and root rot is a common disease in the cultivation of *A. memeranaceus*. After infection, the ground part grows weakly and thinly, the color of the leaves is pale to grayish green. In severe cases, the leaves of the whole plant will be yellow and fall off. At the same time, the underground part becomes rough and brown on the root and stem. *Fusarium oxysporum* is a main pathogen of root rot in *A. memeranaceus*. This worldwide soilborne pathogenic fungus infects with a wide range of hosts, which can cause *Fusarium wilt* in more than 100 species of plants, including melons, solanaceae, bananas, cotton, legumes and flowers.

The incidence of root rot is affected by various factors. Generally, root rot appears at the beginning of May, and becomes serious during mid-July to mid-August. Synthetic fungicides such as carbendazim has been widely used. In agriculture, spray carbendazim powder evenly on the surface under no wind conditions, the control results can be reduced to 47%-56%. Metalaxyl is another fungicide commonly used to control root rot. Although, pesticides have good effects, they caused great damage to the environment. More important, they have negative impact on food security, extensive and repeated use may lead to toxic effects on humans. In recent years, biological agents become emerging, antagonism is a well method. Li et al., constructed a synthetic community that rescues *A. memeranaceus* from root rot disease by activating plant-induced systemic resistance. The *B. atrophaeus SXKF16-1* showed a significant inhibition effect on pathogen causing root rot, which has the potential to be developed as a special biocontrol agent. The emerging nanomaterials are a kind of prevalent antimicrobial method with stable, environmentally friendly, cost-efficient characteristic. More and more studies showed its advantages over chemical pesticides. Ag NPs with high stability and low volatility has a long history of application, exhibits excellent antifungal effects on fungi. ZnO NPs is one of most widely used nanomaterials with high biocompatibility, good chemical stability, and low toxicity, which exhibits attractive antimicrobial properties due to its increased specific surface area and is a promising biosafety material. ZnO NPs has muti-effects, such as promotes plant growth, helps cope with stress, induces resistance genes and antioxidant enzymes. $Fe_3O_4$ NPs also has a good antibacterial effect due to the reactive oxygen species together with superoxide radicals and singlet oxygen. $Fe_3O_4$ NPs can improve plant immunity and act as plant growth promoter.

At present, there are few studies on the application of nanomaterials against *F. oxysporum* in *A. memeranaceus*. Meanwhile, natural and nontoxic biological agents have good antifungal effects. We aimed to screen a kind of composited biological nanomaterial that inhibit root rot, as well as explore the metabolism of *A. memeranaceus* and antifungal mechanism. In this study, we found the multifunctional ZnO-*S. cerevisiae* with good antifungal activity is a promising alternative to traditional antifungal agents and has great potential in the protection of *A. memeranaceus* (see Fig. 1).

## 2 EXPERIMENTAL SECTION

2.1 Materials The seeds of *Astragalus membranaceus* (Fisch.) Bge. var. mongholicus (Bge) Hsiao (*A. membranaceus*) were collected from Inner Mongolia, China. *F. oxysporum* was purchased from CICC (China Center Of Industrial Culture Collection). Pesticides are mainly composed of metalaxyl (6%) and hymexazol (24%).

2.2 Cultivation of hydroponic seedlings The cultivation of *A. membranaceus* is referred to Liu et al.,. The sterilized seeds of *A. membranaceus* were germinated in Murashige and Skoog (MS) medium supplemented with 30 g/L sucrose, and 7 g/L agar to induce seedlings. After 2 weeks of induction, seedlings were subsequently transferred to flasks containing liquid 3/4 B5 medium supple-mented with 1 mg/L IBA, 0.4 mg/L KT and 30 g/L sucrose for suspension cultures. The cultures were maintained at 25℃ on a gyratory shaker at 100 rpm.

2.3 Preparation and characterization of ZnO-*S. cerevisiae*

2.3.1 $Fe_3O_4$ NPs A certain amount (the molar ratio of $Fe^{2+}$, $Fe^{3+}$ and $OH^-$ is 1.00 : 1.00 : 6.00) of ferric salt ($FeCl_2 \cdot 4H_2O$) and trivalent ferric salt ($FeCl_3 \cdot 6H_2O$) is mixed into the flask, and then 28% (mass fraction) of $NH_3 \cdot H_2O$ is added to the flask vigorously stirred by water bath at 30℃ and 1 000 r/min. After the color changes from orange-red to black, continue stirring for 15 min to complete the reaction. Then centrifuge, wash repeatedly with distilled water until pH=7.0, remove the supernatants and dry in a vacuum at 60℃ for 24 h, and then grind to obtain magnetic $Fe_3O_4$ NPs.

2.3.2 The cell wall of *S. cerevisiae* The cell wall of *S. cerevisiae* is obtained by taking 50 μL from a frozen storage tube and culturing it in Potato Dextrose Agar (PDA) medium at 28℃ for two days, and then centrifuging it to obtain principate at 4℃ at 9 000 r/min for 5 min.

2.3.3 Composited NPs 1.5 g yeast is soaked in a 100 mL

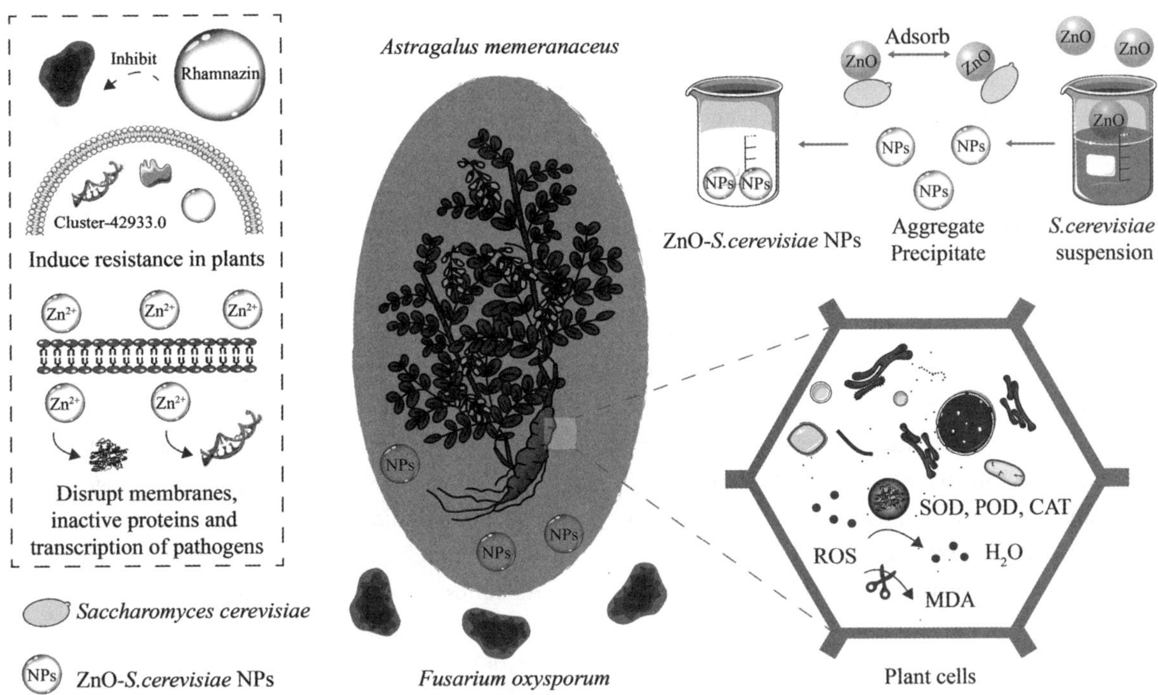


**Fig. 1 Introduction ZnO-*S. cerevisiae* can decompose ROS into $H_2O$ by increasing the activity of SOD and CAT of *Astragalus memeranaceus*, and prevent conversion into the harmful MDA. On the other hand, ZnO-*S. cerevisiae* disrupts the expression of genes related to normal physiological activities of *Fusarium oxysporum*. It can also induce resistance of *A. memeranaceus*, such as Cluster-42933.0, and promote the secretion of antifungal metabolites, such as rhamnazin**

CAT, catalase; MDA, malondialdehyde; POD, peroxidase; ROS, reactive oxygen species; SOD, Superoxide dismutase.

beaker for 5 h with distilled water to obtain the yeast suspension, and adjust the pH to 5.0. A certain amount of nanomaterials is added to a unit amount of deionized water, oscillated evenly, then treated under 40 KHZ ultrasonic wave to relieve agglomerate, and the particles are smaller and more dispersed in deionized water. Nanomaterials are ultrasonically dispersed in the suspension of *S. cerevisiae* and electrically stirred at room temperature for 30 min. NPs on the yeast cells adsorb each other, rapidly aggregate and precipitate. The supernatant is poured and centrifuged (8 000 r/min) for 30 min to obtain composited nanomaterials.

2.3.4 Optimization With other experimental conditions remained, the obtained 0.04, 0.06, 0.08, 0.10, and 0.12 mol nanomaterials are ultrasonically dispersed in the suspension of *S. cerevisiae* and electrically stirred at room temperature for 30 min.

With other experimental conditions unchanged, the obtained 0.1 mol nanomaterials are ultrasonically dispersed in the suspension of *S. cerevisiae* and electrically stirred at room temperature for 10, 20, 30, 40, and 50 min.

NPs on the yeast cells adsorb each other, rapidly aggregate and precipitate. The supernatant is poured and centrifuged (8 000 r/min) for 30 min to obtain composited nanomaterials. 1 g NPs is placed in 3 mL cuvettes and 2 mL of deionized water is added. The deposition is observed every 10 min until 30 min. Then water solubility test is undergone.

2.4 Investigation of antifungal activity In vitro investigation of antifungal activity: NPs are added respectively to PDA to achieve the final concentration of 0 mg/mL, 2 mg/mL, 4 mg/mL, 6 mg/mL, 8 mg/mL, and 10 mg/mL Then pour it into disposable petri dishes. After cooling and solidifying, inoculate the bacteria with a punch. The zone of inhibition is measured after 3 days.

In vivo investigation of antifungal activity: after cultivation for 14 days, 50 μL *F. oxysporum* with an OD value of 0.6 ~ 0.8 and 200 μL NPs with different concentrations are added at the same time. The plants are cultured for 7 days and observed every other day. According to the percentage of disease on the leaves, the severity is visually recorded every other day, and is divided into 0 - 20 grades, with an increase of 5% for each grade, where 0 represents no lesions and 20 represents 100% lesions. Disease index is calculated according to the following formula:

$$\text{Disease index} = \frac{\sum(N \times S)}{totalN \times thehighestS} \times 100\%$$

Note: N represents plant number, S represents disease scale.

The material is harvested on the 7th day for subsequent determination.

2.5 Growth of A. membranaceus seedlings To investigate the growth of infected *A. membranaceus* after treatment of ZnO-*S. cerevisiae*, we determined length, weight and content on the 7th day.

2.5.1 Astragaloside IV content Preparation of reference solution: take an appropriate amount of astragaloside IV reference solution, accurately weigh it, and add 80% methanol to make a solution containing 0.5 mg/mL Preparation of test solution: take about 1 g of the powder (passing through No. 4 sieve), weigh it precisely, put it into a conical flask with stopper, add precisely 50 mL of 80% methanol solution containing 4% concentrated ammonia test solution (take 4 mL of concentrated ammonia test solution, add 80% methanol to 100 mL, shake well), close the stopper, weigh it, heat and reflux for 1 h, cool it, weigh it again, and use 80% methanol solution containing 4% concentrated ammonia test solution to make up the lost weight. The residue is dissolved in 80% methanol and transferred to a 5 mL volumetric flask. Add 80% methanol to the scale. Shake well, filter and take the filtrate. Octadecylsilane bonded silica gel was used as filler and acetonitrile: water (32 : 68) was used as the mobile phase. The temperature of the drift tube is 110℃ and the gas flow rate is 2.8 L/min.

2.5.2 Chlorophyll content 0.2 g fresh leaves were cut into pieces and immersed into 30 mL ethanol: acetone (1 : 1) for chlorophyll extraction. and then determine the absorbance after the material turns white. After incubation overnight at room temperature in the dark, the absorbances of the chlorophyll extracts at 663 nm and 645 nm were measured. The chlorophyll content was expressed as mg per gram of fresh weight (mg/g) and calculated using the equations given by Wintermans et al.

2.6 Lipid peroxidation and antioxidant enzyme activities To investigate the influence of ZnO-*S. cerevisiae* on infected *A. memeranaceus*, we detected the activity of the antioxidant enzyme. The content of malondialdehyde (MDA) and the activities of antioxidant enzymes were measured according to previous reports. Fresh samples (0.3 g) from each treatment were ground with liquid nitrogen and homogenized in 3 mL of 50 mmol/L phosphate buffer solution (PBS, pH 7.8) for the enzyme extraction or in 3 mL of 10% trichloroacetic (TCA) solution for the MDA extraction. The supernatants were collected by centrifugation at 8 000×g for 10 min at 4℃ as raw extraction. The activities of superoxide dismutase (SOD), peroxidase (POD), catalase (CAT) and the content of MDA were measured using a UV/Vis spectrophotometer. For the accuracy, three repetitive samples from each treatment were measured. The UV/Vis spectrophotometer was calibrated before the measurement.

2.7 Comparative analysis of (differentially expressed genes) DEGs To explore the potential antifungal mechanism, we compare the transcriptome data from *F. oxysporum* with that treated with ZnO-*S. cerevisiae*. And compare the transcriptome data from *A. memeranaceus* infected by *F. oxysporum* with that treated with ZnO-*S. cerevisiae*. Differential expression analyses of two conditions per group were performed using the DESeq2 R package. The cDNA libraries were sequenced on the Illumina sequencing platform by Metware Biotechnology Co., Ltd. (Wuhan, China).

2.8 Comparative analysis of essential metabolites To explore the potential antifungal metabolites, we compare the metabolome data from *A. memeranaceus* infected by *F. oxysporum* with that treated with ZnO-*S. cerevisiae*. Differential expression analyses of two conditions per group were performed using the DESeq2 R package.

2.9 Conjoint analysis DEGs of *F. oxysporum* underwent multi-omics association analysis with up-regulated metabolites to reveal the potential mechanism of how antifungal metabolites inhibit pathogens. Thus, establish potential pathways involved in metabolites-pathogen.

Mothur software was used to calculate the Spearman rank correlation coefficient between transcriptomic data and metabolomics data. According to the result of correlation coefficient matrix *_rho_dm.txt (rho correlation coefficient is between −1 and 1, when −1<rho<0, they are negatively correlated. When 0 < rho < 1, they are positively correlated. When rho=0, there is no correlation between them), and correlation verification result *_*P*.values_dm.txt (*P*-value is the correlation test value of them, the lower the *P*-value, the higher the accuracy of the verification results), R software is used to draw heat maps.

2.10 Structure activity relationship of metabolites against F. oxysporum The up-regulated metabolites of *A. memeranaceus* were docked with the down-regulated proteins of related genes in the transcriptome of pathogens.

2.10.1 Construction of experimental related protein database According to the transcriptome of pathogens, potential pathogenic proteins were screened. Proteins were screened based on resolution and whether exists a complex of protein and ligand or not. Their 3D crystal structures with original substrate were downloaded from the RCSB Protein Data Bank (https://www.rcsb.org). 3D crystal structures were imported into Chimera 1.12, water molecules and other ligands were deleted. The 3D structures of receptors and ligands were exported respectively. The separated receptors were introduced into Auto-DockTools 1.5.6, and the polar hydrogen and charge were added to the receptors. A box was set for each receptor at the position where the ligand used to be.

2.10.2 Preparation of active compounds The main ingredients were drawn by ChemBio 3D 14.0.0.117, and energy minimization was set for each molecule.

2.10.3 Molecular docking The molecular docking between the active compounds and the target proteins was simulated. The box for each protein was set at the position where the original ligand of the protein used to be, and molecular docking was performed by the AutoDock 4.2 program with the application of the highest score and Lamarckian genetic algorithm principle. The grid maps generated using the AutoGrid module are 40 * 40 * 40 points, which are separated by 0.375 Å along the x-, y- and z-axis. To evaluate strong interaction between protein and ligand, −7 kcal/mol is considered the threshold value. The binding energy of natural protein substrates and −7 kcal/mol were used as thresholds respectively to evaluate the binding strength of small molecules and proteins. The interactions such as hydrogen bond, π-π interaction, hydrophobic interaction and salt bridge between the active compounds and target proteins were analyzed and drawn by Chimera 1.12.

2.10.4 Molecular network construction According to the docking results, the binding energies obtained by simulated molecular docking for the natural substrates or a reported inhibitor of the selected proteins were used as thresholds. Small molecules with better binding energy than the natural substrates are considered to interact with the protein. The molecule-target interaction network diagram was constructed.

2.11 Statistical analysis All data are presented as the means ± standard deviation (SD). The statistical significance of all data was analyzed using SPSS 19 software. Differences between groups were determined using a one-way analysis of variance (ANOVA) and compared using Duncan's test at the $P<0.05$ level.

## 3 RESULTS AND DISCUSSION

3.1 Preparation and characterization of ZnO-*S. cerevisiae* As shown in Fig. 2A, the synthesized $Fe_3O_4$ NPs were characterized with a good particle size of 248.5 nm. The cell wall of *S. cerevisiae* was characterized by a large particle size, and the analytical quality was still good for biological materials (Fig. 2B). The particle size of ZnO was 1 841 nm (Fig. 2C). The synthesized ZnO-*S. cerevisiae* were characterized. After optimizing the content of ZnO NPs and stirring time, the particle size of the ZnO-*S. cerevisiae* was 562.1 nm when 0.12 mol ZnO NPs was added per 1.5 g *S. cerevisiae* for 10 min (Fig. 2D, F and G). ZnO NPs is an adaptable material that has large specific area and good compatibility. Therefore, ZnO NPs with strong adsorption can be uniformly adsorbed on the *S. cerevisiae*. The adsorption between ZnO NPs caused composited material to flocculate and precipitate in an aqueous solution.

3.2 Antifungal activity of ZnO-*S. cerevisiae* against *F. oxysporum* The NPs were screened by antifungal inhibition test. Astragaloside IV has no significant antifungal effect, and increases the diameter of the antifungal zone, which may be used as the carbon source of pathogens. This indicated that *A. memeranaceus* could not inhibit the growth of pathogens by itself, which excluded the interference of astragaloside IV in subsequent tests. Subsequently, the antifungal activity of NPs was tested. As shown in Fig. 3A and C, it was found that $Fe_3O_4$ had no significant antifungal effect, while ZnO NPs inhibits *F. oxysporum*. Previous studies revealed that ZnO NPs shows significant antifungal activity toward other fungi, such as *Alternaria alternata*, *Rhizopus stolonifer*. As a safe biological material, *S. cerevisiae* were demonstrated that have antimicrobial effects. As shown in Fig. 3A and C, *S. cerevisiae* also has antifungal properties. The composite ZnO-*S. cerevisiae* exhibited ideal antifungal activity at different concentrations, among which the high concentration of NPs had the same effect as the positive control (commercial pesticide for pathogens in agriculture).

The water solubility of materials was investigated. Although the antifungal effect of ZnO NPs is good, its water solubility is poor. As shown in Fig. 3B, individual ZnO NPs gradually precipitated to the bottom, and finally all sank to the bottom within 30 min. Despite the deposition, most of the ZnO-*S. cerevisiae* were still suspended in the cuvette after 30 min.

ZnO NPs as a zinc fertilizer has been studied and applied to promote plants growth. It was reported that ZnO NPs can help *Alfalfa* seedlings alleviate heat-induced morpho-physiological and ultrastructural damages. ZnO NPs can also be used to protect plants from disease. For example, protect rice from rice blast by inhibiting *M. oryzae*. Then the bacteriostatic effect on plants was investigated.

The antifungal inhibition test of the plant was investigated. As shown in Fig. 4, on the 3rd day, the CK group appeared cloudy, on the 5th day, more pathogens appeared, and finally on the 7th day, the bottle was full of pathogens. After adding ZnO-*S. cerevisiae*, the group was more clarified on the 3rd day, some pathogens appeared on the 5th day, and the contamination of the bottle on the 7th day was lighter than that of the CK. To be more specific, at the beginning, 0 - 8 mg/mL are clear, because of the high concentration, few composited materials suspended in solution at 10 mg/mL. On the 3rd day, the treat groups are clearer than the control, among them, the disease index of 4 mg/mL is the most serious, while the other group is the lighter. On the 5th day, pathogens gradually grew, visible colony appeared at the 10 mg/mL, while the disease index of other treatment groups were less serious. On the 7th day, most groups were full of pathogens, among them, the group at 10 mg/mL was the most serious, while, the disease index

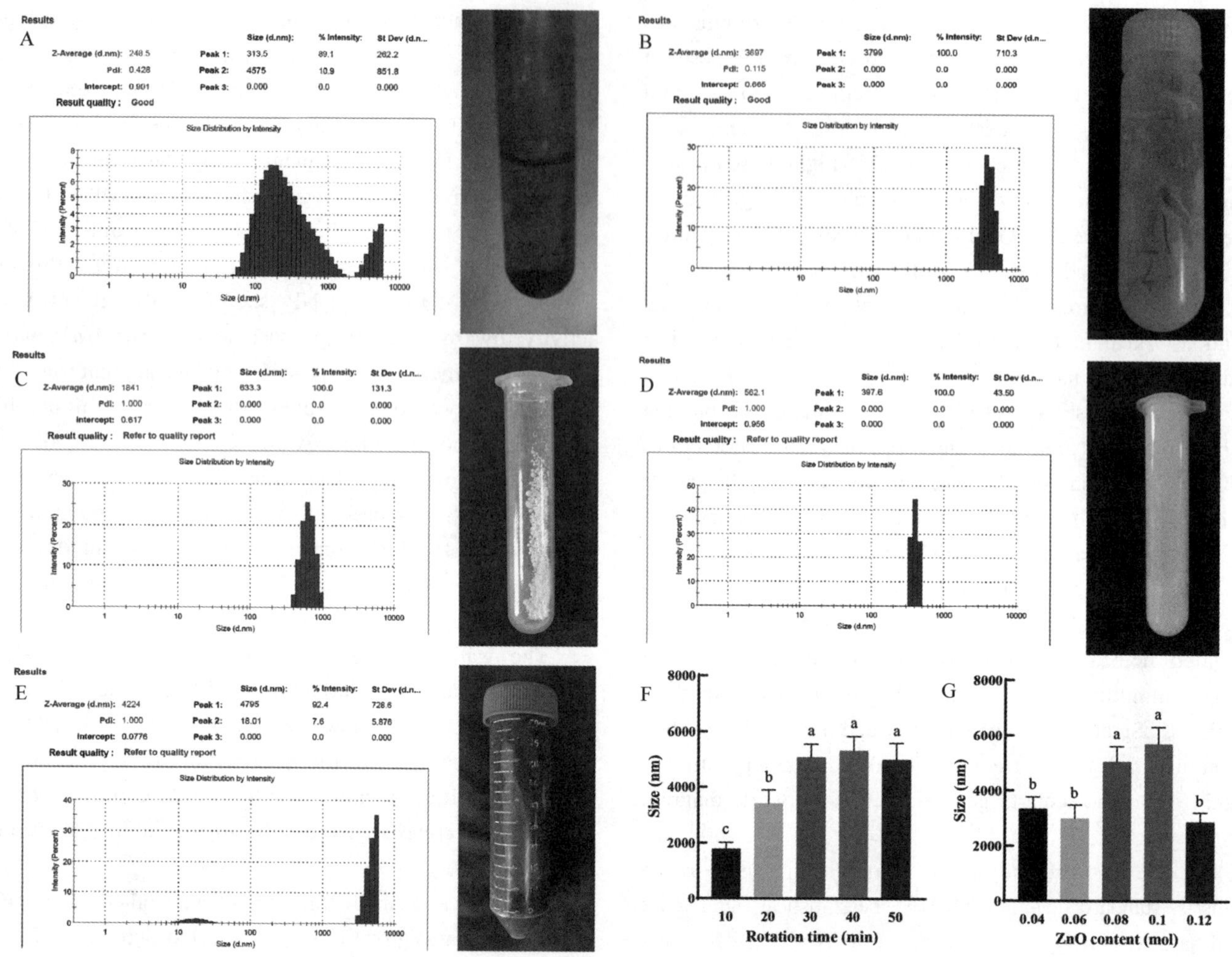


**Fig. 2 Preparation and characterization of materials**

(A) Particle size of $Fe_3O_4$. (B) Particle size of *S. cerevisiae*. (C) Particle size of ZnO. (D) Particle size of ZnO-*S. cerevisiae*. (E) Particle size of $Fe_3O_4$-*S. cerevisiae*. (F) Optimization of rotation time. (G) Optimization of the content of ZnO. The columns marked with the same letter do not differ significantly ($P>0.05$).

of 8 mg/mL was the lightest. These result indicates that the NPs can inhibit the development of *F. oxysporum*.

3.3 Effect of ZnO-*S. cerevisiae* on infected A. memeranaceus growth Zn is essential for plant growth and development. It plays an important role in various physiological processes. ZnO not only supplies $Zn^{2+}$ for plants, but also helps plants cope with stress. ZnO NPs can improve plant growth and decrease Cd accumulation by modulating oxidative stress and expression levels of sucrose and metal-transporter genes. Besides, ZnO NPs has direct antifungal activity against *M. oryzae* by inhibiting the formation of conidia and appressorium. Meanwhile, induces ROS accumulation and defense-related genes.

As shown in Fig. 5, through the physiological indexes of plants, we can find that the negative impact of pathogens on plant growth is alleviated after the addition of NPs. ZnO NPs in vivo exhibited antifungal activity against *F. oxysporum*. and prompted plants growth. *S. cerevisiae* can also promote plants growth by solubilisation of nutrients, synthesis of active compounds, enhancement of chlorophyll. The total length of plants is longer than control, which is potentially induced by material. ZnO-*S. cerevisiae* also improved weight of root, which protected plants from root rot. ZnO NPs exhibits the potential to be used as fertilizer to promote plants weight accumulation. The weight of leaves was significantly enhanced. The chlorophyll rose in treatment group underlying ZnO-mediated plant growth, which decreased with dose at 2 - 6 mg/mL, increased at 6 - 10 mg/mL. This tendency is consistency with weight of leaf. The above results indicated that the good antifungal effect of NPs is at high concentrations, which is consistent with the previous experimental conclusion. Compared with the CK, the content and productivity of astragaloside IV was significantly higher after treatment of ZnO-*S. cerevisiae*. As exogenous stimulation, ZnO NPs promote plant metabolism, especially the expression of genes related to secondary

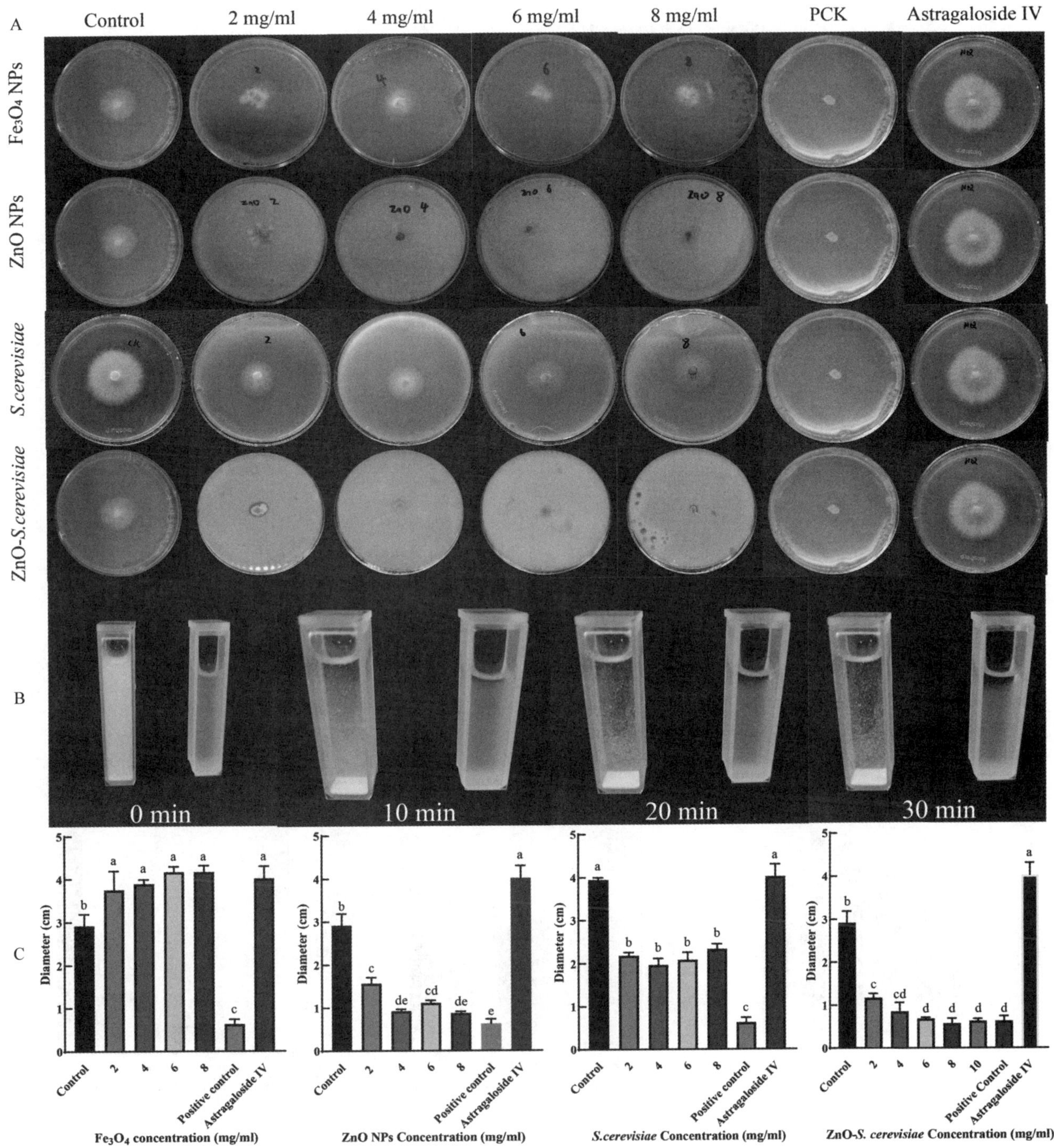


**Fig. 3 In vitro investigation of antifungal activity**

(A) Screen NPs from left to right, control, 2 mg/mL, 4 mg/mL, 6 mg/mL, 8 mg/mL NPs, PCK (pesticide), Astragaloside IV. (B) Water solubility test; left: ZnO NPs, right: ZnO-*S. cerevisiae*. (C) Inhibition zone diameters at different concentrations. The columns marked with the same letter do not differ significantly ($P > 0.05$).

metabolism. The increase accumulation of astragaloside IV in *A. memeranaceus* is curial for the application in agriculture. In conclusion, ZnO-*S. cerevisiae* can not only enhance antifungal activity, but also be used as a fertilizer to promote the accumulation of astragaloside IV.

The toxicity impact of the synthesized materials are crucial for evaluating the safety and ecological consequences of materials. *S. cerevisiae* is a generally recognized as safe (GRAS) microorganism in food. As an emerging material, the safety of ZnO NPs has been widely investigated, which were present within the plant as ions. ZnO NPs may be helpful for people suffer from Zn malnutrition by increasing Zn biofortification in cereals. However, it should point out that excessive application exhibit toxic effects on plants in a dose-dependent manner. The particle size could be a crucial factor in toxicity. The toxicity can be increased to wheat

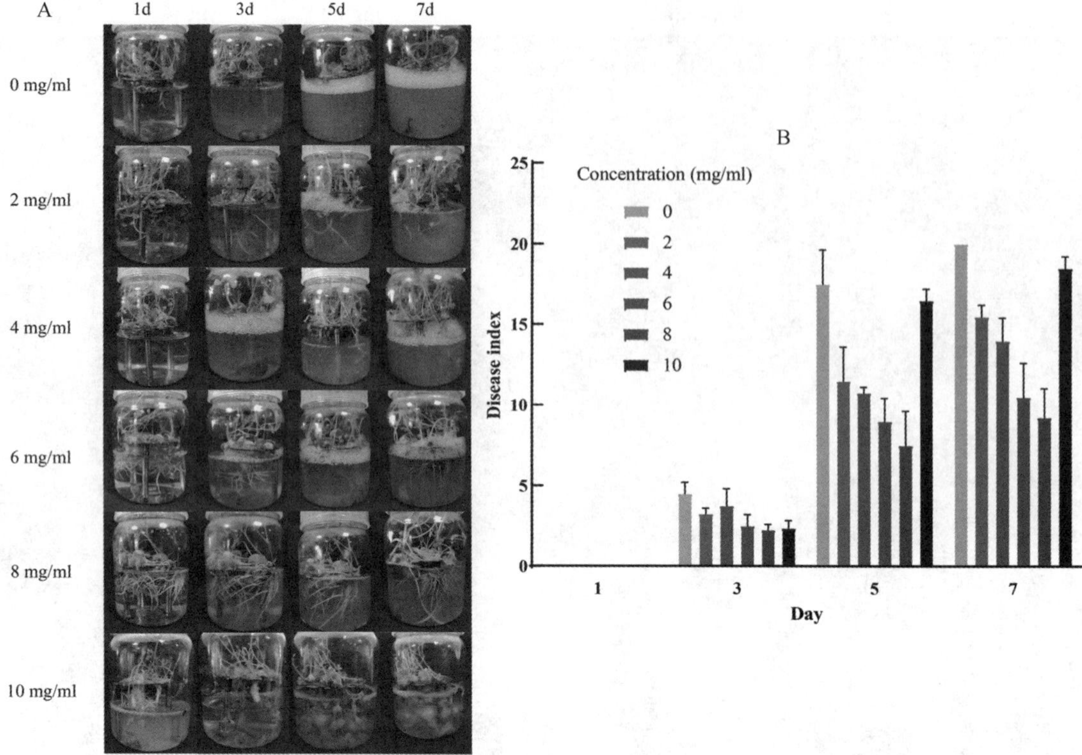


**Fig. 4 Disease severity of detached *A. memeranaceus* treated with ZnO-*S. cerevisiae***

(A) Hydroponic seedlings at 0 mg/mL, 2 mg/mL, 4 mg/mL, 6 mg/mL, 8 mg/mL, 10 mg/mL every other day. (B) Disease index at different concentrations every other day. All experiments were performed in triplicate. The columns marked with the same letter do not differ significantly ($P>0.05$).

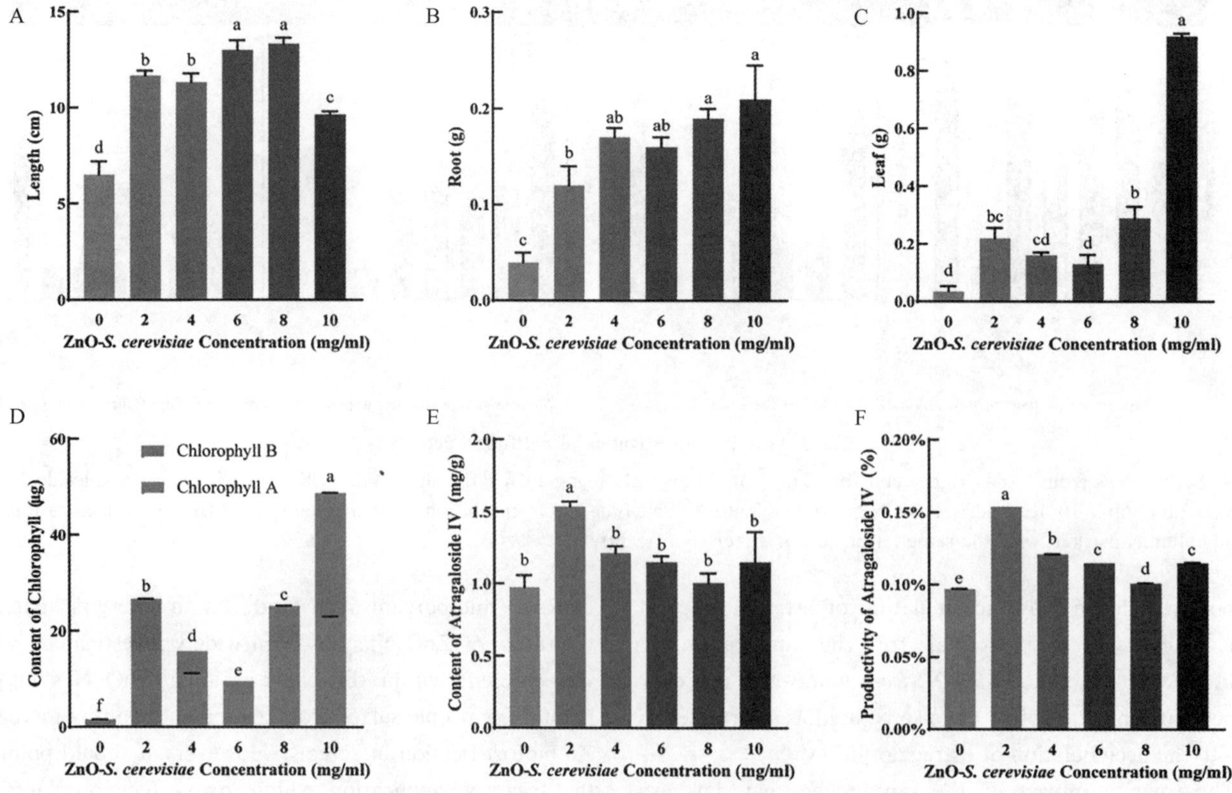


**Fig. 5 Effect of ZnO-*S. cerevisiae* on *A. memeranaceus* growth**

(A) Length. (B) Mass of root (wet weight). (C) Mass of leave (wet weight). (D) Content of chlorophyll. (E) Content of Atragaloside IV. (F) Productivity of Astragaloside IV. The columns marked with the same letter do not differ significantly ($P>0.05$).

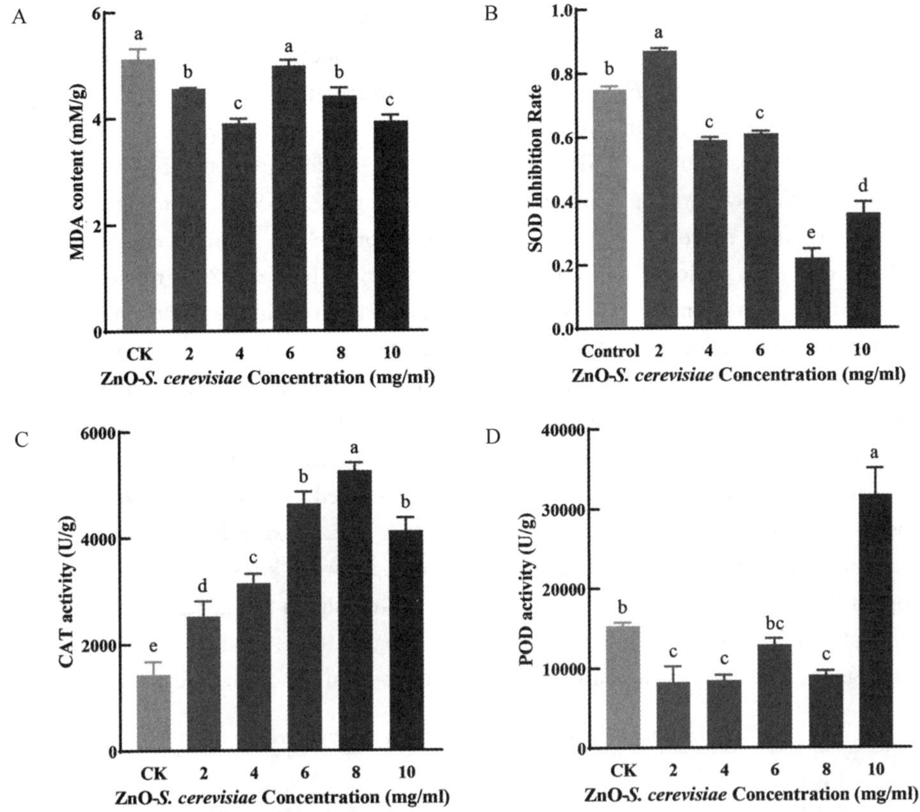


**Fig. 6 MDA content and SOD, POD, CAT activities of ZnO-*S. cerevisiae*-treated *A. memeranaceus* seedlings**

(A) MDA content. (B) SOD inhibition rate. (C) CAT activity. (D) POD activity. The columns marked with the same letter do not differ significantly ($P>0.05$).

upon co-exposure to phenanthrene.

In conclusion, ZnO-*S. cerevisiae* has a certain antifungal effect, and the growth of *A. membranaceus* is improved. Under high concentrations, the proliferation of pathogens was inhibited and the plan growth was good (length, wet weight, chlorophyll). Meanwhile, the content and yield of astragaloside IV were significantly improved compared with control.

3.4 Enhancement of biochemical defense system in infected A. membranaceus seedlings by ZnO-*S. cerevisiae*

ROS is commonly used to estimate oxidative stress levels. In response, plants regulate various antioxidant enzymes to clear ROS, which relieve oxidative damage. The excessive ROS can cause oxidative damage in plant cells, leading to the accumulation of MDA and the destruction of the antioxidant defense system. MDA is a kind of aldehyde produced in the process of lipid peroxidation caused by free radicals, and the content can reflect the degree of damage caused by adversity. As shown in Fig. 6A, MDA content in the control group was significantly higher, which damaged the biofilm greatly. ZnO-*S. cerevisiae* reduced MDA content, thus alleviating the injury normally induced by pathogens.

SOD is an important antioxidant enzyme in living organisms and helps eliminate free radicals. SOD inhibition rate decreased significantly under NPs, which indicates that there was a large amount of SOD in plants to remove harmful substances. The activity of SOD at 4 - 10 mg/mL is higher than control group, and reached maximum at 8 mg/mL. CAT is one of the key enzymes in the biological defense system, which clears hydrogen peroxide in some tissues to protect cells. Compared with control group, the activity of CAT is much higher, especially at 8 mg/mL, which is correspond with the antifungal assay. Therefore, plants may improve the activity of CAT to inhibit pathogens. POD is a kind of oxidase widely present in various animals, plants and microorganisms, which uses $H_2O_2$ as an electron acceptor to oxidize phenols or amines directly. POD can eliminate the toxicity of hydrogen peroxide and phenolamines. The content of POD at 2 - 8 mg/mL group was much lower than that in CK. The decrease in POD might be due to the increasing rate the other antioxidant enzymes.

In conclusion, the SOD and CAT is more active at high concentration, reaching the maximum at 8 mg/mL, corresponding to former experiment. This may be related to antifungal activity. It suggested that ZnO-*S. cerevisiae* induced the defense system of plants by improving the activities of antioxidant enzymes and reduced MDA content to alleviate the harmful impact imposed by pathogens. ZnO-*S. cerevisiae* can not only reduce the toxicity of pathogens, but also help plants improve their resistance to biological stress.

3.5 Multi-omic profiling reveals potential antifungal mechanism

3.5.1 Transcriptomic profiles of *F. oxysporum* influenced by ZnO-*S. cerevisiae* At present, there are three popular antimicrobial mechanisms of ZnO NPs, $Zn^{2+}$ ions denaturate the protein, photocatalytic properties and the hydrogen peroxide of the reaction destroys the membrane and wall of the cell. We explored the molecular basis of *F. oxysporum* being antagonized by ZnO-*S. cerevisiae*. Based on the revelation of lineage-specific (LS) genomic regions in *F. oxysporum*, the gene expression differences of *F. oxysporum* were analyzed by transcriptome sequencing (treated and untreated with ZnO-*S. cerevisiae*). There were 940 up-regulated genes and 810 down-regulated genes. The 15 genes with the largest multiples of difference were displayed using radar maps, detailed information are shown in Table 1. Top 50 log2FoldChange up-regulated and down-regulated differential genes are showed in Fig. S1C.

The down-regulated genes of *F. oxysporum* are related to the physiological activities, as shown in Table 1. FOYG_01035 (annotated by K14709) is a member of the zinc-iron permease family for zinc uptake. FOYG_14219 (annotated by K03448) is involved in the transport of small molecules. FOYG_09069 (annotated by K08139) is responsible for sugar transport. ZnO-*S. cerevisiae* may disrupt the these gene of transporters to inhibit *F. oxysporum*. FOYG_09068 (annotated by K22992) is related to cytochrome P450. P450 plays a key role in the pathogenesis of the fungus, which may be pathogenic genes. ZnO-*S. cerevisiae* may also have influence on metabolism, such as FOYG_09069 and FOYG_02169 (annotated by K22315), which is a key enzyme in the process of glucose metabolism. In addition, some genes were up-regulated, as shown in Table 1. The expression of FOYG_01992 in *F. oxysporum* was increased (annotated by K00276) to cope with stress. Therefore, ZnO-*S. cerevisiae* may down-regulated the genes involved in the normal growth of pathogens to inhibit pathogens, such as transport, metabolism, and down-regulated pathogenic genes.

**Table 1 Differential genes from *F. oxysporum***

| Genes | Regulation | KEGG | KOG |
|---|---|---|---|
| FOYG_08886 | Up | — | — |
| FOYG_01992 | | K00276 primary-amine oxidase | Copper amine oxidase |
| FOYG_15732 | | — | — |
| FOYG_00286 | | K14338 cytochrome P450/NADPH-cytochrome P450 reductase | Cytochrome P450 |
| FOYG_08983 | | — | — |
| FOYG_11942 | | | |
| FOYG_15251 | | | |
| FOYG_12750 | | K19356 lytic cellulose monooxygenase (C1-hydroxylating) | |
| FOYG_14219 | Down | K03448 MFS transporter, ACS family, pantothenate transporter | Permease of the major facilitator superfamily |
| FOYG_09068 | | K22992 cytochrome P450 family 628 | Cytochrome P450 CYP3/CYP5/CYP6/CYP9 subfamilies |
| FOYG_01035 | | K14709 solute carrier family 39 (zinc transporter), member 1/2/3 | $Fe^{2+}$/$Zn^{2+}$ regulated transporter |
| FOYG_02169 | | K22315 sedoheptulose-bisphosphatase | Phosphoglycerate mutase |
| FOYG_12764 | | — | — |
| FOYG_08847 | | — | Monocarboxylate transporter |
| FOYG_09069 | | K08139 MFS transporter, SP family, sugar:$H^+$ symporter | Predicted transporter (major facilitator superfamily) |

ACS, acyl-CoA synthetase; MFS, major facilitator superfamily; SP, Sugar Porter family.

3.5.2 Transcriptomic profiles of infected A. membranaceus influenced by ZnO-*S. cerevisiae* Meanwhile, we analyzed the differential gene expression of *A. membranaceus* cultured with *F. oxysporum*, treated or untreated with ZnO-*S. cerevisiae* by transcriptome sequencing (RNA-seq). There were 10 730 up-regulated genes and 769 down-regulated genes. As shown in Fig. S2B, the 15 genes with the largest multiples of difference were displayed using radar maps. The up-regulated and down-regulated differential genes are showed in Fig. S2D, displayed top 50 log2FoldChange respectively.

ZnO can protect plants from disease by inducing expression of defense-related genes. ZnO-*S. cerevisiae* may enhance the resistance genes of *A. memeranaceus* to fight against pathogens. Among the up-regulated genes, Cluster-42933.0 was annotated as K13430 Serine/threonine-protein kinase PBS1, which is a typical participant in the plant disease immune response. The expression is shown in Fig. S2C. The genes related to transcription factors may be crucial in the plant defense. By screening candidate *Fusarium wilt*-resistance genes from pumpkin, ethylene-responsive transcription factor and germin-like protein were identified as resistance genes. Hence, analysis of the transcriptome can identify the resistance gene in the defense against *F. oxysporum*, such as ethylene-responsive transcription factor (Cluster-45694.0) and germin-like protein (Cluster-39375.9). The expression of genes about Cluster-45694.0 and Cluster-39375.9 are shown in Fig. S2C.

3.5.3 Comparative analysis of essential metabolites in A. membranaceus We analyzed metabolomics of plants to clarify possible metabolic mechanism. There were 12 up-regulated metabolites and 13 down-regulated metabolites. As shown in Fig. S3, the 10 metabolites with the largest multiples of difference were displayed using radar maps.

Several metabolites have been significantly enhanced, as shown in Fig. S3C. These metabolites may be crucial for plants to inhibit pathogens. For example, histamine acts as neurotransmitters (NTs) in plants. ZnO-*S. cerevisiae* may improve antimicrobial metabolites to inhibit pathogens. As a flavonoid compound, rhamnazin was found as anti-bacterial agents. Rhamnazin from *Combretum erythrophyllum* had good activity against *Vibrio cholerae* and *Enterococcus faecalis*. Apart from acting as photosynthetic intermediate of plants, dihydroxyacetone phosphate (DHAP) can mediate production of glycerol to glycerol-3-phosphate (G3P), which contributes to resistance against *Colletotrichum higginsianum*. L-Proline also plays an important role in plants to cope with stress, especially protects plants from disease, such as *F. oxysporum*. ZnO-*S. cerevisiae* may up-regulate histamine, rhamnazin, DHAP and L-Proline of *A. membranaceus* to inhibit pathogen.

3.5.4 Conjoint analysis The potential antifungal metabolites in plants were associated with genes of the pathogen. The results were screened with the largest correlation coefficient and $P<0.05$ to find out the possible antifungal mechanism.

As shown in Table 2, the significant up-regulated metabolites (Rhamnazin, 5′-methoxybilobetin, Histamine, 5,8-Dihydroxyflavanone, Pelargonidin-3,5-O-diglucoside) may inhibit the expression of enzymes and transport of small molecules (FOYG_13104 annotated by K03448). L-Proline, 1-Amino-1-cyclobutane-carboxylic-acid, DHAP down-regulated the expression of FOYG_09069, FOYG_09068, FOYG_02169. These genes are related to transporter and metabolism,

**Table 2 Conjoint analysis of metabolome (plant)-transcriptome (pathogen)**

| Metabolites | Genes | Function |
|---|---|---|
| Rhamnazin | | |
| 5′-methoxybilobetin Histamine | FOYG_13104 | K03448 MFS transporter, ACS family, pantothenate transporter |
| 5,8-Dihydroxyflavanone | FOYG_09672 | K01443 N-acetylglucosamine-6-phosphate deacetylase |
| Pelargonidin-3,5-O-diglucoside | FOYG_12137 | K00274 monoamine oxidase |
| L-Proline | | |
| | FOYG_15430 | K00387 sulfite oxidase |
| | FOYG_13254 | K11153 retinol dehydrogenase 12 |
| | FOYG_10372 | K13333 lysophospholipase |
| | FOYG_02308 | K14454 aspartate aminotransferase, cytoplasmic |
| | FOYG_09257 | K03448 MFS transporter, ACS family, pantothenate transporter) |
| | FOYG_15803 | K15745 phytoene desaturase (3,4-didehydrolycopene-forming) |
| 1-Amino-1-cyclobutane-carboxylic-acid | FOYG_14169 | K20465 oxysterol-binding protein-related protein 9/10/11 |
| | FOYG_14603 | K22134 MFS transporter, DHA2 family, glioxin efflux transporter |
| DHAP | FOYG_13974 | K15388 cytochrome P450 monooxygenase |
| | FOYG_08637 | K14709 solute carrier family 39 (zinc transporter), member 1/2/3 |
| | FOYG_01758 | K22438 *trans*-aconitate 3-methyltransferase |
| | FOYG_09069 | K08139 MFS transporter, SP family, sugar:$H^+$ symporter |
| | FOYG_09068 | K22992 cytochrome P450 family 628 |
| | FOYG_02169 | K22315 sedoheptulose-bisphosphatase |

(Continued)

| Metabolites | Genes | Function |
|---|---|---|
| 4-Ethylbenzoic acid | | |
| | FOYG_13813 | K17742 sorbose reductase |
| | FOYG_01037 | K19787 carnosine N-methyltransferase |
| | FOYG_02625 | K07238 zinc transporter, ZIP family |
| Tricin-7-O-(2″-feruloyl) glucoside | FOYG_13392 | K01569 oxalate decarboxylase |
| 6-O-Caffeoylarbutin | FOYG_00854 | K14709 solute carrier family 39 (zinc transporter), member 1/2/3 |
| 4-Methylazetidine-2-Carboxylic | FOYG_02307 | K02510 4-hydroxy-2-oxoheptane-dioate aldolase |
| acid | FOYG_04280 | K00942 guanylate kinase |
| | FOYG_09897 | K03635 molybdopterin synthase catalytic subunit |
| | FOYG_01035 | K14709 solute carrier family 39 (zinc transporter), member 1/2/3 |
| | FOYG_12764 | — |

$P<0.05$ and results was screened with largest correlation.

**Table 3 Conjoint analysis of transcriptome (plant)-metabolome (plant) ($P<0.05$)**

| Metabolites | Genes | Function of genes |
|---|---|---|
| L-Proline | Cluster-23150.1 | K14018 phospholipase A-2-activating protein |
| DHAP | Cluster-61354.6 | K00083 cinnamyl-alcohol dehydrogenase |
| | Cluster-45694.0 | K09286 EREBP-like factor |
| Rhamnazin | Cluster-53588.1 | K17065 dynamin 1-like protein |
| 5,8-Dihydroxyflavanone | Cluster-35951.0 | K22683 aspartyl protease family protein |
| 6-O-Caffeoylarbutin | Cluster-57876.2 | K20628 expansin |
| 1-Amino-1-cyclobutane-carboxylic-acid | Cluster-44627.7 | K05894 12-oxophytodienoic acid reductase |
| Histamine | Cluster-30663.23 | |
| Pelargonidin-3,5-O-diglucoside | | |
| Tricin-7-O-(2″-feruloyl) glucoside | Cluster-42933.0 | K13430 serine/threonine-protein kinase PBS1 |
| Tricin-7-O-(2″-feruloyl) glucoside | Cluster-57876.1 | K19589 release factor glutamine methyltransferase |
| 4-Ethylbenzoic acid | | |
| 5′-methoxybilobetin | | |
| 4-Methylazetidine-2-Carboxylic acid | | |
| 4-Methylazetidine-2-Carboxylic acid | Cluster-39375.9 | Putative germin-like protein 2-1 |

which are important genes mentioned in Section 3.5.1. The zinc transporter related to FOYG_01035 was negative correlation with 4-Ethylbenzoic acid, Tricin-7-O-(2″-feruloyl)glucoside, 6-O-Caffeoylarbutin, 4-Methylazetidine-2-Carboxylic acid. In conclusion, the significantly up-regulated metabolites may inhibit enzymes, zinc and MSF transporter of pathogens.

The significantly up-regulated metabolites were associated with genes of plants in the transcriptome, as shown in Table 3. The potential resistance genes of plants (Cluster-42933.0, Cluster-45694.0 and Cluster-39375.9 as mentioned in Section 3.5.2) promote the secretion of suggested antifungal metabolites. Cluster-42933.0 promotes Tricin-7-O-(2″-feruloyl) glucoside. Cluster-45694.0 promotes DHAP. Cluster-39375.9 promotes 4-Methylazetidine-2-Carboxylic acid. Meanwhile, Cluster-57876.1 (annotated by release factor glutamine methyltransferase) is up-regulated to promote the accumulation of Tricin-7-O-(2″-feruloyl) glucoside, 4-Ethylbenzoic acid, 5′-methoxybilobetin and 4-Methylazetidine-2-Carboxylic acid. These may be the mechanism for plants to up-regulate resistance genes to secretes antifungal metabolites.

In conclusion, we proposed potential antifungal pathway, as shown in Fig. 7. ZnO-*S. cerevisiae* up-regulated Cluster-42933.0, Cluster-45694.0 and Cluster-39375.9 to promote the secretion of antifungal metabolites, such as Tricin-7-O-(2″-feruloyl) glucoside, DHAP and 4-Methylazetidine-2-Carboxylic acid, then inhibited the expression of genes related to physiological activity in pathogens. Tricin-7-O-(2″-feruloyl) glucoside, 4-Ethylbenzoic acid, 5′-methoxybilobetin, 4-Methylazetidine-2-Carboxylic acid were up-regulated by Cluster-57876.1 to disrupt transport of zinc in pathogens.

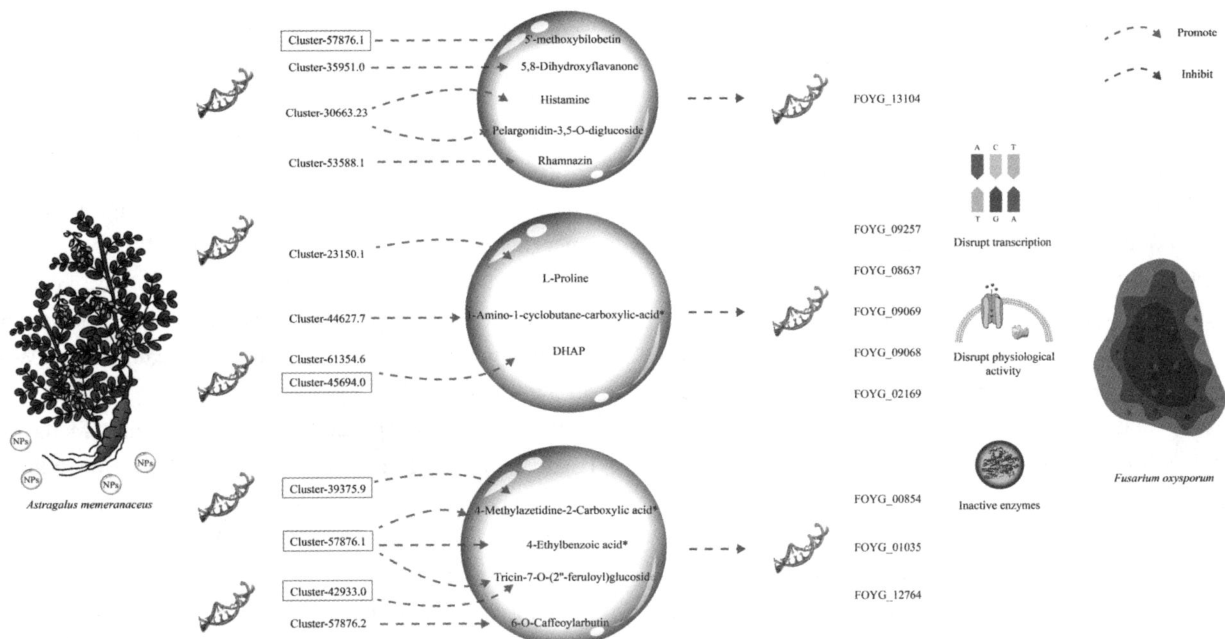


**Fig. 7 ZnO-*S. cerevisiae* up-regulated genes of *A. memeranaceus*, promoted the secretion of related metabolites to inhibit genes of the pathogen The red boxes represent the genes mentioned in detail below. (For interpretation of the references to color in this figure legend, the reader is referred to the web version of this article)**

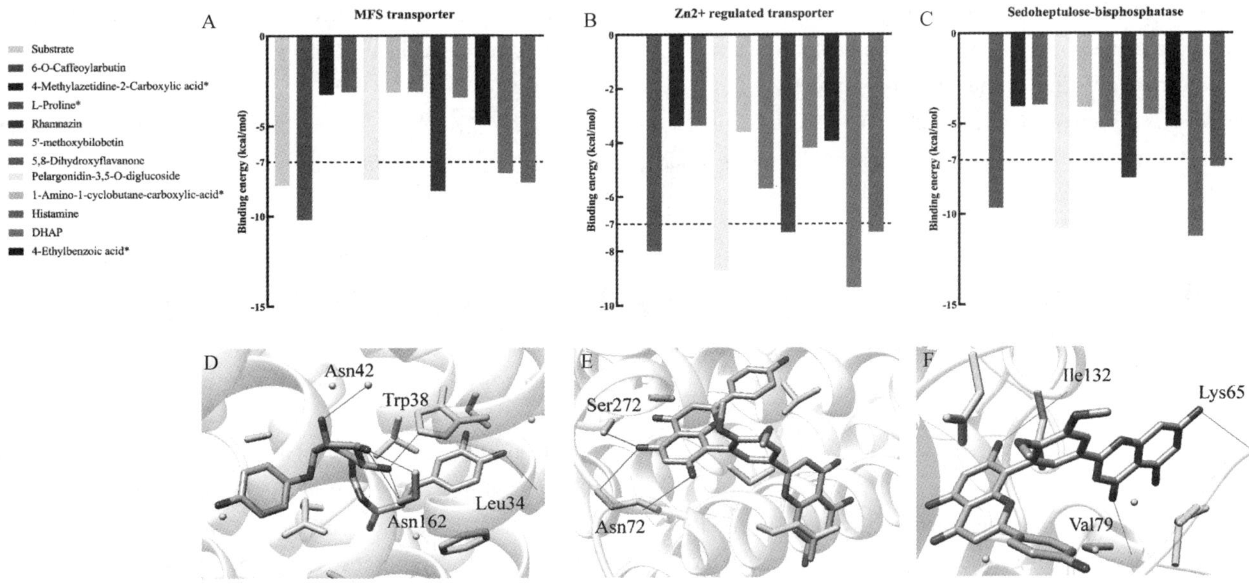


**Fig. 8 Binding conformation and energy of up-regulated metabolites at the active site of potential proteins of pathogens**

(A) The binding energy of MFS transporter and metabolites. (B) The binding energy of $Zn^{2+}$ regulated transporter and metabolites. (C) The binding energy of Sedoheptulose-bisphosphatase and metabolites. (D) The binding conformation of 6-O-Caffeoylarbutin and MFS transporter. (E) The binding conformation of 5′-methoxybilobetin and $Zn^{2+}$ regulated transporter. (F) The binding conformation of 5′-methoxybilobetin and Sedoheptulose-bisphosphatase.

3.5.5 Structure activity relationship of metabolites against *F. oxysporum* Up-regulated metabolites were selected for molecular docking with the down-regulated targets of the pathogen. PDB ID: 7z6m was selected for $Zn^{2+}$ regulated transporter, PDB ID: 3o7q was selected for MFS transporter, sedoheptulose-bisphosphatase based on PDB ID: 4ir8. As shown in Fig. 8 A, 6-O-Caffeoylarbutin and rhamnazin binds to the target protein well as the threshold of substrate, which may inhibit the transport of small molecules. 6-O-Caffeoylarbutin formed six hydrogen bonds with the MFS transporter, Trp38, Asn42 and Asn162 formed hydrogen bonds with three hydroxyl groups on the ring. Leu34 formed hydrogen bond with phenol group. Meanwhile, Trp38 formed $\pi$-$\pi$ interaction with benzene ring to strengthen the interaction. As for $Zn^{2+}$ regulated transporter and sedoheptulose-bisphosphatase, 6-O-Caffeoylarbutin, Pelargonidin-3, 5-O-diglucoside, Rhamnazin, 5′-methoxybilobetin and 5, 8-Dihydroxyflavanone formed strong interaction, as shown in Fig. 8B and C. They inhibited the pathogens by disrupting zinc transporter and glucose metabolism. 5′-methoxybilobetin binds with $Zn^{2+}$ regulated transporter tightly, Asn72 and Ser272 formed hydrogen bonds on the benzene ring, and Arg73 enhanced interaction with π-π interaction. 5′-methoxybilobetin also has tight relationship with sedoheptulose-bisphosphatase, Lys65, Val79 and Ile132 formed hydrogen bonds with phenolic group. 6-O-Caffeoylarbutin, Pelargonidin-3, 5-O-diglucoside and 5′-methoxybilobetin are potential crucial metabolites for the inhibition mechanism.

## 4 CONCLUSION

We prepared ZnO-*S. cerevisiae*, which is a new material with stable, environmentally friendly, cost-efficient characteristic. On the one hand, ZnO-*S. cerevisiae* shows good antifungal activity for *F. oxysporum*. Helping *A. memeranaceus* decomposes ROS through the synergistic action of SOD, CAT and other enzymes, reduces the accumulation of MDA, especially at high concentrations. We also figured out the potential antifungal mechanism, ZnO-*S. cerevisiae* induced the gene highly expressed in *A. memeranaceus*, such as Cluster-42933.0, Cluster-45694.0, Cluster-39375.9, etc. Then the antifungal metabolites, such as 5′-methoxybilobetin and 6-O-Caffeoylarbutin, were improved to inhibit glucose metabolism, MFS and zinc transporter of pathogens. Therefore, multifunctional ZnO-*S. cerevisiae* is a potential material, that can enhance antifungal activity, promote growth and induce resistance. The ZnO-*S. cerevisiae* can be applied in agriculture as an emerging fertilizer to prevent root rot in the future.

CRediT authorship contribution statement Yaowu Su: Data curation, Investigation, Methodology, Project administration, Resources, Software, Validation, Visualization, Writing-original draft, Writing-review & editing. Wenqi Yang: Methodology, Conceptualization. Rubing Wang: Methodology. Huanyu Zhang: Formal analysis. Jie Meng: Writing-review & editing. Hongyan Jing: Writing-review & editing. Guoqi Zhang: Writing-review & editing. Juan Wang: Conceptualization, Funding acquisition, Investigation, Supervision. Lanping Guo: Conceptualization, Funding acquisition. Wenyuan Gao: Conceptualization, Funding acquisition, Supervision, Writing-review & editing.

Declaration of competing interest The authors declare that they have no known competing financial interests or personal relationships that could have appeared to influence the work reported in this paper.

[苏尧兀, 郭兰萍, 王娟, 等. Chemical Engineering Journal, 2024,486:149958.]

# IMP: bridging the gap for medicinal plant genomics

## 1 INTRODUCTION

Medicinal plants have been historically revered for their therapeutic properties and have played a significant role in ethnomedicine and traditional medicine. Their diverse applications in treating ailments such as tumors, inflammation and oxidative stress have garnered considerable attention. Moreover, medicinal plants possess a unique ability to produce complex natural products, making them valuable sources for modern drug discovery. Notably, well-known drugs like artemisinin and salicylic acid have been derived from these botanical treasures. However, relying solely on medicinal plants for natural product drugs is unsustainable, necessitating a deeper understanding of their biosynthetic pathways and the exploration of alternative resources.

Advancements in genomics and transcriptomics have revolutionized research in model plants and important crop species. Yet, genomic studies of medicinal plants have lagged, limiting our knowledge of their molecular makeup. While existing web service databases such as Ensembl, GOLD, TAIR, RGI, MPOD, TCMPG, Phytozome have been valuable resources for biosynthesis and functional studies, they fall short in providing comprehensive gene annotations and tabular formatted gene expression data for medicinal plants. Consequently, effective utilization of medicinal plant genomics remains hindered. Furthermore, a critical need exists for comparative analysis of gene sequences, structures and functional annotations, especially pertaining to gene expression profiles across different organs, developmental stages and diverse treatments. Such analyses are essential for identifying functional genes and assembling metabolic pathways unique to medicinal plants. Unfortunately, no existing database comprehensively addresses these requirements, leaving a gap in our understanding of the intricate metabolic pathways within medicinal plants.

To address these pressing challenges and bridge the gap in medicinal plant genomics, we present the Integrated Medicinal Plantomics (IMP) platform. IMP is a freely accessible database that seamlessly integrates genomic and transcriptomic data for 84 medicinal plants or plants with medicinal benefits, encompassing a vast repository of 8 565 672 genes. Here, the term 'plants with medicinal benefits' refers to species, such as *Cocos nucifera*, *Fagopyrum tataricum* and *Ulmus parvifolia*, which, while not exclusively considered as medicinal plants, do have medicinal usages. The comprehensive nature of this resource overcomes the scarcity of publicly available gene annotations for most medicinal plant genomes, facilitating cross-study comparisons based on unified gene IDs. IMP offers an array of powerful analysis modules, including tools for gene annotations, sequences, structures, functions, distributions and expressions. These modules are designed to handle the volume and complexity of omics data, enabling researchers to explore and analyze medicinal plant genomics efficiently and effectively.

By providing a one-stop mode for data access and analysis, IMP aims to become an invaluable resource in molecular pharmacognosy and synthetic biology medicine research. Researchers can leverage IMP's integrated features to gain a deeper understanding of molecular metabolic pathways within medicinal plants or plants with medicinal benefits. This knowledge, in turn, can fuel advancements in synthetic biology and drug discovery, while also inspiring future investigations into the potential applications of medicinal plants in modern medicine.

In this paper, we present a detailed description of the IMP platform, its data sources, gene annotation pipeline and implementation. We also showcase the various analysis modules and provide case studies to demonstrate the platform's functionality and potential in advancing medicinal plant genomics research.

## 2 MATERIALS AND METHODS

2.1 Data sources Genome assembly data were collected from the National Center for Biotechnology Information (NCBI) and the National Genomics Data Center (NGDC) for 84 medicinal plants including 104 G bases (Supplementary Table S1). Among them, 48 genomes are assembled at the chromosome or pseudo-chromosome level. RNA-seq data from these medicinal plants were collected from the NCBI SRA database and NGDC GSA database (Supplementary Table S1). The dataset includes genome assemblies of well-known medicinal herbs such as *Panax ginseng*, *Artemisia annua*, *Salvia miltiorrhiza*, *Dendrobium huoshanense*, *Tripterygium wilfordii* and *Zingiber officinale*. We meticulously processed and analyzed these datasets to extract relevant information for further analysis.

2.2 Overview of the systematic gene annotation pipeline To construct high-quality gene annotations for medicinal plant genomes, we developed a comprehensive gene anno-tation pipeline (Figure 1). The pipeline integrates three ap-proaches: *ab initio* gene prediction, homology-protein-based gene prediction and RNA-seq-based gene prediction. *Ab ini-tio* gene prediction utilized Braker2 (v2.1.6), ProtH-int (v2.6.0) and AUGUSTUS (v3.4.0). Homology-protein-based gene prediction employed GenomeThreader (v1.7.1) to predict genes based on known homologous protein sequences. RNA-seq-based gene prediction data involved mapping RNA-seq reads to the genome using STAR (v2.7.10a) and assembling transcripts using StringTie (v2.2.1). TransDecoder (v5.5.0) (https://github.com/TransDecoder) was employed to predict the coding se-quences (CDS) of optimal transcripts.

We integrated the three types of gene model evidence using EVidenceModeler (v1.1.1) to obtain comprehensive gene sets. PASA (v2.5.2) was then employed to optimize the gene structure, and the final gene sets were saved in the Generic Feature Format (GFF) files. Functional annotation of the genes was performed using EggNOG (v2.1.5) and PFAM to generate gene ontology (GO) and Kyoto Encyclopedia of Genes and Genomes (KEGG) annotations. Additionally, we pseudo-mapped the RNA-seq data to the respective genomes and gene annotations using salmon (v1.7.0) (36) to get the gene expression value in reads count and TPM (transcripts per million).

2.3 Database implementation IMP was implemented as a web application using Javascript and HTML for front-end development. The core JavaScript libraries used include Vue.js (https://vuejs.org) for the main frame, vis.js (https://visjs.org) for network display, plotly.js (https://plotly.com/), echarts (https://echarts.apache.org), D3.js (https://d3js.org/), igv.js, BlasterJS for interactive charts. The backend data preprocessing and analysis were conducted using the high-level web framework Django (https://www.djangoproject.com). To enable efficient data retrieval, we incorporated the Elasticsearch for efficient data retrieval in the global search function. The Mysql open-source data management system and hdf5-based file index system were utilized for saving and accessing table data. For sequence alignment of genes and proteins, we used NCBI BLAST (v.2.13.0+) and MAFFT (v7.490). Primers are designed based on Primer3 and EMBOSS toolkits. Gene set enrichment analysis is based on R package fgsea.

## 3 RESULTS

3.1 Overview of IMP

3.1.1 Genome data The database currently provides high-quality genome as-semblies for 84 medicinal plants,

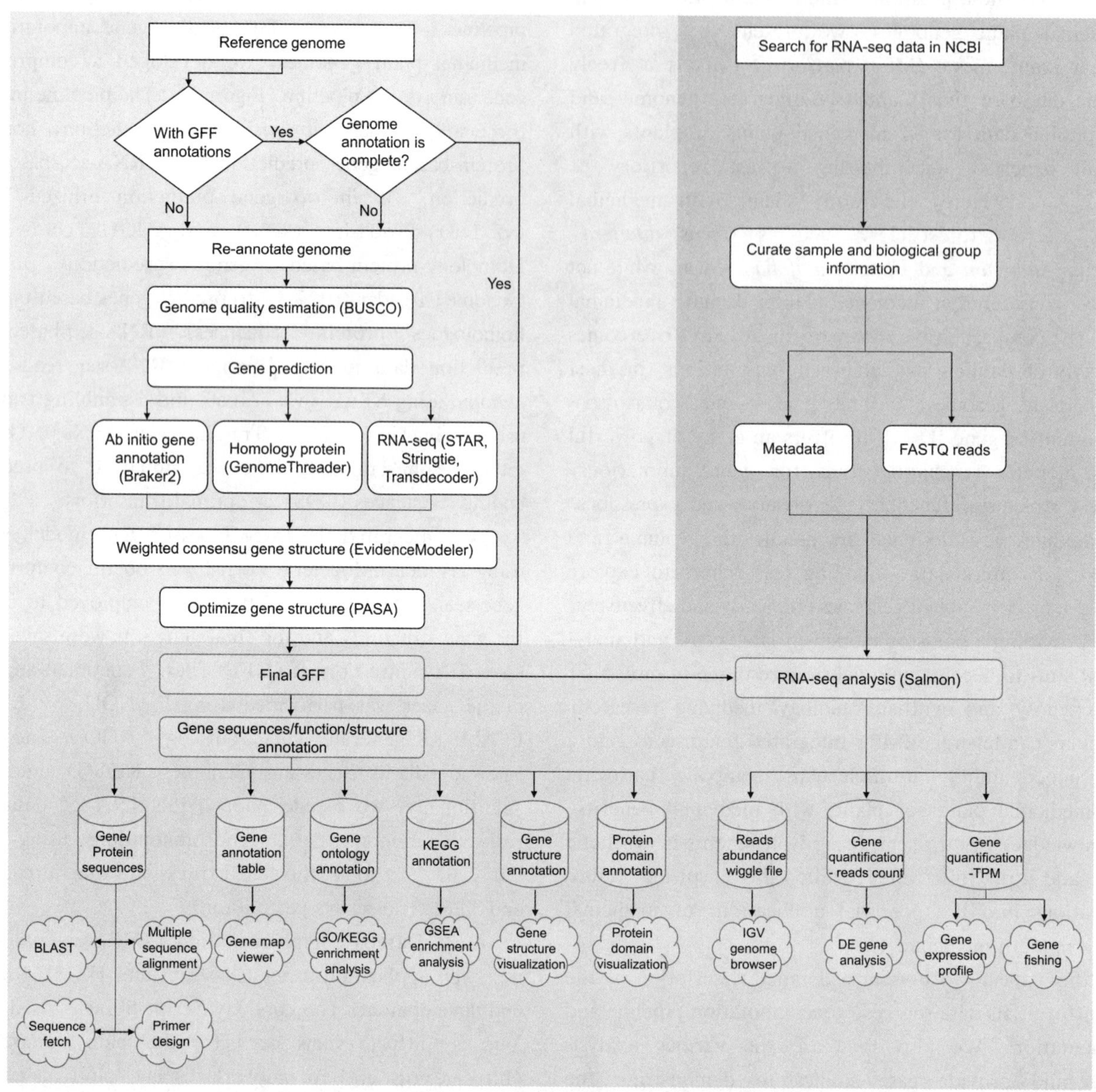


**Figure 1 Overview of data processing steps and function modules of IMP**

The green background section represents the gene annotation pipeline responsible for generating unified gene annotations in GFF format. The blue background section depicts the gene quantification pipeline, responsible for generating gene expression profiles. The pink background section illustrates data storage and the related function modules available in IMP.

encompassing a total of 8 565 672 genes. Additionally, IMP includes 27 890 Gene Ontology terms, 7 320 PFAM domains and 258 KEGG pathways. Researchers could freely download these genome and gene annotation files to conduct in-house analysis for self-generated omics data. The resulting gene lists could be utilized to extract sequences, annotations or perform functional enrichment analysis in IMP, making data exploration and comparisons as straightforward as researchers focusing on model organisms. This integration of unified gene IDs as ENSEMBL IDs or ENTREZ IDs facilitates seamless results publication and cross-study comparisons.

3.1.2 Transcriptome data A curated collection of 2 156 transcriptome sequencing samples is available, encompassing various organs/tissues, such as seed, root, stem, leaf, flower, fruit, callus, calyx and cortex, at different developmental stages (Supplementary Table S1). These samples cover a wide range of biological and abiotic stimulations, including methyl jasmonate, salt, drought, light, fungal infection, etc. Researchers can effortlessly extract and visualize these data on IMP based on their specific research needs. The platform's interactive features enable the postulation of potential functional genes and metabolic pathways based on expression profiles.

3.1.3 Function modules The IMP platform comprises several distinct portals: the home page (main search function) (Supplementary Figure 1), browse page (lists of all species and all genes) (Supplementary Figure 2), tools section (with 10 tools for exploring gene annotations, sequences, structures, functions, distributions and expressions) (Supplementary Figure 1), statistics page (lists of all transcriptome samples) (Supplementary Figure 3), IGV browser (for browsing omics profiles and gene annotations), download page (providing lists of genome/gene/protein sequences in fasta format, gene annotations in GFF format, gene expression TPM matrix) (Supplementary Figure 4), feedback page (for user-driven data submissions) and help (offering tutorials for using IMP). The Browse page in IMP provides researchers with an opportunity to browse all included species, presented through interactive summary pie charts and a table showcasing the basic assembly information of all species. By clicking on the *Species* name column, researchers can access comprehensive information about a specific species and explore all gene lists related to this species (Supplementary Figure 5). Each function module offers specific tools and analyses, empowering researchers with comprehensive data exploration and analysis capabilities.

3.1.4 Interactive plots All visualization results in IMP are generated in an interactive mode. Users could conveniently hover over each point or region in the plot to access detailed data information in the hover box. The platform also offers an interactive toolkit that allows users to fine-tune some visualization styles such as adjusting picture height, paddings, color theme for heatmaps, bar/line plots and filtering enriched functional terms for visualization (Supplementary Figure 6). Moreover, researchers could download the interactive plots in SVG format, facilitating easy modifications for use in publication.

3.1.5 Fast access by searching gene IDs, function descriptions, or pathways The home page features a user-friendly global index-based search function that allows users to quickly access individual genes or gene sets. By searching genes by IDs, function descriptions, or pathways, users can obtain a list of matched genes with related annotation information, like descriptions, GO terms/IDs, KEGG pathway terms/IDs (Supplementary Figure 7). By simply clicking on gene names, users could access detailed gene information, including essential annotation details, sequence information, expression profiles, gene structure maps and protein functional domain maps (Supplementary Figure 6). The basic annotation information comprises gene locus, transcript locus, gene description, GO term names, KEGG pathways, KEGG KO names and COG categories. Furthermore, users can effortlessly navigate to the corresponding database by clicking on GO term names, KEGG pathways or KEGG KO names. For added convenience, the sequence information section allows researchers to copy or download gene, CDS, promoter and protein sequences for further analysis. In addition, the expression profile section vividly displays the expression status of genes, facilitating the exploration of gene expression patterns across different tissues, organs, developmental stages, or treatments, with customizable parameters. The gene structure section shows the distribution of 5′UTR, start codon, CDS, stop codon and 3′UTR regions along genes or transcripts, while the protein functional domain map section illustrates the distribution of predicted PFAM domains along proteins. Researchers can obtain detailed descriptions of each domain by clicking on them, leading to the InterPro database. Notably, researchers can simultaneously select multiple genes and effortlessly send them to 7 analysis modules including Gene expression profiles (for examining the expression patterns of selected genes), GO/KEGG enrichment analysis (for functional enrichment analysis of selected genes), Gene map viewer (for visualizing their distributions along chromosomes/scaffolds), Sequences fetch (for downloading related sequences in FASTA format), Primer design (for designing primers for cloning genes or cDNA), Gene fishing (for identifying more genes with similar expression profiles) and Multiple sequence alignments (for checking sequence conservation) (Supplementary Figure 7).

3.2 Data mining using 10 analysis modules

3.2.1 Integrated description of 10 analysis modules The IMP platform offers a comprehensive set of 10 analysis modules (Figure 2) to empower researchers with efficient data exploration and interpretation. These user-friendly tools can be directly accessed or conveniently cross-linked, providing flexibility and ease of use. By inputting gene IDs, function descriptions, or pathway annotations, users can swiftly generate lists of matched genes for further investigation. Users could select multiple genes and send them to:

3.2.1.1 Gene expression profile module This module allows researchers to compare transcriptome profiles of selected genes across various organs or treatment conditions, facilitating the screening of vital functional genes in one or several datasets. The comparative analysis results are presented through diverse visualizations, including bar/line plots, boxplots, heatmaps or scatter-plot matrices (splom plots) (Figure 2A).

3.2.1.2 Gene fishing module To identify additional genes with similar expression patterns that may function together or share similar functions, researchers can use the Gene Fishing module. The module computes the Spearman correlation value between selected genes and the entire gene

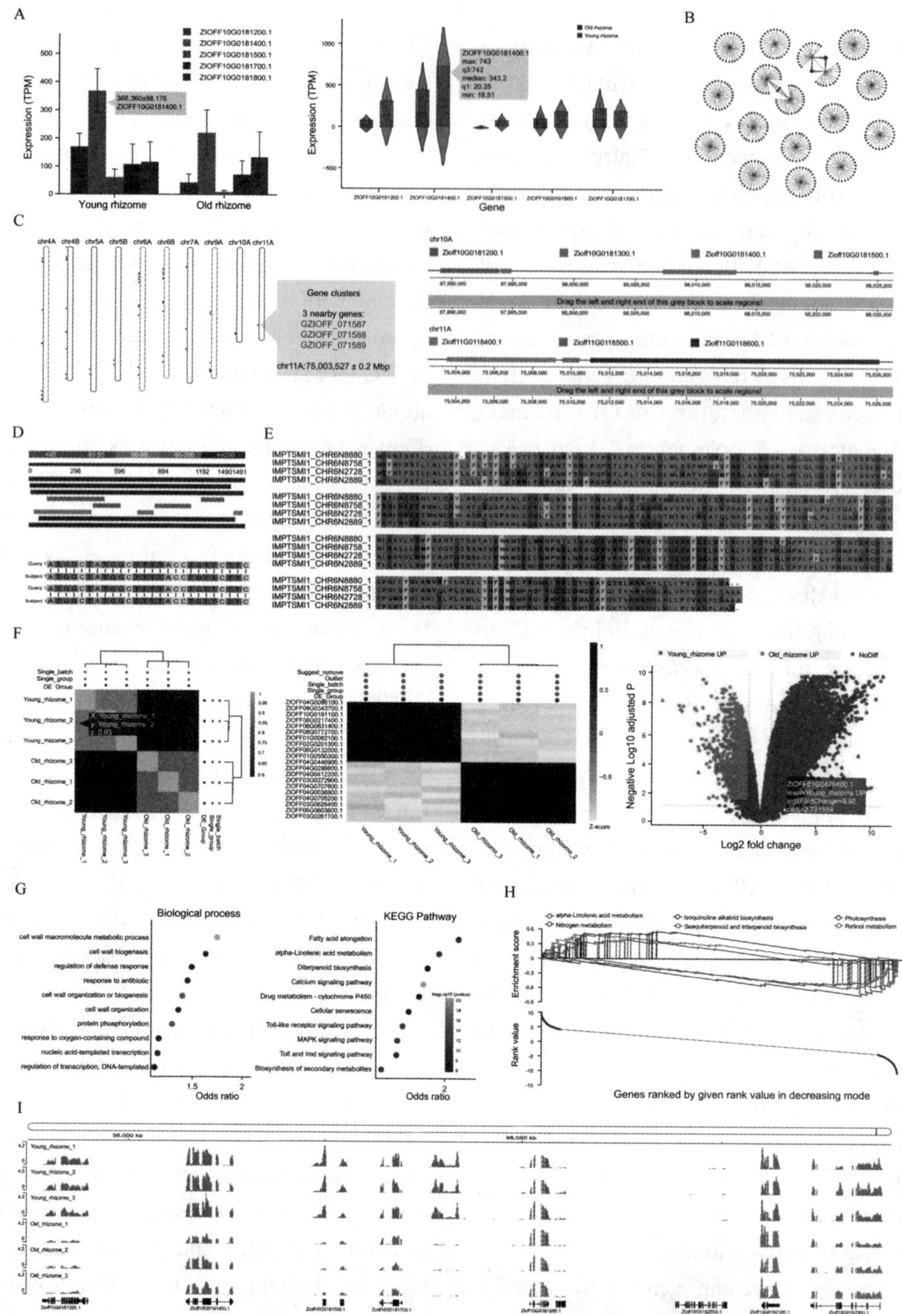


**Figure 2　Demo results of functional modules in IMP**

(A) Bar plot (mean value±standard error of the mean) and violin plot showing expression values of searched genes in given datasets. The upper and lower edges of boxes in violin plots represent the 75th and 25th percentiles, respectively. The upper and lower whiskers extend to data no more than 1.5×the interquartile range from the top and bottom of the box. (B) Gene co-expression correlation networks. In this network plot, blue points represent input genes, while brown points represent genes with significant correlations with respective input genes. Please note that only up to 500 edges are visualized in the network plots. Full results can be browsed online or downloaded. (C) Gene map viewer showing genome-wide distributions of searching genes at the whole chromosome level (left) and local chromosome sub-region level (right). In the left panel, red rectangles represent single genes, while green rectangles represent genes located within 0.2 Mbp. Clicking each gene will redirect to the IGV genome browser. The right panel shows local chromosome regions covering only the target genes. Dragging each end of the grey block allows zooming in/out for viewing regions. (D) BLAST (Basic Local Alignment Search Tool) for sequences match. Four programs (blastn, blastp, blastx, tblastn) and two types of outputs (NCBI-like HTML outputs and table outputs) were designed to facilitate more flexible usages. (E) Multiple sequence alignment visualization. Several colour themes for nucleotides and amino acids are provided. Users have the option to customize the alignment length of each row to generate suitable visualization effects. (F) Representative results for differentially expressed (DE) gene analysis module. The first heatmap shows sample correlation plots for the in-silico-designed projects. Colourful points represent the biological group information of all samples. The second heatmap represents relative gene expression values of the top 20 differentially expressed genes between the two groups. The third volcano plot shows the distribution of all DE genes, with mouse-over information displaying gene names and related details. (G) Bubble plots showing representative enriched gene ontology terms (biological process). Colours represent the enrichment *P*-value computed using Fisher's exact test with the Benjamini-Hochberg procedure for multiple testing correction. (H) Gene set enrichment analysis (GSEA) results. Each line represents one enriched KEGG pathway. Mouse-over information displays gene names, the corresponding NES values and FDR (false discovery rate) values. (I) IGV genome browser showing gene annotations and RNA-seq reads abundance profiles. Samples in each group are color-coded. Positive strand genes are represented in blue, while negative strand genes are represented in brown. Coding exons are depicted by blocks connected by the thinnest lines representing introns. The 5′ and 3′ untranslated regions (UTRs) are displayed as thinner blocks on both ends of genes. RNA-seq reads abundances are normalized as reads per million (RPM).

pool in IMP, presenting significantly correlated genes in a visually informative correlation network. Users can customize visualization attributes to generate suitable correlation networks (Figure 2B).

3.2.1.3 Gene map viewer module The Gene Map Viewer module allows researchers to examine if selected genes could form gene clusters which is an important clue for postulating specific metabolite pathways. Researchers could easily explore gene distributions along chromosomes/scaffolds in two modes: the Annotation mode provides a bird's-eye view of genome-wide gene distributions (Figure 2C, left), while the Overlay mode offers a more detailed focus on gene distribution patterns (Figure 2C, right).

3.2.1.4 BLAST module This module enables researchers to compare selected genes' homology hits within or across other species for functional comparison. The module provides results in standard NCBI formats, including HTML format with pairwise sequence alignments for matching status verification and a table format for id-mapping purposes (Figure 2D). Given that different gene ids used in various experiments or literature are common in non-model plant research, a sequence-based search module is highly useful.

3.2.1.5 Multiple sequence alignments module This module assists researchers in identifying conserved catalyzing sites crucial for metabolite synthesis (Figure 2E).

3.2.1.6 Sequences fetch module With the Sequences Fetch module, researchers can conveniently download related sequences (gene, CDS, protein, promoter se-quences) for further analysis for one or several genes.

3.2.1.7 Primer design module The Primer Design module aids researchers in generating primers for experimental verification.

In addition to the individual modules, researchers can utilize the modules collectively for *in-silico* projects aimed at elucidating valuable component synthetic pathways through cross-organ or along-inducing comparisons, as exemplified by the DE gene analysis model (Figure 2F). Identified differentially expressed genes can be further subjected to GO/KEGG enrichment analysis (Fisher's exact test-based enrichment analysis) (Figure 2G) and Gene Set Enrichment Analysis (Figure 2H). The IGV genome browser serves as a valuable tool for visualizing gene annotations and RNA-seq reads abundance profiles (Figure 2I), enabling researchers to identify alternatively spliced transcripts, and new genes, or integrate omics data for comprehensive analyses.

3.2.2 Case study To illustrate the practical utility of IMP, we present a case study where we identified two syntenic gene clusters comprising 10 genes involved in the tanshinone biosynthesis of our previous work. By feeding the coding sequences of these 10 genes into the BLAST module, we obtained 10 perfect matches (Supplementary Figure 8). This process showed the classical usage of linking foreign genes to unified IDs in IMP. Leveraging these matched IDs, researchers can explore the diverse functions of these genes, accessing detailed annotation, function, structure, domain and expression information in IMP.

Moreover, selecting all these genes and utilizing the Gene Map Viewer module generates a cluster view of these genes along *Salvia miltiorrhiza* chr6 (Supplementary Figure 9). The previously identified CYP450 gene cluster is located at the start of chr6, while the CYP450 - CPS cluster is situated at the end of chr6. Further analysis using the Multiple Sequence Alignments module provides MSA profiles, revealing consensus sites crucial for gene catalytic function (Supplementary Figure 10). Through these 3 modules in IMP, we seamlessly reappeared two main parts of our previous work.

## 4 DISCUSSION

In conclusion, our IMP (Integrated Medicinal Plantomics) platform represents a significant advancement in bridging the gap for medicinal plant genomics. By providing freely accessible gene annotations and tabular formatted gene expression data for 84 high-quality genome assemblies and 2156 transcriptome sequencing samples, IMP offers a one-stop mode for users to examine gene annotations, sequences, structures, functions, distributions and expressions. Additionally, all these data could be freely downloaded for *in-house* omics analysis like transcriptome, genome, epigenome, epi-transcriptome data. This comprehensive resource will play a vital role in enhancing the understanding of molecular metabolic pathways in medicinal plants, thereby driving advancements in synthetic biology and facilitating the exploration of natural sources for drug discovery and drug production.

The IMP platform is designed to cater to the needs of researchers focusing on medicinal plants and offers a range of interactive tools for data visualization and analysis. The integrated 10 analysis modules enable researchers to explore gene expression patterns, perform functional enrichment analysis and identify potential functional genes and metabolic pathways. Moreover, our database will continue to evolve as more medicinal plant genomes and omics data become available, making it the most data-rich platform in the field.

As we move forward, we plan to expand the IMP platform by incorporating more types of omics data and adding additional analysis features. Our goal is to continue providing a valuable resource for researchers in the fields of molecular pharmacognosy and synthetic biology medicine, fostering new discoveries and advancements in the study of medicinal plants or plants with medicinal benefits and their potential applications in medicine.

［陈同，杨莓，黄璐琦，等. Nucleic Acids Research，2024，52：D1347－D1354.］

# Comparisons of wild and cultivated American ginseng (*Panax quinquefolius* L.) genomes provide insights into changes in root growth and metabolism during domestication

American ginseng (*Panax quinquefolius* L.) originated in the forests of North America and was introduced to China over 40 years ago. Cultivated *P. quinquefolius* in China had fewer lateral roots and significantly decreased ginsenoside Rg1 content compared to wild American varieties, both of which determines quality and yield of *P. quinquefolius* (Figure S1).

To explore genetic basis to alterations in both root morphology and specialized metabolite production, we firstly sequenced and assembled the chromosome-level *P. quinquefolius* genome of wild American varieties by PacBio SMRT sequencing, 10× Genomics sequencing and chromatin conformation capture technology (Appendix S1; Appendix S2), and further analysed gene family expansion and contraction in *P. quinquefolius* and *P. ginseng* (fewer lateral roots) genomes compared to *P. notoginseng* (more lateral roots). As a result, there were 84 expanded gene families (1 159 genes) shared by *P. quinquefolius* and *P. ginseng* compared to *P. notoginseng* (Figure S2; Table S1). Compared to *P. notoginseng*, there were significant expansions of the gene families incorporating 1, 3-β-glucan synthase, cellulose synthase, expansin (EXP) and shikimate O-hydroxycinnamoyl transferase in *P. quinquefolius*, with increases of 28, 29, 14 and nine members, respectively, which are thought to participate cell wall synthesis, formation of cell wall skeleton, cell extension, hypothesizing that regulation of the cell wall composition and structure contribute to specific root morphology formation during *P. quinquefolius* speciation.

To identify genes that played key roles in altering *P. quinquefolius* root morphology after its introduction to China, whole-genome resequencing was performed in 23 wild and 30 cultivated samples. Principal component analysis (PCA) and population structure analysis at $K=2$ clustered the analysed accessions into two main groups (16 wild individuals; 30 cultivated and seven wild individuals) (Figure 1b,c; Figure S3), and linkage disequilibrium analysis showed that the cultivated population decayed more slowly than the wild population (Figure S3). To identify key selective signatures contributing to genetic changes in cultivated *P. quinquefolius*, we analysed selective sweep regions using the top 5% of the pairwise Wright's *F* statistics and genetic diversities. This yielded 263 and 397 positively selected genes (PSGs) in the wild and cultivated populations, respectively (Table S2; Table S3).

Through comparative transcriptomic analysis of *P. quinquefolius* roots and leaves, we further analysed expression levels of PSGs to identify potentially functionally important variations during *P. quinquefolius* domestication. Twenty-one of the 397 PSGs in the cultivated population shown in Figure S3 were expressed at significantly higher levels in the roots compared to leaves (Table S4). Two positively selected differential expressed genes were related to cell wall development: an EXP gene (*Pq17G51776*; $\log_2(FC)=5.23$, $p.adj=3.16e^{-09}$) and a beta-galactosidase gene (*Pq06G18190*; $\log_2(FC)=3.45$, $p.adj=2.97e^{-10}$) (Figure S4; Table S4; Figure S6), which were involved in cell wall extension and cell wall degradation, respectively. These results supported the hypothesis that cell wall regulation was at the core of variations in *P. quinquefolius* root morphology.

We also found that two peroxidase genes (*Pq17G50742* and *Pq17G50721*), two isoflavone reductase genes (*Pq23G66278* and *Pq23G66277*) and a β-galactosidase gene (*Pq16G47641*) were positively selected in wild *P. quinquefolius* and highly expressed in the root (Figure S4; Table S5). It is reported that isoflavone reductase and peroxidase enhance plant resistance to biotic and osmotic stress, implying their importance for wild *P. quinquefolius* adaption to environmental stress. Peroxidases strengthen cell wall mechanical properties, and β-galactosidase degrade cell wall polysaccharides, both of which counteract EXP activities. This could explain the key role of EXPs in cultivated populations but the importance of peroxidase and β-galactosidase in wild populations as determined from the selective sweep analysis.

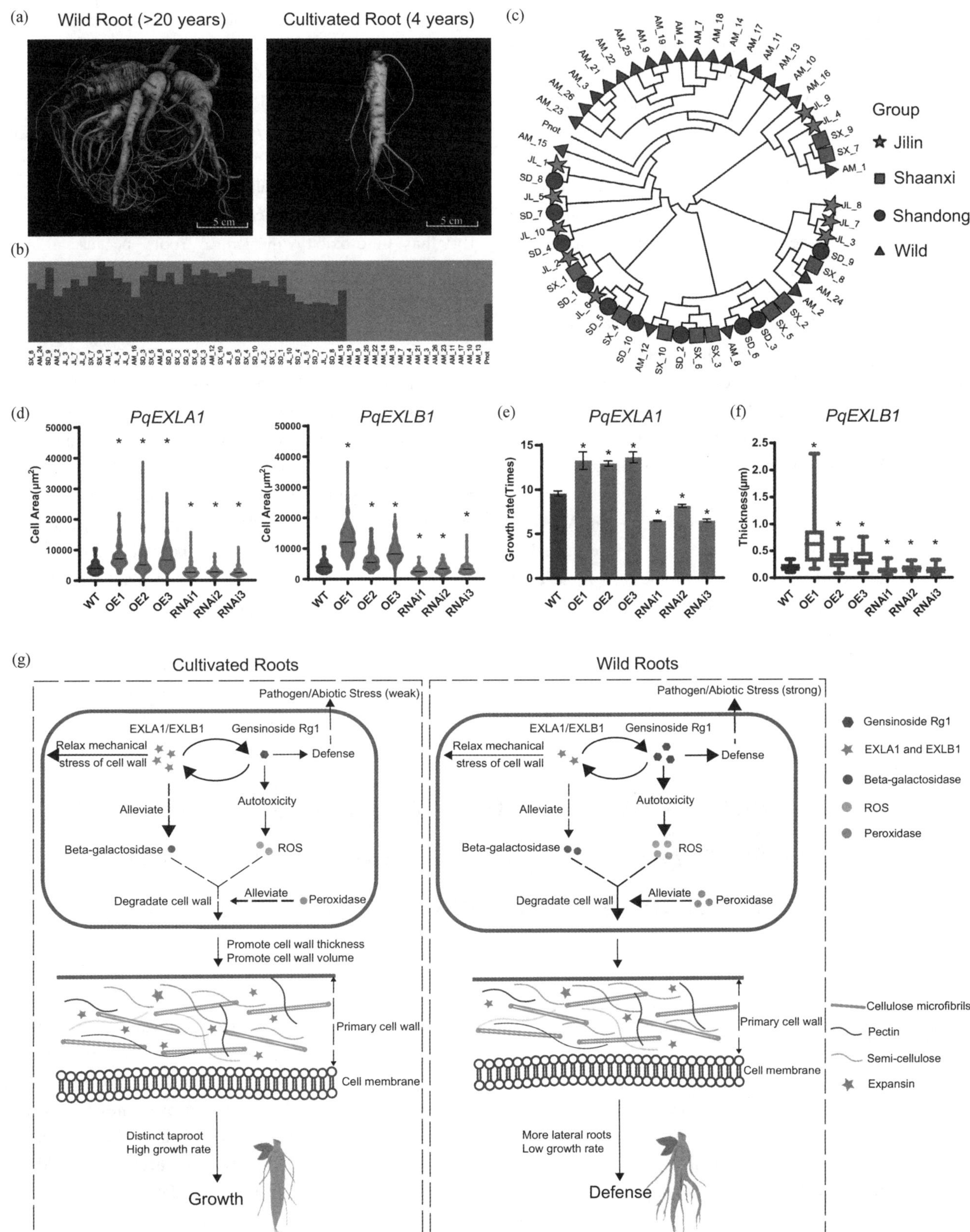


**Figure 1 Expansins mediate the balance between plant requirements for growth and defence processes in wild and cultivated *Panax quinquefolius***

(a) Root morphology in wild and cultivated *P. quinquefolius* plants. (b) Population structure analysis of wild and cultivated accessions at $K=2$. (c) Phylogenetic tree showing relationships between wild and cultivated individuals. (d) Cell volume of transgenic cells in suspension as visualized with a stereo-microscope. (e) Growth rates of transgenic *PqEXLA1*-OE and *PqEXLA1*-RNAi calli. (f) Cell wall thickness in transgenic *PqEXLB1*-OE and *PqEXLB1*-RNAi calli as visualized with electron microscopy. (g) Schematic diagram of growth and defence balance in *P. quinquefolius*.

EXPs serve to relax stress generated in the cell wall and improve extensibility, contributing to root growth. We identified a total of 65 EXP genes in the newly assembled genome and classified them into four subfamilies: the 44 α-expansins (EXPAs), the 14 β-expansins (EXPBs), the two expansin-like As (EXLAs) and the five expansin-like Bs (EXLBs) (Figure S5; Table S6). Positive selection of *PqEXLB5* (*Pq17G51776*) in cultivated populations may indicate that the EXL gene subfamilies significantly contributed to genetic changes that led to differences in *P. quinquefolius* root morphology after introduction (Figure S3).

To further determine the function of EXLA and EXLB gene subfamilies, we constructed overexpression (OE) and RNA interference (RNAi) knockdown vectors for seven EXL genes: *PqEXLA1*, *PqEXLA2* and *PqEXLB1* - *PqEXLB5* (Figure S7). Compared with wild *P. quinquefolius* calli, *PqEXLA1* - OE showed a significant increase in cell volume (73.7%) and rate of tissue growth (38.7%), while which significantly decreased 31.3% and 26.7% in *PqEXLA1* - RNAi calli (Figure 1d, e; Figure S8). Interestingly, *PqEXLB1* - OE calli significantly promote cell volume (111.9%) and cell wall thickness (120.2%), while which were significant reduced in *PqEXLB1* - RNAi calli, compared to wild-type (Figure 1d, f; Figure S9). These results indicated that *PqEXLA1* (*Pq21G63567*) promoted tissue growth by increasing cell volume and *PqEXLB1* (*Pq23G66132*) mediated regulation of cell wall thickness.

Compared to wild calli, Rg1 levels were significantly decreased in *PqEXLA1* - OE and *PqEXLB1* - OE calli but increased in *PqEXLA1* - RNAi and *PqEXLB1* - RNAi calli (Figure S5), and the *PqEXLA1* - RNAi calli showed significant up-regulation of seven Rg1 biosynthesis genes (Figure S5). These results showed that *PqEXLA1* and *PqEXLB1* affected Rg1 accumulation in *P. quinquefolius*. Rg1 has autotoxicity in *Panax* roots because it causes overaccumulation of reactive oxygen species (ROS) and cell wall degradation. In wild *P. quinquefolius*, the high Rg1 contents are expected to cause ROS overaccumulation, which would require alleviation by antioxidants. This is consistent with our finding that two peroxidase genes (*Pq17G50742* and *Pq17G50721*) were under positive selection in the wild population. Previous studies have revealed that ginsenosides may function as defensive compounds, which explains the retention of high Rg1 levels in wild *P. quinquefolius* despite the autotoxicity. Our results thus position *PqEXLA1* and *PqEXLB1* as hub genes that affects both cell growth and Rg1 accumulation, ultimately balancing the plant's requirements for growth and defence (Figure 1g).

［王正鹏，黄璐琦，袁媛，等. Plant Biotechnology Journal, 2024, 27(7): 1-3.］

# The upstream central module of AaBBX21-AaHY5-AaCOP1 regulates light-mediated artemisinin biosynthesis in *Artemisia annua* L.

## 1 INTRODUCTION

Malaria is a severe global epidemic. It caused 608,000 deaths in 2022. Artemisinin is a sesquiterpene lactone synthesized in the glandular secretory trichomes (GSTs) of the traditional Chinese medicinal plant *Artemisia annua* L., which has an irreplaceable function for malaria treatment. Since the conversion of artemisinic acid to artemisinin is significantly more difficult and costly than the extraction of artemisinin from *A. annua* plants, artemisinin of plant origin is still the main market source of artemisinin so far. However, the content of artemisinin is accounting for only 0.1%-1% of the dry weight of wild-type *A. annua* leaves in the natural environment. The biosynthesis pathway of artemisinin has been largely resolved through the efforts of previous researchers. Briefly, precursor for terpene biosynthesis farnesyl diphosphate (FPP) was firstly produced by isopentenyl pyrophosphate (IPP) and dimethylallyl pyrophosphate (DMAPP) catalysed by farnesyl diphosphate synthase (FPS). Then, FPP can be catalyzed into dihydroartemisinic acid (DHAA) and artemisinic acid (AA) by amorpha-4, 11-diene synthase (ADS), cytochrome P450 monooxygenase (CYP71AV1), cytochrome P450 reductase (CPR), alcohol dehydrogenase 1 (ADH1), D11(13)-double bond reductase (DBR2) and aldehyde dehydrogenase 1 (ALDH1) in turn. *ADS*, *CYP71AV1*, *DBR2* and *ALDH1* are four key rate-limiting enzyme genes in the artemisinin pathway and highly express specifically in GSTs. Finally, a photo-oxidation reaction can converse DHAA to artemisinin and AA to arteannuin B, respectively.

As a secondary metabolite, the biosynthesis of artemisinin is strongly influenced by various hormones and environmental signals. Transcription factors in artemisinin biosynthesis responded to these signals and formed a complex transcriptional regulatory network. Light is a essential environmental factor that impacts the growth, development and metabolism of plants. Recent research showed that white light, blue light, red light and UV-B can all promote the biosynthesis of artemisinin. *AaADS*, *AaCYP71AV1*, *AaDBR2*, and *AaALDH1* in the artemisinin-specific pathway significantly increased after exposure to light in transcript level. At present, the light-regulatory mechanism of artemisinin biosynthesis have been preliminarily studied. The basic leucine zipper transcription factor ELONGATED HYPOCOTYL 5 (HY5) was a dominant protein in the downstream regulation of plant light signaling. HY5 in *Artemisia annua* has been identified and was verified to promote artemisinin biosynthesis by directly binding to the promoter of *AaGSW1*. In addition, *AaMYB108* and *AaWRKY9* were verified to be directly bound by AaHY5 and positively regulate artemisinin biosynthesis through the light-dependent JA signaling pathway. Numerous genes including artemisinin biosynthesis-related genes such as *AaWRKY14* and *AaWRKY17* were identified located downstream AaHY5 using a protoplast-based transient expression ChIP-seq system, indicating the potential key role of AaHY5 in the upstream of the artemisinin biosynthesis regulatory network. Moreover, An R2R3 - MYB, AaMYB15, was induced by dark conditions and inhibited artemisinin biosynthesis by directly binding to the *AaORA* promoter.

Plants involved in the response to light signals via wavelength-specific photoreceptors, such as phytochromes (PHYs), cryptochromes (CRYs) and UV-B resistance locus 8 (UVR8). When exposed to light, these photoreceptors can interfere with the activity of CONSTITUTIVE PHOTOMORPHOGENIC 1 - SUPPRESSOR OF PHYA - 105 (COP1 - SPA) E3 ubiquitin ligase complex through protein interaction, allowing the accumulation of downstream transcription factors HY5 and B-box containing proteins (BBXs) that interact with COP1. COP1-HY5-BBXs modules play important roles in mediating light signal transduction in plants. AtBBX21/AtBBX22 in *Arabidopsis* can regulate HY5-controlled genes expression to promote seedlings photomorphogenesis and undergo COP1-mediated degradation in darkness. HY5 is usually thought to be a DNA-binding transcription factor, and AtBBX20/21/22 are essential partners for HY5-dependent modulation of hypocotyl elongation, anthocyanin accumulation and transcriptional regulation. More recently, HY5-BBXs module has been also elaborated in light-mediated secondary metabolism which mainly focuses on anthocyanin biosynthesis. PpBBX16, PpBBX18 and PpBBX21 antagonistically regulate pear fruit anthocyanin accumulation by interacting with PpHY5. In addition, high light-induced PtrBBX23 and UV-B-induced MdBBX22 can both interact with HY5 to regulate procyanidins and anthocyanin biosynthesis. However, the function of HY5-BBXs module in terpenoids biosynthesis has not been reported.

In this study, we identified the B-box protein AaBBX21, the interactor of AaHY5, as a positive regulator of artemisinin biosynthetic pathway. AaBBX21 and AaHY5 could form a complex via direct protein interaction to activate the downstream transcription factors *AaGSW1*, *AaMYB108*, and *AaORA*. AaHY5 functions as a scaffold to bind the promoters while AaBBX21 acts as a transcription activator in the complex. In addition, the E3 ubiquitin ligase AaCOP1 interacts with both AaHY5 and AaBBX21 and reduces the protein levels of both in darkness, disrupting the ability of the complex to promote the biosynthesis of artemisinin. Our study revealed the upstream core module of AaBBX21-AaHY5-AaCOP1 to regulate the light-mediated biosynthesis of artemisinin in *A. annua*.

## 2 RESULTS

AaBBX21 interacts with AaHY5, a core regulator in light-mediated artemisinin biosynthesis HY5 is a key transcription factor in the light signaling pathway, and AaHY5 in *A. annua* can act on downstream transcription factors such as *AaGSW1*, *AaMYB108* and *AaWRKY9* to positively promote artemisinin biosynthesis. The expression of four key enzyme genes (*AaADS*, *AaCYP71AV1*, *AaDBR2* and *AaALDH1*) and four transcription factors (*AaGSW1*, *AaMYB108*, *AaWRKY9* and *AaORA*) were significantly up-regulated in the *AaHY5* over-expressing lines but down-regulated when *AaHY5* was interfered with by RNAi (Figure S1A), suggesting the complexity underlying the regulatory mechanism of AaHY5 on artemisinin biosynthesis. Intriguingly, Dual-LUC showed that AaHY5 alone could only activate the promoter of *AaGSW1*, but not the promoters of the other genes (Figure S1B), suggesting the presence of unknown regulators that function cooperatively with AaHY5 to promote the expression of downstream genes and the accumulation of artemisinin.

To identify potential proteins interacting with AaHY5, we used AaHY5 as a bait to screen the cDNA library of *A. annua*. Interestingly, we found that AA1629300 (AaBBX20) and AA533110 (AaBBX21) could interact with AaHY5. Both proteins possess B-box domains, Recent studies have demonstrated the potential role of B-box (BBX) transcription factors in regulating plant secondary metabolism. Phylogenetic analysis showed that most of the BBX proteins related to secondary metabolism are in group

IV (mainly homologous genes of AtBBX20/21/22/23/24 in *Arabidopsis* (Figure S2A). Based on the expression of group IV *AaBBX* genes in trichomes (Figure S2B) and our previous publication, we examined the interaction of potential AaBBX proteins involved in artemisinin biosynthesis with AaHY5. Yeast two-hybrid (Y2H) assay confirmed that only the homologous genes of AtBBX22 in the AaBBXs family, AaBBX20 and AaBBX21, can interact with AaHY5 (Figure S2C). Furthermore, the expression pattern of *AaBBX21* was highly similar to the genes encoding key enzymes and transcription factors in the artemisinin biosynthetic pathway, suggesting the potential role of AaBBX21 in artemisinin biosynthesis (Figure S2D).

Subsequent Y2H assay demonstrated that AaBBX21 protein interacts with the bZIP domain of AaHY5 through its B-box2 domain (Figure 1A and Figure S3). In addition, Co-immunoprecipitation (Co-IP) (Figure 1B), luciferase complementation assay (LCA) (Figure 1C), and bimolecular fluorescence complementation assay (BiFC) (Figure 1D) were conducted to further confirmed the interaction between AaBBX21 and AaHY5 (Figure 1). Taken together, AaBBX21 is a homoloug of AtBBX22 (Figure S4) that interacts with AaHY5 *in vivo* and *in vitro* showing a high expression level in trichomes. These data suggest that AaBBX21 may be the key regulator that assists AaHY5 in regulating artemisinin biosynthesis.

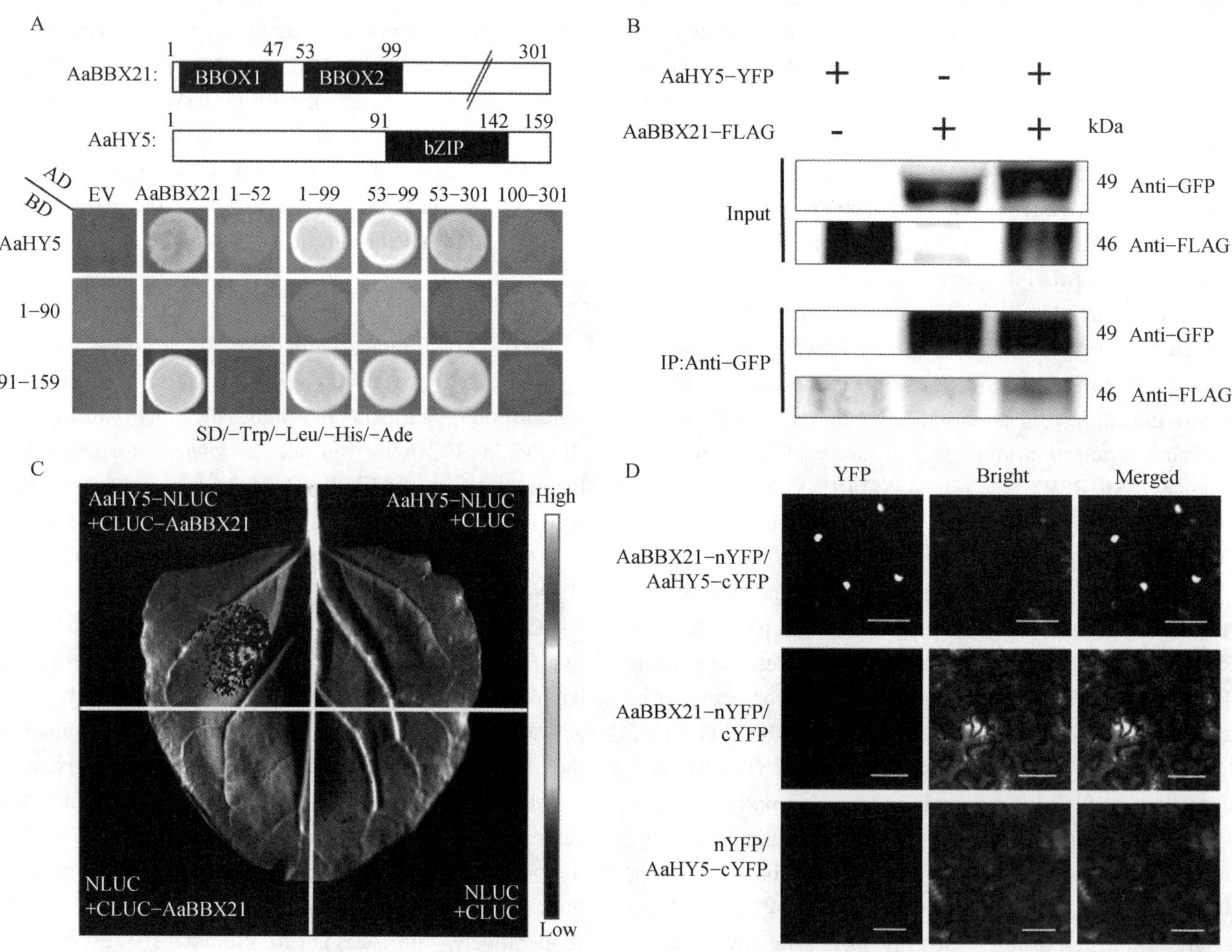


**Figure 1 AaBBX21 interacts with AaHY5 *in vivo* and *in vitro***

(A) Yeast two hybrid assay confirmed that AaBBX21 interacts with AaHY5 in yeast cells. Transformed AH109 yeast cells were resuspended with $ddH_2O$ and then spotted on SD-Trp/-Leu/-His/-Ade plates for detecting the protein interaction. (B) Co-IP in tobacco leaves verified that AaBBX21 and AaHY5 form a complex. AaHY5 - YFP and AaBBX21-Flag proteins were co-expressed in tobacco, and the total proteins were extracted followed by incubation with anti-GFP antibody. Proteins by co-immunoprecipitation were detected by Western Blot using anti-Flag antibody. (C) BiFC assay to verify the interactions between AaBBX21 and AaHY5 proteins in tobacco cells. the AaBBX21 protein was fused to the N-terminal of the YFP fluorescent protein (AaBBX21 - nYFP), and the AaHY5 protein was fused to the C-terminal of the YFP fluorescent protein (AaHY5 - cYFP). The scale bar=50 μm. (D) LCA in tobacco leaves verified that AaBBX21 interacts with the AaHY5 protein. the AaHY5 protein is fused to the N-terminal of the LUC protein (AaHY5 - nLUC), and the AaBBX21 protein is fused to the C-terminal of the LUC protein (AaHY5 - cLUC).

Expression pattern of *AaBBX21* Artemisinin is mainly generated by glandular secretory trichomes (GSTs) in the young tissues. qRT-PCR results showed that *AaBBX21* showed constitutive expression in root, stem, flower, leaf, shoot, bud and trichome of *A. annua* plant (Figure 2A). It is worth noting that the relative expression of *AaBBX21* was highest in trichome, which was 16 - 37 times higher than that in other tissues. The transcript level of AaBBX21 exhibited a tendency to initially decrease and subsequently increase with the age of the leaves. (Figure 2B&C). These results indicated that AaBBX21 is a transcription factor that is dominantly expressed in trichome. In addition, the YFP signals in tobacco epidermal cells showed that AaBBX21 was exclusively localized in nucleus while YFP protein was strongly expressed in all parts of the cells (Figure 2D&E), which is consistent with the role of AaBBX21 as a transcription factor.

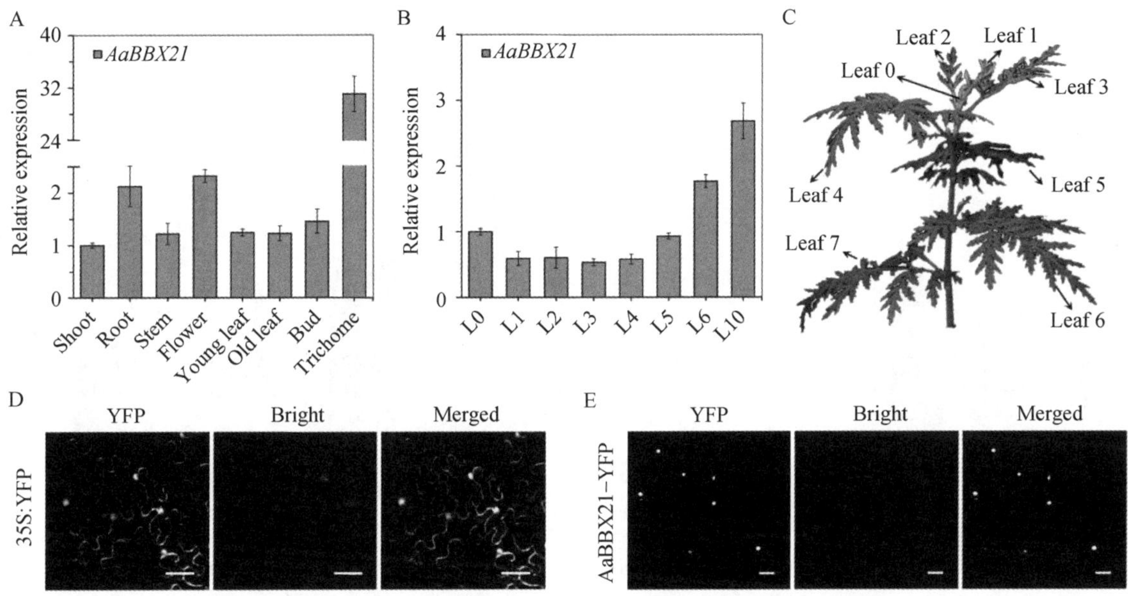


**Figure 2 Expression pattern and subcellular localization of AaBBX21**

(A) The relative expression levels of *AaBBX21* measured by qRT - PCR in different organs (B - C) The relative expression levels of AaBBX21 measured by qRT - PCR in different leaves. Data are mean ± SD of 3 independent biological replicates. (D - E) Subcellular localization of YFP and YFP-fused AaBBX21 proteins. The yellow fluorescent protein signals were observed by confocal laser microscopy after 48 h (24 h dark and 24 h light condition) of incubation. Bar=50 μm.

AaBBX21 is a positive and indirect regulator in artemisinin biosynthesis To confirm the biological function of AaBBX21 in artemisinin biosynthesis, we generated *AaBBX21* over-expressing (OE) and anti-sense (Anti) transgenic *A. annua* plants (Figure S5). OE-*AaBBX21* lines (11#, 23# and 26#) and Anti-*AaBBX21* lines (7#, 8# and 14#) were selected in this study for phenotypic analysis. Our findings revealed that as the expression level of *AaBBX21* increased by 1.74 - 1.86 fold, the artemisinin content also rose by 36.8%- 60.8% compared to wild-type plants (Figure 3A&B). Conversely, a reduction in AaBBX21 expression to 0.45 - 0.68 fold led to a decrease in artemisinin content by 31%- 36% (Figure 3D&E). To further investigate the changes in artemisinin content of transgenic plants, we continued to examine the transcript levels of 4 key enzymes in artemisinin biosynthetic pathway (*AaADS*, *AaCYP71AV1*, *AaDBR2* and *AaALDH1*), along with 4 important transcription factors involved in light-mediated artemisinin biosynthesis (*AaGSW1*, *AaMYB108*, *AaORA* and *AaWRKY9*). Results showed that AaBBX21 can positively regulate the transcript levels of 7 candidate genes, except *AaWRKY9* (Figure 3C&F). These results demonstrated that AaBBX21 is a positive regulator of the artemisinin biosynthesis pathway.

With an effort to elucidate the mechanism of AaBBX21 regulating artemisinin biosynthesis, Dual-LUC assays were performed to scrutinize the relationship between AaBBX21 and the promoter activities of key enzymes genes and transcription factors (Figure 4A). As shown in Figure 4B, AaBBX21 was able to strongly activate the promoters of seven genes except *AaWRKY9*, which was consistent with the results in Figure 3C&F. Since BBX family members mainly bind G-box *cis*-acting elements on the promoters of downstream genes to exercise transcriptional regulatory function, we analyzed a total of 40 G-box elements on the promoters of the above eight genes using the PlantCARE (Figure 4C). To investigate whether AaBBX21 can directly binds to the promoters, yeast one-hybrid assay was performed. However, AaBBX21 could not bind to any of 40

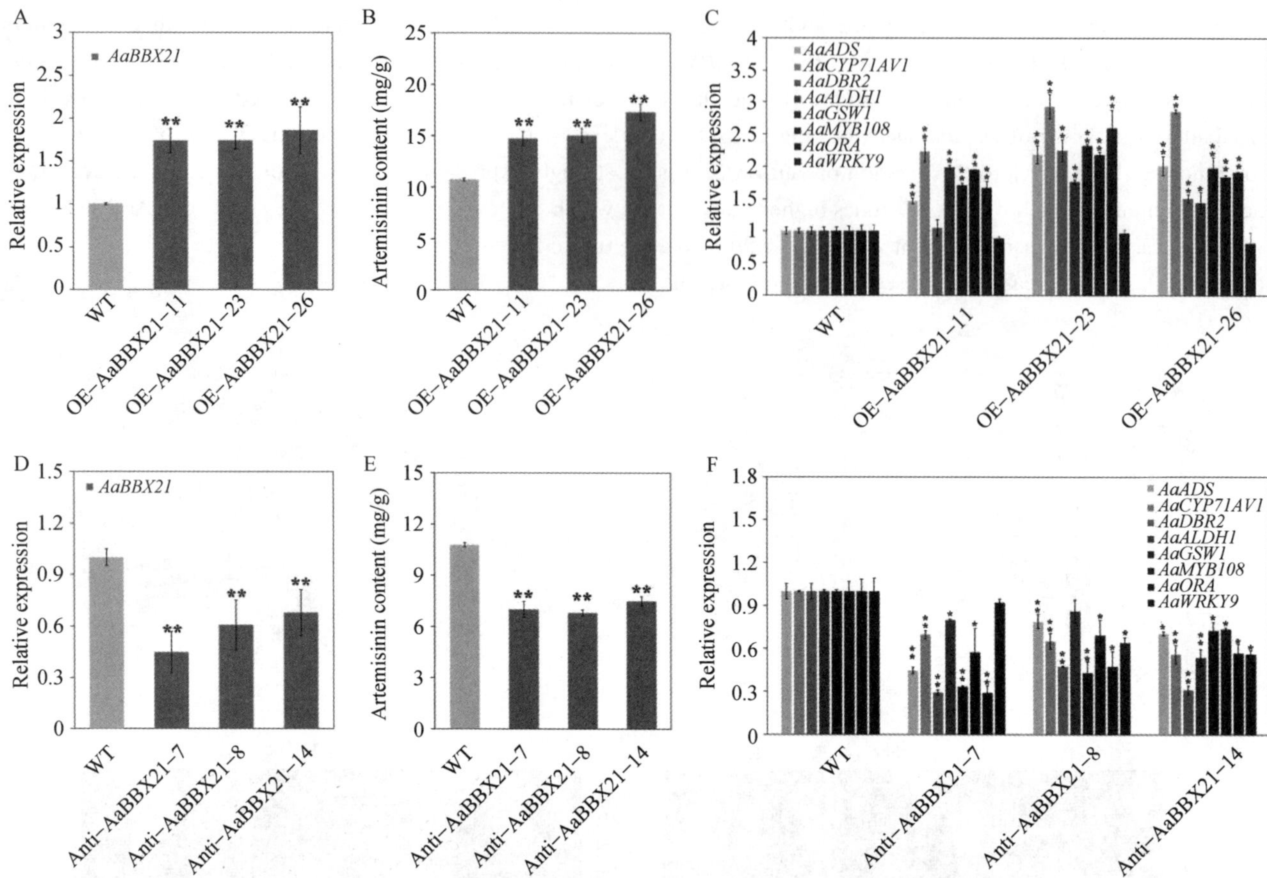


**Figure 3 AaBBX21 positively regulates artemisinin biosynthesis in transgenic *A. annua***

(A, D) Relative expression level of *AaBBX21* in OE-AaBBX21 transgenic *A. annua* plants lines 11＃, 23＃ and 26＃, Anti-AaBBX21 transgenic *A. annua* plants lines 7＃, 8＃ and 14＃, and wild-type (WT) *A. annua* plants leaves. (B, E) Artemisinin content in *AaBBX21* transgenic and wild-type (WT) *A. annua* plants. (C, F) Relative expression level of key enzyme genes *AaADS*, *AaCYP71AV1*, *AaDBR2*, *AaALDH1*, and transcription factors *AaGSW1*, *AaMYB108*, *AaORA* and *AaWRKY9* in AaBBX21 transgenic and wild-type (WT) *A. annua* plants. The asterisk indicates a significant difference between relative gene expression level or artemisinin content of *AaBBX21* transgenic and wild-type (WT) *A. annua* plants (* $P<0.05$, ** $P<0.01$, Student's t-test). Data are mean±SD of 3 independent biological replicates.

G-box elements (Figure 4D). This observation suggests that AaBBX21's role in promoting artemisinin biosynthesis relies on scaffold proteins that can bind to the promoters and subsequently recruit AaBBX21 to function as an activator.

AaBBX21 enhances the activation ability of AaHY5 in artemisinin biosynthesis  Our results suggested that both AaHY5 and AaBBX21 cannot individually function in regulating artemisinin biosynthesis. AaBBX21 can activate but lacks the ability to bind to promoters of downstream genes. Interestingly, yeast one-hybrid (Y1H) assay and electrophoretic mobility shift assay (EMSA) data showed that the AaHY5 can directly bind G-box1/3/5/6 on the *AaGSW1* promoter and G-box4 on the *AaMYB108* promoter (Figure 5A - G). Considering the interaction between AaHY5 and AaBBX21, it is plausible to hypothesize a model where AaHY5 and AaBBX21 function cooperatively to regulate artemisinin biosynthesis.

To test our hypothesis, we first carried out EMSA experiment and found that co-incubating AaBBX21 and AaHY5 proteins together with the probes did not impact AaHY5's binding activity to the target promoter, showing that AaBBX21 does not function by enhancing the binding ability of AaHY5 to *AaGSW1* and *AaMYB108* promoters (Figure S6). Subsequently, we transiently co-expressed AaBBX21 and AaHY5 proteins in tobacco leaves to investigate the activation effect of the AaBBX21 - AaHY5 complex on *AaGSW1* and *AaMYB108*. The Dual-LUC assay demonstrated a significant increase in the activation activity of AaHY5 on the *AaGSW1* and *AaMYB108* promoters when AaBBX21 was introduced (Figure 5H). Moreover, *AaORA*, a crucial positive regulator in artemisinin biosynthesis located downstream of AaGSW1, was also regulated by both AaHY5 and AaBBX21. These findings align with the expression levels of *AaGSW1*, *AaMYB108*, and *AaORA* in *AaBBX21* (Figure 3C&3F) and *AaHY5* (Figure S1) transgenic *A. annua* plants. Overall, our results suggest that AaBBX21

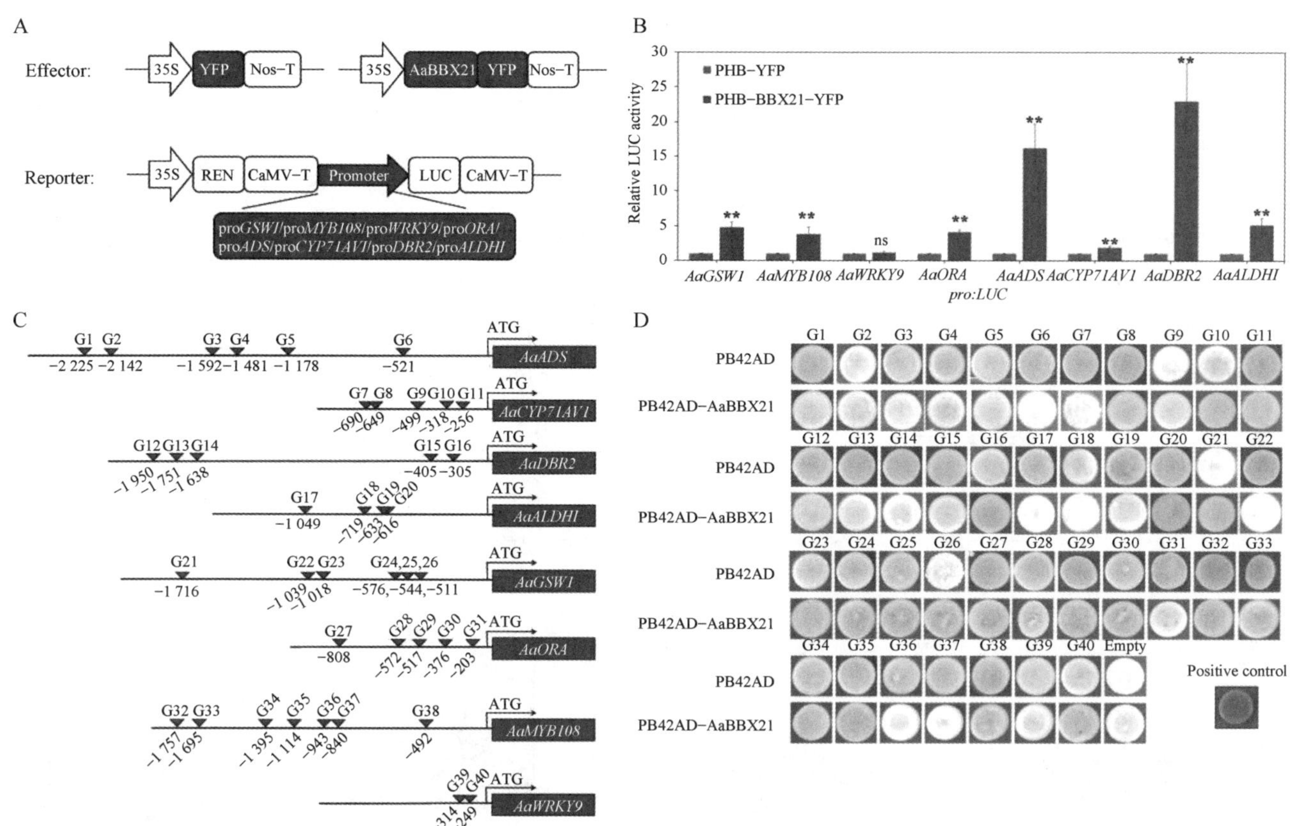


**Figure 4 AaBBX21 indirectly activates artemisinin biosynthesis-related gene promoters**

(A) The schematic representation of the effectors and reporters used in the Dual-LUC assays. (B) Effects of *AaGSW1*, *AaMYB108*, *AaWRKY9*, *AaORA*, *AaADS*, *AaCYP71AV1*, *AaDBR2* and *AaALDH1* gene promoters activities by AaBBX21 in Dual-LUC assay. The empty YFP effector without any gene attached was used as a negative control, and its LUC/REN ratio was set to 1. The strengths of activities are represented by the relative LUC activity. The asterisk indicate a significant difference in the relative LUC between AaBBX21 and the negative control YFP (* $P<0.05$, ** $P<0.01$, Student's t-test). Data are mean±SD of 3 independent biological replicates. (C) Schematic diagram of *AaADS*, *AaCYP71AV1*, *AaDBR2*, *AaALDH1*, *AaGSW1*, *AaORA*, *AaMYB108* and *AaWRKY9* promoters. The blue triangles represent the positions of the potential G-box (G1 - 40). The numbers indicate the distance from the "ATG". (D) Yeast one-hybrid assay showed that AaBBX21 does not directly bind any promoter G-boxes elements of downstream artemisinin biosynthesis-related genes. EGY48A yeast expressing pB42AD - AaBBX21 and pLacZ-3× G-boxes were grown on SD/-Ura/-Trp medium (20 mg/L X-β-gal). "empty", negative control.

interacts with AaHY5, acting as a transcription activator to enhance AaH Y5's activation ability in artemisinin biosynthesis.

AaCOP1 attenuates the function of AaBBX21-AaHY5 complex in darkness  Previous studies have confirmed that light can promote artemisinin biosynthesis pathway. Our transcriptomic data and quantitative PCR experiments demonstrated that light promotes the expression of key artemisinin pathway genes and positive transcription factors, while darkness represses their transcript levels, including *AaBBX21* and *AaHY5* (Figure S7&S8). COP1, the core inhibitor in light signaling pathways, is an E3 ubiquitin ligase that ubiquitinates its interacting proteins for degradation by the 26S proteasome pathway. Light signal can trigger the protection of COP1-interacting proteins from degradation and maintained at high levels. Y2H, BiFC and LCA verified that both AaHY5 and AaBBX21 can interact with AaCOP1 (Figure 6). COP1 typically interacts with the VP motifs through its WD40 domain and then ubiquitinates the interacting proteins for subsequent degradation by the 26S proteasome. AaBBX21 harbours three VP motifs and AaHY5 has only one single VP motif in the C-terminal, respectively (Figure 6A). Our Y2H data showed that any of the VPs is required for AaCOP1 to interact with AaHY5 and AaBBX21 (Figure 6B). Furthermore, AaCOP1 interacts with AaBBX21 through its WD-40 domain and the C-terminus of AaBBX21 (Figure 6C).

To investigate whether AaCOP1 protein can degrade AaBBX21 and AaHY5 in darkness, we transiently expressed AaCOP1, AaHY5 and AaBBX21 in tobacco leaves, and sampled them after 2 days in constant darkness. Western blot showed that the protein levels of AaBBX21 and AaHY5 decreased when AaCOP1 protein was co-expressed, demonstrating that the present of AaCOP1 can reduce the protein levels of AaBBX21 or AaHY5. Moreover, the 26S proteasome inhibitor MG132 could recover the protein levels

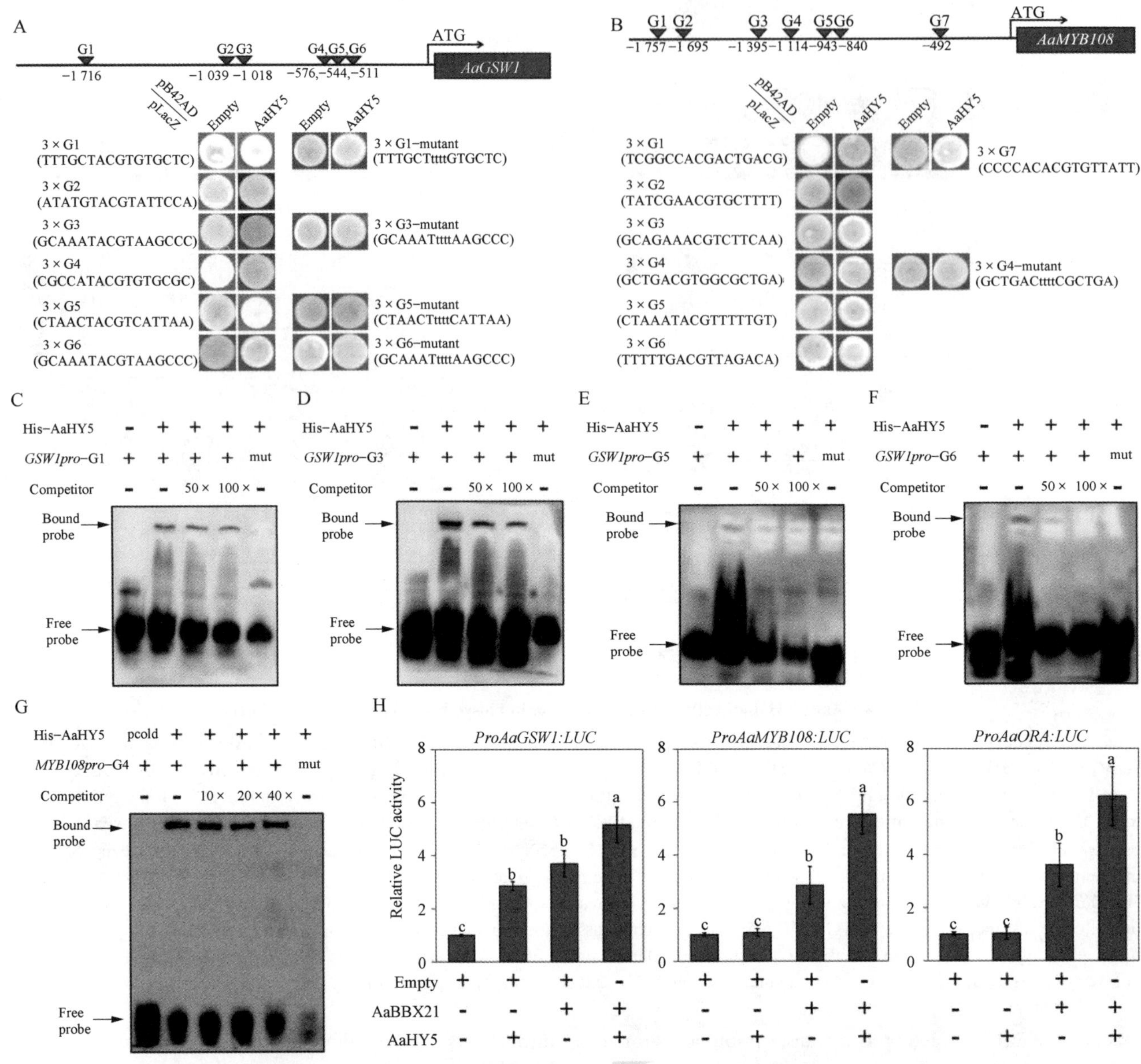


**Figure 5 AaBBX21 protein enhances the transcriptional activation ability of AaHY5**

(A-B) Yeast one-hybrid assay between AaHY5 and G-boxes on the promoters of *AaGSW1* and *AaMYB108*. Schematic diagram of the *AaGSW1* and *AaMYB108* promoters. The blue triangles represent the positions of the potential G-box. The numbers indicate the distance from the "ATG". AaHY5 can directly bind to G-box1/3/5/6 on *AaGSW1* promoters and the G-box4 on *AaMYB108* promoters. EGY48A yeast expressing pB42AD-AaHY5 and pLacZ-3×G-boxes were grown on SD/-Ura/-Trp medium (20 mg/L X-β-gal). (C-G) Electrophoretic mobility shift assay (EMSA) showed that the AaHY5 protein binds to G-box1/3/5/6 on *AaGSW1* promoters and the G-box4 on *AaMYB108* promoters. The groups of no protein added and mutant probes served as negative controls. Unlabeled probes served as competitor and 50× and 100× represent the multiplicity of competitor relative to labeled probes. (H) AaBBX21 and AaHY5 synergistically activate the promoters of *AaGSW1*, *AaMYB108* and *AaORA*. Different lowercase letters represent significant differences in relative LUC activity for different groups by Student's t-test ($P<0.05$). Values are given as means±SD from 3 biological replicates.

of AaBBX21 or AaHY5, suggesting that it is the COP1-mediated 26S proteasome degradation pathway that degrades AaBBX21 and AaHY5 in darkness (Figure 7A&B).

Since AaBBX21 and AaHY5 formed a protein complex to cooperatively regulate artemisinin biosynthesis, we investigated whether AaCOP1 attenuated the function of AaBBX21-AaHY5 complex. The LCA revealed a significant reduction in the interaction between AaBBX21 and AaHY5 in darkness when AaCOP1 was present. However, under light conditions, the interaction between AaBBX21 and AaHY5

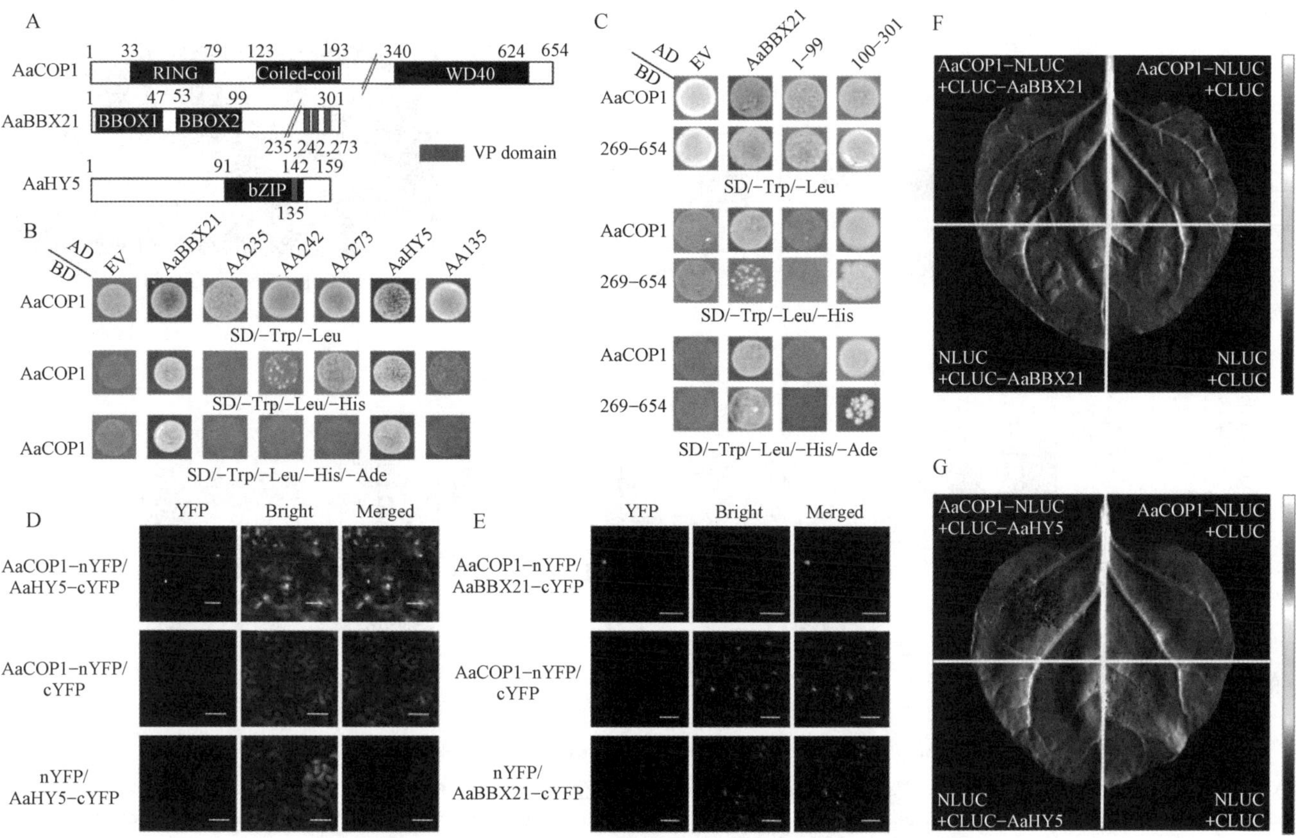

**Figure 6 AaBBX21 and AaHY5 both physically interact with AaCOP1**

(A) Schematic diagram of protein domain of AaCOP1, AaBBX21 and AaHY5. (B) Y2H confirmed that AaBBX21 and AaHY5 interact with AaCOP1 via their C-terminal VP motifs. Transformed AH109 yeast cells were resuspended with dd$H_2O$ and then spotted on SD-Trp/-Leu plates for detecting the successful transformation and on SD-Trp/-Leu/-His/-Ade plates for detecting the protein interaction. (C) Y2H confirmed that AaBBX21 protein interact with WD-40 domain of AaCOP1 via its C-terminal. AaHY5. (D, F) BiFC assay to verify the interactions between AaBBX21 (AaHY5) proteins and AaCOP1 in tobacco cells. the AaCOP1 protein was fused to the N-terminal of the YFP fluorescent protein (AaCOP1-nYFP), and the AaBBX21 (AaHY5) protein was fused to the C-terminal of the YFP fluorescent protein. The scale bar =50 μm. (E, G) LCA in tobacco leaves verified that AaBBX21 and AaHY5 interacts with the AaCOP1 protein. the AaCOP1 protein is fused to the N-terminal of the LUC protein (AaCOP1-nLUC), and the AaBBX21 and AaHY5 protein is fused to the C-terminal of the LUC protein (AaBBX21-cLUC and AaHY5-cLUC).

maintained a relatively high level even in the presence of AaCOP1, suggesting that AaCOP1's inhibition of the AaBBX21-AaHY5 interaction occurs specifically in the dark (Figure 7E). To further investigate whether AaCOP1 impairs the activation of AaBBX21-AaHY5 complex on downstream genes in the darkness, a Dual-LUC assay was conducted to assess the impact of AaCOP1, AaHY5 and AaBBX21 on the promoters of *AaGSW1* (Figure 7F), *AaMYB108* (Figure 7G), and *AaORA* (Figure 7H). AaCOP1 protein alone had no impact on the promoter activities. AaBBX21-AaHY5 complex could strongly activate the promoter activities of *AaGSW1*, *AaMYB108* and *AaORA*. However, when *AaHY5*, *AaBBX21* and *AaCOP1* were co-expressed, the promoter activities significantly decreased, indicating that AaCOP1 weakened the activation ability of the AaBBX21-AaHY5 complex. Additionally, MG132 could recover the function of AaHY5-AaBBX21.

In conclusion, our data demonstrated that AaCOP1 can degrade AaHY5 and AaBBX21, affecting their interactions in darkness and thereby weakening the activation effects of the complex on the transcription factors AaGSW1, AaMYB108 and AaORA. This results in a substantial decrease in their transcript levels, ultimately leading to low artemisinin content.

## 3 DISCUSSION

Artemisinin-based combination therapies (ACTs) are recommended by the World Health Organization as the best method for anti-malaria in almost all malaria-endemic countries. Currently, *A. annua* plants remain the most important source of artemisinin, but artemisinin is at extremely low levels (0.1% - 1%) in wild-type plants. Transcription factor strategies are effective to increase artemisinin content in plants, and so far, many transcription

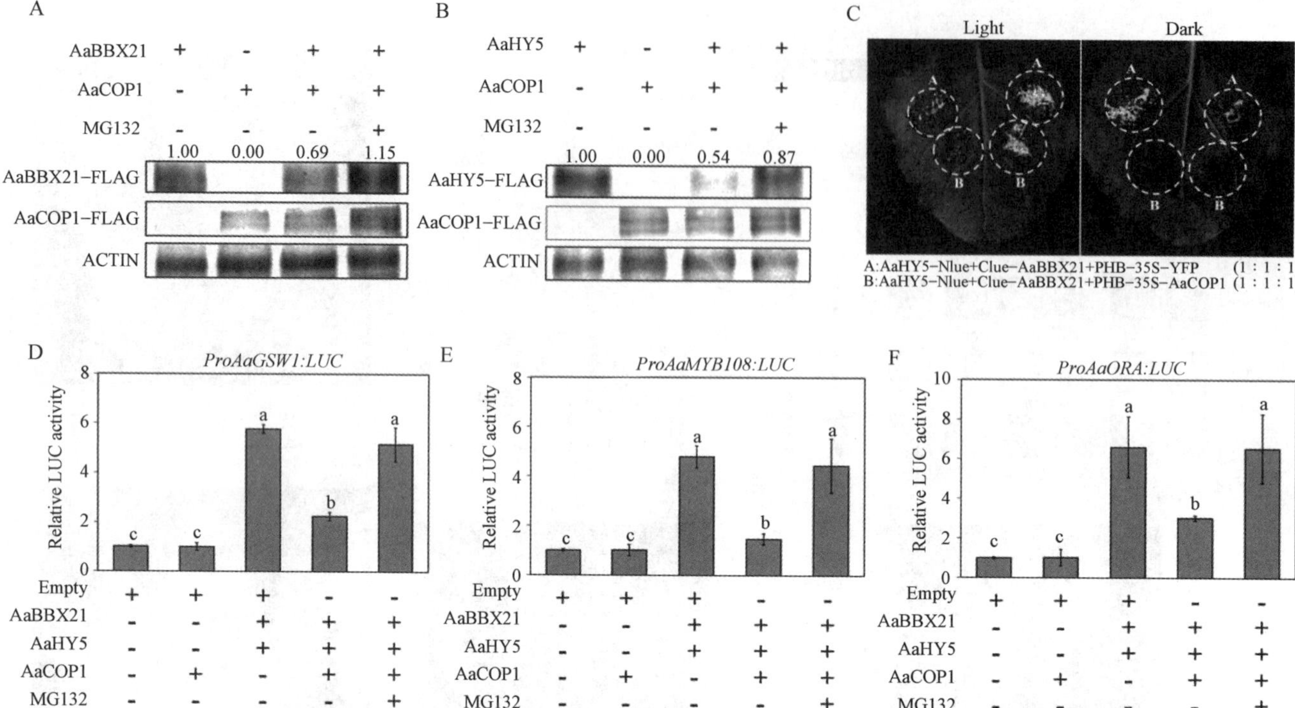


**Figure 7 AaCOP1 impairs the function of AaBBX21 - AaHY5 complex in the dark**

(A - B) AaCOP1 degrades AaBBX21 and AaHY5 via the 26S proteasome pathway in darkness. Changes in protein level of AaBBX21 and AaHY5 proteins in the presence or absence of AaCOP1 protein and proteasome inhibitor MG132 under dark conditions. AaHY5 - Flag (AaBBX21 - Flag) and AaCOP1-Flag were co-transferred into tobacco leaves transiently. After extracting the proteins, western blot with anti-Flag antibody was performed to obtain the changes in the protein level of AaBBX21 and AaHY5 in different groups. The numbers represent the protein contents of AaBBX21, AaHY5 and AaCOP1 relative to β-Actin protein, and the protein content without the expression of AaCOP1 was set to 1. (C) Luciferase complementation assay demonstrated that AaCOP1 weakens protein interactions between AaBBX21 and AaHY5 in darkness. Light treatment: 1 d in the darkness and 1 d in white light, dark treatment: in the darkness for 2 d. (D - F) AaCOP1 weakens the ability of the AaBBX21 - AaHY5 complex to activate downstream gene promoters in darkness. Different lowercase letters represent significant differences in relative LUC activity for different groups by Student's t-test ($P<0.05$). Values are given as means±SD from 3 biological replicates.

factors have been identified and constitute a complex regulatory network of artemisinin biosynthesis. To increase artemisinin content further effectively in *A. annua* plants, it is important to resolve the primary regulatory mechanisms of artemisinin biosynthesis.

Light not only serves as the source of energy for photosynthesis, but also a crucial external environmental factor affecting plant secondary metabolism, which can regulate the biosynthesis of artemisinin. As the central transcription factor in light signaling, HY5 protein could directly bind multiple downstream target gene promoters in plants and thus participate in many light-mediated biological processes. HY5 in *A. annua* has been identified as the positive regulator of artemisinin biosynthesis, and could directly bind to the promoters of downstream transcription factors *AaGSW1* and *AaMYB108* (Figure 5A - 5E). However, our Dual-LUC assay in the tobacco system revealed that AaHY5 was able to exercise a transcriptional activation function to promote *AaGSW1* alone, but was not able to activate *AaMYB108*, indicating that AaHY5 protein could not activate artemisinin biosynthesis pathway independently (Figure S1) and required the assistance of other proteins. Then AaBBX21, a protein encoding B-box domain, was screened for the interacting factor of AaHY5 (Figure 1). Transgenic assay (Figure 3) and Dual-LUC (Figure 4B) further confirmed AaBBX21 could increase the artemisinin content of *A. annua* by activating the artemisinin biosynthesis pathway (Figure 3). Y1H assay indicated AaBBX21 lacked the ability to directly bind the downstream gene promoters (Figure 4D), indicating the activation function of AaBBX21 in artemisinin biosynthesis also need co-factor. Recently, BBXs-HY5 complex was verified to regulate the synthesis of secondary metabolites in plants. AaHY5 and AaBBX21 could form a complex via direct protein interaction to activate downstream transcription factors *AaGSW1*, *AaMYB108* and *AaORA* to promote artemisinin accumulation, in which AaHY5 mainly functioned in binding and AaBBX21 functioned in activating (Figure 5).

Previous study showed that HY5 in *Arabidopsis* did not

possess trans-activity, other activators were needed to accomplish the function of HY5. For example, AtBBX20/21/22 act as essential partners for HY5-dependent modulation of hypocotyl elongation, anthocyanin accumulation and transcriptional regulation. PpHY5 in pear did not possess trans-activity in yeast and tobacco and need BBX family group IV members PpBBX16/18/21 to exercise the function of regulating light-mediated anthocyanin biosynthesis. AaHY5 in *A. annua* also showed weak trans-activity at least when expressed in yeast (Figure S9) and tobacco (Figure S1C), while AaBBX21 possessed strong trans-activity (Figure 4B, Figure S9). Our research further demonstrated that AaBBX21 could enhance the transcriptional activation ability of AaHY5 (Figure 5F), while could not increase the binding capacity (Figure S6). Moreover, evolutionary tree (Figure S2A) showed that the majority of transcription factors that interact with HY5 to regulate light-mediated secondary metabolism are distributed in subgroup IV. Interestingly, only AaBBX21 (the homolog of AtBBX22, Figure S4) both interacted with AaHY5 and showed similar expression patterns in different tissues with key enzymes of artemisinin biosynthesis key enzymes genes as well as transcription factors (Figure S2), suggesting that AaBBX21 is the specific core helper with AaHY5 to exert its function in artemisinin biosynthesis. In addition, our Dual-LUC result in Figure 4B showed that AaBBX21 protein alone could strongly activated the downstream promoters in tobacco system, which may be due to conservation of HY5 in tobacco and *A. annua*.

Furthermore, we investigated deeply into the relationship between AaBBX21-AaHY5 complex and light signal. We found that protein degradation of upstream module is the main reason for the inhibition of artemisinin biosynthesis in darkness. AaCOP1, the crucial E3 ubiquitin ligase in light signal, could interact with both AaBBX21 and AaHY5 via their VP motif (Figure 6). AaCOP1 could attenuate the protein abundance of AaHY5 and AaBBX21 in the dark, and weakened the activation function of complex to *AaGSW1*, *AaMYB108* and *AaORA*, finally inhibiting the artemisinin biosynthetic pathway (Figure 7). Although our results suggested that AaBBX21 - AaHY5 - AaCOP1 is the central upstream regulatory module for light-mediated artemisinin biosynthesis, how light-dark signaling affects AaHY5 and AaBBX21 at the transcription level remains to be further investigated.

In addition to light, plant hormones also had important function in artemisinin biosynthesis, such as jasmonic acid (JA), abscisic acid (ABA), salicylic acid (SA) and ethylene (ETH). When plants received hormonal signals, transcription factors downstream were induced and thus regulated artemisinin biosynthesis. Recently, the crosstalk between JA and ABA in artemisinin biosynthesis regulation was comprehensively investigated, and two transcription factors AabHLH113 and AaTCP15 have significant functions in this pathway. In our study, *AaBBX21* could also be induced by exogenous ABA (Figure S10A) and MeJA (Figure S10B). JA is the most important hormone affecting artemisinin content in *A. annua* plants, and increasing levels of JA led to the degradation of AaJAZ8 via the 26S proteasome pathway, resulting in the release of positive transcription factors related to artemisinin biosynthesis pathway or GSTs initiation. Previous studies have found that the promotion of JA for artemisinin biosynthesis is light-dependent, and we found that AaHY5-interacting core factor AaBBX21 could also interact with the artemisinin repressor AaJAZ8 (Figure S10C), same as the AaWRKY9 and AaMYB108 downstream of AaHY5, which showed the complexity and coordination of the light and JA signal crosstalk in artemisinin biosynthesis. The role of AaBBX21 protein integrating light and JA signals in the regulation of artemisinin biosynthesis needs in-depth exploration in the future.

Taken together, based on our current findings, we propose a working model of AaBBX21 - AaHY5 - AaCOP1 for light-mediated artemisinin biosynthesis in *A. annua* (Figure 8). Briefly, in the absence of light, AaCOP1 interacts with AaHY5 and AaBBX21 and make them degrade by the ubiquitin-26S proteasome pathway, so that downstream positive regulators can not be bound by AaHY5 and their transcription are repressed, resulting in the inhibition of artemisinin biosynthesis pathway and low artemisinin accumulation in darkness. In the light condition, the activity of AaCOP1 protein is inhibited, leading to the release of AaHY5 and AaBBX21. In this case, AaHY5 alone can bind the *AaGSW1* and *AaMYB108* promoters, causing them weakly transcript. However, when AaBBX21 and AaHY5 form a complex via protein interaction, they can largely promote the transcript of *AaGSW1*, *AaMYB108* and *AaORA*, thus strongly activating the artemisinin biosynthesis pathway and eventually causing a high artemisinin accumulation. Our research revealed the upstream central mechanism of artemisinin accumulation under daylight and largely improved the complex regulatory network of artemisinin biosynthesis. The BBX - HY5 - COP1 module can also provide insights into revealing the central regulatory mechanism of terpenoid secondary metabolite biosynthesis in other plants.

## 4 MATERIALS AND METHODS

Plant materials and growth conditions The *A. annua* plant material used in this study is cultivar 'Huhao 1' with high artemisinin content. The seeds were originated in Chongqing and further selected in our laboratory for many

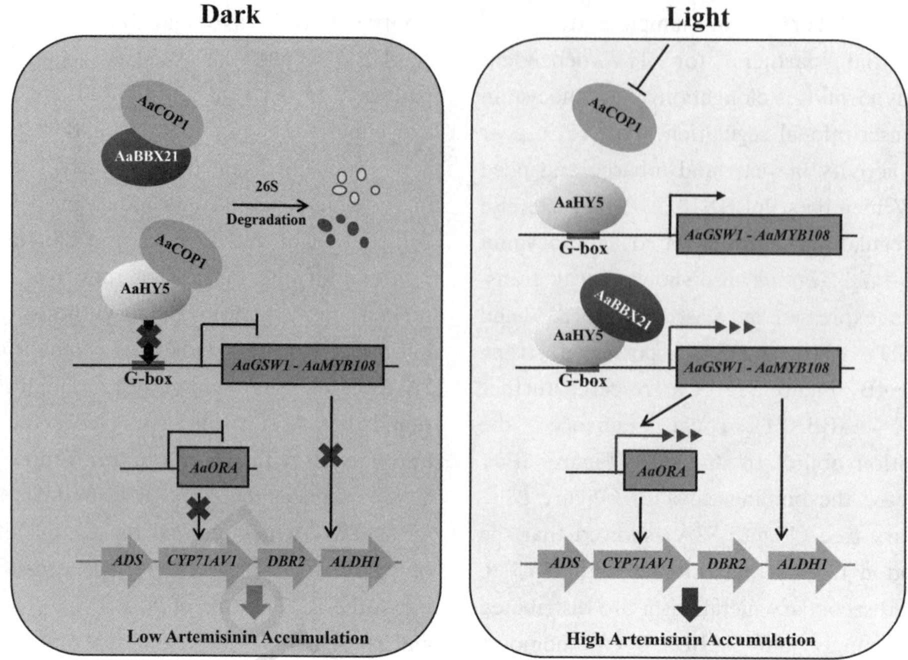


**Figure 8 The working model of the AaHY5 - AaBBX21 - AaCOP1 module**

generations and was used for hormone and light-dark treatments, total RNA and genomic DNA extraction, and stable transformation. The plant material used for transient transformation is *Nicotiana benthamiana*, which belonged to the laboratory's own varieties preserved for many years. *N. benthamiana* plants and *A. annua* seedings were cultured in pots in a growth chamber with 16 h light/8 h dark photoperiod and 65% relative humidity at 25 ± 2 ℃. *AaBBX21* Transgenic and wild-type *A. annua* plants were transplanted into the greenhouse with 24 h light photoperiod for 3 months for further transgenic phenotypic analysis.

Quantitative real-time-PCR analysis  For sampling, young leaves (leaf 1) of *A. annua* plants were collected into a 1.5 mL RNase-free centrifuge tube and frozen in liquid nitrogen. The total RNA was extracted using the OminiPlant RNA Kit (CW Biotech, China). 500 ng RNA for each sample was reverse transcribed using PrimeScript™ RT Master Mix (Takara, Japan) to obtain cDNA templates. Quantitative real-time-PCR assays were conducted using MagicSYBR Mixture (CW Biotech, China). Each analysis was performed with at least three technical and biological replicates. *β-ACTIN* gene was set as a control. The qRT-PCR primer sequences were listed in Table S1. The reaction conditions and procedures of the three assays mentioned were performed following the manufacturer's instructions.

Transformation of *A. annua* plants  The 906 bp full-length *AaBBX21* was cloned by KOD DNA polymerase (Toyobo, Japan) and inserted into the pHB eventual binary vector that used 2 × CaMV35S promoter to generate pHB-AaBBX21 - YFP. A reverse complementary sequence of a non-conserved region on the coding region of *AaBBX21* was inserted into pHB vector to construct *AaBBX21* antisense vector pHB - Anti - AaBBX21. The pHB - AaBBX21 - YFP and pHB - Anti - AaBBX21 vectors were then transferred into *Agrobacterium tumefaciens* strain EHA105 respectively for *A. annua* plant stable transformation as described previously.

Subcellular localization  The coding sequence of *AaBBX21* was cloned into the pHB - X - YFP vector. The pHB - YFP, pHB - AaBBX21 - YFP and P19 vectors were subsequently introduced into the *A. tumefaciens* strain GV3101. pHB - AaBBX21 - YFP/pHB - YFP strains cultured in MS liquid medium ($OD_{600}$ = 0.95) were mixed with P19 strain in a 1 : 1 ratio respectively and were injected into leaves epidermal cells of 4-week-old *N. benthamiana*. After incubation under dark for 1 d and then exposed to light for 1 d, the YFP signals were observed and captured by TCS SP5 - II confocal laser microscopy (Leica Microsystems, Germany).

The Yeast two-hybrid assay (Y2H)  The sequences of *AaBBX21* were inserted into pGADT7 vector and *AaHY5*, *AaCOP1* and *AaJAZ8* into the pGBKT7 vector. Different combinations of pGADT7 recombinant plasmids and pGBKT7 recombinant plasmids were co-transferred into yeast strain AH109, which were cultured on SD/-Leu/-Trp, SD/-Trp/-Leu/-His and SD/-Leu/-Trp/-His/-Ade plates. The protein interaction were detected and observed after 3 - 5 d. The combination of empty pGADT7 vector and recombinant pGBKT7 plasmids were used as negative control. The overlap PCR method was used to replace the amino acid

'VP' with 'AA'.

Bimolecular Fluorescence Complementation (BiFC) The full-length coding sequences of *AaBBX21*, *AaHY5* and *AaCOP1* were inserted into pXY104 (C terminal of YFP, cYFP) and pXY106 (N terminal of YFP, nYFP), and recombinant plasmids were transformed into *A. tumefaciens* strain GV3101. The recombinant plasmids and P19 plasmid strains were co-infiltrated into 4-week-old *N. benthamiana* leaves. *N. benthamiana* plants grew in darkness for 1 d and in light for another 1 d (treated in darkness for 2 d when AaCOP1 protein was present). The YFP signals were observed and captured by TCS SP5 - II confocal laser microscopy (Leica Microsystems, Germany) to detect the protein interaction. The combination of empty pXY104 with pXY106 - AaBBX21/AaHY5/AaCOP1, or pXY104 - AaBBX21/AaHY5/AaCOP1 with empty pXY106 act as the negative control.

Luciferase Complementation Assay (LCA) The full-length coding sequences of *AaBBX21*, *AaHY5* and *AaCOP1* were inserted into pCAMBIA1300 - nLUC (N terminal of LUC) and pCAMBIA1300 - cLUC (C terminal of LUC), and recombinant plasmids were transformed into *A. tumefaciens* strain GV3101 (pSoup - 19). The recombinant plasmids were co-infiltrated into 4-week-old *N. benthamiana* leaves. The treated *N. benthamiana* plants grew in darkness for 1 d and in light for another 1 d (treated in darkness for 2 d when AaCOP1 protein was present). In darkness, Stable-Lite Luciferase Assay System (Vazyme, China) was used for protein lysis and LUC luminescence reaction. The ChemiDoc MP Imaging System (Bio-rad) was applied for observation of LUC luminescence to confirm the interaction strength after 5 min. The combination of empty nLUC with cLUC - AaBBX21/AaHY5/AaCOP1, or AaBBX21/AaHY5/AaCOP1 - nLUC with empty cLUC act as the negative control.

Co-immunoprecipitation (Co-IP) The coding sequences of *AaBBX21* was inserted into the pHB-X-Flag vector, and *AaHY5* was inserted into the pHB-X-YFP vector. Recombinant plasmids were transformed into *A. tumefaciens* strain GV3101. *N. benthamiana* leaves were injected with strain mixtures as shown in Figure 1B. The infiltrated leaves were collected and ground into a crushed powder using liquid nitrogen after incubation under 24 h dark and 24 h light conditions. The total proteins were extracted by lysis buffer [adding protease inhibitors 100 $\mu$mol/L Pefabloc (Sigma-Aldrich, USA), 100 $\mu$mol/L cocktail (Roche, Switzerland), and 50 $\mu$mol/L MG132 (Sigma-Aldrich, USA)]. 10 $\mu$L GFP antibody (GeneScript, China) and 15 $\mu$L protein G beads (GE Healthcare, Bucks, UK) were incubated for 2 h at 4 ℃ for each sample. The total proteins were added into the Protein G and co-incubated for 3 h at 4 ℃. After washing the non-specific proteins in immunoprecipitates for three times, the protein interaction of AaHY5 and AaBBX21 in tobacco were detected by Western Blot using anti-Flag antibody (Sigma-Aldrich, USA) and anti-GFP (AbMart, China).

Dual-luciferase assay (Dual-LUC) The promoters of *AaADS*, *AaCYP71AV1*, *AaDBR2*, *AaALDH1*, *AaGSW1*, *AaMYB108*, *AaORA* and *AaWRKY9* were inserted into pGREENII0800 - LUC vector (reporter). The pHB - AaBBX21 - YFP, pHB - AaHY5 - YFP and pHB - AaCOP1 - YFP plasmids were used as effectors. The reporter mixed with the effector *A. tumefaciens* strain GV3101 (pSoup - 19) and co-infiltrated into 6-week-old *N. benthamiana*. The infiltrated tobacco leaves were sampled after 2 d (1 d under darkness and 1 d under white light). For the assay in Figure 7, plants were cultured under darkness for 2 d after transient expression. On 4 h before sampling, MG132 (100 $\mu$mol/L, dissolved in MS liquid medium) was injected again in the infiltrated area, while others injected equal amounts of DMSO as control. The ratio of LUC/REN were detected using Promega's Dual-Luciferase® Reporter Assay System kit and GloMax 20/20 Luminometer. The LUC/REN ratio of the combination of effector pHB-YFP and reporters were set to 1.

The Yeast one-hybrid assay (Y1H) The full-length coding sequence of *AaBBX21* was inserted into pB42AD vector to construct pB42AD - AaBBX21. Three tandem repeats of 40 G-boxes predicted on promoters of *AaADS*, *AaCYP71AV1*, *AaDBR2*, *AaALDH1*, *AaGSW1*, *AaMYB108*, *AaORA* and *AaWRKY9* were inserted into pLacZ vectors. Different combinations of pB42AD recombinant plasmids and pLacZ recombinant plasmids were co-transferred into yeast strain EGY48A, which were cultured on SD/-Ura/-Trp plates for 3 d. Then the strains were transfer to the SD/-Ura/-Trp medium (20 mg/L X-gal) under darkness. The protein-DNA interaction were detected after 3 - 5 d by observing whether the colonies turn blue. The combination of empty pB42AD vector and recombinant pLacZ plasmids were used as negative control.

Electrophoretic mobility shift assay (EMSA) The coding sequences of *AaBBX21* and *AaHY5* were inserted into pCold-TF vector (TaKaRa, Japan). The pCold-AaHY5, pCold-AaBBX21 and empty pCold-TF vector were transferred into *Escherichia coli* strain Rosetta (DE3) (TransGen Biotech, China). A final concentration of 0.5 $\mu$M Isopropyl-β-d-thiogalactoside (IPTG) was added into the DE3 *E. coli* culture to induce protein expression for 16 h at 16 ℃, and HisSep Nitrilotriacetic Acid Agarose Resin (Yeasen, China) was used for proteins purification. EMSA was performed using the LightShift™ Chemiluminescent EMSA Kit (Thermo, USA) according to manufacturer's instructions. The probes and mutant probes from the promoters of *AaGSW1* and *AaMYB108* were synthesized and labeled with biotin at their 5′ end (Sangon, China).

Measurement of artemisinin content　Fresh leaves from 5-month-old WT and *AaBBX21* transgenic *A. annua* plants in greenhouse were sampled and then dried at 50 ℃ oven for 3 d. The dry leaves were grounded into fine powder and each sample (0.1 g, three technical replicates were performed for each sample) was extracted twice with 1 mL methanol under ultrasound for 30 min. After centrifuging at 12 000 r/min for 10 min, The supernatant was to measure the artemisinin content by high-performance liquid chromatography (HPLC) as described previously. The standard of artemisinin was purchased from Sigma.

Protein degradation assay　The coding sequences of *AaBBX21*, *AaHY5* and *AaCOP1* were inserted into the pHB-X-Flag vector (drove by 2 × CaMV35S promoter). pHB-AaBBX21/AaHY5/AaCOP1-Flag *A. tumefaciens* GV3101 strains were resuspended in in MS liquid medium ($OD_{600}$ = 0.95) and were co-injected into leaves epidermal cells of 6-week-old *N. benthamiana* as the combination shown in Figure 7. *N. benthamiana* plants were cultured under constant darkness for 2 d. 100 μmol/L MG132 (dissolved in MS liquid medium) was injected again in the infiltrated area of leaves 4 h prior to sampling, while others injected equal amounts of DMSO in MS solution as control. Equal sized tobacco leaves were sampled and total protein was extracted and quantified using the Bradford Protein Assay Kit (TaKaRa, Japan). Finally, the protein levels of AaHY5, AaBBX21 and AaCOP1 were detected by Western Blot using anti-Flag (Sigma-Aldrich, USA). β-ACTIN was used as internal reference.

Light and hormone treatment　For light and dark treatment, 2-week-old *A. annua* seedings with uniform and healthy growth status were place in constant darkness or white light for 24 h in advance and then exposed to white light or darkness. For hormone treatment, 14-day-old wild-type *A. annua* seedlings were sprayed with exogenous methyl jasmonate (MeJA) and abscisic acid (ABA) of 100 μmol/L solution. The young leaves (leaf 1) were sampled before treatment (0 h) and several time points after treatment.

Bioinformatics analysis　The protein sequences of 32 AtBBXs were downloaded from the TAIR (The Arabidopsis Information Resource, https://www.arabidopsis.org/). 27 AaBBXs protein sequences were retrieved from the *A. annua* genome database and our previous study. The neighborhood method (NJ) phylogenetic was constructed using MEGA 10.1.8 with 1,000 bootstraps and displayed using TBtools software and *evolview v2* (https://www.evolgenius.info/evolview-v2/# mytrees/). The promoter sequences of *AaADS*, *AaCYP71AV1*, *AaDBR2*, *AaALDH1*, *AaGSW1*, *AaMYB108*, *AaORA* and *AaWRKY9* were submitted to the PlantCARE (https://bioinformatics.psb.ugent.be/webtools/plantcare/html/) to predict *cis*-acting elements.

[贺威智，黎凌，等. Journal of Integrative Plant Biology, 2024, DOI: 10.1111/jipb.13708.]

# Unveiling the regulatory mechanisms of nodules development and quality formation in *Panax notoginseng* using multi-omics and MALDI-MSI

## 1　INTRODUCTION

Root nodular structures play various crucial roles in plant growth and development, and their presence is often associated with the formation of lateral roots (LRs). LRs develop in four sequential stages: LR initiation, formation of lateral root primordia (LRP), LR meristem development, and LR extension, which may be interrupted during any of these stages. Nodular structure formation can be triggered by endogenous phytohormones, which act as key regulators in numerous plant processes including morphogenesis, flowering time, seed germination, senescence and even death, often in response to external environmental cues. Notably, auxin promotes the formation of root primordia while cytokinin inhibits LR development and stimulates the proliferation of cortical cells. Many functional genes involved in auxin and cytokinin biosynthesis such as *IAA*, *CYP735A*, *IPT*, and *CKX* actively participate in the formation of LRs and nodules.

Transcription factors are a class of proteins that bind specifically to *cis*-acting elements in the promoter region of target genes, thereby activating or inhibiting transcription. Several families of transcription factors, including Aux/IAA, MYB, bHLH, ERF, WOX, MADS-box are known to influence the growth and development of LRs and root nodular structures. For example, many members of MYB (SSR1, $HHO_2$, IPN2, MYB73, MYB77, MYB93, and MYBR) and bHLH (PFA, PFB, b HLH1, bHLH2, bHLH48, bHLH68, bHLH112, and bHLHm1) influence root architecture by regulating downstream target gene expression. Notably, MYBs and bHLHs frequently interact, forming protein complexes that execute diverse physiological functions.

*Panax notoginseng*, also named as Sanqi, is highly valued for both its culinary and medicinal applications. Its therapeutic properties are particularly effective for treating cardiovascular and cerebrovascular diseases, inflammation-related chronic conditions, and bruises. Ginsenosides are the main active ingredient and the pivotal index of quality evaluation in *P. notoginseng*, while ginsenoside $Rb_1$, $Rg_1$, notoginsenoside $R_1$ occupying the highest content, and notoginsenoside $R_1$, $R_2$ being the unique ingredients. Nodular structures, also known as nail heads, serve as a distinctive morphological feature for identifying Sanqi. These formations are arranged randomly, typically occurring at the top and occasionally middle of the main root (Fig. 1A). Research concerning these structures is limited, and there have been conflicting conclusions regarding their potential correlation with *P. notoginseng* quality. Additionally, the molecular mechanisms underlying nail head formation are poorly understood and require further investigation. Therefore, studying these structures would provide a basis for developing more effective methods for determine quality and screening *P. notoginseng*.

In this study, we explore various aspects of nail heads, including their structure, environmental influences, molecular mechanisms, regulatory networks, and impacts on *P. notoginseng* quality. Our examination of the morphological features and developmental anatomy reveals the inherent biological nature of the structure, while analysis of ginsenoside and dencichine content in *P. notoginseng* supports a correlation between the structures and plant quality. Gene-level investigations of the regulatory mechanisms in nail head formation were conducted both *in vitro* and *in vivo* by employing imaging mass spectrometry, comparative transcriptome, heterologous function verification, and binding verification. These results suggest that an interaction between PnMYB31/PnMYB78 and PnbHLH31 may regulate the transcription of *PnIAA14*, *PnCYP735A1*, *PnFPS*, and *PnSS*, thereby influencing nail head formation and ginsenoside accumulation in *P. notoginseng*. The findings of this study provide a basis for evaluating *P. notoginseng* suitable for different medication requirements and offer guidance for quality evaluation as well as clinical applications.

## 2 MATERIALS AND METHODS

Plant materials　Fresh *P. notoginseng* were collected from Wenshan county, Yunnan province. *P. notoginseng* of different root weight were purchased from Anhui Tianho Herbal Source Company. *P. notoginseng* possessing different root shapes and different ages were collected from Bozhou medicine market, while dried *P. notoginseng* without transplantation were bought from Panlong town, Yunnan province. Charateristic data of *P. notoginseng* tributed in Qing dynasty (A. D. 1636 to A. D. 1912) was measured in the Palace Museum, Beijing. Main root (PRT), lateral root (PLR) and nail head (PNH) were cut from cleaned fresh *P. notoginseng*, then used immediately. Dried *P. notoginseng* of 40 *tou* (number of *P. notoginseng* contained per 500 g) were divided into PMN (*P. notoginseng* possessing more than 6 nail heads) group and PLN (*P. notoginseng* possessing less than 3 nail heads) group, and stored at room temperature. *Arabidopsis thaliana* mutants of *atiaa14* (SALK_208773c) and *atcyp735a1* (SALK_093028c) were purchased from Arabidopsis Biological Resource Centre.

Determination of nutrient substance　Determination of nutrient substance in PRT, PLR and PNH was performed using starch content assay kit (Solarbio, BC0705), glucose content assay kit (Solarbio, BC2505), plant sucrose content assay kit (Solarbio, BC2465) as well as plant tissue fructose content assay (Solarbio, BC2455), following the manufacturer's instructions.

Determination of ginsenosides and dencichine　Determination of 16 ginsenosides was performed using UPLC-QQQ-MS/MS. 100 mg of the *P. notoginseng* sample was weighed accurately and ultrasonicated in 70% methanol for 3 times, each time for 40 min. The supernatant was collected through centrifugation at 12 000*g* for 10 min, and then diluted with 5 times the 70% methanol before quantification. UPLC-MS/MS analysis is performed on a Waters ACQUITY UPLC I-Class system equipped with a 6 500 Qtrap mass spectrometer (SCIEX Crop., Framinghan, Massachusetts, USA). A ACQUITY BEH C18 column (2.1 mm × 100 mm, 1.7 μm) with a flow rate of 0.4 mL/min at 40 ℃ was used to achieve UPLC separation. Formic acid in acetonitrile (0.1%, *V*/*V*, phase A) and formic acid in water (0.1%, *V*/*V*, phase B) were employed as the mobile phase. The optimized gradient elution was as followed: 0 - 3.5 min, 31%-32% A; 3.5-4 min, 32%-34% A; 4-6 min, 34% A; 6-7 min, 34%-70% A; 7-8 min, 70% A. 1 μL of the solution was injected. Mass spectrometer was performed in a negative ion mode, using multiple reaction monitoring (MRM) mode. Relevant parameters of each analyte were listed in Table S1. The condition of MRM was optimized under the following conditions: curtain gas, 20.0 psi; collision

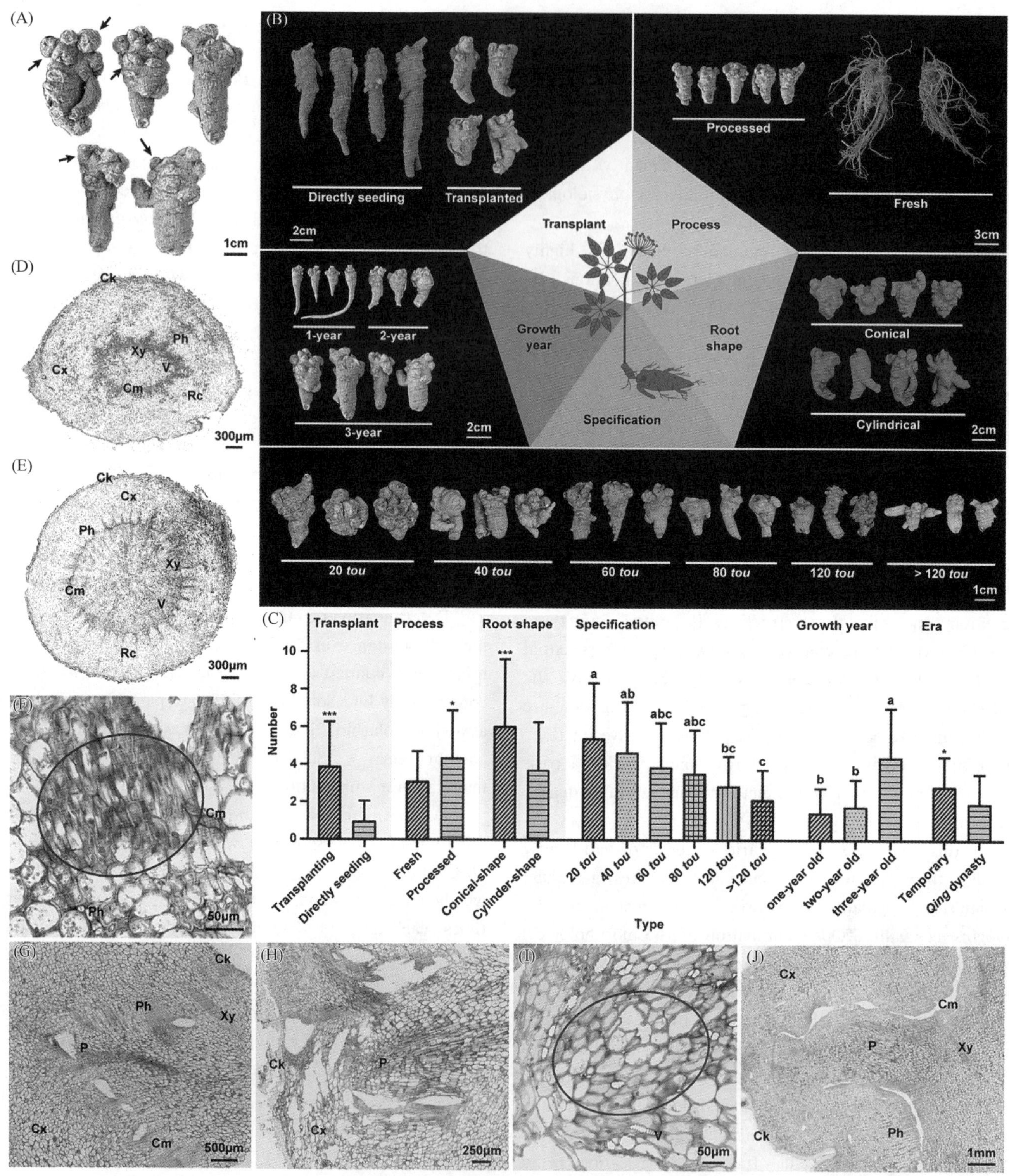


**Fig. 1 Morphological and micrological features of nail heads in *P. notoginseng***

(A) *P. notoginseng* and nail heads on the main root. Nail heads were pointed out by black arrows. (B) *P. notoginseng* of different types. (C) Effect of root weight, root shape, growth year, transplantation, procession and era on number of nail heads. (D) Micrological features of nail head. (E) Micrological features of main root. (F-J) Developmental anatomy during formation of nail head. (F) Cells restoring meristem ability in cambium and phloem. Oval-labelled cells showed a thickened cytoplasm and enlarged nucleus. (G-H) Lateral root primordium-like structure in nail head. (I) The apex of primordium-like structure. Oval-labelled cells showed a thicker cell wall. (J) Micrological structure of mature nail heads. Ck, cork, Cx, cortex, Rc, resin canel, Ph, phloem, Cm, cambium, Xy, xylem, V, vessel, P, primordium. Student's $t$-test was performed for comparison between two groups, $^{*}$, $P<0.05$, and $^{**}$, $P<0.01$. Variance test was performed for comparison more than two groups, with different lowercase letters indicating significant difference between groups ($P<0.05$).

gas, medium; ion spray voltage, −4 500 V; temperature, 550 ℃; ion source gas 1, 16.0 psi; ion source gas 2.0 psi.

Determination of dencichine was performed using UPLC-UV, while extraction of dencichine was carried out as reported previously. Waters ACQUITY-UPLC-I-Class system equipped with a PDA detector was used for dencichine quantitation under a UV wavelength of 213 nm. The mobile phase consisted of phosphate acid in water (0.1%, *V/V*, phase A) and phosphate acid in methanol (0.1%, *V/V*, phase B), a gradient elution of 53% phase A was used at a flow rate as 0.2 mL/min. ACQUITY BEH C18 column (2.1 mm × 100 mm, 1.7 μm) set at 25 ℃ was used for chromatographic seperation. 1 μL of the solution was injected. Information of ginsenosides and dencichine analytical standards were listed in Table S2.

Determination of endogenous phytohormones Quantitation of endogenous phyrohormones was performed using UPLC-QQQ-MS/MS equipped with a ACQUITY BEH C18 column. PRT, PLR and PNH preserved in −80 ℃ were firstly grounded into powder in liquid nitrogen. Extraction of phytohormone was performed as reported previously. The mobile phase was composed of acetonitrile (A) and 0.05% formic acid-water (B). Elution program was as follows: 0–3.5 min, 10% A; 3.5–4 min, 10%–95% A; 4–8 min, 95% A. Flow rate was set as 0.4 mL/min, while column temperature as 40 ℃. The injection volume was 1 μL for each sample. Mass analysis was performed on a 6 500 QTRAP mass spectrometer (SCIEX Crop., Framinghan, Massachusetts, USA). Mass spectrometer was performed in both positive and negative ion mode using multiple reaction monitoring (MRM) mode. Optimized MS/MS parameters of 8 endogenous phytohormones were shown in Table S3. Ion spray voltage was set at −4 500 V for negative mode, and 5 500 V for positive. Turbo spray temperature was 550 ℃, both gas 1 and gas 2 were set at 50 psi. Information of analytical standards were listed in Table S2.

Mass spectrometry imaging of ginsenosides and phytohormones PRT, PLR and PNH were firstly sectioned into 20 μm at −16 ℃ on a Cryostat Microtome 1 860 (Leica Microsystems Nussloch GmbH, Germany). MALDI mass spectrometry imagining of ginsenosides was performed by Create (Beijing) Technology Co., Limited, using a TransMIT AP-SMALDI 10 atmospheric pressure scanning matrix assisted laser desorption ionizing ion source equipped with a Thermo Scientific Q ExactiveTM mass spectrometer.

For mass spectrometry imaging of phytohormone, sections of PRT, PLR and PNH were mounted onto ITO-coated glass slides, followed by matrix coating steps using DAN solution containing 0.1% TFA (ACN: water=7/3, v/v) as matrix at 3.0 mg/mL. The matrix coating was using a $HTX_{TM}$-Sprayer™ matrix sprayer (HTX Technologies, Carrboro, NC) and parameters were set as follows: The flow rate of the sprayer was set to 0.075 mL/min at 60 ℃, and the track speed was set to 1 200 mm/min. The moving distance of the nozzle was 3 mm, the number of spraying cycles was 10 times. MALDI-MS imaging produces were as follow: The *m/z* range of 95–1 200 using Rapiflex MALDI Tissuetyper™ TOF/TOF MS imaging in the negative ion mode analysis. The spatial resolution of the tissue sections is 100 μm, and the repetition rate, frequency, intensity, and global attenuator offset were 1 000 Hz and 5 000 Hz, 70%, and 15% respectively. The obtained mass spectra were analyzed using FlexImaging 5.0 (Bruker Daltonics) and SCiLS Lab2018b soft-ware (Bruker Daltonik GmbH).

Transcriptome analysis and qRT-PCR analysis Transcriptome analysis was performed by Novogene Co. Ltd., Beijing. Three biological duplications of each group were adopted for RNA isolation. Expression level of annotated genes was denoted as FPKM, and differentially expressed genes (DEGs) were obtained by comparing FPKM value among PRT, PLT and PTM. DEGs with padj below 0.05 and log2(FoldChange) greater than 1 were considered.

Total RNAs of PRT, PLR and PNH were extracted following the manufacturer's instructions. cDNA was synthesized from 1 μg total RNA using a Thermo Scientific RevertAid RT Kit (Thermo Scientific, USA). qPCR was performed with TB Green Premix Ex Taq Ⅱ (TaKaRa, Japan) in a Roche LightCycler 480 qPCR System. Three technical replicates and three independent biological experiments were performed in all cases. The relative expression level of each gene was calculated used the $2^{-\Delta\Delta Ct}$ method and normalized against *Pn18s* as an internal reference gene, while *AtACTIN* (AT3G18780) was served as the reference gene in *Arabidopsis thaliana*. Primers used in qPCR analysis were listed in Table S4.

Arabidopsis transformation *Atiaa14* mutant and *atcyp735a1* mutant were identified using primers listed in Table S4. The full length ORF of *PnCYP735A1* and *PnIAA14* was ligated into an overexpression vector *pCAMBIA1300* with a *CaMV35S* promoter. The recombinant plasmids were transferred into *Agrobacterium tumefaciens* GV3101, then infected *A. thaliana* mutant lines by applying the floral dip method. *A. thaliana* accession Columbia (Col-0) was used as wild type.

Subcellular localization The full length ORF of *PnMYB30*, *PnMYB78* and *PnbHLH31* was cloned and subsequently fused to the *pCAMBIA1300* vector in frame with the green fluorescent protein (GFP) gene. The constructs were transferred into *A. tumefaciens* GV3101, and then infiltrated into leaves of *N. benthamiana*. At 48 h after infiltration, the fluorescent signals were visualized using a confocal spectral microscope imagining system

(Leica, German). A nucleus-localized *pCAMBIA1300-SmHY5*-RFP was used as positive control.

Promoter amplification and sequence analysis Promoters of *PnCYP735A1*, *PnIAA14*, *PnCYP716A47*, *PnSS*, *PnDS* and *PnFPS* were amplified from the genomic DNA of *P. notoginseng*, using primers listed in Table S4. Visualization of *cis*-elements in promoter region was performed using online software New PLACE (https://www.dna.affrc.go.jp/PLACE/? action=newplace).

Dual-luciferase assay (Dual-LUC) The dual-luciferase reporter assay was performed in *N. benthamiana* leaves as described previously. Promoters of *PnCYP735A1*, *PnIAA14*, *PnCYP716A47*, *PnSS*, *PnDS* and *PnFPS* were cloned into the *pGreenII 0800* vector, while cDNA of *PnMYB31*, *PnMYB78* and *PnbHLH31* cloned into *pHB-X-YFP* vector. The above engineered *pGREEN0800*-promoters and *pHB*-transcriptional factors strains were co-infiltrated into leaves of *N. benthamiana*. 6 biological replicates for each sample were obtained.

Yeast-one-hybrid (Y1H) and electrophoretic mobility shifts assay (EMSA) Promoters of *PnCYP735A1*, *PnIAA14*, *PnSS* and *PnFPS* were obtained using nested PCR amplification and genome walking according to genomic sequences. The probable binding domains of promoters were firstly inserted into *pAbAi* vector as baits, while coding sequence of full-length *PnMYB31*, *PnMYB78* and *PnbHLH31* constructed into the *pGADT7* vector. The resulting recombinant plasmids were co-transformed into Y1H gold yeast strain. After cultivation on SD/-Ura/-Leu medium with an appropriate concentration of Aureobasidin A (AbA) for 48 h, the positive binding activity was observed. The empty vectors *pGADT7* was used as negative controls.

Prokaryotic expression of the PnMYB31, PnMYB78 and PnbHLH31 fused with maltose binding protein (MBP) was performed at 25 ℃ for 12 h, 30 ℃ for 8 h, and 25 ℃ for 12 h, respectively. Amylose Resin High Flow (NEB, Ipseich, MA, USA) was subsequently used to obtain purified protein. EMSA was performed according to the manufacturer's instructions (Beyotime, Haimen, China).

Biomolecular fluorescence complementation assay (BiFC) The recombinant plasmid *pXY104*-PnMYB31, *pXY104*-PnMYB78 and *pXY106*-PnbHLH31 were generated and transformed into the *A. tumefaciens* strain GV3101. The combination of *pXY104*-PnMYB31 and *pXY106*-PnbHLH31, as well as *pXY104*-PnMYB78 and *pXY106*-PnbHLH31 were infiltrated into leaves of *N. benthamiana*. The yellow fluorescent signal was detected 2 d after infiltration, using a two-photon laser confocal fluorescence microscope (Leica, German).

Luciferase complementation imaging (LCI) The ORFs of PnMYB31 and PnMYB78 were cloned into *pJW771* containing a C-LUC, while the coding region of PnbHLH31 was introduced into *pJW772* vector containing a N-LUC. The LUC activity was measured using a cooled CCD imaging camera (IVIS Spectrum, PerkinElmer, Waltham, MA, USA).

## 3 RESULTS

Nail head formation was associated with lateral roots The morphological features of nail heads on *P. notoginseng* were collected and analyzed to investigate the factors influencing their emergence. It was observed that nail heads in *P. notoginseng* predominantly occurred at the top of the main root near the caudex, displaying a conical or oblate shape (Fig. 1A). Additionally, some nail heads protruded from the middle of the main root. *P. notoginseng* samples were categorized according to root weight, root shape, growth year, and whether they had been transplanted or processed after harvest (Fig. 1B). A higher amount of nail heads were obtained in *P. notoginseng* with a larger root weight, conical root shape, longer growth years, and those that had undergone transplanting during cultivation or processing after harvest (Fig. 1C). Furthermore, the morphological features of modern *P. notoginseng* were compared with thosetributed in Qing dynasty, revealing a contemporary increase in the prevalence of nail heads in roots of equivalent weight (Fig. 1C).

Next, microscopic features and developmental characteristics were analyzed to elucidate the biological nature of nail heads. As shown in Fig. 1D, the structures of PNH contain a broad cortex and cork portion consisting of several layers of flat cells. Resin canals are scattered throughout the phloem, occasionally forming a ring pattern. Vessels in the xylem are arranged radially, with starch granules stored in parenchyma cells. Compared with the main root (Fig. 1E), PNH possess a broader cortex. The microscopic features of nail heads in different developmental stages were also observed. During the initial formation stage, cells in cambium and phloem regained meristematic characteristics such as thickened cytoplasm, an enlarged nucleus, and closely aligned cells, reminiscent of the founder cells in LR primordium (Fig. 1F). As the nodules develop, the founder cells split towards the far axis, gradually forming primordium-like structures with clear stratification (Fig. 1G-1H) and apex cells with thick cell walls (Fig. 1I). These structures finally break through the epidermis (Fig. 1J) to form visible protrusions. This process shares several key similarities with LR development, indicating that nail heads may be a type of stunted LR. We next sought to determine if nail heads are associated with LRs in *P. notoginseng*. Interestingly, we established a weak negative correlation (Table 1), wherein a higher abundance of LRs was always accompanied by fewer nail heads, and vice versa.

**Table 1 Correlation analysis between amount of nail heads and lateral roots**

| | | Lateral roots | Nail heads |
|---|---|---|---|
| Lateral roots | Pearson's correlation coefficient | 1 | −0.230* |
| | Sig. (two-tailed) | \ | 0.040 |
| | Case number | 80 | 80 |

* At level 0.05 (two-tailed), the correlation was significant.

To investigate the potential nutrient storage functionality, we quantified major components such as starch, glucose, sucrose, and fructose in PRT, PLR, and PNH. As shown in Figure S1, starch, glucose, and fructose were highest in PRT, indicating that anil heads possess a weak nutrient storage capacity.

Active component composition was influence by nail heads To discover the relationship between nail heads and active component composition, determination of ginsenosides and dencichine was performed. By employing UPLC-QTRAP-MS/MS, we established a method for simultaneously quantifying 16 ginsenosides, and the verification was provided in Table S5 with the total ion chromatograms (TIC) of standards and samples shown in Fig. S2A and Fig. S2B. PNH was found to contain significantly higher levels of ginsenoside Rb1, Re, Rg1, Rg2, Rg3, Rh1, and Ro compared to PRT, with fold increases of 1.78-, 2.10-, 1.86-, 2.36-, 1.61-, 1.92-, and 2.18-, respectively. Similarly, these ginsenosides levels in PNH were 1.62-, 1.87-, 1.53-, 1.73-, 1.63-, 2.18-, and 1.49-fold higher than in PLR (Fig. 2A). Furthermore, the PMN group exhibited higher content of ginsenoside Rb1 and Rf as well as notoginsenoside $R_1$ and $R_2$ compared to the PLN group, with respective increases of 1.36-, 1.35-, 1.44-, and 1.54 times. This suggests a positive relationship between the ginsenosides content and nail head amount (Fig. 2B). In addition, the content of PPT (protopanaxatriol)-type and PPD (protopanaxadriol)-type ginsenosides was analyzed, indicating a significantly higher content of PPT-type ginsenosides possessed in the PMN group, showing a 1.32-fold increase compared to the PLN group. No significant differences were observed in protopanaxadriol-type (PPD) ginsenosides (Fig. 2C).

As an effective hemostatic agent, we also analyzed the content of dencichine by employing UPLC-UV The verification of the dencichine determination method was provided in Table S6, with chromatogram of standards and samples shown in Fig. S3A and Fig. S3B. Our findings showed no significant differences among root, lateral root, and nail head (Fig. 2D), nor between the PMN and PLN groups (Fig. 2E).

To further investigate the distribution of ginsenosides, MALDI-MSI was performed on PLR and PNH during the early (S1) and middle (S2) developmental stages. As shown in Fig. 2F and Figure S4, ginsenosides $Rb_1$ ($[M+K]^+$, 1147.57) and $Rg_1$ ($[M+K]^+$, 839.45) and notoginsenoside $R_1$ ($[M+K]^+$, 971.50) were distributed throughout the PLR tissue, while ginsenosides Rd/Re ($[M+K]^+$, 985.51) predominantly inhabited the PLR xylem and meristem. During the S1 and S2 stages, Ginsenoside $Rg_1$ and notoginsenoside $R_1$ were distributed throughout the whole nodular structure, while ginsenoside Rd/Re occupied the xylem and primordium of nail heads. Unlike lateral roots, nail heads predominantly accumulated ginsenoside $Rb_1$ in their cortex, potentially explaining the elevated content recorded in these structures.

Auxin, cytokinin and jasmonic acid derivates were highly concentrated during nail head formation To reveal the dynamic distribution patterns of phytohormones during nail head formation, MALDI-MSI was conducted in early-stage tissues. As shown in Fig. 3A, auxin ($[M-H]^-$, 174.18) was predominantly enriched in the primordium of PLR and PNH during the initial stage, with no significant accumulation observed in PRT. JA ($[M-H]^-$, 209.27) was primarily distributed inside the cambium of PRT and the primordium of both PLR and PNH. tZT ($[M-H]^-$, 218.24) was dispersed throughout the PLR, with a high abundance in the primordium, while it mainly distributed in both the cortex and the primordium (A1). In addition, distribution of GA3 ($[M-H]^-$, 345.37) and tZR ($[M-H]^-$, 350.36) in PLR and PNH was detected in another early development sample, with the two phytohormones mainly distributed in cortex of PNH, while no accumulation of tZR in PLR was detected (Figure A2). The sampling diagram of PRT, PLR and PNH groups was shown in Figure A3.

A UPLC-QTRAP-MS/MS method was established to quantify 8 influential phytohormones. Method verification of phytohormone determination was shown in Table S7, while TIC of 8 standard analytes and samples were shown in Fig. S5A and Fig. S5B. As shown in Fig. 3B, the content of tZR in PNH was 3.17 and 2.89-fold higher than in that of PRT and PLR, respectively. PNH also contained a tZT content 1.30-fold higher than PLR. JA derivates accumulated most highly in PNH, indicating that cytokinin and JAs may be crucial for morphogenesis and metabolite accumulation.

PnCYP735A1 and PnIAA14 expressed highest in nail heads inhibited growth of lateral roots Transcriptome sequencing was conducted on PRT, PLR, and PNH to elucidate the molecular mechanisms of nail head formation, while sample

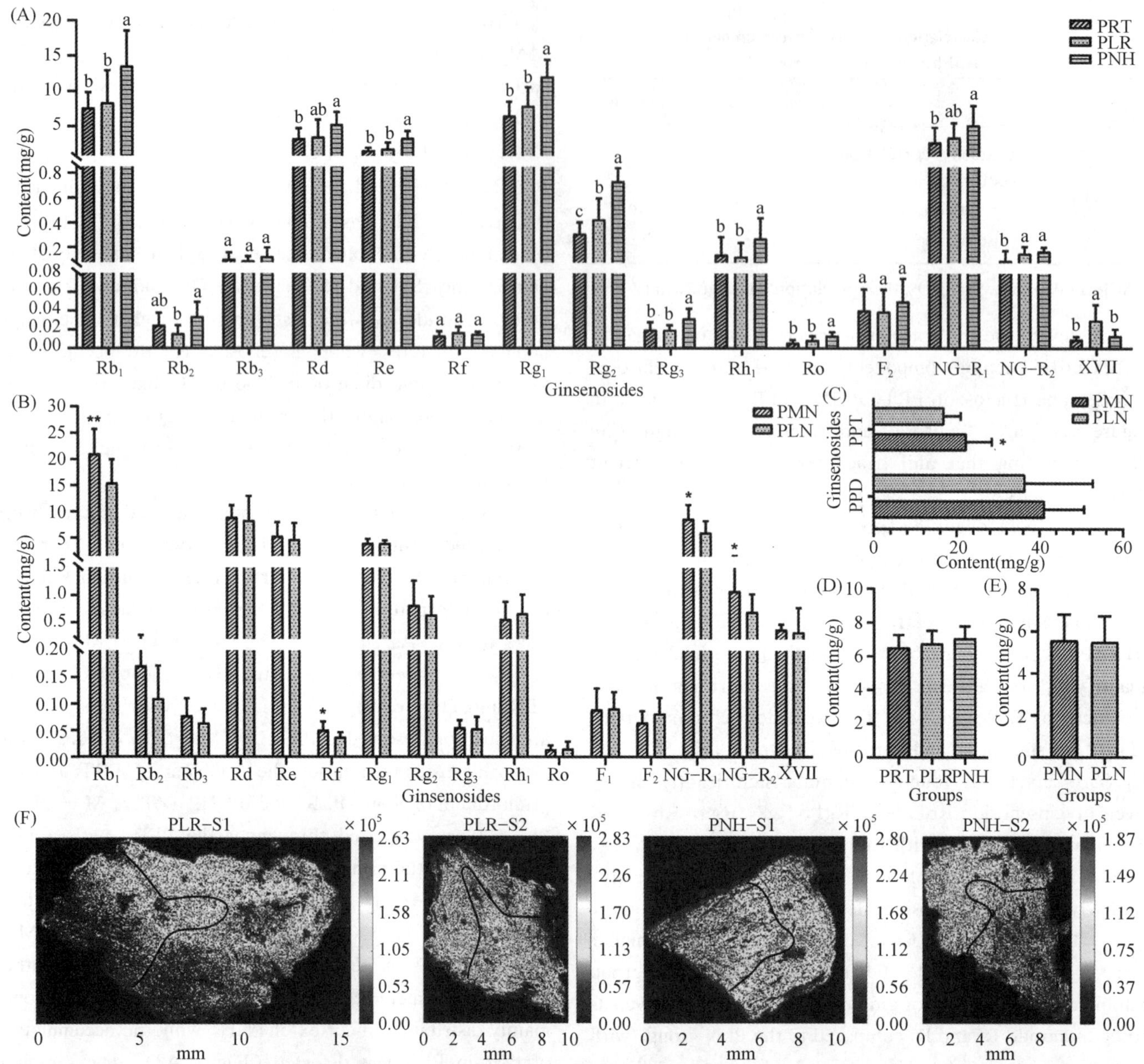

**Fig. 2 Active component composition associated with nail head of *P. notoginseng***

(A) Determination of 16 ginsenosides in PRT, PLR and PNH. (B) Determination of 16 ginsenosides in *P. notoginseng* possessing different amounts of nail heads. (C) Content of PPD-type and PPT-type ginsenosides in PMN and PLN. (D) Determination of dencichine in PRT, PLR and PNH. (E) Determination of dencichine in *P. notoginseng* possessing different amounts of nail heads. (F) MALDI-MSI of ginsenoside $Rb_1$. ($[M+K]^+$, 1 147.60) in lateral root and nail head in *P. notoginseng*. The primordium boundary was represented in the black curve. Student's *t*-test was performed for comparison between two groups, *, $P<0.05$, and **, $P<0.01$. Variance test was performed for comparison more than two groups, with different lowercase letters indicating significant difference between groups ($P<0.05$).

Pearson correlation and data quality control are shown in Figure S6 and Table S8, respectively. A total of 767 DEGs were identified, with 55 displaying up-regulation and the remaining 712 exhibiting down-regulation. DEG distribution was significantly different in PNH compared to both PRT and PLR (Figure S7A-B). GO (Gene Ontology) annotation revealed that in comparison to PRT, the DEGs of PNH were more enriched in processes related to oxidation-reduction reactions. Furthermore, DEGs associated with transportation were enriched in PNH when compared with PLR. The DEGs in both PLR and PRT were predominantly enriched in processes involving catabolism (Table S9). KEGG (Kyoto Encyclopedia of Genes and Genomes) annotation demonstrated that DEGs were primarily enriched in zeatin biosynthesis, phenylpropanoid biosynthesis, plant hormone signal transduction, arachidonic acid metabolism, and glutathione

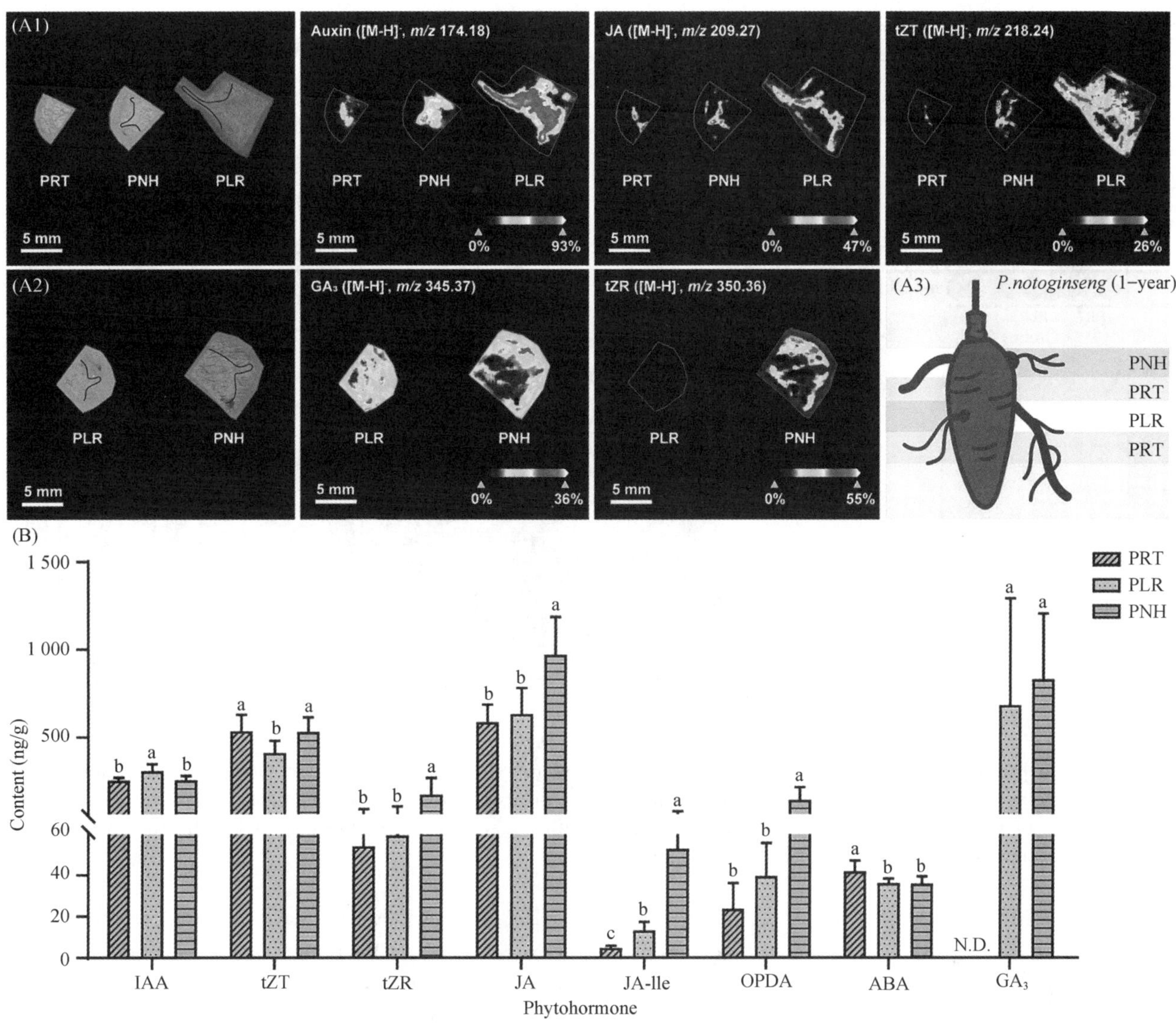


**Fig. 3 Dynamic distribution of endogenous phytohormoyne during nail head formation**

(A1 - A2) MALDI-MSI of endogenous phytohormone in PRT, PLR and PNH of different developing stages. (A3) The sampling diagram of PRT, PLR and PNH groups. (B) Determination of endogenous phytohormone in PRT, PLR and PNH (n=10).

metabolism when comparing PRT to PNH (Figure S7C and Table S10). Additionally, PLR showed higher enrichment of DEGs involved in zeatin biosynthesis when compared to PNH (corrected P-value at 0.001). No DEGs were enriched between PRT and PLR.

Given the crucial role of endogenous phytohormones in regulating root architecture, DEGs related to phytohormone pathways were selectively analyzed. Particular attention was paid to auxin and cytokinin pathways, as they act as key regulators of lateral root and nodular structure development. As displayed in Fig. 4A and Table S11, many genes exhibited high expression levels in PNH and low expression levels in PRT. Notably, several genes involved in zeatin biosynthesis including *CYP735A* (cluster-13244.1166), *IPT* (cluster-13244.1840, cluster-13244.28137, and cluster-13244.11262), and *CKX* (cluster-13244.1701 and cluster-13244.1849) were most highly expressed in PNH, potentially contributing to the high tZT and tZR content in nail heads. Gene expression patterns were verified using real-time quantitative fluorescence PCR. *PnCYP735A1* (cluster-13244.1166) and *PnIAA14* (cluster-13244.1262) showed the highest expression in PNH when compared with PLR and PRT (Fig. 4B).

We furthermore verified the function of *PnIAA14* and *PnCYP735A1*, by overexpressing genes above in mutants of their homologous genes in *A. thaliana* plants. Mutants with *AtIAA14* (AT4G14550) and *AtCYP735A1* (AT5G38450) were firstly obtained and verified using a tri-primer PCR method (Figure S8A). The CDS regions of *PnIAA14* and *PnCYP735A1* were cloned into the pCAM-BIA1300 overexpression vector with a *CaMV35S* promoter. Then, the floral dip method was then used to inoculate the new *atiaa14* and *atcyp735a1* mutants. Four lines of *A. thaliana* were

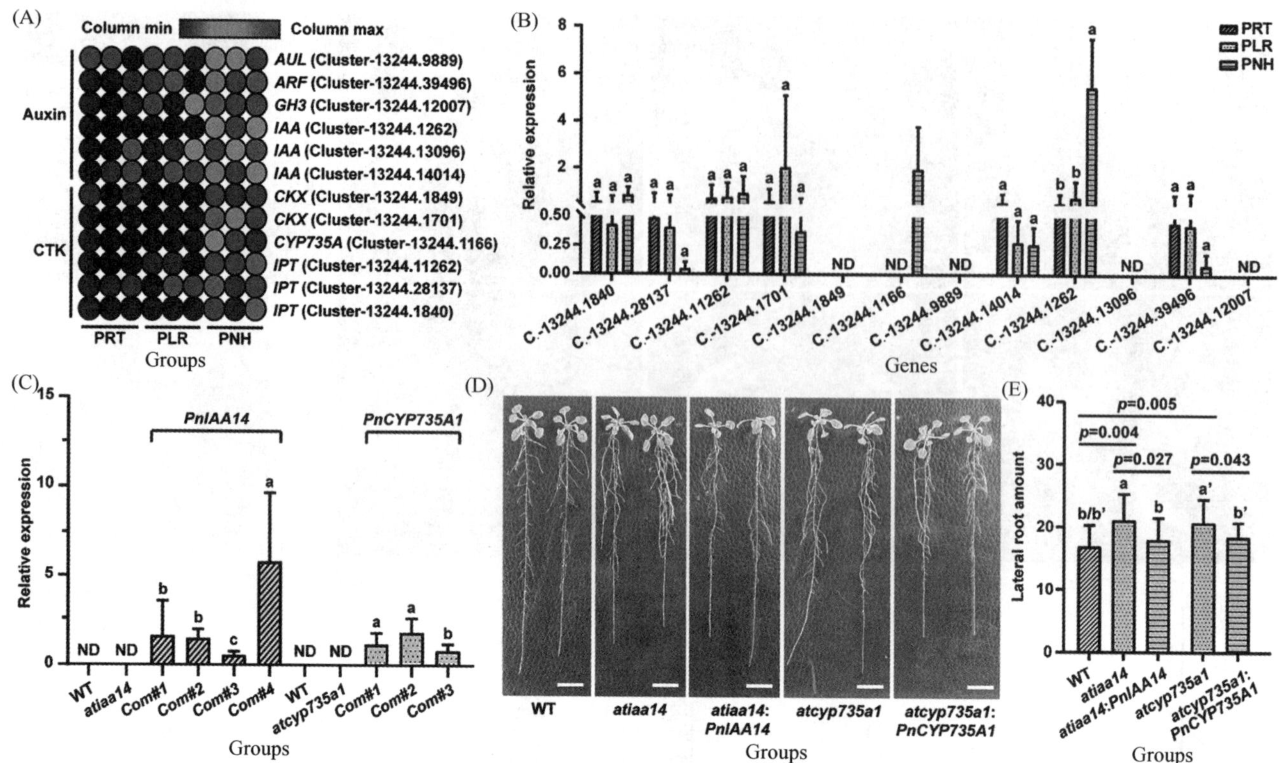

**Fig. 4 Screening and functional verification of *PnIAA14* and *PnCYP735A1***

(A) Expression pattern of DEGs related to phytohormone in transcriptome. (B) qRT-PCR of DEGs related to auxin signal transduction and zeatin biosynthesis (n=3). (C) qRT-PCR of mutant plants transformed with *PnIAA14* and *PnCYP735A1* (n=3). (D) Phenotype of wild type, mutants and mutants transformed with target genes. (E) Numbers of lateral roots in wild type, mutants and mutants transformed with target genes (n=16).

complemented with *PnIAA14*, and three lines were complemented with *PnCYP735A1*. Relatively high expression of *PnIAA14* and *PnCYP735A*1 were observed in *atiaa14*:: *PnIAA14*-Com#4 and *atcyp735a1*::*PnCYP735A1*-Com#2, respectively (Figure S8B and Fig. 4C). When compared with the wild type, *atiaa14* and *atcyp735a1* contained more LRs, while *atiaa14*:: *PnIAA14*-Com # 4 and *atcyp735a1*:: *PnCYP735A1*-Com#2 had an equivalent amount (Fig. 4D - 4E). This indicates that *PnIAA14* and *PnCYP735A1* inhibit LR development.

As secondary metabolites could also serve as inductor regulating root architecture, we explored the effects of ginsenoside $Rb_1$ on nail head formation due to its accumulation in the cortex of the structures. With the increase of ginsenoside $Rb_1$ concentration, both lateral roots numbers and main root length showed increasing first then decreasing tendency (Figure S8C-S8E). However, no significant differences were observed between the WT and the two mutants, indicating that the influence of ginsenoside $Rb_1$ on root architecture is unrelated to *PnIAA14* and *PnCYP735A1*.

PnMYB31, PnMYB78 and PnbHLH31 directly bind to promoters of phytohormone and ginsenosides biosynthetic genes to activate their expression Five MYB and three bHLH transcriptional factors were selected through transcriptomic analysis due to their considerably higher transcriptional levels in PNH (Table S12). A qRT-PCR analysis of these factors revealed a significantly higher expression of cluster-13244. 19973, cluster-13244. 15496, and cluster-13244. 3751 in PNH (Figure S9A). Our sequence analysis suggested that cluster-13244. 19973 and cluster-13244. 15496 possess a conserved R2R3 domain. Additionally, a subgroup 20 specific WxPRL motif was identified in the amino acid sequence of cluster-13244. 19973. Cluster-13244. 3751 contained both a HER motif and a helix-loop-helix region (Figure S9B). A phylogenetic tree constructed with 125 AtMYBs indicated that cluster-13244. 19973 could be categorized into subgroup 20, which is most homologous with AtMYB78. Meanwhile, cluster-13244. 15496 showed great homology with AtMYB31 from subgroup 1 (Figure S9C). Cluster-13244. 3751 shared the closest relationship with AtbHLH31 in sub-group XII and clustered with all 169 AtbHLHs (Figure S9D). Based on these findings, cluster-13244. 19973, cluster-13244. 15496, and dcluster-13244. 3751 were designated as PnMYB78, PnMYB31, and PnbHLH31, respectively. Additionally, both PnMYB31 and PnMYB78 were recognized as members of group C MYB. A subcellular localization test was performed by co-expressing *35Spro*::

*PnMYB78 - GFP*, *35Spro::PnMYB30 - GFP*, and *35Spro::PnbHLH31 - GFP*, along with a nucleus-located *35Spro::SmHY5 - RFP* serving as a marker. The results depicted in Figure S7E demonstrate that PnMYB78 - GFP, PnMYB31 - GFP, and PnbHLH31 - GFP all localized to the nucleus (Figure S9E).

To further investigate the involvement of PnMYB78, PnMYB31, and PnbHLH31 in nail head development and ginsenoside biosynthesis, we firstly screened out functional *PnFPS*, *PnDS*, *PnSS* and *PnCYP716A47* for expressing highest in nail heads (Figure S10A). Promotors sequences of *PnFPS*, *PnDS*, *PnSS*, *PnCYP716A47*, and *PnIAA14*, *PnCYP735A1* participating in nail heads formation were PCR amplified and all were found to contain either an MBS domain or E-box/G-box (Figure S10B). As group C MYB preferring binding to MBSIIG sequence (YACCWAMC), while most bHLH in plant preferring binding to G-box (CACGTG), hence interaction between PnMYB31/PnMYB78 with MBSIIG sequence on the promotor, as well as interaction between PnbHLH31 and G-box on the promotor were studied hereafter.

We next conducted a dual-LUC assay to verify whether the three transcriptional factors target the promotors of genes related to nail head development and ginsenosides biosynthesis in vivo. As shown in Fig. 5A and Figure S11, the detection of LUC luminescence indicated that co-expression with PnMYB31 increased the expression of $proPnSS^{1878}$::*LUC* and $proPnFPS^{1220}$::*LUC* by 3.08- and 2.15-fold, respectively. Additionally, the luminescent activity of $proPnFPS^{1220}$::*LUC*, $proPnCYP735A1^{1675}$::*LUC*, and $proPnIAA14^{1205}$::*LUC* was elevated after introducing *pHB-PnMYB78*, leading to a 1.80-, 17.70-, and 2.07-fold increase compared with an empty vector. However, PnbHLH31 decreased the LUC activity of $proPnIAA14^{1205}$::*LUC* by 0.43-fold. These results uncover major regulatory balancing mechanisms within the plant by indicating that PnMYB31 and PnMYB78 may up-regulate the expression of genes related to ginsenoside biosynthesis and nail head development, while PnbHLH31 may down-regulate the expression of *PnIAA14*.

Yeast one-hybrid and electrophoretic mobility shift (EMSA) assays were further performed to verify whether the promoters $proPnSS^{1878}$, $proPnFPS^{1220}$, $proPnIAA14^{1205}$, and $proPnCYP735A1^{1675}$ can bind specifically with PnMYB31, PnMYB78, and PnbHLH31 in vitro. After introducing *pGADT7-PnMYB31*, *-PnMYB78*, and *-PnbHLH31* into yeast strains containing potential binding domains of the target promoters (Fig. 5B), we found that strains integrating PnbHLH31 with $proPnIAA14^{1205}$*-Gbox*, PnMYB78 with $proPnIAA14^{1205}$*-MBS* Ⅱ *G*, $proPnCYP735A1^{1675}$*-MBS* Ⅱ *G*, and $proPnFPS^{1220}$*-MBS* Ⅱ *G*, PnMYB31 with $proPnFPS^{1220}$*-MBS* Ⅱ *G*, and $proPnSS^{1878}$*-MBS* Ⅱ *G* were able to grow on selective media (Fig. 5C). Our EMSA showed that PnMYB78-MBP was able to bind to the MBS Ⅱ G sequence of $proPnIAA14^{1205}$, $proPnCYP735A1^{1675}$, and $proPnFPS^{1220}$, but failed to bind their mutant probes. PnMYB31-MBP directly binds to the MBS Ⅱ G box of $proPnFPS^{1220}$ and $proPnSS^{1878}$, while PnbHLH31-MBP binds to the G-box of $proPnIAA14^{1205}$ (Fig. 5D).

Previous reports have suggested that MYBs regulating the biosynthesis of secondary metabolites commonly interact with bHLHs. We initially conducted a yeast two-hybrid assay to verify the potential interaction between PnMYB31, PnMYB78, and PnbHLH31. However, autoactivation occurred in the control group during co-culturing with *pGBKT7-PnMYB31/PnMYB78/PnbHLH31* and the *pGADT7* empty vector. Therefore, we chose to validate the interaction using BiFC and LCI assay. YFP fluorescent signals were recorded in the nucleus of leaf epidermal cells co-infected with PnMYB31/PnMYB78 and PnbHLH31 (Fig. 5E), and signal of LUC activity was detected while co-transferring *pJW772*-PnbHLH31 and *pJW771*-PnMYB31/PnMYB78 in the leaves of *N. benthamiana* (Fig. 5F). This analysis indicates that PnMYB31 and PnMYB78 are both capable of interacting with PnbHLH31.

## 4 DISCUSSION

Cytokinin mediates nail head formation by inhibiting the development of lateral roots and promoting cortical cell division Both auxins and cytokinins play important roles in the growth and development of LRs and plant nodular structures. The local accumulation of auxin is a prerequisite for lateral root and root nodule initiation, while cytokinin positively regulates the induction of nodular structures and represses LRs, the cytokinin biosynthesis-related genes also contribute to the morphogenesis. Aux/IAAs function as transcriptional suppressors in the $SCF^{TIR1/AFB}$-Aux/IAA-ARF pathway, and ubiquitination further activates downstream gene expression when sufficient auxin is achieved. As an Aux/IAA-related gene, *AtIAA14* is thought to repress LR formation by interrupting cell cycle progression in the pericycle. In this study, we observed that nail heads with broad cortexes exhibited a local accumulation of auxin in the primordium during the early stages of development. Cytokinin content, however, increased in the cortex along with developmental progression. *PnIAA14* and *PnCYP735A1* expressed highest in nail head also exhibited adverse effect on lateral root growth. Auxin accumulation in primordium is believed to be essential for nail head initiation, which is paired with the inhibitory effects *PnIAA14* and *PnCYP735A1* have on LR growth. These genes also promote cortex division by influencing auxin signal transduction and cytokinin biosynthesis.

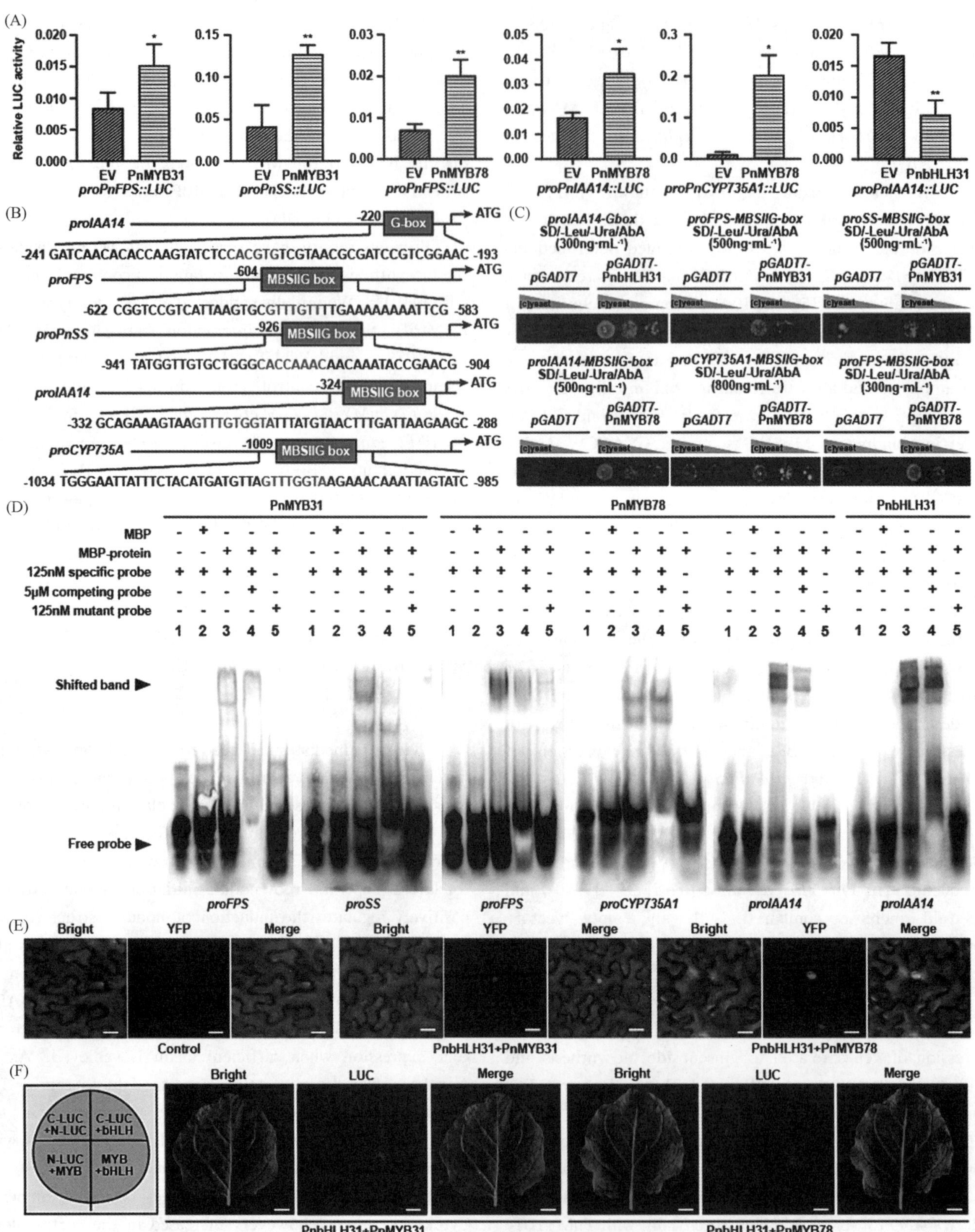

**Fig. 5 Transcriptional regulation of nail head formation and ginsenosides accumulation**

(A) Interaction between PnMYB31, PnMYB78, PnbHLH31 and *proPnFPS*, *proPnSS*, *proPnIAA14*, *proPnCYP735A1* in vivo (n=3). Student's *t*-test was performed, *, $P<0.05$, and **, $P<0.01$. (B) Structural schematics of partial promotor sequences containing MBSⅡG domain or G-box. (C) Y1H assay between PnMYB31, PnMYB78, PnbHLH31 and *PnFPS*, *PnSS*, *PnIAA14*, *PnCYP735A1*. Grey triangles represented dilution factor of the yeast concentration. (D) EMSA between PnMYB31, PnMYB78, PnbHLH31 and *PnFPS*, *PnSS*, *PnIAA14*, *PnCYP735A1*. (E) BiFC assay between PnMYB31/PnMYB78 and PnbHLH31. Horizontal line on the right bottom represented 10 μm. (F) LCI assay between PnMYB31/PnMYB78 and PnbHLH31. Horizontal line on the right bottom represented 1 cm.

Transcription factors coordinately regulates nail heads and quality formation in P. notoginseng  Transcription factors can simultaneously regulate multiple signaling pathways and expression of multiple functional genes, furthermore obtain ability to coordinately mediates morphology and quality formation of plants. It has been reported that PgWOX11 promotes adventitious roots formation in *P. ginseng*, and negatively regulates ginsenosides accumulation by interacting with PgCLE45, while PgMADS41 and PgMADS44 mediates root growth and biosynthesis of ginsenoside Ro in *P. ginseng*. SmSPL6 affects root development and induces phenolic acid biosynthesis, while SmSPL7 inhibits plant growth and phenolic acid accumulation in *Salvia miltiorrhiza*. In this study, PnMYB31-PnbHLH31 and PnMYB78-PnbHLH31 complexes were verified regulating nail heads formation and ginsenosides accumulation by directly binding to the promoter of phytohormone-related and ginsenoside biosynthetic genes, providing evidence for the pivotal role transcription factors play in plant morphology and quality formation.

Composition of active components influenced by nail head presence provides insights into clinical applications  Secondary metabolites potentially function as regulators of root architecture. The biosynthesis of lupeol, the primary active component of *Lotus japonicus*, is associated with *OSC*, which is specifically expressed in root nodules. This gene influences the transcription of *ENOD40*, further regulating the formation of root nodules. Ginsenoside $Rb_1$ and Re regulate branching in *P. ginseng* adventitious roots, while ginsenoside Ro participate in development of adventitious roots through PgMADS41/PgMADS44. In our study, ginsenoside $Rb_1$ was the only PPD-type ginsenoside identified in *P. notoginseng* plants with a high amount of nail heads, and was distributed specificallyin the cortex of nail heads. Induction of ginsenoside $Rb_1$ towards *A. thaliana* revealed an increasing and then decreasing trend alongside both root length and LR amount. The particularly highest content of ginsenoside $Rb_1$ observed in nail heads (roughly 30 μmol/L) might trigger the development of the structures by inhibiting LR development.

PPD-type and PPT-type ginsenosides are divided based on the presence of a hydroxyl substitution on the 6-position carbon of damarane tetracyclic triterpene aglycones. PPD-type ginsenosides reportedly contain central nervous system (CNS) excitation activity and strong anti-oxidative damage function. PPT-type ginsenosides, however, depress CNS and possess strong vasodilation. In this study, *P. notoginseng* plants possessing more nail heads were found to contain higher ginsenoside contents, especially those of the PPT type, indicating better CNS depression and vasodilation. These findings serve as guidance for screening for *P. notoginseng* plants with enhanced blood-activating properties.

## 5 CONCLUSION

Based on the results above, an internal mechanism for nail head formation was also established, that is, auxin promotes LR initiation while *PnIAA14*, *PnCYP735A1* prevent the LR development, and promote cortical cell division by regulating auxin signal transduction and cytokinin biosynthesis. PnMYB31-PnbHLH31 and PnMYB78-PnbHLH31 complexes regulate the formation of these structures by influencing the expression of *PnIAA14* and *PnCYP735A1*. The complexes also increase the accumulation of ginsenosides by binding with the promotors of *PnFPS* and *PnSS*, leading to the increasing content of ginsenosides. Meanwhile, accumulation of ginsenoside $Rb_1$ may also contribute to nail head formation by inhibiting LR growth (Fig. 6). This study elucidates the mechanisms leading to the

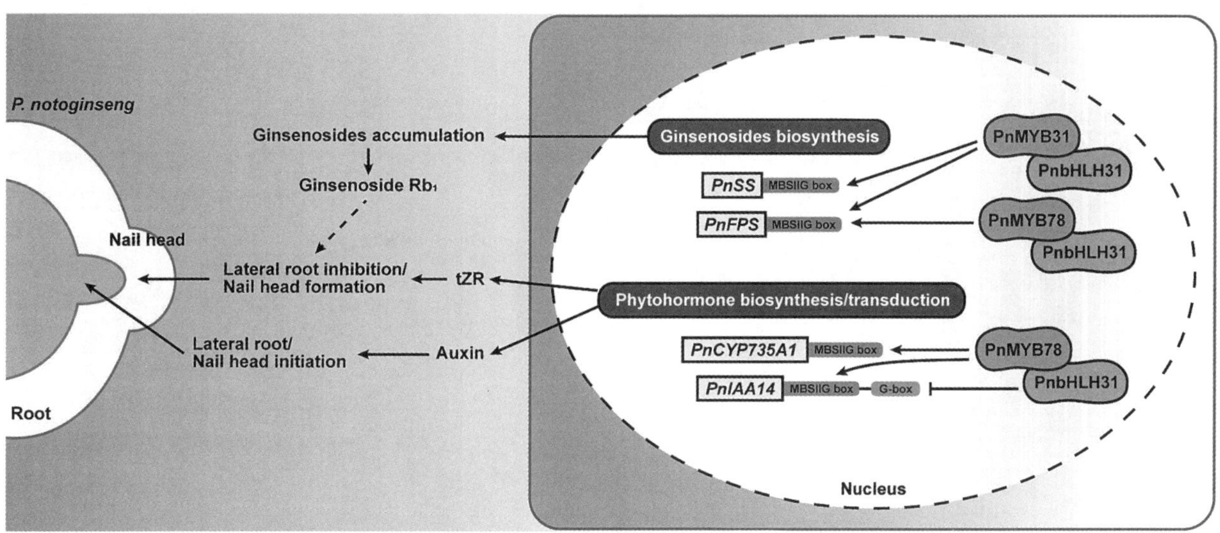


**Fig. 6  A probable regulatory mechanism model for nail head formation in *P. notoginseng***

formation of the characteristic nail heads in *P. notoginseng*. Our findings also verify the influence of these structures on root properties, providing a basis for the evaluation of *P. notoginseng* under different medication requirements.

［虞慕瑶，郑汉，黄璐琦，等. Journal of Advanced Research，2024，DOI：10.1016.］

# 第四篇

# 中药活性成分合成生物学

# 系统生物学方法在药用植物次生代谢产物研究中的应用

次生代谢产物(secondary metabolites)是植物在其生长发育和对环境的适应过程中次生代谢(secondary metabolism)产生的一类小分子有机化合物。这些小分子有机物在植物类群中特异性分布,往往不是细胞正常生命活动所必需的。据估计,植物次生代谢产物在10万种以上,包括萜类、酚类、生物碱、多炔类等。在药用植物中,次生代谢产物通常是新药、新先导化合物、新化学实体的重要来源,是中药的主要活性成分,药材品质的物质基础,是中药现代化研究的重要内容。

目前,对药用植物次生代谢产物的研究多集中在植物化学成分的分离和结构测定,及其生物活性和药理作用等方面。然而,药用植物的次生代谢物往往含量较低,且天然药用植物资源有限,影响了药用植物作为药材的品质控制及其活性成分的开发利用。所以,进行次生代谢产物生物学形成研究,挖掘相关酶基因、信号分子和环境因子等,系统阐释药用成分生物合成途径、信号转导途径、生态学形成机制及它们之间的相互作用显得非常重要。整体了解这些植物代谢的生物学过程,就可以通过构建模型对植物任何特定的基因进行操纵或环境的干扰,从而对植物的功能进行精确地预测,以达到植物资源优化及其可持续利用的目的。系统生物学是继基因组学、蛋白质组学等组学提出之后,首次在分子生物学的知识框架下,从整体层次上研究生命系统的一门新兴科学。与分子生物学集中于研究单独的个体成分不同,系统生物学研究一个生物系统中所有组成成分(基因、mRNA、蛋白质等)的构成,以及在特定条件下这些组分间的相互关系。它是全面探索生物系统的有力工具,其思维与方法在药用植物次生代谢产物的应用,是全面揭示药用植物从基因到次生代谢产物的有效途径。

## 1 药用植物次生代谢产物形成的生物学过程

药用植物次生代谢产物形成的生物学过程非常复杂,受到自身遗传和环境中各种生物和非生物因素的调控。目前,次生代谢物形成和积累的诱导机制存在着多种假说,包括生长-分化平衡(growth-differentiation balance, GDB)假说,碳素-营养平衡(carbon-nutrient balance, CNB)假说,最佳防御(optimum defense, OD)假说,资源获得(resource availability, RA)假说等。从系统生物学的角度,次生代谢物形成是个系统的生物学过程,主要包括环境因子(内、外环境)的刺激,信号转导,基因表达及翻译蛋白酶的催化介导的生物合成3个方面。具体表现为环境因子刺激植物细胞外部的受体,受体活化,活化的受体激活细胞内的信号级联,激活转录因子启动特定基因的表达,基因转录、翻译成对应系列蛋白酶催化形成次生代谢物,见图1。

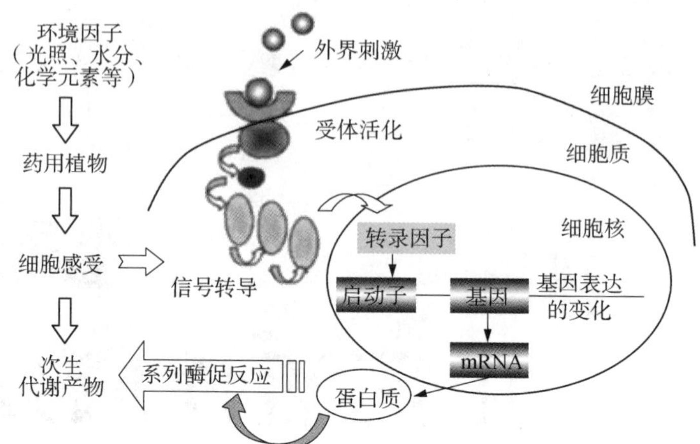


**图1 药用植物次生代谢产物形成的生物学过程**

## 2 系统生物学基本研究方法及技术平台

与分子生物学采取的还原论方法比较,系统生物学是采用系统科学的方法,将生物不是作为孤立的很多部分而是作为整体系统来定量研究。经典的分子生物学研究是一种垂直型的研究,即采用多种手段研究单个基因和蛋白质。首先是在DNA水平上寻找特定的基因,然后通过基因突变、基因剔除等手段研究基因的功能;在此基础上,研究蛋白质的空间结构,蛋白质的修饰以及蛋白质间的相互作用等。基因组学、蛋白质组学和其他各种"组学"则是水平型研究,即以单一的手段同时研究成千上万个基因或蛋白质。而系统生物学的研究方法则是把水平型研究和垂直型研究整合起来,成为一种"三维"的研究。即充分利用各种组学技术,来研究生物系统间分子影响差异,从而外推环境化学在生物系统中作用过程,建立数学模式评估mRNA、蛋白质、代谢水平的变化或差异,阐明整体生物学效应,描述和预测生物功能、表型和行为。

基因组学、转录组学、蛋白质组学、代谢组学、相互作用组学和表型组学构成了系统生物学主要技术与平台。基因组学是对一个物种的所有基因进行基因组作图(包括遗传图、物理图谱、转录图谱),核苷酸序列分析,基因定位和基因功能分析。转录组学常用的分析方法有:差异性显示(differential display)、基因芯片(genechip)、表达序列标签(EST)分析、大规模平行测序技术(MPSS)、cDNA-扩增片段长度多态性(cDNA-AFLP)等。德国科学家Marc Sultan最近利用深测序技术和分析方法(deep sequencing)对于人类转录组的崭新认识,有望进一步在其他物种转录组学研究中运用。双向电泳,质谱技术等为蛋白质组学主要的分离分析方法。代谢组学是药用植物、中医药现代化研究非常重要的手段,常用的分析方法有:核磁共振(NMR)、气相色谱-质谱联用(GC-MS)、液相色谱-质谱联用(LC-MS)、傅立叶质谱(FTMS)和毛细管电泳-质谱联用(CE-MS)等。基因组学、转录组学、蛋白质组学和代谢物组学这几个组学技术分别构成了生物信息传递的多个层次,分别在DNA,mRNA,蛋白质和代谢产物水平检测和鉴别各种分子并研究其功能。相互作用组学系统研究各种分子间的相互作用,发现和鉴别分子途径和网络,绘制生物体的相互作用图谱。表型组学则是生物体基因型和表型的桥梁。

## 3 系统生物学方法在药用植物次生代谢产物研究中的应用

3.1 次生代谢产物生物合成相关基因及其途径研究 生物合成途径是药用植物次生代谢产物研究的核心内容,包含了从基因到生物表型(次生代谢产物)一个非常复杂的生物学过程。经过长期的研究积累,人们对次生代谢途径的主干部分已经基本了解,例如酚类的莽草酸途径,萜类的异戊二烯二磷酸(IPP)途径等。由于次生代谢产物种类繁多,在基本骨架形成之后,往往经过结构修饰生成各种终产物。目前,药用植物中仅有少数次生代谢途径有较深入的认识,如紫杉醇、青蒿素、长春花吲哚生物碱等。而大部分次生代谢途径还有待进一步阐明。

本研究组采用系统生物学的思维和方法,在丹参二萜类次生代谢产物———丹参酮生物合成途径研究中获得系统性结果。采用诱导子刺激,使丹参毛状根产生丹参酮含量上的表型差异,见图2。对具有表型差异的多组材料进行代谢组、蛋白组,以及采用基因芯片进行转录组数据分析。通过多变量分析,筛选到多条与丹参酮次生代谢密切相关的基因片段,并获得全长cDNA。克隆得到的丹参柯巴基焦磷酸合酶(SmCPS)为被子植物中首条(+)-CPP合成酶;类贝壳杉烯合酶(SmKSL)则被鉴定为一种新的二萜合酶,催化(+)-CPP形成新的二萜烯类化合物(miltiradiene),这是一条丹参酮特有的二萜生物合成途径新的分支,并将丹参酮生物合成途径向前推进了2步。

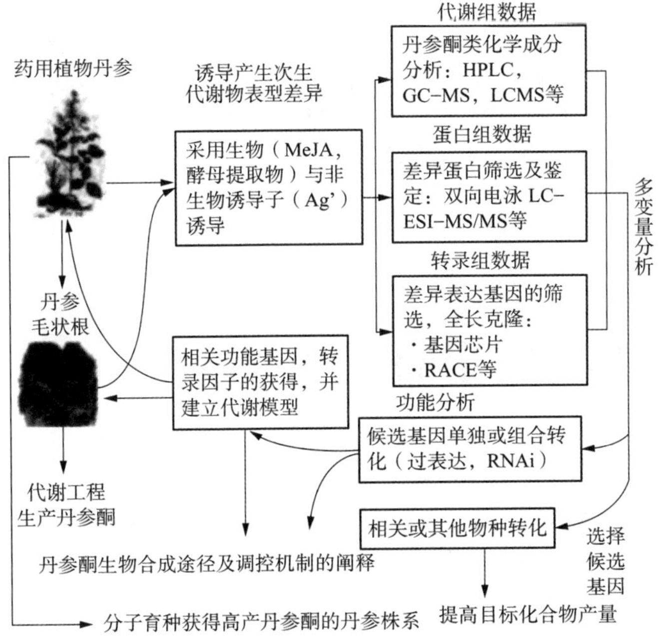


**图2 系统生物学的方法在丹参酮生物合成途径研究中的应用**

3.2 信号因子的挖掘及其信号转导途径的研究 在所用的细胞间通信和细胞受压反应过程中,细胞都从外界接收信号。而这些外部信号被转换成细胞内信号和级联反应。典型的信号包括激素、信息素、热、冷、光、渗透压以及一些物质,如葡萄糖、钾离子、钙离子或cAMP的出现或者浓度变化等。信号转导过程与代谢过程的重要的差异在于:代谢过程主要提供质量的传递,是由一系列催化反应的酶决定;而信号转导过程则是承担着信息的处理与传递。

植物体内次生代谢物质的合成是受细胞内部相关基因调控的一系列复杂的生化反应过程,而环境因素等作为外界刺激因子本身并不直接参与细胞内的次生代谢过程,因此在植物细胞内必然存在着相关的胞内信号分子和相应的信号转导机制来感受并传递外界因子的刺激信号。研究探讨植物细胞中与次生代谢产物合成调控有关的信号分子及信号转导机制将有助于理解植物细胞中次生代谢产物合成的调控规律,为生产实践中提高植物培养细胞的次生物质产量提供理论基础。目前,植物抗病、防御反应等信号转导途径研究比较深入,关于药用植物次生代谢信号转导机制研究仍处在初步探索阶段。徐茂军等在介导连翘细胞生成金丝桃素和银杏细胞中银杏黄酮苷的积累等信号因子及信号转导机制方面研究卓有成效。此外,以建立的金丝桃细胞为材料,在优化细胞培养条件的基础上,发现紫外光(UV-B)辐射作为一种外界环境胁迫因子,在5~30 h内诱发金丝桃细胞中黄酮类物质合成积累,在此基础上,进一步深入研究探讨了UV-B诱发的信号转导机制;认为UV-B处理依赖NO与$H_2O_2$信号分子诱发黄酮类物质的合成积累,且NO与$H_2O_2$在诱发黄酮类物质合成积累中具有的增效作用,是一种新的信号互作用现象;此外,认为NO介导UV-B诱发黄酮类物质合成积累与CHS基因的表达活化有关,而$H_2O_2$与CHS基因的表达活化无关。系统生物学研究最可行的应用是创建细胞调节的详尽模型,焦点集中于特定的各级信号转导和分子,以便系统地深刻理解以机制为基础的药物发现。显然,这是系统生物学思维与方法在次生代谢产物信号转导途径研究中的一些有益探索。植物细胞次生代谢信号调控是一个十分复杂的系统,虽然近年来有关植物细胞次生代谢产物合成信号调控方面的研究取得了一定的进展,但是目前离完全了解植物次生代谢信号转导机制还有很大距离。系统生物学方法的应用,其最终目的是通过寻找使次生代谢产物的表型产生差异的信号分子,高通量分离与植物次生代谢有关的突变体,克隆与次生代谢调节有关的基因并研究其功能,探讨激活转录因子而启动特定基因表达的信号转导途径,从而建立信号因子、基因及代谢产物之间的相互联系和网络,阐明基于次生代谢产物形成和积累的信号转导途径。

3.3 药用植物次生代谢生态学研究 植物在生长过程中会受到各种环境因子的影响甚至胁迫,这些因子包括非生物因子(如光照、温度、土壤、水分、大气等)以及生物因子(如病虫害、食草动物、微生物、人工干扰等)。植物对这些环境因子做出适应性反应,发生在形态结构、生理、生化及基因表达上,其中次生代谢产物是重要的生化调节物质之一,如植物组织中黄酮类、萜类、生物碱、有机酸等浓度在水分亏缺时有不同程度的升高。

植物次生代谢是长期与环境耦合的结果,在提高植物自身保护能力方面发挥重要作用,可以比初生代谢"记录"更多的环境信息。有学者提出植物次生代谢生态学的概念。与化学生态学(chemical ecology)和植物生理生态学(plant physiological ecology)相比,植物次生代谢生态学不仅注重次生代谢产物本身,同时关注环境因子如何诱导这些化合物的产生。因此阐明环境因子如何诱导相关受体活化、基因表达及次生代谢发生的作用机制是植物次生代谢生态学的重要任务。

由于植物次生代谢过程复杂及不同环境因子通常同时影响植物(如干旱与高温往往并存)导致研究生态因子与植物次生代谢之间的关系工作充满挑战。定性描述不能从根本上阐述它们之间的关系,近年来相关研究日益增多,而且正走向定量研究。

在研究中可以通过受控实验手段,采用系统生物学的方法,从信号转导、基因表达、代谢产物等方面来揭示不同外界刺激如何通过受体和细胞内信号转导机制诱导和调控次生代谢。即寻找环境因子、基因及代谢产物之间的相互联系和网络,阐明生态环境如何刺激相关受体活化、启动基因表达,对植株体内次生代谢产物形成和积累诱导作用的生理机制。在这里,可利用以下2种策略来实现这一目标:第一,采用严格控制所考察环境因子(如温度因子)的受控实验,跟踪分析次生代谢过程中关键酶基因的表达,蛋白质(酶)合成及检测次生代谢产物的含量变化,从而正向揭示环境因子与次生代谢之间的关系;第二,通过分析有表型差异植物次生代谢产物的含量及检测相关基因表达,分析可能影响其次生代谢产物积累的环境因子。从而通过反复印证的方式,从次生代谢的角度去解读植物与环境的关系,并且从生态学的角度去认知植物的次生代谢。

3.4 *药用植物次生代谢物的代谢工程研究* 代谢工程主要是通过基因工程的手段改变代谢流或扩展代谢途径和构建新的代谢途径来实现预期目的。近年来,代谢工程研究取得了较大的发展。唐克轩教授课题组将PMT(1,4-丁二胺-氮-甲基转移酶)基因和$H_6H$(莨菪碱6-β-羟化酶)基因共转化莨菪,使转基因莨菪发根中东莨菪碱含量(411 mg/L)比野生型(43 mg/L)提高了9倍,大大提高了莨菪烷类生物碱的合成与积累。美国Jay D Keasling教授等采用一系列的基因调控方法,通过基因工程酵母合成了青蒿素的前体物质—青蒿酸。这是导入单个、多个靶基因或一个完整的代谢途径,使生物体目标代谢物含量增加或产生新的目标物质。

此外,通过反义RNA和RNA干涉等技术降低目标基因的表达水平,从而抑制竞争性代谢途径,改变代谢流和增加目标物质的含量。Allen等研表明,阻断罂粟中产生吗啡的代谢途径,会导致香荔枝碱(reticuline)及其甲酯的积累。

代谢工程的一个新策略是以信号途径和转录因子为调控靶标。对控制多个生物合成基因的转录因子进行修饰,将更有效地调控植物次生代谢以提高特定化合物的积累。比如对长春花二萜类吲哚生物碱生物合成途径上的、具有$AP_2$/ERF功能域的转录因子$ORCA_3$高表达,会导致几种与二萜类吲哚生物碱生物合成相关基因的过量表达以及二萜类吲哚生物碱累积。

药用植物的代谢工程是针对提高某种重要次生代谢物或者其前体的含量的,以期解决药源问题,如果能够用基因工程的方法提高其含量,将具有巨大的经济效益和社会效益。目前,科学家非常重视发展预见性代谢工程,即利用系统生物学的方法来整合代谢组、蛋白组和转录组的分析数据,从而在代谢网络的水平上进行反复的系统模拟,最终得到比较接近真实状态的结果。现有的各种数据库和仪器分析手段已经使这样的系统分析在一定程度上成为可能。

## 4 展望

系统生物学是对生物系统中细胞网络的组分以及各组分间相互作用、高通量全基因组实验技术的应用和计算方法与实验效果的整合的协同研究。用系统生物学的思维和方法来研究药用植物次生代谢物的形成,包括次生代谢物的生源途径、信号分子的信号传递,代谢物的形成和积累与外界环境相互作用的关系,其最大的特点是在还原论基础上的整体性研究,可以充分发掘药用植物次生代谢物生物合成的相关基因、转录因子、信号分子以及环境因子;构建次生代谢物生物合成基因表达调控系统模型,为次生代谢物代谢工程和全面阐释次生代谢物形成的分子机制提供理论基础。并对于系统阐释中药有效成分成因和道地药材形成机制、药用植物资源合理开发利用等具有重要意义。

[黄璐琦,等.中国中药杂志,2010,35(1):8-12.]

# 合成生物学在中药资源可持续利用研究中的应用

药用活性成分是中药的物质基础,随着合成生物学技术在青蒿素、紫杉醇、丹参酮等重要活性成分生物合成研究中的应用,合成生物学用于中药资源可持续利用研究已受到广泛关注。本文从合成生物学的发展及中药资源可持续利用面临的机遇、国内外药用活性成分合成生物学研究现状及进展等方面进行评述,探讨合成生物学在中药资源可持续利用中的应用,并分析发展药用活性成分合成生物学研究的关键环节,展望合成生物学生产将成为中药资源可持续利用中药用活性成分获取的重要途径,是分子生药学学科重点发展领域之一。

## 1 合成生物学的发展及中药资源可持续利用面临的机遇

合成生物学一词最早出现在法国物理化学家Stéphane

Leduc 于 1911 年所著《生命的机理》(*The Mechanism of Life*)一书中，但受限于当时生物学认识水平，合成生物学未得以发展。进入 21 世纪，随着大规模基因组测序技术和序列分析方法的成熟，生命科学研究进入基因组时代。而快速发展的基因工程技术使得人们可以理性地对生物元件进行改造。组学分析技术以及基因工程的发展为合成生物学的产生奠定了基础。于是，学者们开始利用合成生物学构建人工系统执行新的生物学功能。代表性研究是 2000 年《自然》杂志上发表的 2 篇文章：Elowitz 等构建了第一个合成的生物振荡器——压缩振荡子(repressilator)；Gardner 等在大肠杆菌中通过设计基因开关构建了人工双稳态基因调控网络；这两篇论文标志着合成生物学作为一个新的领域正式诞生。近年来，合成生物学进入了一个快速发展时期，被广泛地应用于医药、化工、材料、能源、环境和农业等各个方面，取得了令人瞩目的成果。近年来，重大里程碑式的进展包括微生物全基因组重建和酵母染色体人工合成，以及采用酿酒酵母(*Saccharomyces cerevisiae*)高效生产抗疟疾药物青蒿素关键前体。合成生物学发展从此进入了新的阶段，即由单一生物部件的设计发展到对多种基本部件和模块进行整合，通过多部件或模块之间的协调运作建立复杂系统，从而构建人工系统(包括细胞)行为来实现药物、功能材料及能源替代品的大规模生产。

中药资源多源于药用植物。许多药用植物生长受环境因素影响较大；有些珍稀药材生长缓慢，甚至难以人工种植；大多数药用活性成分在中药材中含量低微，结构复杂，性质不稳定，化学合成困难或产率较低，而直接提取又面临成本高、资源少等。近年来，发展的植物细胞培养技术为生产药用活性化合物提供了一个可行策略，但是，植物细胞培养存在条件苛刻，批次结果相差很大，细胞生长缓慢，产率低下等不足。化学全合成虽然在天然产物合成中有很多成功的案例，但是其产率很低，大多处于实验室水平。实际上，绝大多数中药活性成分分子结构复杂，并且具有多个手性中心，其合成过程涉及多步纯化过程，产率大大降低。

利用生物技术生产有效成分，具有不受气候、病虫害、地理和季节的限制等在内的各种环境因素变化的影响、生产系统规范化、产品生产周期比完整植株短、质量和产量更加稳定的特点，这将可能成为中药材保护性生产的一个新途径。最近，利用合成生物学策略改造天然生产宿主，或者异源宿主，大规模生产药用活性成分，为中药资源可持续利用及中药发展提供了一个崭新的有效策略和发展机遇。加州大学伯克利分校学者与 Amyris 公司合作发表了在酿酒酵母中高效半合成抗疟疾药物青蒿素的结果，青蒿素前体青蒿酸产量达到了 25 g/L，然后经过 4 步化学反应合成了青蒿素，该项研究将微生物半合成青蒿素产业化进程大大向前推进了一步。目前此高效酵母菌株已独家授权给某国际制药公司进行大规模生产。实际上，青蒿素治疗疟疾的物质基础由我国科学家发现，但我们却在利用现代生物技术进行产业化上明显落后于国外同行，反映我们在药用活性成分合成生物学领域研究的不足。所以我们在挖掘我国中药资源的同时，更需要注意发展中药合成生物学，提高中药资源可持续利用并提升其产业化的技术水平。

## 2 药用活性成分合成生物学研究现状及进展

在简单生物，比如大肠杆菌和酿酒酵母中，可以设计由代谢途径和模块组成的生物元件来改变正常的细胞代谢，从而合成人们感兴趣的代谢物，比如中药药用活性成分。与其他中药药用活性成分的合成生物学研究相比，一些植物来源的单体药物的生物合成学研究受到了更广泛的关注。

2.1 青蒿素的合成生物学研究 青蒿素的合成生物学研究是伴随其生物合成途径的逐步阐明而发展起来的。由于从青蒿酸/二氢青蒿酸形成青蒿素的途径不是很清楚，现在通过合成生物学技术制备青蒿素的研究绝大部分采用的都是一种半合成的路线。即通过合成生物学策略制备青蒿素的前体如紫穗槐-4,11-二烯、青蒿酸和二氢青蒿酸，然后通过半合成的方法合成青蒿素。

1972 年，我国科学家在中药材黄花蒿中提取出了抗疟有效成分青蒿素，但植物提取成本高，产量很低，化学方法合成十分困难且成本高昂。加州大学伯克利分校 Keasling 等利用合成生物学技术，对微生物进行工程化操作，实现了青蒿素中间体的微生物合成；他们根据大肠杆菌的密码子偏好性，合成青蒿酸合成酶(ADS)的编码基因、共表达操纵子(编码 DXS、IPPHp、IspA)以及引入异源的酵母菌甲羟戊酸途径，从而提高了青蒿酸的产量。2006 年，该课题组将 ADS 基因插入由 GAL1 启动子控制转录的 pRS435 质粒中，并克隆青蒿的细胞色素 P450 氧化还原酶 CYP71AV1/CPR，通过优化 FPP 生物合成途径使得青蒿酸合成量达到 153 mg/L。如前文所述，通过对代谢途径的不断改造和优化，并发展了化学修饰策略，目前半合成青蒿素的产量已经达到工业化水平。

2.2 紫杉醇的合成生物学研究 紫杉醇是红豆杉次生代谢产生的二萜类物质，具有显著的抗癌效果。但是紫杉醇在自然界中含量极低，化学合成困难，随着合成生物学技术的发展，紫杉醇的生物合成也成了关注的热点。王伟等首次从中国红豆杉中克隆到紫杉烯合酶基因，将其导入酿酒酵母组建了一条紫杉烯生物合成途径，重组菌可以直接产生紫杉醇的前体紫杉烯。Engels 等将紫杉烯合酶转入酿酒酵母细胞中，引入 GGPP 合酶的同工酶(HMG-COA 还原酶)以提高酵母中紫杉二烯前体 GGPP 的合成量，同时抑制宿主酵母中的类固醇竞争途径，研究获得的工程菌 CEN10 紫杉烯的产量达 8.7 mg/L。麻省理工学院 Stephanopoulos 教授团队通过在大肠杆菌中重建紫杉二烯的合成途径，成功获得了这一紫杉醇中间体，以紫杉醇药物中间体紫杉烯生物合成的中间体 IPP 为节点分成 2 个模块：宿主菌自身 MEP 途径合成 IPP 的上游功能模块和异源萜类合成的下游功能模块。通过调控上游和下游模块转化大肠杆菌构建成生物合成紫杉烯的工程菌，紫杉烯的产量提高到 1 020 mg/L。多元模块阐明了紫杉烯合成的非线性代谢流，表明模块间的协调程度不仅影响紫杉烯的产量，还影响工程菌的生长状态、底物甘油消耗、乙酸等副产物积累等。当然通过生物反应器的发酵条件、生长培养基的成分优化可以进一步提高紫杉烯的产量。

2.3 丹参酮的合成生物学研究 丹参酮是我国中药材丹参的活性成分，作者课题组一直致力于解析丹参酮生物合成途径并实现合成生物学异源生产，通过功能基因组学方法首次克隆并鉴定了其合成前体次丹参酮二烯的两个酶SmCPS和SmKSL，并在大肠杆菌中构建了代谢途径，其产量达到了2.5 mg/L。随后Zhou等建立模块途径工程策略，在酵母细胞中快速组装次丹参酮二烯生物合成途径；在此基础上，通过设计模块组合方式，系统考虑途径中涉及的前体供给、限速步骤、底物传输和代谢流分配等问题，对编码SmCPS、SmKSL、法呢基焦磷酸合酶、GGPP合酶和甲羟戊酸还原酶等5个蛋白的基因进行了操作，最优的工程菌株在15 L发酵罐中培养，次丹参酮二烯产量达到365 mg/L。并成功设计开发了一套组合调控酿酒酵母萜类合成途径的功能模块，使次丹参酮二烯产量达到488 mg/L。最近，Guo等利用比较转录组学，利用RNA测序鉴定到了14个与次丹参二烯生物合成相关的CYP450基因；通过建立体外催化反应发现CYP76AH1催化转化次丹参酮二烯合成铁锈醇，然后利用模块途径工程策略将CYP76AH1及CYP还原酶SmCPR1整合到次丹参酮二烯生物合成酵母，工程菌株能合成10.5 mg/L的铁锈醇，并且发现铁锈醇的合成与次丹参酮二烯积累负相关，为进一步解析丹参酮生物合成下游途径以及微生物合成丹参酮打好了基础(图1)。

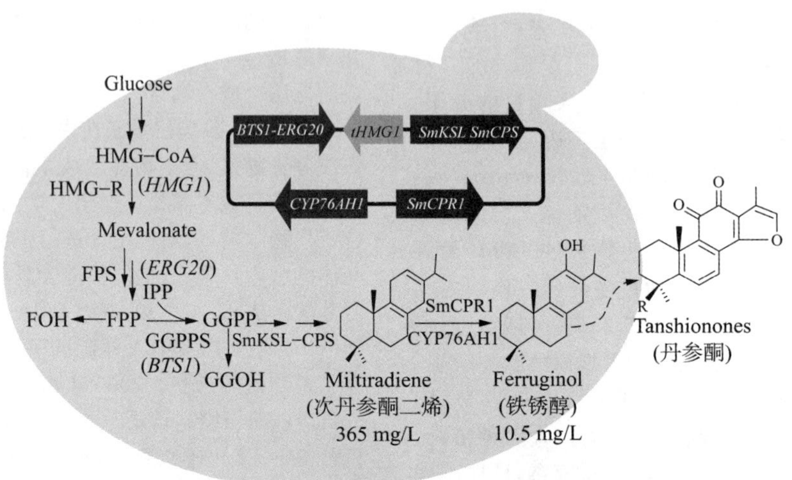


**图1 丹参酮合成生物学研究进展**

2.4 *人参皂苷的合成生物学研究* 目前，人参皂苷生物合成途径的基本框架及相关酶的研究已经取得了较大的进展。目前已从人参和西洋参等人参属植物中克隆到20多个编码人参皂苷生物合成相关酶的基因并进行了功能验证，为通过合成生物学技术生产人参皂苷提供了基本的生物元件，为该研究奠定了较好的基础。最近，我国学者在酿酒酵母中成功构建原人参二醇的生物合成途径，并且发现鲨烯环氧酶在控制三萜化合物的生物合成中起关键作用；在此基础上，通过提高3-羟基-3-甲基戊二酰辅酶A还原酶、法呢烯焦磷酸合酶、鲨烯合成酶和鲨烯环氧酶的活性，将原人参二醇的产量提高了262倍；通过双相发酵工艺优化，最终将原人参二醇的产量提高至1 189 mg/L；该研究为人参皂苷生物合成途径解析和异源生物合成提供了坚实的基础。

2.5 *其他药用活性成分的合成生物学研究* 银杏内酯类(ginkgolides)前体左旋海松二烯(levopimaradiene)，在改造后的大肠杆菌工程菌中达到700 mg/L。此外，赵广荣课题组在构建人工合成途径生产丹参素研究中取得重要进展，实现了以葡萄糖为原料生产丹参素。

这些研究方法和成果为进一步扩大中药药用活性成分合成生物学研究提供很好的示范。

## 3 合成生物学在中药资源可持续利用研究中的应用

合成生物学用于中药资源可持续利用，认为主要研究策略如图2。首先从药用植物中克隆活性成分生物合成途径上的基因；逐一进行功能鉴定并通过基因功能研究解析药用活性成分生物合成途径；然后，参考植物源途径设计并整合异源生物合成途径；将人工设计的途径装载到底盘细胞(大肠杆菌、酵母等)基因组上构建微生物细胞工厂；最后优化发酵条件实现药用活性成分及其中间体的高效发酵生产。自1995年作者提出将分子生物学技术引入中药领域的研究伊始，随着基因组学和转录组学、蛋白质组学、生物信息学等生物技术的不断发展和融合，以中药原物种为研究对象的中药功能基因组学研究，发现大量与次生代谢产物合成与调控相关的基因，既为阐明中药活性成分的生物合成途径奠定了基础，也为中药合成生物学研究提供了丰富的生物元件。基于合成生物学高效、定向地异源生物合成结构复杂多样的中药药用活性成分，将有效地解决许多在中药研究中遇到的难题，同时也将为中药资源的可持续利用提供新策略和技术。

## 4 发展中药活性成分合成生物学研究的关键技术方法分析

4.1 *基因元件的克隆* 基因元件是具有特定功能的氨基酸或者核苷酸序列，它是遗传系统中最简单、最基本的生物积块(BioBrick)，例如启动子、核糖体结合位点、核糖核酸(RNA)、酶编码基因等。随着以中药原物种为研究对象的中药基因组学的发展，将发现大量参与次生代谢产物合成与调控相关的基因，为中药合成生物学研究提供基因元件。但目

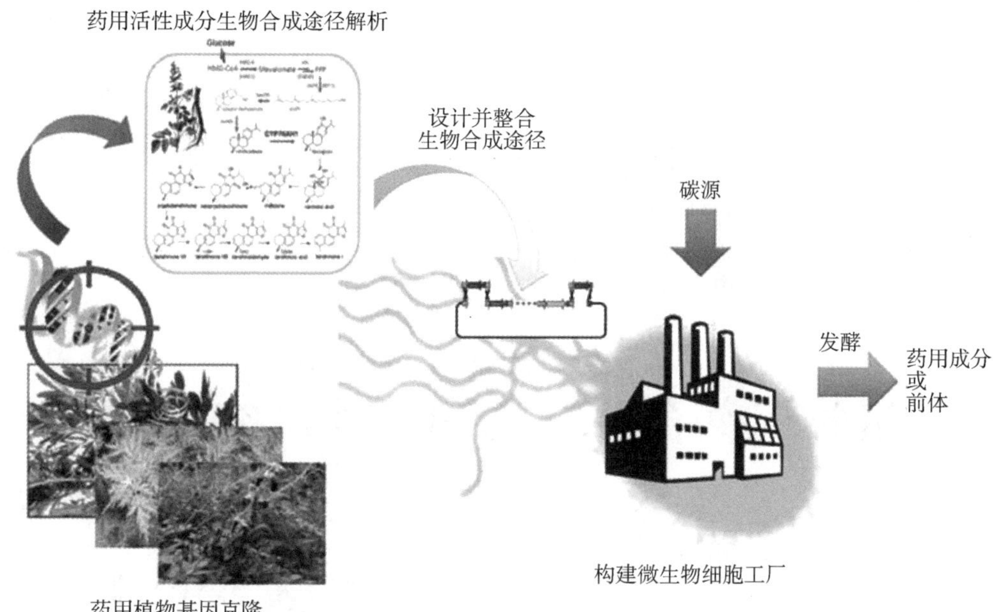


**图 2　合成生物学在中药资源药用活性成分生产中的应用策略**

前，除了紫杉醇、青蒿素、丹参酮、人参皂苷等少数次生代谢途径上基因解析较为清楚外，对于大多数药用活性成分的生物合成途径的了解还非常匮乏。因此，与中药药用活性成分相关基因元件的挖掘和生物合成途径的解析，将是目前中药合成生物学研究的首要任务。

4.2　*底盘细胞的选择与改造*　与普通异源宿主不同的是，用于合成生物学研究的底盘细胞应具备生长快速、遗传操作简单、易于大规模培养、工业化控制简便等特征。近年来被广泛使用的异源合成底盘细胞主要为微生物，如大肠杆菌、酿酒酵母、枯草芽孢杆菌等，随着研究的深入和广泛，具有精细的调控系统、能通过光合作用获得代谢前体物质的植物系统也将被开发为合成某些特定类型化合物的底盘系统，如以烟草细胞构建底盘细胞异源合成青蒿素等代谢物。

4.3　*合成途径构建策略*　目前主要通过两种构建策略在不同的底盘细胞中构建药用活性成分代谢途径。第一种构建策略是药用活性成分固有代谢途径的转移、重构与工程化，这种构建策略是建立在代谢途径的深刻解析的基础之上，是中药合成生物学研究中主要的构建策略，其又可分为 3 个层次：①基于基因工程的原理，只导入药用活性成分生物合成特异途径中的基因，利用底盘细胞中固有的前体供应途径，制备药用活性成分。②基于基因工程原理及模块化设计理念，导入药用活性成分生物合成模块与底物调控模块，通过调控底物的合成，提高目的产物的产量。③基于基因工程原理、模块化设计理念及工程化思想，导入底物合成模块、底物调控模块及药用活性成分生物合成模块，这 3 个模块都由一些可拆卸的"即插即用"的基因元件构成，因此，既可以方便地对模块中的元件进行优化，也能便捷地将这些模块用于其他代谢途径的构建，将众多复杂的生物合成途径演变成可随时拆卸的工程化生物系统。第二种构建策略是全新药用活性成分合成途径的设计、筛选、组装与程序化，这种构建策略是根据药用活性成分的化学结构而设计的一条合成路线。根据这条合成路线从基因数据库中筛选出能参与设计好的合成路线的酶基因，并将这些酶基因导入底盘细胞中，在底盘细胞中组装成一条新的药用活性成分的生物合成路线。

4.4　*合成工艺系统优化*　目前为提高目标产物的产量，需对目标产物代谢途径的上游或下游的生物合成途径进行合成工艺研究，系统优化主要包括 3 个层次：①提高工程菌生物合成途径效率，包括提高前体供应，从而提高进入药用活性成分生物合成途径所需底物的绝对总量，这是提高工程菌产量的主要方式，另外提高目标产物生物合成特异途径中的途径酶效率也是有效策略，即提高单个基因效率和优化平衡整条途径来实现这个目的。主要策略是提高并且平衡代谢途径中各个途径酶的效率，如增加基因拷贝数、对启动子进行修饰、密码子优化、基因替换、调控辅酶数量以及选择不同区室等；或者通过优化或平衡多基因控制的代谢途径增加前体供应。②抑制或下调竞争代谢途径，从而限制或减少流入竞争代谢途径中的代谢流，促使相对更多的底物流入目标产物生物合成的特异途径。③整个代谢系统的平衡和调控：对于代谢途径的平衡优化，主要采用一种基于全局的数学算法和生物信息分析，如代谢流控制分析。对整个细胞进行全转录调控是提高细胞性能的另一个有效策略，通过对细胞全局转录机制的调控改造，不但能增加细胞对产物（中药药用活性成分大多对细胞有一定毒性）耐受性，还有利于整个细胞网络的协调，增加目标产物的合成。

## 5　展望

目前，在我国获取中药药用活性成分主要是从药用植物中直接提取分离，这种获取方式受到植物生长缓慢，需要占用大量土地，易受季节、气候等因素的限制；且有些活性成分在植物中含量极低，需要消耗大量药材；有些属于珍稀濒危植物等。通过合成生物学的设计，实现中药药用活性成分的异源生物合成，其在青蒿素等活性成分研究结果显示出这一技术的巨大优势和应用潜力，也将给传统中药领域的发展注入新的活力。

如前所述，青蒿素的发现表明我国虽然在中药药用活性成分鉴定成果卓著，但在利用现代生物技术进行产业化改进上，尚与国外同行存在一定差距。而且，国外近年来仍然加大其研究力度，2012 年，加拿大启动了名为 PhytoMetaSyn（资助额 1400 万美元）的天然产物人工微生物合成项目，该项目联合了 6 所高校或者研究所，旨在酿酒酵母中合成 6 个高附加值的植物源天然产物。所以发展中药药用活性成分合成生物学研究不仅是中药资源可持续利用发展的需求，还具有重要科学意义和应用价值，保持我国在国际中药研究中的领先地位。可以预见，随着合成生物学的逐渐成熟以及它在传统中药领域应用的深入，合成生物学也必将极大地促进中药领域的发展，成为中药资源可持续利用的重要途径之一。

［黄璐琦，等．药学学报，2014，49(1)：37－43.］

# 植物二萜合酶结构和功能研究进展

二萜类化合物属于天然化合物中种类丰富的一大类群，具有多样的生理功能和工业、医用价值，比如植物激素，光合色素以及作为工业原料和药品使用等。目前，大量的二萜化合物在高等、低等植物，以及真菌、细菌等微生物中被发现报道，如雷公藤甲素、银杏二萜内酯、lepistal 等。二萜化合物结构多样，其初始生物合成源于简单的异戊二烯单元($C_5$)、异戊烯基二磷酸(isopentenyl pyrophosphate, IPP)和其异构体二甲丙烯二磷酸(dimethylallyl pyrophosphate, DMAPP)。4 个 IPP 和 DMAPP 发生 1′－4 缩合反应，从而延伸碳链形成二萜的前体物质香叶基香叶基焦磷酸［(*E*, *E*, *E*,)-geranylgeranyl pyro-phosphate, GGPP, C20］。二萜合酶，又称为二萜环化酶，是一类具有催化链状前体 GGPP 环化，形成二萜环状基本骨架的关键酶。二萜合酶的环化方式决定了二萜化合物的结构和其立体化学多样性；因而，一直以来，国内外学者致力于发现和鉴定新型的二萜合酶；近几年，随着晶体结构学在二萜合酶研究领域的应用，对于一些重要的植物二萜合酶，研究人员已经从蛋白晶体结构角度深入探索，揭示其催化机制和选择性。本文对近年来有关二萜合酶的分类、作用机制，尤其是新近解析的植物二萜合酶蛋白结构、结构与功能关联性等方面进行综述。

## 1 二萜合酶的分类

二萜合酶根据其功能域可分为两大类：Class Ⅰ 类和 Class Ⅱ类。Class Ⅱ类二萜合酶特征功能域是 DXDD，这个富含天冬氨酸的催化功能域在二萜合酶中是保守的；GGPP 在 Class Ⅱ类二萜合酶催化下，选择性地生成带有特殊立体构象的环状烃类结构，如产物柯巴基焦磷酸(copalyl diphosphate, CPP)，目前已知的有 *nor*-CPP、*ent*-CPP、*syn*-CPP 三种不同的构象。而 Class Ⅰ类二萜合酶包含 DDXXD 功能域，可修饰或者重排 Class Ⅱ类二萜合酶的催化产物，进一步环化生成相应的骨架结构(图 1)。在微生物或低等植物中还存在着一类双功能二萜合酶，同时具有 Class Ⅰ和 Class Ⅱ的特征功能域，这种明显的功能域的融合使其同时具有催化两步反应的作用。Kawaide 等发现真菌 Phaeosphaeria sp. L487 中的双功能酶，直接催化 GGPP 生成 KS，参与到赤霉素

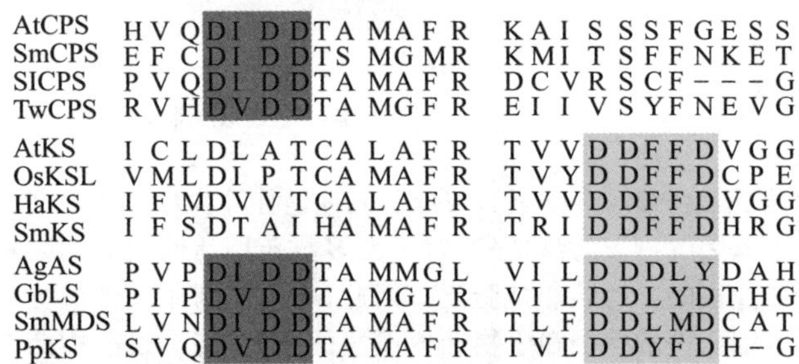


**Figure 1 Clustal W alignment of the amino acid sequences of several Class Ⅰ, Class Ⅱ, and bifunctional diterpene synthases**

Conserved catalytic motifs are highlighted, that is, DXDD and DDXXD. Sequence data: AtCPS, NP_192187.1 | Ent-copalyl diphosphate synthase [*Arabidopsis thaliana*]; SmCPS, ABV57835.1 copalyl diphosphate synthase [*Salvia miltiorrhiza*]; SlCPS, BAA84918.1 copalyl diphosphate synthase [*Solanum lycopersicum*]; TwCPS, AQW38541.1 copalyl diphosphate synthase 4 [*Tripterygium wilfordii*]; AtKS, NP_178064.1 | Ent-kaur-16-ene synthase [*Arabidopsis thaliana*]; OsKSL, Q2QQJ5.2 | KSL10_ORYSJ AltName: Full = Ent-kaurene synthase-like 10; Short = OsKSL10; HaKS, CBL42917.1 kaurene synthase [*Helianthus annuus*]; SmKS, ABV08817.1 kaurene synthase [*Salvia miltiorrhiza*]; AgAS, Q38710.1 | TPSDV_ABIGR AltName: Full = (－)-abieta-7(8), 13(14)-diene synthase; GbLS, AAL09965.1 | AF331704_1 levopimaradiene synthase [*Ginkgo biloba*]; SmMDS, BAL41682.1 miltiradiene synthase [*Selaginellamoellendorffii*]; PpKS, BAF61135.1 ent-kaurene synthase [*Physcomitrella patens*]。

的生物合成途径当中；Hayashi 等在小立碗藓中克隆得到 CPS/KS 双功能酶，同时具有 DVDD 和 DDYFD 功能域；Hall 等研究短叶松和美国黑松中发现其既含有双功能的 Class Ⅰ/Class Ⅱ二萜合酶，又含有单功能的 Class Ⅰ二萜合酶，从系统进化关系上，此单功能的二萜合酶是从双功能的二萜合酶分支进化而来，并非与被子植物的赤霉素途径相关代谢酶归为一类。

## 2 二萜合酶的催化机制

Class Ⅰ类环化酶包含 DDXXD 和(N, D)DXX(S, T)

XXXE 功能域，其催化反应涉及二磷酸基团的初始离子化和碳正离子中间体的形成。功能域中黑体部分氨基酸一般认为是结合 3 个 $Mg^{2+}$，触发底物上二磷酸基团离子化的关键残基。二磷酸基团离子化后，形成活化的碳正离子中间体，然后与双键或者水分子反应，完成环化反应。而 Class Ⅱ类环化酶，如对映柯巴基焦磷酸合酶［*ent*-copalyldiphosphateynthases (CPS)］，包含 DXDD 功能域，天冬氨酸靠近底物 GGPP/CPP 的异戊烯基双键，发生质子化反应形成碳正离子；位于中间位置的天冬氨酸是质子化反应的关键氨基酸。初始质子化后，在异戊烯基碳链上接着进行级联反应，发生多步环化。最终，质子经消除反应形成双键或被亲核基团俘获，结束反应。双功能二萜合酶，如 AgAS(图 1)，催化初始的 GGPP 环化成(+)- CPP，随后离子化环化形成松香烷型二萜骨架。

## 3 植物二萜合酶的功能和系统进化

在植物体内，二萜合酶是二萜类化合物生物合成途径上重要的关键酶，从其催化机制上可以知道它对底物 GGPP ($C_{20}$)有一步或多步环化的功能，包括两环、三环；五元环、六元环、七元环等不同的环状结构，对二萜化合物的多样性有重要的影响力。系统进化树(图 2)显示，二萜合酶的双功能酶位于 Class Ⅰ合酶的相近分支之中，相对更古老一些，主要存在于裸子植物、低等植物和真菌体内。在高等植物体内，Class Ⅰ和 Class Ⅱ二萜合酶虽然是单功能的二萜合酶，但是仍保留有双功能酶相似的 3 个结构，$\alpha$、$\beta$ 和 $\gamma$ 螺旋。一般认为，古老的二萜合酶基因是以双功能酶的形式存在的，在进化过程中，经过不断的复制和亚功能化，导致出现多样的 Class Ⅰ和 Class Ⅱ二萜合酶。在真菌或细菌中，一些仅含有 $\beta\gamma$、$\alpha$ 的二萜合酶被发现之后，进一步证实了二萜合酶进化过程的复制和亚功能化学说(图 3)。

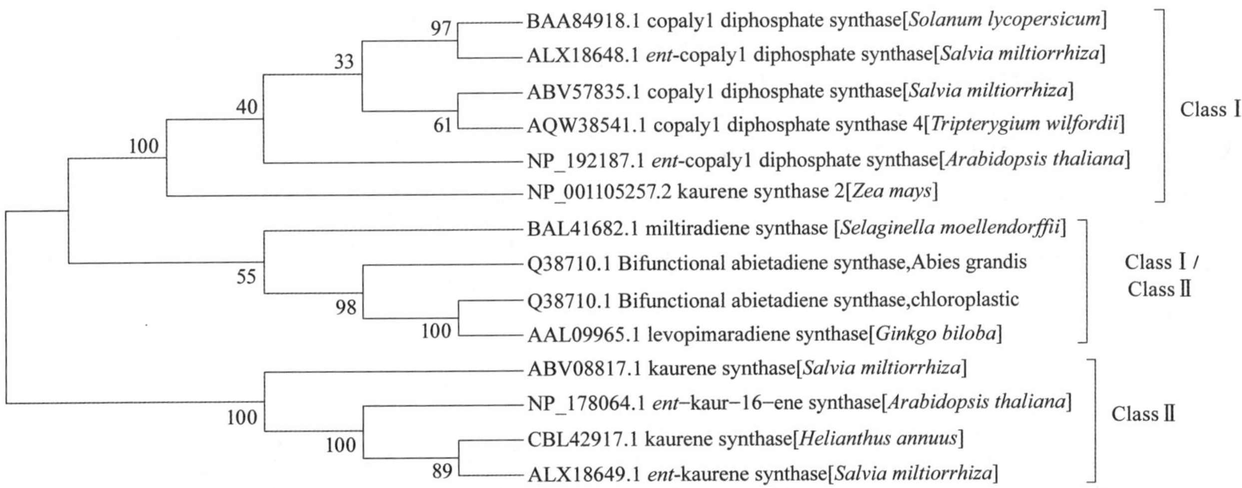


**Figure 2 Phylogenetic analysis of several Class Ⅰ, Class Ⅱ, and bifunctional diterpene synthases**

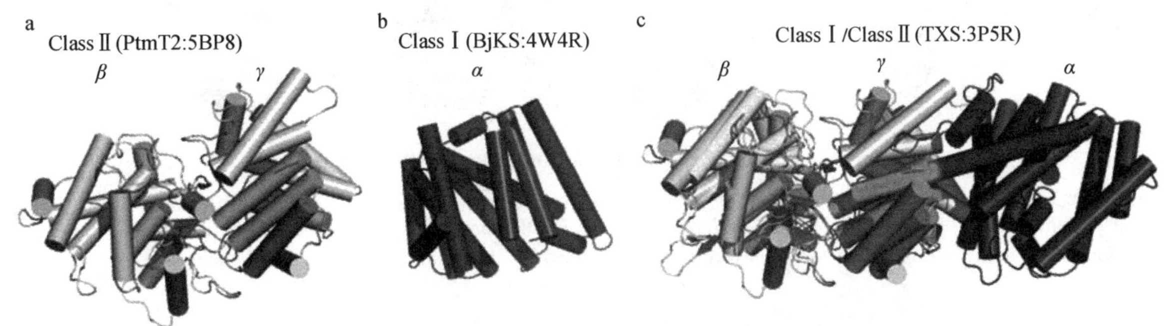


**Figure 3 Superimposition of the overall structure of diterpene synthases**

(a) Overall structure of *ent*-copalyl diphosphate synthase PtmT2 from *Streptomycs platensis* Cb00739 has two domains ($\beta\gamma$; PDB number: 5BP8); (b) Overall structure of *ent*-kaurene synthase (BjKS) from *Bradyrhizobium japonicum* has single domain ($\alpha$; PDB number: 4W4R); (c) Superimposition of BjKS with taxadiene synthase (TAX) from *Taxus brevifolia*. Overall structure of TAX has three domains ($\alpha\beta\gamma$; PDB number: 3P5R).

## 4 植物二萜合酶蛋白结构

二萜合酶的多样功能与其内在的蛋白结构密切相关，从结构生物学和生物化学角度研究二萜合酶蛋白，对解析二萜合酶的催化机制、功能特点、进化关系具有重要意义。随着越来越多的二萜合酶被挖掘并确定功能，在二萜合酶蛋白结构上也有了一些前沿的研究，目前已知有 6 种二萜合酶的结构得到解析(表 1)。

Table 1 Summary of diterpene synthase with crystal structure

| Species | Diterpene synthase | Resolution (Å) |
|---|---|---|
| *Arabidopsis thaliana* | *ent*-Copalyl diphosphate synthase | 2.25,1.55,2.76 |
| *Taxus brevifolia* | Taxadiene synthase | 1.82 |
| Abies grandis | Abietadiene synthase | 2.3 |
| *Streptomyces platensis* CB00739 | *ent*-Copalyl diphosphate synthase | 1.80 |
| *Streptomyces melanosporofaciens* MI614-43F2 | Diterpene cyclase CotB2 | 1.80 |
| *Bradyrhizobium japonicum* | *ent*-Kaurene synthase | 1.9-2.0 |

4.1 拟南芥(*Arabidopsis thaliana*) 拟南芥是植物研究领域常用的模式植物,其萜类合成途径关键酶常有报道,包括倍半萜合酶,二萜合酶 CPS 和 KS 等。Koksal 等对拟南芥中对映柯巴基焦磷酸合酶的结构和催化机制进行研究,分别得到了 AtCPS 蛋白与 GGPP 相似物的复合物晶体,分辨率为 2.25 Å(1 Å=0.1 nm)和 1.55 Å 的晶体(图 4);以及 AtCPS 蛋白与 *ent*-CPP 相似物的复合物晶体,分辨率为 2.76 Å。GGPP 相似物为(*S*)-15-aza-14,15-dihydrogeranyl-geranyl thiolodiphosphate (AGP),与实际的底物相比,在 1 号碳位置,通过硫原子与二磷酸基团连接;14 号由氮原子替代了碳原子,因而与蛋白不发生反应,且与 GGPP 立体化学结构相近。结构解析发现 AtCPS 蛋白具有三个 α-螺旋结构域(α、β 和 γ),但是其只具有催化 GGPP 的单功能酶活性,活性位点位于 β 和 γ 区域的界面,其中 DID[379]D 结构域中的后两个天冬氨酸与 AGP 距离较近(图 4)。而 α 结构域上缺乏和金属离子结合的区域,这是 Class Ⅰ类二萜合酶离子化所必需的;但是功能缺失的 α 结构域在进化中仍保留在拟南芥的二萜合酶基因中。

4.2 红豆杉(*Taxus brevifolia*) 红豆杉科植物含有丰富的二萜类化合物,东北红豆杉、曼地亚红豆杉等均含有几十种紫杉烷二萜类化合物;其中知名而重要的化合物紫杉醇不仅具有促进微管蛋白聚合作用,还在癌症化疗中具有显著的疗效。紫杉醇的第一步关键合成步骤在于异戊烯基底物 GGPP 经紫杉合酶(taxadiene synthase from *Taxus brevifolia*, TbTS)环化,生成 taxa-4(5),11(12)diene。Koksal 等对 TbTS 的蛋白结构进行研究,获得了截短体蛋白与 GGPP 相似物的复合物晶体,分辨率为 1.82 Å;以及 TbTS 截短体蛋白和 FPP 相似物的复合物晶体,分辨率为 2.25 Å。TbTS 晶体结构揭示了蛋白结构域的组成,包括三个 α-螺旋结构域(图 3)。在蛋白的 C 末端,存在 Class Ⅰ二萜环化酶的催化功能域,由两个 α-螺旋结构域组成了一个可以结合底物的活性口袋,在三个金属离子簇下,结合和活化底物 GGPP;而在 N 端,还有另一个插入的结构域,是 Class Ⅱ二萜环化酶的折叠区域,具有启动质子化的功能。TbTS 结构揭示了首个双功能二萜合酶上的两个不同活性功能域值。

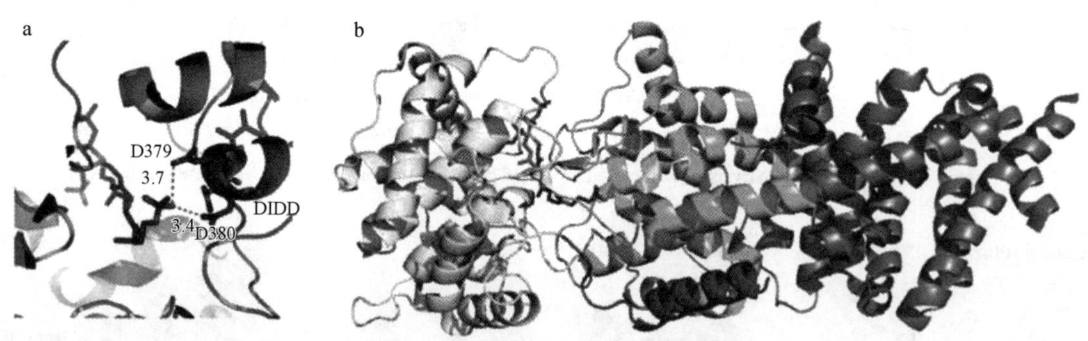


**Figure 4 Binding of AGP at packing interface of AtCPS structure**

(a) Cut away view of the packing interface leading to general acid D379 and D380; (b) Overall structure of *ent*-copalyl diphosphate synthase AtCPS from *Arabidopsis thaliana* Cb00739 (PDB number: 3pya). Color-coded as follows: α domain=blue, β domain=green, γ domain=yellow, N terminal helix=purple, ligand and contiguous acid=magenta.

4.3 巨冷杉(*Abies grandis*) 巨冷杉中同时含有 Class Ⅰ类和 Class Ⅱ类以及双功能二萜合酶。其中,松香二烯合酶,AgAS 是一个双功能的二萜合酶,其晶体结构分辨率为 2.3 Å。AgAS 蛋白由 3 个区域组成(α、β 和 γ),这个组成和单功能二萜合酶,如拟南芥 AtCPS 蛋白的组成相一致。Class Ⅱ类二萜合酶的活性区域的模拟蕴含更多丰富的信息,观察到良好的外部循环迁移。这种"循环"的构象不仅限制了溶剂通道也大大增加了配体进入构象的数量,在基底中存在的"循环"构象中的非生产性底物构象不稳定的状态。此外,这些在 Class Ⅱ类蛋白活性区域的构象变化对主动将底物驱动到提出的过渡状态。AgAS 结构提供了 Class Ⅰ和 Class Ⅱ类二萜合酶的催化反应的分子机制,还对研究植物萜类合酶的进化奠定了基础。

## 5 其他二萜合酶蛋白结构

二萜类化合物是自然界中结构多样的天然产物,然而它在细菌中的分布仍未得到充分研究。大多数植物二萜合酶由 3 个 α 螺旋结构组成(α、β 和 γ),被认为是起源于古老细菌中不连续的 Class Ⅰ类萜类合酶(α)和Ⅱ型萜类合酶(β 和 γ)的融合。细菌起源的 Class Ⅱ类二萜合酶相关结构研究较少,是萜类合酶结构进化中的缺失部分。Jeffery 等研究链霉菌(*Streptomyces platensis* CB00739)中 Class Ⅱ二萜合酶 PtmT2 的晶体结构。PtmT2 具有催化 GGPP 生成对映柯巴基焦磷酸(*ent*-CPP)的功能,并参与了平板霉素和平板素的生物合成。PtmT2 的晶体分辨率为 1.80 Å(图 3)。但是蛋白与底物的复合晶体并未获得,只是通过已有蛋白晶体结构,分子对接预测表明催化 GGPP 过程和关键位点;然后点突变确认了涉及结合 GGPP 二磷酸基团的 K402 位点和 DXXXXE 是潜在的 $Mg^{2+}$ 结合区域。PtmT2 的结构为进一步了解细菌来源的萜类合酶、机制以及在萜类合酶进化过程中的角色奠定了基础。

Tomita 等在 2017 年新得到了黑孢链霉菌(*Streptomyces melanosporofaciens* MI614-43F2)二萜环化酶 CotB2 的晶体结构,其产物较为特殊,是三环二萜结构,5-8-5 稠环骨架结构。晶体结构进一步展现了 GGPP 类似物折叠成独特的 S 形结合在蛋白中。在 GGPP 离子化之前,其周围环绕着疏水性的氨基酸残基,以及几个芳香族和天冬酰胺残基,起到稳定一系列反应中碳阳离子中间体的作用(图 5)。依据结构信息,对 F107、N103、F149、F185、W186、W288 进行多种突变,突变体可生成 7 种新的骨架结构。

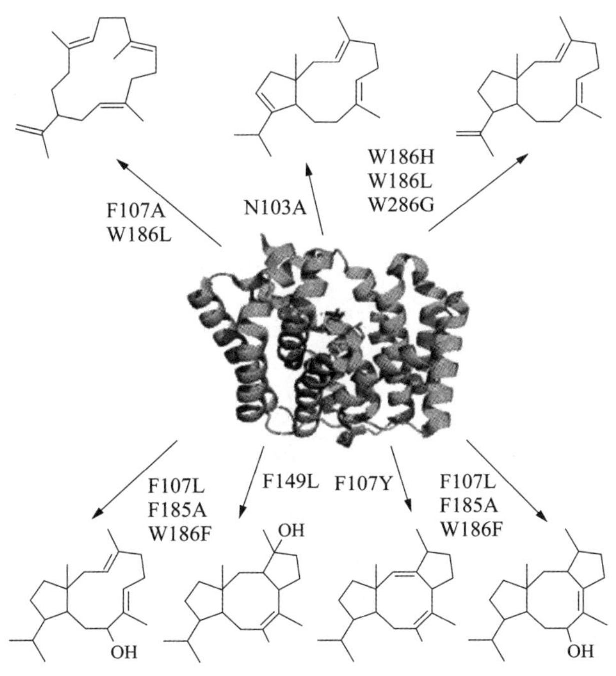


**Figure 5 Active site mutations of cyclooctatenol synthase (CotB2) (PDB number: 4OMG) to generate alternative diterpene products**

大豆根瘤菌(*Bradyrhizobium japonicum*)中存在 Class Ⅰ类二萜环化酶,对映贝壳杉烯合酶(BjKS),BjKS 具有催化对映贝壳杉烯生成贝壳杉烯的功能。目前 BjKS 蛋白已经获得,分辨率为 1.9~2.0 Å。蛋白仅仅由一个 α 螺旋结构组成,这个结果与许多植物二萜环化酶可能来自细菌二萜环化酶一致,BjKS 以二聚体的形式存在,如图 6 所示。BjKS 蛋白的结合口袋是疏水性的,由天冬氨酸和精氨酸这类侧链为芳香基团组成,可以特异性结合底物 GGPP 类似物,而形成的碳正离子由 Leu、Tyr 和 Phe 残基保护;产物类似物 BPH-629 也可特异性结合在此疏水口袋中(图 6)。点突变实验验证 DDXXD 的重要性,同时发现,R204 是高度保守的功能位点,突变后蛋白活性显著降低。

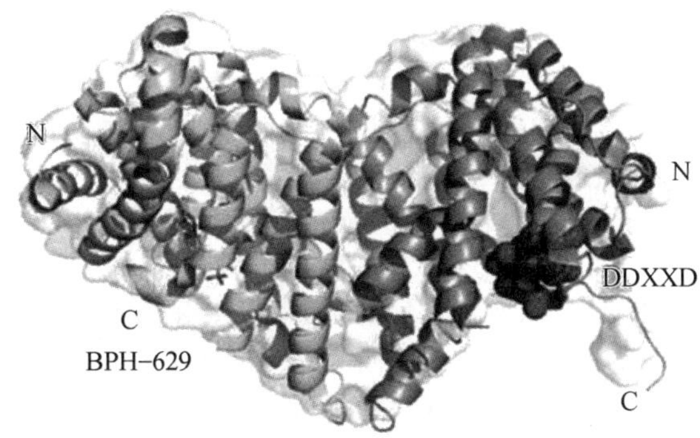


**Figure 6 Dimer structure of *ent*-kaurene synthase from *Bradyrhizobium japonicum***

PDB number: 4W4S WT, the bisphosphonate inhibitor, BPH-629 and the catalytic motifs DDXXD, red are shown。

## 6 问题和展望

二萜合酶的结构多是 α、αβγ、βγ 等模块化结构域组成,其在真菌、裸子植物和被子植物中模块化结构域和分类具有各自的特点。因而,对二萜合酶蛋白的研究尚需要许多新的晶体结构信息。然后,受限于蛋白质晶体的形成、二萜合酶反应的底物和产物小分子的获取,目前得到结构解析的二萜合酶仍然较少,仅为表 1 中的 6 种。随着这一研究热点的持续性拓展,利用合成生物学、化学合成等手段有助于获得底物和产物小分子;此外,利用同位素标记技术,可极大丰富我们对于催化机制的研究,有助于定位行使催化功能的关键氨基酸位点。随着研究人员的深入研究及技术的不断更新,二萜合酶的结构和功能将更多地被探明,二萜合酶在植物进化中的发展规律也将越来越清晰。

二萜类化合物不仅在生物与生物之间相互作用具有重要作用;而且在医学、工业、农业等方面应用广泛。二萜合酶是二萜成分多样性的重要原因,研究这类决定二萜类化合物基本骨架和立体构象的合酶,对于整体研究二萜化合物的生物合成途径以及通过生物工程手段合成二萜化合物具有重要意义和价值。此外,在功能研究上,通过对植物或真菌的二萜环化酶进行活性位点替代和化学策略,可以组合催化多样的类异戊二烯环化反应,对于生物合成已有重大价值化合物和产生新的化合物具有重要意义。

[童宇茹,高伟,黄璐琦. 药学学报,2018,53(8):1195-1201.]

# 基于丹参酮类化合物生源途径的丹参质量标志物研究思路探讨

中药材质量已成为影响中医药现代化进程的重要因素，但由于中药中所含成分复杂多样，且其含量易受产地、种植条件、气候等多种因素影响，因此，如何科学、准确、有效地评价中药材质量已成为中药质量控制体系完整建立的关键前提。丹参 *Salvia miltiorrhiza* Bge. 为唇形科鼠尾草属植物，以根和根茎入药。现代药理学研究表明，丹参具有保护血管内皮细胞、抗心律失常、抗动脉粥样硬化等功效。作为大宗药材，丹参在我国的种植范围十分广泛，受种植条件与地域差异等多种因素的影响，丹参中不同有效成分的含量存在较大差异，导致其质量参差不齐。因此，建立客观、准确且多元的丹参质量评价方法，是构建丹参质量控制体系的关键。2016 年刘昌孝院士首次提出中药质量标志物(Q-markers)这一概念，并在中药质量的物质基础的确定及质量标志物(Q-markers)的提出依据中指出“中药化学成分生物合成途径(生源途径)是化学生物学基础和亲缘学的依据”。目前的丹参质量评价方法大多以丹参中 1 种或几种化学成分的药理活性或含量为选择依据来确定丹参质量标志物，缺少对中药化学活性成分生源途径方面的探究，距 Q-marker 的多元化、完整化的评价标准还有较大差距，因此需要更多的思路与方法去补充与完善丹参质量标志物评价体系。

丹参酮类化合物是由所有二萜的共同前体 GGPP(牻牛儿基牻牛儿基焦磷酸)经过多步生物合成反应生成。已知丹参酮类化合物生源途径见图 1，次丹参酮二烯(miltiradiene)是形成丹参酮类化合物骨架的第一步，铁锈醇(ferruginol)是第一个 CYP450 酶修饰生成的化合物，故这 2 个化合物为丹参酮类化合物生物合成途径上的重要中间体化合物。

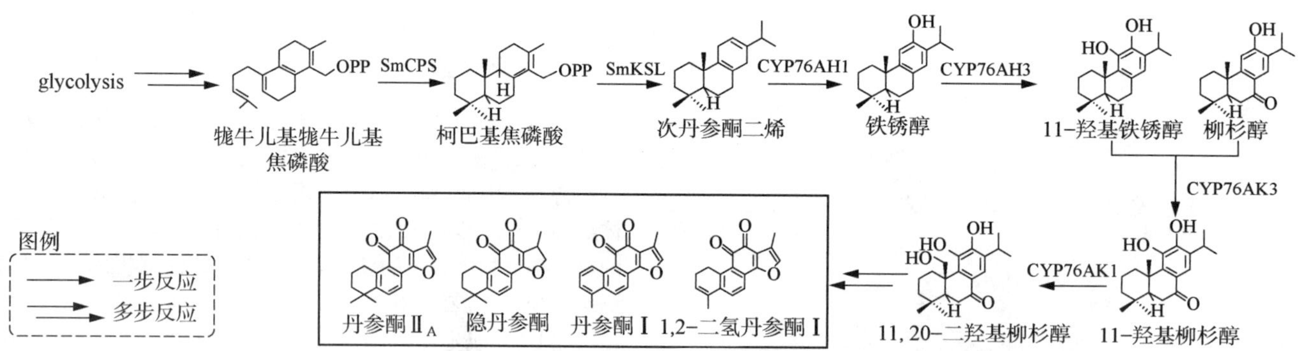


**图 1 丹参酮类化合物生源途径解析现状**

本研究基于中药质量标志物(Q-marker)理论，结合药材质量的可控性与溯源性，从丹参中特有活性成分丹参酮类化合物的生源途径出发，探究丹参酮类化合物含量与其上游基因表达量、中间体化合物(铁锈醇，次丹参酮二烯)含量的潜在关系，从而以新的思路探究中药丹参的质量控制体系，为完善多元化丹参质量标志物体系提供新的研究思路。

## 1 材料

1.1 *丹参毛状根* 丹参毛状根继代培养 6 个月，每 30 日继代 1 批，得到约 100 批毛状根，每批约 4 g。所有毛状根均采用 6,7 - V 毛状根次生代谢产物液体培养基于 25℃，黑暗，120 r/min 的条件下，悬浮培养。

1.2 *丹参药材* 采自河南、河北、山西、四川、甘肃、辽宁、安徽(扦插时间 2018 年 5—7 月，采摘时间 2019 年 4 月)的大田新鲜丹参药材。

1.3 *仪器* U3000 超高效液相色谱系统(赛默飞世尔科技公司)；7000C GC - MS/MS 三重四极杆气质联用仪与样品制备系统(安捷伦公司)；QuantStudio5 荧光定量 PCR 仪(赛默飞世尔科技公司)；1/10 万天平[梅特勒-托利多仪器(上海)有限公司]；超声清洗仪(北京五洲东方科技发展有限公司)。

1.4 *试剂* 色谱纯乙腈、甲醇、异丙醇、正己烷、氯仿(美国 Fisher 公司)；分析纯 $AgNO_3$(沪试，批号 20180830)；酵母提取物(OXOID 公司，批号 2104085 - 02)；TRIzol 试剂；PrimeScript™ RT reagent kit with gDNA eraser(货号 RR047B)；对照品铁锈醇(批号 CFS201801)、丹参酮Ⅱ$_A$(批号 Y20J8C40264)、隐丹参酮(批号 H12O8X45502)、丹参酮Ⅰ(批号 P28D8F51847)和 1,2-二氢丹参酮(上海源叶生物科技有限公司，批号 K11J8B28475)，纯度均≥98%；次丹参酮二烯(由本课题组工程菌发酵制备)。

## 2 方法

### 2.1 毛状根诱导体系的建立

2.1.1 *诱导子配置* 本研究采用酵母提取物与银离子共同诱导(YE＋$Ag^+$ 诱导子)丹参毛状根。YE 诱导子的制备：取 25 g 酵母提取物溶于 125 mL 蒸馏水中，加入 100 mL 无水乙醇，置于 4℃冰箱静置 5 d，除去上清液，下层胶状物质溶于125 mL蒸馏水中，加入无水乙醇（乙醇量达80%）2次沉淀，离心，再将沉淀溶于100 mL蒸馏水中，121 ℃灭菌20 min，冷却后置于4 ℃冰箱备用。$Ag^+$诱导子的制备：取$AgNO_3$ 5.096 g溶于100 mL蒸馏水中，制备得3 mmol/L的$Ag^+$溶液。

2.1.2 毛状根诱导 向培养18 d的丹参毛状根（约4 g）培养基中加入YE+$Ag^+$（YE 1%，$Ag^+$ 0.033%）诱导子进行诱导处理，分别于诱导处理后0、1、2、4、6、9、12、25日取样，每组设置5个生物重复并设置空白对照组（非诱导组）。

2.1.3 实时荧光定量PCR 采用TRIzol法提取丹参毛状根RNA，采用PrimeScript™ RT reagent kit with gDNA eraser进行cDNA反转录，实验操作按产品说明书进行。选择丹参酮类化合物生源途径上*SmCPS*、*SmKSL*、*CYP76AH1* 3条基因为研究对象并设计引物见表1，并测定0、24、48 h的相对表达量。

2.2 色谱条件与质谱条件

2.2.1 UPLC色谱条件 色谱柱Waters ACQUITY UPLC HSS T3（2.1 mm×100 mm，1.8 μm）；流动相为水（A），乙腈（B），乙腈-1%异丙醇（C），梯度洗脱（0～0.5 min，100% A；0.5～2 min，100%～98% A，0%～2% B；2～5 min，98%～90% A，2%～10% B；5～6.5 min，90%～75% A，10%～25% B；6.5～7.5 min，75%～70% A，25%～30% B；7.5～9 min，70%～50% A，30%～50% B；9～19 min，50%～45% A，50%～55% B；19～25 min，45%～40% A，55%～60% B；25～26 min，40%～5% A，60%～0% B，0%～95% C；26～51 min，5% A，95% C）；流速0.5 mL/min；柱温20 ℃；丹参酮$Ⅱ_A$、隐丹参酮、丹参酮Ⅰ、1,2-二氢丹参酮的检测波长设定为254 nm，铁锈醇的检测波长设定为200 nm。

表1 q-RT PCR引物设计

| 引物名称 | 引物序列（5′-3′） |
|---|---|
| SmCPS1-F | CCACATCGCCTTCAGGGAAGAAAT |
| SmCPS1-R | TTTATGCTCGATTTCGCTGCGATCT |
| SmKSL1-F | CTTCCCAAGACAATGCAAAGAT |
| SmKSL1-R | ATTTCCCTCTCACATTATTAGC |
| SmCYP76AH1-F | TCGTGGATGAGTCGGCAAT |
| SmCYP76AH1-R | TGAGTATCTGAGTTCCCT |
| ACTIN-F | AACAGGACCTCAGGGCACC |
| ACTIN-R | TGTCTGGATCGGAGGTTCC |

2.2.2 GC-MS检测次丹参酮二烯色谱条件与质谱条件 气相色谱柱Agilent GC Colums DB-5MS（0.25 mm×15 m，0.10 μm），载气为氦气，色谱条件见表2。

表2 GC-MS色谱条件

| 条件 | 升温速率（℃/min） | 最大值（℃） | 保持时间（min） | 运行时间（min） |
|---|---|---|---|---|
| 初始 | | 100 | 2 | 2 |
| 梯度1 | 40 | 170 | 0 | 5 |
| 梯度2 | 20 | 240 | 0 | 8.5 |
| 梯度3 | 40 | 300 | 1 | 11 |

质谱条件：电离方式采用电子轰击离子源（EI），电子轰击能量为70 eV，扫描范围$m/z$为0～300。使用Mass Hunter软件（美国安捷伦）对进行数据采集和处理。在MRM模式下：碰撞能量为20 eV，溶剂延迟为3 min，将$m/z$ 134用作定量离子，将$m/z$ 65以及$m/z$ 91用作定性离子，停留时间为100 ms，扫描速率为每秒5个循环。

2.3 对照品溶液的制备 精密称取一定量的对照品，制成含丹参酮$Ⅱ_A$ 0.095 mg/mL、隐丹参酮1.35 mg/mL、丹参酮Ⅰ 0.100 mg/mL、1,2-二氢丹参酮0.100 mg/mL、铁锈醇0.237 mg/mL的对照品溶液，4 ℃冷藏保存备用。次丹参酮二烯采用本课题组高产次丹参酮二烯酿酒酵母YJ28发酵提取产物制备而得，制成质量浓度为7.35 mg/mL的甲醇溶液 −20 ℃低温保存备用。

2.4 供试品溶液制备

2.4.1 UPLC样品制备 将样品冷冻干燥48 h，低温粉碎过5号筛。精密称定样品粉末约0.3 g，置具塞锥形瓶中，精密加入甲醇50 mL，密塞，称定质量，超声处理（功率140 W，频率42 kHz）60 min，放冷，补足失重，摇匀，12 000 r/min离心10 min，取上清液，即得（毛状根与药材均用以上方法处理）。

2.4.2 GC-MS样品制备 将样品冷冻干燥48 h，低温粉碎过5号筛。称定样品粉末约0.1 g，置于2 mL EP管中，加入正已烷1.5 mL，超声处理功率140 W，频率42 kHz）5 min，超声结束放冷，继续超声处理5 min，放冷12 000 r/min离心5 min取上清液，即得（毛状根与药材均用以上方法处理）。

2.5 数据处理

2.5.1 毛状根体系实时荧光定量PCR检测 根据实时荧光定量PCR原始检测结果，按照$2^{-\Delta\Delta Ct}$相对定量计算公式，以诱导0 h的毛状根为对照，计算各样品目的基因相对定量结果，见图2。

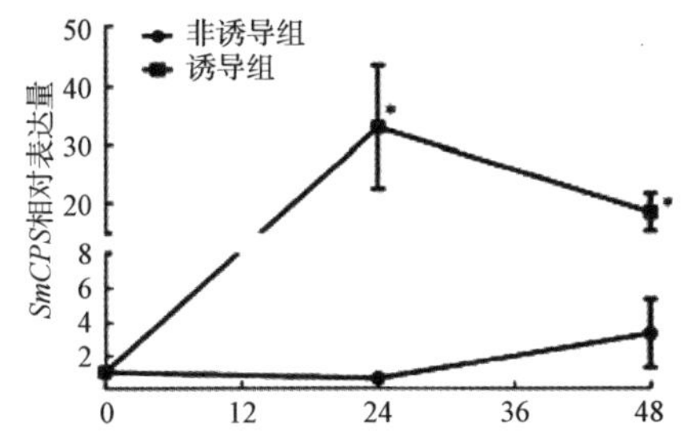

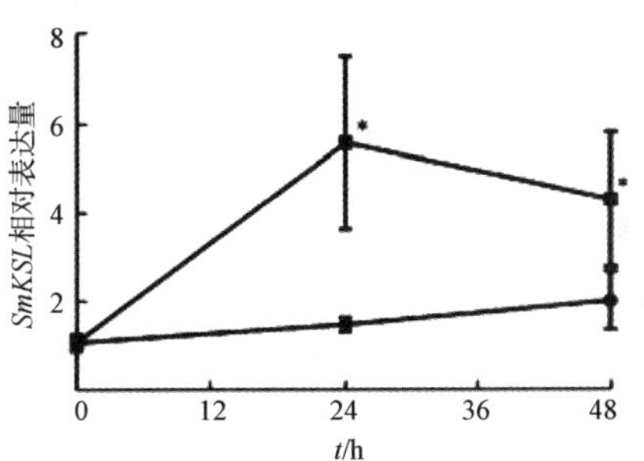

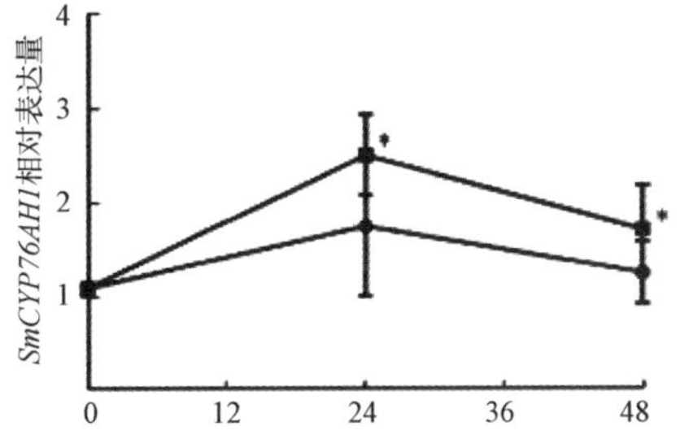


图2 *SmCPS* *SmKSL* *CYP76AH1*基因相对表达量（$n=5$）

* $P<0.05$，差异显著。

采用 SPSS 21 软件进行统计学分析，使用 LSD - $t$ 检验验证诱导前后基因表达量的显著性差异，默认 $\alpha=0.05$，以 $P<0.05$ 为差异具有统计学意义。诱导子可以提高以上3种基因的表达量，且在诱导24 h时表达量到达峰值。

2.5.2 毛状根体系含量测定 毛状根体系中6种化学组分诱导前后的含量变化随时间变化趋势见图3。诱导组丹参毛状根中次丹参酮二烯、铁锈醇和丹参酮类化合物含量较非诱导组中次丹参酮二烯、铁锈醇和丹参酮类化合物含量随时间明显增加。

2.5.3 各地区丹参药材含量测定 对7个省份丹参新鲜药材进行含量测定，检测铁锈醇与丹参酮类化合物含量，见图4。可看出在相同扦插与采收时间内各地大田丹参药材中间体化合物铁锈醇含量与丹参酮类化合物含量的积累趋势是相似的，即在药材中铁锈醇含量相对较高，那么丹参酮类化合物含量相对也较高。

2.5.4 基因表达量与各化合物含量相关性考察 采用 SPSS 21 软件进行统计学分析。首先进行正态性检验，样本量均小于50故参考 S - W 检验结果，若数据符合正态性，则采用 Pearson 相关性分析，若不符合正态性则采用 Spearman 相关分析。

分析非诱导组与诱导组 *SmCPS*、*SmKSL*、*CYP76AH1* 基因前48 h相对表达量与总丹参酮前48 h含量，均不具有正态性，故采用 Spearman 相关分析。非诱导组 *SmCPS*、*SmKSL*、*CYP76AH1* 基因相对表达量与总丹参酮含量相关系数($P<0.05$)分别为 0.164、－0.321、0.661。诱导组 *SmCPS*、*SmKSL*、*CYP76AH1* 基因相对表达量与总丹参酮含量相关系数($P<0.05$)分别为 0.682、0.691、0.491。

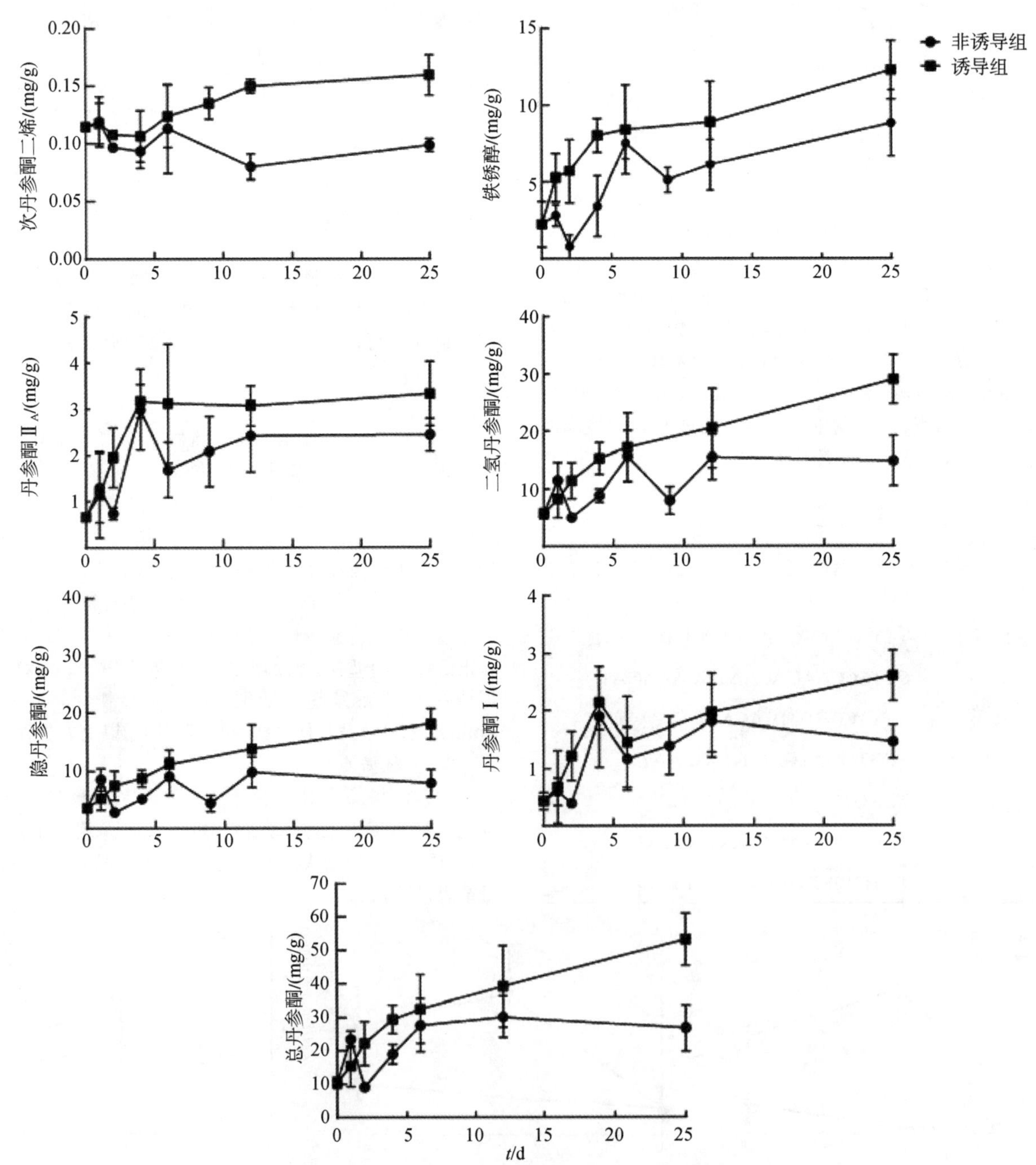


**图3 次丹参酮二烯、铁锈醇、丹参酮 $Ⅱ_A$、二氢丹参酮、隐丹参酮、丹参酮Ⅰ、总丹参酮非诱导组与诱导组积含量($n=5$)**

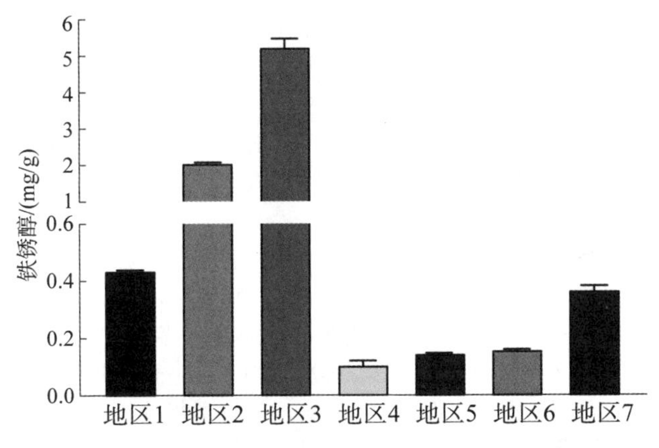


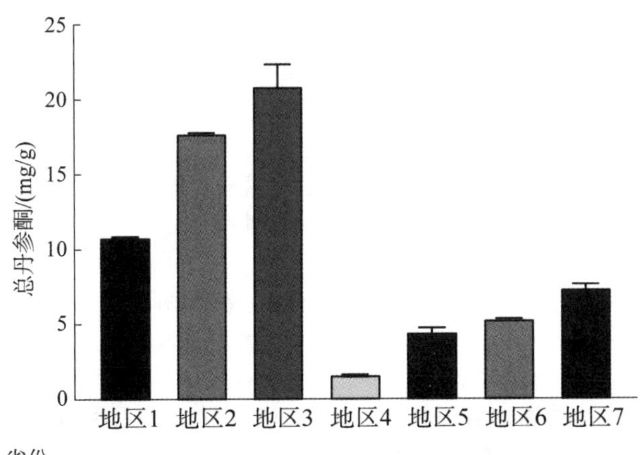


**图4 各省份铁锈醇与丹参酮含量($n=3$)**

省份隐去具体名称。

2.5.5 中间体化合物含量与丹参酮类化合物含量相关性考察 统计方法同2.5.4项下。

分析丹参毛状根诱导组次丹参酮二烯、铁锈醇与总丹参酮含量和非诱导组次丹参酮二烯、铁锈醇与总丹参酮含量,均具有正态性,故采用Pearson相关性分析。诱导组总丹参酮含量与铁锈醇含量相关系数为0.830($P<0.01$);非诱导组总丹参酮含量与中间体铁锈醇含量相关系数为0.577($P<0.01$)。诱导组总丹参酮含量与次丹参酮二烯含量相关系数为0.509($P<0.01$);非诱导组总丹参酮含量与次丹参酮二烯含量相关系数为0.543($P<0.01$)。

分析各省份丹参药材铁锈醇含量与总丹参酮含量无正态性,故采用Spearman相关分析,分析得各省份总丹参酮含量与铁锈醇含量相关系数为0.859($P<0.01$)。因次丹参酮二烯在鲜品药材处理过程中稳定性较差,故本实验未分析次丹参酮二烯含量与总丹参酮含量的统计学关系。

## 3 结论与讨论

本研究通过诱导子对毛状根体系的诱导,使丹参酮类化合物生源途径上3条基因 *SmCPS*、*SmKSL*、*CYP76AH1* 相对表达量上调,同时使得下游丹参酮类化合物含量也相对升高。对丹参毛状根中 *SmCPS*、*SmKSL*、*CYP76AH1* 基因相对表达量与总丹参酮含量进行相关性分析,可以得出这3条基因相对表达量的高低可以一定程度上反映丹参酮含量相对的高低。

毛状根与丹参药材中铁锈醇含量与总丹参酮含量(丹参酮Ⅱ$_A$、隐丹参酮、丹参酮Ⅰ、1,2-二氢丹参酮含量加和)均具有很强的正相关性,铁锈醇含量可一定程度地反映丹参酮化合物的含量,即铁锈醇含量相对较高丹参酮含量也会相对较高。此外,研究在各省份丹参药材中均未检测出次丹参酮二烯,其原因可能与次丹参酮二烯化学性质不稳定和样品处理方式有关,即样品采摘后没及时低温处理而采用常温运输。

综上,在本研究中,丹参中丹参酮类化合物生源途径上重要基因表达量与重要中间体化合物能一定程度上反映下游丹参酮类化合物含量。丹参酮类化合物虽然种类繁多,但拥有相同的生物合成途径,受相同基因调控,同时在生源途径中,它们还拥有共同中间体。所以,将上游基因表达量与中游中间体化合物含量与下游化合物含量关系结合起来,分析其中的规律,以几条基因的表达量或者几种中间体的含量来反映下游一类成分的含量,可以达到"以点带面"的效果。这种方法更加符合整体性思维,也为完善丹参质量标志物体系提供了可能的新研究思路与方法。

[张芮乾,高伟,黄璐琦,等.中国中药杂志,2020,45(13):3098-3103.]

# 植物天然产物途径创建

植物天然产物作为天然产物的重要组成部分,具有抗氧化、抗肿瘤、抗炎、镇痛等诸多活性,广泛应用于医药、化妆品、保健品、调味品、色素等领域,具有非常高的应用价值。1985年,世界卫生组织调查显示约有65%的人口依赖植物来源的药物进行医疗保健,其中大部分来源于植物的特殊代谢产物,包括我们熟知的青蒿素、紫杉醇、丹参酮、穿心莲内酯等。

植物天然产物主要从栽培或野生植物中提取获得,但大多数活性成分在植物的特定组织部位或特定生长阶段积累,且含量较低,如青蒿素含量仅达到干重(DW)的0.1%~1%。一方面受限于植物生长周期以及气候、地理等因素,产量、品质不稳定，难以满足日益增长的需求；另一方面植物中结构类似物多，限制了植物天然产物的分离纯化及其深入发掘利用。近年兴起的合成生物学为植物天然产物的开发应用提供了新的获取方式，通过发掘植物天然产物生物合成关键基因，采用合成生物学策略设计和改造微生物菌株来生产植物天然产物。改造的人工合成细胞能连续、高效地合成特定的植物天然产物，具有低碳、经济和环境友好的特点，是一种极具潜力的资源获取方法。

随着基因组测序、组学分析技术以及基因工程的发展，植物天然产物生物合成研究取得突破进展。2006 年，*Nature* 首次报道了青蒿酸在酿酒酵母中的生物合成；2013 年通过引入植物脱氢酶和细胞色素 CYB5，调节基因表达并采用两相发酵的方法，最终将青蒿酸产量提升至 25 g/L。2015 年，研究人员通过利用来自植物、哺乳动物、细菌和酵母的 20 余种基因，首次实现了阿片类化合物在酵母中的从头合成，完成蒂巴因（6.4 μg/L）和氢可酮（0.3 μg/L）的生物合成，实现复杂代谢途径的微生物转移，是植物天然产物合成生物学的里程碑事件，被评为 *Science* 2015 年度十大科学进展之一。最近由中国科学院天津工业生物技术研究所完成的人工淀粉的从头合成刊登在 *Science* 上，基于计算机途径设计，通过模块化组装和替换，结合三种瓶颈相关酶的蛋白质工程优化，实现人工淀粉的快速合成，其淀粉合成速率是玉米淀粉合成速率的 8.5 倍，为创建新功能的生物系统提供科学基础。这些里程碑工作的报道促进了植物天然产物生物合成以及合成生物学生产的研究和应用。

我国是中药资源大国，据第四次全国中药资源普查显示我国药用植物资源达 12 800 多种，丰富的药用植物资源一方面为我国药物研发提供结构多样的小分子库，另一方面为基础研究、生物合成途径解析、合成生物学和组合生物学提供丰富的酶库。国际植物天然产物合成生物学相关研究以及我国中药资源的传统优势极大地推动了植物来源天然产物的合成途径解析、元件挖掘改造、途径创建和发酵生产的研究与应用。本文在作者前期综述的基础上，进一步对植物天然产物的途径解析和途径创建的整体思路和研究策略进行系统梳理，并对近年来的重要成果、新方法新技术的应用进行总结和展望，为植物天然产物的研究开发利用提供参考（图 1）。

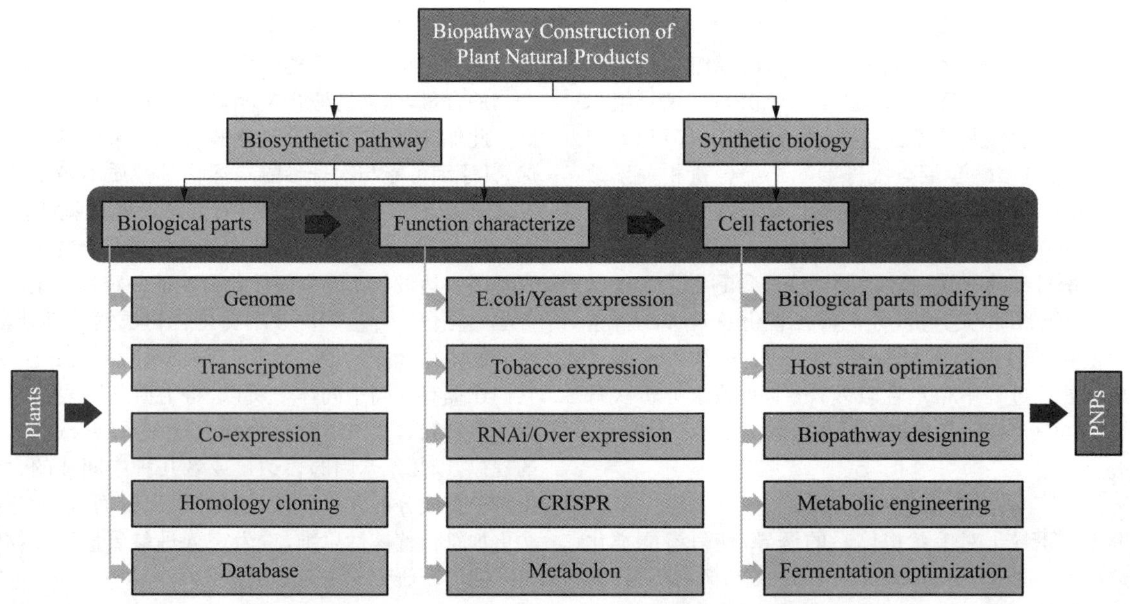

**Figure 1 Biopathway construction of plant natural products**

## 1 植物天然产物生物合成途径及结构修饰酶

1.1 *植物天然产物的主要类型及其生源途径* 植物天然产物主要包括萜类（terpenoids）、生物碱（alkaloids）、苯丙素类化合物（phenylpropanoids）和聚酮（polyketides）等。迄今，超过 22 000 种萜类及其衍生物的化学结构被鉴定，占天然产物总数的 25%～50%，其中包括大家熟知的青蒿素、紫杉醇、丹参酮、人参皂苷等。生物碱类化合物包括多数天然有机化合物中的含氮物质，是天然产物中最大类群化合物之一。目前已知的生物碱有 21 000 多种，根据其基本骨架主要分为吲哚类生物碱、异喹啉类生物碱、有机胺类生物碱、吡啶类生物碱、莨菪烷类生物碱等。常用于临床研究的生物碱有抗肿瘤化合物长春花碱，镇痛化合物吗啡、可待因、延胡索乙素等。苯丙素类化合物是指基本母核具有一个或几个 C6－C3 单元的天然有机化合物类群，通常可分为简单苯丙素类、香豆素类、木脂素和木质素类以及黄酮类等。植物天然产物的生物合成主要以植物初生代谢途径产物为前体，经过一系列的酶催化形成结构多样的天然产物。在植物中，不同类型的天然产物均具有较为保守的前体形成过程，而催化功能多样的结构后修饰酶在植物天然产物的合成中起关键作用。

1.2 *结构后修饰酶* 植物天然产物种类繁多、结构复杂，其上游合成途径较保守，在不同的综述中已有较为详细的阐述。前体经过结构修饰后能显著提高天然产物的活性和成药性，植物中具有良好活性的天然产物多是修饰程度较高、结构复杂的次生代谢产物，在其合成过程中，多是由后修饰酶催化产生的。常见的后修饰酶包括细胞色素 P450(cytochrome P450, P450)、糖基转移酶(glycosyltransferase, GT)、酰基转移酶(acyltransferase, AT)、甲基转移酶(methyltransferase, MT),除此之外酮戊二酸依赖双加氧酶($Fe^{2+}$/2-oxoglutarate-dependent dioxygenase, 2ODD)、黄素腺嘌呤二核苷酸依赖氧化还原酶(flavin adenine dinucleotide-dependent oxidoreductase, FADOX)、脱氢酶(dehydrogenase)、脱羧酶(decarboxylase)和异戊烯基转移酶(prenyltransferase)等在植物天然产物生物合成中亦发挥重要作用。本文主要对广泛参与植物次生代谢途径并且研究较多的 P450、糖基转移酶、酰基转移酶、甲基转移酶等进行总结,为结构后修饰酶的挖掘和功能研究提供参考。

1.2.1 细胞色素 P450 P450 是植物代谢中的最大酶蛋白家族之一,占植物蛋白编码基因的 1%左右,P450 分化与陆生植物的生存进化紧密相关,在初生代谢和次生代谢中均发挥催化作用。植物中参与激素合成或者上游合成途径的 P450 相对较为保守,主要集中在几个家族,而参与次生代谢产物生物合成的 P450 则分化较大,催化产生化学结构的多样性。P450 参与包括羟基化、碳碳偶联、羧化、脱甲基等各种催化反应。对目前已经报道功能的 P450 进行系统进化分析(图 2),结果表明不同植物来源的 P450 主要以基因家族聚类,并且通常情况下,参与结构类似化合物修饰过程的 P450 具有较高的同源性,聚在同一个分支,比如参与紫杉醇生物合成的 P450s 具有 70%同源性;参与丹参酮及鼠尾草酸等类似位点羟基化或者羧化的 P450 大多来自 CYP76 家族。羟基化是 P450 常参与的催化反应,在苄基异喹啉类生物碱(benzylisoquinoline alkaloids, BIAs)生物合成中,P450 被报道参与结构异构化和结构偶联反应。例如来源于日本柳杉(*Cryptomeria japonica*)的 CYP80G2,可催化 *S*-牛心果碱的 C-C 苯酚偶联生成 *S*-紫堇块茎碱;CYP719A 亚家族被鉴定参与分子内偶联反应形成亚甲基二氧桥。此外,P450 还能够催化连续氧化反应、芳香化合物的环氧化反应和胺类及其衍生物的甲基或氨基转移反应等。甘草中的 CYP72A154 能够进行连续 3 步氧化反应,催化甘草酸前体 11-羰基-$\beta$-香树脂醇的 C-30 位成羧基,从而生成甘草次酸。来源于薄荷(*Mentha haplocalyx*)的 CYP71D18 能够催化(+)-(4*R*)-柠檬烯的 C-1、C-2 位置发生环氧化反应,生成顺式-1,2-环氧化物。虽然不同 P450 参与的反应不尽相同,但据目前的研究报道,参与类似反应的 P450 大多具有相对较高的同源性,且随着越来越多的 P450 被鉴定,结合系统进化分析,将为这一重要酶的功能筛选和研究提供更多参考,促进生物合成途径解析。

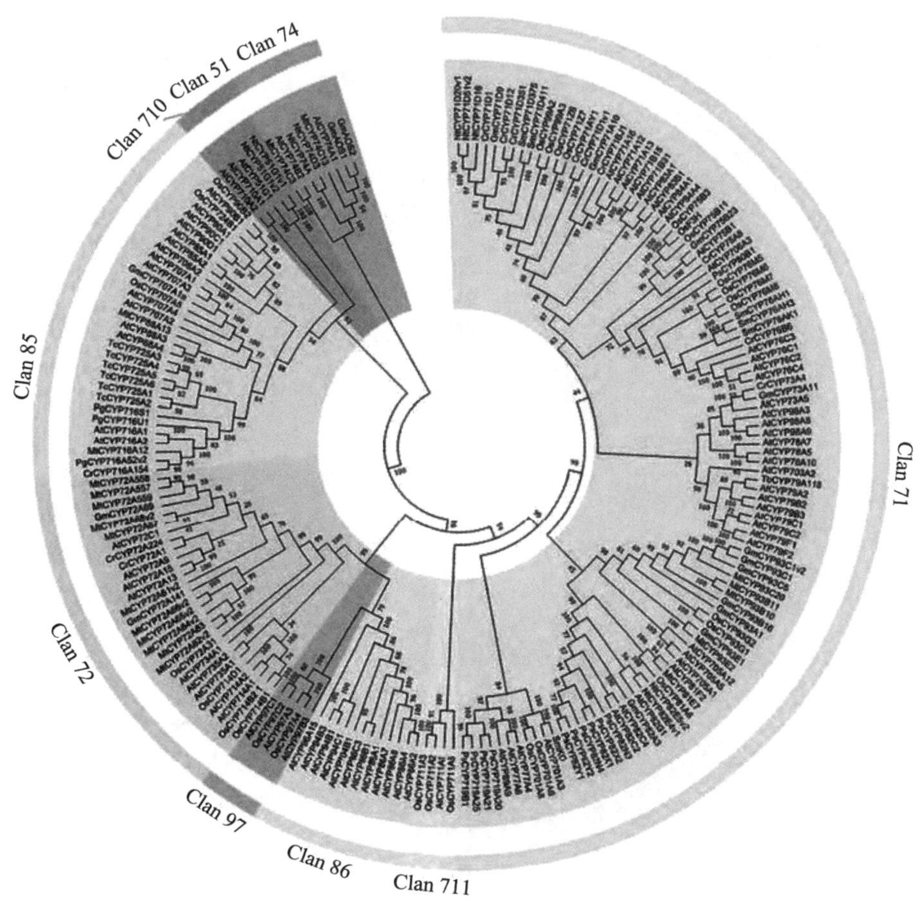


**Figure 2 Phylogenetic analysis of P450s in plant natural product biosynthesis pathway**

P450s from *Arabidopsis thaliana* were employed as references. Sm: *Salviae miltiorrhiae*; Pg: *Panax ginseng*; Mt: *Medicago truncatula*; Tc: *Taxus chinensis*; Cr: *Catharanthus roseus*; Ps: *Papaver somniferum*; Gm: *Glycine max*; Os: *Oryza sativa*; Nt: *Nicotiana tabacum*; At: *Arabidopsis thaliana*. Sequences were downloaded from NCBI or Unipro.

1.2.2 糖基转移酶 糖基转移酶是多基因家族，其中家族1(GT1)最大，称为尿苷二磷酸糖基转移酶(UGT)超家族，主要以UDP-葡萄糖为糖基供体。糖基化反应属于末端修饰，能改变化合物的理化性质，直接或间接影响药用活性，从而影响对活性成分的利用效率和方式。UGT作为植物天然产物生物合成的关键修饰酶，在植物基因组中的扩张和收缩存在种系特异性，在植物次生代谢尤其以黄酮、花青素、三萜类和甾体皂苷类化合物等的结构多样性中起重要作用。近年，随着转录组和基因组数据的大量释放，UGT的研究得以深入开展，从基因功能研究、晶体结构解析、催化机制研究以及蛋白质工程改造等方面均产生了许多突破成果。植物的GT1家族可分为A～R共18个组(group)，不同物种*UGT*基因的总数，在组间的分布均有差异，这也暗示植物GT1家族基因在系统演化过程中的多样性和复杂性。以拟南芥的UGT(不包括两条UGT80家族的UGT)和部分具有代表性且功能明确的植物来源UGT进行系统进化分析，表明功能类似的UGT在系统进化树上通常处于较近的分支(图3)，这为从植物中挖掘糖基转移酶进行结构修饰提供参考和指导。目前糖基化修饰研究最多的是黄酮类化合物，其中*O*-糖基转移酶的研究较为深入。近年不断从植物中克隆获得了一些具有较好活性的*C*-糖基转移酶和*N*-糖基转移酶。北京大学医学部叶敏教授课题组在光果甘草(*Glycyrrhiza glabra*)中鉴定到一条具有双*C*-糖基转移酶GgCGT(UGT708B4)的基因，能够高效催化根皮素发生连续两步的*C*-糖基化反应，生成相应的双碳苷化合物。据报道从多种植物克隆的*C*-糖基转移酶多为UGT708家族，均能催化根皮素或2羟基黄酮的一步或两步的*C*-糖基化。最近，研究人员在银杏(*Ginkgo biloba*)中发现了能够催化IAA和IAA-ASP的*N*-糖基转移酶GbNGT1，完善了生长素的代谢通路和糖基转移酶的功能。除了黄酮类化合物，三萜皂苷类化合物的糖基化包括人参皂苷、三七皂苷、罗汉果甜苷等合成途径中糖基转移酶的研究也较深入。人参皂苷作为人参(*Panax ginseng*)中重要的天然产物，主要是原人参二醇和原人参三醇的糖基化产物。Yan等从人参cDNA中找到第一个糖基转移酶UGTPg1，发现其能够特异性催化原人参二醇的C20位羟基糖基化，并使原人参三醇C20位羟基进行糖基化产生具有生物活性的人参皂苷F1。上海植物生理生态研究所周志华研究员团队随后又从人参中分离得到4个新的糖基转移酶UGTPg100、UGT-Pg101、UGTPg102、UGTPg103，其中UGTPg100能特异性催化原人参二醇的C6位羟基糖基化，生成具有活性的人参皂苷Rh1，UGTPg101催化原人参三醇生成人参皂苷F1，然后从F1生成人参皂苷Rg1。黄酮类化合物以及人参皂苷类生物合成途径糖基转移酶的系统研究能进一步指导其他苯丙素类化合物、三萜皂苷以及甾体皂苷生物合成研究。

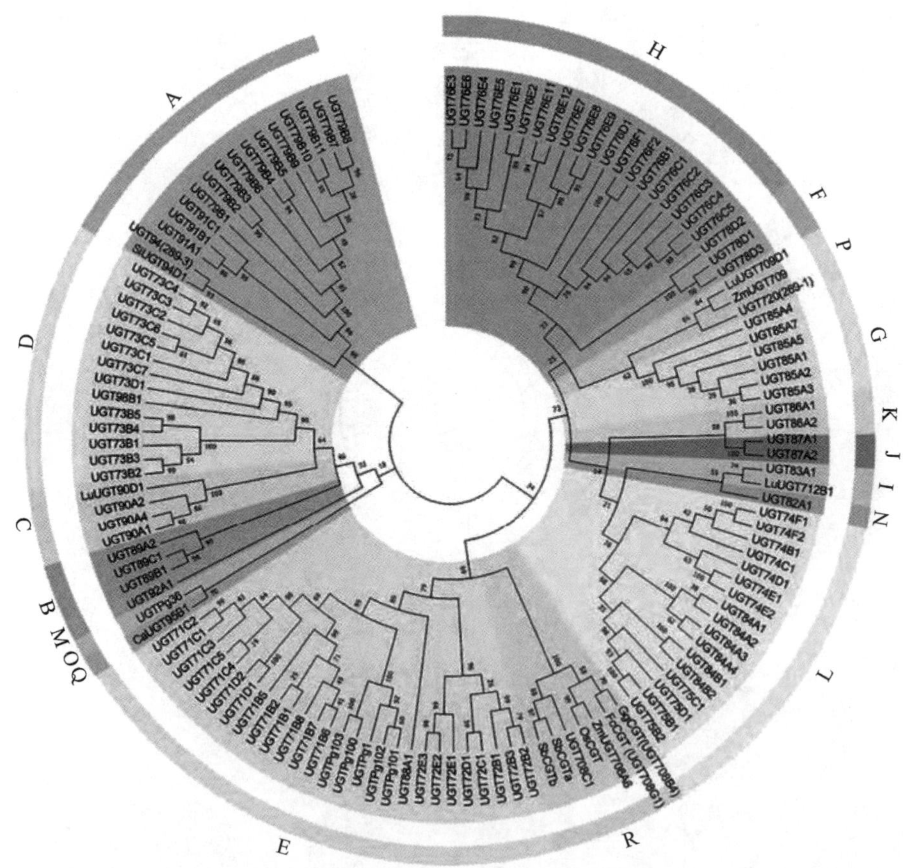


**Figure 3 Phylogenetic analysis of UGTs in plant natural product biosynthesis pathway**

UGTs from *Arabidopsis thaliana* were employed as references. Ca: *Cicer arietinum*; Lu: *Linum usitatissimum*; Si: *Sesamum indicum*; Zm: *Zea mays*; Fc: *Fortunella crassifolia*; Os: *Oryza sativa japonica* group; Pp: *Prunus persica*; Gg: *Glycyrrhiza glabra*; Pg: *Panax ginseng*; Sg: *Siraitia grosvenorii*; Sb: *Scutellaria baicalensis*; At: *Arabidopsis thaliana*. Arabidopsis UGTs was downloaded from the website www. p450. kvl. dk. Other UGTs were downloaded from NCBI or Unipro。

1.2.3 酰基转移酶 植物酰基转移酶包括两大家族：BAHD 酰基转移酶和丝氨酸羧肽酶样(SCPL)酰基转移酶，分别以酰基辅酶 A 硫酯和 1-*O*-*β*-葡萄糖苷为酰基供体。酰基转移酶可修饰多种植物天然产物，包括黄酮类、奎宁酸/莽草酸、萜类、生物碱、醇类、脂类、蔗糖等。药理学研究表明，酰基化修饰能够提高化合物的稳定性和脂溶性，并具有抵御植物病害以及发生应激反应的作用，在植物的生长发育及次生代谢产物的结构修饰、生物活性中均发挥重要作用。Vinorine synthase 是一种乙酰转移酶，在抗心律失常药单萜类吲哚生物碱 ajmaline 的生物合成中起到关键作用，作为 BAHD 超家族中的一员，具有可逆性催化 16-epi-vellosimine 生成 vinoline 的功能。在紫杉醇生物合成过程中，来自红豆杉属植物的 *N*-苯甲酰基转移酶(NDTBT)能够将苯甲酰基团从相应的辅酶 A 硫酯转移到 *N*-debenzoyl-2′-deoxypaclitaxel 中，生成 *N*-苯甲酰基衍生物。NDTBT 具有底物杂泛性，能够催化乙酰基、丁酰基、己酰基与紫杉烷类化合物反应生成对应的酰基取代化合物。在最近的研究中，四川大学张阳教授团队发现菊苣酸的生物合成途径涉及了两大家族酰基转移酶 BAHD 和 SCPL，其中两个胞质中的 BAHD 家族成员 EpHTT 和 EpHQT 分别催化咖啡酰辅酶 A 和酒石酸及奎宁酸反应生成咖啡酰酒石酸和绿原酸，并且当两种产物进入液泡后，会被 SCPL 家族成员 EpCAS 催化，生成菊苣酸和奎宁酸。值得注意的是，EpCAS 酰基供体是绿原酸而不是 SCPL 酰基转移酶常见的酰基供体 1-*O*-*β*-葡萄糖苷，这一发现对 SCPL 家族酰基转移酶的认知具有十分重要的意义。目前酰基化取代在脂肪酰基(乙酰基、丙二酰基、丁酰基、己酰基等)和芳香酰基(肉桂酰基、咖啡酰基、香豆酰基、阿魏酰基等)等天然产物结构修饰中被报道。Wang 等较全面地综述了目前已进行功能研究的植物酰基转移酶，并进行系统进化分析，结果显示目前已报道功能(129 个)的酰基转移酶主要以底物结构聚类，催化同样类型底物的酰基转移酶更倾向于聚在同一个分支，该报道为植物天然产物生物合成中酰基转移酶的筛选和功能研究提供指导。

1.2.4 甲基转移酶 甲基转移酶以 *S*-腺苷甲硫氨酸(*S*-adenosy-*L*-methionine, SAM)为甲基供体，天然产物的甲基化修饰能够改善化合物的稳定性、溶解性和生物活性等，在天然产物药物开发中起重要作用。根据甲基化的靶原子不同，可将甲基转移酶分为氧甲基转移酶(O-MTs)、碳甲基转移酶(C-MTs)、氮甲基转移酶(N-MTs)、硫甲基转移酶(S-MTs)、无机砷甲基转移酶(Cyt19)等，大多数甲基转移酶以底物结构聚类，系统进化分析以及序列的相似性能为酶的功能研究提供初步参考(图 4)。在植物天然产物生物合成中研究较多的是 O-MTs 和 N-MTs，在苄基异喹啉类生物碱生物合成过程中，通过 O-MTs、N-MTs 和 P450 的交替催化产生 *S*-牛心果碱，而 *S*-牛心果碱是吗啡、可待因、诺司卡品、延胡索乙素等 BIAs 的共同前体。暨南大学何蓉蓉教授团队在苦

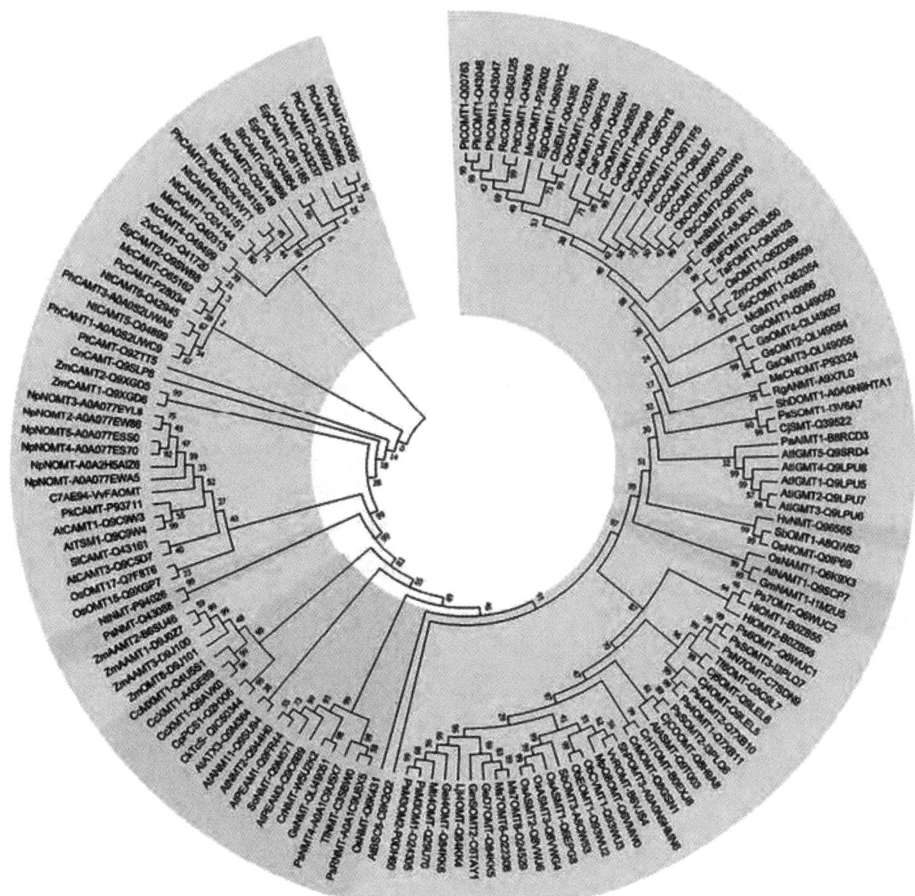

**Figure 4 Phylogenetic analysis of methyltransferase genes in plant natural product biosynthesis pathway**

O-MTs are in blue background. N-MTs are in pink background. Sequences were downloaded from NCBI or Unipro.

茶(*Cammelia assamica*)中找到苦茶碱合成过程中的关键酶 9-*N*-甲基转移酶 CkTcS,并阐明其催化机制,为培育富含苦茶碱的茶叶品种或异源合成苦茶碱奠定理论基础。目前研究人员在甲基转移酶的挖掘和应用方面取得较大进展,实现了如苯丙烷类化合物、生物碱等多种高附加值天然产物的结构修饰,但大多数甲基转移酶具有较强的催化杂泛性,导致副产物产生,使其在工程菌构建中应用受限,因此甲基转移酶的改造提升是其开发利用的重要方向。随着蛋白质工程的逐渐发展以及定向突变和晶体结构的深入研究,将为高效利用甲基转移酶作为生物催化剂提供更有效手段。

## 2 植物天然产物生物合成元件挖掘和功能研究

植物天然产物途径创建的关键是解析生物合成途径,获得催化元件,并根据元件催化特性对其进行适当改造,从而为途径创建提供优质催化元件。植物天然产物的前体合成过程较保守,且研究较透彻,因此其下游合成途径的结构修饰酶的筛选和功能研究是关键。结构后修饰酶大多以基因家族的形式存在于植物基因组中,其生物合成途径中基因的表达相对较弱,因此从庞大组学数据中筛选出候选催化元件,并进行功能研究具有一定的难度,近年相关研究的积累为植物天然产物的生物合成途径解析提供了丰富的案例和参考。

2.1 生物合成途径元件的高效筛选 植物天然产物生物合成途径研究过程中,首要步骤是对基因元件进行挖掘和筛选。随着高通量测序技术的飞速发展,转录组、代谢组、基因组等组学分析为生物元件的挖掘提供数据支持。元件挖掘常用的方法包括基于同源基因克隆和基于差异分析的比较组学筛选,针对未知途径的解析主要依赖于后者,依据不同发育阶段或不同组织部位成分含量差异的特点来筛选与代谢积累相关的候选基因。在研究秋水仙碱生物合成过程中,Nett 等通过代谢组学研究发现嘉兰(*Gloriosa superba*)根茎部分秋水仙碱含量最多,通过比较组学和共表达分析,成功鉴定了 8 个与 *N*-甲酰秋水仙胺生物合成相关的基因,近乎完整地阐释了秋水仙碱的生物合成途径。Ono 等通过分析芝麻(*Sesamum indicum*)6 个生长发育阶段中芝麻素等木脂素类化合物的含量差异,推测在种子发育后期,芝麻素的生物合成才被激活,通过基因表达谱与芝麻素的积累模式分析,找到参与芝麻素生物合成的 *CYP81Q1* 基因。在研究吗啡生物合成途径的最后关键步骤中,Hagel 等将不含吗啡但高含蒂巴因、oripavine 和可待因的罂粟突变品种与 3 个吗啡积累品种进行转录组比较,发现只有一种编码为 2-氧戊二酸/铁(Ⅱ)依赖双加氧酶(*DIOX1*)基因的转录水平在罂粟突变品种中显著低于其他 3 个吗啡积累品种,通过功能研究找到 thebaine 6-O-demethylase(T6ODM)和 codeine O-demethylase(CODM),这是唯一报道的催化 *O*-去甲基化的 2-酮戊二酸/铁(Ⅱ)依赖双加氧酶。这些基于组织表达差异分析、生长发育阶段差异分析、以及品种含量差异分析的基因筛选策略广泛应用于未知功能基因筛选,能够有效缩小候选基因范围,提高研究效率。

当植物受到生物或非生物因子刺激时,会诱导次生代谢途径基因的表达和次生代谢产物的积累。作者课题组利用酵母和银离子诱导丹参(*Salviae miltiorrhiae*)毛状根,导致丹参酮大量积累,同时丹参酮合成相关的上游途径基因表达上调,基于此从比较转录组中筛选到多个参与丹参酮生物合成的 P450 基因,有效推进了丹参酮生物合成途径的解析。Han 等用茉莉酸甲酯诱导人参不定根使人参皂苷积累上调,从上调基因中筛选到 *CYP716A47* 基因,不仅能够在茉莉酸甲酯诱导下被转录激活,还在过表达角鲨烯合酶的转基因人参中被激活,功能鉴定证明 *CYP716A47* 基因具有催化达玛烯二醇氧化生成原人参二醇的功能。有研究发现利用酵母提取物和茉莉酸甲酯分别诱导蒺藜苜蓿(*Medicago truncatula*)毛状根,导致其三萜皂苷积累出现不同响应,30 多种三萜皂苷只有部分受茉莉酸甲酯诱导,这些差异表型为三萜皂苷生物合成途径元件挖掘提供了非常好的筛选材料。

2.2 生物合成途径催化元件功能研究 获得候选基因后,通常利用体外功能研究对其在生物合成途径的催化作用进行分析,较常用的异源表达体系包括基于大肠杆菌和酵母细胞的微生物表达体系、以及近几年在植物天然产物生物合成途径解析中应用较多的烟草表达体系。通过克隆基因全长,在异源体系中表达候选基因蛋白,加入相应底物进行催化并检测,从而确定生物合成途径元件的催化功能。

2.2.1 微生物表达系统应用于生物元件催化功能研究 真核细胞酿酒酵母和原核细胞大肠杆菌是目前常用的微生物表达宿主。大肠杆菌拥有高效的异源蛋白表达效率、异源蛋白含量高、蛋白纯化体系成熟、有适合不同蛋白的商业化表达菌株和载体可选择,并且培养周期短,因此使用更广泛。大多数情况下,包括萜类合酶、糖基转移酶和甲基转移酶等蛋白均能用大肠杆菌进行很好的表达,并进行下一步的体外催化功能研究。有研究者通过改造 P450 基因的膜定位序列,也能实现 P450 在大肠杆菌中的表达和功能研究。但由于 P450 主要定位于植物细胞内质网中,因此用大肠杆菌进行 P450 基因的表达和功能研究仍具有一定的技术难度,大多数情况下很难获得有功能的蛋白,因此利用酿酒酵母来表达 P450 基因是最佳选择。P450 是植物天然产物生物合成中参与度较高的一类酶,参与植物次生代谢的 P450 需要 P450 还原酶或者细胞色素 B5 为其传递电子,因此研究者基于 P450 的异源表达特点,在酿酒酵母染色体上整合了一个来自拟南芥的 P450 还原酶基因(cytochrome P450 reductase, *CPR*),构建了一个专用于植物 P450 表达和功能研究的酿酒酵母菌株 WAT11。目前这个菌株已经广泛用于 P450 基因的表达和功能研究,并且由于酵母表达相对于早期使用的昆虫细胞表达体系操作更简单,基本替代了昆虫细胞表达体系,已被用于丹参酮、雷公藤、苄基异喹啉类生物碱等天然产物生物合成途径的功能基因研究。

2.2.2 烟草表达系统应用于生物元件催化功能研究 除了微生物体系,植物体系尤其是烟草表达体系也是近几年应用较多的植物功能基因异源表达体系。植物固有的光合作用和碳利用机制,可以利用光合作用的还原能力驱动 P450 酶产生化学反应,较微生物宿主表达 P450s 有很大改善。与微生物相比,植物具有蛋白表达和发挥功能的细胞器、辅酶、辅酶因子以及前体物质,更利于植物来源蛋白表达和表达后修饰。烟草作为应用较多的模式植物,其转基因技术体系成熟,自 1989 年第一次用烟草表达抗体,烟草已经成为生产重组蛋白的主要工具，其成熟且简单可行的瞬时表达体系，为植物来源基因的表达和功能研究提供了新的体系。2015 年发表在 Science 的合成依托泊苷苷元的研究中，研究人员在本氏烟草（*Nicotiana benthamiana*）中对桃儿七（*Podophyllum hexandrum*）中的 29 个候选基因进行了组合表达，成功鉴定出 6 个途径催化酶，包括一个酮戊二酸依赖双加氧酶，该双加氧酶能够闭合芳基四氢萘支架的核心环己烷环。Christ 等利用本氏烟草进行基因瞬时表达来筛选重楼（*Paris polyphylla*）和葫芦巴（*Trigonella foenumgraecum*）中的 P450s，成功鉴定出薯蓣皂苷元生物合成的关键 P450 基因。在秋水仙碱生物合成途径的研究中，Nett 等利用本氏烟草对合成途径的甲基转移酶和 P450 进行鉴定，成功在本氏烟草中重构了一条含有 16 个基因的合成路径，实现了从简单氨基酸到 *N*-甲酰秋水仙胺的转化。随着生物合成途径解析的深入，更多酶类型的发现，烟草表达将成为植物来源基因的表达和功能研究更适合的体系。

2.2.3 催化元件的体内功能研究 生物合成元件在植物体内发挥功能是研究植物天然产物形成及调控的基础，但遗传转化体系不成熟限制了如 RNA 干扰、过表达或者 CRISPR/Cas9 等技术的应用。幸运的是随着越来越多的研究关注植物天然产物的合成，不少植物渐渐构建了遗传转化体系，比如丹参、黄花蒿（*Artemisia annua*）、颠茄（*Atropa belladonna*）等。这些遗传转化体系的建立，为药用活性成分生物合成途径的解析提供了技术平台。作者实验室从自交 6 代高度纯合的丹参植株基因组中找到 4 个 CYP71D 候选基因，使用 RNAi 方法将其敲除，获得转基因植株，发现 CYP71Ds-RNAi 植株与野生型植株的根相比表现出明显的橙色表型，进一步的生化研究表明 CYP71Ds 在丹参酮呋喃环形成中发挥重要作用。海军军医大学张磊教授团队利用 CRISPR/Cas9 技术对丹参酚酸类化合物合成途径中的迷迭香酸合成酶（SmRAS）进行编辑，获得突变毛状根，检测发现迷迭香酸和丹酚酸 B 的含量降低，证明 SmRAS 在丹参酚酸类化合物的生物合成途径中发挥重要作用。这些体内功能研究为系统了解植物天然产物代谢网络及调控机制提供支撑，并为植物代谢工程改良奠定基础。

2.3 新技术新方法应用于功能基因筛选和功能研究 计算生物学和合成生物学的发展、基因数据库的扩张以及生物合成途径功能元件的积累为植物天然产物生物合成途径解析提供了新方法和策略。基于合成生物学的植物天然产物途径边解析边重建的方法，解决了代谢中间产物难以获取的问题。次丹参酮二烯作为丹参酮和雷公藤内酯的前体化合物，在植物中含量非常低，难以分离获取，限制了途径的进一步解析，通过构建次丹参酮二烯的酵母工程菌，为下游 P450 功能基因研究提供了底盘和前体，并为途径解析提供了基础平台。除此之外，研究者通过计算生物学的方法从数据库中挖掘天然产物生物合成途径可能的功能元件，通过功能研究和途径重构，实现了阿片类化合物、苄基异喹啉类生物碱等天然产物的生物合成，计算生物学方法的应用能够更精确地获取候选基因并进行功能研究，有效减少工作量、提高筛选效率。

基因组数据和转录组数据的积累、基因合成成本的下降为高通量的自动化筛选提供了数据支撑，已应用于酶的改造和细胞工厂筛选。在采用随机或定向进化的方法提高酶和细胞工厂性能时，突变文库的多样性以及可靠的高通量筛选方法是成败的关键因素。传统的筛选方法如琼脂平板和微孔板筛选法存在无法精准定量或者通量低、操作耗时等缺点，而近年来开发的荧光激活细胞分选（FACS）和液滴微流控分选（DMFS）等超高通量筛选方法，大大提高了筛选通量，可用于酶和细胞工厂定向改造中大容量突变库的筛选。Ma 等开发了一种超高通量双通道液滴微流控筛选系统，每天可筛选多达 107 种酶突变体。基于该系统设计酯酶的对映选择性，以优先生产具有抗炎作用的 profens 对映异构体，在经历五轮定向进化后，从两种荧光信号检测的筛选模式中确定了一种对（*S*）-profens 选择性提高 700 倍的突变体，新系统的应用显著提升了筛选效率。植物天然产物生物合成后修饰酶基因通常以基因家族的形式存在于基因组中，候选基因数量较多，具有普适性的高通量技术的开发应用能够更快推动功能基因的筛选和生物合成途径解析。

## 3 植物天然产物的合成生物学生产

近年来，随着生物合成途径的解析以及合成生物学使能技术的发展，植物天然产物的合成生物学生产逐渐成了生物合成研究的一个重要应用方向。从青蒿素的合成生物学生产到阿片类化合物在酵母中的途径创建，合成生物学为天然产物的研究带来了一场新的革命，为天然产物获取提供了新的方式。在微生物中实现植物天然产物高产需要从元件、途径、细胞三个层面进行系统改造，最后利用发酵工程实现高效生产。

3.1 生物元件的改造 合成生物学元件（biological parts）包括用于调控基因表达的调控元件（启动子、终止子、核糖体结合位点），以及特定功能的结构元件（合成途径中特定的催化酶基因）等。虽然目前紫杉醇、青蒿素、吗啡等植物天然产物生物合成途径的解析取得突破并正在逐步实现合成生物学生产，但对于大多数植物天然产物，其合成生物学产量仍然无法与植物提取相比。途径元件的改造和高效催化是亟需解决的问题，作为研究热点，酶的定向进化和理性改造在催化机制研究以及催化性能提升中发挥重要作用。

3.1.1 利用定向进化提升生物元件催化效率 植物天然产物作为次生代谢产物，在植物中的积累量较低，而受限于次生代谢途径酶的天然特性，相关基因如 P450 或萜类合酶等的表达量低，催化活性弱，其应用进一步受限。定向进化是一种应用广泛的改变酶催化特性的策略，由于其在酶工程领域的重要作用，于 2018 年获得诺贝尔化学奖。定向趋异进化是在定向进化和趋异进化理论上建立的一种重新设计酶催化功能的蛋白质工程学方法，能够将天然蛋白改造成底物专一性各不相同的多种蛋白。中国科学院微生物研究所唐双焱研究员团队利用蛋白质定向趋异进化策略对大肠杆菌单加氧酶 HpaBC 进行了改造，获得了具有酪醇/酪胺羟化酶混杂催化活性的优良突变体 H7，它能够有效减少蛋白质过表达造成的细胞代谢负担，显著提高羟基酪醇生物合成效率，在没有优化发酵条件的情况下，使羟基酪醇产量达到 1 890 mg/L，转化率可达到 82%。定向进化与高通量筛选技术的结合共同提升酶的改造效率。Ellington 团队通过易错 PCR 构建了樟脑诱导型 PCamR/CamR 突变库，筛选出能够特异性响应冰片、芬酚、桉油醇和莰烯等二环单萜的生物传感器，实现了对二环单萜化合物的快速检测，显著提升突变体库的筛选效率，该策略为定向进化在酶改造研究中的应用提供案例。

3.1.2 生物元件的理性设计 对于蛋白质晶体结构、催化机制较清晰的酶，除了利用定向进化产生大量的突变体之外，还可以采用理性设计的方法进行定向改造。天津工业生物技术研究所孙媛霞研究员团队在对罗汉果（*Siraitia grosvenorii*）中糖基转移酶 UGT74AC1 的催化特性和晶体结构认识的基础上，设计一系列突变体，将该酶对三萜类化合物的催化效率提升 100 到 10 000 倍，之后利用优势突变体的体外催化功能合成了一系列新的三萜皂苷化合物。随后孙媛霞研究员团队和孙周通研究员团队合作在罗汉果中发现了一个新的糖基转移酶 UGT74AC2，并采用聚焦理性迭代定点突变（focused rational iterative site-specific mutagenesis, FRISM）的理性设计策略，成功获得催化水飞蓟宾不同位置羟基的突变体，实现了含氮和硫底物的催化功能。定向的进化工程策略以及理性的设计方法可以有目标地改善酶的活性、热稳定性、对底物的亲和力和偏好性，进一步提高从前体到产物的转化效率。

3.2 生物合成途径的设计与优化 植物天然产物途径解析和关键元件的挖掘改造是其合成生物学生产的基础，而在微生物中重构生物合成途径并进行设计和优化是其利用合成生物学高效生产的关键。合成途径长、催化酶类型多是影响产量提高的主要因素，并且部分天然产物存在一定的细胞毒性，导致产量提升困难，因此途径创建和基于细胞整体的代谢流调控对于目标化合物产量提升非常重要。近几年对于天然产物合成生物学菌株改造的策略很多，过表达关键酶基因和抑制竞争途径、蛋白融合或蛋白支架的方法是合成生物学基因工程菌构建的常用手段，最近针对降低代谢物细胞毒性的代谢产物区室化存储、传感器的应用、改善细胞内环境等产量提升策略也发挥越来越重要的作用。

3.2.1 代谢流调控 代谢流调控主要通过调控关键节点基因的表达从而提升目标化合物的产量，包括过表达关键限速酶、降低或沉默竞争途径等。比如 3-羟基-3-甲基戊二酰辅酶 A 还原酶（3-hydroxy-3-methylglutaryl coenzyme A reductase, HMGR）是萜类生物合成的关键限速酶，在工程菌中过表达 *HMGR* 基因的 C-端结构域，能显著提高萜类化合物的产量并提高细胞稳定性，这一策略在青蒿素、丹参酮等天然产物基因工程菌构建中被广泛应用。在单萜生物合成中，Li 等通过将相对较弱的启动子替换为竞争途径元件的启动子，使工程菌中单萜的产量提高了 1.7～21.5 倍。在苯丙素类化合物咖啡酸的工程菌构建中，研究人员通过解除关键前体苯丙氨酸的反馈抑制并敲除竞争途径的关键基因使酵母中的咖啡酸产量提高 2.6 倍。在脂肪酸的合成中，中国科学院青岛能源研究所崔球研究员团队通过过表达脂肪酸前体合成的关键酶 6-磷酸葡萄糖脱氢酶（glucose-6-phosphate dehydrogenase, G6PDH）和乙酰辅酶 A 羧化酶（acetyl-CoA carboxylase, ACC）强化脂肪酸前体供给途径，并且过表达脂肪酸贮存中的关键限速酶二酰基甘油酰基转移酶（diacylglycerol acyltransferase, DGAT），结合弱化产物的竞争途径-脂肪酸合酶途径，最终获得了合成高纯度二十二碳六烯酸（DHA）的细胞工厂（331 mg/g）。虽然基因敲除或过表达等静态调控策略在提高天然产物生物合成的代谢通量方面具有非常有效的作用，但容易引起代谢资源不足从而导致异源细胞生长迟缓。江南大学刘立明教授课题组将稳定期启动子（SPP）和蛋白质降解标签（PDT）与 CRISPR 干扰系统结合，构建了一个动态调控系统，能够根据细胞的生理状态关闭多基因表达，在 5 L 的发酵罐中得到了 21 g/L 的莽草酸。

3.2.2 减少有毒中间体的积累 在异源表达天然产物时，大量外源基因过表达或有毒中间体的积累可能会影响宿主细胞生长，使用动态调控启动子是一种减少或消除有毒中间体积累的有效策略。法呢基焦磷酸（farnesyl diphosphate, FPP）和 3-羟基-3-甲基戊二酰辅酶 A（3-hydroxy-3-methylglutaryl coenzyme A reductase, HMG-CoA）是萜类生物合成中的有毒中间体，Dahl 等通过使用动态调控启动子对有毒中间体进行实时调控，在不使用任何诱导促进剂的情况下，利用两个 FPP 反应促进剂，有效减少有毒中间体的积累，显著提高了基因工程菌中青蒿素前体紫穗槐二烯的产量。上海植物生理生态研究所陈晓亚研究员课题组发现棉花中的糖代谢解毒酶（SPG）在丢失 *N* 端的细胞器定位信号肽和谷胱甘肽（GSH）结合位点后，可以高效催化棉酚生物合成途径中的中间体芳香化且不需要辅因子参与，并且 SPG 可以催化复杂反应，具有潜在的解毒功能，这些酶的发现为新型芳香剂合成提供了新的改造靶点。

3.2.3 代谢物的动态监测 依赖于生物传感器（biosensor）的代谢物动态监测是近年的研究热点，在减少有毒中间体积累、提升目标产物产量中也发挥重要作用。生物传感器依靠对目标代谢物的特异敏感性，可将代谢物的变化信息通过多种信号实时输出，实现动态监测和反馈，从而调节和平衡生物合成途径、提高天然产物产量。通过与高通量筛选相结合能加快代谢途径以及生产菌株的选择过程，是解决异源生产植物天然产物瓶颈的有效方法。Chou 等构建了一个动态控制全基因组突变率的传感器执行器电路，当目标代谢物浓度较低时，突变率增加，在群体中产生多样性，并导致新表型的进化；当目标代谢物浓度增加时，通过反馈调节导致突变率降低，从而降低表型多样性，利用该传感器成功使酪氨酸和番茄红素的产量增加 5 倍和 3 倍。上海交通大学赵心清教授课题组以大肠杆菌木糖激活因子（XylR）及相应结合位点（xylO）为基础构建了突变型木糖传感器，该突变型生物传感器不仅扩大了木糖的浓度检测范围，也可用于 $\beta$-半乳糖苷酶和番茄红素等生物合成途径的木糖诱导表达，为其他生物传感器的设计和进化提供了新见解。目前生物传感器已广泛应用于生物质化学品的合成生物学工程菌构建和产量检测中，相信未来针对天然产物积累或代谢流调控的生物传感器的开发和应用将有效助推天然产物基因工程菌产量提升研究。

3.2.4 亚细胞区室化策略 许多结构复杂的天然产物在微生物的异源合成中含量较低，易产生副反应，这是由于在天然产物生物合成中，部分酶需在特定的亚细胞区室（如细胞质、线粒体、内质网、过氧化物酶体、高尔基体、细胞壁或液泡等）中定位发挥催化活性。亚细胞区室化的优势在于不仅具有独特的生理化学环境、代谢物、酶和辅因子，其细胞质间的物理间隔在消除代谢干扰以及增强区室化途径效率方面也具有良好效果。斯坦福大学 Smolke 课题组在研究托品烷类生物碱的生物合成时，运用亚细胞区室化策略将来自酵母、细菌、植物和动物中的 20 多种酶定位到不同的亚细胞中（包括细胞质、线粒体、过氧化物酶体、液泡等），解决了酶在不同环境中的适配性以及代谢物转运等问题，实现了莨菪碱和东莨菪碱在酵母中的生物合成。单萜类化合物如柠檬酸、冰片等对细胞生长具有较大影响，研究者通过将单萜途径定位至过氧化物酶体，使酵母中单萜的产量提升到胞质表达的 125 倍。该策略也成功应用于人参皂苷以及 BIAs 合成生物学研究中。天津工业生物技术研究所张学礼研究员团队在研究三萜化合物人参皂苷的合成途径时利用脂滴膜蛋白 Pln1p 将定位于内质网中的关键 P450 酶（PPDS）定向到底物（达玛烯二醇-Ⅱ，DD）存储的细胞器脂滴中，使底物 DD 的转化率显著提高，在导入人参皂苷 Compound K 生物合成高效模块后，人参皂苷产量最终滴度达到 5 g/L。去甲乌药碱合酶（NCS）是 BIAs 合成途径的第一个关键酶，但高活性的 NCS 突变体在酿酒酵母细胞质中表达时具有毒性。加利福尼亚大学 Dueber 课题组将 NCS 定位至过氧化物酶体，利用底物和产物在过氧化物酶体膜上的自由流动性，降低了 NCS 细胞毒性，之后进一步模拟脂肪酸诱导过氧化物酶体增殖，将 BIA 产量提高了 74%。除了过氧化物酶体，线粒体工程在工程菌构建中亦有报道。线粒体中含有丰富的乙酰辅酶 A 和氧化还原等价物，是进行萜类化合物生物合成的良好亚细胞区室，但线粒体工程存在代谢负担，会导致细胞生长不良。华东理工大学魏东芝教授课题组在进行角鲨烯的生物合成时在酵母线粒体中引入甲羟戊酸途径并增强细胞质中甲羟戊酸的合成，以此减轻线粒体区室化 MVA 途径引起的代谢负担，促进了细胞生长，最终发酵获得高产角鲨烯 21.1 g/L。植物天然产物合成途径复杂、合成路径长，酶的亚细胞定位或代谢途径的细胞区室化能在一定程度上聚集代谢途径、减少代谢物的交流、抑制竞争途径，实现产量提升。

## 4 展望

合成生物学技术经过 20 余年的发展，在农业、医药、能源、环境等各领域发挥重要作用，是“十四五”期间国家科技前沿重点攻关领域。近期国家发改委与工业和信息化部关于推动原料药产业高质量发展实施方案的通知将合成生物学和生物催化剂作为原料药的先进制造技术创新工程的重点发展任务。结合生物技术、计算机技术与合成生物学在不同层面（酶、途径和细胞）对微生物合成过程进行设计、调控和优化，不仅能够实现植物天然产物的途径创建和微生物生产，而且能够对植物天然产物进行进一步的结构修饰和改造，提升其开发利用价值。与植物天然产物的传统获取方式相比，这种新的资源获取策略以青蒿素、β-榄香烯等为代表的工程菌构建和生产方面的应用，体现其在资源可持续利用、稳定、高效等方面的显著优势，实现了植物天然产物的绿色低碳制造。

植物天然产物生物合成研究一方面为合成生物学生产提供了元件和基础，另一方面通过植物代谢工程也逐渐应用于农业、医药等领域。植物本身含有或编码酶基因，具有类似结构和功能的细胞器、辅酶、辅酶因子以及前体物质，有利于植物来源蛋白表达和翻译后修饰，更适于复杂天然产物生物合成途径的解析以及基于基因编辑技术的药用植物改良，减少可能存在的代谢途径不清晰等造成的困难，并逐渐成了植物天然产物合成生物学生产的方向。比如番茄（*Lycopersicon esculentum*）已被广泛用于如虾青素、单萜、花青素、黄酮醇等天然产物的生产。另外利用本氏烟草作为底盘重构多个天然产物的通路，合成了如长春花碱、鬼臼毒素、红景天苷等天然产物。未来随着植物基因组测序技术的成熟以及基因编辑工具的开发和编辑效率的提升，在植物中以全局代谢网络为基础的代谢途径优化理念和操作的进一步突破，将迎来植物源天然产物途径创建的新时代。

植物天然产物的生物合成及合成生物学研究已取得了突破进展，成了植物天然产物研究的重要方向之一，但是目前仍有许多亟待解决的问题：生物合成途径长、结构修饰酶家族大等因素影响元件筛选和途径解析，许多复杂小分子的生物合成途径仍然未完全解析；即使途径已知，但多个元件组装到一起仍需要克服组件间的协调问题；因此随着途径工程越来越复杂，途径工程的建设和优化过程也是异常艰巨；有些植物天然产物对微生物细胞的增殖有影响，难以实现高产。针对以上问题，理论和技术的发展将不断促进这一领域的发展，植物天然产物的产生是基因组复制和新功能化的结果，由于植物基因组庞大、候选基因多，迫切需要高通量检测技术的开发来配合基因功能研究，从而推动元件的功能筛选；人工智能已应用到药物的筛选和设计，与药物与靶蛋白作用机制类似，生物合成途径酶与底物的互作也符合分子动力学原理，随着 Alphafold2 的应用、量子计算的发展，我们已步入途径计算设计的时期；定向进化、半理性设计的元件改造、底盘驯化、生物传感器、自动化高通量合成生物学工作站等技术的应用，在植物天然产物基因工程菌产量提升上发挥越来越重要的作用；定量合成生物学是合成生物学的前沿，能够实现在基因工程菌中精准地调控、分配和亚细胞区室化生成多组分天然产物，可以预见未来中药复方的合成生物学生产将成为中药创新制剂研发的一种方式。总之，不断增加的科技投入将推动植物天然产物生物合成及合成生物学领域朝着高速、多元化的方向发展。

［刘秀玉，郭娟，黄璐琦，等.药学学报，2021，56(12)：3285-3299.］

# 中药活性成分生物合成研究及应用

中药资源是中药产业和中医药传承发展的基础，是国家的战略性资源。中药活性成分是中药发挥药效的物质基础，也是创新药物的来源，如抗疟药物青蒿素等。第四次全国中药资源普查表明，85%以上的中药来源于药用植物，其中大部分中药活性成分是栽培或野生药用植物的次生代谢产物，在植物的特定组织部位以及特定的生长阶段积累。受气候环境的影响，中药活性成分含量不稳定，且植物中结构类似物多、分离纯化困难等问题，严重制约了中药活性成分的进一步开发利用，因此迫切需要利用现代科技手段寻求新的解决方式。

随着新药开发及中药产业发展对单体活性成分的需求增大，中药资源正面临大宗常用资源短缺、珍稀濒危资源被破坏等诸多问题。国家"十四五"发展规划对社会、经济、环境发展提出了新目标，对中药资源开发利用也提出了新要求，指出绿色可持续发展将是中药资源发展的方向。同时，随着人类基因组测序的完成，生命科学进入了后基因组时代，随之产生的新技术、新方法，如合成生物学、基因编辑、空间组学技术、单细胞测序等推动了中医药现代化和国际化的进程。

中药活性成分主要来源于萜类、生物碱、苯丙素类等植物次生代谢产物，其积累具有较强的时空特异性，比如丹参酮作为丹参的主要活性成分之一，主要在丹参的根中积累。同时这也与中药特定的药用部位以及中药道地性息息相关。因此，研究中药活性成分在药用植物中的合成及调控对探讨中药成药性机制、道地性成因具有重要意义。通过中药活性成分形成机制研究，一方面为利用代谢通路元件在微生物中重构代谢途径，实现高效可控异源生产提供前提，另一方面为药用植物代谢工程改良、药用植物栽培驯化奠定基础。基础研究与开发应用相结合，将成为实现中药资源可持续开发利用的重要途径之一(图 1)。

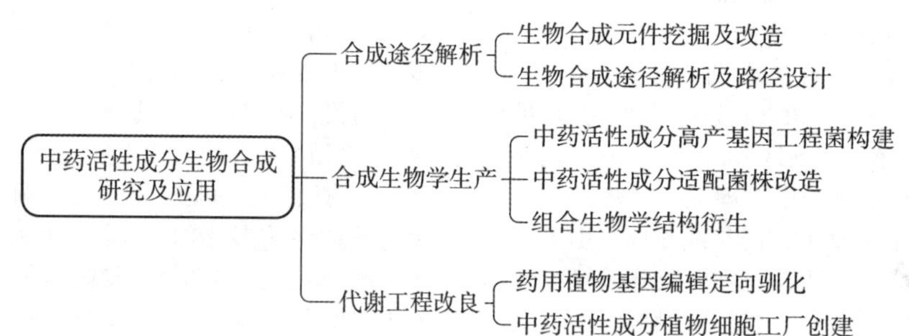


**图 1　中药活性成分生物合成研究及应用方向**

## 1　中药活性成分生物合成途径解析及路径设计

具有明确药理药效作用的中药活性成分主要包括萜类、苯丙素类、生物碱等，比如丹参酮类化合物是二萜、人参皂苷是三萜、黄芩素是苯丙素类、延胡索乙素和汉防己甲素等是苄基异喹啉类生物碱。这些化合物是植物体内主要的次生代谢产物类型，也称为天然产物。据统计，美国食品药品监督管理局(U. S. Food and Drug Administration, FDA)批准上市的药物超过 49.2%与天然产物的结构或信息相关。植物次生代谢产物是不同植物在长期进化过程中为应对不同的环境变化而产生的，与植物的环境适应性密切相关。其中，萜类化合物和苯丙素类广泛存在于不同的科、属、种，生物碱的积累范围相对较窄，比如异喹啉类生物碱仅存在于毛茛目。

植物次生代谢产物的生物合成大体分为上游共同前体形成、下游结构形成及结构修饰三个过程，在植物中以初生代谢产物为前体，通过不同的代谢途径生成，其类型众多、结构复杂。但是这些看似复杂的化学结构间却存在着一定的关联，大多经过一个简短的上游共同前体形成途径生成一些重要的中间体，再在包括细胞色素 P450(cytochrome P450, P450)、糖基转移酶(UDP-glycosyltransferase, UGT)等后修饰酶的催化下生成结构多样的产物。萜类化合物以 3-磷酸甘油醛、乙酰辅酶 A、丙酮酸为前体，通过甲羟戊酸途径(mevalonate pathway, MVA pathway)和位于质体中的甲基赤藓醇-4-磷酸途径(2-C-methyl-D-erythritol-4-phosphate pathway, MEP pathway)产生萜类的共同前体 IPP, DMAPP, GPP, FPP, GGPP 等，不同结构的萜类化合物在植物体内通过萜类合酶(terpene synthase, TPS)、P450、酰基转移酶(acyltransferase, AT)、UGT 等的催化作用生成结构多样的萜类活性成分。苯丙素类化合物主要以 L-苯丙氨酸和 L-酪氨酸为前体，经过短暂的共同途径生成不同类型苯丙素类的中间体，包括 4-香豆酰辅酶 A、查尔酮、黄烷酮、二氢黄酮醇等，其中聚酮合酶(polyketide synthase, PS)、P450、酮戊二酸氧化酶($Fe^{2+}$/2-oxoglutarate-dependent dioxygenases, 2ODD)、UGT、甲基转移酶(methyltransferase, MT)等在产生苯丙素类化合物结构多样性过程中发挥了重要作用。与萜类化合物以及苯丙素类化合物生物合成不同的是，生物碱以不同的氨基酸为前体，比如单萜吲哚生物碱以 L-色氨酸和 GPP 为前体，异喹啉类生物碱以 L-酪氨酸为前体，烟碱和莨菪碱等以鸟氨酸为前体，在生物碱的生物合成过程中，P450、MT、还原酶（reductase）、脱羧酶（decarboxylase）等参与其结构形成和结构修饰过程（图 2）。

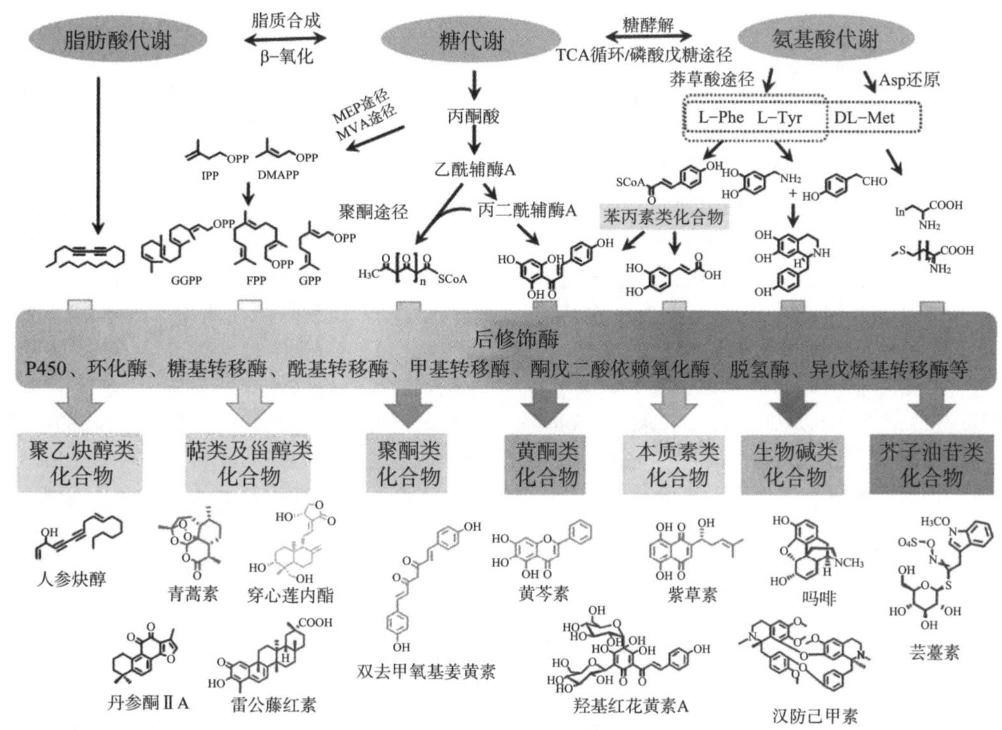


**图 2　中药活性成分生物合成途径**

上游前体形成过程在不同的植物中相对保守，随着基因组测序、转录组测序等技术的提升和成本的下降，上游途径在不同的药用植物中已经研究得很透彻。药用活性成分是这些前体化合物在不同的药用植物中经过不同的结构修饰所产生的活性各异的化合物，这些不同类型的结构修饰是药用植物药效差异的关键。解析其后修饰过程是研究药效物质形成的基础，为合成生物学及代谢工程改良生产药用植物活性成分提供元件和途径。

1.1　*基于组学数据的酶挖掘和功能研究*　中药活性成分生物合成途径十分复杂，往往涉及几个甚至几十个酶的参与。不同于微生物生物合成途径的酶大多在基因组上成簇存在，植物次生代谢途径的基因经过植物基因组的复制和“新功能化”，大多分散在植物基因组中，即使在基因组中成簇，也是在较大的范围内成簇，因此针对植物次生代谢途径生物元件的挖掘具有一定的难度。由于植物次生代谢途径基因大多以基因家族存在，比如在植物次生代谢途径中参与度非常高的细胞色素 P450 酶，在丹参基因组中有 340 个，而参与到丹参酮生物合成途径中的可能不超过 10%，因此对于未有研究过的途径进行分析很大程度上依赖于精确的候选基因筛选。

基因测序技术的加速、检测灵敏度的提升、组学分析技术的发展，为药用植物中活性成分生物合成途径解析提供了更高效的分析筛选手段。大多数情况下，药用活性成分的积累与基因表达成正相关，通过比较组学分析，能有效缩小候选基因范围，获得有效候选基因。以丹参酮为例，丹参酮的积累在丹参毛状根中受生物和非生物因子诱导表达上调，通过对不同诱导时间段的代谢组以及转录组进行比较分析，发现参与丹参酮生物合成的萜类合酶基因表达上调，基于此筛选到 40 个诱导表达上调的 P450 基因，进一步结合时空表达分析，筛选得到可能与丹参酮生物合成相关的多个基因，利用体外酶促结合体内 RNA 干扰研究发现，其中 CYP76AH1, CYP76AH3 和 CYP76AK1 能够催化丹参酮碳骨架结构生成 C 环酮基化的中间代谢产物，CYP71D373 和 CYP71D375 能够催化丹参酮特征五元呋喃环的形成。这种基于比较时空组学分析的基因筛选策略在药用活性成分生物合成研究中应用非常广泛。植物 RNA 干扰或者基于 CRISPR 的基因敲除为候选基因的筛选提供了另一种有效途径，通过对同源性较高的 CYP71D 家族基因型进行 RNA 干扰实验，结果表明，在 RNA 干扰株系中，目标亚基因家族的 4 个基因表达量都有不同程度的下降，代谢物检测发现其中含有呋喃环的丹参酮类化合物积累下调，而不含呋喃环的代谢物显著积累，通过这一方法成功获得丹参酮生物合成途径呋喃环形成的关键催化酶，并且基因组共线性分析也表明，这些基因是丹参属中特有，赋予丹参特有的药效活性。

1.2　*酶改造和定向进化提升酶催化效率*　近年来，中药活性成分尤其是一些具有明确药理活性天然产物的生物合成途径解析广受关注，生物合成途径中有越来越多的生物元件被挖掘，其功能得以解析，为药用植物次生代谢研究提供了思路和方法参考。随着数据的不断增多，越来越多的研究表明，次生代谢途径生物元件具有广泛的催化混杂性，包括底物杂泛性或者催化位点杂泛性，导致植物中次生代谢网络的形成。如穿心莲中的一个糖基转移酶具有非常宽泛的杂泛性，能催化 26 种不同类型的底物（二萜及其衍生物、黄酮类化合物，以及一些简单的芳香族化合物)形成 $O$-、$S$-、$N$-等糖苷。这种催化杂泛性,一方面产生了复杂的药用植物代谢网络,生成结构多样的小分子化合物,但是另一方面,酶的专一性较差影响了目标代谢物的生成和积累,因此基于结构生物学的酶理性结构改造成为近几年的研究热点。通过对丹参酮生物合成途径两个同源性 70% 左右的 P450 进行序列比对分析、分子对接以及点突变改造,成功将两个基因的功能整合至一个 P450 中,显著提升了催化效率。另一方面,酶的改造很大程度上依赖于对酶蛋白结构及其催化机制的了解,通过解析蛋白结构,对关键氨基酸残基进行改造,从而改造酶的催化特性,拓宽其开发应用价值。但是蛋白质组的全面结构解析是后基因组时代的一个重要挑战,截至目前,仅有 35% 的人类蛋白质结构被登记到蛋白质数据库(PDB 数据库),不同蛋白的表达、纯化、数据收集处理还需要克服诸多障碍。所幸的是,2021 年 8 月 DeepMind 公司在其前期工作的基础上公布了 AlphaFold2 人工智能系统及其源代码,其蛋白三级结构预测的准确性和精度进一步提升,在一定程度上解决了一些难以获得晶体的蛋白的建模难题,推动基于结构-功能相关性的结构改造和提升。

自然界中生命无时无刻不在进化发展,但是一个新性状的稳定遗传需要相当长的时间。随着基因工程技术的不断发展,科学家可以通过实验室模拟和加速自然进化,并设计高通量筛选方法来获得目标性状。2018 年,弗朗西斯·阿诺德因酶的定向进化获得诺贝尔化学奖,阿诺德的实验室通过酶的进化演化,产生能够催化自然界不存在的化学反应,利用进化的力量解决化学问题。植物次生代谢的酶在微生物中的表达和功能往往受限,而随着结构生物学和计算生物学的发展,越来越多的酶结构被解析、海量数据集出现、量子化学理论及方法的不断完善、机器学习等人工智能的应用等,人们对酶蛋白序列及其结构与功能关系有了更深入的认识,辅助于计算机的模拟计算可以对酶进行重新设计,并预测突变蛋白的表达、稳定性、活性等特性,通过这样理性的设计计算以及有针对性的建库和筛选,实现了酶的半理性设计。研究者通过利用定向进化技术与晶体结构解析以及理论计算设计的组合,解析了柠檬烯环氧化物水解酶的催化特异性与立体选择性的催化机制;改造了糖基转移酶的区域选择性,将杂泛性糖基转移酶定向改造为具有催化位点特异性的酶。计算生物学和计算化学的发展和应用将为酶的定向进化提速,从而获得目标更明确的酶,以应用到植物天然产物的生成和结构改造中。

1.3 合成途径解析及途径设计 药用活性成分在植物中的合成经过一系列酶的催化产生目标产物,除了人参皂苷、β-榄香烯等部分小分子化合物的完整合成途径已经被解析,大多数药用活性化合物的完整合成途径仍然不明确。青蒿素前体物质青蒿酸虽然已经实现了合成生物学方式的工业化生产,但从青蒿酸到青蒿素的合成过程是否有酶的参与,是哪类酶发挥作用仍然不明确。紫杉醇生物合成的 19 步途径中仍然有多步未被解析,导致合成生物学生产的工作始终无法开展,其生物合成途径的解析备受全球关注。因此在未来一段时间之内,生物合成途径的解析仍然会是中药活性成分生物合成研究应用的瓶颈。转录组和基因组数据提供了丰富的基因元件,全自动克隆挑选系统的应用为高通量筛选提供了平台,但是针对大多数代谢产物的高通量检测技术还非常有限,限制了高通量筛选平台的应用,这是需要重点攻克的难题。随着科技投入的增加,越来越多的课题投入到相关的研究中,这将加快推动该项技术的进步,促进生物合成途径解析速度的提升。

不断产生的组学数据和被验证了功能的基因同时也为计算生物学方法设计生物合成路径提供了数据和基础。2015 年,*Science* 发表了有关阿片类化合物的生物合成途径全解析的文章,涉及 20 多个步骤,研究人员从数据库中挖掘了跨越植物、微生物、动物不同物种的生物元件,完成蒂巴因(thebaine)的 21 步催化过程和氢可酮(hydrocodone)的 23 步催化过程,并在酵母中实现了途径重构,该研究被评为当年十大科学进展,这种复杂代谢途径的解析以及重构被认为是合成生物学的里程碑事件。2021 年,该团队利用计算生物学的方法,基于文献检索、专利检索、计算预测来挖掘活性结构化合物,并预测筛选合成活性结构化合物的高效催化酶,成功完成了四氢巴马汀[($S$)-tetrahydropalmatine]的合成及结构衍生。不断验证的功能基因为计算生物学提供基础数据库,而基于大数据、计算生物学、人工智能相结合的元件筛选、途径解析将在中药活性成分形成机制研究中发挥越来越重要的作用。

由于次生代谢途径中酶的催化混杂性,产生一系列结构类似的化合物,增加了目标化合物分离提取的难度以及生产成本,因此有必要明确植物体内的合成及调控机制。虽然用计算生物学方法在一定程度上能帮助解析药用活性成分的生物合成途径,但是在植物体内,途径解析和代谢网络搭建对了解合成过程以及更好地在植物中调控目标化合物的生成具有重要意义。在异源重构的过程中,正确的路径对于合成生物学途径创建具有重要的参考价值,因此通过元件挖掘,结合植物体内 RNA 干扰、过表达、基因编辑等方法,利用高灵敏检测技术对植物体内代谢物的系统全面分析,解析生物合成途径,能帮助人们更好地了解代谢物的合成及调控,为代谢工程改良以及合成生物学生产提供基础和指导。

## 2 中药活性成分合成生物学生产

中药活性成分在药用植物中大多以次生代谢产物的形式积累,含量相对较低,如人参皂苷作为传统名贵中药人参的主要次生代谢产物,近年来陆续有研究表明,不同结构修饰的人参皂苷类化合物具有多种药理活性,但不同人参皂苷在人参中含量各异。含量低、结构类似物多等问题导致中药活性成分分离纯化困难、获取成本高,在一定程度上限制了中药活性成分的深入开发利用。因此,来源稳定、质量均一的获取方式是中药活性成分深入开发的一个重要前提。近 20 年迅速发展起来的合成生物学为中药活性成分提供了新的、可持续获取的有效策略。通过生物合成途径解析,在微生物中重构中药活性成分的生物合成途径,调控代谢流,优化发酵条件能实现中药活性成分的高效绿色生产。结合合成生物学以及化学转化,研究者们已经实现了青蒿素的细胞工厂生产,酵母中阿片类化合物的生成等里程碑式成果;构建了鼠尾草酸、人参皂苷、大麻素类化合物等的一系列工程菌株,通过在微生物中高效生产中药活性成分或其前体化合物,将有效缓解中医临床用药的压力。

2.1 中药活性成分高产基因工程菌的构建 中药活性成分合成生物学菌株的构建主要是在成分代谢途径清晰的基础上，根据底盘细胞自身的代谢和蛋白修饰特点，在底盘菌内实现已有代谢途径的修饰并引入外源基因进行途径重构。外源基因的引入和底盘细胞的改造修饰使工程菌的生物合成形成相互交错的动态代谢网络，需从整体上对其代谢网络进行引流和调控优化，从而实现目标中药活性成分的高效生物合成。

目前用于中药活性成分合成生物学菌株构建比较常用的底盘细胞有酿酒酵母和大肠杆菌，这两种底盘细胞遗传背景清晰、遗传转化体系成熟、可用操作工具多、生长迅速。但是通常情况下，这些底盘细胞中积累次生代谢产物前体的功能较弱，因此提升前体供给是中药活性成分高产基因工程菌构建的基础。通过筛选多种植物及微生物来源的基因元件，进行高拷贝强启动表达，是中药活性成分工程菌构建的基本策略。另外，过表达反应所需辅酶合成途径，增加其转运效率，补全底盘菌缺陷型，抑制竞争途径等是提高前体积累的常用策略。在松香烷型二萜的前体物质次丹参酮二烯工程菌的构建中，Zhou 等通过过表达萜类上游途径关键酶基因和构建融合蛋白，将丹参酮以及雷公藤内酯的碳骨架结构——次丹参酮二烯的产量提高到 365 mg/L。Hu 等进一步利用 CRISPR/Cas9 技术修饰萜类上游合成途径，敲除竞争支路基因，并筛选多物种来源的松香烷型二萜合酶，将次丹参酮二烯产量提高到 3.5 g/L。

由于一些次生代谢中间产物具有细胞毒性或者存在反馈调节，影响菌体增长和产物积累，通过构建融合蛋白或者蛋白支架，能一定程度上调节代谢流，进而提高产量。左旋龙脑是具有抗炎和镇痛作用的单萜类中药活性成分，冰片基焦磷酸合酶(CbTPS1)是其生物合成途径中的关键合成酶，Ma 等人从梅片树中鉴定出了高度特异性的 CbTPS1，并经过设计截短和添加 Kozak 序列对 CbTPS1 进行改造，同时与 ERG20WW 融合以增强通往 CbTPS1 的代谢流，使左旋龙脑在酵母中的产量提高了 96.33 倍。此外，针对途径中蛋白的动态调控也能防止有毒代谢物的积累，引入可以检测和响应代谢物的传感器，可以有效实现这一动态调控。然而，针对不同代谢物的传感器在很大程度上是未知的。Dahl 等应用全基因组转录阵列来识别响应有毒中间体积累的启动子，利用这些启动子控制中间体的积累，并提高目标产物的最终产量，消除了对昂贵诱导剂的需求，改善了菌体生长情况。

目前，通过微生物生产高价值化合物大多在细胞质中完成，但合成过程多存在竞争途径阻碍目标化合物在细胞质中的有效合成，并且有相当多的中药活性成分具有抗菌活性，导致微生物基因工程菌构建过程中化合物产量提升困难。真核细胞通过利用细胞器隔离生化途径以控制其代谢的复杂性，受此启发，研究者们采用叶绿体、过氧化物酶体、脂滴等亚细胞器作为外源基因表达和蛋白催化的场所。在酵母过氧化物酶体中构建香叶基二磷酸衍生化合物的微工厂，能够使产量较胞质中增加 125 倍，成功将乙酰辅酶 A 转化为具有高商业价值的单萜、单萜吲哚生物碱和大麻素类化合物，使过氧化物酶体工程成为生产类异戊二烯类化合物的有效策略。中国科学院天津工业生物技术研究所与中国中医科学院中药资源中心合作开展人参皂苷酵母工程菌的构建过程中，通过利用脂滴膜蛋白将关键酶靶向至脂滴，在细胞内建立生物反应区室，显著提高了人参皂苷前体 PPD 的生产效率，以三七中人参皂苷 CK 生成模块为例进行转化，获得 CK 产量高达 5 g/L 的工程菌，为稀有人参皂苷的获取提供了高效策略。代谢途径的亚细胞器定位不仅可以避免细胞溶质因子的串扰，还可以将细胞毒性产物隔离，使代谢物底物和产物实现跨过氧化物酶体膜的自由流动，在(*S*)-牛心果碱和下游途径苄基异喹啉生物碱产量提升中取得显著效果，呈现出具有代谢工程所需特征的工程细胞器的潜力。

2.2 适合中药活性成分积累的底盘菌构建 结构后修饰酶通过对天然产物进行修饰，使中药天然成分的结构更加多样，从而提高了成功筛选获得中药活性成分的概率。结构后修饰酶发挥催化功能过程中，需要大量基团供体、辅助因子或在细胞中的特定部位表达等，因此，结构后修饰酶在底盘细胞的高效表达是中药活性成分生物合成研究的重点和难点。在针对中药活性成分底盘菌的构建中，研究者们通过代谢工程提高前体供给，扩展后修饰酶底物谱，增强后修饰酶的立体选择性，提高辅因子产量等方法改良后修饰酶在底盘细胞的表达情况，加速了中药活性成分合成生物学的研究进程。

中药活性成分生物合成后修饰中常见多个 P450 的连续催化反应，据统计 93% 的萜类化合物需要经过 P450 酶的修饰。在中药活性成分底盘菌构建中，常遇到 P450 酶表达稳定性差、辅因子消耗快等问题，是合成生物学研究中尚未有效解决的关键问题。除了针对 P450 蛋白本身进行定向进化改造，缩短催化路径、提高反应效率外，关于辅助因子的研究也为改善其催化效率提供了思路。Liu 等对 P450 蛋白结合的铁血红素的生物合成途径进行工程改造，显著提高了酵母细胞中的铁血红素水平，这是辅助酵母细胞质 P450 蛋白形成催化性结构和发挥功能的潜在策略。NADPH 是大多 P450s 发挥功能的辅助因子，在催化过程中的消耗量极高，其在细胞中的快速再生可以通过 P450s 和醇脱氢酶(alcoholdehydrogenase, ADH)的级联反应实现，这种联合表达策略在天然萜类樟脑的氧化中取得了有效成果，使樟脑的转化率增加了 5 倍。

2.3 组合生物学产生结构衍生化合物 中药天然产物是药物研发的物质基础，但大多数天然产物还需经过提高药效、降低毒性等成药性改造。例如，木脂素五味子丙素具有保肝和降低转氨酶的作用，其结构衍生物联苯双酯的活性强于五味子丙素，因此被开发成新药；进一步将其中一个羧酸酯还原成羟甲基以提高其溶解性，从而被开发成用于降低转氨酶的药物双环醇。基于现代生物催化技术改造中药天然产物，结合合成生物学的绿色低成本生产方式，能有效提升植物天然产物的成药性，推动植物天然产物生物合成和合成生物学生产的转化应用，为中药活性成分的成药性改造提供新的策略。

糖基化通常用于改善苷元的特性，例如溶解度、稳定性和药理活性。丹参酮 $\mathrm{II_A}$ 是一种具有显著抗动脉粥样硬化活性的中药活性化合物，增加其水溶性和生物利用度有助于对其进行成药性开发。通过微生物转化对丹参酮 $\mathrm{II_A}$ 进行糖基化修饰，能够使其在甲醇-水溶液中的溶解度较改造前升高 50 倍，并显著改善其在小鼠体内的口服吸收率。甘草次酸(glycyrrhetnic acid, GA)是一种具有多种药理作用和生物活性的五环三萜疏水苷元，利用大肠杆菌表达系统纯化出GA糖基化的生物催化剂蛋白，将GA转化为相应的GA-3-*O*-单葡萄糖，能使其溶解度和抗菌生物活性显著提高。这表明重组糖基转移酶等蛋白有可能被用作工业和药物用途中糖基化的生物催化剂，用于组合生物学生产活性更优、利用度更佳的结构衍生化合物。甲基化则通常可以改善化合物的脂溶性，从而改善其活性。Cui等利用组合生物学方法和合成生物学相结合，筛选到两个能催化黄芩素甲氧基化的酶，活性研究表明，黄芩素甲氧基化后显著提升其抑制癌细胞生长的活性，且对正常细胞没有毒性，为中药活性成分生物合成研究的应用提供了新思路。

生物合成途径中酶催化的杂泛性导致植物中结构类似产物产生，但结构上的微小差异往往导致化合物活性的消失甚至毒性的产生，并且目标活性化合物与副产物结构和理化性质极为相似，对目标活性产物的提取分离造成了极大的困难，严重阻碍了其原材料的获取和成药开发。合成生物学研究可以在微生物中组装构建目标产物单一合成路径，从而减少副产物的生成。同时，与关键蛋白的定向改造技术相结合，能减轻或去除蛋白催化的杂泛性，在细胞工厂内生产结构单一，提取分离简便的目标活性产物。研究者们利用合成生物学技术成功衍生了结构多样、性质改良的生物活性分子和潜在新药。随着药学、酶学和生物信息学等研究的快速发展，合成生物学技术在新型天然产物的发现、活性天然分子的成药性改良和绿色生产等方面将发挥不可替代的作用。

## 3 代谢工程改良

微生物细胞工厂已实现了诸多中药活性成分的高效合成，但仍然存在高耗能、高耗氧、P450酶表达性差、对次生代谢产物耐受性差等问题。相比之下，植物底盘细胞有其优越性，仅以二氧化碳和水为原料，经光合作用就可合成各种复杂的次生代谢产物，同时，植物底盘细胞本身复杂分区化、不同器官分工协作也为实现复杂人工设计提供了可能。因此药用植物代谢工程成了获得高价值中药活性分子的另一种选择。

代谢工程技术是通过基因工程技术改变代谢流，或扩展、重构代谢途径以获得高产量、高纯度的药用活性成分的方法。有些次生代谢产物药理活性强但毒副作用较大，通过代谢工程技术改善其生物活性，有望制造出具有新的或改进的生物学特性的全新分子。与此同时，考虑到植物体内各种影响目标产物合成与分解的遗传因素、环境因子都可能会影响代谢流中化合物的积累，所以通过基因工程技术对代谢途径进行改造成为代谢工程最有效的手段，目前常用的策略包括增强关键酶的表达或活性，调节调控因子的表达，促进代谢产物的跨膜转运，抑制代谢竞争路径或削弱代谢产物的反馈抑制。

针对酶基因常用的基因工程手段有基因过表达、基因共表达、RNAi、VIGS等。2012年CRISPR/Cas9基因编辑技术的出现，对近10年的生命科学研究及应用产生了深远影响，并获得了2020年的诺贝尔化学奖。2016年，中国科学院遗传与发育生物学研究所高彩霞研究团队在小麦中建立了基于CRISPR/Cas9瞬时表达基因组编辑系统，之后考虑到生物安全问题，又通过体外组装核糖核蛋白复合体RNP建立了全程无外源DNA的基因组编辑系统。2019年报道了一种新型的Cas蛋白（Cas12a/Cpf1）扩展了基因编辑所依赖的Cas蛋白的种类。最近，中国科学家利用基因编辑技术实现了四倍体野生水稻的快速驯化。基因编辑技术的应用缩短了作物的驯化周期，推动了创新作物的诞生，为生长周期长的药用植物提供了技术平台。

3.1 基因编辑定向驯化　基因编辑技术是一种可以精准实现定向遗传改良的现代生物技术，在三大类型（Ⅰ型、Ⅱ型和Ⅲ型）中，Ⅱ型系统CRISPR/Cas9设计简单，并且迅速推广到各种植物的研究中，包括拟南芥、烟草、水稻、小麦、玉米等。一方面用于目标基因的功能研究，另一方面用于优良性状的快速建立。另外，CRISPR/Cas9也可以实现对多个靶位点或多个基因的同时定点修饰。不断更新的基因编辑技术，为遗传操作尚不成熟的药用植物改良提供了诸多的工具和选择。

在次生代谢产物研究方面，CRISPR/Cas9技术主要用于研究植物体外系统的生物合成潜力，通过关闭竞争途径，最终将代谢通量转向目标化合物的生产。通过敲除丹参毛状根*RAS*基因获得的纯合突变体中，迷迭香酸和丹酚酸B含量显著降低，而杂合突变体中含量降低不明显。通过敲除丹参*SmCPS1*基因阻断了GGPP的代谢通量，从而阻断丹参酮的生物合成，由于丹参酮和紫杉醇具有相同的前体（GGPP），研究者们认为GGPP在理论上可以作为其他有价值的二萜生物合成的来源，如紫杉醇。研究者通过敲除罂粟的*4′OMT2*基因使吗啡和蒂巴因含量显著降低，并产生了一种新的苄基异喹啉类生物碱。在定向育种方面，育种家利用连续回交结合分子标记辅助选择策略培育了各种抗性水稻品种，但该策略培育周期长、背景选择随世代提高，进而会因为连锁累赘等导致出现不利表型。近些年，基因编辑技术逐渐被应用于作物的生产实践，该技术可以快速改良作物的农艺性状。2013年，研究者们利用CRISPR技术对水稻香味基因*OsBADH2*进行定点敲除，获得了香稻*osbadh2*突变体，对水稻直链淀粉含量相关基因*OsWaxy*进行定点敲除，创建了糯性水稻资源。基因组编辑CRISPR/Cas9辅助的性状改良与自然驯化相比，具有快速、精准、经济等优点，但需要建立可行的基因组编辑技术体系，获取完整的基因组序列信息以及确定重要农艺性状形成的关键基因及其调控机理。2021年3月，李家洋院士团队联合国内外多家单位研究人员通过组装异源四倍体高秆野生稻基因组，优化遗传转化体系，结合多维基因组学和多靶点精准基因组编辑技术，获得高度显著降低、籽粒长度显著增加的突变体，绘制了异源四倍体野生稻从头驯化的“蓝图”，使作物驯化时间呈现“跳跃式”前进。药用植物栽培种植大多是野生抚育，没有驯化的过程，因此难以形成稳定的品种，基于基因编辑的驯化研究能为药用植物品种构建提供支撑。

3.2 植物细胞工厂构建　生物反应器除了上文提到的大肠杆菌和酵母外，昆虫哺乳动物细胞或植物细胞也常作为生物工厂，用于大规模生产人类使用的疫苗和药用蛋白。从对外源蛋白的加工修饰来说，哺乳动物细胞是较为理想的表达系统，已被应用于数百种药用蛋白的生产，但哺乳动物细胞培养的条件不易掌握，容易污染，所以对资金和技术都有一定的要求。而随着植物基因工程的发展和转基因技术的不断进步，人们已成功实现了植物疫苗和植物源性抗体的表达，植物作为生物反应器已经受到了越来越多的科研机构和商业公司的青睐。

植物生物反应器利用植物细胞、组织、器官或整株植株，大量生产具有重要功能的蛋白质，如疫苗、抗体或次生代谢产物等。相比于以上单细胞培养系统，植物通过光合作用产生能量，代表了未来代谢工程可持续发展的重要方向。植物反应器最大的优势是经济成本低，仅为微生物发酵培养的2%～10%，动物细胞培养生产成本的0.1%～1%。植物的可食性让其表达的医疗或者药用蛋白可以被直接口服，且植物不会携带人类或动物的病原微生物，种植简单，更易大规模生产，但是现阶段很难回答哪种植物作为底盘细胞是最好的。模式植物拟南芥研究基础好且资源极其丰富，是基因组学和基因工程中植物模型的首选，在受控条件下最容易转化和生长，优势十分显著，但它缺乏充足的生物量。因此多数重组蛋白生产的表达系统往往选择生物量相对较大、容易转化且易于操作的模式植物烟草。大量其他植物种类（如水稻、玉米、小麦、大豆、马铃薯、番茄、莴苣和生菜等）也逐渐被用来生产重组蛋白。

目前我国植物生物反应器的研究和利用还主要集中在利用模式植物表达或生产药用蛋白的研究和应用方面，而由于药用植物遗传转化体系不成熟，利用代谢调控及代谢工程等技术对植物进行遗传改造，进而大量生产有用的植物次生代谢产物的研究还相对薄弱。已有的报道仅限于在药用植物组织培养体系中进行代谢调控，或利用烟草等遗传转化成熟的植物作为生物反应器来合成中药活性成分。常用的代谢工程改良策略包括：增强关键酶的表达或活性，调节调控因子的表达，促进代谢产物的跨膜转运，抑制代谢竞争路径或削弱代谢产物的反馈抑制，以及次生代谢物区室化。理论上，单独或者联合使用这些策略，都可以促进药用植物中目标产物的生物合成，提高其产量，但在实际应用中，关键酶基因的过量表达应用较多。例如，2004 年，在药用植物天仙子发状根中同时过表达两个关键酶基因 *PMT* 和 *H6H*，将其中东莨菪碱含量提升到野生对照组的 9 倍，达到了 411 mg/L。将青蒿素代谢途径关键酶基因 *FPS* 导入青蒿中，青蒿素含量提高了 40%。在丹参毛状根中过表达萜类生物合成限速酶 HMGR 基因，其丹参酮含量是对照组的 4.2 倍。抑制代谢竞争路径也能显著提升目标化合物积累，通过下调影响青蒿素生物合成的竞争支路上的关键基因 β-石竹烯合成酶（CPS）、β-法呢基焦磷酸合成酶（BFS）和角鲨烯合成酶（SQS），使青蒿素含量提升达70%。另一方面，利用烟草等遗传转化体系成熟的植物作为异源合成载体生产中药活性成分也有报道，2016 年，Fuentes 等将青蒿素生物合成的核心途径整合到烟草叶绿体基因组中，同时将辅助基因整合到核基因组，最终获得 120 mg/kg 青蒿酸。2019 年，Schultz 等将编码针叶树醇和依托泊苷苷元途径的 16 个基因在烟草叶片中瞬时表达，其去氧鬼臼毒素积累达 4.3 mg/g 干重。虽然目前利用植物生物反应器生产次生代谢产物的例子屈指可数，但随着对重要生物活性代谢物的生物合成所涉及的复杂植物代谢网络的进一步了解，以及对支配次生代谢的调控系统的更深入的了解，植物生物反应器的研究和应用前景将越来越广阔。

## 4 总结与展望

中药活性成分主要是植物次生代谢产物，种类繁多，广泛参与植物的生长、发育和防御等生理过程，对植物自身在复杂环境中的生存和发展起到了重要作用。同时，次生代谢产物向人类提供了大量有用的天然有机化合物，占所有治疗药的1/3 以上。然而，中药活性成分在原植物中含量较低，加之药用植物大多生长缓慢或在实验室条件下无法培养，影响了中药活性成分的开发和利用。随着测序技术、高分辨检测技术、合成生物学技术的发展，通过解析中药活性成分生物合成途径，利用合成生物学方法构建微生物细胞工厂，或者通过代谢工程手段进行遗传改良，为药用活性成分的获取提供了新方式。同时，中药活性成分作为中药发挥药效的物质基础，对其合成及代谢网络的了解，有助于人们更清晰地了解药效形成及道地性形成的机制，推动中医药现代化研究。

从 2006 年报道利用酵母基因工程菌生产青蒿素至今，中药活性成分生物合成及相关研究取得了突破进展，丹参酮（图3）、人参皂苷、雷公藤甲素、乌头碱等中药活性成分生物合成逐渐得以解析。同时，基因组测序手段的提升以及成本的下降，释放了大量用于基因筛选的遗传资源，也为合成生物学相关研究提供了丰富的元件库。然而，现阶段虽然已有大量的研究报道，但是显著性成果屈指可数，具有特殊催化功能的酶的发现及其催化机制的研究依然具有一定的难度，生物合成途径被完全解析的仍然不多。大量数据的积累一方面为酶的筛选以及利用组合成生物学生成结构修饰新产物提供了丰富的元件，但也加大了筛选的难度。因此高通量筛选手段、全自动克隆系统、高通量检测技术等的研发非常有必要。另外，通

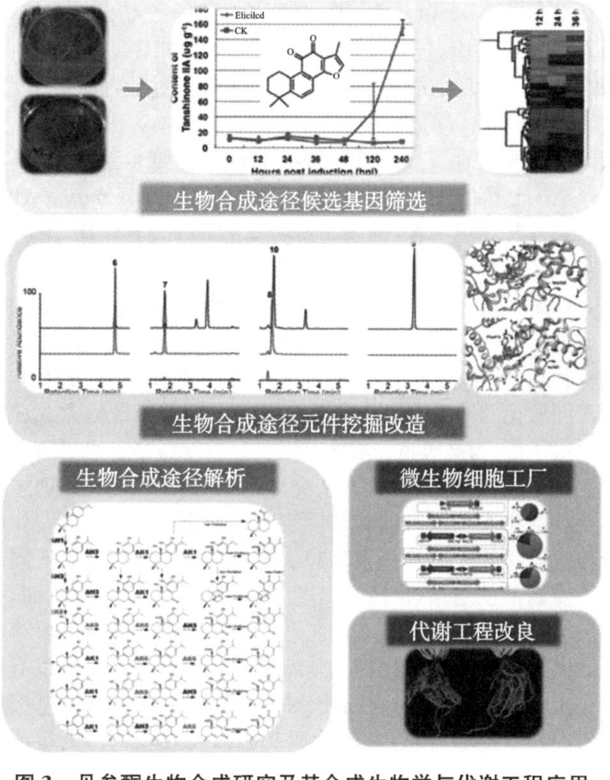


**图 3　丹参酮生物合成研究及其合成生物学与代谢工程应用**

过多组学多维度的比较分析，或者依托人工智能等进行计算设计能有效助推催化酶的筛选和改造。总之，新方法新技术的发展将更快推动中药活性成分生物合成途径的解析。

基于合成生物学技术的微生物基因工程菌的构建已经初显成效，青蒿素、人参皂苷酵母的细胞工厂生产成本已经能与植物提取相抗衡，但对于具有细胞毒性的化合物比如冰片、合成途径冗长的化合物比如吗啡、紫杉醇等，实现微生物生产还有一定的距离。亚细胞器工程、蛋白质工程等对产量的提升有一定成效，另外不断开发应用的新底盘细胞，比如解脂耶氏酵母、甲醇酵母、绿藻等的使用，为中药活性成分细胞工厂构建提供了新的选择。相关底盘基因编辑工具的开发将为在新型底盘细胞中构建中药活性成分合成途径奠定坚实的基础。

药用植物的代谢工程改良是中药活性成分生物合成途径研究的另一个应用方向，但也正是由于植物细胞代谢的特殊性、植物次生代谢途径的复杂性，以及植物生物反应器（植物细胞、组织、器官或植株）的选择问题，建立大规模、可持续的次生代谢产物生产过程，仍有许多瓶颈问题。例如，大多数次生代谢产物的生物合成途径尚未完全解析，已被解析的次生代谢产物的生物合成调控机制尚不十分清楚，合成途径中间体不易获取导致关键基因鉴定受阻等，这些问题都影响着代谢工程研究的进程。药用植物代谢工程改良还面临的另一个挑战是遗传转化和基因编辑难度大，大多数药用植物遗传转化尚未实现，未来基因编辑是植物改良的重要方向，但是建立在遗传转化的基础上，因此加大投入提前技术储备非常必要。更高效基因编辑工具的开发，将为植物底盘的构建以及药用植物代谢工程改造提供技术支持和平台。

中医药是我国古代文明的瑰宝，在新冠疫情防控中发挥重要作用。随着国家对科技投入以及对中医药的重视，越来越多的交叉学科开始关注中医药领域。习近平主席在中国中医科学院成立 60 周年贺信中强调，中医药振兴发展迎来了天时、地利、人和的大好时机。中医药科研工作者唯有抓住机遇、迎接挑战，通过生物技术、生命科学和计算科学等的交叉融合与团队协作，共同促进中医药传承创新发展，共同推动中医药的现代化和国际化。

[马莹，郭娟，黄璐琦，等. 中国科学，2022，52(6)：894－907.]

# 植物质体基因工程调控元件研究进展

质体基因工程的发展历程最早可追溯到 20 世纪 80 年代。1987 年，Daniell 等发现，经 EDTA 体外处理的黄瓜（*Cucumis sativus*）白色体可吸收来自细菌的 *CAT* 基因和蓝藻的 *RuBisCO* 基因，且能够在体内表达这些基因。早期的质体基因工程涉及复杂的质体分离与体外培养过程，操作难度较大，基因枪的出现简化了该操作流程，质体基因工程也由此进入了新的发展阶段。1988 年，Boynton 等将野生型 *atpB* 基因整合至该基因突变型莱茵衣藻（*Chlamydomonas reinhardtii*）的叶绿体基因组中，使莱茵衣藻恢复正常的光合作用功能，首次实现了质体基因工程在单细胞真核生物中的应用。1990 年，Svab 等报道了烟草（*Nicotiana tabacum*）质体基因组的稳定遗传转化，标志着高等植物质体基因工程的开端，此后 Svab 等将壮观霉素抗性基因 *aadA* 靶向整合至烟草质体基因组，得到了同质化的转质体烟草品系并能够以母系遗传的方式稳定遗传给子代，为高等植物质体基因工程的发展奠定了基础。

在过去的一个世纪中，杂交育种是栽培作物获得理想农艺性状的主要手段。随着基因工程的兴起，使得转基因作物较传统栽培作物更易获得理想农艺性状，在提升产量的同时降低农药的使用量，这极大促进了生态农业的发展。然而，大部分转基因作物通过核基因工程实现外源基因的转化，存在外源基因表达量低或生物安全问题。质体基因工程可以有效避免上述情况的发生，在同质化的转质体细胞中，外源基因高达 10 000 个拷贝，可以实现外源基因的高效表达。更重要的是，质体基因组的母系遗传特性能够有效减少或消除外源基因通过花粉逃逸的可能性。

质体(plastid)包括叶绿体、色质体（或称有色体）和白色体，根据内共生学说，质体起源于与真核宿主细胞发生内共生相互作用的蓝细菌，因而质体在基因转录及翻译等方面具有原核特性，且在漫长的进化过程中，大部分原先存在于质体基因组中的基因已转移至细胞核中，仅有少部分基因保留在质体基因组。植物叶绿体基因组是一个大小约为 150 kb 的环状分子，包含 120～130 个基因，其中大部分基因与光合作用或叶绿体基因表达（即编码核糖体的 RNA 和蛋白质亚基、RNA 聚合酶亚基和 tRNA）相关。叶绿体作为植物重要的代谢合成中心，可通过光合作用将太阳能转化为化学能。此外，叶绿体还参与核酸、氨基酸、脂肪酸以及次生代谢产物的生物合成，是植物生长发育过程中重要的细胞器。随着高通量测序技术不断升级迭代，已有越来越多物种的叶绿体基因组信息被揭示，这在一定程度上也促进了质体基因工程的持续发展。随着研究的不断深入，开展质体基因工程的高等植物数量已十分可观，如烟草、拟南芥（*Arabidopsis thaliana*）、马铃薯（*Solanum tuberosum*）、番茄（*Lycopersicon esculentum*）、大豆（*Glycine max*）、莴苣（*Lactuca sativa*）和黄花蒿（*Artemisia annua*）等。相比于其他高等植物物种，烟草具有产量高、质体转化体系成熟、遗传操作简便等优势，且开展以烟草为底盘的质体基因工程研究可以有效降低对食物链的污染，因此烟草已成为当前质体基因工程的模式植物。

由于质体表达系统具有原核表达特性，具备相对独立的区室，拥有丰富的代谢模块，这些特性使质体成为代谢工程及合成生物学的理想受体。截至目前，质体基因工程已广泛应用于性状改良、生物医药以及合成生物学等领域，并取得了丰硕的研究成果。与此同时，质体基因工程也为质体系统的RNA转录调控、蛋白翻译机制、调控元件筛选与鉴定等研究领域提供了帮助。近年来，质体基因工程主要致力于质体转化载体(图1)的设计方案优化(表1)，其中选择稳定且具有高效转录、翻译能力的表达调控元件是实现外源基因高效表达的关键，但外源基因的组成型高效表达会对植物的生长和发育造成代谢负担。为了最大限度地避免这种负面影响，需要采用适当的合成操纵子构建策略实现外源基因在特定时期或空间的表达。因此，本文对质体基因工程的表达调控元件进行了总结，并重点介绍了近5年质体基因工程合成操纵子构建策略的最新研究进展。

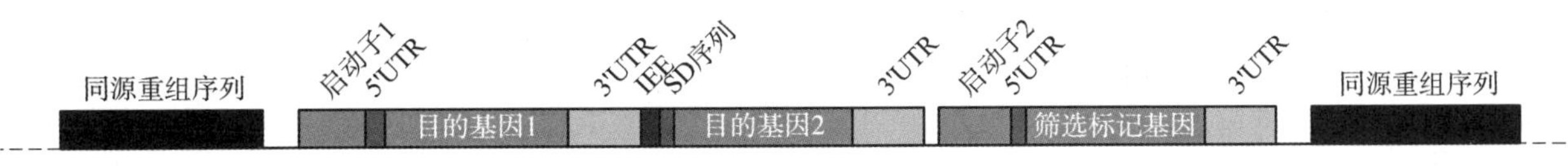


**图1 质体转化载体结构**

黑色方框：左右两侧质体同源重组序列，用于外源蛋白质合成操纵子的定向整合；绿色方框：代表启动子区域；红色方框：5'UTR区域；黄色方框：3'UTR区域。启动子可以是质体启动子或诱导型启动子，用于调控目的基因的表达。当使用IEE元件表达多个基因时，目的基因2前应含有SD(Shine-Dalgarno)序列。

**表1 近5年常用表达调控元件在质体基因工程中的应用**

| 研究内容 | 启动子 | 5'UTR | 3'UTR |
|---|---|---|---|
| 苦瓜(*Momordica charantia*)叶绿体转化载体的构建及其功能评价 | P*psbA* | *psbA* | T*psbA* |
| 可育转质体拟南芥植物的高效培育 | P*rrn*/P*psbA*/P*clp* | *rbcL*/T7*g10*L | T*psbA*/T*atpA*/T*rps16*/T*atpB*/T*rrnB* |
| 适用于拟南芥质体转化的载体及壮观霉素敏感性拟南芥品系的开发 | P*rrn* | *atpB* | T*psbA* |
| 莴苣叶绿体用于生产口服增强型疫苗抗原SARS-CoV-2刺突蛋白 | P*rrn*/P*psbA* | *psbA* | T*rbcL*/T*psbA* |
| RuBisCO的基因工程改良 | P*rbcL* | *rbcL* | T*rps16*/T*rbcL* |
| 药用植物黄花蒿叶绿体遗传转化体系的建立 | P*rrn*/P*psbA* | T7*g10*L/*psbA* | T*psbA*/T*rps16* |
| 揭示质体编码的乙酰辅酶A羧化酶基因对代谢和发育功能的影响 | P*rrn* | | T*psbA* |
| 将复制微型染色体开发为质体基因工程的新工具 | P*rrn*/P*clpP* | T7*g10*L | T*rrnB*/T*psbA* |

## 1 启动子

1.1 *启动子的结构与类型* 高等植物的质体中含有两种类型启动子：PEP(plastid-encoded RNA polymerase)型/NEP(nuclear-encoded RNA polymerases)型，PEP型启动子能够被质体基因组编码的rpoA、rpoB、rpoC1和rpoC2亚基组成的细菌型RNA聚合酶核心识别，在结构上与细菌σ70型启动子非常相似，在−35区和−10区均含有保守序列，因此在大肠杆菌中也能正常发挥作用。NEP型启动子由核基因组编码的噬菌体型RNA聚合酶识别，大多数都包含一个核心的序列基序(YRTA)，与植物线粒体基因组中启动子的共有序列十分相似。从转录水平来看，NEP型启动子的转录效率似乎要弱于PEP型启动子，因此，绝大多数质体转化研究会优先选择PEP型启动子来驱动外源基因的表达。

1.2 *启动子的应用*

1.2.1 *外源基因高效表达* 自从P*rrn*与P*psbA*被应用于质体转化研究以来，这两条启动子已经成为近几十年合成操纵子构建中最常用的两个高效启动子。启动子P*rrn*源自16S rDNA基因，该启动子能够以极高速率驱动核糖体RNA操纵子转录，是高等植物质体转化活性最强的启动子。De Cosa等利用P*rrn*启动子，将*cry2Aa2*细菌操纵子整合至烟草质体基因组，外源蛋白在成熟叶片中的表达量占植物总可溶性蛋白的45.3%，即使在老化的白色叶片中也保持着极为稳定的积累水平(46.1%)。值得注意的是，由于rRNA自身不能够被翻译，故在选用P*rrn*作为启动子时，需要添加适当的翻译起始信号，用以保证外源蛋白的积累。

*psbA*基因在叶绿体中翻译效率最高，且通过改变光照强度能够调控该基因的表达。Boyhan等将胰岛素原叶绿体操纵子分别整合至烟草和莴苣质体基因组，并使用*psbA*基因的启动子P*psbA*驱动胰岛素原叶绿体操纵子的表达。胰岛素原在成熟烟草和莴苣叶片中的积累水平分别占叶片总蛋白(total leaf protein, TLP)的47%和53%，在衰老干燥的莴苣叶片中，胰岛素原的积累水平仍高达约40% TLP。

1.2.2 *植物遗传改良* 在光合作用中，起固定$CO_2$作用的关键酶核酮糖二磷酸羧化酶(Rubisco)是决定碳同化速率的关键酶。通过提高位于叶绿体中的光合酶Rubisco的

$CO_2$ 固定来提高碳同化速率是提升作物产量的有效策略之一。植物 Rubisco 是一种 16 蛋白复合物，由核基因编码的 8 个小亚基 *rbcS* 和叶绿体基因编码的 8 个大亚基 *rbcL* 构成，小亚基与大亚基的相互作用会对 Rubisco 的 $CO_2$ 固定产生影响，因此对其改造包括核转化和质体转化两个方面。Martin-Avila 等首先沉默烟草的核基因 *rbcS*，之后利用烟草内源启动子 P*rbcL*，将 4 种合成操纵子（*rbcL* - *rbcS1*、*rbcL* - *rbcS2*、*rbcL* - *rbcS3* 和 *rbcL* - $rbcS^T$）靶向整合至转基因烟草 RNAi - *rbcS* 的叶绿体基因组，获得 4 种转基因烟草品系，分别表达不同马铃薯 Rubisco 小亚基（叶肉小亚基 pS1、pS2、pS3 以及马铃薯毛状体 $pS^T$ 亚基）组成的植物同源 Rubisco，其中 pS3 亚基降低了 Rubisco 的积累水平，但提高了其羧化比率及羧化效率，$pS^T$ 亚基降低了 Rubisco 的羧化比率及羧化效率，并严重影响了转基因烟草的光合作用及生长发育。通过该研究，作者明确了改善马铃薯 Rubisco 催化作用的小亚基的氨基酸组成，证实优化操纵子设计可以提高外源基因在叶绿体中的表达水平，并为 Rubisco 的基因工程改良提供了有效的生物工程基础。

此外，由于 Rubisco 本质上是一种催化效率低的酶，使用效率更高的外源 Rubisco 取代植物内源 Rubisco，也是提高光合作用效率和作物产量的有效方法。然而，Rubisco 的表达和组装需要分子伴侣，缺乏分子伴侣会阻碍叶绿体中功能性外源 Rubisco 的有效生产。因此，Chen 等利用烟草内源启动子 P*rbcL*，将能够串联表达 *rbcL* 和 *rbcS* 基因的合成操纵子靶向整合至烟草叶绿体基因组，成功在烟草叶绿体中表达了来源于那不勒斯卤硫杆菌（*Halothio-bacillus neapolitanus*）的外源 Rubisco。值得注意的是，转质体烟草能够高效表达功能性的外源 Rubisco16 蛋白复合物，约占野生型烟草 Rubisco 含量的 40%，且不需要外源分子伴侣。外源 Rubisco 显示 2 倍以上的羧化率，并使得转质体烟草与野生型具有相似的自养生长率。这项研究表明，用效率更高的外源 Rubisco 取代植物内源 Rubisco，具有可行性，并为通过 Rubisco 的基因工程改良提升作物光合作用效率和生长率的研究提供技术支撑。

## 2 非质体特异性调控序列

由于质体基因表达受转录后调控，因此 5′UTR 和 3′UTR 对于维持 mRNA 的稳定性及转基因的表达效率尤为重要。迄今为止，已筛选出多条 5′UTR 序列并广泛应用于质体基因工程研究，如 1,5 - 二磷酸核酮糖羧化酶/加氧酶基因（*rbcL*）的 5′UTR、叶绿体 D1 蛋白基因（*psbA*）的 5′UTR、ATP 合酶 β 亚基基因（*atpB*）的 5′UTR 以及来自 T7 噬菌体基因 10 的先导序列 T7*g10*L。近 5 年来，大部分涉及外源蛋白的高效积累的质体转化研究均使用了 T7*g10*L，由于该序列所包含的二级结构以及 SD 序列能够介导外源基因在大肠杆菌中的高效翻译，且众多表达调控元件的组合中，P*rrn* 启动子序列与 5′UTR 序列 T7*g10*L 的组合能够有效保证目标蛋白的表达水平，故使用频率较高。当前应用较为广泛的 3′UTR 序列主要有 *rbcL* 基因的 3′UTR、*psbA* 基因的 3′UTR、*rps16* 基因的 3′UTR 以及来自大肠杆菌 *rrnB* 操纵子的终止序列 *TrrnB*。

2.1 5′UTR 的结构与功能 质体中存在两种翻译方式，二者的区别在于是否具有 SD 序列依赖性。常见的翻译起始方式依赖于 SD 序列，该序列位于起始密码子上游 4～9 个核苷酸的保守区域；另一种翻译起始方式与 SD 序列无关，而是由 mRNA 特异性翻译激活蛋白与 5′UTR 结合并将核糖体 30S 亚基引导至 AUG 起始密码子。基于原核表达系统的翻译机制，通常认为 SD 序列依赖性的翻译效率总体上要高于 SD 序列非依赖性的翻译效率，但目前仍没有相关研究对两种翻译起始方式进行系统比较。

由于 70S 细菌型核糖体是质体中蛋白质的生物合成场所，因此 5′UTR 序列和结构很大程度上决定了 SD 序列依赖性翻译的速率。最近的研究表明，SD 序列与 16S rRNA 3′末端序列结合的强弱与翻译效率有关，并且这种结合会显著影响二级结构稳定的 mRNA 的翻译效率，但对于二级结构稳定性较差的 mRNA 的翻译效率影响较小。因此，结合强度并不是决定 SD 序列依赖性翻译速率的唯一性因素，质体基因的表达主要受到转录后调控的影响。

2.2 5′UTR 的应用

2.2.1 提高重组蛋白表达量 Zhou 等检测了 4 种来自质体转基因的 HIV（human immunodeficiency virus）抗原结合操纵子（*p24*、*Nef*、*p24* - *Nef* 和 *Nef* - *p24*）的表达，其中表达量最高的操纵子将 p24 蛋白序列 N 端与 Nef 蛋白序列 C 端融合，并利用启动子 P*rrn* 与 T7*g10*L 组合驱动，使蛋白产物的积累水平高达植物总蛋白的 40%，是以往常规核转化生产 p24 研究的 100 倍，且 p24 - Nef 融合蛋白的过表达仅对植物表型造成了轻微的影响，该研究揭示了质体基因工程在高水平生产药物蛋白上的巨大潜力。此外，Oey 等使用同样的方式将充分优化后的合成操纵子整合到叶绿体基因组中，使 PlyGBS 裂解酶的表达水平达到了植物总可溶性蛋白的 70% 以上，这是迄今为止在植物中实现的最高外源蛋白表达水平，在叶片发育和衰老过程中该蛋白在叶绿体中仍保持稳定，且蛋白表达量始终维持在较高水平。

2.2.2 提高目标化合物产量 青蒿素是目前治疗疟疾的首选药物，以青蒿素为基础的联合疗法是世界卫生组织推荐的疟疾治疗的最佳疗法。为了满足全世界范围内对青蒿素不断增长的需求，Fuentes 等开发了一种新的合成生物学方法，首先将青蒿酸生物合成的关键酶基因 *FPS*、*ADS*、*CYP71AV1* 以及 *CPR* 整合到叶绿体基因组，进而将影响青蒿酸通量的相关酶基因 *CYB5*、*ADH1*、*ALDH1* 及 *DBR2* 进行核转化，最终获得了青蒿酸含量达 120 mg/kg 鲜重（fresh weight，FW）的烟草品系，该品系所表达的叶绿体操纵子利用莱茵衣藻启动子 CrP*rrn* 和 CrP*psbA*，分别与 T7*g10*L 组合，以多顺反子的形式驱动青蒿酸生物合成途径关键酶基因的表达，实现了将次生代谢产物生物合成途径从原植物向高生物量作物的转移。

2.2.3 研究叶绿体光合作用机制 光系统是由蛋白质和叶绿素等光合色素组成的复合物，是将吸收的太阳能转化为化学能的功能单位，包括光系统Ⅰ（PS Ⅰ）和光系统Ⅱ（PS Ⅱ）。叶绿体 *psbD* 基因编码 PS Ⅱ反应中心 D2 蛋白，细胞核编码的 Nac2 蛋白可与 *psbD* 基因 mRNA 的 5′UTR 特异性结合，二者的相互作用是维持 *psbD* 基因 mRNA 稳定性及 PS Ⅱ反应中心 D2 蛋白正常表达所必需的。Dinc 等将转质体莱茵衣藻 *rps12* 基因的 5′UTR 替换为 *psbD* 基因的 5′UTR，并利用诱导型启动子 MetE 驱动核 *Nac2* 基因的表达。使用维生素对转质体莱茵衣藻进行处理后，MetE 启动子的转录活性被抑制，导致 *rps12* 基因 mRNA 和编码蛋白的水平逐渐下降，进一步抑制了叶绿体的翻译活性；使用维生素处理转质体细胞后的 48～96 h，叶绿素 a 与叶绿素 b 含量的比值显著降低，可变荧光(Fv)与最大荧光(Fm)的比率显著下降，转质体细胞停止生长。此外，转质体细胞低温荧光发射光谱中 PS Ⅰ的发射峰发生了蓝移(blue shift)，与 PS Ⅰ的发射荧光(N700 nm)强度相比，PS Ⅱ的发射荧光(686 nm)强度有所下降。该研究表明，通过在生长培养基中添加维生素对转质体莱茵衣藻的叶绿体翻译进行可逆性抑制，可以用来研究光合复合物在膜中的相对稳定性。

2.3 3′UTR 的结构、功能与应用 质体基因编码区下游的 3′UTR 通常包含一段能够在转录后折叠成稳定茎-环结构的序列，这种结构可以有效避免 3′→5′核糖核酸外切酶对 mRNA 的降解，但不同于真核系统中的终止子或细菌中的终止序列，这种结构在质体中并不具备转录终止功能，而是作为转录加工识别位点以及起到维持转录本稳定性的作用。

此前已有多项研究探究了不同 3′UTR 对叶绿体基因组中报告基因表达的影响。其中 Tangphatsornruang 等比较了不同 3′UTR 对烟草叶绿体中外源基因表达的影响，分别将来自烟草叶绿体基因编码区下游的 T*rbcL*、T*psbA*、T*petD* 和 T*rpoA* 以及大肠杆菌 *rrnB* 操纵子的终止子序列 T*rrnB* 置于绿色荧光蛋白基因(*GFP*)的下游，在含有 P*psbA* - *GFP* - T*rrnB* 操纵子的转质体烟草中 mRNA 的积累水平是含有 T*rbcL* 和 T*rpoA* 操纵子的 4 倍，所有转基因烟草都积累了大约相同水平的 GFP，占总可溶性蛋白的 0.2%，说明翻译受到转录丰度以外其他因素的影响。以上研究表明，3′UTR 会对 RNA 的积累水平产生影响，但对蛋白积累水平的影响有限。

## 3 新型表达调控系统的开发与应用

3.1 多基因共表达调控系统 在设计构建复杂生物合成途径的操纵子时，往往需要将多条途径的相关基因构建至载体上，这可能会重复使用表达调控元件，同时也会提高载体构建的难度。而在质体表达系统中，以单一启动子驱动多条基因的转录较为常见，这种特性为研究人员在质体中构建复杂生物合成途径提供了可能。与细菌以多顺反子为单位直接进行翻译不同，质体中的多顺反子会被加工成单顺反子，但顺反子间的加工是否能够促进操纵子中所有基因的表达仍需进一步研究。

当前比较成熟的构建策略是在合成操纵子序列中添加能够将多顺反子加工形成单顺反子的表达调控元件。Zhou 等首次鉴定出了这种顺反子间表达元件(IEE)，该元件的序列长度仅为 50 bp，位于 *psbT* - *psbH* 基因间隔区，序列中含有 RNA 结合蛋白 HCF107 的识别位点，该元件有效改善了多顺反子中某个顺反子表达水平过低的情况，也为多基因合成操纵子在叶绿体中的表达提供了有效工具。因此在异源生物合成途径的质体转化研究中被广泛使用。

为了避免过度重复使用单一元件，Legen 等测试了 5 个含有五肽重复蛋白(pentatricopeptide repeat，PPR)结合位点的 sRNA 序列，发现其中 5 种 sRNA 能够稳定其下游 *EGFP* 基因的转录本并提高其蛋白的表达水平，说明这些 sRNA 与 IEE 一样能够用于叶绿体多顺反子操纵子的构建。值得注意的是，这种元件与核编码 PPR 蛋白的结合除了会影响多顺反子 mRNA 的加工之外，也可以提高翻译效率和/或影响 mRNA 稳定性，但是这些元件是如何增加外源基因表达的尚不明确。Macedo-Osorio 等测试了来自 *psbB* - *psbT*、*psbN* - *psbH*、*psaC* - *petL*、*petL* - *trnN* 和 *tscA* - *chlN* 叶绿体操纵子的基因间隔区序列，并将这些间隔区序列构建至 *aphA* - *6* - *GFP* 双顺反子操纵子基因之间。尽管所有的转质体细胞系都具有卡那霉素抗性，但只有其中两条间隔区(*psbN* - *psbH* 和 *tscA* - *chlN* 的基因间隔区)序列能够介导细胞系中 *EGFP* 的表达。

3.2 诱导表达调控系统 尽管叶绿体内源强启动子可以实现基因的高效表达，但是随着质体转化研究的不断深入，研究发现某些外源蛋白或异源合成途径在叶绿体中的过度表达可能会对植物本身的生长发育产生负面影响。为了能够精细调控外源基因在叶绿体中的表达水平，就需要开发特异性诱导表达调控元件，这类元件通过特定的物理或化学方式诱导后，不仅能够大幅降低持续表达产生的负面影响，还能根据不同的实验目的和设计需求在特定时间启动或停止外源基因的表达。

3.2.1 核诱导表达调控系统 近年来植物质体基因工程诱导表达调控系统的开发已日趋成熟(表 2)，其中核基因工程诱导表达调控系统动态表达范围高，在未诱导状态下，表达泄漏较少。一种常见的策略是将融合了质体定位信号的外源基因由诱导型或组织特异性启动子驱动在细胞核中表达，该基因编码蛋白与质体基因组内源调控元件特异性结合，进而增强调控元件下游基因的表达。另一种策略是在细胞核中利用诱导型或组织特异性启动子表达可与非质体特异性调控元件结合的外源基因编码蛋白，进而增强调控元件下游基因的表达。

**表 2 近 5 年开发的新型诱导表达调控系统**

| 研究内容 | 启动子 | 5′UTR | 3′UTR |
|---|---|---|---|
| 烟草新型 IEE 的开发 | P*rrn* | T7*g10*L | T*psbA*/T*rbcL*/T*rps16* |
| 莱茵衣藻新型 IEE 的开发 | P*rbcL* | T7*g10*L | T*rbcL* |
| 工程化 PPR 蛋白在新型质体诱导表达调控系统中的应用 | P*rrn*/P*psbA* | *atpB*/*atpH* | T*psbA*/T*rbcL* |
| 工程化 RNA 结合蛋白在新型非绿色质体诱导表达调控系统中的应用 | P*rrn* | *atpB*/*atpH* | T*psbA*/T*rbcL* |

（续表）

| 研究内容 | 启动子 | 5′UTR | 3′UTR |
|---|---|---|---|
| 质体未加工多顺反子中 ORF 独立翻译合成系统的开发 | P*rrn*/P*psbA* | *clp*/*rbcL*/*atpB*/T7*g10*L/*psbA*/*cry9Aa2*/*atpH* | T*psbA* |
| 核编码翻译增强子 TDA1 在莱茵衣藻叶绿体诱导表达调控系统中的应用 | P*rrn* | atpA | |
| 核糖开关质体诱导表达系统在虾青素生物合成中的应用 | T7/P*rrn*/P*psbA* | T7*g10*L/*psbA* | T*psbA*/T*atpA*/T*rps16*/T*rbcL*/T7 T |
| 莱茵衣藻新型温度敏感表达调控系统的开发 | P*psaA* | *psaA* | T*rbcL* |
| 莱茵衣藻维生素可逆性调控系统的开发 | P*psbD*/P*psaA* | *psbD*/*psaA* | T*rbcL*/T*psaD* |

Rojas 等发现，当核基因组编码的 PPR 蛋白被乙醇诱导表达后，能够与叶绿体 mRNA 的 5′UTR 特异性结合，进而稳定 mRNA 的结构，并通过提高翻译效率增强外源基因的表达。Yu 等在此基础上开发了基于此元件的表达调控系统，该系统包含了玉米（*Zea mays*）叶绿体的 PPR10 变体与 *GFP* 基因上游的同源结合位点。由于马铃薯内源 PPR10 蛋白不识别该位点，因此 GFP 在叶片中的表达水平较低。当 PPR10 变体在块茎特异性启动子的驱动下表达时，GFP 的积累水平占总可溶性蛋白的 1.3%，因此，该系统能够增加非光合质体中外源基因的表达，但不会干扰叶片中的叶绿体基因表达。

Rochaix 等建立了 *Nac2* - *psbD* 叶绿体基因诱导表达调控系统，其中铜离子诱导型启动子 Cyc6 驱动核基因 *Nac2* 的表达，该基因编码一种靶向叶绿体的蛋白质，特异性作用于叶绿体 *psbD* 基因的 5′UTR，是保持 *psbD* 基因 mRNA 和光系统Ⅱ稳定性所必需的。当有铜离子存在时，*Nac2* 基因的表达被抑制，导致 *psbD* 基因的 mRNA 稳定性降低，当没有铜离子存在时，*Nac2* 基因发生表达，进而提高了 *psbD* 基因的 mRNA 稳定性及其蛋白的表达水平。通过用 *psbD* 的 5′UTR 替换其他质体基因的 5′UTR，理论上可将这种诱导表达调控系统应用于任何质体基因的表达调控研究。

此外，Carrera-Pacheco 等还开发了用于调控质体表达系统的增强子 TDA1，该增强子由核基因组编码，其 C 端（cTDA1）可通过与 *atpA* 5′UTR 的相互作用促进 *atpA* 的翻译。该研究将诱导型启动子 HSP70A - RBCS2 驱动的 cTDA1 在莱茵衣藻细胞核中表达，将 *atpA* 5′UTR 调控的 *GFP* 基因在莱茵衣藻质体中表达；通过对莱茵衣藻进行特定的热休克及光照处理后，检测到莱茵衣藻中 GFP 的表达水平最高增长了约 1.9 倍，表明 GFP 的表达水平与 cTDA1 的积累水平有关。

3.2.2 质体诱导表达调控系统　质体基因工程可高效表达异源蛋白，避免基因沉默和位置效应，且生物安全性高，但质体诱导表达调控系统需要利用细菌诱导表达调控元件。为此，研究人员开发了一系列能够在质体中进行诱导表达的调控系统。

虾青素（astaxanthin）是迄今为止自然界中最强的天然抗氧化剂，当前已实现了其生物合成途径在转质体种子植物中的异源表达及高水平积累，但虾青素的合成对类异戊二烯前体的消耗限制了叶绿素、类胡萝卜素和植物激素的生物合成，导致转质体植物出现了严重的生长迟缓。因此，在最近的一项研究中，作者利用质体诱导表达调控系统解决了这一问题。该系统利用茶碱依赖性核糖开关，可通过小分子化合物茶碱调控 T7 RNA 聚合酶基因的表达，诱导产生少量的 T7 RNA 聚合酶作用于质体基因组 T7 启动子，在该启动子驱动下的虾青素合成操纵子产生了大量转录本，进一步提高了虾青素的积累水平，且与组成型转质体烟草相比虾青素的含量并未显著减少。更重要的是，诱导型植物与野生型的表型几乎一致，说明该诱导表达调控系统未对植物的正常生长造成影响。

莱茵衣藻叶绿体基因组中不含有终止密码子 TGA，Young 等利用这一特性开发了一种简单的质体诱导表达系统，将 $trnW_{UCA}$ 基因整合至莱茵衣藻的叶绿体基因组，该基因可编码一种对温度敏感的突变体 tRNA，因此，包含 TGA 密码子的外源基因在 P*psaA* 的驱动下表达水平随培养温度的降低而逐渐升高，当温度降低至 15 ℃时表达水平最高，当温度升高至 35 ℃时，蛋白表达水平降至最低或完全不表达。此外，作者还可通过改变转基因内 TGA 密码子的数量来精准调控外源基因的表达水平。该系统为莱茵衣藻的质体基因工程提供了新工具，并能够进一步开发为研究叶绿体中必需基因功能的热抑制系统。

## 4 结语与展望

表达调控元件的选择和组合方式对于质体基因工程研究至关重要，其中启动子决定了转录速率，5′UTR 决定了 mRNA 的翻译效率，3′UTR 主要负责维持 mRNA 的稳定性。值得注意的是，内源表达调控元件的使用虽然在一定程度上可以保证基因的表达水平，但也存在着发生非预期同源重组从而影响蛋白表达水平的可能性。叶绿体基因组中反向重复区的重组会导致插入序列的翻转，这种重组现象也叫作翻转（flip-flop）重组。Rogalski 等在探究烟草质体核糖体蛋白 S18 是否影响细胞存活时，意外发现在叶绿体基因组短反向重复序列发生了两次 flip-flop 重组，这种重组事件的发生使得该研究在使用 *Acc* Ⅰ酶进行限制片段长度多态性分析时，除产生了预计大小为 6 kb 的片段外，还额外产生了大小为 5 kb 的杂交片段。在此基础上，该研究使用限制性内切酶 *Sal* Ⅰ和 *Eco*R Ⅴ进一步证实了这一发现，除产生了预计大小为 9 kb 的片段外，还产生了一个长度明显更小（6.2 kb）的片段。Zhou 等在检测转质体中 HIV 抗原结合操纵子的表达时，发现转质体植物的不同表型与这种非预期同源重组相关。在未发生 flip-flop 重组的情况下，由全长 P*rrn* 驱动 *Nef* 基因的转录，导致了色素缺乏型，即黄色烟草的产生。而 flip-flop 重组事件发生后，由截短的 P*rrn* 启动子驱动 *Nef* 基因的转录，使得该基因的表达水平大幅下降，因此未产生色素缺乏型烟草。为了避免内源调控元件之间发生非预期同源重组，近年来研究者们也在积极开发并使用一些异源调控序列，例如在烟草叶绿体操纵子构建中使用玉米来源的启动子 ZmP*clpP* 和 5′UTR ZmL*atpH*、衣藻来源的启动子 CrP*rrn* 与 3′UTR CrT*rbcL* 以及大肠杆菌来源的 3′UTR T*rrnB*。

利用多基因共表达调控系统可以显著提升异源复杂生化途径引入质体基因组的可行性，但在设计构建多顺反子操纵子时，仍需尽可能避免重复使用单一的 IEE 样元件。此外，在某些情况下，质体中的多顺反子 mRNA 也可以直接作为翻译的模板。Staub 等为了确定在质体中是否存在启动子远端开放阅读框的翻译起始，将不含有启动子的报告基因 *uidA* 整合到了烟草质体基因组 *rbcL* 基因的下游区域后未产生单顺反子 *uidA* mRNA。然而由于 *rbcL* 基因的 3′UTR 转录终止效率较低，产生了包含 *uidA* 基因作为第二个顺反子的多顺反子转录单元，转质体植物中仍能检测到报告基因 *uidA* 编码的产物 GUS 的表达，表明启动子远端顺反子可以在质体中进行有效翻译。Quesada-Vargas 等首次对烟草叶绿体基因组中异源操纵子的转录、转录后和翻译过程进行表征。含有不同异源操纵子（*cry2Aa2* 操纵子、*has* 操纵子、*tps1* 操纵子和 *ctb* 操纵子）的叶绿体转基因系中，转录产物为多顺反子 mRNA。尽管在转质体内缺乏对此类多顺反子 mRNA 的加工，但仍能检测到较高水平的外源蛋白，说明叶绿体可以直接翻译异源多顺反子 mRNA，即使在不存在 3′UTR 的情况下，加工和未加工的异源多顺反子 mRNA 均是稳定的。

经过 30 多年的发展，用于质体转化研究的表达调控元件种类已十分可观，这些元件已基本能够适应绝大多数研究目的及实验设计需求，而关于非绿色组织中质体调控系统的报道仍然较少。此外，利用诱导表达调控系统尽管能够有效降低异源合成所带来的有害影响，实现对质体表达系统的精准调控，但这类系统需要在非诱导状态下避免表达泄露并兼顾更广的动态调节范围，因此需对质体诱导表达调控系统进行更加深入的研究。

［于一凡，赵瑜君，黄璐琦，等. 遗传，2023，45(6)：501－513.］

# 中药活性成分生物合成途径解析研究方法进展

中医药是中国古代医学瑰宝，中药是中医临床诊疗的基石，近年来，中医药在临床治疗中显示出特有的优势，市场对中药材的需求逐渐增大，如何在保障市场需求的同时保护中药资源是目前中医药发展所面临的一大难题。我国中药资源丰富，其中植物药占比 87%。中药植物活性成分包括黄酮类、萜类、生物碱类、苯丙素类化合物等。药用植物的生长受天气、环境、病虫害等影响，中药活性成分的研究和应用也面临着含量低、资源匮乏、化学合成困难、成药性不足等诸多挑战。

合成生物技术的发展为中药活性成分由传统资源保障模式向高效、绿色、可持续工业生产模式转变提供了理论和技术支撑。然而，生物合成途径未知、异源生物合成效率低等关键问题制约中药活性成分的生物合成及应用。挖掘中药活性成分生物合成功能基因，解析复杂生物合成途径，是实现活性成分异源合成的关键，是中药栽培驯化、植物代谢工程改良的基石，除此之外也是道地药材形成遗传成因的重要方面。中药活性成分生物合成途径解析的研究过程可以分为基因元件的筛选、候选元件的功能研究（图 1）。本文将从这 2 个方面系统梳理近年来运用广泛的、有效的，以及新出现的中药活性成分生物合成功能基因的筛选和功能鉴定方法，包括基因元件挖掘、基因的功能验证等，通过该研究为中药活性成分的功能基因研究提供研究思路和技术参考。

## 1　催化元件的筛选挖掘

中药活性成分的生物合成是以初生代谢产物为前体经过一系列的酶催化形成骨架、再在结构后修饰酶的催化下形成结构活性各异的小分子化合物。解析中药活性成分的生物合成过程就是挖掘催化元件的过程。随着高通量测序技术迅速发展，为元件的挖掘提供了大量的数据，怎样从海量的数据中筛选出合成途径的催化元件是关键。基因组学、转录组学、代谢组学、蛋白质组学等组学数据及分析工具的开发，为研究植物中复杂的代谢网络提供了基础和平台。

1.1　转录组学与代谢组学　参与中药活性成分生物合成的基因大多是植物的基因家族，比如广泛参与植物次生代谢合成途径的细胞色素 P450（以下简称 P450）家族占植物基因的 1%。这些家族在植物进化过程中通常会发生扩张或收缩，如在萜类生物合成中 P450 通常会有基因扩张，而在苄基异喹啉生物碱（benzylisoquinoline alkaloid，BIAs）丰富的物种中，通常会有甲基转移酶的扩张。怎样从庞大的基因家族中筛选出参与特殊代谢途径的基因具有一定挑战。中药活性成分通常在植物特殊的生长阶段、特殊的组织器官中积累，并且中药有效成分的积累易受到环境、生物及非生物因子等因素影响，而代谢物水平通常与合成途径催化元件的表达密切相关。因此基于比较转录组和代谢组联合的差异分析以及共表达网络分析为候选基因元件筛选提供了的有效手段。

1.1.1　差异表达分析　中药药用部位与中药活性成分的积累密切相关，中药活性成分的积累与参与其生物合成的催化酶的表达量具有较强的相关性，比如丹参酮主要在丹参 *Salvia miltiorrhiza* 的根中积累，已经鉴定的参与丹参酮生物合成途径的基因在根中的表达量都远高于地上部位。这种基因表达与代谢物积累的相关性有效缩小了中药活性成分的元

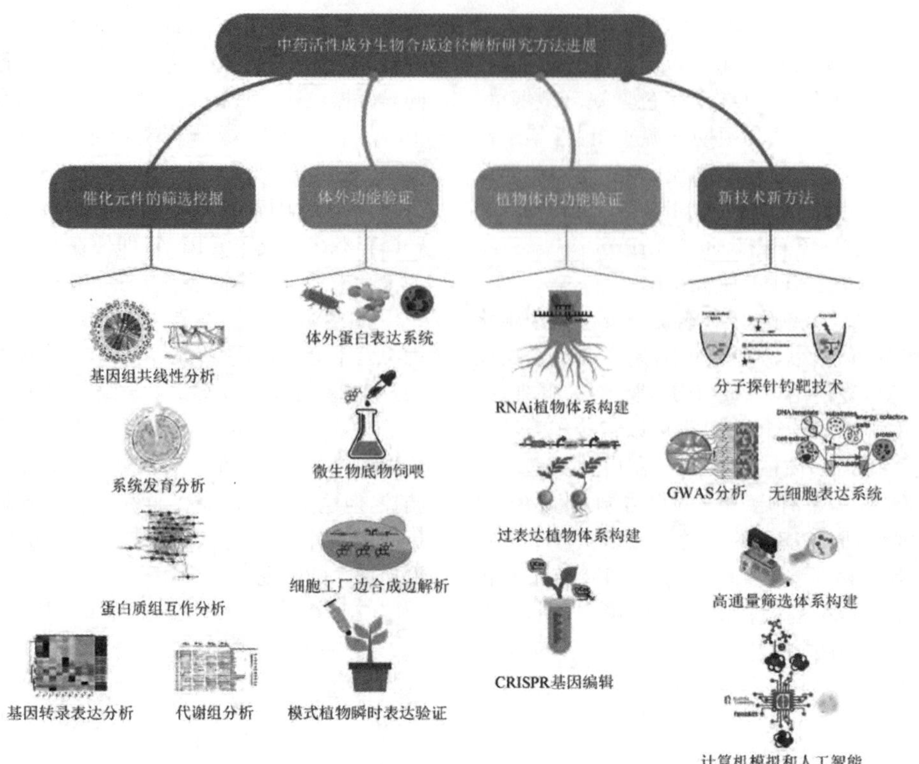


**图1　中药活性成分生物合成途径功能基因研究方法**

件筛选范围。LIU B 等对石仙桃 *Pholidota chinensis* 中根、根茎、假鳞茎等多个器官的转录组和代谢组进行联合分析，筛选差异表达基因和差异积累代谢物，结合同源性分析和共表达分析，获得参与天麻素生物合成的候选糖基转移酶基因。

除了天然的组织特异性积累的特性，通过悬浮细胞或者毛状根等细胞系这些更简单的系统，利用生物或非生物因子进行诱导刺激，能够导致中药活性成分在短期内迅速积累，这是相对于组织表达更有效的筛选手段，同时也可以作为和组织表达互相补充的筛选系统。常见的非生物诱导因子包括茉莉酸、水杨酸及其衍生物等，在药用植物艾 *Artemisia argyi* 中调节活性成分积累的转录因子和雷公藤 *Tripterygium wilfordii* 中参与雷公藤甲素和雷公藤乙素生物合成的 P450 等基因的筛选中起重要作用。生物诱导子来源广泛，包括真菌、细菌、病毒等，能够诱导植物防御机制，积累各种代谢产物。不同类型的诱导子对不同的代谢产物的诱导效果也不同，酵母提取物作为一种常见的生物诱导子，在芹菜素生物合成途径研究中，能显著诱导黄芪属植物 *Astragalus trigonus* 中的查耳酮异构酶 A 的表达上调，提高芹菜素的积累水平；在丹参酮的生物合成研究中，酵母提取物和 $Ag^{+}$ 共同诱导丹参毛状根，能够促使毛状根中丹参酮Ⅱ$_{A}$ 含量在 10 d 内提升约 15 倍。利用丹参毛状根的这一特性，进行比较转录组和代谢组分析，从中筛选并成功验证了丹参酮生物合成途径的 6 个 P450 基因，表明这种简单可控的细胞培养体系在生物合成途径解析中起重要作用。

1.1.2　加权基因共表达网络分析　加权基因共表达网络分析（weighted gene coexpression network analysis, WGCNA）是一种关联性分析，其原理是具有相似表达模式的基因，往往参与同一生物过程，具有潜在联系，这可能是植物在进化过程中形成的规律。ZHENG H 等使用共表达网络分析诱导子处理下的丹参转录组数据，筛选得到具有相同表达模式的功能基因和转录因子。在士的宁的生物合成研究中，HONG B 等分别在马钱子 *Strychnos nux-vomica* 和 *Strychnos* sp. 中运用共表达分析，结合同源性分析和体内外功能验证，筛选并鉴定多个参与士的宁生物合成的 α/β 水解酶和 BAHD 酰基转移酶及中间产物，成功阐明士的宁的生物合成途径。化橘红是化州柚 *Citrus grandis* "Tomentosa"的干燥外果皮，FANR 等对药用化州柚和食用化州柚 2 个品种进行加权共表达网络分析，得到 18 个高度相关的基因模块，再结合转录组和代谢组分析筛选出 25 个黄酮生物合成功能基因和 16 个转录因子作为生物合成途径解析的候选基因元件。

1.2　基因组学　随着基因组测序成本的下降，越来越多的物种基因组数据公布，为利用比较基因组学来筛选催化元件奠定基础。基于基因组图谱，通过对比已知基因和基因组结构和特性，可以了解基因的功能、表达机制以及物种间的遗传进化关系。基因组在生物合成途径解析中的主要运用包括筛选可能的生物合成基因簇、基因家族的扩张和收缩，以及特殊进化导致的独特生物合成途径。通过与不同种属药用植物或模式植物的基因组序列进行比较，能够获得目标药用植物物种中独有的序列，部分独有的基因使该物种产生了独特的中药活性成分。同种属植物基因组内相比较，存在大量的变异和多态性，通过对不同个体与群体比较基因组数据分析，能够缩小候选基因和底物范围，提高基因元件筛选效率，同时为新基因家族功能研究提供参考。如冬凌草 *Isodon rubescens* 基因组中的一系列串联重复的 P450 基因的发现，24 种肉桂属植物全基因组分析得到的肉桂中萜类合酶（terpene synthase, TPS）的筛选。二萜类化合物是唇形科植物的主要活性成分之一，近年来多种唇形科植物的基因组发布和物种间基因共线性分析为二萜类化合物生物合成功能基因挖掘提供了参考。例如，研究者们对药用植物半枝莲 *Scutellaria barbata* 中克罗烷型、药用鼠尾草 *Salvia officinalis* 中松香烷型和美洲紫珠 *Callicarpa americana* 中松香烷、克罗烷型二萜生物合成基因簇进行分析，在生物合成基因簇内挖掘到多个TPS和P450等二萜生物合成途径关键基因，并深入分析了这些基因的功能。中药活性成分生物合成功能基因虽有聚集成基因簇的趋势，但不同于微生物中基因聚集紧密，植物中基因的聚集稍显疏松，通常在较大范围内成簇，且形式多样，基因簇的鉴定有一定的复杂性。信息化的基因组挖掘(genome mining)为功能基因筛选提供新策略，新兴挖掘工具如plantiSMASH、PhytoClust等方便研究者从植物基因组中寻找基因簇。XIONG X 等将红豆杉 *Taxus wallichiana* var. *chinensis* 与其他物种进行同源性分析。与所选物种相比，红豆杉具有多个独特的基因家族，且分别有142、41个家族出现扩张和收缩，表明红豆杉在进化过程中特化形成紫杉醇生物合成途径。进一步研究发现 *CYP725A* 亚家族的扩张在红豆杉紫杉醇生物合成的进化中可能发挥了重要作用，而多个 *CYP725A* 亚家族基因积聚在9号染色体上。成功运用plantiSMASH预测红豆杉基因组9号染色体上的紫杉醇类化合物生物合成相关的潜在基因簇，通过进一步功能研究发现了簇内4个基因 *TS2*、*TS3*、*T5αH1*、*T5αH2* 连续催化二萜前体生成紫杉二烯的生物学功能，该研究也为紫杉醇合成途径的全解析提供基础。

全基因组复制(whole genome duplication，WGD)是被子植物能实现快速进化的主要原因，在植物基因组的全基因组复制或多倍体化后，遗传物质加倍，复制的基因以不同的方式分化，可能导致植物基因组产生新的功能基因、代谢途径或表型特征。迷迭香 *Salvia rosmarinus*、人参 *Panax ginseng* 等均发生1次或多次WGD事件，结合基因组复制后多倍体植物中代谢成分变化，在发生WGD事件的基因中挖掘出大量参与目标代谢成分的TPS和P450等生物合成基因。目前已经在当归 *Angelica sinensis*、香樟 *Cinnamomum camphora*、天师栗 *Aesculus wilsonii*、盾叶薯蓣 *Dioscorea zingiberensis* 等多种药用植物中发现WGD事件并鉴定多个生物合成基因。

1.3 蛋白质组学 蛋白是生物合成途径的直接参与者，虽然植物次生代谢途径催化酶的丰度相对较低，但是随着蛋白质组检测灵敏度的提升，提高了基于蛋白质组的生物合成途径元件筛选的可行性，可用作为比较基因组、转录组、代谢组的补充，应用于生物合成功能基因的筛选。比如川续断 *Dipsacus asper* 在"发汗"过程中三萜皂苷类成分发生显著变化，何华等对续断"发汗"前后差异表达蛋白进行分析，发现参与三萜皂苷结构修饰的P450和糖基转移酶在"发汗"后表达显著下调，通过这些相关性研究能够为进一步的途径解析提供参考。

蛋白质通过与小分子化合物特异性结合发挥作用，化学蛋白质组学是利用与靶蛋白特异性结合的小分子化合物来扰动和探测蛋白质组，从而筛选特定蛋白质。罂粟 *Papaver somniferum* 中的苄基异喹啉类生物碱(BIAs)如吗啡、罂粟碱是其主要活性成分。OZBER N 等研究罂粟BIAs生物合成途径的调控，基于蔗糖密度梯度分离技术对4种化学型罂粟进行蛋白质组学分析，发现2种乳胶蛋白与罂粟主要BIAs发生共沉淀。同源性分析和功能验证实验表明，这些乳胶蛋白属于生物碱结合蛋白家族，参与罂粟生物碱生物合成途径的调控。

不管是基因组、转录组还是蛋白组，都存在自身的局限性，比如基因组能够为系统进化分析提供丰富的数据，但是对于生物合成途径解析信息过于复杂，通过比较转录组能够筛选差异基因，但是需要不同维度的转录组的比较才能更有效地获得候选基因，蛋白组分析灵敏度相对低。因此基于多组学结合的分析将广泛运用于中药活性成分生物合成途径基因元件的筛选。目前通过多种组学分析结合，获取了丹参、人参、雷公藤等中药的活性成分生物合成途径基因元件，并构建多种药用植物功能基因元件库，这些研究不仅为中药活性成分生物合成途径解析奠定基础，也为中药活性化合物的活性改造提供丰富的催化元件。

## 2 体外功能验证

对利用多组学分析筛选得到候选基因进行明确的催化功能研究是生物合成途径解析的关键。参与植物次生代谢途径的基因家族种类繁多，不同基因家族具有不同的特性，可以选择不同的表达体系进行异源表达和功能研究。比如P450酶通常定位于内质网上，且需要P450还原酶为其辅助提供电子，未经过改造的植物P450基因很难在大肠杆菌中进行表达和功能研究，通常选择酵母作为异源表达体系。目前常用的异源表达体系包括大肠杆菌和酵母等微生物体系，以及拟南芥、烟草等植物表达体系等，不同的表达体系各有优缺点。

2.1 微生物体系 微生物因其易得、成本低、便于实验室操作和繁殖快等优点，能够在短时间内表达富集大量蛋白，并且蛋白纯化技术相对成熟，在研究中药活性成分生物合成途径中的运用十分广泛。

2.1.1 体外酶促反应 通过在微生物宿主中表达目的基因，富集和纯化目标蛋白，通过添加底物和反应所需的辅助因子完成酶促反应并检测产物，验证目标蛋白的催化功能是最常用的生物合成基因功能验证方法。研究者们根据不同功能基因表达蛋白的特性，选择合适的表达体系，代表性的原核与真核生物宿主分别为大肠杆菌和酵母菌。

大肠杆菌 *Escherichia coli* 具有繁殖快、易于培养、成本低且操作方便、蛋白产量高等特点，优先选取其作为可溶性蛋白的表达菌种，能高效表达萜类合酶、糖基转移酶、甲基转移酶、2-酮戊二酸依赖性双加氧酶等中药生物合成途径常见的可溶性蛋白，并易于分离纯化进行酶促反应验证。例如延胡索 *Corydalis yanhusuo*、粉防己 *Stephania tetrandra* 中的氧甲基转移酶(*O*-methyltransferases，OMT)等在大肠杆菌中表达获得重组蛋白，研究发现大肠杆菌中表达的OMT极好的还原了该蛋白的催化活性，能够催化多种潜在的BIAs底物。甘草 *Glycyrrhiza uralensis*、菘蓝中的多个糖基转移酶基因，也在大肠杆菌中成功表达。TPS参与多种中药萜类活性成分的生物合成，利用大肠杆菌表达体系，研究者们成功表达了丹参、冬凌草、乌头 *Aconitum carmichaelii*、益母草 *Leonurus japonicus* 等中的TPS，之后通过添加TPS发挥催化功能必需的 $Mg^{2+}$ 进行体外酶促反应，解析其催化功能。

酵母属真核生物，虽然较大肠杆菌相比生长缓慢，蛋白质产量低，但是由于其具有丰富的膜结构细胞器，有利于膜结合蛋白的定位和表达，并且酵母糖基化等蛋白质修饰能力，使得蛋白质的表达更稳定，是研究中药活性成分生物合成途径中膜蛋白基因的重要异源表达宿主。P450 酶是中药活性成分生物合成中的重要结构修饰酶，93%的萜类化合物需要经过 1 个或多个 P450 的修饰，由于其 N 端的内质网膜定位结构，多采用酿酒酵母 *Saccharomyces cerevisiae* 进行异源表达。在二萜、三萜、黄酮、生物碱等多种途径中包含大量 P450 的中药活性成分生物合成功能基因研究中都有使用。研究者们在酿酒酵母中利用诱导型质粒高效表达 P450 蛋白，并通过微粒体提取、全细胞催化等方法验证 P450 蛋白催化功能。相比于酿酒酵母，毕赤酵母 *Pichia pastoris* 具有更高的蛋白表达量，并且蛋白提取纯化过程更为简便。ZIRPEL B 等分别在酿酒酵母、毕赤酵母中异源表达四氢大麻酚酸合酶（$\Delta^9$-tetrahydrocannabinol acid synthase，THCAS），发现毕赤酵母中表达的催化活性要显著高于在酿酒酵母中表达的催化活性，在筛选的最优条件下，毕赤酵母中 THCAS 的活性提高 60 多倍。漆酶被推测为植物中多种二聚化反应过程的重要催化剂，借鉴微生物中漆酶的功能研究方法，中药丹参中丹酚酸类化合物生物合成途径中漆酶的富集和表达均利用了毕赤酵母体系。通常，研究者会使用不同表达体系，来对相同个酶进行研究，以此提高实验的准确性和可信度。CAPUTI L 等将从长春花 *Catharanthus roseus* 中筛选得到 2 个氧化还原酶和 2 个水解酶分别在烟草、大肠杆菌和酿酒酵母中异源表达，以研究其功能。但其中 1 种黄素依赖性氧化还原酶无法在大肠杆菌和酿酒酵母中表达，转而使用毕赤酵母和昆虫草地贪夜蛾 *Spodoptera frugiperda* Sf9 细胞成功实现异源表达，并进行体外酶促实验验证其具有氧化还原功能。

昆虫细胞通过杆状病毒穿梭质粒转染后侵染昆虫细胞获得重组蛋白，与微生物表达体系类似，具有易于放大培养且表达蛋白量高的特点。虽然与微生物表达体系相比培养条件需求稍高，但昆虫细胞体系表达的重组蛋白折叠更为准确，有翻译后修饰（如糖基化等）过程，并且能够较好地表达异源多聚体蛋白。例如 KRAUS P F 等在 Sf9 昆虫细胞中异源表达小檗科植物 *Berberis stolonifera* 中的 *CYP*80，异源表达的蛋白通过酶促反应验证了其作为 C－O 酚偶联酶发挥氧化作用，而不伴随氧结合到产物生物碱中。GESELL A 等发现（*S*）-四氢原小檗碱氧化酶［（*S*）-tetrahydroprotoberberine oxidase，STOX］基因能够在 Sf9 昆虫细胞中异源表达，表达 STOX 蛋白的细胞呈明显黄色，显示出较高的蛋白表达量。

2.1.2 体内催化验证 植物来源功能基因在微生物体内成功表达后，在蛋白的提取过程中很可能存在功能减弱甚至失活，或存在酶促反应条件较难摸索的情况。因此除体外的酶促反应外，可以重构生物合成途径生产底物或人为提供底物在微生物体内进行酶促反应。

人为地提供反应所需底物到目标基因成功表达的微生物培养基中，以适宜条件培养，利用微生物本身的生物环境进行酶促反应并对提取物进行鉴定，可以直观分析并验证基因的功能，阐明生物合成途径。例如 WU F 等研究白花草木樨 *Melilotus albus* 香豆素生物合成途径，筛选得到参与香豆素生物合成的 β－葡萄糖苷酶（β-glucosidase，BGLU）基因簇。在大肠杆菌中异源表达并进行底物饲喂实验，鉴定 *MaBGLU*1 催化东莨菪苷水解生成苷元莨菪亭的生物学功能。糖基转移酶等在大肠杆菌中能顺利表达的植物蛋白也可以用底物饲喂法提高功能验证效率。在酿酒酵母中，基于底物能够成功穿梭细胞膜结构，一些 P450 蛋白也可以通过底物饲喂实验进行功能验证。WANG J 等研究雷公藤 *CYP*81*AM*1 在二萜生物合成中的功能，采用了体外酶促反应和酵母中底物饲喂实验 2 种方法，均能证明 *CYP*81*AM*1 催化生成 15－羟基脱氢枞酸的功能。比较 2 种方法的验证效率，体外催化诱导时间短，但蛋白提取步骤复杂，而底物饲喂法省去蛋白提取和酶促反应步骤，却需要更长的诱导反应时间。

多数中药活性成分生物合成途径冗长复杂，涉及多种酶和中间产物，在解析生物合成途径过程中常面临反应催化酶类型不明确、蛋白底物难以推测和中间体底物极难获取等难题。这种情况就需要进行边合成边解析，模拟生物合成的顺序，逐步推导生物合成过程，最终解析合成途径。由于缺乏松香烷型二萜类化合物前体，SCHELER U 等在酵母中通过边合成边解析的方法，验证了 C－20 氧化酶的基因功能并成功生产鼠尾草酸。在秋水仙碱生物合成途径解析中，NETT R S 等在酵母体系中重构上游生物合成途径，逐步转入多个秋水仙碱生物合成功能基因进行功能验证，彻底阐明秋水仙碱的生物合成途径。

2.2 植物体系 除微生物外，一些植物体系，如拟南芥 *Arabidopsis thaliana*、本氏烟草 *Nicotiana benthamiana* 等也常用于基因的体外瞬时表达，这些模式植物不仅生长周期短，易于培养，还具有瞬时表达操作简便、还原植物蛋白表达环境等优势，解决了部分植物中限速蛋白外源表达难的问题。尤其是烟草作为植物代谢途径催化元件的瞬时异源表达体系，操作简单，近年来在重要的天然产物生物合成途径解析中发挥越来越重要的作用，LAU W 等通过基因元件筛选，利用烟草表达成功解析了抗肿瘤化合物依托泊苷前体的生物合成途径，最近来自英国 John Innes Centre 的 Anne Osbourn 和美国斯坦福大学的 Elizabeth Sattely 实验室合作，利用烟草表达体系鉴定了柠檬苦素生物合成的 22 个酶的催化功能。为研究薯蓣皂苷元的生物合成途径，CHRIST B 等在七叶一枝花 *Paris polyphylla* 和胡卢巴 *Trigonella foenum-graecum* 2 种中草药的转录组中筛选出数个 P450 基因，通过全部共表达后分别减少基因表达逐步缩小目标基因范围。全部 P450 的共同瞬时表达成功异源合成了薯蓣皂苷元，减少部分 P450 表达后，人工模拟基因敲除情况，成功筛选得到薯蓣皂苷元生物合成必须 P450 基因。类似的还有二萜类化合物雷公藤内酯酮的生物合成途径解析过程，利用烟草体系边合成边解析对于酶反应类型复杂多样、途径推测困难的中药活性成分生物合成途径解析和功能基因研究是行之有效的研究方法。烟草表达体系具有高效的瞬时表达体系、植物源的蛋白表达修饰系统、多基因表达兼容的特性，将会在中药活性成分生物合成途径解析中发挥越来越重要的作用。

## 3 植物体内功能验证

除体外功能验证外，为了深入研究功能基因在植物体内的功能，通过构建药用植物的遗传转化体系，利用转基因技术人为干预改变目的基因的表达水平，是体内功能验证的常用手段。常见的方法包括基因沉默、基因过表达和基因敲除等，这些方法技术的应用能够进一步为药用植物的遗传改良提供技术支撑。

3.1 遗传转化体系构建 植物遗传转化体系的建立是通过应用细胞组织培养或种质系统转化技术，在可持续继代的植物培养体系中建立稳定引入外源基因的转化方法，并使其稳定表达与遗传，是开展功能基因植物体内表达验证的基础。目前在药用植物中最常用的遗传转化方法有需要载体介导的农杆菌转化和直接将DNA转入植物细胞的基因枪转化法。现今已有100多种资源植物建立遗传转化体系获得了毛状根，以根部为主要用药部位的植物如丹参、软紫草 *Arnebia euchroma*、人参、地黄 *Rehmannia glutinosa* 等都建立稳定的毛状根、不定根等遗传转化体系，并开展功能基因验证研究。毛状根培养体系的建立不仅能够通过诱导子诱导活性成分快速积累，获得差异转录和差异代谢数据从而筛选功能基因，还可以利用毛状根诱导及其培养方法简单，生长迅速等优势快速获取转基因株系。对于很多极难诱导毛状根的木本、藤本中药植物，可以通过诱导愈伤组织和激素调节获得悬浮细胞体系。目前，研究者们已获得雷公藤、乌头、红花 *Carthamus tinctorius*、栝楼 *Trichosanthes kirilowii* 等药用植物的悬浮细胞体系。由于悬浮细胞体系不均匀、细胞壁增厚较难进行基因转化，因此，使用机械的轰击过程直接将DNA转递到细胞中的基因枪介导法是最快速高效的转化方法。除最常用的叶盘法等外植体侵染诱导法外，直接侵染诱导法（切-浸-芽系统）能够作用于草本、木本和块根植物。直接侵染法可以无需无菌组织培养，使用非常简单的外植体浸润方法即可实现高效转化或基因编辑。多种药用植物如丹参、红豆杉、甘草等建立了转基因植株、毛状根、悬浮细胞等多种遗传转化体系，有利于多种组织培养体系的优势互补，全方位深入开展基因在植物体内的功能研究。

3.2 RNA干扰、过表达与基因编辑 RNA干扰（RNA interference，RNAi）技术已在生物合成功能基因鉴定中广泛运用，如丹参酮生物合成途径中的P450、何首乌糖苷生物合成途径中的糖基转移酶、苦蘵 *Physalis angulata* 活性成分酸浆苦味素生物合成途径中的甾醇异构酶、影响黄花蒿 *Artemisia annua* 青蒿素生物合成的转录因子等。紫草是中医临床常用清热解毒药，具有凉血活血、清热解毒、透疹之功效，紫草素及其衍生物是紫草的主要活性成分，同时也是一种天然色素，致使紫草呈现紫红色。为研究软紫草中紫草素的生物合成途径，WANG S等构建了 *CYP76B74* - RNAi 紫草毛状根体系，RNAi毛状根系颜色明显变淡，紫草素的积累显著减少，证明了 *CYP76B74* 在紫草素生物合成中的关键作用。特征性杂化D环的形成是丹参酮生物合成途径中的关键步骤，D环的形成赋予了丹参中许多丹参酮类化合物的红色、红褐色的显色特征。MA Y等对丹参进行多组学分析，筛选得到4个同家族的P450基因。通过RNAi技术同时降低4个基因的表达水平，几种不具D环的中间体显著积累，最终通过酶促反应被确定为沉默基因蛋白的直接作用底物。这种针对多个目标基因的RNAi实验既缩小了目标基因的筛选范围，也能根据显著的代谢物水平变化快速筛选底物范围。

通过基因过表达（gene overexpression）将目的基因的全长序列构建成质粒载体，通过转化，使基因在人为控制下大量转录翻译，上调目的基因表达水平，可以获得更多表达产物，常与基因沉默、基因敲除等技术联合使用，在研究基因功能时起到相互验证作用，使结果更可靠。在甘草活性成分甘草酸生物合成途径调控功能基因，影响三七植物甾醇生物合成的转录因子，响应脱落酸的丹参酮生物合成调节转录因子等功能基因鉴定中与其他方法共同使用。

植物基因编辑技术是一种可以精准实现定向遗传改造的现代生物技术，CRISPR - Cas9系统设计简单，从模式植物拟南芥、烟草等迅速推广到多种作物和药用植物的功能基因研究及植物代谢工程生产中。CRISPR - Cas9技术可以同时对多个靶点或基因进行精准修饰，为遗传体系建立有待完善的药用植物功能基因研究提供更多选择。为了验证CRISPR - Cas9在非模式植物罂粟中的适用情况，ALAGOZ Y等运用CRISPR - Cas9技术敲除罂粟中BIA生物合成的基因 4′*OMT*2，转基因植株中观察到相关BIA水平显著下降。LIU S等研究丹参转录因子 *SmbHLH*60 功能，使用过表达和CRISPR - Cas9技术构建了 *SmbHLH*60 过表达和敲除转基因毛状根，验证了转录因子 *SmbHLH*60 对丹参酚酸生物合成的负调节作用。此外，在甘草、柴胡 *Bupleurum chinense* 中已运用CRISPR - Cas9体系获得成功编辑目标基因的毛状根系，有望在更多药用植物中开展深入基因功能研究。

## 4 新技术、新方法

由于测序技术的深度和广度不断增加，研究者们从药用植物中获得了海量的基因信息，通过对基因元件的多层次分析后，仍有大量候选基因有待开展功能验证，如何提高筛选速率和精准度是研究者们面临的关键问题。除上述经典的基因筛选和功能验证方法外，一些新方法随着技术的发展也逐步运用到中药活性成分的生物合成研究中，如高通量筛选、分子探针技术等。

4.1 高通量筛选 高通量筛选技术具有高效、微量、快速等特点，在合成生物学菌株筛选和酶突变体筛选研究中发展较为成熟。高通量筛选体系的建立常利用能够快速鉴别的光信号识别系统，将目标蛋白或化合物与显色、荧光、偏振检测信号建立关联，从而在高容量微孔板、流式细胞仪等仪器中进行筛选检测。目前一些微生物中纤维素酶、脂肪酶等的高效筛选已通过高通量筛选技术平台实现。YUAN H等采用常压室温等离子体诱变系统和液滴微流控高通量筛选技术开发了毕赤酵母全细胞进化平台，经过5轮筛选得到的纤维素活性显著增高2倍的高产菌株。QIAO Y等通过基于荧光激活液滴分选的超高通量筛选管道对不同地区样本进行高通量筛选，得到7个属47种产脂肪酶菌株。然而，对于中药活性成分来说，还存在结构复杂导致的标记方法困难、生物合成蛋白表达水平远不如初生代谢酶表达水平、中药活性成分的微生物底盘产量亟待提高等瓶颈问题，高通量筛选体系用于挖掘生物合成途径新基因功能，快速筛选阳性功能蛋白仍有待深入研究和开发。

4.2 分子探针 分子探针多用于临床医学诊疗，辅助对病理过程等进行深入研究。研究者利用基于靶蛋白活性开发的特异化学小分子探针,用于探测具有特定生物合成功能的蛋白质。GAO L 等运用蛋白质组学分析桑 *Morus alba* 中能催化 Diels-Alder 环加成反应的酶,1 种黄素腺嘌呤二核苷酸依赖性酶被筛选为候选酶,命名为桑 Diels-Alder 反应酶(*Morus alba* Diels-Alderase, MaDA)。利用基于生物合成中间体开发的光亲和性探针鉴定出 14 个 MaDA 蛋白,其中 2 个被进一步证实参与环加成反应。该方法简便准确,只需修改生物合成中间体结构,就可运用于一类酶的鉴定,有很好的开发前景。

4.3 *全基因组关联性研究* 全基因组关联性研究(genome-wide association studies, GWAS)在全基因组水平上,对大规模全体样本遗传变异多态性进行检测,对基因型和表型进行统计学分析,从而挖掘与性状变异有关的基因。铁皮石斛以其茎入药,NIU Z 等根据铁皮石斛和 5 个相关物种的性状特征和重测序数据,通过 GWAS 研究发现一种修饰 *MODIFYING WALL LIGNIN*-1 的基因可能参与了铁皮石斛茎的生长。然而,GWAS 存在一定的局限性,如假阳性高,忽略低频突变,只针对单个遗传标记,没有考虑性状可能由多个基因共同决定的情况。为了解决 GWAS 的局限性,更加全面可靠的计算方法有待研究开发,如 GWAS 与蛋白互作网络拓扑结构相结合的组合模型等。

4.4 *无细胞体系* 无细胞蛋白表达系统以外源 mRNA 或 DNA 为蛋白质合成模板,通过人工控制补加蛋白质合成所需的底物和转录、翻译相关蛋白因子等物质,能快速实现目的蛋白质的体外蛋白合成。与传统的体内重组表达系统相比,体外无细胞合成系统具有周期短、表达体系开放、可控、适宜蛋白复合物表达等多种优势。为研究莴苣 *Lactuca sativa* 中五环二萜乙酸酯生物合成途径,CHOI HS 等采用无细胞体系成功表达一种特殊的三萜乙酰转移酶,使用乙酰辅酶 A 作为酰基供体,显示出对多种甾醇的活性。

4.5 *计算模拟和人工智能* 计算机模拟和人工智能是近年来兴起的一项新技术,已经在多领域多学科开展广泛运用。与传统方法相比,计算机模拟虚拟筛选具有高通量、信息化、智能化等优点。目前,LIU Y 等构建了一个综合的植物糖基转移酶数据库(plant UGT database, pUGTdb)以研究底物和糖供体与所表征的糖基转移酶的相互作用机制。基于该数据库,结合计算机模拟和人工智能技术构建了一个网络工具,用于糖基转移酶虚拟筛选和未知糖基转移酶的糖供体预测。可见利用计算模拟预测来进行精确的功能预测,利用高通量筛选来进行功能研究是未来研究中药活性成分生物合成途径解析的重要方向之一。

## 5 展望

一直以来,生物合成途径解析是中药研究领域的重点,但由于缺乏有效的基因元件挖掘手段和基因功能鉴定方法,使得相关途径的解析进展缓慢。一些极有价值的中药活性成分如紫杉醇、丹参酮、雷公藤内酯等的生物合成途径仍未完全阐明。高通量测序技术的发展,使得测序成本下降的同时能获得高精度的植物基因图谱;转录组测序和化学分析手段的升级使得结合基因组、转录组、代谢组和蛋白质组的多组学共表达分析成为可能;大数据信息化时代的到来也让植物全基因组水平分析更加高效准确。目前,以生物合成功能基因为对象开展的多组学、生物信息学、合成生物学等多学科、多角度的研究大大丰富了对中药活性成分生物合成的认识与理解。

随着研究的深入,现有技术手段的局限性日益明显,中药活性成分生物合成研究迫切需要新的方法和思路。一些学者从其他学科中搜寻可以运用于生物合成功能基因研究的方法,如临床病理研究常用的高通量筛选和分子探针技术;在模式植物和农作物中运用广泛的 GWAS 和无细胞蛋白表达系统等。随着计算技术和人工智能的应用,自动化和高通量技术的应用,结合计算模拟虚拟筛选等策略已经应用到了糖基转移酶等比较深入透彻的大基因家族酶的筛选和功能研究,相信随着越来越多的植物次生代谢途径基因功能被解析,将会为计算和模拟提供更可靠的数据支持,为更高效的计算筛选和功能预测奠定基础。通过将这些方法与中药活性成分生物合成研究实际相结合并大胆创新,为中药活性成分生物合成功能基因的研究提供研究模板和新的研究思路。

[史汶龙,马莹,郭娟,等. 中国中药杂志,2023,48(9): 2273-2283.]

# A functional genomics approach to tanshinone biosynthesis provides stereochemical insights

Tanshinones are abietane-type norditerpenoid quinone natural products found in the Chinese medicinal herb *Salvia miltiorrhiza* Bunge. Specifically, they are found as bioactive lipophilic pigments in the intensely red rhizome (root), which is called danshen in Chinese traditional medicine, with records of its use going back millennia. More recently, the predominant and more intensely studied tanshinones Ⅰ (**1**), ⅡA (**2**), and ⅡB (**3**) and cryptotanshinone (**4**) have been isolated and found to have a variety of pharmaceutical activities, including antibacterial, antiinflammatory, and anticancer properties. However, while considered abietane-type diterpenoids, the stereochemistry of the relevant abietadiene olefin intermediate and, hence, other derived biosynthetic intermediates is obscured by the aromatic nature of the identified tanshinones (Figure 1). Resolution of the configuration of this intermediate is a critical step in the characterization of tanshinone biosynthesis.

Tanshinone Ⅰ(1)  Tanshinone ⅡA(2)  Tanshinone ⅡB(3)  Cryptotanshinone (4)

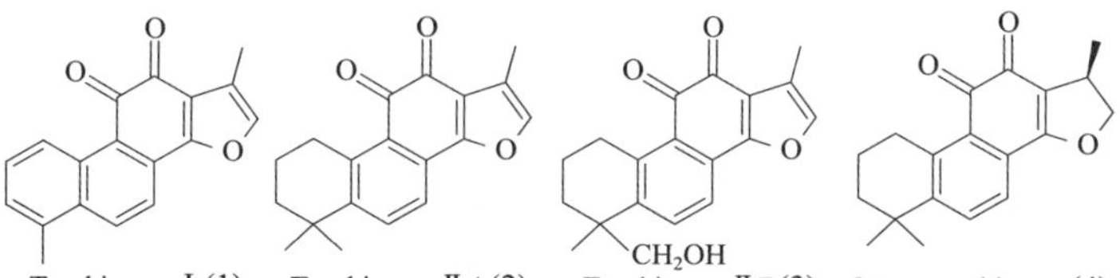

**Figure 1  Major tanshinones(1 - 4) found in *S. miltiorrhiza***

Tanshinones fall into the labdane-related class of diterpenoids, whose biosynthesis is uniquely initiated by a sequential pair of cyclization reactions. The characteristic fused bicyclic hydrocarbon structure is formed from the universal diterpenoid precursor (*E*, *E*, *E*)-geranylgeranyl diphos-phate (GGPP, **5**) in an initial carbon — carbon double-bond protonation-initiated reaction catalyzed by class Ⅱ diterpene cyclases. These typically form labdadienyl/copalyl diphos-phate (CPP), with the corresponding enzymes then termed CPP synthases (CPS). It is at this step that the initial stereochemistry (i.e., of CPP) is established, which is designated by comparison to that of the analogous A/B ring substructure in sterol biosynthesis (i.e., by normal, *ent*, *syn*, or *ent-syn*). Additional stereocenters also are generally formed in the subsequent cyclization and/or rearrangement reaction catalyzed by CPP-specific class Ⅰ diterpene synthases, which are often termed kaurene synthase-like (KSL) because of their similarity to the kaurene synthase found in all higher plants for the requisite biosynthesis of gibberellin phytohormones.

To enable a functional genomics-based approach to tanshinone biosynthesis, a cDNA library was constructed from *S. miltiorrhiza* root tissue. To take advantage of the inducible nature of tanshinone biosynthesis, a microarray chip was manufactured from ~8 700 random cDNA inserts, which ranged in size from 0.5 to 2.5 kb. This was used to compare mRNA levels from induced and control *S. miltiorrhiza* hairy root cultures. Of the clones upregulated by elictor treatment, only one CPS homologue and one KSL homologue were found, both as partial cDNA clones. These also were determined to be the only such homologues in the microarray. Given the importance of the corresponding enzymatic reactions in initiating tanshinone biosynthesis and fixing the stereochemical configuration of the subsequent metabolism, these putative *S. miltiorrhiza* diterpene synthases were chosen for analysis. Thus, the missing sequence for each (SmCPS and SmKSL) was obtained via rapid amplification of the cDNA ends, and the corresponding full-length mRNA sequence was determined.

Plant secondary metabolism, such as tanshinone biosynthesis, is generally regulated by transcriptional control of the genes encoding the relevant enzymes. Thus, both SmCPS and SmKSL seemed likely to be involved in tanshinone biosynthesis because their mRNA levels are increased >2-fold by elicitation, application of a biotic-abiotic combination of the carbohydrate fraction of yeast extract with $Ag^+$, which has previously been shown to induce tanshinone production. This was further examined through application of the plant defense signaling molecule methyl jasmonate (MeJA), which also was found to increase both the mRNA levels of these diterpene synthases and, subsequently, tanshinone ⅡA (**2**) biosynthesis in *S. miltiorrhiza* hairy root cultures (Figure 2). The observed coinduction by two separate treatments and increase in mRNA prior to tanshinone accumulation, similar to the analogous temporal pattern observed with rice labdane-related diterpenoid phytoalexin biosynthesis, indicate that SmCPS and SmKSL may be involved in tanshinone biosynthesis. On this basis, the encoded enzymes were further characterized.

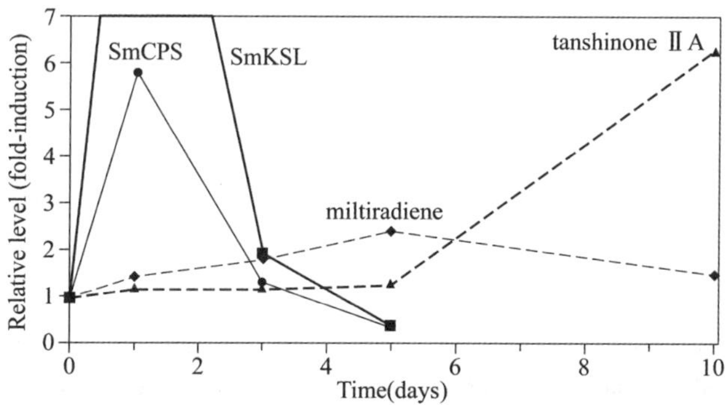


**Figure 2  Relative (fold-induction) levels of SmCPS (squares) and SmKSL (circles, 15-fold at 1 day) mRNA and the amounts of the derived miltiradiene (9, diamonds) and presumably downstream tanshinone ⅡA (2, triangles) found in MeJA treated versus control hairy root cultures of *S. miltiorrhiza***

The SmCPS full-length open reading frame was subcloned into pET32a(+) for recombinant expression in *Escherichia coli* (see the Supporting Information for the Materials and Methods section). This SmCPS construct was expressed and purified, via use of the encoded hexahistidine tag, and then assayed for class Ⅱ diterpene cyclase activity with **5**. The resulting product was enzymatically dephosphorylated for gas chromatography-mass spectrometry (GC - MS) analysis. A comparison to similarly dephosphorylated *ent*- and *syn*- CPP demonstrated that SmCPS-produced CPP of either *ent* or normal stereochemistry (Figure S1 in the Supporting Information). The absolute configuration of the SmCPS-produced CPP was resolved by use of a previously described modular metabolic engineering system, much like that previously described for other class Ⅱ diterpene synthases. In particular, a pseudomature version of SmCPS (i.e., without the plastid targeting prepeptide) was coexpressed with a GGPP synthase and diterpene synthases specific for normal and *ent*- or *syn*-CPP, with the expected diterpene only obtained with the normal CPP specific enzyme. Thus, SmCPS produces CPP of normal stereochemistry (**6**; Scheme 1). Notably, while normal (5*S*, 9*S*, 10*S*) - CPP is transiently formed by the bifunctional diterpene synthases involved in gymnosperm resin acid biosynthesis, SmCPS appears to be the first identified normal CPP specific CPS and the first class Ⅱ diterpene cyclase with this particular stereospecificity from an angiosperm.

**Scheme 1**. SmCPS- and SmKSL-Catalyzed Reactions[a]

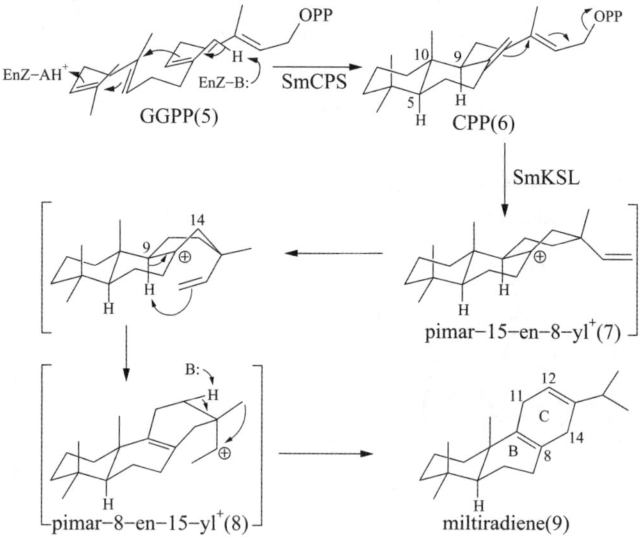

[a] Cyclization of GGPP(**5**) to normal CPP (**6**) catalyzed by SmCPS and subsequent further cyclization and rearrangement of **6** to miltiradiene (**9**). presumably via pimar-15-en-8-yl$^+$ (**7**) and pimar-8-en-15-yl$^+$ (**8**) intermediates, catalyzed by SmKSL.

The catalytic activity of SmKSL was similarly investigated, i.e. first in vitro using recombinant protein expressed from a pET32a(+)-derived construct in *E. coli* and purified via the encoded hexahistidine tag. In coupled assays, this recombinant SmKSL was found to accept the (normal) CPP (**6**) product of SmCPS to produce an unknown diterpene (Figure S2 in the Supporting Information). The identity of this compound was established by use of the same modular metabolic engineering system, much like that described for other novel class Ⅰ diterpene synthases. Specifically, by production of ~5 mg of the SmKSL product derived from **6**, enabling straightforward analysis by NMR (Figures S3 - S8 and Table S1 in the Supporting Information). The structure was assigned using HMBC, HSQC, and COSY data, which demonstrated that this was an abietane-type diterpene, which we propose to name miltiradiene (**9**). Of particular note is the cyclohexa-1,4-diene structure of the distal C ring in **9**, whose double-bond arrangement was evident in the relatively high chemical shifts observed for the protons on the doubly allylic C11 and C14 (i.e., due to deshielding effects), with the presence of only a single methine (i.e., C12) being confirmed by examination of the HSQC data.

While mixtures of abietadienes are produced by some bifunctional diterpene synthases involved in gymnosperm resin acid biosynthesis, SmKSL appears to be the first identified normal CPP specific KSL and the first abietane-type diterpene producing class Ⅰ diterpene synthase of any kind identified from an angiosperm. In addition, the observed 8,12-diene arrangement in **9** presumably requires a distinctly different configuration of the intervening pimar-15-en-8-yl$^+$ (**7**) intermediate in SmKSL, specifically, to enable proton transfer from C9 (Scheme 1) and formation of pimar-8-en-15-yl$^+$ (**8**) rather than proton transfer from C14 to form pimar-8(14)-en-15-yl$^+$, as was previously demonstrated for the bifunctional gymnosperm abietane-type diterpene synthases.

As expected from the inducible nature of the relevant SmCPS and SmKSL, an increase in **9** is observed in *S. miltiorrhiza* hairy root cultures following MeJA treatment (Figure 2). Notably, **9** only transiently accumulates, and its subsequent decrease is inversely related to an increase of tanshinone ⅡA (**2**), suggesting that **9** is an intermediate en route to the tanshinones (**1** - **4**). Given the normal stereochemistry defined by **9**, it seems likely that the previously observed production of ferruginol (**10**) by *S. miltiorrhiza* is also relevant to tanshinone metabolism, and consideration of other identified diterpenoid natural products, specifically miltirone (**11**) and neocryptotanshinone (**12**), enables the proposal of a hypothetical biosynthetic pathway, albeit still incomplete (Scheme 2).

**Scheme 2.** Hypothetical Tanshinone Biosynthetic Pathway

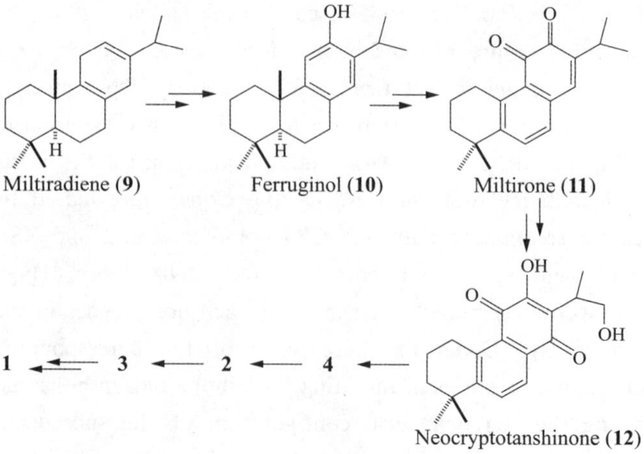

Interestingly, while the bifunctional abietane-type synthases from gymnosperms produce mixtures of conjugated double-bond abietadienes, SmKSL is quite specific in its production of **9**, which is found as > 95% of the total product output. The apposing 1,4-diene arrangement in **9** imposes planarity on the C ring and across the B/C ring bridgehead, just as is found in the aromatic tanshinones and the other identified diterpenoid natural products from *S. miltiorrhiza*. Accordingly, such planarity appears to be imposed early in tanshinone biosynthesis and utilized by the subsequently acting biosynthetic enzymes. Indeed, cyclohexan-1,4-dienes such as that observed in the C ring of **9** are generally considered relatively unstable and will readily aromatize, indicating that **9** is poised for further relevant transformations, specifically aromatization and hydroxylation to form ferruginol(**10**).

Regardless of the exact series of relevant transformations, stereochemical resolution of **9** as a presumably relevant intermediate enables investigation of the critical downstream tanshinone biosynthetic enzymes, which will be further enabled by the molecular tools reported here. Thus, the functional characterization of SmCPS and SmKSL reported here has identified a novel normal stereochemistry specific CPS and subsequently acting miltiradiene synthase (SmKSL) and laid the basis for further investigation of tanshinone biosynthesis.

[高伟，黄璐琦，Reuben J Peters，等. Organic letters，2009,11(22):5170-5173.]

# Modular pathway engineering of diterpenoid synthases and the mevalonic acid pathway for miltiradiene production

## 1 INTRODUCTION

Diterpenoids are 20-carbon terpenoids synthesized from (*E*,*E*,*E*)-geranylgeranyl diphosphate (GGPP) by diterpene synthases/cyclases. Some diterpenoids found in plants possess a wide range of pharmaceutical activities. For example, the paclitaxel, a taxane diterpenoid from *Taxus brevifolia*, is a known antimicrotubule chemotherapy agent for the treatment of cancer. Tanshionones are a group of abietane-type norditerpenoids rich in the Chinese medicinal herb *Salvia miltiorrhiza* (Supporting Information Figure 1), which have demonstrated a variety of biological activities, including antibacterial, antiinflammatory, and anticancer activities. However, the extraction of diterpenoids from plants has been tedious and inefficient, and requires substantial sacrifice of natural resources. Although a number of microorganisms have been engineered to produce isoprenoids as well as their intermediates, the overall efficiency remains low. Further, there are complications that could have adverse effects on the engineered pathway. For example, metabolic flux imbalance, intermediates diffusion, and degradation can decrease the overall efficiency of the engineered pathway. Thus, carefully tuning protein expression levels has been shown to balance the metabolic flux for improving productivity. Artificial protein scaffolds capturing different stoichiometric number of enzymes in proximity have also been used in preventing intermediates loss. These strategies commonly focus on the mevalonic acid (MVA) or methyl-D-erythritol phosphate (MEP) pathways that are at the early stage of terpenoids biosynthesis. However, the conservation and interactions of diterpenoids synthases attracted little attention.

In nature, terpene synthases may contain one, two, or three highly conserved domains: the α domain with a highly α-helical fold containing a conserved DDXXD motif for $Mg^{2+}$-ionization and the βγ domain often containing a catalytic DXDD motif for "protonization-initiated" catalysis. The formation of the core structure of diterpenoids can be catalyzed by a bifunctional synthase or two consecutive enzymes (Figure 1a). The bifunctional synthase such as AgAS contains functional αβγ domains (Figure 1b). In the case of two consecutive enzymes used, the first synthase is a class Ⅱ cyclase containing domains αβγ, but the α domain is a nonfunctional vestige due to the lack of the DDXXD motif. The second synthase is a class Ⅰ enzyme containing either αβγ or αβ domains, but only the α domain is functional, and the β(γ) domain is vestigial due to the lack of the D/E-rich motif and the DXDD motif. No biochemical evidence has been known to support molecular interactions between the two consecutive enzymes, although such interactions are presumably beneficial for efficient substrate channeling in vivo to convert GGPP into diterpenoids.

We have recently demonstrated that in *S. miltiorrhiza* a labdadienyl/copalyl diphosphate synthase (SmCPS) and a kaurene synthase-like (SmKSL) are responsible for the transformation of GGPP into miltiradiene, the key intermediate to the pharmaceutically important compounds tanshinones (Figure 1a). Here, we present the modular

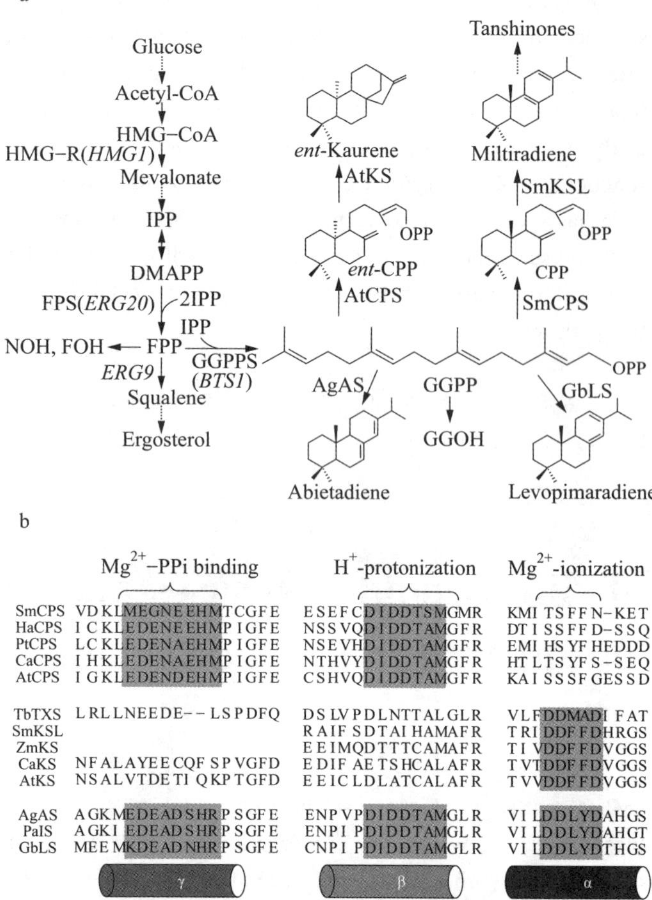


**Figure 1 The diversity and conservedness of diterpenoids biosynthesis**

(a) Schematic representation of the mevalonic acid (MVA) pathway and several diterpenoids biosynthetic pathways. Each solid arrow indicates a biosynthetic reaction step, and dashed arrows indicate the transformation involving multiple-step reactions. Abbreviations: HMG-CoA, 3-hydroxy-3-methylglutaryl coenzyme A; DMAPP, dimethylallyl diphosphate; IPP, isopentenyl pyrophosphate; GGOH, (*E*, *E*, *E*)-geranylgeraniol; CPP, copalyl diphosphate; *ent*-CPP, *ent*-copalyl diphosphate; HMG - R, HMG-coenzyme A reductase (encoded by the *HMG1* gene); FPPS, FPP synthase (*ERG20*); GGPPS, GGPP synthase (*BTS1*); SmCPS, copalyl diphosphate synthase of *S. miltiorrhiza*; SmKSL, kaurene synthase-like of *S. miltiorrhiza*; AtCPS, *ent*-copalyl diphosphate synthase of *Arabidopsis thaliana*; AtKS, kaurene synthase of *A. thaliana*; AgAS, abietadiene synthase of *Abies grandis*; GbLS, Levopimaradiene synthase of *Ginkgo biloba*. (b) Clustal W alignment of several diterpenoid synthases. Conserved catalytic motifs are highlighted, that is, DDxxD in $\alpha$ domain, DxDD in $\beta$ domain, and D/E-rich region in $\gamma$ domain involved in interactions with $Mg^{2+}$ and GGPP.

pathway engineering (MOPE) strategy and its application for a rapid assembling synthetic miltiradiene pathway in the yeast *Saccharomyces cerevisiae*. We analyzed the molecular interactions between SmCPS and SmKSL, and engineered their active sites into close proximity for enhanced metabolic flux channeling to miltiradiene biosynthesis by constructing protein fusions. We show that the fusion of SmCPS and SmKSL, as well as the fusion of BTS1 (GGPP synthase) and ERG20 (farnesyl diphosphate synthase), led to significantly improved miltiradiene production and reduced byproduct accumulation. Our most efficient pathway with the diploid strain YJ2X reached a miltiradiene titer of 365 mg/L in a 15 L bioreactor culture. These results suggested that engineering terpenoids synthases and the precursor supplying enzymes are essential for an efficient heterologous production of terpenoids in *S. cerevisiae*. Moreover, we showed that the fusion of enzymes catalyzing two consecutive reactions within the targeted pathway was in general helpful to improve the effectiveness of the engineered pathway.

## 2 RESULTS

The Interaction between Miltiradiene Synthases in Vivo. Sequence alignment suggested that SmCPS is a class Ⅱ synthase containing $\alpha\beta\gamma$ domains, and SmKSL is a class Ⅰ synthase containing the reserved $Mg^{2+}$-ionization motif DDXXD (Figure 1b). Because the cyclization of GGPP into diterpenoids can be realized by a number of bifunctional synthases, it is inspiring to speculate possible molecular interactions between the two miltiradiene synthases, SmCPS and SmKSL. To test our speculation, we performed coimmunoprecipitation experiments. The lysates of SmCPS-Flag and SmKSL-c-myc coexpressed cells were immunoprecipitated using anti-Flag M2 affinity gel, and then the lysates and eluates were analyzed by immunoblotting using anti-Flag and antimyc antibodies, respectively. Results showed SmKSL-c-myc was coprecipitated with SmCPS-Flag in anti-Flag eluates, indicating a direct interaction between SmCPS and SmKSL (Figure 2). This result suggested that SmCPS and SmKSL may form an enzyme complex in vivo. Although

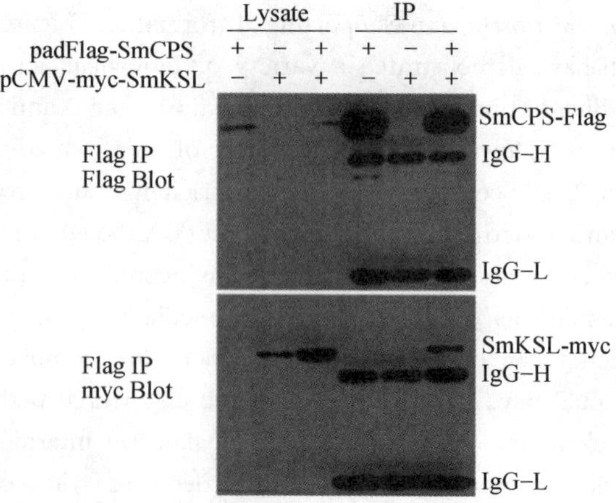


**Figure 2 Sequential immunoprecipitation/immunoblot analysis of molecular interactions between SmCPS and SmKSL**

The lysates of the transfected HEK - 293T containing pad-Flag-SmCPS and/or pCMV-myc-SmKSL were immunoprecipitated using anti-Flag-agarose, and the precipitates were subjected to immunoblot analysis using Flag or c-Myc antibodies. The immuneblot revealed that SmKSL-myc was precipitated with SmCPS-Flag after anti-Flag-agarose immunoprecipitating.

engineering the molecular interactions of diterpenoids synthases has not been demonstrated so far, these results encouraged us to fuse SmCPS and SmKSL for more efficient miltiradiene production (vide infra).

Optimization of the Mevalonate Pathway for Miltiradiene Production. We set up to engineer *S. cerevisiae* for miltiradiene overproduction. As our experiments suggested the presence of molecular interactions between SmCPS and SmKSL, we designed a series of pathway variants having these two proteins fused, hoping to improve productivity (Figure 3a). Our first effort was the transformation of *S. cerevisiae* with the module producing SmCPS and SmKSL (YJ5), or the module producing the fused protein SmCPS - SmKSL (YJ1) or SmKSL - SmCPS (YJ2). However, miltiradiene production was undetectable for all of these three recombinant strains (Figure 3). One might think that SmCPS, SmKSL, and their fusions malfunctioned in yeast, but another possibility might be insufficient precursor supply. Therefore, we decided to make more pathway variants by using the MOPE strategy, which is an improved version of "DNA assembler". In the MOPE strategy, each module was designed to have overlapping ends so that pathways can be generated rapidly in *S. cerevisiae* (Supporting Information Figure 2). We tried to enhance the MVA pathway in the YJ5 background. The modules *ERG20* and *BTS1* were quickly amended, either separately or fused by using the MOPE strategy. When the farnesyl diphosphate (FPP) synthase module *ERG20* was added, the resulting strain YJ6 produced a trace amount of miltiradiene. However, the strain YJ7 expressing the *BTS1* module produced 0.5 mg/L miltiradiene under shake flask culture conditions. Furthermore, the strain YJ8 had both *ERG20* and *BTS1* modules, produced 0.7 mg/L miltiradiene.

Because there are additional pathways consuming FPP (Figure 1a), leading to the synthesis of ergosterol, and FOH, the hydrolysis product of FPP, it is expected to obtain a higher miltiradiene production when the efficiency of the conversion of FPP to GGPP is improved. We reasoned that the fusion of BTS1 and ERG20 might enhance the efficiency of this conversion. Thus, we made two modules that produced fusion proteins ERG20 - BTS1 and BTS1 - ERG20, respectively. While the addition of the *ERG20 - BTS1* module (strain YJ9)

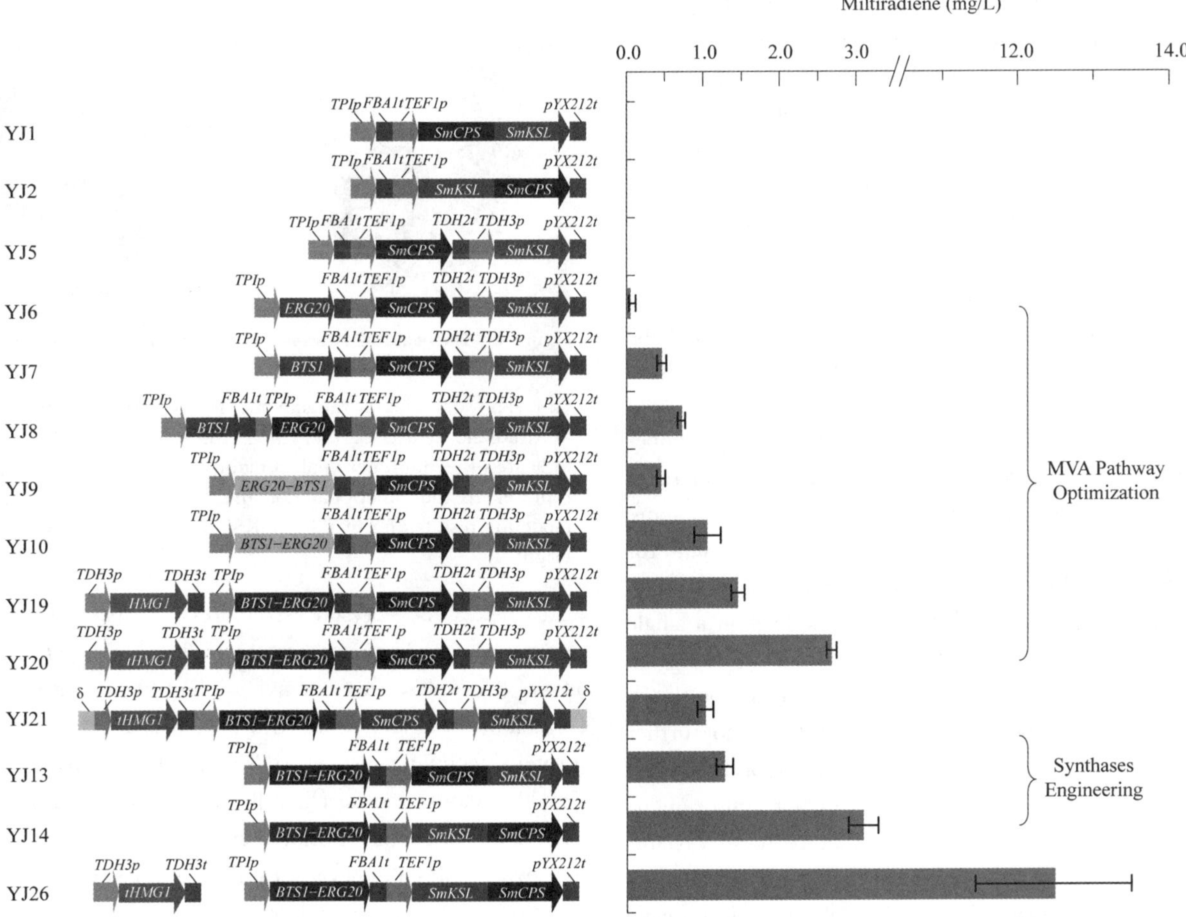


**Figure 3 Miltiradiene production by recombinant yeasts harboring modules overproducing various enzymes**

The strains were cultivated for 48 h in YPD media, and miltiradiene was extracted with equal volume of *n*-hexane. The data represent the averages ± standard deviations of at least three independent clones.

gave a reduced miltiradiene production as compared to that of the strain YJ8, the addition of the *BTS1* - *ERG20* module (strain YJ10) indeed led to an improved miltiradiene production to 1.0 mg/L. Moreover, the strain YJ10 produced less FOH than other strains including the strain YJ9 (Supporting Information Figure 4). These results indicated the presence of BTS1 - ERG20 channeled the FPP flux to miltiradiene production from other FPP-consuming pathways. It should be emphasized that the specific productivity of miltiradiene followed the same trend among these recombinant strains (Supporting Information Figure S3), because these strains had similar growth profiles under shake flask culture conditions.

Another major regulatory control point of the MVA pathway is the formation of MVA from hydroxy-3-methylglutaryl coenzyme A (HMG - CoA) catalyzed by HMG - CoA reductase (HMG) 1 and 2. In *S. cerevisiae*, HMG1 contributes at least 83% of the activity. Early studies showed that the over-expression of the catalytic domain of HMG1 (*tHMG1*) could lead to an improved production of isoprenoids, while a recent report showed the full length version was more effective for the production of prenyl alcohols. We thus examined the capacity of both HMG1 and tHMG1 in this study. Additional expression of *HMG1* in the YJ10 background (YJ19) resulted in a 38% increase in miltiradiene yield, and the expression of *tHMG1* (YJ20) led to a 2.6-fold increase to 2.7 mg/L miltiradiene (Figure 3).

As synthetic pathways integrated into chromosome are considered more stable than episomal plasmid-based systems, we constructed a strain (YJ21) by integrating the optimized module of YJ20 into the chromosome flanked by two selection markers *URA3* and *HIS3* (Supporting Information Figure S2). However, the integrated strain YJ21 produced only 1.1 mg/L miltiradiene, which was lower than that of the strain YJ20. The lower copy number of the integrated pathway might be the main reason for a reduced miltiradiene production. Although there are more than 300 $\delta$ sites on the chromosome of *S. cerevisiae* for integration, it might be difficult to integrate multiple copies of constructs with a recombination of 4 modules in a single transformation experiment. In addition, no selection pressure was applied to enrich strains having multicopy integrations in this study. Developing strategies to further improve integration efficiency should be helpful for the construction of stable strains with higher miltiradiene production capacity. Therefore, all other pathway variants had genes assembled on the plasmid (vide infra).

**Miltiradiene Synthases Engineering.** We next introduced the BTS1 - ERG20 module into the strains with the fused miltiradiene synthases to give the strains YJ13 and YJ14 (Figure 4a). While the combination of BTS1 - ERG20 with SmCPS - SmKSL gave a slightly higher miltiradiene production than that of the Strain YJ10, the combination of BTS1 - ERG20 with SmKSL - SmCPS gave a 2.9-fold increase to 3.1 mg/L. Further, when *tHMG1* was introduced in the YJ14 background, the resulting strain YJ26 produced 12.5 mg/L miltiradiene, which was a 4.0-fold improvement over the parent strain, carrying separate SmCPS and SmKSL. We also observed that the strain YJ26 produced significantly lower GGOH, the hydrolysis product of GGPP, than the strain YJ20 (Supporting Information Figure S6). These results indicated that the fusion SmKSL - SmCPS was advantageous over the fusion SmCPS - SmKSL as well as the two proteins being expressed separately in terms of transforming GGPP into miltiradiene.

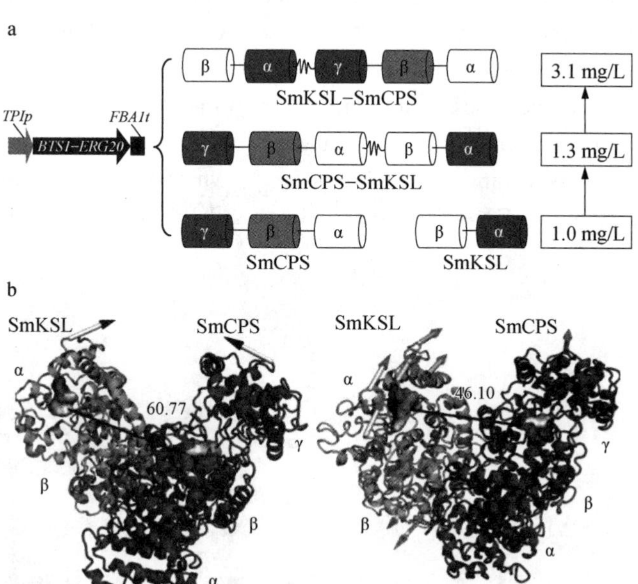


**Figure 4 The modeling structures of the fusion enzymes of miltiradiene synthases**

(a) The domains arrangement in the primary structure of miltiradiene synthases and their fusions. The white columns indicated the nonfunctional domains, and the colorful columns represented the functional domains. (b) Side view of protein modeling results of SmCPS - SmKSL (left) and SmKSL - SmCPS (right).

The X-ray crystal structures of two diterpenoids synthases, taxadiene synthase from *Taxus brevifolia* and the class Ⅱ cyclase ent-copalyl diphosphate synthase from *Arabidopsis thaliana* (AtCPS), have been available recently. Protein modeling using AtCPS as the template showed SmCPS belongs to the class Ⅱ synthase and the active site DXDD motif for $H^+$-initiated cyclization is located between the $\beta\gamma$ domains in the N-terminus (Supporting Information Figure S7). Protein modeling using taxadiene synthase as the template showed the active site of SmKSL is located at the $\alpha$ domain in the C-terminus (Supporting Information Figure S7). It is conceivable that the fusion protein in the SmKSL -

SmCPS format brought the active site of SmCPS and the active $\alpha$ domain of SmCPS closer than that of the SmCPS - SmKSL format (Figure 4a). Indeed, protein modeling showed that active sites in SmKSL - SmCPS have a closer proximity (46.10 Å) than that of SmCPS - SmKSL (60.77 Å). The dynamic behavior derived from normal-mode analysis of these two complexes also showed that the large-scale motion of SmKSL - SmCPS was more favorable for shortening that distance and avoiding the block between two active sites than that of SmCPS - SmKSL (Figure 4b and Supporting Information Figure S7c and d). Therefore, our structural analysis showed protein fusion may bring active sites into a closer proximity, which can be beneficial to miltiradiene production.

Miltiradiene Overproduction by Prototrophic Strains. Because of the *S. cerevisiae* BY4741 background and the presence of pYX212 and p424GPD (HIS) backbone, the above miltiradiene-producing strains remained auxotrophic to leucine and methionine. We further constructed a prototrophic haploid strain YJ28 by complementing the auxotrophic markers *LEU2* and *MET15*. We noticed that *LEU2* and *MET15* complementation improved the cell growth and miltiradiene titer, and that the strain with *LEU2* complementation increased the specific miltiradiene productivity (Figure 5a). The prototrophic strain YJ28 produced 17.9 mg/L miltiradiene in shake flask culture and up to 178 mg/L in 15 L bioreactor culture (Figure 6a), which was significantly higher than the previous data of 2.5 mg/L

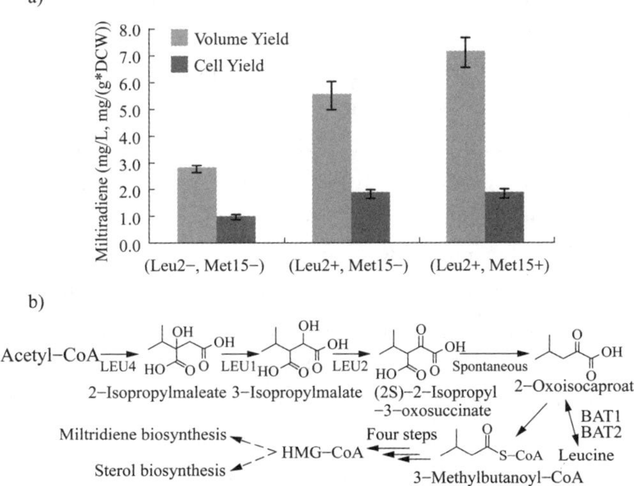


**Figure 5** ***LEU2* complementation improved miltiradiene production**

(a) Miltiradiene production by prototrophic and auxotrophic strains in shake flask cultures. (Leu2 −, Met15 −) represents recombinant strain YJ20 carrying the MVA optimized pathway with methionine and leucine auxotroph, (Leu2 +, Met15 −) represents recombinant strain YJ25 with methionine auxotroph, and (Leu2 +, Met15 +) represents prototrophic strain YJ28. Results are the averages ± standard deviations of four independent clones. (b) The proposed alternative HMG - CoA formation pathway involved in leucine metabolism.

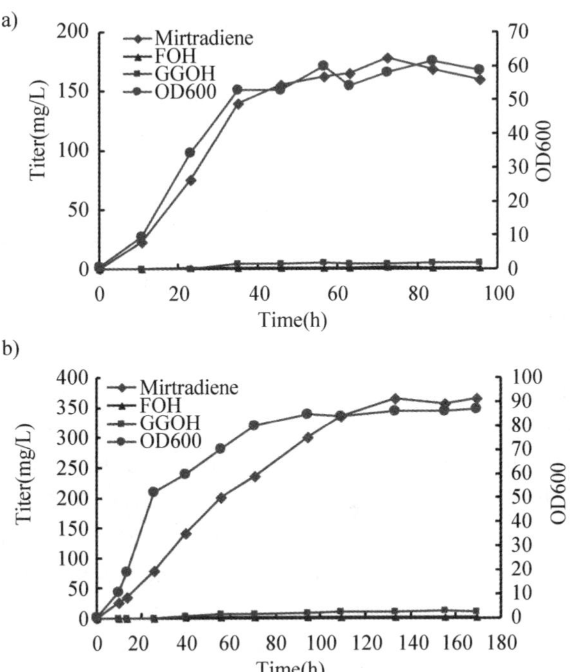


**Figure 6 Fermentation profiles of the prototrophic strain YJ28 (a) and the diploid strain YJ2X (b) in a 15 L stirred-tank bioreactor**

obtained in the recombinant *E. coli* strain. The byproducts FOH and GGOH were only 1.4 and 4.8 mg/L, respectively.

Diploidization is another strategy to improve the productivity due to higher expression levels of heterologous genes and tolerances to various stresses as compared to haploid strains. The prototrophic diploid strain YJ2X, constructed by mating the methionine auxotrophic strain YJ27 and BY4742, produced 22.7 mg/L miltiradiene in shake flask culture conditions, which was slightly higher as compared to the haploid strain YJ28. However, when cultivated in a 15 L bioreactor, YJ2X produced 365 mg/L miltiradiene, which was 2.1-fold higher than that of the YJ28 strain. Again, FOH and GGOH were observed at 1.8 and 10.2 mg/L, respectively (Figure 6b). Because the promoters used in our system were all constitutive, no inducers such as IPTG or galactose were required in the culture media. This feature distinguished our study from those previous reports on isoprenoids production in *E. coli* or yeast, and made it more economical and convenient for a large-scale process.

## 3 DISCUSSION

Early metabolic engineering studies on diterpenoid biosynthesis have been focused on the optimization of the MVA or MEP pathways to increase the precursors supply. When the cyclization step leading to the core structure of diterpenoids is catalyzed by two consecutive enzymes, no information is available in terms of potential molecular interactions between these enzymes. In the case of miltiradiene production from GGPP catalyzed by SmCPS and SmKSL, we observed interactions between them in vivo with coimmunoprecipitation (Figure 2). Such interaction may be biologically significant, because the formation of protein complex could bring active sites into a closer proximity, facilitating more efficient substrate channeling. In other words, it could prevent intermediates from diffusion and degradation by other enzymes. Indeed, the formation of enzyme complexes has been suggested to improve the efficiency of the specific pathways by preventing substrates and intermediates from diffusion and degradation. Recently, several proteomic studies showed that the formation of protein complexes is common and that the interactions between the consecutive enzymes are helpful for substrate channeling. For example, molecular interactions among several enzymes catalyzing the adjacent steps of the tricarboxylic acid cycle in *Bacillus subtilis* were observed for regulating the metabolic fluxes. In human cells, enzymes involved in purine biosynthesis also formed protein complexes. We introduced SmCPS and SmKSL fusions in yeast to improve miltiradiene production, and indeed the fused synthases had better performance. While the pathway variant YJ13 containing the fusion SmCPS - SmKSL only afforded slight improvement as compared to the variant YJ10 with SmCPS and SmKSL being expressed separately, the variant YJ14 contained the reverse fusion SmKSL - SmCPS produced 2.8-fold more miltiradiene (Figure 4). Protein modeling showed that the fusion SmKSL - SmCPS brought the active sites closer than did the fusion SmCPS - SmKSL (Figure 4b). The fact that byproducts GGOH and FOH were less for the variant YJ14 (Supporting Information Figure S6) suggested that GGPP was turned over more efficiently by the fused enzyme SmKSL - SmCPS. As compared to direct evolution of the bifunctional levopimaradiene synthase (LPS) for catalytic activity improvement, engineering the active sites of separate diterpenoid synthases into a close proximity provides another convenient and powerful approach. To test the generality of the approach, we also fused BTS1 and ERG20, enzymes catalyzing the adjacent steps for GGPP production. It turned out that the fusion BTS1 - ERG20 was advantageous over the fusion ERG20 - BTS1 (Supporting Information Figure S4), as the former produced more miltiradiene and less FOH. These results suggested that the fusion BTS1 - ERG20 improved the FPP flux to miltiradiene production. The fusion of enzymes within diterpenoid biosynthetic pathway avoided the loss of intermediates through diffusion, degradation, or conversion by competitive enzymes in multistep metabolic pathways, which was similar to the natural megasynthases systems such as Type Ⅰ polyketide synthase and fatty acid synthase.

It is worth mentioning that the introduction of SmCPS and SmKSL or their fusions into the yeast resulted in no miltiradiene production (Figure 3). These observations may otherwise lead to conclusions that those enzymes were incompetent in yeast, or that those genes were incorrectly expressed. Thanks to the MOPE strategy, we were able to assemble pathway variants by including genes responsible for the formation of metabolites beyond miltiradiene per se. Although the MOPE strategy is technically reminiscent of "DNA assembler" described earlier, the efficiency for the construction of functional modules was substantially improved with one-step SOE PCR. Because all promoter and terminator sequences were purposely included at the termini of each module, the assembled pathway variants essentially had no redundant DNA sequences. Moreover, the MOPE strategy did not limit modules to heterologous genes, as chimeric pathways containing heterologous and endogenous genes were efficiently assembled in this study. Thus, we noticed the overexpression of *ERG20* in the YJ5 background resulted in little improvement in miltiradiene production, which was similar to a number of previous reports on isoprenoids production. However, the expression of *BTS1* resulted in significantly higher miltiradiene production, indicating that GGPP synthesis was the pivotal step to provide extra metabolic flux for miltiradiene production. Similar observations have been documented for the production of other diterpenoids. Early studies showed that the higher level of HMG reductase (HMG1) as well as its catalytic domain tHMG1 were helpful for the isoprenoid biosynthesis. We found that overexpression of both *HMG1* and *tHMG1* in the YJ10 background led to an improved miltiradiene production yield (Figure 3a). However, overexpression of eithor HMG1 (YJ16) or tHMG1 (YJ17) in the YJ5 background produced little miltiradiene (Supporting Information Figure 5). These results indicated in our system that BTS1, but not HMG1, played the most important role in directing the metabolic flux to miltiradiene biosynthesis.

We further constructed the prototrophic haploid strain YJ28 and diploid strain YJ2X, and achieved major improvement in terms of miltiradiene titer at a large-scale culture. The prototrophic haploid strains grew faster and produced more miltiradiene than those auxotrophic strains. Interestingly, the *LEU2* complementation improved the specific miltiradiene productivity, while the *MET15* complementation had no such effect, indicating that leucine supply was beneficial for miltiradiene biosynthesis. It occurred to us that leucine metabolism may be networked with isoprenoid biosynthesis (Figure 5b). A previous report showed that leucine catabolism could lead to the formation of HMG - CoA and the incorporation into sterol in *Leishmania mexicana*. The biosynthesis of leucine produces a precursor 2-oxoisocaproate, and exogenous leucine can be catabolized to this precursor. 2-Oxoisocaproate can be converted into HMG - CoA by a number of enzymes. Therefore, the leucine biosynthetic pathway may be considered as a bypath to facilitate additional HMG-CoA supply. Our observation cautioned one to consider metabolisms beyond the biosynthetic genes and to use leucine prototrophic hosts for a higher isoprenoids production.

In summary, we demonstrated remarkable improvement of miltiradiene productivity by using the MOPE strategy in the construction of flexible pathway variants involving multiple genes in *S. cerevisiae*. Furthermore, protein fusion was shown to be general in directing metabolic flux to focused pathway for the heterologous production of isoprenoids such as miltiradiene. Strategies of pathway assembling in this study should be applicable to engineering microbial hosts for the production of other valuable metabolites.

## 4 EXPERIMENTAL PROCEDURES

Strains, Reagents, and Media. The yeast strains used in this study are listed in Supporting Information Table 1. PrimeStar DNA polymerase, restriction enzymes, and other enzymes were purchased from TaKaRa Bio. Oligonucleotides were purchased from Invitrogen. DNA gel purification and plasmid extraction kits were purchased from Beyotime. Yeast nitrogen base and peptone were products of Difco. Yeast extracts and tryptone were from Oxoid. Amino acids, nucleotides, and agar powder were supplied by Dingguo Biotech. Anti-Flag M2 affinity agarose, mouse Flag antibodies, prenyl alcohols (FOH, GGOH), and other chemicals were purchased from Sigma. Mouse c-Myc antibodies were from Santa Cruz. Enhanced chemoluminescence and PVDF membrane were from Amersham Biosciences. Synthetic dextrose (SD) medium consisted of 20 g/L glucose, 6.7 g/L yeast nitrogen base with $(NH_4)_2SO_4$ and without amino acids. SD containing one or several specific nutrients (20 mg/L uracil, 20 mg/L histidine, 20 mg/L methionine, or 100 mg/L leucine) was used for the corresponding auxotrophic strains cultivation. YPD consisted of 10 g/L yeast extract, 20 g/L peptone, and 20 g/L dextrose. *Escherichia coli* strains were grown at 37 ℃ on Luria-Bertani medium (10 g/L tryptone, 5 g/L yeast extract, 10 g/L NaCl) supplemented with ampicillin (100 ug/mL) if required. Agar plates were made with the corresponding liquid medium supplemented with 15 g/L agar powder. The medium for a large-scale culture using 15 L stirred-tank bioreactor was comprised of 20 g/L glucose, 10 g/L yeast extract, 20 g/L peptone, 10 g/L $(NH_4)_2SO_4$, 1.0 g/L $KH_2PO_4$, 1.0 g/L $MgSO_4 \cdot 7H_2O$, and 1.0 g/L $CaCl_2 \cdot 2H_2O$.

DNA Manipulation. All of the primers used for DNA manipulation were listed in Supporting Information Table 2. The gene expressing modules consisted of a promoter, a structural gene, a terminator, and the promoter of the next module for homologous recombination. The promoter *TPIp* and the terminator *pYX212t* were PCR-amplified from pYX212, which also was used as an expression vector kindly provided by Prof. Ming Yan at Nanjing University of Technology; other prompters (*TEF1p* and TDH3p), terminators (*FBA1t*, *CYC1t* and *ADH2t*), and functional genes (*BTS1*, *ERG20* and *HMG1*) were PCR-amplified from the genomic DNA of *S. cerevisiae* BY4741. *SmCPS* and *SmKSL* were PCR-amplified from the cDNA cloning vectors. The fusion enzymes encoding genes were constructed by inserting a widely used GGGS linker encoding sequence "GGT GGT GGT TCT" between the two corresponding genes. All modules were constructed with the one-step PCR strategy similar to overlap extension PCR. Briefly, purified parts of individual module (promoter, functional gene, terminator, and promoter of next module, molar ratio 1 : 3 : 3 : 1) were mixed in about 100 - 300 ng each, then were added 3 μL of dNTP (2.5 mmol/L each), 5 μL 5×PrimerStar buffer, 1.25 U PrimeSTAR HS DNA polymerase, and $H_2O$ to a total volume of 25 μL, and then it was subjected to PCR amplification with the thermocycle conditions of 95 ℃ for 5 min, 15 cycles of 98 ℃ for 10 s, 68 ℃ for 1 min/kb, and last 68 ℃ for 10 min. Next, 2 μL of unpurified PCR products was taken out as the template and added F- and R-primer and PrimeSTAR HS DNA polymerase and for normal PCR amplification in a total volume of 100 μL according to manufacturer's instructions. The DNA fragments of parts and modules were individually gel-purified from a 0.8% agarose gel. Equal molar amounts of purified individual modules (300 - 500 ng) were mixed and transformed into *S. cerevisiae* with electroporation at 1.5 kV, 10 μF, and 200 Ω in a 0.2 cm gap electroporation cuvette using Eppendorf Eporator (Eppendorf AG, Hamburg, Germany). p424GPD (HIS) used for overexpressing *HMG1* or *tHMG1* was constructed by replacing *TRP1* marker with *HIS3* in p424GPD using RF cloning method as previous described. Next, the *HMG1* or *tHMG1* was cloned to the downstream of the *TDH3p* promoter using RF cloning strategy as mentioned above. The leucine and/or methionine auxotrophic strains were constructed as a previous report. Diploid strain YJ2X was constructed by mating the methionine auxotrophic strain YJ27 and BY4742 as described previously.

Verification of the Assembled Pathways. Selected colonies formed on the plates were cultured in 5 mL of YPD liquid medium at 30 ℃ for 72 h. Cells were collected and disrupted using ethanol-washed glass beads (0.4 g, 0.4 - 0.6 mm). Cell lysates were collected for plasmid extraction using plasmid extraction kit according to manufacturer's instructions. Recovered plasmids were checked by designed PCR procedures to verify the assembled pathways.

Alternatively, positive plasmids were also transformed into *E. coli* DH5α, recovered, digested by the restriction endonuclease Hind Ⅲ, and analyzed by gel electrophoresis.

Extraction and Quantification of Isoprenoids. Miltiradiene samples were purified in house. Briefly, cell pellets of the engineered *S. cerevisiae* were extracted with hexane three times. The hexane phase was pooled and evaporated in vacuum, and the residues were subjected to column chromatography on silica gel eluted with hexane to give miltiradiene with good purity. GC-MS and NMR data of a purified sample were shown (Supporting Information Figures 8-10).

To quantify yields of miltiradiene and prenyl alcohols (FOH, GGOH) of different cultures, 100 mL of hexane was mixed with 100 mL of culture broth (including yeast cells) and vortexed for 30 min. The organic layer was recovered, and concentrated to a final volume of 0.5 mL. The concentrated samples were subjected to GC analysis. The isoprenoids were quantified on the 7890F GC instrument (Techcomp Scientific Instrument Co. Ltd., Shanghai, China) equipped with a flame ionization detector. GC analysis was done with a SE-54 column (30 m×0.25 mm×0.25 μm), and operational conditions were as follows. The carrier gas nitrogen was set at a flow rate of 1.6 mL/min. The oven temperature was first kept constant at 40 ℃ for 10 min, and then increased to 200 ℃ at the increment of 10 ℃/min, and held for 40 min at the final temperature. Temperatures for the injector and the detector were at 250 and 280 ℃, respectively.

Cultivation Procedures for Miltiradiene Production. To determine the performance of recombinant yeast strains, individual clones were transferred into the SC medium lacking the corresponding nutrition and cultivated at 30 ℃, 200 rpm for 48 h. Aliquots were diluted to an initial $OD_{600}$ of 0.05 in 100 mL of YPD medium in 500 mL flasks and grown at 30 ℃, 200 rpm for 48 h. The culture samples were analyzed as described above.

For a larger-scale culture with the 15 L stirred-tank bioreactor (Shanghai Guoqiang Bioengineering Equipment Co. Ltd., Shanghai, China), 6 L of fermentation medium was inoculated at 10 vol % with the preculture of the recombinant yeast prepared in a shake flask at 30℃, 200 rpm for 48 h. The dissolved oxygen, temperature, aeration, and pH were controlled at >40% saturation, 30℃, 1 volume of air per volume of culture per minute and 5.5, respectively. Concentrated glucose solution (100%, wt/vol) was fed periodically to keep the glucose concentration above 1.0 g/L. Dodacane was added to 20% (v/v) of the media volume. Additional yeast extract (10 g/L) and peptone (20 g/L) were fed at 35.2 h for YJ28 growth, and $(NH_4)_2SO_4$ solution (10 g/L) was fed at 39.9 h for YJ2X fermentation. Duplicate culture aliquots were collected periodically to determine glucose concentration, cell density, and miltiradiene content.

Immunoprecipitation Analysis. Transfection cells were cultivated for 48 h, and washed four times with ice-cold PBS buffer. The cells were disrupted at 4 ℃ with sonication (200 W, 2 s sonication and 1 s rest, 30 times) in 1 mL of cell lysis buffer (20 mmol/L HEPES, PH 7.2, 50 mmol/L NaCl, 0.5% TritonX-100, 1 mmol/L NaF, and 1 mmol/L DTT plus protease inhibitors). The lysates were centrifuged for 10 min at 12 000*g* at 4 ℃, and the supernatants were combined with 20 μL of anti-Flag M2 affinity agarose (Sigma) and mixed for 8 h at 4 ℃. The immunoadsorbents were recovered by centrifugation for 5 min at 1 000 *g* in cell lysis buffer and washed two times with NETN buffer (20 mmol/L Tris, 100 mmol/L NaCl, 0.5% NP-40, and 1 mmol/L EDTA plus protease and phosphatase inhibitors, pH 7.5). Next, 50 μL of loading buffer was added to the immunoabsorbents and boiled for 10 min. The eluted samples were subjected to SDS-PAGE and immune-blot analysis as described previously.

Protein Modeling. Detailed computational protein structure modeling methods for SmCPS-SmKSL and SmKSL-SmCPS were described in the figure legend of Supporting Information Figure 7.

## 5 ASSOCIATED CONTENT

Supporting Information　Table S1: *S. cerevisiae* strains used in this study. Table S2: Primers used for part cloning and module construction. Figure S1: Hypothetical tanshinones biosynthetic pathway. Figure S2: Schematic illustration of the modular pathway engineering strategy for rapid pathway construction. Figure S3: The specific miltiradiene titer in recombinant *S. cerevisiae* strains. Figure S4: BTS1-ERG20 fusion decreased FOH level. Figure S5: The BTS1 not the tHMG1 was the key enzyme for miltiradiene production. Figure S6: SmKSL-SmCPS fusion decreased FOH and GGOH levels. Figure S7: The modeling structures of SmCPS and SmKSL. Figure S8: GC-MS of purified miltiradiene from the engineered yeast strain. Figure S9: $^{13}C$ NMR spectra of miltiradiene. Figure S10: $^{1}H$ NMR spectra of miltiradiene. This material is available free of charge via the Internet at http://pubs.acs.org.

[周雍进，黄璐琦，赵宗保，等. Journal of the American Chemical Society, 2012, 134: 3234-3241.]

# CYP76AH1 catalyzes turnover of miltiradiene in tanshinones biosynthesis and enables heterologous production of ferruginol in yeasts

Terpenoids represent a diverse class of secondary metabolites attracting commercial interest due to their use as drugs, fragrances, and alternative fuels. In plants, terpenoids are synthe-sized from two $C_5$ precursors, isopentenyl diphosphate (IPP) and dimethylallyl diphosphate (DMAPP), which are derived via the 1-deoxyxylulose-5-phosphate pathway or the mevalonate pathway. Prenyltransferases then combine DMAPP and IPP to form other building blocks, (*E*)-geranyl pyrophosphate (GPP; $C_{10}$), (*E*, *E*)-farnesyl pyrophosphate (FPP; $C_{15}$), and (*E*, *E*, *E*)-geranylgeranyl pyrophosphate (GGPP; $C_{20}$). These acyclic precursors are transformed by terpene synthases/cyclases, followed by tailoring enzymes to generate compounds with tremendous structure diversities. Thus, over 50, 000 terpenoid compounds have been identified. The most important tailoring process in terpenoid biosynthesis is oxidation/oxygenation, which is largely catalyzed by cytochrome P450 (CYP) enzymes. However, functionally characterizing the role of plant CYP in particular biotransformation step(s) in terpenoid biosynthesis is extremely challenging, because these CYPs normally have high substrate specificity, share low sequence homology, and the encoding genes generally are not physically clustered together with genes responsible for the up-stream enzymatic reactions as found in microbial genomes. For example, despite tremendous efforts during the past two decades to delineate the biosynthetic pathway for the most important diterpenoid, taxol, there are still unresolved steps likely involving transformations catalyzed by CYP. Nonetheless, research continues, and has even intensified, because understanding the molecular basis of terpenoid biosynthesis holds great promise to engineer the native-producing organisms, as well as surrogate microbes, to produce the desired molecules in sufficient quantities for commercial purposes.

Our recent efforts have been focused on the biosynthesis of a group of abietane-type norditerpenoids, tanshinones (Fig. 1), the major lipophilic bioactive components of the rhizome of the Chinese medicinal herb, *Salvia miltiorrhiza* Bunge (Lamiaceae), known as tanshen or danshen. Danshen has been prominently mentioned in discussions of how traditional Chinese medicine might be coupled to a more modern approach. More importantly, tanshinones have been shown to exhibit a variety of biological activities, which includes antibiotic, anti-inflammatory, and antioxidant effects, as well as activity against various aspects of heart disease. Indeed, danshen preparations are in phase Ⅱ clinical trials against cardiovascular disease. Although the production of tanshinones is inducible in *S. miltiorrhiza* hairy roots, the current supply is dependent on field-grown plants, which are subject to variable yields, and genetic modification offers potentially increased yields in either system. However, this requires some understanding of the underlying biosynthetic pathway. Our initial investigations were carried out using a functional genomics approach based on a cDNA microarray using ~4,400 expressed sequence tags (ESTs), generated with traditional sequencing technology. This led to functional identification of two sequentially acting diterpene cyclases, as required for the formation of labdane-related diterpenoids such as the tanshinones: specifically, a class Ⅱ diterpene cyclase, which produces copalyl diphosphate from GGPP, termed CPP synthase (SmCPS), and a subsequently acting class Ⅰ diterpene cyclase, termed *ent*-kaurene synthase-like (SmKSL), which produces the abietane miltiradiene.

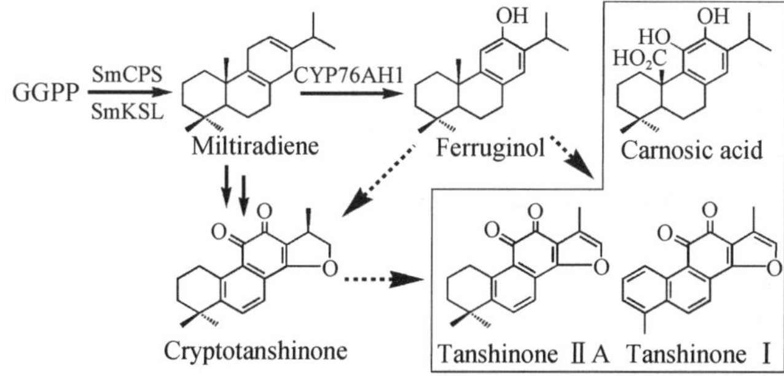


**Fig. 1 Partial pathways for tanshinones biosynthesis and structures for some representative tanshinones. Solid arrows indicate the established relationships, and dashed arrows indicate hypothetical relationships**

Miltiradiene contains a cyclohexa-1,4-diene moiety that imposes a planar configuration on the distal ring, which is suggestively poised for aromatization, as required for the production of tanshinones. Thus, miltiradiene is a potential intermediate in tanshinone biosynthesis, albeit requiring extensive tailoring steps involving oxidation/oxygenation as well as carbon-carbon bond scission (Fig. 1). However, information remains unavailable for structural tailoring miltiradiene and downstream steps of tanshinone biosynthesis at the molecular level. Here we describe results that demonstrate the intermediacy of miltiradiene, at least for late intermediates in the tanshinone biosynthetic pathway, as well as the use of a next-generation sequencing approach to functionally identify a CYP, miltiradiene oxidase CYP76AH1, able to convert miltiradiene to ferruginol. We show that synthetic pathways incorporating CYP76AH1 upon previously engineered *Saccharomyces cerevisiae* enable the production of this elaborated phytoterpenoid up to 10.5 mg/L, providing a platform for further investigation of derived natural products such as the tanshinones.

## 1 RESULTS

Intermediacy of Miltiradiene in Tanshinone Biosynthesis. Whereas the planar conformation of the distal ring in miltiradiene is suggestive, a role for miltiradiene in tanshinone biosynthesis remained hypothetical. This was investigated by stable-isotope labeling. To generate labeled miltiradiene we used a previously developed *Escherichia coli*-based metabolic engineering system that enables coexpression of SmCPS and SmKSL with a GGPP synthase, along with up-regulation of several key enzymes in the endogenous methylerythritol-5-phosphate (MEP)-dependent isoprenoid precursor pathway, as previously described. Accordingly, growth of the resulting recombinant *E. coli* cells in optimized minimal media enabled production of labeled miltiradiene from $^{13}C_6$-glucose. Using this methodology, fully $^{13}$C-labeled miltiradiene was generated, as verified by GC-MS analysis (Fig. 2*A* and *B*).

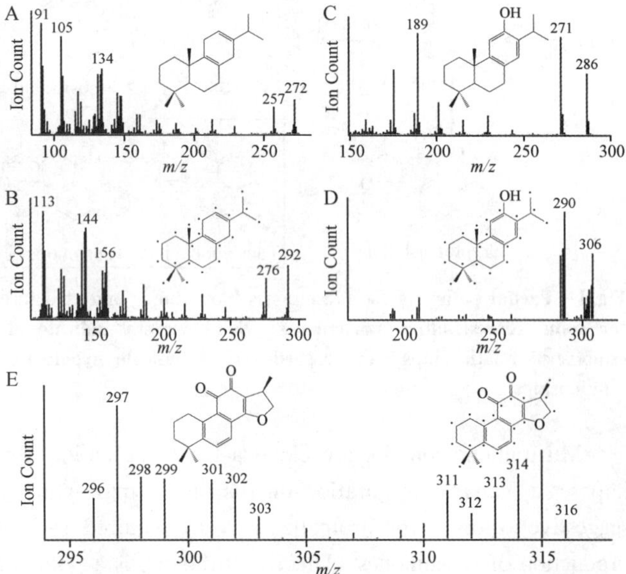

**Fig. 2 Results of stable-isotope labeling experiments. Electrical ionization mass spectra of miltiradiene (*A* and *B*), ferruginol (*C* and *D*), and cryptotanshinone (*E*) from dashen hairy roots fed with unlabeled (*A* and *C*) or $^{13}$C-labeled miltiradiene (*B*, *D*, and *E*)**

To reduce the amount of unlabeled tanshinones, *S. miltiorrhiza* hairy roots were subcultured, with addition of the general CPS inhibitor 2-Isopropyl-4-dimethylamino-5-methylphenyl-1-piperidinecarboxylate methyl Chloride AMO1618, to suppress endogenous production of miltiradiene. Whereas it was possible to observe the incorporation of $^{13}$C-labeled miltiradiene into the oxidized intermediate, ferruginol (Fig. 2*C* and *D*), endogenous production levels were still sufficient to preclude detection of any other fully $^{13}$C-labeled tanshinones (Fig. 1). This confounding endogenous metabolism was further suppressed by addition of the MEP pathway inhibitor, fosmidomycin, as well as AMO1618, along with feeding increased amounts of labeled miltiradiene. Under these conditions, fully $^{13}$C-labeled cryptotanshinone was observed (Fig. 2*E*), demonstrating that the labeled miltiradiene could undergo substantial elaboration and serve as a precursor to compounds found in the late stage of the proposed tanshinone biosynthetic pathway (Fig. 1).

CYP Candidate Gene Discovery. From our previous work with SmCPS and SmKSL, transcription of the encoding genes was clearly increased by induction of hairy root cultures. Such inducible transcription has been shown to extend to the subsequently acting CYPs in other terpenoid biosynthetic pathways. Accordingly, to find candidate CYPs for tanshinone biosynthesis we moved beyond our previously reported EST database and used next-generation sequencing of mRNA from induced hairy roots to generate an extensive transcriptome (accession no. SRX224100), resulting in 25,793 isotigs ranging from 100 to 1,100 nucleotides in length. Analysis of this dataset revealed the presence of ~300 CYP isotigs, close to the numbers of CYPs found in other plant species. Moreover, using an RNA-seq approach to examine the change in transcriptome upon induction with $Ag^+$, 14 CYP genes were selected as initial candidates for investigation on the basis of their significant increase in transcript levels.

Given the accumulation of tanshinones in the rhizome, and previous tissue-specific transcription demonstrated for other diterpenoid metabolism, we hypothesized that tanshinone biosynthetic enzymes would be specifically expressed in the rhizome. Indeed, consistent with previous investigations, quantitative real-time (qRT)-PCR analysis demonstrated that SmCPS and SmKSL mRNA levels were higher in the rhizome than above ground tissues of *S. miltiorrhiza*. Hence, the relative expression of each of the 14 inducible CYPs was similarly analyzed, and transcripts for 6 of the 14 candidate CYPs were found to be more abundant in the rhizome. These 6 CYPs [GenBank accession nos. CYP76AH1 (JX422213), SmCYP-2 (JX422214), SmCYP-10 (JX422215), SmCYP-11 (JX422216), SmCYP-18 (JX422217), and SmCYP-20 (JX422218)] were then cloned to enable biochemical assays using miltiradiene as the substrate. As cytochrome P450 reductases (CPRs) are important to support the activities of CYPs, we also cloned full-length cDNA for two CPRs, SmCPR1 (GenBank accession no. CBX24555) and SmCPR2 (GenBank accession no. JX848592), that were present in our transcriptome. These two CPRs shared 79% nucleotide sequence identities (Fig. S1). Although SmCPR1 had been previously deposited, SmCPR2 seemed to be new.

CYP76AH1 Acts as a Ferruginol Synthase. The ability of these *S. miltiorrhiza* CYPs to react with miltiradiene was examined by recombinant expression in *S. cerevisiae*, followed by in vitro assays using microsomal preparations. Specifically, these six CYPs were expressed in the *S. cerevisiae* WAT11U strain, which expresses a CPR from *Arabidopsis thaliana* (AtCPR1), enabling more efficient reduction of plant CYPs. Microsomal preparations from the resulting recombinant yeasts were then assayed with miltiradiene, in the presence of NADPH, followed by GC-MS analysis. Notably, only one of these CYPs (designated CYP76AH1 by the Cytochrome P450 Nomenclature Committee; GenBank accession no. JX422213), was able to convert miltiradiene to an oxidized derivative (Fig. S2), which was determined to be ferruginol by comparison with an authentic standard (Fig. 3). None of the six CYPs was able to further react with ferruginol under identical assay conditions (Fig. S3). Steady-state kinetic analysis, in the presence of excess NADPH, indicated that CYP76AH1 efficiently catalyzes the conversion of miltiradiene into ferruginol, with $k_{cat}=4.4\pm0.3\ s^{-1}$ and $K_M=13\pm3\ \mu mol/L$ (Fig. 4).

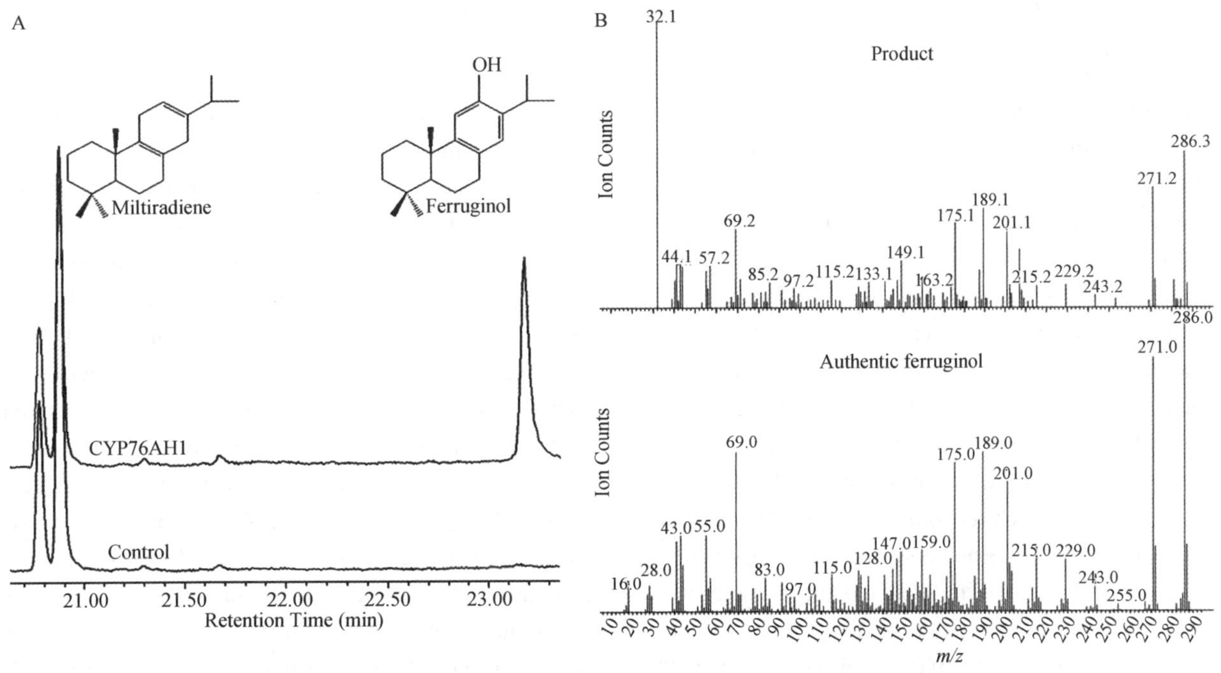


**Fig. 3 Results of in vitro turnover of miltiradiene by CYP76AH1**

(*A*) GC-MS chromatogram of extracts from the reaction containing CYP76AH1 microsomes with NADPH (*Upper* trace) and control (*Lower* trace). (*B*) Mass spectra of the reaction product compared with that of authentic ferruginol.

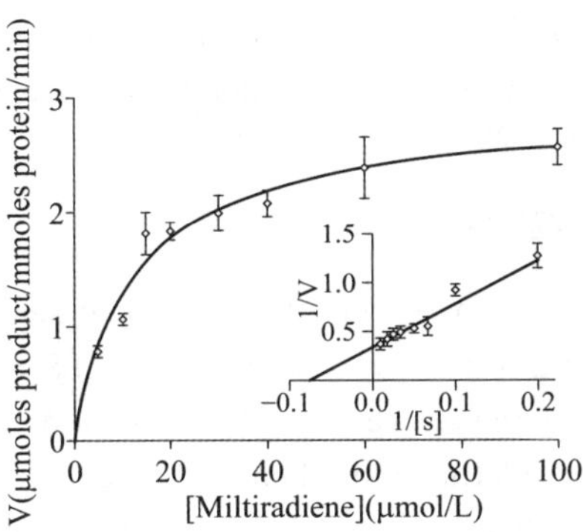


**Fig. 4 Kinetic profile of CYP76AH1. Experimental details are included in *Materials and Methods***

Coincidence of CYP76AH1 Transcription and Ferruginol Accumulation. To further strengthen the relevance of CYP76AH1 to ferruginol and tanshinone biosynthesis, we investigated ferruginol accumulation patterns. It has been reported that ferruginol accumulates along with tanshinones in *S. miltiorrhiza* suspension cells, as well as hairy roots. Tissue-specific analysis of whole plants demonstrated the expected accumulation of ferruginol in the rhizome, whereas none was detected in above-ground tissues, consistent with the *CYP76AH1* transcript accumulation pattern noted above. Moreover, we found that induction of hairy root cultures led to increased levels of ferruginol (Fig. 5*A*), tanshinones (Fig. S4), and *CYP76AH1* transcription (Fig. 5*B*), consistent

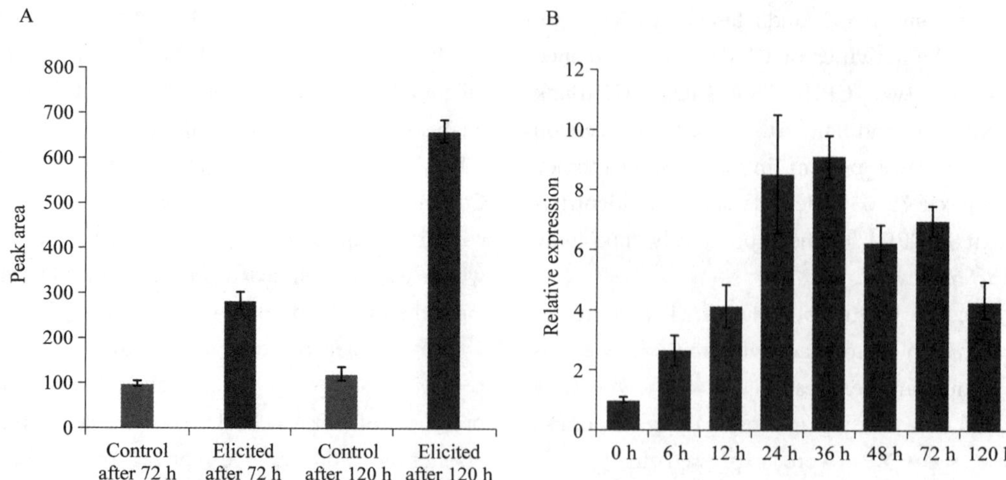


**Fig. 5 Correlation of gene expression of *CYP76AH1* and ferruginol accumulation**

(*A*) Accumulation of ferruginol in hairy roots responding to $Ag^+$ induction. (*B*) Real-time PCR analysis of *CYP76AH1* mRNA level in hairy roots of danshen after exposure to $Ag^+$.

with the hypothesized role for CYP76AH1 in ferruginol and, hence, tanshinone biosynthesis.

Assembling Pathways for Heterologous Ferruginol Production. In previous work, we assembled efficient pathways by using the modular pathway engineering (MOPE) approach and enabled the production of miltiradiene at levels of 365 mg/L in *S. cerevisiae*. This approach was applied here to realize heterologous production of ferruginol by additionally incorporating modules expressing *CYP76AH1* as well as a CPR gene. Initially, a CYP76AH1 (only) module, under the control of the transcription elongation factor 1 (TEF1) promoter, was added to the previously reported miltiradiene production vector, which contained the GGPP synthase (BTS1) and farnesyl diphosphate synthase (ERG20) fusion module BTS1 - ERG20, the tHMG1 module for expressing the catalytic do-main of hydroxy-3-methylglutaryl coenzyme A (tHMG1), and the copalyl diphosphate synthase (SmCPS) and kaurene synthase-like (SmKSL) fusion module SmKSL - SmCPS. The resulting plasmid was transformed into *S. cerevisiae* BY4741 (ML) to give the engineered strain *S. cerevisiae* YJ32 (Fig. 6). However, whereas YJ32 produced considerable amounts of miltiradiene and geranylgeraniol (GGOH, produced by hydrolysis of GGPP), ferruginol was not detected (Fig. 6 and Fig. S5*A*). We hypothesized that the endogenous yeast CPR was incompetent to support the activity of the plant CYP76AH1. Accordingly, we turned to the use of the two *S. miltiorrhiza* CPRs, SmCPR1 and SmCPR2 to support the CYP76AH1 activity. The engineered strains YJ35 and YJ33, containing further assembled SmCPR1 module and SmCPR2 module on plasmid described above in the BY4741(ML), produced ferruginol at a titer of 10.5 and 5.2 mg/L, respectively, after 48 h of shake-flask fermentations. Interestingly, the production of miltiradiene and ferruginol by these strains was inversely correlated (Fig. S5). For example, YJ32 produced no ferruginol, but the highest miltiradiene titer of 5.2 mg/L, whereas YJ35 (contained SmCPR1) produced 10.5 mg/L of ferruginol and only 1.2 mg/L of miltiradiene. These observations indicated that the presence of a phyto-CPR was essential for CYP76AH1 to function in yeast. To further support this idea, the plasmids used for the construction of YJ32 and YJ35 were transformed into WAT11U (28), which harbors a chromosomally integrated copy of *AtCPR1* from *A. thaliana*, leading to engineered strains YJ42 and YJ45, respectively. As expected from our in vitro results described above, YJ42 produced ferruginol at 2.1 mg/L. Interestingly, whereas YJ45 and YJ35 produced equal amounts of ferruginol, YJ45 accumulated significantly higher amounts of miltiradiene than YJ35 (Fig. S5 *C* vs. *D*). These results suggested that WAT11U provided greater metabolic flux to isoprenoid biosynthesis than BY4741 (ML), although the copresence of AtCPR1 and SmCPR1 did not further improve ferruginol production levels. It should be mentioned that the specific ferruginol titers [milligrams per gram of dry cell weight (DCW)] followed similar trends to the volumetric titers (milligrams per liter) among all engineered strains (Fig. S6 vs. Fig. 6).

## 2 DISCUSSION

We have previously reported functional identification of *S. miltiorrhiza* diterpene synthases, SmCPS and SmKSL, which catalyze the conversion of GGPP into the abietane-type diterpene olefin miltiradiene, a potential intermediate in the biosynthesis of the bioactive tanshinones of the important Chinese medicinal herb, danshen. Here we report stable-isotope labeling results that clearly demonstrate that miltiradiene is the precursor to at least two compounds found in the proposed tanshinone biosynthetic pathway, i. e., ferruginol and cryptotanshinone (Fig. 2). The implied formation of (crypto) tanshinones from miltiradiene requires extensive structural elaboration (Fig. S7). To understand the molecular bases of those transformations, we sought to identify the relevant genes, hypothesizing that the transcription of these would be inducible, as previously demonstrated for SmCPS and SmKSL. To provide a comprehensive foundation for these efforts, we undertook a next-generation sequencing-based functional genomics approach, to not only define the *S. miltiorrhiza* transcriptome, but also its transcriptional response to elicitor induction.

Miltiradiene is expected to undergo extensive oxidation, as well as carbon-carbon bond scission, to form diversified metabolites including tanshinones. Given that many of those biological transformations are typically carried out by CYPs, we focused on CYP-encoding genes whose transcription was coregulated with that of *SmCPS* and *SmKSL*, both in induction and rhizome tissue-specific expression patterns. From the six candidate CYPs identified through these criteria, we were able to demonstrate that one, CYP76AH1, readily converts miltiradiene into ferruginol in the presence of CPR1 from *A. thaliana* (Fig. 3). A number of other CYP76 family members have been shown to function in terpenoid biosynthesis. This notably includes four members of the CYP76M subfamily from rice that also function in diterpenoid metabolism, two of which catalyze hydroxylation at C-11 of *ent*-cassadiene, a reaction that exhibits some similarity to the activity shown by CYP76AH1. Kinetic analysis of CYP76AH1 demonstrated not only high catalytic efficiency ($k_{cat}/K_M = 3.4 \times 10^5\ M^{-1} \cdot s^{-1}$), but also a pseudosubstrate binding constant ($K_M$ of $13 \pm 3$ μmol/L) similar to that reported for the CYP76M subfamily members from rice diterpenoid biosynthesis, whose reported $K_M$ values ranged from 2 to 40 μmol/L.

The ferruginol synthase activity exhibited by CYP76AH1 apparently requires a four-electron oxidation cascade. In particular, the production of ferruginol from miltiradiene involves both aromatization and the introduction of an oxygen atom at C-12 (Fig. S8). CYPs are known to catalyze dehydrogenation, as required for aromatization, as well as monooxygenation on a variety of carbon centers. Thus, the catalyzed reaction might follow an aromatization/monooxygenation sequence. Alternatively, the oxygen atom might be incorporated via epoxidation of the C-12, 13 double bond, followed by ring opening and an additional oxidation step en route to ferruginol. Whereas detailed mechanistic insight awaits further biochemical characterization, CYP76AH1 nevertheless represents a unique enzyme that catalyzes a four-electron oxidation cascade on the cyclohexa-1, 4-diene moiety to form a phenol moiety in tanshinone biosynthesis.

Ferruginol is a widespread diterpenoid metabolite, and has been found in the Podocarpaceae, the Cupressaceae, the Lamiaceae, and the Verbenaceae plant families. Notably, a transcriptome recently has become available for the perennial herb rosemary (*Rosmarinus officinalis*; http://medicinalplantgenomics.msu.edu), which also is known to produce ferruginol, and this contains several isotigs that exhibit close homology to CYP76AH1 (~85% nucleotide sequence identity; Fig. S9). Isotig homologs to SmCPS and SmKSL also can be found in the rosemary transcriptome, indicating that our results from investigating tanshinone biosynthesis will be more widely applicable to the metabolism of other plant diterpenoid natural products. Indeed, ferruginol serves as a potential intermediate for the carnosic acid produced by rosemary. In turn, carnosic acid also may be an intermediate in tanshinone biosynthesis (Fig. 1 and Fig. S7). Intriguingly, phylogenetic analysis revealed that four of the remaining five danshen CYPs whose expression pattern matches that of tanshinone accumulation are closely related to CYP99A3 (Fig. S9), which catalyzes the conversion of the C-19 methyl of diterpene momilactone to a carboxylic acid in rice. Particularly given the similar transformations required for tanshinone biosynthesis (e. g., oxidative loss of C-19 and C-20 in formation of tanshinone Ⅰ), these CYPs seem likely to be involved in down-stream transformations for tanshinone biosynthesis. We thus prepared microsome samples from recombinant yeasts harboring these CYP genes and performed reactions using ferruginol as the substrate; however, no product was observed (Fig. S3).

Ferruginol further serves as a bioactive natural product in its own right, and has been shown to exhibit a range of activities similar to that of the tanshinones. Given that it also can be found in *S. miltiorrhiza* rhizomes, ferruginol may contribute to the medicinal effect of danshen. In part based on the potential use of ferruginol itself, we assembled synthetic pathways for microbial production of ferruginol in yeast. Whereas incorporating CYP76AH1 alone into the miltiradiene-producing yeast strain failed to produce ferruginol, yeast strains harboring CYP76AH1 in the presence of plant CPRs from *S. miltiorrhiza* or *A. thaliana* produced ferruginol (Fig. 6). Under flask-shake conditions without process optimization, we achieved a ferruginol titer of 10.5 mg/L, which was comparable to the result obtained in *E. coli* for the production of the first CYP modified taxadiene, taxadien-5α-ol, a precursor to taxol. Furthermore, we expected that it should be possible to significantly increase ferruginol yield via a combination of strain engineering and process optimization.

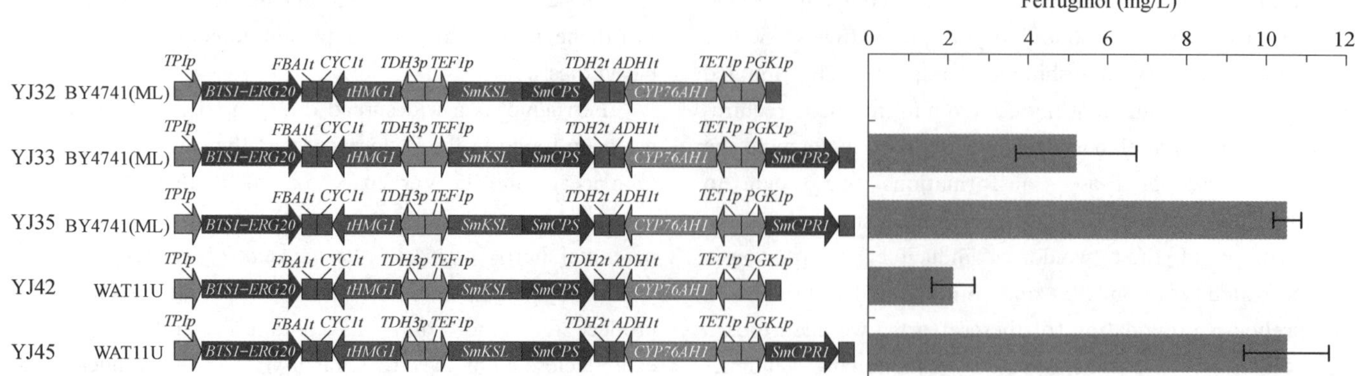


**Fig. 6 Results of the assembled ferruginol production pathways. Yeast strains were cultivated in a ZWY - 1102 shaking incubator (Shanghai Zhicheng) with 100 mL YPD media at 30℃, 200 rpm for 48 h. All data represent the averages±SDs of three independent clones**

In conclusion, here we have established the intermediacy of miltiradiene in the biosynthesis of the bioactive tanshinone diterprenoids from the Chinese medicinal herb *S. miltiorrhiza* (danshen), and used a next-generation sequencing-based approach to functionally identify the relevant ferruginol synthase, CYP76AH1. The results and approaches described here provide a solid foundation for further investigation of not only the biosynthesis of the tanshinones, but that of plant labdane-related diterpenoids more generally. As there is strong interest in microbial production of phytoditerpenoids, our metabolic engineering efforts reported here also will facilitate the construction of such microbial cell factories.

## 3 MATERIALS AND METHODS

Isolation and Quantification of Ferruginol. Analysis of ferruginol levels was carried out much as previously described. Briefly, dried and powered hairy roots were extracted with ethyl acetate, with fivefold concentration of these extracts used for ferruginol quantification by GC analysis. GC analyses were carried out using an Agilent GC7890 system with HP-5 column (320 μm × 0.25 μm × 30 m) and flame ionization detection, with quantification by comparison with an authentic standard for ferruginol, which was obtained from WUXI APPTEC Co.. Samples (1 μL) were injected in splitless mode at 280 ℃. The GC oven temperature was programmed to increase at 6 ℃/min from 150℃ to 220℃, at 3℃/min from 220℃ to 230℃, and at 20℃/min from 230℃ to 280℃.

Isolation of Total RNA and qRT-PCR Analysis. For *CYP76AH1* expression analysis, hairy roots were induced with $Ag^+$, and sampled after 6 h, 12 h, 24 h, 48 h, 72 h, and 120 h. Total RNA was extracted from hairy roots using TRIzol reagent (Invitrogen) following the manufactures' directions. Firststrand cDNA was synthesized with RevertAid First Strand cDNA synthesis Kit (Fermentas) using oligo $(dT)_{18}$ primer. Quantitative real-time PCR was performed using the SYBR Premix Ex Taq (Takara Bio) and an Applied Biosynthesis 7 500 Real-Time machine. The primers used were: 5′-TCGTGGATGAGTCGGCAAT-3′ and 5′-TGAGTATCTGAGTTCCCT-3′. Actin was used as the endogenous control to normalize expression value. At least three independent experiments were performed for each analysis (tissues and time points).

cDNA Cloning and Heterologous Expression of CYP76AH1 in Yeast. The 5′ and 3′ ends of the targeted CYP and SmCPR2 were cloned by RACE (Invitrogen) according to the manufacturer's directions. Full-length cDNA was cloned from cDNA isolated from induced hairy roots 12 h after induction with $Ag^+$, using PrimeStar DNA polymerase (Takara Bio). The ORF region of *CYP76AH1* was subcloned into yeast epitope-tagging vector pESC-His via *EcoR* Ⅰ and *Spe* Ⅰ digestion with PCR amplification using primers shown in Table S1. The pESC-His-CYP76AH1 construct was verified by complete gene sequencing, which was transformed into the yeast strain WAT11U. Transformants were selected on synthetic dropin medium-His (SD-his) containing 20 g/L glucose and grown at 28℃ for 48 h. The resulting recombinant strain was initially grown in SD-His liquid medium with 20 g/L glucose at 28 ℃ for about 48 h to an $OD_{600}$ of 2-3. Cells were centrifuged and washed three times with sterile water to remove any residual glucose. The cells were then resuspended in the yeast peptone galactose (YPL) induction medium (10 g/L yeast extract, 20 g/L bactopeptone, and 20 g/L galactose) and grown over-night at 28 ℃ to induce recombinant protein expression. ORFs of *SmCYP-2*, *SmCYP-10*, *SmCYP-11*, *SmCYP-18*, and *SmCYP-20* were also subcloned into pESC-His as done for *CYP76AH1*, and transformants were generated and confirmed by sequencing.

In Vitro Enzymatic Activity Assay. Miltiradiene samples were prepared using our engineered yeasts as described. Microsomes were prepared as previously described. Microsomal membranes were suspended in storage buffer containing 50 mmol/L Tris · HCl (pH 7.5), 1 mmol/L EDTA, and 20% (vol/vol) glycerol. Initial in vitro hydroxylation assays were conducted in a total volume of 500 μL of 90 mmol/L Tris · HCl (pH 7.5), containing 1 mmol/L NADPH, 500 μg of microsomal protein, and 100 μmol/L miltiradiene. The assays were incubated with shaking for 3 h at 28℃, and the reactions terminated by extraction with an equal volume of ethyl acetate. These extracts were directly analyzed by GC-MS using an Agilent 6890 GC-MS system with an HP-5MS capillary column (250 μm × 0.25 μm × 30 m; J & W Scientific). Analysis was carried out on 4 μL samples with splitless injection at 225 ℃. The GC oven temperature was programmed to increase at 10℃/min from 70℃ to 280℃.

Kinetic Analysis. For kinetic analysis, CYP76AH1 concentration was estimated by measuring the reduced CO-binding difference spectra using an extinction coefficient of 91 $mM^{-1} \cdot cm^{-1}$ as reported. Experiments were carried out using serial concentrations of miltiradiene: 5 μmol/L, 10 μmol/L, 15 μmol/L, 20 μmol/L, 30 μmol/L, 40 μmol/L, 60 μmol/L, and 100 μmol/L, in 1 mL enzyme assays. These also contained 1 mg microsomal protein (0.011 μmol CYP76AH1) in 90 mmol/L Tris · HCl (pH 7.5), with 0.5 mmol/L NADPH along with a regenerating system (consisting of 5 μmol/L FAD, 5 μmol/L FMN, 5 mmol/L glucose-6-phosphate, 0.5 unit/mL glucose-6-phosphate dehydrogenase, and 2 mmol/L DTT). Reactions were initiated by substrate addition, incubated with shaking at 28 ℃ for 30 min, and then terminated by extracting three times with 1 mL of ethyl acetate, with 0.5 μmol/L octadecane as an internal standard. Pooled extracts were completely evaporated under $N_2$ and then dissolved in 50 μL ethyl acetate for quantification by GC analysis, carried out as described above. $K_M$ and $k_{cat}$ values were calculated by nonlinear regression using GraphPad Prism version 5.04, and the data reported are the means ± SD from triplicate analyses.

Engineering Yeasts for Ferruginol Production. The yeast strain BY4741(ML) was constructed by complementing the auxotrophic markers LEU2 (encoding β-isopropylmalate dehydrogenase) and MET15 (encoding O-acetylhomoserine/O-acetylserine sulfhydrylase) in the BY4741 strain as previously described. Synthetic pathways were assembled according to the MOPE strategy, consisted of the previously described BTS1-ERG20 module, overexpressing the fusion protein of GGPP synthase and farnesyl diphosphate synthase, tHMG1 module, overexpressing a truncated hydroxy-3-methylglutaryl reductase, SmKSL - SmCPS module, overexpressing the fused diterpene synthase, along with the CYP76AH1 module, and the SmCPR1 module or the SmCPR2 module described here. The primers used in this work are listed in Table S1. These constructs were transformed into the yeast strains BY4741(ML) or WAT 11U, resulting in strains engineered for ferruginol production (Table S2). Cells were grown in SC medium lacking uracil at 30℃, shaking at 200 rpm for 48 h in a ZWY-1102 shaking incubator (Shanghai Zhicheng), and then transferred to 100 mL of YPD medium in 500 mL flasks to an initial $OD_{600}$ of 0.05, and cultivated for another 48 h. Terpenoid products were extracted as previously described and analyzed by GC using a 7890F system (Techcomp Scientific Instrument Co.) with flame ionization detector, and equipped with an SE-54 column (250 μm × 0.25 μm × 30 m). Column pressure was kept at 0.10 MPa, with 4.5 mL/min carrier gas ($N_2$) flow rate. The injector and detector temperatures were 270 ℃ and 290 ℃, respectively, with oven temperature maximum of 250℃.

Plant Materials, Miltiradiene Labeling, and Feeding Studies. Details of plant materials preparation and analysis; miltiradiene labeling; and the feeding of labeled miltiradiene to freshly subcultured hairy root cultured are given in *SI Materials and Methods*.

[郭娟,赵宗保,黄璐琦,等.PNAS,2013,110(29):12108-12113.]

# Functional divergence of diterpene syntheses in the medicinal plant *Salvia miltiorrhiza*

*Salvia miltiorrhiza*, a Lamiaceae species known as red sage or tanshen, is a traditional Chinese medicinal herb that is described in *Shen Nong Ben Cao Jing*, the oldest classical Chinese herbal book, which dates from between 25 and 220 C.E. The lipophilic pigments from the reddish root and rhizome consist of abietane quinone diterpenoids, largely tanshinone IIA, cryptotanshinone, and tanshinone I. These are highly bioactive. For example, tanshinone IIA exerts vasorelaxative activity, has antiarrhythmic effects, provides protection against ischemia reperfusion injury, and exhibits anticancer activities. In addition, tanshinones have been reported to have a broad spectrum of antimicrobial activities against various plant pathogens, including rice (*Oryza sativa*) blast fungus *Magnaporthe oryzae*. Although tanshinones are mainly accumulated in the roots, trace amounts of tanshinones have been detected in aerial organs as well.

Diterpenoid biosynthesis is initiated by diterpene synthases (diTPSs), which catalyze cyclization and/or rearrangement of the general acyclic precursor (*E*, *E*, *E*)-geranylgeranyl diphosphate (GGPP) to form various hydrocarbon backbone structures that are precursors to more specific families of diterpenoids. Previous work has indicated that tanshinone biosynthesis is initiated by cyclization of GGPP to copalyl diphosphate (CPP) by a CPP synthase (SmCPS1) and subsequent further cyclization to the abietane miltiradiene by a kaurene synthase-like cyclase (SmKSL1), so named for its homology to the *ent*-kaurene synthases (KSs) required for GA plant hormone biosynthesis. Miltiradiene is a precursor to at least cryptotanshinone, and RNA interference (RNAi) knockdown of *SmCPS1* expression reduces tanshinone production, at least in hairy root cultures. The identification of SmCPS1 and SmKSL1 has been followed by that of many related diTPSs from other Lamiaceae plant species. These largely exhibit analogous activity, particularly the CPSs, which produce CPP or the stereochemically related 8α-hydroxy-labd-13*E*-en-15-yl diphosphate (LDPP) rather than the enantiomeric (*ent*) CPP relevant to GA biosynthesis.

To further investigate diterpenoid biosynthesis in *S. miltiorrhiza*, we report here a more thorough characterization of its diTPS family. A previously reported whole-genome shotgun sequencing survey has indicated that there are at least five CPSs, although only two KSL genes in *S. miltiorrhiza* (Supplemental Table S1). Intriguingly, based on a combination of biochemical and genetic (RNAi gene silencing) evidence, we find that these diTPSs nevertheless account for at least four different diterpenoid biosynthetic pathways, each dependent on a unique CPS, with the KS presumably involved in GA biosynthesis seeming to be responsible for alternative diterpenoid metabolism as well. In addition, our studies clarify the evolutionary basis for the observed functional diversity, with investigation of gene structure, positive selection, molecular docking, and mutational analysis used to explore the driving force for the functional divergence of these diTPSs. Moreover, we report metabolomic analysis, also carried out with *SmCPS1* RNAi lines, which enables prediction of the down-stream steps in tanshinone biosynthesis.

## 1 RESULTS

Molecular Analysis of the *S. miltiorrhiza* diTPSs Using the working-draft genome sequences of *S. miltiorrhiza*, we identified seven complementary DNA (cDNA) sequences encoding diTPSs from an inbred line (bh2-7). The deduced amino acid sequences showed that five contain the (D, E) XDD motif required for the protonation-initiated cyclization reactions catalyzed by CPSs and are defined here as SmCPS1 to SmCPS5, while two have the DDXXD motif involved in binding the divalent magnesium ions required for heterolytic cleavage/ionization of the allylic diphosphate ester bond catalyzed by terpene synthases such as KSs and are defined here as SmKSL1 and SmKSL2, respectively (Supplemental Table S1).

Phylogenetic analysis revealed distinct conservation of these diTPSs. SmCPS1 to SmCPS3 cluster with other previously characterized CPSs from the Lamiaceae, all of which (including SmCPS1) produce CPP or the stereochemically analogous LDPP. On the other hand, SmCPS4 and SmCPS5 cluster with CPSs that have been previously shown to produce *ent*-CPP, generally for GA biosynthesis. As previously reported, SmKSL1 has undergone loss of the N-terminal γ-domain usually found in KSLs (although not most other terpene synthases), which has been a characteristic of the KSLs involved in more specialized diterpenoid metabolism from the Lamiaceae. By contrast, SmKSL2 retains the γ-domain and clusters with other dicot KSLs, many of which have been shown to act as KSs involved in GA biosynthesis (Fig. 1).

Biochemical Characterization of the *S. miltiorrhiza* diTPSs To determine the biochemical activity of these diTPSs, in vitro enzyme assays were carried out using crude extracts of recombinantly expressed proteins, separately combining each SmCPS with SmKSL1 or SmKSL2 and feeding GGPP as substrate. As expected, combining SmCPS1 and SmKSL1 led to the previously reported production of miltiradiene. Notably, combining SmCPS2 and SmKSL1 also led to production of miltiradiene (Fig. 2A; Supplemental Fig. S1A). Kinetic analysis indicates that SmCPS1 has both higher affinity ($K_m$=0.54 μmol/L versus 0.95 μmol/L) and activity (>18-fold higher catalytic constant) with GGPP than SmCPS2 (Fig. 2A). Nevertheless, this observation raises the potential for redundancy between SmCPS1 and SmCPS2. No product was observed when either SmCPS1 or SmCPS2 was combined with SmKSL2. No product was observed when SmCPS3 was combined with either SmKSL1 or SmKSL2. Intriguingly, combining SmCPS4 and SmKSL2 led to production of an unknown compound, while combining SmCPS5 and SmKSL2 led to the production of *ent*-kaurene, the diterpene precursor to GAs (Fig. 2A; Supplemental Fig. S1A).

To identify the compound produced by SmCPS4 and SmKSL2, the observed mass spectra was used to search a number of publically available databases, revealing a close match to that of the known diterpenoid 13-epi-manoyl oxide (Supplemental Fig. S1B). This presumably arises from cyclization of LDPP, suggesting that SmCPS4 produces this

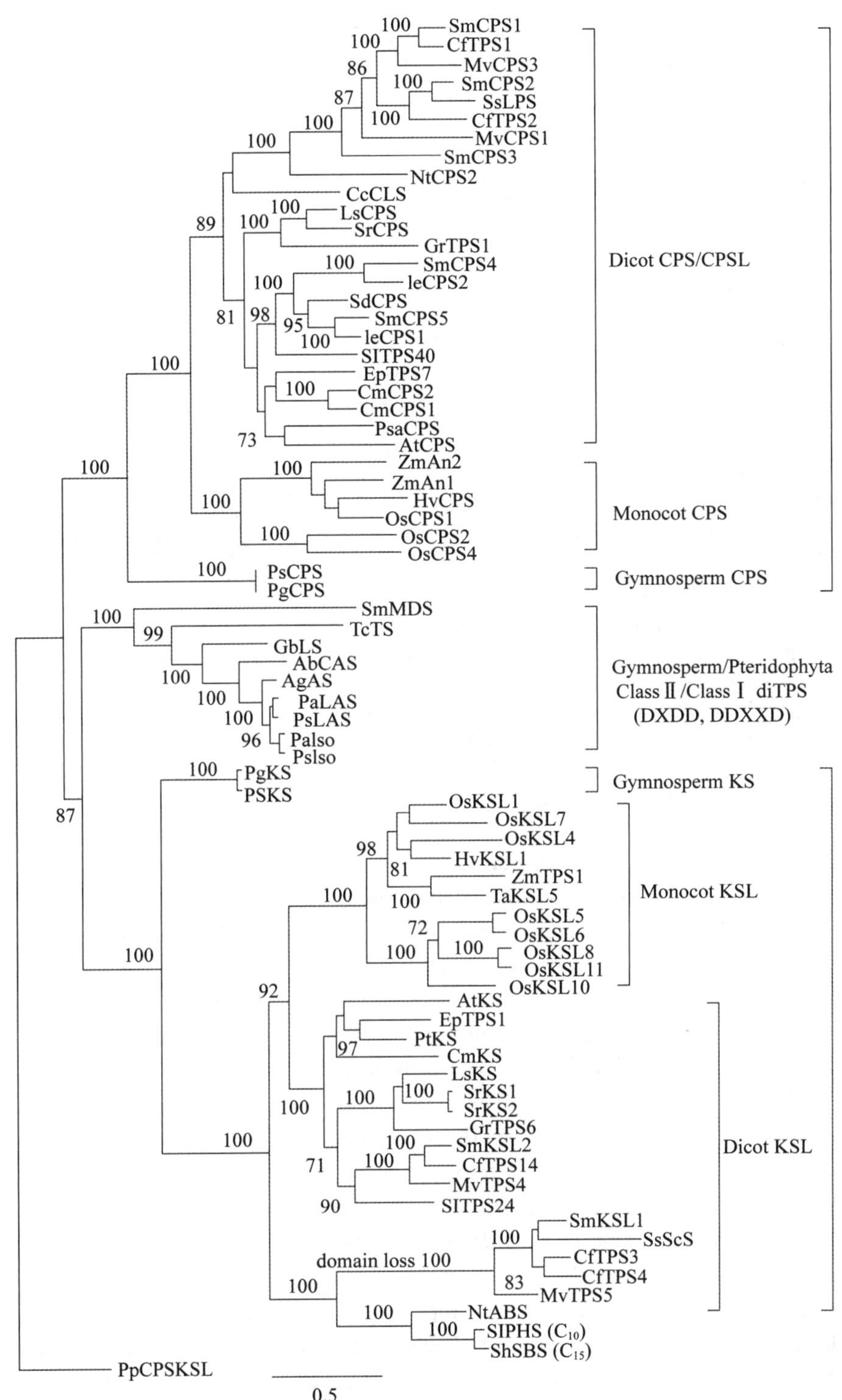


**Figure 1 Phylogeny of diTPS genes in *S. miltiorrhiza*. The phylogenetic relationship was reconstructed using the JTT models by PhyML 3.0 with 68 representative characterized diTPS (Supplemental Table S2)**

Numbers on branches indicate the bootstrap percentage values calculated from 100 bootstrap replicates. *Physcomitrella patens* CPS/kaurene (PpCPSKS) was used as outgroup. Blue lines show diTPS genes involved in more specialized diterpenoid metabolism from Lamiaceae, and red lines show the loss of N-terminal $\gamma$-domain found in KSLs. Red-marked enzymes show diTPS from *S. miltiorrhiza*.

intermediate. However, SmCPS4 is more closely related to *ent*-CPP-producing CPSs rather than the previously characterized LDPP synthases from Lamiaceae, whose products are enantiomeric. Previous mutational analysis has shown that the CPS from Arabidopsis (*Arabidopsis thaliana*) involved in GA metabolism (AtCPS), which then produces *ent*-CPP, can be easily diverted to the production of *ent*-LDPP. Thus, the stereochemistry of the SmCPS4 product was further investigated. Among the previously identified LDPP synthases is one from *Coleus forskohlii*, CfTPS2 (a CPS homolog), and this Lamiaceae species also encodes a subsequently acting KSL, CfTPS3, that reacts with LDPP to produce manoyl oxide. Both SmCPS4 and CfTPS2 reacted with GGPP to produce LDPP, detected as labdenediol by gas chromatography (GC)-mass spectrometry (MS) following dephosphorylation (Fig. 2B; Supplemental Fig. S1B). To determine if these were enantiomeric, CfTPS2 and SmCPS4 were separately incubated with either SmKSL2 or CfTPS3,

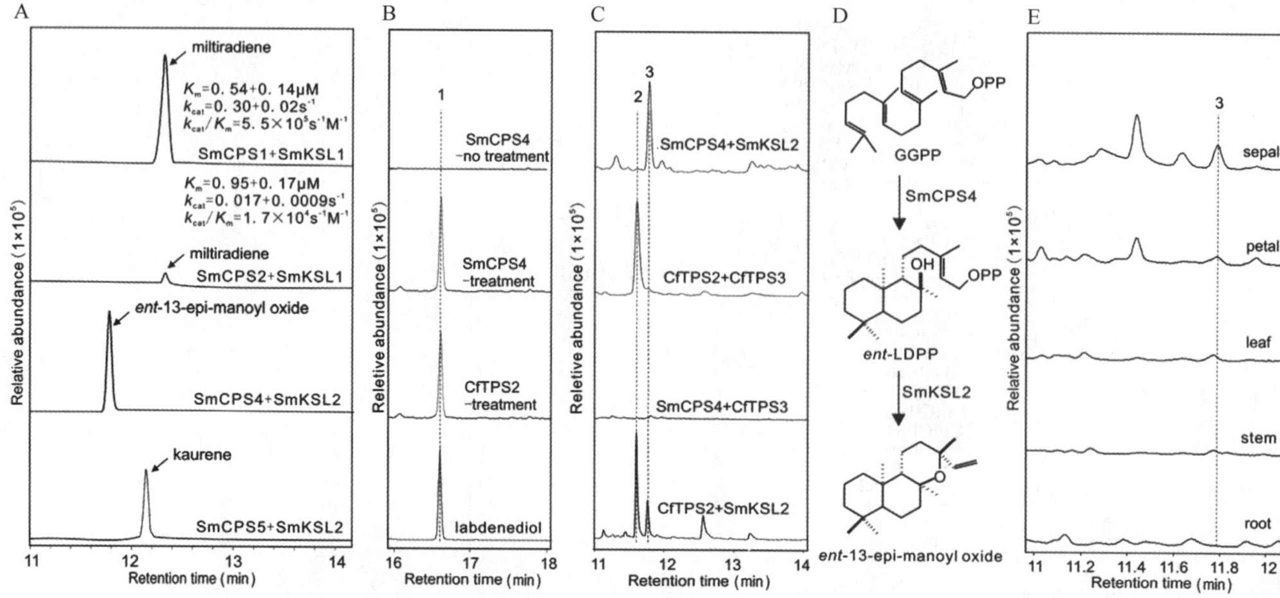


**Figure 2　Functional identification of diTPS in *S. miltiorrhiza***

(A) Total ion chromatography of diterpene products from in vitro assays with kinetic constants of SmCPS1 and SmCPS2. $k_{cat}$, Catalytic constant. (B) Total ion chromatography of the assay with purified SmCPS4 and CfTPS2. The assay product was extracted directly by hexane (no treatment) or after the treatment of alkaline phosphatase (treatment). (C) Total ion chromatography of the assay combines SmCPS4 with SmKSL2, together with the identified enzyme CfTPS2 (CPS) and CfTPS3 (KSL) from *C. forskohlii*. Assays all with 30 μmol/L GGPP as substrate. (D) Proposed pathway to *ent*-13-epi-manoyl oxide in *S. miltiorrhiza*. OH, Hydroxyl; OPP, diphosphate. (E) Total ion chromatography of hexane extracts from different organs in *S. miltiorrhiza*. The compounds are labdenediol (1), manoyl oxide (2), and *ent*-13-epi-manoyl oxide (3).

respectively, and GGPP as substrate. Notably, combining SmCPS4 with CfTPS3 did not lead to the production of manoyl oxide (Fig. 2C). In addition, combining CfTPS2 with SmKSL2 led to predominant production of manoyl oxide with relatively less 13-epi-manoyl oxide (Fig. 2C). These results indicate that SmCPS4 produces *ent*-LDPP (8β-hydroxy-*ent*-CPP). Therefore, the product of SmCPS4 and SmKSL2 appears to be *ent*-13-epi-manoyl oxide (Fig. 2D).

Physiological Roles of *S. miltiorrhiza* diTPSs　The tissue-specific expression pattern of the *S. miltiorrhiza* diTPSs was investigated by quantitative reverse-transcription (qRT)-PCR analysis of various organs, including leaves and roots of 3-d-old seedlings and the root periderm, cortex, and xylem, as well as stem, leaf, sepal, petal, stamen, pistil, and immature seeds of adult plants at the flowering stage (Fig. 3). *SmCPS1* and *SmKSL1* exhibit closely coordinated expression, and their transcripts were found at extremely high levels in the root periderm, consistent with their role in biosynthesis of the tanshinone pigments, which accumulate in this tissue. *SmCPS2* and *SmCPS3* were most highly expressed in seedling leaves, although *SmCPS2* also is highly expressed in the petals of adult plants. *SmCPS4* was most highly expressed in the sepal, and *SmCPS5* was most highly expressed in the stem. *SmKSL2* was most highly expressed in the root xylem, although this was expressed throughout all tissues of adult plants to some extent.

To investigate the diterpenoid natural product arsenal of *S. miltiorrhiza*, both untargeted and targeted metabolomics analyses were carried out using liquid chromatography (LC)-quadrupole time-of-flight (qTOF)-MS and GC-triple quadrupole (QqQ)-MS, respectively. Notably, although *S. miltiorrhiza* has not been previously reported to produce (*ent*-)13-epi-manoyl oxide, this diterpenoid was found here, mainly in sepals, with lower amounts found in petals, leaves, and stems, but not in roots (Fig. 2E; Supplemental Fig. S1B). This tissue-specific accumulation pattern matches *SmCPS4* mRNA expression with a correlation coefficient of 0.97, indicating that the production of *ent*-13-epi-manoyl oxide in *S. miltiorrhiza* depends on expression of *SmCPS4* (as well as the more ubiquitous expression of *SmKSL2*).

As previously reported, tanshinones were found not only in the root and rhizome, but also in aerial tissues of *S. miltiorrhiza*. Given the distinct tissue-specific expression patterns of SmCPS1 and SmCPS2, both of which can produce the relevant CPP intermediate, it seemed possible that these are not redundant but, instead, contribute separately to tanshinone biosynthesis in the roots and aerial tissues, respectively. Moreover, as the only identified *ent*-CPP synthase, it also seemed likely that SmCPS5 is involved in GA metabolism.

Genetic Evidence for Distinct Diterpenoid Pathways in *S. miltiorrhiza*　To further investigate the distinct roles of the various SmCPSs in *S. miltiorrhiza* diterpenoid biosynthesis, RNAi gene silencing was carried out targeting either *SmCPS1* or *SmCPS5* separately. RNAi knockdown of *SmCPS5* (Supplemental Fig. S2A) resulted in dwarf transgenic plants with significantly shorter pinnately compound leaves, shorter and narrower top leaves, and smaller flowers compared with wild-type plants and could be rescued (i.e. normal growth restored) by applying $GA_3$ to the T0 generation plants (Supplemental Fig. S2, B - D). Further, T1 generation plants showed a 3 : 1 segregation ratio for the dwarf phenotype, with severe stunting of shoots as well as dark-green leaves (Supplemental Fig. S2E). These phenotypes are associated with GA deficiency (Margis-Pinheiro et al., 2005), indicating that SmCPS5, presumably together with SmKSL2, function in the GA biosynthetic pathway in *S. miltiorrhiza*.

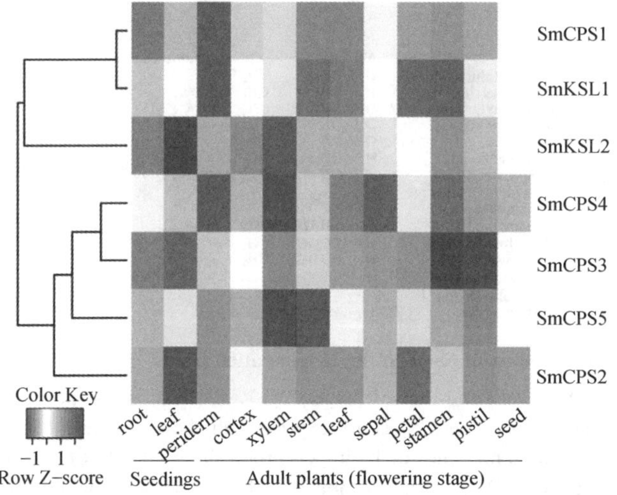


**Figure 3 qRT-PCR analysis of transcript levels of seven diTPS genes in 12 organs including leaves and roots of 3-d-old seedlings, and the root periderm, cortex, and xylem, as well as stem, leaf, sepal, petal, stamen, pistil, and immature seeds of adult plants at the flowering stage**

The expression level was normalized to that of *Actin*. Data are means from three technical replicates of at least three biological replicates.

To investigate the potential redundancy between *SmCPS1* and *SmCPS2*, RNAi targeting *SmCPS1* was carried out, generating five lines exhibiting silencing of approximately 90% (Fig. 4A). These *SmCPS1*-RNAi plants exhibited an obvious white-color root phenotype compared with wild-type roots, which had the characteristic reddish color associated with tanshinones (Fig. 4B). Root-directed metabolite analysis demonstrated that cryptotanshinone, tanshinone IIA, and tanshinone I were dramatically reduced, from 14,465±995, 2,311±13, and 2,010±117 μg/g in wild-type plants to 0.10±0.01, 1.2±0.2, and 14±1 μg/g in the *SmCPS1*-RNAi plants, respectively (Fig. 4C). As a control, the water-soluble polyphenolic acid content of the plants, including lithospermic acid B and rosmarinic acid, also was investigated. The lack of any statistically significant differences between the wild-type and *SmCPS1*-RNAi samples (Fig. 4C) indicates that down-regulation of *SmCPS1* expression specifically affects tanshinone biosynthesis (i.e. this did not interfere with the production of at least these polyphenolic acid metabolites).

Notably, tanshinone levels in the aerial tissues were not affected in the *SmCPS1*-RNAi plants (Table I). Given that *SmCPS2* is predominantly expressed in these tissues (Fig. 3), these results suggest that SmCPS2 mediates tanshinone biosynthesis in aerial organs of *S. miltiorrhiza* independently of the SmCPS1-dependent pathway in the root periderm, such that *SmCPS1* and *SmCPS2* are not redundant.

Metabolomic Analysis Clarifies Tanshinone Biosynthesis

Metabolomics analysis was carried out with not only the wild-type plant roots, but also *SmCPS1*-RNAi plant roots, with LC-electrospray ionization-qTOF-MS revealing 39 and GC-electron impact (EI)-QqQ-MS 19 metabolites with significantly reduced accumulation (i.e. a >2-fold change with $P < 0.05$; Supplemental Tables S3 and S4). On the other hand, four metabolites (by using GC-EI-QqQ-MS) with elevated accumulation also were identified (Supplemental Table S4). By comparison to known compounds, 21 of the metabolites with reduced accumulation in the roots of *SmCPS1*-RNAi plants were identified as diterpenoids, all of which were predominantly accumulated (>94.5%) in the periderm (Fig. 4D; Supplemental Tables S3 and S4). Of the metabolites exhibiting increased accumulation, three were identified as diterpenoids (geranylgeraniol, α-springene, and β-springene), and these were not detected in the periderm, cortex, and xylem of wild-type plant roots (Supplemental Table S4). These compounds presumably appear due to the down-regulation of *SmCPS1*, with accumulation of GGPP leading to hydrolysis to geranylgeraniol, with subsequent dehydration leading to α-springene and β-springene (Fig. 4E).

Of the 21 identified SmCPS1-dependent metabolites, 19 are tanshinones or plausible biosynthetic intermediates, while two are rearranged abietane diterpenoids (i.e. przewalskin and salvisyrianone; Fig. 4E). The 19 tanshinones and biosynthetically relevant metabolites could be further divided into five main groups according to the progressive modification of their carbon skeletons (Fig. 4E). Group I is simply composed of miltiradiene, with its planar cyclohexan-1, 4-diene C ring. Group II compounds are dehydroabietanes, with a characteristic aromatic C ring (i.e. abietatriene, ferruginol, and sugiol). Group III compounds are nor-abietatetraen-11,12-diones, with conversion of the C ring to an ortho-quinone (i.e. keto groups at C-11 and C-12), as well as aromatization of the B ring, along with loss of C-20 (e.g. miltirone and 4-methylene-miltirone). The 11 metabolites comprising group IV all are variously named

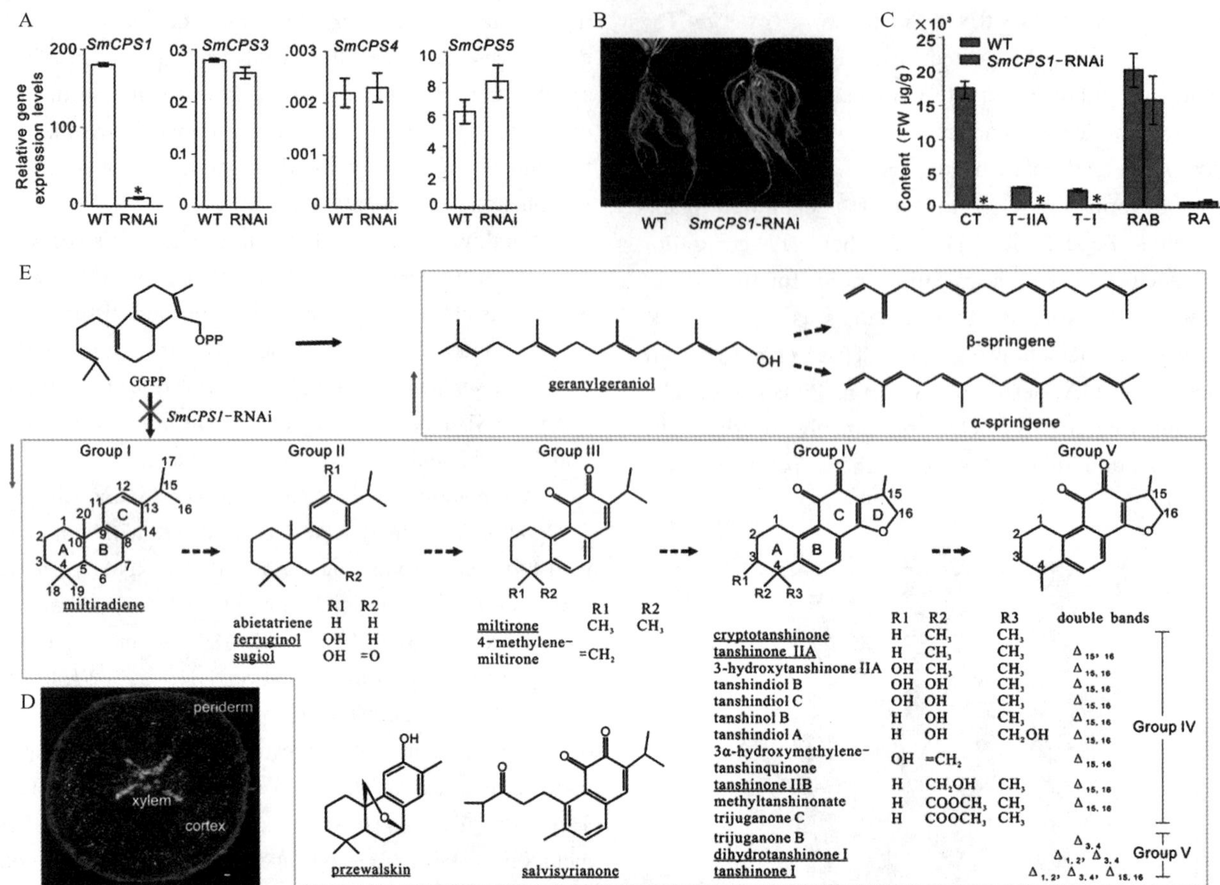


**Figure 4 Phenotype and metabolic profiles caused by down-regulation of *SmCPS1* in T0 generation plants**

(A) qRT-PCR analysis of transcript levels of five *CPS* genes in root of *SmCPS1*-RNAi and the wild type (WT). Expression was normalized to that of *Actin*. The error bars show the SDs from mean value ($n=3$ experiments). *SmCPS2* is not expressed in these samples. (B) The phenotype of down-regulation of *SmCPS1*. (C) Quantitative analysis of five major compounds including cryptotanshinone (CT), tanshinone IIA (T-IIA), tanshinone I (T-I), lithospermic acid B (LAB), and rosmarinic acid (RA) in root of *SmCPS1*-RNAi lines and the wild type. The error bars show the SDs from mean value ($n=3$ experiments). Asterisks indicate significant difference at $P<0.01$ compared with the wild type by Student's *t* test. (D) Cross section of the root. (E) Summary of metabolite flux caused by down-regulation of *SmCPS1*. The red arrow shows the accumulated metabolites, and the blue arrow shows the reduced metabolites in root of *SmCPS1*-RNAi lines compared with the wild type. Underlined metabolites are identified by standard reference. FW, Fresh weight; OH, hydroxyl; OPP, diphosphate; R1, R2, and R3, substituent group. Bar=100 μm.

tanshinones, with addition of the (dihydro) furan ring D. Group V contains three metabolites that have been additionally modified by the loss of one of the geminal methyl groups from the C-4 position, along with the presence of at least one double bond in the A ring.

Positive Selection for Divergent CPS Activity Given the ease with which diTPSs can be diverted to alternative activity, it is not clear what underlies the expanded nature and divergent activity observed in the *S. miltiorrhiza* diTPS family (i.e. selective pressure or genetic drift). Gene structure, specifically the number and placement of introns, has been associated with evolutionary descent in the terpene synthase gene family. Accordingly, the *CPS* and *KSL* genes of *S. miltiorrhiza*, Arabidopsis, and rice can be divided into three groups. Group I genes associated with GA metabolism each have the typical 15 exons and 14 introns for *CPS* genes and 14 exons and 13 introns for *KS* genes (Supplemental Fig. S3), which corresponds to the ancestral plant diTPS gene structure. Group II *CPS/KSL* genes, including *SmCPS1*, *SmCPS3*, *SmCPS4*, *SmKSL1*, *OsCPS2*, *OsCPS4*, *OsKSL5*, *OsKSL6*, *OsKSL8*, and *OsKSL10*, show diverged sequences and genomic architecture. In particular, intron loss relative to the conserved group I genes are often observed. For example, *SmCPS1* has lost the 10th and 12th introns, *SmCPS4* the 5th intron, and *SmCPS3* the first four introns, while *OsCPS2* has lost the 2nd and 3rd introns, and *OsKSL5*, *OsKSL6*, *OsKSL8*, and *OsKSL10* all have lost the last intron (Supplemental Fig. S3). These architecturally divergent group II genes are involved in the biosynthesis of specialized metabolites in *S. miltiorrhiza* and rice. On the other hand, the group III genes *SmCPS2*, *OsKSL4*, and *OsKSL7* exhibit conserved genomic architecture but divergent sequences and functions relative to the group I genes associated with GA biosynthesis (Supplemental Fig. S3).

**Table 1** ***Main compounds detected in aerial part and seedling of the wild type and SmCPS1-RNAi***

| Organ | Concentration[a] | | | | Relative Concentration[b] | | | | | |
|---|---|---|---|---|---|---|---|---|---|---|
| | Cryptotanshinone | | Tanshinone IIA | | Miltirone | | Trijuganone B | | Tanshinone I | |
| | Wild Type | RNAi | Wild Type | RNAi | Wild Type | RNAi | Wild Type | RNAi | Wild Type | RNAi |
| | *ng/g fresh wt* | | | | | | | | | |
| Petal | 0.2 | 0.2 | 2.2 | 2.2 | 12.1 | 12.0 | 19.9 | 20.2 | 10.6 | 11.0 |
| Sepal | 1.2 | 1.2 | 22.1 | 23.0 | 72.2 | 73.0 | 143.0 | 144.4 | 14.4 | 15.0 |
| Young leaf | 0.5 | 0.5 | 7.3 | 7.6 | 25.9 | 26.1 | 67.1 | 68.0 | 13.5 | 13.0 |
| Young root | 0.8 | 0.8 | 8.9 | 9.0 | 61.5 | 62.3 | 59.3 | 60.2 | 20.3 | 21.0 |

[a]The concentration obtained by calibration of standards. [b]The relative concentration obtained by comparison with internal standard umbelliferone.

To investigate whether the observed functional divergence of the CPS genes involved in biosynthesis of the tanshinones and other more specialized labdane-related diterpenoids is a function of positive selection, phylogenetic analysis of the protein-coding DNA sequences of CPS members from an array of angiosperms was carried out. The resulting phylogenetic tree (Fig. 5A) provided the basis for branch site model analysis conducted with the PAML package. This revealed a statistically significant signature for positive selection associated with functional divergence from the production of *ent*-CPP required for GA biosynthesis to the enantiomeric (i.e. normal) CPP involved in production of the tanshinones, as well as stereochemically related LDPP for other more specialized diterpenoid biosynthesis (branch *c*, nonsynonymous to synonymous substitution ratio=5.64, $P<0.01$; Fig. 5, A and B; Supplemental Table S5).

To more closely examine the basis for the observed functional diversification, the analysis was extended to individual codons in SmCPS1 versus SmCPS5. The positively selected sites identified by Bayes Empirical Bayes analysis correspond to Ser-362, Asp-389, Ser-415, and Pro-416 in SmCPS1, which are Trp-364, Ser-391, Thr-416, and Gly-417 in SmCPS5 (Fig. 5C). Models for both SmCPS1 and SmCPS5 were generated and revealed that three of these residues, Ser-362:Trp-364 (S-W) and Ser-415/Pro-416:Thr-416/Gly-417 (SP-TG) are part of the active site cavity, whereas Asp-389: Ser-391 (D-S) is more than 6 Å away from the active site cavity (Supplemental Fig. S4, A and B). Site-directed mutagenesis was performed to swap these residues between SmCPS1 and SmCPS5, except Thr-416 in SmCPS5, as this corresponds to Thr-421 in AtCPS, which has already been reported to be involved in catalysis. Assays using the mutant enzymes reacting with GGPP alone or in combination with SmKSL1 or SmKSL2 showed that the mutant SmCPS1:S362W, in which Ser-362 (S) of SmCPS1 was replaced by the Trp (W) found at the same position in SmCPS5, was more than 100-fold less efficient in the production of CPP, and miltiradiene when assayed with SmKSL1, relative to the wild-type SmCPS1. Moreover, this mutant also did not yield any detectable product when incubated with SmKSL2 and GGPP (Supplemental Fig. S5), indicating that no *ent*-CPP is produced. The mutant SmCPS5:W364S also showed about 80-fold lower efficiency in production of *ent*-CPP, and *ent*-kaurene when assayed with SmKSL2 compared with wild-type SmCPS5. Similarly, this mutant also did not yield any product when incubated with SmKSL1. The other four mutant enzymes SmCPS1: D389S, SmCPS1: P416G, SmCPS5: S391D, and SmCPS5: G417P did not cause significant change in enzymatic activity relative to the parental/wild-type CPSs (Supplemental Fig. S5). Thus, while no change in product stereochemistry was observed, it does seem that the residue corresponding to the S-W position is important for catalysis in both SmCPS1 and SmCPS5 (Supplemental Fig. S4, C and D), despite their difference in product outcome, suggesting that this substitution has a role in enabling the production of normal versus *ent*-CPP and, hence, biosynthesis of the derived tanshinones.

## 2 DISCUSSION

The combined biochemical and genetic work reported here has defined the roles of the diTPS family in *S. miltiorrhiza*. Of the five SmCPSs, while SmCPS3 appears to be inactive, each of the other SmCPSs defines separate diterpenoid pathways. Rather than reflecting redundancy, the similar biochemical activity of SmCPS1 and SmCPS2 is coupled to their distinct roles in tanshinone biosynthesis in the roots versus aerial tissues, respectively. This discovery provides the possibility of using metabolic engineering strategies to enhance the production of tanshinones in aerial organs. Cultivation of the resulting plants could then provide annually renewable source materials for extraction of tanshinones by harvesting aerial tissues without destroying the entire plant.

Both SmCPS1 and SmCPS2 react with GGPP to form

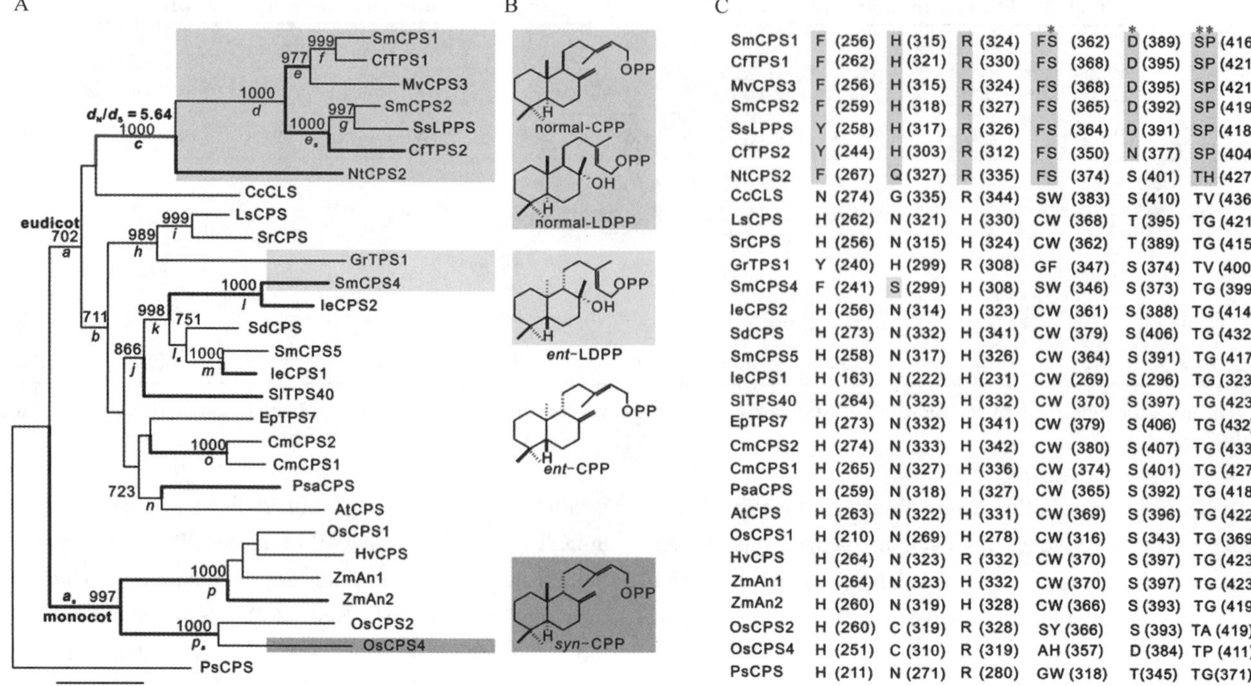


**Figure 5　Molecular evolution of CPS genes**

(A) Bold lines illustrate branches or genes evolved under positive selection with significant statistical support at $P<0.05$ both in branch site model tests 1 and 2. Branch *c* shows the divergence of normal-CPP and normal-LDPP synthase from the *ent*-CPP synthase. $d_N/d_S$, Nonsynonymous to synonymous substitution ratio. (B) Different stereoisomers of CPP and LDPP. (C) Alignment of conserved residues. The asterisks indicate positive selection sites with posterior probability greater than 95% by Bayes Empirical Bayes analysis.

normal CPP in *S. miltiorrhiza*. Our phylogenic analysis indicates that SmCPS1 and SmCPS2 are in the same clade that also contains other CPSs from the Lamiaceae and closely related Solanaceae (Fig. 1) that similarly produce CPP and LDPP with analogous stereochemistry. These CPSs were likely derived from an ancestral CPS that produced *ent*-CPP for GA biosynthesis via early gene duplication and neofunctionalization that occurred at least before the divergence of the Lamiaceae and Solanaceae (Figs. 1 and 5), which has been estimated to have been 64 million years ago (48 - 75 million years). During the evolution of Lamiaceae, two more gene duplication events likely happened, producing SmCPS3 as well as SmCPS1 and SmCPS2, which individually are representative of two more widespread clades (e. g. homologs to both are found in *C. forskohlii*), respectively. SmCPS2 retained the ancestral gene architecture (Supplemental Fig. S3) and exhibits a similar gene expression pattern as the SmCPS5 involved in GA biosynthesis (Fig. 3), whereas SmCPS1 has undergone more divergence, including intron loss (Supplemental Fig. S3) and altered transcriptional regulation (Fig. 3), along with exhibiting significantly higher catalytic activity than SmCPS2. These data suggest that tanshinone biosynthesis may have evolved early in the Lamiaceae, and the gene duplication leading to SmCPS1 and SmCPS2 enabled further localization and up-regulation of tanshinone biosynthesis in root periderm cells in some *Salvia* spp., including *S. miltiorrhiza*. The presence of distinct SmCPS1- and SmCPS2-dependent tanshinone pathways in the root periderm and aerial tissues, respectively, indicates that these labdane-related diterpenoids may play important roles in plant development and in adaptation to different stress conditions, which is a topic worth future investigation.

The ability of SmCPS4 to produce the enantiomeric form of LDPP was suggested by the ability of SmKSL2 to react with both *ent*-CPP (to produce *ent*-kaurene) and this *ent*-LDPP, but not the CPP product of SmCPS1 (or SmCPS2). The observed production of *ent*-13-epimanoyl oxide in *S. miltiorrhiza* then suggests dual function for SmKSL2 (i.e. in GA and this more specialized diterpenoid biosynthesis). Regardless, identification of the ability of SmCPS4 and SmKLS2 provides access to this unique diterpenoid. In addition, the ability of SmCPS4 to produce *ent*-LDPP was presaged by its phylogenetic relationship to *ent*-CPP-producing CPSs. Based on the similar clustering of a previously identified LDPP synthase from *Grindelia robusta*, as well as the ability of a KS to selectively react with its product, it is suggested here that this GrTPS1 may produce *ent*-LDPP (Fig. 2D).

It is interesting to note that certain previously identified residues are consistent with the CPS enzymatic activity observed here. SmCPS5, shown here to play a role in GA biosynthesis, contains the His (His - 326) associated with susceptibility to inhibition by $Mg^{2+}$, which has been suggested to serve a regulatory role in such CPSs. In addition, SmCPS5 contains the His-Asn dyad (His - 258/Asn - 317; Fig. 5C) that has been suggested to act as the catalytic base and is conserved in CPSs that produce *ent*-CPP. By contrast, the *ent*-LDPP-producing SmCPS4 contains a Ser (Ser - 299) in place of the corresponding Asn (Fig. 5C), consistent with the ability of such substitution of smaller residues to enable production of hydroxylated CPP. In addition, the investigation of residues showing signs of positive selection here indicates other positions important for altering stereochemical product outcome, although further experiments are required to determine how many and which residues are required. Nevertheless, altogether, the results reported here suggest that combining phylogenetic relationships with the identity of residues at positions of known catalytic relevance may be predictive for CPS catalytic activity.

## 3 MATERIALS AND METHODS

Plant Materials The *Salvia miltiorrhiza* species has two different flower colors, purple and white. Varieties with purple flowers are distributed throughout China. The variety with white flowers (*S. miltiorrhiza* f. *alba*.) is only found in Shandong Province. *S. miltiorrhiza* f. *alba* is a rare and thus more valuable variety of Danshen. The white flower line bh2 - 7, inbred for 5 generations, was used in our study.

Plant Growth and Culture Conditions bh2 - 7 seeds were surface sterilized with 5% (v/v) sodium hypochlorite and cultured on solid hormone-free Murashige and Skoog basal medium containing 30 g/L Suc and 8 g/L agar. Cultures were maintained at 25℃ under a 16 h-light/8 h-dark photoperiod. Seedlings were transferred to pots filled with soil: vermiculite (3 : 1) mix and grown under the same temperature and light regime in a plant growth room. Dwarf plants of *SmCPS5*-RNAi were sprayed with 150 μmol/L $GA_3$ solution to complement the phenotype in the T0 generation.

Genomic Sequence of diTPS Gene Family Members To show the structural divergence that occurred between *SmCPS1*, *SmCPS3*, and *SmCPS4*, we cloned the full genomic sequence of each gene from bh2 - 7. Cetyl-trimethyl-ammonium bromide method was used to extract the genomic DNA and amplified with specific primers (Supplemental Table S6). Intron/exon structures were predicted using the Gene Structure Display Server.

Gene Expression Analysis Plant samples were harvested and immediately frozen in liquid nitrogen. Total RNA was extracted using a modified cetyl-trimethyl-ammonium bromide protocol and treated with RNase-Free DNase I (Takara) to remove residual genomic DNA. RNA integrity and quality were checked by denaturing gel electrophoresis, and the absence of genomic DNA was confirmed by PCR using primers for *Smactin*, prior to reverse transcription. One to five micrograms of total RNA was reverse transcribed into cDNA using the SuperScript III reverse transcriptase and oligo$(dT)_{12-18}$ primer (Invitrogen), according to the manufacturer's instructions. The synthesized cDNA was then diluted 10-fold. One microliter of this diluted template was used for subsequent qRT-PCR analysis with a total PCR reaction volume of 20 μL. qRT-PCR was performed with a SuperReal PreMix for SYBR Green Kit (TIANGEN) on a Corvett Rotor-Gene 3 000 real-time PCR detection system. All reactions were performed using the following PCR conditions: initial denaturation step of 95 ℃ for 10 min, followed by 40 cycles each of 95℃ for 5 s, 60℃ for 15 s, and 72℃ for 20 s, with a final melting stage from 55℃ to 95℃. A final dissociation step was performed to assess the quality of the amplified product. cDNA from a series of 5-fold dilutions were used for calibration, and the efficiency of the PCR amplifications was found to be in the range of 90% to 110%, which is considered desirable for quantitative PCR. Relative expression levels were calculated as the ratio of the target gene transcript level to the transcript level of the housekeeping gene *Actin* (*Smactin*). Primer specificity was confirmed by direct cloning and sequencing of individual PCR amplification products. qRT-PCR was performed with three technical replicates of at least three biological replicates for each tissue or transformed plant line. The hot map of gene expression data was generated in the *R* software package.

Phylogenetic Analysis Sixty-eight diTPSs with characterized functions were included in the phylogenetic analysis (Supplemental Table S2). To carry out the phylogenic reconstruction, multiple protein sequence alignments were performed with MAFFT version 7.012 employing the E-INS-I method. Maximum likelihood trees were built using PhyML version 3.0. Specifically, PhyML analyses were conducted with the JTT substitution model, four rate substitution categories, and 100 or 1,000 bootstrap replicate analyses. The phylogeny was displayed using FigTree software (http://tree.bio.ed.ac.uk/software/figtree/).

Hairy Root and Plant Transformation for Knockdown of *SmCPS1* and *SmCPS5* by RNAi A 289-bp gene-specific sequence including the 3′ untranslated region of *SmCPS1* and a 399-bp gene-specific sequence in the 3′ end of *SmCPS5* were amplified by PCR using cDNA as a template and then cloned using Gateway technology into the pK7GWIWG (II) binary vector. Positive plasmids of pK7GWIWG-*CPS1* and pK7GWIWG-*CPS5* were identified with sequencing and restriction enzyme analysis and then introduced into *Agrobacterium tumefaciens* strain EHA105 and *Agrobacterium rhizogenes* strain ACCC 10060 by electroporation. Transformation of leaf explants from *S. miltiorrhiza* bh2 - 7 plants was carried out following previously described methods with minor modifications. Single colonies of *A. tumefaciens* strain EHA105 cells harboring the various RNAi vectors were inoculated into 10 mL of liquid Luria-Bertani medium with 50 mg/L spectinomycin and 100 mg/L rifampicin and then grown on a shaker (180 rpm) at 28 ℃ for 16 to 18 h. Cells were collected by centrifugation when the optical density at 600 nm reached 0. 6 and were resuspended in 20 mL of liquid Murashige and Skoog medium. Leaves or petioles were cut into 0. 5-×0. 5-cm pieces discs and precultured for 2 d on Murashige and Skoog basal medium supplemented with 2. 0 mg/L 6-benzyladenine. The discs were then submerged with shaking in a bacterial suspension for 15 min and cocultured on the Murashige and Skoog basal medium for 2 d. The leaf discs were then transferred to selection Murashige and Skoog basal medium supplemented with 2. 0 mg/L 6-benzyladenine, 50 mg/L kanamycin, and 225 mg/L timentin. After two to three rounds of selection (10 d each), the regenerated buds with expression of GFP were transferred to Murashige and Skoog basal medium supplemented with 25 mg/L kanamycin for root formation and elongation. Rooted plantlets were further cultured on Murashige and Skoog basal medium for about 1 month. The plantlets (7 – 8 cm tall, with roots 5 – 6 cm long) were transplanted to soil and vermiculite (3 : 1) and covered by beakers to maintain humidity for 1 week and then gradually hardened off in pots in a greenhouse for further growth.

Hairy root cultures can be successfully obtained with *S. miltiorrhiza*, and we used both hairy root cultures and full plants to analyze the silencing effect of *SmCPS5*. Though hairy root cultures with silencing of *SmCPS5* showed no significant phenotype, we found that it was an easy and fast system to analysis the effect of different silencing vectors. The *A. rhizogenes*-based transformation had a similar procedure as the *A. tumefaciens*-based transformation described above. When the hairy roots were 2 to 3 cm in length, expression of GFP was observed under a fluorescence microscope to identify positive lines. The positive hairy roots were excised and cultured on solid, hormone-free Murashige and Skoog basal medium containing 50 mg/L kanamycin and reduced timentin from 225 mg/L to zero in two or three selection cycles (15 d each). The rapidly growing kanamycin-resistant and GFP-visible lines with no bacterial contamination were then maintained at 25 ℃ in the dark with Murashige and Skoog medium without ammonium nitrate and routinely subcultured every 25 to 30 d.

Metabolomics Profiling Using LC-qTOF-MS and GC-QqQ-MS The metabolomics profiling data were acquired using a combination of two independent analytical platforms. LC-qTOF-MS analysis of methanol extracts was used for global unbiased metabolite detection. GC-QqQ-MS analysis of hexane extracts, optimized for detection of targeted intermediates, was used for the analysis of metabolites that were not readily detectable with the LC-qTOF-MS platform.

For LC-qTOF-MS, fresh plant root samples were frozen in liquid nitrogen and ground to a fine powder under continuous cooling. One hundred milligrams fresh weight of the powder was extracted in 2 mL of methanol, containing an internal standard (umbelliferone, 20 μg/mL). The extracts were sonicated twice for 15 min, centrifuged (1 500*g*) for 10 min, and then filtered through a 0. 2 μm polytetrafluoroethylene syringe filter (Agilent). An aliquot of each filtrate (5 μL) was separated using an Agilent 1 290 Infinity ultra high performance liquid chromatography system consisting of a binary pump, an autosampler, a column temperature controller, and a variable wavelength detector at 285 nm. The chromatography was performed using a ZORBAX RRHD SB-C18 column from Agilent Technologies (2. 1 × 100 mm, 1. 8 μm). The mobile phase consisted of 0. 01% (v/v) formic acid in acetonitrile (A) and water containing 0. 01% (v/v) formic acid (B). A gradient program was used as follows: linear gradient from 10% to 20% A (0 – 5 min), linear gradient from 20% to 40% A (5 – 7 min), linear gradient from 40% to 100% A (7 – 10 min), isocratic at 100% A (10 – 14 min), and linear gradient from 100% to 10% A (14 – 15 min). The mobile phase flow rate was 0. 25 mL/min, and the column temperature was set at 30 ℃. Five reference standard compounds, namely salvianolic B, rosmarinic acid, crypotanshinone, tanshinone IIA, and tanshinone I were dissolved in methanol to create standard curves for use in absolute quantification calculations. To ensure that analytes were in the linear range and to exclude some artifactual peaks, samples were also diluted by 10- and 50-fold and reanalyzed.

MS was performed using an Agilent 6 540 qTOF equipped with an electrospray ionization source operating in positive ion mode. The nebulization gas was set to 40 pounds per square inch. The drying gas was set to 10 L/min at a temperature of 350 ℃, and the sheath gas was set to 11 L/min at a temperature of 350 ℃. The capillary voltage was set to 4,000 V. The qTOF acquisition rate was set to 0. 5 s. For full-scan MS analysis, the spectra were recorded in the range of mass-to-charge ratio ($m/z$) 100 to 1,000. Chromatographic separation, followed by full-scan mass spectra, was performed to record retention time and $m/z$ values of all detectable ions present in the samples.

For GC-QqQ-MS, plant material was lyophilized for 48 h. One hundred milligrams of the lyophilized powder was extracted in 2 mL of hexane that contained two internal standards (tricosane, 6. 5 μg/mL; and tetracosane, 0. 8 μg/mL). The extracts were sonicated twice for 15 min and centrifuged (3 000*g*) for 10 min. The supernatant was evaporated under nitrogen, resuspended in 50 μL of hexanes or derivatized with

80 μL of *N*-methyl-*N*-(trimethylsilyl) trifluoroacetamide and 8 μL of pyridine at 80 ℃ for 40 min, and then analyzed by GC-MS.

GC-MS analyses were performed on an Agilent 7890A GC system connected to an Agilent 7000B triple quadrupole mass spectrometer with EI ionization. A 1 μL portion of the extract was injected in splitless mode onto the column. The column used was a DB-5 ms (30-m×0.25-mm i.d., 0.25-μm film thickness; Agilent J&W Scientific) fused silica capillary column. Helium was used as the carrier gas for GC at a flow rate of 1.0 mL/min. The injector temperature was 280 ℃. The oven program was as follows: 50 ℃ for 2 min, linear ramp at a rate of 20 ℃/min to 200 ℃, and then followed with a linear ramp at a rate of 5 ℃/min to 300 ℃, held at 300 ℃ for 10 min. The transfer line temperature was 280 ℃.

Raw data were processed with Mass Hunter Qualitative Analysis software (Agilent). Mass Profiler Professional (Agilent) software was used to identify significantly different ion features. A series of filtration steps was performed to further filter the initial results. First, only features with abundances above 1,000 ion counts were selected. Second, features were passed through a quality control tolerance window of 0.1% plus 0.15 min and 5 μg/mL plus 2.0 mD chosen for alignment of retention time and $m/z$ values, respectively. Third, features that were not present in all biological replicates of any single sample group were removed. The data were normalized to the detected values for the internal standard peak; GC-QqQ-MS data were normalized to tetracosane. After alignment and normalization of the peaks of each sample, a single data set stored as a matrix was prepared. Fold change values were calculated as the ratio of mean *SmCPS1*-RNAi line feature values compared with the mean values for these features in the wild-type lines. Student's $t$ tests were then used to determine whether each feature was increased or decreased significantly. The aligned data were exported to SIMCA-P + 12.0 for multivariate analyses (partial least-squares discriminant analysis).

Differentially accumulated features detected by LC-qTOF-MS were identified by automatic comparison to a personalized metabolite database established with METLIN software. Seven hundred sixty-two diterpenoids were collected from different *Saliva* spp., among them, 86 tanshinones and biosynthetically related metabolites came from *S. miltiorrhiza*. The putative metabolite peaks were tentatively identified by comparison with MS/MS spectra and reference standard compounds including sugiol, cryptotanshinone, tanshinone IIA, tanshinone IIB, tanshinone I, dihydrotanshinone I, przewalskin, salvisyrianone (BioBiopha), and miltirone (Faces Biochemical). Differentially accumulated features detected by GC-QqQ-MS were compared with the NIST 05 standard mass spectral databases and four reference standard compounds, including geranylgeraniol (Sigma), miltiradiene (Luqi Huang's lab), and ferruginol and sugiol (BioBiopha).

In Vitro Assays For in vitro functional assays, the full coding sequence of *S. miltiorrhiza* diTPS genes with specific restriction enzyme sites (Supplemental Table S6) was cloned into the pGEM-T vector (Promega), digested with corresponding restriction enzymes, and subcloned into the expression plasmid pET32a (Merck) to create pET32-CPSs and pET32-KSLs. AtCPS (AAA53632) and AtKS (AAC39443) were cloned from Arabidopsis (*Arabidopsis thaliana*). CfTPS2 (KF444507) and CfTPS3 (KF444508) were full synthesized. The expression, purification, and kinetic analysis of the recombinant proteins were performed as described previously. The constructs were transformed into Tuner (DE3) or Origami B (DE3) competent cells (Merck). Three to five positive colonies were cultured in Luria-Bertani medium with 50 mg/L carbenicillin, and 0.1 to 0.4 mmol/L isopropyl β-D-thiogalactopyranoside was added to induce the expression of the protein. Subsequently, cell pellets were collected and resuspended in assay buffer (50 mmol/L phosphate, pH 7.4, 10% ($V/V$) glycerol, 2 mmol/L dithiothreitol, and 10 mmol/L $MgCl_2$) and sonicated for 10 s six times on ice. Lysate from the samples was centrifuged at 12 000$g$, and the resulting supernatant was used for the assays. The conversion of GGPP to CPP or LDPP was carried out by incubating 500 μg of pET32-CPS sample protein extract with 20 to 50 μmol/L GGPP (Sigma) in a final volume of 250 μL of assay buffer for 2 to 4 h at 30 ℃. Assay mixtures were hydrolyzed (dephosphorylated) with 75 units of bacterial alkaline phosphatase at pH 8 for 16 h at 37 ℃ to produce hexane-soluble products. GGPP was converted to kaurene, miltiradiene, or manoyl oxide by mixing 250 μg of pET32-CPS protein extract and 250 μg of pET32-KSL protein extraction with 20 to 50 μmol/L of GGPP and incubated for 2 to 4 h at 30 ℃. Assay mixtures were extracted three times with an equal volume of hexane. The hexane fractions were pooled, evaporated under nitrogen, resuspended in 50 μL of hexanes or derivatized with 80 μL of *N*-methyl-*N*-(trimethylsilyl) trifluoroacetamide and 8 μL of pyridine at 80 ℃ for 40 min, and then analyzed by GC-MS. To identify possible products, we obtained and analyzed a series of standard reference compounds including geranylgeraniol (Sigma), geranyllinalool (Sigma), (13*E*)-labda-8α,15-diol (BioBiopha), 13-*epi*-manool (BioBiopha), and sclareol (Sigma).

Purification of Recombinant CPS and KSL Cell pellets were resuspended in 16 mL of protein lysis buffer (50 mmol/L phosphate, pH 7.4, 300 mmol/L NaCl, 10% ($V/V$) glycerol, 10 mmol/L $MgCl_2$, and 20 mmol/L imidazole) and sonicated for 10 s, six times, on ice. Lysate from the samples was centrifuged at 12,000$g$ for 20 min at 4 ℃. The cleared lysate was transferred to prewashed nickel-nitrilotriacetic acid agarose beads and incubated for 30 min at 4 ℃. Thereafter, the nickel-nitrilotriacetic acid agarose beads were rinsed three times with 15 mL of washing buffer (20 mmol/L phosphate, pH 7.4, 300 mmol/L NaCl, and 100 mmol/L imidazole). The tagged protein was then eluted by the addition of 6 mL of elution buffer (20 mmol/L phosphate, pH 7.4, 300 mmol/L NaCl, and 500 mmol/L imidazole) to the bead bed. The buffer of the eluted proteins was then exchanged using a PD-10 column equilibrated with assay buffer (50 mmol/L phosphate, pH 7.4, 10% [v/v] glycerol, 2 mmol/L dithiothreitol, and 10 mmol/L $MgCl_2$). The purified proteins were then identified by SDS-PAGE gel and quantified by Bradford assays (Genstar).

Enzyme Kinetic Analysis of SmCPS1 and SmCPS2 For kinetic assays, 20 nmol/L purified SmCPS1 and SmCPS2 was used, with a 2 min reaction time at 25 ℃. Single-vial assays were used as described above. Assays were completed in triplicate with 0.5 to 20 μmol/L GGPP for SmCPS1 and 0.5 to 8 μmol/L GGPP for SmCPS2. Enzymes were deactivated at the end of the 2 min reactions by incubating the reaction vial at 80 ℃ for 3 min, followed by quenching on ice. Three hundred molar purified SmKSL1 enzyme was then added to the vial in the single-vial assay for another reaction at 30 ℃ for 2 h. Assays were analyzed via GC-QqQ using selected ion monitoring of $m/z$ 57 (for internal standard tetracosane) and $m/z$ 134 for the miltiradiene product. Miltiradiene concentrations were determined relative to the internal standard by using excess SmCPS1 and SmKSL1 in single-vial assays and allowing the reaction to proceed to completion (2 h). Kinetic parameters were determined by nonlinear regression using a Michaelis-Menten model implemented in GraphPad Prism 6.03.

Positive Selection Analysis For molecular evolution analysis, 29 protein-coding DNA sequences for CPSs were used to construct phylogenetic trees, using PhyML3.0 under the general time-reversible nucleotide substitution model with four rate substitution categories. The branches with bootstrap values higher than 700 were used for branch site model tests 1 and 2 in the PAML package to detect whether positive selection had acted on particular amino acid sites within specific lineages. Branch site model uses a maximum-likelihood approach to calculate nonsynonymous to synonymous rate ratios. Likelihood ratio tests were performed, and the values of twice the difference between the log likelihood of different models were posteriorly transformed into exact $P$ values using PAML 4.6. The $\chi^2$ distributions with the degree of freedom=2 and degree of freedom=1, which have been shown to be conservative under conditions of positive selection, were used to perform tests 1 and 2, respectively. Probabilities of sites under positive selection were obtained using Bayesian approaches implemented in PAML.

Homology Modeling, Molecular Docking, and Mutagenesis Homology models were constructed within the SWISS-MODEL Workspace using the automatic alignment algorithm. The crystal structures of CPS from Arabidopsis (Protein Data Bank nos. 3pya and 3pyb) were used as the templates. The ligand docking modeling was performed with AutoDock Vina. Model visualization and binding site analysis were performed using PyMOL (http://www.pymol.org). Mutants were generated by whole-plasmid PCR amplification with overlapping mutagenic primers of the pGEM-T vector (Promega) clones and verified by complete gene sequencing prior to subcloning into the expression vector pET32a (Merck). The resulting constructs were heterologous expressed and analyzed as described above.

Sequence data from this article can be found in the GenBank/EMBL data libraries with the following accession numbers: *SmCPS1* (KC814639), *SmCPS2* (KC814640), *SmCPS3* (KC814641), *SmCPS4* (KP063138), *SmCPS5* (KC814642), and *SmKSL2* (KC814643).

[崔光红, Reuben J Peters, 漆小泉, 等. Plant Physiology, 2015, 169: 1607-1618.]

# Cytochrome P450 promiscuity leads to a bifurcating biosynthetic pathway for tanshinones

## 1 INTRODUCTION

Terpenoids represent the largest group of plant natural products, with over 54,000 structurally defined compounds. Many terpenoids have diverse biological activities and, thus, have been widely used as pharmaceuticals and medicines. For example, artemisinin and taxol are widely used agents in the treatment of malaria and cancer, respectively. Cytochrome P450 (CYP) enzymes are major players in generating the structural diversity of terpenoids, as more than 97% of the terpenoids are oxygenated via the biological activity of CYPs. In fact, CYPs represent the biggest superfamily of enzymes (approximately 1% of all protein encoding genes) in plants. While hydroxylation is the most commonly catalyzed reaction, CYPs can also catalyze many mechanistically more complex reactions. In addition to the typical regio- and stereo-specific hydroxylation reactions, there are increasingly more examples of CYPs exhibiting promiscuity by accepting multiple substrates and/or producing multiple products. The abundance of CYPs in plant genomes, together with their promiscuity, is one of the primary drivers of the chemical diversity of terpenoids. However, this presents daunting challenges to the identification of CYPs associated with the biosynthesis of particular natural products. For example, in the model plant *Arabidopsis thaliana*, more than 70% of CYPs remain functionally uncharacterized. Therefore, functional characterization of plant CYPs is of general interest towards increasing our understanding of plant metabolism, and can provide valuable elements for metabolic engineering.

Tanshinones are a group of abietane *nor*-diterpenoid quinone natural products found in the Chinese medicinal plant *Salvia miltiorrhiza* Bunge (also known as Danshen), which have been widely used in clinical for the treatment of cerebrovascular- and cardiovascular-related diseases. The Fufang Danshen Dripping Pill, with Danshen as one of the major components, is widely used in China. The Pill also has been approved for phase III clinical trials in USA (Clinical Trials. gov Identifier: NCT01659580). There have been more than 40 tanshinones and structurally related compounds identified from Danshen. Studies have demonstrated that various tanshinones, such as tanshinone ⅡA (**1**), cryptotanshinone (**2**) and tanshinone Ⅰ (**3**) (Fig. 1a), have antibacterial, antioxidant, anti-inflammation, and anti-cancer activities. While tanshinones can be extracted from Danshen roots, the ever-growing demand cannot be met by cultivation of Danshen plants. Thus, attempts have been made to improve tanshinones production in Danshen hairy root cultures by enhancing the expression of key enzymes involved in the general isoprenoid/terpenoids precursor biosynthetic pathway. In addition, a synthetic biology approach has been employed to engineer the production of potential intermediates of tanshinone biosynthesis in recombinant *Saccharomyces cerevisiae* (yeast). However, the tanshinone biosynthetic pathway remains incompletely elucidated, particularly the latter modification steps, which impedes the application of such rational approaches to improve access to the tanshinones.

The formation of tanshinones is initiated by cyclization of (*E*, *E*, *E*)-geranylgeranyl diphosphate (GGPP), the general diterpenoid precursor, to the abietane miltiradiene (**4**), which is mediated by two enzymes, SmCPS1 and SmKSL1 (Fig. 1b). To transform **4** into tanshinones, multiple reactions are required, including oxidation, heterocyclization, aromatization and demethylation, all of which fall into the repertoire of known CYP-mediated reactions. We previously demonstrated that **4** is the precursor to tanshinones, and identified a CYP, CYP76AH1, that can produce ferruginol (**5**). In this study, two CYPs (*CYP76AH3* and *CYP76AK1*) were found to exhibit similar transcription profiles as *CYP76AH1* in elicited Danshen hairy roots. Further biochemical analysis and RNA-interference (RNAi) in Danshen hairy root cultures suggested that both CYPs are promiscuous and act sequentially to form a bifurcating pathway for tanshinone biosynthesis. When utilized in engineered yeast, these genes led to the production of six oxygenated diterpenoids, which provide materials for further biological study and the identification of subsequently acting CYPs. Our results further emphasize the utility of such a synthetic biology approach to characterization of plant CYPs, and continued critical examination of the effect of CYP promiscuity on the complex nature of terpenoid biosynthesis.

## 2 MATERIALS AND METHODS

Plant materials and chemicals *S. miltiorrhiza* plants used to analyze organ specific CYP expression were collected in Beijing, China. Ferruginol and sugiol were purchased from BioBioPha (Yunnan, China). Tanshinone I, cryptotanshinone, tanshinone IIA and 11-hydroxy-sugiol were purchased from Chengdu Must Bio-Technology Co., Ltd (Sichuan, China). The purity of these commercial chemicals was >95% (HPLC).

Heterologous expression in yeast and *in vitro* enzymatic activity assay Full-length cDNAs of *CYP76AH3* (Accession No. KR140168) and *CYP76AK1* (Accession No. KR140169) were cloned as previously described, using the primers shown in Table S1. The open reading frame of *CYP76AH3* was sub-cloned into the yeast epitope-tagged vector pESC-His using *BamH*I and *Sal*I restriction sites, yielding pESC-His:: *CYP76AH3*. The open reading frame of *CYP76AK1* was sub-cloned, using *EcoR*I and *Spe*I restriction sites, into plasmid pESC-His and pESC-His:: *CYP76AH3*, yielding pESC-His:: *CYP76AK1* and pESC-His:: *CYP76AH3*/*CYP76AK1*. These plasmids were transformed into the yeast strain WAT11 that enables catalytic activity of plant CYPs by also expressing ATR1 (Urban *et al*., 1997). Yeast cultures were grown and microsomes prepared as described previously.

*In vitro* enzymatic activity assays were performed on a shaking incubator (150 rpm), at 30℃ for 4 hour in 500 μL of 100 mmol/L Tris-HCl, pH 7.5, containing 0.5 mg total microsomal proteins, 500 μmol/L NADPH, along with a

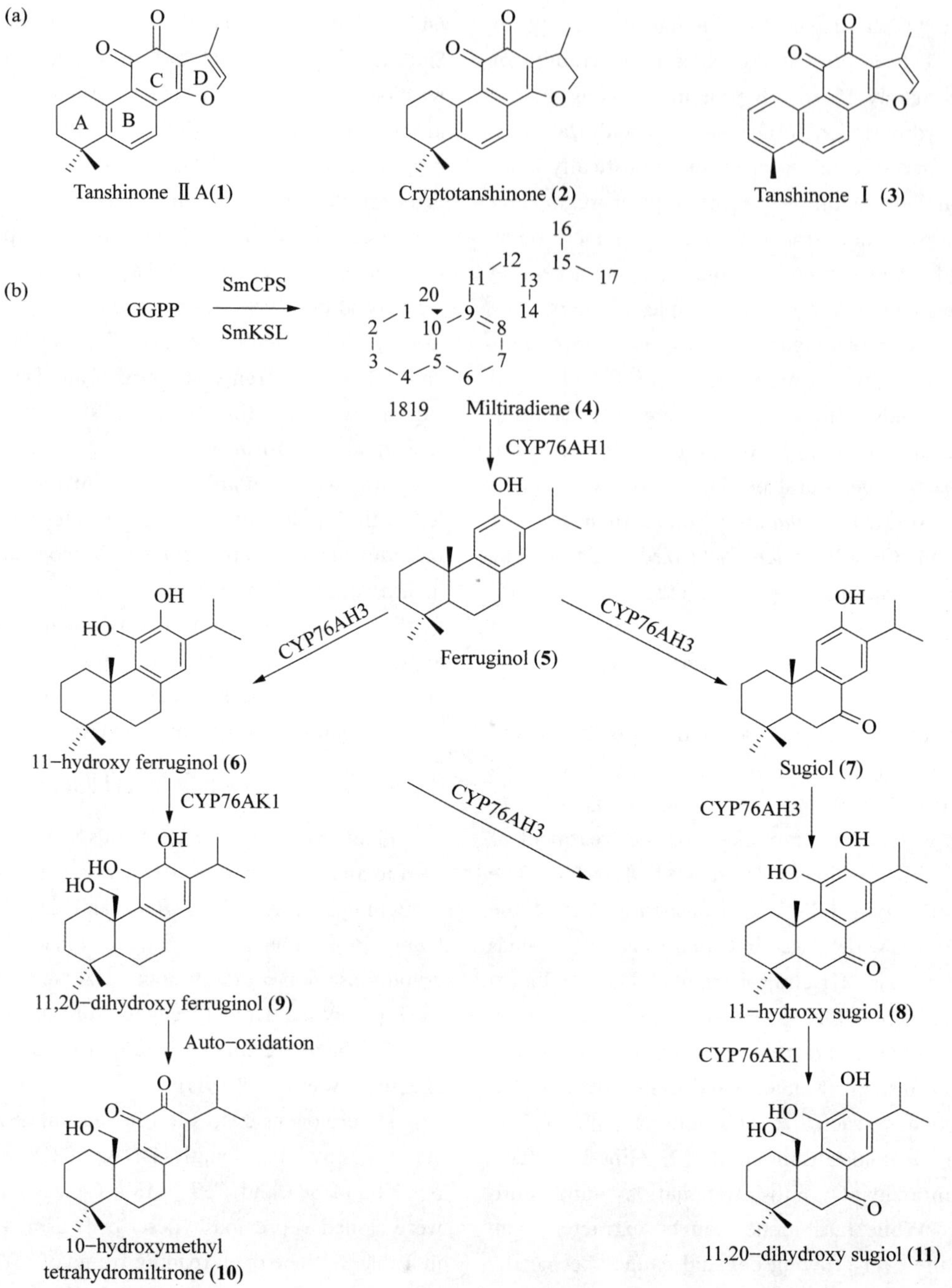

**Fig. 1 Tanshinones and partial biosynthetic pathway in *S. miltiorrhiza***

(a) Representative tanshinones found in *S. miltiorrhiza*. (b) Proposed partial biosynthetic pathway of tanshinones. The red arrow indicates the oxidation reaction catalyzed by the CYP76AH3 enzyme. The blue arrow indicates the oxidation reaction catalyzed by the CYP76AK1 enzyme.

regenerating system (consisting of 5 μmol/L FAD, 5 μmol/L FMN, 5 mmol/L glucose-6-phosphate, 1 Unit/mL glucose-6-phosphate dehydrogenase), and 100 μmol/L of either miltiradiene (**4**), ferruginol (**5**), sugiol (**6**), or 11-hydroxy sugiol (**8**). Reactions were stopped by addition of 500 μL of n-hexane and vortexing. Negative control reactions were carried out with microsomal preparations from recombinant yeast transformed with 'empty' pESC-His.

To produce sufficient amounts of the unknown CYP76AK1 product **11** for chemical structure characterization, these *in vitro* assays were scaled up. Microsomes were prepared from 4 L of yeast expressing *CYP76AK1*. These were used in a 40 mL reaction, with the buffer and NADPH regeneration system described above, and 20 mg of 11-hydroxy-sugiol (**8**) as substrate. The assay was performed on a shaking incubator (150 rpm), at 30 ℃ for 30 h. The incubation products were extracted and **11** purified, using the methods described below, for chemical structure analysis by NMR.

RNA interference in hairy root of Danshen Gene specific fragments of *CYP76AH3* (nucleotides 636～1038) and *CYP76AK1* (nucleotides 651 - 1054) were cloned into the pENTR vector using the Directional TOPO Cloning Kits (Invitrogen) and the primers shown in Table S1, and further sub-cloned into the hpRNA binary vector pK7GWIWG2D using Gateway LR Clonase Enzyme Mix (Invitrogen) to generate RNAi knock-down vectors. Each of these constructs was introduced into *A. rhizogenes* C58C1 via a freeze-thaw transformation method. These recombinant *A. rhizogenes* were then transfected into Danshen leaf explants, using *A. rhizogenes* C58C1 harboring 'empty' pK7GWIWG2D(II) as a negative control, and the resulting transformed explants were used to generate hairy root cultures, as previously described. The transformed hairy root lines were cultured in 1/2 MS solid medium at 25℃ in the dark for 6 - 8 weeks and tissue then collected for qRT-PCR and metabolite analysis, as described below.

Quantitative real-time PCR analysis Total RNA was extracted from *S. miltiorrhiza* or RNAi transformed hairy root cultures using TRIzol reagent (Invitrogen) following the manufactures' directions. First-strand cDNA was synthesized using the PrimeScriptR RT reagent Kit with gDNA Eraser (Takara, Tokyo, Japan). Relative transcript abundance was determined by qRT-PCR using the SYBR Premix Ex Taq II system (Takara, Tokyo, Japan) on an ABI 7 500 instrument (Applied Biosystems, Foster City, CA, USA). The primers used for qRT-PCR analysis are listed in Table S1. The gene for actin was used as the endogenous control. At least three independent experiments were performed for each analysis.

Engineering yeast for production of oxygenated tanshinones intermediates To engineer yeast for production of intermediates from tanshinone biosynthesis, and obtain enough compound for structural characterization, pESC-His:: *CYP76AK1* or pESC-His:: *CYP76AH3/CYP76AK1* were transformed into the ferruginol (**5**) production strain YJ35, using lithium acetate/single-stranded carrier DNA/polyethylene glycol transformation method, to produce the YJ51 and the YJ61 strains (the genotype and characteristics of each of these are listed in Table S2). Transformants were selected on YNB medium containing 20 g/L glucose and grown at 30℃ for 48 h. The recombinant yeast strains were grown in YNB medium containing 2% glucose (YNB/glucose) at 30 ℃, shaking at 250 rpm, for 48 h, then transferred to 50 mL YNB/glucose medium in 250 mL flasks and grown to an initial OD600 of 0.05, and cultivated an additional 12 - 16 h to reach logarithmic phase. Cells were centrifuged and washed twice with sterile water to remove any residual glucose. The cells were then resuspended in 50 mL YNB medium containing 2% galactose (YNB/gal) for induction, and grown for 30 - 72 h to produce diterpenoids.

In order to simplify the fermentation procedure, the inducible promoters in the pESC-His vector were replaced by constitutive promoters from yeast. The constitutive promoters TEF1p and PGK1p were amplified from the genomic DNA of *S. cerevisiae* strain BY4741, and used to replace the GAL10 and GAL1 promoters, respectively, in pESC-His by overlap extension PCR. This replacement resulted in the plasmid pESC-TP. *CYP76AH3* and *CYP76AK1* were sub-cloned downstream of the TEF1p and PGK1p promoter, respectively, using a previously described RF cloning strategy. The resulting pESC-TP:: *CYP76AH3/CYP76AK1* construct was confirmed by PCR screening and sequencing, and then transformed into YJ35, resulting in YJ62 (the genotype and characteristics of which are listed in Table S2).

Strain YJ62 was used for production of oxygenated tanshinones intermediates through fed-batch fermentation. YJ62 was first inoculated into 1 L flask containing 0.2 L YNB medium, and grown at 30 ℃. This starter culture was then transferred to a 5 L fermentor (GS-8000-P, ShanhaiGuangshi, Shanghai, China) containing 2 L YNB medium. Fermentation was carried out at 30 ℃ and 250 rpm. During fermentation, the dissolved oxygen was controlled at >40% saturation, and the pH was controlled and held at 4. Concentrated glucose solution (40%, wt/vol) was fed periodically to keep the glucose concentration above 1.0 g/L. Additional YNB (6.7 g/L) was fed after the initial 30 h of fermentation. The culture was then harvested by extraction after 72 h total fermentation time.

Homology modeling and docking analysis Template selection was carried out by BLAST search of the CYP76AK1 amino acid sequence against the Protein Data Bank (PDB). The CYP76AK1 model was constructed using DISCOVERY STUDIO v2.5 (http://www.accelrys.com). The model with the highest score was validated by PROCHECK.

Compounds **5**,**6**,**7**,**8** were docked into CYP76AK1 using AutoDock 4.0. A grid size of 40×40×40 Å with grid point spacing of 0.375 Å was set for ligand docking. Each compound was subjected to 100 runs of the AutoDock search using the Lamarckian genetic algorithm; all other parameters were set to default values.

Metabolite extraction In vitro enzymatic assays were extracted with an equal volume of n-hexane, which was separated and subjected to GC - MS and LC - MS analysis. Yeast cultures were extracted three times by ultrasonication with an equal volume of n-hexane. After separation, the organic extract was concentrated under vacuum, and the residue resuspended in n-hexane. For isolation of compound **6**, the residue was loaded on silica gel column and eluted with a 20 : 1 mixture of petroleum ether and ethyl acetate (*V/V*). Other diterpenoid products were purified by preparative HPLC, as described below. To determine the content of these compounds in hairy root cultures, approximately 25 mg of lyophilized tissue was extracted three times by ultrasonication in 1 mL methanol, the filtered extract then dried under vacuum, and resuspended in 120 μL acetonitrile for LC - MS analysis, as described below.

LC - MS, GC - MS and NMR analysis GC - MS was carried out using a Trace 1310 series GC with detection via a TSQ8000 MS (Thermo Fisher Scientific Co. Ltd.). Chromatographic separation was performed on a TR - 5 ms column capillary column (30 m×0.25 mm ID DF=0.25 μm; Thermo Fisher Scientific Co. Ltd.). Helium was used as the carrier gas at a constant flow rate of 1 mL/min through the column. The injector temperature was set at 280 ℃. The temperature gradient program was: 50 ℃ (1 min), 50→150℃ at 5 ℃/min, 150→230 ℃ at 20 ℃/min, 230→300 ℃ linear at 30℃/min, 300℃ (5 min). Each run analyzed 1 μL injections of the relevant sample using a 50 : 1 split ratio.

LC - MS was carried out using an Acquity UPLCTM system (Waters Corp., Milford, MA, USA) with an Acquity UPLC BEH C18 column (50×2.1 mm, 1.7 μm). The column temperature was set at 40℃. The flow rate was kept at 500 μL/min. Mobile phases were water (A) and acetonitrile (B). The gradient was as follows: (0～8.0) min, 50%→80% B; (8.0～8.5) min, 80%→100% B; (8.5～11.0) min, 100% B; (11.0～11.5) min, 100%→50% B; (11.4～14.5) min, 50% B. Time-of-flight MS detection was performed with a Xevo G2 - S MS system (Waters Corp., Manchester, UK). The data acquisition range was from 50 - 1 500 Da. The source temperature was set at 100 ℃, and the desolvation temperature was set at 450℃, with desolvation gas flow set at 900 L/h. The lock mass compound used was leucine enkephaline at a concentration 200 pg/μL. The capillary voltage was set at 2.5 KV. The cone voltage was set at 40 V. The collision energy was set as 6 eV for low-energy scan, and 50 - 65 eV ramp for high-energy scan. The instrument was controlled by Masslynx 4.1 software (Waters Corp., Manchester, UK).

Preparative HPLC separation was performed using a Waters 600E - 2487 instrument, using an YMC-Pack ODS - A column (250 mm×20 mm, 5 μm). The mobile phase was a 4 : 6 mixture of water and acetonitrile (*V*/*V*) for compounds **9** and **10**, or a 6 : 4 mixture of water and acetonitrile (*V*/*V*) for compound **11**, in either case run with a flow rate of 6 mL/min.

For chemical structure characterization, $^1$H NMR (400 MHz), $^{13}$C NMR (100 MHz), and 2D - NMR spectra were recorded with a Bruker DRX 400 spectrometer for 11-hydroxy ferruginol (**6**), $^1$H NMR (500 MHz), $^{13}$C NMR (125 MHz), and 2D - NMR spectra were recorded with a Bruker INOVA - 500 spectrometer for 11, 20-dihydroxy ferruginol (**9**) and 10-hydroxymethyltetrahydromiltirone (**10**), $^1$H NMR (600 MHz), $^{13}$C NMR (150 MHz), and 2D - NMR spectra were recorded with a Bruker AVIIIHD - 600 spectrometer for 20-dihydroxy sugiol (**11**). TMS was used as internal standard. The observed chemical shift values were measured in ppm.

## 3 RESULTS

Identification of candidate CYPs Our previous study indicated that the ferruginol synthase, CYP76AH1, is the first CYP responsible for the generation of oxygenated diterpenoids precursors in tanshinone biosynthesis. We also carried out transcriptomic analysis of the elicitation process in Danshen hairy roots culture and found 125 CYPs expressed therein. To identify other CYPs involved in tanshinone biosynthesis, here we carried out further co-expression analysis of this transcriptome dataset (Accession No. SRX224100). It was found that the expression of isotig10614 and isotig05577 was highly correlated with that of *CYP76AH1* (Fig. S1). We cloned the corresponding full-length cDNA for these two isotigs, and identified these as *CYP76AH3* (81% sequence similarity to *CYP76AH1*) and *CYP76AK1* (46% sequence similarity to *CYP76AH1*), which represented promising candidates for further functional analysis.

Biochemical characterization of CYP76AH3 & CYP76AK1 Both CYPs were cloned and expressed in the yeast strain WAT11, which overexpresses the plant CYP reductase ATR1 from *A. thaliana*. Microsomal preparations from the resulting recombinant yeast were used for *in vitro* activity assays with **5** as the substrate. LC - MS analysis of the assay mixtures revealed that CYP76AH3 converted **5** into three compounds, namely, **6**, **7** and **8**, with retention times of 4.75 min, 1.72 min and 1.63 min, respectively (Fig. 2, a - c). Compound **6** had an *m*/*z* of 301.2188 and it was determined to be 11-hydroxyferruginol based on structural analysis by NMR (Fig. S2). The retention times and mass spectra for compounds **7** and **8** matched those of authentic standards for sugiol and 11-hydroxy sugiol, respectively. Moreover, when microsomal preparations from the yeast cells expressing CYP76AH3 were assayed with **6** or **7** as the substrate, **8** was produced (Fig. S3 and Fig. S4). These results indicated that, at least under *in vitro* conditions, CYP76AH3 functioned as a promiscuous enzyme that not only catalyzes hydroxylation at C - 11, but also sequential oxygenation/oxidation reactions at C - 7 to form a keto group.

We then assayed microsomes from the yeast cells co-expressing *CYP76AK1* and *CYP76AH3* with **5** as the substrate. LC - MS analysis revealed the presence of three new compounds, namely, **9**, **10** and **11**, with retention times and *m*/*z* values of 3.31 min and 317.216 2, 1.70 min and 315.195 4, and 1.22 min and 331.194 9, respectively (Fig. 2,

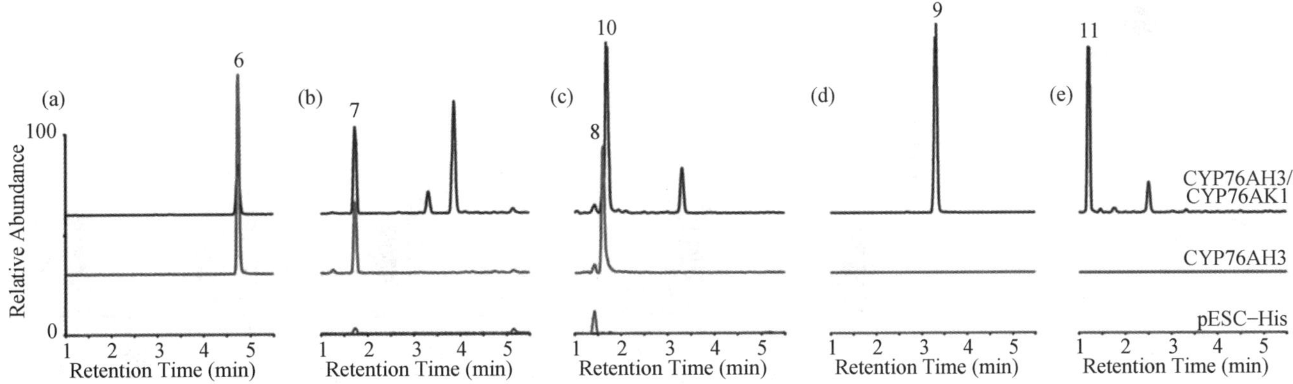


**Fig. 2 LC – MS analysis results of reaction mixtures of 5 catalyzed by yeast microsomes containing CYPs from *S. miltiorrhiza***

(a) The extracted ion current (EIC) chromatogram of 11-hydroxy ferruginol (**6**). (b) The EIC of sugiol (**7**). (c) The EIC of 11-hydroxy sugiol (**8**) and 10-hydroxymethyl tetrahydromiltirone (**10**). (d) The EICs of 11,20-dihydroxy ferruginol (**9**). (e) The EIC of 11,20-dihydroxy sugiol (**11**). The resulting daughter ion mass spectra are shown in Fig. S2, S5, S6, and S8 for compound **6**,**9**,**10**, and **11**, respectively. The green, blue and red lines represent the yeast harboring the plasmid pESC-His, pESC-His::*CYP76AK1* and pESC-His::*CYP76AH3*/*CYP76AK1*, respectively.

c – e). Compound **9** was the major product, and it was determined to be 11, 20-dihydroxy ferruginol based on structural analysis by NMR (Fig. S5). Compound **10** was found to be 10-hydroxymethyl tetrahydromiltirone, again based on structural analysis by NMR (Fig. S6). Compound **9** was unstable under ambient conditions and underwent spontaneous oxidization to **10**. Compounds **9** and **10** were produced when microsomal preparations from yeast cells expressing *CYP76AK1* were assayed with **6** as substrate (Fig. S3). We further assayed microsomal preparations from yeast cells expressing *CYP76AK1* alone with **8** as substrate, and demonstrated that it was efficiently converted into **11** (Fig. S7 and S8). However, no products were found when **4**, **5** or **7** were used as substrate. Accordingly, CYP76AK1 can catalyze hydroxylation at the C – 20 position of the two differentially oxygenated abietanes **6** and **8**. Thus, while CYP76AK1 exhibits some promiscuity, it seems to only react with phenolic abietane diterpenoids that have hydroxy groups at C – 11, as well as C – 12.

Physiological function of CYP76AH3 & CYP76AK1 It is well known that tanshinones accumulate predominantly in the root and rhizome of Danshen. To support physiological roles for CYP76AH3 and CYP76AK1 in tanshinone biosynthesis, we examined the organ specific expression of *CYP76AH3* and *CYP76AK1* by real-time PCR. It was found that the expression of both genes was more abundant in the root than aerial tissues (Fig. 3a), consistent with a role for these two CYPs in the production of tanshinones. In addition, metabolite analysis of Danshen roots by LC – MS revealed the presence of all of the CYP products found here, namely **6** – **11** (Fig. S9), consistent with our in vitro biochemical analyses.

To provide more definitive evidence that CYP76AH3 and CYP76AK1 act in tanshinone biosynthesis, an RNAi approach was used to knock-down expression of the encoding genes in Danshen hairy roots. Unique fragments from each gene were cloned into a previously described RNAi vector, which then expresses self-complementary ‘hairpin’ RNA fragments that induce silencing, and these constructs were used to transfect Danshen leaf explants to produce recombinant hairy root cultures via *Agrobacterium rhizogene*. RT – PCR analysis indicated that the expression of each targeted gene was efficiently suppressed in the transformed hairy root cultures, while those of known similar CYPs were not notably affected (Fig. 3b and Fig. S10). Targeted metabolite analysis indicated that suppression of *CYP76AK1* led to significantly lower levels of tanshinones **1** – **3** (Fig. 3c), as well as the direct CYP76AK1 products **9** and **11** (Fig. 3d). In addition, levels of the CYP76AK1 substrates, **6** and **8**, were slightly increased in this hairy root culture (Fig. 3d). These results indicate that CYP76AK1 functions as a C – 20 hydroxylase for these two intermediates, and the net results suggest a potentially bifurcating pathway in tanshinone biosynthesis. Successful silencing of *CYP76AH3* also was achieved (Fig. 3b), leading to significant reduction in levels of the direct CYP76AH3 products, **6** and **8**, as well as downstream metabolites **9** – **11** (Fig. 3d). This indicates that CYP76AH3 plays a key role in the production of these intermediates. While the levels of tanshinones **1** – **3** were somewhat reduced, this was not statistically significant (Fig. 3c), implying that the reactions catalyzed by CYP76AH3 are not rate limiting in tanshinone biosynthesis.

Homology modeling and docking analysis of CYP76AK1 To gain more insights into the chemo- and regio-selectivity of CYP76AK1, we performed homology modeling and molecular docking with compounds **5** – **8**. The crystal structure of CYP1A2

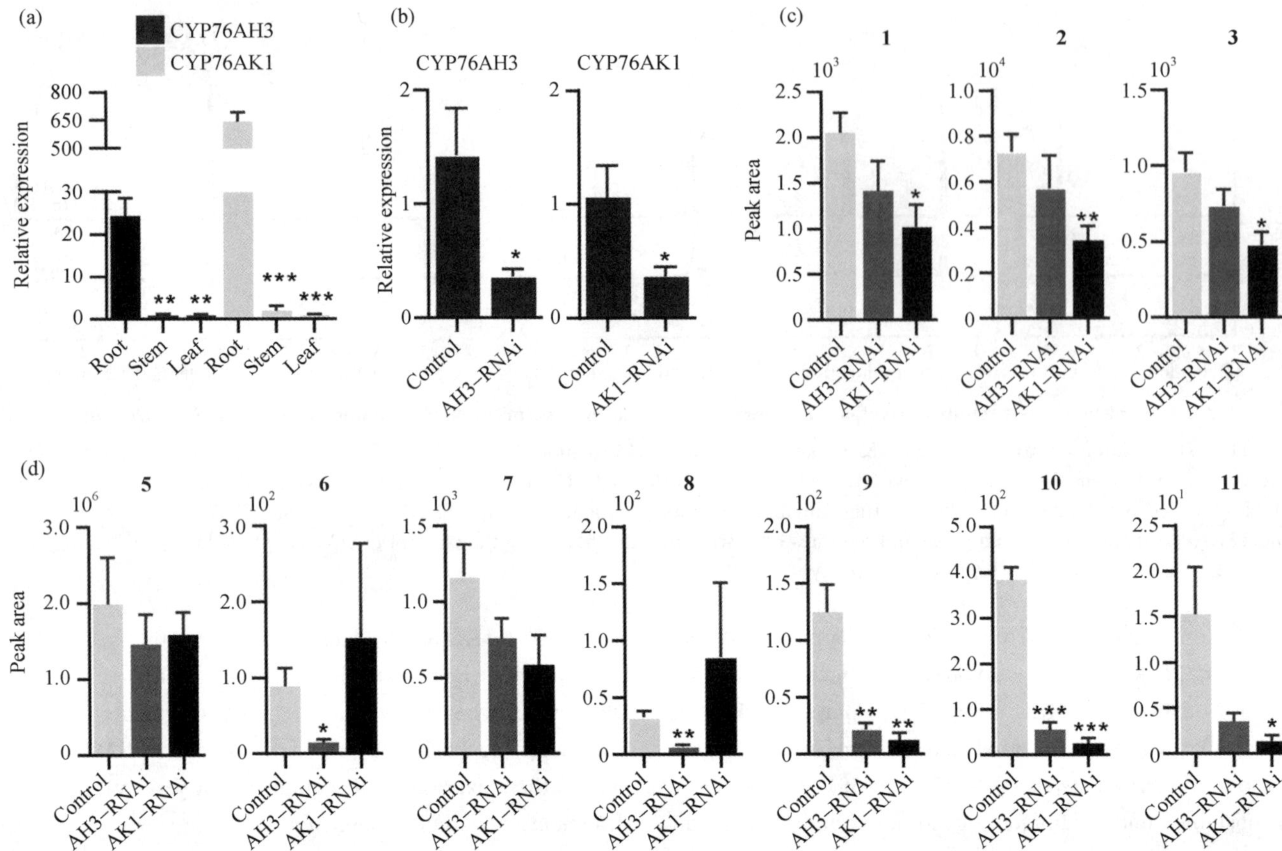


**Fig. 3 The relationship between the expression levels of *CYP76AH3* and *CYP76AK1* and the contents of different terpenoids products**

(a) Expression levels of *CYP76AH3* and *CYP76AK1* in root, stem and leaf of in *S. miltiorrhiza*. (b) Expression levels of *CYP76AH3* and *CYP76AK1* in RNAi down-regulated in *S. miltiorrhiza* hairy roots. (c) Contents of tanshinones **1**, **2** and **3** in RNAi down-regulated in *S. miltiorrhiza* hairy roots. (d) Contents of oxygenated terpenoids intermediates **5**–**11** in RNAi down-regulated in *S. miltiorrhiza* hairy roots. Expression levels were normalized using β-actin as an internal standard. The error bars represent the standard error of means from three independent replications for tissue expression analysis and from 5 to 6 lines for RNAi down-regulated hairy roots. $^{*}P<0.05$, $^{**}P<0.01$ and $^{***}P<0.001$ were determined by an unpaired $t$ test using GraphPad Prism 6.

(code: 2HI4) was selected as the template for homology modeling based on the 44.7% sequence similarity of CYP76AK1 to this human CYP (Fig. S11). As shown in Fig. S12, 88.3% of residues in the homology model are in the most favored region of the Ramachandran plot, with only four outliers in the structure, which suggests that this is a reasonable model for the CYP76AK1 protein structure, and can be used for further structural analysis. Docking results suggested that the distances between the C-20 methyl group in compound **5** and **7** and the catalytic heme iron were 10.8 Å and 9.7 Å, respectively, which are longer than those in the cases of compound **6** and **8** (8.1 Å and 7.0 Å) (Fig. 4). These data are in line with the fact that CYP76AK1 had no activity with **5** and **7**, and to some extent, that the hydroxylation activity with **8** was higher than that with **6**.

Heterologous production of oxygenated tanshinones intermediates in yeast  To further confirm their functions and demonstrate the usefulness of CYP76AH3 and CYP76AK1, these were incorporated into a previously described ferruginol producing yeast strain, YJ35. This strain harbors modules that express a GGPP synthase (BTS1) and farnesyl diphosphate synthase (ERG20) fusion, a SmCPS1 and SmKSL1 fusion, a truncated hydroxy-3-methylglutaryl coenzyme A reductase (tHMG1), and the ferruginol synthase CYP76AH1, as well as the Danshen CYP reductase (SmCPR1). We first incorporated a *CYP76AH3* expression module under the control of the *GAL10* promoter into YJ35 to produce a new strain, YJ51 (Fig. 5a). This YJ51 strain was grown in YNB medium, with glucose as the carbon source, to logarithmic phase, then induced by transferring the cells into medium containing 2% galactose as the carbon source instead. After 72 h, the fermentation broth was extracted with n-hexane. LC-MS analysis of the extracts showed the presence of three diterpenoids, namely, 57.1% (percentage of total diterpenoid peak area) of **6**, 40.6% of **8** and 2.4% of **7** (Fig. 5a). Indeed, it was this strain that provided sufficient amount of **6** for detailed structural characterization by NMR (Fig. S2).

We further added *CYP76AK1* into the *CYP76AH3* expression plasmid, and transformed this into YJ35 to generate the yeast

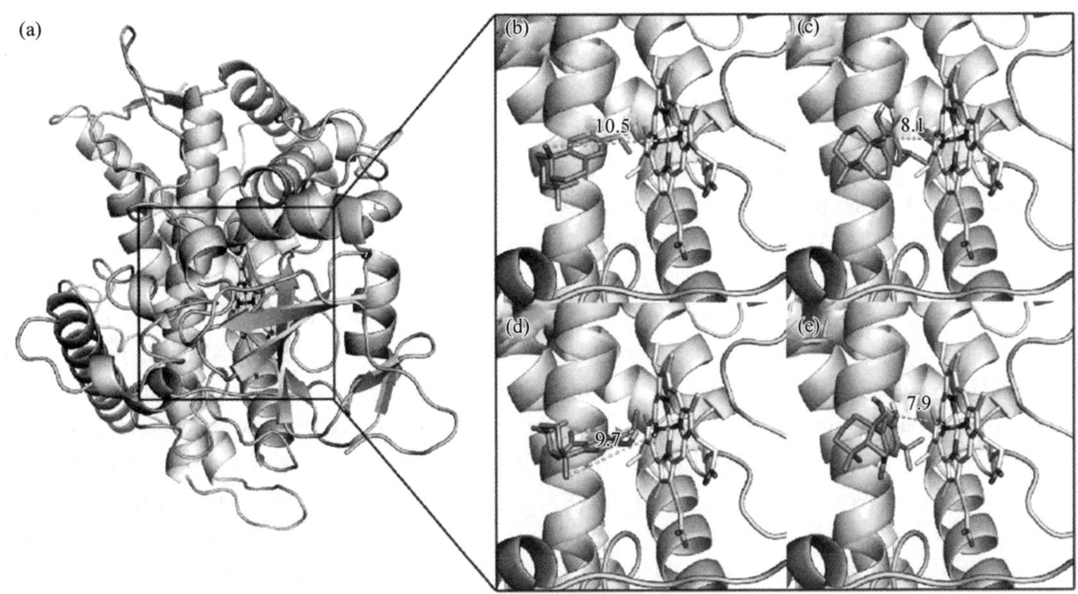


**Fig. 4 Homology modeling and docking analysis of CYP76AK1 from *S. miltiorrhiza***

(a) Homology modeling of CYP76AK1. Docking poses of compound **5** (b), **6** (c), **7** (d), **8** (e). Compound structure is depicted as stick with carbons colored pink and oxygens red. Heme is depicted as stick with carbons colored yellow and iron blue. Distance between C20 and heme iron is indicated by dashed line with the length indicated in Å.

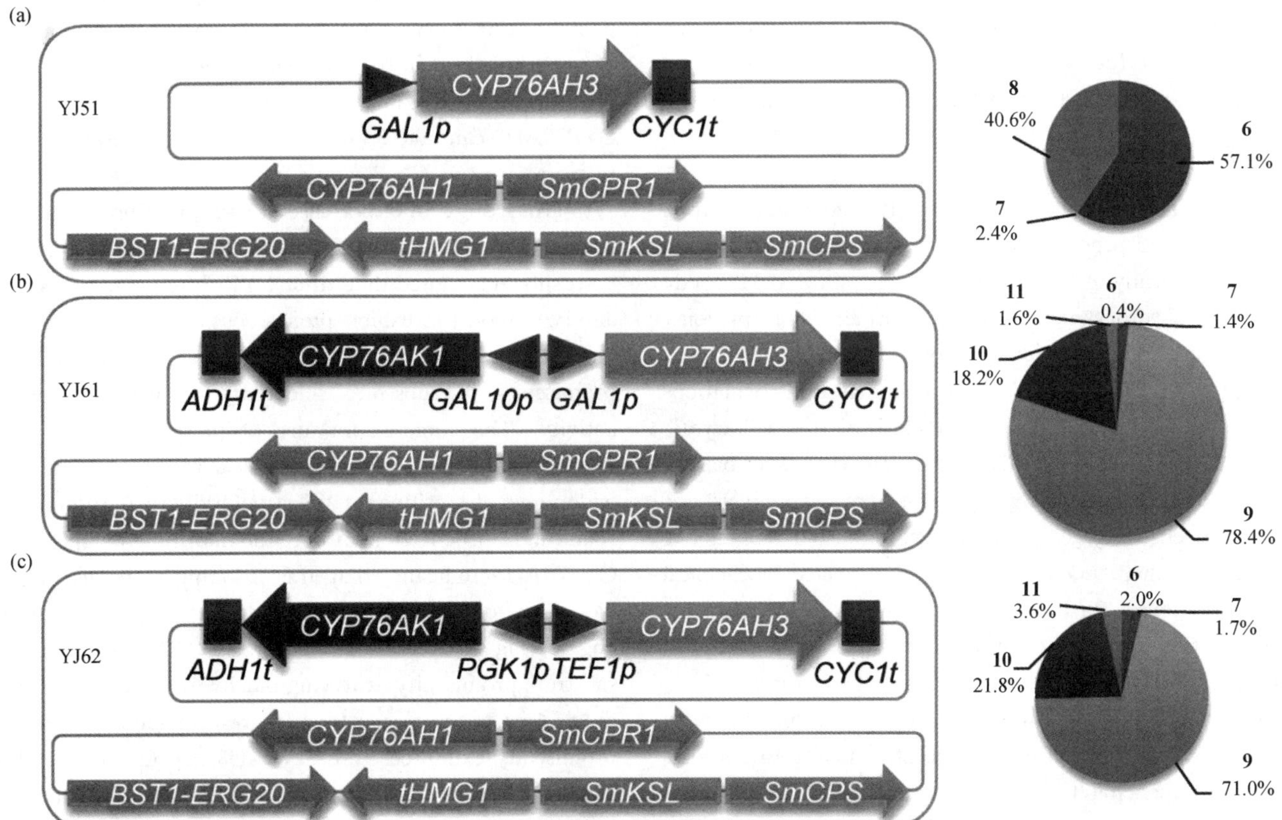


**Fig. 5 Engineered yeasts for the production of oxygenated terpenoids intermediates. YJ35 was constructed previously**

The YJ51 (a) and YJ61 (b) were constructed by transforming pESC-His: : *CYP76AH3* and pESC-His: : *CYP76AH3*/*CYP76AK1* into YJ35, respectively. YJ62 (c) was constructed by replacing the *GAL1* and *GAL10* promoter in pESC-His: : *CYP76AH3*/*CYP76AK1* with the constitutive promoter *TEF1* and *PGK1* and transforming into YJ35. The pie chart and its area represent the percentages of ferruginol derivatives (compounds **6**, **7**, **8**, **9**, **10**, and **11**) and the accumulation of diterpenoids produced in the YJ51 (a), YJ61 (b) and YJ62 (c) after 72 h of shake-flask fermentation at 250 rpm in YNB with galactose for YJ51 and YJ61, and YNB with glucose for YJ62. The data represent the mean value of three independent replications.

strain YJ61 (Fig. 5b). The resulting strain was cultivated, and extracts prepared, as described above for the YJ51 strain. LC-MS analysis indicated that YJ61 produced 78.4% of **9**, 18.2% of **10**, 1.6% of **11**, 1.4% of **7**, and 0.4% of **6** (Fig. 5b), which indicated that most of the intermediates were efficiently converted to the more elaborated compounds **9** and **10**. Again, it was this YJ61 strain that provided sufficient amounts of **9** and **10** for structural characterization by NMR.

The use of the *GAL1p* and *GAL10p* promoters for expressing *CYP76AH3* and *CYP76AK1* required the use of galactose as the carbon source, necessitating a two-stage fermentation process. To avoid this, we replaced these *GAL* promoters with the constitutive promoters *TEF1p* and *PGK1p*. This new expression plasmid was transformed into YJ35 to generate the yeast strain YJ62 (Fig. 5c). When YJ62 was cultivated for 72 h in medium containing glucose as the carbon source, oxygenated diterpenoids were produced with a distribution profile quite similar to that of YJ61, as the peak areas for **9** and **10** were 92.8% of the total. Though total diterpenoid accumulation was lower than with YJ61, the YJ62 strain provides a more straightforward platform for the production of these diterpenoid metabolites, which should facilitate future studies of tanshinone biosynthesis, as well as the biological activity of these diterpenoid metabolites.

## 4 DISCUSSION

CYPs play key roles in producing the tremendous chemical diversity of terpenoids products. These heme-containing enzymes typically insert an oxygen atom into C-H bond, generating a hydroxyl group that enable further transformations, such as oxidation, acylation, methylation and glycosylation. In addition, CYPs can catalyze more unusual transformations as well. However, functional characterization of eukaryotic CYPs remains challenging. This is particularly true in plants, where the CYP superfamily represents approximately 1% of all protein encoding genes. Moreover, terpenoid biosynthetic pathways routinely require multiple CYP-mediated biochemical transformations, further complicating the assignment of their functional roles. For example, the CYPs implicated in catalyzing different steps of taxol biosynthesis share >70% amino acid sequence identity, yet this metabolic pathway remains incompletely elucidated. Recently, thanks to advances in DNA sequencing technology, co-expression analysis has been shown to be useful for identifying pathway-associated CYPs.

As extensively aromatized abietane-type *ortho*-quinone and furan ring containing *nor*-diterpenoids, the tanshinones are formed from the olefinic precursor miltiradiene (**4**) via a series of oxidative transformations. In previous work, we demonstrated that CYP76AH1 produces ferruginol (**5**). To identify CYPs responsible for subsequent steps in tanshinone biosynthesis, we carried out co-expression analysis of the transcriptome dataset to find CYPs whose expression profile matched that of *CYP76AH1* and identified two candidates from the CYP76 family, *CYP76AH3* and *CYP76AK1*. We constructed yeast strains that expressed these CYPs, both separately and together. Using **5** as the substrate, microsomes from the *CYP76AH3* expressing yeast produced three new products, compounds **6** - **8**. When using microsomes that contain both CYPs, three additional products were observed, compounds **9** - **11**. While the structures for **7** and **8** were readily established by comparison with those of authentic standards, the identities of the other four compounds remained elusive. To acquire sufficient amounts of these compounds for structural elucidation, we employed a synthetic biology approach to construct recombinant yeast for heterologous production of **6**, **9** and **10**, while **11** was produced via *in vitro* conversion of **8** at a preparative scale. Critically, RNAi knock-down of *CYP76AH3* and *CYP76AK1* expression in Danshen hairy root cultures afforded results in agreement with the functional assignment based on the biochemical information (*vide ante*). Taken together, these results highlight the utility of this approach towards characterization of CYPs involved in plant terpenoid biosynthesis.

Both CYP76AH3 and CYP76AK1 exhibit promiscuity. CYP76AH3 can take **5** and carry out hydroxylation at C-11 to form **6**, or at C-7, with further oxidation to form the keto group of **7**. In either case, these initial products can be further transformed, via the alternative reaction, to produce **8**. It should be noted that other CYP76 family members have also been shown to exhibit promiscuous activity in diterpenoids biosynthesis, but CYP76AH3 is unique because it shows promiscuity in substrate selectivity as well as catalytic activity. The complex mixture of products observed here suggests that CYP76AH3 may play a role in producing the wide range of tanshinones and structurally related compounds found in Danshen. In addition, the multifunctional nature of CYP76AH3 indicates that this also might be useful as a biocatalyst to produce new diterpenoids — e. g., via metabolic engineering in yeast. By contrast, CYP76AK1 exhibits substrate promiscuity, carrying out hydroxylation at C-20 of either **6** or **8**, to produce **9** or **11**, respectively. Notably, the promiscuity exhibited by CYP76AH3 and CYP76AK1 leads to bifurcation of tanshinone biosynthesis. In particular, the CYP76AH3 products **6** and **8** can be observed in Danshen, serve as substrates for CYP76AK1, and both accumulate upon knocking down *CYP76AK1* expression, which further represses the accumulation of tanshinones. Because of CYP promiscuity, divergent pathways become possible in plants, resulting in additional difficulties for pathway delineation. Such metabolic networks may be advantageous to bypass damages and mutations that may otherwise lead to the breakdown of the biosynthetic process. Perhaps more intriguingly, this also may provide arrays of similar natural products that might interfere with the ability of simple mutations in their molecular targets to escape inhibition.

It is conceivable that both **9** and **11** are precursors to tanshinones, as hydroxylation of C-20 is a necessary step in oxidative removal of this methyl group, as well as the potentially associated aromatization of the B-ring. Indeed, the C－7 keto group in **11** represents further oxidation towards B-ring aromatization. However, the relevance of CYP76AH3 for this transformation is not entirely clear, as knocking down *CYP76AH3* expression has only limited effect on the production of **7**. Consistent with this, C－7 keto containing diterpenoids are accumulated at low levels in the engineered yeast strains, indicating that CYP76AH3 predominantly produces **6**, and has relatively low catalytic activity on **6** and **7**. In addition, knocking down *CYP76AH3* expression only slightly reduces the accumulation of tanshinones, which may reflect a non-rate limiting role for CYP76AH3, and/or some redundancy. Given the presence of multiple CYP76 family members in Danshen, it seems likely that these CYPs may be responsible for C－7 oxidation and/or provide such redundant activity. Regardless, our results indicate that CYP76AK1 plays a key role in tanshinone production, suggesting that overexpression of this might improve yields, which is particularly important as the contents of tanshinones in Danshen are low and vary depending on the place of origin, the harvest season and the traditional processing methods.

In summary, we have functionally identified two CYPs involved in production of tanshiones, and whose promiscuity indicates bifurcation in this biosynthetic process, suggesting it comprises a complex metabolic network. Altogether, we have now identified three CYPs, including the previous reported CYP76AH1, which insert up to four atoms of oxygen into the abietane hydrocarbon intermediate **4** en route to the tanshinones. This represents substantial advancement towards elucidating tanshinone biosynthesis, and enriches our understanding of the complex roles of CYPs in the metabolic networks underlying terpenoid production more generally. Moreover, we have demonstrated that the CYPs identified here can be used in a synthetic biology approach towards heterologous production of tanshinones in yeast. Indeed, the resulting diterpenoids not only provide intermediates for further investigation of tanshinone biosynthesis, but also material for investigation of their own biological activity.

［郭娟，赵宗保，黄璐琦，等. New Phytol，2016，210(2)：525－534.］

# Recent advances in biosynthesis of bioactive compounds in traditional Chinese medicinal plants

## 1 INTRODUCTION

China is rich in plant resources. Of the ～300,000 species of higher plants on the earth, around 10% can be found in China. As in many other countries, people in China have used plants for treatment of diseases for thousands of years. *Compendium of Materia Medica* has been held in high esteem since it was first published in 1593, and this ancient encyclopedia of traditional Chinese medicine (TCM) described more than 1,000 species of plants. Plants produce a wealth of specialized (or secondary) metabolites also known as natural products, which are small molecular weight compounds with enormous structural diversity and show various biological activities. It is estimated that there are approximately 200, 000 secondary metabolites in plant kingdom, which, based on biosynthetic origins, can be classified into three major categories: phenylpropanoids, terpenoids and alkaloids, plus a few other less abundant groups. The usage records of China's ancient medical books, such as *Sheng Nong's Herbal Classic*, *Huang Di's Canon of Medicine* and *Compendium of Materia Medica*, already recognized that plant extracts contain active principles in treating illness and classified them into assumptive, intuitive or largely philosophic categories, such as cold, neutral or hot, toxic or nourishing. Over the past century, hunting the active ingredients has led to important findings, such as artemisinin for malaria, huperzine A for Alzheimer's disease, ephedrine for cold and camptothecin for cancer, which were isolated from *Artemisia annua*, *Huperzia serrata*, *Ephedra sinica*, *Camptotheca acuminate*, respectively. Very recently, tetrandrine, an alkaloid isolated from the TCM plant *Stephania tetrandra* previously used for reducing blood pressure, were reported to have the therapeutic efficacy against Ebola, and celastrol, a triterpene extracted from *Tripterygium Wilfordi*, has the potential as an anti-obesity agent. These findings strongly support that TCMs are the reliable source for new therapies in treatment of lethally epidemic disease and long unsolved disease.

However, multi-classes of natural products are generated by each plant species. In addition, geographic distributions, growth conditions and harvesting seasons could significantly affect chemical compositions of the plant. Whereas one component may act as the active ingredient, the effects of a mixture of many ingredients are often uncertain and this has caused increasing concerns; thus, the traditional practice of herbology has to face the challenges from modern medicine and the manufactures' requirement.

While plant natural products continue to be a prime source for drug discovery and development, supply of these compounds is often curtailed due to limitation of natural resources and/or low contents in plant. The biotechnological platforms, such as metabolic engineering of effective plant and microbial production, are urgently needed to ensure that the supply of bioactive natural products is sustainable and environmentally friendly, rather than at the expense of resource exhaustion. A prerequisite to these solutions is the understanding of the biosynthetic pathways of these specialized metabolites, in particular the cloning and identification of enzymes and the regulatory factors.

In the past two decades, the rapid development in genomics and high-throughput technologies of chemical analysis, in combination with molecular biology tools, has accelerated the research of medicinal plants. In this review, we summarize the recent advances in the elucidation of biosynthetic pathways of secondary metabolites in, not exclusively, TCM plants. Although alkaloids are probably the most important resource for drug discovery and biosynthesis of these amino acid-derived compounds has been investigated intensively, there are, surprisingly to some extent, relatively few studies of alkaloids from TCM plant; thus, this review is emphasized on phenylpropanoids and terpenoids. In addition to enzymes, transcription factors characterized from medicinal plants are also discussed.

## 2 PHENYLPROPANOIDS

Phenylpropanoids, commonly found in plants, are derived from the six-carbon aromatic phenyl group and the three-carbon propene tail, and form a large group of specialized metabolites including monolignols, lignans, flavonoids, phenolic acids and stilbenes. They serve as basic components of a number of structural polymers, as well as floral pigments, scent compounds or signaling molecules to mediate bio-interactions, phytoalexins against herbivores and pathogens, and protective components against ultraviolet light radiation and other abiotic stresses. In many TCM plants, such as the plants of Lamiaceae, Fabaceae (Leguminasae) and Asteraceae, phenylpropanoids are also the bioactive principles (Table 1), which have been shown to act as anti-oxidants, free radical scavengers, anti-inflammatories and anticancer compounds.

The majority of phenylpropanoids are derived from phenylalanine. The first three steps are catalyzed by phenylalanine ammonia lyase (PAL), cinnamate 4-hydroxylase (C4H) and *p*-coumaroyl coenzyme A ligase (4CL), which are commonly referred as "general phenyl-propanoid pathway". The product of 4CL is used as precursor for the biosynthesis of various phenylpropanoids in plants (Fig. 1). Parts of phenylpropanoids are synthesized from L-tyrosine, and the

**Table 1 List of examples of TCM plants rich in phenylpropanoids**

| Plant species | Chinese name in Pin-yin | Family | Representative compounds |
|---|---|---|---|
| *Salvia miltiorrhiza* | Danshen | Lamiaceae | Salvianolic acid A, B and C |
| *Scutellaria baicalensis* | Huangqin | Lamiaceae | Baicalin, wogonin, scutellarin |
| *Glycyrrhiza uralensis* | Gancao | Leguminosae | Liquiritin, isoliquiritin, 7,4′-dihydroxyflavone |
| *Astragalus membranaceus* | Huangqi | Leguminosae | Calycosin-7-glucoside, ononin |
| *Sophora flavescens* | Kushen | Leguminosae | Sophoraflavecromane A, B, C |
| *Sophora tonkinensis* | Shandougen | Leguminosae | Sophoranone, sophoradin |
| *Pueraria lobata* | Ge | Leguminosae | Puerarin, daidzin, genistein |
| *Lonicera japonica* | Jinyinhua | Caprifoliaceae | Chlorogenic acid, luteolin |
| *Dendranthema morifolium* | Juhua | Asteraceae | Chlorogenic acid, acacetin-7-*O*-β-D-glucoside, apigenin-7-*O*-β-D-glucoside, and luteolin-7-*O*-β-D-glucoside |
| *Ginkgo biloba* | Yinxing | Ginkgoaceae | Ginkgetin, isoginkgetin |
| *Epimedium brevicornu* | Yinyanghuo | Berberidaceae | Icariine, icarisid |
| *Isatis indigotica* | Songlan | Brassicaceae | Lariciresinol |

(a)

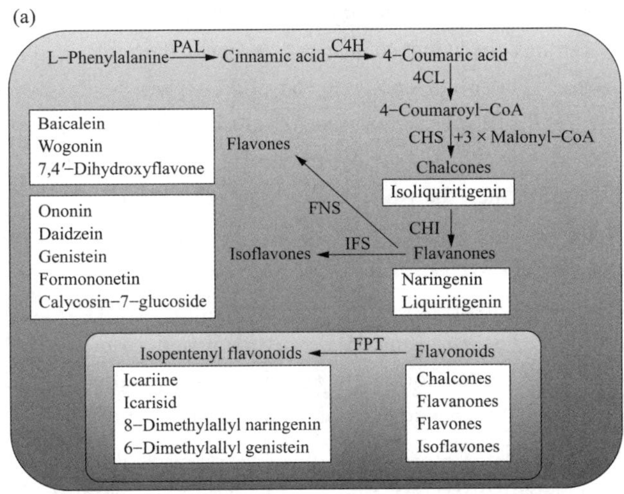


(b)

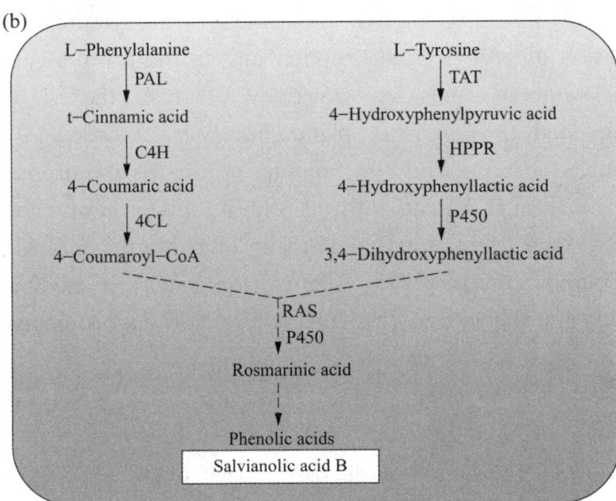


**Fig. 1 (Color online) Biosynthesis of phenylpropanoids in TCM plants**

(a) biosynthesis of flavonoids and isopentenyl flavonoids; (b) formation of phenolic acids from the L-phenylalanine- and the L-tyrosine-derived pathways in *Salvia miltiorrhiza*, a medicinal plant of Lamiaceae. Phenylpropanoids are mainly synthesized from phenylalanine via the "general phenylpropanoid pathway", catalyzed by phenylalanine ammonialyase (PAL), cinnamate 4-hydroxylase (C4H) and p-coumaroyl coenzyme A ligase (4CL). The product of p-coumaroyl-CoA is used for the biosynthesis of flavonoids, isopentenyl flavonoids and phenolic acids. CHS, chalcone synthase; CHI, chalcone isomerase; FNS, flavone synthase; IFS, isoflavone synthase; FPT, flavonoid prenyltransferase; TAT, tyrosine aminotransferase; HPPR, 4-hydroxyphenylpyruvate reductase; RAS, rosmarinic acid synthase; P450, cytochrome P450 monooxygenase. Dotted lines represent multiple enzymatic catalyzed steps.

transformation is more restricted, being mainly limited to members of several families. For instance, 3, 4-dihydroxyphenyllactic acid, one precursor of rosmarinic acid, is synthesized from tyrosine-derived pathway in some species of Lamiaceae, such as *Salvia miltiorrhiza*.

2.1 Flavonoids Flavonoids constitute a highly diverse class of secondary metabolites composed of more than 9,000 structures. They are commonly found in land plants, including all vascular plants and some mosses. Based on the aglycone core, they are generally further grouped into flavanones, flavones, flavonols, isoflavonoids, anthocyanins and proanthocyanidins. All flavonoids are basically derivatives of 1,3-diphenylpropan-1-one (C6 - C3 - C6), which is derived from the condensation of three malonyl-CoA molecules with one *p*-coumaroyl-CoA to form a chalcone intermediate. Chalcone isomerase converts chalcone into flavanones, and respective enzymes transform flavanones to various flavones, isoflavones, dihydorflavonols, flavonols and anthoanidins. Every class of flavanones possesses the compounds with pharmaceutical activity and is widely used in folk medicines.

2.1.1 Flavanones and flavones Two completely different flavone synthase (FNS) proteins have been found to catalyze the biosynthesis of flavones in plants. The first member of the FNS I type was identified from parsley (*Petroselinum crispum*) cell suspension cultures and classified as 2-oxoglutarate-dependent dioxygenase. The FNS I cDNA was then cloned and functionally expressed in yeast, and it shares a high sequence identity to the flavanone 3-β-hydroxylase (FHT). Interestingly, characterized FNS I enzymes appear to be mainly in the family of Apiaceae. Molecular and phylogenetic analysis revealed a gene duplication of FHT, and a subsequent neofunctionalization occurred early in the development of the Apiaceae subfamilies. Formation of most flavones in a wide range of plant species is catalyzed by FNS II, cytochrome P450 proteins of CYP93B subfamily. The FNS II activity was first demonstrated in extract of *Antirrhinum majus* flowers, and the cDNAs were then isolated from other plants, including *Perilla frutescens* (CYP93B6) and *Gentiana triflora*.

*Glycyrrhiza uralensis* is one of the most popular TCM plants and also widely used in food flavoring. Although the sweeting agent of this plant is glycyrrhizin, a triterpenoid saponin, flavanones and flavones are also important components in its root, which include liquiritigenin, isoliquiritigenin and 7,4′-dihydroxyflavone. A P450 enzyme from *Glycyrrhiza echinata*, CYP93B1, was identified as flavanone 2-hydroxylase (F2H), a member of FNS II. The products, 2-hydroxyflavanones, were transformed into flavones in vitro in acid treatment, suggesting that an additional enzyme, probably a dehydratase, was involved in catalyzing the formation of flavones. A full-length cDNA of cytochrome P450 *CYP93C2* was isolated from the elicited *G. echinata* cells, which was shown to encode 2-hydroxyisoflavanone synthase.

The flavones baicalin and wogonoside, as well as their aglycones baicalein and wogonin, represent the dominant flavonoids in *Scutellaria baicalensis*, a perennial species of Lamiaceae and an important herb in Chinese traditional and clinical-orientated medicine. The flavones, such as baicalin and wogonin, are distinct for lacking a 4′-OH group but having a 6-OH group on their A-ring. Genes encoding the upstream enzymes of the pathway, including PAL, C4H, 4CL, chalcone synthase (CHS) and chalcone isomerase (CHI), have been isolated. However, the enzymes committed to the formation of the *S. baicalensis*-type flavones remain unknown. It is also possible that specific enzyme isoforms are involved in the formation of cinnamoyl-CoA. It has been reported that accumulation of these flavones was enhanced by jasmonate (JA) treatment, and a R2R3 - MYB transcription factor, SbMYB8, was found involved in the regulation.

2.1.2 Isoflavones The isoflavones are well studied for their substantial health promoting benefits. They are found mainly in leguminous plants and are the major bioactive ingredients in soybean, *Astragalus*, *Pueraria lobata*. Isoflavones are converted from flavanones by the isoflavone synthase (IFS). By using EST-based approach combined with enzymatic assays, P450s of CYP93C subfamily from soybean were shown to have such activities. Members of this subfamily with IFS activity were also reported in other leguminous plants, such as *Lotus japonicus* and *Trifolium pratense*.

*Astragalus membranaceus*, a species of Fabaceae, has been used in TCM for thousands of years. *Astragaus* is considered an adaptogen because it is believed to help protect the body against stresses, including those of physical, mental or emotional. In China, *Astragalus* has been used to help patients with severe forms of heart disease in relieving symptoms, lowering cholesterol levels and improving heart function. Constituents of the *Astragalus* roots (radix astragali) include polysaccharides, triterpenoids (astragalosides) and isoflavones. Isoflavones such as calycosin-7-glucoside and ononin are considered the important active components in this medicine. Hairy root system of *Astragalus* was developed a long time ago to produce these ingredients. Research at molecular level in this plant is limited, but will help reveal the biosynthetic pathway in this leguminous medicinal plant.

*Pueraria lobata*, also a species of Fabaceae, is commonly known as "kudzu". Puerariae radix, the dried root of the kudzu, has been used in China as herbal medicine for the prevention of cardiovascular disease and rehabilitation of stroke patients. The major secondary metabolites accumulated in kudzu roots are isoflavones, including daidzein, genistein, formononetin and their glucosides Puerarin, among which the 8-*C*-glucoside of daidzein is considered the major active compound. The cooccurrence of both *O*- and *C*-linked glycosides in root is of particular interests and worthy of further investigation. Using a functional genomics approach, He et al. identified enzymes associated with the isoflavone biosynthesis in kudzu roots, including 15 UDP-dependent glycosyltrans-ferases (UGTs), among which one, GT04F14, exhibited the in vitro activity of glycosylation of a wide range of substrates, including coumarins, flavones, flavonols, and isoflavones. The isoflavones are converted region-specifically to their 7-*O*-glucosides, whereas *C*-glycosylation might take place at the 2, 7, 4′-trihydroxyisoflavanone precursor of daidzein, rather than directly on daidzein. Conceivably the intermediate 8-*C*-β-glucopyranosyl-2, 7, 4′-trihydroxy-isoflavanone is converted to puerarin under in vivo conditions by the action of 2-hydroxyisoflavanone dehydratase (HID). A candidate gene encoding HID was identified from the EST library of kudzu root. In addition, a partially purified preparation from kudzu root was shown to have the *C*-glucosyltransferase activity that converted isoliquiritigenin (2′,4′,4-trihydroxychalcone) and UDP-Glc to puerarin.

2.1.3 Isopentenyl flavonoids Prenylation, the addition of prenyl groups, contributes to the diversification of flavonoids, and the occurrence of more than 1, 000 prenylated flavonoids in plants has been recorded. This prenylation represents the coupling process of the aromatic moiety from shikimate pathway and the prenyl (isoprenoid) chain from the isoprenoid pathways. Many prenylated flavonoids were identified as active components in medicinal plants and thus are of particular interests as lead compounds for drugs and functional food ingredients.

Species *Sophora*, family Fabaceae, are widely distributed in Asia. *Sophora flavescens* has a long history of use in China, and the root, known as Ku Shen, is a typical TCM. It is used to dispel heat, dry dampness and eliminate intestinal parasites. It is thus administered in formulas for the treatment of dysentery and jaundice (damp-heat syndromes), edema and dysuria (dampness syndromes), and eczema and pruritis (damp-heat-wind syndromes). The *S. flavescens* prenyltransferase SfN8DT - 1 is the first enzyme identified to be responsible for the prenylation of naringenin at the 8-position, with dimethylallyl diphosphate (DMAPP) as substrate. Later, two new flavonoid prenyltransferases (FPTs) were isolated from *S. flavescens* at the molecular level: one is the isoflavone-specific prenyltransferase (SfG6DT) for the prenylation of the genistein at the 6-position and the other a chalcone-specific prenyltransferase designated as isoliquiritigenin dimethy-lallyltransferase (SfiLDT).

Herba epimedii is prepared from the aerial parts of *Epimedium brevicornum* or *Epimedium sagittatum*, species of Berberidaceae. Herba epimedii contains various bioactive components and has been utilized extensively in China as the tonic and anti-rheumatic herb for thousands of years, and in the treatments of diseases such as impotence, frequency/urgency of urination, coronary heart disease, chronic bronchitis and neurasthenia. The isopentenyl flavonoids icariine and icarisid are the major active compounds; however, their biosynthesis remains poorly understood. Recently, Huang et al. isolated 12 structural genes and two putative transcription factors (TFs) in the flavonoid pathway. Transcriptional analysis revealed that two R2R3-MYB TFs (EsMYBA1 and EsMYBF1), together with a bHLH TF (EsGL3) and WD40 protein (EsTTG1), are probably involved in coordinated regulation of biosynthesis of the anthocyanins and the flavonol-derived bioactive components.

2.2 Phenolic acids *Salvia miltiorrhiza* is a perennial herb in the mint family (Lamiaceae). Its dried root or rhizome is called Danshen in TCM and was recorded in first pharmaceutical monograph *Shennong's Classic of Materia Medica* (A. D. 102 - 200). *S. miltiorrhiza* has been cultivated throughout Eastern Asia and used to prevent and cure cardiovascular, cerebrovascular, hyperlipidemia and acute ischemic stroke diseases. Both the hydrophilic and lipophilic components in *S. miltiorrhiza* are considered active ingredients. The hydrophilic compounds are mainly phenolic acids including rosmarinic acid, salvianolic acid B, lithospermic acid and dihydroxyphenyllactic acid or Danshensu, and they may also function as antioxidative, anti-bacterial and anti-viral reagents.

The biosynthetic pathway for phenolic acids in *S. miltiorrhiza* is distinct and has attracted many interests. Labeling experiments using [ring-(13) C]-phenylalanine suggested two intermediates derived from the phenylalanine-derived general phenylpropanoid pathway and the tyrosine-derived pathway, respectively (Fig. 1): 4-coumaroyl-CoA and 3,4-dihydroxyphenyllactic acid (DHPL), which are coupled by a acyl-CoA-dependent acyltransferase BAHD family enzyme rosmarinic acid synthase (SmRAS) to form 4-coumaroyl-3′, 4′-dihydroxyphenyllactic acid (4C-DHPL). The 3-hydroxyl group is introduced later in the pathway by a P450 monooxygenase (SmCYP98A14) to form rosmarinic acid (RA). This type of P450 was first reported in *Coleus blumei* (Lamiaceae), and it catalyzes the 3-hydroxylation of 4-coumaroyl-3′, 4′-dihydroxyphenyllactate and the 3′-hydroxylation of caffeoyl-4′-hydroxyphenyllactate, in both cases forming rosmarinic acid. Recent genome assembly to search the putative enzymes involved in biosynthesis of phenolics in *S. miltiorrhiza* revealed twenty-nine candidates, among which 15 were predicted in the phenylpropanoid pathway, seven in the tyrosine-derived pathway and six encoding putative hydroxycinnamoyltransferases.

## 3 TERPENOIDS

Terpenoids are formed from sequential assembly of five-carbon building blocks ($C_5H_8$) called isoprene units. Accordingly, single or assemblies of two, three and four units constitute hemiterpenes, monoterpenes, sesquiterpenes and diterpenes, respectively. After the formation of the basic carbon skeletons, subsequent modifications, such as oxidation, reduction, isomerization and conjugation, lead to enormous numbers of structures, which represent the most abundant class of plant specialized metabolites, with more than 36,000 individual compounds.

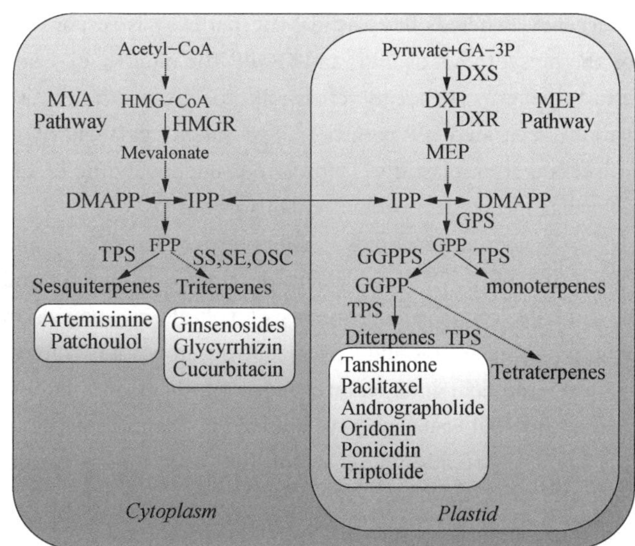


**Fig. 2 (Color online) Biosynthesis of terpenoids in TCM plants**

Terpenoids are synthesized via the cytosol MVA pathway and plastid MEP pathway. Generally, isopentenyl diphosphate (IPP) and dimethylallyl diphosphate (DMAPP) synthesized from the MVA pathway are converted to farnesyl diphosphate (FPP) for the biosynthesis of sesquiterpenoids and triterpenoids, whereas those derived from the MEP pathway contribute to the formation of geranyl diphosphate (GPP) and geranylgeranyl diphosphate (GGPP) for biosynthesis of monoterpenoids, diterpenoids and tetraterpenoids. HMG-CoA, 3-hydroxy-3-methylglutaryl-CoA; MEP, 2-C-methyl-D-erythritol 4-phosphate; GGPP, geranylgeranyl diphosphate; HMGR, 3-hydroxy-3-methylglutaryl-CoA reductase; DXS, 1-deoxy-D-xylu-lose-5-phosphate synthase; DXR, 1-deoxy-D-xylulose-5-phosphate reductoisomerase; GPPS, geranyl diphosphate synthase; GPP, geranyl diphosphate; FPPS, farnesyl diphosphate synthase; GGPPS, geranylgeranyl diphosphate synthase; TPS, terpene synthase; SS, squalene synthase; SE, squalone epoxidase; OSC, oxidosqualene cyclase. Dotted lines represent multiple enzymatic catalyzed steps.

In plant cells, the common precursors of terpenoids, isopentenyl diphosphate (IPP) and dimethylallyl diphosphate (DMAPP) are synthesized via two independent pathways: the cytosolic mevalonic acid (MVA) pathway that starts with the condensation of acetyl-CoA, and the plastid-localized methylerythritol phosphate (MEP) pathway that uses pyruvate and glyceraldehydes 3-phosphate as substrates (Fig. 2). The IPP and DMAPP are condensed into geranyl diphosphate (GPP, $C_{10}$), farnesyl diphosphate (FPP, $C_{15}$) and geranylgeranyl diphosphate (GGPP, $C_{20}$) by the respective prenyltransferases and then converted to terpenes by terpene synthases (TPSs), which catalyze the critical step that determines the structures of terpen skeletons.

Generally, the cytosolic MVA pathway provides the precursor of FPP for the biosynthesis of sesquiterpenes and triterpenes, whereas the plastid MEP pathway is responsible for the biosynthesis of GPP and GGPP for mono-, di-, and tetra-terpenes. Although cross-talk between these two spatially separated IPP pathways is prevalent, particularly in a direction from plastid to cytosol, our understanding of the molecular mechanism behind remains primitive.

3.1 Sesquiterpenoids Monoterpenoids ($C_{10}$) and sesquiterpenoids ($C_{15}$) are widely distributed in plants, and they are the common constituents of volatile compounds in flowers, fruits, stems and leaves, playing important roles in plant-environment interactions, many of them also possess great commercial value and some are used in pharmaceuticals.

3.1.1 Artemisinin One of the most famous plant-sourced medicines is artemisinin, an endoperoxide sesquiterpene lactone isolated from *Artemisia annua* L., an annual herb of Asteraceae. Due to its effectiveness against drug-resistant cerebral malaria, it is the essential component of the combinational therapies recommended by the World Health Organization. It has saved millions of lives globally, especially in developing countries. The 2011 Lasker DeBakey Clinical Research Award and the 2015 Nobel Prize in Physiology or Medicine honor the Chinese scientist Youyou Tu who made the important contribution to the discovery of artemisinin.

As a sesquiterpenoid, artemisinin is believed to be synthesized from the cytosolic MVA pathway. However, a recent report suggested that the MEP pathway may also contribute to its biosynthesis. GPP, which is synthesized in plastids, can be transported to cytoplasm, forming FPP with the addition of another IPP unit. The FPP is converted to the artemisinin skeleton by amorpha-4, 11-diene synthase (ADS), a sesquiterpene synthase, and then oxidated by the cytochrome P450 CYP71AV1. When expressed in *Saccharomyces cerevisiae*, CYP71AV1 catalyzed the continuous oxidation of amorpha-4,11-diene into artemisinic alcohol and artemisinic aldehyde, with significantly increased production of artemisinic acid and artemisinic aldehyde when co-expressed with a cytochrome b5 (CYB5) in yeast. The artemisinic aldehyde Δ11 (13) reductase (Dbr2), a double-bond reductase, catalyzes the formation of dihydroartemisinic aldehyde, which is further converted into dihydroartemisinic acid by aldehyde dehydrogenase 1 (ALDH1). Moreover, an additional alcohol dehydrogenase (ADH1) was also found to be involved in the oxidation of amorpha-4, 11-diene to artemisinic acid, with specificity toward artemisinic alcohol in *A. annua* plants.

Several transcription factors have been shown to participate in the regulation of artemisinin biosynthesis. Two jasmonate responsive AP2/ERF proteins, AaERF1 and AaERF2, were found to up-regulate the transcription of *ADS* and *CYP71AV1* genes, by binding to the CRTDREHVCBF2 (CBF2) and RAV1AAT (RAA) motifs present in their promoters. A WRKY family transcription factor, AaWRKY1, was demonstrated to be capable of binding to the W-box in the *ADS* promoter and involved in the regulation of artemisinin biosynthesis.

A deep sequencing on the transcriptome of *A. annua* to identify genes and markers for fast-track breeding was performed, and a detailed genetic map with nine linkage groups was built. Replicated field trials resulted in a quantitative trait loci (QTL) map that accounts for a significant amount of the variation in key traits controlling artemisinin yield, and positive QTLs in parents of new high-yielding hybrids were enriched, which made it available to convert *A. annua* into a robust crop. Ma et al. recently reported an integrated approach combining metabolomics, transcriptomics and gene function analyses to characterize gene-to-terpene and terpene pathway scenarios in a self-pollinating variety of *A. annua*. Forty-seven genes that mapped to the terpenes biosynthesis pathway were identified by sequence mining, and such metabolites-transcriptome network associated with different tissues is fundamental to metabolic engineering to artemisinin.

3.1.2 Patchoulol Patchouli (*Pogostemon cablin*), a perennial herbaceous species of Lamiaceae, is not only a fragrant plant producing patchouli oil for cosmetics industry, but also a medicinal plant for the treatment of medical ailments, such as removing dampness, relieving summer heat and exterior syndrome, and serving as an anti-emetic and appetite stimulant. The patchouli oil is composed of sesquiterpenoids dominated by (−)-patchoulol. The sesquiterpene synthase, patchoulol synthase, was firstly purified from patchouli leaves by chromatofocusing, anion exchange, gel permeation and hydroxylapatite chromatography. Then, its cDNA was cloned and the recombinant patchoulol synthase was shown to produce patchoulol as the major product, plus at least 13 additional sesquiterpenes.

Patchouli oil in leaves accumulates with plant age: The content is low at juvenile stage and increases during plant growth and reaches a high level in mature plant. The microRNA156 (miR156)-targeted SQUAMOSA promoter binding protein-like (SPL) factors, which function as the major plant age cue in regulating developmental phase transition and flowering, play a key role in the age-dependent progressive up-regulation of the *patchoulol synthase* gene expression, and the patchouli oil biosynthesis. Interestingly, expression of a miR156-resistant form of SPL not only accelerated plant maturation but also promoted patchouli oil production.

3.2 Diterpenoids Certain groups of diterpenoids ($C_{20}$), such as gibberellins, are regulators (phytohormones) of plant growth and development. Many other specialized diterpenoids, like tanshinone from *Salvia miltiorrhiza* and taxol from *Taxus*, are highly valuable in medicine. A few more examples include: stevioside, extracted from *Stevia rebaudiana* of Asteraceae, is a natural sweetest; adenanthin, from the leaves of *Rabdosia adenantha*, induces differentiation of acute promyelocytic leukemia (APL) cells; oridonin, from Lamiaceae plants *Isodon rubescens* and *Isodon amethystoides*, is a potential compound for molecular target-based therapy of leukemia; and triptolide, a highly oxygenated diterpene isolated from *Tripterygium wilfordii*, was shown to have anti-leukemic activity.

3.2.1 Tanshinone Besides the phenolic acids discussed above, tanshinones are another class of active diterpenoid compounds of *S. miltiorrhiza*, which include tanshinone Ⅰ, tanshinone $Ⅱ_A$, cryptotanshinone and dihydrotanshinone Ⅰ. They are all abietane-type derivatives, among which tanshinone $Ⅱ_A$ is considered to be an important bioactive component in protecting cardiovascular system, and tanshinone Ⅰ was reported to be an apoptosis inducer and display anticancer activities.

As diterpenoid compounds, tanshinones are expected to be traced to the plastid MEP pathway, and their biosynthesis starts from the conversion of geranylgeranyl diphosphate (GGPP) to ent-copalyl diphosphate (CPP) and then to miltiradiene. The subsequent extensively structural tailing converts miltiradiene to cryptotanshinone, tanshinone Ⅰ, tanshinone $Ⅱ_A$ or tanshinone IIB.

Based on sequence homology, enzymes shared by other diterpenoid biosynthesis have been characterized. To date, two enzymes specifically committed to the tanshinone biosynthetic pathway have been identified: the kaurene synthase-like (SmKSL), a diterpene synthase that utilizes CPP as substrate to produce miltiradiene, and a P450 monooxygenase CYP76AH1 which transforms miltiradiene to ferruginol, both representing the milestone achievement in the research of TCM plant. Recently, functional divergence of SmCPSs and SmKSLs was reported, which specified the roles of individual CPSs in tanshinone production in different tissues, including SmCPS1 in roots and SmCPS2 in aerial part, and SmCPS4 and SmKSL2 were found to oxidize ent-13-epi-manoyl in floral sepals, and the conserved SmCPS5 involved in the plant growth hormone gibberellin biosynthesis. This study is a typical example of how the evolutionary diversification of diterpenoids in plants in molecular level.

With the rapid development of sequencing technologies, several transcriptome datasets and the draft genome of *S. miltiorrhiza* have been reported. For examples, the cDNA library of whole plant contained 10, 228 ESTs, the transcriptome of nearly entire growing cycle generated by Illumina revealed 56,774 unigenes, and the searching of the draft genome resulted in 40 putative genes encoding enzymes involved in the biosynthesis of universal isoprene precursors of IPP and DMAPP. Genes encoding cytochrome P450 monooxygenases, dehydrogenases and reductases, as well as several groups of transcription factors were predicted to be involved in tanshinone biosynthesis by comparative analysis of transcriptomes generated from different tissues. Recently, next-generation sequencing (NGS) and single-molecule real-time (SMRT) sequencing were combined to generate a more complete/full-length set of *S. miltiorrhiza* transcriptome, which provides a valuable resource for further investigation of tanshinone biosynthesis.

Organ- or tissue-specific patterns are common feature observed in biosynthesis and accumulation of specialized metabolites, as well as the expression patterns of corresponding genes. Tanshinones are actively synthesized and stored in roots, whereas only a low or trace amount was detected in aerial organs like leaves. Moreover, both the accumulation and the expression of the related genes of tanshinones in hairy root cultures can be induced by biotic elicitors, such as the carbohydrate fraction of yeast extract, and phytohormones of salicylic acid and jasmonate. Further investigation can be directed to the characterization of the signaling components and transcription factors that regulate the diterpenoid biosynthesis in *S. miltiorrhiza*.

3.2.2 Taxol (paclitaxel) Taxol (paclitaxel) is a diterpenoid isolated from the bark of *Taxus* trees. The anti-mitotic and cytotoxic properties of taxol are derived from its activity in disrupting normal tubulin dynamics, leading to dysfunction of microtubules. Fourteen enzymes involved in taxol biosynthesis have been identified, they are geranylgeranyl diphosphate synthase, taxadiene synthase, taxadien-5α-ol-*O*-acetyl transferase, taxane 2α-*O*-benzoyltransferase, baccatin III: 3-animo-3phenylpropanoyltransferase, 10-deacetylbacctin III-10-*O*-acetyltransferase, 3′-*N*-debenzoyl-2′-deoxytaxol *N*-benzoyltransferase, taxane 5-alpha hydroxylase, taxane 10-alpha hydroxylase, taxane 13-alpha hydroxylase, taxane 2-alpha hydroxylase, taxane 7-alpha hydroxylase, taxane 14-alpha hydroxylase and phenylalanine aminomutase.

In addition to elucidation of the biosynthetic enzymes, progresses have been made in identification of transcription factors involved in taxol biosynthesis, which include members of the AP2 and WRKY families. A recent report showed that the bHLH transcription factors of TcJAMYC1, TcJAMYC2 and TcJAMYC4 act as negative regulators of taxol biosynthesis *in T. cuspidata* cultured cells.

Due to the extremely low content of taxol (at ppm level) in plant, it requires massive harvesting to obtain sufficient amounts of the drug; thus, productions by total synthesis, semi-synthesis, tissue or cell cultures, endophytic fungal fermentation and more recently metabolic engineering and synthetic biology have attracted great interests. Precursors of taxol biosynthesis have been produced in *Escherichia coli* and *Saccharomyces cerevisiae*, and the integration of parts (modules) of the whole pathway in separate organisms cultured together led to the combination of production of taxadiene in *E. coli* and oxygenation of taxadiene by *S. cerevisiae*.

3.3 Triterpenoids Triterpenoids are cyclization product of squalene which is condensed by two molecules of FPP. In general, triterpenoids are formed from MVA pathway in cytoplasm, as sesquiterpenoids.

3.3.1 Ginsenosides Ginseng, the root of *Panax ginseng*, is one of the oldest traditional medicines and is widely regarded as a tonic in East Asia. The principle bioactive constituents of Ginseng are ginsenosides, a group of tetra- or pentacyclic triterpene glycosides belonging to saponins. The clinical and pharmacological activities of ginsenosides include anti-diabetic, anticancer, anti-amestic hypoglycemic, radioprotective, immunomodulatory, neuroprotective and anti-stress. More than 40 ginsenosides have been isolated from the white and the red ginseng, and they show different biological activities based on their structural differences. Generally, the major pharmacologically active ginsenosides belong to tetracyclic dammarane- and pentacyclic oleanane-type triterpene saponins.

The common precursor of ginsenosides is squalene, which is formed by condensation of two FPPs with squalene synthase (SS). In Ginseng, squalene is converted into dammarenediol-Ⅱ by squalone epoxidase (SE). The cyclization of 2,3-oxidosqualene can result in two different type of triterpenoids: dammarane and oleanane type. Ginsenosides belonging to dammarane-type triterpenoids are biosynthesized from 2,3-oxidosqualene by dammarenediol synthase (DS) to form dammarenediol-Ⅱ, whereas the biosynthesis of oleanane-type ginsenosides is started by β-amyrin synthase (PNY1) that transforms 2,3-oxidosqualene into β-amyrin. SS is considered a rate-limiting enzyme in the pathway and catalyzes the initial biosynthetic step for both steroids and triterpenoids. PgPDR, a member of ABC transporters, was found to be involved in the ginsenosides accumulation upon MeJA induction.

3.3.2 Cucurbitacins Cucurbitacins, conferring a bitter taste in cucurbits such as cucumber, melon, watermelon, squash, and pumpkin, belong to a class of highly oxidized tetracyclic triterpenoids mainly found in the plant of Cucurbitaceae family, in which *Gynostemma pentaphyllum*, *Hemsleya chinesis*, *Siraitia grosvenorii* and *Bolbostemma paniculatum* are well-known TCM plants. Recent studies suggest that cucurbitacins repress cancer cell progression and inhibit neuroblastoma cell proliferation through up-regulation of PETN (phosphatase and tensin homolog). By genome-wide association study based on the genome variation map of 115 diverse cucumber lines, the gene of Csa6G088690 (Bi) encoding oxidosqualene cyclase is found to be correlated to the cucurbitacin C (CuC) biosynthesis. Co-expression and co-regulation studies revealed a 9-gene module responsible for CucC biosynthesis, of which, four enzymes, including Bi, two P450s and one ACT, were characterized. Moreover, two bHLH transcription factors, Bl (bitter leaf) and Bt (bitter fruit), were found to directly regulate the expression of 9-gene module in cucumber leaf and fruit, respectively. During the cucumber domestication, mutations occurred within Bt promoter region which decreased its expression in the fruit tissue which may have been selected and fixed and resulted in nonbitter fruit we eat nowadays.

3.3.3 Glycyrrhizin The roots and stolons of *Glycyrrhiza* plants (*G. uralensis* and *G. glabra*) contain a large amount of oleanane-type triterpenoid glycyrrhizin. It is not only used worldwide as a natural sweetener and flavoring additive due to its sweet taste, but also exhibit a wide range of pharmacological activities, including anti-inflammatory, immunomodulatory, anti-ulcer, anti-allergy, and anti-viral activity.

From *G. glabra*, genes that encode enzymes responsible for triterpene skeleton formation, including the squalene synthase (SS) and β-amyrin synthase (bAS), were isolated. Later biosynthesis steps of glycyrrhizin involve a series of oxidative reactions at positions C－11 and C－30 and glucuronylation of the C－3 hydroxyl group. Enzymes that catalyze the oxidation steps have been found to be cytochrome P450 monooxygenases. One of them, CYP88D6, was characterized to catalyze the sequential two-step oxidation of β-amyrin at C－11 to produce 11-oxo-β-amyrin by both in vitro assay with recombinant protein and co-expression with β-amyrin synthase in yeast. Another P450, CYP72A154, was identified to be responsible for three sequential oxidations at C－30 to transform 11-oxo-β-amyrin to glycyrrhetinic acid, a glycyrrhizin aglycone. Both CYP88D6 and CYP72A154 transcripts were detected in the roots and stolons, but not in the leaves or stems, which is consistent with the accumulation pattern of glycyrrhizin in planta.

## 4 ALKALOIDS

Alkaloids are a group of nitrogen-containing compounds with basic properties, most of which are derivatives of amino acids. Biosynthesis of alkaloids usually starts from modification of amino acids, mostly decar-boxylation or deamination, and undergoes further steps like methylation, hydroxylation and oxidation, and/or coupled with other compounds. There are over 12,000 alkaloids that have been identified from plants. Although widely distributed in plants, they are particularly enriched in certain families, such as Solanaceae, Manispermaceae, Papaveraceae, Berberidaceae and Fabaceae (Table 2).

**Table 2 List of examples of TCM plants rich in terpenoids**

| Plant species | Chinese name in Pin-yin | Family | Representative compounds |
|---|---|---|---|
| *Pogostemon cablin* | Guanghuoxiang | Lamiaceae | Patchoulol |
| *Artemisia annua* | Huanghuahao or Qinghao | Asteraceae | Artemisinine |
| *Salvia miltiorrhiza* | Danshen | Lamiaceae | Tanshinone |
| *Taxus chinensis* | Hongdoushan | Taxaceae | Paclitaxel |
| *Andrographis paniculata* | Chuanxinlian | Acanthaceae | Andrographolide |
| *Isodon rubescens* | Donglingcao | Lamiaceae | Oridonin, ponicidin |
| *Isodon amethystoides* | Xiangchacai | Lamiaceae | Oridonin, ponicidin |
| *Tripterygium wilfordii* | Leigongteng | Celastraceae | Triptolide |
| *Panax ginseng* | Ginsen or Renshen | Araliaceae | Ginsenosides |
| *Panax notoginseng* | Sanqi | Araliaceae | Notoginsenosides |
| *Radix liquiritiae* | Gancao | Fabaceae | Glycyrrhizin |
| *Dioscorea polystachya* | Shuyu | Dioscoreaceae | Dioscin |

**Table 3 List of examples of TCM plants rich in alkaloids**

| Plant species | Chinese name in Pin-yin | Family | Representative compounds |
|---|---|---|---|
| *Camptotheca acuminate* | Xishu | Cornaceae | Camptothecin |
| *Coptis chinensis* | Huanglian | Ranunculaceae | Berberine |
| *Isatis indigotica* | Songlan | Brassicaceae | Isatin, indigotin |
| *Baphicacanthus cusia* | Banlan | Acanthaceae | Isatin, indigotin |

It is noteworthy that the most of alkaloids display bioactivities to certain degrees, often derived from their nitrogen-containing properties. Not surprisingly, alkaloids constitute the major portion of drugs both in history and nowadays. The discovery and isolation of morphine from the opium poppy (*Papaver somniferum*) by Friedrich Sertürner in 1 806 is a milestone in the history of pharmacy. Investigations of biosynthesis of natural alkaloids such as morphinan, vindoline and noscapine have been intensive and led to the complete elucidation of the pathway, and increasing alkaloid biosynthesis in plant through co-expression of enzymes genes was also reported. Unfortunately, although alkaloids with TCM background like camptothecin, higenamine, huperzine A and tetrandrine have been used in pharmacy, reports of their biosynthesis are relatively rare. We list in Table 3 several typical alkaloids in TCM plants, and the relevant references. Various aspects on the alkaloid biosynthesis, regulation and metabolites trafficking can be found in review articles. Without doubt more efforts are needed to study alkaloids in TCM plants to further explore their biological activities and facilitate their usage.

## 5 PERSPECTIVE

Unlike model plant or staple crops, medicinal plants often lack a well-studied genetic background and a high-quality genome sequence. Due to the recently developed high-throughput sequencing technologies, it is possible to generate transcriptomic data of medicinal plants in a short time at an affordable cost. Comparative analysis of chemical constituents, transcriptomes and correlation of spatial and temporal patterns of gene expressions with those of metabolite accumulation have led to the identification of candidate genes of the biosynthesis pathway. GWS combined with metabolomics analysis (mGWAS) provides a powerful platform which screens a large number of accessions simultaneously to understand genetic contributions to the metabolic diversity.

Throughout the history, herbal plants are an integral part of our lives. In addition to curing illness, they are grown in elegant gardens, provide natural fragrance, delicate accessories and stimulate appetite. The biosynthesis of metabolites in medicinal plants is complex and specialized and involves many sequence-similar but functionally diverged enzymes. With the fast development of new technologies of analytical chemistry, bioinformatics and synthetic biology, more and more achievements will be made in this genomic or post-genomic era and bring us better life.

[杨蕾,陈晓亚,等.Science Bulletin, 2016,61(1):3-17.]

# Molecular cloning and functional identification of a cDNA encoding 4-hydroxy-3-methylbut-2-enyl diphosphate reductase from *Tripterygium wilfordii*

## 1 INTRODUCTION

*Tripterygium wilfordii* Hook. F., also known as Lei Gong Teng or thunder god vine, is native to eastern and southern China. This vine-like plant belongs to the Celastraceae family, and has a long history of use in traditional Chinese medicine when treating autoimmune diseases and inflammatory dermatoses, such as psoriasis, erythema nodosum, rheumatoid arthritis, and systemic lupus erythematosus. The research for the medicinal value of *T. wilfordii* has found out that the plant possesses anti-HIV, anti-inflammatory, antitumor, and anti-Parkinsonian effects, which arouses great interest in the field of medicine. The major active compound responsible for its medicinal functions is believed to be triptolide. Currently, only limited information on the biosynthesis of triptolide is available.

Triptolide is a diterpenoid triepoxide derived from isopentenyl diphosphate (IPP) and its isomer dimethylallyl diphosphate (DMAPP). There are two independent pathways leading to the biosynthesis of both IPP and DMAPP localized in different cellular compartments which are the cytosolic mevalonic acid (MVA) pathway and the plastidic 2-*C*-methyl-D-erythritol 4-phosphate (MEP) pathway. While the MVA pathway is responsible for synthesizing sesquiterpenes and triterpenes, the MEP pathway is in charge of the biosynthesis of monoterpenes, diterpenes, and tetraterpenes. As the last enzyme in the MEP pathway for isoprenoid biosynthesis, 4-hydroxy-3-methylbut-2-enyl diphosphate reductase (HDR) catalyzes (*E*)-4-hydroxy-3-methylbut-2-enyl diphosphate (HMBPP) into a mixture of 5 : 1 IPP and DMAPP (Fig. 1). Silencing of *HDR* gene in *Nicotiana benthamiana* can make the isoprenoid-derived chlorophyll and carotenoid pigments decrease to less than 4% of the control plants. And overexpression of *HDR* gene contributes to increasing the production of isoprenoid-derived carotenoid and over-producing taxadiene up to 13-fold of the control group in transgenic *Arabidopsis*, proving its vital role in metabolic regulation of plastidial isoprenoid biosynthesis.

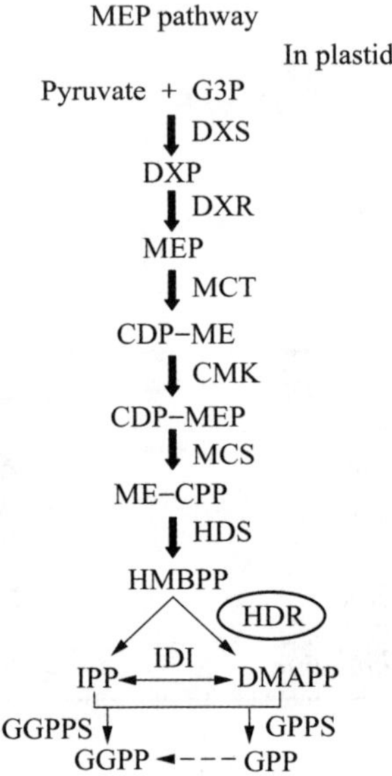


**Figure 1 Schematic MEP pathway for GGPP. Multiple steps are indicated with striped arrows**

G3P, glyceraldehyde 3-P; DXP, deoxyx-ylulose 5-P; MEP, methylerythritol 4-P; CDP-ME, 4-diphosphocytidyl-methylerythritol; CDP-MEP, CDP-ME 2-P; ME-CPP, methylerythritol 2,4-cyclodiphosphate; HMBPP, hydroxymethylbutenyl 4-diphosphate; IPP, isopentenyl diphosphate; DMAPP, dimethylallyl diphosphate; GPP, geranyl diphosphate; GGPP, geranylgeranyl diphosphate. Enzymes are indicated in bold: DXS, DXP synthase; DXR, DXP reductoisomerase; MCT, MEP cytidylyltransferase; CMK, CDP-ME kinase; MCS, ME-cPP synthase; HDS, HMBPP synthase; HDR, HMBPP reductase; IDI, IPP isomerase; GPPS, GPP synthase; GGPPS, GGPP synthase.

Because of the high toxicity, obtaining the effective components from *T. wilfordii* by traditional chemical methods is difficult spending much time and labor. And now the current studies regarding key enzymes of triptolide biosynthesis in *T. wilfordii* are few, and the production of triptolide still cannot be synthesized through biosynthesis methods. Based on the above issues, we present the cloning of full-length *HDR* cDNA of *T. wilfordii* (*TwHDR*) for the first time, proving it having the function of IspH and may acting a role as a potential key enzyme for the biosynthesis of triptolide.

## 2 MATERIALS AND METHODS

2.1 Plant material *T. wilfordii* cell suspensions were cultured in Murashige and Skoog (MS) medium containing 30 g/L sucrose and 8 g/L agar with 0.5 mg/L 2, 4-dichlorophenoxyacetic acid (2, 4-D), 0.1 mg/L kinetin (KT), and 0.5 mg/L indole-3-butytric acid (IBA). All suspension cell cultures were maintained at 25 ± 1 ℃ with shaking by orbital shaker (DZ - 100, Suzhou experimental equipment Co., Ltd., Suzhou, China) at 120 rpm in the dark.

2.2 RNA isolation The 10-day-old *T. wilfordii* suspension cells were treated with MJ for 0, 1, 4, 12, 24, 48 and 72 h at a final concentration of 50 μmol/L. Subsequently, the suspension cells were harvested for RNA isolation. The total RNA was isolated using the cetyltrimethylammonium bromide (CTAB) method.

2.3 Cloning of TwHDR full-length cDNA Total RNA was reverse transcribed into first-stand cDNA with PrimeScript 1st Strand cDNA Synthesis Kit (Takara Biotechnology (Dalian) Co., Ltd., Dalian, China) due to the manufacturer's instruction. The full-length primers were designed based on the transcriptome sequencing data of *T. wilfordii* obtained previously. The prime pairs were as follow: *TwHDR*-F 5′-CTGTTCCAC-GCATTTTTCAACACAG-3′ and *TwHDR*-R 5′-GAGCCTAGAG GTAAAAACTGCGGTC-3′. The product was purified and cloned into the pMD19-T vector (Takara Biotechnology (Dalian) Co., Ltd., Dalian, China). The vector was transformed into *E. coli* DH5α cells and cultured in Luria-Bertani (LB) medium at 37℃ in dark. The positive colonies were sequenced and assembled to verify the correct *TwHDR* insertion.

2.4 Sequence alignment of HDR/IspH proteins The nucleotide sequence was analyzed using Basic Local Alignment Search Tool (BLAST) on the National Center for Biotech-nology Information (NCBI) website. The ORF and amino acid sequence of TwHDR was deduced using the ORF finder. HDR/IspH amino acid sequences from *T. wilfordii*, *Aquilaria sinensi* (AHE93332.1), *Arabidopsis thaliana* (AAN87171.1), *Salvia miltiorrhiza* (AFQ95412.1), *Nicotiana tabacum* (AAD55762.2), *Camptotheca acuminate* (ABI64152.1), *Hevea brasiliensis* (BAF98297.1), *Synechocystis* (WP_010873388.1), *Rhodobacter Capsulatus* (ADE87147), *Aquifex aeolicus* (O67625), and *E. coli* (NP_414570) were aligned with Clustal Omega (http://www.ebi.ac.uk/Tools/msa/clustalo/) and DNAMAN Version 9 (Fig. 2).

2.5 Phylogenetic analysis and homology modeling of Arabidopsis HDR TwHDR and other HDRs downloaded from GenBank were aligned, and the phylogenetic tree was constructed by the neighbor-joining method using MEGA 7.0. The 3-dimensional (3D) structural modeling was predicted by Swiss-Model.

2.6 Functional expression of TwHDR in E. coli hdr mutant The *E. coli hdr* mutant was maintained on LB medium containing 50 μg/mL kanamycin (Kan) and 0.2% (*w*/*v*) arabinose (Ara). Primers 5′-CCTTGGATCCATGG CGATATCTC-3′ and 5′-CCTTGGTAC-CTTACGCTAATT GCAAG-3′ were used to amplify the full-length cDNA of *TwHDR* by PCR. The PCR products were digested with *Bam*HI and *Kpn*I, and ligated to the pQE-30 expression vector (Qiagen, Valencia, CA, USA) which was cut by the same restriction enzymes. The resulting construct pQE-*TwHDR* was transformed into *E. coli hdr* mutant competent cells and selected on LB plates containing 50 μg/mL Kan, 50 μg/mL ampicillin (Amp), and 0.2% (*w*/*v*) Ara. The presence of pQE-*TwHDR* plasmid in surviving colonies was verified. Transformants containing pQE-*TwHDR* plasmids were grown on LB plates containing 50 μg/mL Kan, 50 μg/mL Amp, 0.2% (*w*/*v*) glucose (Glc) and 0.5 mmol/L IPTG to test if the TwHDR protein could complement the *E. coli hdr* mutant. As a control, the empty pQE-30 vector was transformed into the *E. coli hdr* mutant and selected on LB plates containing 50 μg/mL Kan, 50 μg/mL Amp and 0.2% Ara.

2.7 Quantitative real-time PCR Total RNA was used to synthesize the first strand cDNA with TIANScript II RT Kit (Tiangen Biotech (Beijing) Co., Ltd., Beijing, China), according to the manufacturer's protocols. The relative mRNA levels were estimated with the Applied Biosystems 7500 Real Time PCR System (Applied Biosystems, Grand Island, NY, USA) using KAPA SYBR ® FAST qPCR Kit (KAPA Biosystems, Wilmington, MA, USA), and gene expression was quantified with the comparative $C_T$ method (also known as the $2^{-\Delta\Delta CT}$ method). There were three samples in each group and each sample was repeated for three times to insure the credibility of the data. The real-time PCR primers were designed by Primer Premier 5.0 as follows: *β*-actin-F 5′-AGGAACCACCGATCCAGACA-3′, *β*-actin-R 5′-GGTGCCCTGAGGTCCTGTT-3′, *TwHDR* qF 5′-AATGTTACTG-TGAGACTGGCGG-3′ and *TwHDR* qR 5′-GTTGGATTGTGTAT-GATTTCGTTGG-3′.

## 3 RESULTS

3.1 Cloning of full-length cDNA of TwHDR and sequence analysis of TwHDR from T. wilfordii The full-length cDNA of *TwHDR* is 1456 bp containing a 1386 bp ORF (GenBank Accession No. KJ933412.1). The gene encodes a 461-amino-acid protein with a molecular weight of 52.1 kDa and a theoretical isoelectric point of 5.60.

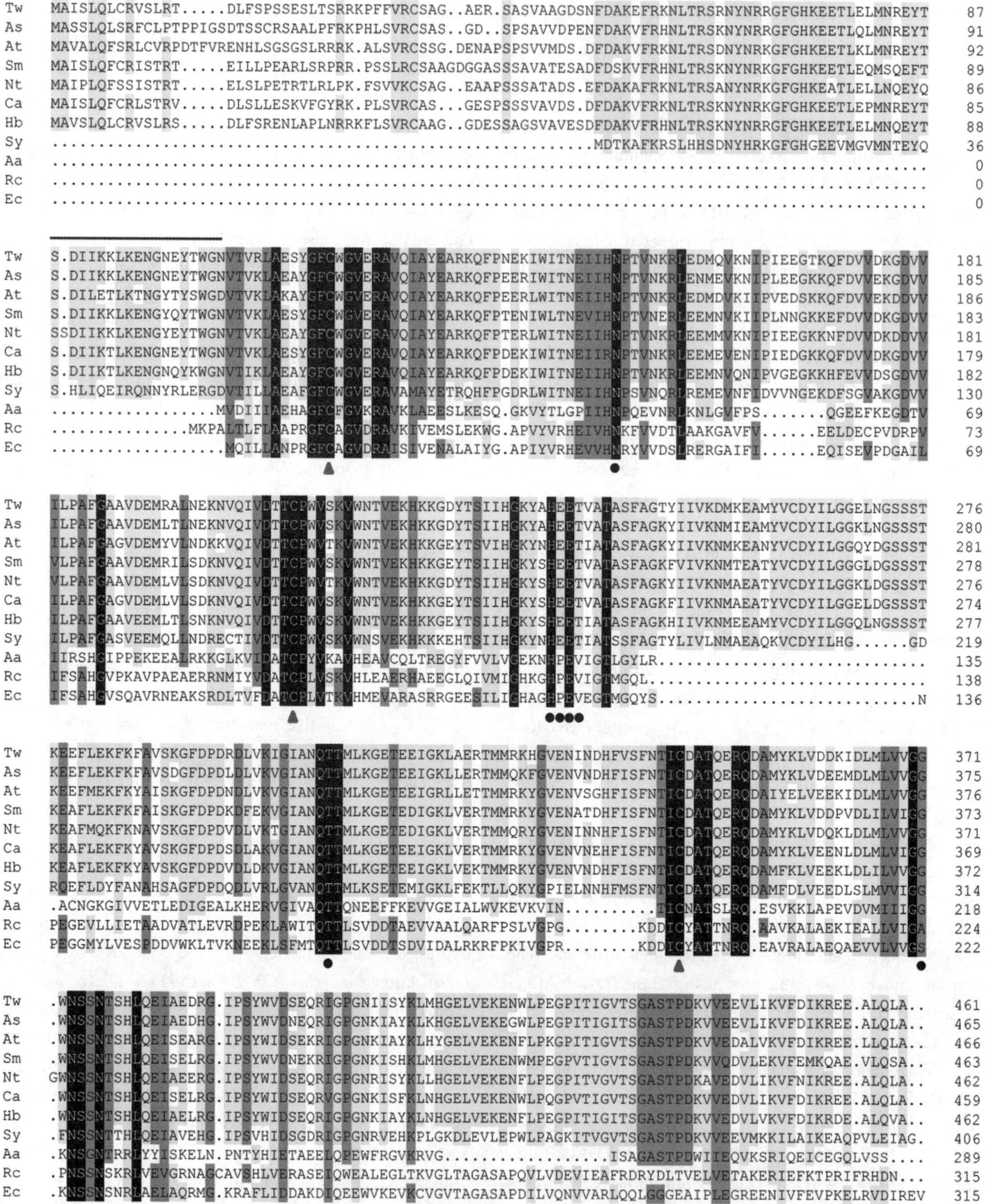


**Figure 2 Amino acid sequence alignment of TwHDR with other plant HDRs and bacterial IspHs**

Tw, *Tripterygium wilfordii*; As, *Aquilaria sinensi*; At, *Arabidopsis thaliana*; Sm, *Salvia miltiorrhiza*; Nt, *Nicotiana tabacum*; Ca, *Camptotheca acuminate*; Hb, *Hevea brasiliensis*; Sy, *Synechocystis* sp. PCC 6 803; Aa, *Aquifex aeolicus*; Rc, *Rhodobacter capsulatus*; Ec, *Escherichia coli*. The NCD among the plants and cyanobacteria is indicated at the top of the alignment. Arrowheads indicate the critical Cys residues that are involved in iron-sulfur cluster formation. Round dots indicate the conserved amino acids near the substrate-binding site.

BLAST result indicated that TwHDR has high homology with many plant HDRs, such as *Aquilaria sinensis* HDR (AsHDR, 85%), *Camptotheca acuminata* HDR (CaHDR, 83%), *H. brasi-liensis* HDR (HbHDR, 82%), *S. miltiorrhiza* HDR (SmHDR, 78%) and *A. thaliana* HDR (AtHDR, 77%). According to the functional domain analysis, TwHDR has the IspH/LYTb domain. The sequence alignment showed that all of *E. coli*, *A. aeolicus* and *Rhodobacter capsulatus* IspHs lacked of a stretch of 53 amino acids in the N-terminus to the cyanobacterial HDR (Fig. 2). And these amino acids are highly conserved in cyanobacteria, *T. wilfordii* and other plants. And beyond the N-terminal con-served domain (NCD), the plant HDR had an extended N-terminal sequence, which was not highly conserved, and it may serve as transit peptides to target plant HDRs.

The *T. wilfordii* IspH domain (amino acid residues 106 - 461, encompassing the bacterial IspH) shares approximately 21.67% identity with the *E. coli* protein. Many amino acid residues found to be critical for *E. coli* and *A. aeolicus* IspHs were also conserved in cyanobacteria and plants including *T. wilfordii*, which may play important roles as iron-sulfur cluster formation and substrate binding. Three conserved cysteine residues of the conserved residues found in TwHDR are present in all HDRs, which might participate in the coordination of the iron-sulfur bridge which might be involved in the catalysis (Fig. 2). And these three cysteine residues have been proved by *E. coli* complementation assays that they are essential for *Arabidopsis* HDR function.

3.2 Phylogenetic analysis and homology modeling for TwHDR The phylogenetic tree was constructed according to the deduced amino acid sequences of TwHDR and other HDRs from different hosts (Fig. 3A). The tree revealed that TwHDR exhibited the highest homology with HDR from *A. sinensis*. All the HDRs selected from the plants clustered together, and the HDRs from eumycophyta clustered together as another sub-branch. The HDRs from bacteria *Salmonella enterica*, *E. coli* and *Shigella flexneri* clustered as a different branch from the branch of plants and eumycophyta. 3D modeling of TwHDR was built by the Swiss-Model used the amino acids 102 - 453 (template: 3dnfB, Seq identity: 29.96%, Fig. 3B).

3.3 T. wilfordii HDR complements the E. coli hdr mutant To further test whether the *T. wilfordii* and *E. coli* HDR proteins are functionally conserved, we performed a complementation assay with a lethal *E. coli* mutant detective in the *HDR* gene (strain MG1655). In *E. coli* *ispH* mutant strain MG1655 *ara* <> *ispH*, the endogenous *ispH* gene was replaced by a kanamycin-resistant cassette and a single copy of *ispH* was present on the chromosome under the control of the $P_{BAD}$ promoter. Since *HDR* gene is essential for survival, the *E. coli hdr* mutant could only grow in the medium containing Ara but not in the medium containing Glc (Fig. 4, left). Upon transformation with the

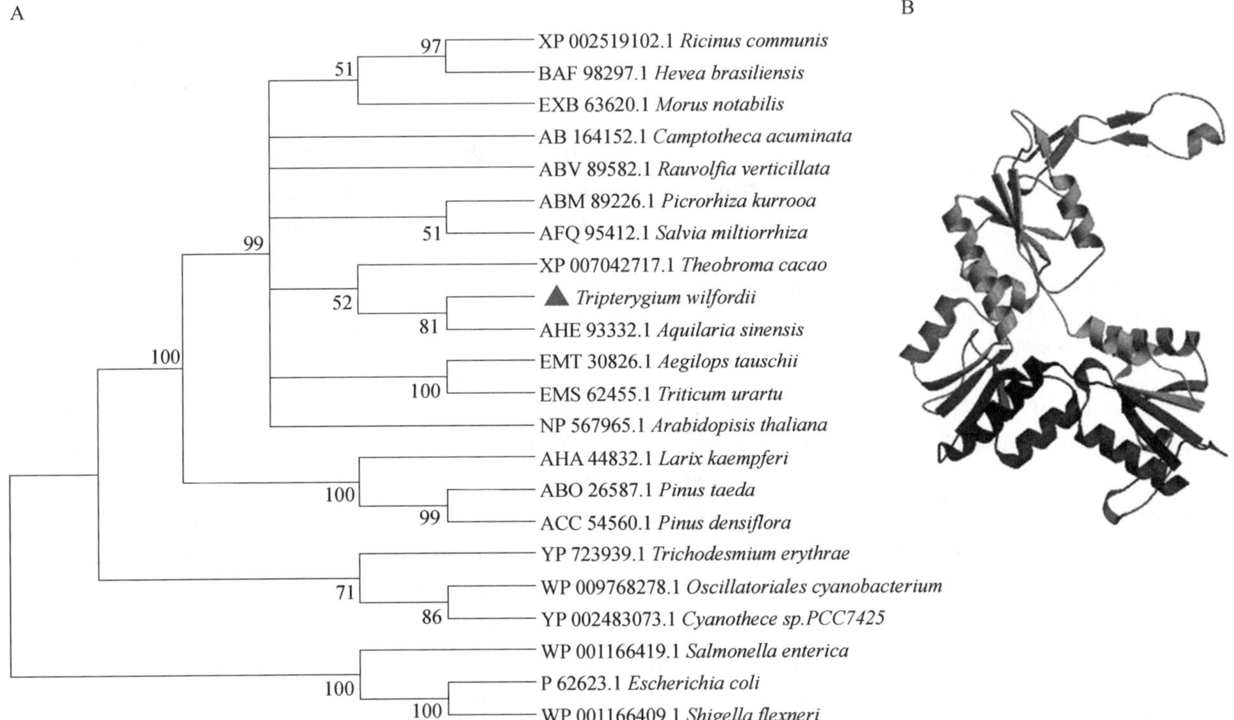


**Figure 3 Phylogenetic tree analysis of the putative TwHDR and other HDRs constructed by the neighbor-joining method (A) and the 3D structure of TwHDR (B)**

constructed vector harboring the *TwHDR* gene ( *pQE-TwHDR* ), the lethal phenotype of the mutant strain was rescued and cells could grow in medium with Glc. The opposite was observed for cells transformed with the empty pQE－30 vector (Fig. 4 right). Therefore, the enzymatic mechanism involved in the synthesis of the isoprenoid precursors between TwHDR and *E. coli* HDR might be similar.

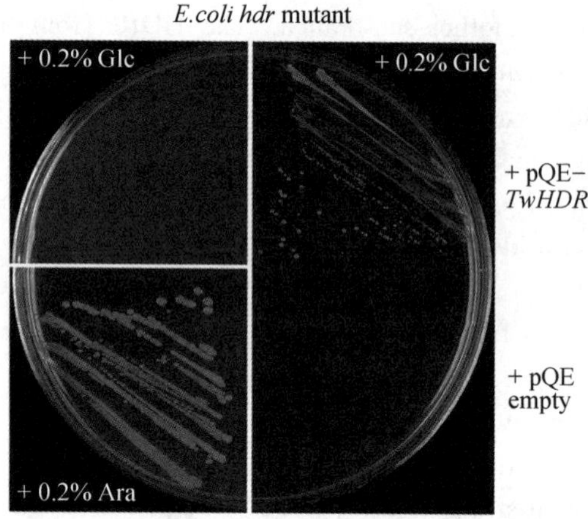


**Figure 4 Complementation of *E. coli hdr* mutant strain MG1655 ara < > HDR**

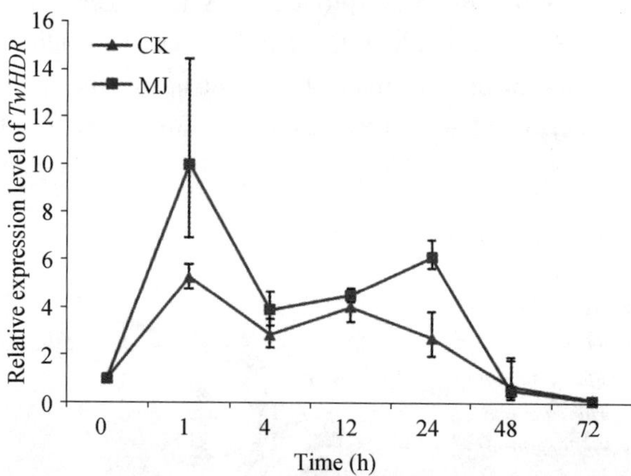


**Figure 5 Expression level of *TwHDR* in suspension cells after methyl-jasmonate ( MJ ) treatment. CK, the control group; MJ, the MJ-induced group**

3.4 Expression of TwHDR in the suspension cells As shown in Fig. 5, quantitative real-time PCR revealed the *TwHDR* expression which was induced by 50 μmol/L MJ in suspension cell cultures. The relative expression level of *TwHDR* in the MJ-induced group peaked at 1 h after the MeJA treatment (9.98 fold of that at the beginning time). After 1 h, the expression level decreased to 3.89 fold at 4 h than at 0 h. From 4 to 24 h, the expression level gradually increased, and it reached up to 6.11 fold at 24 h. And after 24 h it fell down to 10% at 72 h of that at 0 h. At the same time, in the control group, the expression level of *TwHDR* also reached its peak at 1 h. And then it progressively decreased to 13% at 72 h of that at 0 h with only a small increase between 4 and 12 h.

## 4 DISCUSSION

HDR enzyme catalyzes the last step in IPP biosynthesis, playing a key role in terpenoid biosynthesis. Although *HDR* gene has been cloned from many plants, such as *A. thaliana*, *Ginkgo biloba* and *Salvia miltiorrhizae* Bge. G. alba, there is no report on cloning and characterization of the *T. wilfordii* gene encoding HDR. In this study, we examined the biosynthesis pathway of terpenoid in *T. wilfordii* by cloning the *HDR* gene for the first time. *TwHDR* was transformed into a proper *E. coli* mutant strain to verify its function. Furthermore, we also examined the effects of MJ on the expression of *TwHDR*.

Although TwHDR only shares about 21.67% identity with the *E. coli* protein, it was still able to rescue the lethal phenotype of the *E. coli hdr* mutant (as shown in Fig. 4). The *E. coli* IspH protein is a reductase that possesses a dioxygen-sensitive [4Fe－4S] cluster. The result of amino acid sequence alignment has demonstrated that three conserved cysteine residues which may be involved in iron-sulfur cluster formation were conserved in *E. coli* and all plant HDRs including TwHDR ( Fig. 2 ). These results indicate that TwHDR might participate in the coordination of the iron-sulfur bridge. This complementation assay demonstrated that *TwHDR* encodes an active HDR enzyme, with similar enzymatic mechanism in the biosynthesis of IPP and DMAPP.

The expression of *TwHDR* in suspension cells was examined after 1, 4, 12, 24, 48 and 72 h of MJ treatment. The relative expression of *TwHDR* peaked at 1 h. This result indicated that a short-term MJ excitation could activate secondary metabolism MEP pathway and stimulate the plant stress defense system. About the small increase of *TwHDR* expression level between 12 and 24 h, we still cannot find the exact reason. But in the study of wound to jasmonates content in *A. sinensis*, we found the same trend. In that study, the jasmonates peaked at 1 h and then decreased, after 6 h, it increased again and went to the second highest content at 24 h, and then fell again. We speculate that this variation trend may be one way that plant cultures make response to the elicitation, but more study is needed to explain its mechanism. Our results prove that TwHDR is an important enzyme in terpenoid biosynthesis pathway, which may be a good target for engineering active terpenoids in *T. wilfordii*.

Co-expression of a HDR from tomato and a taxadiene synthase from *Taxus baccata* in transgenic *A. thaliana* led to a 13-fold increase in the amount of taxadiene produced. Therefore, it will be an interesting and effective way to improve triptolide content by genetic engineering. The cloning and identification of key enzyme genes in the biosynthesis of active compounds from medicinal plants is important for the analysis of synthesis pathways. Now, more and more enzyme genes in triptolide biosynthesis pathway have been cloned and identified, such as *TwDXS*, *TwDXR*, *TwFPS*, *TwHMGS* and *TwGGPPS*. Our work about cloning and identification of *TwHDR* helps know more about the biosynthesis pathway of terpenoids in *T. wilfordii*. As the biosynthesis pathway of triptolide is still unknown and the transgenic regeneration system of *T. wilfordii* remains unsolved, further studies on *HDR* and the isolation of relevant genes involved in the biosynthesis of terpenoids are still needed, which may provide insights into the production of triptolide in *T. wilfordii*.

## 5 CONCLUSIONS

We analyzed the function of TwHDR after successfully cloned and characterized the full-length *TwHDR* cDNA from *T. wilfordii* for the first time. The combination of cloning, identification, and functional analysis data of TwHDR will offer us more insights into the role of HDR in the MEP pathway and facilitate prospects of triptolide biosynthesis at the molecular level.

[程琪庆，高伟，黄璐琦，等. Acta Pharmaceutica Sinica B, 2017,7(2):208-214.]

# Molecular cloning and functional identification of sterol C24-methyltransferase gene from *Tripterygium wilfordii*

## 1 INTRODUCTION

*Tripterygium wilfordii* Hook. F. is a traditional Chinese medicinal plant that has analgesic and anti-microbial properties, and thus it has been widely used to treat inflammatory diseases. Moreover, recent research showed that *T. wilfordii* could treat immune and tumour diseases.

Isoprenoid compounds are main active ingredients of *T. wilfordii*. Several important enzymes have been cloned and identified for their biosynthetic pathways. The isoprenoid compounds in *T. wilfordii* include sterols, chlorophyll, gibberellin, and a variety of terpenes. Among these, sterols are hydrocarbon derivatives that consist of a four-membered cyclopentanoperhydrophenanthrene ring. Plant sterols are essential components of eukaryotic membranes. They help to maintain membrane integrity and permeability, participate in mammalian, yeast and plant cell endocytosis and production processes, and serve as precursors in the brassinosteroid hormone biosynthesis. In addition, phytosterols can act as signalling molecules in plants, participating in the regulation of various physiological activities, such as photosynthesis, reproduction and immunization. Sterol C24-methyltransferase (SMTs) have been found to play a key role in the synthesis of steroids with its methyltransferase property. The analysis of different amino acid sequences in all the cDNAs suggested that *SMTs* can be separated into two gene families, *SMT1* and *SMT2*. It has been reported that the two compounds play important roles in plant growth and development. The metabolic pathway chart is shown in Fig. 1. It has been

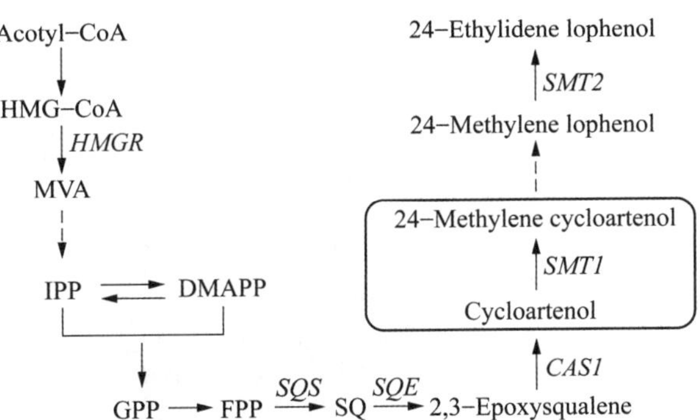


**Figure 1 The biosynthetic pathway of phytosterol involving sterol C24-methyltransferase 1 (*SMT1*) gene and sterol C24-methyltransferase 2 (*SMT2*) gene**

3-Hydroxy-3-methylglutary CoA (HMG-CoA); 3-hydroxy-3-methyl glutaryl coenzyme A reductase (*HMGR*); mevalonate pathway (MVA); isopenteny pyrophosphate (IPP); dimethylally pyrophosphate (DMAPP); gerqnyl pyphosphate (GPP); famesyl pyrophosphate (FPP); squalene synthase (*SQS*); squalene (SQ); squalene epoxidase (*SQE*); cycloartenol synthase 1 (*CAS1*).

indicated that the methylation reactions of cycloartenol and 24-methylene lophenol are cata-lysed by SMT1 and SMT2, respectively. The two gene families are involved in the biosynthesis of 24-methyl and 24-ethyl sterols, respectively. Thus, cloning of the plant *SMT* genes and characterization of the gene products would provide an alternative approach to addressing some of the important questions regarding *SMTs*, such as the C-24 methylation mechanism and developmental regulation of the enzyme.

Molecular cloning of *SMTs* was recently achieved in a

number of higher plant species, including *Astragalus bisulcatus*, *Arabi-dopsis thaliana*, *Oryza sativa*, *Nicotiana tobacum*, *Brassica oleracea*, and *Camellia sinensis*. Until now, no *SMT* gene from *T. wilfordii* has been cloned. In this paper, we report the isolation and identification of a cDNA encoding SMT1 from *T. wilfordii* for the first time. The polypeptide encoded by the *T. wilfordii* cDNA was expressed in *E. coli* and shown to be an active SMT enzyme. The real-time quantitative PCR analysis of *TwSMT1* expression was found to be promoted upon the methyl jasmonate (MeJA) elicitor treatment.

## 2 MATERIALS AND METHODS

2.1 Plant materials Cell suspensions of *T. wilfordii* in the study were cultured in Murashige and Skoog (MS) medium (pH 5.8) containing 2,4-dichlorophenoxyacetic acid (2,4-D, 0.5 mg/L), cytokinin (KT, 0.1 mg/L), indole-3-butytricacid (IBA, 0.5 mg/L), and sucrose (30 g/L), shaking at 120 rpm (Eppendorf, 5810 R, Germany) 25℃ in dark culture and subculture suspension cells (2 g) in the same medium (25 mL) every 20 days. The plants of *T. wilfordii* in the tissue expression analysis were obtained from Fujian province and have grown for seven years.

2.2 Cloning of TwSMT1 from T. wilfordii Total RNA was extracted from *T. wilfordii* suspension cells stored at −70 ℃ using the CTAB-LiCl method. The extract was purified using DNase I (Biolabs, Beijing, China) and an RNA cleaning kit (TIANGEN, Beijing, China) to remove contaminating genomic DNAs.

The purified product was reverse transcribed into first-stand 5′-RACE-Ready cDNA and 3′-RACE-Ready cDNA with the SMART RACE cDNA Amplification Kit (Takara Bio Group, Japan). According to mRNA fragments obtained from the transcription data, specific primers (3′-RACE Primer: 5′-TGGATG-TAGGATGTGGAATCGGTGGA-3′; 5′-RACE Primer: 5′-TTAGGGCCTCAAGGCATTGTCTGG TC-3′) were designed to amplify 5′ and 3′ cDNA, respectively, followed by ligation into the *pEASY*-T3 vector (TransGen Biotech, Beijing, China) and transfer into *E. coli* Trans5α competent cells (TransGen Biotech, Beijing, China). Transformed cells were plated onto Luria-Bertani (LB) solid medium plates containing ampicillin (Amp) and screened

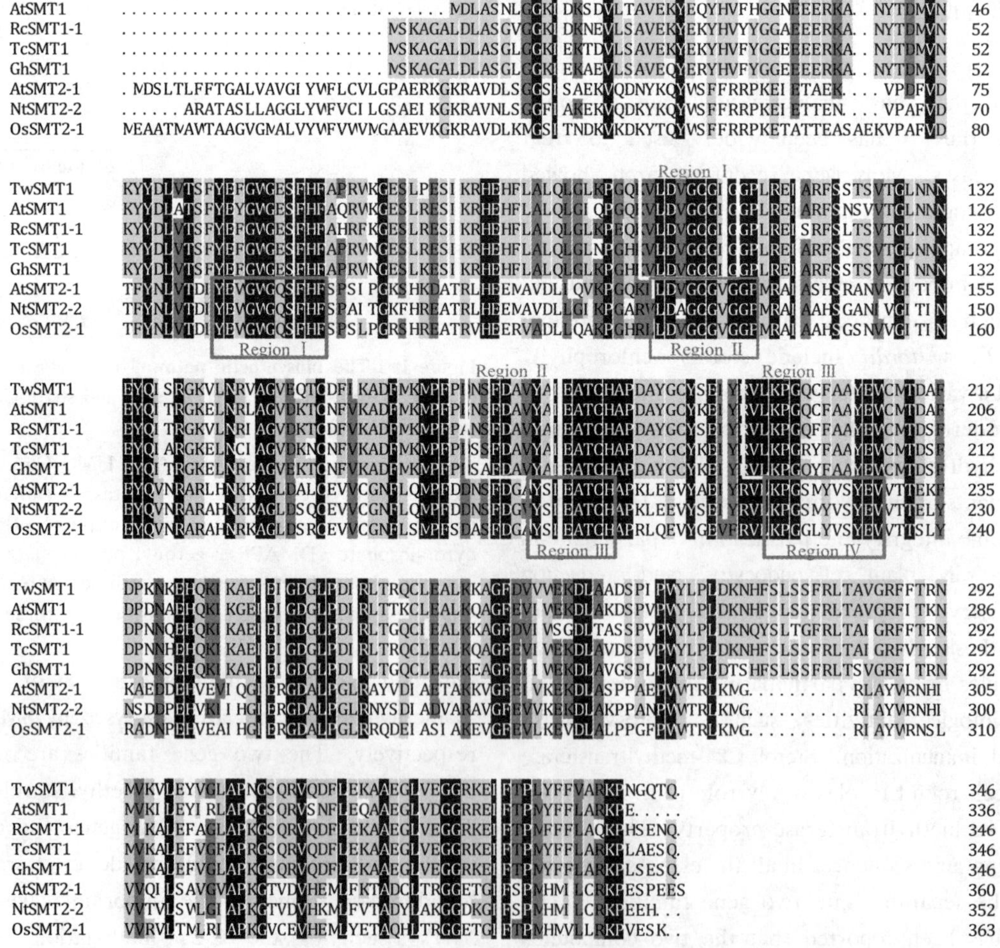

**Figure 2 Sequence alignment of the deduced amino acid sequence of TwSMT1 with those of related proteins**

The three conserved sterol C24-methyltransferase 1 regions and four conserved sterol C24-methyltransferase 2 regions are boxed and numbered with different colours.

using monoclonal colony PCR. Positive bacterial colonies were selected for sequencing to identify and obtain the *TwSMT1* full-length sequence.

2.3 Sequence alignments and phylogenetic analyses The nucleotide and protein sequences were compared using BLAST at the NCBI (http://www.ncbi.NLM.NIH.gov). The ORF was searched using the ORF Finder (www.ncbi.NLM.NIH.gov/Gorf/Gorf.html). The molecular weight (MW) and theoretical isoelectric point (pI) calculations were performed using the Compute pI/MW tool (http://Web.ExPASy.org/compute_pi/). Multi ple sequence alignments were performed using DNAMAN 8.0, and phylogenetic analysis was carried out using MEGA 7.0 software to build evolutionary trees.

2.4 Expression of TwSMT1 in E. coli and purification of recombinant protein Based on the prokaryotic expression vector pMAL-c2X sequence, the restriction endonuclease sites of *Bam*H I and *Xba* I were selected to design primers from which the stop codon (TAA) has been removed to amplify the *TwSMT1* ORF sequence: *TwSMT1*: 5′-CGGGATC-CATGTCGAAGGCTGGGGCGT-3′ (forward) and 5′-GCTCTA-GACTGGGTCTGCCCATTAGGCT-3′ (reverse). According to the instructions of Prime STAR GXL DNA Polymerase (Takara Bio Group, Japan), the PCR reaction conditions were set as follows: 98 ℃ for 3 min; 35 cycles of 98 ℃ for 10 s, 55 ℃ for 15 s, and 68 ℃ for 1 min 20 s; and a final extension at 72 ℃ for 5 min. After the amplified products were purified, both the vector and the purified products were double-digested with corresponding restriction endonucleases; the enzyme-digested products were purified and ligated with T4 DNA ligase, and then transferred into *E. coli* Trans5α competent cells. Transformed cells were cultured in LB solid medium with Amp (100 mg/L) for one night, and then a monoclonal plaque was selected for PCR verification and sequencing to obtain the correct recombinant plaque. The new plasmid extracted from the plaque was named pMAL-c2X-*TwSMT1*.

The recombinant pMAL-c2X-*TwSMT1* was transferred into BL21 (DE3) competent cells along with the same transformation of pMAL-c2X as a control. The detected positive plaques were cultured and induced with 1 mmol/L isopropyl-1-thio-β-D-galac-topyranoside for protein extraction. The extraction procedure was described in Supplementary information, and the purified extract was used for dodecyl sulfate, sodium salt-polyacrylamide gel electrophoresis (SDS-PAGE) detection.

2.5 Enzyme assays To identify *TwSMT1* functions, enzymatic reactions *in vitro* were performed with the purified supplement above using the method reported by Schaeffer et al.. The reaction system contained 0.1 mol/L Tris-HCl (pH 7.5), Tween 80 (0.1%, *W/V*), glycerol

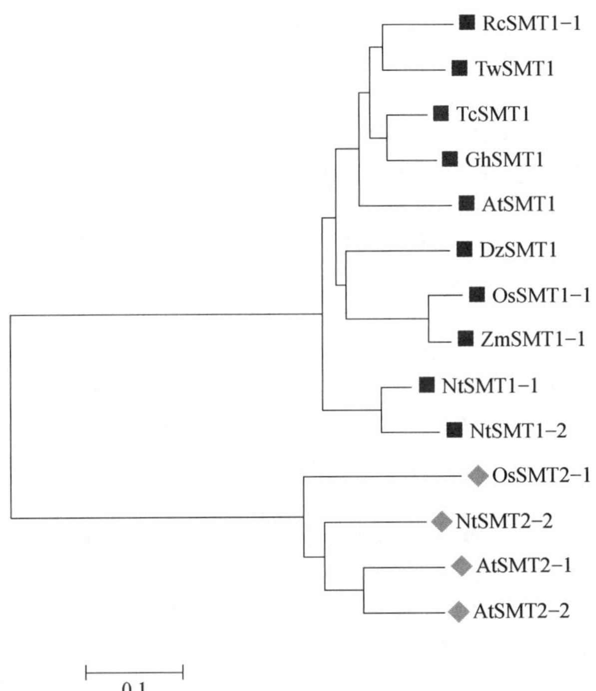


**Figure 3 Phylogenetic tree of the amino acid sequences of sterol C24-methyltransferase from different plants constructed by the neighbour-joining method on MEGA 7.0**

GenBank accession numbers: *Ricinus communis* (RcSMT1-1 AAB62812.1); *Theobroma cacao* (TcSMT1 XP_007052489.1); *Gossypium hirsutum* (GhSMT1 AAZ83345.1); *Arabidopsis thaliana* (AtSMT1 NP_001078579.1); *Dioscorea zingiberensis* (DzSMT1 CBX33151.1); *Oryza sativa* (OsSMT1-1 AAC34988.1); *Zea mays* (ZmSMT1-1 AAB70886.1); *Nicotiana tabacum* (NtSMT1-1 AAC34951.1); *Nicotiana tabacum* (NtSMT1-2 AAC35787.1); *Oryza sativa* (OsSMT2-1 AAC34989.1); *Nicotiana tabacum* (NtSMT2-2 AAB62807.1); *Arabidopsis thaliana* (AtSMT2-1 CAA61966.1); *Arabidopsis thaliana* (AtSMT2-2 AAB62809.1).

(20%, *V/V*), β-mercaptoethanol (1 mmol/L), methyl-3*H*-AdoMet (100 μmol/L), cycloartenol (100 μmol/L) as a substrate, and purified protein (200 μL); the total volume was 500 μL, and the reaction condition was set at 30 ℃ for 45 min and ethanolic KOH (100 μL of 12%, *W/V*) was used as a quenching agent. The sterol compounds in the mixture solution were extracted three times with 600 μL *n*-hexane, combining the supernatant solution and evaporating the solvent with a pressure blowing concentrator, followed by re-dissolving in *n*-hexane (200 μL) for gas chromatography-mass spectrometer (GC-MS) detection.

The GC-MS detection was performed using a Thermo TRACE 1310/TSQ 8000 gas chromatography (splitless; injector temperature 250 ℃) equipped with a DB-5 ms (30 m × 0.25 mm, 0.25 μm) capillary column, and the program condition was set for 1 min at 60 ℃, then increased from 60 to 300 ℃ at a rate of 30 ℃/min, and finally held for 15 min at 300 ℃; the flow rate was 1 mL/min with He as a carrier gas. The mass spectrometry detection range was from

50 to 500 $m/z$.

2.6 Expression analysis of TwSMT1 induced by Methyl Jasmonate MeJA, as an abiotic elicitor, is widely used in tissue expression analysis for its ability to promote content of secondary metabolites. After the suspension cells of *T. wilfordii* were induced by MeJA (50 μmol/L) at 0, 1, 4, 12, 24, 48, 72, and 120 h, total RNA extracted with the CTAB method subsequently was reversely transcribed to obtain cDNA for qRT-PCR analysis. Primers for the housekeeping gene, β-actin, were chosen as described in Tong's paper: β-actin F: 5′-AGGAACCACCGATCCAGACA-3′ and β-actin R: 5′-GGTGCCCTGAGGTCCTGTT-3′. The specific primers (*TwSMT1* F: 5′-TCTAACCGCTGTTGGACGA-3′ and *TwSMT1* R: 5′-CCCTCAACTAACCCCTCTGC-3′) were designed to amplify the fragment of *TwSMT1*. The reaction solutions were prepared according to the manufacturer's protocol from the KAPA SYBR FAST qPCR Kit, and the amplification conditions were 95℃ for 5 min and 40 cycles of 95℃ for 3 s and 60℃ for 33 s. The experiments were repeated three times for biological and technical replicates, respectively, to ensure the authenticity of the data.

2.7 Tissue expression pattern analysis of TwSMT1 Total RNA was extracted from five organs of *T. wilfordii* plants, which were the leaf, stem, phloem, xylem and phellem layer. The purified RNA was reversely transcribed into the First Strand cDNA for relative expression study of *TwSMT1*. The primers for amplifying the housekeeping gene and *TwSMT1*, as well as the reaction condition of RT-PCR were consistent with inducible expression analyses by MeJA, including the operating time.

## 3 RESULTS

3.1 Isolation of the cDNA coding for TwSMT1 and sequence analysis RT-PCR was performed with total RNA from *T. wilfordii*. *TwSMT1* gene fragments were obtained by 3′ rapid amplification of cDNA ends (3′-RACE-PCR) and 5′-RACE-PCR. The full-length cDNA encoding the SMT1 protein was isolated from *T. wilfordii*. The full-length cDNA of *TwSMT1* was 1 530 bp. It had a 1041 bp open reading frame (ORF) encoding a 346-amino-acid polypeptide, with a 177 bp 5′ non-coding-region (NCR) and a 312 bp 3′-NCR including a 19 bp poly (A) tail. The predicted TwSMT1 protein has a calculated molecular mass of 38.99 kDa and a theoretical pI of 6.11 (GenBank accession No. KU885950).

3.2 Comparison of the deduced amino acid sequence of TwSMT1 with other SMTs A Blast search of *TwSMT1* in the NCBI database showed that the deduced amino acid sequence of *TwSMT1* had 75%–86% identity to the SMT1s from *A. thaliana*, *Nicotiana tabacum*, *O sativa*, *Zea mays*, *Ricinus communis*, *Dioscorea zingiberensis*, *Theobroma cacao*, and *Gossypium hirsutum*. Sequence comparison revealed that the deduced amino acid sequence contained three methyltransferase regions identified in diverse sterol C24-methyltransferases. Region I is highly conserved in the protein. Region II contains the invariant central aspartate residue. Region III is located at an interval between the 19-residue C-terminal and region II. The deduced amino acid sequence of *TwSMT1* has 33%–36% identity with the SMT2s from *O. sativa*, *N. tabacum*, and *A. thaliana*. These sequences present highly homologous regions: Region II (IN) LD (A/V)-GCG (V/I) GGP corresponds to the consensus motif described by several authors. Region III IEATCHAP, a second invariant region, is absent in other methyltransferases and is potentially unique for sterol methyltransferases. Those regions marked with boxes suggested that the cDNA of *T. wilfordii* may encode an sterol C24-methyltransferase (Fig. 2).

Comparison of all these amino acid sequences allowed a phylogenetic tree of plant SMTs to be built, which was separated into two main groups (Fig. 3). TwSMT1 clustered with 9 SMT1 sequences and OsSMT2 clustered with 3 SMT2 sequences. Moreover, TwSMT1 and *R. communis* were classified into one cluster. A cluster means that its components had higher homology.

3.3 Functional expression and characterization of TwSMT1 Fig. 4 shows the results of protein expression and GC–MS detection. SDS-PAGE was used to detect purified proteins extracted from BL21 (DE3) strains from which pMAL-c2X or pMAL-c2X-*TwSMT1* was expressed. The electrophoresis results are shown in Fig. 4D. The control vector expressed an MBP-labelled protein with a molecular weight of 42 kDa, whereas owing to the TwSMT1 protein being 39 kDa, the recombinant plasmid expressed the protein at the position of 80 kDa as the sum of the MBP and TwSMT1 proteins. The results suggest that both the *TwSMT1* construct in the pMAL-c2X vector and the empty pMAL-c2X with the MBP label had been successfully expressed in the BL21(DE3) strain, so the extracted protein can be used for further TwSMT1 functional experiments *in vitro*.

The sterol extract from both pMAL-c2X and pMAL-c2X-TwSMT1 in the enzymatic reaction were detected by GC–MS. From the results we can see that, in comparison to a peak of cycloartenol in the pMAL-c2X extract shown in Fig. 4A, a prominent peak whose retention time was 17.96 min was detected in the pMAL-c2X-TwSMT1 protein reaction (Fig. 4B). The experiment was repeated six times, and the same results were obtained. Fig. 4C shows the peak of the predicted product, 24-methylene cycloartenol, which is theoretically SMT1's product when cyclaortenol is the substrate, and it shows the same retention time at 17.96 min as the product in Fig. 4C; thus, they were putatively assigned as the same compound. We then compared the mass spectra

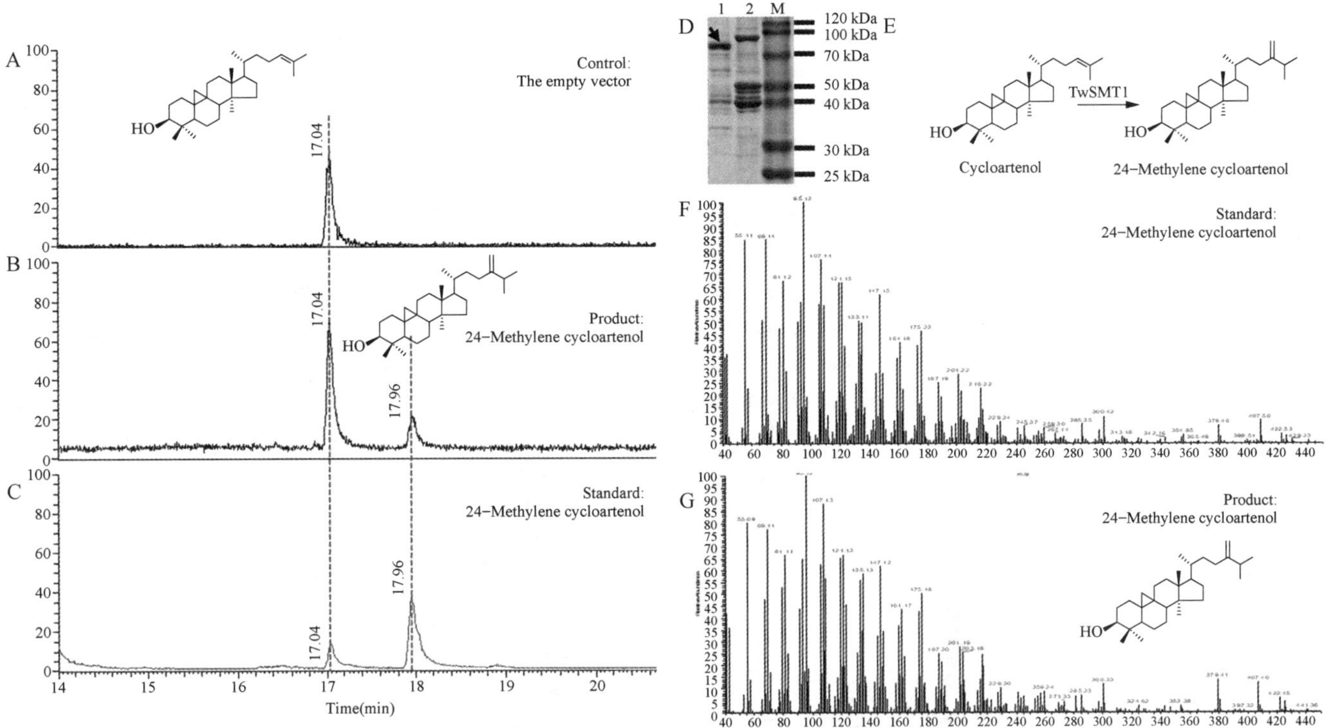


**Figure 4 SDS-PAGE analysis and GC - MS detection results of extract from an enzymatic reaction catalysed by purified pMAL-c2X-TwSMT1 protein and pMAL-c2X protein when using cycloartenol as the substrate**

(A) The peak of extraction in the empty vector protein reaction system; (B) The peak of extraction in the recombinant pMAL-c2X-TwSMT1 protein reaction mixture; (C) A control using a 24-methylene cycloartenol standard; (D) 1: The recombinant pMAL-c2X-TwSMT1 overexpressed by isopropyl-1-thio-$\beta$-D-galactopyranoside (IPTG); 2: the empty pMAL-c2X overexpressed by IPTG; (E) The function of *SMT1* from *T. wilfordii*; (F) Mass spectrogram of the 24-methylene cycloartenol standard; (G) Mass spectrogram of the product catalysed by recombinant TwSMT1 protein.

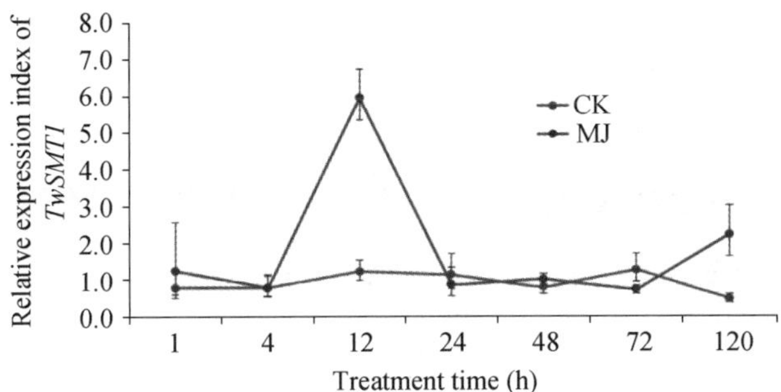


**Figure 5 Expression profile of *TwSMT1* when treated with 1 mmol/L methyl jasmonate (MJ) over 120 h**

RT-PCR analysis was performed using total RNA isolated from suspension cells of *T. Wilfordii*. CK, the control group; MJ, the MJ-induced group.

of the product (Fig. 4G) and the standard (Fig. 4F), and the figures show nearly identical ion peaks, except for a few low intensity peaks. These results demonstrate that TwSMT1 has the function of catalysing the transformation of cycloartenol to 24-methylene cycloartenol, and it is a cycloartenol-C24-methyltransferase.

3.4 Inducible expression of TwSMT1 MeJA has the ability to promote the accumulation of secondary metabolites. From Fig. 5, it is clear that the elicitor MeJA works on the expression level of *TwSMT1*. After the suspension cells were elicited by MeJA, the *TwSMT1* transcript levels have an obvious fluctuation especially at 12 h and it is about four times higher than the blank control group. Afterwards, the curve tends to overlap with the control group and stabilize. The methodology can be used to study sterol content accumulation and other sterol genes through transcriptome data mining.

3.5 Tissue expression pattern of TwSMT1 Fig. 6 shows the relative expression level of *TwSMT1* in different organs. It shows that phellem layer has the highest expression level, which is about ten times higher than the lowest expression in leaf.

## 4 DISCUSSION

The enzyme sterol C24-methyltransferase 1 (SMT1) is involved in the biosynthesis of plant sterol, which plays major roles in plant growth and development. In addition, studies have shown that $\beta$-sitosterol, a phytosterol belonging to the 24-ethyl sterols, has been isolated from *T. wilfordii*, and it has an obvious cholesterol-lowering activity and is widely used in the pharmaceutical industry. In the present study, we have reported the first isolation and characterization of a sterol C24-methyltransferase 1 gene from *T. wilfordii*. The results showed that *TwSMT1* is a 1 530 bp cDNA with a 1 041 bp ORF predicted to encode a 346-amino acid, 38.62 kDa protein. The results also indicated that the *SMT1* obtained belonged to the family of transferases and catalysed the transformation of cycloartenol to 24-methylene cycloartenol. In order to study the inducible expression of *TwSMT1* from cell suspensions upon MeJA, we analysized the changes of real-time PCR in various stages. The results showed that MeJA caused a significant increase in *TwSMT1* levels in *T. wilfordii* cell suspensions. Tissue expression analysis showed *TwSMT1* has a higher expression in velamen compared to other four organs.

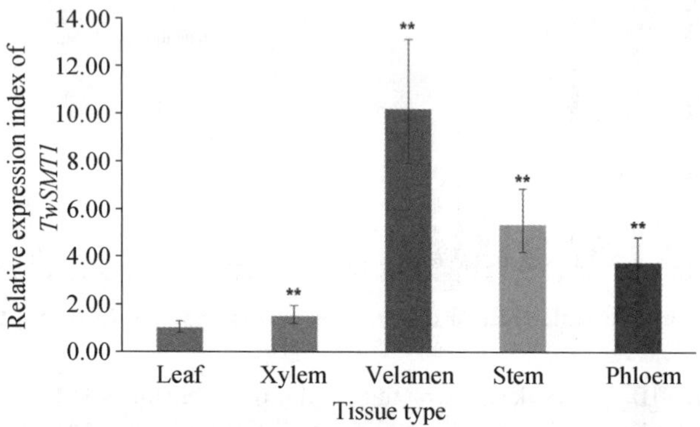


**Figure 6 Tissue expression analysis of *TwSMT1* in the leaf, stem, phloem, xylem and phellem layer of *T. Wilfordii* plants**

The asterisks mean that the difference is acceptable when the values of other organs take leaf as a standard (** $P<0.01$).

Plant sterols play extremely important roles in every stage of plant growth and development. It is important that *SMTs* act on the biosynthesis of plant sterols as many researchers have reported. Researchers often use mutant and enzyme inhibitors to study the functions of plant sterols. Mutants of *SMT1* show abnormal embryoids and cotyledons with different sizes and numbers. This result indicates that plant sterols play a crucial role in the process of embryonic development. Mutants of *SMT1* show cell shrinkage of root epidermis and cortex, stasis phenomenon of the meristem and elongation region cells in the shape of a circle, indicating the importance of sterols in normal growth and development of the roots. The *orc* mutation residing in C－24 *SMT1* shows a position disorder of auxin transmission proteins PIN1 and PIN3, indicating that plant sterols could correct the polarity orientation of proteins.

Sterols play a vital role in the process of eukaryote growth and development. They are not only structural components, but also have important regulatory functions and are precursors for the synthesis of other compounds. Plant sterols participate in almost all processes of plant growth, from the embryo to post-embryonic development. Therefore, they are indispensable to normal plant growth and development. Studies have also shown that consuming more plant sterols can reduce the absorption of cholesterol, and they may be used as therapeutics in the future.

[关红雨，赵瑜君，高伟，等. Acta Pharmaceutica Sinica B, 2017,7(5):603－609.]

# Identification and functional characterization of diterpene synthases for triptolide biosynthesis from *Tripterygium wilfordii*

## 1 INTRODUCTION

*Tripterygium wilfordii* Hook. f., commonly known as Lei Gong Teng in Chinese, has been used medicinally for centuries, mainly to treat rheumatoid arthritis. While the genus *Tripterygium* is known to produce many types of terpenoids, the major bioactive compounds in *T. wilfordii* seem to be diterpenoids, especially triptolide, a triepoxide lactone first identified by Kupchan *et al.*, and related compounds. These natural products have aroused extensive interest due to their broad spectrum of anti-inflammatory, immunosuppressive, anti-cystogenesis and anti-cancer activities. In addition, triptolide exerts effects on central nervous system diseases such as Parkinson's and Alzheimer's. However, these diterpenoids are currently exclusively derived from *Tripterygium* plants with low yields, limiting our ability to investigate and apply these bioactive compounds. Elucidation of the biosynthetic pathways for these complex diterpenoids would enable increased access via metabolic engineering, either in the native plant or using a synthetic biology approach to introduce the pathway into a microbial host.

Triptolide is an abietane-type diterpenoid, which places it in the labdane-related superfamily that is characterized by formation of the underlying hydrocarbon backbone from the general diterpenoid precursor (*E*, *E*, *E*)-geranylgeranyl diphosphate (GGPP) by a sequential pair of cyclization reactions. These are catalyzed firstly by class II diterpene cyclases, which contain a characteristic DxDD motif, and then subsequently acting class I diterpene synthases that contain a separate DDxxD motif instead. Despite their distinct catalytic activity, catalyzed in separate active sites defined by the noted motifs, these enzymes are both members of the terpene synthase (TPS) family, with the class II diterpene cyclases making up the TPS-c subfamily and subsequently acting class I diterpene synthases comprising the TPS-e subfamily.

More specifically, triptolide is presumably produced via initial cyclization of GGPP to copalyl diphosphate (CPP), with subsequent cyclization and rearrangement to an abietane-type diene olefin, which is then further transformed to triptolide. It has been suggested that this proceeds via the aromatized dehydroabietic acid, with subsequent 1, 2-migration of the carboxylic acid (from carbon 4→3) to form the observed *abeo*-abietane backbone. Notably, the cyclohexa-1, 4-diene arrangement of the abietane miltiradiene positions this for aromatization, which readily occurs spontaneously. Thus, miltiradiene is a likely intermediate in triptolide biosynthesis (Figure 1).

Identification of the tissues where the compound of interest is produced and/or conditions that lead to increased accumulation can significantly aid elucidation of the underlying biosynthetic pathway. Consistent with previous results, we have recently developed suspension cell cultures of *T. wilfordii* that produce triptolide and related diterpenoids, as well as the triterpenoid celastrol. Here we report that feeding miltiradiene to these cultures increases triptolide production. In addition, we find that production of triptolide can be induced in these cultures, which are then subjected to RNA sequencing (RNA-seq) to generate a transcriptome. This dataset was mined to discover eight potential (di) terpene synthases which were functionally characterized by subcellular localization and biochemical analysis, revealing two closely related CPP synthases (CPSs), TwTPS7v2 and TwTPS9v2, and a subsequently acting miltiradiene synthase, TwTPS27v2. Critically, RNA interference (RNAi) of *TwTPS7v2* and *TwTPS9v2*, or *TwTPS27v2*, reduced triptolide production, confirming not only the role of miltiradiene as a precursor but also of these diterpene synthases in biosynthesis of this important diterpenoid natural product.

## 2 RESULTS

Suspension cell cultures can be used to illuminate triptolide biosynthetic pathway As previously reported, we have established *T. wilfordii* suspension cell cultures. Critically, these were found to stably produce diterpenoids, particularly including triptolide, over a 3-year period. Briefly, these cultures were grown in defined medium in the dark at 25 ℃ on a rotary shaker and transferred to fresh medium every 18 days, with 2.6-fold increases in the fresh weight of suspension cells over this time (Figure S1). These cultures were found to produce $53 \pm 3\ \mu g/g$ of triptolide in the suspension cells and $4.0 \pm 0.2$ mg/L in the medium (Figure 2c).

To compare the phytochemical complexity of these suspension cell cultures relative to whole plants, extracts from the cells and medium, as well as plant root, stem, leaf and flower tissues, were analyzed by ultra-performance liquid chromatography-quadrupole time-of-flight mass spectrometry (UPLC/Q-TOF MS). The plant samples, especially those from the roots traditionally associated with medicinal use, were largely composed of a variety of alkaloids (e. g. wilforgine and wilforine), with relatively small amounts of diterpenoids, including triptolide. By contrast, the suspension cell cultures appear to selectively accumulate diterpenoids and triterpenoids rather than alkaloids. Indeed, the suspension cultures accumulated triptolide at a higher level than the native plant, and this was particularly prevalent in the medium, which exhibits a relatively simple phytochemical profile that presumably would assist purification of triptolide and/or related diterpenoids. Thus, these cultures represent a potential source of these natural products for commercial production. Perhaps more relevant here, these cultures further provide a system for investigation of the underlying biosynthetic network. For example, potential intermediates such as triptophenolide, triptinin B and triptoquinonide can be readily detected in the suspension cells (Table 1, Figure 2).

Miltiradiene is a precursor to triptolide Notably, miltiradiene, arguably the most likely olefin precursor to triptolide, was detectable in our suspension cell cultures (Figure S2). To further investigate the potential role of miltiradiene in triptolide biosynthesis, this abietane was fed to these cultures, which led to a statistically significant increase in triptolide accumulation relative to control cultures after 5 days (Figure 3). This indicated that miltiradiene does serve as a precursor to triptolide, such that a class I diterpene synthase producing this olefin should be involved in the biosynthesis of these diterpenoids.

Triptolide production is induced by methyl jasmonate Previous work has indicated that the production of (di) terpenoid natural products can be induced by the defense signaling molecule methyl jasmonate (MeJA), which is further useful for co-expression analysis. Indeed, the application of MeJA to *T. wilfordii* cell cultures led to increased production of triptolide, at least in the cells, as measured by UPLC analysis (Figure S3). Elevated levels of triptolide in MeJA-induced relative to control cultures were

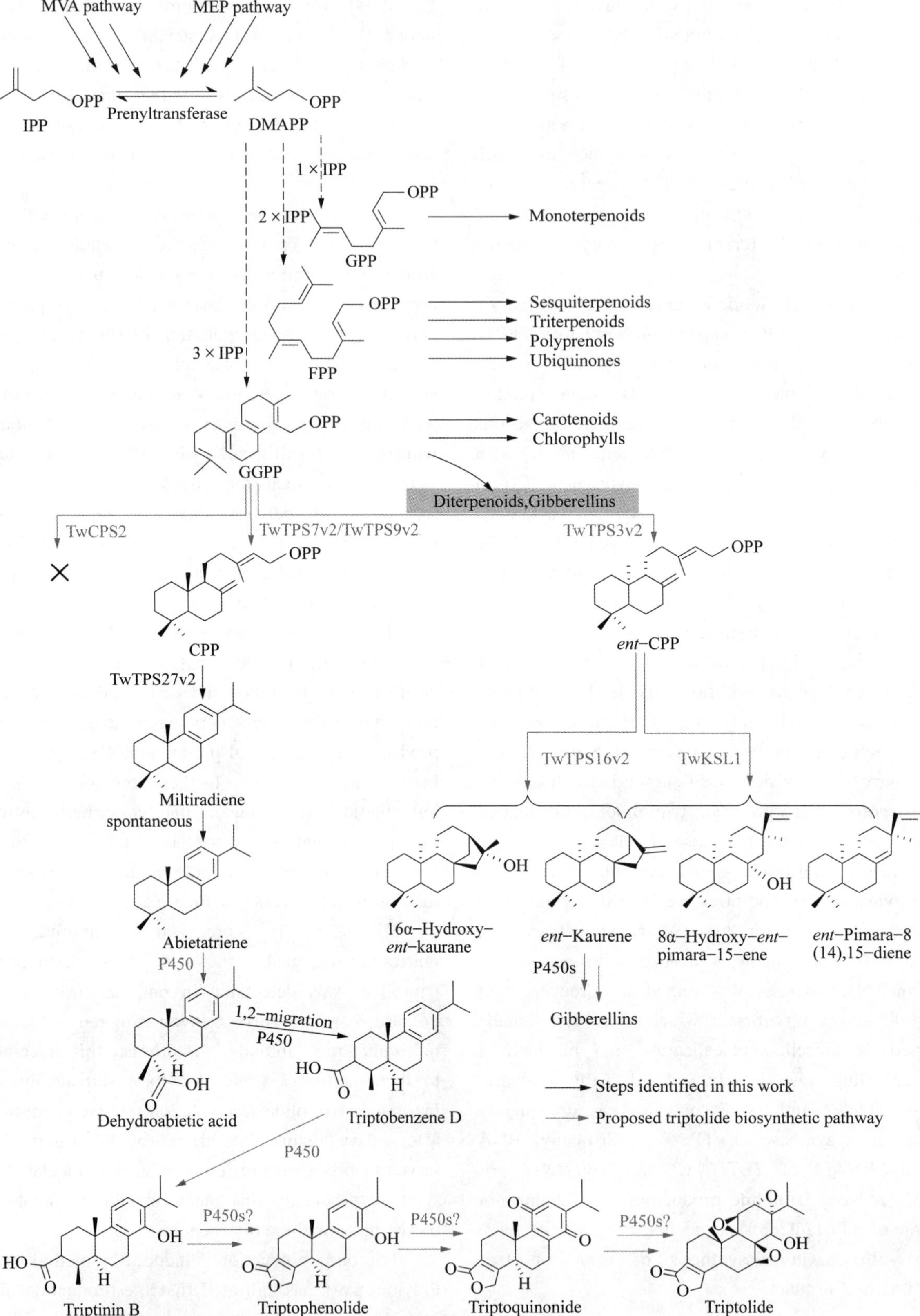


**Figure 1 Diterpenoid biosynthetic network in *Tripterygium wilfordii* as elucidated by the work described here and others**

Colour figure can be viewed at wileyonlinelibrary.com.

evident within 72 h, with even larger differences found at later time points; for example, after 240 h triptolide levels were more than three-fold higher, reaching just over 200 μg/g, in the induced suspension cells (Figure 4). While it seems worth mentioning that the ability to induce higher levels of triptolide may favor the potential use of these suspension

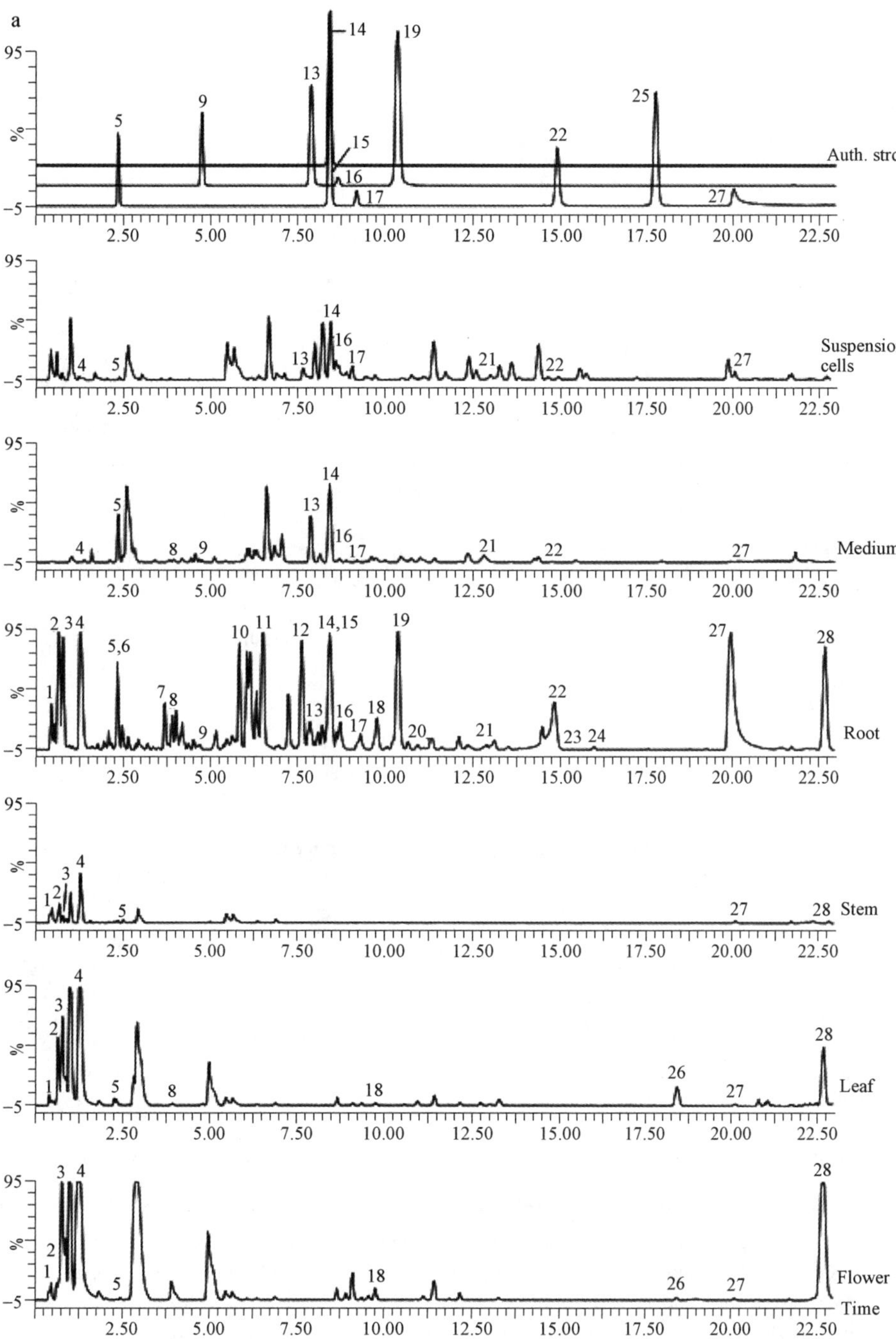


cell cultures for larger-scale production of this and related diterpenoids, here this finding was used to assist elucidation of the underlying biosynthetic network.

Induced transcriptome of *T. wilfordii* Based on the ability of MeJA to increase triptolide production, such induced suspension cells were subjected to deep transcriptome sequencing with the Illumina HiSeq 2000 platform. In total, 12.68 Gb of clean sequence was obtained after adapter-related reads, low-quality reads and reads containing unknown bases were removed from the raw reads (Table S1). A total of 90 801 transcripts were assembled with a mean length of 1 053 bp and an N50 of 1 837 bp (Table S2, Figure S4).

Functional annotation was carried out using multiple databases, specifically Nr (NCBI non-redundant protein sequences), Nt (NCBI non-redundant nucleotide sequences), Pfam (protein family), KOG/COG (clusters of orthologous groups of proteins), Swiss-Prot (a manually annotated and reviewed protein sequence database), KO (KEGG Orthology database) and GO (Gene Ontology). Relevant to triptolide biosynthesis, 27 unigenes potentially involved in such metabolism were found, including eight putative diterpene synthases, defined by falling within either the TPS-c or TPS-e subfamilies (Tables S3 and S4, Figure S5).

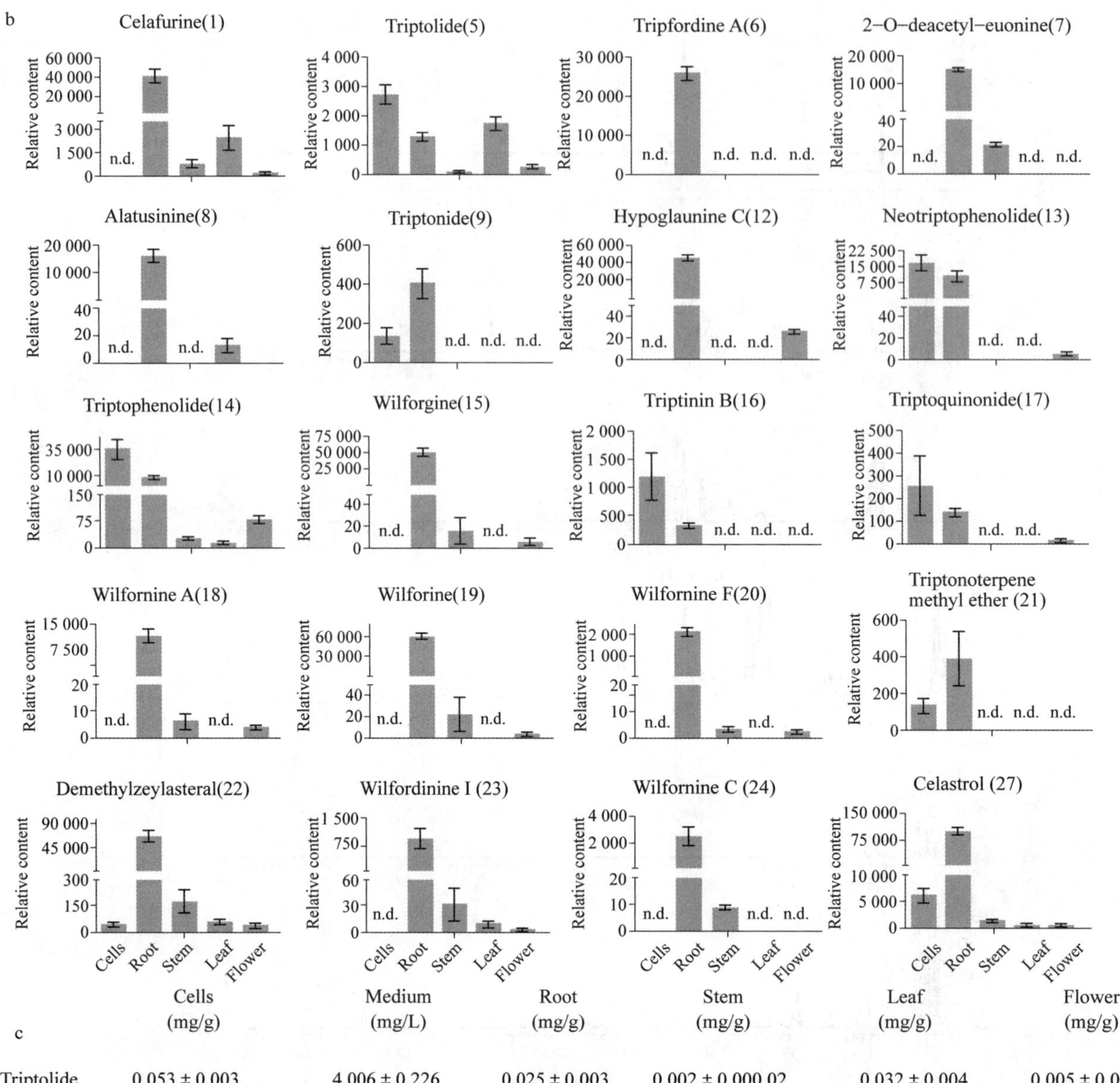


| | Cells (mg/g) | Medium (mg/L) | Root (mg/g) | Stem (mg/g) | Leaf (mg/g) | Flower (mg/g) |
|---|---|---|---|---|---|---|
| Triptolide | 0.053 ± 0.003 | 4.006 ± 0.226 | 0.025 ± 0.003 | 0.002 ± 0.000 02 | 0.032 ± 0.004 | 0.005 ± 0.001 |

**Figure 2　Comparison of extracts from *Tripterygium wilfordii* suspension cells and whole plant organs**

(a) Base peak intensity chromatograms of extracts from suspension culture cells and medium, and plant root, stem, leaf and flower tissues by ultra-performance liquid chromatography-quadrupole time of flight-mass spectrometry. The identities of the metabolite peaks 1－28 are listed in Table 1. (b) Relative content of the identified metabolites from suspension cells, culture medium, root, stem, leaf or flower. (c) Concentrations of triptolide in suspension cells, culture medium, root, stem, leaf or flower. Colour figure can be viewed at wileyonlinelibrary. com.

Cloning of putative diterpene synthases　To demonstrate the utility of the generated transcriptome for elucidation of triptolide biosynthesis, it was hypothesized that the diterpene synthases necessary for formation of miltiradiene should be present, i. e. among those in the transcriptome. Sequence analysis indicated that full-length open reading frames (ORFs) were not present for all eight putative diterpene synthases. Thus, full-length sequences were obtained by 5′ and 3′ rapid amplification of cDNA ends (RACE), also using RNA from induced suspension cells. This eventually led to cloning of cDNA for six distinct full-length diterpene synthases (Table S5).

The obtained putative diterpene synthases were subjected to phylogenetic analysis (Figures 5, S6 and S7). During the course of our studies reports appeared describing similar, although not exactly identical, genes. These are presumably allelic to those identified here and, to be consistent with these recent reports, we utilize nomenclature that reflects these presumed relationships. Four of those found here fall within the TPS-c subfamily and hence were expected to be class II diterpene cyclases. Three appeared to be allelic to previously identified genes and, accordingly, were named *TwTPS7v2*, *TwTPS3v2* and *TwTPS9v2*, while the remaining gene was termed *TwCPS2*. However, in place

**Table 1 Metabolites detected by ultra-performance liquid chromatography-quadrupole time of flight-mass spectrometry in all tissues (root, stem, leaf, and flower) of *Tripterygium wilfordii*, and suspension cells as well as the media**

| Metabolite (no. in Figure 2) | RT[a] (min) | Formula | $[M+H]^+$ Calculated | $[M+H]^+$ Observed | Error (Δp.p.m.) | MS/MS signal patterns (% relative abundance) | Authentic standard confirmed | Tentative ID |
|---|---|---|---|---|---|---|---|---|
| Celafurine (1) | 0.53 | $C_{21}H_{27}O_3N_3$ | 370.2131 | 370.2140 | 2.4 | 370(7.2),317(18.1),305(37.1),287(54.1),263(25.6),179(26.1),139(62.3),127(35.9),100(21.1) | | √ |
| Unknown alkaloid (2) | 0.67 | $C_{20}H_{27}O_2N_5$ | 370.2243 | 370.2270 | 7.3 | 370(11.3),265(3.4),249(5.8),166(9.9),161(16.1),160(100),131(5.6),100(23.9) | | |
| Unknown alkaloid (3) | 0.81 | $C_{21}H_{33}O_5N$ | 380.2437 | 380.2437 | 0 | 380(13.1),275(2.2),259(4.0),188(3.5),176(8.4),161(14.0),105(36.8),100(13.5) | | |
| Unknown alkaloid (4) | 1.30 | $C_{23}H_{35}O_5N$ | 406.2593 | 406.2601 | 2.0 | 406(20.9),301(5.4),258(6.2),188(7.7),161(12.3),160(99.2),131(100),103(13.2) | | |
| Triptolide (5) | 2.35 | $C_{20}H_{24}O_6$ | 361.1651 | 361.1656 | 1.4 | 361(100),279(2.1),250(2.2),201(5.1),157(2.9),145(3.6),108(6.6),105(2.6) | √ | |
| Tripfordine A(6) | 2.35 | $C_{36}H_{45}O_{18}N$ | 780.2715 | 780.2704 | 1.4 | 780(52.2),752(100),734(24.1),674(11.7),632(11.7),204(10.4),194(29.7),176(23.8),158(2.4) | | √ |
| 2-O-deacetyl-euonine (7) | 3.71 | $C_{36}H_{45}O_{17}N$ | 764.2766 | 764.2759 | 0.9 | 764(100),746(51.2),686(16.8),644(8.9),206(72.0),160(2.9) | | √ |
| Alatusinine (8) | 3.92 | $C_{38}H_{47}O_{19}N$ | 822.2821 | 822.2823 | 0.2 | 822(41.3),794(100),776(12.2),674(12.0),250(6.2),194(17.2),176(19.1),160(6.5) | | √ |
| Triptonide (9) | 4.73 | $C_{20}H_{22}O_6$ | 359.1495 | 359.1500 | 1.4 | 359(100),197(1.6),171(2.1),143(3.1),107(3.0) | √ | |
| Unknown alkaloid (10) | 5.85 | $C_{35}H_{46}O_{20}N_3$ | 828.2675 | 828.2670 | 0.6 | 828(43.1),806(100),788(25.9),746(18.8),686(20.6),644(3.6),206(40.6),178(10.2) | | |
| Unknown alkaloid (11) | 6.52 | $C_{35}H_{46}O_{20}N_3$ | 828.2675 | 828.2673 | 0.2 | 828(37.9),806(100),788(50.0),746(48.6),704(14.8),686(12.0),609(5.9),206(21.5),160(6.5) | | |
| Hypoglaunine C (12) | 7.67 | $C_{43}H_{49}O_{19}N$ | 884.2977 | 884.2984 | 0.8 | 884(69.0),856(100),838(15.0),674(12.1),194(11.3),176(14.4),105(6.4) | | √ |
| Neotriptophenolide (13) | 7.88 | $C_{21}H_{26}O_4$ | 343.1909 | 343.1931 | 6.4 | 343(86.4),301(17.8),297(36.9),257(22.3),255(100),240(32.6),205(50.2),177(18.8),163(35.1),137(10.7) | √ | |
| Triptophenolide (14) | 8.44 | $C_{20}H_{24}O_3$ | 313.1804 | 313.1822 | 5.7 | 313(31.0),271(9.7),253(9.1),225(47.8),206(100),178(20.4),133(10.6),106(16.1) | √ | |
| Wilforgine (15) | 8.44 | $C_{41}H_{47}O_{19}N$ | 858.2821 | 858.2871 | 5.8 | 858(100),840(22.3),798(9.4),780(4.8),746(8.3),686(15.4) | √ | |
| Triptinin B (16) | 8.65 | $C_{20}H_{26}O_3$ | 315.1960 | 315.1969 | 2.9 | 297(33.8),279(24.2),269(27.8),255(100),237(47.8),227(41.5),213(34.4),197(29.2),185(38.6),171(78.1),157(34.7),149(40.4),147(48.0),133(39.8),105(12.0) | √ | |

(Continued)

| Metabolite (no. in Figure 2) | RT[a] (min) | Formula | [M+H]+ | | Error (Δp.p.m.) | MS/MS signal patterns (% relative abundance) | Authentic standard confirmed | Tentative ID |
|---|---|---|---|---|---|---|---|---|
| | | | Calculated | Observed | | | | |
| Triptoquinonide (17) | 9.21 | $C_{20}H_{22}O_4$ | 327.1596 | 327.1611 | 4.6 | 327(100),309(6.0),281(77.6),263(24.5),253(24.1),239(62.4),224(17.4),211(18.6),193(15.0),169(16.7),165(12.1),143(6.9),119(7.9),108(5.9) | √ | |
| Wilfornine A (18) | 9.81 | $C_{45}H_{51}O_{20}N$ | 926.3083 | 926.3055 | 3.0 | 926(38.5),804(100),760(11.3),744(6.1),684(6.0),204(6.6) | | √ |
| Wilforine (19) | 10.41 | $C_{43}H_{49}O_{18}N$ | 868.3028 | 868.3049 | 2.4 | 868(100),850(33.6),808(12.6),746(14.6),686(25.2),206(30.7),178(7.1),105(4.8) | √ | |
| Wilfornine F (20) | 10.97 | $C_{41}H_{47}O_{17}N$ | 826.2922 | 826.2901 | 2.5 | 826(74.4),812(100),808(38.6),748(6.6),310(4.7),206(43.4),105(5.6) | | √ |
| Triptonoterpene methyl ether(21) | 12.93 | $C_{21}H_{30}O_3$ | 331.2273 | 331.2281 | 2.4 | 316(17.6),301(16.0),271(21.3),245(21.3),231(19.9),206(59.6),201(27.4),179(100),163(31.5),137(24.6),109(9.0),105(6.2) | | √ |
| Demethylzeylasteral (22) | 14.85 | $C_{29}H_{36}O_6$ | 481.2590 | 481.2603 | 2.7 | 481(100),463(3.2),245(6.5),231(62.1),213(5.0),203(14.4),161(1.5),147(4.5),121(1.8),109(4.6) | √ | |
| Wilfordinine I (23) | 15.41 | $C_{48}H_{51}O_{19}N$ | 946.3134 | 946.3094 | 4.2 | 946(41.0),918(7.8),846(12.7),824(100),764(6.8),746(4.4),625(2.0),204(5.8) | | √ |
| Wilfornine C (24) | 15.97 | $C_{50}H_{53}O_{20}N$ | 988.3239 | 988.3201 | 3.8 | 988(34.1),960(5.5),942(3.9),920(1.9),888(1.8),866(100),848(6.5),822(4.8),806(3.8),788(1.6),764(3.9),746(3.9),204(4.7),105(4.4) | | √ |
| Dehydroabietic acid (25) | 17.76 | $C_{20}H_{28}O_2$ | 301.2168 | 301.2163 | 1.7 | 173(83.1),171(8.0),159(16.7),140(25.4),133(60.1),131(100),106(58.6) | √ | |
| Unknown alkaloid (26) | 18.42 | $C_{34}H_{35}O_9N_4$ | 643.2404 | 643.2399 | 0.8 | 643(100),583(59.2),555(21.5),495(15.2),469(3.1),441(3.0),118(0.9) | | |
| Celastrol (27) | 20.00 | $C_{29}H_{38}O_4$ | 451.2848 | 451.2864 | 3.5 | 451(3.1),215(15.5),202(16.7),201(100),186(7.9),153(11.3),128(8.5),115(7.1) | √ | |
| Unknown alkaloid (28) | 20.69 | $C_{29}H_{42}O_{10}N_4$ | 607.2979 | 607.2989 | 1.6 | 607(100),547(33.2),461(3.7) | | √ |

of the highly conserved DxDD motif, TwCPS2 contains 'DTDC[311]', raising questions about its activity. The two remaining diterpene synthases fall within the TPS-e subfamily, which is anchored by the *ent*-kaurene synthases (KSs) required in vascular plants for metabolism of the gibberellin phytohormone, but also contains derived KS-like (KSL) enzymes. One appeared to be allelic to a previously identified gene, and hence was named *TwTPS16v2*, while the other appeared to be unique, and was named *TwKSL1*.

**Functional characterization of the putative class Ⅱ diterpene cyclases** To determine the function of the putative class Ⅱ diterpene cyclases they were heterologously expressed in *Escherichia coli*, and tested with GGPP as a substrate via *in vitro* cell-free assays. For detection by gas

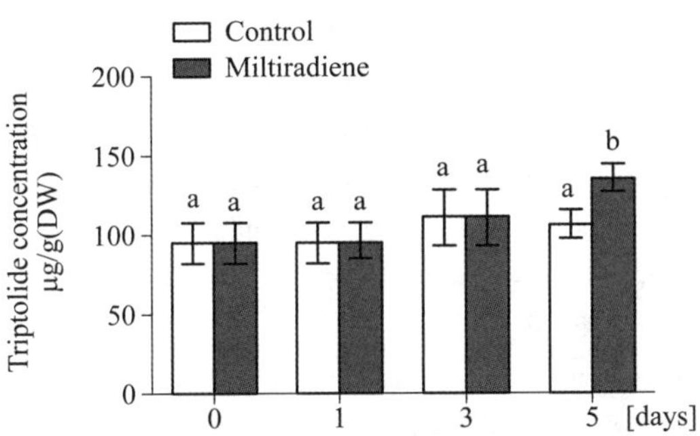


**Figure 3 Triptolide content in suspension cells fed with miltiradiene as measured by ultra-performance liquid chromatography**

The data represent the average ± standard deviation from analysis of at least four independent lines of suspension cell cultures (lettering indicates statistically significant difference from all-by-all comparison using the Student's *t*-test). DW, dry weight.

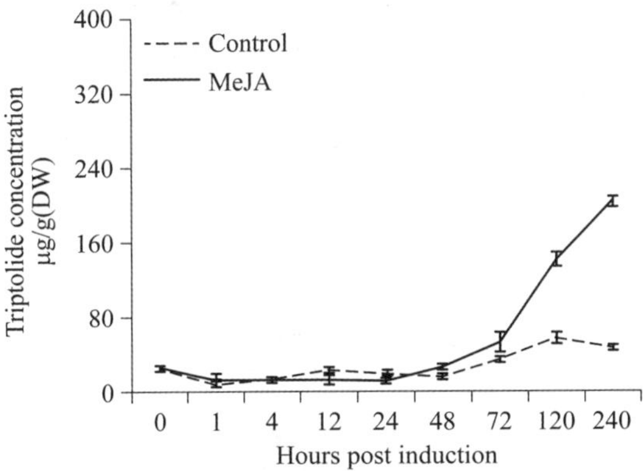


**Figure 4 Accumulation of triptolide in suspension cells induced by methyl jasmonate (MeJA)**

The data represent the average ± standard deviation of at least three independent suspension cell cultures. DW, dry weight.

chromatography-mass spectrometry (GC-MS), phosphatase was added to the assays upon completion to dephosphorylate both the substrate GGPP and any product, such as CPP, yielding geranylgeraniol (GGOH) and copalol, respectively. The production of CPP was detected for TwTPS7v2, TwTPS3v2 and TwTPS9v2 by comparison with the known activity of a CPS from *Salvia miltiorrhiza* (SmCPS1) (Figure 6a); no activity was detected for TwCPS2. Thus, *TwCPS2* appears to be an inactive pseudogene. Both the phylogenetic distance of this from other (functional) members of the TPS-c subfamily, even within the *Tripterygium* genus (Figure 5), and the fact that the lack of activity goes beyond simple loss of the DxDD motif, as correcting this (i.e. by changing C311 to the Asp prototypically found at that position) did not restore any enzymatic activity to TwCPS2, are consistent with this hypothesis.

To determine the absolute stereochemistry of the CPP products of TwTPS7v2, TwTPS3v2 and TwTPS9v2, these were coupled to stereospecific class I diterpene synthases, in particular the miltiradiene synthase from *S. miltiorhiza*,

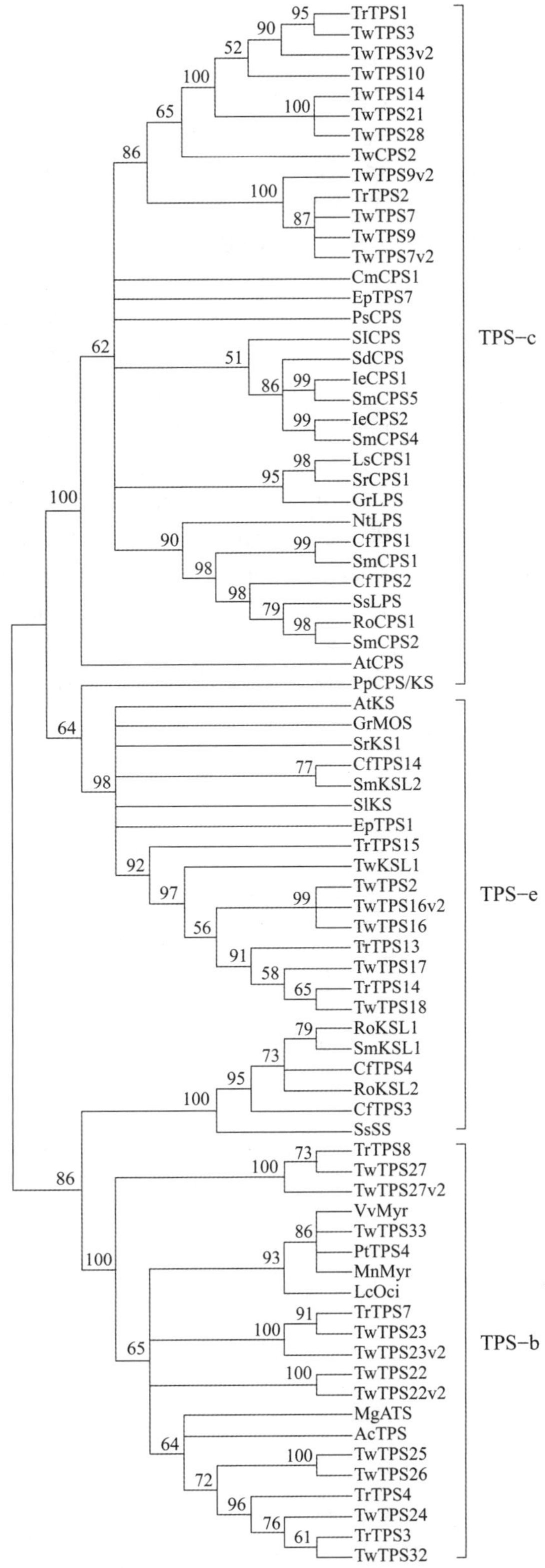


**Figure 5 Phylogenetic tree of *Tripterygium wilfordii* diterpene synthases**

Phylogenetic tree of *Tripterygium wilfordii* diterpene synthases (i.e. those from the TPS-c and TPS-e subfamilies) with representative examples from other species. Abbreviations and NCBI accession numbers are provided in Table S8.

SmMS or KS from *Arabidopsis thaliana*, AtKS, which are specific for CPP or *ent*-CPP, respectively. *In vitro* cell-free assays were carried out in all six possible pairings, with the production of miltiradiene observed in assays with SmMS and either TwTPS7v2 or TwTPS9v2, while *ent*-kaurene was only observed in assays with AtKS and TwTPS3v2 (Figure 6b). Thus, consistent with recently reported work on their allelic variants, both TwTPS7v2 and TwTPS9v2 produce CPP, while TwTPS3v2 produces *ent*-CPP.

Functional characterization of putative class I diterpene synthases To determine the function of the two putative class I diterpene synthases, they were recombinantly expressed in *E. coli* and subjected to *in vitro* cell-free assays in combination with either TwTPS7v2 or TwTPS3v2 (providing CPP or *ent*-CPP, respectively). Neither TwKSL1 nor TwTPS16v2 produced miltiradiene. Instead, both were only active with *ent*-CPP. Consistent with the very recently reported activity of its allelic variant, TwTPS16v2 produced largely 16α-hydroxy-*ent*-kaurane along with small amounts of *ent*-kaurene (Figure S8), which was further confirmed by co-expressing this with TwTPS3v2 in yeast (*Saccharomyces cerevisiae*). TwKSL1 was found to produce a mixture of diterpenes, the major components of which were identified upon incorporation into a modular metabolic engineering system in *E. coli*, and comparison with already characterized enzymes, as *ent*-pimara-8(14),15-diene and small amounts of 8α-hydroxy-*ent*-pimar-15-ene, as well as minor amounts of *ent*-kaurene (Figure 6c).

Interestingly, the production of 16α-hydroxy-*ent*-kaurane has previously been shown to critically depend on the identity of a specific residue, which is conserved as methionine in KSs but is a smaller residue in diterpene synthases that produce 16α-hydroxy-*ent*-kaurane instead, with corresponding site-directed mutagenesis of this residue leading to substantial changes in product outcome. TwTPS16v2 contains an alanine at this position and, consistent with previous reports, substitution of methionine leads to predominant production of *ent*-kaurene, with smaller amounts of 16α-hydroxy-*ent*-kaurane, from *ent*-CPP by the resulting mutant TwTPS16v2:A608M (Figure S8). The result, together with a report identifying

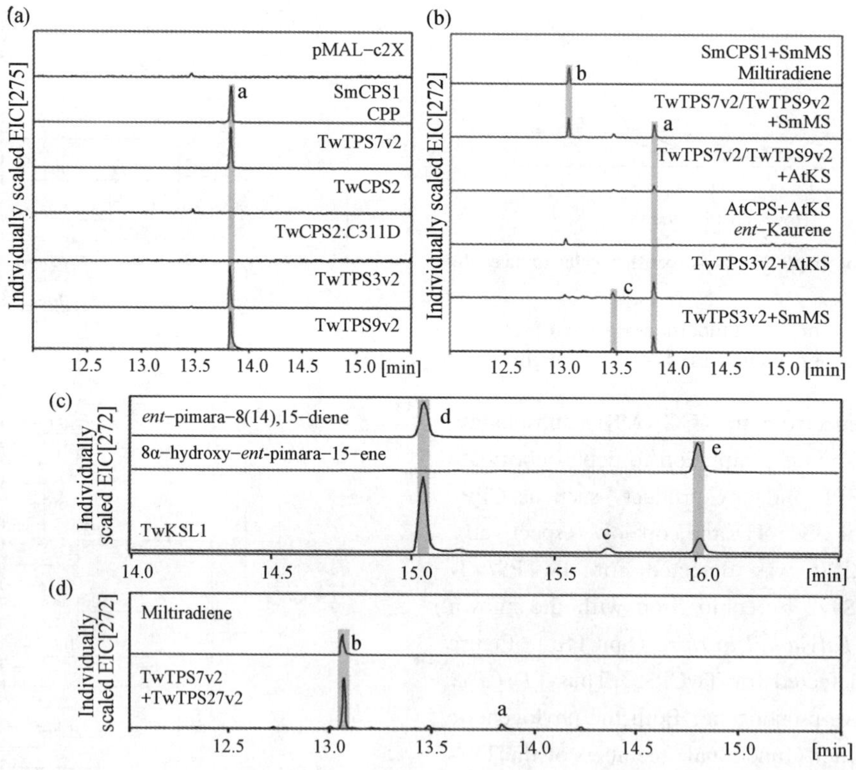


**Figure 6 Gas chromatography-mass spectrometry (GC–MS) analysis of the products from the reactions catalyzed by *Tripterygium wilfordii* (di)terpene synthases *in vitro***

(a) GC–MS analysis of the dephosphorylated reaction products of recombinant *T. wilfordii* (Tw) copalyl diphosphate (CPP) synthases (TwCPSs) with (*E*,*E*,*E*)-geranylgeranyl diphosphate (GGPP) as the substrate, compared with CPP produced by *Salvia miltiorrhiza* (Sm) CPS1, which is detected here as the dephosphory-lated copalol. (b) GC–MS analysis of TwTPS7v2, TwTPS3v2 or TwTPS9v2 coupled with either Sm miltiradiene synthase (SmMS) or Arabidopsis kaurene synthase (AtKS), compared with the miltiradiene or *ent*-kaurene produced by the complementary enzymatic pairs SmCPS1 and SmMS or AtCPS and AtKS, respectively. (c) GC–MS analysis of the TwKSL1 reaction products with *ent*-CPP. (d) GC–MS analysis of the reaction products from TwTPS27v2 and TwTPS7v2 with GGPP. Peaks are lettered as follows: a, (*ent*-)copalol (from dephosphory-lated (*ent*-)CPP); b, miltiradiene; c, *ent*-kaurene; d, *ent*-pimara-8(14),15-diene; e, 8α-hydroxy-*ent*-pimar-15-ene. Colour figure can be viewed at wileyonlinelibrary. com.

two key residues of TwTPS14 and TwTPS21 by Hansen *et al.*, highlights the evolutionary potential of this enzymatic family to drive rapid diversification of plant diterpene biosynthesis through neo-functionalization.

Identification of a miltiradiene synthase  Given the data indicating a role for miltiradiene in triptolide biosynthesis, it was hypothesized that an alternative terpene synthase responsible for its formation must be expressed in the *T. wilfordii* suspension cell cultures. Hence, we screened the transcriptome dataset using the amino acid sequence of the known miltiradiene synthase from *Salvia miltiorrhiza* (SmMS) as the probe sequence (with a cut-off E-value of $<10^{-10}$). In total, six potential terpene synthases were found, including two of the already characterized diterpene synthases, two that fall within the TPS-a subfamily and appear to be sesquiterpene synthases and two that fall within the TPS-b subfamily, which usually indicates that these would be monoterpene synthases (Table S6). However, consistent with a very recent report that appeared during the course of our studies, we also found that one of these, upon recombinant expression in *E. coli* and subsequent *in vitro* cell-free assays in combination with TwTPS7v2, produces miltiradiene (Figure 6d). Given that this TPS appears to be allelic to the previously identified miltiradiene synthase, sharing 98.0% identity, we name this here as TwTPS27v2 to be consistent with that previous report.

Use of TwTPS7v2/TwTPS9v2 and TwTPS27v2 in metabolic engineering  Yeast has been engineered to produce miltiradiene using the relevant diterpene synthases from *S. miltiorrhiza* (SmCPS1 and SmMS), including the use of gene fusions between *SmCPS1* and *SmMS*, which led to increased yield when expressed in the order SmMS-SmCPS1. Here the utility of the relevant diterpene synthases from *T. wilfordii* for similar engineering was investigated. However, the yield from co-expression of TwTPS27v2 with either TwTPS7v2 or TwTPS9v2 in appropriately engineered yeast, which were equivalent to each other (Figure S9A), was not found to be significantly better than that previously reported using SmCPS1 and SmMS. Moreover, fusing TwTPS7v2 and TwTPS27v2, in either orientation actually significantly decreased the yield of miltiradiene to $<5\%$ of that of the strain expressing each of these enzymes separately (Figure S9B). Indeed, unlike SmCPS1 and SmMS, TwTPS7v2 and TwTPS27v2 do not seem to interact, consistent with negative results from yeast two-hybrid assays with these (Figure S10).

Subcellular localization  Given that diterpene biosynthesis is initiated in plastids, separate from the cytosolic location presumed for monoterpene synthases, in order to verify the role of TwTPS27v2 and the other diterpene synthases it seemed worth investigating their subcellular localization. Accordingly, recombinant plasmids containing the ORFs of these genes fused with that for green fluorescent protein (GFP) were transformed into *N. benthamiana* leaves, which were then examined for GFP localization (Figure 7). GFP signals for TwTPS7v2, TwTPS3v2, TwTPS9v2 and

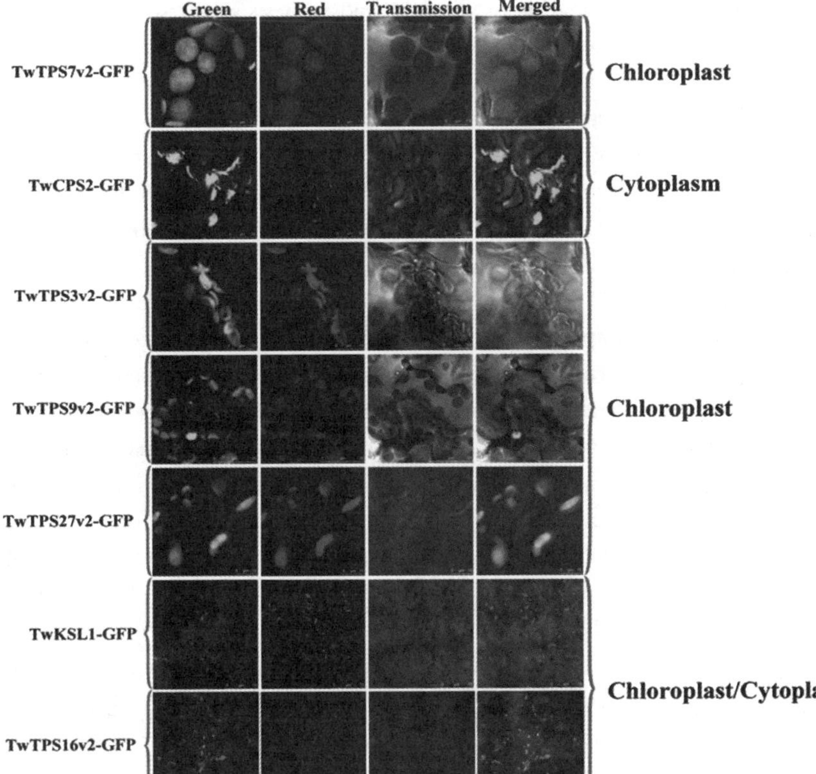


**Figure 7  Subcellular localization of *Tripterygium wilfordii* diterpene synthases with GFP fusion protein in *Nicotiana benthamiana* leaves**

Images were taken with a confocal laser scanning microscope. Green, GFP fluorescence image; Red, chlorophyll autofluorescence image; Transmission, bright-field image; Merged, merger of these images. Bars: 7.5 μm (TwTPS7v2-GFP), 50 μm (TwCPS2-GFP), 10 μm (TwTPS3v2-GFP), 7.5 μm (TwTPS9v2-GFP), 10 μm (TwTPS27v2-GFP), 75 μm (TwKSL1-GFP) and 75 μm (TwTPS16v2-GFP). Colour figure can be viewed at wileyonlinelibrary.-com.

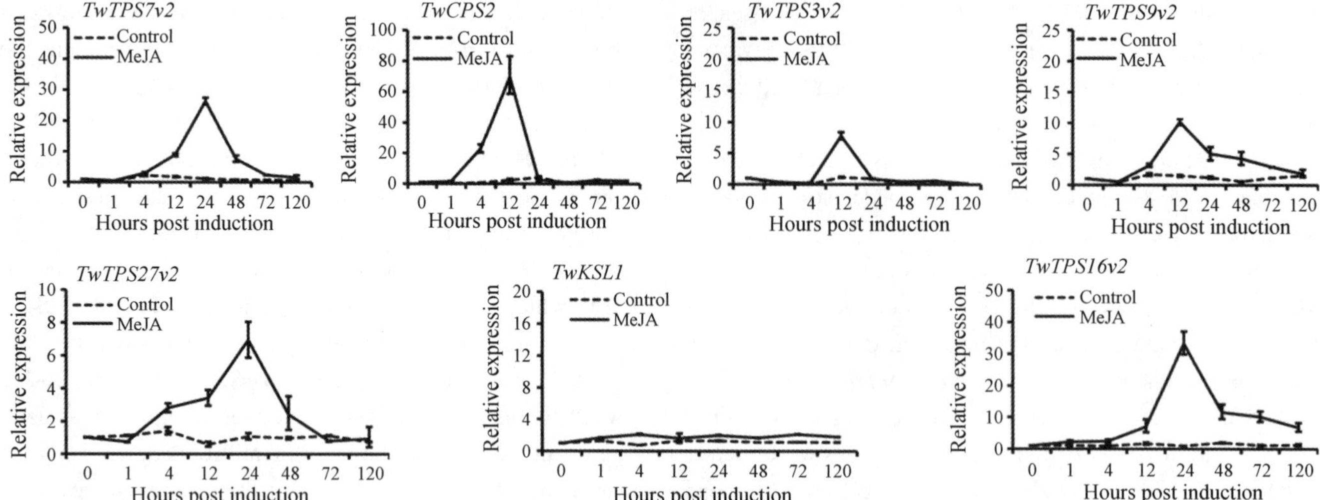


**Figure 8 Relative expression of *Tripterygium wilfordii* diterpene synthases in suspension cells treated with methyl jasmonate (MeJA)**

Key: MeJA, suspension cells treated with 50 μmol/L MeJA; Control, suspension cells treated with carrier solution (dimethyl sulfoxide). The $x$-axis represents the hours after treatment (0,1,4,12,24,48,72,120,240 h).

TwTPS27v2 were mainly found in chloroplasts, while those for TwKSL1 and TwTPS16v2 were found both in chloroplast and cytoplasm, supporting roles for all of these in diterpene biosynthesis. However, consistent with the hypothesis that *TwCPS2* is a non-functional pseudo-gene, the GFP signal for TwCPS2 produced a typical cytoplasmic localization pattern.

Induction of diterpene synthase transcription To further investigate the potential role of the functionally characterized diterpene synthases in triptolide biosynthesis, their transcriptional response to MeJA was investigated. Transcript levels were measured by qRT-PCR in suspension cells after induction with MeJA. This revealed increased levels of mRNA, peaking at 12 or 24 h, for all the diterpene synthases investigated here except TwKSL1 (Figure 8).

RNAi of TwTPS7v2 and TwTPS9v2 or of TwTPS27v2 RNAi was employed with suspension cell cultures to provide more direct evidence of a role in triptolide biosynthesis for TwTPS7v2 and/or TwTPS9v2, as well as TwMS and, hence, miltiradiene. Given the high identity between TwTPS7v2 and TwTPS9v2 (98.5%), both were targeted together using a stretch of identical sequence in the RNAi construct. While this only led to reductions of just over 30% in the transcript level of both *TwTPS7v2* and *TwTPS9v2*, transcript levels for *TwCPS2* and *TwTPS3v2* were not affected, and triptolide accumulation was nevertheless decreased by almost 50% compared with control cultures transformed with the empty vector. When RNAi targeting of *TwTPS27v2* was carried out, the transcript level of *TwTPS27v2* was similarly only reduced by about 30%, with no reduction in the levels of the related TPS-b subfamily members *TwTPS22v2*, *TwTPS23v2*, *TwTPS32* and *TwTPS33*; triptolide accumulation was decreased by about 40% (Figure 9).

## 3 DISCUSSION

The ability of *T. wilfordii* suspension cell cultures to produce valuable terpenoids, particularly the *abeo*-abietane triexpoxide triptolide, has long been appreciated. The suspension cell cultures used here constitutively produce 53±3 μg/g of triptolide in the suspension cells and 4.0±0.2 mg/L in the medium, which is slightly lower than that of recently reported *Tripterygium* adventitious root cultures (90±80 μg/g in the adventitious roots and 4.7±0.9 mg/L in the medium). Here the utility of these cell cultures for investigation of triptolide biosynthesis was first demonstrated by not only finding that miltiradiene can be detected therein but also that feeding this olefin leads to increased accumulation, as well as the presence of several other plausible biosynthetic intermediates. Notably, it was further shown that triptolide biosynthesis can be induced by MeJA in these cultures, which further increases their utility by providing a means for co-expression analysis.

To begin to elucidate triptolide biosynthesis, an RNA-seq approach was taken to generate an induced suspension cell culture transcriptome. The utility of these sequence data was demonstrated by identification of the diterpene synthases involved in production of miltiradiene and, hence, triptolide biosynthesis. These were found to consist of not only the expected class Ⅱ diterpene cyclases that produce CPP, termed here TwTPS7v2 and TwTPS9v2, but also the unusual finding of a subsequently acting class Ⅰ diterpene synthase, TwTPS27v2, which is not from the TPS-e subfamily that typically provides such enzymes in labdane-related diterpenoid biosynthesis, rather being derived from the phylogenetically distinct TPS-b subfamily instead. While similar biochemical characterization has been very recently reported for both

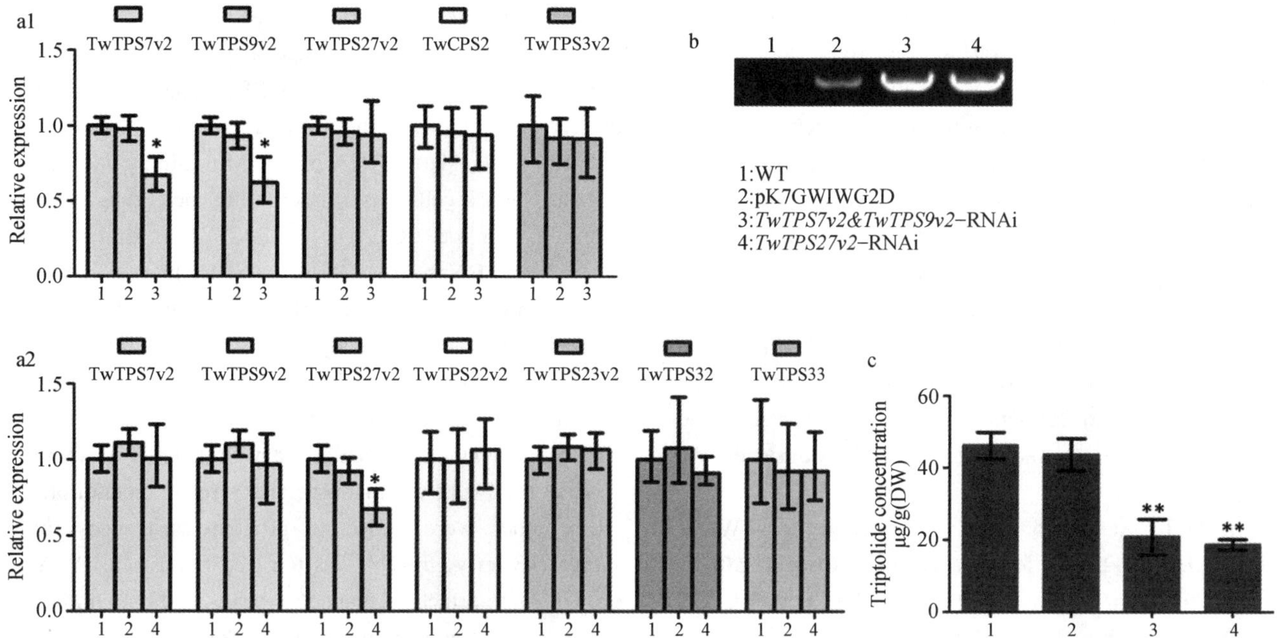


**Figure 9 Relative expression of *TwTPS7v2*, *TwTPS9v2*, *TwTPS27v2*, and closely related terpene synthase genes, as well as triptolide concentration in RNAi suspension cells**

(a1) Relative expression of *TwTPS7v2*, *TwTPS9v2*, *TwTPS27v2*, as well as the related TPS-c subfamily members *TwCPS2* and *TwTPS3v2* in *TwTPS7v2&TwTPS9v2*-RNAi suspension cells. (a2) Relative expression of *TwTPS7v2*, *TwTPS9v2*, and *TwTPS27v2*, as well as related TPS-b subfamily members *TwTPS22v2*, *TwTPS23v2*, *TwTPS32* and *TwTPS33*, in *TwTPS27v2*-RNAi suspension cells. (b) Presence of recombinant RNAi plasmids, as detected by PCR. (c) Triptolide concentration in RNAi suspension cells. The data represent the average±standard deviation of at least four independent lines of suspension cells (* $P<0.05$, ** $P<0.01$). Colour figure can be viewed at wileyonlinelibrary.com.

presumably allelic copies of these *T. wilfordii* diterpene synthases, as well as the orthologs from *T. regelii*, the data reported here go beyond this to unambiguously demonstrate the role of the characterized enzymes in triptolide biosynthesis. Most critically, in addition to showing subcellular localization of these enzymes to the plastid, where such diterpene biosynthesis occurs *in planta*, this includes genetic evidence, with RNAi knock-down of these genes leading to reduced triptolide levels. Thus, it is now clear that *TwTPS7v2*, *TwTPS9v2* and *TwTPS27v2* are involved in triptolide biosynthesis, and these then provide targets for *in planta* metabolic engineering efforts aimed at increasing yields of this valuable natural diterpenoid product. In addition, the unambiguous assignment of miltiradiene as the olefin precursor now enables further investigation of subsequently acting enzymes, such as cytochrome P450 monooxygenases, much as demonstrated in other (di) terpenoid biosynthetic networks, and enabled by the induced transcriptome reported here.

## 4 EXPERIMENTAL PROCEDURES

Plant material, chemicals and reagents The *T. wilfordii* suspension cells were cultured in Murashige and Skoog basal medium containing 0.5 mg/L 2, 4-dichlorophenoxyacetic acid (2,4-D), 0.1 mg/L kinetin (KT), 0.5 mg/L indole-3-buty-tric acid (IBA) and 30 g/L sucrose (pH = 5.8) by incubating in the dark at 25 ℃ on a rotary shaker. After 10 days of cultivation, induced suspension cells were treated with MeJA in carrier solution (dimethyl sulfoxide) at a final concentration of 50 μmol/L, while control cultures were only treated with same volume of carrier solution. *Nicotiana benthamiana* was grown in a greenhouse with a 16-h light/8-h dark cycle. Triptolide, wilforgine and wilforine were purchased from Chengdu Push Bio-Technology Co., Ltd (http://www.push-herbchem.com/en/). Celastrol, demethylzeylasteral and triptonide were purchased from Chengdu Must Bio-Technology Co., Ltd (http://chengdumust.en.china.cn/). Triptophenolide and neotriptophenolide were purchased from Shanghai yuanye Bio-Technology Co., Ltd (http://www.shyuanye.com/). Dehydroabietic acid, triptinin B and triptoquinonide were purchased from BioBioPha Co., Ltd (http://www.biobiopha.com/en). All other reagents were purchased from Merck (http://www.merck.com/).

Metabolite analysis of suspension cell cultures and native plants Solid samples were harvested and homogenized using Retsch MM400 mixer mill (Retsch GmbH, https://www.retsch.com/), and placed in an ultralow-temperature refrigerator at 80 ℃ for at least 4 h prior to freeze drying for 48 h (EYELA FDU-1110, http://www.eyelaworld.com/).

For each sample, aliquots of 50 mg were suspended in 1 mL of 80% (v/v) methanol overnight at room temperature 23 ℃, and then subjected to sonication in an ultrasonic water bath for 60 min. The supernatant was filtered through a 0.22 μm membrane filter (polytetrafluoroethylene) before further analysis. A medium aliquot of suspension cell cultures (generally 7.5 mL) was extracted twice with ethyl acetate (3 mL each time) by thorough mixing for 1 min at room temperature. The organic fractions were pooled and dried using a nitrogen evaporator (Baojingkeji, http://www.zz159.com/). The residue was redissolved in 300 μL of 80% methanol and passed through a 0.22 μm membrane filter prior to injection into the UPLC/Q-TOF MS system for analysis.

The UPLC separation was performed using a Waters Acquity UPLC™ I-Class system (Waters Corp., http://www.waters.com/) with a Waters ACQUITY UPLC HSS T3 analytical column (2.1×100 mm, 1.8 μm) kept at 40 ℃. The mobile phase, consisting of a mixture of 0.1% (v/v) acetic acid in water (A) and acetonitrile (B), was pumped at a flow rate of 0.5 mL/min. The gradient elution was programmed as follows: 0 min at 30% B, 6 min at 45% B, 18 min at 60% B, 23 min at 90% B. The TOF MS experiments were performed using a Xevo G2-S QTOF MS system (Waters Corp.). The experiment was performed in the ESI (+) ionization mode and the data acquisition mode was $MS^E$ continuum. The source and desolvation temperature were 100 ℃ and 450 ℃, respectively, and the desolvation gas flow rate was 900 L/h. The capillary voltage was 0.5 kV and the cone voltage was 40 V. The ramp collision energy was set as 20～40 eV for the high-energy scans. The data acquisition range was 50～1 500 Da. The mass accuracy was maintained using a lock spray with leucine enkephalin (200 pg/μL, 10 μL/min) as the reference [$m/z$ 556.277 1 ESI (+)]. Data analysis was performed using the UNIFI Scientific Information System (Waters Corp.). GC - MS analysis of the diterpene content of suspension cells is provided in the Method S1.

Feeding studies Miltiradiene (13.6 mg) in 200 μL of methanol/DMSO (1/1, v/v) was fed to freshly subcultured suspension cells cultures (about 1 g fresh weight of suspension cells in 10 mL MS media in 50 mL flasks), and cells in the control group were only treated with the same volume of carrier solution. After treatment, the cells were harvested in liquid nitrogen at 0, 1, 3 and 5 days, and the corresponding medium was stored at 4 ℃. All the media (about 10 mL) were extracted twice with ethyl acetate (5 mL each time) and the organic fractions were pooled dried in the 2.0 mL Eppendorf tube as described above. Solid samples were homogenized and freeze dried and about 80 mg was added to the 2.0 mL Eppendorf tube; samples were then extracted with 1.5 mL of 80% (v/v) as described above. The supernatant was filtered through a 0.22 μm membrane filter (polytetrafluoroethylene) for UPLC analysis. Additional details are provided in the Method S2.

RNA-seq Total RNA of the MeJA-induction 12 - 24 - 48 h suspension cells was isolated using the cetyltrimethylammonium bromide (CTAB) method. The total RNA was treated with RNase-free DNase I (NEB, https://www.neb.com/) and purified by a RNA Purification Kit (Tiangen Biotech, http://www.tiangen.com/en/). A total of 3 μg of purified RNA was used as input material for the RNA sample preparations. Sequencing libraries were generated using a NEBNext ® Ultra™ RNA Library Prep Kit for Illumina ® (NEB) following the manufacturer's recommendations, and index codes were added to attribute sequences to each sample. Briefly, mRNA was purified from total RNA using poly-T oligo-attached magnetic beads. Fragmentation was carried out using divalent cations under elevated temperature in NEBNext First Strand Synthesis Reaction Buffer (5×). First-strand cDNA was synthesized using random hexamer primer and M-MuLV Reverse Transcriptase (RNase $H^-$). Second-strand cDNA synthesis was subsequently performed using DNA Polymerase I and RNase H. Remaining overhangs were converted into blunt ends via exonuclease/polymerase activities. After adenylation of 3′ ends of DNA fragments, a NEBNext Adaptor with hairpin loop structure was ligated to prepare for hybridization. In order to preferentially select cDNA fragments of 150～200 bp in length, the library fragments were purified with AMPure XP system (Beckman Coulter, https://www.beckmancoulter.com/). Then 3 μL of USER Enzyme (NEB) was used with size-selected, adaptor-ligated cDNA at 37 ℃ for 15 min followed by 5 min at 95 ℃ before PCR. Then PCR was performed with Phusion High-Fidelity DNA polymerase, Universal PCR primers and Index (X) Primer. Finally, PCR products were purified (AMPure XP system), and library quality was assessed on the Agilent Bioanalyzer 2100 system.

The clustering of the index-coded samples was performed on a cBot Cluster Generation System using TruSeq PE Cluster Kit v3 - cBot - HS (Illumina, https://www.illumina.com/) according to the manufacturer's instructions. After cluster generation, the library preparations were sequenced on an Illumina Hiseq 2 000 platform and paired-end reads were generated. Over 95% of these reads (63 401 185) were judged to be clean and were used for further analysis. The left files (read1 files) from all libraries/samples were pooled into one big left.fq file, and the right files (read2 files) into one big right.fq file. Transcriptome assembly was accomplished based on left.fq and right.fq using Trinity with min_kmer_cov set to 2 by default and all other parameters also set to their default values. Gene function was annotated based on the following databases: Nr, Nt, Pfam, KOG/COG, Swiss-Prot, KO and GO.

RACE and gene cloning Purified RNA was used to synthesize the 3′- or 5′-RACE-ready cDNA with the SMARTer™ RACE cDNA Amplification Kit (Clontech Laboratories, http://www.clontech.com/). To acquire the full-length cDNA sequences it was necessary to perform 3′- and 5′-RACE reactions, which were done following the user's manual and using gene-specific primers based on the corresponding sequences from the *T. wilfordii* transcriptome sequencing dataset (Table S7). The full-length ORFs were cloned by PCR amplification using Pri-meSTAR GXL DNA Polymerase (Takara Biotechnology, http://www.takara-bio.com/), according to the manufacturer's instructions, then ligated into the pMD19-T vector (Takara Biotechnology) and verified by complete sequencing.

Sequence analysis The sequences of the cDNA for *TwTPS7v2*, *TwCPS2*, *TwTPS3v2*, *TwTPS9v2*, *TwTPS27v2*, *TwKSL1* and *TwTPS16v2* were analyzed at NCBI (http://www.ncbi.nlm.nih.gov/). The ORFs and deduced amino acid sequences were determined using the online tool ORF Finder (http://www.ncbi.nlm.nih.gov/gorf/gorf.html) and the ExPASy online tool (http://web.expasy.org/translate/), respectively.

Although none of the *T. wilfordii* diterpene synthases identified here were exactly identical to those recently reported by others, most were similar enough to be allelic and were named accordingly. In particular, given the 96.8%, 98.9%, 99.3%, 98.5% and 98.0% identities (at the amino acid sequence level) to the previously characterized *ent*-CPP synthase TwTPS3, CPP synthases TwTPS7 and TwTPS9, 16α-hydroxy-*ent*-kaurane synthase TwTPS16 and miltiradiene synthase TwTPS27, the corresponding enzymes were named TwTPS3v2, TwTPS7v2, TwTPS9v2, TwTPS16v2 and TwTPS27v2, respectively. By contrast, TwKSL1 shares <95% identity with any of the previously characterized diterpene synthases.

For phylogenetic analysis, amino acid sequences for a variety of diterpene synthases were obtained from the NCBI database (Table S8), and a tree was constructed with the MEGA6 software package using the neighbor-joining method. One thousand bootstrap replicates were performed in each analysis to define the level of confidence support.

Subcellular localization All constructs for *N. benthamiana* transformation were prepared using the E3025 vector, which contains a gene for GFP driven by the 35S promoter; the specific primers are listed in Table S7. The recombinant plasmids containing the ORFs of the targeted diterpene synthase(s) were first transformed into *Agrobacterium tumefaciens* EHA105, then injected to the *N. benthamiana* leaves, with subsequent observation via confocal laser scanning microscopy. Detailed information on subcellular localization analysis is given in the Method S3.

MeJA induction and UPLC analysis After 10 days of cultivation the suspension cells were treated with MeJA in carrier solution (dimethyl sulfoxide) at a final concentration of 50 μmol/L, while cells in the control group were only treated with the same volume of carrier solution. Post-induction cells were harvested in liquid nitrogen after 0, 1, 4, 12, 24, 48, 72, 120 and 240 h. Three samples were prepared for each time point in each group for UPLC analysis. Additional details are provided in the Method S2.

Quantitative RT-PCR analysis The suspension cells harvested for UPLC analysis were also used for real-time gene expression analysis following the procedure previously described. Expression levels were evaluated using the $2^{-\Delta\Delta Ct}$ method based on β-actin as the reference gene, with triplicate measurements from three biological replicates.

Recombinant expression The relevant ORFs were amplified by PCR using PrimeSTAR GXL DNA Polymerase and gene-specific primers (Table S7), then ligated into pMD19-T followed by complete sequencing and subcloning into the N-terminal MBP fusion expression vector pMAL-c2X (NEB). The ORF for *AtKS* was amplified from an *Arabidopsis thaliana* cDNA library and subcloned into the pMAL-c2X vector. *Salvia miltiorrhiza SmCPS1* and *SmMS* ORFs were subcloned into the pET32a(+) vector.

The recombinant plasmids were transformed into *E. coli TransB* (DE3) for heterologous expression using the empty pMAL-c2X vector as a negative control. Cultures (200 mL) were grown in Luria-Bertani (LB) medium (10 g/L Tryptone, 5 g/L yeast extract, 10 g/L NaCl) containing 100 mg/L ampicillin until the optical density of the culture at 600 nm reached 0.6~0.8, then induced with 0.4 mmol/L isopropyl 1-thio-β-D-galactopyranoside (Sigma, http://www.sigmaaldrich.com/) and grown at 16 ℃ for 8 h at 200 rpm. The cell pellets were harvested by centrifugation (3 000 *g*, 20 min, 4 ℃) and resuspended in 5 mL of assay buffer [50 mmol/L HEPES, pH 7.2, 7.5 mmol/L $MgCl_2$, 100 mmol/L KCl, 5 mmol/L DTT and 5% (v/v) glycerol] and lysed by a sonicator on ice. The lysates were centrifuged (12 000 *g*, 30 min, 4 ℃) to produce soluble extracts, which were then concentrated using Amicon Ultra-15 centrifugal filter unit with Ultracel-30 membrane (Merck Millipore, http://www.merckmillipore.com/), according to the manufacturer's instructions.

*In vitro* cell-free assays To determine the catalytic activity of the recombinant proteins, 200 μmol/L GGPP (Sigma-Aldrich) was added to 0.2 mL of recombinant cell-free extracts, incubated for 2 h at 25 ℃ in the dark and then extracted with hexane (3 × 0.5 mL). Residual organic solvent was removed under a stream of $N_2$ before adding

10 units of calf intestinal phosphatase (CIP; NEB), and then incubating for 4 h at 37℃ to allow enzymatic dephosphorylation. A standard for CPP was produced by incubation of SmCPS1 with GGPP for 2 h at 25℃, with dephosphorylation by CIP as above. The dephosphorylated compounds were extracted with hexane (3×0.5 mL), with the organic extracts then completely dried under $N_2$ and the residue dissolved in 60 μL of hexanes for GC-MS analysis.

Coupled assays were performed to determine the stereochemistry of CPP much as previously described. Briefly, assays containing each class II TwTPS and GGPP were preincubated for 2 h at 25℃, at which point equivalent volumes of cell-free extracts from individually expressed diterpene synthases (AtKS, SmMS, TwTPS27v2, TwKSL1 or TwTPS16v2) were added, along with $MgCl_2$ to a final concentration of 10 mmol/L. These reactions were then incubated overnight at room temperature before extraction with hexane (3×0.5 mL) and subsequent GC-MS analysis. Production of 16α-hydroxy-*ent*-kaurane was confirmed by comparison with an authentic sample isolated from gametophores of the moss *Physcomitrella patens*.

Yeast expression To confirm the results of the *in vitro* cell-free assays, the ORFs of single functional class II diterpene cyclases, as well as the functional enzymatic pairings, were PCR-amplified using gene-specific primers (Table S7) then sub-cloned into the yeast epitope-tagging vector pESC-Trp (Agilent Technologies, http://www.agilent.com/) via digestion by the corresponding restriction endonucleases. The resulting plasmids were transformed into the yeast BY-T20 strain (BY4742, *ΔTrp1*, *Trp1*::*HIS3*-$P_{PGK1}$-*BTS1*/*ERG20*-$T_{ADH1}$-$P_{TDH3}$-*SaGGPS*-$T_{TPI1}$-$P_{TEF1}$-*tHMG1*-$T_{CYC1}$), which produces the GGPP substrate, and then enzymatic activity was analyzed much as previously described. Briefly, organic extracts were dried and the residues dissolved in 60 μL of hexanes for GC-MS analysis as described above.

Analysis of TwKSL1 in *E. coli* To identify the products of TwKSL1 it was transferred to pET44a, using the *Bam*HI and *Xho*I restriction sites. This was used for expression in *E. coli* strain C41 OverExpress (Lucigen, http://www.lucigen.com/) also engineered to produce *ent*-CPP, using a previously described modular metabolic engineering system. The resulting recombinant strain was grown in 50 mL of TB media, shaken at 200 rpm, first at 37℃ to approximately $OD_{600}$~0.8, then shifted to 16℃ for 1 h before induction with 1 mmol/L IPTG, following which the culture was further shaken at 16℃ for 3 days. The resulting TwKSL1 products were directly extracted with an equal volume of hexanes, and were then separated, dried under a gentle stream of $N_2$ and the residue resuspended in 500 μL of hexanes, with 1 μL then subjected to GC-MS analysis. Compounds were identified by comparison of the retention time and mass spectra with previously characterized enzymatic products.

Yeast two-hybrid assays To test the interactions of TwTPS27v2 and TwTPS7v2, as well as TwTPS27v2 and TwTPS9v2, TwTPS27v2 was fused with the BD domain in the pGBKT7 vector, and TwTPS7v2 and TwTPS9v2 were individually fused with the AD domain in the pGADT7 vector. Primers used for the constructs are listed in Table S7. To assess protein interactions yeast two-hybrid assays were performed using the yeast strain *S. cerevisiae* AH109, as previously described.

Engineering yeast for miltiradiene production To examine the catalytic efficiency of TwTPS7v2 versus TwTPS9v2, they were both subcloned into the vector pESC-Trp and the resulting vector used for their co-expression in the yeast BY-T20 strain. The induced yeast cells (20 mL, cultivated for 48 h in SD-Trp-His liquid induction medium supplemented with 20 g/L D-galactose) were extracted and analyzed by GC-MS as described above.

To examine the ability of fusion to improve the yield of miltiradiene, TwTPS7v2 was fused with TwTPS27v2. We constructed two modules producing the fused proteins TwTPS27v2-TwTPS7v2 and TwTPS7v2-TwTPS27v2 by inserting a widely used GGGS linker encoded by a 'GGT GGT GGT TCT' sequence, according to the protocol of *pEASY* ®-Uni Seamless Cloning and Assembly Kit (TransGen Biotech, http://www.transbionovo.com/). The recombinant plasmids pESC-Trp::TwTPS7v2/TwTPS27v2, pESC-Trp::TwTPS7v2-TwTPS27v2 and pESC-Trp::TwTPS27v2-TwTPS7v2 were transformed into BY-T20, induced with D-galactose. The products were then analyzed by GC-MS as described above. Linear calibration was performed to calculate the yield of miltiradiene ($R^2$=0.9997).

Site-directed mutagenesis of TwCPS2 and TwTPS16v2 Site-directed mutagenesis of the DXDD motif of TwCPS2 (DTD$\underline{C}^{311}$TAM to DTD$\underline{D}^{311}$TAM) and the active site of TwTPS16v2 (DLLKS$\underline{A}^{608}$LRE to DLLKS$\underline{M}^{608}$LRE) were performed with the relevant pMAL-c2X construct using mutagenic primers (Table S7) and the Fast Mutagenesis System (TransGen Biotech), according to the manufacturer's instructions. Expression and functional characterization of these mutants was carried out as described above.

## 5 RNAi

Vector pK7GWIWG2D (Invitrogen, http://www.invitrogen.com/) was used for RNAi targeting of *TwTPS7v2* and *TwTPS9v2*, or *TwTPS27v2*, in suspension cells. Briefly, fragments of *TwTPS7v2*/*TwTPS9v2* or *TwTPS27v2* were ligated to the vector pK7GWIWG2D using the Gateway cloning system (Invitrogen) and the resulting vectors were transformed into suspension cells.

Suspension cells in the logarithmic growth phase were plated on MS solid medium supplemented with 0.5 mg/L 2,4-D, 0.1 mg/L KT, 0.5 mg/L IBA and 30 g/L sucrose (pH=5.8) and grown for 7 days before bombardment. Then the recombinant plasmids were transformed into the cells using a biolistic gene gun (PDS 100/He, Bio-Rad, http://www.bio-rad.com/). Each transformation was performed twice. The resulting recombinant cells were cultured for 7 days before UPLC analysis. Additional details are provided in the Method S4.

## 6 ACCESSION NUMBERS

The Illumina-derived nucleotide sequences reported in this paper have been submitted to the short-read archive (SRA) at NCBI with the following accession numbers: SRR6001265. Sequence data from this article can be found in the GenBank/EMBL data libraries with the following accession numbers: TwTPS7v2 (AKM28412); TwCPS2 (AKM28413); TwTPS3v2 (AKM28414); TwTPS9v2 (KX931054); TwTPS27v2 (ARQ20737); TwKSL1 (KX931055); TwTPS16v2 (AKM28415).

[苏平,黄璐琦,高伟,等.The Plant Journal, 2018,93:50－65.]

# CYP76B74 catalyzes the 3″-hydroxylation of geranylhydroquinone in shikonin biosynthesis

*Arnebia euchroma*, a perennial herbaceous boraginaceaeous plant, is found in Pamirs, Tian-Shan Mountains, Himalayas, and in western Tibet at an altitudinal range of 3,700 to 4,200 m above sea level. *A. euchroma* is an important commodity in food, cosmetics, and modern pharmaceutical industries, mostly due to its high content of red naphthoquinone pigments (shikonin derivatives) in the root bark (cork layers). Recent studies have demonstrated that shikonin derivatives exhibit diverse biological activities, such as antioxidant, antibacterial, and anticancer activities, which endow them with a high potential for use in drug development.

The naphthoquinone derivatives are a group of prevalent natural products that include juglone, plumbagin, shikonin, lapachol, vitamin K1, vitamin K2, and vitamin K3. Most of their naphthoquinone skeletons are proposed to be generated either by the acetate-malonate pathway involving polyketide synthases, as in the case of fusarubin from *Fusarium fujikuroi*, or the Phe pathway, as for menaquinone biosynthesis. Shikonins, however, are a special subgroup synthesized via the 4-hydroxybenzoic acid/geranyl diphosphate (GPP) pathway with subsequent ring closure reactions (Fig. 1). This special biosynthetic pathway of shikonins represents an expanding understanding of biosynthetic pathways of naphthoquinone derivatives in nature, especially in plants. Confirmation of this route for the formation of the naphthoquinone skeleton would delineate a new metabolic pathway of naphthoquinone derivatives. For these reasons, in vitro biochemical assays and reverse genetics have been employed in the study of shikonin biosynthesis and its regulation.

The first committed step of the shikonin biosynthetic pathway is the condensation of 4-hydroxybenzoic acid and GPP catalyzed by 4-hydroxybenzoate geranyltransferase (also named PGT). After the PGT-catalyzed reaction, little is known about the ring closure reactions that generate the naphthoquinone skeleton. It is generally accepted that the PGT product 3-geranyl-4-hydroxybenzolic acid (GBA) undergoes decarboxylation and hydroxylation of the C-1 position, leading to the generation of geranylhydroquinone (GHQ). After that, hydroxylation of C-3″ of the isoprenoid side chain of GHQ provides the key intermediate 3″-hydroxy-geranylhydroquinone (GHQ-3″-OH) for cyclization to form quinones. The enzyme that catalyzes this reaction, geranylhydroquinone 3″-hydroxylase (GHQ3″H), was once partially purified from the microsomal fraction of nonpigmented *Lithospermum erythrorhizon* suspension cultures and shown to require NADPH and molecular oxygen, suggesting that it is a cytochrome P450 (CYP)-dependent monooxygenase. Until now, the GHQ3″H has never been characterized at the molecular level. The identity, regulation, and phylogeny of the gene encoding this protein remain to be understood.

Previously, we established two types of cultured cells from *A. euchroma* hypocotyls, a red shikonin-proficient (SP) cell line and a white shikonin-deficient cell line, which responded differently to the elicitation by methyl jasmonate. Specialized metabolite contents (shikonins, shikofurans, and phenolic acids) and the expression levels of key enzymatic genes involved in their biosynthesis changed differentially for the two cell lines under elicitation. Here, we performed transcriptome analysis of the two cell lines, combined with in

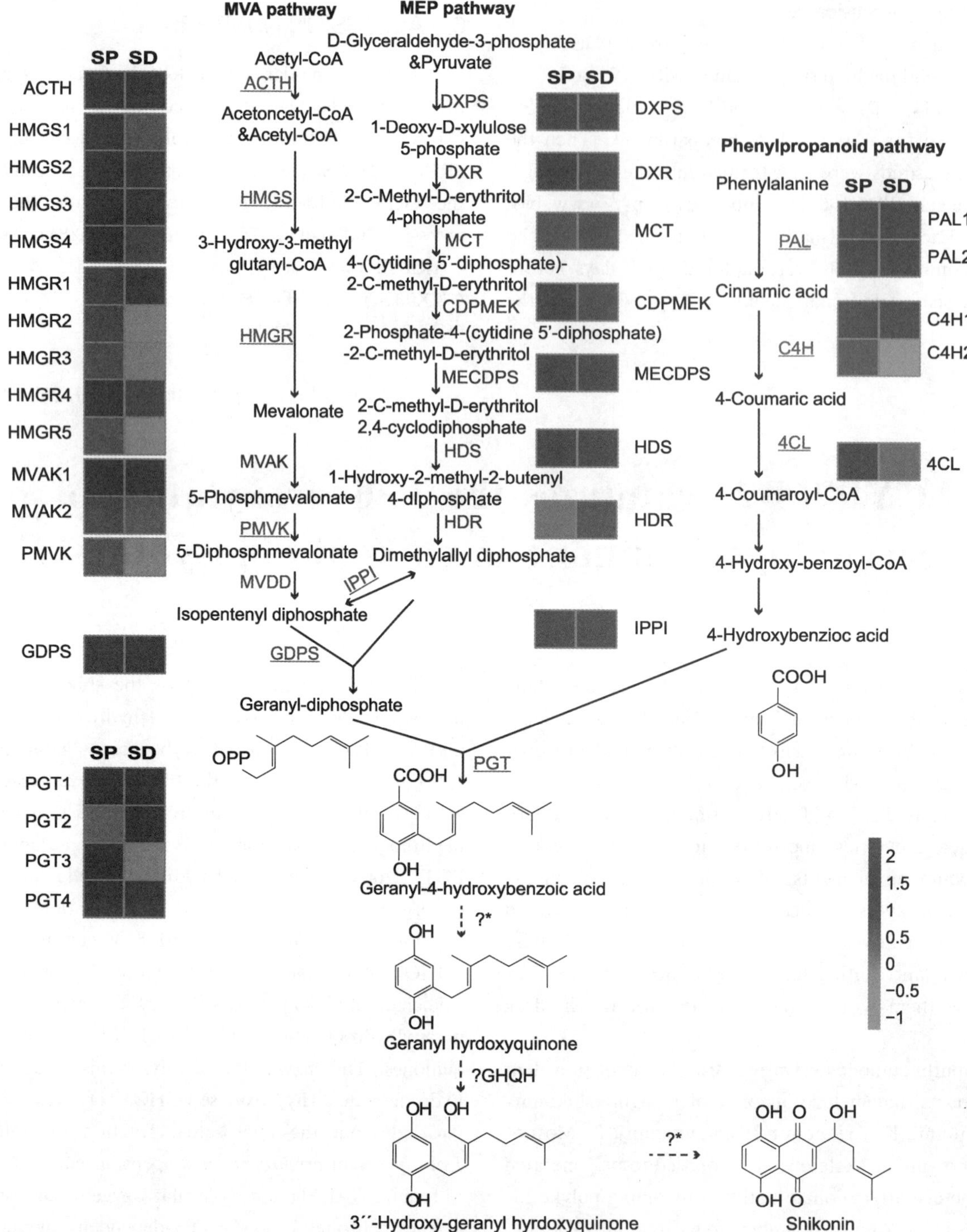


**Figure 1 Expression of unigenes involved in shikonin biosynthesis in shikonin-proficient (SP) and shikonin-deficient (SD) cell lines of *A. euchroma***

Data are from comparative transcriptome analyses of the SP and SD lines. The up-regulated genes in the SP cell line compared with the SD cell line are underlined and marked in red, and genes that are down-regulated or not significantly different are marked in green. Uncharacterized steps are shown with dotted arrows. ? indicates that one step is unknown, and?* indicates that several steps are unknown. MVA, Mevalonate; MEP, 2-*C*-methyl-D-erythritol-4-phosphate; HMGS, 3-hydroxy-3-methylglutaryl-CoA synthase; HMGR, 3-hydroxy-3-methylglutaryl-CoA reductase; MVAK, mevalonate 5-phosphokinase; PMVK, 5-phosphomevalonate phosphokinase; MVDD, mevalonate diphosphate decarboxylase; DXPS, 1-deoxy-D-xylulose-5-phosphate synthase; DXR, 1-deoxy-D-xylulose-5-phosphate reductoisomerase; MCT, 2-*C*-methyl-D-erythritol 4-phosphate cytidylyltransferase; CDPMEK, 4-(cytidine 5′-diphospho)-2-*C*-methyl-D-erythritol 2-phosphokinase; MECDPS, 2-*C*-methyl-D-erythritol 2,4-cyclodiphosphate synthase; HDS, 1-hydroxy-2-methyl-2-butenyl-diphosphate synthase; HDR, 1-hydroxy-2-methyl-2-(*E*)-butenyl-4-diphosphate reductase; IPPI, isopentenyl pyrophosphate isomerase; GDPS, geranyldiphosphate synthase; PAL, phenylalanine ammonia lyase; C4H, cinnamic acid 4-hydroxylase; 4CL, 4-coumaroyl-CoA ligase; PGT, 4-hydroxybenzoate-3-geranyltransferase; GHQH, geranylhydroquinone 3″-hydroxylase.

vitro biochemical assays, subcellular localization analysis, and RNA interference (RNAi), to characterize a candidate CYP gene, *CYP76B74*. Our results indicate that CYP76B74 catalyzes the key 3″-hydroxylation step in the shikonin biosynthetic pathway with high efficiency. The characterization of GHQ3″H paves the way for further exploration of the ring closure reactions generating the naphthoquinone skeleton in Boraginaceae and for the alternative metabolization of GHQ-3″-OH to dihydroechinofuran.

## 1 RESULTS

Discovery of CYP Candidate Genes The differentially expressed transcripts of SP and shikonin-deficient (SD) *A. euchroma* suspension culture cell lines were mined in order to discover possible enzymes involved in shikonin biosynthesis, with a main focus on identifying the GHQ3″H. Two cDNA libraries were prepared from the SP and SD cell lines and then sequenced on an Illumina HiSeq 2000 platform to obtain an overview of genes associated with the shikonin biosynthetic pathway. After raw data filtration and de novo assembly, 103,294 unigenes with N50 length (median length of all nonredundant sequences) of 1,110 bp were generated in the SP library and 100,627 unigenes with N50 length of 1,267 bp were generated in the SD library. From these populations, a total of 121,239 unigenes with N50 length of 1,565 bp were sequenced and bioinformatically processed. The functional annotation of all assembled unigenes was cataloged using six public databases (i.e. Nonredundant Protein Sequence, Nucleotide Sequence, SwissProt, Kyoto Encyclopedia of Genes and Genomes, Clusters of Orthologous Groups of Proteins, and Gene Ontology). As a result, a total of 78,947 unigenes (65.12%) in the SP and SD libraries were annotated in at least one of the above databases.

Based on their annotation, a series of unigenes were found to be related to shikonin biosynthesis according to previous reports (Fig. 1). Most unigenes involved in the shikonin biosynthetic pathway were up-regulated in the SP cell line compared with the SD cell line, such as *HMGR*, *PAL*, and *PGT* genes. This suggested that the transcriptomes could be used to facilitate the discovery of genes involved in the shikonin biosynthetic pathway efficiently based on their coexpression patterns. Additionally, all unigenes related to the mevalonate pathway and the phenylpropanoid pathway were up-regulated, while unigenes related to the methylerythritol 4-phosphate pathway were not. These results support the mevalonate pathway as a preferred route of GPP supply for shikonin biosynthesis in *A. euchroma*.

Coexpression analysis of the transcriptome data set focused on CYP genes whose expression profiles matched those of genes known to encode enzymes that catalyze the early steps of shikonin biosynthesis in an attempt to identify candidates responsible for subse-quent steps. Analysis of the annotated transcriptome data set revealed the presence of approximately 480 *CYP* contigs, which included both full-length and partial cDNA sequences. Analysis of differentially expressed unigenes using a stringent threshold (i.e. $\log_2$[ratio] $\geqslant 1$, false discovery rate $< 0.001$, and maximum [fragments per kilobase per million mapped fragments] $\geqslant 1$) led to the detection of 99 differentially expressed *CYPs*, of which 78 were up-regulated in the SP cell line compared with the SD cell line. This population of *CYP* unigenes was selected for investigation on the basis of their significant increase in transcript levels and integrity of the open reading frame. The search was limited to *CYP* unigenes up-regulated in the SP cell line due to the properties (require NADPH and molecular oxygen) of LeGHQ3″H described by Yamamoto et al., suggesting that it is a CYP-dependent monooxygenase. Unigenes with an open reading frame less than 1,200 bp were abandoned, given the average length of plant *CYPs*. This led to 21 *CYP* candidates that may be involved in shikonin biosynthesis. For each initial candidate, detailed information and BLAST search results are displayed in Supplemental Table S1.

Given the accumulation of shikonin in the root, as well as the previously demonstrated tissue-specific transcription of other secondary metabolites, we hypothesized that shikonin biosynthetic enzymes would be expressed specifically in the root. The relative expression of each of the 21 up-regulated candidates was thus analyzed in the roots and leaves of *A. euchroma* by reverse transcription quantitative PCR (RT-qPCR; Fig. 2). Transcripts for 12 of the 21 candidates were found to be more abundant in the root, four in the leaf, and five showed no significant differential expression. The 12 unigenes showing higher expression in root (framed in Fig. 2) were selected as candidates for further functional screening.

Gene-specific primers were derived and led to the amplification of transcripts from SP cells of *A. euchroma*. The 12 CYP candidates, marked in boldface in Supplemental Table S2, then were cloned to enable further biochemical assays using GHQ as the substrate. The proteins were named based on the standardized CYP nomenclature system (Nelson, 2009; i.e. CYP76A74, CYP706G18, CYP734A49, CYP76A46, CYP82AR1, CYP707A137, CYP73A155, CYP73A64, CYP76A48, CYP76B75, CYP76B74, and CYP88A76).

In Vitro Enzyme Activity Assays for CYP Candidates CYP candidates were heterologously expressed in *Saccharomyces cerevisiae* strain BY - T20 (BY4742). The ability of these CYP candidates to react with GHQ was examined by in vitro assay using microsomal preparations from the resulting recombinant yeast.

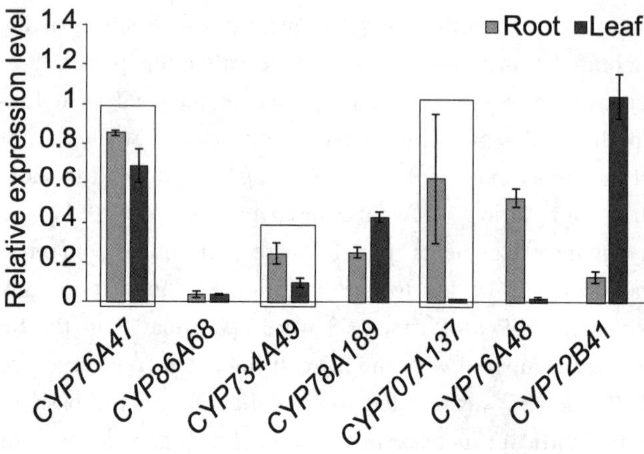


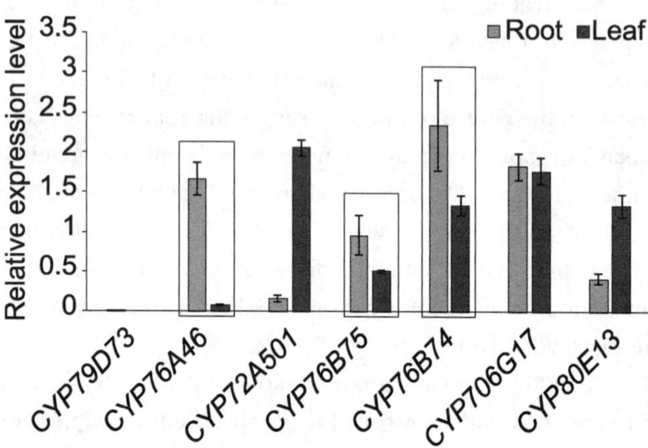


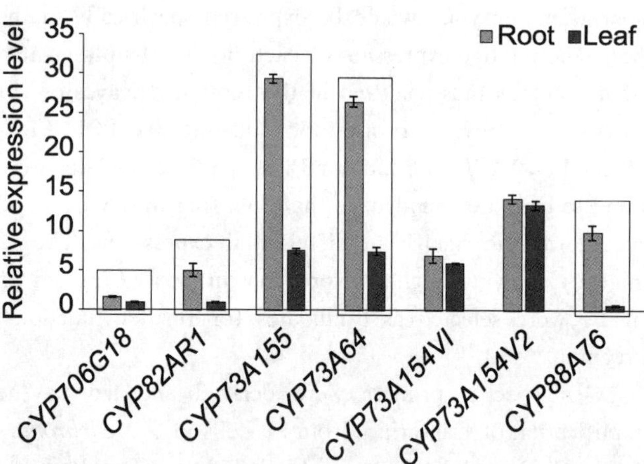


**Figure 2 RT-qPCR analysis of the 21 candidate unigenes in roots and leaves of *A. euchroma***

The error bars in the RT-qPCR results represent SE of three biological replicates consisting of different plants. Unigenes with higher abundance in roots than in leaves are framed.

In the presence of NADPH, only one of the proteins (designated CYP76B74 by the Cytochrome P450 Nomenclature Committee) was found to catalyze the conversion of GHQ to its hydroxide (Fig. 3), as confirmed by liquid chromatography-mass spectrometry (LC-MS). No product formation was found in assays that contained microsomes from yeast cells harboring the empty vector, and none of the other 11 CYPs were able to react with GHQ under the identical assay conditions (Supplemental Fig. S1). After large-scale enzymatic reactions, the oxidized product was purified by preparative HPLC and verified to be GHQ3″H by mass spectrometry and by $^1$H-NMR and $^{13}$C-NMR spectroscopy (Supplemental Figs. S2 and S3).

The results of steady-state kinetic analysis, in the presence of excess NADPH, demonstrated that CYP76B74 efficiently catalyzed the conversion of GHQ to GHQ-3″-OH, with $K_m = 23 \pm 6$ μmol/L and $V_{max} = 8.3 \pm 0.8$ μmol product mmol$^{-1}$ protein min$^{-1}$ (Fig. 4). This $K_m$ is in the same range as the $K_m$ of the CYP76B6 homolog from *Catharanthus roseus* for its substrate geraniol (15.81 μmol/L). These results suggest that GHQ might be the natural substrate of this hydroxylase, CYP76B74, in *A. euchroma*.

The ability of CYP76B74 to react with GBA was assayed under the same conditions used for GHQ (Supplemental Fig. S4). CYP76B74 was found to weakly catalyze the conversion of GBA to its hydroxide. Only a trace amount of hydroxylated GBA can be detected by HPLC, and there was less than 10% of the substrate metabolized when the reaction was left overnight on an incubator shaking at 150 rpm at 28 ℃. Under the same conditions, almost all GHQ was metabolized. Without an authentic reference product, the $K_m$ and $V_{max}$ of recombinant CYP76B74 for GBA were too difficult to determine. This is consistent with the previous findings when microsomes from *L. erythrorhizon* cell suspension cultures were used.

Physiological Function of CYP76B74 in Vivo To provide more definitive evidence for CYP76B74 involvement in shikonin biosynthesis, an RNAi approach was used to knock down its gene expression in *A. euchroma* hairy roots. A less conserved and unique fragment in the upstream coding region (nucleotides 83 – 492 of the cDNA) of *CYP76B74* was cloned into the plant expression vector pK7GWIWG2D(II), which expresses self-complementary hairpin RNA fragments that induce silencing. pK7GWIWG2D-*CYP76B74* and pK7GWIWG2D-control were transfected via *Agro-bacterium rhizogenes* into explants of *A. euchroma* to produce recombinant hairy roots.

Independent hairy root lines generated on plates were transferred to triangular flasks for liquid culture and processed further for gene expression and metabolite analysis. RT-qPCR indicated that the expression of *CYP76B74* was suppressed efficiently in transformed hairy root lines (Fig. 5A). Interestingly, the expression of *AeHMGR*, *Ae4CL*, *AeC4H*, and *AePGT6* involved in shikonin biosynthesis also was repressed in RNAi-*cyp76b74* lines (Supplemental Fig. S5), suggesting a critical role of CYP76B74 in the regulation of shikonin biosynthesis.

Because of shikonin accumulation, the roots and the hairy roots of *A. euchroma* appear red, the characteristic

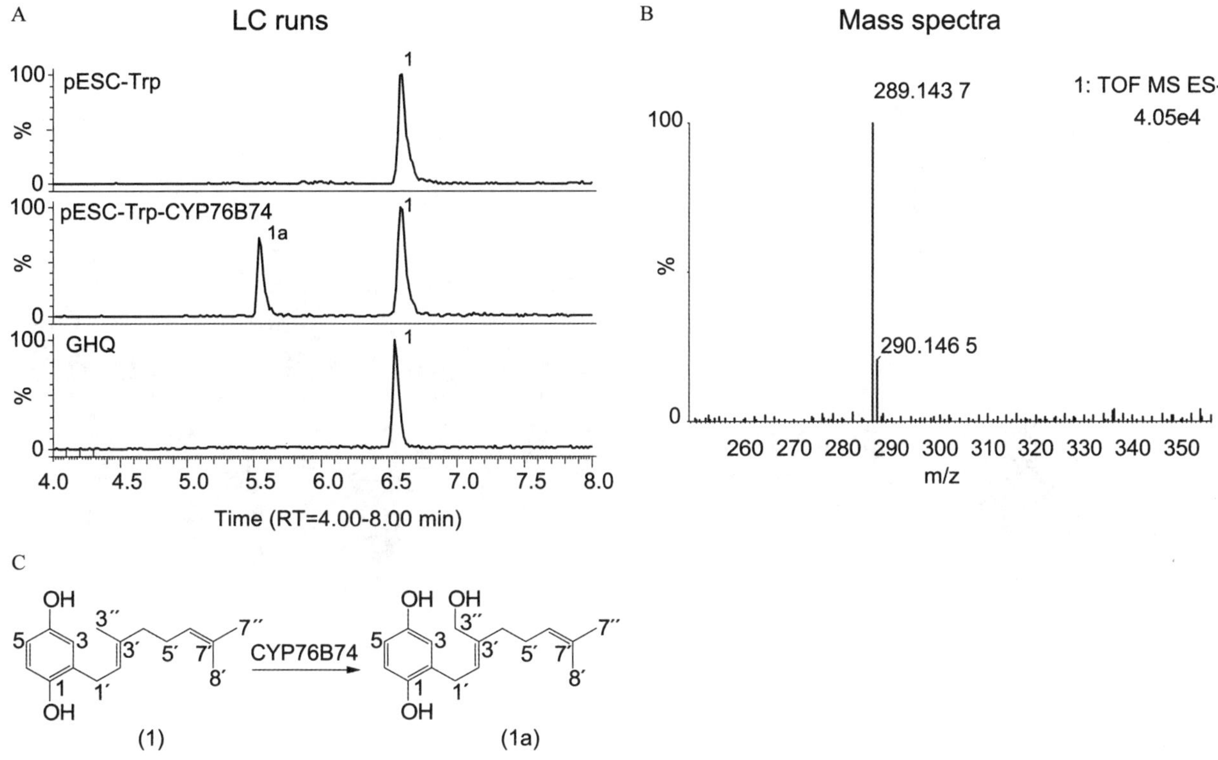


**Figure 3 LC-MS/MS analysis of the recombinant CYP76B74 enzyme assays using GHQ as the substrate. The assay samples were incubated with shaking for 4 h at 28 ℃**

(A) LC-MS chromatograms of extracts from the reaction containing CYP76B74 microsomes with NADPH (pESC-Trp-CYP76B74), empty vector control (pESC-Trp), and microsome-free control (GHQ). (B) Mass spectrum of the reaction product. (C) Direct conversion of GHQ (1) to GHQ-3″-OH (1a).

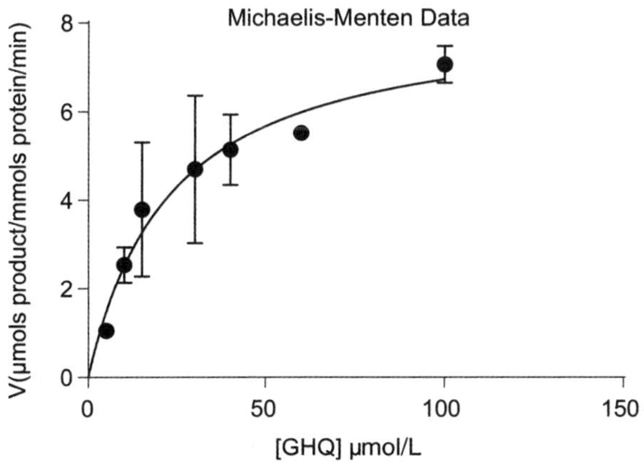


**Figure 4 Kinetic profile of CYP76B74. Experimental details are included in "Materials and Methods"**

The error bars in the kinetics results represent SE of three technical replicates consisting of different reactions.

color of shikonin and its derivatives. The transformed hairy roots grown on plates were observed with a stereoscopic microscope. The readily perceivable color difference between RNAi-*cyp76b74* (Fig. 5Ca) and control lines (Fig. 5Cb) indicated that the accumulation of shikonins was indeed suppressed in RNAi-*cyp76b74* lines. Given the autofluorescence of shikonin derivatives, root tips also were observed using two-photon confocal microscopy. The resulting photomicrographs demonstrated that the accumulation of shikonin derivatives was high in the control lines and almost absent in RNAi-*cyp76b74* lines (Fig. 5C, c–h).

After individual hairy root lines were cultured in liquid medium for 10 d (Fig. 5B), shikonin derivative contents were quantified in root tissues (Fig. 5D) and culture medium (Fig. 5E) by HPLC. Suppression of *CYP76B74* seems to alter the root growth: roots are much shorter, thicker, and have fewer branches, but there is no change in biomass based on the weight of fresh roots, because of its surrounding spongy tissue. The total shikonin content compared with the control decreased about 8-fold in RNAi-*cyp76b74* hairy roots and 9-fold in the culture medium. Among the shikonin derivatives quantified, isovalerylshikonin, isobutyrylshikonin, acetoxylisovalerylshikonin, acetylshikonin, and $\beta$-hydroxyisovalerylshikonin were reduced by an average of about 4- to 7-fold in RNAi-*cyp76b74* hairy roots. And the accumulation of acetoxylisovalerylshikonin was reduced strongly to almost absent by an average of 36-fold in RNAi-*cyp76b74* hairy roots compared with the control and 476-fold in the culture medium. The positive association between the expression of *CYP76B74* and shikonin accumulation thus supports the requirement of this CYP for the production of shikonins in the plant.

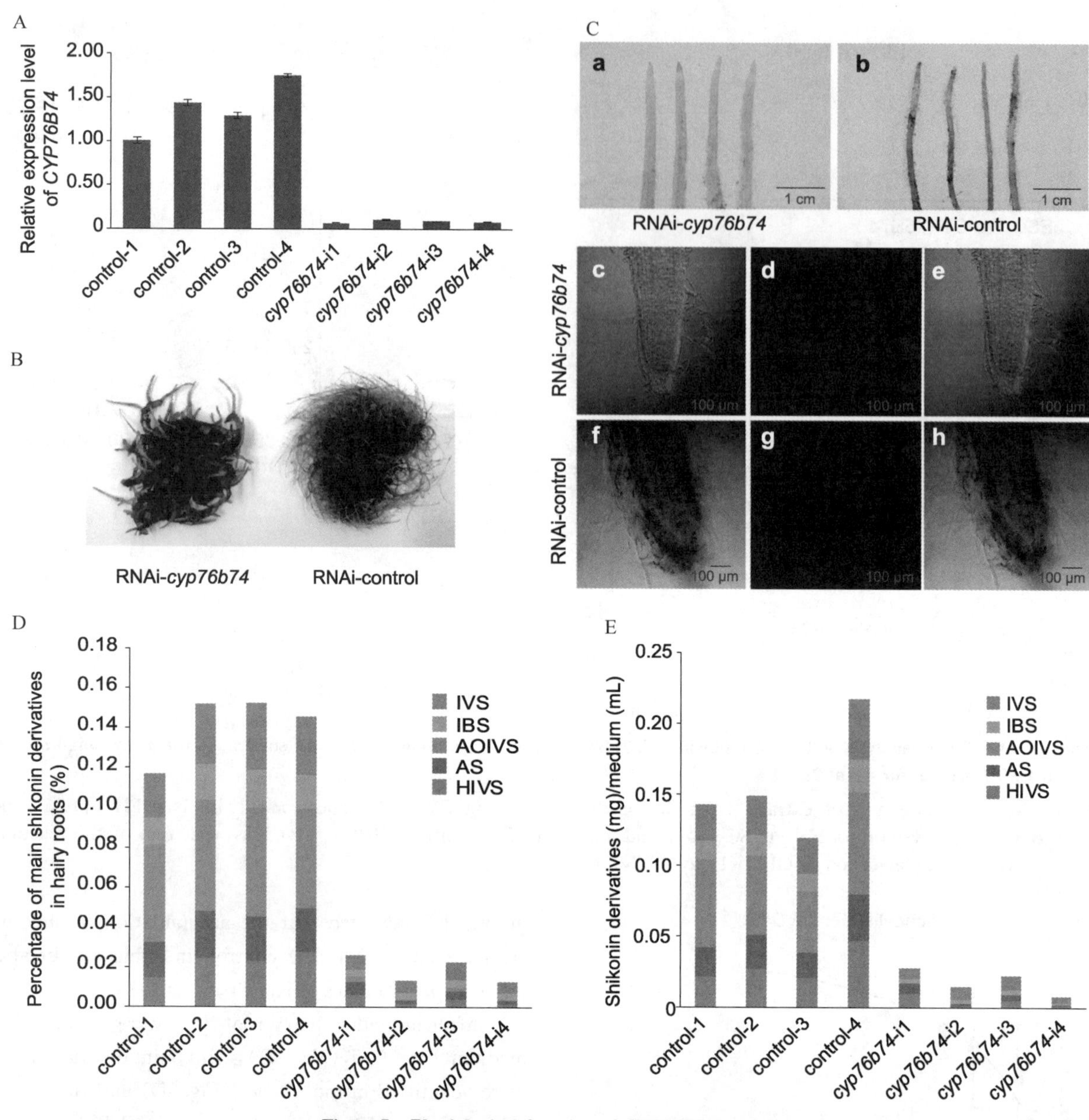


**Figure 5 Physiological function of CYP76B74 in vivo**

(A) Expression levels of *CYP76B74* in hairy roots of the four independent RNAi-*cyp76b74* lines and the control. (B) Phenotypes of RNAi-*cyp76b74* lines and the control cultured for 10 d in liquid medium. (C) Phenotypes of RNAi-*cyp76b74* lines and the control cultured on a plate using a stereoscopic microscope (a and b) and the root tips by two-photon confocal microscopy (c-h). c and f, Bright-field microscopy of root tips; d and g, shikonin autofluorescence field microscopy of root tips; e and h, merged fields of bright-field and shikonin autofluorescence. (D) Percentage of main shikonin derivatives in the dry weight of the four independent RNAi-*cyp76b74* hairy root lines and the control. (E) Contents of main shikonin derivatives in culture medium of the four independent RNAi-*cyp76b74* hairy root lines and the control. IVS, Isovalerylshikonin; IBS, isobutyrylshikonin; AOIVS, acetoxylisovalerylshikonin; AS, acetylshikonin; HIVS, $\beta$-hydroxyisovalerylshikonin.

CYP76B74 Is Anchored to the Endoplasmic Reticulum In silico analysis of CYP76B74 using protein-targeting prediction software (TMHMM) revealed the presence of a 17-amino acid *N*-terminal membrane anchor. Expression of an in-frame fusion of GFP to the N terminus of CYP76B74 under the control of the *Cauliflower mosaic virus* 35S promoter in rice (*Oryza sativa*) protoplasts was used to identify the subcellular localization of the protein (Fig. 6A). The chimeric PIN5:: MKATE protein was used as an endoplasmic reticulum (ER) marker control (Fig. 6B). Image overlay demonstrated identical localization patterns for CYP76B74 and marker proteins, indicating that CYP76B74 is localized to ER membranes (Fig. 6D). Subcellular localization of CYP76B74 is thus consistent with the cytosolic localization of the 4-hydroxybenzoate geranyltransferase in *L. erythrorhizon* cell cultures that generates the expected substrate of the GHQ3″H.

Phylogenetic Analysis of CYP76B74 Using the full-

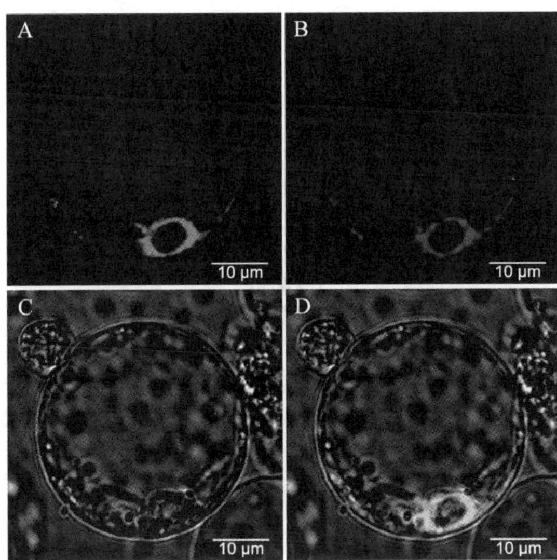


**Figure 6 Subcellular localization of CYP76B74 in rice protoplasts. Protoplasts without chlorophyll were cotransformed with CYP76B74-GFP and PIN5-mKATE, a marker for the endoplasmic reticulum (ER), and examined using confocal microscopy**

(A) Green fluorescence indicates the presence of CYP76B74. (B) Red fluorescence indicates the presence of ER marker protein. (C) Under white light. (D) Overlay of these three images indicates that CYP76B74 localizes to the ER.

length amino acid sequences, a phylogenetic analysis was carried out focused on the evolutionary relationship between CYP76B74 and CYP76 family sequences with CYP71AV1 as an outgroup (Fig. 7). CYP76B74 was used to query the oneKP database (https://db.cngb.org/onekp/search/) in Boraginaceae and de novo assembled transcriptomes of *Arnebia euchroma*, *Echium plantagineum*, and *L. erythrorhizon* with raw RNA sequencing data downloaded from the National Center for Biotechnology Information's Short Read Archive to obtain homologous sequences from Boraginaceae and possibly related taxa. Figure 7 shows sequences from Boraginaceae, which formed a subclade of the larger CYP76B subfamily clade. The other major subclade comprised G10H from various angiosperm species. The resulting neighbor-joining tree confirmed that CYP76B74 evolved specifically in Boraginaceae and belongs to the CYP76B subfamily, which includes CYP76B1 from *Helianthus tuberosus*, CYP76B6 from *C. roseus*, CYP76B10 from *Swertia mussotii*, and CYP76B9 from *Petunia × hybrida*.

## 2 DISCUSSION

Advances in DNA sequencing technology have enabled plant genome-sequencing projects to reveal a vast number of CYPs, leading to the annotation of more than 184,522 sequences in the databases. More than 16,219 CYPs were named and divided into 277 CYP families. CYPs are among the largest plant gene superfamilies and constitute around 1% of all the protein-coding genes in plants. In plants, CYPs play a critical role in secondary metabolic product diversity (e.g. flavonoids, coumarins, alkaloids, terpenoids, and other biological substances). It is a remarkable fact that studies of medicinal plant secondary metabolism genes have shown rapid evolution of *CYPs*, especially the *CYP* genes in a specific down-stream metabolic pathway such as the seco-iridoid pathway from *C. roseus* and the opioid pathway from opium poppies (*Papaver somniferum*). However, the biochemical functions of the majority of CYP proteins remain unknown.

Shikonin and its derivatives are the most abundant naphthoquinones formed in species of the medicinally and economically valuable Boraginaceae. Shikonin biosynthesis was initially proposed to start from geranyl pyrophosphate and 4-hydroxybenzoate, followed by a series of oxidative transformations mediated by the prenylated phenolic GHQ. To identify CYPs that are responsible for the early hydroxylation steps in shikonin biosynthesis, we carried out coexpression analysis using the transcriptomes of SP and SD cell lines and the spatial distribution of candidate gene expression across different organs to find candidates whose expression patterns matched those of known upstream genes in the shikonin biosynthetic pathway. We constructed yeast strains that expressed these CYP candidates. Using GHQ as the substrate, microsomes from the CYP76B74-expressing yeast strain produced GHQ-3″-OH. Furthermore, RNAi knockdown of *CYP76B74* expression in hairy root cultures of *A. euchroma* demonstrated that CYP76B74 was necessary for shikonin biosynthesis. Phylogenetic analysis confirmed that CYP76B74 belongs to the CYP76B subfamily, and subcellular locali-zation indicated that it was anchored to ER membranes. Taken together, the gene identity, regulation, and phylogeny of GHQ3″H was finally elucidated nearly two decades after it was found in *L. erythrorhizon*.

There are currently several CYP76B subfamily members that have been identified, but their physiological functions remain uncertain, except for those of CYP76B6 and CYP76B10, both referred to G10H. The natural substrate of CYP76B1 in the Jerusalem artichoke (*Helianthus tuberosus*) tuber still has not been characterized, and its monoterpenol oxidation activity is low. CYP76B9 was reported to be able to $\omega$-hydroxylate medium-chain fatty acids in vitro, but it has not been confirmed as a physiological function in the plant. In the phylogenetic tree, the CYP76B subfamily is most closely related to the CYP76F subfamily, the members of which catalyze the formation of the santalol and bergamotol components of sandalwood (*Santalum album*) fragrance via santalene and bergamotene hydroxylation at the C-12 position. In the same way, shikonin is hydroxylated on its terpenoid side chain, although not at the terminal position. The involvement of more distantly related CYP76

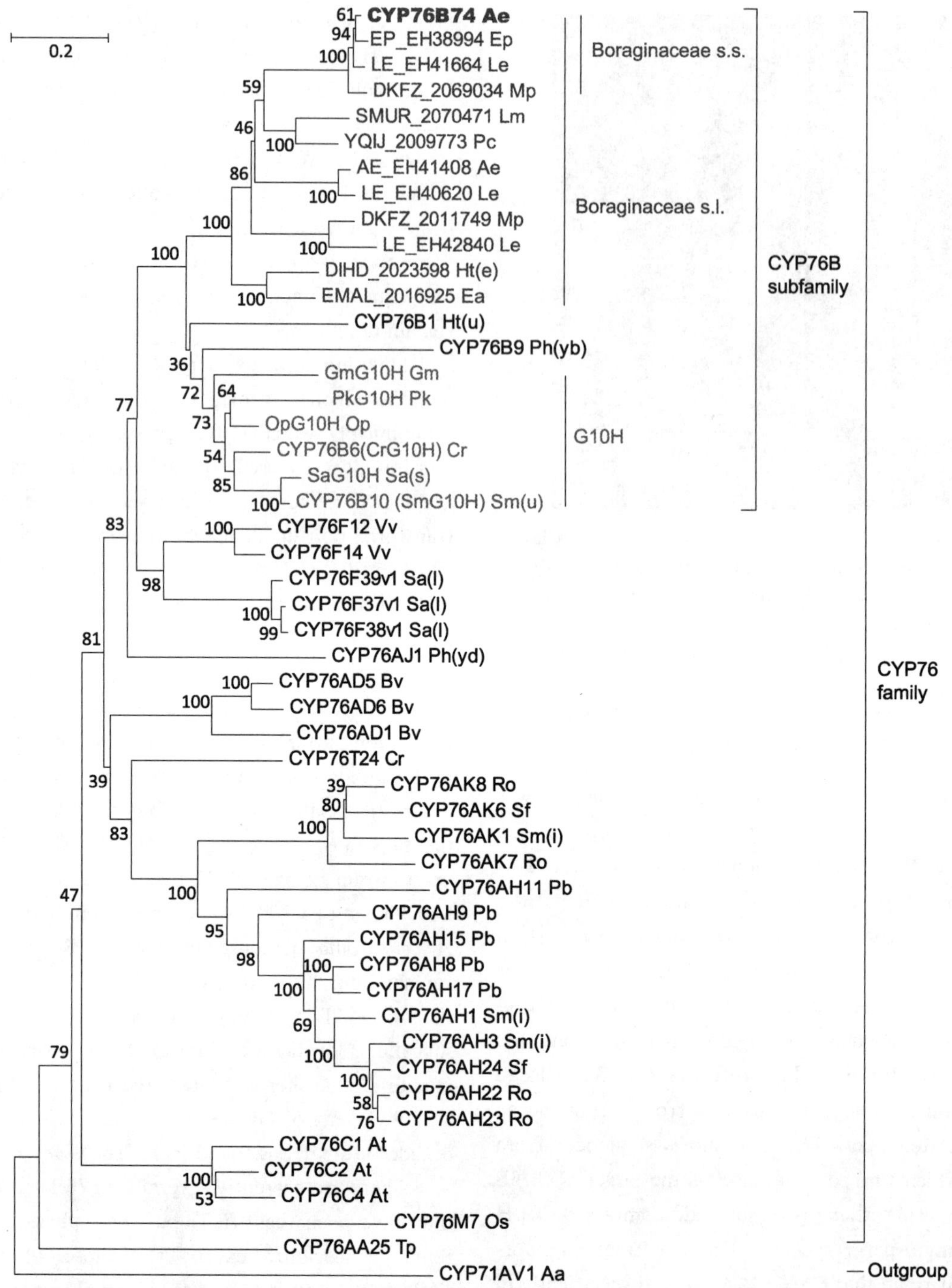


**Figure 7 Phylogenetic analyses of CYP76B74. The neighbor-joining tree was generated using MEGA (version 6) from a multiple protein sequence alignment and illustrates the evolutionary relationship between CYP76B74 and the CYP76 family. Bootstrap values (1,000 repeats) are indicated for each branch of the tree. The scale bar represents 0. 2 amino acid substitutions per site. Known geraniol 10-hydroxylases (G10H) are in pink, protein sequences of Boraginaceae s. l. are in purple, and protein sequences of Boraginaceae s. s. are indicated by red**

Abbreviations for the 28 species used here are as follows: Aa, *Artemisia annua*; Ae, *Arnebia euchroma*; At, *Arabidopsis thaliana*; Bv, *Beta vulgaris*; Cr, *Catharanthus roseus*; Ea, *Ehretia acuminata*; Ep, *Echium plantagineum*; Gm, *Gentiana macrophylla*; Ht(e), *Heliotropium tenellum*; Ht(u), *Helianthus tuberosus*; Le, *Lithospermum erythrorhizon*; Lm, *Lennoa madreporoides*; Mp, *Mertensia paniculata*; Op, *Ophiorrhiza pumila*; Os, *Oryza sativa*; Pb, *Plectranthus barbatus*; Pc, *Phacelia campanularia*; Ph(yb), *Petunia hybrida*; Ph(yd), *Persicaria hydropiper*; Pk, *Picrorhiza kurrooa*; Ro, *Rosmarinus officinalis*; Sa(l), *Santalum album*; Sa(s), *Swertia asarifolia*; Sf, *Salvia fruticosa*; Sm(i), *Salvia miltiorrhiza*; Sm(u), *Swertia mussotii*; Tp, *Thuja plicata*; Vv, *Vitis vinifera*.

family members in isoprenoid metabolism also has been functionally established, for example, for CYP76Cs from Arabidopsis (*Arabidopsis thaliana*) or CYP76Ms from rice. Altogether, our data support a predominant role of CYP76 family members in terpenoid-derived metabolism.

Phylogenetic reconstruction suggests that the group to which CYP76B4 belongs is a single evolutionary subclade of a Boraginaceae-specific clade of CYP76Bs, which most likely are all devoted to the biosynthesis of the same class of compounds (i.e. geranyl-hydroxybenzoic acids). Boraginaceae is one of the few families with uncertain taxonomic status in the APG IV classification system. APG IV recognizes an order, Boraginales, to accommodate the family and considers Boraginales to comprise a single family, Boraginaceae s. l., including Boraginaceae s. s., Codonaceae, Cordiaceae, Ehretiaceae, etc., with *A. euchroma*, *E. plantagineum*, and *L. erythrorhizon* belonging to Boraginaceae s. s. The phylogenetic tree indicated that CYP76B74 evolved specifically in Boraginaceae s. s. Recently, unigenes annotated as G10H, which have a similar function to the GHQ3″H enzyme and belong to the P450 monooxygenase family, have been found up-regulated in red roots compared with green leaves/stems of three Boraginaceae plants (i.e. *L. erythrorhizon*, *A. euchroma*, and *E. plantagineum*). Our results are consistent with this previous work and indicate that CYP76Bs are expanded within Boraginaceae s. s. The fossil record of the Boraginaceae is restricted to the Tertiary starting in the Early Eocene, and the fruit of *Lithospermum dakotense* was dated to the Late Miocene, which was found in Ash Hollow, Bennett, South Dakota. Based on the fossil record, the duplication event leading to the novel activity of CYP76B74 should be dated to the Early Eocene to Late Miocene.

A shikonin biosynthetic pathway has been proposed wherein the cyclization of GHQ-3″-OH to a naphthoquinone skeleton occurs through the oxidation of the C-3″ to an aldehyde group capable of forming the C-C bond with the aromatic-stabilized carbon via an electrophilic reaction. It is important to note that there are many CYP proteins in different pathways catalyzing consecutive oxidations into alcohols, aldehydes, and acids at the same position. Examples of this activity include C20Ox (CYP76AK6 - 8) of *Rosmarinus officinalis* and *Salvia fruticosae*, which ensures sequential oxidation at the C - 20 position leading to miltiradien-20-al, carnosic acid, and pisiferic acid. CYP76C1- and CYP76B6-mediated acyclic monoterpene linalool and geraniol metabolism also has been shown to involve successive oxidation steps. Therefore, we tested yeast-expressed CYP76B74 to determine if it catalyzed the further oxidation of GHQ-3″-OH. However, no further conversion of GHQ-3″-OH was observed. This is consistent with the Michaelis-Menten kinetics observed for CYP76B74 toward GHQ-3″-OH. In the case of the seco-iridoid pathway from *C. roseus*, geraniol 8-hydroxylase (CYP76B6) can catalyze the two consecutive oxidation steps of geraniol to 8-oxogeraniol, while another soluble enzyme, 8-hydroxygeraniol oxidoreductase, was found to catalyze the stepwise conversion of 8-OH-geraniol into 8-oxogeraniol or 8-OH-geranial and then into 8-oxogeranial. Considering the catalytic similarity between CYP76B6 and CYP76B74, we speculated that other CYPs or soluble NADPH-dependent oxidoreductase were oxidizing the allylic primary alcohol at the C-3″ position, as is the case in *C. roseus*. In this study, we also cloned another CYP enzyme belonging to the CYP76B family, CYP76B75, that shares 53% identity with CYP76B74 and 68% identity with G10H from *Ophiorrhiza pumila*. In an analysis of tissue-specific expression, *CYP76B75* was found to be more abundant in the root, similar to *CYP76B74* (Fig. 2). However, when tested via in vitro enzyme activity assay, CYP76B75 showed no catalytic activity toward GHQ or GHQ-3″-OH (Supplemental Fig. S1).

In spite of recent studies regarding the biosynthesis of shikonin and its controlling factors, the site of shikonin biosynthesis in cells is still an open question. Electron microscopy studies suggested that shikonin production was closely associated with the development of elongated rough ER and the subsequent formation of electron-dense vesicles (0.1 - 0.2 picometers), which appeared to transport shikonin derivatives to the outside of the cell wall by a process of exocytosis. However, direct evidence for ER-associated shikonin metabolism remained to be demonstrated. We used protoplast transformation in combination with GFP imaging to localize the GHQ3″H step of shikonin biosynthesis in *A. euchroma*. This approach allowed us to demonstrate that, like most other plant CYP enzymes, CYP76B74 is associated with the ER membranes and may contribute to anchoring the terminal segment of the shikonin metabolism to these membranes. In this study, we also established a direct observation method to observe shikonin localization via two-photon laser confocal microscopy, taking advantage of the spontaneous fluorescence of shikonins. This novel experimental system may enable further biochemical investigation of the kinetics and mechanism of shikonin accumulation and secretion.

In summary, our results conclusively demonstrated that the CYP enzyme CYP76B74 catalyzes the regiospecific C-3″ hydroxylation of GHQ, which is a critical step in the biosynthesis of shikonins, the major active components of Boraginaceae medicinal plants. To date, CYP76B74 is the first CYP enzyme functionally characterized in the shikonin biosynthetic pathway. It will pave the way for the functional investigation of other CYPs potentially involved in shikonin biosynthesis. In addition, the ability to generate GHQ-3″-OH, the CYP76B74 product, will provide an intermediate for testing the next steps of the pathway. We recently established a platform for the production of GBA in yeast. CYP76B74 can now be used in further synthetic biology approaches toward the heterologous production of shikonins in yeast.

## 3 MATERIALS AND METHODS

Plant Materials and Chemicals  The SP and SD suspension culture cell lines were derived from hypocotyls of *Arnebia euchroma* and were grown in improved Linsmaier and Skoog liquid medium as described previously. *A. euchroma* plants for organ-specific expression analysis and seeds for aseptic seedling transformation were collected in Xinjiang, China. GHQ was purchased from WuXi App-Tec. GBA was isolated from engineered yeast in our laboratory. Shikonin derivatives were purchased from Tokyo Chemical Industry. The purity of these chemicals exceeded 95%.

RNA Sequencing and Bioinformatic Processing  The cDNA libraries of SP and SD cells were sequenced on an Illumina HiSeq 2000 platform, and the raw sequencing data were deposited in the National Center for Biotechnology Information's Short Read Archive under accession number SRP137782. The transcriptome was de novo assembled using the Trinity program, and the functional annotation of all assembled unigenes was performed with the Nonredundant Protein Sequence, Nucleotide Sequence, SwissProt, InterPro, Kyoto Encyclopedia of Genes and Genomes, Clusters of Orthologous Groups of Proteins, and Gene Ontology databases successively. The expression level of each unigene was calculated using RNA sequencing quantification analysis with the fragments per kilobase per million mapped fragments method by DESeq2.

Isolation of Total RNA and RT-qPCR Analysis  Total RNA from different tissues and organs of *A. euchroma* was extracted using TRIzol reagent (Invitrogen) following the manufacturer's instructions. After treatment with DNases, samples of total RNA (2 μg) were fractionated on a 1% (w/v) agarose gel in Tris-borate/EDTA buffer and stained with ethidium bromide to analyze RNA integrity and genomic DNA contamination. RNA is considered to be of high quality when the ratio of eukaryotic 28S to 18S band intensity is about 2. First-strand cDNAs were synthesized with the PrimerScript First Strand cDNA Synthesis Kit with random primers and oligo(dT) at the same time (TaKaRa). RT-qPCR was performed using the Power SYBR Green PCR Master Mix (Applied Biosystems) and an Applied Biosystems 7 500 real-time instrument. Real-time PCR was performed as described previously. The primers used are listed in Supplemental Table S3. The 18S rRNA was used as the endogenous control to normalize expression data. At least three independent experiments were performed for each analysis.

cDNA Cloning and Heterologous Expression of CYP Candidates in Yeast  Full-length cDNAs of CYP candidates were cloned from cDNA isolated from SP cells using PrimeStar DNA polymerase (Takara Bio). The open reading frame region of CYP candidates was subcloned into the yeast epitope-tagging vector pESC-Trp by the restriction endonuclease-free cloning method. Primers for PCR amplification are shown in Supplemental Tables S4 and S5. The clones with correct insert were confirmed by sequencing. Constructed expression vectors were transformed into the *Saccharomyces cerevisiae* strain BY-T20, a high-yield diterpene strain derived from BY4742 ($\Delta Trp$-*1*, *Trp-1*::*HIS3*-$P_{PGK1}$-*BTS1*/*ERG20*-$T_{ADH1}$-$P_{TDH3}$-*SaGGPS*-$T_{TPI1}$-$P_{TEF1}$-*tHMG1*-$T_{CYC1}$). The transformants were selected on yeast synthetic dropout medium minus Trp (SD-Trp) containing 20 g/L Glc and grown at 28 ℃ for 48 h. The isolated recombinant strain was initially grown in SD-Trp with 20 g/L Glc at 30 ℃ for about 48 h. Cells were centrifuged and washed with sterile water to remove any residual Glc. Cells then were resuspended in SD-Trp with 20 g/L Gal and grown for 24 h at 30 ℃ to induce recombinant protein expression.

In order to produce a sufficient amount of microsomal protein for kinetic assays of CYP76B74 and a sufficient amount of CYP76B74 product, the fermentation of yeast expressing CYP76B74 was scaled up to 5 L in Minifors (MCGS; GuangShi Bio). Collected cells were homogenized by continuous high-pressure cell disruption (APV2000; APV), and microsomes were prepared by differential centrifugation as described previously. All these procedures were performed at 4 ℃.

In Vitro Enzyme Activity Assay  The in vitro enzyme activity assays with microsomal fractions of yeast expressing CYPs were conducted as described previously. The microsomes were prepared by the glass beads method (Pompon et al., 1996). Microsomes were suspended in storage buffer containing 50 mmol/L Tris-HCl (pH 7.5), 1 mmol/L EDTA, and 20% (v/v) glycerol. Initial in vitro hydroxylation assays were conducted in a total volume of 500 μL of 90 mmol/L Tris-HCl (pH 7.5) containing 250 μg of microsomal protein, 100 μmol/L GHQ, and 0.5 mmol/L NADPH along with a regenerating system (consisting of 5 μmol/L FAD, 5 μmol/L FMN, 5 mmol/L Glc-6-P, 0.5 units of Glc-6-P dehydrogenase, and 2 mmol/L DTT). The assay samples were incubated with shaking for 4 h at 28 ℃, and the reactions were terminated by three extractions with an equal volume of ethyl acetate. The products were dried by $N_2$ and redissolved in methanol for LC-MS analysis. Substrates structurally related to GHQ were assayed under the same conditions except for 100 μmol/L specific substrate in place of GHQ.

In order to produce enough enzymatic product for chemical structure characterization, the enzymatic assay containing the same composition as above was scaled up to 80 mL and performed overnight on an incubator shaking at 150 rpm at 30 ℃. The incubation products were extracted with ethyl acetate, dried by rotary evaporator, and resuspended in methanol. The CYP76B74 product was purified by preparative HPLC for structure characterization by NMR spectroscopy.

Kinetic Analysis For kinetic analysis, the concentration of CYP450 protein was estimated using the reduced CO-binding difference spectra detection kit (GMS18003v. A; Genmed Scientifics). Experiments were carried out against GHQ in serial concentrations of 0, 5, 10, 15, 30, 40, 60, and 100 μmol/L in 1-mL enzyme assays using 1 mg of microsomal protein prepared in the same batch. Enzymatic assay experiments contained the buffer and the NADPH regeneration system described earlier. Reactions were initiated by adding substrate and incubating at 30 ℃ for 30 min with shaking (150 r/min) and terminated by extraction three times with 1 mL of ethyl acetate. The products were dried by $N_2$ and redissolved in methanol for ultra-performance liquid chromatography (UPLC) analysis. $K_m$ and $V_{max}$ values were calculated by nonlinear regression of Michaelis-Menten enzyme kinetics using GraphPad Prism 6, and data reported are means ±SD from triplicate analyses.

A time-series experiment was carried out in a time series of 0, 10, 21, 31, 40, and 50 min to confirm that the 30 min time point for the steady-state kinetics experiments stayed within the linear range of the assay (Supplemental Fig. S6). The enzymatic assay contained the same composition as the kinetic analysis described above with the addition of 100 μmol/L GHQ in the 1 mL enzyme assays, and the products were analyzed using UPLC.

UPLC, LC-MS, and NMR Analyses UPLC was carried out with a Waters Acquity UPLC-PDA system equipped with a Waters C18 1.8 μm 2.1×100 mm T3 HHS column with an absorbance range of 210 to 400 nm. The column temperature was set at 40 ℃. For in vitro enzymatic product determination, the mobile phase comprised acetonitrile (A) and water (0.1% formic acid; B) at 0.5 mL/min with the following gradient program (0 min, 10% A; 4 min, 35% A; 4.3 min, 60% A; 8 min, 72% A; 8.5 min, 98% A; 10.5 min, 98% A; 11 min, 10% A; and 13 min, 10% A). To determine the contents of shikonin derivatives in hairy roots, about 20 mg of lyophilized hairy root was extracted by ultrasonication in 1 mL of methanol. The filtered extract then underwent UPLC analysis with the following gradient program (0 min, 2% A; 1 min, 20% A; 4 min, 25% A; 4.5 min, 75% A; 9.5 min, 75% A; 10 min, 100% A; 11 min, 100% A; 11.5 min, 2% A; and 13.5 min, 2% A).

LC-MS was carried out using an Acquity UPLC system (Waters) with column and separation conditions as described above. Time-of-flight MS detection was performed with a Xevo G2-S MS system (Waters) with the data acquisition range set from 50 to 1 000 D. The source temperature was set at 100 ℃, and the desolvation temperature was set at 450 ℃, with desolvation gas flow at 900 L/h. The lock mass compound used was Leu enkephalin at a concentration of 200 pg/μL. The capillary voltage was set at 2,500 V. The cone voltage was set at 40 V. The collision energy was set as 6 eV for low-energy scan and a ramp from 25 to 40 eV for high-energy scan. The instrument was controlled by MassLynx 4.1 software.

Preparative HPLC separation was performed using an LC-6AD instrument (Shimadzu) with a YMC-Pack ODS-A column (250×10 mm, S-5 μm, 12 nm). The flow rate was kept at 4 mL/min. The mobile phase was a 6 : 4 mixture of water and acetonitrile (V/V). The target fraction was collected manually, identified by UPLC, dried, and resuspended in deuterated chloroform for structural analysis by NMR spectroscopy.

The chemical structure characterization of GHQ and GHQ-3″ OH utilized $^1$H-NMR (400 MHz), $^{13}$C-NMR (100 MHz), and 2D NMR spectra collected on a Bruker DRX 400 spectrometer. Tetramethylsilane was used as the internal standard. The observed chemical shift values are reported in ppm.

RNAi in Hairy Root of *A. euchroma* Gene-specific fragments of *CYP76B74* were cloned into the pENTR vector using the Directional TOPO Cloning Kit (Invitrogen; primers are shown in Supplemental Table S6) and subcloned further into the binary vector pK7GWIWG2D (Ⅱ) using Gateway LR Clonase Enzyme Mix (Invitrogen). Constructs, including a *CYP76B74* RNAi vector and an empty vector used as a negative control, were introduced into *Agrobacterium rhizogenes* C58C1 using the freeze-thaw transformation method. The recombinant *A. rhizogenes* then was transfected into explants of *A. euchroma* as described. In contrast to other plants, only the cotyledons of 2-week-old *A. euchroma* seedlings can be used as explants to generate hairy roots. The transformed hairy root lines were cultured in one-half-strength Murashige and Skoog solid medium without ammonium nitrate at 25 ℃ in the dark for 6 to 8 weeks. The rapidly growing kanamycin-resistant lines in which GFP was visible and that had no bacterial contamination then were maintained at 25 ℃ in the dark with one-half-strength Murashige and Skoog solid medium without ammonium nitrate and routinely subcultured every 10 to 15 d. Tissues then were collected for RT-qPCR, metabolite analysis, and microscopy.

Subcellular Localization of CYP76B74 in Rice Protoplasts A transmembrane helical domain was predicted in the first 40 residues (N-terminal end) of CYP76B74 using TMHMM server analysis (http://www.cbs.dtu.dk/services/TMHMM/).

In order to determine the subcellular localization of

CYP76B74, the complete open reading frame sequence was subcloned into the *Bsa*I/*Eco*31I restriction sites of the pBWA (V) HS-ccdb-GLosgfp plasmid. This fusion expression vector, CYP76B74 - GFP, is driven by the *Cauliflower mosaic virus* 35S promoter. The GFP was codon optimized for high expression in rice (*Oryza sativa*; Genscript).

We also used mKATE, which is a far-red fluorescent protein, fused to PIN5 to stain ER membranes as a control protein for ER targeting [pBWA(V) HS-PIN5-mKATE]. Rice seedlings in plastic pots filled with soil and grown in the dark at 28℃ for 1 to 2 weeks were used for the isolation of leaf protoplasts without chlorophyll. The protoplasts were isolated and transformed as described previously with modifications. The transformed protoplasts were examined with a light microscope as well as a laser confocal microscope (C2 - ER; Nikon). For GFP detection, excitation at 488 nm and detection at 510 nm were used. For mKATE detection, excitation at 588 nm and detection at 635 nm were used. The images acquired from the confocal microscope were processed using NIS-Elements Viewer 4.20.

Microscopy and Confocal Microscopy The phenotype of hairy roots was examined with a stereomicroscope (SZX10; Olympus). *CYP76B74* RNAi-derived hairy roots and the empty vector control were imaged using an LSM 880 (Zeiss) confocal microscope equipped with an AxioObserver. Slides were prepared by the root-tip squashing method. Collected images were processed using Zeiss Efficient Navigation 2 and Adobe Photoshop CS3. Shikonin autofluorescence was detected using a 543-nm excitation wavelength laser and a 568- to 712-nm emission filter for the 640-nm emission wavelength. Fluorescence intensity was analyzed by ImageJ software ($n=3$).

Phylogenetic Sequence Analysis Phylogenetic and molecular evolutionary analyses were conducted using MEGA version 6. Protein sequences were aligned using the MUSCLE program. Phylogenetic relationships were reconstructed by the maximum likelihood method based on the JTT/+G model (five categories) and a bootstrap of 1,000 replicates. All protein sequences used for sequence alignment and phylogenetic tree construction are listed in Supplemental Table S1.

[王升,黄璐琦,等. Plant Physiology, 2019, 179: 402 - 414.]

# Friedelane-type triterpene cyclase in celastrol biosynthesis from *Tripterygium wilfordii* and its application for triterpenes biosynthesis in yeast

## 1 INTRODUCTION

*Tripterygium wilfordii* Hook. F is a medicinal plant known in traditional Chinese medicine as 'Lei gong teng' (also called thunder god vine), the debarked root of which has a long history of use in the treatment of rheumatism and inflammation. Some listed drugs developed from *T. wilfordii* including *Tripterygium* glycoside tablets and Leigongteng tablets, have also been used to treat autoimmune and inflammatory diseases in China since the 1970s. Many pharmacological studies have suggested that *T. wilfordii* extracts can be used to treat tumours, nephrotic syndrome, HIV, Crohn's disease, and a series of autoimmune and inflammatory diseases. These remarkable bioactivities are mainly dependent on the active compounds isolated from *T. wilfordii* such as sesquiterpenoid alkaloids, diterpenoids and triterpenes. Among these components, triptolide and celastrol are thought to be two of the natural products with the greatest potential to be developed into modern drugs. Celastrol is a friedelane-type triterpene that was first isolated from the root of *T. wilfordii*, and was found to be effective in the treatment of inflammatory and autoimmune diseases, Alzheimer's disease and cancer. Interestingly, researchers have also found this compound to be a leptin sensitiser and a promising agent for the treatment of obesity.

Despite considerable pharmaceutical interest, the low celastrol levels, slow growth rate and restricted habitat of this plant have all limited the further study and application of celastrol. To address the above issues, methods have been developed to obtain a sustainable and reliable supply such as cell culture systems and total synthesis. In recent years, metabolic engineering in microorganisms has been shown to be a promising method for the production of high-value natural products. However, the biosynthetic pathway of celastrol remains unknown. The pharmaceutical potential of triptolide has led many researchers to investigate the biosynthetic pathway of this compound, but there have been few reports on the biosynthetic pathway of celastrol.

The common precursors of terpenoids are isopentenyl diphos-phate (IPP) and its isomer dimethylallyl diphosphate (DMAPP) derived from the mevalonate (MVA) pathway and methylerythritol phosphate (MEP) pathway. Celastrol is a friedelane-type triterpene that is synthesised via the MVA pathway. Although the biosynthetic pathway of celastrol is unclear, a potential route (Fig. 1) has been proposed based on reported metabolomic data of triterpenes from *T. wilfordii*. In this pathway, oxidosqualene cyclase (OSC) catalyses the complicated cyclisation of 2,3-oxidosqualene to friedelin, which is further modified by cytochrome P450 to form polpunonic acid and wilforic acid C. After a series of oxidation reactions and rear-rangements, these intermediates are finally transformed to celastrol. The cyclisation of 2,3-oxidosqualene is the first committed step in this unknown pathway and determines the scaffold of celastrol; therefore it is important to determine the OSCs that are responsible for celastrol biosynthesis.

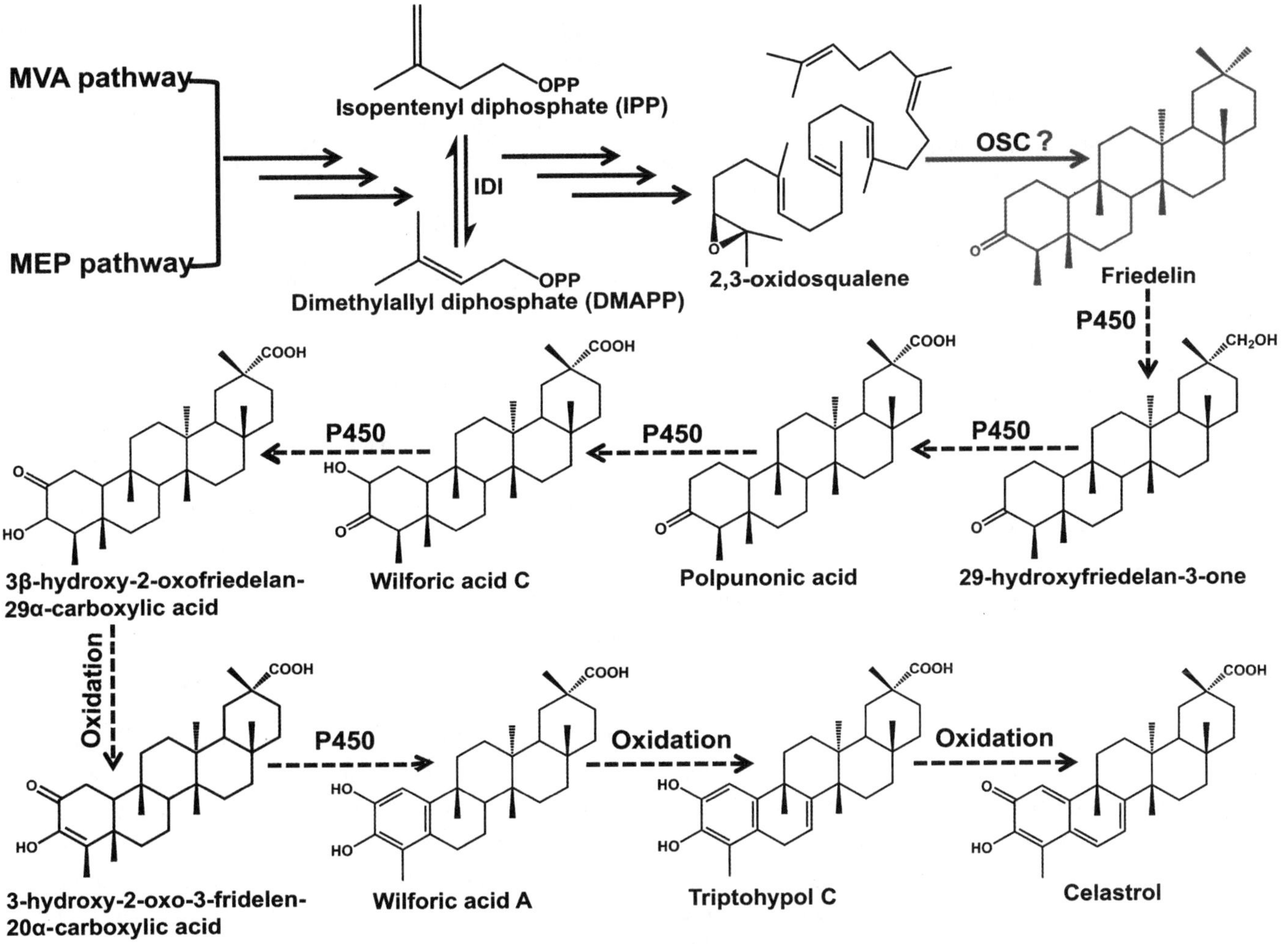

**Fig. 1 Proposed biogenetic pathway for celastrol in *Tripterygium wilfordii***

The red solid arrow indicates a biosynthetic reaction step identified in this study, and each dashed arrow indicates one or multiple proposed step reactions. All triterpenoid intermediates in the proposed pathway have been reported in *T. wilfordii*.

Most triterpene scaffolds are cyclised via the chair-chair-chair (CCC) conformation catalysed by OSC, while sterols are cyclised via chair-boat-chair (CBC) conformation (Fig. 2). The cyclisation of oxidosqualene involved four main steps: first, binding of the substrate and predetermination the ring system; second, initiation of the reaction by protonation of the epoxide; third, cyclisation and rearrangement of carbocation species; and fourth, termination by deprotonation or water capture to yield a final terpene product. More than 200 different triterpene skeletons have been discovered from natural resources or enzymatic reactions. Friedelin is one of the most highly rearranged triterpenes known in plants.

Here, we aimed to identify the OSCs responsible for the biosynthesis of celastrol. Three candidate OSC genes were screened from the transcriptome of *T. wilfordii*. *Tw*OSC1 and *Tw*OSC3 are friedelane-type triterpene cyclases responsible for the biosynthesis of celastrol, while *Tw*OSC2

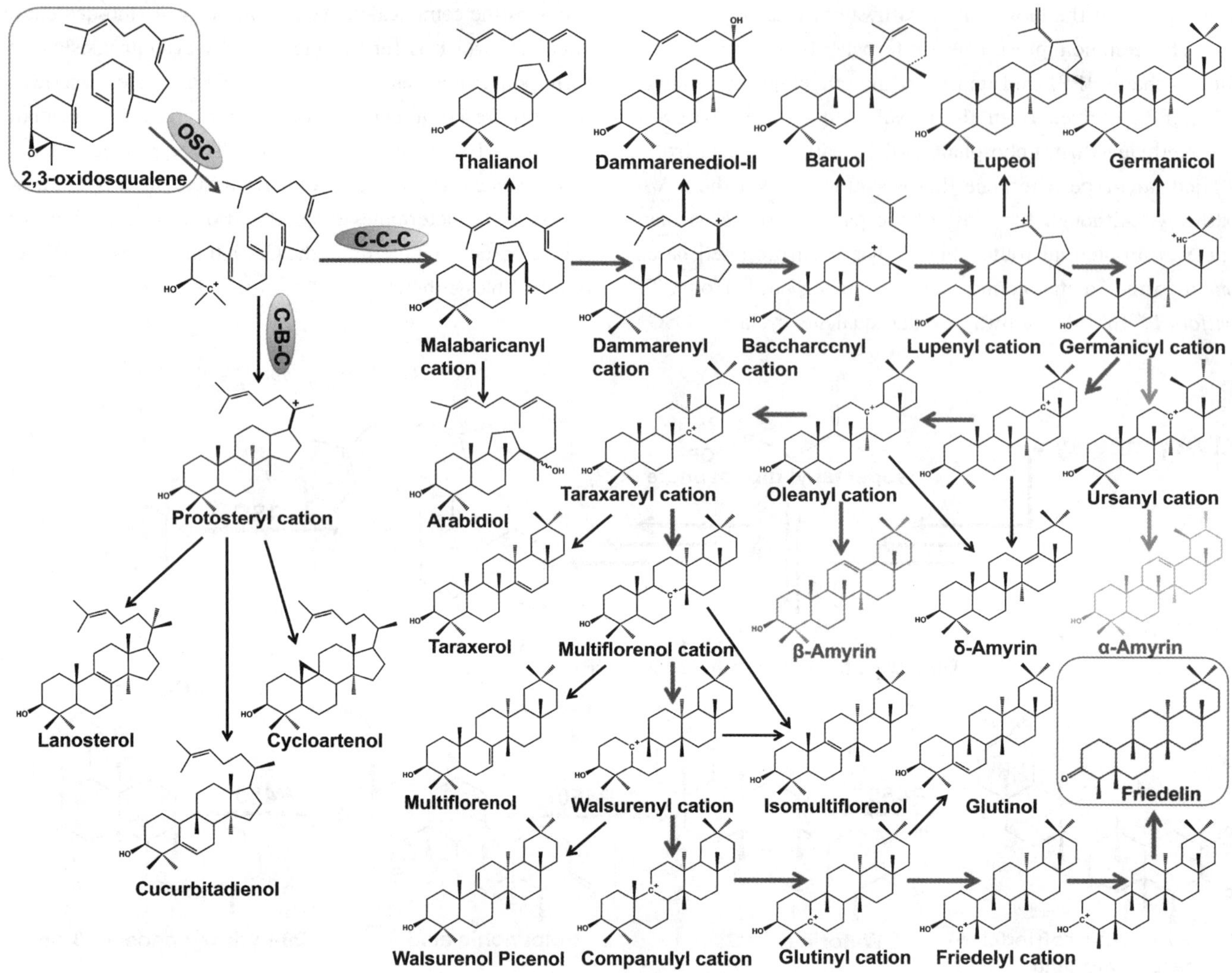


**Fig. 2 Proposed oxidosqualene cyclisation mechanisms**

Friedelin is a most rearranged friedelane-type triterpene found in many plants including *Tripterygium wilfordii*.

is a β-amyrin synthase. Both *Tw*OSC1 and *Tw*OSC3 can cyclise 2,3-oxido-squalene to friedelin as the major product, with β-amyrin and α-amyrin as the minor products. We also showed that friedelin is a precursor of celastrol. In addition, the yield of friedelin in the engineered yeast was also improved using site-directed mutagenesis, the CRISPR/Cas9 system and medium optimisation. Our findings have laid the foundations for exploration of the biosynthetic pathway of celastrol and other friedelane-type triterpenes and have provided insights into the biosynthetic pathways of friedelane-type, oleanane-type and ursane-type triterpenes in *T. wilfordii* and other plants.

## 2 MATERIALS AND METHODS

Plant materials *T. wilfordii* cell suspensions were initiated from calluses of *T. wilfordii* and cultured in Murashige and Skoog (MS) medium containing 30 g/L sucrose with 0.1 mg/L kinetin (KT), 0.5 mg/L 2,4-dichlorophenoxyacetic acid (2,4-D) and 0.5 mg/L indole-3-butyric acid (IBA). These cell suspensions were cultured in the dark at 25 ℃ with rotary shaking at 120 r/min as described previously. Mature *T. wilfordii* plant tissues were collected from the Yongan national forest in Fujian Province, China. Samples of root, stem, leaves and flowers were harvested from three individual plants, and ground in liquid nitrogen using a Retsch MM400 mixer mill (Retsch GmbH, Germany, https://www.retsch.com/) and then stored at −80℃ until use.

RNA isolation, cDNA synthesis and gene cloning Total RNA from *T. wilfordii* suspension cells and plant tissues was isolated using the modified cetyltrimethylammonium bromide (CTAB) method as described previously. Total RNA was purified using an RNA Purification Kit (Tiangen Biotech, Beijing, China). First-strand cDNA was cloned using the SMARTer™ RACE cDNA Amplification Kit (Clontech Laboratories, Mountain View, CA, USA). To mine the candidates, TBLASTN analysis of OSCs in the *T. wilfordii* transcriptome was carried out using BIOEDIT

7.0.9.0. software. Friedelin synthase from *Kalanchoe daigremontiana* (*Kd*FRS, ADK35125) was used as the query sequence. The full-length predicted cDNA sequences of the candidates were obtained from the transcriptome data of *T. wilfordii*. Special primers (Supporting Information Table S1) for cloning the *Tw*OSCs were designed based on the full-length predicted cDNA sequences. The amplification reaction was performed using the Phusion high-fidelity PCR master mix (New England BioLabs, Ipswich, MA, USA) according to the manufac-turer's instructions. The PCR products were purified and ligated into the pEASY - T3 vector, transformed into *E. coli* DH5$\alpha$ cells, and then cultured in Luria-Bertani (LB) medium at 37℃ in the dark. Positive colonies were verified by sequencing.

Sequence and phylogenetic analyses  The open reading frames (ORFs) and amino acid sequences of the *Tw*OSCs were identified using the online tool ORF Finder (http://www.ncbi.nlm.nih.gov/gorf/gorf.html). Multiple sequence alignments were conducted using DNAMAN. INTERPRO (www.ebi.ac.uk/Tools/InterProScan) was used to identify functional domains. The amino acid sequences of OSCs from other species were downloaded from the National Center for Biotechnology Information (NCBI) database and aligned by CLUSTALW. Then, a neighbour-joining tree was built using MEGA6 software via the bootstrap method with 1000 replications.

MeJA-mediated induction of *T. wilfordii* suspension cells  The *T. wilfordii* suspension cells were treated with methyl jasmonate (MeJA) at a final concentration of 50 μmol/L after subculturing. The control group was treated with the same volume of carrier solution. After 0, 4, 8, 12, 24, 48, 72 and 360 h, the suspension cells were harvested in liquid nitrogen and then stored at −80℃ before RNA extraction or ultraperformance liquid chromatography (UPLC) analysis. Four biological duplicates were prepared for each time point in each group.

Quantitative real-time PCR  Total RNA from the treated suspension cells was extracted using the modified CTAB method as described above. First-stand cDNA for quantitative real-time PCR (qRT-PCR) was reverse transcribed from total RNA according to manufacturer's instruction in the FastQuant RT Kit (Tiangen Biotech). qRT-PCRs were performed using gene-specific primers (Table S1) and the KAPA SYBR ® FAST qPCR Kit (KAPA Biosystems, Boston, MA, USA) on an Applied Biosystems QuantStudio 5 real-time PCR System (Applied Biosystems, New York, NY, USA). The PCR conditions were as follows: an initial incubation at 95℃ for 3 min, followed by 45 cycles of 95℃ for 3 s and 60℃ for 30 s and then by a melting curve cycle. Elongation factor 1$\alpha$ (EF1$\alpha$) was used as the reference gene. Relative transcript abundance was evaluated using the $2^{-\Delta\Delta Ct}$ method with triplicate measurements from four biological replicates.

UPLC analysis of celastrol content in induced *T. wilfordii* suspension cells and plant tissues  The *T. wilfordii* suspension cells and powders of plant tissues were stored at −80℃ for at least 4 h before freeze drying for 48 h (Christ Alpha 1 - 2, Osterode am Harz, Germany). Approx. 50 mg of each sample was suspended in 1 ml of 80% (v/v) methanol overnight at room temperature (25℃), and then extracted by sonication in an ultrasonic water bath for 60 min. After centrifugation for 2 min, 10000 g and room temperature, the supernatant was filtered through a 0.22-μm membrane filter (polytetrafluoroethylene) before UPLC analysis.

The analyses were conducted using an Agilent 1290 Infinity II Efficient ultrahigh performance liquid chromatography (UHPLC, Agilent Technologies Inc., Santa Clara, CA, USA) system quipped with a diode array detector (DAD). Chromatographic separation was conducted using a Waters Acquity UPLC HSS T3 analytical column (Milford, MA, USA) (2.1 × 100 mm, 1.8 μm) maintained at 40℃. The mobile phase, consisting of a mixture of 0.1% (v/v) formic acid in water (A) and acetonitrile (C), was pumped at a flow rate of 0.4 mL/min. The gradient programme was 30% C at 0 min, 35% C at 5 - 8 min, 70% C at 15 min, and 90% C at 21 min. The detection wavelength was 425 nm, and ultraviolet (UV) light spectra from 190 to 500 nm were also recorded. The injection volume was 5 μL.

Functional identification in yeast  The ORFs of *Tw*OSCs were amplified and subcloned into the pYES2 expression vector (Invitrogen) separately. The ORFs of *Tw*OSC1 and *Tw*OSC2 were inserted between the *Kpn*I-*Not*I sites of pYES2 via digestion by the corresponding restriction endonucleases. *Tw*OSC3 was inserted between the *Kpn*I-*Bam*HI sites of pYES2 in the same manner. All primers are shown in Table S1. The constructed vectors were transformed into lanosterol synthase-deficient yeast (*Saccharomyces cerevisiae*, purchased from ATCC, cell line number: 4021900, -ERG7, -*ura*) using the Frozen-EZ Yeast Transformation II Kit (Zymo Research, Irvine, CA, USA). The pYES2 vector was transformed into yeast as a control.

The transformants were cultured on solid synthetic complete medium without uracil (SC - Ura) for selection. The positive transformant was then cultured in 20 mL of Sc - Ura medium containing 2% glucose and incubated with shaking at 220 rpm and 30℃ for 2 d. Then, the cells were collected and induced in 20 mL of Sc - Ura medium with 2% galactose in place of glucose and further cultured at 220 rpm and 30℃ for 12 h. After induction, the yeast cells were collected and resuspended in 0.1 mol/L potassium phosphate buffer (pH 7.0) with 2% glucose, and cultured at 220 rpm and 30℃ for 1 d. Finally, the yeast cells were collected and lysed with 10 mL of 20% KOH and 50% EtOH by ultrasonic extraction for 1 h or refluxed for 5 min with 10 mL of 20% KOH and 50% EtOH. The supernatant was extracted with 10 mL of hexane three times. All the extracts were combined and then evaporated by rotary evaporation.

The extracts were dissolved in pyridine and derivatised with *N*-methyl-*N*-(trimethylsilyl) trifluoroacetamide at 70℃ for 1 h. Then, the derived extracts were evaporated under $N_2$ and dissolved in 1 mL trichloromethane (CHCl3) for analysis by gas chromatography and mass spectrometry (GC-MS). The analysis was performed on an Agilent 7000 gas chromatograph (split, 20 : 1; injector temperature, 250℃) with a DB-5 ms (15 m×250 μm×0.1 μm) capillary column. In total, 1 mL of the concentrated organic phase was then injected under an He flow rate of 1 mL/min with a temperature programme of 1 min at 50℃, followed by a gradient from 50 to 260℃ at 50℃/min and then, to 272℃ at 1℃/min with a 4 min held. The ion trap temperature was 230℃. The electron energy was 70 eV. Spectra were recorded in the range of 10-550 *m/z*.

RNAi study A specific 300-500 bp fragment was selected based on the BLAST analysis in *T. wilfordii* transcriptome database (Figs S1, S2) and amplified from the ORF of each *Tw*OSC by specific primers (Table S1) and then inserted into vector pK7GWIWG2D (Invitrogen) using the Gateway cloning system (Invitrogen). The vectors containing each fragment were transformed into *E. coli* and then verified by PCR and sequencing. Resulting vectors were transformed into *T. wilfordii* suspension cells according to Zhao *et al*. Suspension cells in the logarithmic growth phase were plated on MS solid medium (pH=5.8) and grown for 7 d before transformation. The empty vector was transformed into *T. wilfordii* suspension cells as a control, and all samples had five biological duplicates. The transformed cell suspensions were incubated for 7 d on MS medium and then transferred onto selection medium (solid MS medium supplemented with 0.5 mg/L 2,4-D, 0.1 mg/L KT, 0.5 mg/L IBA) supplemented with 100 mg/L kanamycin for selection of transformed cell suspensions. Positive transformed cell suspensions were further inoculated in the selection MS medium for culture growth with shaking. After three generations of screening, the transformed cell suspensions were harvested to measure gene expression and celastrol levels.

Feeding study After subculturing, *T. wilfordii* suspension cells [2 g fresh weight (FW) of suspension cells in 40 mL of MS medium in 100 mL flasks] were further cultured for 10 d and then friedelin (2.77 mg) dissolved in 300 μL ethanol: Tween 80 (1:1, v/v) was added into the culture. The control group was treated with the same volume of carrier solution alone, and each sample set had four biological duplicates. After treatment, the suspension cells were harvested at 0 or 7 d by negative-pressure filtration. Next, the suspension cells were stored at −80℃ for at least 4 h before freeze drying for 48 h. Dried suspension cells (*c*. 50 mg) were extracted with 1.0 mL 80% (*V/V*) methanol as described above. The supernatant was filtered through a 0.22-μm membrane filter (polytetrafluoroethylene) for UPLC analysis.

Molecular docking and site-directed mutagenesis The sequence logo and graphical representation of the DCTAE motif were generated using WEBLOGO 3 (http://weblogo.threeplu sone.com/create.cgi) with default parameters, the alignment of the motif was visualised using DNAMAN. The three-dimensional protein structures of the *Tw*OSCs were created using MODELER 9v11 (Eswar *et al*., 2006) based on the identified crystal structure of human OSC (RCSB Protein Data Bank ID: 1W6K). The three-dimensional protein structures of the *Tw*OSC models are shown in Fig. S3. The product friedelin or substrate 2,3-oxidosqualene was docked with the model structures separately using Sybyl X-1.3 (El Cerrito, CA, USA). Molecular docking was performed as previously described. The docking results were visualised using PYMOL.

Site-directed mutagenesis of the *Tw*OSCs was conducted using the Fast Mutagenesis System (TransGen Biotech, Beijing, China). *Tw*OSC1, *Tw*OSC2 and *Tw*OSC3 mutants were amplified from their templates using specific primers (Table S1). The pYES2 vector containing each *Tw*OSC was used as a template. The constructed mutants were verified by PCR and sequencing. Positive mutants were transformed into lanosterol synthase-deficient yeast and cultured. The products were then extracted and analysed by GC-MS as described above.

Strain construction and fermentation Specific gRNAs targeting *rox1*, *ypl062w* and *yjl064w* were designed by the open-source tool at http://yeastriction.tnw.tudelf t.nl. Single and multiple gRNA expression vectors for *yjl064w*, *ypl062w* and *rox1* were constructed as described previously. The 120-bp repair fragments used for effective repair by the homologous recombination repair machinery were obtained using two complementary single-stranded oligos and an annealing programme: 5 min at 95℃, followed by a gradient from 95℃ to 25℃ at −1℃/min, then to 10℃ and held. For each transformation, the gRNA expression vector containing the gRNA sequence of choice, Cas9 encoding vector and the double-stranded DNA cassette for repair of the double-stranded break were combined and co-transformed into the BY4741 strain; this constructed strain was named strain ZH0.

The squalene synthase (SQS) gene and the catalytic domain of HMG1 (tHMG1) were amplified from *S. cerevisiae* BY4741 genomic DNA and then inserted into the pESC-leu expression vector. Details of all primers used in this experiment are shown in Table S1. After verification by sequencing, this pESC-SQS+tHMG1 vector was transformed into strain ZH0 to obtain strain ZH1. Details of all strains used in this study are shown in Table S2. Vector pYES2-*Tw*OSC1$^{T502E}$ was transformed into strain ZH1, strain BY4741 and a lanosterol synthase-deficient strain. Then, the positive strains were cultured in flasks (300 mL) containing 60 mL of YPD medium at 30 ℃ and 220 rpm for 2 d. Next, the cells were collected and induced in 60 mL of YPG medium at 30 ℃ and 200 rpm for 60 h. The products of the yeast were extracted and analysed as described above.

The high-yield strain containing pYES2-*Tw*OSC1$^{T502E}$ was further cultured in flasks (300 mL) containing 30 mL of optimised yeast extract peptone dextrose (YPD) medium (5% glucose, 1% yeast extract, 3% peptone, 0.8% $KH_2PO_4$, and 0.6% $MgSO_4$), which had been shown in a previous study (Song *et al.*, 2017) to effectively promote rapid propagation of yeast cells. After culturing at 30 ℃ and 220 rpm for 2 d, the cells were collected and induced in 30 mL of optimised yeast extract peptone glycerol (YPG) medium (5% galactose, 1% yeast extract, 3% peptone, 0.8% $KH_2PO_4$, and 0.6% $MgSO_4$) at 30 ℃ and 200 rpm for 60 h. The products of the yeast were extracted and analysed as described above.

## 3 RESULTS

Cloning and sequence analysis of the *Tw*OSCs  In our previous study, we sequenced and reported a transcriptomic library (SRA accession number: SRR6001265) of *T. wilfordii*. Transcripts of OSC candidates were screened via homology-based searches of the transcriptome. Three full-length cDNA sequences of OSCs (*Tw*OSC1, *Tw*OSC2 and *Tw*OSC3) were obtained by polymerase chain reaction and sequencing (GenBank accession nos. KY885467, KY885468 and KY885469). Protein domain analysis showed that all the proteins had a terpenoid cyclase/protein prenyltransferase alpha-alpha toroid domain, but only *Tw*OSC2 had the conserved site of terpene synthase (Fig. S4). Based on the multiple sequence alignments, all three *Tw*OSCs were homologous (average similarity identified as 76.46%) to OSCs in several other species (Fig. S5). The three *Tw*OSCs all hd the conserved region DCTAE of the OSC family, which is associated with substrate binding. The conserved repetitive QW (QXXXXXW) motifs always appear as four to eight repeats in the OSC family and appear as four repeats in the *Tw*OSCs. In addition, the *Tw*OSC2 and *Tw*OSC3 both had the MWCYCR motif, which is predicted to be a highly conserved motif of β-amyrin synthase.

Phylogenetic tree construction  The results of the phylogenetic analysis showed that *Tw*OSC2 differed from *Tw*OSC1 and *Tw*OSC3, which clustered with the previously characterised β-amyrin synthase genes *Ks*bAS, *Hh*bAS and *Ae*bAS (Fig. 3). By contrast, *Tw*OSC1 and *Tw*OSC3 clus-

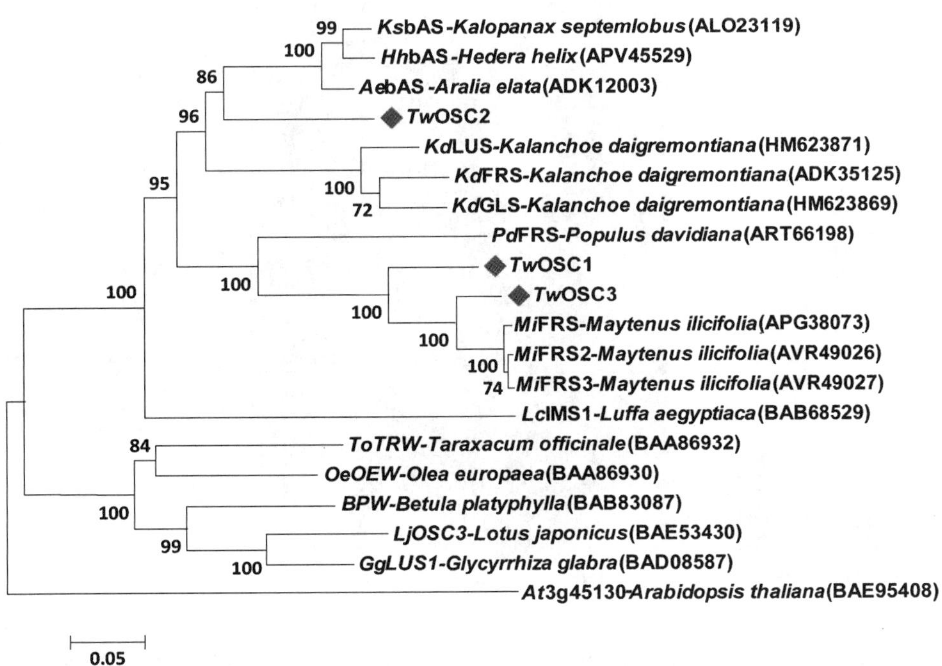


**Fig. 3  Phylogenetic tree of *Tw*OSCs and the characterised oxidosqualene cyclases (OSCs) from other species**

The phylogenetic tree was created using MEGA 6.0 software and the neighbour-joining method. Bootstrap confidence values were obtained based on 1 000 replicates. *Tw*OSCs from *Tripterygium wilfordii* are highlighted with red diamond.

tered with *Mi*FRSs and *Pd*FRS into a clade. As previously described, both *Mi*FRSs and *Pd*FRS were monofunctional friedelin synthases, that can produce friedelin only. Interestingly, there was also a multiproduct friedelin synthase, *Kd*FRS, which could produce friedelin as a major product, taraxerol, and β-amyrin as a minor product. This multiproduct friedelin synthase did not cluster with other friedelin synthases but formed a branch with glutinol and lupeol synthases from *K. daigremontiana* (*Kd*GLS and *Kd*LUS, respectively). These results indicated that *Tw*OSC1 and *Tw*OSC3 were friedelin syn-thases, while *Tw*OSC2 was a β-amyrin synthase.

The transcript levels of the *Tw*OSCs were significantly upregulated after MeJA treatment  MeJA is a plant hormone used in plant defence and many diverse developmental pathways that can increase the levels of plant secondary metabolites by inducing the expression of genes in the biosynthetic pathways of secondary metabolites. In our previous study, we found that MeJA can induce MVA pathway gene expression and accumulation of celastrol in *T. wilfordii* suspension cells. Here, we used real-time PCR to quantify *Tw*OSCs expression after MeJA treatment. We found that the relative expression levels of all three *Tw*OSCs were significantly upregulated; this finding correlated with the accumulation of celastrol (98.16 μg/g in 360 h) after MeJA treatment (Fig. 4a, b). This result showed that all three *Tw*OSCs may be involved in the biosynthesis of triterpene in *T. wilfordii*.

The tissue expression patterns of the *Tw*OSCs were correlated with the celastrol distribution  To determine whether the gene expression levels of the *Tw*OSCs in *T. wilfordii* were correlated with celastrol accumulation, the relative transcript levels of the *Tw*OSCs and the celastrol levels were determined across all established tissues (Figs 4c, d, S6). The relative expression levels of *Tw*OSC2 and *Tw*OSC3 were highest in the root, which was also the tissue with the highest celastrol content (1.87 mg/g DW). The transcript level of *Tw*OSC1 was highest in the leaves, which also exhibited low celastrol levels.

Functional characterisation of *Tw*OSCs in yeast  To

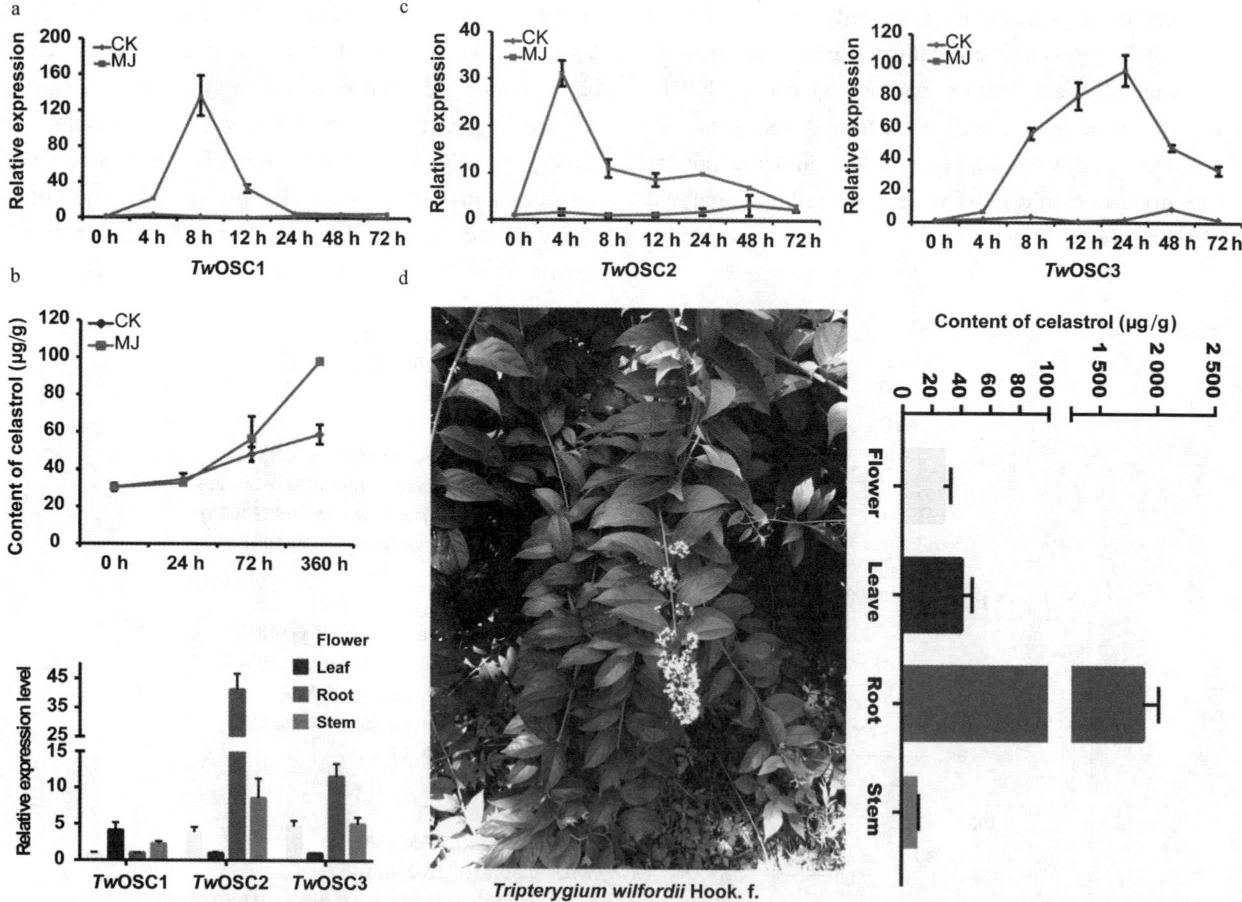


**Fig. 4  Analysis of methyl jasmonate (MeJA)-induced and tissue expression of *Tw*OSCs combined with celastrol distribution**

(a) Relative expression of *Tw*OSCs in the MeJA-induced *Tripterygium wilfordii* suspension cells. CK: control group; MJ: MeJA-treated group. (b) Celastrol content in MeJA-induced *T. wilfordii* suspension cells. CK: control group; MJ: MeJA-treated group. (c) Relative expression of *Tw*OSCs in different *T. wilfordii* tissues. (d) *T. wilfordii* plant and distribution of celastrol in *T. wilfordii*. Error bars represent SDs based on triplicate measurements of at least four biological replicates.

identify the functions of the putative OSCs from *T. wilfordii*, the complete ORFs of all the *Tw*OSCs were subcloned into the pYES2 vector and then transformed into lanosterol synthase-deficient yeast. In parallel, the empty vector was transformed into the yeast mutant to serve as a negative control. After culturing and induction, the metabolite extracts were extracted and analysed by GC - MS. Based on the results of GC analysis (Fig. 5), the extracts from yeast harbouring *Tw*OSC2 contained only one product, which was confirmed to be β-amyrin. Yeast harbouring *Tw*OSC1 and *Tw*OSC3 contained friedelin, β-amyrin and α-amyrin, with friedelin as the major product. The structures of all these products were explained by comparison of the mass spectral characteristics with those of authentic standards (Figs S7 - S9). This result from GC - MS analysis suggested that *Tw*OSC1 and *Tw*OSC3 were multiproduct friedelin synthases and that *Tw*OSC2 was a β-amyrin synthase.

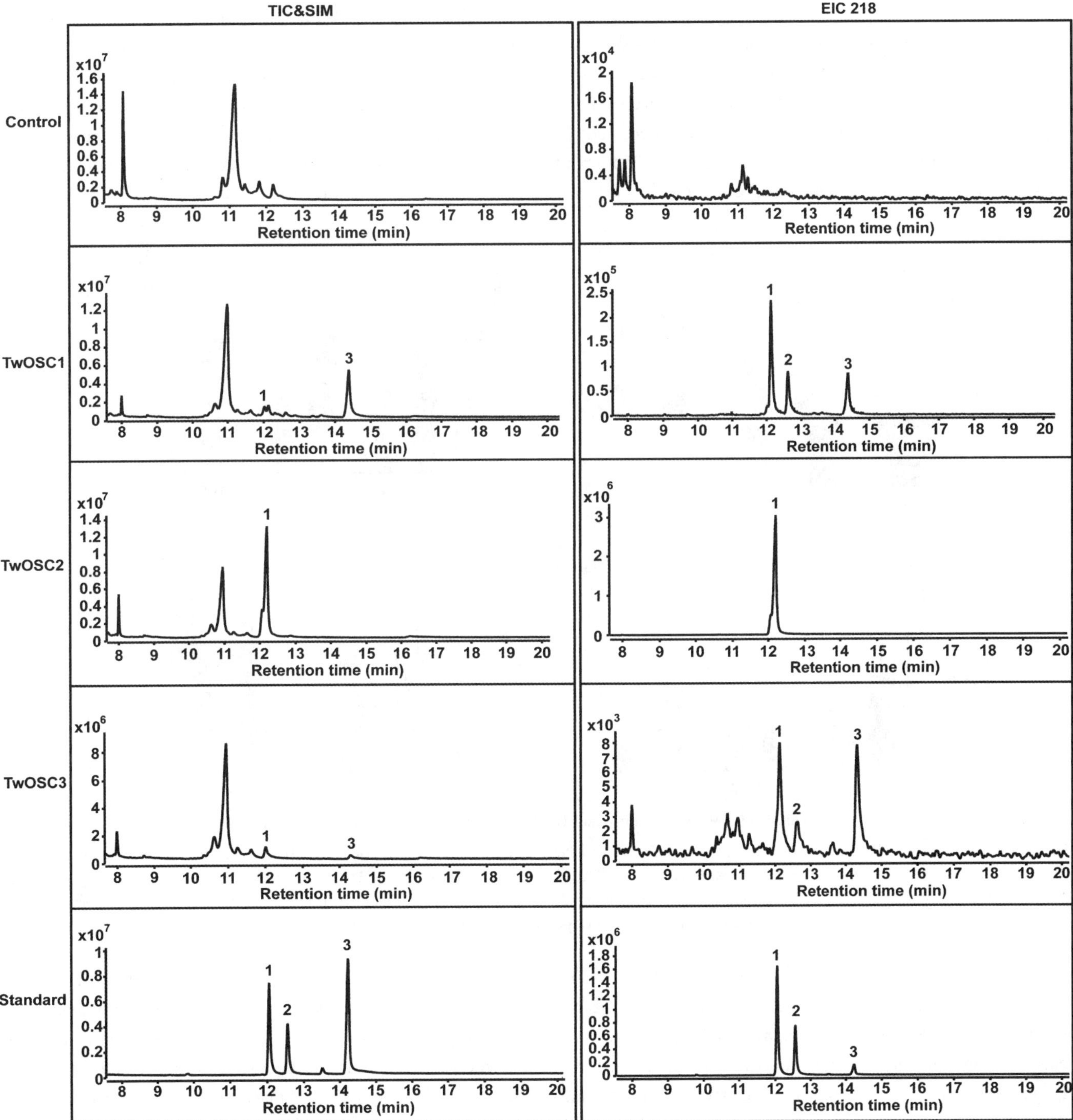


**Fig. 5 Gas chromatography-mass spectrometry (GC - MS) analysis of the products in yeast strains harbouring the *Tw*OSCs from *Tripterygium wilfordii***

Standards: β-amyrin (1), α-amyrin (2), and friedelin (3).

**RNAi identified candidate *Tw*OSCs for biosynthesis of celastrol** To further investigate the *Tw*OSC responsible for the biosynthesis of celastrol, *Tw*OSC1, *Tw*OSC2 and *Tw*OSC3 were selected as candidate genes for the RNA interference (RNAi) study. In our early study, a stable and highly efficient transformation system suitable for *T. wilfordii* cell suspensions was developed based on particle bombardment. Here, we used this transformation system to transform the candidate genes. pK7GWIWG2D (Ⅱ)-*Tw*OSC1, -*Tw*OSC2, -*Tw*OSC3 and the empty vector were separately transformed into *T. wilfordii* cells and screened on MS solid medium with kanamycin. *Tw*OSC1 expression was suppressed by 42.5% and celastrol levels decreased by 32.0% compared with the control. *Tw*OSC3 expression was suppressed by 37.3%, and celastrol levels decreased by 84.2%. By contrast, RNAi suppressed the transcription of *Tw*OSC2 by 47% and increased celastrol levels by 9.5% (Fig. 6a－c). RNAi combined with gene expression analysis and UPLC analysis of celastrol profiles showed that *Tw*OSC1 and *Tw*OSC3 were involved in celastrol biosynthesis and that *Tw*OSC3 may have a stronger effect than *Tw*OSC1 on celastrol biosynthesis.

**Friedelin is a precursor of celastrol** Based on the results of the RNAi study and the observed tissue expression pattern, we determined that *Tw*OSC1 and *Tw*OSC3 were responsible for the biosynthesis of celastrol. GC－MS analysis showed that both *Tw*OSC1 and *Tw*OSC3 can produce friedelin, which is also a friedelane-type triterpene, similar to celastrol. To further investigate the potential role of friedelin in celastrol biosynthesis, we fed friedelin to suspension cell cultures; this process led to a significant increase in celastrol accumulation after 7 d compared with the control groups (Fig. 6d). This finding indicated that friedelin served as a precursor to celastrol.

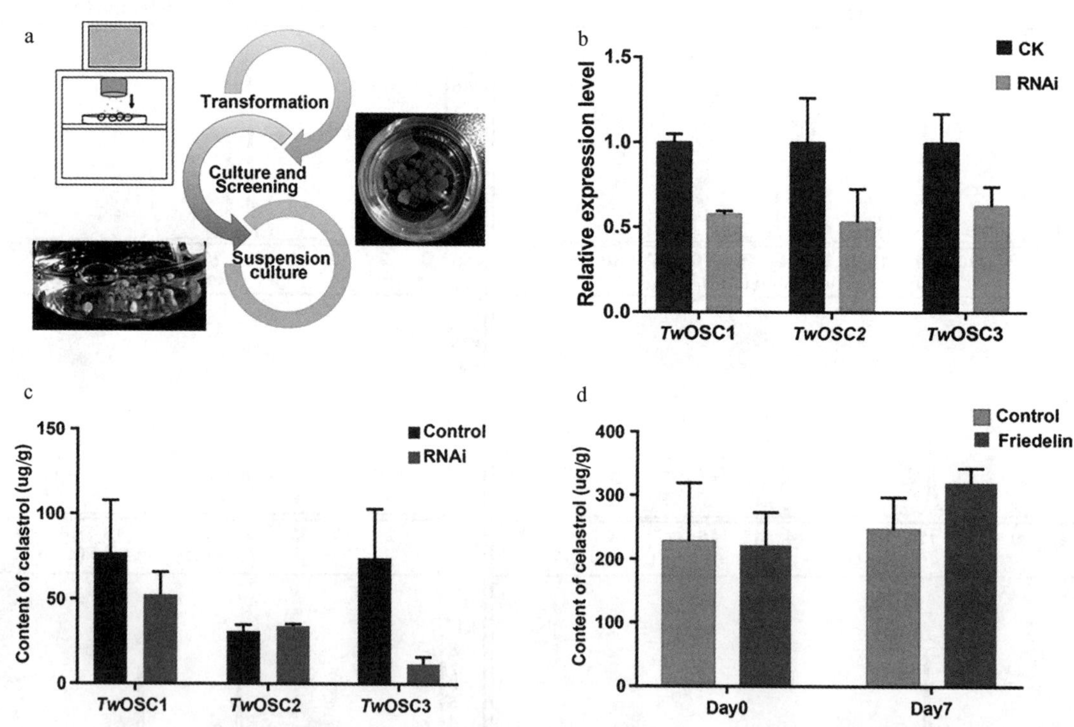


**Fig. 6 Analysis of RNA interference and feeding in *Tripterygium wilfordii* suspension cells**

(a) RNAi process. (b) Relative expression of *Tw*OSCs in the RNAi suspension cells and control suspension cells. (c) Celastrol content in the RNAi suspension cells and control suspension cells. (d) The content of celastrol in the friedelin-feeding group and control group after 0 or 7 d. Student's *t*-test was used to test statistically significant difference of increased celastrol levels between control group and feeding group. The data represent the average±SD of at least four independent lines of suspension cells.

**Site-directed mutagenesis of *Tw*OSC proteins** The reaction catalysed by OSCs is one of the most complicated reactions, and can yield a wide array of triterpene skeletons derived from the same simple substrate 2,3-oxidosqualene. However, the exact mechanism underlying this product diversity remains unknown. Enzymes with a single product and high yield will be helpful for exploration of the subsequent biosynthesis pathway and further commercial application. Therefore, we wanted to identify the crucial amino acids that are involved in the production of friedelin. Recently, Souzamoreira *et al*. found that the amino acid two positions upstream of the DCTAE site in friedelin synthase, usually a leucine (L) residue, was required for friedelin production. Multiple sequence alignment of the friedelin-producing OSCs and molecular docking of *Tw*OSC1 and *Tw*OSC3 showed that the L residue was unique to friedelin-

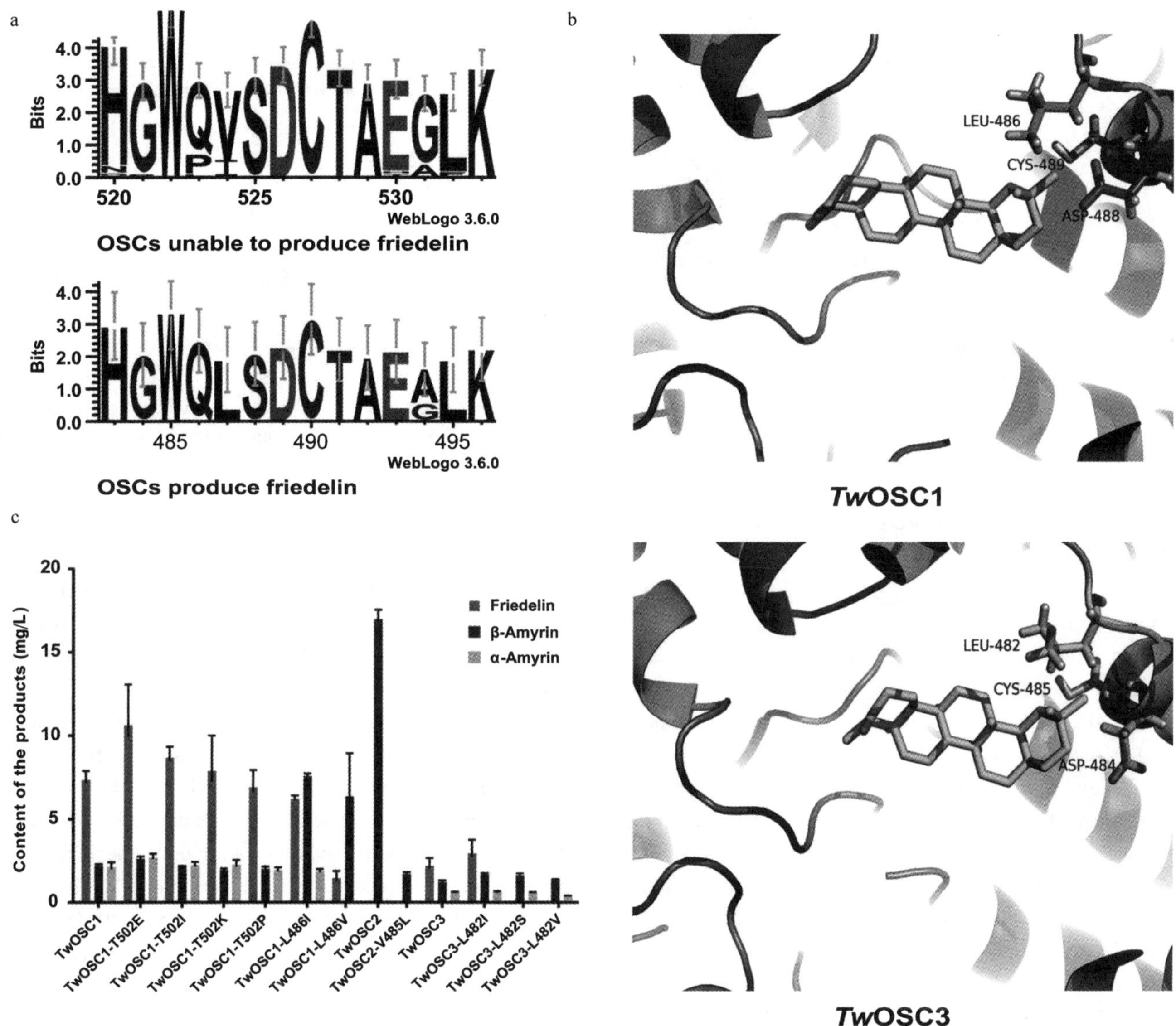


**Fig. 7 Molecular docking and mutagenesis assay of *Tw*OSCs from *Tripterygium wilfordii***

(a) Sequence representation in the DCTAE motifs of *Tw*OSCs. Accession numbers and abbreviations are provided in Supporting Information Table S4. (b) Molecular docking of *Tw*OSC1 and *Tw*OSC3 with friedelin. (c) Product analysis of the mutants. The activities of wild-type and all the mutants are presented as the means±SDs, $n=5$.

producing OSCs and was near the active sites of these enzymes (Fig. 7a, b).

To further investigate this residue in friedelin synthase, we constructed additional mutants by site-directed mutagenesis. Substitution of the L residue with phenylalanine (F), histidine (H), proline (P) or arginine (R) in *Tw*OSC1 and substitution of the L residue with F, P, R, or alanine (A) in *Tw*OSC3 abolished all the products, but substitution of the L residue with valine (V) decreased the production of friedelin and increased the production of β-amyrin. Substitution of the L residue with serine (S) in *Tw*OSC3 also abolished the production of friedelin and increased the production of β-amyrin (Figs S10, S11). Moreover, substitution of the L residue with isoleucine (I) in *Tw*OSC1 and *Tw*OSC3 did affect friedelin production only minimally but increased the production of β-amyrin. In addition, we also constructed a mutant of *Tw*OSC2 to determine whether substitution of the V residue at the same position with L could change the product to friedelin. However, this substitution in *Tw*OSC2 did not lead to friedelin production and decreased the yield of β-amyrin. Fortunately, we found a residue in *Tw*OSC1 (Threonine (T) 502) that could increase the production of friedelin. The best mutant was T502E (glutamic acid), which produced 10.63 mg/L friedelin in a shaker flask culture. The levels of all the products of the *Tw*OSCs and mutants are shown in Fig. 7(c) and Table S3.

Improvement of the yield of friedelin in engineered *S. cerevisiae* To improve the yield of friedelin, two key genes in the triterpene pathway were overexpressed to enhance the metabolic flux towards (3S)-2, 3-oxidosqualene. ERG9 and

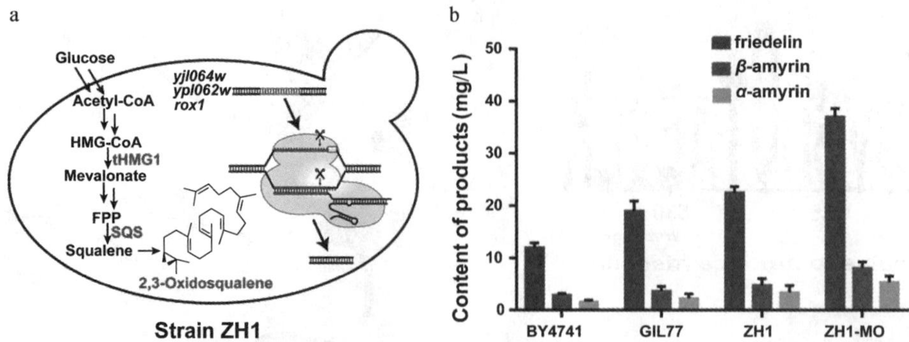


**Fig. 8 Strain construction and friedelin production using *Tw*OSC1$^{T502E}$ from *Tripterygium wilfordii***

(a) A strategy to construct strain ZH1. (b) Levels of products in the three strains containing *Tw*OSC1$^{T502E}$. BY4741 stands for strain BY4741 containing *Tw*OSC1$^{T502E}$; GIL77 stands for the lanosterol synthase-deficient strain containing *Tw*OSC1$^{T502E}$; ZH1 stands for strain ZH1 containing *Tw*OSC1$^{T502E}$; and ZH1 - MO stands for strain ZH1 containing *Tw*OSC1$^{T502E}$ in the optimisation medium. The data are presented as the means±SDs, $n=3$.

tHMG1 from *S. cerevisiae* were separately cloned into the pESC-leu vector then transformed into the yeast BY4741. In addition to overexpressing the key genes in the triterpene pathway, three genes were deleted to further improve friedelin production (Fig. 8a). These genes included a transcriptional regulator, *rox1* and two other genes, namely, *ypl062w* and *yjl064w*. *Rox1* was reported to repress genes in the MVA pathway and ergosterol biosynthesis, while *ypl062w* and *yjl064w* could improve MVA pathway flux when knocked out and especially when combined. When pYES2-*Tw*OSC1$^{T502E}$ was transformed into strain ZH1, strain BY4741 and the lanosterol synthase-deficient strain cultured under the same conditions, the highest yield was 22.52 mg/L in strain ZH1, which was higher than yield in the lanosterol synthase-deficient strain and almost two-fold higher than the yield in the parent strain BY4741 (Fig. 8b). After medium optimisation, the highest yield of strain ZH1 could be improved to 37.07 mg/L. This study is the first on friedelin biosynthesis in engineered yeast with a high yield.

## 4 DISCUSSION

*T. wilfordii* is known to contain a diversity of triterpenes, and celastrol was one of the valuable compounds isolated from *T. wilfordii*. Here, we focussed on the OSCs that were responsible for the main scaffold cyclisation of celastrol. Three OSCs were mined from the transcriptome of *T. wilfordii*. To identify the *Tw*OSC that was responsible for the biosynthesis of celastrol, we tested the expression levels of the OSCs after MeJA treatment and determined the tissue expression patterns of OSCs in *T. wilfordii*. However, these results showed that all three *Tw*OSCs could be induced by MeJA and the tissue expression patterns of these OSCs, except for that of *Tw*OSC1, were correlated with the distribution of celastrol. In a previous study, Corsino *et al*. found that triterpenes, once biosynthesised in the leaves, were translocated to the root bark and further transformed to quinonemethide triterpenoids in the Celastraceae and Hippocrateaceae families. This result indicated that *Tw*OSC1 may also participate in triterpene biosynthesis in the root. Subsequently, functional identification of *Tw*OSCs in lanosterol synthase-deficient yeast revealed that *Tw*OSC1 and *Tw*OSC3 were multiproduct friedelin synthases that could produce friedelin as a major product, and β-amyrin and α-amyrin as minor products. This report is the first to describe simultaneous production of friedelin, β-amyrin and α-amyrin by friedelin synthase. This study also showed that *Tw*OSC2 is a β-amyrin synthase with only one product, β-amyrin, under the experimental conditions. This finding indicated that the common product of both *Tw*OSC1 and *Tw*OSC2 was β-amyrin, belonging to the oleanane-type triterpene family and not the friedelane-type triterpene family. To further identify the roles of the *Tw*OSCs, we performed an RNAi study to suppress gene expression of the *Tw*OSCs. Based on the results of the RNAi study, we determined that decreased expression of *Tw*OSC1 and *Tw*OSC3 can cause a decrease in celastrol levels. This finding indicated that *Tw*OSC1 and *Tw*OSC3 were the genes responsible for celastrol biosynthesis. The feeding study further confirmed that the common product of *Tw*OSC1 and *Tw*OSC3, friedelane-type friedelin, is one precursor of celastrol, and can increase celastrol production.

The mechanistic diversity of OSCs remains intriguing. Although many attempts have been made to study the underlying mechanism, the mechanism of conversion between scaffolds remains poorly understood. Sequence analysis has shown that all three *Tw*OSCs contained terpenoid cyclase/protein prenyltransferase alpha-alpha toroid domains, but only *Tw*OSC2 contained conserved sites of terpene synthase that are rich in aromatic residues, in the C-terminal region. Multiple sequence alignments showed that all these protein contained the conserved DCTAE motif and four conserved repetitive QW motifs. Moreover, *Tw*OSC2 and *Tw*OSC3 both had the MWCYCR motif, which is important for β-amyrin synthase. However, we found that *Tw*OSC1 (containing the IWCYCR motif) as well as *Tw*OSC2 and *Tw*OSC3 could produce β-amyrin. Tetsuo Kushiro *et al*. found that the tryptophan residue in the MWCYCR motif was responsible for the formation of pentacyclic triterpenes and that substitution of this residue with H resulted in the production of tetracyclic dammaradienols. Here, our results suggested that the methionine residue in the MWCYCR motif was not necessary for β-amyrin production.

To identify the key residues involved in functional conversion between friedelin and β-amyrin, we performed site-directed mutagenesis. Our results showed that substitution of L residue (two positions upstream of the DCTAE motif) with F, H, P or R in *Tw*OSC1 and substitution of the L residue with F, P, R, or A in *Tw*OSC3 abolished all the products. From the docking result, we thought that steric hindrance may be the main effect to prevent the reaction in these substitutions (Fig. S12). By contrast, substitution of the L residue with V in *Tw*OSC1 and *Tw*OSC3 decreased the production of friedelin and increased the production of β-amyrin, and substitution of the L residue with S in *Tw*OSC3 also abolished the production of friedelin but increased the production of β-amyrin. Substitution of the L residue with I in *Tw*OSC1 and *Tw*OSC3 affected friedelin production only minimally, but increased β-amyrin production. From the proposed oxidosqualene cyclisation mechanisms, we thought that product diversity depended on the ability to stabilise the cations. Therefore, we thought that these substitutions may allow the enzyme to better stabilise the oleanyl cation, therefore in the reaction blocking the oleanyl cation and generating β-amyrin. Substitution of the V residue with L in *Tw*OSC2 did not lead to friedelin production but decreased the yield of β-amyrin; this also confirmed this inference. This result strongly indicated that the L residue was important for friedelin biosynthesis but was not the only factor influencing friedelin production. In the other *Tw*OSC1 (T502) site, we found that substitution of T with E, I or lysine (K) increased the production of friedelin and substitution with the E residue led to the greatest increase. In a previous study, Thoma *et al*. found that human OSC consisted of two (α/α) barrel domains that were connected by loops and three smaller β-structures. The substrate first entered the active site via channel 1 and then formed the product in the active site. Then, the product was separated from the enzyme by channel 2. The structural model of *Tw*OSC1 showed that residue T502 was located in channel 2 (Fig. S13); therefore we speculated that T502 mutants increased the friedelin yield by influencing release of friedelin from the enzyme.

Biosynthesis of friedelin in yeast with high yields will help reveal the biosynthetic pathway of celastrol and further commercial application. To improve the yield of friedelin in yeast, we constructed an engineered strain by knocking out three downregulated genes and overexpressing two key genes in the triterpene biosynthetic pathway. When the *Tw*OSC1 mutant T502E, with the highest yield, was transformed into the three different strains, strain ZH1 showed the best production capacity with a yield of 22.52 mg/L friedelin, which was almost two-fold higher than that obtained with the parent strain. The lanosterol synthase-deficient yeast was a diploid yeast that lacked one copy of the *ERG1* gene so that it could increase the flux of triterpenoid production by improving accumulation of the common precursor, 2,3-oxidosqualene. Here, we also tested the production of friedelin in this strain, yield was 19.03 mg/L, which was lower than that in strain ZH1. Moreover, we further improved the yield of friedelin in strain ZH1 by optimising the fermentation medium. By a combination of mutagenesis, strain construction and medium optimisation, the highest yield of friedelin was determined to be 37.05 mg/L in a shaker flask culture; this yield was more than five-fold the yield observed for wild-type *Tw*OSC1 (7.35 mg/L).

[周家伟,高伟,等. New Phytologist, 2019,223:722-735.]

# The chromosome-level reference genome assembly for *Panax notoginseng* and insights into ginsenoside biosynthesis

## 1 INTRODUCTION

The Chinese medicine Sanchi is prepared from the dried root and rhizome of *Panax notoginseng* (Burk.) F.H. Chen, a perennial herb that belongs to the Araliaceae ginseng species. Generally, Sanchi is collected and washed before *P. notoginseng* flowers bloom in autumn and is obtained by separating the main root and rhizome after drying. *P.*

notoginseng has a long history of use in China for eliminating congestion and hemostasis and reducing swelling and pain. The brilliant work of the Ming Dynasty, Compendium of Materia Medica (A.D. 1552 - 1578), already described *P. notoginseng*. The medicinal value of *P. notoginseng* arises from the chemical ingredients it contains. To date, the chemical components isolated from *P. notoginseng* include mainly saponins, flavones, sugars, volatile oils, and amino acids. Among these, saponin compounds are the main chemical constituents and are also recognized as the main active ingredients. Modern medical research has shown that saponins from *P. notoginseng* improve myocardial ischemia, protect the liver, defend against cardiovascular disease, lower blood pressure, and improve arteriosclerosis; they also have antithrombotic and anticancer activities. As a rare and valuable medicinal material in China, *P. notoginseng* is also used in various prescriptions, such as capsules, injections, and powders. It is in widespread use, with total annual output values exceeding 70 billion RMB.

To date, the principal means of obtaining saponins has been to extract and isolate them from the original plants; however, the plant saponin content is low, and this process has a low extraction efficiency and is not environmentally friendly. Therefore, reconstruction of the saponin biosynthetic pathway for heterologous production is an alternative method for obtaining these valuable resources. At present, over 80 tetracyclic triterpenoid saponins have been identified from the roots, stems, leaves, flowers, and fruits of *P. notoginseng*, and these saponins can be divided into protopanaxadiol (PPD) and protopanaxatriol (PPT) based on a hydroxyl substitution at the C-6 position of the molecular structure. The biosynthetic pathway of saponins in *P. notoginseng* is divided into four main stages. First, the direct precursors isopentenyl allyl diphosphate (IPP) and dimethylallyl diphosphate (DMAPP) are synthesized by the mevalonate and 2-methyl-D-erythritol-4-phosphate pathways. Second, isopentenyl transferase and terpene synthases catalyze the synthesis of 2, 3-oxidosqualene from IPP and DMAPP. Third, 2, 3-oxidosqualene undergoes cyclization and hydroxylation to form the core structures PPD and PPT. Finally, the formation of various saponins is catalyzed by a number of glycosyltransferases (GTs). The genetic and functional diversity of GTs gives rise to a variety of structurally diverse saponins.

To explore the biosynthetic pathway of ginsenosides, the genome of *P. notoginseng* has been explored and information mined. However, because of sequencing technology limitations, existing genomic information generated from second-generation short-read sequencing is insufficient. Here, we present a high-quality *P. notoginseng* genome obtained using a combination of Illumina, PacBio, and Hi-C (high-throughput chromosome conformation capture) technologies; this is also the first chromosome-level genome of the genus *Panax*. Using comparative genomics, we explored the evolution and whole-genome duplication (WGD) events of *P. notoginseng*. We performed detailed transcriptional analysis and explored gene-level regulatory mechanisms that control the formation of characteristic tubercles, the biosynthesis of saponins at temporal and spatial levels, and the regulation of transcription factors. Combined with genomic analysis, we screened a series of UDP-dependent GT (UGT) candidate genes, five of which were identified as having catalytic functions. Our study provides genetic information for further comprehensive analysis of the saponin biosynthetic pathway and the evolution of the ginseng genus, and also describes useful techniques for the breeding of *P. notoginseng*.

## 2 RESULTS

Genome sequencing, assembly, and annotation

According to the *K*-mer distribution analysis ($K=31$), the estimated size of the *P. notoginseng* genome ($2n=2x=24$ chromosomes) is 2.38 Gb, and the heterozygosity and repeat contents are 0.58% and 69.05%, respectively (Supplemental Figure 1 and Supplemental Table 1). We combined Illumina, PacBio, and Hi-C technologies to sequence and assemble a high-quality, chromosome-level *P. notoginseng* reference genome. A total of 240.22 Gb of Illumina reads, 284.07 Gb of PacBio long reads, and 340.83 Gb of Hi-C data were generated, resulting in ~325.23× coverage of the *P. notoginseng* genome (Supplemental Table 2). The final assembled genome was 2.66 Gb in size and consisted of 219 scaffolds, with a scaffold N50 of 216.47 Mb and a contig N50 of 1.12 Mb (Figure 1 and Table 1). The assembled sequence was then anchored onto 12 pseudochromosomes with lengths of 176.58 - 295.55 Mb. The total length of the pseudochromosomes accounted for 99.89% of the genome sequences, with a scaffold L50 number of 6 (Supplemental Figure 2; Supplemental Table 3). The genome of *P. notoginseng* had a GC content of 34.45% (Supplemental Table 4).

To test the coverage of the *P. notoginseng* genome, the short reads generated from Illumina sequencing were mapped, and 99.82% of these reads could be mapped to the scaffolds with 97.97% overall coverage (Supplemental Table 5). The completeness of the genome assembly was evaluated using BUSCO (Benchmarking Universal Single-Copy Orthologs). Based on BUSCO analysis, 96.6% of plant sets were identified as complete (2 049 out of 2 121 BUSCOs) (Supplemental Table 6). All analyses suggested a high quality of the *P. notoginseng* genome assembly.

Based on a combination of homology-based and *de novo*

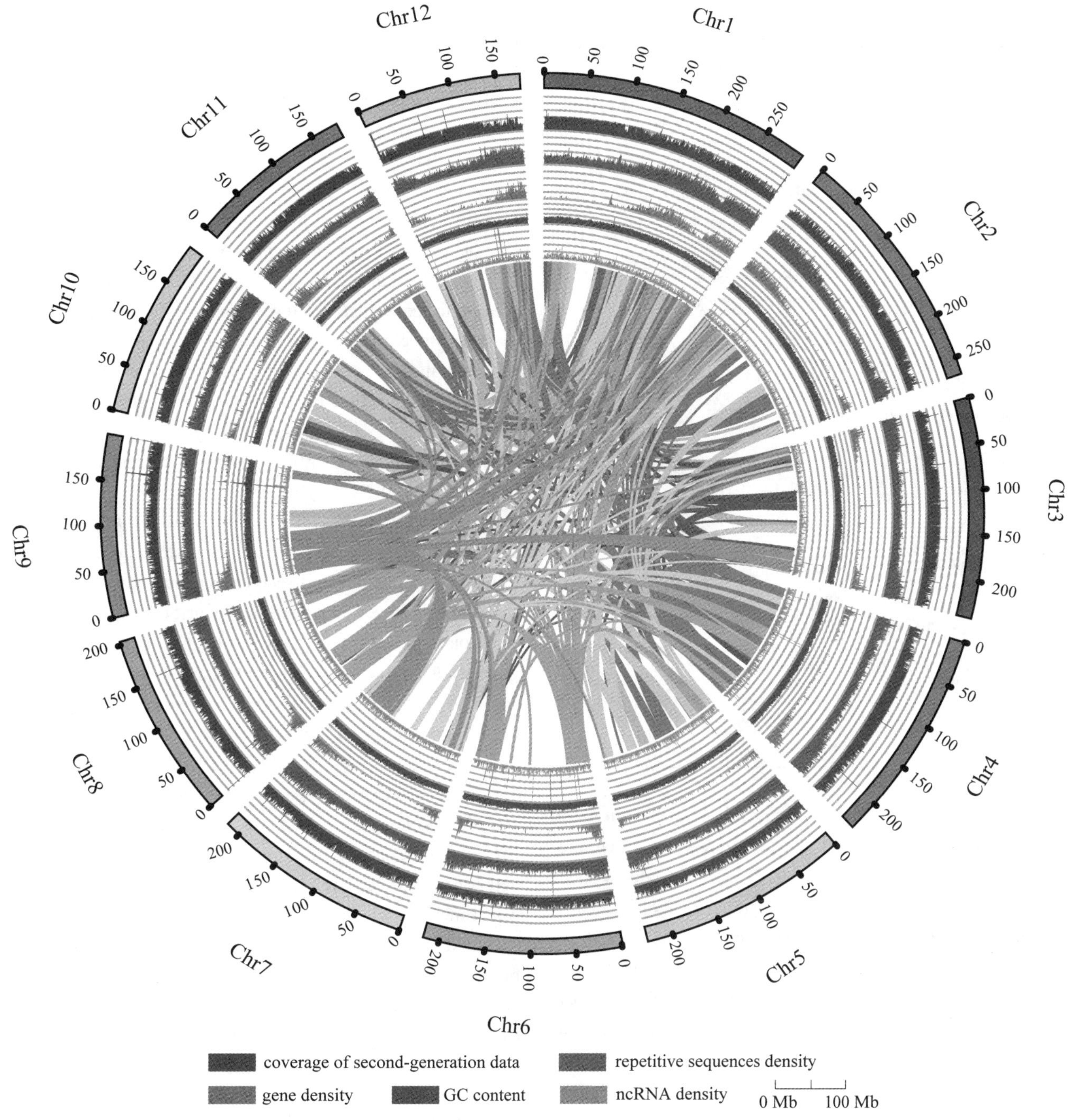


**Figure 1 Genome assembly characterization and chromosome locations of *P. notoginseng***

Landscape of the *P. notoginseng* genome: from outside to inside, chromosome number and length, coverage of second-generation data, density of repetitive sequences, gene density, GC content, noncoding RNA density, and genomic synteny.

approaches, 85.85% of the assembled *P. notoginseng* genome (Supplemental Table 7) consisted of repetitive elements; among them, long terminal repeat (LTR) retrotransposons accounted for the largest proportion and made up 58.88% of the genome (Supplemental Table 8; Supplemental Figure 3A and 3B). Compared with the published reference genome version, there were more predictions of repetitive sequences, a phenomenon that also occurs in other highly repetitive genomes. We compared the predicted repeat sequences with the RepBase database and calculated the degree of difference between them, from which LTR retrotransposons broke out at approximately 8% and an unknown outbreak happened earlier at approximately 5% (Supplemental Figure 3C).

An integrated strategy of *de novo predictions*, *homology-based searches*, *and RNA sequencing* was used to predict the protein-coding genes of the *P. notoginseng* genome. A total of 37 606 genes were annotated, with an average length of 5 059.63 bp and an average exon number per gene of 5.21 (Supplemental Table 9; Supplemental

**Table 1 Summary of the final genome assembly of *P. notoginseng* and comparison with published genomes**

| Items | PN201908 CCMU | 2017pub-1 | 2017pub-2 |
|---|---|---|---|
| Total length of contigs (Gb) | 2.66 | 1.85 | 2.39 |
| Contig N50 | 1.12 Mb | 13.16 kb | 16 kb |
| Longest contig (bp) | 13.35 Mb | 120.91 kb | 199.81 kb |
| Scaffold N50 | 216.47 Mb | 157.81 kb | 96 kb |
| Longest scaffold (bp) | 295.55 Mb | 1.19 Mb | 834.33 kb |
| GC content (%) | 34.45 | 34.85 | 28.65 |
| Number of genes | 37 606 | 34 369 | 36 790 |
| Average gene length (bp) | 5 059.63 | 2 705 | 3 307.48 |
| BUSCO (%) | 96.6 | N | 82.4 |
| Average CDS length (bp) | 1 202.85 | 957 | 942.43 |
| Average exon length (bp) | 231.00 | 251.39 | 211.92 |
| Average exon number per gene | 5.21 | 3.8 | 4.45 |
| Average intron length (bp) | 917.71 | 622.64 | 686.08 |
| Percentage of repeat sequences (%) | 85.85 | 61.31 | 75.94 |
| Percentage of LTR-RTs (%) | 58.88 | 57.41 | 66.72 |

Figure 4). The number of genes was similar to the numbers reported in two articles about the *P. notoginseng* genome published in 2017 (34 369 and 36 790), but other values, such as the average gene length and the average number of exons per gene, have been updated (Supplemental Table 10). Compared with another Araliaceae plant, *Panax ginseng* C. A. Mey (59 352 genes), *P. notoginseng* has a smaller number of genes, which may be related to the subsequent duplication event of *P. ginseng* after the divergence of the two plants. Among the annotated *P. notoginseng* genes, 36 154 (~96.14%) were functionally classified by BLASTing against various functional databases (Supplemental Table 11). We further annotated noncoding RNA genes, obtaining 14 430 microRNA genes, 1 513 transfer RNA (tRNA) genes, 314 ribosomal (rRNA) genes, and 272 small nuclear (snRNA) genes (Supplemental Table 12).

Genome evolution and expansion and contraction of gene families We compared our *P. notoginseng* assembly with sequenced genomes from seven other plants: *P. ginseng*, *Daucus carota* from Apiales, four dicot species (*Arabidopsis thaliana*, *Vitis vinifera*, *Capsicum annuum* L., and *Glycyrrhiza uralensis*), and a monocot, *Oryza sativa*. Based on gene family clustering analysis, 30 874 *P. notoginseng* genes (82.28%) clustered into 15 655 gene families (Supplemental Table 13 and Supplemental Figure 5), which included 7 264 gene families shared by all 8 species and 1 059 families specific to *P. notoginseng* (Supplemental Figure 6). Gene ontology (GO) and KEGG enrichment analysis of these *P. notoginseng*-specific gene families showed that they were mainly involved in a series of biological activities, e. g., mature ribosome assembly, cytosolic part, small-molecule binding, and RNA transport (Supplemental Table 14; Supplemental Figure 7).

We selected 458 single-copy gene families among the 8 species to construct phylogenetic trees. As expected, *P. notoginseng* clustered with another Araliaceae species, *P. ginseng*, and these two species were most closely related to the Apiales family (Figure 2A). We estimated that *P. notoginseng* and *P. ginseng* diverged from the Apiaceae approximately 62.0 million years ago (mya), and *P. notoginseng* and *P. ginseng* diverged around 4.2 mya. These results show that the relationship between *P. notoginseng* and *P. ginseng* is very close, consistent with their very similar morphologies and secondary metabolites.

We compared expanded and contracted gene families in the 8 plant species with their most recent common ancestor. In total, 989 gene families were expanded in *P. notoginseng*, and 1 823 gene families were contracted (Supplemental Figure 8). Compared with *P. ginseng* (6 449), the number of expanded gene families in *P. notoginseng* was significantly smaller, perhaps because *P. ginseng* has experienced one more WGD event than *P. notoginseng*. We performed GO and KEGG enrichment analysis on expanded and contracted gene families in the *P. notoginseng* genome. The functions of the expanded gene families were mainly enriched in GO terms such as transposition, fatty acid biosynthetic process, respiratory chain, and catalytic activity (Supplemental Figure 9; Supplemental Table 15). The functions of the contracted gene families were mainly enriched in GO terms such as protein phosphorylation, protein modification process, β-glucan biosynthetic process, 1,3-β-D-glucan synthase complex, and purine nucleotide binding (Supplemental Table 16). 1, 3-β-D-Glucan is reported to be involved in plant defense against fungi, and contraction in associated gene families may be related to the susceptibility of *P. notoginseng to* fungal pathogens and may explain why it readily develops root rot.

Analysis of WGD and its contribution to terpenoid biosynthesis To study the WGD events that occurred during the evolution of *P. notoginseng*, we first analyzed the 4-fold synonymous third-codon transversion rate (4DTv) (Figure 2B) of syntenic gene pairs. There were two peaks in the 4DTv distribution at approximately 0.16 and 0.50 for all syntenic gene pairs in the *P. notoginseng* genome. The first peak at approximately 0.50 corresponded to the core eudicot

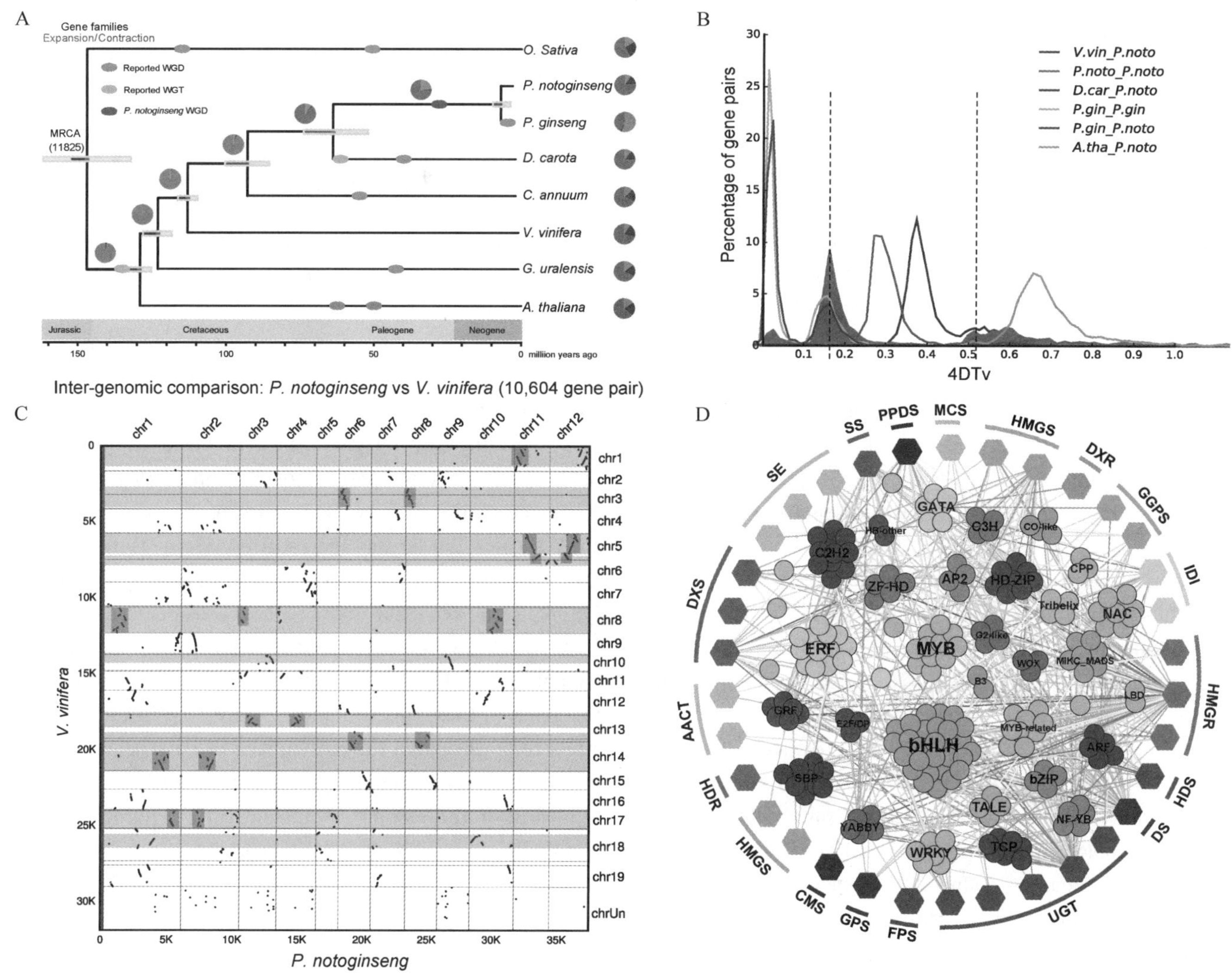


**Figure 2 Genome evolution and transcription factor regulation analysis of *P. notoginseng***

(A) Inferred phylogenetic tree with 458 single-copy genes from eight plant species. Gene family expansions are indicated in green, and gene family contractions are indicated in red. The timings of WGD and whole-genome triplications (WGT) are superimposed on the tree. Divergence times are estimated by maximum likelihood (PAML). (B) Distribution diagram of 4DTv values. The dark green-filled part indicates the 4DTv analysis inside *P. notoginseng*, and the peaks marked by the dotted line indicate where the two WGD events of *P. notoginseng* occurred. (C) Syntenic dot plots show a 2 : 1 chromosomal relationship between the *P. notoginseng* genome and the *V. vinifera* genome. The area in the pink box on each horizontal line represents the collinear block between the two genomes. (D) Correlation analysis of transcription factors with pathway genes. Pathway genes are represented by hexagons and transcription factors by circles. The line indicates the nature of the correlation: red for a positive correlation and blue for a negative correlation. The darker the color, the higher the correlation.

γ triplication event, and the second peak at approximately 0.16 revealed that *P. notoginseng* underwent another WGD event after diverging from *V. vinifera* and *D. carota*. By comparing the *P. notoginseng* genome with the *V. vinifera* genome, we found that 65% of *P. notoginseng* gene models were located in syntenic blocks that corresponded to single *V. vinifera* regions. Meanwhile, 42% of the *V. vinifera* gene models in syntenic blocks had two orthologous regions, and 22% had one orthologous region (Supplemental Figure 10). The results of a genome collinearity analysis between *V. vinifera* and *P. notoginseng* indicated that the WGD event occurred in the *P. notoginseng* genome and that there was a 1 : 2 syntenic relationship between *P. notoginseng* and *V. vinifera* (Figure 2C and Supplemental Figure 11). Based on the distribution of $K_s$ (Supplemental Figure 12) and 4DTv analysis, we calculated that the WGD event occurred approximately 29.6 mya in the ancestor of *P. notoginseng*. Compared with *P. notoginseng*, *P. ginseng* experienced one additional WGD event, and this recent event occurred approximately 1.85 mya after divergence from *P. notoginseng*. The timing of the WGD events was similar to the results of an evolutionary analysis of the *P. ginseng* genome (28 and 2.2 mya), confirming the accuracy of the present results.

Through homologous alignment and a Pfam database search, we identified gene families that were potentially involved in terpenoid biosynthesis in the eight species (Supplemental Table 17). The copy numbers of some gene families in the *P. notoginseng* genome were significantly greater than those in other plant genomes; these included families such as *DXS*, *MCS*, *HDS*, *HDR*, and *SQE*. We also observed that the average copy number of most key enzyme genes in *P. ginseng* was approximately twice that in *P. notoginseng* (Supplemental Figures 13 and 14). We next performed $K_a/K_s$ analysis of these pathway genes to calculate the duplication times of their gene pairs in the *P. notoginseng* genome. The gene pair duplication times were concentrated around the time of the WGD event of *P. notoginseng* (Supplemental Figure 15; Supplemental Table 18), indicating that they may have arisen from the WGD event.

Transcriptome analysis and transcriptional regulation of saponin biosynthesis To further explore the genetic information in *P. notoginseng*, we performed detailed transcriptome sequencing of *P. notoginseng* plants on the basis of the high-quality genome. Samples for transcriptome sequencing were obtained from 1- to 4-year-old *P. notoginseng* plants that were subdivided into root, stem, leaf, flower, rhizome, fibril, periderm, phloem, and tubercle (Supplemental Figures 16 and 17). Data processing (Supplemental Figures 18 and 19; Supplemental Table 19) and related transcriptome analyses, such as alternative splicing event analysis (Supplemental Figure 20; Supplemental Table 20), new transcription prediction, single-nucleotide polymorphism analysis (Supplemental Figure 21; Supplemental Table 21), analysis of gene expression levels (Supplemental Figures 22 and 23), and identification of differentially expressed genes (DEGs) (Supplemental Figure 24; Supplemental Table 22), are detailed in the Supplemental materials.

We further analyzed the regulation of transcription factors in *P. notoginseng*. A total of 2 150 transcription factors from 57 different families (Supplemental Table 23) were identified; we then used correlation analysis to map the gene regulation network (Figure 2D) between terpenoid biosynthetic pathway genes and transcription factors. The transcription factor families that were highly correlated with pathway genes included mainly bHLH, ERF, MYB, WRKY, NAC, and C2H2 transcription factors, as well as other families that play an important role in plant growth and development, stress resistance, and secondary metabolism.

Based on the expression levels of pathway genes (Supplemental Table 24), we explored the secondary metabolism of saponins in *P. notoginseng* plants at the temporal and spatial levels. At the temporal level, we compared the expression patterns of 29 genes from the saponin biosynthesis pathway in the same tissues of 1- to 4-year-old plants. In most tissues, highly expressed genes were concentrated in 3- or 4-year-old tissues, but in the stems, highly expressed genes were mainly concentrated in 1- to 2-year-old tissues (Figure 3). In addition, through comparative transcriptome analysis, we identified 7 792 DEGs that were highly expressed in 3- to 4-year-old plants but poorly expressed in plants of other ages. At the spatial level, we compared gene expression patterns in different tissues of same-aged plants. Except in 1-year-old plants, most of the pathway genes were specifically expressed in flowers, and a few were highly expressed in rhizomes and roots (Supplemental Figure 25).

Analyzing key enzyme genes involved in ginsenoside biosynthesis The biosynthesis of *P. notoginseng* saponins is attributed to the activity of a series of key enzyme genes, among which the largest and most diverse gene families are the CYP450s and the UGTs. Phylogenetic analysis of CYP450s showed that more genes were enriched in the CYP71, CYP72, CYP76, CYP716, and CYP94 superfamilies (Supplemental Figure 26; Supplemental Table 25). Most of the genes in these superfamilies are involved in the oxidative stress response and in the biosynthesis of triterpenes, sterols, indole alkaloids, geraniol iridoid, and so forth.

Most of the saponin compounds in *P. notoginseng* are triterpene glycosides that contain sugar groups, indicating that UGT genes play a vital role in the modification of these saponins. Phylogenetic analysis of 158 UGT genes showed that most were classified into subfamilies, such as UGT73, UGT71, UGT94, UGT91, UGT85, and UGT74 (Figure 4A; Supplemental Table 26). The UGTs encoded by genes in these subfamilies have been reported to catalyze the glycosylation of flavonoids, isoflavones, diterpenes, triterpenes, benzoate, lignans, and other compounds.

We used UGTs involved in terpene biosynthesis as queries to search for homologous UGT candidate genes in the *P. notoginseng* genome and designed primers for cloning (Supplemental Table 27). We ultimately cloned the full lengths of 32 UGT genes (Supplemental Figure 27) and named them *PnUGT1*–*PnUGT32*. Then, by expressing their proteins in *Escherichia coli*, we determined that five of them (*PnUGT1*–*5*) had catalytic functions in the biosynthesis of ginsenosides. We used an *E. coli*-expressed empty vector as the negative control (Supplemental Figure 28). Using PPT and F1 (Monoglycoside; PPT-C20-glucosyl) as substrates, the crude enzyme of gene *PnUGT3* could add a glucosyl group at the C6 position to produce Rh1 (Monoglycoside; PPT-C6-glucosyl) and Rg1 (Diglycoside; PPT-C6-glucosyl, C20-glycosyl), respectively (Figure 4B and Supplemental Figure 29). Its functions are therefore consistent with the functions of UGTPg1 and UGTPg101 from *P. ginseng*, but

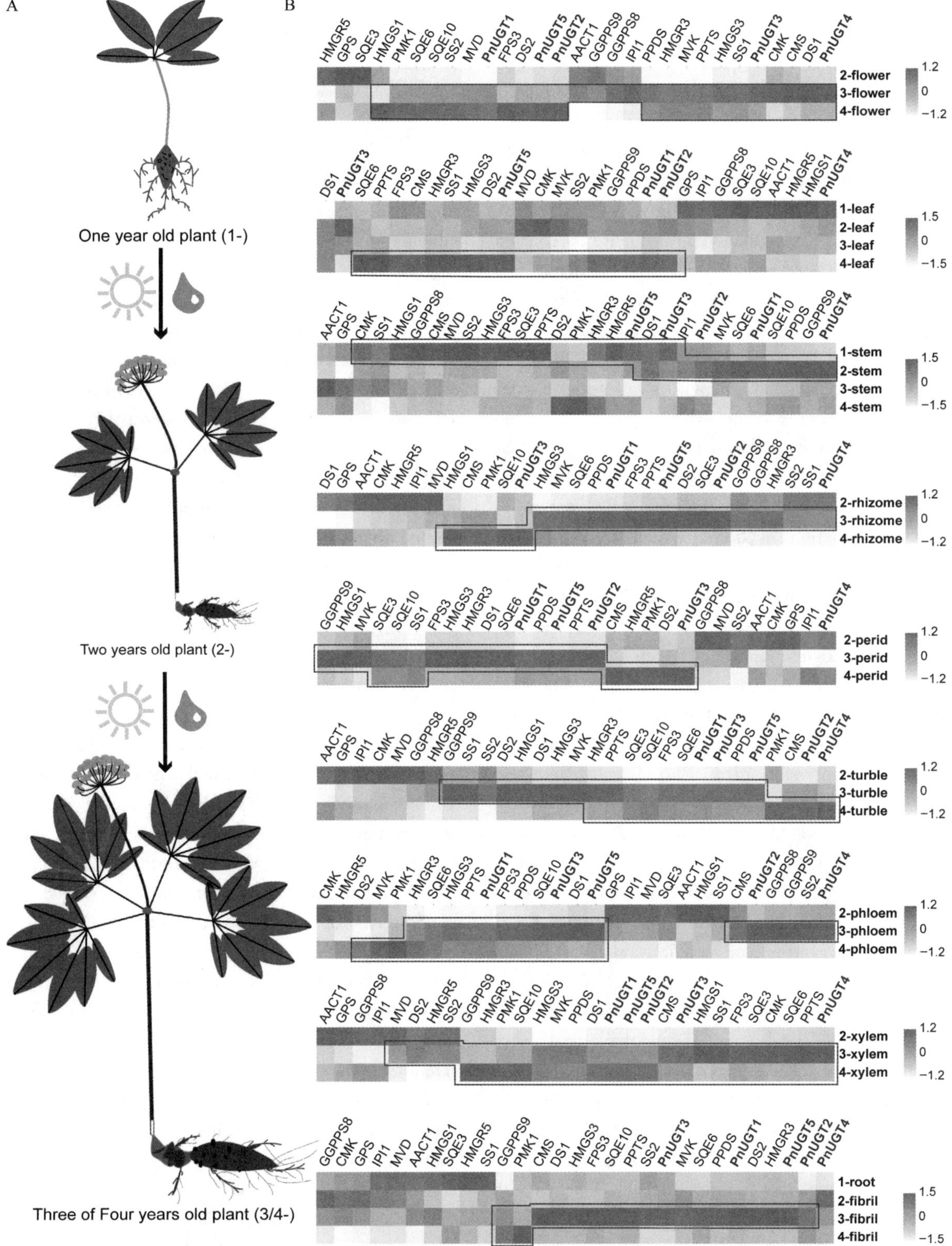


**Figure 3 Temporal expression profile of key enzyme genes in the saponin biosynthesis pathway**

(A) A brief view of the morphological changes in *P. notoginseng* as the years of growth increase during the cultivation process. (B) Temporal expression heatmap of terpenoid biosynthetic pathway genes in *P. notoginseng*. Taking the leaf's heatmap as an example, the Arabic numerals in the label indicate the years of growth; for example, 2-leaf indicates that the sample is the leaf of a 2-year-old *P. notoginseng* plant. Based on the gene expression levels, the pattern of expression change for any one gene can be observed after the data in each column are standardized. The area marked by the red box indicates high gene expression levels. Each heatmap has its own color scale: the higher the expression, the greener the color.

this is a new gene cloned for the first time in *P. notoginseng*. Using PPD and PPT as substrates, the crude enzyme of gene *PnUGT1* could add a glucosyl group at the C20 position to produce CK (Monoglycoside; PPD-C20-glucosyl) and F1 (Monoglycoside; PPT-C20-glucosyl), consistent with the functions of UGTPg100 and UGTPg101 from *P. ginseng*. In addition, PnUGT1 could catalyze the production of ginsenoside F2 (Diglycoside; PPD-C3-glucosyl, C20-glycosyl) from Rh2 (Monoglycoside; PPD-C3-glucosyl) (Figure 4B and Supplemental Figure 30), which is the first reported new function in *P. notoginseng*. The crude enzyme of gene *PnUGT5* could catalyze the production of Rh2 from PPD, and crude enzymes of genes *PnUGT2* and *PnUGT4* could then extend the sugar chain and generate Rg3 (Monoglycoside; PPD-C3-glucosyl-glucosyl) from Rh2 (Figure 4B and Supplemental Figure 31), consistent with the functions of UGTPg45 and UGTPg29 from *P. ginseng*. In addition, the last four genes have also been experimentally shown to perform catalytic functions in *Saccharomyces cerevisiae*.

Besides the more common ginsenoside compounds mentioned above, there are many unique saponins in *P. notoginseng*, such as notoginsenoside R1, notoginsenoside R2, notoginsenoside R4, and notoginsenoside Fc, which have better water solubility and good pharmacological activities (Supplemental Figure 32). To screen out more UGT genes, we conducted weighted gene co-expression network analysis (WGCNA) and expression profile consistency analysis. Through WGCNA, we constructed a correlation network between all genes annotated as UGT in the *P. notoginseng* genome and identified 7 gene modules with strong correlation, including 29 pathway genes and 139 UGT genes (Figure 4C and Supplemental Figure 33). Among them, *PnUGT2* was included in the blue module, and *PnUGT1* and *PnUGT5* were included in the green module. We further analyzed the annotation information and GO enrichment of these candidate UGT genes and found that most were enriched in GO terms such as GO: 0008152 (metabolic process) or GO: 0071555 (cell wall organization) and had different transferase activities (Supplemental Table 28). We then compared the expression patterns of genes in the terpene biosynthesis pathway and identified UGT genes with similar expression patterns. By comparing the expression levels in each transcriptome sample, the expression patterns of key enzyme genes could be divided into three categories (Figure 5): most were highly expressed in flowers, some were highly expressed in roots (each part), and a small number were most highly expressed in leaves (Supplemental Figure 34). A total of 35 UGT genes that were highly expressed and clustered with the pathway genes were screened from the correlation evolution tree (Supplemental Figure 35; Supplemental Table 29). Combining the results of the two analyses above, we identified candidate UGT genes that may be involved in the notoginsenoside biosynthetic pathway, although the specific functions of the encoded enzymes have yet to be experimentally verified.

## 3 DISCUSSION

*P. notoginseng*, one of the most widely used Chinese medicinal plants from the family Araliaceae, is renowned in China and worldwide for its good efficacy. The main active ingredients in *P. notoginseng* are saponins, including higher contents of ginsenoside Rg1, ginsenoside Rb1, and notoginsenoside R1, and other active compounds, such as ginsenoside Rd, ginsenoside Rg3, ginsenoside Re, notoginsenoside R2, and notoginsenoside Fc. The biosynthesis of saponins in *P. notoginseng* has attracted extensive attention from researchers, and some key enzyme genes, such as *HMGR*, *AACT*, *SS*, *PMK*, *MVK*, *IDI*, and *CYP450*, have been identified. However, the complete biosynthetic pathways of unique notoginsenosides have not yet been resolved, and further research and exploration are needed.

Gene mining of high-quality genomic and transcriptomic data can provide resources for further exploration of plant growth and secondary metabolism mechanisms. As early as 2017, two *P. notoginseng* reference genomes were published; however, the quality of these genomes was insufficient because of the limited sequencing capacity at that time. We therefore performed whole-genome sequencing of *P. notoginseng* from Genuine Producing Areas based on third-generation PacBio sequencing technology and used Hi-C technology to construct a high-quality, chromosome-level genome. The assembled genome was 2.66 Gb in size, with a scaffold N50 of 216.47 Mb and a contig N50 of 1.12 Mb. In addition to the depth or accuracy of gene sequencing, this reference genome was greatly improved compared with previous genomes and was resolved to the chromosome level, which can more intuitively reveal the gene distribution and overall genomic landscape.

In addition to *P. notoginseng*, other plants belonging to Araliaceae are used as medicines, including the well-known plants *P. ginseng*, *Panax quinquefolius* L., and *Panax zingiberensis* C. Y. Wu et K. M. Feng. Based on chemotaxonomy, plants of *Panax* L. can be divided into two groups. The chemical composition of the first group mainly comprises dammarane-type tetracyclic triterpenes, and there are obvious similarities in plant morphology, including a short and erect rhizome and a carrot-like fleshy root. In terms of geographical distribution, plants in this group show a characteristic narrow and intermittent distribution, which has been observed in an ancient group of *Panax* plants. Representative plants include *P. notoginseng*, *P. ginseng*, *P. quinquefolius*, and others. The saponins of the second

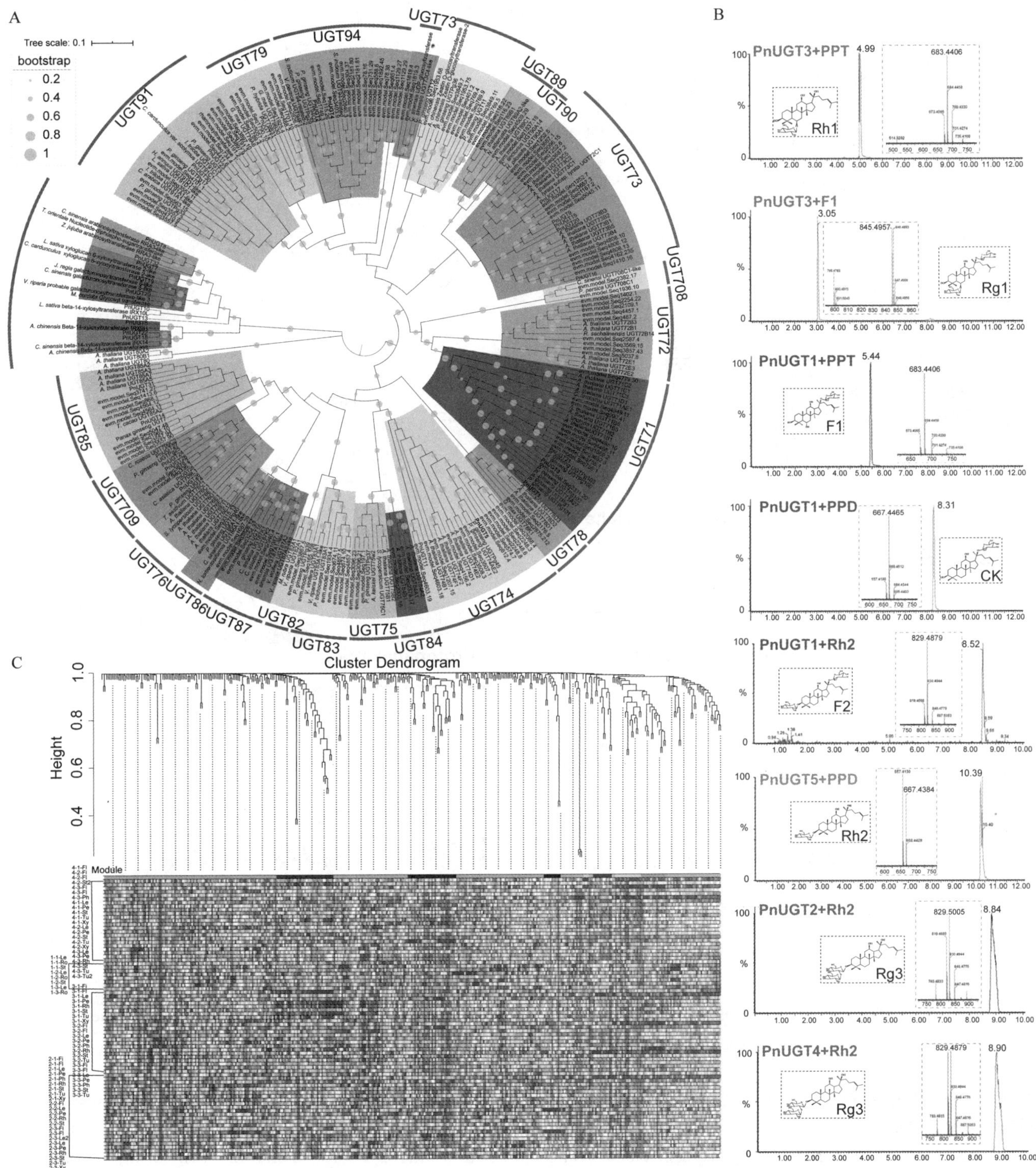


**Figure 4 Screening for candidate UGT genes and functional verification of five UGT genes**

(A) Phylogenetic analysis of UGT genes. The UGT gene families clustered into one clade are represented by different colors. The bootstrap value associated with each branch is represented by a light-purple circle; the larger the radius, the greater the bootstrap value. (B) UPLC/Q-TOF analysis of five functional UGT genes. In catalytic reactions, PnUGT3 uses PPT and F1 as substrates, PnUGT1 uses PPD, PPT, and Rh2 as substrates, PnUGT5 uses PPD as a substrate, and PnUGT2 and PnUGT4 use Rh2 as a substrate to generate corresponding ginsenoside compounds. The chemical structures and characteristic mass spectrum peaks of products from each reaction are displayed in the dashed box of each track. (C) WGCNA analysis of UGT genes.

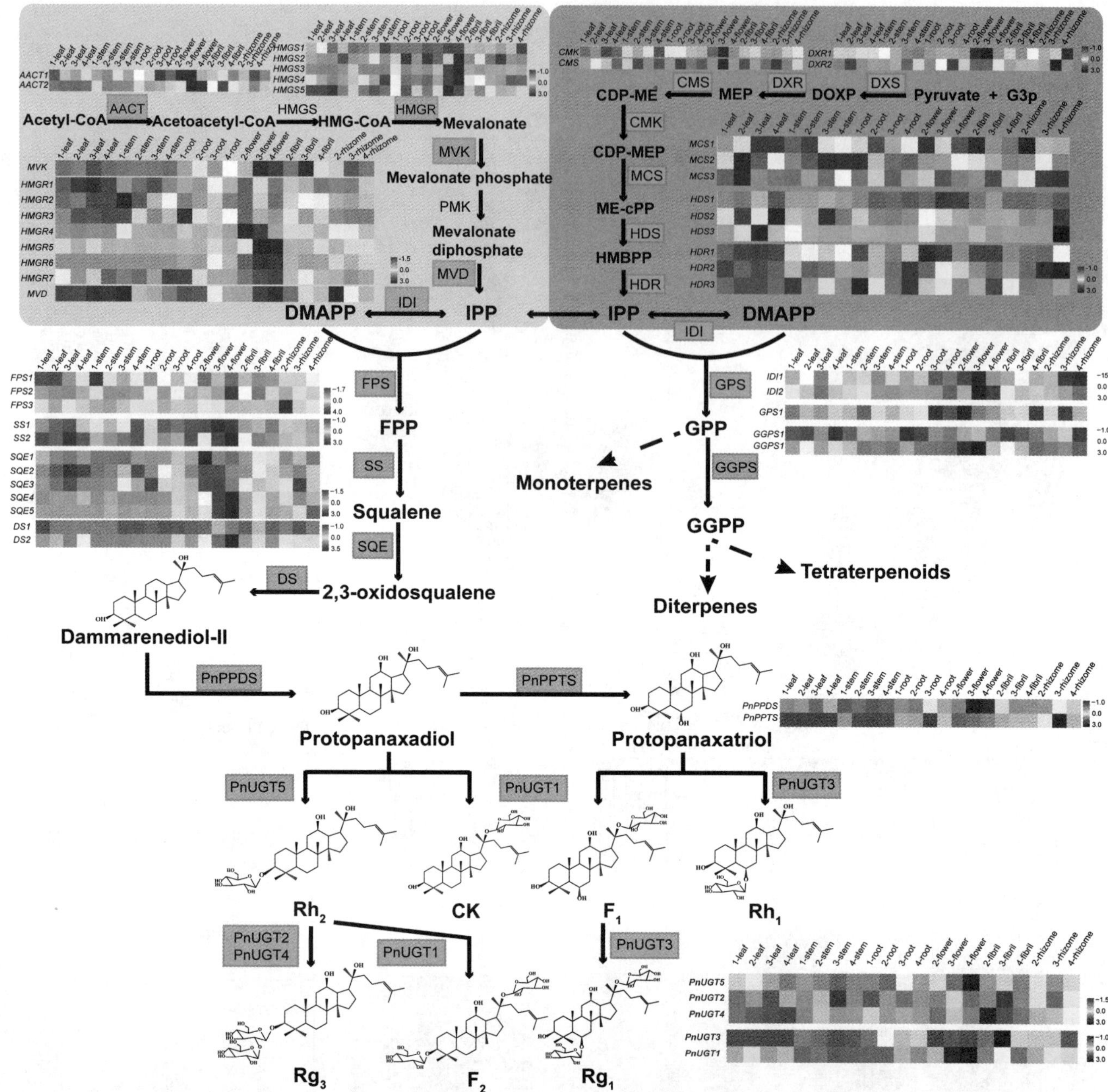


**Figure 5 Overview of the saponin biosynthetic pathway in *P. notoginseng* and expression profiles of key enzyme genes**

The genes in the green box are the UGT genes identified in this study.

group are mainly oleanane-type pentacyclic triterpenes, and their plant morphology includes a long and creeping rhizome and an undeveloped fleshy root. They are distributed over a wide and continuous geographical area and may represent an evolutionary group of *Panax* plants. Representative plants from this group include *P. zingiberensis* C. Y. Wu et K. M. Feng, *P. stipuleanatus* H. T. Tsai et K. M. Feng, *Panax japonicus* (T. Nees) C. A. Mey. and *Panax japonicus* C. A. Mey. var. major (Burk.) C. Y. Wu et K. M. Feng, and others. Based on cytotaxonomy analysis, we found that *Panax* plants had different ploidy types. For example, *P. notoginseng* and *P. japonicus* are diploid, and *P. ginseng* and *P. quinquefolius* are tetraploid, further indicating that *P. notoginseng* is in a relatively primitive evolutionary position among *Panax* plants. By comparing genomes, we found that after diverging from carrots, an independent WGD event occurred in *P. notoginseng*. We then studied the distribution of $K_a/K_s$ values of key enzyme gene pairs in the saponin biosynthesis pathway and found that the WGD event may have contributed to the generation of these gene pairs, directing the metabolic flux toward the production of saponins. Based on the locations of coding genes on the chromosomes, we also found two sets of gene cluster duplication. Notably, upstream HDR, SS, and SE genes and downstream CYP450 and UGT genes that are known to be involved in ginsenoside biosynthesis are close to each other in the *P. notoginseng* genome (Supplemental Figure 36). The gene cluster also contains some UGT and transcription factor genes identified in this study, which are likely to participate in the biosynthesis and regulation of saponins. Compared with *P. notoginseng*, *P. ginseng* experienced one additional WGD event, which was manifested in the larger genome size, more expanded gene families, and multiple copies of key enzyme genes. In summary, we analyzed and explored the genetic information of *P. notoginseng*, one of the more primitive *Panax* plants, laying a solid foundation for subsequent evolutionary research on the genus *Panax*.

In addition, we also established a detailed transcript database of *P. notoginseng* through sequencing and analysis of different tissues from 1- to 4-year-old plants. Through comparative transcriptome analysis, we explored the molecular regulation mechanism of tubercles, a characteristic phenotype of *P. notoginseng*. The associated DEGs were mainly involved in the biosynthesis of plant hormones such as strigolactone, cytokinin, and auxin. The synergistic effects of these phytohormones result in the production of a tubercle phenotype, and further study of the functions of related DEGs will more fully reveal the molecular mechanisms of tubercle formation.

We next explored the saponin biosynthesis pathway in *P. notoginseng* plants at temporal and spatial levels. We compared the expression patterns of saponin biosynthesis genes in the same tissues of 1- to 4-year-old plants and found that most genes in tissues other than stems were highly expressed in 3- or 4-year-old plants. This indicates that as plant age increases, saponin biosynthesis gene expression levels also increase, as does the content of accumulated saponins. The quality of *P. notoginseng* harvested after more than 3 years of growth is therefore optimal, but because of diseases, insect pests, and continuous cropping obstacles, most materials circulated in the market are 3-year-old *P. notoginseng*. At the spatial level, most pathway genes were specifically expressed in flowers, and a few were highly expressed in rhizomes and roots, including the postmodification UGT enzyme genes *PnUGT2*, *PnUGT3*, and *PnUGT4*. These results indicate that saponin compounds or their precursors may be synthesized in the flowers first and then transferred to the roots or further modified in the roots, consistent with a previous report.

The ultimate step in the saponin biosynthesis pathway is glycosylation catalyzed by UGTs. This is the most critical step in determining the structure and pharmacological effects of the compounds, and we therefore focused on identifying candidate UGT genes. First, we conducted a systematic evolutionary analysis of all *P. notoginseng* genes that contained the conserved GT domain. As expected, we obtained five UGT genes that catalyzed the glycosylation of ginsenosides. Second, we performed WGCNA analysis on all genes annotated as UGTs and key enzyme genes of the *P. notoginseng* saponin biosynthetic pathway and screened out seven modules of highly correlated genes. Among these seven modules, two (module blue and module green) contained genes with identified functions, indicating that the genes enriched in these modules were likely to participate in the biosynthesis of saponins. Third, we conducted a consistency analysis of expression profiles and identified 20 UGT genes with high expression levels and expression patterns consistent with those of pathway genes. Combining the results of the two analyses above, we identified candidate UGT genes to lay a foundation for further comprehensive analysis of the complete notoginsenoside biosynthesis pathway.

In summary, we constructed a high-quality, chromosome-level *P. notoginseng* reference genome as a comprehensive genetic inventory for evolutionary phylogenomic studies of *Panax* plants. Using detailed transcriptome data, we explored the molecular mechanism of tubercle formation, investigated the biosynthesis pathway of saponins, and provided many promising candidate genes to fully reveal the biosynthetic pathway of notoginsenosides in *P. notoginseng*.

## 4 MATERIALS AND METHODS

Plant materials, DNA extraction, and library construction Individual plants of *P. notoginseng* (Burk.) F. H. Chen were collected in August 2019 from Wenshan County, Yunnan Province, China (26°49′55″N, 100°3′20″E, 2 630 m above sea level). Fresh and healthy leaves were harvested, immediately frozen in liquid nitrogen, and preserved at −80℃. High-quality genomic DNA was extracted from the *P. notoginseng leaves* using the modified phenol-chloroform isoamyl alcohol extraction method. The quality and quantity of the isolated DNA were assessed using a NanoPhotometer (Implen, CA, USA) and a Qubit 2.0 Fluorometer (Life Technologies, CA, USA). Illumina (350 bp), PacBio, and Hi-C libraries were constructed following the operation guide for each technology.

Genome sequencing, assembly, and quality assessment For PacBio libraries, the whole genome was sequenced on the PacBio Sequel II System based on single-molecule real-time sequencing technology, and 284.07 Gb (~106.79×) of data were obtained. The Illumina library was sequenced on the Illumina HiSeq X Ten platform following standard Illumina protocols. After filtering out adapter sequences and low-quality and duplicated reads, we obtained 231.06 Gb (~86.86×) of clean data. The subreads obtained from PacBio libraries were assembled into contigs using Canu (v1.8), and the consensus genome was polished by referring to the

Illumina reads with BWA (v0.7.9a) and Pilon (v1.22). For Hi-C libraries, Illumina HiSeq X Ten was used for sequencing with PE150, and a total of 340.83 Gb (~128.13×) of data were retained. Finally, based on Hi-C technology using BWA-mem and LACHESIS, the final genome was 2.66 Gb in size, and the contig and scaffold N50 were 1.12 and 216.47 Mb, respectively. We used BUSCO (v3.0.1, default parameters), Illumina reads, and transcriptome mapping to the *P. notoginseng* genome with BWA-mem to confirm the high quality of the assembled genome.

Genome annotation  We used homology-based, *de novo*, and transcriptome-based predictions to predict the protein-coding genes in the *P. notoginseng* genome. The gene sets predicted by various strategies were integrated into a non-redundant and more complete gene set using EVidenceModeler. Gene functional annotation was performed mainly by searching against various functional databases, such as Swiss-Prot, NT (Nucleotide Sequence Database), NR (Non-Redundant Protein Sequence Database), Pfam, eggNOG (Evolutionary Genealogy of Genes: Non-supervised Orthologous Groups), and GO. Repetitive sequences were annotated using an *ab initio* prediction method and a homolog-based approach. We detected noncoding RNA by comparison with known noncoding RNA libraries and Rfam, and we also predicted rRNAs, snRNAs, microRNAs, and so on.

Analysis of genomic evolution and WGD events  We used the OrthoMCL package (1.4) to identify and cluster gene families (clusters) from *P. notoginseng* and seven other plant species: *P. ginseng*, *D. carota*, *V. vinifera*, *C. annuum* L., *G. uralensis*, *A. thaliana*, and *O. sativa*. After gene family clustering, we aligned all 458 single-copy gene protein sequences using MUSCLE and constructed a phylogenetic tree using PhyML. Based on the gene family cluster analysis and after filtering gene families with abnormal gene numbers in individual species, we used the CAFÉ program to identify the expansion and contraction of gene families in each species. To explore the evolution of the *P. notoginseng* genome, we calculated the 4DTv of syntenic blocks and the distribution of synonymous substitutions per synonymous site ($K_s$) to identify WGD events.

Integrated genomic and transcriptomic analysis  One- to four-year-old *P. notoginseng* plants were collected from Wenshan County, Yunnan Province, China. There were three biological replicates for each sample, and samples were taken at least five meters apart. After harvesting, we subdivided the plants into different tissue parts, including the root (xylem), stem, leaf, flower, rhizome, fibril, periderm, phloem, and tubercle. All samples were transported on dry ice, washed with ultrapure water three times, immediately frozen in liquid nitrogen, and stored at −80℃ before RNA extraction. Total RNA was extracted from each tissue using a modified cetyltrimethylammonium bromide method. The RNA purity was checked using a kaiaoK5500 spectrophotometer (Kaiao, Beijing, China), and the RNA integrity and concentration were assessed using the RNA Nano 6000 Assay Kit for the Bioanalyzer 2100 system (Agilent Technologies, CA, USA). cDNA libraries were constructed using the NEBNext Ultra RNA Library Prep Kit for Illumina (New England Biolabs, USA) following the manufacturer's recommendations. After cluster generation, the libraries were sequenced on an Illumina NovaSeq S2 platform, and 150 bp paired-end reads were generated.

Genes encoding key enzymes thought to be involved in the saponin biosynthetic pathway were annotated by BLAST (2.2.28). Their predicted proteins were aligned with the Pfam database using HMMER (3.1b1), and their expression levels in different tissues were obtained from transcriptome data. We used MeV software (4.9.0) to create a heatmap of gene expression and analyze gene expression patterns. In addition, we identified transcription factor genes in the *P. notoginseng* genome by comparison with the PlantTFDB database. We used an R script to calculate the Pearson correlation coefficients between transcription factors and genes in batches and Cytoscape software to draft the correlation map.

Screening and functional verification of candidate UGT genes  Multiple sequence alignments were generated using DNAMAN to visualize the conserved motifs. For phylogenetic tree analysis, the amino acid sequences of UGTs from other species were downloaded from the National Center for Biotechnology Information (NCBI) database and aligned using ClustalW. Then, a neighbor-joining tree was built using MEGA X software with 1000 bootstrap iterations. *P. notoginseng* cDNA was prepared using the PrimeScript 1st Strand cDNA Synthesis Kit (Takara, Dalian, China). After designing primers, we cloned a total of 32 UGT genes, and the PCR products were ligated into the N-terminal MBP fusion expression vector HIS-MBP-pET28a (HIS, histidine; MBP, maltose-binding protein) according to the protocol of the Seamless Cloning Kit (Beyotime, Shanghai, China). We transformed the successfully sequenced positive strains into *E. coli* BL21 (DE3) (Transgen Biotech, Beijing, China) and maintained the cultures in Luria-Bertani liquid medium with kanamycin (50 μg/mL) at 37℃ in a shaking incubator until the optical density at 600 nm reached 0.6 - 0.8. Then, 1 mol/L isopropyl β-D-thiogalactopyranoside was added to a final concentration of 50 μmol/L, and cultures were maintained at 16℃ and 120 rpm for 16 h to allow expression of recombinant proteins. pET28a-transformed *E. coli* BL21 (DE3) cells were treated in parallel as a control. The recombinant cells were harvested by centrifugation at 10 000 *g* and 4 ℃, then resus-pended in 100 mmol/L phosphate buffer (pH 8.0) that contained 1 mmol/L phenylmethanesulfonylfluoride and sonicated in an ice-water bath for 10 min (lysed for 5 s, paused for 5 s). The sample lysates were centrifuged for 20 min at 12 000 *g* and 4 ℃ to separate crude enzymes from cell debris. A UGT activity assay was performed in a total volume of 100 μL that contained 100 mmol/L crude enzyme buffer (pH 8.0), 1 mmol/L UDP-glucose, and 0.1 mmol/L acceptor substrate for 2 h in a 35 ℃ water bath and was terminated by the addition of 200 μL methanol. Precipitated proteins were removed by centrifugation (10 000 *g* for 10 min) and filtered through 0.22 μm filters before injection. Glycosylated products were detected using ultra-high-performance liquid chromatography coupled with quadrupole time-of-flight mass spectrometry (UPLC/Q-TOF-MS, Waters, Milford, MA) using a Waters ACQUITY UPLC HSS T3 analytical column (2.1 × 100 mm, 1.8 μm). Data analysis was performed using MassLynx soft-ware (version 4.1). Standards of saponin compounds and UDP-glucose were purchased from Yuanye Bio-Technology (Shanghai, China). To screen additional candidate UGT genes, we also conducted WGCNA using R and expression profile consistency analysis.

Data availability  The data supporting the findings of this work are available within the paper and its Supplemental Information files. The nucleotide sequencing data for UGT genes identified in this study have been deposited at NCBI GenBank under accession numbers MT551198 to MT551202. The genome sequence data of *P. notoginseng* have been deposited under NCBI Bio-Project number PRJNA658419 https://www.Ncbi.nlm.nih.gov/bioproject/SUB7934826. In addition, the whole-genome sequence data reported in this paper have been deposited in the Genome Warehouse in the National Genomics Data Center, Beijing Institute of Genomics (China National Center for Bioinformation), Chinese Academy of Sciences, under accession number GWHAOSA00000000 and are publicly accessible at https://bigd.big.ac.cn/gsa.

[蒋周倩，黄璐琦，高伟，等. Plant Communications, 2020,2(1):100113.]

# Genome of *Tripterygium wilfordii* and identification of cytochrome P450 involved in triptolide biosynthesis

*Tripterygium wilfordii*, a perennial twining shrub of the Celastrales, has been used medicinally for centuries, mainly to treat rheumatoid arthritis. It has been known to be a rich source of specialized metabolites. Two of these (triptolide and celastrol) are among five natural products high-lighted for their great potential to be developed into pharmaceuticals. Indeed, triptolide has been demonstrated to possess important therapeutic potential with anti-inflammatory, immunosuppressive, and antitumor activities, as well as to exhibit potentially medically relevant activity for central nervous system diseases (e.g. Parkinson's and Alzheimer's diseases). Moreover, several derivatives of triptolide have undergone clinical trials.

Currently, triptolide only can be extracted from *T. wilfordii* with extremely low yields, ranging from 0.000 1% to 0.002% of dry weight biomass, and the plant cannot be cultivated at a large scale as contamination with its pollen renders honey poisonous, which has frequently causes poisoning events in areas where this medicinal plant is cultivated. Although significant efforts have been devoted to improving chemical synthesis, current routes are limited to yields of less than 1.64% due to the structural and stereochemical complexity of triptolide. Accordingly, further investigation of its pharmaceutical utility is severely limited by a shortage of supply. While suspension cultures, tissue cultures, and adventitious root cultures have been investigated as alternative sources of this bioactive diterpenoid, a more promising approach to obtaining such structurally complex natural products is metabolic engineering. This can be attempted in the native plant or accomplished via a synthetic biology strategy, involving reconstitution in a suitably engineered microbial chassis organism, which can establish a sustainable and reliable means of production. However, this latter approach requires elucidation of the relevant biosynthetic pathway.

Triptolide is an abietane-type diterpenoid, produced via initial cyclization of (*E*, *E*, *E*)-geranylgeranyl diphosphate (GGPP) to copalyl diphosphate (CPP), with subsequent cyclization to the abietane-type diene olefin miltiradiene. The 1,4-diene arrangement of the miltiradiene C ring leaves this poised for aromatization, which most likely occurs spontaneously. Along with conversion of carbon-18 (C-18) from a methyl to carboxylic acid, this forms dehydroabietic acid, followed by oxidative 1,2-migration of C-18 (from

C-4→C-3) and further transformation to the phenolic triepoxide triptolide. At present, elucidation of the triptolide pathway relies on transcriptomes, which has only led to identification of the relevant diterpene synthases, namely the relevant CPP synthase (CPS1) and miltiradiene synthase (MS), with subsequently acting enzymes, such as cytochrome P450s (CYPs), involved in further biosynthesis of the highly functionalized triptolide remaining enigmatic. CYPs form the largest family of enzymes in plants, playing manifold roles in their complex metabolism. Indeed, there are still CYP families, defined as phylogenetic clades with < 40% amino acid sequence identity between them, whose function remains unknown, with no biochemical activity yet assigned to any member. Recently, whole-genome sequencing provides a comprehensive genetic resource and has become a practical approach to not only elucidation of natural product biosynthetic pathways, but also insight into their evolution, as well as improvement of their production. Nevertheless, this must be coupled to other information directed more specifically at the natural product of interest.

Here we first present a high-quality reference-grade genome of *T. wilfordii* and show that duplications of triptolide biosynthetic pathway genes are almost all generated by a recent whole-genome triplication event. We then map a gene-to-metabolite network by integrating genomic, transcriptomic, and metabolomic data. Next, we combine the synthetic biology tools, RNAi knock-down, and overexpression to identify a cytochrome P450 (CYP728B70) that can catalyze oxidation of C-18 from a methyl to the acid moiety of dehydroabietic acid in triptolide biosynthesis. This work provides the genomic resource and the candidate genes that may contribute to fully elucidation of the triptolide biosynthetic pathway and consequently lead to heterologous bioproduction.

## 1 RESULTS

Genome assembly and annotation. Based on the k-mer distribution analysis, we estimated the genome size of *T. wilfordii* to be ~365.95 Mb with a high level of heterozygosity (1.95%) and repetition (48.87%), indicating the genome assembly was complicated (Supplementary Fig. 1 and Supplementary Table 1). The genome of *T. wilfordii* was sequenced using PacBio (read length of 60 kb, ~207.10× coverage) and 10X Genomics (~327.23× coverage) (Supplementary Table 2). The total length of the final assembly was 348.38 Mb with 467 contigs and a contig N50 of 4.36 Mb (Supplementary Table 3). Assessment of the completeness of the genome assembly with CEGMA indicated 96.77% coverage of the conserved core eukaryotic genes (Supplementary Table 5), and BUSCO results indicated that the genome was 95.10% complete (Supplementary Table 6). Additionally, 97.06% of the transcriptome can be mapped back to the assembly, further supporting a high level of genome coverage (Supplementary Table 7 and Supplementary Note 1).

**Table 1 Summary of *T. wilfordii* genome assembly and annotation**

| | Number | Size |
|---|---|---|
| Genome assembly | | |
| Total contigs | 467 | 348.38 Mb |
| Contig N50 | 15 | 4.36 Mb |
| Contig N90 | 137 | 265 kb |
| Total scaffolds | 321 | 348.53 Mb |
| Scaffold N50 | 12 | 13.52 Mb |
| Scaffold N90 | 23 | 10.83 Mb |
| Pseudochromosomes | 23 | 315.08 Mb |
| Genome annotation | | |
| Repetitive sequences | 52.36% | 182.52 Mb |
| Noncoding RNAs | 4 235 | 1.12 Mb |
| Protein-coding genes | 28,321 | 109.30 Mb |
| Genes in pseudochromosomes | 28,297 (99.92%) | 109.24 Mb |

The *T. wilfordii* assembly was further refined using high-throughput chromosome conformation capture (Hi-C) data, comprised of 321 scaffolds with a scaffold N50 of 13.52 Mb (Table 1). As a result, 315.08 Mb of the assembly and 99.92% of the genes were distributed across 23 chromosome-level pseudomolecules (Fig. 1a, Table 1 and Supplementary Data 1).

We were able to annotate 28,321 protein-coding genes, with an average sequence length of 3 338 bp, similar to those of other reported plants (Supplementary Tables 8 and 9). On average, each predicted gene contains 5.44 exons with an average sequence length of 228 bp. A total of 182.52 Mb of repetitive elements occupying 52.36% of the *T. wilfordii* genome were annotated (Supplementary Fig. 2 and Supplementary Note 2). The majority of the repeats are long terminal repeats (LTRs) (34.26% of the genome; Supplementary Table 10). Approximately 99.6% of the genes were functionally annotated by similarity searches against homologous sequences and protein domains (Supplementary Table 11). In addition, we identified noncoding RNA (ncRNA) genes, including 2,563 rRNA, 407 tRNA, 373 miRNA, and 892 snRNA genes (Supplementary Table 12). These results further support the completeness of our *T. wilfordii* genome sequence and a schematic representation of the genome is given in Fig. 1a.

Genome evolution contributed to formation of triptolide. To investigate the evolution of *T. wilfordii*, we constructed

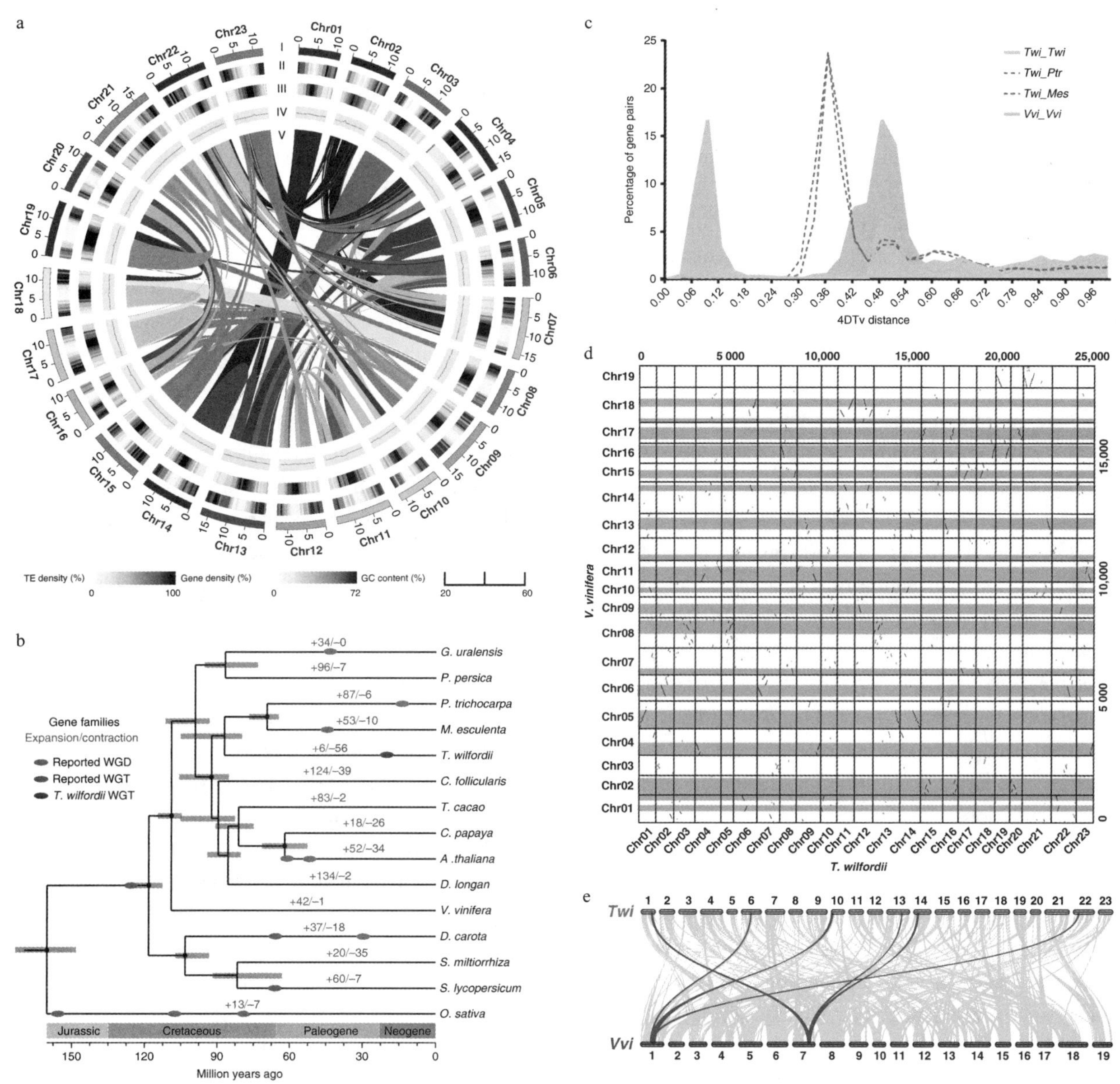


**Fig. 1 Genome evolution of *T. wilfordii***

(a) Distribution of *T. wilfordii* genomic features. (Ⅰ) Circular representation of the pseudomolecule. (Ⅱ-Ⅳ) gene density (500 kb window), percentage of repeats (500 kb window), and GC content (500 kb window). (Ⅴ) Each linking line in the center of the circle connects a pair of homologous genes. (b) Inferred phylogenetic tree with 514 single-copy genes of 15 plant species. Gene family expansions are indicated in green, and gene family contractions are indicated in red. The timing of whole-genome duplication (WGD) and the timing of whole-genome triplication (WGT) are superimposed on the tree. Divergence times are estimated by Maximum Likelihood (PAML). (c) Distribution of 4DTv shown in colored lines as indicated. (d) Syntenic dot plots show a 3-1 chromosomal relationship between *T. wilfordii* genome and *V. vinifera* genome. (e) Macrosynteny between *T. wilfordii* and *V. vinifera* karyotypes. Source data are provided as a Source Data file.

a phylogenetic tree and estimated the divergence times of 15 plant species using 514 single-copy genes (Fig. 1b, Supplementary Fig. 4 and Supplementary Note 3). Phylogenomic analysis showed that *T. wilfordii* was most related to the ancestor of *Manihot esculenta* and *Populus trichocarpa*, with an estimated divergence time of 87.1 million years ago (MYA). Gene family expansion and contraction was examined using CAFÉ (Fig. 1b and Supplementary Note 3). Among the *T. wilfordii*, *P. trichocarpa*, *M. esculenta*, and *Cephalotus follicularis* gene families, a total of 951 genes appeared unique to *T. wilfordii* (Supplementary Fig. 5). Interestingly, Gene Ontology (GO) and Kyoto Encyclopedia of Genes and Genomes (KEGG) analyses found these *T. wilfordii*-specific genes were particularly enriched in the terms terpene synthase, oxidation-reduction process, and plant-pathogen interaction (Supplementary Tables 13 and 14).

The distribution of 4DTv (fourfold degenerate synonymous sites of the third codons) of all gene pairs found in each segment showed two peaks at approximately 0.09 and 0.48 in the *T. wilfordii* genome. The first peak at approximately 0.48 revealed the core eudicot γ triplication event, and the second peak at approximately 0.09 indicated that *T. wilfordii* underwent another whole-genome multiplication event after diverging from *P. trichocarpa* and *M. esculenta* (Fig. 1c). We further compared *T. wilfordii* genome and *Vitis vinifera* genome. 77% of *T. wilfordii* gene models are in syntenic blocks corresponding to one *V. vinifera* region, covering 83% of the *V. vinifera* gene space, among which 35% have three orthologous regions in *T. wilfordii*, 31% have two, and 15% have one (Supplementary Fig. 6). Intergenomic co-linearity analysis was consistent with both the γ-event and another, more specific WGT event for *T. wilfordii*, as indicated by a 1∶3 syntenic relationship between *T. wilfordii* and *V. vinifera* (Fig. 1d, e). The recent WGT event was dated to approximately 21±6 MYA, as indicated by the distribution of synonymous substitutions per synonymous site (*KS*) of syntenic genes in *T. wilfordii* (Supplementary Fig. 7). The recent WGT event occurred in the Paleogene (65 - 23.3 MYA) to Neogene (23.3 - 1.64 MYA) period, which may have enabled *T. wilfordii* to cope better with the markedly changed environment by functional redundancy, mutational robustness, increased evolution rate, and adaptation.

Gene families that may be involved in terpenoid (e.g., triptolide in *T. wilfordii*) biosynthesis were identified in the fifteen reported plant species. The results showed that the copy number of these gene families varied among all examined plant species, with those encoding *DXS*, *GGPPS*, *TPS* and *CYP* exhibiting particularly strong variation (Supplementary Table 18). To further investigate the role of WGT events on triptolide biosynthesis, we carried out phylogenetic analysis of the gene families potentially involved in this pathway, specifically *Ks* calculations for each duplicated gene pair, including those from upstream isoprenoid metabolism (i.e., *ACAT*, *CMK*, *DXS*, *FPS*, *GPS*, *GGPPS*, *HDR*, *HDS*, *HMGR*, *HMGS*, *IDI*, *MCT*, *MVK*, *MVD*, *PMK*) and those more specific to triptolide (i.e., *CPS* and *MS*) (Supplementary Fig. 8 and Supplementary Table 19). We found that duplications of these genes were almost all generated by the recent WGT event (i.e., *ACAT*, *CMK*, *GPS*, *HDR*, *HMGS*, *IDI*, *MVK*, *MVD*, *PMK*, *CPS* and *MS*) (Supplementary Fig. 9), suggesting that the recent WGT event were important to the evolution of triptolide biosynthesis in *T. wilfordii*.

Notably it was found that the *TwCPS1* and *TwMS* genes already known to be involved in triptolide biosynthesis are adjacent to each other in the *T. wilfordii* genome (Supplementary Fig. 10), which is similar to previously identified biosynthetic gene clusters in other plant genomes. However, while the relevant region on chromosome 21 also contains a *CYP* (TW023804.1) that exhibits a similar expression pattern, this is sufficiently distant, including a number of intervening genes clearly unrelated to triptolide biosynthesis, to leave its relevance unclear. Similarly, while there are several nearby transcription factors (TFs), as well as another CPS, these are unlikely to play a role in the production of triptolide.

Integrated transcriptome and metabolome analysis. To gain further insights into triptolide biosynthesis, as well as the organization and regulation of the triptolide pathway, suspension cells induced by methyl jasmonate (MeJA) and seven different tissues were used as the source of transcripts and metabolites (Supplementary Notes 4 and 5). The results showed that triptolide levels in MeJA-induced cells were 3.6-fold higher (relative to control cultures) after 360 h, while the levels of triptophenolide were even higher, 55-fold (Fig. 2). More detailed analysis was focused on a final set of 142 peaks with a mass ratio of 295 - 400, the expected range for diterpenoids (Supplementary Figs. 11 - 14 and Supplementary Note 7). For example, the content of these potentially triptolide-related metabolites was highest in the root bark (Supplementary Figs. 15 and 16). Data sets for these accumulated metabolites and gene expression (including all *CYPs*, *TwCPS1* and *TwMS*) were separately normalized, and correlation network analysis was used to establish gene-to-metabolite coregulation patterns in suspension cells and the various tissues, respectively. The Pearson correlation coefficient between each set of variables (either metabolite or gene) was calculated, including all conditions and time points (Supplementary Data 3 and 4). The correlation network was analyzed by Cytoscape (version 3.6.1), using a correlation coefficient >0.7 as the cutoff (Supplementary Figs. 19 and 20). The utility of the gene-to-metabolite network was verified by the observation that the key genes *TwCPS1* and *TwMS* were both strongly associated with triptolide and triptophenolide. Accordingly, we proceeded under the assumption that the CYP catalyzing the next step to form dehydroabietic acid should similarly be present among such strongly related genes. Indeed, a total of 97 *CYP* genes, of which 57 genes were reasonably well-expressed—i.e., with RPKM>1 (Supplementary Fig. 21 and Supplementary Data 6)—were strongly associated with triptolide in the network. These then are potentially involved in triptolide biosynthesis.

Identification of specific *CYP* genes in *T. wilfordii*. So far, triptolide is found only in *Tripterygium*, indicating that some of the CYPs involved in the biosynthesis of triptolide may be specific to *T. wilfordii*. In order to identify such species-specific CYPs, we annotated a total of 2 335 *CYP* genes in *Arabidopsis thaliana*, *Daucus carota*, *Glycyrrhiza*

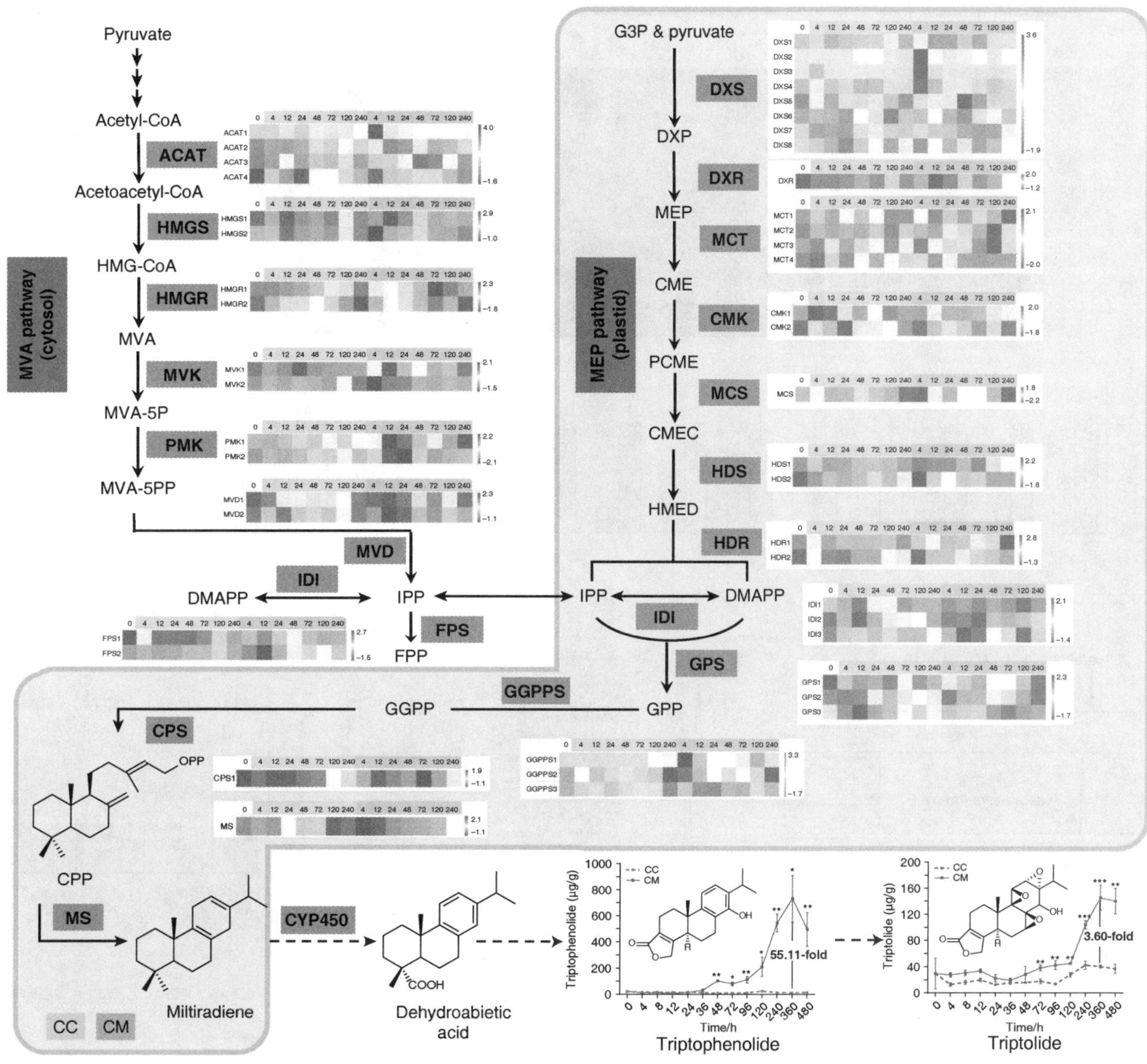


**Fig. 2 Comparative transcriptomic analysis of genes involved in the triptolide biosynthetic pathway**

Suspension cells of *T. wilfordii* were treated with methyl jasmonate and DMSO. 0,4,12,24,48,72,120,240 represent the time points of each sample, CC means the control group of cells, and CM means the group of MJ-treated cells. Heat maps of these genes were plotted using MeV software (version 4.9.0). Error bars, mean±SD ($n=3$ biologically independent samples; $^{*}P<0.05$, $^{**}P<0.01$, $^{***}P<0.001$ by 2-sided Student's $t$ test). Source data are provided as a Source Data file.

*uralensis*, *Prunus persica*, *P. trichocarpa*, *Solanum lycopersicum*, *Salvia miltiorrhiza* and *T. wilfordii* (Supplementary Table 18). We constructed a phylogenetic tree from amino acid sequence alignment of all these CYPs and identified *T. wilfordii* specific CYPs using a cutoff of 55% identity, which indicates separate subfamily assignment. This revealed 22 *T. wilfordii*-specific *CYP* genes (Supplementary Data 5). Interestingly, expression levels of six of these *CYPs* were significantly increased by MeJA induction, and most of these were highly expressed in root bark in which the terpene synthase genes were enriched and most of them were highly expressed (Supplementary Figs. 17, 18 and 22), leading to strong correlation with triptolide and/or triptophenolide.

Functional identification of CYP728B70. Among *CYP* genes correlated with triptolide in the gene-to-metabolite network, as well as those specific to *T. wilfordii*, there were 13 found to express differentially between MeJA-induced and control cells at 4, 12, 24, 48, and 72 h, and/or express differentially between root bark and other tissues (e.g., flower, stem bark, peeled stem, and leaf), and also exhibit highly similar expression patterns as *TwCPS1* and *TwMS*, including high expression levels in root bark (Fig. 3a, Supplementary Fig. 18 and Supplementary Data 6). Among these candidates, TW016590.1 was already previously identified as *ent*-kaurene oxidase, TW012756.1

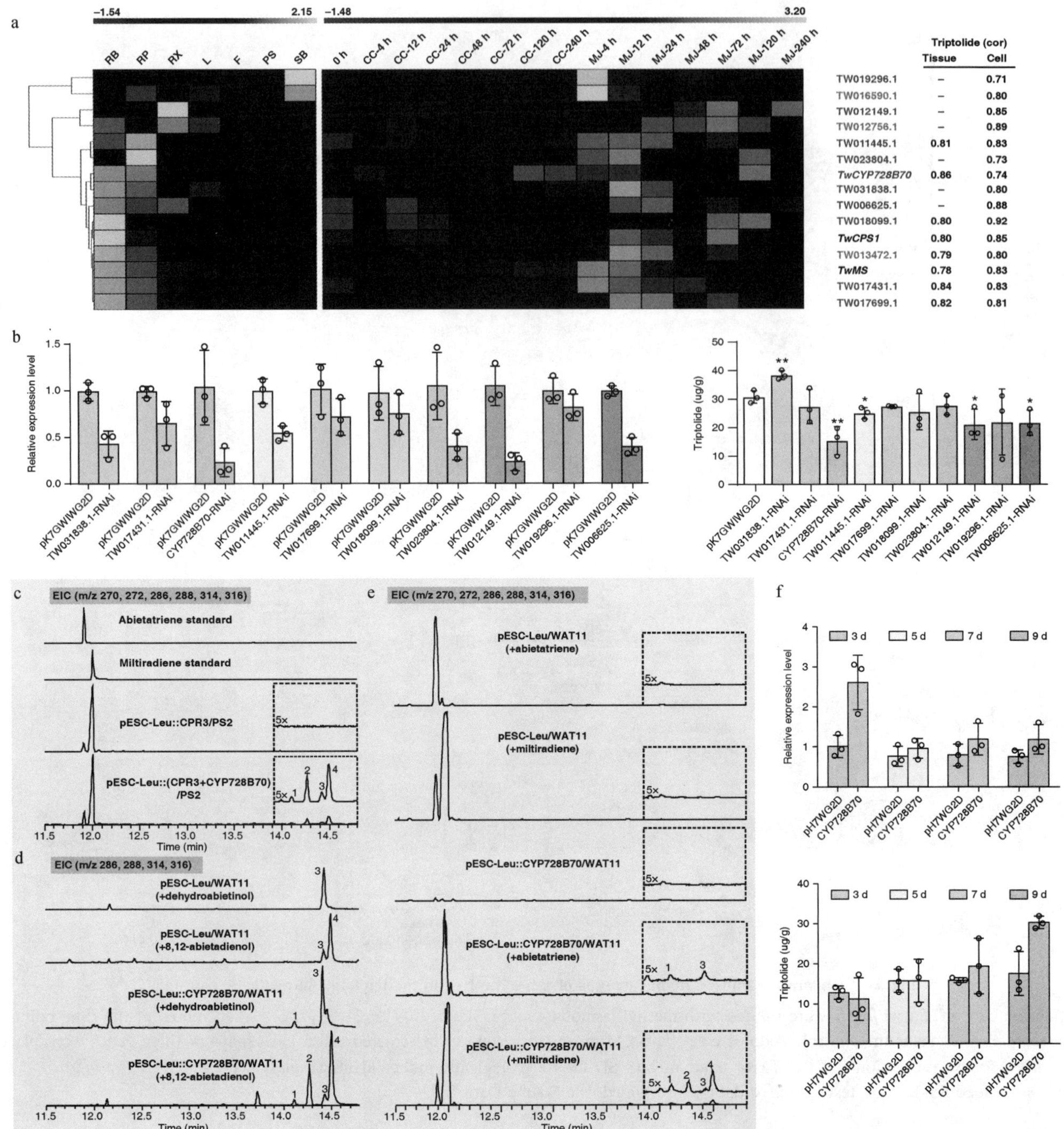

**Fig. 3 *CYP* gene screening and functional identification of CYP728B70**

(a) Hierarchical clustering of RNA-Seq expression data after filtering by expression level. (b) Relative expression of 10 candidate CYPs and triptolide concentration in RNAi suspension cells. (c) Co-expression of CYP728B70 and TwCPR3 in miltiradiene engineering yeast. (d) In vivo transformation of authentic diterpene alcohol substrates to the corresponding alcohols and acids in cultures of yeast cells expressing CYP728B70. (e) In vivo transformation of authentic diterpene substrates to the corresponding alcohols and acids in cultures of yeast cells expressing CYP728B70. (f) Relative expression of *CYP728B70*, as well as triptolide concentration in CYP728B70-overexpressing suspension cells on the 3rd, 5th, 7th, 9th day. Error bars, mean±SD ($n=3$ biologically independent samples; $^{*}P<0.05$, $^{**}P<0.01$ by 2-sided Student's $t$ test). Source data underlying Figs. 3a, b, f are provided as a Source Data file.

was annotated as trans-cinnamate 4-monooxygenase, which is not likely to be involved in terpenoid biosynthesis, while TW017699.1 and TW013472.1 appeared to arise from a relatively recent tandem gene duplication event as their amino acid sequences are 97% identical (Supplementary Data 2), and we chose to only target TW017699.1 directly. Accordingly, we settled on a total of 10 candidates for the follow-up RNAi studies, which were carried out with suspension cell cultures to provide more direct evidence for a role in triptolide biosynthesis for these 10 candidates

(Supplementary Table 20). In 4 RNAi-lines (CYP728B70, TW011445.1, TW012149.1, TW006625.1), the transcript levels of the targeted gene and triptolide accumulation were decreased compared to those in control cultures transformed with an empty vector (Fig. 3b). These four CYPs were co-expressed with the cytochrome P450 reductase 3 (CPR3) in yeast also engineered to produce miltiradiene, as previously described. Gratifyingly, with CYP728B70, which was strongly associated with triptolide in the gene-metabolite network, this led to the formation of four compounds, dehydroabietic acid (abieta-8, 11, 13-trien-18-oic acid, **1**), miltiradienoic acid (abieta-8, 12-dien-18-oic acid, **2**), dehydroabietinol (abieta-8, 11, 13-trien-18-ol, **3**) and miltiradienol (abieta-8, 12-dien-18-ol, **4**), whose structures were identified after purification by $^1H$ NMR and $^{13}C$ NMR (Fig. 3c, Supplementary Figs. 24 – 32 and Supplementary Note 6). To further verify such activity, in vivo assays also were performed, that is, substrate feeding of cultures expressing CYP728B70 in the yeast WAT11 strain that also expresses an Arabidopsis CPR. Compounds **1** – **4** were detected when feeding miltiradiene (abieta-8, 12-diene), while only the derived compounds **1** and **3** were detected when feeding abieta-8, 11, 13-triene. Similarly, compounds **1** and **2** were detected when feeding compound **4** (miltiradienol), while only compound **1** was detected when feeding compound **3** (dehydroabietinol) (Fig. 3d, e). Given that aromatization of the miltiradiene C ring to form abietatriene most likely occurs spontaneously, these results indicate that TwCYP728B70 catalyzes consecutive oxidations at C – 18 of miltiradiene or abietatriene to form the corresponding alcohol and acid derivatives. Although the expected aldehyde intermediate is not observed, this almost certainly also is formed between the alcohol and acid final products.

To further explore the role of CYP728B70 in triptolide biosynthesis, overexpression was employed. This led to a significant increase in transcript level, albeit only by ~1.6-fold compared with the control cultures transformed with the empty vector, on the 3rd day, and it then decreased but was still slightly higher than in the control cultures at later time points. Nevertheless, elevated levels of triptolide in the overexpression line relative to those in the control cultures were evident on the 9th day, reaching just over 30.5 μg/g in the overexpression line, representing an ~70% increase (Fig. 3f). This not only further supports a role for CYP720B70 in triptolide biosynthesis, but also showcases its potential utility for improving production of this valuable diterpenoid in *T. wilfordii*.

To explore the potential functions of the other 9 candidate CYPs, in vitro enzymatic activity assays were performed using the available dehydroabietic acid, triptinin B, triptophenolide and triptoquinonide, all of which are likely intermediates in triptolide biosynthesis (Supplementary Note 7). However, no new compounds were observed, indicating that these CYPs could not catalyze transformation of these intermediates, but does not rule out a role for them in triptolide biosynthesis (i.e., in mediating reactions involving other intermediates) (Supplementary Fig. 33).

## 2 DISCUSSION

Triptolide, a structurally complex phenolic diterpene triepoxide of *T. wilfordii*, has potent antitumor and immunosuppressive activities. Research focusing on its biosynthetic pathway has been stymied, in part, by the absence of a comprehensive genetic accounting. The high-quality reference-grade genome of *T. wilfordii* reported here thus provides a valuable genomic resource for investigation of triptolide biosynthesis, and is, to the best of our knowledge, the first genomic sequence for a plant of the order Celastrales. Accordingly, it further represents a cornerstone for evolutionary phylogenomic studies of not only *T. wilfordii*, but the Celastrales order more generally.

Previous investigations of triptolide biosynthesis relied on transcriptome data, and only identified the relevant diterpene synthases. Herein, we integrated genomic, transcriptomic, and metabolomic data to map a gene-to-metabolite network, screening out 57 *CYP* genes which were potentially involved in triptolide biosynthesis. Then we combined the co-expression patterns, tissue-specificity and inducibility of these candidate genes as well as *T. wilfordii*-specific *CYP* genes for further investigations, resulting in a total of 10 candidates. Through the above analysis, we identified 4 *CYP* genes involved in triptolide biosynthesis, as RNAi knock-down of these led to decreased accumulation of this natural product. Moreover, we successfully characterized the role of CYP728B70, which is responsible for oxidation of C-18 from a methyl to the acid moiety of dehydroabietic acid, in triptolide biosynthesis. As demonstrated here by substrate feeding studies, CYP728B70 exhibits multiple/sequential reactivity in carrying out this transformation in triptolide biosynthesis. Consistent with the limited accumulation of triptolide in *T. wilfordii*, *CYP728B70* exhibits low transcript levels, although it is highest in the root bark where this diterpenoid is primarily found. Notably, over-expression of *CYP728B70* in plant cell cultures led to a significant (~70%) increase in triptolide levels relative to control cultures, indicating that CYP728B70 activity limits triptolide biosynthesis, and demonstrating the utility of the results reported here for improving the yield of this potential pharmaceutical agent.

Perhaps not surprisingly given that CYPs form the largest family of enzymes, there are still CYP families that are completely uncharacterized. Indeed, this included the CYP728 family, which was first observed in *Amborella*, although it has been lost in *Arabidopsis* (Supplementary Fig. 35), and no function has been previously reported for any member of this CYP family. Hence, CYP728B70 appears to be the only one member of this CYP family whose catalytic activity has been identified, and its role in diterpenoid metabolism immediately suggests similar function for other family members. Also, the stepwise carboxylation reaction observed for CYP728B70 is catalytically highly similar to the CYP720B family in conifers that even forms some common products, thus showcasing an intriguing case of independent evolution of these functions in distant plant species. In addition, the other 3 *CYP* genes that affect the biosynthesis of triptolide in the results of RNAi experiment are from *T. wilfordii*-specific CYP (sub-) families. Although we have not identified their catalytic functions, such biochemical characterization will then provide similar insight.

Although some steps in the triptolide biosynthetic pathway still remain unknown, we have provided many promising candidates, including *CYP* genes and metabolites that might constitute yet-unknown intermediates or side products from triptolide biosynthesis. We have also provided many potential TFs that are most likely involved in the regulation of the biosynthesis of triptolide (Supplementary Fig. 34, Supplementary Data 8 - 13 and Supplementary Note 8). Of particular note here is the identification of roles for CYPs from (sub-)families that are specific to *T. wilfordii*, as much of the reported work in such characterization of CYP function in plant natural products biosynthesis has to some extent relied on homology at least at the family, if not sub-family, level.

In addition to our identification of the role of CYP728B70, we used this to engineer yeast for the production of dehydroabietic acid (Fig. 4). This lays the foundation for identification of genes encoding subsequently acting enzymes, and will be invaluable in future investigations of triptolide biosynthesis.

In conclusion, while it is difficult to resolve the biosynthetic pathways of the complex natural products in non-model systems, we have demonstrated here the utility of the multi-omics data, as well as co-expression patterns, tissue-specificity, and inducibility of candidate genes will contribute for such investigations. Interestingly, while genome sequencing found pairing of the genes for the consecutively acting *TwCPS1* and *TwMS* can initiate triptolide biosynthesis, these do not appear to have be co-clustered with genes for later acting enzymes. Nevertheless, the genome sequence reported here provides a comprehensive genetic inventory, which was coupled with the observation that triptolide production is tissue-specific and affected by elicitors, much as found with other plant natural products, to generate gene-to-metabolite networks that can be productively mined. Notably, this approach has led to identification of four relevant CYPs, with the characterized function of CYP728B70 further providing insight into this previously enigmatic CYP family, as well as demonstrating the utility of this approach to increasing the yield of this promising pharmaceutical agent.

## 3 METHODS

Genome sequencing and assembly. A *T. wilfordii* cultivar was used for sequencing (Supplementary Note 1). Genomic DNA was extracted from leaves of *T. wilfordii* using the DNAsecure Plant Kit (TIANGEN) and broken into random fragments. Short-reads libraries were constructed according to the manufacturer's instructions (Illumina, San Diego, CA) and then sequenced on Illumina Hiseq X-ten. For long-read DNA sequencing, 60 kb Single Molecule Real Time (SMRT) long-read library were sequenced on the PacBio Sequel platform (75.79 Gb data, 207-fold coverage of the genome). For 10X Genomics sequencing, a total of 119.75 Gb (327-fold coverage of the genome) data were sequenced on the Illumina Hiseq X-Ten (Supplementary Table 2).

De novo assembly of the long reads from the PacBio SMRT Sequencer was performed using FALCON (https://github.com/PacificBiosciences/FALCON/). To obtain enough corrected reads, the longest coverage of subreads were firstly selected as seed reads to correct sequence errors. Then, error-corrected reads were aligned to each other and assembled into genomic contigs using FALCON with the following parameters: length_cutoff_pr = 10,000, max_diff=95, and max_cov=105. Then, genomic contigs were polished using Quiver, which yielded an assembly with a contig N50 size of 4.36 Mb. The total length of this assembly version was 348.38 Mb. Then, we used BWA-MEM to align the 10X Genomics data to the assembly using default settings. Scaffolding was performed by FragScaff with the barcoded sequencing reads. Last, Pilon was used to perform error correction based on the Illumina sequences, generating a genome with a scaffold N50 size of 6.48 Mb. The total length of this assembly version was 349.91 Mb. Subsequently, the Hi-C sequencing data were aligned to the assembled scaffolds by BWA-mem and the scaffolds were clustered onto chromosomes with LACHESIS (http://shendurelab.github.io/LACHESIS/), the final genome was 348.53 Mb and the contig and scaffold N50 were 4.36 Mb and 13.52 Mb, respectively (Supplementary Tables 3 - 7 and Supplementary Note 1).

Genome annotation. A total of 52.36% repeat sequences in the genome were annotated. Among them, TEs were searched by combining de novo-based and homology-based

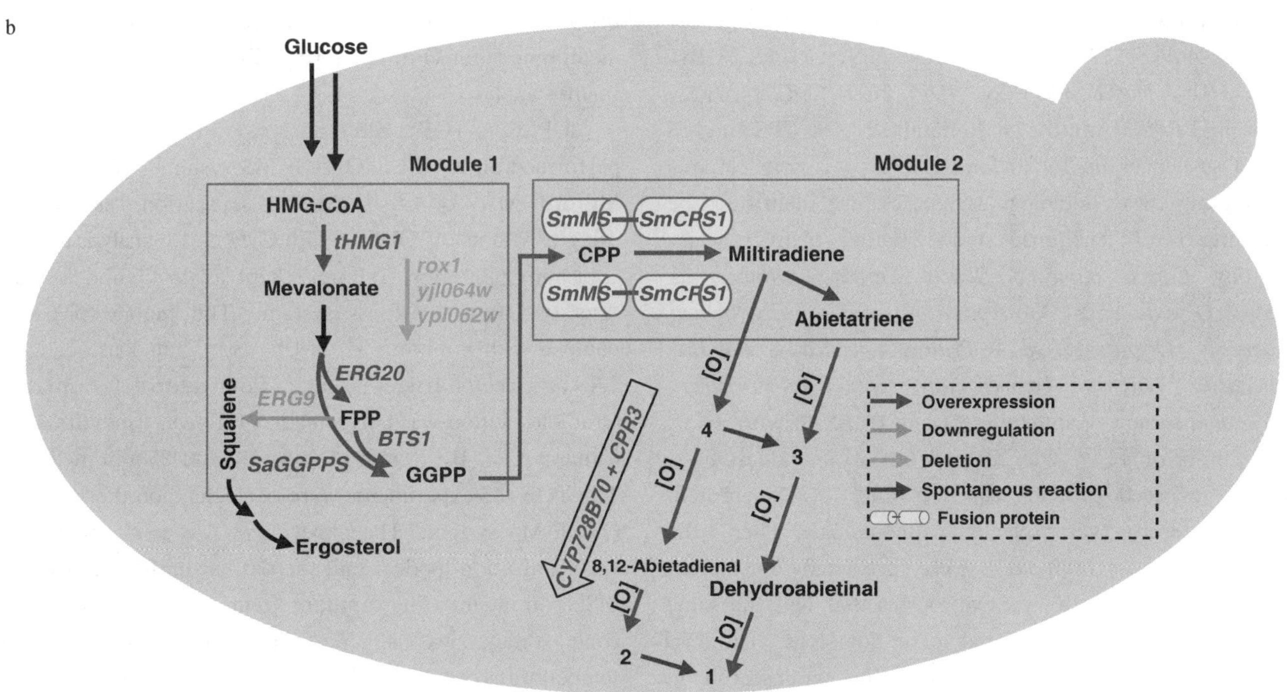


**Fig. 4 Analysis of triptolide pathway and metabolic engineering**

(a) Three reactions presumably catalyzed by CYP728B70 to convert miltiradiene to dehydroabietic acid. (b) Establishing the metabolic pathways in yeast for production of diterpene alcohols and acids. In module 1, *rox1*, *ypl062w*, *yjl06w4* were knocked out, and *ERG9* was down-regulated, and *tHMG1*, *ERG20*, *BTS1*, *SaGGPPS* were overexpressed to improve the production of GGPP. In module 2, double SmMS-SmCPS1 fusion modules were introduced into the yeast chromosome for the production of miltiradiene. Co-expression of TwCYP728B70 and TwCPR3 leads to the observed production of the derived alcohols and acids.

approaches using RepeatModeler (http://www.repeatmasker.org/RepeatModeler/), LTR_FINDER (http://tlife.fudan.edu.cn/ltr_finder/), RepeatScout (http://www.repeatmasker.org/), RepeatMasker (version 3.3.0) (http://www.repeatmasker.org/), and RepeatProteinMask (http://www.repeatmasker.org/). Tandem repeats were detected using Tandem Repeats Finder (TRF) (Supplementary Fig. 2 and Supplementary Table 10). Gene structures were predicted with a combination of homology-based prediction, de novo prediction and transcriptome-based prediction in the genome (Supplementary Fig. 3, Supplementary Tables 8 and 9). We then generated functional assignments of the *T. wilfordii* genes with BLAST in public protein databases, including SwissProt (https://web.expasy.org/docs/swiss-prot_guideline.html), NR, InterPro (V32.0), Pfam (V27.0) and KEGG (https://www.kegg.jp/). Finally, 99.6% of all genes in the genome were predicted to be functional (Supplementary Table 11). Noncoding RNA was predicted using de novo and homology search methods (Supplementary Table 12 and Supplementary Note 2).

Genome evolution. We conducted expansion and contraction analysis using the CAFÉ program (Supplementary Table 15) and identified the positively selected genes in *T. wilfordii* using MUSCLE (Supplementary Tables 16 and 17). To identify the WGD events in the *T. wilfordii* genome, we used McscanX to determine syntenic blocks (regions with at least five genes) and calculated 4DTv for all gene pairs found in each syntenic segment. The synonymous substitution rate (*Ks*) values of *T. wilfordii* syntenic block genes were calculated with the codeml program of the PAML package. We performed synteny analysis on *T. wilfordii* and *V. vinifera* to confirm that *T. wilfordii* had undergone another WGT event.

Evolution of triptolide biosynthesis genes. To investigate the genes involved in triptolide biosynthesis, we first retrieved protein sequences from *Arabidopsis thaliana* genes, including *ACAT*, *CMK*, *DXR*, *DXS*, *FPS*, *GGPPS*, *GPS*, *HDR*, *HDS*, *HMGR*, *HMGS*, *IDI*, *MCT*, *MCS*, *MVK*, *MVD*, and *PMK* from the NCBI database. The CPS and MS protein sequences in *T. wilfordii* were previously cloned. Then, using these homologs as queries, we identified the candidates in *T. wilfordii* and 13 other plant species, including *Carica papaya*, *Daucus carota*, *Dimocarpus longan*, *Glycine max*, *Gossypium raimondii*, *Glycyrrhiza uralensis*, *Oryza sativa*, *Prunus persica*, *Populus trichocarpa*, *Solanum lycopersicum*, *Salvia miltiorrhiza*, *Theobroma cacao*, *Vitis vinifera* using BLASTP with an E-value cutoff of $1e^{-5}$. The aligned hits with at least 50% coverage of seed protein sequences and > 50% protein sequence identity were selected as homologs. Then, the domains of these homologs were predicted by PFAM (http://pfam.xfam.org/). Only genes that had the same protein domain were considered to be homologs. The TPS and CYP450 genes were predicted using hmmsearch in conjunction with the TPS hmm model (PF01397 and PF03936) and CYP450 hmm model (PF00067) from Pfam, respectively. We constructed phylogenetic trees of each identified triptolide biosynthetic gene family from *T. wilfordii* and *Arabidopsis thaliana*. Amino acid sequence alignments of the identified triptolide biosynthetic genes from *T. wilfordii* and *Arabidopsis thaliana* were performed using MUSCLE, and the alignment data were used to construct phylogenetic trees using RAxML with the maximum likelihood method. The timing of the divergence of duplicates in each triptolide biosynthesis gene was estimated based on the calculation of the synonymous substitution rate (Ks) using the codeml program of the PAML package. The calculated *Ks* value was then converted to the divergence time according to $T = Ks/2r$, where r represents a substitution rate of $6.5 \times 10^{-9}$ mutations per site per year for eudicots (Supplementary Table 19). These gene pairs were not adjacent in the distribution of the genome (Supplementary Data 2).

Suspension cell elicitation and sample preparation. It has previously been shown that the application of the plant defence signaling molecule MeJA could increase terpenoid production and affect the transcript levels of the genes involved in the related pathways. Cell samples were harvested at 0, 4, 8, 12, 24, 36, 48, 72, 96, 120, 240, 360, and 480 h after the addition of MeJA and DMSO. Solid samples were homogenized by Mixer Mill MM 400 of Retsch (Retsch GmbH, 42781 Haan, Germany) and stored at −80℃ for at least 4 h prior to freeze drying for 48 h (Alpha 1-2 LDplus, Germany). For each sample, 60 mg aliquots were soaked in 1.5 mL of 80% (v/v) methanol overnight at room temperature and then dissolved in an ultrasonic water bath for 60 min. The supernatant was filtered through a 0.22 μm membrane filter (FitMax Syringe Filter, 13 mm 0.22 μm) for further analysis.

UPLC/Q-TOF MS analysis. All analyses were performed on a UPLC/Q-TOF MS system (Waters Corp., Milford, MA, USA). The UPLC separation was performed using a Waters ACQUITY UPLC HSS T3 analytical column (2.1 mm × 100 mm, 1.8 μm) kept at 40 ℃ and a Waters Acquity UPLC™ I-Class system. The mobile phase was pumped with a mixture of 0.1% (v/v) aqueous acetic acid (A) and acetonitrile (B) at a flow rate of 0.5 mL/min. Gradient elution was performed as follows: 0 min at 30% B, 6 min at 45% B, 18 min at 60% B, and 23 min at 90% B. The TOF MS experiments were performed on the Xevo G2-S QTOF MS system. The experiment was performed in ESI (+) ionization modes, and the data acquisition modes were MSE continuum. The capillary voltage was 0.5 KV, and the cone voltage was 40 V. The source and desolvation temperatures were 100 ℃ and 450 ℃, respectively. The desolvation gas flow was 900 L/h. The ramp collision energy was set as 20-40 eV for the high-energy scans. The MS range of data acquisition was 50-1 500 Da. A lock spray with leucine enkephalin (200 pg/μL, 10 μL/min) was used as the reference [m/z 556.2771 ESI (+)] to maintain the mass accuracy.

Data analysis of metabolic and transcriptional profiles. All mass spectral data were imported into Progenesis QI for data processing, then were grouped and exported to Ezinfo for principal component analysis (PCA). PCA is a very useful statistical method for defining the dimensions of large data sets and identifying significant signals. The data set was log normalized, and PCA and OPLS-DA analyses were performed to determine overall differences in metabolites. An ANOVA with a significance level of $P < 0.01$ and max-fold > 2 was subsequently performed on the doubly filtered peaks to identify metabolites that did not change significantly in response to MeJA treatment. Furthermore, peaks with no fragments were removed.

We selected metabolite peaks and genes including all CYP, CPS1 and MS for network regulation analysis. Both data sets of accumulation of metabolic and gene expression were normalized separately, and correlation network analysis was used to establish gene-to-metabolite coregulation patterns. The Pearson correlation coefficient was calculated by the PCC method in the R platform between each set of variables (either metabolite or gene) across the profiles, and significant positive correlations with $p$-value $< 0.05$ were detected between genes and metabolites. The correlation network was analyzed by the Cytoscape software (version 3.6.1).

Construction of miltiradiene-producing yeast strain. To construct a miltiradiene-producing strain, the corresponding biosynthetic pathway was introduced into yeast. First, the CRISPR/Cas9 system was applied to improve the MVA pathway flux by knocking out three transcriptional regulators (*rox1*, *ypl062w* and *yjl06w4*) and knocking down *erg9* in the yeast BY-T20 strain (BY4742, *ΔTrp1*, *Trp1*::*His3*-$P_{PGK1}$-*BTS1*/*ERG20*-$T_{ADH1}$-$P_{TDH3}$-*SaGGPPS*-$T_{TPI1}$-$P_{TEF1}$-*tHMG1*-$T_{CYC1}$), generating a GGPP-producing yeast strain named BY-HZ16.

The fusion of *SmCPS1* and *SmMS* from *Salvia miltiorrhiza* was reported to possess great potential to synthesize miltiradiene via GGPP. The single or double *SmMS-SmCPS1* fusion module was cloned and integrated into the yeast chromosome by the M2S integration method. Briefly, *SmMS-SmCPS1* was amplified with the addition of a *Bsa*I digestion site and ligated with head-to-head promoters (*pTDH3-pADH1*) into the bi-terminator vector T1-(*tTPI1*-*tPGI1*), resulting in the plasmids T1-(*SmMS-SmCPS1*) and T1-(*SmMS-SmCPS1*)-(*SmMS-SmCPS1*). Two terminators were inserted into the scaffold plasmid, with dedicated homologous arms (L1 and L2) lying on both sides. The integration site *YPRCΔ15* was chosen as the target locus, and *Ura3* was chosen as the selection marker. Each expression cassette with designed to have homologous arms (primers: L1-F/L2-R) was amplified individually. The selection marker module and integration homologous arm module (15Site1-Ura3-L1 and L2-15site2) were also amplified. All the amplified fragments were used to co-transform BY-HZ16 for assembly and integration, and transformants were selected on synthetic dropin medium-Ura-His (SD-Ura-His) containing 20 g/L glucose and 18 g/L agar. Positive transformants were verified by sequencing, yielding the strains PS1 and PS2 (Supplementary Fig. 23). All strains are listed in Supplementary Table 21. All primers used in vector construction are listed in Supplementary Data 7.

*CYP* screening based on the miltiradiene-producing strain. The gene-to-metabolite network analysis and specific-gene analysis in *T. wilfordii* were performed, and 10 highly expressed *CYP* genes were chosen as candidates for investigation. The RNAi results showed that 4 CYPs were most likely to regulate triptolide biosynthesis and were then selected to react with abietane-type diene olefin miltiradiene. First, to simplify the fermentation procedure, the constitutive promoters *pPGK1*-*pTEF2* were cloned into the *BamH*I and *Not*I sites of the pESC-Leu vector to replace the inducible promoters *pGAL1*-*pGAL10*, yielding the plasmid Leu-PT. Second, cytochrome P450 reductase 3 (CPR3) was inserted into the *Not*I site of the plasmid Leu-PT according to the pEASY-Uni Seamless Cloning and Assembly Kit (TransGen Biotech, Beijing, China), resulting in the plasmid Leu-PT-CPR3. Then, each *CYP* gene was introduced into the *BamH*I site of the plasmid Leu-PT-CPR3. All the resulting CYP expression plasmids were individually introduced into strain PS2 following the user manual of the Frozen-EZ Yeast Transformation II KitTM (Zymo Research, USA) for product identification. All primers used for *CYP* gene screening are listed in Supplementary Data 7.

Three colonies were picked for each genotype and used to inoculate 5 mL of synthetic dropin medium -Ura-His-Leu (SD-Ura-His-Leu) containing 20 g/L glucose. The cells were grown in a shaker at 30 ℃ and 230 rpm for 48 h, after which the resulting seed cultures were transferred into fresh medium at a ratio of 1 : 50 and fermented under the same conditions for 3 days. Yeast cells were lysed using a nano homogenizer (AH-1500, ATS Engineering Limited, Canada) and then extracted twice with an equal volume of ethyl acetate. Anhydrous sodium sulfate was added to remove residual water, and the combined organic phases were dried and methylated with (trimethylsilyl) diazomethane (Aladdin Industrial Inc., Shanghai, China). The methylated samples were re-dried and then dissolved in 100 μL of ethyl acetate for gas chromatography-mass spectrometry (GC-MS) using a Thermo TRACE 1310/TSQ 8000 gas chromatograph equipped with a TG-5 MS (30 m × 0.25 mm × 0.25 μm) capillary column. The GC conditions were as follows: the sample (1 μL) was injected in split mode (20 : 1) at 250 ℃ under a He flow rate of 1 mL/min, the GC oven temperature was programmed to rise from an initial 40 ℃ at 20 ℃/min to 200 ℃ and at 15 ℃/min to 250 ℃, then to 270 ℃ at 1.5 ℃/min. The ion trap heating temperature was 250 ℃. The electron energy was 70 eV. Spectra were recorded in the range of 40-500 $m/z$.

In vivo assays for TwCYP728B70 activity. The pESC-Leu::(CPR3+TwCYP728B70) construct was transformed into the yeast strain WAT11, which enables the catalytic activity of plant CYPs by expressing an Arabidopsis CPR.

Transformants were selected on synthetic dropin medium SD-Leu plates containing 20 g/L glucose. The cells were grown in a shaker at 30 ℃ and 230 rpm for 48 h, then transferred into 50 mL of fresh medium at a ratio of 1 : 50 and fermented under the same conditions for 12 h. To confirm engineered yeast strains for oxidative transformation of diterpenoid substrates, miltiradiene, abietatriene, 8, 12-abietadienol, or dehydroabietinol (in methanol) was added to the yeast cultures to final concentrations of 100 μmol/L and fermented for another 48 h. Yeast cells were lysed, extracted twice with an equal volume of ethyl acetate, and methylated before GC - MS analysis, as described above.

RNAi of the candidate *CYP* genes in *T. wilfordii*. The fragments of these 10 candidate *CYP* genes were amplified using Phusion® High-Fidelity DNA Polymerase (New England Biolabs, USA) and inserted into the RNAi vector pK7GWIWG2D according to the Gateway procedure (Invitrogen, USA), and the resulting vectors were verified by complete sequencing.

Suspension cells in the logarithmic growth phase were chose and precultured on Murashige and Skoog (MS) solid medium containing 0.5 mg/L 2,4-D, 0.1 mg/L KT, 0.5 mg/L IBA and 30 g/L sucrose (pH=5.8) for 7 days. Then, the recombinant plasmid DNA mixed with Au microparticles were transformed into the suspension cells through bombardment using a biolistic gene gun (PDS 1 000/He, Bio-Rad). Each transformation was carried out two times. The bombarded suspension cells were cultured for another 7 days before harvesting for qRT-PCR and UPLC analysis.

Overexpression of *TwCYP728B70*. Vector pH7WG2D (Invitrogen) was used to overexpress *TwCYP728B70* in suspension cells following the protocol mentioned above. The resulting recombinant cells were harvested for qRT-PCR and UPLC analysis after being cultured for 3, 5, 7, and 9 days.

Heterologous expression of CYP in yeast and in vitro assays. Each *CYP* gene was inserted into the *BamH*I site of the pESC-Leu vector according to the pEASY-Uni Seamless Cloning and Assembly Kit. The pESC-Leu::CYP construct was verified by complete gene sequencing, which was transformed into the yeast strain WAT11. The cells were grown first in 100 mL of SD-Leu liquid medium with 20 g/L glucose in a shaker at 30 ℃ and 230 rpm to an $OD_{600}$ of 2 - 3. Cells were centrifuged and resuspended in 200 mL of yeast peptone galactose (YPL) induction medium (10 g/L yeast extract, 20 g/L bactopeptone, and 20 g/L galactose) and grown for 12 h at 30 ℃ to induce recombinant protein expression. Microsomes were prepared based on the reported method with some modifications. Briefly, the induced cells were centrifuged (1 914×*g*, 4 ℃, 5 min) and resuspended in 20 mL of TEK buffer (50 mmol/L Tris-HCl, pH 7.4, 1 mmol/L EDTA, 0.1 mol/L KCl), then left at room temperature for 5 min. Cells were centrifuged again (1,914×*g*, 4 ℃, 5 min) and resuspended in 50 mL of TESB buffer (50 mmol/L Tris-HCl, pH 7.4, 1 mmol/L EDTA, 0.6 mol/L sorbitol), then left on ice for 10 min. The cell suspension was lysed for 7 min at 4 ℃ and 12,000 psi using a nano homogenize machine (AH-1500, ATS Engineering Limited, Canada), then centrifuged (17,266×*g*, 4 ℃, 15 min) to collect the supernatant. NaCl (final concentration of 0.15 mol/L) and polyethylene glycol (PEG) − 4 000 (final concentration of 0.1 g/mL) were added to the supernatant, and left on ice for 15 min. The microsomal fractions were collected by centrifugation (17,266×*g*, 4 ℃, 15 min), and resuspended in TEG buffer (50 mmol/L Tris-HCl, pH 7.4, 1 mmol/L EDTA, 20% (v/v) glycerol), which can be kept frozen at −80 ℃ for months.

In vitro enzymatic activity assays were carried out on a shaking incubator (150 rpm) at 30 ℃ for 4 h in 500 μL of 100 mmol/L Tris-HCl, pH 7.5, containing 0.5 mg of total microsomal proteins and 500 μmol/L NADPH, along with a regenerating system (consisting of 5 μmol/L FAD, 5 μmol/L FMN, 5 mmol/L glucose-6-phosphate, 1 unit/mL glucose-6-phosphate dehydrogenase), and 100 μmol/L substrates. Reactions were stopped by the addition of 500 μL of methanol and used for UPLC analysis. Negative control reactions were carried out with microsomal preparations from recombinant yeast transformed with empty pESC-Leu.

Fermentation. To engineer yeast for the production of intermediates involved in triptolide biosynthesis and obtain enough compound for structural characterization, the strain PS2 containing the plasmid Leu-PT-CPR3::TwCYP728B70 was used to inoculate 50 mL of SD-Ura-His-Leu medium in a 250 mL shake flask at 30 ℃ and 230 rpm for 24 h. The entire culture volume was transferred into 500 mL of fresh seed medium and incubated for 24 h, then transferred into 2 mL of fresh seed medium and incubated for another 24 h. The seed medium was then used to inoculate 8 L of fermentation medium in a New Brunswick BioFlo/CelliGen 115 bioreactor (Eppendorf, Germany) with a maximal working volume of 14 L.

The fermentation was performed at 30 ℃. During fermentation, the pH was maintained at 5.0 with the automatic addition of ammonium hydroxide, the agitation rate was kept between 200 and 600 rpm, and the dissolved oxygen was kept above 40%. Concentrated glucose solution (40%, wt/vol) was fed periodically to keep the glucose concentration above 1.0 g/L. Additionally SD-Ura-His-Leu medium was fed after the initial 30 h of fermentation. The culture was then harvested by extraction after 90 h of total fermentation time.

Yeast cells were concentrated to 1 L, then lysed using

the nano homogenizer and then extracted ten times with an equal volume of ethyl acetate. Anhydrous sodium sulfate was added to remove residual water, and the organic fractions were pooled and dried using a Nitrogen Evaporator (Baojingkeji, Henan, China). The yellow oily liquid (15.5 g) was chromatographed on LiChroprep ® Si60 (40 - 63 μm, Merck, MA, USA) with a stepwise gradient of petroleum ether-hexane (v/v, 10 : 1) to obtain the fraction (~500 mL). The fraction was re-dried and then dissolved in 500 μL of acetonitrile. Preparative HPLC was performed on Agilent 1260 Infinity High-Performance Liquid Chromatography System with a Shim-pack GIST C18 (250 × 4.6 mm i. d., 5 μm, SHIMADZU, Kyoto, Japan). The mobile phase, consisting of a mixture of water (A) and acetonitrile (B), was pumped at a flow rate of 1 mL/min and the eluate was monitored at 200 nm. The gradient elution was programmed as follows: 0 min at 65% B, 50 min at 65% B. The injection volume was 20 μL.

**Reporting summary.** Further information on research design is available in the Nature Research Reporting Summary linked to this article.

## 4 DATA AVAILABILITY

The data supporting the findings of this work are available within the paper and its Supplementary Information files. A reporting summary for this Article is available as a Supplementary Information file. The data sets generated and analyzed during this study are available from the corresponding author upon request. The genome sequence data and transcriptome sequence data for *T. wilfordii* have been deposited under NCBI BioProject number PRJNA542587 and the final assembly is available at GenBank under the accession number JAAARO000000000. The source data underlying Figs. 1, 2, 3a, 3b, and 3f are provided as a Source Data file.

Recceived: 28 April 2019; Accepted: 1 February 2020.
Published online: 20 February 2020.

[屠李婵，黄璐琦，高伟，等. Nature Communication, 2020, 11(1): 971.]

# FAD-dependent enzyme-catalysed intermolecular [4+2] cycloaddition in natural product biosynthesis

The Diels-Alder (D - A) reaction, a [4 + 2] cycloaddition between a conjugated diene and a dienophile to yield a cyclohexene skeleton, is one of the most powerful carbon-carbon bond forming reactions in synthetic chemistry. Although putative Diels-Alderases, or [4 + 2] cyclases in the broader sense, have been predicted to be involved in the biosyntheses of many secondary metabolites, only a handful have been identified and characterized, with the majority being multifunctional enzymes. The identification of the first stand-alone [4 + 2] cyclase, SpnF, led to the discovery of other intramolecular [4+2] cyclases from the bio-synthetic pathways of spirotetronate and/or spirotetramate polyketides, decalin-containing polyketide-amino acid hybrids and leporine, as well as intramolecular [6 + 4] cyclases from the bio-synthetic pathway of streptoseomycin, a macrocyclic polyketide. However, no stand-alone intermolecular [4+2] cyclases have been identified to date, even though intermolecular [4+2] cycloadditions have been catalysed by artificial enzymes generated via computational design and immunological selection.

Methylcyclohexene motifs, accessible via D - A reactions, are common in *Moraceae* (mulberry) natural products with a role in Chinese traditional medicine. These natural products display antimicrobial as well as diverse biological activities, such as the inhibition of hypoxia-inducible factor-1 and protein tyrosine phos-phatase 1B. Representative examples that incorporate diverse diene substituents are shown in Fig. 1a. Exogenous substrate feeding and C-labelling experiments in *M. alba* cell cultures indicated the existence of an oxidase to furnish a reactive diene and a putative [4+2] pericyclase to catalyse the intermolecular [4 + 2] cycloaddition (Fig. 1b). We developed a chiral boron-mediated asymmetric D - A reaction for the enantioselective total syntheses of several natural products of this family. A few racemic total syntheses are also reported. Unfortunately, all the existing syntheses failed to achieve high levels of diastereo- and enantioselectivity, a problem that can be addressed chemoenzymatically if the relevant enzymes are isolated and characterized.

Historically, difficulties associated with identifying plant enzymes have slowed their discovery. Unlike in microbes, many biosynthetic genes for secondary metabolites in plants do not occur in gene clusters. In addition, no stand-alone enzymes capable of catalysing intermolecular D - A reactions are known, which makes it difficult to perform homology-based or genome-context-based searches in modern

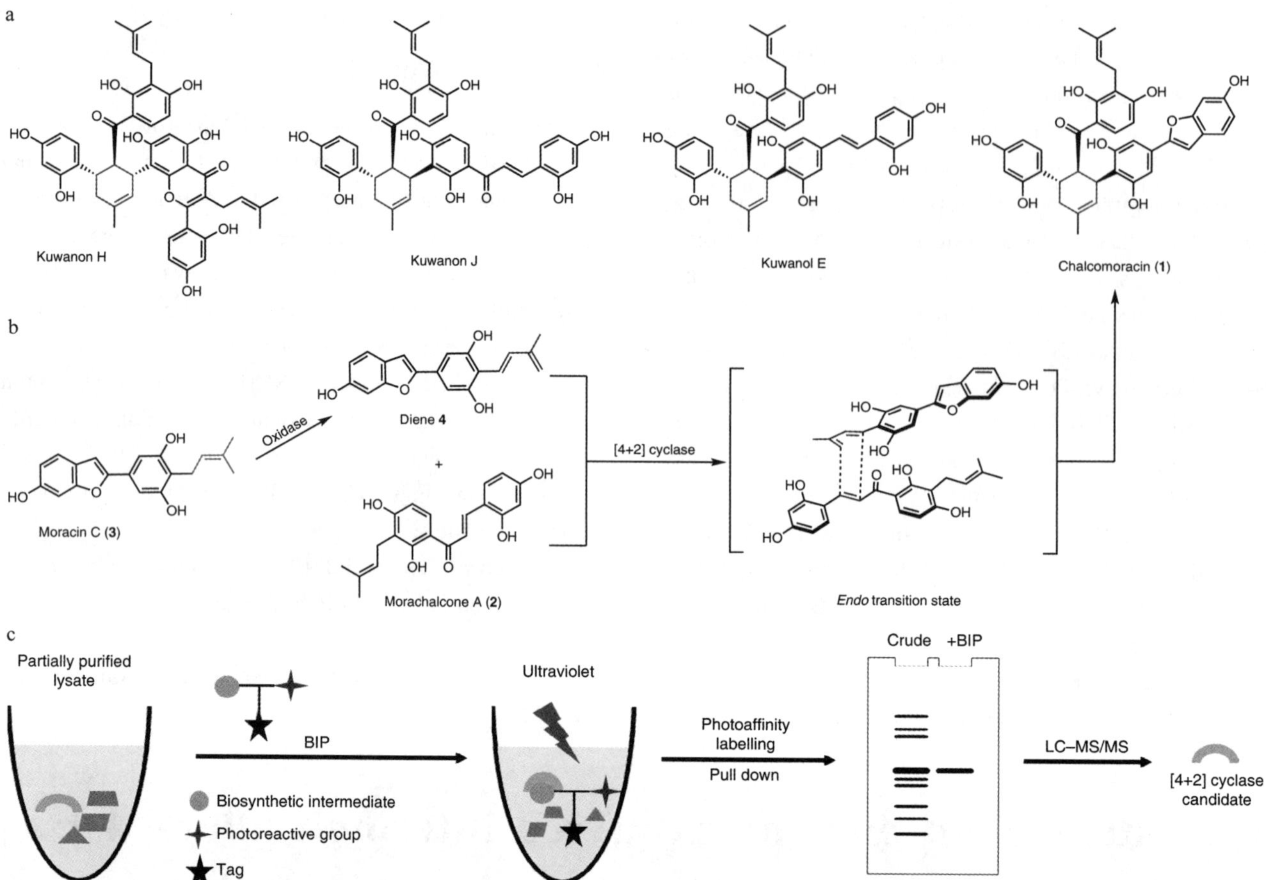


**Fig. 1 Proposed biosynthetic pathway for plant-derived D－A-type natural products and our strategy to identify the hypothetical intermolecular [4＋2] pericyclase**

(a) Representative D－A-type natural products isolated from *Morus* plants. (b) Proposed biosynthetic pathway for D－A-type *Morus* natural products. (c) BIP-based target identification method to identify the putative [4＋2] pericyclase. Using activity-based protein purification, we hoped to enrich the target enzyme(s), which can be more easily identified by using the BIP-based target identification strategy.

biological databases. Both traditional activity-based purification and more modern transcriptomics-enabled methods are used to successfully identify elusive enzymes from plant natural product pathways. However, transcriptomics-enabled methods often require characterized enzymes as bait, as well as gene prediction based on the specialized metabolism for the co-expression analysis, whereas activity-based protein purification entails tedious and lengthy purification processes and often suffers from false negative results. To overcome these challenges, we developed a complementary approach termed 'BIP-based target identification', which reveals unknown biosynthetic enzymes based on substrate binding (Fig. 1c). In our proposal, activity-based protein purification is first used to enrich the target protein(s), which are then subjected to liquid chromatography-mass spectroscopy/mass spectroscopy (LC－MS/MS) proteomics analysis. With this method, possible off-target proteins can be removed, and the abundance of the targeted protein(s) increased to reduce both false positive and false negative results during the photoaffinity labelling and pull-down steps. Hits identified via BIP-based target identification are therefore highly reliable. Transcriptional analysis is then used to narrow down the candidate gene pool for further biochemical and function analysis.

Using the BIP-based method, we identified and functionally characterized the first stand-alone intermolecular Diels-Alderase, *M. alba* Diels-Alderase (MaDA), from *M. alba* cell cultures. MaDA is a flavin adenine dinucleotide (FAD)-dependent oxidase-like Diels-Alderase that demonstrates exceptional catalytic efficiency and broad substrate scope. Density functional theory (DFT) calculations support a concerted but asynchronous D－A mechanism, and preliminary kinetic isotope effect (KIE) studies also show the reaction to be asynchronous in the enzyme. We obtained an X-ray crystal structure of MaDA with FAD covalently bound in (at 2.3 Å resolution), and performed extensive structure-guided mutagenesis to show possible modes of interaction between MaDA and its substrates. *M. alba* moracin C oxidase (MaMO), a FAD-dependent oxidase, was also identified and functionally characterized to catalyse the oxidation of the isoprenyl moiety in moracin C (**3**) into the reactive diene **4**.

## 1 RESULTS AND DISCUSSION

Identification of the oxidase and [4+2] pericyclase Using *M. alba* cell cultures generated from leaves, we identified the major D-A type natural product as chalcomoracin (**1**) (Supplementary Fig. 1). Lysates from the cultures were assayed by incubating with both the putative dienophile morachalone A (**2**) and the diene precursor moracin C (**3**). High-performance liquid chromatography (HPLC) analysis showed that chalcomoracin (**1**) was produced as the major product, alongside an unstable compound subsequently confirmed as diene **4** (Fig. 2a). These observations indicate that an oxidase and an intermolecular [4+2] pericyclase may be involved in the biosynthesis of **1**. Subsequent activity-based protein purification, which consisted of ammonium sulfate (AS) fractionation, hydrophobic interaction chromatography (HIC), ion exchange chromatography (IEC) and size exclusion chromatography (SEC), led to an 11-fold improvement in chalcomoracin (**1**) production (Fig. 2a), suggesting the enrichment of the putative oxidase and [4+2] pericyclase. Incubation of **2** and **3** in the SEC fraction for longer times resulted in increased production of 1, but not diene **4** (Extended Data Fig. 1), which indicates that the [4+2] pericyclase is possibly a different enzyme from the oxidase that has a higher reaction rate. Active fractions obtained by AS precipitation and HIC, IEC and SEC were also resolved by SDS-polyacrylamide gel electrophoresis (SDS-PAGE). We observed one clearly enriched

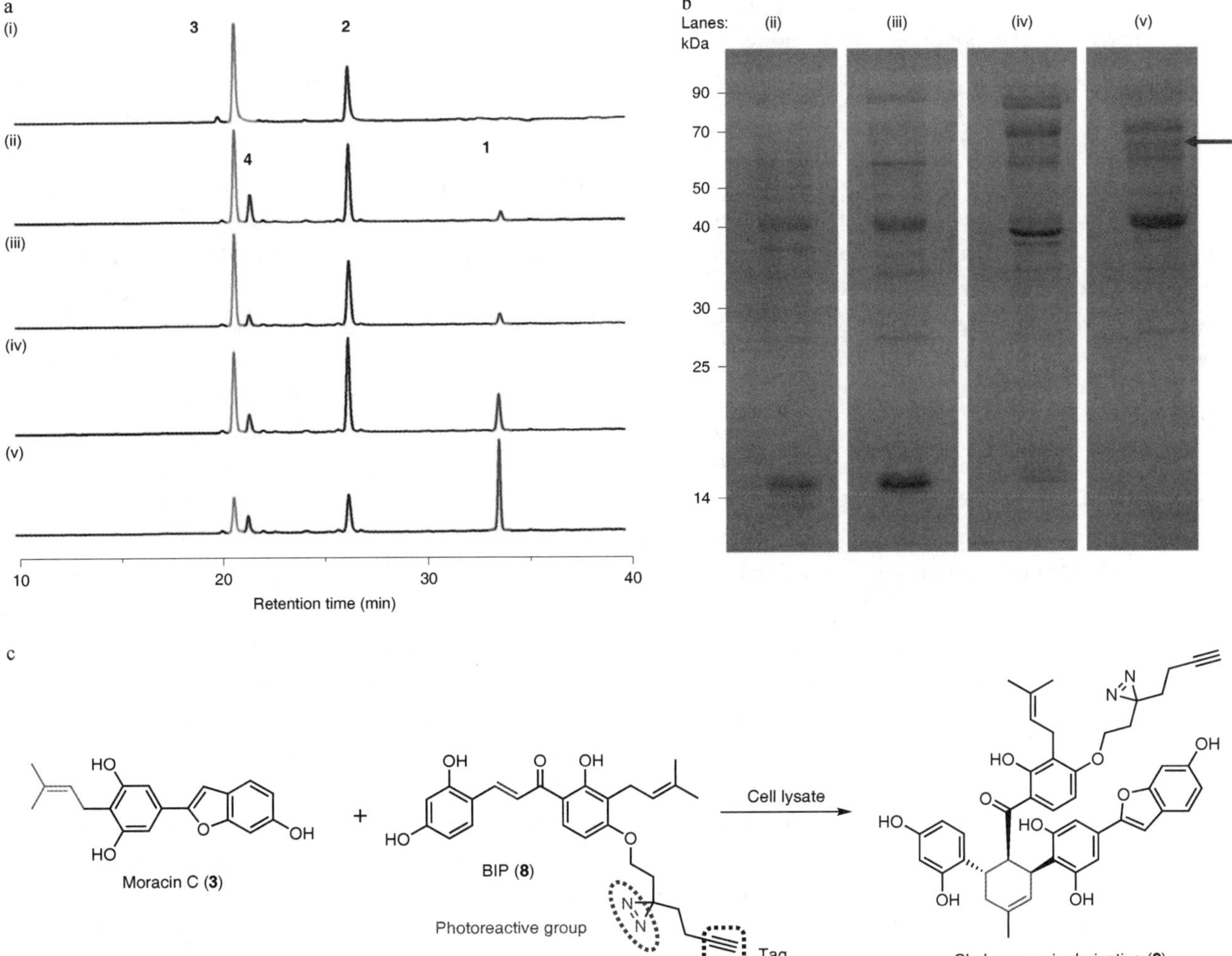


**Fig. 2 Identification of the intermolecular [4+2] pericyclase using activity-based protein purification and BIP-based target identification**

(a) In vitro analysis ($\lambda$ =340 nm) of **2** (100 $\mu$mol/L) and **3** (100 $\mu$mol/L) with 0.1 mg/mL in different protein fractions with the buffer (i), AS fraction (ii), HIC fraction (iii), IEC fraction (iv) and SEC fraction (v). Three experiments were repeated independently with similar results. (b) Approximately 4 $\mu$g of protein was loaded in each lane, and the resolution was achieved using 12% (w/v) acrylamide gel: AS fraction (ii), HIC fraction (iii), IEC fraction (iv) and SEC fraction (v). Three experiments were repeated independently with similar results. (c) Structures of BIP probe **8** and the corresponding chalcomoracin derivative **9**. Probe **8** can be recognized by the putative [4+2] pericyclase and transformed into the [4+2] adduct **9**. After being activated by ultraviolet light (365 nm), the diazirine forms a reactive carbene species that can covalently crosslink with the [4+2] pericyclase in the enzymatic reaction.

band in the SEC fraction with a mobility that corresponded to a molecular mass of ~60 kDa (indicated by the red arrow in Fig. 2b), which possibly contains the oxidase and/or the [4+2] pericyclase. This band was later analysed by a LC-MS/MS proteomics analysis, which suggested that the proteins enriched by activity-based protein purification were berberine bridge enzyme (BBE)-like enzymes (also known as reticuline oxidase-like enzymes) (Supplementary Table 1).

BBE-like enzymes are widely involved in the biosynthesis of bacterial, fungal and plant natural products. PenH, a BBE homologue, is reported to be responsible for the formation of structurally similar dienes in the biosynthesis of fungal natural products. We propose that the BBE-like enzymes in our cell cultures oxidize moracin C (**3**) into diene **4** (Extended Data Fig. 2a) through a similar mechanism, which utilizes $O_2$ and generates $H_2O_2$. Indeed, enzymatic activity was lost in the absence of $O_2$ (Extended Data Fig. 2b), whereas in the presence of $O_2$ (using the SEC fraction as the crude enzyme), $H_2O_2$ was detected as an end product (Extended Data Fig. 2c).

We next used our BIP-based method to reveal the intermolecular [4+2] pericyclase. As diene **4** is unstable under our assay conditions and can also bind to the oxidase, we designed the BIP molecule based on the structure of dienophile **2**. To determine which hydroxyl group in **2** would be suitable for the introduction of a side chain that contained a photoaffinity group and an alkyne tag, we synthesized three derivatives of **2** (**5** - **7**; Extended Data Fig. 3a) and found that 7 showed the best [4+2] activity, comparable to that of 2 (Extended Data Fig. 3b). Based on this result, we synthesized BIP **8**, which gave D - A adduct **9** (Fig. 2c and Extended Data Fig. 3b). We then used **8** in photoaffinity labelling in the SEC fraction, followed by a pull-down assay. One distinctive band with a mobility that corresponded to a molecular mass of ~ 60 kDa, similar in mass to the aforementioned oxidase, was specifically precipitated by the probe in the presence of ultraviolet light (Extended Data Fig. 3c). This band was further excised and subjected to LC-MS/MS proteomics analysis. Interestingly, BBE-like enzymes were identified in this band as among the top 20 possible candidate interacting proteins (Supplementary Table 2), which indicates that the putative [4+2] pericyclase in the *M. alba* cell cultures may also be of this protein family.

We investigated the expression profile of these BBE-like enzymes in our cell cultures. Transcriptome analysis revealed that 14 different transcripts were annotated as BBE-like enzymes or related proteins with the fragments per kilobase of exon per million reads mapped greater than 10 (Supplementary Table 3). We successfully cloned the full-length complementary DNAs (cDNAs) that encoded the top two BBE-like enzymes with a sequence identity of 61.6%, henceforth named MaMO (CL5271.Contig4_ MaL_022) and MaDA (CL1657.Contig4_MaL_022). The deduced protein sequences showed a high sequence similarity with the BBE-type tetrahydrocannabinolic acid (THCA) synthase (47% identity for MaMO and 45% identity for MaDA). Both MaMO and MaDA share the conserved His residue (His115/116) previously shown to undergo covalent binding with FAD. A notable difference, however, was that the other previously reported Cys residue of BBE-like enzymes also known to bind covalently to FAD was present in MaMO (Cys177), but absent in MaDA (Ala178) (Supplementary Fig. 2).

Functional and biochemical characterization of MaMO and MaDA  Next, we successfully expressed MaMO and MaDA in *Komagataella phaffii* and Hi5 insect cells, respectively, and purified them using nickel-charged nitrilotriacetic acid (Ni-NTA) resin chromatography. Solutions with both recombinant MaMO and MaDA appeared yellow in colour, and displayed ultravioletvisible absorption spectra consistent with those of typical flavoproteins (Supplementary Fig. 3). When MaDA was incubated with diene precursor **3**, no product was detected (Extended Data Fig. 4). In contrast, when MaMO was assayed in the same conditions, diene **4** was produced (Fig. 3a), which indicates that MaMO is the oxidase responsible for diene formation. Incubating dieno-phile **2** and diene **4** together with MaDA generated chalcomoracin (**1**) (see Supplementary Information for the high-resolution MS, $^1$H NMR, $^{13}$C NMR and polarimetry characterizations), which shows that MaDA is an intermolecular [4 + 2] pericyclase (Fig. 3b). Comparison with the chemically synthesized racemic **1** confirmed that the product generated by MaDA is optically pure (100% e. e.) and exclusively *endo* (Supplementary Fig. 4). In contrast, when MaMO was incubated with **2** and **3**,**3** was completely converted into diene **4**, whereas neither the oxidation product of **2** nor the D - A product **1** was observed (Extended Data Fig. 4). These observations further demonstrate that MaMO is an oxidase that selectively oxidizes **2** to give diene **4**, whereas MaDA is a stand-alone intermolecular [4 + 2] pericyclase. Biochemical characterization of the two purified recombinant enzymes showed that both enzymes were independent of the divalent cation. The optimal temperature was 50 ℃ for both enzymes, and the optimal pH values were 7.5 and 8.0 for MaMO and MaDA, respectively (Extended Data Fig. 5). We also determined the steady-state kinetic parameters for both MaDA and MaMO (Fig. 3c,d). We found MaDA to be more catalytically efficient ($k_{cat}/K_M$ = 1.97 $\mu M^{-1}s^{-1}$ for dienophile 2) than MaMO ($k_{cat}/K_M$ = 0.19 $\mu M^{-1}s^{-1}$ for 3). As diene **4** is highly unstable (Extended Data Fig. 6), we synthesized a more stable diene analogue **10** and measured

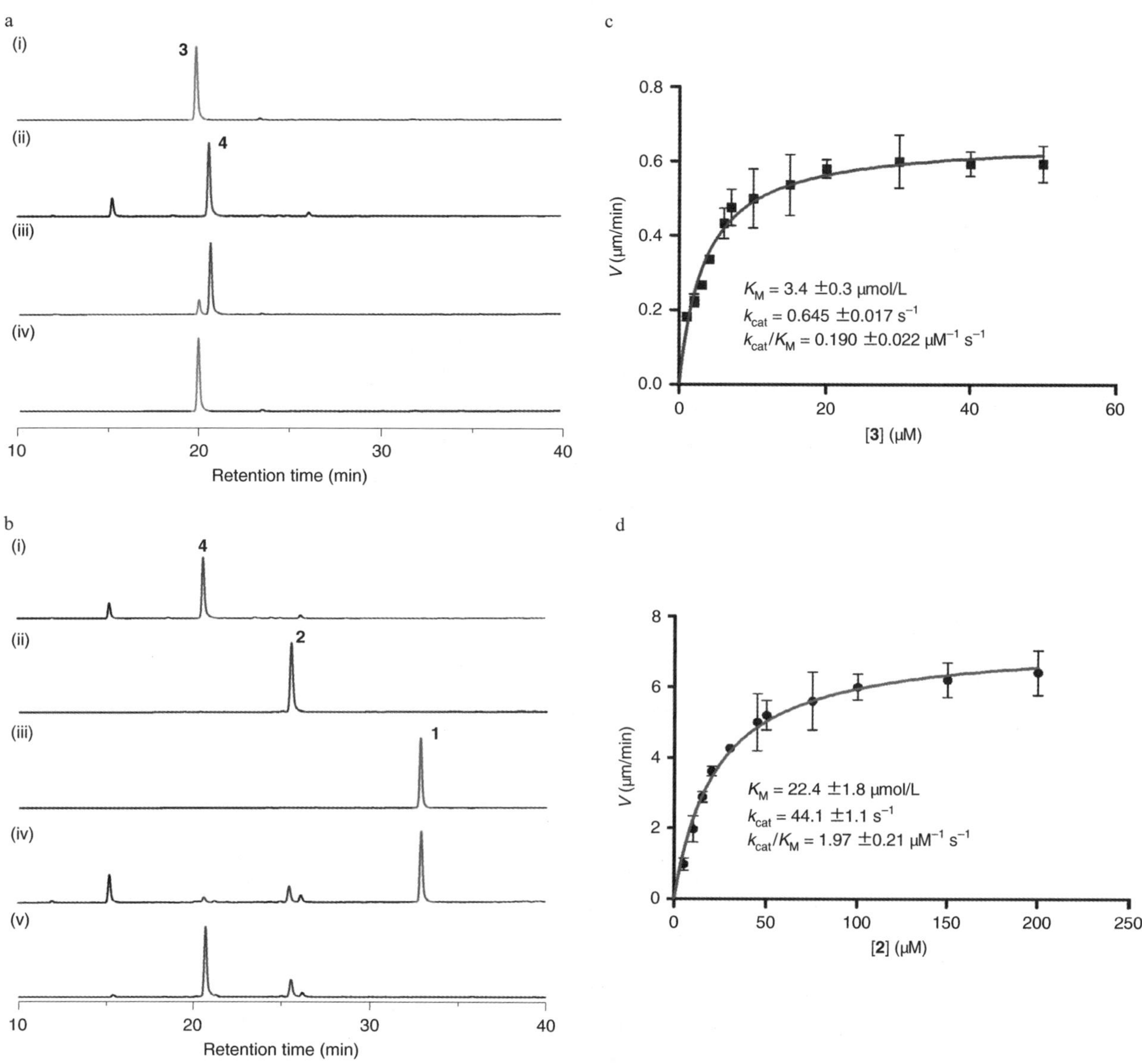


**Fig. 3 Functional and biochemical characterization of MaMO and MaDA**

(a) In vitro analysis ($\lambda$=340 nm) of **3** with 17 nmol/L MaMO for 5 min for standard compound **3** alone (i), standard compound **4** alone (ii), compound **3** with MaMO (iii) and compound **3** with buffer (iv). Three experiments were repeated independently with similar results. (b) In vitro analysis ($\lambda$ =340 nm) of **2** and **4** with 2.7 nmol/L MaDA for 5 min: standard compound **4** alone (i), standard compound **2** alone (ii), standard compound **1** alone (iii), compounds **2** and **4** with MaDA (iv) and compounds **2** and **4** with buffer (v). Three experiments were repeated independently with similar results. (c) Kinetic analysis of MaMO for moracin C (**3**). The reactions were performed with **3** from 1 to 50 μmol/L at pH 8.0 and 50 ℃ in a total volume of 100 μL that contained 17 nmol/L MaMO. (d) Kinetic analysis of MaDA for morachalcone A (**2**). The reactions were performed with **2** from 5 to 200 μmol/L with the saturating diene **4** (1,000 μmol/L) at pH 8.0 and 50℃ in a total volume of 100 μL that contained 2.7 nmol/L MaDA. $K_M$, $k_{cat}$ and $k_{cat}/K_M$ values represent the mean±s.d. of three independent replicates.

the kinetic parameters of MaDA with both diene **10** and dienophile **2** (Extended Data Fig. 7), and found that $k_{cat}/K_M$ for diene **10** and dienophile **2** were 4.04±0.18 mM$^{-1}$ s$^{-1}$ and 10.1±3.8 mM$^{-1}$ s$^{-1}$, respectively.

MaDA is a substrate promiscuous Diels-Alderase To explore the substrate scope and probe the synthetic utility of this novel pericyclase in vitro, three putative diene precursors (**11** - **13**) of D - A products in *M. alba* were synthesized and incubated with dienophile **2**. Six natural and unnatural derivatives (**5** - **7** and **14** - **16**) of **2** as dienophiles were also assayed with diene **4**. LC-MS analysis revealed that MaDA displayed a substrate selectivity for the dienophile, but could react with all of the tested dienes (Fig. 4a), which enabled the incorporation of diverse diene substituents into *Morus* natural products. Efficient chemoenzymatic total syntheses of guangsangon E (**17**), kuwanol E (**18**), kuwanon J (**19**), deoxyartonin I (**20**) and 18″-*O*-methylchalcomoracin (**21**) were accomplished through late-stage enzymatic reactions with a high efficiency (up to 1 873 total turnover number (TTN); Fig. 4b). All the synthesized natural products

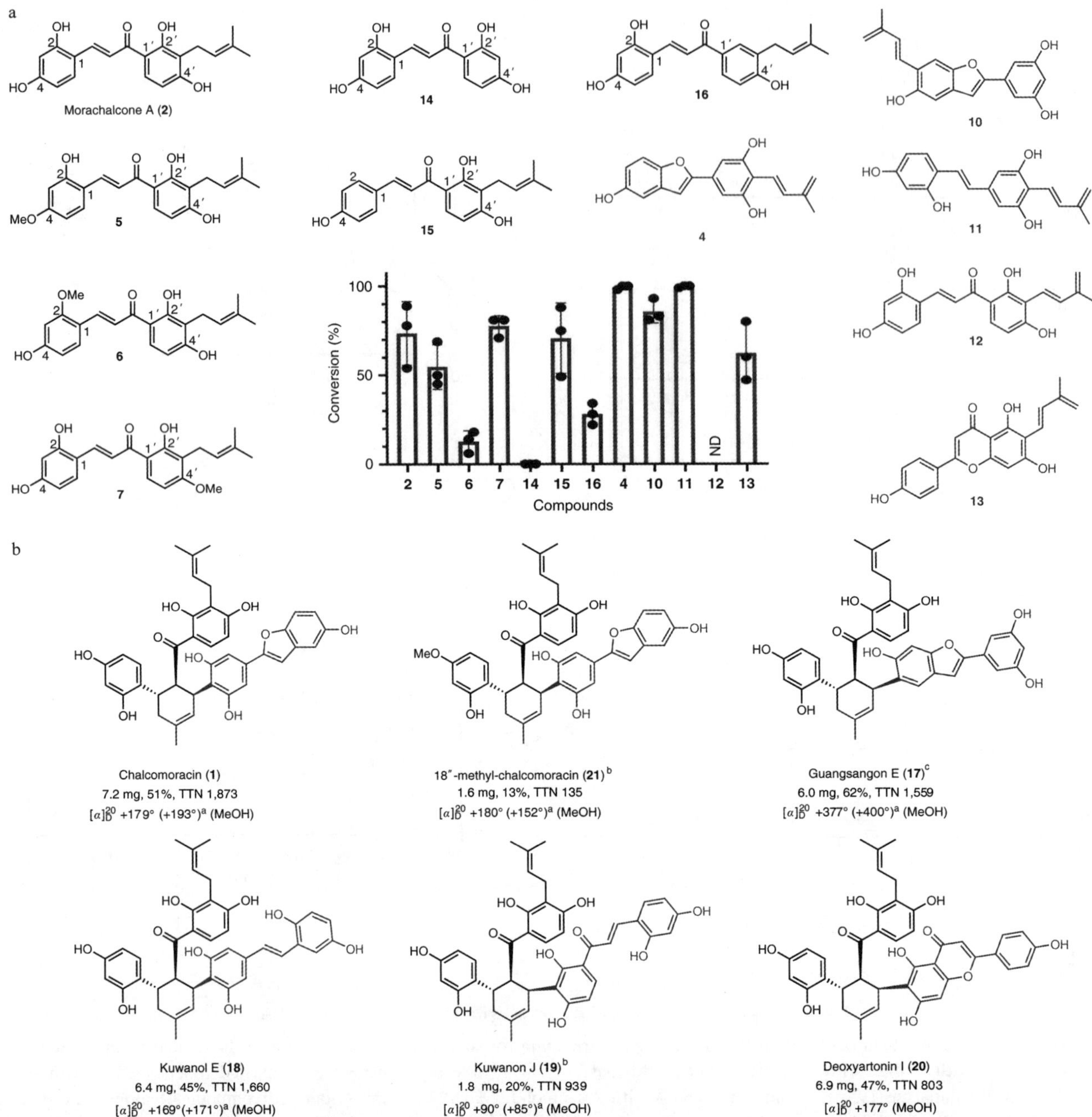


**Fig. 4 Substrate scope of MaDA and the chemoenzymatic synthesis of D－A natural products**

(a) Substrate scope of MaDA. Although the D－A adduct kuwanon J could be detected in a HPLC analysis, diene **12** was too unstable to be detected in a HPLC analysis after incubation at 50℃ for 5 min. Accordingly, the conversion rate of **12** was not determined (ND). Conversion values represent mean±s. d. of three independent replicates. (b) Chemoenzymatic synthesis of various D－A-type natural products by MaDA. Under standard conditions, 0.35 mg of MaDA was used to promote the [4+2] cycloaddition in 100 mL of Tris-HCl buffer (20 mmol/L, pH=8.0). [a]Specific rotation value reported in the literature. [b]The enzymatic reaction was conducted in 150 mL of Tris-HCl buffer with 1.05 mg of MaDA. [c]The enzymatic reaction was conducted in 50 mL of Tris-HCl buffer with 0.35 mg of MaDA. $[\alpha]_D^{20}$, specific rotation at 589 nm (sodium D line) and 20℃.

were characterized by NMR spectroscopy and polarimetry, and the data for synthetic samples fully matched those reported for natural products.

DFT calculation and KIE experiment for the [4+2] cycloaddition reaction  We used DFT calculations to determine the mechanism and intrinsic selectivity of the uncatalysed D－A reaction between **2** and **4**. The lowest-energy D－A transition state (**TS-1**) leads to the *endo* product, and is favoured over the *exo* TS (**TS-2**) by 2.8-3.0 kcal/mol as well as other regioisomers (Fig. 5a and Extended Data Fig. 8a). The geometry of **TS-1** is characteristic of a concerted but asynchronous reaction, with the two forming C-C bonds at 2.03 and 2.69 Å (Fig. 5a). The intramolecular hydrogen bond between O8 and the *ortho*

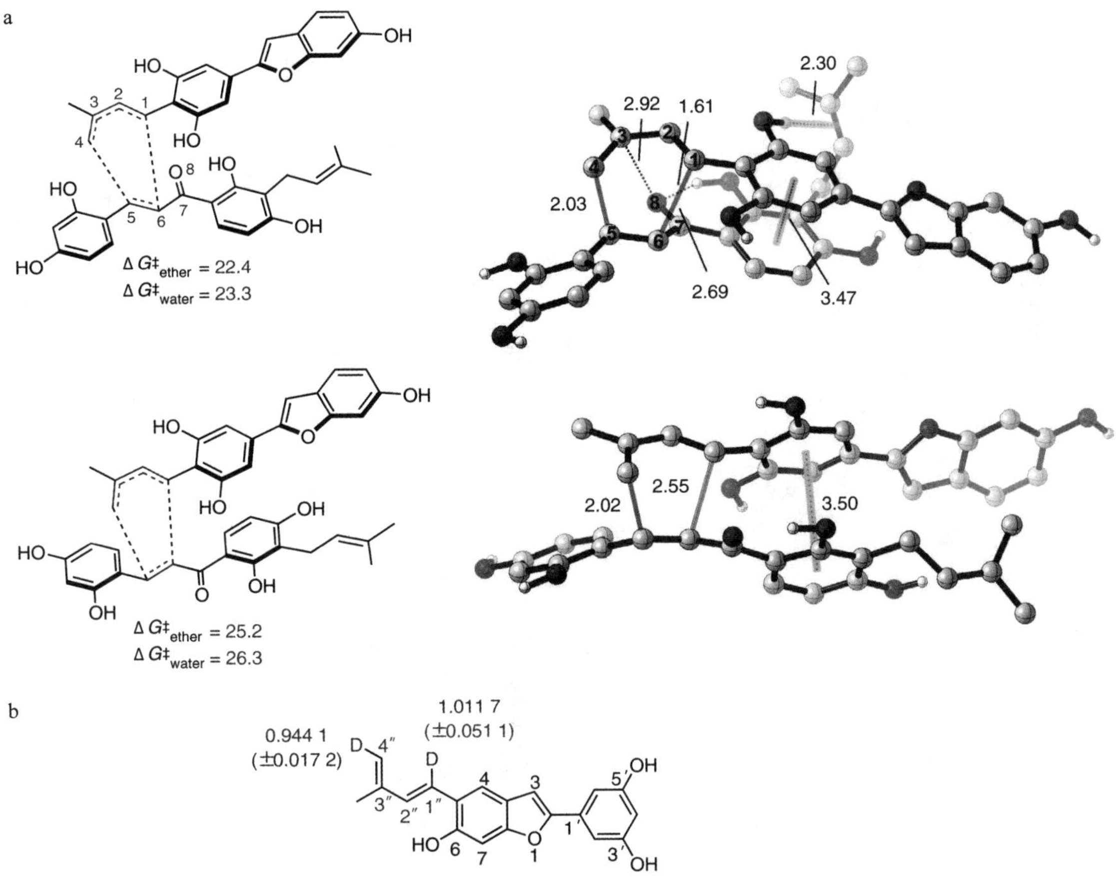


**Fig. 5 DFT calculations and KIE results for the intermolecular [4+2] cycloaddition reaction**

(a) DFT-calculated D - A transition states at the ωB97X - D/6 - 311++G(d, p), CPCM//ωB97X - D/6 - 31G(d) level of theory for *endo* **TS-1** (top) and *exo* **TS-2** (bottom). C-H hydrogens are omitted for clarity. Interatomic distances are in Å. Energies are in kcal/mol. (b) KIE values obtained using two deuterium-labelled diene analogues. The α-secondary deuterium KIE at each site of interest was measured using the method of internal competition in three separate experimental trials. The enzymatic reaction that contained deuterated and non-deuterated diene **10** was quenched at three different timepoints and then the remaining diene **10** from these samples was recovered by preparative HPLC and analysed by MS. Peak integrations of $M + 1$ and $M + 2$ were used to determine the ratios of deuterated/non-deuterated diene **10** in different samples, and these ratios were further used to determine the deuterium KIEs at two different sites of **10**.

hydroxyl group presumably promotes the D - A reaction by lowering the lowest unoccupied molecular orbital energy of the dienophile. The short (2.92 Å) O8 - C3 distance indicates a strong secondary orbital interaction between the O8 lone pair and the antibonding π orbital of the diene (Fig. 5a and Supplementary Fig. 5).

Although the rate of the uncatalysed D - A reaction between **2** and **4** could not be measured due to the instability of **4**, we performed preliminary in-enzyme KIE measurements using a more stable diene analogue (**10**) to obtain insight into the enzyme mechanism. DFT calculations support a similar concerted but asynchronous pathway for the D - A reaction between diene **10** and **2**, with the two forming C - C bonds at 2.05 and 2.69 Å (Extended Data Fig. 8b). Two deuterated derivatives of **10** (**10**-1″D and **10**-4″D) were reacted with **2** in the presence of MaDA to obtain α-secondary KIE values ($k_H/k_D$) of 1.011 7 (0.051 1) and 0.944 1 (±0.017 2), respectively, which provided evidence that an asynchronous D - A pathway was also operational in the enzyme (Fig. 5b).

Interactions between substrates and MaDA To further understand how this intermolecular [4 + 2] cyclization is catalysed by the enzyme, the crystal structure of MaDA was determined at 2.3 Å resolution (Protein Database (PDB) ID 6JQH; Extended Data Fig. 10) using molecular replacement based on the THCA synthase structure (PDB ID 3VTE). Two monomers of MaDA were identified in the asymmetric unit within space group $P2_1$. The overall topology of MaDA is similar to that of THCA synthase (Supplementary Fig. 6), and comprises 26 α-helixes (αA - αZ) and 15 β-strands (β1 - β18), among which 14 α-helixes and 15 β-strands are shown in Fig. 6a. The electron density clearly reveals the presence of FAD, which forms a covalent bond to H116 through the 8α-N1-histidyl-FAD linkage. The flavin moiety of FAD binds to MaDA through hydrogen-bonding interactions with Y192 and Y483, as shown in Fig. 6a. This covalently linked FAD

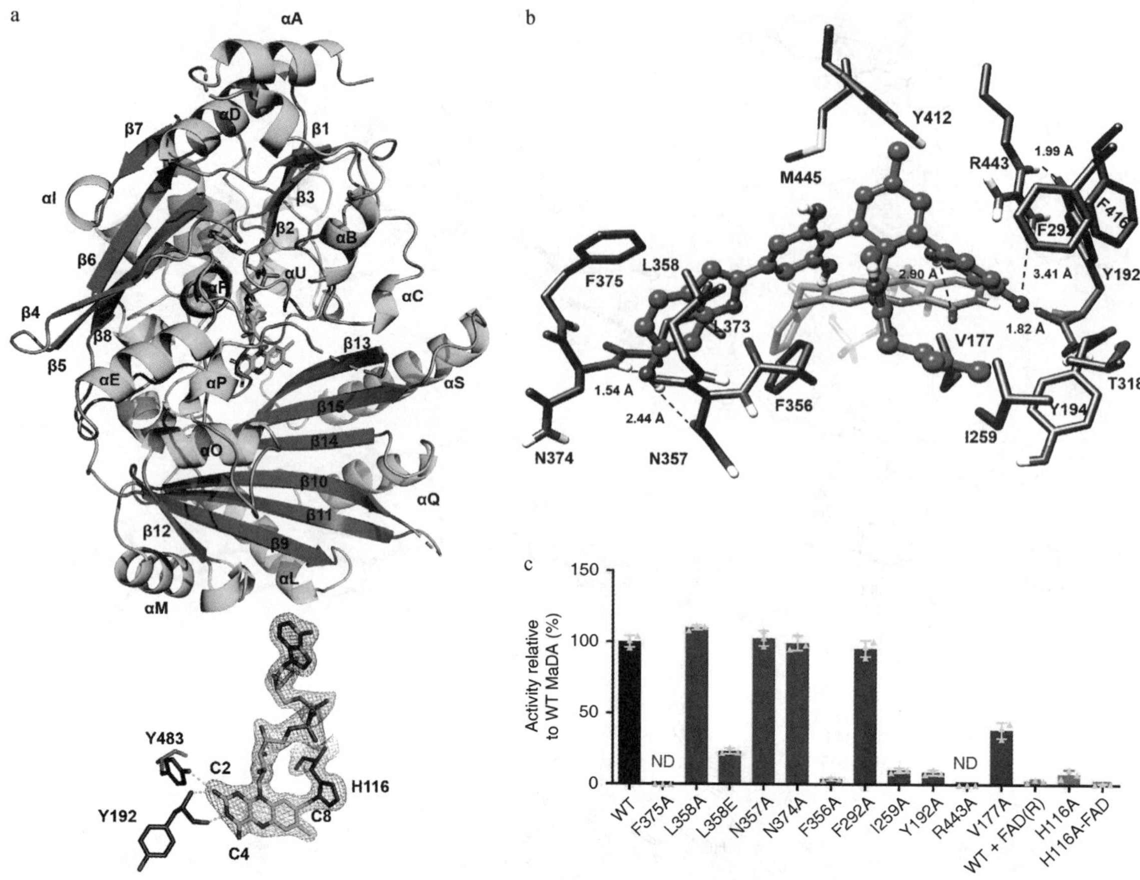


**Fig. 6 Structure, molecular dynamics (MD) simulation and site-directed mutagenesis characterization of MaDA**

(a) Overall structure of MaDA shown in a ribbon model. α-helices, cyan; β-strands, magenta; loops, light pink. The FAD cofactor (green and shown in a stick representation) forms a covalent bond with MaDA, as shown in the 2Fo - Fc electron density map (blue mesh, contoured at the 1.0σ level) for FAD and the covalently bound His116. Residues that form hydrogen bonds with FAD are shown in brown (Y192 and Y483). For amino acids: nitrogen, blue; oxygen, red; carbon, brown. (b) Product **1** docked into a substrate cavity and optimized by 500 ns MD. Stereo views of the docking model show the interactions between **1** (purple) and nearby residues (brown). FAD is shown in green and the hydrogen-bonding interactions are shown as dotted lines. (c) Enzymatic reactions were performed with 2.7 nmol/L MaDA variants and 10 μmol/L of **2** and **4**. Red columns indicate that mutated residues are predicted to interact with **4**, blue columns with **2** and brown columns with FAD. WT+FAD(R), WT with the reduced form of FAD; H116A - FAD, the H116A variant for which non-covalent FAD was removed by adding a 1 mol/L KBr solution. Enzyme activity values represent mean ± s. d. of three independent replicates. ND, activity not detected in the enzymatic assay.

together with one α-helix (αO), four β-strands (β10, β11, β14 and β15) and four loops (residues 175 - 182, 192 - 195, 359 - 367 and 371 - 378) form a large substrate cavity with a volume of 723 Å$^3$ (Supplementary Fig. 6).

Despite numerous attempts, we were not able to obtain a co-crystal structure of MaDA with any native D - A precursors or products, presumably because the remarkably fast kinetics of MaDA limit the possible substrate trapping inside enzyme. To explore possible interactions between MaDA and its substrates, D - A product 1 was docked into MaDA's cavity using UCSF DOCK 3.7, followed by 500 ns MD simulations to relax the protein-ligand binding complex and obtain an energetically favourable binding conformation (Supplementary Fig. 6). It was found that the benzofuran group may interact with F356, N357, L358, L373, N374 and F375 (Fig. 6b). Possible interactions for the dienophile moiety include residues V177, I259, F292, Y192 and R443 (Fig. 6b). Probable hydrogen-bonding interactions include one between the C16″-OH and the C4 carbonyl of the flavin, and an intramolecular hydrogen bond between the C10″-OH and the C8″-carbonyl of **1** (Supplementary Fig. 6), consistent with the DFT calculations. Substrates **2** and **4** were also docked into the MaDA cavity simultaneously (Supplementary Fig. 7). When the two substrates are well positioned by MaDA through numerous interactions, the enone double bond in dienophile **2** and the conjugated diene in **4** are shown to be close enough (3.70 and 3.87 Å, Supplementary Fig. 7) to form the cyclohexene skeleton.

To further probe the involvement of key residues predicted to interact with the substrates by our docking results, we mutated a series of putative binding site residues and compared the D - A catalytic activities of the variants with the wild-type (WT) MaDA (Fig. 6c). The variants F356A, F375A, Y192A and R443A each caused >90% loss of enzymatic activity, which indicates the possible role of these residues in promoting the D-A reaction through $\pi$-$\pi$ stacking and/or hydrogen-bonding interactions. Mutating the bulky hydrophobic residues V177 and I259 to Ala resulted in an ~60 and 90% losses in activity, respectively. The variants N357A and F292A showed little change in catalytic activity. Substitution of L358 with Ala resulted in a slightly higher activity than that the WT MaDA, whereas substitution of the same residue with Glu resulted in an ~80% loss of enzymatic activity. The kinetic characterizations of these MaDA variants (Supplementary Table 4) further support the key roles of these residues for substrate binding and enzyme activity.

To explore the function of the FAD cofactor in MaDA, we reduced MaDA with an excess of sodium dithionite. The reduced MaDA was stable for ~30 minutes (Extended Data Fig. 9a). Reduction of MaDA renders it essentially unable to catalyse the [4+2] cycloaddition (Fig. 6c). When His116 was mutated to Ala to break the covalent linkage between MaDA and FAD, partial loss of FAD was observed through monitoring the absorption change at 450 nm (Extended Data Fig. 9b). This mutation led to dramatically decreased [4+2] activity (Fig. 6c). We conclude that the FAD cofactor is essential for MaDA's catalytic activity in the intermolecular [4+2] cycloaddition, perhaps due to its role in maintaining substrate binding via hydrogen-bonding interaction.

In summary, we identified the enzyme functionally responsible for the intermolecular [4+2] cycloaddition reaction in the biosynthesis of chalcomoracin from *Morus* plants. Since the submission of this article, two new [4+2] cyclases, TiCorS and EupF, were identified from plant and fungi, respectively. TiCorS involves an intramolecular D-A reaction, whereas EupF catalyses the formation of a highly reactive diene that then reacts with a dienophile substrate. These differ from MaDA, which is a stand-alone intermolecular D-A pericyclase that catalyses only the intermolecular D-A reaction; furthermore, MaDA involves a quite different mechanism and outstanding catalytic efficiency. MaMO, the enzyme responsible for the formation of the diene substrate for MaDA, was also functionally characterized. DFT calculations support a concerted, but asynchronous, pericyclic mechanism for the uncatalysed D-A reaction, and preliminary KIE measurements indicate that a similar asynchronous pathway is operational in the enzyme. We show that, due to MaDA's ability to accept a wide scope of diene substrates, a chemoenzymatic total syntheses of many natural products can be accomplished with MaDA. MaDA therefore provides an ideal starting point for future engineering efforts to develop novel intermolecular Diels-Alderases with a versatile catalytic repertoires. Our successful characterization of MaDA highlights the utility of the BIP-based target identification approach as a tool to speed up the discovery of unknown biosynthetic enzymes of plant origin.

## 2 ONLINE CONTENT

Any methods, additional references, Nature Research reporting summaries, source data, extended data, supplementary information, acknowledgements, peer review information; details of author contributions and competing interests; and statements of data and code availability are available at https://doi.org/10.1038/s41557-020-0467-7.

## 3 METHODS

General PCRs were carried out using the standard thermocycling protocols with either TransStart FastPfu DNA Polymerase (Transgene Biotech) or KOD-Plus-Neo (Toyobo) and templates and buffers as specified for each reaction (detailed in the experimental sections below). All the protein quantification was done by the method of Bradford using Protein Assay Dye Reagent Concentrate (Bio-Rad) on protein sample dilutions in MilliQ water. Optical rotations were recorded on a Perkin-Elmer Model-343 digital polarimeter (PerkinElmer. Inc.). The ultraviolet-visible spectra were recorded on Shimadzu UV-3600 Plus UV-VIS-NIR spectrophotometer. Infrared spectra were recorded on a Thermo Fisher FTIR 200 spectrophotometer. NMR spectra were recorded on Varian 400 MHz, Bruker 400 MHz NMR (ARX400) and Bruker 600 MHz AVIIIHD spectrometers at ambient temperature with $CDCl_3$, $CD_3OD$, DMSO-$d_6$ and acetone-$d_6$ as the solvents. Chemical shifts are reported in parts per million and coupling constants are recorded in hertz. High-resolution electrospray ionization (ESI) MS data were measured using an Agilent Technologies 6 520 Accurate-Mass Q-TOF LC/MS spectrometer (Agilent Technologies). The absorption at 450 nmol/L was recorded in a NanoPhotometer (IMPLEN). Photocross-linking experiment was conducted by UVP CL-1000 ultraviolet crosslinker (Analytik Jena) at a wavelength of 365 nm with an intensity of 1,000 W for 1 h.

Chemicals Chemical reagents were purchased from Sigma-Aldrich, J & K Scientific Ltd and Inno Chem Science & Technology Co., Ltd. Moracin C (**3**) and dienophile **15** were purchased from BioBioPha Co., Ltd (Kunming, China). KOD-Plus DNA polymerase was purchased from Toyobo Biotech Co., Ltd. Primer synthesis and DNA sequencing were conducted at the Tsingke Biotech Company. Restriction enzymes and DNA ligase were purchased from Takara Biotechnology Co. Ltd.

Chemical synthesis Chemical synthesis of different dienophiles (**2**, **5**-**8** and **16**), the acetylated precursors of dienes **10**-**13** and deuterated diene **10** are depicted in detail in the Supplementary Information. Dienophile **14** was synthesized according to a literature method.

Chemical analyses The analyses of enzymatic reaction mixtures and the determination of the conversion rates and kinetic parameters were performed on an Agilent 1 200 series HPLC system (Agilent Technologies) coupled with an LCQ Fleet ion trap mass spectrometer (Thermo Electron Corp.) equipped with an ESI source. The LC chromatograph was equipped with a quaternary pump, a diode-array detector, an autosampler, a column compartment and a Shiseido Capcell Pak $C_{18}$ MG III column (250 mm×4.6 mm internal diameter (i.d.), 5 $\mu$m (Shiseido Co., Ltd)). The mobile phase consisted of a gradient elution of solvents A (that is, 0.1% (v/v) formic acid aqueous solution) and B (methanol) at a flow rate of 1.0 mL/min at 30℃. The gradient programmes were 40%-70% B, 0-15 min, 70%-95% B, 15-40 min, 95%-40% B, 40-41 min and 40% B, 41-46 min. For the HPLC-MS analyses, ultrahigh-purity helium was used as the collision gas, and high-purity nitrogen ($N_2$) was used as the nebulizing gas. The optimized ESI source parameters were: sheath gas flow rate, 20 arbitrary units (a.u.); auxiliary gas flow rate, 5 a.u.; spray voltage, 5.0 kV; capillary temperature, 350 ℃; source collision-induced decomposition, 35 V; tube lens offset voltage, −75 V. The spectra were recorded in the 100-1 000 $m/z$ range for a full-scan MS analysis. The split ratio of effluent from the LC to ion source was 2∶1. The data were analysed using XCalibur software.

Activity-guided enzyme purification The reaction mixture, which contained 20 mmol/L Tris-HCl, pH 7.5, 100 $\mu$mol/L morachalcone A (**2**) and 100 $\mu$mol/L moracin C (**3**) as substrates and 9.8 $\mu$g of crude cell lysate in a final volume of 100 $\mu$L was incubated at 30℃ for 1 h. The reactions were terminated by the addition of 200 $\mu$L of ice-cold MeOH and were centrifuged at 15,000 g for 30 min. The supernatants were analysed by HPLC-MS. Chromatography was performed using an ÄKTA prime plus (GE Healthcare). Three parallel assays for enzyme activity were routinely performed.

The fresh *M. alba* cell cultures (200 g) was added into lysis buffer (400 mL) that consisted of 50 mmol/L sodium phosphate, pH 7.4, 1 mmol/L EDTA, 3 mmol/L 2-mercaptoethanol and 100 mmol/L phenylmethanesulfonyl fluoride at a ratio of 1∶100 (v/v) and treated with a Waring blender at 4℃. The mixture was centrifuged at 9,000*g* at 4℃ for 30 min, and solid AS was added to the protein sample to 80% saturation. After gentle agitation at 4℃ for 12 h, the mixture was centrifuged at 9,000*g* at 4℃ for 30 min. The resulting pellet was resuspended in a buffer that contained 20 mmol/L Tris-HCl, pH 7.4, 2 mmol/L EDTA and 3 mmol/L 2-mercaptoethanol, and then centrifuged at 160,000*g* at 4℃ for 2 h. The supernatant was collected and concentrated using a centrifugal concentrator with Amicon Ultra-30K (Millipore), and the resulting solution (AS fraction) was used as a stock solution for the enzymatic assays.

Then, the AS fraction was loaded onto a Hitrap Butyl FF (GE Healthcare) column (5 mL) equilibrated with a 50 mmol/L sodium phosphate buffer, pH 7.0, that contained 1.5 mol/L AS. Protein elution was performed stepwise at a flow rate of 2 mL/min using a 50 mmol/L sodium phosphate buffer, pH 7.0, with a gradient of 0-20 min at 0% ($V/V$), 20-70 min at 20% ($V/V$) and 70-120 min at 100% with respect to the equilibration buffer. the eluted fractions were tested for enzyme activity.

The active fractions (HIC fractions) were pooled, and the buffer was exchanged to 20 mmol/L Tris-HCl, pH 8.0, and loaded onto a HiTrap Q FF (5 mL) column (GE Healthcare) equilibrated with 20 mmol/L Tris-HCl, pH 8.0. Protein elution was performed at a flow rate of 2 mL/min using a buffer that contained 20 mmol/L Tris-HCl, pH 8.0, and 1 mol/L NaCl with a gradient of 0-20 min at 0% ($V/V$), 20-40 min at 10% ($V/V$), 40-60 min at 20% ($V/V$) and 60-100 min at 100% with respect to the loading buffer. The eluted fractions were tested for activity.

The active fractions from HiTrap Q chromatography (the IEC fractions) were concentrated and fractionated using Superdex 200 Increase 10/300 GL columns (GE Healthcare) connected in series. Isocratic protein elution was performed on a $NGC^T$ chromatography system (Bio-Rad) at a flow rate of 0.25 mL/min using a buffer that contained 20 mmol/L Tris-HCl, pH 7.2 and 0.15 mol/L NaCl. the eluted fractions were tested for activity by HPLC to afford the active fraction (SEC fraction).

Photoaffinity labelling and pull down To the PBS buffer (38 $\mu$L) were added 10 $\mu$L of the SEC fraction (1 mg/mL), 1 $\mu$L of **3** (2.5 mmol/L) and 1 $\mu$L of probe **8** (2.5 mmol/L). For the negative control, 1 $\mu$L of DMSO was used instead of probe **8**. The reaction mixture was irradiated at a 365 nm wavelength in ice for 1 h with an intensity of 1,000 W. The resulting mixture was conjugated with a biotin-enrichment tag by click chemistry (1 mmol/L biotin-azide, 1 mmol/L $CuSO_4$, 0.1 mmol/L BTTAA and 10 mmol/L L-ascorbic acid sodium salt for 2 h at room temperature). After conjugation, the proteins were precipitated by adding prechilled acetone (200 $\mu$L). The precipitated mixture was re-dissolved in 50 $\mu$L of PBS buffer that contained 1% SDS, and then added to 500 $\mu$L of PBS. The resulting solution was incubated with 100 $\mu$L of streptavidin agarose (Invitrogen) overnight at 4 ℃. The beads were then washed with PBS (600 $\mu$L) six times and then heated to 95 ℃ for 10 min in the SDS loading buffer. The bead-bound proteins were separated by SDS-PAGE (8%) and visualized by silver staining (Beyotime, P0017S).

LC-MS/MS analysis of proteins The enriched bands in the SEC fraction and the 'pull-down assay' were analysed following the protocol described here. Protein bands on the SDS-PAGE gel were destained and in-gel digested with sequencing-grade trypsin (10 ng/μL trypsin, 50 mmol/L ammonium bicarbonate, pH 8.0) overnight at 37 ℃. Peptides were extracted with 5% formic acid/50% acetonitrile and 0.1% formic acid/75% acetonitrile sequentially and then concentrated to ~20 μL. The extracted peptides were separated by an analytical capillary column (50 μm×10 cm) packed with 5 μm spherical C18 reversed phase material (YMC). A Waters nanoAcquity UPLC system (Waters) was used to generate the HPLC gradient 0%-30% B in 60 min and 30%-70% B in 15 min (A=0.1% formic acid in water and B = 0.1% formic acid in acetonitrile). The eluted peptides were sprayed into an LTQ ORBITRAP Velos mass spectrometer (ThermoFisher Scientific) equipped with a nano-ESI ion source. The mass spectrometer was operated in data-dependent mode with one MS scan followed by ten high-energy collisional dissociation MS/MS scans for each cycle. Database searches were performed on an in-house Mascot server (Matrix Science Ltd) against the proteome of *M. notabilis* (download from the National Center for Biotechnology Information). The search parameters were 10 ppm mass tolerance for the precursor ions, 0.3 Da mass tolerance for the product ions and two missed cleavage sites were allowed for trypsin digestion. Methionine oxidation was set as a variable modification. The search results were filtered with both a peptide significance threshold and an expectation value of less than 0.05. The proteins identified by LC-MS/MS analysis are listed in Supplementary Tables 1 and 2, respectively.

RNA sequencing and cloning of *MaMO* and *MaDA* Ten-day-old *M. alba* cell cultures were treated with 0.1 mmol/L methyl jasmonate for 20 h. After that, the sample was sent to the Beijing Genomics Institute for transcriptome analysis and the total RNA was subsequently extracted from it with an EZNA Plant RNA kit (Omega Bio-tek Inc.) and reverse-transcribed using a SMARTer RACE cDNA Amplification kit (Clontech Inc.). The reverse-transcribed products were subjected to rapid amplification of the cDNA ends (RACE) according to the manufacturer's protocol. The 3′ ends of *MaMO* and *MaDA* were obtained using the primers MaMO-3′GSP and MaDA-3′GSP, respectively. The primer MaMO-3′ GSP was specific for the sequence of Unigene ID CL1657. Contig4 in RNA-sequencing data, and MaDA-3′ GSP was specific for the Unigene ID CL4729. Contig2 sequence. For amplification of the full-length coding sequence of *MaMO*, a forward primer MaMO-Fw and a reverse primer MaMO-Rv were prepared. The full-length *MaDA* coding sequence was acquired using the gene-specific primer pairs MaDA-Fw and MaDA-Rv.

Heterologous expression and purification of *MaMO* The full-length *MaMO* with a C-terminal His tag was obtained by PCR using cDNA as a template with KOD-Plus-Neo (Toyobo) and the primer set MaMO-F/R. The pPIC3.5K (Invitrogen) was double digested using *Eco*RI and *Not*I (Takara Bio Inc.) and purified from agarose gel using Universal DNA Purification Kit (Tiangen Biotech. Co., Ltd). Insertion of *MaMO* into the linearized vector pPIC3.5K was performed with an In-Fusion HD Cloning Kit (Clontech Inc.) according to the manufacturer's protocol. The sequence was confirmed by Sanger sequencing. The expression vector was designed to express the recombinant protein with a C-terminal His tag in *K. phaffii* in the presence of methanol.

The pPIC3.5K expression vector, which contained the full-length *MaMO*, was introduced to *K. phaffii* SMD1168 (Invitrogen) by using a Frozen-EZ Yeast Tarnsformation II kit (Zymo Research). In vivo screening of multiple inserts was performed through the examination of the G418 (Invitrogen)-resistant level for each recombinant. $His^+$ recombinants for *MaMO* (96) were grown to approximately the same cell density by successive inoculations and spotted on yeast extract peptone dextrose plates that contained G418 at final concentrations of 0, 0.25, 0.5, 0.75, 1.0, 1.5, 1.75, 2.0, 3.0 and 4.0 mg/mL. The colonies resistant to G418 at a high concentration were chosen for protein expression. A single colony was inoculated into 50 mL Erlenmeyer flasks, added to 10 mL of BMGY medium that contained 100 mmol/L potassium phosphate buffer, pH 6.0, 1% yeast extract, 2% peptone, 1.34% yeast nitrogen base, $4\times10^{-5}$% biotin and 1% glycerol, and cultivated at 28℃, 220 r/min for 12 h. The cultures were harvested after 12 h and centrifuged at 3,000 g for 5 min to collect the *K. phaffii* strains that harboured the *MaMO* gene. The described strain was precultured in a large volume (1 L) of BMMY medium that contained 100 mmol/L citric acid-sodium citrate buffer, pH 5.5, 1% yeast extract, 2% peptone, 1.34% yeast nitrogen base, $4\times10^{-5}$% biotin and 1% methanol and shaken at 18℃, 100 r/min for 6 days, and protein expression was induced by adding 10 mL of methanol every 24 h. The culture was harvested after 6 days and centrifuged at 6 000*g* at 4 ℃ for 15 min, and the supernatant was concentrated by using a centrifugal concentrator at 4 000*g* at 4 ℃ for 30 min. The protein sample was diluted 20-fold with binding buffer that contained 20 mmol/L phosphate buffer, pH 7.4, 0.5 mol/L NaCl and 20 mmol/L imidazole. The soluble fraction was passed through a 0.45 μmol/L syringe filter unit and the cleared supernatant was immediately applied to 1 mL of Ni-NTA resin (GE) loaded in a column, which was pre-equilibrated with binding buffer. The resin was subsequently eluted with 10 mL (10 column volumes) of binding buffer. Elution was carried out with 10 mL (10 column volumes) of a different gradient elution buffer (20 mmol/L phosphate buffer, 0.5 mol/L NaCl, 50 - 200 mmol/L imidazole, pH 7.4) at a flow rate of 1 mL/min at 4℃. The proteins were concentrated and buffer exchanged to buffer A, which contained 20 mmol/L Tris-HCl buffer, pH 7.4. Protein purity was confirmed by SDS-PAGE to be > 90% (Supplementary Fig. 8). The approximate protein yield for MaMO was 2.0 mg/L and stored at 4℃.

Heterologous expression and purification of *MaDA* The truncated N terminus of *MaDA* without a signal peptide (predicted by PROTTER, http://wlab.ethz.ch/protter/start/) was obtained by PCR using cDNA as the template with KOD-Plus-Neo and primer set MaDA-pInsect-F/R. PI-secSUMOstar was linearized using BamHI-HF (NEB) and XbaI (NEB), and purified from agarose gel using a Universal DNA Purification Kit. A ClonExpress II One Step Cloning Kit (Vazyme Biotech Co., Ltd) was used to generate the MaDA-pI-secSUMOstar construct. The sequence was confirmed by Sanger sequencing and then transformed to DH10Bac competent cells.

*MaDA* was expressed using the Bac-to-Bac system. Recombinant baculoviruses were generated and amplified using the Sf21 insect cells (maintained in the SIM SF medium (Sino Biological Inc.). Recombinant *MaDA* was expressed as a secreted protein in High Five (Hi5) cells with an N-terminal 6×His-SUMO fusion tag. Hi5 cells were infected with recombinant virus (multiplicity of infection of 2) at a density of 1.5 - 2.0×$10^6$ cells m/L. The medium was harvested 48 h after the infection and concentrated using a Hydrosart Ultrafilter (Sartorius), then exchanged into the binding buffer, which contained 25 mmol/L Tris-HCl, pH 8.0 and 200 mmol/L NaCl. The protein was purified using the Ni-NTA resin following same procedure as for *MaMO* and stored at 4℃. The approximate protein yield for MaDA was 3.0 mg/L.

Activity assay, biochemical property and kinetics analyses of MaMO A reaction mixture that contained 20 mmol/L Tris-HCl, pH 8.0, and 100 μmol/L 3 as substrates and 17 nmol/L purified protein in a final volume of 100 μL was incubated at pH 8.0 and 50℃ for 5 min. The reactions were terminated by the addition of 200 μL of ice-cold methanol and were centrifuged at 15,000*g* for 30 min. Supernatants were analysed by analytical reverse-phase HPLC as described above. For quantification, three parallel assays were routinely carried out.

For the investigation on the effects of pH, temperature and divalent metal ions on MaMO activity, enzymatic reactions were performed in reaction buffers with various pH values in the ranges 4.0 - 6.0 (citric acid-sodium citrate buffer), 6.0 - 8.0 ($Na_2HPO_4$ - $NaH_2PO_4$ buffer), 7.0 - 9.0 (Tris-HCl buffer) and 9.0 - 11.0 ($Na_2CO_3$ - $NaHCO_3$ buffer). To assay the optimal reaction temperature, the reactions were incubated at different temperatures (20 - 70℃). To test the necessity of divalent metal ions for MaMO activity, $BaCl_2$, $CaCl_2$, $CoCl_2$, $CuCl_2$, $FeCl_2$, $MnCl_2$, $ZnCl_2$, $NiSO_4$ and EDTA were used individually in a final concentration of 5 mmol/L. All the assays were performed with 17 nmol/L MaMO at 50℃ for 5 min. Aliquots were quenched with 200 μL of ice-cold methanol and centrifuged at 15,000*g* for 30 min. Supernatants were analysed by analytical reverse-phase HPLC as described above.

To determine the kinetic values of **3**, reactions were performed with **3** from 1 to 50 μmol/L at pH 8.0 and 50℃ in a total volume of 100 μL that contained 17 nmol/L MaMO. Aliquots were quenched with 200 μL of ice-cold methanol and centrifuged at 15,000 g for 30 min. Supernatants were analysed by analytical reverse-phase HPLC as described above. Data fitting was performed using GraphPad Prism 8, and $K_M$, $k_{cat}$ and $k_{cat}/K_M$ values represent the mean±s.d. of three independent replicates.

Activity assay and biochemical property analysis of MaDA Diene 4 (10 mmol/L) was generated by hydrolysis *in situ* from the acetylated precursor (for details, see Chemical synthesis in the Supplementary Information). A reaction mixture that contained 20 mmol/L Tris-HCl, pH 8.0, 100 μmol/L, diene **4** and 100 μmol/L **2** as substrates and 2.7 nmol/L purified protein in a final volume of 100 μL was incubated at pH 8.0 and 50℃ for 5 min. The reactions were terminated by the addition of 200 μL of ice-cold methanol and centrifuged at 15,000 g for 30 min. Supernatants were analysed by analytical reverse-phase HPLC as described above. For quantification, three parallel assays were routinely carried out.

For the investigation on the effects of pH, temperature and divalent metal ions on MaDA activity, enzymatic reactions were performed in reaction buffers with various pH values in the ranges 4.0 - 6.0 (citric acid-sodium citrate buffer), 6.0 - 8.0 ($Na_2HPO_4$ - $NaH_2PO_4$ buffer), 7.0 - 9.0 (Tris-HCl buffer) and 9.0 - 11.0 ($Na_2CO_3$ - $NaHCO_3$ buffer). To assay the optimal reaction temperature, the reactions were incubated at different temperatures (20 - 70℃). To test the necessity of divalent metal ions for MaDA activity, $BaCl_2$, $CaCl_2$, $CoCl_2$, $CuCl_2$, $FeCl_2$, $MnCl_2$, $ZnCl_2$, $NiSO_4$ and EDTA were used individually in a final concentration of 5 mmol/L. All the determinations were performed with 2.7 nmol/L MaDA at 50℃ for 5 min. Aliquots were quenched with 200 μL of ice-cold methanol and centrifuged at 15,000*g* for 30 min. Supernatants were analysed by analytical reverse-phase HPLC as described above.

Kinetic analysis of MaDA using 2 as a substrate To determine the kinetic values of **2**, reactions were performed with **2** from 5 to 200 μmol/L with the saturating **4** (1,000 μmol/L) at pH 8.0 and 50℃ in a total volume of 100 μL that contained 2.7 nmol/L MaDA. Aliquots were quenched with 200 μL of ice-cold MeOH and centrifuged at 15,000*g* for 30 min. Supernatants were analysed by analytical reverse-phase

HPLC as described above. Data fitting was performed using GraphPad Prism 8, and $K_M$, $k_{cat}$ and $k_{cat}/K_M$ values represent the mean±s. d. of three independent replicates.

Kinetic analysis of MaDA using diene 10 and dienophile 2 as substrates  To determine the kinetic values of **2**, reactions were performed with **2** (5, 15, 25, 35, 50, 75, 100, 150, 200 and 300 μmol/L) at the saturating **10** (1.5 mmol/L) at pH 8.0 and 50 ℃ in a total volume of 100 μL that contained 270 nmol/L MaDA for 5 min. Meanwhile, to determine the kinetic values of **10**, reactions were performed with 10 (5, 10, 30, 50, 75, 100, 150, 250, 400, 600 and 800 μmol/L) at the saturating **2** (4.0 mmol/L) at pH 8.0 and 50 ℃ in a total volume of 100 μL that contained 270 nmol/L MaDA for 5 min. Aliquots were quenched with 200 μL of ice-cold methanol and centrifuged at 15,000 g for 30 min. Supernatants were analysed by analytical reverse-phase HPLC as described above. Data fitting was performed using GraphPad Prism 8, and $K_M$, $k_{cat}$ and $k_{cat}/K_M$ values represent the mean±s. d. of three independent replicates.

Investigation for the substrate scope of MaDA  Reaction mixtures that contained 20 mmol/L Tris-HCl, pH 8.0, 200 μmol/L diene **4** and 100 μmol/L dienophile **2, 5, 6, 7, 14, 15** or **16** as substrates, 540 nmol/L purified MaDA and 100 μmol/L *p*-methoxyacetophone as the internal standard in a final volume of 100 μL were incubated at 50 ℃ for 5 min. Corresponding negative controls were carried out in the same conditions without adding MaDA. The reactions were terminated by the addition of 200 μL of ice-cold methanol and centrifuged at 15,000*g* for 30 min. Supernatants were analysed by analytical reverse-phase HPLC as described above. The conversion rates of the dienophiles were calculated from the peak areas of each dienophile in the enzymatic reaction mixture and its negative control.

To determine the conversion rates of different dienes, the corresponding precursors were hydrolysed to generate different dienes in situ, following same procedure as for synthesizing **4** (Supplementary Information) and then immediately used in the following assay: reaction mixtures that contained 20 mmol/L Tris-HCl, pH 8.0, 200 μmol/L **2** and 100 μmol/L freshly prepared diene **4, 10, 11, 12** or **13** as the substrates, 540 nmol/L purified MaDA and 100 μmol/L *p*-methoxyacetophone as the internal standard in a final volume of 100 μL was incubated at 50 ℃ for 5 min. The same procedure as that described above was used to calculate the conversion rate of the dienes.

The MaDA-mediated chemoenzymatic syntheses of natural products, that is, chalcomoracin (**1**), guangsangon E (**17**), kuwanol E (**18**), kuwanon J (**19**), deoxyartonin I (**20**) and 18″-*O*-methychalcomoracin (**21**), are described in Supplementary Information.

DFT calculations  DFT computations were performed in Gaussian 09. Molecular geometries were optimized using the ωB97X-D functional and the 6-31G(d) basis set. A pruned (99, 590) grid (specified with the keyword int = ultrafine) was used for optimizations to minimize orientational variations in the evaluation of thermochemical corrections. Frequency calculations were performed at the same level of theory as for geometry optimization to characterize the stationary points as either minima (no imaginary frequencies) or first-order saddle points (one imaginary frequency). Thermal contributions to free energies were calculated from vibrational frequencies using the quasi-rigid rotor-harmonic oscillator approach of Grimme. Intrinsic reaction coordinate calculations were performed to ensure that the first-order saddle points found were true transition states that connected the reactants and the products. Single-point energies were calculated with the ωB97X-D functional and the 6-311++G(d, p) basis set. Solvation effects were incorporated using the CPCM model with diethyl ether or water as the solvent. Molecular structure visualizations were rendered using CYLview. Monte Carlo conformational searches were performed with the Merck molecular force field implemented in Spartan'16 to ensure that the lowest energy conformations were located. The calculated energies (kcal/mol) for DFT-optimized structures are summarized in Supplementary Table 5.

KIE experimental method  The α-secondary deuterium KIE at each site of interest was measured using the method of internal competition in three separate experimental trials. In each trial, site-specifically labelled and unlabelled diene **10** were mixed together (~0.75 mmol/L) in 2 mL of Tris buffer (20 mmol/L, pH = 8.0) that contained 2% DMSO and 0.9 mmol/L dienophile **2**. *p*-Methoxyacetophenone (0.35 mmol/L) was also included in the reaction mixture as an internal standard to standardize the observed ultra-performance liquid chromatography (UPLC) peak integrations. A 0.5 mL aliquot of this pre-enzyme solution was added to 0.5 mL of cold MeCN and stored at −20 ℃ to await HPLC purification of diene **10**. A solution of 132 μmol/L MaDA (7.5 μL) was added to the remaining 1.5 mL of pre-enzyme solution. The reaction mixture was kept at room temperature (~25 ℃) and aliquots were quenched by 0.5 mL of cold MeCN on ice at three different reaction times (less than 7 min). The resulting mixture was immediately centrifuged (12 000 r/min, 10 min) at 4 ℃ to remove MaDA, and analysed at a flow rate of 0.3 mL/min at 40 ℃ by ACQUITY UPLC-MS (Waters, ACQUITY UPLC BEH C18 column, 50 mm×2.1 mm i.d., 1.7 μm) using a gradient elution of water (A) and MeCN (B) to determine the fractions of the reaction. The gradient programmes were 20% B, 0-1 min, 20%-58% B, 1-4 min, 58%-60% B, 4-8 min, 60%-95% B, 8-10 min, 95%-20% B, 10-11 min, and 20% B, 11 - 12 min. A non-enzymatic cycloaddition reaction between 10 and 2 was not observed even at 60℃ for 6 h (Supplementary Fig. 9).

The diene **10** that remained in the four different aliquots was isolated using C18 reversed-phase HPLC (Waters, XBridge pre-C18 OBD, 150 mm × 19 mm i. d., 5 μm) with ultraviolet detection at 280 nmol/L. The column was eluted with water (A) and MeCN (B) using the gradient 30%-40% B, 0-1 min, 40%-64% B, 1-12 min, 64%-66% B, 12-15 min, 66% B, 15-17 min, 66%-95% B, 17-18 min, 95%-30% B, 18-19 min and 30% B, 19-20 min. A solvent blank was run interposed between each HPLC separation to prevent memory effects. The fractions that contained diene **10** were collected and concentrated in vacuo at 30 ℃ to remove the MeCN. The remaining mixtures were lyophilized and re-dissolved in a 1∶1 mixture of MeCN and water (300 μL) for MS analysis.

The MS data of KIE experiments were collected by directly injecting the sample into the mass spectrometer (Waters Vion IMS-QTOF) at a rate of 20 μL/min. Mass spectrometer parameters were: capillary voltage, 3 kV; source temperature, 100 ℃; desolvation temperature, 350 ℃; cone gas, 50 L/h; desolvation gas, 600 L/h; scan time, 1 s. The scan was operated in the ESI positive mode. The lockspray was injected every 2 min using 100 pg/μL leucine encephalin ($[M+H]^+=556.2766\ m/z$). The total runtime was 6 min and signal intensities obtained from 2.5 min to 5.5 min were averaged to obtain a final spectrum for analysis. A solvent blank was injected interposed between each sample to prevent memory effects.

The $M+1$ peak (309.1120 $m/z$) and $M+2$ peak (310.1183 $m/z$) in each sample from the resulting mass spectra were integrated by summing the observed intensities in 0.0023 $m/z$ increments over the entire peaks using Origin 2018 software (Supplementary Fig. 10). These two peak integrations were used to determine the ratio of deuterated/non-deuterated diene **10** in different samples. The equation $KIE=k_H/k_D=\log(1-F)/\log[(1-F)R_{SF}/R_0]$ uses these ratios to determine the deuterium KIE at two different sites of **10**, where $F$ is the fraction of reaction completed, $R_{SF}$ is the ratio of deuterated/non-deuterated diene **10** at fraction $F$ and $R_0$ is the ratio of deuterated/non-deuterated diene **10** in the pre-enzyme fraction. $R_{SF}/R_0$ at different fractions was determined based on the peak integrations. The KIEs of 10-1″D at three different reaction times were 0.9878, 0.9941 and 1.0533, to give an average value of 1.0117±0.0511. The KIEs of 10-4″D at three different reaction times were 0.9550, 0.9310 and 0.9462, to give an average value of 0.9441±0.0172.

Crystallization of MaDA, data collection and structure determination To prepare the protein sample for crystallization, MaDA was digested with tobacco etch virus protease to remove the N-terminal 6×His-SUMO fusion tag. Untagged MaDA was further purified by anion exchange chromatography using a HiTrap Q column, followed by the SEC using a Superdex 200 10/300 GL column. MaDA (59 kDa) existed as a monomer with a molecular weight of ~30 kDa as the SEC indicated (Supplementary Fig. 11). Protein was concentrated to 10 mg/mL. Crystals were grown using a sitting drop vapour diffusion method at 18 ℃. MaDA was crystallized in 0.2 mol/L zinc acetate dihydrate, 0.1 mol/L sodium cacodylate trihydrate, pH 6.5 and 18% PEG8000.

Crystals were cryoprotected in 0.2 mol/L zinc acetate dihydrate, 0.1 mol/L sodium cacodylate trihydrate, pH 6.5, 20% PEG8000 and 20% ethylene glycol, and flash frozen in liquid nitrogen. X-ray diffraction data were collected at the Shanghai Synchrotron Radiation Facility (beamline BL17U) with an X-ray wavelength of 0.9795 Å at a temperature of 100 K. The data were processed using HKL2000 (HKL Research). The structure was solved by a molecular replacement method using Phaser, with the THCA synthase structure (PDB ID 3VTE) as the search model and refined using Coot and Phenix. Of the residues, 96.3% were in the Ramachandran-favoured regions, with 3.3% in the Ramachandran allowed regions and 0.4% as outliers.

The volume of the binding pocket was calculated using the program POVME 2.0. The coordinates of the following atoms were used as centres for POVME inclusion spheres: N5 of the FAD cofactor, CB of the residue Phe359, CB of the residue Phe375 and CB of the residue Phe416. Points were generated in POVME with a grid spacing of 1 Å using inclusion spheres of 9 Å radius around the atom positions. The volume was calculated using the contiguous option (with contiguous seed spheres of radius 4 Å centred at the same coordinates as those of the inclusion spheres).

Computational methods for docking The product chalcomoracin (**1**) or substrates (**2** and **4**) were docked into the binding pocket of MaDA using UCSF DOCK 3.7. The top-ranked 1,000 poses were generated for structural filtering and conformational clustering as previously described. Briefly, the generated docking poses were filtered based on the three types of structural descriptors calculated for each docking pose, namely the number of hydrogen bonds, the number of buried carbon atoms and the hydrophobic contact. For D-A product **1** or substrates **2** and **4**, the unreasonable docking poses were automatically removed if the calculated values of any type of descriptors were below the averaged values throughout the entire conformational ensemble. The docking poses survived from the filtering step were clustered based on Kelley-Gardner-Sutcliffe penalty function, which is cutoff-free, particularly efficient in clustering diverse poses in global space in an unbiased manner to obtain dissimilar docking poses. Then, a more physically rigorous approach (MM-GB/SA) was applied to refine and rescore the survived docking poses.

For the best-scored binding pose, three independent 500 ns MD simulations were further performed with the Desmond software package and three copies of the MD simulations were also carried out for *apo*-MaDA as controls (Supplementary Fig. 12). We used the OPLS-AA 2005 force field parameter set for the protein and ligand and the TIP3P model for water. The system was solvated in a 12 Å cubic water box and neutralizing counterions were added. To mimic the experimental assay conditions, a 0.15 mol/L NaCl salt bath was introduced. The prepared systems were first minimized using 5,000 steps of the steepest descent algorithm and then equilibrated as follows. The system was heated from 0 to 310 K in the NPT ensemble over 100 ps with harmonic restraints of 10.0 kcal $mol^{-1}\cdot Å^{-2}$ on heavy atoms of protein and ligand, and initial velocities sampled from the Boltzmann distribution. Further equilibration was performed at 310 K with harmonic restraints on the protein and ligand starting at 5.0 kcal $mol^{-1}$ $Å^{-2}$ and reduced by 1.0 kcal $mol^{-1}$ $Å^{-2}$ in a stepwise fashion every 1 ns for a total of 5 ns of additional restrained equilibration. Production runs were then made for 50 ns duration in the NPT ensemble. The M-SHAKE algorithm was applied to constrain all the bonds that involved hydrogen atoms with a time step of 2 fs. The short-range electrostatic and Lennard-Jones interactions were cut off at 9 Å. Long-range electrostatic interactions were computed by the particle mesh Ewald method.

Single-site-directed mutagenesis and activity assay of MaDA variants  MaDA variants (H116A, V177A, Y192A, I259A, F292A, F356A, N357A, L358A, L358E, F375A and R443A) were engineered by site-directed mutagenesis (QuikChange, Stratagene) using the primers in Supplementary Table 6. Expression and purification of all these variants were done according to the same protocol described for the WT MaDA.

The enzymatic reactions were performed under optimal conditions with 2.7 nmol/L MaDA and 10 μmol/L **2** and **4**.

Reporting summary  Further information on research design is available in the Nature Research Reporting Summary linked to this article.

## 4 DATA AVAILABILITY

The data that support the findings of this study are available with this article and its Supplementary Information, or are available from the corresponding authors upon reasonable request. The gene sequences of MaDA and MaMO as amplified from cell cultures of *M. alba* are deposited in GenBank, accession no. MK573629 and no. MK573628, respectively. The structural factor and coordinate of MaDA are deposited in the Protein Data Bank under ID 6JQH.

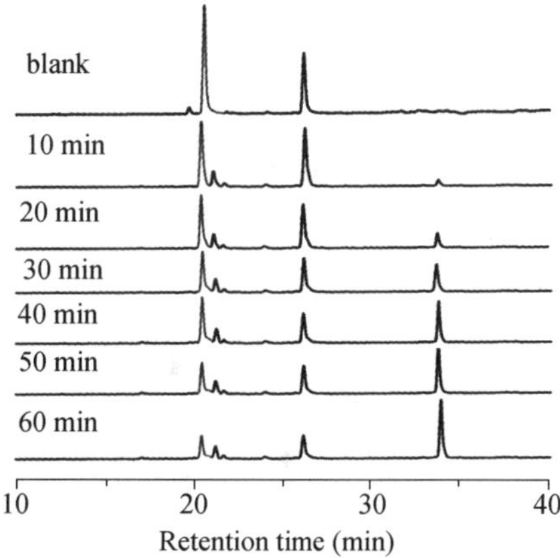


**Extended Data Fig. 1  The time dependent assay using SEC fraction of crude enzyme**

The reaction mixture containing 20 mmol/L Tris-HCl, pH 7.5, 100 mmol/L morachalcone A (**2**), 100 μmol/L moracin C (**3**) as substrates and 9.8 μg of crude cell lysate in a final volume of 100 μL was incubated at 30℃ for 1 h. The reactions were terminated by the addition of 200 μL of ice-cold MeOH and were centrifuged at 15,000 g for 30 min. The supernatants were analysed by the LC/MS. The experiments were repeated three times independently with similar results.

a FAD(ox)  FAD(red)  FAD(ox)

$O_2$  $H_2O_2$

BBE-like enzyme

:B Enz  moracin C (3)  diene 4

proposed mechanism

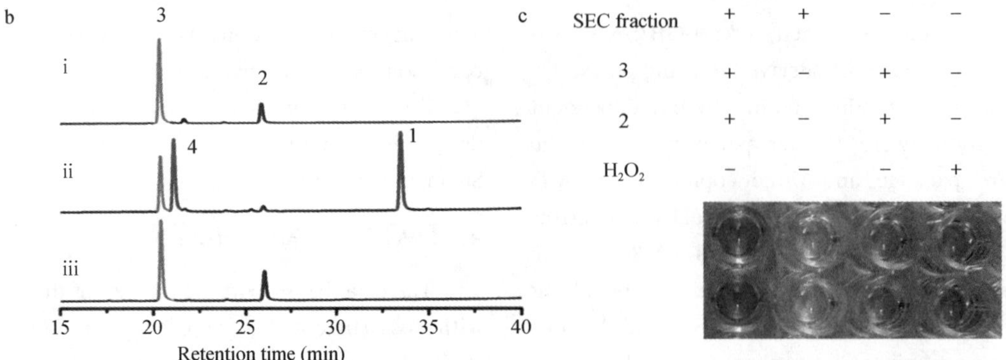


**Extended Data Fig. 2 The evidence suggesting BBE-like enzyme as the putative oxidase**

(a) The proposed mechanism for the formation of diene **4** catalysed by BBE-like enzyme. (b) *In vitro* reaction analysis of **2** and **3** with or without dioxygen using SEC fraction: i) without SEC fraction (negative control), ii) with SEC fraction and dioxygen (positive control), iii) with SEC fraction but without dioxygen. The reaction buffer containing **2** and **3** was degassed in −78 ℃ and charged with argon, and then SEC fraction was added under argon atmosphere at room temperature. The experiments were repeated two times independently with similar results. (c) Detection of hydrogen peroxide using Hydrogen Peroxide Assay Kit (Beyotime, S0038). The purple color indicated the existence of hydrogen peroxide in the reaction buffer. The experiments were repeated three times independently with similar results.

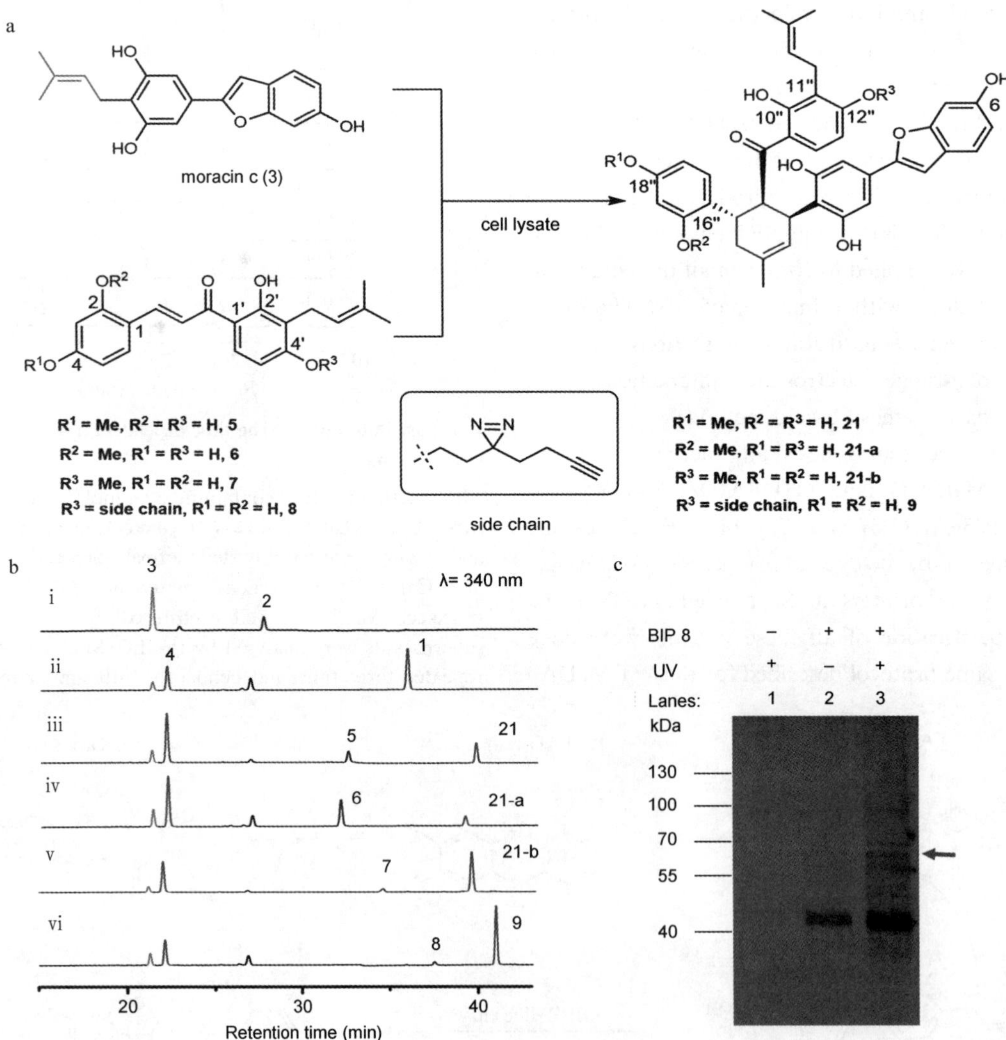


**Extended Data Fig. 3 The activities of the probe 8 and its analogues and the silver staining of pull-down assay using 8 as the photoaffinity probe**

(a) The structures of morachalcone A derivatives and the corresponding chalcomoracin derivatives. (b) *In vitro* analysis using AS fraction (0.25 mg/mL) with different morachalcone A derivatives (100 μmol/L): i) **2** and **3** without the AS fraction, ii) **2** and **3** with the AS fraction, iii) **5** and **3** with the AS fraction, iv) **6** and **3** with the AS fraction, v) **7** and **3** with the AS fraction, vi) **8** and **3** with the AS fraction. The experiments were repeated three times independently with similar results. (c) The SEC fraction was incubated on ice with or without BIP **8** under irradiation of 365 nm UV light or without UV irradiation for 1 h. The following lysates were used for streptavidin-agarose pull-down assays, and the precipitates were resolved by 8% SDS-PAGE, followed by silver staining. The indicated bands were excised and subjected to LC-MS/MS proteomics analysis. The experiments were repeated two times independently with similar results.

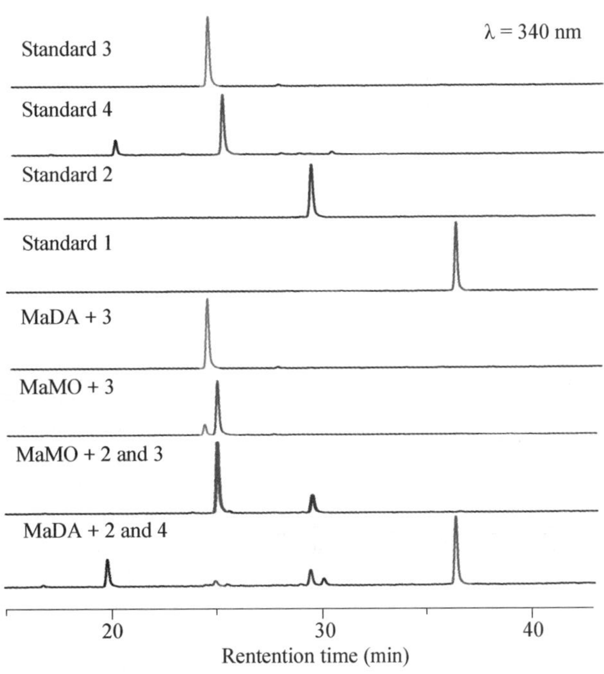


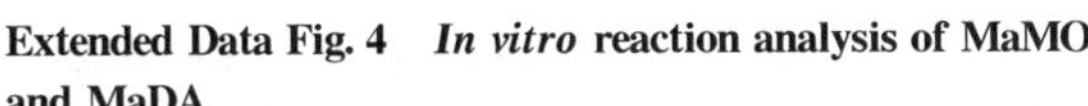

**Extended Data Fig. 4 *In vitro* reaction analysis of MaMO and MaDA**

When MaDA was incubated with **3** alone, no new peak appeared, which revealed the MaDA did not have the oxidative function. In contract, when MaMO was used, diene **4** was formed. On the other hand, when MaMO was incubated with **2** and **3**, **3** was completely transformed to diene **4**, but no chalcomoracin or oxidative product of **2** was observed which indicated MaMO neither oxidized **2** nor catalysed the [4+2] cycloaddition between **2** and **4**. The experiments were repeated three times independently with similar results.

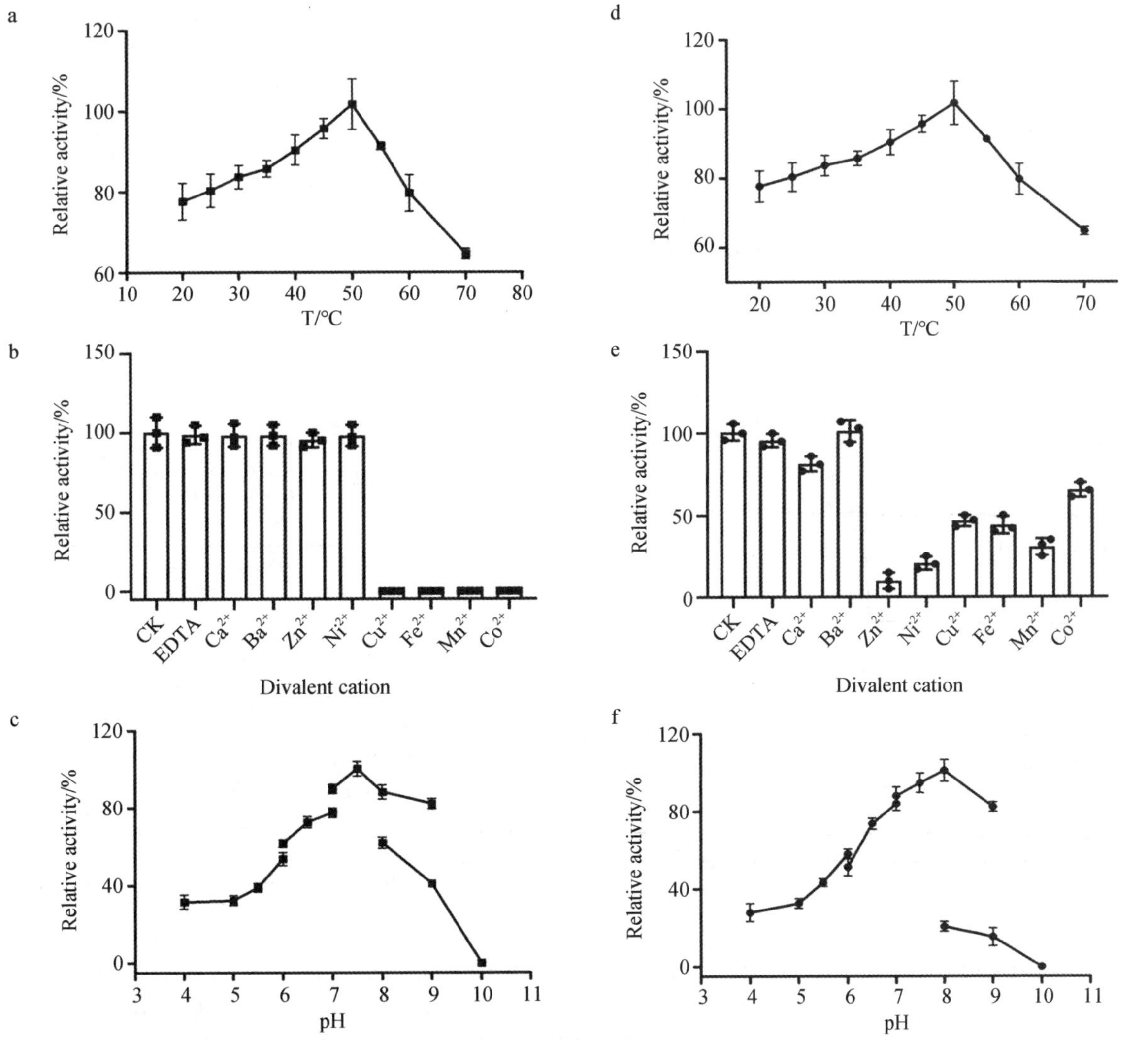

**Extended Data Fig. 5 Effects of pH, temperature and divalent metal ions on the activity of MaMO and MaDA**

(a) Effect of temperature on MaMO's activity. (b) Effect of divalent metal ions on MaMO's activity. (c) Effect of pH value on MaMO's activity. (d) Effect of temperature on MaDA's activity. (e) Effect of divalent metal ions on MaDA's activity. (f) Effect of pH value on MaDA's activity. CK means 'control check'. Enzyme activity values represent mean ± standard deviation (s. d.) of three independent replicates.

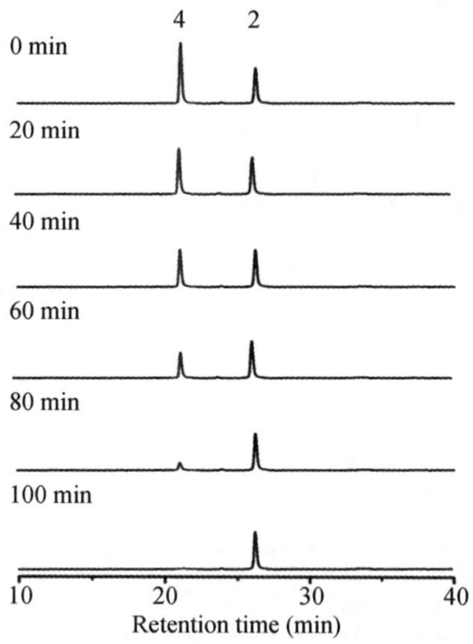


**Extended Data Fig. 6 The time course for the incubation of morachalcone A (2) and 4 without MaDA**

The reaction mixture containing 20 mmol/L Tris-HCl, pH 8.0, 100 $\mu$mol/L morachalcone A (**2**), 100 $\mu$mol/L diene (**4**) as substrates without MaDA in a final volume of 100 $\mu$L was incubated at 50 ℃ for 100 min. The reactions were terminated by the addition of 200 $\mu$L of ice-cold MeOH and were centrifuged at 15,000 g for 30 min. The supernatants were analysed by the LC/MS. The experiments were repeated three times independently with similar results.

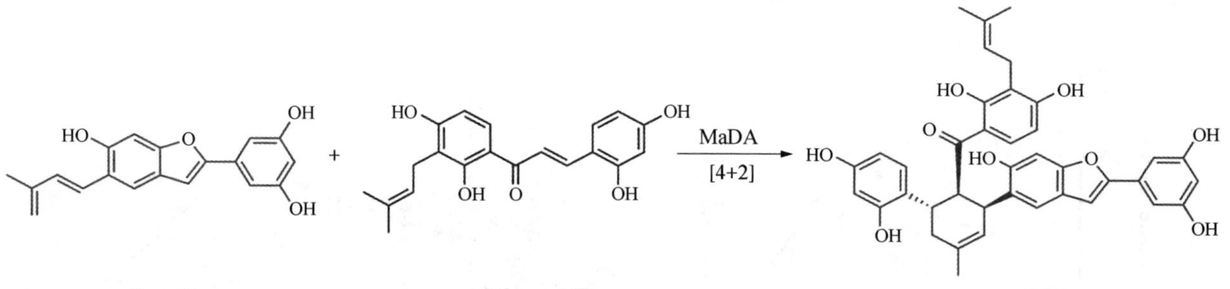


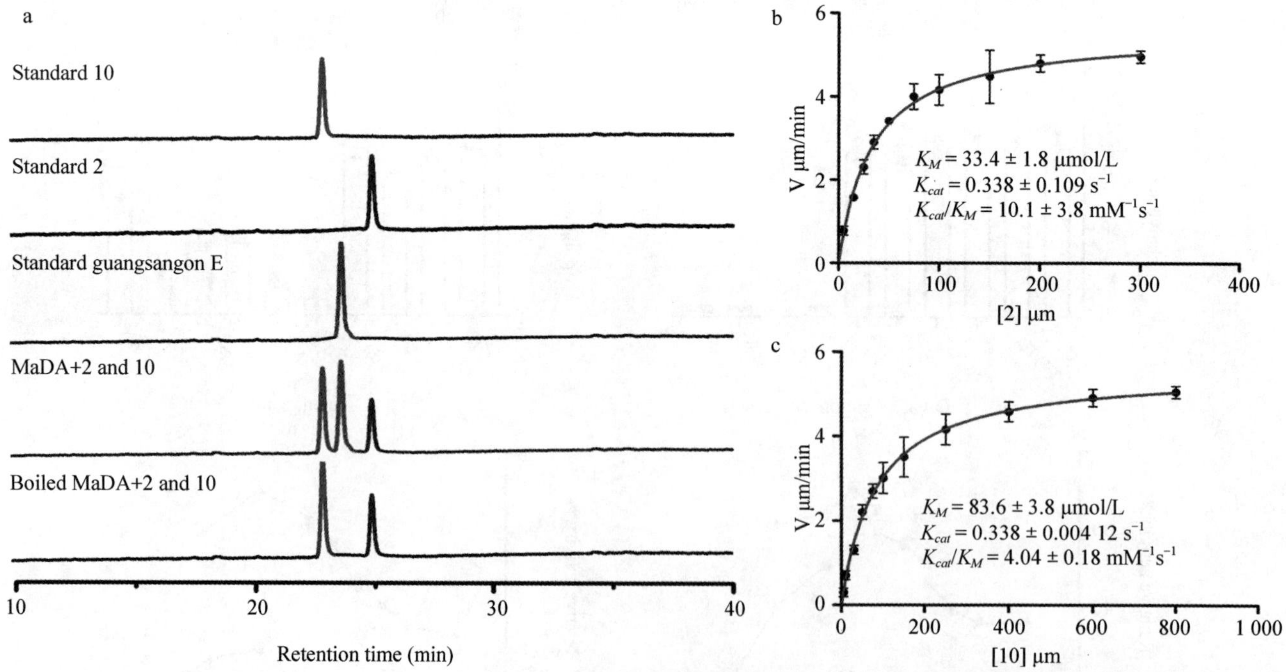


**Extended Data Fig. 7 Determination of the kinetic parameters of MaDA using stable diene 10 and morachalcone A (2)**

(a) Enzymatic assay of 2 and 10 with MaDA. Compounds **2** and **10** were incubated with 270 nmol/L MaDA or boiled MaDA for 5 min. The experiments were repeated three times independently with similar results. (b) Kinetic parameters of MaDA for **2** (5～300 $\mu$mol/L) using **10** (1.5 mmol/L) as diene. (c) Kinetic parameters of MaDA for **10** (5～800 $\mu$mol/L) using **2** (4 mmol/L) as dienophile. $K_M$, $k_{cat}$ and $k_{cat}/K_M$ values represent mean±standard deviation (s.d.) of three independent replicates.

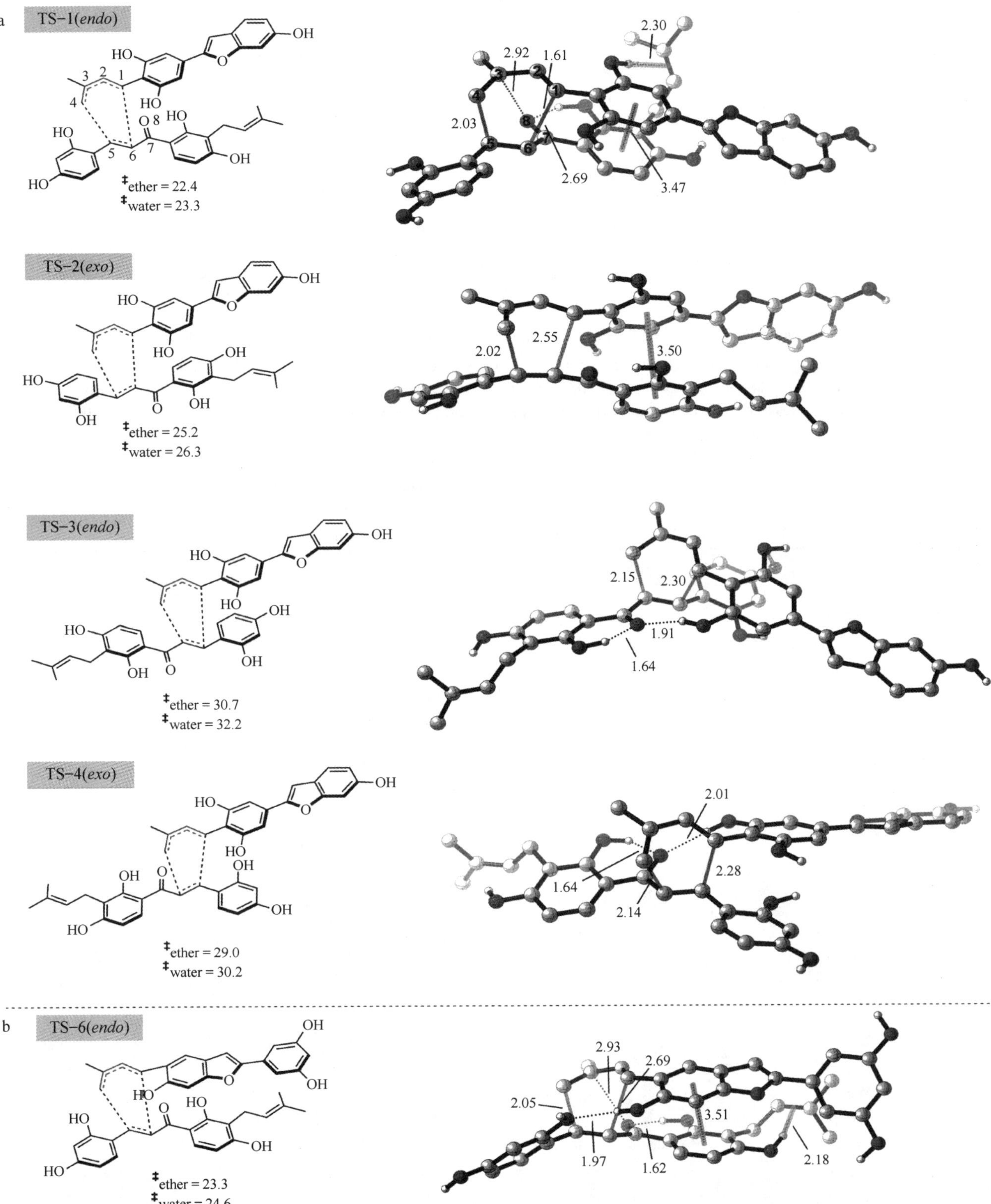


**Extended Data Fig. 8 Calculated transition states of the Diels-Alder reaction between dienophile 2 and dienes 4 or 10**

(a) This data shows the calculated Diels-Alder transition states of Diels-Alder reaction between **2** and **4** leading to the four possible product regio-and stereoisomers. The computed barriers (all with respect to isolated reactants) show that TS-1 is the favored TS, suggesting that the reaction displays intrinsic regio-and stereoselectivity for the experimentally observed product isomer under enzyme catalysis. (b) The DFT calculation supports an endo transition state and a concerted but asynchronous mechanism of the Diels-Alder reaction between **2** and **10**. C-H hydrogen atoms are omitted for clarity. Interatomic distances are in Å. Energies are in kcal/mol.

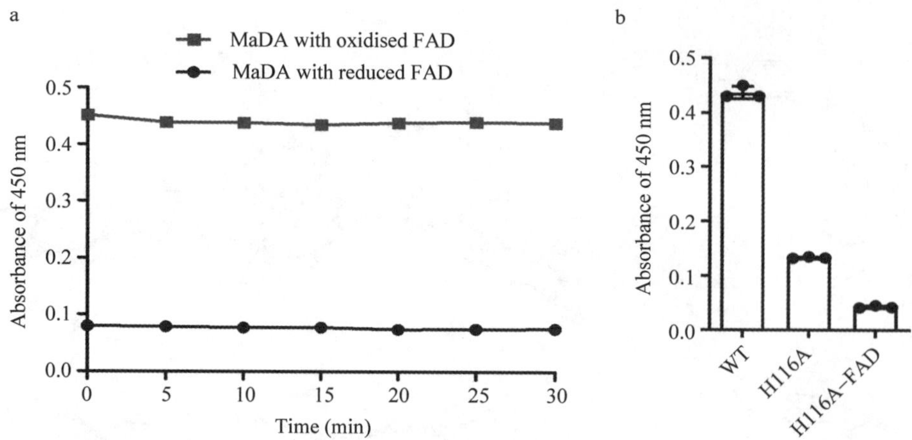


**Extended Data Fig. 9 Different absorbance data of MaDA at 450 nm at different conditions**

(a) The absorbance of MaDA (34 μmol/L) at 450 nm was detected every 5 min with or without adding 6.6 mmol/L sodium dithionite (about 200 eq), indicating the reduced form of MaDA is stable under excess of sodium dithionite for at least 30 minutes. The experiments were repeated three times independently with similar results. (b) The absorbance of 450 nm of $MaDA^{wt}$, $MaDA^{H116A}$ and $MaDA^{H116A}$-FAD were detected at the same protein concentration (34 μmol/L). The $MaDA^{H116A}$ was dialysed in 1 mol/L KBr solution to remove the non-covalent FAD. Absorbance values of 450 nm represent mean±standard deviation (s.d.) of three independent replicates.

**Extended Data Table 1 Data collection and refinement statistics of MaDA - FAD**

| | MaDA |
|---|---|
| **Data collection** | |
| Space group | $P2_1$ |
| Cell dimensions | |
| *a*, *b*, *c* (Å) | 74.66, 115.38, 95.87 |
| α, β, γ (°) | 90, 96.23, 90 |
| Resolution (Å) | 44.0 - 2.30(2.39 - 2.30)* |
| $R_{merge}$ | 0.12(0.59) |
| $I/\sigma I$ | 12.6(4.5) |
| Completeness(%) | 92.1(92.2) |
| Redundancy | 7.0(7.0) |
| **Refinement** | |
| Resolution (Å) | 2.30 |
| No. reflections | 65 799(6 541) |
| $R_{work}/R_{free}$ | 0.186/0.227 |
| No. atoms | |
| Protein | 8 122 |
| Ligand/ion | 106 |
| Water | 473 |
| *B*-factors | 28.8 |
| Protein | 28.5 |
| Ligand/ion | 19.3 |
| Water | 35.8 |
| R.m.s. deviations | |
| Bond lengths (Å) | 0.007 |
| Bond angles (°) | 1.24 |

**Extended Data Fig. 10 Data collection and refinement statistics of MaDA - FAD**

[高磊，王瑞杉，雷晓光，等. Nature Chemistry，2020，12：620 - 628.]

# Engineering chimeric diterpene synthases and isoprenoid biosynthetic pathways enables high-level production of miltiradiene in yeast

## 1 INTRODUCTION

Many diterpenes have valuable pharmaceutical or biological activity, but their structure makes them challenging to be synthesized. According to their main scaffold, diterpenes can be divided into the clerodane, labdane, pimarane, abietane, and kaurane types. All these diterpenes are synthesized from (*E*, *E*, *E*)-geranylgeranyl diphosphate (GGPP), which is derived from isopentenyl diphosphate (IPP) and its isomer dimethylallyl diphosphate (DMAPP) produced via the mevalonate (MVA) pathway or the methylerythritol phosphate (MEP) pathway (Fig. 1). Many of the abietane-type diterpenes are of particular interest and value. This includes triptolide, a bioactive compound isolated from *Tripterygium wilfordii*, the derivatives of which have been evaluated in phase I and II clinical trials, as well as tanshinones, a group of active diterpenoids found in the Chinese medicinal herb danshen (*Salvia miltiorrhiza*), which exhibit diverse pharmacological activities, including cardioprotective, antioxidant and antitumor effects.

In spite of the many promising activities of these diterpenes, their low abundance in natural plant tissues and the tedious and inefficient extraction processes severely limit their further study and application. By contrast, biotechnological production using modified microorganisms is eco-friendly and efficient, already providing sustainable and reliable supplies of many natural compounds, such as artemisinic acid and taxadiene. It is essential in enhancing the supply of their common precursors for high-level production of these diterpenes. Miltiradiene is widely present in medicinal plants and is an important intermediate in the biosynthesis of many abietane diterpenes, such as triptolide, tanshinone, carnosic acid, carnosol and rubesanolides A-D. In our previous study, modxilar pathway engineering of diterpene sjmthases and key enzjones of the MVA pathway in *Saccharomyces cerevisiae* led to a miltiradiene titer of 365 mg/L in a 15 L bioreactor. Then, the production of miltiradiene was further improved to 488 mg/L in fed-batch cultivation by increasing the carbon flux toward FPP and GGPP through plasmidbased overexpression of the key genes involved in the GGPP biosynthetic pathway. However, the titer was still insufficient for industrial production.

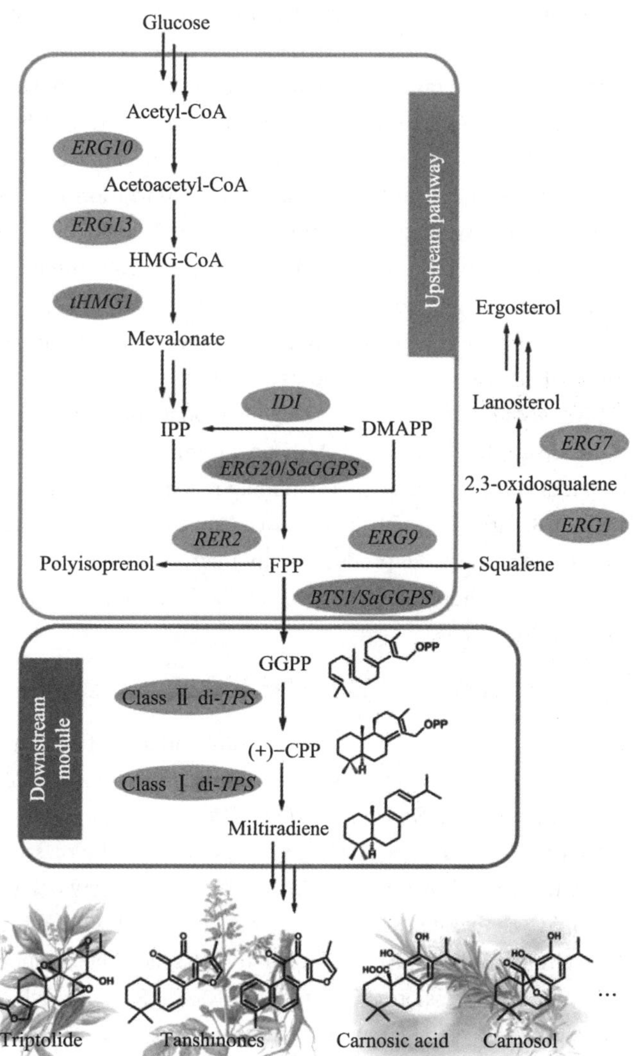


**Fig. 1 The biosynthetic pathway of GGPP and miltiradiene in *S. cerevisiae*. The genes in pink ellipses were overexpressed in BY - T20**

For interpretation of the references to colour in this figure legend, the reader is referred to the Web version of this article.

In the biosynthetic pathway of miltiradiene, class II diterpene synthases, which contain a characteristic DXDD motif, initiate the cyclization of GGPP to (+)-copalyl diphosphate ((+)-CPP), after which the class I diterpene synthases containing a DDXXD motif cyclize and rearrange the (+)-CPP to miltiradiene (Fig. 1). In recent years, more diterpene synthases that catalyze miltiradiene biosynthesis have been identified in different plants, but we are not aware of any publications comparing their ability to produce miltiradiene and the effects of combining different class I and II diterpene synthases. Using recombinant expression of class I and II diterpene synthases from different species, Jia et al. identified 13 previously unknown diterpene products and achieved remarkably high yields with some of the enzyme combinations. In addition, protein modification of key enzymes, including translational fusion and truncation of transit peptides at the N-terminus of the enzymes, is also an effective strategy for increasing the production of terpenes. Jiang et al. improved the geraniol production from trace amounts to 524 mg/L by manipulating the key enzymes geraniol synthase (GES) and famesyl diphosphate synthase (Erg20). It is conceivable that an integrated application of strategies including metabolic pathway optimization of host cells, non-native enzyme combinations, and engineering of diterpene synthases, could lead to a major breakthrough in miltiradiene production.

Here, we further improved the production of miltiradiene by increasing the carbon flux toward GGPP in *S. cerevisiae* and optimizing the gene module of miltiradiene synthases. The final strain with an optimized pathway and efficient miltiradiene synthase module reached a miltiradiene titer of 3.5 g/L in a 5 L bioreactor. Our work offers a good example for terpene production in microbial cell factories and lays a foundation for the biosynthesis of other valuable natural diterpenes.

## 2 MATERIALS AND METHODS

2.1 Strains, plasmids and culture media The initial strain used in this study was BY-T20 (*MATα trp1Δ0 leu2Δ0 ura3Δ0*, *trp1::HIS3-$P_{PGK1}$-BTS1/ERG20-$T_{ADH1}$-$P_{TDH3}$-SaGGPS-$T_{TPI1}$-$P_{TEF1}$-tHMG1-$T_{CYC1}$*, a schematic of strain construction is shown in Fig. S1), which is ultimately derived from *S. cerevisiae* S288C. *E. coli* Transl-Tl (TransGen Biotech, Beijing, China) was used for plasmid amplification. The gRNA expression vector p426-SNR52p-gRNA. CANl. Y-SUP4t (ref. no. 43803) and the Cas9 expression vector p414-*TEF1*p-*Cas9*-*CYC1*t (43802) were purchased from Addgene (http://www.addgene.org/). The vector used for the construction of miltiradiene synthases was pESC-LEU (Cat no. 217452; Agilent Technologies, USA). All the strains and plasmids used in this study are respectively listed in Tables S1 and S2. Synthetic dropout (SD) medium was purchased from Fun-Genome Company (China), and was supplemented with 2% glucose, minus the auxotrophy factors complemented by the propagated plasmids. Yeast extract peptone dextrose (YPD) medium was composed of 1% yeast extract (OXOID, England), 2% peptone (OXOID, England) and 2% glucose.

2.2 Construction of gRNA plasmids and preparation of ds-oligos Specific gRNA sequences targeting *YJL064w*, *YPL062w* and *ROX1* were obtained using an open-source tool http://yeastriction.tnw.tudelft.nl which is specialized for the identification of suitable Cas9 target sites in *S. cerevisiae* strains. Target sequences with highest scores without any 100% identity to other genomic loci were selected. The gRNA sequence targeting the *EGR9* promoter was described in a previous study. All gRNA target sequences used in this study are listed in Table S3. For the assembly of single gRNAs, two reversed *Aar*I recognition sites ($_8$NGCAGGTGNNN NCACCTGCN$_4$) were inserted upstream of the gRNA scaffold by restriction-free cloning based on the p426-*SNR52*p-gRNA. CAN1. Y-*SUP4t* plasmid using the primer pair pUOl-F/R, and the product was re-circularized by ligation. Next, 24 nt gRNA oligos consisting of a 20 nt target sequence and 4 nt 5' overhangs were synthesized. Equal volumes of 100 μm solutions of oligos F and R were mixed and annealed resulting in a double-stranded insert with overhangs at both ends. Then, plasmids expressing single gRNAs were constructed by inserting the double-stranded oligos into the *Aar*I recognition site using Golden Gate assembly (Fig. S2A). Similar to the construction of the single-gRNA plasmids, plasmids expressing multiple gRNAs were efficiently constructed by first inserting two reversed *Aar*I recognition sites into the plasmid with a single gRNA expression cassette, and then amplifying different gRNA fragments using unique primers with different overhangs which were inserted into the *Aar*I cloning site according to the needs of the experiment by Golden Gate assembly (Fig. S2B). The details of the reaction conditions and the primers can be found in the legend of Fig. S2 and Table S4.

The 120 bp double-stranded oligos (ds-oligos) for *YJL064w*, *YPL062w* and *ROX1* knockout were obtained by annealing pairs of complementary single-stranded 120 nt oligos. The repair fragments for *EGR9* knockdown and *UPC2.1* knock-in were amplified by PCR using synthetic DNA sequences as templates. All ds-oligos were purified and then stored at −20 ℃ for further use, and their sequences are listed in Table S5.

2.3 Genome editing in S. cerevisiae using the CRISPR/Cas9 system To obtain a higher genome editing efficiency, the Cas9 expression vector P414-*TRP1*-*TEF1*p-*Cas9*-*CYC1*t was first introduced into BY-T20 using the lithium acetate transformation method according to the directions of the Frozen-EZ Yeast Transformation II Kit. The strain with the Cas9 expression plasmid was named BY-HZ09 and used for the following manipulations. A total of 1 μg of the gRNA expression plasmid was mixed with 1 nmol/L of each corresponding ds-oligo and electroporated into BY-HZ09 at 3.0 kV in a 2 mm gap electroporation cuvette using a

Bio-Rad MicroPulser followed by cultivation on synthetic drop-out medium without tryptophan and uracil at 30 ℃ for 2 - 3 days. After incubation, 5 mutant colonies were selected and genomic DNA was isolated for use as template for PCR of all targeted loci. The isolated genomic DNA of strain BY-T20 was used as negative control. The correct PCR bands were further verified by DNA sequencing. The mutants with desired genotypes were used in the following experiments after removing the gRNA and Cas9 plasmids as described in a previous study.

2.4 Construction of miltiradiene synthase expression plasmids The sequences of miltiradiene sjmthases from 7 plants were downloaded from the National Center for Biotechnology Information (NCBI) database (http://www.ncbi.nlm.nih.gov/gorf/gorf.html), codon-optimized for yeast and ordered as synthetic DNA. The vectors were directly constructed in the yeast strain BY-HZ16 by electroporation as described above. Each miltiradiene synthase fragment had 100 bp overhangs at both ends which were homologous to the linearized eukaryotic pESC-LEU vector. The class II and I di-*TPSs* were inserted into the multiple cloning site 1 (MCS1) and 2 (MCS2), respectively, to be transcribed from the p*GAL10* and p*GAL1* promoter, respectively (Fig. S3).

The fusion-protein expression plasmids were constructed using the same method. The class II di-*TPS CfTPS1* and the class I di-*TPS SmKSL1* were coupled together via the widely used flexible linker GGGS encoding sequence "GGT GGT GGT TCT" and the stop codons of the upstream genes were removed. Additionally, four truncated variants of fusion protein *Sm*KSL1-*Cf*TPS1 were also generated. The truncation 1 named t*Sm*KSL1 - *Cf*TPS1 lacks the transit peptide at the N-terminus of *Sm*KSL1 (M1 - C47), and the truncation 2 t*Sm*KSL1-t*Cf*TPS1 has a further deletion of the transit peptide at the N-terminus of *Cf*TPS1 (M1 - N81). Furthermore, the $\beta$ domain (N48 - S256) away from the active-site of *Sm*KSL1 was removed and the variant was named as *Sm*KSL1$\alpha$-CfTPS1. Similarly, the $\alpha$ domain (D518 - A786) far from the active-site of *Cf*TPS1 was removed and the variant was named as *Sm*KSL1$\alpha$-*Cf*TPS1$\beta\gamma$. All the plasmids encoding the truncated versions were constructed by electroporation using BY-HZ16 as the host strain. After cultured in synthetic drop-out medium without leucine (SD-Leu medium), single clones were selected and plasmids were isolated. The sequence of each variant was verified by specific PCR and sequencing.

2.5 Homology modeling and structural analysis by computational simulation Since the crystal structures of the fusion protein complexes (*Sm*KSL1-*Cf*TPS1 and *Cf*TPS1-*Sm*KSL1) have not been solved, we submitted the sequences to web-based tool I-TASSER (https://zhanglab.ccmb.med.umich.edu/I-TASSER/). To select the models, I-TASSER uses the SPICKER program to cluster all the decoys based on the pair-wise structure similarity, and reports five models which corresponds to the five largest structure clusters. The models were visualized using the versatile molecule model rendering software, PyMOL, and the final models of fusion protein complexes were selected by align to the protein models of *Sm*KSL1 and *Cf*TPS1 which were also predicted using I-TASSER.

The proteins secondary structure and chloroplast transit peptides of *Sm*KSL1 and *Cf*TPS1 were predicted using the web-based tools http://www.compbio.dundee.ac.uk/jpred/index.html and http://www.cbs.dtu.dk/services/ChloroP/. We truncated the transit peptides and domains based on the analysis of protein secondary structure.

2.6 GGOH and miltiradiene fermentation in shake flasks A two-phase extractive fermentation process was performed in this study. For GGOH production, six individual colonies of strain BY-T20 and its mutants were first picked from the agar plates into sterile culture tubes containing 5 mL YPD medium and cultivated at 30 ℃ and 220 rpm for 24 h to the exponential phase. Then, the resulting exponential culture was diluted to an initial $OD_{600}$ of 0.2 in 5 mL of fresh YPD medium and cultivated at 30 ℃ and 220 rpm for 12 h until an $OD_{600}$ of approximately 5.0. Next, aliquots were diluted to an initial $OD_{600}$ of 0.05 in 10 mL medium and cultivated at 30 ℃ and 220 rpm. An extractive *n*-dodecane phase comprising 10% (v/v) of the culture volume was added aseptically after 10 h. The organic layer was harvested for GGOH analysis at 72 h by centrifugation of the fermentation broth at 10,000× g for 1 min, and 10 μL of the *n*-dodecane from each sample were transferred into 990 μL of *n*-hexane (dilution of 1 : 100) in a glass GC vial. The miltiradiene fermentation process was similar to the method mentioned but the medium used here was different because the miltiradiene synthases were expressed from the *D*-galactose-induced promoters p*GAL1* and p*GAL10*. Correspondingly, the medium used for strain activation was SD-Leu with 2.0% glucose and the production medium was replaced with SD-Leu medium containing 1.8% galactose and 0.2% glucose because a small amount of glucose can minimize the lag phase during metabolic adaption to galactose. The organic layer was harvested for miltiradiene analysis after 144 h. Samples and standards were transferred to the gas chromatograph-mass spectrometer (GC-MS) autosampler for qualitative analysis and quantification.

2.7 Fed-batch fermentation for GGOH and miltiradiene production To produce larger amounts of GGOH, strain BY-HZ16 was used for fed-batch fermentation in a 5 L bioreactor (Shanghai Baoxing Bio-Engineering Equipment Co., Ltd., China). Firstly, a single clone was seeded into a

100 mL flask containing 20 mL YPD medium and grown at 30 ℃ and 200 rpm for 24 h. The resulting exponential culture was diluted to an initial $OD_{600}$ of 0.2 in 150 mL of fresh YPD medium and cultivated for another 12 h until the $OD_{600}$ reached approximately 5.0. The seed culture was then used to inoculate a bioreactor containing 1.5 L of optimized YPD medium (OYPD, 5% glucose, 1% yeast extract, 3% peptone, 0.8% $KH_2PO_4$, and 0.6% $MgSO_4$) to an $OD_{600}$ of approximately 0.1. The temperature was set to 30 ℃ and the pH was maintained at 5.5 by the addition of ammonium hydroxide. The dissolved oxygen (DO) concentration was kept above 30% of atmospheric oxygen by adjusting the agitation (300 - 900 rpm) and aeration. Concentrated glucose solution (80%, *W/V*) was fed at an exponential rate to control the glucose concentration below 1 g/L. Additionally, 5×YP mixture (5% yeast extract, 15% peptone) was fed periodically to provide adequate nutrition for cell growth. An extraction phase comprising *n*-dodecane was added to 20% (*V/V*) of the medium volume at 10 h of the fermentation to start the two-phase extractive fermentation. Duplicate culture aliquots were collected periodically to determine cell density and production of GGOH. The miltiradiene fed-batch fermentation was processed in accordance with previous studies. The single clone of BY-HZ70 was activated for two passages in SD-Leu medium with 20 g/L glucose. Minimal medium containing 5 g/L $(NH_4)_2SO_4$, 3 g/L $KH_2PO_4$, 0.5 g/L $MgSO_4 \cdot 7H_2O$, 60 mg/L uracil, 60 mg/L tryptophan, 20 g/L glucose, as well as trace metal and vitamin solutions was used as the initial fermentation medium. The temperature, pH, DO, agitation and aeration were controlled as above. The carbon source was changed into galactose after 6 h. A concentrated galactose solution (60%, *W/V*) and 5×minimal medium were fed to provide adequate carbon source and nutrition for cell growth and miltiradiene production. The galactose and 5 × minimal medium was initially fed with a rate that was exponentially increased to maintain a constant increase of the biomass yield and miltiradiene concentration. After the biomass yield stabilized, the feeding was started once the dissolved oxygen level was higher than 40%. Similarly, 20% (*V/V*) *n*-dodecane was added at 10 h and duplicate culture aliquots were collected systematically to determine the cell density and production of miltiradiene and GGOH. Dry cell weight measurements were performed as reported previously.

2.8 GC-MS analysis of GGOH and miltiradiene For qualitative analysis of GGOH, GC-MS analysis was conducted with an Agilent 7000 gas chromatograph equipped with a DB-5 MS column (15 m×0.25 mm×0,10 μm film thickness) using helium as the carrier gas. The initial oven temperature was set to 100 ℃ for 1 min followed by a 40 ℃/min gradient to 200 ℃, hold for 1 min, and 20 ℃/min gradient to 300 ℃, and a final 1 min hold (total run time 10.5 min). The mass spectrometer was operated in the electron impact (EI) mode at 70 eV in the scan range of 0 - 300 *m/z*. Mass Hunter software (Agilent, USA) was used for data acquisition and processing. Quantification of GGOH was conducted in MRM mode with the same GC conditions, a collision energy of 15 eV, and a solvent delay of 3 min. The dwell time was 150 ms and the scan rate was 3.3 cycles/s. The fragment ions were quantified using 81 m/z as the quantification ion and 41 m/z along with 53 m/z as qualifiers. Calibration standard solutions for the quantification were prepared using authentic GGOH (the purity is 95%, aladdin, China) reference standard (Fig. S4). GC - MS analysis of miltiradiene was conducted using the same instrument and column with the following program: The initial oven temperature was set to 50 ℃ for 2 min followed by a 40 ℃/min gradient to 170 ℃, a 20 ℃/min gradient to 240 ℃, a 40 ℃/min gradient to 300 ℃, and a final 1 min hold (total run time 11 min). The quantification conditions were similar to those of GGOH using the MRM method, whereby 134 *m/z* was used as the quantification ion and 65 *m/z* along with 91 *m/z* were used as qualifiers. The collision energy was 20 eV with 100 ms dwell time, and the scan rate was 5 cycles/s.

## 3 RESULTS AND DISCUSSION

3.1 Pathway modification for GGPP overproduction in S. cerevisiae using the CRISPR/Cas9 system GGPP is the common precursor of diterpenes and its accumulation is essential to the production of downstream products. In *S. cerevisiae*, the 3-hydroxy-3-methyl glutaryl coenzyme A reductase (HMG-R), encoded by the *HMG1* gene is the major rate-limiting enzyme in the MVA pathway, and overexpression of the catalytic domain of *HMG1* (*tHMG1*) led to an improved production of isoprenoids, IPP and DMAPP. The isopentenyl transferase Erg20 condenses IPP and DMAPP to form the linear isopentenyl diphosphate precursor, famesyl diphosphate (FPP). Next, another isopentenyl transferase, Btsl, converts FPP to GGPP. Overexpression of the key genes in the GGPP pathway and modification of culture conditions are widely used strategies to improve GGPP production. However, the metabolic system of *S. cerevisiae* is a complex and precisely regulated network, and combinatorial design of expression cassettes could be helpful for the further accumulation of GGPP. Here, BY-T20, an engineered *S. cerevisiae* with an expression cassette harboring *tHMG1*, the *BTS1-ERG20* fusion protein module and a special gene *SaGGPS*, coding isopentenyl transferase from *Sulfolobus acidocaldarius* that can convert both DMAPP to FPP and FPP to GGPP, and is therefore more efficient than the wild-type yeast was used as the host strain. More comprehensive strategies were applied to achieve a higher titer of GGPP using the CRISPR/Cas9 system. In general, GGPP is nearly undetectable in yeast, and its dephosphorylated derivative (*E*, *E*, *E*)-geranylgeraniol (GGOH) is used as a common and direct reporter of GGPP production instead. Therefore, we measured the GGOH titer to characterize tiie GGPP production capacity of BY-T20 and its mutants.

First, we downregulated the metabolic flux that towards competing pathways. Erg9 is the squalene synthase of *S. cerevisiae*, which converts FPP to squalene. It is the first enzyme in the branching pathway for triterpenoid and ergosterol biosynthesis, and its high expression consumes significant amounts of FPP so that it decreases the precursor supply for GGPP production. Considering that *ERG9* is essential for ergosterol biosynthesis and yeast cannot survive under aerobic conditions in its absence, in this study we repressed the expression of *ERG9* by knocking out the upstream activating sequence (UAS) of its promoter (Fig. S5C). The mutant strain BY-HZ10 showed a significant improvement of the GGOH production from 40.3 to 196.4 mg/L in YPD medium in shake flasks (Fig. 2A, S5 and S6). Additionally, we tried to knock out the *cis*-prenyltransferase gene, *RER2*, because it can competitively convert FPP to polyprenyl compounds in *S. cerevisiae*. However, the mutant strain without *RER2* showed a very low growth rate compared with the other strains, and the editing of this locus was decided against. Schenk et al. reported that yeast cells with a deletion of the *RER2* locus are viable, but defective in protein N-gly-cosylation, which suggested that Rer2 plays an essential role in the normal growth of *S. cerevisiae*.

Next, we manipulated the genes and transcriptional regulators that have impact on the MVA pathway, Roxl (repressor of hypoxia) is a transcriptional regulator that can decrease the accumulation of GGPP by downregulating the expression of genes involved in the ergosterol biosynthesis. Here, we knocked out the open reading frame (ORF) of *ROX1* in BY-T20 (Fig. S5B). The resulting mutant, BY-HZ11, produced 1.96-fold higher GGOH than that of the initial strain (Fig. 2A). To study the combined effect of *ROX1* and *ERG9*, we constructed the strain BY-HZ12, which further improved the GGOH production to 206.9 mg/L (Fig. 2A). It was reported that the yeast strains with deletions of the distant genetic loci *YPL062w* and *YJL064w* showed good plasmid maintenance, high cell density, as well as good titers of bisabolene and carotenoids at the end of production. In this study, the ORFs of *YPL062w* and *YJL064w* were knocked out, resulting in the single knockout strains BY-HZ13 and BY-HZ15 (Fig. 2B), which showed increased GGOH levels of 54.8 and 80.8 mg/L, respectively. Moreover, the GGOH production was significantly improved to 274.7 mg/L in strain BY-HZ16, in which *YPL062w* and *YJL064w* were knocked out simultaneously in the back-groimd of BY-HZ12 (Fig. 2A). Additionally, the uptake control transcriptional regulator, Upc2, enables *S. cerevisiae* to take up external sterols during aerobic cultivation, and its mutant Upc2.1 (G888D) has stronger uptake ability than the wild type. Thus, Upc2.1 was often introduced into engineered yeast to produce specific terpenes of interest in earlier studies. In our work, the ORF of *UPC2.1* was integrated into the *YPL062w* deletion site (Fig. S5C), and the mutant strain BY-HZ17 had a 1.36-fold increase of GGOH titer compared with BY-HZ13. However, when we integrated the *UPC2.1* gene into the strain BY-HZ16, the GGOH production failed to be improved further (BY-HZ18). A possible reason is that the overexpression of *UPC2.1* increased the metabolic burden to the strain due to multiple genetic manipulations. In view of this, we introduced a site-directed mutation (G888D) into the native *UPC2* gene of *S. cerevisiae*, but disappointingly, a back mutation (D888G) was observed in the next generation of the mutant strain (Fig. S7). Leak et al. found that *UPC2.1* mutant yeast had increased sensitivity to metal cations and a reasonable hypothesis is that *UPC2.1* results in a general increase of cellular permeability, which could be indicative of a plasma membrane defect. This phenomenon suggested that Upc2 plays a central role in the cellular homeostasis of *S. cerevisiae*. Among the tested strains, the quadruple mutant BY-HZ16 (*ERG9p*; *ROXl*; *YJL064w*; *YPL062w*) had the highest ability to produce GGPP.

In addition, medium optimization is an effective approach to improve terpene production. Zhou et al. reported that an optimized YPD medium significantly improved the production of friedelin, a triterpene precursor of celastrol. Therefore, we used a medium containing 5% glucose, 1% yeast extract, 3% peptone, 0.8% $KH_2PO_4$, and 0.6% $MgSO_4$ to culture the GGPP high-yield strain BY-HZ16. As shown in Fig. 2B, the optimized YPD medium led to a significant increase of cell density and GGOH production. The highest yield of GGOH in stain BY-HZ16 under shake-flask conditions was 557.2 mg/L, which was 61% higher than in ordinary YPD medium. The optimized YPD medium provided more nutritional components and a suitable pH ($\approx 5.6$) for yeast growth so that a higher cell density was obtained in the same voliime of fermentation medium, which resulted in higher GGOH production. Given this, the optimized YPD medixim was used as the initial medium in fed-batch fermentation of strain BY-HZ16 in a 5 L bioreactor. The GGOH production of the strain reached 2.1 g/L and it kept increasing along with the cell density

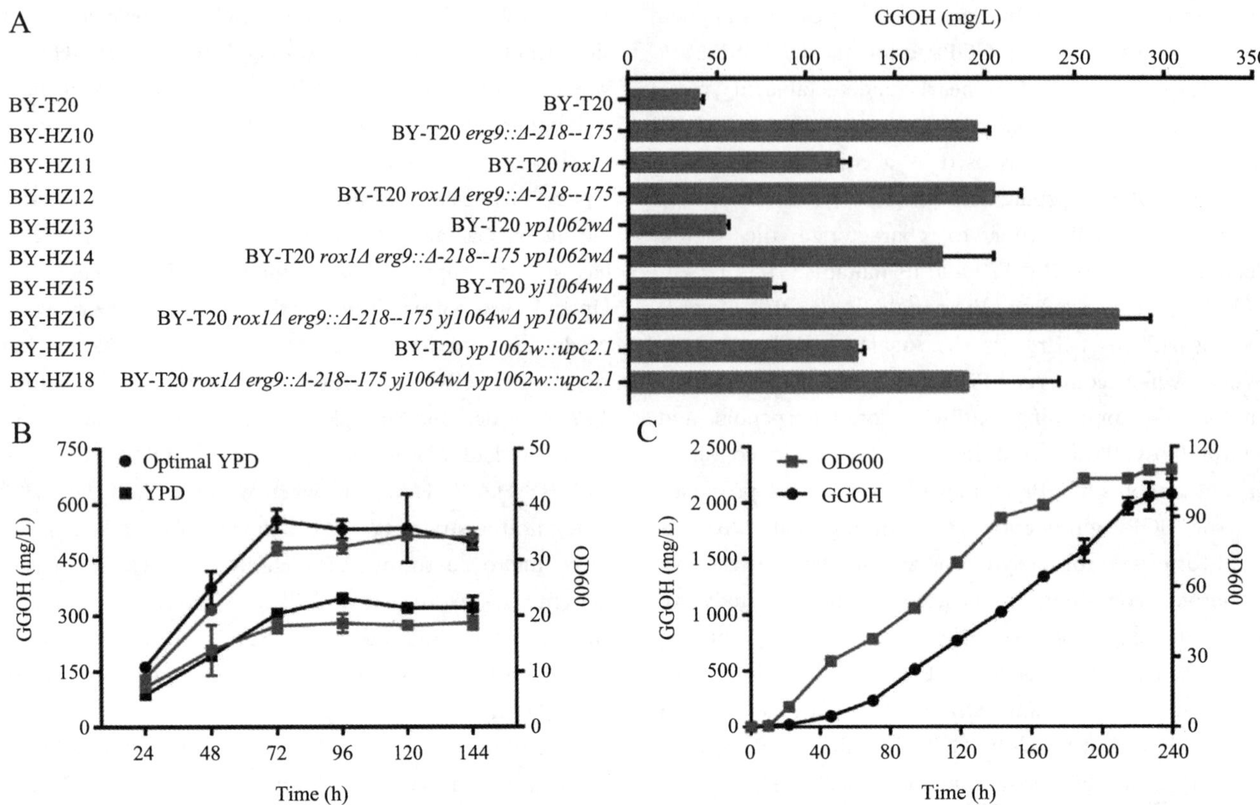


**Fig. 2 The GGOH production of the engineered yeasts**

(A) The genotypes and GGOH levels of the engineered strains. (B) GGOH production of BY-HZ16 cultured in different media. (C) Fed-batch fermentation of the highest GGOH-accumnlating strain BY-HZ 16. The data in (A) and (B) are the averages of 6 biological replicates with error bars representing standard deviations. The data in (C) are the averages of 3 biological replicates with error bars representing standard deviations.

during 10 days of fermentation (Fig. 2C).

In summary, we integrated multiple strategies including overexpression of pathway genes, downregulation of competing pathways, manipulation of transcriptional factors, and optimization of the medium to improve the GGPP production in *S. cerevisiae*. Finally, the mutant strain BY-HZ16 produced 2.1 g/L GGOH in fed-batch fermentation which provided a suitable microbial cell factory for the in-dustrial production of GGOH and laid a foundation for the the overproduction of diterpenes.

3.2 Broad screening of diterpene synthases for high-yield miltiradiene production In addition to the sufficient supply of precursors, the catalytic efficiency of enzymes is another key point for high production of diterpenes. Previous studies showed that screening enzjmies from diverse sources can be an effective strategy to increase the productivity of heterologous pathways in specific hosts. Abietane is the most widespread diterpene skeleton in the family Lamiaceae. The miltiradiene synthases, including *nor*-copalyl diphosphate synthases (CPS) and kaurene synthases-like (KSL), are present in many species of the Lamiaceae, and they share high amino acid sequence similarity with each type of cyclases. Here, 11 miltiradiene synthases, functionally annotated from five representative Lamiaceae plants, including *Salvia miltiorrhiza* (*Sm*CPS1, *Sm*KSL1), *Coleus forskohlii* (*Cf*TPS1, *Cf*TPS3 and *Cf*TPS4), *Marrubium vulgare* (*Mv*CPS3, *Mv*ELS), *Rosmarinus officinalis* (*Ro*CPS1, *Ro*KSL1 and *Ro*KSL2), and *Salvia frudcosa* (*Sf*KSL), whose complete coding sequences can be obtained from the NCBI database were selected as candidates for high-yield miltiradiene synthesis. Additionally, *Tw*CPS1 and the monoterpene synthase, *Tw*MS from the Celastraceae member *Tripterygium wilfordii* were also characterized in terms of miltiradiene production, but they share lower sequence similarity with the miltiradiene synthases of the Lamiaceae. In addition to higher plants, a bifunctional miltiradiene synthase (*Smo*MDS) from the lycophyte *Selaginella moellendorffii* was selected as the final candidate. Among the 14 candidate miltiradiene synthases, *Cf*TPS1, *Sm*CPS1, *Mv*CPS3, *Ro*CPS1 and *Tw*CPS1 are class II diterpene synthases that contain a catalytic "DXDD" motif for the protonation-initiated synthesis of (+)-CPP. *Tw*MS, *Mv*ELS, *Cf*TPS3, *Cf*TPS4, *Ro*KSL1, *Sm*KSL1, *Ro*KSL2 and *Sf*KSL are class I terpene synthases that contain a conserved DDXXD motif for further cyclization of (+)-CPP to miltiradiene. *Smo*MDS contains both active-site motifs

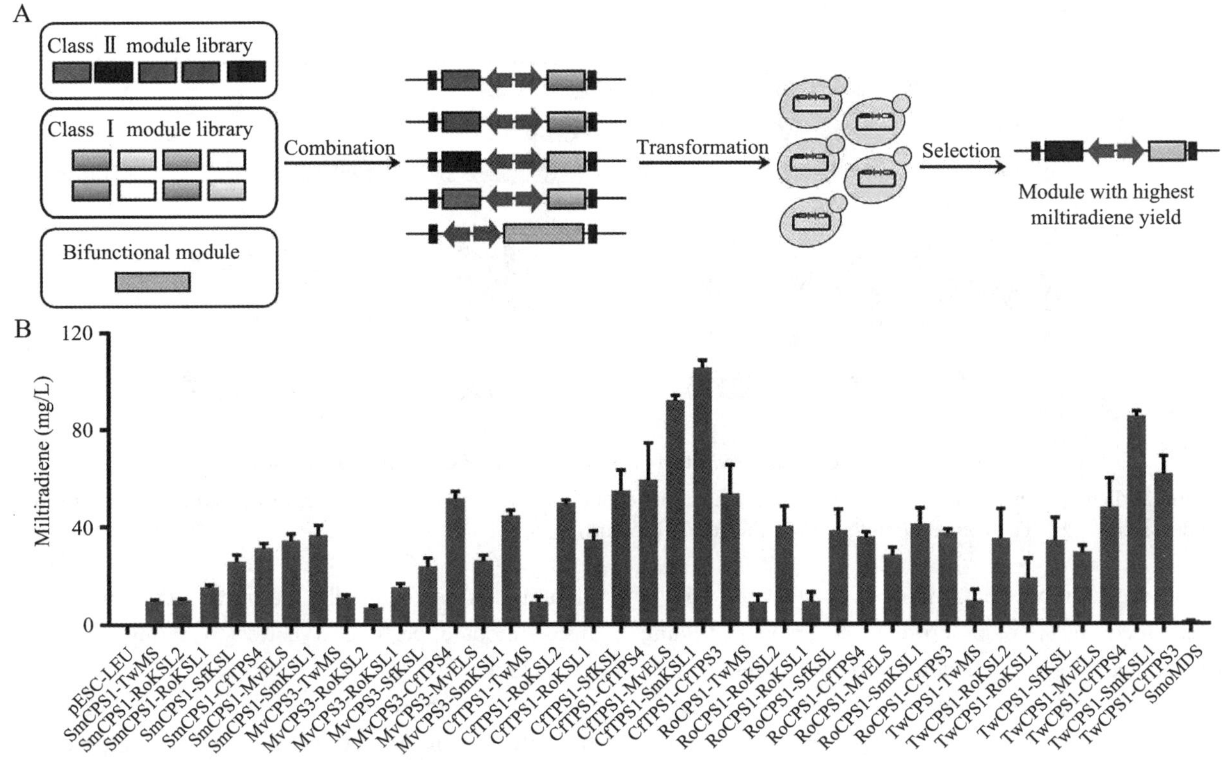


**Fig. 3 The miltiradiene production of different combinations of class Ⅰ and Ⅱ di-*TPSs***

(A) Scheme of selecting the miltiradiene synthase module with, the highest miltiradiene yield. (B) Miltiradiene production by combinations of diterpene synthases from different plants. The data are the averages of 5 biological replicates with error bars representing standard deviations.

and can directly convert GGPP to miltiradiene (Fig. S8). In the following work, we screened the best combinations of class Ⅰ and Ⅱ di-TPSs for high-yield miltiradiene by high-efficiency recombination.

All of the selected di-*TPSs* were codon-optimized and plasmids harboring random combinations of class Ⅰ and Ⅱ di-*TPSs* were introduced into the GGPP high-yield strain BY-HZ16. As illustrated in Fig. 3, 39 miltiradiene-producing strains were constructed and their product titers were investigated by GC-MS analysis (Fig. S9). The results revealed significant differences of miltiradiene production in those strains with different groups of class Ⅰ and Ⅱ di-*TPS*. Among them, strains containing *CfTPS1* exhibited higher miltiradiene production than those with other class Ⅱ di-*TPSs* together with class Ⅰ di-*TPSs* from various plants. Likewise, strains containing *SmKSL1* produced more miltiradiene than those with other class Ⅰ di-*TPSs*, especially when coupled with *CfTPS1* (BY-HZ49). The miltiradiene production of the module consisting of *CfTPS1* and *SmKSL1* was 105.3 mg/L (Fig. 3). By contrast, the class Ⅰ *TPS* from *T. wilfordii* (*TwMS*), showed much lower miltiradiene production with all the tested *CPSs*. Hansen et al. found that *TwMS* is a dose relative of mono-*TPSs* but has a mutant RRx8W motif, and its sequence shares low similarity with other *KSL*s used in this study (Fig. S7). This may be the reason for its low catalytic efficiency in the production of miltiradiene. Furthermore, we also found that the different couples of class Ⅰ and Ⅱ di-*TPSs* produced different miltiradiene titers. For instance, *RoKSL2* had a higher miltiradiene production than *RoKSL1* when coupled with *CfTPS1* and *TwCPS1*, but it was the opposite when coupled with *MvCPS3* and *SmCPS1*. The subtle differences in their protein structures may influence the cooperation between synthases. Surprisingly, the bifunctional enzyme *Smo*MDS produced only trace amounts of miltiradiene in strain BY-HZ16, which might attribute to the enzymatic inhibition of *Smo*MDS by high level of GGPP in BY-HZ16. These results indicated that screening enzymes from different species is an effective strategy for improving the production of miltiradiene as well as other terpenes, and the cooperation between different synthases can influence the efficiency of substrate utilization. This is an important concept for a further enhancement of the heterologous production of terpenes in the future.

3.3 Improving the miltiradiene yield by constructing fusion proteins Fusion proteins generated by fusing two or more genes with a linker region are widely used to enhance the catalytic capacities of enzymes and improve the utilization of substrates between proteins that catalyze sequential steps in a pathway or in which protein-protein

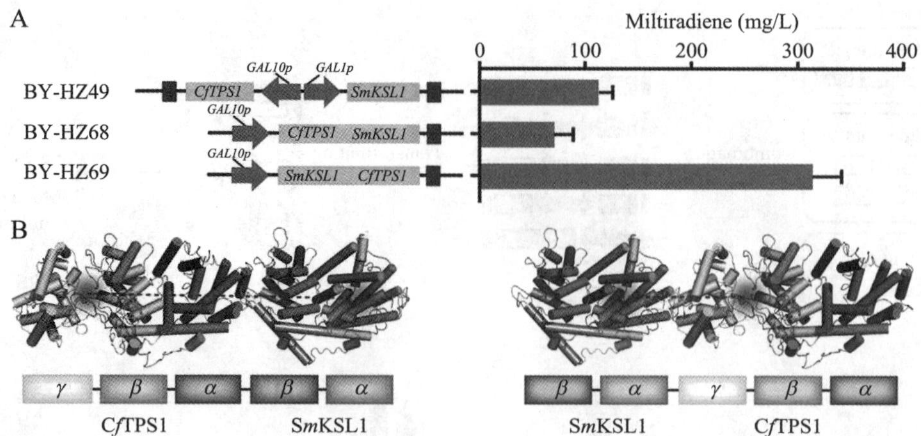


**Fig. 4 The miltiradiene production of fusion proteins of *Cf*TPS1 and *Sm*KSL1**

(A) The miltiradiene production of different fusion proteins. The data are averages of 6 biological replicates with error bars representing standard deviations. (B) The domain architecture of the fusion proteins.

interactions are required for functionality. Flexible linkers are often used in fiission proteins to reduce folding interference, enabling the individual proteins to retain their native activity, and either separate domains spatially or allow them to interact if necessary. Zhou et al. found that the miltiradiene synthases *Sm*CPS1 and *Sm*KSL1 directly interact in *Salvia miltiorrhiza in vivo*. Based on their findings and the sequence alignment of miltiradiene synthases in this study, we speculated that molecular interactions between *Cf*TPS1 and *Sm*KSL1 may exist, too. To test this hypothesis, we fused the proteins *Cf*TPS1 and *Sm*KSL1 in different order using the flexible linker "GGGS". The strain BY-HZ68 expressing the fused module *CfTPS1-SmKSL1* produced 70.5 mg/L miltiradiene, which was lower than the yield of the original separated module (strain BY-HZ49). Nevertheless, the other fused module *SmKSL1-CfTPS1* (strain BY-HZ69) led to 1.81-fold increase of miltiradiene production, which reached 313.4 mg/L (Fig. 4A). This result indicated that the *Sm*KSL1-*Cf*TPS1 fusion is superior to the *Cf*TPS1-*Sm*KSL1 fusion as well as the two proteins being expressed separately in terms of miltiradiene production.

To illustrate the reason for the differences of miltiradiene yield, we produced 3D models of the proteins using the web-based tool I-TASSER. The modeling showed that the class II di-TPS *Cf*TPS1 has an $\alpha\beta\gamma$ domain structure. The active site "DXDD" motif is located between the $\beta$ and $\gamma$ domains at the N-terminus. The class I di-TPS *Sm*KSL1 has an $\alpha\beta$ domain structure, and the active site is located in the $\alpha$ domain at the C-terminus. The schematic diagram of fusion proteins (Fig. 4B) illustrates that the distance between the two active sites of fusion protein *Sm*KSL1-*Cf*TPS1 is shorter than that of *Cf*TPS1-*Sm*KSL1. A closer arrangement of active sites contributes to an increase of the local concentration of intermediates by reducing the spatial diffusion. This may be the reason why the *Sm*KSL1-*Cf*TPS1 fusion module performed better in terms of miltiradiene production.

3.4 Improving miltiradiene production by tailored truncations In order to obtain a higher miltiradiene titer, we engineered the fusion protein by further structure optimization. It is known that many terpene synthases are targeted to plastids in plant, and after the protein has been localized to the plastid, the transit peptides will be hydrolyzed. However, yeast cannot hydrolyze the peptides due to the absence of plastidic transit peptidases, which may affect the catalytic activities of the proteins. Therefore, we truncated the chloroplast transit peptide (M1-C47) at the N-terminus of *Sm*KSL1, and the resulting strain BY-HZ70 showed a significant increase of miltiradiene production to 550.7 mg/L in shake flasks (Fig. 5A). Inspired by this, we further truncated the chloroplast transit peptide located at the N-terminus of *Cf*TPS1 (M1-N81), but the result went contrary to our expectations. The miltiradiene production decreased to 180.5 mg/L (strain BY-HZ71), while the by-product GGOH showed a slight increased production (Fig. 5A and 5C). It is possible that the truncation of the loop between *Sm*KSL1 and *Cf*TPS1 decreased the flexibility of the fusion protein and increased the distance between the two active sites indirectly.

In addition to the transit peptides, we also investigated domaintruncated variants of the fusion protein *Sm*KSL1-*Cf*TPS1. Generally, the *a* domain of class II di-*TPS*s is considered a nonfunctional vestige due to the lack of the DDXXD motif, and the $\beta$ domain of class I di-*TPS*s is considered vestigial due to the lack of the D/E-rich motif and the DXDD motif. Here, we truncated the $\beta$ domain of *Sm*KSL1, resulting in the strain BY-HZ72. However, the resulting protein did not produced miltiradiene, and (+)-copalol, the dephosphorylated derivative of (+)-CPP was

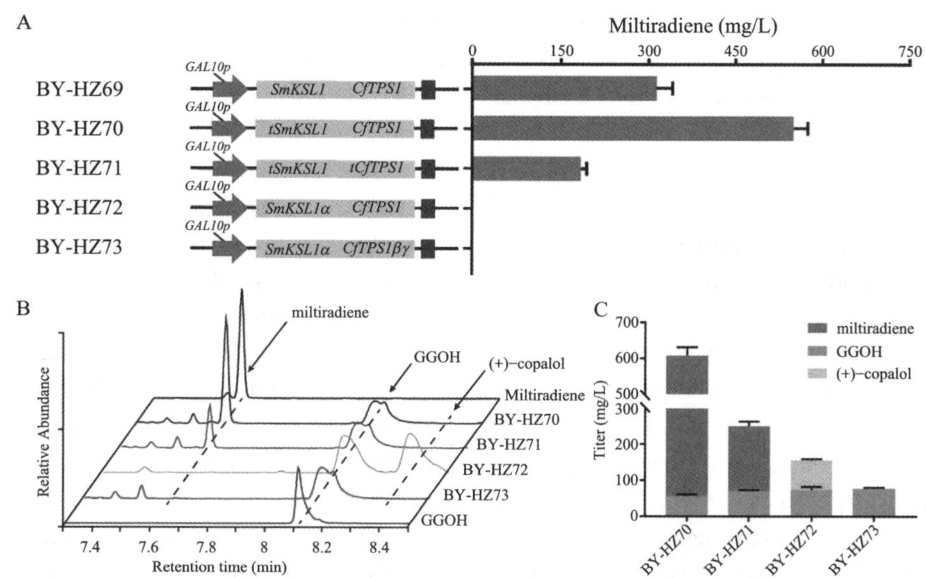


**Fig. 5 The miltiradiene production of strains expressing truncations of the fusion protein *Sm*KSL1-*Cf*TPS1**

(A) The miltiradiene production of strains expressing the truncated variants. The data are averages of 6 biological replicates with error bars reprsenting standard deviations. (B) GC-MS analysis of the fermentation products of strains expressing the truncated fusion proteins. (C) The titer of products in strains expressing the truncated fusion proteins.

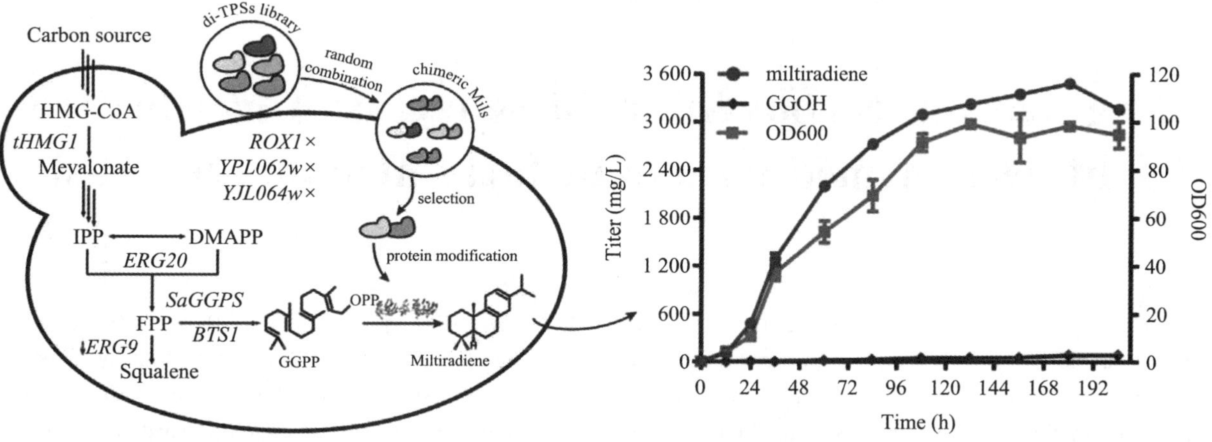


**Fig. 6 Production of miltiradiene in fed-batch fermentation using the engineered strain BY-HZ70 in a 5 L bioreactor**

The data are averages of 3 biological replicates with error bars representing standard deviations.

detected by GC-MS analysis (Fig. 5B, 5C and S10). Similarly, we further truncated the α domain of *Cf*TPS1 but we failed to detect any miltiradiene or (+)-copalol but only the by-product GGOH in the corresponding strain BY-HZ73. These results demonstrate that domains that do not contain active sites can also impact the catalytic function of diterpene synthases and alter the outcome of catalysis, explaining why evolution retained them.

3.5 High-level production of miltiradiene through fed-batch fermentation In an attempt to farther increase the titer of miltiradiene, we cultivated the optimal engineered strain BY-HZ70 in fed-batch fermentation. Minimal medium was used to promote plasmid retention. The strains were seeded into the medium to an initial $OD_{600}$ of 0.1. After 6 h of growth on glucose, the carbon source was replaced with galactose. The process of fed-batch fermentation was controlled as described in previous studies. Time courses of dry cell weight (DCW) and consumed galactose during the fermentation are shown in Fig. S11. As shown in Fig. 6, the biomass started increasing rapidly at 24 h, after the lag phase of metabolic adaption to galactose, and the growth subsequently remained steady until the maximum $OD_{600}$ of 99.3 at 132 h. Production of miltiradiene had a significant positive correlation with biomass, with continuous accumulation until 180 h. The miltiradiene titer reached almost 3.5 g/L. By contrast, we detected only trace amounts of GGOH during the first two days, but it accumulated slowly with the increase of biomass and reached 92.4 mg/L at the end of the fermentation. Compared with shake flask culture, the percentage of the by-product GGOH decreased significantly. Therefore, the fed-batch fermentation efficiently improved the utilization of the precursor GGPP and the process has great potential for the industrial production of miltiradiene.

## 4 CONCLUSIONS

In this study, multiple engineering strategies were applied to increase the supply of GGPP and the production of the important intermediate miltiradiene. We first constructed a series of yeast strains with high GGPP production by combining several strategies based on the CRISPR/Cas9 system. The best strain BY-HZ16 produced 2.1 g/L GGOH in fed-batch fermentation. Then, we took the biosynthesis of miltiradiene as an example to explore more strategies for further improving the production of diterpenes. 14 miltiradiene synthases from 7 species were evaluated. We found that the chimeric diterpene synthase consisting of a fusion of *Cf*TPS1 and *Sm*KSL1 showed the highest efficiency in the conversion of GGPP to miltiradiene in yeast, after which the yield was further improved by protein truncation, reaching a titer of 550.7 mg/L in shake flasks. Finally, this strain produced a miltiradiene titer of 3.5 g/L in a 5 L bioreactor, which is the highest titer in heterologous production reported so far. This work adopted a push and pull strategy for improving miltiradiene production by increasing precursor supply and enhancing the catalytic capacity of diterpene synthases. The strategies combined i) optimization of isoprenoid biosynthetic pathways in the microbial chassis, ii) screening out the optimal module for miltiradiene production from the miltiradiene synthase pool by evaluating their combinational effects, and iii) construction of the chimeric diterpene synthases and truncation of miltiradiene synthases. It lays a solid foundation for the pathway discovery and biosynthesis of active pharmaceutical ingredients, such as triptolide and tanshinones. Moreover, the comprehensive strategies that focus on metabolic pathway optimization of host cells and protein modification of key enzymes could be a good reference for the production of many valuable pharmaceuticals and chemicals.

[胡添源,高伟,等. Metabolic Engineering, 2020,60:87-96.]

# Engineering carboxylic acid reductase for selective synthesis of medium-chain fatty alcohols in yeast

Concerns about climate change drive the scientific community to explore alternative ways to produce renewable biofuels. With straight hydrocarbon chains ranging from C6 to C12, medium-chain fatty alcohols (MCFOHs) are designated as higher alcohols in contrast to lower alcohols, such as butanol, ethanol, and methanol. MCFOHs are considered to be more suitable to substitute the traditional diesel and jet fuels due to their higher energy density, higher cetane number, and lower vapor pressure. MCFOHs are also widely used in surfactants, cosmetics, and plasticizers. Currently, fatty alcohols are synthesized from petrochemical sources or produced from fatty acids (FAs) extracted from oil seeds. A major obstacle with sourcing from oil seeds is the competition with food production by using arable land and deforestation, and there is therefore interest in producing MCFOHs through microbial fermentation, allowing for the utilization of a wide range of feedstocks, including biomass.

In organisms, fatty alcohols are derived from FAs. The bio-synthesis of fatty alcohols can proceed through either fatty aldehyde intermediates via two steps of two-electron reductions or directly from fatty acyl-CoA/ACP via a four-electron reduction. Fatty aldehydes can be generated from 1) activated fatty acyl-CoA/ACP by fatty acyl-CoA/ACP reductase [ACR or AAR] or 2) free FAs by carboxylic acid reductase (CAR). MmCAR from *Mycobacterium marinum* has shown the highest efficiency toward formation of fatty aldehydes that can subsequently be converted to fatty alcohols in a previous study. CARs utilize free FAs as substrates (Fig. 1A), which are usually more abundant than the activated acyl-CoA and acyl-ACP in yeast cells. Moreover, thioesterases hydrolyzing acyl-CoA or acyl-ACP, thus releasing free FAs, can be used not only for controlling the chain length of synthesized FAs but also for increasing the FA synthesis flux, which is restricted by feed-back inhibition mediated by acyl-CoA and acyl-ACP. Therefore, fatty alcohol formation based on free FAs as substrates through CAR enzymes possesses great advantages. Previous studies on engineering the FA synthesis pathway through augmenting the precursor flux and improving FA synthetase (FAS) activity in yeast have generated microbial cells producing substantial amounts of medium-chain FAs (MCFAs) (Fig. 1A), which could be utilized for the synthesis of MCFOHs. In our previous study, an engineered MCFA producing FAS and MmCAR were expressed in yeast

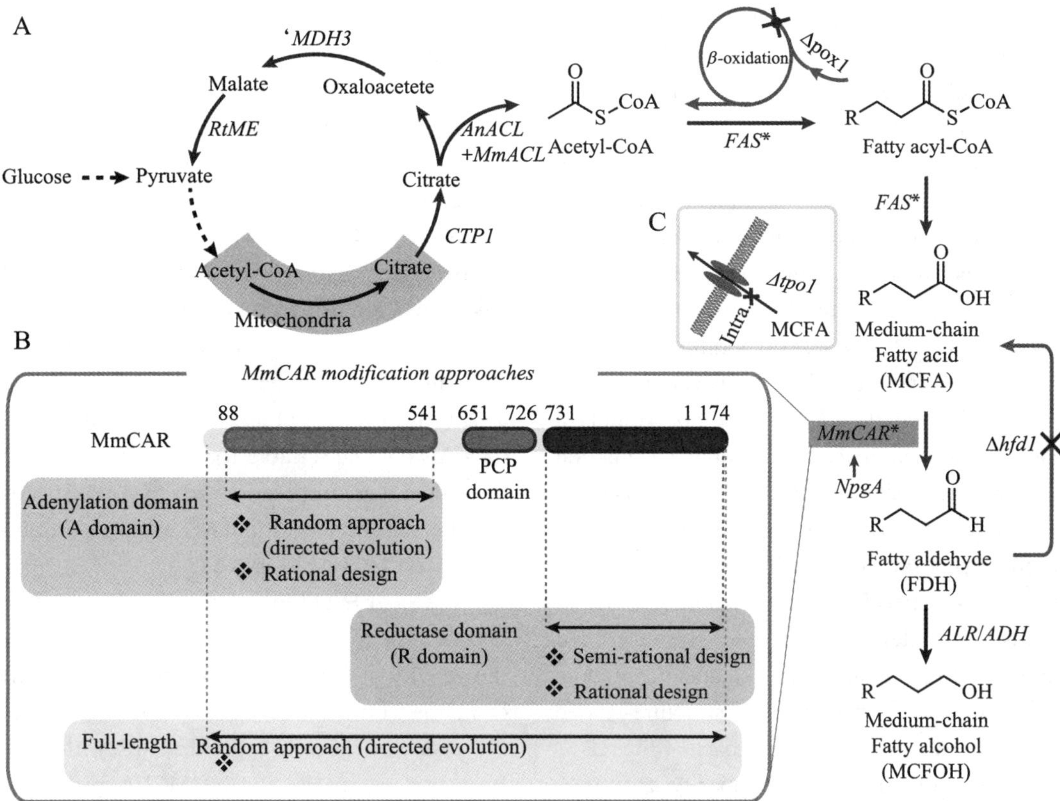


**Fig. 1 Overview of genetic manipulations in yeast enabling selective production of MCFOHs**

(A) Schematic illustration of the pathway engineering strategies in background strain ZWE243. AnACL, ATP-citrate lyase from *Aspergillus nidulans*; Ctp1, mitochondrial citrate transporter; FAS*, engineered en-dogenous fatty acid synthase for MCFAs production; Hfd1, aldehyde dehydrogenase; 'Mdh3, malate dehydrogenase without peroxisomal signal; MmACL, ATP-citrate lyase from *Mus musculus*; MmCAR, carboxylic acid reductase from *Mycobacterium marinum*; NpgA, phosphopantetheinyl transferase from *As-pergillus nidulans*; Pox1, fatty acyl-CoA oxidase; RtME, malic enzyme from *Rhodosporidium toruloides*; The genes encoding 'Mdh3, RtME, MmACL, AnACL, and Ctp1 were overexpressed to increase the acetyl-CoA supply, and *POX1* and *HFD1* genes were deleted to avoid reverse reactions. R represents C3 - C9. (B) MmCAR was modified using diverse approaches. A domain (residues 88 to 541); PCP domain (residues 651 to 728); R domain (residues 731 to 1,174). (C) The predicted MCFA transporter gene *TPO*1 was deleted to prevent the secretion of MCFAs.

to generate aldehyde precursors for alkane synthesis. Substantial quantities of MCFOHs produced by the engineered strain ZW540 (*SI Appendix*, Fig. S1) showed that endogenous alcohol dehydrogenases and aldehyde reductases were able to support a strong down-stream flux toward MCFOH formation. However, a promiscuous CAR enzyme reducing C6 - C18 FAs is not ideal for MCFOH production, as it deprives the cell of C16-C18 long-chain FAs (LCFAs) that are essential for cell growth, and also invests NADPH and ATP in the formation of long-chain by-products. It is therefore of great interest to narrow the substrate spectrum of the enzyme or increase its activity on MCFAs to more specifically produce MCFOHs. Protein engineering of a CAR enzyme would offer the opportunity to change its substrate specificity in the desired direction.

The CAR enzyme consists of an adenylation domain (A domain), a reductase domain (R domain), and a peptidyl carrier protein domain (PCP domain) that links the A domain and R domain (Fig. 1B). A phosphopantetheinyl transferase (PPTases) is required to activate the enzyme by covalently attaching a 4-phosphopantetheine moiety to the PCP domain. The carboxylic group of the FA substrate is converted to the corresponding aldehyde in the presence of $Mg^{2+}$, ATP, and NADPH through a process of two-electron reduction. The A domain exhibits a mechanism of substrate recognition and activation similar to that of the ANL superfamily of adenylating enzymes, where the α-phosphate of ATP is attacked by the carboxylate to generate an AMP-acyl phosphoester. The R domain shows homology to the short-chain dehydrogenases/reductase family whose members commonly exist as subdomains in polyketide synthases (PKSs) and nonribosomal peptide synthases (NRPSs), where they mediate the off-loading of the final products. The R domain of CAR enzymes catalyzes the strict two-electron reduction by consuming one NADPH and releases the corresponding aldehyde.

To change the activity or specificity of an enzyme, different engineering strategies can be chosen that highly depend on the amount of knowledge available on the protein of interest. Random approaches, referred to as directed evolution, with less information being required always rely on the availability of a high-throughput screening method for large libraries of enzyme variants. Smaller libraries are usually generated for rational and semirational approaches that require structural and mechanistic information. The revealed catalytic mechanism and the availability of the enzyme structure provided us with the opportunity to rationally engineer the CAR enzyme. In addition, directed evolution as a powerful tool enables the development of reaction schemes and catalytic mechanisms not found in nature, and could be utilized to access the untapped function of the CAR enzyme using efficient high-throughput selection. In this study, we first developed a high-throughput screening method relying on the detoxification of the toxic MCFAs that proved to be beneficial for selection of efficient MmCAR variants. We designed multiple strategies for comprehensive engineering of MmCAR, including a random approach using directed evolution, a structure-guided semirational design, and a rational approach (Fig. 1B). Measuring the in vivo biotransformation capacity as well as in vitro enzymatic activity on FAs of different chain length showed that some mutants with increased catalytic activities toward MCFAs could be generated and used for the more selective production of MCFOHs. In addition, with enhancing the endogenous MCFA precursor supply through deleting an MCFA transporter (Fig. 1C), a further increase in MCFOH production was achieved. This study demonstrates that engineering key metabolic enzymes can significantly improve the synthesis of the desired product, while reducing by-product formation.

## 1 RESULTS

Growth-Coupled Screening Approach for MmCAR Libraries MCFAs are toxic to yeast cells, the growth of which was significantly reduced by concentrations as low as 1 mmol/L octanoic acid and decanoic acid. However, the toxicity of MCFAs could be exploited for selection of efficient variants of enzymes leading to their detoxification (Fig. 2A). To investigate if MCFOH formation represents a potential detoxification pathway for MCFAs, we first evaluated the cellular toxicity of MCFAs (octanoic acid and decanoic acid) and compared it to the toxicity of the respective fatty alcohols of the same chain length. Strain YJZ03H, which is deficient in both *POX1* and *HFD1*, was used for the toxicity test. Deletion of *POX1* eliminated FA β-oxidation and the deletion of aldehyde dehydrogenase gene *HFD1* was shown to be beneficial for alcohol formation. Next, 0.4 mmol/L (~70 mg/L) of C10 FA or fatty alcohol and 1 mmol/L (~150 mg/L) of C8 FA or fatty alcohol was used to evaluate their toxicity. Results showed that 70 mg/L C10 FA and C10 fatty alcohol were equally toxic to yeast cells (*SI Appendix*, Fig. S2), while the presence of 150 mg/L C8 fatty alcohol allowed cell growth to a much higher final OD than C8 fatty alcohol at the same concentration (Fig. 2B). Correspondingly, expression of MmCAR was beneficial for yeast cell growth at 150 mg/L C8 FA (Fig. 2C), which can be attributed to the detoxifying activity of MmCAR that converts C8 FA to the less toxic C8 fatty alcohol. A further investigation of the detoxification capacity of MmCAR showed that yeast cells containing MmCAR could hardly grow in the presence of 300 mg/L of C8 FA (Fig. 2D), indicating that ~300 mg/L of C8 FA would be suitable for the selection process. Based on these data, we proposed a growth-coupled screening scheme for the selection of MmCAR variants exhibiting a higher activity on MCFAs (Fig. 2A).

Directed Evolution of the Full-Length MmCAR Phosphopantetheinylation undertaken by PPTases is required for the activity of CAR enzymes. We first evaluated the effects of PPTases on the biosynthesis of MCFOH through combined expression of the wild-type MmCAR with different PPTases from various species in the MCFA producing yeast strain ZW2071 (*SI Appendix*, Fig. S3). Among the tested candidates, expression of *NpgA* from *Aspergillus nidulans* resulted in the relatively higher MCFOH titers. *NpgA* was therefore used for all following experiments.

In order to improve the catalytic activity of MmCAR for MCFA conversion, directed evolution was performed by first establishing a random mutagenesis library of the full-length *MmCAR*. The library was cultivated at an increasing concentration of C8 FA from 290 mg/L to 330 mg/L to enrich it for improved enzyme variants. After the enrichment process, single clones were isolated and tested for improved growth on C8 FA. This led to identification of variant M150, whose expression enabled the fastest growth of yeast strain YJZ03H in medium with 330 mg/L C8 FA (*SI Appendix*, Fig. S4A). Sequencing of M150 revealed three amino acid changes compared to the wildtype enzyme. Two of the mutations, D241E and H454R, were located in the A domain of MmCAR, while the mutation L567M was situated between the A domain and PCP domain (Fig. 3A). When expressed in an MCFA-producing yeast strain, M150 enabled a more than 50% increase in MCFOH production compared to the wild-type MmCAR, reaching a titer of 129 mg/L (Fig. 3B). We therefore used M150 as the template for the second round of evolution, from which the efficient variants M7, M9, and M11 were selected on the basis of conferring a superior growth phenotype (*SI Appendix*, Fig. S4B). Although all of these three CAR mutants showed lower in vivo activities on MCFA conversion than M150, two of them still performed better than the wild-type MmCAR in

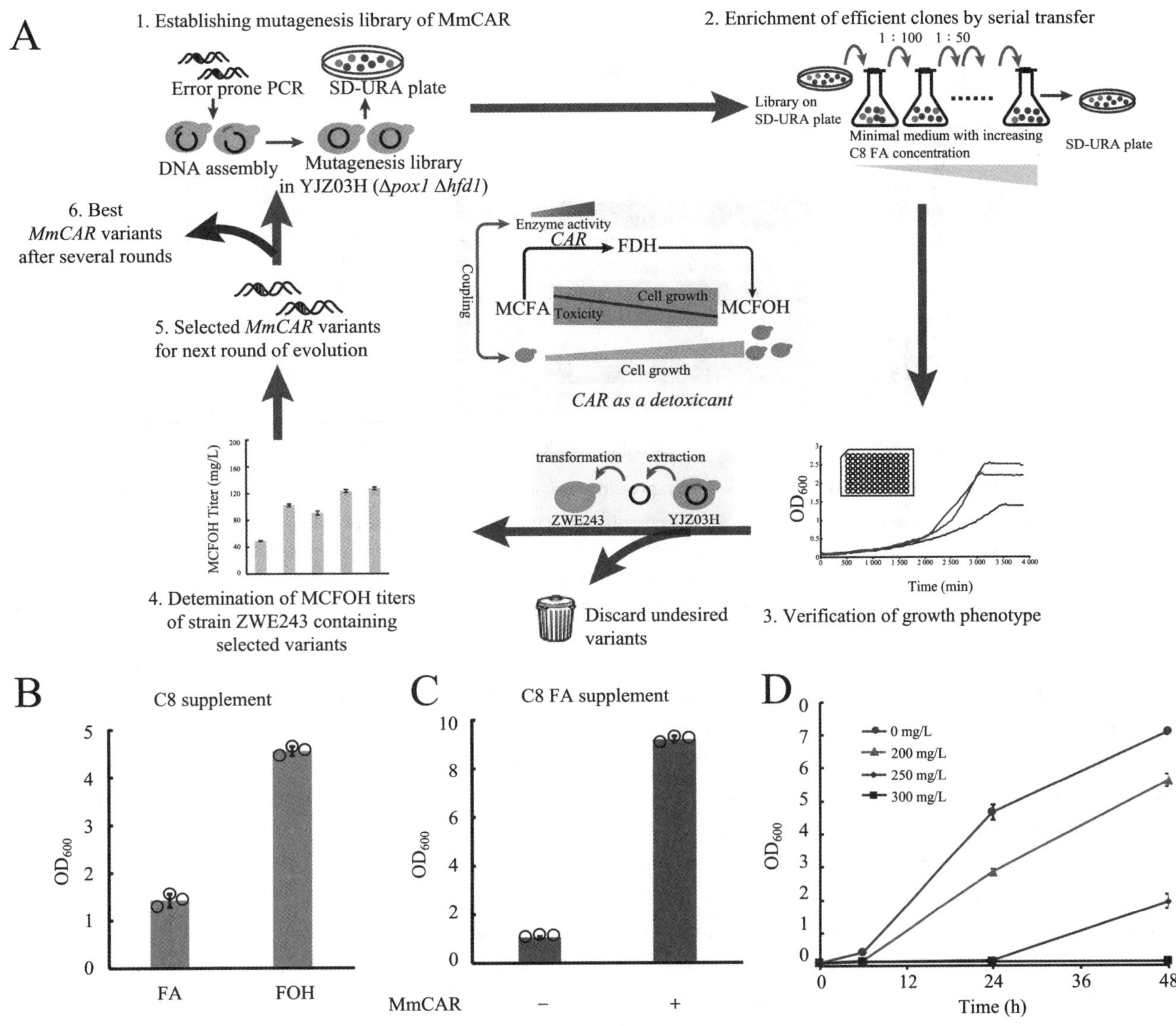


**Fig. 2 Design of the growth-coupled screening approach**

(A) Workflow of the high-throughput screening method coupled to cell growth. (1) Libraries of MmCAR variants expressed from a plasmid were established in yeast strain YJZ03H (*Δpox1 Δhfd1*) via error-prone PCR and homologous recombination. (2) The variants beneficial to cell growth in minimal medium with C8 FA were selected and (3) their growth phenotype was verified using a Bioscreen or Growth Profiler. (4) The variants leading to better growth were tested in the high MCFA-producing strain ZWE243, and (5) the most efficient one was used as the template for the next round of evolution. (B) Comparison of the C8 FA/alcohol toxicity to yeast cells. Strain YJZ03H was cultivated in minimal medium with 150 mg/L of C8 FA/alcohol for 72 h. The final optical density was measured at a wavelength of 600 nm ($OD_{600}$). (C) Growth of yeast strain with or without MmCAR in medium with C8 FAs. Strain YJZ03H carrying an empty vector or plasmid pZW01 harboring wild-type MmCAR was cultivated in minimal medium with 150 mg/L C8 FA. The final $OD_{600}$ was measured after 72 h of cultivation. (D) The effect of MmCAR expression on cell growth at different concentrations of C8 FAs. The yeast strain YJZ03H with pZW01 harboring MmCAR was cultivated in minimal medium with 0 mg/L, 200 mg/L, 250 mg/L, and 300 mg/L C8 FA, respectively. The $OD_{600}$ was measured during the cultivation. The mean±SD of three biological replicates is presented (B, C, and D).

terms of MCFOH production (Fig. 3B). These results clearly demonstrate that our growth-coupled screening was suitable for the selection of CAR variants with improved activity on MCFAs.

Modification of the A Domain  MmCAR is able to reduce diverse aliphatic FAs with chain length ranging from C6 to C18. The broad substrate spectrum of MmCAR is not optimal for MCFOH production, as the generation of long-chain fatty alcohols (LCFOHs) as by-products not only reduces the overall product yield but may also lead to impaired growth as a result of competition for essential LCFAs in yeast cells. According to the catalytic mechanism revealed in a previous study, the volume of the active-site in the A domain could potentially be altered to tailor the substrate specificity of CAR.

Fatty acyl-AMP ligases (FAALs) and fatty acyl-CoA ligases (FACLs) belong to a superfamily of acyl-activating enzymes that activate the carboxyl groups of their substrates

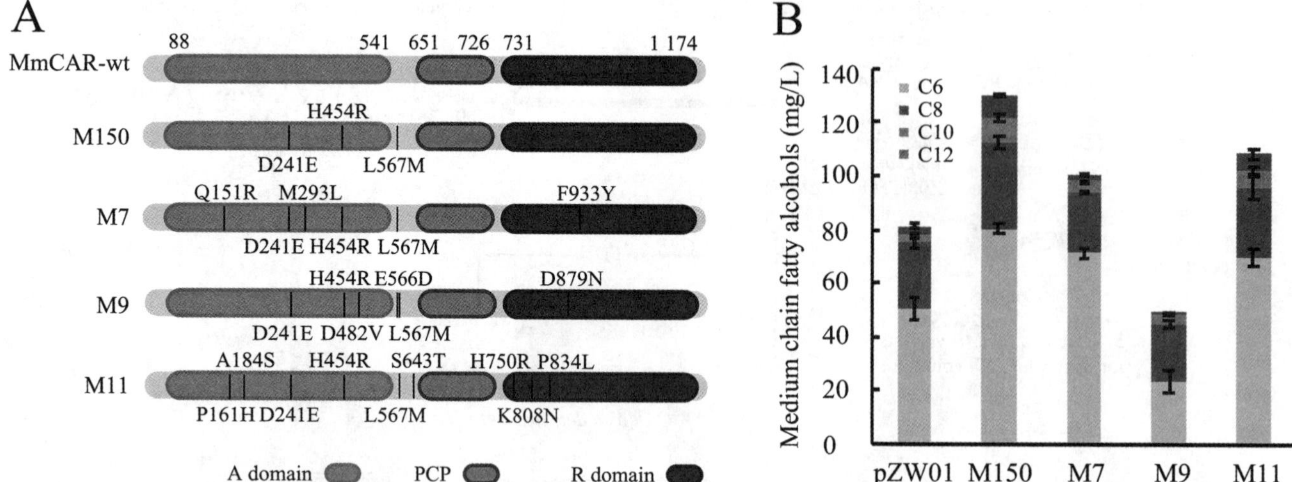


**Fig. 3 The synthesis of MCFOHs in *S. cerevisiae* by expressing variants derived from directed evolution of full-length MmCAR**

(A) Schematic illustration of the mutated MmCARs. (B) Production of MCFOHs in *S. cerevisiae* by enzyme variants derived from two rounds of directed evolution based on full-length MmCAR. pZW01 represents the plasmid containing wild-type MmCAR. M150 represents the variant from the first round of evolution. M7, M9, and M11 represent the variants from the second round of evolution. Strain ZWE243 was used for evaluation, all of the cultivations were performed in minimal medium with histidine for 48 h. The mean±SD of three biological replicates is shown.

to acyl-adenylates and then transfer these to other acceptor groups, thus having a function similar to the A domain of CAR. The FAAL from *Escherichia coli* (PDB ID code 3PBK) containing an acyl-AMP ligand was aligned with the A domain of CAR from *Nocardia iowensis* (NiCAR, PDB ID code 5MSD) to assign the acyl-residing tunnel. A potentially crucial residue S306 (I303 in MmCAR) adjacent to the C11 position was identified (Fig. 4 A and B). A previous study revealed that the mutated proteins FAAL28 (I227W) and FACL13 (T214W), which possessed a bulky tryptophan residue at the position equivalent to I305 in NiCAR and Q302 in MmCAR (Fig. 4B), showed a significant decrease in the activity toward longer acyl chains and an increase in the activity on C10 or C8 FAs. We therefore substituted I303 and Q302 of MmCAR with a tryptophan residue. The strains expressing the MmCAR variants containing the Q302W (AD302) and I303W (AD303) mutations were able to produce 110 mg/L and 129 mg/L of MCFOHs, which was, respectively, 37% and 61% higher than those produced by the strain expressing the wild-type MmCAR (Fig. 4C). Therefore, we speculated that the bulkier tryptophan residue might cause a steric hindrance by which the catalytic pocket of MmCAR was narrowed to result in impaired binding of long-chain acyl groups.

Parallel to the targeted engineering approach, we also engineered the A domain of MmCAR by random mutagenesis (residues 88 to 541) (Fig. 4D). The same workflow as in Fig. 2A was performed by using 290 to 310 mg/L of C8 FA as the enrichment reagent. The best variant AD69 enabled better cell growth (*SI Appendix*, Fig. S5A) and led to a higher production of MCFOHs of 96.9 mg/L, which is a 21% increase compared with that of the wild-type MmCAR (Fig. 4D). Cells expressing the AD10 variant isolated after a second round of evolution (*SI Appendix*, Fig. S5B) produced an approximately equal amount of MCFOHs, which was 102 mg/L (Fig. 4D). Although the total amount of MCFOHs produced by the strain carrying AD10 was not significantly improved compared to the AD69 carrying strain, more C6 and C8 fatty alcohols (around 18%) were produced by the AD10-containing strain, which might indicate that this mutant preferably reduces FAs with a shorter chain length and thereby provided the cells with an increased tolerance toward C8 FA in the medium.

Modification of the R Domain The R domain of MmCAR (residues 731 to 1, 174) enables the enzyme to catalyze a strict two-electron reduction of the acyl-PCP thioester to a fatty aldehyde. This is due to the fact that the conformation adopted by residues 983 to 985 appears to be linked to the position of the smaller substrate-binding domain, which ensures that the reduction cannot proceed beyond the aldehyde product. However, the backbone reorientation of residues 983 to 985 was reported to be able to affect the conformational equilibrium between on- and off-states of the MmCAR R domain. In the active form, the D984 will be positioned pointing away from the nicotinamide and buried within the protein matrix, while in the inactive form, the D984 and the S983 carbonyl group will locate within the nicotinamide binding pocket (Fig. 5A).

MmCAR with an engineered R domain that could reduce free FAs via aldehydes all of the way to fatty alcohols could be beneficial for MCFOH production in yeast. In a previous study, the mutation D998G (equivalent to D984 in

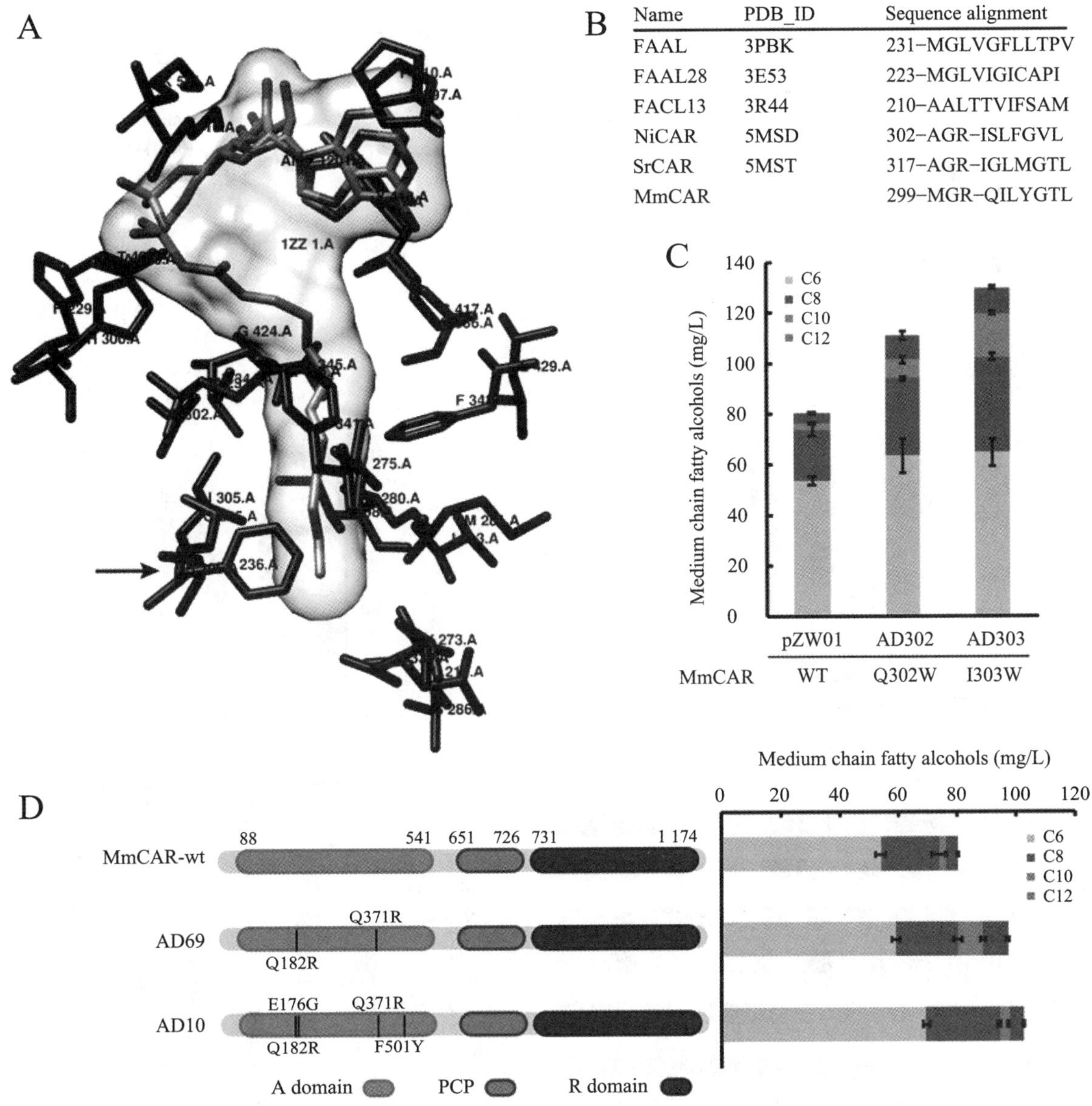

| Name | PDB_ID | Sequence alignment |
|---|---|---|
| FAAL | 3PBK | 231-MGLVGFLLTPV |
| FAAL28 | 3E53 | 223-MGLVIGICAPI |
| FACL13 | 3R44 | 210-AALTTVIFSAM |
| NiCAR | 5MSD | 302-AGR-ISLFGVL |
| SrCAR | 5MST | 317-AGR-IGLMGTL |
| MmCAR | | 299-MGR-QILYGTL |



**Fig. 4 The synthesis of MCFOHs in *S. cerevisiae* by MmCAR variants generated through A domain modifications**

(A) Structure superposition of EcFAAL (PDB ID code 3PBK, in dark red) and the A domain of NiCAR (PDB ID code 5MSD, in dark blue). Residues surrounding the substrate binding pocket are shown in stick representation. The C12 acyl-AMP ligand (gray) is shown in surface representation. The arrow indicates the residues (F236 in EcFAAL and S306 in NiCAR) proximate to C11 of the acyl chain. (B) Structure-based sequence alignment of selected acyl-activating enzymes. Residues crucial for medium-chain carboxylic acid substrates are shown in bold. Production of MCFOHs in *S. cerevisiae* by mutated MmCARs derived from rational design (C) and directed evolution (D) of the A domain, respectively. The schematic illustration of variants from plasmids AD69 and AD10 is shown in d. All variants were assessed in strain ZWE243; all cultivations were performed in minimal medium with histidine for 48 h. The mean±SD of three biological replicates is shown.

MmCAR) (Fig. 5B) in CAR from *Segniliparus rugosus* (SrCAR) led to the formation of alcohol products. However, the same mutation in MmCAR showed a negative effect on MCFOH production in yeast (*SI Appendix*, Fig. S6A). It was reported that the R1339A (equivalent to M985 in MmCAR) (Fig. 5B) mutant of the MxaA R domain from *Stigmatella aurantiaca* exerted significantly increased activities for the reduction of C10 acyl-PCP and C10 aldehyde. After introducing the mutation M985A into MmCAR, we did not observe augmented production of MCFOHs by this mutant (*SI Appendix*, Fig. S6B).

To obtain an engineered R domain free of conformational regulation by C983-M985 or more efficient for reduction of mediumchain substrates, we created a site-directed saturation mutagenesis library targeting residues 983 to 985. Four selected variants (RE5, RE6, RB6 and RF1) (Fig. 5C), which enabled a higher growth rate and final cell mass of yeast cells in medium with 380 mg/L C8 FA (Fig. 5C and *SI Appendix*, Fig. S7), were also beneficial for MCFOH production in yeast (Fig. 5D). Specifically, variant RF1

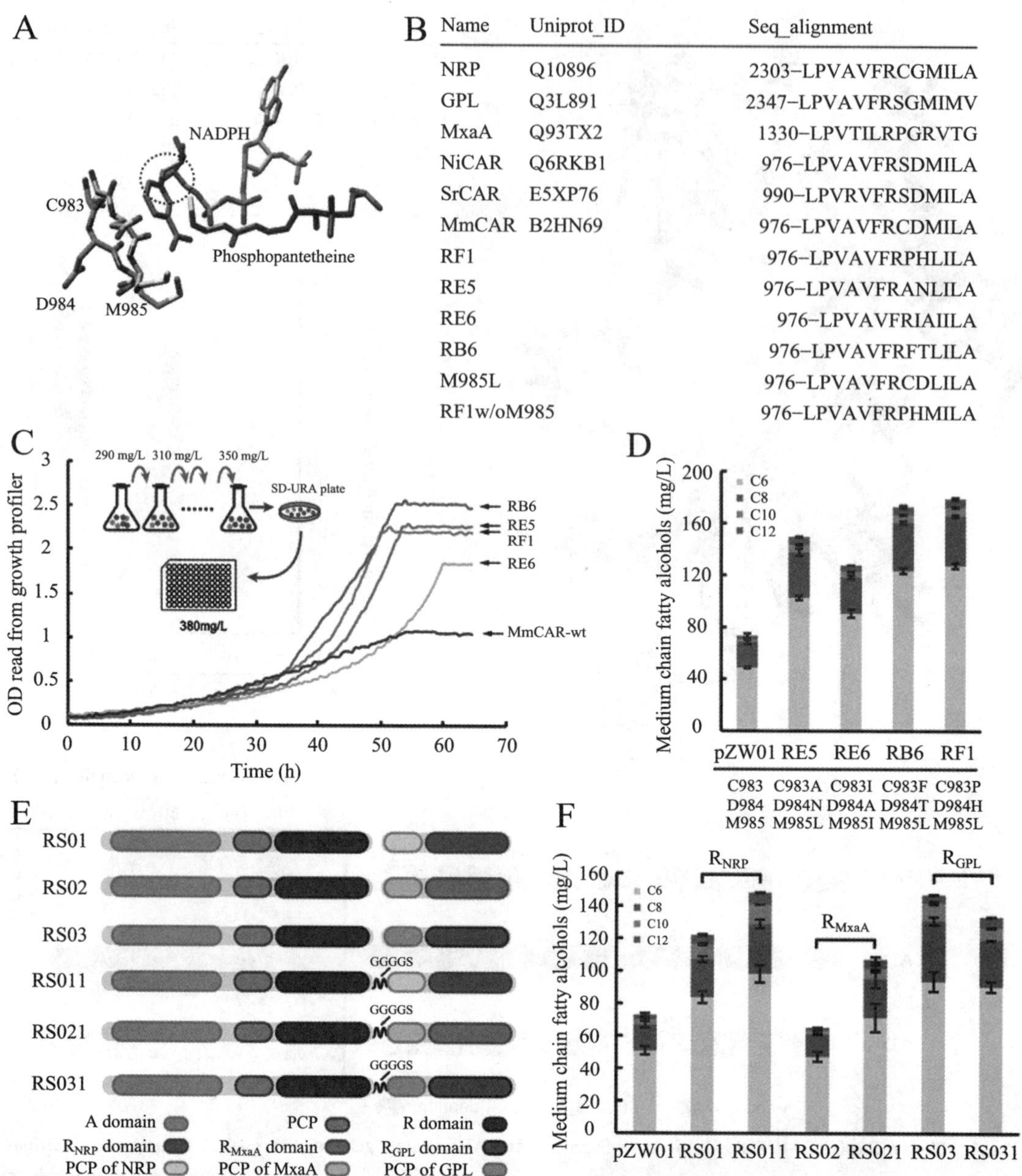


**Fig. 5 The synthesis of MCFOHs in *S. cerevisiae* by MmCAR variants generated through R domain modifications**

(A) The on-and off-states of the R domain determined by the conformation change of C983 - M985. In the active form (cyan), the D984 residue is positioned away from the active center (shown in a dashed ellipse), while in the inactive form (yellow), D984 and the backbone of C983 - M985 occupy the pocket for the nicotinamide moiety of NADPH. (B) Partial sequence alignment of MmCAR, SrCAR, NiCAR, MxaA, GPL, and NRP. (C) Growth curves of strains expressing MmCAR variants selected from the site-directed saturation mutagenesis library. After an enrichment process in the medium with 290 to 350 mg/L C8 FA, the cell growth of selected clones in medium with 380 mg/L C8 FA was monitored by a Growth Profiler. (D and F) Production of MCFOHs in *S. cerevisiae* by mutated MmCAR variants derived from the site-directed mutagenesis library (D) and di-domain expression (F). All plasmids were transformed into ZWE243 for evaluation; all of the cultivations were performed for 48 h in minimal medium with histidine. The mean±SD of three biological replicates is shown. (E) Schematic illustration of the didomain expression constructs. The PCP-R didomains from NRPS enzymes ($R_{GPL}$, $R_{NRP}$, and $R_{MxaA}$) were expressed with MmCAR separately (RS01, RS02, and RS03) or fused with MmCAR via a GGGGS linker (RS11, RS21, and RS31).

containing mutations C983P, D984H, M985L, led to the highest titer of MCFOHs of 178 mg/L, a 2.4-fold increase compared with the wild-type MmCAR (Fig. 5D). A common mutation (M985L or M985I) was found among these four MmCAR variants (Fig. 5B). Therefore, M985L and RF1 without the mutation on M985 (RF1w/o985) variants, which contained either only the M985L mutation or the other two mutations (C983P and D984H) observed in RF1, respectively, were constructed to separately test the effects of these mutations on the enzyme activity. Interestingly, we found that the M985L mutant only led to production of 95.5 mg/L MCFOHs in yeast. The RF1w/o985 variant (Fig. 5B), in contrast, exerted an even slightly stronger effect on MCFOH production than the RF1 mutant (*SI Appendix*, Fig. S8). These results indicated that these two mutations might play a more critical role in RF1 for MCFOH production than M985L.

The comparison based on crystal structures between MmCAR and NRPSs elucidated that they share a high similarity in the structures of the R domains. Nevertheless, some of the R domains from NRPSs differ in their final product determination compared with CARs, as they release alcohols produced through aldehyde intermediates. Three R domains from three NRPS enzymes ($R_{GPL}$, $R_{NRP}$, and $R_{MxaA}$) sharing a high level of identity (~50%) with the R domain of MmCAR (*SI Appendix*, Fig. S9), were reported to catalyze the four-electron reduction of fatty acyl thioesters to the corresponding alcohols. We attempted replacing the MmCAR R domain or PCP-R didomain with the respective domains from NRP, GPL, and MxaA (*SI Appendix*, Figs. S9 and S10) in order to enable a four-electron reduction that could benefit fatty alcohol production. Unfortunately, all of the chimeras seemed to lose their function as no MCFOHs were detected in the yeast strains expressing these constructs. Thus, in order to avoid the potential misfolding of MmCAR, the heterologous PCP-R didomains were introduced into yeast cells through two strategies: 1) Separate expression together with MmCAR or 2) fusion with MmCAR using the flexible linker GGGGS (Fig. 5E). Most of the constructs expressing an additional PCP-R didomains successfully promoted MCFOH production in yeast (Fig. 5F). Among the evaluated variants, the most prominent effect on MCFA conversion was observed for the MmCAR-$R_{NRP}$ fusion (RS011), which enabled production of 148 mg/L MCFOHs (Fig. 5F).

Combination of Modifications Different modifications evaluated above were combined to achieve a more efficient MmCAR variant for MCFOH production in yeast. We combined all of the other beneficial mutations with I303W to ensure a more specific substrate preference toward MCFAs. The highest production of MCFOHs was obtained in strains expressing RF1 + 303, which resulted in production of MCFOHs at a level of 229 mg/L, a 2.8-fold increase over that of the wild-type MmCAR (Fig. 6). Additionally, to enable a further enhancement of MCFOH production, we also incorporated two additional modification (M150 and RS011) into the two best variants RF1 + 303 and RF1w/o985 + 303, respectively. However, none of these combinations reached the MCFOHs levels of RF1+303 (*SI Appendix*, Fig. S11).

Evaluation of Substrate Specificity of MmCAR Variants The strain ZWE243 producing MCFAs provided a platform to evaluate the variants in vivo through measurement of the

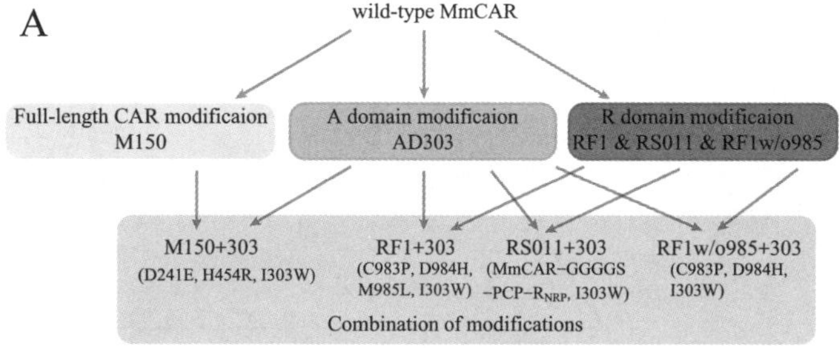


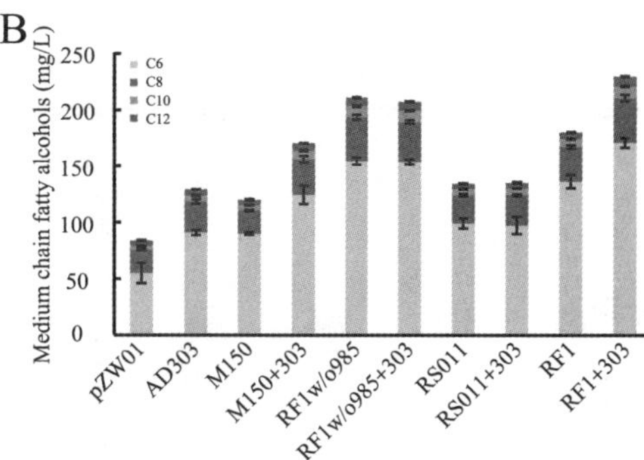


**Fig. 6 The production of MCFOHs in strains with combined modification in MmCAR**

(A) Modifications and changed residues in each enzyme variant. (B) The production of MCFOHs was tested in the strain ZWE243 containing plasmids pZW01, M150, ADD303, M150+303, RF1w/o985, RF1w/o985+303, RS011, RS011+303, RF1, and RF1+303, respectively. All strains were cultivated for 48 h in minimal medium and the final products were quantified by gas chromatography-flame ionization detector (GC-FID); the mean±SD of three biological replicates is presented.

production of MCFOHs. Since this strain generates both LCFAs and MCFAs, the investigation of the profile of intracellular fatty alcohols could therefore represent a complementary assay to interpret the catalytic activities of each enzyme variant. The intracellular fatty alcohols extracted from strains containing the wild-type MmCAR, AD303, M150, and RF1, respectively, were quantified. The GC spectra showed that most of the products were MCFOHs with relatively low amounts of LCFOHs detected (Fig. 7A). We subsequently quantified the intracellular fatty alcohols for each strain and calculated the proportion of each component in the total products. According to the results, the wild-type MmCAR led to a production of 41% of LCFOHs (including C14, C16 : 1, and C16) and 59% of MCFOHs (including C8, C10, and C12) among the intracellular fatty alcohols (Fig. 7B). Compared to the wild-type, all of the other mutant CARs resulted in a higher proportion of MCFAs, 75%, 78%, and 67% of MCFOHs in the strains expressing AD303, RF1, and M150, respectively (Fig. 7 A and B).

To investigate if these MmCAR variants indeed possessed altered substrate preferences, the enzyme activities on FAs of different chain length were measured in crude protein extracts. The crude protein extracted from the strain with

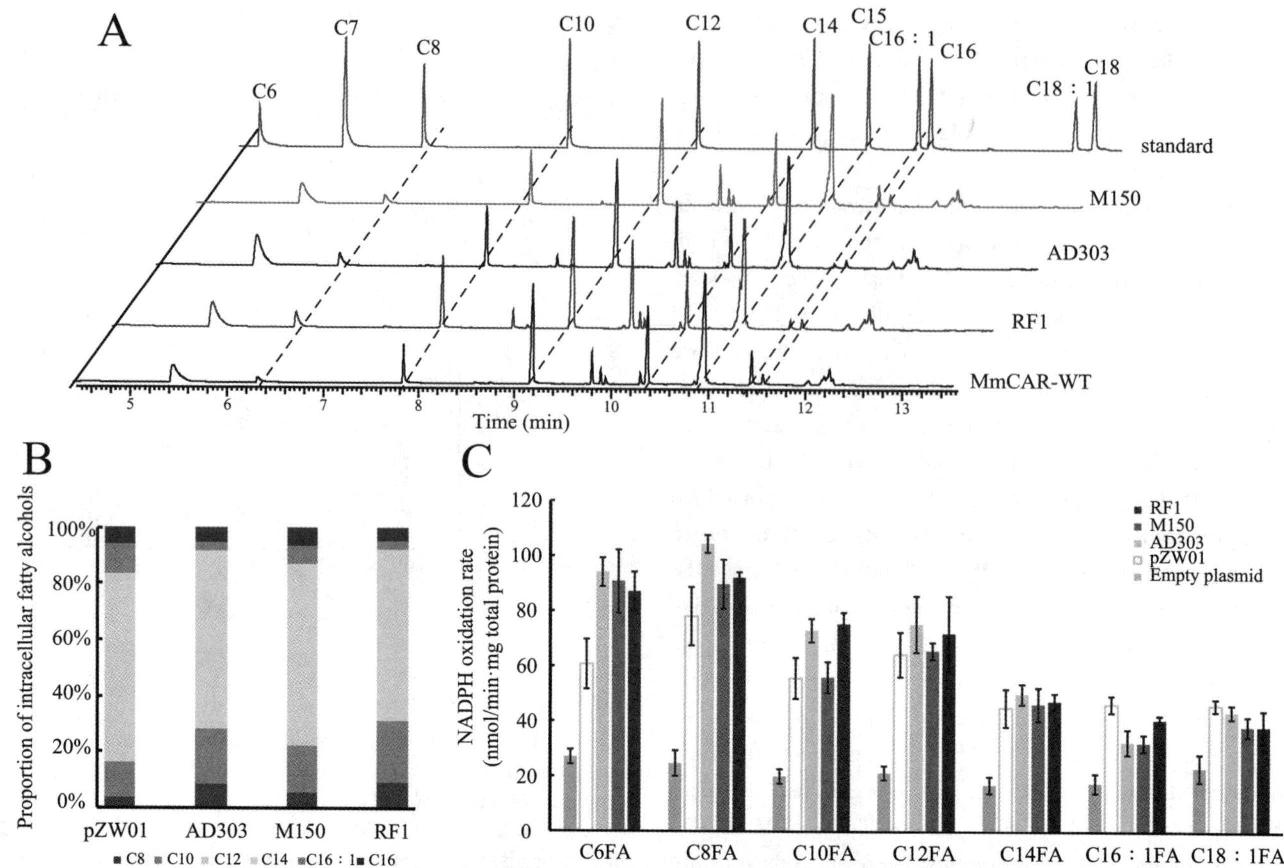


**Fig. 7 Characterization of the substrate specificity of mutated MmCARs**

(A) GC spectra of intracellular fatty alcohols derived from strain ZWE243 with pZW01, M150, AD303, and RF1, respectively. Cultivation was performed for 72 h in minimal medium. (B) Proportion of intracellular fatty alcohols in strain ZWE243 with pZW01, M150, AD303, and RF1, respectively. (C) The NADPH oxidation rate of the crude protein extracted from strain ZWE243 containing RF1, M150, AD303, wild-type CAR and an empty plasmid, respectively, supplemented with different FAs. The samples were taken after cultivation in minimal medium for 24 h. The mean±SD of three biological replicates is presented.

the empty plasmid exerted background NADPH oxidation activity, which was ~23 nmol/(min · mg) total protein and comparatively constant between the different assays. Except for the reduction activity of M150 on C10 FA, which was comparable to that of wild-type MmCAR, all three mutants had improved activities toward C6 - C10 FAs, but comparable or decreased activities toward C12 - C18 FAs (Fig. 7C). Particularly, the I303W mutant showed a roughly twofold increase in activity on C6 FA compared with the wild-type. We therefore compared the kinetic properties between the I303W mutant and wild-type, and observed that, compared with the wild-type, the I303W mutant had a twofold higher $k_{cat}$, albeit a higher $K_m$ value (*SI Appendix*, Fig. S12). These results could partially explain the elevated production of MCFOHs.

Further Increase in MCFOH Production through Deletion of TPO1 The endogenously produced MCFAs were found to be inadequate for MCFOH production in strain ZWE243 containing RF1+303 (*SI Appendix*, Fig. S13); we thus fed the cells with the C8 FA in the medium as the precursor. However, both MCFOH production and cell growth were negatively affected when 100, 200, and 250 mg/L of C8 FAs were added into the medium, respectively (*SI Appendix*, Fig. S14), which might be due to the cellular toxicity caused by high concentrations of C8 FA. Moreover, a bilayer cultivation was conducted through addition of dodecane, but a large amount of the MCFA precursors were captured by the dodecane phase, leading to a low-level production of MCFOHs (*SI Appendix*, Fig. S15).

Tpo1 is a native transporter located on the plasma membrane of yeast that was suggested to contribute to the resistance to polyamines by exporting these substrates. Later, it was identified to confer tolerance against MCFAs as well. In our previous work, an improved Tpo1 variant was able to significantly increase the production of extracellular MCFAs in yeast. We assumed that the deletion of *TPO1* might augment the intracellular MCFA pool by potentially reducing the secretion of MCFAs (Fig. 8A), which would benefit MCFOH synthesis. As expected, upon introducing the *TPO1* deletion, the accumulation of extracellular MCFAs in the resulting strain YH28 was significantly decreased to 109 mg/L compared with the titer of 159 mg/L generated by

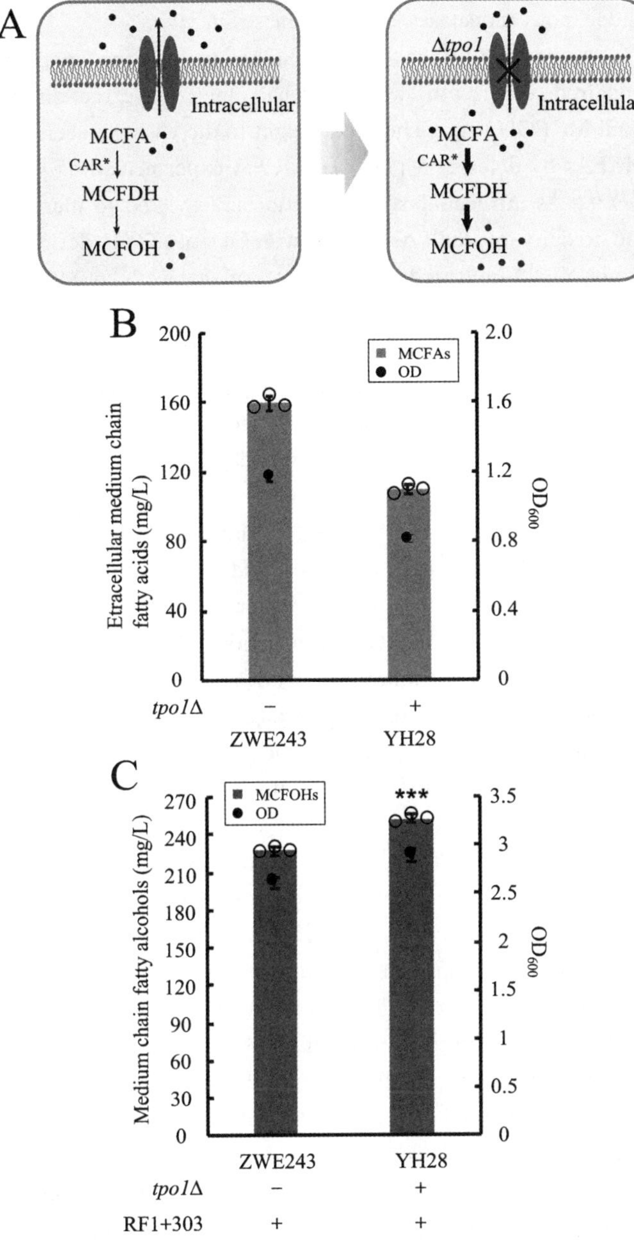


**Fig. 8 The effect of *TPO1* deletion on MCFOH production in *S. cerevisiae***

(A) Schematic illustration of the postulated effect of a *TPO1* deletion. Deleting *TPO1* is assumed to affect MCFA efflux from the cells. With the increased intracellular pool of MCFAs, the flux toward MCFOH production would be enhanced. MCFAs in blue dots, MCFOHs in red dots. MCFDH, medium-chain fatty aldehyde. (B) Production of extracellular MCFAs and final $OD_{600}$ for strains ZWE243 and YH28. Strains were cultivated in minimal medium with histidine and uracil for 48 h. (C) Production of MCFOHs and final $OD_{600}$ for strains ZWE243 and YH28 with RF1 + 303 expression. The strains were cultivated for 48 h in minimal medium with histidine and the final products were quantified by GC-FID. The $P$ value was 0.000 5 (*** $P<0.001$). Statistical analysis was conducted using a Student's $t$ test (one-tailed; two-sample unequal variance). The mean ± SD of three biological replicates is presented in B and C.

the parental strain (Fig. 8B). In line with this, strain YH28 showed a lower final OD, which could result from the inhibitory effect of intracellular MCFAs. Subsequently, the most efficient MmCAR variant RF1 + 303 was introduced into strains ZWE243 and YH28, respectively. As expected, the knockout of *TPO1* led to an ~11% improvement of the final titer of MCFOHs to 252 mg/L, which is around 3.2-fold higher than that of the original strain (ZWE243) harboring wild-type MmCAR (Fig. 8C).

## 2 DISCUSSION

Enlarging the variety of compounds produced by cell factories requires a feasible engineering approach to break the restriction imposed by the native activity of enzymes. Protein engineering has been applied as a powerful tool for fine-tuning enzyme activities, often through the modification of amino acid sequences that are found in nature to expand the borders of biocatalysis. Conferred by protein engineering strategies, such as incorporation of mutations and domain modifications, it was shown that the property of CARs can be improved toward desired functions.

In this study, the MmCAR enzyme was modified to stimulate high-level production of MCFOHs. MmCAR is a relatively large enzyme of ~130 kDa with multiple domains. Thus, we designed different engineering approaches based on the distinct domains. A high-throughput screening method coupled with cell growth was applied, which enabled an efficient selection process for beneficial enzyme variants. We identified several mutations based on directed evolution of the full-length MmCAR that potentially enhanced the catalytic activity toward MCFAs. According to the structural information obtained in a recent study, two of the mutated residues (D241E, H454R) from the best variant M150 are located in the core A domain ($A_{core}$, residues 1 to 510), but on the surface of the A domain, not in the active site. The third mutated residue, L567M, is situated in the mobile domain ($A_{sub}$, residues 511 to 636), whose conformation changes substantially between the adenylation and thiolation states (*SI Appendix*, Fig. S16). Hence, this indicates that these mutations displayed indirect effects on the activity or stability of MmCAR. Although the mechanism of these effects is still unclear, the improved activity of M150 toward shorter chain length substrates, especially C6 FA rather than LCFAs (C16 : 1 and C18 : 1), was confirmed in vitro (Fig. 7C).

Additional efforts of shifting the substrate preference to MCFAs were made through establishing a random mutagenesis library based on only the A domain of MmCAR and rational design to narrow the substrate-binding pocket. Two rounds of evolution were executed, resulting in two CAR variants that benefitted the production of MCFOHs. Four mutations (E176G, Q182R, Q371R, F501Y) were identified in the most-efficient variant, AD10, after the second round of evolution. However, all of them were located on the surface of the $A_{core}$ domain. Although the F517 residue is close to the adenine base of the substrate ATP, the structure analysis showed no involvement of this residue in ATP binding (*SI Appendix*, Fig. S17). It was intriguing that the mutated residues in both M150 and AD10 tended to be on the protein surface and change the charge state, which might influence the protein stability or solubility and also indirectly increase the overall catalytic activity. A smaller space in the substrate-binding pocket would be beneficial for accommodating shorter-chain FA, which was demonstrated in our work by incorporating two tryptophan residues individually substituting two residues (Q302 and I303) close to the binding pocket of the A domain. The best performing mutant, AD303, enabled production of around 130 mg/L of MCFOHs, which was a 1.6-fold increase compared with the wild-type MmCAR, indicating that the rational design directly interfering with the binding pocket was potentially more efficient than the random approach in terms of altering substrate specificity in our study. Similarly, a previous study showed that the rational redesign of CAR enzymes successfully enabled the extension of their reaction scope toward amide synthesis.

Although successful studies on domain exchange in NRPS systems and CAR systems have been reported, replacing the native R or PCP-R domains with the ones from NRPS enzymes sharing high sequence similarity resulted in the complete loss of the activity of MmCAR (*SI Appendix*, Fig. S12), which might be due to an inappropriate domain boundary (*SI Appendix*, Fig. S7) used for domain-swapping, as shown in previous reports on PKS engineering. Thus, in the context of maintaining the biocatalytic activity of MmCAR, we sought to express the heterologous off-loading PCP-R domains without replacing the respective MmCAR domains. The observed positive effect on MCFOH production might be due to the extra aldehyde reductase activity from these off-loading PCP-R domains. In addition, a modification of the native R domain was conducted as well through establishing a site-directed saturation mutagenesis library toward residues 983 to 985. The mutant RF1 showed highest catalytic activity, resulting in a more than twofold increase in MCFOH production compared to the wild-type CAR (Fig. 5C). Consistently, the change in substrate preference to-ward MCFAs was also observed in the enzymatic assay in vitro. Although the positive effect on MCFOH production by the modified residues 983 to 985 has been proven in our study, it was difficult to investigate whether the improvement of the reduction efficiency was conferred by the final product scope being extended to fatty alcohols directly or by other mechanisms, which is due to the complex reaction environment and the presence of other endogenous reductases/dehydrogenases in vivo.

Adding additional MCFA substrates to the medium impaired cell growth, which also had a negative effect on the final MCFOH titer. Thus, we sought to increase intracellular MCFAs by deleting a potential MCFA exporter-coding gene *TPO1*. As intracellular accumulation is expected to increase the toxicity of MCFAs, the lower OD of *TPO1*-deficient strain YH28 indicated that the level of intracellular MCFAs was indeed increased. The successful improvement of MCFOH production in YH28 containing RF1+303 further indicated that the flux toward MCFOH formation was augmented due to the enhanced intracellular substrate level. The cellular toxicity was relieved by the conversion to alcohols, as a higher OD (around 3) was observed for the CAR-expressing strains (Fig. 8C). However, the impaired growth and low final biomass yield resulting from the toxicity of MCFOHs is still a major obstacle for further improvements in MCFOH production. Thus, strategies increasing cellular tolerance against MCFOHs and optimization of the fermentation process through decoupling the cell growth and product formation would be potential future directions in order to obtain further improvements in the production of MCFOHs.

The broad substrate scope of CAR enzymes enables their usage in the bioproduction of diverse aldehydes and alcohols. However, for the production of MCFOHs by microbial cell factories, the substrate promiscuity of CAR enzymes represents an obstacle. Through multiple protein engineering strategies, we succeeded in optimizing MmCAR to significantly enhance MCFOH production to 252 mg/L. Many efforts have been devoted to enable biosynthesis of MCFOHs in yeast cells in previous studies. Targeting a fatty acyl-CoA reductase (TaFAR) to the peroxisomes was demonstrated to be an efficient strategy and resulted in the production of MCFOHs (C10 - C12) in *Saccharomyces cerevisiae* in a dodecane bilayer cultivation (*SI Appendix*, Table S1). However, the C16 fatty alcohol was still the major product (>60%) in this study, for which the substrate preference of TaFAR might be one of the reasons. Our study, on the other hand, provides new insight into MCFOH production. Considering the difference in cultivation conditions, we achieved a significant improvement in both MCFOH titer and yield in minimal medium (*SI Appendix*, Table S1). The catalytic activity of the engineered MmCAR was also investigated both in vitro and in vivo. The efficient reduction of MCFAs by the engineered CAR enzymes will enable the synthesis of versatile aldehyde intermediates with broad applications for further production of, for example, the corresponding alka(e)nes and FA acyl esters. Although CAR enzymes were previously modified by different strategies, this work is unique in comprehensively engineering the CAR enzyme for more selective biosynthesis of MCFOHs. In addition, our engineering strategies may inspire and promote the engineering of other complex multidomain enzymes.

## 3 METHODS

Directed Evolution of Full-Length MmCAR The mutagenesis library of *MmCAR* was constructed by error-prone PCR (GeneMorph II Random Mutagenesis Kit, Agilent Technologies) with a low mutation frequency (0 to 4.5 mutations/kb) using the primers MmCARwm-F/MmCARwm-R. The product was then cotransformed with two backbone fragments of pZW01 into yeast strain YJZ03 (*pox1Δ hfd1Δ*). The primers used for amplification are shown in *SI Appendix*, Table S4. The plasmid-based libraries were established in yeast. The library sizes for the two rounds of evolution were around $6\times10^7$ and $4.5\times10^7$, respectively. All of the colonies from the SD-URA (synthetic complete medium without uracil) plate were all scratched into 20 mL minimal medium with 290 mg/L C8 FA (330 mg/L for the second round). After 24 h, the cells (1 : 100 diluted) were transferred into 20 mL minimal medium with 310 mg/L C8 FAs (350 mg/L for the second round) for 48 h. Then the cells were diluted 1 : 50, and transferred into 20 mL minimal medium with 330 mg/L C8 FA (370 mg/L for the second round) for 48 h. The enriched cells were plated on SD-URA solid medium, and around 60 single colonies were picked randomly into 96-well plate with minimal medium containing 330 mg/L C8 FAs (370 mg/L for the second round). The growth curves were monitored by a Bioscreen C MBR instrument (Growth Profiler 960 was used for the second round). The plasmids from fast-growing colonies were extracted and used to transform strain ZWE243 to determine MCFOH production. The mutant CAR with mutations D241E, H454R, L567M was used as the template for the second round of evolution. The same process was conducted as described above.

Directed Evolution of MmCAR a Domain The random mutagenesis library based on the A domain (residues 88 to 541) of MmCAR was established using error-prone PCR (GeneMorph II Random Mutagenesis Kit) with the low mutation frequency (0 to 4.5 mutations/kb) by primer pair CAR-A-F/CAR-A-R. The primers are listed in *SI Appendix*, Table S4. The wild-type MmCAR was the template for the first round of evolution and the mutant CAR with mutations Q182R; Q371R was used for the second round. The sizes of the two libraries were both around $5\times10^4$. The same workflow for the library enrichment was used as described above, but different concentrations of C8 FA were used, which were 290 mg/L, 300 mg/L, and 310 mg/L for the first round and 310 mg/L, 330 mg/L, and 350 mg/L for the second round. Around 60 single colonies from first round and second round were cultivated in minimal medium with histidine containing 330 mg/L and 370 mg/L C8 FAs, respectively. The growth curves were monitored by a Bioscreen C MBR instrument (Growth Profiler 960 was used for the second round).

Site-Directed Saturation Mutagenesis Library The primers used for establishing the site-directed saturation mutagenesis library based on residues 983 to 985 are listed in *SI Appendix*, Table S4. The same enrichment method was used as described above with concentrations of 290 mg/L, 310 mg/L, 330 mg/L, and 350 mg/L C8 FAs. After isolating the variants on an SD-URA plate, 80 of the colonies were picked to grow in medium with 380 mg/L of C8 FA. Based on the growth curves generated with the help of a Growth Profiler 960, the clones with the highest growth rates were selected.

Enzymatic Assays The yeast cells (50 OD) were harvested after 24 h by centrifuging at $4{,}000\times g$ at 4℃ for 5 min, then washed twice with PBS buffer. After discarding the supernatant, the cells were resuspended in 0.5 mL extraction buffer (50 mmol/L Tris・Cl, 1 mmol/L EDTA, 1 mmol/L KCl, pH 7.5) containing 10 mmol/L DTT and 1% (vol/vol) protease inhibitor. The suspensions were vortexed for 20 s ×5 (5 min intervals on ice) with 300 mg 0.2 to 0.4 mm glass beads. The supernatants of the samples were collected by centrifuging at $20{,}000\times g$ at 0 ℃ for 20 min. Proteins were quantified using a Pierce BCA Protein Assay Kit (ThermoFisher Scientific). The MmCAR activity assay was performed in 96-well microplates; 90 μL reaction mix containing 50 mmol/L Tris・Cl (pH 7.5), 10 mmol/L $MgCl_2$, 1 mmol/L NADPH, 1 mmol/L ATP, and FAs (0.5 mmol/L C10, C12, C14, C16 : 1, C18 : 1 FA, and 5 mmol/L C6, C8 FA) and 10 μL of extracts (5 μg total protein) were mixed to initiate the reaction. Then the reactions were monitored at 340 nm for 30 min at room temperature with a FLUOstar Omega micropate reader (BMG Labtech). The MmCAR activity was defined as NADPH oxidation rate (1 μmol/min) of total protein.

Data Availability All details of strains, plasmids, media, and methods can be found in *SI Appendix*, *SI Materials and Methods*. All data related to this study, including MCFOH production, cell growth in Bioscreen and Growth profiler, and enzymatic assays, can be found in Dataset S1.

[胡雅婷，朱志伟，Jens Nielsen，等. PNAS，2020，117(37):22974 - 22983.]

# Multidimensional engineering of *Saccharomyces cerevisiae* for efficient synthesis of medium-chain fatty acids

Vegetable oils, mostly containing long-chain fatty acid moieties (C16 and C18), are primary feedstocks for the food, oleochemical and biofuel industries. Medium-chain fatty acids (MCFAs; C6 - C12) are desired substrates in many scenarios, such as the production of replacement fuels for gasoline and jet fuels, chemicals for plastics, surfactants and cosmetics. Only a few plant seed oils (coconut and palm kernel oils) contain a high fraction of C12 fatty acid. Their limited annual production due to land, water, fertilizer and climate constraints would not secure the amounts needed, and a further increase in the plantation of oil plants is generally associated with deforestation, which has negative environmental and ecological consequences. Microbial conversion of renewable biomass to MCFAs is a sustainable and promising solution for their production. Moreover, both the mass yield of MCFAs from sugars (Supplementary Table 1) and the selling prices of MCFAs and their derivatives, such as alcohols, are higher than those of long-chain fatty acids, which also makes the synthesis of MCFAs commercially attractive.

MCFAs are rare metabolites in most organisms, which have evolved to predominantly synthesize long-chain fatty acids as precursors for building membranes. As fatty acids are synthesized in forms of either acyl-acyl carrier protein (ACP) or acyl-coenzyme A (CoA), acyl-ACP/CoA thioesterases are key enzymes responsible for controlling the chain length of fatty acids. There has therefore been much interest in producing MCFAs through identification, characterization and engineering of thioesterases specific for MCFA formation. At the same time, a deeper understanding of the chain elongation mechanism of fatty acid synthases (FASs) through biochemical and structural studies has also enabled the manipulation of FAS enzymes to produce MCFAs. Moreover, the reversed β-oxidation, α-keto acid elongation and polyketide synthesis pathways have been employed to synthesize MCFAs. Although the reversed β-oxidation pathway was shown to be more economic for MCFA production because of the higher maximum theoretical yield, the design and deployment of a functional reversed β-oxidation pathway in eukaryotic microbes, such as *Saccharomyces cerevisiae* and *Yarrowia lipolytica*, are still challenging.

Both type II FAS systems present in bacteria and plastids of eukaryotic cells, as well as the reversed β-oxidation pathway, consist of disassociated individual enzymes, while type I FASs (FASIs) from both fungi and bacteria exist as multifunctional polypeptide chains and assemble into barrel-shaped hollow complexes (Fig. 1a, b). All catalytic enzyme domains except the auxiliary phosphopantetheinyl transferase (PPT) domain (or free-standing AcpS) are embedded in an extensive scaffolding matrix to form two reaction chambers, which brings spatial proximity of all catalytic sites for fatty acid elongation. Three tethered ACP domains dwell in each reaction chamber, which secures a high local concentration of ACPs. The elegant architecture of microbial FASI ensures high enzymatic turnover numbers ($k_{cat}$) for fatty acid synthesis, which could be utilized for efficient production of fatty acids, as it has been shown that yeast cells are superior chassis for fatty acid or lipid synthesis. Previously, we have engineered fungal FASIs (fFASIs) by embedding thioesterases into the reaction chambers to release MCFAs, and Gajewski et al. introduced specific point mutations into the ketoacyl synthase, acetyltransferase and malonyl/palmitoyl transferase (MPT) domain of fFASIs for MCFA production (Fig. 1c). Due to the high similarity between bacterial FASI (bFASI) and fFASI, these engineering strategies applied to fFASI might be applicable to bFASI for changing the chain length of fatty acid products. Moreover, fatty acid synthesis is an energy-intensive process and is tightly regulated, while the heterologous bFASI expressed in most microbial chassis is expected to be orthogonal to the respective endogenous FAS systems. It can hence potentially be beneficial to use the deregulated bFASI for oleochemical synthesis in a heterologous host.

However, the toxicity of MCFAs hinders the cellular biocatalysts' ability to efficiently accumulate MCFA products. It is thought that the protonated form of these weak acids can pass across the plasma membrane and dissociate in the cytosol, which leads to a decrease in intracellular pH, and these lipophilic compounds have also been reported to cause membrane leakage. Moreover, the cellular toxicity of MCFAs is enhanced by low pH and the presence of ethanol. It was reported that the C8 and C10 fatty acids at a concentration of ~100 mg/L were able to seriously inhibit cell growth and that the relative order of inhibitory action was hexanoic acid (C6) < octanoic acid (C8) < decanoic acid (C10). Because of the considerably lower solubility of dodecanoic acid (C12), the toxicity of C12 fatty acid is presumably comparative to that of C6 fatty

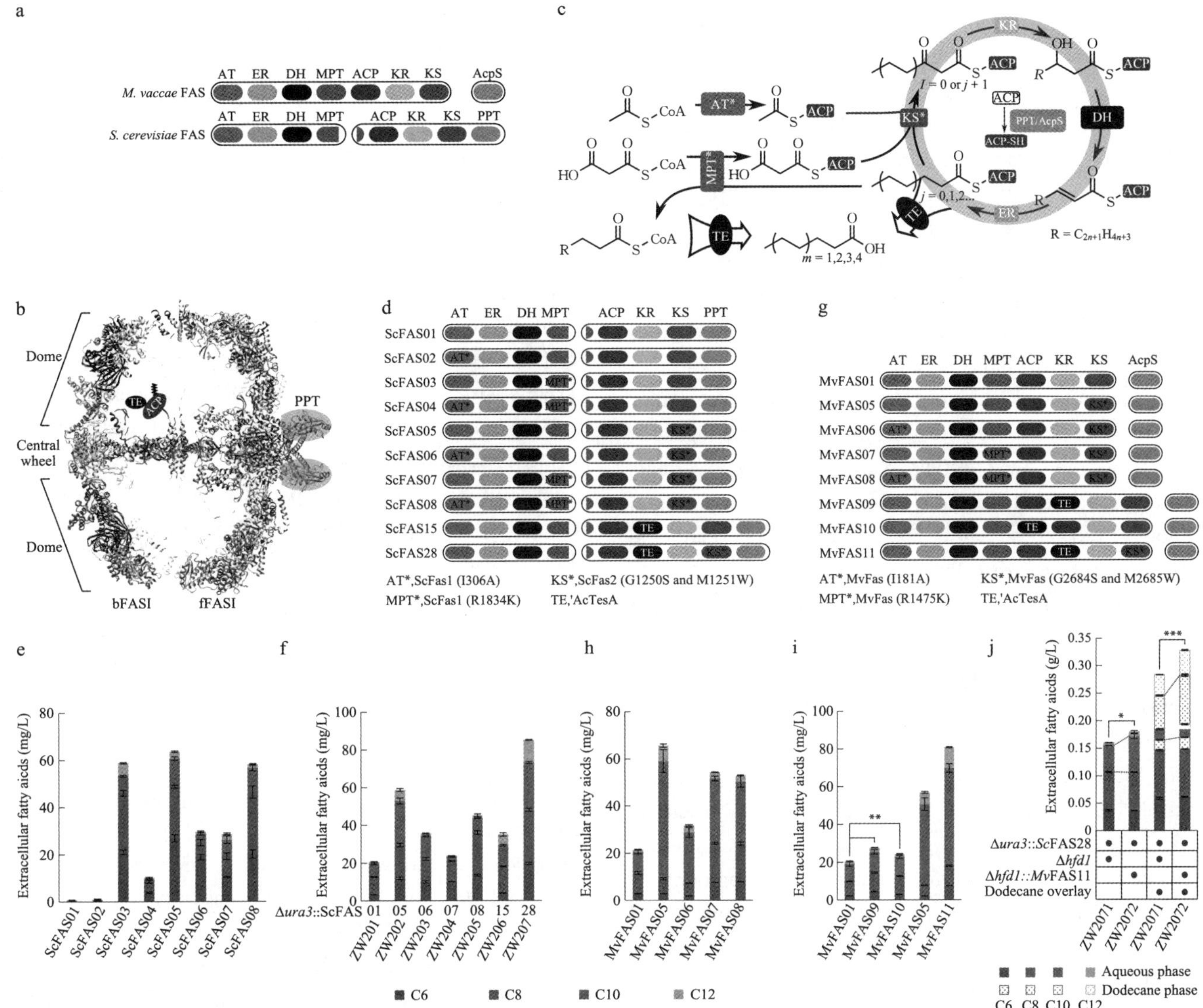

**Fig. 1 Engineering microbial FASI enzymes for MCFA synthesis**

(a) Domain composition of the FASI enzymes from *S. cerevisiae* and *M. vaccae*. AT, acetyltransferase; ER, enoyl reductase; DH, dehydratase; MPT, malonyl/palmitoyl transferase; ACP, acyl carrier protein; KR, ketoacyl reductase; KS, ketoacyl synthase; PPT and AcpS, phosphopantetheinyl transferase. (b) Cross-section of the microbial FASI structure showing the hollow reaction chambers. bFASI from *M. smegmatis* (PDB ID: 4V8L; coloured) and fFASI from *S. cerevisiae* (PDB ID: 3HMJ; grey) are shown. Coloured ribbons show one of the three sets of AT, Er, DH, MPT, Kr and KS domains embedded in the chamber wall. The fused PPT domains (shaded in blue) of fFASI are attached to the barrel-like structure. aCPs located inside the chambers are able to swing around and deliver acyl groups to active centres of enzymatic domains. As ACPs were not determined in the structure model, a schematic representation is shown. Inserted thioesterase (TE) adjacent to ACP could hydrolyse acyl-ACP intermediates and release MCFAs. (c) reactions of fatty acid synthesis. Black arrows indicate reactions manipulated for the synthesis of MCFas. The ACP is activated by the attachment of a phosphopantetheinyl group with a free terminal thiol (-SH). (d,g) Schematics of the engineered *S. cerevisiae* FAS variants (**d**) and *M. vaccae* FAS variants (g). (e,f,h-j) Extracellular fatty acids produced by strains expressing FASI variants. PWY12 (*Δfas1* and *Δfas2*) with plasmids expressing ScFAS variants was cultivated in Delft+Trp medium for 48 h (**e**). The strains integratively expressing ScFAS variants were cultivated in Delft+His+Ura medium for 96 h (**f**). YJZ03 (*Δpox1* and *Δhfd1*) with plasmids expressing MvFAS variants was cultivated in Delft+His medium for 96 h (**h** and **i**). Strains ZW2071 and ZW2072 were cultivated in Delft+Urea+Ura+His medium with or without 15% dodecane overlay for 96 h (**j**). The initial pH of Delft-derived media was adjusted to 6.0 (Supplementary Table 5). At least two independent experiments, started from the cultivation of three or four independent colonies, were performed for each quantification. Error bars represent the standard deviation of more than three biological replicates in a representative measurement. A two-tailed Welch's *t*-test was used to assess the statistical significance between groups (* $P<0.05$; ** $P<0.01$; *** $P<0.001$; sample size: $n \geqslant 3$). Panels **b** and **c** reproduced with permission from ref., Springer Nature America, Inc.

acid. However, the titres of MCFAs currently produced by yeast cells have already approached the inhibitory concentration, so mitigating the toxicity is urgent to increase the production efficiency of MCFAs. Beyond optimizing the cultivation process through, for instance, controlling the medium pH or in situ removal of toxic products, which increases the process costs, improving the cellular resistance against these toxic products is usually beneficial for production. Transporters exporting toxic products out of cells are desired engineering targets because of their potentials on relieving cellular toxicity, reducing the purification cost and the pull effect on the bioconversion pathway. In previous studies, regulating the expression of membrane transporters was shown to increase the tolerance and production of MCFAs. Moreover, through growth-coupled screening of libraries expressing heterologous bacterial efflux pumps, the candidates conferring high resistance against toxic biofuel molecules enabled improved yields of these products. A similar approach was also used to screen random mutagenesis libraries of the AcrB efflux pump, to select variants enhancing the resistance of *E. coli* towards short-chain alcohols. In *S. cerevisiae*, Tpo1 is a plasma membrane transporter involved in cellular resistance against C10 fatty acid. It is therefore possible to use a directed evolution strategy to obtain Tpo1 variants conferring improved tolerance to C10 fatty acid. In addition, adaptive laboratory evolution (ALE) allows the cell to accumulate mutations that are beneficial for cellular resistance. This nonintuitive approach has been widely used to improve tolerance towards stressful environments, including toxic products. Particularly, an evolved *E. coli* strain with increased tolerance to C8 fatty acid produced much higher amounts of fatty acids than the parent strain. Due to the complicated mechanism of tolerance traits, both semi-rational and non-rational approaches taking advantages of the power of evolution are effective strategies for engineering cellular tolerance.

In this work, we first extensively evaluated the abilities of both engineered fFASI from *S. cerevisiae* (ScFAS) and bFASI from *Mycobacterium vaccae* (MvFAS) for MCFA production, and enabled high-level production of MCFAs through the co-expression of both FAS variants. To improve the cellular tolerance, we next engineered the membrane transporter Tpo1 by directed evolution to increase its activity conferring cellular resistance against C10 fatty acid, and also used ALE to obtain strains with higher tolerance towards C8 fatty acid. The highly tolerant strain was then systematically engineered through the deployment of: (1) engineered FASI complexes to control the chain length of fatty acids; (2) enzymes to increase the supply of acetyl-CoA, malonyl-CoA and NADPH precursors; (3) the best Tpo1 variant to improve tolerance; and (4) other manipulations to prevent the re-activation of free fatty acids and the formation of by-products. Under optimized cultivation conditions, the multidimensional engineering of yeast cell factories enabled very efficient production of MCFAs.

## 1 RESULTS

**Engineering FAS enzymes for MCFA production** In our previous study, a heterologous short-chain thioesterase 'AcTesA (from *Acinetobacter baylyi*) was incorporated into three different fFASI systems for MCFA formation. In addition, a modified human FAS whose carboxy-terminal thioesterase domain was replaced with a short-chain thioesterase, TEII, was shown to be able to produce MCFAs. The MCFA production by the *S. cerevisiae* strain YJZ02 deficient in fatty acid β-oxidation (*Δpox1*) and expressing these FAS variants with short-chain thioesterases was compared. The *S. cerevisiae* FAS variant (ScFAS15) was found to be best for MCFA production (Supplementary Fig. 1). We therefore evaluated the insertion of a panel of different thioesterases into the *S. cerevisiae* FAS, as had been done in ScFAS15. However, all of these thioesterases were found to be less effective than 'AcTesA (Supplementary Fig. 2).

Specific mutations in the ketoacyl synthase domain (G1250S and M1251W in Fas2 of *S. cerevisiae*) could contribute to the conformational and steric restriction against long-chain acyl-ACP, and mutations in the acetyltransferase and MPT domains (I306A and R1834K in Fas1 of *S. cerevisiae*, respectively) would presumably alter the substrate loading and product acyl-CoA offloading efficiency. To implement this strategy in our study, seven ScFAS mutants (ScFAS02 - 08; Fig. 1d) were independently constructed and evaluated in the FAS-deficient strain PWY12 carrying deletions of both *FAS1* and *FAS2* genes. As reported earlier, ScFAS02 with a mutated acetyltransferase domain did not produce more MCFAs than the wild-type ScFAS01, and ScFAS03 and ScFAS05 with mutated MPT and ketoacyl synthase domains, respectively, produced substantial quantities of MCFAs. However, combining these mutations (ScFAS04 and ScFAS06 - 08) did not further increase MCFA production (Fig. 1d, e), which was further validated by integrative expression of these FAS variants in the YJZ02 background strain (ZW201 - 205; Fig. 1f). We therefore combined the 'AcTesA thioesterase and the mutated ketoacyl synthase domain in the ScFAS28 variant. Integrative expression of ScFAS28 in ZW207 resulted in the production of 85 ± 2 mg/L MCFAs, which was 45 ± 3% higher than those produced by ZW202 expressing the FAS variant with the mutated ketoacyl synthase domain, and 143±7% higher than those produced by ZW206 with the FAS only containing the thioesterase 'AcTesA (Fig. 1f). This indicated a synergistic effect of the embedded thioesterase and mutated ketoacyl synthase activities.

Among fatty acid synthesis machinery, the FASIs present in the CMN group (that is, *Corynebacteria*, *Mycobacteria* and *Nocardia*) of *Actinobacteria* are multifunctional single-chain

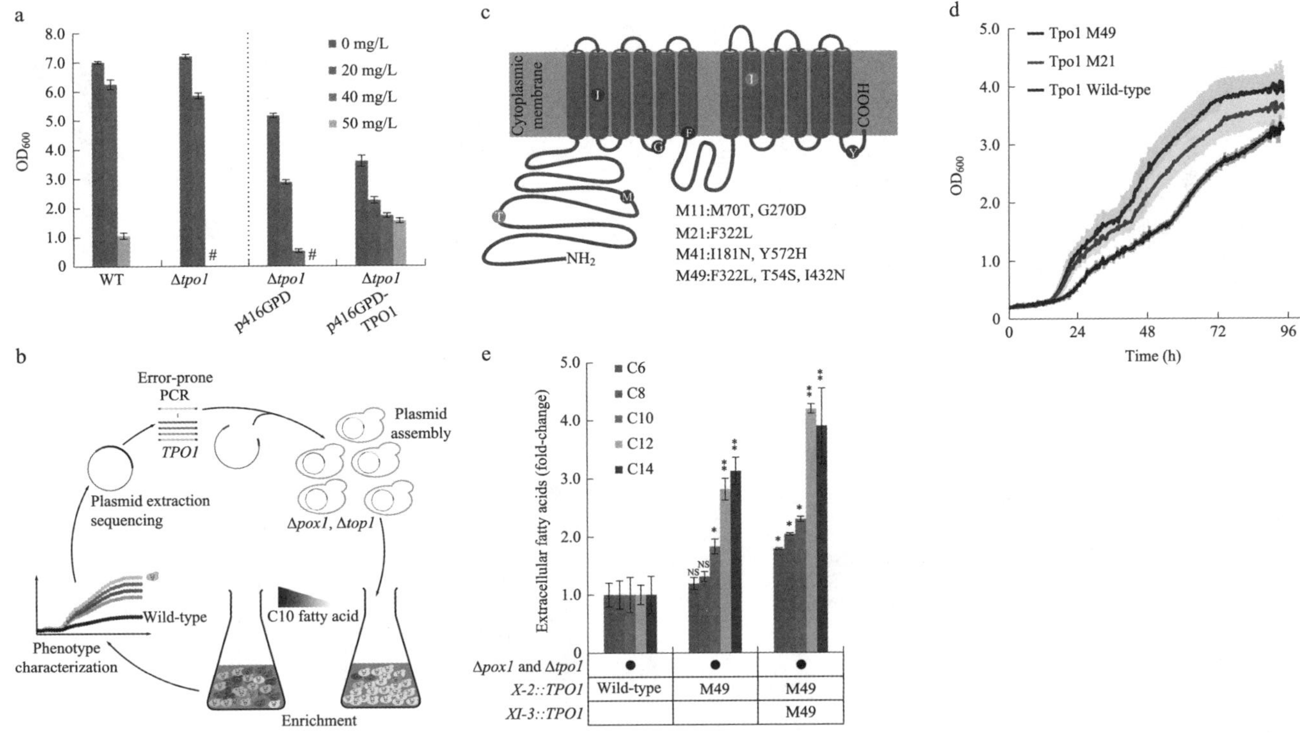


**Fig. 2 Engineering the membrane transporter Tpo1**

(a) Growth phenotype of yeast cells with or without Tpo1 in media with C10 fatty acid as indicated. The $OD_{600}$ of strains cultivated for 72 h is shown. The wild-type strain CEN. PK113 - 5D (WT) and strain YHE01 (*Δtpo1*) were cultivated in CSM medium, while YHE01, with either an empty vector (p416GPD) or a Tpo1-overexpressing plasmid (p416GPD - TPO1), was cultivated in CSM-Ura medium. A hashtag represents no growth. Error bars represent the standard deviation of three biological replicates. (b) Procedures of the directed evolution of Tpo1. (c) Predicted two-dimensional topology of Tpo1. The approximate location of mutated residues is indicated. (d) Growth phenotype of strain YHE02 (*Δpox1* and *Δtpo1*) expressing Tpo1 variants as indicated. The cells were cultivated in CSM-Ura medium with 80 mg/L C10 fatty acid, and the cell density was monitored using a BioLector microreactor. The means (lines) and standard deviations (shaded areas) of three biological replicates are presented. The initial pH of the CSM-derived media was not adjusted (Supplementary Table 5). (e) MCFas produced by strains containing pScFaS28 and expressing wild-type Tpo1 or M49 mutant. The cells were cultivated in Delft medium for 96 h. The two-tailed Welch's $t$-test was used to assess the statistical significance between groups expressing wild-type Tpo1 and the M49 mutant. NS, not significant; * $P<0.01$; ** $P<0.001$ (sample size: $n=4$). Error bars represent standard deviation.

proteins (Fig. 1a and Supplementary Fig. 3). Accompanied by an auxiliary PPT (also named AcpS in bacterial FAS systems), the bFASI is highly similar to the fFASI (Fig. 1a, b). As the bFASI expressed in yeast cells is not subjected to endogenous regulations, it is of great interest to use the orthogonal bFASI for MCFA production. A fused form of the FASI from *M. vaccae* (MvFAS-MvAcpS) was previously expressed in yeast cells for very long-chain fatty acid production. Here, we constructed separate expression cassettes for MvFAS and MvAcpS in plasmid pMvFAS01, and found that MvFAS01 was able to complement the deficiency of endogenous FAS in strain PWY12 (Supplementary Fig. 4a, b), which indicated that MvFAS01 could produce essential fatty acids in yeast. We measured the intracellular and extracellular fatty acids produced by strain PWY12 expressing either MvFAS01 or ScFAS01, and found that MvFAS01 produced substantial quantities of MCFAs (Supplementary Fig. 4c, d). According to the intracellular fatty acid profiles (Supplementary Fig. 5), the major products of strain PWY12 expressing MvFAS01 were long-chain fatty acids (C16 - C18). Moreover, compared with ScFAS01, expression of MvFAS01 in PWY12 led to the production of more intracellular MCFAs and very long-chain fatty acids (C20 - C26), but fewer long-chain fatty acids.

We then sought to engineer MvFAS to generate more MCFAs (Fig. 1g). Similarly, two mutations (G2684S and M2685W, equivalent to G1250S and M1251W in Fas2 from *S. cerevisiae*) were introduced into the ketoacyl synthase domain, and we found that ketoacyl synthase-mutated MvFAS05 also complemented FAS deficiency in PWY12 and led to the production of more MCFAs than wild-type MvFAS01 (Supplementary Fig. 6), showing that the effect of the mutations in MvFAS05 on MCFA formation was consistent with what has been found for fFASI (Fig. 1d, e). Expression of MvFAS05 in strain YJZ03 (*Δpox1* and *Δhfd1*) resulted in the production of 66 ± 8 mg/L extracellular MCFAs, of which approximately 76% were C10 fatty acid, while the expression of wild-type MvFAS01 in YJZ03 only

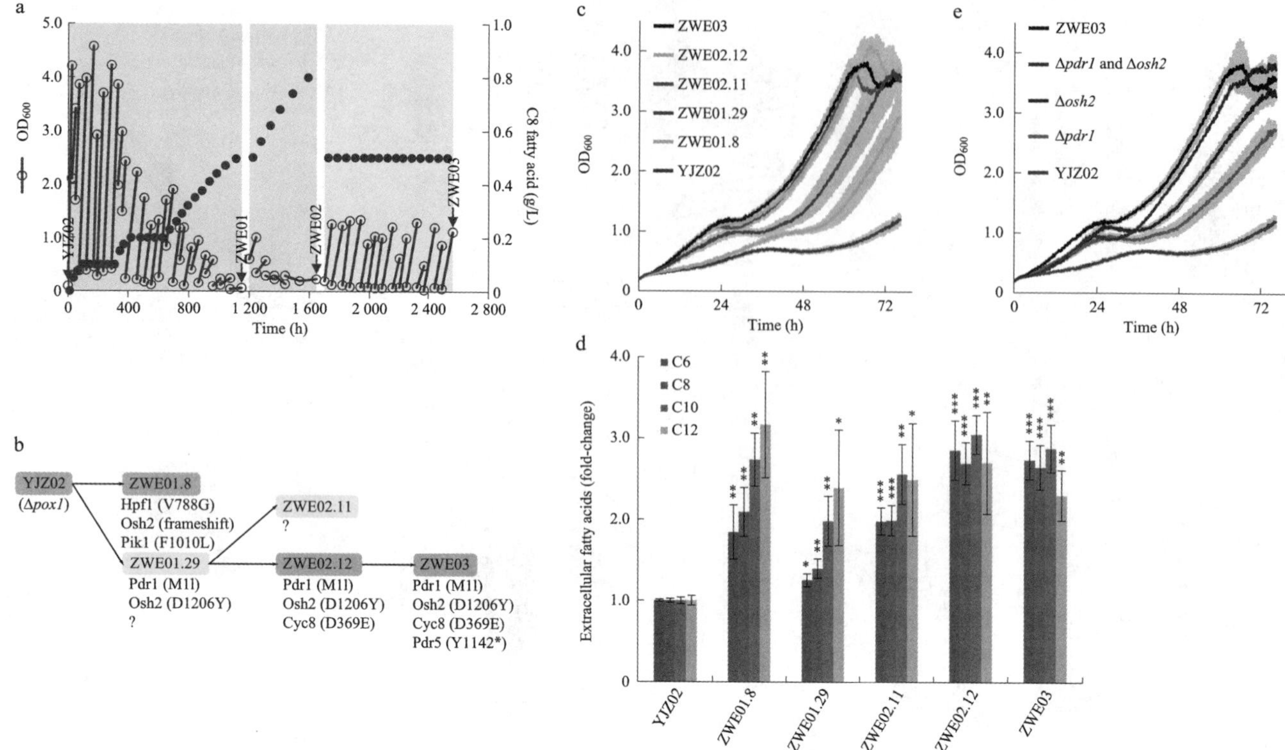

**Fig. 3 improving cell fitness via ALE**

(a) ALE procedure for obtaining C8 fatty acid-resistant strains. Serial cultures of the parent strain YJZ02 (*Δpox1*) were performed in Delft+His+Ura media with C8 fatty acid at the indicated concentrations (right-hand *y* axis). Two colonies (ZWE01.8 and ZWE01.29) were selected from the ZWE01 population, and ZWE01.29 was used for the second stage of ALE. ZWE02.11 and ZWE02.12 were selected from the ZWE02 population. Only one colony (ZWE03) was selected from the ZWE03 population, which was derived from ZWE02.12. (b) Mutations observed in the evolved strains. Arrows indicate the genetic lineage of the strains, and genomes of the strains shaded in pink were sequenced. The question marks represent unknown mutations. (c, e) Growth phenotypes of the evolved strains (**c**) and reverse engineered strains (**e**) in medium with 400 mg/L C8 fatty acid. The cell density was monitored using a BioLector microreactor. The means (lines) and standard deviations (shaded areas) of four biological replicates are presented. (d) MCFAs produced by the parent strain and the evolved strains expressing ScFaS28. Cells were cultivated in the Delft+His medium for 96 h. The two-tailed Welch's *t*-test was used to assess the statistical significance between evolved strain and parent strain ($^{*}P<0.05$; $^{**}P<0.01$; $^{***}P<0.001$; sample size: $n=4$). Error bars represent standard deviation.

resulted in the production of 21 ± 2 mg/L extracellular MCFAs, among which C8 (41 ± 5%) and C10 (42 ± 7%) fatty acids were the major products (Fig. 1h). However, introducing additional mutations into the acetyltransferase domain (MvFAS06), the MPT domain (MvFAS07) or both (MvFAS08) did not improve MCFA production (Fig. 1g, h), which was consistent with what we found for the corresponding ScFAS variants (Fig. 1e, f).

As bFASI assembles into a cage-like structure similar to fFASI, into which heterologous enzymes could be incorporated to tailor the fatty acid products, we also inserted the short-chain-specific thioesterase ′AcTesA into MvFAS in two different contexts (MvFAS09 and MvFAS10; Fig. 1g). From the complementation test (Supplementary Fig. 6), we deduced that both thioesterase-embedded MvFAS variants had fatty acid synthesis activity. Moreover, increased production of MCFAs was observed in strain PWY12 expressing MvFAS09 or MvFAS10, compared with the strain expressing the wild-type MvFAS01 (Supplementary Fig. 6). In addition, we evaluated the in vivo activity of these MvFAS variants in strain YJZ03, and found that MvFAS09- and MvFAS10-expressing strains produced 35 ± 4 and 19 ± 2% more extracellular MCFAs, respectively, than the one expressing the wild-type MvFAS01 (Fig. 1i). This indicated that the context of ACP and thioesterase influenced the activity of releasing medium-chain products, and this was consistent with our previous study, in which the fFASI with thioesterase inserted downstream from ACP (similar to MvFAS09) produced more MCFAs than that with thioesterase inserted upstream from ACP (similar to MvFAS10). After showing that the thioesterase could be embedded into MvFAS to increase MCFA production, we next constructed MvFAS11, which contained the mutated ketoacyl synthase domain and the heterologous thioesterase (Fig. 1g and Supplementary Fig. 6). Expression of MvFAS11 in strain YJZ03 led to the production of 81±1 mg/L MCFAs, which was about 4.0±0.4 times more than the amount produced by the strain expressing wild-type MvFAS01 (Fig. 1i).

To investigate whether co-expression of this engineered bFASI (MvFASI1) with the fFASI variant ScFAS28 has an additive effect on MCFA production, we compared MCFA production of strains ZW2071 (*Δpox1*, *Δhfd1* and *Δura3::ScFAS28*) and ZW2072 (*Δpox1*, *Δhfd1::MvFAS11* and *Δura3::ScFAS28*) under two different cultivation conditions (Fig. 1j). Both strains could produce MCFAs to an extent that was inhibitory to cell growth in regular synthetic media with $(NH_4)_2SO_4$ as the nitrogen source, because acidification of the medium resulting from the assimilation of ammonium elevated the toxicity of MCFAs and promoted growth arrest. We therefore switched to using synthetic media with urea as the nitrogen source (Delft+Urea medium) to stabilize the medium pH during the cultivation. When both strains were cultivated in Delft + Urea + His + Ura medium for 96 h, ZW2072 produced 12.2 ± 0.8% more MCFAs than strain ZW2071. As MvFASI1 preferred to generate C10 fatty acid (Fig. 1h), ZW2072 produced 36±6% more C10 fatty acid compared with ZW2071, which indicated the functionality of MvFASI1 in ZW2072. We found that a dodecane overlay dramatically increased the production of MCFAs by approximately 80% for both strains, indicating that dodecane is an appropriate solvent for in situ extraction of these toxic MCFA products. Similarly, with dodecane addition, ZW2072 produced 15.8±0.3% more total MCFAs and 40 ± 2% more C10 fatty acid than ZW2071. Taken together, both fFASI and bFASI were engineered to generate MCFAs, and simultaneous expression of MvFASI1 and ScFAS28 variants facilitated increased production of MCFAs compared with expression of ScFAS28 alone.

Directed evolution of the transporter Tpo1 The plasma membrane transporter Tpo1 was originally identified as a polyamide transporter, and was later observed to confer resistance of yeast cells to diverse toxic compounds, including C10 fatty acid — the most toxic compound among MCFAs reported. Deletion of *TPO1* resulted in growth arrest in synthetic medium with 50 mg/L of C10 fatty acid, whereas overexpression of *TPO1* from a single-copy plasmid and the *TDH3* promoter (p416GPD vector) restored the resistance against C10 fatty acid (Fig. 2a). We then used directed evolution to obtain a better Tpo1 variant that could potentially enable the yeast cells to have improved tolerance against C10 fatty acid (Fig. 2b). After generation of a random mutagenesis library (~ 8 × $10^4$ mutants) and subsequent enrichment in media with 60 - 90 mg/L C10 fatty acid, three clones expressing Tpo1 mutants (M11, M21 and M41; Fig. 2c and Supplementary Fig. 7a) were selected. The best variant, M21, was used as the template for the second round of directed evolution, and a further-improved variant, M49 (Fig. 2c and Supplementary Fig. 7b), was obtained from the library with 5 × $10^4$ mutants. Expression of M49 and M21 improved cell growth and yielded more cell mass in media with C10 fatty acid, compared with the expression of wild-type Tpo1 (Fig. 2d and Supplementary Fig. 8a). It was shown that the F322L mutation was the major contributor to the phenotype (Supplementary Fig. 7c). Moreover, we found that the M49 mutant improved cell tolerance towards C8 fatty acid as well (Supplementary Fig. 7d). To investigate whether the engineered Tpo1 improved MCFA production, we chromosomally integrated the expression cassettes of wild-type Tpo1 or the M49 variant into strain YHE02 (*pox1Δ* and *tpo1Δ*) and transformed the resultant strains with plasmid pSc-FAS28. Although the C6 and C8 products only slightly increased in the M49-expressing strain, the titres of the other three fatty acids (C10, C12 and C14) produced by the strain expressing the M49 mutant were 0.8 - 2.1-fold higher than the corresponding ones produced by the strain expressing wild-type Tpo1 (Fig. 2e). When two copies of the M49 expression cassettes were integrated, the extracellular fatty acids further increased to 110 ± 2 mg/L, and the titres of each individual product increased by 0.8-3.2-fold (Fig. 2e and Supplementary Fig. 8b). Due to the poor understanding of these major facilitator superfamily transporters, we were unable to deduce the possible roles of the altered amino acid residues. However, it was clearly shown that directed evolution-based transporter engineering can be harnessed to elevate the production levels of chemicals toxic to cells.

Improving cellular resistance against C8 fatty acid by ALE The improvement in cellular resistance against C10 fatty acid through targeted engineering of the Tpo1 transporter was shown to be beneficial for MCFA production (Fig. 2). We then sought to increase cell resistance against C8 fatty acid by ALE, and to obtain additional mutations beneficial for cellular tolerance towards toxic MCFAs. An evolved strain (Lac-4) resistant to a weak acid (lactic acid) was previously obtained by ALE; however, this strain did not have cross-resistance against C8 fatty acid (Supplementary Fig. 9), which led us to establish a new ALE experiment to generate MCFA-tolerant clones. To avoid obtaining tolerant strains with increased activity in MCFA degradation through β-oxidation, we used YJZ02 (*Δpox1*) as the parent strain for ALE. After serially transferring the cells to fresh media containing C8 fatty acid in shake flasks and letting the cells proliferate for more than 100 generations (Fig. 3a), we obtained evolved strains with improved resistance against C8 fatty acid from different stages of the evolution process (Fig. 3b, c and Supplementary Fig. 10a). We evaluated the performance of these evolved strains in terms of MCFA production by introducing the plasmid expressing ScFAS28, and found that they were able to produce more MCFAs (0.3 - 2.2-fold increase for each

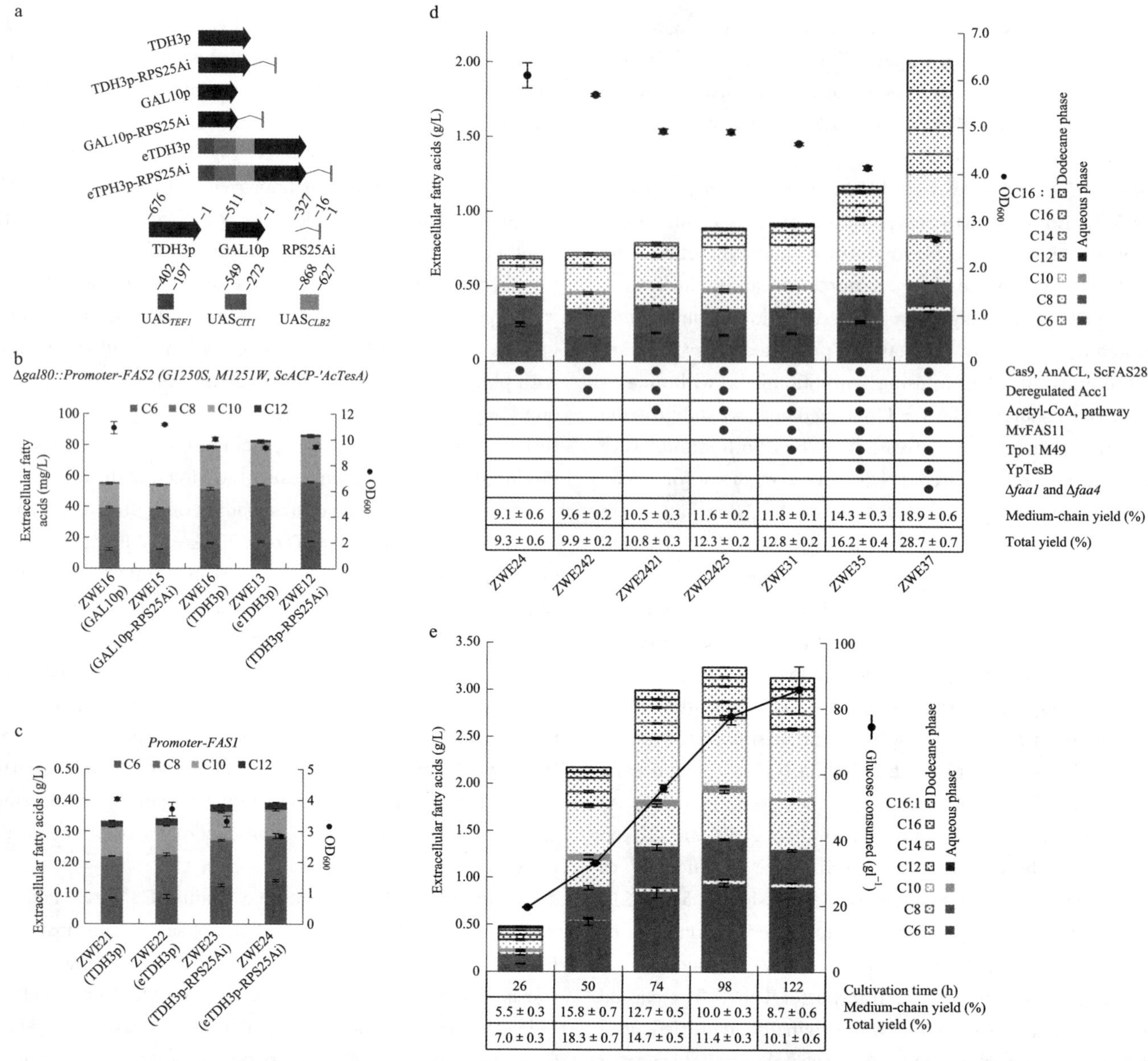


**Fig. 4 MCFAs produced by engineered yeast cell factories**

(a) Structure of promoters used to control the expression of the two subunits of ScFaS28. The numbers indicate the sequence positions. −1 means the nucleotide upstream from the start codon. (b) MCFAs produced by strains expressing the exogenous *FAS2* gene variant under control of the promoters indicated in parentheses. (c) MCFAs produced by strains expressing the endogenous *FAS1* gene by replacing the native *FAS1* promoter with the promoters indicated in parentheses. All of these strains were derived from ZWE12. (d) MCFAs produced by strains with the indicated genetic modifications. A flowchart for the construction of these strains is shown in Supplementary Fig. 14. (e) MCFAs produced by strain ZWE35 during fed-batch cultivation. The cells were cultivated in Delft+Urea+His+Ura media (**b** and **c**) or Delft+Urea+His+Ura media with 15% ($v/v$) dodecane (**d**) for 96 h. The biomass formed (represented as $OD_{600}$; **b**-**d**) and glucose consumed (**e**) are shown. Yield (**d**-**e**) is represented as a percentage of the maximum stoichiometric yield, as calculated in Supplementary Table 1. Error bars (**b**-**e**) represent standard deviation of three or four biological replicates.

individual product) than the parent strain (Fig. 3d and Supplementary Fig. 10b).

We sequenced the genomes of three evolved strains, along with the parent strain YJZ02, to identify genetic mutations that occurred during the ALE process. Seven protein-encoding genes were found to have mutations that altered the protein sequences (Fig. 3b and Supplementary Data 1). Among these genes, *PDR1* encodes a transcription factor regulating multidrug resistance genes. A substitution mutation (Pdr1, M1I) at the start codon of the *PDR1* gene occurred in ZWE01.29 and was passed down to the offspring evolved strains (Fig. 3b and Supplementary Fig. 11). Moreover, one nonsense mutation (Pdr5, Y1142*) in the pleiotropic ABC efflux transporter Pdr5, which is regulated by Pdr1, was identified in ZWE03. This *PDR1* allele (Pdr1, M1I) led to a similar phenotype compared with other alleles (Pdr1, M1*; Pdr1, ΔN181; and Δ*pdr1*) in terms of conferring resistance to C8 fatty acid (Supplementary Fig. 12), which indicated that the mutated Pdr1 (Pdr1, M1I) was a null mutant. Osh2—one of seven members of the oxysterol-binding protein-related proteins (Osh1-Osh7) — has been reported to transport sterols between organelle membranes. A frameshift mutation (Osh2, frameshift) and a substitution mutation (Osh2, D1206Y) were respectively found in two isolates (ZWE01.8 and ZWE01.29) of the ZWE01 population (Fig. 3b and Supplementary Fig. 11). These two mutations probably resulted in loss of function of Osh2, as revealed by structure comparison (Supplementary Fig. 13). As expected, deletion of *OSH2* led to an elevated growth rate in media with C8 fatty acid compared with the parent strain YJZ02, and the level of resistance against C8 fatty acid obtained from deletion of both *OSH2* and *PDR1* was close to that of the final evolved strain ZWE03 (Fig. 3e and Supplementary Fig. 10c), which suggested that the mutations in *OSH2* and *PDR1* were causal for C8 fatty acid resistance.

Engineering yeast cell factories for efficient synthesis of MCFAs To build efficient yeast cells for MCFA production (see the flow-chart for all genetic manipulations in Supplementary Fig. 14), we used the C8 fatty acid-resistant strain ZWE03 as the chassis strain. A *cas9* expression cassette was integrated into the *XI-3* locus of this strain to facilitate genetic engineering via CRISPR-Cas9-mediated genome editing. Two subunits of the acetyl-CoA generating ATP citrate lyase (EC 2.3.3.8) from *Aspergillus nidulans* were expressed under the *GAL1/GAL10* bidirectional promoters to enhance acetyl-CoA supply. Considering that only the Fas2 subunit was modified in the ScFAS28 variant (Fig. 1d), we integrated the *FAS2* gene from ScFAS28 into the *GAL80* locus, thereby inactivating *GAL80* for the autoinduction of *GAL* promoters under glucose-limited conditions. Different promoters (Fig. 4a), including the inducible *GAL10* promoter, the strong constitutive *TDH3* promoter and an enhanced *TDH3* promoter, were evaluated for their control of the expression of the mutated *FAS2* gene. In addition, the intron element from the 5′ UTR of gene *RPS25A* (RPS25Ai) was incorporated into the *GAL10* and *TDH3* promoters, as a previous study had shown that introns in the promoter region could augment the gene expression level. The strain ZWE12, in which the modified *FAS2* gene was expressed under the hybrid *TDH3* promoter containing RPS25Ai, was able to produce 87 ± 1 mg/L extracellular MCFAs (Fig. 4b). We then considered that the amount of Fas1 subunit was probably not sufficient for the FAS complexes, and therefore replaced the promoter of the endogenous *FAS1* gene with the strong *TDH3* promoter or hybrid *TDH3* promoters (Fig. 4c). The MCFA production was elevated by around fourfold; particularly, strain ZWE24 produced 0.39±0.02 g/L MCFAs. However, the high titre of MCFAs resulted in the striking reduction of cell mass yield (Fig. 4b,c). We then used dodecane overlay cultivation for in situ extraction of toxic MCFAs. The total MCFAs from the cell-free aqueous supernatant and the organic phase were 0.70 ± 0.05 g/L for the ZWE24 strain, which is approximately 74% more than that without dodecane overlay. Consistent with this, the cell mass yield also doubled (Fig. 4d), which might resulte from the extraction of toxic products into the dodecane phase.

Acetyl-CoA carboxylase Acc1 is a crucial enzyme for fatty acid synthesis, and its activity is regulated at multiple levels. Phosphorylation of Acc1 by AMP-activated protein kinase (Snf1 in yeast) reduces the activity of Acc1 by up to 90%, and the supposed mechanism is that the phosphorylated Ser1157 residue located in the regulatory loop of the central domain interferes with the Acc1 enzyme dimerization necessary for its activity. Previous attempts at substituting this serine residue with alanine to abolish the phosphorylation regulation resulted in remarkably elevated fatty acid production. Moreover, this manipulation led to increased proportions of long-chain fatty acids (>C16) in yeast cells, and it was also shown that such changes in the fatty acid composition were beneficial for cell resistance against C8 fatty acid stress. We therefore expressed the deregulated Acc1 (S659A and S1157A) through integration of an expression cassette, which was amplified from a previous strain, YT032 (ref.), into strain ZWE12. However, we found that among seven transformants, three contained a back mutation, which resulted in a change of A1157 in the deregulated Acc1 to the serine residue. Besides the genetic instability of the Acc1 mutant (S659A and S1157A), expression of this Acc1 variant also exerted negative effects on MCFA production (Supplementary Fig. 15a,b). As an alternative strategy, the regulatory loop of Acc1 (from residue S1137 to S1170) was replaced with a tetraglycine linker (GGGG) to block the phosphorylation modification, as this loop-deleted Acc1 mutant (Acc1d) retained a considerable activity similar to wild-type unphosphorylated Acc1 (ref.). We introduced such a mutation into the endogenous Acc1 of strain ZWE24 and found that the resultant strain ZWE241 produced more C10 and C12 fatty acids than the control strain ZWE24, even though it produced less C6 fatty acid. Additional expression of another deregulated Acc1 mutant (Acc1d plus S659A) from the *Δgpd1* locus further changed the relative composition of MCFAs produced (Supplementary Fig. 15c). The increase in the chain length of generated MCFAs reflected the elevated availability of malonyl-CoA, as a higher ratio of malonyl-CoA/acetyl-CoA concentration was reported, promoting FASs to form longer-chain products. Although the deployment of deregulated Acc1 only yielded extracellular MCFAs comparable to the background strain

(Fig. 4d and Supplementary Fig. 15c), these metabolic manipulations were kept in further engineered strains.

We then integrated a heterologous acetyl-CoA- and NADPH-generating pathway, which is crucial for lipid accumulation in oleaginous fungi and has been shown to be beneficial for long-chain fatty acid production. Although we had already deployed the heterologous ATP citrate lyase from *A. nidulans*, introducing this chimeric pathway (hereafter called the Acetyl-CoA pathway), which consists of ATP citrate lyase, malic enzyme, cytosolic malate dehydrogenase and the mitochondrial citrate transporter, into the *Δhfd1* locus resulted in an increase in the yield of MCFAs of ~10% and the production of shorter products (C6 and C8; Supplementary Fig. 16). This also indicated elevation of the acetyl-CoA pool and a decrease in the ratio of the malonyl-CoA/acetyl-CoA concentration. Consistent with the above-mentioned results (Fig. 1h - j), additional overexpression of the orthogonal MvFAS11 from the *Δatf2* locus led to increases of C10, C12 and C14 fatty acids of approximately 30, 10 and 70%, respectively, and an increase in the yield of fatty acids of ~10% (Fig. 4d and Supplementary Fig. 16a). After confirming the functionality of the Tpo1 M49 variant in evolved strains with high tolerance to C8 fatty acids (Supplementary Fig. 17a), we introduced the expression cassette of Tpo1 M49 into the *Δeat1* locus of strain ZWE31. This modification did not improve the MCFA production in cultivation with dodecane overlay (Fig. 4d and Supplementary Fig. 17b) because the toxic products were extracted into the organic phase. However, strain ZWE31 produced 13.0 ± 0.7% more MCFAs than the control strain under cultivation without dodecane overlay (Supplementary Fig. 17c).

The FAS variants expressed already possess the ability to release free fatty acids because of the appended thioesterases (Fig. 1b, c). However, free fatty acids generated by the engineered FAS variants are also readily re-activated by acyl-CoA synthetases and then incorporated into lipids, which would hinder the production and secretion of MCFAs. We therefore sought to further express shortchain thioesterases, or delete the endogenous acyl-CoA synthetases. After evaluation of different free-standing thioesterases for MCFA production (Supplementary Fig. 18), the expression of YpTesB in strain ZWE35 resulted in the production of 1.05 ± 0.02 g/L MCFAs during cultivation in shake flasks, which accounted for 89 ± 3% of the total 1.17 ± 0.03 g/L fatty acids secreted (Fig. 4d). Furthermore, 2.87 ± 0.06 g/L MCFAs were produced by consuming 77 ± 4 g/L glucose during fed-batch cultivations for 98 h (Fig. 4e). Further deletion of the *FAA1* and *FAA4* genes encoding the two predominant acyl-CoA synthetases, whose deficiency in yeast could result in secretion of free fatty acids (also see Supplementary Fig. 18e), led to the production of 2.01 ± 0.05 g/L total fatty acids with an approximate yield of 0.1 g/L glucose consumed, of which 1.39 ± 0.05 g/L was MCFAs (Fig. 4d). The additional production of extracellular long-chain fatty acids (C14 and C16) by this *faa1* and *faa4* deletion strain was consistent with previous works on engineering yeast cell factories for free fatty acid production.

Under the current cultivation condition, we observed that the dodecane could extract most of the fatty acid products (>C10) and part of C8 fatty acid, but had minimal ability to capture C6 fatty acid (Figs. 1j and 4d, e). This could be explained by the different partition coefficients of these fatty acids in a water/dodecane biphasic system, which is highly dependent on the hydrophobicity ($\log[P_{oct/wat}]$) and ionization (pKa and pH) of these fatty acid products. It is also noteworthy that the engineered strains contained other gene deletions (*Δgpd1*, *Δhfd1*, *Δatf2*, *Δeat1* and *Δeeb1*). However, all of these modifications had negligible effects on MCFA production (Supplementary Figs. 15 - 18). The intention of employing these genetic modifications relied on the facts that: (1) deletion of *GPD1* was supposed to limit the loss of carbon flux upstream from acetyl-CoA; and (2) deficiency of aldehyde dehydrogenase Hfd1 and alcohol-O-acyltransferases (Atf2, Eat1 and Eeb1) could prevent undesired reactions during medium-chain alcohol formation (one of the applications of using these platform strains efficiently producing MCFAs).

## 2 DISCUSSION

Compared with their long-chain counterparts, which have been produced in engineered microbes at a considerably high titre and yield, MCFAs are more challenging to produce, as they are not inherent metabolites in most organisms and possess cellular toxicity. Because the fFASI is kinetically more efficient than the type II FAS systems and other FASI enzymes, we modified the endogenous fFASI enzyme to enable MCFA production (Fig. 1d - f). We also engineered and utilized the bFASI from *M. vaccae* to increase the flux towards MCFAs (Fig. 1g - j), as this orthogonal bFASI is expected to be free from regulation in yeast cells. Co-expression of both engineered FASI variants in strain ZW2072 led to the production of 70 and 65 mg/L of C8 and C10 fatty acids, respectively, which could seriously impact cell growth. We therefore used two parallel strategies to increase cellular resistance against MCFAs, and the engineered Tpo1 M49 mutant and evolved strains selected from ALE both exerted abilities to elevate MCFA production (Figs. 2e and 3d). Although Tpo1 is involved in diverse resistance phenotypes of yeast, our attempt to engineer Tpo1 by directed evolution increased its activity conferring improved cellular resistance against C10 and C8 fatty acids.

The complementary ALE strategy was used to obtain other beneficial mutations for improved tolerance to C8 fatty acid. *PDR1* and *OSH2*, which were respectively associated with expression regulation of pleiotropic drug-resistance genes and ergosterol transport between membranes, were identified as highly relevant to C8 fatty acid tolerance. Further understanding of the roles of these mutated alleles on the resistance phenotype (for example, through multi-omics studies) would allow the utilization of these mutations for improved cell factory design. Alternatively, mapping the quantitative trait loci will uncover other causative mutations. Changes in fatty acid composition, especially the increase of oleic acid resulting from the expression of deregulated Acc1, were previously shown to mitigate C8 fatty acid toxicity. We therefore also incorporated Acc1 mutants relieved from Snf1-dependent phosphorylation into our engineered strains (Supplementary Fig. 15). We believe that further integration of rational design and random approaches will constantly increase cell tolerance to MCFAs.

Extensive metabolic engineering of the highly tolerant strain ZWE03 through tuning of the expression of ScFAS subunits, enlarging the precursor supply, deploying the engineered MvFAS11 variant and Tpo1 transporter, as well as preventing re-activation of free fatty acids enabled very efficient production of MCFAs. Particularly, 1.39 g/L MCFAs were produced by the engineered strain ZWE37 (Fig. 4d), displaying a higher titre and yield compared with previous set-ups in yeast cell factories (Supplementary Table 2). Considering that the starting strain YJZ02 only produced about 4 mg/L MCFAs, our engineering endeavours resulted in a more than 250-fold improvement in the titre of MCFAs. Because the engineered strains still hold the unmodifed *FAS2* gene and are able to express native FAS complexes predominantly producing long-chain fatty acids. Moreover, the engineered FAS variants deployed presumably retain residual activities for the synthesis of long-chain fatty acids. The final strain ZWE37, with *faa1*/*faa4* deletion, could secrete substantial quantities of long-chain fatty acids (C14 and C16). The further expression of long-chain acyl-CoA synthetases to reduce the leak of long-chain fatty acids (essential metabolites for cellular growth) will improve the cell mass yield as well as the purity of MCFA products. Process optimizations, such as removal of the inhibitory products by organic solvent overlay and recycling of cells, could further improve MCFA production (as is partially shown in Fig. 4e). In addition, these MCFA-producing platform strains could be engineered to produce a range of medium-chain chemicals.

Yield, titre and rate traits of engineered cell factories are quantitative or complex traits that are determined by cumulative actions of many genes and the environment. Improving these metrics to meet the requirements for industrial production is the most challenging part of developing a novel bioprocess. Here, we applied a multidimensional or systems metabolic engineering approach in yeast cell factories to dramatically increase the production of MCFAs. Similar rational-intuitive and/or rational-random strategies for protein/enzyme engineering, pathway optimization and cellular fitness improvement could also be applicable to other cellular production systems for toxic chemicals.

## 3 METHODS

Strains, plasmids and cultivation conditions All strains, plasmids, guide RNA and codon-optimized genes used in this study are listed in Supplementary Tables 3 and 4. The DNA assembler method or the Gibson assembly cloning kit (New England Biolabs) were used for plasmid construction. The strains used for the directed evolution of the Tpo1 transporter were derived from CEN. PK113 - 5D (*MATa SUC2 MAL2 -8c ura3 - 52*). All other yeast strains were derived from CEN. PK113 - 11C (*MATa SUC2 MAL2 -8c his3Δ1 ura3 -52*). A LiAc/SS carrier DNA/PEG method was used for yeast transformation. The complementation of FAS deficiency in PWY12 (*MATα ura3 leu2 his3 trp1 can1 Δfas1::HIS3 Δfas2::LEU2*) by FAS-expressing plasmids, and integration of FAS-expressing cassettes at the *ura3 -52* locus of the YJZ02 strain were carried out as previously described. CRISPR-Cas9-mediated genome engineering was used for other chromosome-based gene knockouts, promoter replacements and gene integrations, as described previously.

YPD medium (10 g/L yeast extract, 20 g/L peptone and 20 g/L glucose; all from Merck Millipore) was used for regular cultures of yeast strains. YPD + G418 medium containing 200 mg/L G418 (Formedium) was used for the selection of transformants with a *kanMX* cassette. CSM-Ura medium containing 20 g/L glucose, 6.7 g/L yeast nitrogen base without amino acids (YNB; Formedium) and 0.77 g/L complete supplement mixture without uracil (CSM-Ura; Formedium) was used for the selection of transformants prototrophic to uracil. CSM + 5-FOA medium containing 6.7 g/L YNB, 0.79 g/L complete supplement mixture (CSM; Formedium) and 0.8 g/L 5-fluoroorotic acid (5-FOA; Sigma-Aldrich) was used for recycling of the *URA3* marker. Then, 20 g/L agar (Merck Millipore) was added to prepare solid media. The detailed recipes of the media used for each experiment are listed in Supplementary Table 5. When needed, 100 mg/L histidine, uracil and/or tryptophan were added to the media. If not specified, Delft medium with 7.5 g/L $(NH_4)_2SO_4$ as the nitrogen source was used. Modified Delft medium (Delft + Urea), in which $(NH_4)_2SO_4$ was replaced with 2.27 g/L urea and 6.6 g/L $K_2SO_4$, was used for the cultivation of strains producing high amounts of MCFAs. A modified YPD medium with 0.1 mol/L $KH_2PO_4$ (pH 6.5) was used for pre-cultivation of engineered strains growing poorly in synthetic medium. 3 mL dodecane was added to 20 mL liquid media for in situ extraction. CSM-Ura media with decanoic acid (C10) was used for the directed evolution of *TPO1*. Delft+His+Ura medium with octanoic acid (C8) was used for ALE of strain YJZ02. Octanoic acid and decanoic acid dissolved in ethanol were added to the medium. The final concentration of ethanol in the medium was 10 g/L.

Directed evolution of the Tpo1 transporter The wild-type *TPO1* gene amplified from strain CEN. PK113-5D was inserted into vector p416GPD to generate p416GPD-TPO1. The random mutagenesis library of *TPO1* was generated through error-prone PCR using the GeneMorph II Random Mutagenesis Kit (Agilent Technologies) according to the low mutation frequency (0-4.5 mutations per kilobase) protocol. The following two primers (forward primer: 5′-cttttatagttagtcttttttttagttttaaaacaccagaacttagtttcgacggatATGTCGGATCA TTCTCCCATTTC-3′; reverse primer: 5′-catgactcgaggtcgac ggtatcgataagcttgatatcgaattcctgcagcccgggTT AAGCGGCGTA AGCATACTTGG-3′) were used for error-prone PCR and the introduction of 50-base pair overlaps (sequences in lower case) homologous to the p416GPD vector, and the wild-type *TPO1* (p416GPG-TPO1) and M21 variant (p416GPD-TPO1-M21) were used as templates for the first and second round of evolution, respectively. The linearized p416GPD vector (digested by XbaI/BamHI) and purified error-prone PCR fragments were used to transform strain YHE02 (*Δtpo1* and *Δpox1*). Approximately 10 transformants were obtained from each transformation, among which >90% of colonies harboured *TPO1* variants. All colonies washed out from plates were first cultivated in 20 mL CSM-Ura medium with 60 mg/L C10 fatty acid for 24 h. Then, 200 μL of cells were transferred to 20 mL CSM-Ura medium with 80 mg/L C10 fatty acid (90 mg/L for the second round of evolution) and cultivated for 48 h. The cells were then diluted 1 : 25 and grown in CSM-Ura medium with 90 mg/L C10 fatty acid (100 mg/L for the second round of evolution) for 48 h. After that, the cells were spread onto CSM-Ura agar plates. A total of 60 single colonies were picked to grow in CSM-Ura medium with 90 mg/L C10 fatty acid (100 mg/L for colonies from the second round), and the growth curves were monitored using a Bioscreen C MBR instrument (Oy Growth Curves). The plasmids from strains with the highest growth rate were extracted and sequenced to identify mutations. These plasmids were transformed into the fresh host strain YHE02. The growth phenotype of the strain YHE02 expressing *TPO1* variants was evaluated in CSM-Ura media with different concentrations of C10 fatty acid or C8 fatty acid using the BioLector microbioreactor (m2p-labs) or Bioscreen C MBR instrument.

ALE The Delft + His + Ura media with different concentrations of C8 fatty acid (Delft + His + Ura + C8) were prepared by mixing one with 0 mg/L C8 fatty acid and the other with 800 mg/L C8 fatty acid. A single colony of the YJZ02 strain was used for inoculation of 20 mL Delft+His+Ura+0 mg/L C8 medium. After cultivation for 24 h, a proportion of the cells was stored in 15% glycerol at −80℃, and this population was designated as the parent strain. The cells were also serially cultivated in Delft+His+Ura+C8 media, as shown in Fig. 3a. At the end of each stage, the culture broth was spread onto YPD agar plates. Then, 30 colonies from YPD plates were cultivated in media with C8 fatty acid. The cell growth rate was monitored using the Bioscreen C MBR instrument. One or two colonies with the highest growth rate were selected for the next stage of evolution.

Genome sequencing and variant calling The genomic DNA of three evolved strains and the parent strain was extracted as previously described. The libraries, prepared by a KAPA HyperPlus kit (Roche), were sequenced using an Illumina MiSeq system (version 2; 300 cycles; 2×150 base pairs). More than 2 million paired-end reads were obtained for each sample. The variant calling was performed as described, using the CEN. PK113-7D genome as the reference genome. Mutations observed in each sample are listed in Supplementary Data 1. The mutations in the *OSH2* and *PDR1* genes were verified by sequencing PCR fragments derived from these genes.

Shake flask cultivation Single colonies were initially used to inoculate 2 mL liquid media and cultivated for 24 h. The cells were then cultivated in 100 mL shake flasks with 20 mL synthetic media supplemented with 20 g/L glucose, 100 mg/L uracil, histidine and/or tryptophan if needed, and/or 3 mL dodecane overlay. Cells growing poorly in synthetic media (strain ZWE24 and its derivatives) were pre-cultivated in 2 mL rich medium (YPD with 0.1 mol/L $KH_2PO_4$, pH 6.5) for 24 h, and washed twice with the desired synthetic medium before inoculation. The initial optical density at 600 nm ($OD_{600}$) was 0.1. For most experiments, the cultivation in shake flasks was maintained for 96 h because of the constant increase of MCFA production until 96 h, as shown previously. However, the cultivation of strain PWY12 was only sustained for 48 h because this strain does not have *Δpox1* deletion, and longer cultivation would result in degradation of MCFAs as glucose was exhausted and these fatty acids can be used as carbon sources. After cultivation for 48 or 96 h, a proportion of aqueous culture broth (0.5, 2 or 4 mL, depending on product titres) was used and adjusted to 4 mL by adding Milli-Q $H_2O$. Then, 0.5 mL 10% NaCl (*W/V*), 0.5 mL acetic acid (containing heptanoic acid and pentadecanoic acid as internal standards; 70 μg/mL) and

2 mL 1∶1 (*v*/*v*) chloroform-methanol were added, and the samples were processed as previously described to extract extracellular fatty acids in aqueous media. The total fatty acid methyl esters (FAMEs) prepared from lyophilized cells according to a previously described method were used for quantification of intracellular fatty acids. For strains cultivated with dodecane overlay, the culture broth was transferred into extraction tubes (16×100 mm PYREX culture tubes and GPI 15-415 Threaded Screw Cap; Corning) and centrifuged at 1,000*g* for 10 min to separate the aqueous and organic layers. The upper dodecane phase was transferred to clean glass tubes, and 0.5 mL lower aqueous solution free of cells and dodecane was taken for the extraction of fatty acids, as described above. From the upper layer, 200 μL dodecane was mixed with 100 μL hexane with internal standards (heptanoic acid and pentadecanoic acid; 2 mg/mL). Then, 20 μL of the mixture was added to 2 mL boron trifluoride-methanol (14%; Sigma-Aldrich). The methylation reaction was carried out at 60℃ for 60 min. After cooling the tubes at 4℃, 2 mL Milli-Q $H_2O$ was added to the reaction tubes, and then 2 mL hexane was added to extract the FAMEs.

Fed-batch fermentation  Individual colonies of the strain ZWE35 were used initially to inoculate 2 mL rich medium (YPD with 0.1 mol/L $KH_2PO_4$, pH 6.5) and cultivated for 24 h, and the cells were then cultivated in 50 mL rich medium in 250 mL flasks for 24 h. Subsequently, the cells were harvested, washed twice and suspended in the initial medium (Supplementary Table 5) for fed-batch cultivation, before inoculating 1 L bioreactors (DASGIP Parallel Bioreactor System; Eppendorf) with 250 mL initial medium and 50 mL dodecane at an $OD_{600}$ of 0.15. The fedbatch fermentation process was monitored and controlled using the DASware Control 5 software (Eppendorf). The temperature was kept at 30℃, and the pH was maintained at 6.0 by the addition of 4 mol/L KOH and 2 mol/L HCl. The dissolved oxygen was maintained above 70% air saturation through a constant aeration rate (36 SL/h) and an agitation rate of 600 rpm. The feeding of concentrated media was initiated after the depletion of glucose and ethanol (26 h after inoculation) with a feeding function as shown in equation (1), where *v* (mL/h) is the feeding rate and *t* (h) is the inoculation time. Feeding medium I containing 400 g/L glucose (Supplementary Table 5) was used in feeding phase I, while feeding medium II containing 600 g/L glucose (Supplementary Table 5) was used in feeding phases II and III. The fatty acid extraction from the cell-free aqueous supernatant and dodecane phase was the same as that from the shake flask culture.

$$v(t) = \begin{cases} 0 & t < 26\,\text{h};\ \text{batch phase} \\ 0.5 \times 10^{0.05(t-26)} & 26\,\text{h} \leqslant t < 74\,\text{h};\ \text{feeding phase I} \\ 0.167 \times 10^{0.05(t-26)} & 74\,\text{h} \leqslant t < 98\,\text{h};\ \text{feeding phase II} \\ 2 & 98\,\text{h} \leqslant t \leqslant 122\,\text{h};\ \text{feeding phase III} \end{cases} \quad (1)$$

Metabolite quantification  The FAMEs were analysed by gas chromatographymass spectrometry, as described in a previous study, except that the ZB-5MS column (30 m × 0.25 mm × 0.25 μm; Phenomenex) and a modified gas chromatography program (an initial temperature at 40℃ for 2 min, increased to 160℃ at a rate of 40℃/min, then increased to 320℃ at a rate of 20℃/min and held for 1 min) were used for analysis of intracellular total fatty acids, because of the higher boiling points of very long-chain fatty acid methyl esters. The residual glucose was measured as described previously.

Statistics and reproducibility  At least two independent experiments started from the cultivation of three or four colonies were performed for each quantification. The two-tailed Welch's unequal variances *t*-test was used for assessment of statistical significance. If not specified, the mean±uncertainty (related to the 95% confidence interval) is presented. The coverage factor *k*, corresponding to the 95% confidence level from the *t*-distribution table, was used for calculation of the uncertainty.

[朱志伟,胡雅婷,等.Nature Catalysis, 2020,3:64-74.]

# *De novo* biosynthesis of liquiritin in *Saccharomyces cerevisiae*

## 1 INTRODUCTION

As an ancient botanical drug with thousands of years of history, licorice root (Glycyrrhizae Radix et Rhizoma, Gan Cao in Chinese) is a widely used medicine mainly derived from the rare and endangered herb *Glycyrrhiza uralensis* Fisch. It shows preventive and therapeutic effects against a variety of diseases with high safety, and appears in almost all Chinese medicine prescriptions, additional health care products, and even food. In addition to triterpenoids such as glycyrrhizin, *G. uralensis* also contains a large group of flavonoids with strong biological activity. The flavonoids include liquiritigenin (LG), and isoliquiritigenin (Iso-LG), as well as their respective glycoside derivatives liquiritin (LN) and isoliquiritin (Iso-LN). Iso-LG is a chalcone with high content in *G. uralensis*, and also a common natural pigment. In spite of its simple structure, Iso-LG has many significant pharmacological activities such as antiinflammatory, anticancer, antihistamine, antioxidation, antiplatelet agglutination, antiallergy, antivirus and estrogen-like activities. Its glycoside derivative Iso-LN is capable of inhibiting tumor angiogenesis, as well as showing antidepressant effects. LG is a dihydroflavone compound formed by the isomerization of Iso-LG, which can inhibit the proliferation of certain cancer cells and induce apoptosis. Its glycoside derivative LN is the quality indicator component of licorice root as prescribed in Chinese Pharmacopoeia. In addition to inducing apoptosis and autophagy in gastric cancer cells, LN can also fight depression. These observations indicate that *G. uralensis* has good development and application prospects in the treatment of cancer and other diseases. Along with the attention of the cosmetics industry in search of additives from natural sources, it was found that flavonoids in *G. uralensis*, especially the above-mentioned components, can be used for the removal of reactive oxygen species (ROS), as well as the safe and gentle whitening of human skin, and as such has been used by Nivea, Shiseido, YUE-SAI cosmetics, etc.

Due to the enormous market demand, wild *G. uralensis* has been overharvested. Once damaged, the *G. uralensis* population is difficult to recover, and the amount of wild *G. uralensis* in China had been reduced to less than 500,000 tons as early as 2009. In addition to the large reduction of *G. uralensis* production, unsustainable development also led to environmental damage and desertification in the growing area. Coupled with the limitations of chemical synthesis and plant cell culture, sourcing the main flavonoids of *G. uralensis* through heterologous biosynthesis has become an effective strategy for the sustainable development of *G. uralensis* resources. In recent years, engineered strains have been used to produce various natural products of plant origin, including artemisinic acid, ginsenoside, paclitaxel, tanshinone, etoposide aglycone and opioids. As a medicinal plant of great concern, the genome of *G. uralensis* has been sequenced and published, and the biosynthesis pathway of the triterpenoid glycyrrhizin has been fully analyzed. However, the biosynthesis of LN has rarely been investigated, even though it is the main active flavonoid component in *G. uralensis*.

In this study, the key enzyme-coding genes responsible for LN biosynthesis, starting from phenylalanine ammonia-lyase, were screened out by combined genome and transcriptome analysis of *G. uralensis* and known homologous genes in the flavonoid biosynthesis pathway. The obtained LN pathway was recon-structed in yeast to realize the heterologous synthesis of the main flavonoids of *G. uralensis*, including LG, Iso-LG, LN, and Iso-LN, which provides a new method for the production and sustainable utilization of *G. uralensis* flavonoids.

## 2 MATERIALS AND METHODS

2.1 Plant materials and stress treatment  Seeds of *G. uralensis* Fisch., collected in Gansu province, were identified by Prof. Chunsheng Liu (Beijing University of Chinese Medicine, Beijing, China). The seeds were immersed in concentrated sulfuric acid for 70 min, then washed with deionized water and soaked at room temperature for 24 h. The treated seeds were sown in vermiculite and grown for 30 days in an artificial climate box (25℃, cycles of 16 h light:8 h dark). After treatment with 0.5% NaCl or 100 mmol/L methyl jasmonate (MeJA) for 7 days, the treated plants were washed and frozen in liquid nitrogen and stored at −80℃.

2.2 Chemicals  All of the chemical reference substances, including liquiritigenin (CAS: 578-86-9), isoliquiritigenin (CAS: 961-29-5), isoliquiritin (CAS: 5041-81-6), liquiritin (CAS: 551-15-5), phenylalanine (CAS: 63-91-2), cinnamic acid (CAS: 140-10-3), *p*-coumaric (CAS: 501-98-4), malonyl-CoA (CAS: 108347-84-8), coumaroyl-CoA (CAS: 119785-99-8), naringenin chalcone (CAS: 73692-50-9), UDP-glucose (CAS: 28053-08-9), and NADPH (CAS: 2646-71-1), had purity >98% and were commercially available (Sigma—Aldrich, Saint Louis, MO, USA; Yuanye, Shanghai, China).

2.3 Deep Illumina sequencing and transcriptome analysis  Total RNA was extracted from three biological replicates of *G. uralensis* roots using the Plant Easy Spin RNA Miniprep Kit (BIOMIGA, San Diego, CA, USA). A cDNA library was constructed after the RNA samples were qualified by Novogene (Beijing, China), and then sequenced on an HiSeq 4000 platform (Illumina, San Diego, CA, USA). The reference genome of *G. uralensis* (http://ngs-data-archive.psc.riken.jp/Gur-genome/download.pl.) was used for bioinformatic transcriptome analysis, and supplemented gene functions were comprehensively annotated based on the following databases: Nr (NCBI nonredundant protein sequences), Nt (NCBI nonredundant nucleotide sequences), Pfam (protein families), KOG/COG (clusters of orthologous groups of proteins), SwissProt (a manually annotated and reviewed protein sequence database), KEGG (Kyoto encyclopedia of genes and genomes database), GO (gene ontology) and KO (KEGG Orthology). The abundance of unigenes was normalized using the FPKM (Fragments Per Kilobase of exon per Million mapped fragments) values.

According to the annotation, the sequences of seven candidate key functional genes in the flavonoid biosynthesis pathway, including the sequences which encoding phenylalanine ammonialyase (PAL), cinnamate 4-hydroxylase (C4H), 4-coumarate CoA ligase (4CL), chalcone synthase (CHS), chalcone reductase (CHR), chalcone isomerase (CHI) and isoflavonoid 7-*O*-glycosyltransferase (F7GT/UGT), were selected. The homologous sequences of candidate genes were searched against the NCBI database and evolutionary analyses were conducted in MEGA 6.0 (Phoenix, USA) by sampling 1 000 bootstrap replicates. Differential gene expression analysis was performed using HemI 1.0 (Wuhan, China), the abundance of candidate genes was represented by $\log_2$ values of FPKM, and sequences with $\log_2$ FPKM$\leqslant -1$ were assigned as low expression in the samples which were excluded from the statistical data. The full-length cDNAs of the target genes were amplified by PCR using Phusion High-Fidelity PCR Master Mix (BioLabs, Ipswich, USA), and the primers designed based on the transcriptomic data (Supporting Information Table S1).

2.4 Bacterial expression and in vitro characterization The ORFs of *PAL*, *CHS*, *CHR*, *CHI* and *UGT* were individually inserted between the *Kpn*I and *Xho*I restriction sites of pET-32a(+) using the EasyGeno Assembly Cloning kit (Tiangen, Beijing, China), and transferred into *Escherichia coli* BL21 (DE3). All primers used in vector construction are listed in Supporting Information Table S2. Transformants were screened on Luria-Bertani (LB) solid culture medium containing 100 mg/mL ampicillin and single clones were picked for sequencing verification. The recombinant cells were cultured in 200 mL of LB medium containing 100 mg/mL ampicillin at 37℃ to an $OD_{600}$ = 0.6 − 1.0, after which expression was induced by isopropyl β-D-thiogalactoside (IPTG) at a final concentration of 0.2 mmol/L and continued at 16 ℃ for 10 h. The expressing cells were harvested by centrifugation at 8 000 × *g* and 4 ℃, resuspended in 3 mL phosphate buffered solution (pH = 8.0), and disrupted by ultrasonication in an ice-bath. The crude lysate was cleared from cell debris by centrifugation at 12,000 × *g* and 4 ℃ and the supernatant was collected for purification. Recombinant protein was purified using the His-Tagged Protein Purification Kit (soluble protein, CWBIO, Beijing, China), and concentrations were measured using the Enhanced BCA Protein Assay Kit (Beyotime, Shanghai, China) with BSA as the standard.

The 1 mL enzymatic reaction systems contained about 0.5 mmol/L recombinant protein (10 mmol/L phosphate buffer solution, pH = 8.0), 1 mmol/L D, L-dithiothreitol (DTT), and 1 mmol/L substrate. For CHR, an equal amount of recombinant CHS protein with known function and 1 mmol/L NADPH were added to the enzymatic system. 25 mmol/L UDP-glucose was added to the enzymatic reaction system of UGT. The reaction was incubated at 30 ℃ for 10 h and stopped by the addition of 200 μL methanol. The catalytic products were analyzed by HPLC-Q-TOF-MS.

2.5 Yeast expression and in vivo characterization Cytochrome P450 gene *C4H* was expressed in *Saccharomyces cerevisiae* WAT11 using pESC-HIS as expression vector. While the catalytic product of 4CL is unstable, the candidate *4CL* and the *CHS* with known function were co-expressed in WAT11 using the binary vector pESC-LEU as expression vector. The yeast expression vector was constructed using the EasyGeno Assembly Cloning kit (Tiangen, Beijing, China). *C4H* and *CHS* were individually inserted between the *Spe*I and *Not*I sites, and *4CL* was inserted between the *Nhe*I and *BamH*I sites of the *CHS* recombinant vector. The recombinant plasmid was transferred into WAT11 using the Frozen-EZ Yeast Transformation Kit II (Zymo Research, Los Angeles, USA), and transformants were grown on corresponding auxotrophy synthetic medium (SC-His or -Leu) with 2% glucose and 2% agar at 30 ℃ for 4 days. Positive clones were cultivated in the corresponding liquid auxotrophy medium (2% glucose) and shaken at 30 ℃ to an $OD_{600}$ of about 0.8. The 2% glucose medium was exchanged for induction medium containing 2% galactose, and after induction at 30 ℃ and 220 rpm (Honour, Tianjing, China) for 6 h, 20 μmol/L cinnamic acid or coumaric acid was added and the cultivation continued for another 12 h. The fermentation broth was extracted with an equal volume of ethyl acetate three times, and after evaporation of the solvent, the products re-dissolved in methanol and analyzed by HPLC-Q-TOF-MS after passing through a 0.22 μm polytetrafluoroethylene (PTFE) filter.

2.6 HPLC-Q-TOF-MS analysis of catalytic product The catalytic products were analyzed using an Agilent 1 200 HPLC system coupled with an Agilent Q-TOF 6 520 mass spectrometer (Agilent, Santa Clara, CA, USA) equipped with an electrospray ionization (ESI) device. Gradient elution was performed on an Agilent XDB-C18 column (150 mm × 2.1 mm, 3.5 μm) at room temperature with a flow rate of 0.3 mL/min using a linear gradient with water containing 0.1% formic acid (A) and acetonitrile (B) as the mobile phases as follows: 0 - 3 min, 5% B; 3 - 9 min, 25% B; 9 - 11 min, 25%- 55% B; 11 - 14 min, 55%- 95% B; 14 - 27 min, 95% B; 27 - 30 min, 95%- 5% B. The injection volume was 20 μL.

2.7 Quantitative real-time PCR (qRT-PCR) analysis Total RNA was extracted from roots, stems and leaves of *G. uralensis* seedlings, and reverse transcription was done used the PrimeScript™ 1st-Strand cDNA Synthesis Kit (Takara, Dalian, China) according to the manufacturer's instructions. The qRT-PCR was performed using the KAPA SYBR FAST

Universal qPCR Kit (Kapa Biosystems, Boston, MA, USA) with gene-specific primer pairs (Supporting Information Table S3). Three technical replicates and three biological replicates were analyzed for each sample. The relative amounts of the target genes were evaluated based on the relative expression index of mRNA using the $2^{-\Delta\Delta Ct}$ method, with *Guβ-actin* as the reference gene.

2.8 Extraction of main flavonoids from G. uralensis After fully pulverizing in liquid nitrogen, samples comprising about 100 mg of freeze-dried roots, stems or leaves of *G. uralensis* seedlings that were grown for one month were accurately weighed, after which 1 mL 70% ethanol was added and the samples ultrasonically extracted at 30 ℃ for 30 min. The product was centrifuged, and the supernatant was passed through a 0.22 μm PTFE filter for quantitative UPLC - MS analysis.

2.9 Reconstitution of the liquiritin biosynthesis pathway in yeast and product analysis The genes of the *G. uralensis* flavonoid pathway with known function (*GuPAL1*, *GuC4H1*, *Gu4CL1*, *GuCHS1*, *GuCHR1*, *GuCHI1*, and *GuUGT1*) were inserted in different combinations into the binary vector pESC downstream of the GAL1 or GAL10 promoters. The 3′ end of *GuCHS1* was fused to the 5′ end of *GuCHR1 via* the linker sequence GGTGGTGGTTCT (*GuCHS1::GuCHR1*). The constructs were verified by bi-directional sequencing, and the resulting plasmids were used to transform the yeast strain WAT11 using the Frozen-EZ Yeast Transformation kit II (Zymo Research, Los Angeles, CA, USA). The transformants were selected on synthetic dropout plates (SC-His, -Leu, -Trp or -Ura) according to the vector label and the positive yeast clones were cultured in SC medium with 2% glucose at 30 ℃ and 220 rpm (Honour, Tianjing, China), and then harvested and resuspended in SC medium with 2% galactose followed by expression for 36 h. All recombinant yeast strains used in this study are listed in Supporting Information Table S4. 500 μL fermentation broth was taken and mixed with an equal volume of methanol, ultrasonicated for 60 min and centrifuged at 13,400× *g* for 10 min. The supernatant was analyzed by UPLC - MS after passing through a 0.22 μm PTFE filter.

2.10 Fermentation Strain WM4 - 3 was used for the production of liquiritin in fed-batch fermentation. Synthetic dropout medium (SC-His-Leu-Trp-Ura) was used for both seed preparation and the fermentation. The seed culture was prepared by inoculating a 250 mL flask containing 100 mL culture medium with 2% glucose. The cells were grown at 30 ℃ and 250 rpm (Honour, Tianjing, China) for 48 h, and then transferred into 1 L of fresh seed medium and incubated at 30 ℃ and 220 rpm (Honour, Tianjing, China) for 36 h. The resulting seed was harvested and used to inoculate an 11 L New Brunswick™ BioFlo ®/CelliGen ® 115 fermenter (Eppendorf, Hamburg, Germany) containing 6 L of induction medium (SC-His-Leu-Trp-Ura with 2% galactose) to an initial $OD_{600}$ = 1.5 — 2.0. The fermentation was carried out at 30 ℃. The dissolved oxygen concentration (DOC) was kept above 40% and the pH was controlled at 5.0 using automatic addition of ammonium hydroxide. Concentrated synthetic dropout medium (SC-His-Leu-Trp-Ura; 80 g/L total solids) and 40% galactose were automatically fed to the fermenter separately at a rate of 6.25 mL/h from the second day. The fermentation broth was sampled at intervals of 24 h to measure the $OD_{600}$, and an aliquot of 500 μL volume was mixed with an equal volume of methanol, ultrasonicated for 60 min, centrifuged at 13,400× *g* for 10 min, and the supernatant was stored at −20 ℃ until UPLC - MS analysis.

2.11 Quantitative UPLC - MS analysis The separation of 1 μL filtrate was performed using an Agilent ZORBAX RRHD SB - C18 column (100 mm×2.1 mm, 1.8 μm) on an Agilent 1 290 Infinity UPLC system (Agilent, Santa Clara, CA, USA) by gradient elution with a mobile phase comprising 0.1% (*v/v*) formic acid aqueous solution (A) and acetonitrile (B) at a flow rate of 0.3 mL/min. The gradient program was as follows: 0 - 1.0 min, 25% B; 1.0 - 4.0 min, 25% - 90% B; 4.0 - 4.5 min, 90% B; 4.5 - 4.51 min, 90%- 25% B; 4.51 - 5.5 min, 25%. The column temperature was set at 25 ℃.

The analyte was quantified using an AB Sciex LC - MS/MS Qtrap 6 500 mass spectrometer equipped with an electrospray ionization (ESI) source (AB Sciex, Singapore). The multiple reaction monitoring (MRM) scan type was used in the negative scan mode to increase the specificity of the analysis. The mass parameters are listed in Table 1. The software MultiQuant 3.0.1 (AB Sciex, Singapore) was used to perform the data analysis.

**Table 1 MS parameters for the quantification of analytes**

| Component | Q1 Mass (Da) | Q3 Mass (Da) | Declustering potential (V) | Collision energy (V) |
|---|---|---|---|---|
| *p*-Coumaric | 163 | 119 | −60 | −23 |
| acid | | 93 | −60 | −40 |
| Isoliquiritigenin | 255 | 135 | −80 | −21 |
| | | 119 | −80 | −30 |
| Isoliquiritin | 417 | 255 | −180 | −25 |
| | | 135 | −180 | −30 |
| Liquiritigenin | 255 | 119 | −100 | −25 |
| | | 135 | −100 | −20 |
| Liquiritin | 417 | 255 | −70 | −27 |
| | | 135 | −70 | −40 |

2.12 Accession numbers Sequence data from this article can be found in the GenBank database under the following accession numbers: *GuPAL1* (MK341789), *GuC4H1* (MK341785), *Gu4CL1* (MK341782), *GuCHS1* (MK341787), *GuCHR1* (MK341786), *GuCHI1* (MK348532), *GuUGT1* (MK341792); the transcriptome datasets: Gu-CK, SRR8400027; Gu-NaCl, SRR8400026; Gu-MeJA, SRR8468083.

## 3 RESULTS

3.1 Screening of liquiritin pathway genes Water deficiency can increase the yield of LN in the roots of *G. uralensis*, and MeJA is also believed to increase the production of flavonoids. Consequently, deep sequencing of the *G. uralensis* root transcriptome was performed after NaCl- and MeJA-treatment, respectively (Supporting Information Tables S5 and S6). The reference genome of *G. uralensis* was used in combination with the Nr, Nt, Pfam, KOG/COG, SwissProt, KO and GO databases for bioinformatics analysis, and gene functions were comprehensively annotated, and a total of 61 genes that were annotated to encode the seven enzymes required for the biosynthesis of LN were screened from the transcriptome database (Supporting Information Table S7). Hierarchical cluster analysis of the candidate genes revealed that *GuPAL1*, *GuC4H1*, *GuCHS1*, *GuCHR1*, *GuCHR4*, *GuCHI1*, *GuCHI5* and *GuUGT1* had relatively high expression levels in both NaCl- or MeJA-treated and control *G. uralensis*. Furthermore, the treatment, and especially NaCl stress, increased the expression levels of these genes to some extent. The expression level of *Gu4CL1* under NaCl stress was significantly higher than under MeJA stress or in the CK group (Fig. 1). In addition, multiple sequence alignment results showed that GuPAL1, GuC4H1, Gu4CL1, and GuCHS1 were respectively 78%, 92%, 72%, and 85% identical to *Populus* hybrid (*P. trichocarpa* × *P. deltoides*) PAL, *Glycine max* C4H, *Petroslinum crispum* 4CL-2, and *P.* hybrid (*P. trichocarpa* × *P. deltoides*) CHS1, which were commonly used for heterologous synthesis of plant-specific flavones.

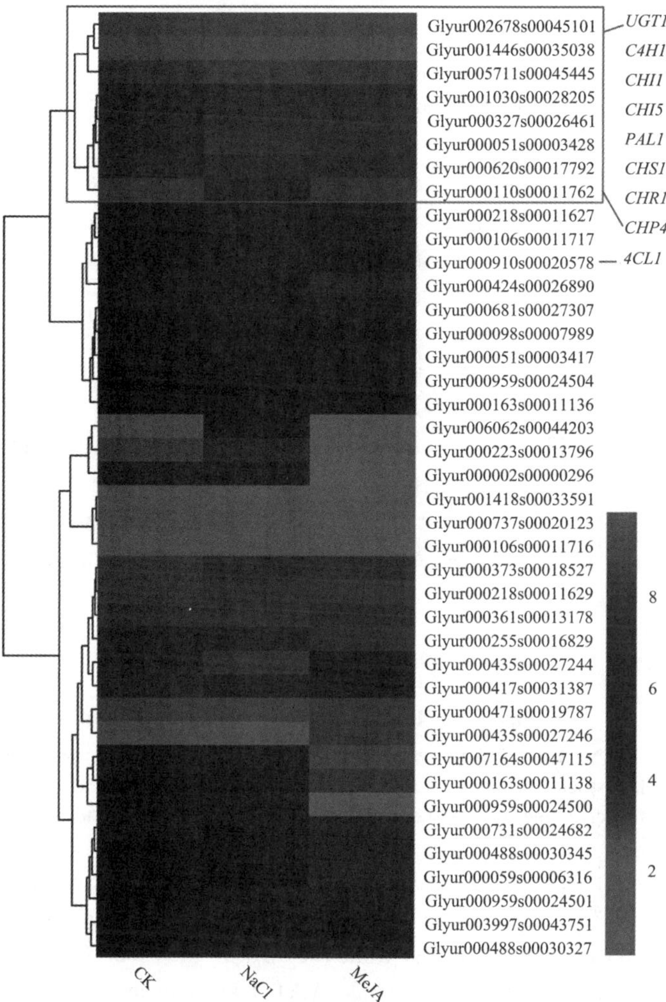


**Figure 1 Hierarchical clustering and corresponding heatmaps of the differentially expressed unigenes across the flavonoid biosynthesis pathway**

CK, control; NaCl, root sample treated with 0.5% NaCl; MeJA, root sample treated with 100 mmol/L MeJA. The heatmap was drawn using HemI 1.0 with log2 values of FPKM (Fragments Per Kilobase of exon per Million mapped fragments) of the candidate genes, and the sequences with $\log_2$ FKPM $\leqslant -1$ were assigned as low expression in the samples which were excluded from the statistical data. Depths of color in the red and green rectangles indicate higher and lower Z-scores ($\log_2$) of the corresponding RNA expression levels. The red font indicates the sequences used for liquiritin pathway reconstruction in yeast.

Subsequently, to screen for the unique CHR and CHI, BLASTX analysis was performed using the NCBI database with the nucleic acid sequences that were annotated as encoding chalcone reductase (or NAD(P)H-dependent 6′-deoxychalcone synthase) and chalcone isomerase, respectively. The sequences with higher identity were used for the neighbor-joining tree construction. Four *CHR* candidate genes were divided into three subgroups in the neighbor-joining tree (Fig. 2A) with GuCHR1, GuCHR2, GuCHR3 belonging to subgroup A, wherein GuCHR1 shares 87% identity to *G. max* CHR5, which had the closest correlation with the accumulation of abundant 5-deoxyisoflavonoids in soybean root. GuCHR4, which is also highly expressed in *G. uralensis*, was clustered in subgroup B with *G. max* CHR4, which previous studies suggested to have no CHR activity for the production of Iso-LG. The eight CHI homologs from *G. uralensis* were classified into four CHI types, whereby GuCHI1 belonged to type II CHIs, which were thought to have the activity of isomerizing Iso-LG into LG, whereas GuCHI5 fell into the type IV subfamily (Fig. 2B).

3.2 Functional characterization of liquiritin pathway enzymes In order to confirm the catalytic function of the enzymes encoded by the candidate genes, *GuPAL1*, *GuCHS1*, *GuCHR1*, *GuCHI1* and *GuUGT1* were expressed

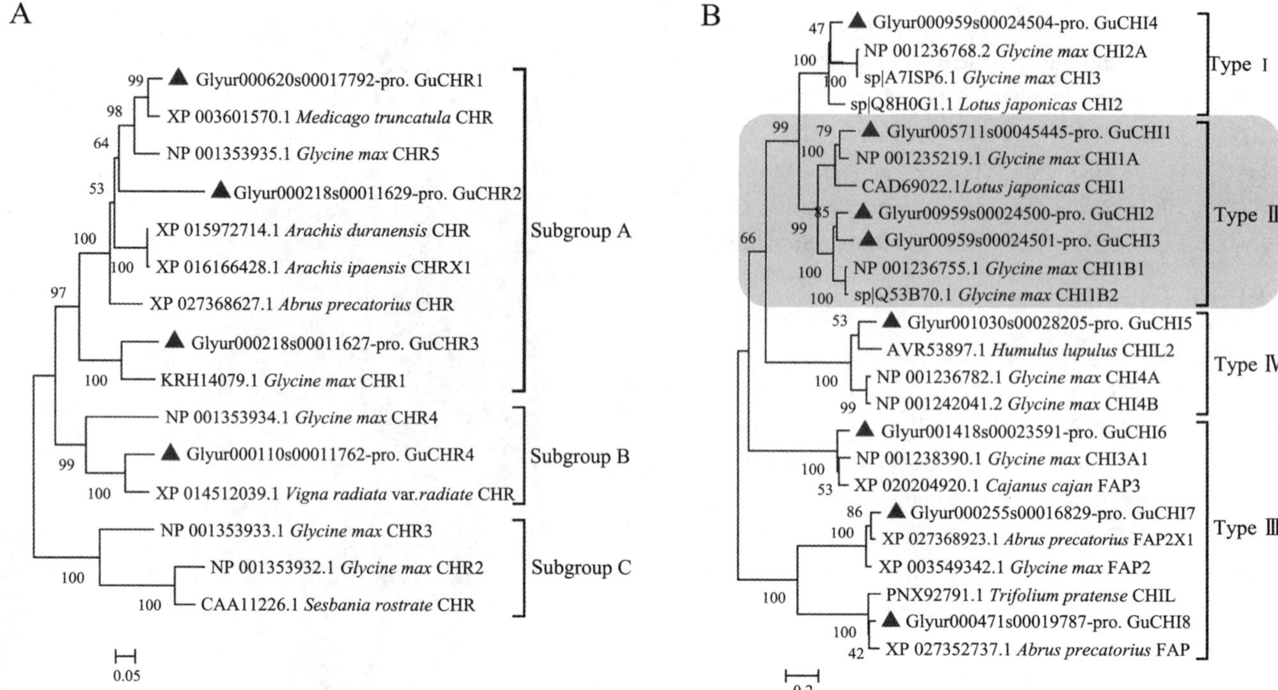


**Figure 2 Phylogenetic analysis of the amino acid sequences of CHR and CHI based on the *G. uralensis* transcriptome**

The evolutionary analyses were conducted in MEGA6.0 using the neighbor-joining method, and the percentage of replicate trees in which the associated taxa clustered together among the 1 000 replicates in the bootstrap test are shown next to the branches. Sequences from the transcriptome were marked with red triangles. Red font indicates the sequences used for liquiritin pathway reconstruction in yeast.

in *E. coli* and the recombinant proteins were extracted and purified (Supporting Information Fig. S1) for *in vitro* enzymatic experiments, while the cytochrome P450 *GuC4H1* was expressed in *S. cerevisiae* WAT11. As indicated by LC-MS, incubation of the staring substrate phenylalanine with GuPAL1 yielded cinnamic acid (Fig. 3B). Similarly, the recombinant yeast harboring *GuC4H1* was able to produce *p*-coumaric acid upon feeding cinnamic acid and galactose (Fig. 3C). In an *in vitro* enzymatic system with coumaroyl-CoA and malonyl-CoA as substrates at a molar ratio of 1:3, naringenin chalcone was produced when only GuCHS1 was added. When the same amount of recombinant GuCHS1 and GuCHR1 proteins and a high concentration of NADPH (1 mmol/L) was added, the production of Iso-LG was also detected in addition to naringenin chalcone (Fig. 3E). As the catalytic product of 4CL was unstable, Gu4CL1 and GuCHS1 were co-expressed in WAT11 using the binary plasmid pESC-LEU as yeast expression vector. Upon feeding with *p*-coumaric acid, naringenin chalcone could also be detected in the culture extracts (Fig. 3D). GuCHI1, which belongs to type II CHIs, was able to isomerize Iso-LG into LG in *in vitro* enzymatic experiments, demonstrating its CHI activity (Fig. 3F). Thus, GuPAL1, GuC4H1, Gu4CL1, GuCHS1, GuCHR1 and GuCHI1 formed a complete biosynthetic pathway of liquiritigenin with phenylalanine as the precursor (Fig. 3A).

In the final step of LN biosynthesis, GuUGT1 was able to produce LN from LG *in vitro* with UDP-glucose as sugar donor (Fig. 3G). The kinetic parameters of GuUGT1, GuUGT2 and GuUGT3, respectively belong to UGT88E, UGT88H and UGT88A subfamilies within the UGT88 family (Supporting Information Fig. S2), were subsequently determined. Not surprisingly, GuUGT1 ($K_m$ 68.17 μmol/L and $V_{max}$ 0.87 μmol/(min · mg)) exhibited a higher maximum activity, and its catalytic efficiency ($V_{max}/K_m$) was also clearly higher (Supporting Information Section 1, Fig. S3 and Table S8). To investigate the structural basis for the binding of LG and UDP-glucose, a homology model was generated for GuUGT1 using the crystal structure of *Arabidopsis thaliana* UGT (PDB ID: 2VCE) with 34% identity as template (Supporting Information Section 2 and Fig. S4). The key residues of *GuUGT1* for liquiritigenin glycosylation (Gly-14 and Gly-277) predicted by molecular docking (Supporting Information Section 3, Tables S9, S10 and Fig. S5) and residue scanning based on simulated mutations (Supporting Information Section 4 and Table S11) were different from those of the known flavonoid glucosyltransferase VvGT1 (His-20 and Asp-119) or isoflavonoid 7-*O*-glycosyltransferase GmIF7GT (Glu-392), which also belong to the UGT88E subfamily.

A comparison was made between the expression profiles of the enzymes whose catalytic functions and flavonoid accumulation in different tissues of *G. uralensis* were characterized. A pattern emerged that indicated that most LN pathway genes were mainly expressed in leaves, except

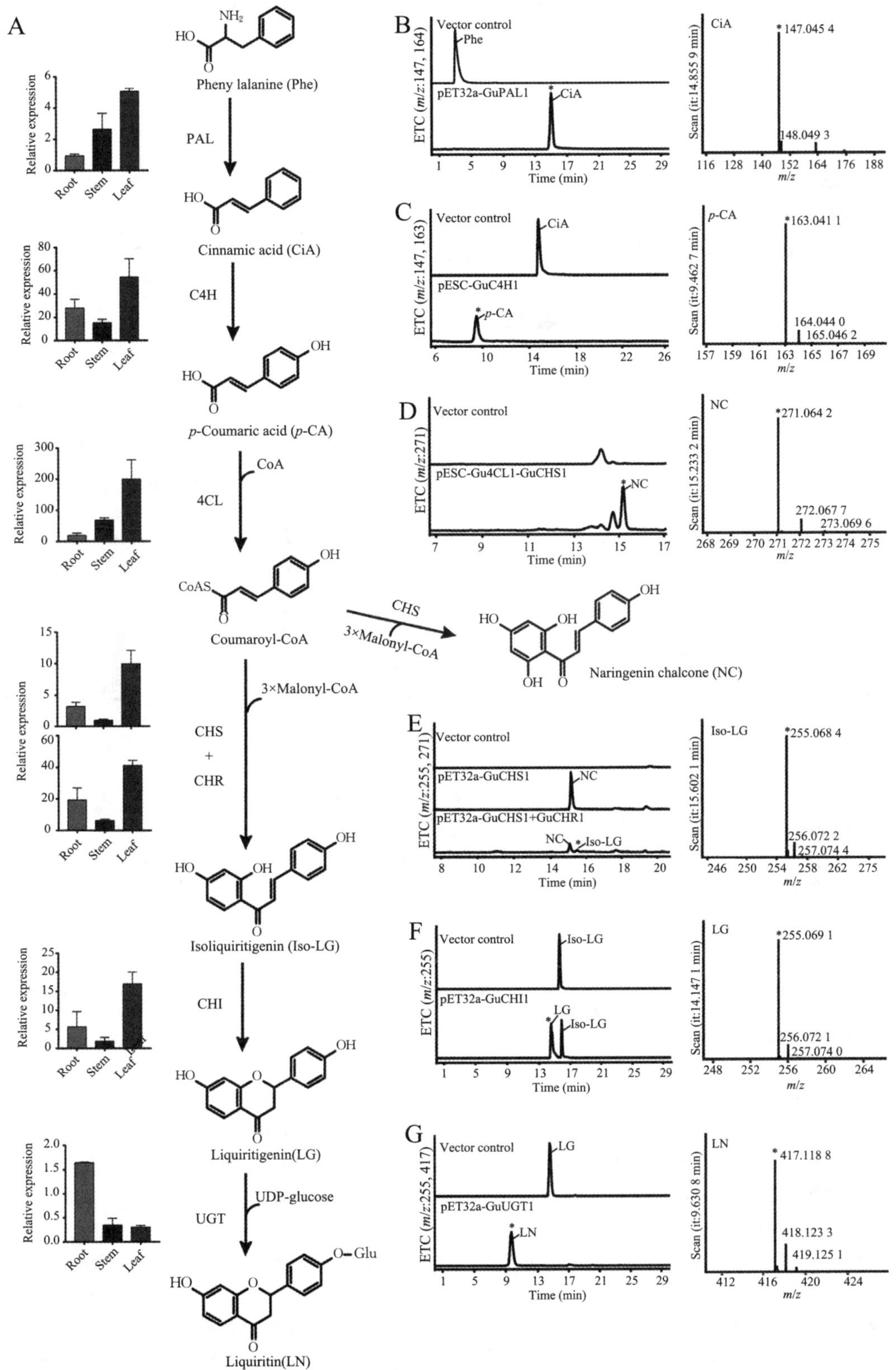


**Figure 3 Analysis of catalytic products of the enzymes encoded by the candidate genes**

(A) The liquiritin biosynthesis pathway of *G. uralensis*, the histogram next to each pathway enzyme name shows relative expression levels of the encoding gene (*GuPAL1*, *GuC4H1*, *Gu4CL1*, *GuCHS1*, *GuCHR1*, *GuCHI1* and *GuUGT1*) in roots, stems and leaves of *G. uralensis* determined by qRT-PCR; (B, E-G) HPLC-Q-TOF-MS profiles of the *in vitro* enzymatic products of recombinant GuPAL1 [B, phenylalanine (Phe) as substrate], GuCHS1 and GuCHR1 (E, coumaroyl-CoA as substrate), GuCHI1 [F, isoliquiritigenin (Iso-LG) as a substrate], GuUGT1 [G, liquiritigenin (LG) as a substrate] expressed in *E. coli* using pET-32a(+) as expression vector; (C, D) HPLC-Q-TOF-MS profiles of the fermentation products of yeast harboring the recombinant vector pESC-GuC4H1 [C, cinnamic acid (CiA) as a substrate] or pESC-Gu4CL1-GuCHS1 [D, *p*-coumaric acid (*p*-CA) as substrate] with external precursor addition. The peaks and mass spectrum of the product indicated by the asterisk, are shown (electron ionization in negative-ion mode, $[M-H]^-$). Extracted-ion chromatogram (EIC) of the analyte, as indicated, at $m/z$ 147,164 (B), $m/z$ 147,163 (C), $m/z$ 271 (D), $m/z$ 255,271 (E), $m/z$ 255 (F), $m/z$ 255,417 (G). All the reactions were performed with empty vector as control.

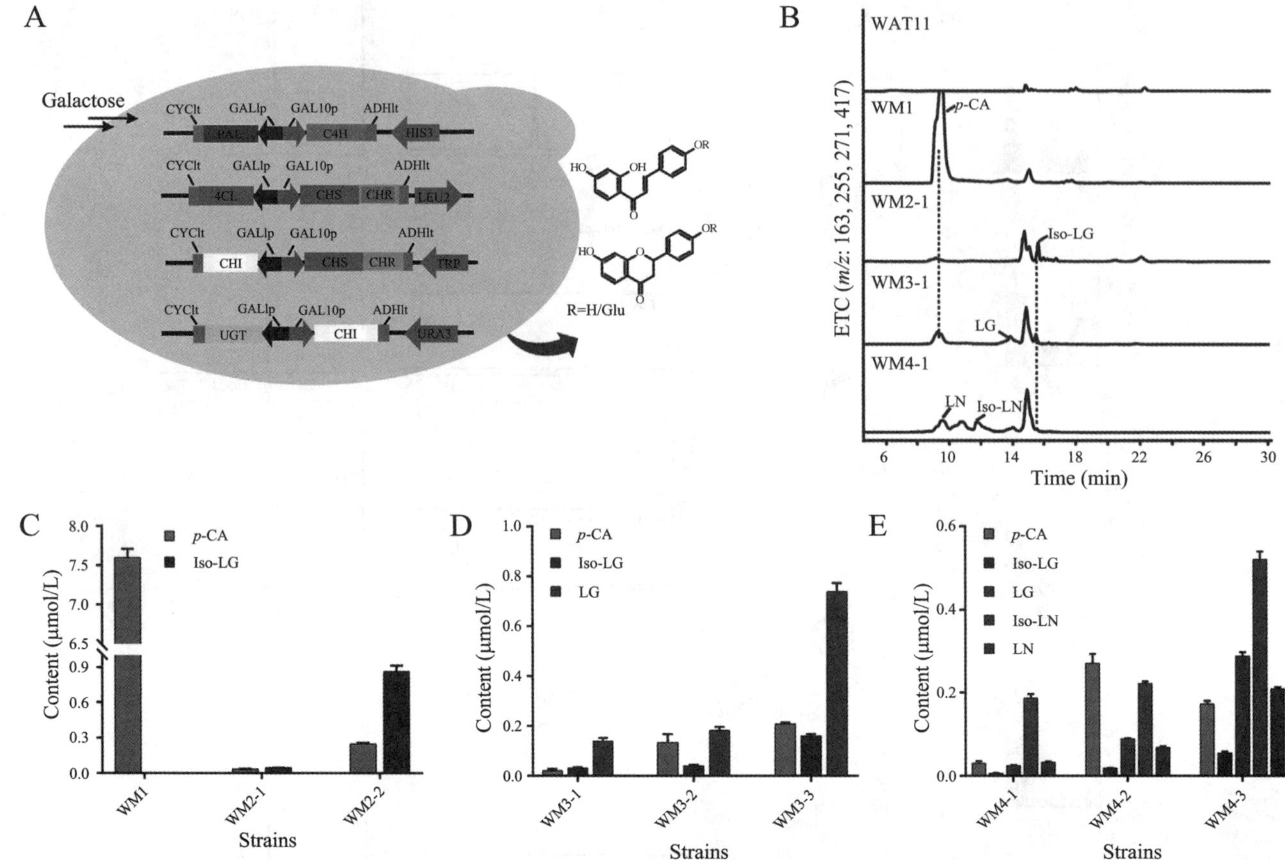


**Figure 4 Reconstitution of the biosynthesis pathway of liquiritin in yeast**

(A) Schematic of the recombinant yeast strain WM4 - 1. (B) Chromatogram of selected ions with $m/z$ 163, 255, 271 and 417 from the fermentation products of the recombinant yeasts using HPLC-Q-TOF-MS; (C) Production of *p*-CA and Iso-LG by yeast stains WM1 (harboring *GuPAL1*, *GuC4H1*), WM2 - 1 (harboring *GuPAL1*, *GuC4H1*, *Gu4CL1*, *GuCHS1*::*GuCHR1*) and WM2 - 2 (*GuCHS1*::*GuCHR1* overexpressed in WM2 - 1); (D) Production of *p*-CA, Iso-LG and LG by yeast stains WM3 - 1 (harboring *GuPAL1*, *GuC4H1*, *Gu4CL1*, *GuCHS1*::*GuCHR1* and *GuCHI1*), WM3 - 2 (*GuCHI1* overexpressed in WM3 - 1) and WM3 - 3 (*GuCHS1*::*GuCHR1* overexpressed in MW3 - 2) after induction with galactose for 36 h; (E) Fermentation products of yeast stains WM4 - 1 (harboring *GuPAL1*, *GuC4H1*, *Gu4CL1*, *GuCHS1*::*GuCHR1*, *GuCHI1* and *GuUGT1*), WM4 - 2 (*GuCHI1* overexpressed in WM4 - 1) and WM4 - 3 (*GuCHS1*::*GuCHR1* overexpressed in WM4 - 2) after induction with galactose in shake flasks. *GuCHS1*::*GuCHR1* represents a construct in which the 3′end of *GuCHS1* was fused to the 5′ end of *GuCHR1* *via* the linker sequence GGTGGTGGTTCT.

for the last UGT responsible for glycosylation, which had the highest relative expression level in the roots (Fig. 3A). However, LG and Iso-LG, as well as their respective glycosylation products LN and Iso-LN are mainly accumulated in the roots (Supporting Information Fig. S6). We therefore inferred that the upstream step of LN synthesis in *G. uralensis* is mainly carried out in the leaves, and aglycones are transferred from the leaves to the roots, followed by glycosylation to form glycosides and accumulation in the roots.

3.3 Heterologous production of G. uralensis flavonoids in yeast  Having demonstrated the catalytic abilities of all the key enzymes in the *G. uralensis* flavonoid biosynthesis pathway *in vitro* or *in vivo*, we attempted to reconstruct the main flavonoid pathway in yeast (Fig. 4A). When *GuPAL1* and *GuC4H1* were simultaneously introduced into *S. cerevisiae* WAT11, harboring the *A. thaliana* NADPH-cytochrome P450 reductase *ATR1*, which provides the reducing equivalents essential for the activity of plant CYP450s such as C4H, the obtained recombinant yeast WM1 was able to produce *p*-coumaric acid under galactose induction (Fig. 4B), and the content of coumaric acid reached 7.59 μmol/L after cultivation for 36 h (Fig. 4C). When the vector carrying *Gu4CL1* and *GuCHS1*::*GuCHR1* was transferred into WM1, a small amount of Iso-LG was detected in the fermentation broth (Fig. 4B, WM2 - 1). Interestingly, Iso-LG was not detected when *GuCHS1* and *GuCHR1* were co-expressed in yeast that was fed with the substrate. After *GuCHI1* and *GuUGT1* were successively transferred to WM2 - 1, strains WM3 - 1 and WM4 - 1 with the capacity to produce LG and LN were respectively obtained (Fig. 4B). Compared with LN, more Iso-LG in WM4 - 1 was glycosylated before isomerization, resulting in 4.7 times higher Iso-LN production than that of LN in shake flasks (Fig. 4E).

3.4 Promoting the production of flavonoids by gene

overexpression To promote the transformation of the upstream metabolites to the downstream flavonoid structure along the liquiritin pathway, we tried to overexpresses the key genes for Iso-LG biosynthesis in the described recombinant strains. The results showed that overexpression of *GuCHS1*::*GuCHR1* significantly increased the synthesis of Iso-LG, and the production of Iso-LG by WM2-2 was increased 18 times compared with WM2-1 (Fig. 4C). To solve the problem of the much lower production of the target product LN than Iso-LN in WM4 - 1, *GuCHI1* was overexpressed in WM3 - 1 and WM4 - 1, after which the yield of LG and LN increased 1.3-fold (Fig. 4D, WM3 - 2) and 2.1-fold (Fig. 4E, WM4 - 2), respectively. Moreover, simultaneous overexpression of *GuCHS1*:: *GuCHR1* and *GuCHI1* increased the LG production of WM3 - 3 5.3-fold compared with WM3 - 1 (Fig. 4D), and the accumulation of LN in WM4 - 3 was 6.4 times higher than in WM4 - 1 (Fig. 4E). In addition, it was found that overexpression of both *GuCHI1* and *GuCHS1*::*GuCHR1* in this yeast system not only increased the production of the downstream products of these enzymes, but also significantly increased the accumulation of the upstream precursor compound *p*-coumaric acid. Additionally, more glycosides (Iso-LN: 89.3%, LN: 90.3%) were secreted into the culture medium, whereas more than 30% of the Iso-LG and LG remained inside the yeast cells (Supporting Information Fig. S7).

3.5 Metabolite accumulation in the fermenter varies with the amount of cells The changes of metabolites in the recombinant yeast strain WM4 - 3 with increasing induction time and biomass were also investigated in the 11 L benchtop fermenter with controlled DOC (> 40%) and pH (5.0) (Fig. 5). In the early stage of fermentation, the upstream pathway accumulated a large amount of *p*-coumaric acid. Subsequently, the metabolites rapidly flowed to the final

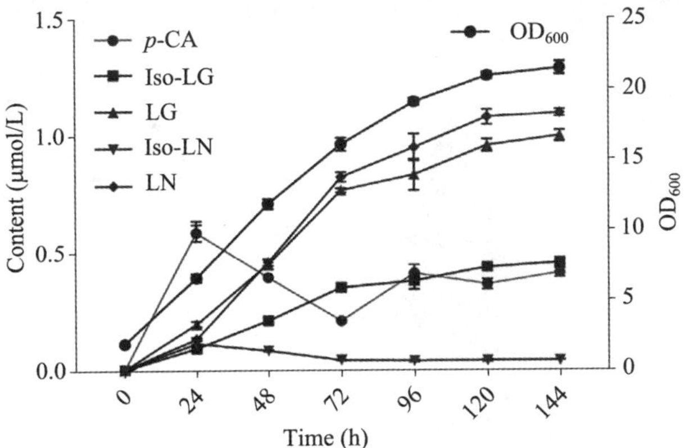


**Figure 5 Cell growth and fermentation products of strain WM4 - 3 in fed-batch fermentation**

The dissolved oxygen concentration (DOC) was kept above 40% and the pH was maintained at 5.0 using automatic addition of ammonium hydroxide. Three replicates were performed for each analysis and the error bars represented the standard deviation (SD).

product after 24 h of fermentation, which was different from the production of a large amount of Iso-LN instead of LN observed in shake flasks (Fig. 4E). At 144 h, the accumulation of LG and LN were respectively reached 1.0 and 1.1 μmol/L. It can be seen that the fermentation conditions can greatly affect the metabolic flow direction, and the potential of this yeast fermentation system can be fully developed in the future *via* metabolic engineering and fermentation optimization.

## 4 DISCUSSION

Flavonoids are an important class of compounds widely found in nature. In addition to their contribution to the gorgeous colors of plants, their enormous medicinal potential has become the most active area of flavonoid research in recent years. With the rapid development of genetic and metabolic engineering, great progress has been made in the analysis of biosynthetic pathways of flavonoids. The complete pathways of plant-specific flavonoids such as quercetin, resveratrol, kaempferol, scutellarin, baicalein and scutellarein have been reconstructed in *S. cerevisiae* or *E. coli*. Some researchers have also expressed a part of the genes encoding the enzymes in the LG biosynthetic pathway from plasmids in *E. coli* or *S. cerevisiae*, and attempted to convert exogenously fed phenylpropanoid acids into 5-deoxyflavonoids such as Iso-LG and LG, but the main fermentation product they obtained was naringenin. In this study, the complete biosynthetic pathway of the main flavonoid of *G. uralensis*, LN, was characterized and reconstructed in *S. cerevisiae*, and achieved the *de novo* biosynthesis of LN using raw materials and cofactors from the endogenous yeast metabolism. This provides a possibility of economically and sustainably producing *G. uralensis* flavonoids through synthetic biology.

The biosynthesis of LN is initiated *via* the general phenylpropanoid metabolism, but the downstream steps of its synthetic pathway leads to the production of 5-deoxyflavonoids (Iso-LG, LG) due to the role of CHR, which is different from the synthetic pathways of quercetin and other 5-hydroxyisoflavonoids. CHR, also known as NADPH-dependent 6′-deoxychalcone syn-thase, can only work with CHS at high concentrations of NADPH (≥0.1 mmol/L) to convert malonyl-CoA and coumaroyl-CoA to synthesize Iso-LG. Otherwise, only naringenin chalcone, the catalytic product of CHS, can be generated. Therefore, in the *in vitro* enzymatic reaction system of CHR, 0.1 mmol/L NADPH was added. Nevertheless, naringenin chalcone still accounted for the main part of the catalytic products in spite of the production of Iso-LG (Fig. 3E). In addition, we also used *S. cerevisiae* WAT11 as a natural NADPH supplier, in which *GuCHS1* and *GuCHR1* were co-expressed, and the precursor compound was fed during fermentation, but no Iso-LG was detected in the extract of the fermentation broth. Although studies have shown that CHR has no obvious interaction with CHS or even other cytoplasmic enzymes in the isoflavone pathway except for IFS, interestingly, the recombinant yeast expressing the fusion of *GuCHS1* and *GuCHR1* was able to produce Iso-LG instead of naringenin chalcone (Fig. 4B). This is in contrast to the LG-producing strain constructed by the Mattheos research team, which produces more by-product, naringenin chalcone, than the target product Iso-LG. The fusion of *GuCHS1* and *GuCHR1* may play a role in shortening the time and distance that the unstable intermediates must traverse from CHS to CHR, which is similar to the immobilization of CHS and CHR recombinant proteins on $Ni^{2+}$-coated beads, which was reported to significantly increase the proportion of deoxygenated products.

In the reconstruction of the LN pathway in yeast, the overexpression of *GuCHI1* significantly increased the yield of *p*-coumaric acid in the upstream pathway even though CHIs have relatively slower kinetics in the conversion of Iso-LG to LG, and overexpression of *GuCHS1*::*GuCHR1* was able to significantly increase the accumulation of both upstream and downstream products (Fig. 4C - E). This phenomenon suggests that there may be an interaction between the different genes of the pathway, or that the downstream product of the LN pathway exerts a positive feedback effect on the upstream pathway. The possible mecha-nisms need further study.

[尹艳,高伟,刘春生,等. Acta Pharmaceutica Sinica B, 2020,10(4):711 - 721.]

# Triptolide: pharmacological spectrum, biosynthesis, chemical synthesis and derivatives

## 1 INTRODUCTION

*Tripterygium wilfordii* Hook. F. is a traditional Chinese medicinal herb, commonly known as "Thunder God Vine" or "Lei Gong Teng" (Figure 1). It is mainly used to treat autoimmune and inflammatory diseases, such as rheumatoid arthritis and systemic lupus erythematosus, and its main active compounds are terpenoids including triptolide and celastrol. Triptolide (Figure 2) is currently considered to be one of the active compounds most likely to translate from traditional to modern medicine.

Triptolide is an important diterpene active compound in *T. wilfordii*. Since 1972, when Kupchan et al. first isolated triptolide and found its significant anti-leukaemic effects, it has also been proven to have significant anti-inflammatory, immunosuppressive, anticancer and other important biological activities (Figure 3). Currently, triptolide is mainly obtained from its extraction from medicinal plants and separation from other compounds. Due to the extremely low content of triptolide in medicinal plants (~66.5 μg/g), chemical extraction and separation are insufficient to meet the needs of industrialization. Triptolide is an abietane-type diterpene with 3 epoxy groups and an α, β-unsaturated five-membered lactone ring structure, which makes the chemical synthesis process challenging and not commercially viable on an industrial scale. Therefore, the current research focus is the biosynthesis of triptolide and its precursor. In recent years, with increasingly intensive study into traditional Chinese medicine (TCM), researchers have developed

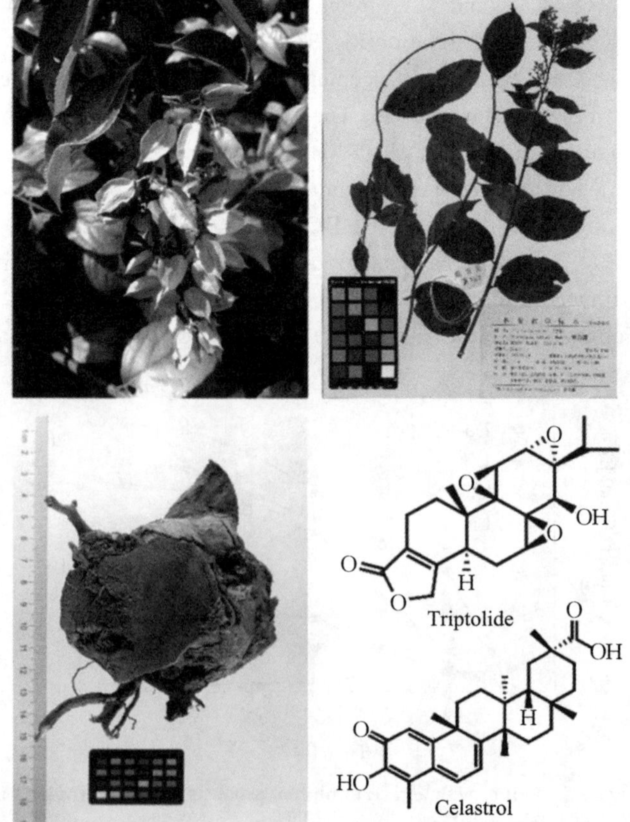


**Figure 1** ***Tripterygium wilfordii*** **and its important active ingredients**

medications based on active compounds such as artemisinin, Taxol and other effective compounds used in TCM. Moreover, artemisinin and paclitaxel are also successful examples of using the principles of synthetic biology used to produce natural products or their precursor compounds at high yields.

In addition, an increasing number of scientific research problems can be solved by interdisciplinary contributions. For example, predicting protein folding structure through AI technology considered among the top ten scientific breakthroughs of *science*. This example provides a reference for scientific researchers seeking breakthroughs of technical bottlenecks. By combining the ideas used in different disciplines to study triptolide, researchers may generate additional novel ideas.

Therefore, to obtain a deeper understanding of triptolide through the combination of multiple disciplinary approaches, we analyzed its biosynthetic pathway. Triptolide and its precursors were efficiently synthesized using the principles of synthetic biology, which laid the foundation for pharmacological research on triptolide, the precursor compounds used in triptolide biosynthesis and triptolide derivatives. This article reviews the research progress on triptolide in terms of its pharmacological activity, biosynthesis, chemical synthesis, and toxicology and discusses recent clinical trials of its derivatives. This review will help researchers better understand all aspects of triptolide and provides constructive suggestions for the further study of triptolide.

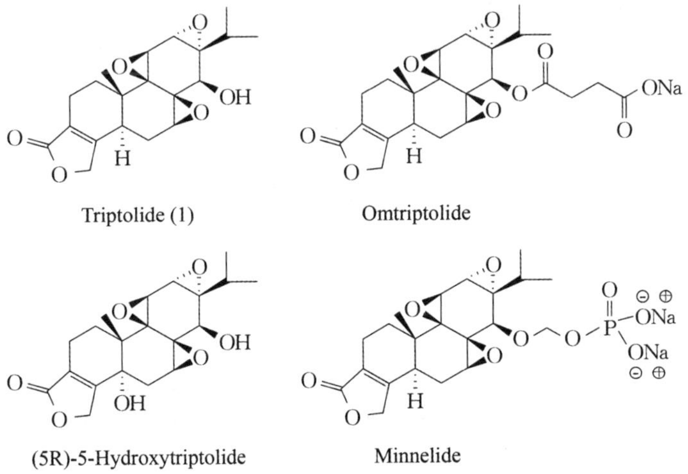

Triptolide (1)

Omtriptolide

(5R)-5-Hydroxytriptolide

Minnelide

**Figure 2 The structures of triptolide (1) and its derivatives**

## 2 BIOLOGICAL FUNCTIONS

2.1 Anti-inflammatory and immunosuppressive effects of triptolide As a TCM herb, *T. wilfordii* has long been used to treat conditions characterized by rheumatism, including rheumatoid arthritis, nephritis and systemic lupus erythematosus. Its main effective component, triptolide, has obvious anti-inflammatory and immunosuppressive effects. Recent studies have shown that triptolide has a positive therapeutic effect on a variety of autoimmune and inflammatory diseases. It not only can induce apoptosis by inhibiting the proliferation of immune cells and inflammation-related cells but can also reduce the release of cytokines and pro-inflammatory mediators, thus inducing anti-inflammatory and immuno-suppressive effects.

2.1.1 Rheumatoid arthritis Rheumatoid arthritis (RA) is an inflammatory, autoimmune disease. Multiple studies have shown that triptolide can be effectively used to treat RA through various mechanisms. These findings suggest that triptolide is one of the main compounds critical for the therapeutic effect of traditional Chinese herbal remedies on RA. The current research on the mechanism of RA treatment with triptolide mainly includes the following aspects: ① Reduction in joint inflammation in RA by inhibiting T cell secretion of inflammatory cytokines. ② amelioration of inflammation in RA by inhibiting angiogenesis at the sites of inflammation. ③ induction of fibroblast apoptosis to inhibit the inflammatory response in RA. ④ reduction in the degree of inflammation by inhibiting multiple signaling pathways (e.g., the TREM1 signaling pathway). ⑤ induction of OCP cell apoptosis by mediating the degradation of clap2, inhibiting OC formation, which has a therapeutic effect on RA.

To study the mechanisms by which triptolide exerts its effects in the treatment of rheumatoid arthritis, network pharmacology and molecular docking were used. Network pharmacology is a new discipline based on the theory of system biology, which analyzes the network of biological system and selects specific signal nodes for multi-target drug molecular design. Molecular docking is a method of drug design based on the characteristics of receptors and the interaction between receptors and drug molecules. First, considering network pharmacology, Yunbin Jiang et al. analyzed the anti-RA active compounds in *T. wilfordii* and concluded that triptolide and celastrol are the key active compounds. The data confirmed that the key molecular mechanism is related to the inhibition of the inflammatory response by inactivating the TNF and NF-κB signaling pathways. Xinqiang Song et al. organized the genes and proteins related to RA in public databases through a creative approach, interpretative phenomenological analysis (IPA). Subsequently, molecular docking was used to predict the binding pockets of the six top candidate triptolide target proteins: CD274, RELA, MCL1, MAPK8, CXCL8 and STAT1. However, network pharmacology is mainly used to analyze big data for predicting potential genes, targets, proteins or signaling pathways. This approach can only provide a certain degree of referent information for the treatment of RA with triptolide. Therefore, researchers need to be cautious and rigorous in the analysis of network

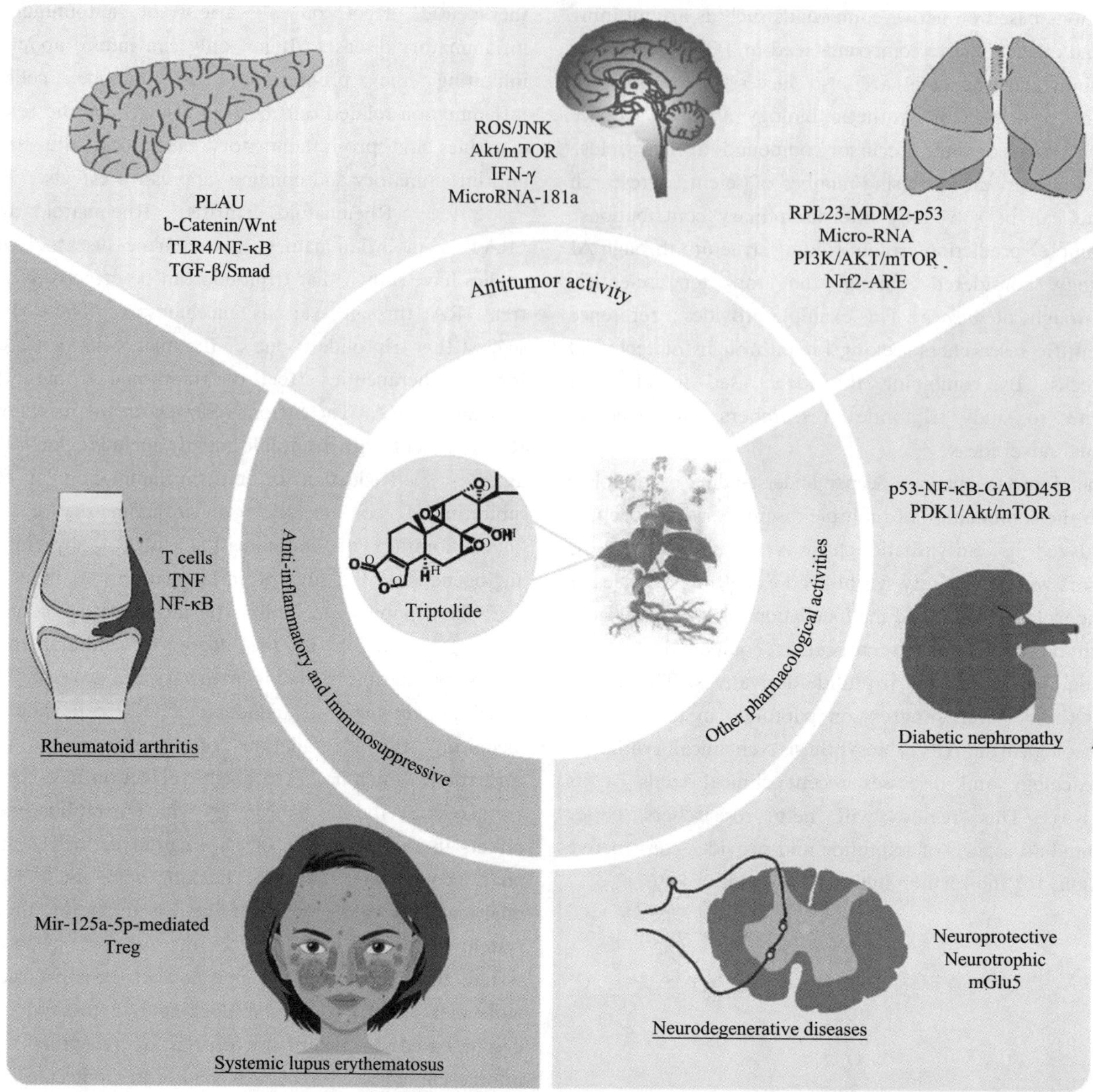


**Figure 3 The pharmacological activity and mechanism of triptolide**

pharmacology results.

Triptolide has a significant therapeutic effect on RA, but due to the own toxicity it induces, the current research hotspot involves technology using nanomaterials to carry triptolide to target the release to the lesion. Studies have shown that the use of poly-γ-glutamic acid-grafted di-tert-butyl L-aspartate hydrochloride (PAT) to prepare a TP-containing nanodrug carrier system can reduce the toxicity of triptolide ensuring the therapeutic effect of triptolide and revealing its potential as an effective drug candidate for RA. The use of amphiphilic pH-sensitive galactosyl dextran-retinal (GDR) nanoparticles to encapsulate triptolide may enhance the anti-inflammatory effect of CIA mouse models. The latest results confirmed that by encapsulating triptolide in the star-shaped amphiphilic block copolymer POSS-PCL-b-PDMAEMA, the constructed pH-sensitive triptolide nanomedicine can achieve significant anti-inflammatory effects at ultra-low doses to treat RA. The use of nanomaterials to carry triptolide has many advantages, such as targeted drug delivery and reduced triptolide dose. Nanomaterials provide effective solutions for accessing the narrow treatment window of triptolide. Nanomaterial carriers are examples of the combination of material chemistry and natural drugs, which in this case was used to address the limitations of triptolide.

2.1.2 Systemic lupus erythematosus Systemic lupus erythematosus (SLE) is a chronic autoimmune inflammatory disease. *T. wilfordii* has been used in the treatment of SLE for centuries, and has achieved remarkable results. Modern research shows that triptolide can alleviate SLE through miR-125a-5p-mediated upregulation of the Treg ratio.

2.1.3 Mechanisms of the anti-inflammatory and immunosuppressive effects of triptolide Research indicates that triptolide exerts its anti-inflammatory and immunosuppressive effects via multiple targets. First, triptolide can regulate signaling pathways, such as by inhibiting the nuclear factor-κB (NF-κB) signaling pathway, or inhibiting the IL-6/signal transducer and transcription 3 (STAT3)-activated signaling pathway and downregulating IL-17. Second, triptolide can inhibit the expression of pro-inflammatory molecules, such as VCAM-1, TGF-β, C3 and CD40. In addition, it can also inhibit myofibroblast infiltration, thereby improving multiple organ fibrosis. With the continuous development of technology, researchers are clarifying the anti-inflammatory and immunosuppressive mechanisms of triptolide at the cellular, molecular and genetic levels.

2.2 Antitumor activity Triptolide has significant, broad-spectrum antitumor and sensitizing effects. In recent years, increasing evidence has shown that triptolide has significant antitumor activity, with potential therapeutic effects on lung cancer, liver cancer, pancreatic cancer and other tumors (Table 1). The antitumor activity of triptolide is reflected in its strong cytotoxicity, which can nullify drug resistance, and inhibit neovascularization and tumor metastasis. Triptolide primarily exerts anticancer effects by inducing apoptosis. In recent years, studies have shown that autophagy and cell senescence are also involved in this process. Triptolide is effective not only in ordinary tumor cells, but also in multidrug resistant cancer cells and some tumor stem cells.

**Table 1 Anticancer effect of triptolide on different cancers**

| Tumor model | Pathway | Mechanism | Cell or animal model |
|---|---|---|---|
| Lung cancer | RPL23-MDM2-p53 | Induce apoptosis, cell cycle arrest and inhibition of cell proliferation | Lung cancer A549 cells (CCL-185™)<br>BALB/cAnNCr-nu/nu mice |
| | Micro-RNA | Reduce cancer cell migration and invasion | H460, A549, and H358 cells<br>Nondiabetic severe combined immune deficiency γ mice |
| | PI3K/AKT/mTOR | Induce apoptosis, inhibition of cell proliferation, glycolysis and energy metabolism | H1299 and NCI-H460 cell |
| | Nrf2-ARE | Enhance cancer cell sensitivity to chemotherapy drugs | Non-small-cell lung cancer (A549)<br>Mouse lung carcinoma 3LL cell<br>liver carcinoma (HepG2) cell |
| Liver cancer | c-Myc/micro-RNA | Induce apoptosis | Liver cancer cell lines SMMC-7721, MHCC-97H, and LM3<br>HepG2 and Hep3B |
| | gene p53 | Inhibit the vitality of cancer cells<br>Induce apoptosis | HepG2 and QSG7701 liver cancer cell |
| Nerve tumor | ROS/JNK<br>Akt/mTOR | Induced G2/M phase arrest, apoptosis, and autophagy | U251, U87-MG and C6 cells<br>BALB/c-nu/nu nude mice |
| | IFN-γ | Inhibits PD-L1 expression<br>Reversing the inhibition of CD4+ T cells by cancer cells | Glioma cell lines, U251-MG, T98G,U87-MG, A172, LN229 and LN18 |
| | MicroRNA-138<br>PI3K/AKT<br>Notch | Induces apoptosis and inhibits cancer cell migration and proliferation | Human medulloblastoma Daoy cells and human embryonic kidney HEK293 cells |
| | MicroRNA-181a<br>p38MAPK<br>NF-κB | Inhibit the proliferation and migration of cancer cells | Human neuroblastoma SH-SY5Y cells |
| Pancreatic cancer | b-Catenin/Wnt | Induces apoptosis of cancer cells | The pancreatic cancer cell line MIA PaCa-2<br>The S2-VP10 cell lines<br>The BxPC-3, Capan-1 and Human pancreatic ductal epithelial cells<br>Genetically engineered KPC ($Kras^{G12D}$, $P53^{R172H}PDX^{Cre}$) mice |
| | TLR4/NF-κB | Enhances the sensitivity of pancreatic cancer PANC-1 cells to GEM | The human pancreatic cancer cell line PANC-1<br>Balb/c nude mice |
| | TGF-β/Smad | Modulate tumor microenvironment<br>Reduces extracellular matrix (ecm) production | The human pancreatic cancer cell line PANC-1<br>Mouse embryonic fibroblast cell line NIH3T3<br>The human pancreatic cancer cell PANC-1-Luc2<br>Pancreatic tumor-bearing nude mice |
| Prostate cancer | Caveolin-1/CD147/MMPs | Inhibition of cancer cell migration and invasion | PC-3 and DU145 human prostate cancer cell |

2.2.1 Lung cancer Lung cancer is a malignancy with some of the highest mortality rates in the world. Studies have shown that triptolide can regulate the ribosomal RPL23-MDM2-p53 signaling pathway to disintegrate the nucleolus and inhibit rRNA synthesis, ultimately inducing cell cycle arrest and apoptosis to inhibit cell proliferation and tumor growth. Reno et al. confirmed that triptolide can change the expression profile of miRNAs in lung cancer cells and inhibit the migration, invasion and metastasis of cancer cells. This research has provided new ideas for the treatment of lung cancer and confirmed that triptolide can be used as a potential lung cancer treatment drug.

Studies have shown that triptolide has a potential therapeutic effect on non-small cell lung cancer (NSCLC). It can induce NSCLC cell apoptosis; downregulate Akt, mTOR and P70S6K phosphorylation levels. At the same time, some researchers found that triptolide can reduce the Wnt signaling pathway, thereby reducing the proliferation of lung cancer cells, tumor formation and metastasis, to treat NSCLC. In addition to its anticancer effect on NSCLC, triptolide can also target the Nrf2 pathway to reduce the chemotherapy resistance of cancer cells, which provides a new potential therapeutic strategy for NSCLC.

At this stage, the combination of triptolide was a hot issue concerning researchers. In one regimen, triptolide is combined with the low-dose anti-inflammatory drug aspirin to prevent lung cancer. Studies have shown that triptolide can activate p53 and inhibit NF - κB at the same time, which has the potential to treat human cancer, and aspirin can improve the efficacy of triptolide. The combination of anticancer drugs and anti-inflammatory drugs may be a promising method for the prevention and treatment of inflammation related cancers (such as lung cancer). In another combination of anticancer drugs, researchers designed lipidpolymer hybrid nanoparticles to serve as a coadministration system. Through *in vivo* and *in vitro* experiments, it was confirmed that the two drugs paclitaxel and triptolide in combination with LPN carriers had a synergistic effect in lung cancer transplantation and exhibited few systemic side effects. There are obvious differences between the two methods. One way is to improve the efficacy of anticancer drugs by inhibiting the pathological process of the cancer response. Another way is to combine different anticancer drugs to form a new drug delivery system, improve the synergy of drugs, and reduce the side effects of drugs and drug resistance.

2.2.2 Liver cancer In hepatocellular carcinoma (HCC), triptolide can inhibit the expression of miR - 17 - 92 and miR - 106b - 25 by inhibiting c-Myc and upregulating their common target genes, thus leading to the death of HCC cells. Moreover, at different concentrations, triptolide was found to induce the phosphorylation of p53 at the serine-15 residue in HepG2 cells. Activating the tumor suppressor gene p53 can induce the apoptosis of liver cancer cells.

Nanomaterial preparation for use with triptolide have consistently been the research focus of scholars. In recent years, researchers have designed galactosylated chitosan TP-nanoparticles (GC - TP - NPs) to induce tumor cell apoptosis by blocking the TNF/NF - κB/BCL2 signaling pathway. These are promising drug candidates that prevent the progression of liver cancer while minimizing systemic toxicity.

2.2.3 Neural tumors Gliomas are common and lethal malignant primary brain tumors that exhibit strong invasion, rapid progression and susceptibility to relapse, leading to a poor prognosis for patients. It has been proven that triptolide not only can inhibit the proliferation of glioma cells and block the cell cycle in the G2/M phase but can also induce apoptosis and protective autophagy. Moreover, triptolide-induced apoptosis and autophagy of glioma cells can inhibit each other. Triptolide can regulate the cell cycle, apoptosis and autophagy by activating ROS/JNK inhibitory functions and the Akt/mTOR signaling pathway. In addition, triptolide can reverse the inhibitory effect of glioma cells on T cells and downregulate the expression of PD - L1 induced by IFN - γ. Therefore, triptolide can be used as an alternative molecule for glioblastoma research and drug development.

Furthermore, triptolide can also achieve anticancer effects by regulating microRNAs. Haifang Zhang et al. found that triptolide can inhibit the PI3K/AKT and Notch pathways, thereby exerting an anticancer effect on medulloblastoma cells. Similarly, studies have shown that triptolide can increase the expression of microRNA-181a, which participates in the proliferation, migration and apoptosis of SH - SY5Y cells, thereby exerting a tumor-suppressing effect.

2.2.4 Pancreatic cancer Triptolide has obvious inhibitory effects on pancreatic cancer. Triptolide, as a super-enhancer (SE) interacting agent, may exhibit its antitumor activity by interfering with cell cross-talk and signal transduction in pancreatic ductal adenocarcinoma.

In addition to inhibiting malignant tumors, triptolide can enhance tumor sensitivity to drugs. For example, triptolide was found to enhance the sensitivity of pancreatic cancer PANC - 1 cells to GEM. Therefore, combined treatment modalities can offer better drug development prospects for pancreatic cancer. Studies have shown that triptolide can activate autophagy and enhance the tumor necrosis factor-related apoptosis-inducing ligand (TRAIL) sensitivity of pancreatic cancer cells. The drug resistance of malignant tumors is a limiting factor in the clinical application of many anticancer drugs. As a broad-spectrum anticancer drug, triptolide can inhibit the drug resistance of cancer cells, which provides a new research idea for the clinical application of triptolide and its derivatives.

In recent years, an increasing number of researchers have used nanotechnology to modify natural products to improve the efficacy of drugs and reduce side effects. For example, silk fibroin nanoparticles loaded with triptolide and celastrol have a certain synergistic effect, which includes reducing cell viability and significantly increasing the cell apoptosis rate, and may be used in a promising treatment strategy for pancreatic cancer. The latest research shows that triptolide can be loaded onto CRPPR peptide-modified tumor-targeting acid-triggered micelles, which can improve the therapeutic effect of triptolide and reduce damage to off-target organs. Therefore, it is believed that nontoxic nanomedicines based on active substances in traditional Chinese herbs have great potential as targeted and adjuvant chemotherapy for pancreatic cancer. Currently, the construction of TCM nanoformulations is providing new choices for antitumor drugs.

2.2.5 Other tumors Triptolide also has antitumor activity in other solid tumors. For example, triptolide inhibits the proliferation, invasion and migration of prostate cancer cells. When shRNA is used to silence the expression of CAV-1, triptolide can reduce the propensity of human prostate cancer cells to migrate and invade tissue. Triptolide inhibits the proliferation, invasion, migration and angiogenesis of oral cancer and oesophageal squamous cell carcinoma (ESCC) cells. Triptolide can trigger the death of colon cancer cells including through apoptosis and *in vitro* experiments indicate that triptolide is effective against colon cancer stem cells (CSCs). In addition, triptolide can reduce tumor-associated macrophage infiltration and inhibit the migration of colon cancer cells. Triptolide is a potent Nrf2 inhibitor that can inhibit the transcriptional activity of Nrf2, leading to the apoptosis of isocitrate dehydrogenase (IDH)-mutant cells, providing an operable strategy for the treatment of malignant tumors with IDH1 mutations. Triptolide can induce the apoptosis of cisplatin-resistant ovarian cancer cells and sensitize them to cisplatin. Various transcription factors, proteins and signaling pathways are involved in the antitumor effects of triptolide, but its anticancer effect is mainly achieved by inducing apoptosis.

In addition to the solid tumors mentioned above, triptolide also has a strong effect on haematological malignancies. Studies indicate that triptolide can induce cell morphological changes and exert cytotoxic effects through G0/G1 phase arrest, as well as induce apoptosis, which may be related to cross talk between components involved in apoptosis and autophagy *in vitro*.

Multidrug resistance (MDR) is the main obstacle to chemotherapy in the treatment of cancer, and triptolide is expected to solve this problem. Triptolide can inhibit the proliferation of A549 lung adenocarcinoma cells resistant to paclitaxel through the MAPK/PI3K/AKT signaling pathway. These studies indicate that triptolide has high-efficiency and broad-spectrum antitumor activity in multidrug resistant tumor cells. Triptolide also plays an important role in certain tumor cells that are resistant to radiotherapy. Triptolide can inhibit the growth and induce the apoptosis of radiotherapy-resistant nasopharyngeal carcinoma cells.

In addition to its roles described in the aforementioned studies, triptolide has an obvious inhibitory effect on the proliferation of pancreatic cancer, ovarian cancer, leukaemia, prostate cancer, lung cancer, liver cancer, colorectal cancer and other tumor cells, showing broad-spectrum antitumor activity. These studies have provided a theoretical basis for the pharmacological activity studies and clinical application of triptolide derivatives. At the same time, the biosynthesis of triptolide can provide a variety of precursor compounds similar to triptolide. Through interdisciplinary biosynthetic studies and pharmacological research, such as those providing precursor compounds of triptolide biosynthesis for functional research, it is possible to identify precursor compounds with anticancer effects and promote the research progress into related topics.

2.2.6 The mechanism of triptolide anticancer effects Triptolide exerts its anticancer effects by influencing apoptosis, senescence, proliferation, invasion, migration, and angiogenesis by regulating multiple signal transduction pathways and gene expression levels, as well as interactions with miRNAs and chaperones. Early studies have shown that triptolide mostly achieves anticancer effects by inducing apoptosis. Current research data show that apoptosis plays a pivotal role in the development of many tumors. The mechanism of triptolide induced apoptosis varies by cell type. In addition to inducing apoptosis, triptolide can also affect the metabolism of tumor cells by reducing cell viability, affecting cell growth and cell cycle arrest. Increasing evidence shows that in addition to the ability of triptolide to induce apoptosis, it can also achieve anticancer effects by inducing autophagy and the combined effects of apoptosis and autophagy. However, the relationship between apoptosis and autophagy is very complicated. Currently, there are three main reported relationships between apoptosis and autophagy: autophagy and apoptosis can cooperate to promote cell death; autophagy and apoptosis can inhibit each other; and autophagy can promote the progression of apoptosis. In addition, autophagy has a dual role in cancer cells. On the one hand, it can provide energy for cells or effective compounds to promote cell survival. On the other hand, excessive autophagy can promote the process of apoptosis. However, the mechanism by which triptolide induces autophagy in cancer cells and the relationship between apoptosis and autophagy have not been clearly elucidated.

In addition to apoptosis and autophagy, cell senescence, which is a form of irreversible cell growth arrest, is related to tumor treatment. Triptolide can inhibit tumor growth by inducing cell senescence. However, research on this effect of triptolide is still relatively limited. As a multitarget anticancer compound, triptolide can also reduce changes in mitochondrial membrane potential and lysosomal membrane permeability (LMP).

Recent research shows that the molecular target of triptolide is the XPB1 subunit of the transcription factor TFIIH. It primarily covalently binds to Cys342 of the XPB1 subunit via the 12, 13-epoxy group, thus inhibiting RNA polymerase Ⅱ-mediated transcription. (Figure 4) It has been reported that triptolide can degrade TFIIH in a CDK7-dependent manner, thereby causing tumor cell death. There are also reports that in multidrug resistant tumor cells,

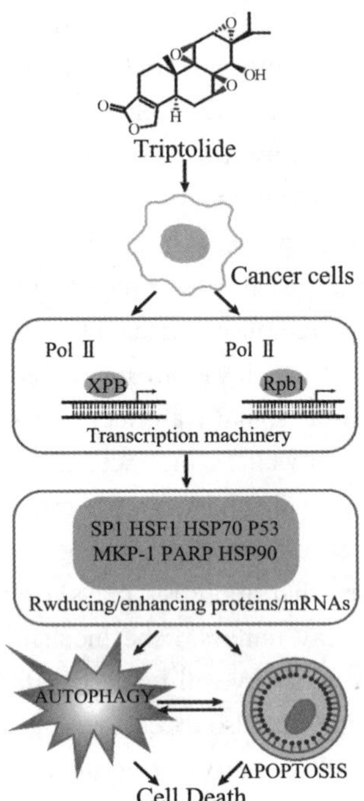


**Figure 4 Mechanism of triptolide induced apoptosis and autophagy**

triptolide achieves antitumor and multidrug resistance effects through cyclin-dependent kinase 7 (CDK7), not XPB. Many other important transcription factors, such as Sp1 and HSF1, are also involved in the survival, development and angiogenesis of tumor cells. Cellular signal transduction pathways such as NF-κB, PI3K/Akt and CaMKK/β-AMPK are also essential for the antitumor activity of triptolide. In tumor cells, triptolide can effectively activate or degrade proapoptotic proteins such as heat shock proteins 90 and 70 (HSP90 and HSP70), caspase-3, caspase-9 and poly-ADP ribose polymerase (PARP).

2.3 Other pharmacological activities In addition to its obvious antitumor, anti-inflammatory and immunosuppressive effects, triptolide has many additional pharmacological effects that are under study. For instance, triptolide has a good effect on some neurodegenerative diseases, and it was found to improve glomerular sclerosis in patients with diabetic nephropathy.

Although the pathogenesis of the most common neurodegenerative diseases such as Alzheimer's disease (AD) and Parkinson's disease (PD) has not been clearly elucidated. Studies have confirmed that triptolide has certain neuroprotective and neurotrophic effects in AD. In addition, triptolide can upregulate mGlu5 to inhibit the activation of microglial cells and induce reactive astrocytes, which in turn protect dopaminergic neurons in a PD model.

Triptolide can inhibit the binding of p53 to the promoter of GADD45B to downregulate its transcription. Inhibiting p53-NF-κB-GADD45B signaling to maintain glomerular barrier function provides new research ideas for the anti-proteinuria effect of triptolide in glomerular diseases. In addition, triptolide may improve the proteinuria of diabetic rats by inhibiting the PDK1/Akt/mTOR pathway. The latest research shows that triptolide can inhibit the PI3K/AKT signaling pathway and the interaction between miR-188-5p and PTEN to treat diabetic nephropathy.

## 3 BIOSYNTHESIS OF TRIPTOLIDE

Following the rapid development of new tools in recent years, synthetic biology has been successfully applied to the production of artemisinin, paclitaxel (Taxol®) and other active compounds isolated from TCM materials. The use of synthetic biology principles to design and modify microbial strains to produce natural active substances has become a very promising method for obtaining sufficient quantities of natural products. This approach is also expected to enable the efficient industrial production of triptolide precursors, triptolide and its derivatives in the future.

3.1 Genomic and transcriptomic studies of *T. wilfordii* To explore the key genes of triptolide biosynthesis, our team analyzed tissue samples of *T. wilfordii* leaves, flowers, stem bark, peeled stem, root bark, root phloem and root xylem, as well as suspensions of cells treated with methyl jasmonate (MeJA) for different times. The samples were classified according to the principle of three biological repeats. The total RNA of each sample was extracted by a modified cetyltrimethylammonium bromide (CTAB) method for sequencing analysis, and finally the transcriptome data were obtained. The results showed that roots and leaves had the highest triptolide content. Therefore, the key genes of triptolide biosynthesis can be screened according to the correlation of their differential expression in different tissues with the triptolide content. Moreover, induction with MeJA increased the content of triptolide in suspension cells. By analysing the expression of genes in suspension cells induced by MeJA at different times, the key genes that regulate triptolide biosynthesis were identified.

In addition, our research team sequenced the genome of *T. wilfordii*. A total of 28 321 protein coding genes were annotated, with an average sequence length of 3 338 bp. On average, each predicted gene contained 5.44 exons, with a total of 182.52 Mb of annotated repeats, accounting for 52.36% of the *T. wilfordii* genome. Based on the genomic data, evolutionary events in the life history of *T. wilfordii* were analyzed. It was found that the most recent WGT events included the duplication of genes in the upstream metabolism of isoprene. These results suggested that recent WGT events are of great significance to the evolution of triptolide biosynthesis.

The genome and transcriptome, as the main tools for screening biosynthetic pathway genes, have some limitations. In the genome, when identifying genes of the same family, it is possible to merge the genes with high similarity into one gene, which is likely to lead to mistakes in the screening process. In the process of cloning target genes, the gene sequence provided by the genome is mainly the open reading frame (ORF) of the gene. Therefore, if the expression level of the gene is low, the target gene may not be identified due to the limitations of the primers. In addition, the gene sequences provided by the transcriptome may have splicing errors or gene sequence deletion problems. Therefore, it is necessary to integrate the gene information provided by the transcriptome and genome for better screening and cloning of target genes.

3.2 Analysis of the upstream terpenoid biosynthesis pathway The carbon backbone of terpenes is mainly formed by condensation of isoprene pyrophosphate (IPP) and dimethylallyl diphosphate (DMAPP). In nature, IPP and DMAPP are synthesized in two different biochemical pathways, the 2*C*-methyl-D-erythritol-4-phosphate (MEP) pathway and the mevalonate (MVA) pathway (Figure 4). Moreover, the MEP and MVA pathways provide precursors for different terpenoids. The MEP pathway mainly produces mono-, di- and tetraterpenes, while the MVA pathway mainly produces sesquiterpenes, sterols, triterpenes and their saponin derivatives.

3.2.1 The mevalonic acid (MVA) pathway The MVA pathway was first discovered by Lynen et al. and elaborated by Newman et al. This pathway mainly produces IPP through a series of 6 enzymatic reactions, as follows: ① The pathway is initiated with acetyl-CoA thiolase (ACAT) catalyzing the formation of acetoacetyl-CoA from two acetyl-CoA units. ② HMG-CoA is generated from acetoacetyl-CoA and a third acetyl-CoA unit catalyzed by 3-hydroxy-3-methylglutaryl-CoA synthase (HMGS). ③ The main regulatory step of the MVA pathway is the reduction of HMG-CoA to mevalonate by HMG-CoA reductase (HMGR) on the surface of the endoplasmic reticulum (ER). ④ Mevalonate is phosphorylated by mevalonate kinase to mevalonate-5-phosphate. ⑤ Subsequently, phosphomevalonate kinase phosphorylates mevalonate-5-phosphate to mevalonate-5-diphosphate. ⑥ The final step of the MVA pathway is the formation of IPP from mevalonate diphosphate by mevalonate diphosphate decarboxylase. IPP can be reversibly isomerized to DMAPP by IPP isomerase (IPI).

Two AACT genes, one HMG gene, two HMGR genes, one MVK gene, one PMK gene and one MVD gene were cloned from *T. wilfordii*. The predicted number of amino acid residues, the ORF sequence, theoretical isoelectric point (pI), molecular weight and the number of genes were analyzed. In addition, some scholars confirmed the gene function by introducing cloned *TwHMGS* into a suitable yeast strain, and then studying the inducible expression and tissue expression patterns.

3.2.2 The 2-C-methyl-d-erythritol-4-phosphate (MEP) pathway In 1999, Rohmer et al. discovered another route for the synthesis of terpenoids, the methylerythritol phosphate (MEP) pathway. This pathway was elucidated by Lichtenthaler et al. and is also called the 1-deoxy-D-xylulose-5-phosphate (DXP) pathway. Under the catalysis of 7 enzymes, D-3-phosphoglyceraldehyde (GAP) and pyruvate are condensed and reduced to produce IPP and DMAPP via the following steps: ① Pyruvate and GAP are condensed to form 1-deoxy-d-xylulose 5-phosphate (DXP) under the catalytic action of DXP synthase (DXS). DXS is a key enzyme that controls the flux of the MEP pathway. ② DXP reductoisomerase (DXR) catalyzes the isomerization of DXP to form MEP. ③ 2-C-methyl-d-erythritol 4-phosphate cytidyltransferase (MCT) activates MEP to form CDP-ME with a cytidine diphosphate linkage at the C4 position. ④ CDP-ME is phosphorylated into CDP-MEP under the action of 4-diphosphocytidyl-2-C-methyl-D-erythritol kinase (CMK). ⑤ Subsequently, MDS cyclizes the activated CDP-MEP to 2-C-methyl-d-erythritol-2,4-cyclodiphosphate (MEcDP). ⑥ MEcDP is reduced to 1-hydroxy-2-methyl-2-(E)-butenyl-4-diphosphate (HMBDP) by 4-hydroxy-3-methylbut-2-enyl diphosphate synthase (HDS). ⑦ In the final step, HMBDP is converted by 4-hydroxy-3-methylbut-2-enyl diphosphate reductase (HDR) to form IPP and DMAPP at a product ratio of approximately 5 : 1. In addition, IPI is also present in plastids, and can catalyze the isomerization of IPP to maintain the optimal ratio of IPP to DMAPP.

Two *TwDXS* and one *TwDXR* gene were cloned from *T. wilfordii*, and the researchers verified their functions through colour complementation experiments. Further overexpression (OE) and RNA-interference experiments confirmed that the expression of *TwDXR* affects the production of triptolide in *T. wilfordii*. The *TwHDR* gene encodes the final enzyme of the MEP pathway, which is very important for regulating isoprene biosynthesis. The function of *TwHDR* was verified by a complementation assay in a mutant strain of *E. coli* with a defective HDR gene, and the expression of *TwHDR* in the cells in suspension was analyzed, and the results contributed to further analysis of the triptolide biosynthesis pathway.

3.3 Analysis of the triptolide biosynthesis pathway. The biosynthesis of triptolide is mainly divided into three steps. The first step encompasses the production of IPP and DMAPP through the MVA and MBP pathways. The second step consists of the formation of geranylgeranyl diphosphate (GGPP) by geranylgeranyl diphosphate synthase (GGPPS), catalyzing the continuous addition of IPP to DMAPP, geranyl pyrophosphate (GPP) and farnesyl pyrophosphate (FPP). In the final step, GGPP is converted to various

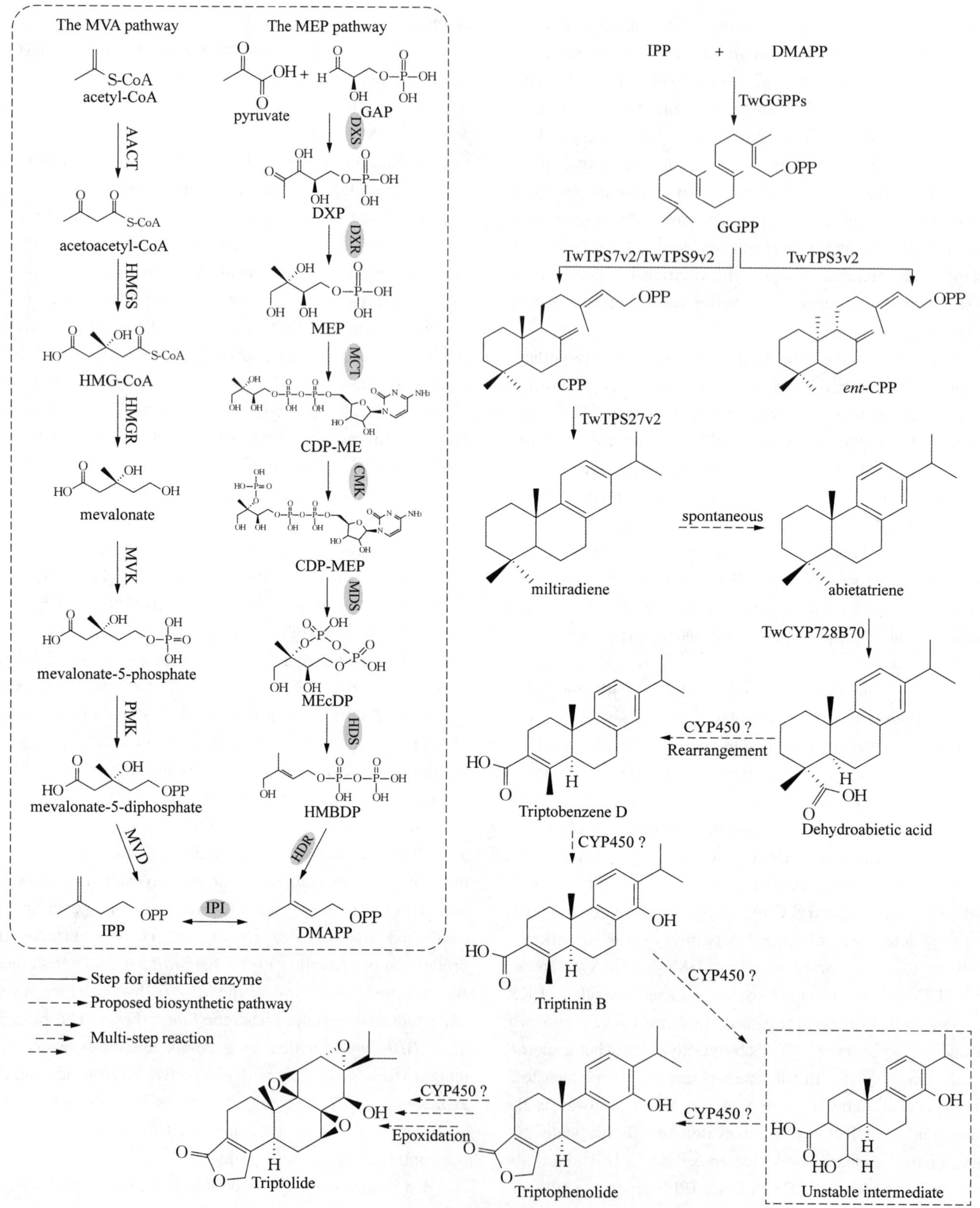


**Figure 5 Analysis of the biosynthetic pathway of triptolide**

The green dashed box shows the common upstream pathways of terpenoids in *T. wilfordii*. The solid arrow and red gene indicate the route of identified function, while the dotted arrow and blue gene indicate the possible route.

terpene intermediates under the catalysis of diterpene synthases (diTPSs), and the intermediates are then modified by different postmodification enzymes to generate the corresponding diterpene products (Figure 5).

GGPPS can catalyze the generation of the common diterpene precursor GGPP and is considered to be one of the key synthetases in the diterpene biosynthesis pathway. Five putative *GGPPS* genes have been cloned from *T. wilfordii*.

The cloned *GGPPS* and *SmCPS/KSL* genes were introduced into E. coli with miltiradiene serving as a marker. Finally, it was determined identified that the proteins encoded by the three *TwGGPPS* exhibited function of GGPPs. By analysing the expression in *TwGGPPS* in MeJA-induced cells in suspension, researchers showed that the accumulation of triptolide is enhanced with the increase of *TwGGPPS1* and *TwGGPPS4* expression, suggesting that these two genes may be the main genes that control triptolide synthesis. The latest research shows that *TwGGPPS8* exhibits an expression pattern similar to that of *TPS7v2*, *TPS9v2* and *TPS27v2*, and the highest transcription levels were found in roots rich in triptolide. Based on this observation, it was speculated that *TwGGPPS8* may be involved in the biosynthesis of triptolide in roots.

After obtaining the common linear diterpene precursor GGPP, researchers further studied the biosynthetic pathway of triptolide. Hansen et al. found that *TwTPS27* coupled with *TwTPS9* converted normal copalyl diphosphate to miltiradiene by screening diterpene synthase family genes in *T. wilfordii*. Su et al. added miltiradiene to the culture medium of suspended cells, and the accumulation of triptolide after 5 days exhibited a statistically significant increase compared with the level in the control group. This is the first evidence that miltiradiene is indeed a precursor of triptolide. Through transcriptome sequencing of cells in suspension induced with MeJA, 8 putative diterpene synthase genes were identified, and 6 full-length diterpene synthase genes were cloned. Using GGPP as a substrate, the functional identification was carried out in *E. coli*, and *TwTPS7v2* and *TwTPS9v2* were confirmed to generate CPP from GGPP. It was confirmed that CPP is a precursor of miltiradiene. The results showed that TwTPS27v2 can catalyze the formation of miltiradiene from CPP, and RNAi experiments showed that decreased expression of *TwTPS7v2*, *TwTPS9v2* and *TwTPS27v2* affects the accumulation of triptolide.

Previous studies had elucidated the biosynthesis of the abietane-type diterpene core skeleton miltiradiene, which laid the foundation for further investigation of cytochrome P450 (CYP450) genes in the downstream synthesis pathway. NADPH-cytochrome P450 reductase acts as the electron donor of CYP450 proteins to support their catalytic function. Four *TwCPR* genes were cloned from *T. wilfordii* and soluble proteins were successfully expressed. The activity of TwCPR enzymes was verified by combining them with kaurene oxidase. The results showed that although *TwCPR3* was expressed at lower levels in certain tissues, it was a more efficient electron donor. Therefore, it was speculated that TwCPR3 is more suitable for the study of other CYP450 monooxygenases in *T. wilfordii*. Studies have reported that CYP720B4 in Sitka spruce (*Picea sitchensis*) can convert miltiradiene to dehydroabietic acid, and it was speculated that dehydroabietic acid may be an important intermediate in the triptolide biosynthesis pathway. The latest research indicates that CYP728B70 is the first CYP450 in the triptolide biosynthesis pathway and that it converts miltiradiene and abietatriene in two consecutive oxidation steps to form the corresponding diterpene alcohol and diterpene acid (dehydroabietic acid) products. Interference and OE analysis indicated that CYP728B70 is involved in triptolide biosynthesis.

Currently, there has been a breakthrough in the understanding of the triptolide biosynthesis pathway, and the first CYP450, *TwCYP728B70*, was discovered. However, there are still many difficulties to be resolved. First, compared with triptolide, the position of the carboxyl group of dehydroabietic acid is problematic. Transfer of the carboxyl group to the three position is an urgent problem for researchers. On the one hand, after decarboxylation, a methyl group may be attached to the third position, and then the three-step oxidation proceeds. On the other hand, there may be an enzyme that can directly transfer the carboxyl group at position 18 to position 3. In addition, the mechanism involved in forming the three epoxy groups in triptolide has not been extensively studied. As suggested in the current literature, CYP450s and dioxygenase may catalyze the formation of these functional groups. Therefore, we hope to solve the problems of carboxyl transfer and epoxy group formation during biosynthesis by combining biosynthesis with chemical synthesis, and ultimately enable the industrial production of triptolide.

3.4 Metabolic engineering for achieving triptolide biosynthesis Studies have shown that the content of triptolide in *T. wilfordii* is low, reaching only 66.5 μg/g. To study triptolide better, researchers used *Agrobacterium rhizogenes* to induce hairy roots from the calli of *T. wilfordii* roots. The concentrations of triptolide in hairy root, callus, adventitious root and natural root samples were 39.98, 1.76, 47.86 and 21.4 μg/g, respectively, and after MeJA induction, the triptolide concentration increased approximately 2-fold. In addition, by optimizing the growth and induction conditions for *T. wilfordii* adventitious root culture, a comparatively large quantity of triptolide was obtained. The yield of triptolide was increased to 648.3 μg per flask by adding inducers XAD - 7 and MeJA and optimizing the growth conditions.

*T. wilfordii* cells in suspension are also important sources of triptolide for research. Suspension cells are also suitable for a variety of experiments, such as RNAi and overexpression studies. In one study, the triptolide concentrations in *T. wilfordii* cells in suspension and culture medium were $53 \pm 3$ μg/g and $4.0 \pm 0.2$ mg/L, respectively.

After 240 h of MeJA induction, the triptolide content was increased 3-fold to 200 μg/g. Furthermore, researchers found that cambial meristematic cells (CMCs) also effectively accumulate triptolide, which has great potential in triptolide biosynthesis research. Studies have shown that CMCs contain triptolide at a concentration of 138.1 μg/g, and after induction with MeJA for 480 h, the content of triptolide can reach 405.1 μg/g. Subsequently, researchers confirmed that MeJA can induce the expression of terpene biosynthesis-related genes in CMCs through real-time reverse transcription-polymerase chain reaction (qRT - PCR). CMCs can therefore be used for the analysis of the triptolide biosynthesis pathway.

3.5 Metabolic engineering of bacteria for triptolide production  Microbial metabolic engineering is a very promising method for obtaining natural products. Miltiradiene is an important intermediate compound of triptolide biosynthesis. The synthesis of miltiradiene by microorganisms is the first step to efficiently produce triptolide. Studies have shown that modular engineering, encompassing the integration of *Sm*CPS and *Sm*KSL together with the integration of BTS1 and ERG20, significantly contributed to the increased output of miltiradiene. Finally, the best synthetic route was introduced into the diploid yeast strain YJ2X, and the resulting engineered strain produced 365 mg/L miltiradiene in a 15 L bioreactor. In addition, Dai et al. increased the yield of miltiradiene to 488 mg/L through various methods, such as overexpression of key enzymes and the use of antibiotic markers to replace auxotrophic markers in plasmids. However, due to the use of antibiotics in the fermentation process to enhance the stability of the plasmid, it cannot be used in large-scale industrial production. Recently, Tianyuan Hu et al. investigated the production capacity of diterpenoid synthases from different species, and selected a class Ⅱ diterpene synthase (di-TPS) *Cf*TPS1 from *Coleus forskohlii* (*Plectranthus barbatus*) and class Ⅰ di-TPS *Sm*KSL1 from *Salvia miltiorrhiza* to use for producing a final titre of miltiradiene of 3.5 g/L in a 5 L bioreactor.

In addition, researchers knocked out *rox1*, *ypl062w*, and *yjl06w4*, downregulated *ERG9*, and overexpressed genes such as *tHMG1* and *ERG20* to increase GGPP production. Subsequently, they introduced double *SmMS* - *SmCPS1* fusion modules to produce miltiradiene and finally co-expressed the *TwCYP728B70* and *TwCPR3* genes to produce dehydroabietic acid. This series of experiments laid the foundation for the subsequent identification of key enzyme-coding genes in the triptolide biosynthesis pathway.

Although a microbial metabolic plant model has been constructed to produce dehydroabietic acid, it is difficult to meet the needs of subsequent research because of its low yield. Currently, there are several ways to improve the yield of synthetic biology: 1. Genes that do not affect the growth of microorganisms are knocked out or weakened in other ways to increase the accumulation of precursor compounds. 2. The yield of target compounds is increased by the overexpression of genes. 3. Genes with the same function but with higher activity are used to replace genes with lower expression or mutation technology is used to identify mutant genes that produce higher yields. 4. Through the technology of protein fusion or substrate channelization, we can connect the active pockets of proteins to improve the yield of target compounds.

## 4 TOTAL SYNTHESIS OF TRIPTOLIDE

Over decades, relatively slow progress has been made toward the goal of total triptolide synthesis, with many of the advancements made attributed the efforts of Berchtold, van Tamelen and Yang. Currently, there are four principal ways to synthesize triptolide: Ⅰ) synthesis from tetralinone, α-abietic acid or α-dehydroabietic acid as starting materials, Ⅱ) synthesis via the Diels-Alder reaction, Ⅲ) synthesis of the core skeleton via a polyene cyclization reaction, and Ⅳ) synthesis via metal catalysis.

As early as 1977, the Berchtold team began research on the total synthesis of triptolide (scheme 1). They used 6-methoxy-1-tetralone (**2**) as the starting material and converted it to tricyclo-enone **3** in 10 steps with a yield of 33%. Then, **3** was transformed into **4** in 5 steps, which laid the foundation for the total synthesis of triptolide. In 1980, the team completely outlined the process of synthesizing racemic triptolide (scheme 2). The reaction is initiated with the alkylation of tetralone (**5**) with 3-(2-iodoethyl) dihydrofuran-2(3H)-one (**6**), and bonds in the product are broken with dimethylamine to form a 1 : 1 enantiomer mixture **7**. The mixture of **8** and **9** is formed by oxidation of **7** with a $CrO_3$.py complex with aldol condensation catalyzed by $Al_2O_3$. To obtain pure compound **10**, the mixture is treated with acid to dehydrate **8**, the aldehyde is reduced with $NaBH_4$ during the acid treatment, and an acid-catalyzed lactonization reaction is performed. The isomerization of **10** catalyzed by methoxide results in compound **11**, which is then oxidized by benzoic acid **11** and demethylated to obtain **12**. Reduction of **12** with $NaBH_4$ provides pure C-7β alcohol (**13**). Finally, triptolide (1, 21%) and 14-epitriptolide (68%) are obtained through an Alder periodate reaction

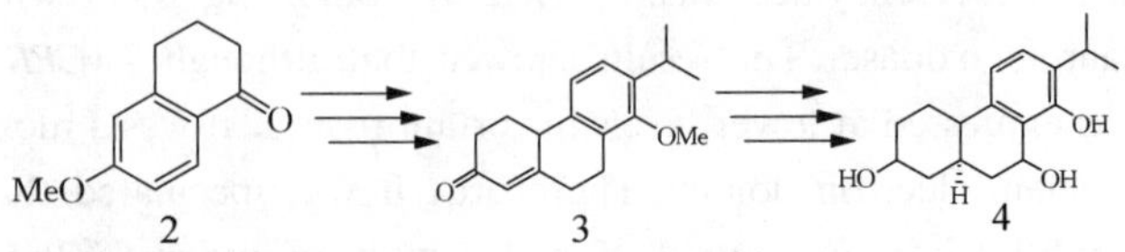

**Scheme 1  Early research on the synthesis of triptolide using 6-methoxy-1-tetraketone (2) as starting material**

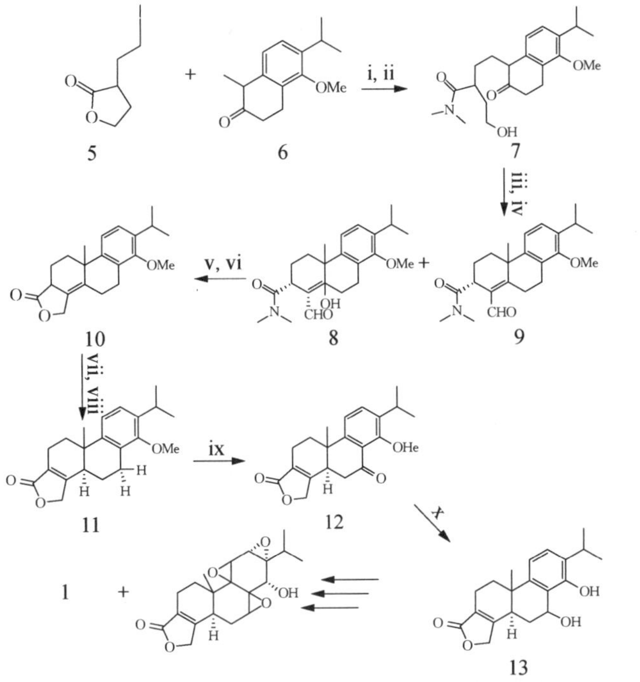

**Scheme 2 Synthesis of triptolide (1) through 5 and 6**

(i) NaH, DMF 25 ℃, 12 h; (ii) $Me_2NH$ 25 ℃, 12 h; (iii) $CrO_3$. py, $CH_2Cl_2$ 25 ℃, 15 min; (iv) grade 3 neutral alumina EtOAc, 25 ℃, 48 h; (v) pTosOH (catalyst) $C_6H_6$, reflux, 2 h; (vi) $NaBH_4$, EtOH, 25 ℃, 2 h aqueous HCl (workup); (vii) $MeO^-$, MeOH 25 ℃, 15 min; (viii) $CrO_3$, HOAc-$H_2O$ (9 : 1) 25 ℃, 6 h; (ix) $BBr_3$, $CH_2Cl_2$ 25 ℃, 10 h; (x) $NaBH_4$, EtOH 25 ℃, 1 h.

($NaIO_4$, 74%), a sequencing m-CPBA oxygenation and basic hydrogen peroxide oxygenation ($H_2O_2/OH^-$) procedure, and sodium borohydride reduction. In summary, the first total synthesis of racemic triptolide was completed from **5** in 16 steps. Although the final yield was low (1.6%), this work undoubtedly laid the foundation for the study of triptolide synthesis.

Later, researchers mostly borrowed from the research ideas of Berchtold et al. The innovation of the synthetic route was mainly focused on different treatment methods of tetralone. However, Li et al. developed a different route to synthesize triptolide in 2014 (scheme 3). The route starts from the hydrogenation of common compound **14**, which is converted to the corresponding Weinreb amide and finally reacts with isopropenyl magnesium bromide to form enol **15**. Compound **15** is then reacted with sodium borohydride in the presence of $CeCl_3$, after which Johnson Claisen rearrangement produces ester **16**. This ester is hydrolysed to form amide **17**, which is then reacted with trimethylsilyl lithium acetylide to obtain acetylene **18**. Compound **18** and 2.5 mol% of (R, R)-**19** are incubated in triethylamine and formic acid for 1.5 h to produce alcohol **20**. Compound **21** is obtained by protecting the hydroxyl group with a *tert*-butyldimethylsilyl ether during the potassium carbonate/methanol repair process and then cleaving the acetylenic

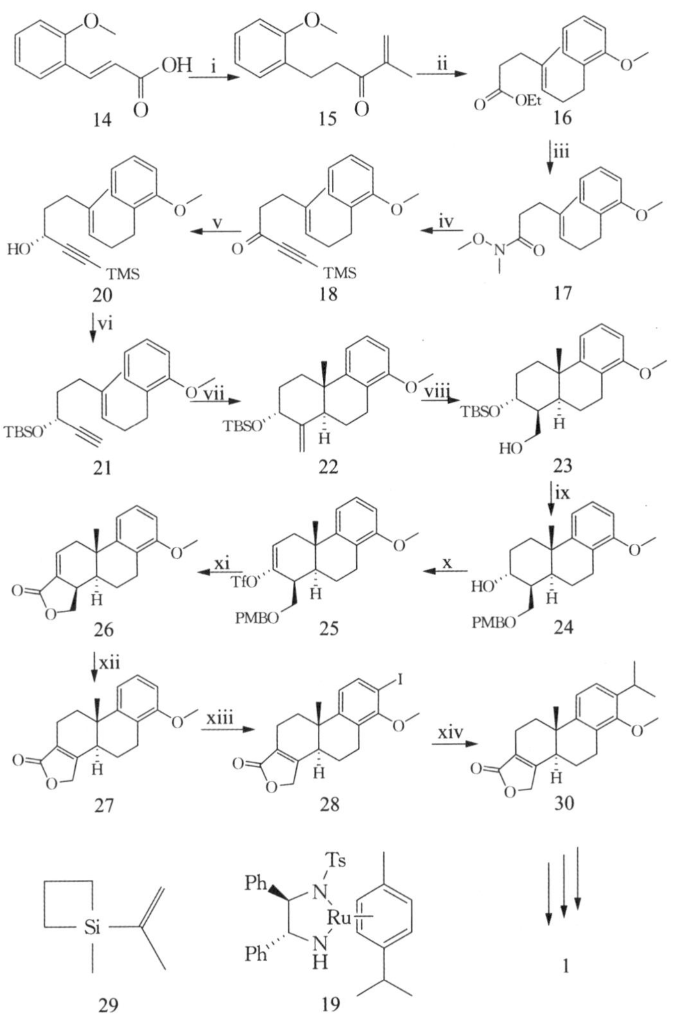

**Scheme 3 Synthesis of triptolide (1) through Compound 14**

(i) $H_2$, Pd/C, NH(OMe)Me · HCl, CDI, Isopropenyl magnesium bromide; (ii) $NaBH_4$, $CeCl_3 \cdot 7H_2O$, $CH_3C(OEt)_3$, $CH_3CH_2COOH$, reflux; (iii) LiOH, NH(OMe)Me · HCl, CDI; (iv) Trimethylsilyl lithium acetylide, −78 ℃ to −20 ℃; (v) compound 19, HCOOH, TEA, THF; (vi) $K_2CO_3$, TBSCI, imidazole; (vii) $InBr_3$ (20%), −20 ℃; (viii) $BH_3$ · THF, $H_2O_2$, 3N NaOH; (ix) NaH, PMBCI, PTSA; (x) Jones reagent, LiHMDS, $Tf_2NPh$, −78 ℃ to rt; (xi) DDQ, CO, $Pd(PPh_3)_4$, $Bu_3N$, LiCl, 80 ℃; (xii) $Rh(PPh_3)_3Cl$, $Et_3SiH$, toluene reflux; (xiii) $I_2$, AgOTf; (xiv) $Pb(dba)_2$, TBAF, compound 29, 5% Pd/C.

trimethylsilyl group. The key to this synthetic pathway is that indium-(Ⅲ) catalyzes the cationic cascade reaction of compound **21**. This reaction proceeds via slow addition of **21** to an intensely stirred suspension of $InBr_3$ in dichloromethane at −20 ℃. Under these conditions, key intermediate **22** is formed as a single isomer. Subsequently, the authors completed the synthesis of the lactone D-ring through a four-step reaction. In the first step, **22** was subjected to hydroboration using a $BH_3$ · THF complex and then oxidized with basic hydrogen peroxide to obtain alcohol **23** as a single isomer. In the second step, PMB ether was formed to protect the free hydroxyl group of alcohol **23**, and then *p*-

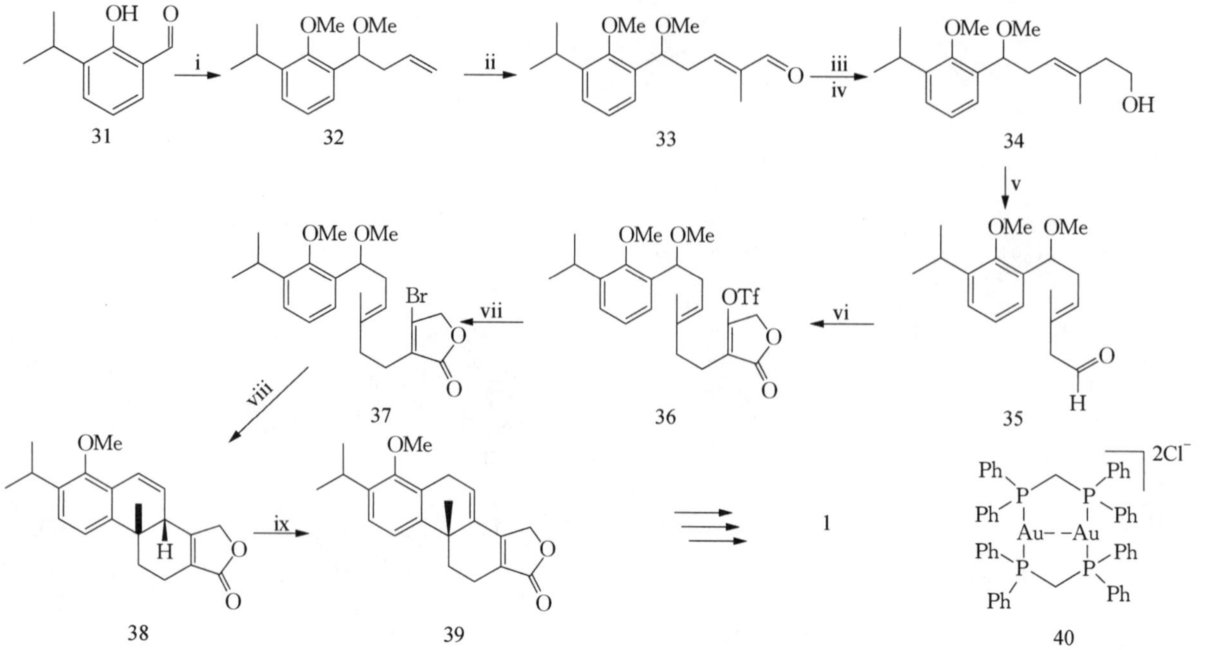

**Scheme 4 Total synthesis of triptolide (1) through simple compound 31**

(i) allylMgBr, THF, $Me_2SO_4$, 70 ℃, 12 h; (ii) Grubbs Ⅱ (1 mol%), CuI (2.5 mol%), Acrolein, $Et_2O$, 40 ℃, 4 h; (iii) $Ph_3PMeI$, KHMDS, THF, 2 h; (iv) $Cy_2BH$, THF, $NaBO_3 \cdot 4H_2O$, 4 h; (v) DMP, $CH_2Cl_2$; (vi) L-proline (5 mol%), tetronic acid, Hantzch ester $CH_2Cl_2$, DIPEA, $Tf_2O$, −78 ℃; (vii) LiBr, THF, 70 ℃, 12 h; (viii) compound 40, $Na_2CO_3$, 365 nm, MeCN, 12 h, $H_2SO_4$, 6 h; (ix) $RuCl_2(PPh_3)_3$, DIPEA, PhMe, 120 ℃, 4 d.

TsOH was used to remove the silyl protecting group to obtain alcohol **24**. The third step is to oxidize **24** with Jones reagent and then convert the resulting carbonyl group to the corresponding trifluorovinyl compound **25**. Finally, the PMB ether of **25** was oxidatively cleaved, and tetracyclic lactone **26** was obtained by palladium-catalyzed carbonylation and *in situ* lactonization. After obtaining intermediate **26**, compound **27** was obtained by reacting 26 with a catalytic concentration of tris (triphenylphosphine)-rhodium and triethylsilane in refluxing toluene. Ortho-iodination of **27** gave intermediate **28**, which was subjected to palladium-catalyzed cross-coupling with 1-methyl-1-(prop-2-enyl) silacyclobutane **29** and then hydrogenated to form triptophenolide methyl ether **30**. Triptophenolide methyl ether, as an important intermediate, has been used in the total synthesis of triptolide many times. The difficulty of this approach is the preparation of optically active propargyl alcohol (R)-**20**. Through several attempts by researchers, the conditions for incubation of **18** and 2.5 mol% of (R,R)-**19** in triethylamine and formic acid for 1.5 h were finally discovered. It is speculated that these conditions may a result of the instability of the trimethylsilyl group in the reaction system. Research mainly utilize $InBr_3$-mediated cationic polyene cyclization and palladium-catalyzed carbonylation with lactone formation, which enables the large-scale synthesis of intermediate **26**.

Recent studies have used dimeric gold complex $[Au_2(dppm)_2]Cl_2$ combined with ultraviolet A (UVA, 365 nm) light irradiation to catalyze the formation of radical intermediates from non-activated bromoalkanes/arenes in a mild photoredox catalysis process (scheme 4). The first step of this reaction is treating aldehyde **31** with allyl magnesium bromide and then adding dimethyl sulfate to obtain allyl **32**. Compound **32** is subjected to a metathesis reaction with methacrolein under the catalytic action of a Grubbs second-generation catalyst and a certain amount of copper iodide to obtain a single isomer of aldehyde **33**. The aldehyde groups of compound **33** are converted to a diene by the Wittig reaction and then to the corresponding primary alcohol **34** by a borohydride/oxidation sequence. Dess Martin oxidation of **34** produces aldehyde **35**, which is subjected to a one-pot proline-catalyzed coupling reaction with tetronic acid in the presence of Hantzsch ester and triflation to afford triflate **36**. The mixture is directly heated with lithium bromide in tetrahydrofuran to obtain bromobutene lactone **37**, which reacts under optimal conditions, followed by treatment with sulfuric acid to obtain tetracycle **38**, and the configuration is confirmed by X-ray analysis. Subsequently, **38** is isomerized using a catalytic amount of $RuCl_2(PPh_3)_3$ and DIPEA in toluene at 120 ℃ to obtain **39**. Finally, the conversion of **39** to triptolide requires 8 more steps. This route can be used to access the important intermediate **39** for triptolide synthesis, which is converted from compound **31** in eight simple steps. However, the difficulty of the entire route is maintaining the optimal conditions for the reaction of bromo-butyrolactone **37**. The researchers finally determined that, vinyl bromide (0.1 mol/L in MeCN), 1 (10 mol%), $Na_2CO_3$ (2 equiv.), subjected to, 365 nm LED light for 12 h at room temperature constituted the best reaction conditions. This study has made important contributions to the large-scale synthesis of polycyclic compounds and can be used in the synthesis of many other terpenoids.

The total synthesis of triptolide mainly includes the following three aspects: i) the synthesis of the tricyclic scaffold; ii) the formation of the butenolide (D-ring), and iii) the construction of the three active epoxy groups. Previous research on the total synthesis of triptolide has solved these three problems in a satisfactory manner and achieved important research results on a laboratory scale. However, in view of the complex chemical structure of triptolide, even as researchers continue to optimize the synthetic pathway and reduce the number of steps required for its total synthesis, the final yield of triptolide remains too low. Therefore, researchers need to make unremitting efforts to develop new approaches for triptolide synthesis.

## 5 TOXICITY OF TRIPTOLIDE

With the increasing clinical application of *T. wilfordii* and triptolide, increasing numbers of studies and clinical case reports indicate that triptolide has serious adverse effects. Currently, triptolide has a narrow therapeutic window and induces serious toxicity and side effects, which limits its clinical application. Considering this information, we have summarized the research progress on the hepatotoxicity, nephrotoxicity, cardiotoxicity and reproductive toxicity of triptolide, hoping to contribute to better clinical prospects of this compound.

5.1 Hepatotoxicity Liver injury is the most common adverse reaction caused by triptolide, and has caused widespread concern. Many studies have been carried out to explain the mechanism of triptolide-induced liver toxicity, mainly focusing on common phenomena such as oxidative stress and inflammation. In recent years, researchers have discovered that mitotic phagocytosis associated with mitochondrial fission may be a new mechanism of induced triptolide hepatotoxicity. Jie Zhao et al. analyzed triptolide-induced changes in the serum and liver metabolome in mice, identified 30 metabolites that were significantly changed, and selected 29 of these metabolites as potential biomarkers related to triptolide-induced hepatotoxicity, with the aim of helping researchers better understand the mechanism of triptolide-induced toxicity. In addition, proteomics and targeted fatty acid analyzes were also used to reveal the mechanism of triptolide hepatotoxicity.

Yan Lu et al. found that triptolide can reduce the transcription of CYP3A, CYP2C9, CYP2C19 and CYP2E1, and the substrate affinity of the proteins leads to liver toxicity. CYP3A is the main isozyme involved in triptolide metabolism; it facilitates the detoxification of triptolide. Experiments show that catalpol (CAT), the main component of *Rehmannia glutinosa*, can increase the expression of detoxification enzymes CYP3A2/4, CYP2C9 and UGT1A6, increase the metabolic transformation of triptolide, and thereby reduce its liver toxicity. Knocking out hepatic cytochrome P450 caused a significant increase in triptolide levels, which aggravated its hepatotoxic effects.

In recent years, researchers have used high-content analysis (HCA) to measure the overall cytotoxicity phenotype of HepG2 cells treated with triptolide and finally confirmed that inhibition of global transcription associated with RNA Ⅱ is the core trigger of hepatotoxicity induced by triptolide. The latest research found that propionate produced by the intestinal flora can promote the protective effect of intestinal flora against triptolide by reducing inflammation levels.

5.2 Nephrotoxicity The nephrotoxicity of triptolide also limits its clinical application. However, the mechanism of this toxicity has not been fully elucidated. Researchers used collagen-induced arthritis (CIA) model rats as the research objects and found that triptolide transport is mediated by OTC2 in rat kidney slices and HEK-293T cells. TNF-$\alpha$ can increase the toxicity of triptolide and regulate the expression and function of OTC2, thus indicating that OCT2 mediates the nephrotoxicity of triptolide *in vitro*.

Wei Huang et al. combined network pharmacology and targeted metabolomics, and identified 61 action targets related to renal toxicity induced by triptolide, including 39 direct targets and 22 indirect targets, and finally confirmed dihydroorotate, thymidine, 2-deoxyinosine, uric acid, adenosine and xanthine as biological markers of renal toxicity. In addition, the purine metabolism pathway, toll like receptor signaling pathway and NF-$\kappa$B signaling pathway play key roles in the nephrotoxicity induced by triptolide.

5.3 Cardiotoxicity Research by Shurong Wang et al. showed that triptolide caused an increase in the expression of more than 108 microRNAs in the heart of male rats by more than twofold and reduced AhR levels in the myocardium and circulation, inducing acute cardiotoxicity. Therefore, circulating AhR levels and microRNA levels can be used as early warning biomarkers for triptolide-induced cardiotoxicity.

Researchers have studied the role of p53 in triptolide-induced cardiotoxicity in H9c2 cells, primary cardiomyocytes, and C57BL/6-derived p53 mouse models. The results showed that Bax, a target protein of p53, leads to important mitochondrial dysfunction and apoptosis in triptolide-induced cardiotoxicity and can block the permeability of the mitochondrial membrane to protect against triptolide-induced myocardial toxicity.

5.4 Reproductive toxicity Triptolide has strong reproductive toxicity, mainly in males. Triptolide can inhibit spermatogenesis and testosterone marker enzymes, reduce sperm count, lower the gonadal index and destroy the testicular microstructure. Bo Ma et al. evaluated the mechanism of triptolide-induced reproductive toxicity and identified possible new biomarkers. They reported that triptolide-mediated downregulation of PPAR caused abnormal testicular lipid and energy metabolism, which led to sperm damage, revealing the mechanism of the reproductive toxicity induced by triptolide.

Recently, researchers analyzed the expression profiles of lncRNAs/circRNAs/mRNAs and revealed the mechanism of the reproductive toxicity induced by triptolide relating to lncRNAs/circRNAs. The results show that triptolide can reduce sperm production, lead to abnormal testicular and sperm morphology, and induce mature sperm dysfunction. After stopping the use of triptolide, male fertility recovery was slow, indicating that triptolide not only destroys germ cells in the testes but also damages epididymal sperm. Data analysis show that the potential mechanism of reproductive toxicity induced by triptolide may involve the interference of genes related to spermatogenesis.

## 6 DERIVATIVES OF TRIPTOLIDE

Although triptolide has strong pharmacological activity, its clinical application is severely restricted due to its poor solubility and bioavailability, and the serious toxicity and side effects it induces, and a narrow therapeutic window. In recent years, researchers have modified the structure of triptolide to increase its water solubility and reduce the toxicity and side effects it induces without affecting its activity. Currently, a variety of triptolide derivatives, such as omtriptolide and minnelide (Figure 6) have been investigated, and some have entered the clinical trial stage (Table 2).

**Table 2 Related research on triptolide and its derivatives**

| Compound | Chemical structure | Aqueous solubility | Pharmacological activity |
|---|---|---|---|
| Triptolide (PG490, LDTT-2) | 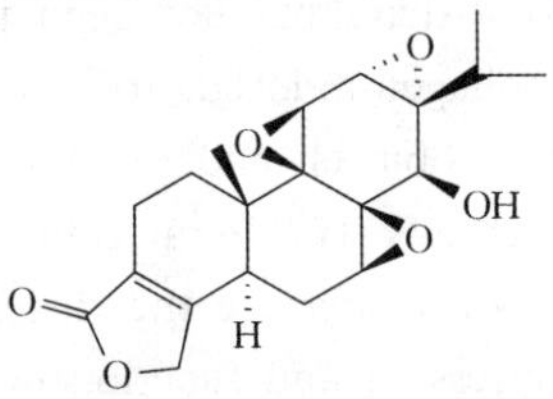 | Poor Solubility | Anti-cancer, anti-inflammatory and immuno-suppression |
| Omtriptolide (PG490-88, F60008) | 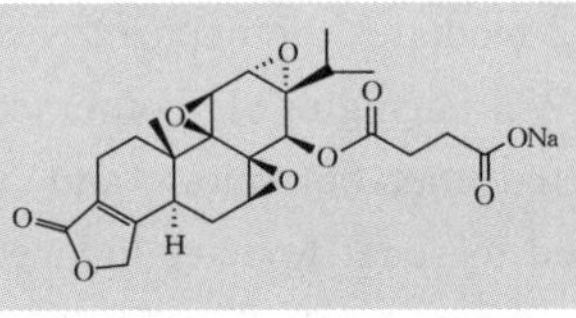 | Soluble | Anti-cancer, immunosuppression, inhibition of pro-inflammatory mediators and cytokines |
| (5R)-5-Hydroxytriptolide (LLDT-8) | 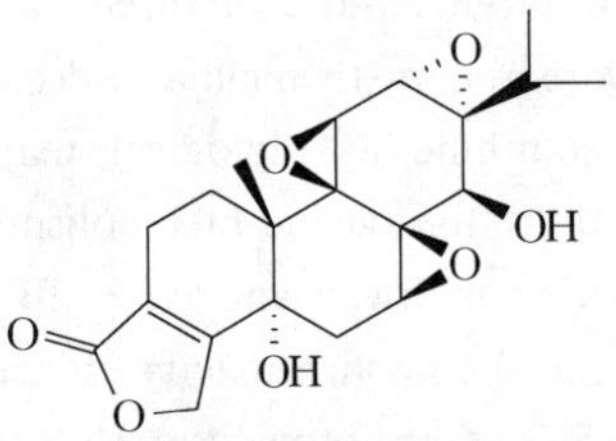 | Soluble | Immunosuppression and anti-inflammatory effects |
| Minnelide | 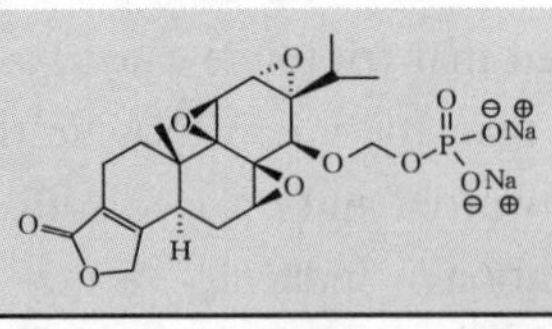 | Soluble | Extensive anti-cancer effects enhance the efficacy of chemotherapy drugs |

6.1 Omtriptolide As early as 1997, researchers designed a new semisynthetic water-soluble derivative, omtriptolide (PG490-88, f60008), by introducing a fatty acid structure into triptolide C-14. Omtriptolide shows immunosuppressive and antitumor activities (scheme 5), and it is currently approved for phase Ⅰ clinical trials of prostate cancer in the United States. Long-term research results show that PG490-88 exhibits cytotoxicity in tumor cell lines, including H23 (NSCLC), HT1080 (fibrosarcoma) and COLO 205 (colon cancer) cells. Studies have shown that when PG490-88 is used alone, it can cause the regression of lung cancer and colon cancer xenograft tumors, and the synergistic effect of PG490-88 and CPT-11 can also cause tumor regression.

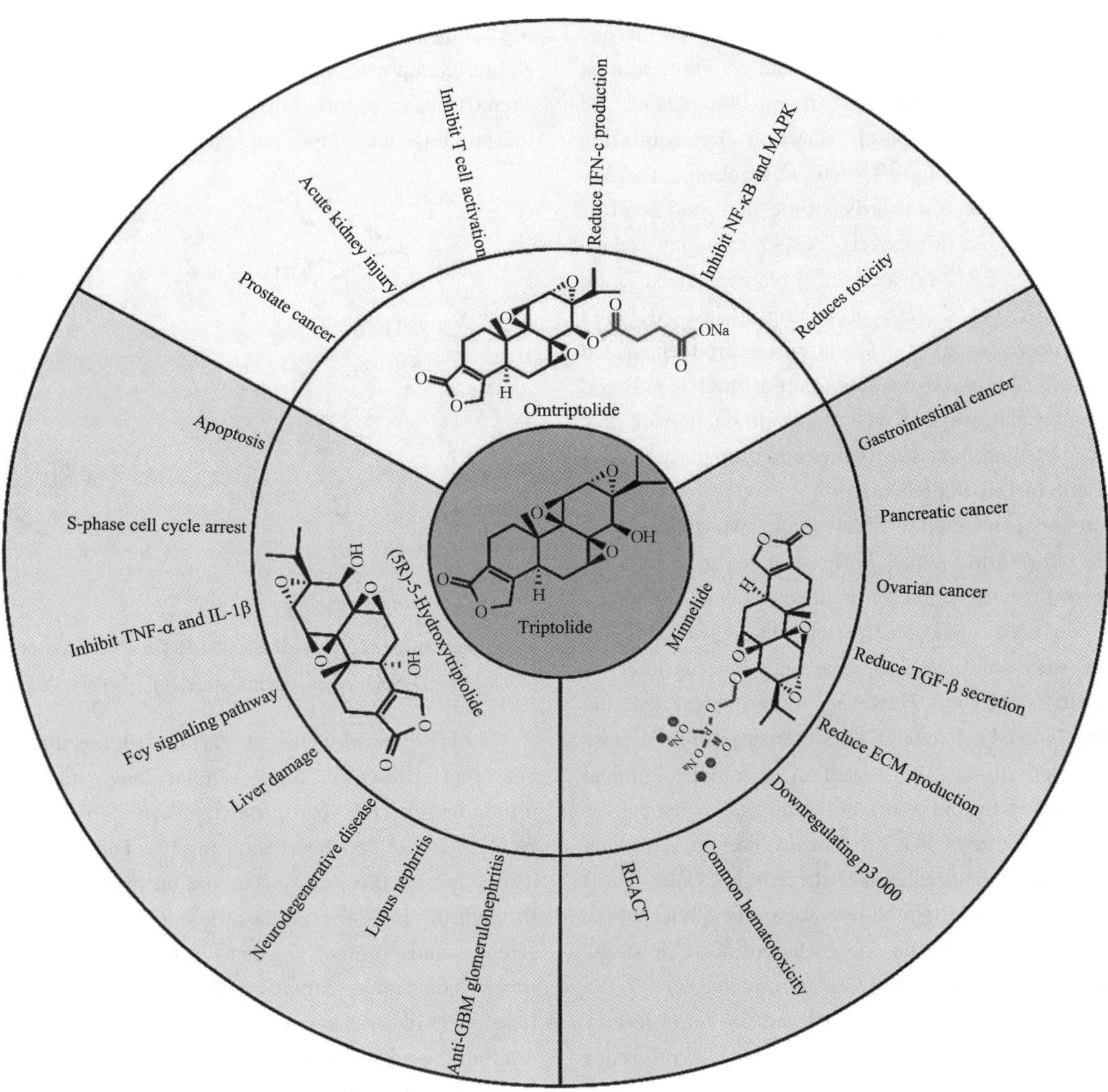


**Figure 6 Common triptolide derivatives and their research contents.**

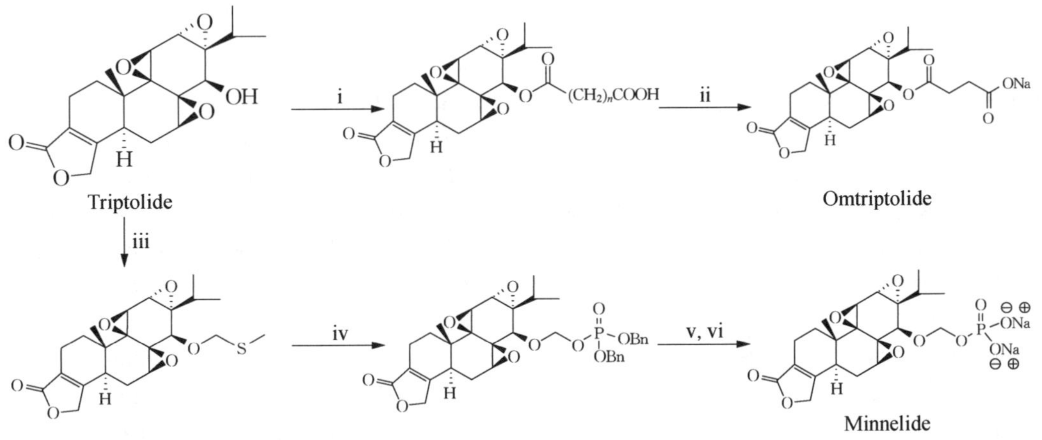

Triptolide

Omtriptolide

Minnelide

**Scheme 5 Total synthesis of Omtriptolide and Minnelide**

(i) $HO_2C(CH_2)_nCO_2H$, DCC/DMAP; (ii) n=2; (iii) $Me_2S$, MeCN, BPO, 2 h; (iv) $CH_2Cl_2$, 4A MS, $(BnO)_2P(O)OH$, NIS, THF; (v) $H_2$, Pb/C, THF; (vi) THF, $Na_2CO_3$.

In recent years, it has been found that PG490 - 88 can reduce the disease progression of kidney disease in various animal models. PG490 - 88 and tacrolimus (Tac) work synergistically to inhibit T cell activation and reduce IFN - c production and NF - AT/NF - jB activity, thereby prolonging the survival time of transplanted kidneys in a monkey model. Some scholars have found that PG490 - 88 can attenuate acute humoural rejection by inhibiting complement activation and T cell infiltration, thereby significantly prolonging the survival time dog models after kidney transplantation. Moreover, PG490 - 88 may reduce the amount of p - ERK released in cisplatin-induced acute kidney injury (AKI), thereby protecting against AKI and acute tubular necrosis (ATN). The latest research confirmed that PG490 - 88 can inhibit the activation of the NF - κB and MAPK signaling pathways as well as the production of pro-inflammatory mediators and cytokines and ultimately plays a protective role in I/R-injured rats.

Researchers conducted a phase Ⅰ and pharmacological study of PG490 - 88 in patients with advanced solid tumors. The adverse reactions were mainly fatigue, nausea, vomiting, diarrhoea, and constipation. The haematological side effects were mild grade 1 anaemia, but no liver or kidney toxicity was found. However, in two cases, the side effects were fatal. One patient died of neutrophilic sepsis, and another patient may have died of a complex clinical syndrome caused by cytokine release. Ultimately, researchers believe that the degree of PG490 - 88 conversion to triptolide in the human body is unpredictable; therefore, PG490 - 88 is not the best derivative of triptolide to use in the clinic. Phase Ⅰ clinical trials were forced to be discontinued in 2009. According to the current experimental results, PG490 - 88 has a strong anticancer effect and reduced liver and kidney toxicity compared to triptolide, which provides a reference for the clinical application of triptolide.

6.2 (5R)-5-Hydroxytriptolide (5R)-5-Hydroxytriptolide (LLDT - 8) is a new triptolide analogue with strong immunosuppressive and anti-inflammatory activity (Scheme 6). Currently, LLDT-8 is being investigated as a low-toxicity immunosuppressive agent in Phase Ⅰ clinical trials for the treatment of RA in China, and the results show that LLDT - 8 can inhibit the production of MMP - 13 and increase the expression of OPG/RANKL through the OPG/RANK/RANK ligand signaling pathway to weaken collagen-induced arthritis (CIA). This experiment used CIA to simulate RA. Early studies have shown that LLDT - 8 may be closely related to anti-inflammatory, antioxidant and cytokine effects and can protect against bleomycin-induced lung fibrosis in mice. Recently, researchers constructed the first lncRNA-TF-mRNA coexpression network, which further explain changes in whole-genome lncRNA and mRNA expression before and after LLDT - 8 treatment. The authors believe that lncRNAs may be biomarkers and targets for LLDT - 8 drug development. At the same time, LLDT - 8 showed a strong anti-inflammatory effect, for example, by regulating the Fcγ signaling pathway to improve anti-GBM glomerulonephritis and inhibiting the expression of renal chemokines to suppress infiltration of kidney immune cells, thereby improving lupus nephritis.

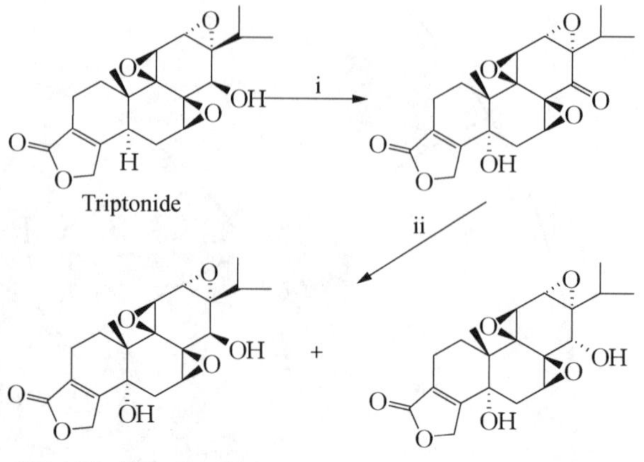

Triptonide

(5R)-5-Hydroxytriptolide

**Scheme 6 Total synthesis of (5R)-5-Hydroxytriptolide**

(i) $SeO_2$, heat reflux 10 h; (ii) $NaBH_4$, 2 h.

LLDT - 8 also has a certain therapeutic effect on neurological diseases. Some scholars have studied the anti-inflammatory and neuroprotective effects of LLDT - 8 on cerebral ischaemia-reperfusion injury. The results show that it may inhibit the neuroinflammation mediated by microglia through the IκB/NF - κB cascade, play an anti-inflammatory effect, and protect against acute cerebral ischaemia-reperfusion injury. Studies have shown that LLDT - 8 can reduce PD-like behaviour and dopaminergic neurodegeneration and neuroinflammation of the nigrostriatal system, providing a new method and entry point for the treatment of PD. LLDT - 8 can effectively inhibit pro-inflammatory factors (TNF - α and IL - 1β) to suppress the NF - κB signaling pathway and thereby reduce neuroinflammation, and it is used to treat neurodegenerative diseases. In addition, LLDT - 8 can also reduce serum alanine aminotransferase (ALT) and aspartate aminotransferase (AST) levels and reduce liver balloon cell formation and macrocystic steatosis, thereby inhibiting liver damage. LLDT - 8 can also regulate the expression levels of stearoyl-CoA desaturase 1 (SCD1) and hepatic peroxisome proliferator-activated receptor α (PPARα), significantly promoting lipid breakdown and inhibiting lipid synthesis.

Clinical trials confirmed that LLDT - 8 has broad-spectrum antitumor activity, inducing S-phase cell cycle arrest and apoptosis. As a novel transcription inhibitor, LLDT - 8 has a potential therapeutic effect on P-glycoprotein-mediated drug-resistant tumors. Researchers used mouse spleen cells for LLDT - 8 cytotoxicity experiments and found that although the inhibitory activity of LLDT - 8 against ConA and LPS cell proliferation was reduced 20-fold and the inhibitory activity against allo-MLR was reduced 14-fold, the toxicity of LLDT-8 was reduced 122-fold compared with triptolide. In addition, data from an acute toxicity study showed that LLDT-8 exhibited a 10-fold reduction in toxicity in mice. Liquid chromatography-tandem mass spectrometry (LC-MS/MS) used for the analysis and characterization and benzylamine chemical derivatization to determine the content of LLDT-8 in human plasma is a more sensitive and reliable quantitative method for studying pharmacokinetics. This method covers a wide linear dynamic range (0.030-100 ng/mL), and within this linear range, it shows better accuracy (RE < 11.7) and precision (RSD < 8.6). Considering current clinical research, LLDT-8 may be a more suitable clinical alternative drug for triptolide. In terms of pharmacological activity, LLDT-8 not only retains the strong immunosuppressive and anti-inflammatory activity of triptolide but also has broad-spectrum antitumor activity. In clinical applications, compared with triptolide, the toxicity of LLDT-8 is greatly reduced.

6.3 Minnelide Minnelide is a water-soluble derivative formed by adding a phosphate group to triptolide, endowing it with a wide range of anticancer effects (Scheme 5). Currently, minnelide has entered Phase Ⅰ clinical trials for gastrointestinal cancer and pancreatic cancer. Studies have shown that minnelide can eliminate colon cancer cells *in vitro*, reduce the growth of primary colon cancer, and metastasize colorectal cancer to the liver *in vivo* and may become a new strategy for the treatment of primary and metastatic colon cancer. A University of Minnesota team found that minnelide reduces CD133+-derived tumor volume and the number of tumor-initiating cells (TICs) in the tumor. This is the first report on the efficacy of minnelide in the syngeneic system of immune tolerance. Subsequently, the group conducted in-depth research and established an *in vitro* model for studying the characteristics of tumor stem cells and tumor-initiating cells and found that minnelide has good prospects in a preclinical evaluation. The team also found that minnelide can deplete extracellular matrix components by depleting hyaluronic acid and collagen to improve drug delivery and survival.

In addition to pancreatic cancer and gastrointestinal cancer, minnelide can also inhibit the activity of NF-κB and prevent metastasis. It effectively reduces the tumor burden and metastasis potential of osteosarcoma, has the least impact on osteoblasts of the tested compounds, and may be developed into a very effective chemotherapy drug for osteosarcoma. Studies have confirmed that minnelide can induce cell death of prostate cancer cells by downregulating AR and its variants. Minnelide can effectively inhibit the proliferation of platinum-sensitive and drug-resistant ovarian cancer cell lines, thereby improving the efficacy of standard chemotherapy, such as carboplatin and paclitaxel. In addition, minnelide combined with an anti-DR5 monoclonal antibody provides a new therapeutic option against metastatic renal cell carcinoma.

In recent years, minnelide has mainly been investigated for the treatment of pancreatic cancer and has entered a phase Ⅱ clinical trial of advanced pancreatic cancer. Minnelide is the fastest developed derivative of triptolide. Clinical trials show that the maximum patient-tolerated dose is 0.2 mg/kg. At this dose, minnelide can induce irreversible CAFs to acquire an inactive state phenotype and reduce TGF-β secretion and ECM production, thereby reducing the proliferation of TECs to cause tumor regression. Minnelide can also inhibit the pro-survival signaling in pancreatic cancer cells by downregulating the expression of p3000 and reducing the transcriptional activity of the HIF-1α transcription complex. Furthermore, minnelide regulates downstream effects by reducing hypoxia and associated signaling.

The results of a phase Ⅰ clinical trial in 27 patients with refractory gastrointestinal cancer (17 pancreas, 7 large intestine and 3 other gastrointestinal tract cancers) showed that the overall treatment effect was good except for haematotoxicity that common among the patients and usually was resolved within 2-3 days after drug withdrawal. Minnelide was administered by intravenous infusion every 28 days on days 1-5, 8-12, and 15-19, with a dose range of 0.16-0.8 mg/$m^2$. However, two patients may have suffered reversible acute cerebellar toxicity (REACT) in a phase Ⅰ clinical trial of minnelide. The patient's imaging scans showed a slight increase in the PLAIR signal and a marked decrease in cerebellar cortical spread. However, the imaging-based findings of another patient indicated a nearly opposite situation: They revealed possible post-reversible encephalopathy syndrome or acute toxic leukoencephalopathy. These results indicate that minnelide may cause potential reversible acute cerebellar toxicity. Therefore, more in-depth research and analysis are needed in the course of clinical trials. The latest research shows that c-myc transcription in AML cells can be inhibited in a range far lower than the equivalent human dose that patients can safely tolerate in phase Ⅰ clinical trials, which leads to cell cycle arrest and apoptosis, thus significantly reducing the burden of leukaemia. After entering the body, minnelide can be rapidly and completely converted into triptolide, which is beneficial for controlling the dosage of the drug, improving its safety and effectiveness.

## 7 CONCLUSIONS AND PROSPECTS

Triptolide is the main active ingredient of the traditional Chinese medicinal herb *T. wilfordii*. It has a unique chemical structure and promising pharmacological activity.

But there are still many challenges in the translation or triptolide from use in traditional to modern drugs, such as poor water solubility, a narrow treatment window, and strong toxicity and side effects. At this stage, the main solution is to modify the different parts of the triptolide structure, such as C－14 hydroxyl group, to obtain derivatives that have improved poor water solubility and fewer and less severe side effects.

In addition, the production of triptolide is also a major challenge. The traditional method for obtaining triptolide cannot meet commercial needs. With good results, research on the total synthesis of triptolide has led to researchers analyzing and optimizing synthetic routes of triptolide. At present, the research on the chemical synthesis of triptolide mainly focuses on the optimization and innovation of synthesis conditions, so as to improve the yield of triptolide. In addition, the use of biosynthetic methods to produce triptolide is the research focus of many groups. Although the biosynthetic pathway of triptolide has not been fully elucidated, the upstream biosynthetic pathway of terpenoids in *T. wilfordii* has been analyzed. Moreover, high-quality genome sequencing and annotation of *T. wilfordii* genes have been completed, laying the foundation for better identification of genes encoding key enzymes in the triptolide biosynthesis pathway.

Many reviews have been focused on triptolide. However, thus far, these reviews have been basically aimed at introducing the research progress of triptolide, such as its anticancer effects, derivative identification and advances in its total chemical synthesis. In this review, triptolide is described in detail from different perspectives such as pharmacological activity and biosynthesis, aiming to provide new ideas for researchers in different disciplines and promote the research progress of triptolide. Currently, the biosynthetic pathway of triptolide has been resolved sufficiently to identify dehydroabietic acid as a key intermediate, and the chemical synthesis of triptolide from dehydroabietic acid has been reported by scholars. This progress suggests that, in the near future research, researchers can combine biosynthesis with chemical synthesis to realize the industrial production of triptolide. Similarly, the combination of pharmacological activity research and synthetic pathway analysis can be used to study the pharmacological activities of intermediates similar to triptolide through synthetic pathways to screen analogues with the rich pharmacological activities of triptolide that induce fewer side effects, such as triptinin B and triptophenolide. For the research of triptolide derivatives, the common derivatization methods include hydroxylation or glycosylation, which may be realized by cytochrome P450 and glycosyltransferase. The analysis of biosynthetic pathways also includes dioxygenase and methyltransferase, which provide more possibilities for the study of triptolide derivatives. In the study of the pharmacological activities of triptolide derivatives and triptolide, many pathways and targets are the same, which can provide more ideas for improving the production of triptolide and its derivatives.

[高杰，黄璐琦，高伟，等. Theranostics, 2021, 11(15): 7199－7221.]

# Versatility in acyltransferase activity completes chicoric acid biosynthesis in purple coneflower

The discovery of America by Columbus changed the world in many ways, particularly through the increased exchange of valuable natural resources. One example was the introduction of *Echinacea*, a genus of herbs native to North America, and used by Native Americans as traditional medicines to treat common colds and infections. Since the 1880s, *Echinacea* extracts have become some of the most popular commercial herbal preparations, and today over 1 000 products containing extracts of *Echinacea* are listed in the Dietary Supplement Label Database (https://dsld.od.nih.gov). The total sales of products from *E. purpurea*, *E. angustifolia*, and *E. pallida*, reached US $120.2 million on the US market alone in 2019 and grew by 90.9% in the first half of 2020, partially due to the COVID－19 pandemic. The main bioactives in *Echinacea* are caffeic acid derivatives (CADs). Chicoric acid is the principal CAD and provides an index for the quality of raw material and commercial preparations of *Echinacea*. Although there isn't sufficient evidence to conclusively establish its functions, chicoric acid has been reported as an potential HIV－1 integrase inhibitor along with other bioactivities including antiviral, anti-inflammatory, glucose and lipid homeostatic, neuroprotective, anti-atherosclerosis, and anti-aging activities. Despite the large number of studies in the potential health benefits of chicoric acid, its biosynthetic pathway remains unclear.

Enzymes that use caffeoyl CoA and *meso*-tartaric acid to

generate mono-*O*-caffeoyl-*meso*-tartrate and add an additional caffeoyl group from caffeoyl CoA to form di-*O*-caffeoyl-*meso*-tartrate were reported in *Equisetum arvense* in 1996, but without identification of the encoding genes. In *Echinacea*, caftaric acid and chicoric acid are L-isomers, which differ from those in *Equisetum arvense* suggesting a distinct biosynthetic pathway. A hydroxycinnamoyl-CoA: tartaric acid hydroxycinnamoyl transferase (HTT) activity synthesizing L-caftaric acid has been reported in *Arachis glabrata*, but without gene information. However, no enzyme activity has yet been described for L-chicoric acid biosynthesis. One of the best-studied CADs is chlorogenic acid. Hydroxycinnamoyl-Coenzyme A: quinate hydroxycinnamoyl transferase (HQT), a BAHD acyltransferase family member, is involved in the biosynthesis of chlorogenic acid in different plant species. Another important acyltransferase group is the serine carboxypeptidase-like (SCPL) family. The major differences between these two families are the acyl donor source and cellular compartment: BAHDs use acyl-CoA thioesters as acyl donors in the cytosol, whereas SCPLs use 1-*O*-β-glucose esters as their acyl donors in the vacuole.

Here we report the elucidation of the chicoric acid biosynthesis pathway in purple coneflower. This pathway involves both BAHD and SCPL acyltransferases. Two BAHD enzymes, EpHTT and EpHQT are responsible for the biosynthesis of caftaric acid and chlorogenic acid in the cytosol, respectively. These two CADs serve as substrates for the generation of chicoric acid in the vacuole by a unique SCPL enzyme. Unlike other SCPLs, this SCPL prefers chlorogenic acid to 1-*O*-caffeoyl β-D-glucose as its acyl donor. Among the species we checked, this chicoric acid biosynthetic route is unique to *Echinacea spp*. and it is likely that chicoric acid biosynthesis in other species evolved by convergent catalytic mechanisms. Our results expand the understanding of acyltransferases and highlight the rapid evolution possible with these types of enzymes.

## 1 RESULTS

EpBAHDs catalyze the synthesis of caftaric acid and chlorogenic acid  Previous studies indicated that purple coneflower (*Echinacea purpurea*) contains much higher levels of chicoric acid than other *Echinacea* species. Metabolic profiling of purple coneflower seedlings revealed the presence of chicoric acid throughout the plant, making it difficult to conduct tissue-specific coexpression analysis to identify biosynthetic genes (Fig. 1). We generated hairy root cultures of purple coneflower and confirmed the presence of chicoric acid (Fig. 1). RNA-seq of hairy roots treated with methyl jasmonate to induce chicoric acid accumulation failed to provide good candidate genes due to the large number of differently expressed genes. As an alternative, we took a traditional biochemical approach and searched for caftaric acid synthase activity as caftaric acid is a likely intermediate (Fig. 1d). Based on the structural similarity of caftaric acid to chlorogenic acid, we investigated whether hydroxycinnamoyl-CoA: tartaric acid hydroxycinnamoyl transferase (HTT) could use caffeoyl CoA as an acyl donor to produce caftaric acid as reported. When tartaric acid and caffeoyl CoA were incubated with a crude protein extract from hairy roots of purple coneflower, we detected the production of caftaric acid, indicating the presence of HTT activity. In addition, the crude protein extract also catalyzed the generation of chlorogenic acid using quinic acid and caffeoyl CoA as substrates, confirming the activity of hydroxycinnamoyl-Coenzyme A: quinate hydroxycinnamoyl transferase (HQT).

We purified HTT activity by ammonium sulfate precipitation and ion-exchange chromatography and found one candidate protein annotated as HQT-like in the fraction with high HTT activity through comparison of peptide mass fingering data to hairy root RNA-seq data (Supplementary Fig. 1a - b). This protein belongs to the BAHD acyltransferase family, which utilize CoA thioesters as acyl donors: BAHD enzymes have two conserved amino acid motifs HXXXD and DFGWG. This HQT-like protein was closely related to the HCT (Hydroxycinnamoyl-Coenzyme A: quinate/shikimate hydroxy-cinnamoyl transferase) clade, with HHLVD and DFGWG motifs (Fig. 2a and Supplementary Fig. 2). In vitro enzyme assays using recombinant protein from *E. coli* confirmed that this enzyme can catalyze the biosynthesis of caftaric acid (Fig. 2b and Supplementary Fig. 3a and 4a - c), and we named it EpHTT. Similarly, in fractions with high HQT activity, we identified another BAHD acyltransferase with classic HTLSD and DFGWG motifs belonging to the HQT clade of BAHD acyltransferases (Fig. 2a, Supplementary Fig. 1a - b and 2), which could catalyze the formation of chlorogenic acid in vitro, and which we named EpHQT (Fig. 2c and Supplementary Fig. 3b and 4d - f). No putative signal peptides were found in the EpHTT or EpHQT sequences. Both EpHTT and EpHQT GFP-tagged proteins were cytosolically localized as reported for other HQTs and showed highest activities at pH 7 (Fig. 2h and Supplementary Fig. 5a - b). Although both enzymes showed promiscuity in their acyl donors, caffeoyl CoA was preferred by both (Supplementary Table 1 - 2). EpHTT differs from HTT activity from perennial peanut which prefers *p*-coumaroyl CoA as its acyl donor. We verified the function of *EpHTT* and *EpHQT* in vivo using both overexpression and gene silencing in hairy roots. When the *EpHTT* gene was overexpressed or silenced, the caftaric acid levels in transgenic hairy roots increased or decreased correspondingly (Fig. 2d, e). Similar results were seen for the *EpHQT* gene, where the contents of chlorogenic acid in the transgenic

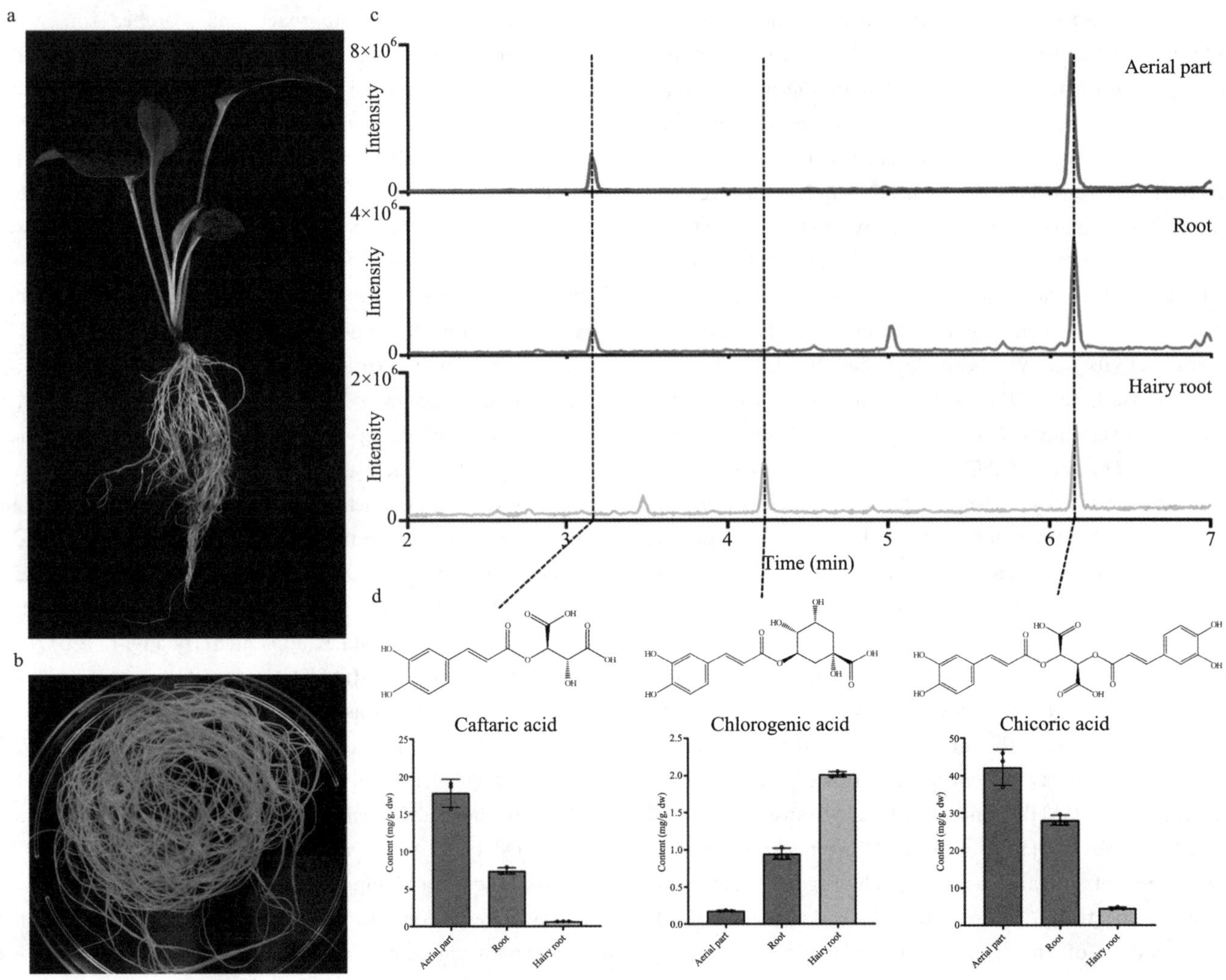


**Fig. 1 Main caffeic acid derivatives in purple coneflower**

(a) Two-month-old seedlings and (b) hairy root cultures of purple coneflower. (c) Total ion chromatograms (TIC) of aerial parts, roots, and hairy root cultures. (d) Main caffeic acid derivatives (CADs) and their abundance. Data are mean±s.d. ($n=3$ biologically independent samples). Source data underlying Fig. 1d are provided as a Source Data file.

hairy roots were correlated positively in the different lines to the expression levels of *EpHQT* (Fig. 2f, g). Our in vitro and in vivo results confirmed that EpHTT and EpHQT are responsible for caftaric acid and chlorogenic acid biosynthesis, respectively in purple coneflower.

Substrate specificities of EpBAHDs Phylogenetic analysis indicated that EpHTT might have evolved from the hydroxycinnamoyl-coenzyme A: shikimate/quinate hydroxycinnamoyl transferase (HCT) clade of BAHD acyltransferases (Fig. 2a). Using AtHCT (AED95744.1) and NtHCT (CAE46932.1) to screen RNA-seq data, we also identified a candidate transcript encoding EpHCT. EpHCT belongs to the HCT clade with conserved HHAAD and DFGWG motifs (Fig. 2a and Supplementary Fig. 2). We confirmed EpHCT function by in vitro enzyme assays which could catalyze the production of *p*-coumaroyl shikimic acid using *p*-coumaroyl CoA and shikimic acid as substrates, and the generation of 5-*O*-caffeoyl shikimic acid using caffeoyl CoA and shikimic acid as substrates (Supplementary Fig. 6). All three BAHD enzymes, EpHTT, EpHQT and EpHCT, showed preferences amongst their potential acyl acceptors (Table 1). EpHTT could use only tartaric acid but not quinic acid nor shikimic acid, EpHQT and EpHCT could use both quinic acid and shikimic acid as acyl acceptors but with significant preferences by EpHQT for quinic acid and by EpHCT for shikimic acid as previously reported (Supplementary Fig. 7). Molecular docking was undertaken based on the structural model for *p*-coumaroyl shikimic acid bound AtHCT (PDB: 5KJU). All three EpBAHDs have similar scaffolds. Compared with EpHQT and EpHCT, EpHTT formed a smaller pocket, that could accommodate only tartaric acid, and not quinic acid and shikimic acid (Supplementary Fig. 8a). Differences between the active pockets of EpHQT and EpHCT appeared critical in determining their acyl acceptor preferences (Supplementary Fig. 8b). In summary, EpHTT has likely evolved from the HCT clade of enzymes, principally through

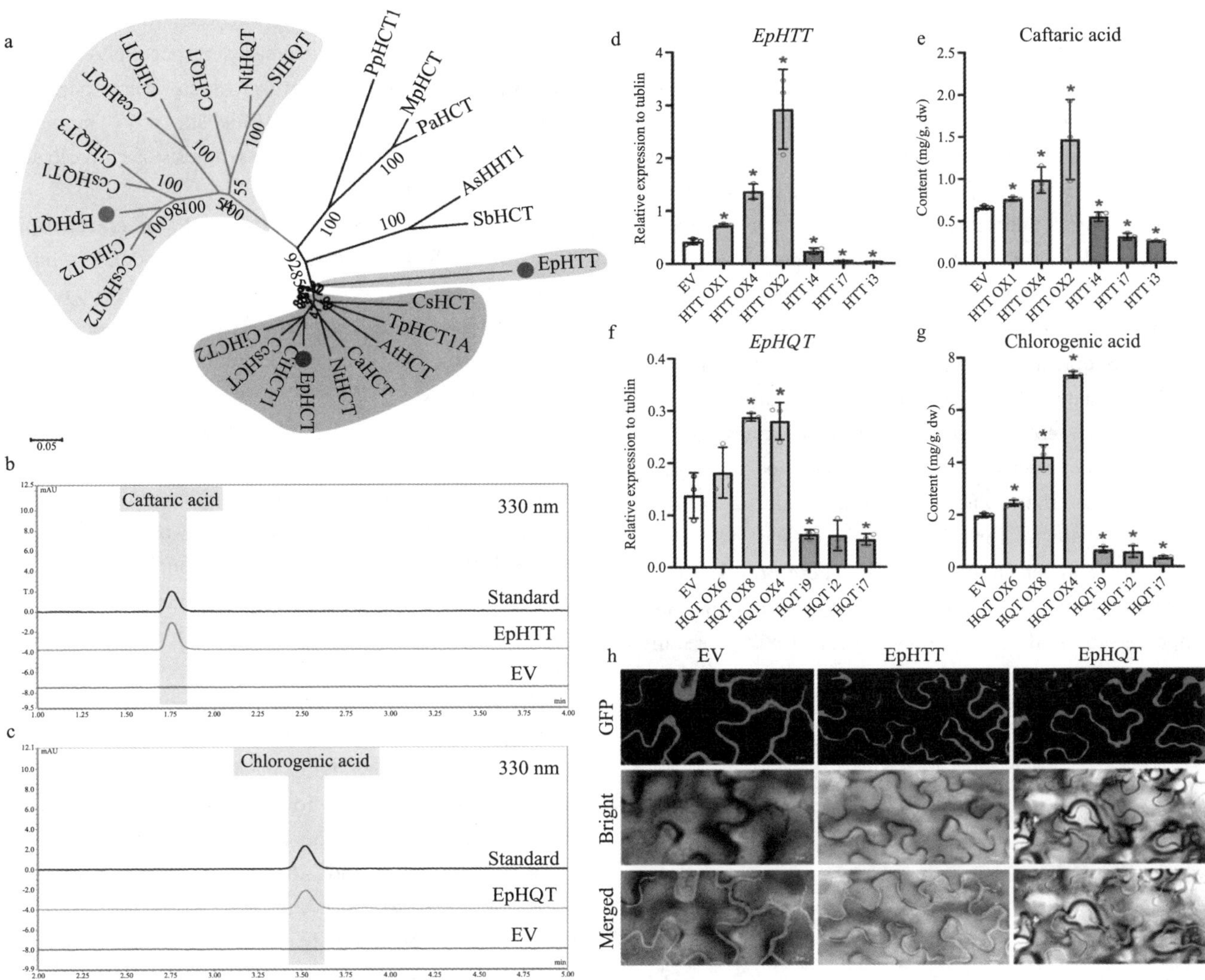


**Fig. 2 Two cytosolic BAHD acyltransferases catalyze the synthesis of caftaric acid and chlorogenic acid**

(a) Phylogenic analysis of EpHTT, EpHQT, and EpHCT with functionally identified BAHDs. GeneBank ID of the proteins used in the tree are listed in methods. The HQT and HCT clades are highlighted in orange and pink, respectively, and EpHTT is highlighted in blue. UPLC detection of caftaric acid and chlorogenic acid production by EpHTT (b) and EpHQT (c), respectively. (d) Relative expression levels of *EpHTT* and (e) caftaric acid contents in transgenic overexpression (OX) and RNAi (i) hairy root lines. (f) Relative expression levels of *EpHQT* and (g) chlorogenic acid contents in transgenic hairy root lines. Data are mean±s. d. ($n=3$ biologically independent samples). * indicates significant difference from empty vector (EV) control line ($P<0.05$) analyzed by two-sided Student's $t$-test. *$P=0.0013$ (HTT OX1), *$P=0.0005$ (HTT OX4), *$P=0.0047$ (HTT OX2), *$P=0.0163$ (HTT i4), *$P=0.0003$ (HTT i7), *$P=0.0002$ (HTT i3) in d; *$P=0.0072$ (HTT OX1), *$P=0.0230$ (HTT OX4), *$P=0.0430$ (HTT OX2), *$P=0.0302$ (HTT i4), *$P=0.0002$ (HTT i7), *$P=0.000008$ (HTT i3) in e; *$P=0.0042$ (HQT OX8), *$P=0.0118$ (HQT OX4), *$P=0.0420$ (HQT i9), *$P=0.0298$ (HQT i7) in f; *$P=0.0053$ (HQT OX6), *$P=0.0013$ (HQT OX8), *$P=0.0000004$ (HQT OX4), *$P=0.0001$ (HQT i9), *$P=0.0005$ (HQT i2), *$P=0.000009$ (HQT i7) in (g). (h) Cytosolic localization of EpHTT and EpHQT in *Nicotiana benthamiana* leaves. Scale bars show 20 μm. This experiment was repeated independently three times with similar results. Source data underlying d-g are provided as a Source Data file.

specialization of its acyl acceptor recognition.

Chicoric acid is synthesized from caftaric acid and chlorogenic acid As suggested by the formation of di-caffeoyl quinic acid in tomato and di-*O*-caffeoyl-*meso*-tartrate in *Equisetum arvense*, we tried to establish a similar in vitro chicoric acid biosynthesis assay. However, neither EpHTT nor crude protein extract could convert caftaric acid or caftaric acid with caffeoyl CoA to chicoric acid (Supplementary Fig. 9a, b). We noticed that decreases in *EpHQT* expression also led to the decline of chicoric acid content in transgenic hairy roots (Supplementary Fig. 9c). Chlorogenic acid has been reported as an acyl donor for the biosynthesis of di-caffeoyl quinic acid by SlHQT, as well as caffeoylglucarate by a GDSL lipase-like acyltransferase in tomato. This suggested that chlorogenic acid might be used as acyl donor in chicoric acid biosynthesis. Consequently, we incubated caftaric acid and chlorogenic acid with a crude protein extract from purple coneflower and detected the formation of chicoric acid. We optimized this assay using acidic and low salt conditions (PBS pH 4.0 without NaCl or

KCl) (Supplementary Fig. 9b). Together, these data suggested that chicoric acid can be synthesized from caftaric acid and chlorogenic acid by a chicoric acid synthase in purple coneflower.

A SCPL enzyme catalyzes the biosynthesis of chicoric acid The activity of chicoric acid synthase was measured and fractions with the highest activities were used for peptide mass fingering (Supplementary Fig. 1c, d). However, peptides of neither BAHDs nor GDSL lipase-like proteins were detected. Instead, we noticed peptides of a Serine carboxypeptidase-like (SCPL) protein were enriched in the fractions (Supplementary Fig. 1e). This protein belongs to the SCPL clade IA which has been reported to have acyltransferase activity (Fig. 3a). In vitro assays indicated that this protein, when expressed and purified from yeast, could catalyze the trans-acylation of caftaric acid by chlorogenic acid to form chicoric acid and quinic acid (Fig. 3b and Supplementary Fig. 10). Therefore, we named this SCPL protein, chicoric acid synthase (EpCAS). Compared to BAHD acyltransferases, EpCAS required longer incubation times for accumulation of its chicoric acid product to become apparent, which is typical of other SCPLs. We determined the kinetic parameters of EpCAS using in vitro enzyme assays and found that EpCAS showed quite low *Kcat* values for its caftaric acid and chlorogenic acid substrates (Supplementary Table 3). Similar to other SCPLs, EpCAS has a conserved vacuolar targeting peptide at its N-terminus (Met1 – His24) (Supplementary Fig. 11). We confirmed that an EpCAS GFP-fusion protein was located in vacuoles, and the enzyme shows highest activity at pH 4 consistent with its vacuolar location (Fig. 3e and Supplementary Fig. 5c). We verified the role of EpCAS in chicoric acid biosynthesis in vivo using hairy roots. When *EpCAS* was overexpressed or silenced, the chicoric acid content was increased or decreased respectively, consistent with *EpCAS* expression levels which were accordingly upregulated or downregulated (Fig. 3c, d). These results showed that EpCAS catalyzes the synthesis of chicoric acid in purple coneflower.

**Table 1 EpBAHD substrate preferences**

| Enzyme | Acyl donors | Acyl acceptors | | |
|---|---|---|---|---|
| | | Tartaric acid | Quinic acid | Shikimic acid |
| EpHTT | Caffeoyl CoA | + | n. d. | n. d. |
| | *p*-Coumaroyl CoA | + | n. d. | n. d. |
| | Feruloyl CoA | + | n. d. | n. d. |
| EpHQT | Caffeoyl CoA | n. d. | + | + |
| | *p*-Coumaroyl CoA | n. d. | + | + |
| | Feruloyl CoA | n. d. | + | n. d. |
| EpHCT | Caffeoyl CoA | n. d. | + | + |
| | *p*-Coumaroyl CoA | n. d. | + | + |
| | Feruloyl CoA | n. d. | n. d. | n. d. |

"+" indicates that the reaction can happen. n. d. means no detection of corresponding products under these experimental conditions.

When the EpCAS was aligned with other functionally characterized SCPL acyltransferases, we found it had the conserved Ser-His-Asp catalytic triad (Supplementary Fig. 12), which is necessary for hydrolysis of peptide bonds by serine proteinase and can be inhibited by phenylmethyl-sulfonyl fluoride (PMSF). Indeed, the in vitro activity of EpCAS was inhibited by PMSF in a dose-dependent manner (Fig. 4a). The significance of the conserved Ser-His-Asp catalytic triad of EpCAS was also confirmed using site-directed mutagenesis. When the Ser180 was replaced by Ala, EpCAS lost acyltransferase activity completely. Mutations converting His430 and Asp374 to alanine also showed significantly lower activities (Fig. 4b). These results demonstrated that the catalytic triad is crucial for the acyl transfer activity. Molecular docking based on the structure of the yeast serine carboxypeptidase (PDB: 1YSC) was used to investigate the catalytic mechanism of EpCAS. The catalytic triad of EpCAS formed the reactive part of the active site, especially Ser180 which could act as a nucleophilic residue and attack the carbonyl C of the chlorogenic acid to form an ester with the caffeic acid intermediate. The ester bond of this complex could be subsequently attacked by caftaric acid and result in the production of chicoric acid (Fig. 4c). Surprisingly, we also detected caffeic acid as a byproduct in the EpCAS reaction (Fig. 3b and Supplementary Fig. 10f – g). An SCPL (1-*O*-sinapoyl-β-D-glucose: L-malate sinapoyl transferase) from *Arabidopsis* has also been reported to have a minor hydrolytic activity producing sinapic acid from 1-*O*-sinapoyl-β-D-glucose (pH 6.0). When EpCAS was mixed with caftaric acid or chlorogenic acid alone (pH 4.0), it cleaved caffeic acid from both these substrates (Supplementary Fig. 13). Another SCPL from *Zea mays*, 1-*O*-(indole-3-acetyl)-β-D-glucose: *myo*-inositol indoleacetyl transferase has also been reported to have hydrolytic activity towards its product. EpCAS could also hydrolyze chicoric acid to release caftaric acid and caffeic acid, but this reaction was irreversible (Supplementary Fig. 13c – d). It seems that the Ser180 of the catalytic triad can attack the ester bond of these caffeic acid esters directly and release minor amounts of caffeic acid.

The substrate specificity of EpCAS Since previous studies have indicated that SCPL acyltransferases use 1-*O*-β-D-glucose esters as their acyl donors, we investigated whether EpCAS could also use 1-*O*-caffeoyl-β-D-glucose as

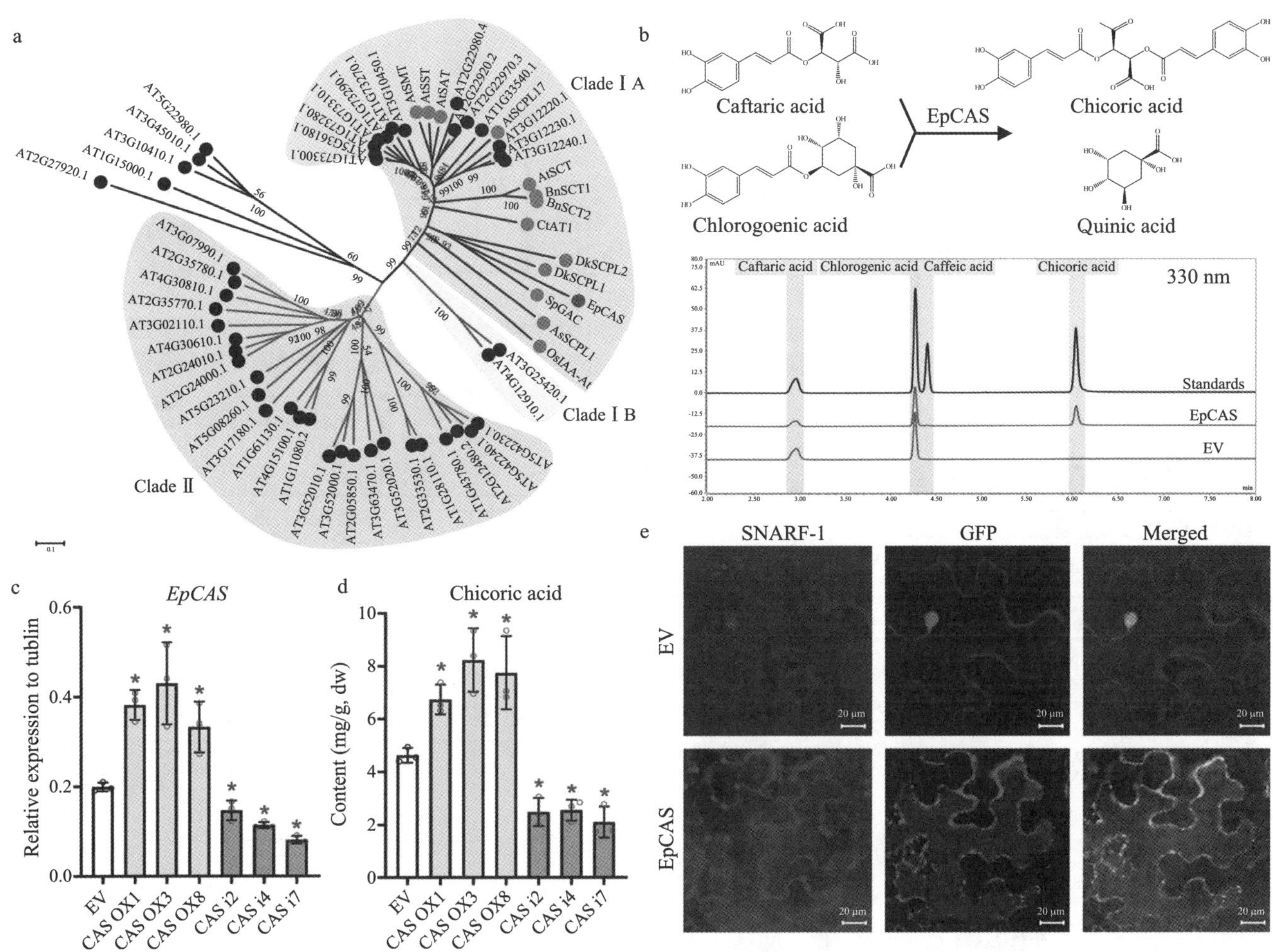


**Fig. 3 A SCPL enzyme catalyzes the biosynthesis of chicoric acid**

(a) Phylogenic analysis of EpCAS together with *Arabidopsis thaliana* and several additional functionally characterized SCPLs. EpCAS is marked in red. SCPLs previously characterized functionally are marked in green. (b) UPLC detection of chicoric acid generated by recombinant EpCAS. (c) Relative expression levels of *EpCAS* and (d) chicoric acid contents in transgenic over expression (OX) and RNAi (i) hairy root lines. Data are mean±s. d. ($n=3$ biologically independent samples). * indicates a significant difference from the empty vector (EV) control line ($P<0.05$) analyzed by two-sided Student's $t$-test. $^*P=0.0008$ (CAS OX1), $^*P=0.0123$ (CAS OX3), $^*P=0.0162$ (CAS OX8), $^*P=0.0187$ (CAS i2), $^*P=0.0002$ (CAS i4), $^*P=0.0001$ (CAS i7) in c; $^*P=0.0045$ (CAS OX1), $^*P=0.0071$ (CAS OX3), $^*P=0.0189$ (CAS OX8), $^*P=0.0034$ (CAS i2), $^*P=0.0017$ (CAS i4), $^*P=0.0025$ (CAS i7) in (d). (e) EpCAS is vacuole-localized in *Nicotiana benthamiana* leaves. The vacuole was visualized by SNARF - 1. Scale bars, 20 μm. This experiment was repeated independently three times with similar results. Source data underlying c and d are provided as a Source Data file.

its acyl donor. When we incubated 1-*O*-caffeoyl-β-D-glucose (Supplementary Fig. 14) with caftaric acid, very little chicoric acid was detected (Supplementary Fig. 15a - b). Compared to chlorogenic acid, the relative activity of EpCAS in using 1-*O*-caffeoyl-β-D-glucose was reduced to 0.67 ± 0.06% (Supplementary Fig. 16a). The in vitro kinetics of EpCAS against 1-*O*-caffeoyl-β-D-glucose compared to chlorogenic acid showed that even though they had comparable *Km* values, the *Kcat* and *Kcat*/*Km* values were much lower for 1-*O*-caffeoyl-β-D-glucose (Supplementary Table 3). Docking results showed that the glucose group of 1-*O*-caffeoyl-β-D-glucose would sink into the inner pocket and hinder the entry of caftaric acid. Although quinic acid and glucose have similar structures, the extra carboxyl group of quinic acid would hinder the entrance of chlorogenic acid to the inner pocket of EpCAS. This difference suggested that quinic acid would be liberated more easily from chlorogenic acid than glucose from 1-*O*-caffeoyl-β-D-glucose, explaining the preference of EpCAS for chlorogenic acid as its acyl donor (Supplementary Fig. 15c). Interestingly, we found that compounds with structures similar to chlorogenic acid (neochlorogenic acid, cryptochlorogenic acid and 5-*O*-caffeoyl shikimic acid) could also be used by EpCAS but with much lower relative activities (<1%) than with chlorogenic acid under identical conditions (Supplementary Fig. 16). These results demonstrated that EpCAS has evolved unique specificity for its acyl donor, distinct from that of other characterized SCPL enzymes in plants. Interestingly, although we could detect very low activity of purified EpCAS enzyme when using 1-*O*-caffeoyl-β-D-glucose as an acyl donor

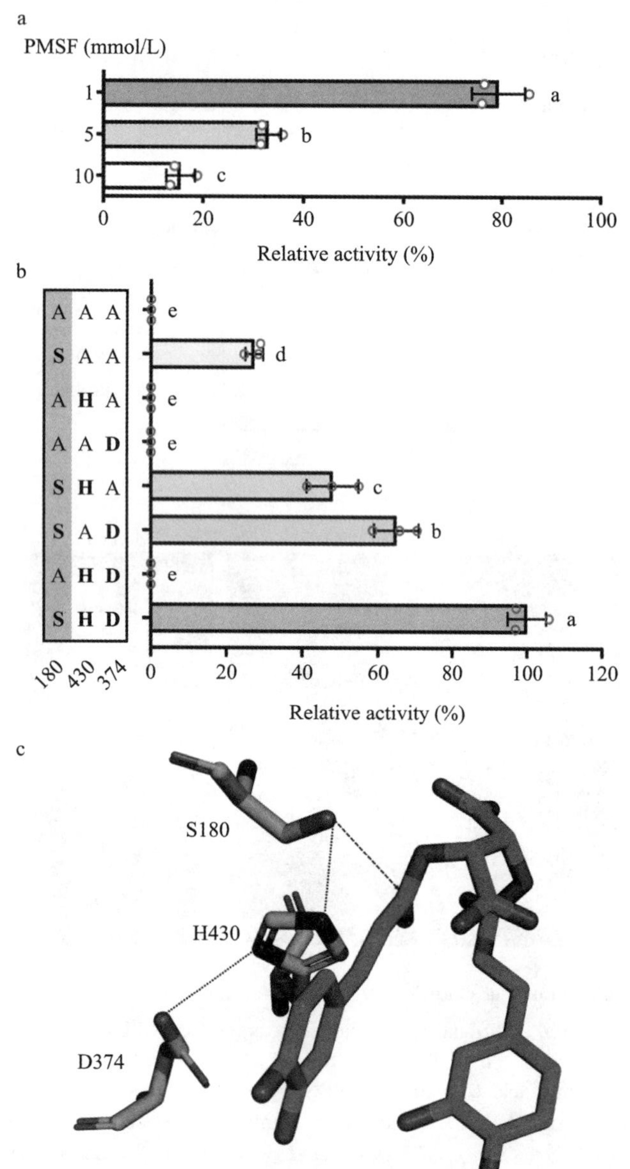


**Fig. 4 The Ser-His-Asp catalytic triad is necessary for the acyltransferase activity of EpCAS**

(a) EpCAS activity was inhibited by Phenylmethylsulfonyl fluoride (PMSF) in a dose-dependent manner. (b) Site-directed mutagenesis of Ser-His-Asp catalytic triad. Ser180 is necessary for the acyltransferase activity of EpCAS. Data are mean ± s. d. ($n = 3$ independent experiments). Different letters in a and b indicate significantly different values at $P < 0.05$ analyzed by one-way ANOVA with Tukey's multiple comparisons test. (c) Molecular docking of Ser-His-Asp catalytic triad with chicoric acid. Source data underlying a and b are provided as a Source Data file.

in vitro, crude protein extracts of purple coneflower could not use 1-*O*-caffeoyl-β-D-glucose as an acyl donor to synthesize caftaric acid, chlorogenic acid or chicoric acid (Supplementary Fig. 17). In addition, we failed to detect any 1-*O*-caffeoyl-β-D-glucose in extracts of purple coneflower (Supplementary Fig. 18). All these results demonstrated that in purple coneflower, EpCAS has evolved specificity for its acyl donor.

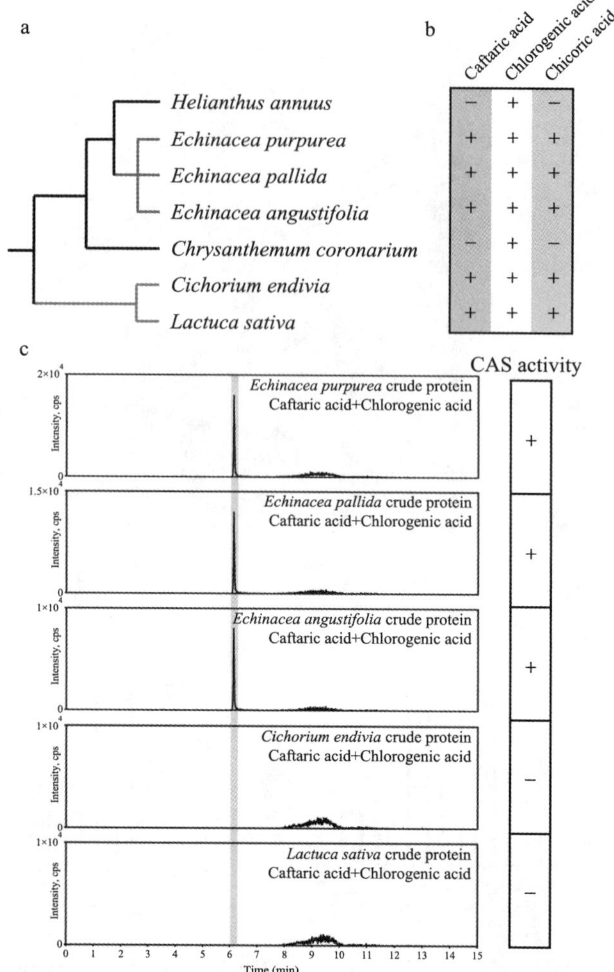


**Fig. 5 Chicoric acid biosynthesis is polyphyletic between different species**

(a) Phylogenetic relationships among several related species. Two *Echinacea* species (*Echinacea pallida* and *Echinacea angustifolia*) and two distantly related species (*Cichorium endivia* and *Lactuca sativa*) containing both substrates (caftaric acid and chlorogenic acid) and chicoric acid; as well as *Helianthus annuus* and *Chysanthemum coronarium*, from two intervening plant lineages which contain only chlorogenic acid were selected for the study of chicoric acid biosynthetic routes. The tree was adopted from NCBI taxonomy (http://lifemap-ncbi.univ-lyon1.fr/). (b) The presence of target compounds in each species. (c) CAS activities from different chicoric acid containing plant crude protein extracts. Only *Echinacea* species can use caftaric acid as an acyl acceptor and chlorogenic acid as an acyl donor to produce chicoric acid.

Chicoric acid biosynthesis is polyphyletic in the plant kingdom So far, over sixty genera and species have been found to contain chicoric acid. To investigate the conservation of EpCAS's unique acyltransferase activity in other chicoric acid producing species, we selected several representative species including: another two *Echinacea* species (*Echinacea pallida* and *Echinacea angustifolia*) and two distantly related species (*Cichorium endivia* and *Lactuca sativa*) known to produce caftaric acid, chlorogenic acid and chicoric acid; as well as *Helianthus annuus* and *Chysanthemum coronarium*, from two different intervening plant lineages which accumulate only chlorogenic acid (Fig. 5a - b and Supplementary Fig. 19). When we incubated crude protein extracts from the other chicoric acid-producing species with caftaric acid and chlorogenic acid, *E. pallida* and *E. angustifolia* crude protein extracts showed CAS activities. However, *Cichorium endivia* and *Lactuca sativa* failed to produce chicoric acid (Fig. 5c). Crude protein extracts from all samples exhibited HQT activities, but *Cichorium endivia* and *Lactuca sativa* crude protein extracts did not show HTT activities agreeing with their lack of CAS activity (Supplementary Fig. 20). In addition, we were unable to find any sequences encoding highly homologous proteins to EpHTT and EpCAS from the *Lactuca sativa* genome or any other public available databases by BLAST, while the BAHD proteins with the HTLSD motif (conserved in HQT-likes proteins) were found. It seems likely that the pathway for chicoric acid biosynthesis catalyzed by HTT and CAS in *Echinacea* species is unique. In other chicoric acid containing species, we conclude that chicoric acid is likely synthesized using different substrates and enzyme activities. Our results support the idea that chicoric acid biosynthesis is polyphyletic and has evolved in different plant lineages by convergence.

**Reconstruction of chicoric acid biosynthesis in *N. benthamiana*** As a proof of concept, we attempted to reconstruct chicoric acid biosynthesis in planta. As *N. benthamiana* leaves produce abundant chlorogenic acid but no tartaric acid, different biosynthetic genes (*EpHTT* and *EpCAS*) and precursor (tartaric acid) combinations were investigated for their ability to produce chicoric acid. Coexpression of *EpHTT* and *EpCAS* and subsequent supplementation with tartaric acid generated chicoric acid verifying the functions of the identified genes and showing that they could be used for engineering chicoric acid production in plant chassis (Fig. 6). Future attempts to scale-up production of chicoric acid could be explored in chassis with a good source of tartaric acid combined with other metabolic engineering tools.

## 2 DISCUSSION

For millennia, humans have used plant specialized metabolites as herbal medicines. During the past two decades, especially in the postgenomic era, strategies such as co-expression and genome mining have been used extensively for metabolic pathway identification. In this study, however, we describe steps in a metabolic pathway identified using traditional biochemistry. While RNA-seq, co-expression analysis and genome mining are becoming more popular approaches, discovery of genuinely novel activities may still be served best by strategies based on characterizing enzyme activities.

We have shown that the biosynthesis of chicoric acid, the major bioactive compound of purple coneflower, involves a two-step process. In the cytosol, two BAHD acyltransferases, EpHTT and EpHQT catalyze the production of caftaric acid and chlorogenic acid intermediates, respectively. Both compounds are transported to the vacuole to form chicoric acid catalyzed by EpCAS (Fig. 7). In purple coneflower, chicoric acid has been reported to be stored in vacuoles, in line with our proposed biosynthetic pathway. Chicoric acid is also present in intercellular spaces and cell walls which may be due to release following cell damage. Like other identified SCPLs, EpCAS prefers acidic conditions and exhibits highest in vitro enzyme activity at pH 4, like SlHQT chlorogenate-chlorogenate transferase activity in vacuoles. EpCAS activity was relatively high (>80% of the maximum) over the pH range of 3.6 to 4.9, which should ensure the production of chicoric acid under vacuolar pH conditions. Based on our results, the biosynthesis of chicoric acid is likely to depend on transport of caftaric acid and chlorogenic acid into the vacuoles, although, to date, no transporters for hydroxycinnamic acid derivatives have been reported. Chlorogenic acid has been reported to be transported into vacuoles by vesicles in *Lonicera japonica* flowers.

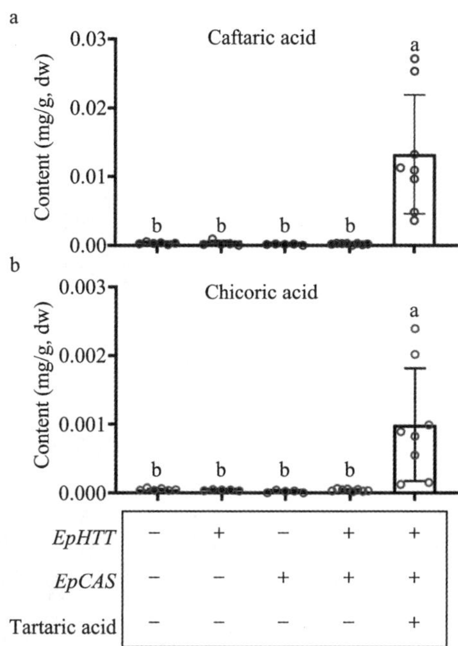


**Fig. 6 Reconstruction of chicoric acid biosynthesis in *Nicotiana benthamiana* leaves**

(a) Caftaric acid and (b) chicoric acid contents of *N. benthamiana* leaves infiltrated with different combinations of genes and precursor. Data are mean ± s. d. ($n$ = 8, 5, 5, 6, 8 biologically independent samples, respectively). Lowercase letters indicate significant differences from each other ($P < 0.05$) analyzed by one-way ANOVA with Tukey's multiple comparisons test. Source data are provided as a Source Data file.

Chicoric acid has been reported to have multiple physiological functions, making it an important target for

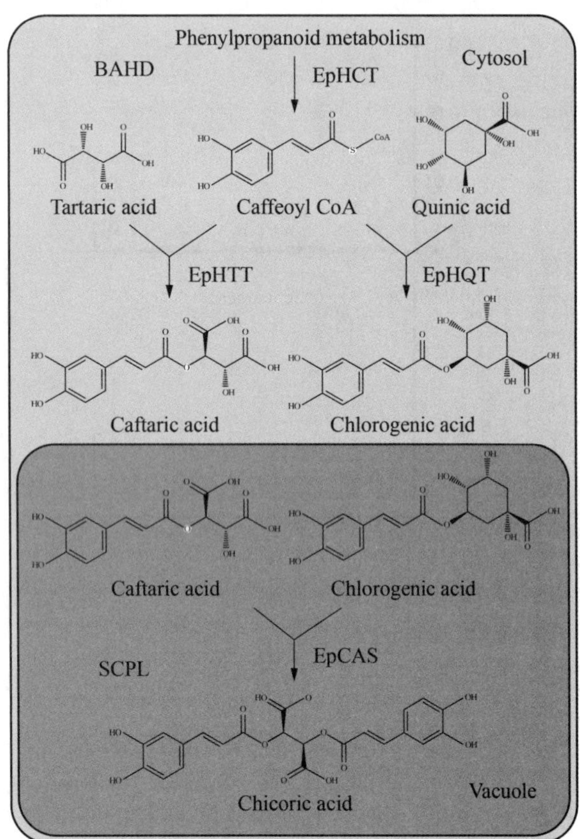


**Fig. 7 Schematic representation of the proposed chicoric acid biosynthetic pathway in purple coneflower**

Two types of acyltransferases distributed in distinct subcellular compartments are involved in the biosynthesis of chicoric acid. In the cytosol, the BAHDs including EpHTT and EpHQT use caffeoyl CoA from phenylpropanoid metabolism as an acyl donor to synthesize caftaric acid and chlorogenic acid, respectively. Both products are then transported into the vacuole. EpCAS, a specialized SCPL acyltransferase, uses chlorogenic acid as its acyl donor instead of 1-*O*-caffeoyl-β-D-glucose and transfers the caffeoyl group to caftaric acid to generate chicoric acid.

synthetic biology. Using *N. benthamiana*, we have successfully reconstituted the chicoric acid biosynthetic pathway. However, due to the absence of tartaric acid, *N. benthamiana* is not the ideal chassis for producing chicoric acid. Since the biosynthesis of tartaric acid has not been fully elucidated, further attempts to reconstruct chicoric acid biosynthesis should be focused on chassis with naturally high tartaric acid contents.

Our results emphasize the flexibility of specialized metabolism in plants, particularly the broad importance of transfer of acyl groups to form specialized bioactives. Unlike other SCPLs, in purple coneflower, EpCAS utilizes chlorogenic acid rather than 1-*O*-caffeoyl β-glucose as its acyl donor. Among the species we tested, this pathway is unique, existing only *Echinacea* species and it is likely that chicoric acid biosynthesis is polyphyletic and has evolved by convergent mechanisms in other plant lineages. Chicoric acid is also vacuole-localized in *Cichorium endivia* where it may be synthesized using caffeoyl CoA as an acyl donor as suggested for *Equisetum arvense*, or produced by modification of other intermediates, such as *p*-coumaroylcaffeoyl tartaric acid. Further research is needed to clarify its biosynthesis in other species. Additionally, it will be interesting to identify the biological functions (if any) of chicoric acid in *Echinacea* and other species. This could help us better understand its evolution and regulation. In summary, our results expand our understanding of acyltransferases in specialized metabolism and highlight the rapid evolution possible with these types of enzymes.

## 3 METHODS

Plant materials  Seeds of *Echinacea purpurea* (No. PI656830) were obtained from United States National Plant Germplasm System. Seeds were pretreated with 40 ℃ water at for 6 h and then grown in sterilized soil in the greenhouse (23 ± 2 ℃, 16 h light/8 h dark). Two-month-old seedings were used for profiling of caffeic acid derivatives. Germination of sterile seedings was conducted as follows: seeds were sterilized with 5% Plant Preservative Mixture (PPM) (Plant Cell Technology, USA) in 3× Murashige and Skoog (MS) basal salt medium for 10 h and washed with sterile water three times. Superfluous water was absorbed with sterile filter paper. The seeds were plated on MS solid medium in the dark (covered with aluminum foil paper) for 2 weeks at 23 ℃ before gemination. Seedings were transferred into an incubator (23℃, 16 h light/8 h dark) and cultivated for one month before hairy root production. *Nicotiana benthamiana* was grown in sterilized soil in a green-house (23± 2 ℃, 16 h light/8 h dark) for subcellular localization and metabolic engineering. *Helianthus annuus*, *Chrysanthemum coronarium*, *Cichorium endivia*, and *Lactuca sativa* were collected from a local supermarket.

Extraction of caffeic acid derivatives  Plant materials were collected and frozen in liquid nitrogen immediately and stored at −80 ℃. On the day of extraction, samples were lyophilized and ground into powder. Ten milligrams dry sample were weighed and extracted with 1 mL 70% methanol (v/v) in an ultrasonic bath (Qsonica 700, USA) with 50% amplitude at 4 ℃, 20 s on 40 s off, for a total of 15 min. Extracts were centrifuged at 5,000× *g* for 10 min at 4 ℃ and the supernatants were collected. The residue was extracted again using the same conditions. The two supernatants were combined and diluted to 2.5 mg/mL (dry material vs. solvent) for analysis using an ultra-performance liquid chromatography-diode array detector (UPLC - DAD) for detection of caffeic acid derivatives (CADs) and 0.5 mg/mL for liquid chromatography-high-resolution mass spectrometry (LC - HRMS) analysis. The extracts were further centrifuged at

20,000 × *g* for 10 min at 4 ℃ and the supernatants were collected and stored at −80 ℃ before analysis.

Qualitative analysis of CADs using LC-HRMS system CADs were qualified based on the comparison of their retention times and mass spectra from samples and standards using LC-HRMS (Nexera UHPLC LC-30A and AB SCIEX qTOF X500R) coupled with a Turbol V™ source and SCIEX OS software (version 1.7). The LC analytical conditions were as follows: samples were separated using a Hypersil Gold C18 column (100 × 2.1 mm, 1.9 μm; Thermo Fisher Scientific, USA) and the column temperature was set at 40 ℃. The flow rate was 0.4 mL/min. The mobile phases were 0.1% formic acid (A) and acetonitrile (B), and the gradient was as follows: 2% B for 0.5 min; 2%-20% B for 5.5 min; 20%-95% B for 4 min; 95% B for 2 min followed by a decrease to 2% B for 0.1 min and re-equilibration of the column for 2.9 min with 2% B. The injection volume was 1.0 μL and the sampler temperature was set at 15 ℃. Mass spectrometry was performed using an electrospray ionization (ESI) source operating with the information-dependent acquisition (IDA) model. The source parameters in negative polarity were as follows: ion source gas 1 : 50 psi; ion source gas 2 : 50 psi; curtain gas: 35 psi; CAD gas: 7; temperature: 450 ℃; spray voltage: −4 500 V; for TOF-MS, the mass range: 100-1 000 Da; declustering potential (DP): −80 V; DP spread: 0; collision energy (CE): −10 V; CE spread: 0; accumulation time: 0.1 s; IDA criteria: small molecule; for TOF-MS/MS, the mass range: 50 https://mpsde3.mpslimited.com/Digicore/DigiEditPage.aspx? FileName=42135245610049141133013 7.xml 1 000 Da; DP: −80 V; DP spread: 0; CE: −40 V; CE spread: 20 V; accumulation time: 0.05 s.

Quantitative analysis of CADs using UPLC-DAD system CAD contents were determined quantitatively using a UPLC-DAD system. Three CAD standards including caftaric acid, chicoric acid and chlorogenic acid were used. Retention times and the UV-vis spectra of standards and samples were compared for confirmation. Quantification was performed on a DIONEX UltiMate 3 000 UHPLC system with Chromeleon software (Thermo Fisher Scientific, USA). Sample separation was performed using a Hypersil Gold C18 column (100 × 2.1 mm, 1.9 μm; Thermo Fisher Scientific, USA), and the column temperature was set at 40 ℃. The mobile phases were 0.1% formic acid water (A) and acetonitrile (B). The gradient was as follows: 2% B for 0.5 min; 2%-14% B for 1 min; 14%-18% B for 5.5 min; 18%-80% B for 2 min; 80% B for 1 min, followed by re-equilibration of the column for 3 min with 2% B. The flow rate was set as 0.5 mL/min and the injection volume was 2.0 μL. The sampler temperature was 10 ℃. UV-vis absorption spectra were recorded online from 190 to 800 nm. Detection was conducted at 330 nm for quantitative purposes. Quantifications were carried out using external standards for calibration curves. The calibration curve coefficients for caftaric acid, chicoric acid, and chlorogenic acid were all above 0.999 9. The results were expressed as mg of each CADs per 1 g dry material.

Generation of *Echinacea purpurea* hairy roots The hairy roots were constructed as previously reported. Briefly, single colonies of pK7WG2R plasmid containing *Agrobactrium rhizogenes* A4 strain were inoculated into 5 mL of tryptone yeast broth (with 10 mmol/L $CaCl_2$, 50 mg/L spectinomycin, and 50 mg/L kanamycin). The cultures were incubated at 28 ℃ overnight with shaking (180 rpm). The cultures were centrifuged for 15 min at 3 000 × *g* at 4 ℃ and resuspended in MS liquid medium containing 200 μmol/L acetosyringone to make infection solution.

Leaf explants from one-month-old *Echinacea purpurea* plants grown on MS medium were scratched by a sterilized knife blade in cold, sterilized water. Explants were immersed in infection solution for 5 min and blotted dry on sterile filter paper. Infected explants were then cocultured on MS medium containing 200 μmol/L acetosyringone at 25 ℃ in the dark for 3 days before moving into MS medium supplemented with cefotaxime (250 mg/L). Hairy roots developed on cut ends of tissue were cultured in fresh 1/2 B5 solid medium (with 250 mg/L cefotaxime) at 25 ℃ in the dark. Hairy root cultures were transferred to fresh solid medium every 3 weeks and maintained as separate independent clones. Elongated root tips were transferred to flasks containing 30 mL of 1/2 B5 liquid medium (250 mg/L cefotaxime) to make liquid cultures, which were subcultured every week.

Methyl jasmonate treatment and RNA-sequencing Empty vector-induced hairy roots were used for methyl jasmonate (MeJA) treatment. Hairy root cultures coming from independent progenitor roots were prepared and part of each independent culture received 100 μmol/L MeJA and the other part was used as the control. The hairy roots were collected after 24 h for RNA-sequencing and after 48 h for profiling of CADs.

Total RNA was extracted using an RNeasy Plant Mini Kit (Qiagen, German). RNA-sequencing was performed using the BGI Illumina-HiSeq2000 platform. Library construction, sequencing, and analysis were carried out by the Beijing Genomic Institute (Shenzhen, China).

Crude protein extracts The plant material was frozen in liquid nitrogen and ground into a fine powder. One gram of powdered material was extracted with 4 mL extraction buffer phosphate buffer saline (PBS: 137 mmol/L NaCl, 2.7 mmol/L KCl, 10 mmol/L $Na_2HPO_4$, and 2 mmol/L $KH_2PO_4$) pH 7.0 containing 10 mmol/L EDTA, 2% PVPP, 5 mmol/L DTT, and 1 × proteinase inhibitor cocktail (product No.: 4693132001, Roche) on ice for 2 h. The mixture was centrifuged at 4℃ at 5,000×g for 10 min. The supernatant was further centrifuged at 4℃ at 15,000×g for 10 min. The supernatant was filtered through a 0.22 μm polyethersulfone (PES) membrane and dialyzed against PBS buffer (pH 7.0) overnight at 4 ℃ refrigeration to remove low molecular weight compounds. The protein concentration was determined using a BCA kit (Sangon Biotech, China).

Assay conditions for BAHD enzymes during protein purification A 100 μL reaction containing PBS buffer (pH 7.0), 20 μL crude protein extract (0.52 μg/μL), 120 μmol/L caffeoyl CoA, and 120 μmol/L tartaric acid or quinic acid was used for EpHTT and EpHQT assays, respectively. The mixture was incubated at 30 ℃ for 30 min and the reaction was stopped by adding 300 μL methanol. The supernatant was collected after centrifugation at 20,000 g at 4 ℃ for 10 min and 2.0 μL was injected for UPLC-DAD analysis. The UPLC conditions were the same as for quantitative analysis of CADs except for the gradient which was isocratic 5% B for 10 min.

Purification of BAHD enzymes First, ammonium sulfate precipitation was used to fractionate crude protein extracts. Following pre-tests, 0%-30%, 30%-40%, 40%-60%, and >60% $(NH_4)_2SO_4$ fractions were collected. After the addition of $(NH_4)_2SO_4$ powder, the mixture was shaken at 4℃ for 1 h and then centrifuged at 20,000 g at 4℃ for 15 min. The supernatant was used for further precipitation and the sedi-ment was resuspended in PBS (pH 7.0). $(NH_4)_2SO_4$ was removed by dialysis against PBS (pH 7.0) at 4 ℃ overnight. During this period, PBS buffer was replaced three times. The enzymes were purified further by FPLC (Fast Protein Liquid Chromatography, ÄKTA, GE Healthcare) coupled with HiTrap Q HP column (GE Healthcare) using a gradient of increasing concentration of NaCl from 0 to 1 mol/L in PBS buffer (pH 7.0). The enzyme activities of fractions were measured, and those fractions with the greatest activity were loaded into SDS-PAGE gels and run for 5 min. When all the samples had entered the separation gel, each lane was cut out and processed for protein MS identification as detailed below.

Protein MS identification Gels segments cut from SDS-PAGE gels were processed for protein MS identification. Peptides were digested by trypsin (Promega) and analyzed using nanoLC-QTOF-MS/MS (Ekspert NanoLC 425 and AB SCIEX Triple TOF 5 600). Peptides were separated using a SiELC ChromXP C18 column (75 μm×15 cm, 3 μm, 120 Å). LC flow rate was set to 0.3 μL/min with phase A (2% acetonitrile, 98% water, 0.1% formic acid) and phase B (98% acetonitrile, 2% water, 0.1% formic acid). Gradients were: 5%-7% B for 1 min, 7%-22% B for 31 min, 32%-38% B for 10 min, 32%-55% B for 7 min, 55%-80% B for 0.5 min, and hold at 80% B for 4.5 min, followed by re-equilibration with 5% B for 10 min. The MS method was as follows: TOF MS: CUR: 30; GS1:12; GS2: 0; IHT: 150; ISVF: 2 300; Mass Range: 300 - 1 250 Da; Accumulation Time: 250 ms. IDA Criteria: 20; TOF MS/MS spectra acquired after each TOF MS scan; Rolling CE was applied. Mass Range: 100 - 1 500 Da; Accumulation Time: 50 ms; CES: 5. Peptides were analyzed with ProteinPilot software and compared with the transcriptome database.

Expression of recombinant BAHD enzymes in *E. coli* and purification Full-length CDS of *EpHTT*, *EpHQT*, and *EpHCT* were amplified from *Echinacea purpurea* hairy root cDNA using primers listed in Supplementary Table 4 and cloned into the pDEST17 plasmid with 6 × His at the N-terminus. The recombinant plasmids were transformed into *E. coli* BL21(DE3) which was grown on LB solid medium (50 μg/mL ampicillin). Overnight cultures were transferred to 200 mL LB liquid medium containing antibiotics until the $OD_{600}$ reached 0.5 - 1.0. Isopropyl β-D-1-thiogalactopyranoside was added to a final concentration of 0.4 mmol/L, and the cultures were grown overnight at 16 ℃ with shaking at 200 rpm. Cells were harvested by centrifugation at 5,000×g for 5 min.

Cells were resuspended in lysis buffer (25 mmol/L Tris-HCl 8.0, 150 mmol/L NaCl, 0.5 mmol/L tris (2-carboxyethyl) phosphine). ATP (1 mmol/L) and PMSF (1 mmol/L) were also added. The cells were broken using a disruptor with 600 bar. After centrifugation at 20,000×g at 4℃ for 30 min, the supernatant was collected. Protein was purified using a $Ni^{2+}$-NTA column (Qiagen) according to the manufacturer's instructions. Imidazole was removed using FPLC coupled with HiTrap Q HP column for purification of enzymes from crude extracts. The protein concentration was determined using a BCA kit (Sangon Biotech, China). Recombinant proteins were stored in PBS (pH 7.0 with 10% glycerol) at −80℃ before use.

Recombinant BAHD activities and kinetics According to our preliminary results, a UPLC based endpoint method was adopted for the determination of kinetics. Standard BAHD in vitro enzyme assays were performed in a 200 μL reaction mix containing PBS buffer (at appropriate pH), acyl-CoA thioesters as the acyl donors, and organic acids as the acyl acceptors. Purified protein (500 ng) was added to start the reaction. The mixture was incubated at 30 ℃ for 30 min. Methanol (300 μL) was added to stop the reaction. After centrifugation at 20,000×g at 4 ℃ for 10 min, the supernatant was collected and analyzed quantitatively using UPLC-DAD under the same conditions used for purification of BAHD activity. The enzyme reaction products were identified using LC-HRMS under the same conditions used for profiling of CADs. Enzyme activity was calculated as production of products and expressed as pkat (pmol/s).

Kinetic parameters were determined from Michaelis-Menten plots using GraphPad Prism software (version 8.01). All in vitro enzyme assays were repeated at least three times.

For investigation of the effects of pH on BAHD activity at different pH values (from 2 to 9), PBS buffers were used in the enzyme assays. 100 μmol/L tartaric acid or quinic acid and 100 μmol/L caffeoyl CoA were used in the enzyme assays. The generation of products was quantified using UPLC.

For kinetic analyses, PBS pH 7.0 was selected as an optimum buffer. The kinetics for the acyl donors of EpHTT were determined using 0.5 mmol/L tartaric acid and caffeoyl CoA (6.25 - 62.5 μmol/L), *p*-coumaroyl CoA (12.5 - 500 μmol/L), feruloyl CoA (25 - 200 μmol/L), respectively. When determining the kinetics for acyl acceptors for EpHTT, different combinations were used, including caffeoyl CoA (50 μmol/L) and tartaric acid (200 - 2 400 μmol/L), *p*-coumaroyl CoA (100 μmol/L) and tartaric acid (500 - 4 000 μmol/L), and feruloyl CoA (100 μmol/L) and tartaric acid (250 - 4 000 μmol/L). Quinic acid was fixed at 1 mmol/L and various acyl-CoA thioesters (caffeoyl CoA (6.25 - 62.5 μmol/L); *p*-coumaroyl CoA (25 - 800 μmol/L) and feruloyl CoA (50 - 400 μmol/L)) were used for the study of the kinetics of EpHQT activity with different acyl donors. The kinetics of EpHQT's activity with different acyl donors were measured using the following combinations: caffeoyl CoA (50 μmol/L) and quinic acid (200 - 2 400 μmol/L), *p*-coumaroyl CoA (100 μmol/L) and quinic acid (250 - 2 000 μmol/L), and feruloyl CoA (100 μmol/L) and quinic acid (1 000 - 5 000 μmol/L). Products including *p*-coumaroylquinic acid, *p*-coumaroyltartaric acid, feruloylquinic acid, and feruloyltartaric acid were identified using LC - HRMS under the same conditions described above. Quantification was based on UPLC - DAD using caftaric acid and chlorogenic acid as references for tartaric acid esters and quinic acid esters, respectively.

For investigating the substrate preferences of BAHDs, acyl-CoA thioesters (100 μmol/L) and organic acids (2 mmol/L) including tartaric acid, quinic acid, and shikimic acid were used. The products were measured with LC - HRMS.

Assay conditions for SCPL enzyme during protein purification  Optimum conditions for SCPL activity were established by pre-tests. Assays were performed in a 200 μL in vitro enzyme reaction containing chlorogenic acid (250 μmol/L), caftaric acid (250 μmol/L), 10 mM $Na_2HPO_4$, and 2 mmol/L $KH_2PO_4$ (pH 4.0). A total of 20 μL crude protein extract (0.4 μg/μL) was added to start the reaction. After incubation at 30 ℃ for 1 h, the reaction was stopped by adding 300 μL methanol. The mixture was centrifuged at 4 ℃ at 20,000 × *g* for 10 min and the supernatant was used for UPLC analysis under the same conditions as described above except the gradients were as follows: 2% B for 0.5 min, 2%- 15% B for 3.5 min, stay 15% B for 3 min, then drop to 2% B in 0.1 min and re-equilibrated with 2% for 2.9 min.

Purification of chicoric acid synthase activity  Similar to the purification of BAHD enzymes, ammonium sulfate precipitation was used to separate chicoric acid synthase activity initially. Following pre-tests, 0% - 20%, 20% - 40%, 40%- 60%, and >60% $(NH_4)_2SO_4$ fractions were used for fractionation. The fractions were prepared and desalted as described for BAHD acyl transferases. The active fraction was separated further by two steps including the use of the same anion exchange column used for BAHD purification and sieve chromatography. Molecular sieve separation was performed on FPLC with Superdex 200 10/300 GL (GE Healthcare) using PBS buffer (pH 7.0). Finally, the active fraction was used for the identification of EpCAS using the protein MS identification method described above.

Recombinant SCPL enzyme expression in *S. cerevisiae* and purification  The full-length cDNA of *EpCAS* was cloned into the pESC-His expression vector with a 6×His tag at the C-terminus using ClonExpress Ⅱ One Step Cloning Kit (Vazyme). *Saccharomyces cerevisiae* BY4741 was used as the host yeast strain. Yeast transformation procedures were conducted using a lithium acetate method and were incubated at 30 ℃. Single colonies were grown on SD dropout media containing 2% dextrose without Histidine (Solarbio) and were picked and then used for purification by inoculation into 15 mL of SD dropout medium containing 2% dextrose. Cells were grown overnight at 30 ℃ on a rotary shaker set at 200 rpm. Cultures were then inoculated in 200 mL of SD dropout media containing 2% dextrose and grown to an $OD_{600}$ of 0.4. All cells were transferred into 200 mL SD dropout medium containing 2% galactose. Yeast cells were grown at 30 ℃ on a rotary shaker for 36 h. The cells were centrifuged at 1 500 × *g* for 5 min at 4 ℃. The supernatant was discarded, and the cells were resuspended in 10 mL of sterile water. Cells were centrifuged at 1 500 × *g* for 5 min at 4 ℃. The supernatant was discarded, and the cell pellets were stored at −80 ℃ for later experiments.

Cells were resuspended in the same volume of Ni - NTA lysis buffer (50 mmol/L $NaH_2PO_4$, 300 mmol/L NaCl and 10 mmol/L imidazole, pH 8.0) and broken using acid-washed glass beads (425 - 600 μm, Sigma) by shaking in a grinding machine (60 Hz, 60 s for 5 times) and then centrifuged at 5,000 × *g* at 4 ℃ for 10 min. The supernatant was collected and further centrifuged at 20,000 × *g* at 4 ℃ for 10 min. After passage through a 0.22 μm PES membrane, the protein was purified using a $Ni^{2+}$ - NTA column (Qiagen) according to the manufacturer's instructions with some modifications. The column was washed using 20 mmol/L imidazole and eluted using pH 4.5 buffer (50 mmol/L $NaH_2PO_4$, 300 mmol/

L NaCl). Protein concentration was determined using a BCA kit (Sangon Biotech, China) and recombinant protein was stored at −80 ℃ before use.

Mutagenesis and expression of EpCAS in *S. cerevisiae* Overlapping gene fragments were separately amplified using *EpCAS* as a template with primers containing the desired single and combined amino acid substitutions. The fragments were simultaneously cloned into pESC-His vector for expression as described above.

Determination of recombinant EpCAS characteristics Standard conditions for EpCAS assays were 100 μL reactions containing chlorogenic acid (200 μmol/L), caftaric acid (100 μmol/L), 10 mmol/L $Na_2HPO_4$, and 2 mmol/L $KH_2PO_3$ (pH 4.0). Protein (1.41 μg) was added to start the reaction. After incubation at 30 ℃ for 12 h (based on pre-experiments), the reaction was stopped by adding 400 μL methanol. The mixture was centrifuged at 4 ℃ at 20,000×*g* for 10 min and the supernatant was used for UPLC-DAD analysis under the same conditions used for the SCPL enzyme assay during purification. Reactions were also analyzed using LC-HRMS by the same method as used for assaying BAHD activities.

For determination of the effects of pH, starting solution (10 mmol/L $Na_2HPO_4$ and 2 mmol/L $KH_2PO_3$) was adjusted into different pH (ranging from pH 1.6 to 10.7) by adding 1 mol/L HCl or 1 mol/L NaOH, and all other procedures were performed using standard conditions. For further identification of EpCAS as an SCPL protein, PMSF at different concentrations including 1, 5, and 10 mmol/L was used to inhibit enzyme activity. For product and substrate degradation assays, 100 μmol/L chicoric acid, 100 μmol/L caftaric acid and 200 μmol/L chlorogenic acid were used. To establish whether caftaric acid and caffeic acid can generate chicoric acid, 100 μmol/L caftaric acid and 200 μmol/L caffeic acid were combined. For kinetic analysis, caftaric acid ranging from 10 to 200 μmol/L was mixed with 200 μmol/L chlorogenic acid and chlorogenic acid ranging from 20 to 200 μmol/L was mixed with 200 μmol/L caftaric acid and assays were incubated with EpCAS for caftaric acid and chlorogenic acid analysis, respectively. For kinetic analysis against 1-*O*-caffeoyl β-D-glucose, caftaric acid 200 μmol/L was mixed with 1-*O*-caffeoyl β-D-glucose ranging from 10 to 400 μmol/L. For the characterization of activities with other acyl donors, 100 μmol/L caftaric acid was mixed with 200 μmol/L candidate donors including chlorogenic acid, 1-*O*-caffeoyl β-D-glucose, neochlorogenic acid, cryptochlorogenic acid and 5-*O*-caffeoylshikimic acid. The products were determined using LC-HRMS and UPLC-DAD. All in vitro enzyme assays were conducted at least three times.

Synthesis of 1-*O*-caffeoyl-β-D-glucose 1-*O*-caffeoyl-β-D-glucose was synthesized according to published methods, and its identity was confirmed using LC-MS and NMR. UV/Vis: $\lambda_{max}$ 330 nm. $^1$H NMR (400 MHz, $CD_3OD$) δ: 7.66 (d, J=16.0 Hz, 1H), 7.06 (s, 1H), 6.97 (d, J=8.4 Hz, 1H), 6.79 (d, J=8.0 Hz, 1H), 6.31 (d, J=16.0 Hz, 1H), 5.58 (d, J=7.6 Hz, 1H), 3.86 (d, J=12.0 Hz, 1H), 3.72-3.68 (m, 1 H), 3.47-3.39 (m, 4H). HRMS (*m/z*): $[M]^-$ calculated. for $C_{15}H_{18}O_9$, 341.087 8; found, 341.088 1 (Supplementary Fig. 12).

Phylogenetic analysis The sequences of BAHD (CcsHCT (AFL93686), CcsHQT1 (CAM84302) and CcsHQT2 (CAR92145) from *Cynara cardunculus var. scolymus*; CiHCT1 (ANN12608), CiHCT2 (ANN12609), CiHQT1 (ANN12610), CiHQT2 (ANN12611), and CiHQT3 (ANN12612) from *Cichorium intybus*; NtHCT (CAD47830) and NtHQT (CAE46932) from *Nicotiana tabacum*; CaHCT (CAJ40778) from *Coffea arabica*; CcHQT (ABO77957) from *Coffea canephora*; TpHCT1A (ACI16630) from *Trifolium pratense*; AtHCT (AED95744) from *Arabidopsis thaliana*; SbHCT (4KE4_A) from *Sorghum bicolor*; AsHHT1 (BAC78633) from *Avena sativa*; CcaHQT (ABK79690) from *Cynara cardunculus var. altilis*; SlHQT (CAE46933) from *Solanum lycopersicum*; MpHCT (AXN55971) from *Marchantia paleacea*; PaHCT (AXN55972) from *Plagiochasma appendiculatum*; CsHCT (AEJ88365) from *Cucumis sativus*; PpHCT1 (AMK38063) from *Physcomitrium patens*) and SCPL (SpGAC (AAF64227) from *Solanum pennellii*; AtSMT (AAF78760), AtSCT (AAK52316), AtSAT (AEC07395), AtSST (AEC07397) and AtSCPL17 (AAS99709) from *Arabidopsis thaliana*; BnSCT1 (AAQ91191) and BnSCT2 (CAM91991) from *Brassica napus*; DkSCPL1 (BAF56655) and DkSCPL2 (BAH89272) from *Diospyros kaki*; CtAT1 (BAF99695) from *Clitoria ternatea*; AsSCPL1 (ACT21078) from *Avena strigosa*; OsIAA-At (EEE56946) from *Oryza sativa*) were obtained from NCBI and other public databases. Amino acid sequences were aligned and the Neighbor-Joining (NJ) trees were built using MEGA6 (Molecular Evolutionary Genetics Analysis version 6.0) with the following parameters: at least 1 000 bootstrap replications, Poisson model, uniform rates and complete deletion.

Subcellular localization Target genes were cloned into pSuper1300-GFP using primers listed in Supplementary Table 4 to create in-frame, C-terminal GFP fusion proteins, and transformed into *Agrobacterium tumefaciens* strain GV3101. Transformed clones were grown on 2 mL LB selective medium (50 mg/L kanamycin, 50 mg/L gentamicin, and 50 mg/L rifampin) for 24 h at 28 ℃ with shaking at 180 rpm. The cultures were transferred to 20 mL LB medium containing antibiotics and grown until the $OD_{600}$ reached 1.0. Cells were harvested and resuspended in infiltration buffer (10 mmol/L MES pH 5.6, 10 mmol/L $MgCl_2$, and 200 μmol/L acetosyringone) and incubated for an additional 2 h in the dark at room temperature. Strains containing target plasmids were infiltrated into the leaves of 4-week-old *Nicotiana benthamiana* plants. The plants were grown in the dark for 24 h (*EpHTT* and *EpHQT*) or 72 h (*EpCAS*) and prepared for microscopic observations. Leaves were cut into small pieces and placed on glass slides and observed with a ZEISS Cell Observer SD Spinning Disk Confocal Microscope. The vacuoles were stained by 10 μmol/L SNARF-1 for 2 h before observation. Detection parameters were as follows: GFP excitation at 488 nm and emission at 500-530 nm, SNARF-1 excitation at 514 nm and emission at 600-700 nm.

Molecular docking The protein 3D structures of BAHD enzymes were modeled using I-TASSER (https://zhanglab.ccmb.med.umich.edu/I-TASSER/) and CISRR. Docking experiments were conducted on CB-Dock based on AutoDock Vina. EpCAS was modeled by SwissModel using SERINE CARBOX-YPEPTIDASE (PDB: IYSC) as template. AutoDock 4.2 was used for docking experiments. Molecular graphics were rendered with PyMOL (version 2.3.2).

Overexpression and RNAi of *BAHDs* and *SCPL* in hairy root cultures *EpHTT*, *EpHQT* and *EpCAS* genes were cloned into plasmid pK7WG2R with a 35 S promoter using Gateway recombination according to the manufacturer's instructions for the overexpression of target genes in hairy roots. Nonhomologous sequences of *EpHTT*, *EpHQT* and *EpCAS* were amplified with the primers listed in Supplementary Table 4 and were cloned into binary hpRNA vector pK7WGIGW2R using Gateway recombination for RNAi. The vectors were introduced into *Agrobacterium rhigogenes* A4 by electroporation. Successful clones were selected on tryptone yeast broth solid medium supplemented with spectinomycin (50 mg/L) and kanamycin (50 mg/L). All other procedures for generation and analysis of hairy roots were as described as above.

Quantitative reverse transcription polymerase chain reaction Total RNA was extracted with an RNeasy Plant Mini Kit (Qiagen). First-strand cDNA was synthesized from 1 μg RNA using a PrimeScript™ RT reagent Kit with gDNA Eraser (Takara). qRT-PCR was performed using a Bio-Rad CFX384 and iTaq Universal One-Step RT-qPCR Kits (Bio-Rad) according to the manufacturer's instructions. Results were calculated using Bio-Rad CFX manager software. Tubulin was used as internal control. The relative expression of genes was calculated using the ΔCt method. The primer pairs for qRT-PCR were designed by Primer3Plus (http://www.primer3plus.com) (Supplementary Table 4) and compared by BLAST analysis to the NCBI database for confirmation of primer specificity.

Reconstruction of chicoric acid biosynthesis in *N. benthamiana* For transient overexpression, *EpHTT* and *EpCAS* were cloned into the destination vector pEAQ-HT-DEST3 using Gateway recombination and transformed into *Agrobacterium tumefaciens* strain GV3101 by electroporation. Single clones with each target construct were transferred into 2 mL LB liquid culture (kanamycin, rifampicin, and gentamicin, 50 mg/L), and the cultures were grown at 28℃ in a shaker at 200 rpm for 1 day. For subculturing, 0.5 mL were transferred into 10 mL LB liquid medium (kanamycin, rifampicin, and gentamicin, 50 mg/L) and cells were grown for 6-8 h until the $OD_{600}$ reached 0.5-0.8. Cells were collected and resuspended in infiltration buffer (10 mmol/L $MgCl_2$, 10 mmol/L MES pH 5.6, and 250 μmol/L acetosyringone) to $OD_{600}=1.0$. The *Agrobacterium tumefaciens* stains with vectors carrying target genes were infiltrated into *Nicotiana benthamiana* leaves by syringe. Substrates (tartaric acid 1 mmol/L, caftaric acid 500 μmol/L) were injected into infiltrated leaves 5 days after inoculation. After 24 h, the leaves were collected for LC-HRMS analysis using the same conditions used for CAD profiling.

Statistical analysis Unless specifically described, all the experiments in this paper were repeated at least three times and results from representative data sets are presented. GraphPad Prism (version 8.02) and Microsoft Excel (version Office 365) was used for the statistical analysis. The statistical evaluations used unpaired *t* tests and one-way analysis of variance (ANOVA) with multiple comparisons, followed by Tukey tests. The results were considered statistically significant at $^*P<0.05$.

Reporting summary Further information on research design is available in the Nature Research Reporting Summary linked to this article.

## 4 DATA AVAILABILITY

Data supporting the findings of this work are available within the paper and its Supplementary Information files. A reporting summary for this Article is available as a Supplementary information file. The datasets and plant materials generated and analyzed during the current study are available from the corresponding author upon request. The sequences of the genes reported in this article have been deposited in NCBI GenBank: EpHTT (MT936803), EpHQT (MT936804), EpHCT (MT936805), and EpCAS (MT936806). The RNA-seq data from MeJA treatment and the control have been deposited in the SRA database of NCBI under accession numbers SRR8935731, SRR8935732, SRR8935733 for MeJA treatments and SRR8937034, SRR8937035, SRR8937036 for controls. The source data underlying Figs. 1d, 2d-g, 3c, 3d, 4a, 4b, and 6, Supplementary Figures 1, 3, 5, 9c, and 16a, as well as Supplementary Tables 1-3 are provided as a Source Data file.

[付饶，张阳，等. Nature Communication，2021，12：1563.]

# Expansion within the CYP71D subfamily drives the heterocyclization of tanshinones synthesis in *Salvia miltiorrhiza*

*Salvia miltiorrhiza* (Danshen in Chinese) is one of the oldest and most important traditional Chinese medicinal herbs. Tanshinones are *nor*-diterpenoids that form the lipophilic bioactive constituents of Danshen (Fig. 1a). More specifically, these are phenolic abietane-type diterpenoids, which are widely found in the Lamiaceae family. The tanshinones are uniquely characterized by the presence of a 14,16-ether D-ring, such as cryptotanshinone (**1**) and 15,16-dihydrotanshinone (**2**). However, this heterocycle is generally further oxidized to form a furan, as found in tanshinone Ⅰ and tanshinone $Ⅱ_A$. Tanshinones and chemically modified derivatives possess broad cardiovascular and cerebrovascular protective actions. For example, the sodium sulfonate of tanshinone $Ⅱ_A$ is widely used in the clinic to treat patients with coronary artery disease. Their pharmaceutical applications also include antioxidant, antibacterial, anti-inflammatory, antitumor, and anti-HIV activities. Structure-activity relationship analysis indicates that the furan or dihydrofuran ring D structure influences pharmacological activities, thus high-lighting the importance of D ring formation.

Due to their medicinal properties, tanshinone biosynthesis has been intensively investigated for over a decade. As labdane-related diterpenoids, tanshinone biosynthesis is initiated by a class Ⅱ diterpene cyclase; mainly the labdadienyl/copalyl diphosphate synthase SmCPS1, with subsequent further cyclization and rearrangement catalyzed by the class Ⅰ diterpene synthase SmKSL1, which produces the abietane miltiradiene. Three relevant cytochromes P450 (CYPs) also have been identified, CYP76AH1, CYP76AH3, and CYP76AK1, which catalyze hydroxylation at carbon-12 (C12), then C11 hydroxylation of the resulting ferruginol and, finally, C20 hydroxylation, respectively. The promiscuity of these CYPs suggests that tanshinone biosynthesis may proceed via a metabolic network (Fig. 1b).

While CYPs prototypically catalyze hydroxylation, these monooxygenases are capable of mediating more complex transformations. Among these, the formation of cyclic ethers is important due to the contribution of these structural features to biological activity. For example, of particular interest here is the formation of the characteristic furan D-ring, which is targeted for the generation of the sulfonated derivative of tanshinone $Ⅱ_A$ that is clinically relevant. However, the biosynthetic origin of this key distinguishing heterocycle in Danshen remains unknown.

Given the widespread production of phenolic abietane-type diterpenoids in the Lamiaceae family, the addition of the D-ring differentiates the tanshinones. It also provides a key point of biosynthetic divergence. The formation of this cyclic ether is expected to be catalyzed by a CYP. However, CYPs form the largest enzymatic family in plants, comprising ~1% of all plant genes. Not surprisingly, the sheer number of CYPs and the diversity of plant metabolism they operate in complicates the assignment of even basic metabolic function of CYPs on the basis of just phylogenetic relationship. Such functional attribution is difficult even within the more closely related CYP families or even subfamilies, which share >40% or >55% amino acid (aa) sequence identity, respectively. For example, members of the CYP71D subfamily function in indole alkaloid and flavonoid, as well as terpenoid biosynthesis. Accordingly, CYPs readily undergo derivation of even basic metabolic function, further increasing the difficulty of identifying the relevant members of the superfamily.

Here, we assemble the genome of line bh2-7, which is derived from *S. miltiorrhiza* var. alba and bred to close to full homozygosity by successive selfings for six generations. Genome analyses reveal an expansion of the CYP71D subfamily. We identify possible roles for three CYP71Ds in catalyzing reactions leading to the formation of the characteristic furan D-ring of tanshinones. Additionally, we discuss the evolutionary origin of tanshinones biosynthesis.

## 1 RESULTS

Genome assembly and annotation  Danshen is highly heterozygous, which hindered genome assembly in previous sequencing efforts. Hence, we selected line bh2-7 for sequencing. Originally derived from *Salvia miltiorrhiza* var. alba, line bh2-7 has been bred close to homozygosity by successive selfings for six generations (Supplementary Fig. 1), with an estimated heterozygosity of 0.43% based on 17-mer depth distribution using 26.73 Gb sequencing reads (Supplementary Fig. 2).

A total of 341.69 Gb of high-quality data were obtained using the Illumina Hiseq2000 platform, along with 30.13 Gb of data using the PacBio RS platform (6.46 kb read length in average) after reads filtering, representing approximately 542.36-fold and 50.21-fold coverage of the predicted Danshen

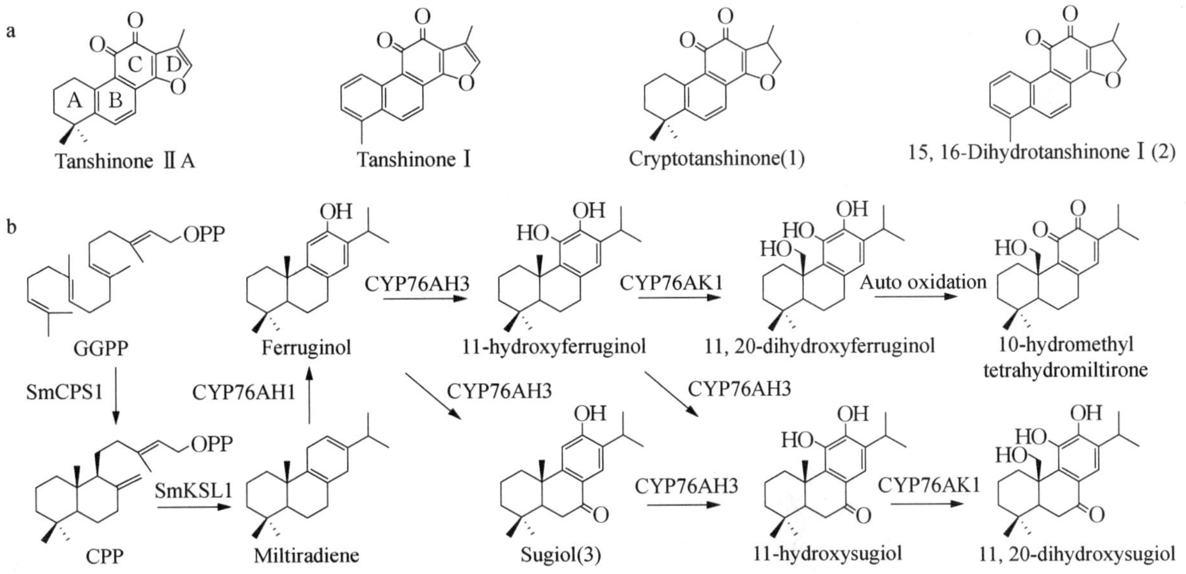

**Fig. 1 Tanshinones and partial biosynthetic pathway in Danshen**

(a) Structures of the major tanshinone constituents of Danshen: tanshinone ⅡA, tanshinone Ⅰ, cryptotanshinone (**1**) and 15, 16-dihydrotanshinone Ⅰ (**2**). (b) Elucidated steps for tanshinone biosynthesis in Danshen.

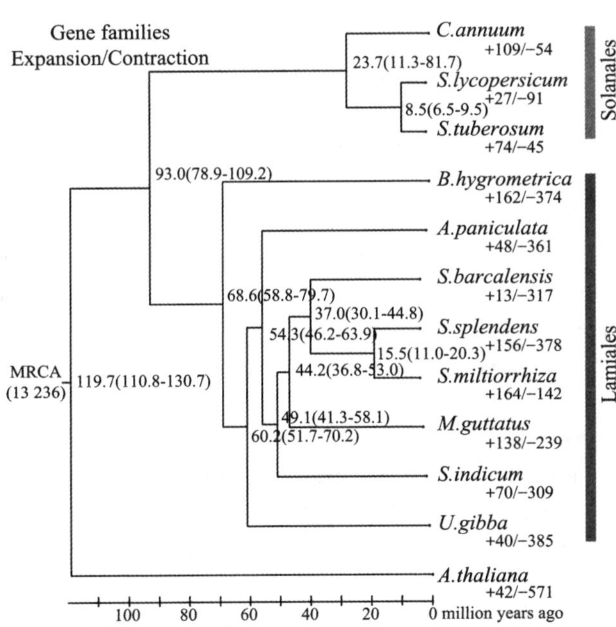


**Fig. 2 Phylogenetic analysis and divergence time estimations among 12 plant species**

The tree was constructed based on 379 single-copy orthologous genes using the maximum likelihood method. Divergence times (Mya) are indicated in black numbers beside the branch nodes. The number of gene-family expansion and contraction events is indicated by green and orange numbers (respectively).

genome (Supplementary Tables 1 and 2). The resulting assembly has a total length of 557 Mb with contig N50 of 505.21 kb and scaffold N50 of 1.26 Mb (Supplementary Table 3). These are approximately 2.7- or 93-fold longer than the previous assemblies of the Danshen genome. The assembly covered about 89% of the genome according to the estimations derived from 17-mer depth distribution (623.58 Mb) (Supplementary Fig. 2) and flow cytometry (622 Mb) (Supplementary Fig. 3). Mapping the original short reads to the draft assembly indicates 97.87% overall coverage (Supplementary Table 4). BUSCO (Benchmarking Universal Single-Copy Orthologs) analysis and ESTs (Expressed sequence tags) mapping implied 91.10% and 99.56% genome completeness in terms of expected gene content, respectively (Supplementary Tables 5 and 6). In addition, 326,420 single nucleotide variations (SNVs) and 32,710 short indels were identified, corresponding to 0.64 SNVs per Kb. This heterozygosity value is 4.3-fold lower than the previous assembly of the Danshen genome. All of the analyses indicate that this line bh2-7-based genome sequence has a relatively high-quality.

A total of 33,760 protein-coding genes with an average transcript length of 2 771 bp were identified through the combination of ab initio, homology-based analyses, and RNA-Seq reads-assisted annotation (Supplementary Table 7). The number of annotated genes was similar to two previously reported Danshen genome assemblies, which reported 30 478 and 34 598 genes. About 81.97% of the genes have homologs in the TrEMBL protein database, and 67.83% can be functionally classified by InterPro. In summary, 83.13% of the genes have either known homologs and/or can be functionally classified (Supplementary Table 8). Regarding non-coding genes, we identified 129 microRNAs, 682 tRNAs, 844 small nuclear RNAs, and 282 rRNA fragments from the assembly (Supplementary Table 9). Repetitive elements accounted for 56.27% of the genome, of which about 46.30% are long terminal repeat (LTR) retrotransposons (Supplementary Table 10).

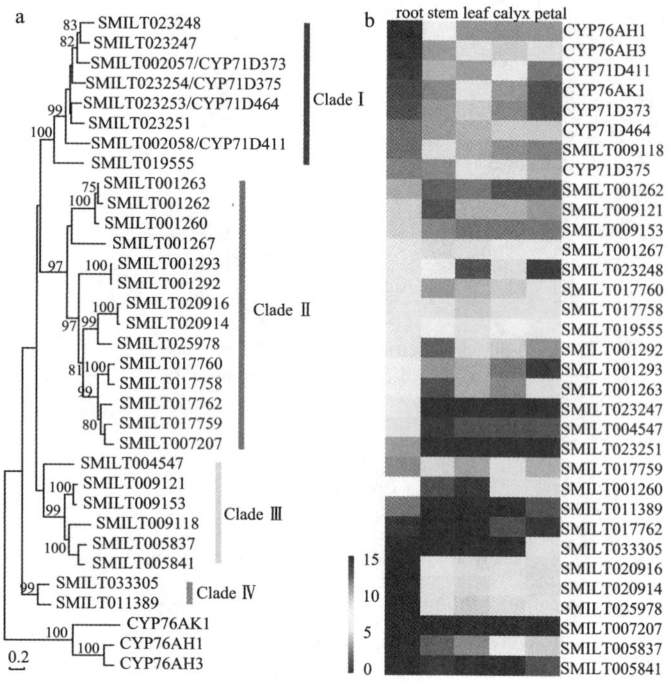


**Fig. 3 Phylogenetic relationship and expression profiles of CYP71D gene family in Danshen genome**

(a) Phylogenetic analysis of Danshen CYP71D subfamily. Maximum likelihood method was used to construct the phylogenetic tree with 1 000 replicate bootstrap support. The tree was rooted with the three CYP76 family members from Danshen previously shown to act in tanshinone biosynthesis. (b) Gene expression heatmap for the Danshen CYP71D subfamily members, as well as three CYP76 family members known to act in tanshinone biosynthesis, displaying relative expression level in root, stem, leaf, calyx, and petal of flowering plants. Source data underlying Fig. 3b are provided as a Source Data file.

Expansion of a clade within the CYP71D subfamily To study expansion and contraction of the gene families, twelve plant species (*Salvia miltiorrhiza*, *Salvia splendens*, *Scutellaria barcalensis*, *Sesamum indicum*, *Andrographis paniculata*, *Mimulus guttatus*, *Boea hygrometrica*, *Utricularia gibba*, *Capsicum annuum*, *Solanum tuberosum*, *Solanum lycopersicum*, and *Arabidopsis thaliana*) were analyzed by CAFE (V2.1) (Fig. 2). The first eight species belong to Lamiales, while *C. annuum*, *S. tuberosum*, and *S. lycopersicum* belong to Solanales, which is closely related to Lamiales, and *A. thaliana* was used as an out-group organism. Of these, only Danshen has been reported to have the ability to produce tanshinones. The analysis indicates that 164 gene families underwent significant expansion and 142 gene families underwent contraction in Danshen (Supplementary Data 1 and 2). The expanded families include CYPs, acyl-transferases, laccases, auxin response factors, genes involving in biosynthesis of salvianolic acid (such as cinnamate 4-hydroxylase, rosmarinic acid synthase, 4-coumarate-CoA ligase). Among these, two expanded (sub)families, Plant_805 (in clade Ⅲ in Fig. 3a) and Plant_13112 (in clade Ⅰ of Fig. 3a), both fall within the CYP71D subfamily that has been reported to play role in terpenoid biosynthesis.

In total, the Danshen genome contained 30 members of the CYP71D subfamily, which were further clustered into four clades (Fig. 3a). Gene structure analysis showed that most of the CYP71D genes in Danshen only have a single intron, consistent with the gene structure of other plant CYP71 clan. Four genes in clade Ⅰ (expansion family Plant_13112, *CYP71D373*, *CYP71D411*, *CYP71D464*, and *CYP71D375*) exhibited their greatest expression levels in roots, and showed similar expression profiles with *CYP76AH1*, *CYP76AH3*, and *CYP76AK1*, which are already known to play roles in tanshinone biosynthesis (Fig. 3b). Thus, these four CYP71Ds were considered to be potential candidate enzymes for tanshinone biosynthesis.

RNAi indicates a role for the CYP71Ds in tanshinone biosynthesis Given that these CYP71Ds are closely related, an RNAi approach targeting a conserved region was utilized to knock down the expression of all four genes. In particular, as *CYP71D411* was the most highly expressed in roots, it was selected as the direct target (Fig. 3b). More precisely, a region of 453 bp (nucleotides 823 - 1 276) was selected, as this exhibited >81% sequence identity with the three other targeted members of the clade, and was <71% identity to the next most closely related SMILT019555 (Supplementary Table 11). Global blast against all of the annotated genes reinforced this specificity; only genes from clade Ⅰ in Fig. 3a have e-values<$1e^{-5}$ (Supplementary Table 12). The targeted fragment was cloned into the binary RNAi vector, pK7GWIWG (Ⅱ) in an inverted-repeat fashion, and *Agrobacterium tumefaciens* was used to transfect Danshen to obtain transgenic plants. After four months of growth in the greenhouse, the *CYP71Ds*-RNAi plants exhibited a distinct orange phenotype in comparison with the wild-type (WT) root, which had the characteristic reddish color associated with tanshinones (Fig. 4a). There were no other obvious phenotypic differences.

To analyze the effect of this RNAi approach, RNA-Seq was carried out to compare the root transcriptomes of *CYP71Ds*-RNAi versus WT plants. As expected, the expression of the four targeted CYP71D subfamily members was significantly decreased in the *CYP71Ds*-RNAi lines, with their mRNA levels exhibiting a > 10-fold reduction compared with WT (Fig. 4b). Other members of the CYP71D subfamily showed trivial expression changes in the *CYP71Ds*-RNAi lines, except for *CYP71D414* (SMILT001293.1), which showed a >6-fold expression increase (Supplementary Table 13). The expression of the five genes known to be involved in tanshinone biosynthesis, *CPS1*, *KSL1*, *CYP76AH1*, *CYP76AH3*, and *CYP76AK1*, also were reduced in *CYP71Ds*-

RNAi lines (Supplementary Table 13). Beyond these genes, there were eight other genes down-regulated, and fifteen genes up-regulated in *CYP71Ds* - RNAi lines relative to WT.

Metabolomic analysis suggests a role for CYP71Ds in heterocyclization  The different root colors illustrated a change in metabolic profile for the *CYP71Ds* - RNAi lines. To characterize this, metabolomic analysis of roots from both *CYP71Ds* - RNAi and WT plants was carried out using LC-electrospray ionization-qTOF - MS and GC-electron impact (EI)-triple quadrupole (QqQ)-MS methods. The LC-qTOF - MS analysis revealed that 24 metabolites showed significantly reduced and 16 metabolites showed significantly elevated accumulation in *CYP71Ds* - RNAi lines compared with WT (Fig. 4c, d; Supplementary Data 3 and 4). The more targeted GC - MS analysis revealed that three known tanshinone biosynthetic intermediates, miltiradiene, abietatriene, and ferruginol, accumulated at higher levels in the *CYP71Ds* - RNAi lines (Supplementary Fig. 4).

A total of 21 out of the 24 metabolites with reduced accumulation in the *CYP71Ds* - RNAi lines could be identified (Supplementary Data 3). Notably, 14 of these metabolites contain a 14, 16-epoxy D-ring (Fig. 4c). For example, the levels of active compounds of Danshen including cryptotanshinone (**1**) and 15,16-dihydrotanshinone Ⅰ (**2**), and tanshinone ⅡA were decreased ~27, ~2, and ~3-fold, respectively. This indicated that the reduced expression of these four CYP71D subfamily members seems to decrease the formation of the characteristic heterocyclic D-ring in the tanshinones. Accordingly, we hypothesized that at least one of the down-regulated CYP71Ds play a role in the heterocyclization required for tanshinone biosynthesis.

Integrating the LC - MS and GC - MS analyses, there were a total of 19 metabolites found to exhibit elevated accumulation in the *CYP71Ds* - RNAi lines. Nine are known or potential intermediates in tanshinone biosynthesis (Fig. 4d and Supplementary Data 4). These included sugiol (**3**), 11-hydroxysugiol, miltirone (**4**) and 10-hydroxymethyl tetrahydromiltirone. Of particular interest, **4** has been predicted to be a key intermediate, as the immediate precursor of **1** and subsequently derived tanshinone ⅡA, and accumulated in ~9-fold higher amounts in *CYP71Ds* - RNAi lines relative to WT. In addition, increases were observed with Ro (**5**), as well as 4-methylenemiltirone (**6**), which similarly do not contain the heterocyclic D-ring, with the content of **5** and **6** increased ~38 and ~3-fold in *CYP71Ds* - RNAi relative to WT plants. Given together, we hypothesized that some of the accumulated diterpenoids in the *CYP71Ds* - RNAi plants might serve as substrates for these CYPs, particularly **4**, **5**, and **6**, which appear to be poised for D-ring heterocyclization.

Biochemical analysis of the targeted CYP71D clade  To investigate the biochemical activity of these CYPs, recombinant expression in yeast (*Saccharomyces cerevisiae*) was employed, as this has proven to be successful for previous such characterization. For this purpose, full-length cDNAs for all four CYP71Ds (*CYP71D373*, *CYP71D375*, *CYP71D411*, and *CYP71D464*) were cloned into the pESC-His expression vector, and the resulting constructs transformed into the WAT11 yeast strain in which the endogenous NADPH - CYP reductase has been replaced by one from *A. thaliana*. In vitro assays were then carried out with microsomal preparations from induced cultures of this recombinant yeast, using **4**,**5**, and **6** as potential substrates. Only CYP71D375 accepts miltirone (**4**) as a substrate, with three products detected (Fig. 5a). The major product was found to reflect mass addition of [M]=13.9789 Da and was identified as the heterocyclic **1** by comparison to an authentic standard, and is labeled as such here—i. e., **1** (Supplementary Fig. 5a). Two minor products also were observed, with the earlier eluting product (**7**) found to have a mass addition of [M]=15.9926 Da, suggesting this was generated by a hydroxylation reaction (Supplementary Fig. 5b). This compound also was detected in Danshen roots, and was determined to be 16-hydroxymiltirone (**7**) by NMR (Supplementary Fig. 6). The remaining minor product (**8**) was found to have a mass addition of [M]=31.9894 Da, and was identified as the known 14, 16-dihydroxy derivative neocrypto-tanshinone (**8**) by comparison to an authentic standard (Supplementary Fig. 5c). These results indicate that CYP71D375 functions to convert **4** to the 14, 16-epoxy heterocyclic derivative **1**, which is consistent with the accumulation of **4** in the *CYP71Ds* - RNAi lines.

When **5** was used as substrate, two products were observed with both CYP71D373 and CYP71D375 (Fig. 5b). The major product was found to have a mass addition of [M]=13.9797 Da, identified as the heterocyclic derivative **2** by comparison to an authentic standard (Supplementary Fig. 7a). Similarly, the mass of the minor product suggests that it was generated by hydroxylation, and was identified as the 16-hydroxy derivative (**9**) by comparison to an authentic standard (Supplementary Fig. 7b).

Only CYP71D375 accepts **6** as a substrate, with two products detected (Fig. 5c). The structure of **10** was inferred based on various sources of information including MS analysis, retention time, compound degradation behavior, known CYP71D375-catalyzed chemistry and chemical logic. On this basis, **10** is speculated to be 16-hydroxy-4-methylenemiltirone. **11** was identified as methylenedihydro-tanshinquinone by comparison to an authentic standard (Supplementary Fig. 7c - d).

The biochemical assays with **4**,**5**, and **6** indicated that CYP71D411 and CYP71D464 are not involved in heterocycliza-

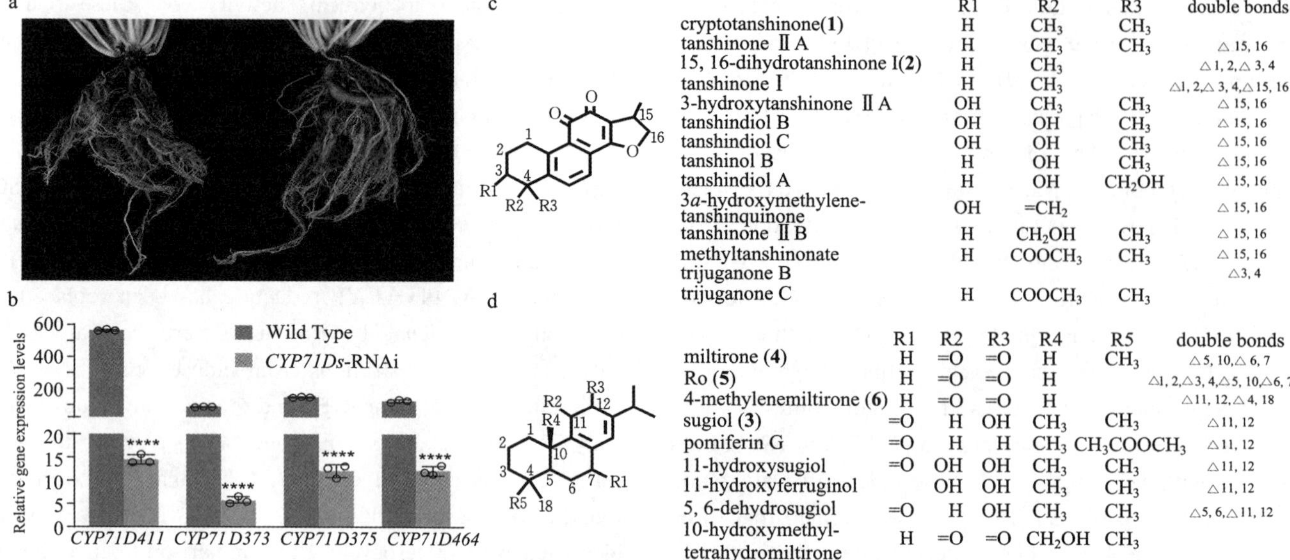


**Fig. 4 Phenotype, expression and metabolite profile changes of *CYP71Ds*-RNAi plants**

(a) Coloration of roots from WT (left) and *CYP71Ds*-RNAi knockdown (right) plants. (b) Relative mRNA levels of the four CYP71D genes in *CYP71Ds*-RNAi and wild-type plants from transcriptome data. Error bars represent standard deviation SD ($n=3$ biologically independent samples; **** $P<0.0001$ by 2-sided Student's $t$ test). (c) Down-regulated tanshinone related diterpenoids in roots of *CYP71Ds*-RNAi relative to WT plants. (d) Up-regulated tanshinone related diterpenoids in roots of *CYP71Ds*-RNAi relative to WT plants. Source data underlying Fig. 4b are provided as a Source Data file.

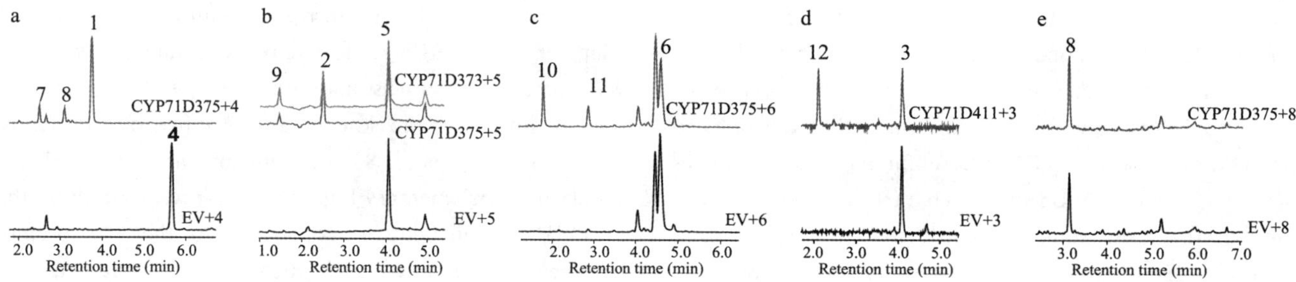


**Fig. 5 Catalytic activity of targeted CYP71D subfamily members with putative tanshinone intermediates accumulating in *CYP71Ds*-RNAi plant roots**

Extracted ion chromatograms showing the in vitro catalytic activity of (a) CYP71D375 with **4**. (b) CYP71D373 and CYP71D375 with **5**. (c) CYP71D375 with **6**. (d) CYP71D411 with **3**. (e) CYP71D375 with **8**. In each case, enzyme-mediated activity is indicated by the green chromatograms (with the relevant enzyme noted), while those for the empty vector (EV) negative control assays are in black.

tion. Conversely, while other compounds that accumulated in RNAi lines also were tested with these four CYP71D subfamily members, no products were detected with CYP71D373, CYP71D375, or CYP71D464. However, CYP71D411 accepts sugiol (**3**) as a substrate, and the mass $[M-H]^- = 315.1947$ of the product was indicative of hydroxylation (Fig. 5d). In order to characterize this product, the enzymatic reaction system was scaled-up to 100 mL to enable purification of sufficient amounts for structural analysis by NMR, which identified this as 20-hydroxysugiol (**12**) (Supplementary Figs. 8－9).

Altogether, these in vitro assays provided biochemical evidence for specific functions of three members of the targeted CYP71D clade in tanshinone biosynthesis. In particular, the results suggest that CYP71D375 and CYP71D373 are important for heterocyclization to form the characteristic D-ring of the tanshinones (Fig. 6a), while CYP71D411 acts as a C20 hydroxylase of **3**.

Biochemical analysis of heterocyclization of miltirone by CYP71D375 The heterocyclization catalyzed by CYP71D375 represents the characteristic step in tanshinone biosynthesis (Fig. 6a). To probe the biochemical mechanism underlying the formation of this cyclic ether, the conversion of **4** to **1** was further investigated here. The presence of the 14, 16-dihydroxylated derivative **8** might suggest that this serves as an intermediate, such that heterocyclization occurs via dehydration. However, when **8** was fed to CYP71D375, product **1** was not observed (Fig. 5e), indicating that heterocyclization is not achieved by dehydration. Accordingly, it seems most likely that CYP71D375 catalyzes cyclic ether formation directly from the 16-hydroxylated derivative **7**, which we hypothesize utilizes the basic CYP free radical

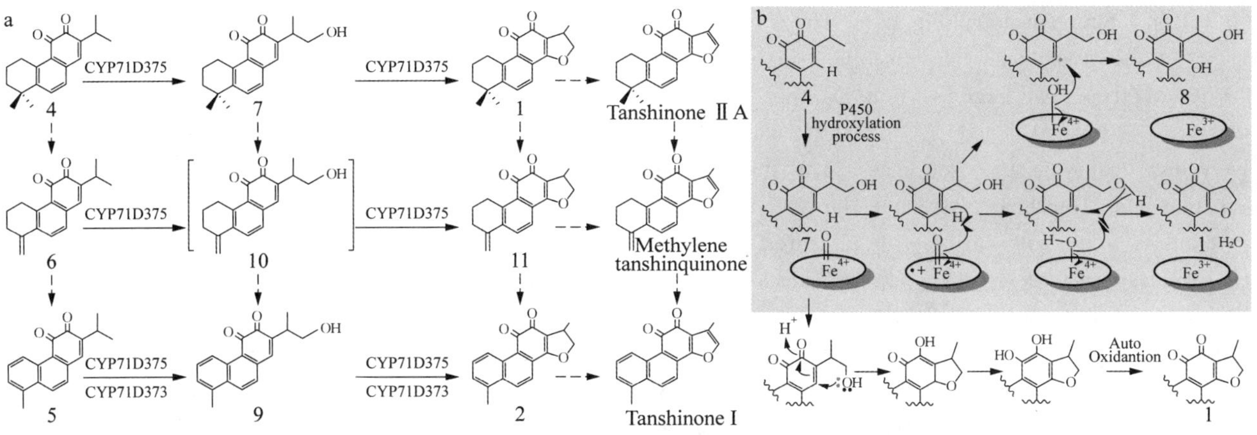

**Fig. 6 Catalytic process analysis of CYP71D373 and CYP71D375**

(a) Role of CYP71D373 and CYP71D375 in forming the characteristic tanshinone D-ring heterocycle in a metabolic grid for tanshinone biosynthesis in Danshen. (b) Proposed reaction mechanisms for heterocyclization of **4** to **1**.

mechanism. Accordingly, following initial hydroxylation of **4** to **7**, CYP71D375 would mediate the prototypical hydrogen abstraction from C14, but the resulting radical would then undergo direct (hetero) cyclization to form **1** (Fig. 6b). However, we cannot rule out alternative mechanisms, such as Michael addition or ketone formation (Supplementary Fig. 10), although we did not find any peaks with molecular weights corresponding to possible intermediates from such mechanisms.

Mutational analysis of heterocyclization of miltirone by CYP71D375 To examine the enzymatic structure-function relationships underlying the heterocyclase activity of CYP71D375, we used protein modeling with substrate docking to guide site-directed mutagenesis. Models of all four CYP71Ds examined here were generated based on the crystal structure reported for CYP76AH1. Miltirone (**4**) was then docked into these CYP71D models, enabling estimation of the proximity of amino acids lining the active site to **4** (Fig. 7a, b). Of particular interest were such residues (within 5 Å of **4**) that substantially differ between CYP71D375, as well as CYP71D373, which can both catalyze heterocyclization, versus CYP71D411 and CYP71D464. From this, five residues were targeted for mutagenesis (Fig. 7c).

These residues were subjected to a series of substitutions in CYP71D375, with a total of 37 mutants constructed, and the effect of these on catalytic function with **4** examined (Fig. 7d). The results indicated that L366 is a key residue, as all mutants at this position lost the ability to react with **4**. Notably, L366 is situated 5 residues after the ExxR-motif in substrate recognition site 5, a position which has been proposed to direct substrateheme interaction in CYPs. Similarly, for A301, a position that also has been suggested to affect substrate-heme interactions, only substitution of the smaller glycine for A301 retained catalytic activity.

Gene clustering contributed to evolution of the tanshinone pathway The results reported above further increase the number of genes associated with tanshinone biosynthesis, with three diterpene synthases, *SmCPS1*, *SmCPS2*, and *SmKSL1*, and now six CYPs, *CYP76AH1*, *CYP76AH3*, *CYP76AK1*, *CYP71D373*, *CYP71D375*, and *CYP71D411*. These nine genes were distributed over five scaffolds (Supplementary Fig. 11). It has previously been reported that *SmCPS2* is co-clustered with *CYP76AH1* and *CYP76AH3*, demonstrating that Danshen contains a biosynthetic gene cluster for tanshinone production. In order to further explore the role of gene clustering in the evolution of tanshinone biosynthesis, Hi-C was employed to assign the assembled scaffolds to chromosome-scale pseudomolecules. Altogether, 1115 scaffolds were anchored to 340 super-scaffolds with N50 of ~73.9 Mb. While falling short of chromosomal definition, we obtained one pseudochromosome (~65 Mb) with remarkably higher inner fragment interactions, defined here as pseudochromosome 6 (Supplementary Fig. 12). This pseudochromosome 6 includes all of the identified genes involved in tanshinone biosynthesis except *CYP76AK1* (Supplementary Fig. 13).

Notably, *SmCPS1*, *SmCPS2*, *SmKSL1*, *CYP76AH1*, and *CYP76AH3* are clustered within a 310 kb region (Supplementary Fig. 13), defining an even larger tanshinone biosynthetic gene cluster in Danshen. This cluster contains a number of potential gene duplicates. For example, *SmCPS1* and *SmCPS2* are the two most closely related class Ⅱ diterpene cyclases in Danshen, with *SmCPS2* predicted to be involved in tanshinone biosynthesis in aerial tissues, while *SmCPS1* is known to play a role in root tanshinone biosynthesis. Similarly, although CYP76AH1 and CYP76AH3 catalyze distinct reactions in tanshinone biosynthesis, these are also quite closely related to each other. In addition, the four CYP71Ds investigated here are also found within a ~160 kb region (Supplementary Fig. 13). To examine the origins of these two gene clusters, we analyzed the collinearity of these two regions from Danshen with *S. splendens*, *S. barcalensis* and *S. indicum*, which have relatively high-quality genome sequences. This comparison showed that the Danshen tanshinone biosynthetic gene cluster exhibits some collinearity with all three of these related species. By contrast, the Danshen CYP71D subfamily gene cluster only exhibits evident collinearity with *S. splendens*, while the orthologous loci in *S. barcalensis* does not contain any members of this subfamily (Supplementary Fig. 14). This then provides an opportunity to investigate the mechanism of diterpenoid diversification in Lamiaceae.

In the collinear region corresponding to the Danshen tanshinone biosynthetic gene cluster, there were three diterpene cyclases/synthases in *S. indicum* and *S. splendens* (albeit these are scattered across two scaffolds in the latter), and seven diterpene cyclases/synthases in *S. barcalensis* (Fig. 8a, b). There are orthologs of *SmCPS1* and *SmCPS2* in the isogenic regions of *S. barcalensis* (*SbTPS3* (Sb06t19660) and *SbTPS5* (Sb06t19680)), and *S. splendens* (*SsTPS2* (Saspl_048790. T1) and *SsTPS3* (Saspl_017770. T1)). But there is only one ortholog *SiTPS1* (rna17299) in *S. indicum* (Fig. 8b). Notably, *SmKSL1* is phylogenetically distinguished by a relatively recent relictual domain loss event. This is still evident in the orthologs from *S. barcalensis* (*SbTPS2*) and *S. splendens* (*SsTPS1*) that is found on the same scaffold as the *SmCPS1* ortholog *SsTPS2*. However, the ortholog in Sesame (*SiTPS2*) exhibits the more ancestral three-domain structure, which suggests that the domain loss event may have occurred prior to the divergence of the *Salvia* and *Scutellaria* genera relative to the *S. indicum* lineage. Intriguingly, although *TPS/CYPs* gene pair are the core components of terpenoid biosynthetic gene clusters, only Danshen and *S. splendens* have *CYPs* in this region (Fig. 8b). Though *S. splendens* has two CYP76AH subfamily members, *SsCYP76AH1.1* (Saspl_017771. T1) and *SsCYP76AH1.2* (Saspl_017768. T1), full-length cDNAs are not evident for these two genes, suggesting that these may be inactive. There is an apparent ortholog of *SsCYP76AH1.1* between *SmCPS1* and *SmKSL1* in the Danshen tanshinone biosynthetic gene cluster, but a premature termination codon indicates that this *SmCYP76AH1.1* is also inactive. In contrast, *S. indicum* and *S. barcalensis* have no CYPs in the corresponding region. Notably, the pair of class Ⅱ diterpene cyclases in this region of the Danshen and *S. splendens* genomes may have originated from *SiTPS1* by tandem duplication, while *CYP76AH1* and *CYP76AH3* seem to have emerged following divergence of the Danshen and *S. splendens* lineages.

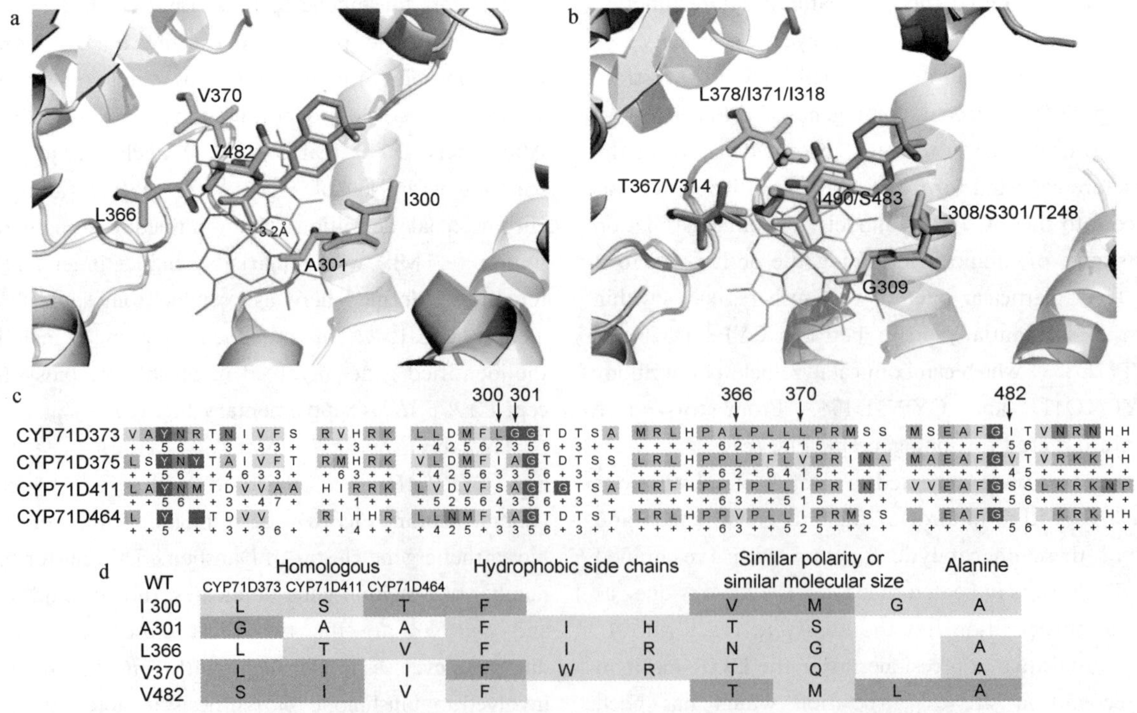


**Fig. 7 Docking analysis and mutation verification of CYP71Ds active sites in catalyzing miltirone**

(a) Docking result for miltirone (pink) in the CYP71D375 model, with side-chains for the targeted residues shown (green). (b) Docking result for miltirone, with side-chains of the targeted residues shown (as indicated), in the models for CYP71D373 (yellow), CYP71D411 (blue) and CYP71D464 (purple). (c) Alignment of the regions around the five proposed distinguishing active site residues. (d) Table indicating positive (green) and negative (blue) impact of CYP71D375 mutations on enzymatic reaction with miltirone.

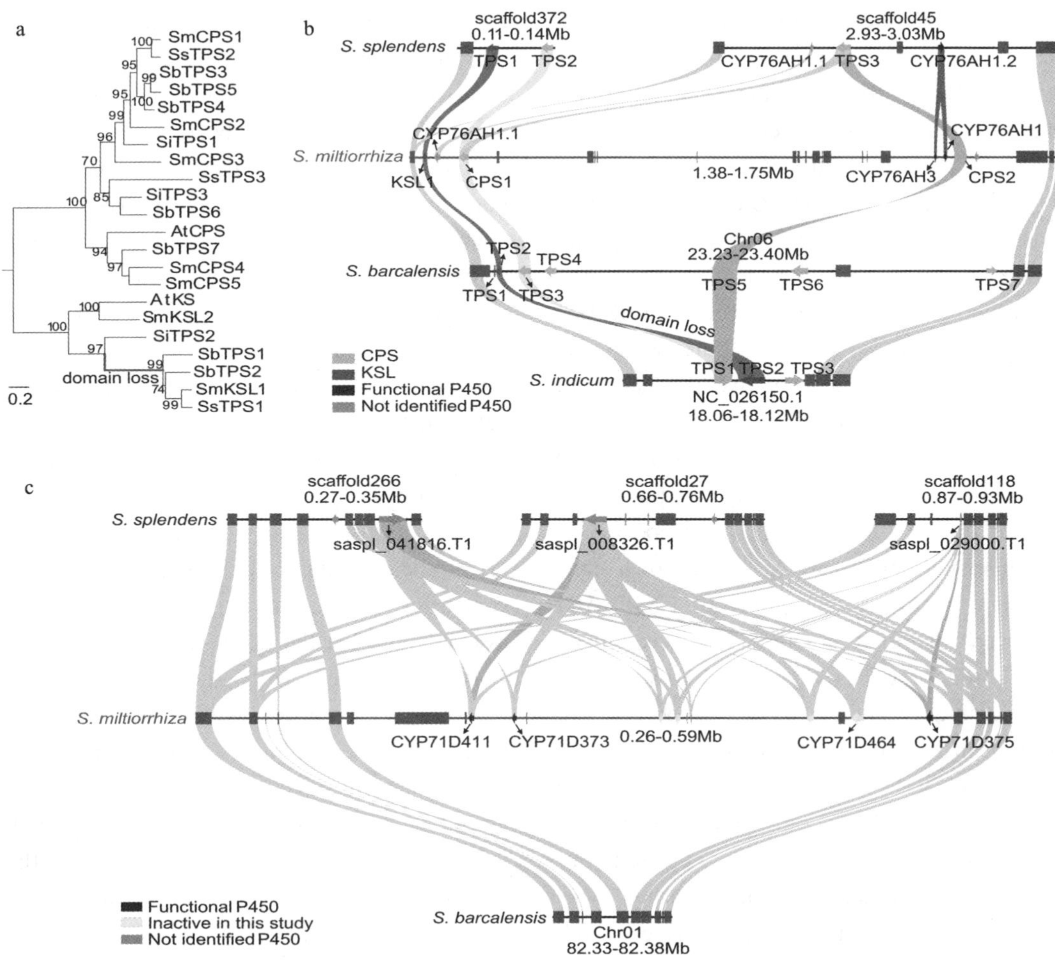

**Fig. 8 Tandem duplication and syntenic analysis of genes involved in tanshinone biosynthesis**

(a) ML phylogeny of diterpene cyclases and synthases from *S. miltiorrhiza* (Sm), *S. splendens* (Sp), *S. baicalensis* (Sb), *S. indicum* (Si) and *A. thaliana* (At). Bootstrap support values (percentages) from 1 000 replicates are shown next to relevant clades. (b) Syntenic analysis of Danshen tanshinone biosynthetic gene cluster by comparison to *S. splendens*, *S. baicalensis* and *S. indicum*. (c) Syntenic analysis of the Danshen CYP71D subfamily gene cluster by comparison to *S. splendens* and *S. baicalensis*. Source data underlying Fig. 8b and c are provided as a Source Data file.

The Danshen CYP71D subfamily gene cluster did not have orthologs in *S. indicum* and *S. barcalensis* (Supplementary Fig. 14). In the case of *S. barcalensis*, while nine genes on pseudochromosome 1 are orthologous to the four upstream and five downstream genes from Danshen, no CYP71D subfamily members are present in this region (Fig. 8c). Three collinear blocks can be found in *S. splendens* (Fig. 8c), each of which contains a CYP71D subfamily member. These are saspl_041816. T1, saspl_008326. T1, and saspl_029000. T1, which seem to be related to the Danshen CYP71D clade targeted here, although full-length cDNAs are not evident for any of these putative *S. splendens* CYP71D subfamily members. Among them, saspl_041816. T1 and saspl_029000. T1 have the highest homology with *CYP71D375*, while saspl_008326. T1 has the highest homology with *CYP71D411*. Thus, this CYP71D clade, which seems to be responsible for heterocyclization to form the D-ring, seems to have emerged in the *Salvia* genus.

## 2 DISCUSSION

Generation of the 14, 16-epoxy D-ring not only distinguishes the tanshinones within the phenolic abietane-type *nor*-diterpenoids found throughout the Lamiaceae family, but also provides pharmaceutical import as the target for sulfonation to generate a clinically relevant derivative. While tanshinone biosynthesis has been investigated for many years, the origin of this heterocycle has remained unknown. Here, we improved upon previously reported draft genomes by sequencing a highly homozygous line of Danshen. This highlighted the expansion of a clade within the CYP71D subfamily, with the expression of four of these found to be tightly correlated with tanshinone biosynthesis. Indeed, our results indicate that at least two of these, CYP71D373 and CYP71D375, play important roles in forming the characteristic 14,16-epoxy D-ring. This is supported by both the observed relative increase in intermediates that do not contain the heterocyclic D-ring in *CYP71Ds* - RNAi plants and recombinant biochemical activity. The promiscuity observed with CYP71D375 further suggests that tanshinone biosynthesis might operate as a metabolic grid, with heterocyclization to form the D-ring occurring after loss of C20 (Fig. 6a). While CYP71D373 and CYP71D375 exhibit partial functional redundancy, the substantial sequence divergence between these (aa sequence identity of ~70%) suggests the presence of selective pressure for the retention of both. Given their differential induction, this may reflect distinct roles in inducible versus constitutive production of tanshinones for *CYP71D373* and *CYP71D375*, respectively.

In contrast, CYP71D411 seems to act as earlier acting C20 hydroxylase. However, this activity overlaps that previously reported for CYP76AK1, which is supported by metabolite accumulation upon RNAi knockdown and biochemical activity. Moreover, a number of CYP76AK1 orthologs have been identified in other Lamiaceae plant species that also produce C20 oxygenated derivatives of phenolic abietane-type diterpenoids, further supporting this functional assignment. While we speculate that the appearance of CYP71D411 was driven by a need for increased flux towards tanshinone biosynthesis, consistent with the notable effect of these pigmented (reddish) diterpenoids on the coloration of the Danshen root periderm, this is purely hypothetical. Regardless, this distinct biochemical activity helped direct mutational analysis of the enzymatic structure-function relationships underlying the heterocyclization activity exhibited by CYP71D375. The results indicate an important role for substrate positioning within the active site, with particularly important roles played by A301 and, especially, L366.

Perhaps more interestingly, the improved genome sequence reported here provides insight into the evolution of both the phenolic abietane-type diterpenoids and tanshinones. It has previously been shown that other Lamiaceae plant species use orthologs of the genes firstly discovered in Danshen to produce 11-hydroxyferruginol—i.e., *SmCPS1*, *SmKSL1*, *CYP76AH1*, and *CYP76AH3*. Notably, these are exactly the genes found in the larger tanshinone biosynthetic gene cluster defined here. Given that collinear regions can be found in *S. splendens*, this might be more accurately termed a ferruginol biosynthetic gene cluster. It seems to have evolved in the lineage that gave rise to the *Salvia* genus, much as recently reported for triterpenoid biosynthetic gene cluster in the *Arabidopsis* genus. Such co-clustering of *CPS*, *KSL*, and a *CYP76AH* subfamily member containing all the genes necessary for the production of ferruginol is consistent with the widespread production of phenolic abietane-type diterpenoids in the *Salvia* genus. More specific to tanshinone production is elucidation of the biosynthetic origins of the characteristic D-ring heterocycle reported here, as the relevant CYP71D clade Ⅰ seems to have been expanded upon, in large part as a tandem gene array, in Danshen. While CYP71D subfamily members are present in the collinear regions of *S. splendens*, given that this species is not thought to produce such heterocyclic D-ring containing abietane diterpenoids, as well as the highly divergent activities observed in this subfamily, we hypothesize that it was neofunctionalization of this clade that led to the observed characteristic 14, 16-epoxidation activity in Danshen. In addition to clade Ⅰ, the CYP71D clade Ⅲ also seems to have been expanded in the Danshen genome, and may play a role in biosynthesis of other characteristic metabolites such as salvianolic acid B.

In conclusion, we sequenced a highly homozygous line of Danshen and substantially improved the genome assembly comparing to the existing ones. The improved genome assembly enabled the discovery of a large biosynthetic gene cluster associated with the early steps in tanshinone biosynthesis. More specifically, this biosynthetic gene cluster enables the production of at least ferruginol, and may be more widespread in *Salvia*, consistent with the broad appearance of such phenolic abietane-type diterpenoids in this genus. By contrast, elucidation of the biosynthetic origins of the D-ring reported here provides insight into the evolution of this characteristic heterocycle. In particular, this seems to have arisen from the expansion of a clade within the CYP71D subfamily that underwent neofunctionalization to catalyze the formation of this 14,16-epoxide. Accordingly, our results provide insight into not only the more specific biosynthetic origins and evolutionary derivation of the medically relevant tanshinones, but also that of the more general phenolic abietane-type diterpenoids, which are more broadly distributed in the Lamiaceae family.

## 3 METHODS

Plant materials and chemicals  In order to reduce heterozygosity, line bh2 - 7, which has been subjected to six cycles of self-pollination, was used in this study. Seedlings of this line were grown in sterile culture, with the shoot tips used for further propagation without hormones. The resulting plant material was used for DNA sequencing and Hi-C library construction. The transformed seedlings were transplanted in a soil: vermiculite (3 : 1) system and grown in a greenhouse under the same temperature and light regime. For RNA sampling, self-pollinated progeny of bh2 - 7 was subjected to low-temperature vernalization outside (February to March), and then moved into greenhouse for flowering. The *CYP71Ds* - RNAi and wild-type plants were grown in the greenhouse for three months before analysis. Tanshinone Ⅰ, tanshinone ⅡA, **1**, **2** and sugiol (**3**) were purchased from Chengdu Must Bio-Technology Co., Ltd (Sichuan, China). Miltirone (**4**), neocryptotanshinone (**8**) and methylenedihydrotanshinquinone (**11**) were purchased from Beijing Rongchengxinde Co., Ltd (Beijing, China). 2-isopropyl-8-methylphenanthrene-3,4-dione (here after Ro, **5**), 4-methylenemiltirone (**6**) and 16-hydroxyRo (**9**) were kindly provided by Prof. Jungui Dai, Prof. Wude Yang, and Prof. Kun Gao, respectively. The purity of these standards was >95%.

Genome sequencing  Genomic DNA was extracted from leaves with a standard CTAB method. DNA purity was verified by spectroscopic analysis with NanoDrop Spectrophotometers (Thermo Scientific). The Illumina paired-end genome library was constructed according to the standard protocol and seven paired-end Illumina WGS libraries were constructed with multiple insert sizes (200 bp, 450 bp, 500 bp, 800 bp, 2 kb, 5 kb, 10 kb, and 20 kb), which were then sequenced on a HiSeq 2 500 platform.

Library construction for PacBio sequencing was carried out using the protocols recommended by the manufacturer. A 20 kb single-molecule read library was constructed, which was then sequenced with a PacBio RSII Sequencer (Pacific Biosciences, USA) using the P6 - C4 chemistry system.

The Hi-C library was prepared following standard procedures by Annoroad Genomics (Beijing, China) following their standard procedure. The sequencing reads were mapped to the draft genome assembly by BWAmem. Then the contigs were clustered onto super-scaffolds with LACHESIS (http://shendurelab.github.io/LACHESIS).

Estimation of genome size  The genome size was measured by flow cytometry according to the protocol described by Dolezel et al.. Briefly, young seedlings were chopped up with a sharp razor blade for about 1 minute in LB01 buffer (15 mmol/L Tris, 2 mmol/L $Na_2EDTA$, 0.5 mmol/L spermine tetrahydrochloride, 80 mmol/L KCl, 20 mmol/L NaCl, 0.1% (v/v) Triton X-100, β-mercaptoethanol to 15 mmol/L; pH 7.5). The homogenate was mixed by pipetting up and down several times, then filtered through a 42-μm nylon mesh into a labeled sample tube. Plant cell nuclei were stained by adding DNA propidium iodide and RNase A at a concentrate of 50 μg/mL. The mixture was gently shaken and incubated on ice before analysis, with occasional shaking to keep in suspension. Two sequenced species, tomato and *Cusumis sativus*, were used to analyze the genome size of Danshen. The genome size was further evaluated by k-mer frequency analysis, based on Illumina short reads using the k-mer Analysis Toolkit (http://www.earlham.ac.uk/kat-tools).

Genome assembly and annotation  Two intermediate assembly versions of the genome were separately generated by DISCOVAR, using the Illumina reads (v0.1), and Falcon (v1.7.4), using the PacBio reads (v0.2). These were then merged using the HABOT (hybrid assembly of third-generation sequencing 2; https://github.com/asarum/HABOT2) software (1gene Corp., Hangzhou, China). A final round of scaffolding and gap filling was performed using Illumina reads to obtain a v1.0 of the Danshen genome. A more detailed protocol of genome assembly methods can be found in Supplementary Method 1.

The gene prediction pipeline used here combined ab initio gene prediction, homologous sequence searching and transcriptome sequence assembly. A detailed description for the prediction of genes, repeat sequences, non-coding RNA and tRNA can be found in Supplementary Method 2.

Genome evolution  Danshen gene evolution was analyzed by identifying orthologous genes from selected species—i.e., *A. thaliana*, *C. annuum*, *S. lycopersicum*, *S. tuberosum*, *B. hygrometrica*, *M. guttatus*, *A. paniculata*, *S. indicum*, *U. gibba*, *S. splendens*, and *S. barcalensis*. Proteins from all selected species were analyzed via all-by-all blastp. Similar gene pairs were then clustered into groups using OrthoMCL (v2.0.2). The single copy orthologous genes were used to construct the phylogenetic tree using the maximum likelihood method in the PhyML (v3.0) software package. More detailed description of gene family and genome evolution analyses can be found in Supplementary Method 3.

The dynamic evolution of gene families was investigated using CAFE software (v2.1, -filter) with a probabilistic graphical model. Finally, gene families with significantly different sizes ($P \leqslant 0.05$) in each species were annotated.

We performed syntenic searches to compare the specific regions containing diTPSs and CYP71Ds from Danshen with the most closely related species, particularly *S. splendens*, *S. barcalensis* and *S. indicum*. Syntenic blocks were assigned via all-by-all BLASP with cutoffs of identity ≥40% and *e*-value ≤ $1e^{-10}$. Synteny comparison was performed using JCVI with LASTAL as sequence alignment tool with default parameters. Microsynteny visualization was drawn using a modified version of JCVI.

Transcriptome analysis and cDNA cloning  For transcriptome analysis, five tissues at the flowering stage (root, stem, leaf, calyx, and petal), together with roots of *CYP71Ds*-RNAi and paired WT, were collected, with three biological replicates for each. Total RNA was extracted using a quick RNA isolation kit (HuaYueYang Biotechology, Beijing, China) according to the manufacturer's instructions. Then the RNA is shipped to the Novogene company (www.novogene.com) for quality estimation, library construction and sequencing. The RNA quality was determined using an Agilent 2100 Bioanalyzer. The cDNA libraries were sequenced on one lane for 151 cycles from each end of the cDNA fragments on a HiSeq 2 500 (Illumina). The full-length cDNA for *CYP71D373*,

*CYP71D375*, *CYP71D411*, and *CYP71D464* were identified based on the genome and transcriptome sequencing data. The open reading frames were further cloned into the pESC-His vector for functional analysis.

Plant transformation for RNAi of CYP71D candidates The region comprising nucleotides 823 – 1 276 from *CYP71D411* was cloned and transferred into the pK7GWIWG (Ⅱ) binary vector using Gateway technology. The resulting pK7GWIWG-CYP71D was introduced into *Agrobacterium tumefaciens* strain EHA105 by electroporation. Cells were cultured to an OD600 of 0.6, and then collected by centrifugation. The cells were resuspended in liquid Murashige and Skoog (MS) medium for genetic transformation. Before transformation, leaves or petioles were cut into disks and precultured for 2 days on MS basal medium supplemented with 2.0 mg/L 6-benzyladenine. The prepared disks were incubated with cell suspension by shaking for 15 min, and then cocultured on MS medium for 2 days. The leaf disks were selected on MS medium supplemented with 2.0 mg/L 6-benzyladenine, 50 mg/L kanamycin, and 225 mg/L timentin. After 2 – 3 rounds of selection (10 days each), the regenerated buds with GFP fluorescence were transferred to MS medium supplemented with 25 mg/L kanamycin for root formation and elongation. Rooted plantlets were cultured on MS medium for about 1 month, then transplanted to soil and vermiculite (3 : 1) and covered by beakers to maintain humidity for 1 week.

Metabolomics profiling using LC – qTOF – MS and GC – QqQ – MS Two independent analytical platforms were employed to acquire and analyze the metabolomic data. Briefly, LC – qTOF – MS analysis of methanol extracts was used for global unbiased metabolite detection. GC-QqQ-MS analysis of hexane extracts was optimized for detection of miltiradiene, abietatriene and ferruginol. LC – qTOF – MS analyses was carried out using an Agilent 1290 Infinity UPLC system with a VWD detector at 285 nm. An Agilent ZORBAX RRHD SB – C18 column (2.1×100 mm, 1.8 μm) was used for chromatographic separation. Mass spectrometry was acquired with an Agilent 6 540 qTOF equipped with an electrospray ionization (ESI) source operating in positive ion mode. For full-scan MS analysis, the data acquisition range of mass-to-charge ratio ($m/z$) was from 100 to 1 000. The nebulization gas was set to 40 pounds per square inch. The flow rate of drying gas and sheath gas was set at 10 L/min and 11 L/min at 350 ℃, respectively. The capillary voltage was set to 4 000 V and the acquisition rate was set at 0.5 s. GC – QqQ – MS analyses were performed on an Agilent 7 890 A GC system with a 7 000B triple quadruple MS detector at electron impact ionization. The column was an Agilent DB-5 ms (30 m×0.25 mm i.d., 0.25 μm film thickness; Agilent J&W Scientific). Helium was used as the carrier gas for GC with a flow rate of 1.0 mL/min. The injector and transfer line temperature was 280 ℃. The following temperature program was used: 50 ℃ for 2 min, then a linear ramp at a rate of 20 ℃/min to 200 ℃ followed by a 5 ℃/min linear ramp to 300 ℃, and held at 300 ℃ for 10 min.

Heterologous expression in yeast and in vitro activity assay The epitope-tagged pESC-His vectors carrying *CYP71D373*, *CYP71D375*, *CYP71D411*, or *CYP71D464* were each transformed into the yeast strain WAT11, which enables catalytic activity of plant CYPs by also expressing the *A. thaliana* NADPH-CYP reductase ATR1. WAT 11 transformed with empty pESC-His was employed as control. TE buffer was prepared with 50 mmol/L Tris-HCl, 1 mmol/L EDTA, pH 7.5. The cells were recovered by centrifugation at 5 000 g for 4 min, resuspended in TEK (0.1 mol/L KCl in TE) to a concentration of 0.5 g wet cells per mL and left at room temperature for 5 min. The cells were again recovered by centrifugation and resuspended in TESB (0.6 mol/L sorbitol in TE). Cells were broken up at 2 – 6 ℃ by a cryogenic homogenizer. After centrifugation at 20 000 g for 20 min, microsomes were precipitated by adding NaCl to the supernatant to a final concentration of 0.15 mol/L and polyethylene glycol PEG4000 to a final concentration of 0.1 g/mL. Pellets were resuspended in TEG (20% (v/v) glycerol in TE). In vitro activity assays were performed in a 500 μL reaction system that included 100 mmol/L Tris-HCl (pH 7.5) and 500 μmol/L NADPH, along with a regenerating system (5 mmol/L glucose-6-phosphate, 1 unit glucose-6-phosphate dehydrogenase, 5 μmol/L FAD, and 5 μmol/L FMN), 0.5 mg microsomal protein, and 100 μmol/L of the substrate. The reactions were incubated at 30 ℃ for 4 hours with shaking, and then extracted with 500 μL of ethyl acetate.

Isolation of products and NMR analysis Dried Danshen root was ground up and the resulting powder (200 g) was soaked in 2 L ethyl acetate overnight, then the mixture homogenized by sonication for 30 minutes. The organic phase was separated, dried, and the residue dissolved in 20 mL acetonitrile for isolation of 16-hydroxymiltirone (**7**). For isolation of sufficient amounts of 20-hydroxysugiol (**12**) for NMR analysis, the in vitro enzymatic reaction system was expanded from 500 μL to 100 mL. The assay was incubated in a shaker at 100 rpm/min for six hours. Ethyl acetate (100 mL) was then added to the assay, followed by sonication for 20 minutes. After centrifugation at 4 000 g for ten minutes, the ethyl acetate layer in the supernatant was collected and dried under nitrogen, then the residue dissolved in 5 mL acetonitrile. Compounds **7** and **12** were purified using a Shimadzu LC – 20AR preparative liquid chromatography system, with a J'sphere ODSM80 column (20×250 mm, 4 μm). The mobile phase for purification of **7** was a 3.5 : 6.5 mixture of water and acetonitrile (v/v), while a 3 : 7 mix of water and acetonitrile (v/v) was used as mobile phase for purification of **12**, with a flow rate of 8 mL/min in each case. For chemical structure characterization, $^{1}H$ NMR (600 MHz), $^{13}C$ NMR (100 MHz), and two-dimensional (2D) NMR spectra were recorded with a Bruker DRX Avance-600 (Bruker Co., Switzerland) NMR spec-trometer. The observed chemical shift values are reported in ppm.

Modeling docking and mutagenesis CYP71D373, CYP71D375, CYP71D411, and CYP71D464 were modeled using SwissModel, with the structure of the most closely related CYP76AH1 (5YLW) serving as the template. The coordinates of the heme protoporphyrin were then inserted in the modeled CYP71D structures from that found in 5YLW. Miltirone was protonated and docked into the structures with AutoDock Vina. Molecular distances were calculated using PyMol (http://www.pymol.org). Substitutions for the selected residues in CYP71D375 were constructed by PCR using the primers listed in Supplementary Table 14.

Reporting summary Further information on research design is available in the Nature Research Reporting Summary linked to this article.

## 4 DATA AVAILABILITY

The data supporting the findings of this work are available within the paper and the Supplementary Information files. A reporting summary for this article is available as a Supplementary Information file. The data sets generated and analyzed during this study are available from the corresponding author upon request. The genome sequence and assembly are available at NCBI BioProject PRJNA682867. The databases of KEGG (http://www.genome.jp/kegg/), Swissprot and TrEMBL (http://www.uniprot.org/), and InterPro (https://www.ebi.ac.uk/interpro/) are used for data analyses in this study. Source data are provided with this paper.

[马莹，郭娟，黄璐琦，等. Nature Communication, 2021, 12:685.]

# Recent progress and new perspectives for diterpenoid biosynthesis in medicinal plants

## 1 INTRODUCTION

Diterpenoids, comprised of four isoprene structural units are derived from (*E*, *E*, *E*)-geranylgeranyl diphosphate (GGPP). In plants, GGPP-derived compounds include the hormone gibberellin (GA) and one of the side chain groups of chlorophyll. In addition to the primary metabolic rate of GGPP, by recruitment from an ancient series of reactions, plants employ GGPP as a substrate to produce large amounts of diterpenoid natural products. These products are not always required for plant growth or development but have important ecological and agronomic functions. They also have a wide range of commercial applications in the cosmetic, food additive, and pharmaceutical industries, among others.

More than 126 different diterpenoid carbon skeletons have been identified that give rise to more than 18,000 compounds (http://dnp.chemnetbase.com). Many oxygenated derivatives of diterpenes have biological activities and some are widely used as important clinical drugs. One of the most famous plant diterpenoids used as a pharmaceutical compound is the blockbuster anticancer drug paclitaxel (tradenames Taxol and Abraxane). Paclitaxel was firstly isolated from *Taxus brevifolia* (Pacific yew). It has excellent anticancer activity and can be used to treat a variety of cancers. In addition to paclitaxel, many other diterpenoids have also been recognized as lead compounds for anticancer drugs such as ingenol mebutate from *Euphorbia peplus*, forskolin from *Coleus forskohlii*, and triptolide from *Tripterygium wilfordii*. Andrographolide is a labdane diterpenoid obtained from *Andrographis paniculata*. In its water-soluble form, andrographolide is the active substance in Xiyanping Injection, a widely used medicine in the development of anti-inflammatory and antiviral agents. Patients are currently being recruited for a clinical trial with this drug for the treatment of acute bronchitis (NCT03132623). Tanshinone $II_A$, extracted from roots of *Salvia miltiorrhiza* Burge, exhibits several medicinally valuable properties, including anti-inflammatory activity, antioxidant activity, and cardiovascular effects. Sodium tanshinone $II_A$ sulfonate, a water-soluble derivative of tanshinone $II_A$, is widely used in the clinic. The complexity and diversity of the structures of diterpenoids result in different biological activities and have become clinically important drugs. Several reviews have described the use of diterpenoids as drugs or lead compounds with anticancer, anti-inflammatory, antibacterial, and other activities.

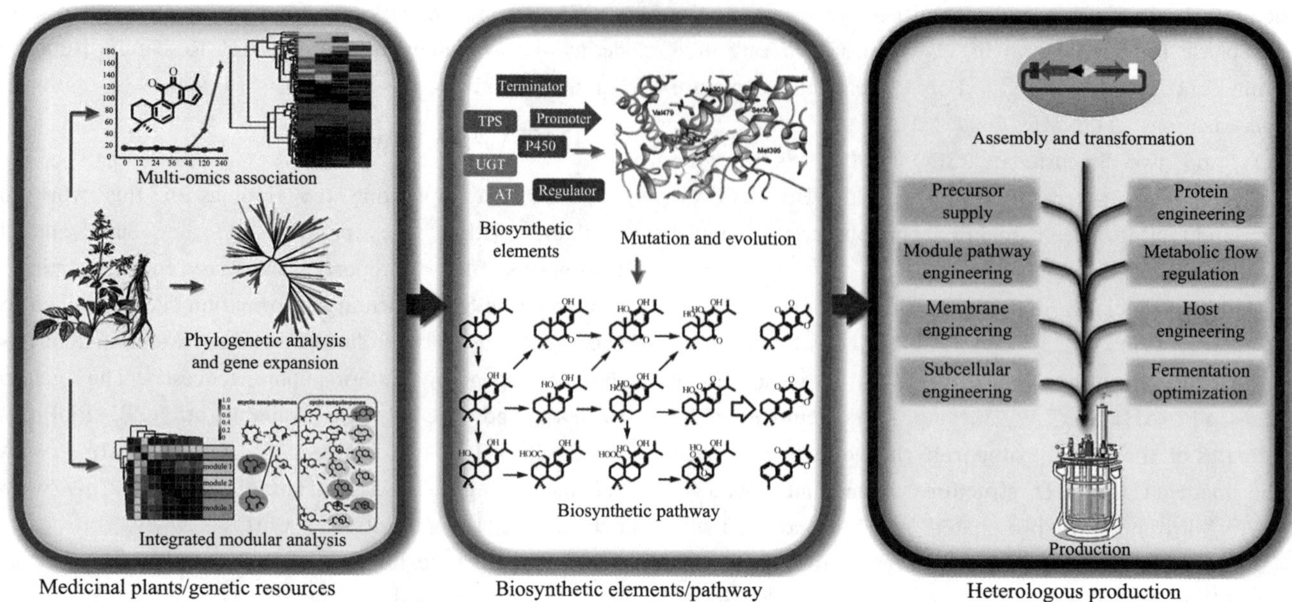


**Figure 1　Overview of biosynthetic pathway analysis of plant diterpenoid and its heterologous production (Color figure can be viewed at wileyonlinelibrary. com)**

One of the most significant challenges of using these compounds is to obtain sufficient quantities and quality for treatment. Diterpenoids accumulate in plants as specialized metabolites at low concentrations and may be produced as varied structural analogs. Traditional extraction and separation methods are inefficient, time-consuming, and costly, which greatly restricts the development of new drugs. Major advances in our understanding of the genes and pathways for biosynthesis of these active compounds are providing new and unprecedented opportunities for metabolic engineering and synthetic biology applications in their production (Figure 1). Several recent reviews have explored different perspectives on diterpenoid biosynthesis. In this review, we focus on the biosynthesis of diterpenoid natural products that have important medicinal activities and which are found in medicinal plants. In particular, we take a close look at two of the most important enzyme families (diterpene synthase and cytochrome P450), as well as recent progress in understanding the biosynthetic pathways of different groups of ringed compounds. The application of synthetic biology and metabolic engineering for diterpenoid production is also considered.

## 2　BIOSYNTHETIC PATHWAY OF DITERPENOIDS

The biosynthesis of diterpenoids can be divided into three steps: the formation of GGPP, the precursor of all diterpenoids; the construction of carbon skeletons of diterpenoids; and the post-synthesis modification of the molecular skeletons. All diterpenoids share similar upstream biosynthetic pathways, which means that the complete formation of GGPP is present within these pathways. Details about this step are available elsewhere. Here, we detail the compounds and biosynthetic reactions that predominantly rely on catalysis by diterpene synthases (diTPSs) and post-modification enzymes, especially cytochrome P450s (P450s or CYPs), for the formation of diterpenoids.

2.1　DiTPSs for the formation of the molecular skeleton of diterpenoids　Diterpene synthase/cyclase is the basis of the structural diversity of diterpenoids. It forms different diterpene compounds through cyclization and/or rearrangement of the central GGPP precursor. In general, diterpenoid biosynthesis can be initiated by either of two distinct enzymes: class Ⅱ diTPSs (copalyl diphosphate synthases-like, CPSLs) or class Ⅰ diTPSs (kaurene synthases-like, KSLs). Diterpenoids resulting from class Ⅱ diTPSs are known as labdane-related diterpenoids, which usually proceed via a bicyclic diphosphate intermediate. Nonlabdane diterpenoids are usually initiated by class Ⅰ diTPSs that react directly with GGPP. The biosynthetic origin and characterization of relevant enzymes can be found in several reviews.

In recent years, some KSL enzymes, such as SsSS from *Salvia sclarea*, have been shown to have substrate promiscuity and can react with nearly all available products of CPSLs. This leads to complex labdane-related enzyme combinations. At the same time, the same specialized metabolite can also be synthesized by enzymes from different subfamilies. The most notable case is the biosynthesis of miltiradiene, a precursor of tanshinones, carnosic acid, and triptolide. In Lamiaceae, miltiradiene is synthesized by a combination of class Ⅱ diTPS CPS1 (TPS-c subfamily) and class Ⅰ diTPS KSL1 (TPS e/f subfamily), while in *T. wilfordii*, a KSL TwTPS-27 in the TPS-b subfamily converts the class Ⅱ diTPS product CPP into miltiradiene. In *Selaginella moellendorffii*, a bifunctional diTPS SmMDS in the TPS-h subfamily directly catalyzes GGPP to miltiradiene. These pathway variations high-light the complex and polyphyletic evolution of diTPS and diterpene skeletal diversity. Here, we place special emphasis on diterpene structures created by combinations of native diTPSs in a given species, that is, excluding diterpenoids produced via nonnative enzyme combinations.

Rapidly developing transcriptome and genome sequencing technologies have been the driving force for the identification of diTPSs. For example, the CPP synthase and miltiradiene synthase in *S. miltiorrhiza* were first identified as diTPSs in Lamiaceae in 2009. In 2018, these types of enzymes were investigated from the leaves of 48 phylogenetically diverse Lamiaceae species using a database-driven approach. This analysis functionally identified 9 Class Ⅱ and 10 Class Ⅰ of diTPSs at the same time. In total, 135 diTPSs from 37 medicinal plants in eleven families were investigated. Twenty species belong to four subfamilies of Lamiaceae, including Ajugoideae, Viticoideae, Lamioideae, and Nepetoideae. Eleven species are from Celastraceae, Euphorbiaceae, Asteraceae, and Pinaceae. The other species are from Iridaceae, Acanthaceae, Oleaceae, Taxaceae, Selaginellaceae, and Ginkgoaceae. Among the 135 diTPSs, 58 belong to Class Ⅱ diTPSs, 72 belong to Class Ⅰ diTPSs, and 5 are bifunctional Class Ⅰ/Class Ⅱ diTPSs (Table S1). These enzymes, combined, give rise to 42 distinct diterpenes, including 15 different skeletons (Figure 2), which we summarize below.

2.1.1 Diterpenoids initiated by monofunctional Class Ⅰ and Class Ⅱ diTPSs Notably, most of the medicinal plants produce labdane-related diterpenoids, whose biosynthesis is initiated by Class Ⅱ diTPSs. 58 CPS enzymes have been reported that can form 11 diphosphate scaffolds: copalyl diphosphate (CPP), *ent*-CPP, *syn*-CPP, 8-α-hydroxy-CPP, 8β-hydroxy-*ent*-CPP, peregrinol diphosphate, labdan-7-13*E*-dienyl diphosphate (*endo*-CPP), *ent*-kolavenyl diphosphate (*ent*-KPP), kolavenyl diphosphate (KPP), 10*R*-labda-8, 13*E*-dienyl diphosphate, and *neo*-cleroda-4(18), 13*E*-dienyl diphosphate (Figure 3A). For these enzymes, 35% produce CPP, and 30% produce *ent*-CPP (necessary for the production of GAs). The largest number of reported CPP synthases are involved in the biosynthesis of widely distributed abietane-type diterpenoids found in the Lamiaceae plant family. Most Lamiaceae species contain this specific enzyme (Table S1).

Eleven of the diphosphate scaffolds are further catalyzed by 63 Class Ⅰ diTPSs to produce 34 diterpenes (Figure 3A). Around half of the KSL enzymes react with *ent*-CPP (54%), 46% react with CPP, 24% react with 8α- hydroxy-CPP and peregrinol diphosphate, and 13% react with 8β-hydroxy-CPP. These diterpenes correspond to nine skeletons, which include bicyclic labdane (Sk1) and clerodane (Sk2); tricyclic abietane (Sk3) and pimarane (Sk4); tetracyclic kaurane (Sk5), atisane (Sk6), trachylobane (Sk7), beyerane (Sk8), and stemodane types (Sk9; Figure 2).

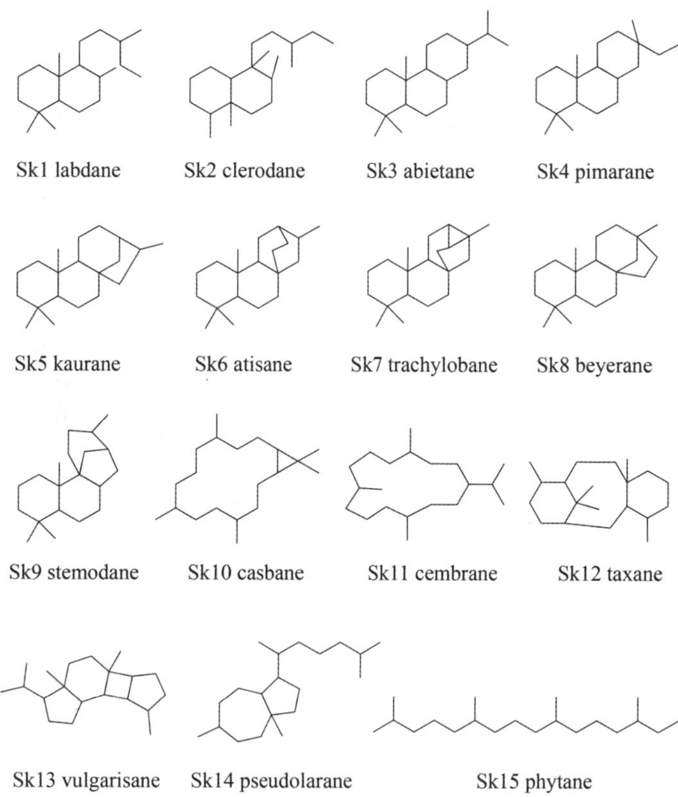


**Figure 2 Diterpene skeletons produced by published diterpene synthases from medicinal plants**

2.1.2 Diterpenoids initiated by bifunctional Class Ⅰ/Class Ⅱ diTPSs Bifunctional diTPSs have been identified in gymnosperms and lycophytes, which are different from the monofunctional diTPS mentioned above. They form five different diterpenes which belong to labdane and abietane skeletons (Figure 3B). Examples of bifunctional diTPSs include abietadiene synthase from *Abies grandis* (AgAS), *cis*-abienol synthase from *Abies balsamea* (AbCAS), levopimaradiene synthase from *Ginkgo biloba* (GbLPS), labda-7, 13*E*-dien-15-ol synthase (SmCPSKSL1), and miltiradiene synthase (SmMDS) from *S. moellendorffii*.

2.1.3 Diterpenoids initiated by Class Ⅰ diTPSs Six nonlabdane diterpene compounds are synthesized directly by Class Ⅰ diTPSs in plants. They are taxa- 4(5), 11(12)-diene, casbene, neocembrene, 11-hydroxyvulgarisane, pseudolaratriene, and geranyllinalool (Figure 3C). Casbene and neocembrene belong to the macrocyclic casbane (Sk10) and cembrane (Sk11) types. The others belong to taxane (Sk12), vulgarisane (Sk13), pseudolarane (Sk14), and phytane (Sk15). The corresponding enzymes include taxadiene synthase in *T. brevifolia* (TbTS), casbene synthases in *Ricinus communis* (RcCAS3), *Euphorbia Esula* (EeTPS2), and *Sapium sebiferum* (SsTPS10); neocembrene synthase in *R. communis* (RcCAS2), 11-hydroxyvulgarisane synthase in *Prunella vulgaris* (PvHVS), pseudolaratriene synthase in *Pseudolarix amabilis* (PxaTPS8), and geranyllinalool synthase in *T. wilfordii* (TwGES1).

In summary, 11 of the diphosphate scaffolds and 42 diterpene compounds have been reported from medicinal plants (Figure 3). Diterpenes with a bicyclic labdane skeleton (Sk1), such as sclareol, and 13*R*-manoyl oxide represent the largest group, accounting for 38%, while 19% have tricyclic pimarane skeletons (Sk4), such as nezukol, sandaracopimaradiene, and so on. Tricyclic abietane (Sk3) and tetracyclic kaurane skeleton (Sk5) account for 9% and 7%, respectively. Abietadiene, miltiradiene, and levopimaradiene belong to the abietane skeleton group. Kaurane skeletons include *ent*-kaurene, *ent*-kaur-15-ene, and 16α-hydroxy-*ent*-kaurene. The biosynthesis of labdane, abietane, and kaurane, together with taxane and macrocyclic diterpenoids are summarized below.

2.2 Post-modification for the formation of diverse diterpenoids

2.2.1 P450-initiated post-modification for the formation of diterpenoids  Formation of diterpene carbon skeleton mediated by diterpene synthase represents the first steps in the biosynthesis of diterpenoids. But diterpenoids with medicinal activity are typically highly oxygenated, with more than 97% of diterpenoids oxygenated at one or more carbon positions to produce active compounds. In plants, the vast majority of terpene oxidation is carried out by cytochrome P450 enzymes. Hydroxylation is the most common reaction catalyzed by P450s, which also allows sequential oxidation and other decoration to occur at a given position. In addition, some unusual reactions such as the generation of C-C double bonds can lead to re-arrangement or closure of the ring to increase the complexity of the diterpenoid structures. In contrast with substrate-specific enzymes, evidence has emerged supporting the catalytic promiscuity of P450s, especially in secondary metabolic pathways. Irreversible reactions and promiscuity of P450s can result in metabolic bifurcation and structural diversity of diterpenoids in plants.

Bathe and Tissier summarized all P450s that have been functionally characterized for their roles in the biosynthesis of diterpenoids up to 2018. They concluded that the known P450s involved in the biosynthesis of plant diterpenoids are dominated by three clans, namely CYP71, CYP72, and CYP85. The most commonly reported enzymes belong to the CYP71 clans, and the majority of these enzymes participate in the biosynthesis of macrocyclic or labdane-related diterpenoids. This is unsurprising since the CYP71 clan represents more than 50% of all plant P450 enzymes. Within the CYP71 clan, the CYP76 family accounts for more than half of the specialized diterpene metabolism, and participates in the metabolism of diterpenoids in both monocotyledonous and dicotyledonous plants. These CYP76s, together with a few from the CYP71 family, play important catalytic roles in the synthesis of labdane diterpenoids. By contrast in gymnosperms, P450s involved in the biosynthesis of labdane diterpenoids were found to be in the CYP720s family of the CYP85 clan. In addition, CYP726As and CYP71Ds from the CYP71 clan reportedly decorate macrocyclic diterpenoid skeletons in Euphorbiaceae, and CYP720s from the CYP85 clan were shown to play essential roles in the biosynthesis of paclitaxel. Only five functionally characterized P450s from the CYP72 clan have thus far been found to inactivate gibberellic acid in plants and catalyze C13-hydroxylation en route to steviol glycoside biosynthesis in *Arabidopsis thaliana*. Though there is no general rule for the function of P450s within such a large family, it could not be ruled out that diterpenoids from one plant family or species are likely to be oxidized by a subfamily of P450s within a taxonomic clade (i.e., CYP76AHs from *Salvia* and *C. forskohlii* catalyze the oxidation of phenolic diterpenoids) suggesting monophyletic evolutionary origins of this activity within a taxonomic clade.

Due to the importance of P450s involved in the biosynthesis of diterpenoids, their functional characterization is essential for biosynthetic pathway analysis. Unlike diterpenoid synthases that use GGPP or its carbon skeletons as substrates, P450 enzymes can act on a considerably different range of substrates, many of which have not been definitively identified. It is the largest family of enzymes in plant metabolism, accounting for around 1% of plant protein-coding genes. The presence of hundreds of P450 enzymes in the plant genome limits the discovery of functional P450 enzymes. In addition, due to a lack of reliable mutant lines for medicinal plants, the recent identification of P450 enzymes mostly relies on comparative transcriptomics and metabolomics from different tissues, cell types, or treatments. Recently, breakthroughs in sequencing technologies have increased the availability of plant genomes for studies. Investigations of multiple plant genomes have revealed that in some natural product pathways, functional genes are clustered in the genome, thus providing an additional means for screening candidate genes. A physical cluster of diterpenoid biosynthetic genes has been found in *R. communis*, including casbene synthases and P450s from the CYP726A subfamily. Evidence of a similar cluster was also found in two other members of the Euphorbiaceae. These results demonstrate the conservation of gene clusters at the higher taxonomic level of the plant family. Gene clusters in

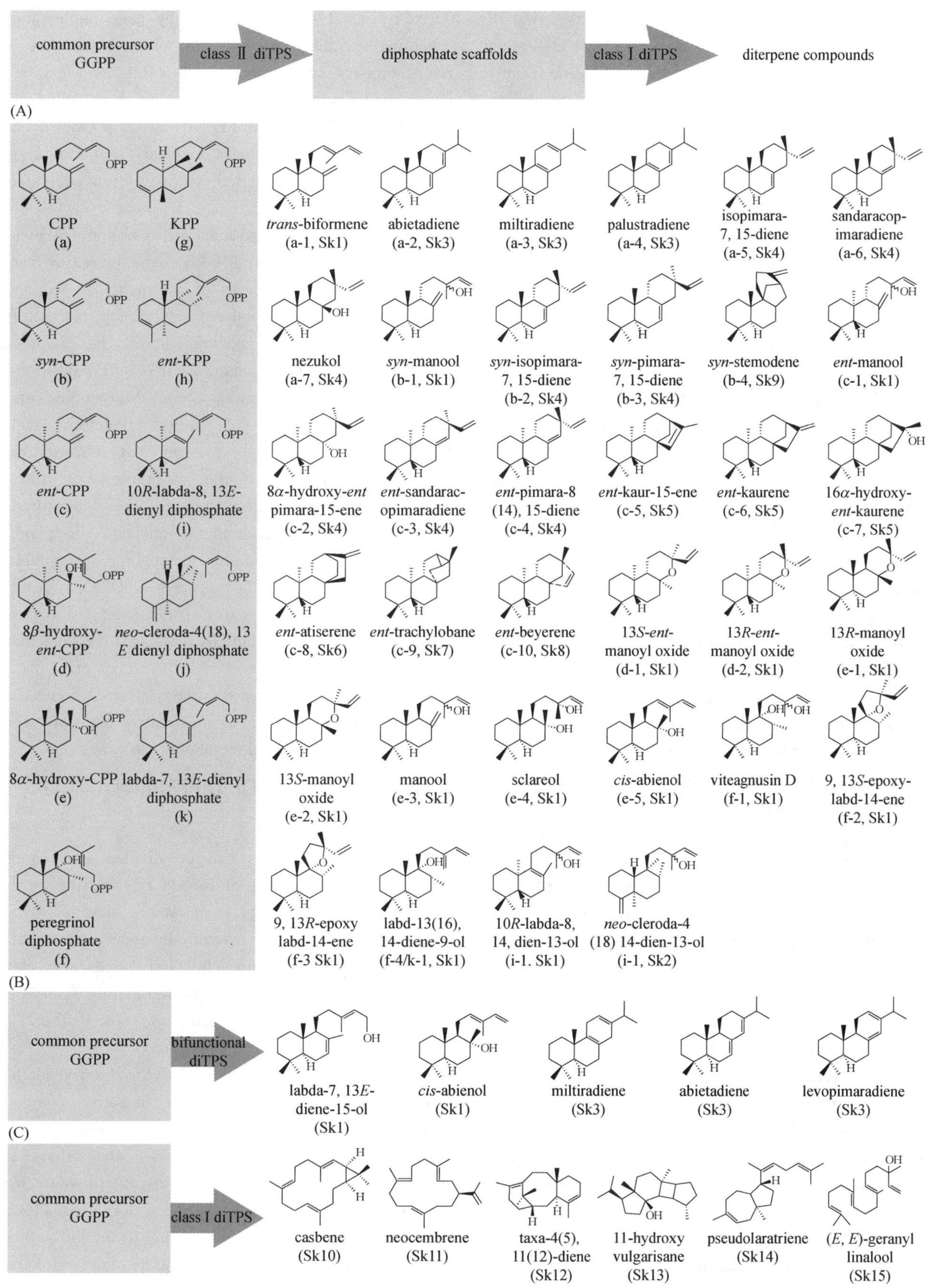


**Figure 3 Diterpenoids produced by natural diTPS combinations in medicinal plants**

(A) Diterpenes initiated by class Ⅱ diTPSs, which first produce eleven diphosphate scaffolds (blue), and are further ionized by class Ⅰ diTPSs to produce 34 diterpene compounds (green). (B) Diterpenes catalyzed by bifunctional diTPSs. (C) Diterpenes catalyzed directly by class Ⅰ diTPSs. The classes of diterpene skeletons (Sk1 - Sk15 in Figure 2), together with their corresponding diphosphate scaffolds (a - f), are shown in brackets [Color figure can be viewed at wileyonlinelibrary. com] the diterpenoid pathway and the coordinated expression of proteins in response to environmental stimuli or elicitation have also been observed. In the genome, gene family expansion and gene clusters of novel P450 multigene subfamilies for secondary metabolic pathways have been observed in certain plant orders, families, or species. This limited distribution suggests that phylogenetic analysis of genes in clusters could facilitate the discovery and characterization of plant P450s involved in highly specialized pathways, although it is worth keeping in mind the possibility that genes encoding P450s may not always be clustered with genes encoding the relevant terpene synthases.

2.2.2 Other enzymes involved in post-modification/decoration of diterpenoid skeletons Most of the active diterpenoids are generated by post-modification/decoration enzymes. P450 is one example of an enzyme that initiates the modification process to produce active compounds or to provide an active site for further modifications. In addition to hydroxylation mediated by P450s, other types of enzymes also play roles in the formation of active compounds, such as glycosyltransferases (GTs), acycosyltransferases (ACTs), and other enzymes related to diterpenoid synthesis.

Glycosylation of secondary metabolites improves the solubility and chemical stability of the compounds. Glycosyltransferases represent a large enzyme family in plants, and play an essential role in the structural diversity of triterpenoids and steroid saponins, but are less commonly reported in the biosynthesis of diterpenoids. Some diterpenoids are glycosylated, and several glycosyltransferases have been shown to be involved in the biosynthesis of neoandrographolide and steviosides. It warrants mention that glycosylation reactions necessary for diterpenoid biosynthesis mostly occur after oxidation, and are typically performed with high catalytic efficiency and substrate promiscuity, such as ApUGT from *A. paniculata*, which can glycosylate 26 natural and synthetic compounds.

Many diterpenoids have acyl/aroyl groups, although until recently, the acyltransferases identified in the diterpenoid biosynthetic pathway have been reported only in the biosynthesis of paclitaxel and forskolin. Plant acyltransferases include two families: the BAHD acyltransferases (named for the first four characterized enzymes) and serine carboxypeptidase-like (SCPL) acyltransferases. The genes involved in paclitaxel and forskolin biosynthesis belong to the BAHD acyltransferases, which constitute a large family of acyl CoA-utilizing enzymes that play important roles in the biosynthesis of a variety of active, acylated natural products. Based on differences in substrate specificity and amino acid sequence, BAHD acyltransferases have been sub-classified into five clades. The five acyltransferases in paclitaxel biosynthesis belong to clade Ⅴ. These genes were likely derived from a common lineage by gene duplication and functionally differentiated in their substrate and regiochemistry specificity, which catalyzes acety/benzoylation of the taxane core and the side chain. Phylogenetic analysis showed that CfACT1 - 8 from *C. forskohlii* belongs to clade Ⅲ, which includes members that can accept a diverse range of hydroxylated substrates using acetyl-CoA as the main acyl donor.

P450-dependent hydroxylation and oxidation, glycosylation, and acyl/aroylation have all been characterized as reactions involved in the biosynthesis of diterpenoids, while other steps, especially enzyme-catalyzed ring-opening, rearrangement, carbon reduction, and polymerization, have apparently complicated catalytic mechanisms that still require further investigation. For example, some diterpenoids undergo carbon reduction of the carbon skeleton, such as tanshinones, which are a group of C20-norabietane diterpenoids. However, the mechanism of the decarboxylation/demethylation step in the biosynthesis of specialized diterpenoids remains unclear. In plant GA biosynthesis, GA20-oxidase, belonging to soluble 2-oxoglutarate-dependent dioxygenases (2ODDs), can decarboxylate C20 diterpenes to C19 diterpenes, and generate biologically active $GA_{20}$ and $GA_9$. While it warrants mention that this process is catalyzed by P450s in bacteria, plant GA biosynthesis by 2ODDs via decarboxylative carbon reduction could nevertheless provide an informative point of reference for analysis of specialized metabolite pathways.

## 3 BIOSYNTHESIS OF DIFFERENT CYCLIC DITERPENOIDS

Diterpene structures can be divided into categories according to the number of carbon rings in the molecule, such as acyclic (chain), monocyclic, bicyclic, tricyclic, tetracyclic, taxane, and macrocyclic types, among others. Natural acyclic and monocyclic diterpenoids are relatively rare in plants. In this section, we mainly focus on the analysis of biosynthetic pathways for other cyclic diterpenoids with medicinal importance.

3.1 Bicyclic diterpenoids Bicyclic diterpenoids include many pharmaceutically important bioactive compounds. Three types of structures have been reported: labdane diterpenoids, clerodane diterpenoids, and others (i.e., ginkgolides). Among them, the biosynthetic route for the labdane diterpenoid forskolin has been elucidated. However, post-modifications performed en route to the biosynthesis of labdane diterpenoids such as andrographolides, ginkgolides, and the clerodane-type diterpenoids still need investigation.

The diterpenoid components found in *C. forskohlii* include labdane-type, pimarane-type, abietane-type, and others. Labdane-type diterpenoids are the most common diterpenoid components, and more than 30 compounds of this type have been isolated from *C. forskohlii*. Forskolin is the major metabolite found exclusively in the cork cells of *C. forskohlii* roots. This compound is used commercially for the treatment of glaucoma, asthma, and several heart ailments. The complex chemical structure of forskolin with a decalin core, a tetrahydropyran ring, five oxidation sites, and eight chiral centers, represents a challenge for classical organic chemical synthesis. Pateraki et al. reported the functional characterization of four CfTPSs via in vitro and *in planta* assays. CfTPS2 catalyzes the formation of forskolin by synthesizing the intermediate 8α-hydroxy-CPP from GGPP, after which 13*R*-manoyl oxide is formed by the action of Class Ⅰ diTPS (CfTPS3) (Figure 4). 13*R*-manoyl oxide is converted into 11-oxo-13*R*-manoyl oxide by CYP76AH8/15/17. This intermediate is further converted into 9-deoxy-7-deacetylforskolin by multifunctional CYP76AH11, which in turn produces 7-deacetylforskolin by CYP76AH16, and finally, CfACT1 - 8 acetylates 7-deacetylforskolin at C7 to obtain forskolin (Figure 4). Co-expression of *CfPOR*, *CYP76AH15*, *CYP76AH11*, *CYP76AH16*, and *CfACT1 - 8* in the yeast strain EFSC4498 (engineered for production of 13*R*-manoyl oxide), resulted in the production of forskolin. The biosynthesis of forskolin is the most fully elucidated pathway for diterpenoid biosynthesis. In addition to CfTPS2 and CfTPS3, involved in the biosynthesis of forskolin, CfTPS1 can catalyze GGPP to CPP (Figure 5), which can be further cyclized by Class Ⅰ diTPS CfTPS3 or CfTPS4 to form miltiradiene, the precursor of abietane diterpenoids in *C. forskohlii*. Miltiradiene can be hydroxylated to ferruginol by CYP76AH15 (Figure 5).

Andrographolides, which accumulate in the stems and leaves of *A. paniculata*, are *ent*-labdane-type diterpenoid lactones with a core formed by a decahydronaphthalene ring as the basic skeleton. *Ent*-CPS was originally thought to synthesize the core structure of andrographolide. Misra et al. cloned two *ApCPSs* from *A. paniculata*. Tissue-specific expression and in vitro analysis indicated that ApCPS2 was potentially involved in the tissue-specific accumulation of *ent*-labdane-related diterpenes. Subsequently, Shen et al. identified another *ent*-CPS (ApCPS1) that catalyzed GGPP conversion to form *ent*-CPP, which was proposed to be the precursor of andrographolides. However, none of these activities have been verified *in planta*. Sun et al. reported a chromosomescale genome sequence of *A. paniculata* and carried out the functional characterization of pairs of Class Ⅰ and Class Ⅱ diTPSs, which revealed the ability to produce diversified labdane-related diterpene scaffolds such as *ent*-CPP and CPP. Thus, ApCPS1 and ApCPS2 have been demonstrated to catalyze GGPP cyclization to form *ent*-CPP which might serve as an intermediate in the biosynthesis of andrographolide, while ApCPS3 produces CPP (Figure 4). The conversion of *ent*-CPP to andrographolide was predicted to be catalyzed by P450s or 2ODDs. However, none of these biosynthetic enzymes have been identified. Based on genome and transcriptome sequencing, Li et al. and Sun et al. identified two UDP-glycosyltransferases (UGTs; ApUGT74 and ApUGT73AU1) from *A. paniculata*, both of which were able to catalyze *O*-glycosylation of andrograpanin, yielding the major active product neoandrographolide (Figure 4).

Ginkgolides are unique compounds isolated from *G. biloba*. They are reported effectively for the treatment of cardiovascular and cerebrovascular diseases and for the protection of the central nervous system. Ginkgolides are bicyclic diterpenoids, the formation of which has been proposed to involve C ring dehydrogenation of the tricyclic skeleton levopimaradiene, followed by oxidization and rearrangement. GGPP is converted to levopimaradiene by the cyclase, levopimaradiene synthase (GbLPS; Figure 4). Schepmann et al. amplified a probe from a cDNA library of ginkgo seedling root tissues using conserved primers for the terpenoid synthase sequence of gymnosperms. A full-length clone, isolated through colony hybridization and rapid amplification of cDNA ends, was predicted to encode a gymnosperm diterpenoid synthase protein similar to other gymnosperm diterpenoid synthases. The protein was functionally characterized as GbLPS by expression in *Escherichia coli*. However, the potentially complicated steps related to oxidation and rearrangement remain unclear.

In addition to these bicyclic diterpenoids, other biosynthetic pathway genes have been reported. *Vitex agnus-castus* L. (Lamiaceae) is a medicinal plant with good curative effects in the treatment of premenstrual syndrome and its main active components are labdane-diterpenoids. CYP76BK1 was identified in *V. agnus-castus* and could catalyze 16-hydroxylation of the diol-diterpenoid, peregrinol, to generate labd-13*Z*-ene-9, 15, 16-triol, which was a potential intermediate in the production of furan-containing and lactone-containing diterpenoids (Figure 4). CYP71AU87 from *Marrubium vulgare* can catalyze the formation of the isomeric products 9, 13-epoxy labd-14-ene-18/19-ol after a continuous reaction by the diterpenoid synthases MvCPS1 and MvELS (Figure 4), and the 9, 13-epoxy labd-14-ene-18/19-ol isomers may be intermediates in the biosynthesis of the diterpenoid marrubiin.

3.2 Tricyclic diterpenoids Tricyclic diterpenoids include abietane-type, pimarane-type, and other diterpenoids (such as totarane from *Podocarpus totara*, daphnane from *Daphne mezereum*, icetexane from *Chamaecyparis pisifera* and *Salvia przewalskii*). Abietanes (including tanshinones, carnosic acid, and triptolide) are the most abundant type of tricyclic terpenoids, and the biosynthetic pathway of which

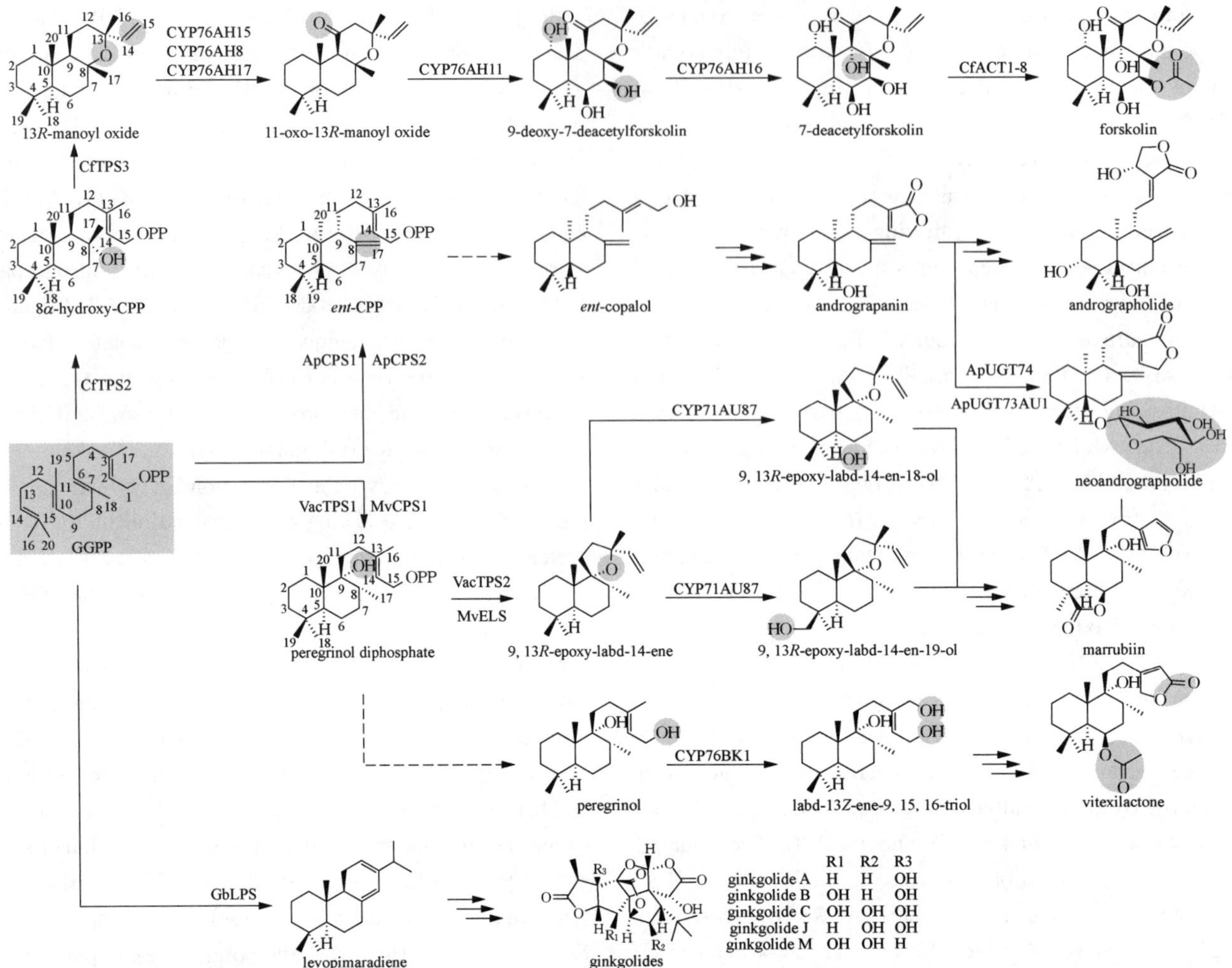


**Figure 4 Biosynthetic pathway of bicyclic diterpenoids (Color figure can be viewed at wileyonlinelibrary. com)**

has been best investigated.

Tanshinone is the active ingredient in Danshen, a widely used traditional Chinese medicine (derived from the rhizome of *S. miltiorrhiza*). These abietane-type diterpenoids show antioxidant, antibacterial, anti-inflammatory, and antitumor effects. In *S. miltiorrhiza*, GGPP can be catalyzed by SmCPS1, followed by SmKSL1 enzymes, to produce miltiradiene (Figure 5). Experiments in which hairy roots of *S. miltiorrhiza* were fed with isotope-labeled miltiradiene demonstrated that the labeled miltiradiene could be decorated to produce isotope-labeled cryptotanshinone, indicating that miltiradiene serves as the carbon skeleton of tanshinone. Guo et al. identified six candidate P450s involved in the biosynthesis of tanshinones based on their co-expression correlated with the accumulation of tanshinones in different tissues. Functional characterization revealed that one of them, designated CYP76AH1, could convert miltiradiene to an oxidized derivative, ferruginol. RNA interference (RNAi) analysis of *CYP76AH1* in hairy roots of *S. miltiorrhiza* showed that CYP76AH1 is a crucial enzyme in the downstream pathway of tanshinone biosynthesis. Based on comparative omics analysis, Guo et al. further identified two tanshinone-modifying enzymes (CYP76AH3 and CYP76AK1), which act sequentially in the biosynthesis of tanshinones. Specifically, CYP76AH3 oxidizes ferruginol at two different carbon sites, while CYP76AK1 hydroxylates the C20 intermediate using two different substrates that are produced by CYP76AH3. Substrate promiscuity of both enzymes can lead to pathway bifurcation en route to tanshinones (Figure 5). Recently, by gene expansion analysis, a P450 tadem gene array was identified. Two of them (CYP71D373 and CYP71D375) were characterized to catalyze hydroxylation and heterocyclization to form the D-ring of tanshinones. Based on genome sequencing and comparative omics data, several promising P450s and 2ODDs have been identified as candidates that complete the final steps in the biosynthetic pathway for these active compounds.

Carnosic acid, carnosol, and pisiferic acid, the main labdane-type diterpenoids in rosemary and various sage species (*Salvia sp.*), show diverse biological and chemical activities, including antioxidative, anticancer, anti-inflammatory, as well as antimicrobial properties. These tricyclic diterpenoids have been proposed as preventive or therapeutic agents for neurodegenerative disorders. In

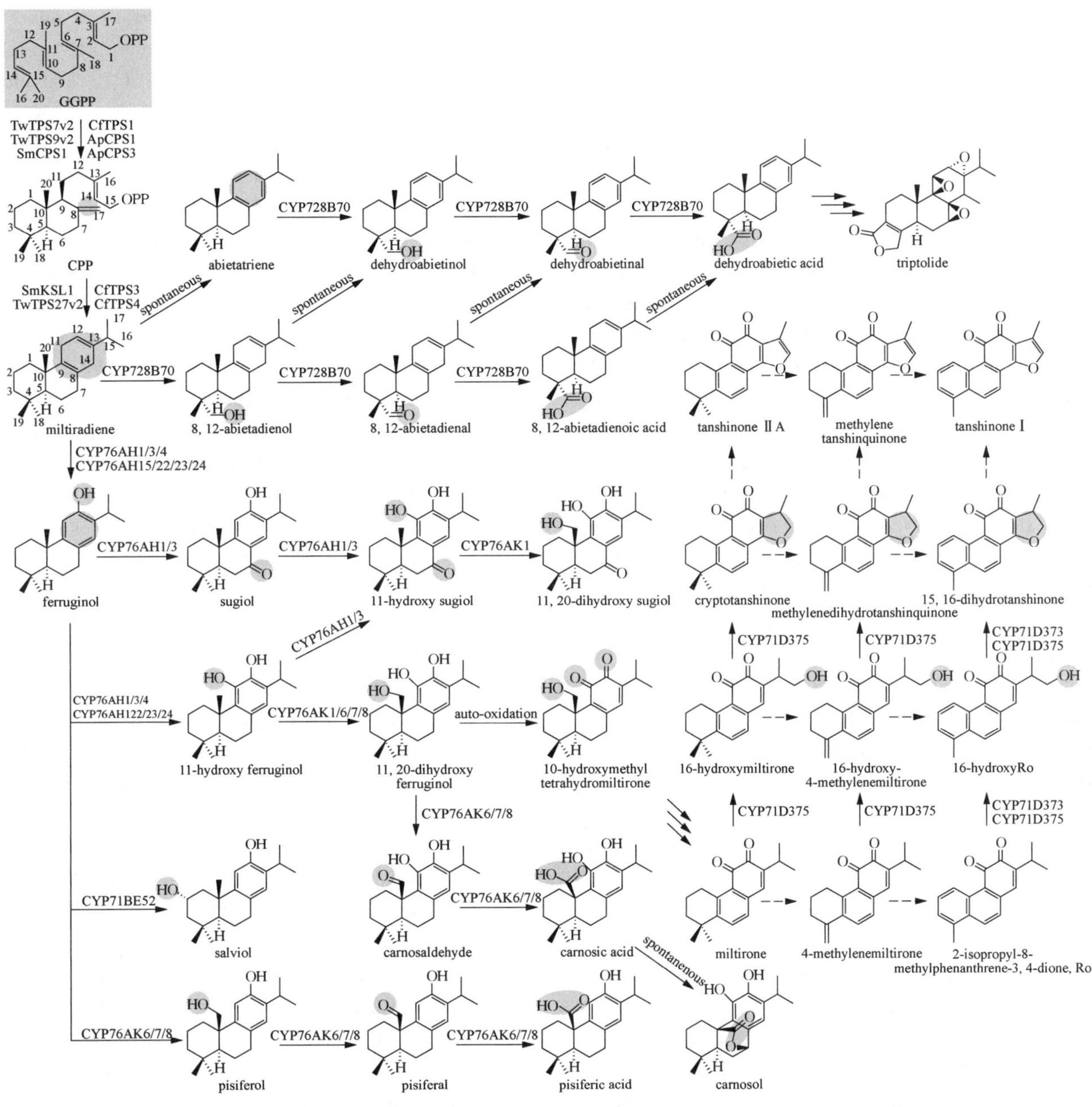


**Figure 5 Biosynthetic pathway of tricyclic diterpenoids (Color figure can be viewed at wileyonlinelibrary. com)**

addition, they are likely intermediates in the biosynthesis of other diterpenoids, such as tanshinones. Similar to the function of CYP76AH3, CYP76AH4 and CYP76AH22 - 24 are also able to produce 11-hydroxy ferruginol. The three sequential C20 oxidations catalyzed by CYP76AK6 - 8 convert 11-hydroxy ferruginol to carnosic acid, which spontaneously oxidizes to carnosol. CYP76AK6 - 8 can also oxidize miltiradiene and ferruginol, the latter leading to pisiferic acid. In *Salvia pomifera*, CYP71BE52 oxidizes ferruginol at position 2$\alpha$ to produce salviol.

*T. wilfordii* has been used medicinally for hundreds of years, mainly for the treatment of rheumatoid arthritis. It is well known that it produces abundant natural metabolites, including triptolide, which has been shown to have therapeutic potential. Triptolide is a diterpenoid epoxide, which possesses antitumor, immunosuppressive, and anti-inflammatory properties. The amount of triptolide in *Tripterygium* plants is extremely low (6 - 16 ng/g), and its chemical synthesis is cumbersome, with low yield. The production capacity for this compound is therefore insufficient to meet large commercial needs, especially for the industrial production of triptolide and its derivatives. Su et al. employed feeding studies in suspension cell cultures that produced triptolide under induction, and showed that miltiradiene is the precursor. Transcriptome analysis of *T. wilfordii* cells identified eight candidate diTPSs. Functional characterization and RNAi analysis indicated that TwTPS7v2 or TwTPS9v2 could use GGPP to produce CPP. CPP was subsequently cyclized to miltiradiene by TwTPS27v2, which spontaneously formed abietatriene. Recently, Tu et al. reported a reference-grade genome of *T. wilfordii*, which is the first genome sequence reported for genus *Euonymus*. Genomic, transcriptomic, and metabolomic data were further integrated to map a correlation network of genes and metabolites, resulting in the identification of four candidate cytochrome P450 genes that potentially related to triptolide biosynthesis. Furthermore, by combining synthetic biology, RNAi, and overexpression, the authors identified CYP728B70, which can catalyze the oxidation of a methyl group to the acid moiety of dehydroabietic acid in the triptolide biosynthesis pathway (Figure 5). The genome sequence and functional characterization of genes encoding diTPSs and P450 enzymes help pave the way to determine the remaining components of the pathway to triptolide.

3.3 Tetracyclic diterpenoids Tetracyclic diterpenoids are distributed widely in higher plants. Tetracyclic diterpenoids can be divided into tetracyclic diterpenoids with a bridged ring at C-8 (i.e., *ent*-kaurane and *ent*-gibberellane types) or C-9 according to the biogenic relationship. *Ent*-kaurane-type compounds, including the promising drug candidates oridonin and eriocalyxin, and the sweetening agents steviol glycosides, represent the most abundant type of tetracyclic diterpenoids.

Steviol glycosides, which are the particularly sweet constituents of *Stevia rebaudiana*, have been confirmed to have nutritional and pharmacological activities. More than 30 steviol glycosides have been reported in stevia leaves, of which stevioside and rebaudioside A are the most abundant and have the best-characterized sweetness profiles. Steviol glycosides are *ent*-kaurane diterpenoids that share the upstream of their biosynthetic pathway with gibberellins, but then diverge from *ent*-kaurenoic acid. The last five steps are specific to steviol glycosides biosynthesis, and are catalyzed by P450 (*ent*-kaurenoic acid 13-hydroxylase, KA13H) and UGTs. *Ent*-kaurenoic acid is hydroxylated by kaurenoic acid 13-hydroxylase (SrKA13H) to generate the aglycone, steviol. In *S. rebaudiana*, glycosylation is catalyzed by SrUGT85C2, and preferentially begins on the C-13 hydroxyl group of the steviol producing steviolmonoside. The follow-up glucosylation occurs on the C-2 hydroxyl group of its C-13 glucose moiety, and is catalyzed by SrUGT91D2 to form steviolbioside. Stevioside is obtained after a SrUGT74G1- catalyzed glucosylation at the C-19 hydroxyl (C-4 carboxylic acid) moiety of steviolbioside, followed by a SrUGT76G1-catalyzed glucosylation at the C-3 hydroxyl group of the C-13 glucose, forming rebaudioside A. Researchers have also established a novel pathway and constructed an *E. coli* strain for the production of steviol glycosides.

The steviol glycoside rubusoside, is produced mainly by the two edible, medicinal plants *Rubus suavissimus* and *Angelica keiskei*, and is the first molecule reported to inhibit both the human fructose transporter GLUT5 and glucose transporter GLUT1. Li et al. found that SrUGT73E1 glycosylate steviol and steviolmonoside on the C-19 hydroxyl group to generate steviol 19-O-β-D-glucopyranoside and rubusoside, respectively. Sun et al. identified six key UGTs in the glycosylation steps of rubusoside synthesis based on transcriptomic analysis of *R. suavissimus* and *A. keiskei* leaf tissues, inter-species evolutionary analysis, gene cloning, and functional characterization. RsUGT75L20, RsUGT75T4, AkUGT75L21, and AkUGT75W2 catalyze the glycosylation on the C-19 hydroxyl group of *ent*-kaurenoic acid, steviol, and steviolmonoside to generate β-D-glucosyl *ent*-kauren-19-oate, steviol 19-*O*-β-D-glucopyranoside, and rubusoside, respectively. Furthermore, RsUGT85A57 and AkUGT85A58 serve as 13-*O*-glycosyltransferases converting steviol 19-*O*-β-D-glucopyranoside to rubusoside. AkUGT85A58 also exhibits substrate flexibility, and can use both steviol and steviol 19-*O*-β-D-glucopyranoside as substrates, similar to SrUGT85C2 (Figure 6). Research on steviol glycoside biosynthesis provides important insights into the potential molecular basis of specific glycosylations in the biosynthesis of diterpenoid glycosides, therefore providing a conceptual framework for the high yield production of important diterpenoid molecules using diterpenoid UGTs.

Oridonin is known for its potent anticancer activity, and has also been shown to serve as a covalent NLRP3 inhibitor with strong anti-inflammasome activity. Jin et al. identified five genes encoding CPS and six genes encoding KSL enzymes by transcriptomic profiling of *Isodon rubescens*. Functional characterization revealed that IrCPS4 and IrCPS5 can convert GGPP to *ent*-CPP. IrKSL5 converted *ent*-CPP to *ent*-kaurene (Figure 3). *Ent*-kaurene is likely to be the carbon skeleton of oridonin and can be modified by P450s. The biosynthetic pathway of this active compound is still ongoing.

3.4 Taxane diterpenoids Taxane diterpenoids represent a special type including more than 650 compounds that are mainly found in *Taxus* and *Austrotaxus*. Paclitaxel, a complex tetracyclic diterpenoid compound produced by *T. brevifolia*, is one of the most important plant natural products in clinical practice, although the full pathway of paclitaxel biosynthesis is still unclear. It has been speculated that conversion of the precursor GGPP to paclitaxel requires 19 enzymatic steps, including eight oxidation steps, five acetyl/aroyl transferase steps, a C4β, C20-epoxidation reaction, a phenylalanine aminomutase step, *N*-benzoylation, and two CoA esterifications.

GGPP is cyclized to taxa-4(5),11(12)-diene (also called taxadiene) by TbTS, forming the tricyclic diterpenoid skeleton

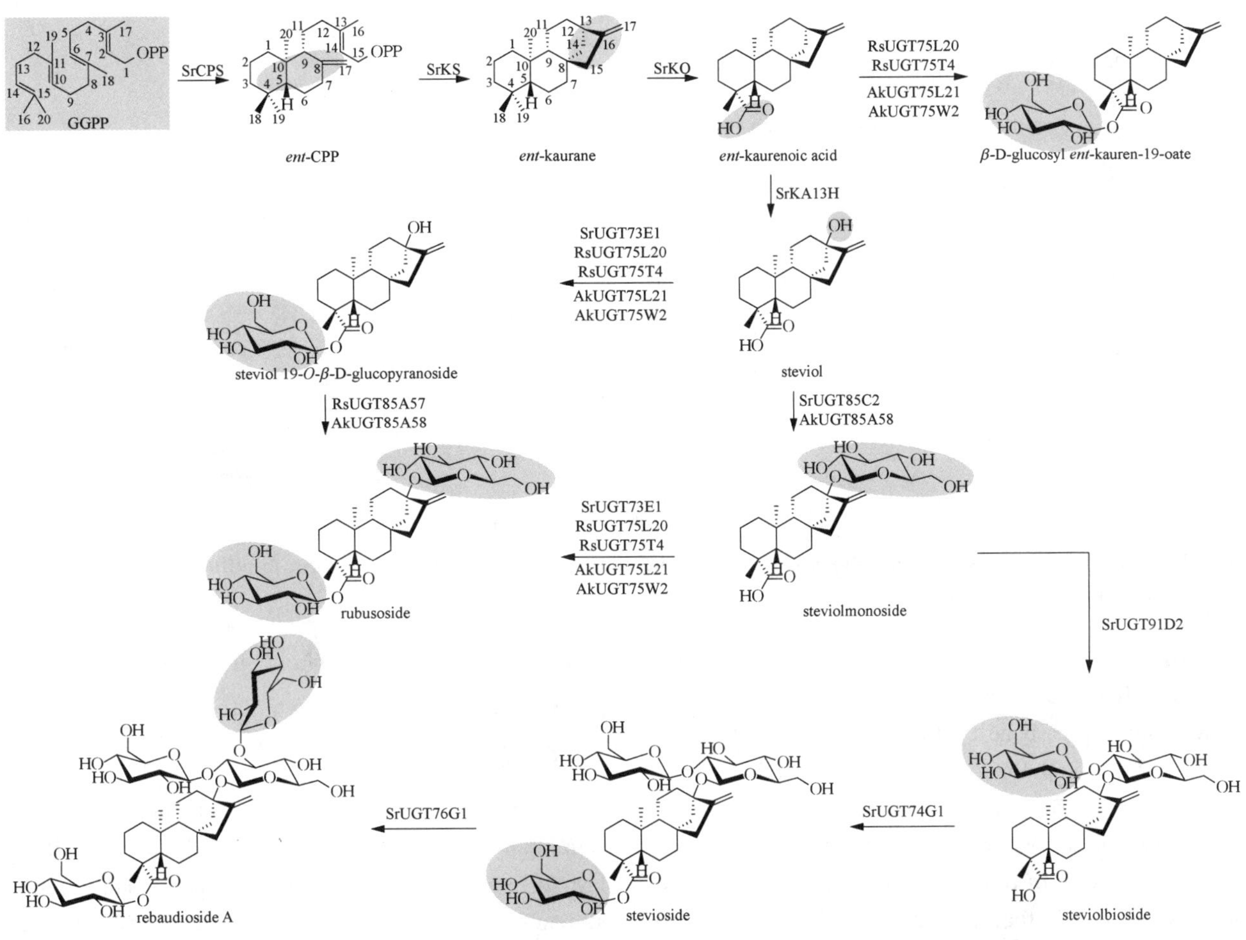


**Figure 6 Biosynthetic pathway of tetracyclic diterpenoids (Color figure can be viewed at wileyonlinelibrary. com)**

of paclitaxel, a reaction which is considered to be the rate-limiting step in paclitaxel synthesis. Baccatin Ⅲ is produced following hydroxylation at C1, C2, C5, C7, C9, C10, and C13; the establishment of the cyclic epoxypropane by linking C4 and C5; acylation at C2, C5, and C10; and ketone formation at C9. Taxadiene is converted by a P450 hydroxylase, CYP725A4 (taxadiene-5α-hydroxylase; T5αOH), into taxa- 4(20),11(12)-dien-5α-ol via hydroxylation at C5 and migration of the carbon double bond. The next reaction, which converts 5α-hydroxytaxane to 2-debenzoyltaxane, remains unclear, but likely entails either a hydroxylation at the 13α position or an acylation at the 5α position of the taxane skeleton of taxa-4(20),11(12)- dien-5α-ol. In the latter case, the intermediate is acetylated by taxadiene-5α-ol-*O*-acetyltransferase (TAT) on the 5α hydroxy group to form taxa-4(20),11(12)-dien-5α-yl acetate, which is then further hydroxylated by a P450 enzyme of the CYP725A1 family, taxane 10β-hydroxylase (T10βOH), to form 5α-acetoxytaxadien-10β-diol. In the former case, the intermediate undergoes hydroxylation at C13 catalyzed by taxane 13α-hydroxylase (T13αH) to generate taxa-4(20), 11(12)-dien-5α, 13α-diol (Figure 7). However, the order of the reactions is not clear for hydroxylation at other sites C1, C2, C4, C7, and C9, the formation of the 4,5-epoxypropane ring, or the acylation of the C2, C5, and C10 hydroxyl groups, and the ketonization at the C9 position. This ambiguity analyzes the biosynthetic pathway for these important compounds challenging. In addition to the formation of diterpenoid taxane core, post-modification of paclitaxel includes the formation of 2-debenzoyltaxan, baccatin Ⅲ, and its C13 side chain, among other steps. Biosynthesis has been comprehensively reviewed by Croteau et al.

3.5 Macrocyclic diterpenoids Macrocyclic diterpenoids are a class of diterpenoids that contain at least a seven-membered or larger carbocyclic ring in their structure. They have been mainly reported in Euphorbiaceae and are usually highly oxygenated and functionalized. Ingenes, lathyranes, jatrophanes, tiglianes, and daphnanes, all diterpenoids from *Euphorbia*, have been the focus of considerable research attention because of their diverse scaffolds and extensive biological activity.

Euphorbia factors and macrocyclic diterpenoids from the seed oil of *E. lathyris*, are the industrial source of macrocyclic diterpenoids such as ingenol mebutate. Casbene, is thought to be the first committed intermediate in the synthesis of the more complex macrocyclic diterpenoids

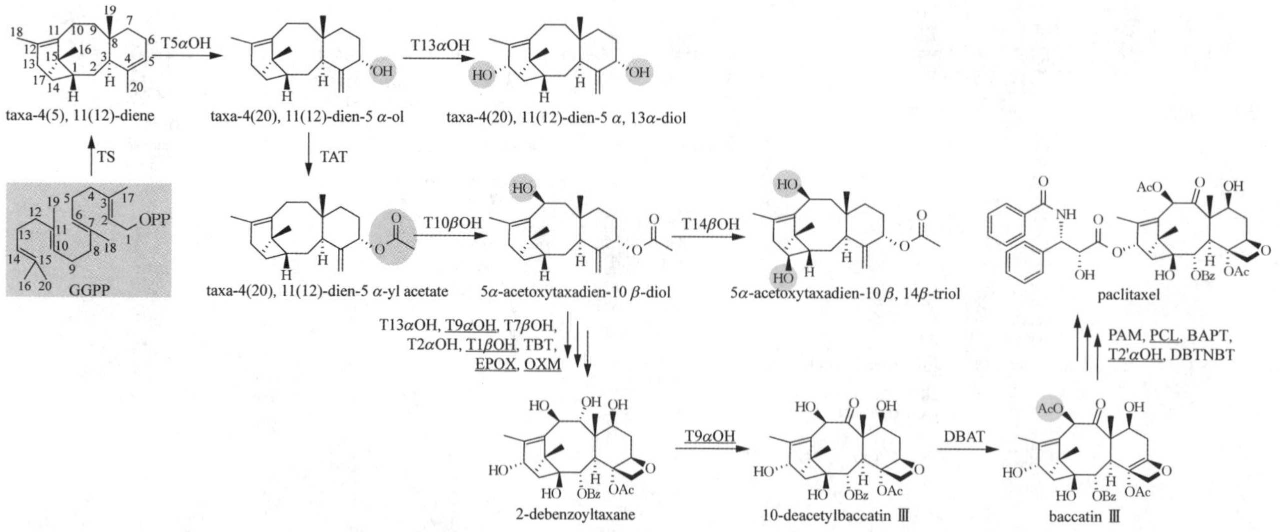

Figure 7 Biosynthetic pathway of taxane diterpenoids. Underline indicates that enzymes have not been identified (Color figure can be viewed at wileyonlinelibrary. com)

found in the *Euphorbia* species. Casbene synthase (CBS) was first identified in *R. communis*. Kirby et al. identified five genes encoding casbene synthases (EeTPS2, HnTPS4, ErTPS6, SsTPS10, and RcCAS3) from five Euphorbiaceae species, *E. esula*, *Hyptis nutans*, *E. resinifera*, *S. sebiferum*, and *R. communis*, respectively. Based on a previous report, as well as lack of other casbene synthase candidates, the authors postulated that casbene was the precursor of ingenols in Euphorbiaceae. Furthermore, a physical cluster of biosynthetic genes from *R. communis* was reported. This gene cluster included genes encoding casbene synthase, neocembrene synthase, P450s from the CYP726A subfamily, and short-chain alcohol dehydrogenases (ADH) that participate in the biosynthesis of macrocyclic diterpenoids. CYP726A14, CYP726A17, and CYP726A18 were shown to catalyze 5-oxidation of casbene to produce 5-keto-casbene, while CYP726A16 used 5-keto-casbene as substrate to catalyze 7,8-epoxidation to form 5-keto-7,8-epoxy-casbene. Neocembrene synthase (RcCAS2) used GGPP as substrate to produce neocembrene, which was further catalyzed by CYP726A15 to produce 5-keto-neocembrene. Transcriptomic analysis of the mature seeds of *E. lathyris* and functional characterization *in planta* by Luo et al. further identified two P450s and an alcohol dehydrogenase (ElADH1) involved in the conversion of casbene to jolkinol C (a probable intermediate in the biosynthesis of ingenol mebutate). In addition, CYP71D445 and CYP726A27 could catalyze 9-oxidation and 5-hydroxylation of casbene, respectively. Coexpression of *ElADH1* with *ElCBS*, *CYP71D445*, and *CYP726A27* in *Nicotiana benthamiana* resulted in subsequent rearrangement and cyclization yielding jolkinol C. Homologs were also identified from *E. peplus* (EpCBS, CYP71D365, CYP726A4, and EpADH1) by comparative transcriptomics of *E. lathyris* with *E. peplus* (Figure 8).

## 4 HETEROLOGOUS PRODUCTION OF DITERPENOIDS

Over the last 50 years, genetic engineering has enabled significant progress in many areas of biology, while in the last 20 years, it has provided several tools needed for systems-based approaches to heterologous production of plant terpenoids. Progress has been made in the design and construction of synthetic biology systems in yeast and *E. coli* that serve as chassis for the production of these compounds. Metabolic engineering in microorganisms can provide a cost-effective alternative for the production of medicinal terpenoids such as artemisinin. Advances in synthetic biology-based production of plant-derived natural products are summarized in detail elsewhere. Using synthetic biology for the production of diterpenoids has lagged behind that of sesquiterpenoids and triterpenoids. Limited expression and catalytic efficiency of functional P450s in microorganisms may be the limiting factors. Below, we discuss recent progress in synthetic biology-based approaches for the synthesis of plant diterpenes as well as some of the remaining obstacles to progress.

4.1 Heterologous production in *E. coli* *E. coli* has been used for the production of diterpenoid carbon skeletons. *E. coli* has a short generation time, suitable for high expression of enzymes, and abundant metabolite production. However, its use has been limited to several active compounds including steviol glycosides, the precursors of paclitaxel, ginkgolides, and sclareol. Ajikumar et al. partitioned the taxadiene metabolic pathway into two biosynthetic modules: the isopentenyl diphosphate (IPP) production module and the skeleton formation module. Systematic multivariate

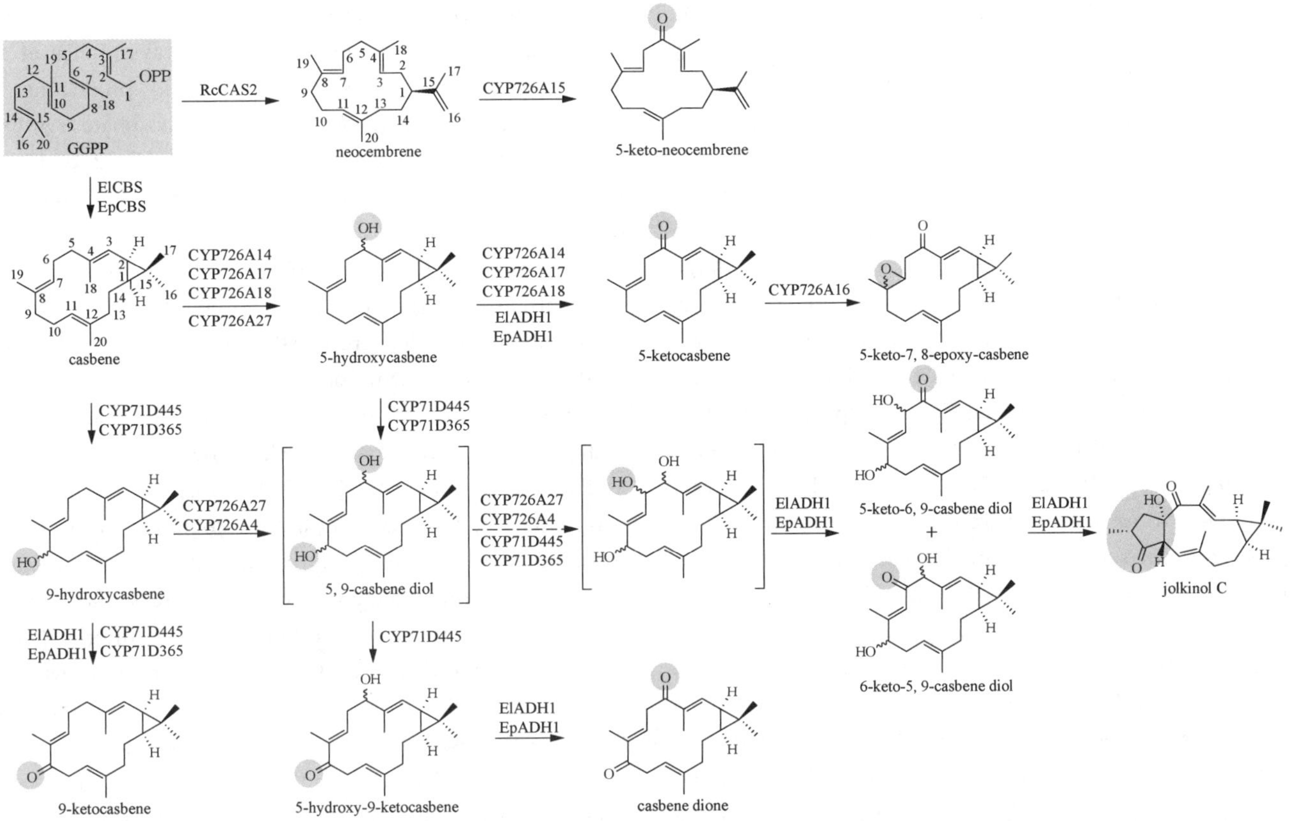

**Figure 8 Biosynthetic pathway of macrocyclic diterpenoids (Color figure can be viewed at wileyonlinelibrary. com)**

analysis was used to determine a balance between the two modules that could maximize the production of taxadiene. This isoprenoid pathway optimization strategy resulted in the metabolic engineering of *E. coli* with a yield of $1.02 \pm 0.08$ g/L taxadiene in fed-batch fermentations. Leonard et al. combined metabolic and protein engineering of the terpenoid biosynthetic pathway for the large-scale production of levopimaradiene, the diterpenoid gateway precursor of ginkgolides. Specifically, this report highlighted the use of protein engineering in reprogramming the rate-limiting nodes for high-level production of commercially important compounds using synthetic biology. Ambergris is a highly prized fragrance ingredient from the intestinal tract of sperm whales. Sclareol can be used as a substrate for the semi-synthesis of the key olfactory components and suitable substitutes for ambergris. Schalk et al. identified the key enzyme responsible for the biosynthesis of sclareol and genetically engineered its production in *E. coli*, resulting in a metabolically engineered strain that produced 1.5 g/L sclareol, which provides a cost-effective route.

The use of *E. coli* for large-scale production of plant diterpenoids in microorganisms was significantly reduced when P450 activity was needed, such as exemplified by paclitaxel and steviol glycosides production. The in-troduction of a plasmid bearing a P450 - CPR fusion disturbed the balance of metabolic flow, resulting in the accumulation of equal amounts of by-product and taxadien-5α-ol (i.e., yields of only $58 \pm 3$ mg/L). Wang et al. constructed a novel pathway including P450s and UGTs for steviol glycosides in *E. coli*. This resulted in generating a strain for production of steviol glycosides with yield of 10.03 mg/L. Low accumulation of decorated diterpenoids in *E. coli* was due mainly to the lack of endoplasmic reticulum, the absence of electron transfer machinery, or the absence of P450 reductase needed for P450 activity in *E. coli*. However, the synthetic biology-engineered production of diterpenoids by microorganisms is always challenged by the multiple steps requiring P450-mediated oxidation and other modifications necessary for the biosynthesis of complex diterpenoids. For example, there are at least eight P450s involved in the biosynthesis of paclitaxel, and at least four P450s are involved in the biosynthesis of tanshinones. In this case, yeast, with its internal membrane system and native mevalonate pathway, has assumed an essential role in the production of diterpenoids.

4.2 Heterologous production in yeast Yeast has also been engineered for the production of plant diterpenoids by metabolic engineering and synthetic biology. Various strategies were employed to improve the diterpenoid yields in yeast. The increased production of diterpenoids in yeast typically relies on overexpression of pathway genes/gene-fusions and accompanying regulatory factors, or knockdown/out of genes that function in competing pathways. Increasing precursor accumulation can be achieved by overexpression of the upstream genes or their fusions (such as the truncated *HMGR*, *DXS*, *IDI*, *ERG8*, *ERG12*, *ERG10*, *ERG19*, and *UPC2.1*, the mutated global regulatory factor in yeast). Overexpression of the *tHMGR-upc2.1* cassette can result in a 33% increase in miltiradiene production in yeast, as well as the accumulation of large amounts of squalene. Coexpression of *HMG1* and the *ERG20*-*BTS1* fusion in yeast produced 138.8 mg/L (*E*, *E*, *E*)-Geranylgeraniol (GGOH) under optimal conditions. Yeast produces IPP and dimethylallyl diphosphate (DMAPP) to synthesize the sterols needed to form the cell membrane, so the majority of IPP and DMAPP flows from FPP (farnesyl diphosphate) to squalene. Therefore, knock-down of *ERG9* expression in the squalene production pathway is a means of improving metabolic flux to GGPP. In addition, heterologous deletion of some genes in the terpenoid production chassis, such as malonyl-CoA: ACP transferase (*mct1*/*MCT1*), the cytoplasmic scaffold protein required for proper activation of the general stress response (*whi2*/*WHI2*), and NADP(+)-dependent glutamate dehydrogenase 1 (*gdh1*/*GDH1*), in the terpenoid production chassis, has resulted in a 9.5-fold increase in production of the forskolin precursor 11-β-hydroxy-manoyl oxide in yeast.

Modular pathway reconstruction has also been frequently used to improve the production of diterpenoids in yeast. applied modular pathway engineering (MOPE) for rapid assembly of a synthetic miltiradiene pathway, which resulted in a remarkable improvement of miltiradiene biosynthesis in yeast. The miltiradiene pathway was divided into three modules: the *SmKSL*-*SmCPS* module, the *BTS1*-*ERG20* module, and the *tHMG1* module, which resulted in miltiradiene yields of 365 mg/L in yeast. further employed comprehensive engineering strategies to improve miltiradiene production in yeast. These strategies include: ① overexpression of the pathway genes. ② downregulation of the metabolic flux for competing pathways. ③ manipulation of the transcriptional regulators (*Rox1*) of the MVA pathway. ④ screening of the highest efficiency diTPS. ⑤ construction of fusion proteins and further structural optimization. This resulted in miltiradiene yields of 3.5 g/L in a 5 L bioreactor, which is the highest titer reported for heterologous production. constructed 51 functional combinations of Class Ⅰ and Class Ⅱ diTPS enzymes in yeast by mimicking the modularity of diterpene biosynthesis in plants, resulting in the synthesis of more than 50 carbon skeletons. This chassis was able to yield 250–370 mg/L of several important diterpene skeletons, including the precursor of forskolin (13*R*-manoyl oxide) at 368±1 mg/L. This chassis strain was further used for the production of forskolin.

Protein engineering could be used to improve the efficiency of enzymes involved in biosynthetic pathways. Ignea et al. established a yeast strain for diterpenoid production by engineering the endogenous farnesyl diphosphate synthase Erg20p to produce GGPP. The fusion of the Erg20p (F96C) with terpene synthase significantly enhanced the production of several diterpenoids, and the chassis could also be used for the elucidation of other biosynthetic pathways. The problems associated with synthetic biology approaches to diterpenoid production are mostly linked to the engineering of P450s. Improvements of activity or stability have been achieved through directed evolution and site-directed mutagenesis to engineer some well-characterized P450s, such as P450BM3. Similarly, CYP76AH15 from *C. forskohlii* was mutated in the SRS1 (substrate recognition site 1) region to improve the efficiency of forskolin production in yeast. The best performing mutant resulted in increased amounts of 11-oxo-manoyl oxide and other pathway intermediates, though the yield of the end-product forskolin was low. The biosynthesis of diterpenoids always involves more than two P450 enzymes, which limits the rate of production. Structural analysis of CYP76AH1 and CYP76AH3 by molecular docking revealed that the amino acids at positions 301 and 479 play essential roles in catalytic efficiency. Mutation of Asp301 and Val479 in CYP76AH1 to glutamic acid (Glu) and phenylalanine (Phe), respectively, as these residues are found in CYP76AH3, resulted in a functionally integrated mutant that could perform the activities of both P450 enzymes. Wong et al. employed a protein tagging strategy to optimize the soluble expression of a target gene and combinatorial P450 screening to improve the production of the precursor of ingenol-3-angelate. The final resultant strain produced ~800 mg/L of jolkinol C. These achievements provide valuable references for synthetic biology approaches to P450 protein engineering for the production of diterpenoids.

Other strategies include altering the subcellular morphology (i.e., endoplasmic reticulum engineering) and enhancing the capacity for product accumulation through host engineering (i.e., engineering synthetic hydrophobic droplets, liquid engineering, and harnessing peroxisomes). More comprehensive engineering strategies should be employed to achieve high-efficiency production of active diterpenoids in yeast, considering the difficulties currently associated with industrial diterpenoid biosynthesis.

4.3 Production of diterpenoids by metabolic engineering or synthetic biology in plants  In addition to *E. coli* and yeast, plants have also been employed for diterpenoid production since they contain plant-specific subcellular compartments and the relevant protein-processing steps. Medicinal plants could be used as homologous chassis for improving the accumulation of target products by metabolic engineering.

Kai et al. co-expressed *SmHMGR* and *SmGGPPS* in transgenic hairy roots of *S. miltiorrhiza* and achieved 4.74-fold higher accumulation of tanshinones in the hairy roots. This approach has also been successfully demonstrated in the production of artemisinin. However, this strategy depends on the susceptibility of medicinal plants to *Agrobacterium*-mediated transformation, although this obstacle may be less of a concern given that susceptibility to *Agrobacterium rhizogenes* is relatively broad, and genetically transformed hairy roots can be easily identified, selected, and cultured.

Transient expression of the genes encoding plant pathway enzymes in model plants like *N. benthamiana* is an alternative for the production of diterpenoids in plant chassis. This approach has been used for synthesizing the precursor of paclitaxel. The researchers used a chloroplast-compartmentalized metabolic engineering strategy that was combined with improved production of terpenoid precursors to produce taxadiene and taxadiene-5α-ol in *N. benthamiana* at 56.6 and 1.3 μg/g, respectively. The use of *N. benthamiana* compared with single-cell organisms for the heterologous production of highly valued diterpenoids by synthetic biology is currently limited due to constraints that warrant further study in the next few years.

## 5 CONCLUSION AND PERSPECTIVES

Plants offer abundant chemical diversity for the development of new drugs. A good example is the discovery of artemisinin by Tu Youyou as a treatment for malaria. Plants can also serve as genetic resources for the production of these compounds by metabolic engineering and synthetic biology. Diterpenoids have a variety of pharmacological activities and many applications in clinical research and drug development. However, the direct extraction of diterpenoids from plants is usually insufficient to meet healthcare needs. The heterologous production of diterpenoids from different hosts offers highly effective alternatives. The yield of target products can be increased by effective design, regulation, and optimization of the microbial synthesis processes at the enzyme, metabolic pathway, and genomic levels. Future progress depends on elucidating and simulating the biosynthetic pathways of diterpenoids and artificially designing and constructing new biological systems with specific physiological functions. The combination of new synthetic technologies and metabolic engineering thus offers considerable potential for the production of diterpenoids.

Many of the crucial details about the complex metabolic pathways that produce diterpenoids in plants have not been established. Therefore, the focus in the next few years will be to mine the principal components of the biosynthetic pathways and reveal the overall pathways in detail. Comparative omics analysis, phylogenetic analysis, and other methods, such as computational tools that can be used to narrow down the candidates from gene families suitable for functional characterization. Heterologous expression systems, which include those of *E. coli*, yeast, and tobacco provide diverse platforms for functional analysis in vitro. However, the key to advancing our understanding of the biosynthetic pathways that lead to diterpenoids will be a more efficient selection of molecular candidates and improved high-throughput approaches that achieve greater functional characterization of the molecules involved.

Many of the genes involved in the biosynthesis of plant natural products have been mined and functionally verified due to rapid advances in DNA and protein sequencing technologies, which has led to an abundance of genetic elements. Advances in our knowledge of biosynthetic pathways can therefore provide more of these elements to facilitate improvements to the industrial synthesis of diterpenoids. Such improvements may involve optimized production through synthetic biology or metabolic engineering. In addition, the catalytic promiscuity of the enzymes encoded by these biosynthetic pathway genes could also be exploited to expand the structural diversity of diterpenoids. In this context, combinatorial biology and synthetic biology could be used to produce new structural modification products.

Catalytic promiscuity can be exploited to produce new derivative products. However, it is a limiting factor in the application of synthetic biology for heterologous production. Enzyme promiscuity can lead to the production of by-products that decrease the yield of the target molecule. The directed evolution of enzymes, or rational design of enzymes combined with site-directed mutagenesis can effectively improve the catalytic efficiency of enzymes. However, this type of approach is based on an understanding of protein structure. A comprehensive understanding of the catalytic mechanisms can help researchers in their efforts to engineer molecules and pathways more effectively, such as the data obtained through X-ray crystallography and NMR structural resolution. However, these processes are technically difficult for some plant enzymes. For example, to date, only two P450 structures are available (CYP76AH1 and CYP74A2) in the Protein Data Bank (https://www.rcsb.org/). These and future structures provide a reference for the directed evolution of P450 enzymes in plants. In addition, sequential enzymes in biosynthetic pathways may be organized as metabolons. Examples include the metabolons involved in flavonoid biosynthesis and cyanogenic glucoside biosynthesis. In such cases, techniques like cryoelectron microscopy require fewer proteins for the structural characterization of the catalytic complex. These core structures provide a basis for structural elucidation of the metabolic complex as well as for the resolution of catalytic processes and mechanisms.

Future directions for research into the biosynthesis of diterpenoids will make use of different approaches. The search for new chassis that can produce these compounds will include analyses of biosynthetic pathways, heterologous production using synthetic biology, or metabolic engineering of single-cell microorganisms, as well as similar studies in more complex higher plants. Mining for genetic elements and assembly of synthetic pathways form the basis of metabolite production using synthetic biology. Pathway optimization and improvement of overall cell performance are crucial to improving the subsequent production processes. Accurate and dynamic regulation of the overall synthetic pathways can optimize the direction of metabolic flow. The production capacity of the chassis cells can be improved by endoplasmic reticulum engineering, cell membrane modifications, construction and utilization of subcellular organelles, mixed-culture fermentations of strains harboring complex metabolic pathways, and other novel approaches. In addition, the development of computational technologies such as AlphaFold, as well as improvements in computational speed through advances in quantum computing, should provide strategies that offer greater precision in the regulatory control of metabolic flow. New computational tools could also be used to design catalytic steps, mine or design similar enzymes with improved features, and develop novel metabolic engineering strategies. Advances of this type promise to open considerable new opportunities to produce plant natural products through a detailed understanding of the salient biosynthetic pathways and rapid developments in synthetic biology.

[胡志敏，郭娟，黄璐琦，等. Medicinal Research Reviews，2021，41：2971－2997.]

# Functional identification of the terpene synthase family involved in diterpenoid alkaloids biosynthesis in *Aconitum carmichaelii*

## 1 INTRODUCTION

*Aconitum carmichaelii* Debx. is a traditional herb belonging to Ranunculaceae. Its principal and lateral roots after processed, named “wu tou” and “fu zi” respectively, are its most commonly used components in traditional Chinese medicine (Fig. 1), and have been used for the treatment of pain, rheumatics, heart failure, colds, diarrhea, beriberi, and edema for 2000 years. Diterpenoid alkaloids (DAs) are believed to be the predominant bioactive compounds in *A. carmichaelii*, with over 100 isolated. $C_{19}$-diterpenoid alkaloids, which contain unusual 6,7,5,6 carbon skeletons, are both the dominant bioactive and toxic constituents in *A. carmichaelii*. The most toxic compounds are aconitine, mesaconitine, and hypaconitine, characterized by acetyl and benzoyl esters (Fig. 1C), while alcohol amine-DAs are the primary bioactive compounds and exhibit reduced toxicity. In addition to the $C_{19}$-type, several $C_{18}$-and $C_{20}$-DAs have also been found in *A. carmichaelii*, such as vilmorrianine D, songorine, napelline, atisine (Fig. 1C) and aconicarmissulfonine A: linked to significant analgesic activity.

DAs, whether $C_{18}$, $C_{19}$, or $C_{20}$, are all presumed to be derived from the kaurane and atisane diterpenoid families. That is, $C_{20}$ atisane and kaurane serve as biosynthetic precursors to $C_{18}$-and $C_{19}$-DAs, a mechanism proven by total synthesis. Thereby, the biosynthesis of DAs undergoes two principal phases. First, is the formation of the $C_{20}$ diterpene skeleton by terpene synthase (TPS): the universal precursor geranylgeranyl pyrophosphate (GGPP) is cyclized by class Ⅱ diterpene synthase (copalyl-diphosphate synthase, CPS) to produce *ent*-copalyl diphosphate (*ent*-CPP), then undergoes further cyclization or rearrangement by class Ⅰ diterpene synthase (kaurene synthase-like, KSL) to form *ent*-kaurene or *ent*-atiserene. Second, is the insertion of the nitrogen into the mature diterpene scaffolds to form $C_{20}$-DAs, *e. g.*, atisine and napelline (Fig. 1C), which then undergo further development leading to the terminus $C_{18}$- or $C_{19}$-DAs. Historically, the specific enzymes and biosynthetic pathways in the plant have garnered substantially less interest than the total synthesis of these compounds: from 1963 to 2018, 24 different DAs have identified *via* total synthesis. One of the few key mechanistic finding has been that L-serine may serve as the nitrogen source of atisine-type DAs.

Recently, several RNAsequencing (RNA-seq) approaches using the Illumina platform have analyzed the transcriptome of *A. carmichaelii* and *Aconitum heterophyllum*. Many candidate genes, such as terpenoid-related enzymes, monooxygenases, methyltransferases, and BAHD acyltransferases (named according to the first four identified enzymes of the family: BEAT, benzylalcohol *O*-acetyltransferase; AHCT, anthocyanin *O*-hydroxycinnamoyltransferase; HCBT, anthrani-

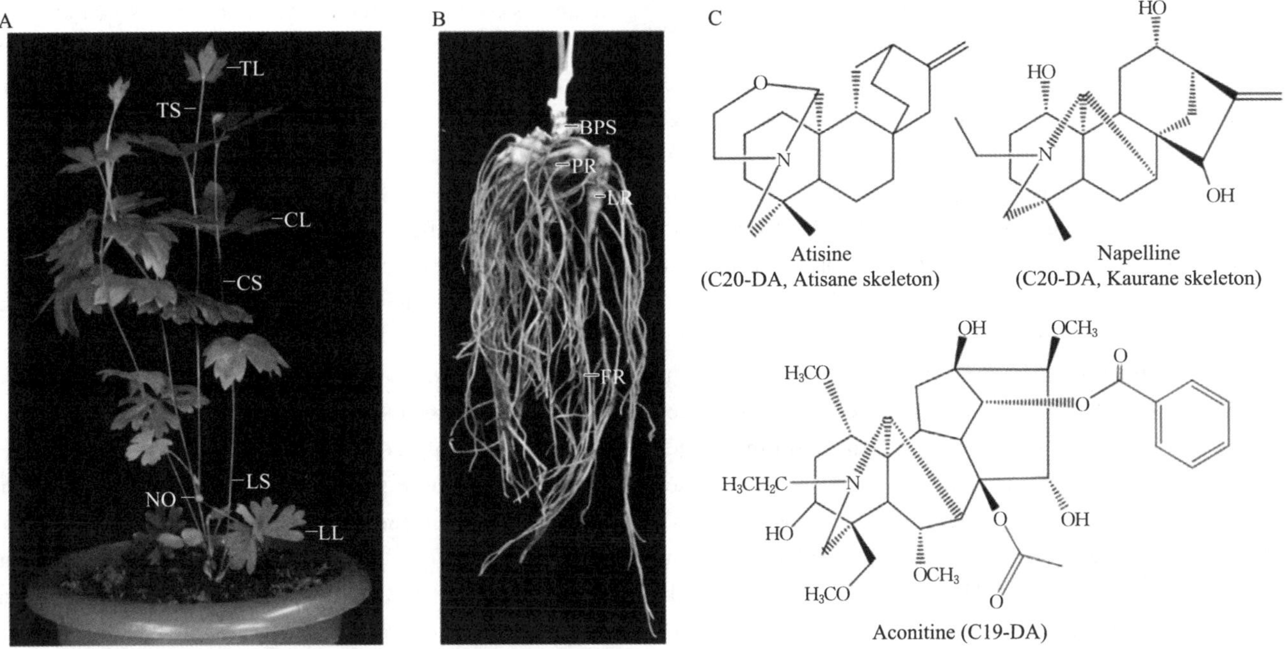


**Figure 1 The plant shows tissues used in this study for sequencing and the characteristic DAs in *A. carmichaelii***

The four-month-old plant (A) and roots (B) of *A. carmichaelii* in the greenhouse. (C) The characteristic skeleton of DAs in *A. carmichaelii*. PR, principal root; LR, lateral root; FR, fibrous root; BPS, basal part of the stem; TL, Top leaf; CL, central leaf; LF, lower leaf; TS, Top stem; CS, central stem; LS, lower stem, NO, nodular like organs.

late *N*-hydroxycinnamoyl/benzoyltransferase; DAT, deacetylvindoline 4-*O*-acetyltransferase) related to DAs biosynthesis have been identified. However, the limitations of short-read sequencing results in the vast majority of isotigs not representing full-length cDNA sequences, and none of these candidates have yet been functionally identified through *in vivo* or *in vitro* analysis.

In addition to being initiated by class Ⅱ diterpene synthase, diterpenes can also be initiated by class Ⅰ diterpene synthase, such as taxa-4(5), 11(12)-diene, casbene, and pseudolaratriene. Meanwhile, there are case reports that in addition to the TPS-c (*e.g.*, CPS) and TPS-e/f (*e.g.*, KSL) subfamily genes, the TPS-a and TPS-b subfamily genes have also been linked to diterpene biosynthesis. This suggests that $C_{19}$-DAs backbones could be synthesized by unexpected enzymes. Accordingly, identifying all the TPS family genes from the whole transcriptome is a critical step in understanding the therapeutic agents of *A. carmichaelii*.

Single-molecule real-time (SMRT) sequencing provides reads>10 kb and up to 60 kb (PacBio, Menlo Park, CA, USA 2016), enabling more complete and even full-length transcriptome data. Herein, we combined full-length isoform sequencing (Iso-seq) and RNA-seq technology to obtain a more reliable *A. carmichaelii* transcriptome. Combined with PCR cloning, we finally identified 19 TPS genes in *A. carmichaelii* and five alternative splicing isoforms. *In vivo* and *in vitro* assay identified 14 functional TPS genes, which establish biosynthetic routes to the diterpene scaffolds *ent*-atiserene, *ent*-kaurene, and *ent*-13-*epi*-sandaracopimaradie, clarifying the molecular basis for *A. carmichaelii* DAs biosynthesis.

## 2 MATERIALS AND METHODS

2.1 Plant material *A. carmichaelii* was acquired from Jiangyou, Sichuan Province, which is the genuine location for "wu tou" and "fu zi" material, in June 2018. The plant was grown in a greenhouse until February 2019. Then, 7 lateral roots from the same plant were divided and planted in separate flowerpots. These were then grown in a greenhouse at 25 (±2℃) under a 16 h-light/8 h-dark cycle provided by a white fluorescent lamp (3 000 lux). After 4 months growth, 3 plants with similar conditions were selected for the study. Different tissues were collected and immediately frozen in liquid nitrogen for further study.

2.2 RNA extraction Total RNA was extracted using an RNA isolation kit (HuaYueYang Biotechnology, Beijing, China) following the manufacturer's instruction. The integrity and concentration of total RNA was monitored using 1.0% agarose gel electrophoresis and NanoDrop ND-100 (NanoDrop Technologies, DE, USA). The electrophoretogram is shown in Supporting Information Fig. S1. The Agilent Bioanalyzer 2100 system (Agilent Technologies, CA, USA) was further used to assess the quality of extracted RNA.

2.3 Iso-seq and RNA-seq library construction and sequencing Due to the relatively high DAs content in the top leaves, principal roots, and lateral roots, to perform Iso-seq we mixed RNA from these three tissues together; concurrently, 13 tissues from three biological replicates were used for RNA-seq. The library construction for Iso-seq was described in Supporting Information Fig. S2. Briefly, mRNA was isolated from total RNA and converted into full-length cDNA using a SMARTer PCR cDNA Synthesis Kit (Clontech, CA, USA). Then, cDNA amplification was performed *via* an advantage 2 PCR kit (Clontech). After purification, size selection using a BluePippin Size selection system was performed (Sage Science, MA, USA) to enrich fragments longer than 4 kb. Then, an equal molar ratio mixed library of enriched fragments with those not processed by size selection was constructed using a SMRTbell Template Prep kit (Pacific Biosciences, CA, USA). The libraries' quality was assessed by Agilent Bioanalyzer 2 100 system (Agilent Technologies, CA, USA) and Qubit fuorometer 2.0 (Life Technologies, CA, USA) before sequencing. To prepare the libraries for sequencing, sequencing primer was annealed and polymerase was added to the primer annealed template. Subsequently, the polymerase-bound template was bonded to MagBeads and sequenced on a PacBio RS Ⅱ instrument (Novogene company, www.novogene.com).

RNA-seq was performed according to the standard protocol. Briefly, mRNA was converted into library templates using a Tru-Seq RNA Sample Prep Kit v2 (Illumina, San Diego, CA, USA). The cDNA libraries were then sequenced from each end of the cDNA fragments on a HiSeq 2 500 (Illumina).

2.4 Full-length transcript data processing and annotation The SMRT-Analysis software package SMRTlink v7.0 (Pacfic Biosciences) was used for Iso-seq data analysis. Briefly, low-quality reads (<50 bp) were first removed to obtain subreads. The subreads were then classified into circular consensus sequence (CCS) and non-CCS subreads using a ToFu pipeline (Pacific Biosciences). If the sequence contained a 3′ and 5′ primer or a poly (A) tail, the read was then used to obtain the full-length non-chimeric read (FLNC). Redundant FLNCs from same transcripts were discarded to form the consensus reads. The consensus reads were then polished with arrow software, and sequencing errors were further corrected using Illumina reads from the 13 different tissues *via* LoRDEC. Lastly, the redundant transcripts were removed *via* CD-HIT software. The resultant transcripts then underwent the standard annotation process using 7 databases: Nr, Nt, Pfam, KOG/COG, Swiss-prot, KEGG, and GO.

2.5 Cloning, sequence alignment, and phylogenetic analysis of TPS genes 1 μg of total RNA from 5 tissues were reverse transcribed into cDNA using the PrimerScript™ RT reagent kit with gDNA eraser (TaKaRa Corp., Dalian, China) according to the manufacturer's instructions. TPS genes were then amplified with specific primers (Supporting Information Table S1) and cloned into a pET32 plasmid (Merck) with a seamless cloning kit (TransGen Biotech, Beijing, China). TPS alignment was represented using CLC Sequence viewer 7 (Qiagen, Denmark) software. The previously identified 51 diTPSs (Supporting Information Table S2) together with TPS from *Arabidopsis thaliana* were used to construct the maximum likelihood phylogenetic tree using MEGA 6.0.

2.6 In vitro assays The functions of the AcTPSs were tested *via in vitro* assays as has been previously described. AcTPSs were analyzed alone or coupled with others, and an appropriate substrate supply. Briefly, recombinant plasmids were expressed in *Escherichia coli* Transetta (DE3). The crude proteins were then affinity-purified and individually assayed *via* GPP, FPP, GGPP, and CPP. CPP was obtained by incubating 200 μL of the purified ZmCPS2 enzymes with 20—50 μmol/L GGPP (Sigma) for 3 h at 30 ℃. AcCPS function was estimated using the GGPP substrate; AcKSL function was assessed *via* the GGPP and CPP substrates; the other TPSs were tested with all possible substrates, respectively. Nine known enzymes, ZmCPS2 (Genbank: NM_001111787), IrCPS4 (KU180502), SmCPS1 (KC814639), SmKSL1 (EF635966), IrKSL4 (KX580633), IrKLS5 (KX580634), EpTPS23 (KP889108), OsKSL10 (DQ823355) and MsTPS1 (MH626616) were used as controls. Different enzymes were mixed with equal volume, typically 300 μL each, in a 2 mL vial. After incubation for 2—4 h at 30℃, an equal volume of hexane was used to extract the terpene product. The hexane extracts were dried under a gentle stream of $N_2$, and the residue suspended in 100 μL hexane. 1 μL was later subjected to GC-MS analysis.

2.7 Metabolic engineering of diterpenes in E. coli A previously reported modular metabolic engineering system was used in our study. Briefly, the plasmid pIRS overexpressed IDI and DXR, which are key genes from endogenous isoprenoid precursor pathway. The plasmid pGG-ZmCPS2 contained a pseudomature GGPS from *Abies grandis* and ZmCPS2/An2 from maize, which have been designed to efficiently produce GGPP and CPP, respectively. These two plasmids, together with pET32-AcKSLs, were transfected into an *E. coli* C41 overexpression strain (Lucigen). The recombinant cultures were grown in 30 mL TB medium (pH 7.0), with appropriate antibiotics, in 100 mL flasks. These cultures were grown at 37 ℃ till $OD_{600}$ reached 0.7. The temperature was then dropped to 16 ℃ for 0.5 h prior to induction with 1 mmol/L isopropylthiogalactoside (IPTG), followed by supplementation with 40 mmol/L pyruvate and 1 mmol/L $MgCl_2$. The induced cultures were grown for additional 48～72 h, then 3 mL of the cultures were used for extraction with an equal volume of hexane. The extraction process was the same in the *in vitro* assays.

2.8 Terpene product analysis by GC - MS chromatography GC - MS analysis was carried on a Thermo TRACE 1 310 gas chromatograph with a TSQ8000 mass detector (Thermo Fisher Scientific) in electron ionization mode. A capillary column TR-5 ms (30 mm × 0.25 mm ID; DF = 0.25 μm; Thermo Fisher Scientific) was used with a 1.0 mL/min helium flow rate. The temperature program was as follows: initial column oven temp 50 ℃, maintained for 2 min followed by a linear ramp at 40 ℃/min to 210 ℃; linear ramp at 5 ℃/min to 250 ℃; linear ramp at 40 ℃/min to 300 ℃, with a 5 min hold at 300 ℃. The ion trap temperature was 280 ℃. The terpenes were identified by a comparison of retention time and mass spectra to previously characterized enzymatic products or authentic standards.

2.9 DiTPS gene expression analysis The expression of diTPS genes were obtained by two means: RNA-seq and qPCR analysis. For the RNA-seq, bowtie2 in RSEM software was used to map RNA-seq reads from the 13 tissues to the SMRT-based reference transcriptome. The read counts were then transformed to FPKM values to determine the gene expression levels of all identified genes. For qPCR analysis, 5 RNA extracts from the fibrous root, principal root, lateral root, leaf, and stem, respectively, were synthesized into cDNA by PrimerScript™ RT reagent kit with a gDNA eraser (TaKaRa Corp.). A SYBR Green kit (TaKaRa Corp.) for quantitative real-time polymerase chain reaction (qPCR) was applied to a ABI7500 real-time PCR detection system according to the manufactory's instructions. The primers sequences are listed in Table S1. Primer specificity was assessed by agarose gel and melting curve analysis. The results were normalized with the housekeeping gene *Actin*. Relative expression levels were calculated as the mean of three technical replicates of three biological replicates.

2.10 GenBank accessions The full-length transcriptome reported in this paper has been deposited in China National Center for Bioinformation under accession number CRA003781, which is publicly accessible for all researchers at http://bigd.big.ac.cn/gsa. GenBank accession numbers for the functional terpene synthases described in this paper are AcCPS1 (MW478118), AcCPS2 - 1 (MW478119), AcCPS2 - 2 (MW478120), AcCPS2 - 3 (MW478121), AcKSL2 - 1 (MW478123), AcKSL2 - 2 (MW478124), AcKSL3 - 1 (MW478125), AcKSL 3 - 2 (MW478126), AcTPS3 (MW478129) and AcTPS4 (MW478130). The sequences of different isoforms and *E. coli* codon optimized AcKSL1 were listed in Supporting Information isoform.seq.

## 3 RESULTS

3.1 Full-length transcriptome sequencing using Iso-seq and RNA-seq platforms Due to the relatively high DAs content in the top leaves, principal root, and lateral root, we mixed RNA from these together tissues for Iso-seq. Concurrently, 13 tissues from differing spatial locations (Fig. 1A and B) were sequenced on an Illumina HiSeq 2 000 platform to quantify gene/isoform expression levels and correct the Iso-seq reads. Utilizing 40.86 Gb sequenced data, we obtained 37,182,436 subreads (Supporting Information Table S3). The Iso-seq subreads' length distribution was shown in Supporting Information Fig. S3. From the subreads we extracted 983,658 circular consensus sequence (CCS) reads. Subsequent trimming, assembly, filtering, classification, and clustering revealed that 52.95% were full-length reads, indicated by the detection of poly (A) or 3′ and 5′ sequences (Supporting Information Table S4). These were then used in the construction of full-length non-chimeric sequences (FLNCs), which ranged from 72 to 12,220 bp, with a 2 023 bp average. The cDNA N50 values were determined to be 2 612 bp. Of 520,860 full-length cDNAs, 48,240 polished, high-quality, isoform consensus reads were filtered out using arrow software. After isoform-level clustering, next generation short sequencing (Illumina) was performed for error correction, with redundant sequences removed *via* CD-HIT software, and 21,087 unigenes were generated for *A. carmichaelii*: average length 1991 bp, N50 value 2 446 bp (Supporting Information Fig. S4). The N50 obtained in this study is 3-fold higher than previously reported (830 bp and 844 bp), providing a novel opportunity to identify all TPS genes involved in DAs biosynthesis.

3.2 Identification of A. carmichaelii terpene synthases To identify the *A. carmichaelii* TPS gene family, the above obtained unigenes were annotated using seven databases: Nr, Nt, Pfam, KOG/COG, Swiss-prot, KEGG, and GO (Supporting Information Fig. S5). We also mined the data using BLAST analysis against the enzymes like casbene and neocembrene synthases, which are responsible for macrocyclic or unusual skeleton formation. In addition, for genes with unpredictable lengths we used BLAST analysis against the reported transcriptome database.

A total of 19 TPS unigenes were identified, of which 14 represented full-length sequences (Supporting Information Table S5). The remaining 5 represented alternative splicing events. Transcript13827 (1 617 bp), transcript12676 (1 443 bp) and transcript12546 (567 bp) had a 515 bp overlap (Supporting Information Fig. S6). The integration of transcript13827 and transcript12676 forms a common full-length CPS gene (average 2 400 bp), annotated as *AcCPS1*. It was verified by polymerase chain reaction (PCR) amplification from the cDNA of fibrous root. At the same time, we obtained an isoform *AcCPS1a*, which had 98.70% sequence similarity with *AcCPS1* (Supporting Information

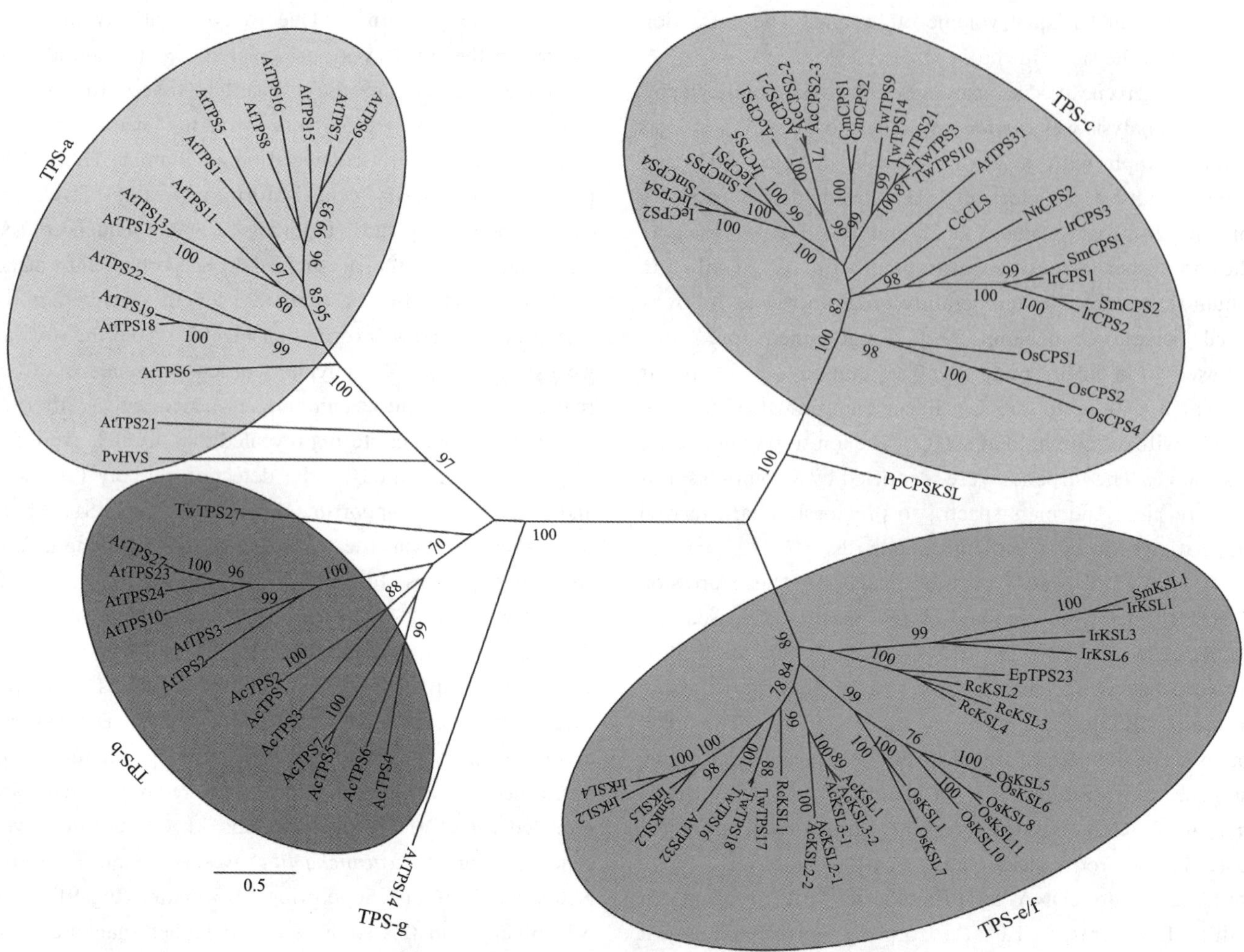


**Figure 2 Phylogeny of *A. carmichaelii* terpene synthases**

The maximum likelihood tree was reconstructed using MEGA6.0. Numbers on branches indicate the bootstrap percentage values calculated from 1000 bootstrap replicates. TPSs from representative characterized subfamily genes are shown in Table S6. *Physcomitrella patens* copalyl diphosphate synthase/kaurene (PpCPSKS) was used as outgroup.

Fig. S7). We further used specific primers to clone the three alternative splicing isoforms. We got the expected PCR product of transcript13827 and transcript12676, while didn't obtain any PCR product when using the specific primers of transcript12546. After sequenced the individual clones, we found nine of the transcript12676 clones were the same, which was nearly identical with *AcCPS1* except the 11 nucleotides at the beginning of "ATG". However, the condition was much more complexed for the clones from transcript13827. There were 37 nucleotide variations among the six clones and divided into three types. Four of them had the same sequence with *AcCPS1a*, clone-3-12 was identical with *AcCPS1* except two nucleotide variations. Clone-4-12 was more different from the others. Sixteen nucleotides belonged to *AcCPS1a*, 8 nucleotides belonged to *AcCPS1*, and the other 13 nucleotides were different from both of them (Fig. S7). But all the six clones didn't contain the 34 bp deletion compared with *AcCPS1*, thus made them didn't have the open reading frame except clone-4-12, which occasionally had a nucleotide deletion at the 3′-terminar stop codon (Fig. S7). Thus, we finally obtained two full-length *AcCPS1* isoforms, *AcCPS1* and *AcCPS1a*, together with two alternative splicing isoforms including transcript12676 and clone-4-12 from transcript13827.

Transcript11709 was 2 247 bp, which was a little shorter than the common KSL genes (average 2 400 bp). When blast against the reported transcriptome data we further got a full-length KSL gene with a 2 454 bp open reading frame, which was annotated as *AcKSL1*. Further *AcKSL1* and the transcript11709 were cloned from the cDNA of basal part of the stem. The process of cloning is not smooth for *AcKSL1* (more than five times and from different organs); however, the cloning of transcript11709 was much easier. After sequencing, we got four isoforms of transcript11709. Clone-1-15 was identical with *AcKSL1* besides the early termination. Clone-6-2 and clone-6-5 were extremely identical beside a three nucleotides insertion for clone-6-5 at the positon of 123 bp, and they had about 97% sequence similarity with clone-

1-15. Clone-1-8 is much more different from others, with about 94.7% sequence similarity with *AcKSL1*. At the same time, the stop codon of clone-1-8 mutated into "GGA", which resulted in the absence of a complete open reading frame (Supporting Information Fig. S8). Thus, we further got one full-length *AcKSL1* and three alternative splicing isoforms, clone-1-15, clone-6-2 and clone-6-5 of transcript11709. Transcript26960 was identical with the full-length transcript20586, annotated as *AcTPS7*, from 498 to 1 743 bp; we thus didn't design primers to clone the transcript26960.

At the process of cloning the other genes from cDNA, we further obtained two more isoforms of *AcCPS2-3*. They have more than 98.6% sequence similarity with *AcCPS2-3* (Supporting Information Fig. S9). In summary, we cloned all the genes from various tissues except transcript19787 (*AcTPS2*). It has 98.09% sequence identity with *AcTPS1*, and the main difference was in the 3′ terminal stop codon (Supporting Information Fig. S10). Finally, we obtained 19 TPS genes and five alternative splicing isoforms from a single *A. carmichaelii* plant (Supporting Information Table S6). We further blast these TPS genes against the previously reported transcriptome, it showed that nearly all genes except *AcTPS4* could found corresponding unigenes with similarity higher than 92% (Supporting Information Table S7). However, all these unigenes didn't represent the full-length cDNAs except TR36313 | c0 _ g1 _ i1, which corresponded to *AcTPS2*. Unigene TR48214|c4_g1_i1 had the highest similarity with *AcKSL3-1* (98%), while when using *AcKSL1* and *AcKSL3-2* as the query, the result also to be TR48214|c4_g1_i1 with similarity of 92%. These results demon-strated that the Pacbio full-length platform enabled an in-depth investigation of the TPS gene families in *A. carmichaelii*. In order to make the result clear, the following analysis mainly focused on 16 TPS genes which had identical sequence with the transcriptome data (Table S6), and generally didn't contain various isoforms cloned by PCR, unless otherwise specified.

3.3 Phylogenetic relationship of A. carmichaelii terpene synthases We further categorized the 16 TPS genes by signature sequence motif analysis and phylogenetic comparison with TPS families from *A. thaliana* and 51 previously identified related functional diTPS (Fig. 2). The presence of the catalytic DXDD motif in combination with a close phylogenetic relationship to known TPSs of the TPS-c clade, illustrated that 4 TPS genes were linked to class Ⅱ diTPS: AcCPS1 and AcCPS2-1 through AcCPS2-3 (Supporting Information Fig. S11). These 4 enzymes formed a single group, which differs from class Ⅱ diTPS in other species (*i.e.*, *Salvia miltiorrhiza* and *Isodon rubescens*) where class Ⅱ diTPS usually form two distinct groups. AcCPS1 shares ~64% identity with AcCPS2-1 through AcCPS2-3, and the 3 AcCPS2s share >87% sequence identity. Due to the high consistency of AcCPS2s, we speculate that they may come from duplication in a single chromosome or from a similar allele of different chromosomes, given that *A. carmichaelii* has been reported to be a polyploidy plant. The close relationship found between CmCPS1 and CmCPS2, and other CPSs in *S. miltiorrhiza* and *I. rubescens* that have been linked to *ent*-CPP production indicates that AcCPS1 and AcCPS2s are *ent*-CPP synthases.

The 12 remaining candidate genes were designated as class I TPS, according to the presence of the conserved DDXXD motif (Fig. S11). Of these TPSs, 5 were clustered with diTPSs from the TPS-e/f clade: AcKSL1, AcKSL2-1, AcKSL2-2, AcKSL3-1, and AcKSL3-2 (Fig. 2). Their 5 respective enzymes were also clustered together. AcKSL1 shares ~63% identity with AcKSL2-1 and AcKSL2-2, and ~85% identity with AcKSL3-1 and AcKSL3-2. AcKSL2-1 and AcKSL2-2 share 98% sequence identity, while AcKSL3-1 and AcKSL3-2 share 92% sequence identity, again suggesting they are allelic variants or from tandem duplicates. The other 7 TPSs, AcTPS1 to AcTPS7, were determined to be within the TPS-b subfamily. Most of the characterized TPSs in this subfamily are monoterpene synthases or isoprene synthases. AcTPS1 and AcTPS2 share 98% identity, AcTPS5 and AcTPS7 share 87%, and the others share a substantially lower sequence identity (~40%). This clade included TwTPS27, whose function is corollary to diTPS and can convert copalyl diphosphate to miltiradiene in *Tripterygium wilfordii*. These results indicate that all these TPS candidates have the potential to be involved in *A. carmichaelii* DAs biosynthesis.

3.4 Functional characterization of class Ⅱ terpene synthases from A. carmichaelii Based on the full-length transcriptome sequencing, we cloned all the *AcCPSs* from *A. carmichaelii*, including seven full-length *AcCPSs* and two alternative splicing isoforms of *AcCPS1* (Table S6). We then functionally characterized these *AcCPSs* through *in vitro* assays with recombinant proteins expressed *via E. coli* (Supporting Information Fig. S12). We first separately incubated the AcCPSs with GGPP to compare with the results from *ent*-CPP synthase ZmCPS2 of *Zea mays*. All enzymes except the two alternative splicing isoforms yielded a product with identical retention time and mass spectra to the product of ZmCPS2 after dephosphorylation (Fig. 3A and B), indicating that the primary product of these AcCPSs is CPP.

To further investigate the stereochemistry of the CPP products, these enzymes were coupled to stereospecific class I diterpene synthases, such as SmKSL1 (specific to normal-CPP) and IrKLS5 (specific to *ent*-CPP). Reactions where

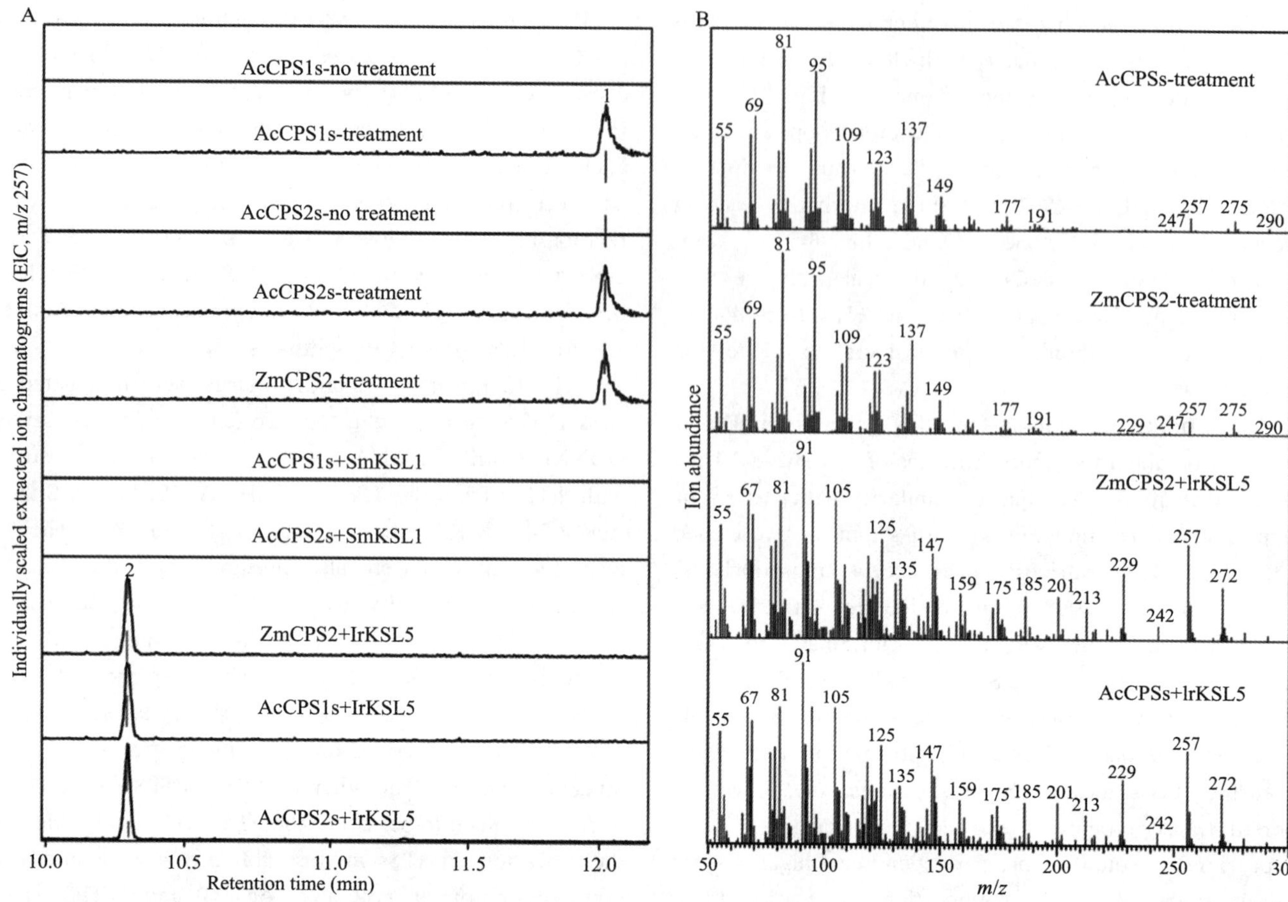


**Figure 3 GC-MS analysis of AcCPSs reaction products obtained from *in vitro* assays**

(A) Extracted ion chromatograms (EIC) of $m/z$ 257 with AcCPS1s and AcCPS2s alone or in combination with IrKSL5 (specific to *ent*-CPP) or SmKSL1 (specific to *normal*-CPP) with GGPP as the substrate. "Treatment" indicates the dephosphorylation of the product of CPS with Alkaline Phosphatase. (B) EI mass spectra of the dephosphorylated product of AcCPSs and ZmCPS2 and of the product of AcCPSs and ZmCPS2 combination with IrKSL5. (1) copalol. (2) *ent*-kaurene.

AcCPSs were coupled with IrKLS5 resulted in the formation of *ent*-kaurene, while no product was evolved when they were coupled with SmKSL1 (Fig. 3A). That all AcCPSs could produce *ent*-CPP indicates their involvement in *A. carmichaelii* DAs biosynthesis.

3.5 Functional characterization of class I terpene synthases from A. carmichaelii We cloned 14 class I TPS genes for functional identification except *AcTPS2*, which included 5 *KSLs*: *AcKSL1*, *AcKSL2-1*, *AcKSL2-2*, *AcKSL3-1* and *AcKSL3-2*, and 6 TPS-b subfamily genes: *AcTPS1*, *AcTPS3* through *AcTPS7*, together with three alternative splicing isoforms of *AcKSL1*. Having identified only the *ent*-CPP activity of the 7 AcCPSs, we first identified the products of the 5 class I diTPS AcKSLs and three alternative splicing isoforms of AcKSL1 in combination with *ent*-CPP synthase (AcCPS2-1). When GGPP was used as the substrate, AcKSL2-1 and AcKSL2-2 turned *ent*-CPP into *ent*-atiserene, a result identical to IrCPS4 in combination with IrKSL4 in *I. rubescens*; AcKSL3-1 produced *ent*-kaurene, identical to the product of IrCPS4 coupled with IrKLS5, and AcKSL3-2 coupled with AcCPS2-1 produced a product similar to *ent*-sandaracopimaradie (Fig. 4). We further synthesized two known *ent*-sandaracopimaradie synthases, EpTPS23 from *Euphorbia peplus* and OsKSL10 from *Oryza sativa*, along with sandaracopimaradie synthase (MsTPS1) from *Mentha Spicata* to verify the product stereochemistry of AcKSL3-2. When AcKSL3-2, EpTPS23, and OsKSL10 were respectively combined with AcCPS2-1, the product mass spectra of AcKSL3-2 revealed to be identical to the products of EpTPS23 and OsKSL10, though its retention time was ~0.8 min earlier (Fig. 4). While sandaracopimaradie, the product of MsTPS1 combined with normal-CPP synthase (SmCPS1 from *S. miltiorrhiza*), had exactly the same retention time and mass spectra with the product of EpTPS23/OsKSL10. These results confirmed that the product of MsTPS1 with normal-CPP and EpTPS23/OsKSL10 with *ent*-CPP were enantiomers, while the product of AcKSL3-2 was the C-13 epimer of the product of EpTPS23/OsKSL10, due to the fact that they all originated from *ent*-CPP. Thus, the product of AcKSL3-2 was assigned to be *ent*-13-*epi*-sandaracopimaradie.

Due to the poor protein expression of AcKSL1 and its

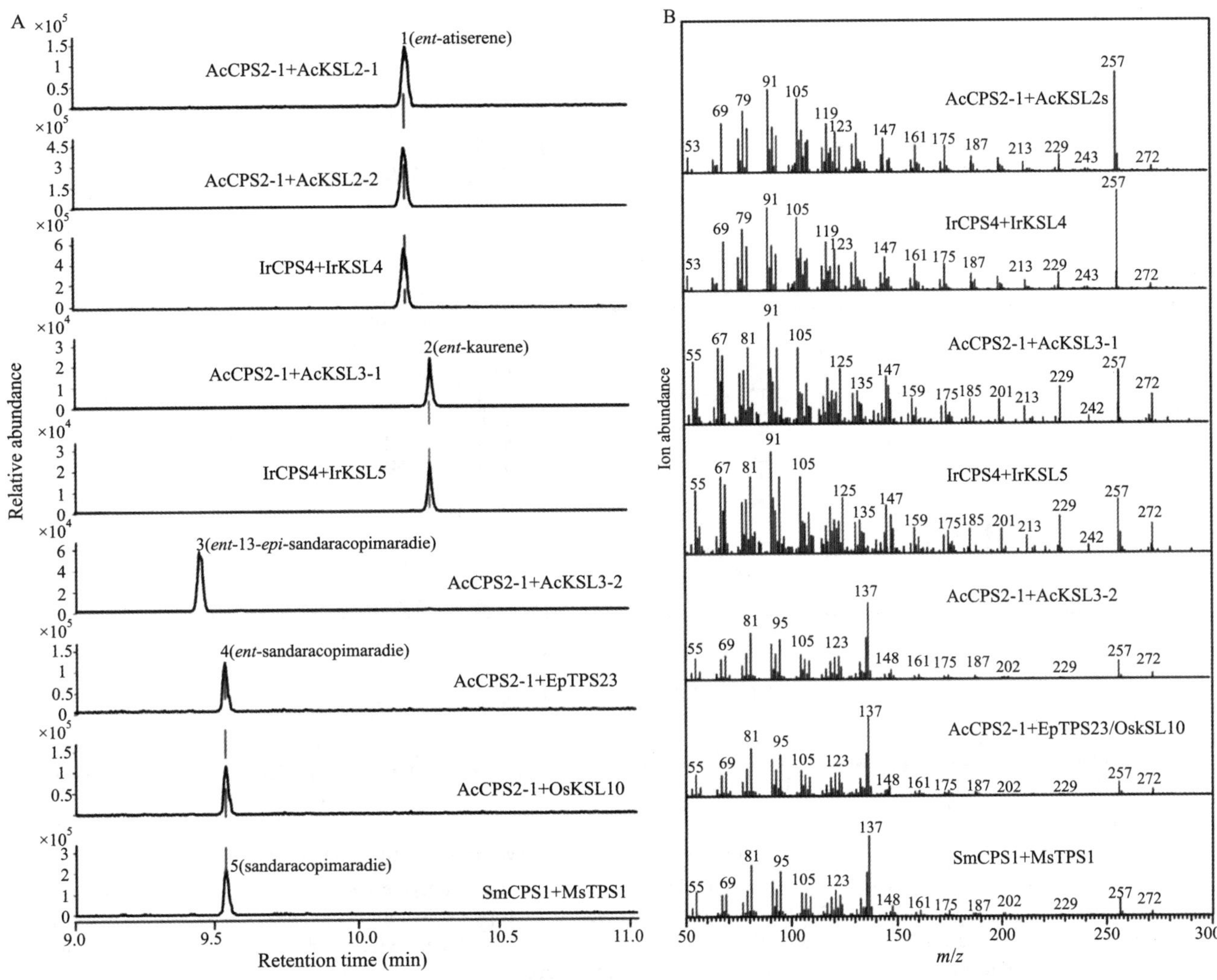


**Figure 4 GC-MS analysis of AcKSLs reaction products obtained from *in vitro* assays**

(A) EIC of $m/z$ 257 of AcCPS2-1 and SmCPS1 in combination with different KSLs. The enzymes SmCPS1, IrCPS4, IrKSL4, IrKSL5, EpTPS23, OsKSL10 and MsTPS1 were used as controls. (B) EI mass spectra of the product of AcCPS2-1, IrCPS4 and SmCPS1 in combination with different KSLs. (1) *ent*-atiserene. (2) *ent*-kaurene. (3) *ent*-13-*epi*-sandaracopimaradie. (4) *ent*-sandaracopimaradie. (5) sandaracopimaradie.

three alternative splicing isoforms in *E. coli*, we could not identify its function *in vitro*. Therefore, we used a highly efficient diterpene modular metabolic engineering system to further verify the function of all 8 of the KSLs. Three vectors, pIRS, pGG-ZmCPS2, and pET32-AcKSLs, were transfected into the C41 over-expressing strain of *E. coli*. After incubation for 72 h the product was analyzed by GC-MS. The results of AcKSL2s and AcKSL3-1 were analogous to the above *in vitro* assays. AcKSL3-2 produced two other products in addition to *ent*-13-*epi*-sandaracopimaradie: one was *ent*-kaurene at 10.30 min based on the same retention time and mass spectra with the product of AcKSL3-1. The other product at 10.75 min showed to be an unidentified diterpene. *Ent*-atiserene was produced by the *E. coli* codon optimized AcKSL1, which had identical retention time and mass spectra with the products of AcKSL2s (Fig. 5). No obvious products were produced by the none codon optimized AcKSL1 and its three alternative splicing isoforms.

To investigate whether class I TPS genes have the capacity to produce diterpenes from GGPP, we first incubated all the recombinant class I TPS with GGPP. No product was formulated in these experiments (Supporting Information Fig. S13). We next incubated the 6 TPS-b enzymes with GGPP and AcCPS2-1, but again no products were formed. We thus conclude that in *A. carmichaelii*, DAs are only produced by the combination of the TPS-c and TPSe/f subfamily genes. In order to identify the function of the TPS-b genes, we incubated them with FPP and GPP, respectively. Our results showed that two genes, AcTPS3 and AcTPS4, generated a product similar to farnesene with FPP, which was identified to be $\alpha$-farnesene with authentic standard $\beta$-farnesene and $\beta$-disabolene (Fig. S13), illustrating they are sesquiterpene synthases. The others showed no enzymatic activity *in vitro* assay though AcTPS1 and AcTPS6

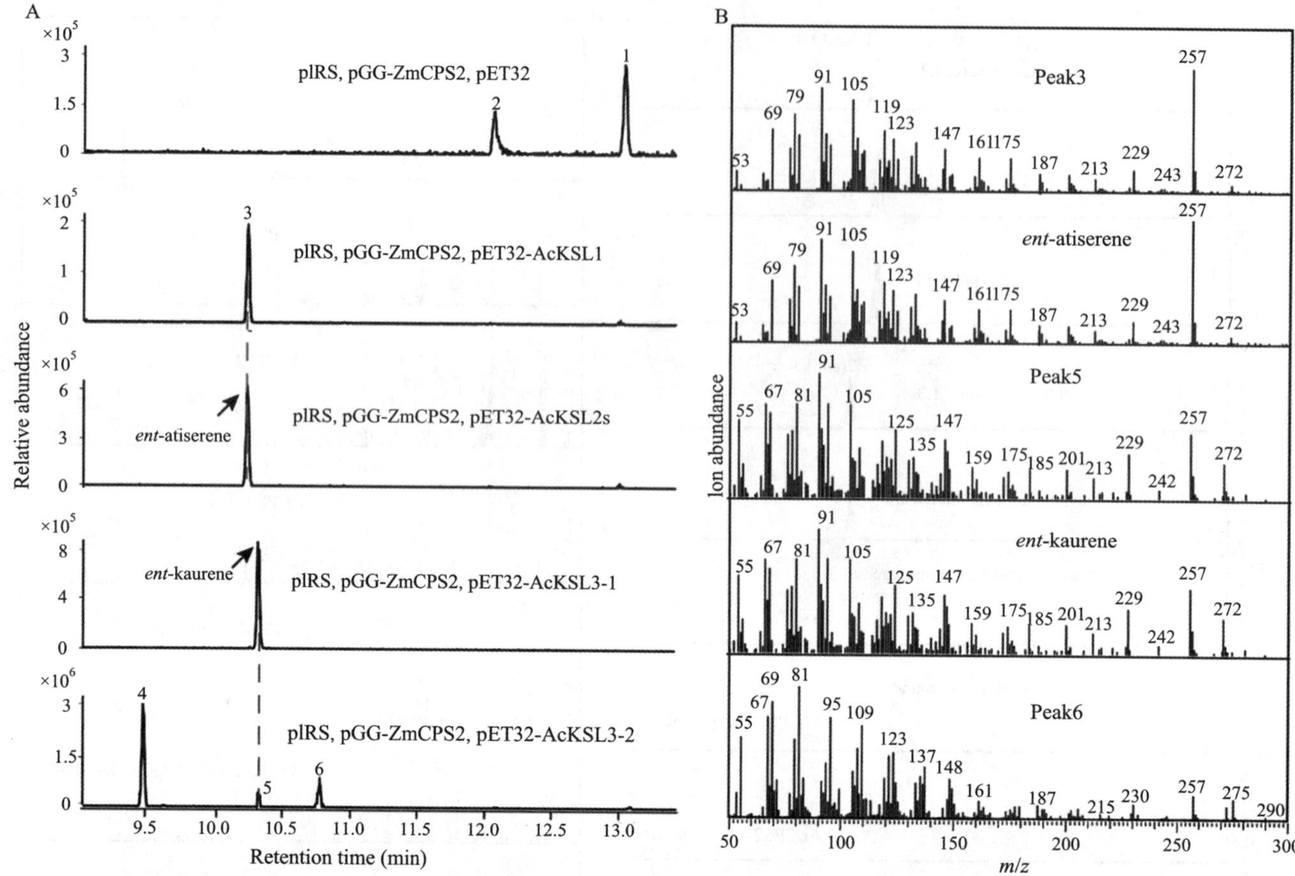


**Figure 5 GC - MS analysis of extracts from *E. coli* engineered for diterpene production**

(A) EIC of $m/z$ 257 with pIRS, pGG-ZmCPS2 in combination with AcKSLs. The empty vector pET32, together with pIRS and pGG-ZmCPS2 was used as the negative control, which produces the hydrolysis products geranylgeraniol and copalol. (B) EI mass spectra of the product of codon optimized AcKSL1 and the two other products of AcKSL3-2. (1) geranylgeraniol. (2) copalol. (3) *ent*-atiserene. (4) *ent*-13-*epi*-sandaracopimaradie. (5) *ent*-kaurene. (6) unidentified diterpene.

had high quality of recombinant proteins (Fig. S12).

3.6 Gene expression patterns of A. carmichaelii terpene synthases In order to investigate the potential physiological roles of the candidate *TPSs*, we performed RNA sequencing across 13 tissues based on spatial location. Six were underground tissues: principal root, fibrous root, cortex, phloem and xylem from lateral root, and the basal part of the stem; and seven were aerial tissues: the top, central, and lower parts of the leaf and stem respectively, and the nodular like organs in the stem (Fig. 1A and B).

Thirteen tissues were able to be differentiated into two groups according to their spatial locations, with the aerial tissues forming one group and the underground tissues the other, illustrating that the expression of TPS genes indeed has a spatial difference (Fig. 6A). The 16 TPS genes formed 3 groups: group Ⅰ included 3 *AcCPS2*s, *AcKSL1*, and *AcKSL3-2*, all of which had similar moderate expression levels in across all tissues; group Ⅱ included 4 TPS-b subfamily genes (*AcTPS1*, *AcTPS2*, *AcTPS3*, and *AcTPS6*) and *AcKSL3-1*, which had relatively high expression levels in the aerial leaf and stem; and group Ⅲ included *AcKSL2-1*, *AcKSL2-2*, *AcCPS1* and 3 TPS-b subfamily genes (*AcTPS4*, *AcTPS5*, and *AcTPS7*), with relatively high expression in the underground tissues, especially for *AcKSL2-1* and *AcKSL2-2*. Notably, *AcCPS1* had specifically high expression levels in the fibrous root samples.

In order evaluate the expression levels from RNA-seq, we further evaluated the mRNA transcription levels of 4 diTPSs in the principal root, lateral root, fibrous root, stem, and leaves by qPCR (Fig. 6B). The results were in agreement with the RNA-seq data: *AcCPS1* was specifically expressed in the fibrous root; *AcCPS2-1* had relatively high expression levels in all tissues; *AcKSL2-1* showed relatively high expression level in principal and lateral root, but lower expression level in stem and leaves; and *AcKSL1* had relative low expression levels in all the tissues.

## 4 DISCUSSION

Diterpenoid alkaloids (DAs) are the most well-known medicinal compounds of *Aconitum*. Most previous studies have focused on phytochemical composition and pharmaceutical usage of DAs, and significantly less research has gone into

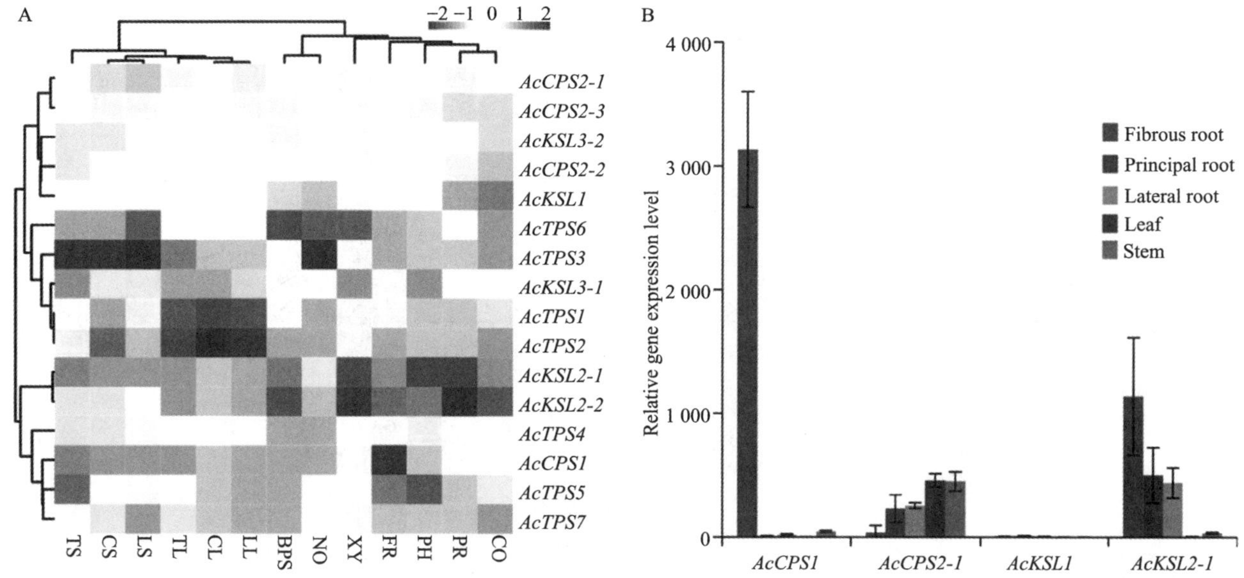


**Figure 6 The gene expression patterns of TPS in *A. carmichaelii***

(A) Heat map of 13 spatial tissues obtained by RNA-seq: PR, principal root; FR, fibrous root; CO, cortex; PH, phloem; CY, Xylem; BPS, basal part of the stem; TL, top leaf; CL, central leaf; LL, lower leaf; TS, top stem; CS, central stem; LS, lower stem, NO, nodular like organs. (B) qPCR analysis of 4 diTPSs in 5 tissues. The FKPM values in A and relative expression levels in B were obtained from 3 biological replicates.

the molecular biology of DAs formation in *Aconitum*. To better understand the molecular basis for the complex biosynthesis of DAs; herein, we applied Pacbio full-length transcriptome in conjunction with RNA-seq and PCR cloning to mine for the TPS family and their potential roles, searching specifically for enzymes involved in DAs metabolism. Using this combination approach, we identified 19 TPS genes and five alternative splicing isoforms in *A. carmichaelii*. The diTPS, excepting the alternative splicing isoforms, were functionally identified using *in vitro* and *in vivo* diterpene metabolic engineering system. Using *in vitro* assays—with GPP, FPP, and GGPP as substrates—we eliminated the potential involvement of the TPS-b subfamily in DAs biosynthesis, and established biosynthetic routes to the diterpene scaffolds *ent*-atiserene, *ent*-kaurene, and *ent*-13-*epi*-sandaracopimaradie (Fig. 7) based on 12 diTPS genes, clarifying the molecular basis for *A. carmichaelii* DAs biosynthesis.

The AcTPSs found in the TPS-c and TPS-e/f subfamilies cluster together, analogous to the diTPS found in *T. wilfordii*, indicating a recent evolutionary event may responsible to the emergence of different classes of diterpene scaffolds. All of the class II diTPS genes proved to be *ent*-CPP synthase, which is accord with the common view that *ent*-CPP is the only intermediate involved in *A. carmichaelii* DAs biosynthesis. Notably, AcCPS1 is specifically expressed in the fibrous root, as verified by RNA-seq and qPCR analysis, raising interesting questions about its function that necessitate further study. Due to their relatively high expression levels in underground tissues, AcKSL2-1 and AcKSL2-2 are presumed to be the key enzymes involved in DAs biosynthesis. If this is the case, the product of AcKSL2s, *ent*-atiserene, would be the only precursor for atisane-skeleton $C_{20}$-DAs, such as the atisine-, denudatine-, hetidine-, hetisine- or vakognavine-types, which is agreement with the previous hypothetical biosynthetic pathway based on chemical structure. Besides AcKSL2s, AcKSL1 also identified to be an *ent*-aitiserene synthase in *A. carmichaelii*. The relative low expression level of *AcKSL1* in different tissues (Fig. 6) and the close phylogenic relationship with *ent*-kaurene synthase (AcKSL3-1) (Fig. 2) illustrated AcKSL1 might be the ancestral enzyme for atisane-skeleton $C_{20}$-DAs biosynthesis, and AcKSL2s undergone a functional divergence from AcKSL1, which shed light on the evolutionary origin of $C_{20}$-DAs biosynthesis. The product of AcKSL3-1 was *ent*-kaurene, which would be the precursor for the biosynthesis of gibberellin and napelline-type $C_{20}$-DAs. The product of AcKSL3-2 was found to be *ent*-13-*epi*-sandaracopimaradiene, making it the first enzyme to be identified to synthesize this diterpene. Other *ent*-sandaracopimaradiene-like compound derivatives have been isolated from several species including rice, *Kaempferia galanga*, and *Guarea rhophalocarpa*; however, it has not reported previously in *Aconitum*. On the other hand, beside *ent*-13-*epi*-sandaracopimaradiene, it also produced *ent*-kaurene and another unknown diterpene in the engineered *E. coli*. Further study into the chemistry and metabolic fate of these diterpenes *in planta* will be needed to fully elucidate its role. Collectively, AcCPS1, AcCPS2s, AcKSL1, AcKSL2s, and AcKSL3-1 appear to be responsible for all the known $C_{20}$-DAs biosynthesis in *A. carmichaelii*.

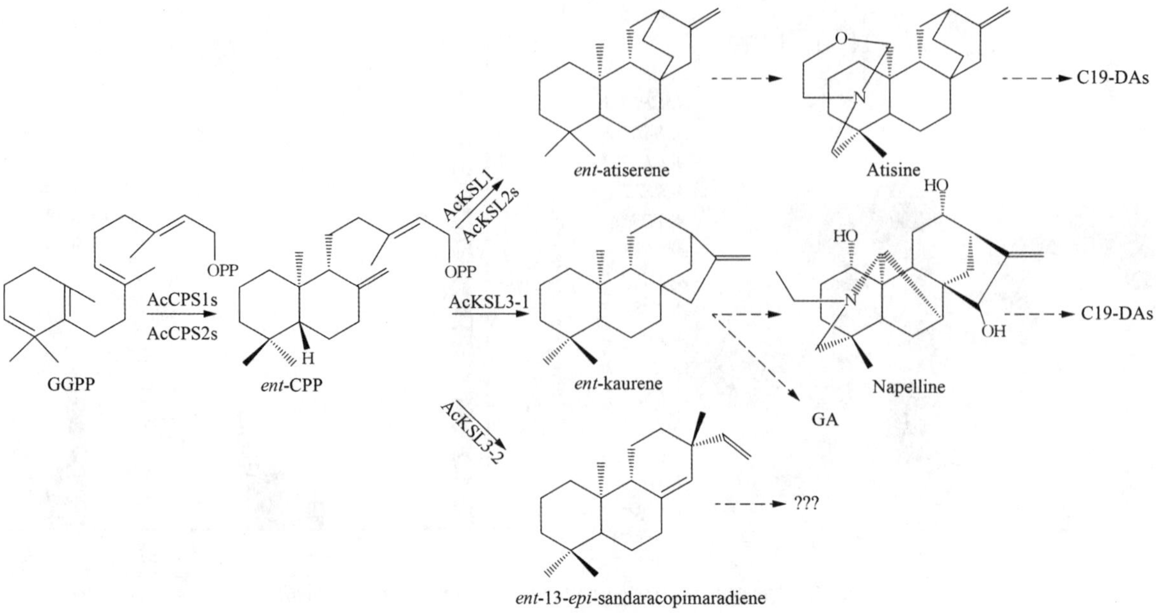

**Figure 7 The proposed diterpenoid biosynthesis in *A. carmichaelii***

Twelve identified diterpene synthases, and their corresponding reactions are indicated, along with the possible biosynthetic downstream DAs. Dashed arrows indicate multiple enzymatic reactions.

Many secondary metabolites are synthesized in highly specific tissues, such as tanshinones and forskolin in the roots. More specifically, tanshinones are synthesized in the root periderm of *S. miltiorrhiza* and forskolin is synthesized in the root cork of *Coleus forskohlii*. Accordingly, the diTPS involved in their biosynthesis have specific, high expression levels in these organs. In our recent study focused on DAs metabolites in different species, we found that despite the principal and lateral root being considered the primary medicinal components of *A. carmichaelii*, the characteristic DAs including aconitine, mesaconitine and hypaconitine have a relatively high content in stem and leaves as well. Indeed, when total DAs content was assessed, the top leaves contained the highest DAs content. It is therefore difficult isolate which enzyme or substrate is responsible for the large array of $C_{19}$-DAs biosynthetic pathways of *A. carmichaelii* based on gene expression patterns and metabolite locations alone. Due to the high expression levels of AcKSL2s, we postulate that the atisine type $C_{20}$-DAs are the main precursor for $C_{19}$-DAs; however, further proof by RNA interference using microprojectile bombardment (gene gun) or virus-induced gene silencing technology to knock down AcKSLs gene expression *in planta* or through isotope labeling analysis is needed.

The Pacbio isoform sequencing offered information about alternative splicing transcripts. In terpene synthase, there were few reports about functional alternative splicing transcripts. In *S. miltiorrhiza*, the kaurene synthase like gene *SmKSL1* and several genes involved in production of isoprenoid precursors were reported to exhibit alternative splicing without functional identification. In *I. rubescens*, the alternative splicing IrKLS3a was identified to alter the product outcome. IrKSL3 produced miltiradiene, while IrKSL3a produced isopimaradiene and miltiradiene. Here, we identified two alternative splicing transcripts of *AcCPS1* and three of *AcKSL1* in *A. carmichaelii*. However, none were identified to be functional genes. Compared with the full-length gene, clone-4-12 from transcript13827 lost $\alpha$ domain of CPS, while transcript12676 lost $\gamma$ and partial $\beta$ domain, thus it is reasonable for them to lose diTPS functions. However, we are surprised by the loss of function of AcKSL1 and its three alternative splicing transcripts *in vitro*. This was partly due to the low solubility of recombinant protein in prokaryotic expression, after codon optimized of *E. coli* for AcKSL1, we finally identified its function in the highly efficient diterpene modular metabolic engineering system, indicating we should attempt more platforms such as by transient expression of these genes in *Nicotiana benthamiana* to characterize their functions.

In conclusion, by combining full-length Iso-seq and RNA-seq we obtained a robust *A. carmichaelii* transcriptome and identified all the TPS family genes involved in *A. carmichaelii* DAs biosynthesis. While not conclusive, our results highlight the atisine type $C_{20}$-DAs as the predominate precursor of the medicinal $C_{19}$-DAs, clarify the biosynthetic pathway for $C_{20}$-DAs in *A. carmichaelii*, and pave the way for further exploration of $C_{19}$-DAs biosynthesis pathway in *Aconitum*.

[毛柳英,崔光红,黄璐琦,等.Acta Pharmaceutica Sinica B,2021,11(10):3310-3321.]

# Structure-based engineering of substrate specificity for pinoresinol-lariciresinol reductases

Lignans are a major group of secondary metabolites in plants. This family has numerous biological effects in humans (e. g., anticancer, antiviral, antioxidant, and immunosuppression) owing to their structural diversity—nearly 2000 distinct lignans have been reported. For example, the furofuran lignans such as kandelisesquilignan A/B and terminaloside K have antioxidant effects. The dibenzylbutyrolactone lignans including arctigenin, traxillagenin, arctiin, traxillaside, and their glycosides have neuroprotective activities. Finally, the aryltetralin lignan podophyllotoxin is the precursor for the semi-synthesis of anticancer drugs such as etoposide.

Lignans biosynthesis starts with the coupling of two coniferyl alcohols by an oxidase (laccase or peroxidase) with the aid of a dirigent protein to form pinoresinol. Pinoresinol/lariciresinol reductase (PLR), an NADPH-dependent reductase, converts pinoresinol to lariciresinol and subsequently to secoisolariciresinol. Because the reductive steps that give rise to lariciresinol and secoisolariciresinol represent entry points for the biosynthesis of the lignan subclasses furofurans, dibenzylbutane, dibenzylbutyrolactone, and aryltetrahydronaphthalene, PLR is regarded as a pivotal enzyme that contributes to lignan structural diversity. Moreover, variation in both the composition and accumulation of lignans among different plant species, organs, and developmental stages can be ascribed, at least in part, to the characteristics of reactions catalyzed by PLRs as well as their expression patterns. Therefore, characterization of the catalytic mechanisms of PLRs—especially their substrate selectivity— is particularly crucial for understanding the molecular basis of the remarkable diversity of both chemical structures and biological activities of lignans.

The substrate selectivity of PLRs has attracted considerable attention. Most PLRs that have been characterized reduce both pinoresinol and lariciresinol efficiently to produce lariciresinol and secoisolariciresinol, respectively. Known exceptions are *Arabidopsis thaliana* reductases that have substrate preference for pinoresinol, but only weak (*At*PrR1) or no activity (*At*PrR2) toward lariciresinol and are thus named pinoresinol reductases (PrRs). A recent study indicated that the L174I mutant of *Camellia sinensis* PLR1 (*Cs*PLR1) loses the capacity to reduce pinoresinol and specifically catalyzes the conversion of lariciresinol to secoisolariciresinol, but the underlying mechanism is unclear. The three-dimensional structure of *Thuja plicata* PLR1 (*Tp*PLR1) has been elucidated and indicates that K138 is responsible for the basic catalysis, because the mutant K138A lacks the ability to convert pinoresinol. However, the apo structure does not provide sufficient information to interpret the substrate-selective mechanism of PLRs/PrRs.

Phylogenetic analysis of PLRs/PrRs from different species has revealed that *Isatis indigotica* PLR1 (*Ii*PLR1), a key enzyme involved in lariciresinol biosynthesis, has the closest relationship to *At*PrRs with a high level of amino-acid sequence identity (> 80%) and is grouped with *At*PrR2, which cannot utilize lariciresinol as substrate (Fig. 1). Interestingly, in contrast to *At*PrRs that has substrate preference for pinoresinol, *Ii*PLR1 from *I. indigotica* (family Cruciferae, same as *A. thaliana*) can reduce both pinoresinol and lariciresinol efficiently with comparable $k_{cat}/K_m$ values. The finding that *Ii*PLR1/*At*PrRs, which differ in substrate selectivity, are clustered together suggests that substrate specificity is independent of sequence conservation among PLRs/PrRs. Therefore, the amino-acid residues responsible for PLR/PrR substrate selectivity are difficult to determine merely through sequence analysis, and thus structural information on PLR/PrR enzymes is vital—as are data concerning how these two enzyme types can utilize two different substrates.

In the present work, we compare crystal structures of *Ii*PLR1, *At*PrR1, and *At*PrR2 and identify residues that may be responsible for the observed substrate selectivity of PLRs and PrRs. Mutagenesis of these residues alters the substrate specificities for pinoresinol and lariciresinol. For example, mutagenesis of *Ii*PLR1 successfully eliminates the second reaction that converts lariciresinol to secoisolariciresinol, leading to a high accumulation of the pharmaceutically valuable compound lariciresinol. Our study will enable the synthesis of lignans with diverse chemical structures and bioactivities by biotechnological means or by enzyme-assisted chemistry.

## 1 RESULTS

**Characterization of *Ii*PLR1, *At*PrR1, and *At*PrR2 crystal structures** To understand both the catalytic mechanism of

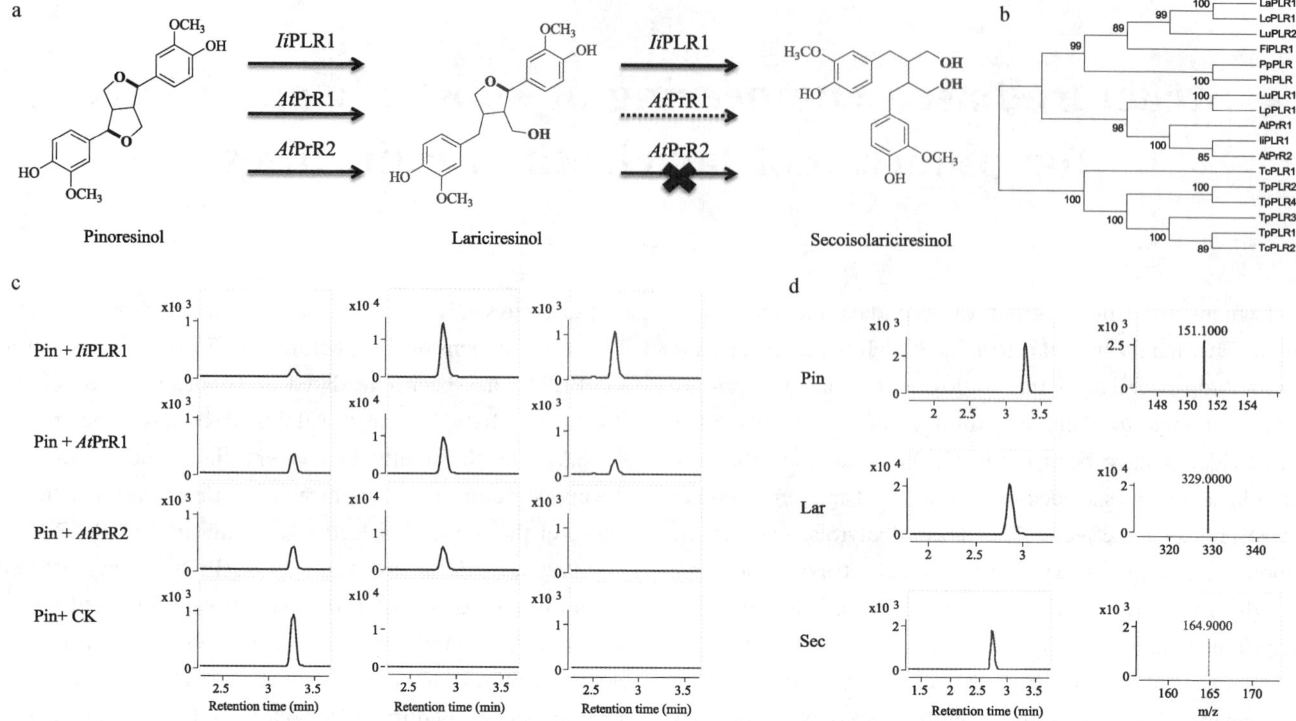


**Fig. 1 Biochemical assays for *Ii*PLR1 and *At*PrRs function**

(a) *Ii*PLR1 efficiently catalyzes the conversion of pinoresinol into lariciresinol and also catalyzes the conversion of lariciresinol into secoisolariciresinol. In contrast, *At*PrR1/2 exhibit a substrate preference for pinoresinol, yet exhibit only weak activity (*At*PrR1) or no activity (*At*PrR2) for lariciresinol. (b) Phylogenetic tree of PLRs/PrRs from different species. (c) Conversion of pinoresinol into lariciresinol and then into secoisolariciresinol by recombinant *Ii*PLR1, *At*PrR1, and *At*PrR2. The reaction products were analyzed by LC-MS. (d) Chromatograms for pinoresinol, lariciresinol, and secoisolariciresinol are denoted in black, blue, and red, respectively.

PLR and the mechanism underlying the substrate specificity of PLRs/PrRs, we chose *Ii*PLR1, *At*PrR1, and *At*PrR2 for a structure study. The crystal structures were captured in the apo, substrate-bound and/or product-bound forms (Table 1). We found that, for all 16 structures we solved, each enzyme adopts a similar head-to-tail dimer conformation (Fig. 2a and Supplementary Fig. 1), strongly suggesting that each PLR/PrR functions as a homodimer, consistent with the literature that *Tp*PLR1 exists as a dimeric entity in solution.

Taking the structure of *Ii*PLR1_NAP_+PIN for the purpose of a detailed description, each protomer contains two domains, namely the N-terminal NADPH binding domain (NBD) and the C-terminal substrate binding domain (SBD). The NBD comprises seven β-strands (β1 - 6, β8) surrounded by six α-helices (α1 - 5, α7), whereas the SBD comprises two β-strands (β7, β9) with five small α-helices (α6, α8 - 11). A large groove is formed between NBD and SBD (Fig. 2a). This groove can be roughly divided into two parts—the positively charged part that associates with the NBD and the hydrophobic part that associates with the SBD. The substrates or products can be clearly defined within the groove (Fig. 2a and Supplementary Fig. 2). Several regions (α5 loop, α9-helix, and α9 loop) are partially disordered both in the *Ii*PLR1_apo and *Ii*PLR1_NAP structures, for which the differences can be characterized by a RMSD of 0.287 Å, whereas the β4 loop is well defined in the apo structure (Fig. 2b). Intriguingly, the β4 loop is well defined in the *At*PrR1_NAP structure but disordered in the *At*PrR1/2_apo structures (Supplementary Fig. 3). These structural differences suggest that the loops are somewhat flexible, and act as a switch to control the binding of NADPH and release of $NADP^+$. Moreover, the β2 loop moves slightly towards $NADP^+$ in the *Ii*PLR1_NAP structure, catering to the entry of the coenzyme (Fig. 2b). $NADP^+$ forms strong hydrogen bonds and hydrophobic interactions with residues within the groove (Fig. 2c), among which the GXXGXXG motif (considered as the conserved NADPH-binding motif) binds the phosphate and deoxyribose groups, and residues Ala164, Cys165 together with Phe166 fix the position of the catalytically active nicotinamide group. Residue Lys144, which corresponds to the previously reported Lys138 in *Tp*PLR1 that serves as the general base for catalysis, forms direct hydrogen bonds with $NADP^+$ in *Ii*PLR1_apo and *Ii*PLR1_NAP.

Catalytic mechanism of PLR based on its homodimeration

The dimers of *Ii*PLR1_NAP and *Ii*PLR1_NAP_+PIN have similar structures, as suggested by a RMSD of 0.362 Å,

**Table 1 The crystal structure information of *Ii*PLR1, *At*PrR1, and *At*PrR2 proteins in their apo, NADP+ and substrate/product binding forms**

| | apo | $NADP^+$ | $NADP^+$ | | $NADP^+$ | | $NADP^+$ | |
|---|---|---|---|---|---|---|---|---|
| | | | (+)-Pinoresinol | (−)-Pinoresinol | (+)-Lariciresinol | (−)-Lariciresinol | (+)-Secoisolariciresinol | (−)-Secoisolariciresinol |
| *Ii*PLR1 | *Ii*PLR_apo 2.7Å | *Ii*PLR1_NAP 2.4Å | *Ii*PLR1_NAP_+PIN 2.3Å | *Ii*PLR1_NAP_-PIN 2.1Å | — | *Ii*PLR1_NAP_-LAR 2.2Å | *Ii*PLR1_NAP_+SEC 2.3Å | *Ii*PLR1_NAP_-SEC 2.6Å |
| *At*PrR1 | *At*PrR1_apo 2.8Å | *At*PrR1_NAP 2.0Å | *At*PrR1_NAP_+PIN 2.0Å | *At*PrR1_NAP_-PIN 2.5Å | *At*PrR1_NAP_+LAR 1.8Å | *At*PrR1_NAP_-LAR 2.5Å | — | *At*PrR1_NAP_-SEC 2.0Å |
| *At*PrR2 | *At*PrR2_apo 2.0Å | — | *At*PrR2_NAP_+PIN 1.6Å | — | — | — | — | — |

indeed, even the $NADP^+$ moieties could be aligned almost in the same position (Fig. 2d). Both β4 loops are disordered, further implying their flexibility, but β2 loop and α10-helix from neighboring molecules of *Ii*PLR1_NAP_+PIN dimer make contacts with and stabilize the substrate (Fig. 2d, e). Similar conformational changes of β2 loop and α10-helix can be seen by comparing the structure of *At*PrR1_NAP_+PIN with that of *At*PrR1_NAP and the structure of *At*PrR2_NAP_+PIN with that of *At*PrR2_apo (Supplementary Fig. 4a, b). (+)-Pinoresinol is inserted as a straight chain deep into the hydrophobic groove, for which the hydrophilic ends are stabilized through the formation of hydrogen bonds with main-chain atoms of Met125 and Gly178, and the hydrophobic region is surrounded by a series of hydrophobic groups (Fig. 2e). The inner 2-methoxy-phenol group of (+)-pinoresinol forms a sandwich-like π-π stack comprising the nicotinamide head of $NADP^+$ and Phe166. Two furan rings in the middle are surrounded by Tyr169 and Phe170 from α6-helix and by His276 and Phe277 from α10-helix. The outer 2-methoxy-phenol group is coordinated by Phe277 and Val46 of β2 loop from a neighboring protomer, which is distant from the $NADP^+$ and (+)-pinoresinol of the protomer (Fig. 2a, c, e). Further, Lys144 is far away from the furan rings, indicating that it may not participate in catalysis directly. Based on this structure analysis, we propose that both the entry and exit of NADPH are controlled by the β4 loop of *Ii*PLR1. Once one molecule of (+)-pinoresinol is captured by the narrow hydrophobic groove, each protomer forces the prepositioning of the α10-helix and β2 loop in the other protomer, resulting in tight binding of the substrate. This allows H: transfer from the NADPH to the proximal furan ring of the substrate to produce one molecule of (+)-lariciresinol.

Regarding the mechanism of the second catalytic step, we further compared the structures of *Ii*PLR1_NAP_+PIN, *Ii*PLR1_NAP_-LAR and *Ii*PLR1_NAP_-SEC, which revealed a similar mode for substrate/product binding (Fig. 2f). Furthermore, Leu46 (corresponding to Val46 in *Ii*PLR1), His276 and Phe277 of *At*PrR1 are positioned similar to the corresponding residues of *Ii*PLR1 to effect substrate binding or product release, except that the β4 loops cover the substrate/product, which are disordered in the *Ii*PLR1 structures (Fig. 2d and Supplementary Fig. 4a, c, d). The importance of Val46 for catalysis in *Ii*PLR1 is underscored by data from a mutational analysis (Fig. 2g). Mutation of Val46 to Ala improved the conversion of pinoresinol to lariciresinol by ~16%, and the subsequent conversion to secoisolariciresinol was greatly reduced. The *Ii*PLR1 mutant V46L had little ability to catalyze the conversion of lariciresinol to secoisolariciresinol. These data suggest that *Ii*PLR1 undergoes substrate-induced conformational changes upon homodimerization to achieve catalysis, and the principle of catalytic reactions using lariciresinol as substrate (second step) appears to be like that using pinoresinol as substrate (first step).

Mechanism underlying the substrate selectivity of PLR/PrR A previous study reported that the recombinant *At*PrR1 can only weakly reduce lariciresinol whereas *At*PrR2 lacks activity, which is in sharp contrast to all known PLRs. To determine the mechanism underlying this difference in substrate specificity, we confirmed the relative lack of activity for *At*PrR1/2 (Fig. 1) and then carried out a structure analysis of *Ii*PLR1, *At*PrR1, and *At*PrR2. Each of *Ii*PLR1_NAP_+PIN/*At*PrR1_NAP_+PIN/*At*PrR2_NAP_+PIN forms a homodimer, and superimposition of the protomers among the three complexes revealed RMSDs of 0.374, 0.365, and 0.308 Å, respectively (Fig. 3a, c and Supplementary Fig. 1). In contrast to *Ii*PLR1_NAP_+PIN, the β4 loops of *At*PrR1_NAP_+PIN and *At*PrR2_NAP_+PIN can be clearly identified (Fig. 3 and Supplementary Fig. 4). These well-defined loops twist as an "8" shape and cover both the NADP+-binding and substrate-binding grooves. Within the twisted loop, His93 and His97 "grasp" helices α5 and α10, while Val92 and Phe94 interact directly with (+)-pinoresinol; Arg95 strongly interacts with $NADP^+$ as well as each of the GXXGXXG motif and α2-helix from

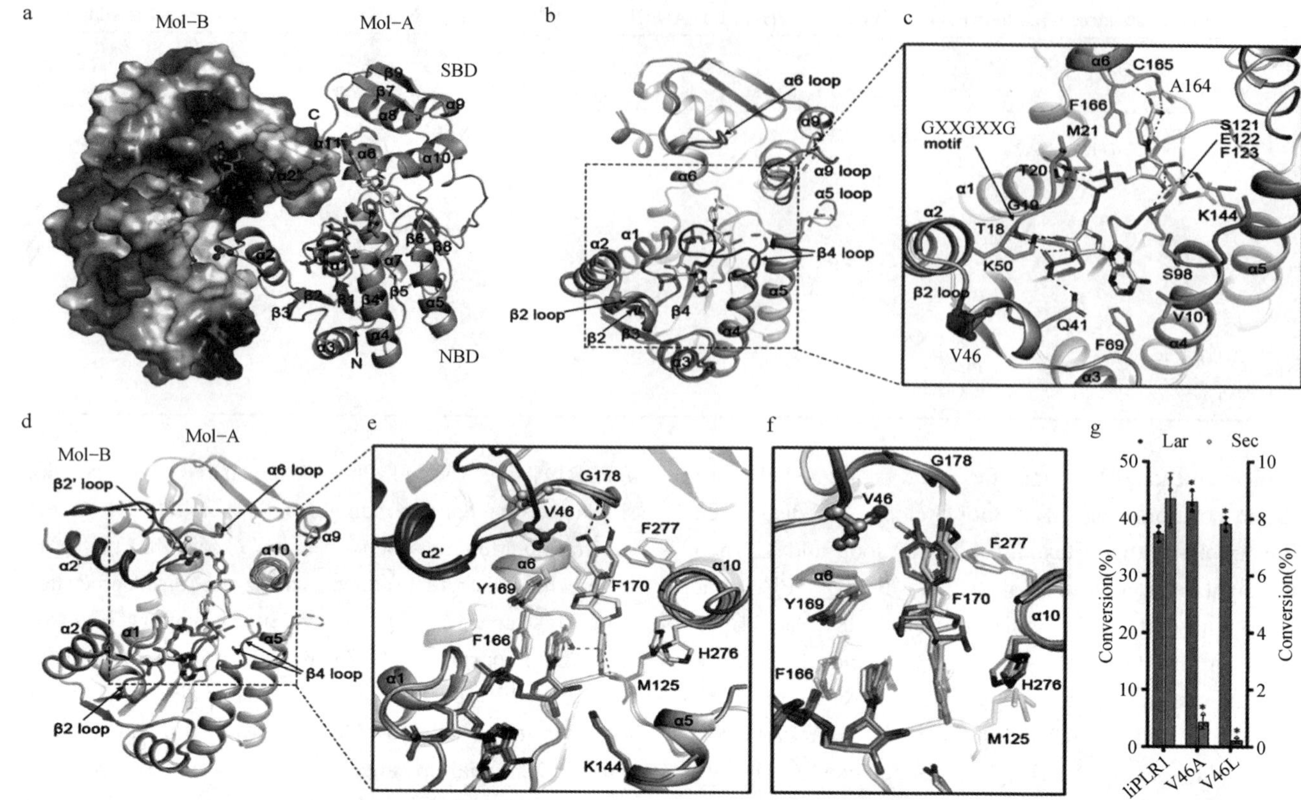


**Fig. 2 Structural mechanism of continuous catalytic reactions by *Ii*PLR1 based on homodimerization**

(a) Dimer formation of *Ii*PLR1_NAP_+PIN. Mol-A is shown as cartoon model, with its NBD and SBD colored in light blue and green cyan, respectively. Mol-B is represented as an electrostatic-surface model, on which blue and red colors represent positive and negative charges, respectively. $NADP^+$ and (+)-pinoresinol are shown as sticks and colored in orange and yellow, respectively. (b) Conformational changes were assessed by comparing monomer structures of *Ii*PLR1_apo (gray) and *Ii*PLR1_NAP (light orange). The $NADP^+$ bound to *Ii*PLR1_NAP is colored gray. The β4 loops of *Ii*PLR1_apo and *Ii*PLR1_NAP are highlighted as purple and green, respectively. (c) Zoom-in view of the NADPH-binding groove of *Ii*PLR1_NAP. Residues interacting with $NADP^+$ are colored cyan. The conserved GXXGXXG motif is indicated. Residue Val46 involved in dimer formation and substrate binding is shown as a ball- and-stick model and colored magenta. Dotted lines denote possible hydrogen bonds. (d) Structure comparison of *Ii*PLR1_NAP_+PIN and *Ii*PLR1_NAP. Mol-Bs of *Ii*PLR1_NAP_+PIN and *Ii*PLR1_NAP, Val46s in *Ii*PLR1_NAP_+PIN, and *Ii*PLR1_NAP are colored in marine, orange, magenta, and light yellow, respectively. (e) Zoom-in view of the substrate-binding groove. Residues of Mol-As in *Ii*PLR1_NAP_+PIN and *Ii*PLR1_NAP are colored green cyan (or light blue) and light yellow, respectively. (f) Structural comparation of the substrate/product-binding grooves in *Ii*PLR1_NAP_+PIN, *Ii*PLR1_NAP_-LAR (blue white), and *Ii*PLR1_NAP_-SEC (smudge). The cartoons are generated by PyMOL. (g) Enzyme assays for wild-type *Ii*PLR1 and its mutants V46A and V46L. Data are mean±s. d. ($n=3$ independent experiments). Asterisk* indicates significant difference from the wild-type enzyme ($P<0.05$) analyzed by one-way ANOVA with Tukey's multiple comparisons test. Source data underlying Fig. 2g are provided as a Source Data file.

neighboring protomer of the dimer. Similar β4 loops are also observed in all other *At*PrR1 substrate/product-bound structures, whereas each β4 loop is disordered in the corresponding *Ii*PLR1 structures, which indicates that the β4 loop may participate in substrate selectivity and, hence, catalysis.

We further explored why the loops behaved differently between *Ii*PLR1 and the *At*PrRs. The amino acid sequences of the β4 loops in the three proteins are quite similar (Supplementary Fig. 5), but the residue corresponding to Ser98 at the C-terminal end of the loop in *Ii*PLR1 is replaced as Asn98 in *At*PrR1/2. Combining the sequence and structural data, the difference can be explained reasonably as follows: the serine side chain is short enough to remain beneath the guanine group of NADPH, whereas the asparagine side chain cannot do so owing to steric hindrance. Consequently, the asparagine lies nearly vertical to the guanine group and points upward in the structure shown in Fig. 3b, d, and thus the swing of the β4 loop is limited in the *At*PrR1_NAP structure. As substrate enters the catalytic site, β4 loop can fold and cover the substrate-binding groove (Fig. 3b, d and Supplementary Figs. 3b and 4a). Besides the β4 loop, Val46 in *Ii*PLR1 is replaced with Leu46 in *At*PrR1, which has the effect of compressing the substrate-binding pocket. Although Val46 is unchanged in *At*PrR2, the α2-helix and β2 loop from the neighboring protomer move closer to the substrate upon its entry at the catalytic site, further condensing the pocket. The relative movement of dimers between *At*PrR2 and *Ii*PLR1 (as suggested by

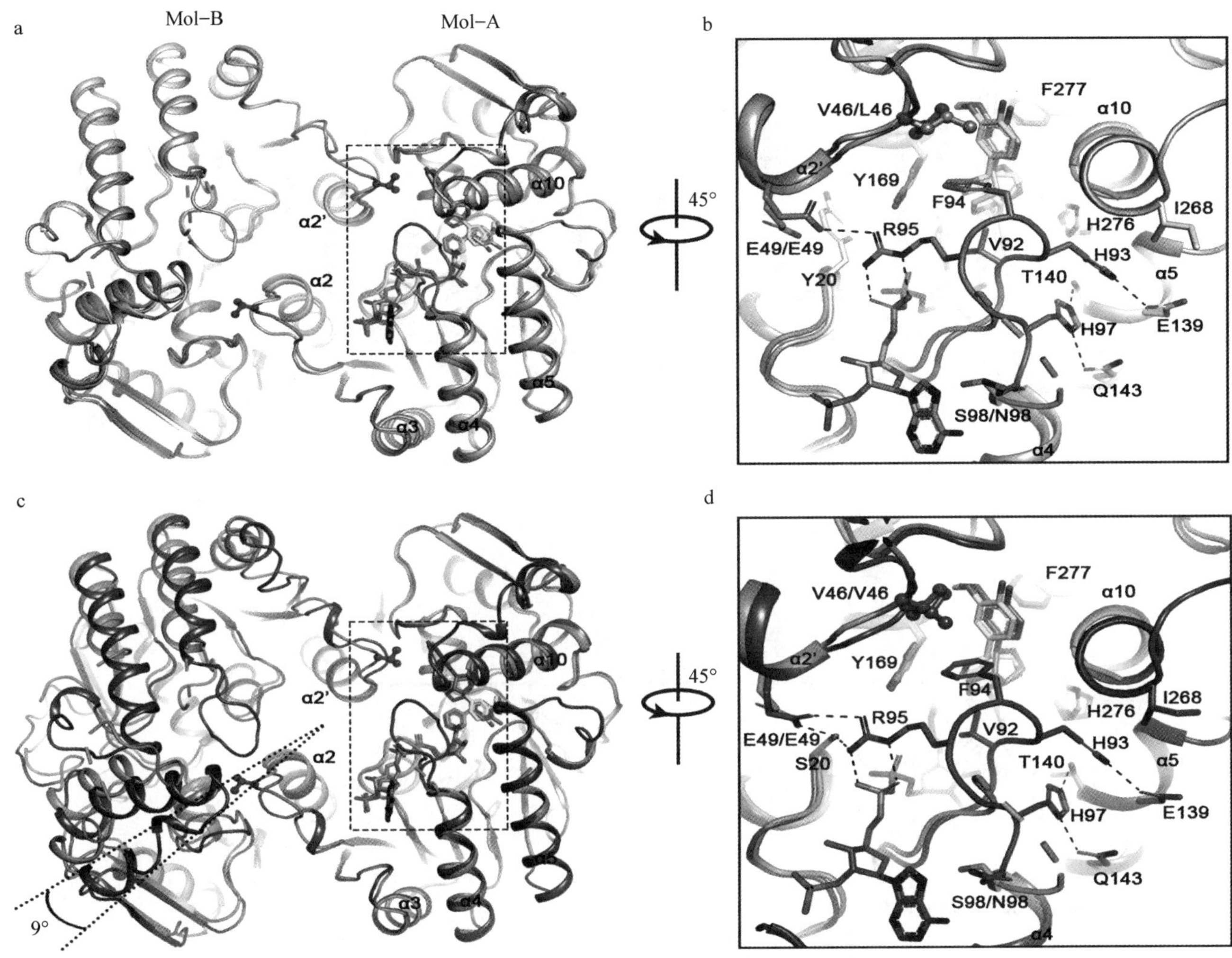


**Fig. 3 Structural differences among *Ii*PLR1, *At*PrR1, and *At*PrR2 indicating different catalytic capacities**

(a) Structural alignment of dimerized *Ii*PLR1_NAP_+PIN (green cyan) and *At*PrR1_NAP_+PIN (light gray). (b) Zoom-in view of dashed box in **a**. The β4 loop of *At*PrR1_NAP_+PIN is highlighted in orange. (c) Structural alignment of dimerized *Ii*PLR1_NAP_+PIN (green cyan) and *At*PrR2_NAP_+PIN (slate blue). (d) Zoom-in view of the dashed box in **c**. The β4 loop of *At*PrR2_NAP_+PIN is highlighted in magenta. For brevity, $NADP^+$ and some residues in *Ii*PLR1 are hidden. The cartoons are generated by PyMOL.

the ~9° shift shown in Fig. 3c) could be induced by different dimer orientations. Two molecules of the dimer exhibit relative torsion in *At*PrR2, and consequently, Val46 is forced deeper into the substrate-binding pocket compared with what occurs in *Ii*PLR1. Therefore, the entrance and orientation of the substrate in *At*PrR1/2 is more tightly controlled than in *Ii*PLR1.

Mutagenesis-based alteration of the substrate selectivity

Based on the structural analysis of *Ii*PLR1, *At*PrR1 and *At*PrR2, the importance of the candidate amino acids controlling substrate specificity was verified through site-directed mutagenesis. Enzy-matic assays using pinoresinol as substrate revealed that the *Ii*PLR1 mutations including V46A, V46L, S98A, S98H, and S98N somewhat enhanced the conversion rate of lariciresinol while significantly reduced that of secoisolariciresinol, and mutants V46A, S98A, and S98H had > 40% conversion rates for lariciresinol (Fig. 4a), suggesting that residues 46 and 98 are critical for the substrate preference. Taking V46A as an example for the kinetic analysis, its $K_m$ value for pinoresinol (29.4 ± 1.62 μmol/L) is comparable with that for lariciresinol (26.5 ± 0.60 μmol/L), however its $V_{max}$ for pinoresinol (3.22 ± 0.68 μmol/L/min) is 140-fold higher than that for lariciresinol (0.023 ± 0.001 3 μmol/L/min), and its $k_{cat}/K_m$ for pinoresinol (3.88 ± 0.65 $\mu M^{-1}$ $min^{-1}$) is 126-fold higher than that for lariciresinol (0.031 ± 0.002 $\mu M^{-1}$ $min^{-1}$) (Table 2). Compared with wild-type *Ii*PLR1, the activity of mutant V46A towards pinoresinol increases 4-fold, whereas that towards lar-iciresinol decreases 98% with regard to $k_{cat}/K_m$ values. These results indicate mutant V46A enhances catalytic efficiency for the first reaction but dramatically eliminates the second reaction. Consistent with the data for *Ii*PLR1, *At*PrR1 mutants L46A and L46V could enhance the conversion rate of lariciresinol and partially reduce that of secoisolariciresinol (Fig. 4a), which confirmed the importance of these two sites in substrate binding and

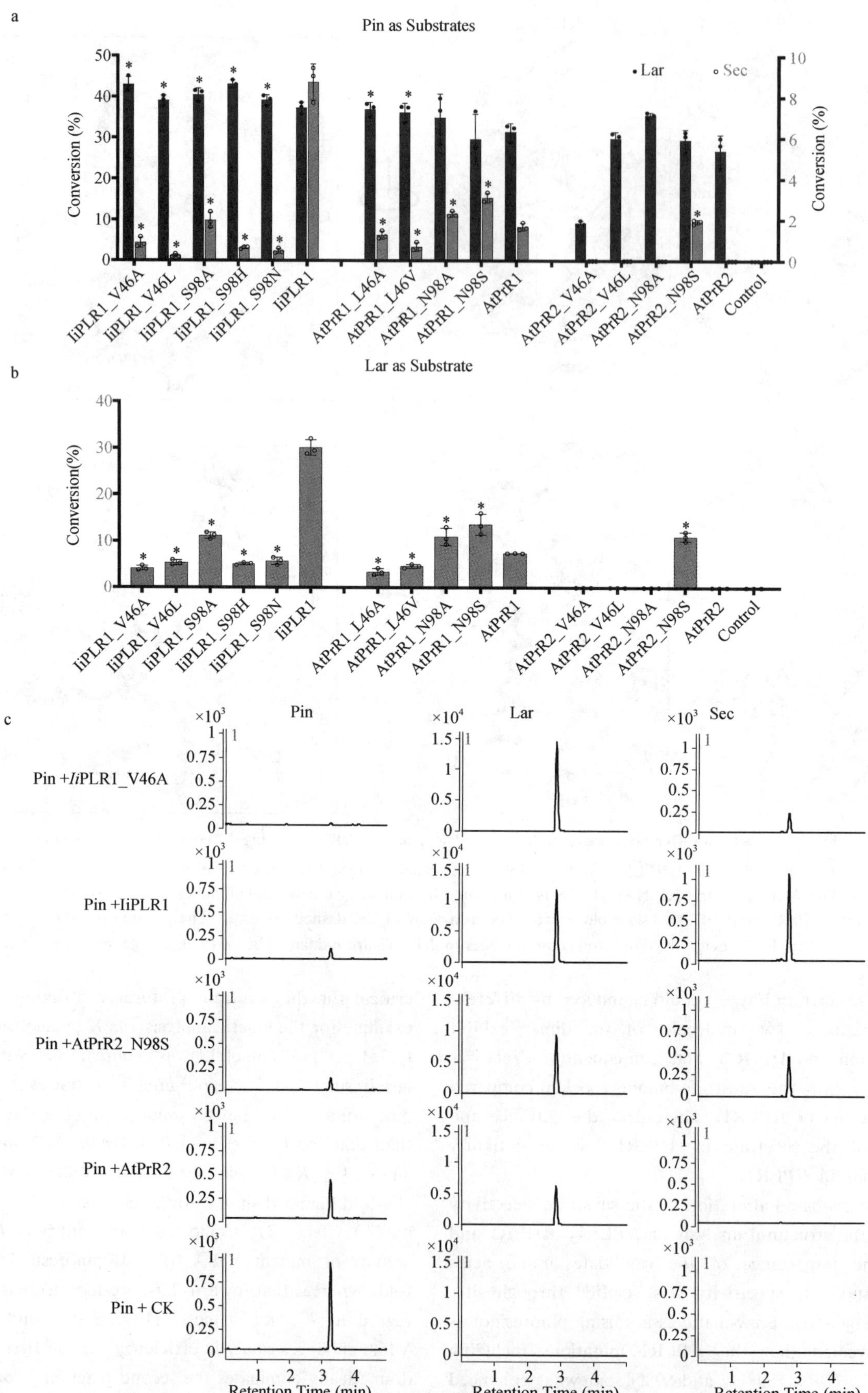


**Fig. 4 Percent conversion of pinoresinol to lariciresinol and subsequently to secoisolariciresinol by mutants of *Ii*PLR1, *At*PrR1 and *At*PrR2**

(a) Conversion of pinoresinol into lariciresinol and subsequently to secoisolariciresinol. (b) Conversion of lariciresinol into secoisolariciresinol. Data are mean±s. d. ($n$=3 independent experiments). Asterisk (*) indicates significant difference from the wild-type enzyme ($P<0.05$) analyzed by one-way ANOVA with Tukey's multiple comparisons test. Source data underlying Fig. 4a, b are provided as a Source Data file. (c) LC-MS determination of the products as catalyzed by *Ii*PLR1, *Ii*PLR1_V46A, *At*PrR2 and *At*PrR2_N98S.

**Table 2 Kinetic properties of *Ii*PLR1_V46A**

| Substrate | $K_m$ (μmol/L) | $V_{max}$ (μmol/L/min) | $k_{cat}$ ($min^{-1}$) | $k_{cat}/K_m$ ($\mu M^{-1}$ $min^{-1}$) |
|---|---|---|---|---|
| (±)-pinoresinol | 29.4±1.62 | 3.22±0.68 | 114.7±24.1 | 3.88±0.65 |
| (±)-lariciresinol | 26.5±0.60 | 0.023±0.0013 | 0.81±0.045 | 0.031±0.002 |

Data are expressed as mean±s.d. with three independent experiments. Source data are provided as a Source Data file.

product release thus in catalysis. As expected, mutants N98A and N98S in *At*PrR1 had increased activity for secoisolariciresinol production compared with wild type (Fig. 4a), strongly implying that residue 98 controls the swing of the β4 loop, which affects substrate binding and catalysis. Interestingly, *At*PrR2 mutant N98S could utilize lariciresinol to produce secoisolariciresinol, with a conversion rate of 1.91%, in contrast to the wild type which lacks this activity (Fig. 4a). Other *At*PrR2 mutants, including V46A, V46L, and N98A, varied in their activities for pinoresinol, as indicated by the relative rates of conversion to lariciresinol (Fig. 4a). Similar results were obtained for conversion of lariciresinol to secoisolariciresinol (Fig. 4b). Altogether, the structure-guided mutagenesis indeed could switch the substrate specificity of PLR/PrR, e.g., the *Ii*PLR1 mutant V46A had increased preference for pinoresinol but little catalytic activity for lariciresinol, whereas the *At*PrR2 mutant N98S gained the activity to catalyze the conversion of lariciresinol to secoisolariciresinol (Fig. 4c).

Taking structure and enzymology data together, we proposed a three-step catalytic mechanism for PLR based on its homodimerization. First, the protomers of dimeric PLRs recruit free NADPH through the very flexible β4 loop. Second, pinoresinol binds into one protomer via the substrate-binding groove, and the other protomer of the homodimer helps stabilize the substrate. Subsequently, pinoresinol receives H: from NADPH and be reduced to lariciresinol released later. Third, free lariciresinol is bound by another reductive PLR molecule and fixed by another homodimer, and then the lariciresinol is reduced to secoisolariciresinol and finally released (Fig. 5 and Supplementary Movie 1).

Importantly, the PrRs have more strict requirements for the binding and orientation of lariciresinol compared with PLRs, so PrRs cannot efficiently carry out the third step (Fig. 5). Hence, the substrate-specificity mechanism of PLRs/PrRs could be that residues located around the substrate-binding pocket and within the loop, together with residues that promote homodimerization, form the appropriate hydrophobic environment for binding a specific substrate.

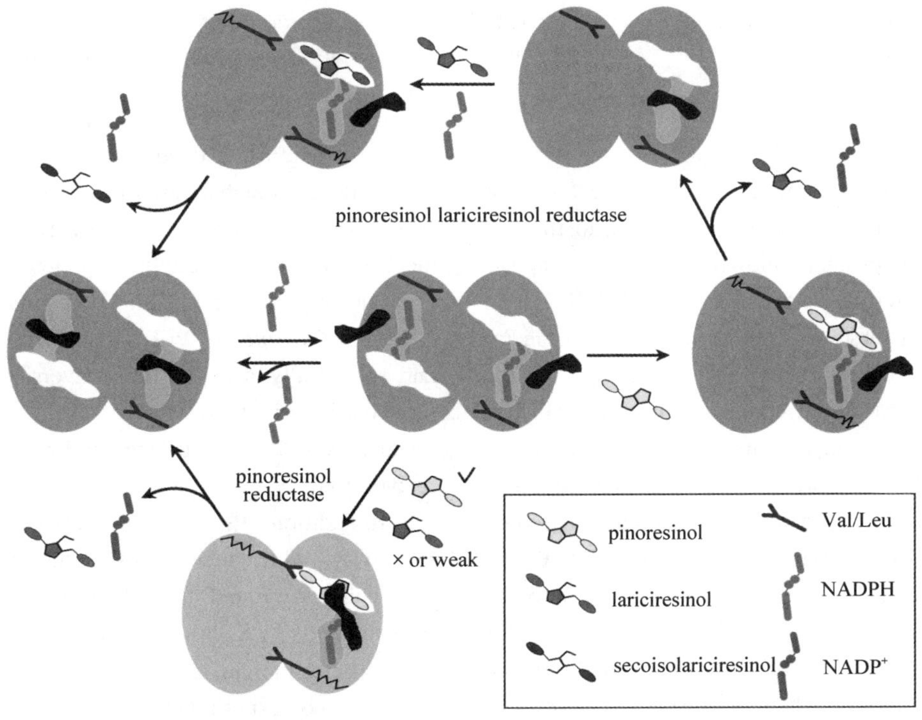


**Fig. 5 Model depicting the catalytic processes of PLRs and PrRs**

The blue dumbbell-shaped objects represent switches composed of β4 loops. A movie showing how the enzymes change conformation throughout a single round of catalysis can be found in Supplementary Movie 1.

**Mutation increases lariciresinol and reduces secoisolariciresinol production in vivo** Enzymatic assays indicated that certain *Ii*PLR1 mutants had increased activity for producing lariciresinol from pinoresinol in vitro (Fig. 4). Therefore, these *Ii*PLR1 mutant genes were selected for lariciresinol production using pinoresinol-producing *E. coli*. Because matairesinol, which is derived from secoisolariciresinol, is detectable only when CueO (multicopper oxidase), PLR and SDH (secoisolariciresinol dehydrogenase) are individually expressed in cells, each of wild-type *Ii*PLR1 and its mutants were co-cultured in pinoresinol-producing *E. coli*. Consistent with the enzyme assay results, *Ii*PLR1_V46A produced the greatest amount of lariciresinol (997.79 mg/L compared with 936.14 mg/L for wild-type). However, mutants V46L, S98A, S98H, and S98N were not as efficient as wild-type cells at producing lariciresinol, which was opposite to the results from in vitro enzyme assays. This may reflect the potential effects of complex metabolic networks and feedback mechanisms in vivo, which are not relevant to in vitro enzyme assays. Moreover, the provision of NADPH is tightly regulated in prokaryotic systems, which also may influence the activity of PLRs.

Notably, all the *Ii*PLR mutants produced significantly less secoisolariciresinol than wild-type cells, i.e., by 22.7%~52.5%; in particular, *Ii*PLR_V46A produced 46.4% less secoisolariciresinol than wild type (Fig. 6). These results paralleled those obtained in vitro with the *Ii*PLR1 mutants in which there was elimination of the second catalytic step, i.e., the conversion of lariciresinol to secoisolariciresinol (Fig. 4). Taken together, our results establish a promising route for the production of lariciresinol by synthetic biology strategies, and mutant *Ii*PLR_V46A mutant would be a good candidate for use in the large-scale production of the pharmaceutically valuable compound lariciresinol.

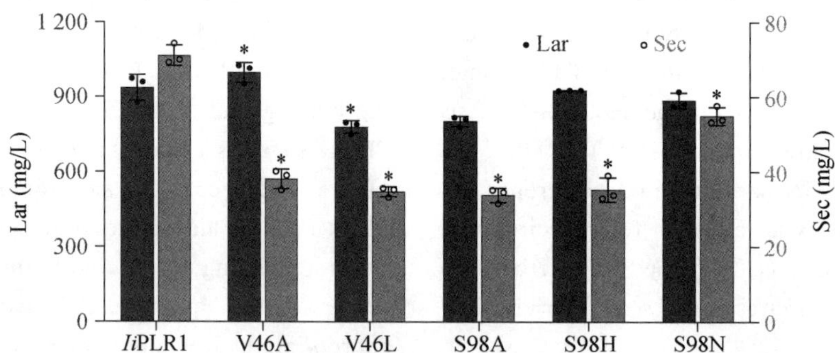


**Fig. 6 Lariciresinol production through co-culture of different strains harboring a plasmid encoding *Ii*PLR1 or its single-site mutants with pinoresinol-producing cells**

Data are mean±s.d. ($n=3$ independent experiments). Asterisk (*) indicates significant difference from the wild-type enzyme ($P<0.05$) analyzed by one-way ANOVA with Tukey's multiple comparisons test. Source data are provided as a Source Data file.

## 2 DISCUSSION

The molecular mechanism of substrate selectivity of PLR/PrR has attracted particular interest owing to the key role of these enzymes in lignan biosynthesis. However, the lack of structural results—especially for PLRs/PrRs in complex with different substrates—has limited our understanding of the mechanism underlying enzyme specificity. In the present study, we characterized crystal structures of *Ii*PLR1, *At*PrR1, and *At*PrR2 in complex with their various substrates. Several residues participating in substrate binding and catalysis were identified either directly or indirectly based on structural analysis, and these residues were validated by enzyme assays. All these data provide solid evidence to explore the mechanistic basis of substrate selectivity for PLRs/PrRs. Besides residues 46 and 98 in *Ii*PLR1 and *At*PrRs that we identified as being critical for binding and catalysis, residues Phe166, Tyr169, Phe170, His276, and Phe277 within the substrate-binding groove were also strongly correlated with enhanced substrate binding and catalysis. We further deduced that any residue in PLRs/PrRs around the hydrophobic groove or affecting homodimerization may impact the conformation of the active site, thereby dictating substrate selectivity (Supplementary Figs. 5 and 6). Consequently, it is not difficult to understand why mutant L174I of *C. sinensis* PLR1 can hardly reduce pinoresinol and specifically catalyze the conversion of lariciresinol to secoisolariciresinol, i.e., because Leu174 points directly toward Tyr163 and thus may indirectly promote substrate recognition.

In addition, PLRs also display substrate stereochemical selectivity, which contributes to the enantiomeric diversity of lignans. We found this to be true for *Ii*PLR1, which gave comparable $k_{cat}/K_m$ values for both (±)-pinoresinol and (±)-lariciresinol in the range of 0.9 - 1.6 $\mu M^{-1}$ $min^{-1}$, although no experiments with respect to the enantio-specificity of this enzyme have been performed. Despite past research on this topic, however, the mechanism underlying the substrate stereochemical selectivity of PLRs remains unclear. Comparison of the enantiospecifically opposite PLRs *Tp*PLR1 and *Tp*PLR2 suggests that F164, V268, and L272 in *Tp*PLR1 contribute to the catalysis of (−)-pinoresinol, whereas L164, G268, and F272 in *Tp*PLR2 prefer to bind (+)-pinoresinol. Nevertheless, site-directed mutagenesis carried out in flax indicates that these positions are insufficient to determine enantiospecificity. Based on amino-acid sequence and structural analyses, it seems that residues Phe94 and Phe277 in *Ii*PLR1/*At*PrR1 may act in concert to determine the enantiospecificity of PLRs (Supplementary Fig. 6). These two residues are highly conserved in PLRs that have no enantiospecificity, whereas Ile94 and Tyr277 are present in PLRs that have a strict substrate preference for (+)-pinoresinol. Moreover, in *Linum usitatissimum* PLR1 (*Lu*PLR1), which has strict enantiospecificity for (−)-pinoresinol, a leucine residue is deleted as are two other residues on β4 loop (corresponding to the β4 loop of *Ii*PLR1, where Phe94 is located). Unfortunately, we could not obtain sufficient amounts of the enantiomerically pure substrates to carry out the experiments necessary to establish the enantio-selectivity.

Nature uses a dazzling array of enzymes to produce diverse natural products. However, some modifications are challenging to control because the relative lack of substrate specificity often generates undesired byproducts. *Ii*PLR1 plays an important role in the biotechnological production of lariciresinol, which represents the most important component for the antibacterial, antiviral, and the immune-regulatory effects of the traditional Chinese medicine Radix Isatidis. The fact that *Ii*PLR1 can efficiently utilize both pinoresinol and lariciresinol as substrates suggests that the biosynthetic efficiency towards the pharmaceutically valuable compound lariciresinol in Radix Isatidis has been hampered by the relatively low substrate specificity of *Ii*PLR1. In our present work, structure-guided mutagenesis successfully switched the substrate specificity of *Ii*PLR1, leading to overproduction of lariciresinol and reduced production of secoisolariciresinol by *E. coli*. Our study provides insight into the molecular mechanism underlying the substrate specificity of PLRs/PrRs, and paves the way for the manufacture of lariciresinol through microbial fermentation. Moreover, this work suggests the possibility of using targeted mutagenesis of *Ii*PLR to improve the efficiency of synthesizing bioactive compounds in *I. indigotica* using gene-editing technologies.

## 3 METHODS

Phylogenic analysis of plant PLRs Phylogenetic relationships were analyzed using the maximum likelihood method with the pairwise deletion option in MEGA 6.06. Tree reliability was estimated using a bootstrap analysis of 1 000 replicates. Plant PLR amino-acid sequences used in the phylogenic analysis were retrieved from GenBank, including *Tp*PLR1 (AAF63507.1), *Tp*PLR2 (AAF63508.1), *Tp*PLR3 (AAF63509.1), *Tp*PLR4 (AAF63510.1), *Pp*PLR (AHL21381.1), *La*PLR1 (CAH60857.1), *Lu*PLR1 (CAH60858.1), *Lu*PLR2 (ABW24501.1), *Lp*PLR1 (ABM68630.1), *Lc*PLR1 (ABW86959.1), *Ph*PLR (ACF71492.1), *Tc*PLR1 (AZL88516.1), *Tc*PLR2 (AZL88517.1), *Fi*PLR1 (AAC49608.1), *Ii*PLR1 (AEA42007.1), *At*PrR1 (NP_174490.1), and *At*PrR2 (NP_193102.1).

Heterologous expression of *Ii*PLR1, *At*PrR1, and *At*PrR2 in *E. coli* Total RNA was extracted from leaves of wild-type *I. indigotica* or *A. thaliana* using TRIzol Reagent (GIBCO BRL). The mRNA was reverse transcribed with oligo dT to generate cDNA as a template for PCR. Full-length cDNA sequences of *Ii*PLR1 (GenBank accession no. JF264893), *At*PrR1 (AY065214) and *At*PrR2 (BT002882) were cloned into pET-duet-1 (Novagen, USA) to generate *Ii*PLR1-pET, *At*PrR1-pET, and *At*PrR2-pET, respectively. The primers used are listed in Supplementary Table 1. *E. coli* Rosetta (DE3) cells were transformed with purified plasmid DNA and then grown at 37 ℃ to an $OD_{600}$ of 0.8. Then, protein expression was induced by adding 0.5 mmol/L isopropyl β-D-thiogalactoside (IPTG, final concentration) with incubation overnight at 16 ℃. Cells were collected, resuspended in buffer A (20 mmol/L Tris-HCl pH 8.0, 100 mmol/L NaCl), and lysed with a French press. The lysate was centrifuged at 20,000 × *g* for 45 min, and the supernatant was applied to a Ni-NTA column equilibrated with buffer A supplemented with 25 mmol/L imidazole. Bound protein was eluted using buffer A containing 250 mmol/L imidazole and was concentrated for further purification on a Superdex-200 column equilibrated with buffer A. Protein purity was assessed by SDS-PAGE (12% polyacrylamide), and protein concentration was determined by the Bradford method.

Crystallization, data collection, and structure determination The full-length *Ii*PLR1/*At*PrR1/*At*PrR2 were purified as described above and concentrated to 5 ~ 10 mg/mL for crystallization. Aliquots of each concentrated protein sample were mixed 1 : 1 with reservoir solution, and crystals were grown at 20 or 4 ℃ in one week using the sitting-drop vapor-diffusion method. For co-crystals, protein was combined with $NADP^+$ at a 1 : 5 molar ratio, and protein with $NADP^+$ and substrate/product at a 1 : 5 : 10 molar ratio. For reservoir solutions, *Ii*PLR1 apo and co-crystals were grown with 0.2 mol/L sodium citrate tribasic, 0.1 mol/L sodium citrate/citric acid, pH 4.0 and 20% polyethylene glycol (PEG) 3 350; *At*PrR1 apo crystals were grown in 0.2

mol/L lithium chloride, 20% w/v PEG 3 350; *At*PrR1_NAP, *At*PrR1_-NAP_+PIN, *At*PrR1_NAP_+LAR and *At*PrR1_NAP_-SEC were grown in 0.2 M sodium fluoride, 20% w/v PEG 3 350; *At*PrR1_NAP_-PIN and *At*PrR1_NAP_-LAR crystals were grown in 0.2 M sodium malonate, pH 6.0, 20% w/v PEG 3 350; *At*PrR2 apo crystals were grown in 0.2 M magnesium chloride, 0.1 M sodium HEPES, pH 7.5 and 25% PEG 3 350; *At*PrR2_NAP_+PIN crystals were grown in 2.1 M DL malic acid, pH 7.0. The crystals were cryoprotected by serial transfers into reservoir solutions supplemented with 30% (v/v) glycerol and then flash-cooled in liquid nitrogen. Data collections were performed at the BL17U1 and BL19U1 beamline of the Shanghai Synchrotron Radiation Facility. The data were processed with HKL3000, and the initial phase was determined by molecular replacement with Phenix using the crystal structure of *Tp*PLR1 (PDB ID: 1QYD [https://doi.org/10.2210/pdb1qyd/pdb]) as a template. The structure models were firstly auto-built in Coot and then refined by iterative rounds of manual adjustment with Coot and refinement with Phenix. The statistics of data collection and structure refinement are shown in Supplementary Tables 2 - 5.

Site-directed mutagenesis of *Ii*PLR1, *At*PrR1, and *At*PrR2 and enzymatic assays  Single-site mutagenesis was achieved through one-step PCR, and mutants were verified with Sanger sequencing. All primers are listed in Supplementary Table 1. After expression and purification of recombinant enzymes under the aforementioned conditions, the results for the enzyme assays for mutants were compared with those for wild-type recombinant *Ii*PLR1, *At*PrR1, and *At*PrR2 as follows.

Enzyme activity assays were conducted strictly according to our previous work. Assay mixtures (1 mL) consisted of TG buffer (50 mM Tris-HCl, 10% [w/v] glycerol, pH 7.0), 150 μM NADPH], 100 μM pinoresinol, or 100 μM lariciresinol and 5 μg of purified protein. Assays without a fusion protein were used as controls. Protein, buffer, and substrate were pre-incubated for 5 min at 30 ℃, and each reaction was initiated by addition of NADPH and terminated after 30 min by addition of 300 μL ethyl acetate. Each assay mixture was extracted with ethyl acetate (3×300 μL total). The combined ethyl acetate phases were dried under vacuum, and the residue was dissolved in 1 mL methanol. Conversion rate was then determined. The content of pinoresinol, lariciresinol and secoisolariciresinol was determined by LC-MS using a triple-quadrupole mass spectrometer (Model 6 410, Agilent, Santa Clara, CA) following our published methods. MassHunter Qualitative Analysis B.06.00 was used for the data analysis. The selected transitions of $m/z$ were 357→151 for pinoresinol, 359→329 for lariciresinol, and 361→164 for secoisolariciresinol. All standards were purchased from Sigma-Aldrich (St. Louis, MO).

For determination of $V_{max}$ and $K_m$ values for *Ii*PLR1_V46A, 10 different concentrations of substrate (pinoresinol or lariciresinol; 5 - 200 μM) and 1 μg purified protein were used. Samples were incubated at 30 ℃ for 5 min (during which substrate consumption was ≤10%). Samples without protein were used as controls. The rate of substrate consumption was calculated for kinetic analysis. $V_{max}$ and $K_m$ values were determined from Lineweaver-Burk plots, and $k_{cat}$ was determined by dividing $V_{max}$ by the enzyme concentration.

Bioconversion  For the production of lariciresinol, biotransformation was divided into two modules, namely the accumulation and conversion of the precursor, pinoresinol. *E. coli* strain strOpr2 carrying plasmid pET28a-Prx02-PsVAO was used to produce pinoresinol, whereas *E. coli* BL21(DE3) carrying a plasmid encoding *Ii*PLR1 or its mutants was used for conversion of pinoresinol to lariciresinol. These *E. coli* strains were cultured in LB medium at 37 ℃ with shaking (220 rpm) for 12 h as seed cultures, and then a 2% seed culture was transferred to a 250-mL shaker flask containing 25 mL TB medium. After culturing for 2 - 2.5 h at 37 ℃ and 220 rpm, 500 μM IPTG (final concentration) was added to the medium with continued cultivation for 12 h at 25 ℃ and 220 rpm. These cells were used for pinoresionol accumulation and conversion, respectively. Cells from *E. coli* strain strOpr2 were harvested by centrifugation at 4 ℃ and 3 724 × *g* for 30 min and then resuspended in phosphate-buffered saline (pH 7.0) to adjust the $OD_{600}$ value to 20. Then 0.15% (v/v) eugenol was added into 15 mL of the resuspension at 0, 1, 3, 5, and 7 h for pinoresinol accumulation (20 ℃, 220 rpm). At 9 h, 15 ml of a culture of *E. coli* expressing *Ii*PLR1 and each mutant ($OD_{600}$ = 20) was added to determine the conversion of pinoresinol to lariciresinol (25 ℃, 220 rpm), and samples were taken after 20 h. The concentration of each of lariciresinol and secoisolariciresinol was determined by HPLC.

Statistical analysis  All the experiments in this paper were repeated at least three times and results from representative data sets are presented. GraphPad Prism (version 9.1.0) was used for the statistical analysis. The statistical evaluations used one-way analysis of variance (ANOVA) with multiple comparisons, followed by Tukey tests. The results were considered statistically significant at $^{*}P<0.05$.

Reporting summary  Further information on research design is available in the Nature Research Reporting Summary linked to this article.

## 4 DATA AVAILABILITY

Data supporting the findings of this work are available within the paper and its Supplementary Information files.

The atomic coordinates and structure factors for the structures have been deposited in the Protein Data Bank with accession codes 7CS2 (Apo structure of dimeric *Ii*PLR1), 7CS3 (*Ii*PLR1 with $NADP^+$), 7CS4 (*Ii*PLR1 with $NADP^+$ and (+)pinoresinol), 7CS5 (*Ii*PLR1 with $NADP^+$ and (−) pinoresinol), 7CS6 (*Ii*PLR1 with $NADP^+$ and (−) lariciresinol), 7CS7 (*Ii*PLR1 with $NADP^+$ and (+) secoisolariciresinol), 7CS8 (*Ii*PLR1 with $NADP^+$ and (−) secoisolariciresinol), 7CS9 (*At*PrR1 in apo form), 7CSA (*At*PrR1 with $NADP^+$), 7CSB (*At*PrR1 with $NADP^+$ and (+) pinoresinol), 7CSC (*At*PrR1 with $NADP^+$ and (−) pinoresinol), 7CSD (*At*PrR1 with $NADP^+$ and (+) lariciresinol), 7CSE (*At*PrR1 with $NADP^+$ and (−) lariciresinol), 7CSF (*At*PrR1 with $NADP^+$ and (−) secoisolariciresinol), 7CSG (*At*PrR2 in apo form), 7CSH (*At*PrR2 with $NADP^+$ and (+) pinoresinol). The initial phase was determined by molecular replacement using the crystal structure of *Tp*PLR1 (PDB ID: 1QYD [https://doi.org/10.2210/pdb1qyd/pdb]) as a template. The source data underlying Figs. 2g, 4a, b, and 6, as well as Table 2 are provided as a Source Data file. All data generated and analyzed during the current study are available from the corresponding authors upon reasonable request. A reporting summary for this Article is available as a Supplementary Information file. Source data are provided with this paper.

[肖莹，张鹏，陈万生，等. Nature Communications, 2021, 12:2828.]

# Gene delivery strategies for therapeutic proteins production in plants: emerging opportunities and challenges

## 1 INTRODUCTION

Recombinant protein therapeutics have revolutionized modern medicine and are widely used to treat diseases such as diabetes, anemia, hepatitis and cancer. To date, therapeutic recombinant proteins range from vaccines, antibodies, and antibody derivatives to cytokines, growth hormones, interleukins, and interferons. The demand for these recombinant proteins is growing rapidly, which has led to a severe shortage in manufacturing. Conventional extraction of proteins from their natural sources is complicated and expensive. However, proteins from human or animal sources pose viral infection risk and limitations including high cost, low scalability, unsatisfactory safety and protein authenticity. Fig. 1A shows the basic scheme of protein production *via* mammalian, plant, and microbial cells.

The choice of production host for recombinant protein is dependent primarily on the post-translational modifications, which are often required for proper assembly and functionality. Bacterial cells, such as *Escherichia coli* (*E. coli*), lack the machinery to perform necessary post-translational modifications. Mammalian cells provide full post-translational machinery. However, their handling, media, and fermentation requirements are significant and low titre production is kept a challenge. Therefore, simple and inexpensive systems that allow the large-scale production of safe recombinant proteins are desirable. At present, plant bioreactors, such as "Molecular Farming", have become useful biosynthesis platforms for natural products, including triptolide, triptophenolide, celastrol, ginsenosides, and shikonin. Molecular farming by using plant cells or intact plants has practical, economical, and safety advantages when compared with conventional systems. Plants take precedence over microbial or eukaryotic expression systems because they do not foster any microbial, zoonotic pathogens, or oncogenic DNA sequences. Moreover, they can produce proteins with relatively low cost, easier large-scale cultivation and economical advantage when compared with traditional fermentation methods. However, there are limitations linked with the use of transgenic intact plants as a bioproduction platform, such as the risk of contamination from field-grown habitats, exorbitant downstream processing expense, prolonged production timespans, less consistency in product yield, and purification complexity.

The use of plant cells to produce proteins has recently gained attention. Undifferentiated plant calluses can be separated and propagated under a controlled liquid medium environment. They are therefore frequently used as the stable sources of plant suspension cells. Suspension cells grow rapidly, improve the continuity of recombinant protein production, and simplify separation and purification. Furthermore, culturing in a controllable fermenter avoids biotic or abiotic stress and reduces the occurrence of post-transcriptional silence. Previously, over 100 recombinant proteins have been produced in different plant species (Fig. 1B). For example, scientists have successfully introduced the human growth hormone gene into tobacco to obtain the recombinant hormone protein. Additionally, many recombinant antibodies,

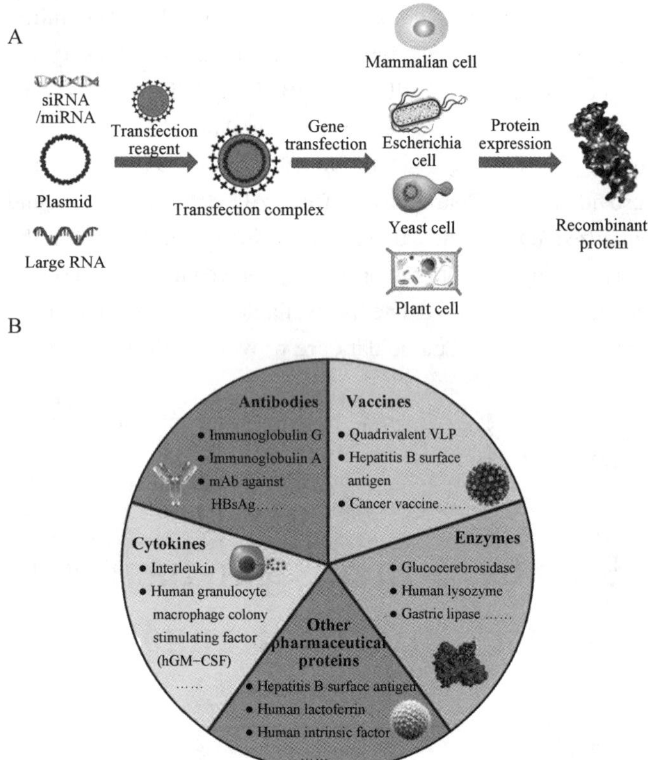


**Fig. 1 Common gene expression platforms for protein production and therapeutic proteins derived from genetic recombinant plant**

(A) Gene expression systems developed for protein production. Plasmid DNA, siRNA, miRNA and other nucleic acids form transfection complexes with delivering reagents. The complexes integrate the target gene into the host cell to express the therapeutic protein. At present, commonly used host cells include mammalian cells, plant cells, *E. coli*, and yeast cells. (B) Plant cells produce therapeutic proteins, including antibodies, vaccines, enzymes and cytokines.

vaccines, enzymes, and cytokines have been expressed in transgenic plants, such as lettuce, tomato, carrot, soybean, potato, alfalfa, rice and maize. The first commercial production of a plant-made pharmaceutical protein is glucocerebrosidase, which was expressed in carrot cells and developed by Protalix. This was approved by the US Food and Drug Administration in 2012 to treat Gaucher's disease and its price remained cheaper than that of drugs from natural sources. Subsequently, plant-made pharmaceutical proteins, such as CaroRX™ for caries prevention, vaccines for hepatitis B treatment, and the human growth factor, Dermokine™ have been approved for marketing. To date, a vast number of protein-based drugs from plants has entered clinical trials. Researches into plant cell bioreactors remains vital.

Plant cell-based platforms are able to produce therapeutic recombinant proteins with accurate post-translational modification. In addition, they offer the benefits of intrinsic safety and lower production cost. Cross contamination with human or zoonotic pathogen has received significant consideration after Genzyme ®, the commercial Gaucher disease therapeutic derived from Chinese Hamster Ovary (CHO) cell. It experienced an interruption in their production due to the infection of calicivirus from their production cell line. In contrast, plant cells do not harbour any known human pathogens, reducing the regulatory and environmental issues required for plant cell-based protein production. Furthermore, plant cells have relatively rapid doubling times and can be grown in simple synthetic media using conventional bioreactors. Taken together, plant cells are appropriate platforms that integrate the merits of the intact plant and microbial fermentation system, namely the "Protein Factory".

In this review, the technological basis of Molecular Farming for protein production *via* whole plant or plant cells are introduced, including the illustration of biological, physical, and chemical technologies for plant genetic engineering. Furthermore, we address the constraints that hinder this technology from reaching its full potential. Moreover, we discuss the design concepts, superiorities, and potential research directions of non-viral nanovector-based gene delivery strategies to plant cells.

## 2 GENETIC RECOMBINATION STRATEGIES FOR PLANT COMPONENTS

The plant cell-based production of recombinant proteins can be divided into three steps: establishment of transgenic suspension cell lines, scale-up culture in the bioreactor, and downstream purification of recombinant proteins (Fig. 2).

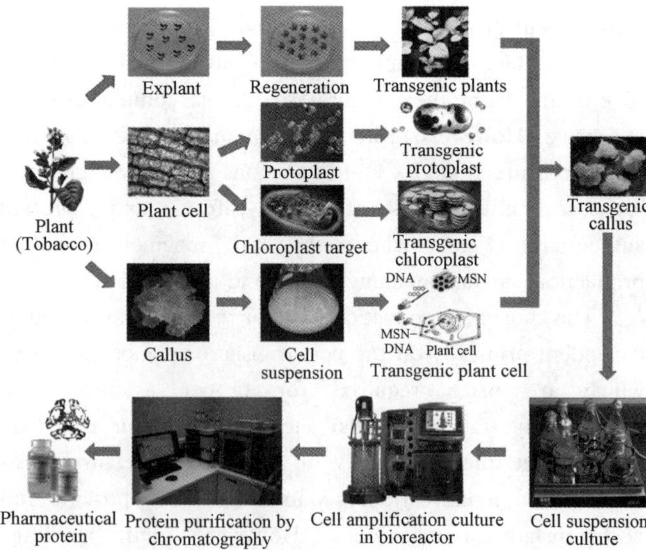


**Fig. 2 Schematic illustration of plant component uses to produce pharmaceutical proteins**

Production suspension cell lines are established from transgenic explants, plant calluses, or cells. After scale-up cultures in the bioreactor, target proteins are produced *via* downstream purification.

An ideal plant cell culture bioreactor system for large scale foreign protein production should possess the following features: 1) ease of genetic manipulation by either stable or transient transfection; 2) high protein expression capacity; 3) low endogenous proteolytic activity; 4) high product stability in the heterologous expression environment (inside and outside of the cells); 5) low concentrations of secondary metabolites that may cause changes in the protein structures, biological properties and/or complicated down streaming process; 6) post-translational modification capability, uniform glycosylation pattern, and regular protein folding; and 7) homogeneous dispersion in a bioreactor.

2.1 Biological strategies for gene recombination in plant components One of the most important steps in plant cell-based protein production is to transform plant cells efficiently. Consequently, the success of genetic transfection is dependent on the employed methods. Various methods have been explored to obtain high gene transfection efficiency in plant cells. Biological methods achieve transfection by viral or bacterial infection and physical methods achieve transfection *via* physical tools. These have solved many problems associated with transgenic plant use and generate a substantial amount of therapeutic proteins (Table 1), however, their further application is currently limited.

**Table 1 Pharmaceutical proteins produced by plant components transfected with biological or physical methods**

| Strategies | Transaction target | Produced proteins | Applications | Transfection efficiency |
|---|---|---|---|---|
| *Agrobacterium* meditated transfection | *W. somnifera* hairy roots | Globular adiponectin | Obesity | Transformation efficiency >70% |
| | Rapeseed (*Brassica napus L.*) seeds | Hemagglutinin-neuraminidase-fusion (HN-F) antigen | Newcastle disease | 45.55 μg HN-F/ seed |
| | *N. benthamiana* leaf disks | Endostatin | Tumor | 3.6 μg endostatin /g total soluble proteins (TSPs) |
| | Broccoli explants | Early secretory antigenic target of M. tuberculosis | Tuberculosis | 5 mg target protein /g TSPs |
| | *N. benthamiana* explants | Adalimumab | Autoimmune and inflammation | 8.5 mg adalimumab/kg fresh leaf. |
| Virus meditated transfection | *N. benthamiana* leaves | Alpha(1)-Microglobulin ($A_1M$-$NB_1$) | Oxidative damage | 50 mg $A_1M$-$NB_1$ /kg fresh leaf |
| | *N. benthamiana* leaves | Human mature interferon γ (mIFNγ) | Rheumatoid arthritis | 209 ± 7 mg mIFNγ /kg cell fresh weight |
| | *N. benthamiana* leaves | Fusion protein lhmlt | Cancer | 42μg lhmlt /mL TSPs solution |
| | *N. benthamiana* leaves | Human myoglobin | Myocardial Injury | 210mg myoglobin /kg fresh leaf tissue |
| Micro projectile bombardment | Tobacco leaves | Interferon-γ | Tuberculosis | 4.2 mg interferon-γ /g TSPs |
| | Tobacco leaves | Proinsulin | Diabetes mellitus type 1 | 2 mg proinsulin /g TSPs |
| | Tobacco leaves | Human tissue-type plasminogen activator(tPA) | Cardiovascular diseases | 31 μg tPA /100 mg leaf tissues. |
| Electroporation | *Chlorella vulgaris* cells | Bovine lactoferrin N-lobe | Iron deficiency anemia | Transformation efficiency two orders of magnitude higher than the glass beads method |

2.1.1 Agrobacterium meditated transfection *Agrobacterium* meditated transfection is the earliest method used in plant transgenesis and remains the most widely used method for plant genetic modification. When virulent strains of *Agrobacterium* infect plant cells, they transfer one or more DNA segments from Tumor inducing (Ti) or Root inducing (Ri) plasmids into host plant cells. Based on these characteristics, the target gene is connected with T-DNA, and then the plant cells can be infected by *Agrobacterium* to achieve gene transfection (Fig. 3A). To date, most pharmaceutical proteins produced by plants are transfected *via Agro-bacterium tumefaciens*. Dehdashti et al. successfully expressed globular adiponectin (gAd) in the hairy root culture of *Withania Somnifera* with *A. tumefaciens* and its yield was 5.1 times higher than gAd produced from *E. coli*. Additionally, Tzvi et al. achieved stable expression of adalimumab *via* co-incubation of *A. tumefaciens* with tobacco leaf sections, which was as effective as commercially available CHO-derived adalimumab (Humira). *Agrobacterium* transfection has low operating cost and simple transfection protocols, however, it is bound by species-range limitations and its inability to execute DNA- and transgene-free editing. Further, *Agrobacterium* contamination during transfection has been noted, inappropriate bacterial concentration and infection times cause plant cell invasion and explant adherence, which can lead to cell death and toxicity. These problems prevent the further application of *Agro-bacterium* in plant transgenes.

2.1.2 Virus-meditated transfection Plant virus-mediated transfection is a widely exploited technique in which a

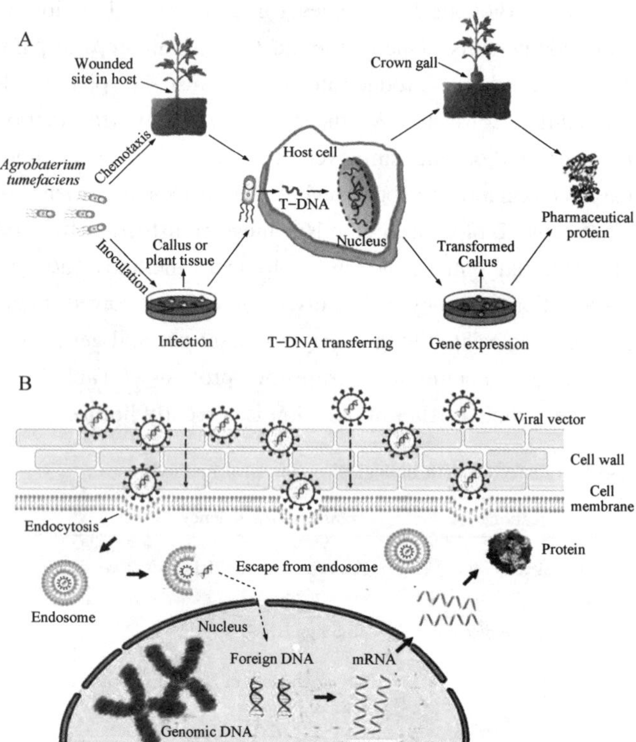


**Fig. 3 Biological methods for gene transfection in plants**

(A) *Agrobacterium*-meditated transfection in plant cells, calluses, and tissues. (B) Virus-meditated transfection in plant cells.

target gene is introduced into the plant virus genome through gene replacement, insertion, or complementation. Next, the virus is used as a vector to introduce the target gene into the recipient cell *via* virus infection (Fig. 3B). The *tobacco mosaic virus* (TMV) was the first exploited virus, which led to the production of a diverse range of proteins of interest. This technique is better than the *Agrobacterium* mediated method because it has high efficiency, shorter production time, and no species-range limitations. Recently, Jiang et al. have enhanced the secretion and solubility of bioactive human mature interferon-γ in TMV by combining a native *N. benthamiana* extensin secretory signal with pKB19. This was an expression system derived from bamboo mosaic virus. Compared with the traditional viral vector systems, the yield was increased by 2.5 times. However, virus-meditated transfection has low stability and the size of the inserted or replaced foreign gene is limited by the viral vector. Moreover, some modified plant viral vectors can spread to other parts of the plant over long distance after formation in inoculated leaves, which causes host plant pathogenesis. These problems have hindered the application and development of viral vectors.

2.2 Physical strategies for gene recombination in plant components

2.2.1 Gene gun-based micro-projectile bombardment Micro-projectile bombardment is executed by introducing DNA into intact cells and tissues by accelerating microparticles driven at high speed through a gene gun. Next, accelerated particles traverse the cell wall and nucleus membrane (Fig. 4A). In the nucleus, exogenous DNA fragments are liberated and may be integrated into chromosomal DNA through illegitimate or homologous recombination, which depends exclusively on cellular components. Shahla et al. successfully introduced interferon-γ into tobacco chloroplast DNA by gene gun-mediated transformation, and reported that protein expression was higher than that compared with nuclear-transformed plants. Similarly, the gene gun supported the transformation of therapeutic proteins, such as proinsulin and human tissue type plasminogen activator. The main advantages of particle bombardment lie in the wide range of target receptors and no host restriction. However, its high cost of application and risks of exogenous gene inactivation and silencing during transfection remain unresolved.

2.2.2 Microinjection Microinjection employs microinjector to directly insert foreign DNA into the cytoplasm or nucleus of recipient cells (Fig. 4C). This method was first used for protoplasts. It had been developed for DNA direct injection in powder (pollen injection), egg cells (zygote injection), and ovaries (ovary injection). Martin et al. successfully injected the neomycin phosphotransferase II gene into the nucleus of tobacco mesophyll protoplasts by microinjection technology, and confirmed that the foreign gene was transmitted to the next generation in the Mendelian fashion. The wide applicability of this method to a variety of plants means that it is an important tool with significant plant transfection potential.

2.2.3 Electroporation Electroporation is a simple and convenient method that directly electroporates walled plant tissues or cells to introduce foreign DNA. The cell membrane is a capacitor with a resting membrane potential of approximately 100 mv. Briefly, an increasing external electric field (V) will break the cell membrane down to form micropores. The opening of micropores leads to nucleic acid perforation from cytoplasm to the nucleus and integration into the chromosome. Electroporation does not puncture cell walls. Therefore, it is often exploited as an auxiliary means for gene delivery. For example, Jungmo et al. successfully perforated the cell wall of *Chlorella vulgaris via* electroporation to introduce the pCAMBIA1304 vector containing the target gene into its nucleus DNA. This achieved bovine lactoferrin N-lobe expression. The micropores produced by electroporation are reversible when compared with gene gun-based technology, which improves the survival rate of plant cells (Fig. 4D). However, the transfection efficiency has not been increased.

2.2.4 The pollen-tube pathway method The pollen-tube pathway method was first proposed in 1983 by exploiting

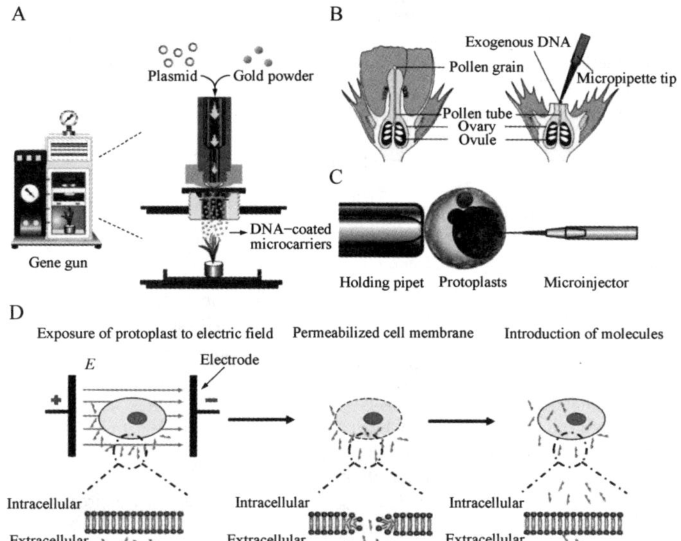


**Fig. 4 Physical methods for gene transfection in plants**

(A) Micro projectile bombardment. (B) Pollen-tube pathway method. (C) Micro-injection. (D) Electroporation.

the germplasm cells of the plant's own reproductive system. Its principle is to use pollen tube channels to introduce foreign DNA into the embryo sac and transform egg cells, zygotes, or early embryonic cells that do not yet have normal cell walls (Fig. 4B). At present, this method is used to improve breed crops. Few report assesses its value in the production of pharmaceutical proteins. Kanghua et al. used the plasmid containing green fluorescent protein (GFP) and β-glucuronidase (GUS) genes to study the transgenic technology of *Dendrobium officinale* using this method. They revealed that exogenous GFP and GUS gene fragments could be detected in almost all the transformed materials. In addition, using the pollen-tube pathway method as a transformation technology can achieve higher transformation efficiency when compared with *Agrobacterium*. Therefore, this method could produce plant-made pharmaceutical proteins in the future. Taken together, this method has a simple and convenient process that uses the natural reproductive process without the need for subsequent tissue culture and regeneration. However, there are limitations, such as a working time limited by the flowering period and difficulties in operating crops with small flowers.

In conclusion, the delivery of biomolecules to plant cells *via* rigid cell walls remains a bottleneck for efficient plant genetic transfection. Currently, there is few delivery tool that can transfer biomolecules into plant cells and each tool has considerable limitations. Biological transgenic methods have certain restrictions, such as species limitations and foreign DNA size limitations. Similarly, physical methods will cause inevitable damage to host cells and biomolecules, which may affect the subsequent transfection. Therefore, the development of a method without restriction on species transfection and does not damage target DNA remains the focus of plant genetic modification studies.

### 2.3 Nanoparticle-based plant transfection strategies

Previously, scientists have sought to chemically link target genes with nanocarriers or encapsulate them in carriers to achieve gene delivery. Various nano-delivery platforms, including the nanoscaled graphene oxide, noble metal nanoparticles, nanomicelles, synthetic and biological vesicles, have been developed for gene delivery. Mechanistically, as the size of nanomaterials decrease, their specific surface area and energy increase rapidly. This generates a large number of dangling and unsaturated bonds, which leads to many chemically active sites. These active sites easily interact with organics or genes to achieve high loading efficiency and produce stable synthetic gene vectors. Accordingly, the synthetic nanovectors are universal platforms for delivering genes to plant cells because they do not induce physical damage or potential infection to cells or protoplasts. In addition, nanocarriers can protect DNA from enzymatic degradation or denaturation. Therefore, focus on nanocarriers as an alternative tool for plant cells transformation has increased.

Multiple nanocarriers can deliver genes into plants, including cationic polymers represented by polyethyleneimine (PEI) and chitosan, phospholipids, and inorganic nanomaterials (Table 2). To date, nanoparticles for plant genetic recombination are composed of carbon, metal, dendrimers, or composite materials, which can transfer DNA into targeted cells to confer stable incorporation and fast transgene expression. Nanoparticles offer efficient conjugation with biomolecules owing to their electronic, optical, and catalytic traits. Additionally, they shield embedded DNA sequences by virtue of a greater surface area and porous design. The post-conjugation of engineered nanoparticles with a gene of interest is ensured by the identification and adsorption on the plant cell membrane. Following this, gene-conjugated nanoparticles are endocytosed. For example, mesoporous nanoparticles with ends crowned with gold nanoparticles that are laden with a gene of interest and chemical inducer can be successfully endocytosed into maize plant cells. Next, an uncrowning stimulus can be exploited to break the bonds holding the gold nanoparticles to the mesoporous nanoparticles, which elicits the cargo and induces the desired gene expression.

2.3.1 Liposomes Studies have reported that liposomes can mediate plant transgenes effectively since 1985. Liposomes are artificial vesicles with external lipid bilayers and internal water layers. The bilayer membrane is fused with the protoplast membrane to facilitate exogenous DNA endocytosis into the cytoplasm, followed by the nucleus to

**Table 2 Applications of nanocarriers in gene delivery to plant components**

| Carriers | Foreign gene | Conjugation | Transfection target | Method | Transfection efficiency |
|---|---|---|---|---|---|
| PEI | GFP plasmid DNA (pDNA) | Electrostatic adsorption | Arabidopsis protoplasts | Co-incubation | 65% |
| PEI | pDNA | Electrostatic adsorption | Saffron cells | Co-incubation | Increased by 2 times under ultrasound |
| Chitosan | GFP pDNA | Electrostatic adsorption | Arabidopsis protoplasts | Co-incubation | 1% |
| Chitosan | GFP pDNA | Electrostatic adsorption | Onion skins | Gene gun | 8% |
| Cadmium selenide- chitosan nanoparticles | GFP pDNA | Electrostatic adsorption | Jatropha calluses | Co-incubation | Successfully express GFP |
| Single-walled carbon nanotubes | ss DNA | π bond stacking | Tobacco BY-2 cells | Co-incubation | 80% |
| PEI-modified carbon nanotubes | Cy3–DNA | Electrostatic adsorption | *N. benthamiana* Mesophyll cells | Leaf injection penetration | 62% |
| Chitosan-modified carbon nanotubes | YFP pDNA | Electrostatic adsorption | Arugula Mesophyll cell chloroplasts | Localized infiltration | 47% |
| PEI-modified triferric oxide nanoparticles | GUS pDNA | Electrostatic adsorption | Cotton pollens | Pollen magnetofection | Successfully express GFP |
| Triethylene glycol modified mesoporous silicon-gold particles | GFP pDNA | Electrostatic adsorption | Tobacco leaves and corn calluses | Gene gun | GFP transient expression |
| Nano-silicon plating gold powder | GFP pDNA | Electrostatic adsorption | Onion skin, tobacco and corn leaves | Gene gun | 76% |
| Calcium phosphate nanoparticles | GUS pDNA | Internal embedding | Mustard cotyledon hypocotyls | Co-incubation | 80.7% |
| Layered double hydroxides | GUS ds RNA | Internal embedding | *N. tabacum* leaves | Spray on the leaves | Successfully express GUS dsRNA |

Yellow fluorescent protein (YFP); Double-stranded RNA (dsRNA); Single-stranded DNA (ssDNA).

achieve target gene expression. This method is minimally cytotoxic and effective in protecting DNA from nuclease degradation. Moreover, it offers a high transfection rate for plant RNA. However, based on its principle, it is only suitable for protoplasts, and difficult to transform intact cells with cell walls.

2.3.2 Polymeric nanoparticles Polyethyleneimine (PEI) is a positively charged cationic polymer that binds to plasmid DNAs (pDNAs) by electrostatic adsorption. After the PEI/pDNAs complex is endocytosed, exogenous protons flow in and a large volume of water inflow causes the endocytic vesicle to lyse and release the PEI/pDNAs complexes through the nucleus membrane into the nucleus. Based on this process, gene transfection is accomplished. Ying et al. fabricated the PEI/pDNAs composites by exploiting the adhering nature of PEI to attach the plant expression plasmid, pCMl205-GFPn. Consequently, plasmids harbouring GFP were expressed in Arabidopsis with a transfection rate of 65%. PEI is a well-recognized plant transfection vector, however, its ability to enter walled plant cells are yet to be elucidated.

2.3.3 Chitosan nanoparticles Chitosan is the derivative product of the natural polysaccharide, chitin. This confers the nano gene carrier system, which has been extensively investigated in biomedicine due to its biocompatibility, biodegradability, strong solubility, and non-toxicity. Yu et al. prepared chitosan/pDNAs nanocomplexes using chitosan as a gene vector. Further, they directly transformed GFP into Arabidopsis protoplasts. However, the transfection efficiency was very low and the nanocomplexes were toxic. Wang et al. prepared chitosan nanoparticles using a cross-linking method. After adsorbing pDNAs by electrostatic action, onion cells were transformed using the gene gun-based method. They observed that 8% of the cells were successfully transformed and expressed the target gene. Interestingly, chitosan nanoparticles could improve the germination of plant seeds, such as cucumber, maize, and chili. It was hypothesized that chitosan formed an excellent semi-permeable coating on the surface of seeds, which retained the moisture of seeds and absorbed the soil moisture. This enhanced their germination rate. Additionally, chitosan had a strong inhibitory effect on the seed microflora, which might be another hypothesis for promoting early seed germination. Chitosan can be chemically and biologically modified to improve the specificity of its gene transfer as a natural high molecular polymer. It retains a strong potential to be developed into a new type of eco-friendly plant genetically engineered-mediating substance.

2.3.4 Carbon nanotubes A carbon nanotube (CNT) is a nanomaterial with a high ratio of diameter length, large payload capacity, and rich functional surface chemistry. CNTs have strong cell membrane penetration and functional modification. Additionally, drugs or nucleic acids can be delivered *via* surface adsorption or macromolecules loading in the cavity tube of CNTs. They are regarded as the most promising gene carriers in future endeavours. The effects of

CNTs on the seed germination and seedling growth are concentration- and species-dependent. At a concentration of 1 000 mg/L, multi-walled carbon nanotubes (MWCNTs) had no effect on the germination process of courgettes and carrots. However, at a concentration of 10~40 mg/L, they significantly enhanced tomato seed germination and seedling growth. The promoting effect of MWCNTs was due to their ability to penetrate the seed coat and promote water uptake. In addition, Cañas et al. compared the effects of single-walled carbon nanotubes (SWCNTs) on plant root growth. They observed that this was species-dependent. There was no effect in cabbages and carrots, but inhibition in tomatoes, and promotion in onions and cucumber seedlings. Therefore, the optimal use conditions of CNT should be verified before actual application.

Liu et al. prepared fluorescein isothiocyanate (FITC)-labelled SWCNTs and observed that it could enter tobacco BY-2 cells and was distributed throughout the cytoplasm. For the first time, they demonstrated the ability of carbon nanotubes to traverse across plant cell walls and cell membranes. Gozde et al. have shown the development and optimization of dialysis and electrostatic grafting methods to load DNA plasmids or linear amplicons onto high aspect ratio CNTs. They confirmed the feasibility and tested the efficacy of this platform by delivering reporter GFP pDNA constructs into mature tobacco, arugula, wheat and cotton leaves, and arugula protoplasts, and obtained strong functional transgenic protein expression. Seon et al. recently invented a novel SWNT-chitosan based pH-mediated gene delivery platform for chloroplast transgene delivery to solve the outcrossing issues of nuclear genome transfection. According to the lipid exchange envelope penetration model, chitosan-wrapped SWNTs could carry the target gene through the cell wall and into the plant cells. Meanwhile, based on the pH difference of the different partitions of plant cells, the primary amines of chitosan achieved targeted hydrolysis to deliver the target gene to the chloroplast. This selective nanoparticle-mediated chloroplast transgene delivery platform was simple, easy to perform, cost-effective, implementable to mature plants across different species, and did not require specialized or expensive equipment. Therefore, it had widespread applications in plant bioengineering and plant biology studies.

2.3.5 Magnetic nanoparticles The magnetic transfection technique employs magnetic nanoparticles (MNPs) combined with DNA, which are transfected into cells under the influence of an external magnetic field. This method has been applied widely in animal cell transfection. Zhao et al. developed a pollen magnetic transfection technique to avoid the hindrance of plant cell walls to foreign genes by delivering genes to pollen, which had 5~10 μm apertures in its cell wall. In this system, positively charged, PEI-coated $Fe_3O_4$ MNPs were used as DNA carriers to bind and condense with DNA to form MNP-DNA complexes. After mixing MNP-DNA complexes with pollen, a magnetic field was then applied to direct the MNP-DNA complexes into the pollen through the apertures before pollination. Transgenic plants were obtained after kanamycin screening from transformed seeds. Exogenous DNAs had been successfully integrated, effectively expressed, and stably inherited in plants. However, Barrena et al. reported that $Fe_3O_4$ nanoparticles inhibited the germination of cucumber and lettuce seeds and reduced the elongation of primary roots. In this case, the small size of nanoparticles (7.6 nm) could be more easily absorbed by the roots during plant growth. Following this, excess iron (Fe) would be highly reactive and toxic due to reactive oxygen species (ROS) overproduction *via* the Fenton reaction. In summary, pollen magnetofection technology is convenient and fast, because it does not require tissue culture and prominently diminishes the duration cost. However, the potential toxicity of magnetic nanoparticles and pollen specificity associated with pollen magnetic-based transfection technology require further improvement.

2.3.6 Mesoporous silicon nanoparticles Silicon is an important element in plant formation, thereby silicon-based materials have good plant biocompatibility. Dequan et al. investigated the effects of mesoporous silicon nanoparticles (MSNs) on the growth and development of wheat and lupin under controlled conditions. They found that when mature wheat seeds were treated with 500 and 2 000 mg/L MSN, their germination significantly improved. Furthermore, the germination of lupin seeds exposed to 1 000 mg/L MSNs was significantly enhanced. The ability of MSNs to penetrate the seed coat while supporting water uptake may explain this phenomenon. However, further research was required to elucidate the exact mechanism. In addition, they did not promote plant root elongation in two experimental plants. MSNs are one of the most popular plant gene nanocarriers. They can efficiently introduce foreign genes into different plant tissues and achieve expression *via* gene gun. In 2007, Torney et al. first used triethylene glycol-modified mesoporous silicon encapsulating gold particles to deliver GFP pDNAs, which were electrostatically adsorbed onto mesoporous silicon. Following this, Ortigosa et al. fixated gold powder particles onto the surface of mesoporous silicon *via* multiple electroplating methods and attached the pDNAs with electrostatic adsorption to bombard the walled onion epidermis with a gene gun. Using this method, the transfection rate was enhanced to $>76\%$ when compared with the MSN system reported by Tony. Notably, gold-plated MSNs have been used for the biolistic gene gun to deliver the Cre-recombinase, a kind of tool for the site-specific recombination, and finally reached a transfection efficiency of 20%. This demonstrated the ability of MSNs to deliver the hybrid pDNAs-proteins for gene editing. Taken together, these studies highlight that MSNs can be used as highly biosafety nano-vehicles not only to efficiently deliver DNA into plants, but also to achieve targeted gene editing, which can aid further investigation of plant genomics and gene function as well as improvement of crop species.

2.3.7 Gold nanoparticles  Gold is used in diverse applications, including gene delivery, due to its inactive nature, ease of synthesis, and high functionalization ability. In 2013, Hao et al. synthesized magnetic gold nanoparticles (mGNPs) of uniform size and morphology, and covalently bound FITC molecules to their surface. Driven by an external magnetic field, FITC-labelled nanoparticles had a delivery efficiency of 95% in canola protoplasts and walled cells. This indicated the great potential of mGNPs in plant gene transfection. In 2015, Hitomi et al. fabricated a conical-shaped gold microneedle array using the template-synthesis method, which then coated with pDNAs. The microneedles punctured the cell surface of *Chlamydomonas reinhardtii* to facilitate DNA endocytosis into the cytoplasm. Cell viability tests showed that the plant cells remained viable after being punctured and the genes were successfully expressed. Furthermore, the application of gold nanoparticles in certain crops had beneficial effects. Treatment of cucumber and lettuce seeds with a solution containing 62 μg/mL Au nanoparticles for 7 days promoted the seed germination. Similar results were shown after immersing pearl millet in 20—50 μg/mL of Au nanoparticles for 2 h. These results indicated that gold microneedles held immense potential as a low-toxic gene delivery platform for microalgae, and perhaps for plant cells.

2.3.8 Calcium phosphate nanoparticles  Calcium phosphate (CaP) is found in human physiological tissues. CaP nanoparticles are widely acknowledged for gene delivery in animal cells due to their good biocompatibility and low immunogenicity. In 2002, Sone et al. produced micrometre-sized calcium alginate beads that encapsulated pDNAs. Approximately ten-fold higher GFP expression was observed after 24 h incubation using the bio-beads treatment when compared with the conventional method of using a naked pDNAs solution. Following this, Naqvis et al. developed the ultra-small-pore calcium phosphate nanoparticles that encapsulated a binary vector using the GUS reporter gene to transfect the hypocotyl. GUS delivered by CaPs successfully entered the nucleus and expressed with a conversion rate reaching 80.7%. This demonstrated that CaP nanoparticles could be efficiently applied in plant cell transfection.

2.3.9 Clay nanosheets  Layered double hydroxides (LDHs) are a classic anionic layered compound composed of positively charged structural units. Anions or neutral molecules are freely movable between layers to compensate for charge balance. Based on its strong anion exchange capacity, it can insert negatively charged biomolecules such as DNAs into it by substitution to form a gene carrier. In 2017, Neena et al. used LDH nanosheets to deliver dsRNAs into mature plants. dsRNA was loaded onto LDH and converted into a spray. Gene transfection was achieved by spraying onto the leaf surface. This demonstrated that LDH nanosheets protected dsRNA from RNase degradation and environmental conditions such as rain and sunlight. At the same time, this nanocarrier could be dissolved by the carbonic acid, which was formed from $CO_2$ and the water film on the leaf surface, allowing a stable release of dsRNAs. LDH nanosheets provide a novel way of gene transfection, however, the delivery mechanism remains unexplored.

To date, nanodelivery systems have made significant progress in the field of plant transgenic recombination. Practically, the size of foreign gene inserted or replaced in the plant virus vector is limited by the vector itself, making it feasible for the expression small gene fragments alone. If the expression of large gene fragments is required, *Agrobacterium* transformation or physical methods are used. These methods can achieve transfection, however, there are some obstacles at the application level. *Agrobacterium* transfection is restricted by the host and can only transfect dicotyledonous plants. The pollen tube passage must be carried out during the flowering period of plants, and methods such as gene gun, electroporation, and microinjection require expensive equipment and complicated operation steps. As the gene delivery platforms, nanocarriers have no restriction on transfection target and are less toxic. They can carry nucleic acids of the same size carried by physical equipments with more convenient operating conditions and low cost (Table 3). Nanocarriers can be designed as the 'rocket' loaded with external genes (Fig. 5A, B) to be delivered to a specific site of plant cells, calluses, and intact plants for targeting transfection (Fig. 5C). Plant cells contain multiple organelles with highly polyploid genomes, therefore, the structural optimization of nanocarriers (such as pH-mediated and targeted peptide modification) to achieve plastid and mitochondrial targeting can increase the expression of target gene. For plant callus delivery, combining the nanodelivery platform with a gene gun or ultrasound can render stably expressed transgenic plants (Fig. 5D). Similarly, through leaf injection, nanocarriers can realise gene transfer in mature intact plants without the aid of external chemical or mechanical force (Fig. 5E). These results demonstrate the great potential of nano-technology and physical technique combination as novel strategies in plant genetic transfection.

## 3 MECHANISMS OF NANOPARTICLES MEDIATED GENE DELIVERY IN PLANT CELLS

The successful penetration of nanoparticle into plants requires either apoplastic (occurs exterior to plasmalemma) or symplastic (occurs interior to plasmalemma and adjacent cells cytoplasm) transport. The symplastic transport pathway is the primary route for the uptake and further translocation of nanoparticles in plant cells. Nanoparticles must be taken up by the plant cells and traverse the plasmalemma to adopt the symplastic pathway. Next, nanoparticles must traverse an array of chemical and physiological barriers that have size exclusion limits. The plant cell wall poses the first barrier. Its intrinsic pore diameter ranges from 5 to 20 nm and serves as a size exclusion limit. However, the maximum nanoparticles size dimension permitted by plant cells for uptake and translocation usually lies within the range of 40–50 nm. Multiple mechanisms are exploited to account for this, such as nanoparticle-meditated endocytosis, pore formation, plasmodesmata, transport proteins, and ion channels.

Nanoparticles are internalized into cells during endocytosis *via* the formation of a cavity-like structure around nanoparticles with a phospholipid bilayer. The resultant vesicles can translocate into various cell compartments (Fig. 6). In addition to this, the pore formation mechanism is induced by nanoparticle disruption in the plasmalemma in a similar fashion to cell wall penetration. After successful pore enlargement and formation, nanoparticles can easily arrive in the cytoplasm, avoiding any entrapment or organelle encapsulation. Another passage for nanoparticles to enter plant cells is *via* plasmodesmata, which is the exclusive channel traversing cell walls. It facilitates the translocation of materials between plant cells with a size exclusion limit of 3–50 nm. Moreover, nanoparticles can also cross cellular barriers by adhering to surrounding transport proteins, including plasma membrane proteins, such as aquaporins, which could perform as the vehicles for internalisation into the cell cytoplasm. However, their miniscule pore size sets constraints for nanoparticle penetration, unless this can be altered. Lastly, ion channels, despite having a very small pore size (1 nm), may be a po-tential passage for nanoparticle internalisation, however, they will be subjected to vital modifications. Among these mechanisms, endocytosis seems to be the best route to deliver nanoparticles into a specific organelle and helpful in evading endosomes and other lytic organelles. In addition, the chemical composition, morphology type, and surface coating of nanoparticles may influence the nature and extent of its internalisation and translocation in plant cells.

**Table 3 DNA/RNA delivery capabilities of current transfection technologies for plant components**

| Categories | Delivery strategies | Transaction targets | Cargo types | Cargo size (approximately) |
|---|---|---|---|---|
| Biological transfection methods | *Agrobacterium* meditated transfection | Cells, explants and seeds | pDNA | 15 kb |
| | Virus meditated transfection | Leaves | pDNA, small interfering RNA (siRNA), miRNA | 1.5 kb |
| Physical transfection methods | Micro-projectile bombardment | Cells and tissues | pDNA, siRNA, miRNA | 15 kb |
| | Microinjection | Protoplasts | pDNA | 15 kb |
| | Electroporation | Cells and protoplasts | pDNA, siRNA, miRNA | 15 kb |
| | Pollen-tube pathway method | Sperms and eggs | pDNA | 15 kb |
| Nanoparticles based transfection methods | Liposome | Protoplasts | pDNA, RNA | 5 000 bp (5 kb) |
| | Polymeric nanoparticles | Cells | pDNA, ssDNA, siRNA, miRNA | 5 000 bp (5 kb) |
| | Chitosan nanoparticles | Cells and protoplasts | pDNA | 12 kb |
| | Carbon nanotube | Cells and leaves | ssDNA, siRNA, pDNA | 5 kb |
| | Magnetic nanoparticles | Cells and protoplasts | pDNA | 15 kb |
| | Mesoporous silicon nanoparticles | Cells and tissues | pDNA | 15 kb |
| | Gold nanoparticles | Cells and embryos | pDNA | 11.5 kb |
| | Calcium phosphate nanoparticles | Cells | pDNA | 15 kb |
| | Clay nanosheets | Leaves | miRNA, dsRNA, pDNA | 15 kb |

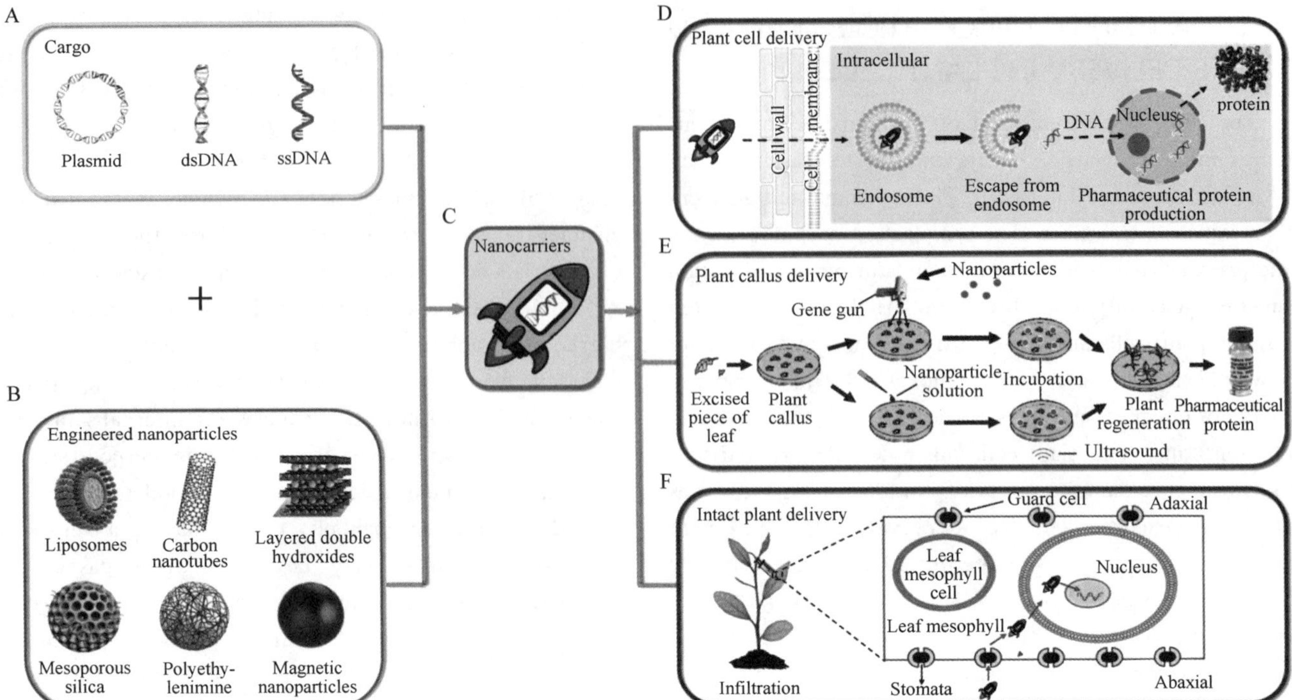


**Fig. 5 Schematic representation of the applications of nanovectors in plant-derived pharmaceutical protein production**

(A) Engineering nanoparticles as carriers for delivery of exogenous cargos, (B) including pDNAs, double-strand DNAs (dsDNAs) and ssDNAs. (C) Nanoparticles used as vectors for gene delivery to plant cells. (D) Nanoparticles used as DNA vectors for gene delivery to plant calluses. (E) Nanoparticles used as DNA vectors for gene delivery to intact plants.

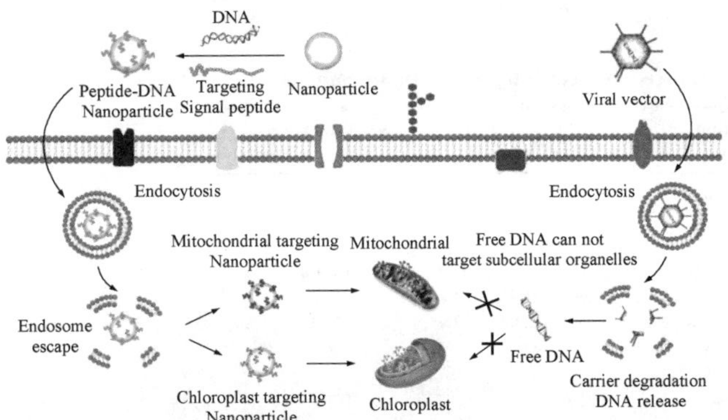


**Fig. 6 Schematic diagram of nanoparticles used as DNA vector targeting plant subcellular organelles**

Nanoparticles transport DNA to plant subcellular organelles, such as mitochondria or chloroplasts, by connecting specific targeting signal peptides. By contrast, viral DNA vectors do not achieve similar targeting functions.

## 4 COMBINED STRATEGIES FOR GENE DELIVERY IN PLANT COMPONENTS

Nanomaterials have been used as carriers for gene delivery to mammalian cells *in vitro* & *in vivo* for many years, however, researches into plant gene delivery are relatively new, due to the plant cell wall constraints. Furthermore, the uptake and transport of nanoparticles throughout plant tissue are limited by pore diameters, setting size exclusion for various tissues and organs. Plasma and nuclear membranes pose additional barriers to delivery where cytosolic or nuclear localisation is necessary to affect gene function. The development of a hybrid strategy using nanomaterials and physical techniques, such as ultrasound or sonication, may boost the transfection efficiency of nanovectors in plant cells. Use of the PEI/DNAs complex and sonication has a synergistic effect on DNA transmission to saffron cells. The hybrid utilisation of ultrasound and PEI nanoparticles increase the transfection efficiency of saffron cells by up to two times more than those obtained by PEI or ultrasound separately. Moreover, nanomaterials act as gene carriers, protect genes from lysosomes, and allow target genes to enter the nucleus through the nucleus membrane in this hybrid system. Furthermore, the physical methods assist the perforation of nanocarriers through plant cell walls. Laser microbeam aspiration and ultrasound mediation produce holes in the cell wall. Reversible pore formation means that cells can heal automatically after a brief duration without affecting subsequent growth. Nanogene delivery using this hybrid technique exploits laser microbeams or ultrasound to permit the carrier entry into the cell *via* a channel, which improves delivery efficiency. Meanwhile, cell wall perforation resolves any restrictions on the choice of nanomaterials. This methodology enables the exploitation of certain nanomaterials that cannot enter the cells as gene carriers but exhibit low toxicity. Some studies have reported that the combination of nanocarriers and ultrasound can improve the transfection efficiency of nanocarriers in animals *via* ultrasound targeted microbubble destruction. Based on this, it may be feasible to use nanotechnology and physical methods to deliver genes into plants. Rajesh et al. have recently reported the use of a disposable polymer microneedle patch. Plant DNA can be extracted within one minute after attaching the patch to its leaves. This highlights that microneedles are a promising tool to deliver the DNAs/RNAs into the plant cells. Microneedle-based technology can deliver nanoparticles into plant cells more conveniently by circumventing a series of operations, such as plant cell extraction. Similarly, while the microneedles are attached to the leaves, this process can be assisted by ultrasound or laser stimulation to improve transfection efficiency. In short, the development of appropriate physical methods to assist nanocarriers can produce a multiplier effect for gene delivery.

## 5 STRATEGIES FOR EDITING SPECIFIC PLANT GENES

With the advancement of gene delivery technologies, genetic engineering can now introduce target genes into plants *via* a series of transgenic methods. However, most of these transgenic technologies cannot perform specific plant gene editing. The host genome site where the transgene is inserted into is random, which may cause redundant mutation due to the disruption of active plant genes. In order to solve above-mentioned problems, targeted gene editing tools such as homologous recombination (HR), zinc finger nucleases (ZFNs), transcription activator-like effector nucleases (TALENs), and clustered regularly interspaced short palindrome repeats (CRISPRs) have been utilized for the gene editing in plants. Especially, HR introduces foreign genes into the chromosomes of recipient cells, because there is a sequence homologous to the introduced gene at this locus. Through single or double exchange, new gene fragment can replace original gene fragment to achieve the gene editing purpose. However, HR is often accompanied by non-homologous end joining (NHEJ). NHEJ will force the two DNA ends to be connected to each other, reducing the probability of correct insertion of the target gene and resulting in insufficient HR efficiency. Blocking the NHEJ may be a good strategy, but studies have reported that there may be independent end joining pathways in plants. When single NHEJ factors were knocked out, the DNA transfection efficiency was slightly reduced. So far, no convincing research has been published to improve the efficiency of HR by blocking the NHEJ. However, as engineered nuclease technology matures, it has gradually become a new direction to improve plant gene targeting.

ZFNs are artificial restriction enzymes. They are developed by linking the zinc-finger DNA binding domain that recognizes a specific DNA sequence with the restriction enzyme *Fok* Ⅰ, which cuts DNA or nuclease domain through peptide bonds. The zinc finger domain $Cys_2$-$His_2$ designed at the N-terminus can recognize new DNA sequences in complex genomes, thereby manipulate ZFNs for precisely editing of the endogenous gene loci in eukaryotic organisms. To deliver ZFNs into cells, electroporation is usually used. At present, ZFNs have achieved targeted plant mutagenesis such as heat-shock promoter, stress response regulator and ABA INSENSITIVE$_4$ in Arabidopsis. In addition, ZFNs are also used to edit endogenous genes in maize, tobacco, bread wheat and soybeans. However, it is worth noting that if the Zinc Finger domain is inaccurately specific for the target site or the target is not unique in the eukaryotic genome, the engineered nuclease will be off-target and inactivated.

TALENs are developed by fusing transcription activator-like effectors (TALEs) to the catalytic domain of Fok Ⅰ endonuclease. As an alternative to ZFNs, the structures are similar to ZFNs, including the non-specific nuclease domain of Fok1 and a customizable DNA binding domain. Currently, TALENs have been frequently used as the choice of engineered nucleases in human cell lines and animal species, but due to the long generation time in plants, the application of these enzymes in plants is scarce. However, in 2012, Li et al. used TALENs for targeted mutations within the ALS gene of transformed tobacco protoplasts. The efficiency of gene targeting as high as 14%. Recently, the TALENs technology has realized glycol-engineering and monoclonal antibody production in tobacco, which demonstrated that TALENs might be a very effective tool for targeted gene editing in plants.

The latest tool for gene targeting is based on the enhanced efficiency of the CRISPR/CRISPR-associated (Cas) type Ⅱ prokaryotic system. CRISPR forms a part of bacterial and archaeal adaptive immunity against viruses and plasmids in the form of immune memories from previous infections. The expression of these sequences results in small non-coding RNAs or interfering CRISPR RNAs (crRNAs), which in turn guide the Cas9 endonucleases to the target sequence, thereby cutting them. CRISPR/Cas9 has been used to manipulate eukaryotic genomes such as human cells, zebrafish, yeast and mice. This revolutionary technology has also been used in plants to raise grain weight and increase the blast resistance to improve rice productivity. Recently, with the widespread application of nanodelivery platforms in the field of plant research, the combination of CRISPR and nanotechnology has emerged. Liu et al. successfully delivered Cas9/guide RNA ribonucleoprotein complex into tobacco cv. BY-2 protoplasts by using two lipofection reagents, Lipofectamine 3 000 and RNAiMAX. Finally, they achieved the the best transfection efficiency of 66% and 48%, respectively. Sun et al. used pepper B2 as the test material, combined magnetic nanoparticles and CRISPR/Cas9-carrying plasmids at a mass ratio of 1 : 1, and introduced the nano-mixture into pollen through a magnetic plate under the action of a magnetic field. The results showed that the average transfection efficiency was about 63.70%. What's more, Khromov et al. combined functionalized chitosan nanoparticles with CRISPR/Cas9, delivered them into the potato meristem by means of vacuum infiltration, and successfully edited the StPDS gene. Although the nano-platform technology for delivering CRISPR/Cas9 has just started, its development can solve the problems caused by traditional delivery methods. With the rapid development of delivery methods, it is imperative to successfully transform the CRISPR/Cas9 technology into agricultural applications and major improvements can be anticipated.

## 6 OUTLOOK

Traditional bacterial fermentation and mammalian cell production have been unable to meet the supply of market demand for pharmaceutical proteins. Coupled with the safety and production cost of expression systems, a cheaper and safer protein synthesis platform is urgently needed. The advantages of a plant expression system lie in its lower investment and operating costs, and DNA sequences that are not pathogenic to humans and animals. Furthermore, plant suspension cell bioreactors have a shorter protein production cycle, simple production conditions, and downstream post-translational modification capabilities when compared with the whole-plant system. This indicates the significant potential for processing factories that replace bacteria and mammals.

The most serious problem encountered by plant factories in the production of pharmaceutical proteins is the low protein expression that cannot meet the requirements of commercial production. Protein yield mainly depends on the expression degree of the foreign protein and the expression ability of the host. The construction of plasmid is essential to increase the target protein expression. Furthermore, tissue-specific or inducible promoters are advantageous. For example, the expression efficiency of the CaMV 35S promoter in dicot plants is higher than in monocot plants, while Actin and Ubi promoters are more suitable for monocot plants. It is necessary to select plant-preferred codons according to their degeneracy to make full use of the tRNA in the host plant. In addition, the use of specific regulatory sequences, such as the tobacco etch virus 5′ untranslated guide sequence, as a translation enhancer can improve expression efficiency.

The choice of host is crucial for plant protein production. Currently, higher plant chloroplasts are becoming an ideal host for foreign gene expression based on their characteristics. The chloroplast genome is separate from the nuclear genome and highly polyploidy, therefore, chloroplast transformation can lead to extremely high levels of protein production by introducing thousands of foreign genes in each plant cell. Accumulating evidences show that multiple approaches can ensure the correct folding of proteins in chloroplasts and eliminate the misfolded proteins in time, which maintains the stability of organelle proteins during the production of pharmaceutical proteins by plants. In addition, the maternal inheritance of chloroplast genomes in mostly higher plants leads to restrictions in transgenic hybridisation. This makes the introduced foreign genes safer and more stable. Therefore, targeting chloroplasts is an alternative strategy to improve protein production. At present, the most commonly used method modifies the localisation signal sequence on the foreign gene to create an expressed foreign protein transport to the chloroplast. For example, Yoshizumi et al. connected DNA with the Arabidopsis chloroplast-targeted polypeptide, AtOEP34, through a polycationic DNA binding domain (KH), and successfully achieved the targeted delivery of chloroplast genome. Interestingly, Seon et al. designed a pH-mediated CNT vector by taking advantage of the difference in pH between the chloroplast and cytoplasm. This directed the reporter gene YFP into the chloroplast and achieved transient expression. Therefore, the targeted delivery of chloroplasts can be achieved by structural modifications to nanocarriers.

High-yield protein processing plants depend on efficient gene delivery methods. Currently, nanodelivery platforms have relatively mature applications in mammalian cells, but they remain in infancy in plant gene delivery. Several studies have reported that the expression of reporter genes in plant cells is achieved through nanodelivery vectors and it has a higher efficiency than conventional methods. In a reported case, it was found that the gene gun based transfection method would lead to variable tissue penetration depth, depending on the plant species and tissue types. Plants with thicker tissues tend to have lower transfection efficiency. However, using nanocarriers can overcome this challenge, and achieve stable and uniform gene expression in the plant species and tissues of different types. At the same time, the strategy based on nanocarriers can not only reduce cell damage and increase the success rate of transfection, but also express the target gene in dicotyledonous and monocotyledonous plants, effectively solving the problem that conventional transgenic methods only transfect limited species. In addition, the results showed that *Agrobacterium* transformation method could integrate the target gene into the plant genomic DNA during the transfection process, which would cause genetic pollution in the subsequent passage of plants. However, there was no gene integration for gene delivery with the nanocarriers, which fitted well with the global demands of non-integrative and/or DNA-free plant genetic transformation approaches. Therefore, nanocarriers are expected to be developed into the major vectors for carrying functional plasmids into plant cells for many applications such as the production of pharmaceutical proteins. Besides that, nanocarriers also have the advantage in allowing simple coupling chemistry to carry other biomolecular cargoes, such as ZFNs, TALENs, and CRISPR/Cas9 to achieve the targeted editing of plant genes. Additionally, gene-assisted delivery systems (such as laser and ultrasound generation systems) are worth development. Nanocarriers can carry more functional genes into plant cells when mediated by laser microbeams and ultrasound. This can promote the production of diversified pharmaceutical proteins.

In summary, nanomaterials have come to prominence as gene carriers in plant transgenics. We believe that further research will highlight the significant potential of nanomaterials to become a universal plant gene delivery platform and progress protein production. To date, the mechanism by which foreign genes are integrated into plant genomes remains unclear, therefore, elucidating the entry mechanism of nano-materials, improving transfection efficiency, and establishing an efficient nanocarrier plant transfection system are challenges to be solved. For the ultimate goal of achieving economically feasible yields of pharmaceutical proteins that are structurally and functionally equivalent to their native counterparts, bioengineering-based systematic and concerted research efforts will be critical to the success of any plant cell culture protein production platform.

[彭丽华,黄璐琦,等. Biotechnology Advance, 2022,54: 107845.]

# Biosynthesis, total synthesis, and pharmacological activities of aryltetralin-type lignan podophyllotoxin and its derivatives

## 1 INTRODUCTION

PTOX, a type of aryltetralin-type lignan, was first discovered in the plant *P. peltatum* and its structure was clarified by W. Borsche and J. Niemann in 1932. PTOX is considered a potent anti-cancer agent and occupies a unique and significant place among lignan natural products through chemical structural modification. Etoposide (VP-16) and teniposide (VM-26), the typical glycosyl derivatives of PTOX commonly used in the clinic, exert significant effects on the treatment of almost all types of cancer cells. Since the 1980s, dozens of PTOXs anti-cancer drugs targeting lung cancer, leukemia, lymphatic cancer, breast cancer, testicular cancer, glioma, and other multiple human cancers have entered clinical phases Ⅰ-Ⅲ. The natural drug deoxypodophyllotoxin (DPT) and its injection, a new class Ⅰ anti-cancer drug, won the approval for phase Ⅰ drug clinical research issued by the National Medical Products Administration in China in 2017. Indeed, because of the potential therapeutic effects and special chemical structure, PTOX has attracted the interest of numerous scholars. To develop it into a clinical drug, it is necessary to solve the challenges of resources and production, elucidating the molecular mechanism of its pharmacological effects, as well as clinical trials. In this review, we will discuss the research progress and development trends of PTOX in biosynthesis, total synthesis, and pharmacological activities, which may cause the attention of many researchers in the fields of synthetic biology, chemistry, pharmacology, clinical research, *etc*.

Currently, extracting from plants such as *Sinopodophyllum hexandrum* (Royle) Ying, *P. peltatum* from Podophylloideae (Berberidaceae, Ranunculales) is the main method to obtain natural PTOXs. However, with the recklessly extensive excavation of medicinal natural resources, wild *S. hexandrum* has become an endangered species. Biotechnological strategies, such as endophytic fungus culture, have also become feasible alternatives at present.

In recent years, with the sequencing of plant genomes and transcriptomes such as *Tripterygium wilfordii*, *Taxus chinensis*, and *Panax notoginseng*, the biosynthetic pathways of many star compounds such as triptolide, celastrol, and paclitaxel have been gradually revealed, bringing the hope for the heterologous synthesis of these natural compounds by using biotechnological strategies such as the microbial cell factories or plant chassis. Nowadays, the technology of synthetic biology has achieved some inspiring results, some precursors such as artemisinin (25 g/L), taxadiene (1 g/L), and miltiradiene (3.5 g/L) have realized gram-scale production. Therefore, the key to realizing the heterologous biosynthesis of PTOX is to identify its biosynthetic pathway genes. By 2019, the biosynthetic pathway of PTOX and its derivatives have almost been revealed, making it possible for heterologous biosynthesis of pathway intermediates. For example, using the late-stage biosynthetic precursor DPT has realized milligram-scale production, both in *Escherichia coli* and plant classis. The upstream compounds caffeic acid (CaA) and ferulic acid (FA) were achieved in gram-level production ($5.5 \pm 0.2$ g/L CaA, $3.8 \pm 0.3$ g/L FA) in microbial cell factories by engineering cofactor supply and recycling. Moreover, the catalytic mechanism of pathway enzymes, such as dirigent proteins (DIRs), secoisolariciresinol dehydrogenase (SDH), and deoxypodophyllotoxin synthase (DPS) have been revealed, enhancing understanding of a growing number of biochemical transformations.

Chemical synthesis is another effective approach to producing PTOXs. The first reported in 1966, the original chemical total synthesis product is basically racemic compounds. At present, methods such as Friedel-Crafts alkylation and metallic ion catalytic strategies have been able to strictly control the chirality of compounds and have been gradually developed for commercial use. Some chemo-enzymatic synthesis of PTOXs, which combine the advantages of efficiency and extension of chemical synthesis and stereo-selectivity and precision of biosynthesis, have been reported with the knowledge of biosynthetic pathway, making it possible to form enantiomeric products through concise routes.

The structure of PTOX contains five rings (A - E) and four consecutive chiral centers (C1 - C4), which exert strong pharmacological activities in cancer cells by inhibiting microtubule assembly and type Ⅱ topoisomerase (TOP2) degradation. The research and development of PTOX new drugs is a hot spot around the world, impelling researchers to design and synthesize derivatives with less cytotoxicity and drug resistance through structural modification, as well as separation from natural plants. In these efforts, anti-cancer types, activities, and mechanisms of different structurally modified compounds have been revealed, providing more basis for the clinical application of these potent drugs. Moreover, the insecticidal and antiviral activities of PTOX can also be improved by structural modification.

In this review, we will focus on the recent advances in biosynthesis, total synthesis, and pharmacological activities of PTOX and its derivatives. We believe it will be meaningful work and might arouse the interest of many biologists, chemists, pharmacologists, and clinical researchers, providing references for related studies on PTOXs.

## 2 BIOSYNTHESIS

2.1 Upstream pathway The upstream pathway of PTOXs involves multiple routes starting from L-phenylalanine and L-tyrosine to coniferyl alcohol (CA) (Fig. 1). This phenylpropanoid pathway is one of the main universal ways to synthesize secondary metabolite phenols in plants, such as flavonoids, lignan, and coumarins. Phenylalanine ammonia-lyase (PAL) is involved in the first committed step of phenylpropanoid pathway, catalysing the deamination of L-phenylalanine to produce cinnamic acid, which is subsequently hydroxylated at the C - 4 positions *via* a cytochrome P450 monooxygenase cinnamate 4-hydroxylase (C4H) to generate *p*-coumaric acid. Another pathway to generate *p*-coumaric acid involves catalysis by tyrosine ammonia-lyase (TAL) to directly transform L-tyrosine into *p*-coumaric acid.

Due to the need for lignan synthases from different families to form a variety of bioactive lignans, the pathway from *p*-coumaric acid to CA is complex and about ten enzymes are involved, including 4-coumarate-CoA ligase (4CL), coumarate 3-hydroxylase (C3H), cinnamoyl-CoA reductase (CCR), caffeate 3-*O*-methyltransferase (COMT), caffeoyl aldehyde 3-*O*-methyltransferase (CCoAOMT), cinnamyl alcohol dehydrogenase (CAD), hydroxycinnamoyl-CoA: shikimate/quinate hydroxycinnamoyl transferase (HCT) and *p*-coumaroyl quinate/shikimate 3′-hydroxylase (C3′H).

The main pathway utilizes C3H, 4CL, CCR, *O*-methyltransferase (OMT), and CAD to realize corresponding hydroxylation, enzymization, deenzymization, methylation, and dehydrogenation. CoA ligation of 4-coumaric acid is essential for the 3-hydroxylation of coumarate. 4CL, the main branch point enzyme in phenylpropanoid biosynthesis, converts various hydroxycinnamic acids into CoA esters and contributes to the channelizing flux of different lignan structures, which include constituent monolignol derivatives, namely H, G, and S. Yi Li *et al*. found that four isoforms of 4CL in *Arabidopsis thaliana* have overlapping yet distinct roles in phenylpropanoid metabolism, in which 4CL3 plays a distinct role in the flavonoid pathway while 4CL1, 2, and 4 are more closely related to lignifying process. Jin *et al*. found that *Piper nigrum* 4CL isoforms Pn4CL3 show higher catalytic efficiency towards 3, 4-methylenedioxy-cinnamic and piperic acid, suggesting its specific role in piperine biosynthesis. These results indicate that 4CL is the basis of the diversity of lignan. HCT and C3′H regulate the other collateral pathway between *p*-coumaroyl CoA and feruloyl CoA. HCT is a key metabolic entry point for the synthesis of the most important lignan monomers. It has substrate promiscuity, thus involving a two step catalyses of the CA pathway. The reactions of the shikimate shunt involve the forward "$HCT_{For}$" and reverse "$HCT_{Rev}$" enzymes. $HCT_{For}$ catalysed, the shikimatation of *p*-coumaroyl CoA; the products were then hydroxylated by C3′H to generate caffeoyl quinate and caffeoyl shikimate, which metabolised

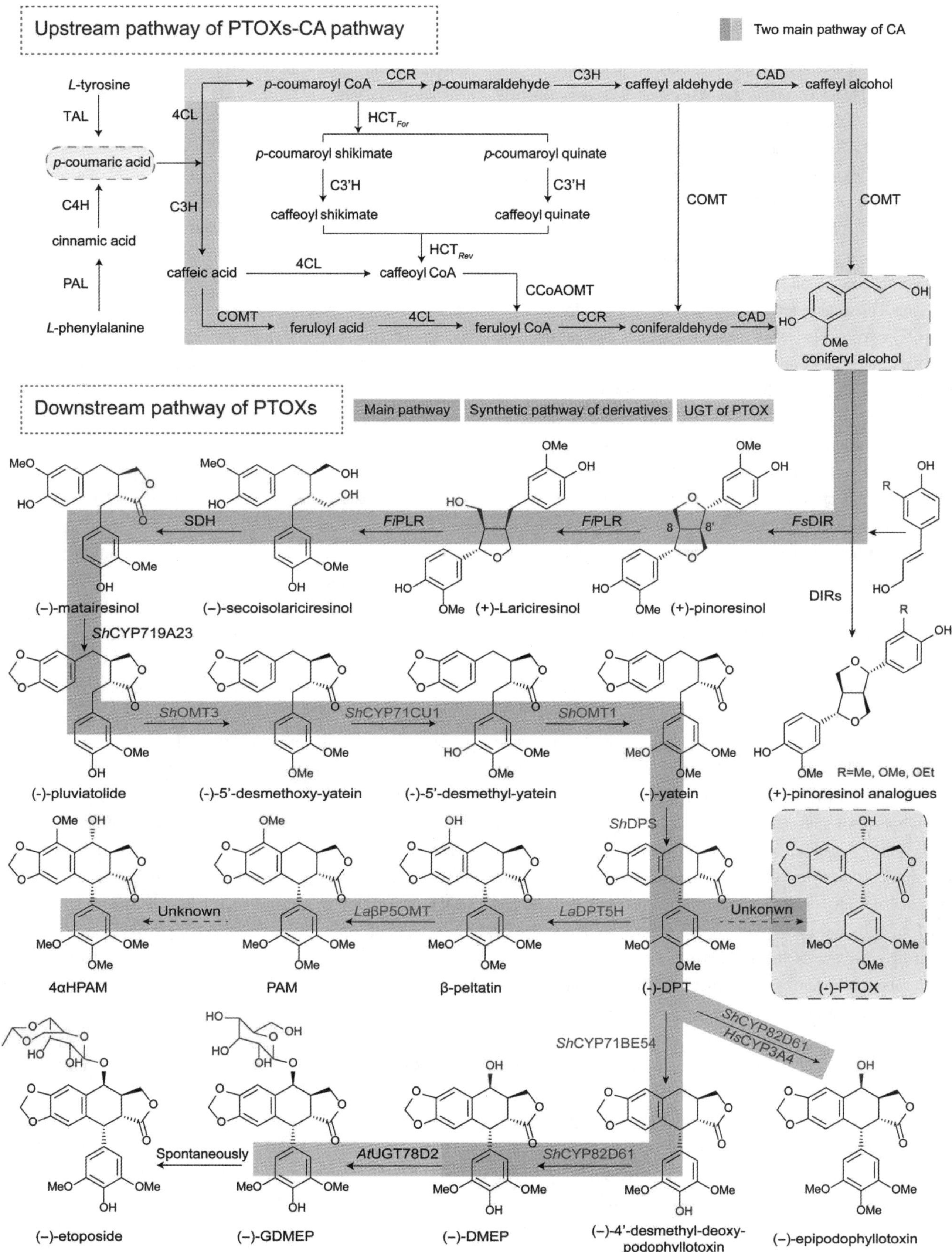


**Fig. 1 Biosynthetic pathway of PTOXs**

*p*-coumaroyl quinate and *p*-coumaroyl shikimate with the same efficiency. $HCT_{Rev}$ returns the CoA back and produces the same compound caffeoyl-CoA.

So far, the upstream pathway of PTOX has been

clarified. It produces CA to participate in the subsequent synthesis steps.

2.2 Downstream pathway The initial step of the downstream pathway starts from CA and is subsequently catalysed by dirigent proteins (DIRs) to produce pinoresinol. DIRs play a crucial role in the biosynthesis of distinct complex classes of bioactive natural plant phenolics such as lignan and aromatic terpenoid and impart stereo-selectivity to phenoxy radical coupling reactions. The accurately regioselective and enantioselective coupling of two monolignols controlled by DIRs is the key step to generating PTOX and its analogues. In 1997, Davin firstly found a 78 kD protein from *Forsythia suspensa*, which determined the specificity of the bimolecular phenoxy radical coupling reaction, and described this new class of proteins as dirigent proteins. Due to the lack of a catalytically active (oxidative) center, the functional mechanism of DIRs is presumed to involve the capture of *E*-CA-derived free-radical intermediates, with consequent stereoselective coupling to generate 8- and 8′-linked lignan (+)-pinoresinol. In 2016, Raphael revealed the crystal structure of (−)-pinoresinol forming DIR6 from *A. thaliana* (AtDIR6), which had an eight-stranded antiparallel β-barrel that forms a trimer with spatially well-separated cavities for substrate binding. The binding cavities are two-lobed, exhibiting two opposing pockets, in which the propionyl side chains face each other for radical-radical coupling, and stereo selectively yielded (+)- or (−)-pinoresinol determined by the exact positioning of the side chains. In 2021, DIR, in combination with a laccase, was proven to utilize two different achiral monomers to generate (+)-pinoresinol analogues, with structures of three new bonds and four stereocenters, which provides vise biocatalytic routes to difficult-to-access non-natural lignan analogues and etoposide derivatives. What is more, DIR has been found to enhance plant resistance as well due to its regulating activities of lignan biosynthesis.

Pinoresinol-lariciresinol reductase (PLR) is an enzyme that catalyses the conversion of (+)-pinoresinol to (−)-secoisolariciresinol. This process involves two isoforms firstly demonstrated from *Forsythia intermedia*. The molecules are catalysed sequentially, NADPH-dependently, and stereo-specificly. One step converted (+)-pinoresinol into (+)-lariciresinol, while the other utilized the intermediate to give (−)-secoisolariciresinol. By using abiotic stress and RNA interference treatments, researchers found that the expression level of *PLR1* from *Linum usitatissimum* or *Isatis indigotica* contributed greatly to the content of lignan, especially lariciresinol.

The resulting (−)-secoisolariciresinol was enantiospecifically dehydrogenated into 8−8′-lignan (−)-matairesinol *via* the NAD(H)-dependent SDH. In 2005, Buhyun revealed the crystal structures of apo-form and binary/ternary complexes of podophyllum SDH to clarify the functional mechanism of this enzyme. As a homotetramer, its overall monomeric structure is similar to a NAD(H)-dependent short-chain dehydrogenases/ reductases, with a highly conserved catalytic triad (Ser153, Tyr167, and Lys171) adjacent to both NAD(+) and substrate molecules.

According to massively parallel sequencing of transcriptomes and subsequent bioinformatics analyses of the corresponding assemblies, two cytochrome P450s monooxygenases, CYP719A23 from *S. hexandrum* and CYP719A24 from *P. peltatum*, were proven to be capable of converting (−)-matairesinol into (−)-pluviatolide by catalysing the methylenedioxy bridge formation. Further experiments indicated that these two enzymes did not act on other possible substrates tested.

By the year 2015, Lau *et al*. identified six pathway enzymes from transcriptome information of *S. hexandrum*, including three hydroxylase CYP71CU1, CYP71BE54, and CYP82D61, two *O*-methyltransferase pluviatolide *O*-methyltransferase (OMT3) and 5′-desmethyl-yatein *O*-methyltransferase (OMT1), and DPS, a 2-oxoglutarate-dependent (Fe/2OG) oxygenase that closes the core cyclohexane ring to complete the tetracyclic core. By co-expressing four previous genes and six late-stage genes in tobacco, (−)-pluviatolide was converted into the etoposide aglycone, (−)-4′-desmethyl-epipodophyllotoxin [(−)-DMEP], which is not only a type-Ⅱ topoisomerase inhibitor but also an intermediate for the semi-synthesis of etoposide from PTOX. These results provide a more direct precursor for the synthesis of etoposide and a strategy for PTOX demethylation. In 2021, Tang *et al*. elucidated the mechanism underlying the regio- and stereo-selectivity of DPS cyclization event and found that it differs from a prior proposal of on-pathway benzylic hydroxylation, the DPS-catalysed cyclization was likely related to the formation of a benzylic carbocation, adding an understanding of the biotransformation process.

To this day, the direct pathway of PTOX, which adds an α-OH at the C−4 position, still remains unknown. In 1995, Uden found that the cell suspensions of *S. hexandrum* could accumulate PTOX and its β-D-glucoside when fed DPT, however, he did not identify the enzyme. In the process of searching for the biosynthetic pathway of PTOX, the pathway of collateral compounds has been gradually clarified. Using genetic information from *Linum album*, DPT was hydroxylated at the C−5 position by deoxypodophyllotoxin 5-hydroxylase (DPT5H) and converted into β-peltatin, which was subsequently methylated by β-peltatin 5-*O*-methyltransferase (βP5OMT) to produce β-peltatin-A-methylether (PAM). However, the α-hydroxylation of PAM at the C－4 position [producing 4-hydroxy-PAM (4HPAM)], which may be the same enzyme as DPT 4α-hydroxylase, has not been verified. Researchers assumed the enzyme might be a dioxygenase or peroxidase, rather than a cytochrome P450. What is more, the recombinant human cytochrome P450 CYP3A4, the same catalysing function as *Sh*CYP82D61, could stereo-selectively convert DPT into (－)-epi-podophyllotoxin, which has β-OH at the C－4 position compared with PTOX (Fig. 1).

2.3 Glycosylation The natural glycosides of PTOXs from Podophyllum mainly contain eight compounds, including podophyllotoxin 4-*O*-β-D-glucopyranoside, 4′-demethylpodophyllotoxin 4-*O*-β-D-glucopyranoside, epipodophyllotoxin 4-*O*-β-D-glucopyranosyl-(1→6)-β-D-glucopyranoside, 4′-demethyl-picropodophyllo-toxin 4-*O*-β-D-glucopyranoside (4DPG), 4′-demethyl-epipodophyllotoxin 4-*O*-β-D-glucopyranoside, 4′-demethyl-deoxypodophyllotoxin 4-*O*-β-D-glucopyranoside, sinolignan A (6″-acetyl-podophyllo-toxin-4-*O*-β-D-glucopyranoside), sinolignan B (4′-demethyl-pic-ropodophyllotoxin-4-*O*-β-D-glucopyranosyl-(1→6)-β-D-glucopyr-anoside). As is known, glycosylation could enhance the solubility of drugs, recognize membrane proteins and modify protein structures. Some PTOX glycosides have entered clinical applications, such as etoposide, which are not only a semi-synthetic derivative of PTOX but also exists in plants with a low content. The extracted ingredient 4′-demethyl-deoxypodophyllotoxin 4-*O*-β-D-glucopyranoside also exerted a potent activity against breast cancer. Therefore, glycosides may become promising anticancer ingredients, and studies on UDP-dependent-glycosyltransferases (UGTs) have important scientific significance and may become a hot spot for future studies. However, since the genome of *S. hexandrum* belongs to the super genome, it is hard to be sequenced and there is little information about the UGTs of PTOXs. In 2008, Berim found a series of 4-*O*-glucosyltransferase from *Linum nodiflorum* suspension cell culture, these enzymes catalysed PTOX and its 5-methoxy derivative to the corresponding glycosides. Based on the total biosynthetic pathway of DMEP, researchers further found that UGT78D2 from *A. thaliana* could catalyse (－)-DMEP to directly produce the glycosylated precursor of etoposide, 4-*O*-β-D-glucopyranoside of DMEP [(－)-GDMEP]. Some essential amino acid residues surrounding the putative substrate entrances have been found as well, which relate to substrate specificity and high *O*-glucosyltransferase activity to (－)-DMEP (Fig. 1).

2.4 Synthetic biology Due to over-exploitation for medicinal purposes and health protection, natural resources of PTOXs, especially *S. hexandrum* are on the verge of extinction. *In vitro* culture for the effcient regeneration and production of PTOXs has become a newly developed alternative approach and an important research priority.

In 2019, Schultz transiently expressed sixteen pathway-related genes from *S. hexandrum* in tobacco, including both upstream and downstream pathway enzymes. By engineering the supply of CA, this system resulted in the accumulation of up to 4.3 mg/g dry plant weight (－)-DPT. It is the longest pathway reconstruction of natural products in a plant class and provides novel access to valuable precursors of the chemotherapeutic etoposide.

Since insuffcient CA supply may limit the production of PTOXs, constructing CA-producing stains may become a promising strategy for producing PTOXs and intermediates. In 2020, Yang *et al*. chose a pathway from multiple routes for CA biosynthesis containing fewer phenylpropanoid aldehydes, which are toxic to *Saccharomyces cerevisiae*. However, the production of CA by reconstructing seven pathway genes in yeast [TAL from *Herpetosiphon aurantiacus*, 4-hydroxyphenylacetate 3-monooxygenase (HpaB) from *Pseudomonas aeruginosa*, flavin reductase (HpaC) from *E. coli*, COMT1, 4CL5, CCR1 and CAD5 from *A. thaliana*], respectively, is still far from the expectation. Further, Chen overexpressed 3-deoxy-D-arabino-heptulosonate-7-phosphate synthase mutant ($ARO4^{K229L}$), chorismate mutase mutant ($ARO7^{G229S}$), prephenate dehydrogenase (TYR1) and glucose-6-phosphate 1-dehydrogenase (ZWF1) from *S. cerevisiae*, which regulates the biosynthesis of tyrosine and regeneration of the cofactor NADPH, respectively. After 72 h fed-batch fermentation, the content of CA reached 201.1±13.6 mg/L in a 5 L fermenter.

In 2021, Davide *et al*. sequentially biotransformed common higher-lignan (＋)-pinoresinol to (－)-pluviatolide, a crossroad intermediate channelling the biosynthetic pathway to (－)-PTOX, *via* four enzymes, three of which were related to a biosynthetic pathway, while the other ensured P450 activity. By using an *E. coli* strain, PLR from *F. intermedia* (FiPLR), SDH from *Podophyllum pleianthum* (PpSDH), CYP719A23 from *S. hexandrum* and an NADPH-dependent cytochrome P450 reductase (CPR) from *A. thaliana* (ATR2) eciently convert (＋)-pinoresinol, and enantiopure (－)-pluviatolide isolated was at a concentration of 137 mg/L (ee ≥99%). The next year, they mined pathway genes from *S. hexandrum* and established a five-step multi-enzyme cascade biotransforming (－)-matairesinol to (－)-DPT in *E. coli* with the assistance of ATR2. Using a two-cell approach, this cascade yielded 78 mg/L (－)-DPT with 98% conversion. Further, they extended the previous cascade with the co-expression of *Sh*CYP82D61, which converted (－)-DPT into (－)-epipodophyllotoxin. This six-step strategy produced 8.3 mg/L (－)-epipodophyllotoxin with 10% conversion.

Besides enzyme engineering and pathway optimization

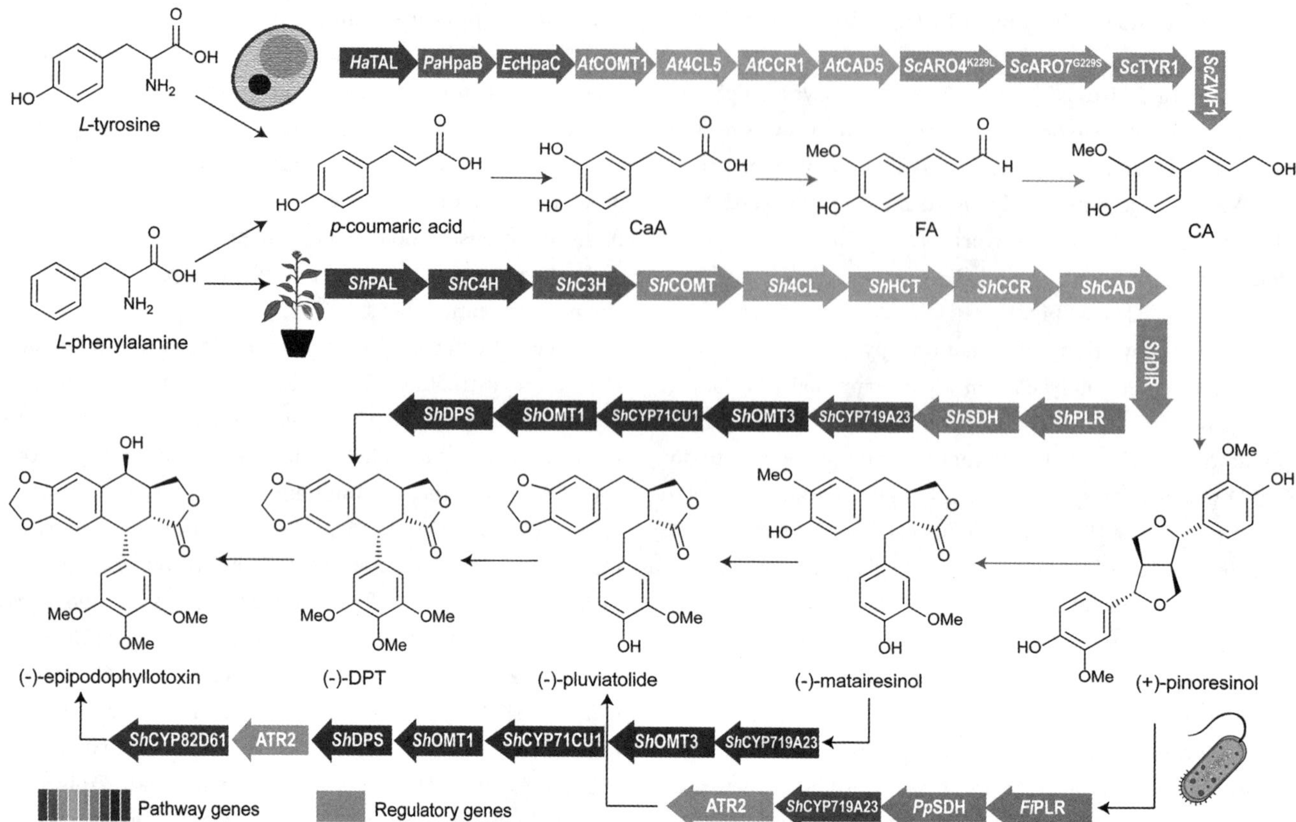


**Fig. 2 Synthetic biology of PTOXs**

*in vitro*, engineering the supply and recycling of cofactors, which participate in many intracellular metabolic processes and reactions, is also a feasible way to enhance PTOX production. In 2022, on the basis of pathway optimization in yeast *S. cerevisiae*, Chen *et al*. manipulated biosynthesis, compartmentalization, and recycling of two cofactors, NADPH and *S*-adenosyl-L-methion (SAM), which participate in redox reactions and methylation reactions, respectively. The production of the phenylpropane pathway intermediates CaA (5.5±0.2 g/L) and FA (3.8±0.3 g/L) reached gram-level production in the fedbatch fermentation, which has a considerable production potential at present (Fig. 2).

## 3 TOTAL SYNTHESIS

Since PTOXs are extracted from natural resources, it is difficult to meet the market demand, and the productive potentials of heterologous synthesis are far from being achieved. Total synthesis has become a powerful means for sustainable production because of its special structure (heavily oxygenated aromatic core, four contiguous chiral centers, pseudoaxial ring E, and facile epimerization at C2 and C4), and PTOX has attracted the attention of chemists and biochemists. A subtle change in aromatic ring substitution patterns can cause changes in pharmacological activities. Therefore, stereospecific synthesis of (−)- PTOX is of great significance to maintain its activity. At present, the correct stereocenter formation can be achieved quickly by metallic ion-catalyzed chemical or chemoenzymatic methods, greatly promoting the application of PTOX and its derivatives.

3.1 Chemical synthesis In 2008, Daniel *et al*. reported a six-step synthesis method of (−)-PTOX (**1**), which involved the rapid synthesis of the tetracyclic core through intramolecular $Fe^{3+}$-catalysed arylation and did not require group-protection (Scheme 1). Through the aldol reaction between Taniguchi lactone (**2**) and aldehyde (**3**), researchers successfully synthesized compound (**4**) containing a stereocenter on lactone. Although the diastereoselectivity of **4** was low (dr=52 : 48), it did not affect the reaction process. Subsequently, 1,3-benzodioxole and its derivatives were screened, and catalytic conditions were optimized for inter-molecular Friedel-Crafts alkylation. $FeCl_3$ was selected to catalyze the reaction of sesamol (**5**) with **4**, resulting in alcohol (**6**) with high diastereoselectivity and almost quantitative yield (99%, dr=6 : 94). Transformed from **6b**, triflate (**7**) was converted by the Heck reaction into the cyclization product olefin (**8**), which successfully generated the target product (−)-PTOX by dihydroxylation and periodate cleavage. The overall yield was 35%. Compared with former strategies, this method combines several fragments to obtain the PTOX skeleton by tandem conjugate addition in a short sequence and high yield, and only needs slight modifications to obtain target ingredients with excellent

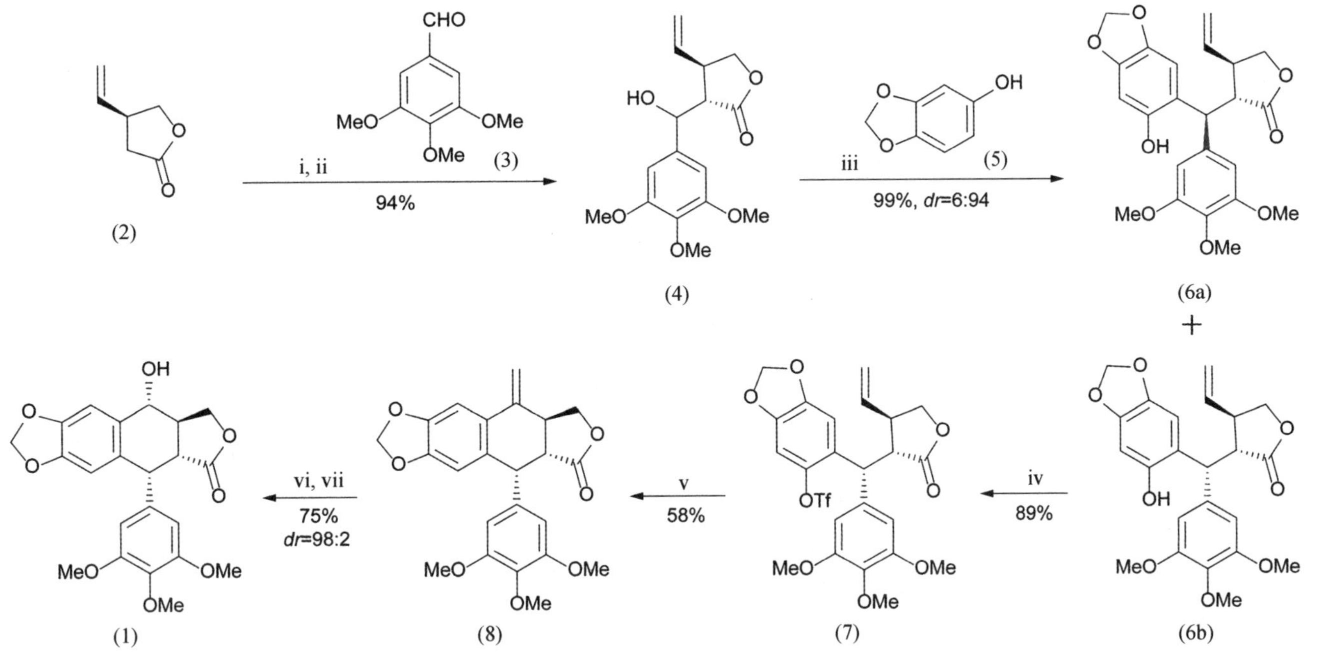

**Scheme 1 Chemical synthesis of (−)-PTOX from Daniel *et al*.**

(i) Lithium diisopropylamide (LDA, 1.1 equiv.), THF, −78℃, 30 min; (ii) 4 (1.1 equiv.), −78℃, 3 h; (iii) $FeCl_3$, $CH_2Cl_2$, 20℃, 1 h; (iv) $Tf_2O$ (1.5 equiv., Tf = trifluoromethanesulfonyl), $NEt_3$ (2 equiv.), $CH_2Cl_2$, 0℃, 1 h; (v) $Pd(OAc)_2$ (10 mol%), $PPh_3$ (0.3 equiv.), $K_2CO_3$ (3 equiv.), MeCN, 80℃, 20 h; (vi) $OsO_4$ (5 mol%), NMO (3 equiv.), $CH_2Cl_2$, 20℃, 4 h, then $NaIO_4$ (2 equiv.), 30 min; (vii) $LiAlH(O\textit{t}Bu)_3$ (10 equiv.), $Et_2O$, −78 to 20℃, 18 h.

stereoselectivity.

In 2018, Xiao *et al*. innovatively used stereoselective nickel-catalyzed cascade cyclization to realize the asymmetric synthesis of (−)-PTOX and its derivatives on the basis of conventional synthesis schemes such as the conjugate addition route and γ-lactone route (Scheme 2). The initial compound 6-bromopiperonal (**9**) extended the carbon chain with the assistance of triethyl phosphonoacetate through Horner-Wads-worth-Emmons (HWE) olefination. The generated ester reacted with pivaloyl chloride after saponification to form acyl chloride, which introduced a chiral auxiliary (*S*)-4-phenyl-2-oxazolidinone to generate α, β-unsaturated acyl oxazolidinone (**10**) (94%). The key asymmetric conjugate addition reaction was achieved by the subjection of an arylcopper(I) reagent *in situ* on the reaction product of a compound with (3, 4, 5-trimethoxyphenyl)-magnesium bromide. The yield of compound (**11**) with excellent diastereocontrol was 80% (dr=97 : 3). Then, **11** removed the chiral auxiliary mediated by $NaBH_4$ to generate the corresponding alcohol, followed by oxidation and acetylation to generate acetal (**12**) (88%), which produced β-elimination in the mixture of TMSOTf and DIPEA to provide enol ether (**13**) as a *Z*/*E* mixture in 67% (85% brsm). Under the treatment of 2, 4, 6-tetrabromo-2, 5-cyclohexadienone (TBCD) in $CH_2Cl_2$ at 0℃, the key site-selective bromination of enol ether at the double bond occurred, generating β-bromoacetals (**14**) with pseudoboat conformation and half-chair conformation (76%, dr=1.2 : 1) as substrates for subsequent Ni-catalyzed tandem reductive cyclization. Through a series of oxidation reactions, Ni-catalyzed products *cis*-THN[2,3-c] furan (**15**) and *trans*-THN[2,3-c] furan (**16**) can generate the natural ingredients (−)-PTOX and its derivatives. The acetal moiety in β-bromoacetals was initially hydrolyzed and subsequently oxidized to give lactol intermediate, (+)-DPT (**17**) and (+)-isoDPT (**18**). Under the enolization/quenching conditions (LDA, THF, −78℃ then glacial acetic acid), (+)-DPT was epimerized at the C-2 position to generate (−)-DPT (**19**). Labile bromide, which was obtained after radical bromination under visible-light irradiation, was hydrolysed during column chromatography on silica gel to produce (−)-epipodophyllotoxin (**20**) with regio- and stereo-selectivity, and the yield was 81%. In order to obtain (−)-PTOX with α-hydroxyl configuration, (−)-epipodophyllotoxin was oxidated first [generated (−)-podophyllotoxone (**21**), PDC in $CH_2Cl_2$] and subsequently stereospecifically reduced (L-selectride in THF at −78℃) to generate natural product (−)-PTOX. However, the same method cannot be used in (+)-isoDPT. Finally, researchers refer to methods from Meyers in 1988, which opened the ring of γ-lactone and constituted a formal synthesis of (−)-picropodophyllotoxin (**22**).

3.2 Chemoenzymatic synthesis  At present, the stereoselective closure of C ring is still the main bottleneck

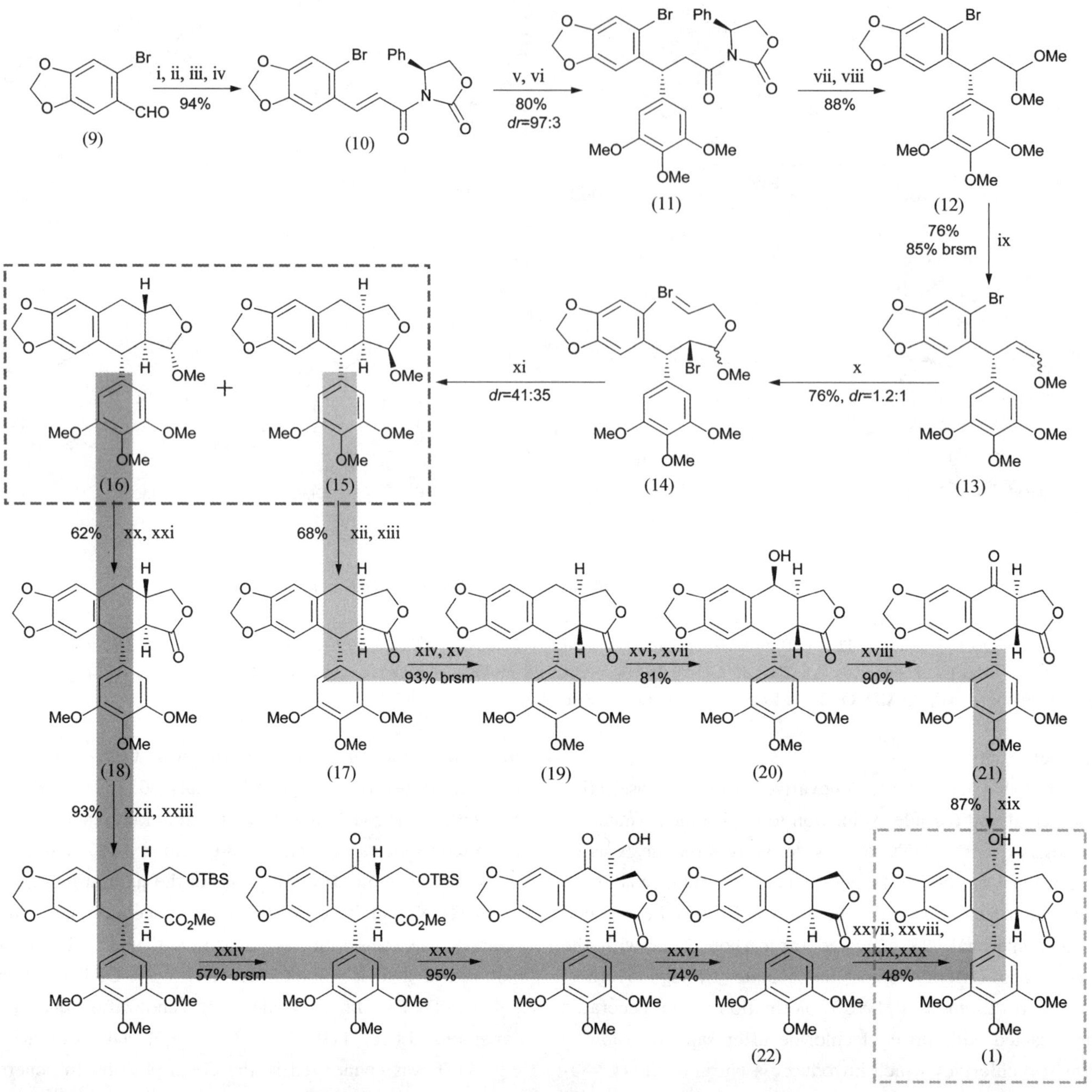

**Scheme 2 Chemical synthesis of (−)-PTOX and related lignans from Xiao *et al*.**

(i) $(EtO)_2P(O)CH_2CO_2Et$; (ii) NaOH; (iii) PivCl; (iv) (*S*)-4-phenyl-2-oxazolidinone; (v) 3, 4, 5-$(OMe)_3$PhMgBr, (vi) CuBr · $SMe_2$, THF, −48 to 0℃; (vii) $NaBH_4$; (viii) PCC, $CH(OMe)_3$; (ix) TMSOTf, DIPEA, $CH_2Cl_2$, −25℃ to RT; (x) TBCD, allyl alcohol, $CH_2Cl_2$, 0℃; (xi) Zn (1.5 equiv.), Nicl$_2$ · DME (30 mol%), ethyl crotonate (90 mol%), pyridine, DMA, RT, 4 h; (xii) HCl; (xiii) PCC; (xiv) LDA, THF, −78℃; (xv) HOAc; (xvi) NBS, hν, 1, 4-dioxane; (xvii) silica gel; (xviii) PDC, $CH_2Cl_2$; (xix) L-selectride, THF, −78℃; (xx) HCl; (xxi) PCC; (xxii) $H_2SO_4$, MeOH, reflux; (xxiii) TBSCl; (xxiv) $CrO_3$, 3, 5-DMP, $CH_2Cl_2$; (xxv) HCHO, NaOH; (xxvi) PhMe, 210℃, 36 h, then −78℃; (xxvii) LiAl(*t*-BuO)$_3$H, THF; (xxviii) 2, 6-lutidine, $CH_2Cl_2$, TMSOTf, 0℃, 4 h; (xxix) LiHMTS, THF, −78℃; (xxx) $Et_3HNF$, MeCN, RT, 72 h.

for asymmetric synthesis. Although some problems have been solved through expensive reagents or catalysts, synthetic biology strategies also provide conditions for heterologous synthesis, butyrolactone moiety and substitution on aromatic rings take several steps in biosynthesis. Chemo-enzymatic strategy, which combines the advantages of chemical total synthesis and biosynthesis, provides a new method for asymmetric synthesis.

In 2019, Mattia *et al*. envisaged a tandem conjugate addition route for rapid synthesis (**23** - **26**) of the racemic product *rac*-yatein (**28**), followed by selective cyclization by dioxygenase DPS to realize biocatalytic kinetic resolution and obtain a tetracyclic core of (−)-PTOX. However, the DPS-catalyzed production of *rac*-yatein occurred through an enantiodivergent reaction, making it difficult to purify intermediates. Therefore, researchers hypothesized that the

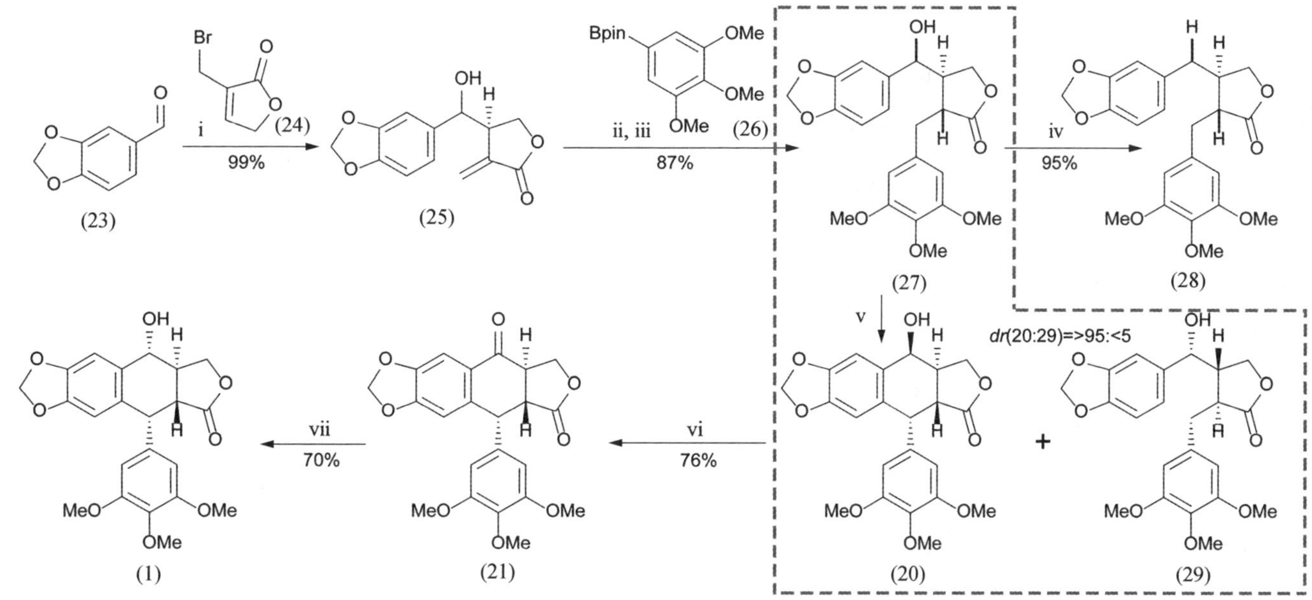

**Scheme 3 Chemoenzymatic synthesis of (−)-PTOX from Mattia *et al.***

(i) Zn, $NH_4Cl$, **24**, toluene/DME, RT; (ii) $[(Rhcod)Cl]_2$, $Et_3N$, **26**; (iii) 1,4-dioxane, $H_2O$, 70 ℃, 3 h; (iv) Pd/C, $H_2$, $HClO_4$, MeOH, 6 h; (v) DPS, $Fe^{2+}$, Na ascorbate TRIS buffer (pH=7.4), 18 ℃; (vi) DMP, $CH_2Cl_2$, RT, 16 h; (vii) L-selectride, THF, −78 ℃, 2 h.

addition of a chiral center in the northern benzylic position can improve product specificity. *rac*-Hydroxyyatein (**27**), a dibenzylbutyrolactone with a hydroxyl group in the north, generated a C ring-unclosed product (+)-hydroxyyatein (**29**) and epipodophyllotoxin (**20**) when catalysed by soluble DPS enzyme. Referring to previous methods, epipodophyllotoxin was accurately converted into (−)-PTOX with correct conformation through two steps (Scheme 3).

Subsequently, Li *et al*. used an asymmetric chemoenzymatic synthesis method to rapidly generate the absolute stereochemistry configuration precursor, which was subsequently catalyzed by enzyme DPS for the closure of the C ring to form the stereospecific compound (−)-DPT. This strategy provides a concise method for the subsequent synthesis of aryltetralintype lignans. Compared with the previous study, this method did not require a kinetic resolution process to deal with racemic compounds, which is a more efficient way to synthesize (−)-PTOX (Scheme 4). Researchers first used the oxidative enolate coupling methodology to couple oxazolidinone (**30**) with an ester (**31**) to form a single diastereomer dibenzylbutyrolactone (**32**) as the natural substrate of the DPS enzyme. Then, they used chaperones GroEL and GroES to optimize the soluble expression level of the DPS enzyme, leading **32** to completely transform into (−)-DPS (**19**). The titer yield was more than 3 g/L. By using $CrO_3$ for oxidation and L-selectride for reduction, (−)-DPS was converted into ketones and (−)-PTOX (**1**), respectively. The overall yield of this five-step chemoenzymatic method for the rapid synthesis of (−)-PTOX reached 28%.

Furthermore, this method was successfully applied to other aryltetralin-type lignans. By comparing the conversion rates of different substrates (**33a**-**c**, **34a**-**d**), it was found that the trimethoxybenzene moiety was crucial to the C-C coupling of the C ring (**19**,**35d**, **35e**). The conversion of the 1,2-dimethoxy motif into the 1,2-methylenedioxy bridge (**19** *versus* **35a**, **35b** *versus* **35c**) would significantly reduced the conversion efficiency.

## 4 PHARMACOLOGICAL ACTIVITIES

### 4.1 Anti-cancer activity

4.1.1 Anti-cancer mechanism of PTOXs. The molecular mechanism of PTOXs in anti-cancer activity is mainly reflected in its effects on inducing cancer cells apoptosis and autophagy (Fig. 3).

Firstly, PTOXs affect microtubule assembly and nucleoside transport to block cell mitosis. From Loike's perspective, both PTOX and etoposide can inhibit the uptake of thymine and uracil to cells, thereby inhibiting the synthesis of DNA, RNA, and protein. However, these two compounds have different effects on microtubule assembly. Etoposide, which contains glycosyl, does not inhibit polymerization while PTOX does because of its spindle poisons. Further studies suggest that PTOX may destroy the spindle organization and affect the arrangement of chromosomes in the middle of the first mitosis. Joseph summarized previous studies and found that the reason for etoposide's inhibiting activity of DNA synthesis is related to the inhibition of the mitotic cycle, especially at the stage of

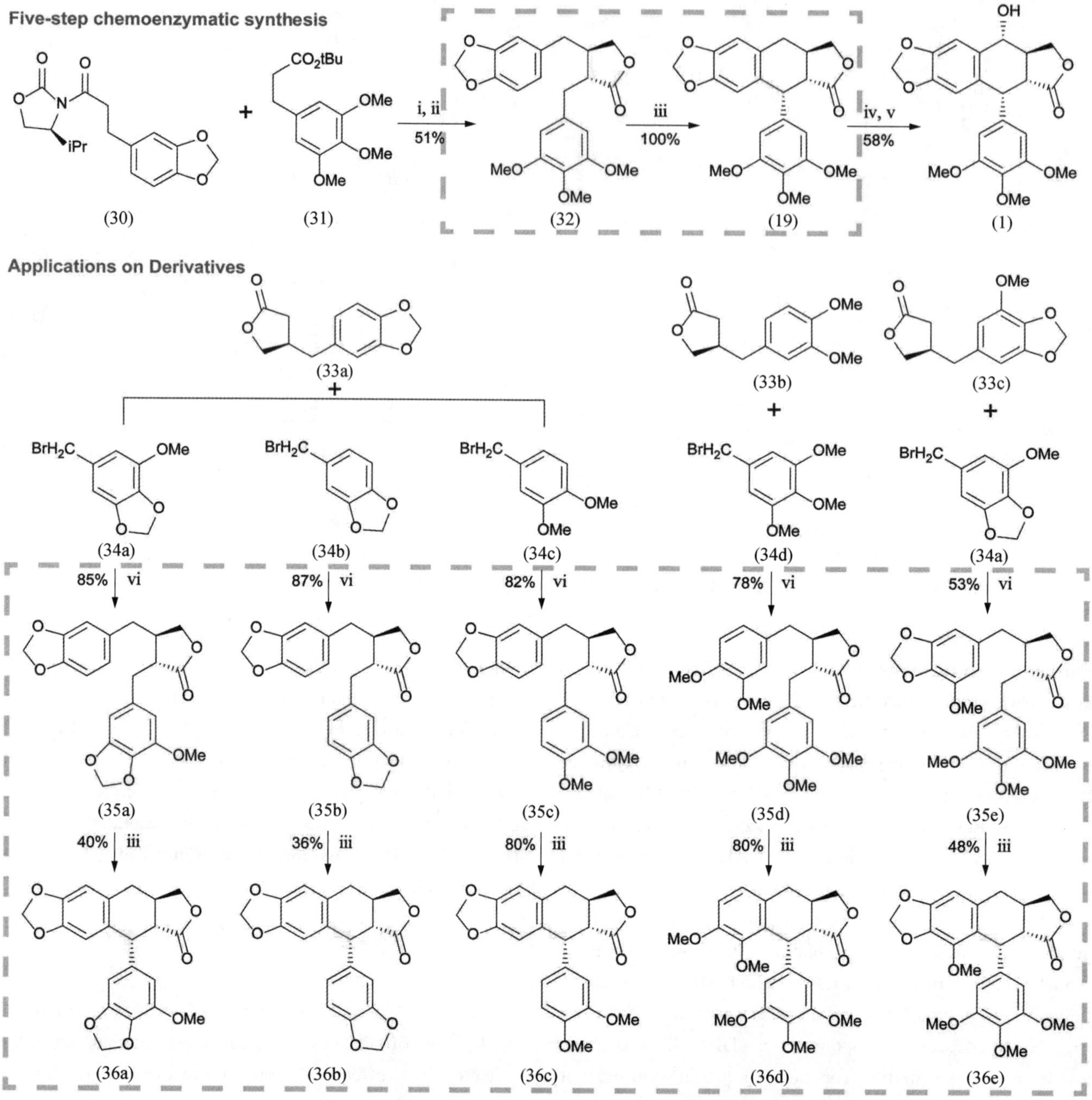

Five-step chemoenzymatic synthesis

Applications on Derivatives

**Scheme 4 Chemoenzymatic synthesis of (−)-PTOX and related lignans from Li *et al*.**

(i) LDA, $Cu^{2+}$; (ii) $LiBH_4$, DBU, Δ; (iii) $O_2$, $Fe^{2+}$, αKG, DPS; (iv) $CrO_3$, 3,5-DMP; (v) L-selectride; (vi) LHMDS.

late S and G2.

Secondly, PTOXs kill cancerous cells by inhibiting type II topoisomerases (TOP2s), increasing the steady-state level of DNA-TOP2s-drug cleavage complexes to promote the formation of cytotoxic DNA lesions, inducing double-stranded breaks and eventually restraining the rapid proliferation of cancer cells. However, this activity occurs only after conformational changes and the introduction of sugar groups, the PTOX itself is not a TOP2 inhibitor. Meanwhile, the cytotoxicity of the improved PTOXs is significantly reduced because the formed complexes will degrade with the disappearance of the drugs. To further explain the three-dimensional structural basis of the drug actions and resistance, researchers determined the high-resolution crystal structure, which revealed the detailed interplay between the enzyme, the DNA, and etoposide, suggesting that the drug stabilizes the cleavage complex in part by disfavoring the relegation of cleaved DNA ends *via* decoupling of the key catalytic residues. This result provides molecular insights for observed structure-activity relationships and strategies for producing isoform-specific TOP2-targeting drugs.

4.1.2 PTOX and its derivatives as anti-cancer drugs. Since the 1980s, dozens of PTOXs anti-cancer drugs targeting

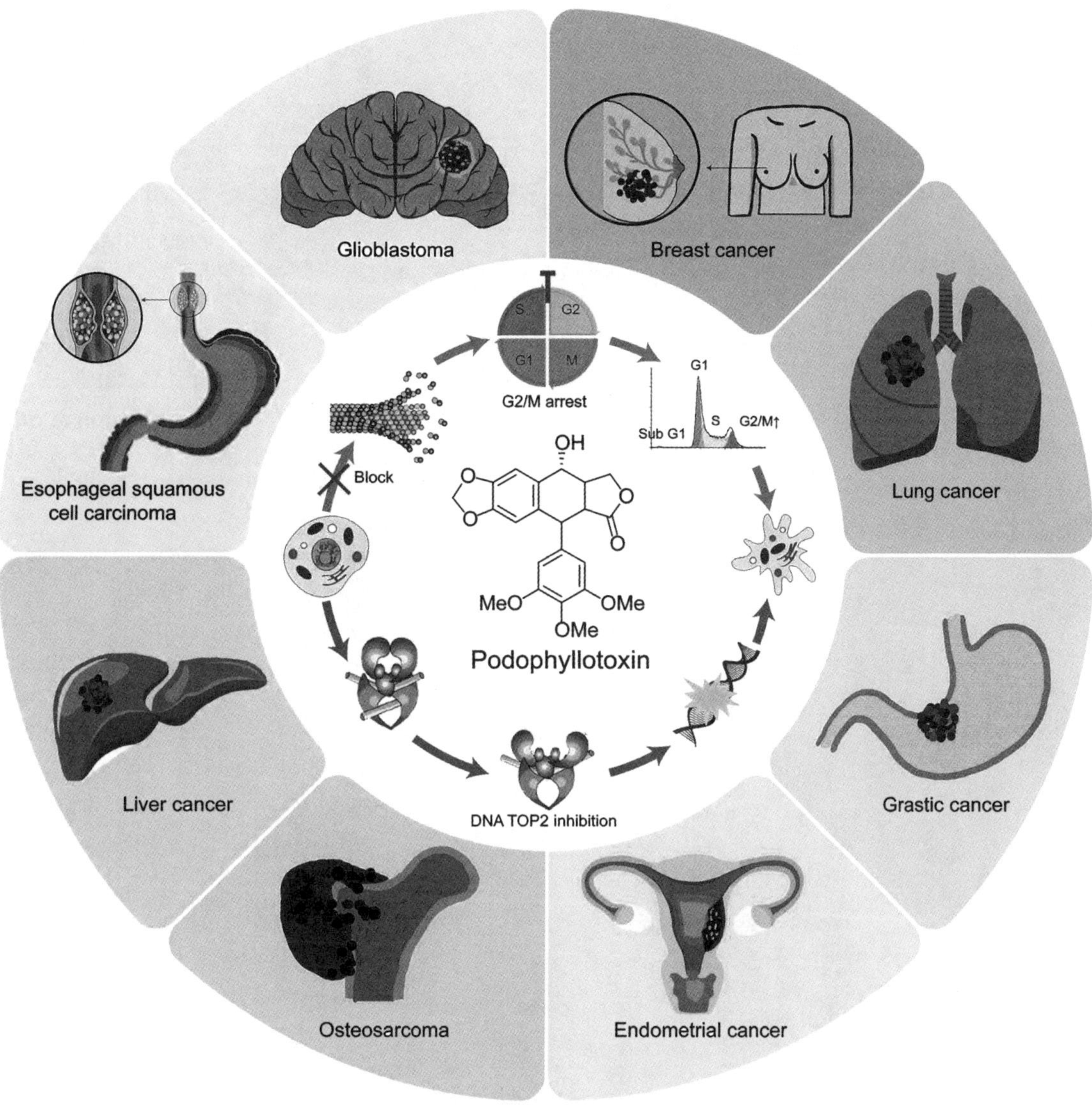


**Fig. 3 Pharmacological activity mechanism and anticancer types of PTOXs**

breast cancer, gastric cancer, lung cancer, endometrial cancer, glioblastoma, leukemia cancer, liver cancer, colorectal cancer, osteosarcoma, esophageal squamous cell carcinoma (ESCC) and other multiple human cancers have entered clinical phases I-III (Fig. 3). These compounds are obtained by structural modification of PTOX. Designing and synthesizing derivatives with lower cytotoxicity and drug resistance through structural modification of PTOX, as well as extracts from natural plants have always been a research hotspot (Fig. 4 and Table 1).

PTOX (**1**) is often used as a precursor of clinical drugs because of its strong cytotoxicity. As a toxic and polycyclic antimitotic agent isolated primarily from the rhizome of the plant *S. hexandrum*, this agent is formulated for topical applications. In 2021, Lee evaluated the anticancer mechanism of PTOX on human colorectal cancer and found that it could induce cell cycle arrest in the G2/M phase and apoptosis through the p38 MAPK signalling pathway by upregulating reactive oxygen species (ROS) in HCT116 cells. However, more applications of PTOX deal with its structural derivatives.

DPT (**19**) is a natural ingredient and is only different from PTOX at the C-4 position. DPT is used as a precursor for the semi-synthesis of the cytostatic drugs etoposide phosphate and teniposide. As a new class I anti-cancer drug, it plays an important role in a variety of cancers and won the approval for phase I-III drug clinical research issued by the National Medical Products Administration in China in 2017. In 2013, Jiang found that the anti-cancer activity of DPT may have been related to the ideal anti-cancer target blood vessels. They found that DPT exerts both anti-angiogenesis and vascular disruption activities, making it become a promising new anticancer drug. In the same year, Jung investigated the effect of DPT in autophagy and mammalian target of rapamycin (mTOR) signalling as an anti-cancer action in breast cancer cells and found DPT decreased the levels of phosphorylated Akt and mTORC1, followed by inhibition of the cell growth. Further research found that the

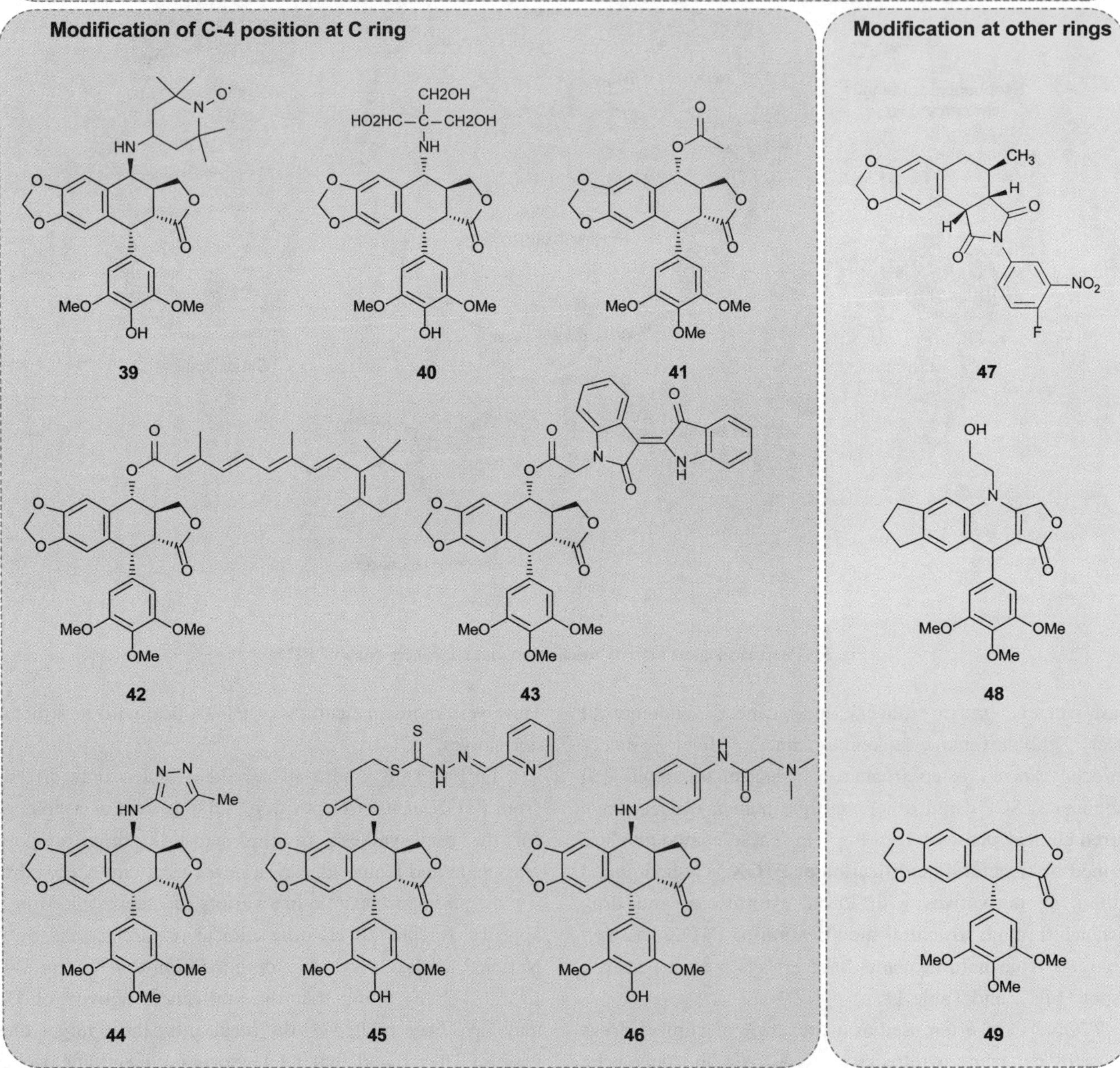


**Fig. 4 Structure of PTOX and its derivatives as anti-cancer drugs**

DPT is a potent inducer of caspase-dependent programmed cell death (apoptosis) in malignant MB231 breast cancer cells by inhibiting cell survival pathways mediated by the MAPK/ERK and NF-κB signalling pathways. DPT could also be a novel chemotherapeutic for human gastric cancer. In 2015, Wang found that DPT inhibited gastric cancer cell proliferation and induced G2/M cell cycle arrest accompanied by an increase in apoptotic cell death. These activities were mediated by caspase pathways. To prevent glioblastoma progression, in 2019, Wang found that the DPT

**Table 1 Mechanism of PTOX and its derivatives in the treatment of different types of cancer**

| Name | Anti-cancer type | Signaling pathway | Mechanism |
|---|---|---|---|
| PTOX (**1**) | Colorectal cancer | p38/MAPK | Induce G2/M cell cycle arrest and apoptosis |
| DPT (**19**) | Breast cancer | Akt/mTOR MAPK/ERK & NF-κB | Induce cell apoptosis |
| | Gastric cancer | Caspase-dependent | Induce G2/M cell cycle arrest and apoptosis |
| | Glioblastoma | PI3K/Akt & BAX/Bcl-2 | Induce G1/S cell cycle arrest |
| | ESCC | AKT/ERK | Induce G2/M cell cycle arrest and apoptosis |
| | NSCLC | EGFR/MET | Induce cell apoptosis |
| PPP (**37**) | Endometrial cancer | PI3K/Akt | Inhibited cell proliferation |
| | ESCC | (JNK)/p38 | Induce G2/M cell cycle arrest and apoptosis |
| | Colorectal cancer | p38/MAPK | Induce G1 cell cycle arrest and apoptosis |
| 4′-Demethyl-deoxy-podophyllotoxin -4-*O*-β-D-glucopyranoside (**38**) | Breast cancer | Chk-2 | Induce mitotic catastrophe and G2/M cell cycle arrest |
| GP7 (**39**) | Leukemia cancer | Caspase-3-dependent or -independent | Induce apoptosis of DNA fragmentation |
| | Osteosarcoma | Caspase-independent or caspase-9-dependent | Induce S cell cycle arrest and apoptosis |
| | Gastric cancer | Caspase-3-dependent | Inhibits cell proliferation |
| 4-*N*-Tris(hydroxymethyl) methylaminomethane -4-deoxy-4′-demethyl-epipodophyllotoxin (**40**) | Gastric cancer | ATM/ATR | Inhibit TOP2 and induce cell apoptosis |
| PA (**41**) | NSCLC | ROS/p38/caspase & EGFR-p38/ ERK-CREB-1/STAT3-EMT | Induce G2/M cell cycle arrest, apoptosis, inhibited microtubule polymerization |
| ATRA conjugate with PTOX (**42**) | Gastric cancer | Caspase-3, -8 and -9 ERK1/2 & AKT | Induces cell cycle arrest and apoptosis |
| Podophyllotoxin–indirubin hybrid (**43**) | Leukemia cancer | JNK/AKT | Induce G2 cell cycle arrest, apoptosis and disrupt microtubule organization |
| OAMDP (**44**) | Liver cancer | Bax, caspase-9, caspase-3 Bcl-2, *p*-Akt & MAPK | Induce S or G2/M cell cycle arrest and apoptosis |
| 2-Pyridinealdehyde hydra-zone dithiocarbamate *S*-propionate PTOX ester (**45**) | Liver cancer | PI3K/Akt/mTOR | Inhibit TOP2 and induce cell apoptosis |
| SU212 (**46**) | Breast cancer | AMPK | Induce mitotic phase arrest and apoptosis |
| Compound A398 (**47**) | Leukemia cancer | MAPKs & Bcl-2 | Induce cell apoptosis |
| XWL-1-48 (**48**) | Liver cancer | PI3K/Akt/Mdm2 | Trigger DNA damage and induce S cell cycle arrest |
| | Breast cancer | ATM/p53/p21 PI3K/Akt/Mdm2 | Induce S cell cycle arrest and mitochondrial apoptosis |
| APP (**49**) | NSCLC | Caspase-3, -8 and -9 | Induces cell cycle arrest and apoptosis |

suppressed cellular viability by inducing cell cycle arrest at the G1/S phase by targeting the PI3K/Akt-mediated signalling pathways as well as the apoptosis regulator BAX/Bcl-2. In 2020, Kwak found the DPT-induced G2/M phase arrest and apoptosis of ESCC cells by inhibiting the epidermal growth factor receptor (EGFR) mediated AKT/ERK signalling pathway. To overcome the resistance to inhibitors of the epidermal growth factor receptor (EGFR), which is related to the hepatocyte growth factor receptor MET, for targeted therapy of cancer. In 2021, Kim used DPT to treat non-small cell lung cancer (NSCLC) and found that DPT could suppress the expression of *p*-EGFR and p-MET as well as their downs treat proteins *p*-ErbB3, *p*-AKT, and *p*-ERK, and induced high ROS generation.

Picropodophyllotoxin (PPP, **37**), the epimer of PTOX, is a cyclolignan alkaloid found in the mayapple plant family (*P. peltatum*), and a small-molecule inhibitor of the insulin-like growth factor 1 receptor (IGF1R) with potential antineoplastic activity. PPP showed anti-cancer activity during the growth and development of endometrial cancer, the molecular mechanism is related to the down-regulation of IGF - IR phosphorylation and inhibiting cell proliferation *via* the PI3K/Akt signalling pathway. In 2020, Kwak found that PPP showed the potential apoptotic effect on ESCC cells by the activation of the c-Jun N-terminal kinase (JNK)/p38 signalling pathways and the generation of ROS, which induced G2/M phase cell cycle arrest and annexin V-stained cell apoptosis. Moreover, Lee found that PPP could also induce G1 arrest and apoptosis in human colorectal cancer cells *via* ROS generation and activation of the p38 MAPK signalling pathway.

Zilla extracted 4′-demethyl-deoxypodophyllotoxin 4-*O*-β-D-glucopyranoside (**38**) from the root of *S. hexandrum* in 2014 and found this glycoside analogue augmented the apoptotic cascades in MCF - 7 breast cancer cells by destabilizing the microtubular protein tubulin and inducing mitotic catastrophe and G2/M cell cycle arrest, exhibiting better antiproliferative and ROS generating activity than its aglycone. The potential anticancer activities may relate to the Chk-2 signalling pathway.

Besides the natural ingredients of PTOX, the major target for structural modification to produce more efficient products or drugs with better pressure resistance is at the C-4 position of the C ring.

4-[4″-(2″, 2″, 6″, 6″-Tetramethyl-1″-piperidinyloxy) amino]-4′-demethyl-epipodophyllotoxin (GP7) (**39**), the semi-synthesized derivative of PTOX, exhibits lower sub-chronic toxicity compared to etoposide. In 2004, GP7 was used to treat human leukemia cancer by inducing caspase-3-dependent or-independent activation, which was related to the apoptotic DNA fragmentation of cancer cells. In 2013, Yang found that GP7 had an apoptosis-inducing effect on osteosarcoma cells. Differing from etoposide, GP7 arrested the cell cycle in the S phase rather than in the G2/M phase. The mechanism of apoptosis induction may be mediated by caspase-independent or caspase-9-dependent pathway. In 2017, Yang found that the inhibitory effect of GP7 on the proliferation of human gastric cancer cells was higher than that of etoposide. The mechanism is mediated by a mitochondrial pathway with caspase-3-dependent BID cleavage.

In 2014, Xiao designed an amination derivative of PTOX named 4-*N*-tris (hydroxymethyl) methylaminomethane-4-deoxy-4′-demethyl-epipodophyllotoxin (**40**), which significantly improved the anti-cancer activities in many cancer cell lines compared to etoposide. This potent drug could diminish the relaxation reaction TOP2 DNA decatenation and induce apoptosis of gastric cancer cells by breaking DNA double-strand and activating ATM/ATR signalling pathways.

Podophyllotoxin acetate (PA) (**41**), a naturally occurring derivative of PTOX, shows strong anti-cancer activity, especially against NSCLC cells. In 2015, Choi found PA-induced cell cycle arrest at the G2/M phase due to the inhibition of microtubule polymerization. The PA-induced activation of DNA damage, ER stress, and autophagy also lead to apoptotic cell death. Further research found that PA could enhance apoptosis of NSCLC induced by γ-ionizing radiation (IR) by increasing the production of ROS, inducing phosphorylation of p38, suppressing phosphorylation of extracellular-signal-regulated kinase (ERK), and activating caspase-3, -8, and -9 (ROS/p38/caspase pathway). What is more, PA could block the EGFR-p38/ERK-CREB-1/STAT3-EMT pathway to inhibit IR-induced invasion/migration of cancer cells.

All-trans retinoic acid (ATRA) is a promising compound that regulates many biological processes, such as cell differentiation, reproduction, and regulation of the immune system. The structural modifications of ARTA were reported to have the potential to kill various cancers. In 2017, Zhang designed and synthesized a novel ATRA conjugate with PTOX (**42**), which triggered cell cycle arrest, induced apoptosis of gastric cancer cells *via* caspase-3, -8, and -9, and inhibited the ERK1/2 and AKT signalling pathway.

In 2018, Wang synthesized the PTOX-indirubin hybrid (**43**), which significantly induced apoptosis and cell cycle arrest at the G2 phase *via* JNK/AKT signalling pathway and disrupted the microtubule organization, to overcome cancer drug resistance. This compound might be a promising agent for the treatment of drug-resistant leukemia cancer.

The same year, Ren found a novel derivative 4β-(1,3,4-oxadiazole-2-amino-5-methyl)-4-deoxypodophyllotoxin (OAMDP) (**44**) that could cause cell cycle arrest at the S or G2/M phase and apoptosis of liver cancer cells HepG2 cells. OAMDP regulates many signalling pathways such as Bax, caspase-9, caspase-3, Bcl-2, *p*-Akt, and MAPK, making it possible become a novel anti-cancer agent.

TOP2 inhibitor, combined with a metal ion chelator, could achieve the goal of both inhibiting cancer cell growth *via* TOP2 inhibition and inactivating metalloproteinase by chelation. In 2019, Li chose dithiocarbamates as a metal ion chelator to synthesize a novel PTOX derivative 2-pyridinealdehyde hydrazone dithiocarbamate *S*-propionate PTOX ester (**45**), which revealed the anti-cancer activity in liver cancer cells through multiple pathways including alterations in apoptosis, autophagy, and the PI3K/Akt/mTOR signalling pathway.

AMP-activated protein kinase (AMPK) signalling pathway is a well-known pathway related to cell-cycle arrest and protein reduction. In 2021, Tailor reported a novel aza-podophyllotoxin derivative named SU212 (**46**). This potential drug, which is highly potent and relatively safe, induces mitotic phase arrest and apoptosis of triple-negative breast cancer cells by directly activating the AMPK pathway.

Although there are few structural modifications on other rings, there are still relevant reports.

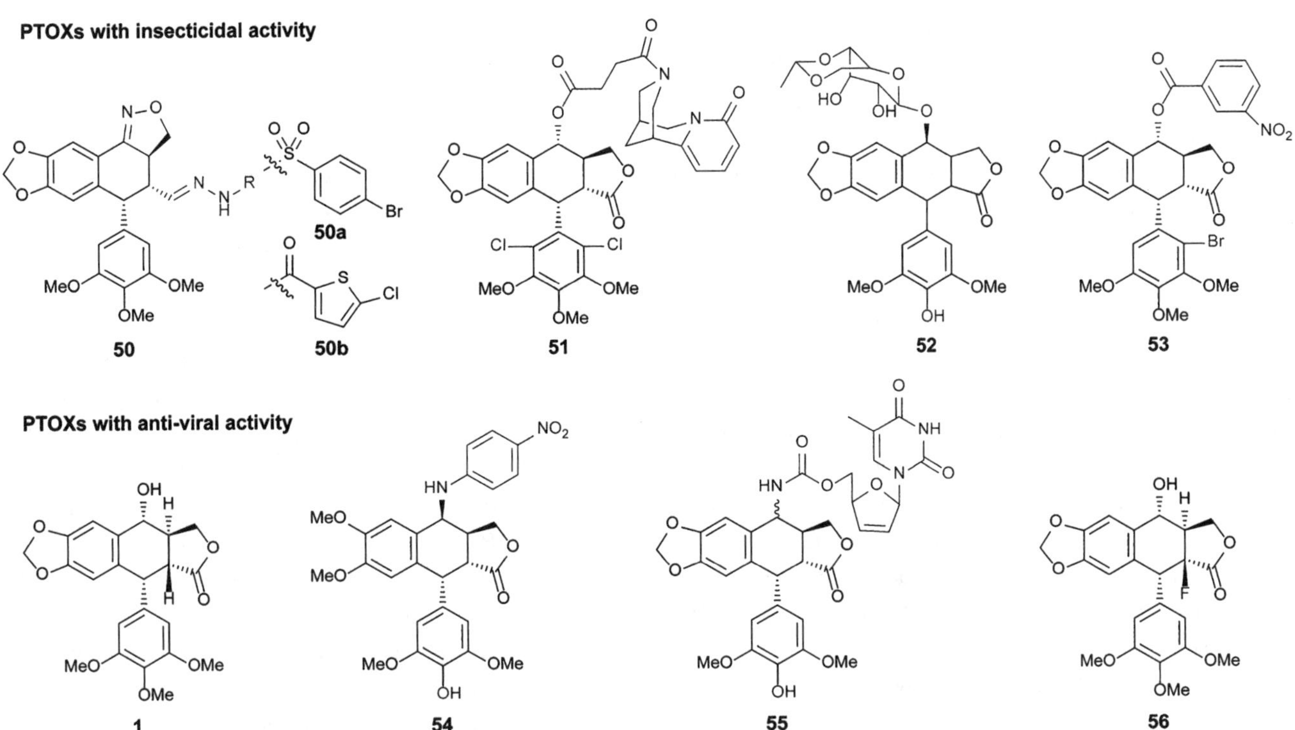


**Fig. 5 Insecticidal activity and anti-viral activity of PTOXs**

In 2014, Silveira found that the candidate anticancer PTOXs, compound A398 (**47**), was cytotoxic to human leukemia cells. The mechanism involves the inhibition of MAPKs and Bcl-2 to induce apoptosis through the activation of intrinsic and extrinsic death pathways.

GL-331 is a semisynthetic TOP2 inhibitor that is less cytotoxic than etoposide. GL-331 induces apoptotic cell death through the activation of protein tyrosine phosphatases. XWL-1-48 (**48**) is more potent than its congener GL331. As a new orally PTOX derivative, XWL-1-48 inhibits TOP2 activities through two strong hydrogen bonds and potential $\pi-\pi$ interactions. In 2017, Wang found XWL-1-48 suppressed liver cancer survival by triggering DNA damage, arresting the cell cycle at the S phase and blocking the PI3K/Akt/Mdm2 pathway. Furthermore, they found that the anti-cancer mechanism of XWL-1-48 in breast cancer included triggering the generation of ROS and DNA damage through the ATM/p53/p21 pathway, inducing S-phase arrest and mitochondrial apoptosis, and blocking the PI3K/Akt/Mdm2 pathway to enhance Mdm2 degradation.

To enhance PA activity, in 2018, Choi identified a novel derivative named β-apopicropodophyllin (APP) (**49**). As a strong anti-cancer agent, APP caused disruption of microtubule polymerization and DNA damage, leading to cell cycle arrest of NSCLC. Meanwhile, caspase-3, -8 and -9 were activated, which provided evidence for APP-induced apoptosis.

4.2 Insecticidal activity PTOX and its derivatives are natural-product-based insecticide candidates, which may have a high value-added application to natural plants in agriculture (Fig. 5).

In 2014, Wang synthesized a series of novel hydrazone derivatives of PTOX, which were natural and could be isolated from the roots and rhizomes of Podophyllum species and also evaluated as insecticidal agents. Compounds (**50a**-**b**) showed potent insecticidal activities with final mortality rates greater than 60%. This provides an idea for the search for pesticides from natural sources. In 2021, Zhang prepared a series of twin compounds (**51**) from two natural products PTOX and cytisine, which modified PTOX at the C-4 position, and exhibited >2-fold potent insecticidal activity of PTOX against armyworm.

*Aedes aegypti* carries several viruses of public health importance, including the dengue virus. Dengue is the most rapidly spreading mosquito-borne viral disease in the world. Prevention and control of dengue mainly rely on mosquito control as there is no antiviral treatment or WHO-approved vaccine. In 2021, Daniele found that TOP2 mRNA is expressed at all stages of mosquito development, and concentrated along the ovarian follicular cells as well as in the region of the follicles. The treatment with the drug etoposide (**52**), a classic inhibitor of TOP2, could result in a 30%-40% decrease in survival with persisting larvae and pupae presenting incomplete development, as well as morphological abnormalities. Also, approximately 50% of the treated larvae did not reach the pupal stage.

Some derivatives exhibit growth inhibitory activity against some insect pests, resulting in malformed moths with vestigial wings. In 2022, Sun found a new derivative (**53**) that resulted in 22.1% of malformed moths with vestigial wings but also significantly decreased the fecundity of vestigial-winged female moths in the P generation. This mechanism may be related to the suppression of insulin receptor 1 (InR1) mRNA level, and block tyrosine phosphorylation of InR1.

4.3 Anti-viral activity PTOX and its derivatives are also powerful drugs for the treatment of viral diseases (Fig. 5).

Since 1948, PTOX (**1**) has become the most effective drug in the clinic to treat the disease so far after being proven to be able to treat condyloma acuminatum, which is a sexually transmitted disease caused by human papillomavirus (HPV) infection. Considering the tolerance and clinical efficacy, 0.5% PTOX cream is more efficacious than 0.3% because of its mild and tolerable side effects. In 2013, Massip found that etoposide induced apoptosis of HPV-positive carcinoma HeLa cell line by activating p53 transcription through the E2F1 pathway.

Molluscum contagiosum is a self-limiting benign skin disease, which is caused by the molluscum contagiosum virus (MCV), which mainly influences children and young adults. In 1994, Syed found that response to the trial medications appeared to be directly proportional to the concentration of PTOX, and the 0.5% PTOX cream preparation was more efficacious than the 0.3% incorporation considering the clinical efficacy and tolerance. What is more, PTOX was considered a topical chemical treatment in the 2020 European guidelines on the management of genital molluscum contagiosum.

The modified PTOX derivatives demonstrated significant anti-HIV-1 activity. Researchers found that *para*-substitution on the 4β-aniline and an opened A-ring coupled with 4′-demethylation compounds (**54**) enhanced anti-HIV activity. Further-more, 4β-amide group substitution coupled with 4′-demethylation resulted in a compound (**55**) with better anti-HIV-1 activity. Non-Hodgkin lymphoma is one of the AIDS-related cancers, this activity has been applied in the therapy of HIV-associated lymphoma.

What is more, PTOXs have inhibitory effects on the herpes simplex virus (HSV). Nishiyama found the etoposide may inhibit viral DNA synthesis by impairing the function of host cell TOP2 to kill virus. Van Vliet found that a synthesized compound 2-fluoropodophyllotoxin (**56**) showed unusual 10-fold selectivity for HSV-2 compared to HSV-1. Cheema enhanced the anti-cancer eiffcacy of low-dose etoposide with oncolytic HSV in human glioblastoma stem cell xenografts thus providing prospects for anti-virus and anti-cancer drugs.

## 5 CONCLUSIONS

According to the database from the Global Cancer Observatory (GCO), the estimated number of new cancer cases is nearly 20 million people and there were 9.96 million deaths in 2020, including 1.8 million lung cancer deaths, far exceeding other cancer types and ranking first in cancer deaths. The number of new breast cancer patients released by the International Cancer Research Institute (IARC) in 2020 was 2 260 000, which even officially replaced lung cancer and became the world's leading cancer incidence rate. Thus, it is of great importance to accelerate the progress of cancer treatment. Medical plants, which contain natural products with excellent therapeutic effects, have broad prospects for clinical application. For example, alkaloid vincristine from *Catharanthus roseus* (L.) G. Don has excellent outcomes when treated with standard-risk B-lymphoblastic leukemia and large B-cell lymphoma in the clinic. Paclitaxel, combined with Trastuzumab and Carboplatin, has good curative effects in phase Ⅲ clinical trials of HER2-positive breast cancer and advanced endometrial cancer, respectively.

Up to now, about 60 types of aryltetralin-type lignans have been found in *S. hexandrum*, among which PTOX is the most concerned compound by scholars. Etoposide and teniposide, the semi-synthesized derivatives of PTOX, show extensive pharmacological activities, among which the anticancer activity is the most significant. Using a series of cancer cell lines, researchers found the anticancer molecular mechanisms, such as PI3K/Akt, (JNK)/p38, Bax-dependent, ROS/p38/caspase, and EGFR-p38/ERK-CREB-1/STAT3-EMT signaling pathways. Based on these signaling pathways, these drugs induce the apoptosis and autophagy of cancer cells by affecting microtubule assembly and nucleoside transport and inhibiting TOP2. What is more, the natural drug DPT and its injection, a new class Ⅰ anti-cancer drug, won the approval for phase Ⅰ drug clinical research issued by the National Medical Products Administration in China in 2017, which further proved the development prospect of natural PTOX drugs.

However, the lack of large amounts of PTOX presents an obstacle to transforming PTOX into clinical therapeutics. *S. hexandrum*, one of the common natural resources containing the maximum content of PTOX, grows in harsh plateau areas with chilling temperature, high altitude, and strong ultraviolet light, contributing to the extremely low plant reservation. Currently, the biosynthetic pathways of DPT and DMEP, the direct precursor of etoposide, have been fully revealed, providing a scientific basis for the heterologous synthesis of PTOXs. Some intermediates, such as CA, (−)-pluviatolide, and DPT have realized a heterologous milligram-scale production by using synthetic biological strategies. However, no plant of Podophylloideae (Berberidaceae) has completed genome analysis so far and the genome size of the main source plant *S. hexandrum* is too big (~16 G) to be sequenced. Therefore, the key process, which involves an oxidase gene catalyzed α-hydroxylation at the C-4 position, has not been found and identified due to the lack of important bioinformatics information from the genome scale. Future research in synthetic biology requires a focus on genome analysis and transcriptome information to mine candidate genes. In this process, more transcription factors and regulatory genes related to the biosynthesis of PTOXs and the collateral pathway can also be screened.

Structure-optimized derivatives of PTOX exert the diversity of anticancer activities, which reduce the toxicity and side effects of drugs compared to PTOX. The mechanisms, anti-cancer types, and activities are strongly influenced by substitution groups. C-4 is the major position for the structural modification of PTOXs. For example, sugar hybrids of PTOX show low side effects thus forming various drugs with excellent anticancer activities. The five-membered nitrogen azoles can also provide valuable anticancer agents. Some azole hybrids show far higher anti-cancer activities than that of etoposide by causing cell cycle arrest at the G2/M phase and inducing apoptosis of cancer cells. Therefore, current studies on the pharmacological activities of PTOX and its derivatives provide good references and significance for future chemical semi-synthetic PTOX drugs.

All the information shows the advantages of PTOX as a precursor of existing and future anticancer drugs with more efficiency, strong drug resistance, and fewer side effects. However, the scarcity of medicinal plant resources and incomplete pathway analysis still restrict the research of these important compounds. Similarly, due to its own cytotoxicity, the hepatorenal toxicity and nervous system toxicity caused by PTOX drugs still need to be improved. Nowadays, NK611, GL331, TOP53, and other modified compounds have entered the clinical phase Ⅰ-Ⅲ experiments. In the future, more new PTOX drugs will undergo clinical trials for the benefit of humans.

[沈思雨，黄璐琦，高伟，等. Natural Product Reports, 2022,39:1856-1875.]

# Diterpene synthases from *Leonurus japonicus* elucidate epoxy-bridge formation of spiro-labdane diterpenoids

## 1 INTRODUCTION

Over 18,000 diterpenoids compounds have been identified, many with important biological activities, and these have emerged as innovative lead compounds for development of modern drugs. An intriguing group of diter-penoids are labdanes containing an oxy group at C9, with those containing a spiro-9,13-epoxy ring providing a particularly distinct structural feature. A considerable number of these diterpenoids have strong biological activity, such as the anticancer activity of LS-1/2, analgesic and anti-diabetic activity of marrubiin, and anti-platelet aggregation and coagulant activity exhibited by prehispanolone and related spiro-epoxy-labdane diterpenoids. This type of diterpenoid is prevalent in the genera *Leonorus*, *Otostegia*, *Ballota*, and *Marrubium* from the Lamiaceae plant family. Spiro-epoxy-labdane diterpenoids are particularly common in the genus *Leonorus*, with about 70 spiro-epoxy-labdane diterpenoids having been identified from these plant species.

The C9-oxy group of these labdane diterpenoids seems to generally stem from addition of water during initial (bi) cyclization of the general diterpenoids precursor (*E*, *E*, *E*)-geranyl-geranyl diphosphate (GGPP) catalyzed by a class Ⅱ diterpene cyclase. These enzymes utilize a conserved DxDD motif to catalyze a protonation-initiated carbocation cascade reaction with GGPP that forms a decalin bicycle, initially labda-13-en-8-yl$^+$ diphosphate. Deprotonation of this carbocationic intermediate at the neighboring methyl generates labda-8(17),13-dien-15-yl diphosphate, which has been termed copalyl diphosphate (CPP), with enzymes producing this termed CPP synthases (CPSs). CPP can be produced in various stereoisomeric forms, with that defined as the *enantiomeric* form, *ent*-CPP (**1**), produced by all vascular plants as a necessary precursor for gibberellin (GA) phytohormone biosynthesis. However, particularly relevant here, this carbocationic intermediate also can undergo a 1,2-hydride shift from C9 to C8, with addition of water to the ensuing carbocation at C9 prior to concluding deprotonation, to yield 9α-hydroxy-labda-13-en-15-yl diphosphate, which has been termed peregrinol diphosphate (PPP, **3**).

Class Ⅱ diterpene cyclase products such as *ent*-CPP and PPP are generally further reacted upon by more prototypical class Ⅰ terpene synthases (TPSs). Class Ⅰ TPSs are characterized by DDxxD and DTE/NSE motifs that chelate trio of divalent metal ion co-factors that assist lysis of the allylic diphosphate ester to initiate another carbocationic cascade leading to cyclization and/or rearrangement, and that also can include the addition of water prior to concluding deprotonation. Those that act on class II diterpene cyclase products almost invariably arise from the TPS-e subfamily, which is anchored by the requisite member for production of *ent*-kaurene (2) from *ent*-CPP for GA biosynthesis, then termed kaurene synthases (KSs). Again of relevance here, it is notable that a number of class I diterpene synthases (diTPSs) that catalyze further cyclization of CPP, involving addition of the 8(17)-ene to the initially formed 13-yl tertiary allylic carbocation (such as KSs), have been shown to efficiently (hetero) cyclize the stereochemically relevant C8 hydroxylated variant (i.e. 8-hydroxy-labda-13-ene-15-yl diphosphate), forming the 8, 13-epoxy derivative manoyl oxide with high stereoselectivity. With regards to nomenclature, due to an ancestral fusion event, class II diterpene cyclases are con-sidered members of the TPS family, typically falling within the TPC-c subfamily in angiosperms. Thus, these and the subsequently acting class I TPSs are both termed diTPSs.

Arguably somewhat surprisingly, while previous studies found that PPP is produced quite specifically by the relevant class II diTPSs, subsequent production of 9, 13-epoxy-labda-14-ene (**4**) is catalyzed much less selectively by the relevant class I diTPSs. In particular, all those identified to date produce not only a mixture of the two C13 epimers of this spiro-epoxy, but generally also the *exo*-ene and/or tertiary alcohol derivatives stemming from deprotonation, either immediately of the neighboring methyl or following the addition of water to the initially generated 13-yl tertiary allylic carbocation, generating labda-13(16), 14-dien-9α-ol (**5**) or viteagnusin D (**6**), respectively (Figure 1A). Examples of such enzymes are found throughout the Lamiaceae plant family, as originally reported from *Marrubium vulgare*, with MvCPS1 producing PPP (**3**), which 9, 13-epoxy-labda-14-ene synthase (MvELS) further converts to a mixture, largely 9, 13*S*-epoxy-labda-14-ene (**4b**), but with significant amounts of the 13*R* epimer (**4a**) as well as **5**. Similar catalytic promiscuity in product outcome is observed with class I diTPSs from *Ajuga reptans* (ArTPS3), *Leonotis leonurus* (LlTPS4), *Perovskia atriplicifolia* (PaTPS3), *Salvia officinalis* (SoTPS1), and *Origanum majorana* (OmTPS5), while another from this species (OmTPS4) exhibits additional promiscuity and yields all four products, and yet another (OmTPS3) produces largely **4a** along with significant amounts of **4b**, with one from *Prunella vulgaris* (PvTPS1) producing an analogous epimeric mix along with substantial amounts of **5**. Class I TPSs from *Vitex agnus-castus* also react with PPP, with one (VacTPS2) predominantly producing **4a** along with significant amounts of **6**, while another (VacTPS6) produces largely **5** along with an equimolar mixture of **4a** and **4b**. There are class I TPSs that react with **3** much more selectively to produce either **5**, such as one from *Mentha spicata* (MsTPS1) and another from the bacterium *Kitasatospora griseola* (KgTS), or **6**, such as the sclareol synthase from *Salvia sclarea* (SsSS). *L. japonicus* is a perennial medicinal shrub of the mint family (Lamiaceae) that has been utilized in Asia for over 1,800 years and has a wide range of pharmacological activities. More than 60 C9-oxy containing labdane diterpenoids have been isolated from this plant, and 38 exhibit a spiro-9,13-epoxy ring, including examples derived from both 13*R*- and 13*S*-epimers. Given the prevalent nature of these diterpenoids in *L. japonicus*, it was expected that investigation of this species would help further elucidate such spiro-9,13-epoxy-labdane diterpenoid biosynthesis. In this study, a transcriptome was generated for *L. japonicus*, from which seven diTPSs, four class II and three class I diTPSs, were identified. These LjTPSs were biochemically characterized, and structure-function investigation carried out with the 9,13-epoxy-labda-14-ene producing LjTPS6, leading to identification of a critical residue. Notably, this enabled identification of LjTPS6: I420G as providing catalytic efficient and selective production of 9, 13*S*-epoxy-labda-14-ene (**4b**). Altogether this report provides a strong foundation for future investigation of the biosynthesis of derived diterpenoids in *L. japonicus*.

## 2 RESULTS

Accumulation of diterpenoids in *L. japonicus* More than 60 C9-oxy containing labdane diterpenoids (e.g. 9,13-epoxylabdane diterpenoids) have been reported in *L. japonicus*. Given that only 11 authentic standards were available, in order to analyze tissue-specific accumulation of diterpenoids in *L. japonicus* a $m/z$ mass fragmentation library (DLJ library) was constructed from the results of previous studies. The diterpenoid profile of the root, stem and leaf of *L. japonicus* were analyzed using ultra performance liquid chromatography coupled with quadrupole time of flight mass spectrometry (UPLC-Q/TOF-MS), with comparison to the available authentic standards and searches of the DLJ library assisted by the UNIFI information system. In particular, the $[M+H]^+$, $[M+Na]^+$, and $[M+K]^+$ adducts were observed and analyzed (Supplemental Table S1). While only galeopsin could be identified by comparison to an authentic standard, 10 other diterpenoids were identified by UNIFI software matching to the DLJ library. All of these identified diterpenoids were mainly accumulated in leaves, and five (including galeopsin) were C9-oxy containing labdane diterpenoids. This relatively high accumulation of C9-oxy diterpenoids in leaves was consistent with the leaf-specific expression pattern of the rele-

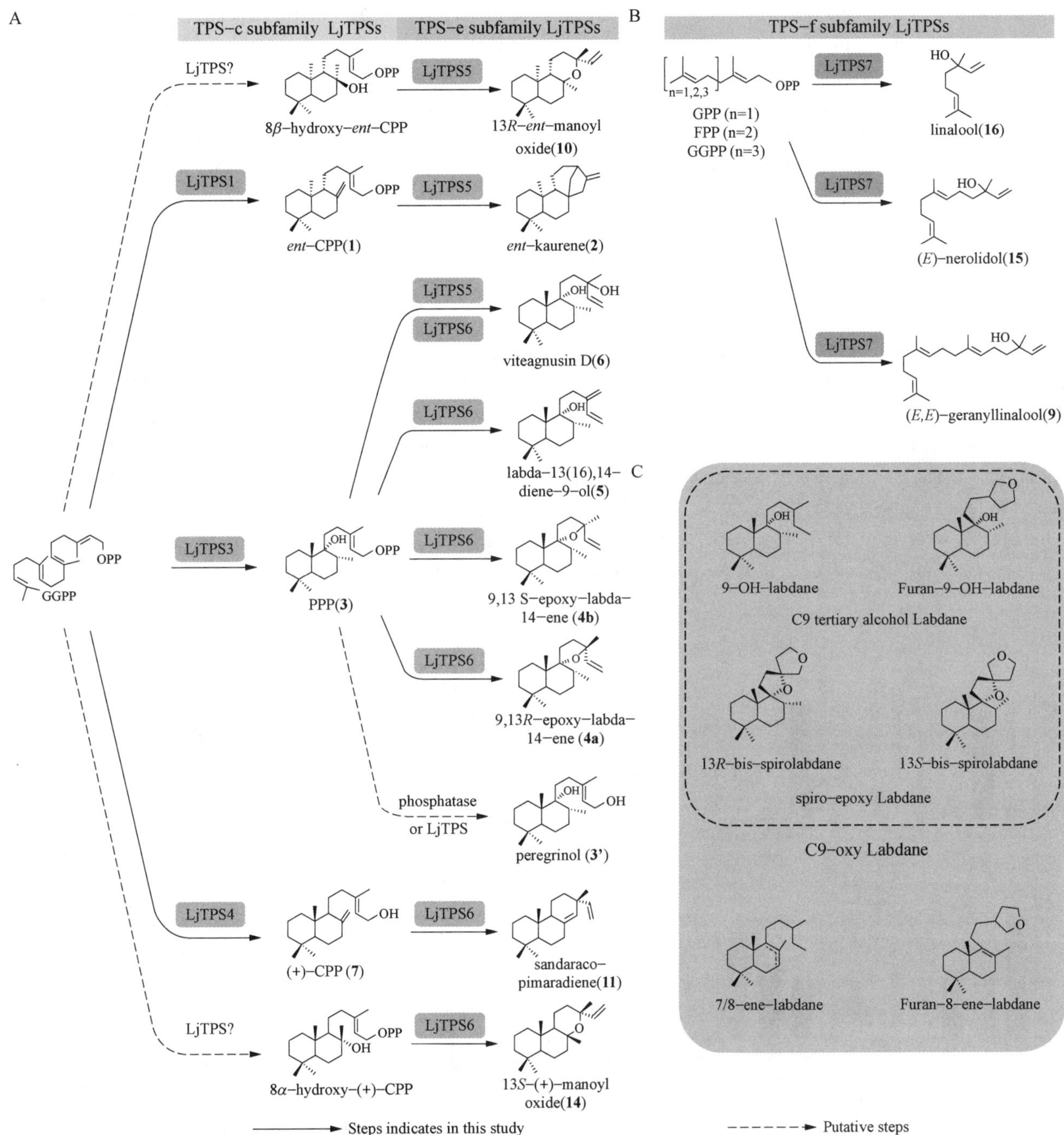


**Figure 1 The diTPSs in the diterpenoid biosynthetic pathway, along with their possible downstream natural products in *L. japonicus***

(A and B) Catalytic function of *L. japonicus* diTPSs. diTPSs in boxes were characterized in this study. (A) Catalytic function of TPS-c and TPS-e subfamily LjTPSs. (B) Catalytic function of TPS-f subfamily LjTPSs. (C) Diterpene scaffolds found in *L. japonicus*. Geranylgeranyl diphosphate (GGPP), farnesyl diphosphate (FPP), geranyl diphosphate (GPP), copalyl diphosphate (CPP) and peregrinol diphosphate (PPP).

vant class II diterpene synthase LjTPS3 (see below).

Identification of multiple diTPSs in an *L. japonicus* transcriptome To enable investigation of diterpenoid biosynthesis in *L. japonicus*, RNA from root, leaf, and stem, from three independent individuals, was extracted and utilized to generate a transcriptome for this medicinal herb. Briefly, a nonnormalized complementary DNA (cDNA) library was prepared from separated and mixed RNA from different tissues of *L. japonicus*, and sequenced using the Illumina novaseq6000 platforms. A total of 279,710,836 reads were obtained. The Trinity de novo assembler found 133,725 contigs with an average length of 1,119 bp, and lengths varying from 201 to 15,425 bp (Accession number: RPJCA, CRA004698).

Homology searches and annotation information of this *L. japonicus* transcriptome revealed seven diTPSs (designated

LjTPS1 to LjTPS7) (Supplemental Table S2), of which six (excluding LjTPS2) had full-length Open Reading Frames (ORFs). To understand the physiological roles of the candidate diTPS in *L. japonicus*, the transcript levels in various organs, including root, stem, and leaf were show by the Reads Per Kilobase Million (FPKM) value (Figure 2A). This reveals that all candidates are expressed in all tissues, with the exception of LjTPS3. Three LjTPSs (e.g. LjTPS4, LjTPS5, and LjTPS6) had higher transcript levels in root, and two (e.g. LjTPS1 and LjTPS7) in stem, with only LjTPS3 specifically expressed in leaves. To verify these expression profiles, LjTPS transcripts in leaf, stem, and root were quantified using reverse transcription quantitative PCR (RT-qPCR). The expression profiles of LjTPSs by RT-qPCR are similar to that from the transcriptome, with the exception of LjTPS4, which was found to be more highly expressed in leaf (Figure 2A).

Six LjTPSs were used for phylogenetic analysis with a representative set of TPSs. Three of these putative diTPSs contained the DDxD motif (LjTPS1, LjTPS3, and LjTPS4) and were clustered in the TPS-c subfamily with the class II diTPS of other plants (Figure 2B). The other three putative diTPSs (LjTPS5, LjTPS6, and LjTPS7) were tentatively identified as Class I diTPSs based on the conserved DDxxD and NSE/DTE motifs, and fell within the TPS-e/f subfamily (Figure 2B; Supplemental Figure S1). LjTPS1 and LjTPS5 clustered with the known *ent*-CPSs (e.g. VacTPS5 and IrCPS5) and *ent*-EKSs (e.g. MvEKS and VacTPS4), suggesting roles in GA biosynthesis. LjTPS3 was grouped with the three known PPP synthases (e.g. LlTPS1, MvCPS1, and VacTPS1). LjTPS6 was clustered with multiple diTPS that can react with PPP. This suggested that LjTPS3 and LjTPS6 are involved in the synthesis of C9 oxidized diterpenoids in *L. japonicus*. LjTPS4 was most closely related to CPSs that produce CPP of normal stereochemistry (e.g. MvCPS3, IrCPS1, and CfTPS1), which also is widespread in the Lamiaceae plant family. Finally, LjTPS7 falls within the TPS-f subfamily, members

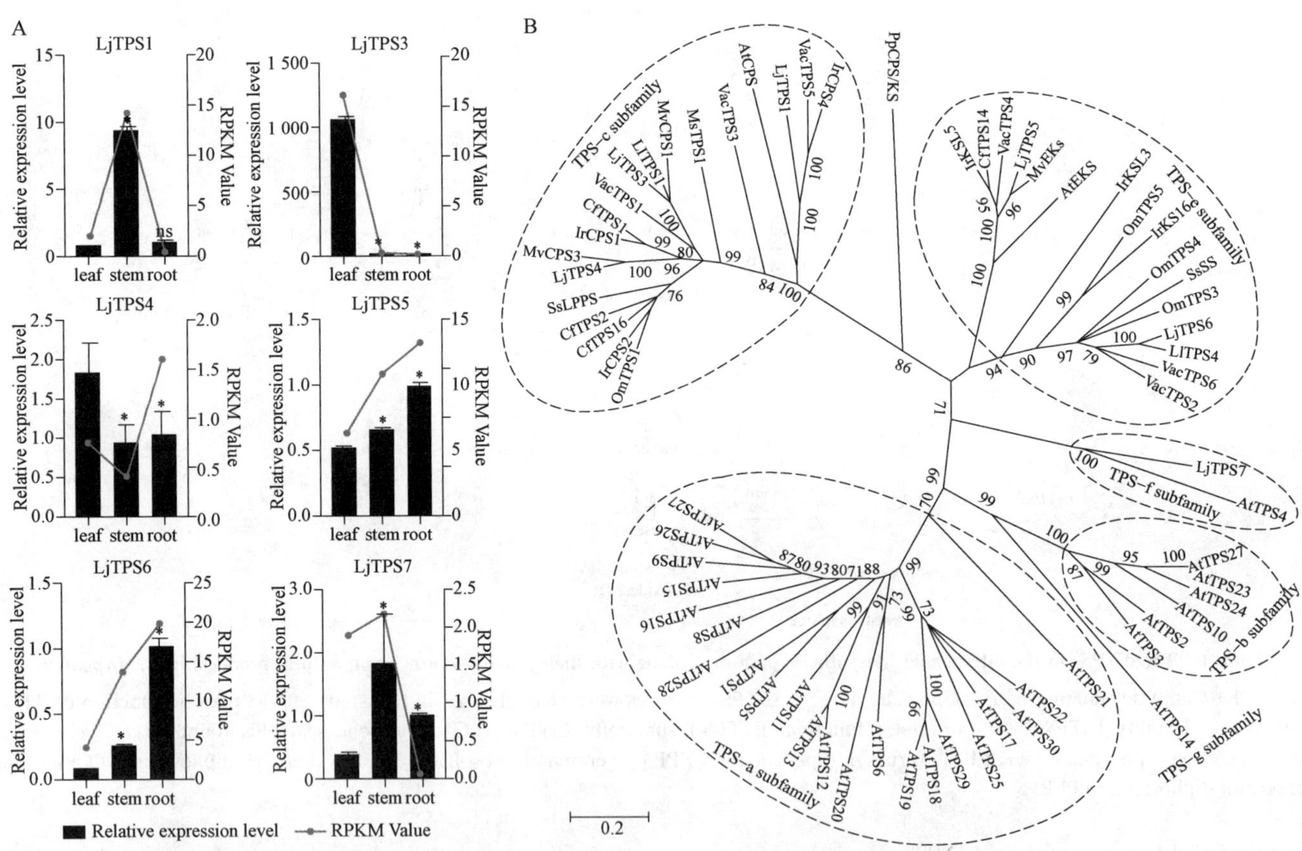


**Figure 2 Phylogenetic analysis of diTPSs from *L. japonicus* and relative expression of *diTPSs* in different tissues**

(A) Relative expression level of *L. japonicus* diTPSs. Relative expression level of *L. japonicus diTPSs* in leaf, stem, and root by RT-qPCR and the reads per kilobase million value from the *L. japonicus* transcriptome. The expression level was normalized to that of actin, and the error bars show the SDs from mean value ($n = 3$). Statistically significant differences between the transcript levels of leaf and stem or root based on a Student's $t$-test ($P < 0.05$). (B) Phylogeny of *L. japonicus* diTPSs. Constructed using the NJ algorithm with a representative set of TPSs (Supplemental Table S3). The tree is drawn to scale, with branch lengths in the same units as those of the evolutionary distances used to infer the phylogenetic tree. Bootstrap values (1,000 replicates, shown if >70%) are given. PpCPS/KS was used as outgroup. Red-marked enzymes show diTPSs from *L. japoni-cus* in this study.

of which often play a role in homoterpene biosynthesis.

### Functional characterization of putative class II LjTPSs

For functional characterization of the three class II diTPSs (LjTPS1, LjTPS3, and LjTPS4), these were heterologously expressed in *Escherichia coli* with a C-terminal 3His epitope tag. Crude recombinant proteins were assayed *in vitro* with GGPP, and subsequent dephosphorylation carried out to enable extraction and analysis of the reaction products by GC-MS. When compared to the products of known CPSs, LjTPS1 and LjTPS4 were found to produce CPP (Figure 3). To determine the absolute stereochemistry of their products LjTPS1 and LjTPS4 were incorporated into coupled assays. In particular, with class I diTPSs specific for either *ent*-or normal CPP, either the KS from Arabidopsis (*Arabidopsis thaliana*) (AtKS) or miltiradiene synthase from *Salvia miltiorrhiza*, respectively. These assays were compared with those utilizing CPSs of known stereochemistry. In this manner, LjTPS1 was shown to produce *ent*-CPP (**1**) (Figure 3A), while LjTPS4 produced normal CPP (**7**) (Figure 3C). LjTPS3 was shown to produce PPP (**3**), as evidenced by the analogous mixture of products as observed with MvCPS1—that is, upon dephosphorylation to peregrinol (**3′**), there is spontaneous formation of a small amount of a mixture of the C13 epimers of 9,13-epoxy-labda-14-ene (Figure **4A** and **4B**). The latter two products were identified by comparison to coupled assays with a class I diTPS that produces **5** (KgTS) and **6** (SsSS), respectively, with equivalent results from assays with either MvCPS1 or LjTPS3 (Figure 1A). Thus, LjTPS3 is a PPP synthase.

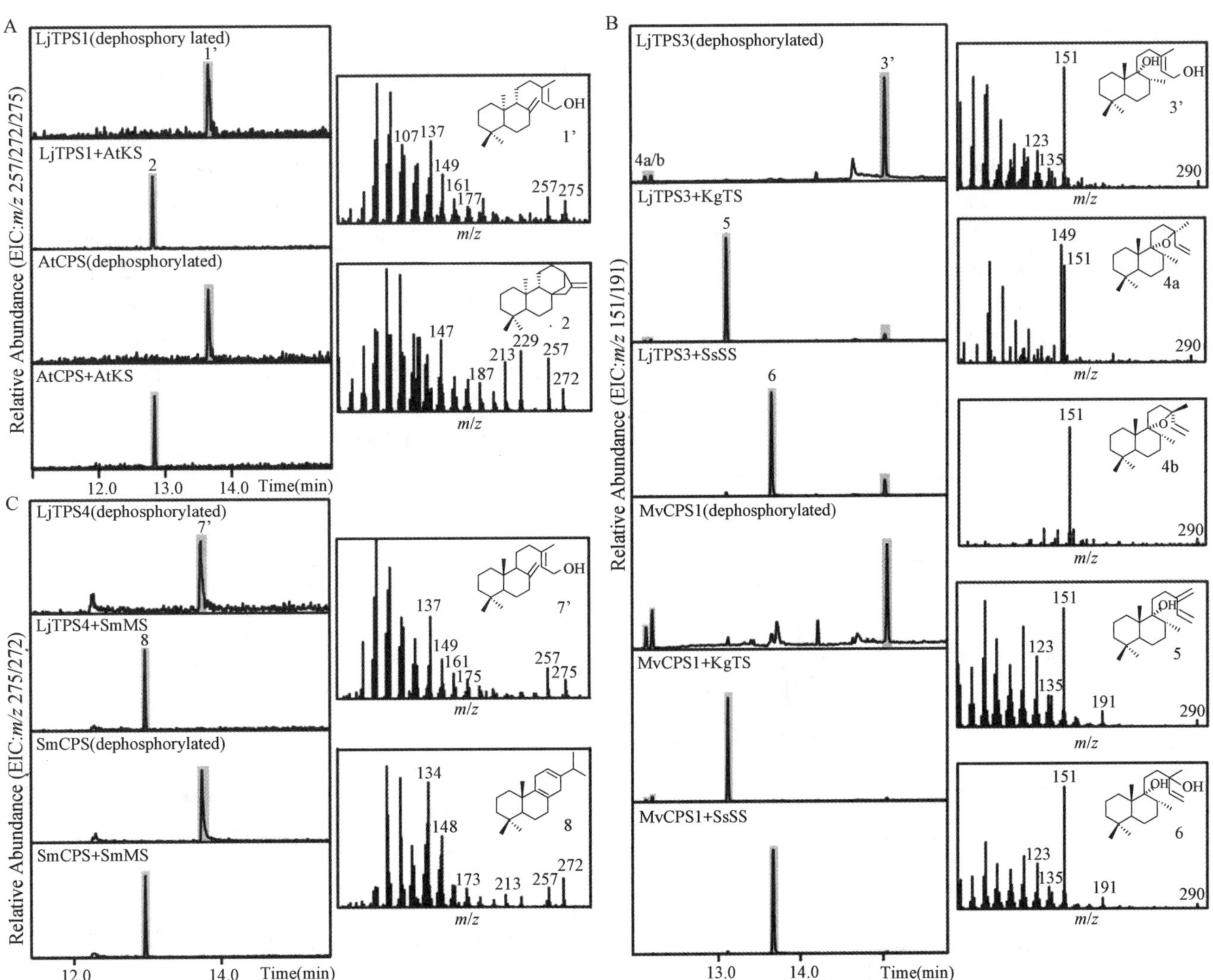


**Figure 3 GC-MS analysis of *L. japonicus* Class II diterpene cyclases with comparison to known diTPSs from *in vitro* assays**

(A-C) Extracted ion chromatograms (EICs) of the dephosphorylated reaction products obtained by Class II LjTPSs and known cyclases, or the products obtained by coupling with class I diTPSs with known substrate stereospecificity. (A) Dephosphorylated products from LjTPS1, *A. thaliana* (At) copalyl diphos-phate synthase (AtCPS), or either coupled with At KS (AtKS). (B) Dephosphorylated reaction products obtained by LjTPS3, *Marrubium vulgare* (Mv) copalyl diphosphate synthase (MvCPS1), or either coupled with *Kitasatospora griseola* (Kg) terpene synthase (KgTS) or *Salvia sclarea* (Ss) sclareol synthase (SsSS). (C) Dephosphorylated reaction products obtained by LjTPS4, *Salvia miltiorrhiza* (Sm) copalyl diphosphate synthase (SmCPS), or either coupled with Sm miltiradiene synthase.

Functional characterization of putative class I diTPSs For the functional characterization of the three class I diTPSs (LjTPS5, LjTPS6, and LjTPS7), these also were heterologously expressed in *E. coli* with a C-terminal 3His epitope tag, and the crude recombinant proteins used for *in vitro* assays, in the case of LjTPS5 and LjTPS6 these were coupled with various class II diTPSs. By comparison to the known activity of the *ent*-CPP producing AtCPS and AtKS, LjTPS5 was shown to produce *ent*-kaurene (**2**) when coupled with either AtCPS or LjTPS1 (Figure 4A). Thus, LjTPS5 was identified as a KS, presumably involved in GA biosynthesis in *L. japonicus*. On the other hand, LjTPS6 was found to react with PPP (**3**), as produced by either MvCPS or LjTPS3, and produce largely labda-13(16),14-dien-9α-ol (**5**), along with smaller amounts of viteagnusin D (**6**) and a mixture of the C13 epimers of 9,13-epoxy-labda-14-ene (**4**), with somewhat more of 13*S* (**4b**) than 13*R* (**4a**) (Figures 1, A and 4, B). Accordingly, LjTPS6 appears to be a catalytically promiscuous labda-13(16), 14-diene-9-ol synthase that may enable production of C9-oxy containing labdanes in *L. japonicus* more generally. In contrast, LjTPS7 was found to react directly with GGPP, producing (*E*,*E*)-geranyllinalool (Figure 4C).

Substrate specificity of class I LjTPSs Many diTPSs exhibit substrate promiscuity, particularly class I diTPSs that react with a variety of class II diTPS products to yield distinct diterpenoid skeletons as described by previous studies. To investigate the substrate promiscuity of class I LjTPSs in *L. japonicus*, these were each co-expressed with the previously described set of 12 catalytically distinct class II diTPSs in a modular metabolic engineering system. Both LjTPS5 and LjTPS6 displayed catalytic activity when combined with two other class II diTPSs. In particular, LjTPS5 could functionally couple with MvCPS1 (producing PPP) and AtCPS:H263A (producing 8β-hydroxy-*ent*-CPP) to produce viteagnusin D (**6**) and 13*R*-*ent*-manoyl oxide (**10**) (respectively), as identified by comparison to previously identified diTPS products (Figures 1, A, 5, A, and B). LjTPS6 was active in combination with AgAS:D621A (producing normal CPP) and NgCLS (producing 8α-hydroxy-CPP). LjTPS6 coverts normal CPP largely to sandaracopimaradiene (**11**), and two by-products, the oxygenated diterpene nezukol (**12**) and an unidentified product (**13**), again with product identification by comparison to known diTPS products (Figure 5C). Similarly, LjTPS6 was found to convert 8α-hydroxy-CPP to 13*R*-manoyl oxide (**14**) (Figures 1, A and 5, D).

No product was found upon co-expression of LjTPS7 with this set of class II diTPSs. However, previous studies reported that most geranyllinalool synthases can react with isoprenyl diphosphate precursors of other chain lengths (e.g. (*E*, *E*)-farnesyl diphosphate [FPP, C15] and (*E*)-geranyl diphosphate [GPP, C10]). Thus, LjTPS7 assayed *in vitro* with either FPP or GPP as substrates. The results revealed that LjTPS7 could also react with FPP to produce nerolidol (**15**), and GPP to produce linalool (**16**) (Figures 1, B, 5, E and F). Thus, LjTPS7 is capable of producing tertiary alcohols of varied isoprenoid chain length in *L. japonicus*.

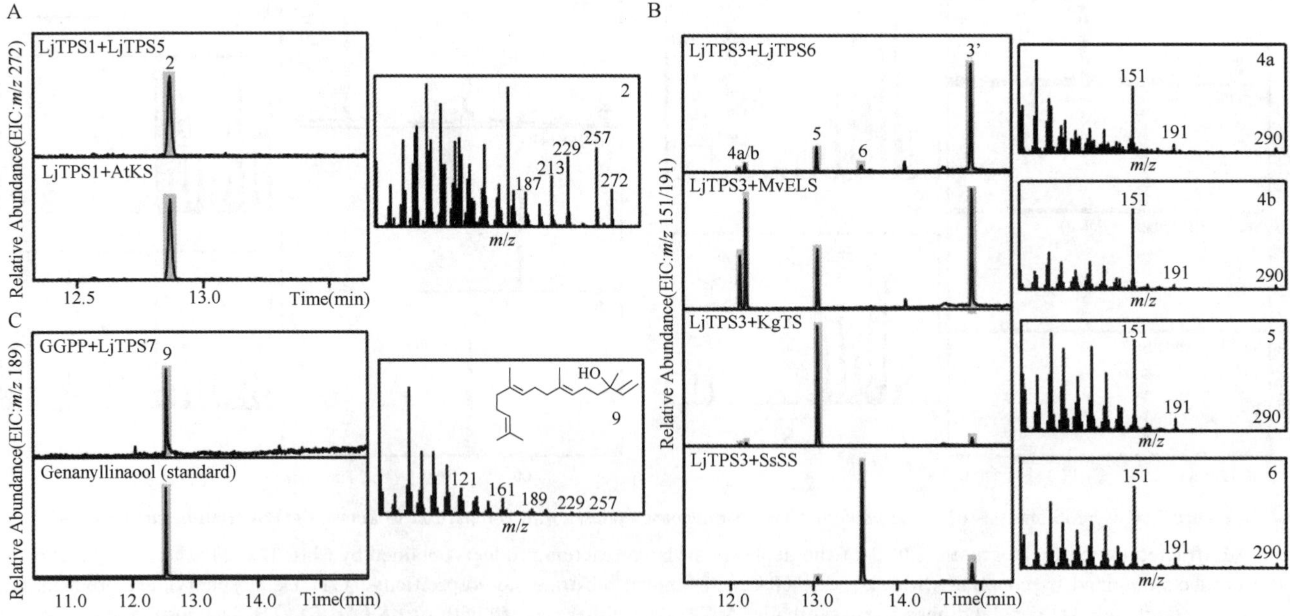


**Figure 4 GC–MS analysis of *L. japonicus* class I terpene synthase products from (coupled) *in vitro* assays**

(A–C) EICs of the products obtained by class I LjTPSs and identified synthases coupled with class II TPSs *in vitro*. (A) LjTPSS or AtKS coupled with LjTPS1 (producing *ent*-CPP). (B) LjTPS6, KgTS, SsSS, and MvELS coupled with LjTPS3 (producing PPP). (C) LjTPS7 with GGPP as substrate.

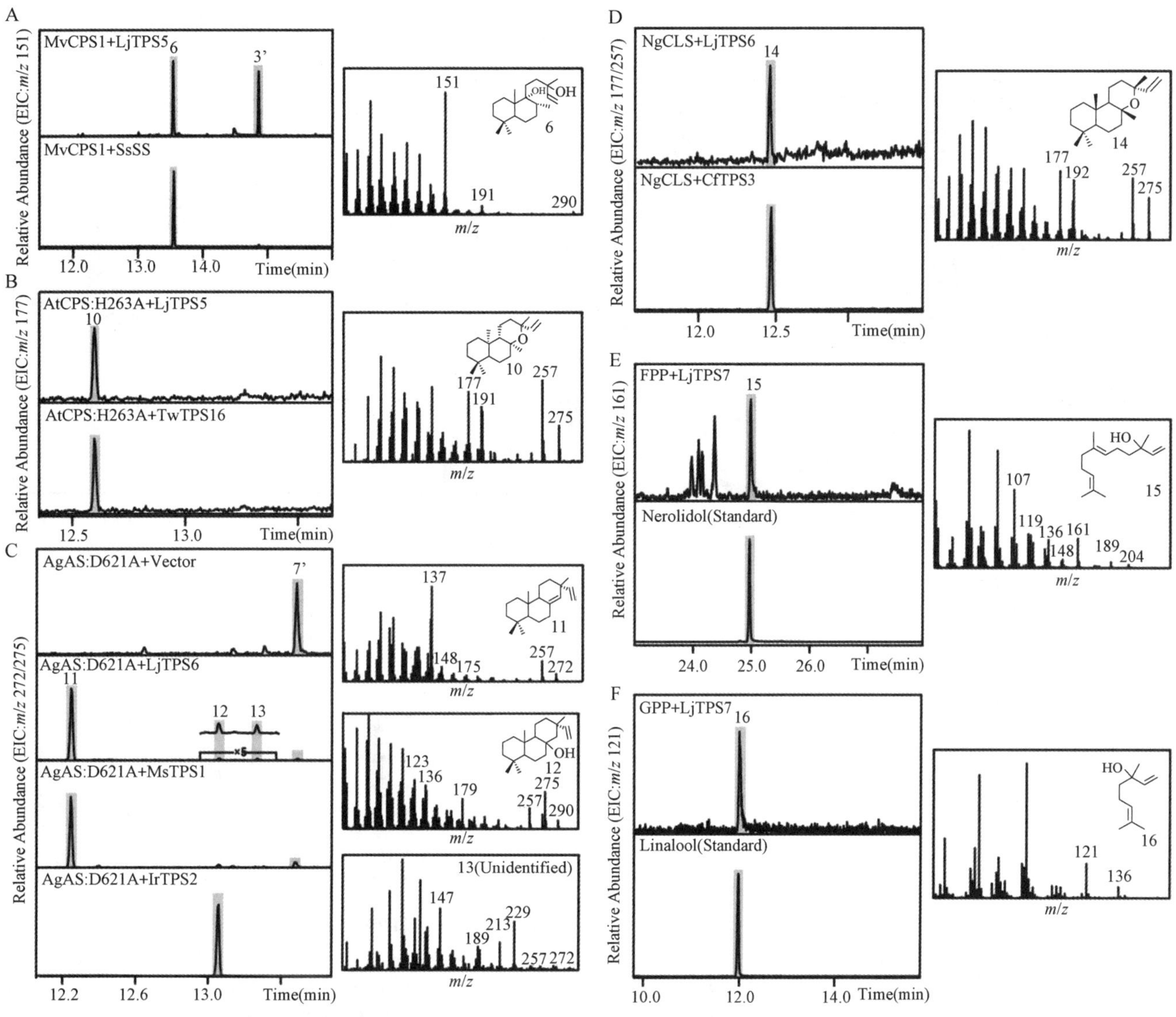


**Figure 5 Diterpenes produced by class I LjTPSs with alternative substrates *in vivo* or *in vitro***

(A-D) The EIC of the product(s) obtained with LjTPS5 or LjTPS6 coupled with other class II diTPS in a previously described metabolic engineering system, termed here *in vivo*. (A) LjTPS5 or SsSS coupled with MvCPS1 (producing PPP) *in vivo*. (B) LjTPS5 or TwTPS16 coupled with AtCPS: H263A (producing 8β-hydroxy-*ent*-CPP) *in vivo*. (C) LjTPS6 or CfTPS3 coupled with NgCLS (producing 8α-hydroxy-CPP) *in vivo*. (D) LjTPS6 or *Isodon rubescens* TPS2 (IrTPS2), *Mentha spicata* TPS1 (MsTPS1) coupled with AgAS: D621 (producing (+)-CPP) *in vivo*. E and F, The EICs of the product obtained by LjTPS7 with FPP or GPP as substrate *in vitro*. (E) LjTPS7 with FPP as substrate *in vitro*. (F) LjTPS7 with GPP as substrate *in vitro*.

Single residue mutation switches the catalytic specificity of LjTPS6 LjTPS6 produces a mixture of products from PPP (**3**), much as reported for related class I diTPSs—for example, LlTPS4, OmTPS3, OmTPS5, and MvELS. Notably, it has been previously shown that sin-gle residue changes can dramatically alter product outcome in diTPSs. Given the interest in spiro-9,13-epoxy-labdane diterpenoids, it was hypothesized that single residue mutations in LjTPS6 may impart more specificity for such heterocyclization. Among such diTPSs OmTPS3 was the most specific, albeit still producing both C13 epimers. Thus, LjTPS6 was aligned with these related diTPSs, and its protein structure modeled, with the hallmark DDxxD and DTE/NSE motifs used to define the active site cavity into which PPP was docked. This led to identification of two candidate sites for mutagenesis in LjTPS6, T315, and I420, for which the residues found in the related diTPSs were substituted (Figure 6, A and B). These mutants were characterizing by co-expression with MvCPS1 in the modular metabolic engineering system. Notably, mutation of I420 but not T315 can substantially increase the specificity of LjTPS6 product outcome with PPP as substrate. In particular, substitution of either Asn or Val for I420 led to production of only the 13*S* epimer (**4b**) of 9,13-epoxy-labda-14-ene, with the **4a**, **5**, or **6** also produced by the wild-type (WT) enzyme no longer observed (Figure 6C).

It also has been reported that replacement of the key

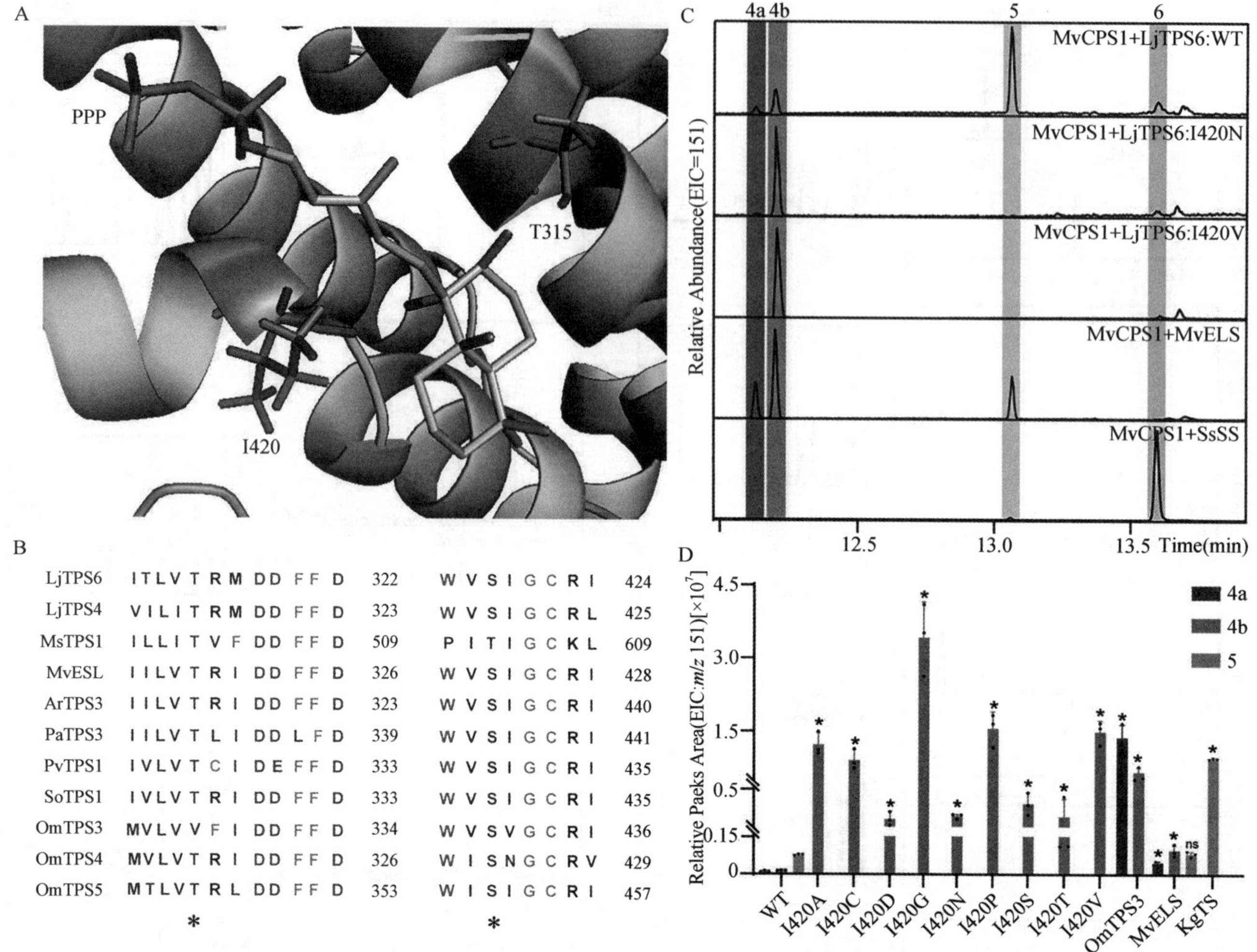


**Figure 6 Single residue mutations affect the products of LjTPS6 with PPP**

(A) Homology modeling and docking with PPP as ligand. (B) Multiple sequence alignments of LjTPS6 with related diTPSs. (C) EIC of the products obtained by LjTPS6: I420V/N coupled with MvCPS1 (producing PPP) *in vivo*. (D) Relative peak area of diterpenes produced by LjTPS6 mutants with PPP as the substrates, and the error bars show the SDs from mean value ($n=3$). Statistically significant differences between the product abundance of LjTPS6 mutants and LjTPS6 WT based on a Student's $t$-test ($P<0.05$).

residue by different amino acid can have distinct effects on diTPSs activity. Thus, saturation mutagenesis was carried out at residue 420, revealing that substitution with seven other amino acids (A/C/D/G/P/S/T) can increase LjTPS6 catalytic specificity, similarly imparting selective production of **4b**, albeit with varied catalytic efficiency. The activity of LjTPS6 mutants with nonpolar amino acid substitution (i.e. Ala, Gly, Val, and Pro) was higher than those with polar amino acids (i.e. Cys, Asp, Asn, Ser, and Thr) (Figure 6d). Strikingly, LjTPS6: I420G was found to not only selectively produce **4b** but also exhibit the highest catalytic efficiency.

To determine if changes at I420 altered reactivity with alternative substrates these LjTPS6 mutants also were tested with normal CPP and 8α-hydroxy-CPP using the modular metabolic engineering system (i.e. via co-expression with AgAS: D21A and NgCLS). The results indicated that these changes also affect reactivity with these substrates (Figure 7). Eight of these LjTPS6: I420 mutants (A/C/G/N/P/S/T/V) reacted with normal CPP to produce the *endo* olefin derivative *trans*-biformene (**17**) (Figure 7, a and b), and with 8α-hydroxy-CPP to produce 13*S*-manoyl oxide (**13b**) as well as the same 13*R* epimer selectively produced by WT (Figure 7, c and d)

## 3 DISCUSSION

Here, an *L. japonicus* transcriptome was generated, enabling identification of six diTPSs, which were then functionally characterized, elucidating the relevant enzymes for diterpenoid metabolism in this medicinal plant. In addition to the *ent*-CPP synthase (LjTPS1) and subsequently acting *ent*-KS (LjTPS5) required for GA phytohormone biosynthesis, diTPSs that act in more specialized diterpenoid biosynthesis also were identified. One of these serves as a geranyllinalool synthase (LjTPS7), suggesting the possibility that *L. japonicus* produces homoterpenes, which are often involved in tritrophic plant-(insect herbivore)-predator/parasitoid

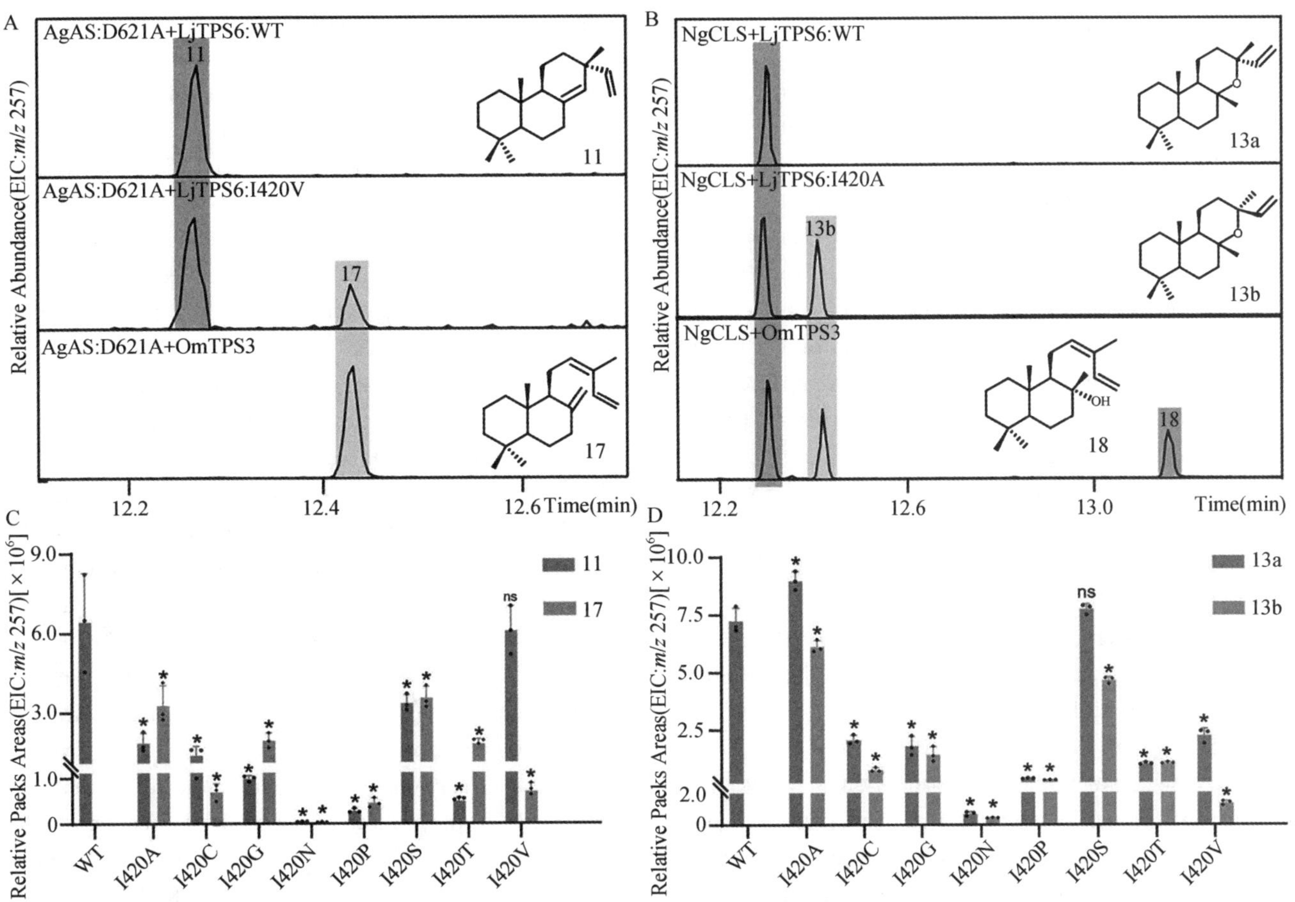


**Figure 7 GC-MS analysis of extracts from *in vivo* assay of LjTPS6:I420 mutants coupled with AgAS:D621 or NgCLS**

(A and B) EICs of the products obtained by LjTPS6:I420V coupled with (A) AgAS:D621A (producing (+)-CPP) or (B) NgCLS (producing 8$\alpha$-hydroxy-CPP) *in vivo*. (C and D) Relative area of product peaks obtained from LjTPS6:I420 with (C) AgAS:D621A or (D) NgCLS A *in vivo*, and the error bars show the SDs from mean value ($n=3$). Statistically significant differences between the product abundance of LjTPS6 mutants and LjTPS6 WT based on a Student's $t$-test ($P<0.05$).

interactions. In addition, these include another class II diTPS that produces normal CPP (LjTPS4), as well as one that produces a C9 hydroxylated derivative, PPP (LjTPS3). The final class I diTPS (LjTPS6) reacts with both normal CPP and PPP, producing sandaracopimaradiene and a mixture of C9-oxy derivatives, respectively (Figure 1, A and B). While *L. japonicus* is not known to produce any sandaracopimaradiene-derived diterpenoids, these results encourage further examination for such natural products. The gene expression and metabolites analysis showed that only LjTPS3 has a close relationship with C9-oxy diterpenoids distribution, which was mainly accumulated in aerial parts (Figure 2A), consistent with a role for LjTPS3 in C9-oxy diterpenoids biosynthesis in *L. japonicas*.

Despite the preponderance of derived diterpenoids in this plant, LjTPS6 does not primarily produce 9,13-epoxy-labda-14-ene. While similar observations have been made for other class I diTPSs from related plant species that also produce such diterpenoids, this catalytic promiscuity complicates both further biosynthetic investigations, as well as use of these enzymes for metabolic engineering directed at specific production of derived diterpenoids. Further elucidation of biosynthesis is additionally complicated by the often-observed promiscuity of the subsequently acting cytochrome P450 monooxygenases. For example, currently only MvCYP71AU87 has been identified as acting on 9,13-epoxy-labda-14-ene, but catalyzes hydroxylation of either of the C4 *geminal* methyl substituents to yield C18 or C19 hydroxylated products. Notably, while a diTPS has been found to specifically produce 9,13-epoxy-labda-14-ene (**4a** and **4b**; OmTPS3), this yields significant amounts of both C13 epimers. Thus, the enzymatic engineering undertaken here that resolves this key issue, stereospecifically producing the 13*S* epimer (**4b**), with LjTPS6:I420G further exhibiting strong catalytic efficiency as well, provides a key reagent for further studies of the biosynthesis of derived bioactive diterpenoids. Together with the *L. japonicus* transcriptome generated here, there is now a strong foundation for such biosynthetic investigations, which are expected to enable access to important diterpenoids such as prehispanolone and similar spiro-9,13*S*-epoxy ring containing diterpenoids that exhibit anti-platelet and anti-coagulant properties.

## 4 MATERIALS AND METHODS

Plant materials, RNA isolation, and cDNA synthesis The plants of *L. japonicus* were received from Nanjing, Jiangsu, China (store at −80 ℃). Three plants of similar conditions were selected and divided into three parts (root, stem, and leaf) and stored at −80℃. Total RNA was extracted from these organs using a Quick RNA Isolation Kit (HuaYueYang Biotechnology, Beijing, China) following the manufacturer's instructions. The integrity and concentration of total RNA were detected by 1.0% (*w*/*v*) agarose gel electrophoresis and NanoDrop ND-3000 (Thermo NanoDrop, Wisconsin, USA). A PrimeScript RT Reagent Kit with gDNA Eraser (Takara Bio., Dalian, USA) was used to re-verse transcribed into cDNA with 1 μg of total RNA from three tissues.

Transcriptome sequencing, de novo assembly, and annotation Total RNA from *L. japonicus* tissues (e.g. leaf, root, and stem) was extracted using a Quick RNA Isolation Kit (HuaYueYang biotechnology, Beijing, China) and the integrity checked using a 2,100 RNA Nano 6,000 Assay Kit (Agilent Technologies, Palo Alto, CA, USA) following the manufacturer's instructions. RNA was prepared for sequencing using Illumina TruSeq sample preparation kit version 2 (Illumina, San Diego, CA, USA). The fragments were sequenced with paired ends (2×150 bp) on a Illumina NovaSeq6000 (Illumina San Diego, CA, USA) by the Annoroad Gene Tech. Co., Ltd, Beijing, China. A total 279 million raw reads were generated. Adapter sequences were removed from raw reads and reads were trimmed at the ends to Q30, using the fastq-mcf tool from ea-utils (https://github.com/Expression Analysis/ea-utils). Processed reads were de novo assembled and estimated using the Trinity (Trinity Release version 2.4.0) pipeline according to guide-lines in the published protocols, resulting in a total of 133,725 assembled putative transcripts. ORFs were predicted by TransDecoder. Trinotate was used for the functional annotation of unigenes and ORFs to known sequence data (BLAST + /SwissProt), protein domain identification (HMMER/PFAM), protein signal peptide and transmembrane domain prediction (singalP/tmHMM), and comparison to currently current annotation databases (EMBL Uniprot eggNOG/GO Pathways databases).

LjTPSs screening in *L. japonicus* and bioinformatic analysis The genes were filtered according to their transcriptome information to comprehensively identify *TPS* genes in *L. japonicus*. The nucleotide and deduced amino acid sequences were analyzed, and the BLASTP tool on the NCBI online database (http://www.ncbi.nlm.nih.gov/) was used to compare the sequences. Multiple sequence alignment was implemented by ClustalW software, and MEGA version 7.0 software was used to construct a phylogenetic tree using the neighbor-joining (NJ) method (bootstrap = 1,000).

Cloning of LjTPS coding sequences According to the transcriptome sequence information, specific primers were developed to amplify the LjTPS ORFs (the primers are listed in Supplemental Table S4). A GeneJET Gel Extraction Kit (Thermo Scientific, San Jose, CA, USA) was used to purify the PCR products, after which the products were cloned into a T-Vector (pEASY-Blunt Zero Simple Vector) (TransGen, Beijing, China), which was subsequently transformed into *E. coli* DH5α (Covin Biosciences, Beijing, China) competent cells. Sangon Biotech (Shanghai) Co., Ltd. isolated the rebuilt plasmids and sequenced their nucleotides.

Functional characterization of LjTPSs The ORF regions of the *LjTPS*s were subcloned into a pET-32a (+) (EMD Biosciences, Novagen) expression vector via PCR amplification with a pEASY-Uni Seamless Cloning and Assembly Kit (TransGen, Beijing, China), and the amplicons were digested with BamH I restriction enzymes (New England Biolab, Ipswich, MA, USA) (the primers are listed in Supplemental Table S4). The verified vectors were subsequently transformed into *Rosetta* (DE3) *in vitro*. The biochemical functional characterization of LjTPS was performed as the follows: the 500 μL reaction volume contained 200 μL solution of the crude enzyme, 50 mmol/L HEPES buffer (pH 7.5), 100 mmol/L KCl, 7.5 mmol/L $MgCl_2$, 1 mmol/L DTT, 5% glycine, 40 μmol/L GPP, FPP, GGPP, or couple with class I diTPS. Class II LjTPSs were estimated with 40 μmol/L GGPP as a substrate for 8 h at 30 ℃, class I LjTPSs were estimated with GPP, FPP, GGPP, or couple with class I diTPS. The *in vitro* products were hydrolyzed for 10 h at 30 ℃ using two units of calf intestinal alkaline phosphatase and two units of potato apyrase in hydrolysis buffer (100 mmol/L Tris-HCl, pH 9.5), and extracted thrice using an equal volume of n-hexane. The extracts were dried with N2 and dissolved in 100 μL n-hexane for GC-MS analysis. The substrate specificity of class Ⅰ LjTPSs were coupled with the reported 12 class Ⅱ diTPSs in the *E. coli* OverExpress C41 strain (Lucigen, Middleton, WI, USA), using the previously developed modular metabolic engineering system, which can produce 12 different substrates of class Ⅰ diTPSs.

The products of diTPSs analysis by GC-MS The GC-MS analysis was performed by a Trace 1310 instrument equipped with a TSQ 8000 mass detector and then separated by a TG-5 MS column (30 m×0.25 mm I.D., DF = 0.25 μm; Thermo Scientific, USA). Helium was used as a carrier gas at a flow rate of 1.0 min/mL. The oven program was as follows: 50℃ for 2 min, an increase of 20℃/min to 300℃, and then holding for 10 min (for GGPP as substrate), or 50℃ for 2 min, an increase of 5℃/min to 150℃ holding for 5 min, an increase of 10℃/min to 220℃ and holding for 2 min, an increase of 30 ℃/min to 300 ℃ and holding for 5 min (for GPP as substrate), or 50℃ for 2 min, an increase of 8℃/min to 250℃, an increase of 10℃/min to 320℃ and then holding for 10 min (for FPP as substrate). The ion trap temperature was 250℃, and the scan range was 40 – 450 *m/z*.

Metabolite analysis of *L. japonicus* by UPLC – Q/TOF – MS For metabolite analyses, 100 mg finely powdered tissues of *L. japonicus* were ultrasound extracted with 0.5 mL methanol (contain 50 μg/mL Andrographolide as internal standard) at 25℃ for 1 h, and then centrifuged at 12,000*g* for 15 min at room temperature, and three independent experiments of the tissues were performed for each analysis. The supernatant was directly analyzed by UPLC – Q/TOF – MS. UPLC – Q/TOF – MS was carried out using an Acquity UPLC system (Waters Corp., Milford, MA, USA) with an Acquity UPLC BEH C18 column (50×2.1 mm, 1.7 μm). The column temperature was set at 40℃. The flow rate was kept at 400 μL/min. Mobile phases were water (with 0.1% Formic acid)(A) and acetonitrile (B). The gradient was as follows: 0 – 8 min, 5%– 20% B; 8 – 16 min, 20%– 100% B; 16 – 21 min, 100% B; 21 – 21.5 min, 100%– 5% B; 21.5 – 24.5 min, 5% B. Time-of-flight MS detection was performed with a Xevo G2-S MS system (Waters Corp., Manchester, UK). The data acquisition range was from 50 to 1,000 Da. The source temperature was set at 100℃, and the desolvation temperature was set at 450 ℃, with desolvation gas flow set at 900 L/h. The lock mass compound used was leucine enkephalin at a concentration 200 pg/μL. The capillary voltage was set at 2.0 kV. The cone voltage was set at 500 V. The collision energy was set as 6 eV for a low-energy scan, with a 35 – 60 eV ramp for a high-energy scan. The instrument was controlled by MassLynx version 4.1 software (Waters Corp., Milford, MA, USA).

RT-qPCR Total RNA was extracted from *L. japonicus* tissues using a Quick RNA Isolation Kit (HuaYueYang Biotechnology, Beijing, China) following the manufacturer's instructions. First-strand cDNA was synthesized using the PrimeScript RT Reagent Kit with gDNA Eraser (Takara Bio., Dalian, USA). Relative transcript abundance was determined by RT-qPCR using the TransStart Top Green qPCR SuperMix (TransGen Biotech, Beijing, China) on a Roche LightCycler480 (Roche, Basel, Switzerland). The primers used for RT-qPCR analysis are listed in Supplemental Table S4. The gene for actin was used as the endogenous control. At least three independent experiments were performed for each analysis.

Molecular docking and site-directed mutagenesis Within SWISS – MODEL Workspace, homology modeling was utilized to create the three-dimensional structure of LjTPS6. After searching the PDB (https://www.rcsb.org/) for templates based on alternate sequence alignments, templates were chosen based on their GMQW values, and multiple models were generated using the chosen templates. To relate sequence position, a multiple sequence alignment was created using the sequences. The PHENIX suite's elBow algorithm was used to refine the substrate. Molecular docking was used to model LjTPS6 and its substrates (CPP, PPP, and 8-hydroxy-CPP). AutoDock4 was used to perform docking calculations, as previously stated. The results of this docking were shown by PyMOL.

The mutations of the LjTPS6 were cloned into a pET – 32a (+) expression vector via PCR amplification with a pEASY – Uni Seamless Cloning and Assembly Kit (TransGen, Beijing, China), the primers were digested with BamH I restriction enzymes (New England Biolab, USA) and shown in Supplemental Table S4. Using the previously described modular metabolic engineering system, functional assessment of LjTPS6 mutations was coupled with MvCPS1, AgAS:D621A, and NgCLS in the *E. coli* Over Express C41 strain (Lucigen).

[王健,崔光红,黄璐琦,等.Plant Physiology, 2022,189: 99 – 111.]

# Engineering of triterpene metabolism and overexpression of the lignin biosynthesis gene *PAL* promotes ginsenoside $Rg_3$ accumulation in ginseng plant chassis

## 1 INTRODUCTION

The ginsenoside $Rg_3$ has extensive pharmacological properties, most notably anti-cancer effects. Shenyi capsules, the first class I Chinese medicine monomer anti-cancer drug independently developed in China, contain $Rg_3$ as a primary component. At present, the main source of $Rg_3$ production is field cultivation of *Panax* plants, such as *Panax ginseng* (ginseng); however, this poses problems, such as deforestation, pesticide residues, and heavy metal pollution. Moreover, the yield of $Rg_3$ from *Panax* plants is limited, with only about 0.03 mg per gram of raw material. Thus, direct extraction of the ginsenoside $Rg_3$ from cultivated *P. ginseng* cannot meet the increasing market demand.

Recent studies have identified the route of $Rg_3$ biosynthesis in *Panax* plants. The mevalonate (MVA) pathway catalyzing the conversion of glucose to farnesyl diphosphate (FPP) is the starting point of ginsenoside biosynthesis. Squalene synthase (SS) and squalene epoxidase (SE) then transform FPP into 2, 3-oxidosqualene, an important precursor of sterols and saponins that can be cyclized to form dammarenediol by dammarenediol synthase (DS). Next, the cytochrome P450 enzyme CYP716A47 catalyzes the formation of protopanaxadiol from dammarenediol. Protopanaxadiol can be either glycosylated into $Rh_2$ via UGTPg45 or transformed into protopanaxatriol by CYP716A53v2. The ginsenoside $Rg_3$ is then biosynthesized through glycosylation of $Rh_2$ by UGTPg29 and Pq3-O-UGT2. Therefore, reconstruction of the $Rg_3$ biosynthesis pathway in a cell factory, such as yeast, is a feasible and potentially effective strategy to obtain high yields of $Rg_3$. Recently, a ginsenoside $Rg_3$ yield of 2.7 mg/g was obtained from metabolically engineered yeast. Compared with the use of yeast and other cell factories, the use of plant chassis has the advantages of low toxicity and high biosafety for the production of bioactive compounds, cost-effectiveness, environmental friendliness, and potential for large-scale agricultural production.

Plant metabolic engineering has been successfully used to improve the production of bioactive components such as diterpenoid jolkinol C, tropane alkaloids, momilactone B, and taxanes. Plant metabolic engineering has benefits for environmental protection and agriculture. Plants can absorb pollutants and greenhouse gases from the environment and can be engineered to increase their resistance to diseases and insect pests, reducing the use of pesticides, and to increase their content and ratio of nutritional substances. Because the ginsenoside $Rg_3$ is naturally produced in *P. ginseng* plants, engineering the *P. ginseng* chassis is a promising approach for the production of $Rg_3$ in high yield.

Reconstruction of the biosynthesis pathway and overexpression of essential genes are the main strategies for the production of bioactive compounds via exogenous systems. However, when using a plant system, other strategies may also be feasible, such as blocking the branch flux of unwanted products and controlling related signal pathways. Protopanaxatriol, the key precursor of protopanaxatriol-type ginsenosides, is the oxidation product of protopanaxadiol, produced in a reaction catalyzed by CYP716A53v2, and is thus the product of a competing pathway with respect to the protopanaxadiol-type ginsenoside $Rg_3$. Knocking down *CYP716A53v2* might therefore be an effective way to improve $Rg_3$ production in *P. ginseng*. Furthermore, $Rg_3$ accumulates abundantly within the root xylem, which has a high lignin content; therefore, phenylalanine ammonia lyase (PAL), the first enzyme in the lignin biosynthesis pathway, could affect xylem structure by changing lignin biosynthesis. Indeed, overexpression of *PAL* in sweet potato has been reported to stimulate secondary xylem cell expansion in stems and promote chlorogenic acid biosynthesis. The effect of PAL on ginsenoside accumulation has not been reported, but we speculated that overexpression of *PAL* could contribute to $Rg_3$ accumulation.

In this study, we therefore combined multiple modules, including engineering of triterpene metabolism and overexpression of *PAL*, for high-yield production of the protopanaxadiol-type ginsenoside $Rg_3$ in a *P. ginseng* chassis. First, we used a semi-rational design to improve the enzymatic efficiency of Pq3-O-UGT2 in regard to $Rh_2$. Second, we applied clustered regularly interspaced palindromic repeats (CRISPR)/CRISPR-associated protein 9 (Cas9) editing to knock down the branch pathway of protopanaxatriol-type ginsenoside biosynthesis to enhance the metabolic flux of $Rg_3$. We also examined the function of PAL in lignin biosynthesis and ginsenoside accumulation in *P. ginseng*. Based on our results, we combined overexpression of *SE*, the optimized *Pq3-O-UGT2*, and *PAL* with CRISPR/Cas9 knockdown of *CYP716A53v2* in *P. ginseng* to improve ginsenoside accumulation. The high-yield system established here may provide an effective platform for the large-scale production of $Rg_3$ in a *P. ginseng* chassis.

## 2 RESULTS

Pq3-O-UGT2 was screened as target gene  Many genes are involved in the biosynthesis of $Rg_3$ in *Panax* plants (Figure 1). To find target genes that could be modified to improve $Rg_3$ production in *P. ginseng*, we treated *P. ginseng* and *P. quinquefolium* root cultures with a jasmonate (JA) elicitor and analyzed the correlation between $Rg_3$ and genes involved in biosynthesis of $Rg_3$ (Figure 2A). The expression levels of *Pq3-O-UGT2* and *UGTPg29* had a significant positive correlation ($P < 0.01$) with $Rg_3$ concentration, which is consistent with the function of Pq3-O-UGT2 and UGTPg29 in catalyzing $Rh_2$ into $Rg_3$. There was also a strong positive correlation ($P < 0.01$) between *SE* expression and $Rg_3$ concentration, suggesting that *SE* is a key gene in $Rg_3$ biosynthesis. Furthermore, there was a negative correlation ($P < 0.05$) between *CYP716A53v2* expression

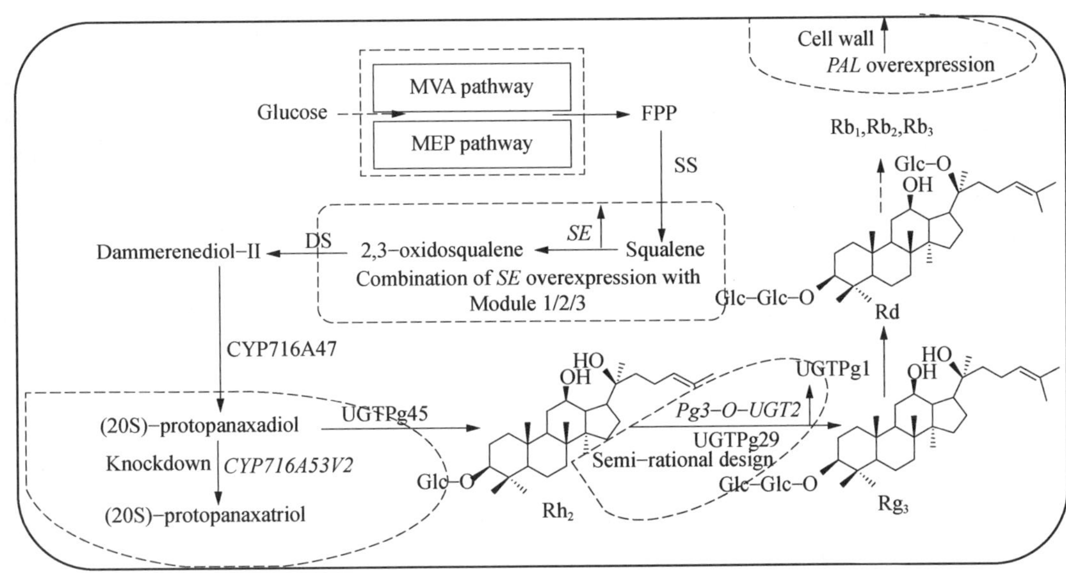


**Figure 1 Strategy of improving ginsenoside $Rg_3$ content**

The biosynthesis pathway of $Rg_3$ and strategies used in this study to improve the content of $Rg_3$ are shown. The genes with identified functions are colored in blue. The genes (SE and Pq3 - O - UGT2) overexpressed in this study are indicated with green arrows. CYP716A53v2 is colored in gray to indicate that it was knocked down. FPP, farnesyl diphosphate; SS, squalene synthase; SE, squalene epoxidase; DS, dammarenediol synthase; CYP716A47, CYP716A53v2, cytochrome P450 monooxygenase; PgUGT74AE2, UGTPg45, UGTPg29, UGTPg1, Pq3 - O - UGT2, UDP-glycosyltransferase.

and $Rg_3$ concentration (Figure 2A; Table S1), consistent with the function of CYP716A53v2 in diverting protopanaxadiol into protopanaxatriol. These data suggest that overexpression of *Pq3 - O - UGT2*, *UGTPg29*, and *SE*, as well as knockdown or knockout of *CYP716A53v2*, might contribute to higher concentrations of $Rg_3$ in *P. ginseng* root cultures.

Since Pq3 - O - UGT2 and UGTPg29 have a similar function of catalyzing $Rh_2$ into $Rg_3$, we compared their enzyme activity and affinity to $Rh_2$ to determine which was a better target for achieving high $Rg_3$ production. In the enzyme activity assay, Pq3 - O - UGT2 showed a slightly higher catalytic efficiency ($k_{cat}/K_M$ value); ($2.51 \times 10^5$/mol/L/s) than UGTPg29 ($2.07 \times 10^5$/mol/L/s) (Figure 2B; Table S2). Furthermore, Pq3 - O - UGT2 exhibited a lower $K_M$ (20.53 μmol/L) value for $Rh_2$ than for UGTPg29 (42.53 μmol/L), indicating a stronger affinity for $Rh_2$ as substrate. We also applied SPR (surface plasmon resonance) analysis to detect the binding affinity between Pq3 - O - UGT2 or UGTPg29 and $Rh_2$. The binding affinity (equilibrium dissociation constant, $K_d$) of Pq3 - O - UGT2 to ginsenoside $Rh_2$ was 14.31 μmol/L (Figure 2C), slightly stronger than that of UGTPg29 (19.83 μmol/L; Figure 2D). Thus, Pq3 - O - UGT2 was a better target than UGTPg29 for increasing the biosynthesis of ginsenoside $Rg_3$.

**Semi-rational design to improve the catalytic activity of Pq3 - O - UGT2** We further tried to enhance the enzymatic activity of Pq3 - O - UGT2 in catalyzing the glycosylation of $Rh_2$ through protein engineering. Since the structure of Pq3 - O - UGT2 has not been resolved, we built its model with known plant UGT (UDP-glycosyltransferase) structures for a semi-rational design. UGT74AC1 from *Siraitia grosvenorii* catalyzes the transfer of glucose to triterpene, a large sugar acceptor similar to $Rh_2$, and it has been successfully engineered to obtain a $10^4$-fold improvement in catalytic efficiency. We built the model of Pq3 - O - UGT2 using the structure of UGT74AC1 as a template. Through structure alignment of Pq3 - O - UGT2 and UGT74AC1, we mapped the seven key residues that are mutated in engineered UGT74AC1 onto Pq3 - O - UGT2 (Figure 3A). All seven residues are located in the N-terminal domain that binds the sugar receptor $Rh_2$. Among them, four Pq3 - O - UGT2 residues (Q30, S49, I50, and H85) are distinct, so we mutated the gene to match the changes in UGT74AC1, resulting in Pq3 - O - UGT2 with Q30H, S49R/I50M, and H85Y substitutions.

We determined the catalytic kinetic parameters of wild-type and mutant Pq3 - O - UGT2 to check whether the mutations improved the enzyme's catalytic activity (Tables 1, S3). Compared with that of the wild-type enzyme ($5.13 \pm 0.31$/s), the $k_{cat}$ value of each mutant enzyme showed a slight increase, of 1.78 -, 1.90 -, and 1.65-fold in the Q30H, S49R/I50M, and H85Y mutants, respectively. However, the $k_{cat}/K_M$ value of the Q30H mutant enzyme was lower than that of the wild-type enzyme. We therefore combined the two remaining mutations, S49R/I50M and H85Y, to construct a three-point mutation, and found that the $k_{cat}/K_M$ value of the resultant S49R/I50M/H85Y mutant

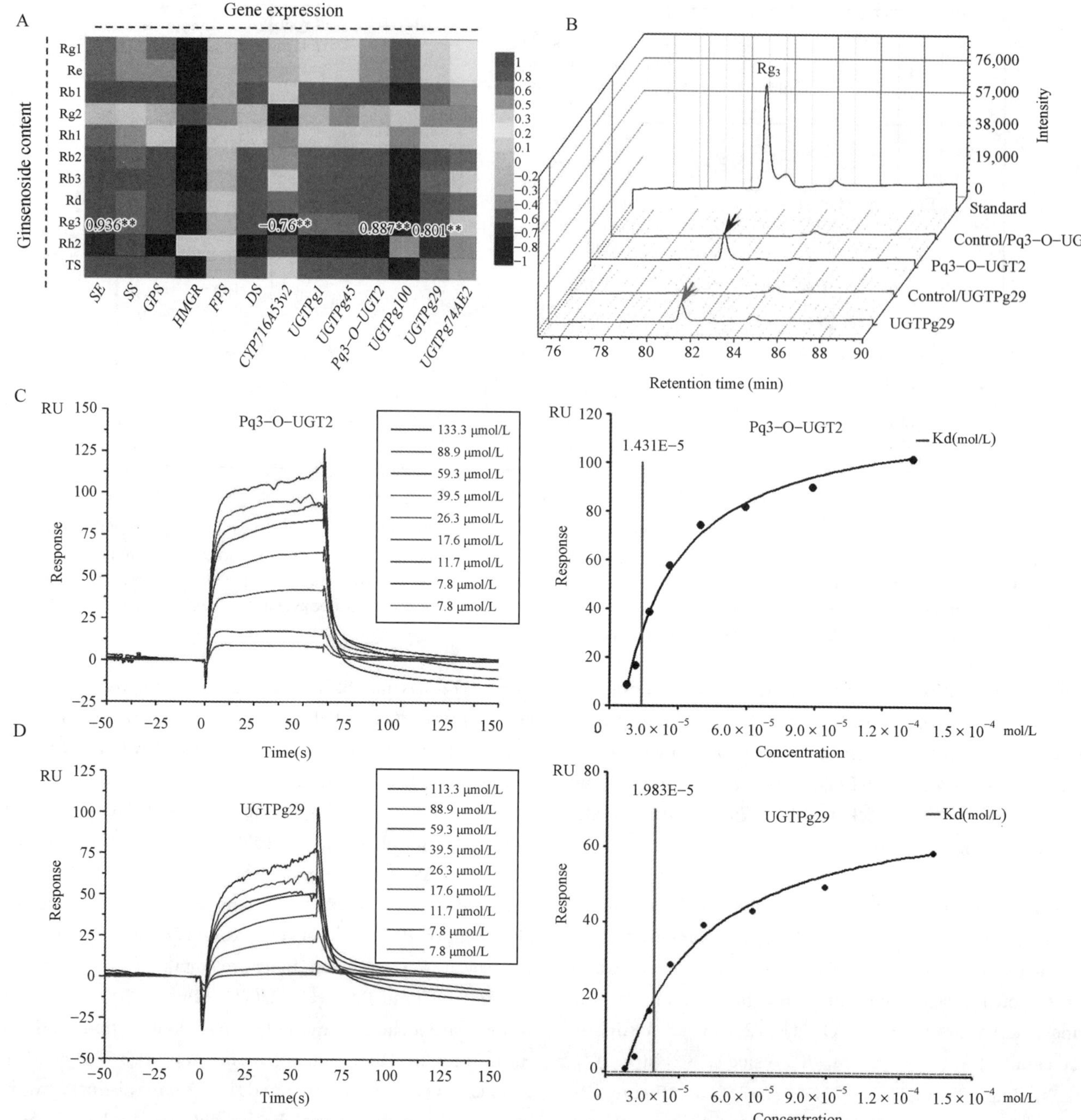


**Figure 2　Identification and analysis of key genes and enzymes involved in $Rg_3$ biosynthesis**

(**A**) Pearson's correlation analysis between relative expression level of ginsenoside biosynthesis genes and ginsenoside content in root cultures of *Panax quinquefolium* or *P. ginseng* under jasmonate (JA) induction. Pq-O-UGT2 gene came from root cultures of *P. quinquefolium*, other genes came from root cultures of *P. ginseng*. Data represent mean values ± *SE* of three replicates. * $P<0.05$, ** $P<0.01$, the significance of Pearson's correlation coefficients. (**B**) High-performance liquid chromatography analysis of the conversion of ginsenoside $Rh_2$ to $Rg_3$ catalyzed by Pq-O-UGT2 and UGTPg29. (**C, D**) Surface plasmon resonance (SPR) analysis of the interaction between Pq-O-UGT2 or UGTPg29 and $Rh_2$. Pq-O-UGT2 and $UGTPg_2 9$ were immobilized on a CM5 chip, and $Rh_2$ at the indicated concentrations flowed over the chip. SPR response curves are shown on the left. The data were analyzed through kinetics fitting with a 1 : 1 binding model and shown on the right.

enzyme was 1.3-fold greater than that of the wild-type, corresponding to a higher catalytic efficiency than those of the S49R/I50M and H85Y enzymes. We also tried to engineer Pq3-O-UGT2 based on sequence consensus. The plant secondary product glycosyltransferase (PSPG) motif is a highly conserved motif in plant UGTs and plays an important role in binding the sugar donor UDP-glycan. We created mutants of several residues in the PSPG motif of Pq3-O-UGT2 (S339N, L358A, A355P, and I341L/A342T) to match the most conserved residues in the consensus on the

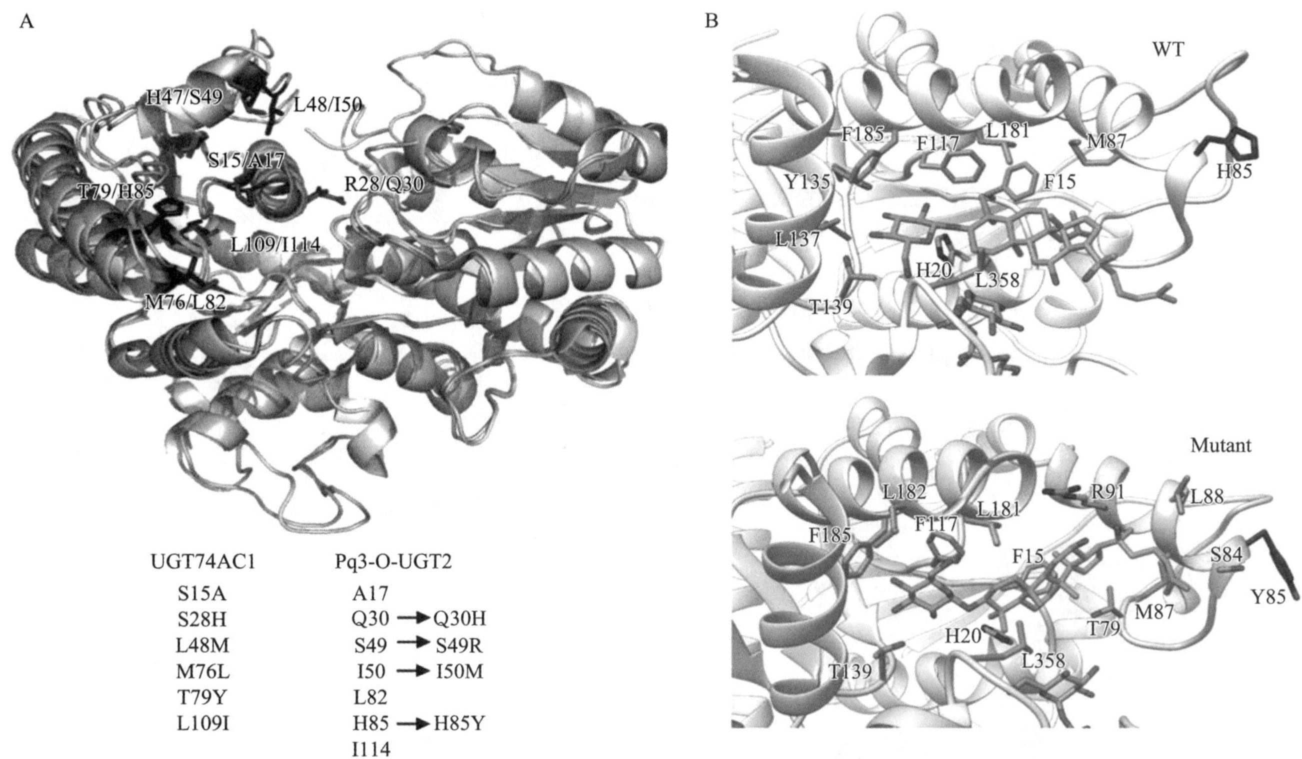


**Figure 3 Semi-rational design of Pq3 - O - UGT2**

(**A**) The structure model of Pq3 - O - UGT2 is superimposed onto crystal structure of UGT74AC1 (PDB: 6L8Z). The mutant residues of engineered UGT74AC1 and corresponding residues of Pq3 - O - UGT2 are indicated. Mutations designed in this study are shown at the bottom. (**B**) Catalytic conformations of Pq3 - O - UGT2 (WT)- UDPG - $Rh_2$ (top) and Pq3 - O - UGT2 (S49R/I50M/H85Y, Mutant)- UDPG - $Rh_2$ (bottom) after molecular dynamics simulations. $Rh_2$ and uridine diphosphate glucose (UDPG) are shown in orange and dim gray, respectively. Residues in $Rh_2$ binding pocket are shown in light blue. His85 in wild-type (WT) and Y85 in Mutant are shown in dark blue. Hydrogen bonds are indicated with magenta dash line.

**Table 1 Enzymatic kinetics parameters of Pq3 - O - UGT2 and its mutants to $Rh_2$**

| | $V_{max}$ (nmol/L/s) | $K_m$ (μmol/L) | $K_{cat}$ (/s) | $K_{cat}/K_m$ (/mol/L/s) |
|---|---|---|---|---|
| Pq3 - O - UGT2 - WT | 102±6 | 20.46±1.51 | 5.13±0.31 | 25.0733±13.782 |
| Q30H | 182±9 | 47.31±3.46 | 9.12±0.65 | 19.2876±17.702 |
| S49R/I50M | 166±6 | 36.50±2.31 | 9.77±0.58 | 26.7687±12.168 |
| H85Y | 160±8 | 33.21±2.22 | 8.46±0.32 | 25.4837±9.360 |
| S49R/I50M/H85Y(Mut) | 130±5 | 23.47±1.53 | 7.67±0.64 | 32.7075±11.665 |

Data represent mean values ±*SD* of three replicates; each experiment was repeated twice.

basis of the S49R/I50M/H85Y mutation (Figure S1). However, these mutations resulted in lower catalytic efficiency compared with the S49R/I50M/H85Y triple mutation (Table S3). Since the S49R/I50M/H85Y mutant enzyme had the highest catalytic efficiency among the variants tested, we used this mutant for the biosynthesis of ginsenoside $Rg_3$ in *P. ginseng* chassis.

We also ran a molecular dynamics simulation to analyze possible conformational changes induced by the S49R/I50M/H85Y mutations (Figures 3B, S2). Although the three mutation sites are outside the ligand-binding pocket, they cause conformational changes to the pocket. The molec-ular dynamics simulation indicated that the helix where H85 resides differed slightly in conformation between the wild-type and mutant enzymes, leading to a longer binding pocket in the mutant that accommodates the whole $Rh_2$ molecule. In contrast, in the wild-type enzyme, the hydrophobic tail of $Rh_2$ was outside of the binding pocket. Moreover, R91 in the mutant enzyme interacted with $Rh_2$ via hydrogen bonds. Both of these differences seemed likely to contribute to the greater catalytic activity of the triple mutant enzyme.

CRISPR/Cas9 knockdown of the branch pathway promotes ginsenoside $Rg_3$ biosynthesis To decrease side-products of protopanaxatriol-type ginsenoside biosynthesis and promote

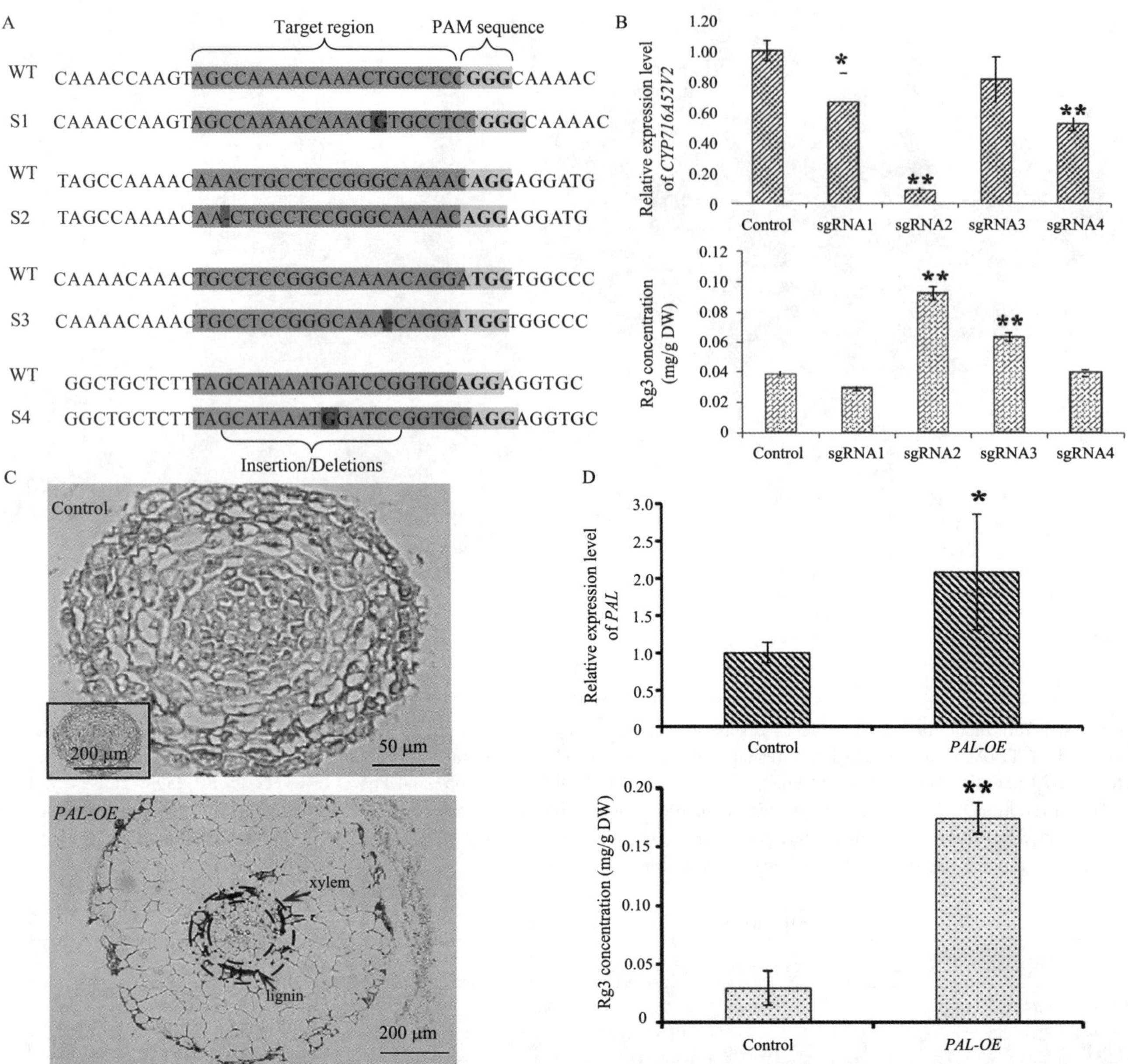


**Figure 4 Clustered regularly interspaced palindromic repeats (CRISPR)/CRISPR-associated protein 9 (Cas9) system targeting CYP716A53v2 and characterization of genetically transformed ginseng roots (GTGRs) with phenylalanine ammonia-lyase gene overexpression (PAL - OE)**

(**A**) Four mutant sequences were identified from transient GTGRs of *Panax ginseng*. Single guide RNA (sgRNA) targets of CYP716A53v2 are indicated by red font and sequence changes by blue font (insertion) or dashes (deletion). The protospacer-adjacent motifs (PAM) are represented in bold font. (**B**) Gene expression of CYP716A53v2 and ginsenoside $Rg_3$ content (mg/g fry weight (DW)) in transient GTGRs of *P. ginseng*. Statistical analysis was performed by Duncan's multiple range test using the SPSS statistic 16.0 software (SPSS Inc., Chicago, IL, USA). The error bars indicate the data of three biological replicates. $^*P<0.05$, $^{**}P<0.01$, significant differences between experimental group and control group, respectively. (**C**) The deposition of lignin in GTGRs by phloroglucinol staining. (**D**) PAL expression level and ginsenoside $Rg_3$ content (mg/g DW) in GTGRs with PAL overexpression. Statistical analysis was performed by Duncan's multiple range test using the SPSS statistic 16.0 software (SPSS Inc., Chicago, IL, USA). The error bars indicate the data of three biological replicates. $^*P<0.05$, $^{**}P<0.01$, significant differences between experimental group and control group, respectively.

the metabolic flux of the protopanaxadiol-type ginsenoside $Rg_3$, we used the CRISPR/Cas9 editing system to knock down *CYP716A53v2*. We constructed four single guide RNAs (sgRNAs) targeting *CYP716A53v2* and transformed each of them, along with *Cas9*, into *P. ginseng* root. Sequencing of the resulting four groups of plants with genetically transformed ginseng root (GTGR) revealed guanine (G) insertions due to sgRNA1 and sgRNA4 and adenine (A) deletions due to sgRNA2 and sgRNA3 in the *CYP716A53v2* gene (Figure 4A). In these GTGR root cultures (RCs), the expression of *CYP716A53v2* was suppressed and the $Rg_3$ content was significantly increased (Figure 4B). The expression of

*CYP716A53v2* in the sgRNA2-transformed plants was significantly decreased (to 0.08 times that of the control group), and the corresponding $Rg_3$ content significantly increased to 2.39 times higher than that of the control group (Figure 4B). These results confirmed the successful application of the CRISPR/Cas9 system in *P. ginseng* root and revealed that knockdown of *CYP716A53v2* indeed enhances $Rg_3$ content. Based on these results, we chose CRISPR/Cas9 with sgRNA2 for use in the following experiments.

Overexpression of PAL, a xylem structure gene, contributes to $Rg_3$ accumulation The ginsenoside $Rg_3$ is abundant in the xylem and pith of the root. *PAL* is a xylem structural gene, and its overexpression substantially increased lignin development and xylem cell expansion in *P. ginseng* RCs, causing the roots of *PAL* overexpression (*PAL* - OE) plants to be thicker than those of control plants (Figure 4C). A transient expression assay showed that the expression level of *PAL* was 2.63-fold higher in *PAL* - OE RCs than in control RCs (Figure 4D). *PAL* overexpression increased the expression level of *Pq*3 - *O* - *UGT*2, which was 3.73-fold higher in *PAL* - OE RCs than in control RCs (Figure 5B). Correspondingly, the content of ginsenoside $Rg_3$ was 6.19-fold higher in *PAL* - OE RCs than in control RCs (Figure 5F). The content of the ginsenoside $Rg_3$ in *PAL* - OE RCs was also higher than that in *SE* - OE and *Pq3* - *O* - *UGT2* - mutant (Mut) - OE RCs. These results indicate that *PAL* overexpression can change the structure of xylem and significantly increase $Rg_3$ accumulation in *P. ginseng* roots.

Co-expression of multiple genes in a transient GTGR system To further improve $Rg_3$ accumulation, we combined the coexpression of added *SE*, *Pq3* - *O* - *UGT2* - Mut, and *PAL* with the CRISPR/Cas9 mutations of *CYP716A53v2* (Figures 5, S3). At the C-terminal end of the overexpressed genes, we added a green fluorescent protein (GFP) tag to check the transfection efficiency. No green fluorescence was evident in wild-type *P. ginseng* RCs (Figure 5A). By contrast, in the GTGR RCs transiently overexpressing multiple genes, green fluorescence could be visualized. Furthermore, the gene expression levels of *SE*, *Pq3* - *O* - *UGT2*, *PAL*, and *CYP716A53v2* in these RCs indicated that the genes had successfully integrated into the genomes of the *P. ginseng* RCs (Figure 5B-E). The gene expression level of *Pq3* - *O* - *UGT2* in the *Pq3* - *O* - *UGT2* - Mut - OE RCs was 3.18-fold higher than that in the control RCs. In the *Pq3* - *O* - *UGT2* - Mut&*SE* - OE RCs, the *Pq3* - *O* - *UGT2* expression level was further improved (6.44-fold). In the *PAL*&*Pq2* - *O* - *UGT2* - Mut&*SE* - OE&sgRNA2 RCs, the *Pq3* - *O* - *UGT2* expression level was 11.68-fold higher than that in the control RCs. The gene expression levels of *SE* and *PAL* in the corresponding RCs showed similar patterns to those of *Pq3* - *O* - *UGT2*. However, combining *SE* and *PAL* overexpression resulted in a reduced amount of $Rg_3$ compared to overexpressing either gene alone. The *CYP716A53v2* expression level in the other overexpression RCs showed a certain degree of variance, while it was significantly lower in *PAL*&*Pq2* - *O* - *UGT2* - Mut&*SE* - OE& sgRNA2 RCs than in the control RCs. The ginsenoside $Rg_3$ contents in the *PAL* - OE (0.18 mg/g dry weight (DW)) and *PAL*&*Pq2* - *O* - *UGT2* - Mut&*SE* - OE RCs (0.18 mg/g DW) were significantly higher than that in the controll (pCambia1300) RCs (0.03 mg/g DW) and *Pq3* - *O* - *UGT2* - Mut - OE (0.05 mg/g DW) system. In the *PAL*&*Pq2* - *O* - *UGT2* - Mut&*SE* - OE&sgRNA2 RCs, the ginsenoside $Rg_3$ content was up to 0.27 mg/g DW, which was 9.10 times as high as in the control RCs (Figure 5F).

GTGR system screening and treatment for high $Rg_3$ yield To obtain stable GTGRs, we performed resistance screening in solid selective medium. After 3 to 4 weeks, GTGRs developed new branches (Figure 6A - J), which we transferred into liquid selective medium for scale-up cultivation. We then performed a polymerase chain reaction (PCR) assay to further verify positive GTGR roots by measuring *rolB* and kanamycin resistance genes. The *rolB* and kanamycin resistance genes were detected in all of the GTGR RCs (Figure 6K), indicating successful establishment of the overexpression systems. When we combined this with JA treatment, and chemical and heat treatment, the content of ginsenoside $Rg_3$ in the GTGR system of *PAL*&*Pq2* - *O* - *UGT2* - Mut&*SE* - OE&sgRNA2 was up to 7.0±0.4 mg/g DW (Figure 6M, rightmost dark blue bar), which was about 10.08 times/8.51 times higher than those in the control groups (Figure 6M, black bar (0.69±0.02 mg/g DW) and red bar (0.82±0.02 mg/g DW)) and 21.12 times higher than in wild-type RCs (0.33±0.03 mg/g DW) (Figure S4; Table 2). JA treatment, and chemical and heat treatment were previously established as effective means to improve ginsenoside content. In this study, we successfully established a new genetically based protocol to obtain a GTGR system with high ginsenoside $Rg_3$ accumulation (Figure 6l). Furthermore, the $Rg_3$ glycosylation products, ginsenosides $Rb_1$, $Rb_2$, $Rb_3$, and Rd, were mostly transformed to $Rg_3$ in these different processing groups (Table 2)

## 3 DISCUSSION

The metabolic engineering of plant chassis is a potential green production method with the advantages of low toxicity, renewable raw materials, environmental friendliness, and high biosafety. It has been successfully used to construct production systems of diterpenoid jolkinol C, tropane alkaloids, momilactone B, and taxanes. Ginsenoside $Rg_3$ is an important bioactive component in the traditional Chinese medicine plant *P. ginseng*. It has many functions in human

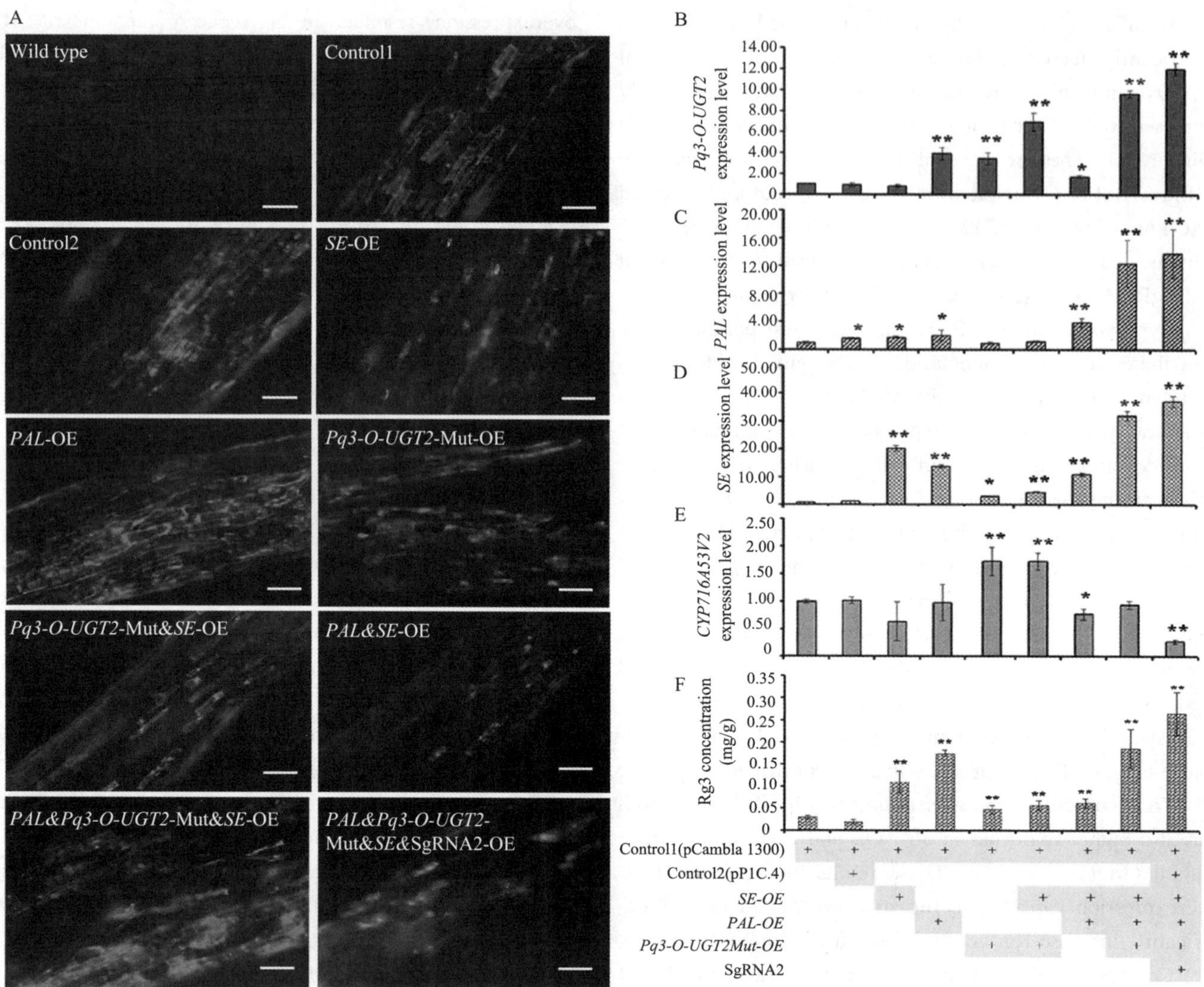


**Figure 5 Transient coexpression of multiple genes in genetically transformed ginseng root (GTGR) system of *Panax ginseng***

(**A**) Fluorescence signal of transient overexpression of multiple genes in GTGR system of *P*. *ginseng*. Scale bar, 200 μm. (**B**-**E**) Relative gene expression level in transient GTGR system of *P*. *ginseng*. Statistical analysis was performed by Duncan's multiple range test using the SPSS statistic 16.0 software (SPSS Inc., Chicago, IL, USA). The error bars indicate the data of three biological replicates. * $P<0.05$, ** $P<0.01$, significant differences between experimental group and control group, respectively. (**F**) Ginsenoside $Rg_3$ content (mg/g dry weight (DW)) in transient GTGR system of *P*. *ginseng*. Statistical analysis was performed by Duncan's multiple range test using the SPSS statistic 16.0 software (SPSS Inc., Chicago, IL, USA). The error bars indicate the data of three biological replicates. * $P<0.05$, ** $P<0.01$, significant differences between experimental group and control group, respectively.

health, such as anti-tumor and anti-cancer effects, and thus is of great interest to the pharmacy industry. Since traditional methods of $Rg_3$ production have many limitations and cannot meet the substantial market demand for the compound, a method for the biosynthesis of $Rg_3$ in yeast factories has been developed and proven to be effective in improving yields. However, *P*. *ginseng* tissue cultures could provide a more efficient chassis for $Rg_3$ production given the relatively good adaptation of enzymes in plant compared to yeast fermentation. In this study, we therefore sought to increase the yield of $Rg_3$ in *P*. *ginseng* plants through a multi-module strategy (Figure 1).

To achieve this, we first analyzed the key genes involved in $Rg_3$ biosynthesis. Correlation analysis is usually performed to determine the potential relationships between different genes and target compounds. *SE* is an upstream synthetic gene in triterpenoid biosynthesis, and its protein product has been reported to be a rate-limiting enzyme. Overexpression of *SE* can thus boost triterpenoid production in plants and yeast. In hairy root lines of *Cucurbita pepo* with *CpSE2* overexpression, the production of cucurbitacin E was increased by two-fold compared with that in control lines. The high correlation between *SE* and $Rg_3$ in our correlation analysis indicated that *SE* overexpression could contribute to ginsenoside biosynthesis. Indeed, when we overexpressed *SE*, $Rg_3$ production was greatly improved (Figures 5F, 6M).

The ginsenoside $Rg_3$ is a protopanaxadiol-type ginsenoside that is synthesized by the glycosylation of ginsenoside $Rh_2$

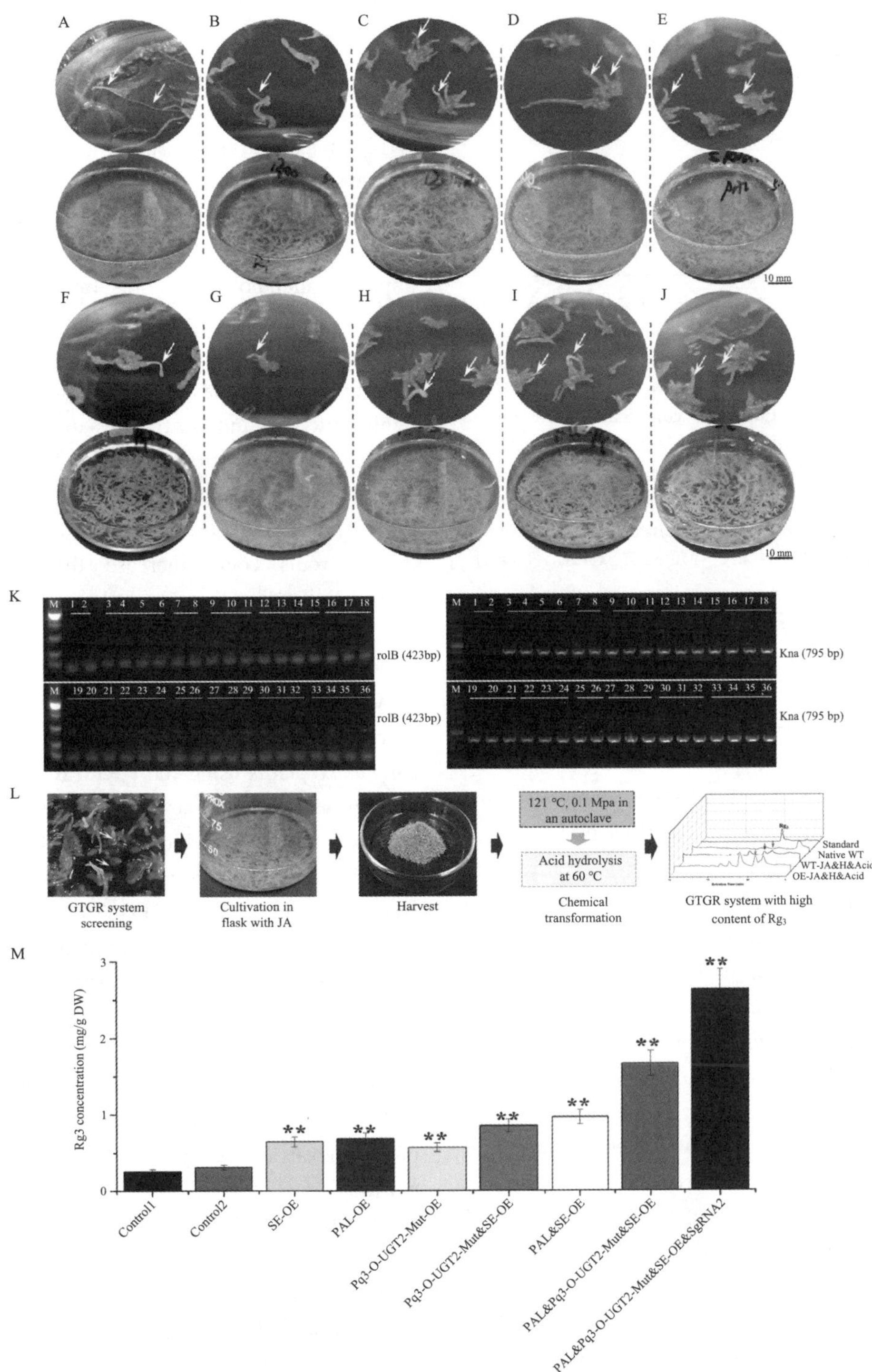


**Figure 6 Characterization of genetically transformed ginseng root (GTGR) system**

(**A**-**J**) Kanamycin resistant GTGRs formation (arrows) on solid selective medium (Up). Subcultivation of kanamycin resistant GTGRs in liquid selective medium (Down). (A) wild-type; (B) control1 (pCambia1300); (C) control2 (pCambia1300&pP1C.4); (D) squalene epoxidase (SE) overexpression (OE); (E) PAL-OE; (F) Pq3-O-UGT2-Mut-OE; (G) Pq3-O-UGT2-Mut&SE-OE; (H) PAL&SE-OE; (I) PAL&Pq3-O-UGT2-Mut&SE-OE; (J) PAL&Pq3-O-UGT2-Mut&SE&SgRNA2-OE. Scale bar =10 mm. (**K**) Representative polymerase chain reaction analysis of the rolB and kanamycin resistance (Kna) gene in GTGR systems. M, DL-5000 Marker; 1 to 2, the wild-type root cultures (RCs); 3 to 6, control1 (pCambia1300); 7 to 8, control2 (pCambia1300&pP1C.4); 9 to 11, SE-OE; 12 to 15, phenylalanine ammonia lyase (PAL)-OE; 16 to 18, Pq3-O-UGT2-Mut-OE; 19 to 21, Pq3-O-UGT2-Mut&SE-OE; 22 to 23, PAL&SE-OE; 24 to 26, PAL&Pq3-O-UGT2-Mut&SE-OE; 27 to 30, PAL&Pq3-O-UGT2-Mut&SE&SgRNA2-OE. (**L**) Scheme of chemical treatment to obtain high ginsenoside $Rg_3$ yield with GTGR system. Positive GTGR systems were transferred into liquid selective medium with jasmonate (JA) and cultured for 7 d. The harvested roots were treated in an autoclave (121 ℃, 0.1 Mpa), and then the supernatant was hydrolyzed by lactic acid at 60 ℃ for further improving ginsenosides content. (**M**) Ginsenoside $Rg_3$ content (mg/g dry weight) in GTGR systems of *Panax ginseng* after JA and chemical transformation treatment. control1 (pCambia1300), control2 (pCambia1300&pP1C.4). Statistical analysis was performed by Duncan's multiple range test using the SPSS statistic 16.0 software (SPSS Inc., Chicago, IL, USA). The error bars indicate the data of three biological replicates. $^{*}P<0.05$, $^{**}P<0.01$, significant differences between experimental group and control group, respectively.

**Table 2 The ginsenosides content in root cultures with different processing**

| Group | Ginsenosides content (mg/g DW) | | | | |
|---|---|---|---|---|---|
| | $Rb_1$ | $Rb_2$ | $Rb_3$ | Rd | $Rg_3$ |
| WT - H&Acid | n.d. | n.d. | n.d. | n.d. | 0.33±0.03 |
| WT - JA&H&Acid | n.d. | n.d. | n.d. | 0.10±0.01 | 0.69±0.02 |
| OE - JA&H&Acid | n.d. | n.d. | n.d. | n.d. | 7.0±0.1 |

DW, dry weight; WT, control, wild-type root culture; JA, plant materials were treated with jasmonate for 7 d; H, heat, plant materials were treated in 121 ℃, 0.1 Mpa for 40 min; n.d., not detected; acid, lactic acid, plant materials were treated in 0.1% lactic acid at 60 ℃ for 5 h; OE, the genetically transformed ginseng root system of combination the overexpression of squalene epoxidase (SE), Pq3 - O - UGT2, phenylalanine ammonia lyase 1 (PAL1) and the clustered regularly interspaced palindromic repeats (CRISPR)/CRISPR-associated protein 9 (Cas9) system of CYP716A53v2 (PAL&Pq2 - O - UGT2 - Mut&SE - OE&sgRNA2).

catalyzed by UGTPg29 and Pq3 - O - UGT2. The fact that $Rg_3$ content is more strongly correlated with *Pq3 - O - UGT2* expression than with *UGTPg29* expression suggested that Pq3 - O - UGT2 could be a more efficient UGT in ginsenoside $Rg_3$ biosynthesis. We also analyzed the functions of these two enzymes in $Rg_3$ production using *in vitro* enzymatic as-says. The higher $k_{cat}/K_M$ value of UGT71L2 compared with Pq3 - O - UGT2 with salicyl-7-benzoate as substrate indicated that UGT71L2 is more efficient in glycosylating salicyl-7- benzoate. In contrast, we found here that for the conversion of $Rh_2$ to $Rg_3$, Pq3 - O - UGT2 showed a higher $k_{cat}/K_M$ value than UGTPg29, indicating that it is a more efficient catalyst in this reaction. Thus, we chose to use Pq3 - O - UGT2 for $Rg_3$ biosynthesis.

To improve the enzymatic activity of Pq3 - O - UGT2, we used a semi-rational design and mutagenesis. Among all known plant UGTs, UGT74AC1 has the substrate closest in structure to $Rh_2$, and the sequence of UGT74AC1 has previously been optimized through directed evolution to obtain up to $4.17 \times 10^4$-fold improvement in catalytic efficiency. We took advantage of this knowledge, supposing that the mutations that increased the catalytic efficiency of UGT74AC1 might also work for Pq3 - O - UGT2, and designed three corresponding mutations. Indeed, all three substitutions, Q30H, S49R/I50M, and H85Y, resulted in improved $k_{cat}$ values, and the combination of S49R/I50M and H85Y improved the $k_{cat}/K_M$ value by 1.3-fold (Table 1). Even though the improvement was not great, it was substantial and comparable to the effect achieved through the directed evolution of UGTPg45, by which the $k_{cat}/K_M$ value was improved from 0.07 to 0.11 (mmol/s). Thus, we used the *Pq3 - O - UGT2* mutant (S49R/I50M/H85Y) for high-yield production of $Rg_3$.

The ginsenoside $Rg_3$ has been detected in the xylem and pith of *P. ginseng*. Plant xylem contains abundant lignin, which can be observed by phloroglucinol staining. PAL, as the first enzyme in the lignin biosynthesis pathway, can affect xylem structure by changing lignin biosynthesis. Overexpression of *PAL* stimulates secondary xylem cell expansion in stems and promotes the biosynthesis of chlorogenic acid in *Ipomoea batatas* (L.) Lam. In this study, we improved metabolite contents by regulating plant morphological structure. The xylem in transverse sections of *P. ginseng* RCs overexpressing *PAL* was significantly thicker, indicating that PAL plays an important role in the formation of lignin in xylem and contributes to ginsenoside $Rg_3$ accumulation. Although some lignin is biosynthesized, ginsenosides are the main secondary metabolites of *P. ginseng*. Due to the increase in tissues and cells that synthesize saponins, thicker roots could increase the biosynthesis of $Rg_3$, eventually leading to an overall increase in $Rg_3$ content.

In recent years, the CRISPR/Cas9 system has been effectively utilized in plants to verify gene functions and improve target compounds by targeted mutagenesis. However, before this study there was no successful transgenic system for *Panax* plants using the CRISPR/Cas9 system to achieve high ginsenoside production. CRISPR/Cas9 editing can be used to promote the biosynthesis of target compounds by knocking down branch biosynthesis pathways. For example, lycopene epsilon-cyclase (LCYε) catalyzes the biosynthesis of $\alpha$ - carotene, which is a branch biosynthesis pathway of $\beta$ - carotene. CRISPR/Cas9 editing was used to modify the *LCYε* gene, and the modified lines showed a significant reduction in $\alpha$ - carotene content with a concomitant increase in $\beta$ - carotene levels. $Rg_3$ is a protopanaxadiol-type ginsenoside, and CYP716A53v2 participates in the biosynthesis of protopanaxatriol-type ginsenosides and belongs to a branch pathway of $Rg_3$. Therefore, in this study, we successfully applied the CRISPR/Cas9 system to *P. ginseng* to knock down the expression of *CYP716A53v2*. The decreased expression of *CYP716A53v2* increased the biosynthesis of $Rg_3$, as expected. Even though sequence changes were detected with *CYP716A53v2*, its expression could still be detected. This is because *P. ginseng* is a tetraploid plant, meaning that unaltered copies still remain in the genome. The transgenic lines constructed with sgRNA2 and sgRNA3 contained base deletions of the *CYP716A53v2* gene. In a previous study, nucleotide deletions resulted in amino acid deletions in the conserved MIR domain of BnC09. TT8b in *Brassica napus* L.. Nucleotide deletions may also have changed the amino acids of the conserved domain and altered the function of CYP716A53v2 in this study.

The expression of one gene can be influenced by that of other genes. The *Pq3 - O - UGT2* expression level in the *Pq3 - O - UGT2*-Mut&*SE*-OE system was higher than that in the

*Pq3-O-UGT2*-Mut-OE system, indicating that upstream *SE* overexpression promotes the accumulation of the ginsenoside $Rg_3$ precursor. In the *PAL&Pq3-O-UGT2*- Mut&*SE*-OE& sgRNA2 GTGR RCs, the *Pq3-O-UGT2* expression level was further improved, which may be the result of the knockdown of *CYP716A53v2* and decreased protopanaxatriol-type ginsenoside biosynthesis, which then promoted protopanaxadiol-type ginsenoside ($Rg_3$, Rd, etc.) biosynthesis. Both *SE* and *PAL* had similar expression patterns to *Pq3-O-UGT2*. In the *SE*-OE and *PAL*-OE RCs, the content of ginsenoside $Rg_3$ was significantly higher than that in the control and *Pq3-O-UGT2*-Mut-OE RCs. SE is a rate-limiting enzyme; thus, *SE* overexpression can effectively increase ginsenoside biosynthesis. PAL plays an important role in the formation of lignin in xylem; therefore, *PAL* overexpression likely increased the accumulation of ginsenoside $Rg_3$, which could explain why it promoted $Rg_3$ accumulation in this study. However, combining *SE* and *PAL* overexpression led to a reduced amount of $Rg_3$ compared to the overexpression of each gene alone. This may be attributable to the short transient expression time or to interference between the co-expression of *SE* and *PAL*. In summary, the overexpression of key genes combined with CRISPR/Cas9 knockdown of *CYP716A53v2* is an effective strategy to improve ginsenoside $Rg_3$ biosynthesis.

The *Agrobacterium*-mediated transgenic system is a powerful tool for obtaining stable systems for high yields of target compounds. In transgenic hairy root lines of *Ophiorrhiza pumila*, co-overexpression of genes encoding geraniol-10-hydroxylase and strictosidine synthase improved the accumulation of camptothecin. Furthermore, *rolB*, *rolC*, and the kanamycin resistance genes are important target genes for verifying successful and positive transgenic systems. JA treatment and chemical transformation processing are widely used to enrich ginsenosides. In this study, we used JA treatment to induce ginsenoside accumulation. Chemical transformation by heating and hydrolysis with lactic acid can improve the generation of ginsenoside $Rg_3$ from ginsenoside $Rb_1$, $Rb_2$, $Rb_3$, and Rd. Rd, which is the glycosylation product of ginsenoside $Rg_3$, could be further glycosylated to biosynthesize ginsenoside $Rb_1$, $Rb_2$, and $Rb_3$. The final ginsenoside $Rg_3$ content in the 500 mL flasks in this study was up to $7.0 \pm 0.4$ mg/g DW (83.64 mg/L), which is 2.58 times higher than a previously reported yield (2.7 mg/g) in metabolically engineered yeast. In a recent study, the diterpenoid jolkinol C, momilactone B, and taxanes were synthesized in the chassis of a model plant, *Nicotiana benthamiana*. The content of tropane alkaloids was improved by the plant biosynthesis system in *Atropa belladonna*. In the future, bioreactor cultures and parameter optimization should be performed to further improve the ginsenoside $Rg_3$ yield. The high-production plant chassis for producing ginsenoside $Rg_3$ established via engineering of triterpene metabolism and overexpression of the lignin biosynthesis gene *PAL* in this study resulted in an $Rg_3$ content 21.12-fold higher that in wild-type *P. ginseng*, providing a proof of concept for this potential platform as a means to improve accumulation of ginsenosides.

## 4 MATERIALS AND METHODS

Plant materials, culture, and treatment  Root cultures of *Panax ginseng* and *Panax quinquefolium* were induced and subcultured according to a procedure described in a previous study. The callus was induced from fresh cultivated roots of *P. ginseng* and *P. quinquefolium*. RCs were further induced from callus and then subcultured on medium with their corresponding phytohormone. JA (0, 1, and 5 mg/L) was added to 28-d-old RCs. After treatment for 7 d, RCs were harvested, and the expression levels of functional genes involved in the biosynthetic pathway of ginsenosides and the ginsenoside content were analyzed.

RNA isolation, cDNA production, and molecular cloning  Total RNA and first-strand complementary DNAs (cDNAs) were isolated and prepared from RCs of *P. ginseng* and *P. quinquefolium* according to a previous study. The coding sequences (CDS) of candidate genes (*Pq3-O-UGT2* from *P. quinquefolium*, and *UGTPg29*, *SE*, and *PAL* from *P. ginseng*) were amplified from cDNA with PCR using gene-specific primers (Table S4). A Spark Seamless Cloning Kit (Beijing, China) was used to ligate PCR amplicons into base vectors. *Pq3-O-UGT2* and *UGTPg29* were inserted into the NcoI site of a pET28a vector to construct the plasmids pET28a-*Pq3-O-UGT2* and pET28a-*UGTPg29* for recombinant protein production in *Escherichia coli*. pCambia1300-eGFP, a binary vector, was chosen for over-expression of multiple genes (*Pq3-O-UGT2*, *SE*, and *PAL*) and protein production in transgenic plants.

Enzyme activity assay, kinetic analysis, and SPR analysis of Pq3-O-UGT2 and UGTPg29  For preparation of the recombinant proteins, pET28a-*Pq3-O-UGT2* and pET28a-*UGTPg29* were transformed into *E. coli* BL21 (DE3). The recombinant *E. coli* BL21 (DE3) strains were cultured in Luria-Bertani (LB) medium (50 mg/L kanamycin) at 37℃ and 200 r/min until the optical density at 600 nm ($OD_{600}$) absorbance reached 0.6 - 0.8. Protein expression was induced with 0.5 mmol/L isopropyl-β-D-thiogalactopyranoside (IPTG) at 18 ℃ for 18 h. The cells were harvested by centrifugation and resuspended in phosphate buffer (pH 8.0, 100 mmol/L) supplemented with 1 mmol/L phenylmethylsulfonyl fluoride and then disrupted with a JY92-IIN Ultrasonic Cell Disruption System (UCDS, Xinzhi, Ningbo, China). The cell debris was removed by centrifugation at $\times 12,000 \times g$ for 20 min. The supernatant containing the target protein was loaded onto a nickel-nitrilotriacetic acid-agarose column and purified using a 25 - 200 mmol/L imidazole gradient.

Enzymatic assays (100 μL) of recombinant proteins were conducted with 0.5 mmol/L ginsenoside $Rh_2$, 5 mmol/L UDP-glucose, 100 mmol/L phosphate buffer (pH 7.5), 1% Tween-20, and 0.02 μg of purified recombinant proteins. The mixture was incubated for 6 h at 37℃. An equal volume of methanol was added to terminate the reactions. The reactants were subsequently centrifuged at $\times 10,000 \times g$ for 5 min and directly analyzed by high-performance liquid chromatography.

Kinetic studies (100 μL) of recombinant proteins toward ginsenoside $Rh_2$ were conducted with purified recombinant proteins (100 ng), 100 mmol/L phosphate buffer (pH 7.5), 1% Tween-20, 5 mmol/L UDP-glucose, and varying concentrations of ginsenoside $Rh_2$ (50, 100, 200, 400, 500, and 600 μmol/L). The mixtures were reacted at 37℃ for 15 min and terminated by adding an equal volume of methanol. All the subsequent steps were performed as described above. The kinetic parameters were calculated by nonlinear regression analysis using the software of GraphPad Prism 5.0.

SPR analysis was performed using the Biacore S200 system to analyze the interactions between Pq3 - O - UGT2, UGTPg29, and their sugar acceptor (ginsenoside $Rh_2$). Experimental parameters were set as previously described.

Homology modeling and molecular dynamics simulation For semi-rational design, the model of Pq3 - O - UGT2 was built using UGT74AC1 (PDB ID: 6L8Z) as a template with I-TASSER. The obtained model was checked and validated with the ProCheck program. For molecular dynamics simulation, the models of wild-type and mutant Pq3 - O - UGT2 were generated with AlphaFold2. Ligand docking and molecular dynamics simulation were performed with YASARA v17.4.17. All atoms were energy- minimized with the AMBER14 force field. During simulation, the environment of the protein-ligand complex was set to physiological conditions (0.9% NaCl, pH 7.4). Isothermal and isobaric conditions of 298 K and 1 atm were maintained. Approximate 60-ns simulation was conducted for both wild-type and mutant Pq3 - O - UGT2.

Site-directed mutagenesis Initially, three mutations, H85Y, Q30H, and S49R/I50M, were introduced into *Pq3 - O - UGT2* by site-directed mutagenesis using the primers listed in Table S5. To construct each mutation, a 50-μL PCR system containing 100 ng pET28a - *Pq3 - O - UGT2* plasmid as a template, 0.15 μmol/L forward and reverse primers, and 2 × Es Taq MasterMix (KANGWEI Tech, Beijing, China) was mixed well and subjected to a 32-cycle PCR reaction. Then, 10 μL of PCR product was digested in DpnI at 37℃ for 2 h to remove the template and then transformed into DH5α competent cells. The resulting clones were confirmed to be correct mutants by sequencing. To construct the three-point mutation S49R/I50M/H85Y, a similar method was used in which the template was changed to the S49R/I50M plasmid and the primers were H85Y mutagenesis primers. To construct S49R/I50M/H85Y-based mutations (S49R/I50M/H85Y/S339N, S49R/I50M/H85Y/L358A, S49R/I50M/H85Y/A355P, and S49R/I50M/H85Y/I341L/A342T), the S49R/I50M/H85Y plasmid was used as a PCR template.

Design of sgRNA and assembly of the CRISPR/Cas9 construct The sequence of *CYP716A53v2* was input into the online tool CRISPOR (https://zlab.bio/guide-design-resources) to find potential Cas9 target sites, and the output target sites were selected for designing target sgRNAs based on their location in the gene and off-target possibilities. The CRISPR/Cas9 system was constructed following the manual of CRISPR/Cas9 pP1C.4 Vector with DNA Recombinase (GP0144, Genloci, China).

*Agrobacterium*-mediated transient gene expression analysis and GTGR system screening For plant expression, the binary vector was digested with the restriction endonuclease BamHI and then was ligated to PCR amplicons of target genes using a Spark Seamless Cloning Kit. After transformation into *Agrobacterium*, positive clones were identified by PCR analysis and confirmed by sequencing. *Agrobacterium tumefaciens* C58C1 cells containing the transgene construct (control1 (pCambia1300), control2 (pCambia1300&pP1C.4), *SE* - OS, *PAL* - OE, *Pq3 - O - UGT2* - Mut - OE, *Pq3 - O - UGT2* - Mut&*SE* - OE, *PAL*&*SE* - OE, *PAL*&*Pq3 - O - UGT2* - Mut&*SE* - OE, or *PAL*&*Pq3 - O - UGT2* - Mut&*SE*&SgRNA2 - OE) were grown to a target OD ($OD_{600}$ of 0.8) in 200 mL of LB medium (10 g/L tryptone, 5 g/L yeast extract, 10 g/L NaCl). For co-expression of multiple genes, individual *A. tumefaciens* cultures containing the unique transgene construct were grown to a higher OD, so that each individual culture in the mixed cultures was present at a concentration equivalent to an $OD_{600}$ of 0.8. Vacuum infiltration of RCs of *P. ginseng* was performed by dipping plants into LB medium (200 μmol/L acetosyringone plus *A. tumefaciens*) in a degassing chamber at 0.08 MPa for 10 min. The RCs were washed twice with sterile water and then transferred onto coculture medium (Murashige and Skoog (MS) basal medium supplemented with 3% sucrose, pH 5.8). Two days later, explants were partially harvested for fluorescence observation, transient gene expression tests, and ginsenoside content analysis. The remaining explants were transferred onto selective medium (MS medium supplemented with 5 mg/L indolebutyric acid (IBA), 3% sucrose, pH 5.8) with 50 mg/L kanamycin until resistant GTGRs were generated. The quantitative PRD (qPCR) reaction was performed following a method from a previous study. *ACTB* was used as a reference gene. Each reaction was conducted with three biological replicates. The primers of genes used in qPCR are shown in Table S6. Genomic DNA was extracted from 45-d-old GTGRs using a One-Tube Plant DNAout Kit (TIANDZ, China). The kanamycin resistance gene (*Kna*) and *rolB* gene were also checked using primers Kna-F/Kna-R and rolB-F/rolB-R listed in Table S4. The contents of ginsenoside $Rg_3$, $Rb_1$, $Rb_2$, and $Rb_3$ were determined.

Fluorescence observation and histochemical staining of lignin The coding regions without the stop codons of *PAL* and other target genes were inserted into the BamHI site of the pCAMBIA1300-eGFP vector using a Spark Multi-Seamless Cloning Kit (AK0602, Spark, China, Beijing) to generate their corresponding overexpression systems and determine subcellular localization. The primers used for subcloning are listed in Table S4. These recombinant vectors were transformed into *A. tumefaciens* C58C1 for transient expression. Transient expression was visualized using a confocal laser scanning microscope (Nikon, Japan) as previously described.

Microscopy preparations for lignin observation were performed according to a previous study with slight modifications. Transverse sections were cut at 5 mm of fresh and newly developed RCs from the root tip using a microtome Leica RM2235 (Wetzlar, Germany). The sections were stained with 4% phloroglucinol (dissolved in 95% (v/v) ethanol) for 10 min and then treated with 9% (w/v) hydrochloric acid for 5 min, after which the sections on glass slides were observed using a Leica ICC50W (Wetzlar, Germany) microscope.

Jasmonate treatment and chemical transformation Positive GTGRs were transferred in selective medium (MS medium supplemented with 5 mg/L IBA, 3% sucrose, pH 5.8) with 50 mg/L kanamycin for rapid propagation. JA (5 mg/L) was added to the 28-d-old resistant GTGRs to improve the ginsenoside content. After treatment for 7 d, the roots were harvested for further post- processing.

Dry GTGR samples (5 mg/L) were transferred into 100-mL flasks with 20 mL distilled water, which were autoclaved (121 ℃, 0.1 Mpa) for 40 min following a previous study. The supernatant was hydrolyzed by lactic acid at 60 ℃ for 5 h. Then, ginsenosides were extracted following a previous study and quantified.

Determination of ginsenoside content The samples were prepared following a previous study and used for ginsenoside quantitation. A Shimadzu LC-2 030C prominence system (Shimadzu, Kyoto, Japan) with a Kromasil $C_{18}$ (4.6 × 250 mm, 5 μm) column was used to determine ginsenoside content at a wavelength of 203 nm. The mobile phase was composed of water (A) and $CH_3CN$ (C), and the flow rate was 1.0 mL/min. The column was kept at 35 ℃, and the linear gradient was as follows: 0 - 35 min, 20% C; 35 - 40 min, 20%- 30% C; 40 - 50 min, 30%- 31% C; 50 - 60 min, 31%- 32% C; 60 - 70 min, 32% - 45% C; 70 - 100 min, 45%- 60% C; 100 - 110 min, 60% C; 110 - 111 min, 60%- 20% C; 111 - 120 min, 20% C. The sample injection volume was 20 μL. The ginsenosides ($Rg_1$, Re, Rf, $Rb_1$, $Rg_2$, $Rh_1$, Rc, $Rb_2$, $Rb_3$, Rd, $Rg_3$, and $Rh_2$) were identified and quantified using 0.2 mg/L of standards (from the National Institute for the Pharmaceutical and Biological Products, Beijing, China). All analyses were performed with three replications.

Statistical analysis Significant differences were determined with Duncan's multiple range test using SPSS v16.0 (SPSS Inc., Chicago, IL, USA) as previously described. Pearson's correlation coefficient (*r*) analysis was carried out to assess the correlation between gene expression levels and ginsenoside content. The significance of Pearson's correlation coefficients was evaluated at the $P<0.05$ level according to a previous study. All analyses were performed with three replications.

[姚陆，王娟，高文远，等. Journal of Integrative Plant Biology，2022,64(9):1739 - 1754.]

# Functional and structural dissection of a plant steroid 3 - *O* - glycosyltransferase facilitated the engineering enhancement of sugar donor promiscuity

## 1 INTRODUCTION

Natural products are major sources for drug and lead compound discovery, and a large number of present-day drugs are derived from natural sources. Cardiotonic steroids (CTSs) constitute an important class of natural products including cardenolides and bufadienolides, which have been well known for their medicinal importance. Digoxin has been used as a remedy for congestive heart failure for over 200 years. Both ouabain and digoxin were shown as broad-spectrum potential senolytics. CTSs are also involved in a variety of pharmacological activities, such as neuroinflammatory, antitumor, immunomodulatory, and antiviral activities. However, clinical application of CTSs is limited due to poor solubility and severe cardiotoxicity. The structure-function relationship study indicated that glycosylation at the C-3 position of the CTS could significantly reduce its cardiotoxicity. Moreover, various glycosyl groups were proven to be associated with the diverse bioactivities of CTSs. Thus, the pharmaceutical applications of CTSs may be broadened by increasing the specific 3-*O*-glycosylation and expanding the diversity of the glycosyl moieties.

Chemical glycosylation of CTSs is restricted by poor regio- and stereoselectivity, low yield, and tedious protection/deprotection steps of the CTS functional groups. In contrast, enzymatic glycosylation mediated by glycosyltransferases (GTs) showed great advantages of high efficiency and regiospecificity. GTs transfer the sugar moiety from donor sugar to an acceptor. Until now, there are 114 GT (EC 2.4.x.y) families classified on the amino acid sequences (CAZY, http://www.cazy.org/). Many UDP-glycosyltransferases (UGT) from the GT1 family were found in the biosynthesis pathways of natural products. In the past few years, mining and characterization of plant and microbial UGTs have made great progress. However, only several steroid 3-*O*-glycosyltransferases (S3GTs) were identified, including the microbial UGT OleD and YjiC1, which were reported with low catalytic efficiency, narrow spectra of the substrates, and poor regioselectivity toward CTS. The plant UGTs UGT74AN1 and UGT74AN3 from the UGT74AN subfamily were thought to contribute to the biosynthesis of CTS 3-*O*-glycosides. UGT74AN1 is a permissive GT identified from *Asclepias curassavica* and exhibited robust capabilities of the regiospecific C-3 glycosylation of CTSs. UGT74AN3 from *Catharanthus roseus* showed catalytic efficiency toward eight structurally different CTSs and phenolic compounds. Nevertheless, both UGT74AN1 and UGT74AN3 only accept UDP-Glc as the main sugar donor. Although UGT74AN1 could take UDP-GlcNAc as a sugar donor, the utilization rate is extremely low (Figure S1). Glycosyltransferases with substrate and sugar donor promiscuity as promising biocatalysts have great potential in drug discovery. For instance, OleD, MiCGTb, Sb3GT1, and GgCGT could recognize various types of natural products and could also utilize various sugar donors such as UDP-Glc, UDP-Xyl, and UDP-Gal. Therefore, a novel S3GT with both substrate and sugar donor promiscuity is desired.

The enzyme structure is pivotal to understand catalytic mechanisms and guide rational engineering. Crystal structures of a few plant UGTs have been solved, including flavonoid OGTs (UGT89C1, UGT78K6, UGT74AC2, VvGT1, UGT85H2, and UGT78G1), flavonoid CGTs (TcCGT1, GgCGT, UGT708C1, LpCGTa, LpCGTb, SbCGTa, SbCGTb, and ZmCGTa), benzophenone CGT (MiCGT), terpenoid GTs (UGT71G1, Os79, UGT76G1, UGT74AC1, and OsUGT91C1), polyphenol GTs (PaGT2

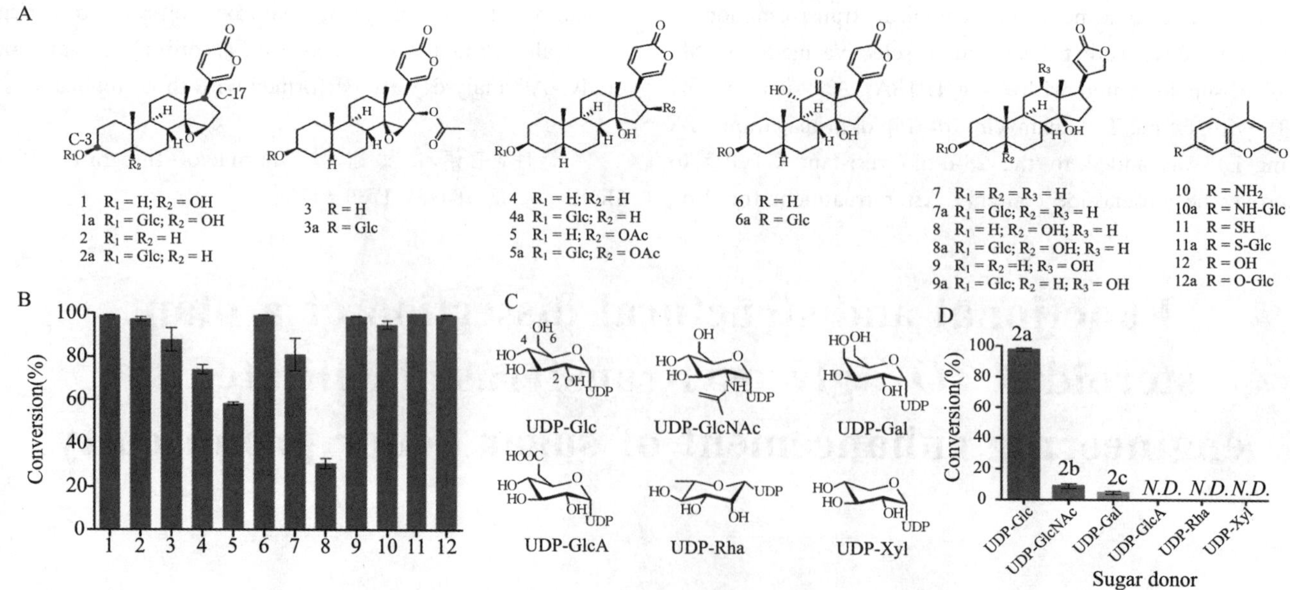


**Figure 1 Substrate and sugar donor specificity of UGT74AN2**

(A) Structures of 1-12 and their 3-*O*-glycosylated products and (B) conversion rates of the glycosylated products catalyzed by UGT74AN2. Compound numbers correspond to the structures listed in panel A. (C) Structures of various sugar donors and (D) conversion rates of the glycosylated products (2a, 2b, and 2c) using resibufogenin (2) as the substrate. ND, no products detected.

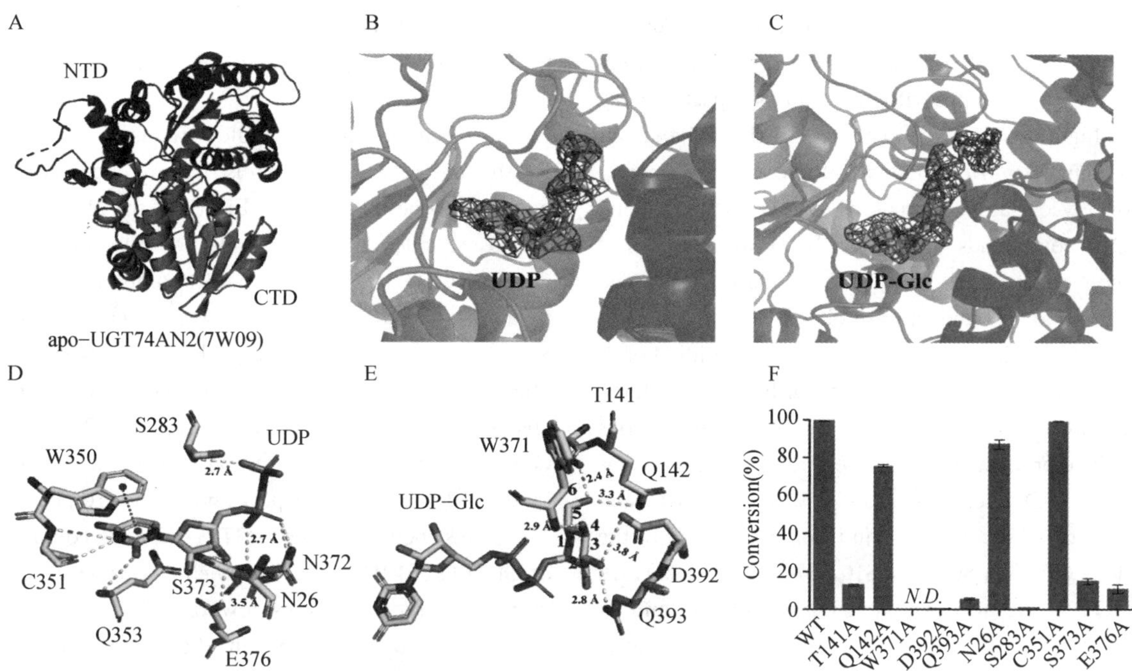


**Figure 2 Sugar donor recognition and preference of UGT74AN2**

(A) Overall three-dimensional structure of apo-UGT74AN2 with the highlighted NTD (blue) and CTD (magenta). (B, C) Sugar donors in the structures of UGT74AN2 complexed with UDP (B) or UDP - Glc (C) are shown in the $2F_o - F_c$ electron density maps contoured at 1.5$\sigma$. (D, E) Interactions between UGT74AN2 and UDP (D) or the glucose moiety of UDP - Glc (E). Hydrogen bonds are represented by yellow dashed lines. $\pi$-stacking interaction is shown in a red dashed line. (F) Conversion rates of UGT74AN2 and the mutants, using resibufogenin (**2**) as the substrate and UDP - Glc as the sugar donor.

and PaGT3), alkaloid GT (PtUGT1), xenobiotics GT (UGT72B1), and salicylic acid GT (UGT74AF2). However, none of these GTs could take CTS as the substrate. No structure is available for deciphering the enzymatic glycosylation of CTSs. Although the apo form structure of the microbial UGT OleD was determined, it did not provide many mechanistic details. Thus, mechanisms of the plant S3GT for the CTS recognition and catalysis remain unclear.

In recent years, several protein engineering strategies, such as directed evolution, focused rational iterative site-specific mutagenesis (FRISM), and domain shuffling, have been explored to increase the substrate promiscuity and regiose-lectivity of plant UGTs. The structure-based rational and semirational engineering have also been successfully applied to broaden sugar donor flexibility of several UGTs, such as UGT78H2. However, relatively limited success was achieved in expanding the sugar donor promiscuity of plant UGTs. It is likely because the sugar donor binding pocket of plant UGTs contains a plant secondary product glycosyltransferase (PSPG) motif, which is evolutionarily conserved.

Herein, we reported steroid 3 - O - glycosyltransferase UGT74AN2 from the cardenolide producing plant *Calotropis gigantea*, catalyzing 3 - O - glycosylation of CTS with high regiospecificity. The crystal structures of UGT74AN2 were determined in the apo form and in complexes with UDP, UDP - Glc, UDP/resibufogenin (**2**), UDP/bufalin (**4**), UDP/digitoxigenin (**7**), and UDP/digitoxigenin 3 - O -$\beta$-D-glucoside (**7a**) (Figure S2). These structures provided a molecular basis for understanding the sugar donor/acceptor recognition and catalytic mechanisms of S3GTs. Furthermore, a mutant of UGT74AN2 was designed and confirmed with elevated catalytic efficiency and improved sugar donor promiscuity.

## 2 RESULTS AND DISCUSSION

2.1 Functional Characterization of UGT74AN2 *C. gigantea* is a worldwide popular medicinal herb with good capability of producing a wide variety of CTS glycosides. The phylogenetic analysis showed that UGT74AN2 from *C. gigantea* (GenBank accession No. MF942417.1) was grouped with two other characterized plant S3GTs (UGT74AN1 and UGT74AN3) into the same clade of the UGT74AN subfamily (Figure S3), indicating that UGT74AN2 is a predicated steroid GT. To investigate the steroid substrate spectrum of UGT74AN2, nine structurally diverse CTS aglycones (**1** - **9**) and three simple aromatics (**10** - **12**) were tested for catalytic activity using UDP - Glc as a sugar donor (Figure 1A). The purified UGT74AN2 enzyme (final protein purity > 90%), which was heterogeneously expressed in *Escherichia coli* followed by the purification using the Ni-NTA affinity and size-exclusion chromatography (Figure S4), was used in the assay with the heat-inactivated enzyme as a negative control. The enzymatic products were further analyzed using high-performance liquid chromatography (HPLC) and liquid chromatography-mass spectrometry (LC-MS) (Figures S5 - S13). The results showed that all tested CTS aglycones were individually converted into a single major glycosylated product by UGT74AN2, among which six CTS compounds (**1** - **3**, **6**, **7**, **9**) were catalyzed with high conversion rates (> 85%) (Figure 1B). The products **2a**, **3a**, **4a**, **6a**, and **7a** were obtained by preparative-scale reactions. For all of the products, the glycosidic bonds were shown in the $\beta$ configuration, according to the large coupling constants ($J = 7.8$ Hz) of the anomeric protons (Table S1). The product structures were further identified as the CTS 3-$O$-$\beta$-D-glucosides by LC-MS, $^1$H NMR, and $^{13}$C NMR spectroscopic analysis and comparison with the published data (Figures S6 - S8, S10, S11, S14 - S23). In addition, UGT74AN2 also exhibited remarkable *N*- and *S*-glycosylation catalytic activities on a few simple aromatics (**10** - **12**) with conversion rates over 95% (Figures 1B and S24 - S26). Furthermore, 15 additional substrates, including flavonoids (**13** - **21**), chalcones (**22**, **23**), stilbene (**24**), curcuminoid (**25**), terpenoid (**26**), and xanthone (**27**), were selected to test the substrate promiscuity of UGT74AN2. All of these compounds could be glycosylated by UGT74AN2 (Figures S27 - S29). In contrast to the glycosylated cardiotonic steroids, a majority of the tested flavonoids were glycosylated by UGT74AN2 with poor regioselectivity and consequently converted into heterogeneous products. UGT74AN2 exhibited a $K_m$ value of 10.38 μmol/L for **2**, and the corresponding $K_{cat}/K_m$ value was 1.58 $mM^{-1} \cdot s^{-1}$. It indicated that UGT74AN2 shows a high affinity toward cardiotonic steroids (Figure S30).

To explore the sugar donor promiscuity of UGT74AN2, six sugar donors including UDP-Glc, UDP-Gal, UDP-GlcNAc, UDP-GlcA, UDP-Rha, and UDP-Xyl were tested using resibufogenin (**2**) as an acceptor, respectively (Figure 1C). UGT74AN2 was shown with a significant preference for UDP-Glc as a sugar donor with a high conversion rate (>98%) (Figure 1D). Unlike the other characterized plant steroid GTs, UGT74AN2 possessed glycosylation catalytic activities using UDP-GlcNAc or UDP-Gal as a sugar donor, although the conversion rates were relatively low (13% for UDP-GlcNAc, 6% for UDP-Gal) (Figures S31 and S32). It suggested that the stereo configuration of the C-2 and C-4 groups on the sugar scaffold might be relevant to the sugar donor preference of UGT74AN2. Since UGT74AN2 did not accept UDP-GlcA, UDP-Xyl, or UDP-Rha as sugar donors, the existence of the 6-hydroxyl groups on the sugar moiety of the donor might be essential for its recognition and binding by UGT74AN2.

2.2 Overall Structure of UGT74AN2 The crystal structure of UGT74AN2 in the apo form was determined in the space group $P2_1$ with only one molecule in an asymmetric unit at a resolution of 1.95 Å (Table S2A). UGT74AN2 exhibits a canonical GT-B fold structure, consisting of two Rossmann-like $\beta/\alpha/\beta$ domains that are connected by a hinge linker (residues 234 - 260). Either of the N-terminal domain (NTD, residues 1 - 233 and 460 - 476) and the C-terminal domain (CTD, residues 261 - 459) comprises a core region of parallel $\beta$ strands surrounded by $\alpha$ helices (Figures 2A and S33). The two domains are packed very tightly facing each other, forming a deep cleft in between. Similar to the other glycosyltransferases in the GT-B superfamily, the NTD and CTD domains are mainly responsible for the recognition and binding of the sugar acceptor and donor, respectively.

The structure of apo-UGT74AN2 was compared to that of OleD (PDB ID: 4M60), which is a bacterial GT showing limited catalytic activities toward CTSs. The two proteins share about 15% identity in the protein sequences. The superimpositions between the equivalent C$\alpha$ atoms of the overall structures, NTD or CTD resulted in the root-mean-square deviations (rmsd) of 2.96, 2.52, and 1.75 Å, respectively (Table S3 and Figure S34A - C). UGT74AN2 shares the highest structural similarity with UGT74F2 (PDB: 5U6M, sequence identity about 40%), which is a salicylic acid glycosyltransferase from *Arabidopsis thaliana*. The rmsd values of the superimpositions between the equivalent C$\alpha$ atoms of the overall structures, NTD or CTD are 1.45, 1.50, and 0.85 Å, respectively (Table S3 and Figure S34D - F). The structure of apo-UGT74AN2 was also superimposed with several other structurally characterized plant UGTs; the rmsd values of the NTD superimpositions (in a range of 1.45 - 2.89 Å) are relatively higher than those of the CTD superimpositions (in a range of 0.85 - 1.64 Å) (Table S3). The high similarity of the CTD structures is likely due to the existence of a conserved PSPG motif, which is responsible for the sugar donor binding of plant UGTs. The NTD structure contains an acceptor binding site, accommodating structurally diverse substrates, and hence exhibits slightly more structural variance than CTD. These structural comparisons indicated that the substrate recognition of UGT74AN2 is likely different from that of the bacterial and other known plant UGTs.

2.3 Sugar Donor Recognition and Preference of UGT74AN2 The crystal structures of UGT74AN2 in complex with UDP or UDP-Glc were solved at resolutions of 2.04 and 2.15 Å, respectively (Table S2A). The structures of UGT74AN2 in the presence of UDP or UDP-Glc were almost the same (rmsd of 0.17). The molecule of UDP or UDP-Glc was placed into the obvious electron densities within a long and narrow tunnel buried in UGT74AN2. The interactions between UGT74AN2 and the

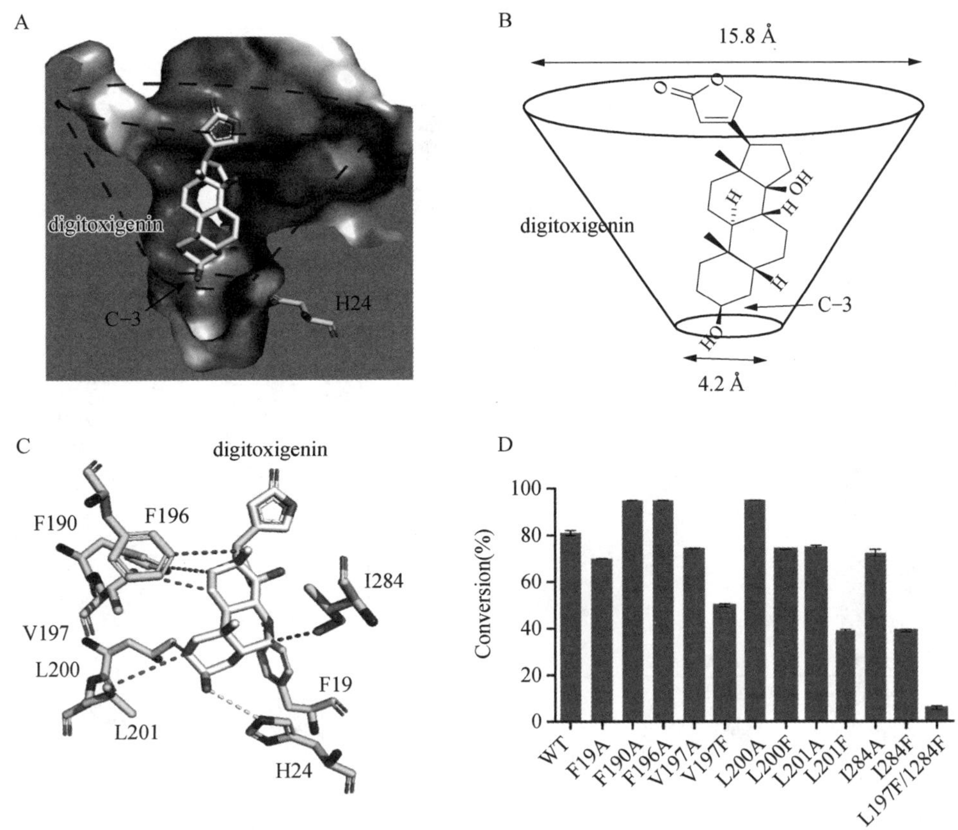


**Figure 3 Cardiotonic steroid recognition of UGT74AN2**

(A) Surface view of the *V*-shaped hydrophobic pocket of UGT74AN2. (B) Diagram of the *V*-shaped pocket with digitoxigenin inside. The top and bottom diameters are labeled. (C) Interaction between UGT74AN2 and digitoxigenin. The hydrogen bonds are represented by yellow dashed lines. The hydrophobic interactions are shown as magenta dashes. (D) Conversion rates of UGT74AN2 and its mutants, using digitoxigenin (**7**) as the substrate and UDP - Glc as the sugar donor.

sugar donor were examined in detail (Figure 2B - E and Table S4). UDP mainly interacts with the residues in the PSPG motif via hydrogen bonds and $\pi$-stacking interaction. The mutagenesis study further confirmed that the residues C351, S373, E376, and S283 are critical for the sugar donor binding of UGT74AN2 (Figure 2F).

Interaction between glycosyltransferase and the sugar moiety accounts for the sugar donor preference. The 3-/4-/ and 6-hydroxyl groups of the glucose moiety form hydrogen bonds with the D392, Q393, W371, T141, and Q142 residues of UGT74AN2 (Figure 2E and Table S4). The sequence alignment indicated that D392, Q393, W371, and T141 are highly conserved among the plant UGTs with UDP - Glc preference (Figure S35). The alanine mutation of these residues resulted in the nearly abolished glycosylation of the substrate (Figure 2F). To explore the sugar donor preference of UGT74AN2, the molecules of UDP - Gal and UDP - GlcNAc were modeled into the sugar donor binding site using the UGT74AN2/UDP - Glc structure as a template (Figure S36). The 4-hydroxyl group of the galactose moiety of UDP - Gal points in a direction away from W371, which prevents it from forming a strong hydrogen bond with UGT74AN2. In the case of UGT74AN2/UDP - GlcNAc, the *N*-acetyl group of the GlcNAc unit causes large steric hindrance with UGT74AN2 in contrast to that of the 2-hydroxyl group of the Glc unit. These findings explained that UGT74AN2 prefers UDP - Glc as the major sugar donor. The low conversion rates for UDP - Gal and UDP - GlcNAc likely resulted from the weak interaction and possible steric hindrance between UGT74AN2 and the sugar donors.

2.4 Cardiotonic Steroid Recognition of UGT74AN2

The structures of UGT74AN2 in complexes with three different substrates including UDP/resibufogenin (**2**), UDP/bufalin (**4**), and UDP/digitoxigenin (**7**) were obtained at the resolutions in a range of 2.10 - 2.30 Å (Table S2B and Figure S37). These complex structures revealed that the CTS compounds bind to UGT74AN2 in a spacious hydrophobic pocket formed by the residues F19, F190, F196, V197, L200, L201, and I284 (Figure 3A - C). A mutagenesis study was performed to test the roles of these residues related to the catalytic activities of UGT74AN2 using compound **2** as a sugar acceptor (Figure 3D). The alanine mutations only conferred marginal changes of the glycosylation activities of UGT74AN2. In contrast, most of the phenylalanine mutants, especially V197F, I284F, and V197F/I284F, showed significant decreases in their glycosylation capabilities. It could be reasoned

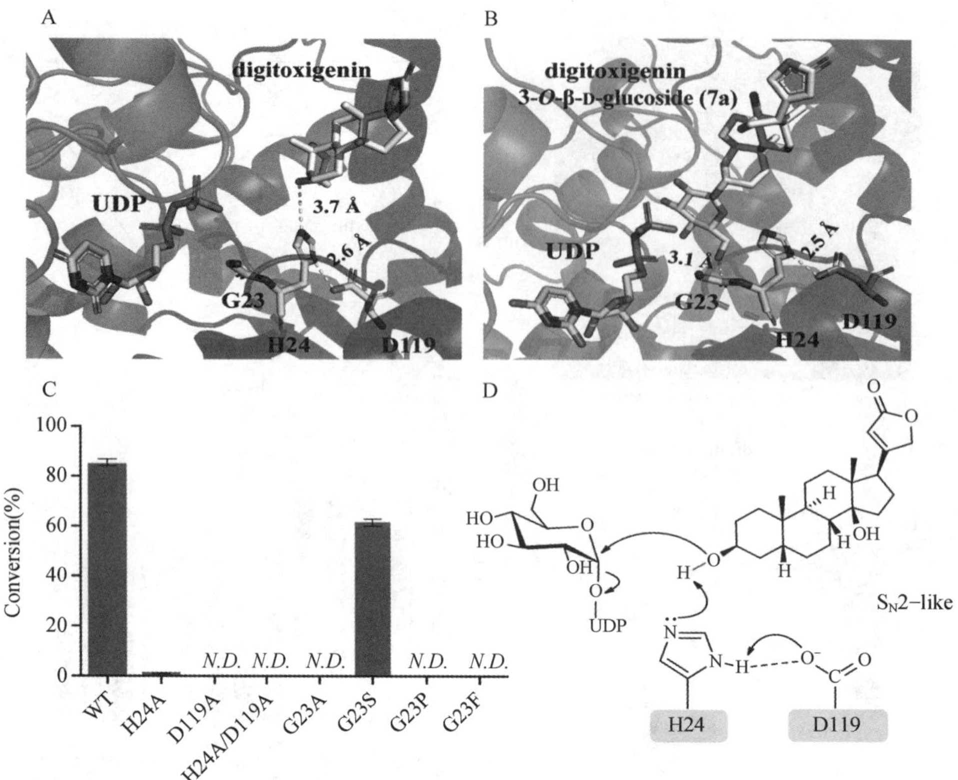


**Figure 4 Catalytic mechanism of UGT74AN2**

(A, B) Catalytic dyads in the structures of UGT74AN2/UDP/digitoxigenin (7) (A) and UGT74AN2/UDP/digitoxigenin 3 - *O* -*β*-D-glucoside (**7a**) (B). The hydrogen bonds are represented by yellow dashed lines. (C) Conversion rates of UGT74AN2 and its mutants, using **7** as the substrate and UDP - Glc as the sugar donor. (D) Proposed catalytic mechanism of UGT74AN2.

that the large hydrophobic side chains of the introduced phenylalanine mutations greatly blocked the binding of the steroid substrates and thus hampered the enzymatic activities.

The substrate-binding pocket of UGT74AN2 is distinctive *V*-shaped, which is different from other plant UGTs. The pocket entrance has a wide opening with a diameter of around 15. 8 Å, while the bottom of the pocket is relatively narrow (about 4. 2 Å in diameter) (Figure 3B). The pocket volume is about 2 212. 89 Å, which could easily accommodate various substrates. Furthermore, it is found that the *V*-shaped pocket restricts the 3-hydroxyl group of the CTS substrates (**2**, **4**, and **7**) facing toward the bottom of the pocket and forming hydrogen bonds with the critical catalytic residue His24 that is located right below (Figures 3A and S38). Therefore, although UGT74AN2 could tolerate structurally diverse CTSs, it still presented the specific glycosylation at the C - 3 position of the CTS.

2. 5 Catalytic Mechanism of UGT74AN2 Several UGT structures were reported previously, revealing a catalytic dyad that was formed by the highly conserved His and Asp near the acceptor binding pocket (Figure S35) and was critical for initiating catalytic reactions. The corresponding residues were identified as His24 and Asp119 in UGT74AN2. In the structure of UGT74AN2/UDP/**7**, the His24 residue forms hydrogen bonds with the 3-hydroxyl group of digitoxigenin and the side chain of Asp119. Similar interactions were also detected in the UGT74AN2/UDP/**2** and UGT74AN2/UDP/**4** complexes (Figures 4A and S39). The alanine mutations of His24 and Asp119 lead to the complete loss of the catalytic activities (Figure 4C), confirming that the conserved catalytic dyad (His-Asp) is essential for UGT74AN2 to function. It is likely that UGT74AN2 adopts a direct displacement $S_N$2-like mechanism to form a glycosidic bond (Figure 4D). In short, the His24 residue serves as the catalytic base and detaches a proton from the 3-hydroxyl group of the CTS substrate, facilitating nucleophiles to attack the anomeric carbon of UDP - Glc, which leads to formation of 3 - *O* - glycoside products. The Asp119 residue balances the charge after the proton detachment by interacting with His24.

To identify more key residues in the catalytic center, the crystal structure of UGT74AN2 complexed with the glycosylated product, digitoxigenin 3 - *O* - *β*-D-glucoside (**7a**), was solved at a resolution of 2. 45 Å (Table S2B and Figure S37). In the structure of UGT74AN2/UDP/**7a**, the Gly23 residue is located near the catalytic dyad within the interaction interfaces between UGT74AN2 and **7a** (Figure 4B). Almost no glycosylated product was detected in the

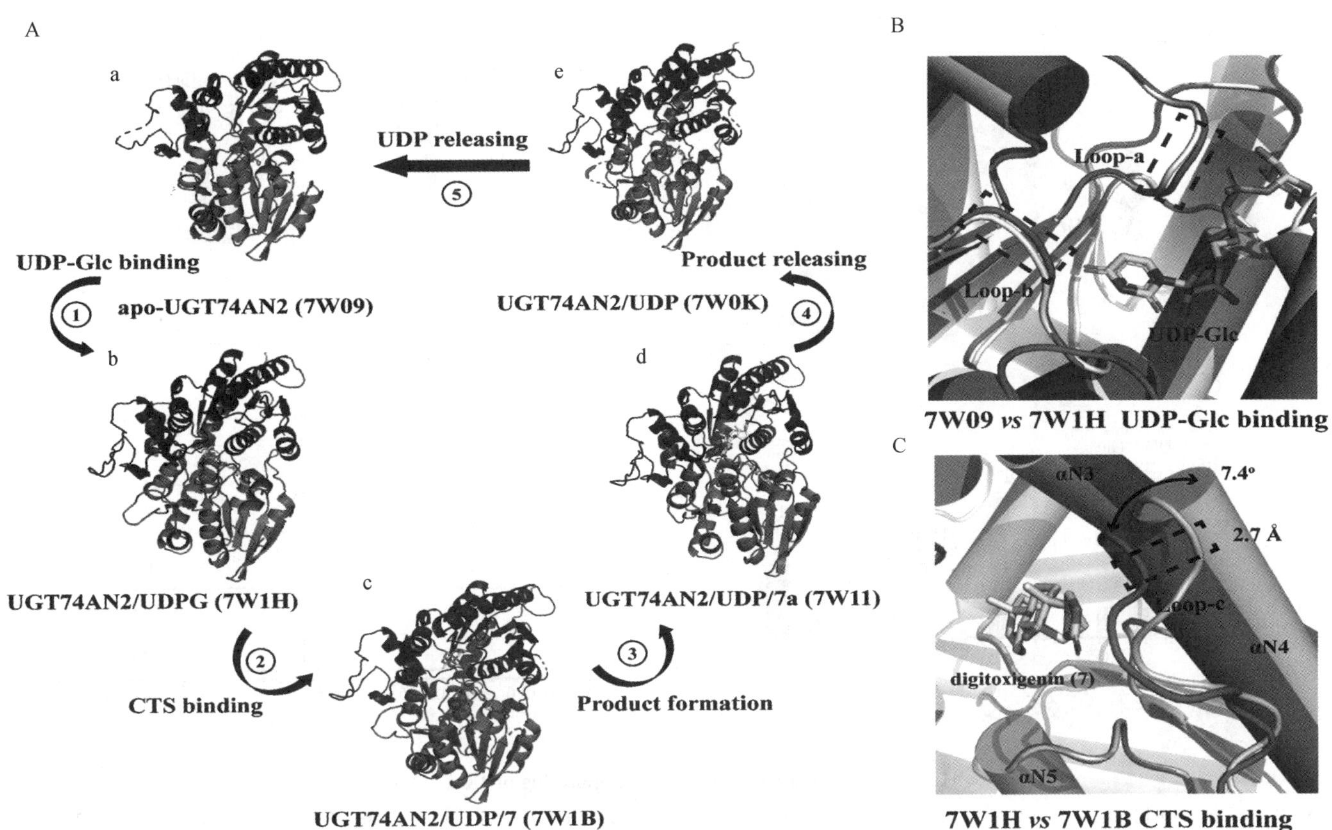


**Figure 5 Schematic diagram for the catalytic glycosylation process of UGT74AN2**

(A) Five-step workflow of UGT74AN2 is marked with black circled numbers (①-⑤). (B) Structure superimposition between apo-UGT74AN2 (white) and UGT74AN2/UDP - Glc (red). Loop-a and Loop-b are highlighted using the black dashed rectangles. (C) Structure superimposition between UGT74AN2/UDP - Glc (red) and UGT74AN2/UDP/digitoxigenin (wheat). Loop-c is indicated in a black dashed rectangle.

enzymatic reaction of the G23A mutant, indicating that Gly23 of UGT74AN2 is critical for function (Figure 4C). The sequence alignment suggested that Gly23 is actually conserved among the plant UGTs, further supporting the importance of this specific residue (Figure S35). Considering the location of Gly23, the abolishment of the catalytic activity is possibly due to the alanine mutation of Gly23, restricting the movement of its neighbor residue His24, as well as the flank helix N$\alpha$2 (residues 23 - 37) and a flexible loop (residues 17 - 22). To further test this hypothesis, Gly23 was replaced with the flexible residue (Ser) and the rigid residues (Pro and Phe), respectively. The results showed that the glycosylation activities of the UGT74AN2 mutants G23F and G23P were completely abolished, while G23S still maintained about 80% catalytic activity. (Figure 4C) Thus, the moderate structural flexibility of the key residue His24 and its nearby architecture is likely crucial for facilitating the catalytic processes to be completed in the reaction center of UGT74AN2. In addition, Gly23 may also help to stabilize the glycosylated products by forming hydrogen bonds with the sugar hydroxyl groups of the products after the catalytic reaction is over.

2.6 Structural Basis of the UGT74AN2 Workflow It is still a challenge of obtaining the enzyme structures complexed with different substrates and products, which are necessary for dissecting the sequential catalytic statuses of GTs during the whole glycosylation process. The crystal structures of UGT74AN2 were captured almost in a full set of activity states, including the apo, donor-bound, substrate-bound, product-bound, and product release forms. A five-step workflow of UGT74AN2 was proposed based on the structural and functional findings (Figure 5A). The apo form of UGT74AN2 is in the initial conformation for processing glycosylation. The first step is to recognize and bind the sugar donor. The structures of apo-UGT74AN2 and UGT74AN2/UDP - Glc were compared. The loop-a (residues 281 - 285) and loop-b (residues 348 - 352) of the CTD underwent a slight shift upon the binding of UDP - Glc (Figure 5B). The NTD conformation stayed unchanged during this process. The second step is the recognition and binding of the substrate. It was unable to capture the structure of UGT74AN2 in the presence of both UDP - Glc and the substrate because this intermediate complex was extremely unstable. The structures of UGT74AN2/UDP/substrates were obtained instead. The binding of the substrate had a subtle effect on the CTD, whereas an obvious change was observed

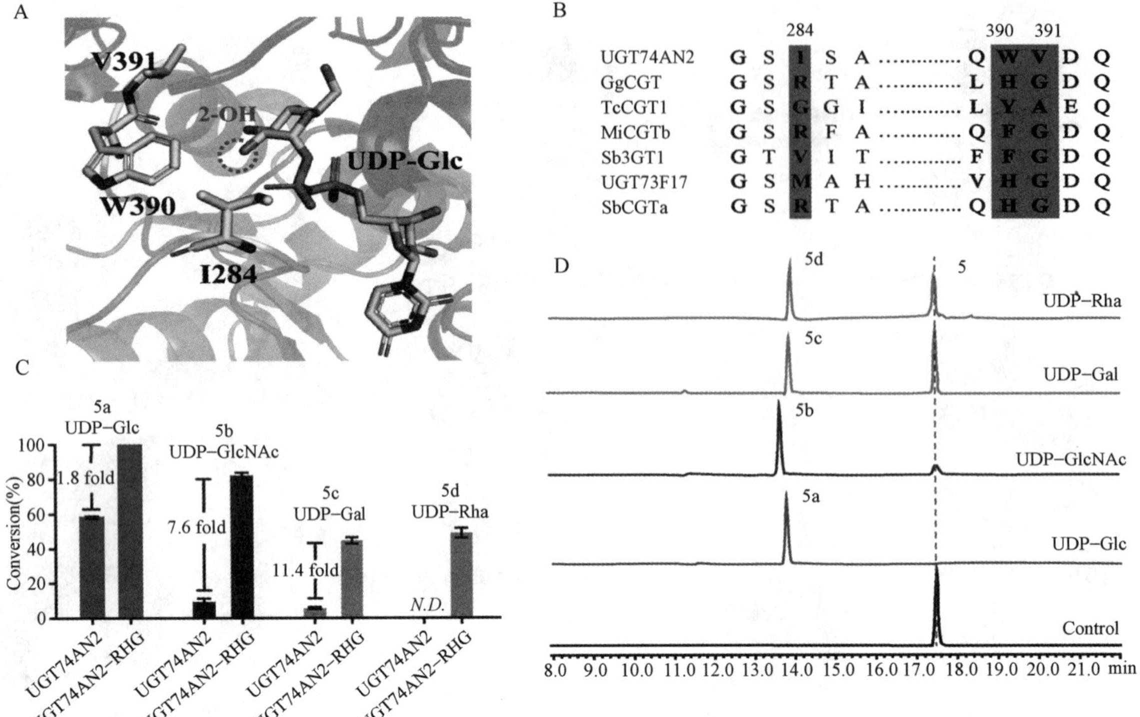


**Figure 6 Structure/sequence-based engineering of UGT74AN2**

(A) Three key residues around the 2-hydroxyl group of the glucose moiety of UDP - Glc; (B) sequence alignment between UGT74AN2 with other plant UGTs known with sugar donor promiscuity; (C) comparison of the conversion rates for different sugar donors catalyzed by UGT74AN2 and UGT74AN2 I284R/W390H/V391G, using bufotalin (**5**) as the substrate; and (D) HPLC analysis of the enzymatic reaction products catalyzed by UGT74AN2 I284R/W390H/V391G using UDP - Glc, UDP - GlcNAc, UDP - Gal, and UDP - Rha as sugar donors.

in the NTD. The Nα4 helix (residues 81 - 106) and the loop-c (residues 73 - 81) underwent an approximate rotation of 7.4° and a swing of ~2.4 Å, respectively (Figure 5C). The movements resulted in a wide-opened entrance of the hydrophobic pocket for efficient access to the substrates. Since the overall conformation of UGT74AN2/UDP/**7a** is very alike to that of UGT74AN2/UDP/**7**, no significant changes were captured during the third step of the product formation. This is probably due to the fast catalytic reaction rate and unstable intermediate status. The fourth step is to release the glycosylated product. Compared to UGT74AN2/UDP/7a, the Nα4 helix and loop-c in the structure of UGT74AN2/UDP were restored to the same positions as found in UGT74AN2/UDP - Glc. The last step is the release of UDP. By comparing the structures of UGT74AN2/UDP and apo-UGT74AN2, it was found that UGT74AN2 returned to its initial conformation after minor changes and prepared for the next round of the catalytic reaction. During the entire glycosylation event mediated by UGT74AN2, the Nα4 helix and loop-c were conferred with an important role by guarding the entry/exit of substrates and products.

2.7 Engineering Improvement of the Sugar Donor Promiscuity of UGT74AN2 Recent studies have demonstrated the bioactivity significance of CTS 3 - *O* - glycosides. For example, **6a** and **7a** were shown as potential inhibitors with enhanced affinity and selectivity for the α2 isoform of $Na^+/K^+$ - ATPase, which could be an ideal drug target for treating the congestive heart failure; **3a** and **6a** were shown with reduced toxicity compared with the corresponding aglycones in the zebrafish model. Furthermore, a subtle variation of the sugar moiety at the C - 3 position of CTSs also greatly affected their bioactivities. To this extent, protein engineering of UGT74AN2 may contribute to generating more diverse CTS 3 - *O* - glycosides for drug discovery. Although UGT74AN2 was shown with certain promiscuity for sugar donors, the catalytic activities for the sugar donor UDP - GlcNAc and UDP - Gal were still rather weak. To improve the sugar donor promiscuity, a structure/sequence-based rational design of UGT74AN2 was employed. The preference of the sugar donor is primarily controlled by numerous hydrogen bonds formed between sugar donors and GTs. The plant flavonoid UGT GgCGT, was proven with great sugar donor promiscuity, which could accept UDP - Glc, UDP - GlcNAc, UDP-Ara, UDP - Xyl, and UDP - Gal as the sugar donors. The molecular interactions between the sugar donors and the glycosyltransferase were closely examined and compared side by side for GgCGT and UGT74AN2. It was revealed that an important hydrogen bond formed between the 2-hydroxyl group of the sugar moiety of the donor and arginine of GgCGT was not found in the case of UGT74AN2 because the corresponding residue for arginine was isoleucine (I284) in UGT74AN2 (Figure 6B). Two residues, tryptophan (W390) and valine (V391), were identified near the 2-hydroxyl group of UDP - Glc in the structure of UGT74AN2/UDP - Glc, which may cause steric hindrance with the *N*-acetyl group, preventing UDP - GlcNAc from binding (Figure 6A). The sequence alignment among the plant UGTs with sugar donor promiscuity further showed that the residues in these UGTs corresponding to the W390 and V391 positions of UGT74AN2 are histidine (H) and glycine (G), respectively (Figure 6B). Compared with tryptophan and valine, histidine and glycine have smaller side chains or no side chains, resulting in less steric hindrance. Therefore, the abovementioned findings led to the rational design of a triple mutant, UGT74AN2 I284R/W390H/V391G, which hypothetically forms a hydrogen bond with the 2-hydroxyl group of various sugar moieties while weakening steric hindrance. To evaluate the sugar donor promiscuity of UGT74AN2 I284R/W390H/V391G, bufotalin (**5**) with a relatively low conversion rate was chosen as a substrate to test its catalytic activities. The conversion rate of the triple mutant is approximately 1.8-fold that of the wild type using UDP - Glc as the sugar donor. UGT74AN2 I284R/W390H/V391G showed a sharp increase in catalytic activities for UDP - GlcNAc (7.6-fold) and UDP - Gal (11.4-fold) as the sugar donors in comparison to wild type. Furthermore, the triple mutant could take UDP-Rha as a supplemented sugar donor with a conversion rate of around 55%. (Figures 6C, D and S40 - S43) Thus, the mutant UGT74AN2 I284R/W390H/V391G has significant potential in creating glycosyl diversities of the CTS, which would benefit the screen for safer cardiotonic products.

## 3 CONCLUSIONS

In summary, we identified plant steroid 3 - *O* - glycosyltransferase, UGT74AN2, from the medicinal plant *C. gigantea*. UGT74AN2 could regiospecifically catalyze 3 - *O* - glycosylation of cardiotonic steroids and accept UDP - Glc, UDP - GlcNAc, and UDP - Gal as the sugar donors. Crystal structures of the UGT74AN2 complexes revealed the key residues of UGT74AN2 in charge of the sugar donor recognition and preference and a unique *V*-shaped hydrophobic pocket responsible for the CTS recognition and regiospecificity. The catalytic dyad (His24-Asp119) and the conserved residue Gly23 are essential for the catalytic reaction of glycosylation. A workflow of UGT74AN2 was proposed, indicating that the N$\alpha$4 helix and loop-c control the entry/exit of the substrate and the product during the whole process of glycosylation reactions. Moreover, structure/sequence-based engineering resulted in the success of obtaining a triple mutant, UGT74AN2 I284R/W390H/V391G, which showed remark-ably broader sugar donor promiscuity and higher catalytic activities compared to the wild-type UGT74AN2 and other known plant steroid GTs. Taken together, these results provided mechanistic insights into CTS 3 - *O* - glycoslation and a potentially powerful biocatalyst for synthesizing variant CTS 3 - *O* - glycosides that are of great interest for drug discovery.

## 4 EXPERIMENTAL SECTION

4.1 Chemicals and Reagents Substrates **1** - **6** and **13** - **27** were purchased from Baoji Chenguang Biotechnology Co, Ltd. (Baoji, China) Compounds **7** - **12**, UDP - Glc, UDP - Gal, UDP-Rha, UDP - GlcA, UDP - GlcNAc, and UDP - Xyl, were purchased from Shanghai YuanYe Biotechnology Co, Ltd. (Shanghai, China). Compounds **2a** and **7a** were gifted from Prof. Ren-wang Jiang (Jinan University). Crystallization screening kits were purchased from Hampton Research (Laguna Niguel, CA). All other chemicals and reagents were purchased from Sigma-Aldrich (St. Louis, MO) unless otherwise specified.

4.2 Phylogenetic Analysis. The phylogenetic tree was constructed with the neighbor-joining method using MEGA-X online software (https://www.megasoftware.net/).

4.3 Expression and Purification of UGT74AN2. The full-length gene of UGT74AN2 (GenBank: MF942417.1) from *C. gigantea* was cloned into the pET28a (+) vector (Novagen) with an N-terminal hexa-His tag and a thrombin cleavage site. The recombinant plasmid was transformed into *E. coli* Rosetta (DE3) (Novagen) for heterologous expression. The colonies were picked from the agar plate, and cultured in 20 mL of an LB medium (1% tryptone, 5% yeast extract, 5% NaCl) containing 50 μg/mL kanamycin at 37 ℃ and 220 rpm overnight. The cultures were 1 : 100 diluted into 2 L of the LB medium supplemented with 50 μg/mL kanamycin and shaken at 37 ℃ and 220 rpm until $OD_{600}$ reached ~0.6. The cultures were then induced with 0.4 mmol/L isopropyl 1-thio-$\beta$-D-galactopyranoside (IPTG) and further grown at 18 ℃ for 20 h. The cells were harvested by centrifugation (SORVALL LYNX 4000, Thermo Scientific) at 5000 rpm for 15 min and washed with buffer A (20 mmol/L Tris - HCl pH 8.0, 500 mmol/L NaCl). The cell pellets were resuspended in 50 mL of buffer A supplemented with 1 μg/mL DNase I and 2.5 mmol/L $MgCl_2$ and disrupted by a high-pressure homogenizer (EmulsiFlex-C3, AVESTIN, Canada) at 12000 psi. The cell debris was removed by centrifugation at 12000 r/min for 45 min. The supernatant was loaded to a gravity column with 5 mL of Ni-NTA affinity resins (GenScript, Nanjing, China). The column was washed with 10 CV (column volume) of buffer B (20 mmol/L Tris - HCl pH 8.0, 500 mmol/L NaCl, 20 mmol/L imidazole) and eluted with 2 CV of buffer C (20 mmol/L Tris - HCl pH 8.0, 500 mmol/L NaCl, 300 mmol/L imidazole). The eluted protein was purified by gel filtration using a HiLoad 16/600 Superdex 75 column (GE Healthcare) and exchanged into buffer D (20 mmol/L Tris - HCl pH 8.0, 150 mmol/L NaCl, 1 mmol/L dithiothreitol (DTT), 5% glycerol). The target protein was pooled and incubated with thrombin at 4 ℃ for 12 h to remove the His tag. The digestion mixture was reloaded into the Ni - NTA affinity column. The tag-free protein was eluted from the resin with 1 CV of buffer D (20 mmol/L Tris - HCl pH 8.0, 500 mmol/L NaCl, 10 mmol/L imidazole). The eluted protein was further purified by passing through a HiLoad 16/600 Superdex 75 column (GE healthcare) and exchanged into buffer E (20 mmol/L Tris - HCl pH 8.0, 100 mmol/L NaCl, 1 mmol/L DTT). The peak fractions containing UGT74AN2 were collected and checked by 10% sodium dodecyl sulfate-polyacrylamide gel electrophoresis (SDS-PAGE). Finally, the purified protein was concentrated to 5 - 10 mg/mL using an Amicon Ultra-30 K (Millipore), flash-frozen in the liquid nitrogen, and kept at −80 ℃ for future uses.

4.4 Site-Directed Mutagenesis Site-directed mutagenesis of UGT74AN2 was performed by the polymerase chain reaction (PCR) with primers designed to generate the desired mutations (Table S5). The wild-type pET28a-UGT74AN2 plasmid was used as a PCR template. PCR was set up using a Phanta Max Super-Fidelity DNA Polymerase (Vazyme, Nanjing, China) in a Biorad C1 000 Thermal Cycler. After digestion of the template DNA with *Dpn*I (Thermo Scientific), the PCR products were transformed into the DH5a competent cell. All of the mutations were confirmed by the plasmid sequencing (Tsingke Biotechnology Co., Ltd.). The mutant proteins were purified following the same procedures used for the wild type.

4.5 Enzyme Activity Assay The glycosylation activity assay was performed in 100 μL of a reaction mixture containing 1 mmol/L different substrates, 4 mmol/L UDP-sugar, 5 mmol/L $MgCl_2$, 50 mmol/L Tris - HCl (pH 8.0), and 50 μg of purified enzyme (UGT74AN2 or the mutants). The reactions were incubated at 37 ℃ for 1 h and then stopped by adding 100 μL of methanol. The reactions were centrifuged at 12 000*g* for 30 min. The supernatant was filtered through a 0.45 μm microporous membrane and analyzed by HPLC and LC - MS. The HPLC analysis was performed on a Shimadzu-LC - 20AT (Japan) with an Ultimate XB-C18 column (4.6 mm × 250 mm I.D., 5 μm, Welch Materials, Inc., China) at a flow rate of 0.8 mL/min, using the mobile phase of (A) 0.1% formic acid in deionized $H_2O$ and (B) 100% $CH_3CN$. The gradient settings for separating the glycosylated products and substrates were 0 - 20 min 10% B to 100% B, 20 - 25 min 100% B to 100% B, 25 - 28 min 100% B to 10% B, and 28 - 35 min 10% B to 10% B. The glycosylated products were further confirmed using an LTQ XL Orbitrap mass spectrometer (Thermo Fisher Scientific Inc.) The MS/MS analysis was carried out in a positive ionization mode with 35% relative collision energy. The conversion rate was determined by HPLC and calculated by dividing the integrated peak area of the glycosylated product by the sum of peak areas of the glycosylated product and the remaining substrate. All experiments were performed in triplicate.

4.6 Determination of Kinetic Parameters Kinetic parameters of UGT74AN2 were determined using resibufogenin (**2**) as a substrate in the reactions with a final volume of 50 μL, consisting of 50 mmol/L Tris - HCl (pH 8.0), 5 mmol/L $MgCl_2$, 340 ng of purified UGT74AN2, 10 mmol/L UDP - Glc, and different concentrations of resibufogenin (5, 10, 15, 20, 40, 80 μmol/L). After incubating at 37 ℃ for 30 min, all of the reactions were quenched with 50 μL of MeOH and centrifuged at 12 000 rpm for 30 min. The supernatants were analyzed by HPLC as described above. All experiments were performed in triplicate ($n = 3$). The values of $K_m$ and $K_{cat}/K_m$ were calculated using the Michaelis-Menten plot.

4.7 Scaled-Up Reactions **2a**, **3a**, **4a**, **6a**, and **7a** were synthesized by preparative-scale reactions. The scaled-up reactions with a final volume of 10 - 20 mL, consisting of a buffer solution (50 mmol/L Tris - HCl, pH 8.0), 5 - 10 mg of aglycones (dissolved in dimethylsulfoxide, DMSO), 10 - 20 mg of UDP-Glc, and 5 - 10 mg of purified UGT74AN2, were performed at 37 ℃ overnight. The products were purified by semipreparative HPLC and dissolved in methanol-$d_4$ for the determination of the NMR spectra.

4.8 Protein Crystallization The purified UGT74AN2 (5 mg/mL) with or without 2.5 mM UDP was incubated with 1 mM CTAB at 4 ℃ for 30 min before the set up of the crystallization trays. Lamellar crystals of apo-UGT74AN2 were observed at 18 ℃ within 2 d using the hanging drop vapor diffusion method by mixing 1 μL of protein with 1 μL of the reservoir solution (0.1 mol/L sodium chloride, 0.1 mol/L MES (pH 6.5), and 18% (*W*/*V*) PEG 3 350). The crystals of UGT74AN2/UDP were obtained in the reservoir solution containing 0.1 mol/L sodium acetate, 0.1 mol/L Bis-Tris (pH 6.5), and 18% (*W*/*V*) PEG 3 350. The crystals of UGT74AN2/UDP-Glc were obtained by soaking the UGT74AN2 crystals with 10 mmol/L UDP-Glc in the mother liquor for 20 min. The crystals of UGT74AN2/UDP/substrates (**2**, **4**, and **7**) were obtained by soaking the UGT74AN2/UDP crystals with 2 mmol/L substrates in the mother liquor for 24 h. The crystals of UGT74AN2/UDP/the glycosylated product (**7a**) were obtained by soaking the UGT74AN2/UDP crystals with 5 mmol/L **7a** in the mother liquor for 48 h. All crystals were harvested in the same reservoir solution supplemented with 20% glycerol as a cryoprotectant and flash-frozen in the liquid nitrogen.

4.9 Data Collection and Structure Determination The crystallographic data sets were collected on the beamlines 18U1 and 19U1 at the Shanghai Synchrotron Radiation Facility (SSRF) (Table S2). The diffraction images were processed using XDS and HKL 3 000. The structure of UGT74AN2 was solved by molecular replacement using a Phaser from the CCP4 suite. The structure of UGT74AC1, a triterpene glycosyltransferase from *Siraitia grosvenorii* (PDB code: 6L8Z, 40% sequence identity with UGT74AN2), was used as a searching model. The model of UGT74AN2 was built initially using AutoBuild and manually using Coot. The iterative refinement and structure validation were done using Phenix.

4.10 Structure Analysis Protein-ligand interaction profiler and PyMOL (The PyMOL Molecular Graphics System, Version 2.0 Schrödinger, LLC) were used to visualize the models and produce the figures. Sequence alignments were created using Clustal Omega and ESPript. Structures were superimposed using the Structure Similarity Matching (SSM) server.

4.11 Molecular Docking The molecule of UDP-GlcNAc or UDP-Gal was docked into the structure of UGT74AN2 using Autodock 4.0. The structure of UGT74AN2/UDP-Glc was used as a template.

[黄伟，龙凤，等. ACS Catalysis, 2022, 12: 2927-2937.]

# Engineering cofactor supply and recycling to drive phenolic acid biosynthesis in yeast

In the past decade, the development of synthetic biology and metabolic engineering has facilitated the harnessing of yeast for de novo biosynthesis of complex natural products, such as artemisinic acid, cannabinoids and alkaloids. Enzyme and pathway engineering have been extensively used to enhance biosynthetic efficiency. However, natural product titers remain to be largely improved. For example, the opioid titer from an engineered yeast cell factory was less than 1 μg/L (ref.). Some key enzymes often require special cofactors to maintain high activity and insufficient cofactor supply may cause metabolic obstruction during natural product biosynthesis. In particular, expression of heterologous enzymes in yeast may suffer from insufficient or deficient cofactor supply due to the different cellular environments between yeast and the natural host.

Cofactor is an organic compound that is required for numerous intracellular metabolic processes and reactions. Although the two most common redox cofactors, $NAD(P)^+$ and NAD(P)H, have been extensively manipulated for improving cellular performance, engineering other relatively rare cofactors to improve biosynthesis efficiency remains a challenge due to the complex nature of cofactor metabolism and the lack of necessary information to do so. *S*-adenosyl-L-methion (SAM) acts as an essential methyl donor in many methylation reactions catalyzed by SAM-dependent methyltransferases. The regeneration and methyl transfer of SAM are completed through the methyl cycle. However, successful cases of SAM engineering for enhancing methylation efficiency in yeast are rare, possibly owing to the complex feedback regulation of the methyl cycle and sulfur assimilation. Furthermore, cofactor biosynthesis in eukaryotic cells is distributed in suborganelles to couple compartmentalized cellular metabolism in the native hosts, which might limit the efficiency of reconstructed biosynthetic pathways in yeast. Flavin cofactors $FMN(H_2)$ and $FAD(H_2)$[(reduced) flavin adenine dinucleotide] play an important role in maintaining the mitochondrial redox homeostasis in yeast. It is generally believed that riboflavin is synthesized in the cytosol and then transported to the mitochondria for the synthesis of the other two active forms of flavin, $FMN(H_2)$ and $FAD(H_2)$ (ref.). The $FAD(H_2)$ concentration in mitochondria is more than ten times higher than that in the cytosol, and the total NAD(H) level is at least 20 times higher than that of $FAD(H_2)$ in *S. cerevisiae*. $FAD(H_2)$ usually forms an electron transport chain with NAD(P)H to perform a complete redox function. Therefore, $FAD(H_2)$-dependent catalytic reactions in the cytosol may be relatively inefficient and engineering cofactor supply should be helpful for improving the biosynthesis of molecules that involves cofactors.

Lignans, such as medicinal podophyllotoxin, silibinin, rosmarinic acid and clemastanin B, are widely used as pharmaceutical agents (Extended Data Fig. 1). Phenolic acids, such as caffeic acid (CaA) and ferulic acid (FA), are core precursors of these complex lignan chemicals and themselves can also serve as pharmaceuticals. The biosynthesis of phenolic acids requires many cofactors (Fig. 1 and Extended Data Fig. 2), furthermore enhancing the difficulty of efficient biosynthesis in yeast. CaA synthesis in plants requires

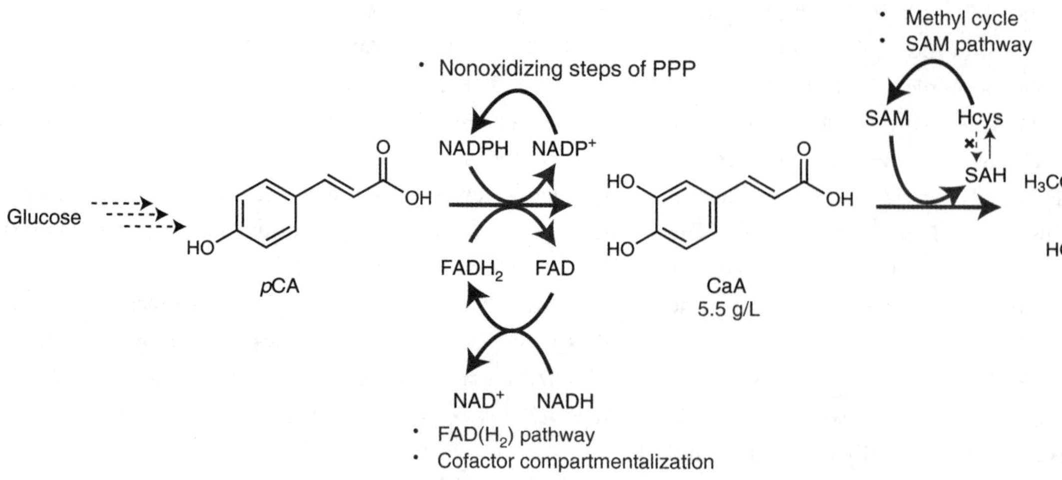

**Fig. 1 Biosynthesis of CaA and FA requires numerous cofactors**

NADPH and FAD($H_2$) play a crucial role in CaA biosynthesis, while SAM is the methyl donor for FA biosynthesis from CaA methylation. The reversible nonoxidizing steps of the PPP were rewired to regenerate NADPH for CaA biosynthesis. FAD($H_2$) supply and compartmentalization were rate-limiting steps during high levels of CaA synthesis. Reversing the thermodynamic equilibrium of Sahl and enhancing SAM biosynthesis improved the CaA methylation for FA biosynthesis. These tailored cofactor engineering strategies enabled the highest microbial production of CaA (5.5±0.2 g/L) and FA (3.8±0.3 g/L). NADP(H), (reduced) nicotinamide-adenine dinucleotide phosphate; NAD(H), reduced nicotinamide-adenine dinucleotide. The dotted lines indicate multiple biosynthetic steps.

multiple steps of oxidation and esterification, and occurs at low efficiency. An alternative pathway catalyzed by bacteria-coupled enzymes HpaB (FAD-dependent 4-hydroxyphenylacetate-3-monooxygenase) and HpaC (NADH-flavin oxidoreductase) is considered to be a feasible route for CaA synthesis in yeast. In this process, the electrons are transferred from NADH to FAD through HpaC to form $FADH_2$, which is further captured by HpaB to oxidize *p*-coumaric acid (*p*CA) in the presence of oxygen. Thus, cytosolic FAD($H_2$) might be a rate-limiting step in the electron transfer of CaA biosynthesis. Also, NADPH (reduced icotinamide adenine dinucleotide phosphate) regeneration is important for Cyp function to synthesize the precursor *p*CA, which has been shown through strengthening the oxidation steps of the pentose phosphate pathway (PPP). Furthermore, SAM is important for the methylation step of FA biosynthesis catalyzed by the SAM-dependent *O*-methyltransferase (Omt). Taken together, this would suggest that cofactor engineering has great potential in improving the biosynthesis of CaA and FA in yeast.

Herein, we developed tailored engineering strategies for enhancing, relocating and/or recycling $FADH_2$, SAM and NADPH, which substantially improved the production of CaA and FA to 5.5±0.2 and 3.8±0.3 g/L, respectively (Fig. 1). Our observation shows that cofactor engineering can drive metabolic flux toward natural product biosynthesis.

## 1 RESULTS

Engineering the biosynthesis of CaA and FA in yeast. We designed CaA/FA biosynthetic pathways by using *p*CA as a precursor, which can be synthesized from condensation of two precursors, phosphoenolpyruvate (PEP) and erythrose-4-phosphate (E4P), through the aromatic amino acid biosynthesis pathway (Fig. 2a, Extended Data Fig. 2 and Supplementary Fig. 1 for more strain information). PEP derived from glycolysis and E4P derived from the PPP are important metabolites in glucose catabolism for cell growth. To relieve the metabolic burden, a galactose regulatory (GAL) system based on a *GAL80* knock-out was adopted (Supplementary Fig. 2a), which enables repression of exogenous genes under the control of galactose metabolism related promoters ($P_{GAL1}$, $P_{GAL7}$ and $P_{GAL10}$) at high glucose concentration during growth phase. Conversely, exogenous genes are expressed at low glucose concentration during production phase (Supplementary Fig. 2b).

To produce a considerable concentration of precursor *p*CA by increasing phenylpropanoid flux, the feedback-insensitive 3-deoxy-D-arabino-heptulosonate-7-phosphate (DAHP) synthase $Aro4^{K229L}$, chorismate mutase $Aro7^{G141S}$ and *Escherichia coli* shikimate kinase II (aroL) were introduced along with the deletion of phenylpyruvate decarboxylase *ARO10* (Extended Data Fig. 3a). Then, a tyrosine derived pathway was constructed by expressing a *Flavobacterium johnsoniae* tyrosine ammonia lyase (*Fj*Tal) together with the deletion of pyruvate decarboxylase *PDC5*, which enabled *p*CA production of 23.1±2.7 mg/L in the engineered strain RB2 (Extended Data Fig. 3b). Furthermore, a phenylalanine derived pathway was constructed by expressing a *Sorghum bicolor* phenylalanine ammonia lyase (*Sb*Pal1), an *Arabidopsis thaliana* cytochrome P450 reductase (*At*Cpr1) together with an identified Cyp complex (containing *Populus trichocarpa*

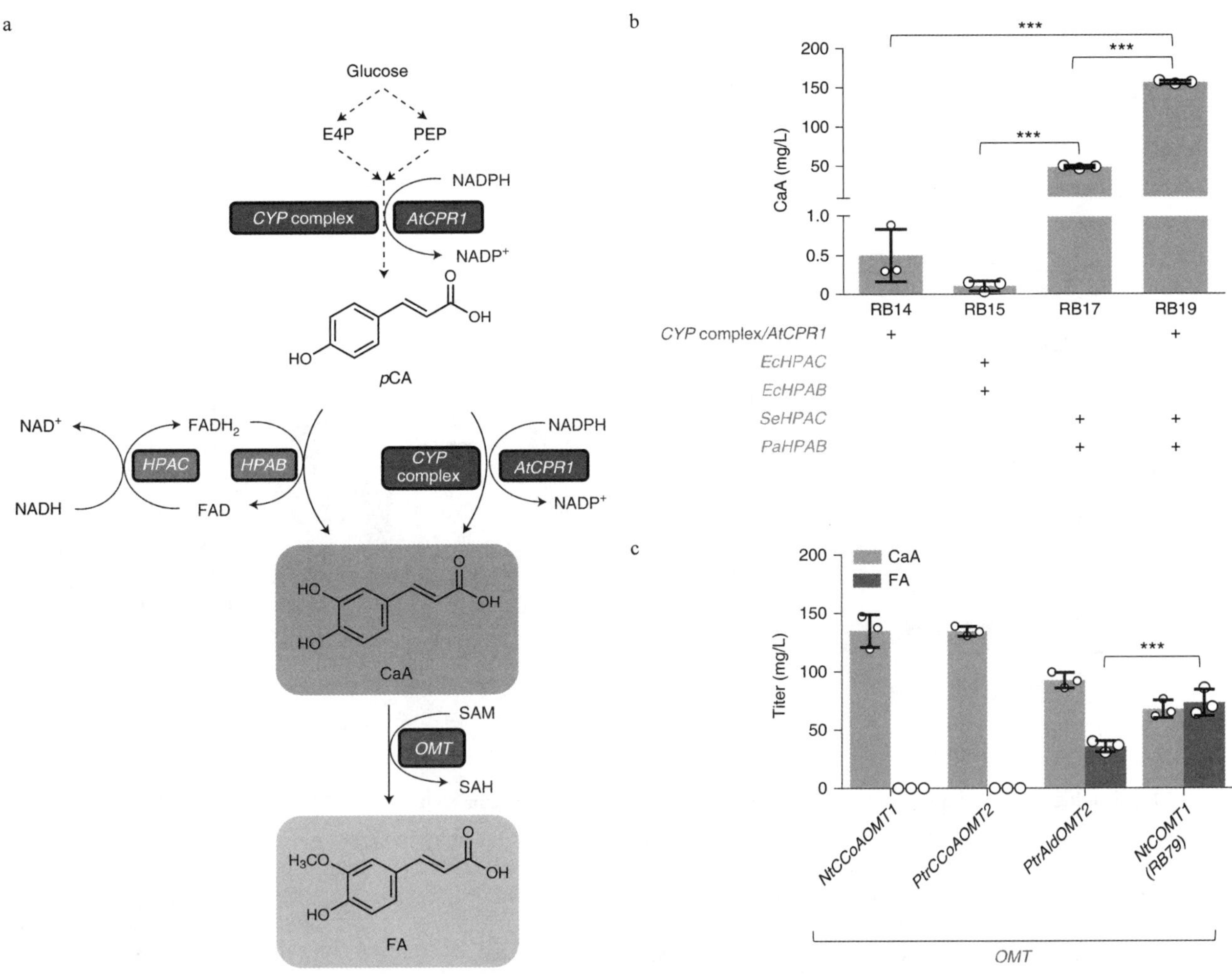


**Fig. 2 Construction of CaA/FA biosynthetic pathways in yeast**

(a) Overview of yeast metabolic pathway for phenolic acid biosynthesis. Plant-derived pathway consisting of *P. trichocarpa CYP* complex (*PtrC4H1* + *PtrC4H2* + *PtrC3H* encoding *P. trichocarpa* coumarate-3-hydroxylase and cinnamic acid hydroxylase 1/2) and *AtCPR1* (encoding *A. thaliana* cytochrome P450 reductase) are shown in blue. Bacteria-derived pathway consisting of *HPAB* (encoding $FADH_2$-dependent 4-hydroxyphenylacetate 3-monooxygenase) and *HPAC* (encoding NADH-dependent flavin oxidoreductase) are shown in green. The FA biosynthetic pathway catalyzed by Omt is shown in pink. All cofactors are shown in red. The dotted lines indicate multiple biosynthetic steps. (b) CaA production by engineered strains with the combination of both plant and bacterial biosynthetic pathways. *PaHPAB* encodes *P. aeruginosa* HpaB; *SeHPAC* encodes *S. enterica* HpaC; *EcHPAB* encodes *E. coli* HpaB; *EcHPAC* encodes *E. coli* HpaC. (c) Screening *O*-methyltransferase genes for FA production. *NtCCoAOMT1* and *PtrCCoAOMT2* encode caffeoyl-CoA O-methyltransferases from *N. tabacum* and *P. trichocarpa*, respectively; *PtrAldOMT2* encodes *P. trichocarpa* 5-hydroxyconiferaldehyde *O*-methyltransferase 2; *NtCOMT1* encodes *N. tabacum* CaA *O*-methyltransferase 1. Yeast cells were grown in defined minimal medium containing 20 g/L glucose and cultures were extracted after 96 h of growth for phenolic acid quantification. All data represent the mean of $n = 3$ biologically independent samples and error bars show standard deviation. Statistical analysis was carried out by using Student's *t*-test (one-tailed; two-sample unequal variance; * $P<0.05$, ** $P<0.01$, *** $P<0.001$). These methods for fermentation and extraction were used for all subsequent experiments unless otherwise stated.

cinnamic acid hydroxylase, *Ptr*C4h2 and *Ptr*C4h1, and coumarate-3-hydroxylase, *Ptr*C3h3). The resulting strain RB14 produced 130.8 ± 17.0 mg/L of *p*CA in shake-flask cultivation (Extended Data Fig. 3b). Notably, coexpression of *Ptr*C3h3, *Ptr*C4h1 and *Ptr*C4h2 (strain RB14) had a 90% increase in *p*CA production compared to strain RB13 that only expressed *Ptr*C4h2 (Extended Data Fig. 3c), which may be attributed to the protein-protein interaction for improved catalytic efficiency.

It is reported that C3h can convert *p*CA to CaA in plants, however, the trace amount of CaA in strain RB14 (Fig. 2b) suggested that the low efficiency of this plant-derived pathway in yeast. We thus searched for alternative pathways of CaA biosynthesis from *p*CA. Bacterial *Ec*HpaB and *Ec*HpaC produce considerable CaA in *E. coli*, which, however, did not work efficiently in yeast (strain RB15, Fig. 2b). Fortunately, the combination of *Pseudomonas aeruginosa Pa*HpaB and *Salmonella enterica Se*HpaC, enabled a CaA production of 48.3 ± 1.1 mg/L in strain RB17, which was 439-fold higher than that of strain RB15

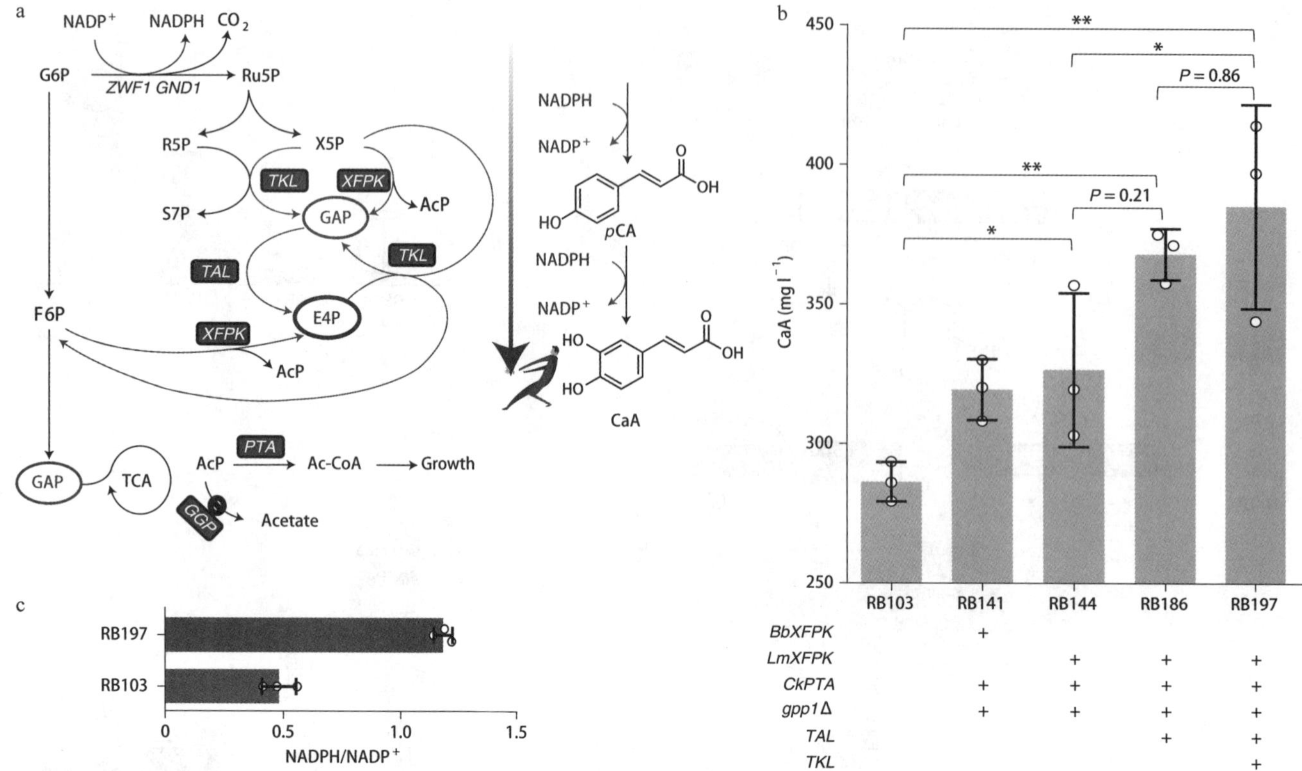


**Fig. 3 Engineering NADPH regeneration for CaA production by pulling nonoxidizing steps of the PPP during glucose-limited conditions**

(a) Schematic overview of pulling the PPP for the regeneration of NADPH, which consists of overexpressing *XFPK* (encoding phosphoketolase), *TAL* (encoding transaldolase), *TKL* (encoding transketolase), *PTA* (encoding phosphotransacetylase) and deleting *GPP1* (encoding GAP phosphatase), in the CaA-producing strain RB103. This strategy couples NADPH regeneration with enhancing the supply of precursor E4P. G6P, glucose-6-phosphate; F6P, fructose 6-phosphate; Ru5P, ribulose 5-phosphate; R5P, ribose 5-phosphate; X5P, xylose 5-phosphate; S7P, sedoheptulose 7-phosphate; AcP, acetyl-phosphate; Ac-CoA, acetyl-CoA; TCA, tricarboxylic acid cycle. (b) CaA production by engineering the nonoxidizing steps of the PPP. (c) Cellular $NADPH/NADP^+$ ratios in the engineered *S. cerevisiae* strains, the samples for NADP(H) quantification were harvested at 36 h. *BbXFPK* encodes *Bifidobacterium breve* phosphoketolase; *LmXFPK* encodes *L. mesenteroides* phosphoketolase; *CkPTA* encodes *C. kluyveri* phosphotransacetylase. All data represent the mean of $n = 3$ biologically independent samples and error bars show standard deviation. Statistical analysis was carried out by using Student's *t*-test (one-tailed; two-sample unequal variance; * $P<0.05$, ** $P<0.01$, *** $P<0.001$).

(Fig. 2b). Considering HpaC supplies $FADH_2$ for HpaB, we constructed an HpaB - HpaC fusion protein (RB18 and RB16) to enhance $FADH_2$ channeling; however, it resulted in a lower CaA production (Extended Data Fig. 4b, c), which might have been caused by the frequent steric hindrance of the protein structure. Finally, we reconstructed the Cyp complex and the HpaBC pair (individually expressing HpaB and HpaC) in the *p*CA overproduction background, which enabled a CaA production of 157.5±1.2 mg/L in strain RB19 (Fig. 2b).

The synthesis of FA from CaA can be accomplished via a single orthodiphenol-*O*-methyltransferase (Omt). However, the substrate range of Omt in lignan biosynthesis is broad and complicated, such as CaA *O*-methyltransferase (Comt), 5-hydroxyconiferaldehyde *O*-methyltransferase (AldOmt) and caffeoyl-CoA O-methyltrans ferase (CCoAOmt). To select highly efficient Omts for FA synthesis in *S. cerevisiae*, four Omts were randomly selected and individually introduced into the RB19 background. Comt1 from *Nicotiana tabacum* (*Nt*Comt1) and AldOmt2 from *P. trichocarpa* (*Ptr*AldOmt2) showed activity toward CaA, and *Nt*Comt1 produced the highest concentration of FA of 73.1 ± 5.6 mg/L by converting half of the CaA (strain RB79, Fig. 2c).

Engineering NADPH supply. The plant-derived CaA pathway requires a large amount of NADPH as a crucial cofactor of electron transfer conduit in the Cyp system (Fig. 2a). We speculated that enhancing the NADPH supply could increase CaA biosynthesis in yeast. Considering that the higher CaA yield requires more NADPH, we thus introduced the upstream genes *ARO1-3* (encoding shikimate dehydrogenase, chorismate synthase and DAHP synthase) together with *PHA2* and *MtPDH1* into the strains RB19 for higher precursor supply (Extended Data Fig. 4d). The engineered strain, RB103, produced 286.3 ± 4.1 mg/L of CaA and should require higher NADPH regeneration.

PPP is the main source of NADPH, and is commonly engineered for NADPH regeneration by overexpressing the key genes encoding glucose-6-phosphate dehydrogenase (Zwf1)

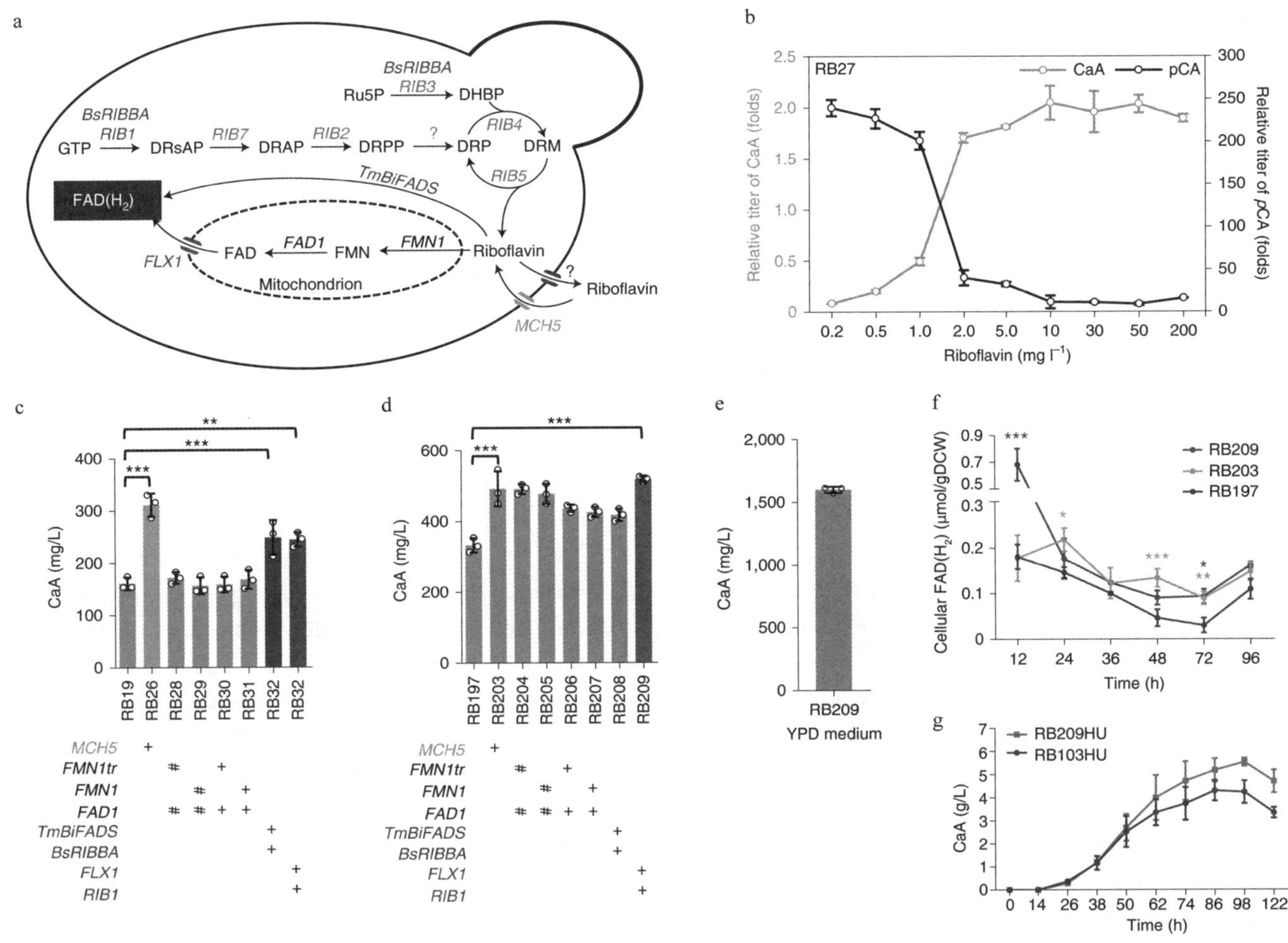


**Fig. 4 Manipulation of $FADH_2$ biosynthesis and relocation for enhancing CaA production.**

(a) Schematic illustration of the engineered $FADH_2$ biosynthesis and transport in yeast. Riboflavin is synthesized from GTP and Ru5P through several enzymes: GTP cyclohydrolase II (*RIB1*); 2,5-diamino-6-ribitylamino-4(3H)-pyrimidinone 5′-phosphate (DRAP) deaminase (*RIB2*); 3,4-dihydroxy-2-butanone-4-phosphate (DHBP) synthase (*RIB3*); lumazine synthase (*RIB4*); riboflavin synthase (*RIB5*); 2,5-diamino-6-ribosylamino-4(3H)-pyrimidinone 5′-phosphate (DRsAP) reductasein (*RIB7*). Riboflavin is exported by unknown transporters (marked as '?') and also imported by a riboflavin transporter (*MCH5*). Riboflavin is transported into the mitochondria for FAD synthesis through the riboflavin kinase *Fmn1* and the FAD synthetase *Fad1*. The mitochondrial FAD is exported to the cytosol by a mitochondrial FAD exporter (encoded by *FLX1*). *B. subtilis BsRIBBA* encoding bifunctional DHBP synthase/GTP cyclohydrolase II and *T. maritima TmBiFADS* encoding bifunctional riboflavin kinase/FAD synthase were used for alternative FAD biosynthesis. DRPP, 5-diamino-6-ribitylamino-2,4(1H, 3H)-pyrimidinedione 5′-phosphate; DRP, 5-diamino-6-ribitylamino-2,4(1H, 3H)-pyrimidinedione; DRM, 6,7-dimethyl-8-ribityllumazine. (b) Relative titers of CaA in strain RB27 were normalized to reference strain RB19 with addition of riboflavin. (c,d) $FADH_2$ engineering for CaA production in the engineered CaA low-producing strain RB19 (**c**) and in the CaA high-producing strain RB197 (**d**). *FMN1* was truncated as *FMN1tr* according to the predicted transit peptide cleavage site. The # indicates expression under strong constitutive promoters ($P_{tHXT7}$ and $P_{TDH3}$). (e) CaA production by the best engineered strain RB209 when cultured in YPD medium. (f) Time courses of cellular $FAD(H_2)$ level of strain RB197, RB203 and RB209. Statistics are comparing the two red-toned strains to the blue strain. μmol/gDCW refers to the number of moles of cofactor per gram of dry cell weight (DCW). (g) CaA production by fed-batch fermentation of the prototrophic strain RB209HU and control strain RB103HU under glucose-limited conditions. All data represent the mean of $n = 3$ independent biological samples and error bars show standard deviation. Statistical analysis was carried out by using Student's $t$-test (one-tailed; two-sample unequal variance; $^{*}P<0.05$, $^{**}P<0.01$, $^{***}P<0.001$).

and 6-phosphogluconate dehydrogenase (Gnd1) (Fig. 3a). Previously, metabolic flux analysis (MFA) suggested that *ZWF1* and *GND1* expression were not rate-limiting steps during glucose-limited conditions (production phase in this study), but downstream reversible steps. Therefore, we tried to pull the PPP flux for NADPH regeneration by overexpressing the downstream genes of PPP (Fig. 3a). Phosphoketolase (Xfpk) is able to split xylose 5-phosphate (X5P) and/or fructose 6-phosphate (F6P) into acetyl-phosphate and glyceraldehyde-3-phosphate (GAP)/E4P. Furthermore, acetyl-phosphate can be efficiently converted to acetyl-CoA for growth by phosphotransacetylase (Pta) with the deletion of GAP phosphatase (Gpp1). Thus, combinatorial overexpression of *XFPK* and *PTA* may not only strengthen the PPP downstream for NADPH regeneration, but also enhance E4P supply for aromatic biosynthesis. To validate our strategy, two Xfpks showing different activities toward the substrates X5P and F6P were tested and were found to substantially improve CaA production (Fig. 3b). In particular, expression of *Leuconostoc mesenteroides LmXFPK* and *Clostridium kluyveri CkPTA* in a *gpp1Δ* strain resulted in a CaA titer of 326.7±15.9 mg/L (strain RB144), 20% higher than that of the control strain RB103. We also combined the Xfpk/Pta with overexpression of the native transaldolase (Tal) to further drag flux toward E4P (strain RB186) and NADPH regeneration, which enabled an extra 12.7% improvement in CaA production (368.1±5.3 mg/L) compared with strain RB144. Finally, overexpressing a transketolase gene *TKL* increased CaA production by 5% (385.2±36.52 mg/L) in the high-production strain RB197 compared with the parental strain RB186. Taken together, NADPH regeneration strategies achieved a 45% increase in CaA titer compared with the initial strain RB103. Consistently, NADPH/$NADP^+$ ratio was 46% higher in strain RB197 than that of strain RB103 (Fig. 3c). These results indicate that enhancing NADPH regeneration through the nonoxidizing steps of PPP is beneficial for CaA synthesis.

FAD engineering to increase CaA production. As shown in Fig. 2a, the bacterial CaA biosynthetic pathway consumes a large amount of cytosolic $FADH_2$ and disrupts intracellular $FADH_2$/FAD homeostasis. In yeast, precursor riboflavin is synthesized through multiple step reactions in the cytosol (Fig. 4a), and then imported into the mitochondria for FAD biosynthesis by the monofunctional riboflavin kinase Fmn1 and FAD synthase Fad1. In *S. cerevisiae*, cytosolic FAD ($H_2$) is shown to be much lower than that in the mitochondria, so we speculated that FAD($H_2$) supply might limit CaA biosynthesis in the cytosol. Thus, we tried to engineer the biosynthesis and relocation of FAD($H_2$) for improving the supply of cytosolic FAD($H_2$).

To predict the potential of the FAD($H_2$) engineering strategy to increase CaA production, we first constructed a riboflavin auxotrophic *rib4Δ* strain together with riboflavin transporter gene *MCH5* overexpression in strain RB19. The resulting strain RB27 was able to grow in minimal medium with external riboflavin addition. CaA production was improved with the incremental addition of exogenous riboflavin and reached the highest level with the addition of 10 mg/L riboflavin (Fig. 4b). Consistently, *p*CA accumulation negatively correlated with CaA titer, suggesting that enhancing the supply of FAD ($H_2$) precursor riboflavin substantially improved CaA biosynthesis. We further engineered FAD ($H_2$) synthesis using three strategies: ① strengthening native FAD($H_2$) biosynthesis. ② constructing bacterial FAD($H_2$) biosynthesis in the cytosol. ③ manipulating export of mitochondrial riboflavin and FAD ($H_2$) to the cytosol (Fig. 4a). Overexpressing cytosolic Rib1 (to strengthen the first rate-limiting step of the FAD($H_2$) pathway) and Flx1 (to export mitochondrial FAD into the cytosol) resulted in a 51.7% improvement of CaA titer (244.4±13.8 mg/L) in strain RB33 compared to the control strain RB19 (Fig. 4c). Yeast Rib1 is allosterically inhibited by FAD($H_2$), but the bifunctional bacterial RibBA with guanosine triphosphate (GTP) cyclohydrolase II activity and 3, 4-dihydroxy-2-butanone-4-phosphate synthase activity shows no such inhibition. Furthermore, it has been reported that bifunctional riboflavin kinase/FAD synthase (BiFads) is the last step in bacterial FAD biosynthesis. We thus combinatorically expressed *Bacillus subtilis BsRIBBA* and *Thermotoga maritima TmBiFADS* for construction of a chimeric cytosolic FAD($H_2$) pathway, which improved CaA production by 54% in strain RB32 (248.2±33.0 mg/L). Overexpression of the transporter gene *MCH5* alone increased CaA production by 93% in strain RB26 (311.0±22.3 mg/L). However, overexpression of endogenous mitochondrial *FMN1* and *FAD1* did not display a positive effect on CaA production (strain RB28, RB29, RB30 and RB31), which suggests that Fad1 and Fmn1 are not limiting enzymes in this case. Additionally, combined overexpression of *MCH5* with other strategies did not further improve CaA production (Extended Data Fig. 5), possibly owing to inhibition of FAD($H_2$) biosynthesis or disturbance of cofactor homeostasis due to excess riboflavin uptake.

Next, we explored the applicability of these strategies in the CaA high-producing strain RB197 with enhanced NADPH supply, which theoretically requires more $FADH_2$ (Fig. 4d). Similarly, overexpression of *MCH5* substantially improved CaA biosynthesis by 48% in strain RB203 (492.1±49.2 mg/L) compared to the parental strain RB197. For the strategies that did not display a positive effect in the low CaA production strain RB19, all increased CaA production in this genetic background (RB204, RB205, RB206 and RB207). Strong constitutive promoters ($P_{tHXT7}$ and $P_{TDH3}$) driving expression had slightly higher CaA production than those with GAL promoters (RB204 versus RB206, RB205 versus RB207, Fig. 4d), suggesting that a continuous supply of FAD($H_2$) was beneficial for CaA production in a precursor enhanced strain. In particular, expression of *FLX1* and *RIB1* resulted in highest CaA titer of 518.0±8.4 mg/L in strain RB209, representing a 56% increase compared with strain RB197. It is worthy to mention that cultivation of strain RB209 in YPD (yeast, peptone, dextrose) media resulted much higher CaA production of 1.60±0.02 g/L (Fig. 4e). It further indicates that the supply of cofactors NADPH and FAD is of great value in the synthesis of CaA. Cofactor quantification showed

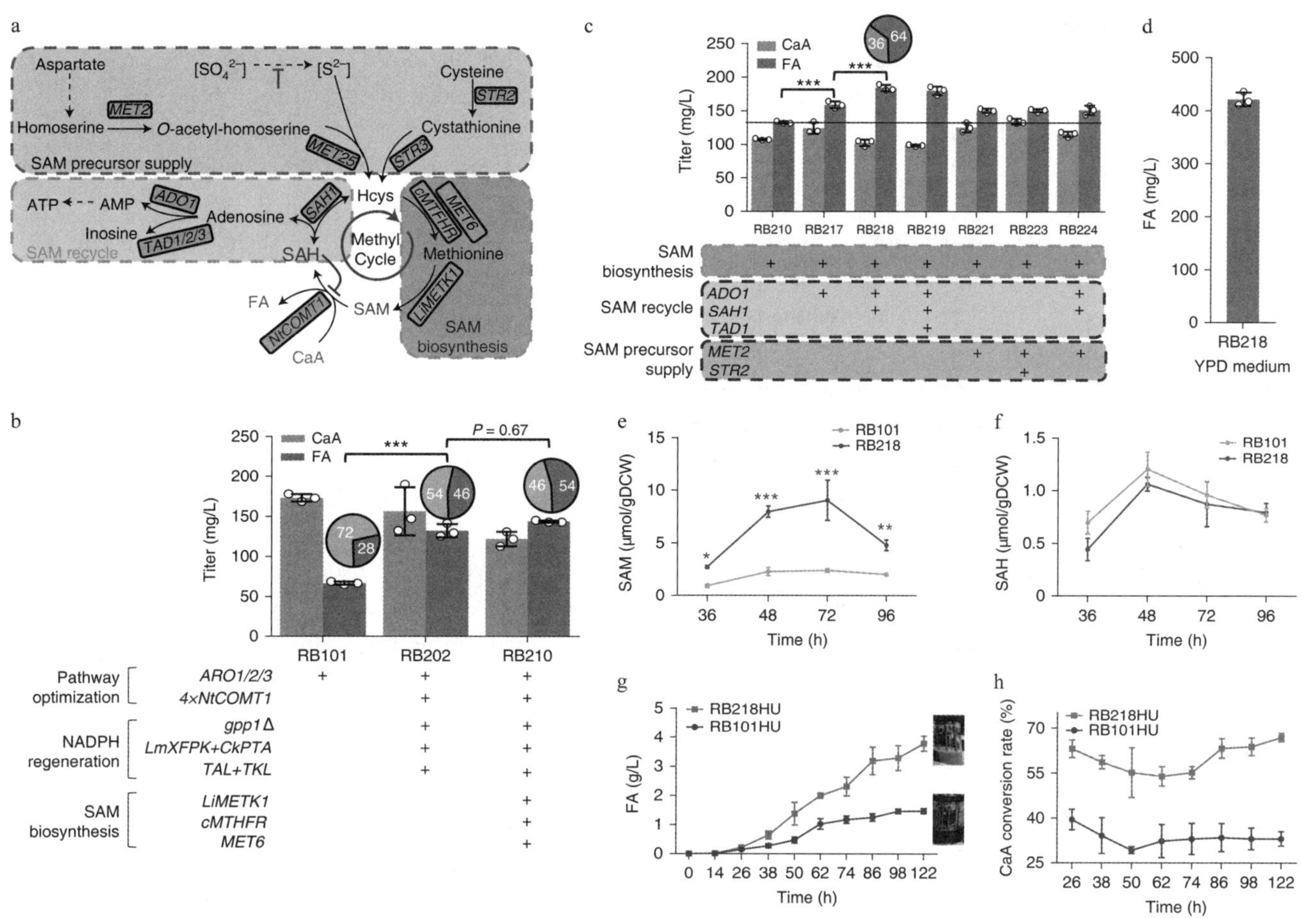


**Fig. 5 Engineering SAM biosynthesis and recycling for FA production**

(a) Schematic illustration of engineering SAM metabolism. The pathways surrounded by different colored rectangles correspond to the engineering strategies in **b** and **c**. Dashed arrows represent multi-step reactions and two-headed arrows represent reversible reactions. The red circular arrow represents the methyl cycle after optimization. *ADO1* encoding adenosine kinase 1, *TAD1* - *3* encoding adenosine deaminase 1 - 3, *SAH1* encoding SAH hydrolase, *MET2* encoding L-homoserine-*O*-acetyltransferase, *STR2* encoding cystathionine gamma-synthase, *MET25* encoding *O*-acetyl homoserine-*O*-acetyl serine sulfhydrylase, *STR3* encoding cystathionine beta-lyase, *LiMETK1* encoding *Leishmania infantum* *S*-adenosylmethionine synthetases, *MET6* encoding methionine synthase, *cMTHFR* encoding chemeric Mthfr. SAM, *S*-adenosylmethionine; 5, 10-$CH_2$-THF, 5,10-methylene tetrahydrogen folic acid; ATP, adenosine triphosphate. (b) Enhancing SAM biosynthesis improved FA titer and CaA conversion under sufficient supply of substrate CaA and *NtCOMT1* overexpression. Pathway optimization, NADPH regeneration and enhancing SAM biosynthesis were combined to improve FA production and CaA conversion. Pie charts show the proportions of CaA and FA. 4 × *NtCOMT1* represents four copies of *NtCOMT1*. Other abbreviations can be found in the Fig. 3 legend. (c) Combined engineering of SAM recycling, biosynthesis, and its precursor supply further improved FA production and CaA conversion. (d) FA production by the best engineered strain RB218 when cultured in YPD medium. (e,f) Cellular SAM (e) and SAH (f) of engineered strain RB218 and control strain RB101. μmol/gDCW refers to the number of moles of cofactor per gram of dry cell weight (DCW). (g) FA production by fed-batch fermentation of prototrophic strains RB101HU and RB218HU under glucose-limited conditions. (h) CaA conversion rates during the fed-batch fermentation. The glucose feeding was started at 12 h. All data represent the mean of $n=3$ independent biological samples and error bars show standard deviation. Statistical analysis was carried out by using Student's $t$-test (one-tailed; two-sample unequal variance; * $P<0.05$, ** $P<0.01$, *** $P<0.001$).

that cellular FAD($H_2$) was significantly higher in both strain RB209 and RB203, compared to reference strain RB197 (Fig. 4f). The cellular FMN($H_2$) and riboflavin were also enhanced in strain RB209 (Extended Data Fig. 6), suggesting that our cofactor engineering strategies successfully enhanced cellular FAD($H_2$) level and further improved CaA production. Accumulation of the intermediates of CaA biosynthesis such as shikimate, phenylalanine and tyrosine was lower in stain RB209 compared with RB103 (Supplementary Fig. 3), suggesting that the FAD($H_2$) engineering successfully drove the metabolic flux toward CaA biosynthesis.

To simplify the composition and reduce the cost of medium, we constructed the prototrophic strains RB103HU and RB209HU (in situ integration of the *HIS3* and *URA3* genes in the corresponding auxotrophic strains RB103 and RB209) for fed-batch fermentation. Strain RB209HU had the highest CaA titer of 5.5 ± 0.2 g/L at 98 h, which was 31% higher than that of strain RB103HU (4.2 ± 0.5 g/L)

(Fig. 4g). To our knowledge, this is the highest CaA titer reported in yeast using minimal medium. MFA analysis showed metabolic flux was redirected to cofactor regeneration (NADPH and $FADH_2$) in strain RB209HU compared with control strain RB103HU (Extended Data Fig. 7), which was supposed to be sufficient to support the 35% increase in carbon flux toward CaA synthesis. These data indicate that enhancing cofactor supply may play an important role in driving natural product biosynthesis when the metabolic flux is elevated.

SAM engineering to increase FA production. SAM serves as the methyl donor in many methyl transfer reactions and enhancing SAM supply may improve FA production in the case of excess accumulation of precursor CaA. Although metabolic engineering for SAM production has been extensively explored, there are few reports on engineering SAM supply for promoting the synthesis of natural products due to the complexity of SAM metabolism. Enhancing the expression of the rate-liming enzyme methionine adenosyltransferase (Mat) is considered to be the primary strategy for increasing SAM supply. Additionally, relieving feedback inhibition of the NADPH-dependent methylenetetrahydrofolate reductase (Mthfr) by SAM may also elevate SAM levels by increasing the supply of the methyl donor 5-methyl-tetrahydrofolate ($CH_3$ - THF) in methionine biosynthesis. Finally, methionine feeding might drive SAM biosynthesis as *S. cerevisiae* is capable of methionine uptake (Fig. 5a). Unfortunately, all strategies mentioned above were not successful in increasing FA titer in strain RB79 (Extended Data Fig. 8a, b), although they have been previously shown to increase SAM levels.

We speculated that the rate-limiting steps in FA synthesis under the current condition in the strain RB79 may not be the SAM supply, but the insufficient supply of substrate CaA or *NtCOMT1* expression. The results supported our hypothesis that enhancing the supply of substrate CaA may result in higher FA yields in RB101 and RB119, although this is very limited (Extended Data Fig. 8c). We further investigated the enhancement of *NtCOMT1* expression by expressing 2 - 4 copies under of the control of $P_{GAL}$ or strong constitutive promoters, and found that four copies under the control of $P_{GAL}$ improved the CaA conversion rate by 150%, increased from 20% of RB119 to 50% of RB187 (CaA conversion rate = (CaA mol/(CaA+FA) mol) × 100%, Extended Data Fig. 8d). Finally, expression of the four *NtCOMT1* copies together with the NADPH regeneration strategy resulted in an FA titer of 132.1 ± 8.2 mg/L (RB202), representing a 98% increase compared with strain RB101. These results validated our hypothesis that before regulating SAM biosynthesis, insufficient supply of substrate CaA and low expression of *NtCOMT1* are rate-limiting steps of FA synthesis.

The low CaA conversion rate (46%) in strain RB202 suggested that the SAM supply might become the rate-limiting step under the relatively high levels of CaA synthesis. As expected, enhancing SAM biosynthesis by expressing *LiMETK1*, *cMTHFR* (chimeric *MTHFR*) and *MET6* in strain RB202 led to an FA production of 143.7 ± 1.3 mg/L in strain RB210, a slight enhancement (9%) compared with strain RB202 (Fig. 5b). Notably, the conversion of CaA increased from 46 to 54%, although it was still low. These results indicate that increasing the SAM level alone is not sufficient to improve CaA conversion.

It has been reported that *S*-adenosy-L-homocysteine (SAH), a by-product of transmethylation, is a potent inhibitor of Omt activity. Thus, enhancing SAH degradation might relieve the inhibition of *Nt*Comt1 and improve FA biosynthesis (Fig. 5a). In yeast, SAH hydrolase (Sah1) is the only enzyme capable of SAH degradation by producing homocysteine (Hcys) and adenosine. However, the thermodynamic equilibrium of Sah1 favors the direction of SAH synthesis in vivo. Therefore, continuous consumption of adenosine and Hcys might pull SAH hydrolysis in vivo. Adenosine kinase (Ado1) and adenosine deaminase (Tad1 - 3) are potential enzymes for increasing the consumption of adenosine, and this strategy may help to push Hcys back into the methyl cycle. As expected, a designed SAH consuming pathway that contains the two genes, *ADO1* and *SAH1*, lead to a 39% increase in FA production (184.2 ± 4.6 mg/L) with a 64% conversion of CaA in RB218 (Fig. 5c). Further expression of *TAD1* in strain RB219 did not have a notable effect on FA production, which suggested that introducing *SAH1* together with *ADO1* is sufficient to consume adenosine and redirect flux to Hcys. We also tried a heterologous autoinducers pathway for SAH consumption by expressing *E. coli EcMTNN* (NP_414701.1) encoding a 5′-methylthioadenosine/*S*-adenosylhomocysteine (SAH) nucleosidase and *EcLUXS* (NP_417172.1) encoding a *S*-ribosylhomocysteine lyase. *Ec*MtnN is able to convert SAH to *S*-ribosyl-L-homocysteine, which further leads to the autoinducer-2 biosynthesis by *Ec*LuxS, which could, theoretically, consume SAH (Supplementary Fig. 4a). However, this strategy did not promote FA synthesis, but instead increased CaA production by 84% (strain RB213) compared with strain RB210 (Supplementary Fig. 4b). To further enhance the supply of Hcys, the cysteine and aspartate pathways were engineered to improve the entrance flux into the methyl circle. Overexpression of the rate-limiting genes *MET2* and *TYR2* (strains RB221 and RB223) moderately improved FA production by 13 and 14%, respectively. However, these strategies did not result in a further increase of FA biosynthesis when combined with the SAM recycle strategy (RB224, Fig. 5c). Taken together, SAM engineering (184.2 ± 4.6 mg/L in strain RB218) dramatically improved FA production by 180% compared with the initial strain RB101, and CaA conversion was also enhanced from 28 to 64%. Strain RB218 was also tested in YPD medium and produced a higher FA titer of 421.8±12.9 mg $l^{-1}$ (Fig. 5d and Table 1). Cofactor analysis showed that SAM engineered strain RB218 had much higher SAM level and lower SAH accumulation compared with control strain RB101 (Fig. 5e, f and Extended Data Fig. 9). Metabolite analysis showed that strain RB218 had much lower accumulation of intermediates of FA biosynthesis pathway (Supplementary Fig. 5), which again suggested that SAM engineering drove the metabolic flux toward FA biosynthesis.

To evaluate the production potential, the cofactor-engineered FA producing strains were also cultivated in fed-batch fermentation under a glucose-limited feeding strategy. The best prototrophic strain RB218HU (in situ integration of the *HIS3* and *URA3* gene in the corresponding auxotrophic strain RB218) produced 3.8±0.3 g/L of FA, representing a 150% improvement over the reference strain RB101HU (1.5 ± 0.1 g/L), and the highest titer reported in the literature so far (Fig. 5g). The accumulation of FA in the culture medium resulted in a change in the color of the medium from dark brown (CaA) to yellow (FA). The final glucose consumption of 97.0±1.7 g at 122 h and the highest optical density ($OD_{600}$) of 67.3±5.9 at 74 h were detected with the strain RB218HU (Supplementary Fig. 6). The CaA conversion rate of the strain RB218HU was elevated to 67%, a 103% improvement over the strain RB101HU (33%) (Fig. 5g). Furthermore, MFA study showed that higher metabolic flux was directed to methyl cycle in strain RB218HU compared with RB101HU, which improved the rate-limiting step of FA synthesis (Extended Data Fig. 10). These results indicate that SAM engineering offers a more substantial effect on FA production and application potential in the fed-batch fermentation compared with shake-flask cultivations (Fig. 5c).

## 2 DISCUSSION

Enhanced metabolic flux toward overproduction in yeast cell factory might perturb cofactor equilibrium since many enzymes consume considerable amounts of cofactor to ensure their activity. Exogenous addition of cofactors may limit large-scale industrial applications due to their instability and high cost. Furthermore, cells are unable to directly uptake some cofactors from the medium due to permeability issues. More importantly, the state of equilibrium of many cofactors is dynamic and tightly regulated in the cell, and cannot be easily modulated through metabolic enhancement. Thus, proper cofactor engineering should be helpful for maintaining the high enzyme activity required for efficient natural product biosynthesis in yeast.

Current cofactor engineering focuses primarily on the regulation of the redox pairs $NAD^+$/NADH and $NADP^+$/NADPH. However, more than 20 known cofactors play essential roles in numerous intracellular metabolic processes and reactions in various ways. Different cofactors have distinct characteristics and require specific strategies for improving their bio-catalysis efficiency. In this work, we successfully demonstrated the important roles of three of the most common cofactors (NADPH, $FADH_2$ and SAM) in bio-production and developed tailor-made cofactor engineering strategies for improving the production of phenolic acids in *S. cerevisiae* (Table 1).

**Table 1 Phenolic acid production in yeast and *E. coli***

| Products | Host | Cultivation condition[a] | Titers (g/L) | Yield[b] (mg/g glucose) | Ref. |
|---|---|---|---|---|---|
| CaA | *S. cerevisiae* | Shake flask, MYPD | 0.01 | 0.3[b] | 52 |
| | *S. cerevisiae* | Shake flask, YPD | 0.03 | 1.4[b] | 15 |
| | *S. cerevisiae* | Shake flask, YPD | 0.57 | 28.5[b] | 53 |
| | *E. coli* | Shake flask, MM, 20 mg $l^{-1}$ phenylalanine | 0.05 | ND[c] | 54 |
| | *E. coli* | Shake flask, MM, 20 mg $l^{-1}$ phenylalanine | 0.79 | ND[c] | 55 |
| | *S. cerevisiae* | Shake flask, MM | 0.52 | 26.0 | This study |
| | *S. cerevisiae* | Shake flask, YPD | 1.60 | 80.0[b] | This study |
| | *S. cerevisiae* | Fed-batch, MM, glucose feeding | 5.52 | 31.8 | This study |
| FA | *S. cerevisiae* | Shake flask, YPD | 0.04 | 2.0[b] | 15 |
| | *S. cerevisiae* | Shake flask, MM | 0.18 | 9.0 | This study |
| | *S. cerevisiae* | Shake flask, YPD | 0.42 | 21.0[b] | This study |
| | *S. cerevisiae* | Fed-batch, MM, glucose feeding | 3.8 | 17.1 | This study |

[a] MM, minimal media; YPD, complex medium containing 20 g/L peptone, 10 g/L yeast extract and 20 g/L glucose; MYPD, YPD medium containing 40 g/L glucose [b] These data, only used for comparing the biosynthesis efficiency under the same condition, cannot reflect the real yield from glucose since YPD containing yeast extract and peptone, which can be used for product synthesis. [c] ND, not detected.

NADPH regeneration is beneficial for CaA biosynthesis from the NADPH-dependent Cyp pathway. Previous studies mainly enhanced the oxidative steps of PPP by overexpressing corresponding genes, such as *ZWF1* and *GND1* (ref.). However, it has been reported that metabolic flux through Zwf1 and Gnd1 is already more than 50%–80% under glucose-limiting conditions (production phase in this study). As such, we enhanced the nonoxidative steps of the PPP pathway for pulling metabolic flux toward PPP for NADPH regeneration, which significantly improved CaA production by 35% ($385.3 \pm 36.52$ mg/L in RB197 comparing to $286.3 \pm 7.1$ mg/L in RB103). These results indicate that NADPH engineering strategies can vary with culture conditions.

Heterologous expression of enzymes derived from other species in yeast will likely suffer from insufficient or deficient cofactor supply, due to the different cellular environment between yeast and the natural host. In eukaryotic organisms, cellular metabolism and their corresponding cofactors are often compartmentalized in different suborganelles. We observed that the bacterial phenolic hydroxylase pair HpaB/HpaC had an insufficient supply of cofactor $FADH_2$ for CaA biosynthesis in the yeast cytosol. FAD($H_2$) serves as electron transmitter between NADH and the HpaB/HpaC pathway in CaA biosynthesis. This might be explained by previous observations that cytosolic NAD(H) levels are more than 20-fold higher than FAD($H_2$) in *S. cerevisiae*. Compared with NADPH, regulation of the FAD($H_2$) supply is more complex since the FAD($H_2$) biosynthetic pathways are distributed in different cellular compartments (cytosol and mitochondrion) and are also tightly correlated with the respiratory chain. Our results demonstrated that engineering FAD($H_2$) biosynthesis and mitochondrial exportation were beneficial for CaA biosynthesis, suggesting that more attention should be paid to cofactor compartmentalization, in addition to the metabolic pathways, for improving the performance of cell biocatalysts. Recycling extracellular riboflavin for FAD($H_2$) biosynthesis was a key process for increasing CaA production in a CaA low-producing strain, while exporting mitochondrial FAD($H_2$) to the cytosol drove the most CaA production in a CaA high-producing strain. These data indicate that FAD($H_2$) levels should be carefully regulated for coupling the capacity of CaA biosynthesis, which can avoid the perturbation of $FADH_2$/FAD homeostasis. It is worthy to mention that the CaA production of our best strain RB209 was 181% higher than that of previously engineered yeast strain (Fig. 4e and Table 1). Even with the relatively low efficient Cyp complex pathway (Fig. 2b), cofactor engineering substantially improved CaA production, which further demonstrated that enhanced the supply of cofactor NADPH and $FADH_2$ was beneficial for biosynthesis of CaA. It should be noted that sustained small increases of cofactor level resulted in much higher improvements of product biosynthesis (Fig. 4f and Extended Data Fig. 6).

Although improving SAM supply increased catalytic efficiency of the SAM-dependent Omt in *E. coli*, it did not improve FA production in our engineered yeast strain harboring the *NtCOMT1* gene (Extended Data Fig. 8). In yeast, the synthesis of SAM and sulfur-containing amino acids is strictly regulated by the Cbf1-Met4-Met28 complex, which is repressed by the addition of methionine or SAM. Alternatively, we accelerated the methyl cycle by redirecting the reversible reaction catalyzed by Sah1 and removing the inhibition of SAH, which substantially improved CaA conversion and FA production. On SAM recycling, elevating SAM levels further improved FA production as the accelerated methyl cycle could consume SAH rapidly and alleviate SAH/SAM-mediated repression (Fig. 5c). The increased SAM/SAH ratio (Extended Data Fig. 9) further confirmed that reducing the accumulation level of SAH was much more helpful in strengthening the SAM-mediated methylation in yeast.

Due to the complicated regulation, enhancing the cofactor biosynthesis and supply not always help to improve the product biosynthesis. Just like in this study, blindly enhancing the biosynthesis of SAM and FAD failed to improve the production of phenolic acids. Alternatively, FAD relocation and SAM recycling were much more helpful for biosynthesis of CaA and FA, respectively. Different cofactors have their unique characteristics of feedback regulation, organelle localization and rate-limiting steps, thus, it should carefully design the cofactor engineering strategies to cope with the cellular metabolic state.

In summary, we have demonstrated the important role of the cofactors NADPH, $FADH_2$ and SAM in natural product biosynthesis and developed tailored cofactor engineering strategies, which enabled the highest production of FA and CaA in the yeast cell factory (Table 1). The engineered strains can be used as a chassis cell for the biosynthesis of aromatic-derived pharmaceuticals, such as clemastanin B and nutraceutical vanillin. Cofactor engineering, in addition to pathway engineering, presents a promising strategy for improving the biosynthesis of complex molecules.

## 3 METHODS

Yeast strains and reagents. *S. cerevisiae* strain CEN. PK113-11C* (*MATa*, *SUC2*, *MAL2-8c*, *his3Δ*, *ura3Δ*, *gal80Δ*, *XI5*::($P_{TEF}$-*CAS9*-$T_{CYC1}$) derived from CEN. PK113-11C (*MATa*, *SUC2*, *MAL2-8c*, *his3Δ1*, *ura3Δ-52*) was used as the background strain for all genetic manipulations and strain construction. The constructed strains are listed in the Supplementary Table 1. The engineering strategy and the flowcharts of yeast strain construction are shown in Extended

Data Fig. 2 and Supplementary Fig. 1. PrimeStar DNA polymerase was purchased from TAKARA Bio-tek and was used for gene amplification using designed primers (Supplementary Data 1). DNA gel purification and plasmid extraction kits were purchased from Omega Bio-tek. All chemical standards were purchased from Sigma-Aldrich unless stated otherwise.

Genetic engineering. All gene overexpression cassettes, consisting of a promoter, a target gene, a terminator and a block of the next cassette for homologous recombination, were constructed by overlapping extension PCR (Supplementary Data 2). The expression vectors of all codon-optimized enzyme were synthesized by Sangon Bio-tek (Supplementary Data 3). Other native promoters, genes and terminators were cloned from genomic DNA of *E. coli* DH5α and *S. cerevisiae* CEN.PK113-11C.

All overexpression cassettes were integrated into their designated chromosomal loci to provide a stable and high-level expression of heterologous genes (Supplementary Data 4). The gel purified overexpression cassettes and a guide RNA (gRNA) plasmid were cotransformed into the CEN.PK113-11C* for cassette knock-in by the CRISPR-Cas9 method as previously reported. The CRISPR-Cas9 web tool CHOPCHOP was used to select two specific gRNAs for each selected genomic locus (Supplementary Data 4). Taking the example of the targeted integration of ($T_{PRM9}$ > *PtrC4H2*-$Sc^{OPT1}$ < $P_{GAL10/1}$ > *PtrC4H1*-$Sc^{OPT1}$ < $T_{PYK}$) + ($P_{GAL7}$ > *PtrC3H3*-$Sc^{OPT1}$ < $T_{DIT1}$) at *XII4* locus in strain RB14, the whole pathway was divided into two fragments: (1) XII4up-$T_{PRM9}$-(*PtrC4H2*-$Sc^{OPT1}$)-$P_{GAL10/1}$-(*PtrC4H1*-$Sc^{OPT1}$)-$T_{PYK}$ and (2) $T_{PYK}$-$P_{GAL7}$-(*PtrC3H3*-$Sc^{OPT1}$)-$T_{DIT1}$-XII4dw. In detail, the upstream locus arm XII4up with 30-40 bp of next block as a homologous arm was amplified from genomic DNA and defined as XII4up < $T_{PRM9}$. Similarly, all arm-containing blocks $T_{PRM9}$, $T_{PRM9}$ > *PtrC4H2*-$Sc^{OPT1}$ < $P_{GAL10/1}$, $P_{GAL10/1}$, $P_{GAL10/1}$ > *PtrC4H1*-$Sc^{OPT1}$ < $T_{PYK}$ and $T_{PYK}$ were amplified and used for the assembly of fragment I through overlapping extension PCR. Fragment II was assembled using the same methods. Then, cotransformation of equimolar amounts of purified fragments I and II (50-100 ng per kb) with the gRNA plasmid into *S. cerevisiae* was conducted according to the described protocol and transformants were selected on plates containing solid synthetic medium (SD) added with 0.02 g/L histidine (SD + histidine). Clones were verified by colony PCR and sequencing. Subsequently, verified clones were cultivated overnight in SD + histidine liquid medium and then plated on solid medium containing SD + histidine + uracil + FOA (1 g/L, 5-fluoroorotic acid) to loop out the gRNA vectors and recycle the *URA3* marker. For gene deletion, 500 ng of a fusion consisting of roughly 500 bp sequences homologous to upstream and downstream regions of the chromosomal target site was used for the homologous repair of the genome break introduced by cleavage of the Cas9 nuclease.

Strain cultivation. Yeast cells were normally cultivated in YPD media containing 20 g/L glucose, 20 g/L peptone and 10 g/L yeast extract. Strains containing *URA3*- and/or *HIS3*-based plasmids/cassettes were selected on SD media (6.7 g/L yeast nitrogen base without amino acids and 20 g/L glucose) without uracil or L-histidine, respectively. The *URA3* maker plasmid was removed on SD + uracil (0.02 g/L) + FOA plates.

Shake flask batch fermentations for production of phenolic acids were performed in 20 mL of minimal medium (Delft-D) containing 2.5 g/L $(NH_4)_2SO_4$, 14.4 g/L $KH_2PO_4$, 0.5 g/L $MgSO_4 \cdot 7H_2O$, 20 g/L glucose, 2 mL of trace metal and 1 mL of vitamin solutions (Delft-D medium) supplemented with 40 mg/L histidine and/or 60 mg/L uracil if needed. Cultures were inoculated at an initial $OD_{600}$ of 0.1 in 50 mL flasks and cultivated at 200 r/min, 30 ℃ for 96 h.

The *HIS3* and *URA3* genes were reinserted into their original genomic locations to construct prototrophic strains for fed-batch fermentations. Bioreactor cultivations for phenolic acid production were performed in 1.2 L vessels using the DasGip Parallel Bioreactors System (Eppendorf). The initial fermentation was started in 0.25 L of Delft-D medium. The fed-batch fermentations used in this study were performed as previously described.

Metabolite extraction and quantification. Syringic acid was predissolved in ethyl acetate (0.2 g/L) as an internal standard. Then, 1 mL of culture broth from shake-flask batch fermentation was vortexed thoroughly with 1 mL of syringic acid solution twice. The extractions were merged, dried and resuspended in 0.5 mL of methanol. Before analysis, the extract solution was filtered through a 0.2 μm organic membrane. Extraction of the fed-batch fermentation samples was performed as previously described. All extracted samples were quantified by high-performance liquid chromatography (HPLC). Briefly, 1 mL of sample was analyzed on a LC-2030 HPLC (Shimadzu) equipped with a Poroshell 120 EC-C18 column (2.7 μm, 3 × 100 mm) (Agilent) connected to a photodiode array detector. Samples were analyzed by a gradient method with two solvents: 0.05% formic acid (A) and acetonitrile with 0.05% formic acid (B). The key analysis parameters are listed in Supplementary Table 2 and a representative chromatograph of the standards is shown in Supplementary Fig. 7. LabSolutions LC Workstation v.5 was used for liquid chromatography data analysis.

The method of extracting and analyzing FAD($H_2$), FMN($H_2$) and riboflavin was designed and performed according to the procedure described in reference (Supplementary

Table 3). Cellular NADPH/$NADP^+$ were quantified using the CheKine $NADP^+$/NADPH assay kit (catalog no. WST-8; Abbkine). Cells from 36 h cultures were centrifuged and resuspended in cold PBS buffer to an $OD_{600}$ of 10. Samples were individually extracted with the NADPH or $NADP^+$ extraction buffers and all subsequent steps were performed according to the manufacturer's instructions. The intracellular amount of SAM and SAH was determined by HPLC-tandem mass spectrometry (Agilent) in positive ion mode using a Poroshell 120 EC - C18 column (2.7 μm, 3 × 100 mm, Agilent) at 0.2 mL/min and 30 ℃ as previously described. Water containing 0.05% trifluoroacetic acid and 3% methanol was used as the mobile phase.

After being centrifuged (3, 000g, 4 ℃, 3 min), collected cells were broken and extracted by ultrasound in methanol-chloroform (50%, *V*/*V*) solution. The upper extract was dried and redissolved in 50% acetonitrile. An Agilent 1290 Infinity II UHPLC system coupled to a 6470A Triple Quadrupole mass spectrometer and a ThermoFisher Q Exactive Hybrid Quadrupole-Orbitrap Mass Spectrometer in heated electrospray ionization negative mode were together used for analysis of different intermediates. Method details are listed in Supplementary Table 4.

MFA. The latest genome-scale metabolic model of *S. cerevisiae* Yeast8 (ref.) was extended by adding heterologous pathways, which was subsequently used to generate strain-specific models for various strains (RB103HU, RB209HU, RB101HU and RB218HU) by blocking corresponding reactions. To simulate flux distributions, flux balance analysis was carried out using various strain-specific models constrained by experimentally measured glucose uptake, ethanol production, CaA and FA production rates with the objective function of growth maximization (Supplementary Table 5). Model construction and simulations were performed in MATLAB with the COBRA toolbox (Supplementary Data 5, 6 and 7).

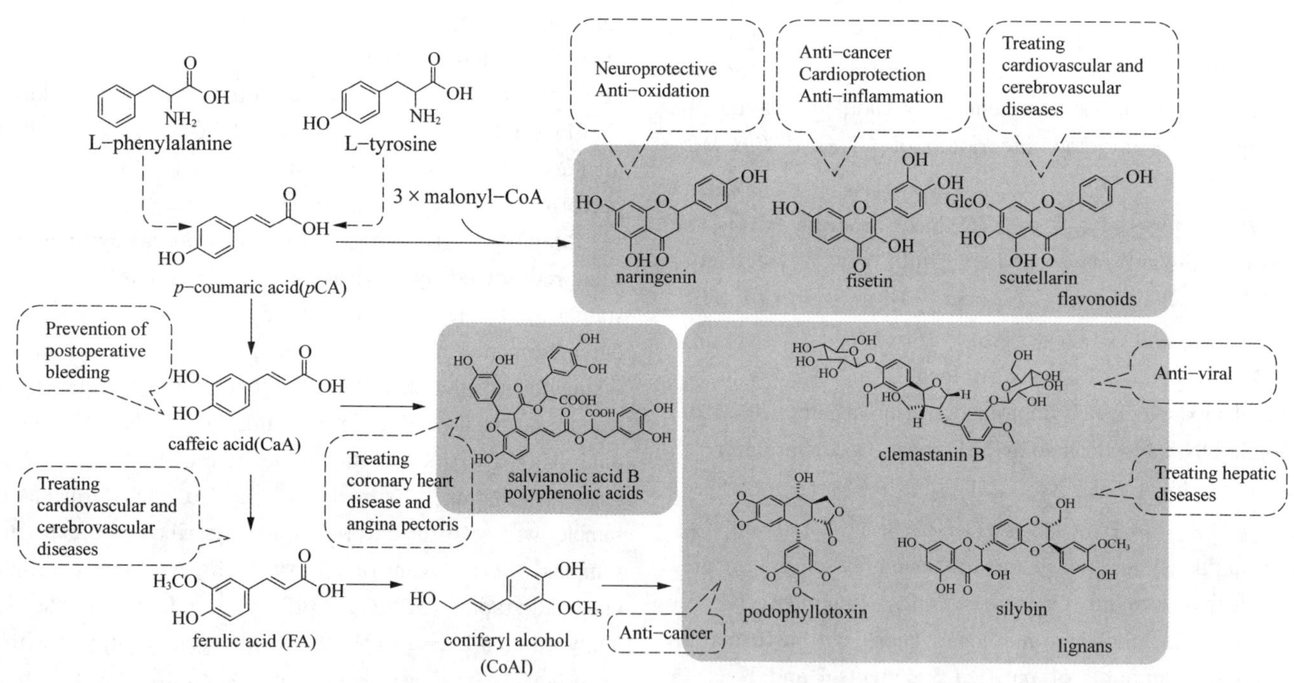


**Extended Data Fig. 1 Biosynthesis of phenolic acids and their derivatives**

Structures of *p*CA-(green), CaA-(orange) and FA-derived (pink) natural products, and their pharmaceutical properties.

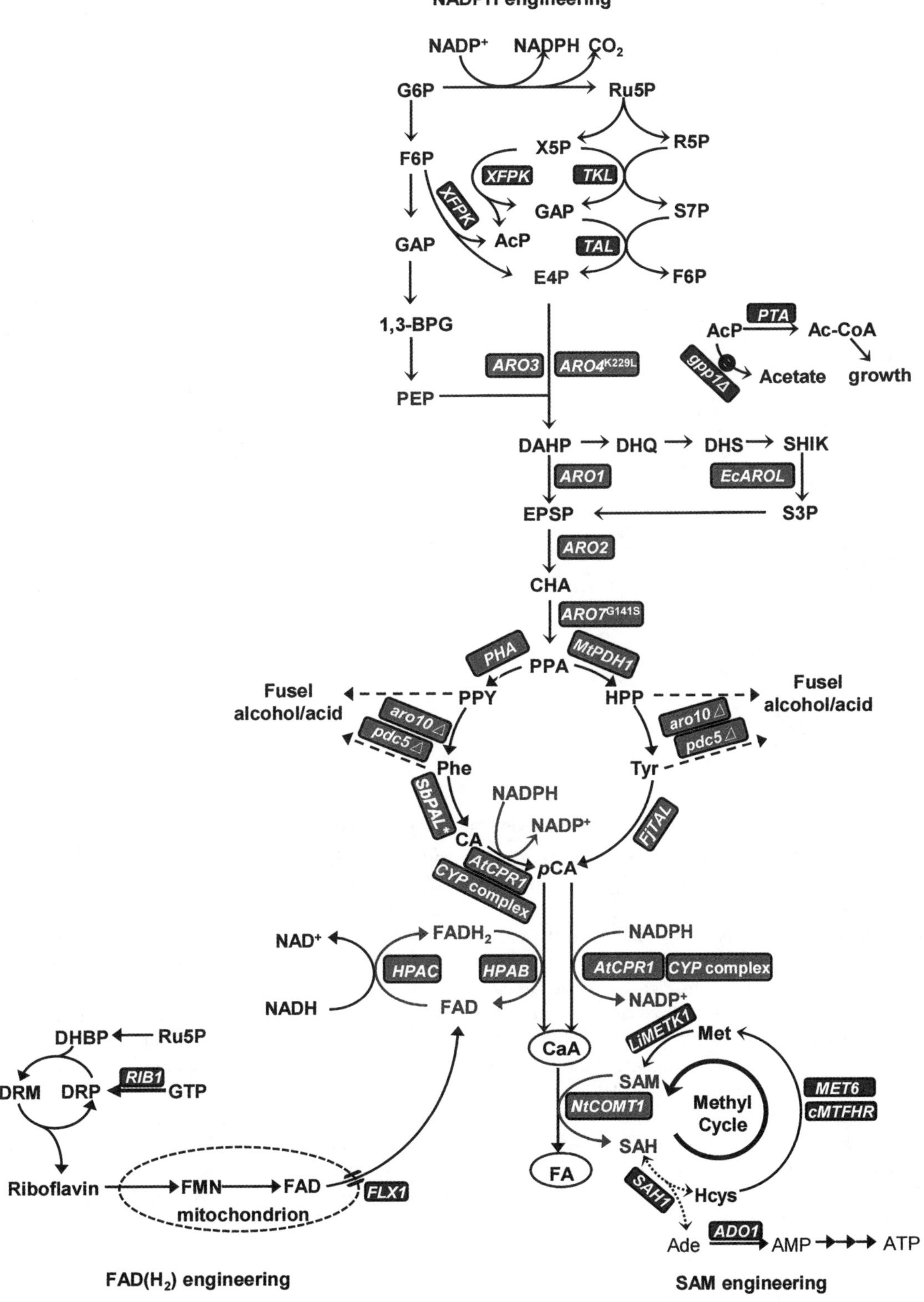


**Extended Data Fig. 2 Engineering strategies for improving the production of CaA and FA**

The engineered gene targets for pathway optimization were marked as golden and the cofactor engineering was marked as blue. See Fig. 2 and Fig. 3 legends regarding abbreviations of other metabolites.

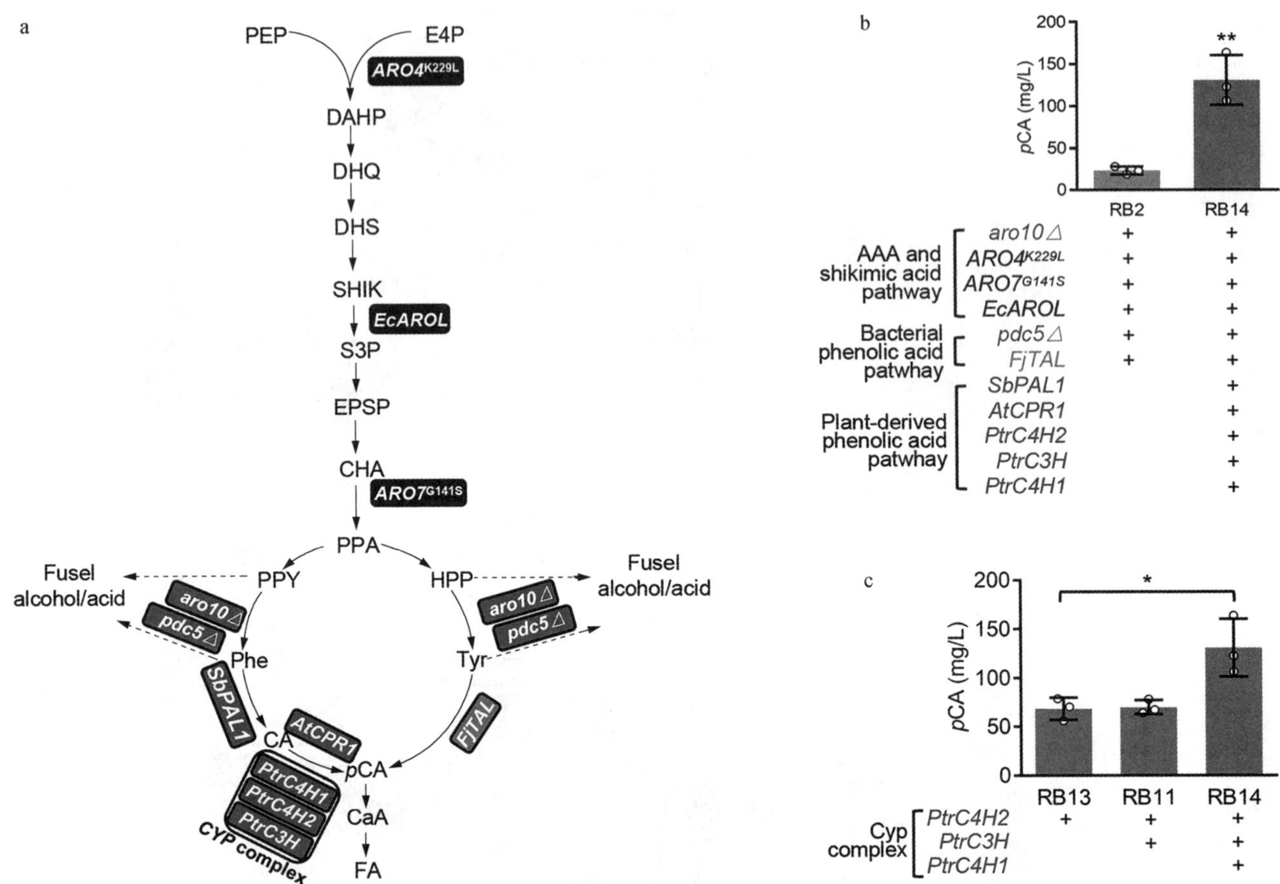


**Extended Data Fig. 3 Engineering the biosynthesis of precursor *p*CA in yeast**

(a) Overview of the engineered metabolic pathway for *p*CA biosynthesis. Optimization of the shikimic acid and aromatic amino acid (AAA) pathways together with the introduction of bacteria- and plant-derived phenolic acid pathways were used for *p*CA production. *ARO10* encoding phenylpyruvate decarboxylase, *PDC5* encoding pyruvate decarboxylase, *ARO4* encoding 3-deoxy-D-arabino-heptulosonate-7-phosphate (DAHP) synthase, *ARO7* encoding chorismate mutase, *EcAROL* encoding *E. coli* shikimate kinase II, *FjTAL* encoding *Flavobacterium johnsoniae* tyrosine ammonia lyase, *SbPAL1* encoding *Isatis indigotica* phenylalanine ammonia lyase 1, *AtCPR1* encoding *Arabidopsis thaliana* cytochrome P450 reductase, *PtrC4H1/2* encoding *Populus trichocarpa* cinnamic acid hydroxylase 1/2, *PtrC3H* encoding *P. trichocarpa* coumarate-3-hydroxylase, *CYP* complex consisting of *PtrC4H1* + *PtrC4H2* + *PtrC3H*. PEP, phosphoenolpyruvate; DHQ, 3-dehydroquinate; DHS, 3-dehydro-shikimate; SHIK, shikimate; S3P, shikimate-3-phosphate; EPSP, 5-enolpyruvyl-shikimate-3-phosphate; CHA, chorismic acid; PPA, prephenate; PPY, phenylpyruvate; HPP, para-hydroxy-phenylpyruvate; Phe, phenylalanine; Tyr, tyrosine; CA, cinnamic acid; *p*CA, coumaric acid; CaA, caffeic acid; FA, ferulic acid. (b) Production of *p*CA in yeast. (c) Introduction of the *CYP* complex further improved *p*CA biosynthesis. All data represent the mean of n = 3 independent biological samples and error bars show standard deviation. All data represent the mean of n = 3 independent biological samples and error bars show standard deviation. Statistical analysis was performed by using Student's *t* test (one-tailed; two-sample unequal variance; * $P<0.05$, ** $P<0.01$, *** $P<0.001$).

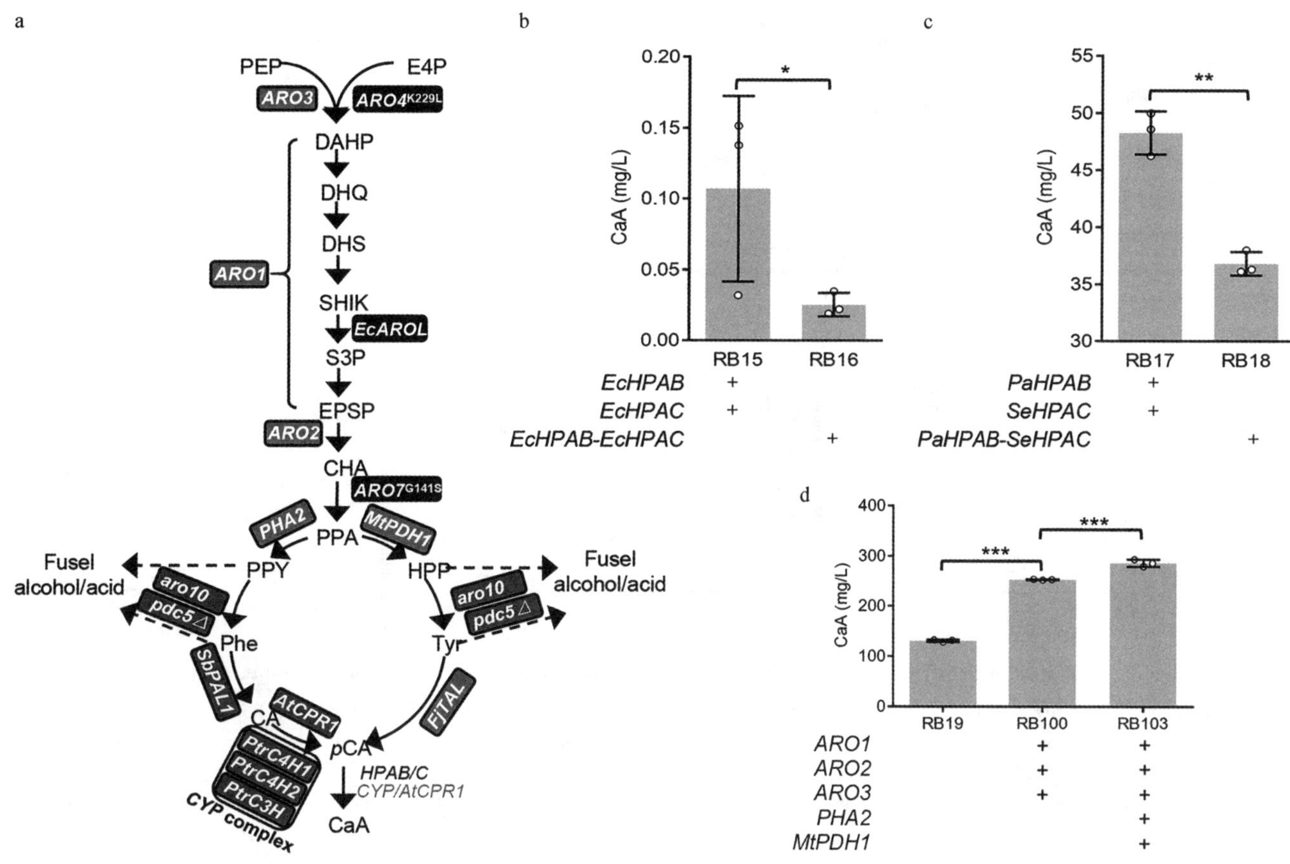


**Extended Data Fig. 4 Optimization of HPAB/C and the shikimic acid pathway for CaA production**

(a) Overview of the yeast metabolic pathway for CaA biosynthesis. *ARO1* encoding shikimate dehydrogenase, *ARO2* encoding chorismate synthase, *ARO3* encoding DAHP synthase, *MtPDH1* encoding *Medicago truncatula* prephenate dehydrogenase, *PHA2* encoding *S. cerevisiae* prephenate dehydratase 2. See Supplementary Fig. 5 legend regarding other abbreviations. The fusion *EcHPAB-EcHPAC* (**b**) and *PaHPAB-SeHPAC* (**c**) result in a negative effect on CaA production. *PaHPAB*, encoding *Pseudomonas aeruginosa* HpaB; *SeHPAC*, encoding *Salmonella enterica* HpaC; *EcHPAB*: encoding *E. coli* HpaB; *EcHPAC*: encoding *E. coli* HpaC. (d) Further optimization of the shikimic acid pathway increased CaA titers with the CYP system. Cells were grown in defined minimal medium containing 20 g/L glucose and cultures were extracted after 96 h of growth for phenolic acid detection. All data represent the mean of n = 3 independent biological samples and error bars show standard deviation. All data represent the mean of n = 3 independent biological samples and error bars show standard deviation. Statistical analysis was performed by using Student's *t* test (one-tailed; two-sample unequal variance; * $P<0.05$, ** $P<0.01$, *** $P<0.001$).

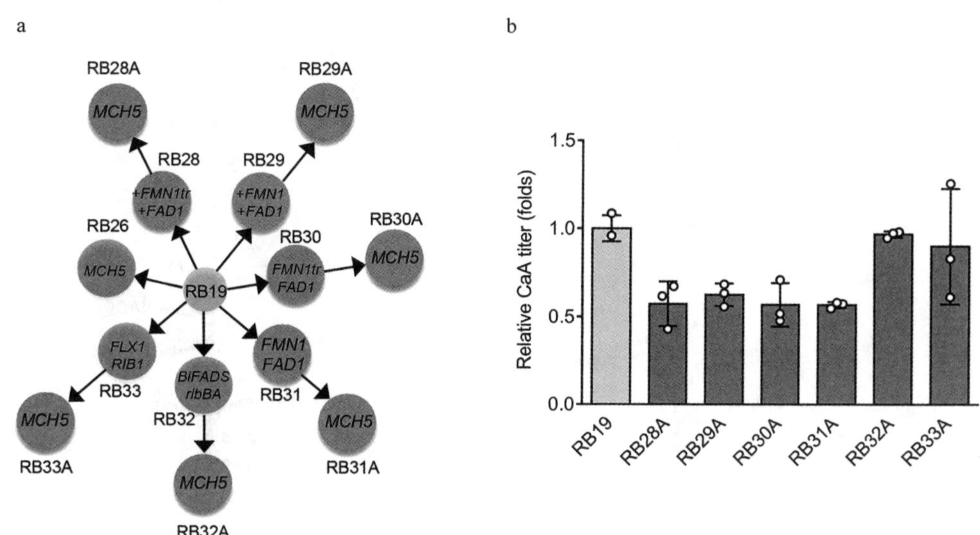


**Extended Data Fig. 5 Effect of combining *MCH5* overexpression with $FADH_2$ strategies on CaA production**

(a) Schematic illustration of the combinations of $FADH_2$ strategies. See Fig. 4 legend regarding abbreviations. (+) indicates expression under strong constitutive promoters. Strain RB19 is the reference strain for regulating $FADH_2$. (b) Relative titers of engineered strains normalized to the titers of reference strain RB19. All data represent the mean of n = 3 independent biological samples and error bars show standard deviation.

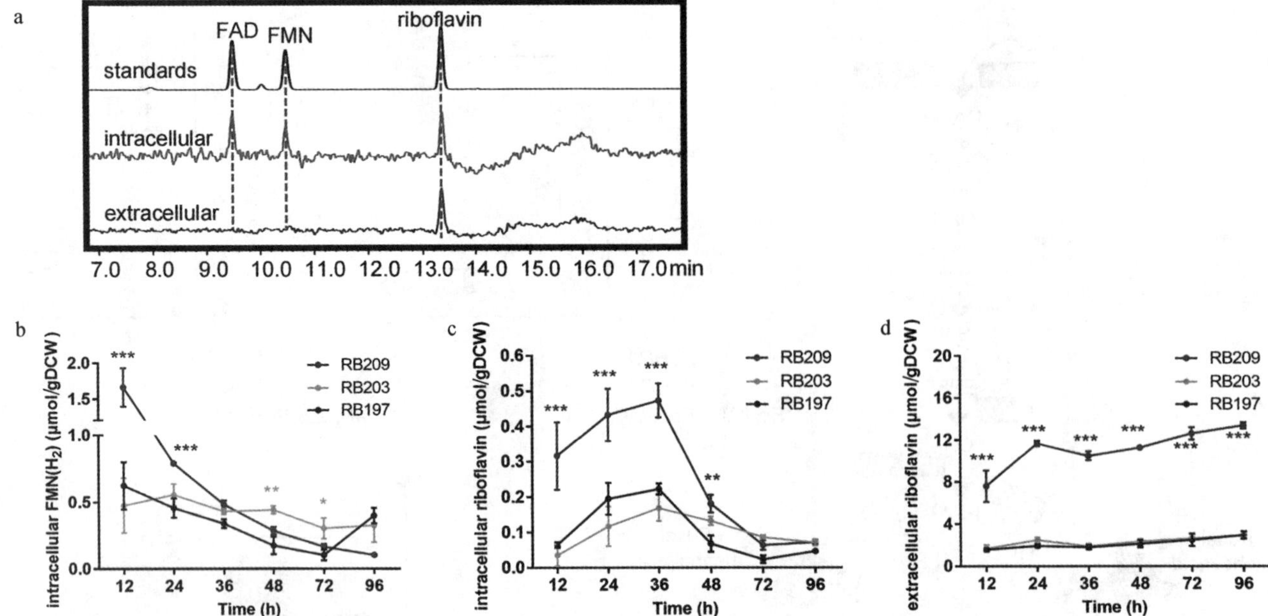


**Extended Data Fig. 6 Quantification of flavin derived cofactors in CaA producing strains.**

(a) Representative chromatographs of standards and samples. Total concentration of intracellular FMN($H_2$) (**b**) intracellular riboflavin (**c**) and extracellular riboflavin (**d**) was detected at different time points. μmol/gDCW refers to the number of moles of cofactor per gram of dry cell weight (DCW). All strains were grown at 30℃ in 20 mL of Delft-D medium containing 20 g/L glucose with an initial $OD_{600}$ of 0.1. All data represent the mean of n = 3 independent biological samples and error bars show standard deviation. Statistical analysis was performed by using Student's *t* test (one-tailed; two-sample unequal variance; * $P<0.05$, ** $P<0.01$, *** $P<0.001$).

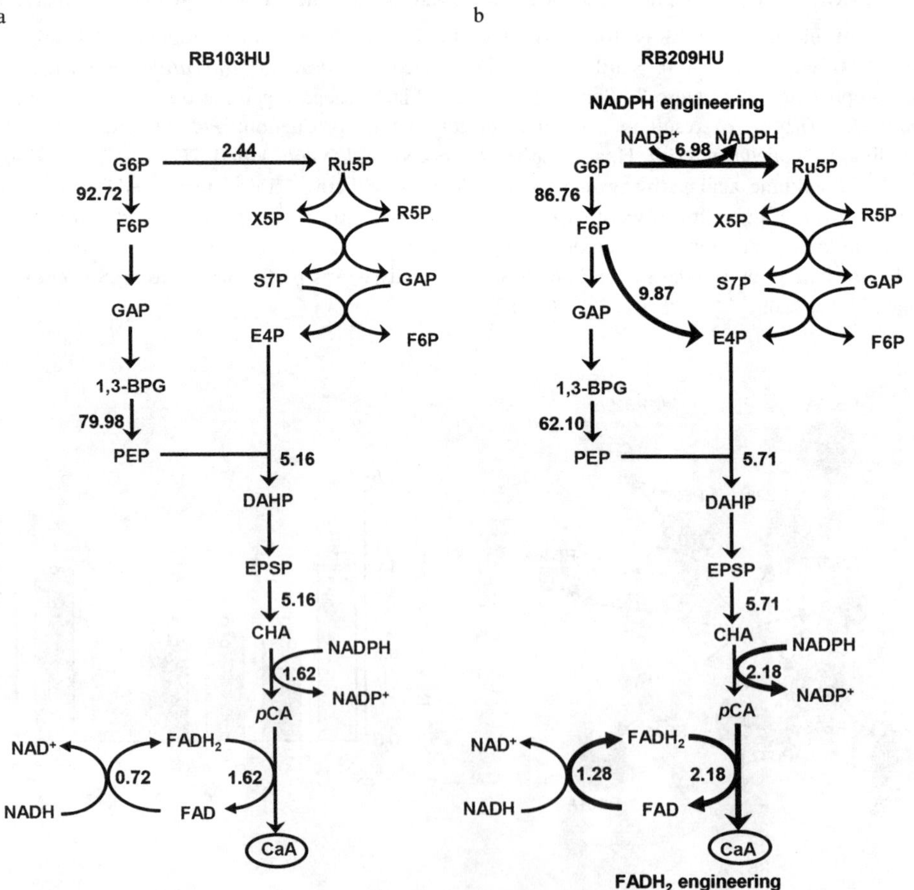


**Extended Data Fig. 7 Metabolic flux analysis (MFA) in the CaA producer RB209HU (right, with cofactor-engineering strategy) and RB103HU (left, without cofactor-engineering strategy)**

Based on MFA, the fluxes to the different products were represented relative to the uptake of 100 mmol of glucose. Cofactor-related pathways is highlighted in blue. 1,3 BPG, 1,3-biphosphoglycerate. See Fig. 2 and Fig. 3 legends regarding abbreviations of other metabolites.

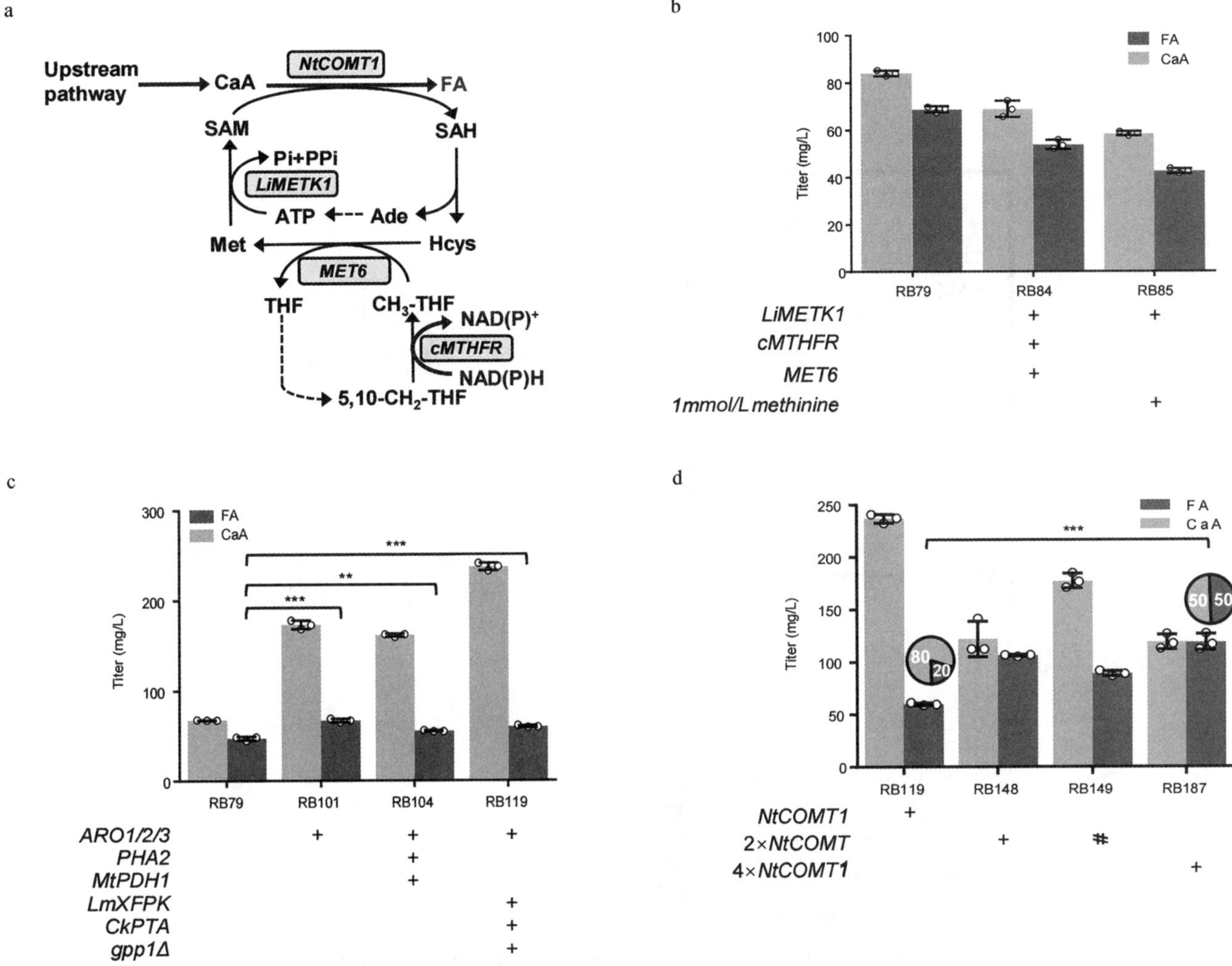


**Extended Data Fig. 8 Cofactor engineering and pathway optimization for FA production**

(a) Schematic illustration of the SAM cycle. *LiMETK1* encoding *Leishmania infantum* S-adenosylmethionine synthetases, *MET6* encoding *S. cerevisiae* methionine synthase, *cMTHFR* encoding chemeric methylenetetrahydrofolate reductase. SAM, S-adenosylmethionine; Met, methionine; Hcys, homocysteine; SAH, S-adenosylhomocysteine; $CH_3$ - THF, 5-methyl tetrahydrogen folic acid; 5, 10 - $CH_2$ - THF, 5, 10-methylene tetrahydrogen folic acid; ATP, adenosine triphosphate. (b) Overexpression of the SAM pathway reduced phenolic acid titers. (c) Enhancing CaA biosynthesis improved FA production. *ARO1* encoding shikimate dehydrogenase, *ARO2* encoding chorismate synthase, *ARO3* encoding DAHP synthase, *MtPDH1* encoding *Medicago truncatula* prephenate dehydrogenase, *PHA2* encoding *S. cerevisiae* prephenate dehydratase 2, *LmXFPK*, encoding *Leuconostoc mesenteroides* phosphoketolase; *CkPTA*, encoding *Clostridium kluyveri* phosphotransacetylase. *gpp1Δ* indicates deletion of *GPP1* (encoding GAP phosphatase). (d) Overexpression of *NtCOMT1* using multiple gene copies under of the control of $P_{GAL}$ or strong constitutive promoters improved FA production and the CaA conversion rate. The # indicates expression under strong constitutive promoters ($P_{tHXT7}$ and $P_{TDH3}$). All data represent the mean of n = 3 independent biological samples and error bars show standard deviation. All data represent the mean of n = 3 independent biological samples and error bars show standard deviation. Statistical analysis was performed by using Student's *t* test (one-tailed; two-sample unequal variance; * $P<0.05$, ** $P<0.01$, *** $P<0.001$).

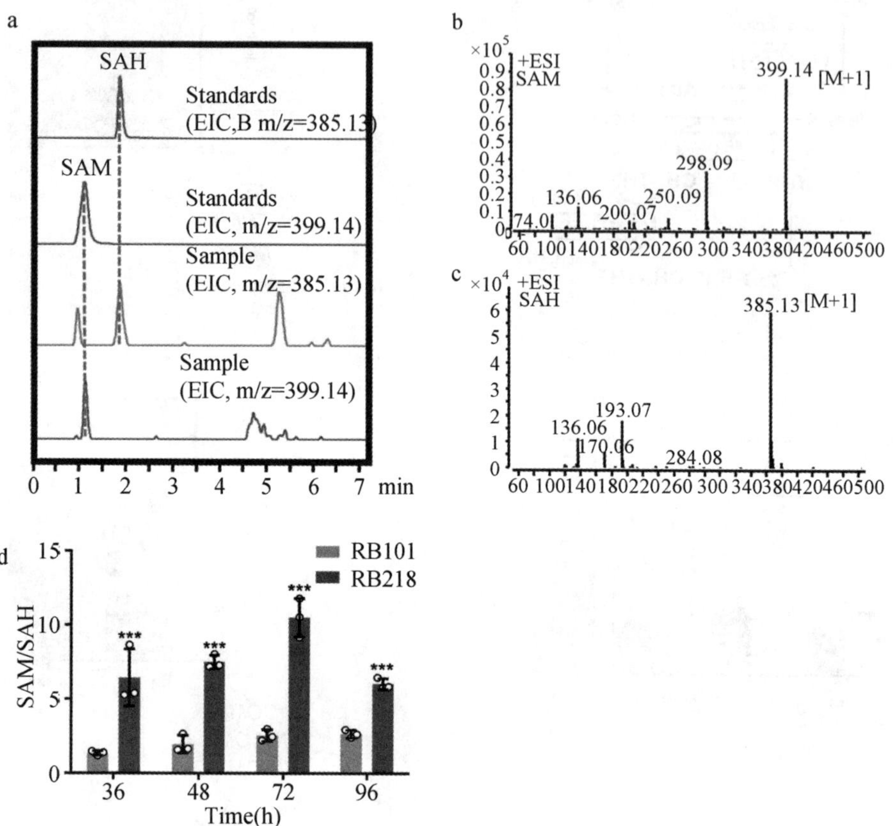


**Extended Data Fig. 9 Quantification of cellular SAM and SAH in FA producing strains**

(a) Representative chromatographs of standards and samples. Corresponding mass spectra of SAM (b) and SAH (c). (d) Cellular SAM/SAH ratios were detected at different time points. All strains were grown at 30 ℃ in 20 mL of Delft-D medium containing 20 g/L glucose. All data represent the mean of n = 3 independent biological samples and error bars show standard deviation. Statistical analysis was performed by using Student's *t* test (one-tailed; two-sample unequal variance; $^{*}P<0.05$, $^{**}P<0.01$, $^{***}P<0.001$).

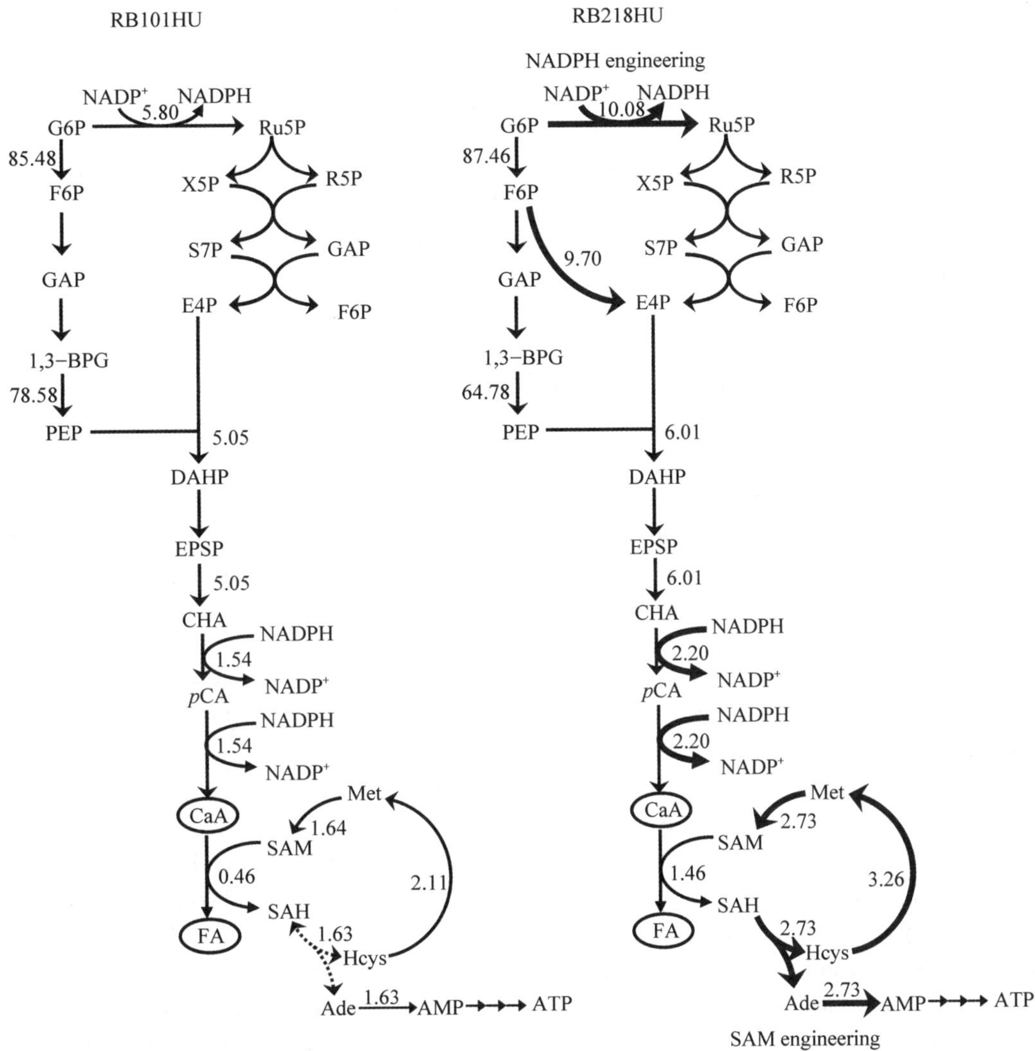


**Extended Data Fig. 10 Metabolic flux analysis (MFA) of the FA producer RB218HU (right, with cofactor-engineering strategy) and RB101HU (left, without cofactor-engineering strategy)**

Based on MFA, the fluxes to the different products were represented relative to the uptake of 100 mmol of glucose. Cofactor-related pathways is highlighted in blue. See Fig. 2 and Fig. 3 legends regarding abbreviations of other metabolites.

[陈瑞兵，张磊，周雍进，等. Nature Chemical Biology，2022，(8)：520－529.]

# Revealing evolution of tropane alkaloid biosynthesis by analyzing two genomes in the Solanaceae family

Solanaceae is one of the largest families of Angiosperm plants and includes economically important species such as tomatoes, potatoes, and eggplants. In addition to cultivated species, several species have also attracted considerable interest due to their lethal toxicity and medicinal value, such as *Atropa belladonna* L., *Hyoscyamus niger* L., and *Datura stramonium* L. These plants have been used globally as poisons, hallucinogens, and anesthetic agents for a long time in both the New and Old Worlds, as their usage can be traced back to ancient Egypt in 1 500 BC. The main pharmacological substances in those plants are hyoscyamine and scopolamine. They are still utilized to treat neuromuscular disorders such as Parkinson's disease or used as anesthetics and analgesics, and antidotes to nerve agent, which are listed in the Model

Lists of Essential Medicines by the World Health Organization. Hyoscyamine and scopolamine are tropane alkaloids (TAs), which are widespread in some distantly related plant families, including Solanaceae, Erythroxylaceae, Euphorbiaceae, Rhizoporaceae, and Convolvulaceae. The scattered distribution of TAs along the Eudicots branch is considered as the result of convergent evolution.

TAs are characterized by an 8-azabicyclo octane core skeleton containing a cycloheptane ring with a nitrogen bridge. There is a diverse class of ~300 specialized TAs, which may have evolved in response to strong natural selection. Structurally, almost all TAs are esters of various organic acids, including tropic, benzoic, cinnamic, isovaleric, and tiglic acids conjugated to hydroxylated tropane derivatives. However, not all TAs have defined physiological activity. TAs used as medicinal substances are therefore termed medicinal tropane alkaloids (mTAs), especially anticholinergic hyoscyamine and scopolamine in the Solanaceae.

After more than a century of research, it was not until 2020 that the complete biosynthetic route of hyoscyamine and scopolamine was clarified. Thirteen enzymes are involved in the biosynthesis of scopolamine from two starting amino acid precursors, ornithine and phenylalanine. The complete biosynthetic pathway of mTAs can be divided into three modules (see below): Ⅰ, biosynthesis of the core structure of TAs, tropine; Ⅱ, biosynthesis of the tropyl moiety; and Ⅲ, modification followed by condensation of tropine and tropyl. In the module Ⅰ, ornithine decarboxylase (ODC), putrescine *N*-methyl-transferase (PMT), *N*-methylputrescine oxidase (MPO), type Ⅲ polyketide synthase (PYKS), tropinone synthase (CYP82M3), and tropine reductase (TRI) are involved. In module Ⅱ, biosynthesis of the tropyl moiety, aromatic amino acid aminotransferase 4 (AT4), phenylpyruvic acid reductase (PPAR), and phenyllactate UDP-glycosyltransferase (UGT1) leads to the production of phenyllactylglucose. Subsequently, in module Ⅲ, the tropine esterification of phenyllactylglucose is catalyzed by littorine synthase (LS), leading to the production of littorine, which was successively modified by littorine mutase (CYP80F1), hyoscyamine dehydrogenase (HDH), and hyoscyamine 6$\beta$-hydroxylase (H6H) to generate scopolamine. Modules Ⅰ and Ⅱ were termed upstream pathways; module Ⅲ was termed the downstream pathway and the mTAs-specific pathway. All the identified enzymes leading to the production of hyoscyamine, and scopolamine are dominantly expressed in the roots, especially the secondary roots, of mTAs-producing plants, such as *A. belladonna* and *D. stramonium*. In addition to scopolamine, norhyoscyamine, resulting from the *N*-demethylation of hyoscyamine, has also been identified in mTAs-producing species in Solanaceae, such as the *Anthrocercis albi-cans* × *Duboisia myoporoides* hybrid and *Datura innoxia*. Norhyoscyamine is an important intermediate that produces ipratropium bromide, an anticholinergic drug used in the control of symptoms related to bronchospasm in chronic obstructive pulmonary disease (COPD) and asthma. However, there is still limited information on the enzymes that convert hyoscyamine to norhyoscyamine.

Although the chemical and enzymatic routes of scopolamine production have been identified and used for scopolamine biosynthesis in yeast, the complete biosynthesis route has not been revealed in any species. Different mTAs producing plants were used by different research groups to elucidate each reaction step. In the 1990s, Hashimoto and coworkers identified the enzymes and the corresponding genes of PMT, MPO, TRI, and H6H mainly in *D. stramonium*, *H. niger*, and *Nicotiana tabacum*. Subsequently, in the 2 000s, a few inde-pendent research groups identified the other genes mainly in *A. belladonna* and *D. stramonium*. The most intensively studied species in relation to the biosynthetic pathway of mTAs is *A. belladonna*, in which all the genes participating in scopolamine biosynthesis have been identified except *MPO* and *TRI*. In another well-known mTAs-producing plant, *D. stramonium*, only a few genes involved in mTAs biosynthesis have been reported, including *PMT*, *TRI*, *HDH*, and *H6H*. *A. belladonna* and *D. stramonium* belong to two main tribes that produce mTAs, Hyoscyameae (including *Atropa*, *Anisodus*, and other genera) and Daturaeae (including *Datura*, *Brugmansia*, and other genera), respectively, which belong to two early-diverging clades. Interestingly, the distribution centers of Atropa and Datura are quite different; Atropa is distributed exclusively in Eurasia, while Datura is mainly distributed in the New World. Thus, whether the same biosynthetic genes are employed by *A. belladonna* and *D. stramonium* to produce the same mTAs remains unclear. Furthermore, how homologous genes among distant species in the Solanaceae family evolved to produce tropine, the chemical foundation of TAs that are widely distributed in this family, has not yet been determined.

In this work, we present two chromosome-level genomes of two medicinal plants (*A. belladonna* and *D. stramonium*) of Solanaceae, which not only provide insights into the diversification of TAs biosynthetic pathway but also provide valuable bioinformatic and genetic resources that could be used to enhance the production of mTAs by genetic engineering of plants or microbes. By employing phylo-genetic analysis along with synteny analysis, we find that the biosynthetic pathway of TAs is highly conserved in Solanaceae, at least in module Ⅰ and Ⅱ. Moreover, we uncover a conserved gene cluster for tropine biosynthesis, composed of *TRI* and *CYP82M3*. Combined with *TRI* expansion driven by tandem duplication and/or whole-genome triplication (WGT), this gene cluster provides a basis for inferring the widespread distribution of TAs in this family. Nevertheless, the loss of the mTAs-specific genes, *LS* and *CYP80F1*, shapes the uneven distribution of mTAs in the Solanaceae. Furthermore, we identify a cytochrome P450 gene that catalyzes the *N*-demethylation of hyoscyamine to generate norhyoscyamine. These findings contribute to our understanding of the evolution of TAs in Solanaceae and will be valuable for metabolic engineering of mTAs.

## 1 RESULTS

Genome sequencing, assembly, and annotation of two species Using *K*-mer analysis with short reads (Supplementary Fig. 1), the genome size of *A. belladonna* was estimated to be ~1.65 Gb and that of *D. stramonium* was estimated to be ~1.80 Gb, and the heterozygosity calculated as 0.39% and 0.5%, respectively. We generated 170.64 Gb (~107 × coverage) of Oxford Nanopore Technologies (ONT) long reads from *A. belladonna* and 828.66 Gb (~460 × coverage) of PacBio long reads from *D. stramonium* using the CCS model, which was subsequently corrected to 52.47 Gb (~29.15 × coverage) of high-fidelity (HiFi) reads (Table 1). We used these data to produce draft genome assemblies. The assemblies were polished using Illumina short reads (*A. belladonna*: 53.88 Gb; *D. stramonium*: 145.27 Gb) and then further improved to a chromosome-level assembly with Hi-C data (*A. bella-donna*: 244.16 Gb; *D. stramonium*: 320.93 Gb) (Supplementary Tables 1 and 2). The final assembly of the *A. belladonna* genome was ~1.59 Gb, with a contig N50 size of 3.03 Mb and scaffold N50 size of 42.83 Mb, for which 99.50% of the sequences were anchored onto 36 pseudochromosomes (Supplementary Fig. 2a and Supplementary Table 3). The *D. stramonium* genome size was ~1.84 Gb, with a contig N50 size of 105.17 Mb, a scaffold N50 size of 156.09 Mb, 97.42% of the sequences anchored onto 12 pseudochromosomes (Supplementary Fig. 2b), and average pseudochromosome length of 149.77 Mb, among the pseudochromosomes, the shortest was 82.81 Mb (LG12), and the longest was 236.94 Mb (LG01) (Supplementary Fig. 2b and Supplementary Table 4). More than 99.63 and 99.94% of the genomic regions could be covered by short reads in the two species, indicating a high level of continuity of the assembly (Supplementary Fig. 3 and Supplementary Table 2).

Based on de novo and homology-based predictions and transcriptome data, 70,209 (*A. belladonna*) and 32,037 (*D. stramonium*) protein-coding genes were predicted with average lengths of 4,802 and 3 913 bp, and average coding sequence (CDS) lengths of 1 156 and 1 127 bp, respectively, and 98.9% of complete conserved homologs was observed in

**Table 1 Summary of *A. belladonna* and *D. stramonium* genome assembly and annotation**

| Sequencing | *A. belladonna* | *D. stramonium* |
|---|---|---|
| Raw bases from WGS-Illumina (Gb) | 53.88 | 145.27 |
| Raw bases from WGS-Nanopore (Gb) | 170.64 | / |
| Raw bases from WGS-PacBio (Gb) | / | 828.66 |
| HiFi (Gb) | / | 52.47 |
| Raw bases from Hi-C (Gb) | 244.16 | 320.93 |
| **Assembly** | | |
| Number of contigs | 1 753 | 1 298 |
| Assembled genome size (bp) | 1,595,075,802 | 1,844,831,445 |
| Contig N50 (Mb) | 3.03 | 105.17 |
| Scaffold N50 (Mb) | 42.83 | 156.09 |
| Average Scaffold length (bp) | 1,468,823 | 1,503,559 |
| GC content (%) | 33.86 | 39.16 |
| Anchorage to chromosomes (%) | 99.50 | 97.42 |
| Complete BUSCOs (%) | 98.9 | 98.9 |
| **Annotation** | | |
| Percentage of repeat sequences (%) | 64.72 | 82.98 |
| LTR rate (%) | 43.14 | 66.16 |
| Number of predicted genes | 70,209 | 32,037 |
| Average gene length (bp) | 4 801.59 | 3 913.23 |
| Average CDS length (bp) | 1 155.96 | 1 127.27 |
| Average exon length (bp) | 288.83 | 235.26 |
| Average intron length (bp) | 756.68 | 734.77 |

the two species based on BUSCO analysis (Table 1; Supplementary Tables 5 - 8). The spatial distribution of these protein-coding genes along the pseudochromosomes was uneven, with higher densities located at the ends of the chromosomal arms (Fig. 1). Comparison of gene structure with that of other species revealed that the average length and numbers of exons and introns were similar, while the gene length of *D. stramonium* was slightly shorter than that of *A. belladonna* (Supplementary Table 9). Moreover, 96.22 and 88.74% of all predicted protein-coding genes were annotated by at least one database (that is, SwissProt, TrEMBL, KOG, NR, GO, or KEGG) for *A. belladonna* and *D. stramonium*, respectively (Supplementary Table 10). In addition, 9 333 and 27 434 noncoding RNA (ncRNA) genes were detected in the *A. belladonna* and *D. stramonium* genomes, yielding 437 and 173 microRNA (miRNA) genes, 2 344 and 4 880 transfer RNA (tRNA) genes, 3 715 and 9 326 small nuclear RNA (snRNA) genes and 2 837 and 13 055 ribosomal RNA (rRNA) genes, respectively

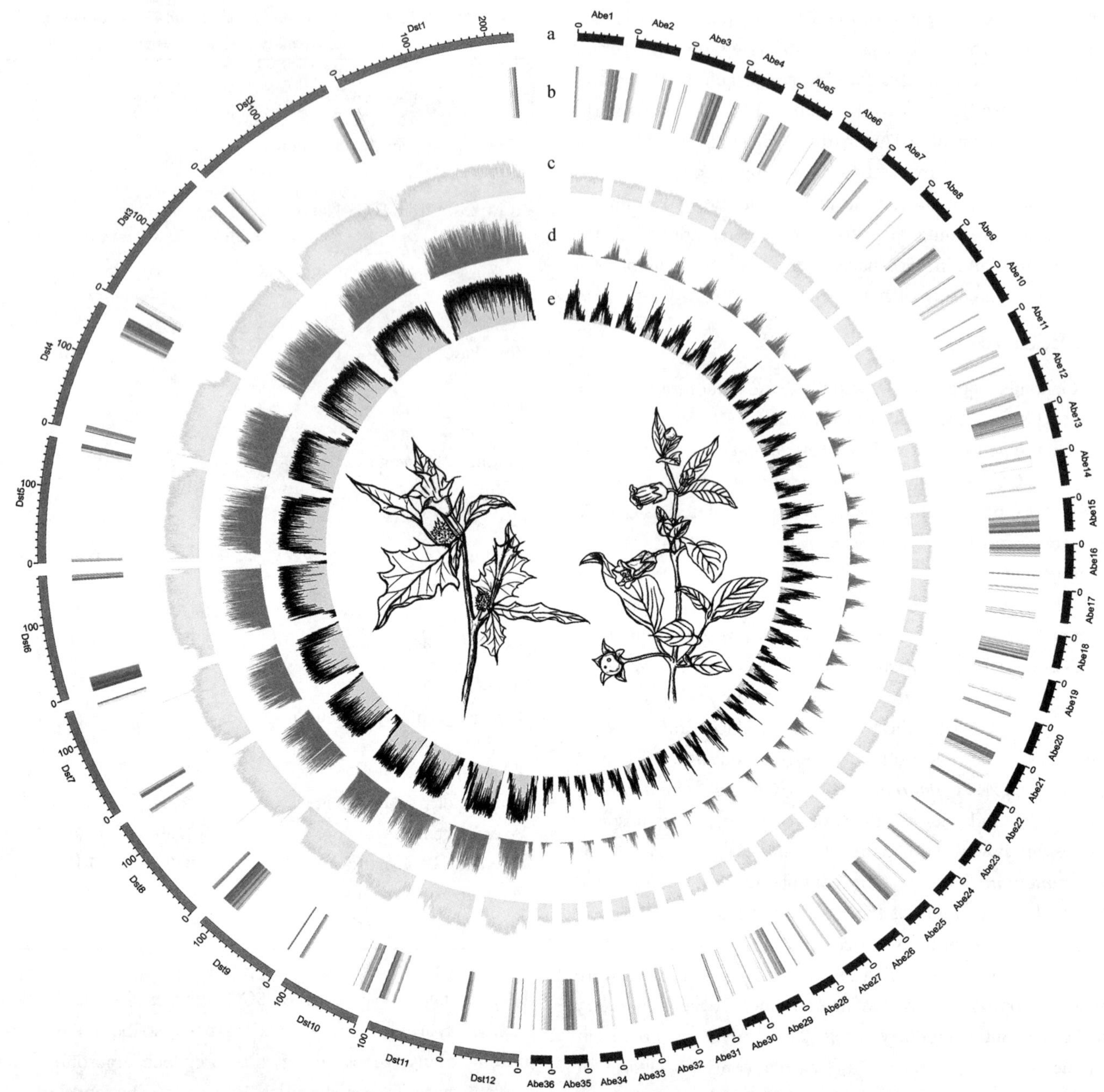


**Fig. 1 An overview of the genomic features of *A. belladonna* and *D. stramonium***

(a) The genomic landscape of the 36 *A. belladonna* pseudochromosomes (right) and 12 *D. stramonium* pseudochromosomes (left). All density information was counted in nonoverlapping 1-Mb windows. (b) Gene density. (c) Guanine-cytosine (GC) content. (d) The distribution of Copia-type retrotransposons. (e) The distribution of Gypsy-type retrotransposons.

(Supplementary Table 11). Finally, the percentage of predicted repetitive elements was much higher in the genome of *D. stramonium*, 64.72% versus 82.98%, respectively (Table 1; Supplementary Tables 12 - 14).

We further sequenced 43.53 Gb of PacBio full-length cDNA data for *Lycium chinense*. After preprocessing by removing redundant reads from the generated data, 25,777 full-length transcripts were obtained (Supplementary Table 15). A total of 25,263 transcripts (genes) were identified in six databases: 24,761 in Nr, 24,925 in NT, 19,603 in GO, 13,567 in KEGG, 11,387 in KOG, 20,800 in SwissProt (Supplementary Table 16), and 72% of complete conserved homologs was observed by BUSCO analysis (Supplementary Table 17).

Comparative genomic and phylogenomic analyses We clustered the annotated genes into gene families among *A. belladonna*, *D. stramonium*, and the other 10 species. A total of 318, 352 genes from 12 species, including eight Solanaceae species, potato (*Solanum tuberosum*), tomato (*Solanum lycopersicum*), tobacco (*Nicotiana tabacum*), hot pepper (*Capsicum annuum*), eggplant (*Solanum melongena*), petunia (*Petunia axillaris*), and four other angiosperms

(Supplementary Table 18), were clustered into 37,515 gene families with an average of eight genes per family (Supplementary Table 19). A total of 43,921 *A. belladonna* genes were clustered into 23, 879 gene families, and 26, 109 *D. stramonium* genes were clustered into 20,328 gene families, which included 1 172, and 657 specific families, respectively (Supplementary Fig. 4).

We selected 207 single-copy gene families among the 13 species (adding the full-length transcriptome data of *L. chinense*) to construct the phylogenetic tree, which showed that *A. belladonna* and *L. chinense* belong to a clade, while *D. stramonium*, *C. annuum*, *S. melongena*, *S. lycopersicum*, and *S. tuberosum* belong to the other clade. Based on molecular clock analysis, we estimated that *Petunia axillaris* diverged from the Solanaceae species ~43 million years ago (Mya) (33 - 56 Mya), *D. stramonium* diverged from the clade composed of *A. belladonna* and *L. chinense* ~28 Mya (23 - 37 Mya), and *A. belladonna* diverged from *L. chinense* ~24 Mya (18 - 31 Mya) (Fig. 2a).

We conducted expansion and contraction analysis based on the constructed phylogenetic tree and discovered 11,684 expanded and 1 022 contracted families in *A. belladonna* compared with 1 579 expanded and 5 282 contracted families in *D. stramonium* (Fig. 2a). The GO enrichment analysis of the expanded gene families of *A. belladonna* suggested that these genes were enriched in "ATPase-coupled cation transmembrane transporter activity," "cellular nitrogen compound biosynthetic processes," and "regulation of flavonoid biosynthetic processes." The expanded gene families in *D. stramonium* were enriched in "oxidoreductase activity," "acting on NAD(P)H," "NADH dehydrogenase (ubiquinone) activity," "response to stimulus," and "defense response" (Supplementary Fig. 5; Supplementary Data 1, 2). KEGG functional enrichment analysis of the expanded gene families demonstrated that they were mainly assigned to "plant-pathogen interactions," "energy metabolism," "sesquiterpenoid and triterpenoid biosynthesis," and "flavonoid biosynthesis" (Supplementary Fig. 6; Supplementary Tables 20, 21).

**Two different forces drive genome size variation in *A. belladonna* and *D. stramonium*** Genome sizes vary widely across the Solanaceae, ranging from ~900 Mb in tomato to 4.5 Gb in tobacco and even larger in the Cyphomandra genus. The proliferation of repetitive elements, especially the Gypsy family, was regarded as the main cause for the expansion of genomes of species in the Solanaceae family. The genome sizes of *A. belladonna* and *D. stramonium* were larger than those of tomato and potato. To infer the driving force of the genome variation in *A. belladonna*, we used the distribution of synonymous substitution rates per gene ($K_S$) between collinear paralogous genes to identify whole-genome duplication events based on the assumption that the number of silent substitutions per site between two homologous sequences increases in a relatively linear manner with time. We selected a range of species for the comparative genomic investigation and assessment of polyploidization events in *A. belladonna* and *D. stramonium*: *S. lycopersicum*, *C. annuum*, *S. tuberosum*, and *S. melongena* as representatives of the Solanaceae, and *V. vinifera*, which represents the closest modern chromosome relative of the ancestral eudicot karyotype (AEK) with seven protochromosomes. By con-structing the distribution of $K_S$ within each genome, we detected three and two polyploidization events in the genomes of *A. belladonna* and *D. stramonium*, respectively. The distribution of the reciprocal best hit (RBH) gene pair $K_S$ values exhibited a peak at ~ 0.55 in the Solanaceae species (*A. belladonna*, *D. stramonium*, *S. lycopersicum*, and *S. melongena*), further confirming the recent alpha WGT event common to all Solanaceae species. According to the relative times estimated by $K_S$ change, the Solanaceae species shared the older gamma paleopolyploidy event with other higher eudicots (Fig. 2b). Indeed, 716 syntenic blocks containing 28,463 paralogous gene pairs, were identified in the *A. belladonna* genome and the RBH paralog $K_S$ value distribution showed a peak at ~0.125 - 0.130, corresponding to another WGT event that occurred at ~17.50 - 18.20 MYA in *A. belladonna* after its split from other closely related species (Fig. 2b).

Synteny analyses between the genomes of *A. belladonna*, *D. stramonium*, and *V. vinifera* also showed clear evidence of another recent WGT event for *A. belladonna*. For each genomic region in *V. vinifera*, we typically found three matching regions in *D. stramonium* with a similar level of divergence and identified 3 : 1 syntenic depth ratios in the *A. belladonna*-*D. stramonium* genome comparison (Fig. 2c; Supplementary Figs. 7 - 9).

Given that the genome size of *D. stramonium* was ~ 250 Mb larger than the *A. belladonna* genome, we investigated the evolution of LTR retrotransposons and their potential contribution to the growth of the two species' genomes. We identified 832 Mb and 1,290 Mb (52.17% and 69.91%, respectively) of sequences in the assembled *A. belladonna* and *D. stramonium* genomes as transposable elements (TEs) (Supplementary Tables 13 and 14). The predominant type of TE was LTR elements, which represented ~ 667 and 1 221 Mb (more than 64.65 and 79.73%, respectively) of the total repetitive sequence in the two genomes. Among the LTRs, most were Gypsy elements, which accounted for 38.92% and 72.91% of the total repetitive sequences in *A. belladonna* and *D. stramonium*, respectively, followed by Copia elements (22.57 and 5.17%, respectively) (Fig. 1d, e; Supplementary Fig. 10a;

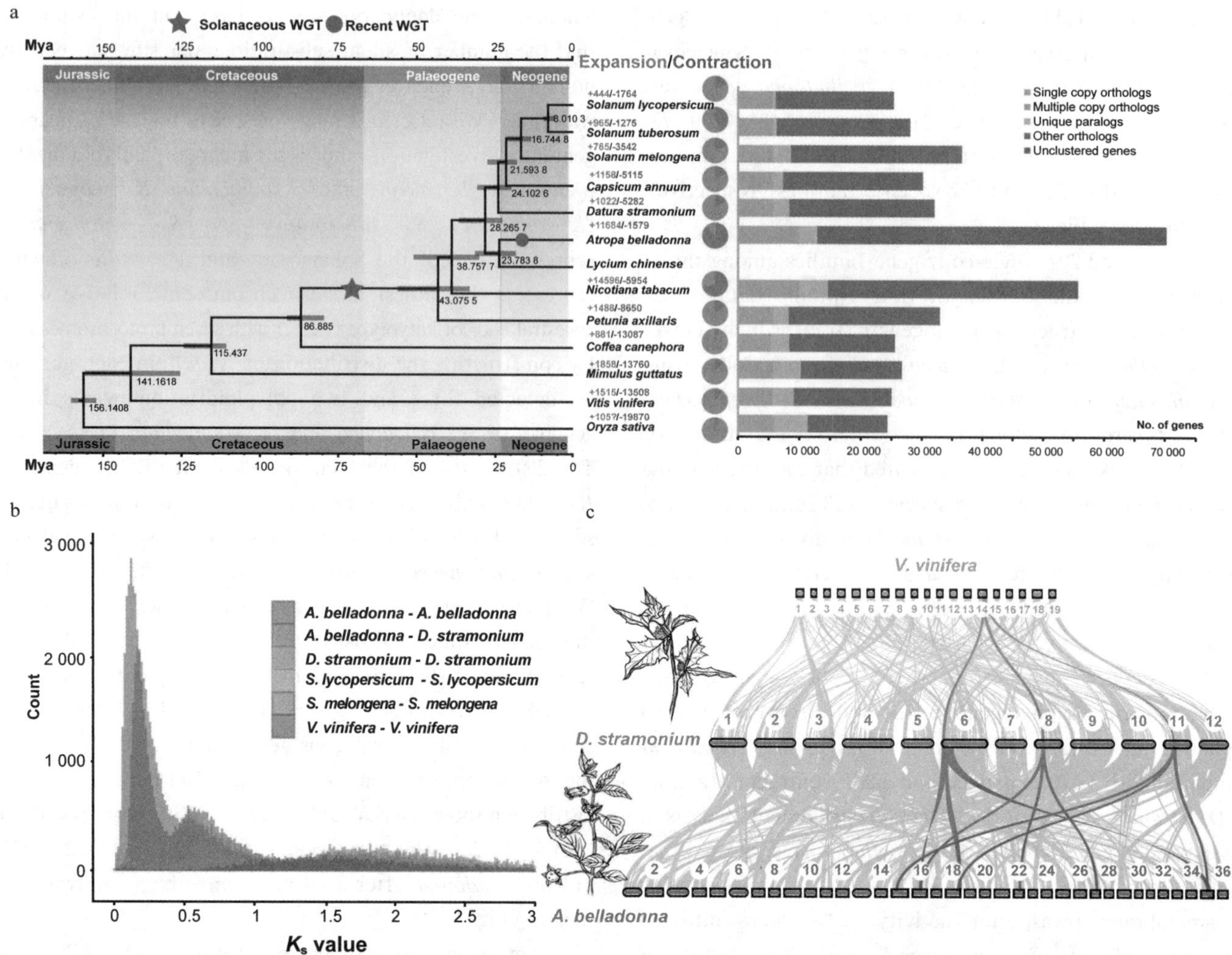


**Fig. 2 Phylogenetic relationships and divergence times among 13 species**

(a) Phylogenetic tree of *A. belladonna*, *D. stramonium*, and *L. chinense* along with 10 other plants. Gene families of the *A. belladonna*, *D. stramonium*, and other sequenced genomes are shown on the right. All branch bootstrap values are out of 100. Gene family expansions are indicated in orange, and gene family contractions are indicated in gray; the corresponding proportions of total changes are shown using the same colors in the pie charts. The estimated divergence time (million years ago, Mya) is indicated at each node; bars are the 95% highest posterior density (HPD). Circles in orange represent recent whole-genome duplication events. (b) *Ks* values revealed a recent WGT event during the evolution of *A. belladonna*, a WGT event shared by Solanaceae species, and a WGT event shared by Solanaceae species and *V. vinifera*. (c) Collinearity between *A. belladonna*, *D. stramonium*, and *V. vinifera* chromosomes. The collinearity pattern shows that a typical ancestral region in the *V. vinifera* genome can be traced to three regions in the *D. stramonium* genome and nine regions in the *A. belladonna* genome. Gray wedges in the background indicate syntenic blocks spanning more than 15 genes between the genomes.

Supplementary Tables 13, 14). We then estimated the times of the LTR-RT burst in the two genomes, and the results suggested that the timing of the main LTR-RT burst was earlier in *A. belladonna* (~2.0 Mya, Supplementary Fig. 10b, c) while *D. stramonium* exhibited many more recent LTR-RT bursts (~0.6 Mya, Supplementary Fig. 10d, e).

*D. stramonium* and *A. belladonna* employ a conserved biosynthetic pathway to produce mTAs Given that both *D. stramonium* and *A. belladonna* produce mTAs, it is of interest to investigate whether *D. stramonium* employs the same biosynthetic pathway as *A. belladonna* to produce mTAs. To this end, we first elucidated the TAs biosynthetic pathway by transgenic and biochemical approaches in *A. belladonna* to identify *MPO* and *TRI*, which are the only two uncharacterized TAs biosynthetic genes in this species. The oxidative deamination of *N*-methylputrescine is a key step in TAs biosynthesis, and this reaction may be catalyzed by *N*-methylputrescine oxidase (MPO). However, the gene encoding MPO has not been characterized in TAs-producing plants. We retrieved three putative MPOs, EVM0017027.2, EVM0068072.1, and EVM0064643.2, using BLASTP search in which MPO from tobacco was used as a query. However, we cloned only two of them from *A. belladonna*, *EVM0017027.2* and *EVM0068072.1*, which were named

*AbMPO1* and *AbMPO2*, respectively. *AbMPO1* was highly expressed in the roots of *A. belladonna*, while *AbMPO2* was predominantly expressed in above-ground tissues (Supplementary Fig. 11a). Suppressing the expression of *AbMPO1* but not *AbMPO2* significantly decreased the contents of hyoscyamine and scopolamine in hairy root cultures of *A. belladonna* (Fig. 3b and Supplementary Fig. 11). Thus, AbMPO1 is the primary functional MPO involved in mTAs biosynthesis in *A. belladonna*. We also identified the TRI in *A. belladonna* via in vitro TRI enzyme activity assays (see below). Subsequently, we used the functionally characterized genes of *A. belladonna* as seeds to retrieve all homologous genes across nine Solanaceae for each gene family involved in TAs/mTAs biosynthesis. By constructing the phylogenetic trees of each family at each step (Supplementary Figs. 12 - 23), we defined the well-supported subfamily containing the functionally tested sequence as the most likely mTAs-related group at each step. Subsequently, we determined the mTAs biosynthetic genes of each species and constructed phylogenetic relationships of all homologs across all species for each subfamily (Supplementary Figs. 24, 25). Most of the genes in the upstream pathway of mTAs biosynthesis were multicopy and conserved across Solanaceae, for which the phylogenetic relationships were consistent with the interspecific relationships. Moreover, the results of microsynteny analysis were consistent with the results of phylogenetic analysis. All genes in modules I and II showed a very high degree of synteny across Solanaceae with high sequence similarity except PPAR (Fig. 3a; Supplementary Figs. 26 - 38). Recently, a widespread alternative trans-cinnamic acid (CA) formation pathway in plants was reported. Two PPARs from tea plants were also found to transform phenylpyruvic acid into phenyllactic acid. Thus, we hypothesized that this enzyme is also widely distributed across Solanaceae and is unlikely to be a bottleneck in the biosynthesis of phenyllactylglucose. To test this hypothesis, we characterized the function of PPARs from *A. belladonna*, *D. stramonium*, *P. axillaris*, *S. lycopersicum*, and *C. annuum* by in vitro enzymatic assays. Consistent with our speculation, all the tested PPARs transformed phenylpyruvic acid into phenyllactic acid (Fig. 3c; Supplementary Fig. 39; Supplementary Table 22). Taken together, the identified scopolamine biosynthetic genes and results of phylogenetic analysis combined with microsynteny analysis revealed the conservation of phenyllactylglucose and tropine biosynthetic genes in Solanaceae species.

Interestingly, the phylogenetic analysis showed that the *TRI*, *LS*, *CYP80F1*, *HDH*, and *H6H* genes of *A. belladonna* and *D. stramonium* are clustered on one branch and divergent from related genes in other Solanaceae species without mTAs (Supplementary Figs. 24, 25). The sequence similarity of the *TRI*, *LS*, *CYP80F1*, *HDH*, and *H6H* genes between *A. belladonna* and *D. stramonium* were likewise dramatically higher than those between *A. belladonna* and other species (Supplementary Fig. 40). Furthermore, the microsynteny analysis showed that the *LS*, *CYP80F1*, and *HDH* genes in *A. belladonna* have syntenic genes only in *D. stramonium* (Fig. 3a; Supplementary Figs. 34 - 37). The integrated evidence of multiple resources from synteny analysis, phylogeny analysis and sequence alignments indicated that *D. stramonium* employs the same biosynthetic route as *A. belladonna* to produce mTAs, although the two species belong to distant genera.

Using RNA-Seq reads generated from tissues in two species with mTAs, we further examined the expression of all the genes identified above. The results showed that at least one mTAs-related gene identified at each biosynthesis step was highly expressed in the roots of *A. belladonna* and *D. stramonium* (Fig. 3d). The high levels of hyoscyamine and scopolamine in the roots of *A. belladonna* and *D. stramonium* are likely attributable to the constant and high expression of these genes. To examine the coexpression of the pathway-related genes more broadly, we constructed weighted gene coexpression networks by WGCNA using all differentially expressed genes in *A. belladonna*, obtaining seven clusters (Supplementary Fig. 41, Supplementary Data 3 - 9). Remarkably, the identified probable mTAs genes are classified into 'blue module' and are highly expressed in root tissues with other related genes (Supplementary Figs. 42, 43b). The GO enrichment analysis of these 'blue module genes' suggested that they are enriched in the "tropane alkaloid biosynthetic process," "tropane alkaloid metabolic process," "alkaloid metabolic process," "oxidoreductase activity, acting on peroxide as acceptor," and "peroxidase activity" (Supplementary Fig. 43a).

The evolution of gene clusters correlates with the widespread distribution of TAs across Solanaceae Given the wide distribution of TAs across Solanaceae and the high conservation of tropine biosynthetic genes, we further examined the chromosomal positions of those genes (Supplementary Figs. 44, 45; Supplementary Tables 23, 24) and found that *CYP82M3* and *TRI* genes were clustered in representative genomes of Solanaceae species except tobacco (Fig. 4a). CYP82M3 catalyzes the formation of tropinone; TRI subsequently reduces tropinone to produce tropine, the core structure of TAs, which has been documented in many Solanaceae species. We speculated that the evolution of this gene cluster contributed to the widespread distribution of tropine in this family. Moreover, this gene cluster cannot be identified in the most distantly related species in our analysis, *Ipomoea triloba* (Convolvulaceae). We proposed that the recruitment of *CYP82M3* and *TRI* occurred after

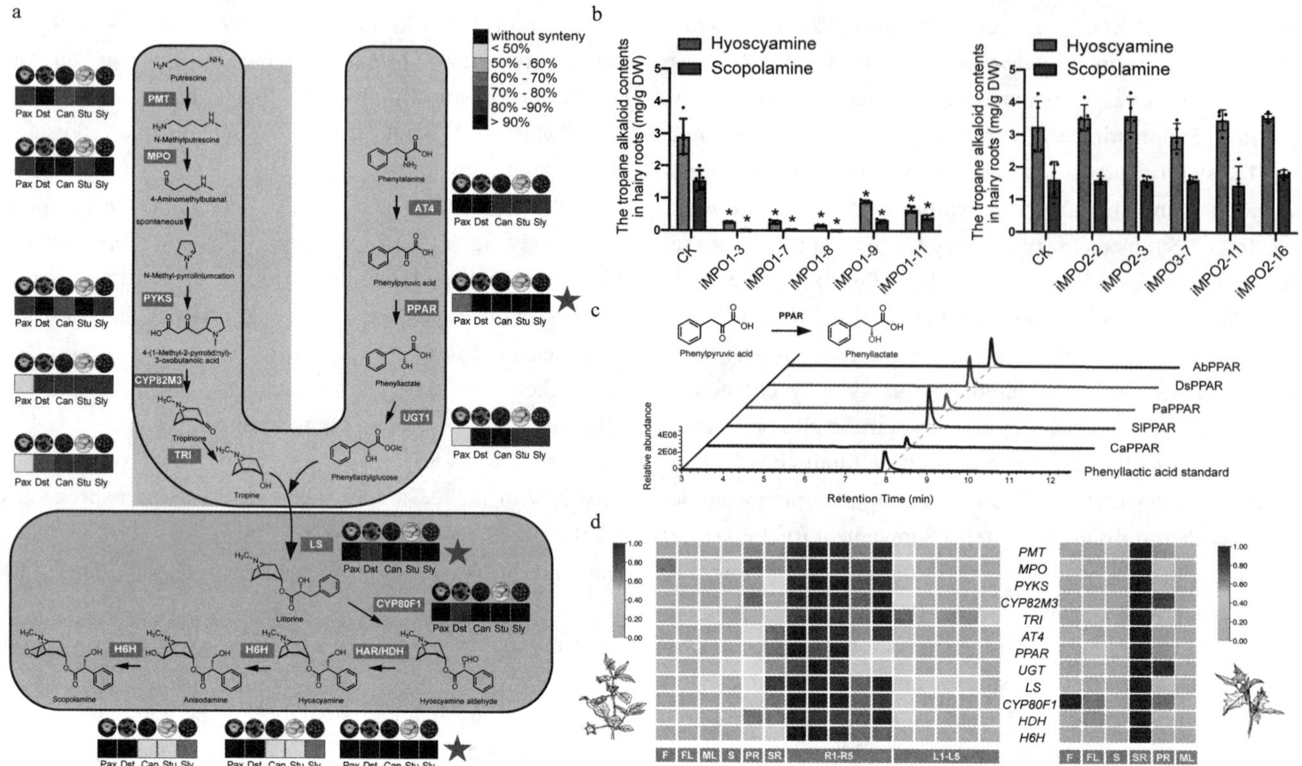


**Fig. 3 Biosynthetic pathway of medicinal tropane alkaloids (mTAs)**

(a) Schematic representation of the medicinal tropane alkaloid biosynthetic pathway. Light green represents module I, including PMT putrescine *N*-methyltransferase, MPO *N*-methylputrescine oxidase, PYKS type III polyketide synthase, CYP82M3 tropinone synthase, and TRI tropinone reductase I. Light blue represents module II, including AT4 aromatic amino acid aminotransferase 4, PPAR phenylpyruvic acid reductase, and UGT1 phenyllactate UDP-glycosyltransferase. Light red represents module III, including LS littorine synthase, CYP80F1 littorine mutase, HDH hyoscyamine dehydrogenase, and H6H hyoscyamine 6β-hydroxylase. Pax, *P. axillaris*; Dst, *D. stramonium*; Can, *C. annuum*; Stu, *S. tubersoum*; Sly, *S. lycopersicum*. (b) The functional characterization of MPOs from *A. belladonna* by RNA interference in hairy roots. Left, the hyoscyamine and scopolamine contents in AbMPO1 - RNAi root cultures. Right, the hyoscyamine and scopolamine contents in AbMPO2 - RNAi root cultures. CK, control root cultures. iMPO1, hairy root cultures with *AbMPO1* RNAi. iMPO2, hairy root cultures with *AbMPO2* RNAi. DW, dry weight. The data are presented as means values +/− s.d. ($n = 5$ biologically independent samples). ∗, represents a significant difference from control line (CK) at the levels of $P<0.01$ as determined by two-sided Student's *t*-test. For hyoscyamine contents, $^*P = 0.0000$ (iMPO1 - 3), $^*P = 0.0000$ (iMPO1 - 7), $^*P = 0.0000$ (iMPO1 - 8), $^*P = 0.0000$ (iMPO1 - 9), and $^*P = 0.0000$ (iMPO1 - 11). For scopolamine contents, $^*P = 0.0000$ (iMPO1 - 3), $*P = 0.0000$ (iMPO1 - 7), $*P = 0.0000$ (iMPO1 - 8), $*P = 0.0000$ (iMPO1 - 9), and $^*P = 0.0000$ (iMPO1 - 11). (c) Extracted ion chromatograms showing the in vitro catalytic activity of five purified recombinant PPARs from *P. axillaris* (PaPPAR, Peaxi162Scf00071g00082.1), *A. belladonna* (AbPPAR, EVM0020147.2), *D. stramonium* (DsPPAR, DstT013938.1), *C. annuum* (CaPPAR, XM_016708230.2), and *S. lycopersicum* (SlPPAR, XM_004229823.4) with phenylpyruvic acid (PPA) used as a substrate. The blue dotted line represents the retention time of phenyllactic acid, the product of PPAR. (d) Gene expression profiles (in normalized TPMs) of different tissues in two species are presented in the heatmap alongside the gene names (F fruit, FL flower, L mature leaf, S stem, PR primary root, SR secondary roots, R1-R5 the roots of *A. belladonna* at five different development stages, L1 - L5 the young leaves of *A. belladonna* at five different development stages). Source data underlying **b** and **d** are provided as a Source Data file.

the ancient WGT event in Solanaceae because no intraspecies synteny region was found in any analyzed species except *A. belladonna*, in which a recent WGT event occurred (Fig. 4a).

We noticed that only one *CYP82M3* gene existed in the gene cluster across Solanaceae; nevertheless, *TRI* underwent tandem duplication (in *C. annuum* and *D. stramonium*) and/or duplication caused by WGT in *A. belladonna* (Fig. 4a). This led us to hypothesize that the duplication of *TRI* contributed to the distribution of tropine biosynthesis in Solanaceae species. To test this hypothesis, we first tested for tropine in the species and detected it in *C. annuum*, *A. belladonna* and *D. stramonium* but not in *P. axillaris*, *S. lycopersicum*, and *S. tuberosum* (Fig. 4b). Moreover, the duplicated *TRI* genes showed a high diversity of tissue expression patterns, while all the *CYP82M3* genes in the species investigated in this study were predominantly expressed in the root (Fig. 3d; Supplementary Fig. 46). Contrary to the result in non-TAs-producing species, at least one TRI gene was highly expressed in the roots of TAs-producing species, suggesting that the subfunctionalization of *TRI* occurred after its duplication. Biochemical assays further confirmed that the plants with *TRI* duplications har-

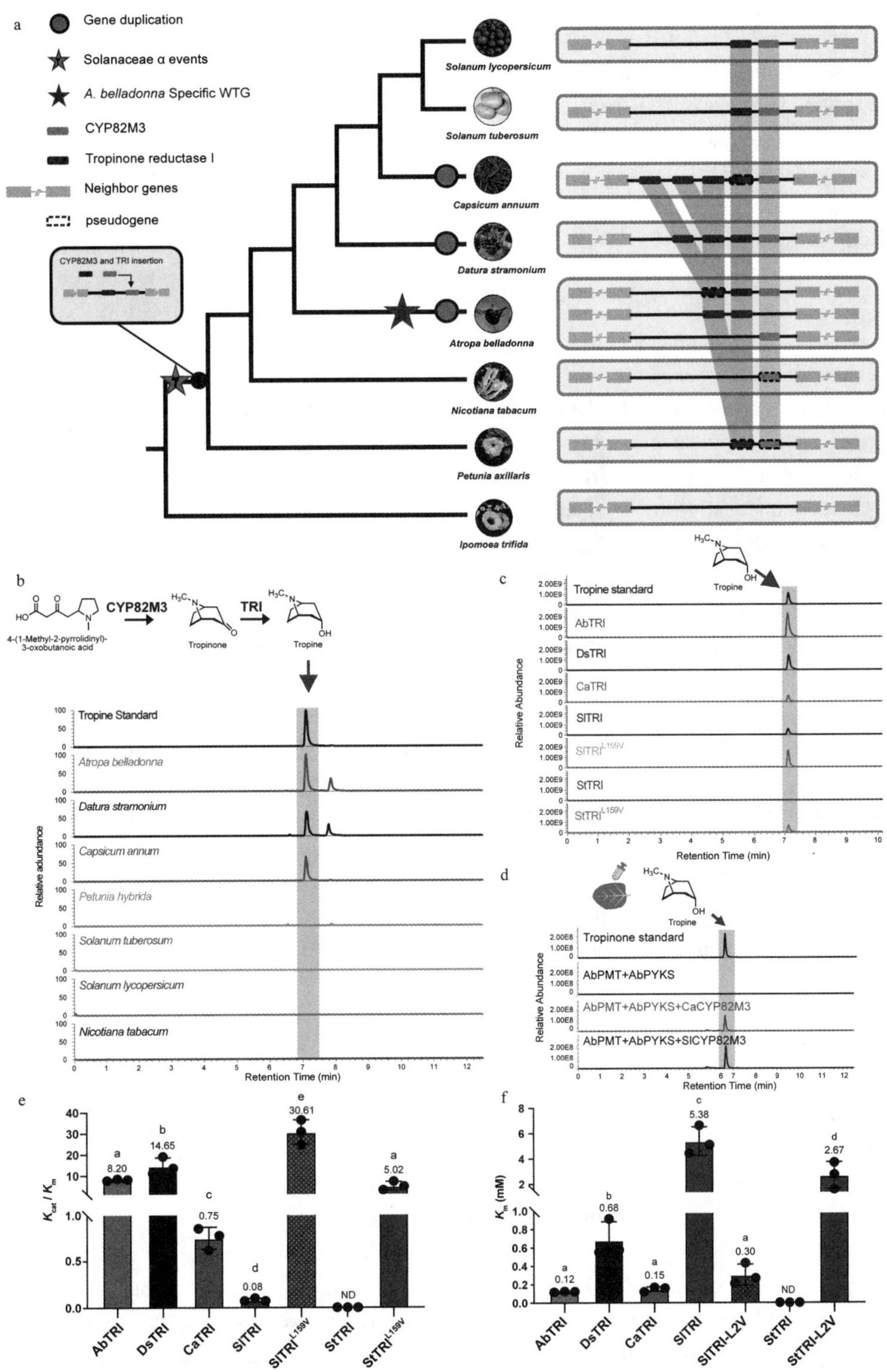


**Fig. 4 The evolution of the tropine gene cluster is associated with tropine diversity across the Solanaceae family**

(a) The tropine gene cluster syntenic regions of seven Solanaceae species and the outgroup species *Ipomea trifida* (Convolvulaceae). Genes encoding TRI are indicated in the red rectangle, and genes encoding CYP82M3 are indicated in the green rectangle. (b) Analysis of tropine in plants by combined LC/MS. The roots, stems and leaves of plants were analyzed for the detection of tropine. The extracted ion chromatograms of tropine are high-lighted in red. (c) Extracted ion chromatograms showing the in vitro activity of seven purified recombinant TRIs from *A. belladonna* (AbTRI), *D. stramonium* (DsTRI), *C. annuum* (CaTRI), *S. lycopersicum* (SlTRI), *S. tubersoum* (StTRI), $SlTRI^{L169V}$, and $StTRI^{L169V}$ with tropinone used as substrate. (d) Extracted ion chromatograms showing the in vivo activity of CaCYP82M3 and SlCYP82M3 in tobacco leaves. (e, f) The evaluation of enzymatic kinetics on five wild-type TRIs and two mutants by $K_{cat}/K_m$ values (**e**) or by $K_m$ values (**f**). The raw Michaelis-Menten curves of these TRIs for the NADPH-dependent reduction reaction of tropinone are presented in Fig. S31. The data are presented as means values +/− s. d. ($n$ = 3 biologically independent samples). Different letters in (e) and (f) indicate significantly different values compared with each other at $P < 0.05$ analyzed by two-sided Student's $t$-test. ND not detectable. Source data underlying (e) and (f) are provided as a Source Data file.

bored at least one functional *TRI* with tropinone reductase activity (Fig. 4c). However, in contrast with the result that we could not detect tropine in tomato, TRI from tomato also showed TRI activity. This prompted us to conduct further enzymatic kinetic analysis of TRI from plants with *TRI* duplication (*A. belladonna*, *D. stramonium*, and *C. annuum*) and without *TRI* duplication (*S. lycopersicum*). The $K_{cat}/K_m$ value of SlTRI was dramatically low, only ~0.01, 0.006, and 0.11 of that of AbTRI, DsTRI, and CaTRI, respectively (Fig. 4d; Supplementary Fig. 47). Moreover, the $K_m$ value of SlTRI was ~43.56, 7.88, and 36.09 times greater than that of AbTRI, DsTRI, and CaTRI, respectively (Fig. 4e; Supplementary Fig. 47). The enzymatic kinetic analysis indicated that the catalytic efficiency of SlTRI is dramatically lower than that of AbTRI, DsTRI, and CaTRI. Since the crystal structures of DsTRI have been resolved, we compared the amino acid sequences of TRIs from these five species, especially the ten residues that were predicted to contact with tropinone. Only one of the ten residues could be correlated with the low or null catalytic efficiency of SlTRI and StTRI (Supplementary Fig. 48). $Val^{168}$ was conserved across the TAs-producing species but substituted by $Leu^{159}$ in SlTRI and StTRI. Consequently, we analyzed the enzymatic kinetics of $SlTRI^{L159V}$ and $StTRI^{L159V}$. The $K_{cat}/K_m$ value of $SlTRI^{L159V}$ increased, followed by a decrease in the $K_m$ value (Fig. 4c - f; Supplementary Fig. 47). More significantly, the $StTRI^{L159V}$ gained the ability to catalyze tropinone to tropine (Fig. 4c - f, Supplementary Fig. 47). In addition, we tested the function of CYP82M3 from *C. annuum* and *S. lycopersicum* in tobacco leaves. Both CaCYP82M3 and SlCYP82M3 transformed 4-(1-methyl-2-pyrrodinyl)-3-oxobutanoic acid into tropinone when they were coexpressed with AbPMT and AbPYKS in tobacco leaves, indicating that the enzyme activity of CYP82M3 was conserved in Solanaceae and that the failure to detect tropine in tomato was not because of the functional defficiency of CYP82M3 (Fig. 4d). Together, these results suggested that the genes involved in the two important tropine biosynthetic steps were arranged in a gene cluster that is conserved across Solanaceae. The subfunctionalization of *TRI* after its duplication promoted higher expression levels in roots and more robust TRI enzymatic activity.

Evolution of mTAs biosynthetic pathway-specific genes

Although TAs are widely distributed across Solanaceae, mTAs, such as hyoscyamine and scopolamine, can be detected only in limited tribes, especially in Daturaeae and Hyoscyameae. Compared with upstream pathway genes that were conserved in Solanaceae, mTAs biosynthetic pathway-specific genes, such as *LS*, *CYP80F1*, and *HAR*, from the two mTAs producing species, *A. belladonna* and *D. stramonium*, formed a clade clearly distinct from other homologs of the species without mTAs (Supplementary Fig. 25). Consistently, we observed littorine, the direct product of LS, only in *A. belladonna* and *D. stramonium* (Fig. 5a). We speculated that the functional LS only existed in Daturaeae and Hyoscyameae. To test this hypothesis, we carried out relative enzyme activity assays of three LS homologs in *D. stramonium* (DsLS), *A. belladonna* (AbLS), and *L. chinense* (LcLS) by expressing them transiently in tobacco leaves together with AbUGT1, which converts phenyllactate into phenyllactylglucose used as substrate. After infiltration with phenyllactate and tropine, we detected littorine in tobacco leaves expressing DsLS and AbLS but not in those expressing LcLS. This suggested that both DsLS and AbLS have LS activity (Fig. 5b, c). In addition, DsLS had significantly higher enzyme activity than AbLS in our test, suggesting that DsLS is a better candidate for engineering mTAs in plants or in yeast (Fig. 5c). To understand *LS* gene evolution, we employed microsynteny analysis, which revealed that the syntenic region of *LS* in *A. belladonna* showed a high degree of synteny among all tested species, but *LS* genes were dramatically absent in *P. axillaris*, *C. annuum*, *S. lycopersicum*, and *S. tuberosum* (Supplementary Fig. 34). Interestingly, by performing more detailed sequence analysis, we found that the portion of the *AbLS* promoter region was highly conserved in all the tested non-mTAs-producing species, and even the first two exons could be detected in *Iochroma cyaneum*, a species in Physalideae, with high similarity (Supplementary Figs. 34, 35). Combining the results of microsynteny analysis with those of phylogeny analysis, sequence alignments and enzyme activity assays led to the hypothesis that mTAs biosynthetic genes have been lost in non-mTAs-producing species. To address this, we further investigated the microsynteny of *CYP80F1*. Consistent with the observation for *LS*, the genomic region in which *CYP80F1* is located also showed a high degree of synteny among the tested species and *CYP80F1* was absent in non-mTAs-producing species again (Fig. 5d). Nevertheless, a syntenic *CYP80F1* homolog was detected in petunia. Moreover, two traces of the first exon of *CYP80F1* and a trace of the second exon of *CYP80F1* were detected in the syntenic region of *C. annuum* and *S. tuberosum*, respectively (Fig. 5d). Thus, our evidence suggested that the gene loss in non-mTAs-producing tribes contributed to the limited distribution of mTAs in Solanaceae.

A cytochrome P450 in the CYP82M subfamily accounts for the *N*-demethylation of hyoscyamine  Although the biosynthesis of hyoscyamine and scopolamine has been resolved, the enzymes modifying them have not been reported. Norhyoscyamine, the product of *N*-demethylation of hyoscyamine, was identified in many mTAs-producing species, such as *A. myoporoides*, *A. pannosa* and *A. walcottii*

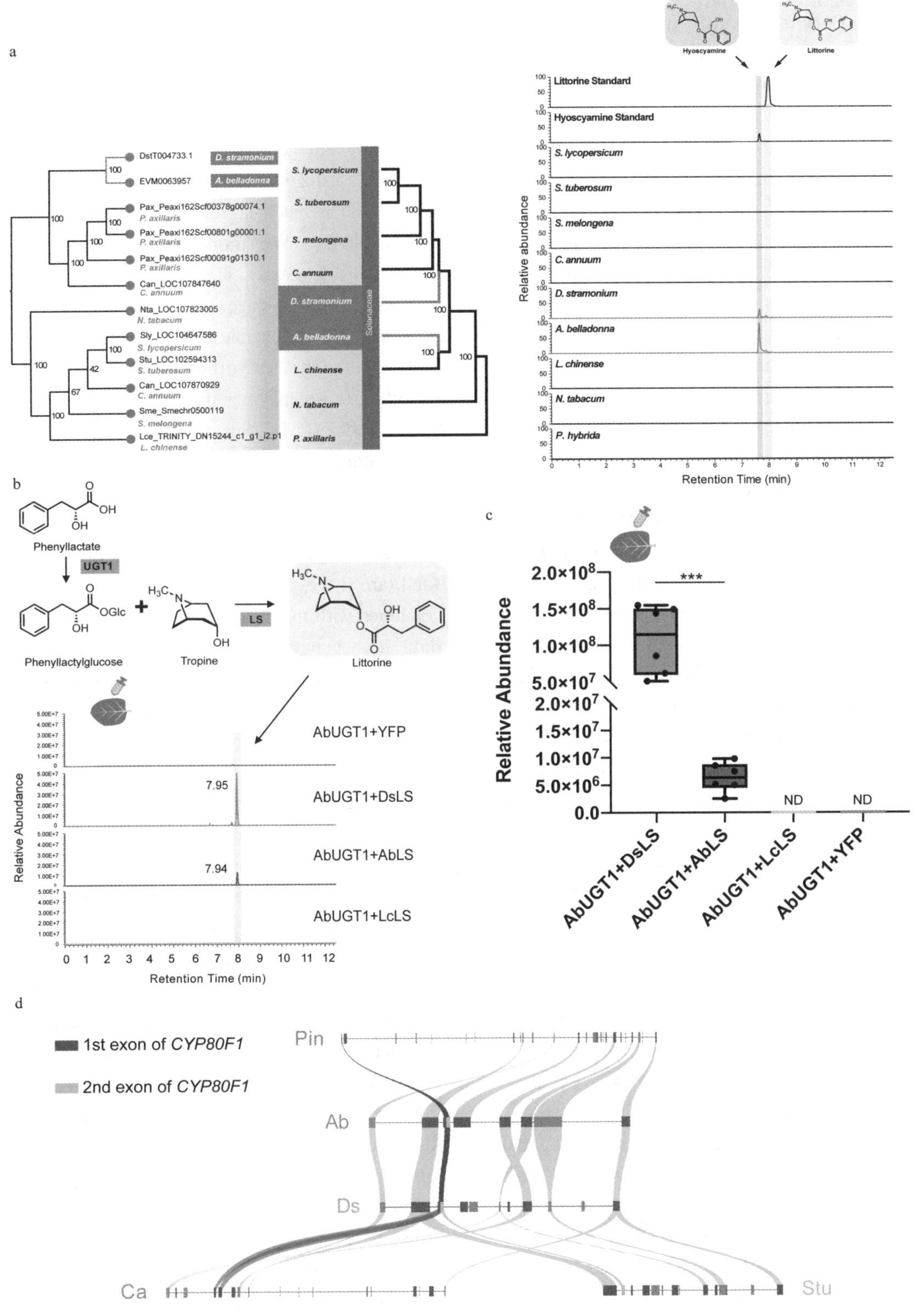


**Fig. 5 The evolution of mTAs-specific genes**

(a) Left, the gene tree of *LS* genes and species tree of nine Solanaceae species; right, the extracted ion chromatograms of hyoscyamine (light red) and littorine (light yellow). The roots, stems, and leaves of plants were analyzed for the detection of hyoscyamine and littorine by UPLC-MS. (b) Extracted ion chromatograms showing the in vivo activity of three LS form *A. belladonna* (AbLS), *D. stramonium* (DsLS) and *L. chinense* (LcLS) by coexpressing AbUGT, which converted phenyllactate into phenyllactylglucose in tobacco leaves; phenyllactate and tropine were used as substrates by coinfiltration into tobacco leaves. (c) The relative LS activity of AbLS and DsLS. For the boxplot ($n = 6$ biologically independent samples), the centerline, median; box limits, upper and lower quartiles; whiskers, data range. *** represented significant difference analyzed by two-sided Student's $t$-test at the level of $P < 0.001$. *** $P = 0.0004$ (AbUGT1+DsLS compared with AbUGT1 + AbLS). ND not detectable. (d) Synteny analysis of the *CYP80F1* gene in different tribes. Pin, *P. inflata*; Ab, *A. belladonna*; Ds, *D. stramonium*; Ca, *C. annuum*; Stu, *S. tuberosum*. Syntenic pieces of *CYP80F1* are highlighted in red. The red rectangle on the chromosome represents the first exon of *CYP80F1*; the light blue rectangle on the chromosome represents the second exon of *CYP80F1*. Source data underlying (c) is provided as a Source Data file.

in *Anthotroche*, *Datura arborea* in *Datura* and the *Anthrocercis albicans* × *Duboisia myoporoides* hybrid. To characterize the enzymes involved in the *N*-demethylation of hyoscyamine, we first measured the contents of norhyoscyamine in different tissues of *A. belladonna*. Consistent with the distribution of hyoscyamine, norhyoscyamine was predominantly distributed in the roots of *A. belladonna*, especially in the primary roots (Fig. 6a, b). Because members of the CYP82 subfamily from tobacco convert nicotine to nornicotine by *N*-demethylation, we first retrieved all *CYP* genes using hidden Markov model-based conserved motif searches in *A. belladonna* and *D. stramonium* (Fig. 6c). By building a phylogenetic tree of CYPs in *A. belladonna*, *D. stramonium* and *Arabidopsis*, we found that eight CYPs from *A. belladonna*, including two AbCYP82M3s, were clustered in the CYP82M clade. Further coexpression analysis revealed that one member, *EVM0022661.2*, was highly coexpressed with *AbCYP82M3*s in the primary root and secondary root of *A. belladonna*. To test the enzymatic function of EVM0022661.2, we cloned *EVM0022661.2* and expressed it transiently in *N. benthamiana* leaves. After infiltration with hyoscyamine as the substrate, norhyoscyamine was detected in tobacco leaves expressing EVM0022661.2 (Fig. 6e), suggesting that EVM0022661.2 has hyoscyamine *N*-demethylase activity. To further verify the activity of EVM0022661.2, we expressed EVM0022661.2 in yeast and the corresponding *N*-demethylase activity was assayed in yeast microsomes (Fig. 6f). Norhyoscyamine was readily detected in assays containing microsomes isolated from yeast expressing EVM0022661.2 and hyoscyamine. To validate the function of EVM0022661.2 in plants, we overexpressed it in the hairy roots of *A. belladonna* (Supplementary Fig. 49). The norhyoscyamine levels in *EVM0022661.2* overexpression lines significantly increased by ~2.09-fold to ~5.70-fold, compared with those in vector control lines (Fig. 6g). Furthermore, we applied the CRISPR/Cas9 system to generate mutants of the *EVM0022661.2* gene in the hairy roots of *A. belladonna* (Supplementary Fig. 49). When *EVM0022661.2* was edited, the norhyoscyamine level decreased to ~17% to ~26% of that in vector control lines (Fig. 6h). Taken together, our data provide evidence that the production of norhyoscyamine is catalyzed by EVM0022661.2.

## 2 DISCUSSION

Some species in the family Solanaceae are of great value to human, such as tomato and potato, while others produce such lethal toxic compounds that they are given ominous names, such as *A. belladonna*, which is also called deadly nightshade. Given that most sequenced genomes in the Solanaceae are from crops, the high-quality genomes of the two medical plants presented here have provided a great opportunity to gain a complete understanding of the evolution of the mTAs biosynthetic pathway. Based on the high-quality genome sequence, we identified an additional WGT event for *A. belladonna* after its split from *L. chinensis*. The genome size of *A. belladonna* is smaller than that of *D. stramonium*; however, the gene number in *A. belladonna* is much larger than that in *D. stramonium* due to polyploidy. We found that extreme TE amplification (especially of Gypsy TEs) in *D. stramonium* caused this increase in genome size.

Although the chemical and enzymatic routes of hyoscyamine and scopolamine biosynthesis have been clarified, the genes encoding those enzymes have not all been characterized in a single species. In the present work, we elucidated the hyoscyamine and scopolamine biosynthetic pathways by functional identification of *MPO* and *TRI* from *A. belladonna*. Thus, the mTAs biosynthetic genes of *A. belladonna* have been functionally characterized, which will facilitate the exploration of mTAs evolution. Furthermore, combined with the high-quality genome, abundant transcriptome data, easy genetic manipulation, and easy virus-induced gene silencing, it also makes *A. belladonna* an ideal reference species for studying the further modification of mTAs, transcriptional regulation, and biosynthesis of other mTAs. Correspondingly, we characterized a *N*-demethylase in *A. belladonna* that converts hyoscyamine to norhyoscyamine (Fig. 6). However, trace amounts of norhyoscyamine were detected when we performed an *N*-demethylation activity test in transient expression assay in tobacco leaves and in yeast microsomes (Fig. 6d, e). This may be due to non-specific enzyme catalysis because *N*-demethylation of TAs might be a general mechanism to detoxify metabolites, even in mammals. Consistently, norhyoscyamine was also detected in the engineered hyoscyamine-producing yeast strains. Furthermore, two CYPs from humans, HsCYP2C19 and HsCYP2D6, involved in the *N*-demethylation of hyoscyamine were identified. Considering the distant relationship between humans and *A. belladonna* and the low identity between HsCYP2C19/HsCYP2D6 and EVM0022661.2 (lower than 25%, Supplementary Fig. 50), we speculate that the similar function of *N*-demethylation of hyoscyamine is the consequence of convergent evolution.

Solanaceae species produce diverse types of TAs in addition to hyoscyamine and scopolamine. However, the genetic basis of the broad distribution of TAs across Solanaceae remains unclear. Using the abundant genomic data for the Solanaceae family, we explored the evolution of the biosynthesis of tropine, the core structural component of TAs. Through phylogenetic analysis, microsynteny analysis, and in vivo/in vitro enzymatic assays, we provided a clear evolutionary landscape of TAs biosynthesis in the Solanaceae

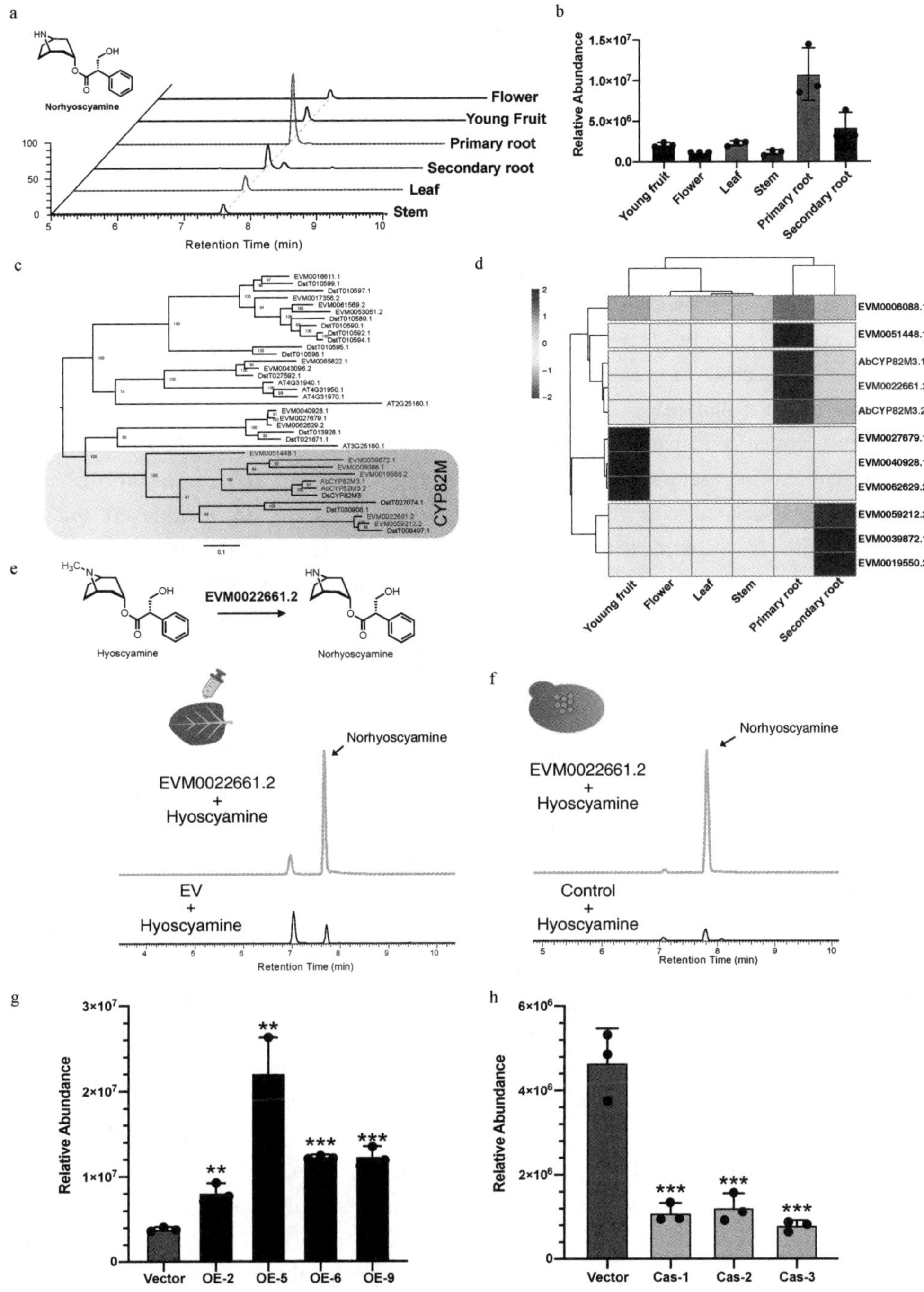


**Fig. 6 Characterization of the *N*-demethylase of hyoscyamine in *A. belladonna***

(a) Analysis of norhyoscyamine content in different tissues of *A. belladonna* by UPLC-MS. The light blue line represents the retention time of norhyoscyamine. (b) The relative abundance of norhyoscyamine in different tissues of *A. belladonna*. The data are presented as means values +/− s. d. ($n = 3$ biologically independent samples). (c) The maximum-likelihood tree of the CYP82 subfamily in *A. belladonna*, *D. stramonium* and *A. thaliana*. The CYP82M clade is highlighted. The bootstrap support value ($n = 1000$) is shown on the branch. (d) The coexpression analysis of CYP82M family members in different tissues of *A. belladonna*. The expression values are scaled as TPM. (e) Functional identification of the *N*-demethylase activity of EVM0022661. 2 by tobacco transient expression assays. Extracted ion chromatograms showing the in vivo *N*-demethylase activity of EVM0022661. 2 in tobacco leaves. Hyoscyamine was used as a substrate by infiltrating tobacco leaves. (f) Functional identification of the *N*-demethylase activity of EVM0022661. 2 using microsomes extracted from a yeast strain expressing EVM0022661. 2; the untransformed yeast strain was used as a negative control. (g) The relative abundance of norhyoscyamine in the EVM0022661. 2 overexpressed *A. belladonna* hairy roots. The data are presented as means values +/− s. d. (n = 3 biologically independent samples). ** represents significant difference from control line (Vector) analyzed by two-sided Student's *t*-test at the level of $P < 0.01$. *** represents significant difference from control line (Vector) analyzed by two-sided Student's *t*-test at the level of $P < 0.001$. ** $P = 0.0030$ (OE-2), ** $P = 0.0016$ (OE-5), *** $P = 0.0000$ (OE-6), *** $P = 0.0003$ (OE-9). (h) The relative abundance of norhyoscyamine in the EVM0022661. 2 genome-edited *A. belladonna* hairy roots. The data are presented as means values +/− s. d. ($n = 3$ biologically independent samples). *** represents significant difference from control line (Vector) analyzed by two-sided Student's *t*-test at the level of $P < 0.01$. *** $P = 0.0018$ (Cas-1), *** $P = 0.0024$ (Cas-2), *** $P = 0.0012$ (Cas-3). Source data underlying (b, d, g) and (h) are provided as a Source Data file.

family. Our results suggested that the biosynthetic genes of tropine are conserved across this family. Interestingly, tropine was detected in hot pepper, a popular vegetable and source of capsaicin. Although the poisonousness of tropine has not been reported, we cannot exclude the possibility that tropine in hot pepper can be converted into physiologically toxic compounds. Furthermore, we identified a conserved gene cluster comprising *CYP82M3* and *TRI* in Solanaceae. Recently, much evidence has indicated that the gene cluster is more common than previously thought, especially in the biosynthesis of plant natural products, such as morphinan, thalianol and momilactones. In Solanaceae, Itkin et al. reported a conserved gene cluster contributing to steroidal glycoalkaloid (SGA) biosynthesis in potato and tomato; Fan et al. reported a gene cluster associated with medium chain acyl sugar biosynthesis, which was located next to the SGAs gene cluster, implying that this mechanism might be prevalent in this family and helping to elucidate the biosynthesis and evolution of other secondary metabolisms in Solanaceae. By linking the TRI-CYP82M3 gene cluster genotype and tropine phenotype, we found that this gene cluster cannot ensure tropine production (Fig. 4), which is contracted with the synchronization of the gene cluster genotype and metabolite pheno-type observed in other species. Both tomato and potato contain this gene cluster, but tropine was not detected in them (Fig. 4b). In contrast, tropine production is associated with the duplication of *TRI*, suggesting that more powerful TRI with higher tropinone reductase activity and more specific expression in roots emerged through TRI duplication in some genera (Fig. 3). However, we cannot exclude the possibility that the duplication of TRI occurred in Solanoideae and has since been lost in some genera in Solaneae. In *Physalis floridana*, a species belonging to Physaleae, also has a duplicated TRI in its TRI-CYP82M3 gene cluster (Supplementary Fig. 51). Furthermore, it is very likely that *Physalis floridana* contains TAs as well because *Physalis peruviana*, another species in the *Physalis* genus, contains tropine. It would be interesting to investigate TAs content and biosynthesis in *P. floridana* in the future. Regarding the retained *TRI* in tomato and potato, one possibility is that they are undergoing nonfunctionalization or pseudogenization, similar to what happened to *LS* and *CYP80F1* in *C. annuum*. Nevertheless, we cannot reject the speculation that *TRI*s in tomato and potato have undergone neofunctionalization and may have distinct biochemical activities by gaining novel enzymatic functions that have not been identified. Taken together, our findings indicated that gene clusters combined with gene duplication underlie the widespread distribution of tropine in Solanaceae.

Regarding the specific esterification and consequent modification of tropine to produce scopolamine in two distant genera, our results support previous findings that these two species (representatives of Daturaeae and Hyoscyameae) do not comprise a monophyletic clade (Fig. 2a). It is likely that the biosynthesis of mTAs appeared more than once, even in the same family, because of convergent evolution. The microsynteny analysis rejected this hypothesis, although the results of phylogenetic analysis and sequence alignments supported it. First, the genomic region *LS* showed a high degree of synteny across Solanaceae, even in *Petunia*, which is not included in the "x= 12" clade; the nucleotide sequence identity between *AbLS* and *DsLS* is as high as ~89%, and the functional *LS* of the two species are syntenic (Supplementary Figs. 34, 40). Second, a portion of the *AbLS* promoter region can be traced to the corresponding syntenic region of species in *Petunia*, *Capsicum*, *Solanum*, and *Iochroma*. Even the first two exons of *AbLS* can be found in the syntenic region of *Iochroma cyaneum* (Fig. 5d; Supplementary Figs. 34, 35). Moreover, the microsynteny analysis of *CYP80F1* provides more evidence. Similar to the *LS* gene, the genomic blocks of the *CYP80F1* gene likewise showed a high degree of synteny across Solanaceae, whereas only *DsCYP80F1* and *AbCYP80F1* were syntenic. Nevertheless, two exons of *CYP80F1* from *A. belladonna* can be found in hot pepper and tomato. All the evidence related to *LS* and *CYP80F1* indicates that the mTAs biosynthesis pathway might exist in the early diverging Solanaceae ancestor, probably before the *P. axillaris* speciation event, and gene loss led to the uneven distribution of mTAs in Solanaceae. Although evolutionary innovation by neo-functionalization or subfunctionalization through gene duplication has been reported in many species, a perspective of gene loss as a pervasive source of genetic change that causes phenotypic diversity has been proposed since the burst of high-quality genome sequencing (reviewed by Albalat et al.). The pervasiveness of gene loss in most life forms suggests that gene loss would be a general force that affects all organisms. For instance, the biased loss of the wingless (*Wnt*) gene, a key regulator involved in animal cell fate determination during tissue differentiation, in different animal taxa contributes to the varying shapes of animals. In Solanaceae, the loss of *AN2* leads to white flowers in *P. axillaris*, which might change its pollinators. Similarly, the asymmetric loss of medium chain acyl sugar biosynthesis genes also determined the distribution of medium chain acyl sugar in Solanaceae.

## 3 METHODS

Plant materials *A. belladonna* and *D. stramonium* were grown in a greenhouse at 24℃ under a light period of 16-h light/8-h dark. The fresh leaves were collected to exact high-quality genomic DNA for genome sequencing. Fresh leaves of *Lycium chinense* were collected from Anning District,

Gansu Province, for high-throughput full-length sequencing. For transcriptome sequencing, tissues of *A. belladonna* and *D. stramonium* were sampled, including leaf, stem, flower, fruit, primary roots, and secondary roots tissues. To validate the TAs and mTAs contents in *S. lycopersicum*, *S. tuberosum*, *S. melongena*, *C. annuum*, *L. chinense*, *N. tabacum*, and *P. hybrida*, we cultured those plants in our greenhouse at 24 ℃ under a light period of 16-h light/8-h dark. To perform transient expression assays in tobacco leaves, the *Nicotiana benthamiana* were grown in the greenhouse at 28℃ under a light period of 16-h light/8-h dark.

Genome sequencing For Nanopore sequencing of *A. belladonna*, high-quality genomic DNA was extracted from young leaves using the cetyltrimethylammonium bromide (CTAB) method and purified by a QIAGEN DNA purification kit. For each Nanopore library, high-quality genomic DNA fragments (> 20 kb) were selected using BluePippin and used to construct long-read libraries following the protocols for the ONT platform (https://nanoporetech.com). The libraries were sequenced using GRIDION X5 (v 9.4.1; Oxford Nanopore Technologies) with 22 nanopore flow cells and the SQK-LSK108 sequencing kit. Base-calling of the raw nanopore reads was performed using the Oxford Nanopore base caller GUPPY (v 3.2.2; Oxford Nanopore Technologies) with default parameters.

For circular consensus sequencing of *D. stramonium*, high-quality genomic DNA was isolated from young leaves of *D. stramonium* using the CTAB method. A 15 kb DNA SMRTbell library was constructed following the protocol for the PacBio Sequel2 platform and the circular consensus sequencing (CCS) was performed; these sequencing reads are known as highly accurate long reads, or HiFi reads.

For Illumina sequencing of *A. belladonna* and *D. stramonium*, genomic DNA was extracted from young leaves using the CTAB method and broken into random fragments. Short-read libraries of *A. belladonna* and *D. stramonium* were constructed according to Illumina's standard protocol, and paired-end reads (2 × 150 bp) were sequenced on an Illumina HiSeq X Ten platform.

To construct Hi-C libraries, young leaves of *A. belladonna* and *D. stramonium* were fixed in 1% formaldehyde for crosslinking. Cells were lysed using a Dounce homogenizer and digested using the *Hin*d III restriction enzyme. The DNA ends were filled and labeled with biotin and the filled-in *Hin*d III sites were ligated to form *Nhe* I sites. Complexes containing the biotin-labeled ligation products were purified and sheared, and the biotinylated Hi-C ligation products were pulled down and used to construct Illumina sequencing libraries.

Genome size estimation Genome size was estimated by *K*-mer frequency distribution analysis (genome Size= *K*-mer_num/Peak_depth). First, the short reads were filtered using fastp (v 0.19.4) with default parameters. Subsequently, the *K*-mers were counted using Jellyfish (v 2.2.10) with the parameter "-C -m 51 -s 10000000000 -t 50". The output file was then used as input for GenomeScope to estimate the genome size with default parameters. The frequency distribution of 17-mers is based on the genome characteristics and in the light of the pattern of Poisson distribution.

Genome assembly To assemble the contigs of *A. belladonna*, the ONT reads were first corrected and trimmed using Nextdenovo (v2.0-beta.1) (parameters: read_cuoff = 1k, seed_cutoff = 28k, blocksize = 8 g) (https://github.com/Nextomics/NextDenovo.git). The corrected ONT reads were directly assembled using SMARTDENOVO (v 1.0.0) with default para-meters. (https://omictools.com/smartdenovo-tool). The assembled contigs were polished four times by Pilon (v 1.18) and NextPolish (v 1.0.5) with default parameters, using 53.88 Gb (34×) of Illumina short reads, to yield high-quality contigs of *A. belladonna*.

To primarily assemble the genome of *D. stramonium*, a total of 828.66 Gb of raw PacBio subreads were filtered and corrected using the pbccs pipeline with default parameters (https://github.com/PacificBiosciences/ccs). The resulting CCS reads were subjected to hifiasm (v 0.14) for de novo assembly with default parameters (https://github.com/chhylp123/hifiasm). We corrected the primary contigs with the Pilon (v 1.18) program with default parameters using 145.27 Gb (79×) of Illumina paired-end reads. BWA (v 0.7.10-r789) and SAMtools (v 1.9) were used for read alignment and SAM/BAM format conversion.

Chromosomal genome construction Hi-C Pro (v 2.11.4) was used to validate paired-end reads with default parameters. Draft contigs were clustered and ordered into chromosomes following intrachromosomal interactions estimated by LACHESIS (v 1.0.0). Validated paired-end reads were also used to calculate interchromosomal interactions to analyze chromosome territories. The contigs were further independently assembled into scaffolds using SLR (v 1.0.0, https://github.com/luojunwei/SLR) and SALSA (v 2.2) to validate the accuracy of the LACHESIS assembly with default parameters. To assess the completeness of *A. belladonna* and *D. stramonium*, we performed Benchmarking Universal Single-Copy Orthologs (BUSCO, v 5.3.2) analysis against embryophyta_odb10 (release Sep 2020) with default parameters.

Annotation of genome sequences To enable better parallel computation and accelerate the annotation of repetitive sequences, we used the scaffolds rather than the chromosome-level genome assembly. Tandem repeats and TEs were predicted separately. Tandem repeats were identified using Tandem Repeats Finder (v 4.0.9), which was implemented with 'Match = 2, Mismatch = 7, Delta = 7, PM = 80, PI = 10, Minscore = 50 and MaxPeriod = 2000'. Then, for TE identification, a combination of homology-based and de novo approaches were mainly used. We first used RepeatMasker (v 4.0.5) (http://www.repeatmasker.org) with the Repbase TE library and RepeatProteinMasker (v 1.36) with the TE protein database to search for homologous repeat sequences in the genome with default parameters. Then, de novo-based identification was performed by RepeatModeler (v 1.0.9) (http://www.repeatmasker.org/RepeatModeler.html) and LTR_FINDER (v 1.0.6) with default parameters to predict the repeat element boundaries and family relationships from genome data. Finally, all repeat identification results from different software were integrated with redundancy elimination as the final repeat annotation results. We applied the same protocol to annotate the genome sequences of *A. belladonna* and *D. stramonium* for further comparison.

Three complementary methods incorporated in the MAKER pipeline (v 2.31.9) were employed to predict the high-quality protein-coding genes: homology-based, de novo, and transcriptome-based predictions. In homology-based predictions, protein sequences of six species (*A. thaliana*, *S. tuberosum*, *S. lycopersicum*, *C. annuum*, *N. tabacum*, *S. pennellii*, and *S. melongena*) were downloaded from the Phytozome database (https://phytozome.jgi.doe.gov/pz/portal.html) and aligned to the repeat-masked genomes of two species by BLASTN with an E-value cutoff of 1e-5, and gene models were defined using GeMoMa (v 1.3.1) with default parameters. The aligned sequence and candidate genomic regions were corrected and optimized by Gene-Wise (v 2.4.1) with default parameters to further predict the exact structure of the protein-coding gene. For de novo prediction, 3 000 full-length genes were randomly selected from the homology-based prediction results to train gene models of the two species. Four de novo prediction programs, including Augustus (v 3.2.1), GlimmerHMM (v 3.0.4), Genscan (v 1.1), and SNAP (v 2006-07-28), were utilized with *A. belladonna* and *D. stramonium* gene models for de novo prediction with default parameters. Genes with coding sequences < 150 bp were discarded. For transcriptome-based predictions, we first performed end-trimming by SeqClean (http://www.tigr.org/tdb/tgi/software) for transcriptome assembly. Then, all transcript sequences from different tissues (flowers, leaves, stems, fruits, primary roots, and secondary roots) were aligned to the genome by the PASA pipeline (v 2.1.0) with default parameters, and TransDecoder (v 3.0.0, https://github.com/TransDecoder) was used to produce the annotation file. All predictions of gene models from the above approaches were finally integrated using EVidenceModeler software (EVM; v 1.1.1) with default parameters to generate consensus gene sets. The completeness of the gene sets was evaluated for both species with BUSCO (v 5.3.2) against embryophyta_odb10.

Noncoding RNAs (ncRNAs) and functional annotation  Noncoding RNAs and small RNAs were annotated by alignment to the Rfam and miRNA databases using INFERNAL (v 1.1.2) and BLASTN with default parameters, respectively. The tRNA genes were identified using the tRNAscan-SE software (v 2.0) with default parameters. rRNA fragments were predicted by alignment to rRNA sequences based on BLASTN analysis (E-value of 1e-10). Functional annotations of the predicted protein-coding genes were performed (E-value of 1e-5) against publicly available protein databases including KEGG, SwissProt, NR databases, and InterPro. InterProScan (v 4.8) and HMMER (v 3.3) were used to query the InterPro and Pfam databases to identify the protein domain, respectively. Then, GO terms were assigned by the Blast2GO pipeline (v 3.1.3) with default parameters. GO enrichment and KEGG pathway analysis were performed using an online platform, OmicShare (https://www.omicshare.com/).

Identification and classification of TEs  Long terminal repeat retrotransposons (LTR-RTs) were initially identified using LTRFinder (v 1.02) and LTRharvest (v 1.5.10). LTR_retriever (v 3.0) was then used to filter out false LTR-RTs using structural and sequence features of target site duplications, terminal motifs, and LTR-RT Pfam domains with default parameters. Finally, LTR-RTs were annotated by RepeatMasker using the constructed nonredundant LTR-RT library and intact LTR insertion time provided by LTR_retriever. The identification parameters were as follows: for LTR-harvest, overlaps best -seed 20-minlenltr 100-maxlenltr 2 000-mindistltr 3 000-maxdistltr 25 000-similar 85-mintsd 4-maxtsd 20-motif tgca-motifmis 1-vic 60-xdrop 5-mat 2-mis-2-ins-3-del-3, and for LTR-finder:-D 15 000-d 1 000-L 7 000-l 100-p 20-C-M 0.9. The two datasets were integrated to remove false positives using the LTR-retriever package. The insertion time was estimated using the formula

$$T = Ks/2r \tag{1}$$

where *Ks* is the divergence rate and *r* ($3.48 \times 10^{-9}$) is the substitution rate.

Genome evolution analysis  To clarify the phylogenetic relationships of *A. belladonna*, *D. stramonium*, and *Lycium chinense*, we selected 10 additional species for analyses of WGD events. The homologous groups among all 13 species were identified using the OrthoMCL (v 2.0.9) method. The homologous clusters were obtained using the Markov graph clustering (MCL; v 14.137) algorithm, through an all-vs-all sequence similarity search by BLASTP (v 2.2.29) with an E-value cutoff of 1e-3. Then we extracted single-copy homologous genes from OrthoMCL results. Protein sequences were aligned by MAFFT (v 7.407) and Gblocks (v 0.91b) with default parameters to extract conserved sites of multiple sequence alignment results and construct a phylogenetic tree by RAxML (v 8.1.13) with the GTRGAMMA model for amino acid sequences and *Oryza sativa* as the outgroup. Then, 1000 bootstrap analyses were performed to test the robustness of each branch. To estimate the divergence time, we extracted the 4-fold sites from the 229 homolog pairs and estimated the divergence time using MCMCTree in the PAML (v 4.9e) package with the "relaxed-clock (clock = 2)" model and "F84" model. The divergence times of *Vitis vinifera* and *Oryza sativa* (mean: 160.0 Mya, std dev: 4.0) obtained from the TimeTree database (http://www.timetree.org) were applied to calibrate the divergence times. CAFE (v 3.1) was used to identify expansions and contractions of gene families with default parameters following divergence predicted by the phylogenetic tree with a probabilistic graphical model. A conditional *P* value was calculated for each gene family, and families with conditional *P* values $< 0.05$ were considered to have had a significantly accelerated rate of expansion or contraction.

Genome synteny and whole-genome duplication (WGD) event analysis The distribution of synonymous substitutions per site (*Ks*) within paralogs was used to examine the most recent WGD event in *A. belladonna* and *D. stramonium*. For intergenomic comparison, we compared the *A. belladonna* and *D. stramonium* genomes with those of five other species (eggplant, tobacco, tomato, grape, and pepper) or with themselves. The homologs between these species were identified using MCScanX (v 11-13-2012). Subsequently, the *Ks* substitution rates of the gene pairs in syntenic blocks were calculated. Finally, we illustrated the *Ks* distribution and generated dot plots of homologous blocks using MCScanX. *Ks* values between colinear genes were estimated using the CodeML approach as implemented in the PAML package. Finally, we illustrated the *Ks* distribution and created dot plots of homologous blocks using MCScanX. The CIRCOS (v 0.69.6) software was used to visualize gene density, GC content, repeat content, and gene synteny on individual pseudochromosomes.

RNA-seq sequencing and gene coexpression analysis Total RNA was extracted using a RNeasy Plus Mini Kit (Qiagen). Then mRNA isolation, fragmentation, and purification were performed using a TruSeq RNA Library Prep Kit v.2 (Illumina, San Diego, CA, USA). The libraries were sequenced using the Illumina NextSeq 500 platform. Raw RNA-seq data (Supplementary Table 25) were trimmed using TRIMMOMATIC (v 0.39). Cleaned reads were mapped to genome assembly guided by gene annotation models using HISAT2 (v 2.0.5) with default parameters. The read counts and transcripts per million (TPM) values for each gene was performed by StringTie (v 1.3.3b). After then the read counts and TPM values were filtered using the sva R package (v 3.11) to decrease batch effects and hidden variables. Differentially expressed genes (DEGs) were detected using DESeq2 (v 1.27.12) based on absolute log 2 transformed fold-change values $> 2$ and a *P* value of 0.05 after applying the Benjamini-Hochberg correction.

To identify relationships between differentially expressed genes, we performed weighted gene coexpression analysis with the R package WGCNA (v. 1.69). All R packages were run in version 3.1 of R. The expression data were prefiltered using the built-in quality control function. A signed coexpression network was constructed using a soft-thresholding power of 8 and default parameters. The only exception was the mergeCutHeight parameter, controlling the minimum distance between coexpression clusters, which was set to 0.25. Finally, we obtained 30 clusters for these genes. Then we used Cytoscape (v 3.5.1) to display the network. Network statistics were calculated using Network Analyzer in Cytoscape.

Full-length RNA sequencing and analysis of *L. chinense* The total RNA of young *L. chinense* leaves was extracted using the RNeasy Plus Mini Kit (Qiagen). RNA quality was analyzed using the Plant RNA Nano assay of a 2,100 Bioanalyzer (Agilent). PacBio library preparation and sequencing were performed according to the Iso-Seq protocol by Pacific Biosciences. Sequencing was performed on the PacBio RSII System. PacBio ROIs were processed using PacBio's Iso-seq ToFU tool and PacBio SMRT Analysis (v 5.1) with default settings. Then, we classified the reads into full-length and non-full-length reads by ToFU pbtranscript classify with default parameters, and the full-length reads were clustered and error corrected using ToFU pbtranscript cluster with default settings. The full-length sequences generated by ToFU were then clustered by CD-HIT (v 4.8.1) to remove redundancy furthermore. Subsequently, putative coding regions were predicted using TransDecoder.

Identification of genes involved in mTAs biosynthesis According to our previous studies, we downloaded first-generation sequencing data of the key enzymes in the TAs biosynthetic pathway from the National Center for Biotechnology Information (NCBI) database. We annotated the key enzyme genes by BLAST (v 2.2.28) and aligned them with the Pfam database by HMMER (v 3.3) with default parameters in *A. belladonna*, *D. stramonium*, and eight other Solanaceae species.

*MPO* RNA interference transgenic hairy root establishment and tropane alkaloid content analysis The 521-bp fragment of *AbMPO1* (*EVM0017027.2*) and *AbMPO2* (*EVM0068072.1*) was amplified and inserted into the RNA interference vector pHannibal, generating AbMPO1-RNAi and AbMPO2-RNAi cassettes. Thereafter, the cassettes were inserted into the plant expression vector pBIN19 and then transferred into *Agrobacterium tumefaciens* strain C58C1, which was used to infect leaf explants obtained from 4-week-old *A. belladonna* plants to initiate root cultures on MS medium. Five independent positive transformants were selected, and the relative expression levels of *AbMPO1* and *AbMPO2* were measured by qRT-PCR (Supplementary Fig. 11). The contents of tropane alkaloids in hairy root cultures were analyzed by high-performance liquid chromatography (HPLC). The HPLC system was a Shimadzu LC-20 A instrument (Shimadzu Corp., Kyoto, Japan), and the detector was the photo-diode array. The detecting wavelength was 226 nm. The mobile phase consisted of $CH_3CN$: 20 mmol/L $NH_4OAc$ (11 : 89, *V/V*), and the $NH_4OAc$ solution included 0.1% EtOAc (pH 4.0). To exact the alkaloids, 200 mg fine powdered dry hairy roots were immersed in the exaction buffer (chloroform/methanol/17% ammonia, 15 : 5 : 1, *V/V/V*) over night, and then the filtered exaction buffer was evaporated at 40 ℃. The dried samples were dissolved in 5 ml of chloroform. Subsequently, 2 mL $H_2SO_4$ (0.5 mol/L) was added to extract the alkaloid into the aqueous phase, which was transferred into a 10 mL EP tube. 1.5 mL of ammonia (17%) and 2 mL chloroform was added in and then the chloroform phase was transferred into a beaker and placed in an oven at 40 ℃ to evaporate the chloroform. The dryness was dissolved in 1 mL methanol. After centrifugation at 13 000 × *g* for 5 min, the supernatant was used for HPLC analysis. All the primers used in the functional characterization of MPO are listed in Supplementary Table 26.

Quantification of tropane alkaloids by UPLC-MS To quantify tropane alkaloids by ultra-high-performance liquid chromatography coupled mass spectrometry (UPLC-MS), the plant samples were lyophilized and ground into a fine powder. One milliliter of extraction buffer containing 20% methanol, and 0.1% formic acid was added to 25 mg of each sample powder. After centrifugation at 13 000 × *g* for 5 min, the supernatant was used for UPLC-MS analysis.

We detected the littorine, hyoscyamine, scopolamine, and nor-hyoscyamine by a Thermo Scientific UltiMate 3 000 UPLC system with a Thermo Scientific Q Exactive Orbitrap LC-MS instrument. A 3 μL volume of each extract was analyzed using a Hypersil GOLD C18 column (2.1 mm × 100 mm, 1.9 μm) obtained from Thermo Scientific (Pittsburgh, PA, USA). Measurements of littorine, hyoscyamine, scopolamine, and norhyoscyamine were taken using electron spray ionization (ESI) in positive ion mode and full MS mode. The instrument parameters were as follows: source voltage of 3.0 kV; capillary temperature of 350 ℃; S-lens RF level of 50; and auxiliary gas heater temperature of 350 ℃. To detect phenyllactate, the same UPLC-MS system and a Symmetry C18 Column with the mobile phases added 0.02% formic acid and instrument parameters were used, but a 3 μL volume of each extract was separated and detected using ESI in negative ion mode and full MS mode. To detect tropinone and tropine, the same UPLC-MS system with the same instrument parameters was used, but a 3 μL volume of each extract was separated by an ACQUITY UPLC BEH HILIC column (2.1 mm × 100 mm, 1.7 μm) obtained from Waters (Milford, MA, USA), and detected using ESI in positive ion mode and full MS mode.

PPAR enzyme activity assay To perform the PPAR activity assays, the coding sequences of *PPAR*s were cloned from the corresponding species and inserted into the protein expression vector pET28a. Recombinant His-tagged PPARs were purified using HisPur Ni-NTA resin. The purified PPARs (20 μg) were incubated with 2 mM phenylpyruvic acid in reaction buffer (500 μL) containing 2 mmol/L NADPH in 50 mmol/L potassium phosphate (pH 8.0) at 30 ℃ for 2 h, while boiled enzyme was used as a negative control. The products were detected by UPLC-MS as described in the above section on quantification of tropane alkaloids by UPLC-MS. The enzymatic kinetics of PPARs were determined for 1 h at pH 8.0. The 250 μL reaction buffer containing 20 μg of PPAR protein, 2 mmol/L NADPH+, and phenylpyruvic acid (0.1 - 14 mmol/L) for the determination of $K_m$ values in 0.1 mol/L Tris-HCl buffer (pH 8.0). The kinetic constants were calculated with a nonlinear regression of the Michaelis-Menten equation using OriginPro (v 8.0, OriginLab). All assays were repeated three times, and mean values with standard deviations are reported. All the primers used for cloning *PPAR*s and constructing protein expression plasmids are listed in Supplementary Table 27.

LS enzyme activity assay To evaluate the activity of the LS enzyme, *AbUGT1* from *A. belladonna* and *LS* from different plants were transiently expressed in *N. benthamiana* leaves. First, the full-length CDSs of *AbUGT1*, *DsLS*, *AbLS*, and *LcLS* were cloned into the transient expression vector pEAQ-HT using the restriction enzymes *Age*I and *Xho*I to generate pEAQ-AbUGT1, pEAQ-DsLS, pEAQ-AbLS, and pEAQ-LcLS, respectively. Subsequently, they were independently transformed into *Agrobacterium* GV3101. Ten milliliters of overnight cultured engineered *Agrobacterium* were centrifuged, and the pellets were resuspended in liquid MS medium containing 10 mmol/L MES, 10 mmol/L $MgCl_2$, and 150 mmol/L acetosyringone to an OD600 of 0.5-0.6. Tobacco leaves were infiltrated with resuspension by using a 1 mL needleless syringe. Four days later, tobacco leaves were infiltrated with substrate solution containing 1 mmol/L tropine and 1 mmol/L phenyllactate. Finally, tobacco leaves infiltrated with substrates were harvested for metabolite analysis after 24 h. Each group had six biological replicates. The littorine was quantified by UPLC-MS as described in the above section on quantification of tropane alkaloids by UPLC-MS. The primers used for cloning *LS*s and constructing overexpression plasmids are listed in Supplementary Table 28.

In vitro TRI enzyme activity assay To characterize the activity of TRI from *A. belladonna*, *D. stramonium*, *C. annuum*, *S. lycopersicum* and *S. tuberosum*, we cloned the coding sequence of *TRI*s from the cDNA of those plants and inserted it into the protein expression vector pET28a. Recombinant His-tagged TRIs were purified using HisPur Ni-NTA resin. To detect the products of TRIs, His-tagged TRIs (5 μg) were incubated with tropinone (100 mmol/L) in the presence of NADPH (200 μmol/L) for 2 h at 30 ℃. Subsequently, the reaction products were extracted and analyzed by UPLC-MS as described in the above section on quantification of tropane alkaloids by UPLC-MS. We detected the activity of TRI by measuring NADPH + $H^+$ consumption, substituted with the direct product tropine, using a spectrophotometer (U3010, HITACHI, Japan) at 340 nm and 30 ℃. Then, 1 mL samples containing 20 μg of TRI protein, 200 μmol/L NADPH + $H^+$, and tropinone (0.01 - 30 mmol/L for the determination of $K_m$ values, as the concentration range of each substrate needed to be adjusted according to the results of enzymatic assays), and 0.1 mol/L potassium phosphate to yield pH 6.4. Data were collected during the initial linear phase of the enzyme reaction to calculate the kinetic parameters. The kinetic constants were calculated with a nonlinear regression of the Michaelis-Menten equation using OriginPro (v 8.0, OriginLab). All assays were repeated three times, and mean values with standard deviations are reported. The primers used for *TRI*s cloning and constructing protein expression plasmids are listed in Supplementary Table 29.

CYP82M3 enzyme activity assay To characterize the activity of CYP82M3, the CDSs of *CYP82M3* from *C. annuum* and *S. lycopersicum* were cloned and inserted into the transient expression vector pEAQ-HT, generating pEAQ-CaCYP82M3 and pEAQ-SlCYP82M3. The CDSs of *AbPMT* and *AbPYKS* were cloned from *A. belladonna* and inserted into pEAQ-HT as well to generate pEAQ-AbPMT and pEAQ-AbPYKS, which provided the substrates of CYP82M3. Subsequently, those vectors were transferred into *Agro-bacterium* GV3101, and then the resulting *Agrobacterium* were infiltrated into tobacco leaves. Four days later, infiltrated tobacco leaves were harvested to detect tropinone by UPLC-MS as described in the above section on quantification of tropane alkaloids by UPLC-MS. The primers used for *CYP82M3* cloning and constructing overexpression plasmids are listed in Supplementary Table 30.

*N*-demethylase activity assay To evaluate the *N*-demethylase activity of EVM0022661.2, methods similar to those described above for LS enzyme activity assays were employed. The CDS of *EVM0022661.2* was amplified from *A. belladonna* and inserted into the pEAQ-HT vector. Subsequently, EVM0022661.2 was transiently expressed in the tobacco leaves and hyoscyamine was infiltrated and used as a substrate after four days. To perform the in vitro *N*-demethylase activity, the CDS of *EVM0022661.2* was inserted into the yeast expression vector pYES2 and transformed into the yeast strain WAT11. An untransformed yeast strain was used as the negative control. The yeast cells were collected by centrifugation and the generated pellets were resuspended twice in TEK (50 mmol/L Tris-HCl, pH 7.4, 1 mmol/L EDTA, 0.1 mol/L KCl) and TESB (50 mmol/L Tris-HCl, pH 7.4, 1 mmol/L EDTA, 0.6 mol/L sorbitol) buffers. Subsequently, the pellets were broken up by a cryogenic homogenizer and the precipitated micro-some pellets were collected by further centrifugation. Consequently, 0.5 mg of resuspended microsomal protein and 100 μmol/L hyoscyamine were included with the reaction buffer (500 μL) at 30 ℃ for 2 h. The detection method of norhyoscyamine was the same as that of hyoscyamine, as described in the above section on quantification of tropane alkaloids by UPLC-MS.

*EVM0022661.2* overexpressed and genome-edited transgenic hairy root establishment To overexpress *EVM0022661.2*, the CDS of *EVM0022661.2* was cloned and inserted into the plasmid pBI121, generating plasmid EVM0022661.2-pBI121. To edit *EVM0022661.2* in the hairy root of *A. belladonna* via CRISPR technology, a 20-bp fragment of the *EVM0022661.2* was used as the targeting sequence for genome editing (Supplementary Fig. 49). Subsequently, the synthesized primers containing targeting sequence was inserted into the p1300-Cas9N vector to generate the genome editing plasmid Cas9N-EVM0022661.2. The constructed plasmids, EVM0022661.2-pBI121 and Cas9N-EVM0022661.2, were then transferred into *Agrobacterium tumefaciens* strain C58C1. The hairy root of *A. belladonna* was established and cultured as described in the above section on *MPO* RNA interference transgenic hairy root establishment and tropane alkaloid content analysis. The primers used for *EVM0022661.2* cloning and constructing plasmids for overexpression and genome edition are listed in Supplementary Table 31.

[张芳源，廖志华，等. Nature Communication，2023，14：1446.]

# Structural and mechanistic insights into the precise product synthesis by a bifunctional miltiradiene synthase

## 1 INTRODUCTION

Diterpenes constitute a large family of natural products. According to backbone structure, diterpenes can be categorized as abietanes, pimaranes, kaurenes, labdanes and fusicoccanes. Diterpenes are diverse in structure and stereochemistry, especially abietane-type diterpenes, thereby providing abundant sources for drug discovery. Triptolide and its analogues exhibit anticancer activity in multiple cancers, including pancreatic cancer, breast cancer and glioma. The anti-ulcer agent ecabet sodium is a dehydroabietic acid derivative prepared from pine resin. Carnosol, an abietane-type diterpene, exhibits anti-inflammatory and anticancer activities. Due to its high medical value, different approaches to synthesize abietane-type diterpenes have been explored. When focusing on the chemical synthesis or the enzymatic reaction of therapeutic natural products, we face an interesting question regarding the mechanisms by which the synthetic process selects a particular isomer of a complex molecule. Considering that the cyclization reactions catalysed by diterpene synthases (diTPSs) show high substrate selectivity and product stereospecificity, diTPSs have become a good target system for structural and functional studies to answer this question.

The diversity of diterpenes derived from the (*E*, *E*, *E*)-geranylgeranyl diphosphate (GGPP) precursor is determined by stereochemically controlled class II and class I diTPS combinations. The enzymatic synthesis of miltiradiene, the key backbone precursor of abietane-type diterpenes, has attracted considerable attentions. Usually, miltiradiene is synthesized through a two-step cyclization reaction that includes sequential conversion of GGPP *via* (+)-copalyl diphosphate (CPP) to miltiradiene. Recently, monofunctional class II diTPS and class I diTPS for biosynthetic miltiradiene have been isolated from seven angiosperm plants. In one case, however, a bifunctional diTPS with two independent active sites (class II/class I) was discovered in *Selaginella moellendorffii* (*S. moellendorffii* miltiradiene synthase, *Sm*MDS). Previously, we applied modular pathway and chimeric diTPS engineering attempts for the high production of miltiradiene in yeast. However, few reports on the structural mechanism of diTPSs can provide structural basis for directed enzyme evolution.

To date, the crystal structure of only three plant diTPSs has been reported, namely monofunctional taxadiene synthase from *Taxus brevifolia* (*Tb*TS), monofunctional *ent*-copalyl diphosphate synthase from *Arabidopsis thaliana* (*At*CPS) and bifunctional abietadiene synthase from *Abies grandis* (*Ag*AS). Compared to abietadiene, levopimaradiene and neoabietadiene (multiple conjugated double-bond products of *Ag*AS), miltiradiene contains the specific cyclohexa-1, 4-diene structure of the distal ring. The apo-state structure of *Ag*AS from gymnosperms has been determined and provides the inferred structure-function relationships underlying mixture abietadienes. The bifunctional diTPS *Ag*AS produces multiple abietane-type products, but *Sm*MDS strictly converts GGPP to dominant miltiradiene with characteristic double bonds (>95% of total products). Thus, we focused on the structure-function catalytic mechanisms to produce diverse abietane backbones and the precise control over carbocation intermediates in the reaction.

Here, through sequence alignment of *Sm*MDS and other class II and class I diTPSs, by site-directed mutagenesis, we identified E690 mutagenesis leads to multiproduct sandaracopimaradiene and miltiradiene. We further determined the apo-state and GGPP-bound state crystal structures of *Sm*MDS, providing the possible catalytic structural mechanism of the bifunctional active pockets and the transportation of (+)-CPP. Our findings are a good example of the intermediate product transport mode in a bifunctional diTPS and the mechanisms by which *Sm*MDS control the fate of carbocations to generate a single product.

## 2 RESULTS

Sandaracopimaradiene supports the conformation of intermediate pimar-15-en-8-yl$^{+}$ Bifunctional *Sm*MDS catalyses protonation-initiated cyclization of GGPP to (+)-CPP and converts (+)-CPP to miltiradiene based on ionization-initiated cyclization (Figure 1a). *Sm*MDS showed high homology with *Ag*AS (identity = 38.36%), isopimaradiene synthase from *Picea abies* (*Pa*ISO, identity = 38.67%) and the levopimaradiene/abietadiene synthase from *Picea abies* (*Pa*LAS, identity = 37.84%). All of these enzymes are bifunctional class II/class I diTPSs that share the same intermediate (+)-CPP. *Ag*AS and *Pa*LAS convert (+)-CPP to multiple products that have the same abietane-type skeleton as miltiradiene, while *Pa*ISO produces the single pimarane-type product isopimaradiene. We focused on the

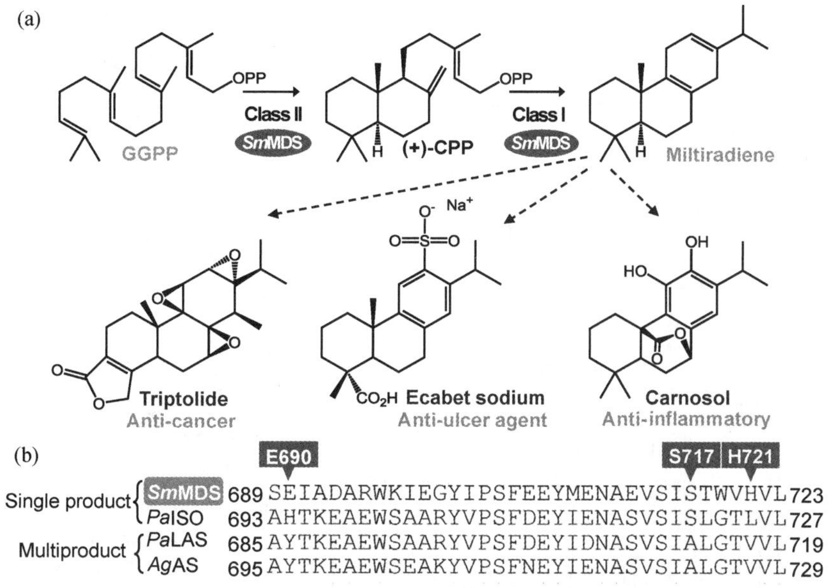

**Figure 1 The biosynthesis pathway of bioactive abietane-type diterpenes with miltiradiene as the precursor (a) and sequence alignment of diterpene synthases (b)**

(a) *Sm*MDS catalyses GGPP to (+)-CPP in class II active site and (+)-CPP to miltiradiene in class I active site. Miltiradiene is the precursor of triptolide, ecabet sodium and carnosol. (b) Sequence alignment of single product diterpene synthases *Sm*MDS and *Pa*ISO and multiproduct diterpene synthases *Pa*LAS and *Ag*AS. The amino acids E690, S717 and H721 in *Sm*MDS are labelled.

relationship between amino acid specificity and product complexity and analysed the sequence alignment to delineate the amino acid differences in the second active site that determine product diversity. Three crucial residues, namely E690, S717 and H721, which are unique in *Sm*MDS and *Pa*ISO, are most likely to modulate product diversity. Compared to key residues in multiproduct diTPSs, E690, S717 and H721 were special in *Sm*MDS, while these positions were occupied by tyrosine, alanine and valine in *Ag*AS and *Pa*LAS (Figure 1b).

The enzyme activity of the E690Y mutant decreased significantly. After extending the reaction time and adding more substrates, the E690Y mutant produced no detectable products. Previous research reported that the *Pa*ISO: H694Y mutation resulted in a slight amount of the products sandaracopimaradiene and isopimaradiene. We hypothesized that the outcome alteration was derived from the replacement of carboxyl groups with hydroxyl groups in the side chain, whereas the enzyme inactivity of *Sm*MDS: E690Y may be caused by too long side chain. Then, we constructed a slightly shorter hydroxylated side chain mutant, E690S, and found that it exhibited partial enzyme activity. Moreover, E690S can also convert GGPP to a new product, sandaracopimaradiene, which was identified by comparing the mass spectra of GC-MS results with previously characterized enzyme products (Figures 2a and S1).

To investigate different amino acid substitution effects on E690, we further performed saturation mutagenesis experiments (Figure 2b). E690Q, which has similar side chain length with WT, had the highest enzyme activity in all of the mutants. E690 mutants that have hydrophobic side chain, namely E690I, E690L, E690V and E690M, all had lower enzyme activity, or no enzyme activity (E690A). E690T, E690C and E690N, which have similar polar neutral side chains to E690S, produced sandaracopimaradiene and miltiradiene. Besides, E690G and E690H were also multiproduct mutants that produce sandaracopimaradiene and miltiradiene. Other too long or special side chain substitutions, that were E690W, E690R, E690F, E690K and E690P, all had no detectable products. Surprisingly, similar property but shorter side chain substitution, E690D, totally abolished its enzyme activity. These results highlighted the importance of residue E690 and also shed light on the rational enzyme design focusing on amino acid property and length.

*Ag*AS: A723S leads to pimaradiene production, while both *Pa*LAS: A713S and *Pa*ISO: S721A result in isopimaradiene and sandaracopimaradiene. The enzyme activity of *Sm*MDS: S717A was almost the same as that of *Sm*MDS and produce only miltiradiene, as well as that of *Sm*MDS: S717G (Figure 2b). Single mutant *Sm*MDS: S721V totally abolished its enzyme activity (Figure 2b). The catalytic activity of the double mutant *Sm*MDS: S717A/H721V was reduced. After extending the reaction time and adding more substrates, S717A/H721V catalysed GGPP to form a series of small products with a molecular ion peak at m/z 272 (Figure S2).

The *Sm*MDS: E690S and similar polar neutral side chain amino acid substitutions indicate that *Sm*MDS catalysed (+)-CPP to generate the pimar-15-en-8-yl$^+$ intermediate,

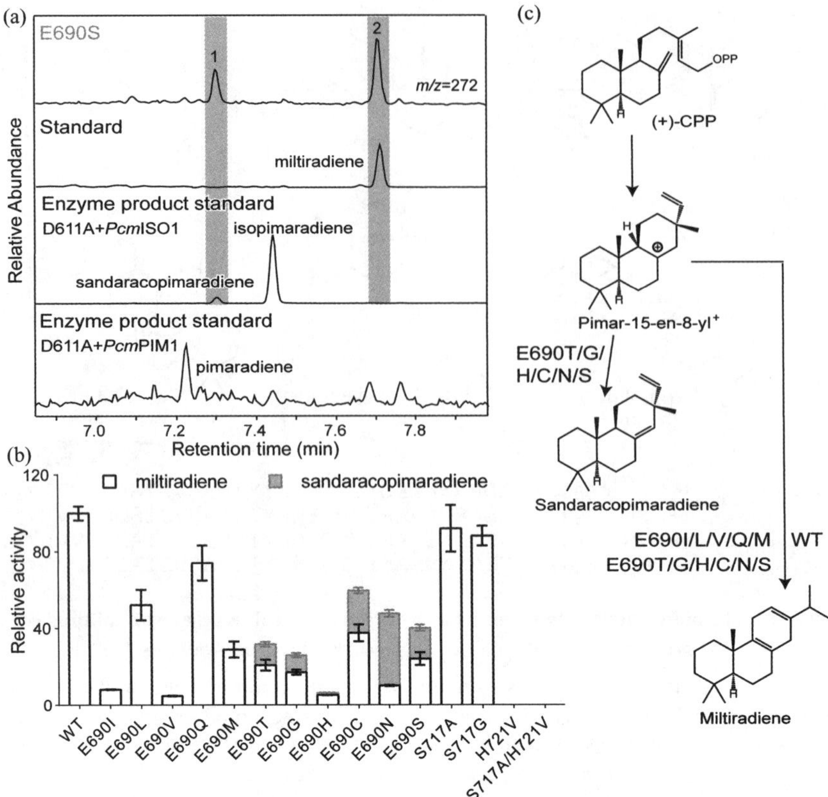


**Figure 2 Effects of E690 and related residue substitutions on *Sm*MDS production outcome**

(a) Extracted ion chromatograms (*m*/*z* 272) from GC-MS analysis of the standard miltiradiene and products formed by E690S, D611A+*Pcm*ISO1 and D611A+*Pcm*PIM1. The enzyme products of D611A+*Pcm*ISO1 and D611A+*Pcm*PIM1 present authentic standards of sandaracopimaradiene, isopimaradiene and pimaradiene. (b) Relative activity of different mutants of *Sm*MDS. (c) Pimar-15-en-8-yl$^+$ is the proposed intermediate in the biosynthesis pathway of abietane-type diterpenes. E690T, E690G, E690H, E690C, E690N and E690S (E690T/G/H/C/N/S) catalyse (+)-CPP to sandaracopimaradiene and miltiradiene. E690I, E690L, E690V, E690Q and E690M (E690I/L/V/Q/M) catalyse (+)-CPP to miltiradiene.

and deprotonation of the carbocation resulted in sandaracopimaradiene (Figure 2c). E690 determines the abietane-type transformation of miltiradiene. The single mutation effect of S717 did not seem obvious in *Sm*MDS, while the double mutant S717A/H721V resulted in small alterations. These results made us consider what the choreographed reaction process is and how specific amino acids participate in and affect the reaction. Meantime, we solved the crystal structure of *Sm*MDS and attempted to reveal the mechanism of tricycle diterpene formation.

Overall structure and functional analysis of *Sm*MDS First, we solved the crystal structure of *Sm*MDS in its apo state (Table S1). The crystal structure contains residues 94-867 and an additional LEHHHHHH tag at the C-terminus. The enzyme with the truncation of the N-terminal residues 1-93 retains catalytic activity (Figure S3) and adopts the classical $\alpha\beta\gamma$ module of plant diTPSs (Figure 3a). We superposed the *Sm*MDS structure with three available plant diTPS structures, which showed RMSD values for Cα of 2.1, 1.8 and 1.6 Å for monofunctional *Tb*TS, monofunctional *At*CPS and bifunctional *Ag*AS, respectively, suggesting that they all have a similar overall architecture (Figures S4d,e,h, S5 and S6; Robert and Gouet, 2014).

To obtain the binding states of *Sm*MDS, we soaked crystals of *Sm*MDS and different mutants with the substrate GGPP and/or miltiradiene. Fortunately, we observed the density for GGPP in a WT structure named as *Sm*MDS$^{4h}$, whose crystal were soaked with GGPP for 4 h (Table S1). *Sm*MDS and *Sm*MDS$^{4h}$ structures differed in the conformation of amino acids around the two active pockets, especially in the class I active pocket (Figure S4a, b). In the *Sm*MDS structure, α33 (residues 839-844) showed strong electron density, and the downstream residues 845-850 were not modelled in the structure because of weak electron density. In the *Sm*MDS$^{4h}$ structure, the density of residues 839-850 was not present. This region is predicted to adopt a loop conformation as the corresponding region in *Tb*TS (Figure S4c). Deletion of residues 841-867 from *Sm*MDS (*Sm*MDS$^{1-840}$) significantly impaired *Sm*MDS activity, while the *Sm*MDS$^{1-846}$ truncation retained enzyme activity (Figure S3), suggesting that residues 841-846 play an important role in maintaining enzyme activity. Based on the structures, we propose that residues 840 - 850 form a flexible loop that may turn to the class I active site during the class I active site reaction.

Structure analysis of class II active site The entrance of class II active site is separated into two tunnels by Thr270 (Figure 3b). We name the tunnel between residues Glu221 and Thr270 as tunnel **1**, while the tunnel between Thr270 and Phe425 as tunnel **2**. In the apo state, we observed a continuous rope-shaped density occupies part of the class II active site and the tunnel **2**, which we assume to be a small molecule from the cell extract. While in the *Sm*MDS$^{4h}$ structure, the continuous rope-shaped density becomes weaker and moved from the active cavity to tunnel **1** (Figure S7). Using Ligand_identification wizard from PHENIX, the rope-shape density was predicted to be corresponding to a nonaethylene glycol (2PE) molecule which was constructed in many crystal structures as a exogenous molecule from *Escherichia coli*. Thus, we temporarily construct 2PE molecule, which fits the electron density well (Figure 3c,d). Besides, substrate GGPP can be modelled in the class II active site of *Sm*MDS$^{4h}$ structure perfectly, in which the pyrophosphate group has the occupancy of 0.5 (Figure 3d).

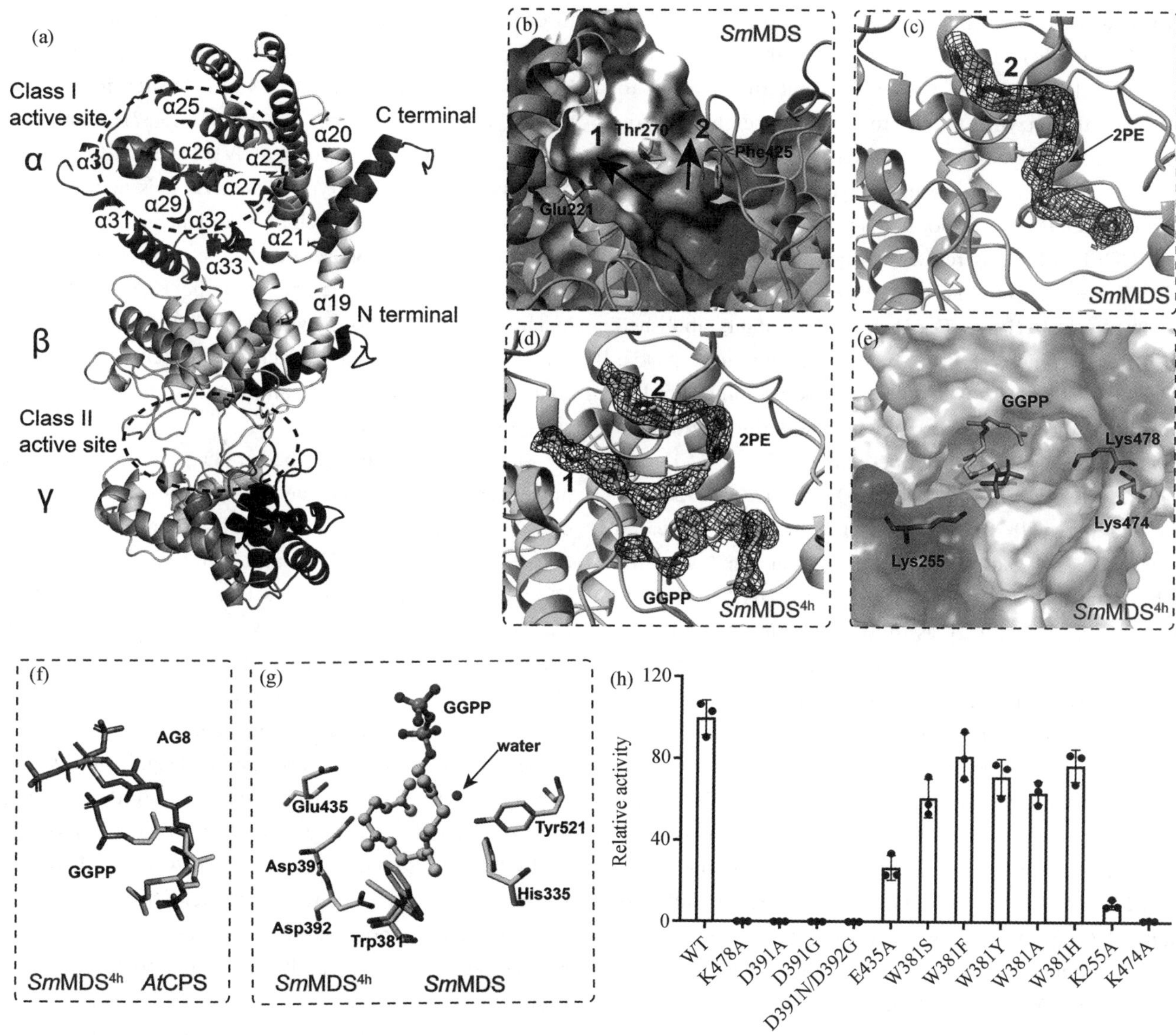


**Figure 3 The overall structure of *Sm*MDS and class II active site**

(a) The structure of *Sm*MDS is coloured in a rainbow mode. The active sites are indicated by circles. (b) Class II active site entrance is separated into two tunnels. *Sm*MDS is coloured violet. (c, d) The 2Fo-Fc map of GGPP and 2PE when constructed in structure (sigma level = 0.6). *Sm*MDS is coloured violet and *Sm*MDS$^{4h}$ is coloured lime green. (e) The protein surface electrostatic potential map of class II active site from *Sm*MDS$^{4h}$ structure. GGPP and key residues are shown as sticks. The red is for negative potential, white at zero, and blue is for positive. (f) Structure comparison of GGPP from *Sm*MDS$^{4h}$ (lime green) and substrate analogue AG8 from *At*CPS (PDB ID: 3PYA, slate). (g) Key residues in the class II active site. Side chain of Trp381 in *Sm*MDS is shown in violet. (h) The relative activity of key residue mutants around the class II active site. All reaction times were limited to comparing relative activities.

In the previously reported structure of *At*CPS in complex with the GGPP analogue AG8, the class II active site was shown to be relatively narrow than that of *Sm*MDS, mainly because of that loop 457 – 468 in the *At*CPS structure is in a more compact conformation than loop 468 – 479 in the *Sm*MDS structure (Figures S4g and S5). The distinct pocket sizes of *At*CPS and *Sm*MDS may correlate with the mechanism by which GGPP is catalysed to different enantiomers of *ent*-CPP and CPP. The substrate analogue AG8 in *At*CPS is located in a limited space, and the phosphate part has dual conformations (Figure 3f). In *Sm*MDS$^{4h}$ structure, the pyrophosphate is predicted flexible and the constructed part interacts with the density that 2PE is located (Figure 3d). Lys478 contributes to the only positive part in the class II active pocket and mutating Lys478 to alanine lost the enzyme activity totally (Figure 3e, h). So, we infer that the dynamic pyrophosphate of *Sm*MDS could possibly interact with Lys478 in catalytic process.

The DXDD motif is located in the isoprene terminal part of GGPP. Mutating residues around the isoprene part of GGPP affected the enzyme activity differently (Figure 3g, h). D391A, D391G and D391N/D392G mutants abolished the entire enzyme activity. E435A mutant had partial enzyme activity. In *Ag*AS, the tyrosine-histidine dyad is speculated as the catalytic base in which mutating histidine to alanine produced hydroxylated derivatives of CPP (Criswell *et al.*, 2012; Mafu *et al.*, 2015; Potter *et al.*, 2014). After soaking with GGPP, a water molecule appeared between Tyr521 and His335, other than the predicted possible catalytic base dyad (Tyr273 and His335), which indicates that Tyr521 may assist the possible catalytic base dyad in *Sm*MDS catalysing process (Figure 3g).

Compared to the class II active site in the two previously solved structures, the most significant change site is Trp381 (Figure 3g). Trp381 is not strictly conserved (Figure S5). The corresponding residue in a CPS from *Salvia miltiorrhiza* is serine, and serine substitution of tryptophan reduced its catalytic activity by more than 100-fold in the production of (+)-CPP. While in *Sm*MDS, the enzyme activities of mutants W381F, W381Y, W381H, W381S and even W381A were all decreased slightly, indicating that W381 is replaceable in *Sm*MDS (Figure 3h). We found that two positively charged residues, Lys255 and Lys474, are highly conserved among CPSs but exhibit considerably different conformations in the *Sm*MDS structure compared to those in the *At*CPS and *Ag*AS structures (Figures 3e and S5). The two residues are located at the entrance of the class II active site, and mutating either residue affected the enzyme activity to different degrees (Figure 3e, h). On the basis of these results, we propose that in addition to the residues located in the pocket, other residues near the pocket entrance influence catalysis. Residues K255 and K474 may assist substrate entry into the class II active pocket by interacting with pyrophosphate.

Produced CPP leaves from a channel The class II active site is located at the $\beta\gamma$ interface. Mutating residues around the pocket, such as Lys478, Asp391 and Asp392 can influence the enzyme activity. The K478A mutant almost lost its enzyme activity entirely. In addition, by analysing *Sm*MDS structure, we found a relatively continuous channel that is close to K478 (Figure 4a). The channel is composed of a narrow part and a broad part with lengths of 17 and 22 Å, respectively, with the exit at the $\alpha\beta$ interface. We predict that (+)-CPP leaves the class II active pocket through this channel. To validate the internal channel, we mutated three residues within this putative channel, namely Leu437, Lys820 and Arg824. L437 is located in the narrow part of the channel, and the mutant L437R retained low activity (Figure 4b, approximately 12% activity relative to the activity of the wild-type protein). This may be because arginine has a longer side chain than leucine, and the longer side chain is able to block the channel. For K820, which is located at the channel exit, both the K820A and K820G mutants lost part of its enzyme activity (Figure 4b). R824A completely lost the catalytic activity, which perhaps led to a completely blocked channel and almost decreased the entire catalytic ability (Figure 4b).

To further investigate whether this channel is functionally important, we compared the miltiradiene-producing activity of wild-type *Sm*MDS with that of a mixture of two mutated *Sm*MDS proteins, D391A and D611A. As D391A and D611A possess class I and class II activity, respectively, the D391A and D611A mutant mixture can recover the whole enzyme activity if the newly produced (+)-CPP enters the class I active site *via* free diffusion (Figure S3). Our results showed that compared to the enzyme activity of the *Sm*MDS, this mutant mixture exhibited significantly reduced enzyme activity (Figure 4b). Interestingly, the R824G and D611A mutant mixture restored catalytic ability of the *Sm*MDS in the same level as the D391A and D611A mutant mixture did. Thus, we infer that after (+)-CPP leaves the channel, it may move towards the class I active site *via* a surface route that is currently unclear but probably lined with positively charged residues. This observation is distinct from the previously reported bifunctional *Ag*AS, where the CPP intermediate is transferred between class II and class I active sites *via* free diffusion. On the basis of these observations, we propose that the structural integration of $\alpha$ and $\beta\gamma$ modules endows *Sm*MDS with a higher miltiradiene-producing efficiency, probably by means of forming an internal transportation route between the two active sites. Notably, in a previous study, a fusion of kaurene synthase-like (KSL) and CPS from *Salvia miltiorrhiza* significantly

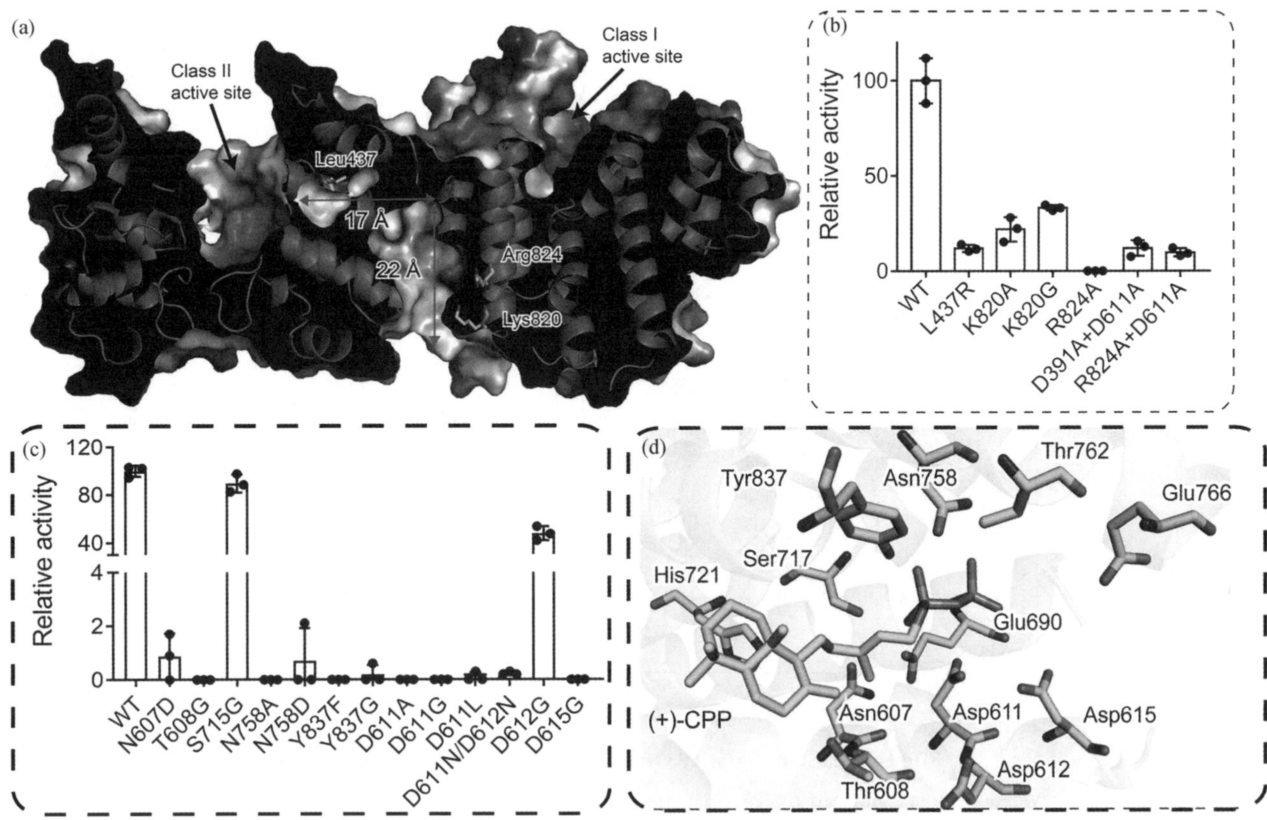


**Figure 4 (+)-CPP channel and the class I active site of *Sm*MDS**

(a) Section view of the channel surface electrostatic potential map in *Sm*MDS$^{4h}$. The red is for negative potential, white at zero, and blue is for positive. (b) Relative activity of mutants related to the channel. All reaction times were limited to comparing the relative activity. (c) Site-directed mutagenesis analysis of key residues involved in the cyclization of (+)-CPP to miltiradiene. All reaction times were limited to comparing the relative activity. (d) The molecular docking results of (+)-CPP (coloured cyan) to the class I active site of *Sm*MDS$^{4h}$. Key residues related to the cyclization reaction are labelled.

increased miltiradiene production in an engineered yeast strain. Therefore, the detailed structural information of the channel of bifunctional *Sm*MDS may provide a basis for designing and optimizing a fusion protein comprising both class I and class II diTPSs activities.

The structural mechanism of converting (+)-CPP to the single product miltiradiene In the *Sm*MDS$^{4h}$ structure, the position of $\alpha$-helixes surrounding the class I active site appears to be tilted to active pocket, which may be caused by enzymatic reaction after soaking with GGPP (Figure S4a, b). In the *Sm*MDS$^{4h}$ structure, $\alpha$29, $\alpha$30 and $\alpha$31 turn to the active site, which facilitates the binding of one magnesium ion by the residues in the conserved motif of **N**$^{758}$**DXXT**$^{762}$**XXXE**$^{766}$ (the bold residues). The bold residues in the conserved motif **D**$^{611}$**DXXD**$^{615}$ bind another two magnesium ions, thus stabilizing the pyrophosphate group. Mutating the residues that bind magnesium ions completely abolished the enzyme activity (Figure 4c).

The diterpene cyclization reaction can be divided into a series of carbocation intermediates that are catalysed by nearby residues or water molecules. To better understand the mechanism of the class I active site reaction, we docked (+)-CPP and miltiradiene with *Sm*MDS$^{4h}$ structure using AutoDockTools and AutoDock Vina software (Figures 4d and S8). SmMDS protein were co-crystallized with miltiradiene. Interestingly, in both *Sm*MDS and *Sm*MDS$^{4h}$ structures, miltiradiene-like residual density was observed in the class I active site, and its position matched to that of the docked ring structures of (+)-CPP and miltiradiene (Figure S8), thus supporting the docking results.

Around (+)-CPP, we found E690, S717, H721, and other key residues (Figures 4d and S8). Targeted mutagenesis of these residues showed that a single residue substitution can alter the product outcome. The T608G mutant exhibited a falling of enzyme activity compared to the enzyme activity of wild-type *Sm*MDS. After extending the reaction time and adding more substrates, T608G produced a mixture of diterpene products, namely, miltiradiene and (+)-copalol (Figures 5a, b and S9a). As the single mutation resulted in multiple products, we hypothesized that (+)-CPP was converted to a (+)-copal-15-yl$^+$ intermediate and that water-assisted deprotonation of this carbocation resulted in the product (+)-copalol (Figure 5b).

Multiple sequence alignment of Class I diTPSs that use

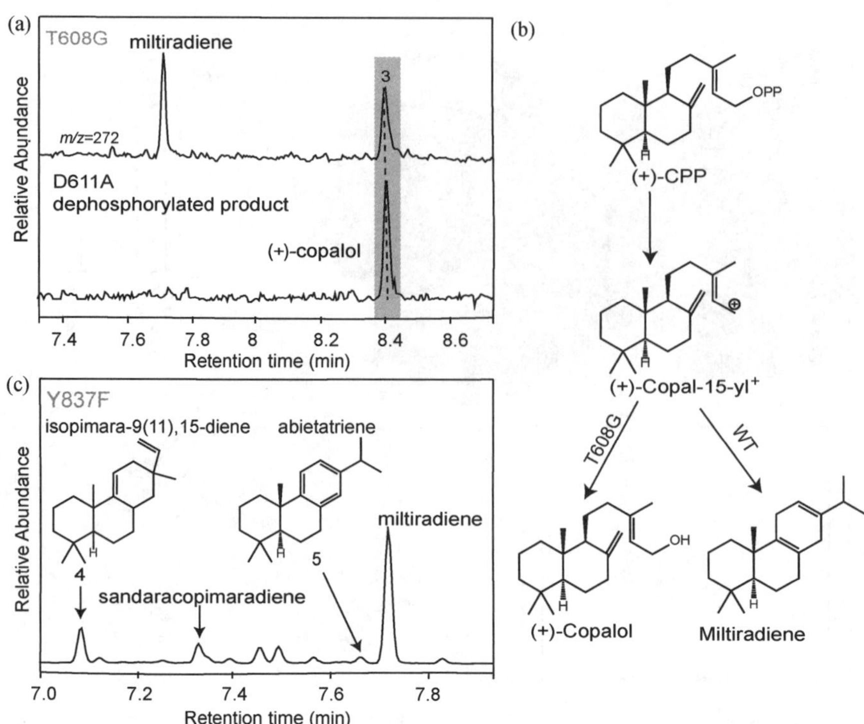


**Figure 5 Effects of the T608G and Y837F mutations on the *Sm*MDS product outcome**

(a) GC-MS analysis of enzymatic products formed by T608G. (b) (+)-Copal-15-yl$^+$ is the proposed intermediate in the biosynthesis pathway of abietane-type diterpenes. T608G catalyses (+)-CPP to (+)-copalol. (c) GC-MS analysis of enzymatic products formed by Y837F.

(+)-CPP as substrate showed that Y837 is a highly conserved residue (Figure S6). Both the Y837F and Y837G mutations decreased the enzyme activity of *Sm*MDS (Figure 4c). After extending the reaction time and adding more substrates, Y837G produced no products, whereas Y837F generated a mixture of diterpene products with a molecular ion peak at $m/z$ 272. The mixture of products was identified to be sandaracopimaradiene, miltiradiene and two other products (Figures 5c and S9b; namely peak4 and peak5). The yield of the compound corresponding to peak 4 was too low to prepare, so we investigated it using gas chromatography quadrupole time-of-flight (GC-Q/TOF). The results showed that its spectrum matched that of isopimara-9 (11),15-diene in the National Institute of Standards and Technology (NIST) library. The compound corresponding to peak 5 was identified to be aromatic abietatriene by comparing the mass spectra with prepared abietatriene (Figure S10). Abietatriene is assumedly derived from miltiradiene spontaneously, but Y837F catalysed GGPP to produce it in small amounts. We hypothesized that the hydroxyl group of the conserved Y837 stabilized intermediate carbocations during cyclization. When phenylalanine was substituted for Y837 (Y837F), the interacting status between the protein and carbocations was destabilized, resulting in multiple diterpene products.

The functional identification of mutants reveals that copal-15-yl$^+$ and pimar-15-en-8-yl$^+$ are key intermediates in the class I active site, which are quenched to (+)-copalol and sandaracopimaradiene, respectively. Based on structural and mutagenesis analyses, we proposed a structural mechanism model in which key residues stabilize intermediate carbocations during the cyclization of (+)-CPP to miltiradiene (Figure 6). The model described five intermediates (**1** – **5**) in the catalytic process. At the beginning of the catalysis reaction, the class I active site utilizes a trinuclear metal cluster triggering the ionization of the isoprenoid substrate (+)-CPP, resulting in the loss of diphosphate abstraction. The ionization of (+)-CPP leads to an allyl cation that can be drawn with two mesomeric structures, namely copal-15-yl$^+$ (intermediate **1**) and intermediate **2**. Then, the carbocation transfers to form the pimar-15-en-8-yl$^+$ (the intermediate **3**). Subsequently, the specific C8-C9 double bond formed at intermediate **4**, with the participation of Y837, S717, H721 and E690. Moreover, based on our molecular docking results, both E690 and Y837 are located at the newly formed ring of miltiradiene and may participate in the final 1, 2-methyl migration of intermediate **4** to intermediate **5**.

## 3 DISCUSSION

Here, we successfully determined the *apo* and GGPP-bound state crystal structures of *Sm*MDS and explored the precise control over copal-15-yl$^+$ and pimar-15-en-8-yl$^+$ intermediates in the presence of enzyme and further demonstrated

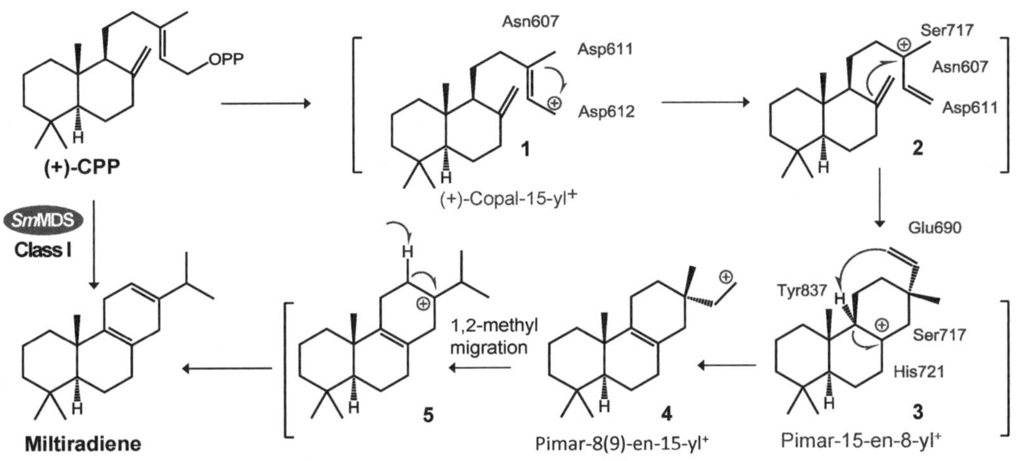

**Figure 6 Cyclization mechanism of (+)-CPP to miltiradiene at the *Sm*MDS class I active site**

*Sm*MDS catalyses (+)-CPP to miltiradiene through five intermediates, namely, intermediate **1**–**5**. (+)-Copal-15-yl$^+$ (**1**) and pimar-15-en-8-yl$^+$ (**3**) are marked blue. Curved arrows show movement of electrons. The positions of amino acid residues were drawn according to the docking results.

an effective transport mode of (+)-CPP. As described for multiple sequential post-transition-state bifurcations, the inferred pimar-15-en-8-yl$^+$ rearrangement mechanisms in the absence of enzymes have significant implications for ensuing selectivity prediction and controlling biosynthesis of complex organic reactions in general. Early mechanistic work by Ravn *et al*. demonstrated the intermediacy of pimar-15-en-8-yl$^+$ (intermediate **3**) in the cyclization of (+)-CPP to a mixture of abietadiene double-bond isomers catalysed by *Ag*AS. From the intramolecular proton transfer perspective, later work by Wilderman and Peters suggested that a shift from intermediate **3** to isopimar-8(14)-en-15-yl$^+$ was needed. However, here we demonstrate that copal-15-yl$^+$ is an intermediate derived from the cleavage of the (+)-CPP diphosphate group, while pimar-15-en-8-yl$^+$ (intermediate **3**) is the intermediate between (+)-CPP and miltiradiene. Among them, an inferred shift from the intermediate **3** to pimar-8(9)-en-15-yl$^+$ (intermediate **4**) provides an intermediate for the subsequent intramolecular proton transfer. *Sm*MDS:T608G produced (+)-copalol as a minor component of its product output, indicating that (+)-copalol is a potential stable intermediate. Further site-directed mutagenesis of N607 and T608 around (+)-copalol suggested that a pair of charged N607 and T608 stabilizes the formation of the copal-15-yl cation intermediate. Furthermore, *Sm*MDS:E690S and similar polar neutral side chain mutants lead to two isomeric products, sandaracopimaradiene and miltiradiene. Mutagenesis of residues E690, S717, H721 and Y837 around sandaracopimaradiene explained the catalysis mechanism of the C ring stereocentre in the pimar-15-en-8-yl$^+$ cation intermediate. We inferred that another pair of charged S717 and H721 assists in regulating the transition state. Compared to other diTPSs with multiple products, *Sm*MDS specifically has more charged amino acids in the class I active site, which perhaps produce a single product, miltiradiene, in such an enzymatic reaction (Figures 1 and S6).

In the field of metabolic engineering, perhaps one of the most arduous is controlling metabolic flux distributions, that is, how to make a particular biosynthesis route when other metabolic routes competitively share the same precursors. The biosynthesis of miltiradiene is an example facing this situation. Miltiradiene is an important precursor in the biosynthesis of tanshinones, triptolides and resin acids. Importantly, the characteristic cyclohexa-1,4-diene structure of the C ring in miltiradiene is rare in other abietane-related diterpenes. Through chimeric fusion proteins of class II and class I diTPSs, more metabolic flux of (+)-CPP flowed to class I diTPS, and, as a result, the production of miltiradiene was improved, reaching a highest miltiradiene titre of 3.5 g/L in a 5-L bioreactor. The modular architecture of chimeric fusion proteins is $\beta\alpha$ and $\gamma\beta\alpha$ (bold is the active domain); however, we directly found an inner channel in *Sm*MDS with an active $\alpha\beta\gamma$ domain. This natural strategy makes (+)-CPP metabolic flux concentrated and quick, generating more miltiradiene. The production of miltiradiene and no other competitive products from (+)-CPP is undoubtedly significant to *S. moellendorffii*. The accepted hypothesis is that plant diTPSs evolved from archaea by fusion of the $\alpha$ and $\beta\gamma$ enzymes. *S. moellendorffii* belongs to an ancient lineage, namely lycophyte, which diverged shortly after land plants evolved vascular tissues. The $\alpha\beta\gamma$ architecture of *Sm*MDS may support this hypothesis from the perspective of early vascular plants.

In summary, we described the X-ray crystal structures of *Sm*MDS in apo and GGPP-bound state. They are first reported structures of a bifunctional diTPS that produces only a single product. Furthermore, we proposed a catalytic mechanism taking into account the individual contributions of key active site residues. Structural and mutagenesis analyses show that copal-15-yl$^+$ and pimar-15-en-8-yl$^+$ are intermediates between (+)-CPP and miltiradiene. The associated molecular docking demonstrates that several key amino acid residues, such as E690, Y837, S717 and H721, precisely control intermediates and exhibit unique enzymatic selectivity. Moreover, we observed an inner channel that assisted (+)-CPP transportation, which may prevent the competition from other enzymes using (+)-CPP as a substrate in plant. Our findings advance the structural determinants of product specificity in class I active site and the transport mode of (+)-CPP in bifunctional diTPSs, providing an effective strategy for the biosynthesis of high-value bioactive diterpenes.

## 4 EXPERIMENTAL PROCEDURES

Strains, plasmid and reagents All the *E. coli* strains and plasmids are listed in Table S2. Phusion High-Fidelity DNA Polymerase for polymerase chain reaction (PCR) was purchased from New England Biolabs (Ipswich, MA).

Preparation of miltiradiene and abietatriene The YJ28 strain was used to obtain the compound miltiradiene and abietatriene. Single colonies were grown in 50 mL of YPD liquid medium (1% yeast extract, 2% peptone, and 2% glucose) in a 250 mL shake flask at 30 ℃ and 230 rpm for 48 h. The entire culture volume was transferred into 500 mL of fresh seed medium and incubated for 24 h and then transferred into 2 L of fresh seed medium and incubated for another 24 h. The seed medium was used to inoculate 8 L of fermentation medium in a New Brunswick BioFlo/CelliGen 115 bioreactor (Eppendorf, Hamburg, Germany) with a maximal working volume of 14 L. Fermentation was performed at 30 ℃. During fermentation, the pH was maintained at 4.0 with the automatic addition of ammonium hydroxide, the agitation rate was kept at 250 rpm, and the dissolved oxygen was kept above 40%. Concentrated glucose solution (40%, wt/vol) was fed periodically to keep the glucose concentration above 1.0 g/L. Additional YPD medium was fed after the initial 30 h of fermentation. The culture was then harvested by extraction after 96 h of total fermentation time.

Yeast cell suspensions were concentrated at 1 L, lysed using a nano homogenizer machine (AH-1500; ATS Engineering Limited, Brampton, ON, Canada) and extracted 10 times using an equal volume of hexane. Organic fractions were pooled and dried using a nitrogen evaporator (Baojingkeji, Henan, China) and then dissolved in 10 mL of methanol before purification using preparative liquid chromatography. High-performance liquid chromatography (HPLC) separation was performed using a SHIMADZU LC-20AR (Kyoto, Japan) with a YMC HPLC column (YMC-Pack ODS-A, 250×20 mm L.D., S-5 μm, 12 nm). The mobile phase, consisting of a mixture of water (A) and methanol (B), was pumped at a flow rate of 8 mL/min. The injection volume was 500 μL. The gradient elution was 100% B from 0 to 50 min.

Protein expression and purification The coding sequence of the miltiradiene synthase gene from *S. moellendorffii* was optimized for expression in *E. coli*. The full and truncated fragments were amplified by PCR and inserted into the pET-24a plasmid using the *Xho*I and *Nde*I restriction sites. The plasmids were transformed into *E. coli* BL21-(DE3) competent cells (TransGen Biotech, Beijing, China). The bacteria were grown at 37 ℃ to an optimal density at 600 nm ($OD_{600}$) of 0.8-1.0 and cooled to 16 ℃. After adding 0.2 mM isopropyl-1-thio-β-D-galactopyranoside, the induction continued by shaking for 16-20 h. Cells were harvested by centrifugation and then resuspended in lysis buffer containing 20 mmol/L Tris-HCl (pH 8.0), 250 mmol/L NaCl and 20 mmol/L imidazole. Bacteria were disrupted using an automatic cryogenic crusher and separated by centrifugation. Protein supernatant was loaded to a pre-equilibrated Ni-affinity chromatography column. The *Sm*MDS protein with a His tag at the C-terminus was washed with lysis buffer containing 50, 100 and 300 mmol/L imidazole. Selected fractions were concentrated using an Amicon Ultra-15 concentrator (Merck KGaA, Darmstadt, Germany). The concentrated protein was applied to a Resource Q column (GE Healthcare, Chicago, Illinois, USA) with buffer A containing 20 mmol/L Tris-HCl (pH 8.0), 10 mmol/L NaCl, 5 mmol/L $MgCl_2$, and 2 mmol/L dithiothreitol and buffer B containing 20 mmol/L Tris-HCl (pH 8.0), 1 mol/L NaCl, 5 mmol/L $MgCl_2$ and 2 mmol/L dithiothreitol. Finally, the protein was purified using Superdex™200 HR 10/300 gel filtration (GE Healthcare) with buffer containing 20 mmol/L Tris-HCl (pH 8.0), 200 mmol/L NaCl, 5 mmol/L $MgCl_2$ and 2 mmol/L dithiothreitol. The full-length diTPS from *Pinus contorta* that catalyses (+)-CPP to isopimaradiene and sandaracopimaradiene (*Pcm*ISO1) and a diTPS from *P. contorta* that catalyses (+)-CPP to pimaradiene (*Pcm*PIM1) with a His tag at N-terminus were purified by a Ni-affinity chromatography column.

Crystallization and data collection The *Sm*MDS protein was concentrated at 8 mg/mL (with 2 mmol/L miltiradiene) for crystal screening. *Sm*MDS crystals were grown at 16 ℃ by the hanging drop method using 1 μL of protein, 0.8 μL reservoir buffer and 0.2 μL of crystal seeds. The reservoir contains 0.1 mol/L MES (pH 6.5) and 22% (*V/V*) poly (ethylene glycol) methyl ether (PEG 2 000 MME). To obtain crystals of the *Sm*MDS-GGPP complex, 0.2 μL of

20 mmol/L GGPP was added to the hanging drop to a final concentration of 2 mmol/L, and the crystals were soaked for different times. Finally, crystals were dehydrated using reservoir solution containing 10% glycerol (v/v) before flash freezing in liquid nitrogen for data collection.

X-ray diffraction data were collected on beamlines BL18U and BL19U at the Shanghai Synchrotron Radiation Facility (SSRF). *Sm*MDS and *Sm*MDS$^{4h}$ diffraction data were processed with HKL2000.

Structure determination The crystal belonged to the space group $P2_12_12_1$, and the phase was determined by the molecular replacement (MR) method using the *Ag*AS structure (PDB ID: 3S9V). Electron density maps were calculated by PHENIX. Model building was performed using Coot and refined with PHENIX. The structures of CPP, copalol and sandaracopimaradiene were downloaded from the PubChem website, and the. cif files were generated using PHENIX. The final structure was analysed by PHENIX. Data collection and refinement statistics are presented in Table S1.

Site-directed mutagenesis Mutants were constructed by PCR using an overlap extension strategy with pET-24a-truncated *Sm*MDS (90 - 867) as a template. Following PCR, *Dpn*I was used to digest the wild-type template. The digested product was then transformed into *E. coli* DH5α chemically competent cells. The mutants were verified by sequencing.

Enzyme activity assays *In vitro* enzyme activity assays were performed in a 100 μL reaction system containing 50 μg of purified enzymes and 2.5 μg of GGPP (Sigma Aldrich, St. Louis, Missouri, USA) for 2 h at 16 ℃, except for assays with the E690A, T608, S717A and Y837G mutants, which required more substrates and extended incubation times to detect products (10 μg of GGPP for 24 h). The reaction mixture was then extracted three times with a threefold volume of n-hexanes, followed by GC - MS analysis, which was carried out on a DB-5MS column (15 m×0.25 mm×0.10 μm film thickness) using helium as a carrier gas. The initial oven temperature was set at 50 ℃ for 2 min followed by a 40 ℃/min gradient to 170 ℃, and 20 ℃/min gradient to 240℃, 40℃/min gradient to 300℃ and held at 300℃ for 1 min.

Mutant product identification The product of the first active site remains as diphosphate, so calf intestinal (CIP) alkaline phosphatase (New England Biolabs) was used to hydrolyse phosphate. The dephosphorylation product copalol was also determined using GC - MS analysis. After verification of the product, miltiradiene and copalol were quantified by GC-MS analysis. Miltiradiene was extracted and prepared from the fermentation product of strain YJ28. We also obtained abietatriene, the spontaneously oxidized product of miltiradiene.

*Pcm*ISO1 (NCBI accession numbers: JQ240314), a diTPS from *P. contorta*, catalyses (+)-CPP to isopimaradiene and sandaracopimaradiene. *Pcm*PIM1 (NCBI accession numbers: JQ240316), a diterpene synthase from *Pinus contorta*, catalyses (+)-CPP to pimaradiene. The sequences of *Pcm*ISO1 and *Pcm*PIM1 were synthesized by Shanghai Generay Biotech Co., Ltd., Shanghai, China. Since the D611A mutant generates (+)-CPP when co-incubated with GGPP, the catalytic products of the *Pcm*ISO1 and D611A mixture when co-incubated with GGPP are isopimaradiene and sandaracopimaradiene. Pimaradiene is the product of the *Pcm*PIM1 and D611A mixture with GGPP as the substrate.

[童宇菇,高伟,黄璐琦,等. Plant Biotechnology Journal, 2023,21:165 - 175.]

# Elucidation of the 1-phenethylisoquinoline pathway from an endemic conifer *Cephalotaxus hainanensis*

Phenylethylisoquinoline alkaloids (PIAs) are crucial secondary metabolites with high pharmacological potential, especially against cancer, inflammation, and cardio-cerebro-vascular disease. Their medicinal impact is illustrated by well-known compounds, e.g., colchicine. The PIA homoharringtonine (HHT, *SI Appendix*, Fig. S1) has been approved by the US Food and Drug Administration for the therapy of chronic myeloid leukemia. The great potential of PIAs is constrained by their sporadic occurrence to the conifer genus *Cephalotaxus*, the monocot family *Colchicaceae*, and the dicot genus *Phelline*. For instance, HHT is uniquely found in *Cephalotaxus* which is endemic to East Asia. Although HHT has been generated by chemical synthesis, extraction from plants has remained the only commercial source of HHT. Since several species of this genus, for instance *Cephalotaxus hainanensis*, have been shifted to the verge of extinction, sustainable alternatives, safeguarding biodiversity, are urgently needed. However, semisynthetic strategies, such as metabolic engineering of microbes, are hampered by the fact that the biosynthesis mechanism of these PIAs has remained largely elusive.

A nearly complete reconstruction of colchicine biosynthesis has been achieved recently, which can be used as template for PIA biosynthesis in general, for all the PIAs share a common precursor, the 1-phenethylisoquinoline scaffold **15** (Fig. 1 and *SI Appendix*, Figs. S2 and S3). Starting from this biogenetic intermediate **15**, nine newly identified enzymes can generate *N*-Formyldemecolcine, a precursor of colchicine. Moreover, a CYP71D12 protein, an α/β hydrolase protein, and a *N*-acetyltransferase superfamily protein were shown to be involved in colchicine biosynthesis. However, the pathway leading to this crucial precursor **15** has remained elusive, although a plausible upstream pathway for this PIA was proposed and reconstructed in *Nicotiana benthamiana* using nine enzymes from *Gloriosa superba*, *Coptis japonica*, and *Beta vulgaris*.

Isotope tracing experiments suggest that the PIA scaffold **15** derives from both, phenylalanine and tyrosine, which means that a part of the pathway is shared with that of benzylisoquinoline alkaloids (BIAs). The two pathways diverge from the precursor for the PIA and BIA scaffold, respectively (Fig. 1 and *SI Appendix*, Fig. S4). In case of BIAs, (*S*)-norcoclaurine synthase (NCS) joins dopamine with 4-hydroxyphenylacetylaldehyde (4-HPAA) by a Pictet-Spengler condensation, while for PIAs, dopamine is fused with 4-HDCA. Considering the structural similarity of 4-HPAA and 4-HDCA, we assumed that their biosynthesis might be similar, and the fusion into the 1-phenethylisoquinoline scaffold should also be achieved by a similar enzymatic Pictet-Spengler condensation driven by an NCS-like protein. This notion is supported by the fact that PIAs can also be produced in *N. benthamiana* upon expression of a NCS from *C. japonica*. However, it has remained unclear, how phenylalanine is converted into 4-HDCA, and which enzyme is responsible for the condensation in plants capable of PIA biosynthesis.

## 1 RESULTS AND DISCUSSION

A Novel Pr10 Enzyme was Screened Out and Identified.

The attempt to find homologs of the *Cj*NCS in the transcriptomes of *G. superba* or *C. hainanensis* (NCBI accession no. SRX12392777) did not lead to any candidate, indicating that, in those species, the Pictet-Spengler condensation might be driven by enzymes that derive from a convergent evolution. This assumption is supported by the fact that strictosidine synthase, that catalyzes the Pictet-Spengler condensation in the tetrahydroindole alkaloid pathway by joining tryptamine with secologanin, lacks homology with NCS. Since the gymnosperm *C. hainanensis* and the dicot *C. japonica* have diverged almost 400 Mya, and this condensation step occurs sporadically, dispersed over several, unrelated taxa, homology is not to be expected, anyway. We, therefore, changed the strategy, focusing on crucial features of three-dimensional structure rather than on overall sequence homology in the first place. The substrate of the putative Pictet-Spengler enzyme in *C. hainanensis* (4-HDCA) differs from 4-HPAA, the substrate of NCS, only by a reduction of one carbon in the side chain of the phenolic ring. Since NCS belongs to the pathogenesis-related 10/Bet v1 proteins, we inferred that the unknown

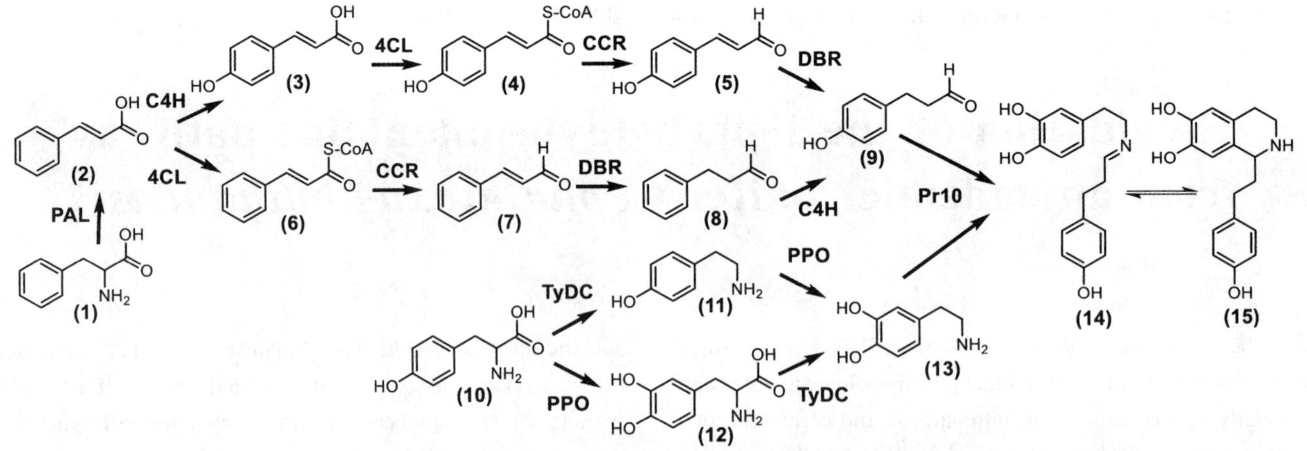

**Fig. 1 Proposed upstream biosynthesis pathway of PIAs**

Compounds: 1) L-phenylalanine; 2) cinnamic acid; 3) *p*-coumaric acid; 4) *p*-coumaroyl-CoA; 5) *p*-coumaroyl aldehyde; 6) cinnamoyl-CoA; 7) cinnamaldehyde; 8) phenylpropyl aldehyde; 9) 4-hydroxydihydrocinnamaldehyde (4-HDCA); 10) L-tyrosine; 11) tyramine; 12) L-DOPA; 13) dopamine; 14) 6,7-dihydroxy-1-(4-hydroxyphenylethyl)-1,2,3,4-tetrahydroisoquinoline intermediate; 15) 6,7-dihydroxy-1-(4-hydroxyphenylethyl)-1,2,3,4-tetrahydroisoquinoline (1-phenethylisoquinoline scaffold). Enzymes: PAL, phenylalanine ammonia-lyase; C4H, cinnamate 4-hydroxylase; 4CL, 4-coumarate CoA ligase; DBR, NADPH-dependent double-bond reductases; CCR, cinnamoyl-CoA reductase; TyDC/DODC, tyrosine/DOPA decarboxylase; PPO, polyphenoloxidase; Pr10, pathogenesis-related 10/Bet v1 proteins (*Ch*PSS).

enzyme might be a member of the same protein family. In fact, we could identify 32 candidates from our recently constructed *C. hainanensis* transcriptome (*SI Appendix*, Figs. S5 and S6) that qualified as Pr10-like proteins, among those we found 22 members of the Pr10/Bet v1 family (*SI Appendix*, Table S1).

To filter out the most relevant candidate for the Pictet-Spengler reaction, we made use of a working model that had been developed for the NCS from *Thalictrum flavum* (a member of the Ranunculaceae) based on quantum chemical calculations, crystal structures inferred from X-ray diffraction, as well as in vitro assays using recombinant enzyme tailored by site-specific mutagenesis. These studies identified a glycine-rich loop, which is conserved in all identified NCSs, connecting the β2 and β3 sheets, and linked with enzymatic activity. Furthermore, a highly conserved motif in β-sheet 4 was predicted to be crucial for the activity (*SI Appendix*, Fig. S7). Among the Pr10/Bet v1 candidates, only six were found to exhibit this glycine-rich loop motif (*SI Appendix*, Fig. S8). Thus, these six proteins represented the most likely candidates for the putative Pictet-Spengler enzyme responsible for the formation of the PIA backbone and were scrutinized further by heterologous expression in *Escherichia coli*. After feeding the substrates, dopamine and 4-HDCA, only one of these candidates converted the substrates into a product, which dis-played a $[M+H]^+$ ion peak at a m/z 286.143 19 (Fig. 2 *A* and *B*) diagnostic for the phenethylisoquinoline backbone. Although this enzyme shows only 17% identity with *Tf*NCS, it seems to mediate phenethylisoquinoline scaffold synthesis in *C. hainanensis* and was, therefore, named phenethylisoquinoline scaffold synthase (*Ch*PSS). The identification of intermediate **15** from the leaves of *C. hainanensis* supports a role for this intermediate in the biosynthesis of HHT (*SI Appendix*, Fig. S9). To further linked the recombinant enzyme activity with the actual activity in the plant itself, we extracted the crude protein of leaves of *C. hainanensis*, after adding the precursors **9** and **13**, and we detected the product **15** (*SI Appendix*, Fig. S10).

Exploring the Catalytic Mechanism of *Ch*PSS. As next step, we tried to get insight into the mechanism, by which *Ch*PSS is mediating the formation of the PIA scaffold. We were not successful in generating crystals from the recombinant protein, despite testing several thousands of conditions. Therefore, we modeled the 3D structure of *Ch*PSS using colabalphafold2 (*SI Appendix*, Fig. S11). The model obtained for *Ch*PSS predicted a strong overlap with that for *Tf*NCS, implying they may have a similar catalytic mechanism. Both proteins consist of three alpha helices and seven beta strands, enclosing a cavity. We decided, therefore, to use site-directed mutagenesis of potentially crucial amino acids to assess the effect on the in vitro activity of *Ch*PSS. A crucial tyrosine residue at position 108 in *Tf*NCS was conserved among all four known NCSs (*SI Appendix*, Fig. S7 and Fig. 2C) and had been shown to be essential for enzymatic function. While this tyrosine is missing in the corresponding position of *Ch*PSS β-sheet 4 (*SI Appendix*, Fig. S7 and Fig. 2C), we wondered whether a tyrosine in the neighborhood of the glycine-rich loop and also associated with a β-sheet might be functionally equivalent. These criteria were met by Tyr86 of *Ch*PSS (Fig. 2C). When we mutated this tyrosine to alanine, the in vitro activity decreased significantly to 8% compared with the wild-type protein (Fig. 2D and *SI Appendix*, Figs. S12 - S14). Likewise, a lysine (Lys122) plays a key role for the cyclization driven by *Tf*NCS. However, it was also missed in *Ch*PSS (Fig. 2C). In contrast, we identified the key amino acid residues corresponding to Glu110 and Asp141 of *Tf*NCS. When we mutated Glu70 in *Ch*PSS located in the above-mentioned conserved charge pattern in β-sheet 4 into alanine, a more substantial decrease of activity to 26% was achieved (Fig. 2D and *SI Appendix*, Figs. S12 - S14) (13). Another Lewis acid residue, Asp122, also turned out to be crucial to maintain its activity, because mutant E91A nearly lost the activity, while mutating it to another Lewis acid glutamic acid (D122E), ~21% activity remained (Fig. 2D and *SI Appendix*, Figs. S12 - S14). In summary, the implications from the model for *Ch*PSS based on the *Tf*NCS template were not totally met by the experimental results; however, some key residues with potential similar function with that of *Tf*NCS were identified, implying a similar catalytic process may be governed by these residues (*SI Appendix*, Fig. S15). The observed disparity between the two enzymes has to be seen along with the lacking phylogenetic relationship between the two classes of enzymes (*SI Appendix*, Figs. S16 and S17). Thus, it seems that their function (Pictet-Spengler condensation) has been acquired by convergent evolution. While the low sequence identity does not rule out the possibility of a common ancestor for these proteins, a deeper insight into structural aspects of these quite divergent enzymes might help to pinpoint structural requirements of functionality that might act on the background of a poor of even missing overall similarity.

In the next step, we investigated the substrate specificity of recombinantly expressed *Ch*PSS. Interestingly, the enzyme also accepted 4-HPAA and dopamine to produce (*S*)-norcoclaurine reported by the diagnostic m/z peak at 272.127 53 (Fig. 2 E and F). In addition, we were able to confirm the stereoselectivity of *Ch*PSS toward **15** by CD spectroscopy. These results are in good accordance with findings on *Cj*NCS, where a pure (*S*)-enantiomer was found (*SI Appendix*, Fig. S18). Thus, *Ch*PSS, in addition to its function

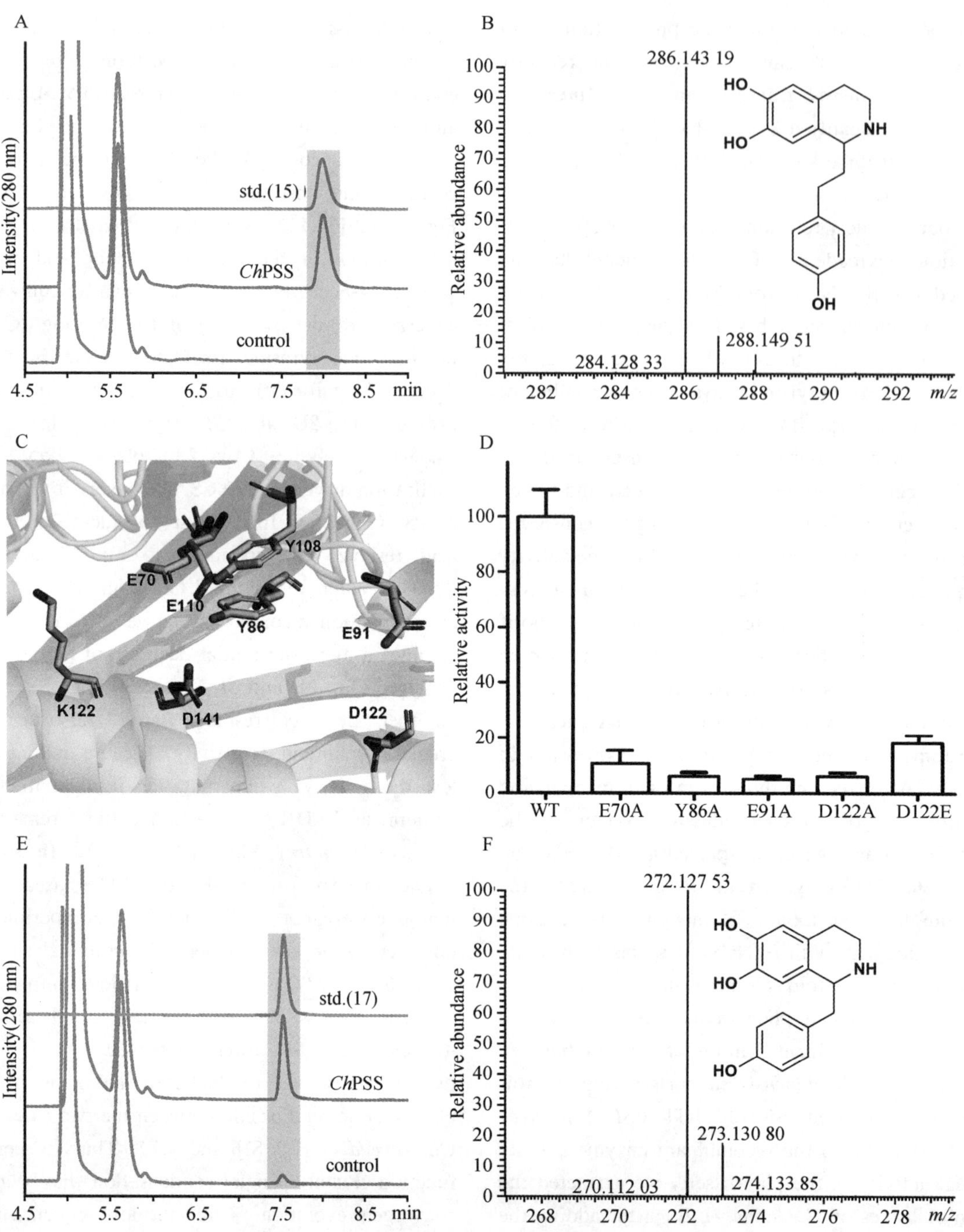


**Fig. 2 Identification of *Ch*PSS**

(A) The activity of *Ch*PSS was detected by feeding compounds **9** and **13** with 10 μg purified protein. A weak spontaneous reaction was detected in the control. (B) The reaction product of *Ch*PSS was confirmed by LC-MS (m/z 286.143 19). (C) The superposed structures of *Ch*PSS (blue) with *Tf*NCS (green) and their key amino acid residues. (D) The relative activity of wild type and mutants of *Ch*PSS was detected by HPLC. The reaction system containing 5 mmol/L dopamine, 2.5 mmol/L 4-HDCA in 50 mmol/L HEPES (5 mmol/L ascorbate sodium, pH 7.0). The reaction product **15** was detected. The results were displayed as mean±SD of three biological replicates, and the spontaneous activity was deducted from every measurement. (E) The activity of *Ch*PSS was detected by feeding compounds 4-HPAA (**16**) and **13**. A weak spontaneous reaction was also detected in the control. (F) The reaction product of *Ch*PSS was confirmed by LC-MS (m/z 272.127).

in PIA biosynthesis, was able to act as NCS. While this broad substrate promiscuity was to be expected from the large catalytic cavity (Fig. 2C and *SI Appendix*, Fig. S11), (16, 22), this observation accentuates the question, how specificity is brought about. The fact that the enzymes from *G*. *superba* and *C*. *hainanensis* generate PIAs, while their counterparts from opium poppy and *C*. *japonica* produce BIAs, had remained elusive. When the catalytic cavities are permissive and not homologous, it might be substrate availability that delineates the biosynthesis of PIAs (deriving from dopamine and 4-HDCA) and BIAs (deriving from dopamine and 4-HPAA). Isotope trace analysis had shown that these substrates derive from phenylalanine and tyrosine, respectively (Fig. 1). However, so far, the details for 4-HPAA and 4-HDCA biosynthesis as well as for the origin of dopamine have remained unclear in both BIA and PIA accumulating plants.

Elucidation of the Biosynthetic Pathway for Dopamine. Decarboxylation of tyrosine by the aromatic amino acid decarboxylase (AAADC) and subsequent hydroxylation by the cytochrome P450 family protein CYP71AD6 seem to be crucial for the synthesis of BIAs, as well as for the production of betanin in *B. vulgaris*. For this reason, we searched for *Ch*AAADC candidates. We were able to identify one AAADC candidate (*Ch*TyDC1) and demonstrated that this enzyme was able to decarboxylate both tyrosine and L-DOPA as substrate (*SI Appendix*, Fig. S19). Our findings are consistent with the data from other plants, where AAADC was shown to accept both tyrosine (generating tyramine) and L-DOPA (generating dopamine) as well (*SI Appendix*, Fig. S20). Since a CYP71AD family protein with a hydroxylase function, present in red beet, qualified as candidate for the subsequent hydroxylation, we searched the transcriptome of *C. hainanensis* for potential homologs but did not identify any member of the CYP71AD family. However, this kind of hydroxylase seems also to be absent from other plants that accumulate BIAs. Searching for alternatives, we wondered, whether a polyphenol oxidase (PPO) might bridge the gap, for it was reported that silencing of PPO in *Juglans regia* led to accumulation of tyramine, the direct precursor of dopamine. Since PPOs generally catalyze the oxidation of aromatic rings, which has also been proposed for colchicine biosynthesis, we tested the hypothesis that a PPO may exert a similar function in *C. hainanensis*. In fact, we identified two candidates from the *C. hainanensis* transcriptome, and one of them, *Ch*PPO1, was able to generate L-DOPA after feeding tyrosine (Fig. 3A). The same protein was also able to form dopamine after feeding tyramine (Fig. 3B). Thus, *Ch*PPO1 qualifies as the elusive aromatic hydroxylase (Fig. 3). Furthermore, when we co-expressed recombinantly, under the same bacterial promoter, *Ch*TyDC1 and *Ch*PPO1 (Fig. 3C), we achieved the complete biosynthesis of dopamine after feeding tyrosine (Fig. 3C and D). Therefore, PPO might function as a hydroxylase in the biosynthesis of dopamine in our PIA-producing plant, which is in good accordance with the role suggested for this enzyme in colchicine biosynthesis.

Elucidation of the Biosynthetic Pathway for 4-HDCA. The next open issue was the formation of 4-HPAA and 4-HDCA. The two compounds differ mainly by a C-atom in the aliphatic chain of 4-HDCA. This structural difference might be crucial for channeling the metabolic flow between BIAs and PIAs (*SI Appendix*, Fig. S4), but it is not clear, how 4-HDCA is generated. To resolve this uncertainty in the pathway, we used information from colchicine biosynthesis and labeling experiments in cephalotaxine biosynthesis as template for two concurrent models of 4-HDCA from phenylalanine (Fig. 1 and *SI Appendix*, Fig. S21) that were also congruent with the early pathways proposed for *G. superba* and other PIA-producing plants. The difference between these concurrent schemes for 4-HDCA biosynthesis is the position of hydroxylation within this pathway. We, therefore, tested the possibility of a "hydroxylation-first" and a "hydroxylation-last" model. In the hydroxylation-first model, **2** is hydroxylated by C4H and then converted by 4CL and CCR to form **5**. Here, the sequence of reactions would be shared with the pathway leading to monolignols, which would also be consistent with our in vitro enzymatic reaction (Fig. 4 A and B and *SI Appendix*, Figs. S22 – S25). We found that *Ch*C4H1 – 3 behaved as to be expected from the hydroxylation-first model. More importantly, however, feeding compound **8** did not yield 4-HDCA for none of the four C4H members (Fig. 4C), falsifying a central implication predicted by the hydroxylation-last model. The reduction of the double bound in **5** to form **9** would represent the point where PIA biosynthesis diverges from lignin biosynthesis. For the PIA accumulator *G. superba*, an alkenal reductase has been described recently, and the search for double-bond reductases (DBR) in the transcriptome of *C. hainanensis* recovered five candidates. In fact, two of them, *Ch*DBR2 and *Ch*DBR3, were able to convert **5** to **9** in vitro (Fig. 4 D and E). In contrast, none of the five *Ch*DBRs was able to convert **7** to **8** (Fig. 4F), which imply the hydroxylation-last model is infeasible, even though that 4CL and CCR are able to accept **2** and **6** as substrates to form **7** (*SI Appendix*, Fig. S25).

In conclusion, using a combination of pathway modeling, mining the *Cephalotaxus* transcriptome, and experimental verification of recombinantly expressed candidates by precursor feeding in vitro, we could construct the pathway leading to the first committed compound in PIA biosynthesis. A novel member of the Pr10/Bet v1 family were identified as the key enzyme driving the Pictet-Spengler condensation to give rise to the 1-phenethylisoquinoline scaffold (Fig. 2). In addition, we could pinpoint DBR as crucial step, where the PIA precursor 4-HDCA diverges from the early lignin pathway. We proved that the hydroxylation of cinnamic acid (hydroxylation-first) as a necessary step to deliver the substrate for DBR to produce 4-HDCA (Fig. 4D). To what extent DBRs define, whether a given plant accumulates PIAs or their 4-HPAA derived counterparts, the BIAs, remains to be investigated. This work provides an important stepstone for the subsequent analysis and biotechnological application of cephalotaxine biosynthesis, which is expected to differ

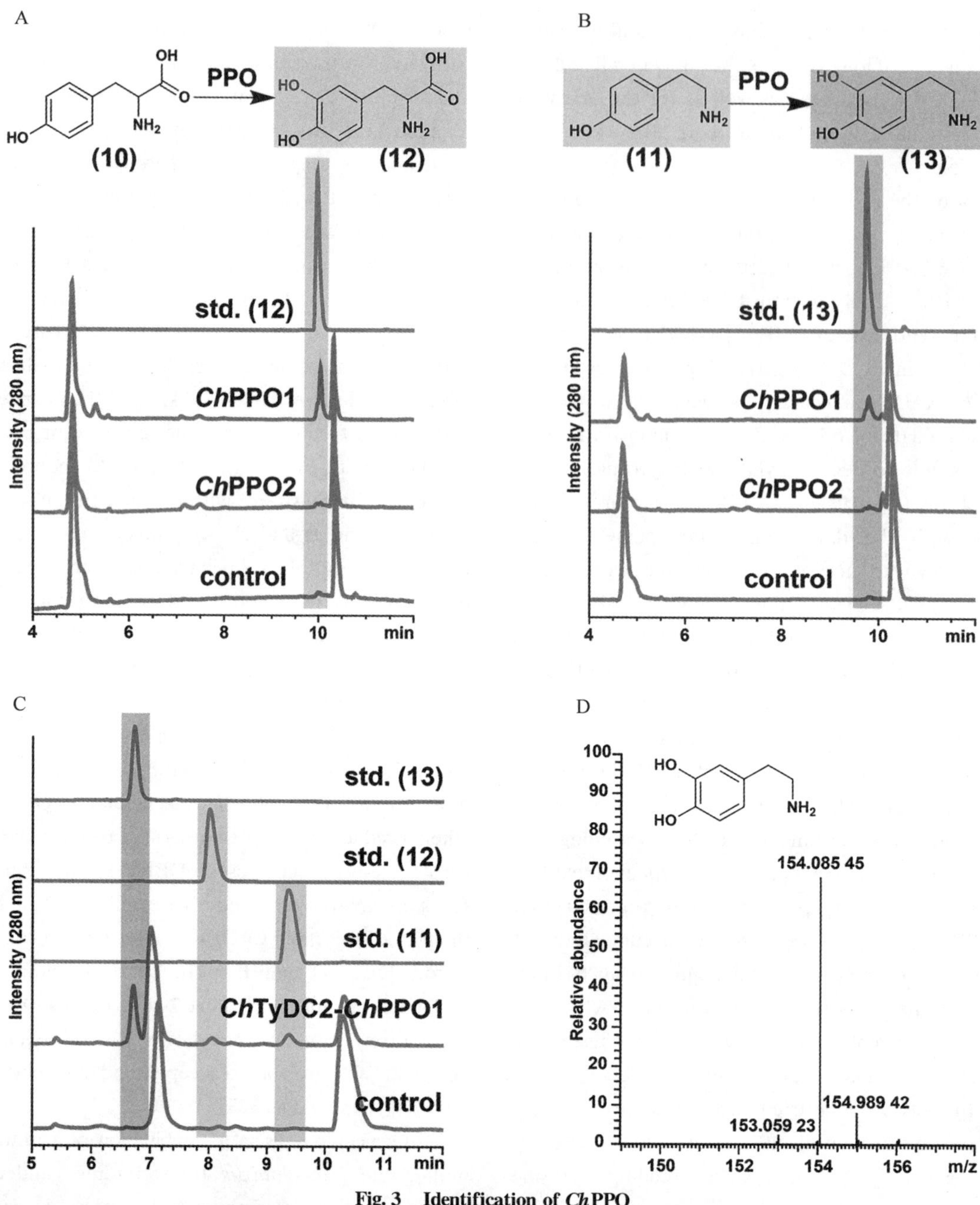


**Fig. 3 Identification of *Ch*PPO**

(A) The activity of *Ch*PPO was detected by feeding L-tyrosine **10** with 10 μg purified protein. (B) The activity of *Ch*PPO was detected by feeding tyramine **11**. Sample without PPO protein was used as control. (C) The activity of *Ch*PPO1 was further confirmed by using co-expression of *Ch*TyDC1 which was detected in HPLC. The intermediates **12** and **13** were detected. (D) The catalytic product of *Ch*TyDC1-PPO1, dopamine, was confirmed by LC-MS (m/z 154.085 45).

considerably from the alkaloid pathways that have already been constructed in other plants.

## 2 MATERIALS AND METHODS

Plant Materials and c-DNA Preparation. Plant materials of *C. hainanensis* were collected from Jianfengling in Ledong, Hainan, China (18°75′N, 108°85′E). Needle leaf, phloem, and root samples were harvested, then immediately frozen in liquid nitrogen and stored at −80 ℃ until use. Total RNA was extracted using the RNAprep Pure Kit (TIANGEN) according to the manufacturer's instructions. The quality and quantity of total RNA were measured by a NanoPhotometer NP50 (Implen). Then, PrimeScript™ RT Master Mix (Takara) was employed to perpetrate c-DNA template for gene clone and expression analysis.

Chemicals, Strains, and Enzymes. Compounds **1** to **13** were purchased from Sinoreagent (https://www.sinoreagent.com/), Bidepharm (https://www.bidepharm.com/), Aladdin (https://www.aladdin-e.com/), and Sigma-Aldrich (https://www.sigmaaldrich.cn/CN/zh). Compound **15** was synthesized by Wuxi Apptec (https://www.wuxiapptec.com/zh-cn), and the NMR and LC-MS data are listed in *SI*

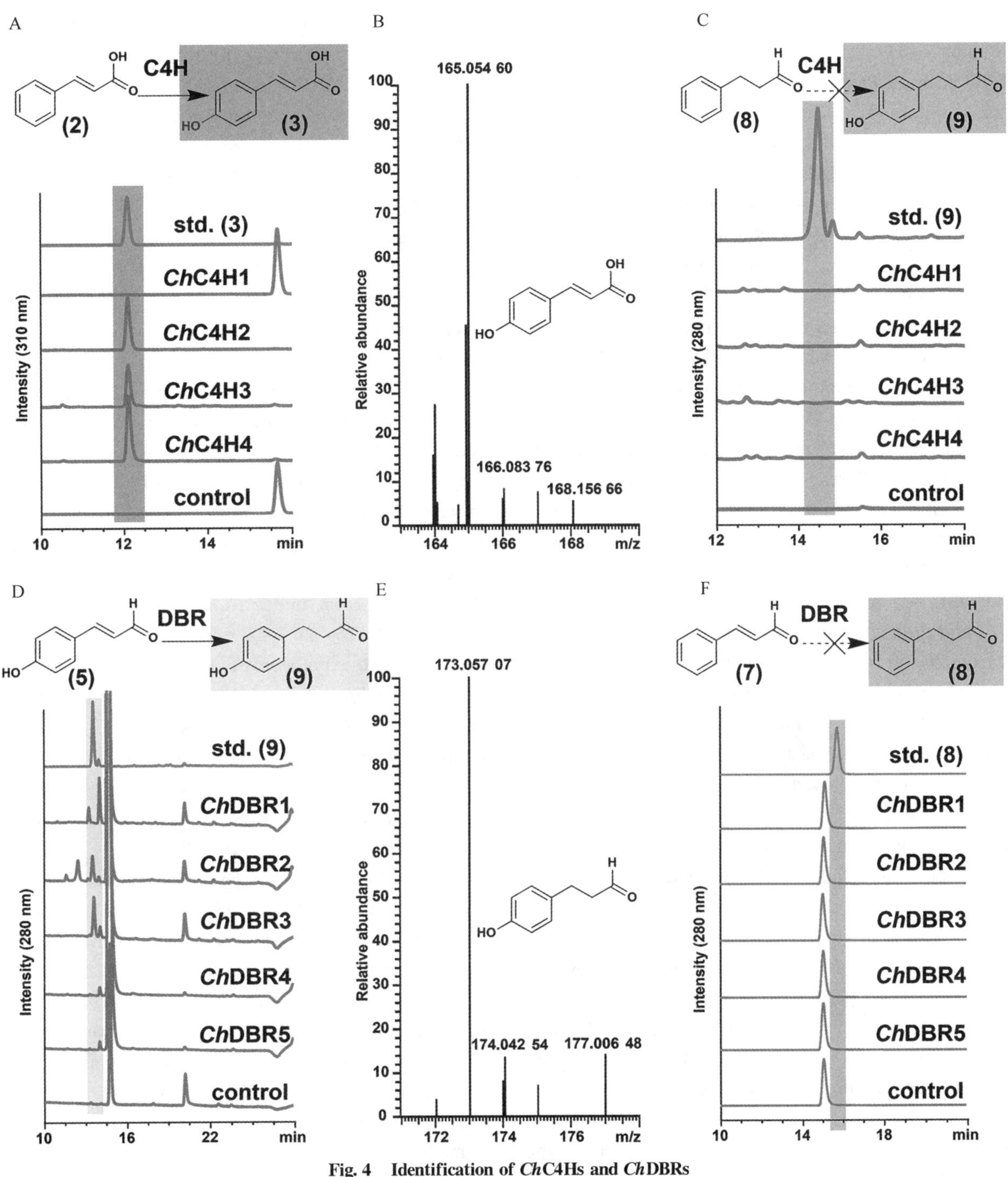


**Fig. 4 Identification of *Ch*C4Hs and *Ch*DBRs**

(A) The activity of *Ch*C4Hs was detected by HPLC. *Ch*C4H1 - 3 could catalyze **2** to form **3**, while *Ch*C4H4 has no function to **2**. (B) The catalytic product of **3** was further confirmed by LC-MS (m/z 165.054 60). (C) The catalytic activity of *Ch*C4Hs was detected by HPLC after feeding compound **8**. These results indicated that the hydroxylation-last routine could not be realized. (D) The activity of *Ch*DBRs was detected by HPLC. *Ch*DBR2 and 3 could catalyze **5** to form **9**, while *Ch*DBR1, 4, and 5 have no function to **5**. (E) The catalytic product of **9** was further confirmed by LC-MS in $[M+Na]^+$ mode (m/z 173.057 07). (F) The catalytic activity of *Ch*DBRs was detected by HPLC after feeding compound **7**. These results also indicated that the hydroxylation-last routine could not be realized.

*Appendix*, Figs. S2 and S3. Compound **16** was synthesized according to the previously report. The compatible vectors pET28a, pYeDP60, and pCDFDuet-1 (Novagen) were used to express multiple genes. *E. coli* Top10 competent cells were used for plasmid amplification and isolation in the vectors construct process. *E. coli* BL21 (DE3) containing the corresponding expression vectors was used for all protein expression except *Ch*C4Hs were expressed by *Saccharomyces cerevisiae* WAT 11. PrimeSTAR® Max DNA Polymerase (Takara) that used for PCR amplification, all other enzymes used for cloning were purchased from New England Biolabs (NEB). PCR products and Plasmid DNA were purified according to the procedure of E. Z. N. A. ® Gel Extraction Kit and Plasmid mini Kit (Omega BIO-TEK).

SMRT Library Preparation, Sequencing, and Analysis. For Iso-Seq library construction, the c-DNA was prepared from five whole seedlings including leaves, roots, twigs, and barks by using of the SMARTer PCR c-DNA Synthesis Kit (Takara), and the full-length transcriptome was achieved by Iso-Seq method performed by Novagene Co., Ltd. Size fractionation and selection (non-fractionation and >4 kb) were performed using the Blue Pippin Size Selection System protocol as described by Pacific Biosciences (PN 100-092-800-03). Sequence data were processed using the SMRTlink 5.1 software, and circular consensus sequence (CCS) was generated from subread BAM files. A total of 18.17 Gb of clean data and 785,720,100 polymerase reads were obtained. A total of 962,965 CCS reads were generated, with a total of 16,598,265 subreads from 8 SMRT cells of non-normalized bins (0.5 to 2.5 kb, 2 to 3.5 kb, 3 to 6 kb, and 5 to 10 kb) and normalized bins (0.5 to 2.5 kb and 2 to 3.5 kb), including 581,486 (60%) full-length reads and 381 479 (40%) non-full-length reads. The length of CCS reads ranged from 200 bp to 8 900 bp. Additional nucleotide errors in consensus reads were corrected using the Illumina RNA-seq data with the software LoRDEC. Any redundancy in corrected consensus reads was removed by CD-HIT to obtain final transcripts for the subsequent analysis. Finally, a total of 282 151 transcripts were obtained. Gene function was annotated based on seven databases (NR, NT, Pfam, KOG/COG, Swiss-port, KO and GO, *SI Appendix*, Figs. S5 and S6). BLAST (setting the e-value threshold to $10^{-10}$), Diamond BLASTX (setting the e-value to threshold to $10^{-10}$), and Hmmscan software were used in NT, NR/KOG/Swiss-Prot/KEGG, and Pfam database analysis, respectively.

Gene mining and Selection. Experiments with $^{14}C$- and $^{3}H$-labeled compounds show that both, tyrosine and phenylalanine, are the precursors of PIAs, and this also had been confirmed by recent work. However, the elusive 3′-hydroxylase on **10** or **11** renders the exact order of the upstream PIA biosynthetic pathway unclear. Even though *Bv*CYP76AD5 and *Cj*NCS had been suggested to complement the pathway, neither the true homologues, nor the order of the reactions is understood. Hence, we used a model for the upstream PIA pathway to focus on the hydroxylase and NCS-like protein (Fig. 1). Based on this metabolic-flux analysis, we can propose that eight enzymes should be sufficient to catalyze this part, which allowed to select candidate genes from our functionally annotated full-length transcriptome dataset. As a result, in total 309 transcripts were selected, including 120 transcripts for PAL genes, 27 for C4H genes, 15 for 4CL genes, 62 for CCR genes, 28 for DBR genes, 20 for TyDC genes, five for PPO genes, and 32 for Pr10/Bet v1 genes. Because the SMRT sequencing platform allows for obtaining the full-length CDS with complete ORFs, we finally screened out 30 genes sequences with complete ORFs after removing repetitive and redundant transcripts (*SI Appendix*, Tables S1 and S2). The sequences used in this study were listed in *SI Appendix*, Table S6.

Cloning of Candidate Genes. All candidate genes were amplified from a c-DNA pooled from leaf, phloem and root of *C. hainanensis*. The purified amplicons were then inserted into the corresponding expression vectors using in-fusion cloning (Clontech). The genes of C4H were inserted into pYeDP60 vector between *BamH I* and *EcoR I* sites. All the other genes were inserted into pET28a vector between *Nde I* and *EcoR I* restriction sites, except for *Ch*PSS that was inserted between *Nco I* and *Xho I* sites. To obtain a co-expression construct combining TyDC and PPO, the DNA fragment containing the PPO1 coding sequence, T7 promoter region, and RBS was amplified with primers PPO-F-SacI and PPO-R-XhoI from pET28a-*Ch*PPO1 and inserted into the linearized pET28a-*Ch*TyDC2 to generate pET28a-TyDC2+PPO1. For co-expression of 4CL and CCR, *Ch*4CL2 and *Ch*CCR1 coding sequences were obtained using primers 4CL2-F-NcoI/4CL2-R-BamHI and CCR1-F-NdeI/CCR1-R-EcoRV, respectively, and cloned into pCDFDuet-1 between the *NcoI* /*BamH I* and *Nde I* /*EcoR V* sites, giving rise to the vector pCDFDuet-4CL2+CCR1. All primers used in this study are listed in *SI Appendix*, Table S3.

Heterologous Expression of C4H in Yeast. The reconstructed plasmid pYe-DP60-C4H was transformed into the *S. cerevisiae* strain WAT11, and positive transformants were screened on solid plates of SC-U (SC dropout medium without uracil) containing 20 g/L glucose. Positive clones were incubated under shaking at 30℃ until the $OD_{600}$ reached to 2. The cells were then spun down and the sediment washed several times with $ddH_2O$ to remove residual glucose. Subsequently, the sediment was resuspended in SC-U medium containing 20 g/L galactose to induce expression of the target protein. As substrates, cinnamic acid or phenylpropyl aldehyde was added to a final concentration of 100 μmol/L to the resuspended cells and then incubated at 28℃ for 12 h. After collection of the cells, they were resuspended in 2 mL methanol and then ultrasonicated twice for 30 min, collecting the supernatant for HPLC-MS analysis.

Heterologous Expression and Purification of Candidate Proteins in *E. coli*. All the inserts were transformed into *E. coli* BL21 (DE3) by the heat shock method and then selected on LB plates containing 50 mg/L kanamycin. After sequencing, positive single colonies were inoculated separately into LB medium containing 50 mg/L kanamycin for seed culture. Then, the overnight culture was inoculated into an appropriate volume of LB medium containing 50 mg/L kanamycin and grown at 37 ℃ until a $OD_{600}$ of 0.6, before inducing with 0.5 mmol/L isopropyl-β-D-thiogalactoside (IPTG) at 25 ℃ and 180 rpm. After incubation for additional 16 to 20 h, the culture was spun down at 5,000 rpm for 10 min at 4 ℃. Then, the pellet was resuspended in lysis buffer containing 20 mmol/L HEPES, 500 mmol/L NaCl, 20 mmol/L imidazole, and 10% ( V/V ) glycerol. The suspension was homogenized in by ultrasonication, and then the homogenate was collected at 25 000 rpm at 4 ℃. The supernatant was purified on a Ni-NTA column, and purity and molecular weight of the fusion proteins were verified by SDS-PAGE and nanodrop 2 000 ultramicro-spectrophotometer ( *SI Appendix*, Fig. S12). The *Ch*PSS proteins were further purified on AKTA™ pure protein purification system by using Hitrap Q and Superdex 200 Increase 10/300 GL columns ( *SI Appendix*, Fig. S12). The purified protein was concentrated and dialyzed against storage buffer ( 20 mmol/L HEPES, 200 mmol/L NaCl, and 20% ( V/V ) glycerol) and then stored at −80 ℃ till analysis.

Structure Prediction. The model prediction of *Ch*PSS was conducted using colabAlphaFold2 which is released on the GitHub by DeepMind. We also adopt auto dock vina to dispose the interaction between the *Ch*PSS and two ligands ( dopamine, 4-HDCA ). Finally, we adopt open sourced PyMOL to show the track and the binding mode of the *Ch*PSS and two ligands.

In Vitro Characterization and Screening of Recombinant Candidate Genes. If not specified otherwise, reaction conditions and detection procedures were as specified in *SI Appendix*, Tables S4 and S5, respectively. All the reactions were conducted in 30 ℃ for 30 min, while, for *Ch*PSS, temperature was raised to 45 ℃. Reactions were stopped by transfer of the reaction mix on ice. The con-ditions had been adjusted based on extensive preparatory studies exploring different reaction and detection conditions, with special focus on detection of L-DOPA and dopamine by HPLC. For co-expression active assays of pET28a-TyDC2 + PPO1 and pCDFDuet-4CL2+CCR1, after 8 h of IPTG induction, the culture was centrifuged, the supernatant was discarded, cell pellet was re-suspended in 100 mmol/L tris base buffer at pH 7.5. Then, the corresponding substrates were added to the mixture in 30 ℃ for about 8 h. Kinetic assays were performed under the same conditions as routine activity assays ( 10 μg protein and reaction at 45 ℃ for 30 min ) and kinetic parameters determined by varying substrate concentrations while maintaining other reactants at saturation ( same concentrations as in routine activity assays ). Kinetic constants were calculated by nonlinear regression analysis (Origin 8; OriginLab Corp).

For products identification, the samples were diluted by 500 μL acetonitrile and analyzed by UPLC-MS/MS after filtering through a 0.22 μm filter membrane. UPLC was performed at a flow rate of 0.3 mL/min in solvent A (98% [V/V] acetonitrile, 2% [V/V] water, and 0.2% formic acid) and solvent B (2% [V/V] acetonitrile, 98% [V/V] water, and 0.2% formic acid ) using an InfinityLab Poroshell 120 EC-C18 column ( 2.1 × 100 mm, 2.7 μm particle size; Agilent Technologies). The gradient elution program is as follows: 5% solvent A, 0 to 1.5 min; 50% solvent A, 1.5 to 2 min; 95% solvent A, 2 to 2.5 min; 100% solvent A, 2.5 to 3 min; 95% solvent A, 3 to 4 min; 50% solvent A, 4 to 5 min; 95% solvent A, 5 to 6 min.

For collecting of all MS data, the Exactive™ Plus Orbitrap Mass Spectrometer ( ThermoFisher Scientific™ ) equipped with an electrospray ionization (ESI) probe inlet was used. The signal was achieved in positive ion mode with ESI. Ions were generated and focused using an ESI voltage of 4.0 kV; sheath gas (nitrogen) flow rate, 40 arb; aux/sweep gas (nitrogen) flow rate, 15 arb; capillary temperature, 350 ℃.

[乔飞,赵玉戍,等. PNAS, 2023,120(1):e2209339120.]

# Discovery, structure, and mechanism of the (*R*, *S*)-norcoclaurine synthase for the chiral synthesis of benzylisoquinoline alkaloids

## 1 INTRODUCTION

Stereochemistry has captivated humanity since its inception by the French microbiologist and chemist Louis Pasteur, retaining its relevance as a complex subject in the 21st century. Its profound implications in pharmacy, life sciences, and physics have spurred interest in understanding its origins, formation, functions, and effect on the three-dimensional nature of human society. However, synthesizing chiral molecules, especially those with multiple chiral centers, poses considerable challenges. For instance, commercial chemical syntheses of analgesics such as morphine and codeine, along with their subclasses, have been hindered owing to the five inherent asymmetric carbons. Plants are deemed to be the greatest chemists and various compounds of particular configuration were created, whereas the underlying mechanisms of plants to synthesize chiral-specific compounds remain largely undeciphered. One representative example is benzylisoquinoline alkaloids (BIAs), a diverse group of natural compounds with significant pharmacological activities and biological effects. While most BIAs in nature are recognized as (*S*)-enantiomers, numerous (*R*)-enantiospecific BIAs, including morphine and its derivatives, are also abundant in certain species such as opium poppy and lotus (*Nelumbo nucifera*). Considering that chiral-specific BIAs have attracted continuous attention for their role in drug discovery and development, understanding of underlying mechanisms of chiral control is helpful in developing a biotechnological strategy for their production.

Recently, a reticuline epimerase was demonstrated to be instrumental in converting (*S*)-reticuline to (*R*)-reticuline (STORR, Figure S1), facilitating the biosynthetic pathway research of opioids, such as thebaine and morphine. Further analysis of the opium poppy genome revealed that gene duplication, rearrangement, and fusion events influence the evolution of STORR, enabling it to produce specific (*R*)-enantiomers of metabolic products. However, the chirality-determining mechanism of (*R*)-enantiopreference in opium poppy and the biosynthetic mechanism of (*R*)-enantiospecific BIAs in other species have not yet been reported. The first committed step in the biosynthesis of BIAs is the enantioselective Pictet-Spengler (PS) condensation between dopamine and 4-hydroxyphenylacetaldehyde (4-HPAA, Figure S2). This step is catalyzed by norcoclaurine synthase (NCS), and the formed norcoclaurine constitutes the central precursor for the biosynthesis of the structurally diverse BIAs. In the NCS-catalyzed PS reaction, it has been demonstrated that the iminium intermediate is the divergence point of the pathways leading to (*S*)- and (*R*)-enantiomers of norcoclaurine (Figure S2). The (*E*)/(*Z*) configuration of the iminium and the position of the dopamine phenol ring relative to the iminium decide whether the *Re*- or *Si*-face of the C=N double bond will be attacked. Hence, NCS is theoretically the first enzyme to introduce a unique chiral carbon center by producing (*R*)-stereochemical configuration precursors, such as the skeleton molecule (*R*)-norcoclaurine. Nevertheless, all of the NCSs isolated from the opium poppy and other related members of plants, such as Ranunculales, were all characterized as (*S*)-enantiospecific, and correspondingly, most BIAs found in nature were characterized as (*S*)-enantiomers. Considering the importance of chiral compounds, especially the (*R*)-stereochemistry in medicine, the origins of the stereochemistry of BIAs are worth investigating.

The sacred lotus, an ancient aquatic plant (Figure S3), boasts widespread use in Ayurvedic and traditional Chinese medicine to treat dysentery, arrhythmia, and inflammation. Interestingly, many BIAs found in lotus were identified to be (*R*)-enantiospecific, which is contrary to the fact that BIAs in nature are mostly (*S*)-enantiomers. Despite considerable progress in characterizing the biosynthetic pathways of BIAs in alkaloid-producing plants such as the opium poppy and *Coptis chinensis* have been made, the biosynthesis of BIAs in the sacred lotus remains largely uncharted (Figure S1). Key BIA intermediates in the sacred lotus, such as (*R*)-pronuciferine and (*R*)-glaziovine, are suggested to be synthesized from (*R*)-norcoclaurine through specific *O*-methyltransferase (OMT), *N*-methyltransferase (NMT), and cytochrome P450 proteins. Recently, it was demonstrated that OMT from *N. nucifera* (*Nn*OMT1/5) and *Nn*CYP80Q1 (or *Nn*CYP80G) play significant roles in the biosynthesis of lotus BIAs. However, the exact biosynthetic mechanisms of lotus BIAs, particularly the origins of (*R*)-enantiospecific alkaloids and the chiral controlling mechanism, remain unknown.

In this study, through genome mining and *in vitro* functional validation, we characterized five lotus NCSs capable of producing (*R*/*S*)-enantiomers of norcoclaurine, which is responsible for the origin of the stereochemistry of compounds in lotus. We determined the crystal structure of *Nn*NCS1 by crystallographic methods and subsequently clarified its potential reaction mechanism and enantioselectivity using quantum chemical calculations. This process revealed that the Glu72 and Lys84 residues function as general base/acid groups during catalysis and that the Tyr40 residue is proposed to play a significant role in controlling enantioselectivity. Guided by the derived mechanism, the single-point mutations of residues situated around the active pocket, namely, Ile43, Leu60, and Phe101, resulted in an (*R*)-enantiopreference of the enzyme. This study makes a significant contribution to the existing literature as it unravels the previously obscure pathway of (*R*)-BIA biosynthesis and will provide a valuable enzymological tool for synthesizing chiral molecules.

## 2 RESULTS AND DISCUSSION

Identification of NCSs from Lotus. To probe the (*R*)-enantiomer source of BIAs in lotus, we initially focused on the function of *Nn*NCS, which theoretically creates the first chiral carbon atom in the BIAs skeleton through Pictet-Spengler condensation. The prevalence of (*R*)-enantiospecific BIAs in the lotus suggests that certain candidate genes, such as NCS, might contribute (*R*)-configuration chiral carbon.

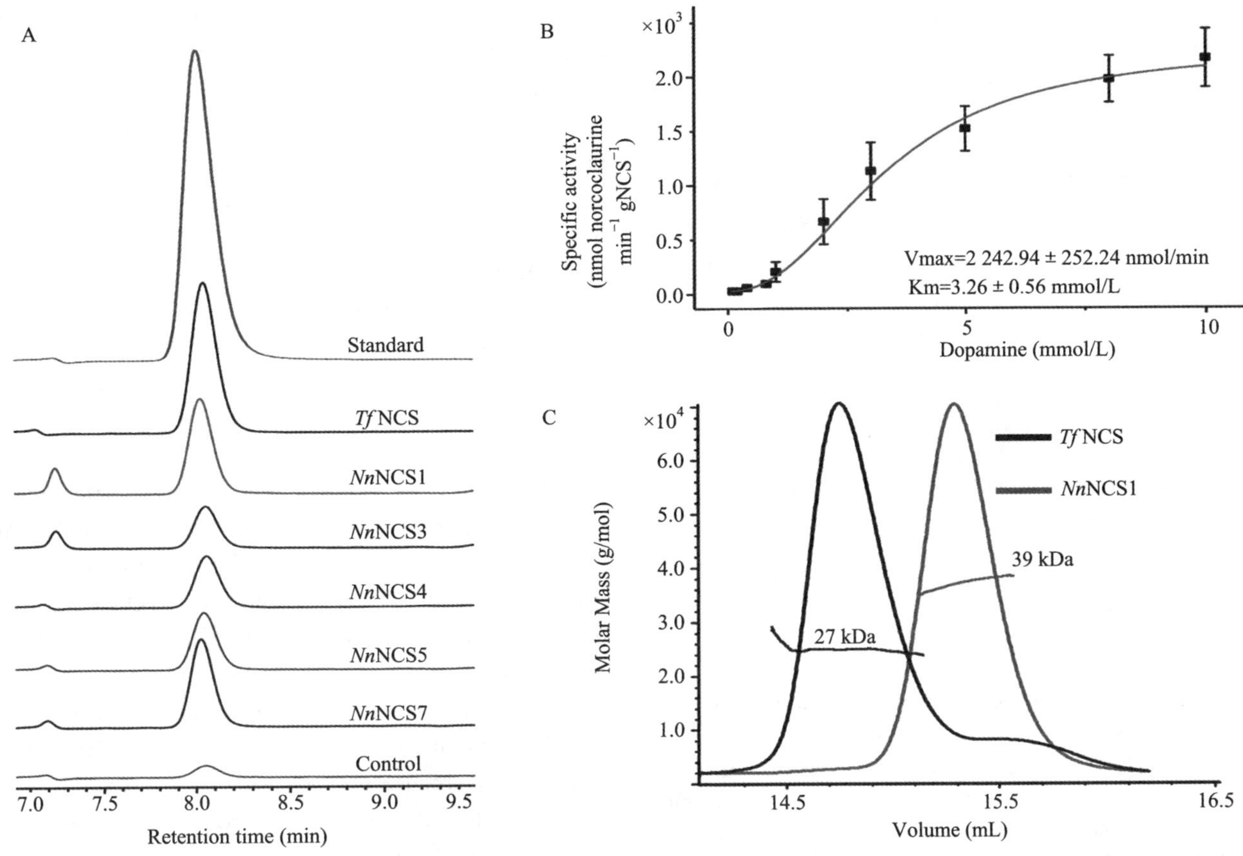


**Figure 1 Functional verification of *Nn*NCSs**

(A) High-performance liquid chromatography (HPLC) assay of enzymatic products detected by a UV spectrum under 280 nm. The curves in different colors represent different enzymatic products using different proteins. "Standard" is short for (*R*/*S*)-norcoclaurine standard, "*Tf*NCS" is the positive control using NCS isolated from *Thalictrum flavum*, "Control" indicates a negative control without enzymes, "*Nn*NCS1, 3, 4, 5, and 7" are five NCS homologues identified in *N. nucifera*. (B) Enzymatic kinetic analysis of *Nn*NCS1. The concentration of dopamine varies from 0 to 10 mmol/L and the concentration of 4-HPAA was fixed at 1 mmol/L. Each reaction was repeated three times ($n = 3$). The fitted curve is calculated by a logistic equation based on the homotropic effect of dopamine and NCS protein interaction, and specific activity refers to the amount of norcoclaurine produced by 1 g of *Nn*NCS1 within a minute. The figure is the same as Figure S9C. (C) Size-exclusion chromatography with multiangle light scattering detection analyses of *Nn*NCS1 (marked in pink) and *Tf*NCS (marked in black). The molecular weight of each protein was 39 and 27 kDa, respectively.

Upon analyzing the reported lotus genome, we identified seven genes potentially encoding NCS, two of which were pseudogenes (*Nn*NCS2, *Nn*NCS6). We successfully cloned and synthesized five genuine *Nn*NCS genes. They all belong to the PR-10 family with the conserved glycine-rich loop region "GDGTVGT" and the conserved catalytic residues Lys84 and Glu72, suggesting potential NCS activity (Figures S4 and S5).

We employed a prokaryotic expression system for protein purification and subsequent activity testing. The results indicated that *Nn*NCS1, *Nn*NCS3, *Nn*NCS4, *Nn*NCS5, and *Nn*NCS7 all possess the capability to condense dopamine with 4-HPAA to form the BIAs skeleton, although *Nn*NCS3 exhibited significantly lower activity compared to the others (Figures 1A, S6, and S7). Furthermore, we hypothesized about the potential aldehyde substrate compatibility of *Nn*NCSs. Besides 4-HPAA, 4-methyloxylphenylaceticaldehyde (4-MOPAA), 4-hydroxydihydrocinnamoyl aldehyde (4-HDCA), and other substrate analogues could potentially serve as substrates for *Nn*NCSs (Figure S8). This largely aligns with the known wide-ranging aldehyde substrate adaptability of NCSs from other plants.

We then utilized *Nn*NCS1 to examine its enzymatic properties, given its impressive catalytic activity. Our findings revealed optimal performance at 43 ℃ with a pH of 8.0 (Figure S9A, B). Kinetic analyses of the two substrates were also conducted. Interestingly, the enzymatic kinetic characteristic of *Nn*NCS1 toward dopamine exhibited a distinct sigmoidal curve (Figure S9C), signifying a homotropic effect with an $n_H$ value of 1.56 (Figure 1B). Conversely, thebaine synthase (THS) and NCSs isolated from *Thalictrum flavum* (*Tf*NCS) demonstrated noncooperative effects on dopamine and conformed to Michaelis-Menten kinetics. These outcomes suggest that different PR-10 proteins exhibit varying catalytic behaviors, largely attributable to PR-10 proteins assembling into diverse forms in nature to acquire

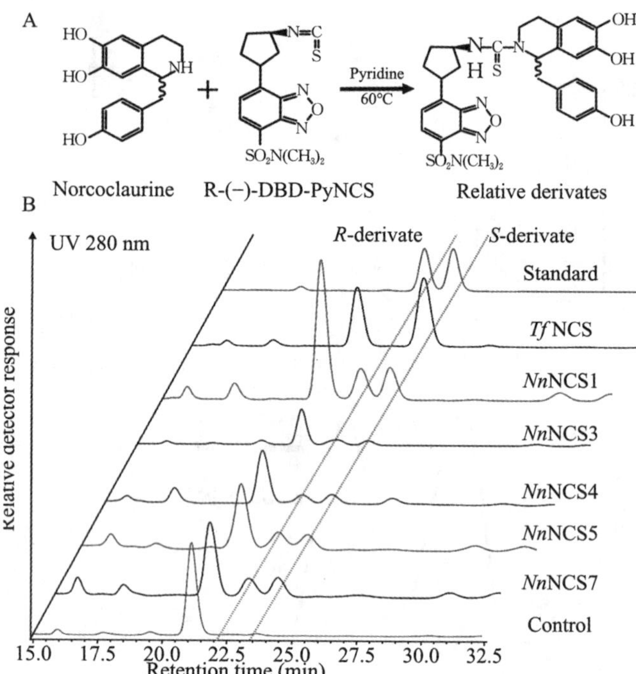


**Figure 2 Configuration assay of the norcoclaurine produced by *Nn*NCSs using precolumn derivatization**

(A) The chemical reaction equation for the precolumn derivatization process that produces diastereoisomeric derivates from norcoclaurine enantiomers. The reaction uses 1% (v/v) pyridine and 10 mM *R*-(−)-DBD-PyNCS in acetonitrile, incubated at 60 ℃ in a water bath for 1 h. (B) HPLC assay of the diastereoisomeric derivatives detected by UV spectrum under 280 nm. The (*R*)-derivate exhibits a retention time shorter than that of the (*S*)-derivate. Precolumn derivatization products of racemic standard norcoclaurine, NCS isolated from *T. flavum*, negative control without enzymes, and five NCS homologues identified in *N. nucifera* are short for Standard, *Tf*NCS, Control, and *Nn*NCS1, 3, 4, 5, and 7, respectively. The major species eluted at ~21.0 min is 4-HPAA. "*R*-derivate" indicated (*R*)-norcoclaurine and exhibits a retention time at ~22.0 min. "*S*-derivate" indicated (*S*)-norcoclaurine and exhibits a retention time of ~23.5 min.

variable functions. According to size-exclusion chromatography with multiangle light scattering detection (SEC-MALS) analysis, *Nn*NCS1 appears as a homodimer in solution, whereas *Tf*NCS is a monomer (Figure 1C). Nevertheless, all resolved *Tf*NCS structures showed similar crystal packing to form asymmetric dimers, leading us to speculate that the divergent catalytic behaviors of *Nn*NCS and *Tf*NCS could be ascribed to differences in their active site structures.

Stereochemical Attributes of *Nn*NCSs. We subsequently probed the stereochemical attributes of *Nn*NCSs employing the precolumn derivatization method. The outcomes were consistent with expectations: all of the identified *Nn*NCSs exhibited nearly equal production of (*R*)- and (*S*)-enantiomers, but the activities of *Nn*NCS3, 4, and 5 detected by UV spectrum in liquid chromatography were somewhat lower (Figure 2). This finding illuminates the origin of (*R*)-enantiospecific BIAs in lotus, which starkly contrasts with the biosynthetic mechanism of (*R*)-enantiomers reported in the opium poppy, necessitating an additional CYP450-oxidoreductase fusion protein. This alternate source of (*R*)-enantiomers also contravenes the prevailing view that BIAs metabolism has a monophyletic origin across all angiosperms (Figure S4). Considering the unique evolutionary position of *N. nucifera* among angiosperms, we hypothesized that ubiquitously distributed (*S*)-preferred NCS is a product of selective evolution over time. Consequently, we cloned the NCS from *Gnetum montanum* (*Gm*NCS), an ancient gymnosperm rich in BIAs, and examined its stereochemical properties. Despite the majority of products being identified as (*S*)-configured, one *Gm*NCS demonstrated slight (*R*)-enantioselectivity (Figure S10). We hereby demonstrate that the production of (*R*)-conformers is not exclusive in nature, and its mechanisms may differ from those of STORR. While we have established that *Nn*NCS plays a critical role in the production of the (*R*)-enantiomer, the reason why the majority of alkaloids in the lotus are characterized as (*R*)-enantiomers remains unclear. Given that *Nn*NCSs have been identified to produce norcoclaurine in a racemic form, we postulated that at least one enzyme acts as a filter in the biosynthesis of lotus BIAs. This enzyme selectively accepts the (*R*)-enantiomer of the precursors, or accepts both (*S*)- and (*R*)-enantiomers but yields only the (*R*)-product (Figure S11). Additional evidence is needed to corroborate the aforementioned hypothesis. This hypothesis was tested on *Nn*OMTs, but the results were disappointing. All of the *Nn*OMTs, along with OMTs previously studied in other plants, either lack stereospecificity or exhibit strict (*S*)-stereospecificity. However, one recent work reported that one CYP80G could stereospecifically convert (*R*)-*N*-methylcoclaurine to the proaporphine alkaloid glaziovine, which is a good evidence for our hypothesis above.

Crystal Structure of *Nn*NCS1. The identification of NCS clarifies the previously elusive origin of the (*R*)-enantiomer in lotus BIAs. This discovery lays the groundwork for the future biosynthesis of (*R*)-BIAs, such as morphine (Figure S1). However, the mechanism by which NCS catalyzes racnorcoclaurine formation remains poorly understood. This knowledge gap is exacerbated by the distinct origin of *Nn*NCSs compared to other identified NCSs (Figure S4), which may lead to diverse functions. To explore the intriguing stereochemistry of *Nn*NCS, we solved the crystallographic structure of *Nn*NCS1 at 1.7 Å resolution (Table S1). The overall structure reveals that *Nn*NCS1 forms homodimers in the crystal lattice, bearing characteristic features of the PR-10 family proteins (Figures 3A and S12, Table S2). The *Nn*NCS1 dimer is chiefly formed by interactions between residues $\beta1$ and $\alpha3$ in the

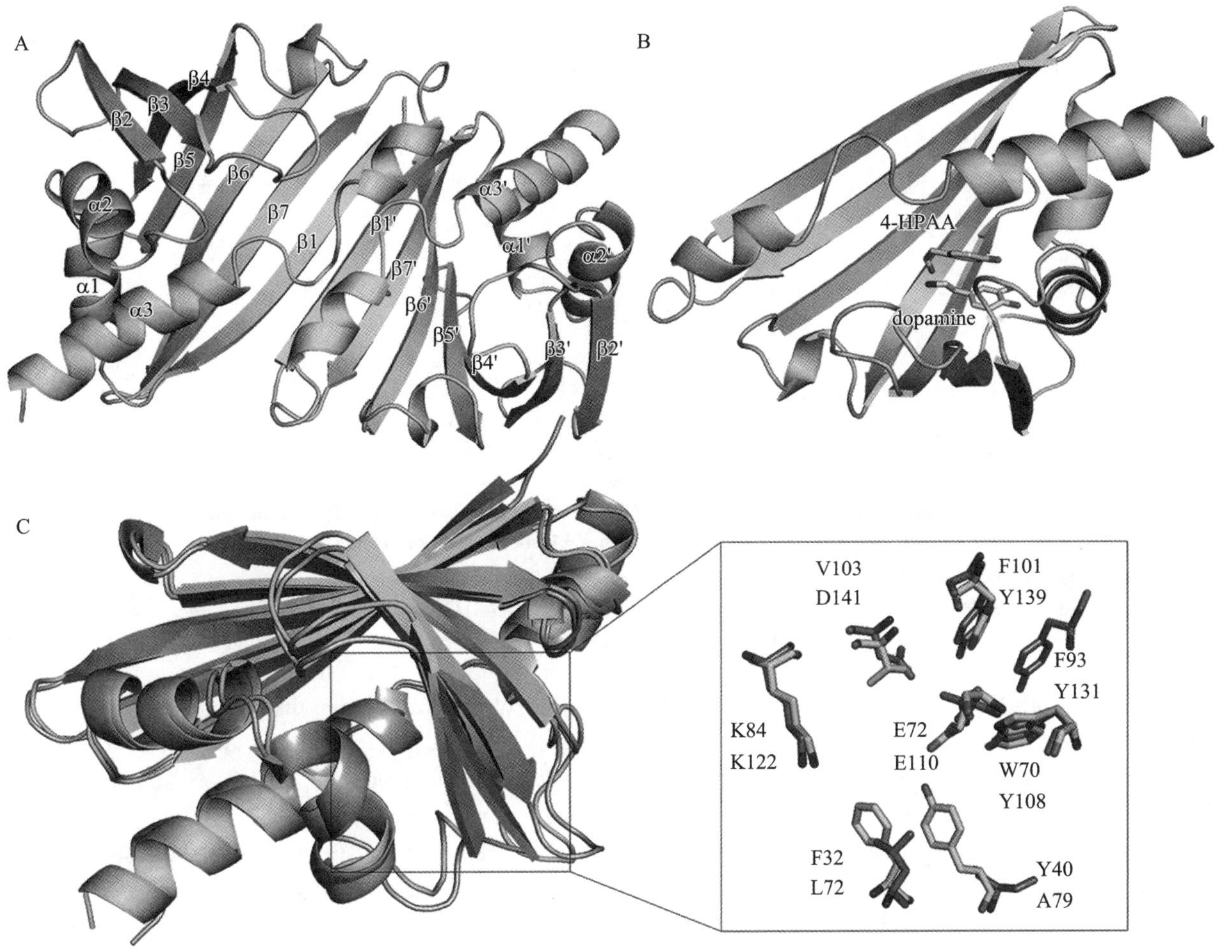


**Figure 3 Structural analysis of *Nn*NCS1**

(A) Dimeric structure of *Nn*NCS1, with one subunit colored cyan and the other green. Labels indicate secondary structures. (B) Complex structure of *Nn*NCS1 docked with 4-HPAA and dopamine. The ligands are displayed as white sticks. (C) Comparison of monomeric structures between *Nn*NCS1 (green) and *Tf*NCS (light blue; PDB ID: 5N8Q). Differences in the active pocket amino acid residues are emphasized in a close-up view and labeled.

two subunits (Figure S13). Each monomer is composed of seven-stranded antiparallel $\beta$-sheets and three $\alpha$-helices (Figure 3B). The edges of the $\beta$-sheet are defined by strands $\beta1$ and $\beta7$, separated by two consecutive short helices, $\alpha1$ and $\alpha2$. Strands $\beta2$ - $\beta7$ are interconnected by five hairpin loops, drawing $\beta7$ back into the proximity with $\beta1$. The helices $\alpha1$ and $\alpha2$ form a V-shaped brace for the C-terminal part of long helix $\alpha3$.

Additionally, C-terminal helix $\alpha3$ is shaped by two helical segments connected by an extended stretch (residues 136 - 141). This helix structure varies among PR-10 proteins, the inserted coil structure in this helix potentially being a common feature of NCSs and the inserting coli structure in this helix may be a common feature of NCSs. Each monomer shows a traversable cavity extending through the protein matrix to form a long tunnel, which could be the substrate-binding site (Figure S14). This cavity is primarily formed by hydrophobic amino acid residues and can be accessed via several openings. The wider opening is formed by a sequence of hydrophobic residues with Pro65, Trp70, Phe93, and Phe101 side chains situated at the entrance. The smaller opening of the catalytic tunnel is positioned beside His79 and Lys84 and is accessible to solvents. We compared the crystal structures of *Nn*NCS1 and *Tf*NCS to discern the causes of their different enantiopreferences and specifically investigate why *Nn*NCS1 produces both (*R*)- and (*S*)-enantiomers. First, these two proteins exhibit different patterns of dimer organization (Figure S14). Although the general structures of the two enzymes are similar, their active site structures differ (Figure 3C). Key residues in *Tf*NCS, namely, Glu110, Lys122, and Asp141, have been proven vital for enzymatic activity as a general acid-base group in the reaction. Their counter-parts in *Nn*NCS1 are Glu72, Lys84, and Val103, respectively. The negatively charged residue in *Tf*NCS at site 141 (Asp) is replaced by a neutral residue at the corresponding site 103 (Val) in *Nn*NCS1. The active site of *Nn*NCS1 contains more aromatic residues than that of *Tf*NCS. The residues corresponding to Phe32 and Tyr40 in *Nn*NCS1 are smaller aliphatic residues

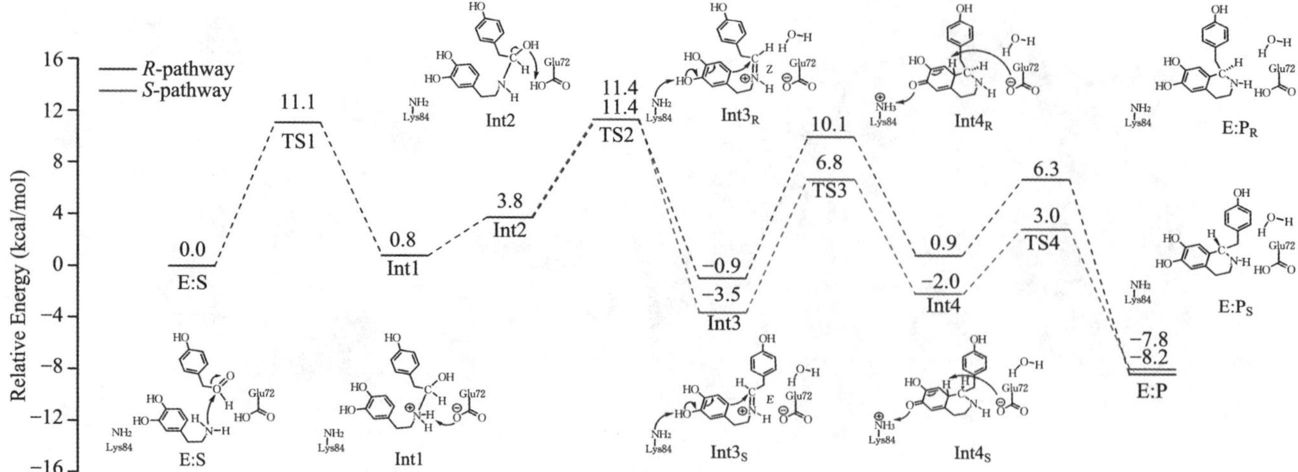


**Figure 4 Calculated energy profiles of *Nn*NCS1 for the lowest-energy pathways, leading to the formation of (*R*)-and (*S*)-products, including scheme illustrations of key intermediates**

The (*R*)- and (*S*)-pathways are colored in blue and red, respectively. The quantum chemical cluster approach was utilized, with calculations performed at the B3LYP-D3BJ/6-311+G(2d,2p) //B3LYP-D3BJ/6-31G(d,p) level. Reported energies are those from the large basis set, corrected for zero-point energy (ZPE) and solvation effects.

compared to Leu72 and Ala79 in *Tf*NCS, respectively. We theorized that the variation of key residues surrounding the pocket in these two enzymes could result in different substrate-binding patterns, leading to diverse orientations of iminium intermediates and, consequently, differing enantiopreferences.

Reaction Mechanism of *Nn*NCS1. To verify our hypothesis, we performed quantum chemical calculations and site-directed mutagenesis experiments. These were designed to examine the reaction mechanism of *Nn*NCS1, delineate the roles of key residues in catalysis, and identify the factors that influence enantiopreference. The fact that the two natural substrates of NCS enzymes bind to the enzyme in a random order, but the chemical reaction follows a dopamine-first mechanism, has been substantiated by experimental and computational studies. Therefore, we considered only the dopamine-first binding mode and corresponding mechanism in this study. The two substrates, dopamine and 4-HPAA, were manually added to the active site model, which was designed based on the crystal structure of the apoenzyme (*Nn*NCS1) that we solved in this study. Numerous enzyme-substrates complexes, featuring diverse conformations and rotamers of both the substrates and the active site residues, were optimized, and their energies were evaluated. The optimized structure of the lowest-energy complex is shown in Figure S15, while others are depicted in Figure S16. The enzyme-substrates complexes with relatively low energies were used to investigate the chemical steps of the reaction, and the pathway with the lowest barriers is presented in the following discussion (Figure 4). The optimized structures of the intermediates and transition states involved in the lowest-energy pathway are shown in Figures S17 - S20. For each species in this pathway, different structures were considered in the calculations to ensure that the lowest-energy conformations were obtained. The reported results therefore represent the most favorable reaction pathway, connecting the lowest-energy structures for each species.

In the optimized structure of the lowest-energy enzyme-substrates complex of *Nn*NCS1 (**E : S** in Figure S15), the amino group of the dopamine substrate was neutral, while Glu72 was protonated. This contrasts with *Tf*NCS, in which the equivalent Glu110 is protonated, while dopamine is positively charged. The discrepancy can be largely ascribed to the proximity of Asp141 to Glu110 in *Tf*NCS, a circumstance absent in *Nn*NCS1. Moreover, due to the differences in amino acids at structurally equivalent positions, such as Val103 and Trp70 in *Nn*NCS versus Asp141 and Phe108 in *Tf*NCS, unique hydrogen bond networks and steric effects are introduced between the substrates and the residues. Consequently, the substrates bound in different orientations in the two enzymes (see Figure S21 for an overlay of E : S of *Nn*NCS1 with that of *Tf*NCS from the previous study).

The subsequent mechanistic study demonstrated that the reaction mechanism of *Nn*NCS1 (Figure 4) closely mirrors that of *Tf*NCS in the sequences of bond formation and cleavage. The reaction commences with the formation of a C—N bond between the two substrates (**E : S** to **Int1** via **TS1**) and proceeds with a barrier-less proton transfer process from the substrate's amino group to Glu72 (**Int1** to **Int2**). For this step, the corresponding transition state could be located by geometry optimization in the gas phase (Figure S18). However, after the addition of the solvation and ZPE corrections to the large basis set energies, the final energy of the transition state was slightly lower than that of the connecting intermediate **Int2** (Table S3).

Subsequently, the pathway diverges because ($Z$)- and ($E$)-iminium intermediates (**Int3**$_R$ and **Int3**$_S$) are generated through the following dehydration. As the dopamine phenol ring is located at similar positions in two intermediates, the ($E$)/($Z$) configuration of the iminium decides whether the *Re*- or *Si*-face of the C=N double bond will be attacked, leading to the formation of different enantiomers of norcoclaurine. Interestingly, the formations of intermediates with two configurations have identical energy barriers (**TS2**$_R$ and **TS2**$_S$, 11.4 kcal/mol, Figure 4). The succeeding cyclization step (**Int3** to **Int4** via **TS3**) was calculated to have similar energies: 11.0 kcal/mol for **TS3**$_R$ and 10.3 kcal/mol for **TS3**$_S$ relative to those of **Int3**$_R$ and **Int3**$_S$, respectively (Figure 4). This cyclization reaction was facilitated by Lys84, which accepts a proton from the phenol group of the dopamine moiety. Interestingly, as shown in Figure 4, the energy difference in the cyclized intermediates (**Int4**$_R$ and **Int4**$_S$, 2.9 kcal/mol) is very similar to those of the iminium intermediates (**Int3**$_R$ and **Int3**$_S$, 2.6 kcal/mol) and the transition states of cyclization (**TS3**$_R$ and **TS3**$_S$, 2.6 kcal/mol). As the large substituent on the six-membered ring in the equatorial position is inherently more favored, these similar energy differences indicate that effects have been developed in the cyclized intermediate to disfavor **Int4**$_S$ and to favor **Int4**$_R$. Detailed structural analysis of the optimized structures showed that it can be attributed to the steric effects from the active site residues in the ($S$)-pathway, such as the Tyr40, Ile43, Ile58, and Leu60 residues.

The cyclized intermediate was then deprotonated by Glu72, a process that has barriers of 5.4 and 5.0 kcal/mol for **TS4**$_R$ and **TS4**$_S$ relative to **Int4**$_R$ and **Int4**$_S$, respectively. Owing to the fact that the steric effects between the active site residues and the substrates in the ($S$)-pathway are maintained, the deprotonation step in the ($S$)-pathway is less exothermic than that in the ($R$)-pathway. Consequently, the **E**:**P**$_R$ and **E**:**P**$_S$ bear very similar energies, namely, 8.2 and 7.8 kcal/mol lower than that of **E**:**S**, respectively (Figure 4). As illustrated in Figure 4, the dehydration step is rate-limiting for the ($R$)- and ($S$)-pathways, and the calculated energy barriers (corresponding transition states **TS2**$_R$ and **TS2**$_S$) are identically matched. Therefore, the calculations precisely mimic the experimentally observed racemic products.

Rational Design of *Nn*NCS1 for ($R$)-Enantiopreference. From a mechanistic perspective, the nonenantioselective outcome of *Nn*NCS1 is a compelling observation since the enantioselectivity of the NCS reaction is largely determined by the position of the sizable substituent on the newly formed six-membered ring during the reaction. This was demonstrated in the previous study on *Tf*NCS, where the typically favored equatorial position of the large substituent led to the formation of the experimentally observed ($S$)-norcoclaurine. Therefore, a detailed analysis of the optimized structures would provide explanation for the interesting shift of the enantiopreference from complete ($S$)-selectivity in *Tf*NCS to nonselectivity in *Nn*NCS1, and also important information for the rational design of *Nn*NCS1 for ($R$)-enantiopreference. In this section, the transition state geometries of the dehydration step and the cyclization step, which have similar barriers (Figure 4), are analyzed to guide the design of mutants with ($R$)-enantiopreference.

Upon examining the optimized structures of the selectivity-determining **TS2**$_R$ and **TS2**$_S$, we identified that introducing an extra hydrogen bond to the phenolic hydroxyl group of the substrate could stabilize **TS2**$_R$ more than **TS2**$_S$, improving ($R$)-enantioselectivity. To verify this hypothesis, we targeted and replaced the Phe101 residue with tyrosine. The F101Y mutant exhibited ($R$)-selectivity (19.16% ee, Figure S23 and Table S4).

Structural comparison reveals considerable differences in substrate orientations within the active sites between *Nn*NCS1 and *Tf*NCS. These differences are attributed to the replacement of Tyr40 in *Nn*NCS1 and Ala79 in *Tf*NCS at the structurally equivalent position, with Tyr40 introducing a greater steric effect with the substrate (Figures S21 and S22). In particular, the presence of Tyr40 in *Nn*NCS1 causes the 4-hydroxybenzyl substituent to exhibit a high level of steric interaction with Tyr40 in **TS3**$_S$ but not in **TS3**$_R$ (Figure S19). Consequently, the formation of ($S$)-cyclic amine intermediates is not favored over the ($R$)-form. From these observations, we conclude that Tyr40 is a pivotal residue that influences the enantioselectivity of *Nn*NCS1. This finding was supported by experimental mutation analysis, where substituting Tyr40 with a much smaller alanine residue resulted in ($S$)-selectivity (about −28.73% ee, Figure S23 and Table S4). However, when we mutated the corresponding residues in *Tf*NCS, none of them have significant activities to produce ($R$)-enantiomers (Table S5). Furthermore, in **TS3**$_S$, the 4-hydroxybenzyl substituent encounters steric effects from several residues, including Ile43, Ile58, and Leu60. Hence, we hypothesized that replacing these amino acids with larger ones would intensify the steric effect and consequently deter the ($S$)-preference of the reaction. Subsequently, nine mutants were designed and evaluated experimentally (I43K/L/W, I58K/W/Y, and L60F/K/W in Figure S23). Among them, four mutants demonstrated ($R$)-enantioselectivity (up to 35.68% ee, Table S4). Future research could involve further mutagenesis at these positions, exploring amino acids possessing even larger side chains, or performing combined mutagenesis.

## 3 CONCLUSIONS

NCS catalyzes the production of the first chiral compound,

norcoclaurine, in the biosynthetic pathway of BIAs. In this study, we identified five NCS homologues from *N. nucifera* capable of producing a mix of (*R*/*S*)-enantiomers of norcoclaurine. This finding presents the first example of NCSs that can facilitate the formation of (*R*)-norcoclaurine. Drawing on the crystal structure determined in this study, we utilized quantum chemical calculations to examine the detailed reaction mechanism of *Nn*NCS1. We determined that Glu72 and Lys84 act as crucial general acid-base groups in the proton transfer processes during catalysis, and Tyr40 emerged as the key residue controlling enantioselectivity. Guided by these calculation results, we rationally designed single-point mutations of Ile43, Leu60, and Phe101, leading to the acquisition of mutants with an (*R*)-enantiopreference. This research offers valuable insights for future studies focused on the synthetic biology of chiral BIAs.

## 4 MATERIALS AND METHODS

Isolation of Targeted Genes. Lotus petals, leaves, petioles, and embryos were collected from the medicinal botanical garden of the China Pharmaceutical University (118.83E, 31.95N). Total RNA was extracted using RN52-EASYspin kit (Aidlab, Beijing, China), and total cDNA was prepared immediately using PrimeScript II first Strand cDNA Synthesis Kit (TaKaRa, Dalian, China) and stored at −20 ℃. Gene sequences of *Nn*NCSs were downloaded from the NCBI genome database (https://www.ncbi.nlm.nih.gov/), including *Nn*NCS1 (KT963033), *Nn*NCS3 (KT963034), *Nn*NCS4 (KT963035), *Nn*NCS5 (KU234431), *Nn*NCS7 (KU234432).

Genes were cloned by polymerase chain reaction (PCR) using PrimeSTAR Max DNA Polymerase (TaKaRa, Dalian, China). The PCR products were confirmed by agarose gel electrophoresis. The recombinant vectors were sequenced by General Biol company (General Biol, Chuzhou, China) and compared with sequences from the genome by DNAman software (https://www.lynnon.com/). Two genes were synthesized by General Biol, including *Nn*NCS5 and *Tf*NCS.

Chemicals. Chemicals including dopamine, 4-MOPAA, 4-HDCA, 3,4-dihydroxybenzaldehyde, *R*-(−)-4-(*N*, *N*-dimethylaminosulfonyl)-7-(3-isothiocyanatopyrrolidin-1-yl)-2,1,3-benzoxadiazole (*R*-(−)-DBD-PyNCS), and norcoclaurine were all purchased from Sigma-Aldrich (Sigma-Aldrich, St. Louis, MO, USA).

4-HPAA was prepared through the demethylation of 4-methoxyphenaldehyde (Figure S24A). For details, 4-methoxyphenaldehyde (0.5 mmol/L, 1.0 equiv) was added to dry dichloromethane (5.0 mL), and boron tribromide (2.0 equiv) was added at 0 ℃. The mixture was stirred at 0 ℃ for 4 h, then 5.0 mL of water was added, and the aqueous layer was extracted three times with 10 mL of DCM. The combined organic layer was washed three times with 10 mL of brine, dried over anhydrous sodium sulfate, filtered, and concentrated to obtain the crude product as a yellow oil. The crude mixture was purified by column chromatography with a petroleum ether/ethyl acetate (5 : 1) eluent to obtain the target compound. Prepared 4-HPAA was confirmed by NMR (Figure S24B, C) method and the data are shown as follows: $^{1}$H NMR (500 MHz, Acetone-$d_6$) $\delta$ 9.67 (t, $J$ = 2.3 Hz, 1H), 8.31 (s, 1H), 7.10 (d, $J$ = 8.5 Hz, 2H), 6.83 (d, $J$ = 8.5 Hz, 2H), 3.61 (d, $J$ = 2.3 Hz, 2H); $^{13}$C NMR (125 MHz, Acetone-$d_6$) $\delta$ 199.21, 156.57, 130.73, 123.25, 115.58, 49.15.

Protein Expression and Purification. *Nn*NCSs were cloned into the pET-28a vector (Novagen) with the 6× His fusion tag at the C-terminus. *Tf*NCS were constructed into the pET-29a vector (Novagen) with a 6× His fusion tag at the C-terminus. All expression vectors are constructed using ClonExpress II One Step Cloning Kit (Vazyme, Nanjing, China). The vectors containing NCSs were transformed into *Escherichia coli* BL21(DE3) competence cells, respectively. Monoclonal cells were cultured in Luria-Bertani medium containing 50 mg/mL kanamycin at 37 ℃ and 180 rpm until $OD_{600}$ reached 0.6. After overnight induction with 0.5 mM isopropyl 1-thio-$\beta$-galactopyranoside (IPTG) at 20 ℃, the bacteria cells were collected by centrifugation and resuspended in buffer A (20 mmol/L HEPES, 500 mmol/L NaCl, 20 mmol/L imidazole, 10% (v/v) glycerol, pH 7.5). The following operations were all carried out under 4 ℃. Suspended bacteria were lysed by ultrasonic and protein-containing supernatant was isolated by centrifugation of 12,000 rpm. Crude NCS proteins were purified using the Ni-NTA column (Smart Lifesciences, Changzhou, China). The resin was prebalanced with buffer A before crude protein supernatant was loaded into the column. The resin was washed with buffer A to wash off the impurities. The targeted protein was eluted by buffer B (20 mmol/L HEPES, 500 mmol/L NaCl, 10% (v/v) glycerol, 300 mmol/L imidazole, pH 7.5). Then, the purified protein was concentrated through the ultrafilter MRCPRT010 (Sigma-Aldrich, St. Louis, MO, USA) and dialyzed with buffer A twice to reduce the concentration of imidazole and improve protein stability. Primary purified proteins were analyzed by SDS-PAGE. For crystallization, *Nn*NCS1 was further purified using protein purification system SDL-030-F2 (SePure Instruments Co., Ltd., Suzhou, China) with buffer C (20 mmol/L HEPES, 150 mmol/L NaCl, pH 7.5). The purified proteins were concentrated and stored at −80 ℃ until use.

Size-Exclusion Chromatography with Multiangle Light Scattering Detection. Size-exclusion chromatography with multiangle light scattering detection (SEC-MALS) was performed according to the previously reported method at the National Facility for Protein Science in Shanghai (NFPS). A Superdex 200 Increase 10/300 GL column (Cytiva, Shanghai, China) was used for MALS analysis and equilibrated with a buffer containing 20 mmol/L HEPES pH 7.5 and 150 mmol/L NaCl until the baseline was stable. Next, 100 μL of the protein solution (2 mg/mL) was injected and loaded onto the column. A Detector-11the (refractive-index-corrected scattering angle at 90°) was used to detect the sample. The results were analyzed by using Astra software (Wyatt Technology Corporation, Beijing, China).

Site-Directed Mutagenesis of *Nn*NCS1. Site-directed mutagenesis experiments were conducted using the rolling circle replication method. The pET-28a vector harboring the *Nn*NCS1 segment was used as the template. After PCR amplification, the products were digested with the *Dpn* I restriction endonuclease to remove origin templates and then transformed into *E. coli* DH5α cells. The plasmids from positive strains were extracted for sequencing. Positive plasmids were subsequently transferred to *E. coli* BL21 (DE3). The mutant proteins were expressed and purified as described for wild-type proteins.

Purified mutant proteins were used to analyze both the catalytic activity and optical rotation of their products. Reaction cocktails of mutant proteins were the same as wild-type ones. Each series of reactions contains one group of *Nn*NCS1 wild-type as positive control and protein-free cocktail as negative control, each group contains six independent cocktails but also equal cocktails of 100 μL, after the reaction, the six equal cocktails were mixed, and 100 μL of the mixture was isolated and further used for activity verification compared to the area peak in HPLC of wild-type. The other 500 μL of the mixture was used for enantiomer detection following the method mentioned below.

Enzymatic Activity Assays of *Nn*NCSs. All NCS proteins were heterologously expressed in the *E. coli* strain with a C-terminal $His_6$ tag. The primary 100 μL assay system contained 50 mmol/L HEPES buffer pH 7.0, 2 mmol/L dopamine, 1 mmol/L ascorbate, 2 mmol/L 4-HPAA, and 150 μg of purified proteins. Assay cocktails were mixed well and incubated at 45 ℃ for 30 min, then the reaction was terminated by the addition of 20 μL of 1 mol/L HCl to denature the protein. Assay cocktails were centrifuged at 12,000 rpm for 10 min, and 10 μL of the supernatant was injected into the HPLC system and electrospray ionization mass spectrometry (ESI-MS) equipment for analysis (Figure S7). The LC condition was as follows: 0.1% HCOOH aqueous solution-acetonitrile 15 : 85 (v/v) 0.5 mL/min gradient elution in a Hedera C18 - 24.6 * 250 mm 5 μm column (Hanbon, Huaian, China) detected at 280 nm, with Shimadzu LC-2010AT (Shimadzu, Tokyo, Japan). ESI-MS method followed as positive mode, spray voltage 3.7 kV, 40Arb Sheath gas, 15Arb aux gas, 320 ℃ capillary temperature, scan range selected within 50 - 500 *m/z*, with a Thermo Scientific/Exactive Plus equipment.

Enzyme Kinetic and Substrate Specificity Analysis of *Nn*NCSs. Assays for optimum pH, temperature, and enzyme kinetic study were based on the original condensation of dopamine and 4-HPAA. The optimum pH assay cocktail ingredients are the same as mentioned above except the buffer was replaced with 50 mmol/L citrate buffer for pH 5.5 - 6.5, 50 mmol/L HEPES buffer for pH 7.0 to 8.5, and 50 mmol/L glycine-NaOH buffer for pH 9.0. The reaction proceeded in a 45 ℃ water bath for 30 min and was stopped by cooling down on ice while 100 μL of methanol was added. The optimum temperature reactions were run in the PCR equipment, and the temperature was selected from 30 to 55 and 5 ℃ between each gradient. Among them the optimum temperature was located from 40 to 45 ℃, so another gradient from 37 to 45 ℃ with an interval of 2 ℃ was tested, and the termination of the reaction was the same as the optimum pH assay.

We studied the kinetic function of *Nn*NCS1 with dopamine and 4-HPAA, respectively. The kinetic curve of dopamine was measured by variant concentrations of dopamine from 0.1 to 10 mmol/L with a constant concentration of 4-HPAA for 2 mmol/L. The cocktail used the optimum pH and temperature studied previously, and the reaction was initiated by adding *Nn*NCS1 and lasted for 10 min to prevent the error caused by depleted dopamine. Each cocktail of the concentration gradient was repeated three times and their peak area analyzed by HPLC was collected and further processed by OriginPro software (https://www.originlab.com/). The kinetic curve of 4-HPAA was measured by the same approach as dopamine. Kinetic parameters were analyzed by fitting initial velocity to the Michaelis-Menten (4-HPAA) and Logistic (dopamine) kinetic equations, respectively.

Other aldehydes that are similar to 4-HPAA and amines similar to dopamine were tested as substrates to test the substrate specificity of *Nn*NCS1. 4-HPAA or dopamine of the reaction cocktail was substituted by the following compounds, while other ingredients and the reaction conditions remained unchanged: aldehydes include p-hydroxybenzaldehyde, benzaldehyde, 4-HDCA, methylglyoxal, 4-MOPAA, and acetophenone; amines include levodopa, tyramine, and tryptamine. Liquid chromatography-mass spectrometry (LC - MS) was utilized to analyze the existence of deduced products of each substrate based on the Pictet-Spengler formula.

Detection of Enantiomers. To separate and detect the (*R*)- and (*S*)-norcoclaurine, a reported precolumn derivatization method was utilized. For details, five enzymatic reaction cocktails (100 μL) were prepared according to the previous assay method. The cocktails were then gathered and extracted by 500 μL of ethyl acetate three times to remove dopamine and hydrophilic impurities. The organic phase was collected and distilled with a rotary evaporator. The remaining solid was dissolved in 50 μL of acetonitrile. Precolumn derivatization was achieved by mixing an equal volume of the product-acetonitrile solution, 3% pyridine acetonitrile solution, and 30 mmol/L *R*-(−)-DBD-PyNCS acetonitrile solution, then heating at 60 ℃ for 60 min. Precolumn derivates were analyzed by HPLC using an isocratic elution containing 0.2% HCOOH aqueous solution-methanol-acetonitrile (45 : 30 : 35), 0.5 mL/min, for 120 min; the detector wavelength was selected at 280 nm.

The proportion of (*R*)- and (*S*)-norcoclaurine was indicated by enantiomer excess (ee%) and it was calculated by the following formula: ee = ([*R*] − [*S*])/([*R*] + [*S*]) × 100% ([*R*] and [*S*] stand for the contents of each isomer). The ee value of the enantiomer is selected as 0%, and when the proportion of (*R*)-norcoclaurine increases, the ee value tends to be positive, and contrary for (*S*)-norcoclaurine. *Tf*NCS was used as a negative control because it can form only form (*S*)-norcoclaurine.

Crystallization, X-ray Diffraction, and Structure Data Construction of *Nn*NCS1. The crystallization method was selected as sitting-drop vapor diffusion at 16 ℃. The drip plate, cyroloop, adhesive tape, and other crystallization equipment were purchased from FAstal BioTech (Fastal BioTech, Shanghai, China), and the reagents were purchased from Sigma-Aldrich. Purified *Nn*NCS1 proteins at a concentration of 20 mg/mL were mixed with an equal volume of reservoir solution containing 8% (v/v) polyethylene glycol 3 350, 12.8 mmol/L $(NH_4)_2SO_4$, and 10 mmol/L betaine hydrochloride. Then, the Sessile drop plate was covered by adhesive tape and incubated in a 16 ℃ cabinet. Diffraction-quality crystals appeared within 3 − 5 days. The protein crystals were then picked up by cyroloop, washed with antifreeze liquid, and frozen in liquid nitrogen immediately.

The X-ray diffraction data were collected at Shanghai Synchrotron Radiation Facility (SSRF) beamline BL19U1. All data were indexed, integrated, and scaled by XDSgui and replaced by the structure of *Tf*NCS (PDB ID: 5N8Q) by Phenix 1.18.2 molecular replacement. Refinement of the coordinate was carried out by cooperation of Phenix 1.18.2 Refinement and Wincoot0.6. Resolved protein structure is observed by PyMOL 2.3 (http://www.pymol.org/).

DFT Calculations. *Active Site Model*. The cluster model was designed based on the crystal structure of the *Nn*NCS1 (PDB ID: 8HO2), and the substrates dopamine and 4-hydroxyphenylacetaldehyde were added to the model manually. The model consists of the two substrates and the residues that contribute to the assembly of the active site, namely, Tyr23, Ser24, Leu28, Pro29, Phe32, Met36, Val39, Tyr40, Ile43, Leu56, Ile58, Leu60, Trp70, Glu72, Phe74, Lys84, Val86, Gln88, Phe93, Phe101, Val103, Phe105, Thr121, Asn140, Leu141, Gly143, Ala144, and Ala145. The total sizes of the active site model are 414 atoms, and the overall charge is 0. The amino acid residues in the active site model were truncated, and the truncated carbons and a number of hydrogen atoms were kept fixed at their crystallographic positions to avoid unrealistic movements during geometry optimizations (Figure S15). For clarity, these fixations are not indicated in other figures, but the same atoms are indeed fixed. This coordinate-fixing protocol is very important to avoid large unrealistic movements of the various groups at the active site. Given the size of the active site model and the fact that the fixations were made at the edge of the active site model, enough flexibility can be granted to the active site residues to adjust the geometries along the reaction. The protonation state of Glu72 warrants a comment here. In the initial structure of all of the considered enzyme-substrates complexes for *Nn*NCS1, Glu72 was modeled in the deprotonated state, following the set for the equivalent residue in the previous study on *Tf*NCS. However, during geometry optimization, a spontaneous proton transfer from the protonated amino group of the dopamine substrate to Glu72 takes place, leading to a structure in which both dopamine and Glu72 are in their neutral forms.

*Technical Details*. All of the calculations were performed using the Gaussian 16 program with the B3LYP − D3(BJ) density functional method. The geometry optimizations were carried out with the 6 − 31G(d, p) basis set. Single-point energies were calculated at the same level of theory using the SMD solvation model with $\varepsilon = 4$ to estimate the surrounding effects, and zero-point energies (ZPE) were obtained by performing frequency calculations also at the same level. To get more accurate energies, the single-point calculations were performed at a higher-level basis set 6 − 311+G(2d,2p) on the basis of the optimized structures. The presented energies in this work are single-point energies at the large basis set (which include dispersion effects) corrected for ZPE and solvation effects. The quantum chemical cluster approach used in the present study has been successfully applied to solve the mechanistic problem of enzymatic reactions, and recently to reproduce and rationalize the enantioselectivity, especially for another NCS enzyme (*Tf*NCS).

[张李博，张士清，赵玉成，等. ACS Catalysis, 2023, 13: 15164 − 15174.]

# MALDI imaging assisted discovery of a di-*O*-glycosyltransferase from *Platycodon grandiflorum root*

## 1 INTRODUCTION

*Platycodon grandiflorum* is an herbaceous perennial plant belonging to the family *Campanulaceae* and has been used as a food and medicine since ancient times. Modern research has confirmed its various pharmacological properties, such as anti-inflammatory, antitumor, anti-obesity, and cognitionenhancing activities. Oleanane-type triterpenoid saponins (OTSs) are pharmaceutically active saponins isolated from the root of *P. grandiflorum*, predominantly including platycodigenin-type aglycones, such as platycodin D (PD), platycodin $D_3$ ($PD_3$) and platycoside E (PE). These three saponins share a common platycodigenin skeleton and an identical sugar side chain attached to C28 of the aglycone, only differing from each other in the number of glycosyl units attached to the hydroxy group at the C3 position.

In general, obtaining large amounts of pure OTSs by using traditional solvent extraction from plant materials is difficult due to their low content and interference from complex sample matrixes, resulting in high costs of production and environmental contamination. Chemical total or semisynthesis of natural products is challenging and has some disadvantages, such as side reactions, low regioselectivity, and low yield. Synthetic biology has emerged as a vital environmentally friendly alternative for efficiently producing glycosylated triterpenoids through the introduction of various glycosyltransferase (GT) genes from plants into microorganisms, contributing to expedited development of heterologous production of target compounds. Therefore, numerous efforts have been made to decipher the biosynthetic pathway of OTSs and discover the corresponding GTs to produce OTSs. The enzymatic biotransformation of PE to PD through intermediate $PD_3$ using fungal extracellular $\beta$-glucosidases has been investigated, whereas the pathway for biosynthesis of PE is still unknown.

Over the last two decades, next-generation sequencing (NGS) has led to an exponential increase in the amount of genomic data available for medicinal plants. However, a quantum leap in sequence data does not necessarily lead to a rapid increase in pace with the identification of key enzymes responsible to produce bioactive natural products. One possible reason might be the omission of the spatial dependence of the consequences of the gene at the tissue level. Specialized tissues in plants have unique anatomical features, which can be attributed to differential gene expression and metabolite distributions. Increasing evidence confirmed that the spatial distribution patterns of plant secondary metabolites were well correlated with the localization of associated gene expression. Therefore, starting with the accurate localization of metabolites in tissues would provide important clues for the readout of region-specific gene expression profiles. However, the spatial distribution of secondary metabolites in plant tissues is often lost because tissue homogenization is required prior to liquid chromatography- or gas chromatography-mass spectrometry (LC/GC-MS) analysis.

As a label-free imaging technique with high molecular coverage and sensitivity, matrix-assisted laser desorption/ionization mass spectrometry imaging (MALDI MSI) has been used to visualize the spatial distribution of various secondary metabolites in medicinal plant tissues. MALDI MSI can provide crucial clues in deciphering the metabolic pathways of natural products, but analysts have rarely attempted to exploit spatial clues obtained from MALDI MSI to establish the metabolite-gene expression relationship. Herein, we reported a strategy to mine candidate GT genes from the root of *P. grandiflorum* by combining MALDI MSI, transcriptome, and phylogenetic analysis. MALDI MSI was first performed on root tissues to visualize the spatial distribution of saponins and identify the region of interest (ROI). Subsequently, RNA sequencing was performed on individual ROI to generate the region-specific transcriptome readouts. Consequently, nine differentially expressed GT genes involved in saponin biosynthesis were identified, and a di-*O*-glycosyltransferase PgGT1, which can catalyze a two-step glycosylation reaction on PD to synthesize PE, was discovered and characterized from *P. grandiflorum* root. Furthermore, the substrate promiscuity, sugar donor specificity, and structure-function relationships of PgGT1 were also elucidated.

## 2 RESULTS AND DISCUSSION

Initially, the spatial distribution patterns of various metabolites in *P. grandiflorum* root were unraveled by MALDI MSI. Among various saponins, the spatial distribution patterns of three structurally consecutive saponins, namely PD, $PD_3$, and PE, exhibited both similarities and differences (Figure 1A). From the overlaid ion image, a major differ-

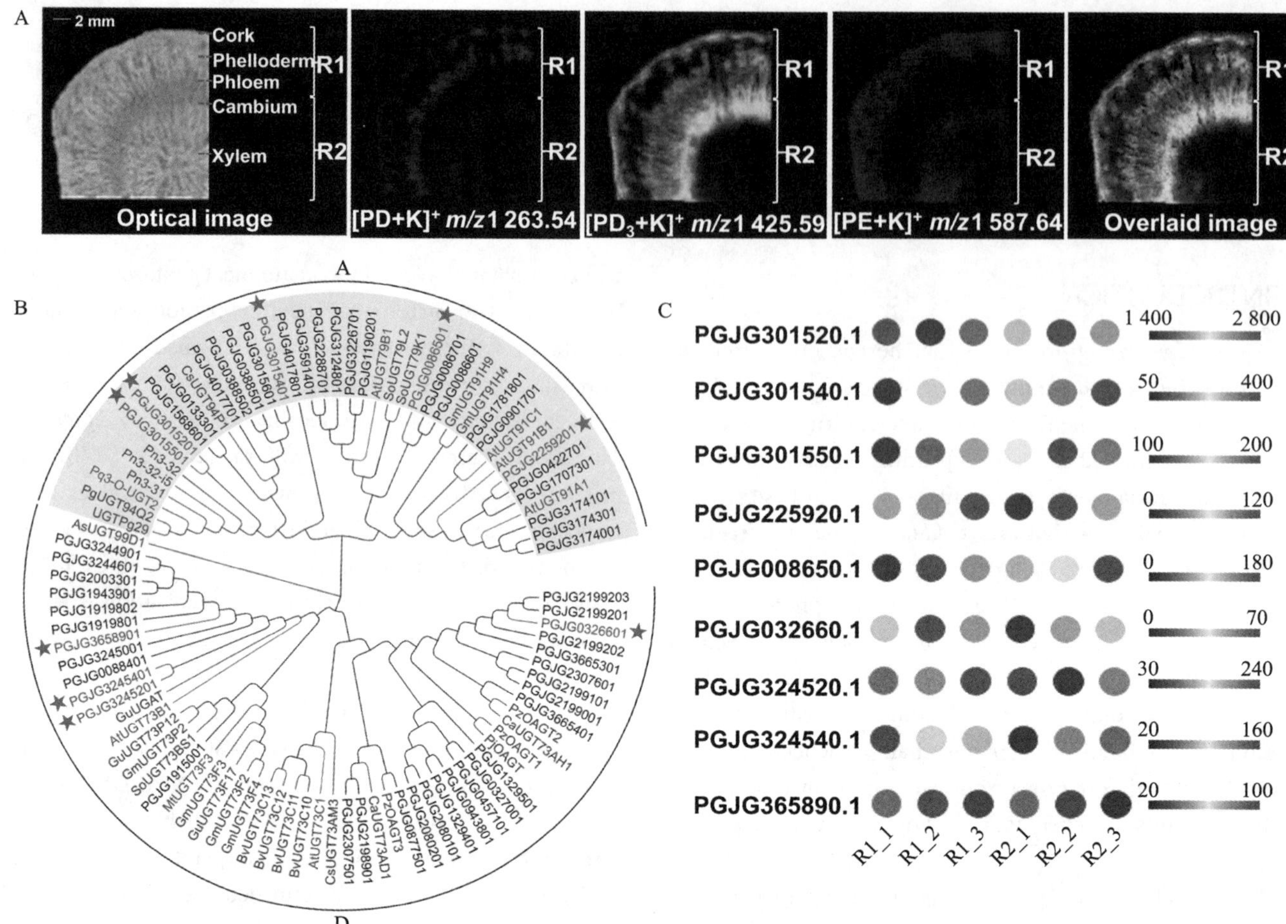


**Figure 1 Region-specific screening of GT genes from *P. grandiflorum* root**

(A) Optical image of root section and MALDI images of selected saponin ions, including $[PD+K]^+$ ($m/z$1 263.54), $[PD_3+K]^+$ ($m/z$ 1 425.59), $[PE+K]^+$ ($m/z$ 1 587.64), and the overlaid ion image of these three ions. The mass accuracy was better than 2 ppm, and a bin width of $m/z = \pm 5$ ppm was used for image generation. Detailed parameters can be found in the Supporting Information. (B) Phylogenetic tree of candidate UGTs (black) from *P. grandiflorum* with characterized UGTs derived from the group A and D. AtUGTs are indicated in green, and the nine PgGTs with high expression levels are indicated in red and marked with a red star. Other known UGTs are indicated in purple. A detailed list is available in Table S1. (C) The individual gene expression heatmap of nine highly expressed PgGTs in R1 and R2 regions.

ence in spatial distribution could be observed between the xylem (R2) and tissues outside of the xylem (R1), which were segmented by the cambium layer. Therefore, enzymes that catalyzed the conversion of these three saponins might be differentially expressed between R1 and R2 regions.

On the other hand, the publicly available genome (SPEA00000000) was analyzed using the Hidden Markov Model (HMM), and 194 PgGTs were found in the whole genome of *P. grandiflorum*. Phylogenetic analysis was performed on a dataset consisting of these 194 PgGTs and the full-length amino acid sequences of GTs derived from other species (Table S1 and Figure S1). The results revealed the presence of 18 distinct groups (A - R) of UDP-sugar-dependent glycosyltransferases (UGTs) based on the phylogeny of *P. grandiflorum*. It was particularly noteworthy that 26 and 31 members were classified into group A and group D, respectively (Figure 1B), which have been reported to play roles in transferring sugar moieties to the biosynthetic intermediate of saponins. Thereafter, PgGTs in groups A and D were selected for further study. Unfortunately, as shown in Figure S2, the differential expression of GT genes could not be easily obtained via the bulk analysis of RNA-seq data from eight different integrated tissues (leaves, stems, roots, petals, sepals, pistils, stamens, and seeds) (SRR8712510 - SRR8712517), as well as RNA-seq data from 12 h, 24 h, and 48 h methyl jasmonate-treated and 12 h control seedlings (SRR8712518 - SRR8712529). Therefore, according to the results of MAL - DI MSI, the root section was manually divided into R1 and R2 regions as shown in Figure 1, and the RNA-seq analysis (SRR22045622 - SRR22045627) of R1 and R2 were performed for the screening of differentially expressed genes, respectively. Interestingly, differentially expressed GT genes were readily obtained from R1 and R2 regions (Figure S2), and nine differential PgGT genes expressed at a high level (FPKM≥20) in groups A and D were targeted (Figure 1C). Among them, three PgGT genes (PGJG301520.1, PGJG301540.1, and PGJG301550.1) expressed at higher levels in the R2 region were chosen as high-priority candidate genes since they might be involved in the conversion of target saponins. Compared to traditional bulk RNA-Seq analysis, our screening strategy demonstrated high efficiency and convenience in identifying the differentially expressed genes.

To validate the biochemical activity in vitro, full-length cDNAs of these screened genes were cloned using the designed primers (Table S2) and overexpressed in *Escherichia coli* BL21 (DE3) strain. The catalytic activities of three high-priority candidate PgGTs were first tested using uridine 5′-diphosphate glucose (UDP - Glc) as the sugar donor and PD as the sugar acceptor. Similarly, the other six candidate PgGTs were also cloned but no catalytic activity to PD was observed. LC - MS results showed that among three high-priority candidate PgGTs, only PGJG301540.1 could catalyze PD to form two products (Figures 2A and 2B). Convincingly, a more polar product **3** was presented as the major product. The $[M-H]^-$ ion of product **3** appeared at $m/z$ 1 547.5, which was 324 Da greater than that of PD. The MS/MS spectra of product **3** showed characteristic fragment ions at $m/z$ 1005.4, $m/z$ 1223.4, $m/z$ 1385.5, and $m/z$ 1415.5, indicating the addition of two glucosyl moieties to PD (Figure 2C). Product **3** was further purified from a prepara-tive-scale reaction and identified as PE by nuclear magnetic resonance (NMR) analyses (See Supporting Information). Intermediate product **2** was identified as $PD_3$ through comparison with the MS/MS profile of an authentic standard (Figure 2D). As shown in Figure 2E, PGJG301540.1 showed high conversion efficiency (96.6%) in the catalyzation of $PD_3$ to PE. Consequently, this novel GT gene (PGJG301540.1) discovered from *P. grandiflorum*, containing an open reading frame of 1 392 bp which could encode a protein of 463 amino acids was named PgGT1 (GenBank accession no. OP626755), and designated as UGT94U4 according to the UGT Nomenclature Committee. The protein sequence of PgGT1 was compared with five known GTs belonging to the UGT94 family (Table S3 and Figure S3). The sequence analysis revealed that PgGT1 shared approximately 56% sequence identity with these five GTs and belongs to the CAZy GT1 family.

The recombinant plasmid pET-32a (+)-PgGT1 was constructed and introduced into *E. coli* BL21 (DE3) for heterologous expression. Overexpressed PgGT1 was purified using Ni-NTA affinity chromatography (Figure S4). The biochemical properties of PgGT1 were investigated using $PD_3$ as the acceptor and UDP - Glc as the sugar donor. As a result, PgGT1 exhibited its maximum catalytic activity at pH 6.0 (50 mmol/L $NaH_2PO_4$ - $Na_2HPO_4$) (Figure S5A) and 42 ℃ (Figure S5B), and it was also independent of divalent metal ions (Figure S5C). The di-*O*-glycosylation reaction catalyzed by PgGT1 was a continuous two-step pathway. The first step (PD to $PD_3$) was completed within 10 minutes, resulting in difficulty in determining the kinetic parameters (Figure 2E). The apparent $K_m$ value for the second step ($PD_3$ to PE) was 64.16 μmol/L and the $K_{cat}$ value was 1.97 $s^{-1}$ (Figure S6). To our knowledge, PgGT1 is the first reported OTS glycosyltransferase discovered from *P. grandiflorum*, capable of the attachment of two β-1, 6-linked glucosyl residues sequentially to the glucosyl residue at the C3 position of PD to synthesize PE.

A small library consisting of 25 OTSs was then applied for substrate screening using UDP - Glc as the sugar donor (Figures 3 and S7). High-performance liquid chromatography (HPLC) methods used in this study were presented in Table S4 and the detailed information on substrates catalyzed by PgGT1 was presented in Table S5. It was particularly noteworthy that PgGT1 could not only catalyze the two-step glycosylation pathway from PD (**1**) to PE (**3**) but also convert polygalacin D (**4**) into platycoside D (**4b**) (Figure 3A). PgGT1 could also catalyze mono-*O*-glycosylation of $PD_3$(**2**), macranthoidin A (**5**), and macranthoidin B (**6**), respectively (Figure 3A). Moreover, PgGT1 could convert macranthoidin A (**5**) into a new compound **6a** via the catalyzation of the sequential addition of two glucoses to the glucosyl chain attached to the C3 position of macranthoidin A, albeit with a low yield. The identity of compound **6a** and other final products was verified by LC - MS and NMR (See Supporting Information). For other 20 substrates, PgGT1 showed virtually no catalytic activity. Interestingly, the catalytic reactions driven by PgGT1 mainly occurred at the branched glycoside at the C3 position for all five oleanane-type substrates in which the terminal ester at the C28 position was occupied by the saccharide side chains. When the branched-chain saccharides at the C3 position were all glucosyl moieties, the catalytic reactions occurred at 6′- OH of glucose. In contrast to most saponin GTs, PgGT1 showed relatively high substrate specificity. The structural alterations of sugar chains at C3 and C28 in the substrates could lead to the loss of catalytic activity, as exemplified by **1** vs. **8** and **2** vs. **10** (Figure 3B and C). For oleanane-type substrates without the sugar side chains at both C3 and C28 positions such as platicodigenin (**11**) or with only one sugar chain at C3 position such as macrantho-side B (**25**), PgGT1 did not show catalytic activity (Figure 3C).

Six sugar donors including UDP-glucose (UDP - Glc), UDP-xylose (UDP - Xyl), UDP-galactose (UDP - Gal), UDP-rhamnose (UDP - Rha), UDP - *N*-acetylglucosamine (UDP - GlcNAc), and UDP-glucuronic acid (UDP - GlcA)

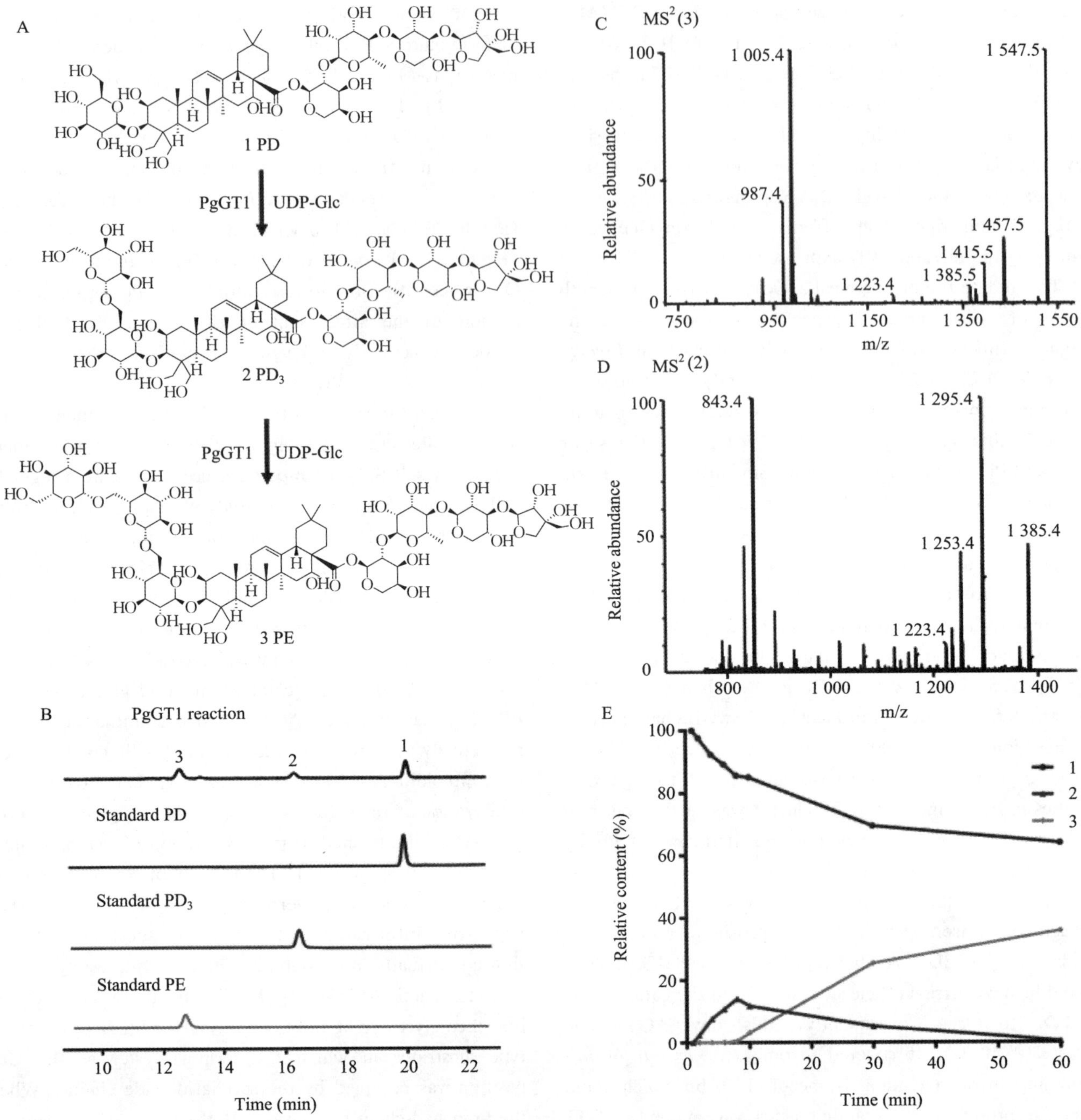


**Figure 2 Di-*O*-glycosylation of PD catalyzed by PgGT1**

(A) Two-step glycosylation of PD (**1**) to $PD_3$ (**2**) and PE (**3**) in sequence. (B) LC-MS for the determination of enzymatic reactions. (C) MS/MS spectrum of product **3**. (D) MS/MS spectrum of product **2**. (E) Monitoring enzymatic conversions by LC-MS.

were selected to evaluate the sugar donor specificity of PgGT1 (Figures 4A and S8). Among them, PgGT1 showed a significant preference for UDP-Glc with a high conversion rate (96.6%), followed by UDP-Xyl (16%) and UDP-GlcNAc (0.6%) (Figure 4B) when $PD_3$ was used as the substrate. However, no reaction product was detected in the presence of UDP-Gal, UDP-Rha, and UDP-GlcA. These results indicated that PgGT1 preferentially selected UDP-Glc as the sugar donor.

To further estimate the molecular basis for the sugar donor specificity of PgGT1, molecular docking was performed on PgGT1 and UDP-Glc to identify the crucial amino acid residues. As shown in Figures 4C and D, UDP-Glc is almost completely buried in a long, narrow channel mainly within the C-terminal domain of PgGT1 where it interacts with amino acids of the PSPG motif. Docking results indicated that W332 formed $\pi-\pi$ interactions with the uridine ring of UDP. Two hydrogen bonds were formed from S273 to both hydroxy hydrogen atoms of the ribose. In addition, W353 formed a hydrogen bond with the phosphate

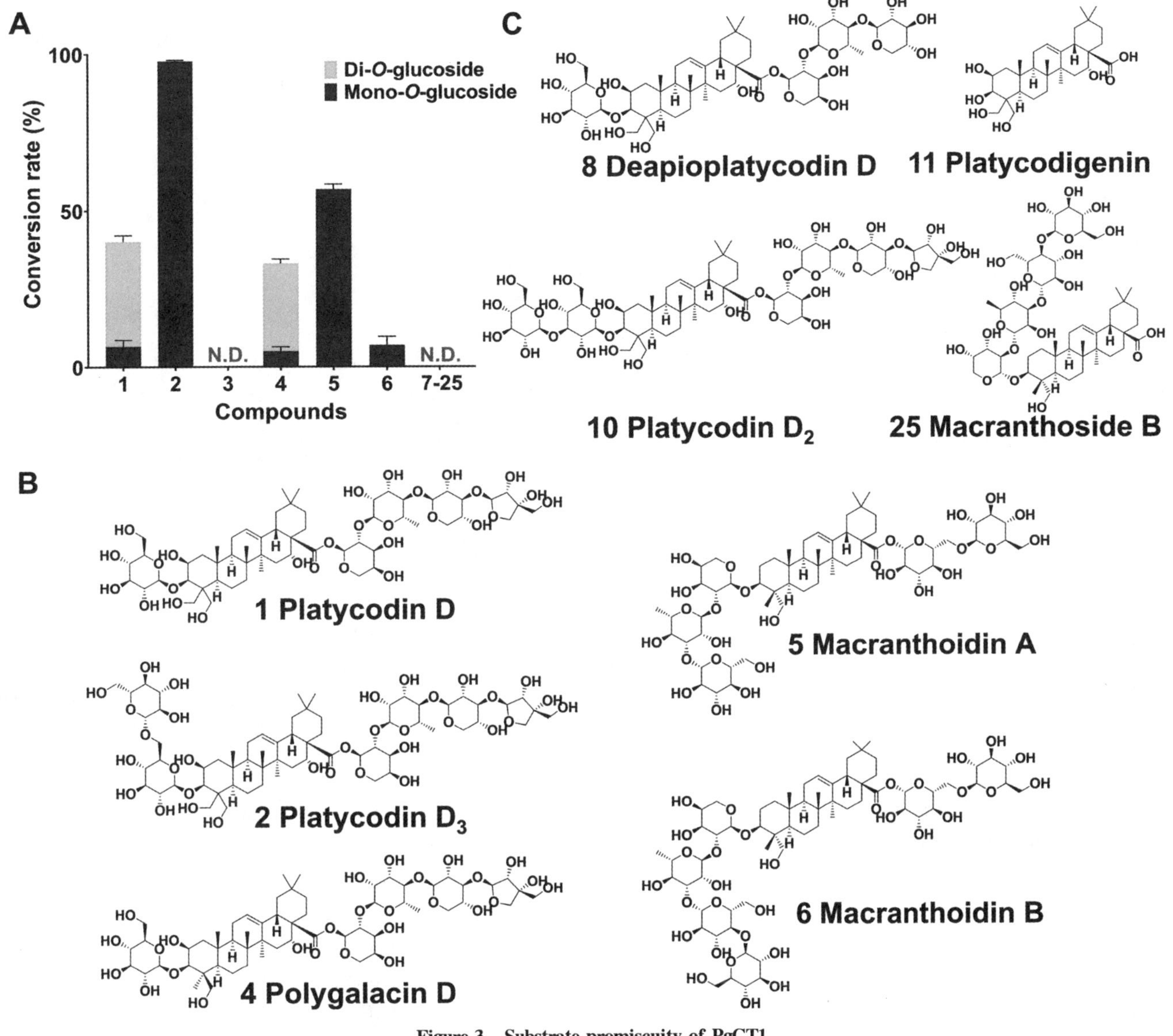


**Figure 3 Substrate promiscuity of PgGT1**

(A) Conversion rate of 25 candidate substrates catalyzed by PgGT1. (B) Structures of reactive substrates: **1**, **2**, **4**, **5**, and **6**. (C) Structures of partly unreactive substrates: **8**, **10**, **11**, and **25**. N.D.: not detectable.

residue close to the glucose, whereas H350 formed a hydrogen bond with the phosphate residue close to the ribose. It was noteworthy that D374 and Q375 were hydrogen-bonded to the C4-OH and C3-OH of the glucose residue, respectively, suggesting that the stereo-configuration of 4-OH and 3-OH played essential roles in the catalytic efficiency. Moreover, N122 was hydrogen-bonded to the C6-OH group of glucose and E274 was hydrogen-bonded to the C2-OH group respectively. The exchange of N122 and E274 by alanine resulted in the loss of enzymatic activity (Figure 5). These results indicated the UDP-sugar specificity of PgGT1 depended on the different spatial arrangement of the hydroxy groups at the carbohydrate structures. The stereochemistry of the C2-OH, C3-OH, C4-OH, and C6-OH determined the glucose specificity of PgGT1.

To examine the enzymatic structure-function relationships, Robetta modeling of three-dimensional protein structure was applied to provide further insights into the structural basis of PgGT1. Molecular docking of PgGT1/UDP - Glc/PD and PgGT1/UDP - Glc/$PD_3$ were performed respectively to obtain possible conformations and orientations of the substrates in the binding pocket. The docking site on PgGT1 was defined by establishing a grid box with a default grid spacing, centered at the position of the substrate. The docked conformations of PD and $PD_3$ with the lowest estimated binding energy were chosen for molecular dynamics (MD) simulation. The results from the MD simulation suggested that the protein structures were stable in the binding pocket within 50 ns (Figure S9). The RMSD and $R_g$ values of PD_PgGT1 system were higher than those of $PD_3$_PgGT1 system in a period of 30 - 40 ns of the simulation time (Figure S9). These results indicated that the latter system

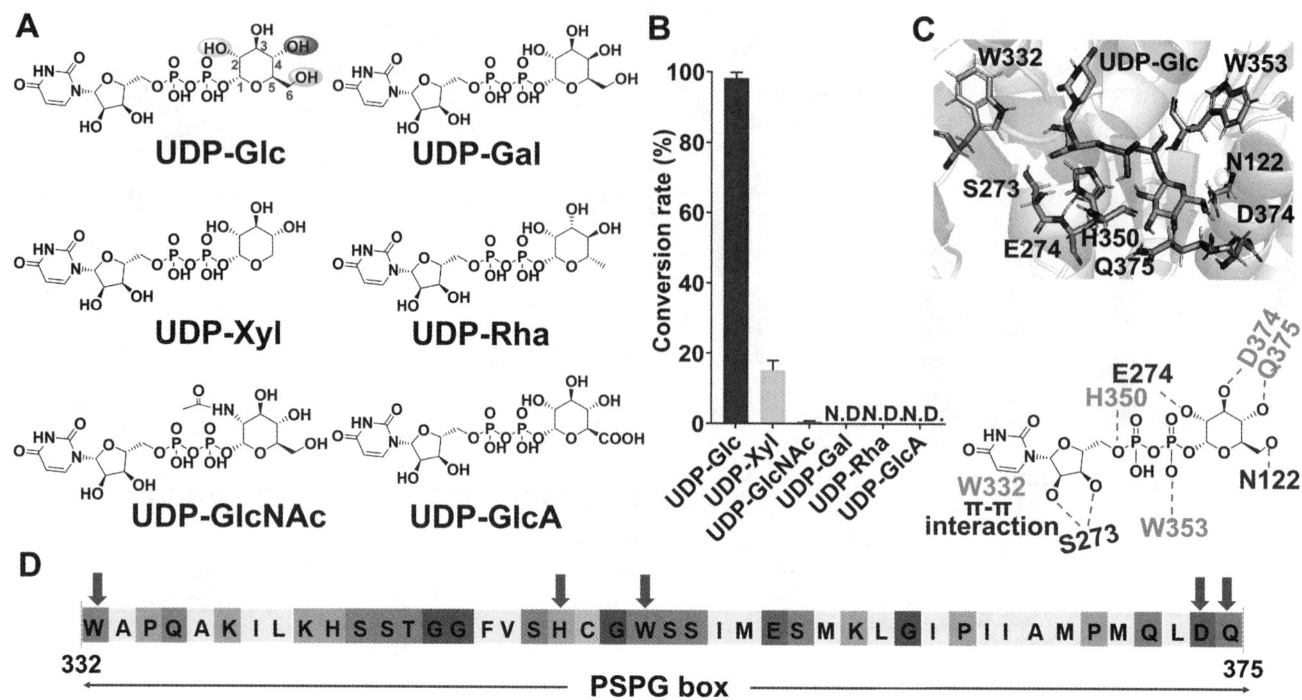


**Figure 4 Determination of sugar donor specificity of PgGT1**

(A) Structures of six sugar donors. (B) Conversion rates of six different sugar donors catalyzed by PgGT1 with $PD_3$ as the sugar acceptor. (C) Molecular docking of PgGT1/UDP - Glc. Top: The key residues and substrate molecules are shown as sticks. Bottom: Hydrogen bonds are indicated by yellow broken lines. (D) The conserved protein sequence of the PSPG box. The key residues mentioned above are marked with red arrows.

has lower and more stable motility than the former system, which is consistent with the specificity of PgGT1 towards $PD_3$.

The surrounding residues within 5.0 Å of substrates were selected and six of them were targeted for site-directed mutagenesis. A total of 25 mutants were constructed in which these six residues were subjected to a series of substitutions at PgGT1. Primers for site-directed mutagenesis were presented in Table S6, and the effects of these mutations on the catalytic function of PD and $PD_3$ were examined (Figures 5 and S10 - S15). The docking models of PgGT1/UDP - Glc/substrate suggested that the terminal hydroxy group of S273 was hydrogen-bonded to the C2-OH and C3-OH of ribose, and the terminal carboxyl group of E274 was hydrogen-bonded to the C2-OH of glucose. Additionally, H350 was hydrogen-bonded to the phosphate residue close to the ribose of UDP. These residues were considered to be the key residues that contributed significantly to the stabilization of glucose and positioning of the glucose for the optimal orientation of glycosylation sites. Consistently, mutations at S273, E274, and H350 drastically decreased or even abolished the *O*-glycosylation activity of PgGT1. Only the substitution of H350 with structurally similar tryptophan could retain the catalytic activity. Notably, residues R179 and W353 mainly influenced the catalytic activity towards di-*O*-glycosylation of PD since mutations at R179H, W353A, and W353G could retain the catalytic activity towards the mono-*O*-glycosylation of $PD_3$. Moreover, structural analyses of PgGT1/UDP - Glc and PgGT1/UDP - Glc/substrate revealed that N122 was linked to the C6-OH of glucose, and the C28 sugar moiety of the substrate located near N122. When N122 was substituted by other amino acids with a long side chain, such as glutamine, the *O*-glycosylation activity of PgGT1 decreased remarkably. The above evidence indicated that the residues S273, E274, and H350 played important roles in stabilizing and optimizing the orientation of the glucose donor for the glycosylation reaction. The mutations at R179 and W353 mainly influenced the catalytic activity towards di-*O*-glycosylation of PD and N122 was an essential residue that provides a spacious binding pocket for the substrate.

## 3 CONCLUSION

In our proof-of-concept study, a promising MALDI MSI assisted gene mining strategy was developed to efficiently screen functional genes responsible for the synthesis of bioactive saponins in *P. grandiflorum* root. By following this strategy, which combined MALDI MSI, transcriptome, and phylogenetic analysis, PgGT1 was discovered and characterized from the root of *P. grandiflorum* for the first time. Correspondingly, the unknown pathway for the biosynthesis of PE from PD was elucidated. PgGT1 could

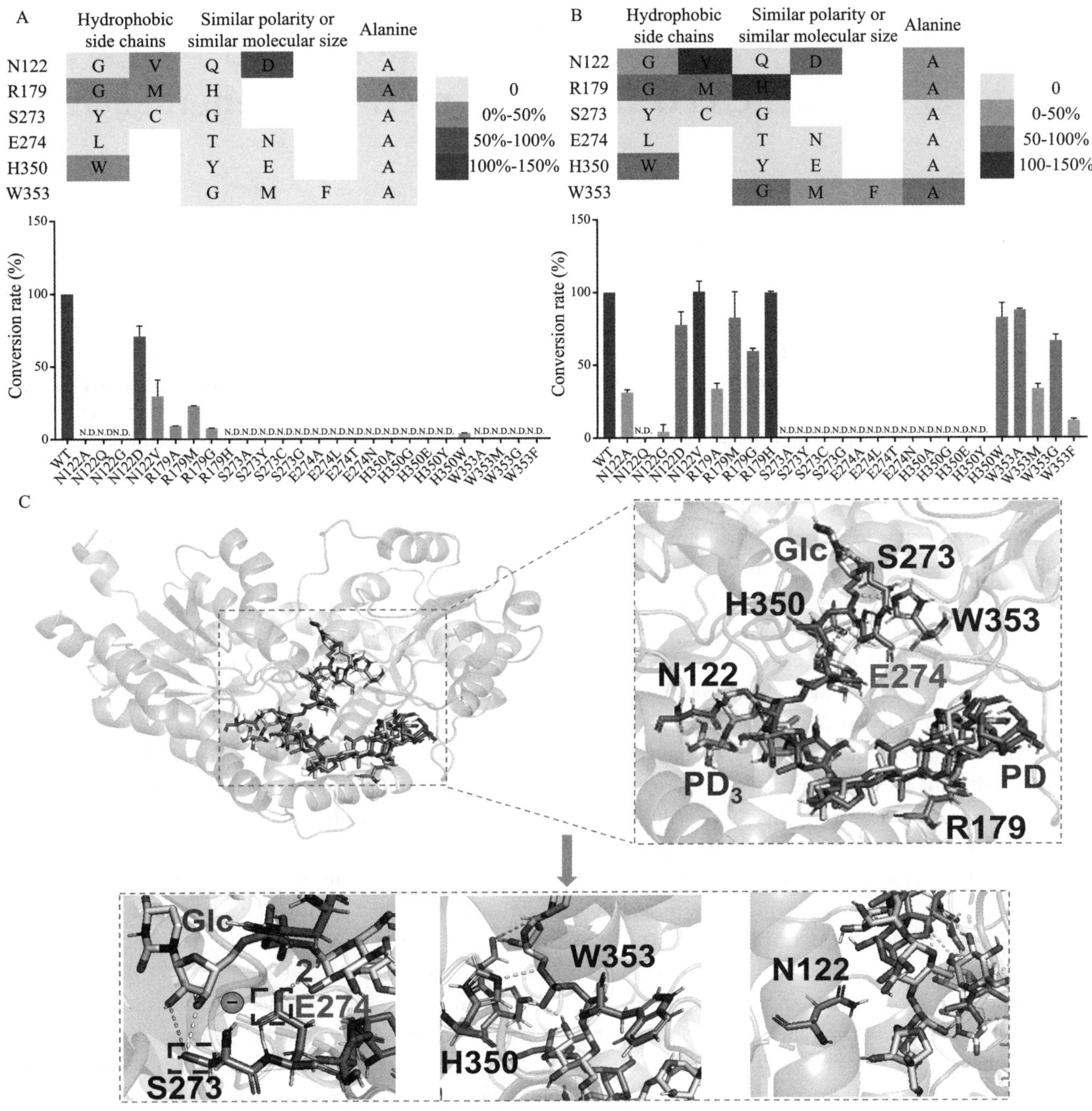


**Figure 5　Structural comparison and structure-guided mutagenesis of PgGT1**

(A) Comparison of catalytic activities of wild-type (WT) PgGT1 and its mutants towards di-$O$-glycosylation of PD and (B) mono-$O$-glycosylation of $PD_3$. (C) Structural model of PgGT1/UDP－Glc-docked PD and $PD_3$. The key residues and substrate molecules are shown as sticks.

efficiently drive a two-step di-$O$-glycosylation reaction that converts PD into PE. PgGT1 has relatively high substrate specificity as reflected in the conservation of structural features. The lack and alteration of sugar side chains at C3 and C28 positions could lead to the loss of catalytic activity. The C2-OH, C3-OH, C4-OH, and C6-OH configurations determined the glucose specificity of PgGT1. Site-directed mutagenesis studies suggested that residues S273, E274, and H350 played an important role in stabilizing the sugar donor and optimizing its orientation. We believe this strategy is a fast and efficient way of screening differential expression of genes from a huge quantity of information and connecting the metabolites with their biosynthetic gene clusters. This study could also inspire future advancement in the industrial biotransformation of bioactive PE.

［汤维维，陆续，李彬，等. Agewandte Chemie-International Edition，2023，62：e202301309.］

# Cytochrome P450s in plant terpenoid biosynthesis: discovery, characterization and metabolic engineering

## 1 INTRODUCTION

Terpenoids, as the largest family of natural products with over 70,000 known compounds (http://dnp.chemnetbase.com), have numerous valuable uses in the fields of medicine, agriculture, cosmetics and food. The triterpenoids glycyrrhizin and mogroside V, as well as the diterpenoid stevioside can be used as sweetening agents. The acyclic monoterpenoid nerol is a fragrance ingredient that is widely used in toiletries, perfumed soaps and fine fragrances. Moreover, many bioactive terpenoids or their precursors are important pharmaceuticals for the treatment of diseases. The famous anti-malarial agent artemisinin, which has saved millions of patients and earned its discoverer the Nobel Prize in 2015, is an endoperoxide sesquiterpene lactone. The triterpene saponins ginsenosides have pharmacological effects on: the central nervous, endocrine, cardiovascular and immune systems. The diterpenoids tanshinones have antibacterial, antioxidant, anti-inflammatory, and anti-tumor properties.

Terpenoids as secondary metabolites are usually present at very low concentrations in the original wild-type species. For example, the average taxol concentration in the bark of *Taxus baccata* trees is about 0.055 8%, the artemisinin content of *Artemisia annua* ranges from 0.003% to 0.21%, and the anti-inflammatory triptolide content in *Tripterygium wilfordii* only 0.000 1 - 0.002% of dry weight biomass. Direct extraction and separation from the original species not only requires high technology inputs with low efficiency, but is also unfriendly to the environment. Meanwhile, terpenoids usually contain a large number of chiral centers and complex structures, which makes them very challenging to obtain by chemical synthesis. In this regard, modern biotechnology based on fully elucidated biosynthetic pathways is considered to be a promising way for terpenoids production.

According to the number of basic isoprene (C5) units, terpenoids can be classified as: monoterpenes (C10), sesquiterpenes (C15), diterpenes (C20), triterpenes (C30), etc. The plant terpenoid biosynthetic pathway can be divided into four phases (Figure 1): C5 precursor generation, linear precursor formation, core skeleton cyclization, and functional decoration. In the first phase, the C5 precursors isopentenyl diphosphate (IPP) and its isomer dimethylallyl diphosphate (DMAPP) are produced through the cytoplasmic mevalonate (MVA) pathway and the plastidic 2-*C*-methyl-D-erythritol 4-phosphate (MEP) pathway. Notably, IPP is transmitted through the plastidic membrane, thereby playing a role in connecting the MVA and MEP pathways. In the second phase, DMAPP condenses with different amounts of IPP to form linear precursors such as: geranyl diphosphate (GPP, C10), farnesyl diphosphate (FPP, C15), and geranylgeranyl diphosphate (GGPP, C20). In addition, triterpene linear precursor 2,3-oxidosqualene (2,3 - OSQ) is synthesized from two molecules of FPP in a reaction catalyzed by squalene synthase (SQS) and squalene epoxidase (SQLE). Subsequently, the linear precursor is cyclized to form the core skeleton by terpene synthase (TPS). In the final phase, the functionalization process involving cytochrome P450s (oxidation of $>97\%$ terpenoids) is an important factor in generating the large number and structural diversity of terpenoids.

P450s are ubiquitous in the genomes of plants, animals, bacteria, fungi, and other organisms. These heme-thiolate proteins undergo monooxygenation reactions in the presence of molecular oxygen and reduced cellular cofactors, exerting: hydroxylation, epoxidation, isomerization, carbon-carbon bond cleavage, etc.. It is the largest enzyme family in nature, with over 184,522 plant-derived P450s identified to date, divided into 227 CYP families. These P450s are involved in important functionalization processes in the terpenoid biosynthetic pathway and modify the catalytic products of TPSs (Table 1, for more comprehensive information, see Supplementary Table S1). CYP88D6 from *Glycyrrhiza uralensis* catalyzes the oxidation of β-amyrin at the C - 11 site in two consecutive steps to produce 11-oxo-β-amyrin, after which CYP72A154 catalyzes the sequential three-step oxidation of 11-oxo-β-amyrin at the C - 30 site to produce glycyrrhetinic acid. In the ginsenosides biosynthetic pathway of *Panax ginseng*, CYP716A47 and CYP716A53v2 separately catalyze hydroxylations at the C - 12 and C - 6 positions for the formation of protopanaxatriol through dammarenediol-II. The precursor of abietane-type diterpene tanshinones, ferruginol is generated from miltiradiene in a reaction catalyzed by CYP76AH1, after which it is further converted by CYP76AH3 and CYP76AK1 to form 11,20-dihydroxy ferruginol and 11,20-dihydroxy sugiol in *Salvia miltiorrhiza*.

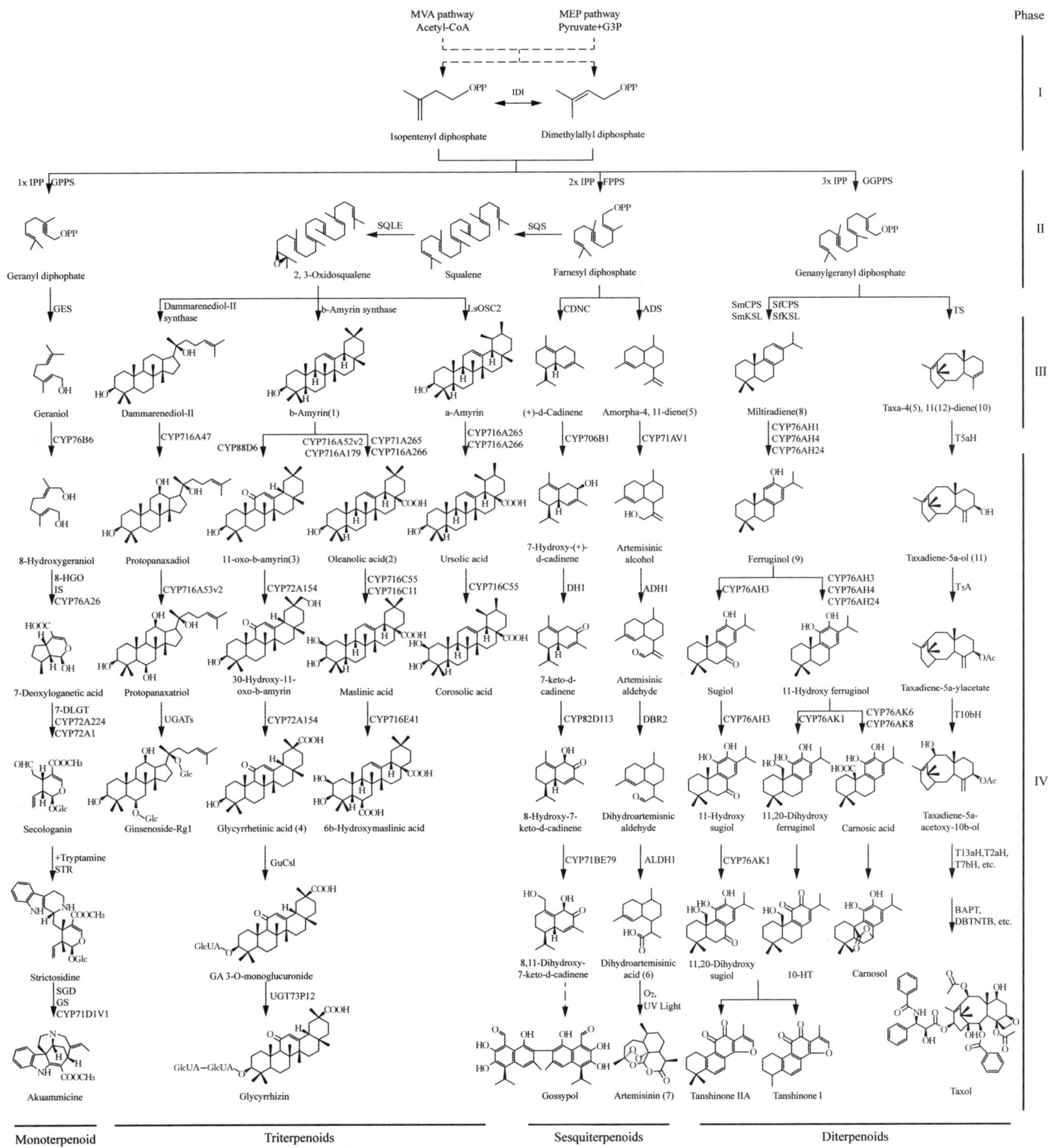


**Figure 1 The biosynthetic pathways of plant terpenoids, highlighting the functionalization process catalyzed by cytochrome P450s**

Different colors indicate P450s involved in different species-derived terpenoids, including monoterpenoid akuammicine (*Catharanthus roseus*), the sesquiterpenoids gossypol (*Gossypium hirsutum*) and artemisinin (*Artemisia annua*), the diterpenoids tanshinones (*Salvia miltiorrhiza*), carnosol (*S. fruticosa*), and taxol (*Taxus baccata*), as well as the triterpenoids ginsenosides (*Panax ginseng*), glycyrrhizin (*Glycyrrhiza uralensis*), maslinic acid, and corosolic acid (*Lagerstroemia speciosa*). Terpenoid biosynthetic pathways can be divided into four phases: C5 precursor generation, linear precursor formation, core skeleton cyclization, and functional decoration. A single solid arrow represents a one-step reaction, and a dotted arrow represents a multi-step reaction.

To date, a large number of P450s have been verified to participate in terpenoid biosynthesis, but there remain many P450s that decorate important functional steps which have not been discovered and functionally characterized, limiting the development of biotechnological production. Therefore, we system-atically introduce the recent biotech approaches on how to discover and characterize terpenoid-related P450s, review their scope of application, as well as appropriate metabolic engineering strategies for industrial production.

**Table 1 Cytochrome P450s involve in plant terpenoid biosynthesis. More information in Supplementary Table S1**

| P450 | Function | Substrates | P450 | Function | Substrates |
|---|---|---|---|---|---|
| **Triterpenoids** | | | | | |
| CYP71A16 | C-23 oxidase | Marneral, marnerol | CYP716A14v2 | Amyrin 3-hydroxy oxidase | α-amyrin, β-amyrin |
| CYP71BQ4 | C-21 hydroxylation | Dihydroniloticin | CYP716A15 | Multifunctional 28-oxidase | α-amyrin, β-amyrin, lupeol |
| CYP71BQ5 | C-21 hydroxylation | Dihydroniloticin | CYP716A17 | Multifunctional 28-oxidase | α-amyrin, β-amyrin, lupeol |
| CYP71CD1 | C-23 hydroxylation | Tirucalla-7, 24-dien-3β-ol | CYP716A44 | Amyrin 28-oxidase | α-amyrin, β-amyrin |
| CYP71CD2 | C-23 hydroxylation | Tirucalla-7, 24-dien-3β-ol | CYP716A46 | Amyrin 28-oxidase | α-amyrin, β-amyrin |
| CYP71D353 | C-20 hydroxylupeol oxidase | 20-hydroxylupeol | CYP716A47 | Dammarenediol 12-hydroxylase | Dammarenediol-ll |
| CYP81AQ19 | Cucurbitadienol 23-hydroxylase | Cucurbitadienol | CYP716A51 | Multifunctional 28-oxidase | α-amyrin, β-amyrin, lupeol |
| CYP81Q58 | Cucurbitadienol 19, 25-hydroxylase | Deacetyl-cucurbitadienol | CYP716A52v2 | β-amyrin, 28-oxidase | β-amyrin |
| CYP93E1 | Multifunctional 24-hydroxylase | β-amyrin, sopohradiol | CYP716A53v2 | Protopanaxadiol 6-hydroxylase | Protopanaxadiol |
| CYP93E2 | β-amyrin 24-hydroxylase | β-amyrin | CYP716A75 | β-amyrin 28-oxidase | β-amyrin |
| CYP93E3 | β-amyrin 24-hydroxylase | β-amyrin | CYP716A78 | Multifunctional 28-oxidase | α-amyrin, β-amyrin, lupeol |
| CYP93E4 | β-amyrin 24-hydroxylase | β-amyrin | CYP716A79 | Multifunctional 28-oxidase | α-amyrin, β-amyrin, lupeol |
| CYP93E5 | β-amyrin 24-hydroxylase | β-amyrin | CYP716A80 | Multifunctional 28-oxidase | α-amyrin, β-amyrin, lupeol |
| CYP93E6 | β-amyrin 24-hydroxylase | β-amyrin | CYP716A81 | Multifunctional 28-oxidase | α-amyrin, β-amyrin, lupeol |
| CYP93E7 | β-amyrin 24-hydroxylase | β-amyrin | CYP716A83 | β-amyrin C-28 oxidase | β-amyrin |
| CYP93E8 | β-amyrin 24-hydroxylase | β-amyrin | CYP716A86 | β-amyrin C-28 oxidase | β-amyrin |
| CYP93E9 | β-amyrin 24-hydroxylase | β-amyrin | CYP716A94 | β-amyrin C-28 oxidase | β-amyrin |
| CYP712K1 | C-29 carboxylation | Friedelin | CYP716A140 | Multifunctional 28-oxidase | β-amyrin, 16-hydroxy β-amyrin, 12, 13α-epoxy β-amyrin |
| CYP712K2 | C-29 carboxylation | Friedelin | CYP716A140v2 | β-amyrin 28-oxidase | β-amyrin |
| CYP712K3 | C-29 carboxylation | Friedelin | CYP716A141 | multifunctional oxidase | β-amyrin; Oleanolic acid; 16β-hydroxy β-amyrin |
| CYP712K4 | C-29 carboxylation | Friedelin | CYP716A155 | Multifunctional 28-oxidase | α-amyrin, β-amyrin, lupeol |
| CYP72A61v2 | 24-hydroxy β-amyrin 22-oxidase | 24-hydroxy β-amyrin | CYP716A179 | Multifunctional 29-oxidase | α-amyrin, β-amyrin, lupeol |
| CYP72A63 | Multifunctional 30-oxidase | 11-oxo- β-amyrin, β-amyrin | CYP716A180 | Lupeol 28-oxidase | Lupeol |
| CYP72A67 | Multifunctional 2β-hydroxylase | Oleanolic acid, hederagenin | CYP716A244 | β-amyrin 28-oxidase | β-amyrin |
| CYP72A68 | Multifunctional 23-hydroxylase | Oleanolic acid, Bayogenin | CYP716A252 | β-amyrin 28-oxidase | β-amyrin |
| CYP72A68v2 | Oleanolic acid 23-hydroxylase | Oleanolic acid | CYP716A253 | β-amyrin 28-oxidase | β-amyrin |
| CYP72A154 | 11-oxo-β-amyrin 30-oxidase | 11-oxo-β-amyrin | CYP716A254 | β-amyrin 28-oxidase | β-amyrin |
| CYP72A397 | Oleanolic acid 23-hydroxylase | Oleanolic acid | CYP716A265 | Multifunctional 28-oxidase | α-amyrin, β-amyrin, lupeol |
| CYP72A552 | C-23 hydroxylation | Oleanolic acid | CYP716A266 | Multifunctional 28-oxidase | α-amyrin, β-amyrin, lupeol |
| CYP714E19 | Multifunctional 23-oxidase | ursolic acid, oleanolic acid | CYP716AL1 | Multifunctional 28-oxidase | α-amyrin, β-amyrin, lupeol |
| CYP749A63 | C-2α oxidase | Ursolic acid, oleanolic acid, betulinic acid | CYP716C11 | Oleanolic acid 2α-hydroxylase | Oleanolic acid |
| CYP87D16 | Amyrin 16α-hydroxylase | β-amyrin | CYP716C49 | Oleanolic acid 2α-hydroxylase | Oleanolic acid |
| CYP87D20 | C11 carbonylase and C20 hydroxylase | Cucurbitadienol | CYP716C55 | Multifunctional 2α-hydroxylase | Ursolic acid, oleanolic acid |
| CYP88A60 | Cucurbitadienol 19-hydroxylase | Cucurbitadienol | CYP716E22 | Amyrin 6-hydroxylase | α-amyrin, β-amyrin |
| CYP88D6 | β-amyrin 11-oxidase | β-amyrin | CYP716E26 | α-amyrin 6β-hydroxylase | α-amyrin |
| CYP88L2 | Cucurbitadienol 19-hydroxylase | Cucurbitadienol | CYP716E41 | Maslinic acid 6β-hydroxylase | Maslinic acid |
| CYP88L7 | Cucurbitadienol 19-hydroxylase | Cucurbitadienol | CYP716S5 | Oleanolic acid oxidase | Oleanolic acid |
| CYP88L8 | Cucurbitadienol 7β-hydroxylase | Cucurbitadienol | CYP716Y1 | Amyrin 16α-hydroxylase | α-amyrin, β-amyrin |

(Continued)

| P450 | Function | Substrates | P450 | Function | Substrates |
|---|---|---|---|---|---|
| CYP708A2 | Thalianol 7β-oxidase | Thalianol | CYP51A2 | Sterol 14-demethylase | Obtusifoliol |
| CYP716A1 | β-amyrin 28-oxidase | β-amyrin | CYP51G1 | Sterol 14-demethylase | Obtusifoliol |
| CYP716A12 | β-amyrin 28-oxidase | β-amyrin | CYP51H10 | 12,13β-epoxidation | β-amyrin |
| **Diterpenoids** | | | | | |
| CYP71AU87 | C-18&19 hydroxylation | 9,13-epoxy-labd-14-ene | CYP701A8 | Multifunctional 3α-hydroxylase | *ent*-sandaracopimaradiene, *ent*-cassadiene, *ent*-kaurene |
| CYP71BE52 | Ferruginol 2α-oxidase | Ferruginol | CYP701A9 | Kaurene oxidase (KO) | *ent*-kaurene |
| CYP71BN1 | Lycosantalene oxidase | Lycosantalene | CYP701B1 | Kaurene oxidase (KO) | *ent*-kaurene |
| CYP71D16 | α-cembratrieneol hydroxylase | Cembratriene-ol | CYP726A14 | Casbene oxidase | Casbene |
| CYP71D353 | C-20 hydroxylation | Dihydro-lupeol | CYP726A15 | Neocembrene-5-oxidase | neocembrene |
| CYP71D365 | Casbene-9-oxidase | Casbene | CYP726A16 | C-7,8-epoxidation | 5-keto-casbene |
| CYP71D381 | Forskolin biosynthesis | 13R-manoyl oxide | CYP726A17 | Casbene-5-oxidase | Casbene |
| CYP71D445 | Casbene-9-oxidase | Casbene | CYP726A18 | Casbene-5-oxidase | Casbene |
| CYP71D495 | Casbene-9-oxidase | Casbene | CYP726A19 | Casbene-5-oxidase | Casbene |
| CYP71Z6 | *ent*-isokaurene C2/C3-hydroxylase | *ent*-isokaurene | CYP726A20 | Casbene 5,6-oxidase | Casbene |
| CYP71Z7 | *ent*-cassadiene hydroxylase | *ent*-cassa-12,15-diene | CYP726A27 | Casbene oxidase | Casbene |
| CYP76AH1 | Ferruginol synthase | Miltiradiene | CYP726A35 | Casbene 5,6-oxidase | Casbene |
| CYP76AH3 | Hydroxyferruginol synthase | Ferruginol | CYP72A9 | GA 13-hydroxylation | $GA_4$ and $GA_9$ |
| CYP76AH4 | Multifunctional oxidase | Abietatriene; 13R-manoyl oxide | CYP72A552 | C-23 hydroxylation | Oleanolic acid |
| CYP76AH8 | Forskolin biosynthesis | 13R-manoyl oxide | CYP714A1 | C16-carboxylation | $GA_{12}$ |
| CYP76AH11 | Forskolin biosynthesis | 13R-manoyl oxide | CYP714A2 | GA 13-hydroxylation | $GA_{12}$ |
| CYP76AH15 | Forskolin biosynthesis | 13R-manoyl oxide | CYP714B1 | Gibberellin 13-oxidase | $GA_{12}$ |
| CYP76AH16 | Forskolin biosynthesis | 13R-manoyl oxide | CYP714B2 | gibberellin 13-oxidase | $GA_{12}$ |
| CYP76AH17 | Forskolin biosynthesis | 13R-manoyl oxide | CYP714D1 | 16α,17-epoxidase | $GA_9$, $GA_{12}$ |
| CYP76AH18 | Forskolin biosynthesis | 13R-manoyl oxide | CYP88A | *ent*-kaurenoic acid oxidase | *ent*-kaurenoic acid |
| CYP76AH22 | Ferruginol synthases | Miltiradiene | CYP88A2 | *ent*-kaurenoic acid oxidase | *ent*-kaurenoic acid |
| CYP76AH23 | Ferruginol synthases | Miltiradiene | CYP88A3 | *ent*-kaurenoic acid oxidase | *ent*-kaurenoic acid |
| CYP76AH24 | Labdane skeleton 11/12-oxidase | Miltiradiene, abietatriene, ferruginol, manoyl oxide | CYP88A4 | *ent*-kaurenoic acid oxidase | *ent*-kaurenoic acid |
| CYP76AH24 | Ferruginol synthases | Miltiradiene | CYP88A5 | *ent*-kaurenoic acid oxidase | *ent*-kaurenoic acid |
| CYP76AH24 | ferruginol synthases | Miltiradiene | CYP88A6 | *ent*-kaurenoic acid oxidase | *ent*-kaurenoic acid |
| CYP76AK1 | Multifunctional 20-oxidase | 11-Hydroxy ferruginol, 11-Hydroxy Sugiol | CYP88A7 | *ent*-kaurenoic acid oxidase | *ent*-kaurenoic acid |
| CYP76AK6 | Multifunctional 20-oxidase | 11-Hydroxy ferruginol, ferruginol, miltiradiene | CYP720B1 | Abietadienol/abietadienal oxidase | abietadienol, abietadienal, levopimaradienol, isopimara-7, 15-dienol, isopimara-7, 15-dienal, dehydroabietadienol, dehydroabietadienal |
| CYP76AK7 | Miltiradien 20-oxidase | Miltiradiene | CYP720B2 | Hydroxyl abietene oxidase | 13-hydroxy-8(14)-abietene |
| CYP76AK8 | Multifunctional 20-oxidase | 11-hydroxy ferruginol, ferruginol, miltiradiene | CYP720B4 | Diterpene C-18 oxidase | Multi-resin olefin |
| CYP76BK1 | C-16 hydroxylase | Peregrinol | CYP720B5 | Diterpene C-18 oxidase | Multi-resin olefin |

(Continued)

| P450 | Function | Substrates | P450 | Function | Substrates |
|---|---|---|---|---|---|
| CYP76M5 | Oryzalexin synthase | *ent*-sandaracopimaradien-3β-ol | CYP720B7 | Diterpene C-18 oxidase | Multi-resin olefin |
| CYP76M6 | Oryzalexin E synthase | *ent*-sandaracopimaradiene, *syn*-stemodene; ent-sandaracopimaradien-3β-ol | CYP720B12 | Hydroxyl abietene oxidase | 13-hydroxy-8(14)-abietene |
| CYP76M7 | *ent*-cassadiene 11α-hydroxylase | *ent*-cassadiene | CYP725A1 | Taxoid 10β-hydroxylase | taxadien-5α-yl acetate |
| CYP76M8 | Multifunctional oxidase | Synpimaradiene, *ent*-pimaradiene, *ent*-sandaracopimaradiene, *ent*-isokaurene, *ent*-kaurene, *ent*-cassadien | CYP725A2 | Taxoid 13α-hydroxylase | Taxadien-5α-ol |
| CYP99A3 | Pimaradiene oxidase | *syn*-pimara-7, 15-diene; *syn*-stemod-13(17)-ene | CYP725A3 | Taxoid 14β-hydroxylase | Taxadien-5α-acetoxy-10β-ol |
| CYP701A | Kaurene oxidase (KO) | *ent*-kaurene | CYP725A4 | Taxadiene-5α-hydroxylase | Taxadiene |
| CYP701A1 | Kaurene oxidase (KO) | *ent*-kaurene | CYP725A5 | Taxoid 7β-hydroxylase | Taxusin |
| CYP701A3 | Kaurene oxidase (KO) | *ent*-kaurene | CYP725A6 | Taxoid 2α-hydroxylase | Taxusin |
| CYP701A5 | Kaurene oxidase (KO) | *ent*-kaurene | CYP728B70 | C-18 oxidase | Miltiradiene |
| CYP701A6 | Kaurene oxidase (KO) | *ent*-kaurene | CYP97C27 | C-18 hydroxylation | Geranylgeraniol |
| **Sesquiterpenoids** | | | | | |
| CYP71AV1 | Amorpha-4,11-diene 12-hydroxylase | Amorpha-4,11-diene | CYP71D20 | 5-epiaristolochene 1,3-dihydroxylase | 5-Epiaristolochene |
| CYP71AV2 | Germacrene A oxidase | Germacrene A | CYP71D55 | Premnaspirodiene oxygenase | Premnaspirodiene |
| CYP71AV8 | (+)-valencene oxidase | (+)-valencene | CYP71DD6 | Eupatolide synthase | 8β-hydroxy germacrene A acid |
| CYP71BA1 | C-8 hydroxylation | α-humulene | CYP71DJ1 | Valerena-4,7(11)-diene oxidase | Valerena-4,7(11)-diene |
| CYP71BE5 | α-guaiene 2-oxidase | α-guaiene | CYP71Z18 | (S)-β-macrocarpene 15-oxidase | (S)-β-Macrocarpene |
| CYP71BE79 | 8-hydroxy-7-keto-δ-cadinene 8-hydroxylase | 8-hydroxy-7-keto-δ-cadinene | CYP76AE2 | C-12 hydroxylation | Epikunzeaol |
| CYP71BL1 | Germacrene A acid 8β hydroxylase | Germacrene A acid | CYP76AE4 | C-8 hydroxylation | Epikunzeaol |
| CYP71BL2 | Costunolide synthase | Germacrene A acid | CYP82D113 | 7-keto-δ-cadinene 8-hydroxylase | 7-keto-δ-Cadinene |
| CYP71BL3 | Costunolide synthase | Germacrene A acid | CYP706B1 | (+)-δ-cadinene 7-hydroxylase | (+)-δ-cadinene |
| CYP71BL6 | C-8α,β hydroxylation | Germacrene A acid | CYP706M1 | Valencene oxidase | (+)-valencene |
| Monoterpenoids | | | | | |
| CYP71B31 | Linalool oxidase | Linalool | CYP76B6 | Geraniol 8-hydroxylase | Geraniol |
| CYP71D12 | Tabersonine 16-hydroxylase | Tabersonine | CYP76C1 | Linalool oxidase | Linalool |
| CYP71D13 | Limonene oxidase | (−)-4S-limonene | CYP76C2 | Linalool oxidase | Linalool |
| CYP71D15 | Limonene oxidase | (−)-4S-limonene | CYP76C3 | Linalool oxidase | Linalool |
| CYP71D18 | Limonene oxidase | (−)-4S-limonene | CYP76C4 | Linalool oxidase | Linalool |
| CYP71D174 | Limonene oxidase | (−)-4S-limonene | CYP750B1 | C-3 hydroxylase | (+)-sabinene |
| CYP71D351 | Tabersonine 16-hydroxylase | Tabersonine | CYP72A1 | Secologanin synthase | Loganic acid |
| CYP76A26 | 7-deoxyloganetic acid synthase | Iridodial/nepetalactol | CYP72A224 | 7-deoxyloganic acid 7-hydroxylase | 7-deoxyloganic acid |

## 2 DISCOVERY OF TERPENOID-RELATED P450s

Based on the rapid development of sequencing technology combined with multi-omics, four biotech approaches are introduced for accelerating the discovery of candidate terpenoid-related P450s from the plant gene kingdom (Figure 2(A); Table 2).

Multi-omics technology The rapid development of multi-omics technologies such as: genomics, transcriptomics, proteomics, and metabolomics, enabled a deeper understanding of genes, and provided a powerful method for mining candidate P450s. At present, the P450 sequences encoded in the genomes of: *Oryza sativa*, *Arabidopsis thaliana*, *P. ginseng*, and other plants, have been determined (http://drnelson.uthsc.edu/cytochromeP450.html), which undoubtedly expands the P450 candidate pool. However, the workload of functional research on each P450 is huge and difficult to complete currently, the transcriptome analysis of cells grown under different induction conditions, physiological states, or plant tissues, combined with metabolomics or proteomics, dramatically reduce the candidate P450 population. In one study, the contents of major pentacyclic triterpenes were analyzed in leaves that varied in color from green to red. The red leaves that accumulated higher concentrations of ursane and oleanane were selected as the best leaf materials for RNA-seq analysis. Treatment of whole plants or cell cultures with elicitors leads to the tran-scriptional activation of terpenoid biosynthetic genes, and can be used as an optional tool for filtering candidate genes. Transcriptomic analysis of *Centella asiatica* leaves elicited by methyl jasmonate (MeJA) uncovered four P450s which were highly expressed in response to MeJA treatment, in accordance with the accumulation patterns of the ursane-type triterpene saponins asiaticoside. An integrated MeJA-induced metabolome and proteome approach revealed the enhanced levels of enzymes (terpene skeleton enzymes, P450s and 3β-hydroxysterioid dehydrogenase), and the metabolic changes in *Physalis angulata* L., which provided a pre-liminary understanding of the regulatory mechanisms underlying MeJA induction.

Homologous sequence screening Genome and transcriptome sequencing provides abundant sequence information for classification and nomenclature of P450s. Homologous sequences generally have similar functions, which can be used to explore new functional P450s. To discover genes in the pentacyclic triterpene biosynthetic pathway of *Lagerstroemia speciosa*, eight P450s with homology to known functional CYP716s and CYP72As (C-2α hydroxylation and C-28 oxidation) were chosen as potential candidates for function research. The same method was used for querying sequences with similarity to members of the CYP76 family that are specific for diterpenoids in *Vitex agnus-castus*. Another generic homology-based approach, based on the highly conserved PERF motif in the region surrounding the heme binding and invariant cysteine residue, was used to clone three new taxoid oxygenase genes from *Taxus* sp.. It should be noted that the catalytic ability of P450 isozymes that catalyze the same reaction are diverse. Unigene25647 from *G. uralensis* with 97% amino acid similarity to the homologous CYP88D6, was used to replace CYP88D6 due to a 1.94-fold increase of 11-oxo-β-amyrin production. In the subsequent downstream C-30 oxidation process, under the optimized coupling efficiency of P450 and cytochrome P450 reductase (CPR), the titer of glycyrrhetinic acid catalyzed by CYP72A63 of *Medicago truncatula* was 2.15 times that of licorice CYP72A154. A phylogenetic tree is a manifestation of sequence homology and its clustering shows the evolutionary relationship between different sequences. Phylogenetic comparisons between *A. thaliana*, *Cucumis sativus* and *Melia azedarach* assisted in classifying 9 *M. azedarach* P450s from the CYP71 family, including 7 enzymes that were phylogenetically distinct from the other two species, were selected as candidate genes to elucidate the early steps in limonoid biosynthesis. To identify species-specific P450s involved in triptolide biosynthesis (only found in *Tripterygium*), a phylogenetic tree with 2 335 P450 amino acid sequences from eight species was constructed, which revealed 22 *Tripterygium*-specific P450s for follow-up functional studies.

Gene co-expression analysis Co-expression analysis is one of the most powerful approaches for the initial discovery of functional associated genes from massive transcriptome data. The similar profiles in transcriptional gene expression may suggest the potential linkage of biological function between the genes. *CYP71DJ1* exhibited highest similarity to the tissue expression profile of valerena-4, 7 (11)-diene synthase (*VoVDS*), and it could hydroxylate the catalytic product of VoVDS in valerenic acid biosynthesis. An expression heatmap of *Arabidopsis* P450s co-expressed with seven monoterpene synthases (monoTPS) in 29 various organs and tissues was built to retrieve potential P450s involved in the metabolism of monoterpenoids. The strongest correlation coefficients of two monoTPS (TPS10 and TPS14) and two P450s belonged to the CYP71 clan (CYP76C3 and CYP71B31) mainly expressed in flowers, and were subsequently chosen for functional investigations. In addition, the expression profiles of pathway genes are usually similar to the accumulation pattern of metabolites, which was confirmed in *TpGAS*, *TpGAO*, *TpCOS*, and *TpPTS* genes of *Tanacetum parthenium* and parthenolide accumulation. Downstream P450s with similar expression patterns during six different stages of ovary development were detected, after which 27 P450s from the CYP71 family were further

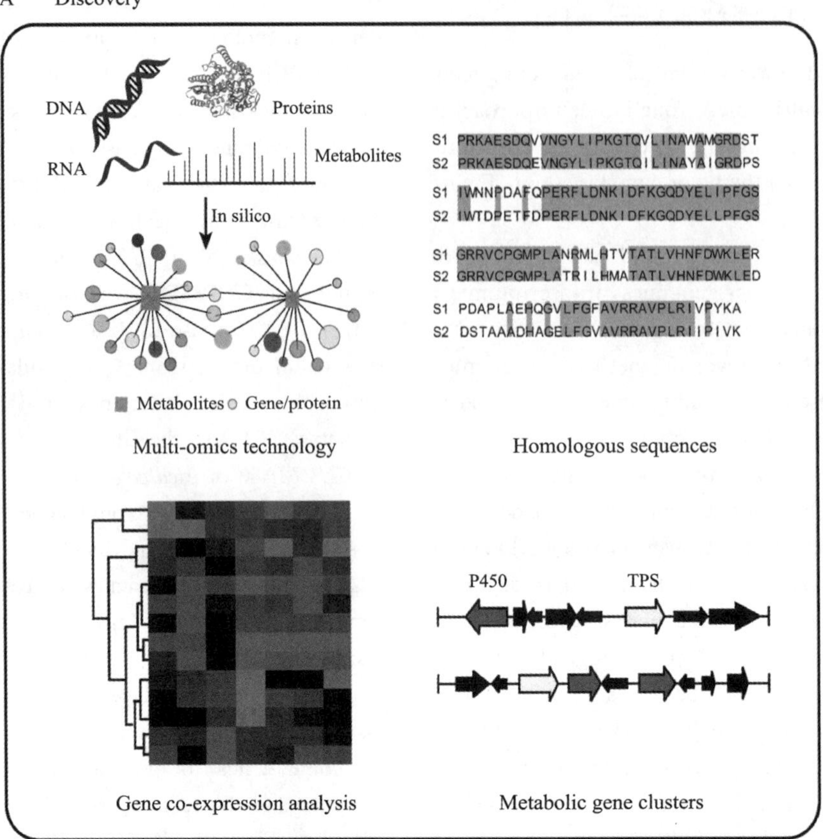


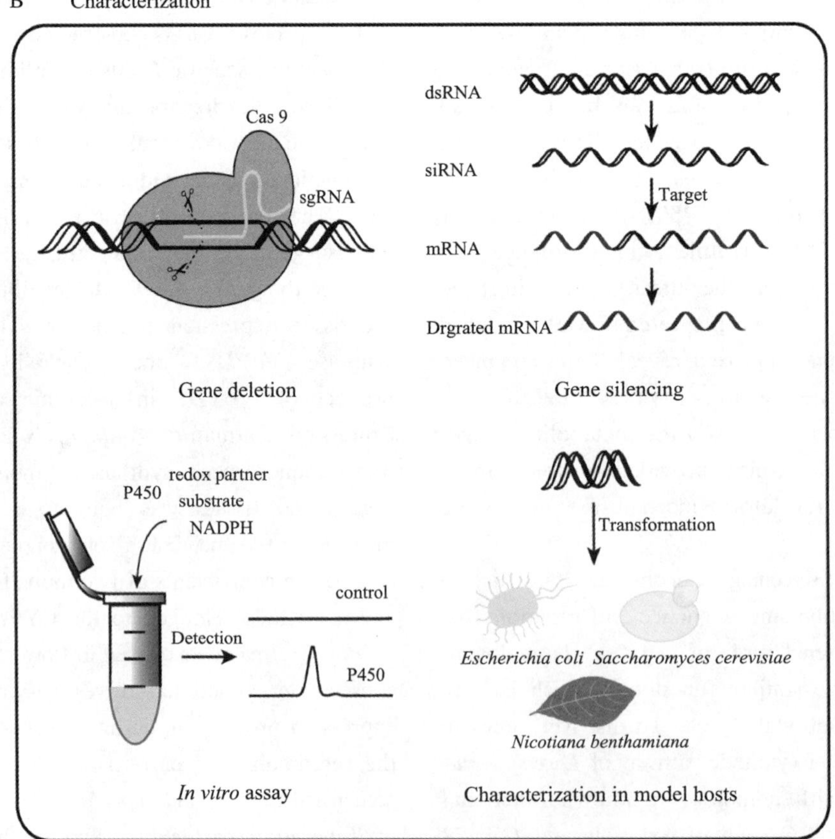


**Figure 2 Schematic diagrams of the available biotech approaches for the discovery and functional characterization of P450s involved in plant terpenoid biosynthesis**

dsRNA, double-stranded RNA; sgRNA, single guide RNA; siRNA, small interfering RNA.

**Table 2 Representative examples of the discovery and functional characterization of terpenoid-related P450s**

| Approach | Organism(s) | Enzyme(s) | Function | Substrate |
|---|---|---|---|---|
| **Discovery** | | | | |
| Multi-omics technology | *Lagerstroemia speciosa* | CYP716C55 | C-2α hydroxylation | Pentacyclic triterpenoids |
| | *Tripterygium wilfordii* | CYP728B70 | C-18 carboxylation | Miltiradiene |
| Homology sequences screening | *Maytenus ilicifolia* | CYP712K4 | C-29 carboxylation | Friedelin |
| | *Melia azedarach* | CYP71CD2, CYP71BQ5 | C-3 hydroxylation | Tirucalla-7,24-dien-3β-ol, dihydroniloticin |
| Gene co-expression analysis | *Valeriana officinalis* | CYP71DJ1 | Angular methyl hydroxylation | Valerena-4,7(11)-diene |
| | *Centella asiatica* | CYP714E19 | C-23 hydroxylation | Oleanolic acid, ursolic acid |
| Metabolic gene clusters | *Arabidopsis thaliana* | CYP72A9 | GA 13-hydroxylation | $GA_4$ and $GA_9$ |
| | *Barbarea vulgaris* | CYP72A552 | C-23 hydroxylation | Oleanolic acid |
| **Functional** Characterization | | | | |
| Gene deletion | *Lotus japonicus* | CYP93E1 | C-24 hydroxylation | β-amyrin |
| | *Arabidopsis thaliana* | CYP96A15 | midchain alkane hydroxylation | Midchain alkane |
| Gene silencing | *Gossypium hirsutum* | CYP706B1; CYP82D113 | C-7 hydroxylation; C-8 hydroxylation | (+)-δ-cadinene; 7-keto-δ-cadinene |
| | *Salvia miltiorrhiza* | CYP76AK1 | C-20 hydroxylation | 11-hydroxy ferruginol |
| *In vitro* assay | *Saccharomyces cerevisiae* (*Picea sitchensis*) | CYP720B4 | C-18 carboxylation | Resin olefin |
| | *Escherichia coli* (*Croton stellatopilosus*) | CYP97C27 | C-18 hydroxylation | Geranylgeraniol |
| Functional characterization in model hosts | *Saccharomyces cerevisiae* (*Inula hupehensis*) | CYP71BL6 | C-8α&β hydroxylation | Germacrene A acid |
| | *Nicotiana benthamiana* (*Marrubium vulgare*) | CYP71AU87 | C-18&19 hydroxylation | 9,13-epoxy-labd-14-ene |

analyzed. Jasmonates (JAs) are plant hormones that induce biosynthesis of terpenoids by JAs-responsive transcription factors: MYB, MYC, WRKY, etc., activate the biosynthetic gene promoters. The expression of *OSC2*, *BAS* and four candidate P450s in *A. annua* "Meise" treated with different hormones (JA, cytokinin 6-benzylaminopurine, and gibberellic acid) revealed that only *CYP716A14v2* was co-induced with *OSC2* and *BAS*, and it further led to the characterization of CYP716A14v2 in the biosynthetic pathway of triterpenes with a carbonyl group at position C-3 after OSC2 cyclization. Therefore, the co-expression phenomenon of TPS and candidate genes can be used as an indicator for discovery candidate P450 for further functional characterization.

Metabolic gene clusters As the genomics technology assembled to the chromo-somal level, gene clusters are constantly being discovered, and they are beneficial for gene co-regulation and synergistic function, which enable rapid stress response and are linked during heredity. It is reported that gene clusters are likely to be assembled by gene recruitment from elsewhere in the plant genome through: gene duplication, neofunctionalization and genome reorganization. Research on the function of eight tandem duplicated CYP72As in the *A. thaliana* gene cluster *GFPPS-sesTPS-P450* on chromosome (Chr) 3, demonstrated that CYP72A9 catalyzed the 13-hydrox-ylation of bioactive gibberellins. Similar to *A. thaliana*, a tandem repeat in *Barbarea vulgaris* was identified that co-localized to a region on pseudomolecule 7 containing eight tandem duplicated *CYP72As*, of which 3 orthologous pairs between two species were arranged at the same end of the tandem array. However, in the opposite direction. Nonorthologous CYP72A552, located at the other end, oxidized C-23 of oleanolic acid to generate hederagenin. In addition, the functions of these physically linked genes are often related and have similar expression patterns. A 150 kb biosynthetic gene cluster discovered from the bryophyte *Calohypnum plumiforme* genome that contained: *CYP970A14*, *CYP964A1*, and *CpDTC1/HpDTC1* and dehydrogenase momilactone A synthase (*CpMAS*) tandem arrangement. These four genes were orthologs of the: *OsCPS4*, *OsKSL4*, *OsCYP99A2/3*, and *OsMAS* in *O. sativa* cluster that sequentially catalyzed GGPP to momilactone A and expressed significant increase under $CuCl_2$ and chitosan treatment. In *Arabidopsis*, CYP706A3 oxidized the products of TPS11, only 5 kb apart on Chr5, and these two clustered genes were tightly co-expressed in floral tissues, upon anthesis and during floral bud development. *AMY2* (OSC), *CYP88D5*, and *CYP71D353*, which co-located on Chr3 of *Lotus japonicas*, were highly co-expressed in hormone-treated plants during root and nodule development, and under various environmental stresses. Nevertheless, the expression of CYP76AHs incomplete follows the expression of co-clustered CPSs in *S. miltiorrhiza TPS/CYP* gene clusters. *CYP76AH12* was equally expressed in both roots and leaves, when it was clustered with the root-specific *SmCPS1* and *CYP76AH13*. In addition, *CYP76AH1* and *CYP76AH3* were differentially expressed in roots, despite were clustered with the leave-specific *SmCPS2* and *CYP76AH28P*.

## 3 CHARACTERIZATION OF P450S INVOLVED IN TERPENOID BIOSYNTHESIS

Characterization of P450 function is an important prerequisite for the production of terpenoids in synthetic biology. In this section, we summarize four commonly applied biotech approaches used to characterize the function of terpenoid-related P450s and exemplify their usage and shortcomings (Figure 2(B); Table 2).

Gene deletion  Gene deletion is usually operated in native plants with the clear genetic background and reliable genetic manipulation techniques, which is one of the effective ways to directly characterize gene function by studying the metabolic profiles of mutants. Stem wax of T-DNA insertional strains carrying the mutant allele *cyp96a15* was found to have less secondary alcohols and ketones than the *Arabidopsis* wild-type (WT), verified that the CYP96A15 was a midchain alkane hydroxylase and involved in wax biosynthesis. The third-generation genome editing technology of the clustered regularly interspaced short palindromic repeat (CRISPR)/CRISPR-associated protein 9 (Cas9) system is used to introduce site-specific double-stranded DNA break gene knock-outs. This versatile, simple and powerful platform for genome engineering, with large number of available vectors, provides the possibility of plant P450 functional characterization. When *CYP716A51* was knocked out in the transgenic hairy roots, oleanolic acid and betulinic acid were eliminated. In addition, the *cyp93e1*-mutant *Lotus retrotransposon 1*-tagged lines completely lost the production of soyasapogenols and soyasaponin I. The direct product disappearance indicates the roles of P450 *via* loss-of-function analysis *in planta*. However, the current CRISPR-Cas9 application of P450 is mainly in bacteria, fungi and mammals, and there is little research on plants which is probably due to the mysterious genome and immature genetic manipulation in P450 native plants.

Gene silencing  Compared with gene deletion, which is completely dependent on the genome, gene silencing is an effective alternative approach for characterizing P450. It also relies on mature genetic transformation systems to operate in native plant, and can adopt virus-induced gene silencing (VIGS) and RNA interference (RNAi) to play a role in post-transcriptional gene silencing to characterize enzyme functions and putative location in the biosynthetic pathways through metabolites distinction. Gas chromatography-mass spectrometry (GC-MS) of silenced-gene cotton leaves indicated that the substrate of VIGS-*CYP706B1* was (+)-δ-cadinene $m/z$ 204, that of alcohol dehydrogenase VIGS-*DH1* was 7-hydroxy-(+)-δ-cadinene $m/z$ 220, and that of VIGS-*CYP82D113* was 7-keto-δ-cadinene $m/z$ 218. The substrate accumulated by VIGS-treated enzyme was the product of the previous enzyme, indicating that the three genes CYP706B1, DH1 and CYP82D113 catalyzed sequential three-step reaction. *Agrobacterium rhizogenes*-mediated hairy root transformation has been used as a biotechnological tool to discover the function of metabolic enzymes in various plant species by RNAi. Unique fragments from *CYP76AH3* and *CYP76AK1* were cloned into the pK7GWIWG2D RNAi vector to express self-complementary "hairpin" RNA fragments. Targeted metabolite analysis indicated that inhibition of both *CYP76AK1* and *CYP76AH3* led to a significant decrease in the content of tanshinone intermediates and final products. Genegun-mediated *CYP728B70*-RNAi also hindered the biosynthesis of triptolide, characterizing its role in triptolide biosynthetic pathway.

In vitro assay  The *in vitro* enzymatic assay can overcome complex plant transformation techniques and plant slow growth rates when expressing plant-derived P450. It has the advantages of simple operation, reliable results, and is not being affected by intracellular factors. The reaction requires P450 protein, its redox partner CPR, substrate and in the presence of nicotinamide adenine dinucleotide phosphate (NADPH), ferredoxin and ferredoxin reductase together with oxygen molecules. Liquid chromatography-MS identified the reaction product of CYP82D113-enriched yeast microsomes, substrate 7-keto-δ-cadinene and NADPH, and found that CYP82D113 hydroxylated substrate to generate 8-hydroxy-7-keto-δ-cadinene. This *in vitro* system, which only has to replace different P450 enzymes to facilitate large-scale detection of P450, found that only CYP720B1 from both *Pinus banksiana* and *P. contorta* and CYP720B4 from *Picea sitchensis* among 14 CYP720Bs in the conifer genomes could catalyze 24 diterpene resin acid precursors. In addition, prokaryotically expressed proteins can also be employed to successfully characterize the function of P450 *in vitro*. The mixed reaction contained *Croton stellatopilosus*-derived

CYP97C27 and CPR proteins extracted from *Escherichia coli*, geranylgeraniol (GGOH) and NADPH, and the formation of the product plaunotol (18-OH GGOH) showed a time dependence. The P450 pro-tein use for *in vitro* study needs to be soluble and stable. In addition, proteins that cannot be properly folded and expressed, and substrates that are difficult to obtain directly, also present difficulties to achieve.

Functional characterization in model hosts The model hosts, with clear genomic sequences, well-manipulated genetic tools and natural terpenoid precursor biosynthesis, become tractable hosts for functional characterization of plant-derived P450 functional characterization. *Saccharomyces cerevisiae* (baker's yeast), *Nicotiana benthamiana*, *E. coli*, etc., enable to: directly provide natural reaction substrates and cofactors, only transform heterologous genes (P450s and TPSs), CPR (sometimes required), avoid protein inactivation *in vitro*, and accurately and simply characterize gene function for those that cannot be genetically manipulated species.

Functional characterization in eukaryotic *S. cerevisiae* Eukaryotic *S. cerevisiae* has: a relatively complex subcellular structure (e. g., endoplasmic reticulum, ER), low native P450 content, clearly studied metabolism and mature, stable genetic tools, and has been used in plant-derived P450 research for 30 years. Due to its ability to produce heterologous proteins with high catalytic activity, yeast is an ideal microbial host for the heterologous expression of plant-derived terpene P450, especially the triterpene P450 that can utilize the natural MVA pathway. Three functional CYP716s (CYP716A83, CYP716C11, and CYP716E41) found in *C. asiatica* transcriptome were heterologously co-expressed in engineered *S. cerevisiae* with GgBAS, MTR1, and finally yielded 6β-Hydroxymaslinic acid. CYP71BL6 from *Inula hupehensis* was co-expressed with TPS in the WAT11 strain, and the previously reported lettuce costunolide synthase CYP71BL2 and no p450 served as control. Surprisingly, CYP71BL6 did not exhibit the same catalytic product as CYP71BL2 of the same subfamily to produce costunolide, but instead generated 8α- and 8β-hydroxyl germacrene A acids, and only 8α-configuration spontaneously lactonized to the 12, 8α-sesquiterpene lactone inunolide, indicating a non-stereoselective cytochrome P450 and speculating 8β-hydroxylation might occur before the C12 triple oxidation in nature. This approach, based on self-gen-erated substrates from engineered yeast for characterizing functional P450 *in vivo*, has the advantage of being more time- and labor-saving. By replacing the terpene skeleton decoration module, it was found that CYP76AH24 oxidized miltiradiene to ferruginol, and then CYP76AK6 oxidized ferruginol to carnosic acid. In another branch, CYP71BE52 catalyzed oxidation of ferruginol at position 2α, giving rise to salviol, one of the major diterpenes of *S. pomifera*.

Functional characterization in eukaryotic *N.* benthamiana Plants as photoautotrophic organisms have advantages such as: the use of carbon dioxide as a carbon source, light-driven biosynthesis, and grow in greenhouses. In addition, the protein translation, post-translational modification and protein targeting transit peptides (TPs) are conserved between plants, thereby eliminating some of the problems encountered when trying to express plant genes in microbial hosts. An established *Agrobacterium*-mediated transient co-expression assays in dicotyledonous tobacco was used to co-express *CYP71AU87* from *Marrubium vulgare* with *MvCPS1* and *MvELS*, which revealed its hydroxylation activity in 9, 13-epoxy-labd-14-ene to yield two isomeric products 9,13-epoxy labd-14-ene-18-ol and 9,13-epoxy labd-14-ene-19-ol. 1 : 1 : 1 mixed *A. tumefaciens* carrying *AttHMGR*, *TITPS* and *CYP76AE4* infiltrated tobacco leaves. Product detection after 5 days showed that CYP76AE4 hydroxylated epikunzeaol at C – 8 to generate tovarol. The co-expression of multiple P450 genes probably occur as sequential reactions, or even unexpected new products. The co-expression of *AiOSC1* from *Azadirachta indica* and *MaCYP71CD2* from *Melia azedarach* resulted in partial consumption substrate tirucalla-7, 24-dien-3β-ol, and introduced a C23-OH and an epoxide at the C24 – 25 alkene. Co-expression of *AiOSC1* and *MaCYP71BQ5* consumed fractional substrate and added a single C21 – OH. When the three genes were co-expressed, it showed that the substrate was completely consumed, and this new product did not correspond to the prediction of MaCYP71CD2 and MaCYP71BQ5 working together, but spontaneously formed a hemiacetal ring by nucleophilic attack of C21, thereby forming protolimonoid melianol. In general, most research work uses mutual verification between fungi and plant hosts.

Functional characterization in prokaryotic host The interaction between membrane-bound P450s, that receive two NADPH electrons from membrane-anch-ored CPR, usually occurs in the ER, and *E. coli* clearly lacks such compartmentalization, accompanying translational incompatibility of the membrane signal modules. Using prokaryotic hosts inevitably leads to difficulties in the expression of plant-derived P450, including: gene expression, protein post-translational modification, etc., which are determinative for valid folding and full functionality of P450 proteins. Nevertheless, it is feasible that *E. coli* be engineered to produce terpenoids, and paclitaxel P450 is one of the most successful representatives of plant-derived P450 expression. N-terminal transmembrane (TM) engineering and fusional chimera At24T5αOH-tTCPR successfully carried out taxadiene conversion to taxadien-5α-ol and the byproduct 5 (12)-oxa-3 (11)-cyclotaxane (OCT). Using endogenous

MVA pathway to provide FPP, optimizing the P450 N-terminal membrane anchor and choosing redox partner CPR strategies, has successfully produced artemisinin precursor artemisinic acid and gossypol precursor 8-hydroxycadinene in *E. coli*, details of which are summarized in Section **"Engineering terpenoid-related P450s."**

## 4 ENGINEERING TERPENOID-RELATED P450S

The shortcomings of membrane-bound P450s, such as: low stability, narrow substrate spectrum, incorrect heterologous folding and localization, dependence on redox partners, and electron uncoupling, limit the efficiency of terpenoid metabolic engineering. Moreover, the reactive oxygen species (ROS) generated due to the partial electron transfer leads to heterologous host cell death. In this section, we summarize the metabolic engineering strategies for overcoming these bottlenecks of P450-based biocatalysis, improving P450 expression and increasing the biosynthesis yield of ter-penoids *via*: protein engineering, optimization of redox partners and chassis cell engineering, and elaborate on the metabolic engineering in plants and yeast (Figure 3; Table 3).

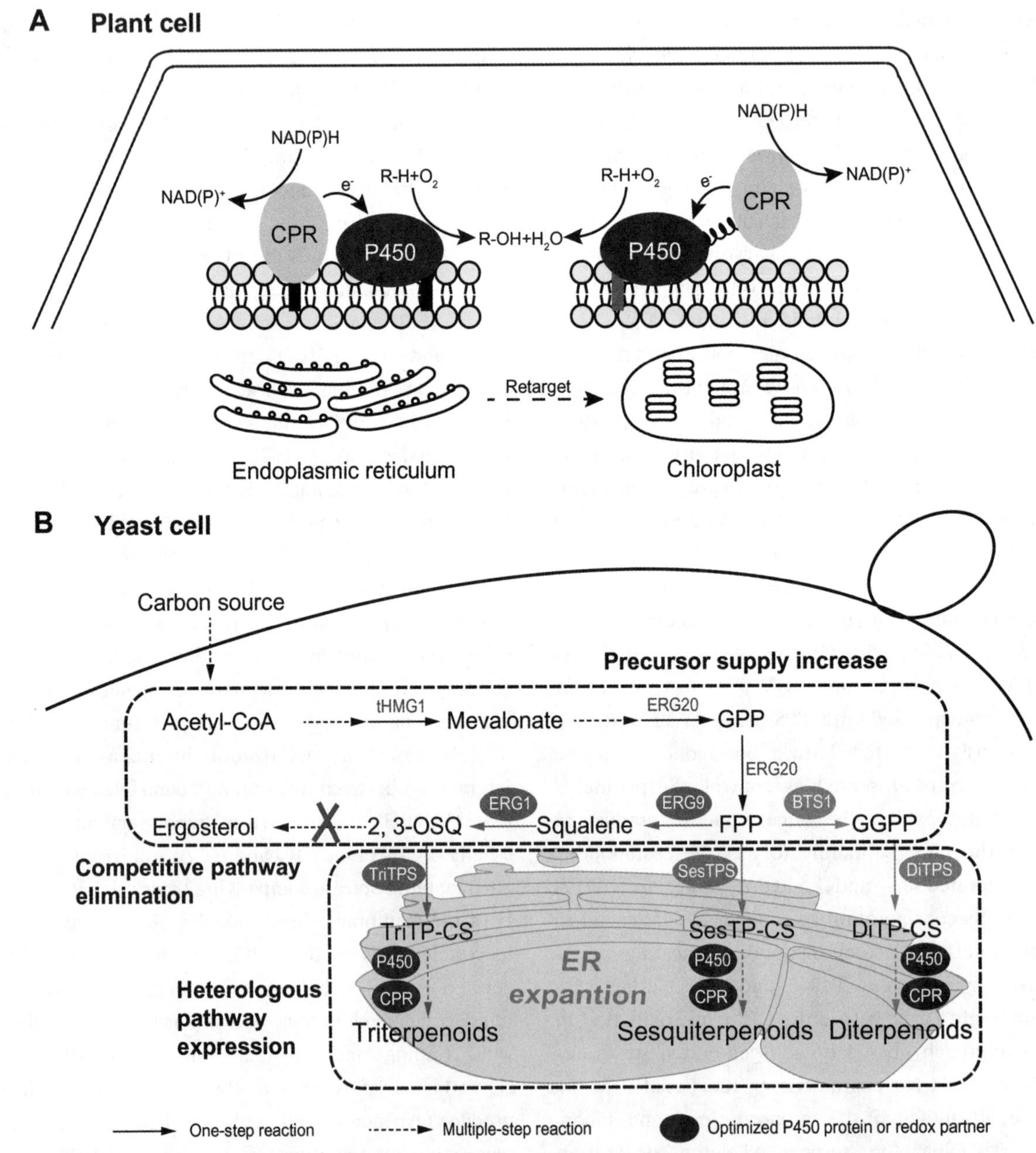


**Figure 3 Biotech approaches for improving the metabolic engineering production of terpenoids**

(A) Schematic diagrams of protein engineering and redox partner optimization in plant cell. (B) Chassis cell engineering in yeast. Simple metabolic pathways and rate-limiting enzymes for the biosynthesis of various terpenoids, including sesquiterpenoids (blue), diterpenoids (orange) and triterpenoids (green). 2,3-OSQ, 2,3-oxidosqualene; BTS1, geranylgeranyl diphosphate synthase; CS, core structure; ER, endoplasmic reticulum; ERG1, squalene epoxidase; ERG9, squalene synthase; ERG20, farnesyl pyrophosphate synthase; FPP, farnesyl pyrophosphate; GGPP, geranylgeranyl pyrophosphate; GPP, geranyl pyrophosphate; tHMG1, truncated 3-hydroxy-3-methylglutaryl-CoA reductase.

**Table 3 Representative examples of metabolic engineering approaches for terpenoid-related P450**

| Limitation | Organism(s) | Enzyme(s) | Engineering | Subclassification |
|---|---|---|---|---|
| Low catalytic efficiency | *Coleus forskohlii* | CYP76AH15 | Protein engineering | Directed Evolution |
| Low main product ratio | *Nicotiana tabacum* | CYP71D20 | | Directed Evolution |
| Low solubility and stability | *Arabidopsis thaliana* | CYP71A16 | | N-terminal modification |
| Limitations of electron transfer rate | *Glycyrrhiza uralensis* | CYP72A154 | Optimization of redox partners | Optimal CPR screen |
| Electron uncoupling | *Taxus brevifolia* | CYP725A4 | | Fusion P450 and CPR |
| Weak heterologous gene expression | *Panax ginseng* | CYP716A47 | Chassis cells engineering | Endoplasmic reticulum expansion |
| Low catalytic substrate content | *Salvia miltiorrhiza* | CYP76AH1 | | Precursor supply optimization |

Protein engineering

Protein engineering for expression of plant-derived P450s

Plant-derived P450s are usually localized at the membranes by the N-terminal membrane-anchoring region contains: TM domains, TPs, signal peptide (SP), etc., which limits their solubility and heterologous expression. To increase the water solubility and stability, the N-terminal domain of P450 is often truncated or modified. Heterologous expression of N-terminally truncated CYP71A16, with a deletion of the initial 74 amino acids and His6-tag insertion, increased P450 expression in *E. coli*, and added the possibility to apply purification methods *in vitro*. The localization of proteins was changed by fusion with TP or SP. In the process of heterologous production of artemisinin in tobacco, targeting the *ADS* gene to mitochondria by fused cox4 mitochondrial SP increased the production of precursor amorphadiene. To avoid cytosol hindering precursor generation and precursor glycosylation, *DBR2* gene was targeted to glycosylation-free chloroplasts by the rbcS1 TP, and *AaCPR* and *CYP71AV1* used chloroplast TP. Another study truncated TM regions of T5αOH and *Taxus* CPR, and MALLLAVF derived from bovine P450 was added to the N-terminus of T5αOH to enhance its expression and located in bacterial plasma membrane. It is worth noting that truncation is not always effective and requires assays to verify protein activity. In another study, 17, 26, 31, and 43 amino acid residues of the *Panax* protopanaxadiol synthase (PPDS or CYP716A47) were individually truncated. However, only 31tPPDS had PPDS activity, which was lower than that of WT PPDS. Further co-expression with 46tATR1 led to a complete loss of PPDS function.

Protein engineering for improvement of products Appropriate protein engineering can improve the affinity of P450s for target substrates, expand the substrate scopes, and change the product structures and profiles. Directed evolution (Nobel Prize in 2018) is an effective approach to change the chemical configuration of P450s and improve the efficiency of the enzyme to obtain a desired ratio of products by sequence alignment to find potential mutation sites and engineering of protein substrate recognition sites (SRS). For example, biosynthesis of glycyrrhetinic acid (ratio of 29%) accompany with licorice triterpenoids glycyrrhetol (45.2%, the rate-limiting step of consecutive oxidation at C-30), glycyrrhetaldehyde and 29-OH by-product. Molecular docking exhibited hydrophilic C30-hydroxyl and was pushed away from the heme-Fe due to the hydrophobic force of threonine (T338) methyl. Controlling the catalytic property of CYP72A63, mutant T338S kept proton delivery activity while decreasing the hydrophobicity slightly, pulled C30-hydroxyl closer to the heme-Fe and pushed away the C-29 methyl, result 94.2% glycyrrhetinic acid which was 7.1-folds higher than WT. The same approach screened the four differential sites within the active pockets of homologous CYP76AH1 and CYP76AH3, revealing that CYP76AH1$^{D301E, V479F}$ could assemble all the functions of two enzymes and significantly enhance production of: 11-hydroxy ferruginol, sugiol, and 11-hydroxy sugiol in yeast. Its enzymatic mechanism was further confirmed by classical molecular dynamic simulations, metadynamics, and DFT calculations, which provide valuable guidance for rational protein engineering.

Optimization of redox partners

Screen the best paired redox partner Redox partners sequentially transfer two electrons from NAD(P)H and the electrons shuttle through the flavin adenine dinucleotide (FAD) and flavin mononucleotide (FMN) domains to the P450 heme-iron reactive center to activate substrate oxygenation. Therefore, optimization of protein-protein interactions between P450 and its cognate redox partner to enhance the electron transfer efficiency can mitigate the poor coupling of P450 systems and increase terpenoid production. To achieve efficient pairing between P450 and its partner, different CPRs were introduced into engineered yeast expressing GgbAS and MtCYP716A12, showed that coupling efficiency was in the order MtCPR > GuCPR > LjCPR > AtCPR. Much research confirms that the optimal combination generally comes from the same species, two

P450s Uni25647 and CYP72A154 with GuCPR1 (the best electron transfer ability of six different species) for glycyrrhetinic acid, VvCYP716A15 and VvCPR for betulinic acid production. Furthermore, cytochrome *b*5 (CYB5) can provide electrons to its interacting partner P450, enhancing the P450's enzymatic activity. Expression of AaCYB5 increased the production of artemisinic aldehyde, leading to a 40% increase of total sesquiterpene production. When GuCYB5 was introduced into engineered yeast, the glycyrrhetinic acid concentration reached 545 μg/L, which was about 8-fold higher than before. Additionally, carbon flux was successfully channeled toward triterpenoid biosynthesis rather than the competitive sterol pathway.

P450-CPR fusional chimera The physical fusion of P450 and CPR to mediate the effective P450/CPR interaction, reduces the distance between active pockets and improve the efficiency of electron transfer. In engineered *E. coli*, a translational fusion of T5αOH with TCPR was highly efficient in carrying out the first oxidation step, resulting in more than 98% taxadiene conversion to taxadien-5α-ol, as the electron transfer usually takes place in the ER, and physical fusion breaks the barrier of bacteria that lack such compartmentalization. PPDS and 46tATR1 were fused using three different lengths linkers. Compared with the non-fusion group, all yeast strains expressing fusion proteins showed an increase in the amount of products, regardless of the linker length. Although functional in many cases, it is worth noting that the fusion approach is not always effective. For example, CYP716A180 was fused with CPR using four linkers: GGGS, GSG, GGGGS, or EAAAK (rigid linker). When CYP716A180 was fused to the N-terminus of the CPR, the production of betulinic acid declined in all cases compared with the non-fusion control. However, fusion with C-terminus of the CPRs barely produced triterpenoids in *Yarrowia lipolytica* (oleaginous yeast). This physical combination may hinder the optimal protein-protein interactions, eliminate the flexibility of P450/CPR ratio, and adjust the ratio to 1∶1. Generally, the appraisal ratio between P450 and CPR in membrane is 15∶1 in order to ensure efficient electrons transfer from CPR to P450s *in planta*. Furthermore, the chimeric construct prevents the natural phenomenon shared by CPR, and the complete biosynthetic pathway contains multiple P450s. Obviously, maintaining normal terpenoid biosynthesis requires more genetic manipulations for each physical link.

Chassis cell engineering

Subcellular organelle optimization of chassis cells The ER provides a microenvironment that optimizes accurate and efficient manufacture of P450, and its volume is the key determinant of protein folding ability. This section introduces three approaches of expanding ER. First, overexpressing *INO2* (a transcription factor for lipid biosynthesis) led to an increased capacity to synthesize heterologous or endogenous ER-associated proteins, resulting in a significantly 8-fold increase in CYP716A47-mediated bioconversion of protopanaxadiol yield of 12.1 mg/L. The transcriptome analysis demonstrated that carbon metabolism changed toward increasing glucose uptake when ER expansion was induced and ER-resident chaperones were overexpressed to ensure the production of biologically active properly folded proteins. Another approach dramatically amplifies ER by disruption of the phosphatidic acid phosphatase-encoding *PAH1* gene, thereby stimulating the production of recombinant proteins and ultimately increasing the accumulation of medicagenic acid by 6-fold to 27.1 mg/L. Yeast engineered for heterologous biosynthesis by knocking out *PAH1* also showed an increased yield of friedelin, the substrate of CYP712K4. The third approach Ice2p is a type III membrane protein with eight predicted TM domains that play essential roles in: ER localization, intracellular zinc homeostasis and neutral lipid transport. AtCPR was prone to degradation in the Δ*ice2* knockout strain, while Ice2 overexpression stabilized AtCPR levels and improved (+)-valencene hydroxylation to trans-nootkatol by 40%-50%.

Precursor supply optimization of chassis cells Chassis cell engineering requires not only expanding the ER to obtain more active proteins, but also increasing the accumulation of precursors to provide sufficient substrates for P450. The optimal genes from six species of: bacteria, fungi and plants were introduced to reconstruct the MVA pathway in engineered *E. coli*. After site-directed mutagenesis and adjustment of the translation initiation rate to overproduce mevalonate, the FAB80 promoter accelerated midstream biosynthesis and simultaneously co-expressed SlNPPS and MsLS in the downstream pathway. The final limonene yield was greatly increased to 1.29 g/L in shake flask cultures. This evaluated the ability for diterpene synthases (diTPS) from multiple species to produce miltiradiene, the substrate of both CYP76AH1 and CYP728B70, and yielded an optimal chimeric miltiradiene synthase, consisting of class II diTPS CfTPS1 from *C. forskohlii* and class I diTPS SmKSL1, which showed the highest efficiency for miltiradiene production in yeast, with a yield of 3.5 g/L in a bioreactor.

Metabolic engineering strategies in yeast Metabolic engineering in yeast, which relies on multimodular strategies to: increase precursor supply, express heterologous pathways, eliminate competitive pathways, and ultimately achieve a high yield of target products, has been demonstrated as a promising strategy for sustainable green biosynthesis and successfully produce many pharmacological terpenoids or their precursors.

The toolbox for engineering of *S. cerevisiae* generally

includes overexpressing the MVA pathway: truncated forms of the rate-limiting enzyme 3-hydroxy-3-methyl-glutaryl-CoA reductase (*tHMG1*), farnesyl pyrophosphate synthase (*ERG20*), as well as the corresponding TPS, squalene synthase (*ERG9*) and squalene epoxidase (*ERG1*) for triterpenoids, geranylgeranyl diphosphate synthase (*BTS1*) for diterpenoids. In the construction of yeast cell factories, CaCYP716C49 was further introduced into the betulinic acid producing strain, which expressed the optimal VvCYP716A15 and VvCPR pair, and integrated with *ERG20*, *ERG9*, and *ERG1*, which finally led to the production of 22.7 mg/L alphitolic acid. In another study, overexpressed the MVA pathway and then optimized AtSQS2 and AtSQLE2 as well as SmFPS to enhance 2, 3-OSQ. In the betulinic acid module, the CYP716A155 from *Rosmarinus officinalis* and AtLUP were optimized and two copies introduced, which increased production to 1.5 g/L. In addition, methyl-β-cyclodextrin has been successfully shown to stimulate the production of triterpenoids in the metabolic engineering yeast platform.

Engineering for the production of the diterpenoid tanshinone precursor included three modules: tHMG1, fusion of SmCPS-SmKSL, and fusion of BTS1-ERG20 in a diploid strain. Further, integrating CYP76AH1 and SmCPR1 increased ferruginol production to 10.5 mg/L. The P450-oxidized miltiradiene product was produced using a modular strategy. In module 1, providing *GGPP*, *tHMG1*, *ERG20*, *BTS1*, and *SaGGPPS* were overexpressed, *rox1*, *ypl062w*, and *yjl06w4* were knocked out, and *ERG9* was down-regulated. In module 2, achieving miltiradiene production, a double *SmMS-SmCPS1* chimera was introduced into the yeast chromosome. The co-expression of *CYP728B70* and *TwCPR3* in module 3 led to the production of dehydroabietic acid and derivatives.

Multiple studies have shown heterologous production of natural terpenoids causes cell death due to their inherent toxicity, especially the P450-mediated functionalization processes produce oxygenated products that are generally more toxic than the corresponding olefin. The recombinant CYP71D51v2 and ATR biocatalyzed (+)-valencene to production of β-nootkatol and nootkatone. However, the bioconversion efficiency showed opposite to substrate concentration, due to the toxicity of the accumulation of β-nootkatol in yeast endomembranes. Some improvement measures for solving the biological toxicity in fermentation were introduced, for example: appropriate structural modification (e.g., glycosylation), the compartmentalization balanced transport strategy, accelerated the bioconversion to nontoxic products, or optimized the fermentation processes and used two-phase fermentation to absorb the products out of the cell.

Metabolic engineering strategies in plant hosts Because of their native MVA and MEP pathways, cofactors and CPRs, photoautotrophic plants are promising, effective and economical hosts for the metabolic engineering production of P450-decorated terpenoids. For instance, the functional yeast MVA pathway was genetically transformed into the chloroplast of homoplastomic plants (e.g., tobacco). The vector was sequentially transformed containing IDI, FPPS from *E. coli* with modified dihydroartemisinic acid (DHAA) biosynthetic genes *DBR2*, *AaCPR*, and *CYP71AV1* were targeted to chloroplasts, and the ADS gene was targeted to mitochondria into the nuclear. This balanced compartmentalization approach to the heterologous production of artemisinin used three cellular compartments (cytosol, chloroplast, and mitochondria), and biosynthesis of artemisinin 0.8 mg/g and DHAA 0.15 mg/g. Moreover, oral delivery of these metabolic engineering tobacco leaves was considerably better than pure artemisinin by *in vitro* and *in vivo* antimalarial efficacy studies, which fully proved the effectiveness and safety of the heterologous artemisinin production. In another study, co-expression of TS and the new chimera TP (TS)/tT5αOH/tCPR (fused with TS chloroplastic SP) significantly increased the taxadiene 5α-ol to 0.90 μg/g FW. Due to further integration with isoprenoid precursor supply enhancement strategy (DXS-GGPPS overexpression), the accumulation was further increased to 1.3 μg/g FW.

Compared to the established yeast platforms, plants are generally not regarded as the first-choice for terpenoid production due to their difficulties in: stable transformation, complicated metabolic network, time consumption, and challenges in industrial scale production. Nevertheless, *Physcomitrella patens* with fully sequenced genome, the haploid life cycle and efficient homologous recombination had become an attractive photosynthetic chassis for terpenoid industrial production. All five artemisinin biosynthetic pathway genes (*ADS*, *CYP71AV1*, *ADH1*, *DBR2*, and *ALDH1*) were transformed into the moss genome using *in vivo* homologous recombination, and a high initial production of 0.21 mg/g DW artemisinin was observed after 3 days of cultivation. The knock-out of endogenous enzymes in *P. patens*, which expressed similar activity to that of the artemisinin biosynthetic pathway in *A. annua*, inhibited the conversion of amorpha-4, 11-diene to artemisinic acid and stimulated the flux to dihydroartemisinic aldehyde which could improve the yield of artemisinin. In addition, using the moss platform for light-driven produce, sesquiterpenoids patchoulol reached 1.34 mg/g DW, diterpenoid sclareol reached 2.84 mg/g DW, and 0.05% tissue FW of taxa-4(5), 11(12)-diene. Moreover, the triterpenoids betulin and lupeol were successfully produced by introducing three plant enzymes, LjOSC from *Lotus japonicus*, and *M. truncatula*

CYP716A12 together with its CPR into the photosynthetic eukaryotic microalgae *Phaeodactylum tricornutum*.

These bioengineering plant-based chassis, which use light as an energy source and can be scaled up for industrial production of non-native terpenoids, are potentially more cost effective than other carbon supplemented biotechnological platforms and gradually develop as alternative heterologous production hosts.

In this section, we discuss general strategies for engineering terpenoid-related P450, indeed, metabolic engineering is a global regulation that needs to be controlled by "point-line-plane," which can be detailed in the literatures.

## 5 CONCLUSIONS AND PERSPECTIVES

Evolving technological advancements have improved our ability to discover, characterize and metabolic engineer of P450s and their redox partners, and break through the low-yield limitations in the original plants to heterologously biosynthesize pharmacological complex terpenoids, thereby greatly reducing the pressure on plant resources and alleviating clinical supply short-age. With the development and popularization of sequencing technology, the plant genomes have been fully parsed, and the combined application of multiomics provides the sequence, expression and location information of P450s, so that through biotech approaches such as homologous sequences, gene co-expression and physically linked gene clusters, with the identified functional genes to discover and narrow down the scope of candidate P450s.

Gene deletion, which is highly dependent on genetic manipulation, is currently mainly used in *Arabidopsis* and other plant hosts with a clear genetic background. In comparison, gene silencing with high operability is an alternative biotech approach to study the role of P450 in native plants, however, the lower expression level of P450 also limits the operation. Therefore, for plants without genetic transformation systems, *in vitro* assay and intractable hosts are more suitable for functional characterization of plant-derived P450s. Furthermore, utilization of protein engineering, optimization of redox partners, and chassis cell engineering approaches to ensure correct folding and expression of P450, improve protein activity and stability, and ultimately increase the production of terpenoids in metabolic engineering. Currently using the discovery, characterization and metabolic engineering approaches, we have discussed in this review, many important medicinal terpenoids have been successfully produced in heterologous hosts with high yields (Table 4).

**Table 4 Metabolic engineering strategies to produce plant-derived terpenoids with P450 participation**

| Final products | Host | P450 involved | Strategies | Titer |
|---|---|---|---|---|
| **Triterpenoids** | | | | |
| Glycyrrhetinic acid | *S. cerevisiae* | β-amyrin 11-oxidase (97% similar to CYP88D6), CYP72A63 | 4.2.1/4.4 | 18.9 mg/L* |
| Protopanaxadiol | *S. cerevisiae* | CYP716A47 | 4.2.2/4.3.2 | 11 020 mg/L* |
| Maslinic acid | *S. cerevisiae* | CYP716A15, CYP716C49 | 4.2.1/4.3.2 | 384.3 mg/L* |
| Corosolic acid | *S. cerevisiae* | CYP716A15, CYP716C49 | 4.2.1/4.3.2 | 141.0 mg/L* |
| Alphitolic acid | *S. cerevisiae* | CYP716A15, CYP716C49 | 4.2.1/4.3.2 | 22.7 mg/L* |
| Polpunonic acid | *S. cerevisiae* | CYP712K1 - 3 | 4.4 | 1.4 mg/L |
| Oleanolic acid | *S. cerevisiae* | CYP716A12 | 4.2.1/4.3.2/4.4 | 606.9 mg/L* |
| Betulinic acid | *S. cerevisiae* | CYP716A155 | 4.3.2/4.4 | 1 000 mg/L* |
| Betulinic acid | *Y. lipolytica* | CYP716A180 | 4.2.1/4.2.2 | 51.9 mg/L |
| **Diterpenoids** | | | | |
| Carnosic acid | *S. cerevisiae* | CYP76AH22, CYP76AK8 | 4.4 | 2.7 mg/L |
| Taxadiene-5α-ol and other oxygenated taxanes | *E. coli* | CYP725A4 | 4.1.1 | 570 mg/L* |
| Taxadiene-5α-ol | *N. benthamiana* | CYP725A4 | 4.1.1/4.3.2 | 1.3 μg/g FW |
| Forskolin | *S. cerevisiae* | CYPAH15 | 4.1.2 | 0.7 mg/L |
| Ferruginol | *S. cerevisiae* | CYP76AH1 | 4.3.2/4.4 | 10.5 mg/L |
| 18-hydroxy-miltiradiene | *S. cerevisiae* | CYP720B1 | 4.1.2/4.4 | 69.0 mg/L |
| 19-hydroxy-miltiradiene | *S. cerevisiae* | CYP720B1 | 4.1.2/4.4 | 9.6 mg/L |
| 3β-hydroxy-manool | *S. cerevisiae* | CYP720B1 | 4.1.2/4.4 | 13.8 mg/L |
| **Sesquiterpenoids** | | | | |
| (+)-nootkatone | *S. cerevisiae* | CYP71D55 | 4.1.2/4.3.2 | 59.78 mg/L |
| Zerumbone | *S. cerevisiae* | CYP71BA1 | 4.2.1/4.3.1/4.3.2 | 40 mg/L* |

(Continued)

| Final products | Host | P450 involved | Strategies | Titer |
|---|---|---|---|---|
| Valerenic acid | *S. cerevisiae* | CYP71DJ1 | 4.2.1 | 4 mg/L |
| Artemisinic acid | *S. cerevisiae* | CYP71AV1 | 4.2.1/4.4 | 25 000 mg/L* |
| Artemisinin | *N. tabacum* | CYP71AV1 | 4.1.1/4.5 | 0.8 mg/g DW |
| Artemisinin | *P. patens* | CYP71AV1 | 4.5 | 0.21 mg/g DW |
| **Monoterpenoids** | | | | |
| Pyrethric acid | *N. benthamiana* | CYP71NBZ1 | 4.5 | 24.0 μg/g FW |

* Large volume bioreactor. The strategies are the metabolic engineering strategies in the Section "Engineering terpenoid-related P450s."

Individual functional characterization of those P450 candidate genes that have been scaled down by discovery approaches are still time-consuming. Novel multiple engineering strategies for bi-directional promoters with broad expression levels, ratios and different regulation profiles, should be developed, alleviating the restricting of mono-directional promoters to multi-gene co-expression capabilities, thereby constructing gene pools to characterize P450 functions on a large-scale. In addition, biotechnology innovative machine-based high-throughput technology assists *in vitro* rapidly characterize P450 by changing the substrate or enzyme variables.

P450-related metabolic engineering opens a door for the industrial production of low-yield terpenoids in natural plants. Utilization of the yeast platform, artificially using high-efficiency P450 isozymes from different species to integrate the complete biosynthetic pathway can greatly increase the yield of target products, and even "combinatorial biosynthesis" approach to produce unnaturally active terpenoids, which had been confirmed available in triterpenoids. The other direction is to fully understand the relationships between protein sequence, structure and function, and redesign the P450 through directed evolution or enzymatic engineering to have the desired characteristics, thereby changing the substrate specificity so that the neofunctional P450 variant can accept the original uncatalyzed substrate and generate the designed products. Based on all the above knowledge, the machine learning applications in systems metabolic engineering allow efficient development of high performing microbial strains for the sustainable production.

Photosynthesis in plants converts solar energy into ATP and NADPH for primary metabolism. However, it usually produces more than actually required. Using these excess NADPH as electrons to supply the plant-derived P450 reaction will save more energy. Retargeting and co-localization of the fusion of P450 with ferredoxin or the biosynthetic pathway enzymes (including P450, UGT, etc.) in the chloroplast thylakoid membrane, using photosynthetic electron transfer, can reduce the loss of intermediates and significantly improve product yield, by passing the involvement of CPR and poor coupling of P450 system, and CPR optimization. This light-driven approach is currently successfully applied in cyanogenic glucoside dhurrin and can be extended to terpenoid biosynthesis in the future.

[张逸风，黄璐琦，高伟，等. Critical Reviews in Biotechnology, 2023,43(1):1-21.]

# Tandemly duplicated CYP82Ds catalyze 14-hydroxylation in triptolide biosynthesis and precursor production in *Saccharomyces cerevisiae*

*Tripterygium wilfordii* Hook. F., a medicinal plant also known as Lei Gong Teng, has been used in China for >500 years (Ming dynasty, AD 1 476) for the treatment of autoimmune diseases, and modern pharmacological studies have shown its extensive antitumor, anti-inflammatory, and immunosuppressive effects. The root is the main medicinal part of *T. wilfordii* and contains up to 415 chemical components, including terpenoids and alkaloids. Among this rich treasure trove of compounds, triptolide (**1**) is undoubtedly an important contributor to pharmaceutical properties.

Triptolide, an 18(4 → 3) *abeo*-abietane diterpenoid with a tri-epoxy group and $\alpha$, $\beta$-unsaturated lactone moiety (Fig. 1a), has been designed with multiple structure-based artificial derivatives, particularly through carbon-14 (C-14) modifications, which have been implemented to improve its water solubility, and some of the generated compounds have entered clinical trials (ClinicalTrials. gov), leading to a tremendous demand for triptolide. However, the content of **1** in its native plant is only 139 ng · $g^{-1}$ dry weight, and the chemical synthesis approach exhibits low synthesis efficiency and multiple steps due to the stereo-chemical complexity of its structure (e.g., three epoxy groups, unsaturated lactone, and nine chiral centers). Although the cambial meristematic cells of plant tissue culture technology have increased the yield to 138.1 $\mu$g · $g^{-1}$, synthetic biology strategies based on elucidating the biosynthetic pathway appear to be a more promising, sustainable, and alternative method and have been successfully applied to achieve heterologous acquisition of potential intermediates and analog triptonide in microorganisms. In contrast, natural products such as tripdiolide (**2**), triptolidenol (**3**) and triptriolide (**4**), which have the same 18(4 → 3) *abeo*-abietane skeleton and similar biosynthetic pathways as **1** (Fig. 1a), also have multiple pharmaceutical properties. Elucidating the biosynthetic pathway of **1** will ultimately lead to pharmaceutical, economic and environmental benefits.

The core skeleton cyclization and functional decoration in the biosynthesis of **1** are initiated by two types of diterpene synthases, class II TwTPS7 (v2) and class I TwTPS27 (v2), which cyclize geranylgeranyl diphosphate (GGPP) to produce olefin miltiradiene (**5**) and catalyze double-bond rearrangement on the C-ring for spontaneous conversion to stable aromatized abietatriene (**6**), and CYP728B70 then catalyzes carboxylation at C-18 to generate dehydroabietic acid (**7**). However, the multiple downstream steps from **7** to **1** remain enigmatic and are mainly divided into C-14 hydroxylation, C-18, 19 lactonization, and triepoxidation processes. According to the proposed biosynthetic pathway (Fig. 1b), cytochrome P450s (CYPs) with hydroxylation, epoxidation, and isomerization functions are highly likely to contribute to the biosynthesis of **1**, which has been shown to consist of a minimal set of four biosynthetic components of CYPs for the heterologous production of triptonide.

Here, we reveal that CYP82D274 and CYP82D263 in tandem duplicated CYP82Ds catalyze the C-14 hydroxylation grid in the biosynthesis of **1** through genetic manipulation in native plant cells and functional characterization in a heterologous host. The two CYP82Ds can also transform the aromatization of **5** and promote the production of the rate-limiting **7**. In vivo assays and kinetic parameters indicate that CYP82D274 prefers to catalyze **7** in the pathway and thereby

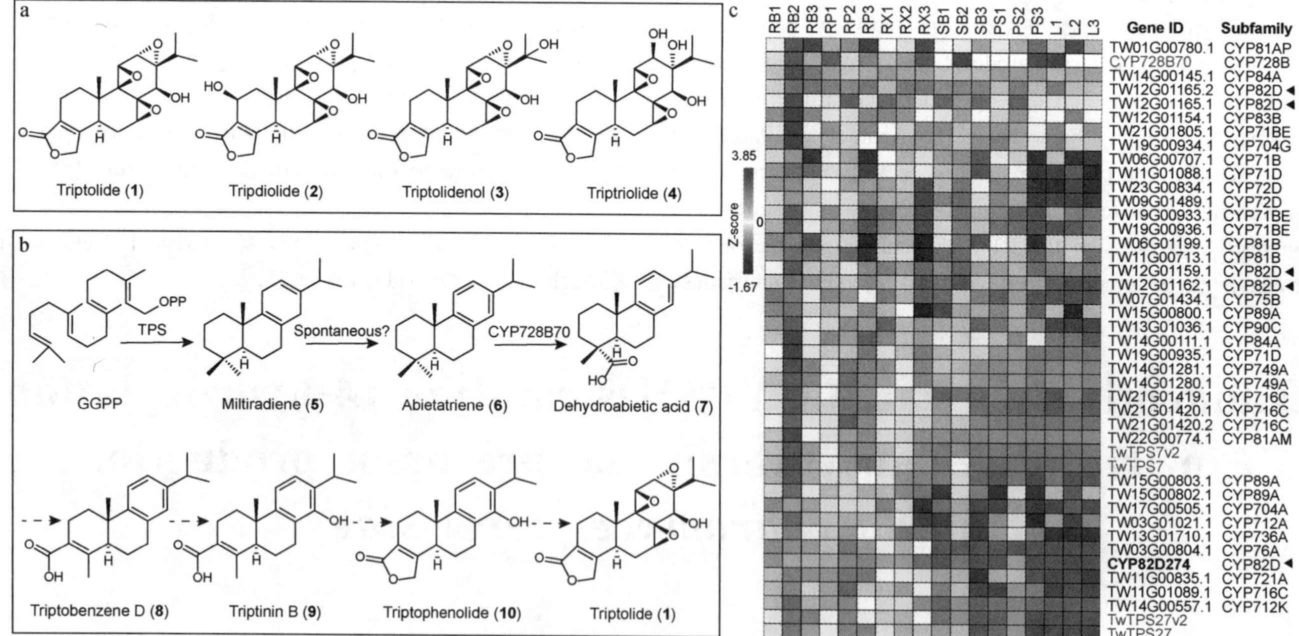


**Fig. 1 Bioactive metabolites in *Tripterygium wilfordii* and biosynthesis of triptolide.**

(a) Structures of major bioactive diterpenoids of *T. wilfordii*. (b) Proposed triptolide biosynthetic pathway. A solid arrow represents an identified reaction, and a dotted arrow indicates an unknown pathway. GGPP: Geranylgeranyl diphosphate. (c) Coexpression profiles of CYPs with genes in the triptolide biosynthetic pathway. *TwTPS7 (v2)*, *TwTPS27 (v2)* and *CYP728B70* are marked in red. The black triangles indicate CYP82D subfamily genes that cluster with identified functional genes. The gene ID of *CYP82D274* is TW12G01155.1. Root periderm (RB), root phloem (RP), root xylem (RX), stem vascular bundle (PS), stem periderm (SB), and leaf (L). Source data are provided as a Source Data file.

advance the biosynthesis of **1**. The intermediate 14-hydroxy-dehydroabietic acid (**11**) is successfully biosynthesized de novo in *Saccharomyces cerevisiae*. This study provides a systematic introduction to C－14 hydroxylases from evolutionary hypotheses and functional characterization to heterologous biosynthesis and thus paves the way for elucidation of the biosynthetic pathway of **1** and other 14-hydroxyl labdane-/abietane-type secondary metabolites.

## 1 RESULTS

Screening of candidate CYPs involved in triptolide biosynthesis Pathway genes undertake the biosynthesis of secondary metabolites together, and these genes often exhibit similar expression patterns; therefore, coexpression analysis is one of the most powerful approaches for the initial screening of functional-associated genes from massive transcriptome data. To identify the CYP gene encoding the enzyme responsible for the biosynthesis of **1**, we analyzed 416 CYPs in the *T. wilfordii* transcriptome (NCBI SRA accession SRP199495) of different plant tissues for expression correlation with previously characterized biosynthetic genes, including *TwTPS7* (*v2*), *TwTPS27* (*v2*) and *CYP728B70*. The expression profiles in the heatmap were grouped into 67 clusters, and 38 genes from 16 CYP families, including CYP71, CYP72, CYP76, and CYP82, exhibited the same pattern of root periderm-specific high expression and clustered with identified functional genes (Fig. 1c). Notably, the most numerous genes, TW12G01155.1 (*CYP82D274*), TW12G01159.1, TW12G01162.1, TW12G01165.1, and TW12G01165.2, belonged to the CYP82D subfamily, whose family is reportedly involved in terpenoid biosynthesis. The genes belonging to the CYP82D subfamily were selected as candidate CYPs for further analysis.

Tandem duplication of CYP82Ds and analysis of their transcriptional expression A chromosomal localization analysis of all CYP82D genes revealed that they were localized at Chr06, Chr08, Chr11, Chr12, Chr15, and Chr19. Further local BLAST analysis of the whole genome using the nucleic acid and amino acid sequences of CYP82D genes revealed a tandem duplication gene cluster at Chr12 containing 11 complete CYP82D genes, which had a length of 133 kb with 4 additional incomplete CYP82D gene residues (Fig. 2a). This tandem duplication of CYP82Ds occurred in dynamic chromosomal regions enriched in transposable elements (TEs) and was presumably generated by the duplication and rearrangement of long terminal repeat (LTR) elements of retro-transposons within chromosomes. A phylogenetic analysis of orthologous CYP82D genes (Fig. 2b) indicated that all TwCYP82Ds clustered into six clades, and the duplication event and neofunctionalization of Clade I and Clade II appeared to have occurred at 26.52 MYA, which was comparable to the timing of the *T. wilfordii* whole-genome triplication (WGT) event. The synonymous substitution rate (*Ks*) values of orthologous CYP82D genes indicated that the specific expansion of the CYP82D genes occurred via tandem duplication (Supplementary Data 1).

Heatmap analysis of the genes in Clade I and Clade II with known functional genes *TwTPS7* (*v2*), *TwTPS27* (*v2*), and *CYP728B70* as well as the content of **1** was achieved by combining the transcriptomic data and metabolite analysis (Supplementary Fig. 1). **1** exhibited a distribution pattern of root periderm and leaf tissue-specific expression. *CYP82D274* and TW12G01165.1 in Clade I showed the same high expression pattern in root tissues as the previously characterized genes, whereas *CYP82D263* in Clade II showed high expression in the root periderm, stem periderm, and leaves. TW12G01158.1 was highly expressed in the stem periderm and leaves, particularly the stem periderm. In addition, TW12G01156.1 and TW12G01157.1 were not detected and were supposedly selectively silenced by gene redun-dancy during evolution. In particular, TW08G01036.1 (*CYP82D213*) exhibited root peridermal-specific expression, and CYP82D213 is reportedly involved in the final step of the analog triptonide biosynthetic pathway. The transcriptional expression of the other five complete CYP82D genes of this tandem duplication gene cluster was also analyzed. In Clade V, TW12G01162.1 was highly expressed in the root and stem periderm, whereas TW12G01159.1 had a base deletion at position 44 in the coding region, causing termination of protein translation at position 26. TW12G01164.1 in Clade VI was highly expressed in the stem periderm, whereas the expression of TW12G01161.1 and TW12G01163.1 was too low to be detected.

CYP82D274 and CYP82D263 catalyze C－14 hydroxylation of dehydroabietic acid Among the CYP82D genes discovered from the transcriptomes, 11 were cloned (Supplementary Table 1). To investigate the biochemical activity of the CYPs, these 11 CYP82Ds were integrated into the plasmid pESC-LEU expressing both CYP and cytochrome P450 oxidoreductase 3 from *T. wilfordii* (TwPOR3) and then transformed into the yeast strain BY4741. Substrate feeding has been proven to be effective in yeast fermentation; thus, the intermediate **7** was fed into the cultures, and the fermentation products were extracted. Among 11 CYP82Ds, CYP82D274 and CYP82D263 accepted **7** as a substrate with the same three products at *m*/*z* 330 (Fig. 3a and Supplementary Fig. 2). The major product **11** was enriched and identified as 14-hydroxydehydroabietic acid (**11**), which was independently confirmed by $^{1}H$, $^{13}C$, HSQC, $^{1}H-^{1}H$ COSY, and NOESY NMR analyses (powder purity 98.23%) (Supplementary Figs. 3－7 and Supplementary Note 1). The additional minor product **13** was identified as 15-hydroxy-dehydroabietic acid

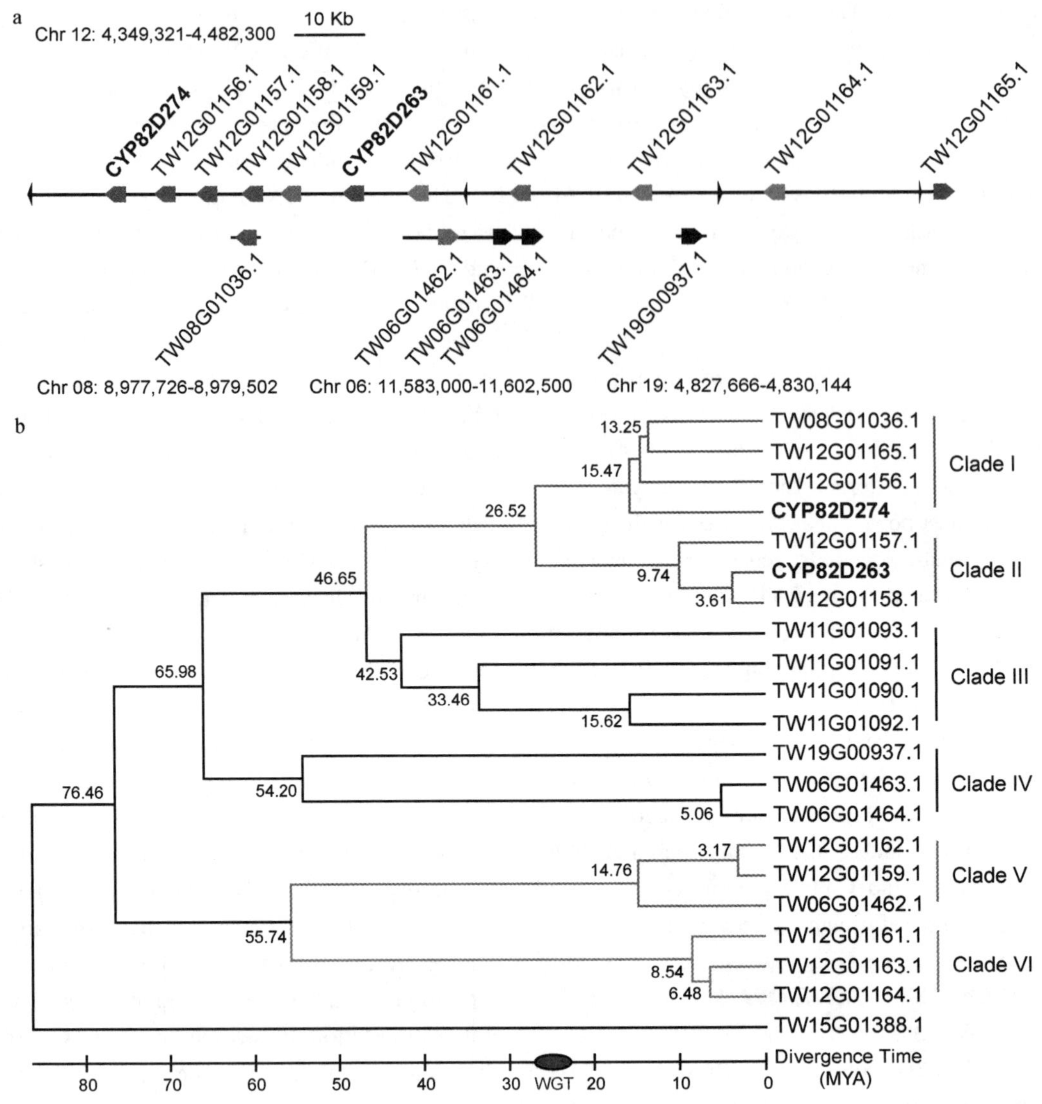


**Fig. 2 Chromosomal localization and evolutionary analysis of the CYP82D genes**

(a) Chromosomal localization of the 133-kb tandem duplicated CYP82Ds on Chr12 encoding 11 complete genes. The same color indicates orthologous CYP82D genes and the small triangles represent the incomplete gene residues. (b) Phylogenetic analysis of the TwCYP82D genes. The phylogenetic tree was constructed based on the maximum likelihood method (1 000 bootstraps). The numbers represent the predicted divergence time and WGT indicates the whole-genome triplication event of *T. wilfordii*.

upon comparison to the authentic standard (Supplementary Fig. 8). And further optimization of the GC-MS detection by increasing the MS resolution revealed that CYP82D274 and CYP82D263 catalyzed the production of another byproduct, 12-hydroxy-dehydroabietic acid (**18**), which is isomeric with **11** and has identical MS fragments (Supplementary Fig. 9). Altogether, CYP82D274 and CYP82D263 can catalyze **7** to produce **11** by inducing C-14 hydroxylation (Fig. 3b), albeit with promiscuity (C-12, C-15, etc.).

As resulted by in vitro enzyme assays, both CYP82D274 and CYP82D263 could exhibit their major 14-hydroxylase functions and generated **11** in the presence of TwPOR3, NADPH, substrate **7**, and cofactors (Fig. 3a). The $K_m$ values of CYP82D274 and CYP82D263 were $0.99 \pm 0.17\ \mu M$ and $8.42 \pm 1.89\ \mu M$, respectively, at the optimal reaction time (Fig. 3c and Supplementary Fig. 10a). These steady-state kinetic parameters indicated that CYP82D274 was significantly superior to CYP82D263 in terms of substrate affinity and catalytic efficacy.

*CYP82D274* and *CYP82D263* are involved in triptolide biosynthesis  To further investigate the definitive role of *CYP82D274* and *CYP82D263* in **1** biosynthesis, RNA interference (RNAi) was utilized to knock down the expression of these two genes in *T. wilfordii* suspension cells. All TwCYP82D nucleic acid sequences in the genome showed a high identity of 69.61%, mainly between CYP82D274 and CYP82D263, with 81.41% concordance. We specifically selected a 459-bp (nucleotides 459 - 917) fragment of *CYP82D274* and a 498-bp (nucleotides 373 - 870) fragment of *CYP82D263* to construct the binary vector

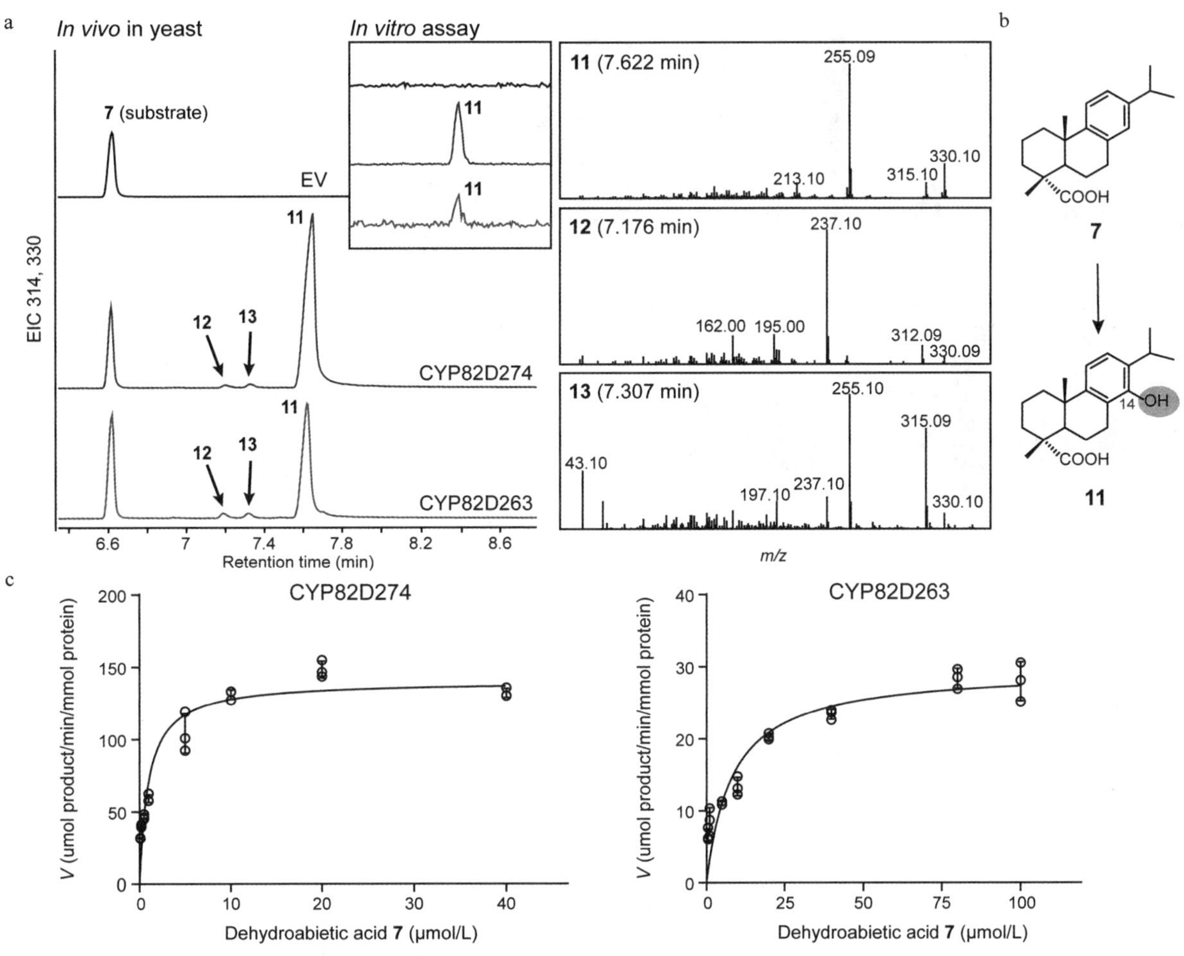


**Fig. 3 Functional characterization of CYP82D274 and CYP82D263**

(a) GC-MS analysis of methylated products of CYP82D274 and CYP82D263 catalyzing dehydroabietic acid (**7**) in vivo or in vitro. Empty vector (EV) denotes yeast transformed with an empty vector without CYP. (b) Catalytic process in (a). (c) Kinetic profiles of CYP82D274 and CYP82D263 catalyzing **7** in vitro. The quantification of **11** was based on the standard curve $y = 0.7336x - 0.014$ ($R^2 = 0.9994$) obtained by LC-TQ-MS/MS. The concentration of CYPs was estimated by measuring the reduced CO-difference spectrum. Kinetic parameters were calculated by nonlinear regression analysis using the Michaelis-Menten model. Data are presented as mean values ± standard deviation SD from three biological independent replicates, and the black circles represent the individual data points. Source data are provided as a Source Data file.

pK7GWIWG2D (II) and transformed them into suspension cells by plasmid bombardment. The electrophoretic bands of the vector-specific fragment indicated successful transformation (Supplementary Fig. 11a), and detection of the expression of *CYP82D274* and *CYP82D263* showed that they were targeted for disruption as expected (Fig. 4d). Metabolite profiling revealed that the inhibition rate of **1** was 60.37% and a considerable reduction in the accumulation of triptophenolide (**10**), triptobenzene D (**8**) and the direct product **11** in the *CYP82D274*-RNAi cell lines (Fig. 4d and Supplementary Data 2). In particular, the expression of *CYP728B70*, *TwTPS27* (*v2*), and *TwTPS7* (*v2*) exhibited opposing changes, which were hypothesized to be intergenic feedback regulation. In the *CYP82D263*-RNAi cell lines, three metabolites, **1**, **10** and **8**, were significantly decreased. Furthermore, based on the inhibition rates of individual metabolites, we observed stronger inhibition of metabolites in *CYP82D274*-RNAi and *CYP82D263*-RNAi as the pathway progressed downstream, suggesting a cascade accumulation of metabolites.

*CYP82D274* and *CYP82D263* were also specifically overexpressed in plant cells, as evidenced by electrophoretic bands and gene expression (Supplementary Fig. 11). Targeted metabolite analysis indicated that the overexpression of *CYP82D274* and *CYP82D263* resulted in a significant increase in the accumulation of **1** and **10** as well as the direct product **11** (Fig. 4e and Supplementary Data 3). The results of these in vivo assays suggested that CYP82D274 and CYP82D263 are involved in **1** biosynthesis as 14-hydroxylases.

14-Hydroxy-dehydroabietic acid is a precursor of triptolide To provide direct evidence showing whether **11** is implicated in **1** biosynthesis, mass spectrometry imaging and metabolite analysis were employed. Previous studies found that **1** exhibits a build-up property specific to root periderm

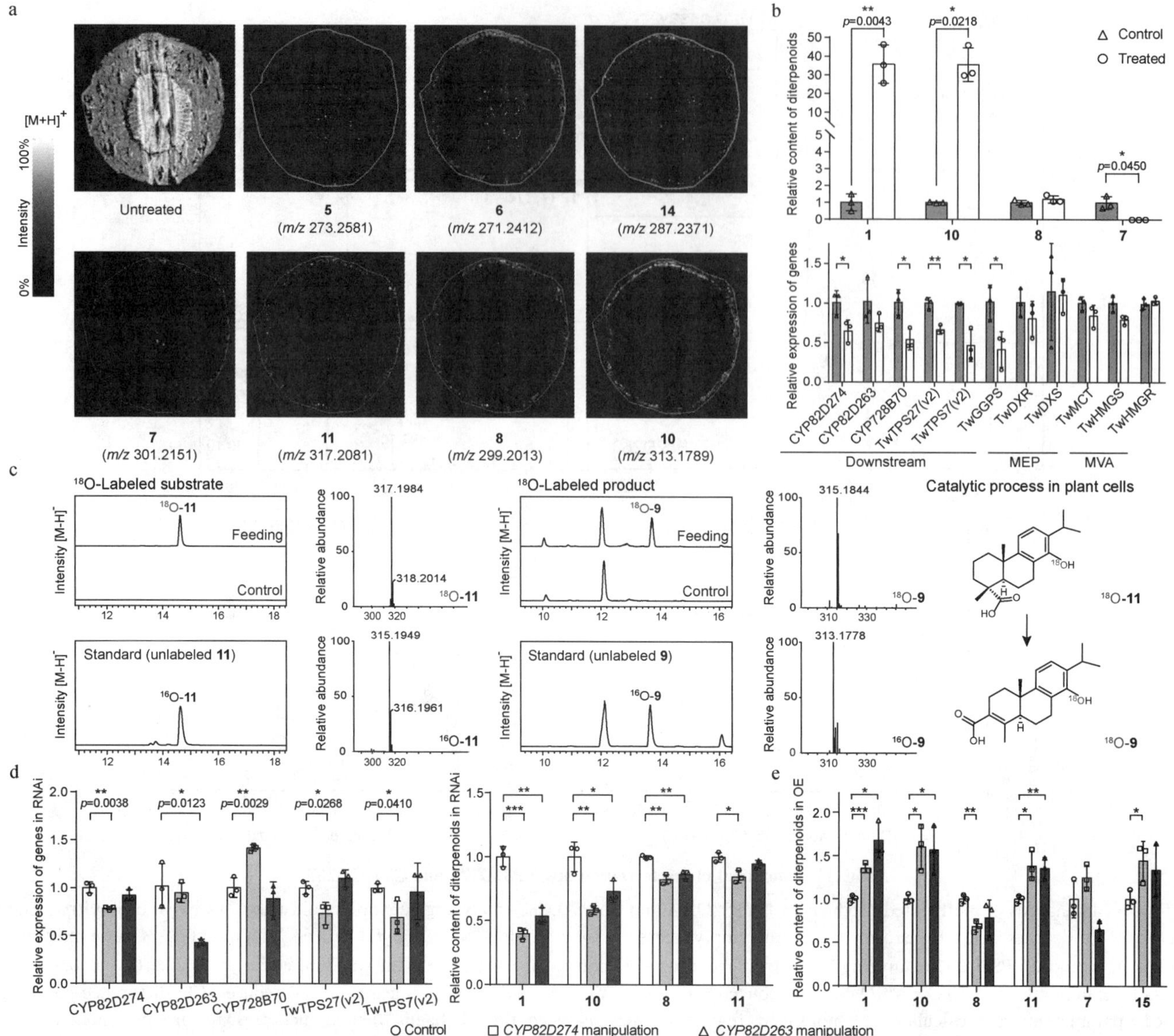


**Fig. 4 Intermediates and genes involved in triptolide biosynthesis**

(a) MALDI - MSI analysis of the distribution of triptolide intermediates in *T. wilfordii* root tissue. DHB was used as a matrix for metabolite imaging in the positive ion mode. The colors represent the intensity percentage, and each image is independent. (b) Relative content of diterpenoids and relative quantification of gene expression in 14-hydroxy-dehydroabietic acid (**11**)-fed cell lines. Cells that were not fed **11** served as a negative control. *P*-values of genes with significant differences in expression between groups were 0.0375, 0.0178, 0.0031, 0.0448, and 0.0294 in that order. (c) Metabolite analysis of $^{18}$O-labeled **11**-treated cell samples. $^{18}$O-**11** was fed to *T. wilfordii* suspension cells that inhibited the biosynthesis of precursors, and wild-type (WT) and unlabeled **11**-treated cells were used as negative controls. $^{18}$O-**11** was converted into $^{18}$O-triptinin B (**9**) in plant cells, and the mass spectra of labeled versus unlabeled metabolites are provided. (d) Relative content of diterpenoids and relative gene expression in *CYP82D274* and *CYP82D263* RNAi cell lines. **e** Relative content of diterpenoids in *CYP82D274*- and *CYP82D263*-overexpressing cell lines. The cell lines bombarded with corresponding empty vectors served as controls in **d** and **e**, and significant differences (*P*-values) in metabolites between the groups are shown in Supplementary Data 2 and 3. (b, d, e) The relative quantification of each metabolite was calculated by dividing each sample by the average content of the control group. The relative expression of genes was determined by the $2^{-\Delta\Delta Ct}$ method. *EFLα* was designated as the housekeeping gene, and the corresponding control group was assigned as the reference sample. Data are presented as mean values±SD ($n$ = 3 biologically independent replicates). *** $P<0.001$, ** $P<0.01$ and * $P<0.05$ determined by two-sided Student's $t$ test. Source data are provided as a Source Data file.

tissues (Supplementary Fig. 1). The distribution of metabolites in fresh roots was investigated in a targeted manner using MALDI - TOF - MS, and the acquainted intermediates **6** and **10** were found to accumulate within the periderm (Fig. 4a). In addition, the putative intermediates **7** and **8**, including the compound **11** discovered in this study, with carboxyl groups also displayed a high distribution in the periderm region, elucidating their spatial correlation. However, **1** was not available for MALDI - MS imaging due to the extremely low content of the compound, the choice of medium, the ionic pattern, and the competition of surrounding ions for laser ionization possibilities.

In combination with the abovementioned tissue distribution pattern of the intermediates, we fed **11** to *T. wilfordii* suspension cell cultures and found that the contents of **1** and **10** were elevated 35.73 and 35.60 times, respectively, compared with the levels in the negative control (Fig. 4b and Supplementary Data 4). Moreover, the catalytic substrate **7** of CYP82D274 and CYP82D263 was markedly reduced. The results further showed that all downstream pathway genes known to be involved in **1** biosynthesis (*CYP82D274*, *CYP82D263*, *CYP728B70*, *TwTPS27* (*v2*), *TwTPS7* (*v2*), and *TwGGPS*) showed reductions in expression to 0.42 - 0.76-fold in different proportions but did not affect genes involved in the upstream MVA and MEP pathways (Fig. 4b). To ensure that the abovementioned changes in metabolites were caused by **11**, stable isotope labeling was employed for more in-depth analysis. The use of the MEP inhibitor fosmidomycin and the use of the gene gun to suppress *TwTPS7* (*v2*) and *TwTPS27* (*v2*) inhibited the biosynthesis of precursors, whereas the elicitor subsequently increased the expression of downstream genes, as revealed when $^{18}$**O-11** was fed to the cells. Although the native metabolic pathway was not completely inhibited and endogenous **1** and **10** interfered with the determination of isotopically labeled products, we still found the peak of $^{18}$O-labeled triptinin B (**9**) (Fig. 4c), which could be further lactonized by CYP71BE to generate the expected intermediate **10**. The above-described results indicated that **11**, which has a carboxyl group, serves as a pre-cursor in the late stage of **1** biosynthesis.

**CYP82D274 and CYP82D263 catalyze the hydroxylation and aromatization of multiple substrates** When *CYP82D274* and *CYP82D263* were overexpressed, a 0.69-fold decrease in **8** and a 1.45-fold increase in ferruginol (**15**) were also observed, which appeared to indicate other catalytic processes played by these two genes (Fig. 4e and Supplementary Data 3). The fermentation of yeast strains harboring CYP82D274 or CYP82D263 and subsequent incubation with the intermediate **8** revealed that CYP82D274 generated three hydroxylated products with a charge of $m/z + 16$ (Fig. 5a). The retention time and mass spectral fragmentation for the major product matched the authentic standard for the derivatization of **9** (Supplementary Fig. 12), indicating that CYP82D274 played a C-14 hydroxylation role in catalyzing the formation of **9** from **8**. In addition, the incubation of substrate **5** further gave rise to two different ratios of C-14 and C-12 hydroxylated products (Fig. 5b and Supplementary Fig. 13). For CYP82D274, the major product **14** was identified to be 14-hydroxy-abietatriene with small amounts of **15** (12-hydroxy-abieta-triene or ferruginol, Supplementary Fig. 14). For CYP82D263, **5** was converted into the hydroxylated major product **15** accompanied by trace amounts of **14**.

Double bond rearrangement in the C-ring of olefin **5** to yield stable aromatized **6** has been repeatedly reported to be a spontaneous reaction process. In our study, we transformed plasmids into engineered yeast BY-PS2, which could self-produce **5** as a substrate. The presence of a double peak for **5** and **6** in CYP82D274 and CYP82D263 compared with the single peak for **5** in the EV (Fig. 5b) indicated that CYP82D274 and CYP82D263 were capable of catalyzing the aromatization of **5** to generate **6**. Nevertheless, we demonstrated the existence of spontaneous reactions with small amounts of **6** (Fig. 5c), and if the yield of **6** in the EV was regarded to be 1.00, the relative yield of **6** in CYP82D274 was 180.09 and that in CYP82D263 was 23.89. This finding suggested that CYP82D274 and CYP82D263 can specifically and effectively catalyze the aromatization of **5**, whereas other genes in the same CYP82D subfamily cannot (Supplementary Fig. 15).

Based on these results, we conclude that CYP82D274 and CYP82D263 catalyze important hydroxylation and aromatization processes and contribute to the biosynthesis of **1** through multiple pathways (Fig. 5d).

**CYP82D274 creates a metabolic grid in triptolide biosynthesis** In the previous section, we revealed that the wide substrate range of CYP82D274 enabled the simultaneous catalysis of different substrates, and CYP728B70 catalyzes the reaction of **5** to generate **7**. By feeding strains harboring CYP728B70 with **14**, the fermentation products were detected to contain both abietatriene-14,18-diol (a CYP728B70 catalyzed intermediate, **19**) and **11** (Supplementary Fig. 16), suggesting that the biosynthetic pathway is not a linear and specific pathway but rather that the products are generated via multiple pathways together through a metabolic grid, a phenomenon that has also been found in forskolin and tanshinones.

In the face of a metabolic grid with multiple substrates, the substrate affinity and catalytic efficiency of the enzymes are quite different and can be reffected by kinetic parameters. We found that the $K_m$ values of CYP82D274 and CYP82D263 for catalyzing **7** equaled $0.99 \pm 0.17$ μM and $8.42 \pm 1.89$ μM (Fig. 3c), indicating their higher sensitivity to **7**. We also carried out microsomal experiments with CYP82D274 and CYP82D263 in the presence of NADPH, a redox partner, cofactors, and the substrates **5** and **8**. The results showed that only CYP82D274 could catalyze **5** to produce small amounts of **14** with a $K_m$ of $47.30 \pm 12.98$ μM (Supplementary Fig. 10b), but the target product was not detected under the conditions of catalytic **8** or CYP82D263-

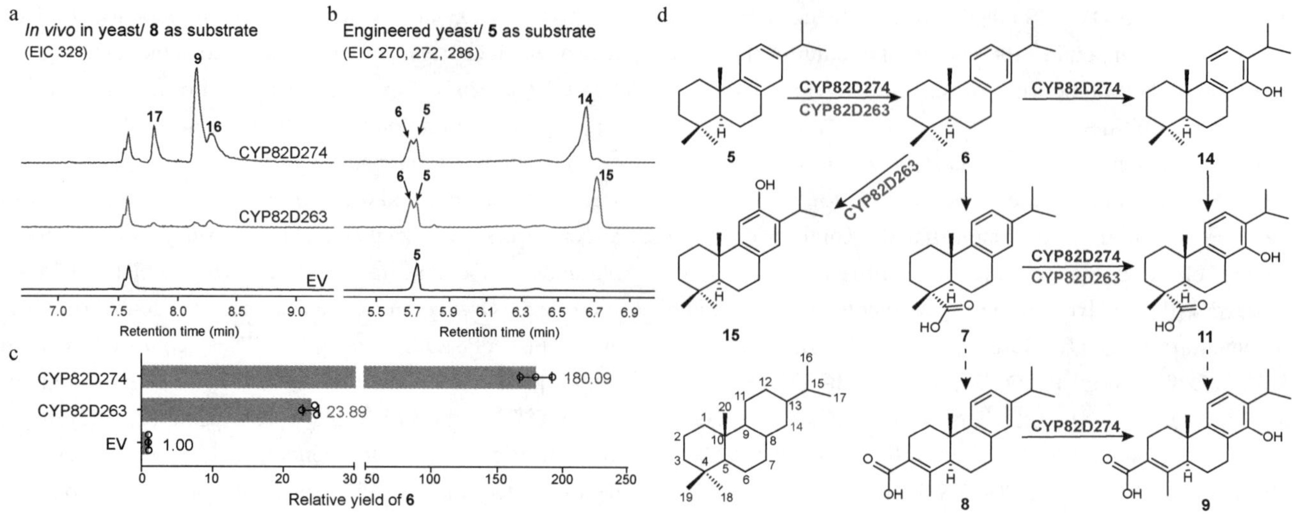


**Fig. 5 Metabolic grid of C-14 hydroxylation and aromatization**

(a) GC-MS analysis of methylated products with triptobenzene D (**8**) as the substrate. (b) GC-MS analysis of the catalytic products of miltiradiene (**5**) in engineered yeast. The mass spectrum results are shown in Supplementary Figs. 12 and 13. (c) Relative yield of abietatriene (**6**) in spontaneous, CYP82D274 and CYP82D263 cultures. Data are presented as mean values ± SD ($n = 3$ biologically independent replicates). (d) Catalytic process of the CYP82D274 and CYP82D263 metabolic grid for triptolide (**1**) biosynthesis. A solid arrow represents an identified reaction, and a dotted arrow indicates an unknown reaction. Source data are provided as a Source Data file.

catalyzed **5**. In addition, the $V_{max}$ values of CYP82D274 for catalyzing **7** and **5** were 140.30 ± 5.10 μmol of product · $min^{-1}$ · (mmol of protein)$^{-1}$ and 44.08 ± 6.13 μmol of product · $min^{-1}$ · (mmol of protein)$^{-1}$, these kinetic parameters indicated that CYP82D274 has a higher preference for substrate **7**.

De novo biosynthesis of 14-hydroxy-dehydroabietic acid in yeast To further address the unknown biosynthetic pathway of **1**, self-produced engineered yeast was first constructed to provide sufficient amounts of the precursor **11** for gene mining. CYP82D274 and CYP82D263 were coexpressed with CYP728B70, suggesting that yeast is capable of expressing multiple CYPs simultaneously to produce **11** (Fig. 6a and Supplementary Fig. 17). To achieve a high yield of **11**, three functional modules were designed and investigated for optimization. Multispecies-derived diterpene synthases confirmed that tSmKSL1-CfTPS1 (the fusion of truncated *ent*-kaurene synthase-like 1 from *Salvia miltiorrhiza* and terpene synthase from *Coleus forskohlii*) was the most efficient **5** biosynthase. The GGPP high-yielding strain BY-HZ16, tSmKSL1-CfTPS1 (module I) and the more active CYP82D274 (module III) were selected for the production of **11**. In this section, we utilized synthetic biology strategies for the optimization of genetic elements and chassis strains.

The optimization of protein-protein interactions between CYP and its redox partner POR to enhance the electron transfer efficiency can alleviate the poor coupling of CYP systems and increase terpenoid production. Because module II (generation of **7**) acted as a rate-limiting step hindering the final product yield, this module was first optimized for the genetic elements. Comparison of the yields from multiple species sources revealed that native POR generally exhibits the highest efficiency of electron transfer. Twelve enzyme combinations (Supplementary Table 2) with truncated or nontruncated CYP728B70 and representative TwPORs (without TwPOR2, a high identity of 98.73% with TwPOR1) were transformed into the BY-ZY1 strain. LC-MS/MS quantification of the yield of **11** showed that TwPOR3 and TwPOR4 with intact CYP728B70 had the highest yields among the combinations, presumably due to differences in the electron transfer capacity associated with the phylogenetic clade of POR (Supplementary Fig. 18). None of the six combinations with truncated TwPORs detected the final product, suggesting that the intact transmembrane domain is essential for electron transfer. In addition, truncated CYP728B70 showed reduced yields, indicating that the complete transit peptides are important for peptide translocation and folding. TwPOR3, which is more biostable, was selected as the electron shuttle with a yield of **11** equal to 2.23 μg/L (Fig. 6b). Further replacement of CYP728B70 with CYP720B4 from *Picea sitchensis* resulted in a 17.10-fold increase in the yield to 49.43 μg/L (Fig. 6b).

Subsequently, optimization of the chassis strain was performed. Chromosome integration and diploidization are promising strategies to improve heterologous gene stability and expression levels and thus enhancing the fermentation ability. We introduced the optimal genes (i.e., *tSmKSL1-CfTPS1*, *CYP82D274* or mutants, *CYP720B4*, and *TwPOR3*) into the diploid strain BY-ZY2D (Supplementary Table 3)

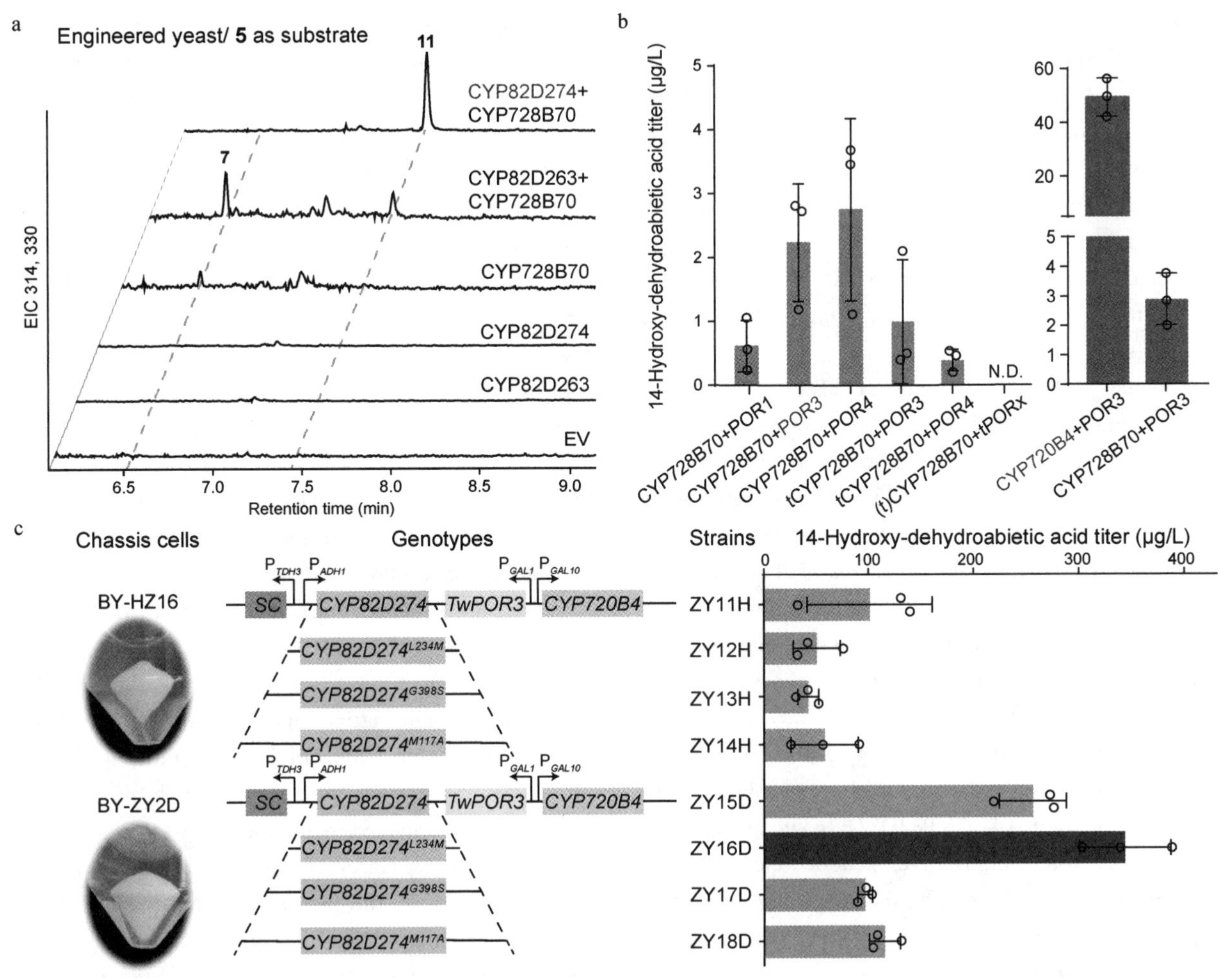


**Fig. 6 De novo biosynthesis of 14-hydroxy-dehydroabietic acid (11) in yeast**

(a) GC - MS analysis of methylated products in CYP82D274 and CYP82D263 coexpressed with CYP728B70. (b) Screening for optimal combinations of CYP and TwPOR. Optimal genes are marked in red. N. D. indicates not detected. (c) Yield of **11** in the engineered strains. The images show the biomass of haploid and diploid strains under the same culture conditions. The genotype schematic is shown in the figure, and detailed information is provided in Supplementary Table 3. Data are presented as mean values±SD ($n$ = 3 biologically independent replicates). Source data are provided as a Source Data file.

and haploid strain BY - HZ16. Diploid strains have higher cell growth rates, cell yields, and tolerances to various stresses than haploid strains. In this study, we quantitatively inoculated different haploid and diploid strains and confirmed that the diploid strains exhibited ~2 - 3 times more biomass than the haploids under identical fermentation conditions (Fig. 6c). The diploid strain BY - ZY16D, in which *tSmKSL1-CfTPS1* and *CYP82D247*$^{L234M}$ were integrated into the yeast chromosome and which carried an inducible plasmid pESC-LEU: : (*CYP720B4* + *TwPOR3*), had the highest yield among the compared strains, and the yield of **11** equaled 343. 87 μg · $L^{-1}$, which was 1. 34 times ($P < 0.05$) higher than that of the WT BY - ZY15D strain and 6. 78 times ($P < 0.01$) higher than that of the haploid strain BY - ZY12H of the same genotype (Fig. 6c).

## 2 DISCUSSION

Triptolide (**1**) is largely insoluble in aqueous solvents; however, chemical structure-bioactivity correlation analyses indicate that the characteristic hydrogen bond at the C - 14 position is the key functional group for its antitumor effect by selective alkylation of thiol groups of enzyme-mediated tumor growth. Further modification of the C - 14 position, which was the earliest and most diverse target, is effective not only for increasing its water solubility but also for enhancing its antitumor activity and lower toxicity; as a result, various compounds, e. g. , minnelide (ClinicalTrials. gov: NCT03129139) and 14-succinyl triptolide sodium salt (PG490-88), have entered clinical trials. The biosynthetic pathway of **1** in native plants has advanced to the first step in skeleton modification after several years. In this study, we revealed the mechanism for 14-hydroxylation formation and demon-strated the involvement of carboxyl groups in the biosynthetic pathway of **1**. CYP82D274 and CYP82D263 act as 14-hydroxylases to catalyze the metabolic grid in **1** biosynthesis and exhibit better affinity and catalytic efficiency for multiple intermediates toward **7** (Fig. 5d). Previous pharmacological studies on the chemical synthesis of **11**, the main product of CYP82D274 catalyzing **7**, have shown its small level of cytotoxic activity, particularly in human acute T-cell leukemia. Using synthetic biology strategies, the intermediate **11** was successfully produced in yeast with a shake flask yield of 343.87 $\mu g \cdot L^{-1}$ to not only obtain pharmacologically active products in an environmentally friendly manner but also facilitate the mining of enigmatic pathway genes.

In particular, CYP82D274 and CYP82D263 can catalyze the aromatization of **5** to yield **6** (Fig. 5), a process that was previously reported as a spontaneous reaction, which results in the wide-spread presence of tanshinones, carnosic acid, carnosol, and other labdane- or abietane-type diterpenoids. We have demonstrated that functionalized CYP82D274 and CYP82D263 could increase the yield of the rate-limiting enzyme and thus the heterologous production of final products (Fig. 6a). It is reasonable to believe that the introduction of CYP82D274 and CYP82D263 in other **5**-derived metabolic pathways could effectively improve access to the target products. Furthermore, the extensive C－14 hydroxylation function of CYP82D274 could effectively provide the necessary alternative genetic element and synthetic precursors for these pharmacologically important natural products and derivatives, for instance, gerardianin A from *Isodon lophanthoides*.

CYP82D274 and CYP82D263 identified in this study are located on a tandem duplication gene cluster on Chr12 containing 11 CYP82D subfamily genes (Fig. 2a), presumably arising from LTRs of the retrotransposon (Class I element) generated by intrachromosomal replication rearrangements. According to the evolutionary divergence, the following hypothesis is proposed. In Clade I, the first duplication of neofunctional CYP82D produced CYP82D274, and gene duplication and transfer of TW08G01036.1 (CYP82D213) via transposon from Chr12 to Chr08 then occurred; in addition, the duplication of CYP82D274 produced TW12G01156.1, which then duplicated to generate TW12G01165.1 rearrangement at the other end of the tandem array. CYP82D213 reportedly undertakes the triepoxidation function in the last step of triptonide, indicating that it underwent neofunctionalization after separation from CYP82D274. In Clade II, the duplication order follows TW12G01157.1, TW12G01158.1 and CYP82D263 (Supplementary Fig. 19).

Genes in the CYP82D subfamily are commonly found in flavonoid biosynthesis. SbCYP82D1.1 in *Scutellaria baicalensis* functions as a flavone 6-hydroxylase (F6H) in catalyzing chrysin, whereas SbCYP82D2 acts as a flavone 8-hydroxylase (F8H). A comparison of eight orthologous gene pairs of CYP82Ds in the genomes of *S. barbata* and *S. baicalensis* revealed the presence of the F6H tandem gene clusters *SbaiCYP82D1*-*SbaiCYP82D7*-*SbaiCYP82D8* and *SbarCYP82D1*-*SbarCYP82D6*-*SbarCYP82D8* on Chr06 in both species, with chromosomal localization distances of <30 kb. In particular, CYP82D8 showed interspecies gene synteny, indicating conserved and species-specific gene evolution. In addition to flavonoids, CYP82Ds have been reported to be involved in the biosynthesis of furanocoumarin isopimpinellin, lignan (－)－4′-desmethylepipodophyllotoxin, and sesquiterpenoid gossypol. Both CYP82D213 and the two CYP82D genes reported in the present study are involved in diterpenoids biosynthesis, and the construction of a phylogenetic tree with different functions (Fig. 7) revealed a clear phylogenetic differentiation of CYP82Ds involved in different types of compounds, which can also be used to guide future directions of research on CYP82Ds of unknown function.

Recently, a minimal set of four genes from the CYP71BE and CYP82D subfamilies required for the formation of triptonide from **5** was reported, and these undoubtedly constitute an alternative and simple way to bypass the carboxylation step and obtain triptonide in heterologous hosts. However, whether it is an absolute biosynthetic pathway or a branched metabolic pathway in its native plants remains unclear. Here, we confirmed the involvement of carboxyl groups in the biosynthetic pathway of **1** via plant cell experiments. From the current perspective, C－18 carboxyl generation is the rate-limiting step responsible for the extremely low levels of **1** in *T. wilfordii*, and the *Tripterygium* genus contains many active natural products with carboxyl or carbonyl groups at C－18 or C－19. Improving protein activity is essential for improving the yield of carboxyl-related metabolites. The mechanism of carboxyl shift also needs to be explored for the biosynthesis of **1**.

In conclusion, our study revealed the key enzymes for the C－14 hydroxylation metabolic grid of **1**, characterized the hydroxylation and aromatization functions of tandemly duplicated CYP82D274 and CYP82D263, and successfully achieved the de novo biosynthesis of precursor **11** in yeast. The elucidation of the formation mechanism of C－14 hydroxylation not only provides important genetic elements for the synthetic biology production of **1** but is also useful for revealing the biosynthetic pathways of other labdane-type compounds with C－14 hydroxylation.

## 3 METHODS

Plant materials and chemicals *T. wilfordii* suspension cells were cultured in Murashige & Skoog (MS) with vitamins (Caisson Lab, USA) medium containing 30 $g \cdot L^{-1}$ sucrose with 0.5 mg/L indole-3-butyric acid (IBA), 0.5 mg/L 2,4-dichlorophenoxyacetic acid (2,4－D) and 0.1 mg/L kinetin (KT), and the final pH was adjusted to 5.8. Suspension cells

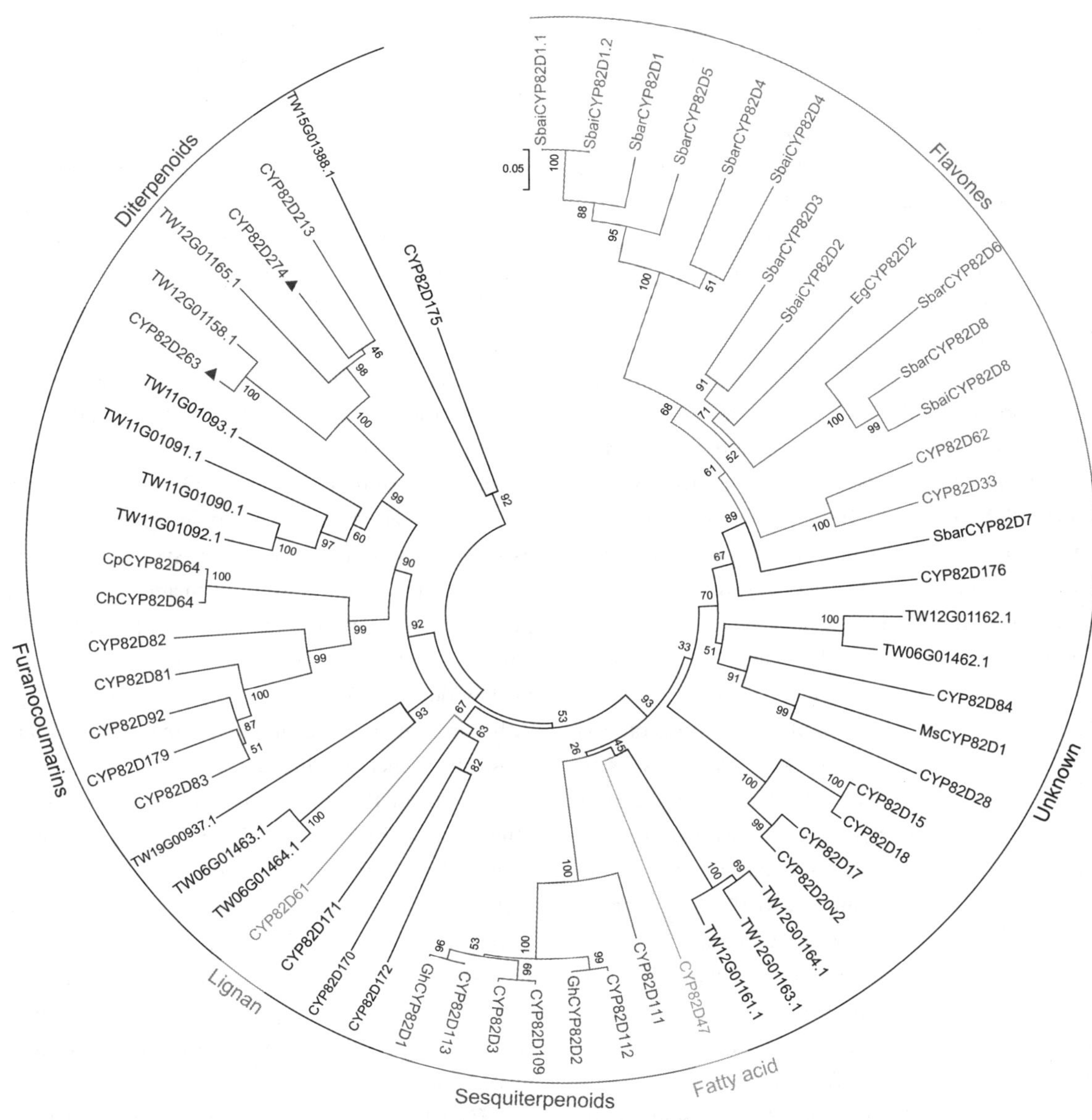


**Fig. 7 Phylogenetic analysis of CYP82Ds**

A total of 61 CYP82Ds from flavonoids, furanocoumarins, lignan, fatty acid, sesquiterpenoids, diterpenoids, etc., were included and indicated by different colors. Phylogenetic analysis was performed using MEGA 6.0 software with maximum likelihood method (1 000 bootstraps). The two functional CYP82Ds in this study are marked with red triangles. The GenBank accession numbers are provided in Supplementary Data 6.

were grown at 25 ℃ in darkness with shaking at 120 rpm. A total of seven four-year-old *T. wilfordii* plants (No. 164 - 170) were collected from Taoyuan Town, Datian County, Sanming City, Fujian, China. The geographic coordinates were E117°31′44″, N25°49′29″, and the altitude was 908 m. The chemical standards **7**, **10**, and **13** were purchased from Shanghai Yuanye BioTechnology Co., Ltd. (Shanghai, China), and **9** and **15** were procured from BioBioPha Co., Ltd. (Yunnan, China). Compound **8** was kindly provided by Prof. Fei Li from Kunming Institute of Botany, Chinese Academy of Sciences, and **5**, **6**, **11**, and **14** were isolated from enriched fermentation products.

Strains, vectors and media The initial yeast strain used in this study was BY-HZ16 (*MAT*α; *trp1Δ0*; *leu2Δ0*; *lys2Δ0*; *ura3Δ0*; *rox1Δ*; *yjl064wΔ*; *ypl062wΔ*; *erg9*::Δ-218-175; *trp1*::*HIS3*-$P_{PGK1}$-*BTS1*/*ERG20*-$T_{ADH1}$-$P_{TDH3}$-*SaGGPS*-$T_{TPI1}$-$P_{TEF1}$-*tHMG1*-$T_{CYC1}$). The engineered yeast strains are listed in Supplementary Table 3. *Escherichia coli* Trans1-T1 (TransGen Biotech, China) was used for cloning and plasmid construction. The shuttle vectors were pESC-LEU, pESC-TRP (Agilent Technologies, USA), and pYES2 (Invitrogen, USA). Synthetic dropout (SD) medium (FunGenome, China) was selected according to the auxotroph and carried plasmids. Yeast extract peptone dextrose (YPD) and YPL media were composed of 1% yeast extract, 2% peptone (OXOID, UK), and 2% D-(+)-glucose (Glc, Sigma-Aldrich, USA) for YPD or 2% D-(+)-galactose (Gal, Inalco S.p. A, Italy) for YPL.

Chromosome location and evolution analysis of CYP82Ds To obtain more chromosome information on CYP82Ds, BioEdit software (version 7.0.9.0) was used to search the open reading frame (ORF) of CYP82Ds from the whole genome through the local BLAST function. A sequence with a 'blastn' identity greater than or equal to 99% was regarded as one gene, and genes with similarity greater than 50% were recorded. Each CYP82D was ultimately identified by chromosome localization. A phylogenetic analysis was performed using MEGA 6.0 software to align the CYP82D sequences using ClustalW function, and the maximum likelihood method (1 000 bootstraps) was used to build a phylogenetic tree. A total of 3n different sites were removed, and the online conversion ALTER (http://www.sing-group.org/ALTER/) and KaKs_Calculator 2.0 software were used to calculate the nonsynonymous substitution rates (*Ka*), synonymous substitution rates (*Ks*), and *Ka*/*Ks* in the Linux operating environment.

Candidate CYPs screening and cloning CYPs were obtained from the PFAM database and annotated as cytochrome P450 (PF00067). A heatmap of gene expression was generated using MultiExperiment Viewer (MeV, version 4.9.0) and Java 8 software. The RPKM reads of the root periderm, root phloem, root xylem, stem vascular bundle, stem periderm, and leaf originated from previous tissue transcriptomes (NCBI SRA number SRP199495, Supplementary Fig. 20), and the data were normalized and processed by hierarchical cluster analysis with Pearson correlation. CYPs with gene expression profiles similar to those of *TwTPS7* (*v2*), *TwTPS27* (*v2*), and *CYP728B70* were selected as candidate CYPs for further analysis. The candidate CYPs were amplified using 2 × Phusion High-Fidelity PCR Master Mix (New England Biolabs, USA) and cDNA of *T. wilfordii* root as the template, which was consistent with the transcriptome after complete sequencing (Supplementary Data 5).

Heterologous expression and functional characterization in yeast Candidate CYPs were integrated into the high-copy plasmid pESC-LEU expressing TwPOR3 from the GAL1 promoter and CYP from the GAL10 promoter (Supplementary Data 5). The recombinant plasmids were transformed into the yeast strain BY4741, and pESC-LEU with *TwPOR3* was employed as an empty vector control. For the in vivo assay, SD medium without tyrosine and leucine (SD-Trp-Leu) and 2% Glc was used to select positive strains, and 2% Gal was added to 20 mL of SD-Trp-Leu for the fermentation of fresh cells in a shaker at 30 ℃ and 200 rpm for 12 h. After the feeding of **7** or **8** to a final concentration of 50 μM, the resulting mixture was fermented for another 48 - 60 h, and ultrasonic extraction of fermentation products with an equal volume of ethyl acetate was then performed twice for 1 h each time. For the in vitro assay, microsomes were extracted according to the following experimental procedure. The base buffer TE (pH 7.5) consisted of 50 mM Tris-HCl and 1 mM EDTA. Cells were collected by centrifugation at 4 000 × *g* for 3 min, resuspended in TEK (0.1 M KCl in TE), and left at room temperature for 10 min. The cells were collected again by centrifugation and resuspended in pre-cooled TESB (0.6 M sorbitol in TE). The cells were completely crushed using a cryogenic homogenizer (ATS, Canada) for 3 - 5 cycles. After centrifugation at 12,000 × *g* for 15 min, the microsomes were precipitated by adding NaCl at a final concentration of 0.15 M and polyethylene glycol PEG4000 at a final concentration of 0.1 g · $mL^{-1}$ to the supernatant. The pellets were resuspended in TEG (20% (v/v) glycerol in TE) for preservation and catalytic reactions. The enzymatic assay was performed in a 500-μL system containing 100 mM Tris-HCl (pH 7.5), 1 mM nicotinamide adenine dinucleotide phosphate (NADPH), 4 mM glucose-6-phosphate, 1 unit of glucose-6-phosphate dehydrogenase, 5 μM flavin mononucleotide, 5 μM flavin adenine dinucleotide, 1 mM dithiothreitol, 0.5 mg of microsomal protein, and 100 μM substrate, which was incubated for 20 h at 30 ℃ with shaking at 100 rpm in the dark and then extracted with 500 μL of ethyl acetate three times. The organic phases of both the in vivo and in vitro samples were dried, reconstituted with methanol and then derivatized with trimethylsilyl diazomethane (Tokyo Chemical Industry, Japan). The methylated samples were dissolved with ethyl acetate for GC-TQ-MS/MS analysis. For the **5**-catalyzed reaction, the plasmid was transformed into engineered yeast BY-PS2 (Supplementary Table 3).

Enrichment, isolation, and NMR analysis of the product Strains containing the pESC-LEU::(*CYP82D274* + *TwPOR3*) plasmid were inoculated into 500 mL of SD-Trp-Leu + 2% Glc fluid medium and grown at 30 ℃ and 200 rpm to an $OD_{600}$ of ~10. The cells were collected by centrifugation, evenly distributed into twenty 2-L flasks containing 500 mL of YPL and 100 μM substrate **7**, and then fermented at 30 ℃ and 200 rpm for 72 h. Then, 15 - 20 g of HP2MGL resin (Mitsubishi, Japan) was added to each flask in a sterile environment, and the fermentation product was extracted in a shaker at 200 rpm for another 24 h.

Ten liters of fermentation broth was centrifuged at 4 000 × *g* for 5 min, and the yeast cells and resin were collected and dried in an oven at 40 ℃. Eight times the volume of anhydrous methanol was added, and the catalytic product was extracted by ultrasonication at low temperature for 30 min. The solids were repeatedly extracted until the anhydrous methanol extract was colorless. The extracts were filtered to remove the resin and cell residues and evaporated under a vacuum at 40 ℃. The products were dissolved with

4 mL of chromatography-grade methanol and sampled into a Gilson 281 semipreparative HPLC connected to an H322 pump, GX-281 autosampler, 156 dual wavelength UV detector, and Trilution LC 2.1 workstation. An Xtimate C18 column (30 mm × 75 mm × 3.0 μm, Welch) with 0.1% trifluoroacetic acid-water (mobile phase A) and acetonitrile (mobile phase B) was used. Gradient elution was started with 50% B and then increased to 100% B over 8.0 min, the flow rate was set to 25 mL·min$^{-1}$, and the injection volume was 500 μL. The product fractions were collected at 7.4-7.8 min and freeze-dried. Three milligrams of product powder was weighed precisely and fully dissolved in 500 μL of deuterated acetone ($C_3D_6O$, InnoChem, China). For chemical structure characterization, $^1H$-NMR (800 M), $^{13}C$-NMR (200 M), NOESY, HSQC, and $^1H$-$^1H$ COSY were analyzed using a Bruker Avance III HD (Bruker BioSpin, Germany). MestReNova 14 software was used to analyze the data.

Kinetic analysis The CYP concentration was estimated by measuring the reduced carbon monoxide difference spectrum using an extinction coefficient (450 versus 490 nm) of 91 mM$^{-1}$·cm$^{-1}$. Incubation times from 0.5 to 8h were used. The $K_m$ values were determined using serial concentrations from 0.1 to 100 μmol/L for **7** and 5 to 80 μM for **5** in 300-μL enzyme assays. These also contained ~0.4 mg of microsomal protein, Tris-HCl (pH 7.5), NADPH, and the regenerating system mentioned above. The reactions were initiated by substrate addition and incubated with shaking at 30℃ for 30 min in the dark. Extraction was then terminated three times with 300 μL of ethyl acetate, and the extracts were completely dried with a vacuum concentrator (Eppendorf Concentrator plus, Germany). The product **11** was quantified using 100 μL of methanol dissolved for LC-TQ-MS/MS analysis, and the product **14** was dissolved in 100 μL of ethyl acetate for quantification by GC-MS. The $K_m$ values were calculated by nonlinear regression using GraphPad Prism version 7.

Gene overexpression and RNA interference in suspension cells The specific fragments of *CYP82D274* and *CYP82D263* were chosen via multiple sequence alignment of all CYP82D nucleic acid sequences in *T. wilfordii*. The specific fragments (Supplementary Data 5) were inserted into the pH7WG2D (for OE) and pK7GWIWG2D (for RNAi) binary vectors. Using the developed gene gun technology, recombinant plasmids were transformed into suspension cells that had been precultured for 7 days and then cultured for another 7 days to collect samples. RNA extraction and reverse transcription were performed using Total RNA Extraction Kit (Promega, China) and FastQuant RT Kit (Tiangen Biotech, China), and gene expression was detected using qRT-PCR (Supplementary Data 5). Twenty milligrams of freeze-dried sample powder was precisely weighed, soaked in 1 mL of 80% (v/v) methanol overnight at 4℃, and subjected to ultrasonication at 40 kHz for 1 h at 25℃. After centrifugation at 13,000 × g for 10 min, the supernatant was filtered through a 0.22-μm PTFE microporous membrane to obtain the samples for Q Exactive HF LC-MS/MS.

Metabolite feeding studies The substrate feeding was performed by soaking 0.2 g of suspension cells with 1 mL of MS medium containing 0.8 mM **11** for 7 days before sampling, and the negative control was soaked using an equal volume of MS liquid. For stable isotope labeling assay, $^{18}O$-**11** was obtained by expanding the above microsomal assay system to 600 mL and completely replacing $^{16}O_2$ with $^{18}O_2$ (purity > 97%) before the addition of substrate **7**, and after 1 h of reaction, an equal volume of ethyl acetate was extracted three times and then subjected to product enrichment and isolation. The purified $^{18}O$-**11** was determined by LC-qTOF-MS. After gene gun bombardment of *TwTPS7*&*TwTPS27*-RNAi (Supplementary Data 5) for 5 days, ~0.2 g of cells were soaked in 1 mL of MS medium with 0.4 mM $^{18}O$-**11** and 100 μM fosmidomycin for 5 days and then sampled after 2 days of induction with 50 μM methyl jasmonate. Equal concentrations of unlabeled **11** with identical treatment and WT cells were used as controls. Three biological replicates of each group were included in the experiment. The metabolite extraction was performed as described above, with Q Exactive HF LC-MS/MS for quantitative assays and LC-qTOF-MS for qualitative assays.

Yeast engineering For CYP coexpression, the recombinant plasmids pESC-LEU::(-*CYP82Ds* + *TwPOR3*) and pESC-TRP::(*CYP728B70* + *TwPOR3*) were chemically transformed into the yeast strain BY-PS2 together or separately. A corresponding auxotrophic medium was employed for selection and fermentation, and products were extracted with ethyl acetate and detected via GC-MS. For the screening of CYP and POR combinations, the recombinant plasmid pYES2::($P_{TDH3}$-*tSmKSL1*-*CfTPS1*-$T_{TPI1}$-$P_{ADH1}$-*CYP82D274*-$T_{PGI}$) was constructed (Supplementary Data 5) using BY-HZ16 strain homologous recombination to generate the BY-ZY1 strain. Truncated transit peptides (50 amino acids at the N-terminus predicted by TargetP Server v2.0) or complete CYP728B70 was constructed at multiple cloning site (MCS) 1, and a truncated transmembrane domain (67 amino acids for TwPOR1 and 46 amino acids for TwPOR3 and TwPOR4, predicted by TMHMM Server v2.0) or complete TwPOR was integrated at MCS2 of pESC-LEU (Supplementary Data 5). Twelve enzyme combinations (Supplementary Table 2) were transformed into the BY-ZY1 strain. For optimization of the chassis strain, the haploid strains BY4741H (Supplementary Table 3) and BY-HZ16 were inoculated in the respective media and incubated at 30℃ and 200 rpm for 24 h. The two strains were mixed in

SD - His - Trp supplemented with 2% Glc liquid medium at an equal OD and cocultured for another 24 h. After centrifugation, the cells were collected and coated on SD - His - Trp with 2% Glc solid plates and incubated at 30 ℃ for 72 h, and the monoclonal strains were selected. The newly constructed diploid strain was identified and named BY - ZY2D. The *tSmKSL1* - *CfTPS1* and *CYP82D274* (or mutants) modules were cloned and integrated into the haploid strain BY - HZ16 and diploid strain BY - ZY2D chromosome *YPRCΔ15* locus by the modularized two-step chromosome integration technique using *Ura3* as a selection marker (Supplementary Fig. 21 and Supplementary Data 5). Subsequently, pESC-LEU::(*CYP720B4* + *TwPOR3*) was chemically transformed to generate BY - ZY11H to ZY14H (haploid strains) and BY - ZY15D to ZY18D (diploid strains) (Supplementary Table 3). For quantitative inoculation, the seed strain was transferred into 20 mL of fresh medium with a quantitative OD of 0.1, and three biological replicates of each group were included in the experiment. The product was extracted with an equal volume of n-hexane and dissolved in 100 μL of methanol for LC - TQ - MS/MS.

## 4 MALDI-MSI

Matrix-assisted laser desorption/ionization-mass spectrometry imaging (MALDI - MSI) is a label-free technique used for tissue sample imaging that allows the localization of known or unknown biological molecules in a spatial region within subcellular compartments. The sample is rasterized while a laser is used as a stationary ionization source, and the mass spectrum is utilized for recording and converting the ion signal intensity and then drawing the XY coordinate, enabling the spatial distribution of the ion of interest for visualization. High-coverage MALDI - MSI was employed to map the target molecules in the root of *T. wilfordii*. The fresh root was flash-frozen in liquid nitrogen and then maintained at −80 ℃ for over 8 h. The root tissue was cryosectioned into 20-μm sections on a cryostat microtome (CM3050S, Leica Biosystems, Germany) in a −20 ℃ environment and attached to the conductive side of an indium tin oxide (ITO)-coated glass slide (Bruker, Germany). The glass slide was kept in a vacuum desiccator and dried for 30 min. Then, 2,5-dihydroxybenzoic acid (DHB) was selected as the matrix under the positive ion mode after the pre-experiment and was sprayed evenly on the surface of the slide by an HTX™-Sprayer (HTX Technologies, USA). MALDI - MSI was conducted with a timsTOF fleX™ mass spectrometer (Bruker), and the parameter settings were as follows. The laser frequency and accumulated shots were set to 10,000 Hz and 500 shots, respectively, the spatial resolution was 50 μm, and the target profile was 18.70 μm. The raw mass spectra data were acquired over the $m/z$ range of 200 - 1 000. A Bruker SCiLS Lab 2020a instrument and MetaboScape software were used to analyze the MALDI imaging data and visualize the $m/z$ values.

GC - TQ - MS/MS  GC - TQ - MS/MS was performed on an Agilent 7890B GC system equipped with a 7 000 C GC/MS Triple Quad. For the DB-5MS (15 m × 0.25 mm × 0.1 μm) capillary column, splitless injection was performed at 250 ℃. The GC oven temperature was adjusted according to the following program: an initial temperature of 50 ℃ was maintained for 1 min, followed by an increase to 200 ℃ at a rate of 40 ℃ · $min^{-1}$, an increase to 240 ℃ at a rate of 20 ℃ · $min^{-1}$, an increase to 246 ℃ at a rate of 1.5 ℃ · $min^{-1}$, and an increase to 300 ℃ at a rate of 40 ℃ · $min^{-1}$, with the final temperature being maintained for 3 min. For the DB - 5MS (30 m × 0.25 mm × 0.1 μm) column, the oven temperature program was as follows: 50 ℃ isothermal for 1 min, increased to 240 ℃ at 50 ℃ · $min^{-1}$, increased to 255 ℃ at 1.5 ℃ · $min^{-1}$, increased to 300 ℃ at 50 ℃ · $min^{-1}$ and maintained at the final temperature for 1 min. Helium was used as the carrier gas at a flow rate of 1 mL · $min^{-1}$. The inlet temperature was set to 300 ℃, the ion trap temperature was 250 ℃, the electron energy was 70 eV, and the spectra were recorded over a range of 10 - 400 $m/z$. Qualitative Analysis software (B.07.00) was used for data analysis.

LC - TQ - MS/MS  LC - TQ - MS/MS was performed with an Agilent 1 290 Infinity LC tandem QTRAP 6 500 MS (AB SCIEX). We used an ACQUITY UPLC HSS T3 column (2.1 mm × 100 mm × 1.8 μm, Waters) with 0.1% formic acid-water as mobile phase A and acetonitrile as mobile phase B. A flow rate of 0.3 mL · $min^{-1}$ was used, and the gradient program was as follows: 0 - 1 min, 40% B; 2 - 3 min, 90% B; and 5 - 6 min, 40% B. In each run, 3 μL of the sample was analyzed, and the column temperature was 40 ℃. The quantitative ions for multiple reaction monitoring (MRM) *11* were 315 and 269 $m/z$.

Q Exactive HF LC - MS/MS  Q Exactive HF LC - MS/MS (Thermo Scientific) was performed on an ACQUITY UPLC HSS T3 column (2.1 mm × 100 mm × 1.8 μm, Waters) with 0.1% formic acid-water as mobile phase A and acetonitrile as mobile phase B. A flow rate of 0.4 mL/min was used, and the gradient program was as follows: 0 - 4 min, 30%-34% B; 4 - 8 min, 34%-52% B; 8 - 12 min, 52% B; 12 - 23 min, 52%-77% B; and 23 - 26 min, 90% B. In each run, 2 μL of the sample was analyzed, and the column temperature was 40 ℃. When the parent ion quantification method was applied, either positive or negative ion mode was used for different metabolites.

LC - qTOF - MS  LC - qTOF - MS (Waters) was performed on an ACQUITY UPLC HSS T3 column (2.1 mm ×

100 mm × 1.8 μm, Waters) with 0.1% formic acid-water as mobile phase A and acetonitrile as mobile phase B. The gradient program was as follows: 0 – 0.5 min, 20% B; 0.5 – 21 min, 20%- 85% B; 21 – 23 min, 85%- 100% B; 23 – 26 min, 100% B; 26 – 27 min, linear decrease from 100% to 20% B; and 27 – 30 min, isocratic 20% B. The flow rate was set at 0.4 mL/min. Mass spectra were acquired in positive/negative ion mode over a scan range of $m/z$ 50 – 1200 with a scan time of 0.2 s. The MS settings were as follows: resolution analyzer mode; normal dynamic range; ramp collision energy 10 – 50 V; cone voltage 40 V. MassLynx v4.2 was used for data analysis.

qRT – PCR Primers (Supplementary Data 5), cDNA, and reagents were added according to the TransStart Top Green qPCR SuperMix (TransGen Biotech) instructions. QuantStudio5 (Applied Biosystems) was employed to assay the expression of genes, and each reaction was repeated three times. The mixed reagents were first activated for 30 s at 94 ℃, and then denaturation occurred for 5 s at 94 ℃, followed by annealing for 15 s at 56 ℃ and extension for 10 s at 72 ℃. This proce-dure was repeated for 45 cycles, followed by the dissociation stage. *EFLα* (Supplementary Data 5) was used as the housekeeping reference gene. The relative expression of genes was analyzed using the $2^{-\Delta\Delta Ct}$ method.

[张逸风，高伟，黄璐琦，等. Nature Communications, 2023,14:875.]

# Functional divergence of CYP76AKs shapes the chemodiversity of abietane-type diterpenoids in genus *Salvia*

Plant-derived natural products are a valuable resource for pharmacological research and the development of health-related products, and their structural diversity is related to various biological activities. Both Taxol, a diterpenoid alkaloid obtained from *Taxus chinensis* (Pilg.) Rehder, and Artemisinin, a sesquiterpenoid derived from *Artemisia annua* L., have received a great deal of attention worldwide due to their exceptional anticancer and antimalarial effects, respectively. Because of the high demands for natural products, approaches for obtaining specific compounds via metabolic engineering have become a major trend, necessitating the elucidation of biosynthetic pathways and the identification of key genes involved in these pathways.

Most natural products obtained from plants are specialized metabolites. However, elucidating a biosynthetic pathway is limited when the pathway is complex and includes multiple steps, making it challenging to identify the relevant genes. Generally, the emergence of plant specialized metabolites is an evolved defense mechanism that protects plants against a barrage of biotic and abiotic stresses, with chemical diversity reffected in the diversity of their skeletons and chemical modifications. In general, similar skeletons are derived from similar biosynthetic pathways within homologous plants. However, natural products based on the same skeletons with various chemical modifications (e.g., glycosylation, methylation, hydroxylation, acylation, prenylation) are diverse within species. Such structural modifications play important roles in how plants respond to changes in the external environment for their growth and development.

Given the rapid advancements in recent omics technologies, it is now possible to trace evolutionary origin, distribution, and composition of metabolites on lineage scale, and shed light on their ancient or novel functions, as well as the emergence and radiation of their biosynthetic pathways over time. For instance, the Mint Plant Genome Project has made significant contributions in this regard, by investigating the distribution patterns of volatile terpenoids in the Lamiaceae family, and exploring the radiations of the iridoid pathway across various lineages. They have also brought insights into the mechanisms behind the loss and subsequent re-evolution of nepetalactone biosynthesis in the *Nepeta* lineage. Another highly representative instance is the origin of morphinan in genus *Papaver* (Papaveraceae). By tracing the fusion events of *STORR* gene among *Papaver* genomes, and correlated whole-genome duplications (WGDs), chromosomal rearrangements, and subgenome evolution, the innovation of this specialized metabolite was demonstrated. Therefore, establishing the genetic mechanism for the formation of natural product diversity across species is of great importance for understanding the pathways, providing synthetic elements for metabolic engineering and molecular breeding.

Tanshinones and carnosic acid-related compounds are specialized abietane-type diterpenoids (ATDs) in Lamiaceae. Tanshinones were originally identified from *Salvia miltiorrhiza* Bunge and have been utilized for the treatment of coronary artery disease, angina pectoris, and myocardial infarction. Carnosic acid and its derivatives found in *Salvia officinalis* L. have strong antioxidant, antiparasitic, antitumor, antifungal, antiadipogenic, and antibacterial activities. The specific biosynthesis of these ATDs initiates from the biosynthesis of their common precursor, miltiradiene, catalyzing by copalyl diphosphate synthase (CPS) and kaurene synthase-like (KSL). In *S. miltiorrhiza*, CYP76AH1 catalyzes oxidation of miltiradiene at C-12 to form ferruginol. Besides, other members of CYP76AH subfamily can catalyze oxidation of miltiradiene at C-7, -11, and -12 to generate a metabolite array with diverse modification on ATD rings. CYP76AK subfamily further promotes the specificity and diversity of ATDs in *Salvia*. CYP76AK6 from *S. officinalis*, *Salvia fruticosa* Mill. and *Salvia pomifera* L., CYP76AK7 and CYP76AK8 from *Salvia rosmarinus* Schleid convert 11-hydroxyferruginol into carnosic acid by generating a carboxyl group at C-20, whereas CYP76AK1 from *S. miltiorrhiza* only executes hydroxylation at C-20 to generate an alcohol group. This suggests that functional diversity of CYP76AKs may contribute to presence of different types of ATDs in various *Salvia* species. In addition, it is worth noting that the oxidation pattern pre-sent on the C-20 position could also play a crucial role in the formation of miltirone, the key precursor to tanshinones. This may involve the demethylation process (resulting in the loss of C-20) and the aroma-tization of ring B, which remain unresolved catalytic steps in the pathway (Supplementary Fig. 1). Therefore, a lineage-wide character-ization of ATDs distribution, functions of CYP76AKs, as well as the relevant evolutionary events would be necessary for revealing the tanshinone biosynthesis pathway. Furthermore, in the case of evolution of CYP family in plants, the dynamic of CYP76AKs would provide insight into the interplay between function divergence and genome evolution in the evolution of CYP76AK clan.

*Salvia* L. (Lamiaceae, Nepetoideae) is the largest genus in the mint family comprising ca. 1 000 species, and it includes several culturally and economically important species that are used as tradi-tional herbs (e.g., *S. miltiorrhiza* and *S. officinalis*), fragrance (e.g., *Salvia sclarea* L.), ornamentals (e.g., *Salvia splendens* Sellow ex Wied-Neuw.), and functional foods (e.g., *Salvia hispanica* L.). *Salvia* has a cosmopolitan distribution consisted of three species diversity centers: Central-South America (ca. 500 species), Southwest Asia-Mediterranean (ca. 250 species), and East Asia (ca. 100 species). *Salvia* is known for having a rich variety of ATDs, making it a suitable model genus to investigate the evolutionary origins of ATDs diversity. Tanshinones primarily accumulate in *S. miltiorrhiza*, *Salvia przewalskii* Maxim., and *Salvia yunnanensis* C. H. Wright, whereas carnosic acid-related metabolites have been found in European sage species such as *S. officinalis*, *S. fruticosa*, and *S. pomifera*. It is, however, unclear whether the metabolic differences represent an isolated event or a consistent variation caused by clade differentiation within the genus. Thus, the overall correlated pattern between chemical diversity and genetic diversity based on a robust phylogeny of the genus is the basis support for investigating ATDs formation in this economically important genus.

Here, we combined the concepts of phylogenetic reconstruction, metabolome analysis, pathway analyses, and evolutionary mechanisms to characterize 71 *Salvia* species to investigate the molecular and evolutionary mechanisms that resulted in ATDs diversity in the genus. Our metabolome analysis revealed the distribution of ATDs in this genus, and in vitro enzyme activity assays were then performed to investigate the mechanisms by which the CYP76AK subfamily is involved in ATDs biosynthesis. In addition, an evolutionary model of the CYP76AK subfamily was proposed based on comparative geno-mics, phylogenetic analyses, and the enzymology of reconstructed ancestral biosynthetic enzymes. Our results suggest that the evolution of the CYP76AK family may have played a major role for the chemical diversity of ATDs in *Salvia*.

## 1 RESULTS

Phylogenetic relationships within *Salvia* To characterize chemical diversity and phylogenetic relationships within the genus *Salvia*, 77 species, including six outgroups (*Melissa officinalis* L., *Mentha spicata* L., *Clinopodium polycephalum* (Vaniot) C. Y. Wu & S. J. Hsuan, *Origanum vulgare* L., *Nepeta cataria* L., and *Pru-nella vulgaris* L.), were sampled for analyses (Supplementary Data 1), covering the main geographic distribution areas (America, West Asia, Europe, and East Asia) of the genus except Africa. In total, we generated 72 new transcriptomes, from mixed cDNA libraries of leaves and roots, resulting in an average of 40,876 transcripts representing 38.2 Mb per species (Supplementary Data 1). In addition to three published transcriptomes (*M. officinalis*, *M. spicata*, and *O. vulgare*) and two genomes (*S. miltiorrhiza* and *N. cataria*), 77 nuclear gene sets were obtained for our analyses. Five sets of orthologous groups (OGs), composing of 2 178, 1 532, 1 169, 512, and 130 orthologous genes, respectively, were applied to reconstruct *Salvia* phylogeny using a coalescent method through a multi-step procedure with consideration for alignment length, species coverage, and other factors (Fig. 1; Supplementary Figs. 2-6). Monophyly of the genus *Salvia* and six subgenera (*Calosphace*, *Audibertia*, *Glutinaria*, *Sclarea*, "*Heterosphace*", and *Salvia*) were maximally supported (bootstrap support [BS] = 100%; Fig. 1; Supplementary Figs. 2-6). Consistent with previous phylogeny studies, the genus was split into three successive major clades (Clade I, II, and IV) that reffected their

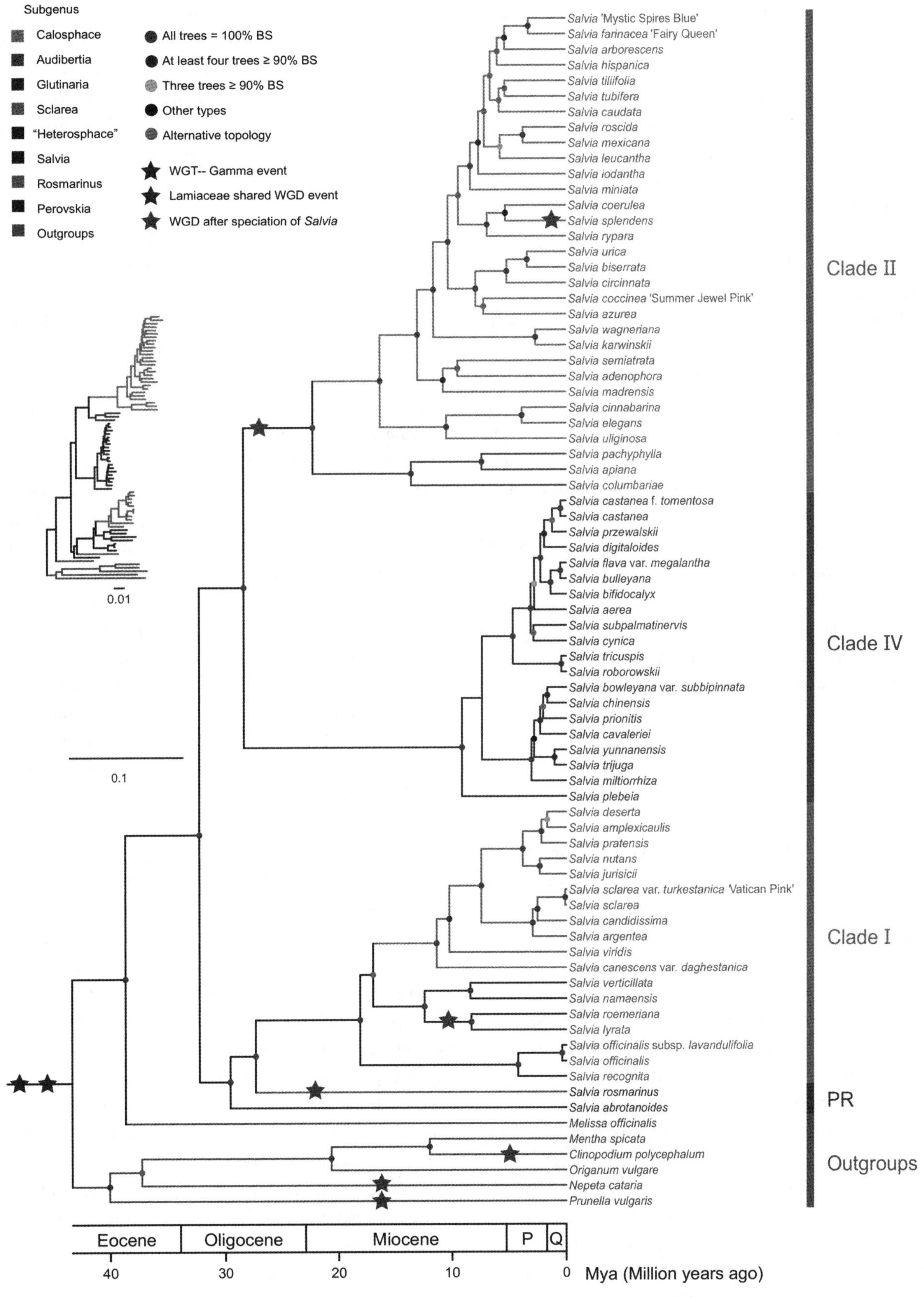


**Fig. 1 Phylogenetic relationships of *Salvia* estimated by Astral using five gene sets**

Five levels of bootstrap values are denoted with red, blue, yellow, black, and green solid circles. Green solid circles indicate alternative topologies for the node among the five trees (see Supplementary Figs. 2 – 6). Species belonging to the same subgenus are marked with the same branch color. Species names are shown to the right of the tree, and clades are indicated on the far right and highlighted with colored labels. Colored solid stars denote genome duplication identified in this study. Mya million years ago, P Pliocene, Q Quaternary, WGD whole-genome duplication, WGT whole-genome triplication. PR subgenera *Perovskia* and *Rosmarinus*. Source data are provided as a Source Data file.

geographic distribution, which could be roughly divided into Eurasia, America, and East Asia. *Salvia abrotanoides* (Kar.) Sytsma and *S. rosmarinus*, belonging to subgenera *Perovskia* and *Rosmarinus* (PR), are sister to Clade I. Thus, the phylogeny of *Salvia* provided well-supported grouping for further lineage-wide metabolic profiling.

According to the tree constructed from 130 OGs concatenations for all taxa with four fossils as calibration points, the evolutionary timescale of *Salvia* lineages was further estimated (Fig. 1, Supplementary Fig. 7). Our chronogram illustrated the origin of the genus *Salvia* could be dated to the Late Eocene (~38.1 million years ago, Mya) to the Middle Oligocene (~26.1 Mya), for the crown group of *Salvia* were estimated to occurred at ~32.1 Mya with a 95% credible interval (CI) of 26.1 - 38.1. Shortly after that, the crown group of Clade I, *Rosmarinus*, and *Perovskia* might have occurred at ~29.5 Mya (95% CI: 23.7 - 35.2). In parallel, the node containing both Clade II and Clade IV might originate at ~28.2 Mya (95% CI: 22.7-33.8). Subsequently, Clade II and Clade IV were estimated to diverge at ~22.1 Mya (95% CI: 17.6 - 27.0) and ~9.1 Mya (95% CI: 6.7 - 11.8), respectively.

Based on the transcriptomes and genome datasets in hand, we also identified whole-genome duplication (WGD) events among *Salvia* species according to synonymous substitutions per site ($K_S$) among paralogous gene pairs (Fig. 1; Supplementary Fig. 8). First, two previously known WGD events, the gamma event shared by core eudicots ($K_S$ = 2.27 in average) and Lamiaceae shared WGD event ($K_S$ = 1.18 in average), were confirmed on our sampling scale. We didn't find a common WGD event among the whole *Salvia* genus, however, we identified a lineage-shared WGD ($K_S$ = 0.30 on average) in Clade II. In addition, some individual species seemed to have undergone unique WGD events, i. e., *S. splendens*, *Salvia lyrata* L., and *Salvia roemeriana* Scheele.

Chemical diversity and distribution of ATDs in *Salvia*

Understanding the relevancy between chemical diversity and genetic information is essential for the elucidation of biosynthetic pathways and the mining of functional genes. The roots and leaves of 71 *Salvia* species were prepared and analyzed using a liquid chromatography-mass spectrometry (LC - MS)-based metabolomics approach. Total ion current (TIC) chromatograms revealed that phenolic acids and ATDs were the main metabolites in both roots and leaves of *Salvia* (Supplementary Figs. 9 - 24). After peak detection, alignment and normalization using the MS-DIAL tools, the resultant feature tables were split into two tables based on the accumulation level of phenolic acids and ATDs and imported into SIMCA-P for the investigation of which classification of metabolites closely associated with the evolution of *Salvia* (Supplementary Data 2 - 7). ATDs accumulation in roots and leaves led to discernible division among the four clades using principal component analysis (PCA) when compared with phenolic acids, particularly the clustering results in the positive ion mode (Supplementary Figs. 25 and 26), which was consistent with the phylogenetic analysis results (Fig. 1).

In Fig. 2a, the 36 most prevalent ATDs were identified in both roots and leaves from the 71 *Salvia* species and were classified into five groups (A - E) based on structural characteristics. Reference standards and diagnostic neutral losses were used to identify the chemical modifications of rings and methyl groups at C-20 (Supplementary Data 8 and Figs. 27 - 31). Figure 2b depicts the accumulation patterns of the 36 ATDs in the 71 *Salvia* species, as well as the relationships between chemical modifications and organ specificity. Hydroxylation and carbonylation on the rings were the common reactions in the ATD biosynthetic pathways that occur in all four clades of *Salvia*. The accumulation of 20-keto and 20-carboxyl ATDs displayed species specificity in Clade I, II, and PR. Furthermore, strong organ specificity found in carboxylated and epoxide derivatives, such as carnosic acid and carnosol, were detected only in leaves of individual species from Clade I, II, and PR. In contrast to other ATDs with 20 carbon atoms, tanshinones (group B) had a greater ionic response in the positive ion mode and specifically accumulated in roots. Thus, although ATD chemical diversity was derived from various chemical modifications of rings and methyl groups, the accumulation pattern and organ specificity were correlated with specific methyl group modifications. Miltirone (Compound 6 in Fig. 2), the key precursor of tanshinone synthesis, was present in all clades and is formed by the unclear reactions of coupled demethylating C-20 and aromatizing ring B based on 11-hydroxyferruginol. However, more-diverse tanshinones formed by subsequent heterocyclization, demethylation, and aromatization are present only in Clade IV. Thus, C - 20 is a potentially critical position: when the rings and methyl groups at C-20 are modified by varied substitutions, it correlates with the formation of diverse ATD characteristic structures and promotes species and organ specificity in *Salvia*.

Catalytic divergence of CYP76AK subfamily  As the oxidation pattern on C - 20 might bring the divergence of ATDs across the *Salvia* lineages. Thus, CYP76AK, a Lamiaceae-specific CYP subfamily that was previously discovered to catalyze the C - 20 oxidation, might have shaped such metabolic diversity. To examine the enzyme activity across the CYP76AKs, all *CYP76AK* genes were annotated from the 71 transcriptomes we generated to study their phylogenetic relationship first. A total of 185 putative

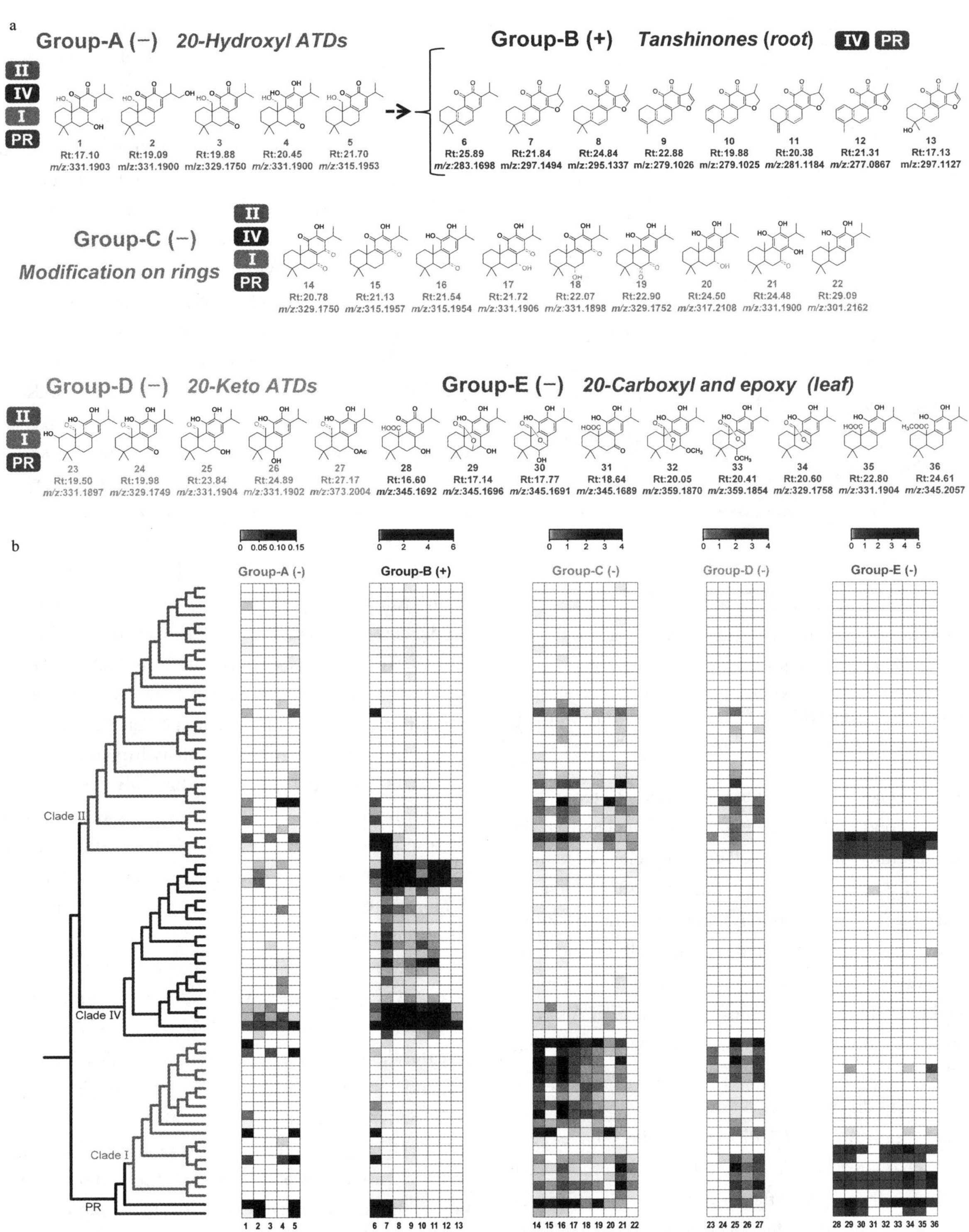

**Fig. 2 Chemical diversity and distribution of ATDs in *Salvia*. The most prevalent ATDs identified by LC-MS in both roots and leaves from *Salvia***

(a) Thirty-six ATDs were divided into five groups based on different structural characteristics. ATDs in groups A, C, D, and E (which accumulated specifically in leaves) exhibited higher intensities in the negative ion mode, and ATDs in group B (which accumulated specifically in roots) exhibited higher intensities in the positive ion mode. 1: 7, 20-Dihydroxyabietaquinone; 2: 16, 20-Dihydroxyabietaquinone; 3: 7-Keto, 20-hydroxyabietaquinone; 4: 11, 20-Dihydroxysugiol; 5: 20-Hydroxyabietaquinone; 6: Miltirone; 7: Cryptotanshinone; 8: Tanshinone IIA; 9: 1, 2-Dihydrotanshinquinone; 10: Dihydrotanshinone I; 11: Methylenetanshinquinone; 12: Tanshinone I; 13: Przewaquinone C; 14: 7-Keto-royleanone; 15: Royleanone; 16: 11-Hydroxysugiol; 17: 7-Hydroxyroyleanone; 18: 6-Hydroxyroyleanone; 19: 6-Keto-11-hydroxysugiol; 20: 7, 11-Dihydroxyferruginol; 21: 11, 14-Dihydroxysugiol; 22: 11-Hydroxyferruginol; 23: 20-Keto-2, 11-dihydroxyferruginol; 24: 20-Keto-11-hydroxysugiol; 25: 20-Keto-7-hydroxyferruginol; 26: 20-Keto-6-hydroxyferruginol; 27: 20-Keto-7-acetyferruginol; 28: 7-Hydroxy-20-carboxyabietaquinone; 29: 7-Hydroxyisocarnosol; 30: 6-Hydroxycarnosol; 31: 7-Keto-carnosic acid; 32: 7-Methoxycarnosol; 33: 6-Methoxycarnosol; 34: Carnosol; 35: Carnosic acid; 36: Methyl carnosate. (b) Distribution patterns of the 36 ATDs in 71 *Salvia* species. PR, subgenera *Perovskia* and *Rosmarinus*. Source data are provided as a Source Data file.

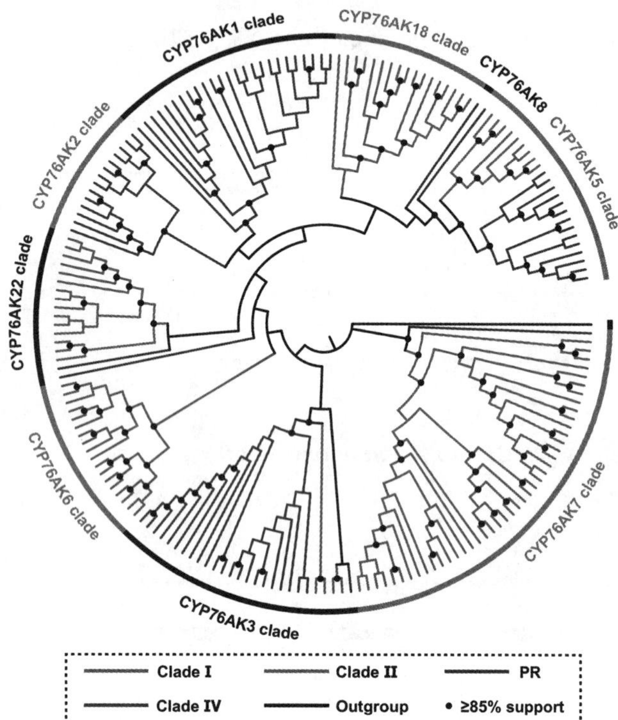


**Fig. 3 Cladogram of the CYP76AK subfamily members**

The branch color represents the lineage to which the species containing these CYP76AK genes belong. See Supplementary Fig. 32 for the annotated phylogram. PR, subgenera *Perovskia* and *Rosmarinus*. Source data are provided as a Source Data file.

full-length sequences were obtained and used to generate a maximum likelihood (ML) tree (Fig. 3), which classified the CYP76AK subfamily into nine well-resolved clades (namely CYP76AK1, 2, 3, 5, 6, 7, 8, 18, and 22; Supplementary Data 9 and Fig. 32) with broadly taxonomic distribution. CYP76AK6s were unique to Clade I, as well as the only CYP76AK clade in this lineage. CYP76AK7, 22, 18 were specific to the Clade II lineage. Meanwhile, CYP76AK1, 2, and 3 were basically specific for the Clade IV lineage. Besides, CYP76AK3, 7, 8, and 22 genes were also annotated from the transcriptomes of PR.

Till now, only a few CYP76AK members have been functionally characterized. To investigate whether each clade exhibits divergent catalytic properties, in total sixteen CYP76AKs, covering all clades, were selected for in vitro functional investigation using yeast microsome expression system. Two substrates, 11-hydroxyferruginol and 11-hydroxysugiol were tested to elucidate the oxidation patterns on C - 20. Because 11-hydroxyferruginol was not commercially available, SmCYP76AH3 was introduced into the yeast strain WAT11 to transfer ferruginol into 11-hydroxyferruginol as the source of substrate (Fig. 4a). The sequential oxidation products were analyzed using LC-MS according to their MS features (Supplementary Fig. 33). When using 11-hydroxyferruginol as substrate, two products (11, 20-dihydroxyferruginol and carnosic acid) were produced, representing the products for hydroxylation and carboxylation on C - 20. Among the CYP76AKs we tested, no products were observed for SmCYP76AK3 and 5. SmCYP76AK2, SpCYP76AK22, and ScCYP76AK18 exhibited hydroxylation activity, and only ScCYP76AK18 had subsequent carboxylation activity. Taken together with the previously functional descriptions on CYP76AK1, 6, 7, and 8, we assume that CYP76AKs exhibit three distinct catalytic properties towards 11-hydroxyferruginol, i. e., CYP76AK1, 2, and 22 can only exhibit hydroxylation of C - 20, whereas CYP76AK6, 7, 8, and 18 had the further oxidation properties to produce carnosic acid. Besides 11-hydroxyferruginol, SmCYP76AK1 was able to convert 11-hydroxysugiol into 11, 20-dihydroxysugiol. To test if other CYP76AK clades have promiscuities as well, 11-hydroxysugiol was fed into the microsomes preparations expressing each selected CYP76AK (Fig. 4b). As a result, all CYP76AKs except CYP76AK3 and 5 were capable of catalyzed C - 20 oxidation of 11-hydroxysugiol. Different from using 11-hydroxyferruginol as substrate, 20-keto products were detected in the products of CYP76AK6, 7, 8, and 18. In addition, carboxylated products (7-keto-carnosic acid was purified and identified by nuclear magnetic resonance (NMR), Supplementary Fig. 34) were obtained in turn. Consistent with the 11-hydroxyferruginol feeding groups, CYP76AK1, 2, and 22 only exhibited one-step oxidation to produce 11, 20-dihydroxysugiol. In addition, we also selected complementary CYP76AKs from each clade for confirmation of function (Supplementary Fig. 35), demonstrating that CYP76AKs from the same clade had consistent functions.

Collectively, CYP76AKs appear to perform three types of catalytic properties, while adhering distinct phylogenetic divergence (Fig. 4c): i: CYP76AK7, 6, 18, and 8 were able to catalytic successive oxidation on C - 20; ii: CYP76AK1, 2, and 22 only exhibited the hydroxylation step; iii: CYP76AK3 and 5 showed no catalytic ability to both 11-hydroxyferruginol and 11-hydroxysugiol. To further take comprehensive consideration of the catalytic properties, phylogenetic relationship of CYP76AK subfamily, and the ATDs distribution, there appears to be a strong correlation between the function divergence of CYP76AKs and species-specific accumulation of ATDs among different *Salvia* lineages. For instance, 20-keto products as 20-keto-11-hydroxysugiol were specifically generated by CYP76AK6, 7, 8, and 18. Correspondingly, such 20-keto ATDs were restricted to Clade I, II, in addition to the PR (Fig. 2), which were consistent with the distribution of CYP76AK clades, i. e., CYP76AK6 might contribute for Clade I, CYP76AK7 and 8 in Clade II of the genus.

Organ constraint transcriptional patterns of CYP76AK

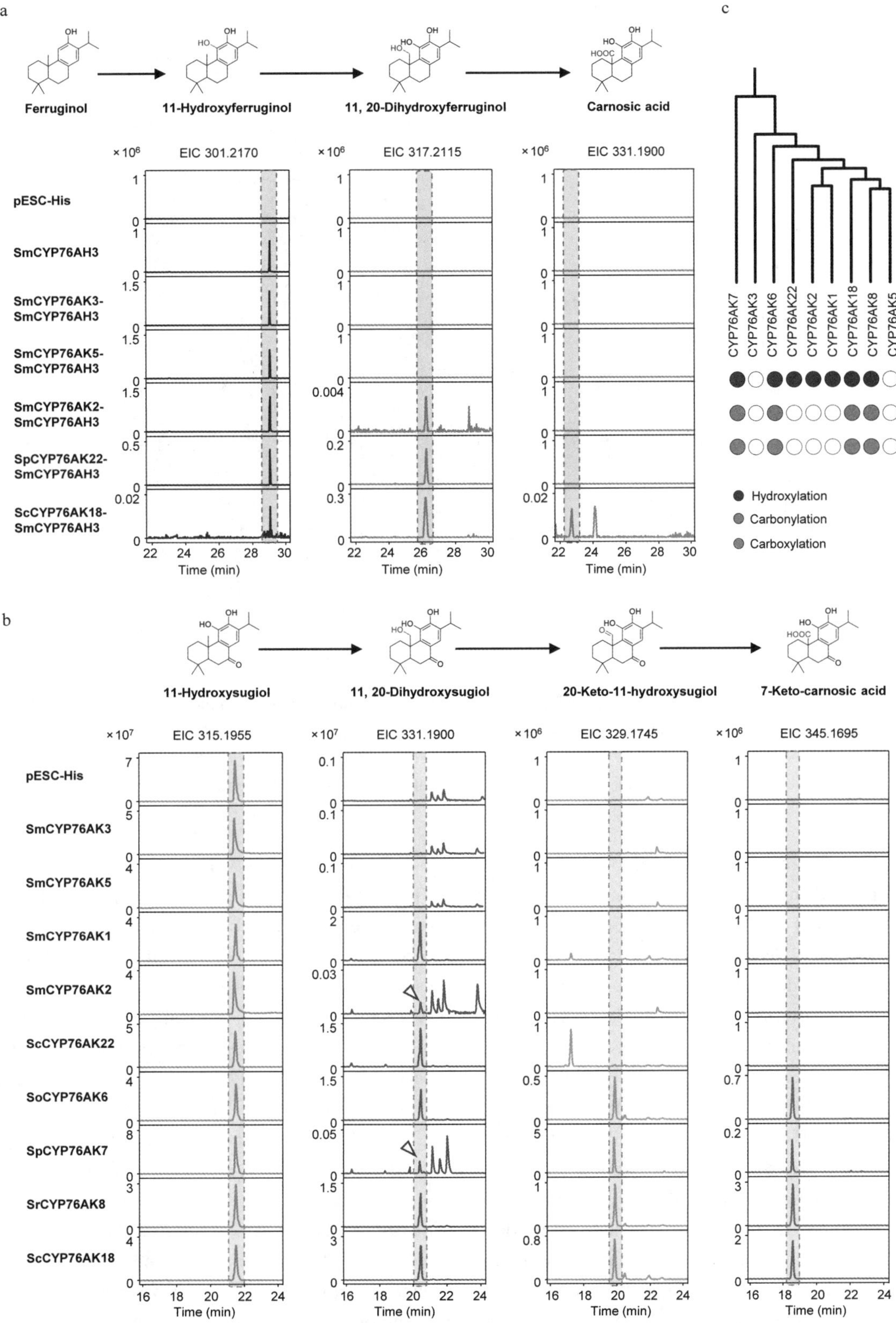


**Fig. 4 Catalytic activity of targeted CYP76AK subfamily members with two substrates**

(a) Extracted ion chromatogram (EIC) analysis of the CYP76AK catalytic reaction products in vitro with 11-hydroxyferruginol. To obtain 11-hydroxyferruginol, all plasmids contained SmCYP76AH3, which converts ferruginol to 11-hydroxyferruginol. A sample with only SmCYP76AH3 protein functioned as the negative control. Peaks corresponding to potential products are indicated by the m/z value of 11, 20-dihydroxyferruginol (*m/z* 317.211 5), and carnosic acid (*m/z* 331.190 0). (b) EIC overlays showing in vitro catalytic activity of CYP76AKs with 11-hydroxysugiol. The sample with the empty vector (pESC-His) functioned as the negative control. Peaks corresponding to potential products are indicated by the *m/z* value of 11, 20-dihydroxysugiol (*m/z* 331.190 0), 20-keto-11-hydroxysugiol (*m/z* 329.174 5), and 7-keto-carnosic acid (*m/z* 345.169 5). (c) Enzyme activity summary of CYP76AKs.

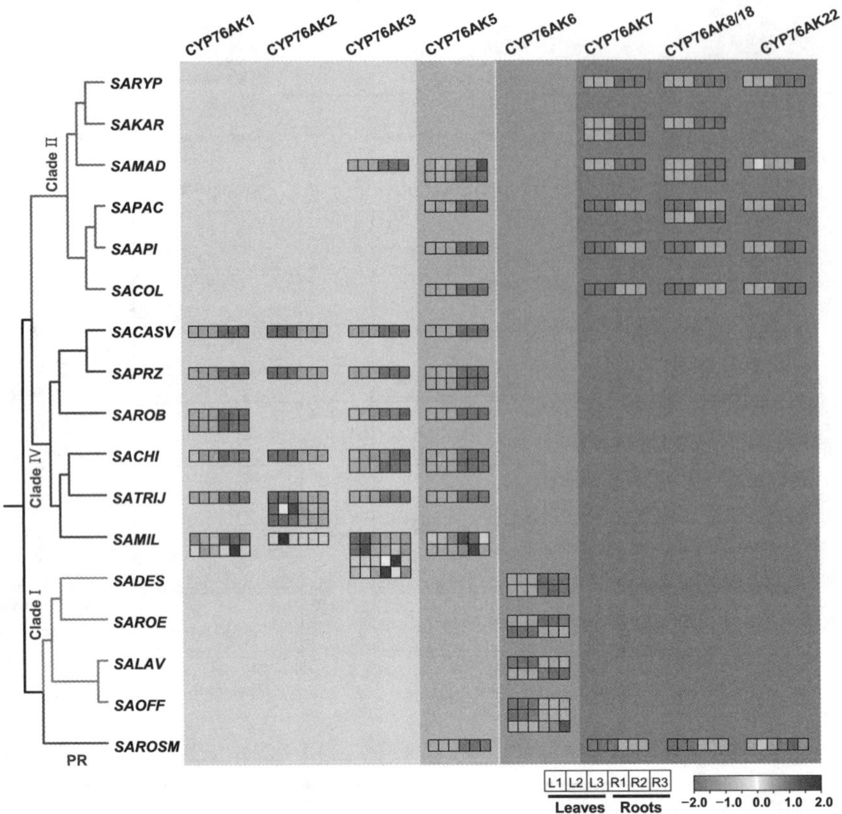


**Fig. 5 Expression profiles of the CYP76AK subfamily members in Salvia**

Gene expression heatmap for CYP76AK subfamily members from representative species of each branch of Salvia, displaying the relative expression levels in leaves (L) and roots (R). The heatmap shows three biological replicates, each plotted individually. Expression values represent Z score-transformed log (TPM + 1) values. Species abbreviations can be found in Supplementary Data 1. Source data are provided as a Source Data file.

genes provided further evidence for their contributions to ATDs diversity. Using RNA sequencing, we tested transcription patterns of CYP76AK genes in leaves and roots from seventeen selected *Salvia* species (Fig. 5), revealing their distribution according to lineages and diverse organ-specific expression patterns. Generally, *CYP76AK* genes belonging to the same clade had identical transcription pattern, and presented identical organ distribution to corresponding metabolites in the lineage. For instance, in Clade IV and Clade II, respectively, CYP76AK1 and 22 exclusively catalyzed the C－20 hydroxylation with root-specific expression, demonstrating their distinct role in the production of tanshinones. In contrast, 20-carboxyl products such as carnosic acid were specifically accumulated in the leaves in the basal lineages of Clade I and Clade II, respectively, which were most likely due to the organ-specific expression of CYP76AK6, 7, 8, and 18 in leaves of corresponding *Salvia* species. It should be noted that although CYP76AK3 and 5 did not demonstrate activity towards the tested substrates in our study, substantial transcription levels were found in the roots of the relevant *Salvia* species, indicating their unrevealed catalytic functions towards other unidentified substrates.

Evolution of the ATDs biosynthetic pathway in *Salvia*

The above phylogenetic, metabolic, and catalytic functional studies revealed that this distinct metabolic divergence was accompanied by the evolution of the CYP76AK subfamily in each *Salvia* lineage. To trace the evolutionary route of the ATDs pathway in *Salvia*, comparative genome analysis and reconstruction of ancestral genes and metabolic traits were performed. Currently, there are six *Salvia* genomes available, enable us to investigate the evolutionary history of *CYP76AK* genes in the majority of *Salvia* lineages. These are *S. rosmarinus* (PR), *S. officinalis* (Clade I), *S. miltiorrhiza* and *Salvia bowleyana* Dunn (Clade IV), *S. hispanica* (North American lineage of Clade II), and *S. splendens* (South American lineage of Clade II). First, microsynteny blocks were investigated to determine the evolutionary history of CYP76AKs (Fig. 6a). Conserved syntenic regions containing CYP76AKs were observed in all studied genomes and were not located in the known gene cluster related to diterpenoid biosynthesis. Two duplicated regions were present in the *N. cataria* genome, allowing the tracing of the ancestor of CYP76AK genes before the speciation of *Salvia*. Meanwhile, duplication of the region was discovered that showed an obvious correlation with the

WGD event of each genome. For *N. cataria* and *S. rosmarinus*, the duplication was probably produced by their unique WGD events. In the *S. hispanica* genome, the duplication was related to the Clade II-common WGD. Subsequently, *S. splendens* experienced another unique WGD event, which eventually resulted in a genome with four duplicated regions. Thus, the discovery of the syntenic regions and their duplication events suggested that this region contained ancestral CYP76AKs in the genome of the *Salvia* ancestor. Along with genome evolution, CYP76AK originated and evolved into divergent clades in different *Salvia* lineages. In the phylogeny of both CYP76AKs (Fig. 3) and *Salvia*, CYP76AK7 and 22 might have emerged first in the ancestor of the *Salvia* lineages as shown in the *S. rosmarinus* genome, and subsequent duplication events then led to CYP76AK8 (*S. rosmarinus*) and CYP76AK18 (Clade II). In taxa that have not undergone WGD events, CYP76AK is separated into CYP76AK1 (Clade IV) and CYP76AK6 (Clade I). In addition, no collinearity relationship for CYP76AK2, 3, and 5 were discovered among all *Salvia* genomes (Supplementary Data 10). Their emergence might have been caused by unique duplication events in certain species or lineages (e. g., segmental and transposon-mediated duplication).

In consideration of the functional differences among CYP76AKs within the context of their evolutionary histories, the divergence of catalytic activity at C-20 seemed to represent a taxonomic loss of function rather than a neofunctionalization. Thus, ancestral gene reconstruction and function validation were performed. Based on the phylogeny of CYP76AKs, six branch nodes were selected for ancestral enzyme resurrection (Fig. 6b, Supplementary Data 11). The ancestral enzyme corresponding to each of these nodes was expressed in yeast and functionally confirmed using 11-hydroxyferruginol and 11-hydroxysugiol as the substrates. Consistent with expectations, all CYP76AK ancestors exhibited hydroxylation, carbonylation, and carboxylation at C-20 of both 11-hydroxyferruginol and 11-hydroxysugiol, as each oxidation product was produced by each CYP76AK ancestor (Fig. 6c, d). Node 6 represented the most ancestral CYP76AK protein, which exhibited a complete oxidation function, indicating that such catalytic trait of CYP76AKs had already been acquired when the CYP76AK subfamily initially emerged in *Salvia*. Node 3 (ancestor of CYP76AK1, 2, 5, 8, 18, and 22) and Node 2 (ancestor of CYP76AK1, 2, 5, 8, and 18) also exhibited complete oxidation capacities toward C-20, implying that CYP76AK1, 2, and 22 (only performing hydroxylation) lose the carboxylation activity. CYP76AK3 and 5 showed no catalytic activity with any of the substrates assessed (Fig. 4), suggesting that CYPs in the two clades experienced complete loss of activity towards the tested substrates. They might undergo pseudogenization or have catalytic activities towards other unknown substrates.

Considering the evolutionary history of CYP76AKs in *Salvia*, the metabolic diversity of ATDs appears to represent a pathway loss rather than metabolic innovation. Thus, ancestral phenotype reconstruction (APR) was performed according to the realistic chemical traits in each taxon to predict the chemical traits of their common ancestors (Supplementary Fig. 36). The abilities to produce carnosic acid, tanshinone, or 20-keto ATDs were considered as key traits. APRs for the early speciation nodes of the *Salvia* phylogeny (PR and Clade I, II, and IV) were indicated to produce all types of ATDs, implying that the ancestor of *Salvia* most likely produced all ATDs. With the speciation of *Salvia*, this chemical trait was retained in PR (*S. rosmarinus*) and the North American taxa in the Clade II lineage, but it was partially lost in other lineages. Loss of activity at the clade level was observed in the evolutionary history of CYP76AKs, thus suggesting a major cause for the metabolic diversity among lineages. To model how the evolution of activity of CYP76AKs directed ATDs diversity, the chronology of all CYP76AKs was further assessed (Supplementary Fig. 37). The CYP76AK clades that originated from the ancestral syntenic segments were presented (Fig. 6e, f). The chronology revealed that the MRCA of CYP76AK (~76.4 Mya) was present at a time much earlier than the first divergence between CYP76AK7 and the other clades (~45.1 Mya). Each clade emerged at the time of, or just after, the speciation of its corresponding lineages. For example, CYP76AK6 might have emerged along with the speciation of Clade I (~20.4 Mya). Moreover, the loss of activity of CYP76AK22 (~26.3 Mya) and CYP76AK1 (~7.9 Mya) occurred after the speciation of *S. rosmarinus* (~27.2 Mya) and Clade IV (~9.1 Mya), respectively.

Based on the catalytic traits, lineage distribution, and transcriptional pattern of each CYP76AK clade, the gene contributing to ATDs biosynthesis in a particular lineage can be determined. CYP76AK7 was found in *S. rosmarinus* and Clade II, thus contributing to carnosic acid biosynthesis in the aerial parts of the corresponding lineage. However, CYP76AK7 might also be responsible for the accumulation of 20-keto ATDs in roots of species in the South American taxa of Clade II. CYP76AK6 was present only in Clade I; thus, it might enable the biosynthesis of carnosic acid-related metabolites and 20-keto ATDs in specific organs. CYP76AK22 was retained in *S. rosmarinus* and Clade II and is expressed only in roots where it is responsible for tanshinone accumulation. Meanwhile, CYP76AK1 contributed to tanshinone biosynthesis only in Clade IV. In addition, CYP76AK8/18 shared a similar distribution to CYP76AK22 and might

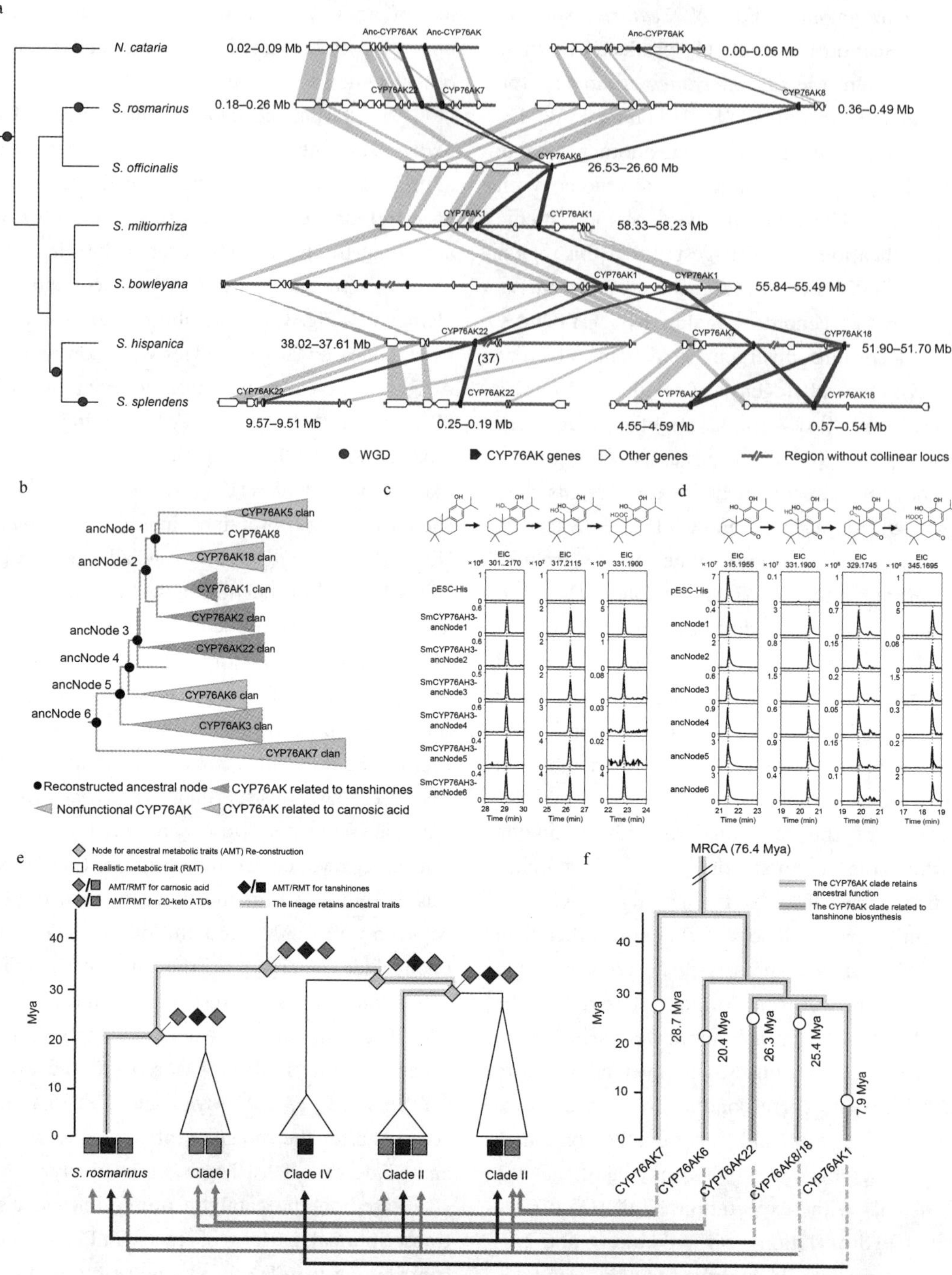


**Fig. 6 Evolution of the CYP76AK subfamily**

(a) Syntenic relationships among *CYP76AK* genes in *Salvia* genomes revealed the divergence of CYP76AK clades. The phylogenetic tree in the left panel represents the phylogeny of six *Salvia* species with *N. cataria* as the outgroup. WGD events are indicated by red dots. Micro-synteny of *CYP76AK* genes in the synteny blocks. Red polygons show syntenic relationships between *CYP76AK* genes, and gray polygons show other genes. Anc-CYP76AK, Ancestral *CYP76AK* gene. (b) Reconstruction of ancestral CYP76AK proteins. Ancestral nodes (ancNodes) 1 - 6 show the resurrected enzyme of each major branch point of the CYP76AK phylogenetic tree. Functional characters of each branch are distinguished by different colors. (c, d) Ancestral function of CYP76AKs. Extracted ion chromatograms (EICs) showing in vitro catalytic activity of each ancestral CYP76AK using 11-hydroxyferruginol and 11-hydroxysugiol as the substrate, respectively. (e) Evolution of ATDs biosynthesis in *Salvia*. The phylogenetic tree shows the speciation of the clades of *Salvia*, and the diamonds represent the predicted ancestral metabolic traits for each speciation node. Square frames represent the realistic metabolic traits of each *Salvia* clade as shown in Fig. 3. Green, red, and light blue represent the existence of carnosic acid, tanshinones, and 20-keto ATDs, respectively. The time scale on the left reffects the time of speciation for each clade. Branches highlighted in light blue indicate clades in which the ancestral metabolic traits have been retained. (f) Chronology of *CYP76AK* genes. The phylogenetic tree represents the evolution of CYP76AK clades according to the MCMCtree model. The speciation time for each clade is labeled. Branches high-lighted in blue indicate CYP76AK clades that have retained their ancestral catalytic functions, and branches highlighted in red indicate clades that have undergone a loss of function. The arrows at the bottom indicate the CYP76AK clade that contributes to producing the type of ATDs in the corresponding lineage. Green, red, and indigo gray arrows indicate the biosynthesis of carnosic acid, tanshinones, and 20-keto ATDs, respectively. Source data are provided as a Source Data file.

perform hydroxylation and carbonylation in roots for the biosynthesis of 20-keto ATDs. Overall, previous studies on the metabolic evolution of ATDs and our findings concerning the functional divergence of the CYP76AK subfamily support a model of metabolic diversity in *Salvia* lineages based on loss of activity.

## 2 DISCUSSION

In this study, we combined lineage-wide phylogeny, metabolic profiling, genomic comparison, and enzyme function evolution analyses to illustrate how ATDs divergence in the genus *Salvia*. Our metabolic profiling for ATDs provides the model for ATDs pathway evolution and serves as an example of chemical diversity in plants due to the loss of activities of catalytic enzymes.

Previous phylogenetic reconstructions of *Salvia* were mainly based on ribosomal, mitochondrial, and chloroplast genes, with a few protein-coding nuclear genes having been used in the phylogeny of *Salvia* at the family level. Uniparental heritability of organellar genes, as well as gene recombination and transformation in the plastid genome, has resulted in phylogenetic reconstruction biases and inaccuracies. In contrast, nuclear genes have many advantages, such as their large numbers and parental inheritance. The use of the thoroughly evaluated nuclear gene sets can provide evidence for robust and well-supported deep angiosperm lineages. Here, we presented phylogenetic analysis of *Salvia* based on large-scale nuclear genes, obtained from transcriptome sequencing with the largest sampling scale for *Salvia* lineage to date, to infer infrageneric relationships within the genus. Consistent with previous studies, *S. abrotanoides* and *S. rosmarinus* formed a clade with *Salvia* species, whereas *M. officinalis* acted as a sister clade.

Morphologically, the traditionally defined genus *Salvia* is distinct from other genera of Lamiaceae in that two of its fertile stamens are separated by a significantly elongated connective tissue. However, molecular phylogenetic studies expanded *Salvia* to include other genera (i.e., *Dorystaechas*, *Meriandra*, *Perovskia*, *Rosmarinus*, and *Zhumeria*). Here, although representatives of "*Rosmarinus*" and "*Perovskia*" formed a sister group to Clade I (Fig. 1), the metabolic traits for ATDs and catalytic properties of CYP76AKs in two subgenera are distinctly different from that of Clade I. Thus, the above findings could provide new insights from more aspects into the taxonomic attribu-tion of *Dorystaechas*, *Meriandra*, and *Zhumeria*.

CYPs oxidize the hydrocarbon skeleton generated by terpenoid synthase during plant terpenoid biosynthesis, while chemical modifications include hydroxylation, continuous oxidation, ring rearrangement, and heterocyclization also occur. These reactions greatly increase the structural diversity of terpenoids, while providing anchor points for future moiety modifications. Therefore, CYPs are considered the key factors for the diversity of plant terpenoids. According to our metabolome analyses, ATDs with modified rings (group C) showed no specific accumulation in all clades and were produced by functional genes such as CYP76AH subfamily, which is able to carry out carbonylation at C-7 of ring B. In contrast to the modifications carried out by the CYP76AH, the chemical modifications at C-20 are driven by the diverse CYP76AK family, which is responsible for the accumulation and organ specificity of ATDs in *Salvia*. According to Figs. 2 and 5, the *CYP76AK1* gene was highly expressed in roots of taxa in Clade IV and produces 20-hydroxyl ATDs (group A), the accumulation patterns of which were similar to those of miltirone, especially for the 7, 20-dihydroxyabietaquinone (compound 1), 7-keto-20-hydroxyabietaquinone (compound 3), and 20-hydroxyabietaquinone (compound 5), which is speculated that the 20-hydroxyl ATDs are the primary precursors for miltirone synthesis. Being similar to CYP76AK1, CYP76AK22 was also found to produce hydroxylated derivatives at C-20 for miltirone synthesis in individual species from Clade II and PR, and had high transcriptional level in roots as well (Fig. 5). Contrary to Clade I, species fall into Clade II as *S. pachyphylla*, *S. apiana*, and *S. columbariae* produce cryptotanshinone. The production of cryptotanshinone (Compound 7; Fig. 2) by the CYP71D family acting on miltirone for the heterocyclization of ring D showed that Clade II species had a more comprehensive tanshinone biosynthetic pathway than species in Clade I (Fig. 2). However, most downstream tanshinones were more abundant in Clade IV, indicating that ATDs biosynthesis in Clade IV consisted predominantly of tanshinone synthesis (group B). This was also the possible reason why the common ATDs with 20 carbon atoms (group C) in Clade I and II accumulated to higher levels (Fig. 2). In addition, the subsequent aromatization of ring A requires functioning genes for hydroxylation at C-18 or -19, which were exclusively expressed in Clade IV. Besides, a side product of SmCYP76AK1 and ScCYP76AK22 was detected when 11-hydroxysugiol was used as the substrate (time = 17.25 min; Fig. 4b), which was tentatively identified as 6-hydroxy-7-ketoabietaquinone (Supplementary Fig. 38). This side function might contribute to the ATDs with hydroxyl group at C-6 in Clade II (Compound 18) and IV (Compound 18, 26, and 30). Correspondingly, the enzymes response for C-6 oxidation in Clade I and PR still need to be explored.

Apart from the significance of CYP76AK1 and CYP76AK22 for the synthesis of 20-hydroxyl ATDs and tanshinones, the unique accumu-lation of 20-keto ATDs (group D) in Clade I, II, and PR was based on the specific expression of CYP76AK6, 7, and 8/18. Whereas CYP76AK6 was uniquely expressed in

Clade I, CYP76AK7 and 8/18 were expressed in Clade II and PR, and performed similar activities of hydroxylation, carbonylation, and carboxylation at C-20 in the in vitro enzyme activity assays (Fig. 4). In the enzyme activity assays, the 20-carboxyl derivatives, such as carnosic acid (Compound 35), were also found to spontaneously oxidize 20-epoxy ATDs such as carnosol (Compound 34) (Supplementary Fig. 39). However, species with higher expression of CYP76AK6, 7, or 8/18 in leaves, such as *S. officinalis* in Clade I, *S. columbariae* in Clade II, and *S. rosmarinus* in PR, were the few species with both 20-carboxyl and 20-epoxy ATDs (group E) in leaves (Figs. 2 and 5). Such species-specific accumulation of carnosic acid-related metabolites may be related to the ability to withstand the harsh climatic conditions in the Mediterranean habitat. Leaves from these species showed higher expression of CYP76AKs than roots, which might be related to the specific localization of 20-carboxyl and 20-epoxy ATDs in the chloroplasts of photosynthetic green organs. Carnosic acid was previously speculated to be a potential intermediate for demethylation (C-20), leading to the formation of a heterocyclic bridge between C-20 and C-7. This, in turn, suggested that the carboxylic acid group on the C-20 may be responsible for aromatization of ring B, ultimately resulting in the production of miltirone. However, the accumulation of carnosic acid was strict to certain organs and species, this indicates that it cannot serve as a precursor for tanshinones. Instead, hydroxylation (C-20) catalyzed by CYP76AK1 and 22 demonstrates a stronger correlation with subsequent demethylation and aromatization due to its co-existence and similar accumulation pattern with tanshinones in Clade IV. This represents a significant step in the mechanistic investigation of the formation process of tan-shinones, specifically in understanding the mechanisms of demethylation and aromatization. Thus, the variable expression of distinct CYP76AKs between evolutionary clades might direct the evolution of ATD biosynthesis pathway, resulting in the specific production of ATDs in *Salvia*, such as tanshinones and carnosic acid-related metabolites.

In addition, based solely on the in vitro activity evidence of CYP76AK, we cannot rule out the possibility of other enzymes participating in the consecutive oxidation of ATDs. Similar to the artemisinin biosynthetic pathway, although in vitro evidence shows that CYP71AV1 can catalyze the consecutive oxidation of amorpha-4, -11-diene on C-12 to form artemisinic aldehyde and artemisinic acid, other enzymes such as alcohol dehydrogenase (ADH1) and artemisinic aldehyde dehydrogenase (ALDH1) are also involved in the last two oxidation steps in glandular trichome cells of *Artemisia annua*. This also suggests the possibility of the involvement of other enzymes, in addition to CYP76AK, in the C-20 oxidation of ATDs in *Salvia*, which requires further in vivo functional studies of CYP76AKs and the discovery of new enzymes.

It is the activity loss of CYP76AKs rather than neofunctionalization that has driven the diversity of ATDs in the genus *Salvia*. The differentiation and expansion of CYP76AKs caused by WGD events have not resulted in neofunctionalizations as in previous cases but rather in a loss of activities in corresponding taxa (Fig. 6). It is interesting to note that the loss of activity has also triggered changes in structural characteristics and distribution patterns that result in metabolic diversity, such as the production of tanshinones and carnosic acid derivatives. Contrary to most cases, which have assumed that functional innovation is what leads to metabolic diversity, the results from this study suggest that the loss of activities may also act as the key factor for metabolic diversity.

On the other hand, with respect to the functional divergence, CYP76AKs also exhibit distinct transcriptional patterns, which even-tually lead to the completely opposite organ-specific accumulation of carnosic acid derivatives and tanshinones. On the basis of this, we speculate that the physiological and ecological functions of these metabolites may be connected to the metabolic divergence present in this genus. For instance, carnosic acid and carnosol are mainly accumulated in the chloroplasts of green tissues, thereby providing a unique and effective antioxidant mechanism in the photosynthetic tissues of these plants. The carnosic acid-based protection mechanism is proved to be crucial for enabling *Salvia* species to withstand harsh climatic conditions, whereas tanshinones may be involved in the interaction between roots and the microorganisms in the surrounding soil.

Furthermore, the distinct transcription patterns of each CYP76AK clade represented another aspect of function evolution. Their organ-specific patterns are not independent, but are accompanied by other catalytic genes involved in carnosic acid derivatives and tanshinones biosynthesis as *KSL*s, *CYP76AH*s, and *CYP71D*s. In the meantime, such patterns are maintained in different *Salvia* lineages, thus, raising the question about the origin of their organ-specific transcriptions as a further research topic. To summarize, ATD differentiation in *Salvia* provides a complete model involving multiple species, gene families, metabolic diversity, and ecological evolution, making it an ideal research object for the genetic mechanisms responsible for chemical diversity in plants.

## 3 METHODS

Plant materials  Most recent molecular phylogenetic studies support the presence of 11 subclades in the genus *Salvia* (subg. *Audibertia*, subg. *Calosphace*, subg. *Dorystaechas*, subg. *Glutinaria*, subg. *Heterosphace*, subg. *Meriandra*, subg. *Perovskia*, subg. *Rosmarinus*, subg. *Salvia*, subg. *Sclarea*, and subg. *Zhumeria*). A phylogenetic tree of *Salvia* was constructed to obtain a sampling scheme to analyze chemical diversity among these species (Supplementary Data 1). In total, 71 species from three major distribution centers for this genus representing 8 out of the 11 recognized subclades of *Salvia* were sampled. Six species (*M. officinalis*, *M. spicata*, *C. polycephalum*, *O. vulgare*, *N. cataria*, and *P. vulgaris*) from other Mentheae tribes were selected as outgroups. To obtain sufficient materials for both transcriptome and chemical analyses, samples were collected at the vegetative or flowering stages. Three organs (roots, stems, and leaves) were collected at the vegetative stage and four organs (roots, stems, leaves, and flowers) at the flowering stage. To permit sampling of the same tissue type for transcriptome and chemical analyses, tissues from each organ were ground into a fine powder and divided into aliquots.

RNA isolation, transcriptome sequencing, assembly, annotation, and analysis In order to obtain more comprehensive transcripts, a mixed organ strategy for library construction was performed, by which the transcript database generated was used for phylogenetic studies. For transcription profiling, libraries for individual leaves and roots from representative plants in each clade were generated (i.e., *S. rypara*, *S. karwinskii*, *S. madrensis*, *S. pachyphylla*, *S. apiana* and *S. columbariae* from Clade II; *S. castanea f. tomentosa*, *S. przewalskii*, *S. roborowskii*, *S. chinensis*, *S. trijuga*, *S. miltiorrhiza* from Clade IV; *S. deserta*, *S. roemeriana*, *S. officinalis* subsp. *lavandulifolia*, *S. officinalis* from Clade I; *S. rosmarinus* from PR). Total RNA was isolated using the TransZol Plus RNA Kit (TransGen Biotech, Beijing, China). The cDNA libraries were prepared using the Illumina TruSeq RNA Sample Preparation Kit (Illumina, San Diego, CA, USA) and were sequenced on an Illumina NovaSeq 6 000 sequencer, generating 2 × 150-bp paired-end reads. Reads were assessed and trimmed by fastp (https://github.com/OpenGene/fastp) with default parameters. The transcript assemblies were generated using Trinity assembler. For the transcriptome annotation, all transcripts were searched against the *Arabidopsis thaliana* proteome, SwissProt, and Pfam databases using BLASTX, BLASTP, and HMMER v3.1b2 with an e-value cutoff of 1E-5, respectively. The gene expression values (transcripts per million reads [TPM]) were calculated by RSEM software. Essentially, differential expression analysis was performed using DESeq2 with $p$ adjust $<0.05$ and $|\log2FC| \geqslant 1$ as the threshold. The gene heatmaps were generated using TBtools (https://github.com/CJ-Chen/TBtools) with the Heatmap Illustrator function.

Orthologous identification, single/low-copy gene selection, and phylogeny construction All assembled transcripts were filtered to retain the longest transcript isoforms, and the protein sequences were further predicted using TransDecoder v5.5.0. Orthologous groups were constructed with OrthoFinder v2.5.4 using TransDecoder-predicted protein sequences from all 77 species. Considering that fragmented assembly, incorrect assembly, insufficient informative sites, and other factors might result in biased inferences, the five gene sets including four low-copy gene sets, i.e., 2,178 OGs, 1,532 OGs, 1,169 OGs, and 512 OGs, and one single-copy gene set, i.e., 130 OGs, were extracted for the construction of phylogenetic tree. The resulting protein sequences from single/low-copy gene sets were aligned with MAFFT v7.487 using the default settings, and poorly aligned regions were trimmed by TrimAl v1.4. rev15. The phylogenetic tree of each orthologous from individual OGs was constructed using RAxML-NG v1.0.3 with 100 replicates under the JTT + I + G4 model. Then, Astral v5.6 was used to concatenate the phylogeny trees for each of the five OG sets with 100 replicates from RAxML to obtain the BS values of all nodes. In addition, 130 OGs were concatenated into a supermatrix, and the final phylogenetic relationship was reconstructed using RAxML-NG v1.0.3 with 1 000 replicates under the JTT + I + G4 model. Among all 77 species, *M. officinalis*, *M. spicata*, *C. polycephalum*, *O. vulgare*, *N. cataria*, and *P. vulgaris* were chosen as the outgroups.

Divergence time estimation MCMCTree in the PAML package v4.9 was employed for Bayesian inference of divergent time estimation of candidate species. The topology of candidate species from ML reconstruction with the concatenated 130 OGs was used as the input tree. The resulting nucleotide sequences with codon substitution models were aligned and trimmed with MAFFT v7.487 and the "backtrans" parameter of TrimAl v1.4. rev15. Firstly, the branch lengths and overall substitution rate (rgene gamma) were measured using the BASEML program in the PAML package v4.9 under the GTR + G model. Secondly, the divergent time was estimated using MCMCtree, and the parameters of burn-in, sampfreq, and nSample were set to 500,000, 150, and 10,000, respectively. The divergence time of candidate *Salvia* species was estimated based on the following fossil age constraints: 11 - 27 Mya for the divergent of *C. polycephalum* and *M. spicata*, and 21 - 47 Mya for the divergent between *M. officinalis* and the other outgroups, i.e., *N. cataria*, *C. polycephalum*, *M. spicata*, *O. vulgare*, and *P. vulgaris*. Lastly, multiple iterations of MCMCTree estimation made the deviation of divergent time $<0.1\%$.

WGD events identification $K_S$-based age distributions for paralogs of all candidate species were constructed using the "wgd" pipeline. Briefly, the paralogs for each species were identified using the Diamond v0.9.18.119 sequence similarity search tool with an E-value cutoff of 1E-10. The paralogous gene families were clustered using the Markov cluster algorithm. The genes within each paralogous gene family were aligned using MAFFT v7.487 with the default parameters, respectively. The $K_S$ values of all paralogous gene pairs within one gene family were measured using the CodeML program in the PAML package v4.9. $K_S$ values were subsequently node-weighted to correct for the redundancy with the phylogenetic tree construction for each family using FastTree v2.1.7. The $K_S$ aging distribution of paralogs of all tested species is shown in the gray bars of Supplementary Fig. 7.

Given the different substitution rates of all tested species, the species-shared or specific WGD events were further adjusted using a $K_S$-based tree. Here, 130 single-copy genes from OrthoFinder v2.5.4 for all tested species were used to calculate the branch lengths of phylogeny in the $K_S$ unit using the CodeML program in the PAML package v4.9 with a free-ratio model.

CYP76AK sequences, phylogenetic analyses, and molecular dating analysis The genes with the Pfam domain of PF00067 were identified as CYP450 family members. Seven known CYP76AK genes (*SmCYP76AK1*: KR140169.1, *S. miltiorrhiza*; *SmCYP76AK2*: KP337688.1, *S. miltiorrhiza*; *SmCYP76AK3*: KP337689.1, *S. miltiorrhiza*; *SfCYP76AK6*: KX431218.1, *S. fruticosa*; *SpCYP76AK6*: KT157045.1, *S. pomifera*; *SrCYP76AK7*: KX431219.1, *S. rosmarinus*; and *SrCYP76AK8*: KX431220.1, *S. rosmarinus*) were downloaded from the NCBI database as a local CYP76AK data-base. BLASTP searches were performed to identify the corresponding *CYP76AK* genes with an E-value cutoff of 1E－5. The protein sequences of the selected *CYP450* genes that encoded proteins of ≥466 amino acids were aligned and trimmed using MAFFT v7.487 and TrimAl v1.4.rev15, respectively. The phylogeny of *CYP76AK* genes was inferred using *CYP76AH1* gene as outgroup via ModelTest-NG v0.1.7 and RAxML-NG v1.0.376. For *CYP450* genes that encoded proteins of <466 amino acids, BLASTP searches were used to classify the candidate genes.

According to the phylogenetic tree above, the molecular dating of CYP76AKs from different species was analyzed using MCMCTREE of the PAML package v4.9 under the GTR + G model (model = 7) with 500 000 iterations and 150 sample frequencies, following 500 000 iterations as burn-in. The substitution rate, i.e., rgene gamma was calculated as G (1, 5.95) using BASEML of the PAML package v4.9. The crown node of two single-copy gene families (i.e., CYP76AK3 and 22) and two species-specific gene families (i.e., CYP76AK1 and 6) were used to estimate the divergent time of each node. We used the following age constraints for each estimation procedure: a minimum and maximum age of 23.7 and 35.2 Mya for the crown node of CYP76AK3 (the divergence time of *S. abrotanoides* and other species); a minimum and maximum age of 21.8 and 32.9 Mya for the crown node of CYP76AK22 (the divergence time of *S. rosmarinus* and others); a minimum and maximum age of 14.3 and 22.5 Mya for the crown node of CYP76AK6 (the divergence time of Clade I and others); a minimum and maximum age of 6.7 and 11.8 Mya for the crown node of CYP76AK1 (the diver-gence time of Clade IV and others).

Collinearity analysis of CYP76AK members Synteny blocks between each pair of candidate species (*N. cataria*, *S. rosmarinus*, *S. miltiorrhiza*, *S. bowleyana*, *S. hispanica*, and *S. splendens*) were performed using MCScan (Python version). The targeted CYP76AKs or neighboring genes were chosen as seeds to search for synteny blocks of conserved evolution.

Reconstructions of ancestral sequences and traits Using the matched sequence file, phylogenetic tree file, and config-ured control file, the JTT + GAMMA model of the CodeML program in the PAML package v4.9 was used to estimate the hypothetical ancestor sequence of CYP76AK subfamily members. The regions with alignment gaps were analyzed by the parsimony method to determine the ancestral residue base. The estimated ancestral genes were then synthesized and codon-optimized for functional identification in *S. cerevisiae*.

Based on the metabolic results and literature research, the species composition types of *Salvia* were coded. The component types are coded into 6 states: none (A); TAs (B); 20-keto ATDs (C); TAs and 20-keto ATDs (D); CAs and 20-keto ATDs (E); TAs, CAs, and 20-keto ATDs (F). Taking the evolutionary tree (ML) with branch length infor-mation as the input tree, Statistical Dispersal-Vicariance Analysis (SDIVA) from Reconstruct Ancestral State in Phylogenies (RASP) software was used to infer ancestral states of component types and calculate phylogenetic signals.

Chemical standards Chemical standards were purchased from Shanghai Standard Technology Co., Ltd. (Shanghai, China). The other chemicals and reagents were purchased as follows: acetonitrile and methanol (HPLC grade; Merck, Darmstadt, Germany), warfarin (Sigma-Aldrich, Madrid, Spain), chloroform (Sinopharm Chemical Reagent, Shanghai, China), leucine encephalin (Waters, Milford, MA, USA), pure distilled water (Watsons Water, Hong Kong, China), and formic acid (HPLC grade; Fisher Sci-entific, Fairlawn, NJ, USA).

Extraction and analysis of ATDs by UPLC－QTOF－MS Each plant was separated into root and leaf samples, with three biological replicates. All samples were ground into a fine powder, and 10 mg prepared powder was extracted with 1 mL of 70% methanol (v/v) containing warfarin (5 μg/mL) as the internal reference for 1 h in an ultrasonic bath (53 kHz, 350 W) at 4 ℃. After centrifuging at 12,000 × *g* at 4 ℃ for 30 min, the supernatant was used for UHPLC-QTOF-MS analysis.

An Acquity UPLC system (Waters, Milford, MA, USA) coupled with a Xevo G2-XS QTOF mass spectrometer (Waters, Milford, MA, USA) was used for the metabolic analysis. The samples were first separated using an Acquity UPLC T3 column (2.1 mm × 100 mm, 1.8 μm). The column temperature was kept constant at 40 ℃, and the flow rate was 0.40 mL/min with an injection volume of 1.0 μL. The mobile phases for gradient elution consisted of 0.1% (v/v) formic acid/water (solvent A) and 0.1% (v/v) formic acid/acetonitrile (solvent B). The elution gradients were 98 - 80% A over 0 - 7 min, 80 - 78% A over 7 - 11 min, 78 - 40% A over 11 - 20 min, 40 - 35% A over 20 - 25 min, 25 - 28 min at 35% A, 35 - 5% A over 28 - 30 min, 30 - 33 min at 5% A, and final re-equilibration at 98% A for 5 min.

A Xevo G2 - XS with an electrospray ionization source was used to collect MS data. MS was performed in both positive ion and negative ion modes under 30 V cone voltage, with a capillary voltage of 3.0 kV (positive ion mode) or 2.5 kV (negative ion mode). The desolvation temperature was set at 450 ℃ with a desolvation gas flow rate of 600 L/h, and the source temperature was set at 150 ℃ with a cone gas flow rate of 50 L/h. All data were collected in the $MS^E$ mode, with the following parameters: $MS^E$ range, 50-1 200 *m*/*z*; $MS^E$ low energy, 6 eV; and $MS^E$ high energy, 15 - 30 eV. To calibrate the instrument, a sodium formate solution (0.5 mM) was used. Continuous acquisition of leucine enkephalin was used as an external standard for mass correction. All data were viewed in MassLynx v4.2 (Waters, Milford, MA, USA).

Processing of metabolomics data The raw data were first converted to the analysis base file (ABF Converter; https://www.reifycs.com/AbfConverter/) format before being imported into the MS-DIAL v4.60 software. The parameter settings were as follows: the tolerances for MS1 and MS2 were 0.01 Da and 0.02 Da, respectively. The mass range of MS1 and MS/MS was set between 100 and 1 000, with the MS/MS amplitude cutoff at 800. The retention time range was set between 1.0 and 29.5 min, with a retention time tolerance of 0.15 min. The width of the mass slice was 0.1 Da. Adduct types such as $[M-H]^-$, $[M+HCOO]^-$, $[M+Na-2H]^-$, $[M+K-2H]^-$, $[2M-H]^-$, and $[2M+FA-H]^-$ were selected for the negative ion mode. $[M+H]^+$, $[M+Na]^+$, $[M+K]^+$, $[M+NH4]^+$, and $[2M+H]^+$ were selected for the positive ion mode. Each of the obtained feature tables was split into two peak tables based on the retention time ranges, which were according to the accumulation level of phenolic acids (1.0 - 18.5 min for both root and leaf samples) and ATDs (16.5 - 29.5 min for root samples; 14.0 - 29.5 min for leaf samples). Normalized metabolomics data were imported into SIMCA - P 14.1 (Umetrics AB, Umea, Sweden) to conduct the chemometric analysis.

Heterologous expression in yeast and yeast microsome isolation Based on the genome and transcriptome sequencing data, all candidate CYP76AK genes were identified and cloned using the primers shown in Supplementary Data 12. The open reading frames were further subcloned into the epitope-tagged vector pESC-His using *Eco*R I and *Not* I restriction sites for expression in the WAT11 yeast strain, which contains *A. thaliana* NADPH - CYP reductase ATR1. WAT11 transformed with empty pESC - His was employed as control. Transformants were cultured on SD dropout medium (-His) and grown at 28 ℃ for 72 h. A single positive colony was initially grown in 5 mL of SD-His liquid medium for about 24 h at 28 ℃ in a shaking incubator (200 rpm). The culture was then used to inoculate 250 mL of fresh SD-His liquid medium for another 24 h at 28 ℃ with shaking. Cells were then collected and washed three times with sterile water and yeast extract peptone dextrose medium with 2% galactose (YPL). Cells were then induced with YPL with shaking for 16 h at 28 ℃. Tris - EDTA buffer solution was prepared with 50 mM Tris - HCl and 1 mM EDTA at pH 7.4. Cells were recovered and transferred to a 50 mL tube by centrifugation at 7 000×g for 5 min and were resuspended in 25 mL of TEK buffer (0.1 mol/L KCl in TE buffer). Cells were then left at room temperature for 5 min and were again recovered and resuspended in pre-chilled TESB (0.6 M sorbitol in TE). All steps were then performed at 4 ℃. Cells were lysed at 4 - 6 ℃ by a low-temperature ultra-high-pressure continuous-flow cell disrupter. The procedure was repeated three times. The tube was then centrifuged at 12 000 × *g* for 30 min, and the supernatant was transferred to tubes containing 10 mL polyethylene glycol (PEG)-NaCl (PEG4000 and 0.15 mol/L NaCl). The tube was again centrifuged at 12 000 × *g* for 30 min. The supernatant was discarded, and the pellet was resuspended in TEG buffer (5% [v/v] glycerol in TE buffer).

In vitro activity assays Activity assays were performed in a 1.5 mL microtube using 500 μL of TE buffer (pH 7.5) that included 0.5 mg total microsomal proteins, 300 μmol/L NADPH, 50 μmol/L of substrate, and a regenerating system (2.5 μmol/L FAD, 2.5 μmol/L FMN, 1 mmol/L DTT, 2 mmol/L glucose-6-phosphate, and 2 U glucose-6-phosphate dehydrogenase). The reaction mixtures were incubated at 28 ℃ for 16 h in a shaking incubator (200 r/min) and then were extracted with 500 μL of ethyl acetate three times with vortexing. After centrifugation at 12,000 × *g* for 10 min, the organic phase was transferred to fresh microtubes, concentrated under a vacuum, and resuspended in 200 μL methanol for LC-MS analysis.

［胡佳栋，陈军峰，陈万生，等. Nature Communications，2023，14：4696.］

# Natural products of pentacyclic triterpenoids: from discovery to heterologous biosynthesis

## 1 INTRODUCTION

Pentacyclic triterpenoids are important natural secondary metabolites that are connected by six isoprene units with the closed pentacyclic ring as the parent and can be divided into various types according to their different aglycones. Pentacyclic triterpenoids are not only involved in plant communication, defense, and sensory regulation but also have a wide range of pharmacological effects and important biological activities. The amount of pentacyclic triterpenoid resources in the diet is closely related to human health, and thus the wide development and application of pentacyclic triterpenoids are necessary. Pentacyclic triterpenoids are mainly synthesized *via* the mevalonate (MVA) pathway in the cytoplasm and methylerythritol phosphate (MEP) pathway in the plastid. Currently, the main recognized pathway to synthesize triterpenoid sapogenins is the MVA pathway, in which squalene is transformed into 2,3-oxidosqualene under the action of squalene epoxidase (*SE*), serving as the precursor of pentacyclic triterpenoids and key enzyme of this reaction. OSC can catalyze the cyclization of 2, 3-oxidosqualene to generate more than 100 triterpenoids with different carbon skeletons. Higher plants have evolved multiple OSCs that are involved in the biosynthesis of triterpenoid saponins of different types. OSC can catalyze the reaction of 2,3-oxidosqualene to complete the cyclization *via* protonation, cyclization, rearrangement and deprotonation, thereby generating the precursor of triterpenoid saponins. OSC mainly catalyzes the generation of four types of pentacyclic triterpene skeletons, namely α-amyrin, β-amyrin, lupeol, and friedelin. Oleanane-type is the main variant of pentacyclic triterpenoid saponins, the biosynthesis of which is completed by β-amyrin synthase (βAS). CYP450s such as CYP716As undergo continuous oxidation to generate oleanolic acid, which is further modified by UDP-glycosyltransferase (UGT) to generate a variety of triterpene saponins. The biosynthetic pathway of triterpenoid saponins involves certain sequential enzymatic reactions, mainly involving three types of enzymes: OSCs, CYPs and UGTs, which all exist in the form of moderate or large gene families with dozens or hundreds of members in plants.

The biosynthesis of triterpenoid saponins is affected by the genetic manipulation of the above-mentioned pathway gene. An increased content of triterpenoid saponins can be achieved by overexpressing key enzyme genes in the biosynthetic pathway or silencing genes in a competitive metabolic pathway. Studies have shown that the biosynthesis of triterpene saponins in *Panax ginseng* and other plants can be regulated by the over-expression of 3-hydroxy-3-methylglutaryl-coenzyme A (CoA) reductase (*HMGR*), farnesyl pyrophosphate synthase (*FPS*), squalene synthase (*SS*) and squalene epoxidase (*SE*) genes, or down-regulation of competing pathways by CRISPRi or RNAi interference. Transcription factors (TFs) play an important role in regulating the biosynthesis of triterpenoid saponins, which can simultaneously control the expression of multiple key genes during the biosynthesis of plant secondary metabolites. At present, four main types of TF families have been reported to regulate the biosynthesis of plant triterpenoids, including APETALA2/ethylene responsive factors (AP2/ERFs), basic helix-loop-helix (bHLH), WRKYs, and basic region/leucine zipper motifs (bZIPs). However, there are a few studies on the regulation of triterpenoid saponin biosynthesis by TFs, while their transcriptional regulations need to be further explored. In addition, studies have shown that microRNA (miRNA) is one of the main regulators in the formation of plant secondary metabolites. However, experimental evidence for miRNA regulating the biosynthesis of pentacyclic triterpenoids has been less reported. The target gene of miRNA and its molecular mechanism in controlling the biosynthesis of plant triterpenoid saponins are not clear, and thus still require further research and exploration.

With the development of synthetic biology and metabolic engineering, the heterologous synthesis of plant natural products is emerging as an alternative for the massive production of these high-value compounds. By importing the biosynthetic pathway of natural products into heterologous hosts such as *Saccharomyces cerevisiae* and *Escherichia coli*, with a clear genetic background and simple genetic manipulation, the synthesis of specific target natural products can be achieved *via* simple fermentation technology. The heterologous biosynthesis of natural products has many advantages including rapid growth, simple nutritional requirements, mature and reliable genetic operation methods, and convenient modification of genes or metabolic pathways. Primary or secondary metabolic products of different types, sources, and biological activities have been successfully synthesized in various heterologous hosts. Therefore, heterologous biosynthesis has a promising future and is expected to become the mainstream method for the large-scale production of valuable natural products.

In this review, we systematically summarize and analyze the classification, distribution, structural characteristics, and bioactivity of pentacyclic triterpenoids. Furthermore, we discuss the biosynthetic pathways, transcriptional regulations and the recent progress in the heterologous synthesis of pentacyclic triterpenoids *via* plant chassis and microbial cell factories. Also, we analyze the distinctions between heterologous plants and microbial cell factories for the biosynthesis of pentacyclic triterpenoids. Subsequently, we propose potential strategies to improve the accumulation of triterpenoid saponins, aiming to provide a reference for their large-scale synthesis, development and application. Finally, we also present some prospects for the biosynthesis of natural products such as triterpenoid saponins *via* plant chassis and microbial cell factories, aiming to offer new insights for the future biomanufacturing of natural products.

## 2 STRUCTURE, DISTRIBUTION AND BIOACTIVITY OF PENTACYCLIC TRITERPENOIDS

2.1 Structural characteristics Pentacyclic triterpenoids are composed of 6 isoprene units, and their basic skeleton contains 30 carbon atoms. According to the different aglycones, pentacyclic triterpenoids can be mainly divided into four categories including oleanane, ursane, lupane and friedelane (Fig. 1). Some other type of skeletons such as fernane and isofernane, hopane and isohopane have also been found.

Oleanane-type triterpenoid saponins are also known as β-amyrin-derived pentacyclic triterpenoids, whose basic skeleton is a five-ring parent nucleus of polyhydropinene. In the case of the five rings of the basic skeleton, A/B, B/C, and C/D are all *trans*, only D/E is *cis*, and there are 8 methyl groups on the parent nucleus, of which C-8, C-10, and C-17 are β-type, while C-14 belongs to α-type. These compounds are widely distributed in the plant kingdom, which exist as plant secondary metabolites in the free state and the combined state of saponins and triterpene esters, and oleanolic acid, glycyrrhizic acid, saikosaponin, maslinic acid, esculentoside, and polygalacic acid are their typical representatives.

Ursane-type pentacyclic riterpenoids are also known as α-amyrin-derived pentacyclic triterpenoids, most of which are derivatives of ursolic acid, and they have five six-membered rings in their structure, where the A/B, B/C and C/D rings are all *trans*, and the D/E rings are mostly *cis*. Ursane and oleanane are isomers of each other, where the difference in their structure is that the methyl group at the C-20 position on the ring is transferred to the C-19 position, and only the methyl position on the E-ring is different. Ursane-type pentacyclic triterpenoids mainly exist in the form of free state or glycosides in plants such as *Rosa laevigata*, *Ilex chinensis*, *Centella asiatica*, and *Sanguisorba officinalis* and other plants.

There are four six-membered rings and one five-membered ring in the structure of lupane, where the isopropyl group at the C-19 position on the E-ring is substituted by the α-configuration. Besides, the A/B, B/C, C/D and D/E rings are all arranged in the *trans* configuration. To date, the research on the bioactivity of lupane-type pentacyclic triterpenoids mainly focuses on betulinic acid, betulin, lupeol, and betulonic acid.

Friedelane is derived from oleanane through methyl translocation, and its structural feature is that the condensed methods of the A/B, B/C and C/D rings are all *trans*, while the D/E ring is *cis*. There are 8 methyl groups on the parent nucleus, among which there is a geminal dimethyl group at the C-20 position. Besides, the methyl groups of C-4, C-5, C-9, C-14 and C-17 are all in the β-configuration, while the methyl group of C-13 is the α-configuration. Tripterygone and celastrol isolated from *Tripterygium wilfordii* belong to friedelane. Moreover, the tingenone contained in *Euonymus* plants and the pristimerin contained in *Celastrus orbiculatus* also belong to friedelane-type pentacyclic triterpenoids.

Fernane and isofernane are isomers of lupane, whose substituents on the E-ring are at the C-22 position, and the horn methyl at the C-8 position is transferred to the C-13 position. Arundoin and fernenol belong to fernane-type pentacyclic triterpenoids, and their C-13 methyl group is in the α-configuration, while the C-14 methyl group is in the β-configuration. In addition, cylindrin belongs to the isofernane type, and contrary to arundoin and fernenol, its C-13 methyl group is in the β-configuration, which the C-14 methyl group is in the α-configuration.

Hopane and isohopane are both isomers of fernane, where both C-14 and C-18 have angular methyl groups, which are their typical structural characteristics. The E-ring of the hopane-type pentacyclic triterpenoids is a five-membered carbocyclic ring, and the C-21 position of the E-

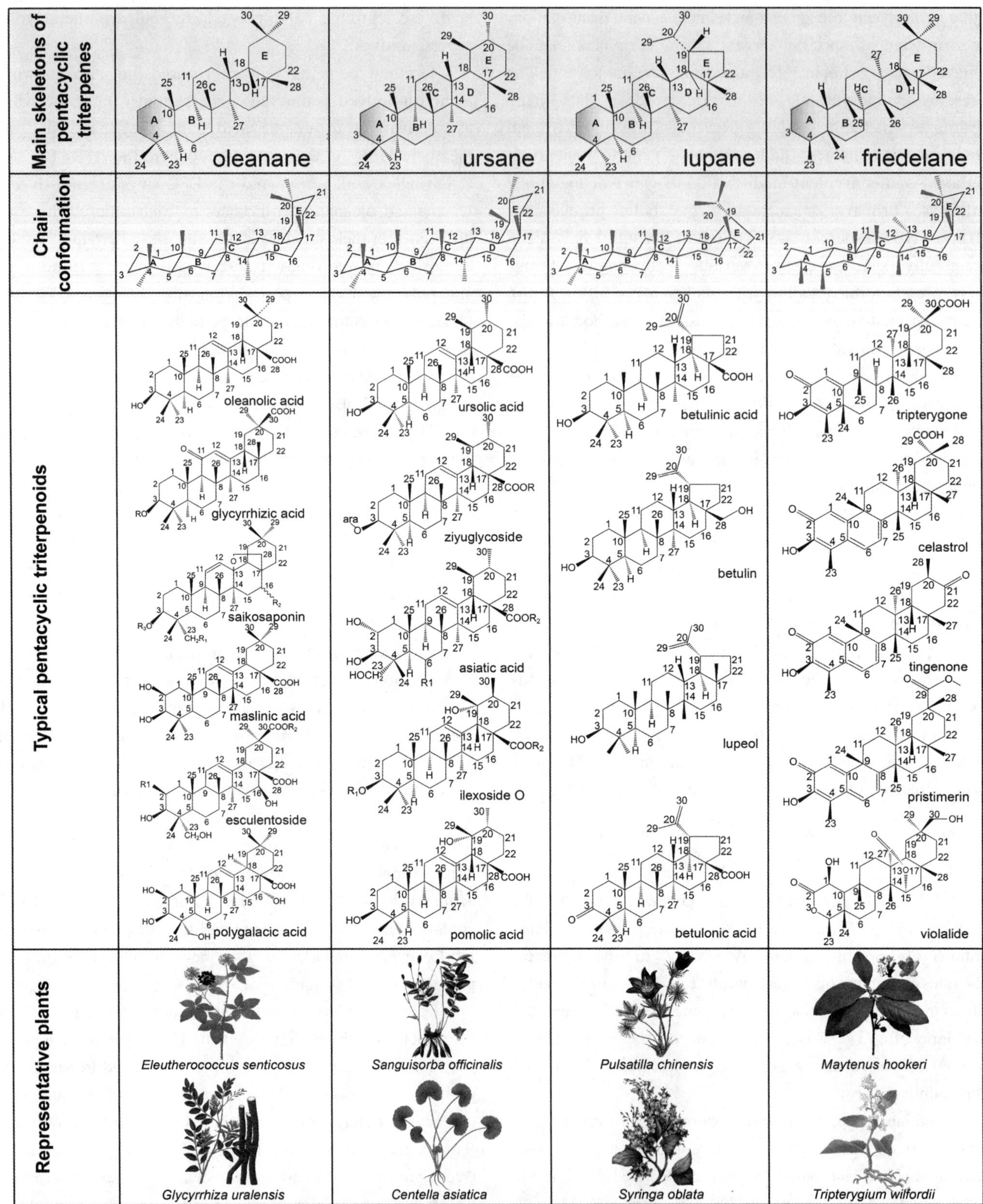


**Fig. 1 Main classification and structures of pentacyclic triterpenoids**

ring is substituted by isopropyl group. For the basic skeleton, their A/B, B/C, C/D and D/E rings are all *trans*-condensed. The C-21 isopropyl group of the isohopane type is the β-configuration, whereas that in the hopane type is the α-configuration. Currently, hopane-7 β-ol has been isolated from *Gomphrena globosa*, hydroxyhopanone- and hopane-type pentacyclic triterpenoids have been found in *Aquilaria sinensis*. Besides, the diplotene of hopane-type pentacyclic triterpenoids was found in *Pyrrosia lingua*, *Polytrichum commune* and *Drynaria roosii*.

Furthermore, pentacyclic triterpenoids also include triterpenoids whose C-ring is a seven-membered ring, such as lycoclavanin and lycoclavanol in *Lycopodium clavatum*. However, this type of pentacyclic triterpenoid has been rarely discovered and reported.

2.2 Distribution in nature Triterpenes and their saponins are the second largest secondary metabolites in nature, with a total of more than 20 000. Pentacyclic triterpenoids, as an important member of triterpenoids, are widely distributed and diverse in nature, which exist in higher plants, fungi, pteridophytes, monocotyledons, dicotyledons and marine organisms, especially in dicotyledons. In the plant kingdom, pentacyclic triterpenoids are mainly distributed in Araliaceae, Leguminosae, Compositae, Aesculaceae, Polygalaceae, Oleaceae, Akebiaceae, Cucurbitaceae, Euphorbiaceae, Campanulaceae, Caryophyllaceae, Poaceae and other plants (Fig. 2).

2.2.1 Pentacyclic triterpenoids in monocotyledons. Pentacyclic triterpenoids are widely distributed in monocotyledonous plants, such as the lupane-type compounds and oleanolic acid contained in *Cyperus rotundus* of Cyperaceae, pentacyclic triterpenoid orysatinol contained in *Oryza sativa* of Poaceae, friedelin and cylindrin contained in *Coix lachryma*-jobi, arundoin, cylindrin and fernenol contained in *Imperata cylindrica*, and the abundant ursolic acid contained in the leaves of Bambusoideae. Besides, two oleanane-type triterpenoid saponins called azafrine are distributed in *Crocus sativus* of Iridaceae. In addition, they are distributed in the lupeols contained in *Acorus tatarinowii* of Araceae and *Curcuma phaeocaulis* of Zingiberaceae, as well as the friedelin contained in *Commelina communis* of Commelinaceae.

2.2.2 Pentacyclic triterpenoids in dicotyledons. Pentacyclic triterpenoids are widely distributed in dicotyledons, where *Eleutherococcus senticosus*, *P. ginseng*, *Panax quiquefolium*, *Aralia elata*, *Panax notoginseng*, and *Schefflera arboricola* in Araliaceae and *Glycyrrhiza uralensis*, *Astragalus membranaceus*, *Albizia julibrissin*, *Pueraria lobata*, and *Herba Abri* in

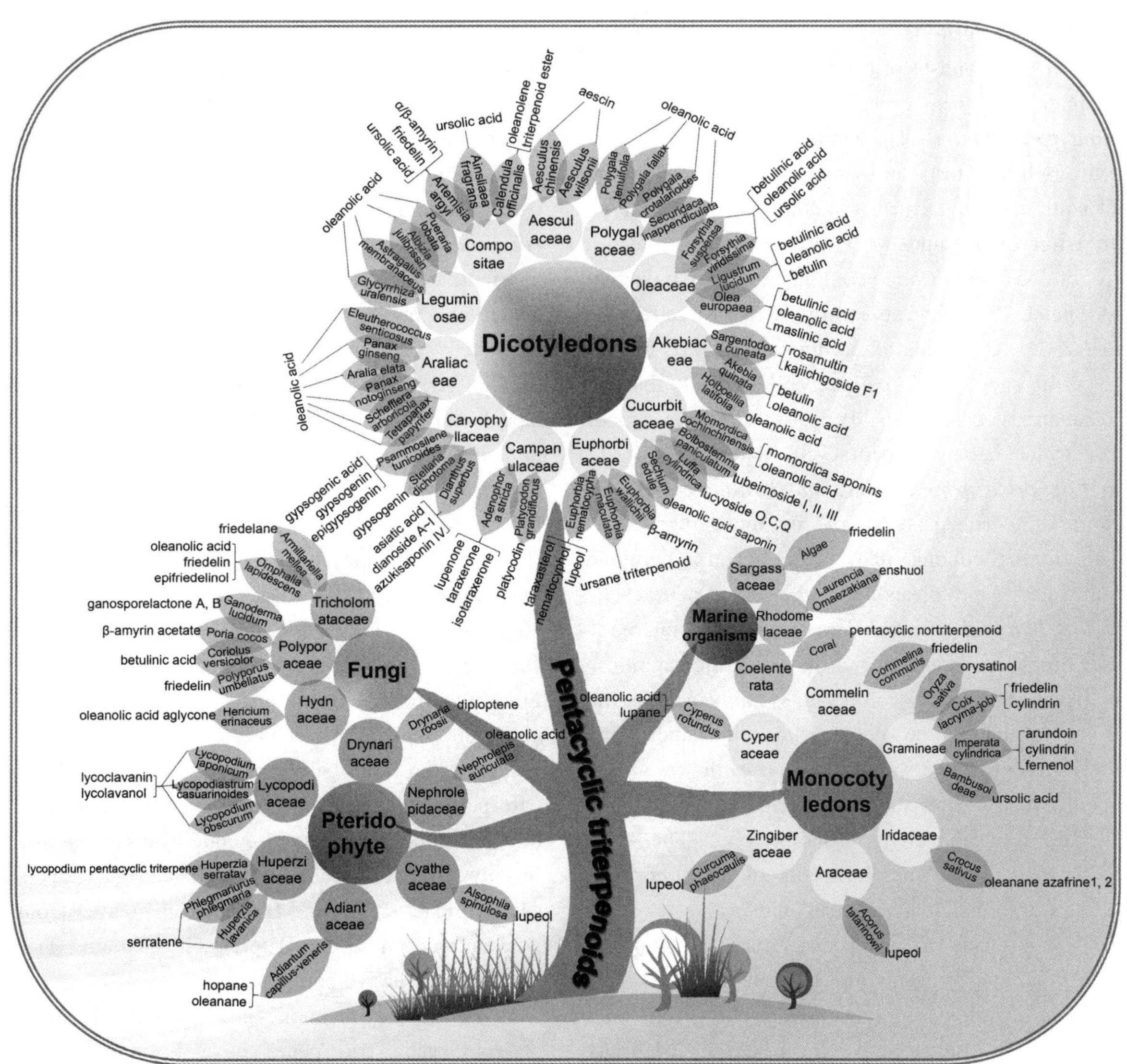


Fig. 2 Main distribution of pentacyclic triterpenoids in nature

Leguminosae are rich in oleanolic acid. *Artemisia argyi* in Compositae contains α-amyrin, β-amyrin, friedelin and ursolic acid. *Calendula officinalis* contains oleanene-type triterpenoid esters, and *Ainsliaea fragrans* contains ursolic acid. The seeds of *Aesculus chinensis* in Aesculaceae mainly contain pentacyclic triterpenoid saponins such as aescine, isoaescine, esculin and deacylated aescine. Both *Aesculus wilsonii* and *Aesculus chekiangensis* are rich in aescine. In the case of Polygalaceae, *Polygala tenuifolia*, *Polygala fallax*, *Polygala crotalarioides*, and *Securidaca inappendiculata* all contain oleanolic acid. *Forsythia suspensa* and *Forsythia viridissima* in Oleaceae contain betulinic acid, oleanolic acid and ursolic acid. *Ligustrum lucidum* contains betulinic acid, oleanolic acid and betulin, and the triterpenoids in *Olea europaea* are mainly pentacyclic triterpenoids, including betulinic acid, oleanolic acid and maslinic acid. *Sargentodoxa cuneata* in Akebiaceae is rich in rosamultin and kajiichigoside F1. The cane of *Akebia quinata* contains pentacyclic triterpenoids such as betulin and oleanolic acid. The fresh peel of *Holboellia latifolia* is rich in oleanolic acid. Tubeimosides Ⅰ, Ⅱ, and Ⅲ of traditional Chinese medicine are all oleanane-type pentacyclic triterpenoid saponins in *Bolbostemma paniculatum*. The fruits and leaves of *Luffa cylindrica* are rich in triterpenoid saponins, the lucyosides O, C, and Q contained in its leaves belong to oleanane-type pentacyclic triterpenoid saponins. The roots, stems, leaves and fruits of *Sechium edule* contain saponin bioactive substances. Unlike Cucurbitaceae, which is rich in tetracyclic triterpenoids, the terpenoids of *Sechium edule* are mainly oleanane-type saponins. *Euphorbia wallichii* in Euphorbiaceae contains oleanane-type β-amyrin. Taraxastrol, nematocyphol and lupeol, which belong to pentacyclic triterpenoids, are present in *Euphorbia nematocypha*. *Phyllanthus emblica* is rich in pentacyclic triterpenoids, and its active ingredients such as β-amyrone, betulonic acid, lupeol acetate, betulinic acid, ursolic acid, and oleanolic acid are all pentacyclic triterpenoids. *Platycodon grandiflorus* in Campanulaceae, traditional Chinese medicine, is rich in triterpene saponins. As one of its main bioactive components, platycodin is the derivative of oleanane-type pentacyclic triterpene. The triterpenoids present in the roots of *Adenophora stricta* are mostly pentacyclic triterpenoids, including lupenone, taraxerone and isooleanane-type isotaraxerone. The main medicinal components of the dry roots of *Psammosilene tunicoides* in Caryophyllaceae are saponins, and its roots contain multiple oleanane-type compounds, such as gypsogenic acid, gypsogenin, epigypsogenin and 16-isoquillaic acid. The root of *Stellaria dichotoma* contains pentacyclic triterpenoid gypsogenin. The anti-tumor active ingredient in *Dianthus superbus* is the pentacyclic triterpenoid asiatic acid. In addition, *D. superbus* also contains dianosides A, B, C, D, E, F, G, H, and I, and azukisaponin Ⅳ, all of which are pentacyclic triterpenoid saponins.

2.2.3 Pentacyclic triterpenoids in pteridophyte. Pteridophytes, also known as ceterach, are a group of spore plants with the highest level of evolution, which generally contain triterpenoids, mainly belonging to hopane- and fernane-type pentacyclic triterpenoids in nature. There are about 12 000 species of pteridophyte in the world, which are widely distributed all over the world, especially in tropical and subtropical areas, and most of them are geophilous, lithophytic, and epiphytic, while only a few are hygroscopic or aquatic. In addition, they prefer a damp and warm environment. There are about 2 600 species of pteridophyte belonging to 231 genera in 63 families in China, which are mainly distributed in provinces and regions south of the Yangtze River, and remarkably, there are more than 1 500 species in Yunnan province alone. In the case of Lycopodiaceae, *L. japonicum*, *L. casuarinoides* and *L. obscurum* all contain pentacyclic triterpenoids such as lycoclavanin and lycolavanol. Thus far, more than 30 triterpenoids have been isolated and identified from *Huperzia serrata* in Huperziaceae, most of which are lycopodium pentacyclic triterpenoids, and the C-rings are a seven-membered ring structure. Serratene pentacyclic triterpenes are both found in *Phlegmariurus phlegmaria* and *Huperzia javanica*. There are many types of triterpenoids distributed in *Adiantum capillusveneris* of Adiantaceae, which are mainly hopane-type and a few oleanane-type pentacyclic triterpenoids. *Alsophila spinulosa* in Cyatheaceae is rich in terpenoids, and pentacyclic triterpenoids such as lupeol have been identified. Moreover, *Nephrolepis cordifolia* in Nephrolepidaceae contains oleanolic acid, and *Drynaria roosii* in Drynariaceae contains diploptene, which belongs to hopane-type pentacyclic triterpene.

2.2.4 Pentacyclic triterpenoids in fungi. There are more than 120 000 species of fungi, which are composed of a large group of lower organisms with wide distribution and varieties in nature. Among them, the medicinal fungi in Eumycota are the most distributed, and currently there are about 300 known medicinal fungi. Most of the terpenes isolated from fungi belong to sesquiterpenes, diterpenes and triterpenes, among which triterpenes are important products in the metabolic process of fungi. The *Ganoderma lucidum* in Polyporaceae contains more than 100 triterpenoids, and ganosporelactones A and B (Fig. 3A) isolated from its spore powder are pentacyclic triterpenoid lactones. Triterpenoids are the main active components of *Poria cocos*. At present, β-amyrin acetate, oleanolic acid and 3-*O*-acetyloleanolic acid of pentacyclic triterpenes have been isolated from the sclerotia and mycelium of *Poria cocos*. Studies revealed that *Coriolus versicolor* contains pentacyclic triterpenoid betulinic

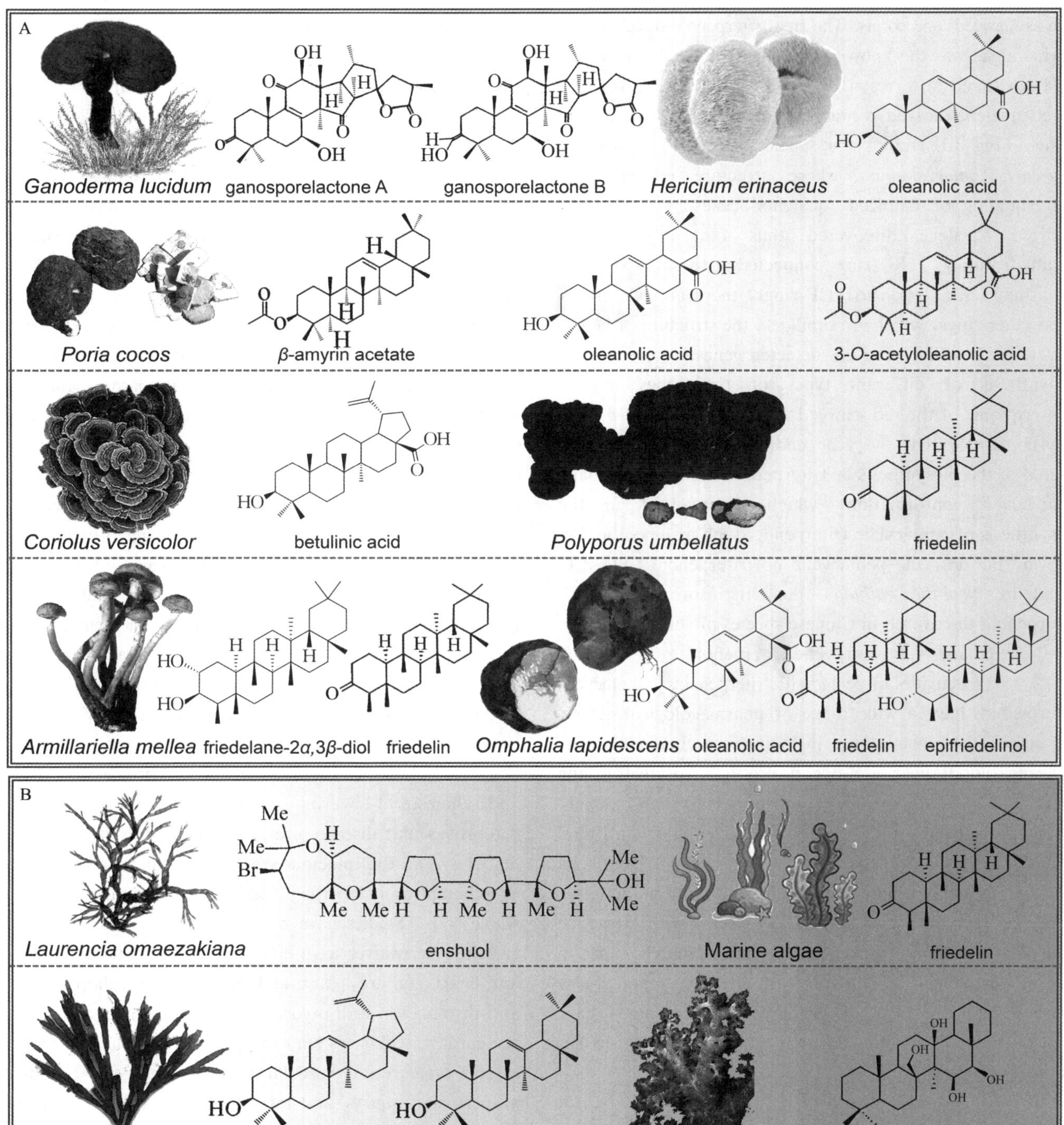


**Fig. 3 Chemical structures of pentacyclic triterpenoids in fungi and marine organisms**

(A) Fungi; (B) marine organisms.

acid, and the friedelin of friedelane-type pentacyclic triterpenoid was also isolated from *Polyporus umbellatus*. *Armillariella mellea* is a medicinal and edible fungus in Tricholomataceae, which contains many friedelane-type pentacyclic triterpenoids such as friedelane-2α, 3β-diol (Fig. 3A) and friedelin. The sclerotia of *Omphalia lapidescens* is rich in pentacyclic triterpenoids such as oleanolic acid, friedelin and epifriedelinol (Fig. 3A). Additionally, a variety of pentacyclic triterpenoids with oleanolic acid as aglycone has been identified in the culture of *Hericium erinaceus* in Hydnaceae.

2.2.5 Pentacyclic triterpenoids in marine organisms. Terpenoids are important components of marine bioactive substances, which are widely distributed in marine organisms, such as corals, sponges, coelenterates, molluscs, seaweed and other marine organisms. Among the marine natural products, terpenoids are the most widely distributed, accounting for about 40%, but the number and types of triterpenoids are scarce and only rarely studied in organisms such as seaweeds and corals. The first triterpenoid discovered in marine algae was the known component of friedelin, which has been found in terrestrial plants. Matsuo *et al*. found a novel squalene-derived pentacyclic triterpene alcohol called enshuol (Fig. 3B) from a new species of the red algal genus *Laurencia omaezakiana*, whose structure enriches the understanding of oxidized squalene because most of the oxidized squalene discovered thus far only contain tetrahydrofuran (THF) rings connected at the 2,5-position. In enshuol, in addition to THF rings, there are two *trans*-fused ether rings, which are similar to the structure of ladder polyether. De Oliveira *et al*. detected genes involved in the biosynthesis of different types of triterpenes in the transcriptome of the red seaweed *Laurencia dendroidea*, and they confirmed that the gene coding lupeol synthase 1 is related to the biosynthesis of triterpenes with a "chair-chair-chair-boat" conformation, which is involved in the biosynthesis of pentacyclic triterpenes, such as lupeol and β-amyrin. Besides, the pentacyclic nortriterpenoid (Fig. 3B) found in *Nephthea albida*, the first soft coral with triterpenoid discovered in Chinese species of soft corals, is a novel oleanolane-type pentacyclic triterpenoid.

2.3 Bioactivities of pentacyclic triterpenoids Pentacyclic triterpenoids have a wide range of pharmacological effects and significant bioactivities, including immunomodulatory, lowering blood sugar and blood pressure, protecting the liver, and anti-inflammatory, anti-bacterial, anti-oxidant, anti-cardiovascular and cerebrovascular, and anti-viral activities (Fig. 4). Some pentacyclic triterpenoids have been reported to exhibit anti-tumor cell proliferation activity, induce cell apoptosis and anti-AIDS effects, with attractive clinical application prospects and a hot research topic in natural medicinal chemistry. In recent years, new pharmacological effects of pentacyclic triterpenoids have been discovered, and the research on their mechanism has gradually deepened.

2.3.1 Anti-inflammatory, anti-bacterial, anti-oxidant and immunomodulatory. Numerous studies have shown that most pentacyclic triterpenoids have anti-inflammatory effects, and thus have been used in clinic. Oleanolic acid mainly exists in the form of glycosides in Chinese herbal medicine and has various bioactivities such as anti-inflammatory and anti-bacterial. Martín *et al*. proved that oleanolic acid is effective for the treatment of Th1 cell-mediated inflammatory diseases. Zhang *et al*. found that glycyrrhizic acid can effectively reduce the severity of Coxsackievirus B3 (CVB3)-induced myocarditis and may serve as a new treatment for viral myocarditis. Saikosaponin has strong anti-inflammatory activity, and *in vivo* studies have shown that it can effectively alleviate inflammatory diseases, reduce the expression of pro-inflammatory cytokines, and exert anti-inflammatory effects mainly by inhibiting the nuclear factor-κB (NF-κB) signaling pathway. Besides, saikosaponin has intense anti-oxidant activity, which can significantly reduce the levels of oxygen free radicals and malondialdehyde, the product of lipid peroxidation, and enhance the activities of anti-oxidant enzymes such as superoxide dismutase, catalase and glutathione peroxidase. The anti-oxidant effect of saikosaponin may be related to the activation of the nuclear TF NF-E2-related factor 2 (Nrf2) signal pathway. Ursolic acid, mainly in the form of free or glycosides in *Ligustrum lucidum*, *Arctostaphylos uva-ursi*, *Prunella vulgaris*, *Eriobotrya japonica* and other plants, has various pharmacological effects and activities such as anti-inflammatory, inhibiting apoptosis, immunomodulation, anti-scarring and promoting the repair of damaged neurons. It also has significant anti-oxidant function and is widely used in the fields of medicine and cosmetics. Lupeol widely exists in the seed epidermis of *Lupinus micranthus*, the leaves of *Verbena officinalis* and the latex of *Ficus carica* trees, which has anti-inflammatory, analgesic and anti-allergy effects. Lupeol can exert a protective effect on lipopolysaccharide-induced neuroinflammation by activating the P38-MAPK and JNK pathways and has potential efficacy in the treatment of various neuroinflammatory diseases. Ginsenosides have many effects such as anti-fatigue, anti-tumor, anti-aging, and anti-oxidant.

2.3.2 Anti-cardiovascular and cerebrovascular disease and cholesterol-lowering effects. Cardiovascular and cerebrovascular diseases are mainly caused by hypertension, diabetes, and dyslipidemia syndrome, which are manifested as ischemic or hemorrhagic lesions in the brain, heart and whole body. Studies have found that pentacyclic triterpenoids and their derivatives have effects on anti-myocardial ischemia, anti-heart failure, anti-arrhythmia, anti-atherosclerosis, anti-thrombosis, anti-myocardial hypertrophy and fibrosis in the cardiovascular system. In addition, they have protective effects on cerebral vascular ischemia injury and ischemiareperfusion injury, and inhibit cerebral neuron apoptosis. Oleanane-type and ursane-type compounds have relatively noticeable therapeutic effects for the above-mentioned diseases. Oleanolic acid, glycyrrhizic acid, glycyrrhetinic acid, hederagenin, maslinic acid, and rotundic acid are oleanane-type pentacyclic triterpenoids that mainly used against cardiovascular and cerebrovascular diseases. Ursolic acid, asiatic acid, asiaticoside and corosolic acid are ursane-type pentacyclic triterpenoids with anti-cardiovascular and cerebrovascular pharmacological effects. It was found that the degree of atherosclerosis was improved when apolipoprotein E-deficient mice induced by a high-fat diet were treated with a new pentacyclic triterpenoid called ilexgenin A.

The saponins contained in Medicago plants are mainly oleanane-type pentacyclic triterpenes, namely alfalfa saponins,

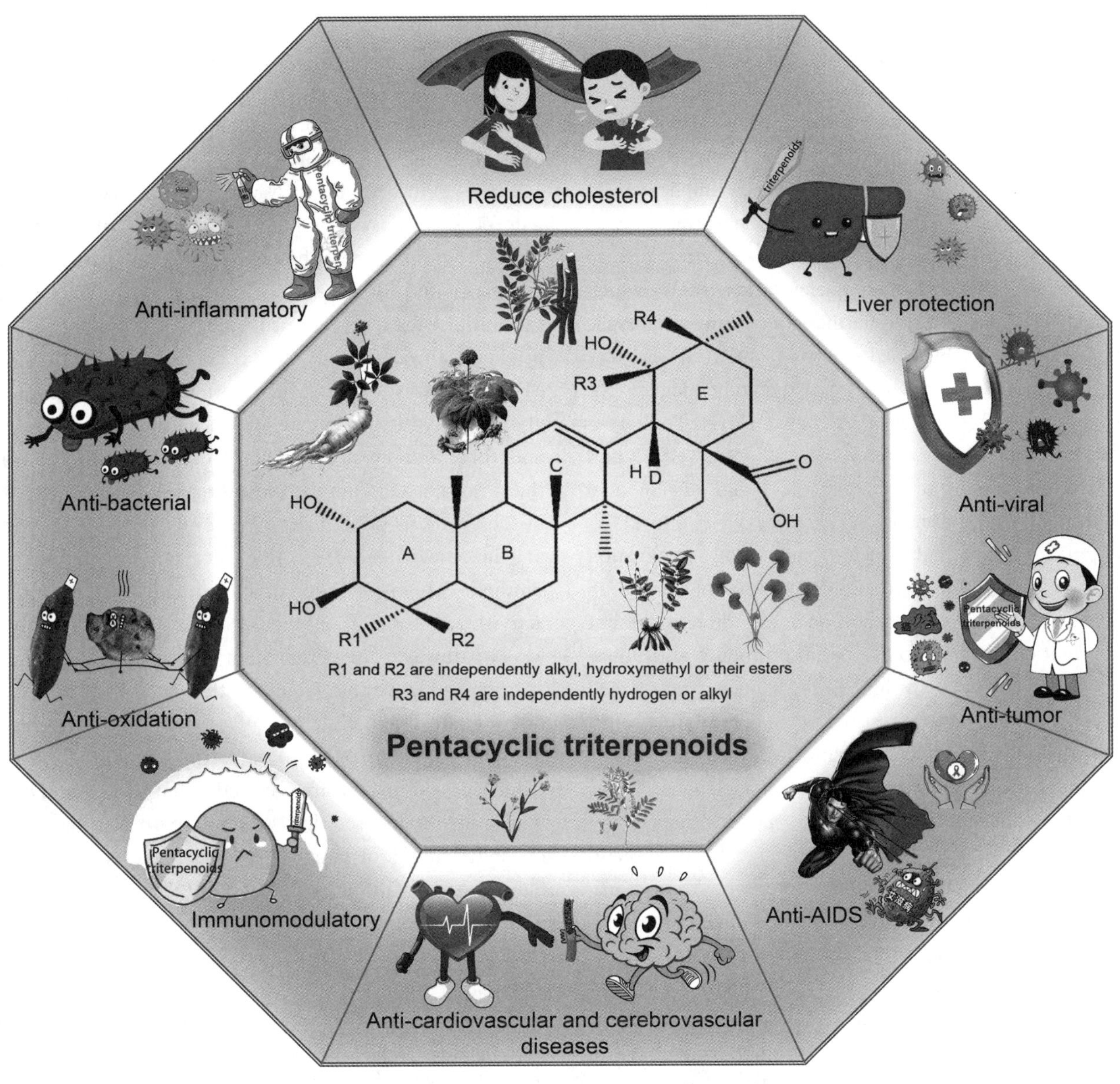


Fig. 4 Bioactivities of pentacyclic triterpenoids

which can improve the production performance of animals, have an excellent cholesterol-lowering effect, and can enhance the immunity of animals and reduce blood lipids. Fan *et al*. added alfalfa saponins in the diets of laying hens, which effectively reduced the cholesterol concentrations in the eggs, and thus they concluded that dietary alfalfa saponins can affect cholesterol metabolism by up-regulating the expression of the ATP-binding cassette transporters G5 and G8 in hens, and that alfalfa additive is a potential agent for reducing cholesterol concentrations.

2.3.3 Liver protection, anti-viral and anti-tumor bioactivities. Recent studies have shown that oleanane-type and ursane-type pentacyclic triterpenoids have good anti-hepatic injury activity, which can rapidly repair the necrotic area and reduce the inflammatory response of liver tissue by promoting the regeneration of liver cells, inhibiting the proliferation of collagen fibers and other ways, playing a role in liver protection. At present, oleanolic acid and glycyrrhizinic acid are used as liver protective drugs in the clinical treatment of infections acute icteric hepatitis, viral and chronic persistent hepatitis. Oleanane-type pentacyclic triterpenoids 1 - 3 of *Callicarpa nudiflora* have significant hepatoprotective activity against D-galactosamine-induced toxicity of WB - F344 rat hepatic epithelial stem cells. Currently, most anti-tumor drugs have specific damage effects on the liver. However, ursolic acid not only can fight against tumors but also significantly and rapidly reduce alanine aminotransferase, eliminate gangrene, enhance the appetite, fight liver fibrosis and restore liver function with the characteristics of rapid effect, a short course of treatment and stable effect, which makes up for the deficiency of anti-tumor drugs and is expected to be further developed as anti-cancer drugs, especially anti-liver cancer drugs.

Pentacyclic triterpenes and their derivatives and analogues

play a vital role in the field of anti-viral medicine. In recent years, with the emergence of toxic side effects and drug resistance of traditional anti-viral drugs, the anti-viral activity of pentacyclic triterpenoids with low toxicity and novel mechanism has attracted extensive attention from researchers. Certain pentacyclic triterpenoids have been implicated in influenza virus, hepatitis B virus (HBV), hepatitis C virus (HCV), HIV, SARS coronavirus, corona virus disease (COVID)-19 (ref.) and other nucleic acid viruses, which have sound inhibitory effects. Furthermore, some pentacyclic triterpenoids even show broad-spectrum anti-viral activity, such as betulinic acid, which has different degrees of inhibition on HIV, influenza A virus (H1N1), herpes simplex virus (HSV), respiratory syncytial virus (RSV) and CVB. The derivatives of oleanolic acid and ursolic acid inhibit the entry of influenza A (H5N1) virus into cells, showing the unique advantages and good application prospects of pentacyclic triterpenoids in anti-viral drugs.

Pentacyclic triterpenoids not only can directly inhibit the proliferation of tumor cells, but also produce anti-tumor activity by enhancing body immunity, inducing tumor cell apoptosis, reversing drug resistance and exhibiting anti-angiogenesis activity. Ursolic acid has good anti-tumor activity and certain inhibitory effects on melanoma, liver cancer, lung cancer, rectal cancer, gastric cancer and prostate cancer. It can act on various signal pathways to induce tumor cell apoptosis and differentiation. Yang *et al*. synthesized 19 betulin derivatives, among which compounds 3a-3d and 5 exhibited apparent anti-tumor activity.

Pentacyclic triterpenoids have the above-mentioned pharmacological effects and biological activities, which have brought a new era in the treatment of stubborn diseases in human beings. However, the research on pentacyclic triterpenoids is mainly limited to the cell level and animal experiments and lack of clinical research data. Meanwhile, its therapeutic development is still in its infancy, and the pharmacological mechanism has not been clarified. Moreover, pentacyclic triterpenoids have low polarity and bioavailability, which limit their clinical application. However, pentacyclic triterpenoids have attractive prospects in clinical application. With the expansion of research and technological innovation, it is believed that they will be widely used in clinical treatments in the future.

## 3 BIOSYNTHETIC PATHWAYS AND TRANSCRIPTIONAL REGULATION OF PENTACYCLIC TRITERPENOIDS

The biosynthetic pathway of pentacyclic triterpenoids has attracted interest from many scientists, which reasonable progress achieved in recent years. Determining the key enzyme genes involved in triterpenoid biosynthetic pathway, TFs, miR-NAs and their synergy in pentacyclic triterpene biosynthesis, and artificially transforming the key enzyme genes and making them highly expressed in hosts provide genetic parts for the future heterologous large-scale production of pentacyclic triterpenoids.

3.1 Phylogenetic analysis of key enzymes in pentacyclic triterpenoid biosynthesis  Pentacyclic triterpenoids are synthesized in plants through the MVA pathway in the cytoplasm and MEP pathway in the plastid. Acetyl CoA is the initial substrate, and isopentenyl diphosphate (IPP) is produced through a six-step condensation reaction in the MVA pathway. The MEP pathway uses pyruvate and glyceraldehyde 3-phosphate (G3P) as starting substrates and undergoes a seven-step reaction to synthesize IPP, which is then transported from the plastid to cytoplasm to participate in the synthesis of terpenes. However, despite the existence of the mevalonate-free IPP biosynthetic pathway, the synthesis of many isoprenoids with important biological activities still relies on the MVA pathway. Notably, the MVA pathway plays a dominant role in the biosynthesis of triterpenoid saponins. Under the action of isopentenyl diphosphate isomerase (IDI), IPP and dimethylallyl pyrophosphate (DMAPP) are interconverted, and the triterpenes in plants are derived from IPP and DMAPP, which are condensed into geranyl pyrophosphate (GPP) under the action of geranyl pyrophosphate synthase (GPS). Subsequently, GPP is catalyzed by *FPS* and a second IPP unit is added to generate farnesyl pyrophosphate (FPP). Then, the two FPPs are condensed by *SS* to form squalene, which is epoxidated to 2,3-oxidosqualene under the action of *SE*. Subsequently, 2,3-oxidosqualene is cyclized by OSC to form various tetracyclic and pentacyclic triterpenoid skeletons. Then, these skeletons rely on CYP and UGT with uridine modification such as oxidation, replacement, hydroxylation and glycosylation, and finally produce various pentacyclic triterpenoids. The biosynthetic pathway of pentacyclic triterpenes is shown in Fig. 5.

3.1.1 Phylogenetic analysis of OSCs.  OSC is the first ratelimiting enzyme in the downstream synthetic stage of triterpenoid saponins, which can catalyze the formation of sterols and triterpenoid precursors from 2,3-oxidosqualene. Meanwhile, OSC is the key enzyme and branch point of this reaction, which is also a key step to generate diverse triterpenoid products. 2,3-Oxidosqualene is cyclized by OSC to generate a variety of triterpenoids with different carbon skeletons, and this cyclization process is completed through a series of protonation, cyclization, rearrangement and deprotonation reactions to form diverse triterpene skeletons. The structural diversity of the triterpene skeleton may be related to the flexible and changeable core site of the related enzymes, where a change in one amino acid sequence in the

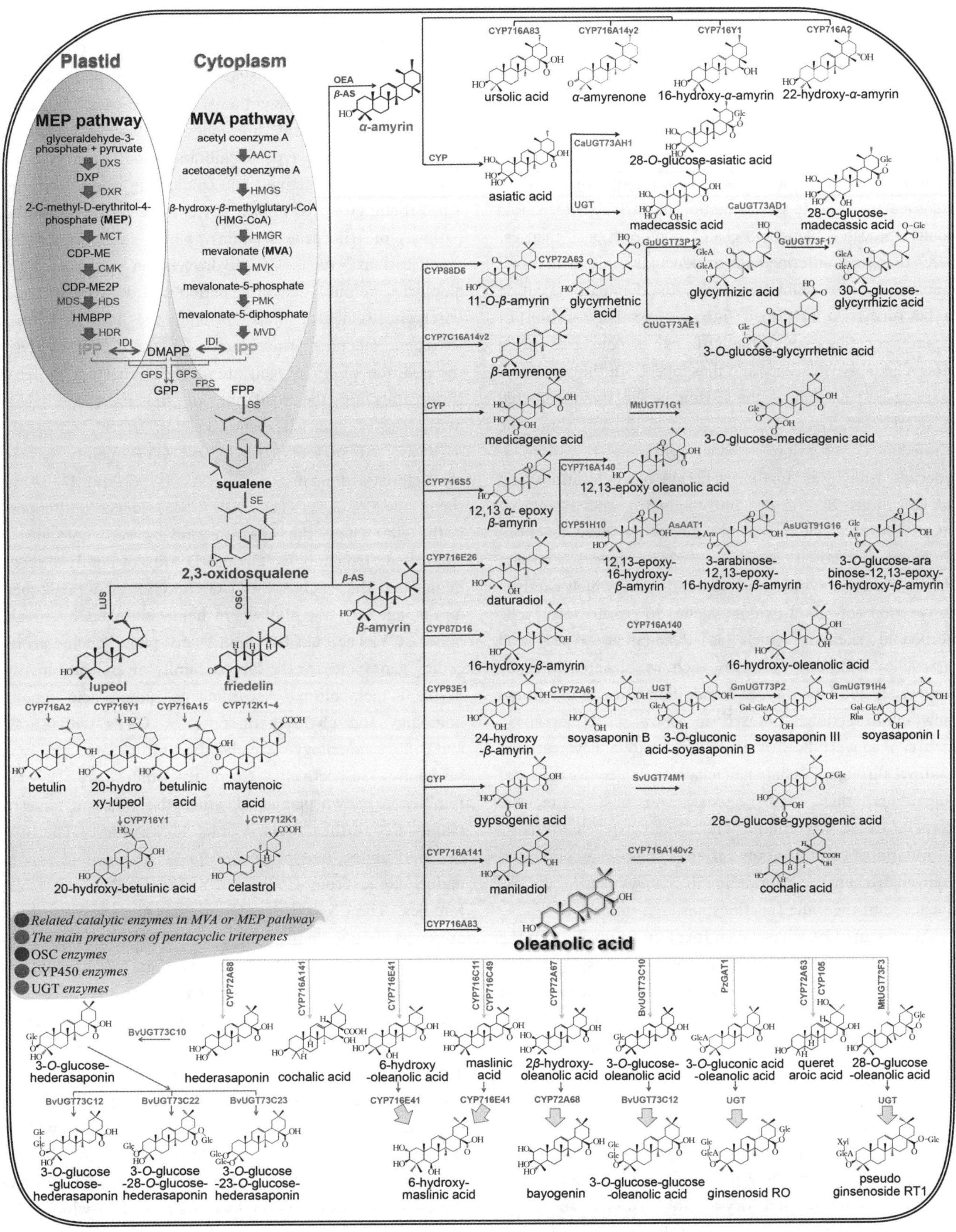


**Fig. 5 Biosynthetic pathway of pentacyclic triterpenoids in plants**

Abbreviations not explained in the main text: AACT, acetoacetyl-CoA thiolase; HMGS: 3-hydroxy-3-methyl glutaryl coenzyme A synthase; HMGR: 3-hydroxy-3-methyl glutaryl coenzyme A reductase; MVK: mevalonate kinase; PMK: phosphomevalonate kinase; MVD: mevalonate 5-diphosphate decarboxylase; DXS: 1-deoxy-D-xylulose-5-phosphate-synthase; DXP: 1-deoxy-D-xylulose-5-phosphate; DXR: 1-deoxy-D-xylulose-5-phosphate reductase; MCT: 2-*C*-methyl-D-erythritol-4-phosphate cytidylyltransferase; CMK: 4-(cytidine-5′-diphospho)-2-*C*-methyl-D-erythritol kinase; MDS: 2-*C*-methyl-D-erythritol-2, 4-cyclodiphosphate synthase; HDS: 1-hydroxy-2-methyl-2-*E*-butenyl-4-diphosphate synthase; HMBPP: (*E*) 4-hydroxy-3-methyl-but-2-enyl-pyrophosphate; HDR: 1-hydroxy-2 methy-3-*E*-butenyl-4-diphosphate reductase.

OSC may lead to formation of different products.

Studies have shown that more than 100 triterpene skeletons have been produced by the divergent evolution of OSCs in plants. Most pentacyclic triterpene skeletons and dammarane-type tetracyclic triterpene skeletons are formed by dammarenyl cations in the 'chair-chair-chair (C-C-C)' conformation, such as lupeol and β-amyrin. 2, 3-Oxidosqualene leads to the formation of various triterpenoid saponins through 'chair-chair-chair' conformational changes, where the first intermediate product in this process is dammarenyl cation. Simultaneously, the dammarenyl cation can be further transformed into a tirucallanyl cation or baccharenyl cation, where the latter can be converted into a pentacyclic lupanyl cation, and thus lupeol. In the process of reopening and expanding the E-ring in the five-membered ring of the lupanyl cation into a six-membered ring, the intermediate cyclization product germanicyl cation is produced, which can further generate oleanyl cations and ursanyl cations to convert into β-amyrin and α-amyrin, respectively. The main enzymes mediating these reactions are dammarenediol-Ⅱ synthase (DS), lupeol synthase (LUS), α-amyrin synthase (αAS) and βAS, which catalyze the reaction of 2, 3-oxidosqualene to form tetracyclic triterpenoid skeletons such as dammarane type, and pentacyclic triterpene skeletons such as oleanolane type, ursane type, and lupine type. In addition, Xue *et al*. found a new multifunctional OsOSC7 in *Oryza sativa* japonica, which can convert 2, 3-oxidosqualene into a new cationic orysatinyl through a 'chair-half chair-chair' conformational change, and then further generate a new pentacyclic triterpene called orysatinol. The 'chair-half chair-chair' conformational change is between the 'chair-boat-chair' and 'chair-chair-chair' conformational change, and the OSC sequence with the same functions has high similarity.

At present, OSCs have been found to be involved in the biosynthesis of pentacyclic triterpenes in many species. We collected 96 OSC genes from related studies on various plant pentacyclic triterpenes, constructed a phylogenetic tree based on their protein sequences, and compared their catalytic products, as shown in Fig. 6 and Table 1. Accordingly, OSCs mainly catalyze the formation of four different pentacyclic triterpene precursors, namely, β-amyrin, α-amyrin, lupeol and friedelin, in addition to germanicol, taraxasterol, taraxerol, δ-amyrin, multiflorenol, isomultiflorenol, isoarborinol, glutinol, orysatinol, and orysaspirol. Among them, β-amyrin products are the most widely distributed, indicating that β-amyrin occupies a dominant position among the products of pentacyclic triterpenes catalyzed by OSCs. The OSCs with different functions, such as αAS, βAS, LUS, and FRS, are clustered on different branches of the phylogenetic tree (Fig. 6), which further indicates that OSCs with the same function have high sequence similarity.

3.1.2 Phylogenetic analysis of CYPs. CYPs belong to a large family of enzyme proteins in plants, mainly involved in the biosynthesis of terpenes, alkaloids, phenylpropanes, plant hormones and other substances, which are a kind type membrane binding protein with extensive catalytic activity and conducting iron porphyrin as a prosthetic group. CYP is a key enzyme in the biosynthetic pathway of triterpene saponins, which catalyzes structural modifications such as hydroxylation, carboxylation, aldehyde, ketone, dehydrogenation and dehydration of the triterpene skeleton, thus forming the intermediates of triterpene saponins. The common feature of CYP catalysis is the addition of an oxygen atom to the reactant molecule, thus catalyzing the oxidation of the inert methyl and methylene of the triterpene skeleton in the downstream pathway. At present, the typical CYP mainly has four characteristic domains, *i.e.*, A, B, C and D. Among them, the (A/G) GX(D/E)T(T/S) sequence on domain A is the site where the substrate and oxygen molecules are connected. Domains B, C, and D are covalently linked to heme, and the PFG(A/S/V) GRRXC(P/A/V)G sequence on domain D is the site where heme is linked by covalent bonds. CYPs account for about 1% of plant genome protein-coding genes and are the largest family of enzymes involved in plant metabolism. According to amino acid sequence homology and phylogenetic criteria, CYPs with $>40\%$ and $>55\%$ homology were classified in the same family and subfamily, respectively. Currently, there are 127 CYP families in known plants, of which the CYPs in terrestrial plants are further divided into 11 families. The CYPs involved in the biosynthesis of plant triterpenoid saponins mainly come from CYP51, CYP71, CYP72 and CYP85 families. The CYP716 family enzymes in the CYP85 family are considered to be the main contributors to the biosynthetic diversity of dicotyledons, and members of its subfamily CYP716A/-C/-E/-Y are mainly involved in the oxidation of the pentacyclic triterpene skeleton in dicotyledons. CYP450s have a large number of members, strong substrate specificity, and low sequence similarity, and the physical properties of the expressed products are very similar and difficult to separate, which greatly deepens the difficulty in analyzing their biotransformation steps. At present, more than 70 types of CYP450s that modify the pentacyclic triterpene skeleton in plants have been identified, most of which belong to the CYP716 family, and CYP87, CYP88 and CYP93 are also involved in the modification of pentacyclic triterpenes. Studies have shown that the CYP51H subfamily from the CYP51 family is exclusively responsible for the modification of the pentacyclic triterpene skeleton in monocotyledons. CYP51H10 of *Avena sativa* catalyzes the C12-C13 β-epoxidation

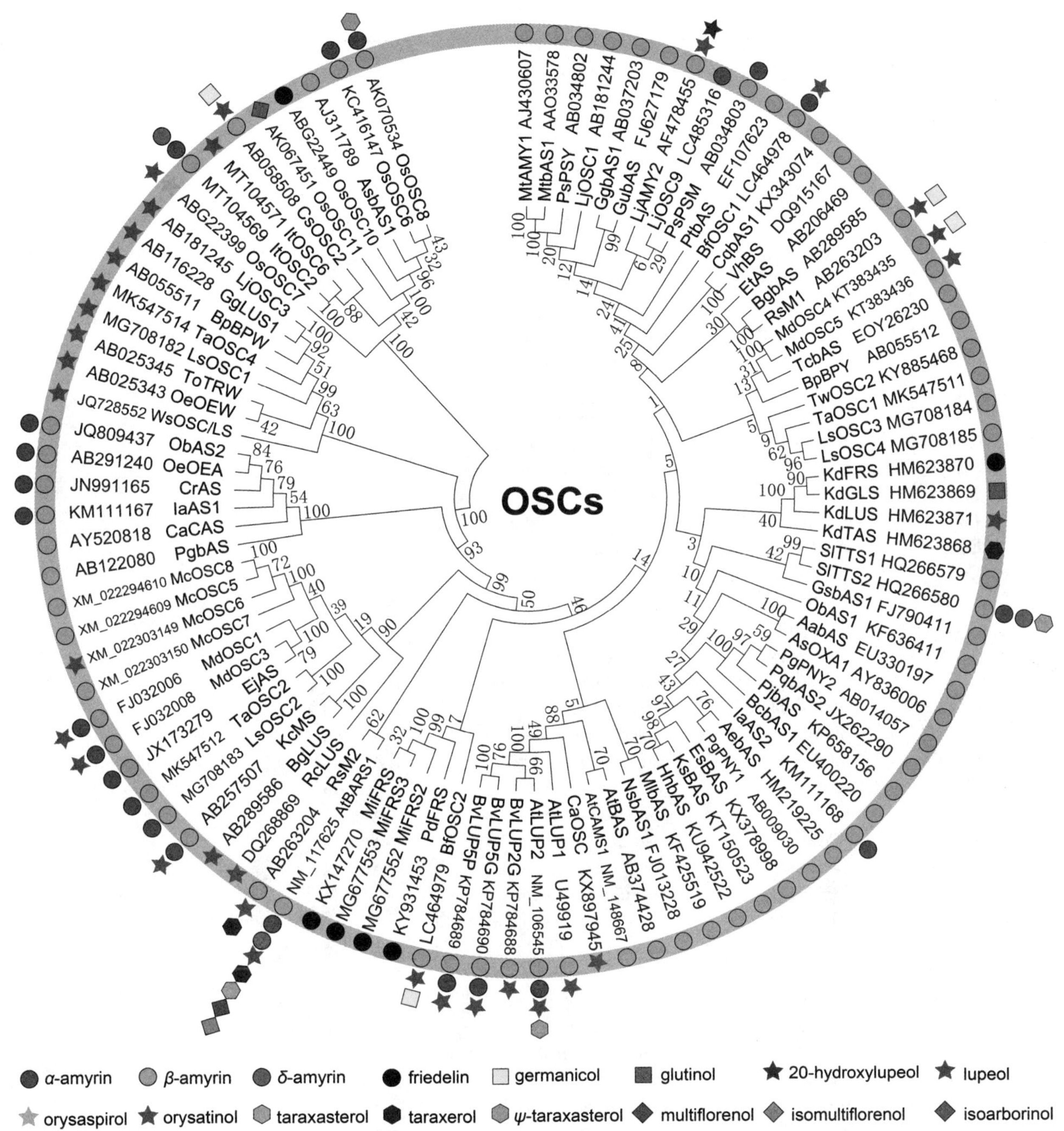


**Fig. 6 Phylogenetic tree of OSCs involved in pentacyclic triterpenoid biosynthesis**

The MUSCLE method in the MEGA6.0 software was used to align the amino acid sequences of OSCs, the maximum likelihood method was then used to construct the phylogenetic tree, and the Bootstrap value was set to 1000. The catalytic products, references and other detailed information of OSCs are shown in Table 1. Black text represents OSC proteins, blue text is the corresponding protein accession numbers in NCBI, and the small colored shapes represent the corresponding catalytic products.

**Table 1 Related *OSC* genes for pentacyclic triterpenoid biosynthesis**

| Category | *OSC* genes | GenBank ID | Organisms | Catalytic products |
|---|---|---|---|---|
| AS | *LjOSC9* | LC485316 | *Lotus japonicus* | α-Amyrin |
| | *CrAS* | JN991165 | *Catharanthus roseus* | α-Amyrin, β-amyrin |
| | *EjAS* | JX173279 | *Eriobotrya japonica* | α-Amyrin, β-amyrin |
| | *IaAS1* | KM111167 | *Ilex asprella* | α-Amyrin, β-amyrin |
| | *OeOEA* | AB291240 | *Olea europaea* | α-Amyrin, β-amyrin |
| | *IaAS2* | KM111168 | *Ilex asprella* | α-Amyrin, β-amyrin |
| | *LsOSC2* | MG708183 | *Lagerstroemia speciosa* | α-Amyrin, β-amyrin |

(Continued)

| Category | *OSC* genes | GenBank ID | Organisms | Catalytic products |
|---|---|---|---|---|
| | *TaOSC2* | MK547512 | *Terminalia arjuna* | α-Amyrin，β-amyrin |
| | *PsPSM* | AB034803 | *Pisum sativum* | α-Amyrin，β-amyrin |
| | *ObAS2* | JQ809437 | *Ocimum basilicum* | α-Amyrin，β-amyrin |
| | *OsOSC6* | KC416147 | *Oryza sativa* | α-Amyrin，β-amyrin |
| | *ItOSC2* | MT104569 | *Iris tectorum* | α-Amyrin，β-amyrin，δ-amyrin |
| βAS | *AebAS* | HM219225 | *Aralia elata* | β-Amyrin |
| | *AsbAS1* | AJ311789 | *Avena strigosa* | β-Amyrin |
| | *AtBAS* | AB374428 | *Arabidopsis thaliana* | β-Amyrin |
| | *AtCAMS1* | NM_148667 | *Arabidopsis thaliana* | β-Amyrin |
| | *BgbAS* | AB289585 | *Bruguiera gymnorhiza* | β-Amyrin |
| | *BpBPY* | AB055512 | *Betula platyphylla* | β-Amyrin |
| | *CaCAS* | AY520818 | *Centella asiatica* | β-Amyrin |
| | *CqbAS1* | KX343074 | *Chenopodium quinoa* | β-Amyrin |
| | *EsBAS* | KX378998 | *Eleutherococcus senticosus* | β-Amyrin |
| | *TcbAS* | EOY26230 | *Theobroma cacao* | β-Amyrin |
| | *TwOSC2* | KY885468 | *Tripterygium wilfordii* | β-Amyrin |
| | *EtAS* | AB206469 | *Euphorbia tirucalli* | β-Amyrin |
| | *GgbAS1* | AB037203 | *Glycyrrhiza glabra* | β-Amyrin |
| | *GubAS* | FJ627179 | *Glycyrrhiza uralensis* | β-Amyrin |
| | *AabAS* | EU330197 | *Artemisia annua* | β-Amyrin |
| | *AsOXA1* | AY836006 | *Aster sedifolius* | β-Amyrin |
| | *KsBAS* | KT150523 | *Kalopanax septemlobus* | β-Amyrin |
| | *LjOSC1* | AB181244 | *Lotus japonicus* | β-Amyrin |
| | *LsOSC3* | MG708184 | *Lagerstroemia speciosa* | β-Amyrin |
| | *LsOSC4* | MG708185 | *Lagerstroemia speciosa* | β-Amyrin |
| | *MtAMY1* | AJ430607 | *Medicago truncatula* | β-Amyrin |
| | *MlbAS* | KF425519 | *Maesa lanceolata* | β-Amyrin |
| | *MtbAS1* | AAO33578 | *Medicago truncatula* | β-Amyrin |
| | *NsbAS1* | FJ013228 | *Nigella sativa* | β-Amyrin |
| | *ObAS1* | KF636411 | *Ocimum basilicum* | β-Amyrin |
| | *PgbAS* | AB122080 | *Panax ginseng* | β-Amyrin |
| | *PgPNY1* | AB009030 | *Panax ginseng* | β-Amyrin |
| | *PgPNY2* | AB014057 | *Panax ginseng* | β-Amyrin |
| | *BcbAS1* | EU400220 | *Bupleurum chinense* | β-Amyrin |
| | *HhbAS* | KU942522 | *Hedera helix* | β-Amyrin |
| | *PqbAS2* | JX262290 | *Panax quinquefolius* | β-Amyrin |
| | *PsPSY* | AB034802 | *Pisum sativum* | β-Amyrin |
| | *PtbAS* | EF107623 | *Polygala tenuifolia* | β-Amyrin |
| | *PjbAS* | KP658156 | *Panax japonicus* | β-Amyrin |
| | *SlTTS1* | HQ266579 | *Solanum lycopersicum* | β-Amyrin |
| | *GsbAS1* | FJ790411 | *Gentiana straminea* | β-Amyrin |
| | *TaOSC1* | MK547511 | *Terminalia arjuna* | β-Amyrin |
| | *VhBS* | DQ915167 | *Vaccaria hispanica* | β-Amyrin |
| | *McOSC5* | XM_022294609 | *Momordica charantia* | β-Amyrin |
| | *McOSC7* | XM_022303150 | *Momordica charantia* | β-Amyrin |
| | *McOSC8* | XM_022294610 | *Momordica charantia* | β-Amyrin |
| LuS | *ItOSC6* | MT104571 | *Iris tectorum* | Lupeol |
| | *LjOSC3* | AB181245 | *Lotus japonicus* | Lupeol |
| | *CaOSC* | KX897945 | *Cleome arabica* | Lupeol |
| | *LsOSC1* | MG708182 | *Lagerstroemia speciosa* | Lupeol |
| | *TaOSC4* | MK547514 | *Terminalia arjuna* | Lupeol |
| | *ToTRW* | AB025345 | *Taraxacum officinale* | Lupeol |
| | *WsOSC/LS* | JQ728552 | *Withania somnifera* | Lupeol |
| | *McOSC6* | XM_022303149 | *Momordica charantia* | Lupeol |

(Continued)

| Category | *OSC* genes | GenBank ID | Organisms | Catalytic products |
|---|---|---|---|---|
| | *RcLUS* | DQ268869 | *Ricinus communis* | Lupeol |
| | *OeOEW* | AB025343 | *Olea europaea* | Lupeol |
| | *BgLUS* | AB289586 | *Bruguiera gymnorhiza* | Lupeol |
| | *BpBPW* | AB055511 | *Betula platyphylla* | Lupeol |
| | *GgLUS1* | AB116228 | *Glycyrrhiza glabra* | Lupeol |
| | *KdLUS* | HM623871 | *Kalanchoe daigremontiana* | Lupeol |
| FRS | *MiFRS3* | MG677553 | *Maytenus ilicifolia* | Friedelin |
| | *MiFRS2* | MG677552 | *Maytenus ilicifolia* | Friedelin |
| | *MiFRS* | KX147270 | *Maytenus ilicifolia* | Friedelin |
| | *PdFRS* | KY931453 | *Populus davidiana* | Friedelin |
| | *KdFRS* | HM623870 | *Kalanchoe daigremontiana* | Friedelin |
| | *OsOSC10* | ABG22449 | *Oryza sativa* | Friedelin |
| Others | *MdOSC1* | FJ032006 | *Malus domestica* | α-Amyrin, β-amyrin, lupeol |
| | *MdOSC3* | FJ032008 | *Malus domestica* | α-Amyrin, β-amyrin, lupeol |
| | *BfOSC1* | LC464978 | *Bauhinia forficata* | α-Amyrin, β-amyrin, lupeol |
| | *BvLUP5G* | KP784690 | *Barbarea vulgaris* | α-Amyrin, β-amyrin, lupeol |
| | *BvLUP5P* | KP784689 | *Barbarea vulgaris* | α-Amyrin, β-amyrin, lupeol |
| | *KcMS* | AB257507 | *Kandelia candel* | α-Amyrin, β-amyrin, lupeol |
| | *BvLUP2G* | KP784688 | *Barbarea vulgaris* | β-Amyrin, lupeol |
| | *AtLUP1* | U49919 | *Arabidopsis thaliana* | β-Amyrin, lupeol |
| | *MdOSC5* | KT383436 | *Malus domestica* | β-Amyrin, lupeol |
| | *BfOSC2* | LC464979 | *Bauhinia forficata* | β-Amyrin, lupeol, germanicol |
| | *CsOSC2* | AB058508 | *Costus speciosus* | β-Amyrin, lupeol, germanicol |
| | *MdOSC4* | KT383435 | *Malus domestica* | β-Amyrin, lupeol, germanicol |
| | *RsM1* | AB263203 | *Rhizophora stylosa* | β-Amyrin, lupeol, germanicol |
| | *AtLUP2* | NM_106545 | *Arabidopsis thaliana* | α-Amyrin, β-amyrin, lupeol, taraxasterol |
| | *LjAMY2* | AF478455 | *Lotus japonicus* | β-Amyrin, lupeol, 20-hydroxylupeol |
| | *RsM2* | AB263204 | *Rhizophora stylosa* | β-Amyrin, lupeol, taraxerol |
| | *KdTAS* | HM623868 | *Kalanchoe daigremontiana* | Taraxerol |
| | *AtBARS1* | NM_117625 | *Arabidopsis thaliana* | α-Amyrin, β-amyrin, δ-amyrin, multiflorenol, isomultiflorenol, taraxerol, taraxasterol, lupeol |
| | *SlTTS2* | HQ266580 | *Solanum lycopersicum* | α-Amyrin, β-amyrin, δ-amyrin, taraxasterol |
| | *OsOSC8* | AK070534 | *Oryza sativa* | α-Amyrin, β-amyrin, ψ-taraxasterol |
| | *OsOSC11* | AK067451 | *Oryza sativa* | Isoarborinol |
| | *KdGLS* | HM623869 | *Kalanchoe daigremontiana* | Glutinol |
| | *OsOSC7* | ABG22399 | *Oryza sativa* | Orysatinol, orysaspirol |

on the C-ring and β-hydroxylation of the C16 position on the D-ring of β-amyrin, and finally forms an intermediate in the biosynthetic pathway of oat albumin, namely 12,13 β-epoxy-16 β-hydroxy-β-amyrin. In addition, studies also found that CYP93E in the CYP71 family, CYP72A in the CYP72 family and CYP88D subfamily members in the CYP85 family are closely related to the oxidation of the triterpene skeleton in legumes. The members of the CYP72A subfamily are also commonly involved in the biosynthesis of pentacyclic triterpenes, and CYP72As of *Medicago sativa* and *G. uralensis* are involved in the biosynthesis of legume-specific pentacyclic triterpenes. For instance, thus far, four CYP72A subfamily members, *i. e.*, CYP72A61, CYP72A63, CYP72A67 and CYP72A68, of *M. sativa* and one CYP72A subfamily member, *i.e.*, CYP72A154 of *G. uralensis* have been reported to be involved in the oxidation of the oleanane pentacyclic triterpene skeleton. CYP88D6 is an enzyme associated with the biosynthesis of glycyrrhizinic acid, and CYP88D6 catalyzes the sequential 2-step oxidation of the C-11 position of β-amyrin to generate 11-oxo-β-amyrin, the substrate of CYP72A154. The CYP93E subfamily members are also involved in the biosynthesis of triterpene saponins in legumes. CYP93E1 of *Glycine max* was the first to be identified as a C24-hydroxylase, which converts β-aromaticinol and sophorodiol to 24-hydroxy-β-amyrin and soyasapogenol B, respectively. Currently, 9 CYP93Es (CYP93E1-9) have been identified from 8 types of legumes, all of which have C24-hydroxylase activity. At present, there are approximately 20 CYP716A family members characterized by C28-oxidase activity of amyrin or lupeol, and most of these CYP716As

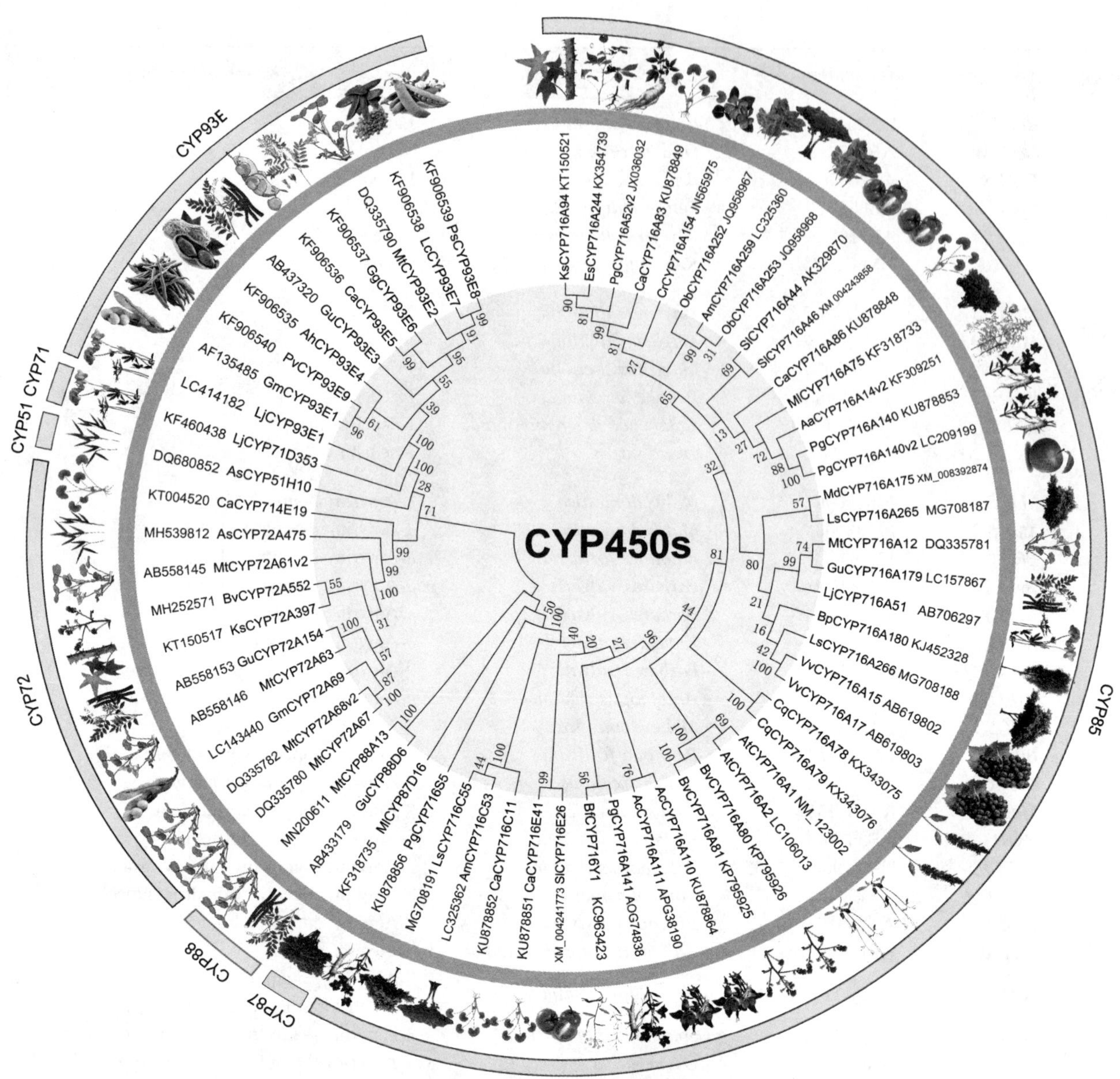


**Fig. 7 Phylogenetic tree of CYP450s involved in pentacyclic triterpenoid biosynthesis**

The MUSCLE method in the MEGA6.0 software was used to align the amino acid sequences of CYP450s, the maximum likelihood method was then used to construct the phylogenetic tree, and the Bootstrap value was set to 1 000. The catalytic substrates, catalytic products, references and other detailed information of CYP450s are shown in Table 2.

catalyze continuous three-step oxidation reactions of the amyrin or lupeol skeleton, resulting in the successive formation of hydroxyl, aldehyde and carboxyl groups at the C-28 position. Fukushima *et al*. revealed that the CYP716A12 of *Medicago truncatula* is a multifunctional oxidase for the biosynthesis of triterpenoids. Consequently, the oleanolic acid of the yeast expression product was obtained when CYP716A12 from *M. truncatula*, βAS and CYP450 reductase from *Lotus corniculatus* were co-expressed in yeast. CYP716A12 was identified as a β-amyrin-C28 oxidase that modified β-amyrin to oleanolic acid. Carelli *et al*. also confirmed this catalytic pathway. Yeast expression experiments confirmed that CYP716A12 can also catalyze the oxidation of α-amyrin-C28 to form ursolic acid, and catalyze the oxidation of lupeol-C28 to form betulinic acid. Tamura *et al*. revealed that CYP716A179 is a multifunctional enzyme, and its heterologous expression in yeast engineering strain showed that CYP716A179 is a C-28 oxidase, which can oxidize the C-28 position of α-amyrin, β-amyrin and lupeol to generate ursolic acid, oleanolic acid and betulinic acid, respectively. Han *et al*. conducted a functional study on CYP716A52v2 through a yeast expression system and found that it possessed β-amyrin C-28 oxidase activity and could oxidize the C-28 position of β-amyrin to generate oleanolic acid.

With the development of metabolome, transcriptome and genomics, many CYP members have been identified in plants. We collected 65 CYPs related to pentacyclic triterpenes in a variety of plants and constructed a phylogenetic tree according to their protein sequence (Fig. 7). Subsequently, their evolution was analyzed, where the clustering results confirmed the above-mentioned CYP family classification characteristics, and most of the CYPs were classified into the CYP85 family, and some CYP450s were classified in the CYP72, CYP93E, CYP71, CYP51, CYP87 and CYP88 family. Although the classification of CYP can only represent the phylogenetic relationship, which is not necessarily related to its function, we found through various analyses that the catalytic substrates, catalytic products and reaction types of the same CYP family members are similar according to Table 2. For instance, the catalytic substrates of the CYP71 family members are mostly β-amyrin and 24-hydroxy-β-amyrin, while the catalytic products are mostly 24-hydroxy-β-amyrin and 24-carboxy-β-amyrin, and the reaction types are mostly C－24-hydroxy and C－24 oxidation, indicating that the CYPs distributed on same branches of the phylogenetic tree may have similar functions.

3.1.3 Phylogenetic analysis of UGTs. Skeleton glycosylation is the key modification reaction during the biosynthesis of pentacyclic triterpenes, which is achieved by UGTs. Triterpene glycosylation catalyzed by UGTs is generally considered to be the last step in the biosynthesis of triterpenoid saponins, which is a key link in the diversity and bioactivities of triterpenoid saponins. Glycosylation reactions are catalyzed by GTs, which transfer glycosyl groups from activated donor molecules to acceptor molecules to generate a rich variety of glycosides. GTs are divided into 114 families (GT1－GT114) according to the UGT sequence similarity, specificity of the catalytic substrate, stereochemical structure of the catalytic product, and carbohydrate active enzyme database (CAZy). GTs involved in plant secondary metabolism are mainly distributed in the GT1 family, which contains the largest number of glycosyltransferases. The glycosyl donor of the GT1 family is a nucleoside diphosphate sugar (NDP-sugar), and the donor molecules of UGT mainly include uridine diphosphate (UDP)-glucose, UDP-glucuronic acid, UDP-rhamnose, and UDP-xylose. The amino acid sequence identity between members of the same UGT family is higher than 40%, while the identity between members of the same subfamily is higher than 60%. Although the sequence homology is not high, typical plant secondary metabolic UGTs have similar structural domains, possessing the plant secondary product glycosyltransferase (PSPG) motif, which is the substrate-binding region in UGTs.

With the continuous development of high-throughput sequencing, *de novo* sequencing and other technologies, an increasing number of UGT sequences have been discovered, but only a few UGTs in plants have been cloned and identified. At present, more than 50 types of UGTs involved in the modification of plant pentacyclic triterpenes have been identified in plants, which are mainly distributed in the UGT71, UGT73, UGT74, UGT85, UGT91 and UGT94 families. Studies have shown most UGTs members of the UGT73 family are involved in the glycosylation modification of pentacyclic triterpenes, dominating the glycosyl transfer at the C－3, C－23 and C－28 positions of oleanolic acid, hederasaponin, *etc*. A comprehensive gene expression cluster analysis identified that the glycosyltransferase UGT73F3 in *M. truncatula* can catalyze the carboxy glucosylation at the C－28 position of hederasaponin and oleanolic acid, of which the catalytic activity at C28－COOH of hederasaponin is the strongest.

It was found that the sequence identity of UGT73F17 in *G. uralensis* and UGT73F1 of isoflavone glucosyltransferase in *G. echinata* was 71%, which catalyzed the glycosylation at C30－COOH of glycyrrhizic acid to generate licorice saponin A3. Besides, UGT73F17 also possessed certain substrate heterogeneity, but it had strict regioselectivity and only glycosylated the C30－/C29－COOH of pentacyclic triterpenes or their saponins. Integrative analysis of the transcriptional and metabolic profiles of *M. truncatula* confirmed that the glycosyltransferase UGT73K1 can catalyze the glucose glycosylation at the C－3 and C－28 positions of hederasaponin, as well as the glucose glycosylation of soyasaponin at the C－3, C－22 and C-23 positions. Sayama *et al*. revealed that the glycosyltransferases UGT73F4 and UGT73F2 of soybean sequentially transfer glycosyl from UDP-xylose and UDP-glucosyl to C－22 position of soyasaponin A to generate 22-*O*-xylose-glucose-soysaponin A.

We collected 41 pentacyclic triterpene-related UGTs or related genes with UGT activity in a variety of plants and used their proteins to construct a phylogenetic tree, as shown in Fig. 8. The analysis showed that 41 glycosyltransferases or related enzymes involved in the post-modification are mainly distributed in the UGT73, GT2, UGT74, UGT91, UGT71, and UGT99 families. It is worth noting that AsTG1 is not a member of the UGT family, but a glycosidase belonging to GH1, which is the first glycosidase with terpenoid glycosyltransferase activity found in plants. The UGTs of different families are distributed on different branches of the phylogenetic tree and have similar functions. For example, most members of the UGT73 family have glucose glycosylation activity at the C－3 or C－28 position. Moreover, the UGTs distributed in the different families may have the same regioselectivity, and different UGTs may have the same function at the same position on different substrates. However, UGTs have a large degree of substrate confusion in plants, and it is a very complicated process to determine the specificity of the glycosyl donors and acceptors and the catalytic activity of UGTs. Therefore, it is still not accurate to predict the biological function of UGTs only

**Table 2 Related *CYP* genes for pentacyclic triterpenoid biosynthesis**

| Category | *CYP* genes | GenBank ID | Organisms | Substrates | Reactions | Catalytic products |
|---|---|---|---|---|---|---|
| CYP51 | *AsCYP51H10* | DQ680852 | *Avena strigosa* | β-Amyrin | C12，C13β-epoxy，C16β-hydroxy | 12,13β-Epoxy-16β-hydroxy-β-amyrin |
| CYP71 | *LjCYP71D353* | KF460438 | *Lotus japonicus* | Dihydro-lupeol，20-hydroxy-lupeol | C-20-hydroxy，C-28 oxidation | 20-Hydroxy-lupeol/20-hydroxy-betulinic acid |
| | *LjCYP93E1* | LC414182 | *Lotus japonicus* | β-Amyrin | C-24-hydroxy | 24-Hydroxy-β-amyrin |
| | *GmCYP93E1* | AF135485 | *Glycine max* | β-Amyrin/24-hydroxy-β-amyrin/sophoradiol | C-24-hydroxy/C-24 oxidation | 24-Hydroxy-β-amyrin，24-carboxy-β-amyrin，soyasapogenol B |
| | *MtCYP93E2* | DQ335790 | *Medicago truncatula* | β-Amyrin | C-24-hydroxy | 24-Hydroxy-β-amyrin |
| | *GuCYP93E3* | AB437320 | *Glycyrrhiza uralensis* | β-Amyrin/24-hydroxy-β-amyrin | C-24-hydroxy/C-24 oxidation | 24-Hydroxy-β-amyrin/24-carboxy-β-amyrin |
| | *AhCYP93E4* | KF906535 | *Arachis hypogaea* | β-Amyrin/24-hydroxy-β-amyrin | C-24-hydroxy/C-24 oxidation | 24-Hydroxy-β-amyrin/24-carboxy-β-amyrin |
| | *CaCYP93E5* | KF906536 | *Cicer arietinum* | β-Amyrin/24-hydroxy-β-amyrin | C-24-hydroxy/C-24 oxidation | 24-Hydroxy-β-amyrin/24-carboxy-β-amyrin |
| | *GaCYP93E6* | KF906537 | *Glycyrrhiza glabra* | β-Amyrin/24-hydroxy-β-amyrin | C-24-hydroxy/C-24 oxidation | 24-Hydroxy-β-amyrin/24-carboxy-β-amyrin |
| | *LcCYP93E7* | KF906538 | *Lens culinaris* | β-Amyrin | C-24-hydroxy | 24-Hydroxy-β-amyrin |
| | *PsCYP93E8* | KF906539 | *Pisum sativum* | β-Amyrin/24-hydroxy-β-amyrin | C-24-hydroxy/C-24 oxidation | 24-Hydroxy-β-amyrin/24-carboxy-β-amyrin |
| | *MlCYP87D16* | KF318735 | *Maesa lanceolata* | β-Amyrin | C-16α-hydroxy | 16α-Hydroxy-β-amyrin |
| | *PvCYP93E9* | KF906540 | *Phaseolus vulgaris* | β-Amyrin/24-hydroxy-β-amyrin | C-24-hydroxy/C-24 oxidation | 24-Hydroxy-β-amyrin/24-carboxy-β-amyrin |
| CYP72 | *MtCYP72A67* | DQ335780 | *Medicago truncatula* | Oleanolic acid/hederagenin/gypsogenic acid/gypsogenin | C-2β-hydroxy | 2β-Hydroxy-oleanolic acid/bayogenin/medicagenic acid |
| | *MtCYP72A61v2* | AB558145 | *Medicago truncatula* | 24-Hydroxy-β-amyrin | C-22β-hydroxy | Soyasapogenol B |
| | *GmCYP72A69* | LC143440 | *Glycine max* | Soyasapogenol B | C-21β-hydroxy | Soyasapogenol A |
| | *AsCYP72A475* | MH539812 | *Avena strigosa* | 12,13β-Epoxy，16β-hydroxy-β-amyrin | C-21β-hydroxy | 12,13β-Epoxy，16β，21β-dihydroxy-β-amyrin |
| | *MtCYP72A63* | AB558146 | *Medicago truncatula* | β-Amyrin | C-30 oxidation | 11-Deoxoglycyrrhetinic acid |
| | *GuCYP72A154* | AB558153 | *Glycyrrhiza uralensis* | β-Amyrin/11-oxo-β-amyrin | C-30 oxidation | 30-Hydroxy-β-amyrin/glycyrrhetinic acid |
| | *MtCYP72A68v2* | DQ335782 | *Medicago truncatula* | Oleanolic acid | C-23 oxidation | Gypsogenic acid |
| | *KsCYP72A397* | KT150517 | *Kalopanax septemlobus* | Oleanolic acid | C-23-hydroxy | Hederagenin |
| | *BvCYP72A552* | MH252571 | *Barbarea vulgaris* | Oleanolic acid | C-23-hydroxy | Hederagenin |
| | *CaCYP714E19* | KT004520 | *Centella asiatica* | Oleanolic acid/ursolic acid | C-23-hydroxy | Hederagenin/23-hydroxy ursolic acid |
| CYP85 | *AtCYP716A1* | NM_123002 | *Arabidopsis thaliana* | α-Amyrin/β-amyrin/lupeol | C-28 oxidation | Ursolic acid/oleanolic acid/betulinic acid |
| | *MtCYP716A12* | DQ335781 | *Medicago truncatula* | α-Amyrin/β-amyrin/lupeol | C-28 oxidation | Ursolic acid/oleanolic acid/betulinic acid |

(Continued)

| Category | *CYP* genes | GenBank ID | Organisms | Substrates | Reactions | Catalytic products |
|---|---|---|---|---|---|---|
| | *VvCYP716A15* | AB619802 | *Vitis vinifera* | α-Amyrin/β-amyrin/lupeol | C-28 oxidation | Ursolic acid/oleanolic acid/betulinic acid |
| | *LjCYP716A51* | AB706297 | *Lotus japonicus* | α-Amyrin/β-amyrin/lupeol | C-28 oxidation | Ursolic acid/oleanolic acid/betulinic acid |
| | *CrCYP716A154* | JN565975 | *Catharanthus roseus* | α-Amyrin/β-amyrin/lupeol | C-28 oxidation | Ursolic acid/oleanolic acid/betulinic acid |
| | *MdCYP716A175* | XM_008392874 | *Malus domestica* | α-Amyrin/β-amyrin/lupeol | C-28 oxidation | Ursolic acid/oleanolic acid/betulinic acid |
| | *LsCYP716A265* | MG708187 | *Lagerstroemia speciosa* | α-Amyrin/β-amyrin/lupeol | C-28 oxidation | Ursolic acid/oleanolic acid/betulinic acid |
| | *LsCYP716A266* | MG708188 | *Lagerstroemia speciosa* | α-Amyrin/β-amyrin/lupeol | C-28 oxidation | Ursolic acid/oleanolic acid/betulinic acid |
| | *AtCYP716A2* | LC106013 | *Arabidopsis thaliana* | α-Amyrin/β-amyrin/lupeol | C-16/C-22α/C-28-hydroxy | 22α-Hydroxy-α-amyrin/22α-hydroxy-β-amyrin/16-hydroxy-β-amyrin/betulin |
| | *GuCYP716A179* | LC157867 | *Glycyrrhiza uralensis* | α-Amyrin/β-amyrin/lupeol | C-28 oxidation/C-22α-hydroxy | Ursolic acid/oleanolic acid/betulinic acid |
| | *AmCYP716A259* | LC325360 | *Avicennia marina* | α-Amyrin/β-amyrin/lupeol | C-28 oxidation | Ursolic acid/oleanolic acid/betulinic acid |
| | *PgCYP716A140* | KU878853 | *Platycodon grandiflorus* | β-Amyrin/16β-hydroxy-β-amyrin/12,13α-epoxy-β-amyrin | C-28 oxidation | Oleanolic acid/16β-hydroxyoleanolic acid/12,13α-epoxy-oleanolic acid |
| | *AaCYP716A14v2* | KF309251 | *Artemisia annua* | α-Amyrin/β-amyrin/δ-amyrin | C-3 oxidation | α-Amyrone/β-amyrone/δ-amyrone |
| | *SlCYP716A44* | AK329870 | *Solanum lycopersicum* | α-Amyrin/β-amyrin | C-28 oxidation | Ursolic acid/oleanolic acid |
| | *SlCYP716A46* | XM_004243858 | *Solanum lycopersicum* | α-Amyrin/β-amyrin | C-28 oxidation | Ursolic acid/oleanolic acid |
| | *CaCYP716A83* | KU878849 | *Centella asiatica* | α-Amyrin/β-amyrin | C-28 oxidation | Ursolic acid/oleanolic acid |
| | *CaCYP716A86* | KU878848 | *Centella asiatica* | α-Amyrin/β-amyrin | C-28 oxidation | Ursolic acid/oleanolic acid |
| | *ObCYP716A252* | JQ958967 | *Ocimum basilicum* | α-Amyrin/β-amyrin | C-28 oxidation | Ursolic acid/oleanolic acid |
| | *ObCYP716A253* | JQ958968 | *Ocimum basilicum* | α-Amyrin/β-amyrin | C-28 oxidation | Ursolic acid/oleanolic acid |
| | *BvCYP716A80* | KP795926 | *Barbarea vulgaris* | β-Amyrin/lupeol | C-28 oxidation | Oleanolic acid/betulinic acid |
| | *BvCYP716A81* | KP795925 | *Barbarea vulgaris* | β-Amyrin/lupeol | C-28 oxidation | Oleanolic acid/betulinic acid |
| | *PgCYP716A141* | AOG74838 | *Platycodon grandiflorus* | β-Amyrin | C-16β-hydroxy, C-28 oxidation | Oleanolic acid, maniladiol, cochalic acid |
| | *BpCYP716A180* | KJ452328 | *Betula platyphylla* | Lupeol | C-28 oxidation | Betulinic acid |
| | *VvCYP716A17* | AB619803 | *Vitis vinifera* | β-Amyrin | C-28 oxidation | Oleanolic acid |
| | *PgCYP716A52v2* | JX036032 | *Panax ginseng* | β-Amyrin | C-28 oxidation | Oleanolic acid |
| | *MlCYP716A75* | KF318733 | *Maesa lanceolata* | β-Amyrin | C-28 oxidation | Oleanolic acid |
| | *CqCYP716A78* | KX343075 | *Chenopodium quinoa* | β-Amyrin | C-28 oxidation | Oleanolic acid |
| | *CqCYP716A79* | KX343076 | *Chenopodium quinoa* | β-Amyrin | C-28 oxidation | Oleanolic acid |
| | *KsCYP716A94* | KT150521 | *Kalopanax septemlobus* | β-Amyrin | C-28 oxidation | Oleanolic acid |
| | *AcCYP716A110* | KU878864 | *Aquilegia coerulea* | β-Amyrin | C-28 oxidation | Oleanolic acid |
| | *PgCYP716A140v2* | LC209199 | *Platycodon grandiflorus* | β-Amyrin | C-28 oxidation | Oleanolic acid |
| | *EsCYP716A244* | KX354739 | *Eleutherococcus senticosus* | β-Amyrin | C-28 oxidation | Oleanolic acid |
| | *AcCYP716A111* | KY047600 | *Aquilegia coerulea* | β-Amyrin | C-16 β-hydroxy | 16β-Hydroxy-β-amyrin |

(Continued)

| Category | *CYP* genes | GenBank ID | Organisms | Substrates | Reactions | Catalytic products |
|---|---|---|---|---|---|---|
| | *CaCYP716C11* | KU878852 | *Centella asiatica* | Ursolic acid/oleanolic acid/6β-hydroxy-oleanolic acid | C-2 α-hydroxy | Corosolic acid/maslinic acid/6β-hydroxy-maslinic acid |
| | *AmCYP716C53* | LC325362 | *Avicennia marina* | Oleanolic acid/ursolic acid | C-2 α-hydroxy | Maslinic acid/corosolic acid |
| | *LsCYP716C55* | MG708191 | *Lagerstroemia speciosa* | Ursolic acid/oleanolic acid | C-2 α-hydroxy | Corosolic acid/maslinic acid |
| | *SlCYP716E26* | XM_004241773 | *Solanum lycopersicum* | α-Amyrin/β-amyrin | C-6 β-hydroxy | 6β-Hydroxy-α-amyrin/daturadiol |
| | *CaCYP716E41* | KU878851 | *Centella asiatica* | Ursolic acid/oleanolic acid/maslinic acid | C-6 β-hydroxy | 6β-Hydroxy-ursolic acid/6β-hydroxy-oleanolic acid/6β-hydroxy-maslinic acid |
| | *PgCYP716S5* | KU878856 | *Platycodon grandiflorus* | β-Amyrin/oleanolic acid | C-12,13α-epoxy | 12,13α-Epoxy-β-amyrin/12,13α-epoxy-oleanolic acid |
| | *BfCYP716Y1* | KC963423 | *Bupleurum falcatum* | α-Amyrin/β-amyrin | C-16α-hydroxy | 16α-Hydroxy-α-amyrin/16α-hydroxy-β-amyrin |
| | *GuCYP88D6* | AB433179 | *Glycyrrhiza uralensis* | β-Amyrin | C-11 oxidation | 11-Oxo-β-amyrin |
| | *MtCYP88A13* | MN200611 | *Medicago truncatula* | Medicagenic acid | C-16 α-hydroxy | Zanhic acid |

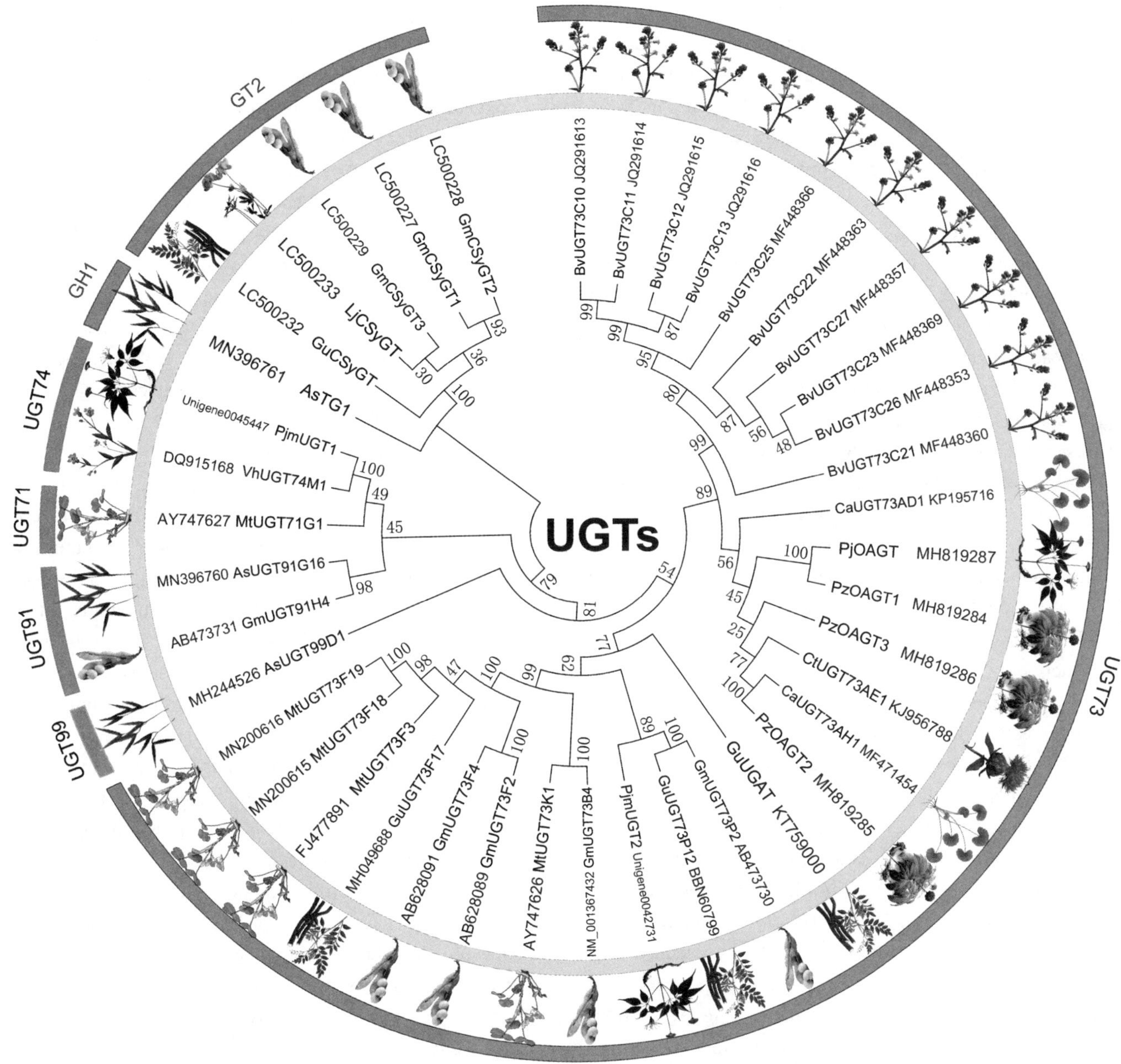


**Fig. 8 Phylogenetic tree of UGTs or enzymes with UGT activity involved in pentacyclic triterpenoid biosynthesis**

The MUSCLE method in the MEGA6.0 software was used to align the amino acid sequences of UGTs, the maximum likelihood method was then used to construct the phylogenetic tree, and the Bootstrap value was set to 1000. The catalytic substrates, catalytic products, references and other detailed information of UGTs are shown in Table 3. AsTG1 is not a member of the UGT family, but a glycosidase of GH1 with UGT activity. GuCSyGT, GmCSyGT1 - 3, and LjCSyGT are the cellulose synthase superfamily-derived glycosyltransferases of the GT2 family.

through phylogenetic analysis and *in vitro* biochemical research.

3.2 Functional analysis of the key enzymes in the biosynthesis of pentacyclic triterpenoids The biosynthetic pathway of triterpene saponins includes more than 20 consecutive enzymatic reactions, among which the upstream and midstream metabolic pathways from acetyl coenzyme A to 2,3-oxidosqualene have been clearly studied (Fig. 5). The key enzymes studied in this process mainly include *HMGR*, *FPS*, *SS*, and *SE*. However, the downstream metabolic pathways of triterpene saponin biosynthesis from OSCs, CYPs and UGTs to the final step of triterpene saponin formation have diverse functions in different plants. The mechanism is relatively complex and needs further exploration.

3.2.1 Functional analysis of OSCs. OSCs, as the first rate-limiting enzyme in the downstream synthetic stage of pentacyclic triterpene saponins, guide the cyclization of 2, 3-oxidosqualene to generate pentacyclic triterpene skeletons, which are further modified by CYP450s, UGTs and other enzymes to finally form a variety of pentacyclic triterpenoids. Currently, numerous OSC genes have been isolated and identified from a variety of plants.

We collected, sorted and summarized the GenBank accession numbers, organisms, catalytic products and other detailed information of the 96 identified *OSC* genes in Table 1, which demonstrates that the catalytic products of the *OSC* gene mainly include α-amyrin, β-amyrin, lupeol, friedelin, germanicol, taraxasterol, taraxerol, δ-amyrin, isoarborinol, and glutinol. In addition, a new multifunctional *OsOSC7* gene was discovered in *Oryza sativa* japonica, which could can 2,3-oxidosqualene into a new cationic orysatinyl through a 'chair-half chair-chair' conformational change, and then further generate a new pentacyclic triterpene called orysatinol.

3.2.2 Functional analysis of CYPs. CYPs are the largest enzyme family in plant metabolism and the key enzymes in the biosynthetic pathway of pentacyclic triterpene saponins, catalyzing the structural modification of the basic skeleton of pentacyclic triterpenes to generate the intermediates. The CYP450 genes that specifically regulate the biosynthesis of triterpene saponins are mainly distributed in the CYP51, CYP71, CYP72, and CYP85 families. The AsCYP51H10 enzyme gene of *Avena sativa* is a multifunctional CYP gene capable of modifying the C- and D-rings of the pentacyclic triterpene skeletons to generate 12, 13β-epoxy-3β and 16β-dihydroxy-oleanane, which is essential for the biosynthesis of oleanane-type pentacyclic triterpene saponins. The LjCYP71D353 gene of *Lotus japonicus* has the function of oxidizing lupane-type pentacyclic triterpenes, and catalyzes the hydroxylation of dihydrolupeol at the C-20 position to generate 20-hydroxylupeol. Meanwhile, LjCYP71D353 was also confirmed to generate 20-hydroxybetulinic acid by sequentially oxidizing the C-28 position of 20-hydroxylupeol in three steps. The BvCYP72A522 gene of *Barbarea vulgaris* has been confirmed by *in vitro* enzymatic reaction to catalyze the hydroxylation of oleanolic acid at the C-23 position. Owing to the complexity of the plant CYP450 enzyme catalytic reaction, the catalytic mechanism of CYP450 on pentacyclic triterpenoids has not been clarified. Besides, CYP450s in plants exist in the form of the gene superfamily, and their expression products are similar, which makes it difficult to isolate and purify them using traditional reverse genetics research methods.

We collected, sorted and summarized the GenBank accession numbers, catalytic substrates, catalytic products and other detailed information of the 65 identified CYP450 genes in Table 2. According to this table, the catalytic substrates of the CYP450 gene mainly include β-amyrin, 16β/24-hydroxy-β-amyrin, oleanolic acid, ursolic acid, 12, 13β-epoxy, α-amyrin, and lupeol, and the main catalytic products are oleanolic acid, ursolic acid, betulinic acid, 24-hydroxy-β-amyrin, 24-carboxy-β-amyrin, maslinic acid, corosolic acid, hederagenin, and soyasapogenol A and B. Moreover, the main reactions caused by CYP450 genes involve C-28 oxidation, C-24 oxidation, C-23 hydroxylation, C-24 hydroxylation, C-2α hydroxylation, and C-6β hydroxylation.

3.2.3 Functional analysis of UGTs. The glycosylation of pentacyclic triterpene catalyzed by UGTs is generally considered to be the last step in the biosynthesis of pentacyclic triterpenes and the key link in the diversity and bioactivity of pentacyclic triterpene saponins. The *UGT* gene belongs to the supergene family with diverse type and high specificity in organisms. Typical triterpene saponins contain 2-5 glycogens, usually forming glycans at the C-3 or C-28 positions of saponins, and there are also glycosylated triterpenoid saponins at the C-4, C-16, C-20, C-21, C-22 and C-23 positions. UGTs catalyze the connection of activated glycogens to different receptor molecules *in vivo*, and participate in various regulatory and metabolic pathways in plants by activating, inhibiting or regulating the solubility of a series of compounds. It was found that the *GuUGAT* gene in *G. uralensis* is co-expressed with amyrin synthase. *In vitro* experiments showed that *GuUGAT* could continuously catalyze the glucuronidated group added at C3-1 and C3-2 positions of glycyrrhetinic acid to finally generate glycyrrhizin. The catalytic activity of UGTs mostly comes from the *in vitro* catalysis of genes and heterologous expression products of *Escherichia coli* or yeast strains, which indicates that their catalytic substrates are diverse and complex. However, the *in vivo* activity characteristics of UGTs and the regulation of gene expression have rarely been reported. Thus, the substrates catalyzed by UGTs and their regulatory functions in the biosynthesis of pentacyclic triterpenes need to be further explored and verified.

We collected, sorted and summarized the GenBank accession numbers, catalytic substrates, catalytic products and other detailed information of the 41 *UGT*-related genes currently identified in Table 3. According to this table, the catalytic substrates of *UGT* genes mainly include β-amyrin, UDP-Glc, UDP-GlcA, oleanolic acid, betulinic acid, medicagenic acid, soyasapogenol A and B, asiatic acid, madecassic acid, hederagenin, 3-Glc-oleanolic acid, and glycyrrhetinic acid, and the main catalytic products are 3-Glc-β-amyrin, 3-Glc-oleanolic acid, 3-Glc-betulinic acid, 28-Glc-betulinic acid, 3-Glc-hederagenin, 3-Glc-28-Glc-oleanolic acid, 3-Glc-hederagenin, 3-Glc-medicagenic acid, oleanolic acid, and 3-*O*-glucoronide. Moreover, the main reactions caused by *UGT* genes involve C-28 glycosylation, C-3 glycosylation, C-22 glycosylation, C3 GlcA, and C3 Glc.

3.3 Transcriptional regulations of pentacyclic triterpenoids The accumulation of triterpenoid saponins in plants is often

**Table 3 *UGT*-related genes for pentacyclic triterpenoid biosynthesis**

| Category | UGT genes | GenBank ID | Organisms | Substrates | Reactions | Catalytic products |
|---|---|---|---|---|---|---|
| UGT71 | *MtUGT71G1* | AY747627 | *Medicago truncatula* | Medicagenic acid, UDP-Glc | Glycosylation | Medicagenic acid-Glc |
| UGT73 | *CaUGT73AD1* | KP195716 | *Centella asiatica* | Asiatic acid/madecassic acid, UDP-Glc | C-28β glycosylation | 28β-Glc-asiatic acid, 28β-Glc-madecassic acid |
| | *CtUGT73AE1* | KJ956788 | *Carthamus tinctorius* | Glycyrrhetinic acid, UDP-Glc | O/S/N glycosylation | Glycyrrhizin |
| | *CaUGT73AH1* | MF471454 | *Centella asiatica* | Asiatic acid, UDP-Glc | C-28 glycosylation | 28-Glc-asiatic acid |
| | *BvUGT73C10* | JQ291613 | *Barbarea vulgaris* | β-Amyrin/oleanolic acid/betulinic acid/hederagenin/3-Glc-oleanolic acid, UDP-Glc | C-3/C-28 glycosylation | 3-Glc-β-amyrin/3-Glc-oleanolic acid/3-Glc-betulinic acid/28-Glc-betulinic acid/3-Glc-hederagenin/3-Glc-28-Glc-oleanolic acid |
| | *BvUGT73C11* | JQ291614 | *Barbarea vulgaris* | β-Amyrin/oleanolic acid/betulinic acid/hederagenin, UDP-Glc | C-3/C-28 glycosylation | 3-Glc-β-amyrin/3-Glc-oleanolic acid/3-Glc-betulinic acid/3-Glc-hederagenin/28-Glc-betulinic acid |
| | *BvUGT73C12* | JQ291615 | *Barbarea vulgaris* | β-Amyrin/oleanolic acid/betulinic acid/hederagenin/3-Glc-oleanolic acid, 3-Glc-hederagenin, UDP-Glc | C-3/C-28 glycosylation | 3-Glc-β-amyrin/3-Glc-oleanolic acid/3-Glc-betulinic acid/28-Glc-betulinic acid/3-Glc-hederagenin/3-Glc-28-Glc-oleanolic acid/3-Glc-28-Glc-hederagenin/3-Glc-28-Glc-hederagenin/3-Glc-28-Glc-betulinic acid |
| | *BvUGT73C13* | JQ291616 | *Barbarea vulgaris* | β-Amyrin/oleanolic acid/betulinic acid/hederagenin/3-Glc-oleanolic-acid/3-Glc-hederagenin, UDP-Glc | C-3/C-28 glycosylation | 3-Glc-β-amyrin/3-Glc-oleanolic acid/3-Glc-betulinic acid/28-Glc-betulinic acid/3-Glc-hederagenin/3-Glc-28-Glc-oleanolic acid/3-Glc-28-Glc-betulinic acid |
| | *BvUGT73C22* | MF448363 | *Barbarea vulgaris* | Oleanolic acid/hederagenin, UDP-Glc | C-3/C-28 glycosylation | 3-Glc-oleanolic acid/3-Glc-28-Gle-oleanolic acid/3-Glc-28-Glc-hederagenin/28-Glchederagenin/28-Glc-oleanolic acid |
| | *BvUGT73C23* | MF448369 | *Barbarea vulgaris* | Oleanolic acid/hederagenin, UDP-Glc | C-3/C-28 glycosylation | 3-Glc-oleanolic acid/3-Glc-28-Glc-oleanolic acid/3-Glchederagenin/3-Glc-28-GlcHederagenin/3-glc-23-glchederagenin |
| | *BvUGT73C25* | MF448366 | *Barbarea vulgaris* | Oleanolic acid/hederagenin, UDP-Glc | C-3/C-23/C-28 glycosylation | 3-Glc-oleanolic acid/3-Glc-28-Glc-oleanolic acid/3-Glchederagenin/3-glc-23-glc-hederagenin |
| | *BvUGT73C21* | MF448360 | *Barbarea vulgaris* | Oleanolic acid/hederagenin, UDP-Glc | C-3 glycosylation | 3-Glc-oleanolic acid/3-Glc-hederagenin |
| | *BvUGT73C26* | MF448353 | *Barbarea vulgaris* | Oleanolic acid/hederagenin, UDP-Glc | C-3 glycosylation | 3-Glc-oleanolic acid/3-Glc-hederagenin |
| | *BvUGT73C27* | MF448357 | *Barbarea vulgaris* | Oleanolic acid/hederagenin, UDP-Glc | C-3 glycosylation | 3-Glc-oleanolic acid/3-Glc-hederagenin |
| | *MtUGT73F18* | MN200615 | *Medicago truncatula* | Medicagenic acid | C-3 glycosylation | 3-Glc-medicagenic acid |
| | *MtUGT73F19* | MN200616 | *Medicago truncatula* | Medicagenic acid/gypsogenic acid | C-3 glycosylation | 3-Glc-medicagenic acid/3-Glc-gypsogenic acid |
| | *PjOAGT* | MH819287 | *Panax japonicus* | Oleanolic acid, UDP-GlcA | C-3 glycosylation | Oleanolic acid, 3-*O*-glucoronide |
| | *PzOAGT1* | MH819284 | *Panax zingiberensis* | Oleanolic acid, UDP-GlcA | C-3 glycosylation | Oleanolic acid, 3-*O*-glucoronide |

(Continued)

| Category | *UGT* genes | GenBank ID | Organisms | Substrates | Reactions | Catalytic products |
|---|---|---|---|---|---|---|
| | *PzOAGT2* | MH819285 | *Panax zingiberensis* | Oleanolic acid, UDP-GlcA | C-3 glycosylation | Oleanolic acid, 3-*O*-glucoronide |
| | *PzOAGT3* | MH819286 | *Panax zingiberensis* | Oleanolic acid, UDP-GlcA | C-3 glycosylation | Oleanolic acid, 3-*O*-glucoronide |
| | *GuUGAT* | KT759000 | *Glycyrrhiza uralensis* | Glycyrrhetinic acid/3-GlcA-glycyrrhetinic acid, UDP-GlcA | C-3 glycosylation | 3-GlcA-glycyrrhetinic acid/glycyrrhizin |
| | *GmUGT73F2* | AB628089 | *Glycine max* | Saponin A0-gα, UDP-Glc | C-22 glycosylation | Saponin Ab |
| | *MtUGT73F3* | FJ477891 | *Medicago truncatula* | Hederagenin/soyasapogenol A/soyasapogenol B/bayogenin/medicagenic acid, UDP-Glc | C-28/C-3 glycosylation | Hederagenin-C28-*O*-Glc/soyasapogenol A-Glc/soyasapogenol B-Glc/bayogeninC28-*O*-Glc/medicagenic acid-C28-*O*-Glc |
| | *GmUGT73F4* | AB628091 | *Glycine max* | Saponin A0-αg, UDP-Xyl | C-22 glycosylation | Saponin Aa |
| | *GmUGT73B4* | NM_001367432 | *Glycine max* | Soyasapogenol B/soyasaponin I, UDP-Glc/UDP-Gal | C-22 glycosylation | 22-Glc-soyasapogenol B, 22-Gal-soyasapogenol B, 22-Glc-soyasaponin I, 22-Gal-soyasaponin I |
| | *GuUGT73F17* | MH049688 | *Glycyrrhiza uralensis* | Glycyrrhizin, UDP-Glc | C-30/C-29 glycosylation | Licorice-saponin A3 |
| | *MtUGT73K1* | AY747626 | *Medicago truncatula* | Hederagenin/soyasapogenol B/soyasapogenol E, UDP-Glc | Glycosylation | Hederagenin-Glc, soyasapogenol B-Glc, soyasapogenol *E*-Glc |
| | *GmUGT73P2* | AB473730 | *Glycine max* | Soyasapogenol B/3-*O*-glucuronide, UDP-Gal | C-3 glycosylation | Soyasaponin III |
| | *GuUGT73P12* | BBN60799 | *Glycyrrhiza uralensis* | 3-*O*-gluconic acid-glycyrrhetinic acid | C3-2 GlcA | Glycyrrhizin, glycyrrhetinic acid 3-*O*-monoglucuronide |
| | *PjmUGT2* | Unigene 0042731 | *Panax japonicus* | Oleanolic acid 3-*O*-β-D-glucuronide and chikusetsusaponin IVa | C-28 glycosylation | Zingibroside R1, ginsenoside Ro |
| UGT74 | *PjmUGT1* | Unigene 0045447 | *Panax japonicus* | Oleanolic acid 3-*O*-β-D-glucuronide and zingibroside R1 | C-28 glycosylation | Chikusetsusaponin IVa, ginsenoside Ro |
| | *VhUGT74M1* | DQ915168 | *Vaccaria hispanica* | Gypsogenic acid/betulinic acid/hederagenin/ypsogenin/echinocystic acid/16α-hydroxygypsogenic acid/quillaic acid, UDP-Glc | C-28 glycosylation | 28-Glc-gypsogenic acid/28-Glc-betulinic acid/28-Glchederagenin/28-Glc-gypsogenin/28-Glc-echinocystic acid/28-Glc-16α-29-hydroxygypsogenic acid/28-Glcquillaic acid |
| UGT91 | *AsUGT91G16* | MN396760 | *Avena strigosa* | 3-*O*-arabinose-12, 13-epoxy-16β-hydroxy-β-amyrin | C3-2 Glc | 3β-{[β-D-glucopyranosyl-(1 → 2)-α-L-arabinopyranosyl]oxy}-12, 13β-epoxy, 16β-hydroxy-β-amyrin |
| | *GmUGT91H4* | AB473731 | *Glycine max* | Soyasaponin III, UDP-Rha | C-3 glycosylation | Soyasaponin I |
| UGT99 | *AsUGT99D1*/*AsAAT1* | MH244526 | *Avena strigosa* | 12,13β-Epoxy-16β-hydroxy-β-amyrin | C3-1 Ara | Bisdeglucosyl avenacin A-1 |

(Continued)

| Category | *UGT* genes | GenBank ID | Organisms | Substrates | Reactions | Catalytic products |
|---|---|---|---|---|---|---|
| GH1 | *AsTG1* | MN396761 | *Avena strigosa* | 3-*O*-Arabinose-glucose-12,13-epoxy-16β-hydroxy-β-amyrin | C3-3 Glc | 3β-{[β-D-glucopyranosyl-(1 → 2)-[β-D-glucopyranosyl-(1→4)]-α-L-arabinopyranosyl]oxy}-12-keto,16β-hydroxy-β-amyrin |
| GT2 | *GuCSyGT* | LC500232 | *Glycyrrhiza uralensis* | Glycyrrhetinic acid, soyasapogenol A, soyasapogenol B | C3 GlcA | Glycyrrhetinic acid-3-*O*-monoglucuronide, soyasapogenol A-3-*O*-monoglucuronide, soyasapogenol B-3-*O*-monoglucuronide |
| | *LjCSyGT* | LC500233 | *Lotus japonicus* | Glycyrrhetinic acid, soyasapogenol A, soyasapogenol B | C3 GlcA | Glycyrrhetinic acid-3-*O*-monoglucuronide, soyasapogenol A-3-*O*-monoglucuronide, soyasapogenol B-3-*O*-monoglucuronide |
| | *GmCSyGT1* | LC500227 | *Glycine max* | Glycyrrhetinic acid, soyasapogenol A, soyasapogenol B | C3 GlcA | Glycyrrhetinic acid-3-*O*-monoglucuronide, soyasapogenol A-3-*O*-monoglucuronide, Soyasapogenol B-3-*O*-monoglucuronide |
| | *GmCSyGT2* | LC500228 | *Glycine max* | Glycyrrhetinic acid, soyasapogenol A, soyasapogenol B | C3 GlcA | Glycyrrhetinic acid-3-*O*-monoglucuronide, soyasapogenol A-3-*O*-monoglucuronide, Soyasapogenol B-3-*O*-monoglucuronide |
| | *GmCSyGT3* | LC500229 | *Glycine max* | Glycyrrhetinic acid, soyasapogenol A, soyasapogenol B | C3 GlcA | Glycyrrhetinic acid-3-*O*-monoglucuronide, Soyasapogenol A-3-*O*-monoglucuronide, Soyasapogenol B-3-*O*-monoglucuronide |

influenced by their growth environment. Environmental factors such as light, temperature, humidity, salt, soil and exogenous plant hormone elicitors such as methyl jasmonate (MeJA), salicylic acid (SA), auxin, abscisic acid (ABA) and gibberellin (GA) are common influencing factors. After plants are stressed by environmental factors and elicitors, the differential expression of key rate-limiting enzyme genes such as *HMGR*, *FPS*, *SS*, and *SE* in the body increases the accumulation of secondary metabolites to respond to stress and reduce the damage to the plants. In this process, transcription factors (TFs) activate or inhibit the expression of key rate-limiting enzyme genes by binding to their promoters, thereby affecting the accumulation of triterpenoid saponins. Besides, miRNAs target key rate-limiting enzyme genes or TFs at the post-transcriptional level through splicing and translation control or other modes of action, and ultimately regulate the biosynthesis of pentacyclic triterpenoids.

3.3.1 Elicitors and environmental factors. *HMGR*, as the first important rate-limiting enzyme and important regulatory site in the MVA pathway, plays an important role in the biosynthesis of triterpene saponins in medicinal plants. Wang *et al*. revealed the ultrahigh production of oleanolic acid in the shoot of *Achyranthes bidentata* of 371.8 mg $L^{-1}$, a 5.4-fold increase compared to the control after 2 days treatment of 0.2 mM MeJA, while the *AbHMGR* gene was expressed at a higher level, which suggested that oleanolic acid production may be the result of the up-regulated expression of *AbHMGR*. Additionally, auxin, SA, and GA were also reported to regulate the *HMGR* gene, thus affecting the biosynthesis of pentacyclic triterpenoids. *FPS* is a key enzyme that regulates the synthesis of terpenoid precursors such as IPP and DMAPP in the MVA pathway. The *FPS* gene is not only an important rate-limiting enzyme gene in the synthesis of triterpenes, but also guides the flow direction of carbon and precursors. Yin *et al*. revealed that the expression of *BpFPS* in birch leaves and bark promoted an increase in the squalene content of triterpenoid precursor, thus achieving a significant increase in betulinic acid, oleanolic acid and betulin content. *SS* catalyzes FPP to synthesize squalene (SQ), which is a key step in the biosynthesis of triterpene saponins. *SS* has a strong regulatory function in the biosynthesis of triterpene saponins and phytosterols. The treatment of MeJA on the adventitious roots of *P. ginseng* can induce the up-regulation of *SS* gene expression, which proceeds to the next step to significantly enhance the expression levels of *SE* and *βAS* genes. Furthermore, SA, cold stress and shading percentage were verified to affect the accumulation of pentacyclic triterpenoids by regulating the *SS* gene. *SE*, as one of the key enzymes in the biosynthetic pathway of triterpene saponins, catalyzes the epoxidation of SQ by inserting an oxygen source between C=C to generate 2,3-oxidosqualene. Su *et al*. found that the total saponin content dramatically increased (up to 2.49-fold) with the addition of 5 mg $L^{-1}$ SA in hairy roots for 1 day compared to the control. Furthermore, MeJA and fungal elicitor could regulate the expression of the *SE* gene, thereby influencing the biosynthesis of triterpene saponins.

3.3.2 Regulation by transcription factors. TFs, also known as trans-acting factors, can simultaneously participate in the expression and regulation of multiple key genes in terpenoid metabolism-related gene clusters. Thus, TFs are an ideal strategy for microbial cell factories to enhance the efficiency of the target compound synthesis. It is worth noting that there are different TF systems in plants and microorganisms. Studying the functions of key TFs in terpenoid synthesis is of great significance for further elucidating the biosynthetic pathway of pentacyclic triterpenoids. Currently, there are mainly six TF families reported to be related to terpenoid metabolism in plants, including AP2/ERF, bHLH, WRKY, bZIP, MYB and NAC (NAM, ATAF1/2, and CUC2). Among them, AP2/ERF, bHLH, WRKY, bZIP, and MYB have been reported to mainly regulate the biosynthesis of plant triterpenoids.

Besides the above-mentioned elements, miRNA plays an important role in the post-transcriptional regulation of key enzyme genes in the biosynthesis of pentacyclic triterpenoids. miRNA mainly regulates the expression of target genes through splicing and translation control. Besides, they are the main biological factors that regulate the production of secondary metabolites in many plants and play an important role in regulating the biosynthesis and decomposition of secondary metabolites in plants. miRNA can only bind to a special site in the untranslated region at the 3′ end of its target gene, thereby further inhibiting the expression of genes that play a regulatory role in the translation process. miRNA generally affects the biosynthesis of plant triterpenoid saponins by regulating the expression of rate-limiting enzyme genes in the MVA pathway, as reported in previous studies. Therefore, it is also crucial to study the post-transcriptional regulation of miRNAs on key enzyme genes and related TFs in the biosynthesis of triterpenoid saponins.

However, the research on the relationship among miRNA, key enzyme genes and TFs in the MVA pathway for regulating the biosynthesis of pentacyclic triterpenoids is still in its infancy. Thus far, there have been few reports on this regulatory mechanism, and only functional predictions have been made. With the rapid development of high-throughput sequencing technology and bioinformatics, more and more plant miRNAs have been predicted, and the regulation of miRNAs in the biosynthesis of triterpenoids is becoming a hot spot, with broad research space in the future.

## 4 STRATEGIES FOR INCREASING THE ACCUMULATION OF TRITERPENOID SAPONINS *VIA* HETEROLOGOUS BIOSYNTHESIS

Most pentacyclic triterpenoids come from valuable, rare and slow-growing plants, which are difficult to directly extract from plants. Also, due to their structural complexity with multiple chiral centers, the steps for their chemical synthesis are inefficient, costly and highly toxic, making it difficult to achieve their mass production. Accordingly, heterologous plants have become an important way to synthesize target products, which overcome the synthetic problems. As the production chassis of plant natural products, plants have many natural advantages, such as photosynthesis system, extremely rich enzyme library (cytochrome P450) and the existence of various cell compartments, which can decompose the complete pathway into independent components, and simultaneously optimize the conditions such as reactions and precursor compounds in each cell compartment. Although the transformation of metabolic engineering technology in plants can increase the output of target natural products, this method also suffers from many drawbacks such as long cycle, high cost and low efficiency. Microbial cell factories have gradually become a new method for the efficient synthesis of natural products, presenting a way for the large-scale and industrialization of pentacyclic triterpenoids. The synthesis of target products by heterologous hosts of *E. coli* and *S. cerevisiae* has many advantages, such as rapid growth, short cycle, simple nutritional requirements, easy extraction and separation, and mature and reliable genetic manipulation methods. Terpenoids, flavonoids, alkaloids and other primary or secondary metabolites from different sources such as plants, fungi and symbiotic microorganisms have been successfully biosynthesized in heterologous hosts. Recently, with the development of synthetic biology, major breakthroughs have been made in the heterologous biosynthesis of pentacyclic triterpenoids. For instance, pentacyclic triterpenoids such as oleanolic acid, taraxasterol, soyasaponins Ⅰ and Ⅲ, 3-*O*-glucose-oleanolic acid, 3-*O*-glucose-glycyrrhetinic acid and calenduloside E have been successfully synthesized in *Nicotiana benthamiana*, *Nicotiana tabacum*, *E. coli* and *S. cerevisiae*.

The use of synthetic biology to produce natural products with medicinal value has received increasing attention. Heterologous biosynthesis brings opportunities and strong support for the large-scale production and sustainable supply of natural products. However, it is still a challenging task to achieve an industrialized yield of target products through heterologous synthesis. Elucidating the key enzyme reaction mechanism responsible for the formation of unique chemical structures and bioactive centers is the core content of natural product biosynthesis, while the key enzyme reaction mechanism in the biosynthetic pathway of some natural products remains unascertained. Meanwhile, chassis cells are very complex systems, and the introduction of exogenous pathways will cause a series of reactions in the chassis system, including growth rate regulation, heat shock response, stress response, and stringent response, which will lead to the instability of plasmid, cell lysis and changes in the cellular genetic information, resulting in the inability to synthesize the target product or extremely low yield. Therefore, based on the existing research results, we propose some optimization strategies to improve the biosynthetic yield of natural products and modify and optimize biosynthetic pathways, regulatory factors, exogenous metabolic pathways, feature elements, chassis cell systems, fermentation conditions, *etc.*, to achieve a high yield of the target products. The heterologous biosynthetic pathways of pentacyclic triterpenoid saponins are presented in Fig. 9.

### 4.1 Host selection for heterologous biosynthesis

When choosing a heterologous host, factors such as the host metabolism and the feasibility of using genetic technology in the heterologous host should be considered, and similarity between gene expression and cellular environment is conducive for better adaptation to the remodeling of heterologous metabolic pathways. Heterologous plant expression systems can produce correctly folded active enzymes and utilize light energy to biosynthesize natural products, but plant metabolic systems are more complex than microorganisms, which is not easy to scale up industrially for cell culture and is difficult for large-scale production. With the development of synthetic biology, the reconstruction of important plant metabolic pathways in microorganisms has become a research hotspot. Microbial *de novo* synthesis or semi-synthesis of various natural products has been achieved through metabolic pathway optimization, candidate gene library screening, gene function identification, multifactorial expression regulation, *etc*. At present, the hosts of heterologous biosynthesis mainly include heterologous plants, *E. coli*, *S. cerevisiae* and *Pichia pastoris*. The selection of the heterologous host is an important link in the heterologous biosynthesis of natural products.

**4.1.1 Plant cells as the chassis.** The biosynthetic pathways of most plant natural substances are complex and include many membrane-bound proteins that require special intracellular infrastructure, which make it challenging to transfer this synthetic mechanism to other organisms. Compared with microbial hosts, heterologous plant hosts exhibit a more similar microenvironment to the host plant in terms of heterologous protein expression and have similar core metabolic pathways, which provide a natural supply of precursors for downstream biosynthetic pathways. However,

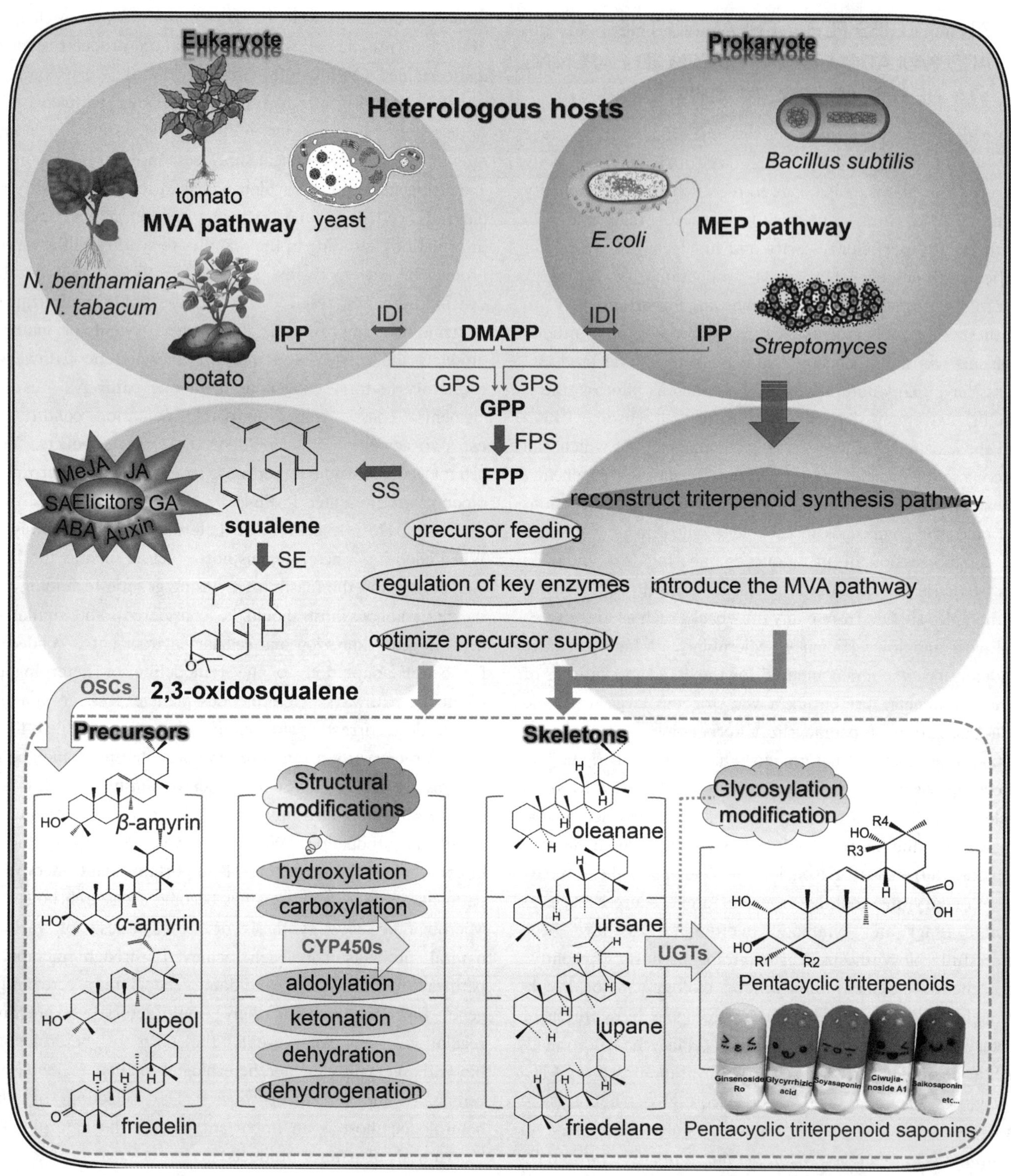


**Fig. 9 Heterologous biosynthetic pathway of pentacyclic triterpenoid saponins**

heterologous plant expression systems have long production cycles, often lack robust and well-established genome engineering methods, and exhibit complex metabolite backgrounds, which may lead to difficulties in isolating target phytochemicals. Most plant hosts are genetically intractable, and there are no mature molecular biology tools to express heterologous genes. Therefore, only a few heterologous model plants are commonly used for the production of natural products.

*N. tabacum* and *N. benthamiana* are often used as heterologous plant hosts to synthesize natural products. *N. benthamiana* is the most common heterologous plant, and its leaves have large biomass and relatively mature genetic transformation, which are suitable for bioreactors to produce compounds with medicinal value. Thus far, a variety of natural products have been produced in *N. benthamiana* by transient co-expression. Stephenson *et al*. described a detailed protocol for the rapid (5 days) preparative-scale production of about 15 pentacyclic triterpenoids, such as β-amyrin and oleanolic acid, in *N. benthamiana* utilizing this powerful plant-based platform, and they previously isolated yields of β-amyrin derivatives from their combinatorial biosynthetic experiments ranging from 0.12 to 3.87 mg $g^{-1}$ of dry leaf powder in *N. benthamiana*. Choi *et al*. revealed that the ectopic expression of both the *LsOSC1* and *LsTAT1* genes in yeast and *N. tabacum* could produce pentacyclic triterpenoids, such as taraxasterol acetate, ψ-taraxasterol acetate, β-amyrin acetate, and α-amyrin acetate. Han *et al*. established the heterologous production of multiple pentacyclic triterpenes in transgenic *N. tabacum* by over-expressing the *TcOSC1* gene from *Taraxacum coreanum*. All the lines of transgenic *N. tabacum* produced five new triterpenes, namely, taraxasterol, ψ-taraxasterol, δ-amyrin, β-amyrin, and α-amyrin, with the total amount of triterpenes ranging from 401.3 to 617.7 μg/g DW in the leaves of all the Tr4 transgenic lines. Today, many biosynthetic pathways have been recreated in *N. tabacum* and *N. benthamiana* for the synthesis of various compounds, including sesquiterpenes, monoterpenes, diterpenes, and flavonoids. In addition, as a well-studied model organism with relatively well-established molecular biology techniques, tomato has been used to produce taxadiene, a biosynthetic precursor of the anti-cancer agent paclitaxel (taxol). Moreover, *Solanum tuberosum*, *Cichorium intybus*, *Lactuca sativa*, and *Physcomitrella patens* are also used as hosts for the heterologous expression of the target products. However, there are few reports on the heterologous synthesis of pentacyclic triterpenoids from other plants besides *N. tabacum* and *N. benthamiana*.

Compared with heterologous microorganisms, due to the challenges encountered in engineering plant transformation, the strength of plants as the chassis for the production of natural products is largely underestimated. Plant hosts have many natural advantages, such as the photosynthesis system, extremely rich enzyme library, and various cell compartments, whih are better than microorganisms. Therefore, employing plants as the chassis has great potential for production and application and using plant synthetic biology to realize the rapid and sustainable production of high-value plant natural products shows the important role and great potential of plant chassis in industrial production. We speculate that the plant chassis as a sustainable heterologous host will be an important way to synthesize natural products in the future.

4.1.2 Eukaryotic microbes as the chassis. *S. cerevisiae* functions a model eukaryotic cell that not only has the characteristics of fast reproduction, easy culture and convenient genetic engineering operation of prokaryotes, but also has the functions of protein processing and post-translational modification of eukaryotes. In particular, compared with *E. coli*, *S. cerevisiae* is more suitable for the functional expression of the plant CYP450 protein. Besides, *S. cerevisiae* also has many advantages such as high stress resistance, high substrate tolerance, and strong metabolic capacity, and thus has unique advantages as a heterologous synthetic host for natural products. In addition, its genetic background is relatively clear, and its genetic manipulation has been systematized and standardized, making it easy to perform heterologous synthesis. Li *et al*. reconstituted the whole biosynthetic pathway of tunicosaponin aglycones in *S. cerevisiae* by transforming the platform strain BY-bAS with the *CYP716A262* and *CYP716A567* genes, and the resulting strain could produce 146.84 and 314.01 mg/L of gypsogenin and quillaic acid, respectively. Yu *et al*. obtained the highest yield of α-amyrin in engineered *S. cerevisiae* by remodeling αAS MdOSC1 and expanding the storage pool. The yield of α-amyrin increased to 11-fold higher than that of the control.

However, the conventional expression system of *S. cerevisiae* has some problems, such as low fermentation density, poor protein secretion ability, lack of strong promoter, and side effects that may be caused by excessive glycosylation modification, which has been gradually replaced by new yeast hosts, especially *P. pastoris* in recent years.

*P. pastoris* is a new type of eukaryotic expression system developed in recent years, which uses methanol as the only energy and carbon source, contains a unique and powerful promoter of alcohol oxidase gene (AOX), and possesses low culture cost and easy separation of products. Meanwhile, methanol can strictly regulate the expression of exogenous genes. In addition, the exogenous protein genes of *P. pastoris* are genetically stable and the exogenous genes can be integrated into the *P. pastoris* genome in a high copy number, which is not easy to be lost and can be highly expressed in strains. As a eukaryotic expression system, *P. pastoris* has the subcellular structure of eukaryotes and post-translational modification processing functions such as glycosylation, fatty acylation, and protein phosphorylation. Lu *et al*. provided an effective strategy to enhance metabolites by *P. pastoris* treatment in adventitious roots of *G. uralensis*. In their study, the highest concentration of glycyrrhizic acid (0.62 mg/g) and glycyrrhetinic acid (0.29 mg/g) was obtained in 200 mg/L of *P. pastoris*, which was 3.89-fold and 2.42-fold greater than the control group, respectively. Liu *et al*. successfully constructed a dammarenediol-Ⅱ producing *P. pastoris* strain by introducing *PgDDS* from *P. ginseng* to *P. pastoris*. By increasing the expression of *ERG1* and downregulating the expression of *ERG7*, the yield of dammarenediol-Ⅱ increased from 0.03 to 0.736 mg/g dry cell weight (DCW). Finally, the yield of dammarenediol-Ⅱ reached up to 1.073 mg/g DCW by adding extra supplementation of 0.5 g/L squalene to the culture medium. However, the *P. pastoris* system also has some defects, such as the existence of aggregates, internal degradation, glycosylation of exogenous proteins, and incomplete processing of signal peptides, which bring certain difficulties in the synthesis of the target products.

4.1.3 Prokaryotic microbes as the chassis. As a model microorganism, *E. coli* has a clear genetic background, mature and reliable genetic manipulation methods, rapid growth, and a short fermentation period (2 to 3 days). The simple relatively linear terpenoid synthetic pathway does not substantially avoid triterpenoid precursors. However, the preference of *E. coli* for codon usage is very different from that of eukaryotes, which limits its application in heterologous synthesis to a certain extent. Li *et al*. reconstructed the synthetic pathway of dammarediol, the key precursor of ginsenosides in *E. coli*, and realized the heterologous *de novo* synthesis of tetracyclic triterpenoid dammarediol in a yield of 8.63 mg/L. At present, there are few reports on the heterologous biosynthesis of triterpenoids in *E. coli*. Reconstructing the triterpenoid biosynthetic pathway by means of genetic transformation, introduction of exogenous MVA pathway and regulatory elements, and increasing the supply of precursors will promote the efficient biosynthesis of triterpenoid precursors in *E. coli*.

*B. subtilis* has been used as a model strain and excellent chassis cell for studying bacterial genetics and cell metabolism owing to its clear physiological and biochemical characteristics, simple genetic operation, strong secretion and expression ability, convenient culture and fermentation, *etc*. *B. subtilis*, as a heterologous host, can secrete recombinant proteins extracellularly, and it has no special preference for codon usage, which makes it better to express genes from eukaryotes, and it can secrete the synthesized proteins directly into the medium. Furthermore, *B. subtilis* grows faster, which is conducive to shorten the product synthetic cycle. At present, there is a set of mature and reliable molecular biology tools for the genetic and metabolic engineering of *B. subtilis*. A variety of natural products can be biosynthesized by *B. subtilis*, which functions as natural producer of some terpenoids. However, *B. subtilis* has certain drawbacks, and one of the bottlenecks is the lack of stable plasmid vectors for introducing exogenous genes or gene clusters into cells. Meanwhile, there are some problems such as the toxicity and high price of inducers, which limit the application potential of *B. subtilis* in industrial production. Shen *et al*. semi-synthesized five glycyrrhetinic acid derivatives *via* a series of chemical reactions, which were selected as substrates for biotransformation and yielded 13 metabolites in *B. subtilis*. Recently, some important progress has been achieved in the biosynthesis of natural products using *B. subtilis*. However, there are few reports on the biosynthesis of triterpenoids from *B. subtilis*, which needs further breakthroughs.

Compared with eukaryotic hosts, *E. coli* lacks post transcriptional modification, endoplasmic reticulum and auxiliary P450 reductase, which makes it difficult to functionally express plant-derived CYP450. More efforts will be required to address the functional expression of plant-derived genes. Similar to *E. coli*, the functional expression of plant-derived CYP450 needs to be solved before realizing *B. subtilis* as a promising host for pentacyclic triterpenoid overproduction. Besides, most of the enzymes involved in the biosynthesis of triterpenoids are membrane-bound, such OSCs and CYPs, which is a central problem regarding their production in prokaryotes, lacking suitable membrane systems.

4.1.4 Other heterologous hosts as the chassis. In addition to the above-mentioned hosts, *Streptomyces* is also one of the commonly used hosts for heterologous synthesis, which can produce anti-bacterial, anti-fungal, antibiotics and a wide range of bioactive substances such as immunosuppressants and anti-cancer agents. Moreover, it possesses the precursor metabolic pathways of these classes of natural products and is one of the ideal hosts for the heterologous synthesis of natural products. The terpene compound botryococcene has been expressed in several microorganisms, and the yield obtained in *Streptomyces* was 212±20 mg $L^{-1}$ (ref.) compared with 60 mg $L^{-1}$ in yeast. Thus, the natural biological elements, modification systems, and antibiotic resistance-tolerance systems in *Streptomyces* comprise a substantial advantage for natural product discovery and overexpression. Ghimire *et al*. cloned genes encoding enzymes with sequence similarity to hopanoid biosynthetic enzymes of the hopanoid (hop) gene cluster from *Streptomyces peucetius* ATCC 27 952 and transformed them into *Streptomyces venezuelae* YJ028. Finally, the pentacyclic triterpenoid lipid, namely, hopene, was successfully synthesized *via* the YJ028 strain. At present, some *Streptomyces* strains such as *S. coelicolor*, *S. erythraea*, and *S. avermitilis* have completed whole genome sequencing and established standard genetic manipulation procedures, which facilitate the heterologous synthesis of natural products. However, the defects of *Streptomyces*, such as slow growth, complex life history and relatively difficult genetic manipulation, must also be considered in determining whether it can be selected as a heterologous host.

In addition to *Streptomyces*, other microorganisms have currently been used as hosts for the heterologous synthesis of natural products, such as *Pseudomonas*, *Sorangium cellulosum* and *Myxococcus xanthus*. In the case of fungi, *Aspergillus niger*, *Aspergillus nidulans*, *etc*. function as heterologous hosts, but few related studies have been reported on triterpene saponins thus far.

4.2 Mining and optimizing feature elements The biosynthetic pathways of natural products are usually relatively complex, including multiple key enzymes and regulatory genes, and the key enzyme reactions and regulation mechanisms are the core content of natural product biosynthesis. Identifying and optimizing the key gene elements in the biosynthetic pathway of plant natural products is the core and mainstream of applying synthetic biology technology to modernize the production mode of natural products. Promoter replacement, optimization of the gene copy number, and codon usage are commonly employed to improve gene expression. In recent years, these methods have been applied in the pathway optimization of many natural products.

4.2.1 Promoter modification. The promoter structure will affect its affinity with RNA polymerase, thus affecting the transcription efficiency of the promoter to the gene, and the intensity of the promoter determines the transcriptional intensity of the structural genes. Studies have shown that the modification of the promoter, such as mutating it, changing the length of its sequence and replacing it with a stronger promoter, can regulate the expression efficiency of related enzyme genes in the metabolic pathway. Lu *et al*. revealed that the multifunctional amyrin synthase gene (*CrMAS*) from *Catharanthus roseus* was controlled by PGK1 and GAL1 promoters. ScLCZ03 and ScLCZ06 of *S. cerevisiae* strains were generated by the introduction of *CrMAS* genes into the chromosomes of the *S. cerevisiae* strain WTE at the rDNA sites, and the ScLCZ03 strain produced 1.51 g/L α-amyrin and 0.46 mg/L β-amyrin, while the ScLCZ06 strain accumulated 5.64 mg/L α-amyrin and 1.64 mg/L β-amyrin, which indicated that the GAL1 promoter is more beneficial for amyrin production than the PGK1 promoter. Therefore, the use of the GAL1 promoter is a strategy to increase the accumulation of pentacyclic triterpenoids. Li *et al*. developed a biosynthetic method to produce soyasapo-genol B by expressing βAS derived from *G. glabra* in *S. cerevisiae* and adopting several different types of promoters to regulate the expression of key genes in the MVA pathway. Ultimately, this increased the yield of β-amyrin to 17.6 mg/L, which was 25-fold greater than that produced in the original strain L01 (0.68 mg/L).

4.2.2 Modulating gene copies. During the heterologous biosynthesis of terpenoids, it is an important method to enhance the product expression by modulating the multi-copy target genes. Increasing the copy number of genes by cloning them into multi-copy expression plasmid is one of the most commonly used tools to regulate the expression of heterologous genes in the chassis system, which can promote the high-level expression of genes. It is worth noting that the best optimization effect can be achieved only when the plasmid copy number is within a reasonable range due to the metabolic bottlenecks that arise from imbalances in the pathway flux. Furthermore, the use of multi-copy genes to overexpress ratelimiting enzyme genes often imposes a metabolic burden on bacteria, and the plasmids are unstable and easily lost, whereas the direct regulation of genes in the genome can avoid these problems. Li *et al*. performed multi-copy expression of MVA pathway-related genes with homologous recombination, and they overexpressed *ERG1*, *ERG9*, and *ERG20* genes together with *t1HMG1* at multiple copies of the zeta locus to obtain the YL-OA4-7 strain. Finally, the maximum oleanolic acid production (92.1 mg/L) was achieved with YL-OA7, corresponding to a 5.65-fold increase from the level achieved with *Y. lipolytica*. Besides, compared with rDNA sites, the integration efficiency of the zeta sites significantly improved, and the effect was more obvious with an increase in recombinant fragments. In recent years, some new technologies have been developed to competently solve the problems caused by multi-copy genes. Shi *et al*. developed a simple Di-CRISPR (delta integration CRISPR-Cas) platform for the high-efficiency, single-step, markerless, multi-copy chromosomal integration of full biochemical pathways in *S. cerevisiae*. They harnessed the CRISPR-Cas system to specifically generate double stranded breaks (DSBs) at the delta sites in the chromosomes of *S. cerevisiae* to increase homologous recombination efficiency, which enabled the single-step, multi-copy and markerless integration of DNA constructs ranging from 8 kb to 24 kb with high efficiencies. Bourgeois *et al*. developed a simple and highly characterized CRISPR-Cas9 integration system called the Landing Pad (LP) System for multi-copy gene integration in *S. cerevisiae*, which introduced a series of synthetic DNA LPs in the *S. cerevisiae* genome to act as sites for high-level gene integration and improved the efficiency of multicopy gene integration. LPs facilitate multicopy gene integration in a single transformation, thus providing precise control of the DNA copy number. Wang *et al*. revealed that a large number of tandem duplications occurred in the triterpenoid saponin-modifying enzyme genes in the genome of *Aralia elata*, resulting in the accumulation of rich and diverse pentacyclic triterpenoid saponins. They *de novo* synthesized more than 13 pentacyclic triterpenoid aralosides with different structures through the heterologous biosynthetic pathway using *S. cerevisiae* as the chassis cells, which facilitated the heterologous bioproduction of aralosides.

4.2.3 Codon optimization. Codon optimization strategies mainly include codon preference, codon coordination, codon sensitivity, and adjustment of gene sequences. Codon preference is the most commonly used codon optimization strategy at present, which mainly replaces the donor codon with the synonymous codon with the highest frequency in the host genome and uses the most abundant codon in the host to encode the amino acids in the optimized sequence. Adopting host-preferred codons and reducing or avoiding the use of rare codons are important means to improve the heterologous expression level of key enzyme genes in biosynthetic pathways. Codon coordination mainly involves replacing the donor codon with the codon most frequently used in the host and using a codon with similar frequency to encode the protein, which has a significant impact on the economy of the enzyme industrial production process and can markedly reduce the production cost. Choosing the appropriate frequency of codons is the key factor for the successful expression of active proteins. Codon sensitivity refers to the strength of tRNA binding to amino acids in the absence of amino acids in cells. At present, the optimization strategy using codon sensitivity has not been popularized. Qiao *et al*. engineered the triterpene pathway in *E. coli* BL21(DE3) and two different *S. cerevisiae* background, WAT11 and EPY300, by recruiting three codon-optimized lupeol pathway genes from different organisms. Finally, the engineered strains based on EPY300, named ECHHOe, processed the best lupeol-producing ability with the maximum lupeol titer being 200.1 mg/L at 30℃ in a 72 h-flask culture, which is the highest amount of lupeol obtained by a microbial system thus far. Arnesen *et al*. engineered oleaginous yeast *Y. lipolytica* to produce three valuable plant pentacyclic triterpenoids (asiatic, madecassic, and arjunolic acids) by fermentation. Further expression of the codon-optimized CaCYP714E19p based on the codon usage of highly expressed genes (KsCYP72A397_IhOP) resulted in the formation of 4.4 mg/g DCW arjunolic acid efficiently.

4.3 System-level optimization of chassis cells Chassis cells, as the carrier of biosynthetic pathway expression, provide the initial parts for the synthesis of natural products, which determine the substrate and metabolic flux of biosynthesis, while the substrate and metabolic flux determine the characteristic and yield of natural product synthesis. Chassis cells are often one of the determinants of heterologous expression efficiency, and thus their selection and modification are also important considerations for the construction of natural product biosynthetic pathways. The remodeling and optimization of chassis cells mainly involve the simplification and optimization of the genome, control and optimization of the metabolic flux, transformation of regulatory factors, and remodeling and utilization of subcellular compartments. Selecting appropriate chassis cells according to the actual biosynthetic pathway and optimizing the enzymes and regulatory factors of their metabolic process are the key to improving the yield of heterologous expression of target products. The biosynthesis and storage of complex natural products are characterized across many types of subcellular compartments, such as mitochondria, endoplasmic reticulum, lipid droplets, vacuoles, and even across different tissues and organs. The remodeling and utilization of specific subcellular compartments of chassis cells have broad application prospects in improving the synthetic efficiency of microbial cell factories.

4.3.1 Genome reduction of chassis cells. Appropriate genome reduction will provide ideal chassis cells for the heterologous biosynthesis of important natural products, which enables the optimization of cellular metabolic pathways, not only improving the cell utilization efficiency of the substrate and energy and better tolerating the metabolic burden of various enzymes and metabolites, but also better maintaining the exogenous gene network and greatly improving the predictability and controllability of cell physiological performance. The deletion of non-essential genes unrelated to the synthesis of target products in heterologous microbial hosts, such as the gene cluster-related genes of secondary metabolites, transposons, and inserted sequence genes, can improve the genetic stability of cells and reduce the metabolic burden. Drawing support from CRISPR/Cas9 technology, multiple automated genome engineering, homologous recombination based on site-specific recombinase and other genome editing technologies, arbitrary multiple sites can be synchronously modified in the genome to realize the transformation of chassis cells.

The classic strategy for the simplification and optimization of chassis cells is the Cre/LoxP gene recombination system, where the main principle of this method is to use Cre recombinase to specifically recognize the LoxP site and mediate its recombination. The Cre/LoxP system is highly adaptable and has a wide range of applications, but the introduced LoxP site will be left after it mediates recombination. Therefore, when multiple non-consecutive gene editing is required, its application is limited by the design of LoxP sites. For yeast genome editing, homologous recombination and Cre/Lox-mediated integration have largely been replaced by the CRISPR/Cas9 system, which is still being improved to facilitate and accelerate DNA assembly and genome manipulation. Compared with the Cre/LoxP system, the CRISPR/Cas9 system is more flexible in selecting targets and is easier to design and operate for discontinuous multi-segment knockouts. The principle of CRISPR/Cas9-mediated gene deletion is that the Cas9 protein recognizes specific PAM sites under the action of single guide RNA (sgRNA), and then recombines. Cobb *et al*. used the CRISPR/Cas9 system to knockout DNA of 20 bp to 30 kb with an efficiency of 70% to 100%. Gao *et al*. employed a combined strategy with the integration of endogenous pathway genes in the genome of *S. cerevisiae* and knockout of inhibiting genes by CRISPR/Cas9 technology, which successfully engineered multiple strains. After introducing the efficient *TwOSC1*, all strains with genetic integration showed a 3.0 - 6.8-fold increase in friedelin production compared with the BY4741 strain. Bicalho *et al*. produced maytenoic acid by the expression of the *MiFRS* gene of *Maytenus ilicifolia* in *N. benthamiana* leaves and *S. cerevisiae* strain engineered using CRISPR/Cas9. Also, they transiently expressed *CYP712K4* in combination with *tHMGR1* and *MiFRS4* into *N. benthamiana* to increase the accumulation of friedelin for $0.43 \pm 0.16$ mg $g^{-1}$ DW. Besides, they added methyl-β-cyclodextrin (MβCD) to the cultivation medium and knocked out the *PAH1* gene using CRISPR/Cas9 in *S. cerevisiae*, which increased the yield of friedelin to $2.27 \pm 0.32$ mg/L. Zhou *et al*. reconstructed the biosynthetic pathway of friedelin by CRISPR/Cas9 and expressed the *TwOSC1* and *TwOSC3* genes in *S. cerevisiae*. With the protein modification and medium optimization, the friedelin content reached 37.07 mg/L. Hansen *et al*. revealed that CYP712K1, CYP712K2, and CYP712K3 can effectively oxidize friedelin to form 29-hydroxy-friedelin and polpunonic acid in *S. cerevisiae*. Subsequently, the AM254 yeast strain was constructed by deleting the *UBC7* gene, which afforded a five-fold increase in friedelin titer. Shortly afterwards, they further introduced the CYP712K1 enzyme into yeast, and heterologously synthesized 1.4 mg/L polpunonic acid.

4.3.2 Control of metabolic flux and modification of regulatory factors. The balance optimization of metabolic pathways is an important link in the heterologous biosynthetic pathway, and regulatory factors control the expression of multiple key gene enzymes in the synthetic pathway. At present, the control of metabolic flux and the transformation of regulatory factors are mostly achieved by editing the original genes, regulating TFs and introducing new gene elements.

In addition to increasing the expression of exogenous genes, up-regulating the expression of endogenous genes in the host or introducing strong promoter elements can also increase the biosynthesis of the target products. Zhao *et al*. constructed a novel pathway for the biosynthesis of oleanolic acid in *S. cerevisiae*. The cellular galactose regulatory network was reconstructed by knocking out the galactose metabolic genes *GAL80* and *GAL1* to improve the transcriptional efficiency of the heterologous genes. Finally, the *HMGR*, *SS* and *OSC* genes were further overexpressed, increasing the oleanolic acid production to $186.1 \pm 12.4$ mg/L in the shake flask. Krokida *et al*. revealed 20-hydroxy lupeol and 20-hydroxy betulinic acid were biosynthesized when AMY2 (OSC enzyme) oxidized by CYP71D353 at the C-20 and C-28 positions, respectively, was transiently expressed in *N. benthamiana* leaves by agroinfiltration. Qiao *et al*. heterologously expressed the *LUS* gene *OeLUP* in *S. cerevisiae* to achieve the heterologous synthesis of lupeol alcohol. Dai *et al*. expressed *CYP716C49* from *Crataegus pinnatifida* in *S. cerevisiae* to synthesize betulinic acid and alphitolic acid from scratch, and the yield of alphitolic acid reached 23 mg/L. Sun *et al*. coexpressed lupeol synthase *AtLUP1*, P450 enzyme *CYP716A12* and reductase *AtCPR1*, which come from *Arabidopsis* in *Y. lipolytica*, and successfully achieved the heterologous synthesis of betulinic acid with a yield of 0.32 mg/L. Subsequently, the P450 enzyme was fused and expressed with its truncated reductase, and the key genes of the upstream MVA pathway were overexpressed to increase the yield to 9.41 mg/L. Finally, the yield of betulinic acid reached 16.98 mg/L through glycerol fermentation. In addition, regulating TFs in heterologous metabolic pathway can strengthen the metabolic pathway of the target products. The overexpression of TFs can activate a series of related endogenous key genes in the synthetic pathway, enhance the synthesis of metabolites, and finally increase the yield of target products. Besides the targeted regulation, the transcription regulation strategy was employed by overexpressing *UPC2-1* (a global TF gene of yeast ergosterol synthesis). The incorporation of the targeted and global transcription regulation strategy increased the yield of ginsenoside CK by 5-fold, which reached up to 1 mg/L. Zhang *et al*. reconstructed the promoters with the binding site of *UPC2* and reconstructed the galactose regulatory network to promote the gene expression in *S. cerevisiae*. Ultimately, the β-amyrin titer increased 65-fold and the oleanonic acid titer increased 6.8-fold.

Down-regulation or blocking of competing metabolic pathways can limit or reduce the supply of substrates flowing into competing metabolic pathways, thereby maintaining the abundance of important precursors or intermediates in chassis cells, which can be achieved through silencing of negative regulators or the use of a weak promoter to inhibit competing metabolic pathways to obtain more precursors, facilitating the redistribution of pathway fluxes. Bröker *et al*. developed a new heterologous platform for the production of pentacyclic triterpenes in *S. cerevisiae* based on a combinatorial engineering strategy involving the overexpression of the MVA pathway gene *ERG13* in *S. cerevisiae*, the knockout of negative regulator *ROX1* gene, and the suppression of a competing pathway, resulting in a push-and-pull strategy to enhance the metabolic flux in the system. Finally, they increased the yield of lupeol by 127-fold. Zhang *et al*. developed a strategy to enhance the triterpene efflux through manipulation of lipid components in *Y. lipolytica* by overexpressing the *OLE1* gene and disturbing the *PAH1* and *DGK1 genes*. The highest lupeol production was achieved, where the titer in the organic phase reached 381.67 mg/L and the total production was 411.72 mg/L in the shake flasks, exhibiting a 33.2-fold improvement over the initial strain.

4.3.3 Remodeling and utilization of subcellular compartments in chassis cells. During the heterologous biosynthesis of natural products, their enzymes, cofactors and intermediates often have compartmental distribution in heterologous hosts, which have gradually become the key limiting factors in the creation and application of efficient heterologous biosynthetic systems. *S. cerevisiae* contains various subcellular compartments, each of which provides a unique physiological environment and is considered to be one of the best choices for the heterologous synthesis of complex natural products. Therefore, the remodeling and utilization of specific subcellular compartments play an important role in improving the synthetic efficiency of microbial cell factories. Protopanaxadiol synthase (PPDs), the key P450 enzyme in the ginsenoside biosynthetic pathway, is usually considered to be located in the endoplasmic reticulum and is not in the same reaction zone chamber with its substrate damanediol II (DD). The compartmentalized segregation of PPDS and its substrates DDs in ginsenoside-engineered bacteria may be an important factor affecting the catalytic efficiency of the pathway. To verify and utilize this inference, Dai *et al*. extracted and analyzed lipid droplets from engineered cells of *S. cerevisiae* and found that multiple intermediate metabolites in ginsenoside biosynthesis were abundantly stored in yeast lipid droplets. Meanwhile, the fluorescence localization of each key enzyme in the pathway was carried out, which revealed that the key PPDS in the pathway was mainly localized on the endoplasmic reticulum, thus confirming the inference that the reaction substrate and the enzyme were compartmentalized in the heterologous engineered bacteria. Based on this, the lipid droplet membrane protein Pln1p was further utilized to target the PPDS located in the endoplasmic reticulum to the storage organelle lipid droplets of DD, which reconstructed a new reaction zone chamber for the enzymatic reaction. Consequently, the production efficiency of protopanaxadiol (PPD) was significantly improved, and the substrate conversion rate reached 86%. Wang *et al*. introduced Pn3-29, a high-efficiency biosynthetic module of ginsenoside compound K (CK) excavated from the medicinal plant *P. notoginseng*, into a chassis strain with a high yield of PPD, and the results showed that the maximum titer of ginsenoside CK obtained by the engineering strain in a 5 L bioreactor reached 5 g/L.

4.4 Precursor supply, pathway regulation and reconstruction for heterologous biosynthesis As is known, heterologous hosts do not produce or rarely produce the desired target products, and the introduction of exogenous synthetic pathways will inevitably increase the metabolic burden of the host. The synthetic process of many terpenoids is complex and diverse, and there are multi-step chemical reactions. Thus, effectively improving the supply level of precursors to meet the synthesis of downstream natural products is challenge. The choice of precursor pathway and the supply of precursors are two key issues in the heterologous biosynthesis of natural products. At present, the supply of precursor compounds is mainly improved by modifying and regulating the endogenous metabolic pathway of microorganisms, especially eukaryotes, or introducing heterologous metabolic pathways.

4.4.1 Modifying and regulating endogenous metabolic pathways to increase the precursor supply. Although terpenoids have different structures and functions, they are all derived from C5 precursor compounds, namely IPP and DMAPP, which are the common precursors for the biosynthesis of terpenoids, and in most cases, they can be interconverted by the isomerase encoded by the *IDI* gene. DMAPP condenses with one or more IPPs to produce the precursor compounds of isopentenyl diphosphate, and these precursor skeletons undergo a series of cyclization, methylation, acetylation, rearrangement and other reactions to generate various end-products of terpenoids. Given that IPP and DMAPP are synthesized through the MVA pathway or MEP pathway, theoretically increasing the supply of precursor compounds can also increase the production of IPP and DAMPP. Acetyl-CoA is the direct precursor of the MVA pathway, which has been intensively studied in the metabolic process of *S. cerevisiae* in recent years. Acetyl-CoA is produced in the nucleus, cytoplasm, mitochondria and peroxisomes of *S. cerevisiae*, but only acetyl-CoA in the cytoplasm can be used to synthesize terpenoids. The precursor molecules of the MEP pathway are pyruvate and G3P, and their ratio is an important factor affecting the production of terpenoids by cells dependent on the MEP pathway.

For increasing the supply of precursor compounds, engineering and modulating microbial endogenous metabolic pathways to increase the expression of rate-limiting enzyme genes are the effective methods. For the MVA pathway, *HMGR* is the first rate-limiting enzyme in this pathway, and the overexpression of the *HMGR* gene can increase the synthesis of downstream natural products. The rate-limiting enzymes in the MEP pathway mainly include DXS, DXR and IDI. DXS catalyzes pyruvate and G3P to generate DXP, which is the first rate-limiting step in the synthesis of plant terpenoids, and the overexpression of the *DXS* gene can promote the accumulation of downstream terpenoids. DXR is the second rate-limiting enzyme of the MEP pathway and catalyzes the formation of MEP from DXP. The conversion between IPP and DMAPP is completed by IPP isomerase, namely IDI. The overexpression of rate-limiting enzyme genes such as *DXS*, *DXR* and *IDI* can successfully increase the amount of metabolic precursor compounds, thereby increasing the yield of the target products. An insufficient supply of UDP-glucose is a common problem that limits the high yield of heterologous synthetic saponins in microbial cell factories. Wang *et al*. combined the strategy of 'open source and cut expenditure', where on the one hand, it systematically strengthened the synthetic pathway of UDP-glucose in cells. On the other hand, it strengthened the UDP-glucose supply level of the PPD high-yield yeast chassis constructed by the team in the early stage by weakening the consumption pathway of UDP-glucose in the cells, and finally the yield of ginsenoside CK increased to 5.7 g/L. Jin *et al*. applied a multi-modular strategy to systematically improve the biosynthesis of betulinic acid and related triterpenoids in *Y. lipolytica*. They selected two optimal betulinic acid-producing strains, and then overexpressed the *ERG1*, *ERG9*, and *HMG1* genes of the MVA module in the two strains, which dramatically increased the production of betulinic acid and resulted in a strain (YLJCC56) that exhibited the highest betulinic acid yield of 51.87 ± 2.77 mg/L. Lu *et al*. overexpressed *HMG-CoA*, *ERG20*, and exogenous *SE* of *Candida albicans* ERG1 in *S. cerevisiae* to enhance the supply of the precursor squalene. They integrated amyrin synthase from *Catharanthus roseus*, screened and optimized promoters with different strengths, and combined P450 enzymes from *M. sativa* and *C. roseus* with CPR from *Arabidopsis* and L. *corniculatus* for screening. Ultimately, the optimal combination of the P450 enzyme of *M. sativa* and CPR of *Arabidopsis* was determined, and the yield of oleanolic acid obtained by fed-batch fermentation was 155.58 mg/L. Yu *et al*. constructed the α*AS* gene *MdOSC1* in *S. cerevisiae*, while increasing the supply of the precursor substance 2,3-oxidosqualene, and the results of shake flask fermentation showed that the yield of α-amyrin reached 11.97 ± 0.61 mg/L, which was 5.8-times higher than the previously reported highest yield. Soon afterwards, by engineering the *MdOSC1* gene and expanding its intracellular storage pool, high yields of α-amyrin of greater than 1.1 g/L were achieved in fed-batch fermentation.

4.4.2 Regulation techniques of metabolic engineering.

The main purpose of metabolic engineering research is to efficiently synthesize target products by modifying the metabolic network of strains. New cells can be created through the introduction, knockout or meticulous regulation of enzyme genes in metabolic networks, and the conversion of cheap raw materials into valuable target products is the main focus of current metabolic engineering and synthetic biology research. The heterologous biosynthetic pathway from raw materials to target products often includes dozens of enzymatic reactions. Thus, to maximize the synthesis of target products, the commonly used strategies of metabolic engineering are mainly overexpressing and optimizing key enzyme genes in the product synthetic pathway, knocking out the by-product generation pathway, and releasing the inhibition of product synthesis. Specifically, the synthesis of metabolites can be enhanced by means of increasing the expression of upstream encoding rate-limiting enzymes or multiple key enzyme genes of the target pathway to ensure the sufficient supply of precursors, knocking out or inhibiting the key enzyme genes involved in the branch competition or degradation metabolic pathway of the target product to avoid the degradation of the target metabolite or the formation of intermediate and by-products, and overexpressing the TFs to activate a series of related endogenous key genes in the synthetic pathway. It is worth noting that the above-mentioned methods can be comprehensively combined to maximize the synthesis of the target product.

Li *et al*. constructed an engineered yeast strain by introducing three genes, *IaAO1*, *IaAO4* and *IaCPR*, isolated from *Ilex asprella* into *S. cerevisiae*, which can produce C-23 hydroxyl ursane-type triterpenoid derivatives efficiently by metabolic engineering. To achieve the heterologous biosynthesis of pentacyclic triterpenoids, Sandeep *et al*. coexpressed *LsOSC1* and *CYP716A265* genes in the leaves of *N. benthamiana*, and they successfully synthesized betulinic acid. Meanwhile, corosolic acid and maslinic acid were produced by the coexpression of *LsOSC2*, *CYP716A265* and *CYP716C55* genes. Likewise, the coexpression of *LsOSC4*, *CYP716A265* and *CYP716C55* genes also produced maslinic acid in *N. benthamiana* leaves. Reed *et al*. revealed that the accumulation of heterogenous triterpene products β-amyrin can be increased several folds by the co-expression of an N-terminal-truncated, feedback-insensitive form of *tHMGR* in *N. benthamiana*. Surprisingly, Lee *et al*. revealed that the overexpression of *BCCP* linked to *truncated HMG-CoA reductase* (*tHMGR*) by a cleavable peptide 2A showed a 6-fold increase of C30 β-amyrin, reaching 9.8 mg $g^{-1}$ DW in *N. benthamiana*. Moses *et al*. implemented the galactose-induced expression of *tHMG1* and *GgbAS* in *S. cerevisiae*, which biosynthesized β-amyrin with a yield of 3.20 ± 0.09 mg/L. Geisler *et al*. coexpressed *βAS* and *AsCYP51H10* genes in *N. benthamiana* leaves, and approximately 20 mg of β-amyrin was purified from 17 g DW of AsbAS1-AsCyp51H10 coinfiltrated plant material (1.18 mg/g DW). Soon after, Reed *et al*. revealed that the inclusion of a feedback insensi-tive form of HMG-CoA reductase in their coinfiltration experiments increased the yields of simple and oxidized triterpenes, namely, β-amyrin by 4-10 fold (4.72-11.8 mg/g DW). Khakimov *et al*. revealed that the combinatorial expression of lupeol synthase genes (*LUPs*) and *CYP716As* in *N. benthamiana* produced oleanolic, ursolic and betulinic acids, but at highly varying levels. The highest accumulation was observed for ursolic acids under the combination of *LUP5* and *CYP716A80*. Han *et al*. overexpressed the *TcOSC1* gene *of Taraxacum coreanum* in *N. tabacum*, and all lines of transgenic *N. tabacum* produced five new triterpenes, namely, taraxasterol, ψ-taraxasterol, δ-amyrin, β-amyrin, and α-amyrin.

The main bottleneck of metabolic engineering research is the complexity of the cellular metabolic network. With the rapid development of genome sequencing technology, the types of enzymes encoded by the genome and the chemical reactions that occur can be quickly determined through genome annotation information, thus forming a biological metabolic network model. Metabolic network models and computational design methods based on metabolic network models provide new strategies for synthetic biology and metabolic engineering. In recent years, the concept and method of dynamic metabolic engineering have been proposed, that is, the dynamic regulation of gene expression and activity, thus avoiding the accumulation or deficiency of intermediate metabolites and meeting the differentiated needs of metabolic flux distribution at different stages. Through the metabolic network model and dynamic metabolic engineering, researchers can choose appropriate exogenous genes to construct new pathways to realize the synthesis of new products from scratch, and can also use gene circuits to correlate the changes in the state and environment during cell fermentation and culture with the expression of specific genes, thus achieving the precise balance of metabolic activity, making cells adapt to different goals, and maintaining the optimal state, thereby maximizing the synthesis of the target product.

4.4.3 Introducing heterologous MVA pathway. To achieve the synthesis and accumulation of a large number of target products, in addition to modifying the endogenous metabolic pathways of microorganisms, the most commonly used strategy is to express multiple heterologous proteins or introduce heterologous metabolic pathways to increase the supply of IPP and DMAPP, which can make the heterologous metabolic pathway not controlled by the regulation mechanism of bacterial endogenous metabolic networks. In recent years, break-throughs have been made in the synthesis of terpenoids based on the heterologous MVA pathway. Due to the lack of glycosylation pathways for the biosynthesis of UDP-xylose in yeast, Li *et al*. heterologously expressed the *Arabidopsis*-derived UDP-xylose synthetic modules AtUGD1 and AtUXS and co-expressed the newly identified transglycosylation enzyme called PgUGT94Q13, successfully synthesizing notoginsenoside R1 in a high-yield Rg1 yeast chassis with a yield of 1.62 g/L. Meanwhile, in the yeast chassis with high protopanaxatriol yield, a cell factory with high-yield notoginsenoside R2 was constructed by co-expressing the UDP-xylose synthetic module, *i. e.*, glycosyltransferases PgUGT94Q13 and PgUGT71A54, and its yield was 1.25 g/L. Moreover, isoprene, sabinene, pinene, geraniol, β-caryophyllene and other terpenoids were successfully synthesized in microorganisms by introducing heterologous metabolic pathways.

Although the expression of heterologous metabolic pathways can effectively increase the amount of precursor compounds due to the lack of regulation of heterologous metabolic pathways by microorganisms, it may cause the imbalance of metabolic flux and accumulate toxic intermediates in cells, resulting in some negative effects. When the MVA pathway is heterologously expressed in *E. coli*, the intermediate product HMG-CoA accumulates, which is toxic to cells, thus inhibiting bacterial growth. After the overexpression of *tHMGR*, the consumption rate of HMG-CoA increased and the bacterial growth rate returned to the same level as that of wild-type bacteria. Therefore, to further improve the yield of terpenoids, it is necessary to adjust the expression level of various genes to balance the overall metabolic flux.

4.5 Cell engineering techniques In addition to totipotency, plant cells are biosynthetically totipotent, each of which retains all the genetic information and has the ability to synthesize secondary metabolites. In recent years, great progress has been made in the application of cell culture to produce natural products, and the reactor for culturing plant cells has been expanded from 1 to 30 L on an experimental scale to thousands of litres on an industrial scale. The utilization of cell culture to produce natural products has great economic potential and is becoming an important development direction in modern production technology. At present, the main ways to obtain plant natural products by means of cell engineering are cell culture, micropropagation technology and plant bioreactors.

4.5.1 Cell culture. Cell culture has the advantages of stability, high efficiency, and easy control. Besides, the cultured cells have the ability to synthesize plant natural products. Therefore, plant cell culture is an important source to obtain rare pentacyclic triterpene saponins and other natural products. At present, some triterpenoid saponins, such as ginsenosides, alfalfa saponins, and esculentoside, have been successfully obtained by establishing a suspension cell culture system. During cell engineering, the synthesis and accumulation of plant natural products can be effectively regulated by changing the culture conditions. For instance, the biosynthesis of triterpenoid saponins in the cell culture system can be regulated by changing the conditions or adding elicitors such as hormones. The secondary metabolic synthetic pathway of terpenoids is mainly regulated by the signal transduction pathway of JA, and MeJA has a selective induction effect on the secondary metabolic pathway. Scholz *et al*. revealed that the contents of hederasaponin and *Kalopanax* saponin I in *Nigella sativa* increased by 12 times compared with the control after the treatment of 100 μmol/L MeJA. Exogenous inducers increased the content of triterpenoid saponins by regulating the expression of the key enzyme genes or TFs. MeJA can induced the up-regulation of *FPS*, *SS*, and *SE* genes in the triterpene synthetic pathway of *Betula platyphylla* plants and their cells. Meanwhile, these genes in the triterpene synthetic pathway could be regulated by bHLH and MYB TFs, which were induced by MeJA. The biosynthetic steps of natural products are complicated, and adding intermediate metabolites or bypass inhibitors to the culture medium can greatly improve the yield of natural products.

4.5.2 Micropropagation technology and plant bioreactor. Micropropagation involves the use of plant organs, tissues, cells or protoplasts as explants to regenerate plants under *in vitro* culture conditions, which is the most widely used and effective technology in tissue culture production. In the process of plant micropropagation, hormones can not only regulate the growth and development of plants, but also regulate the biosynthesis of saponins, but the effect of this regulation is closely related to the types of hormones and the biosynthetic pathways of natural products. During the micropropagation of *Centella asiatica*, the addition of cytokinin TDZ significantly increased the total glycoside content of *C. asiatica*, while the addition of auxin 2,4-D decreased the accumulation of asiaticosides. Micropropagation technology is an important method for the rapid propagation of plants, and the combination of heterologous plant synthesis and micropropagation technology provides a new strategy for improving the yield of the target products, which will promote the biosynthesis of natural products to be more efficient, productive and convenient.

The utilization of bioreactors to culture plant cells, tissues and organs in large quantities or on a large scale to produce triterpenoid saponins is a hot research topic at present. Plant bioreactors are developing rapidly, which have been enlarged from a few liters to more than ten tons. Recently, there have been many reports on the use of small bioreactors to culture adventitious roots, hairy roots and embryogenic cells of traditional medicinal plants. Han *et al.* adopted a 17 L air-lift bioreactor to culture suspension cells of *P. notoginseng*, and the dry mass of cells and the production of saponins reached the maximum value of 24 g/L and 91 mg/L, respectively, after 15 days of culture. Paek *et al.* gradually expanded the culture from small-scale cultivation in air-lift bioreactors, and finally reached a scale of more than 10 tons in the root bioreactor cultivation of *P. ginseng*, realizing the industrialization of *P. ginseng* root cultivation. Wu *et al.* used a 5 L balloon-type foam bioreactor to culture the adventitious roots of *Astragalus membranaceus*, and the initial inoculation amount was 30 g fresh mass. After 40 days of culture, the fresh mass of the harvested adventitious roots reached 540 g, and the accumulation of saponins was 3.4 mg/g, which was almost the same as the amount of saponins in 3 year-old *Astragalus* root (3.6 mg/g). Kochan *et al.* selected a 10 L nutrient spray bioreactor to culture the hairy roots of *P. quinquefolium*, and the initial inoculation amount was 27 g of fresh mass. After 30 days of culture, the amount of harvested hairy roots was 5-times higher than the initial inoculation amount, and the accumulation of ginsenosides reached 6 mg/g. Cao *et al.* developed a tissue culture system for the adventitious roots of *P. ginseng*, from solid culture to liquid culture, and then to air-lift reactor culture, the reactor of ginseng adventitious root was gradually scaled up to 10 L. Furthermore, induced by MeJA, the accumulation of active substances was basically the same as that of 5 year-old wild *P. ginseng*.

4.6 Regulation techniques of enzyme engineering and fermentation engineering

4.6.1 Regulation techniques of enzyme engineering. With the development of synthetic biology, enzyme engineering is an indispensable research field for heterologous biosynthesis. As one of the important basic disciplines of synthetic biology, enzyme engineering has also ushered in new development opportunities. The discovery of microbial enzymes, the analysis of enzyme structure and function, the transformation and design of enzymes will provide further technical support for the development of synthetic biology. The physical and chemical structure of enzymes, which can affect their catalytic rate, stability, specificity, and cofactor requirements, exhibit some deficiencies due to an installed heterologous or artificial *de novo* biosynthetic pathway. As is known, plant P450s are critical enzymes for generating triterpene chemodiversity by catalyzing the site-specific oxidation of the triterpene skeleton. However, heterologously expressing P450s in microorganisms showed poor chemical and regional selectivity, which limited the efficient biosynthesis of related natural products. Sun *et al.* identified the key residues that influenced the P450-substrate hydrophobic interaction in controlling the chemo- and regio- selectivity of the enzyme and engineered the enzyme toward selectivity oxidation to hydroxyl and carboxylic acid. Besides, tuning the redox partner of P450 led to selective production of glycyrrhetaldehyde, a good starting point for further modification. They also revealed that controlling the catalytic property of plant P450s is of great use in the biosynthesis of desired licorice triterpenoids, which can be used in the biosynthesis of other terpenoid natural products. Soon after, Li *et al.* used *Y. lipolytica* as the host, combined with the strategy of fusion expression of the P450 enzyme and CPR, to increase the production of oleanolic acid to 540.7 mg/L, which greatly improved the yield of oleanolic acid. Fanani *et al.* identified two amino acid residues, namely Leu149 and Leu398, that controlled C-30 product regioselectivity and contributed to the chemodiversity of triterpenes accumulated in legumes and increase in the production of high-value triterpene compounds, which were further confirmed by the mutagenesis of CYP72A154 homologs from glycyrrhizin-producing species, functional phylogenomic analyses, and comparison of corresponding residues of C-30 oxidase homologs in other legumes. Zhang *et al*. mined candidate *GTs* of ginseng, namely, *PgCSyGT1*, *PgUGT18* and *PgUGT8*. Subsequently, they integrated these *GTs* in combinations in the *S*. *cerevisiae* genome and realized the *de novo* biosynthesis of oleanane-type ginsenosides with a yield of 1.41 μg/L ginsenoside Ro in the shake flasks. Wu *et al*. successfully induced the transformation of betulin to betulinic acid by co-expressing the *CYP716A12* gene from *M*. *truncatula* and ATR1 from *Arabidopsis* in *S*. *cerevisiae*. Eventu-ally, the optimal yield of betulinic acid reached 18.70%. After optimization, the yield and conversion rate of betulin increased by 83.97% and 136.39%, respectively. Romsuk *et al*. established a method called the 'Tsukuba system' for producing oleanolic acid in substantial quantities *via* the heterologous expression of pathway enzymes, and the product yields of β-amyrin, oleanolic acid and maslinic acid significantly improved compared with the previously reported yield in *N*. *benthamiana leaves*. Lu *et al*. introduced oxidosqualene cyclase (CrMAS), CYP450 oxidase and CPR from different plant sources into *S*. *cerevisiae* and successfully achieved the heterologous synthesis of ursolic acid and oleanolic acid. Dai *et al*. identified the P450 enzyme gene *CYP716C49* from *Crataegus pinnatifida* and expressed it heterologously in *S*. *cerevisiae*, and successfully synthesized corosolic, maslinic, and alphitolic acid in yields of 141, 384 and 23 mg/L, respectively. Li and Zhang heterologously expressed *LUS1* from *Arabidopsis* and CYP450 oxidase (*CrAO*) from *Catharanthus roseus* in *S*. *cerevisiae*, realizing the heterologous synthesis of betulinic acid. Dai *et al*. discovered a new P450 enzyme CYP716C49 from *Crataegus pinnatifida* and heterologously expressed this enzyme gene in *S*. *cerevisiae*-producing strains of oleanolic acid to achieve the *de novo* synthesis of maslinic acid with a final yield of 384 mg/L. Zhu *et al*. successfully obtained the P450 enzyme Uni25647 and its reductase with stronger specificity and higher activity from *M*. *sativa* and *G*. *uralensis*, and optimized the synthetic pathway of glycyrrhetinic acid in *S*. *cerevisiae*, causing the yield of glycyrrhetinic acid to reach 18.9 mg/L in a 5 L fermentor.

Although there have been numerous studies on the biosynthetic pathways of triterpenoid saponins, the specific steps of their synthesis have not been elucidated due to the complexity of the structures and types of multi-gene family enzymes involved in their middle and downstream synthesis. Clarifying the key enzyme genes and their synergy in the biosynthetic pathway of triterpenoid saponins and regulating and modifying the level of key enzyme genes are the core contents of the application of enzyme engineering in triterpenoid heterologous biosynthesis.

4.6.2 Fermentation engineering techniques. Microbial fermentation engineering is based on the achievements of genetic engineering, metabolic engineering, enzyme engineering, cell engineering, synthetic biology and other technologies with respect to the fermentation process. Microbial fermentation engineering is the most widely used technology in modern bioengineering technology. At present, it is widely used in heterologous biosynthesis, which greatly promotes the development of the heterologous synthesis of natural products. Since the 1970s, the development of biological engineering technologies such as genetic engineering and cell engineering has brought fermentation engineering into the stage of directional breeding. At the end of the 20th century and the first 20 years of the 21st century, the rapid development of biotechnology began to reshape the world. The technological innovations of predictability, re-engineering, regulation, bionics, regeneration and creation, biological storage, high-energy cells and human-computer interaction provide an important foundation for the development of fermentation engineering in the new era. Based on the principles of synthetic biology, it can be used for the large-scale production of natural products with the help of microbial fermentation engineering by designing and transforming dominant microbial strains into heterologous and high-yield chassis cells. Microbial fermentation engineering provides a new strategy for the heterologous and efficient synthesis of target products. On the one hand, biosynthetic gene clusters silenced in the original host can be activated by reconfiguring the biosynthetic pathway of the target compounds in chassis cells. On the other hand, under the guidance of synthetic biology, the biological elements can be redesigned, integrated and assembled, and the newly introduced metabolic pathway is adapted to the original metabolic pathway of the host in the chassis cell to form a new metabolic network, thereby providing sufficient precursor supply for the synthesis of the target product, finally achieving the high yield, high conversion, high efficiency and low cost heterologous biosynthesis of natural products. Czarnotta *et al*. re-engineered the reported betulinic acid pathway in *S*. *cerevisiae* and used this novel strain to develop efficient fermentation and product purification methods. The beneficial effect of excess ethanol was further exploited in nitrogen-limited resting cell fermentations, finally yielding a betulinic acid concentration of 182 mg/L and total triterpenoid concentration of 854 mg/L. Ni *et al*. developed a CRISPRi method by constructing a multi-gRNA plasmid to down-regulate seven genes simultaneously in *S*.

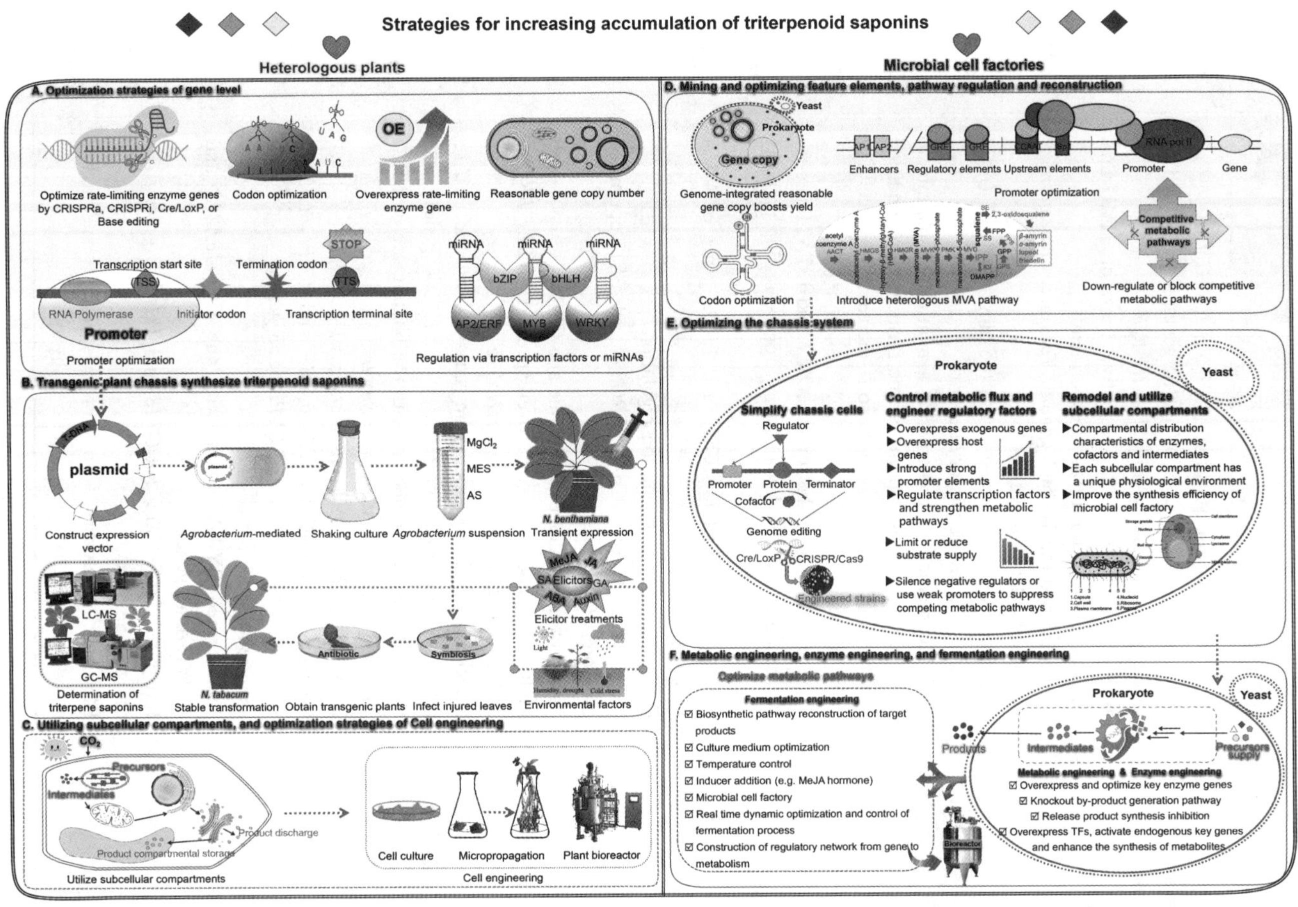


**Fig. 10 Strategies for increasing the accumulation of triterpenoid saponins**

*cerevisiae*. They optimized the fermentation condition including pH, inoculum size, initial glucose concentration and feed of glucose or ethanol, and increased extracellular transportation by supplying methyl-β-cyclodextrin. Ultimately, the β-amyrin concentration of the engineered strain SGibSdCg increased by 44.3% compared with the parent strain SGib, achieving 156.7 mg/L, which was the highest concentration of β-amyrin reported in yeast.

In the 21st century, some core connotations of fermentation engineering technology have changed. The construction and improvement of the microbial cell factory have replaced the previous improvement of fermentation microbial strains, and the optimization of the fermentation process and dynamic control have replaced the previous optimization of the fermentation process. In addition, it also includes high-throughput screening technology of fermentation strain, rapid gene editing assembly and expression regulation technology, microreactor and combinatorial optimization technology, transformation and precise regulation of microbial cell system, process reengineering technology of typical fermentation products, real-time dynamic optimization and control of fermentation process based on multi-parameter detection analysis and omics technology. Microbial fermentation engineering is taking a new approach to deliver 'fresh blood' and vitality for heterologous biosynthesis.

The strategies for increasing the accumulation of triterpenoid saponins are shown as Fig. 10.

4.7 Current status of heterologous biosynthesis in pentacyclic triterpenoids The heterologous biosynthesis of pentacyclic triterpenoids has achieved significant breakthroughs in recent years. We summarized the research status of four main types of pentacyclic triterpenes, namely, oleanane, ursane, lupane and friedelane, *via* heterologous biosynthesis, and analyzed their existing problems and deficiencies.

Most of oleanane-type pentacyclic triterpenoids are formed through the subsequent modification of β-amyrin generated from 2,3-oxidosqualene under the catalytic reaction of OSC. The main heterologous biosynthetic host of oleanane is *S. cerevisiae*. Over the years, the heterologous plant *N. benthamiana* has been successively reported on the synthesis of pentacyclic triterpenoids. The heterologous biosynthesis of oleanane has made important progress, and oleanolic acid, glycyrrhetinic acid, and maslinic acid have been successfully synthesized in heterolo-gous hosts, as presented in Table 4. However, most of them have problems such as low activity and poor specificity, resulting in many by-products and low yield. With the continuous in-depth analysis of the terpenoid pathway and the gradual optimization of chassis

**Table 4 Heterologous biosynthetic levels of pentacyclic triterpenoids**

| Categories | Products | Yields | Heterologous hosts | Strategies | Year |
|---|---|---|---|---|---|
| Oleanane-type | β-Amyrin | 3.20±0.09 mg/L | *S. cerevisiae* | Galactose-induced expression of *tHMG1* and *GgbAS* | 2014 |
| | β-Amyrin | 1.18 mg/g DW | *N. benthamiana* | Co-expressed *βAS* and *AsCYP51H10* genes | 2013 |
| | β-Amyrin | 9.8 mg/g DW | *N. benthamiana* | Overexpressed of *BCCP* linked to *tHMGR* | 2019 |
| | β-Amyrin | 4.72 - 11.8 mg/g DW | *N. benthamiana* | Inclusion of a feedback insensitive form of HMG-CoA reductase in the coinfiltration experiments | 2017 |
| | β-Amyrin | — | *N. tabacum* | Overexpressed the *TcOSC1* gene of *Taraxacum coreanum* | 2022 |
| | β-Amyrin | 1.64 mg/L | *S. cerevisiae* | Adopted GAL1 promoter | 2018 |
| | β-Amyrin | Increased 65-fold | *S. cerevisiae* | Reconstructed the promoters with the binding site of *UPC2* and the galactose regulatory network | 2015 |
| | β-Amyrin | 156.7 mg/L (increased by 44.3%) | *S. cerevisiae* | CRISPRi method by constructing a multigRNA plasmid to down-regulate genes; optimized the fermentation condition and feed of glucose or ethanol; increased extracellular transportation | 2019 |
| | β-Amyrin acetate | — | *N. tabacum*, *S. cerevisiae* | Ectopic expression of both the *LsOSC1* and *LsTAT1* genes | 2022 |
| | β-Amyrin, oleanolic acid, maslinic acid | Increased 13.1-fold | *N. benthamiana* | A method called 'Tsukuba system' for expressing pathway enzymes | 2022 |
| | Oleanolic acid | 186.1 mg/L | *S. cerevisiae* | Overexpressed *tHMG1*, *ERG1* and *ERG9* genes of MVA pathway | 2017 |
| | Oleanolic acid | 606.9 mg/L | *S. cerevisiae* | Optimization of fermentation regulation | 2017 |
| | Oleanolic acid | 155.58 mg/L | *S. cerevisiae* | Overexpressed *HMG-CoA*, *ERG20* and *SE*; optimized promoters | 2018 |
| | Oleanolic acid | 540.7 mg/L | *Y. lipolytica* | Fusion expression of P450 enzyme and CPR | 2020 |
| | Oleanolic acid | 92.1 mg/L (5.65-fold) | *Y. lipolytica* | Multi-copy gene expression; overexpressed *ERG1*, *ERG9*, and *ERG20* genes along with *t1HMG1* | 2020 |
| | Oleanolic acid | 186.1±12.4 mg/L | *S. cerevisiae* | Knocked out galactose metabolic genes *GAL80* and *GAL1*; further overexpressed the *HMGR*, *SS* and *OSC* genes | 2018 |
| | Oleanonic acid | 6.8-fold | *S. cerevisiae* | Reconstructed the promoters with the binding site of *UPC2* and the galactose regulatory network | 2015 |
| | Maslinic acid | 384 mg/L | *S. cerevisiae* | Expressed *CYP716C49* from *Crataegus pinnatifida* | 2019 |
| | Maslinic acid | — | *N. benthamiana* | Co-expressed *LsOSC2*, *CYP716A265* and *CYP716C55* or *LsOSC4*, *CYP716A265* and *CYP716C55* genes | 2019 |
| | Germanicol | — | *N. benthamiana* | Transient expression of *MdOSC4* | 2016 |
| | Gypsogenin | 146.84 mg/L | *S. cerevisiae* | Transformed BY-bAS strain with the *CYP716A262* and *CYP716A567* genes | 2021 |
| | Ginsenoside Ro | 1.41 μg/L | *S. cerevisiae* | Integrated *PgCSyGT1*, *PgUGT18* and *PgUGT8 genes from* the ginseng | 2022 |
| | Glycyrrhetinic acid | 18.9 mg/L | *S. cerevisiae* | P450 and its reductase with stronger specificity and higher activity; optimized the synthetic pathway | 2018 |

(Continued)

| Categories | Products | Yields | Heterologous hosts | Strategies | Year |
|---|---|---|---|---|---|
| | Quillaic acid | 314.01 mg/L | *S. cerevisiae* | Transformed BY-bAS strain with the *CYP716A262 and CYP716A567* genes | 2021 |
| | Arjunolic acid | 4.4 mg/g DCW | *Y. lipolytica* | Expressed a codon-optimized CaCYP714E19p based on codon usage of highly expressed genes (KsCYP72A397_IhOP) | 2022 |
| | Soyasapogenol B | 17.6 mg/L (25-fold higher) | *S. cerevisiae* | Expressed *βAS* derived from *G. glabra*; adopted several different types of promoters | 2021 |
| | 13 Pentacyclic triterpenoid aralosides | Rich and diverse | *S. cerevisiae* | Large number of tandem duplications of triterpenoid saponin-modifying enzyme genes in the genome | 2022 |
| Ursane-type | α-Amyrin | 11.97±0.61 mg/L | *S. cerevisiae* | Constructed *MdOSC1* into *S. cerevisiae*; increasing the supply of the precursors | 2018 |
| | α-Amyrin | 1.1 g/L | *S. cerevisiae* | Engineered the *MdOSC1* gene and expanding its intracellular storage pool | 2020 |
| | α-Amyrin | 11-Fold higher | *S. cerevisiae* | Remodeling αAS MdOSC1 and expanding the storage pool | 2020 |
| | α-Amyrin | 5.64 mg/L | *S. cerevisiae* | Adopted GAL1 promoter | 2018 |
| | Ursolic acid | High level | *N. benthamiana* | Combinatorial expression of *LUP5* and *CYP716A80* | 2015 |
| | Ursolic acid | — | *S. cerevisiae* | Introduced CrMAS, CYP450 oxidase and CPR | 2018 |
| | Corosolic acid | 141 mg/L | *S. cerevisiae* | Expressed *CYP716C49* from *Crataegus pinnatifida* | 2019 |
| | Corosolic acid | — | *N. benthamiana* | Coexpression of *LsOSC2*, *CYP716A265* and *CYP716C55* genes | 2019 |
| | Taraxasterol | 149.3 and 266.1 μg/g DW | *N. tabacum* | Overexpressing the *TcOSC1* gene of *Taraxacum coreanum* | 2022 |
| | Taraxasterol, ψ-taraxasterol, α-amyrin | — | *N. tabacum* | Overexpressed the *TcOSC1* gene of *Taraxacum coreanum* | 2022 |
| | ψ-Taraxasterol acetate, α-amyrin acetate | — | *N. tabacum*, *S. Cerevisiae* | Ectopic expression of both the *LsOSC1* and *LsTAT1* genes | 2022 |
| | ψ-Taraxasterol, α-amyrin | — | *N. tabacum* | Overexpressing the *TcOSC1* gene of *Taraxacum coreanum* | 2022 |
| | C-23 hydroxyl ursane-type triterpenoid derivatives | — | *S. cerevisiae* | Introducing three genes *IaAO1*, *IaAO4* and *IaCPR that isolated from Ilex asprella* | 2022 |
| Lupane-type | Betulinic acid | Increased by 136.39% | *S. cerevisiae* | Co-expressing *CYP716A12* gene from *M. truncatula* and ATR1 from *Arabidopsis* | 2017 |
| | Betulinic acid | — | *S. cerevisiae* | Expressed *LUS1* from *Arabidopsis and CrAO* from *Catharanthus roseus* | 2014 |
| | Betulinic acid | 0.32 mg/L | *Y. lipolytica* | Co-expressed *AtLUP1*, *CYP716A12* and reductase *AtCPR1* that come from *Arabidopsis* | 2019 |
| | Betulinic acid | 9.41 mg/L | *Y. lipolytica* | Fused and expressed P450 enzyme genes with its truncated reductase, and overexpressed the key genes of the upstream MVA pathway | 2019 |
| | Betulinic acid | 16.98 mg/L | *Y. lipolytica* | Glycerol fermentation | 2019 |

(Continued)

| Categories | Products | Yields | Heterologous hosts | Strategies | Year |
|---|---|---|---|---|---|
| | 20-Hydroxy betulinic acid | — | *N. benthamiana* | Transiently expressed *AMY2* (*OSC* gene) oxidized by CYP71D353 | 2013 |
| | Betulinic acid | — | *N. benthamiana* | Coexpressed *LsOSC1* and *CYP716A265* genes | 2019 |
| | Betulinic acid | 51.87±2.77 mg/L | *Y. lipolytica* | A multimodular strategy: selected optimal betulinic acid-producing strains, overexpressed the *ERG1*, *ERG9*, and *HMG1* genes of MVA module | 2019 |
| | Betulinic acid | 182 mg/L | *S. cerevisiae* | Re-engineered the reported betulinic acid pathway; further exploited excess ethanol in nitrogen-limited resting cell fermentations | 2017 |
| | Lupeol | 200.1 mg/L | *S. cerevisiae* | Recruiting the codon-optimized three lupeol pathway genes | 2019 |
| | Lupeol | Increased 127-fold | *S. cerevisiae* | A combinatorial engineering strategy: overexpressed *ERG13* genes, the knockout of negative regulators *ROX1* gene, suppression of a competing pathway | 2018 |
| | Lupeol | 411.72 mg/L (33.2-fold) | *Y. lipolytica* | Overexpressing the *OLE1* gene and disturbing *PAH1* and *DGK1 genes* | 2020 |
| | 20-Hydroxy lupeol | — | *N. benthamiana* | Transiently expressed *AMY2* (*OSC* gene) oxidized by CYP71D353 | 2013 |
| | Alphitolic acid | 23 mg/L | *S. cerevisiae* | Expressed *CYP716C49* from *Crataegus pinnatifida* | 2019 |
| | Lupeol alcohol | — | *S. cerevisiae* | Expressed the *LUS* gene *OeLUP* | 2018 |
| Friedelane-type | Friedelin | 37.07 mg/L | *S. cerevisiae* | Expressed *TwOSC1* and *TwOSC3* genes; reconstructed the biosynthetic pathway of friedelin by CRISPR/Cas9; protein modification and medium optimization | 2019 |
| | Friedelin | 0.43±0.16 mg/g DW | *N. benthamiana* | Transiently expressed CYP712K4 in combination with *tHMGR1* and *MiFRS4* | 2019 |
| | Friedelin | 2.27±0.32 mg/L | *S. cerevisiae* | Using methyl-β-cyclodextrin (MβCD) in the cultivation medium; knocking out *PAH1* using CRISPR/Cas9 | 2019 |
| | Friedelin | Increase 5-fold | *S. cerevisiae* | Deleting the *UBC7* gene | 2020 |
| | Friedelin | Increase 3.0 - 6.8-fold | *S. cerevisiae* | A combined strategy with integration of endogenous pathway genes and knocking out of inhibiting genes by CRISPR/Cas9 technology | 2022 |
| | 29-Hydroxy-friedelin | — | *S. cerevisiae* | Expressed *CYP712K1*, *CYP712K2*, and *CYP712K3* to oxidize friedelin | 2020 |
| | Maytenoic acid | — | *N. benthamiana* | CYP712K4 catalyzes the oxidation of friedelin at the C-29 position | 2019 |
| | Maytenoic acid | — | *S. cerevisiae* | CYP712K4 catalyzes the oxidation of friedelin at the C-29 position | 2019 |
| | Polpunonic acid | — | *S. cerevisiae* | Expressed *CYP712K1*, *CYP712K2*, and *CYP712K3* to oxidize friedelin | 2020 |
| | Polpunonic acid | 1.4 mg/L | *S. cerevisiae* | Introduced the CYP712K1 enzyme into yeast | 2020 |

cells and metabolic pathway, the category and yield of oleanane-type pentacyclic triterpenoids will be significantly expanded and improved, respectively.

In the terpenoid metabolic pathway, the formation reaction of 2, 3-oxidosqualene is catalyzed by OSC to generate α-amyrin, which functions as a precursor of ursane-type pentacyclic triterpenes. Subsequently, α-amyrin was modified by glycosyla-tion, acylation, redox reaction and other modifications to form a variety of ursane-type pentacyclic triterpenoids with various structures and functions, and the representative compounds mainly include ursolic acid, asiatic acid, ziyuglycoside, and taraxasterol. Currently, the functional mechanism of CYP450 enzymes related to asiatic acid, ziyuglycoside and other compounds has not been fully clarified, and the modification process of various glycosyl groups also has not been elucidated, which hinder the study of the heterologous biosynthesis of ursane. Given that the structures of ursane and oleanane are similar, the enzymes in some heterologous synthetic pathways can be used universally, and they can refer to each other in the natural synthetic pathways of various compounds. Ursane-type pentacyclic triterpenoids will have great development potential and space in the future.

Lupane-type pentacyclic triterpenes were synthesized from the catalytic reaction of 2,3-oxidosqualene *via* LUS to produce lupeol, which was subsequently modified based on the lupeol structure. The representative compounds mainly include lupeol, betulinic acid, and betulin. At present, there are several reports on the heterologous biosynthesis of lupane-type pentacyclic triterpenoids, and their yields are at a relatively low level. With the in-depth analysis of the biosynthetic pathway, more and more lupane-type pentacyclic triterpenoids will be produced on a large scale through heterologous plants or microbial cell factories in the future.

Friedelane-type pentacyclic triterpenoids were synthesized by various modifications and structural derivation of friedelane evolved from oleanene methyl translocation, and their representative compounds mainly include friedelin, tripterygone, celastrol, and maytenoic acid. Currently, some studies on the heterologous synthesis of friedelane *via* *N. benthamiana* and yeast have been, but its biosynthetic levels are still deficient. Besides, the functional mechanism of the CYP enzyme and the modification process of multiple glycosyl groups have not been clarified, which restricts their heterologous synthesis, and thus further in-depth research is still required.

We compared the heterologous biosynthetic levels of four different types of pentacyclic triterpenoids, including the above-mentioned research cases, summarized in Table 4. According to this table, we can find that *S. cerevisiae* is the most commonly used host for the heterologous biosynthesis of pentacyclic triterpenoids, and there are still relatively few studies on the biosynthesis of pentacyclic triterpenoids *via* heterologous plants. In terms of synthetic levels, the heterologous syntheses of microbial cell factories and *N. benthamiana* have their own characteristics. Due to their different measurement units, it is difficult to see obvious differences, which should be compared comprehensively based on the raw material cost, labor cost, and other aspects. Generally, microbial cell factories consume various raw materials, while heterologous plants mainly rely on light energy to produce pentacyclic triterpenoids. At present, the biosynthesis of some pentacyclic triterpenoids has reached a relatively high level, but there is still a gap between that and their large-scale production. Moreover, the types and total amounts of pentacyclic triterpenoids involved in heterologous biosynthesis are still insufficient to meet the relatively low cost needs of human beings. Thus, it is still necessary to carry out and optimize new strategies like those mentioned above to improve the efficiency of biosynthesis and the accumulation of natural products.

## 5 CONCLUSIONS AND FUTURE PERSPECTIVES

5.1 Conclusions Pentacyclic triterpenoids, as natural active substances, have extensive pharmacological effects and important biological activities, and play an important role in lowering the blood sugar, protecting the liver, and anti-inflammatory, anti-oxidation, anti-fatigue, anti-virus and anti-cancer activities. Pentacyclic triterpenoids are widely distributed in nature and diverse, which exist in monocotyledons, dicotyledons, pteridophyta, fungi and marine organisms. We systematically summarized the classification, distribution, structural characteristics, and bioactivity of pentacyclic triterpenoids, and analyzed the regulation of key enzyme genes, namely, *OSC*, *CYP450*, *UGT*, *HMGR*, *FPS*, *SS* and *SE*, in the biosynthesis of pentacyclic triterpene saponins, aiming to provide a reference for heterologous biosynthesis *via* plant chassis. OSC catalyzes the formation of the basic skeleton of pentacyclic triterpenes, which is the key enzyme to produce diverse triterpene products. CYP catalyzes the structural modification of the triterpene skeleton, such as hydroxylation, carboxylation, aldehydeylation, ketonation, dehydrogenation and dehydration, to form the intermediates of triterpene saponins. The intermediates of triterpene saponins were glycosylated by UGTs to produce different types of triterpenoid saponins, which is the key link in the formation of the diversity and biological activities of triterpenoid saponins. The differential expression of key rate-limiting enzyme genes, namely, *HMGR*, *FPS*, *SS* and *SE*, in the biosynthetic pathway of triterpenes responds to environmental factors and elicitors such as light, temperature, humidity, salt, soil, MeJA, SA, ABA, GA, and auxin, regulating the biosynthesis of triterpenoid saponins in plants. During this process, TFs activate or inhibit the expression of these key rate-limiting enzyme genes by binding to their promoters, thus affecting the accumulation of triterpenoid saponins. Additionally, miRNAs target these key rate-limiting enzyme genes or TFs at the post-transcriptional level through splicing and translation control or other modes of action, and ultimately regulate the accumulation of pentacyclic triterpenoids. We presented a general analysis and summarized the transcriptional regulation model of pentacyclic triterpenoids associated with environmental factors, elicitors, the key rate-limiting enzyme genes (*HMGR*, *FPS*, *SS* and *SE*), TFs (AP2/ERF, bHLH, WRKY, bZIP and MYB) and miRNAs, which can provide reference for clarifying this complex transcriptional regulation mechanism. Heterologous biosynthesis has gradually become a new method for the efficient synthesis of natural products. At present, the hosts of heterologous biosynthesis mainly include heterologous plants, *S. cerevisiae*, *P. pastoris*, and *E. coli*. Utilizing synthetic biology technology by means of introducing regulatory elements, artificially transforming the metabolic flux and regulation of heterologous hosts, optimizing culture conditions and establishing general high-throughput screening methods contributes to reconstructing the triterpene biosynthetic pathway in heterologous hosts. Subsequently, through the engineering transformation of the biosynthetic pathway of the chassis cell precursor, global metabolic network and product transportation, a high and stable yield of the target product can be realized. We comprehensively discussed the characteristics of the heterologous synthesis of heterologous plants and microbial cell factories, which can provide an important reference for the selection and application of heterologous hosts. Meanwhile, we summarized the research progress and heterologous synthetic level of four main types of pentacyclic triterpenoids, *i.e.*, oleanane-type, ursane-type, lupane-type and friedelane-type, *via* the plant chassis and microbial cell factories. Based on the existing research results, we proposed optimization strategies to improve the biosynthesis and accumulation of triterpene saponins. We proposed and optimized the biosynthetic pathway, regulatory factors, exogenous metabolic pathway, chassis cell system and fermentation conditions, and used the regulation technologies such as metabolic engineering, enzyme engineering, cell engineering and fermentation engineering to improve the accumulation of the target products and realize the large-scale and efficient production of triterpenoid saponins.

At present, the research on the biosynthetic pathway of triterpenoid saponins mainly focuses on the discovery of key enzyme genes in the post-modification stage of triterpenoid saponin biosynthesis. The functions of some P450 oxidases and glycosyltransferases in plants are still unknown, and the specific catalytic process, structural modification and transcriptional regulation mechanism of key enzymes are still less studied. In addition, the cognition of the biosynthetic pathway of triterpenoid saponins is still not systematic and comprehensive. Heterologous biosynthesis has the advantages of short cycle, high efficiency, simple nutritional requirements, easy extraction and separation, and mature and reliable genetic operation methods, which provide an important pathway for the large-scale and efficient production of triterpenoid saponins. However, the introduction of heterologous biosynthetic pathways and the modification of microbial metabolic pathways can lead to imbalances in metabolic flux and accumulation of toxic intermediates in cells, resulting in some negative effects. Furthermore, some key enzymes have poor heterologous expression ability and low activity in microorganisms. Also, screening key enzymes with strong specificity and high catalytic activity is also a key issue in heterologous biosynthesis at this stage. The single species and insufficient supply of UDP glycosyl donors in microbial cells also limit the production of pentacyclic triterpenoid saponins. The biosynthesis of natural products completed by microbial cell factories often encounters low yields and low titers. Accordingly, an effective way to address these bottlenecks is to design genetic biosensors to monitor and regulate the biosynthesis of the target natural products, but this approach is still in its infancy, which needs to be further improved. Moreover, currently it is still a challenging task to achieve the industrialized production of pentacyclic triterpenoids through heterologous biosynthesis.

5.2 Future perspectives Synthetic biology has developed rapidly in recent years and has become an important way to solve the problems of source, scale and sustainable supply of pentacyclic triterpenoids. There are many types of pentacyclic triterpenoids with complex and diverse structures. Although triterpenoid saponins share a common precursor synthetic pathway, the post-modification stage is highly specific and diverse. Therefore, it is imperative to explore the biosynthetic pathway and regulatory mechanism of pentacyclic triterpenoid saponins. The biosynthetic pathway of triterpenoid saponins includes more than 20 consecutive enzymatic reactions, among which the upper and middle metabolic pathways from acetyl-CoA to 2,3-oxidosqualene have been clearly studied. However, the downstream metabolic biosynthetic pathways of triterpenoid saponin from 2,3-oxidosqualene to the final triterpenoid saponins have their own rules in different plants, and the functions and pathways of some key enzyme have not yet been clarified. For a long time, triterpenoids originated from the formation of squalene from two molecules of FPP catalyzed by squalene synthase, and further oxidized to form 2,3-oxidosqualene. However, surprisingly, Tao *et al*.

utilized efficient microbial chassis and artificial intelligence strategies to overturn the long-standing inherent cognition that all triterpenoids were synthesized with squalene as the only starting unit, and found that a number of triterpenoids can be catalyzed by type I terpenoid synthases, namely TvTS and MpM, which belong to non-squalene synthase, filling the cognitive gap in the diversity of natural product synthetic mechanisms of this huge group and greatly expanding the space for the in-depth mining and accurate discovery of new triterpenoids.

Drawing support from modern synthetic biology, the heterologous biosynthesis of pentacyclic triterpenoids has shown great application potential. Meanwhile, with the large-scale development of metabolomic and genomic analysis technologies in medicinal plants and the advent of the post-genomic era, more synthetic pathways of secondary metabolism of triterpenoids will be analyzed more comprehensively. The enzymatic structure modification and application of endoplasmic reticulum engineering can improve the expression ability and catalytic activity of plant-derived enzymes in microbial hosts. The problem of insufficient coenzymes and donors can be solved by optimizing the metabolic flux direction of the host through synthetic biology. Besides, it is expected that the problem of product cytotoxicity to the host with be solved through host selection and organelle regional production. Meanwhile, the development of synthetic biology will also provide a series of suitable chassis cells for the functional identification of related genes, which will greatly promote the development of the heterologous biosynthesis of triterpenoid saponins towards a large scale and industrialization.

In the few past decades, the development of synthetic biology and the study of heterologous synthesis of terpenoids have provided researchers with a relatively complete genetic manipulation platform and some high-yield triterpenoid chassis cells. To further optimize the chassis cells and meet the needs of the large-scale synthesis of numerous complex terpenoids, more rational design methods and more powerful genetic manipulation platforms need to be developed, such as pathway kinetic analysis and efficient chromosome editing technology. After realizing the respective optimization of cell functional elements or modules, it is necessary to propose engineering means from the system level to solve the adaptation problem between modules, and finally construct various efficient, stable and controllable heterologous biosynthetic cell factories of pentacyclic triterpenoids. The application of the cross-fusion strategy of biosynthetic and chemical synthesis will be a new trend in the total synthesis of natural products. By building a microbial cell factory, combining genetic engineering and bioengineering technology, the metabolic pathway of biologically active substances is constructed in microorganisms, thus producing a large amount of valuable natural active substances through microorganisms. Utilizing multiomics and big data to explore the functional genes of the biosynthetic pathway of bioactive substances and study the metabolic regulation network, constructing the regulatory network from gene to metabolism, and applying functional genomics technologies, such as VIGS, RNAi and CRISPR/Cas9 to non-model plants, will help to clarify the regulatory mechanism for the biosynthesis of biologically active substances. In addition, it will be a new development trend in this field to integrate artificial intelligence technology with synthetic biology to realize the intelligence, economization, automation and efficiency of total biological synthesis. The breakthrough of computer-aided design, whole gene and even genome synthesis will make the biosynthetic industry enter the industrial development of engineering and design. The transformation, design and even re-synthesis of life processes or organisms through synthetic biology not only can provide a research system for basic biological research, but also provide new solutions for biomedicine, environmental energy, biomaterials and other industries, thereby promoting a new wave of technological revolution.

[李艳林,袁吉锋,薛哲勇,等. Natural Product Reports, 2023,40:1303-1353.]

# Progress and prospect: biosynthesis of plant natural products based on plant chassis

## 1 INTRODUCTION

Plants serve as a crucial source of natural drug resources and are widely used in China's traditional Chinese medicine system. Issues surrounding public health safety, as well as resource conservation and development, have garnered increased attention in recent years. Consequently, the exploration of plant products with pharmacological effects, along with the cultivation and identification of authentic medicinal plants, has gained prominence. Plant natural products are predominantly secondary metabolites that are not essential for plant growth and reproduction. They face barriers such as spatial and temporal accumulation specificity and species specificity, resulting in scarce natural product content. Therefore, the limited accumulation of natural medicinal products in plants poses a significant challenge for commercial applications.

Synthetic biology is an emerging interdisciplinary field that combines systems biology with genetic engineering technology to construct artificial biocatalytic systems according to human design. The discipline follows the "design-build-test-learn" process, which begins with selecting and designing chassis cells, analyzing and reconstructing specific metabolic pathways, and discovering and assembling biological elements to produce substances and materials essential for society. As a result, synthetic biology can help address fundamental social issues such as fuel and energy scarcity, food crop shortages, and the medical drug shortage by meeting the supply and demand of basic materials in the global market.

The synthesis of natural plant products currently involves plant tissue extraction or chemical synthesis, but the application of synthetic biology can provide an alternative approach. Plant natural product synthesis is mainly carried out in either a microbial or plant chassis, with the latter possessing several advantages. Plants offer a finely compartmentalized cellular structure, which supports the proper functioning of membrane-localized exogenous enzymes, particularly cytochrome P450 (CYP450) enzymes. In terms of species relationship, plant chassis are better suited for expressing exogenous genes from plant species compared to microbial chassis. The synthesis of natural products in plants frequently entails multiple biochemical reaction steps and the involvement of active enzymes, some of which are absent in microbial chassis. Consequently, this may require additional genes and hinder the attainment of target products. Additionally, plant chassis possess a comprehensive post-translational modification system for structurally modifying natural products, ensuring the functionality of heterologous proteins. By synthesizing and accumulating natural products within the plant chassis, the costs associated with cultivation environment, transportation, and preservation can be significantly reduced. While there have been successful examples of producing active natural products in microbial cell factories (C. Q.), a fundamental difference lies in the mechanism of transgenesis between the two. Plant chassis can integrate exogenous genes into the host genome more stably, allowing these genes to be inherited by the next generation. In contrast, prokaryotic chassis normally rely on recombinant plasmids that exist independently of the host genome and may be lost during culture, resulting in the loss of exogenous genes (Fig. 1). Furthermore, while some metabolic synthetic genes from plants can be transformed into microbial and heterologous plant cells, product synthesis may only be successful in the plant chassis. Therefore, the development of plant synthetic biology is necessary. Here we compare and contrast the advantages and disadvantages of different plant and microbial chassis (Table 1).

This paper aims to examine the mechanisms of efficient heterologous and native accumulation of natural active products in plants, commencing from the plant chassis. Furthermore, it will explore the enabling technologies that have facilitated the recent development of synthetic biology in plants, as well as the strategies and methods to overcome the current limitations in product accumulation, thereby providing a substantial material basis for energy, pharmaceuticals, food, agriculture and industry.

## 2 SYNTHESIS OF NATURAL PRODUCTS IN PLANT CHASSIS

Plant chassis have recently been utilized in fields of energy synthesis, pharmaceutical development, food processing, and environmental monitoring. Natural products can be classified into three major groups, including terpenoids, alkaloids and phenols. This paper provides examples of both heterologous and native synthesis of these natural products using plant chassis (Table 2).

2.1 Terpenoids  Terpenoids are a major class of secondary metabolites in plants. They are synthesized through the 2-*C*-methyl-D-erythritol-4-phosphate pathway in the plastid, using pyruvate and Acetyl-CoA as substrates to form dimethylallyl diphosphate (DMAPP), and through the mevalonate pathway in the cytoplasm, where isopentenyl diphosphate (IPP) is formed. DMAPP and IPP then combine in different molecular ratios (1 : 1, 2 : 1, 3 : 1) to form precursors, which branch into different synthetic pathways and result in different terpenoids. Based on the number of isoprene units they contain, terpenoids can be classified as monoterpenes, sesquiterpenes, diterpenes, triterpenes, and so on. Terpenoids exhibit a wide range of pharmacological and biological activities. For example, monoterpenes such as geraniol, limonene, and peppermint oil have been shown to possess antibacterial, anti-inflammatory, analgesic, anticancer, and antioxidant effects. Diterpenoids, including tanshinone, paclitaxel, and cosbene, have demonstrated antioxidant, anticancer, and antiviral activities. Triterpenoids such as ginsenoside, diosgenin, and withanolide have been found to have anticancer, antidiabetic, and neuroprotective effects. Finally, tetraterpenoids like β-carotene and canthaxanthin have shown anticancer, antibacterial, and anti-neurodegenerative properties.

Despite their significance, the accumulation of terpenoids in plants is typically low. For example, the artemisinin in

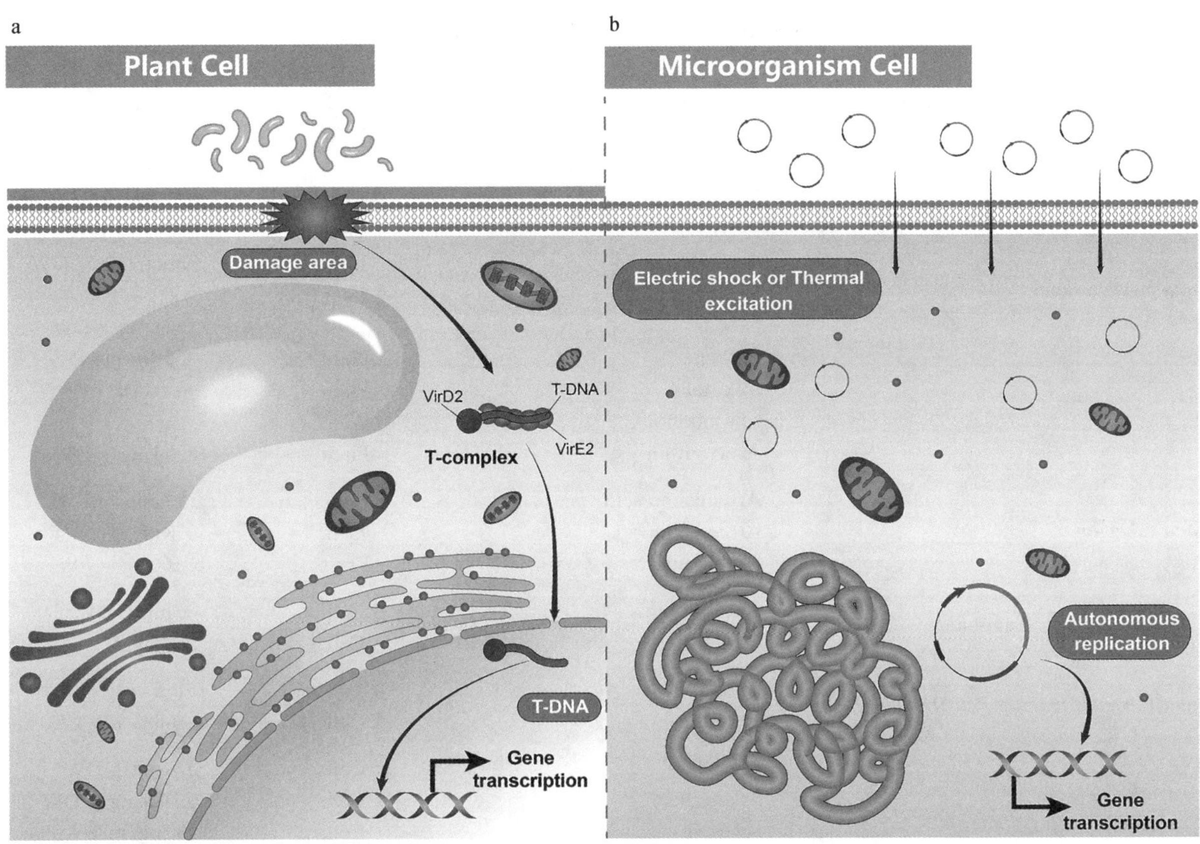


**Fig. 1 Comparison between plant cells and microbial cells in terms of exogenous gene expression patterns**

(a) The accompanying image demonstrates the process by which Agrobacterium enters a plant cell through a wound surface and utilizes its own and related protein molecules within the host cell (e. g. , Vir gene series and transporter proteins) to target the T-DNA complex to the nucleus, followed by the active transport of this complex into the nucleus where it integrates into the plant chromosome. Subsequently, the expression of T-DNA is controlled by the expression of the genome. Vir, Virulence protein; T-complex, VirD2/T-strand/VirE2 complex. (b) The image on the right illustrates how microbial cells are subjected to physicochemical effects, such as electric shock, heat, and chemicals, that create gaps in the cell membrane. These gaps provide a pathway for exogenous gene vectors to enter the cell, where they are expressed independently of the host genome with the assistance of the host cell.

**Table 1 Comparison of various chassis cells in synthetic biology**

| Comparative items | | Chassis Types | | | | |
|---|---|---|---|---|---|---|
| | | Higher plant | Hairy root | Eukaryotic | Prokaryote | Photosynthetic Microbe |
| Cellular gene level | Easy genetic engineering manipulation | × | × | √ | √ | √ |
| | Clear genetic background | × | × | √ | √ | × |
| | High efficiency of gene conversion | × | × | √ | √ | √ |
| Cellular structure level | Compartmentalization of the Cellular structure | √ | √ | √ | × | × |
| | Membrane structures facilitating the binding of CYPs | √ | √ | √ | × | × |
| | High cellular antitoxicity | √ | √ | √ | × | × |
| Cell culture level | Short growth period | × | √ | √ | √ | √ |
| | Low cultivation difficulty | × | √ | √ | √ | √ |
| | Low cost of cultivation | √ | √ | × | × | √ |
| | Autotrophism | √ | √ | × | × | √ |
| | High light energy utilization | √ | × | × | × | √ |
| Product application level | Ease of storage and use of products | √ | √ | × | × | × |
| | Strong ability to produce natural products of plant | √ | √ | √ | × | × |
| | Simple downstream extraction and purification | × | √ | √ | √ | √ |
| | High biosecurity | √ | √ | √ | × | × |
| | Heterologous product diversification | √ | √ | × | × | × |

In the table, √ indicates that the function is available, and × indicates that the function is not available or is partially available.

**Table 2 Production of natural products in different plant chassis**

| Categorys | Products | Tissue | Product yields |
|---|---|---|---|
| *Nicotiana benthamiana* | Taxadien<br>Taxadiene-5α-ol<br>Omega-3 fatty acid<br>Lycopene<br>Artemisinin<br>Diterpenoids<br>Crocins<br>Casbene<br>Jolkinol C<br>Epi-jolkinol C<br>Astaxanthin | Leaf<br>Leaf<br>Leaf<br>Leaf<br>Leaf<br>Leaf<br>Leaf<br>Plant<br>Plant<br>Plant<br>Plant | 56.6 μg/g FW<br>1.3 μg/g FW<br>—<br>150 μg/g DW<br>about 3 ng/g DW<br>—<br>1.61 mg/g DW<br>3.9 μg/mg DW<br>—<br>—<br>0.99 mg/g DW |
| *Nicotiana tabacum* | Artemisinic acid<br>Artemisinin<br>Flavonoids | Leaf<br>Cell<br>Fruit | 120 mg/kg FW<br>0.8 mg/g DW<br>1 100 μg/g FW |
| *Nicotiana tabacum* cv. Samsun | Anthocyanins<br>Geraniol | Cell<br>Cell | 30 mg/g DW<br>5.2 mg/L |
| *Nicotiana tabacum L. cv. Petit Havana SR1* | Geraniol<br>Taxadiene | Hairy root<br>Cell | 31.3 μg/g DW<br>0.05% FW of tissue |
| *Physcomitrella patens* | Patchoulol<br>β-Santalene<br>Sclareol | Cell<br>Cell<br>Cell | 0.8 mg/g DW<br>0.035 mg/g DW<br>280 μg/g DW |
| *Arabidopsis thaliana* | Cyanidin 3-O-glucoside<br>DHA<br>Carotenoid<br>Taxadiene | Cell<br>Seed<br>Seed<br>Hairy root | 90 mg/L<br>15.1 of seed oil<br>10-fold of control<br>600 ng/g DW |
| *Silybum marianum* | T-resveratrol | Cell | 12 mg/L |
| *Camelina sativa* | DHA | Seed | 12.4% of seed oil |
| *Brassica napus* | DHA | Seed | 3.7% of Canola oil |
| *Oryza sativa* | Provitamin A | Seed | 2 μg/g |
| *Glycine max* | Phytosterol<br>Vitamin D3 | Seed<br>Fruit | 3.8 μg/g DW<br>0.3 μg/g DW |
| *Solanum lycopersicum* | Lutein<br>Linolenic acid | Fruit<br>Fruit | 422.6 μg/g DW<br>about 100 μg/g FW |
| *Citrus paradise* | Crocetin | Fruit | 9.88 μg/g DW |
| *Lemna minor* | Stigmasterol | Plant | 1 600 mg/kg FW |
| *Panax ginseng* C. A. Meyer | Taxadiene<br>Ginsenoside Rg3 | Hairy root<br>Hairy root | 15.9 μg/g DW<br>7.0 mg/g DW |
| *Centella asiatica* | Triterpenoids | Hairy root | 60.25 mg/g DW |
| *A. membranaceus* | Astragaloside | Hairy root | 5.5 mg/g DW |
| *Pelargonium sidoides* | Coumarin | Hairy root | 427.37 μg/g DW |
| *Hyoscyamus reticulatus* | Hyoscyamine<br>Scopolamine | Hairy root<br>Hairy root | 140.15 μg/g FW<br>67.71 μg/g FW |
| *Salvia Miltiorrhiza* | Salvianolic acid B | Hairy root | 1.43-fold of control |
| *Atropa belladonna* | Scopolamine | Hairy root | — |

*Artemisia annua* accounts for only 0.1 - 1.0% of its dry weight, and the biomass of tanshinone in the roots of *Salvia miltiorrhiza* is only 0.1 mg/g. Similarly, paclitaxel is found in only 0.01% of the bark of *Taxus wallichiana*.

It is clear that many natural products accumulate in insignificant amounts in their native plants. Even the chemical synthesis of natural products presents several issues, including chiral carbon-induced enantiomeric toxicity, residual chemical reagent toxicity during down-stream processing, and cost-yield imbalances. Therefore, the use of plants as a chassis for synthetic biology has gained significant attention as a means of producing terpenoids.

2.1.1 Monoterpenes Monoterpene compounds are composed of two isoprene units and can be classified as acyclic, monocyclic, bicyclic, and tricyclic structures. Monoterpenoids naturally exist as volatile oils. However, the traditional method of extracting chemicals from plant tissues causes the destruction of natural plant resources, leading to a loss of biodiversity. Therefore, efficient plant chassis are preferred for environmental, efficiency, and cost reasons. Moreover, plant chassis offer certain advantages in the synthesis and extraction of such compounds. Firstly, the plant chassis inherently hosts numerous secondary metabolic pathways capable of autonomously synthesizing volatile products. Consequently, these compounds can be generated within the plant chassis more naturally, circumventing the need for reconstructing or adapting synthetic pathways, as in microbial platforms. Secondly, the plant chassis exhibits a capacity for synthesizing an extensive array of plant-derived natural volatile products through its intrinsic secondary metabolic pathways, thus fostering a more varied product portfolio. Thirdly, distinct cellular compartments within the plant chassis, such as chloroplasts, possess the inherent capability to synthesize specific categories of volatile components. Lastly, the plant chassis' innate competence to naturally synthesize and stabilize the storage of volatile components contributes to heightened product stability and purity. Geraniol is essential in aromatherapy and widely used in spicery and pharmaceutical applications. Geraniol and other plant essential oils have significant development and utilization value. In a market analysis report, the Newsijie Industry Research Center predicted that the domestic demand for geraniol will reach 1,000 t in the next five years, which indicates considerable potential for developing an efficient plant synthesis platform for geraniol production. Nikolay Vasilev et al. combined the tobacco cell suspension culture technique with an orthogonal array experimental design to demonstrate that sucrose, liquid medium volume, and inoculum volume positively promote geraniol production in tobacco cells, obtaining 5.2 mg/L geraniol in shake flasks over a 12-day period. Soheil S Mahmoud et al. introduced limonene synthase and limonene 3-hydroxylase in *Mentha* × *piperita* and found that co-inhibition of limonene 3-hydroxylase resulted in high accumulation of limonene.

2.1.2 Sesquiterpenes Sesquiterpene compounds, which consist of three isoprene units, are the most abundant group of terpenes, exhibiting acyclic, monocyclic, bicyclic, tricyclic and tetracyclic structures. Although both sesquiterpenes and monoterpenes exist as volatile oils, sesquiterpenes generally have higher boiling points. The main representative substances are artemisinin, patchoulol and parthenolide. Artemisinin has been a potent anti-malarial agent since its discovery, and further research on this substance has shown considerable promise in the fight against leukemia, the treatment of systemic lupus erythematosus and some allergic diseases. Scientists from three different groups have obtained high accumulations of artemisinin in different plant chassis to address the current shortage of artemisinin in some regions of the world. The effect of parthenolide in relieving headaches and migraines is better than that of common analgesic and anti-inflammatory drugs, such as aspirin. This natural product has miraculous effects on glioblastoma, and parthenolide is also able to fight against the disruption of host immune response by COVID - 19. However, it is in short supply in clinical and daily life, and there is an urgent need to use synthetic biology to address this dilemma. Farzaneh Pourianezhad et al. studied parthenolide and parthenolide synthase using the hairy root culture technique in combination with the use of elicitors. Finally, the content of parthenolide reached 0.05 mg/g dry weight, with the highest expression of parthenolide synthase under the combination of 2.5 mg/L yeast extract and 100 μM methyl jasmonate induction.

2.1.3 Diterpenes Diterpenoids are a class of natural products composed of four isoprene units, with a subgroup of oxygenated derivatives having significant research and production importance in medicinal applications. Paclitaxel, tanshinone compounds, and casbene are among the most well-known substances in this group. Despite the increasing market demand and price of paclitaxel, its synthesis and production have been insufficient due to its widespread use as an anticancer agent. Therefore, there is an urgent need for a platform that enables efficient synthesis of paclitaxel-like compounds, and tobacco is a promising host. For instance, Jianhua Li et al. employed a chloroplast compartmentalized metabolic engineering strategy and overexpression of isoprene precursors to achieve 56.6 μg/g fresh weight and 1.3 μg/g fresh weight of paclitaxel intermediates, taxadiene and taxadiene-5α-ol, in *Nicotiana benthamiana* leaves. Casbene is a crucial precursor for many medicinally active products in Euphorbiaceae. The chemical synthesis of casbene is challenging, so plant synthetic biology could offer an alternative approach. For instance, Edith C. F. Forestier et al. heterologously expressed 1-deoxy-D-xylulose 5-phosphate synthase (DXS), 4-hydroxy-3-methylbut-2-enyl diphosphate reductase (HDR), and geranylgeranyl diphosphate synthase (GGPPS) from *Arabidopsis thaliana* and casbene synthase from *Jatropha curcas* in tobacco, resulting in a 410% higher yield of casbene than the transformed tobacco lines only expressing casbene synthase. This indicates that the supply of precursors required for secondary metabolite synthesis plays a crucial role in their accumulation, and highlights the importance of studying the silencing and inhibition of related bypass metabolic pathways.

2.1.4 Triterpenes Triterpenoids are a group of natural products composed of six isoprene units, which are divided into two types: tetracyclic triterpenes and pentacyclic triterpenes. They often combine with sugars to form glycosides or lactones in plants. Representative substances of this group include ginsenosides, diosgenins, and withanolides. Ginsenosides, for instance, are a class of derivatives with various medicinal values, such as anti-cancer and cancer metastasis inhibition effects. To improve the yield of ginsenoside Rg3, Lu Yao et al. optimized the ginseng root plant chassis by overexpressing key enzyme genes, CRISPR/Cas9 gene editing to knock out bypass enzyme genes, and rational point mutation of the protein structural domain of key heterologous glycosyltransferases. This resulted in an 83.6 mg/L yield of ginsenoside Rg3 in a shake flask culture environment, which was 21.12-fold higher than that of wild-type plants. Diosgenin, on the other hand, has significant effects in anti-angina and the treatment of atherosclerosis, making it an ideal precursor for semi-synthetic steroid hormone drugs. Thus, the advancement of its application in synthetic biology and the analysis of synthetic pathways will greatly reduce the environmental pollution problems associated with the traditional acid hydrolysis extraction of diosgenin. Bastien Christ et al. investigated and resolved the key catalytic steps of the diosgenin synthesis pathway in two plants, *Paris polyphylla* and *Trigonella foenum-graecum*, revealing the significance of spiroketalization and providing valuable insights into the production of diosgenin and its derivatives in heterologous hosts. Additionally, Xue Yin et al. developed a *Nicotiana benthamiana* platform to produce diosgenin with mg grade yield through co-expressing several sterol pathway genes.

2.1.5 Tetraterpenes Triterpenoids are a class of compounds composed of eight isoprene units and can be classified into carotenoids, which contain only carbon and hydrogen atoms, and luteins, which contain additional oxygen-containing functional groups. Astaxanthin and lycopene are representative compounds belonging to the lutein and carotenoid categories, respectively. Astaxanthin is a powerful natural antioxidant widely used in the food, pharmaceutical, and cosmetic industries, but its production mainly relies on natural or artificially cultured *Haematococcus Pluvialis*, which requires harsh growth conditions. Therefore, synthetic biology presents a promising platform for convenient and large-scale astaxanthin production. Qinlong Zhu et al. successfully reconstituted astaxanthin synthesis in rice seeds using a heterologous plant with a minimal number of exogenous gene combinations, demonstrating that the plant chassis has certain advantages over the microbial chassis. Lycopene is also a potent antioxidant, and its demand has been growing rapidly in recent years, with an estimated international market value exceeding $200 million in the next five years. Synthetic biology can be used to achieve efficient production of lycopene. Eszter Majer et al. used tobacco as a heterologous plant chassis and combined the tobacco etch virus vector with three bacterial phytoene synthases. This approach not only shortened the lycopene synthesis pathway but also led to a 10% share of lycopene in the total carotenoid content, which was monitored with a novel visualization perspective.

2.2 Alkaloids Alkaloids are a group of alkaline organic compounds that contain nitrogen and possess complex cyclic structural features with significant biological activity. They are an essential class of secondary metabolites in herbal medicine, which can be categorized into various types based on their core parent nuclei structures, such as isoquinolines, quinolines, indoles, and piperidines. The diverse chemical structures of alkaloids also provide them with numerous medicinal properties, including anticancer, neuronal modulation, smoking withdrawal, antimalarial, hypoglycemic, and anti-ulcer effects.

Amino acids, such as lysine, tyrosine, and tryptophan, serve as precursors for the synthesis of alkaloids, some of which are derived from amino acid derivatives combined with precursors of terpenoid and steroid synthesis, producing various types of alkaloids. The majority of alkaloids are synthesized via the shikimic acid pathway, which generates aromatic amino acids that are required for alkaloid synthesis. For instance, thebaine synthesis begins with erythrose-4-phosphate (E4P) in the pentose phosphate pathway and phosphoenol-pyruvate in the glycolytic pathway, leading to the formation of 3-deoxy-D-arabino-heptulosonate-7-phosphate (DAHP) and then shikimic acid. The process uses tryptophan, which is produced by the shikimic acid pathway, as a precursor for the final production of thebaine. Although alkaloids are mostly present in higher dicotyledons, their low expression levels in native plants remain a problem. For example, hyoscyamine and scopolamine accumulate in less than 1% of both root and leaf tissues of *Datura arborea*, and the amount of berberine in *Coptis chinensis* does not exceed 60 mg/g. Vinblastine in *Catharanthus roseus* is also extremely scarce, and conventional cultivation methods cannot meet the market demand for this type of anticancer natural product.

The development and application of synthetic biology in alkaloids is at an imminent stage. To provide widespread, inexpensive, and convenient access to medically active alkaloids such as vinblastine, hyoscyamine, and thebaine is essential for meeting the needs of people in less developed areas. For example, betalain, an efficient methyl donor that can prevent the formation of fatty liver, was synthesized by Guy Polturak et al. in *Nicotiana tabacum* using a CYP450 enzyme, CYP76AD6, and transcriptome analysis of two different species, which provided insights into the heterologous plant synthesis of betalain. Hyoscyamine, a class of anticholinergic substances used clinically for anesthesia, analgesia, and detoxification of phosphorus-containing pesticide poisoning, can be directly produced using a plant synthetic biology platform. Lingjiang Zeng et al. obtained recombinant plants with high hyoscyamine by knocking down hyoscyamine 6β-hydroxylase (AbH6H) using the native plant *Atropa belladonna* as the plant chassis, simplifying the extraction, isolation, and purification of tropane alkaloids. Vinca alkaloids, such as vinblastine and vincristine, are essential in treating malignant tumors, especially leukemia. However, these drugs are mainly extracted from plants, leading to shortages in clinical practice. Using a synthetic biology platform to analyze and heterologously produce these substances can significantly alleviate this supply shortage. Lorenzo Caputi et al. explored the synthetic pathway of vinblastine, identified two key enzymes catalyzing the intermediate metabolites of this class of alkaloids, stemmadenine, and made the heterologous development of vinblastine possible Colchicine, the preferred medicinal ingredient in gouty arthritis, as well as some dermatological and cardiovascular diseases, accumulates sparsely in native plants. Therefore, Ryan S Nett et al. synthesized N-formyldemecolcine, an important precursor of colchicine, in tobacco plants using simple aromatic amino acids supported by a multi-omics analysis. This approach provides a possibility to explore natural product synthesis pathways without knowing the relevant synthetic genes and the whole genome Although current reports suggest that nicotine may lack medicinal value, recent studies have found that small amounts of pure nicotine have anti-aging, anti-inflammatory, and neuroprotective effects in humans. Moreover, with the increasing global sales of pure nicotine due to the widespread use of e-cigarettes, it is necessary to improve the yield of nicotine and simplify the extraction and purification process. Bo Zhao et al. treated the NUP1 enzyme in the tobacco hairy root chassis, releasing more nicotine into the medium and simplifying the extraction and purification process while enhancing the yield of natural products.

### 2.3 Phenols

**2.3.1 Phenylpropanoids and flavonoids** Phenylpropanoids are substances with a phenol structure, consisting of single or multiple C6 - C3 repeating units with three straight-chain carbons attached to the benzene ring. They can be classified into five categories based on the number of C6 - C3 or C6 - C3 - C6 units, namely simple phenylpropanoids, coumarins, lignans, lignins, and special flavonoids. Phenylpropanoids exhibit various medicinal properties, such as treating Alzheimer's disease, antibacterial, antidepressant, antioxidant, antithrombotic, and anti-inflammatory activities.

The synthesis pathways of phenylpropanoids and flavonoids are similar to those of alkaloids, as they all depend on the shikimic acid pathway for the supply of precursors. However, unlike alkaloids, these two pathways either use aromatic amino acids directly as the only precursors after passing through the shikimic acid pathway or polymerize with different precursors (such as Malonyl-CoA) to form down-stream secondary metabolites. Anthocyanins, a major group of phenylpropanoids responsible for the bright colors of flowers, fruits, and plants, also accumulate in negligible amounts, with less than 10 mg/g of anthocyanin content found in fruits such as apples and sweet oranges (W. F.). For instance, the biomass of podophyllotoxin in *Callitris drummondii* callus was only 1.56%, and even with the use of tobacco heterologous production, the yield remained low.

Anthocyanins are bioactive compounds with many health benefits, including protecting and improving vision, making them ideal candidates for development and use as adaptogens. In a study by Yuan Zong et al., the *AN2* gene was investigated for its role in promoting the synthesis and expression of anthocyanins in two *Lycium* species using tobacco plant chassis, which could help in the selection and breeding of better crops. Flavonoids, another class of adaptogens, are commonly used in the clinical treatment of cardiovascular and cerebrovascular disorders, but the individual plants themselves contain only small amounts. Zahra Gharari et al. increased the yield of flavonoids, including chrysin, wogonin, and baicalein, in *Scutellaria bornmuelleri* hairy root chassis by 9.15, 10.56, and 13.25-fold, respectively, using elicitor treatment combined with transcription factor over-expression. Peipei Zhang et al. used multiple CRISPR/Cas9 gene editing techniques to modify soybean plant chassis and increase the content of isoflavonoid compounds in the crop, demonstrating qualitative improvement in flavonoids and soybean mosaic virus resistance. Coumarin derivatives have various applications in the pharmaceutical, cosmetic, and food industries as anticoagulants, fluorescent fuels, fragrance fixing agents, and food flavoring agents. Coumarin is an economically important natural product and a promising precursor for synthetic biology. To this end, Zeynab Yousefian et al. used an elicitor to induce the production of coumarin in *Pelargonium sidoides* hairy roots, yielding a natural product with a biomass of 9.6 g fresh weight and the plant itself with a fresh weight of 32.68 g.

2.3.2 Tannins and quinones Tannins, and quinones are essential secondary metabolites in plants. Tannins are known for their complex polyphenolic structures and can be classified into hydrolyzed and condensed tannins. Quinones, on the other hand, have unsaturated cyclic diketone structures and can be categorized into benzoquinone, naphthoquinone, phenanthrenequinone, and anthraquinone. Although these secondary metabolites have different structures, they share some medicinal activities, including anti-cancer, antioxidant, anti-bacterial, and preventive and therapeutic effects against certain diseases.

The synthesis of secondary metabolites is reliant on specific metabolic pathways, such as the shikimic acid pathway, mevalonate pathway, and phenylpropane pathway. For instance, phenylpropanoids, flavonoids, and alkaloids require the metabolic substrates synthesized by the shikimic acid pathway as a source for replenishing their own synthetic pathways, whereas the synthetic pathways of tannins and quinones also depend on the shikimic acid pathway. This highlights the dialectical unity between the whole and the parts of biological organisms, underscoring the ingenious connection between the labor and cooperation of organisms.

The heterologous synthetic biology of the two types of secondary metabolites discussed in the above is relatively understudied, despite their significant roles in food, medicine, industry, agriculture, and energy. Synthetic biology can help adjust the supply and demand of related products in the market and discover more potent natural active products. Proanthocyanidins are potent antioxidants with numerous pharmacological effects, including the ability to clean up oxygen radicals. Zhongzhiyue Jin et al. studied the role and function of *MYB* transcription factors in 46 different sainfoin leaves under transcriptome analysis and overexpressed them in heterologous chassis of alfalfa plants to finally obtain alfalfa hairy root strains with high proanthocyanidin production (Z. Z. Y.). Shikonin is a naphthoquinone compound with significant cosmetic and skin repair effects, but its isolation and purification in the traditional extraction process is very difficult and expensive. Synthetic biology can improve the accumulation of active products and help express shikonin heterologously when the synthetic pathway is unclear. Thiti Suttiyut et al. investigated the synthesis and accumulation of shikonin in *Lithospermum erythrorhizon* by using hairy roots and RNAi technology and found that the expression of shikonin is spatially specific by silencing the GPPS enzyme gene, revealing that the Mevalonate pathway in the cytoplasm is one of the primary pathways for shikonin synthesis.

## 3 TYPES AND CHARACTERISTICS OF PLANT CHASSIS

As synthetic biology advances, the number and diversity of available chassis cells continue to increase. However, the selection of the appropriate chassis has become a topic of intense debate. In synthetic biology, the choice of host cells for natural product production is often more critical than the optimization strategies employed to transform the cells. Additionally, a comparison between plant and microbial chassis reveals that plant-based hosts offer several advantages, including lower culture costs, more sophisticated protein modification, advanced gene regulation mechanisms, and enhanced biosafety. Therefore, this paper high-lights the characteristics of several commonly used plant-based chassis and their respective applications (Fig. 2).

3.1 Leaf The leaf is a crucial organ in plants for photosynthesis, respiration, and transpiration, and contains the most chloroplasts of all land plant organs, making it a hub for organic compound synthesis and distribution. Leaves can synthesize various natural secondary metabolites, such as terpenoids, polyphenols, and flavonoids. In particular, tobacco, a model plant, has a significant advantage in terms of leaf biomass percentage among many plants. In recent years, tobacco leaves have played an irreplaceable role in transient expression of plant synthetic biology, making it a highly utilized and developed chassis.

*N. benthamiana* belongs to the Solanaceae family and was originally utilized for medicinal and cigarette manufacturing purposes. However, with the advancements in multi-omics analysis of its genome, transcriptome, and metabolome, it has been recognized for its large biomass, short growth cycle, and heterozygous polyploid nature. These attributes have earned it the reputation of being a "molecular biology studio." This plant has become a model for implementing genetic engineering techniques and discovering new biological phenomena, such as nuclear and plastid transformation, intercellular gene and genome transfer, homology-dependent gene silencing, and male reproduction. Additionally, *N. benthamiana*'s status as a "non-crop" plant makes it a promising candidate for the production of commodities like pharmaceutical chemicals, fuels, and industrial materials without competing with food and feed supplies. However, as a eukaryotic organism, *N. benthamiana* possesses complex and diverse metabolic pathways, which may interfere with the orthogonality of heterologous gene pathways and affect the expression and accumulation of heterologous genes. Furthermore, the lack of precursor substrates in the expression of some heterologous pathways poses another challenge that needs to be addressed by substrate feeding or co-transformation

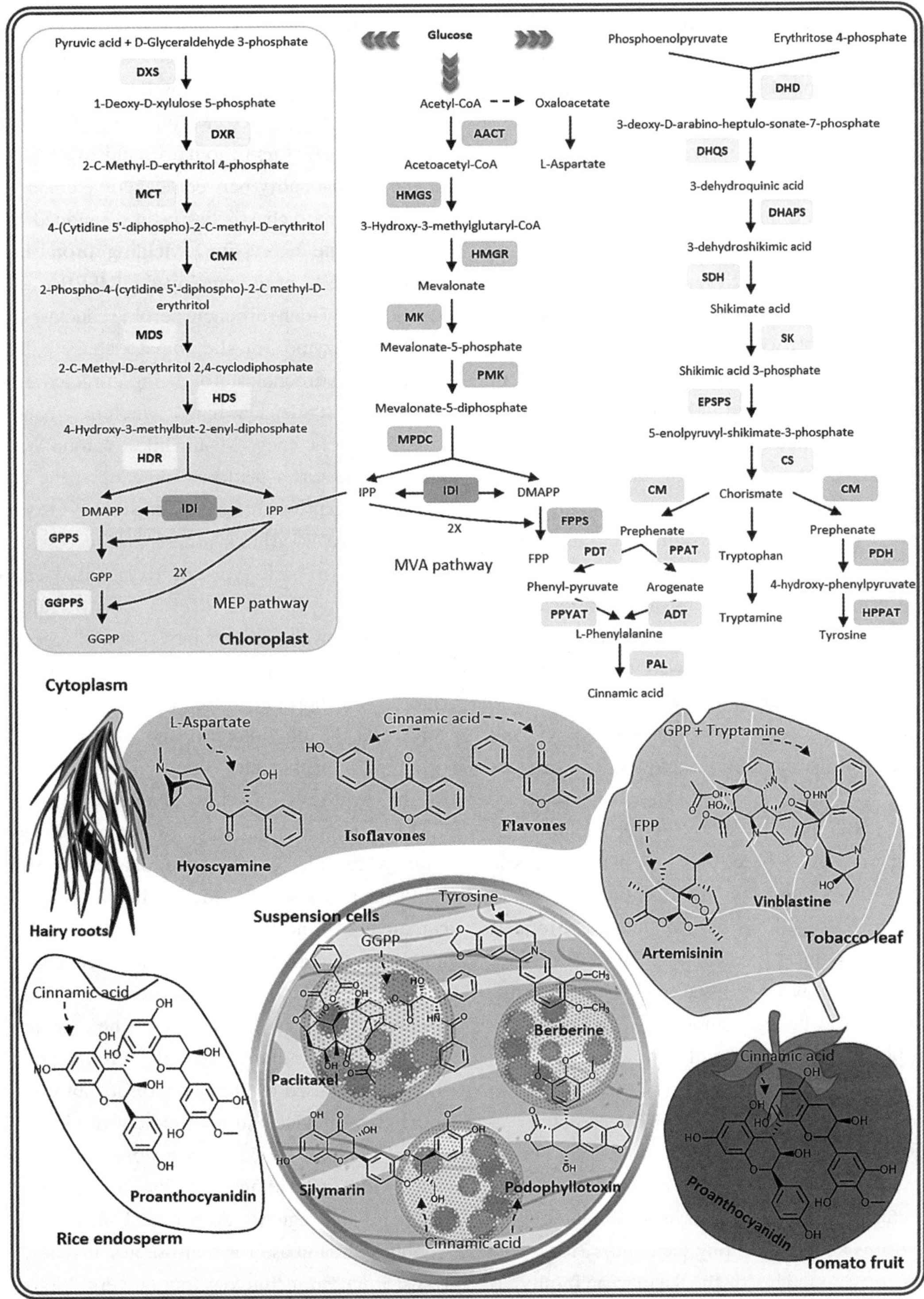


**Fig. 2 Progress in synthesizing natural products from different plant chassis. Compounds in different plant chassis indicate representative substances synthesized using the chassis**

DXS, 1-deoxy-D-xylulose 5-phosphate synthase; DXR, 1deoxy-D-xylulose 5-phosphate reductoisomerase; MCT, 2-*C*-methyl-D-erythritol 4-phosphate cytidylyltransferase; CMK, 4-(cytidine 5″ diphospho)-2-Cmethyl-D-erythritol kinase; MDS, 2-*C*-methyl-D-erythritol 2, 4-cyclodiphosphate synthase; HDS, 4-hydroxy-3-methylbut-2-enyl-diphosphate synthase; HDR, 4-hydroxy-3-methylbut-2-enyl diphosphate reductase; IDI, isopentenyl diphosphate isomerase; GPPS, geranyl diphosphate synthase; GGPPS, geranylgeranyl diphosphate synthase; AACT, acetyl-CoA acetyltransferase; HMGS, hydroxymethylglutaryl-CoA synthase; HMGR, 3-hydroxy-3-methylglutaryl-CoA reductase; MK, mevalonate kinase; PMK, phosphomevalonate kinase; MPDC, MVA diphosphate decarboxylase; FPPS, farnesyl diphosphate synthase; DHD, dehydroquinate dehydratase; DHQS, 3-dehydroquinate synthase; DHAPS, 3-deoxy-D-arabino-heptulosonate7-phosphatesynthase; SDH, shikimate dehydrogenase; SK, shikimate kinase; EPSPS, 5-enolypyruvylshikimate 3-phosphate synthase; CS, chorismate synthase; CM, chorismate mutase; PDT, prephenate dehydratase; PPAT, prephenate aminotransferase; PPYAT, phenylpyruvate aminotransferase; ADT, arogenate dehydratase; PAL, phenylalanine ammonialyase; PDH, prephenate dehydrogenase; HPPAT, 4-hydroxyphenylpyruvate aminotransferase. DMAPP, dimethylallyl diphosphate; GPP, geranyl pyrophosphate; GGPP, geranylgeranyl pyrophosphate; IPP, isopentenyl pyrophosphate; FPP, farnesyl pyrophosphate.

of enzymes related to the precursor pathway.

In recent years, *N. benthamiana* has been increasingly utilized as a chassis for synthetic biology in combination with Agrobacterium-mediated transient transfection. This approach enables faster, more efficient and safer production of natural products. For instance, Xue Yin et al. employed the tobacco plant chassis together with transient transfection technology, precursor substrate overexpression, and stepwise screening strategy to establish a complete pathway from cycloartenol to cholesterol. They built a platform for efficient heterologous accumulation of cholesterol, which was over 11 times higher than the control, and further developed a plant chassis for heterologous production of diosgenin. This study demonstrated the crucial role of plant chassis and transient transfection technology in uncovering little-known natural product synthesis pathways. Similarly, Jianhua Li et al. achieved efficient heterologous production of taxadiene and taxadiene-5α-ol in chloroplasts of *N. benthamiana* chassis by enhancing the expression of isoprene precursor substrates and localizing *TS*, *T5αH* and *CPR* genes from the Taxol synthesis pathway to the same space (plastids) This showed that short-term production and efficient storage of scarce natural products is now possible. Edith C F Forestier et al. combined stable and transient genetic transformation techniques to produce jolkinol C in *N. benthamiana* chassis. This approach remedied the gap caused by the lack of substrate accumulation of terpenoid precursors in tobacco as a plant chassis. Therefore, *N. benthamiana* plays an essential facilitating role in the heterologous synthesis of plant natural products and the elucidation of natural product synthesis pathways.

3.2 Fruit The fruit is a vital tissue organ in angiosperms, comprising mainly of the pericarp and seeds, and playing a crucial role in plant propagation and reproduction. Most fruits contain varying colors, making them rich in anthocyanins and carotenoids. *Solanum lycopersicum*, a model plant, exhibits a high seed and fruit set rate in above-ground parts, and its sturdy, multi-colored fruits make it a common plant chassis used in plant synthetic biology for producing adaptogens and gene editing techniques.

*S. lycopersicum*, a member of the Solanaceae family, is a widely cultivated fruit and vegetable with high nutritional value and a rich source of vitamins. Its strong genetic transformation system and diverse genetic germplasm resources make it a popular chassis for plant synthetic biology, and with the availability of the tomato genome sequences, quantitative trait locus databases, genetic maps, and mutant phenotype libraries, its potential uses go beyond heterologous synthesis of specific vitamins or anthocyanins. Furthermore, the abundance of metabolites in tomato, especially in the phenylpropanoid pathway, suggests that precursor substrates for certain metabolic pathways are readily available in this chassis. This compensates for the limitation of insufficient precursor substrates in tobacco. However, like the tobacco chassis, tomato also has complex metabolic pathways, and the heterologous expression of exogenous genes or transcription factors in tomato requires careful consideration of the orthogonality between genetic elements.

The tomato chassis has been developed for gene editing and transgene expression, yielding promising results. For instance, Jie Li et al. employed CRISPR-Cas9 technology to knock out 7-dehydrocholesterol reductase, a cholesterol synthesis enzyme, in the tomato chassis. This resulted in more 7-dehydrocholesterol being directed towards vitamin D3 synthesis under UV light, which may benefit people with vitamin B deficiency. Meanwhile, Yanjun Wu et al. used the tomato chassis as a platform for synthesizing natural products. They overexpressed four endogenous enzymes related to lutein and zeax-anthin synthesis and successfully accumulated high levels of both types of oxygenated carotenoids while also extending the shelf life of tomato fruits after harvest. This work provides insights into fruit and vegetable preservation and could reduce the use of chemical preservatives in the future. Furthermore, Emmanuel Rezende Naves et al. compared the physiological and biochemical properties and genomes of pepper and tomato and found many similarities in the synthesis of capsaicinoids. They proposed using TALEs technology and promoter-directed substitution strategy to enhance transcriptional activity of capsaicinoid synthesis genes in tomato, leading to stable production of capsaicinoid on the tomato platform. These examples highlight the advantages of plant chassis over microbial chassis in heterologous expression of plant-based natural product synthesis pathways. The tomato chassis, in particular, is suitable for the production of secondary metabolites based on the phenylpropanoid pathway due to its short growth cycle and high biological yield.

3.3 Seed Rice (*Oryza sativa*) is a crucial food crop worldwide, providing a major food source in numerous countries and regions. As a model plant, rice boasts a well-established database for multi-omics analysis, mature genetic transformation technology, and diverse biological germplasm resources. Additionally, target products expressed in rice can maintain long-term stability and undergo correct protein modification, whereas natural products expressed in rice seeds have high affinity and can reduce the cost of downstream material extraction and purification. Nevertheless, rice has inherent limitations as a chassis for genetic modification. Transgenic or gene editing operations may compromise the safety of this essential food crop. Furthermore, the lengthy growth cycle of rice renders it susceptible to abiotic stresses, and the degradation mechanism of certain substances in rice seeds remains unknown, leading to the synthesis of natural products that are incompatible with rice seeds.

Rice has become a widely used chassis in synthetic biology. Its applications span a spectrum that includes the effective expression of adaptogens, high-throughput screening for the elucidation and enhancement of plant secondary metabolic pathways, and the heterologous expression of biologically active natural products with pharmaceutical relevance. For instance, Yongsheng Tian et al. introduced six yeast enzyme genes related to riboflavin synthesis into rice endosperm as a chassis, resulting in more than four times higher riboflavin accumulation than the control. The modified rice maintained normal growth, nutritional quality, and yield. Changfu Zhu et al. used rice callus as a platform for carotenoid production, where a endosperm-specific promoter was employed to regulate exogenous gene expression, achieving the synthesis and accumulation of the product without affecting normal plant growth. This indicates that inducible promoter-regulated expression is more suitable for plant chassis than universal constitutive promoter regulation. Hyeon Baek et al. enriched resveratrol accumulation in rice by using maize Ubi promoter to regulate the expression of heterologous *AhSTS1* gene and performing stepwise phenotypic analysis, which resulted in 19 μg/g of resveratrol in rice seeds. Animal tests clearly demonstrated the effect of this transgenic rice in regulating blood pressure and antioxidants, indicating its potential to prevent or treat related diseases through diet alone. However, although rice is an important food crop and a well-established model plant with a developed database of multi-omics analysis, mature genetic transformation technology, and diverse biological germplasm resources, its application in synthetic biology is limited due to safety concerns as a food source and its long growth cycle. Moreover, the degradation mechanism of some substances in rice seeds is not well understood, which can result in the synthesis of natural products not suitable for rice seeds. Therefore, although rice can be a useful platform for biofortified heterologous synthesis, its application to products in the fields of energy, chemicals, and pharmaceuticals may not be recommended.

3.4 Suspension cell Plant suspension cells are a class of dedifferentiated, homogeneous cells that float in culture media and serve as a primary synthetic biology platform for heterologous production of natural products. Compared to whole plants, plant suspension cells offer several advantages, including large-scale culture potential, a fast growth rate, independence from environmental factors, and no biotic stress infringement. Moreover, when compared to microbial chassis, plant suspension cells have unique characteristics, such as a separated cell structure, *CYP450s* and their reduction enzymes, and a complete protein modification system. In recent years, due to advancements in bioreactors, the commercial use of plant suspension cells has become increasingly common. However, there are also some limitations associated with cell culture. Firstly, high aseptic conditions are necessary for the technology. Secondly, the culture process requires the input of a carbon source or precursor material, which may increase costs. Lastly, unstable cell transformation can occur, particularly in non-model plants whose genetics are not well understood.

Plant suspension cells constitute one of the extensively utilized categories of chassis in plant synthetic biology. Primarily employed as a production platform, they facilitate the proficient synthesis and accumulation of valuable endogenous natural products. The enriched cultivation mode in fermenters offers superior access to the desired compounds compared to conventional cultivation practices within the industry. For example, Homare Tabata et al. utilized *Taxus* suspension cells as a platform and combined biotic and abiotic elicitors to regulate the effect, ultimately achieving 295 mg/L of taxol compound in high-density fermentation culture. Xiaohui Wang et al., after resolving the synthesis of 2-(2-Phenylethyl) chromones, a unique component of agarwood, used *Aquilaria sinensis* callus as suspension culture cells and employed gene editing techniques in combination with precursor feeding methods to successfully reduce the content of the chromones in the chassis, providing a crucial theoretical foundation for the production of valuable Chinese herbs and spices using heterologous plants. Alexander Mehring et al., based on a comparison of cambial meristematic cells of *Ocimum basilicum* with dedifferentiated cells, found that the former showed an overwhelming advantage in the production of triterpenoids, with oleanolic acid and ursolic acid content 232.3% and 192.44% higher than the control, respectively. This indicates the significant role of developing various types of plant stem cells for the synthesis and accumulation of heterologous natural products by relevant plant suspension cells. In conclusion, plant suspension cells have a wide range of applications in the energy, pharmaceutical, chemical, and food industries. However, the commercial application of this technology is currently focused more on enhancing secondary metabolites in the native synthetic pathway, and there is still a long way to go for heterologous biosynthesis of plant suspension cells. Additionally, plant suspension cell culture has some limitations, including the requirement for high aseptic conditions, the cost of carbon source or precursor materials, and the potential for unstable cell transformation in non-model plants with poorly understood genetics.

3.5 Hairy root Hairy root tissue, initially a plant lesion induced by microbes, has been discovered to possess some similarities to plant root tissue. In some cases, hairy roots even exhibit a stronger metabolic synthesis capacity and a shorter product accumulation cycle than plant root tissue. Moreover, hairy root chassis cells offer several advantages in synthetic biology, such as being hormone autotrophic, having good genetic stability, and being low-cost to culture. However, the hairy root culture system also faces some challenges. For instance, there is no universal plant chassis cell, which makes it difficult to induce hairy roots in some plants. Additionally, the culture system tends to agglomerate.

The advantages of the hairy root chassis outweigh the limitations. It has been extensively used for the production of various natural products and has become a well-established and efficient platform for plant synthetic biology. Hairy root culture technology enables the production of terpenoids, alkaloids, phenylpropanoids, flavonoids, and other natural products and secondary metabolites. Additionally, this platform facilitates the analysis and reconstruction of synthetic pathways and the rapid characterization of related genes. In summary, the hairy roots chassis is not only suitable for the heterologous synthesis of diverse natural products but also holds promise as one of the most significant synthetic biology platforms in the future.

## 4 ENABLING TECHNOLOGY ON PLANT CHASSIS

The term "enabling" is not yet universally defined, but it generally refers to a category of multidisciplinary technologies with multiple applications developed to achieve specific purposes. In the field of synthetic biology, enabling technologies are defined as a series of techniques developed to improve human welfare, including gene cloning, gene editing, tissue culture, and gene transformation, with diverse applications in agriculture, medicine, environment, energy, pharmaceuticals, and light and heavy industries. As the synthetic biology of plants continues to evolve, novel techniques and tools are being developed. Gene editing is a prime example of such a technology. Therefore, this section provides a summary of the molecular biology techniques that have contributed to the development of plant synthetic biology to its present state.

4.1 DNA synthesis and assembly DNA synthesis techniques can be categorized into three types: columnar oligonucleotide synthesis, microarray DNA synthesis, and enzymatic DNA synthesis. Chemical synthesis is used in the first two techniques, while the third technique relies on biosynthesis without the need for DNA templates. Unlike DNA synthesis that occurs cyclically in living organisms through unwinding, single-strand extension, double-strand formation, and helix formation, in vitro chemical DNA synthesis follows a different principle. It involves designing a nucleotide sequence, attaching the first single nucleotide to a specific medium, and synthesizing bases in the direction of the 3′ end to the 5′ end until a single-stranded oligonucleotide sequence of the desired length is synthesized. This is the basic workflow of the original DNA synthesizer. However, technological advancements have led to the development of a new, environmentally friendly and stable technique for the in vitro synthesis of biological DNA known as enzymatic DNA synthesis. This technique involves the formation of crosslinks with dNTP using terminal deoxynucleotidyl transferase (*TdT*) without the need for a DNA template, followed by nucleotide chain extension. Due to its outstanding advantages, many DNA synthesis techniques based on enzymatic DNA synthesis have been developed, including the yeast in vivo DNA synthesis method and the ligation-mediated DNA synthesis method.

DNA synthesis and assembly are crucial to synthetic biology as they enable the construction of modular elements, such as functional genes, regulatory elements, reporter genes, and biosensor elements. Several techniques have been developed for DNA assembly, including nonenzyme-dependent DNA assembly (e.g., EFC and TPA technology), homologous recombinant DNA assembly (e.g., TAR technology, CasHRA technology, and *Cre/loxP*-mediated DNA in vivo assembly), and seamless DNA assembly techniques (e.g., Gibson assembly technology, SLIC assembly technology, and Golden Gate technique). The Golden Gate technique uses IIS-type restriction endonucleases to produce four-base overhangs for easy ligation of gene sequences into the vector. The Gibson technique uses in vitro multi-fragment ligation, while *Cre/loxP*-mediated DNA assembly utilizes recombinase to recombine two *loxP* sites, which can result in deletion, inversion, or exchange of gene fragments. The TPA technology uses PCR to achieve multi-segment concatenation with homologous arm interactions between fragments. Among these techniques, the Golden Gate technique and *Cre/loxP*-mediated DNA in vivo assembly technique are the most popular.

Progress in DNA synthesis and assembly technologies, pivotal in plant synthetic biology, equips the field with potent tools. The former enables accurate synthesis of genes of varying lengths, while the latter streamlines the precise and expeditious assembly of multiple genes into the ultimate "container." The maturation of the latter technique fosters enhanced precision and swiftness in amalgamating multiple genes into the final construct. As both technologies continually advance, prospects expand for metabolic engineering of high-value compounds, gene analysis within pathways, high-throughput screening of advantageous mutations, and in vitro full-length construction of intricate metabolic pathways.

4.2 Gene editing Gene editing technologies have had a significant impact on synthetic biology in plant chassis, particularly in enhancing the accumulation of terpenoids, phenols, and alkaloids, natural products of native origin. Zinc finger nuclease, transcription activator-like effector nucleases, CRISPR/Cas9, and LEAPER™ RNA single-base editing technology are some of the key gene editing techniques utilized in this field. TALENs are a gene editing method that involves TALE proteins recognizing specific target sequences and *Fok* I restriction enzymes. By combining different TALE proteins, the target fragment can be specifically identified and bound in the host genome, and the dimeric FokI restriction enzyme can then digest it. On the other hand, ZFNs are similar to TALENs, but they consist of a class of zinc finger proteins and FokI restriction enzymes that recognize three bases, which affects the binding of the rest of the front and back ends, making TALENs a more suitable platform. CRISPR/Cas9 is a DNA editing technology that enhances the accuracy of the editing site by the dual recognition and binding of sgRNA and PAM sequences. Compared to ZFNs and TALENs, it is more effective. LEAPER, unlike the previous three techniques, is an RNA editing technology that relies on reversible single-base editing, using a circ-arRNA with sequence recognition specificity to change the gene without introducing large molecular weight protein molecules. This circumvents the problem of heterologous protein expression and transport in the host cell. In summary, while the first two techniques use the binding of the restriction enzyme *Fok* I to specific recognition proteins, CRISPR/Cas9 relies on the binding of a nucleic acid sequence to a Cas9 protein, which cleaves a specific gene fragment under the dual effect of nucleic acid sequence complementarity and PAM sequence recognition. LEAPER is a reversible editing method derived from the consideration of the effect of exogenous gene introduction (transgenesis) on the host.

In recent years, a diverse array of prominent CRISPR/Cas systems has arisen, categorized into CRISPR/Cas12, CRISPR/Cas13, CRISPR/Cas10, and CRISPR/Cas14 based on Cas protein structure and functionality. Among these, CRISPR/Cas13 predominantly operates at the RNA level, encompassing RNA editing, RNA interference, and virus detection. Conversely, the remaining three CRISPR systems are primarily geared towards genomic DNA sequences of the host. These encompass gene editing (S.), expression regulation of coding genes (S.), and virus detection. Notably, another gene editing technique, Prime Editing (PE), has emerged as distinct from CRISPR/Cas9 due to its independence from supplementary DNA templates and the absence of double-stranded breaks at target DNA sites. However, PE's application in plant synthetic biology remains relatively infrequent. This partly stems from its novelty, the notably low editing efficiency within plant cells (0.03%–21.8%), and its current emphasis on monocotyledonous plants. Application of PE in dicotyledonous plants remains scant in the literature.

Gene editing technology has introduced significant prospects and challenges to plant synthetic biology, particularly with the advent of CRISPR/Cas9 methodology. The implications of gene editing encompass: (1) modulation of primary metabolic pathways within plants; (2) enhancement of plant resilience against biotic and abiotic stresses; (3) exploration of the intricate mechanisms governing plant interactions with soil microorganisms; (4) augmentation of both yield and quality of valuable plant compounds; (5) validation of the functionality of artificially hypothesized candidate genes in plants; (6) identification of advantageous mutants within diverse plant mutant populations through directed evolution, among other possibilities.

4.3 Agrobacterium-mediated organs transformation

The hairy root culture system is a widely used method for plant genetic transformation. This technique is achieved by infecting the plant with a specific type of *Agrobacterium* containing a root-inducing plasmid (Ri) with a T-DNA region that encodes relevant phytohormone and opine synthesis genes. Upon integration of the T-DNA into the plant chromosome, genes in the T-DNA region are expressed, leading to the proliferation of tissue cells in the infected part of the plant, resulting in the formation of root-like tissue. Hairy roots have several advantages, including the ability to synthesize secondary metabolites comparable to the original plant, producing natural products or intermediates that the original plant does not have, faster growth rate, independence from exogenous hormones, and stable inheritance of the transformed genes. Hairy roots culture systems have seen significant progress in recent years in the field of plant synthetic biology, including the induction of new hairy roots tissue systems and the development of large reactors for mature hairy roots systems, highlighting their potential as a plant chassis.

The hairy root culture system is a widely used form of gene delivery in nuclear genome genetic transformation, while transient transfection is a more rapid and less manipulative method of transgenesis. Transient transfection mainly involves the action of *Agrobacterium tumefaciens*, which contains tumor-inducing plasmids (Ti) that produce tumor-like tissue in the infected part of the plant. This technique is commonly used for validation experiments, such as subcellular localization of gene expression, nucleic acid-nucleic acid interactions, and nucleic acid-protein interactions, owing to its simplicity, high expression efficiency, lack of screening gene involvement, and biosafety. However, unlike hairy root stable transformation, transient transfection lacks stable heritability, which has prevented its use for trait improvement in plants such as crops and flowers, but it can respond to sudden pandemics and replenish clinically important protein formulations in the short term. Recent breakthrough production of recombinant protein COVID - 19 vaccines on heterologous plants exemplifies the efficacy of this technique.

Hence, the *Agrobacterium*-mediated transformation technology, as a pivotal tool within the realm of plant synthetic biology, offers researchers an expansive terrain for advancement and an array of research opportunities. To begin with, this technology exhibits remarkable efficiency, enabling the stable integration of exogenous genes into plant cells within a relatively brief timeframe, thereby swiftly generating a sizable population of transgenic plants. Furthermore, its applicability spans across diverse plant species, encompassing both economically significant crops and model plants, affording researchers a versatile spectrum of choices in selecting appropriate plant chassis aligned with research goals and requisites. Moreover, exogenous genes introduced through this method tend to exhibit stability within the plant genome, facilitating integration and inheritance across generations, ensuring research sustainability and the potential for multigenerational propagation. Notably, Agrobacterium-mediated transformation technology finds utility not only in gene expression and functional validation but also extends its reach to metabolic engineering, pharmaceutical exploration, and the cultivation of pest-resistant strains, thereby blazing a novel trail in the exploration and practical application of plant synthetic biology.

4.4 Plant chromosome engineering The Plant Artificial Chromosome (PAC) technique allows for the manipulation of plant chromosomes to add, subtract, or replace parts according to human preferences. It consists of three key elements: the primary replication sequence, the centromere, and the telomere. The primary replication sequence initiates chromosome replication, the centromere ensures proper chromosome separation, and the telomere closes chromosome ends, maintaining stability. The technique involves two parts: first, the introduction of target gene and telomere sequences into one chromosome to create a plant artificial chromosome, and second, the introduction of Crease gene sequence into another chromosome to mediate homologous recombination between two different chromosomes, resulting in a recombinant plant artificial chromosome with exogenous target gene expression. Compared to plasmids and adenoviruses, PAC technology can carry large gene segments and integrate numerous identical or different gene fragments. Additionally, PAC technology can circumvent issues of chromosomal genetic chain reactions that occur in traditional breeding efforts. Telomere-mediated truncation of chromosomes in plants and the creation of engineered mini-chromosomes is an example of plant chromosome engineering.

Compared to exogenous gene expression in microbial chassis cells, exogenous gene expression in plant chassis cells involves the plant's own genome, resulting in the integration of exogenous genes into the plant genome in the form of T-DNA and their subsequent expression along with the plant genome. This integration process is prone to several problems, such as (1) the randomness of T-DNA integration sites, (2) the instability of T - DNA integration after expression, (3) the negative impact of T-DNA integration on gene expression, and (4) the gene load of T - DNA carrying exogenous genes, among others. Artificial plant chromosomes provide a solution to these problems. On the one hand, the use of artificial plant chromosomes makes the introduction of exogenous genes more directional, minimizing the loss of exogenous genes and their effect on the expression of other genes. It also excludes non-target gene sequences (partial backbone sequences of vectors) and reduces gene redundancy. On the other hand, artificial plant chromosome technology overcomes the problem of target gene loading on the transformation medium and enables the transformation of ultra-long chain gene sequences in the plant host at one time, compared with Agrobacterium-mediated transformation and gene gun transformation method. James A Birchler et al. showed the use of telomere-mediated chromosome technology to form artificial mini-chromosomes and combined mini-chromosome with double haploid (DH) technology, achieving the maximum stacked transformation of multiple exogenous genes into the target plant, even if the plant is transformed with minimal efficiency in conventional gene transformation. Lili Hou et al. used plant artificial chromosomes to introduce a phage *Bxb1* and *Cre* recombinase system-mediated multigene transformation approach in tobacco, which enables the purposeful addition of exogenous genes to characteristic chromosomal sites and also the insertion of specific recombination sites on defective chromosomes to reverse the repair of damaged chromosomes, thereby restoring the original environmental resistance and metabolite production of the defective precious plant. Despite the difficulties inherent in applying plant chromosome engineering technology in practice, such as the large genome contained in plants and the more complex chromosome behavior, it offers a broad prospect and development space for plant chromosome engineering research since plant centromere sequences cannot maintain the stability of chromosomes and Spindle once they are reintroduced into plant cells after passing through microbial hosts.

## 5 PLANT CHASSIS OPTIMIZATION STRATEGY

The natural product yield obtained through single or multiple gene transformations in heterologous plants is sometimes substantial. However, this is only the lower limit of heterologous synthesis of natural products, especially when compared to the minimal content of secondary metabolites in native plants. To further increase the biomass of natural products in both heterologous and native plants, one or more plant chassis optimization approaches can be combined to achieve greater than 100% product accumulation. The expression of transgenes in plant synthetic biology is influenced by various host cell factors. These factors include internal factors such as preferential selection of codons in each species, transcription factors, cis-acting elements regulating gene expression, regulation of metabolic flow in the synthesis pathway, compartmentalized localization of enzymes, and improvement of transporter proteins, as well as external factors such as exogenous elicitor treatment and bioreactor culture. Exploiting these factors can lead to unexpected results.

5.1 Codon optimization Codons, playing a crucial role in orchestrating the translation of genetic information into functional proteins, serve as a linchpin bridging nucleic acid and amino acid conversions. However, despite their universal presence across species, individual codons display variability in their usage, thereby giving rise to distinct codon preferences. To enhance gene expression efficiency, codon optimization strategies have been ingeniously designed within the realm of plant synthetic biology. The primary purpose of these strategies is to strategically modify the codon usage patterns within a gene sequence, aligning them with the specific preferences of the host organism (Fig. 3a). For example, Chuang Wei et al. involved the development of an adenine base editor that integrates nuclear localization signals alongside codon optimization techniques. This novel fusion yields a heightened efficacy in generating pure strains within primary transformants, surpassing the conventional ABEmax system. Of notable significance, this tool exhibits remarkable editing efficiency for rice, making it particularly well-suited for the modification of pathways within the rice chassis. Furthermore, codon optimization's potential is manifest in addressing challenges within specific metabolic pathways. Guillaume N Menard et al. harnessed this technique to mitigate the issue of Sinapine accumulation in *Camelina sativa*. Their strategic optimization of codon usage facilitated the enzyme's heightened substrate specificity for sinapic acid. Combined with the judicious regulation of the phenylpropanoid metabolic pathway's flow division, this approach enabled the conversion of Sinapine to 4-vinyl phenol (4 - VP) derivatives, culminating in 4 - VP biosynthesis. This illustrative case underscores the transformative potential of codon optimization, highlighting its capacity to enhance specific enzyme performance within organisms and subsequently empowering plants to catalyze the transformation or degradation of harmful substances present within the soil environment. However, few examples of heterologous synthesis of bacterial genes in plants have been reported, with more reports of heterologous expression of plant genes in model microorganisms. This indicates that there is still a lot of room for the development of plant synthetic biology.

5.2 Regulation of transcription factors and cis-acting elements Transcription factors are pivotal proteins that orchestrate gene expression by binding to gene promoters, either directly or indirectly, thus recruiting RNA polymerase and subsequently modulating down-stream gene activity, either positively or negatively. Concurrently, cis-acting elements, akin to berthing sites for various molecules, including proteins, RNA molecules, and signaling molecules, function as DNA sequences that intricately regulate gene expression. The purpose of these regulatory mechanisms is to precisely control the temporal and spatial expression of genes, enabling organisms to adapt to various environmental and stress. A strategic approach to modifying gene expression involves the deliberate manipulation of transcription factors and cis-acting elements. Changing the concentration of transcription factors within a cell can amplify the expression of the target gene. This augmentation can be further magnified by coupling it with the deployment of robust promoters or enhancers (Fig. 3b). For instance, Jiafa Wang et al. unveiled the potential of transcription factor regulation. By repressing specific *NF - YB* genes within the transcription factor complex, they demonstrated the capacity to induce the formation of pink-hued fruits, thereby shedding light on the role of flavonoid biosynthesis within tomatoes. Similarly, Yuqing He et al. embarked on a meticulous exploration of the interplay between phosphorus (Pi) stress and anthocyanin accumulation pathways within *Arabidopsis thaliana*. Through meticulous investigation, they ascertained the mode of action of three distinct transcription factors, namely *SYG1*, *Pho81 and XPR1* (*SPX 4*), *PHOSPHATE STARVATION RESPONSE1* (*PHR1*), and *PRODUCTION OF ANTHOCYANIN PIGMENTS1* (*PAP1*).

5.3 Metabolic flow control Organisms have a myriad of intricate metabolic pathways. These pathways interplay by either fostering, inhibiting, co-inhibiting, co-promoting, or antagonizing each other, collectively contributing to the maintenance of the organism's internal homeostatic equilibrium. In the field of plant synthetic biology, how to clarify the relationship between metabolic pathways and thus promote the accumulation of natural product content in the host has become the one of most concerned issue. Metabolic engineering is the primary method employed to exert control over divergent metabolic pathways. Gene editing techniques are harnessed to deactivate pertinent enzyme genes within these pathways. This intervention redirects the flow of precursor metabolites towards the "favorable" metabolic trajectory, consequently augmenting the targeted product's accumulation. Moreover, directed evolution techniques are employed to manipulate specific enzyme molecules with

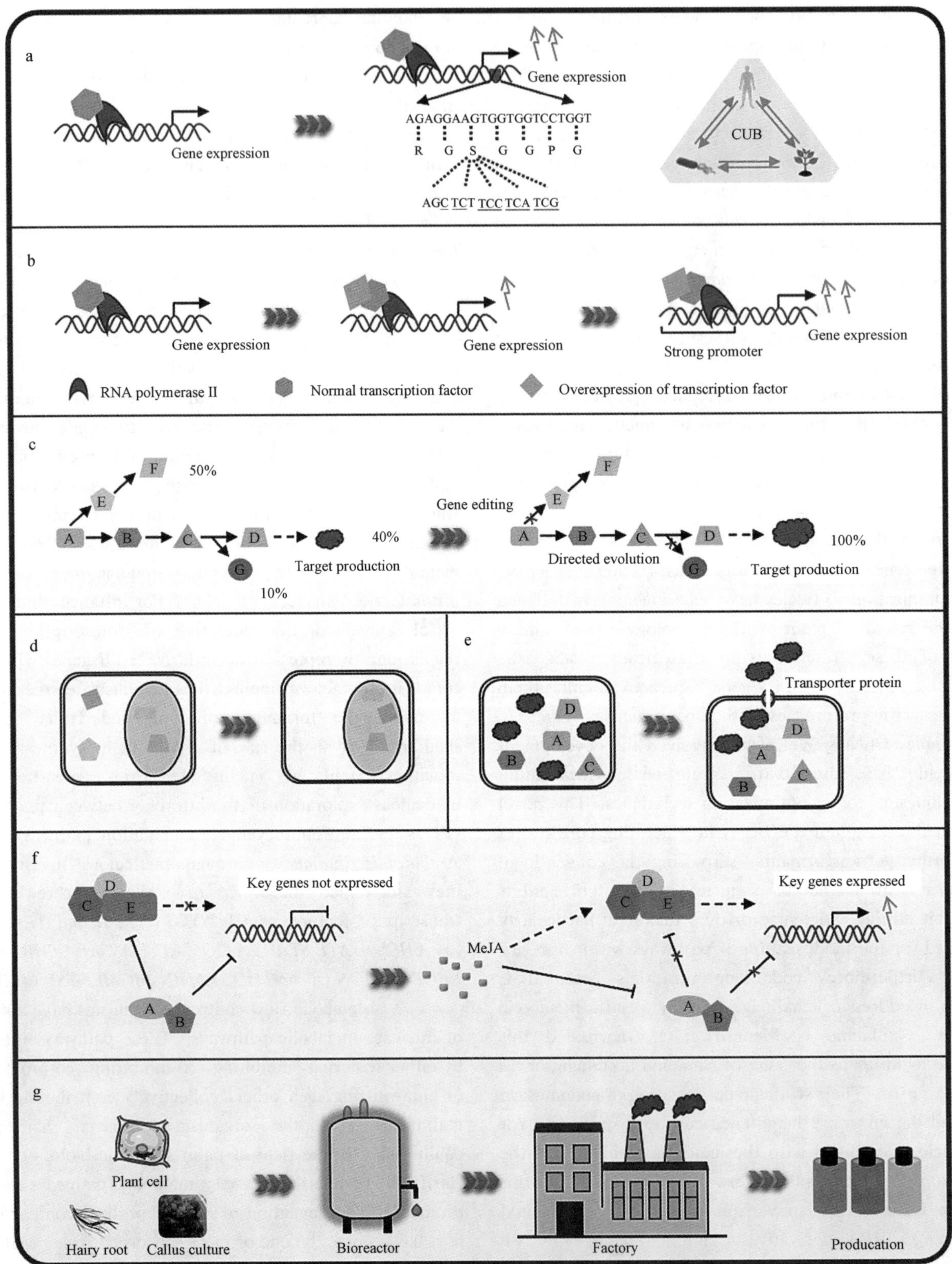


**Fig. 3 Chassis optimization strategies in plant synthetic biology**

(a) Codon optimization, in which the expression of target genes is enhanced by changing codons that are used more frequently. Cub indicates codon preference. (b) Transcription factor and promoter regulation, where the expression level of target genes is further enhanced by the use of the two alone or in combination. (c) Metabolic flow regulation, in which the production of target product in a metabolic pathway is gradually idealized through gene editing and directed evolution. (d) Enzyme compartmentalization, which directs enzymes of the same metabolic pathway to localize in the same space by altering the enzyme's signal peptide. (e) Transporter protein regulation, which increases the number of transporter proteins in the target cell to circumvent product cytotoxicity as well as to expand product production capacity. (f) Elicitor treatment, where the expression pattern of different transcription factors in plant cells changes under methyl jasmonate treatment. (g) Bioreactor culture, where bioreactor enrichment culture of the target cell chassis is employed thereby allowing the accumulation and synthesis of the target product to be idealized.

"omnivorous" properties. This strategic alteration renders the enzyme molecule more adaptable to diverse reaction substrates, thereby curbing or eradicating the loss of precursors through unwanted side reactions (Fig. 3c). For example, Lu Yao et al. employed this approach to enhance ginsenoside production within the ginseng plant chassis. By knockout of a specific *CYP450* gene within the ginsenoside synthesis pathway, they managed to curtail pathway divergence, thereby boosting the metabolic flow towards ginsenoside accumulation. This methodological integration showcases the multifaceted nature of metabolic flow regulation, high-lighting its potential to fine-tune and enhance metabolic pathways for optimal product yield.

5.4 Compartmentalized localization of enzymes and improvement of transporter proteins The biosynthetic pathways operating within plant cells comprise intricate networks, where each metabolite synthesized through these pathways acquires a distinct spatial localization within the cell. This spatial arrangement significantly influences their synthesis and accumulation within the host cell chassis. For instance: ① metabolites generated within a specific organelle tend to readily engage the synthetic pathways of that locale due to the prevalent co-localization of requisite enzymes and cofactors within the same organelle. ② The compartmentalized localization of enzymes not only segregates distinct reactions but also establishes specialized microenvironments favoring specific biosynthetic pathways, thereby bolstering the yield of target metabolites. ③ The distribution of precursor substrates and metabolic intermediates spatially further impacts substrate availability for biosynthetic reactions, thus influencing pathway flux and ultimate metabolite production. ④ The introduction of heterologously expressed metabolites could potentially exert cytotoxic effects on the host chassis; strategically altering spatial localization effectively mitigates these toxic influences, preserving cell growth and viability (Fig. 3d). For instance, Jianhua Li et al. ingeniously modified signal peptide localization sequences to co-localize three enzyme genes along the paclitaxel synthesis pathway within the chloroplasts of tobacco leaves. This approach not only mitigated the negative impact of intermediate substances during translocation but also significantly elevated the content of taxadien and taxadiene-5α-ol in the heterologous plant chassis. Zheng et al. conducted a heterologous transformation, introducing three carotenoid enzyme genes sourced from *Neurospora crassa* into distinct plant chassis—tobacco, *Arabidopsis thaliana*, and citrus. Alongside this, they overexpressed the *tHMGR* precursor genes. The results of their intervention were the accumulation of phytoene, γ-carotenoids, β-carotenoids, and torulene. Remarkably, their revelation of carotenoid storage within lipid droplets in citrus's healing tissues laid the groundwork for synthesizing and accumulating other potentially hazardous heterologous compounds. Engineered compartmentalized enzyme targeting not only effectively mitigates the adverse impacts of exogenous products on host cells but also optimizes the augmentation of specific natural products within native producers by modulating plant physiological pathways. For example, Wang et al. pursued the targeted localization of four enzyme genes (*OsGLO1*, *EcCAT*, *EcGCL*, *EcTSR*) linked to the GCGT photorespiratory pathway within the chloroplasts of rice, a chosen plant chassis. This precise manipulation induced elevated carbon dioxide concentrations within the chloroplasts, subsequently enhancing the organism's photosynthetic capacity. As a result, this strategy significantly amplified biomass production and seed yield in GCGT transgenic rice. These compartmentalized enzyme targeting approaches represent a remarkable leap forward in harnessing the host's physiological compartments to maximize product yields and alleviate the adverse effects of exogenous compounds, underscoring their pivotal role in advancing the field of plant synthetic biology.

Transporter proteins play a pivotal role in the cellular transport of substances across membranes, spanning various essential life processes such as metabolism, nutrient acquisition, and adaptation to the environment. Given their significance, enhancing relevant transporter proteins within plants can hold the potential to amplify the synthesis rate of secondary metabolites and channel these metabolites to specific desired locations. This strategic improvement can, for instance, result in the exocytosis of heterologously expressed products into the culture medium, indirectly mitigating their potential toxicity to tissue cells. This approach leverages the controlled release and replenishment of the culture medium, facilitating the sustainable production of target substances and thereby augmenting overall production efficiency (Fig. 3e). For instance, Guopeng Miao et al. employed RNAi technology to silence the expression of the *TwMDR1* transporter gene in *Tripterygium wilfordii* Hook. f. suspension cells. This strategic yielded a significant reduction in the content of related alkaloids within the plant cells. This reduction, in turn, facilitated downstream processes such as extraction and purification of the target natural product. Critically, this approach averted the issue of excessive alkaloid accumulation, thereby sidestepping potential toxicity concerns associated with such buildup. By utilizing transporter protein manipulation, we can use this powerful tool to optimize the synthesis, accumulation, and directed movement of secondary metabolites, leading to enhanced product yields.

5.5 Elicitor modulation and bioreactor culture The phenotype of a species is largely contingent on both its genetic makeup and the influence of the surrounding environment. This intrinsic connection between plant growth, biomass accumulation, and environmental conditions underscores the potential for optimizing plant chassis by harnessing external factors, including the introduction of hormones, inorganic ions, and elicitors that trigger signal transduction, thereby orchestrating the expression of pertinent compounds within the plant (Fig. 3f). Additionally, the cultivation of plant tissues or cells in bioreactors under carefully controlled growth conditions, characterized by enriched nutrients, optimal oxygen supply, and ample light, offers a pivotal avenue for this optimization (Fig. 3g). Elicitors, operating as positive regulators, align seamlessly with the principles of sustainable scientific practices. These molecules exclusively serve as signal agents, activating specific factors within plant cells. When the elicitors disappeared or decreased, their positive regulatory effects disappeared. For instance, employing yeast extract as a bioinducer, Wei Zhou et al. successfully harnessed the exogenous addition of yeast extract to the *S. miltiorrhiza* hairy root plant chassis as a signaling molecule for *SCR1* transcription factor. This method culminated in the downstream enhancement of gene expression and efficient tanshinone accumulation. In a separate study, Abdulwadood Shakir Mahmood Alsoufi et al. treated *Calendula officinalis* hairy roots with two substances, jasmonic acid and chitosan, respectively, highlighting the superior regulatory effects of jasmonic acid over chitosan. Under hormone induction, oleanolic acid saponin content in hairy roots escalated 20-fold compared to controls, coupled with augmented extracellular secretion of this substance. Similarly, Arti Sharma et al. stimulated *Withania somnifera* seedlings with jasmonic acid in vitro, orchestrating the upregulation of withanolide and stigmasterol synthesis and accumulation via *WsMYC2*. This yielded notable withanolide accumulation at the protein level. Ahmad Faizal et al. embraced the hairy roots of *Talinum paniculatum* as a chassis, introducing two phytohormones, methyl jasmonate and salicylic acid, into a liquid culture environment. This yielded hairy roots with 1.5-fold and 1.3-fold higher total ginsenoside levels compared to controls. Mingyuan Yuan et al. delved into the impact of phytohormones, jasmonic acid, and abscisic acid, on *Artemisia annua*, culminating in a substantial increase in *AabHLH113*. This transcription factor elevation effectively promoted gene expression in the artemisinin synthesis pathway, resulting in more than twofold amplified artemisinin and dihydroartemisinic acid biomass. Furthermore, Zhihua Song et al. showcased how melatonin treatment of *Cajanus cajan* enhanced resistance to external abiotic stresses while augmenting flavonoid accumulation, notably luteolin. The increased expression of the *F3′H* gene and its transcription factor *CcPCL1* in the phenylpropanoid pathway substantiated the heightened flavonoid accumulation. Beyond these effects, elicitors find derivative applications, including biosensor development and recombinant inducible plasmid construction. In parallel, the utilization of bioreactors has grown indispensable for many commercial applications involving plant chassis. Bioreactors confer several advantages over traditional planting methods, notably the ability to achieve maximal yield with minimal floor space, provision of an ideal growth environment for plant tissues or cells, reduced demands for human and material resources, and shorter growth cycles for tissues or cells. Nguyen Huu Nhan et al. harnessed plant tissue cell culture techniques to enhance the yield of the natural active product Eurycomanone in *Eurycoma longifolia*. The induced MS medium yielded a higher product yield in a shorter time frame compared to control conditions. Plant cells, callus, or hairy root tissues can be effectively employed as culture materials within bioreactors to manufacture specific substances and process products. Furthermore, plants themselves can serve as proficient bioreactors.

## 6 CHALLENGES AND FUTURE PERSPECTIVE

Plants, the producers of ecosystems, contain many types of active substances, and only a handful of functional plants have been explored and discovered by researchers. However, the contradiction between the lack of resources and the backward exploitation and production methods has made many plant species endangered, such as some *taxus* genus plants, *Adiantum nelumboides* and *Victoria amazonica*. Many efforts have been taken in the conservation of plant germplasm resources (establishment of ecological reserves, biodiversity hotspots, migratory culture, etc.), but they have not been met in terms of resources, and the filling of this gap will likely affect the survival of other plant species. If the cycle will continue, the number of endangered plants will continue to increase, so scientific researchers urgently need to find a strategy for the efficient production of plant natural products. Synthetic biology can address this environmental paradox at its root. Synthetic biology relying on plant host (chassis) cells not only allows for efficient heterologous expression and accumulation of plant-based natural products, but also enhances the biomass of endogenous plant natural products in combination with various chassis optimization strategies, thus avoiding conventional harvesting and conserving biodiversity.

The field of synthetic biology employs a range of organisms, from prokaryotes to eukaryotes, with common prokaryotic platforms including *Escherichia coli* and cyanobacteria, while common eukaryotic platforms include *Saccharomyces cerevisiae*, *Arabidopsis thaliana*, tobacco, and ginseng (hairy roots). Both types of platforms are essential for the expression and accumulation of plant natural products. Taxol, artemisinin, ginsenosides, and hyoscyamine, as well as their intermediates, have been successfully produced in both types of platforms, but higher yields have generally been observed in prokaryotic platforms. For example, recombinant *E. coli* fermentation cultures have produced up to 1.02 g/L of taxadiene while heterologous tobacco chassis produced the same product at 56.6 μg/g fresh weight. The difference in yield can be attributed to the operational maturity and development of enabling technologies in both platforms. Presently, when compared to microbial chassis, plant-based platforms might entail higher production costs in certain facets. The cultivation of plants demands substantial land, water, and nutrient resources. The extraction of target products from plants, especially when intricately embedded in their tissues, can be challenging. Furthermore, biosynthesized products within plant chassis commonly share finite nutrients and resources, potentially posing a challenge to balance biomass and overall performance. Additionally, divergent plant characteristics and growth conditions across diverse geographical contexts can arise. Nonetheless, chassis optimization is achievable via modifications, such as gene editing or genetic engineering. By enhancing parameters like growth rate, yield, product storage locations, precursor substrate distribution, and resistance, production and natural product extraction costs from plants can be mitigated. Although eukaryotic platforms, especially plants, are currently underestimated, prokaryotic platforms are also limited by structural barriers such as cells without compartmentalized compartments, cells unable to accommodate larger plant natural products, toxicity of plant natural products, and poor enzyme activity of plant origin. Therefore, the technical and cognitive issues facing eukaryotic platforms are worthy of further exploration and research.

The application of synthetic biology extends beyond the synthesis of plant-based natural products, and has the potential to advance several fields in the near future. In agriculture, synthetic biology could enhance food crops to resist biotic or abiotic stress, decrease accumulation of heavy metals, increase growth and biomass, and more. In landscape architecture, it could enable flower coloring and matching, among other possibilities. In pharmaceuticals and medicine, synthetic biology has potential for drug production, disease treatment and diagnosis, and drug-resistant bacteria elimination. In the field of energy and environmental protection, synthetic biology could modify soil and develop non-renewable energy substitutes. Therefore, synthetic biology offers numerous potential platforms and systems to advance a variety of fields, marking a golden age for the field.

[林俊杰,薛哲勇,杨东风,等. Biotechnology Advances, 2023,69:108266.]

# Structural and catalytic insight into the unique pentacyclic triterpene synthase TwOSC

## 1 INTRODUCTION

Pentacyclic triterpenoids (PTs) are widely distributed in higher plants and exhibit a wide range of bioactivities, such as antitumor, anti-inflammatory, and antiviral activity. Recent studies have identified PTs as vaccine adjuvants to boost the immune response. Similar to all 2,3-oxidosqualene-derived triterpenoids, the first step in PT synthesis is the cyclization of the linear substrate (3*S*)-2,3-oxidosqualene to form PT skeletons, which is catalyzed by oxidosqualene cyclases (OSCs). The putative mechanism of OSCs involves protonation of the (3*S*)-2,3-oxidosqualene epoxide ring, followed by a series of ring formation and rearrangement reactions, and finally, deprotonation or water capture to terminate the reaction. OSCs catalyze one of nature's most complex polycyclization reactions, which have been extensively studied.

Phylogenetic analysis suggests that PT oxidosqualene cyclases are derived from the ancestral lanosterol synthase-like enzymes. Additionally, PTs derived from 2,3-oxidosqualene are widespread in dicots but almost absent in other organisms. The crystal structure of human oxidosqualene cyclase (hOSC) has been used to elucidate the mechanism of the tetracyclic triterpenoid lanosterol. However, the reaction process of PTs involves additional complex cyclization and rearrangement steps compared with that of lanosterol. Currently, no plant OSC structures have been identified; thus, studies on their catalytic mechanisms rely only on predictive models generated via computational approaches. In addition, extensive mutagenesis research has suggested that almost a single residue can alter the function of plant OSCs. To gain comprehensive insights into the catalytic mechanism of PT formation, it is crucial to determine the structure of plant OSCs.

Oxidosqualene cyclase from *Tripterygium wilfordii* Hook. f (TwOSC) produces friedelin and two other minor products, $\beta$-amyrin and $\alpha$-amyrin. TwOSC undergoes one of the most rearrangement steps to produce friedelin. The cation moves from the C2 position of the substrate to the other side of the skeleton to form the lupyl cation and returns to the C3 position for deprotonation, forming friedelin through nine-step rearrangements. We referred to this interesting phenomenon as the "Cation Shuttle-Run (CSR) mechanism." Stage 1 (CSR carbocation-go) presents the cascades cyclization steps and initial rearrangement reaction from 2, 3-oxidosqualene to lupyl cation. Stage 2 (CSR carbocation-return) refers to the sequential methyl/hydride-shift steps (Figure S1a). The carbocation-go stage has been well described, and the carbocation-return stage is closely associated with PT formation, which requires further study. A high number of $\beta$-amyrin synthases found in nature seems to favor the formation of $\beta$-amyrin. Among the putative

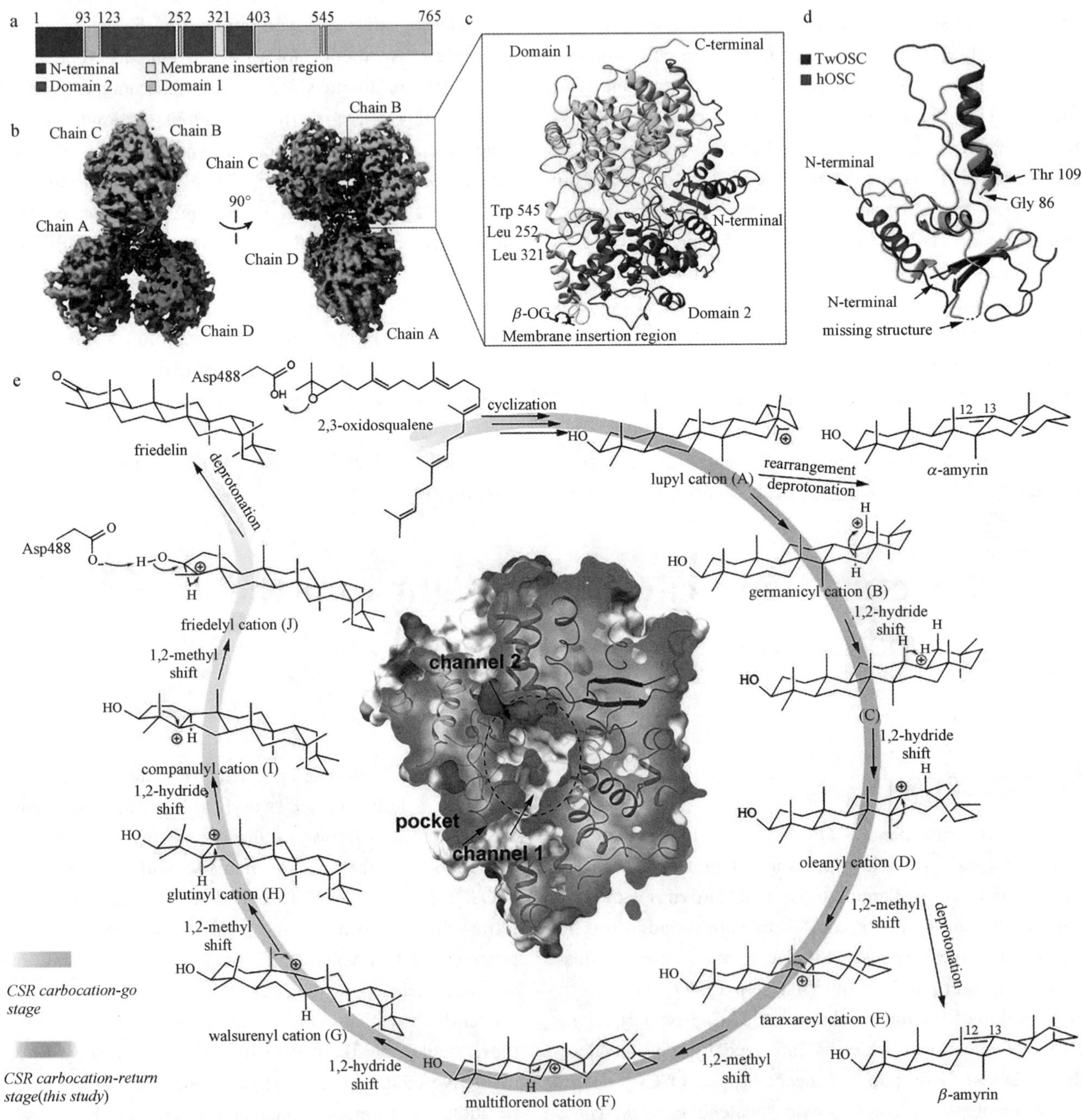


**Figure 1** (a) Domain organization of TwOSC. The names of the structural domains and the range of amino acids comprising them are indicated. The N-terminal region is colored royal blue. Domain 1 is colored light green. Domain 2 is colored forest green. The membrane insertion region is colored yellow. (b) Two views of the density map of the TwOSC tetramer. Chains A, B, C, and D are colored lime green, cyan, orange-yellow, and salmon, respectively. (c) Cartoon representation of TwOSC monomer, which is composed of the N-terminal region, domain 1, domain 2, and the membrane insertion region. $\beta$ - OG is shown in blue, while other domains are colored as shown in (a). (d) Comparison of the N-terminal regions of TwOSC and hOSC, which are colored royal blue and violet, respectively. (e) The protein surface representation displays the substrate channel and pocket, while the peripheral Scheme shows the catalytic mechanism of TwOSC, including the deprotonation of intermediates A, D, and J to form three products: $\alpha$-amyrin, $\beta$-amyrin, and friedelin, respectively.

intermediates in Figure 1e (state E-J), more rearrangement mechanisms are involved in the formation of friedelin, which we referred to as the "CSR mechanism," involving intermediates and catalytic mechanisms that remain elusive. Early termination of CSR produces other PT scaffolds, such as $\beta$-amyrin, taraxerol, and multiflorenol. Thus, understanding the CSR mechanism is crucial for unraveling the formation mechanism of PTs.

Herein, we report the cryogenic electron microscopy (cryo-EM) structure of the TwOSC tetramer and perform quantum mechanics/molecular mechanics (QM/MM) simulations to probe the CSR mechanism and investigate intermediate interactions. Based on the cryo-EM structure and theoretical calculations, we identified key sites that regulate the intriguing nine-step CSR cascade arrangement. Finally, semirational design and mutation by evolution (MbyE) were used to increase the catalytic activity of TwOSC to expand their applications.

## 2 RESULTS AND DISCUSSION

Overall structure of TwOSC  TwOSC, consisting of 765 amino acids, was analyzed to explore the complex reactions organized by plant triterpenoid synthases from a structural perspective (Figure 1a). We determined the cryo-EM structure of the full-length TwOSC at an overall resolution of 4.75 Å, while the resolution of the active site reached up to 4.4 Å (Table 1 and Figure S2). The density of amino acids in the structure was clear, especially in the active site where the side chains exhibited clear densities (Supplementary Figures S2d and S3). The overall structure of TwOSC displayed a tetrameric composition labeled as chains A, B, C, and D (Figure 1b). The structure of TwOSC can be divided into three parts, namely the N-terminal, domain 1, and domain 2 (Figure 1a, c). TwOSC is a peripheral membrane protein, and its membrane insertion region is in domain 2, composed of a flat plane formed by loop$^{251-253}$, $\alpha$-helix $\alpha 12$ (residues 320-343), and $3_{10}$-helix $\eta 3$ (residues 545-549; Figure 1c and Figure S4a). In the tetrameric structure, the membrane insertion region was located in the middle of the entire structure and detergent $\beta$-OG was constructed with a clear density (Figure 1c).

The overall structure of the TwOSC monomer was similar to that of human oxidosqualene cyclase (hOSC) and squalene-hopene cyclase from *Alicyclobacillus acidocaldarius* (SHC). However, compared with hOSC, TwOSC had a complete N-terminal density, starting at the $\beta$-sheets and ending at the helix structure, whereas the N-terminal structure of hOSC was discontinuous, and the $\beta$-sheets were in the middle of the structure (Figure 1d). Similar to hOSC and SHC, domains 1 and 2 of TwOSC were also composed of an inner-outer ring of $\alpha/\alpha$ barrel domains; the active site

**Table 1 Cryo-EM data collection, refinement, and validation statistics**

| | TwOSC tetramer |
|---|---|
| | EMD-35996, PDB: 8J5Z |
| **Data collection and processing** | |
| Magnification | 22500X |
| Voltage (kV) | 300 |
| Electron exposure (e/Å$^2$) | 60 |
| Defocus range ($\mu$m) | -1.5 to -2.3 |
| Pixel size (Å) | 1.07 |
| Symmetry imposed | C2 |
| Micrographs collected (No.) | 3097 |
| Particles used (No.) | 32698 |
| Map Resolution (global Å) | 4.75 |
| FSC 0.5 (unmasked/masked) | 6.97/5.75 |
| FSC 0.143 (unmasked/masked) | 4.23/4.19 |
| Map sharpening B factor (Å$^2$) | -230.641 |
| **Refinement** | |
| Model Composition | |
| Chains | 4 |
| Residues (aa) | 3056 |
| Ligands (No.) | 4 |
| B factors (Å$^2$) | |
| Protein | 131.38 |
| Ligand | 143.91 |
| R.m.s. deviations | |
| Bond lengths (Å) | 0.002 |
| Bond angles (°) | 0.460 |
| **Validation** | |
| Molprobity score | 2.15 |
| Clashscore | 6.20 |
| Poor rotamers (%) | 3.96 |
| Ramachandran plot | |
| Favored (%) | 94.88 |
| Allowed (%) | 5.12 |
| Disallowed (%) | 0.00 |

Model statistics were generated using Phenix comprehensive validation (cryo-EM).

was located between two domains (Figure 1e and Figure S4b, c). There were two channels near the active site, with the entrance (channel 1) to which is located in the channel formed by the membrane insertion region (Figure 1e).

QM/MM simulations of CSR  To illustrate the enzyme catalytic mechanism of TwOSC, hybrid QM/MM calculations were performed to probe the reaction pathway from the lupyl cation (A) to friedelin (Figures 1e and 2a). First, a 5-6 expansion reaction with lupyl cation occurred, yielding germanicyl cation (B) with a low energy barrier (1.8 kcal/mol) and exothermicity (-2.0 kcal/mol). Then, state C was generated through 1, 2 hydrogen transfer with a significant heat release (-13.4 kcal/mol). Subsequently, each step from C to J state (friedelyl cation) was endothermic, except for the transition from the taraxareyl (state E) to multiflorenol cation (state F). In this regard, most carbocations transferred in CSR cascade reactions were kinetically achievable but thermodynamically unfavorable. Nevertheless, two aspects should be noted: first, kinetically, the initial cyclization step is rate-limited, and more or less heat release for the cyclization reaction is usually expected, easily overcoming the barrier for CSR (22.3 kcal/mol; Figure S1b); second, thermodynamically, the CSR reaction was terminated by a subsequent deprotonation reaction with a general base (D488), which had no energy barrier and released abundant heat (−46.3 kcal/mol), making the entire enzymatic catalysis exoenergetic. Compared to the previously proposed mechanism, our calculations indicated the infeasibility of carbocation transfer from C5 (state I) to the C3 position, owing to the electron-withdrawn effect caused by the hydroxyl group. Instead, we found that a carbocation located at the C4 position is preferable for state J. Although multistep endothermic reactions are extremely rare in the formation of terpenoids, a continuous three-step endothermic reaction has been reported during the cyclization process by a diterpenoid cyclase. It is worth noting that the entire reaction process is still in an exothermic state, which is consistent with our results. In this context, the QM/MM-mapped relative energy profile of the reaction (Figure 2a) validated the hypothesized complete catalytic process (Figure 1e) from the linear substrate to the final friedelin.

The final product friedelin obtained from the QM/MM scan exhibited an all-chair (c-c-c-c-c) conformation (Figure 1e). However, the X-ray structure of friedelin shows a chair-chair-chair-boat-boat (c-c-c-b-b) conformation. To investigate the conformational difference of friedelin in the enzyme environment, further calculations were performed. We observed that the initial c-c-c-b-b conformation spontaneously converted to c-c-c-c-c conformation after about eight ps in the QM/MM MD trajectory of c-c-c-b-b-friedelin-OSC complex (Figure S5). Additionally, we were unable to obtain the c-c-c-b-b conformation for intermediates B to J during the QM/MM scan. Therefore, the presence of friedelin with a c-c-c-c-c conformation, as captured in this QM/MM study, is rational. Furthermore, we calculated the energy difference between c-c-c-b-b and c-c-c-c-c conformers in PCM water implicit solvent. The energy of the c-c-c-c-c conformation is only 0.22 kJ/mol higher than the c-c-c-b-b conformation (Figure S6). This suggests that the product friedelin could partially transform into a c-c-c-b-b conformation upon released from the the enzyme pocket into the solvent environment. However, the ring where the carbocation was located presented a boat conformation temporarily for intermediates D to J (Figure 1e). When the carbocation left the ring, it caused a shift to a chair conformation. A similar conformational change has also been detected in previous QM/MM studies of carbocation cascade mechanisms for lupyl cation in the enzyme environment and pure QM calculations of friedelin in the gas phase. The detailed conformational change could not be straightforwardly explained by the current static QM/MM scan, but a more meticulous and computationally expensive QM/MM MD simulation is required.

We found that the reaction relative energy potential of the CSR cascade reaction increased from state C to J and descended for the carbocation ($C^+$) rearrangement reaction, as reported in previous studies of several OSCs. To determine the details of the unique CSR cascade rearrangement reaction, we compared the binding poses of intermediates D–I and found that the stabilization effect for these intermediates was primarily due to aromatic residues Y262, F477, F731, W615, and W420 (Figure S7). In particular, the orientation of aromatic residues was unfavorable for establishing cation-π interactions, elongating the distances between the aromatic residues and cation in state E, compared with those in other intermediates. Nevertheless, it had a significant endothermic effect on all CSR cascade rearrangement reactions, particularly the methyl shift from the companulyl cation (state I) to friedelyl cation (state J), which is thermodynamically unfavorable (+6.8 kcal/mol). This raises the question of why such a thermodynamically unfavorable process could occur.

To reveal the intrinsic working mechanism of the enzyme driving this remarkable CSR reaction, an electrostatic potential map of the active pocket of the enzyme with a lupyl cation was constructed (Figure 2b). The pocket region around the A ring and cation had a negative electrostatic potential, which could stabilize the lupyl cation and drive the carbocation ($C^+$) shift to the A ring for good electrostatic complementarity. However, the electrostatic potential of the pocket contour along the cation transfer path (black arrow in Figure 2b) was substantially positive, indicating electrostatic repulsion, resulting in endothermicity from states C to I. In view of the entire catalytic cycle, we deduced that the pent-up energy from the cyclization reaction was largely stored as electrostatic potential energy in the enzyme pocket and ultimately released when the reactive carbocation was quenched by deprotonation to the neutral product friedelin (Figure S8). To summarize the enzymatic catalysis, the TwOSC enzyme utilizes a sophisticated energy-delay-releasing mechanism to drive such a CSR-driven triterpenoid skeleton rearrangement with the longest (nine steps) known reaction pathway.

Key residues regulating the CSR reaction  Based on the above QM/MM study of the TwOSC enzyme, computational modeling on several OSC enzymes was used to determine the

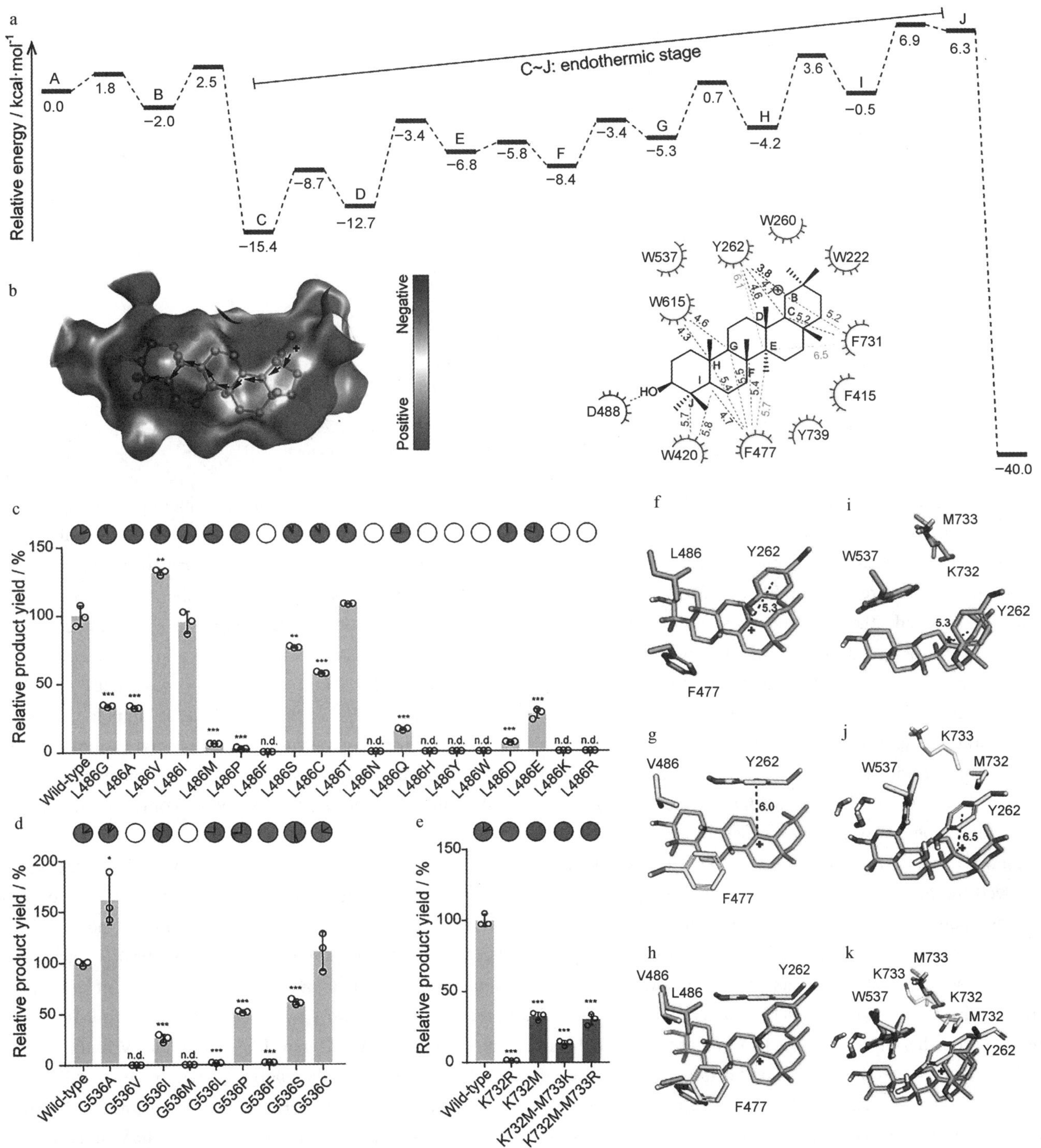

**Figure 2** (a) Reaction energy profiles from lupyl cation to product friedelin in the wild-type TwOSC (the entire QM/MM scan energy curve is shown in Figure 1b). The cyan amino acids indicate the aromatic amino acids in the pocket, while the red amino acids indicate the key amino acids involved in protonation and deprotonation. The number indicates the distance of the amino acid from the carbocation in Å. (b) The electrostatic potential map of TwOSC. The substrate, colored green, represents the lupyl cation. The pathway of carbocation transfer is shown as black arrows. (c-e) Mutation results of L486, G546 (d), and K732-M733 sites. The pie chart above the bar shows the proportion of the product, with orange representing friedelin, green representing $\beta$-amyrin, and blue representing $\alpha$-amyrin. (f-k) Differences in the active site pose after 100 ns of MD: (f) wild-type TwOSC; (g) L486V mutant; (h) alignment of wild type (green) and L486V model (yellow); (i) wild-type TwOSC; (j) K732M-M733K mutant; (k) alignment of wild type (green) and K732M-M733K model (yellow).

key residues responsible for the CSR reaction. We established a database containing $\beta$-amyrin synthase ($\beta$AS), $\alpha$-amyrin synthase ($\alpha$AS), and friedelin synthase (FRS) and found that 88.7% of the residues in the active pocket of TwOSC were highly conserved. Of the residues, 60.2% were completely conserved, and 28.5% were highly conserved. Surprisingly, three sites, L486, G536, and K732-M733 dyad, were highly correlated with friedelin synthase (Figure S9). After

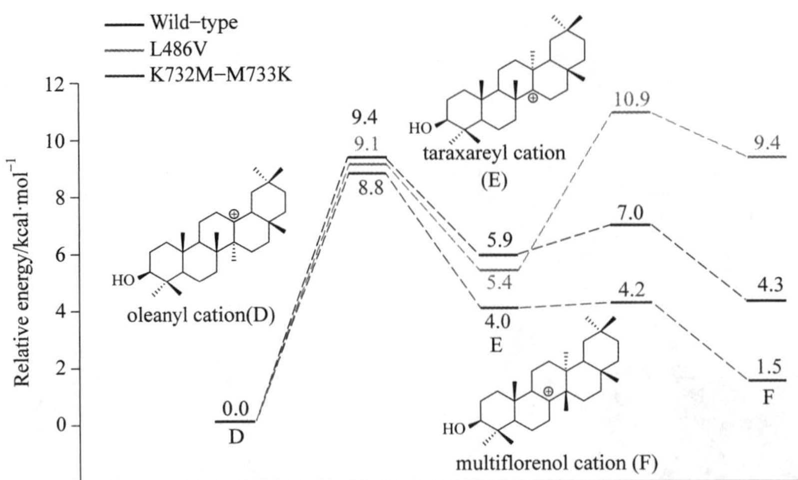


**Figure 3 Reaction energy profiles from oleanyl cation (state D) to multiflorenol cation (state F) in the wild-type, L486V mutant, and K732M - M733K mutant**

multiple sequence alignment analyses of AS ($\beta$AS and $\alpha$AS) and FRS, we found that L486 in FRS was a Leu residue, while that in AS was a Val residue. At the G536 site, Gly was in the FRS, whereas Ala and Ile were in the AS. For the K732 - M733 dyad, the Lys-Met dyad was in FRS and the Met-Lys or Met-Arg dyad was in AS (Figure S10). Mutation experiments were performed to investigate the roles of these three sites in friedelin synthesis (Figure 2c - e).

Saturation experiments at the L486 site showed that the variants were detrimental to friedelin production, suggesting that Leu is the optimal amino acid for friedelin synthesis. Meanwhile, some variants were beneficial for $\beta$-amyrin production, especially the L486V variant, which also improved the total product flux. The steric bulk at position 486 was essential for TwOSC function; mutants with a large steric bulk were inactivated (Figure 2c). Saturation experiments at site 536 showed that most mutants lost their activity, indicating that G536 is susceptible to TwOSC function. Furthermore, the G536A mutant increased the friedelin yield (Figure 2d). The G536A mutant showed improved catalytic efficiency without altering the products ratio, which did not seem to influence the CSR mechanism. Interestingly, the dyad K732-M733, composed of a hydrophobic Met residue and a charged Lys or Arg residue, was M-K in FRS, whereas it was K-M in $\beta$AS and $\alpha$AS. The K732R mutant almost lost its activity; only a small amount of friedelin was detected, and the K732M mutant transferred TwOSC function to $\beta$AS. Notably, the $\beta$-amyrin yield of the K732M mutant was higher than that of the wild-type. When the positions of the hydrophobic and charged residues were shifted, no friedelin was detected, and only $\beta$-amyrin was produced (Figure 2e). These results suggest that the Lys residue at position 732 is essential for friedelin formation and that the Met residue is beneficial for $\beta$-amyrin synthesis.

To explain the mutation experimental results, QM/MM and 100 ns MM molecular dynamics (MD) simulations of these mutated systems were performed to elucidate the regulatory mechanisms caused by the mutations. For the L486V variant model (Figure 2f - h), as the residue 486 was close to the catalytic site and might alter the side chain orientation of F477 and Y262, we propose that changing the orientation of F477 and Y262 will impair subsequent reactions, forming an intermediate oleanyl cation (state D). The relative energy profile of the reaction mapped by the QM/MM scan for the L486V model confirmed our hypothesis (Figure 3).

Methyl-transfer yielding taraxareyl cation (state E) had a similar energy barrier (9.1 kcal/mol) and endothermic effect (+ 5.4 kcal/mol) to the wild-type model (energy barrier is 9.4 kcal/mol and endothermic heat 5.9 kcal/mol). This indicates that orientation had little effect on this reaction step. However, subsequent methyl transfer to yield multiflorenol cation (state F) for the L486V mutant became challenging because the energy barrier of the L486V mutant increased to 5.5 kcal/mol, whereas it was only 1.1 kcal/mol for the wild-type. The reaction of the L486V mutant became endothermic (+4.0 kcal /mol), whereas it was thermodynamically more feasible for wild-type, with a heat release of 1.6 kcal/mol. We also confirmed that the endothermic effect of yielding intermediate F in the L486V mutant, contrary to the wild-type, was mainly attributed to the change in F477 orientation (Figure S11). In comparison to the wild-type, the L486V mutation increased the survival time of intermediate D and expanded the options of the branching route to yield $\beta$-amyrin (Figure 1e) according to the reaction relative energy profile (Figure 3). This was consistent with the experimental finding that the L486V variant increased the production of $\beta$-amyrin and decreased that of friedelin.

Regarding the K732M - M733K mutant, the reactions from intermediate D to E occurred easily, as shown in Figure 3, crossing an energy barrier of 8.8 kcal/mol, which was comparable to that of the wild-type and the L486V mutant. Differently, the conversion from intermediate E to F was a nearly no energy barrier reaction (0.2 kcal/mol) and showed favorable thermodynamical features. This failed to explain the loss of TwOSC activity by the K732M - M733K double mutation, indicating that the QM/MM scan calculation might not be applicable for capturing the circum-stances caused by the K732M - M733K mutation. We realized that residues K732/M733 were far from the active site, and the conformational dynamics induced by the double mutation cannot be ignored; however, static QM/MM calculations, even for QM/MM MD simulations, cannot capture this conformational change. Thus, we performed a 100 ns MM MD simulation to detect the effect of the K732M - M733K double mutation and found that water enters the active pocket as a result of the orientation change of W537 and Y262 (Figure 2i - k), particularly the water molecule forming a hydrogen bond with Y262. Y262 could serve as a general base to extract the hydrogen of the oleanyl cation to prematurely quench carbocation, thereby producing β-amyrin in advance. Furthermore, additional water molecules entering the active pocket destroy the hydrophobic environment, which is essential for carbocation transfer reactions, leading to an overall decrease in enzyme activity of the K732M - M733K mutant.

Semirational design of TwOSC Protein engineering in OSCs is hindered by the lack of a high-throughput screening system, thereby limiting the use of deep mutational scanning for directed evolution. Never-theless, the OSC family contains a large amount of sequence information in its database, and amino acid variation is a virtual mirror of protein evolution and function, which has potential applications in OSC engineering.

In this study, we used the MbyE method to extend the mutation search space to the entire amino acid sequence of TwOSC. First, we established a dataset of 198 amino acid sequences of OSCs that produce tetra- or pentacyclic skeletons from the NCBI database, including lanosterol synthases, cycloartenol synthases, lupeol synthase, αAS, βAS, FRS (Table S1).

Phylogenetic tree analysis revealed that OSCs with the same function grouped, indicating a strong correlation between sequence and function (Figure S12). We then analyzed the conservation of amino acids and the frequency of variants among the homologs at each amino acid of TwOSC using the local DeMaSk software. Amino acid conservation reflects the importance of the site for protein function, and variant frequency indicates whether the variant can be accommodated at the site in other homologs with similar functions.

Among the 765 sites of TwOSC, 69 sites showed a potential increase in activity after residue replacement (Figure 4a). These sites were scattered outside the active pocket, which could be related to the high amino acid conservation of the OSC pockets. For each of these sites, the mutant with the highest predicted activity was selected for further testing (Figures 4b, c). Interestingly, we found three mutants with significantly increased activity, namely N11S, V59I, and R669K, all of which were in the outer loops of TwOSC (Figure S13). Furthermore, we performed saturation mutation experiments at these three sites and found that N11S, V59I, and R669K mutations exhibited the highest activities (Figure S14). We also performed combinatorial double mutations on the N11S, N11A, V59I, V59S, and R669K mutants identified in the saturation mutation experiment and showed promising activity and found no double mutants with higher activity than the N11S and V59I mutants (Figure S15).

We combined the out-pocket mutants N11S and V59I with the in-pocket mutants G536A, L486V, and K732M to generate mutants that efficiently produced friedelin and β-amyrin and L486V mutant with the K732M mutant, both of which are beneficial for β-amyrin production, to determine possible synergistic effects. The results showed that the V59I-G536A mutant slightly increased the friedelin yield compared with the V59I mutant. The friedelin yield of the N11S - G536A mutant was lower than that of the N11S mutant. Thus, the N11S mutant achieved the highest yield of friedelin by producing 507% friedelin compared with the wild-type (Figure 5a). The N11S - L486V, N11S - K732M, and V59I - L486V mutants significantly increased the yield of β-amyrin. Surprisingly, the L486 - K732M mutant improved the yield of β-amyrin by a remarkable 21 200% and 348% compared with the wild-type and GgbAS1, respectively (Figure 5b). We introduced N11S/V59I into L486V-K732M to generate a triple mutation. The mutant V59I-L486V-K732M showed the highest titer of β-amyrin (21 700%) compared with the wild-type (Figure 5b).

Mutations in residues that directly interact with the substrate alter the product profile or even cause a loss of function. However, except for a few mutants with low activity and whose product ratios changed due to detection limit errors, most mutants did not affect the product ratio of TwOSC (Figure 4b, c). This suggests that these sites do not have a significant impact on the core CSR mechanism of TwOSC. Moreover, the sites that showed increased activity were in the outer loop of TwOSC, suggesting that the catalytic efficiency of TwOSC may be altered by regulating the rigidity of the outer loops. This finding is consistent with

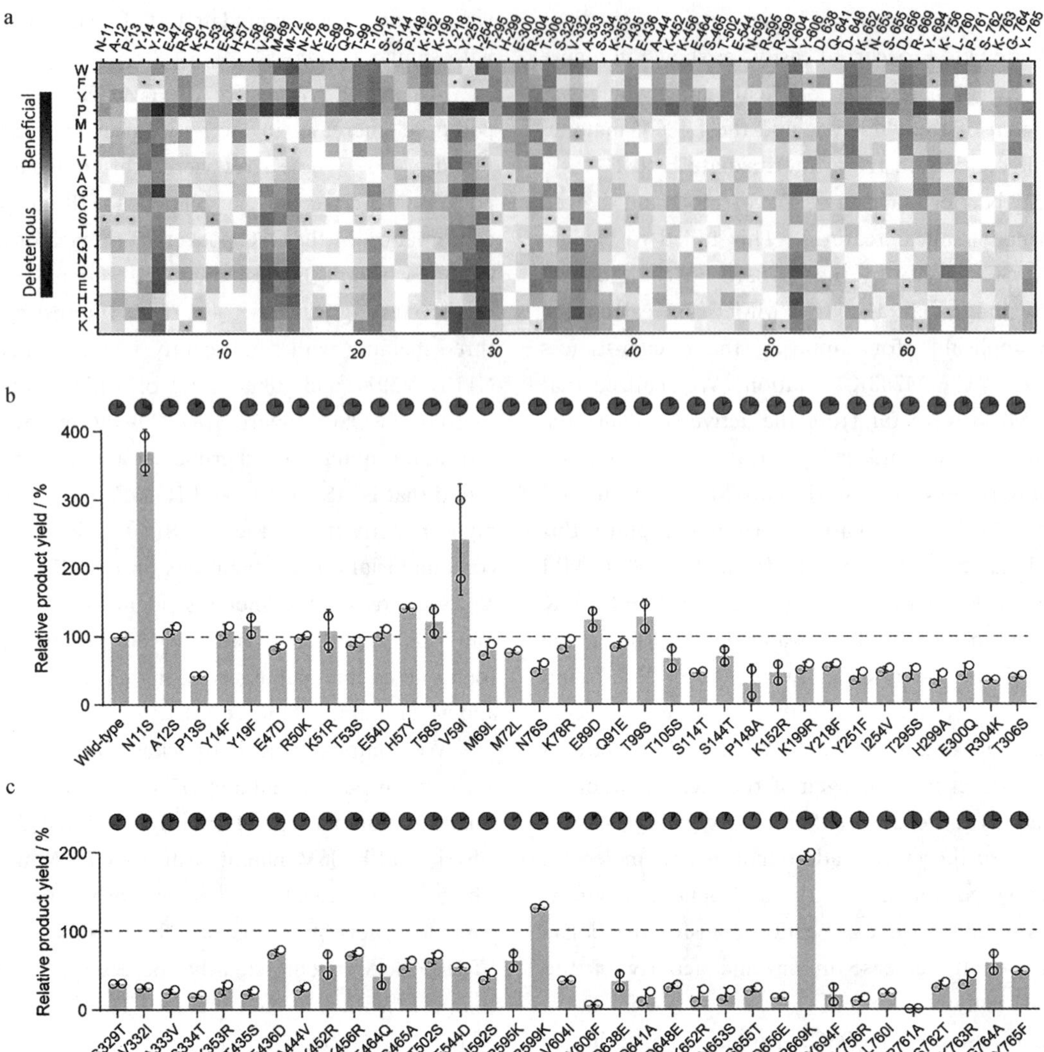

**Figure 4** (a) Potential activity-enhancing loci from DeMaSk analysis. Red indicates mutations predicted to be activity-enhancing, blue indicates deleterious mutants, and the site marked with an asterisk represents the mutant with the highest predicted activity for each site. (b, c) Product assay results for mutants with the highest predicted activity at each site. The pie chart above shows the proportion of product, with orange representing friedelin, green representing $\beta$-amyrin, and blue representing $\alpha$-amyrin.

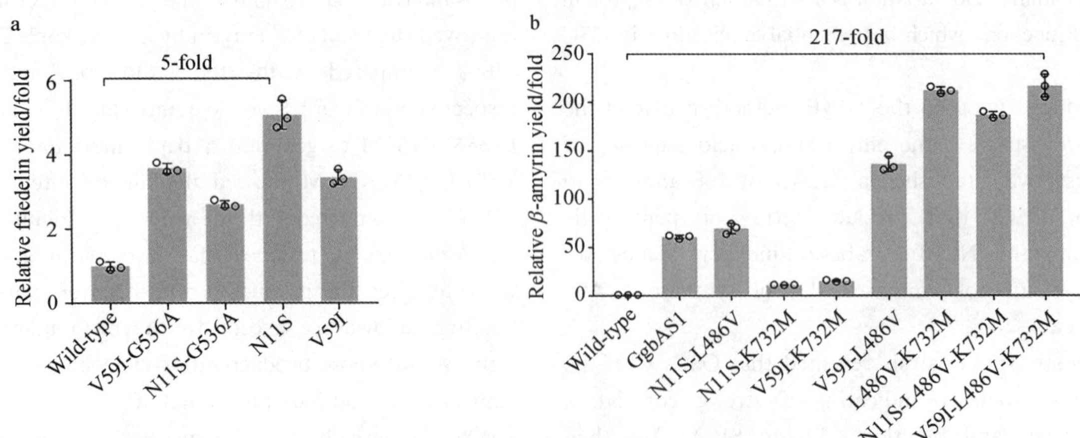

**Figure 5 Results of mutations in amino acid combinations in the periphery and in the pocket**

(a) Friedelin production. (b) $\beta$-Amyrin production.

a report on an ancestral diterpene cyclase. In addition, the mutants screened using the MbyE method typically retained their activity (Figure 4b, c) and had an advantage in saturation mutation experiments (Figure S14). Notably,

N11S and V59I were both located at the N-terminus and exhibited greater activity than R669K, suggesting that the N-terminus is important for OSC function, consistent with previous findings.

## 3 CONCLUSION

In this study, we determined the cryo-EM structure of the TwOSC tetramer. Based on this structure, we performed mutation experiments and hybrid QM/MM calculations to illustrate the CSR mechanism of TwOSC and found that three sites, G536, L486, and the K732 - M733 dyad, were crucial for PT skeleton generation. Moreover, we semirationally designed the TwOSC using the MbyE method and generated two variants, V59I - L486V - K732M and N11S, which significantly increased the yields of $\beta$-amyrin and friedelin, respectively. Our study uncovered the underlying CSR mechanism of the TwOSC enzyme catalysis and proposed a new strategy for the semirational design of other OSCs to promote PT biosynthesis.

[骆云峰，黄璐琦，童宇茹，等. Angewandte Chemie-International Edition, 2023, 62: e202313429.]

# From functional plasticity of two diterpene synthases (IrTPS2/IrKSL3a) to enzyme evolution

As retrieved from TeroKit, there are more than 24,000 known diterpenoid natural products, of which approximately 18,000 are from plants. Currently, about 200 diterpene synthases (diTPSs), which are the essential enzymes for constructing the carbon skeletons of diterpenoids, have been identified. The diTPSs fall into two distinct classes. The class I diTPSs catalyze ionization of the allylic diphosphate ester bond in their substrate to initiate carbocation formation, just as with other terpene synthases. This can occur with the general diterpenoid precursor ($E$, $E$, $E$)-geranylgeranyl diphosphate (GGPP), such as in the synthesis of taxadiene, a precursor of the anticancer medication Taxol. By contrast, class II diTPSs catalyze protonation-initiated carbocation formation in bicyclization of GGPP to products such as *ent*-copalyl diphosphate (*ent*-CPP), followed by subsequent reaction with a class I diTPS, as seen in the synthesis of kaurene, a precursor in the biosynthesis of the plant hormone gibberellin. The enzymes that catalyze this two-step process are known as copalyl diphosphate synthase (CPS) and kaurene synthase (KS), respectively, with other such diterpenoids termed labdane-related based on the eponymous hydrocarbon back-bone of CPP.

Gene duplication and neo-functionalization of CPSs and KSs has led to alternative functions, with class II diTPSs producing more than ten bicyclic products and subsequently acting class I diTPSs, generally derived from KS and termed KS-like (KSL), producing dozens of diterpenes currently known. An early example of such functional divergence are CPSs from the Lamiaceae (mint) plant family, which form a conserved clade generally producing CPP of normal (9S, 10S) stereochemistry (hereafter (+)-CPP) or the hydroxylated derivative (+)-labda-13-en-8-ol diphosphate (LPP). Accordingly, lineage-specific KSLs from the Lamiaceae react with (+)-CPP or (+)-LPP to produce the hydrocarbon backbones for a large array of specialized metabolites such as tanshinone, forskolin, or sclareol with potential pharmaceutical or perfume usages. KSLs in this lineage have usually undergone loss of the N-terminal ($\gamma$) domain. However, the evolution of these KSLs from the ancestral KS, or KSLs acting on *ent*-CPP for specialized metabolism instead, remains largely unknown.

Pimaranes and abietanes are the most widely distributed diterpenoids produced by KSLs from Lamiaceae. A summary from TeroKit showed that these two skeletons are usually decorated, with hydroxylation being the most common (Figure 1a). The hydroxylation is usually mediated by cytochrome P450s, and only a few natural or mutated diTPSs that directly form hydroxylated products have been reported. An interesting case is the two KSLs from *Isodon rubescens*, IrKSL3a previously reported by us, and IrTPS2 reported by Zerbe. Despite sharing 98% sequence identity and using the same substrate (+)-CPP, IrKSL3a only produces the olefin isopimaradiene (**1**), whereas IrTPS2 produces the hydroxylated nezukol (**2**). It has been previously reported that the replacement of a key alanine (at position 523) with isoleucine in IrTPS2 completely altered the product outcome from hydroxylated nezukol to isopimaradiene. Similar single residue switches altering product outcomes have also been reported in KS(L)s and other diTPSs. However, the limited crystal structures for diTPSs, with none reported for angiosperm KSLs, impedes our understanding of how these enzymes quench their final carbocation intermediate and further evolved to produce distinct skeletons.

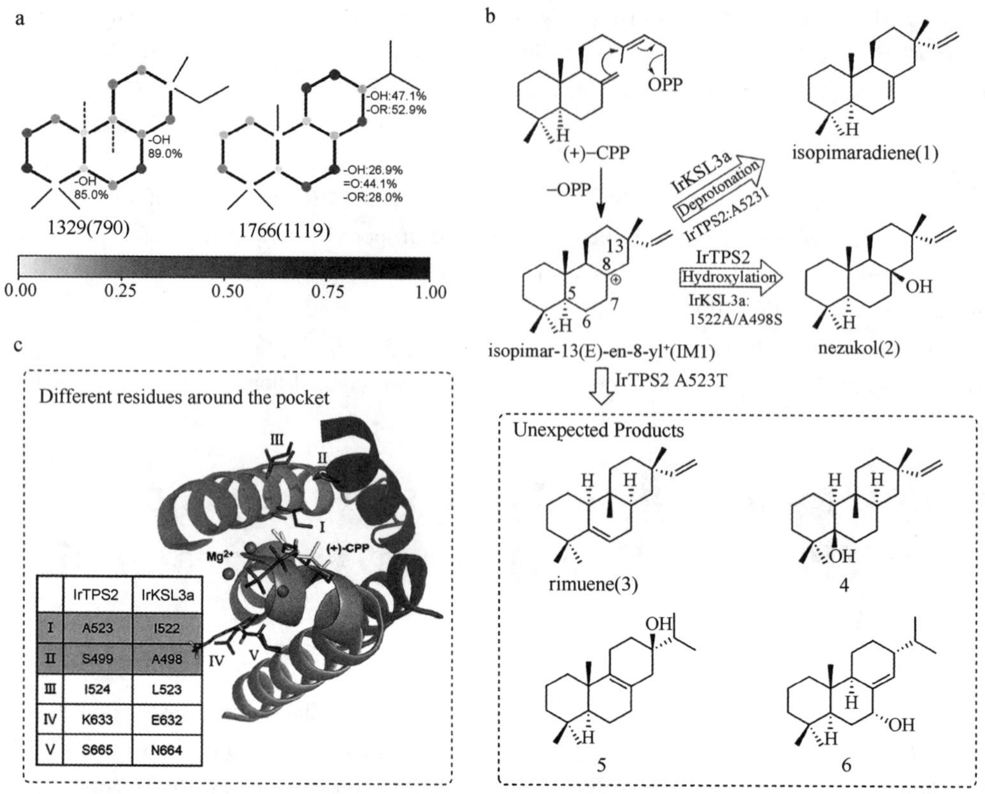


**Figure 1 Chemoinformatics statistical analysis, product generation schematic, and pocket structure alignment**

(a) Statistical analysis of the presented skeletal types of diterpenoid natural products. The darker the color, the higher the frequency of oxidative modification (percentages provide the proportion of the indicated type of modification in the known derivatives). The numbers underneath indicate the number of known diterpenoids and in parentheses, those from plants. The two dashed lines in the first skeleton represent the potential occurrence of methyl migration. (b) Scheme for the reactions leading to the main products of IrTPS2 and IrKSL3a as well as several unexpected products also observed here. (c) Structural differences between IrKSL3a and IrTPS2 (note the slight difference in residue numbering between IrTPS2 versus IrTPS3a is due to a single amino acid insertion/deletion).

Investigation of TPS structure-function relationships is an active area of study. For example, our previous work with TPSs revealed the crucial role of a water molecule in the selinadiene synthase SdS, in which the water forms hydrogen bonds with the main chain and then serves dual roles as both general base and acid to facilitate proton transfer. This emphasizes the role played by water molecules and hydrogen-bonding networks in the regulation of enzyme catalysis not only in TPSs but also in other types of enzymes.

In this work, we reveal the enzymatic structure-function relationship underlying hydroxylation versus deprotonation in IrTPS2 and IrKSL3a. From our work, besides products **1** and **2**, four additional products, three new hydroxylated diterpenes, and two rosane-type diterpenes can be generated (Figure 1b). Inspired by these molecular insights, we also discuss the potential of these insights for the rational redesign of the product outcome and the evolution of diterpene synthases in the Lamiaceae.

## 1 RESULTS AND DISCUSSION

Product Specificities of IrTPS2 and IrKSL3a Determined by a Key Residue Sequence alignment reveals only 16 differences between IrTPS2 and IrKSL3a (Figure S1). The three-dimensional superposition of their modeled structures further revealed that only five of the 16 different amino acid residues are located near the active site pocket (Figure 1c). In particular, only residues 523 and 499 (referring to residue number in IrTPS2) are located on the inside of one of the $\alpha$-helices that line the cavity (i.e., near the substrate), while the other three amino acid residues are on the outside of these helices. Nonetheless, all five distinct amino acids (Figure 1c) in IrTPS2 were substituted by the corresponding amino acids from IrKSL3a and their impact on the product profile was determined. As previously reported, the IrTPS2: A523I enzyme variant switches product outcome, yielding almost exclusively **1** (Figure 2a). By contrast, the other four substitutions did not alter product outcomes (Figure S2). It has been previously hypothesized that the residue at position 523 is likely a gatekeeper, with the steric hindrance of isoleucine preventing water from entering this portion of the active pocket, thereby preventing addition—i. e., to yield hydroxylated product **2**—leading to direct deprotonation yielding olefinic product **1** instead.

To test this mechanistic hypothesis, leucine, with a steric

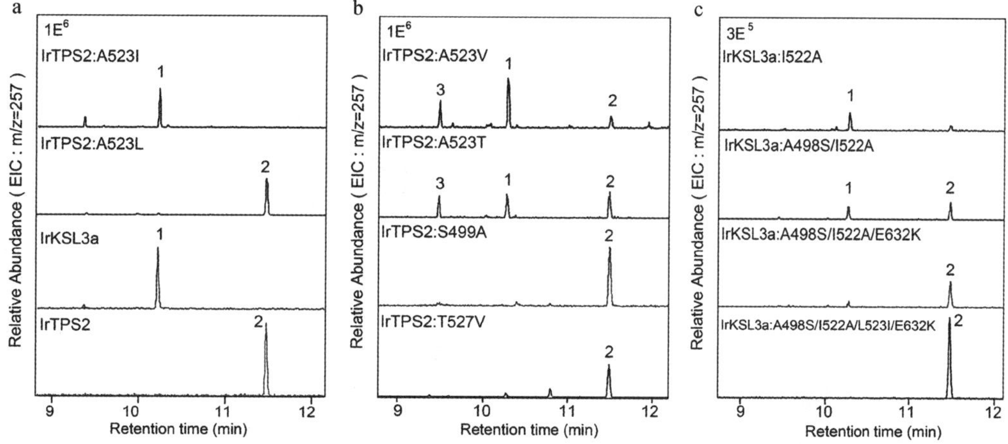


**Figure 2 Products distribution of wild-type and enzyme variants**

(a) Replacement of the Ala residue at position 523 in IrTPS2 with bulky side chains of comparable size, Ile and Leu, results in contrasting effects on product outcome. (b) The presence of a $\beta$-methyl containing side-chain has a considerable influence on the formation of **1**, as well as the appearance of additional products, such as rimuene (3), while aliphatic replacement of S499 and T527, which hydrogen bond the relevant water, decreases the yield of **2**. (c) Reengineering IrKSL3a to achieve selective production of **2** requires multiple mutations.

effect similar to that of isoleucine, was utilized. However, IrTPS2: A523L continued to produce the hydroxylated **2** (Figure 2a). This raises a very interesting question as to why very different product distributions are detected upon substitution with these highly similar amino acids (I and L). We also carried out the reverse mutational analysis, i. e., the five differing sites in IrKSL3a were replaced with the corresponding sites from IrTPS2. Interestingly, none of these substitutions appreciably altered the product distribution, as the mutants continued to largely produce **1**, with some exhibiting a loss of activity (e. g., IrKSL3a: I522A; see Figure S2). All of these findings indicate that this residue, A523 in IrTPS2/I522 in IrKSL3a, is key to the distinct product specificity of these two KSLs, but the underlying mechanism is not the previously proposed simple steric hindrance. Accordingly, we further investigated the enzymatic structure-function relationship underlying the different product specificities for IrKSL3a and IrTPS2.

Presence of a Water-Binding Dyad Sensitive to a Neighboring $\beta$-Methyl. To further investigate this enzymatic structure-function relationship, the (+)- CPP substrate was docked into the modeled wild-type and mutants along with the trio of divalent magnesium ($Mg^{2+}$) cofactors, and dozens of nanosecond classical molecular dynamics (MD) simulations that include solvent (water) were performed. Cluster analysis was performed for all these MD trajectories, and a representative structure for each system was extracted. Subsequent QM/MM optimization and QM/MM MD were conducted to test the stability of the hydrogen-bonding network, as shown in Figure 3 and described below. For wild-type IrTPS2, T527, and S499 both hydrogen-bond a water molecule located near (~4 Å) the relevant carbon-8 (C8). We hypothesize it is this water that adds to the C8 carbocation, with deprotonation of the resulting alkyloxonium then yielding hydroxylated product **2**.

Although there is only a slight difference in the positioning of a methyl group in the side chain, a comparison of IrTPS2: A523I with IrTPS2: A523L found that this leads to a very significant structural difference (Figure 3). Our simulations revealed that the water site in IrTPS2: A523I was occupied by the $\beta$-methyl of I523, which displaces the water molecule that presumably quenches the C8 carbocation intermediate. By contrast, despite occupying equivalent volumes, the substituted leucine in IrTPS2: A523L is oriented away from the substrate, allowing a water molecule to bind to T527 and S499, as observed in MD and QM/MM MD simulations. These results are consistent with the hypothesis that the presence or absence of water near C8 determines if a hydroxylated product is formed, matching the experimental investigation, in which IrTPS2: A523I no longer leads to product **2**, while IrTPS2: A523L still does (Figure 2a).

To investigate the importance of a $\beta$-methyl group more generally, the same computational protocols were also performed on the A523T and A523V variants of IrTPS2. Consistent with an influential role for $\beta$-methyl, both substitutions were found to hamper the binding of a water molecule to T527 and S499. This prediction was validated by the observed change in product outcome (Figure 2b, Figure S3a and Table S1), as the proportion of **2** was significantly decreased (57.1% reduction) with IrTPS2: A523V and IrTPS2: A523T (33.6% reduction) relative to IrTPS2: A523L. Meanwhile, more product **1** was found with these two IrTPS2 mutants, and this even became the main product of IrTPS2: A523V, with both also producing another olefin (i.e., from direct deprotonation of a carbocation intermediate rather than the addition of water). It should be noted that

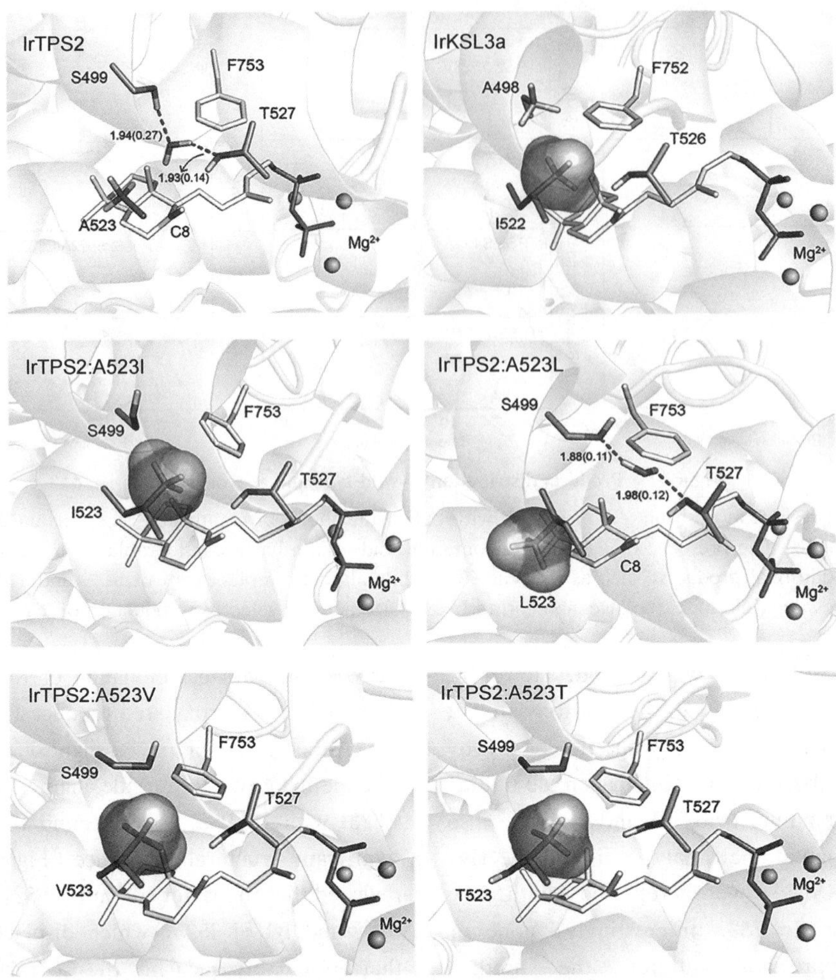


**Figure 3 Comparison of the residues at the same site around the active pocket, as captured from QM/MM MD, with the van der Waals surface (drawn in cyan) of methyl that hampers water binding**

Modeled active site for indicated enzyme (variant) including the (+)- CPP substrate. Bold blue numbers represent the average distance, with standard deviation in parentheses.

the amount of product **2** is relatively higher with IrTPS2: A523T, which could be related to the hydroxyl group of threonine, which can form a metastable hydrogen bond with S499, allowing an alternative orientation wherein the β-methyl no longer completely blocks the binding of a water molecule (Figure S4). This would further be consistent with the more important role of T527 indicated by the continued selective production of **2** by IrTPS2:S499A (Figure 2b).

Moreover, at the A523 site, an additional set of substitutions with various residues (all without a β-methyl) were constructed. As expected, no significant production of **1** was observed with most of these variants (Figure S5). It is noteworthy that with the A523N mutant, where there is no β-methyl group, we still detected a noticeable amount of product **1**. This observation was further elucidated by MD simulations, which indicate that the carboxamide group on the side-chain substitutes for the water, hydrogen bonding to both S499 and T527 (Figure S6). We also constructed two mutants, IrTPS2: T527V and IrTPS2: S499A, that differ from wild-type IrTPS2 only in a lack of hydroxyl at the corresponding locations. As expected, the yield of product **2** was significantly reduced (62.0 and 13.7%, respectively) in these two mutants relative to wild-type IrTPS2 (Figure 2b, Figure S3a and Table S1). The reduction in yield highlighted the importance of the hydrogen bonding by Ser499 and Thr527 in positioning a water molecule for addition and the subsequent production of **2**.

While the A523I mutation has a profound effect on IrTPS2, the converse mutation in IrKSL3a (I522A) led to only a very small amount of product **2**, while the amount of product **1** was greatly reduced (Figure 2c). In other words, the function of IrKSL3a was not fully reversed by this change. We hypothesized that this is due to residue 498 in IrKSL3a being an alanine instead of the serine that hydrogen bonds the relevant water in IrTPS2 (S499). To investigate this hypothesis, we added the A498S mutation to construct IrKSL3a:A498S/I522A. The results showed that this double mutant more selectively produced **2**, with a significantly increased yield, which was about 7.9-fold higher than seen with the IrKSL3a: I522A single mutant (Figure 2c, Figure S3b and Table S1). Nevertheless, IrKSL3a: A498S/I522A still produces modest amounts of **1** and less of **2** than wild-type IrTPS2. In order to fully convert IrKSL3a activity, additional mutational changes to the other distinct active-site residues found in IrTPS2 were made and tested, revealing that the triple-substituted variant IrKSL3a: A498S/I522A/E632K and quadruple-substituted variant IrKSL3a: A498S/I522A/E632K/L523I more selectively produce **2**, with the latter found to be particularly efficient (Figure 2c). It should be noted that even the quintuple-substituted variant IrKSL3a: A498S/I522A/E632K/L523I/N664S still produces less **2** than IrTPS2 (Figure S3b, Table S1), which indicates that residues outside the active site still affect enzyme function.

Notably, one of the tested doubly substituted variants, IrKSL3a:I522T/E632K, was found to make four additional products, all apparently unknown diterpenes. Further testing, using a previously described modular metabolic engineering system in *E. coli*, demonstrated these were also made by IrTPS2: A522T, albeit in smaller amounts (Figure S7). Accordingly, cultures expressing this IrKSL3a: I522T/E632K in *E. coli* also engineered to produce (+)-CPP were scaled up, and the novel products were extracted. NMR structural analysis (Table S2; Figures S8 - S31) revealed that these were the known olefin rimuene (rosa-5,15-diene, **3**), and three hydroxylated products (Figure S32). One of these is derived from the same rearrangement of the isopimar-13(*E*)-en-8-yl carbocation formed by initial cyclization as for **3**—i.e., a series of 1,2-hydride (C9 → C8), methyl (C10 → C9) and hydride (C5 → C10) shifts—before the addition of water and deprotonation forms the observed rosa-15-en-5-ol (**4**). The other two are abietanes, requiring proton shifts to C16 with an accompanying 1,2-methyl (C13 → C15) shift. Water is immediately added to the resulting abietaen-13-yl carbocation to produce the observed abieta-8-en-13*β*-ol (**5**). By contrast, some rearrangement is required to generate the final abieta-8(14)-en-7-yl carbocation to which water is added to yield the observed abieta-8(14)-en-7*α*-ol (**6**). These last three appear to be novel compounds, and **3**, **5**, and **6** exhibit structural similarities to 13-*epi*-5, 15-rosadien-3*α*, 11*β*-diol, lophanic acid/rubesanolide D and 7*α*, 9*α*, 13*α*-trihydroxyabiet individually, which have previously been reported as active ingredients with antibacterial or anti-inflammatory effects (Figure S32).

Regardless, these experimental and computational results indicate that the hydrogen bonding capacity provided by S499 and T527 is required for the production of **2** in IrTPS2, along with the absence of a *β*-methyl-containing residue at position 523. Indeed, IrKSL3a, which originally generated **1**, can be engineered to generate **2** by mutation of these key amino acid residues and can be fully converted to IrTPS2-like catalytic function by further substitution of active site residues to those found in IrTPS2 (IrKSL3a: A498S/I522A/E632 K/L523I).

Quenching Mechanism in IrTPS2 and IrKSL3a. To further investigate the addition of water catalyzed by IrTPS2, hybrid quantum mechanical/molecular mechanical (QM/MM) free energy calculations were employed (Figure 4a). For this purpose, (+)-CPP was replaced with the relevant isopimar-13(*E*)-en-8-yl carbocation reactant, as well as released inorganic pyrophosphate coproduct and accompanying trio of $Mg^{2+}$ to generate the first intermediate state (IM1). The resulting free energy curve shows that the process of water addition is very facile since it is exothermic (~11.7 kcal/mol heat release) and has almost no energy barrier. With the help of the cation-polar interaction with the C8 carbocation, the above-mentioned water molecule (Wat, as shown in Figure 4a), ligated by S499 and T527, gradually approaches the carbocation reactant (from 3.0 to 2.1 Å) along the reaction coordinate. At the transition state (TS), the hydrogen bonding distance between T527 and Wat is 1.9 Å, shorter than the hydrogen bonding distance in the IM1 state (2.6 Å), while the hydrogen bonding distance between S499 and Wat is significantly increased (from 2.2 to 3.1 Å). The transition to the TS is almost barrier-free and thus kinetically very favorable, while the reaction is thermodynamically driven by the increased stability of the alkyloxonium reactant formed by the addition of water, representing the second intermediate state (IM2). This mainly reflects the formation of the C - O bond, and stabilization by continued hydrogen bonding to S499 (4.1 Å) and, especially, T527 (1.4 Å), which likely serves as the catalytic base, as has been seen with other TPSs. Regardless, considering that S499 only loosely binds the water while T527 maintains strong hydrogen bonding throughout the process, T527 appears to be more important than S499 in the formation of hydroxylated products such as **2**, consistent with the experimental results. Intriguingly, the sequence alignment of Lamiaceae diterpene synthases (Figure S33) shows that T527 is more conserved, suggesting that a threonine at this position is important.

We also performed QM/MM calculations to examine the formation of product **1** by direct deprotonation of the isopimar-13(*E*)-en-8-yl carbocation in wild-type IrKSL3a (Figure 4b). The modeled structure indicates that the T526 hydroxy is the only functional group close enough to carry out deprotonation (Figure S34). While this is usually considered to be a very weak general base, and such side-chains were previously assumed to stabilize carbocations by dipole interaction, it has been more recently appreciated that the higher $pK_a$ for protonated alcohols (which range from

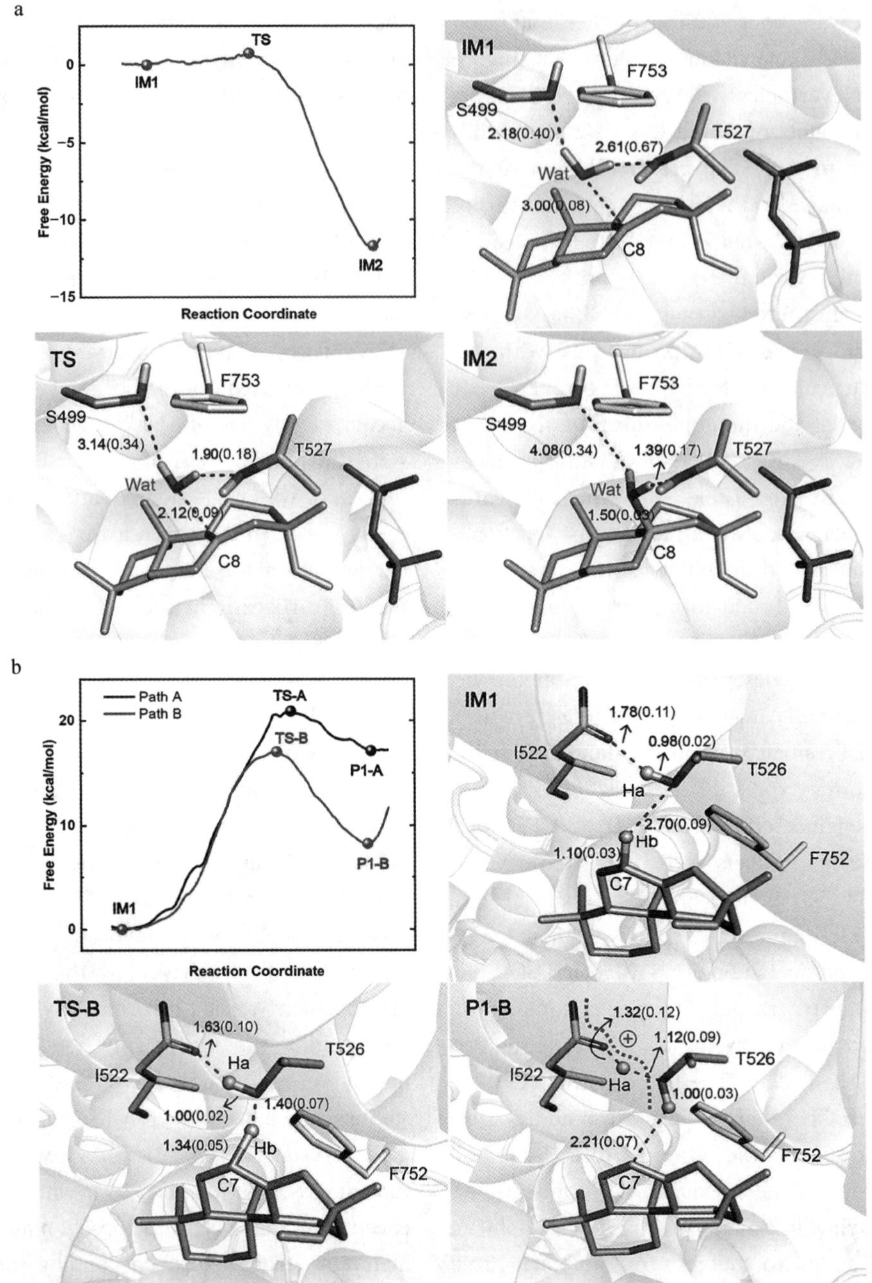


**Figure 4 QM/MM predicted reaction-free energy profiles and representative structures for the quenching reaction in IrTPS2 (a) and IrKSL3a (b)**

Modeled active site for indicated intermediate with key interactions shown. Bold blue numbers represent the average distance, with standard deviation in parentheses.

−1 to −4) relative to carbocations (< −10) indicate such activity may be widespread. While the initial QM/MM free energy calculation suggests the energy barrier to such deprotonation is about 20.9 kcal/mol and a large amount of endothermy (~17.1 kcal/mol) is required for the production of **1** by deprotonation using T526 (Figure 4b, path A), a more energetically reasonable alternative exists (Figure 4b, path B). In particular, we found that the amide bond between I522 and L523 can form a hydrogen bond with T526, which correctly orients the hydroxyl for deprotonation in IM1 and the TS, as well as enhances the basicity of T526 by stabilizing its protonated form (P1 - B). Inclusion of this portion of the peptide backbone in the QM/MM free energy calculation led to the shown path B (Figure 4b), which led to reduction to only a 17.0 kcal of energy barrier and slight endothermicity (~8.1 kcal/mol). Such use of an amino acid backbone carbonyl in the deprotonation catalyzed by terpene synthases is supported by our previous report. Furthermore, mutational analysis indicates that substituting T526 with other amino acids significantly decreases the catalytic activity (Figure S35).

Extended Engineering of Nezukol Production. To determine if the key residue change identified here (i.e., the amino acid corresponding to IrTPS2: A523) was more

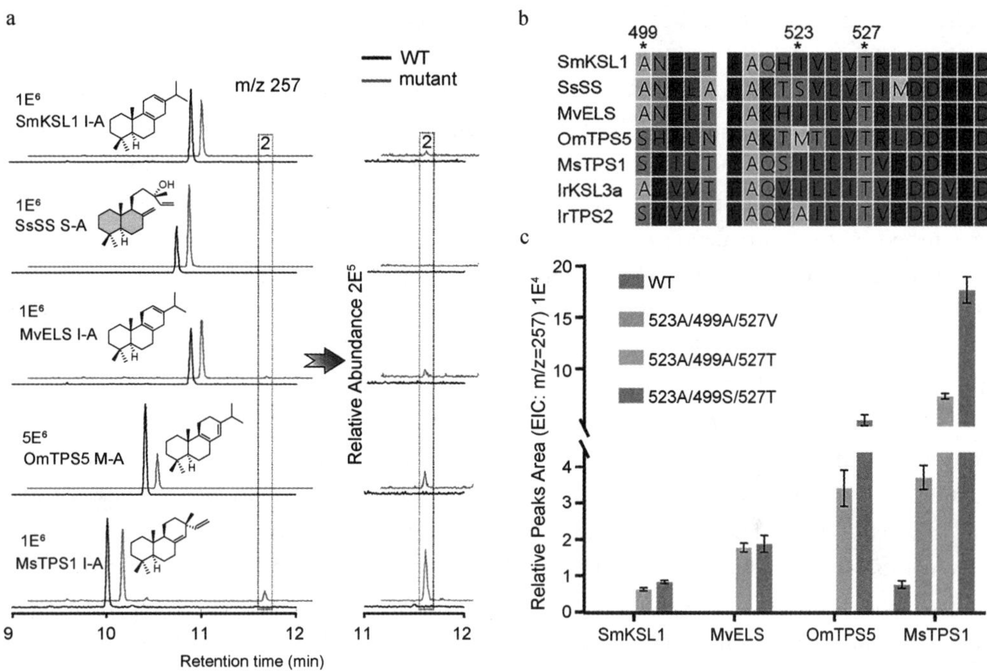


**Figure 5 Examination of the identified three key residues in other homologous class I diTPSs**

(a) Substituting the amino acid at position 523 to alanine eliminated steric hindrance and resulted in the detection of product **2** in all cases except for SsSS. (b) Partial sequence alignment between IrKSL3a, IrTPS2, and other homologous enzymes. (c) Incremental addition of hydrogen bonding capacity led to a progressive increase in the yield of product **2** (amino acid numbering refers to that in IrTPS2).

widely applicable, we performed site-directed mutation of the homologous proteins MsTPS1, OmTPS5, MvELS, SsSS, and SmKSL1 from different Lamiaceae species (Figure S36) to obtain the variants MsTPS1: I509A, OmTPS5: M353A, MvELS: I326A, SsSS: S333A, and SmKSL1: I338A. Our results (Figure 5a) showed that the hydroxylated product **2** was detectable in all variants except SsSS:S333A, which may reflect the fact that SsSS does not naturally catalyze cyclization (i.e., to the necessary pimarenyl carbocation). Of the enzyme variants that produce the hydroxylated **2**, their yield decreases in the order MsTPS1: I509A > OmTPS5: M353A > MvELS: I326A > SmKSL1: I338A. Notably, their yield of **2** is correlated with homology with IrTPS2, the higher the sequence identity the larger the output of **2**.

To investigate the roles of the two water-binding residues (i.e., S499 and T527 in IrTPS2), the relevant residues were changed in the four single-substituted variants mentioned above: MsTPS1, OmTPS5, MvELS, and SmKSL1. Given the conservation of T527 noted above, this was substituted with valine in all four, while S499 was conserved in MsTPS1 and OmTPS5, so substituted with alanine, and the alanine at this position in MvELS and SmKSL1 changed to serine (Figure 5b). Consistent with the importance of T527 shown above, substitution with valine was sufficient to block production of the hydroxylated product **2** other than that in MsTPS1, where small amounts of **2** were still observed (Figure 5c). In contrast, changing the alanine to serine in MvELS and SmKSL1 had minimal effect, and, although the converse substitution of alanine for S499 in OmTPS5 and MsTPS1 did reduce the amount of **2**, this was a relatively moderate effect (<3-fold, see Figure 5c).

These results further highlight the importance of the three residues identified here in the production of **2**. However, their effect is clearly further dependent on additional factors, as highlighted by the significant correlations between homology and the amount of **2** resulting from the introduction of the associated residues (i.e., S499, A523, and T527). Indeed, even almost identical IrKSL3a requires additional mutations to exhibit selective and efficient production of **2**. This demonstrates that the evolution of the unusual hydroxylation function in IrTPS2 required multiple changes/steps.

## 2 CONCLUSIONS

Here, we show that the ability of a previously identified alanine to isoleucine switch in IrTPS2 to block the production of **2** (i.e., the addition of water) depends on the presence of a $\beta$-methyl containing side-chain. Building on this finding, we employed molecular modeling of IrTPS2 and the very closely related IrKSL3a, with subsequent molecular dynamics analysis and QM/MM calculations to identify two residues, S499 and T527, that position the relevant water molecule for addition to the pimaren-8-yl carbocation formed by initial cyclization to produce **2**. QM/MM analysis highlighted T527 as most likely serving as the catalytic base in both IrTPS2 and IrKSL3a. The importance of these two residues was verified by additional mutagenesis, which also revealed that further changes were required to fully convert IrKSL3a to IrTPS2 activity (i.e., the selective and efficient production of **2**). Notably, certain variants were found to yield novel products, demonstrating not only the broader effects of these altered residues but also selective pressure for the production of **2** more specifically. The evolutionary implications of our results were further tested by the introduction of these key residues into more distantly related class I diTPSs, which further emphasized the importance of genetic/enzymatic context. Specifically, the three key residues (corresponding to the residue site 523/499/527 in IrTPS2) require other epistatic changes within the enzyme in order to effectively introduce the addition of water, to reshape the function. The apparent complexity of such alteration in product outcome for class I diTPSs shown here (and implied in previous studies) contrasts with the single residue changes that efficiently impart the addition of water in class II diTPSs. We speculate this may reflect the hypothesized use of the pyrophosphate coproduct as the catalytic base in class I terpene synthases. Regardless, such complexity is consistent with the relative rarity of class I diterpene synthases that add water, despite the essentially invariable need to incorporate such hydroxyl groups to provide solubility as well as hydrogen binding potential for specificity in the construction of bioactive terpenoids, and provides an intriguing challenge for future engineering efforts with this important family of biosynthetic enzymes.

## 3 METHODS

Structure Preparation Due to the lack of available crystal structures for IrTPS2 and IrKSL3a, we employed Alpha-Fold2 to predict their structures. Among the predicted structures, we selected the one with the highest rank for further modeling for each. The Ramachandran plots for these two structures are presented in Figure S37. The predicted structures lacked the essential trinuclear magnesium cluster necessary for catalysis. To rectify this, we manually incorporated the cluster into the active sites by referring to the crystal structure of *Aspergillus terreus* aristolochene synthase (PDB entry: 4KUX), which possesses an intact magnesium cluster. Enzyme variants were constructed using the PyMOL program (http://pymol. sourceforge. net/). After preparing these structures, molecular docking of the substrate (+)-CPP to the enzymes was performed using Autodock vina software. The docking poses were manually verified to exclude any implausible conformations. The optimal pose for each system was utilized as the initial structure for subsequent classical molecular dynamics (MD) simulations.

Classical MD Simulations The Amber FF99SB force field was used for the protein, while the TIP3P model was employed for the solvent waters. The restrained electrostatic potential (RESP) charges of the ligand were calculated at the HF/6-31(G)* level using the Gaussian 16 package. The substrate was described by the Amber GAFF force field. MD simulations were performed using the AMBER20 software, with periodic boundary conditions and cubic models applied to all systems. The initial coordinates and topology files were generated with the tleap module implemented in AMBER20. Sodium ions were added to each system to neutralize the charges. Routine minimizations were applied to each system, starting with the solvent molecules, followed by the side chain of the protein, and finally all atoms. After minimization, each system was gradually heated from 0 to 300 K under the NVT ensemble, followed by a 100 ps NPT ensemble density equilibration at 300 K and a pressure of 1.0 atm. Subsequently, a 30 ns NVT ensemble production MD simulation with a time step of 2 fs was performed for each model. All systems achieved stability (Figure S38). The trajectories obtained by MD were used for cluster analysis. General restraints were applied to the $PP_i$ group and $Mg^{2+}$ cluster because of the known poor treatment of metal-ligand coordination interactions. The SHAKE algorithm was used to constrain the hydrogens during MD simulations, and a cutoff of 12 Å was set for both van der Waals and electrostatic interactions.

QM/MM Simulations. Our QM/MM calculations incorporate nine models (referenced in Table S3). The first six models were designed to evaluate the stability of the hydrogen-bonding network observed in classical MD simulations. The remaining three models were employed to compute the free energy associated with the key reaction steps. For the first set of models, the initial structures were extracted from classical MD clustering, which were then subjected to QM/MM optimization followed by 5 ps of QM/MM MD simulations. For the last three models, in addition to the aforementioned procedures, QM/MM potential energy scan (PES) and QM/MM umbrella sampling were conducted. The initial structures used for the QM/MM scan were extracted from the classical MD trajectories. Then the (+)-CPP substrate was replaced by the carbocation IM1, along with the $PP_i$ coproduct, because the well-known understanding that water molecules involved in quenching carbocations are in place prior to the initiation of the reaction, as the time scale of the reaction is much shorter than required for conformational adjustment of enzyme (and water molecules). In addition, the focus of this work is on product differentiation after carbocation IM1. Following the substitution of ligands, the structure was allowed to relax briefly under the molecular force field prior to initiating the standard QM/MM calculations. For all models, water molecules beyond 30 Å from the C8 atom of the substrate were deleted. For the selection of the QM region for each model, refer to Table S3. All atoms in the QM subsystem were treated using the M06 - 2X/6 - 31 G(d) method, which has been widely used in our previous research. The QM/MM boundary was treated using the improved pseudo approach. The Amber FF99SB force field was used for the MM subsystem, as in previous classical MD simulations. The spherical boundary condition was employed for each model, with atoms more than 30 Å from the spherical center being fixed. A 12 Å cutoff was employed for van der Waals interactions and 18 Å for electrostatic interactions. The system temperature was controlled by the Langevin thermostat method at 300 K, and the Newton equation of motion was integrated by the Beeman algorithm during the QM/MM MD simulations. These equilibrated structures were used to map out the PES curves with the reaction coordinate driving method. Definitions of reaction coordinates, potential energy curves, variations in key distances with respect to the reaction coordinates, and the key distance evolution during the QM/MM simulations can be found in Figures S39 - S49. After scanning the reaction path, we divided it into several windows. Then the MM subsystem was further equilibrated for 500 ps at the MM level, with the QM subsystem fixed for each window. Finally, each window was subjected to QM/MM MD umbrella sampling for at least 10 ps with a time step of 1 fs. The weighted histogram analysis method (WHAM) method was employed to calculate the free energy profiles with data collected from the umbrella sampling processes. All QM/MM calculations were performed using the modified QChem and Tinker programs developed by Prof. Yingkai Zhang's group (http://www.nyu.edu/projects/yzhang/). A similar QM/MM protocol had also been employed in our previous studies of other TPSs.

Mutant Construction. The *IrKSL3a* and *SmKSL1* constructs used here were those previously cloned into pET32a (Merck, Kenilworth, NJ, USA). Genes for *IrTPS2*, *MsTPS1*, *OmTPS5*, *SsSS*, and *MvELS* were synthesized and optimized by Genscript and also cloned into pET32a, utilizing its N-terminal 6 × His-tag. Site-directed mutagenesis was performed via PCR using the primers in Table S4. Each mutant was verified by complete gene sequencing.

In Vitro Assays The recombinant plasmid was transformed into *Escherichia coli* Transetta (DE3). Three colonies were cultured in LB medium with 50 mg/L carbenicillin, grown at 37 ℃ to an optical density of 0.8, then 0.4 mmol/L isopropyl-*b*-D-thiogalactopyranoside (IPTG) was added to induce the expression of the protein for 16 h at 16 ℃. Subsequently, cell pellets were collected and resuspended in assay buffer (50 mmol/L Phosphate buffer, pH 7.4, 10% glycerol, 2 mmol/L DTT, and 10 mmol/L $MgCl_2$) and sonicated six times for 10 s on ice. Lysate from the samples was centrifuged at 12,000 × *g* for 20 min at 4 ℃. The proteins were purified using nickel-nitrilotriacetic acid agarose beads following the method previously described. Every KSL (WT or variant) was performed in 3 replicates and obtained the corresponding purified proteins. The concentration of the purified protein was detected by the Bradford Protein Quantification Kit (Trans Gen Biotech) and then adjusted to 0.2 mg/mL using an assay buffer. SmCPS1 (KC814639) from *Salvia miltiorrhiza* was used in this study to produce (+)-CPP. The KLSs and variants were assayed in combination with SmCPS1. 200 μL of the purified SmCPS1 and KSL (WT or variant) were incubated with 50 μmol/L (*E*, *E*, *E*)-geranylgeranyl diphosphate (GGPP) (Sigma-Aldrich) for 4 h at 30 ℃ in the dark. Assay mixtures were extracted three times with an equal volume of hexane which contained tetracosane ($C_{24}H_{50}$) as the internal standard. The hexane fractions were pooled, evaporated under nitrogen, resuspended in 100 μL of hexane, and then analyzed by GC-MS.

GC-MS Analysis. The assay was carried out using a Trace 1310 series GC with a TSQ8000 MS detector (Thermo Fisher Scientific Co. Ltd.). A TR-5 ms capillary column (30 m × 0.25 mm i.d.; DF = 0.25 μm; Thermo Fisher Scientific) was used for GC-MS analysis. Separation of the injected sample (1 μL) was achieved with a Helium flow rate of 1 mL/min with a temperature program of 2 min at 50 ℃, followed by a gradient from 50 to 210 ℃ at 40 ℃ $min^{-1}$, then 5 ℃/min to 250 and 40 ℃/min to 300 ℃, and then held at 300 ℃ for 5 min. Products **1** and **2** were identified by comparison of retention time and mass spectra to those known for the wild-type IrTPS2 and IrKSL3a. The peak area of different enzymatic products was normalized to that of the internal standard (tetracosane) to eliminate bias during sample preparation.

Isolation of Products and NMR Analysis. To identify the unexpected products, a previously developed metabolic engineering system was utilized. The plasmids pIRS and pGG-AgAS:D621A were transfected into *E. coli* C41 to obtain an efficient (+)-CPP producing strain. The pET32-IrK-SL3a:I523T/E633K construct was transfected into this strain to accumulate the target products. The recombinant cultures were grown in 400 mL of TB medium (pH 7.0), with appropriate antibiotics, in 1 L flasks. These cultures were grown at 37 ℃ until $OD_{600}$ reached 0.5 - 1.0. The temperature was then dropped to 20 ℃ for 0.5 h prior to induction with 1 mmol/L IPTG, followed by supplementation with 40 mmol/L pyruvate and 1 mmol/L $MgCl_2$. The induced cultures were grown for an additional 72 h. In order to isolate sufficient amounts of the target products, 10 L of induced cultures were collected. These cultures were concentrated to 1 L before breaking up by a high-pressure homogenizer (ATS Engineering). Then these cultures were extracted with an equal volume of hexanes 10 - 15 times. The organic phases were concentrated by a rotary evaporation apparatus, and then the compounds were purified by preparative liquid chromatography. For chemical structure characterization, $^1$H NMR (600 MHz), $^{13}$C NMR (100 MHz), and two-dimensional (2D) NMR spectra were collected on a Bruker DRX Avance - 600 (Bruker Co., Switzerland) NMR spectrometer for products **3** - **6**.

[靳保龙，崔光红，黄璐琦，等. ACS Catalysis，2024，14：2959 - 2970.]

# Versatile CYP98A enzymes catalyse *meta*-hydroxylation reveals diversity of salvianolic acids biosynthesis

## 1 INTRODUCTION

Salvianolic acids (SA), such as rosmarinic acid (RA), danshensu (DSS), and their derivative salvianolic acid B (SAB), widely existed in Lamiaceae and Boraginaceae families. In addition, it has been described sporadically presented in other species, including Apiaceae, Rubiaceae, Araliaceae, ferns, and hornworts. Due to multifaceted medicinal properties and potential for treating various diseases, SA has garnered particular attention. For instance, RA is known for its anti-oxidant and neuro-protective effects. STAT3 and NF-κB signalling pathways can be repressed by RA to play anti-inflammatory roles in many diseases' treatment. DSS has a series of pharmacological activities such as anti-oxidants, anti-inflammatory properties, anti-fibrotic effects, anti-myocardial ischemia properties, and improves cardiovascular function. Some derivatives of DSS have shown the potential to ameliorate acute liver injury and colitis. Moreover, RA and DSS are direct substrates of SAB; the most effective substances among water-soluble SA possess significant bioactivities, including anti-inflammatory, anti-apoptotic, and anti-fibrotic effects, and beneficial effects on cardiovascular and cerebrovascular diseases, which is driving global attention to SA biosynthesis elucidation.

Reported biosynthesis pathway of SA is nonlinear and diverging-converging, consisting of two parallel pathways derived from the phenylalanine and tyrosine pathways. The acyl donor of 4-coumaroyl-CoA (4C-CoA) from phenylpropanoid-derived pathway and 4-hydroxyphenyllactic acid (4-HPL) as the acyl acceptor from tyrosine-derived pathway are catalysed by rosmarinic acid synthase (RAS) to synthesize 4-coumaroyl-4′-hydroxyphenyllactic acid (4C - 4′- HPL). The CYP98A (Cytochrome P450 98A) family enzymes catalyse the hydroxylation at C - 3 or C - 3′ position of aromatic rings to yield RA and then catalysed by laccase family to biosynthesize SAB.

Among the SA biosynthesis pathway elucidation studies reported in many species, DSS has been recognized as a unique metabolic intermediate that only exists in *Salvia miltiorrhiza*. However, in our recent study, several acyl donors and acceptors included DSS as well as their ester-forming products like 4C-4′-HPL, 4-coumaroyl-3′, 4′-dihydroxyphenyllactic acid (4C-3′,4′-DHPL), and caffeoyl-4′-hydroxyphenyllatic acid (Ca-4′-HPL) all were determined in SA-rich plants extraction samples, which indicated previous recognition to SA biosynthesis is insufficient (Figure 1a, Figure S1). Roles of other acyl donors and acceptors as well as function of catalytic enzymes to patriciate SA biosynthesis have been ignored for a long time. The focus question on SA biosynthesis is whether different acyl donors and acceptors are connected by RAS to form several precursors of RA and then hydroxylated at C - 3 and C - 3′ of the aromatic ring by different CYP98A members. Furthermore, an enzyme that catalyses DSS biosynthesis from 4-HPL has not been elucidated in plants, and the RA structure containing the DSS scaffold provides insight into DSS generation. Based on CYP98A members can catalyse the hydroxylation of Ca-4′-HPL at C - 3′, this family of enzymes was speculated to be responsible for DSS generation.

CYP98A is an enzyme belonging to the cytochrome P450 family that catalyses the *meta*-hydroxylation of *p*-coumarate derivatives, an essential step in the entry of the lignin branch of the phenylpropanoid network. This *meta*-hydroxylation reaction usually involves the esterification of *p*-coumarate with quinic, shikimic, or phenyllactic acids. CYP98A family enzymes play a vital role in phenylpropanoid and lignin biosynthesis pathways, the function of which is not limited to the direct synthesis of caffeoyl ester derivatives but has a significant impact on plant growth and development. A previous study revealed that a complex evolutionary process occurred in the CYP98A family that acquired new functions involved in pollen development in plants. Other studies have demonstrated that CYP98A family members respond to small molecules such as salicylic acid derivatives and isonicotinic

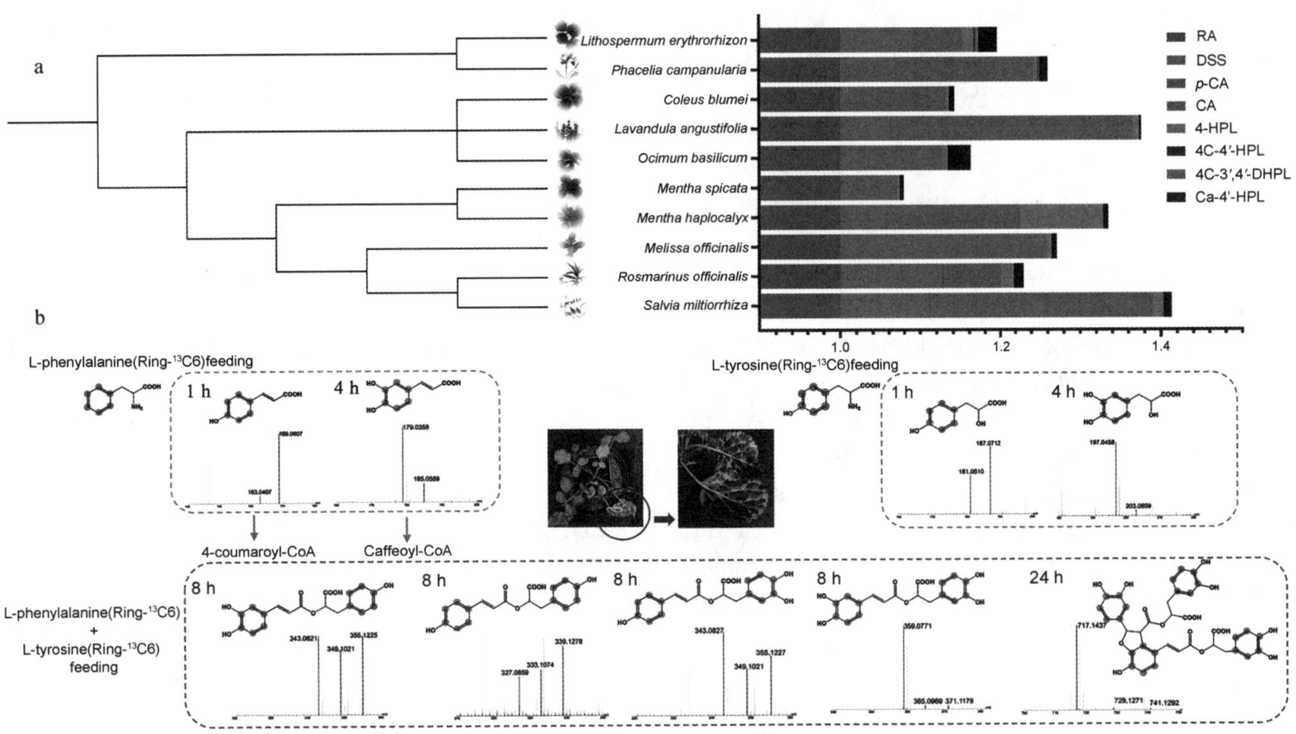


**Figure 1 SA are widely distributed in Lamiaceae as well as Boraginaceae plants and the biosynthesis pathway of SA was verified by isotope-labelled feeding studies**

(a) Different acyl donors and acceptors as well as their ester-forming products exist extensively in RA-abundant species. The content of SA determined by UHPLC-MS/MS in these plants was used for comparisons. The ratio of each component was proportional to the content of RA. The phylogenetic tree indicates the evolutionary relationship of representative Lamiaceae and Boraginaceae plants. DSS accumulation was higher in the clade including *Rosmarinus officinalis*, *Melissa officinalis*, and *S. miltiorrhiza*. (b) UPLC-Q-TOF/MS analysis of SA after feeding of isotope-labelled L-phenylalanine and L-tyrosine to 3-month-old *S. miltiorrhiza*. Exogenously fed isotope-labelled L-phenylalanine and L-tyrosine were successfully incorporated into different SA structures. Mass fragmentation spectra $[M-H]^-$ for SA are shown in blue line and isotope-labelled SA are shown in red lines.

acids, and the expression levels of the corresponding genes are highly increased after UV-C treatment, indicating that CYP98A enzymes might participate in plant abiotic responses.

For Lamiaceae and Boraginaceae plants, studies about CYP98A family enzymes concentrate on their catalytic characteristics in SA biosynthesis (Figure S2). Several CYP98 enzymes are involved in determining the substitution patterns of aromatic rings. Among Boraginaceae species, *Le*CYP98A6 catalyses the C-3 hydroxylation of 4C-4′-HPL to form Ca-4′-HPL in *Lithospermum erythrorhizon*. *Pc*CYP98A112 specifically catalyses C-3 hydroxylation, and *Pc*CYP98A113 catalyses C-3′ hydroxylation of the 4C-4′-HPL in *Phacelia campanularia* (desert bells). However, in representative Lamiaceae *Coleus blumei*, *Cb*CYP98A14 catalyses the hydroxylation of C-3 and C-3′ of 4C-4′-HPL to synthesize RA simultaneously. These reactions indicate different catalytic preferences for the CYP98A family in different species. As the final hydroxylase in RA generation, *Sm*CYP98A14 plays a significant role in RNA antisense experiments in *S. miltiorrhiza*, in which RA decreases dramatically in hairy roots after *Sm*CYP98A14 is repressed. Based on metabolic flow analysis, *Sm*CYP98A14 was speculated to hydroxylate the C-3 of 4C-3′,4′-DHPL to produce RA but lack enzyme catalytic evidence.

In recent years, researchers have synthesized SA in *Escherichia coli* and *Saccharomyces cerevisiae*, and several heterologous enzymes have been selected to reconstruct the SA pathway. For instance, 4-hydroxyphenylpyruvic acid (4-HPPA) is catalysed to 4-HPL by *D-LDH* from *Lactobacillus pentosus*, and 4-HPL is catalysed by 4-hydroxyphenylacetate 3-hydroxylase complex (*Echpa*BC) from *E. coli* to generate DSS. Due to the lack of comprehensive knowledge of key enzymes, only few plants enzymes have been applied in synthetic biology studies. With the development of synthetic biology and metabolic regulation methods to increase the yield of SA, it is essential to gain insight into the molecular mechanisms of SA biosynthesis and determine the function of CYP98A enzymes.

Here, after figuring out the distribution diversity of SA in different species, isotope-labelled feeding experiment showing different acyl donors and acceptors participate in SA biosynthesis. *S. miltiorrhiza*, an important medicinal plant rich in SA, used to explore the diversity of SA biosynthesis pathway and DSS formation mechanism, relying on *Sm*RAS and *Sm*CYP98A enzyme functional studies. Different acyl donors and acceptors were catalysed by *Sm*RAS to form precursors of RA. Two *Sm*CYP98A family members, *Sm*CYP98A14 and *Sm*CYP98A75, are responsible for the C-3 and C-3′ hydroxylation of these precursors to generate RA. *Sm*CYP98A75 preferentially catalyses C-3′ hydroxylation of Ca-4′-HPL, while *Sm*CYP98A14 preferentially catalyses C-3 hydroxylation of 4C-3′,4′-DHPL. Notably, *Sm*CYP98A75 is verified to participate in DSS generation. Simultaneous knockout of both enzymes using CRISPR/Cas9 editing technology resulted in a significant decrease in SA accumulation, and the overexpression of *Sm*CYP98A14 and *Sm*CYP98A75 increased the content of SA. Our study deepens the understanding of SA biosynthesis diversity in SA-abundant species and versatility of CYP98A enzymes catalytic preference in *meta*-hydroxylation reactions. Moreover, CYP98A enzymes are ideal metabolic engineering targets to elevate SA content.

## 2 MATERIALS AND METHODS

Plant materials and growth conditions The *S. miltiorrhiza* cultivar used in this study was '*S. miltiorrhiza* f. alba'; it has stable RA and SAB contents and was gifted from the Institute of Botany, the Chinese Academy of Science.

Chemicals 4C-4′-HPL, 4C-3′,4′-DHPL, Ca-4′-HPL, *p*-coumaroyl shikimic acid (*p*CSA), *p*-coumaroyl quinate (*p*CQ), caffeoyl shikimic acid (CSA), and chlorogenic acid (CGA) were purchased from DeSiTe Biological Technology Co., Ltd (China, Chengdu). DSS, 4-HPL, 4-HPPA, 4-coumaric acid (*p*CA), caffeic acid (CA), RA, and SAB were purchased from Macklin Biochemical Technology Co. Ltd. L-phenylalanine (Ring-$^{13}$C6) and L-tyrosine (Ring-$^{13}$C6) were purchased from Cambridge Isotope Laboratories, Inc.

Metabolomic profiling and enzyme catalytic assays analysis The products of the catalytic reaction and the extracts of the different plant species samples were analysed using an ACQUITY UPLC system coupled to a Xevo G2-XS QToF mass spectrometer (Waters), which was equipped with an electrospray ionization source. The conditions for the UPLC-Q-TOF/MS analysis were set as previously described. Mass-to-charge ratio (m/z) values are listed in Table S2.

The content of SA in *S. miltiorrhiza*, other Lamiaceae and Boraginaceae plants, and the kinetic parameters of CYP98A enzymes were determined using high-performance liquid chromatography-tandem mass spectrometry (UHPLC-MS/MS) analysis on an Agilent 1 200-6 460 LC/MS. The conditions for the UHPLC-MS/MS analysis were set as previously described. Quantitation was performed in multiple-reaction monitoring (MRM) mode, the MRM parameters are listed in Table S3.

Feeding experiment For feeding experiment in *S. miltiorrhiza*, L-phenylalanine (Ring-$^{13}$C6) and L-tyrosine (Ring-$^{13}$C6) were dissolved to 1 mmol/L. The solution was infiltrated into 2-3 months old *S. miltiorrhiza* leaves. Infiltrated leaves were harvested at 1, 2, 3, 6, 8, 12 and 24 h after infiltration. For feeding experiment in Lamiaceae and Boraginaceae plants used in this study, cut-stem plants were placed into a glass bottle and then supplied with stable isotope-labelled L-phenylalanine and L-tyrosine solution (0.5 mmol/L). Leaves and roots of each plant were collected after two weeks, and metabolites were extracted and determined using UPLC-Q-TOF/MS.

Sequence and phylogenetic analysis of *Sm*CYP98A genes The amino acid sequences of CYP98A enzymes from different species, including *Sm*CYP98A75 (AJD25229), *Sm*CYP98A76 (AJD25230), *Sm*CYP98A77 (AJD25231), and *Sm*CYP98A14 (also termed *Sm*CYP98A78, ADP00279), were obtained from the *S. miltiorrhiza* genome database (PRJNA682867) and were subjected to sequence alignment analysis using the ClustalX2 software. To analyse the phylogenetic relationships of CYP98A family enzymes, neighbour-joining (NJ) trees were constructed using the MEGA X software with the following parameters: at least 1 000 bootstrap replications, Poisson model, uniform rates, and complete deletion.

*Sm*CYP98A enzymes cloning and quantitative analysis in different organs To obtain the real sequences of *Sm*CYP98A, total RNA mixtures from different *S. miltiorrhiza* roots, stems, leaves, and flowers were extracted using the EasyPure Plant RNA Kit (Transgen, China) following the manufacturer's protocol. Reverse transcription reactions were performed with TransScript One-Step RT-PCR SuperMix Kit (Transgen) using 1 μg of total RNA with an oligo-dT primer at 45 ℃ for 30 min. Next, 1 μL of cDNA was used as a template to amplify *SmCYP98A75*, *SmCYP98A76*, *SmCYP98A77*, and *SmCYP98A14* genes using the primers listed in Table S1. Quantitative real-time (qRT)-PCR was performed on a ROCHE LightCycler96 instrument using TransStart Top Green qPCR SuperMix (Transgen) to detect the expression levels of these four enzymes in different organs using the primers listed in Table S1. The relative expression levels were calculated by using the $2^{-\Delta\Delta Ct}$ method.

Recombinant *Sm*RAS enzyme expression in *E. coli* and purification *SmRAS* were cloned into *Bam*H1 and *Not*I restriction sites of pGEX-4T-1 vector and transformed into the *E. coli* BL21(DE3) strain. The strain was grown in LB medium at 37 ℃ as above to an $OD_{600}$ of 0.4-0.8, followed by induction of expression with 0.5 mmol/L IPTG at 16 ℃ and 80 rpm for 14 h. The cells were harvested by centrifugation (5 000 ***g***, 15 min), suspended in PBS buffer, and lysed at 4 ℃ with an ultra-high pressure continuous flow cell disrupter (JNBIO, Guangzhou, China). Lysate was clarified by centrifugation at 15 000×***g*** for 30 min at 4 ℃ and affinity-purified immediately with protein purification column. The GSTrap HP (GE Healthcare Life Science) glutathione Stransferase tagged protein column was used for *Sm*RAS purification. The affinity purification was proceeded on AKTA Pure FPLC (GE Healthcare Life Science). The purified proteins were concentrated to 500 μL using 50 kDa Amicon Ultra-15 centrifugal filter units with Ultracel-10 membrane (Millipore) and concentrations of protein were determined photometrically according to the method of Bradford with bovine serum albumin as the standard.

Recombinant *Sm*CYP98A enzymes expression in *S. cerevisiae* and purification *Sm*CYP98A75, *Sm*CYP98A76, *Sm*CYP98A77, and *Sm*CYP98A14 were cloned into *Eco*RI and *Bam*HI restriction sites of the pYEDP60 vector. The constructed expression vectors were then transformed into *S. cerevisiae* WAT11 cells. Each strain was grown at 30 ℃ in YPGE medium (10 g/L yeast extract, 10 g/L peptone, 5 g/L glucose, and 3% (v/v) ethanol) to $OD_{600}$ of 2.7 and then added 20 g/L galactose to induce expression till to $OD_{600}$ of 4.0. Cells were harvested by centrifugation (2 000 × **g**, 5 min), suspended in TEK buffer (0.1 mol/L KCl, 50 mmol/L Tris-HCl, 1 mmol/L EDTA), and incubated for 5 min. Cells were resuspended using TESB buffer (0.6 mol/L sorbitol, 50 mmol/L Tris-HCl, 1 mmol/L EDTA) and lysed at 4 ℃ with an ultra-high pressure continuous flow cell disrupter. PEG4000-NaCl solution was added to the supernatant, and the mixture was agitated slightly for 15 min at 4 ℃ before centrifugation at 12 000 × **g** for 30 min. The pellet was resuspended in TEG buffer (50 mmol/L Tris-HCl, 1 mmol/L EDTA, 10% (v/v) glycerol) and stored at −80 ℃.

Determination of characteristics of recombinant *Sm*RAS and *Sm*CYP98A enzymes To identify the products of acyl-CoA donors and acceptors catalysed by *Sm*RAS, 2 mmol/L 4-HPL or DSS was added to 4C-CoA or Ca-CoA with 2 nmol *Sm*RAS.

The standard system for *Sm*CYP98A enzyme catalytic reaction was a 100 μL reaction containing 1 mol/L DTT, 1 mol/L glucose-6-phosphate, 1 U glucose-6-phosphate dehydrogenase, 1 mmol/L flavin adenine dinucleotide (FAD), 1 mmol/L flavin mononucleotide (FMN), and 0.5 mol/L NADPH. Hundred microlitres of thawed microsomes was added to 1 mmol/L substrate of 4C-4′-HPL, 4C-3′,4′-DHPL, Ca-4′-HPL, *p*CQ, and *p*CSA to start the reaction. The reaction was incubated at room temperature for 30 min and quenched by the addition of 10 μL 10 mol/L acetic acid. The reaction products were extracted three times with ethyl acetate and evaporated under a vacuum. The residues were redissolved in 500 μL MeOH-0.1% acetic acid (1 : 1) and subjected to UPLC-Q-TOF/MS analysis.

Kinetic parameters of *Sm*CYP98A enzymes were determined in a total volume of 200 μL of 0.1 mol/L pH 7.5 Tris/HCl buffer. The reaction system contained 1 mol/L DTT, 1 mol/L glucose-6-phosphate, 1 U glucose-6-phosphate dehydrogenase, 1 mmol/L FAD, 1 mmol/L FMN, and 0.5 mol/L NADPH. Assays were routinely incubated at 30 ℃ for 5 min with shaking at 1 000 rpm and stopped by addition of 500 μL ethyl acetate and cooling on ice. Proteins were quantified according to the method of Bradford using bovine serum albumin as the standard.

Subcellular localization analysis *Sm*CYP98A75 and *Sm*CYP98A14 were cloned into the pEAQ-GFP vector using *Xho*I and *Age*I restriction sites to construct in-frame C-terminal GFP fusion proteins using the primers listed in Table S1. *At*ROP10 (NM_114673), which is located in the cytomembrane and *At*RIP1 (NM_112362.4), which is located in the mitochondria, were selected as organelle markers. The constructed vectors were transformed into GV3101. *A. tumefaciens* strains are grown in kanamycin-resistant YEB medium (50 mg/L kanamycin, 5 g/L beef extract, 1 g/L yeast extract, 5 g/L peptone, 5 g/L sucrose, and 4 g/L $MgSO_4 \cdot 7H_2O$) until the $OD_{600}$ reached 0.6. The cells were harvested and resuspended in infiltration buffer (10 mmol/L $MgCl_2$, 10 mmol/L MES, and 200 μmol/L acetosyringone) and incubated for an additional 2 h in the dark at room temperature. Strains containing the target plasmids were infiltrated into the leaves of 6-week-old *Nicotiana benthamiana*. Leaves near the injection site were cut into small pieces and observed using a Leica TCS SP5 laser confocal scanning microscope (Leica Microsystems, Germany) at an excitation wavelength of 488 nm and an emission wavelength of 520-548 nm.

Generation of *Sm*CYP98A overexpression and editing of *S. miltiorrhiza* hairy roots For *Sm*CYP98A75 and *Sm*CYP98A14 single or dual CRISPR/Cas9 editing vector construction, sgRNAs for the two enzymes were designed based on CHOPCHOP online tools. A pair of oligos was synthesized and annealed to form a 20 bp DNA fragment. For single-target editing vector construction, the sgRNAs of *Sm*CYP98A75 and *Sm*CYP98A14 were cloned into the intermediate construct psgR-Cas9-At (gifted by Jiankang Zhu lab) using *Bbs*I restriction sites, respectively. For dual-target-editing vector construction, the cassette containing *At*U6 and the sgRNA of *Sm*CYP98A75 was amplified with *Kpn*I and *EcoR*I restriction sites and subcloned into the constructed *Sm*CYP98A14-psgR-Cas9-At vector. Finally, the intermediate CRISPR/Cas9 vectors were subcloned into *pCAMBIA*1 300 plant expression vector for transformation. To overexpress *Sm*CYP98A75 or *Sm*CYP98A14 genes, the full-length *Sm*CYP98A75 or *Sm*CYP98A14 was constructed into a binary PHB-myc vector driven by a 35S promoter to construct OE-*Sm*CYP98A75 and OE-*Sm*CYP98A14 overexpression vectors using homologous recombination, respectively. All primers used in the constructed vector are listed in Table S1.

After verifying the resulting constructs, the constructed CRISPR/Cas9 vector and overexpression vector were transferred into *A. tumefaciens* strain C58C1. Transgenic hairy roots were obtained using the leaf-disc method. Explants of *S. miltiorrhiza* leaves were infected with the engineered C58C1 strains and placed on 1/2 MS solid medium in the dark for 2 days. The explants were then transferred to 1/2 MS solid medium supplemented with 250 mg/mL cephalosporin and transferred to gradually decreasing concentrations (200 mg/mL and 150 mg/mL) of cephalosporin every 2 weeks. DNA from monoclonal hairy roots was extracted, and the *rol*B and *HPT* genes were amplified using specific primers to identify positive lines. Positive hairy roots were cultured in shaker flasks for propagation. CRISPR/Cas9 transgenic hairy roots were genotyped by Sanger sequencing of gene-specific PCR products amplified using the primers listed in Table S1.

Reconstitution of the RA pathway in *N. benthamiana* Full-length cDNAs of *At*4CL, *At*HPPR, *Sm*RAS, *Sm*CYP98A75, and *Sm*CYP98A14 were cloned into pEAQ-HT and transformed into *A. tumefaciens* strain GV3101. *A. tumefaciens* harbouring the constructed vectors were grown overnight at 28 ℃ in YEB medium. The cells were collected by centrifugation, washed, and resuspended in infiltration buffer to $OD_{600}$ reached 0.4 and incubated for 2 h at room temperature. The solution was infiltrated into 4 - 5 -weeks-old *N. benthamiana* leaves. Infiltrated leaves were harvested at 4 days after infiltration and metabolites were extracted and analysed like catalytic reaction by UPLC - Q - TOF/MS analysis as described above.

Homology modelling The structural models were generated online using SWISS - MODEL (https://swissmodel.expasy.org) based on the crystal structure of *Sm*CYP76AH1 (PDB code: 5YLW for *Sm*CYP98A14 and *Sm*CYP98A75) from *S. miltiorrhiza* and cinnamate 4-hydroxylase (C4H1) from *Sorghum bicolor* (PDB code: 6VBY for *Cb*CYP98A14). The three-dimensional figures were visualized and analysed in the program PyMOL (http://www.pymol.org). CAVER (http://loschmidt.chemi.muni.cz/caver/) was used to explore the channels from active sites to protein surfaces.

Molecular docking The models for 4C - 4′- HPL, 4C - 3′,4′- DHPL, and Ca - 4′- HPL were drawn in ChemDraw 22.0 and generated in Chem3D. The three-dimensional structures of *Sm*CYP98A14, *Sm*CYP98A75, and *Cb*CYP98A14 were prepared using AutoDock Tools 1.5.7 and then were used in the AutoDock Vina calculation. The results were returned after calculation, and the appropriate conformers possessing a binding energy for *Sm*CYP98A14, *Sm*CYP98A75, and *Cb*CYP98A14 structures. The docked conformers were visualized and analysed in PyMOL.

Statistical analysis All enzyme catalytic experiments were repeated at least three times, and the results were analysed using GraphPad Prism. Unpaired *t*-tests and one-way analyses of variance (ANOVA) were used for statistical evaluation.

## 3 RESULTS

Feeding experiment to validate the biosynthesis pathway of SA in Lamiaceae and Boraginaceae plants Di *et al*. have elucidated the phenylalanine-derived pathway of *S. miltiorrhiza* using isotope-labelled L-phenylalanine. However, the tyrosine-derived pathway in *S. miltiorrhiza* has never been reported, and whether DSS participates in SA biosynthesis remains unknown. Additionally, different acyl donors and acceptors as well as their ester-forming products all occur in SA-rich plants, which suggests that SA biosynthesis is diverse and our hypothesis should be verified on the basis of isotope-labelled feeding experiments. The solution we used contained isotope-labelled L-phenylalanine and L-tyrosine, and was infiltrated into 3 months old *S. miltiorrhiza* leaves. SA were extracted from collected leaves at different points in time and analysed using UPLC - Q - TOF/MS. Moreover, other Lamiaceae and Boraginaceae stem-cut plants were placed into a glass bottle and then supplied with stable isotope-labelled L-phenylalanine and L-tyrosine solution (0.5 mmol/L) and including *C. blumei*, *Lavandula angustifolia*, *Mentha haplocalyx*, *Rosmarinus officinalis*, *Ocimum basilicum*, *L. erythrorhizon*, and *P. campanularia*.

Labelled and non-labelled SA were detected by monitoring $[M-H]^-$ ions with mass-to-charge ratio (m/z) values (Table S2). In *S. miltiorrhiza*-infiltrated leaves, labelled *p*-CA and CA were identified in the L-phenylalanine feeding group and labelled 4 - HPL as well as DSS were successively detected in the L-tyrosine feeding group. In addition, RA and its precursors, including 4C - 4′- HPL, 4C - 3′,4′- DHPL, and Ca - 4′- HPL, as well as SAB were all labelled in different feeding groups (Figure 1b). In other Lamiaceae and Boraginaceae plants feeding experiments, labelled *p*-CA, CA, 4 - HPL, DSS, 4C - 4′- HPL, 4C - 3′, 4′- DHPL, Ca - 4′- HPL, and RA were detected (Figure S3). These results verified our speculation that different acyl donors, including 4C-CoA and Ca-CoA and acyl acceptors containing 4-HPL and DSS are involved in SA formation. The SA biosynthesis pathway is diverse and various.

Characteristics of *Sm*CYP98A enzymes in *S. miltiorrhiza* Four enzymes belonging to the *Sm*CYP98A subfamily were identified from the genome database of *S. miltiorrhiza*. Based on specific primers directed against putative *Sm*CYP98A enzymes, these four enzymes were cloned. The open reading frame nucleotide lengths of *SmCYP98A75*, *SmCYP98A76*, *SmCY P98A77*, and *SmCYP98A14*

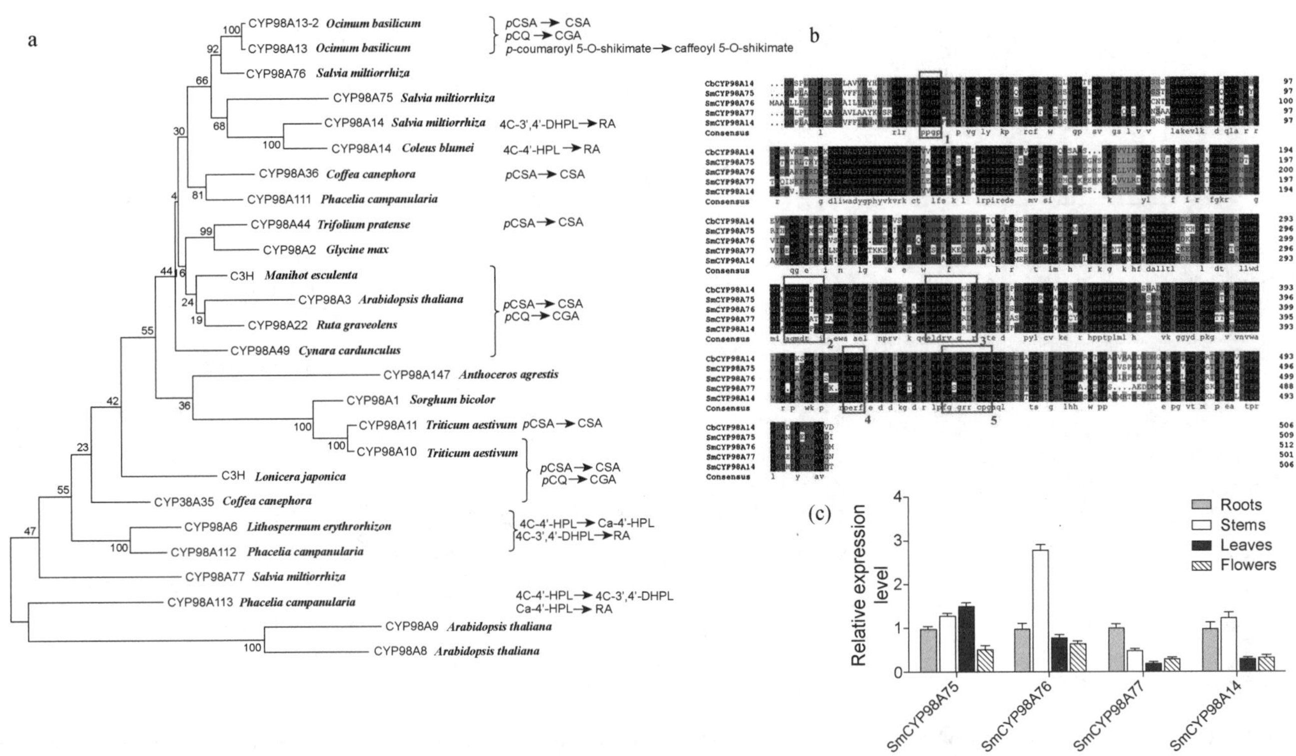


**Figure 2 Sequence analysis, expression pattern study, and phylogeny of *Sm*CYP98A enzyme with other function-known CYP98A members**

(a) Protein sequences used in the analysis include CYP98A enzymes from *S. miltiorrhiza*, *Arabidopsis thaliana* (OAP09214.1/*At*CYP98A3, OAP19075.1/*At*CYP98A8 and OAP16063.1/*At*CYP98A9), *Coffea canephora* *p*-coumaroyl 3′-hydroxylase (ABB83676.1/*Cc*CYP98A35, ABB83677.1/*Cc*CYP98A36), *Cynara cardunculus* *p*-coumaroyl ester 3′-hydroxylase (ACO25188.1/*Cc*CYP98A49), *L. erythrorhizon* (BAC44836.1/*Le*CYP98A6), *p*-coumaroyl ester 3′-hydroxylase (AGQ48118.1/*Lj*C3H), *Manihot esculenta* *p*-coumaroyl shikimate/quinate 3′-hydroxylase (UWV81047.1/*Me*C3H), *O. basilicum* *p*-coumaroyl shikimate 3′-hydroxylase (AAL99200.1/*Ob*CYP98A13-1, AAL99201.1/*Ob*CYP98A13-2), *Phacelia campanularia* (QDF44409.1/*Pc*CYP98A111/*p*-coumaroyl shikimate 3′-hydroxylase, QDF44410.1/*Pc*CYP98A112/4-coumaroyl-3-(3,4-dihydroxyphenyl) lactate 3′-hydroxylase, QDF44411.1/*Pc*CYP98A113/caffeoyl-3-(4-hydroxyphenyl)lactate 3-hydroxylase), *Ruta graveolens* (AEG19446.1, *Rg*CYP98A22), *Triticum aestivum* (CAE47489.1/*Ta*CYP98A10, CAE47490.1/*Ta*CYP98A11), *Trifolium pratense* p-coumaroyl-shikimate 3′-hydroxylase (ACV91106.1/*Tp*CYP98A44), *Glycine max* (NP_001235563.1/*Gm*CYP98A2), *Anthoceros agrestis* (MT119883/*Aa*CYP98A147) and *S. bicolor* (AAC39316.1/*Sb*CYP98A1). The NJ method was used to study the evolutionary history. The percentages of replicate trees in the bootstrap test (1 000 replicates) are shown next to the branches. The tree is drawn to scale, with branch lengths in the same units as those of the evolutionary distances used to construct the phylogenetic tree. The function of enzymes was listed on the right of NJ-tree. (b) Compared the amino acid sequences encoded by the four *Sm*CYP98As and *Cb*CYP98A14. Sequence alignments were performed with the ClustalW. Black boxes enclose amino acids that are identical in the four *Sm*CYP98As and are common with *Cb*CYP98A14. The P450-conserved domains are marked with red rectangles: (1): Proline-rich membrane hinge (PPGP), (2): I-helix involved in oxygen binding and activation (A/G-G-X-E/D-T-T/S), (3): ERR triade (E-X-X-R-R), (4): Clade signature (PERF), and (5): Heme-binding region (F-X-X-G-X-F-X-C-X-G). (c) Expression level of four identified *Sm*CYP98A enzymes in *S. miltiorrhiza* roots, stems, leaves, and flowers.

were 1 527, 1 536, 1 524, and 1 524 bp, respectively. The four *Sm*CYP98A enzyme genes are distributed unevenly among the 3 Lachesis groups of *S. miltiorrhiza* genome. *SmCYP98A75* and *SmCYP98A14* were located in the same cluster in Lachesis group 7, which indicated *SmCYP98A75* and *SmCYP98A14* may have functional relevance (Figure S4).

*Sm*CYP98A family enzymes catalyse the *meta*-hydroxylation of hydroxycinnamic acid ester to form RA, indicating that they belong to the family of 4-coumaroyl ester 3-hydroxylase (C3H). The amino acid sequences of C3H from different species were used to construct NJ trees using the MEGA X program to analyse the phylogenetic relationship between *Sm*CYP98A enzymes and C3H (Figure 2a). The results suggested that *Sm*CYP98A75 shares more significant sequence homology with *Sm*CYP98A14 and *Cb*CYP98A14. Two other CYP98A members from *S. miltiorrhiza* (*Sm*CYP98A76 and *Sm*CYP98A77) constituted different clusters; *Sm*CYP98A76 shows high sequence similarity to *Ob*CYP98A13 of sweet basil (*O. basilicum*), which *meta* hydroxylates *p*CSA and *p*CQ into its caffeoyl derivative. However, *Sm*CYP98A77 shares a low sequence homology with other CYP98A members. The amino acid sequences of the four *Sm*CYP98A enzymes contained several characteristic motifs of P450 monooxygenases, such as the PERF motif, heme-binding cysteine motif, and threonine-containing binding pocket (Figure 2b).

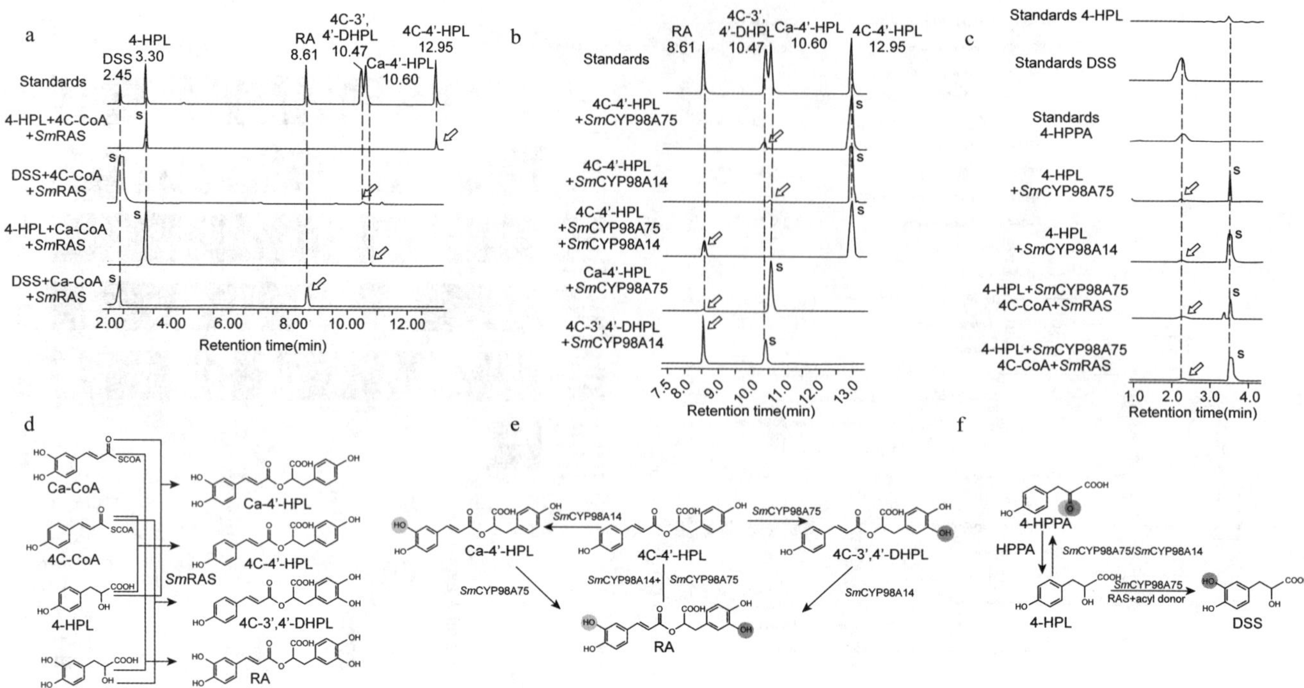


**Figure 3 UPLC-Q-TOF/MS profiles of *Sm*RAS and *Sm*CYP98A enzymes-catalysed reactions in SA biosynthesis. *Sm*RAS as well as yeast microsomes containing *Sm*CYP98A75 and *Sm*CYP98A14 were incubated with the substrates indicated**

(a) Reactions of recombinant *Sm*RAS enzyme assays using different acyl donors and acceptors as substrates. (b) Reactions of recombinant *Sm*CYP98A75 and *Sm*CYP98A14 enzymes assays using 4C-4'-HPL, 4C-3',4'-DHPL, Ca-4'-HPL as substrates. (c) Reactions of recombinant *Sm*CYP98A75 and *Sm*CYP98A14 enzymes assays using 4-HPL as substrates versus reaction system addition with *Sm*RAS and acyl donor participation. (d) Scheme showing the steps of acyl donors and acceptors ester-forming reactions *in vitro* by the recombinant *Sm*RAS. (e) Scheme showing the steps of RA and its precursors synthesized *in vitro* by the recombinant *Sm*CYP98A75 and *Sm*CYP98A14. (f) Scheme showing the steps of DSS and 4-HPPA synthesized *in vitro* by the recombinant *Sm*CYP98A75 and *Sm*CYP98A14. The blue circle indicated the catalytic position of *Sm*CYP98A75, and the red circle indicated the catalytic position of *Sm*CYP98A14. 'S' represented the substrate used in reactions and the bold arrow indicates the product of each catalysis assay.

To analyse the expression profiles of the four *Sm*CYP98A enzymes in *S. miltiorrhiza*, tissues from different organs, including roots, stems, leaves, and flowers, were collected. The results showed that both genes were expressed in all organs and that the expression level of *Sm*CYP98A75 was high in flowers and leaves; that of *Sm*CYP98A76 was high in stems; that of *Sm*CYP98A77 was high in flowers and leaves, and that of *Sm*CYP98A14 was high in roots (Figure 2c). SA is mainly accumulated in leaves and roots, and the high expression level of *Sm*CYP98A enzymes in these two organs indicates that they may participate in SA biosynthesis.

*Sm*RAS catalyse the precursors of RA formation Several acyl donors and acceptors as well as their ester-forming products such as 4C-4'-HPL, 4C-3',4'-DHPL, and Ca-4'-HPL were determined in SA-rich plants, which indicated that RAS may play a key role in forming RA and its precursors. Therefore, it is essential to verify the catalytic activities of *Sm*RAS in catalysing different acyl donors and acceptors.

The ORF of *SmRAS* was cloned into pGEX-4T-1 vector and heterologously expressed as GST fusion protein in *E. coli*. The cells were ruptured and the crude protein were purified by affinity chromatography. To test the substrate specificity, the *Sm*RAS was incubated with combinations of acyl-CoA donors (4C-CoA and Ca-CoA) and acyl acceptor substrates (4-HPL and DSS), which existed in the rosmarinic acid biosynthesis in *S. miltiorrhiza*. The reaction mixture was detected by UPLC-Q-TOF/MS to analyse the products. The result showed that *Sm*RAS catalysed the 4C-CoA and Ca-CoA with 4-HPL and DSS to form 4C-4'-HPL, 4C-3',4'-DHPL, Ca-4'-HPL, and RA (Figure 3a, d, Figure S5).

*Sm*CYP98A75 and *Sm*CYP98A14 participate in the biosynthesis of RA The coding sequences of *Sm*CYP98A75, *Sm*CYP98A76, *Sm*CYP98A77, and *Sm*CYP98A14 were ligated into the pYEDP60 vector and transformed into yeast WAT 11 strain co-expressed *At*CPR (NM_118585.4). Purified yeast microsomes containing recombinant P450s was used to conduct characterization assays against three substrates including 4C-4'-HPL, 4C-3',4'-DHPL and Ca-4'-HPL. The products were analysed using UPLC-Q-TOF/MS. The results showed *Sm*CYP98A75 could convert 4C-4'-HPL to 4C-3',4'-DHPL, and Ca-4'-HPL to RA, demonstrating that *Sm*CYP98A75 catalysed the C-3' hydroxylation of the acyl acceptor-derived phenolic ring. *Sm*CYP98A14 could catalyse 4C-4′-HPL to Ca-4′-HPL, 4C-3′,4′-DHPL to RA; however, it cannot directly convert 4C-4′-HPL into RA, indicating that *Sm*CYP98A14 catalyses C-3 hydroxylation of aromatic ring derived from acyl donor. Additionally, 4C-4′-HPL was catalysed to RA when *Sm*CYP98A75 and *Sm*CYP98A14 were present in the reaction system, suggesting that *Sm*CYP98A75 and *Sm*CYP98A14 participate in the biosynthesis of RA (Figure 3b, e, Figure S6a-e). Furthermore, *Sm*CYP98A76 and *Sm*CYP98A77 lacked activity in the aforementioned catalytic reactions. Negative control assays with boiled enzymes failed to produce enzymatic products from all substrates (Figure S6f); similarly, yeast microsomes harbouring the empty plasmid did not generate products.

Purified recombinant proteins were analysed to assess their substrate specificity and catalytic properties, which helped validate the enzymatic properties of CYP98A proteins. For kinetic analysis of CYP98A enzymes, 4C-3′,4′-DHPL, and Ca-4′-HPL were used as substrates in different concentration ranges (30-300 μmol/L). Purified enzyme (100 μg) was incubated in reaction mixtures as described above. Kinetic parameters were calculated by the accumulation of products in the Lineweaver-Burk plot. The kinetic properties of *Sm*CYP98A75, *Sm*CYP98A14, and *Cb*CYP98A14 were determined by analysing the linear range of the enzymatic reaction and are listed in Table S4. The results indicated that *Sm*CYP98A14 had an effect on the *meta*-hydroxylation of 4C-3′,4′-DHPL. The *K*m values of *Sm*CYP98A75 with Ca-4′-HPL and 4C-3′,4′-DHPL were 43.51 and 677.55 μmol/L, respectively, while the $K_{cat}$ values were 0.10 and 0.01 $min^{-1}$, respectively, which indicated that *Sm*CYP98A75 preferentially catalyses C-3′ hydroxylation of Ca-4′-HPL but hardly C-3 hydroxylation of 4C-3′,4′-DHPL. The catalytic characteristic of *Cb*CYP98A14 was similar to that of *Sm*CYP98A14.

Additionally, *Sm*CYP98A75, *Sm*CYP98A76, *Sm*CYP98A77, and *Sm*CYP98A14 were tested for their *meta*-hydroxylation ability of *p*CQ and *p*CSA. However, the four enzymes were unable to convert *p*CQ to CGA or catalyse *p*CSA to CSA (Figure S7).

*Sm*CYP98A75 participate in biosynthesis of DSS Based on the assays of *Sm*CYP98A75, which is responsible for C-3′ hydroxylation of the acyl acceptor moiety in RA biosynthesis, *Sm*CYP98A enzymes may play a significant role in DSS formation in *S. miltiorrhiza*. Therefore, *Sm*CYP98A proteins were further tested using 4-HPL as a substrate. When *Sm*CYP98A75 or *Sm*CYP98A14 were incubated with 4-HPL, 4-HPPA was detected in the product, demonstrating that the two enzymes exhibited the ability to directly oxidize the side chain hydroxyl group of 4-HPL to a ketone. However, DSS was not detected in either of the reaction systems. Considering that the real internal biosynthetic environment is complex and includes many metabolic fluxes and catalysing enzymes, acyl donors and *Sm*RAS were added to the reaction system to simulate DSS biosynthesis in *S. miltiorrhiza*. After incubation with *Sm*RAS and 4C-CoA or Ca-CoA, DSS was produced only in the reaction catalysed by *Sm*CYP98A75 (Figure 3c, f, Figure S8a-g). However, when *Sm*RAS, acyl donors, or *Sm*CYP98A75 were absent or altered, DSS formation was not observed in the reaction system (Figure S8h).

*In vivo* function of *Sm*CYP98A75 and *Sm*CYP98A14 in *S. miltiorrhiza* To further investigate the functions of *Sm*CYP98A75 and *Sm*CYP98A14 in SA biosynthesis, we generated *Sm*CYP98A75 and *Sm*CYP98A14 single and double mutants using CRISPR/Cas9 technology. Three homozygous lines were identified in each transgenic hairy root line and used to analyse SA accumulation (Figure 4a,b). Compared to the WT and empty vector lines, CRISPR/Cas9 editing lines showed lower SA accumulation. DSS, RA, and SAB levels were decreased in *SmCYP98A75* and *SmCYP98A14* mutant lines; the DSS content in *SmCYP98A75* knockout lines almost could not be detected. RA was reduced to 0.43 mg/g DW and 0.004 mg/g DW in line *CR-14 # 3* and line *CR-75/14 # 1* compared with 7.63 mg/g in the wild line. SAB was decreased to 2.32 mg/g DW and 2.31 mg/g DW in line *CR-14 # 1* and line *CR-75/14 # 2* compared with 3.45 mg/g in the WT line. Compared to *SmCYP98A75* or *SmCYP98A14* single mutant lines, double mutants of the enzymes resulted in lower SA content in transgenic hairy roots. The accumulation of DSS and RA was almost undetectable and SAB decreased by 34% compared with WT lines, indicating that both CYP98A members play significant roles in SA biosynthesis (Figure 4c-e). We detected the expression levels of key enzymes in the SA biosynthetic pathway, including *SmPAL*, *SmC4H*, *Sm4CL*, *SmTAT*, *SmHPPR*, and *SmRAS* in the edited hairy roots. The results showed that the transcript levels of *SmPAL*, *SmC4H*, *SmTAT*, and *SmRAS* were decreased dramatically in *SmCYP98A75* and *SmCYP98A14* single mutant lines and double mutant lines, compared with the levels in the empty vector (Figure S9a-c).

To further evaluate the functions of *Sm*CYP98A75 and *Sm*CYP98A14 in SA biosynthesis, *Sm*CYP98A75 or *Sm*CYP98A14 was overexpressed in transgenic hairy roots. The *A. rhizogenes* strain C58C1 containing *Sm*CYP98A75- or *Sm*CYP98A14- overexpressing plasmids with a Myc tag was used to generate two enzyme-overexpressing lines. Compared to the WT and empty vector lines, *Sm*CYP98A75 and *Sm*CYP98A14 overexpression lines showed higher SA accumulation. The contents of DSS, RA, and SAB increased

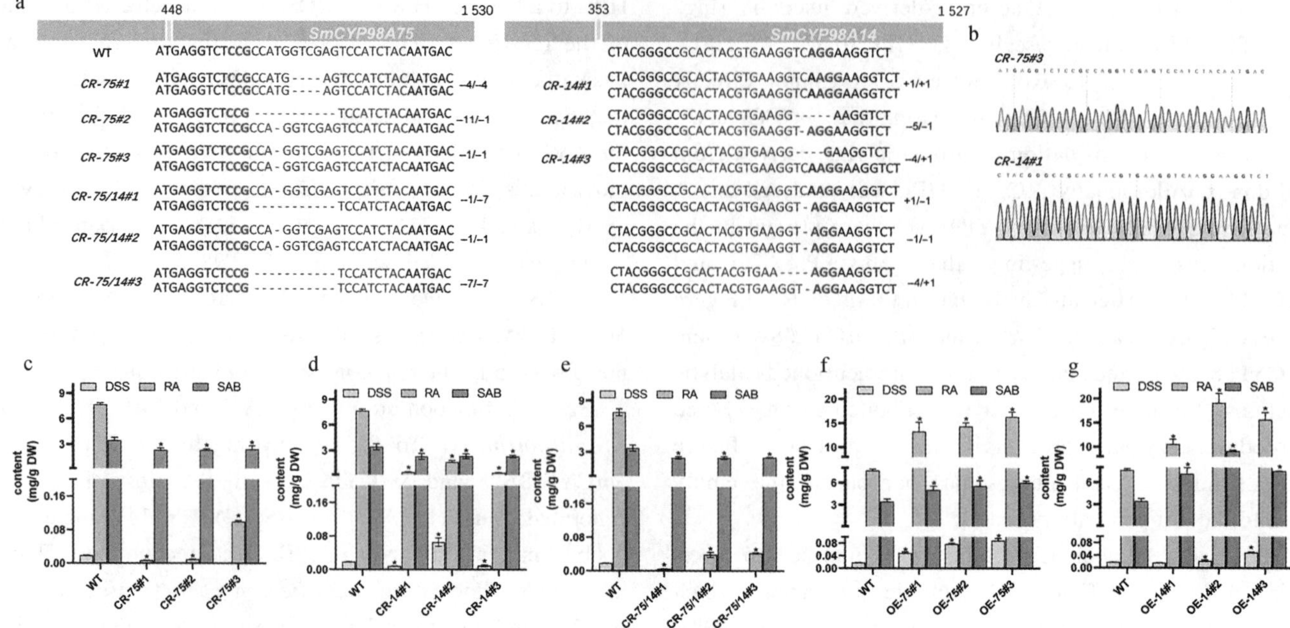


**Figure 4 Determination of SA from *Sm*CYP98A75 and *Sm*CYP98A14 knockout and overexpression transgenic hairy root**

(a) *Sm*CYP98A mutation introduced by CRISPR-Cas9 and schematic diagram showing the *Sm*CYP98A75 and *Sm*CYP98A14 structure as well as editing sites. Deletions are shown with dashed lines, and insertions are shown in purple colour. (b) CRISPR/Cas9-introduced *Sm*CYP98A75 and *Sm*CYP98A14 representative mutation chromatography, as determined by Sanger sequencing after PCR amplification. (c) The content of SA in *Sm*CYP98A75-knockout lines. (d) The content of SA in *Sm*CYP98A75-knockout lines. (e) The content of SA in *Sm*CYP98A75 and *Sm*CYP98A14 in dual-targets mutant lines. (f) The content of SA in *Sm*CYP98A75 overexpression lines. *Sm*CYP98A14 overexpression lines. (g) The content of SA in *Sm*CYP98A14 overexpression lines. Data are presented as means ± SD of three biological replicates. Asterisk indicates a significant difference compared to the corresponding control lines with $^{*}P < 0.05$ (Student's *t*-test).

in *SmCYP98A75*- or *SmCYP98A14*-overexpressed lines, indicating that these enzymes could be metabolic regulation targets to increase SA content. The amount of DSS increased from 0.018 mg/g DW in the wild-type line to 0.077 and 0.049 mg/g in lines *75-OE#2* and *14-OE#3*, respectively. RA was increased to 16.33 mg/g DW and 19.14 mg/g DW in lines *75OE#3* and *14-OE#2* compared to 7.63 mg/g in the wild line. SAB was raised to 6.01 mg/g DW and 9.18 mg/g DW in lines *75-OE#3* and *14-OE#2* compared with 3.45 mg/g in the WT line (Figure 4f, g). Furthermore, the expression levels of *Sm*CYP98A75, *Sm*CYP98A14, and key enzymes in the SA biosynthesis pathway in overexpression lines were confirmed using RT-qPCR. The results showed that the transcript levels of *SmPAL*, *SmC4H*, *SmTAT*, and *SmRAS* were increased in *SmCYP98A75* overexpressed lines and *SmCYP98A14* overexpressed lines, compared to levels in WT lines (Figure S9d, e).

Subcellular localizations of *Sm*CYP98A75 and *Sm*CYP98A14 To study the localization patterns of *Sm*CYP98A75 and *Sm*CYP98A14 at the subcellular level, *Sm*CYP98A75-GFP and *Sm*CYP98A14-GFP fusion proteins were constructed and transiently expressed in leaves of *N. benthamiana* by infiltration. The results demonstrated that fluorescent signals of *Sm*CYP98A75-GFP and *Sm*CYP98A14-GFP fusion proteins were observed in the cytomembrane and mitochondria under light conditions, which was consistent with the CYP protein localization characteristics. Additionally, the localization pattern of *Cb*CYP98A14-GFP was in accordance with two *Sm*CYP98A enzymes (Figure S10).

*In vivo* reconstruction of the RA biosynthesis in *N. benthamiana* To verify the function of CYP98A enzymes in planta, *At*4CL, *At*HPPR, *Sm*RAS, *Sm*CYP98A75, and *Sm*CYP98A14 in pEAQ-HT vectors were inoculated into leaves of *N. benthamiana* to determine whether together they could reconstitute entire pathway to synthesis RA (Figure S11a). Compared with the control group infiltrated with pEAQ-GFP vector, there is clearly a novel peak identical to the RA standard, which indicated RA was heterologous and successful biosynthesis in *N. benthamiana* (Figure S11b, c).

Structural recognition in *Sm*CYP98A75 and *Sm*CYP98A14 Variations in *Sm*CYP98A75 and *Sm*CYP98A14 substrate specificities provided an opportunity to investigate the structural features involved in substrate recognition and metabolism. Homology modelling was performed using the online SWISS-MODEL server based on the crystal structure of *Sm*CYP76AH1 (PDB code: 5YLW) from *S. miltiorrhiza*. The overall structure models of *Sm*CYP98A75 and *Sm*CYP98A14

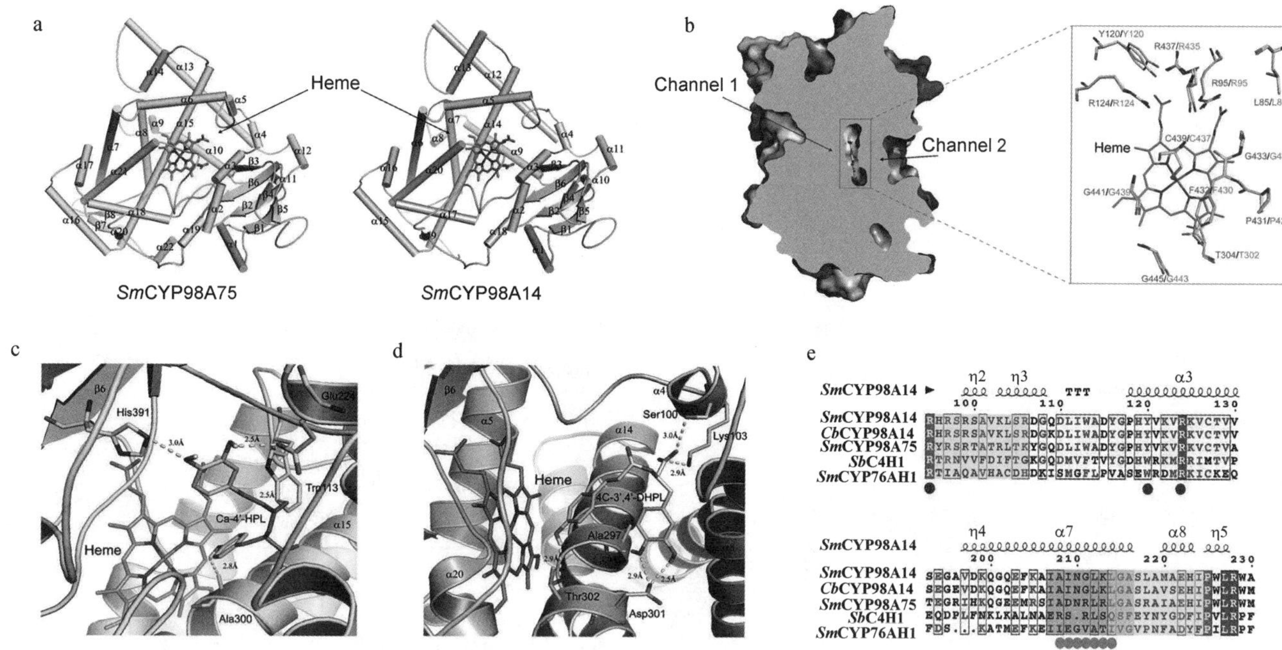


**Figure 5 Structural analysis of *Sm*CYP98A75 and *Sm*CYP98A14**

(a) Overall structure of *Sm*CYP98A75 and *Sm*CYP98A14. The cofactor Heme is shown as sticks in *Sm*CYP98A75 (aquamarine) and *Sm*CYP98A14 (wheat). (b) Channels in the structure of *Sm*CYP98A75 and *Sm*CYP98A14. The electrostatic surface of *Sm*CYP98A75 and *Sm*CYP98A14 and the two substrate channels are shown and labelled. Blue and red colours represent positive and negative charges, respectively. Red and blue arrows indicate the hypothetical channels for substrate and water, respectively. The residues binding to Heme are shown as sticks (*Sm*CYP98A75, aquamarine; *Sm*CYP98A14, wheat). (c) Interactions of Ca - 4′- HPL and *Sm*CYP98A75 in the active pocket. Yellow dashes indicate H-bonds, and the residues involved in interactions are shown as sticks and labelled. Heme is shown as sticks and coloured salmon. (d) Interactions of 4C - 3′, 4′- DHPL and *Sm*CYP98A14 in the active pocket. Heme was shown as sticks and coloured deep orange. (e) Two key motifs for substrate recognition. The substrate selection region is shaded in cyan, the substrate binding motif is shaded in green.

were highly similar. The R. M. S. D. value between *Sm*CYP98A75 and *Sm*CYP98A14 was 0.163, indicating that substrate recognition and metabolism of the two *Sm*CYP98As were conserved. The overall structure models of *Sm*CYP98A75 contained 22 α-helixes and 8 β-strands, and the overall structure models of *Sm*CYP98A14 contained 20 α-helixes and 6 β-strands (Figure 5a). The *Cb*CYP98A14 structure model contained 20 α-helixes and 6 β-strands, which were highly similar to those of *Sm*CYP98A14 (Figure S12a). The Heme molecule was observed to bind to the active pocket of two *Sm*CYP98As in the structure models. It was stabilized at the right place through multiple interactions with the residues inside the pocket. The Heme-surrounded motif and key catalytic amino acids of the two *Sm*CYP98As and *Cb*CYP98A14 were highly conserved (Figure 5b, Figure S12b). Based on superposition with known P450s, channel 1 might accommodate substrate access and product, and channel 2 was likely to enable water and proton access for the Heme.

The most significant recognition was that *Sm*CYP98A75 and *Sm*CYP98A14 catalyse C - 3′ and C - 3 hydroxylation of RA aromatic rings, respectively. In addition, DSS was only detected in the reaction system with *Sm*CYP98A75 rather than in that with *Sm*CYP98A14. To explore the underlying molecular mechanism for the selectivity of the two *Sm*CYP98As, molecular docking was performed. The Ca - 4′ - HPL molecule was observed to bind to the active pocket of *Sm*CYP98A75, with a binding energy of −8.4 kcal/mol. It was stabilized at the right place through multiple interactions with the key residues His391, Glu224, Trp113, and Ala300 in the pocket (Figure 5c). The 4C - 3′, 4′- DHPL molecule in the active pocket of *Sm*CYP98A14 with a binding energy of −7.5 kcal/mol and was stabilized by multiple interactions with the residues Asp301, Thr302, Ala297, Ser100, and Lys103 in the pocket (Figure 5d). The regions with key residues sited were highly conserved in the multiple sequence alignment of CYPs, which in turn suggested that these regions are relevant to substrate recognition (Figure 5e, Figure S13). Moreover, two key motifs that Glu224 (*Sm*CYP98A75), Ser100, and Lys103 (*Sm*CYP98A14) located were identified as substrate selection and binding regions (F/G loop in *Sb*C4H1). Interestingly, the residues of two key motifs in *Sm*CYP98A14 and *Cb*CYP98A14 were almost similar, which suggested that the two proteins might have the same substrate selection preference (Figure 5e). The 4C - 4′- HPL and 4C - 3′, 4′- DHPL molecules in the active pocket of *Sm*CYP98A14 with binding energies of

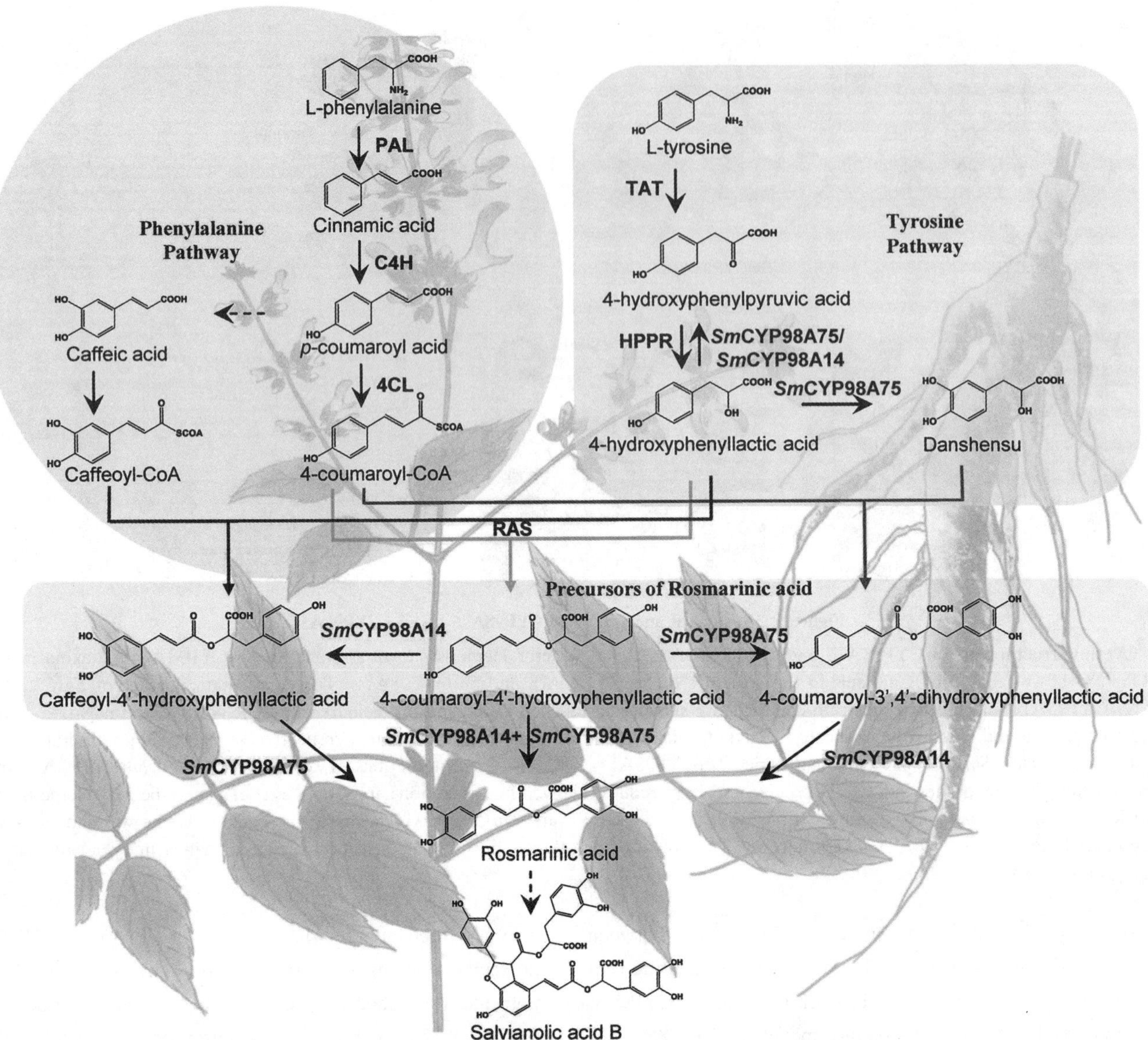


**Figure 6 The biosynthesis pathway of SA in *S. miltiorrhiza* verified in this study**

Different acyl donors from phenylalanine pathway as well as acyl acceptors from tyrosine pathway are synthesized by *Sm*RAS to generate precursors of RA. *Sm*CYP98A14 and *Sm*CYP98A75 catalyse the hydroxylation at C-3 or C-3′ of aromatic rings to yield RA. dash lines indicate the reaction has been characterized, but the enzyme has not been identified. 4CL, 4-coumaric acid coenzyme A ligase; HPPR, hydroxyphenylpyruvic acid reductase; PAL, L-phenylalanine ammonia-lyase; TAT, L-tyrosine aminotransferase.

−6.5 and −6.8 kcal/mol, were stabilized by multiple interactions with the residue Thr301, Ala297, Trp113, Ala101, etc. (Figure S12c,d).

## 4 DISCUSSION

SA show great potential in multiple food as well as medical industry applications, which is driving global attention to SA generation. The biosynthesis pathway of SA has been reported in several species, almost all studies considered that only one acyl donor and acceptor participate in SA formation. Our research highlights that various acyl donors and acceptors are involved in ester-forming reactions and CYP98A enzymes are responsible for different *meta*-hydroxylation in SA biosynthesis. Here, we take *S. miltiorrhiza* as an example, to elucidate the diversity of SA biosynthesis (Figure 6). Our study substantially deepens understanding of the SA even in phenolic acid biosynthesis pathway and enhances our capacity to overcome the synthetic biology challenges of engineering complex SA with diverse pharmacological activities.

RA biosynthesis is deverse and needs different CYP98A members' participation  According to previous studies, CYP98A family members participate in RA generation and catalyse two *meta*-hydroxylation steps to biosynthesize RA, but catalysis reactions are different in diverse species.

In *C. blumei*, *Cb*CYP98A14 was reported as a bifunctional enzyme capable of hydroxylating C-3 and C-3′ of 4C-4′-HPL; Based on previous experiment, *Cb*CYP98A14 catalyed 4C-3′,4′-DHPL, and Ca-4′-HPL to form RA. However, this finding has to be interpreted with caution due to the absence of well-grounded assays that employ 4C－4′－HPL as the substrate. In our study, we tested the activity of *Cb*CYP98A14 and calculated enzyme kinetic parameters with different substrates. The results showed that the catalytic characteristic of *Cb*CYP98A14 was similar to that of *Sm*CYP98A14, which is responsible for the *meta*-hydroxylation of 4C－3′,4′-DHPL. Molecular docking was used to simulate a pocket of *Cb*CYP98A14 with different precursors of RA, and docking results demonstrated that the key motif residues of *Cb*CYP98A14 were also similar to those of *Sm*CYP98A14. This suggested that the two enzymes might have identical substrate selection preference, which is in accordance with our *in vitro* enzyme assay. Combined with isotope-labelled feeding experiment, we speculate that other *Cb*CYP98A enzymes involved in SA biosynthesis in *C. blumei* exist.

For other representative Lamiaceae plants, *Sm*CYP98A14 has been the only *Sm*CYP98A family enzyme speculated to catalyse 4C－3′,4′－DHPL in *S. miltiorrhiza*, but *in vitro* enzyme assays are lacking. Our study verified that *Sm*CYP98A14 and *Sm*CYP98A75 both participate in SA biosynthesis and are responsible for *meta*-hydroxylation of different moieties to form RA.

In *P. campanularia* (Boraginaceae), *Pc*CYP98A112 and *Pc*CYP98A113 catalyse two *meta*-hydroxylation steps to generate RA. Therefore, the evolution of the SA biosynthesis pathway between Lamiaceae and Boraginaceae families only slightly varied based on the currently avaliable evidences.

Nevertheless, in our present study, we found the existence of two *Sm*CYP98A enzymes responsible for RA formation in *S. miltiorrhiza*. Three RA precursors all determined in the extraction of SA-rich species compared with isotope-labelled feeding assays showed that SA biosynthesis in both Lamiaceae and Boraginaceae species is diverse and involves different acyl donors and acceptors participation. This is the first study to resolve two regioselective P450s that catalyse two *meta*-hydroxylations in SA biosynthesis in Lamiaceae. We provide a reference for SA and phenolic acids metabolism studies in other Lamiaceae plants.

*Sm*CYP98A75 is the first characterized enzyme in the plant kingdom to participate in DSS biosynthesis DSS, effective in treating several diseases, has significant potential in the biomedical industry. Notably, the enzyme that catalyses DSS formation is still unknown, and no 3-hydroxylase using 4-HPL as substrate *in planta* has been reported. Based on our RA biosynthesis study, *Sm*CYP98A75 is responsible for C－3′ hydroxylation of the acyl acceptor moiety in RA biosynthesis, which indicates that the *Sm*CYP98A family may play a significant role in DSS formation in *S. miltiorrhiza*.

After identifying the respective full-length sequences of *Sm*CYP98A members, the first attempt of expression in *S. cerevisiae* was not successful; 4－HPPA rather than DSS was detected in the reaction system containing the active protein of *Sm*CYP98A75 or *Sm*CYP98A14, which indicated that *Sm*CYP98A75 and *Sm*CYP98A14 oxidize the hydroxyl group of the 4－HPL lateral chain to the ketone group. We speculated that DSS was not generated in the reaction system because DSS biosynthesis in *S. miltiorrhiza* is a biological process needing several enzymes. Therefore, *Sm*RAS and acyl donors, 4C－CoA and Ca-CoA, were attempted to added into assay system to simulate DSS biosynthesis in plants. The results demonstrated that when *Sm*RAS and acyl donors were present in the reaction, *Sm*CYP98A75 catalysed *meta*-hydroxylation of 4-HPL to generate DSS.

Our results suggested that *Sm*CYP98A75-mediated molecular oxygen activation catalyses 4-HPL generation via 4-HPPA or DSS. However, in the absence of an acyl donor, *Sm*CYP98A75 tends to oxidize the hydroxyl group of the 4-HPL lateral chain to a ketone group other than *meta*-hydroxylation of the benzene ring. When *Sm*RAS and acyl donors were present in the reaction system, which simulated the real environment of *S. miltiorrhiza*, the hydroxyl group of the 4-HPL lateral chain was inclined to esterify, and DSS was generated by *Sm*CYP98A75.

The direct introduction of a hydroxyl group into the aromatic C-H bond is challenging due to low reactivity of aromatic C－H bonds and product selectivity. *Sm*CYP98A75 catalyses *meta*-hydroxylation of 4－HPL and directly introduces hydroxyl groups into aromatic rings, giving light to similar ortho-benzene hydroxylation reactions.

Biotechnological application DSS and RA are representative SA in *S. miltiorrhiza* used in the food, cosmetic, and pharmaceutical industries. Currently, the production of RA and DSS is based on plant extraction under high temperatures and pressure or chemical synthesis methods (with undesirable by-product generation under harsh reaction conditions), which is an environmentally hazardous and expensive process. Therefore, an environmentally sustainable and economical DSS and RA biosynthesis solution must be considered. Synthetic biology offers a valuable tool for obtaining large amounts of SA. Identifying *Sm*CYP98A75 and *Sm*CYP98A14 helps refine and expand our knowledge of the SA biosynthesis pathway in *S. miltiorrhiza*, even in Lamiaceae and Boraginaceae plants.

[周正，张磊，陈万生，等. Plant Biotechnology Journal, 2024, DOI:10.1111/pbl.14284.]

# Enhanced precision and efficiency in metabolic regulation: compartmentalized metabolic engineering

## 1 INTRODUCTION

With advancements in technologies like cellular factories and metabolic engineering, the production of biofuels, commodity chemicals and natural products has become feasible with improved cost-effectiveness and efficiency by utilizing model strains or plant cell factories. Nonetheless, these approaches still face certain limitations, including cofactor imbalance, resource competition, toxic side effects resulting from product accumulation and the complexity of multi-enzyme catalysis. In such instances, the strategic implementation of cellular compartmentalization in bioproduction emerges as a pivotal approach.

In cellular systems, a considerable portion of metabolic pathways is confined to specific regions within the cell. Cellular compartmentalization serves as a mechanism employed by cells to regulate their cellular signaling, and metabolic processes in a spatial manner. Traditional cellular compartments are closed structures surrounded by monolayer or bilayer phospholipid membranes, mostly present in eukaryotic organisms. Various intercellular potential of hydrogen, cofactors and enzyme systems, etc. provide suitable metabolic sites for biosynthetic pathways. They are more mature compartments in terms of development and application. In recent years, with the development of bacterial microcompartments (BMCs) and membraneless organelles (MLOs), the new membraneless compartments formed by protein assemblies or phase separations have complemented the concept. These compartments provide possibility for precise metabolic regulation in prokaryotes that lack membrane systems. Inspired by this, compartmentalized metabolic engineering was developed to assign enzymes or intermediates, etc. involved in part or the whole metabolic pathway in metabolic engineering to appropriate compartments for more precise and efficient metabolism and production.

This review comprehensively summarizes the field of compartmentalized metabolic engineering. First, compartmentalized production can be achieved through strategies such as encapsulation of key enzymes, modulation of compartment morphology and copy factors, and multicompartment association. Different membranous compartments and emerging BMCs and MLOs provide options for precise and efficient production of different compounds in different hosts. Finally, the challenges and countermeasures of compartmentalized metabolic engineering are discussed and the prospects for development are outlined.

## 2 COMPARTMENTALIZED STRATEGIES

2.1 Encapsulating key enzymes  The most common strategy for compartmentalized metabolic engineering is to encapsulate key enzymes of specific pathways in targeted compartments for more precise and efficient production. This is mainly achieved through peptide-peptide interactions of proteins, using tools such as signal peptides (SPs), encapsulated peptides (EPs) and protein covalent coupling systems (Fig. 1A).

In eukaryotes, SPs are the most commonly used tools. The majority of SPs of the same type have a common amino acid sequence. Fusing the SPs to the N- or C-terminus of cargo proteins allows them to be recognized by the signal recognition particles of the corresponding compartments, thus enabling encapsulation. Currently, SPs targeting compartments such as the mitochondria, peroxisome and endoplasmic reticulum (ER) are employed as model tools for compartmentalization. In prokaryotes, the primary method for protein localization to bacterial microcompartments involves the use of EPs. EPs typically consist of 15 - 20 amino acids located at the C-terminus of BMC shell proteins. They interact with specific short helical regions present on the shell proteins. Homologous EPs that specifically target various types of microcompartments have been identified. Furthermore, novel molecular toolkits can be employed to generate functional and innocuous SPs and EPs de novo.

In addition, protein covalent tags have been widely employed for protein assembly, and the encapsulation of proteases in BMCs and the formation of multi-enzyme complexes in MLOs can be achieved through covalent peptide-peptide interactions of protein tags. The SnoopTag/SnoopCatcher system is not cross-reactive with the SpyTag/SpyCatcher system, and they can encapsulate multiple enzymes simultaneously. In particular, SpyTag and SnoopTag are incorporated into the BMC shells, while their corresponding structural domains (SpyCatcher and SnoopCatcher) are incorporated into the heterologous protein cargo. The interaction between the structural domains results in a covalent linkage between the proteins, which enables a more stable encapsulation, improves the reaction performance, and reduces the catalyst loading.

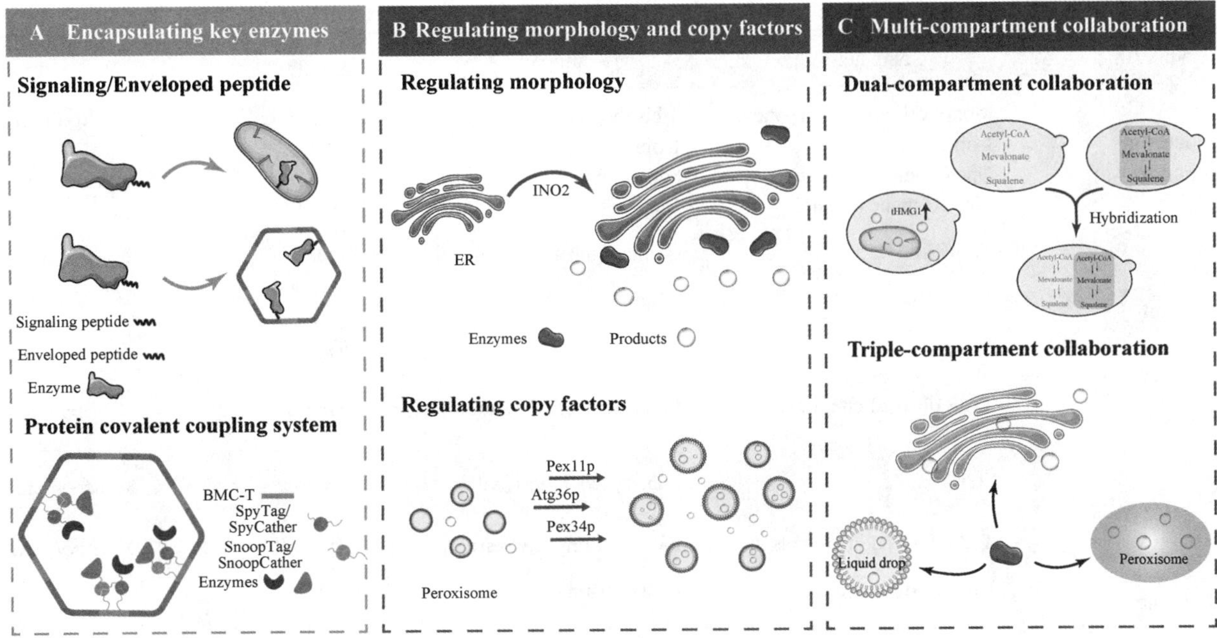


**Fig. 1 Compartmentalization strategies**

(A) Encapsulating key enzyme. The targeting of key enzymes to membranous compartments or BMCs can be achieved by fusion SPs or EPs. Protein covalent systems are attached to protein scaffolds and cargo proteins, respectively, and encapsulation can be achieved through covalent forces. (B) Regulate compartment morphology and replication factors by modulation of the corresponding genes. (C) Multi-compartment collaboration can be divided into dual-compartment collaboration and triple-compartment collaboration. Dual compartments can be achieved through overexpression of rate-limiting enzyme and yeast hybridization in the cytoplasm.

2.2 Regulating compartment morphology and copy factors The efficacy of compartmentalized metabolic engineering is intricately linked to the physiological state of cell compartments, which play a crucial role in determining their storage capacity and the catalytic efficiency of associated enzymes. Therefore, regulating the size and number of cellular compartments provides an effective strategy to enhance protein synthesis within compartments and alleviate metabolic constraints caused by limited enzyme abundance (Fig. 1B). Presently, the predominant strategy entails the precise regulation of genes accountable for organelle growth, development and dynamics.

ER plays a pivotal role as the site for protein synthesis, providing a dynamic and efficient environment for the folding of proteins destined for secretion and for a variety of cellular compartments and membranes. Spatial expansion of the ER by overexpression of the key ER size regulator INO2/ICE2 or knockdown of PAH1 encoding phosphatidic acid phosphatase or the lipid-regulated gene OPI1 enhances synthesis and folding of endoplasmic reticulum protein. Expression of the genes encoding peroxisome-population-regulated proteins (Pex11p, Pex34p) and autophagy-related protein (Atg36p) was genetically engineered to increase peroxisome copy factors and size. FLD1 (one of the FLD mutants) regulate the cellular dynamics of lipid droplets (LDs), and deletion of FLD1 in *Saccharomyces cerevisiae* (*S. cerevisiae*) increases lipid levels, LD clustering and expanded LD formation.

2.3 Multi-compartment collaboration Most metabolic pathways in eukaryotes typically span multiple subcellular compartments. The integration of multiple compartments, while ensuring separation from competing metabolic pathways, simultaneously allows for optimal utilization of cofactors and intermediates within each compartment and mitigates cytotoxicity due to the accumulation of excessive intermediates in the single compartment (Fig. 1C). Currently, the approach of multi-compartment collaborative production has been widely used to enhance in lipid and terpene production (Table 1).

For the compartmental co-production of terpenoids, the mevalonate (MVA) pathway is usually dual-regulated in the mitochondria or peroxisome and cytoplasm. This regulation alleviates the metabolic burden of a single compartment, thereby promoting healthy cell growth and efficient terpenoid production. As a rate-limiting enzyme in the MVA pathway, the catalytic product of truncated HMG1 (tHMG1), mevalonate, plays an important role in DNA synthesis and repair. Furthermore, the expression of the tHMG1 alleviates the metabolic stress induced by the toxic effects of the phosphorylated metabolites, mevalonate-5-P and mevalonate-5-PP, on mitochondria. Consequently, the overexpression of tHMG1 in the cytoplasm not only promotes cell growth but also significantly increases precursor supply and coordinates two independent MVA pathways, mitochondrial and cytoplasmic. In

**Table 1 Progress in Co-production of Compounds using Multiple Compartments**

| Compartment | Compound type | Compound | Output | Host |
|---|---|---|---|---|
| Mitochondrion Cytoplasm | Monocyclic sesquiterpenoid | α-bisabolene | ~ 1 058 mg/L | *Y. lipolytica* |
| | Isoprene | Isoprene | 2 527 mg/L | |
| | Open chain triterpene | Squalene | ~ 21 g/L | *S. cerevisiae* |
| | Monoterpene alcohol | Linalool | ~ 23 mg/L | |
| Peroxisome Cytoplasm | Terpenoid | Cannabigerol | 138 mg/L | *S. cerevisiae* |
| | | α-humulene | ~ 1 727 mg/L<br>~ 22 g/L | *Y. lipolytica* |
| | | α-farnesene | ~ 2.6 g/L | *P. pastoris* |
| ER peroxisome | TAG derived chemicals | Fatty acid ethyl esters | ~ 136 mg/L | *Y. lipolytica* |
| ER LD | Sterol | 7-Dehydrocholesterol | ~ 361 mg/L | *S. cerevisiae* |
| LD ER peroxisome | TAG derived chemicals | Fatty acid methyl esters | ~ 1 645 mg/L | *Y. lipolytica* |
| | Unsaturated terpenes | Astaxanthin | 858 mg/L | |
| Chloroplast nucleus Mitochondrion | Sesquiterpene lactones | Artemisinin | ~0.8 mg/g dry weight | *N. benthamiana* |

addition, hybrid strains have gained widespread recognition for their superior stress tolerance compared to haploid strains. Dual-engineered diploid strains obtained by crossing two single-compartment engineered haploids exhibited enhanced stress resistance and robust cell growth.

The strategy of three-compartment co-production has proven successful in the synthesis of lipophilic compounds, particularly triacylglycerol derivatives. ER serves as the primary site for synthesizing substances such as triacylglycerols (TAGs). Synthetic lipophilic derivatives, including TAGs, are primarily transported to LD storage, subsequently mobilized by lipase to convert fatty acids within the peroxisome, thereby initiating β-oxidation. The peroxisome functions as a hydrophobic chamber and also a storage site for lipophilic compounds. Consequently, the integration of the ER, LD and peroxisome enables the optimal utilization of precursors, facilitating the efficient synthesis of target lipophilic compounds. This novel approach represents an innovative strategy for biosynthesizing lipid-derived chemicals.

## 3 APPLICATIONS

3.1 Membranous compartment Membranous compartments are predominant in eukaryotes and feature phospholipid membranes. Eukaryotes exhibit conserved organelles, each offering a unique chemical and physical environment with specific metabolite, enzyme and cofactor compositions. These compartments provide conducive conditions for distinct metabolic pathways. Moreover, they serve as a temporary storage site for substrates and reduces the metabolic burden of cell growth. Therefore, membranous compartments are optimal sites for performing compartmentalized metabolic regulation.

To achieve optimal results in compartmentalized metabolic engineering, it is critical to select the appropriate target compartment for specific metabolic pathways and host cells. The potential adverse physiological conditions and limited availability of cofactors or pre-cursors have detrimental effects on enzyme activity. Mitochondria and peroxisomes, the most well-established compartments used in compartmentalized metabolic engineering, have been widely used for the production of various metabolites. In recent years, there has been a great deal of interest in LDs due to their storage properties and suitability for the production of lipophilic products. Furthermore, chloroplasts, which are unique cellular compartments exclusive to photosynthetic organisms, serve as effective platforms for the production of natural plant metabolites. Fig. 2 illustrates the detailed progress regarding the production of various types of metabolites by different membranous compartments.

3.1.1 Mitochondrion compartment Mitochondria are vital subcellular compartments in eukaryotic cells and have significant advantages in compartmentalized production, with high redox potentials, abundance of adenosine 5′-triphosphate (ATP) and acetoacetyl coenzyme A. Recent studies have demonstrated the potential of mitochondria for the production of terpenoids, organic acids and branched alcohols.

Targeting MVA pathway to mitochondria is a favorable method for the synthesis of terpenoids. The yield of terpenoid production can be effectively enhanced by increasing precursor utilization and availability. For instance, overexpression of

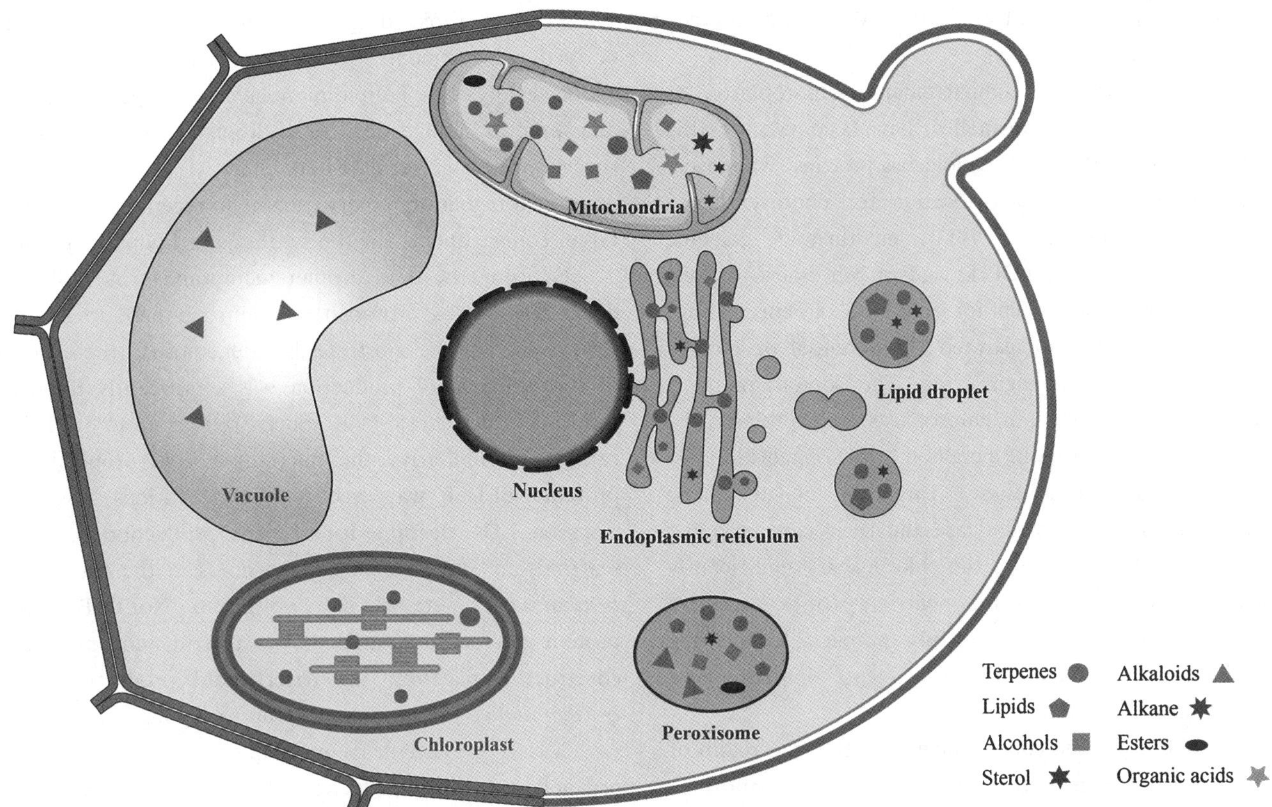


**Fig. 2 Cumulative advances in compartmentalized metabolic engineering within membranous compartments**

Mitochondria, ERs and peroxisomes are the most applied compartments and have been used for the production of terpenes, alcohols and esters, in addition to mitochondria for the production of organic acids and peroxisomes for the production of alkaloids. LDs are mostly used for the production of esters, sterols and other nonpolar substances. Chloroplasts are mainly used for the production of terpene-activated natural products and vesicles are used mainly for the production of alkaloids.

genes such as encoding acetoacetyl-CoA thiolase, mevalonate kinase, and tHMG1 in *S. cerevisiae* can promote the utilization of precursors by mitochondria to reach the highest value of eukaryotic engineered isoprene production (2 527 mg/L).

Fatty acid-derived chemicals, including fatty alcohols, alkanes and alkenes, can freely diffuse between subcellular compartments. Therefore, the de novo biosynthesis pathway of fatty acids and the β-oxidation pathway can be successfully transplanted into mitochondrial compartments. To overcome the limitations imposed by subcellular partitioning of isobutanol pathway enzymes in yeast, the isobutanol synthesis pathway was expressed in mitochondria by introducing cytoplasmic enzymes into the mitochondria. This modification led to a remarkable 260% increase in isobutanol production in *S. cerevisiae*. Mitochondria have also proven to be well-suited for 3-hydroxypropionate (3-HP) synthesis through the malonyl-CoA pathway, with a record-breaking 3-HP production of 71 g/L in *S. cerevisiae*. Furthermore, mitochondria serve as suitable compartments for the production of organic acids and organic acid salts. Targeting aconitase and *cis*-aconitate decarboxylase to the mitochondrial chambers of *Aspergillus niger* significantly resulted in a 14 – 24-fold increase in the production of itaconic acid. By manipulating the genes encoding mitochondrial carriers, improvements in Tricarboxylic acid cycle intermediates can be achieved. A citric acid titer of 97 g/L was achieved in *Yarrowia lipolytica* (*Y. lipolytica*) by identifying and characterizing citrate mitochondrial vectors.

3.1.2 Endoplasmic reticulum compartment ER expansion can lead to increased abundance of ER-associated enzymes and consequential improvement in metabolic capacity. The overexpression of INO2, the key regulator of ER size, resulted in a 71-fold increase in squalene production (634 mg/L) in *S. cerevisiae* by expanding the endoplasmic reticulum. The disruption of PAH1 resulted in a significant expansion of the ER, which resulted in an 8-, 6- and 16-fold increase in the accumulation of β-amyrin, its oxidized derivative pharmacophoric acid and its glucosylated version pharmacophoric-28-O-glucoside in *S. cerevisiae*.

ER is a key organelle for the synthesis of protein and acts as a central hub within the cell, connecting with various other membranous organelles. Recent studies have revealed that the ER can also interact and cooperate with MLOs. Besides the conventional secretory and translocon pathways, proteins can be transported in co-ordination with MLOs, such as ribonucleoprotein complexes. Furthermore, the ER serves as a platform for the formation of MLOs and is crucial in their division.

3.1.3 Chloroplast compartment Chloroplasts, as semi-autonomous genetic organelles, have become a versatile platform for the synthesis of heterologous proteins. Moreover, chloroplasts are the primary location for photosynthesis, promoting the synthesis of ATP, nicotinamide adenine dinucleotide phosphate (NADPH) and carbohydrates, making them an attractive compartment for plant metabolic engineering. Recent studies have demonstrated the potential of chloroplasts in plant metabolic engineering. The isoprene pathway was successfully reshaped in chloroplasts by expressing the MVA pathway, resulting in increased levels of mevalonate, carotenoids and artemisinin. Targeting of taxadiene synthase, taxadiene-5α-hydroxylase and their corresponding cytochrome P450 reductase to the chloroplasts, significantly reduced transmembrane spatial barriers for consecutive catalytic reactions. This successful approach led to the synthesis of taxadiene-5α-ol (0.9 μg/g) in *Nicotiana benthamiana* (*N. benthamiana*).

3.1.4 Peroxisome compartment Within the realm of cellular lipid metabolism, peroxisomes occupy a central role, serving as the principal locus for fatty acid β-oxidation. They represent suitable compartments for the production of biofuels like fatty alcohols, alkanes and olefins, as well as for the synthesis of biodegradable plastics such as polyhydroxybutyrate. Additionally, peroxisomes participate in the synthesis and removal of hydrogen peroxide, β-oxidation of fatty acids, and the generation of acetyl-CoA pools. The peroxisomal NADP-dependent isocitrate dehydrogenase isoenzyme maintains a redox state within the compartment by providing the essential substrate and cofactor NADPH for terpene biosynthesis. Furthermore, peroxisomes function as dynamic storage chambers for hydrophobic terpenes, making them a suitable choice for compartmentalized terpene production. Introducing the complete MVA pathway into peroxisomes facilitates the generation of geranyl pyrophosphate (GPP) and farnesyl pyrophosphate (FPP) pools, enabling the synthesis of a wide array of monoterpenes and sesquiterpenes. Moreover, peroxisomes play a crucial role as essential cellular compartments in penicillin-producing strains.

Peroxisomes are non-essential for cell growth and have minimal impact on cell state, making them suitable for accommodating exogenous pathways and alloenzymes that produce cytotoxic intermediates and products. Nortropic clathrate synthase (*NCS*) is a key rate-limiting enzyme in the benzylisoquinoline alkaloid biosynthetic pathway, and its cytoplasmic expression is toxic to *S. cerevisiae*. Efficient targeting of toxic *NCS* to peroxisomes through compartmentalization strategies can reduce *NCS* toxicity and enhance the (S)-reticular titer.

3.1.5 Lipid droplet compartmen LDs are ER-derived compartments consisting of neutral lipid aggregates surrounded by phospholipid monolayers and specific proteins, and serve as storage sites for hydrophobic substances such as triacylglycer-ols, sterol esters and terpenes. As newly developed regulatory compartments in recent years, they are target compartments for the synthesis of lipophilic products.

By using the lipid droplet membrane protein Pln1p to direct ER-located protopanaxsaponin synthase to LDs, the storage site for the substrate damalenediol-II, the efficiency of protopanaxadiol production was significantly improved, resulting in ginsenoside CK concentrations up to 5 g/L in *S. cerevisiae*. Similarly, the microalgal lipid droplet surface protein NoLDSP was used to anchor various biosynthetic steps on LDs, leading to efficient production of terpene scaffolds and functionalized terpenoids in the transient *N. benthamiana* system. The optimized NoLDSP scaffold protein can be retargeted to the plastid and employed to construct a platform for triterpenoid production in *N. benthamiana*, yielding squalene up to 0.6 mg/g FW.

3.1.6 Vacuole compartment As the largest organelles in mature cells, vacuoles store organic metabolites and participate in the transport or synthesis of various substances within cells, such as alkaloids and artemisinin. Consequently, vacuoles are potential compartments for the selective synthesis of compound.

Tropine alkaloids (TAs) extracted from *Solanaceae* are nerve conduction inhibitors used in the treatment of neuromuscular diseases. Protein engineering techniques demonstrated the vacuolar compartment expression of acyltransferases from the serine carboxypeptidase-like protein family of plant origin, leading to the successful biosynthesis of hyoscyamine and scopolamine in *S. cerevisiae*. However, the accumulation of the product is limited by vesicular transport. To increase TA production in engineered *S. cerevisiae*, the transporters *Atropa belladonna* purine uptake permease-like 1 and lactose permease-like 1 facilitate vacuolar export and cellular reuptake of littorine and hyoscyamine. Additionally, by targeting a heteromethyl halosylmethionase to *S. cerevisiae* vacuoles and utilizing the halide ion pool and the cofactor S-adenosylmethionine, the production of methyl iodide was increased by 1.5 times.

3.2 Membraneless compartment In contrast to traditional membranous organelles composed of phospholipid membranes, membraneless compartments are emerging which represent the most significant and promising cell compartments for the future. In this context, membraneless compartments are defined as "cellular compartments without phospholipid boundaries". These compartments primarily encompass protein-coated BMCs and MLOs formed via Liquid-liquid phase separation (LLPS), expanding the development of compartmentalized metabolic engineering.

3.2.1 Bacterial microcompartments In contrast to the phospholipid membrane of eukaryotic cells, BMCs represent prokaryotic organelles that consist of a protein shell acting as a semipermeable barrier. Various types of BMCs have been extensively studied, including carboxysomes involved in carbon dioxide ($CO_2$) fixation, as well as metabolic BMCs associated with the breakdown of compounds like 1, 2-propylene glycol (Pdu), ethanolamine (Eut) and choline. Engineering BMCs can be constructed to facilitate metabolic production by modifying the BMC shells and applying BMC recombination techniques. BMCs, in combination with programming, modeling and cargo encapsulation strategies, provide ideal compartments for re-engineering biological processes. By spatially organizing biosynthetic pathways and controlling the transport of small molecules between catalytic enzymes, BMCs can reduce metabolic crosstalk and facilitate compartmentalized metabolic engineering. This makes them highly promising for the production of small molecules.

3.2.1.1 Carboxysome. Carboxysomes, the first discovered anabolic BMCs, are important in photosynthetic carbon fixation and serve as fixation organelles in cyanobacteria and various chemoautotrophs. The intrinsically disordered protein CsoS2, which is highly conserved, has been demonstrated to serve as a hub that connects the shell to the cargo Rubisco in vitro. This facilitates the efficient formation of α-carboxysomes and provides the basis for the artificial construction of carboxysomes. By expressing genes encoding carboxysome proteins, large and complete carboxysome shells can be constructed in model microorganisms, which is an important reference value for prokaryotes to carry out partitioned biosynthesis.

Hydrogen-producing nanoreactor with catalytic functions was established in *Escherichia coli* (*E. coli*) by using the C-terminal of CsoS2 as the EP to encapsulate [FeFe]-hydrogenase (HydA) and its partner ferredoxin, as well as ferredoxin NADP-redox enzyme, in a self-assembled carboxysome. The encapsulation of the shell and the specific microenvironment within the reactor promote the enhancement of catalytic activity in HydA and exhibit notable tolerance towards the resulting catalyst, ultimately leading to improved hydrogen production. Moreover, carboxysomes have the broad applicability across different species. When the nine carboxysome genetic components from *Proteobacteria* were introduced into tobacco chloroplasts, chloroplast-expressed carboxysomes were produced with structural and functional integrity comparable to natural carboxysomes.

3.2.1.2 Metabolic bacterial microcompartments. The $B_{12}$-dependent Eut and Pdu metabolosomes from *Salmonella typhimurium* represent the most extensively studied metabolic BMCs. The catabolic pathway commences with the conversion of the compound to an aldehyde intermediate by a characterized enzyme. This highly reactive intermediate is activated or reduced to metabolites for ATP generation or cofactor recycling by enzymatic reactions. The toxic intermediate propionaldehyde can be isolated and its toxicity mitigated by its proteosome chelation. The local concentration of propionaldehyde can also be increased by chelation to enhance pathway flux, and effective enzyme concentrations and specialized cofactor libraries for multistep metabolic reactions can be maintained to improve reaction efficiency. Compositional and engineering models have been proposed for both metabolites. Heterologous enzymes and pathways can be successfully encapsulated in metabolizing BMCs and enable compartmentalized metabolic production of the products by EPs or protein-interacting systems.

Currently, Pdu BMCs are most commonly utilized for production purposes. On the one hand, they can be employed to construct bio-reactors for production. Pdu EPs were utilized to target glycerol dehydrogenase, dihydroxyacetone kinase, methylglyoxal synthase and 1,2-propanediol oxidoreductase to recombinant Pdu BMCs, thereby enhancing 1, 2-propanediol production in *E. coli*. A recombinant ethanol-producing bioreactor was constructed in *E. coli* using the EP P18 to require pyruvate decarboxylase and alcohol dehydrogenase for ethanol production and targeting and encapsulating them into the shell of Pdu BMCs. In contrast, Pdu BMCs can serve as storage compartments. Liang et al. targeted polyphosphate kinase to Pdu BMCs for the purpose of increasing polyphosphate formation and stabilizing the storage of polyphosphates within the cellular compartment. This has potential applications in removing biophosphates from wastewater.

3.2.1.3 Engineering bacterial microcompartments. In contrast to natural BMCs, engineered BMCs are more capable of being reliably, specifically and independently applied to prokaryotic compartmentalized produc-tion. They serve as the basis for future large-scale applications of BMCs. The structure and function of BMCs are inherently modular. A model of the basic structure of BMC shells from *Haliangium ochraceum* informs the rational design of engineered microcompartments. The structural redundancy of BMCs allows for the creation of channels for different metabolites to pass through the shells. Additionally, the use of different convex binding surfaces of different shell proteins enables the immobilization and spatial organization of encapsulated enzymes. This provides the foundation for the design of engineered BMCs and nanobioreactors, which offer an optimal platform for compartmentalized production of prokaryotes.

A multi-enzymatic and modular formate-oxidizing BMC was engineered in *E. coli*, paving the way for a new class of engineered BMCs for compound production. The engineered

BMC provides a well-defined environment with a private cofactor coenzyme A that efficiently cycles between encapsulated enzymes. The SpyTag/Spy-Catcher and SnoopTag/SnoopCatcher systems were employed to specifically covalently target two active key enzymes (pyruvate formate lyase and active phosphotransacetylase) to the inner protein shell for the production of pyruvate. Future research endeavors to develop self-assembled, catalytically programmable and genetically transferable BMCs, aiming to provide a versatile and convenient biological tool for compound production within BMCs.

3.2.2 Membraneless organelles MLOs represent a novel paradigm in cell compartmentalization. The spontaneous condensation and formation of LLPS of a number of macromolecules (disordered proteins and RNAs) is the basis for the MLOs formation in the cell. MLOs exhibit remarkable dynamics and fluidity, allowing for the exchange of components across their boundaries with the surrounding environment. Utilizing interaction-driven self-assembly within MLOs, a powerful tool for compartmentalized metabolic engineering can be developed, enabling the design of multi-enzyme biosynthesis systems. Different cargo proteins can be recruited into synthetic MLOs by fusing directly to disordered proteins or by co-operating with different protein interaction motifs, improving the efficiency of multi-enzyme biocatalysis. MLO-mediated multi-enzyme synthesis systems have the potential to increase metabolite yields. Co-assembly of the enzymes isopentenyl-diphosphate delta-isomerase (Idi) and α-far-nesyl diphosphate synthase (IspA), which are involved in the terpene biosynthesis pathway, into MLOs resulted in an increase in FPP titer more than 50% by employing the high-affinity peptide-peptide interaction pair RIAD-RIDD (Fig. 3A).

The choice of protein scaffolds is extremely important for the construction of MLOs, and the arginine/glycine-rich RGG structural domain (derived from the disordered P granule protein LAF-1) has been shown to serve as an ideal protein scaffold for the synthesis of MLOs. Building upon this work, modular MLOs for the production of α-farnesene were successfully engineered in *E. coli*. Furthermore, Wan et al. investigated the versatility of the RGG domain in mediating the formation of MLOs. By utilizing this domain, de novo biosynthesis of 2′-fucosyllactose (2′-FL) was achieved within MLOs (Fig. 3B). These studies highlight the high degree of versatility, tunability and programmability of MLOs, as well as the potential of modular design in synthesis pathways. They supply a novel approach for the biosynthesis of valuable chemicals using functional compartments in prokaryotic hosts.

In addition, MLOs offer the advantage of encapsulating intermediates, thereby protecting unstable molecules and

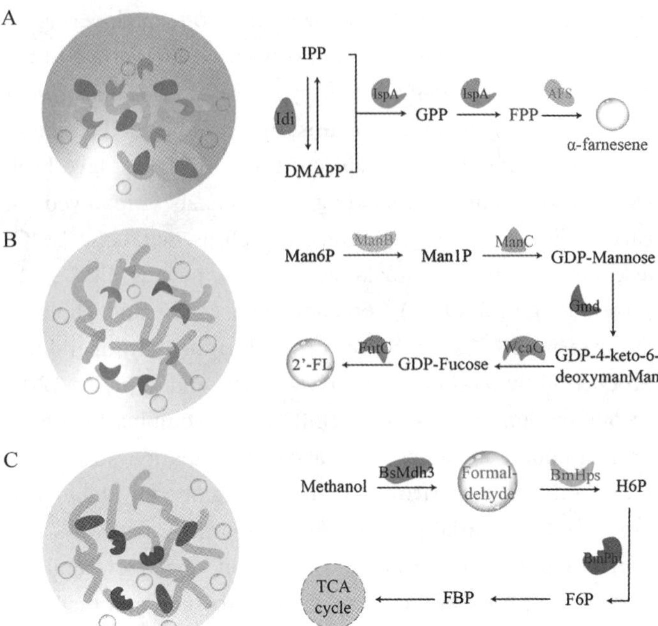


**Fig. 3 Application of MLOs**

(A) Production of FPP and α-farnesene. (B) Production of 2′-FL. (C) Encapsulation of harmful substance formaldehyde. Isopentenyl diphosphate, IPP; dimethylallyl pyrophosphate, DMAPP; mannose-6-phosphate, α-farnesene synthase, AFS; Man6P; phosphomannomutase, ManB; mannose 1-phosphate, Man1P; α-d-mannose-1-phosphate guanyltransferase, ManC; GDP-d-mannose-4, 6-dehydratase, Gmd; GDP-l-fucose synthetase, WcaG; fucosyltransferases, FutC; methanol dehydrogenase, BsMdh3; hexulose phosphate synthase, BmHps; 6-phospho-3-hexuloisomerase, BmPhi.

effectively isolating toxic metabolites. MLOs constructed in *S. cerevisiae* by artificial intrinsically disordered protein enhanced methanol assimilation by mitigating formaldehyde toxicity and increased n-butanol production by redirecting metabolic flux from oxidative to non-oxidative glycolysis (Fig. 3C). This provides a strategy for improving the efficiency synthesis of fine chemicals in *S. cerevisiae*.

## 4 ISSUES AND SOLUTIONS

While compartmentalized metabolic engineering has been progress, it still faces several challenges. These include metabolic burden, limitations in membraneless compartments, unclear subcellular localization of enzymes and restrictions in host selection. The feasible solutions to solve the related problems are proposed to further realize more precise and efficient metabolic production (Fig. 4).

4.1 Metabolic burden Metabolic burden poses a significant limitation in compartmentalized metabolic engineering, particularly in organelles. They have inherent limitations on maximum protein load and metabolite storage capacity. Excessive accumulation of products or by-products can lead to toxicity, which directly impact the efficiency of compartmentalized metabolic engineering. Regarding their

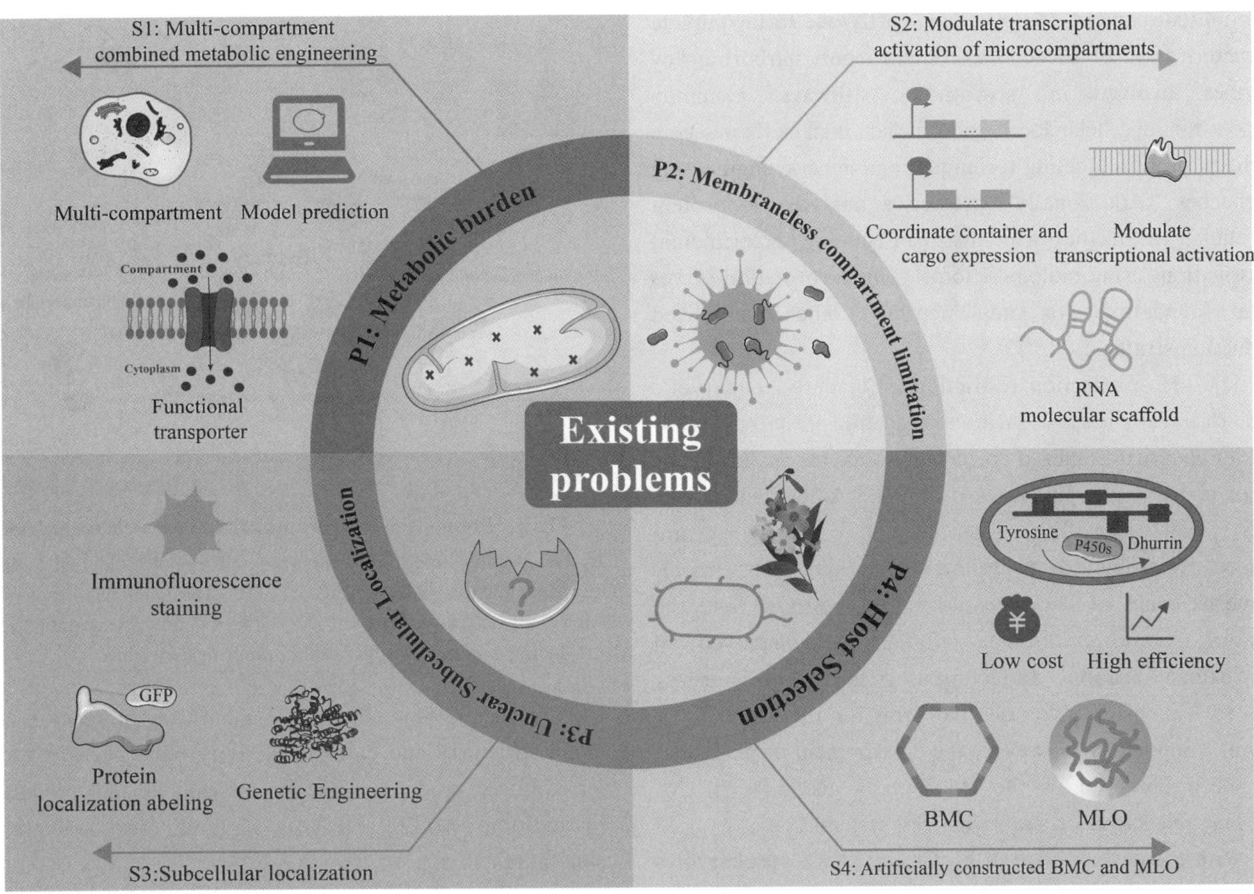


**Fig. 4 Existing problems and solutions in compartmentalized metabolic engineering**

P1: Metabolic burden, which can be mitigated by multi-compartment collaboration, uncovering functional transporters and model predictions; P2: The membraneless compartment limitation, which is primarily the encapsulation problem, can be alleviated by regulating the transcriptional activation of the microcavity and coordinating the expression of microcavity and heterotrimeric cargo proteins; P3: Unclear subcellular localization of enzymes, which can be solved by immunofluorescence staining, protein labeling techniques and genetic engineering; P4: Host selection restriction, which can be overcome by artificially constructing universal compartments. The labels P1-P4 represent the problems, and S1 - S4 represent the solutions.

solutions, studies have been conducted to mitigate them using strategies such as joint metabolic engineering of multiple compartments, strain hybridization and exploration of transporter proteins.

The development of a comprehensive metabolic model for cells offers a valuable tool for predicting protein expression constraints and compartment allocation in compartmentalized metabolic engineering. Comprehensive models of eukaryotic compartmentalization have been developed to reveal the conditional dependencies, activities and protein concentration constraints specific to different compartments. This model contributes to the prediction of each compartment's adaptation to metabolism following regulatory intervention.

4.2 Membraneless compartment limitation The membraneless compartment has shown promising potential. However, its research is in its infancy, leading to several challenges. One crucial challenge is the development of efficient encapsulation strategies to enhance cargo loading. Current strategies exhibit low efficiency, with the risk of encapsulation leakage and susceptibility to aggregation. Additionally, the binding mechanism between EPs and the compartment shell remains incompletely understood. To tackle this, two strategies can be employed: modulating the transcriptional activation of microcompartments and coordinating the expression of micro-compartments and allosteric cargo proteins.

The internal physical and chemical environments of bacteria and eukaryotic cells differ significantly, and proteins from eukaryotic MLOs tend to form solid precipitates in bacteria. To overcome this challenge, a synthetic RNA molecular architecture called Transcriptionally Engineered Addressable RNA Solvents was designed, which enables the programming of spatiotemporal regulation to recruit proteins and achieve synthetic organelles in bacteria.

4.3 Unclear subcellular localization of enzymes To date, the application of compartmentalization in compound production is mostly limited to terpenoids, a few branched alcohols and certain organic acids within membrane compartments.

This limited scope of compounds is partly due to incomplete characterization of subcellular compartments harboring key enzymes involved in biosynthetic pathways. Common methods for subcellular localization include immunofluorescence staining, protein labeling techniques and genetic engineering approaches. Additionally, predictive analysis of protein subcellular localization can assist in guiding experimental investigations using biological tools. This information serves as a foundation for implementing compartmentalized production strategies.

4.4 Host selection restriction Currently, eukaryotic hosts, particularly single-celled microorganisms, are predominantly used for compartmentalized production, while the application of higher plants and prokaryotes is limited. Among eukaryotic hosts, yeast, especially *S. cerevisiae* and *Y. lipolytica*, are the most commonly used compartmentalized hosts. Furthermore, the peroxisomes of *Pichia pastoris* (*P. pastoris*) and the LDs of *Rhodosporidium toruloides* are employed in compartmentalization. In comparison to microorganisms, plant systems offer favorable platforms for the synthesis of natural compounds. However, the development of plants has only been observed in the chloroplasts and LDs of *N. benthamiana* leaves or suspension cell systems.

With the development of BMCs and MLOs, prokaryotes are gradually being used for compartmentalized metabolic engineering. *E. coli*, as a widely studied model organism, serves as an ideal host for membraneless compartment production, in which artificially constructed BMCs and MLOs have been used for the production of small molecules and terpenoids, which is gradually matured and patterned.

## 5 PROSPECTS

5.1 Functional and versatile engineering tools One promising direction in compartmentalized metabolic engineering is the the development of functional, versatile and model biological tools (Fig. 5A). These tools include the manual development of engineered compartments (engineered organelles, BMSs and MLOs), efficient and versatile compartmentalization strategies, and convenient production platforms.

5.2 Drug screening The utilization of microbial synthetic cellular compartments provides a novel platform for drug discovery (Fig. 5B). Synthetic organelles not only enhance the targeting specificity of multiple drugs but also significantly reduce the production of metabolic byproducts to levels below detectable thresholds. LLPS-based drug screening is a rapidly growing area of research.

5.3 Nanobioreactor Self-assembly techniques are currently being used to construct nanobioreactors, which has become a research focus (Fig. 5C). BMCs represent protein macromolecule nanobioreactors with diameters ranging from

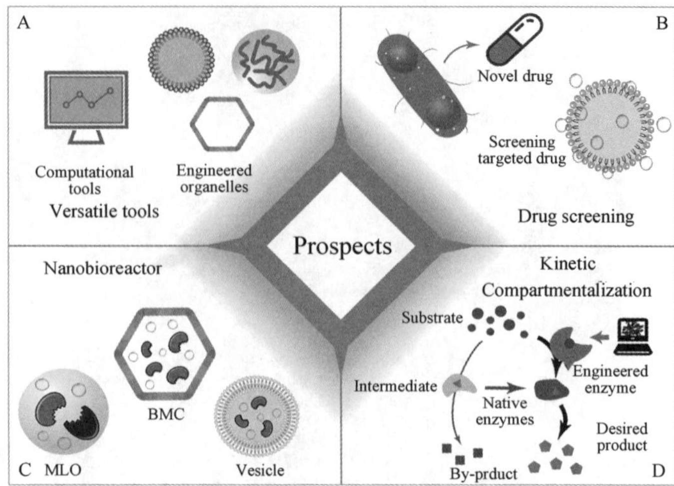


**Fig. 5 Prospects of compartmentalized metabolic engineering**

(A) Developing functional, versatile and model biological tools; (B) Drug screening using MLOs or vesicles; (C) Designing nanoreactors using BMCs, MLOs or vesicles; (D) Kinetic compartmentalization by introducing kinetically separated competing reactions.

100 nm to 150 nm, and novel nanoscale bioreactors with intact structures and catalytic activity have been developed for hydrogen production and recombinant ethanol production. In addition, MLOs and vesicles have great potential as nanobioreactors.

5.4 Kinetic compartmentalization Compartmentalized metabolic engineering involves more than just spatial segregation. Achieving kinetic compartmentalization based on the properties of enzymatic reactions can overcome the limitations of spatial compartmentalization, providing a new direction for compartmentalized metabolism. In most prokaryotes, simultaneous reactions involving multiple substrates within a single space are primarily governed by the kinetic properties of the enzyme. Approximately 40%-50% of enzymes with characterized functions exhibit promiscuity towards multiple substrates, with 10% - 20% of these enzymes capable of facilitating continuous reactions. The kinetic compartmentalization of the metabolic reaction can be achieved by designing and screening the modification of suitable hybrid enzymes and introducing kinetically separated competing reactions, which can increase the substrate availability and improve the productivity (Fig. 5D).

## 6 CONCLUSION

Due to the limitations of metabolic engineering, compartmentalization has emerged. This review comprehensively summarizes the strategies and applications of compartmentalized metabolic engineering, and further discusses the challenges and prospects. Eukaryotes mainly target membranous compartments. The development of BMCs and MLOs offers new opportunities for compartmentalized metabolic production in prokaryotes. Compartmentalized metabolic engineering is crucial for achieving more precise and efficient production of target compounds.

## CREDIT AUTHORSHIP CONTRIBUTION STATEMENT

Rubing Wang: Writing-review & editing, Writing-original draft, Investigation. Yaowu Su: Writing-review & editing, Writing-original draft. Wenqi Yang: Writing-review & editing, Investigation. Huanyu Zhang: Investigation. Juan Wang: Writing-review & editing, Project administration, Funding acquisition. Wenyuan Gao: Supervision, Project administration, Funding acquisition.

[王如冰，王娟，高文远，等. Bioresource Techrology, 2024,402:130786.]

# Substrate promiscuity, crystal structure, and application of a plant UDP - glycosyltransferase UGT74AN3

## 1 INTRODUCTION

Natural products (NPs) have a wide range of biological activities and are an important source of drug discovery, occupying a core place in the history of drug development. However, a large number of NPs still face serious obstacles in the drug development process, such as poor solubility, stability, and oral bioavailability. Glycosylation is one of the most common and important modifications of NPs in nature, contributing to the structural diversity and pharmacological activity of NPs. Therefore, glycosylation is widely recognized as an effective modification strategy that could lead to discovering more new drugs from NPs. Glycosylation is the process of transferring sugar moieties from sugar donors, such as an activated nucleoside diphosphate sugar (NDP-sugar), to acceptors to form glycosides. In contrast to using chemical synthesis and isolation to obtain active glycoside molecules, glycosylation reactions mediated by glycosyltransferases possess multiple advantages including mild reaction conditions, high efficiency, environmental friendliness, and high selectivity. In recent years, enzymatic glycosylation of NPs by uridine diphosphate-dependent glycosyltransferases (UGTs) from plants has attracted a lot of attention from researchers.

Plant UGTs are a class of enzymes found in plant cells that have the ability to transfer various glycosyl groups to substrate molecules, hence altering their biological activity and characteristics. Many bioactive compounds, including alka-loids, saponins, and steroids, are produced by the catalysis of plant UGTs. The glycosylation process generally occurs at functional groups such as hydroxyl, amino, carboxyl, thiol groups or even carbon atoms of the substrate molecules, and the resulting glycosylated relatives could be endowed with reduced toxicity and enhanced biological activity. In addition, the use of plant UGTs also allows the synthesis of non-natural products, which are new natural active substances with different activities and potencies from the original compounds. Therefore, the study of plant UGTs and the glycosylation of NPs has potential applications for the development of new drugs.

In recent years, an increasing number of functionally specific plant UGTs have been identified and applied to the enzymatic synthesis of various NP glycosides. For example, SbCGTa/b has been used for the synthesis of the (iso) schaftoside, TcCGT1 has been used for the synthesis of orientin and vitexin, and UGT76G1 has been used for the synthesis of rebaudioside M, and so on. Although great progress has been made in the identification and characterization of UGTs, the majority of the reported plant UGTs show relatively narrow substrate spectra and strict substrate selectivity, which limits their use in creating the glycosylated derivatives of NPs. Plant UGTs with substrate promiscuity are generally considered to be effective catalysts for the glycosylation of NPs and have the potential for practical applications. Recently, a few plant *C*-glycosyltransferases (CGTs) with substrate promiscuity have been reported, e.g., MiCGT, TcCGT1, and GgCGT, which mainly catalyze the formation of C - C glycosidic bonds. Several *O*-glycosyltransferases (OGTs) with moderate substrate promiscuity have been reported, but they still show significant substrate preferences. For example, Sb3GT1 prefers to glycosylate flavonoid compounds and UGT71BD1 prefers to recognize aromatic glycosides. Moreover, the structural basis for substrate promiscuity of plant UGTs is still unclear. Since the first crystal structure of the plant UGT UGT71G1 was solved, the crystal structures of 27 plant UGTs have been reported. Among these structures, most of the promiscuous UGTs have been reported in the apo form or as binary complexes with UDP. Only a few promiscuous UGTs have been reported with bound substrates in the ternary complexes, such as the structures of GgCGT complexed with UDP/phloretin or UDP/nothofagin. The limited structural information

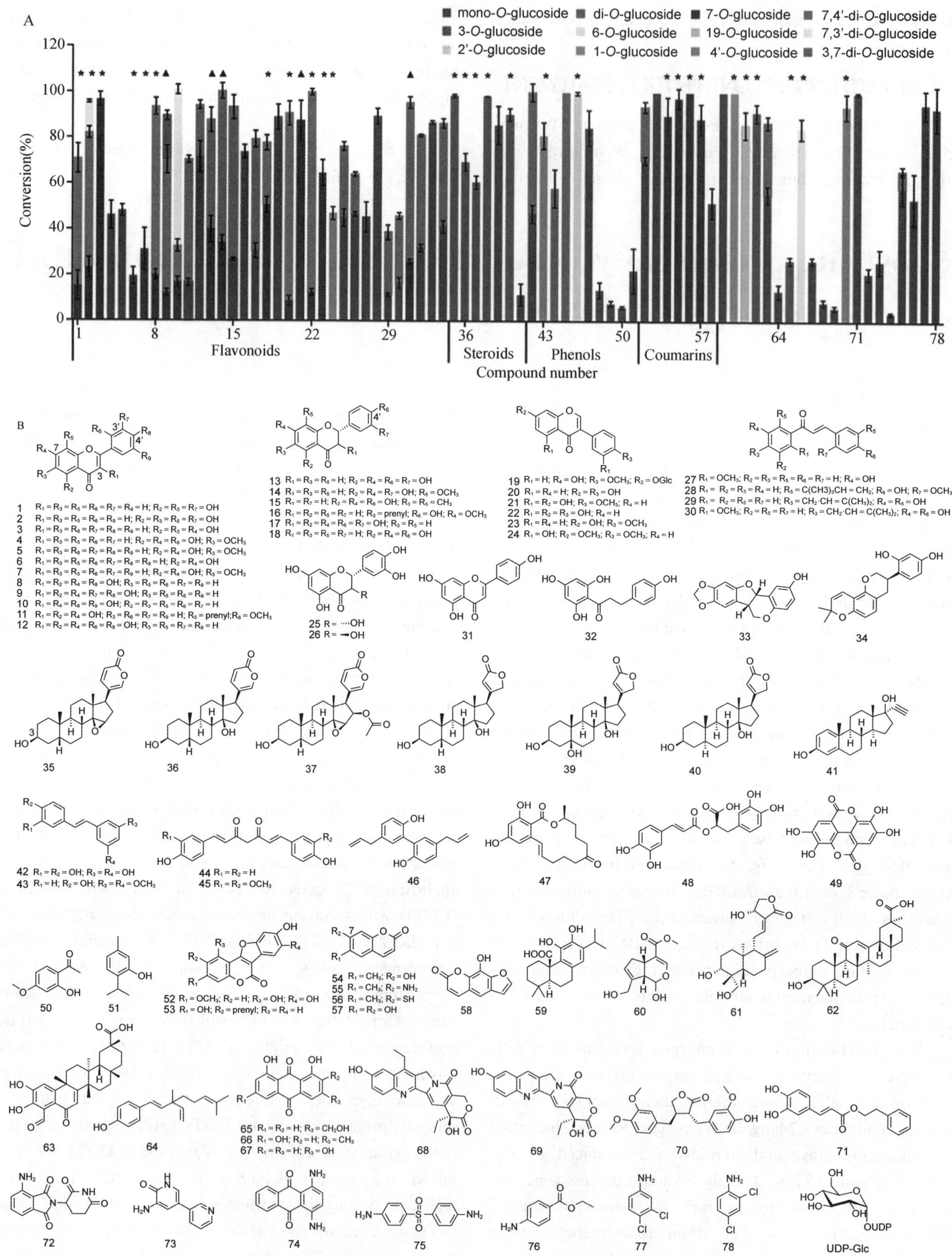


**Figure 1 Substrate promiscuity of UGT74AN3**

(A) Percentage conversion rates of the glycosylated products for various substrates **1** - **78**, using UDP - Glc as the sugar donor. The bar colors represent the different types of glycosylated products for each substrate. The products purified and identified by NMR were labeled with the asterisks (＊). The products labeled with the symbols (▲) were identified by comparing with reference standards. (B) Structures of the compounds (**1** - **78**) catalyzed by UGT74AN3.

about the promiscuous UGT complexes does not provide many mechanistic details of substrate promiscuity. Therefore, it is necessary to identify plant UGTs with high substrate promiscuity in practice and reveal the structural basis of substrate promiscuity in plant UGTs.

UGT74AN3 is a plant UGT from *Catharanthus roseus* that exhibited capabilities for glycosylation of cardiotonic steroids and phenolic compounds. Herein, we further explored the substrate promiscuity of UGT74AN3, finding that it displayed high sugar acceptor-donor promiscuity. We determined the crystal structures of UGT74AN3/UDP in complex with different NPs and revealed the structural basis of its substrate promiscuity. Furthermore, to expand the glycosylation application of UGT74AN3, we established and optimized a UDP-Glc biorecycling system by coupling UGT74AN3 with plant sucrose synthase, which was successfully applied to produce glycosides of several different types of NPs.

## 2 RESULTS AND DISCUSSION

2.1 Probing the Substrate Promiscuity of UGT74AN3. To systematically explore the substrate promiscuity and synthetic utility of UGT74AN3 to glycosylate drug-like scaffolds, an acceptor library of 92 representatives with structurally diverse natural or unnatural compounds was tested using UDP-Glc as the sugar donor and the purified recombinant UGT74AN3 as the enzyme catalyst (Figure S1). All of the reaction mixtures were analyzed by liquid chromatography coupled with mass spectrometry (LC-MS). UGT74AN3 exhibited unprecedented high catalytic promiscuity could *O*-glycosylate 78 of 92 tested substrates (Figures 1 and S2 and Table S1), including 35 flavonoids (**1**-**35**), 7 steroids (**35**-**41**), 10 phenols (**42**-**51**), 7 coumarins (**52**-**58**), 6 terpenoids (**59**-**64**), 3 anthraquinones (**65**-**67**), 2 alkaloids (**68**-**69**), 1 lignan (**70**), 1 phenylpropanoid (**71**), and 7 simple aromatic amino compounds (**72**-**78**). High percentage conversion rates (>80%) were observed for 48 out of 78 substrates (Figures S3-S80). When the flavonoids simultaneously present with 7-OH and 4′-OH were used as the substrates (**1**-**2**, **8**-**10**, **12**-**13**, **15**, **18**, **20**, **22**, **25**-**26**, and **29**-**32**), at least two products were generated by UGT74AN3 and the di-*O*-glucoside is the main product. As for the substrates of steroids with multiple hydroxyl groups, UGT74AN3 exhibited catalytic consistency, generating only a mono-*O*-glycoside product. The glycosylation of phenols, coumarins, and terpenoids by UGT74AN3 produced mostly mono-*O*-glycosides with a few exceptions of di-*O*-glycosides, likely because most of the tested substrates only contain a single hydroxyl group (**43**, **50**-**51**, **54**-**56**, and **58**). UGT74AN3 exhibited *S*-glycosylation activity. The mass spectrum of **56a** yielded a fragment ion ($[M-Glc+H]^+$) at $m/z$ 193.0312, and the $^1H$ and $^{13}C$ NMR spectra further revealed the chemical structure of **56a** as 4-methylcoumarin 7-*S*-β-D-glucoside (Figures S58, S81, and S82). UGT74AN3 also showed substrate promiscuity for *N*-glycosylation toward 8 aromatic amine compounds with various structural features (**55**, **72**-**78**), among which pomalidomide (**72**) and amrinone (**73**) are clinically used to treat multiple myeloma and heart failure, respectively. Although a few promiscuous OGTs from plants or microorganisms have been reported, their substrate acceptance rates, e.g., UGT74AN1 with 77% (53 out of the 69 tested compounds), OleD (ASP) with 52% (71 out of the 135 tested compounds) and MhGT1 with 77% (72 out of the 93 tested compounds), are much lower than that of UGT74AN3 (with 85%, 78 out of the 92 tested compounds). To the best of our knowledge, the substrate promiscuity of UGT74AN3 as an *O*-glycosyl is the most diverse known to date.

To further confirm the catalytic characteristics of UGT74AN3, 7 di-*O*-glucosides (**1b**, **2b**, **2c**, **8b**, **18b**, **20b**, and **22b**) and 27 mono-*O*-glucosides were purified, and their structures were unambiguously identified by $^1H$ NMR, $^{13}C$ NMR, and HMBC spectroscopic analyses. The structures of **9a**, **9c**, **13a**, **14a**, and **21a** were identified by comparing with reference standards (Figures S81-S169). All of the *O*-glycosides contain a β-glycosidic bond, which was indicated by the large coupling constants ($J$ = 7.2-8.1 Hz) of the anomeric protons (Table S2). UGT74AN3 exhibits a certain regioselectivity for the C-7 OH and C-4′ OH of flavonoids. In the presence of 7-OH or 4′-OH individually, the substrates were glycosylated to produce 7-*O*-glucosides (**3a**, **6a**, **7a**, and **23a**) or 4′-*O*-glucosides (**24a**), respectively. In the simultaneous presence of 7-OH and 4′-OH, the substrates were first catalyzed to produce 7-*O*-glycosides (**1a**, **2a**, **8a**, **18a**, **20a**, and **22a**), and the subsequent 4′-OH glycosylation resulted in the main products of 7,4′-di-*O* glycosides (**1b**, **2b**, **8b**, **18b**, **20b**, and **22b**). Very limited plant GTs were found capable of sequentially glycosylation of the flavonoids on 7-OH and 4′-OH. Unlike that the recently reported flavonoid 7, 4′-di-*O*-glycosyltransferase (ZjOGT3) initially produces a 4′-*O*-glucoside, the initial product of UGT74AN3 was determined to be a 7-*O*-glucoside by time-course experiments (Figure S170). It is noteworthy that UGT74AN3 is not strictly regioselective for the 7-OH and 4′-OH of flavonoids and also exhibits weak 3-OH and 3′-OH activity, e.g., the structures of **2c** and **9c** were identified as 7,3′-di-*O* glucoside and 3,7-di-*O*-glucoside, respectively. UGT74AN3 exhibits strict regioselectivity for the 3-OH of steroids, capable of catalyzing the generation of a 3-*O*-glycoside (**35a**, **36a**, **38a**, and **40a**) from diverse structural steroids. For coumarins, their glycosylation by UGT74AN3 occurs at 7-OH to produce 7-*O*-glycosides (**55a**, **56a**, and **57a**). For anthraquinones,

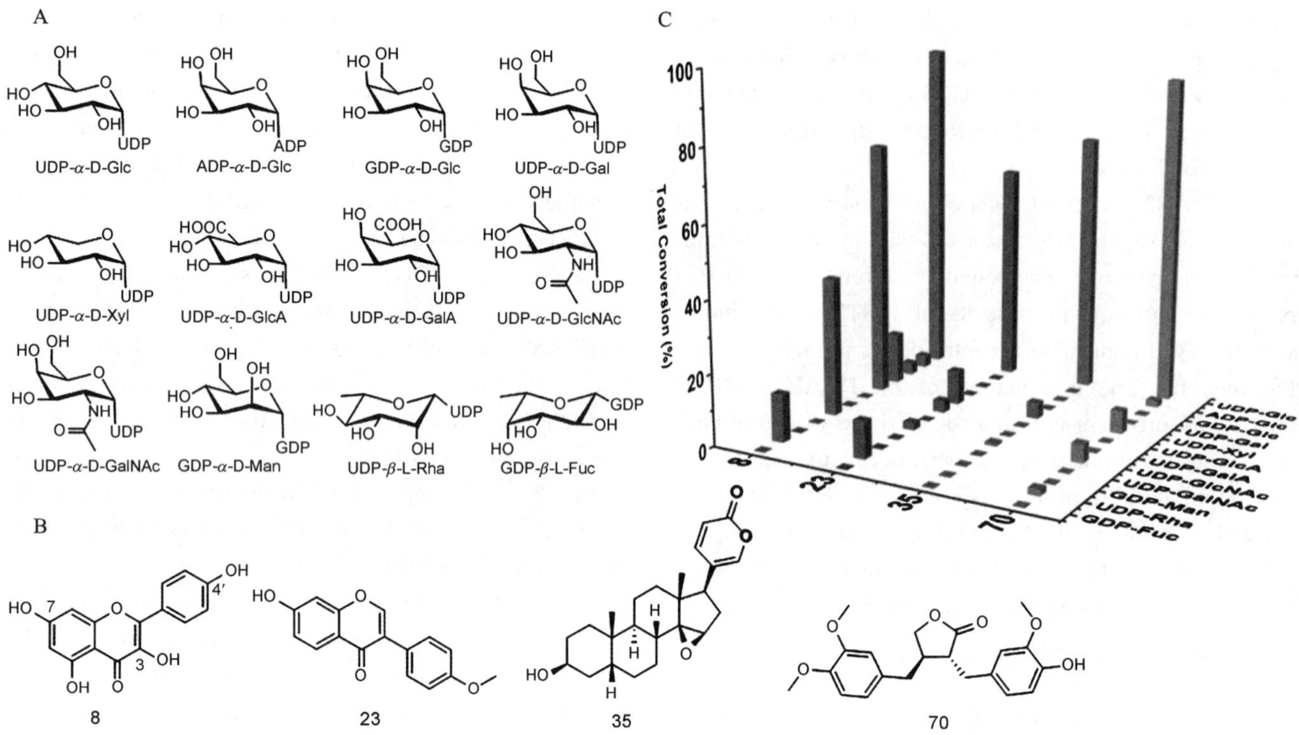


**Figure 2 Sugar donor promiscuity of UGT74AN3**

(A) Structures of different sugar donors. (B) Structures of four representative substrates. (C) Percentage conversion rates of the glycosylated products using different sugar donors and four substrates.

glycosylation by UGT74AN3 occurs at 3 - OH or 6 - OH, yielding 3-*O*-glycoside (**65a**) or 6-*O*-glycoside (**66a**). Moreover, for some substrates with only a single hydroxyl group, the structures of the glycosylated products were identified by MS/MS spectrometry. Overall, a total of 50 products were structurally characterized (Figure S171 and Table S3). These results suggested that UGT74AN3 is a promising and potentially applicable enzyme for the efficient synthesis of glycosides with different structures.

2.2 Exploring the Sugar Donor Promiscuity of UGT74AN3. To explore the sugar donor promiscuity of UGT74AN3, we tested 11 NDP-sugar donors other than UDP - Glc, including ADP - Glc, GDP-Glc, UDP - Gal, GDP-Xyl, UDP - GlcA, UDP - GalA, UDP - GlcNAc, UDP - GalNAc, GDP - Man, UDP - L - Rha, and GDP - L - Fuc, and four substrates including kaempferol (**8**), formononetin (**23**), resibufogenin (**35**), and arctiin (**70**) were selected as the sugar acceptors (Figure 2A, B). The results showed that UGT74AN3 exhibited preferences but high promiscuity for sugar donors (Figures 2C and S172 - S186). When the substrates **23**, **35**, and **70** were employed, UGT74AN3 demonstrated a significant preference for UDP - Glc with percentage conversion rate in a range of 61.0% - 92.0%, whereas low percentage conversion rate (0.7% - 10.3%) were observed using UDP - Xyl, UDP - GlcNAc, UDP - GlcA, or UDP-Rha as the sugar donors. UGT74AN3 still exhibited a noticeable preference for UDP - Glc (percentage conversion rate of 95.0%) when compound **8** was the substrate, but its capability of utilizing UDP - GlcNAc (percentage conversion rate of 38.9%) and UDP - Xyl (percentage conversion rate of 71.6%) was much higher compared to using **23**, **35**, and **70** as the substrates. These findings suggest that UGT74AN3 is a sugar donor promiscuous and selective plant UGT and that the sugar donor promiscuity is greatly influenced by the type of substrates.

2.3 Crystal Structure of UGT74AN3/UDP and Recognition of the Sugar Donor. To reveal the molecular mechanism underlying the promiscuity of UGT74AN3, we determined the structure of UGT74AN3 using X-ray crystallography. To obtain high-quality crystals, we truncated the first 10 residues at the N-terminus of UGT74AN3 that were computationally predicted to be disordered in the structure (Figure S187). The resulting recombinant protein UGT74AN3$_{11\text{-}474}$ showed the same catalytic activity as the full-length protein (Figures S188 and S189). When demon-strating the crystal structures, UGT74AN3$_{11\text{-}474}$ is always referred to as "UGT74AN3" unless otherwise stated. The crystal structure of the binary complex UGT74AN3/UDP was solved at a resolution of 1.86 Å (PDB ID: 8INA) (Figures S190 and S191 and Table S4A). UGT74AN3 exhibits typical GT - B fold structural features containing two $\beta$, $\alpha$, and $\beta$ Rossmann-like domains that face each other and pack tightly together. The N-terminal domain (NTD, residues 11 - 236 and 457 - 474) and C-terminal domain (CTD, residues 274 - 456) are connected by

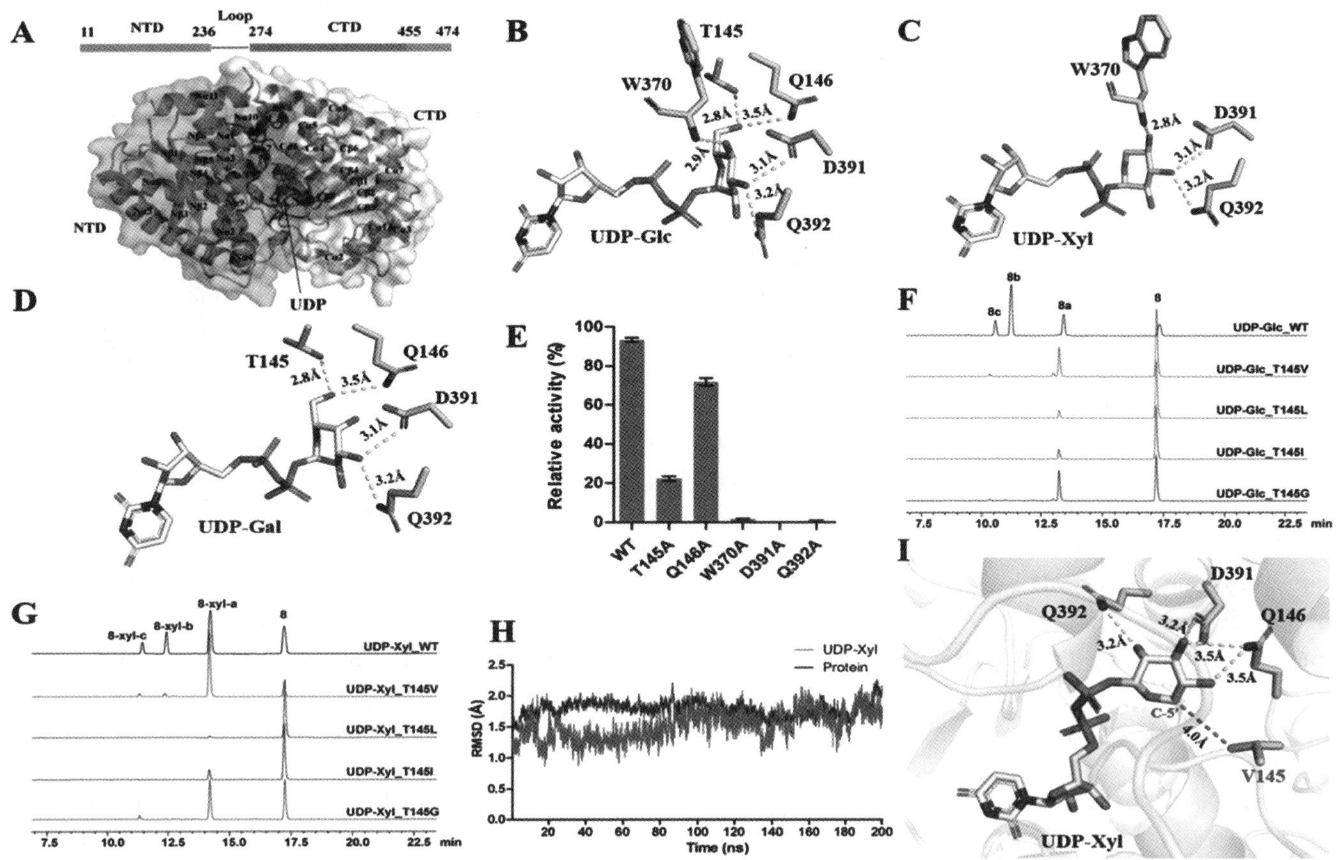


**Figure 3 Crystal structure of UGT74AN3/UDP and recognition of the sugar donors**

(A) Structural features of UGT74AN3/UDP. The N-terminal domain (NTD) and C-terminal domain (CTD) are colored cyan and gray, respectively. The ligand UDP is shown as sticks and the deep cleft for ligand binding is highlighted in red. (B - D) Interactions between UGT74AN3 and the glucose moiety of UDP - Glc (B), and the xylose moiety of UDP - Xyl (C), and the galactose moiety of UDP - Gal (D), respectively. Hydrogen bonds are represented by yellow dashed lines with the corresponding atomic distances labeled. (E) The relative catalytic activities of the UGT74AN3 mutants (related to sugar donor recognition) using **8** as the substrate and UDP - Glc as the sugar donor. (F, G) HPLC analysis of the products of UGT74AN3 and the T145-related mutants using **8** and UDP - Glc (F) or UDP - Xyl (G). (H) Time evolution of the RMSD for the heavy atoms of protein backbone and UDP - Xyl in dynamic simulation. (I) Interactions between the UGT74AN3-T145V and the xylose moiety of UDP - Xyl. The hydrophobic interaction is shown as magenta dashes.

a flexible loop region (237 - 273). The NTD containing 13 $\alpha$-helices and 6 $\beta$-sheets and the CTD containing 9 $\alpha$-helices and 6 $\beta$-sheets are generally accountable for binding the sugar acceptors and sugar donors, respectively (Figure 3A). According to the DALI server analysis, the structure of UGT74AN3 is highly similar to the structures of UGT74AN2 (PDB: 7W0K), UGT74F2 (PDB: 5U6N), Os79 (PDB: 5TMB), and UGT74AC1 (PDB: 6L8X), with the C$\alpha$ root-mean-square deviations (RMSDs) ranging from 1.2 to 2.2 Å (Figure S192 and Table S5).

The residue interaction with the sugar moiety of UDP-sugar is a key factor for the sugar donor selectivity and promiscuity of plant UGTs. To investigate the sugar donor selectivity of UGT74AN3, the models of UGT74AN3/UDP - Glc, UGT74AN3/UDP - Xyl, and UGT74AN3/UDP - Gal were established by molecular docking based on the structure of UGT74AN3/UDP. Structural analysis showed that the glucose moiety of UDP - Glc forms hydrogen bonds with T145, Q146, W370, D391, and Q392 of UGT74AN3 (Figure 3B). Compared to UDP - Glc, the 4-OH of the galactose moiety in UDP - Gal points at the opposite direction, which prevents it from forming a hydrogen bond with W370 of UGT74AN3 (Figure 3C). The absence of the 5-hydroxymethyl group in the xylose moiety in UDP - Xyl resulted in its inability to form hydrogen bonds with T145 and Q146 of UGT74AN3 (Figure 3D). These findings may explain that UGT74AN3 prefers UDP - Glc as the major sugar donor over the others. The relative catalytic activity of the mutants Q146A and T145A was reduced to 70 and 20%, respectively. The mutants W370A, D391A, and Q392A almost lost all of the catalytic activities (Figure 3E). Based on these findings, attempts were made to alter the sugar donor specificity of UGT74AN3 by mutations. T145 and W370 were selected for further mutagenesis analysis, and kaempferol (**8**) was used as the substrate to test the activity of all mutants. Different mutants of T145/(V/L/I/G) are all shown with substantially enhanced regioselectivity for the 7-OH of the kaempferol (**8**), but with significantly reduce in their ability of utilizing UDP - Glc (Figure 3F). Among these T145 mutants, the percentage conversion rate of T145V utilizing UDP - Xyl was most improved, from 71.6 to 93.2% (Figure 3G). Furthermore, the T145V mutant has a broadly enhanced ability to utilize UDP - Xyl to glycosylate other types of substrates (Figure S193). To gain in-depth insights into the mechanism of the altered sugar donor specificity of UGT7AN3-T145V, the model of UGT7AN3 - T145V/UDP - Xyl was built and analyzed by 200 ns molecular dynamics (MD) simulation (Figure 3H). The results show that nonpolar valine (V145) forms a hydrophobic interaction with the C - 5′ atom of the xylose in UDP - Xyl during the MD simulations (Figure 3I). In contrast, the 5-hydroxymethyl group of glucose is unable to form a hydrogen bond with valine. Therefore, UGT74AN3 - T145V prefers UDP - Xyl as the sugar donor.

2.4 Crystal Structures of UGT74AN3/UDP in Complex with Different Substrates. To further explore structural basis of the substrate promiscuity of UGT74AN3, 32 substrates with high percentage conversion rate (>85%) were selected to screen the ternary complex structures of UGT74AN3 by cocrystallization or crystal soaking. The crystal structures of UGT74AN3/UDP/**35**, UGT74AN3/UDP/**36**, UGT74AN3/UDP/**38**, UGT74AN3/UDP/**40**, and UGT74AN3/UDP/**42** were solved at the resolutions in a range of 1.85 - 2.30 Å (Figure S191 and Table S4). Interestingly, the ligands **35**, **36**, **38**, and **40** are all cardiotonic steroids (CTs), which are easily visualized in good electron densities of the complex structures (Figure 4A - D). The ligand **42** belongs to the phenols, and the electron density of **42** is relatively poorer compared to those of CTs (Figure 4E). A great effort has been made to obtain crystal structures of UGT74AN3 complexed with other types of NPs, but this has been without any success. To determine the substrate affinity of UGT74AN3 for various substrates, kinetic analyses were performed using UDP - Glc as the sugar donor. The $K_M$ values of UGT74AN3 for **35**, **38**, and **42** were $0.019 \pm 0.003$, $0.029 \pm 0.005$, and $0.078 \pm 0.010$ mmol/L, respectively (Figure 4F). UGT74AN3 showed the highest affinity for CTs compared with other types of substrates (Figure S194 and Table S6). These results suggest that the native substrate for UGT74AN3 may be CTs, which might explain our failure in obtaining the structure of UGT74AN3 in complex with other low affinity substrates.

Structural analysis revealed that UGT74AN3 has a unique U-shaped substrate binding pocket consisting of a series of residues, including F20, H16, H25, M84, E85, M88, D123, S125, Q146, F193, V200, L204, Q207, L288, L297, W361, W389, A390, and D391, with an inner diameter of about 12.4 Å (measured between its widest points, from A22 to V200), and a depth of about 17.9 Å (from E85 to S125) (Figure 4G - I). Unlike other plant GTs with hydrophobic substrate-binding pockets, the residues that make up the pocket of UGT74AN3 contain a relatively large number of hydrophilic residues in addition to hydrophobic residues. This feature facilitates formation of the rich interactions between UGT74AN3 and various substrates and guarantees the regioselectivity of UGT74AN3 toward different substrates in the way that substrates with different properties could be stabilized with different binding poses. For example, the weakly polar substrates **35**, **36**, **38**, and **40** are stabilized in the pocket mainly by their interactions with hydrophobic residues (Figure 4J - M), whereas the polyhydroxylated substrate **42**, is stabilized in the pocket by forming hydrogen bonding interactions with hydrophilic residues (Figure 4N). Moreover, the pocket volume of UGT74AN3 is about 1 176 $Å^3$, which is larger than that of most of the plant GTs with available substrate bound structures (Table S7). These structural features may ensure that substrates with different sizes smoothly enter and are stabilized in the pocket of UGT74NA3 and provide intrinsic support for the substrate promiscuity of UGT74AN3.

To identify the key residues of UGT74AN3 involved in the substrate binding, we examined the interactions between the substrates and binding pockets were examined. The residues F20, I81, E85, F193, L203, V200, L297, and W389 form hydrophobic interactions with the CTs in general, and Q146 forms an extra weak hydrogen bond with **38** (Figure 4J - M). The residues H16 and W361 forms hydrogen bond with **42**, and L288 form hydrophobic interactions with the **42** (Figure 4N). Structure-based site-directed mutagenesis of these residues was designed, followed by an enzymatic activity test of the UGT74AN3 mutant using **35** or **42** as the substrate and UDP - Glc as the sugar donor. The catalytic activities of the mutants F20A, V200A, and L297A were significantly reduced, probably due to disruption of the hydrophobic environment of the substrate binding pocket, which hampers the binding of the CTs in the pocket (Figure 4R). The mutant H16A showed lower enzymatic activities than the wild type due to the blockage of hydrogen bond formation (Figure 4S). The mutants I81A, F193A, L203A, and W389A showed higher enzymatic activities than the wild type, likely causing the reduced steric hindrance within the binding pocket in the presence of shortened side chains or more facilitating entry/exit of the substrate/product in the pocket (Figure 4R). Moreover, the capability of the highest relative activity mutant, F193A, to glycosylate other substrates was further

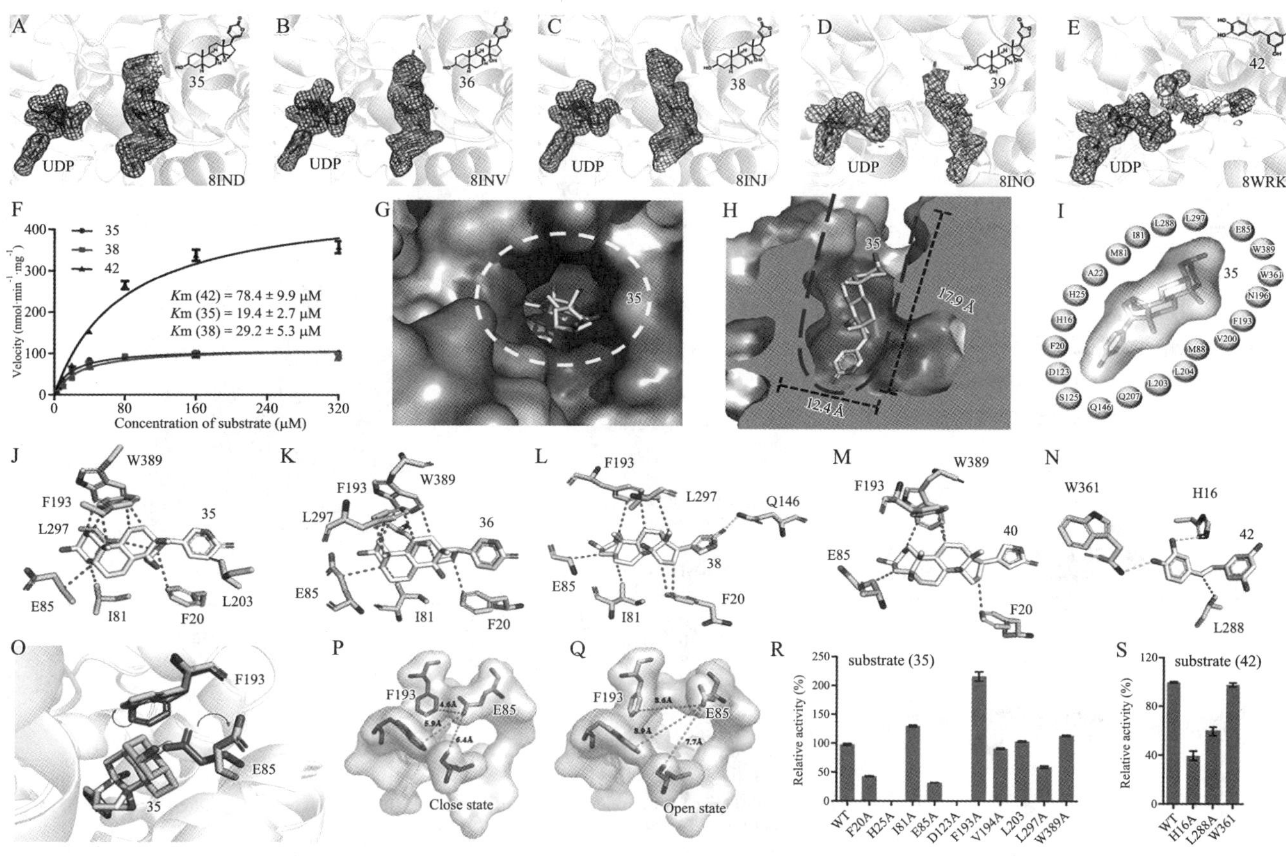


**Figure 4 Structural basis for the substrate binding of UGT74AN3**

(A-E) The substrates **35**, **36**, **38**, **40**, and **42** in the complex structures of UGT74AN3/UDP are enlarged and shown in the $F_o - F_c$ omit electron density maps contoured at 2.0 $\sigma$. (F) Kinetic parameters for UGT74AN3. **35**, **38**, and **42** were used as substrates, and UDP-Glc was used as sugar donor. (G) The substrate **35** is bound within a hydrophobic pocket of UGT74AN3, which is colored based on hydrophobicity. The entrance is marked with a yellow dashed circle. (H) The cross-section and diagram of the U-shaped hydrophobic pocket of UGT74AN3 with substrate **35** inside. The maximum diameter and height are labeled in black-colored fonts. (I) The key amino acid residues that make up the U-shaped pocket. (J-N) Interactions between UGT74AN3 and **35**, **36**, **38**, **40**, and **42**, respectively. The hydrophobic interactions are shown as magenta dashes. The hydrogen bonds are represented by yellow dashed lines. (O) The structure superimposition was between UGT74AN3/UDP and UGT74AN3/UDP/**35**. In the structure of UGT74AN3/UDP, residues F139 and E85 are represented with purple sticks, while in the structure of UGT74AN3/UDP/**35**, they are represented with cyan sticks. (P, Q) The conformation of F193 and E85 at the entrance of the substrate binding pocket of UGT74AN3 in the closed state (P) and in the open state (Q). (R, S) The relative catalytic activities of UGT74AN3 and its mutants were obtained using **35** (R) or **42** (S) as the substrate and UDP-Glc as the sugar donor.

examined. Compared to the wild type, F193A showed enhanced catalytic activity for all 14 substrates that were selected (Figure S195).

To discover the conformational changes of UGT74AN3 induced by the substrate binding, the structures of UGT74AN3/UDP were compared with those of four ternary complexes, respectively. Two distinct conformations were adopted by the two residues E85 and F193, which are located near the entrance of the substrate binding pocket of UGT74AN3 (Figure 4O). In the absence of the substrate, the carboxyl side chain of E85 and the benzene ring side chain of F193 are close to each other, resulting in a narrow entrance to the pocket. This conformation is considered to be a "closed" state (Figure 4P). When the substrate is bound, the side chains of the two residues swing oppositely away from each other, and the entrance of the pocket becomes wider, which is considered an "open" state (Figure 4Q). These results indicated that E85 and F193 might serve as the gatekeepers of UGT74AN3 to control substrate binding. The mutagenesis analysis also showed that E85A and F193A have a great effect on the UGT74AN3 catalytic activity (Figure 4R). To probe the functions of E85 and F193 in depth, extremely rigid residue proline was used to replace E85 and F193, respectively. The catalytic activities of mutant E85P and F193P were both significantly reduced, and the double mutant E85P/F193P activity was nearly completely lost (Figure S196). Due to the fact that E85 locates at the top end of the pocket and on the surface of the protein, its hydrophilicity is essential for protein stabilization. E85 was mutated into basic residues (D, H, K) and hydrophobic residues (L, F), respectively. E85H and E85K maintained the same catalytic activity as the wild type, whereas the relative

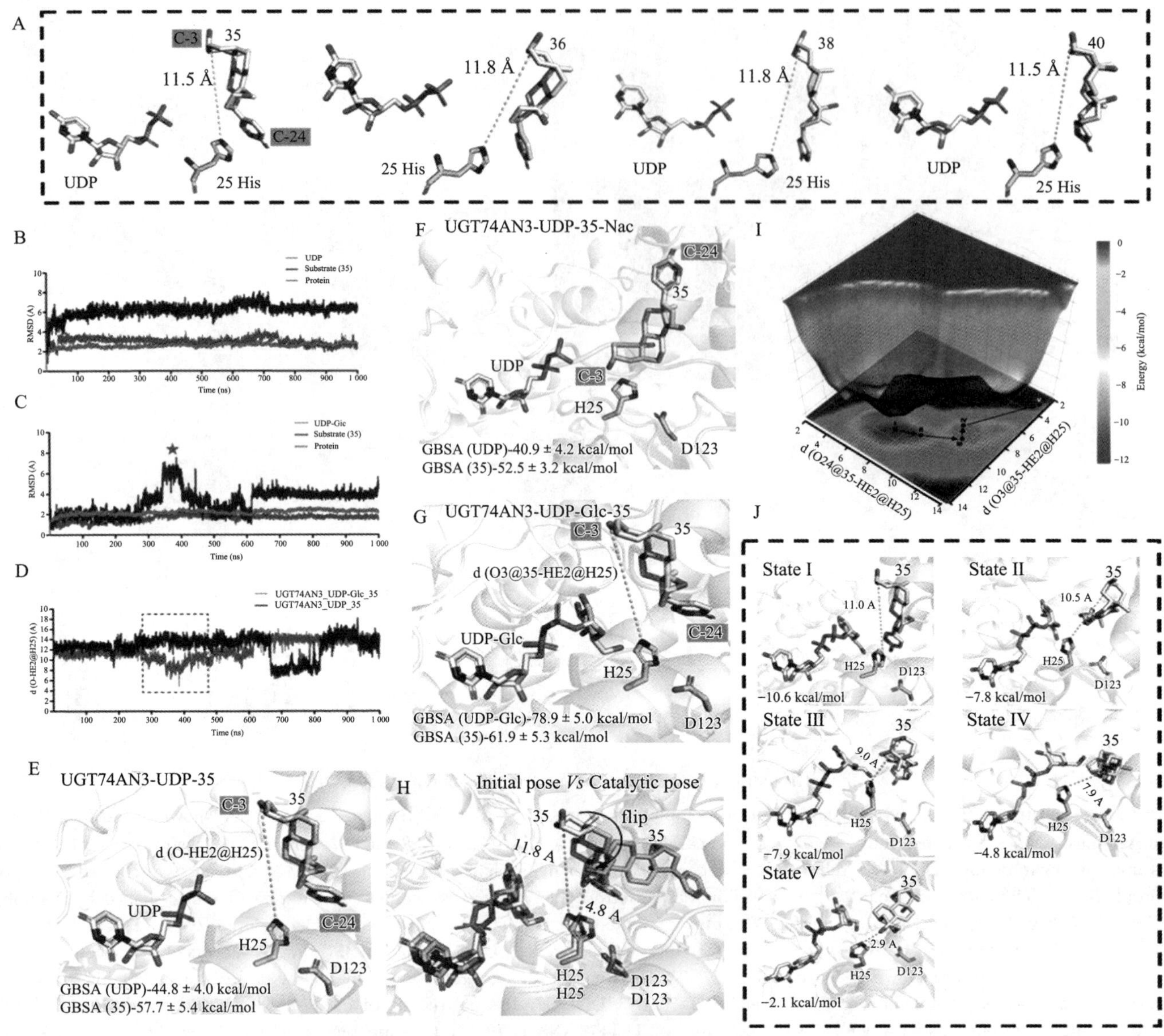


**Figure 5　Unusual substrate binding mode of UGT74AN3**

(A) Binding mode of CTs **35**, **36**, **38**, and **40** in the structures of UGT74AN3, respectively. (B,C) RMSD for the heavy atoms of protein backbone, UDP or UDP-Glc, and substrate (**35**) in the UGT74AN3-UDP-**35** (B) and UGT74AN3-UDP-Glc-**35** (C) simulation systems, respectively. (D) Distance between the hydrogen atom (HE2) of the imidazole ring of H25 and the oxygen atom at the C-3 position of **35** during 1 000 ns MD simulation for the ternary complex UGT74AN3-UDP-**35** and UGT74AN3-UDP-Glc-**35**. (E-H) The complex structure models and MM/GBSA binding free energy of UGT74AN3-UDP-**35** (E), UGT74AN3-UDP-**35**-Nac (F), and UGT74AN3-UDP-Glc-**35** (G). (H) Structural superposition of the initial and catalytic conformations. The ligan is shown as a yellow stick in the initial conformation and as a green stick in the catalytic conformation. (I) The free energy profile obtained from the MetaMD simulation of the ternary complex UGT74AN3-UDP-Glc-**35**. (J) The free energies of five representative metastable states in the **35** binding process.

activities of E85F and E85L were reduced to 48.0 and 40.5%, respectively (Figure S196). F193 was replaced with the same type residues but with different side-chain sizes (W, V). The relative activity of F193W was significantly reduced to 57.8%, and the relative activity of mutant F193V was increased to 140.5% (Figure S196). These results suggest that the main purpose of the swinging of E85 and F193 is to enlarge the pocket diameter and reduce the spatial steric hindrance for facilitating substrate entry into the pocket, and that E85 may also play a role in stabilizing the surface charge of the protein.

2.5　Unusual Substrate Binding Mode of UGT74AN3. Previous studies have shown that GT-B type plant UGTs usually obey the classical inverse catalytic mechanism ($S_N2$-like), in which a highly conserved catalytic dyad, His-Asp, is essential for initiating the reaction. The corresponding residues in UGT74AN3 were mapped as H25 and D123 (Figure S197). Similar to other UGTs, the H25-D123 dyad of UGT74AN3 was located in the catalytic core in the neighborhood of the substrate (Figure S198). The mutants

H25A and D123A were completely devoid of catalytic activity (Figure 4R), confirming that the catalytic dyad (His-Asp) is essential for the function of UGT74AN3. UGT74AN3 likely adopts a $S_N2$-like mechanism to form *O*-glycosidic bonds. Interestingly, an unusual binding mode of the CTs was identified in the structure of UGT74AN3. The glycosylation site of 3 - OH for the CTs is far away from the catalytic residue His25 with a distance of about 11.8 Å (Figure 5A). The structure of UGT74AN2 was deciphered by our group, which also formed complexes with CTs. However, the 3 - OH of CTs was only 3 - 4 Å away from the catalytic residue His24 of UGT74AN2 and formed hydrogen bonds with His24 (Figure S199). The structural comparison showed that the binding directions of CTs in the substrate pockets of UGT74AN3 and UGT74AN2 were completely opposite (Figure S200). The distance between the glycosylation site and the catalytic histidine residue was all within 6 Å in the other plant UGT complexes (Figure S201). By superimposing the four complex structures, the spatial location of the bound substrates is nearly identical, and a molecule of Tris is found between UDP and the substrate. To examine the effect of Tris on the binding poses of CTs, the complex structure of UGT74AN3/UDP/**35**_No_Tris was solved at a resolution of 1.85 Å under conditions with the reagent Tris completely avoided (Figure S191 and Table S4B). Structural comparison analysis revealed that the binding pose of **35** in the complex structure was fully identical (Figure S202). Thus, Tris has no effect on the binding mode of CTs in UGT74AN3. To the best of our knowledge, this unique substrate binding mode is captured for the first time in the structural study of plant UGTs. Although the binding mode of CTs in the hydrophobic pocket of UGT74AN3 is not optimal for the catalytic reactions in terms of its spatial distance, the hydrophobic pocket of UGT74AN3 is large enough to allow CTs to move and flip throughout the catalytic reaction.

To reveal the unique binding mechanism of CTs in UGT74AN3 and to draw the complete conformational changes, molecular docking, MD simulation, and metadynamics (MetaMD) simulation were used to analyze the UGT74AN3 complexes. The complex models of UGT74AN3 - UDP - **35**, UGT74AN3 - UDP - **35** - Nac (**35** ideal near-attack conformation obtained by docking), and UGT74AN3 - UDP - Glc - **35** (obtained by docking based on the crystal structure) were prepared separately for 1 000 ns MD analysis (Figures 5B - D and S203). The MM/GBSA (molecular mechanics with generalized Born and surface area solvation) binding free energy of **35** in UGT74AN3 - UDP - **35** is 5.2 kcal/mol lower than that in UGT74AN3 - UDP - **35** - Nac (Figure 5E, F). This result indicates that the special binding conformation of **35** in UGT74AN3 is more stable than the catalytic conformation in the presence of UDP. In fact, most of the protein crystals will favor a more stable conformation during their formation process, which could be the reason why the unusual binding conformation of **35** could be captured. Although the MM/GBSA binding free energy of **35** is 4.2 kcal/mol lower in UGT74AN3 - UDP - Glc - **35** than in UGT74AN3 - UDP - **35**, during the simulation, **35** swings much more dramatically in UGT74AN3 - UDP - Glc - **35**, with a swing scale close to 7 Å (Figure 5C, E, G). This suggests that UDP - Glc, the real sugar donor of UGT74AN3, can induce **35** to undergo a significant conformational change. During the 1 000 ns simulation of UGT74AN3 - UDP - Glc - **35**, the key reaction coordinate, *d* (O3 - HE2@H25) [the distance between the hydrogen atom (HE2) of the imidazole ring of H25 and the oxygen atom (O) at the C - 3 position of **35**] undergoes a dramatic change. At 385.4 ns, *d* (O3 @ **35**-HE2 @ H25) reaches a minimum of 4.8 Å (Figure 5D). Compared to the initial model, the binding conformation of the substrate in the pocket changes drastically, completing the move and flip and being in the catalytic conformation (Figure 5H). These results indicate that it is possible for **35** to complete the reaction by conformational flip in the pocket of UGT74AN3. To trace the process of the conformational change of **35** in the pocket, the movement of the ligand was also sampled by MetaMD simulation, in which the movement of key reaction coordinates was enhanced by the biased potential. Five metastable states were identified in the binding process of **35** and the energy barrier for all conformational changes is only —8.5 kcal/mol (Figure 5I). The five conformations were placed on the potential energy surface, showing the complete free energy landscape of **35** flipping in the pocket (Figure 5J). Based on the MetaMD simulation, we propose that the catalytic process of the substrate **35** may be initialed from the starting binding conformation (**I**), after which **35** gradually moves backward and flips toward the catalytic residue H25 (**II** - **IV**). Finally, it adopts an ideal catalytic conformation (**V**) to complete the reaction (Figure 5J). This may provide new insights into our understanding of the catalytic processes of promiscuous plant UGTs.

2.6 Establishment and Optimization of a UDP - Glc Biorecycling System. Despite the multiple advantages of promiscuous UGTs in their applications of glycosylation modification of NPs, high cost of the active sugar donor UDP - Glc has limited the use of glycosyltransferases on a broad scale. Sucrose synthase (SuSy) is a type of enzyme capable of effectively generating UDP - Glc from inexpensive sucrose and UDP. To fully exploit the potential for UGT74AN3 in the cost-effective production of active NP glycosides, a UDP - Glc biorecycling system by coupling UGT74AN3 with *At*SuSy, a sucrose synthase derived from *Arabidopsis thaliana*, was constructed (Figure 6A). The recombinant *At*SuSy with a molecular weight of 92 kDa, was

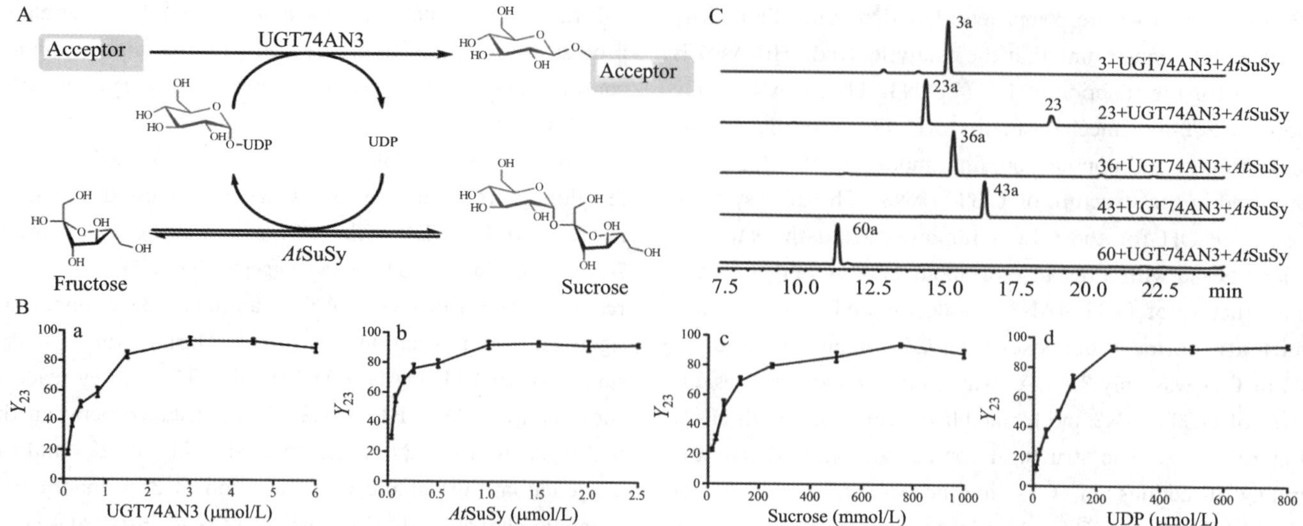


**Figure 6 Catalytic reaction of UGT74AN3 using a UDP - Glc biorecycling system**

(A) Scheme of the cascade reaction of UGT74AN3 coupled with the sucrose synthase *At*SuSy aimed for recycling UDP - Glc. (B) Optimization of the UDP - Glc biorecycling reaction conditions including: concentration of *At*SuSy (a), concentration of UGT74AN3 (b), concentration of sucrose (c), and concentration of UDP (d). (C) HPLC analysis of the glycosylation reaction products using five different substrates to test the UDP - Glc biorecycling system.

purified by Ni - NTA affinity chromatography (Figure S188). The coupling reaction system was initially set up using formononetin (**23**) as the substrate with UDP and sucrose supplemented in the presence of the two purified enzymes. $Y_{23}$ denotes the conversion rate of formononetin. The reaction was further optimized by adjusting both enzyme concentrations and UDP and sucrose concentration (Figure 6B). The highest $Y_{23}$ value was obtained when 3 μmol/L UGT74AN3 was used. With a fixed concentration of UGT74AN3 (3 μmol/L) and gradually increasing concentrations of *At*SuSy, an increase of the $Y_{23}$ value was observed accordingly until *At*SuSy reached a concentration of 1 μmol/L. Therefore, 3 μmol/L UGT74AN3 and 1 μmol/L *At*SuSy were fixed for further optimization of the other parameters in the cascade reaction. As the supply of UDP - Glc significantly impacted the glycosylation reaction, the amounts of sucrose and UDP were also tuned for the reaction. When the sucrose concentration was gradually raised from 50 mmol/L, $Y_{23}$ achieved a maximum with about 750 mmol/L sucrose and any additional input of sucrose afterward indeed reduced $Y_{23}$. Similarly, it was found that $Y_{23}$ reached its peak in the presence of 250 μmol/L UDP. As a result, 750 mmol/L sucrose and 250 μmol/L UDP were used for the UGT74AN3 - *At*SuSy coupling reaction. A series of NPs with different backbones including flavonoid (**3**), steroids (**35**), polyphenols (**43**), and terpenoids (**60**) were selected to test the feasibility of the coupling system. The results showed that the UGT74AN3 - *At*SuSy coupling system could efficiently glycosylate all of the above tested substrates (Figure 6C). The establishment of this coupling biorecycling glycosylation system expands the application scope of UGT74AN3 and greatly exploits its potential in the field of synthetic biology.

## 3 CONCLUSIONS

In summary, the catalytic function of UGT74AN3 was explored in depth. UGT74AN3 exhibited high promiscuity of both acceptor and sugar donors, capable of glycosylating 78 natural/non-natural structurally diverse substrates and utilizing six sugar donors. Besides its O-glycosylation activity, UGT74AN3 also exhibited *S*-glycosylation activity and certain *N*-glycosylation promiscuity. We determined the binary complex structure of UGT74AN3/UDP and five ternary complex structures of UGT74AN3/UDP/**35**, UGT74AN3/UDP/**36**, UGT74AN3/UDP/**38**, UGT74AN3/UDP/**40**, and UGT74AN3/UDP/**42**. Structure-based mutant design of T145V achieves a shift in the preference of UGT74AN3 for sugar donors from UDP - Glc to UDP - Xyl. Crystal structures of the UGT74AN3 complexes revealed a broad U-type substrate binding pocket as the structural basis for its promiscuity of catalytic function. The structural comparisons revealed that the key residues E85 and F193 near the entrance of the substrate binding pocket likely play critical roles as gatekeepers during the entry/exit of the substrate. Meanwhile, a rare substrate binding mode of CTs was captured in the ternary structure of UGT74AN3. MD simulations and binding free energy calculations explain the formation of the unique binding poses of the CTs, and they reveal the possible mechanisms of processing the CTs by moving and flipping them in the UGT74AN3 pocket to complete the reaction. These findings enrich the structural information on plant UGTs and provide new insights into the understanding of the catalytic process of plant promiscuous UGTs. Finally, UGT74AN3 was successfully coupled with the sucrose synthase *At*SuSy to set up a UDP-Glc biorecycling glycosylation system, which was further validated using various NPs as the substrates for its catalytic and cost efficiency. These results provide a basis for structural and functional studies of promiscuous plant UGTs and establish an efficient, economical, and green enzymatic strategy for the preparation of valuable glycosides, which has important theoretical and application values.

## 4 EXPERIMENTAL SECTION

4.1 Chemicals and Reagents. All of the substrates used in this study were purchased from Aladdin Biochemical Corporation (Shanghai, China), YuanYe Biotechnology (Shanghai, China), and Chengguang Biotechnology (Baoji, China). UDP-Glc, ADP-Glc, GDP-Glc, UDP-Gal, UDP-Xyl, UDP-GlcA, UDP-GalA, UDP-GlcNAc, UDP-GalNAc, GDP-Man, UDP-L-Rha, and GDP-L-Fuc were purchased from Angfei Biotechnology (Guangzhou, China). All crystallization reagents were purchased from Hampton Research (Laguna Niguel, CA, USA). Acetonitrile and formic acid of HPLC grade were purchased from Thermo Fisher Scientific (Waltham, MA, USA). Phanta Max Super-Fidelity DNA Polymerase was purchased from Vazyme Biotechnology (Nanjing, China). *Dpn*I, *Hin*dIII, and *Nde*I were purchased from Takara Biotechnology (Japan). DMSO-$d_6$ and methol-$d_4$ were purchased from Energy Chemistry (Anhui, China). All NMR spectra of purified glycosylation products in this study were recorded using a Bruker Avance III-600 NMR spectrometer (Bruker, Billerica, MA, USA). All other chemicals and reagents were purchased from Sigma-Aldrich (St. Louis, MO, USA) unless otherwise specified.

4.2 Expression and Purification of UGT74AN3 and Mutants. The recombinant plasmid of pET28a-UGT74AN3 was constructed previously for the expression of the full-length protein. For crystallization purposes, the construct of pET28a-UGT74AN3$_{11\text{-}474}$ was obtained for the expression of a truncated protein with the N-terminal first ten amino acids removed. Expression and purification of UGT74AN3 and UGT74AN3$_{11\text{-}474}$ followed the methods reported in our previous work. All proteins were concentrated to 5 mg/mL using Amicon Ultra-30k (Millipore, USA), flash-frozen in liquid nitrogen, and kept at −80 ℃ for future use. The site-directed mutagenesis of *UGT74AN3* was performed by the polymerase chain reaction (PCR) amplification with designed primers (Table S3) using the wild-type pET28a-UGT74AN3 plasmid as the template, followed by the *Dpn*I digestion of the template DNA. The PCR products were then transformed into *Escherichia coli* DH5a, and the *UGT74AN3* mutations were confirmed by plasmid sequencing.

4.3 Cloning, Expression, and Purification of *At*SuSy. The coding region of *At*SuSy (NP_192137.1) was amplified from the cDNA of *A. thaliana* using the gene-specific primers (Table S1) and subsequently cloned into the pET28a vector with an N-terminal hexa-His tag. The recombinant plasmid of pET28a-*At*SuSy was transformed into *E. coli* Rosetta (DE3) for protein expression. Some colonies were picked and inoculated into 80 mL of LB medium containing 50 μg/mL kanamycin grown at 37 ℃ and 220 rpm overnight. The cultures were transferred into 8 L of LB medium with 50 μg/mL kanamycin at 37 ℃ and 220 rpm until the $OD_{600}$ reached 0.6. The protein expression was then induced with 0.2 mmol/L IPTG at 16 ℃, 180 rpm for 20 h. The cell pellets were harvested by centrifugation at 6 000 rpm for 10 min and resuspended in 100 mL of lysis buffer (20 mmol/L Tris-HCl pH 8.0, 150 mmol/L NaCl, 10% glycerol). The cells were disrupted by an EmulsiFlex-C3 high-pressure homogenizer, and the supernatant containing the target protein was obtained by centrifugation at 12,000 rpm for 45 min at 4 ℃. The supernatant was then loaded onto the pre-equilibrated Ni-NTA column, washed with 10 CV washing buffer (20 mmol/L Tris-HCl pH 8.0, 150 mmol/L NaCl, 20 mmol/L imidazole, 10% glycerol), and eluted in the elution buffer (20 mmol/L Tris-HCl pH 8.0, 150 mmol/L NaCl, 150 mmol/L imidazole, and 10% glycerol). The fractions containing target protein were collected and concentrated to ~2 mL using an Amicon Ultra-50k centrifugal filter. The target protein was further purified by size-exclusion chromatography using a Superdex 200 Increase 10/300 GL column (GE Healthcare) in the stock buffer (20 mmol/L Tris-HCl pH 8.0, 150 mmol/L NaCl, 5% glycerol). The purified recombinant protein of *At*SuSy was concentrated to 5 mg/mL and stored at −80 ℃.

4.4 Enzyme Activity Assay of UGT74AN3. To explore the substrate promiscuity of UGT74AN3, different sugar acceptors (**1**-**92**) were tested. The glycosylation reactions were performed in a final volume of 100 μL, containing 50 mmol/L Tris-HCl buffer (pH 8.0), 1 mmol/L acceptors, 4 mmol/L UDP-sugar, and 25 μg of purified UGT74AN3. The reactions were incubated at 37 ℃ for 2 h and then terminated by adding 100 μL of ice-cold methanol. To investigate the sugar donor specificity of UGT74AN3, diverse sugar donors were tested using kaempferol (**8**), formononetin (**23**), resibufogenin (**35**), and arctiin (**70**) as the substrates, respectively. All the reaction supernatants were collected by centrifugation at 12,000*g* for 30 min, then filtered through a 0.45 μm microporous membrane, and subjected to the HPLC and LC-MS analysis.

4.5 Preparative-Scale Reactions. A semipreparative scale reaction was performed at 37 ℃ for 2 h in a final volume of 25 mL containing 50 mmol/L Tris-HCl (pH 8.0), 1 mmol/L aglycones (dissolved in DMSO), 4 mmol/L UDP-Glc, and 250 μg/mL purified UGT74AN3. The glycosylation reaction was stopped by adding 50 mL of methanol and then centrifuged at 12 000*g* for 30 min. The glycosylated products were purified using a Shimadzu-LC-20AT HPLC system coupled with a reverse-phase COSMOSIL 5C18-MS-II (250 mm × 10 mm, 5 μm) and characterized by HR-ESI-MS and nuclear magnetic resonance (NMR) spectroscopy.

4.6 Crystallization, Data Collection, and Structure Determination. The purified truncated UGT74AN3 (5 mg/mL) was incubated with 2.5 mmol/L UDP at 4 ℃ for 30 min before the setup of crystallization trays. The crystals of UGT74AN3/UDP were observed within 3-4 d using the hanging drop vapor diffusion method by mixing 0.6 μL of protein with 0.6 μL of the reservoir solution [0.2 mol/L potassium nitrate, 0.1 mol/L Hepes (pH 7.0), and 28% (w/v) PEG 2 000 MME] at 18 ℃. The crystals of UGT74AN3/UDP/substrates (**35**, **36**, **38**, **40**, and **42**) were obtained by soaking the UGT74AN3/UDP crystals with 2 mmol/L substrates in the mother liquor for 24 h. Crystals of UGT74AN3-UDP-**35**_No_Tris were obtained after several attempts by replacing all of the Tris in the purification and crystallization processes with Hepes. All crystals were harvested in the same reservoir solution supplemented with 20% glycerol as the cryoprotectant and flash-frozen in liquid nitrogen. The X-ray diffraction data sets were collected on the beamlines 19U1 at the Shanghai Synchrotron Radiation Facility (SSRF). The diffraction images were processed using XDS. The structure of UGT74AN3/UDP was solved by molecular replacement using Phenix. The structure of UGT74AN2, a steroid glycosyltransferase from *Calotropis gigantea* (PDB code: 7W09, 59% sequence identity with UGT74AN3), was used as the searching model. The model of UGT74AN3/UDP was built initially using AutoBuild and manually using Coot. The iterative refinement and structure validation were done using Phenix. Structural visualization analysis was performed using the protein-ligand interaction profiler and PyMOL (the PyMOL Molecular Graphics System, Version 2.0 Schrödinger, LLC).

4.7 Kinetic Studies of UGT74AN3. An assay containing 50 mmol/L Tris-HCl (pH 7.8), 2.4 μg of purified UGT74AN3, 10 mmol/L saturating UDP-Glc, and varying concentrations of the substrate (2.5-640 μmol/L) was conducted in a final volume of 100 μL. The reactions were incubated at pH 8.0 and 35 ℃ 10 min. The reactions were quenched, centrifuged, and analyzed by HPLC as described above. The $K_M$ values were calculated by following the Lineweaver-Burk plot method.

4.8 Molecular Dynamics System Preparation. The initial structures of UGT74AN3 were prepared using the Protein-Preparation-Wizard module of the Schrödinger Suite (version 2021-4) by adding hydrogen atoms and assigning proper types to atoms and bonds. According to the PROPKA3 prediction and protein environment, histidine 14, 31, 78, 134, 156, and 401 were double protonated, while H25 and the resting histidine residues (H358 and H367) were protonated at the δ- and ε-positions, respectively. The missing loops in the solved crystal structures of UGT74AN3 were modeled by the Prime homology modeling module. UDP-Glc was modeled by using the coordinates from the prealigned UGT74AN2/UDP-Glc structure (PDB code: 7W1H). Accordingly, a new complex with a manually adjusted conformation orienting the 3-OH close to H25 was prepared, which is named the "Nac" (near-attacked) conformation.

4.9 Molecular Dynamics Simulations. The MD simulations for the UGT74AN3/UDP/**35**, UGT74AN3/UDP/**35**-Nac, and UGT74AN3/UDP-Glc/**35** systems were carried out using the Desmond MD package (implemented in Schrödinger Suite, version 2021-4) with the OPLS4 force field for all the atoms. A 10.0 Å buffering area to the protein-ligand complex was used for solvating the system with about 15,480 TIP3P water molecules. Counter ions ($Na^+/Cl^-$) were placed into the solvent to neutralize and increase the salt concentration to 0.15 mol/L. The Nose-Hoover chain thermostat and Martyna-Tobias-Klein barostat were used for maintaining of temperature (~303.15 K) and pressure (1.0 atm). System is energy-minimized and equilibrated using the default procedures before the 1 μs production simulation. VMD (visual molecular dynamics, version 1.9.4-a55) and the in-house python scripts were used to analysis the simulation results.

4.10 Binding Free Energy Calculations. The MM/GBSA (molecular mechanics, the generalized Born model, and solvent accessibility) binding free energies were calculated by the Prime module with the OPLS4 force field and the VSGB (variable dielectric surface generalized Born) solvent model. The final binding free energies were averaged from 200 snapshots evenly extracted from the 400-500 ns trajectories. Per-residue contributions to the total MM/GBSA binding free energies were calculated using the in-house python script.

4.11 Metadynamics Simulation. The movement of **35** was sampled with a metadynamics simulation. To trace conformational change, the distance between HE2 of H25 and the O3 of **35** [*d*(O3@**35**-HE2@H25)], as well as the distance between the C-**24** carbonyl of **35** and the HE2 of H25 [*d*(O24@**35**-HE2@H25)] were defined as two independent collective variables (CVs). The grid's boundary was set to 2.0 Å (lower boundary) and 14.0 Å (upper boundary), and the grid width was set to 0.2 Å. The hill weight and hill width were set to 0.01 and 1.0, respectively.

Metadynamics simulations were performed using NAMD 2.

4.12 UDP - Glc-free Glycosylation Reaction of UGT74AN3. A cascade reaction system was established by coupling UGT74AN3 with *At*SuSy in a total volume of 100 μL, containing 50 mmol/L Tris-HCl (pH 8.0), 1 mmol/L acceptor, 750 mmol/L sucrose, 0.25 mmol/L UDP, 3 μmol/L purified UGT74AN3, and 1 μmol/L purified *At*SuSy. The reaction was conducted at 37 ℃ for 6 h and then stopped by adding 200 μL of methanol. The supernatants were collected by centrifugation at 12,000 *g* for 30 min and analyzed by HPLC - MS.

4.13 HPLC and LC - MS Analysis. The HPLC analysis was performed on the Shimadzu - LC - 20AT (Japan) with an Ultimate XB - C18 column (4.6 mm × 250 mm I.D., 5 μm, Welch Materials, Inc., China) at a flow rate of 0.8 mL/min, using the mobile phase of (A) 0.1% formic acid in deionized $H_2O$ and (B) 100% $CH_3CN$. The gradient settings for separating the glycosylated products and substrates were 0 - 20 min 10 to 100% B, 20 - 25 min 100 to 100% B, 25 - 28 min 100 to 10% B, and 28 - 35 min 10 to 10% B. The glycosylated products were further confirmed by the LTQ XL Orbitrap mass spectrometer (Thermo Fisher Scientific Inc.) The MS/MS analysis was carried out in the positive ionization mode with 35% relative collision energy. The percentage conversion rate was determined by HPLC and calculated by dividing the integrated peak area of the glycosylated product by the sum of the peak areas of the glycosylated product and the remaining substrate. The relative percentage conversion rate was determined by the percentage conversion rate of mutant dividing the percentage conversion rate of WT. All experiments were performed in triplicate.

[黄伟,龙凤,等. ACS Catalysis, 2024,14:475 - 488.]

# A chromosome-level genome assembly reveals that a bipartite gene cluster formed via an inverted duplication controls monoterpenoid biosynthesis in *Schizonepeta tenuifolia*

## 1 INTRODUCTION

Plants interact with their environment through the production, sequestration, and emission of organic molecules. Specialized metabolites are taxon restricted and can vary both between and within species, with potential roles in ecological adaptation. For a subset of metabolite pathways, genes encoding biosynthetic enzymes can be found in biosynthetic gene clusters (BGCs), genomic regions where multiple non-homologous pathway genes are adjacent. BGCs may persist due to enhanced co-regulation of clustered pathways, or due to the suppression of recombination that could unlink a polygenic trait, or some combination of the two. The explanation as to why certain pathways are in BGCs, whereas some are not, remains unclear, as does their specific contribution to the remarkable variation of plant chemistry. Practically, BGCs can aid in the discovery of biosynthetic enzymes that can have use for synthetic biology and biocatalysis.

Highly aromatic plants gain their specific odor through the accumulation and emission of volatile terpenoids, often 10-carbon monoterpenoids. These compounds have ecological roles in repelling herbivores and attracting pollinators, and are major components of commercially available fragrances and flavors. Many monoterpenoids are bioactive, which is reflected in the traditional medicinal use of aromatic plants and in the use of purified monoterpenes in pharmaceutical formulations. Elucidation of monoterpenoid pathways and identification of their constituent enzymes can provide access to valuable compounds and feedstocks via plant-based, biocatalytic, and synthetic biology approaches.

Members of the mint family (Lamiaceae), especially those from the large subclade (same to traditional subfamily) Nepetoideae, are rich in monoterpenes, and include many culinary and medicinal herbs, and plants harvested for their essential oils. These include the medicinal herb *Schizonepeta tenuifolia* (Benth.) Briq. (Japanese catnip), which is native to China, Korea, and Japan, and is used in traditional medicine for its proposed immunomodulatory, anti-inflammatory, and anti-viral properties. The major component in its essential oil is pulegone, a monoterpene with a *p*-menthane structure (Figure 1A).

Plants from the closely related genus *Mentha* also produce *p*-menthane compounds, though in the opposite enantiomeric series (Figure 1A). This stereochemical divergence is caused by the selectivity of the initial limonene synthase (LS) catalyzed step: LSs from *Mentha* spp. produce (−)-limonene, whereas LS from *S. tenuifolia* produces (+)-limonene. Recently, a transcriptome for *S. tenuifolia* has enabled identification and characterization of downstream

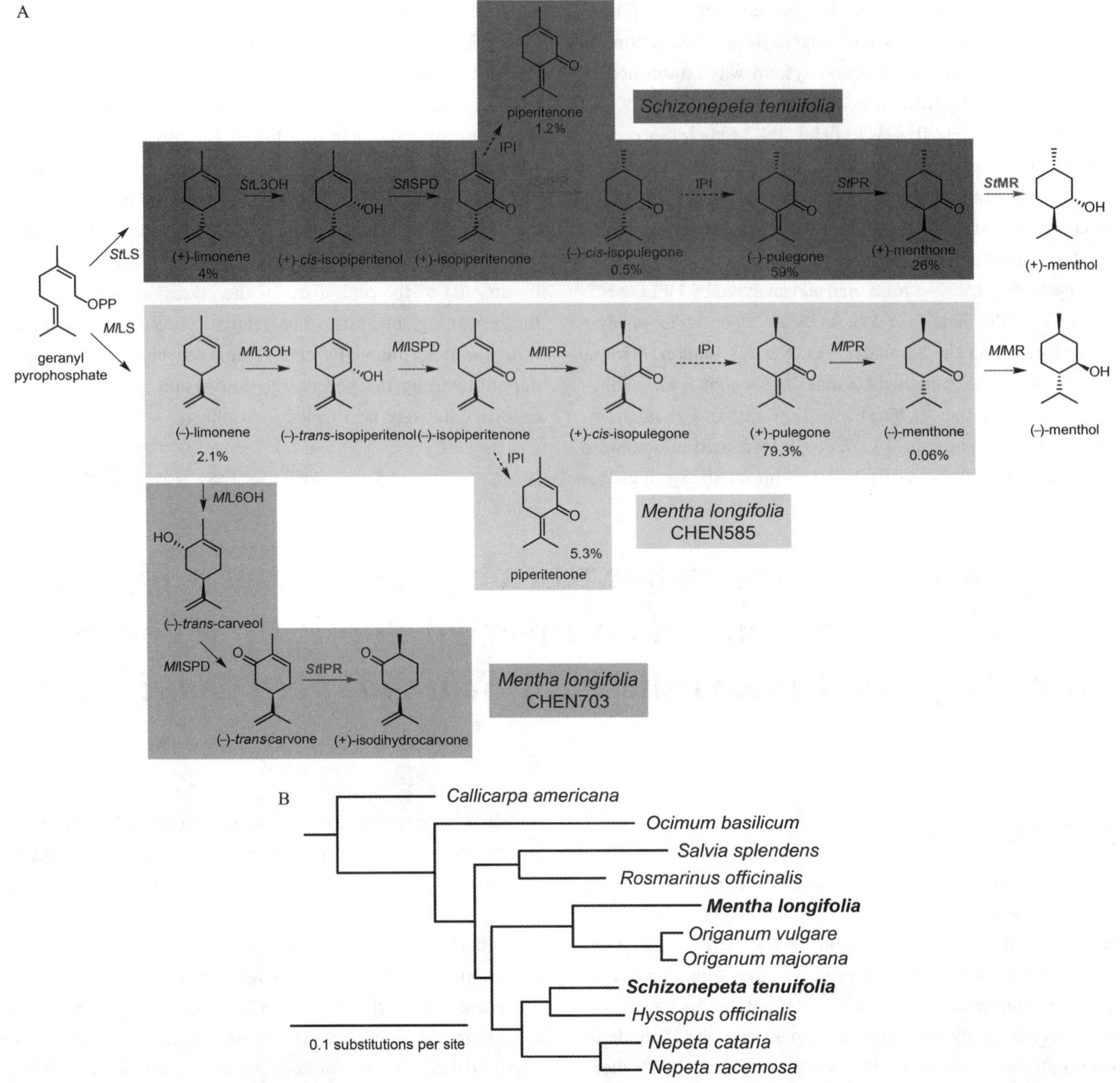


**Figure 1 Monoterpene biosynthesis in *Schizonepeta tenuifolia***

(A) Overview of *p*-menthane monoterpene structures and their biosynthesis in *S. tenuifolia* and *Mentha longifolia*. The boxes indicate *p*-menthane biosynthesis in *S. tenuifolia* and *M. longifolia* CHEN585 and CHEN703 varietals. Percentages under *S. tenuifolia* compounds represent relative abundance in essential oil, those under *M. longifolia* compounds represent relative abundance of monoterpenoid content. Dotted arrow indicates the reaction is unknown. Red text/arrows are reactions described for the first time in this manuscript. LS, limonene synthase; L3OH, limonene 3-hydroxylase; L6OH, limonene-6-hydroxylase; ISPD, isopiperitenone dehydrogenase; IPR, isopiperitenone reductase; PR, pulegone reductase; MR, menthone reductase. (B) Maximum likelihood species tree of selected mint family species in the Nepetoideae, with *Callicarpa americana* used as a non-Nepetoideae outgroup. Tree inference was based on a supermatrix alignment of single-copy genes and was inferred using iQ-Tree. All branches show 100% support as judged by 1 000X SH-aLRT and UltraFast Boostrapping replicates.

enzymes active in *p*-menthane biosynthesis through comparison with well characterized *Mentha* enzymes. For known steps in the *Mentha* pathway up to menthone, a closely related homolog was identified in *S. tenuifolia* and shown to be active. The exception to this is isopulegone isomerase, which is unknown in both pathways, and isopiperitenone reductase (IPR), which is described in *Mentha* but no active homolog could be identified in *S. tenuifolia* transcriptomes.

In this work, we set out to elucidate the genetic, genomic, and enzymatic basis for *p*-menthane biosynthesis in *S. tenuifolia*. We assembled a chromosome-scale genome that revealed a monoterpenoid BGC with a unique bipartite structure. In addition to known pathway genes, this BGC contains genes encoding the missing IPR. This old yellow enzyme (OYE) evolved convergently to the short chain reductase that catalyzes the equivalent step in *Mentha* spp. Comparison with related species' genomes showed that the BGC was assembled uniquely in the *S. tenuifolia* lineage through recruitment of genes into a region enriched in monoterpene synthases, and later gained its unique bipartite structure via a duplication-inversion event. This work provides an example of gene discovery through BGCs and highlights how phylogenomic analysis can reveal the origins of BGCs in dynamic genomic neighborhoods.

## 2 RESULTS

*Schizonepeta tenuifolia* genome, phylogenetic placement, and ancient whole-genome duplication To obtain an *S. tenuifolia* genome assembly, we combined PacBio (80.68 Gb), DNBSEQ (67.57 Gb), and Hi-C sequencing reads (102.96 Gb) into a 762 Mb (contig N50 length = 1.37 Mb, scaffold N50 length = 101 Mb) assembly, of which 696 Mb were mapped onto six pseudomolecules (Supplemental Figure 1 and Supplemental Tables 1, 2, and 3). A total of 30 283 protein-coding genes supported by the Illumina RNA-seq reads was annotated, and 91% of these were functionally annotated (Supplemental Table 4). The BUSCO score, which assesses genome completeness, was 94.5% (Supplemental Table 5).

*S. tenuifolia* is considered synonymous to *Nepeta tenuifolia* Benth. by some sources. As an understanding of the phylogenetic placement of species is important for effective interpretation of comparative genomic analysis, we set out to confirm the phylogenetic placement of *S. tenuifolia* within Lamiaceae, especially its relationship to species of *Nepeta* L. To do this, we inferred a molecular phylogeny using a set of species that had high-quality, well-annotated genomes. We only included species from Nepetoideae, except *Callicarpa americana* L., an early diverging lineage within Lamiaceae, which acted as an outgroup. *Schizonepeta tenuifolia* was recovered as a sister to *Hyssopus officinalis* L., which together were sister to two *Nepeta* spp. (Figure 1B). This topology supports previous morphology- and DNA-based phylogenetic results that placed *Schizonepeta* within Nepetinae but not within *Nepeta*. Thus, until contrary phylogenetic evidence based on broader sampling within *Nepetinae* becomes available, we recognize *S. tenuifolia* as a distinct lineage and, for convenience, use the name proposed by Briquet (1896) to distinguish this taxon from other species recognized within *Nepeta*.

Given the widespread but asymmetrical levels of gene duplication and ancient whole-genome duplication (WGD) (polyploidy) reported in Lamiaceae and their potential impacts on chemical evolution, we investigated ancient WGDs in Nepetinae using the newly available genomes for *S. tenuifolia* and three additional species (i.e., *H. officinalis*, *Nepeta cataria* L., *N. racemosa* Lam. subsp. *racemosa*. [syn. *N. mussinii* Spreng.]). Distributions of estimates of synonymous substitutions per synonymous site ($K_S$) among pairs of paralogous sequences present in *S. tenuifolia* revealed no unique events. The four genomes showed similar patterns, each with two punctuated episodes of large-scale gene duplication characterizing putative WGDs at $K_S \simeq 0.1-0.2$ and 1 (Supplemental Figure 2 and Supplemental Table 6), respectively, corroborating previously reported estimates for Nepetinae based on transcriptome data.

Bipartite BGC for *p*-menthane biosynthesis Examination of the genome sequence revealed that certain genes encoding enzymes involved in the biosynthesis of *p*-menthane monoterpenoids were present in a bipartite BGC on chromosome 6 (Figure 2A). The cluster contains copies of genes encoding the previously characterized enzymes LS and limonene 3-hydroxylase (L3OH), as well a gene with 92% nucleotide identity (nt id) to the previously described isopiperitenol dehydrogenase (*ISPD*) (Supplemental Figures 3 - 5). The BGC features two regions separated by 260 kb. The 5′ region features *LS1* (Sch000026966) and *L3OHv1* (Sch000028184) separated by a gene annotated as 12-oxophytodienoate reductase, a member of the OYE family (Sch000024746, *OYE1v1*) (Supplemental Figure 6). Just upstream of *LS1* are two uncharacterized monoterpene synthases and two cytochrome P450s. The 3′ BGC contains *ISPD1* (Sch000027339), three intervening genes and then *L3OHv2* (Sch000028415) and *LS2* (Sch000026106), separated by two copies of *OYE* (Sch000027597, *OYE1v2*; Sch000025300, *OYE1v3*).

There is a degree of symmetry across the unusual bipartite cluster, with the *LS1* - *OYE1v1* - *L3OHv1* sequence in the 5′ region reflected in the *L3OHv2* - *OYE1v2* - *OYE1v3* - *LS2* sequence in the 3′ region. Alongside the reversal of the *LS* and *L3OH* gene order, the gene orientations are also mirrored. Furthermore, the paralogs are also remarkably similar: the *L3OH* nucleotide coding sequences are identical, as are the three copies of *OYE1*. The two *LS* paralogs have 98% nt id, with all changes occurring at the N terminus, within the first 9% of the sequence's length (Supplemental Figure 3).

To assess the possibility of an assembly error causing the unusual symmetric bipartite BGC, we re-mapped PacBio reads onto all assembled pseudomolecules, and then extracted the top 10% of the longest reads mapping to the BGC region. The mapping shows good coverage over the whole region (> 50 ×) (Figure 2B). Remarkably, the whole region is spanned by just two long reads, and the boundary between these reads has good coverage. This indicates that the BGC is not an assembly error but a real feature of the genome sequence.

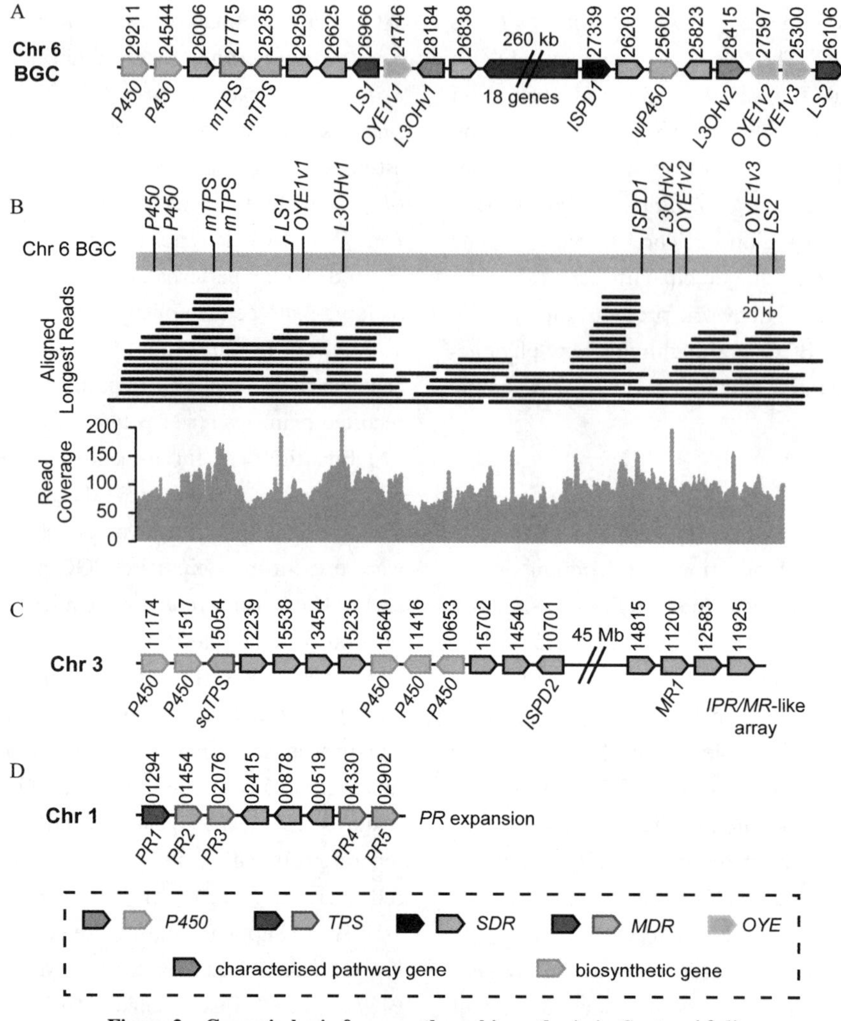


**Figure 2 Genomic basis for *p*-methane biosynthesis in *S. tenuifolia***

(**A**) Chromosome 6 bipartite biosynthetic gene cluster (BGC). Functional annotations or assigned names noted below gene symbols; gene index number noted above (with Sch0000 removed). (**B**) Re-mapped PacBio reads onto the chromosome 6 BGC to assess assembly quality. (**C**) Chromosome 3 containing biosynthetic generich region including *ISPD* and *L3OH* homologs. An *IPR*/*MR*-like array is also present. (**D**) Chromosome 1 *PR* array. Genes colored by protein family. Color outline/gray interior represents uncharacterized biosynthetic genes and color fill refers to characterized pathway genes. *ISPD*, isopiperitone dehydrogenase; *L3OH*, limonene 3-hydroxylase; *LS*, limonene synthase; *PR*, pulgeone reductase; *IPR*, isopiperitenone reductase; *MR*, menthone reductase; *P450*, Cytochrome P450; *TPS*, terpene synthase (sq, sesqui-; m, mono-); *SDR*, short-chain dehydrogenase/reductase; *MDR*, medium chain reductase; *OYE*, old yellow enzyme.

The genes contained in functional BGCs typically demonstrate coordinated expression across different tissues and treatments. Using RNA-seq, we examined gene expression across different tissues (seedlings, leaves, or roots), ages (10, 20, or 35 days), and treatments (0, 100, or 300 μmol/L methyl jasmonate). Compared with genes in the wider chromosomal region, the genes in the bipartite cluster co-express (Figure 3). This indicates that they are under similar regulatory control and are functionally related, supporting the identification of this region as a functional *p*-menthane BGC.

Biosynthetic regions outside the BGC  Genes with connection to the *p*-menthane pathway were also found in other genomic locations. Most notably, a region on chromosome 3 highly enriched in biosynthetic genes including P450s and an *ISPD* paralog (*ISPD2*, Sch000010701) (Figure 2C). Curiously, the previously characterized *StISPD* is more closely related to this chromosome 3 *ISPD2* (98% nt id) than it is to the chromosome 6 *ISPD1* (92% nt id) (Supplemental Figure 5). Another *ISPD* paralog (*ISPD3*, Sch000024019) is present on unplaced scaffold 59 and has 83% nt id with the previous reported *StISPD*.

The genome also features two arrays of reductases potentially connected to *p*-menthane biosynthesis. Chromosome 3 features a tandem array of four short-chain dehydrogenase/reductases (*SDRs*), with homology to *Mentha IPRs* and menthone/isomenthone reductases (*MR*) (Figure 2C and Supplemental Figure 7). On chromosome 1 is an array of five closely related (80% nt id) pulegone reductase (*PR*) homologs, with one of these (Sch000001294, *PR1*) being identical to the previously characterized *StPR* gene (Figure

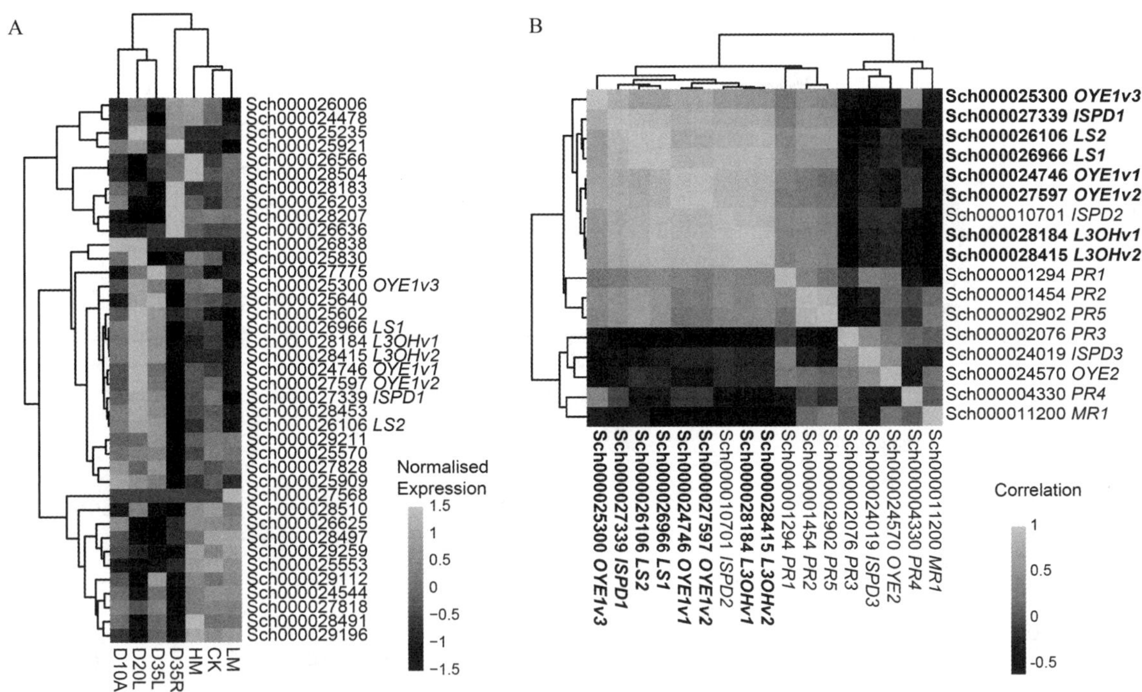


**Figure 3 Coordinated expression of $p$-menthane biosynthesis genes in BGC**

(**A**) Expression levels of genes in the chromosome 6 synteny block encapsulating the BGC region. Heatmap clustered by hierarchical clustering (relationships shown with dendrogram). Conditions: D10A, 10-day-old aerial tissues; D20L, 20-day-old leaves; D35L, 35-day-old leaves; D35R, 35-day-old roots; HM, high methyl jasmonate-treated leaves; LM, low methyl jasmonate-treated leaves; CK, untreated leaves. RNA-seq experiments conducted as biological triplicate and values averaged and normalized. (**B**) Expression correlation of $p$-menthane pathway genes and homologs. Heatmap of pairwise Pearson correlation coefficients calculated from normalized gene expression from RNA-seq experiments, clustered by hierarchical clustering (relationships shown with dendrogram). BGC genes shown in bold.

2D and Supplemental Figure 8).

Experimental validation of gene activity and function

To validate the function of the genes associated with $p$-menthane biosynthesis, we characterized them through recombinant protein assays and virus-induced gene silencing (VIGS) (Supplemental Tables 7 and 8). The two full-length LSs found encoded in the BGC were expressed in *Escherichia coli* and demonstrated limonene formation from GPP (Figure 4A). The previously described *St*LS has 99% and 97% amino acid identity with LS1 and LS2, respectively, so this result was expected. Suppressing the expression of *LS* genes using VIGS led to a significant reduction of limonene and pulegone, validating its role in the pathway (Figure 4B and Supplemental Figure 9A).

The L3OHs encoded by the BGC genes *L3OHv1* and *L3OHv2* are identical to each other and to previously characterized *St*L3OH (CYP71D544). We confirmed their activity, hydroxylation of limonene to *cis*-isopiperitenol, using yeast feeding assays (Figure 4C). VIGS targeting both *L3OH*s confirmed their role in the pathway as reduction in gene expression led to accumulation of limonene and reduction of pulegone compared with the empty vector control (Figure 4D and Supplemental Figure 9B).

The enzyme encoded by *ISPD1* (Sch000027339), was characterized using recombinant expression in *E. coli*. This enzyme was active on isopiperitenol, forming isopiperitenone in the presence of $NAD^+$ (Figure 4E). We targeted the gene expression using VIGS but were only able to knock down gene expression by around 50% (Supplemental Figure 9C). Consequently, we saw no notable changes to the concentration of the majority of compounds in the $p$-methane pathway. However, we did observe a new peak emerge in the chromatogram, corresponding to isopiperitenol, the substrate of ISPD (Figure 4F). With less ISPD present, the rate of isopiperitenol consumption appears to have decreased and it has accumulated. The combination of activity, expression, and VIGS data support that, in the specific plant investigated here, the clustered *ISPD1* is the active gene in the $p$-menthane pathway.

The PR from *S. tenuifolia*, catalyzing reduction of (−)-pulegone to (+)-menthone and (−)-isomenthone, is a member of the medium chain dehydrogenase family and has been previously characterized. On the genome, there is a tandem array of *PR* paralogs (Figure 2D and Supplemental Figure 8). We investigated their activity using recombinant expression in *E. coli*. PR1 (Sch000001294) is identical to the previously described enzyme, and was able to reduce pulegone to menthone (Supplemental Figure 10A). Enzymes encoded by the paralogous genes *PR2* (Sch000001454) and

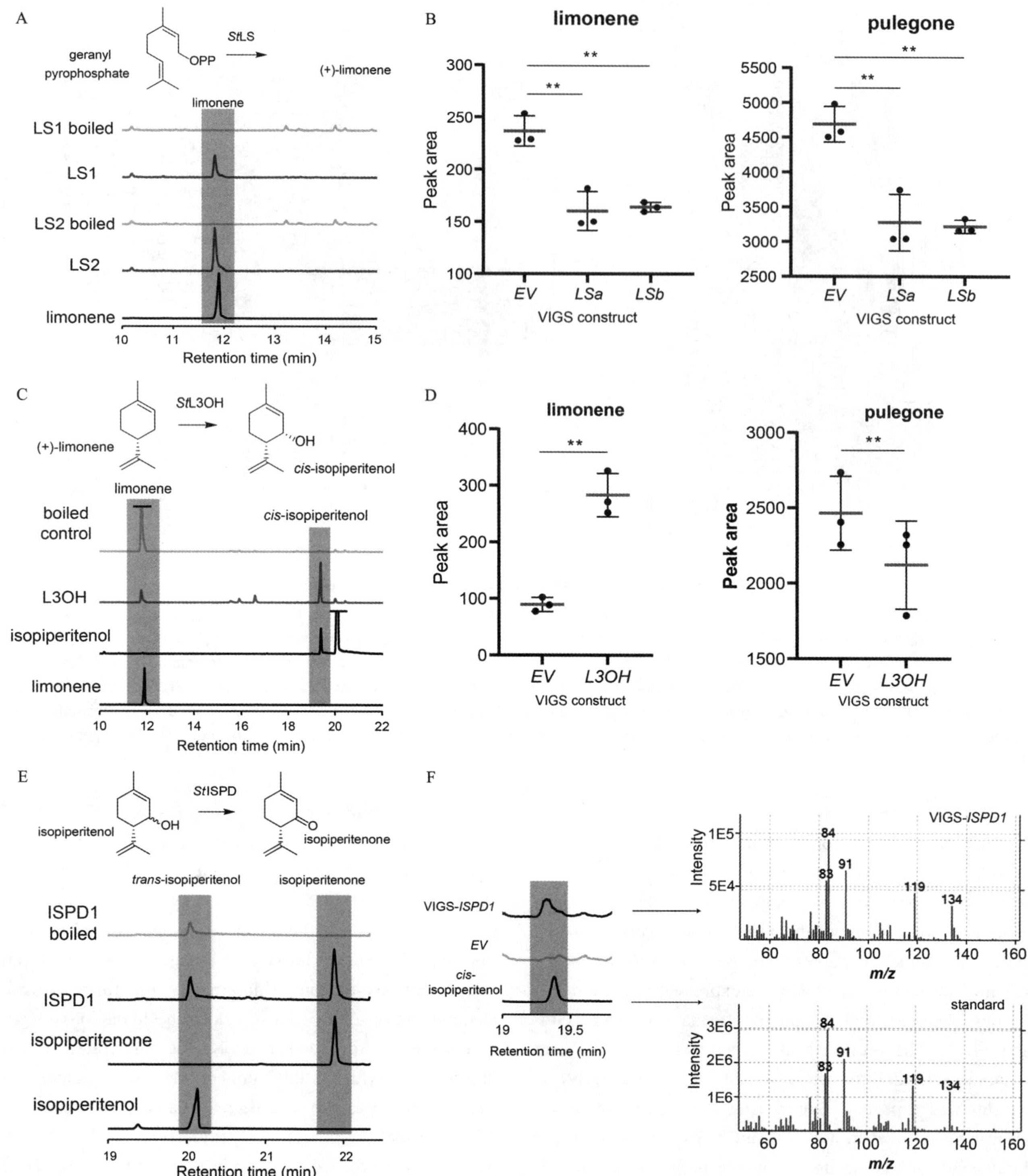


**Figure 4 Validation of biosynthetic pathway steps**

(**A**) Limonene synthase (LS) enzyme activities, converting geranyl pyrophosphate to limonene. (**B**) Metabolite content of VIGS silenced leaves measured by GC-MS. Two different regions for *LS* silencing were used (LSa and LSb). (**C**) Limonene 3-hydroxylase (L3OH) enzyme activity, converting (+)-limonene to *cis*-isopiperitenol, with additional NADPH. The isopiperitenol standard consists of two isomers, the *trans* major component, and *cis* minor component. (**D**) Metabolite content of VIGS silenced leaves with *L3OH* silencing construct. (**E**) Isopiperitenol dehydrogenase (ISPD) enzyme activity. The isopiperitenol substrate consists of a *trans* major isomer and *cis* minor isomer. $NAD^+$ was added to the reaction. (**F**) Metabolite content of leaves silenced with *ISPD* targeting construct. A peak corresponding to *cis*-isopiperitenol emerges in silenced plants. Electron impact (EI) spectrum of isopiperitenol standard (inset, bottom) matches the new peak in the VIGS-ISPD silenced plants (inset, top). Significance tests are one-tailed *t*-tests ($^*p<0.05$, $^{**}p<0.01$), EV, empty vector. qRT-PCRs to verify silencing are found in Supplemental Figure 9, and details of regions targeted in Supplemental Figures 3-5. Chromatograms of standards have been scaled for ease of comparison. All chromatogram traces are total ion chromatograms (TICs). Peak identities were verified using EI spectral matches to standards and NIST library.

*PR5* (Sch000002902) were also examined and made the same products.

In *Mentha*, the reduction of isopiperitenone to pulegone is catalyzed by IPR, a NADPH-dependent member of the SDR family. The IPRs are closely related to (−)-menthone: (+)-neomenthol dehydrogenase enzymes (MR). Unlike other pathway steps, no clear ortholog to *Mentha IPR* could be found in the *S. tenuifolia* transcriptome; searching the genome also failed to yield close orthologs. Genes homologous to *Mentha IPR/MR* were found in an array of four genes on chromosome 6, which shared 67%–88% nt id (Supplemental Figure 7). The enzyme encoded by the most highly expressed gene (*MR1*, Sch000011200) was produced recombinantly in *E. coli* and tested with NADPH and various substrates. No products could be detected with isopiperitenone or pulegone (Supplemental Figure 10B and 10C). However, the enzyme was able to reduce menthone to produce menthol, despite menthol not being a known naturally occurring compound in *S. tenuifolia* (Supplemental Figure 10D).

Discovery of an old yellow enzyme as an isopiperitenone reductase With the key candidate enzymes for IPR failing to show expected activity, we searched for other enzymes capable of catalyzing the reaction. We had noted the presence of the three identical copies of *OYE1* in the BGC. OYEs are flavin-dependent reductases known for their ability to reduce the double bond of an α,β-unsaturated carbonyl (1,4- or Michael reduction). The IPR reaction is of the same reaction class. The BGC localization and enzyme class led us to suspect that the *OYE* genes encoded the missing IPR.

We cloned *OYE1* and tested it using recombinant expression in *E. coli*. The purified enzyme was capable of reducing isopiperitenone to isopulegone in the presence of NADPH (Figure 5A). We also examined a closely related paralog, *OYE2* (Sch000024570), also on chromosome 6 but not in the cluster. The *OYE2* enzyme product has 69% amino acid identity to OYE1 and is also able to act as an IPR (Figure 5A). We also tested OYEs for activity with piperitenone, but failed to see activity (Supplemental Figure 10E), and with carvone, which was successfully turned over by OYE1 (Supplemental Figure 10F).

The function of *OYE1* paralogs in the *p*-menthane biosynthetic pathway is supported by their co-expression with other pathway genes (Figure 3). In contrast, *OYE2* does not share a similar expression pattern (Figure 3B). To further validate the *in planta* role of *OYE*s, we targeted them with VIGS silencing. We examined three VIGS constructs, one targeting *OYE1*, another targeting *OYE2*, and a hybrid construct combining both genes (Supplemental Figure 6 and Supplemental Table 8). Due to the high identity of the genes, off-target silencing was observed and the specific

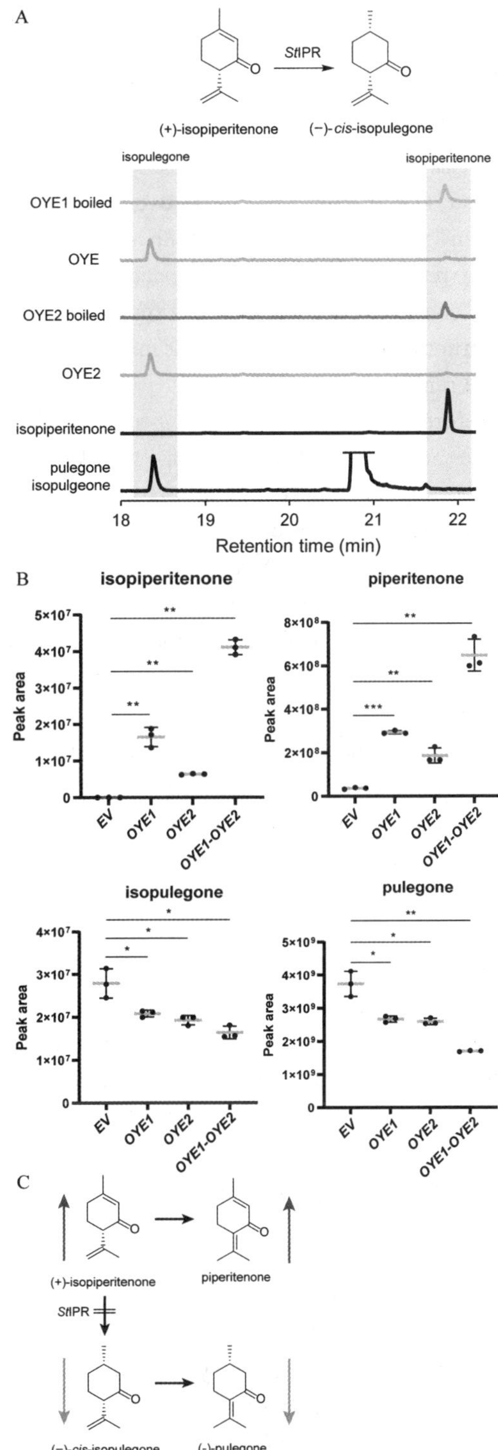


**Figure 5 Activity of the isopiperitenone reductase from *S. tenuifolia***

(**A**) IPR enzyme activity catalyzed OYEs, with addition of NADPH. Chromatograms of standards have been scaled for ease of comparison. All peak identities were verified using EI spectral matches to standards and NIST library. (**B**) Metabolite content of VIGS silenced leaves, with IPR silencing constructs. Significance tests are one-tailed *t*-tests (* $P<0.05$, ** $P<0.01$, *** $P<0.001$). EV, empty vector. qRT-PCR to verify silencing is found in Supplemental Figure 9, and details of regions targeted on Supplemental Figure 6. (**C**) Schematic of effect of VIGS silencing of IPR. When the IPR reaction is blocked the substrate and its shunt product piperitenone increases, and the product isopulegone and its downstream product pulegone decreases.

contributions of *OYE1* and *OYE2* could not be resolved with this method (Supplemental Figure 9D), although co-expression supports *OYE1*s as the active pathway genes (Figure 3). Nevertheless, with all constructs we observed an increase in isopiperitenone and a reduction in isopulegone, the substrate and the product, respectively. We also saw a decrease in pulegone, a downstream product, and an increase in piperitonone, a shunt product (Figure 5B and 5C). The combination of *in vitro*, expression, and VIGS data confirm that the OYEs act as IPRs in *S. tenuifolia*, and these were renamed accordingly.

Therefore, unlike the other *p*-menthane pathway genes, the *StIPR* is not homologous to *Mentha* genes. Instead, *Mentha* and *S. tenuifolia* have evolved an IPR enzyme convergently from different enzyme families, SDR and OYE, respectively. While convergence in plant biosynthetic pathways is not rare, it is more typically found as parallel evolution, where the enzymes originate from the same families. The result highlights the power of BGC analysis for gene discovery.

Phylogenomic analysis of the BGC and related regions

To examine the evolutionary origin of the *S. tenuifolia* BGC and *p*-menthane pathway, we compared the *S. tenuifolia* genome with other Lamiaceae genomes (Supplemental Tables 9 and 10). Synteny analysis revealed that, in other species, the region syntenic to the *S. tenuifolia* bipartite BGC contains monoterpene synthase genes (*mTPS*), including putative *LS*s, but lacks any evidence of *L3OH*, *ISPD*, and *OYE* (Figure 6A and 6B). This indicates that the *p*-menthane BGC is unique to the *S. tenuifolia* lineage, emerging in a locus already rich in monoterpene synthases. The BGC emerged in the *S. tenuifolia* lineage through the recruitment of pathway genes.

In *S. tenuifolia*, the two *LS* paralogs flank a region of approximately 300 kb, with the two parts of the BGC at either end. Compared with other genomes, this whole region is inverted in *S. tenuifolia*, with the boundaries of the inversion approximately marked by *LS1* and *LS2*. Despite some gene gain/loss within each lineage, the inversion is clearly marked by reversal of gene order and orientation in *S. tenuifolia* compared with other genomes (Figure 6A and Supplemental Figure 11). The monoterpene synthase content shows variation between species, with *H. officinalis* only having a single *mTPS* copy in the region, *N. cataria* and *Mentha longifolia* (L.) Huds. having two copies flanking the region, and *N. racemosa* containing three *mTPS*s but on one side of the syntenic region. Phylogenomic analysis of the *mTPS*s in this region shows syntenic *mTPS* orthologs are present in the early diverging Lamiaceae species, *C. americana* (Figure 6B and Supplemental Figure 11). The locus therefore appears to be a region associated with monoterpene diversity across the Lamiaceae, with variation caused by sequence changes in *mTPS*s alongside local duplications.

The *S. tenuifolia* chromosome 3 region described above (Figure 2C), which contains paralogs of *L3OH* and *ISPD*, lies on the edge of a larger region containing many *P450* and *TPS* genes (Supplemental Figure 12). This region corresponds to a diterpenoid-related BGC described in multiple Lamiaceae species. Combined phylogenetic and synteny analysis indicates that the *L3OH* paralog (CYP71) duplications in this region predate the *S. tenuifolia* lineage (Supplemental Figures 12 and 13A). For example, closely related genes are found in syntenic locations in *H. officinalis* and *N. cataria*. In contrast, no other genomes contain syntenic *ISPD* homologs, indicating that the *ISPD2* gene was introduced into this region uniquely in the *S. tenuifolia* lineage (Supplemental Figures 12 and 13B).

There is no syntenic region to the chr 3 diterpenoid BGC or *L3OH/ISPD* region in the *M. longifolia* genome. Furthermore, the *mTPS*s in the region syntenic to the *S. tenuifolia* chr 6 BGC are uncharacterized *LS*-like paralogs with 77% nucleotide identity compared with the bone fide *M. longifolia LS* (Figure 6A and 6B). Instead, the active *L3OH* and *LS* in *M. longifolia* can be found as duplicated gene pairs on chr 5 (Figure 6C), in a region that has no syntenic relationship to *S. tenuifolia* chr 6 BGC or chr 3 *L3OH/ISPD*s. The *M. longifolia LS*s therefore have originated from a dispersed duplication, which moved them from the *mTPS*/BGC syntenic region to chr 5 where they formed gene pairs (Figure 6B and 6C). Based on this it appears that the genomic association of *L3OH* and *LS* occurred independently in *S. tenuifolia* and *M. longifolia* (Figure 7). This is an unusual example of the convergent evolution of genome structures, essentially independent evolution of collinearity.

## 3 DISCUSSION

This work demonstrates how genomics can enhance our understanding of plant specialized metabolism, aiding biosynthetic gene discovery and revealing the evolutionary origins of line-age-specific pathways. While the majority of the genes in the *S. tenuifolia* pulegone pathway had previously been described based on homology to *Mentha* spp. enzymes, the *IPR* was missing. The chromosome-level *S. tenuifolia* genome assembly revealed the presence of a monoterpenoid-related BGC. Alongside the known pathway genes *LS*, *L3OH*, and *ISPD*, the cluster contained copies of a gene encoding an *OYE*. This gene, which has no homology to the *Mentha IPR* (Supplemental Figure 14), was shown to encode the missing IPR through *in vitro* (enzyme assays) and *in vivo* (VIGS) methods (Figure 5).

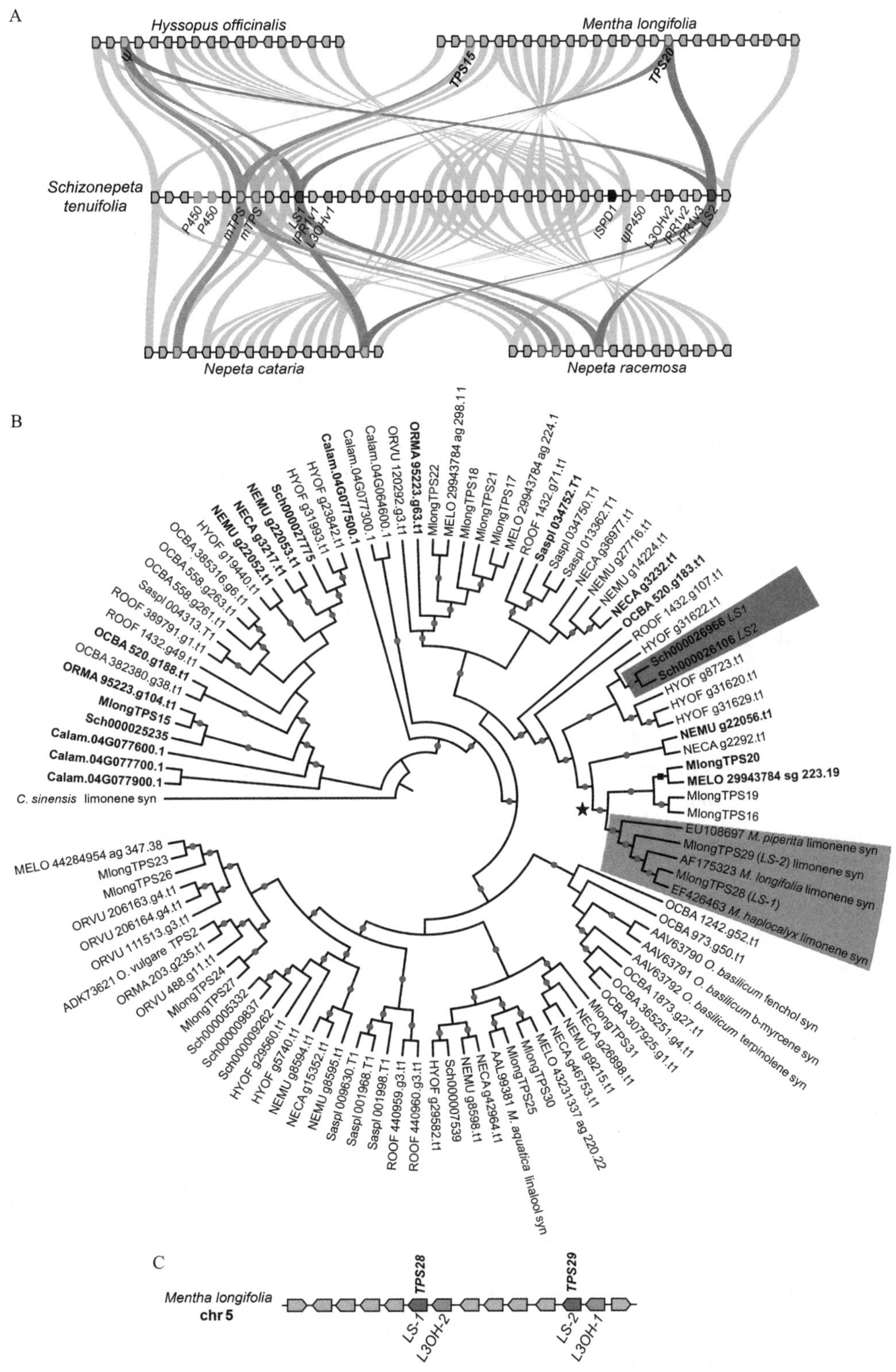


**Figure 6 Phylogenomic analysis of BGC in *S. tenuifolia***

(**A**) Syntenic analysis of BGC. Collinearity (synteny) analysis of bipartite BGC compared with other high-quality Lamiaceae genomes. Lines indicate homologous genes. Colored lines are monoterpene synthases. Gene size and space has been normalized. Note the lack of *L3OH*, *IPR*, and *ISPD* homologs in other genomes indicating unique assembly of the BGC in *S. tenuifolia*. Also, note the relative inversion of the region between the two BGC regions. (**B**) Limonene synthase maximum likelihood phylogenetic tree, depicted as a cladogram without branch lengths. All genes in chr 6 BGC syntenic region are in bold (A) and Supplemental Figure 11. The *S. tenuifolia LS* paralogs are in a colored box. The characterized *Mentha LS* genes found as gene pairs (C) are in a colored box. The star shows a dispersed duplication in *M. longifolia* leading to non-syntenic *LS*s (C). Circles show branches with >85% and >95% support as judged by 1 000X SH-aLRT and UltraFast Boostrapping replicates, respectively. See Supplemental Tables 9 and 10 for sources of genes and acronyms. (**C**) Duplicated *p*-menthane biosynthesis gene pairs in *M. longifolia* genome. These appear unique to *Mentha* spp. and therefore independently assembled compared with the *S. tenuifolia* BGC.

The presence of non-homologous IPRs in *M. longifolia* and *S. tenuifolia* is an example of convergent evolution, with the two lineages evolving enzymes from different superfamilies to catalyze the same reaction. This stands in contrast to the preceding pathway enzymes, LS, L3OH, and ISPD, which are very closely related in the two lineages (Figure 6B and Supplemental Figure 13). These enzyme pairs would be considered true orthologs if the common ancestor of *M. longifolia* and *S. tenuifolia* had a similar monoterpenoid pathway. Indeed, closely related Lamiaceae species are also rich in monoterpenoids derived from limonene, including *Agastache rugosa* (Fisch. & C. A. Mey.) Kuntze, which also produces pulegone. However, the monoterpenoid pathways in *Mentha* spp. and *S. tenuifolia* are of the opposite enantiomeric series set by LS (Figure 1A). Kinetic analysis of *p*-menthane enzymes from *Mentha* × *piperita* L. and *S. tenuifolia* indicate that they (with the exception of L3OH) are more active (i.e., higher $k_{cat}/K_m$) with the substrate enantiomers derived from their pathway. However, whether these homologs are derived from convergent, parallel, or divergent evolution has not yet been determined.

The BGC containing the first four steps of pulegone biosynthesis has an unusual bipartite structure, with the core cluster (*LS*, *L3OH*, and *IPR1*) duplicated and separated by over 260 kb. *ISPD* appears only once, indicating it is a late acquisition to the BGC, possibly occurring after the duplication. While this bipartite BGC structure has not be described previously, similar BGC structures are known. For example, split BGCs, spread over multiple loci, have been described, such as momilactone biosynthesis in rice. Large, relatively diffuse BGCs are also known, such as the 260 kb taxol-associated locus in *Taxus* genomes, sitting in a wider 72 Mb biosynthetically rich region. Duplicated BGCs have also been described in polyploids, such as the nepetalactone BGC in *N. cataria*, although these would occur on separate chromosomes.

The duplication of the *S. tenuifolia* monoterpenoid BGC appears to be relatively recent, judging by the near-identical nature of genes in the two regions (Supplemental Figures 3, 4, and 6). A BGC duplication may initially be advantageous through a dosage effect, although eventually one BGC copy may decay or diversify in a manner akin to gene duplication. While it appears that genes in both regions of the BGC co-express and contribute to *p*-menthane biosynthesis, some paralogs (i.e., *L3OH*s, *IPR1*s) are so similar it is challenging to determine the exact contribution of each specific gene using the methods employed here (VIGS, qRT-PCR, and RNA-seq). Ultimately, genome editing may be required to examine each gene specifically.

Comparisons with related genomes indicate the BGC structure arose through an inverted duplication (Figures 6A and 7). Inversions as a mechanism of BGC growth has recently been described in *Arabidopsis*. Intriguingly, chromosomal inversions are also a feature of supergenes, loci that are similar to BGCs in that they contain multiple genes contributing to a specific adaptive trait. Inversions in supergenes are proposed to be a mechanism for suppressing recombination and fixing genes in adaptive proximity.

The mechanism of the inverted duplication is unknown. Inversions can occur via ectopic recombination of homologous sequences at different loci, inverting the region between the break-points. However, this would not account for the duplication. Transposable elements (TEs) may be involved, either serving as homologous sequences for recombination breakpoints, or perhaps as active partners in the rearrangement. There are indeed plenty of both DNA and RNA TE signatures in the BGC, although it is not known if they are enriched or active in this region (Supplemental Figure 15).

The phylogenomic comparison highlights the importance of particular biosynthetic genomic "hotspot" regions across a multiple lineages and pathways. The *S. tenuifolia* BGC formed around *LS* which was present in a region enriched in *mTPS*. This region is found across the Lamiaceae and originates from a *mTPS* tandem expansion, as seen in *C. americana* (Supplemental Figures 11 and Figure 6B). Furthermore, *L3OH* and *ISPD* paralogs are found in a chr 3 region which is highly enriched in other *TPS* and *P450* genes, and where a diterpene BGC resides in closely related species (Supplemental Figure 12). The link between the chr 5 BGC and chr 3 biosynthetic region points toward genomes containing multiple biosynthetic hotspots that exchange genetic material.

In the *M. longifolia* lineage, rather than receiving genes into the *LS* locus to build a BGC, instead a *LS* has undergone a dispersed duplication into chr 5, alongside *L3OH* (Figure 6B, 6C, and 7). This *LS-L3OH* gene pair has then undergone a duplication. However, no other pathway genes are present in this locus so it cannot be strictly termed a BGC. The genomic association of *LS* and *L3OH* in *M. longifolia* and *S. tenuifolia* are independent events. This is an example of the convergent, or parallel, evolution of gene order. The convergent evolution of a BGC has previously been described, with a bryophyte and rice independently evolving a momilactone BGC.

This work highlights the role of BGCs in plant specialized meta-bolism. We identified a BGC for *p*-menthane biosynthesis in *S. tenuifolia*, enabled by a high-quality genome assembly. BGC genes' involvement in pulegone biosynthesis was verified by co-expression and VIGS. Enzyme activities were verified by re-combinant expression and enzyme assays. We discovered a missing *p*-menthane biosynthesis pathway gene in the BGC: an *IPR* from the OYE family. The BGC has an

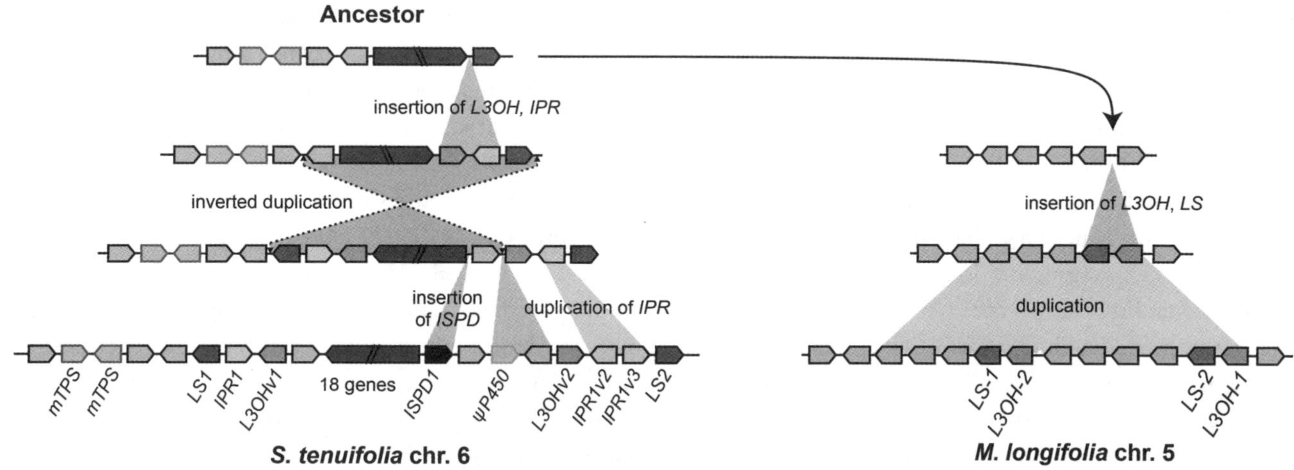


**Figure 7 Proposed evolutionary origin of *S. tenuifolia* bipartite BGC and *M. longifolia* duplicated gene pairs**

Based on the syntenic and phylogenetic analysis, we propose the origins of *p*-menthane-related genome structures in the *S. tenuifolia* and *M. longifolia* lineages. In the *S. tenuifolia* lineage, genes encoding *L3OH* (blue) and *IPR* (from old yellow enzyme family, yellow) were inserted into a region containing monoterpene synthases (red) to form a *p*-menthane BGC. An inverted duplication of the region led to its development into a bipartite BGC. Subsequently *ISPD* moved into the cluster and *IPR* underwent tandem duplication. In contrast, in the *Mentha longifolia* lineage, *LS* and *L3OH* inserted into a non-syntenic region to form a gene pair. A five-gene region containing the gene pair underwent segmental duplication.

unprecedented "bipartite" structure, which, through comparative phylogenomics, appeared to be formed through an inverted duplication. We identified two examples of convergent evolution between the *M. longifolia* and *S. tenuifolia* lineages, at the enzymatic (independent origin of IPRs) and genomic level (independent *LS* and *L3OH* associations in non-syntenic regions). The Lamiaceae (mint family), has large chemical diversity; species with cultural, medicinal and economic importance; and relatively manageable genome sizes and cultivation. This makes it an excellent model for examining metabolic evolution in plants. Such studies reveal how genomes, enzymes, and metabolism have co-evolved to provide the rich chemistry of the natural world.

## 4 METHODS

Genome assembly　The *S. tenuifolia* genome was assembled using reads from PacBio, DNBseq, and Hi-C. Details are available as supplemental methods. The BGC was identified by first finding the genes corresponding to previously described *S. tenuifolia* pathway enzymes using sequence similarity. Then, using genome position annotations (as described in the genome GFF file), the genomic position of the pathway genes, both in the context of a chromosome and relative to each other, were determined.

Chemicals　Commercially available monoterpene standards, (−)-limonene (CAS: 5989-54-8, Sigma-Aldrich), (+)-limonene (CAS: 5989-27-5, Sigma-Aldrich), (−)-pulegone (CAS: 3391-90-0, Sigma-Aldrich), (+)-pulegone (CAS: 89-82-7, Sigma-Aldrich), (−)-menthone (CAS: 14073-97-3, Sigma-Aldrich), (+)-menthone (CAS: 3391-87-5, Sigma-Aldrich), (−)-menthol (CAS: 2216-51-5, shyuanye), (+)-menthol (CAS: 25356-60-2, shyuanye), (−)-isomenthone (CAS: 18309-28-9, Toronto Research Chemicals), (+)-isomenthone (CAS: 1196-31-2, ZZSRM), and camphor (CAS: 76-22-2, Macklin) were used for annotation peak or normalization. Isopiperitenol and isopiperitenone was synthesized as described previously. D-Glucose 6-phosphate disodium salt hydrate (CAS: 3671-99-6, Solarbio), G-6PDH (CAS: 9001-40-5, shyuanye), NADPH tetrasodium salt hydrate (CAS: 2646-71-1, shyuanye), $NAD^+$ (CAS: 53-84-9, shyuanye), methanol (CAS: 67-56-1, shhuishi), n-hexane (CAS: 110-54-3, yonghuachem), D-Sorbitol (CAS: 50-70-4, shyuanye), NaCl (CAS: 50-70-4, qschem), glycerol (CAS: 56-82-5, shhuishi), and $KH_2PO_4$ (CAS: 7778-77-0, nanjingchem) were used for enzyme expression and enzyme assays.

Plant growth conditions　*S. tenuifolia* seeds were obtained from Hebei province, China. They were grown in a growth incubator under 100001× intensity and 50% humidity with 16/8 h light/dark photoperiod at 25 ℃. Plant tissues were carefully removed, immediately snap-frozen in liquid nitrogen, and stored at −80 ℃ for RNA extraction.

Gene cloning and enzyme expression　Total RNA was extracted using a FastPure Plant Total RNA Isolation Kit (Polysaccharides/Polyphenolics-rich) (Vazyme Biotech, Nanjing, China). cDNA libraries were formed from young leaf RNA using a HiScript III 1st Strand cDNA Synthesis Kit (+gDNA wiper) according to kit instructions. Single-strand cDNA was used as the template for PCR amplification of the target cDNA with 2× PrimeSTAR Max DNA Polymerase (Takara, Japan) and gene-specific primers designed based on annotated results from the transcriptome database. The PCR products were separated using the GeneJET Gel Extraction Kit (Thermo Scientific), and the purified DNA fragment was subcloned into the pCE2TA/Blunt-Zero vector (Vazyme Biotech) for sequencing. The primers and vectors used for cloning and expressing are listed in Supplemental Table 7. All cloned and subcloned genes were sequenced by Sanger Sequencing (Sangon Biotech, Shanghai, China). The gene model sequence of Sch000024570 was different to the cloned *OYE2* as it had an extended N terminus and extra inserted exon.

Single colonies were used to inoculate LB medium (5 mL) containing 100 ng/L kanamycin. The culture (1 mL) was transferred into 100 mL of the same medium and continued to grow at 37 ℃ to reach an $OD_{600}$ of approximately 1.0. Protein expression was induced by adding isopropyl β-thiogalactopyranoside to a final concentration of 1 mmol/L. After 24 h incubation at 16 ℃, the cells were harvested by centrifugation (15 min at 4 ℃ and 5 000 rpm). The cells were resuspended in 5 mL lysis buffer containing 10 mmol/L Tris-HCl (pH 8.0), 200 mmol/L NaCl, and 5% (v/v) glycerine. The suspension was transferred to an ultrasonic cell disruptor system and ultrasonically disrupted for 25 s each with 35 s on ice between disruptions. The mixture was centrifuged (30 min, 4 ℃, 12 000 rpm) and the supernatant was carefully collected as crude protein.

Then, 2 ml of Ni-NTA Sefinose (TM) Resin 6FF (C600033, BBI) was taken into a centrifuge tube, centrifuged (4 ℃, 3 000 rpm, 2 min) and the supernatant was carefully discarded. Four milliliters of Binding/Wash Buffer (10 mmol/L imidazole, NaCl, $NaH_2PO_4 \cdot 2H_2O$ [pH 7.9 - 8.1]) (C600303 - 0500, BBI) was added and shaken at 4 ℃ for 30 min to make Binding/Wash Buffer and resin completely homogenous, and the supernatant was discarded by centrifugation (4 ℃, 3 000 rpm, 2 min). The His-tagged crude protein (Sch000025300 and Sch000024570) (2 mL) was mixed with Binding/Wash Buffer (2 mL). The mixture was added to the resin and shaken at 4 ℃ for 30 min. The resin was collected by centrifugation (4 ℃, 3 000 rpm, 2 min) and supernatant removed. The pellet was washed by repeated addition of 4 mL of Binding/Wash Buffer followed by centrifugation (4 ℃, 3 000 rpm, 2 min) until the supernatant elution had an absorbance at 280 nm close to the baseline. The resin was eluted with 2 mL of Elution Buffer (250 mmol/L imidazole, NaCl, $NaH_2PO_4 \cdot 2H_2O$ [pH 7.9 - 8.1]) (C600304 - 0500, BBI), and the supernatant was collected by centrifugation (4 ℃, 3 000 rpm, 2 min). This step was repeated twice, and the supernatants were the purified enzyme protein. SDS-polyacrylamide gel electrophoresis and spectrophotometric analysis (absorbance at 280 nm) were used to check purity and approximate quantity of protein. The crude and purified enzyme protein were stored at −20 ℃ until required for further enzyme activity testing.

For eukaryotic expression of *NtL3OH*, the plasmid pYeDP60-L3OH was introduced into *Saccharomyces cerevisiae* WAT11 using a transformation kit (Frozen-EZ Yeast Transformation II Kit, Zymo Research). The empty vector was used as control. The transformation mixture was plated on SGI medium containing 20 g/L glucose, 6.7 g/L yeast nitrogen base without amino acids, 1 g/L bactocasamino acids (Difco), 15 g/L agar, and 40 mg/L DL-tryptophan. A single colony from SGI medium was grown in 50 ml of SGI liquid medium at 30 ℃ for 12 h. The cells were centrifuged at 1 630 *g* for 5 min and resuspended in SGI medium containing 20 g/L galactose. The suspension was diluted to an $OD_{600}$ of 0.4 and induced at 16 ℃ for 12 h.

Enzyme assays  For NADPH-dependent reduction reactions, the reaction (0.4 mL) consisted of buffer B (50 mmol/L $KH_2PO_4$, 10% sorbitol, 1 mmol/L DTT [pH 7.5]), containing 20 μmol/L substrate, 10 mmol/L NADPH tetrasodium salt hydrate, 6 mmol/L glucose-6-phosphate, 20 U glucose-6-phosphate dehydrogenase (Solarbio), and 50 μL protein extract. For NAD-dependent reduction reactions, 10 mmol/L NAD was used instead of NADPH, and no glucose-6-phosphate or glucose-6-phosphate dehydrogenase was added. For Sch000025300 and Sch000024570, purified enzyme was used in place of protein extract, whereas all other reductase/dehydrogenase reactions were conducted with protein lysate. n-Hexane (0.2 mL) was added on the top of the reaction solution. Reaction was carried out at 31 ℃ for 16 h with slow stirring. The reaction was terminated by placing the reaction vial at − 80 ℃ for 2 h. The upper organic phase was transferred into a new 2 ml glass vial containing a conical glass insert, which was then analyzed by GC - MS.

Activities of L3OH enzymes were determined using yeast feeding assays. Limonene solution was added to the culture to a final concentration of 0.2 mmol/L. The reaction was stopped by sonication for 15 min after 12 h incubation. The products from each reaction were extracted with 200 μL n-hexane. After the enzyme reactions, the glass vial was placed in a freezer (−80 ℃) for 2 h and the upper organic phase was transformed into a new 2 ml glass vial containing a conical glass insert (while the still frozen aqueous phase of the original glass vial was discarded). Negative controls were generated by heating the reconstitution for 5 min at 100 ℃.

GC - MS and chiral-GC method  Gas chromatography-mass spectrometry (GC - MS) was performed using a 6890N GC interfaced with 5973 inert MS instrument (Agilent Technologies, Santa Clara, CA) and chromatographic column (Agilent, 19091S - 433 - HP - 5 ms, 30 m × 250 μm ×

0.25 μm). Helium was used as the carrier gas at a linear velocity of 1.2 mL/min. The injector temperature was kept at 220 ℃. Mass spectra were recorded in electron impact ionization mode at 70 eV. The quadrupole mass detector, ion source, and transfer line temperatures were set, respectively, at 150 ℃, 230 ℃, and 280 ℃. The MS was selected ion monitoring mode was used for the identification and quantification of analytes. The GC - MS procedure for enzyme assays was maintained at 50 ℃ for 3 min, elevated to 90 ℃ at 3 ℃/min, and then raised to 150 ℃ at 5 ℃/min. The injection volume was 1.0 μL and splitless. The GC - MS procedure for VIGS was maintained at 50 ℃ for 3 min, elevated to 90 ℃ at 3 ℃/min, then raised to 150 ℃ at 5 ℃/min, and raised to 220 ℃ at 10 ℃/min, and maintained at 220 ℃ for 5 min. The injection volume was 1.0 μl and splitless.

VIGS assay Fragments of open reading frames encoding *S. tenuifolia* phytoene desaturase (460 bp) were amplified with PrimeSTAR Max DNA Polymerase. The target genes were similarly amplified from *S. tenuifolia* cDNA and inserted in pTRV2 vector at EcoRI and SacI sites with a ClonExpress II One Step Cloning Kit (https://www.vazyme.com/product/81.html). The plasmid was transformed into *E. coli* DH5a (Vazyme Biotech). The recombinant plasmid was purified using a GeneJET Plasmid Miniprep Kit and verified by sequencing, using pTRV2 vector-specific primers (Supplemental Table 8). The vectors pTRV1 and pTRV2 target genes were introduced into the Agrobacterium strain *GV3101*, and resuspended in infiltration medium (10 mmol/L $MgCl_2$, 10 mmol/L MES, 200 μmol/L acetosyringone) and adjusted to an $OD_{600}$ of 1.0. Strains harboring pTRV2 constructs were then mixed in a 1 : 1 ratio with strains harboring pTRV1 with dark activation at room temperature for 3 h and then injected into the cotyledons of 30 10-day-old *S. tenuifolia* seedlings. The plants were placed in the dark for 24 h and then incubated at 25 ℃ with a 16 h/8 h light/dark cycle. As experimental controls, the empty vectors pTRV1 and pTRV2 were injected. The *phytoene desaturase* gene was used as a marker of the silencing effect. At about 3 weeks post-injection, the leaves were collected for analysis. Transformants were screened by PCR with the pTRV2 vector-specific primers to ensure that the cultures contained the expected construct. Then, the metabolites were extracted with 2 mL n-hexane including camphor as an internal standard (final concentration at 30 ng/μL) from 0.2 g fresh leaves, after leaf samples were frozen in liquid nitrogen and pulverized with a tissue grinder. VIGS experiments were conducted with three biological replicates for initial screening experiments.

Gene expression and essential oil measurement RNA samples were extracted using a FastPure Plant Total RNA Isolation Kit (Polysaccharides/Polyphenolics-rich) (Vazyme Biotech), and aliquots of 0.5 μg of total RNA were used in reverse transcriptase reactions with the HiScript III 1st Stand cDNA Synthesis Kit (+gDNA wiper) (Vazyme Biotech). The qRT-PCR reactions were performed in triplicate on a QuantStudio 3 Real-Time PCR Systems (Thermo Fisher Scientific, Waltham, MA) using ChamQ Universal SYBR qPCR (Vazyme Biotech). *St*Actin was the reference gene, and the relative expression levels are $2^{-\Delta Ct}$ values of target compared with actin, and then normalized to the average value of empty vector negative control. All the primers used in the qRT - PCR are listed in Supplemental Table 8. Metabolite identification was achieved by comparison with the chromatographic retention and electron impact mass spectrum characteristics of authentic standards. The peak areas of the compounds were corrected by internal standard and then the relative content of the substance can be calculated. Three biological repeats were measured for each sample and significant differences were determined by one-tailed *t*-tests.

RNA extraction, sequencing, and expression analyses Arial tissue of 10-day-old seedlings, leaves of 20-day-old plants, leaves and roots of 35-day-old plants, and leaves treated with methyl jasmonate (0, 100, and 300 μmol/L) were collected and frozen in liquid nitrogen. Total RNA was extracted from different tissues using TRIzol reagent (Sigma). Sequencing libraries were generated using a NEBNext Ultra RNA Library Prep Kit for Illumina (NEB) following the manufacturer's recommendations and index codes were added to attribute sequences to each sample, in which the mRNA was purified from total RNA using poly-T oligo-attached magnetic beads, and PCR products were purified (AMPure XP system) and library quality was assessed on the Agilent Bioanalyzer 2100 system. The clustering of the index-coded samples was performed on a cBot Cluster Generation System using TruSeq PE Cluster Kit v3-cBot-HS (Illumina). After cluster generation, the library preparations were sequenced on an Illumina HiSeq platform and paired-end reads were generated.

Adapters and low-quality reads were removed from the raw reads followed by quality assessment using FastQC (https://www.bioinformatics.babraham.ac.uk/projects/fastqc/). Reads were aligned using STAR v2.7.10a with the number of reads counted using the "quantMode" option. MultiQC was used to assess the quality of the STAR alignments. Reads per gene count (counts for unstranded RNA-seq) were concatenated into a single matrix and genes with no expression removed. The DESeq2 (release 3.15) R package was used to normalize the counts data based on library size followed by variance stabilization. Co-expression analyses were performed using the CoExpNetViz application within Cytoscape v3.9.1 and GraphBio.

Syntenic relationships  Interspecies syntenic blocks were identified using the mcscan pipeline of the JCVI suite. Pairwise orthologs to *S. tenuifolia* were identified in full mode using default settings. Macrosyntenic blocks were identified using the default settings. Microsyntenic regions were identified using default settings with a maximum of six iterations to ensure that possible genome duplications were identified.

Orthogroups, single-copy gene discovery, and phylogenetics  Orthogroups were identified with OrthoFinder using the protein sequences accompanied with each of the genomes. Where protein sequences were not provided, the CDS regions were extracted from the genome sequences using available GFF annotations. Exonic regions were concatenated and the longest ORF translated using Geneious Prime. Single-copy genes were identified with MarkerMiner v1.2 using default settings and the *A. thaliana* reference. Codon alignments of GOIs and nucleotide alignments of single-copy genes were performed using MAFFT L-INS-i. Alignments were iteratively curated and initial trees inferred using FastTree in Geneious Prime. Gaps were removed for single-copy alignments using trimAl and individual alignments concatenated into a supermatrix. Maximum likelihood trees were inferred using IQ-Tree 2 with ModelFinder, ultrafast bootstraps (UFBoot2, X1000), and SH-aLRT supports (X1000). Partitioning was performed for the single-copy supermatrix. Gene trees were visualized using iTOL 6.3.2.

Ancient WGSs  Ancient WGD events were inferred from estimates of divergence at synonymous sites ($K_S$) among paralogous gene pairs present in the genomes of *S. tenuifolia*, *H. officinalis*, *N. cataria*, and *N. racemosa*. The DupPipe pipeline was used with its default settings to analyze coding sequences representing the longest isoforms of genes filtered from high-confidence (HC) gene sets. For *S. tenuifolia*, the HC gene set included coding sequences representing the longest open reading frames predicted by TransDecoder that had detectable expression and an InterProScan annotation. For the remaining genomes, coding sequences representing the longest isoform of each gene were filtered from existing HC gene sets downloaded from Dryad (https://doi.org/10.5061/dryad.88tj450). The analyses followed a workflow used previously with Lamiaceae. Peaks in the observed $K_S$ distribution for each species were identified with Gaussian mixture models, as implemented with the mixtools R package, and corroborated with results from a SiZer analysis.

TEs  TEs were predicted using EDTA with the -anno and -evaluate options selected. The *S. tenuifolia* CDS were specified and gene regions were excluded from the prediction using the BED annotation for the CDS regions. Predicted TEs were extracted using the *getfasta* tool from the BEDTools suite. The default parameters of the search workflow of MMseqs2 were used to align scaffold_6 extracted TEs to the *S. tenuifolia* TE library. Intergenic coordinates were used to subset TEs for genomic regions of interest. The percentage identity, e value, and bit scores were used as edge weights to construct homology networks in Cytoscape v3.7.2. The kpPlotDensity function of karyoploteR was used to visualize TE density and genomic positions for the Scaffold 6 BGC. TE densities were calculated using a sliding window of 5 000 bp.

Long-read coverage on the BGC  Minimap2 was used to re-map PacBio reads to assembled scaffolds. BEDTools was used to extract the coordinates of the top 10% longest reads mapping to the BGC region and visualized using the kpPlotRegions function of karyoploteR. Read coverage of reads longer than 4 000 bp was visualized with kpPlotCoverage function karyoploteR.

[刘潺潺，吴启南，等. Molecular Plant，2023，16：1-16.]

# Comparative genomics reveals the diversification of triterpenoid biosynthesis and origin of ocotillol-type triterpenes in *Panax*

## 1 INTRODUCTION

Plants have evolved to synthesize a diverse array of metabolites that play essential roles in various biological processes. The adaptivity derived from these metabolites has driven the evolution of plants and even their interactors. For decades, biologists have been intrigued by the evolutionary mechanism underlying the diversification of metabolite biosynthesis in the plant kingdom. Gene duplication is proposed to be the major force driving the evolution of metabolite biosynthesis: relaxed from functional constraints, one duplicate can accumulate mutations. In most cases, such mutations will result in gene loss, but some may be fixed owing to selective advantages conferred by their altered function, whether neofunctionalization, subfunctionaliza-tion, or specialization. These novelties in function or expression pattern would gradually reshape the biosynthetic pathway for metabolites. In land plants, pervasive whole-genome duplications (WGDs) or polyploidizations serve as the primary sources of gene duplicates. These frequent WGDs are thought to have a key causal role in species diversification, phenotypic evolution, and chemical diversification in both gymnosperm and angiosperm lineages. The causal linkage between WGDs and diversification of metabolite biosynthesis, although supported on a theoretical basis, remains to be rigorously tested.

Triterpenoids are one of the most diverse metabolites present in plants. Their biosynthesis is catalyzed by enzymes known as oxidosqualene cyclases (OSCs), which can cyclize the precursors 2, 3-oxidosqualene and 2, 3; 22, 23-dioxidosqualene. Two different types of substrate conformation exist during the cyclization process: the chair-boat-chair (CBC) conformation and the chair-chair-chair (CCC) conformation. Sterols, including cycloartenol and lanosterol, are produced via CBC folding, whereas triterpenes are produced via CCC folding. Based on the catalytic products, plant OSCs can be broadly classified into cycloartenol synthase (CAS), lanosterol synthase (LAS), lupeol synthase (LUS), β-amyrin synthase, and other multifunctional triterpene synthases (bAS and other mTTSs). Sterols function as important membrane components and also as plant hormones that regulate growth and development. The "nonessential" triterpenes are considered to have more specialized functions in plant defense and microbiome interactions. Genomic screening of the Viridiplantae phylogeny revealed that angiosperms are a hotspot of OSC diversification. Both divergent and convergent evolutionary processes are thought to have influenced the evolution of OSCs, and it is generally accepted that expansion of OSCs has been driven mainly by tandem duplications and that the triterpene synthases of eudicots likely originated from LAS rather than CAS. However, the impact of WGDs on the diversification of OSCs and the corresponding evolutionary trajectory remain unresolved.

The genus *Panax* L. (Araliaceae), which contains seven well-defined species and one species complex, is one of the most medicinally important plant genera. The pharmaceutical activities of *Panax* species have been attributed mainly to ginsenosides (glycosylated triterpenoids). Biochemical approaches have revealed a wide variety of triterpenoids in *Panax* species, including the dammarane, α/β-amyrin, and ocotillol types. To date, OSC genes responsible for synthesis of dammarane-type triterpenes have been reported for several *Panax* species, but the biosynthetic pathway of ocotillol-type triterpenes remains unclear. As one *Panax* species with high medicinal value, *Panax vietnamensis* var. *fuscidiscus* is widely cultivated in Yunnan, China. The high content of ocotillol-type saponins in *P. vietnamensis* var. *fuscidiscus* make it a suitable model for exploring the mechanism of ocotillol-type triterpene biosynthesis. *Panax* species have experienced several rounds of WGD in their evolutionary history, but whether extra WGDs have occurred in the common ancestor of all Apiales species after the γ whole-genome triplication (WGT) remains a topic of controversy. Regardless of disputes about WGD history, genomic and phytochemical evidence indicates that the evolution of triterpenoid biosynthesis in *Panax* species is likely to have been affected by WGDs. The diversity of triterpenoids and the presence of WGDs in *Panax* species make this genus a suitable model for examining the effects of WGDs on the evolution and diversification of OSCs.

Here we report a high-quality chromosome-level assembly for *P. vietnamensis* var. *fuscidiscus*, together with an improved assembly for *Panax notoginseng*. We found that WGDs have occurred independently in Araliaceae and Apiaceae species rather than being shared by Apiales. Comparative genomics revealed that the diversification of triterpenoid biosynthesis was promoted mainly by WGDs and tandem duplications. Notably, the dammarenediol-II synthases (DDSs) in *Panax* species were functionally character-ized as mTTSs. These *Panax* DDS genes originated from the specialization of one OSC gene duplicate produced by the Pg-β WGD. Our findings systematically reveal how gene duplication drives the diversification of triterpenoid biosynthesis in plants and reveal the origin of ocotillol-type triterpenes in *Panax* species.

## 2 RESULTS

*Panax* genome sequencing, assembly, and annotation

PacBio long reads were used to build a *de novo* assembly for *P. vietnamensis* var. *fuscidiscus* (Supplemental Figure 1A). This preliminary assembly was polished with Illumina short reads and scaffolded using Hi-C technology. The final chromosome-level assembly of *P. vietnamensis* var. *fuscidiscus* spans 1.73 Gb, with a scaffold N50 of 144.08 Mb (Supplemental Table 1). The largest 12 scaffolds, which correspond to the karyotype of *P. vietnamensis* var. *fuscidiscus* (2n = 2x = 24), covered 91.04% of the assembly (1.57 Gb) (Supplemental Figures 1B, 2A). The size of the pseudochromosomes is close to the flow cytometry (1.61 Gb) and k-mer-based estimates (1.43 Gb) (Supplemental Figure 3A; Supplemental Tables 2, 3). To evaluate the quality of the *P. vietnamensis* var. *fuscidiscus* genome, 229.47 Gb of the Illumina short reads (132.64×) were mapped to the assembly. The mapping

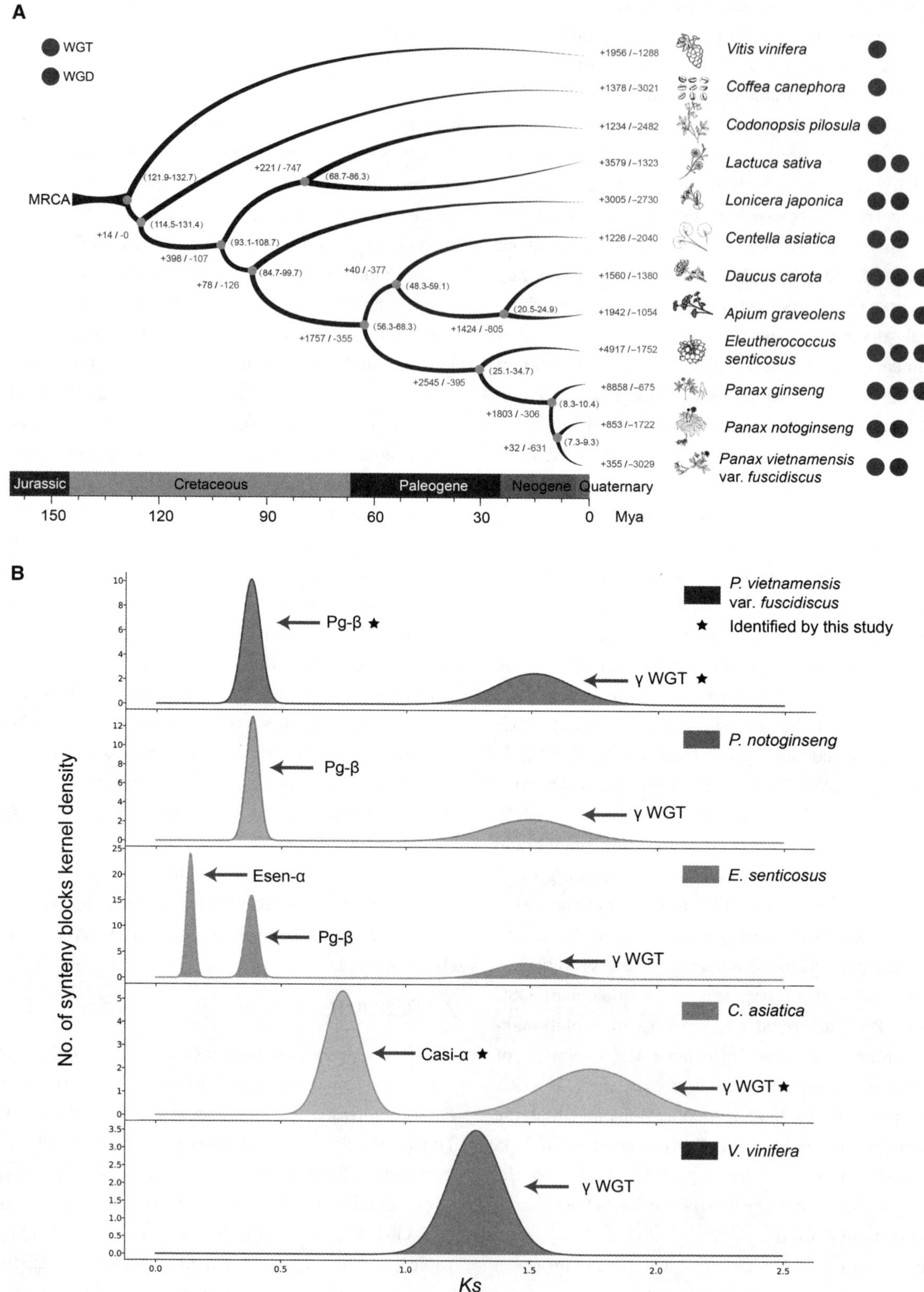


**Figure 1 Evolutionary analysis of *P. vietnamensis* var. *fuscidiscus***

(A) Species tree for 12 eudicots including *P. vietnamensis* var. *fuscidiscus*. Numbers in parentheses indicate estimated divergence times in Mya with 95% confidence intervals. Expansion and contraction of gene families are indicated with plus and minus signs. Whole-genome duplications (WGDs) and whole-genome triplications (WGTs) in each species are shown in blue/red circles. MRCA, most recent common ancestor. (B) *Ks* distribution of intraspecific collinear blocks. *Ks* peaks of polyploidizations are labeled for each species. Esen, *E. senticosus*; Casi, *C. asiatica*.

rate of properly paired reads and genome coverage rate were 94.47% and 97.40%, respectively (Supplemental Table 4). We annotated 36454 protein-coding genes in the *P. vietnamensis* var. *fuscidiscus* genome, with an average gene length of 6166.47 bp (Supplemental Table 5). A total of 33570 (92.09%) predicted genes could be functionally annotated (Supplemental Table 6). Benchmarking Universal Single-Copy Orthologs (BUSCO) completeness of the assembly and annotated genes were 95.3% and 92.6% (Supplemental Figure 3B; Supplemental Table 7). The reported genome assembly size for *P. vietnamensis* Ha *et* Grushv. (2n = 2x = 24) is 3.00 Gb, which is 1.73-fold larger than the genome size of *P. vietnamensis* var. *fuscidiscus*. Thus, *P. vietnamensis* var. *fuscidiscus* is likely to be an independent species rather than a variety of *P. vietnamensis* Ha *et* Grushv. If not, *P. vietnamensis* var. *fuscidiscus* is still worth studying for its different genome size compared with *P. vietnamensis* Ha *et* Grushv. and well-developed biosynthetic modules based on *P. vietnamensis* var. *fuscidiscus*.

We also provide an improved chromosome-level assembly of *P. notoginseng* (2n = 2x = 24) created using a previous contiglevel assembly (Supplemental Table 8). More sequences (94.29%) were anchored to the 12 pseudochromosomes compared with the previous assembly (86.87%) (Supplemental Figure 2B). We annotated 36747 protein-coding genes in the updated *P. notoginseng* genome, 92.79% of which were functionally annotated (Supplemental Tables 5 and 9). BUSCO analysis suggested 97.5% and 93.3% completeness of the updated *P. notoginseng* assembly and annotated genes (Supplemental Figure 3B; Supplemental Table 7).

Species-specific LTR expansion produced genome size variation in *Panax* Repetitive elements constitute 86.79% and 88.18% of the *P. vietnamensis* var. *fuscidiscus* and *P. notoginseng* assemblies. LTR - RTs are the most abundant type of transposable elements (TEs) in both *Panax species*, accounting for 78.94% and 80.66% of the *P. vietnamensis* var. *fuscidiscus* and *P. notoginseng* assemblies. Among the LTR - RTs in *P. vietnamensis* var. *fuscidiscus*, Gypsy elements (54.52% of the genome) are far more abundant than Copia elements (5.67%). A similar phenomenon was observed in the *P. notoginseng* genome, with Gypsy and Copia elements accounting for 55.49% and 4.55% of the genome. DNA transposons are the second most abundant type of TE and constitute 2.90% and 3.13% of the *P. vietnamensis* var. *fuscidiscus* and *P. notoginseng* genomes (Supplemental Tables 10 and 11). Based on intact LTR - RTs (21251 in *P. vietnamensis* var. *fuscidiscus* and 24899 in *P. notoginseng*), we estimated the insertion times for LTR-RTs. *P. vietnamensis* var. *fuscidiscus* was found to have experienced a more recent burst of LTRs compared with *P. notoginseng* (Supplemental Figure 4). Clade-level classification of TEs revealed that the numbers of several Gypsy-clade elements (mainly Tekay, Ogre, and Athila) are much higher in *P. notoginseng* than in *P. vietnamensis* var. *fuscidiscus* (Supplemental Tables 12 and 13). These results indicate that *P. notoginseng* experienced a more intense expansion of LTR insertions compared with *P. vietnamensis* var. *fuscidiscus* after their divergence; the difference in genome sizes between the two *Panax* species (~680 Mb) can be attributed mainly to the more intense expansion of LTRs in *P. notoginseng* (LTR size difference, ~609 Mb).

Phylogenomics and evolution of *P. vietnamensis* var. *fuscidiscus* To study the evolutionary history of *Panax* species, we first performed gene family analysis using 12 eudicots: *Vitis vinifera*, *Coffea canephora*, *Codonopsis pilosula*, *Lactuca sativa*, *Lonicera japonica*, *Centella asiatica*, *Daucus carota*, *Apium graveolens*, *Eleutherococcus senticosus*, *Panax ginseng*, *P. notoginseng*, and *P. vietnamensis* var. *fuscidiscus*. A total of 30074 ortholog groups, harboring 93.1% of all the studied genes, were identified for the 12 species, and 168 groups are presented as single-copy orthogroups (Supplemental Figure 5A; Supplemental Table 14). Investigation of gene families in *P. vietnamensis* var. *fuscidiscus* and five other Apiales species suggested that *P. vietnamensis* var. *fuscidiscus* and *P. notoginseng* contain 436 and 673 unique gene families, respectively (Supplemental Figure 5B).

Single-copy orthogroups were used to construct maximum likelihood (ML) phylogenetic trees. The species trees inferred by the concatenation method and coalescence-based phylogenetic anal-ysis are identical and well supported (Supplemental Figure 6A and 6B). *P. vietnamensis* var. *fuscidiscus* is placed as a sister lineage to *P. notoginseng* rather than *P. ginseng*, consistent with a *Panax* phylogeny based on chloroplast genomes and ribosomal DNA. Divergence times were estimated using MCMCTree with time calibrations. The estimated divergence between Araliaceae and Apiaceae occurred ~56.3 - 68.3 million years ago (Mya). In the *Panax* genus, the speciation of *P. ginseng* occurred first (~8.3 - 10.4 Mya), followed by the divergence of *P. vietnamensis* var. *fuscidiscus* and *P. notoginseng* (7.3 - 9.3 Mya) (Figure 1A). We also noted the early divergence of *C. asiatica* in the family Apiaceae, which occurred approximately 48.3 - 59.1 Mya, validating the basal group position of *C. asiatica* in Apiaceae.

Finally, we estimated the expansion and contraction of gene families during the phylogenetic history of the 12 species using the resolved species tree. In *P. vietnamensis* var. *fuscidiscus*, 355 gene families had undergone expansion, whereas 3029 gene families had undergone contraction ($P <$

0.05) (Figure 1A). Expanded gene families in *P. vietnamensis* var. *fuscidiscus* showed functional enrichment in sesquiterpenoid and triterpenoid biosynthesis ($P < 0.05$) (Supplemental Figure 7A; 7B, Supplemental Tables 15 and 16).

Polyploidization history in Apiales Polyploidizations in Apiales were systematically characterized to study their impact on the evolution of triterpenoid biosynthesis. The *V. vinifera* genome was used as an outgroup because only one polyploidization event (γ WGT) occurred during its evolution. We inferred WGDs and speciation events by examining the synonymous substitutions per synonymous site (*Ks*) of collinear gene pairs and intra/interspecific syntenic relationships. Two clear peaks were observed in the *Ks* distribution of intraspecific collinear gene pairs for *P. vietnamensis* var. *fuscidiscus*, suggesting an extra round of WGD after the γ WGT (Figure 1B). Interspecific synteny comparison between genomes of *P. vietnamensis* var. *fuscidiscus* and *V. vinifera* revealed that for each genomic region in *V. vinifera*, there are up to six syntenic matches in *P. vietnamensis* var. *fuscidiscus*, validating the extra round of WGD in the latter species (Supplemental Figure 8). In addition to recent peaks attributed to speciation, extra peaks were detected in the *Ks* distribution of collinear gene pairs between *P. vietnamensis* var. *fuscidiscus* and the other two Araliaceae species (*P. notoginseng* and *E. senticosus*) (Supplemental Figure 9). The ancient peaks indicate the shared γ WGT, and the relatively young peaks may represent the Pg-β WGD, which is presumed to be shared by Araliaceae species. The *Ks* peak values for the Pg-β WGD and the γ WGT are nearly identical in the three Araliaceae species, suggesting little variation in evolutionary rates among Araliaceae. Synteny comparisons of the updated *P. notoginseng* assembly with that of *E. senticosus* showed exactly 1 : 2 ratios for the best-matched regions in the largest 12 pseudochromosomes, validating the high quality of the updated *P. notoginseng* assembly compared with an older version (Supplemental Figure 10A and 10B). *C. asiatica* experienced two WGDs according to our analysis (Figure 1B). The *Ks* distribution of interspecific collinear gene pairs between *C. asiatica* and *P. vietnamensis* var. *fuscidiscus* showed two peaks, which correspond to speciation (~0.53) and the shared γ WGT (~1.63) (Supplemental Table 17). The absence of additional peaks suggested that the younger WGDs in Apiaceae and Araliaceae may have occurred independently after their speciation (Figure 2A).

To examine Apiales evolution with greater resolution, we performed synteny-based phylogenetic analysis. Five species (*V. vinifera*, *C. asiatica*, *E. senticosus*, *P. notoginseng*, and *P. vietnamensis* var. *fuscidiscus*) that exhibit a well-preserved ancestral eudicot karyotype (AEK) were selected for the analysis. Using the AEK and the *V. vinifera* genome as references, collinear regions were partitioned into different copies for each species with consideration of WGDs (Supplemental Figures 11 - 15; Supplemental Table 18). Based on 2 255 collinear gene pairs (23 821 genes), ASTRAL produced a phylogenetic tree for the five species with a normalized quartet score of 0.814 6. The topology of the synteny-based species tree provides solid evidence that the Pg-β WGD occurred independently in Araliaceae and was shared by Araliaceae species (Figure 2B and Supplemental Figure 16). Interestingly, the collinear subsets for *C. asiatica* in all three lineages produced by the γ WGT did not form sister groups but split successively instead. This suggested that the relatively recent WGD in *C. asiatica* may have been induced by an ancient hybridization.

Evolution of OSCs was mainly promoted by WGDs and tandem duplications

Previous studies have suggested that OSCs for sterol biosynthesis in Eukarya have a bacterial origin and that plant OSCs have likely undergone divergent evolution, with triterpene biosynthesis derived from sterol biosynthesis. Thus CAS likely served as the foundation of OSC evolution. Here, we performed phylogenetic and comparative genomics analyses to clarify the evolution of OSCs in plants. Nine species (*Amborella trichopoda*, *Aristolochia fimbriata*, *V. vinifera*, *C. asiatica*, *E. senticosus*, *P. ginseng*, *P. vietnamensis* var. *fuscidiscus*, *P. notoginseng*, and *Panax quinquefolius*) were included in the analysis, including six Apiales species selected for their diversity in triterpenoid biosynthesis and well-characterized phylogenetic history. We included *A. trichopoda* (ANA-grade) and *A. fimbriata* (Magnoliids) in the analysis for their absence of WGD since the emergence of flowering plants. First, we performed genome-wide identification of OSCs based on conserved protein domains. For *P. quinquefolius*, which lacks a reference assembly, one DDS was used (Supplemental Table 19). In contrast to the abundant OSC genes in eudicots, we identified only one putative OSC in *A. trichopoda* and two putative OSCs in *A. fimbriata*, implying an important role for WGDs in the expansion of OSCs. An ML phylogenetic tree was built for the identified putative OSCs using codon alignments (Figure 4A). On the basis of conserved motifs (Supplemental Figure 17) and phylogenetic relationships with functionally characterized OSCs, the OSCs were classified into putative functional groups (CAS, LAS, LUS, and bAS and other mTTSs). Functionally characterized DDSs from *Panax* species were nested within bAS and other mTTSs, indicating their close phylogenetic relationship. We also noticed that members of bAS and other mTTSs were recovered in two lineages (group I and group II) with high support, suggesting their distinct origins.

The distribution pattern of OSCs on the synteny-based

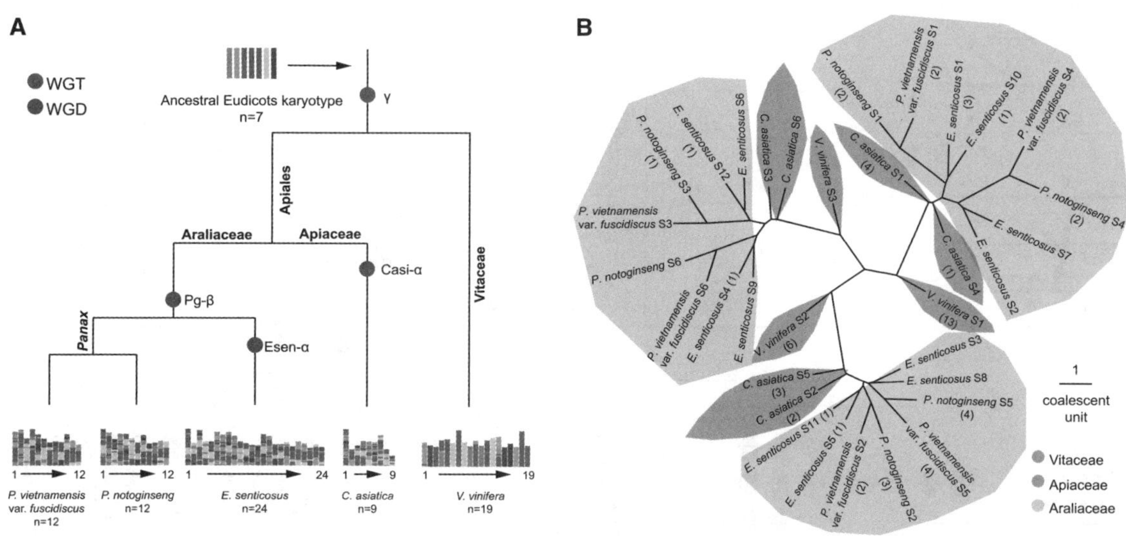


**Figure 2 Inference of polyploidization and speciation history in Apiales**

(A) The inferred phylogeny of Apiales species with placement of polyploidizations. Karyotypes were painted in seven colors, corresponding to the seven ancestral eudicot chromosomes. (B) Synteny-based coalescent species tree showing independent WGDs in Apiaceae and Araliaceae. Genomes were classified into collinear subsets based on polyploidization history (denoted with S). Branch lengths are shown in coalescent units. Because the ASTRAL tree leaves the branch length of terminal branches empty, the lengths of terminal branches were all set to one. Numbers in parentheses represent the number of putative OSC genes.

species tree suggested that the expansion of OSCs was affected by WGDs (Figure 2B). In addition, the scarcity of OSCs on the lineage leading to *V. vinifera* S3 indicated that gene loss or translocation events had occurred before speciation. We next performed inter/intraspecific synteny analysis to investigate the evolutionary trajectory of OSCs with differentiation of paralogous and orthologous syntenic regions produced by polyploidizations and speciation. Intraspecific synteny comparisons revealed OSCs produced from recent WGDs (Casi-α and Pg-β WGD) in Apiales species (Supplemental Figure 18). In *P. vietnamensis* var. *fuscidiscus*, no direct syntenic relationship was found for *PvOSC7* (DDS gene) and *PvOSC6* (bAS and other mTTSs), yet both genes were located on highly syntenic chromosomal regions produced by the Pg-β WGD. The same phenomena were also observed in *P. notoginseng* between *PnOSC5* (bAS and other mTTSs) and the tandemly-duplicated *PnOSC6*/*PnOSC7* (DDS genes) (Supplemental Figure 18). Thus, we speculate that DDS in *Panax* species likely originated from neofunctionalization of a group I bAS and other mTTS copy produced from the Pg-β WGD. We observed only one syntenic relationship between *VvOSC12* (from chromosome [chr] 9) and *VvOSC9* (from chr 10) in *V. vinifera*. Considering the fact that OSCs in grape are found on only three chromosomes (chr 9, 10, 11) and that chr 9, chr 11, and a part of chr 4 were produced by the γ WGT, grape OSCs from chr 9, 10, and 11 are likely to share the same origin. After the γ WGT, a chromosomal region harboring OSCs in chr 4 was translocated to chr 10. This assumption was verified by interspecific synteny comparisons between *V. vinifera* and Apiales species, in which the grape CASs *VvOSC7* (from chr 11) and *VvOSC1* (from chr 9) showed syntenic relationships with the same *P. vietnamensis* var. *fuscidiscus* CAS, *PvOSC1* (Figure 3). We also compared OSC syntenic relationships of *P. vietnamensis* var. *fuscidiscus* and *V. vinifera* with species with non-duplicated genomes (*A. trichopoda* and *A. fimbriata*). The CASs produced by the Pg-β WGD (*PvOSC3* and *PvOSC1*) and an LAS (*PvOSC4*) from *P. vietnamensis* var. *fuscidiscus* showed clear syntenic relationships with OSC genes from *A. trichopoda* (*AtOSC1*) and *A. fimbriata* (*AfOSC1* and *AfOSC2*). A syntenic relationship was also found between grape *VvOSC7* and *A. trichopoda AtOSC1* (Figure 3). Such conservation was even detected between *A. trichopoda* and the gymnosperm *Welwitschia mirabilis* (Figure 3), demonstrating that CAS genes are spatially conserved in higher plants.

With the above information, we deduced the evolutionary trajectory of OSCs (Figure 3). OSCs were conserved for sterol biosynthesis during the early stages of plant evolution, as only CASs were found in the genomes of lower plants. Following the emergence of angiosperms, one CAS duplicate (possibly produced by tandem duplication) may have diversified to give rise to LAS through neofunctionalization. The absence of LAS in *Amborella* suggests that the duplication probably occurred after *Amborella* speciation. The chromosomal region harboring CAS and LAS was

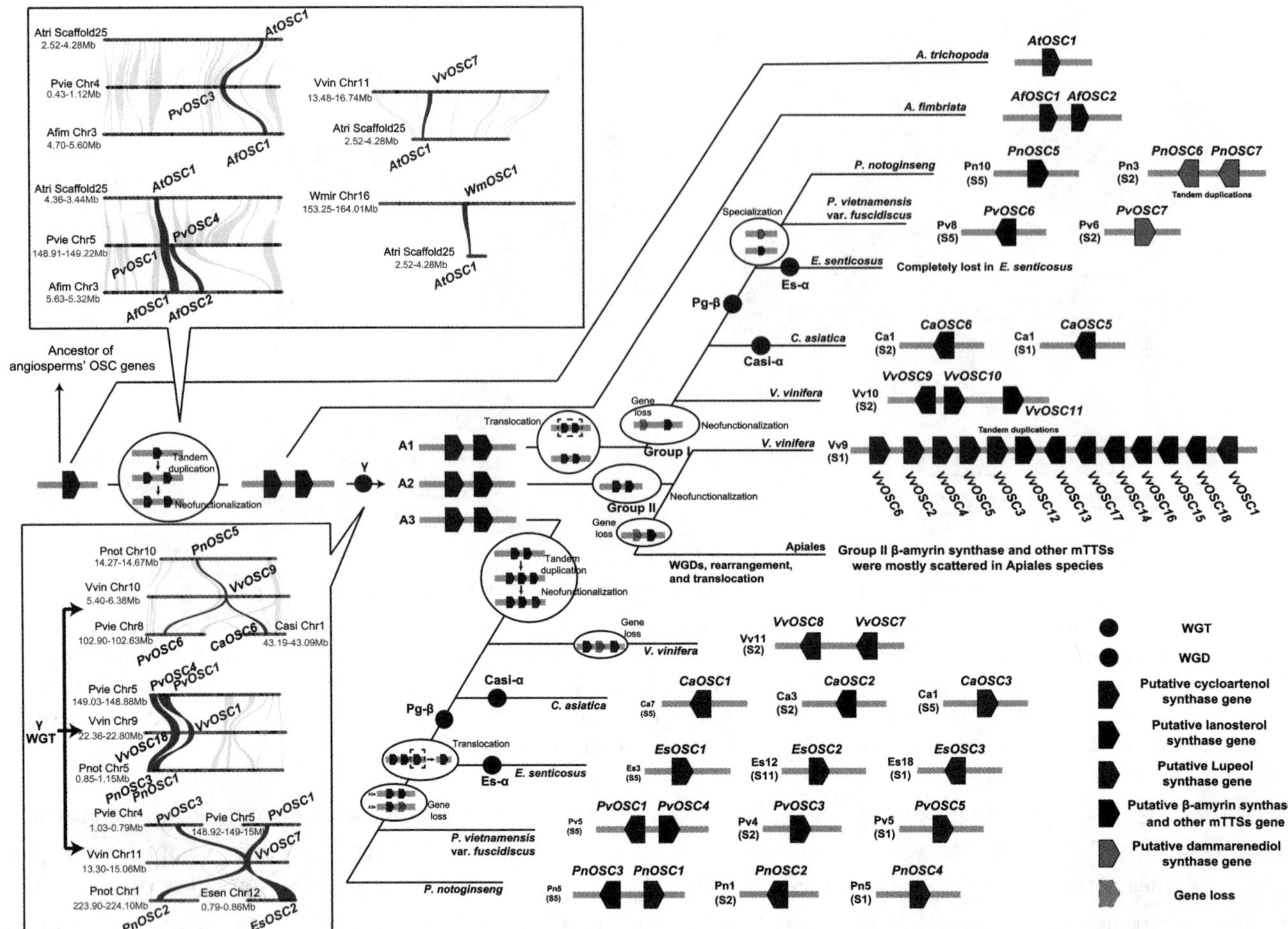


**Figure 3 The inferred evolutionary trajectory of OSC genes in plants**

Polyploidizations are shown with blue and red circles. Pentagons with a solid border represent OSC genes. Gene loss is shown by pentagons with a dashed border. Interspecific micro-syntenic relationships of putative OSC genes are shown in boxes. Direct collinear relationships between putative OSC genes are highlighted in green (Vvin, *V. vinifera*; Pvie, *P. vietnamensis* var. *fuscidiscus*; Pnot, *P. notoginseng*; Atri, *A. trichopoda*; Afim, *A. fimbriata*; Wmir, *W. mirabilis*). Inferred gene duplication, neofunctionalization, translocation, and loss are highlighted in circles.

triplicated into three copies by the γ WGT (A1 - 3). Several changes were inferred for the triplicated copies. Before the speciation of grape and Apiales, A1 experienced translocation followed by functional diversification of LAS to group I bAS and other mTTSs. The newly formed group I bAS and other mTTSs was duplicated by the Pg-β WGD, with one copy then neofunctionalizing to DDS in the ancestor of extant *Panax* species. For A2, neofunctionalization of LAS gave rise to group II bAS and other mTTSs. In the lineage leading to Apiales, CAS was lost, and the group II bAS and other mTTSs was likely affected by reshuffling, resulting in a non-syntenic distribution pattern. By contrast, CAS and group II bAS and other mTTSs were retained and proliferated through tandem duplications in grape. LUS may have been produced by neofunctionalization of a tandemly duplicated copy of LAS in A3 before the speciation of grape and Apiales. In the Apiales lineage, the LUS probably experienced translocation, as no syntenic relationships were found between LUS and other OSCs.

**Functional characterization revealed the origin of ocotillol-type triterpenes in *Panax*** To verify the proposed Pg-β origin of DDSs in *Panax* species, we performed functional analysis to determine the catalytic activities of each tested OSC. Nine OSC genes (five from group I bAS and other mTTS clades and four from the DDS clade) were selected for the analysis (Figure 4B). The OSC genes were heterologously expressed in mutant yeast strain GIL77, which was engineered to accumulate the precursor oxidosqualene. The products were identified through GC - MS and NMR (Supplemental Figures 19 - 26; Supplemental Tables 20 and 21). Nine products were identified for every OSC from group I bAS and other mTTSs. For PvOSC6, PgOSC9, PnOSC5, and CaOSC5, α-amyrin, β-amyrin, ψ-taraxasterol, and 3-epicabraleadiol were identified as the main products,

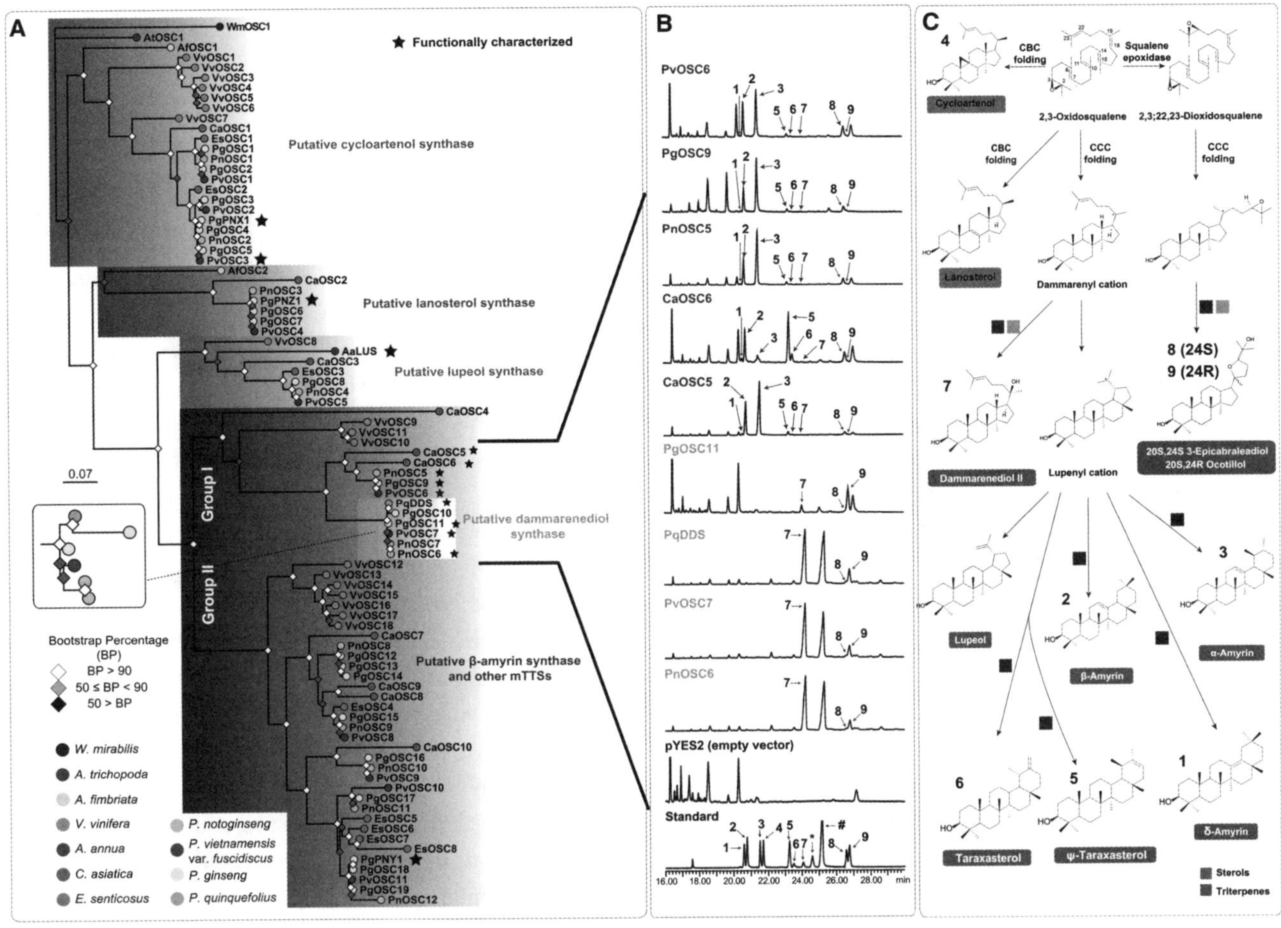


**Figure 4 Phylogenetic analysis and functional characterization of OSCs**

(A) ML phylogenetic tree of OSCs based on codon alignments. Bootstraps are shown as colored squares at each node, and species are shown as colored circles at each terminal branch. (B) Functional characterization of nine OSCs using heterologous expression. The asterisk (*) and hash (#) in the total ion chromatograms (TICs) represent the epoxydammaranes mono-trimethylsilyl ether and dammarenediol-II mono-trimethylsilyl ether, respectively. 1, δ-amyrin; 2, β-amyrin; 3, α-amyrin; 4, cycloartenol; 5, ψ-taraxasterol; 6, taraxasterol; 7, dammarenediol-II; 8, 20S,24S-3-epicabraleadiol; 9, 20S,24R-ocotillol. (C) Schematic for triterpenoid biosynthesis with sterols highlighted in blue and triterpenes highlighted in red. Compound numbers correspond to the numbers in TICs from (B). Colored squares indicate functions of enzymes in (B).

with trace amounts of δ-amyrin, taraxasterol, dammarenediol-II, ocotillol, and an unidentified product. The product profile of CaOSC6 was slightly different, with an increased proportion of ψ-taraxasterol and a decrease in α-amyrin content (Figures 4B, 4C, and 27; Supplemental Table 22). In a recent study, CaOSC5 was functionally characterized as a multifunctional OSC producing δ-amyrin, α-amyrin, β-amyrin, ψ-taraxasterol, taraxasterol, and an unidentified product in a ratio of 1 : 67 : 26 : 4 : 1 : 1. The previously reported catalytic activities of CaOSC5 are highly consistent with our results, except for the weak ability to produce dammarane-type triterpenes (dammarenediol-II, ocotillol, and 3-epicabraleadiol) identified in our study. Surprisingly, ocotillol and 3-epicabraleadiol were also detected in addition to dammarenediol-II as catalytic products of DDSs from *Panax* species (PgOSC11, PqDDS, PvOSC7, and PnOSC6) (Figure 4B and Supplemental Figure 27; Supplemental Table 22). This multifunctional nature of DDSs in *Panax* species has not previously been reported. We also noted that PgOSC11 produces mainly ocotillol, whereas the other DDSs predominantly produce dammarenediol-II. These findings validate our assumption that DDS in *Panax* species originated from a duplicate of a group I bAS and other mTTSs produced from a WGD. After the Pg-β WGD, one copy of group I bAS and other mTTSs retained its original function (similar to homologs in *C. asiatica*), whereas the other copy experienced neofunctionalization. Judging by the catalytic products, this neofunctionalization should be viewed as a specialization process: from a generalist ancestor to a more specialized state.

Selective forces underlying evolution of OSCs According to their deduced evolutionary trajectory, OSC genes have experienced several rounds of independent neofunctionalization and specialization events. It is expected that the diversifications occurred under various selection pressures. To characterize the selective forces driving the evolution of OSC genes, we performed various branch-specific tests.

Branch-site unrestricted statistical test for episodic diversification (BUSTED) analysis found evidence (likelihood ratio test [LRT], $P < 0.05$) of gene-wide episodic diversifying selection on at least one site on at least one branch in the phylogeny (Supplemental Figure 28). Adaptive branch-site random effects likelihood (aBSREL) and mixed effects model of evolution (MEME) were then used to determine the exact lineages and sites that were under positive selection. With *a priori* knowledge that CAS genes serve as a blueprint for functional diversification of OSCs, CAS lineages were labeled as background in the branch-site analysis. Analysis with aBSREL found evidence of episodic diversifying selection on 20 out of 159 branches in the tested phylogeny (LRT, $P \leqslant 0.05$), with only four in the CAS and LAS clades and the rest distributed in lineages leading to LUS, bAS and other mTTSs, and DDS (Supplemental Figure 29). The fact that almost all of the CAS genes were under negative or neutral selection could be explained by the importance of their cycloartenol product, which is the precursor for almost all plant sterols and plays an essential role in plant developmental processes. Notably, episodic diversifying selection was detected on internal branches leading to LUS and group I/II bAS and other mTTSs (nodes 3 - 5), in which the major neofunctionalization of OSCs occurred (Supplemental Figure 29). This indicates that the diversification of sterol biosynthesis toward triterpene biosynthesis in core eudicots was driven by episodic positive selection, possibly due to the better adaptability conferred by the triterpene products. Notably, the specialization of DDS from group I bAS and other mTTSs in *Panax* species was predicted to be under neutral or negative selection. This could be explained by trade-offs during specialization: for an enzyme in the generalist state, specialization toward certain functions requires a decrease in the rest. In most cases, reduced promiscuity was shaped by negative selection.

MEME found evidence of episodic diversifying selection at 84 sites ($P < 0.05$) (Supplemental Figure 30A). Most of these sites were located near the N/C terminus and the putative active center (Supplemental Figure 30B). Residues from several function-related motifs were found to be under episodic positive selection. For the motif M(W/L)C(Y/H)CR, which has been proposed to stabilize tetracyclic or pentacyclic intermediates, the second site (W/L) was identified as being under episodic positive selection. Motif Y410, which has been proposed to play an important role in ceiling formation of the active center or in D-ring formation, was also under diversifying selection. The site is conserved as Y in CBC-folding OSCs and F in CCC-folding OSCs. These results provide insights into the evolution of OSCs at the molecular level.

## 3 DISCUSSION

The discovered evolutionary trajectories for triterpenoid biosynthesis demonstrate the prominent role of gene duplication in creating a diverse array of triterpenoids in plants. WGDs and tandem duplications are the main forces driving the diversification of OSCs. An ancient tandem duplication of CAS during the early evolution of angiosperms may have given rise to LAS. This event possibly predates the emergence of Nymphaeales species, given the presence of LAS orthologs in *Nymphaea colorata*. The expansion and diversification of OSCs in core eudicots were attributed mainly to the γ WGT, with subsequent neofunctionalization occurring in the LAS triplicates. Specifically, triterpene synthases in core eudicots originated from independent neofunctionalization of LAS copies. This finding supports the hypothesis that eudicot triterpene biosynthesis derives from LAS rather than CAS. Indeed, experimental evidence suggested that LAS can supplement the biosynthesis of phytosterols in plants. However, the methyl jasmonate/bacteria-induced regulatory mechanism and tissue-specific expression pattern of LAS suggest its similarity to triterpene synthases. The altered regulation and expression pattern of LAS may represent the initial step toward triterpene biosynthesis. Major angiosperm lineages such as monocots also exhibit great potential for the synthesis of various triterpenes; thus, the revealed γ WGT origin of triterpene biosynthesis in core eudicots suggests convergent evolution in OSC diversification in addition to the prevalent divergent evolution. We also revealed that group I and group II bAS and other mTTSs in eudicots originated from different LAS copies, thus explaining their distant phylogenetic relationship. A recent study of the evolutionary path of OSC genes based on phylogenetic trees inferred several major duplication events for OSC genes, including one ancient duplication event generating the CAS and LAS lineages and another three separate duplication events generating triterpene synthase (LUS and bAS). Our results show that the former ancient duplication event was likely caused by tandem duplication of the ancestral OSC gene, whereas the latter three duplication events actually resulted from a single duplication event, the γ WGT. This finding also demonstrates the limitations of using only phylogenetic trees when inferring the evolutionary paths of genes.

Dammarane-type and ocotillol-type triterpenes are abundant mainly in *Panax* species. Several *Panax* DDS genes have been functionally characterized as producing dammarenediol-II, but the genes responsible for synthesizing ocotillol-type triterpenes remain unclear. Our analysis revealed the origin of the DDS gene family in *Panax* species and its multifunctional nature. Future studies using site-directed mutagenesis and crystal structure analysis may provide insight into the reaction mechanism that underlies the shift in product profile of these OSCs.

In principle, reshaping of metabolite biosynthesis after gene duplication is strongly affected by selection. Our results suggest that most of the WGD-derived OSC gene copies were lost during evolution, possibly owing to accumulation of negative mutations under relaxed selection pressure. However, some OSC duplicates acquired altered functions through mutations, which were then fixed by fitting ecological opportunities. This scenario was illustrated by the effect of episodic diversifying selection on neofunctionalization of LAS copies toward triterpene synthases in core eudicots. Such functional innovations of duplicates are not always driven by positive selection. In ancestral lineages of *Panax* species, one group I bAS and mTTS copy (which mainly produced amyrin) that derived from the Pg-β WGD experienced functional specialization under negative/neutral selection, eventually giving rise to DDS. The absence of positive selection might be explained by the trade-off in catalytic activities between amyrin-type and dammarane-type triterpenes. Accordingly, it should be noted that the absence of positive selection during the creation of novelties does not necessarily indicate a lack of improvement in adaptivity.

In summary, the revealed origin and evolutionary history of triterpenoid biosynthesis in angiosperms provide insight into how gene duplication can drive the diversification of metabolite biosynthesis. In plants, triterpenoids are often further modified by tailoring enzymes (e.g., cytochrome P450s, glycosyltransferases, and acyltransferases). Studies have suggested that genes for OSCs and tailoring enzymes are likely functionally co-opted by gene duplication, resulting in diversification in gene regulation and expression patterns for triterpenoid biosynthesis. Future studies on the interactions between these tailoring enzymes and OSCs and their origins will deepen our understanding of the evolution of metabolite biosynthesis.

## 4 METHODS

Genome sequencing and assembly  Plant samples of *P. vietnamensis* var. *fuscidiscus* were collected from individuals cultivated in Jinping County, Yunnan, China. Fresh leaves, stems, and roots were stored in liquid nitrogen and sent to Novogene for sequencing (Beijing, China). High-molecular-weight genomic DNA was extracted from leaves using the cetyltrimethylammonium bromide (CTAB) method and purified with a QIAGEN Genomic Kit (Qiagen, USA). For long-read sequencing, 20-kb SMRTbell libraries were generated and sequenced on the PacBio Sequel platform. This produced ~67.7 × PacBio long reads. We also generated ~132.6 × Illumina short reads. Four libraries with an insert size of 300 bp were prepared and sequenced on the Illumina HiSeq 2 000 platform (Illumina, San Diego, CA, USA). High-throughput chromosome conformation capture (Hi-C) libraries were prepared and sequenced on the Illumina HiSeq 4 000 platform. In brief, chromatin was cross-linked with formaldehyde and digested with the restriction enzyme *DpnII* before sequencing. For the purpose of gene prediction, total RNA was isolated from leaves, stems, and roots using the RNAprep Pure Plant Kit (TIANGEN). RNA libraries with an insert size of 300 bp were generated and sequenced on the Illumina HiSeq 2 000 platform (Supplemental Table 23).

The genome size of *P. vietnamensis* var. *fuscidiscus* was estimated using flow cytometry (BD FACSCalibur) and GenomeScope (v2.0) with kmer frequencies counted from 132.6 × Illumina reads using Jellyfish (v2.2.10). The PacBio reads were assembled using NextDenovo (v2.4.0) (https://github.com/Nextomics/NextDenovo), followed by two rounds of polishing with NextPolish (v1.3.1). After removing allelic contigs using Purge Haplotigs (v1.1.1), we performed scaffolding using Juicer (v1.6.2) and the three-dimensional (3D) *de novo* assembly (3D-DNA) pipeline. Mis-joins were manually corrected on the basis of Hi-C contact signals. For transcriptome assembly, raw reads were trimmed with fastp (v0.20.1) and assembled using Trinity (v2.11.0).

The quality of the genome assemblies was evaluated using BUSCO (v5.1.2) with dataset eudicots_odb10. We also mapped Illumina reads to the genome using BWA-MEM (v0.7.12) and calculated the mapping statistics using SAMtools (v1.9).

Genome annotation  We used LTR_FINDER_parallel (v1.1) and LTRharvest (v1.0) to predict long terminal repeat retrotransposons (LTR-RTs). The identified LTR-RT candidates were passed to LTR_retriever (v2.8) to filter out the false positives and generate a genome LTR assembly index (LAI). Only intact LTRs were retained for insertion time estimation. The equation $T = K/2\mu$ was used for time estimation, where K is the LTR divergence rate and $\mu$ is the neutral mutation rate ($1.3 \times 10^{-8}$ mutations per site per year). We also used RepeatModeler (v2.0) to detect novel repeat sequences. Repetitive elements generated by LTR_retriever and RepeatModeler were fed to RepeatMasker (v4.0.9) (http://www.repeatmasker.org) for *de novo* prediction. For evidence-based methods, repetitive elements were predicted using RepeatMasker and RepeatProteinMask (v4.0.9) (http://www.repeatmasker.org) with Repbase (v24.06) as the reference. The tandem repeats were annotated using Tandem Repeat Finder (v4.09). The predicted LTR-RTs were further classified by TEsorter (v1. 2. 5) with REXdb Viridiplantae (v2. 2).

Gene structures were predicted using a combination of *ab initio*-, homology-, and transcript-based methods. GenScan (v1. 0), GlimmerHMM (v3. 0. 3), geneid (v1. 4. 4), Augustus (v3. 2. 2), and SNAP (v1. 0) were used for *ab initio* prediction of protein-coding genes. For the homology-based method, proteomes of *A. thaliana*, *V. vinifera*, *E. senticosus*, *D. carota*, and *P. ginseng* were searched against the genomes using TBLASTN (v2. 2. 29+) with $1e^{-5}$ as the cutoff e-value. Gene models were predicted by GenomeThreader (v1. 7. 3) using the above hits. For the transcript-based method, Program to Assemble Spliced Alignments (PASA) (v2. 4. 1) was used for gene prediction by comparing Trinity transcripts with genomes. Finally, all gene models were integrated using EVidenceModeler (v1. 1. 1) and updated with PASA. Functional annotation was performed with eggNOG-mapper (v2. 1. 7) by searching the eggNOG database (v5. 0. 2) (Viridiplantae-33090) using DIAMOND (v2. 0. 14).

Phylogenomics and evolutionary analysis Orthogroups were identified using OrthoFinder (v2. 5. 4) based on protein sequences of 12 species (Supplemental Table 24). The Venn diagram was visualized using Evenn.

Species trees were inferred based on single-copy orthogroups. Protein sequences from each single-copy orthogroup of 12 species were extracted and aligned using MAFFT (v7. 475). Then, the protein alignments were converted to codon alignments using PAL2NAL (v14). Poorly aligned regions from codon alignments were trimmed using trimAl (v2. rev0). For the concatenation-based method, an ML phylogenetic tree was built based on concatenated codon alignments using IQ-TREE (v2. 0. 3) with the best-fit substitution model determined using ModelFinder. Branch supports were estimated using 1 000 replicates with ultrafast bootstrap approximation (UFBoot2). For the coalescent-based method, a species tree was estimated using ASTRAL (v5. 7. 7) based on ML trees produced from IQ-TREE. We estimated species diver-gence times using MCMCTree from the PAML package (v 4. 9j) with molecular clock and nucleotide substitution set as correlated rates and JC69 model. The MCMC process was run for 100 000 iterations with a burn-in of 50 000 and a sam-pling frequency of five. The tree was calibrated with the following constraints: divergence time of *D. carota* and *A. graveolens* (~22 - 37 Mya), divergence time of Araliaceae and Apiaceae (~45 - 70 Mya), and divergence time of *V. vinifera* and the other studied species (~111 - 131 Mya). Phylogenetic trees were visualized using FigTree (v1. 4. 4) (http://tree. bio. ed. ac. uk/software/figtree/).

Changes in gene family size during species evolution were estimated using CAFE (v5). Gene Ontology (GO) and Kyoto Encyclopedia of Genes and Genomes (KEGG) enrichment analyses of gene families were performed using clusterProfiler (v4. 2. 2) and TBtools (v1. 098685), respectively, with *P* values adjusted by the Benjamini and Hochberg method.

WGD and speciation analysis The WGDI toolkit (v0. 5. 1) was used to detect WGD and speciation events. First, BLASTP (v2. 2. 29+) was used to search for homologs with a $1e^{-5}$ cutoff e-value. Collinear genes were identified by WGDI on the basis of the identified homologs using the parameter -icl. *Ks* values of collinear gene pairs were then calculated using the YN00 program from the PAML package with the Nei-Gojobori method. The median *Ks* values of inter/intraspecific collinear blocks were fitted using Gaussian kernel density estimation with the parameter -pf. The intraspecific syntenic relationships within *P. vietnamensis* var. *fuscidiscus*, together with the GC content, TE density, and gene density, were visualized using Circos (v0. 69 - 9).

Synteny-based phylogenetic analysis was used to infer the WGD and speciation history. On the basis of the similarity and completeness of inter/intraspecific syntenic blocks, syntenic regions were assigned to WGD-related putative sets for *V. vinifera*, *C. asiatica*, *E. senticosus*, *P. notoginseng*, and *P. vietnamensis* var. *fuscidiscus* with parameters -bi and -a. Collinear genes from the characterized sets were extracted and used to construct ML phylogenetic trees separately using IQ - TREE. Collinear gene pairs encompassing genes from all studied species were retained for ASTRAL analysis.

Inferring evolutionary trajectories of OSC genes Putative OSCs were identified using HMMER (v3. 1b2) by searching with the squalene-hopene cyclase N-terminal domain (PF13249) and C-terminal domain (PF13243) from Pfam (v35. 0) with the parameter -cut_tc. Sequences that contained both domains were retained for analysis. For phylogenetic analysis, protein sequences of the putative OSCs were aligned using MAFFT. The protein alignments were converted to codon alignments by PAL2NAL, followed by trimming with trimAl. IQ-TREE was used to construct an ML phylogenetic tree for the putative OSCs. The tree and motifs were visualized using the R packages ggtree (v2. 4. 1) and ggmsa (v1. 0. 0) (http://yulab-smu. top/ggmsa/). To assist with classification of putative OSCs, sequences of functionally characterized OSCs were downloaded from NCBI and included in the analysis. One *P. vietnamensis* var. *fuscidiscus* OSC (PvOSC3) was also functionally characterized (Supplemental Figure 31). For synteny-based analysis, the syntenic relationships among putative OSC genes were identified with WGDI. We used JCVI utility libraries (v1. 1. 23) to visualize the micro-synteny of OSCs.

Functional characterization of OSCs Nucleotide coding sequences of putative OSC genes were synthesized and ligated into the yeast expression vector pYES2 (Invitrogen) under the control of the *GAL1* promotor by GeneCreate (Wuhan, China). Vectors carrying putative OSC genes were transformed into DH5α competent cells. The resulting plasmid DNAs were transformed into the mutant yeast strain GIL77 by the lithium acetate/single-stranded carrier DNA/PEG method. Yeast strains transformed with the empty vector were used as controls. Yeast strains were incubated in synthetic medium containing ergosterol (20 μg $ml^{-1}$), hemin chloride (13 μg $ml^{-1}$), and Tween 80 (5 μg $ml^{-1}$) for 3 days followed by 48-h Gal induction and another 24-h incubation. Cells were harvested and refluxed in 20% KOH/50% EtOH for 10 min and extracted with petroleum ether three times. The organic phase was concentrated *in vacuo*. Gas chromatography-mass spectrometry (GC-MS) analysis was performed using an Agilent 7890A and Agilent 6540 Accurate-Mass Q-TOF (Santa Clara, USA). NMR analysis was performed on a Bruker AV 600 MHz spectrometer (Billerica, USA) (see supporting information Methods S1).

Selection analysis　The codon alignments and ML phylogenetic tree for putative OSCs from the previous step were used for selection analysis. We used HYPHY (v2.5.32) (http://hyphy.org/) to perform the BUSTED, aBSREL, and MEME analyses. The 3D protein structure of *P. ginseng* CAS was downloaded from UniProt with identifier AF-O82139-F1 (predicted by AlphaFold). PyMOL was used for visualization of protein structures (The PyMOL Molecular Graphics System, Version 2.5, Schrödinger, LLC.).

[杨子江，李晓波，杨生超，等. Plant Communications, 2023,4:100591.]

# Comparative genomics of the medicinal plants *Lonicera macranthoides* and *L. japonica* provides insight into genus genome evolution and hederagenin-based saponin biosynthesis

## 1 INTRODUCTION

The honeysuckle has been one of the most widely used herbs in traditional Chinese medicine (TCM) for more than a thousand years. Its usage for human health benefit was first recorded in the *Tang Materia Medica* (*Tang Ben Cao*) dating as far back as the year 659. In TCM theory, the honeysuckle flower is described as having sweet taste, a cold property, and a link with the channels of the lungs, heart, and stomach. TCM practitioners use the honeysuckle for treatments of a variety of health conditions, including heat-related illnesses, viral respiratory infections, skin diseases, and inflammation. The honeysuckle flowers have played a significant role in preventing and treating viral diseases, such as the SARS coronavirus and influenza. These flowers are a major ingredient in an herbal prescription called Yinqiaosan, which has been demonstrated to be as efficacious as oseltamivir in the treatment of human H1N1 influenza. Recently, herbal formulations containing the honeysuckle flowers, such as Lianhua Qingwen Capsules, Toujie Quwen Granules, and Jinhua Qinggan Granules contributed immensely to the management of COVID-19 in China. Additionally, honeysuckle flower is also authorized as a functional food, and is widely used in herbal teas to reduce the effect of summer heat on human body temperature and relieve sore throat.

The honeysuckle belongs to the genus *Lonicera* that is composed of approximately 100 species of shrubs and climbers in the Caprifoliaceae family. Among these species, *Lonicera japonica* (LJ) and *L. macranthoides* (LM) are widely used as medicinal plant sources of honeysuckle flowers. Dried flower buds and flowers of LJ have been officially recorded as “Jinyinhua” since the 1963 Edition of the Chinese Pharmacopoeia. LJ is also listed as a dietary supplement in the United States Pharmacopoeia and the National Formulary. LM was first recorded in the 2005 Edition of the Chinese Pharmacopoeia as a major plant source of “Shanyinhua” and independently from LJ (Jinyinhua). The functions and indications of these two *Lonicera* species, as captured in the Chinese Pharmacopoeia, are nearly equivalent. In the latest 2020 Edition of Chinese Pharmacopoeia, Jinyinhua is one of the composition elements in approximately 92 TCM prescriptions, and Shanyinhua is present in 14 TCM prescriptions. However, uncertainty remains as to which one provides better efficacies in specific formulations. Consequently, there is an urgent need for comprehensive comparisons between the two *Lonicera* species regarding their genome sequences, secondary metabolite compositions and abundances, pharmacological activities, and clinical efficacies. Such comparisons will promote a better understanding of the two herbs, facilitate governmental regulations, and lead to safer clinical use.

The hederagenin-based saponins with notable examples,

such as macranthoidin B, dipsacoside B, and macranthoidin A, have been shown to have strong antiviral activities. The biosynthetic pathway of the hederagenin-based saponins involves three main stages: the initial stage, the triterpenoid skeletal construction stage, and the glycosylation stage. In the biosynthetic process, squalene cyclooxygenase, β-Amyrin synthase, and oleanolic acid synthase (OAS) are the key enzymes for the construction of the triterpenoid saponin skeleton. Cytochrome P450s and UDP-glycosyltransferases (UGTs) are the key enzymes in the triterpenoid modification process. Recently, genomic studies have been applied to exploring the biosynthesis of secondary metabolites, such as carotenoids, triterpenes, wogonin, and triptolide. The biosynthesis of the hederagenin-based saponins has been partly documented in *Staphylococcus aureus* and Ilex specie plants. However, the key genes, including those involved in the biosynthesis of oleanolic acid, hederagenin, and hederagenin-based saponins, remain largely unexplored in LM.

Here, we report a comprehensive comparison of the metabolomes, genomes, and transcriptomes of LM and LJ, with the aim of providing insights into their genome evolution, and mechanistic explanation for their differential secondary metabolite production. We also provide evidence through heterologous expression in *N. benthamiana*, protein purification, and enzyme activity analyses to support the assertion that LmOAS1 and LmUGT73P1 play important roles in oleanolic acid and α-hederin production, respectively, in LM. Furthermore, we identified key amino acids involved in the enzymatic activities of LmOAS1 and LmUGT73P1, laying a foundation for large-scale bioproduction of the hederagenin-based saponins.

## 2 RESULTS

Metabolomic comparison between LM and LJ  A total of 12 batches of LM and 22 batches of LJ were collected from different places in China. Since LM and LJ belong to the same genus (i.e., *Lonicera*), the morphology of their dried flower buds is very similar (Figure 1a), with a few exceptions. For example, filamentous hairs are commonly abundant on the surface of LJ flower buds but absent on LM flower buds (Figure S1). A liquid chromatography-quadrupole time of flight-mass spectrometer (LC-QTOF-MS/MS) was employed for metabolome analysis of dried flower buds of LM and LJ. The total ion chromatograms showed similar chemical profiles between the two herbs within the retention time of 0-30 min (Figure 1b; Figure S2). Thereafter, LM notably displayed abundant secondary metabolites within 30-50 min (Figure 1b). Principal component analysis indicated a clear separation between LM and LJ in terms of secondary metabolite production (Figure S3). By comparing precursor and fragment ions of the bud samples with reference compounds and previous reports, 36 compounds (peak numbers, **1**-**36**) were identified in both LJ and LM, including 10 flavonoids, 10 iridoids, 14 organic acids, and 2 saponins. Importantly, LM presented seven (peak numbers, **37**-**43**) high-abundant hederagenin-based saponins that were absent in LJ (Figure 1b, Data S1). A heatmap based on peak abundance clearly demonstrated that the contents of flavonoids and iridoids were higher in LJ than in LM, while organic acids and saponins were much more abundant in LM (Figure 1c). We then focused on the quantification of nine hederagenin-based saponins, including macranthoidin B (peak number, **35**), macranthoside A (peak number, **36**), dipsacoside B (peak number, **37**), asperosaponin VI (peak number, **38**), macranthoside (peak number, **39**), H-hederin (peak number, **40**), α-hederin (peak number, **41**), cauloside A (peak number, **42**), and hederagenin (peak number, **43**). Noticeably, LM buds contained an average of 86.01 mg/g hederagenin-based saponins, while LJ buds only had trace amounts of these saponins, as low as 0.045 mg/g (Figure 1d). Macranthoidin B, macranthoside A and dipsacoside B were the major saponins in LM at the average amounts of 72.81, 5.71 and 6.90 mg/g, respectively (Figure 1d).

Construction of the LM genome  Genome sequence and assembly of LM were generated using the sequencing data obtained from Illumina and PacBio platforms. Using k-mer frequency analysis of the Illumina sequencing reads, the genome size of LM was estimated in 888.36 Mb with a relatively high level of heterozygosity (1.44%) and with a content of 52.6% of high copy number DNA repetitive sequences (Figure S4, Table S1). To construct the genome sequence of LM, the datasets generated by short-read Illumina sequencing, long-range PacBio sequencing, and chromatin conformation capture (Hi-C) sequencing were integrated. We obtained 56.74 Gb of short reads sequences, 107.89 Gb of long reads, and 121.35 Gb of Hi-C data (~64×, ~121×, and ~140×, respectively), representing a total of ~325-fold coverage of the estimated LM genome size (Tables S1-S3). The full-length assembly of LM was 818.38 Mb, including 1 609 contigs, a 1.1 Mb contig N50, and 82.4 Mb scaffold N50 (Table S4). From the total assembled genome, 811.06 Mb (99.11%) were anchored onto nine pseudo-chromosomes, of which 741.75 Mb (91.45%) were oriented (Tables S5 and S6). The chromosomal interaction signal was strong (Figure S5), indicating that the quality of Hi-C assembly was high. Evaluation of the genome completeness indicated 94.98% coverage of the conserved core eukaryotic genes by the Core Eukaryotic Genes Mapping Approach (CEGMA) analysis (Table S7), and 94.36% coverage of plant-specific conserved genes by the Benchmarking Universal Single-Copy Orthologs

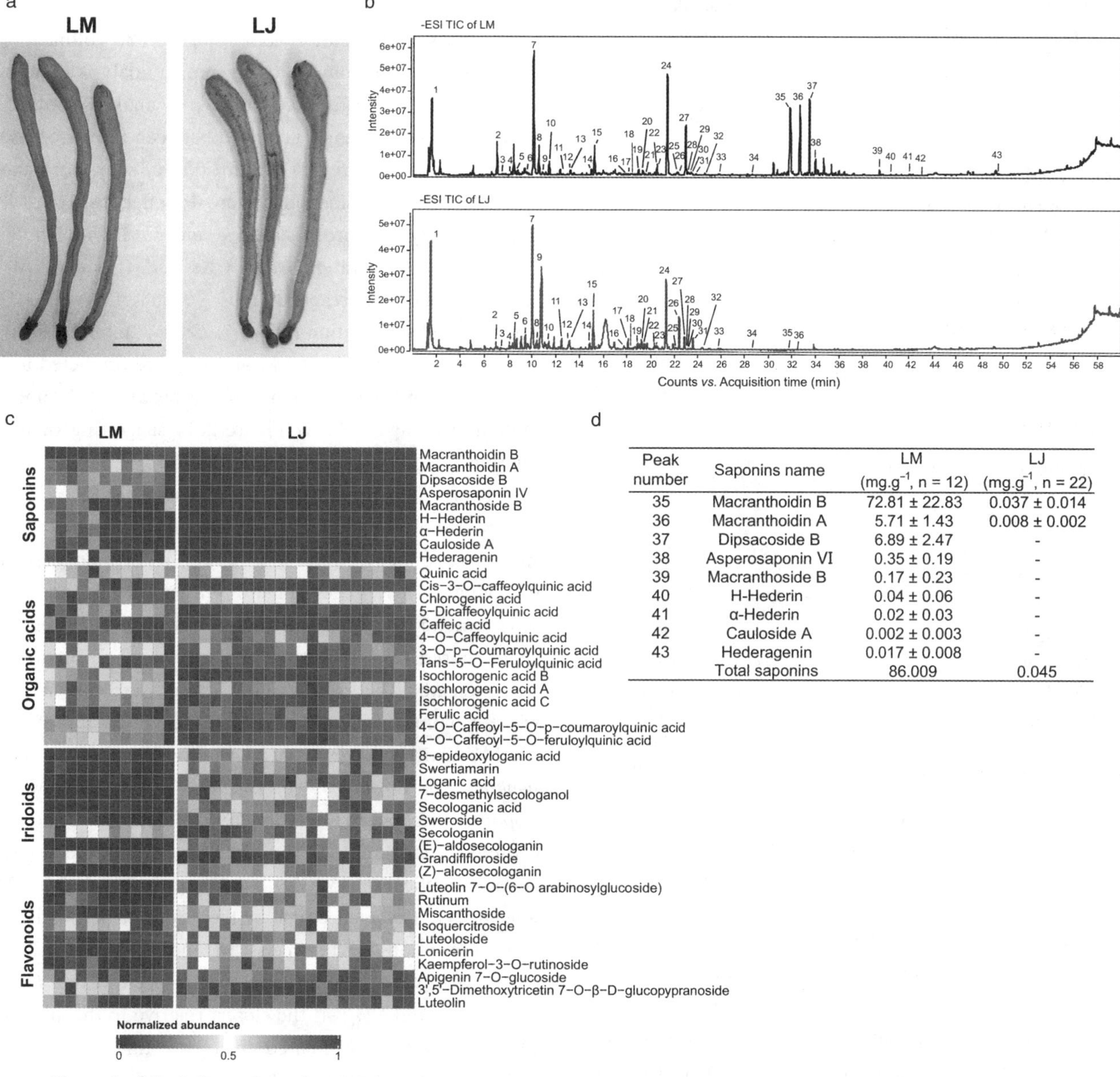


| Peak number | Saponins name | LM (mg.g$^{-1}$, n = 12) | LJ (mg.g$^{-1}$, n = 22) |
|---|---|---|---|
| 35 | Macranthoidin B | 72.81 ± 22.83 | 0.037 ± 0.014 |
| 36 | Macranthoidin A | 5.71 ± 1.43 | 0.008 ± 0.002 |
| 37 | Dipsacoside B | 6.89 ± 2.47 | - |
| 38 | Asperosaponin VI | 0.35 ± 0.19 | - |
| 39 | Macranthoside B | 0.17 ± 0.23 | - |
| 40 | H-Hederin | 0.04 ± 0.06 | - |
| 41 | α-Hederin | 0.02 ± 0.03 | - |
| 42 | Cauloside A | 0.002 ± 0.003 | - |
| 43 | Hederagenin | 0.017 ± 0.008 | - |
| | Total saponins | 86.009 | 0.045 |

**Figure 1 Metabolome comparison between the dried flower buds of *Lonicera macranthoides* (LM) and *L. japonica* (LJ)**

(a) Macroscopic characteristics of dried flower buds of LM and LJ. Scale bars: 0.5 cm. (b) Total ion chromatograms (TIC) of LM and LJ by liquid chromatography-quadrupole time of flight-mass spectrometry (LC–QTOF–MS) in electrospray ionization (ESI) negative ion mode. Peaks 1–36 are common components present in both LM and LJ. Peaks 37–43 are only detected in LM. (c) Heatmap of the 43 identified compounds in 12 batches of LM and 22 batches of LJ. These compounds were classified into four main chemical groups including 10 flavonoids, 10 iridoids, 14 organic acids, and nine saponins. Each compound was displayed by min-max normalization of peak abundance. Colours from blue to red indicate concentrations of compounds from low to high. (d) The average content of each hederagenin-based saponin in 12 batches of LM and 22 batches of LJ.

(BUSCO) analysis (Table S8). Additionally, 94.89% of the short-read sequences could be mapped back to the assembly of long reads (Table S9).

Using the assembly data, we performed genome annotation and identified a total of 40 097 protein-coding genes with an average sequence length of 5 231 bp per gene (Table S10, Figure S6). Approximately 97.9% of the genes were annotated based on a sequence blast against homologous sequences and protein domains (Table S11). On average, every predicted gene contained 5.44 exons with an average length of 295.5 bp per exon (Table S12). In total, 492.05 Mb repetitive elements representing 60.11% genome sequences were identified (Table 1; Table S13). Like most plant genomes, the predominant types of transposable elements were long terminal repeat retrotransposons (18.79% gypsy and 18.48% copia retroelements) and large retrotransposon derivatives (14.47%; Table S13). A schematic outline of the genome construction is given in Figure 2a.

Comparison of LM and LJ genomes for evolutionary study of *Lonicera* genus Comparisons were made between

**Table 1 Global statistics for assembly and annotation of *Lonicera japonica* and *L. macranthoides* genomes**

| | *L. japonica* | *L. macranthoides* |
|---|---|---|
| Length | | |
| Total length, Mb | 903.8 | 818.4 |
| Chromosome length, Mb | 843.2 | 811.1 |
| Unplaced length, Mb | 60.6 | 7.3 |
| Scaffold number | | |
| Total scaffold number | 145 | 293 |
| Chromosome number | 9 | 9 |
| Unplaced scaffold number | 136 | 284 |
| Scaffold N50 length, Mb | 84.4 | 82.4 |
| Transposable elements (TEs) | | |
| TE quantity, Mb (% of genome) | 526 (58.2%) | 547 (60.11%) |
| Genome annotation | | |
| Protein-coding genes | 33 939 | 40 097 |
| Average gene length, bp | 3 527.9 | 5 231.4 |
| Exon number | 157 099 | 218 179 |
| Exon length, Mb | 38.0 | 64.5 |
| Average exon length, bp | 241.7 | 295.5 |
| Intron number | 123 160 | 178 082 |
| Intron length, Mb | 81.7 | 145.2 |
| Average intron length, bp | 663.9 | 815.8 |
| Gene density (Genes/Mb) | 37.55% | 48.99% |

Genome information, including gene structure, scaffold numbers, transposable elements, and gene densities counted in *L. japonica* and *L. macranthoides*.

our assembled LM genome and the reported LJ genome, revealing a slightly smaller genome size for LM (818.4 Mb) than for LJ (903.8 Mb; Table 1). LM contained a total of 9 chromosomes at a length of 811.1 Mb, compared with 843.2 Mb for nine chromosomes of LJ (Table 1). The number of protein coding genes for LM was 40 097 with a gene density (total gene number/genome size) of 48.99%, which was greater than the 33 939 genes and 37.55% density for LJ (Table 1). The average gene length was 5 231.4 bp in LM and 3 527.9 bp in LJ (Table 1). LM contained higher number and larger length of introns (Table 1). Among the annotated genes, LM and LJ shared 17 134 common orthologous groups (25 311 genes in LM and 27 426 genes in LJ; Figure 2b). The sequence similarities for the common orthologous genes between LM and LJ averaged 96.13% (median 97.5%) at the DNA level and 96.39% (median 97.8%) at the protein level (Figure 2c). A total of 12 946 genes corresponding to 905 orthologous groups were specifically present in LM and absent in LJ (Figure 2b; Table S14). Kyoto Encyclopedia of Genes and Genomes (KEGG) enrichment analysis showed that LM-specific genes were mainly attributed to protein kinases, tRNA biogenesis, and sesquiterpene/triterpenoid biosynthesis (Figure S7). In total, 155 syntenic blocks containing 16 625 collinear genes were found in the comparative genomic analysis of LM and LJ (Data S2). Intergenomic co-linearity analysis showed that most genes were linearly arranged between the chromosomes of LM and LJ (Figure 2d). Interestingly, some chromosome inversions and translocations were found between LM and LJ, especially on chromosomes 7 and 8 (Figure 2d). The synonymous substitution rate (Ks) distribution of the collinear gene pairs reached 0.015 - 0.035 (Data S2). Using the universal substitution rate of $7.7\times10^{-9}$ mutations per site per year, the genomes of LM and LJ were predicted to have diverged from their common ancestor between 1.30 and 2.27 million years ago (MYA; Figure 2e), suggesting their close relation.

To further investigate the evolution of the *Lonicera* genus, orthologous groups from LM, LJ, and 11 other plant species were analysed, producing 31 618 orthologous groups involving 404 827 genes (Figure S8, Tables S15 and S16). A phylogenetic tree was constructed based on 231 single-copy genes shared by the 13 analysed species. The phylogenetic tree indicated that LM and LJ shared a common gamma whole-genome triplication (γ-WGT) event at approximately 120 MYA with *Daucus carota*, *Lactuca sativa*, *Chrysanthemum nankingense*, *Solanum lycopersicum*, *Tripterygium wilfordii*, *Populus trichocarpa*, *Arabidopsis thaliana*, and *Vitis vinifera*. Importantly, LM and LJ displayed a special whole-genome duplication (WGD) event approximately 54.5 MYA (Figure 2f). Divergence time by the phylogenetic tree indicated a sister relationship between LM and LJ (Figure 2f). In comparison with 11 additional plant species, the *Lonicera* genus (LM and LJ) was the closest relative to the ancestor of *D. carota* with an estimated divergence time of 71.2 MYA, and a secondary linkage to Asteraceae species *C. nankingense* and *L. sativa* with a divergence period around 75 MYA (Figure 2f). The Ks distributions of paralogous genes further confirmed a WGD and a γ-WGT event in the *Lonicera* genus, a γ-WGT event in *V. vinifera*, and Dc-α, Dc-β, and γ-WGT events in *D. carota* (Figure S9). Distributions of logarithmic Ks values showed that the Ks peak values were 0.83 for LM and 0.85 for LJ (Figures S10 and S11), also indicating a special WGD event at approximately 53.9 - 55.2 MYA for the *Lonicera* genus (Figure 2f). Intergenomic co-linearity (Figure S12) and gene-block (Figure S13) analyses indicated a double gene syntenic relationship for the *Lonicera* genus compared with *V. vinifera*.

Genome-based transcriptomics identifies biosynthetic genes for hederagenin-based saponins  Metabolome analysis have clearly shown a considerably higher level of the hederagenin-based saponins in LM compared with LJ. We then centered on identifying the gene families involved in the

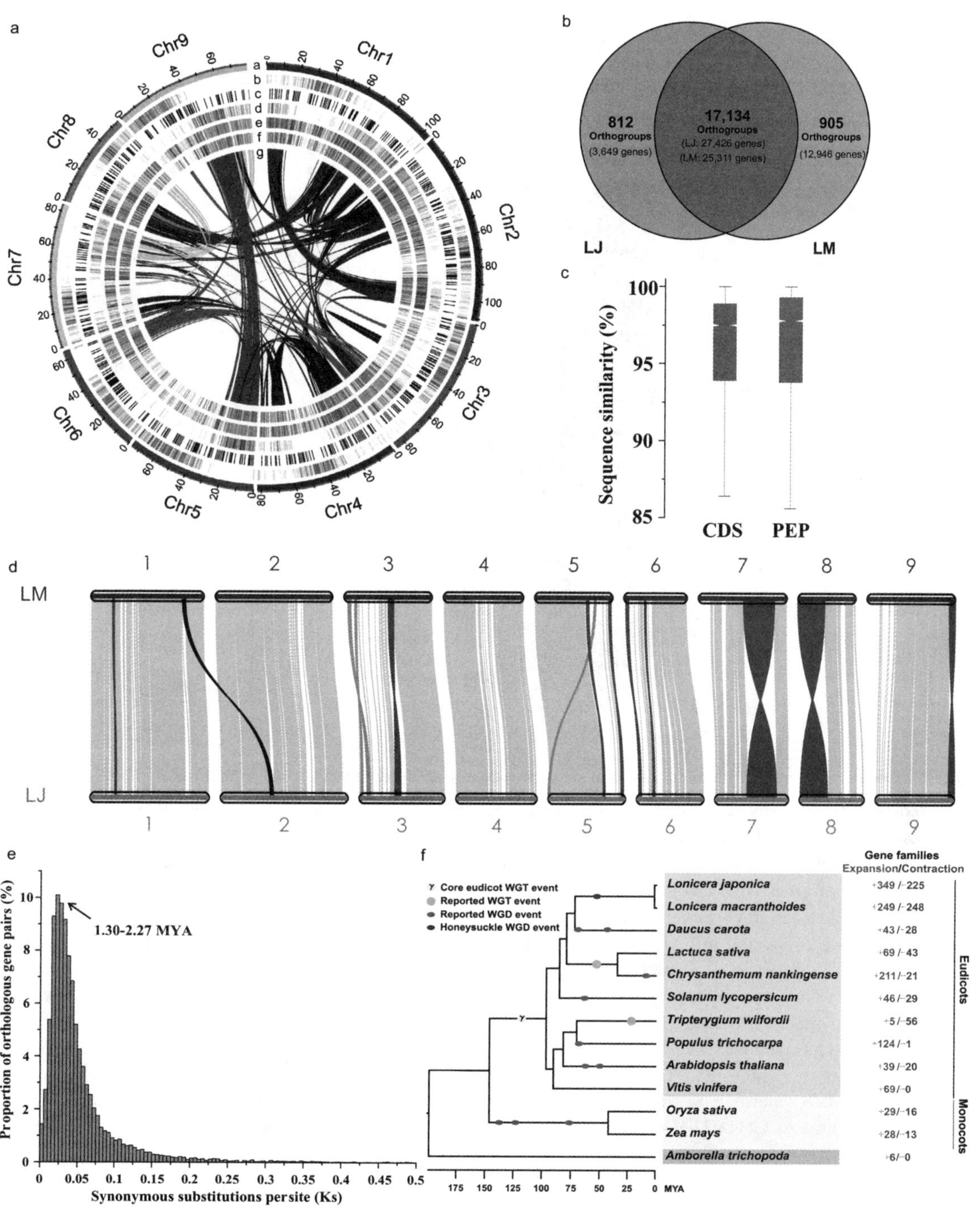


**Figure 2 Construction of the *Lonicera macranthoides* (LM) genome and its comparison with the *L. japonica* (LJ) genome**

(a) Global view of the LM genome. a, The nine pseudo-chromosomes (Chr1–Chr9). (b) Transposable element density. (c) The density of repeat sequence. (d) Gene density (500 kb window), (d–f) INDEL polymorphism density (500 kb window), and SNP density (500 kb window). (g) Linking lines in the center of the circle correspond to pairs of homologous genes. (b) Venn diagram analysis of orthologous groups and genes between LM and LJ. (c) CDS and PEP similarity of orthologous genes between LM and LJ. Error bars indicates the max-min sequence similarity of orthologous genes. (d) Macrosynteny visualization between LM and LJ. The syntenic block in grey indicates a collinearity of genes between LM and LJ, red blocks represent intra-chromosomal inversion, and the blocks in orange and blue indicate intra-chromosomal translocation and inter-chromosomal translocation. (e) Estimation of divergence time (MYA) between LM and LJ using orthologous gene pairs within collinear blocks. (f) Phylogenetic analysis and whole genome duplication events of LM and LJ. The inferred phylogenetic tree was constructed using 231 common single-copy genes in LM, LJ, and other 11 plant species (*Daucus carota*, *Lactuca sativa*, *Chrysanthemum nankingense*, *Solanum lycopersicum*, *Tripterygium wilfordii*, *Populus trichocarpa*, *Arabidopsis thaliana*, *Vitis vinifera*, *Zea mays*, *Oryza sativa*, and *Amborella trichopoda*). Gene family expansions are indicated in green, and gene family contractions are indicated in red. The timing of WGD and WGT are superimposed on the tree. Divergence times are estimated by maximum likelihood. γ represents the gamma triplication event. CDS, coding sequence; INDEL, insertion and deletion; MYA, million years ago; PEP, peptide; SNP, single nucleotide polymorphism; WGD, whole-genome duplication; WGT, whole-genome triplication.

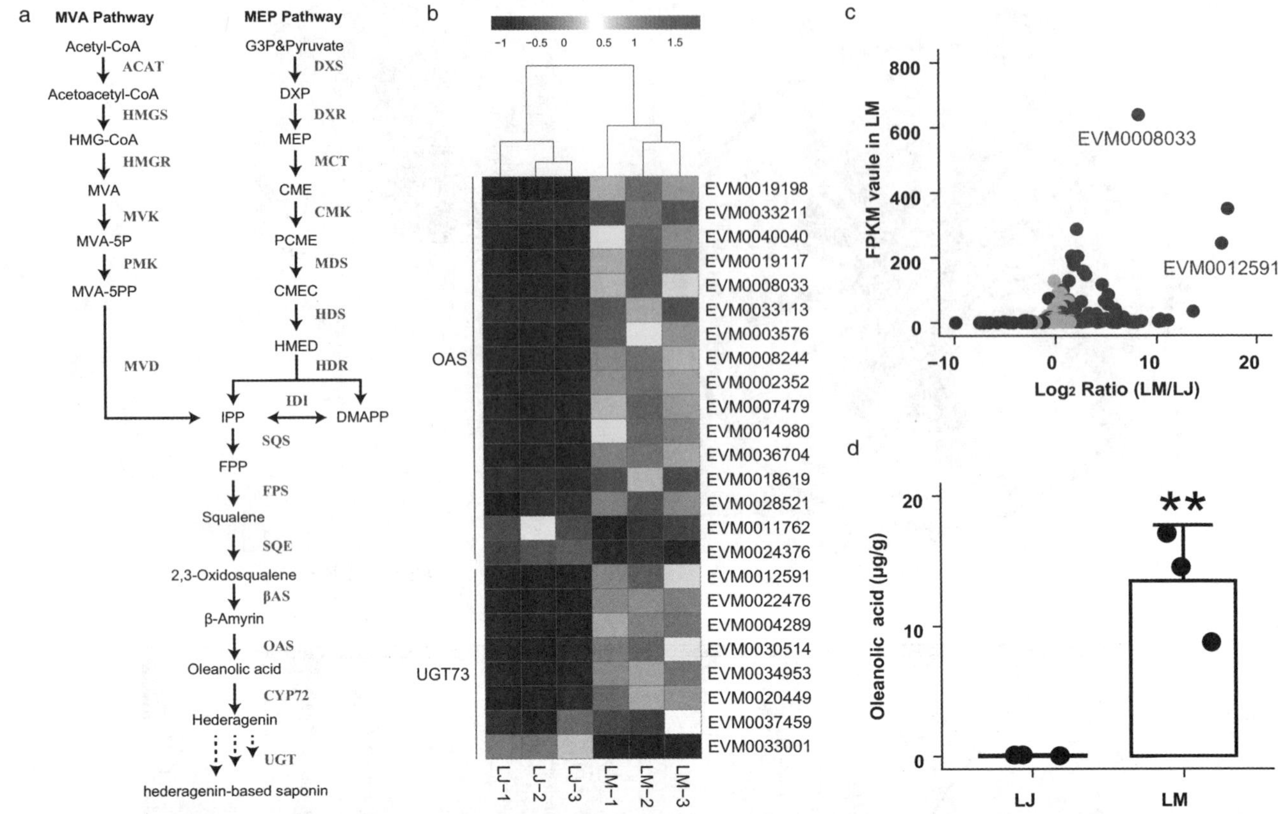


**Figure 3 Comparative transcriptomic analysis of genes involved in the hederagenin-based saponin biosynthetic pathway.**

(a) The potential biosynthetic pathway of the hederagenin-based saponin. The dotted line indicates unidentified steps. (b) Heatmap of differentially expressed genes involved in the hederagenin-based saponin biosynthetic pathway in LM and LJ. Each gene was displayed by $\log_2$ normalization of Fragments Per Kilobase of exon model per Million mapped fragments (FPKM) values. Colours from blue to red indicate the expression level of genes from low to high. (c) Volcano plot of genes involved in the biosynthetic pathways of hederagenin-based saponins. The red circle means highly expressed genes in LM, blue circle indicates highly expressed genes in LJ, and the grey circle shows genes have similar-level expression in LM and LJ. (d) The content of oleanolic acid in LM and LJ. ACAT, acetoacetyl-CoA thiolase; CMK, 4-(cytidine-5-diphospho)-2-C-methyl-D-erythritol kinase; DXR, 1-deoxy-D-xylulose-5-phosphate reductase; DXS, 1-deoxy-D-xylulose-5-phosphate-synthase; FPS, farnesyldiphosphate synthase; HDR, 1-hydroxy-2-methy-3-E-butenyl-4-diphosphate reductase; HDS, 1-hydroxy-2-methyl-2-E-butenyl-4-diphosphate synthase; HMGR, 3-hydroxy-3-methyl glutaryl coenzyme A reductase; HMGS, 3-hydroxy-3-methyl glutaryl coenzyme A synthase; IDI, isopentenyl diphosphate isomerase; MCT, 2-C-methyl-D-erythritol-4-phosphate cytidylyltransferase; MDS, 2-C-methyl-D-erythritol-2, 4-cyclodiphosphate synthase; MVD, mevalonate 5-diphosphatcdecarboxylase; MVK, mevalonate kinase; OAS, oleanolic acid synthase; PMK, phosphomevalonate kinase; SQE, squalene epoxidase; SQS, squalene synthase; UGT, UDP-glycosyltransferase; βAS, beta-amyrin synthase.

biosynthetic pathway of the hederagenin-based saponins. The hederagenin-based saponins are mainly derived from methylerythritol phosphate or mevalonic acid pathways, an enzymatic process that consists of more than 20 steps (Figure 3a). Unexpectedly, LJ and LM displayed comparable copy numbers of saponin-biosynthetic genes (Table S17). As a further characterization, we performed comparative transcriptomics. A total of 5 211 genes showed higher transcript levels in LM than in LJ with the change ratio $> 2$ and adjusted $P < 0.05$ (Data S3). In contrast, 3 308 genes were less expressed in LM than in LJ with the change ratio $< 0.5$ and adjusted $P < 0.05$ (Data S3). Among these differentially expressed genes (DEGs), 98 might be involved in the hederagenin-based saponin biosynthesis (Data S4). As expected, 71 of 98 DEGs were more highly expressed in LM than in LJ (Figure 3b; Figure S14). Among them, most of the genes belonging to the *UGT* family, such as those of *UGT74* and *UGT85* subfamilies, were more highly expressed in LM than in LJ (Figure S14). It is worth noting that the transcript levels of an OAS-encoding gene (*EVM0008033*) and a UGT73-encoding gene (*EVM0012591*) were extremely high in LM, but their expression levels were almost undetectable in LJ (Figure 3c). In addition, the upstream genes, such as those encoding farnesyldiphosphate synthase, squalene synthase, and squalene epoxidase, had higher transcript abundance in LM than in LJ (Data S4). In line with this finding, oleanolic acid, an indispensable precursor of hederagenin-based saponins, was predominantly higher in

LM than that in LJ (Figure 3d).

LmOAS1 catalyses β-Amyrin to oleanolic acid *EVM0008033* (named as *LmOAS1*), a highly expressed OAS-encoding gene in LM, was cloned to confirm the step of oleanolic acid formation (Figure 4a). Results showed that protein extracted from yeast strains expressing *LmOAS1* could effectively produce oleanolic acid from β-Amyrin by adding a carboxyl group at the C-28 position (Figure 4b). To identify the key amino acids for sustaining the enzymatic activity of LmOAS1, molecular docking and mutation assays were performed. The docking experiment identified that the amino acid regions 145-150, 340-355 and 435-441 were around the binding pocket. The amino acid region 145-150 including K145, P146, E147, A148, L149 and R150, positioned in non-conserved sequences, were chosen for mutation assay (Figure 4c; Figure S15). Residues P146, A148 and L149 were mutated into amino acids with opposite polarity. Residues K145, E147 and R150 were mutated into amino acids with opposite pH. Results showed that mutation of E147 did not affect the enzyme activity, whereas mutations of K145E, P146S, and A148S reduced the enzyme activity (Figure 4d). Importantly, mutations of L149G and R150N resulted in complete losses of enzyme activity (Figure 4d). In addition, the amino acids at 1-26 were predicted to be the transmembrane motif of LmOAS1 (Figure 4e, f). *In vitro* enzymatic assay showed that when the 1-26 amino acids were removed, the catalytic activity of LmOAS1 to produce oleanolic acid was lost (Figure 4g). The collinearity analysis indicated that the *LmOAS1* was expanded to two copies (*EVM0033113* and *EVM0008033*) on chromosome 5 of LM compared to its collinear gene (*Lj5A798G50*) in LJ (Figure 4h).

LmUGT73P1 catalyses cauloside A to α-hederin Next, *EVM0012591*, a highly expressed UGT-encoding gene in LM, was also cloned to confirm the key step of glycosylation (Figure 5a). We renamed EVM0012591 to LmUGT73P1 because of its high homology to the UGT73P2 from *Glycine max* and a common putative secondary plant glycosyltransferase (PSPG) motif in the C-terminus (Figure S16). Using nickel-nitrilotriacetic acid (Ni-NTA) affinity chromatography, the recombinant protein expressed in the *Escherichia coli* was purified and verified by SDS-PAGE (Figure S17). Three possible substrates, including oleanolic acid, hederagenin, and cauloside A, were separately incubated with LmUGT73P1 and sugar donors containing uridine 5-diphosphate arabinose (UDP-Ara), uridine 5-diphosphate glucose (UDP-Glc), or uridine 5-diphosphate rhamnose (UDP-Rha). We did not observe any products when oleanolic acid or hederagenin was added as the substrate (Figure S18). However, when cauloside A was used as the substrate, LmUGT73P1 could effectively transfer a Rha residue into cauloside A, forming the expected product α-hederin (Figure 5b; Figure S19). For further *in vivo* confirmation, *LmUGT73P1* was transiently expressed in the leaves of *Nicotiana benthamiana* using cauloside A as the substrate. As expected, LmUGT73P1 effectively catalysed the conversion of cauloside A to α-hederin in *N. benthamiana* by adding a Rha residue (Figure S20). The catalytic efficiency of LmUGT73P1 was calculated, and the $K_m$ value was found to be 32.96 μM (Figure 5c).

To identify the key amino acids for LmUGT73P1 enzymatic activity, molecular docking and mutation assays were then performed. The amino acid residues, including S53, E83, K258, E312, T330, and V338, around the binding pocket were changed into alanine using single-site mutation (Figure 5d). Results showed that mutations of S53A, K258A, E312A, T330A, or V338A did not significantly affect the enzymatic activity of LmUGT73P1, whereas mutation of E83A noticeably reduced its enzymatic activity (Figure 5e). The collinearity analysis indicated that the *LmUGT73P1* was expanded to two copies (*EVM0009409* and *EVM0012591*) on chromosome 4 of LM, while its collinear gene *Lj4C768T0* in LJ has a single copy (Figure 5f).

## 3 DISCUSSION

LM and LJ are two of the most widely used plant source of the honeysuckle flowers among the various *Lonicera* species. In this work, we performed a comprehensive comparison between LM and LJ in terms of their metabolome, genome, and transcriptome. The major findings included the followings: (i) quantitative analysis that showed that LM buds contained 2000-fold higher level of hederagenin-based saponins than LJ buds; (ii) the assembly and annotation of a reference-grade genome of LM, which provides insights into the evolution of the *Lonicera* genus and divergence of LM with LJ; (iii) Genome-based transcriptomic analysis that revealed that most of the genes involved in the hederagenin-based saponin biosynthesis had much higher expression levels in LM than in LJ; and (iv) identification of *LmOAS1*, an OAS-encoding gene, and *LmUGT73P1*, an UGT-encoding gene that encode the enzymes responsible for the biosynthesis of oleanolic acid from β-Amyrin and the conversion of cauloside A to α-hederin, respectively; (v) discovery of an interesting phenomenon, the so-called 'neighbourhood replication' of *LmOAS1* and *LmUGT73P1* in LM genome in comparison with their collinear genes in LJ.

More specifically, qualitative and quantitative analyses were performed to compare the chemical compositions of LM and LJ. Belonging to the same genus (*Lonicera*), LM and LJ present similar morphological characteristics as well as common secondary metabolites. A total of 43 major chemical constituents belonging to four groups of compounds (flavonoids, iridoids, organic acids, and saponins) were

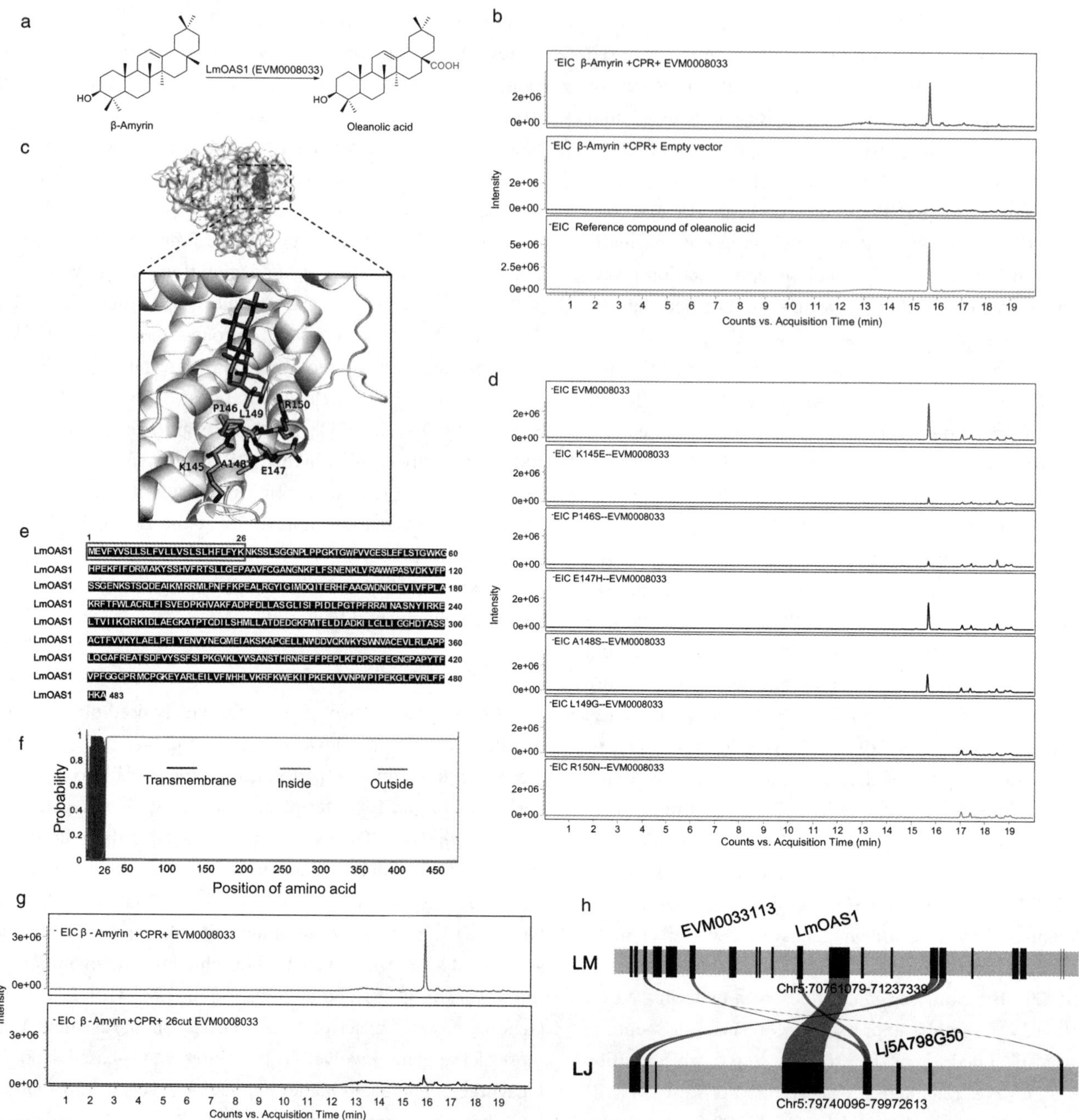


**Figure 4 Functional identification of LmOAS1**

(a) Schematic diagram of reaction from β-Amyrin to oleanolic acid. (b) *In vitro* assay of LmOAS1 in the catalysis of β-Amyrin to oleanolic acid. Extracted ion chromatogram of the product, oleanolic acid ($m/z$ 455.35) was shown. (c) Overview of LmOAS1 model docked with β-Amyrin. β-Amyrin is shown in brown and the mutated amino acids around the binding pocket were marked with green and blue. The image was produced by Pymol. (d) The effect of amino acid site-mutation on LmOAS1 enzyme activity. (e) Sequence alignment of LmOAS1 (EVM0008033). (f) Transmembrane motif predication of LmOAS1. Transmembrane domain of LmOAS1 was predicted using TMHMM server version 2.0. The purple colour indicates transmembrane motif, pink colour means outside sequence of cell membrane, and green colour shows sequence inside cell membrane. (g) The effect of the cutting 1-26 amino acids on LmOAS1 enzyme activity. (h) The colinearity relationship of *LmOAS1*, between *Lonicera macranthoides* (LM) and *L. japonica* (LJ). The syntenic blocks are connected by grey lines. The syntenic target genes are connected by yellow lines. Extracted ion chromatogram of product, oleanolic acid (m/z 455.35) was shown. *OAS*, *oleanolic acid synthase*.

characterized in LM, of which 36 were shared by LJ. In the herbal market, LJ is usually adulterated with LM because of a 10-fold price difference. It should be noted that the two herbs displayed marked differences in their chemical profiles. A remarkable feature shown in this work, as well as in previous reports, is that the hederagenin-based saponins are approximately 2 000-fold higher in LM (86.01 mg/g) than in LJ (0.045 mg/g). Macranthoidin B, the most abundant hederagenin-based saponin,

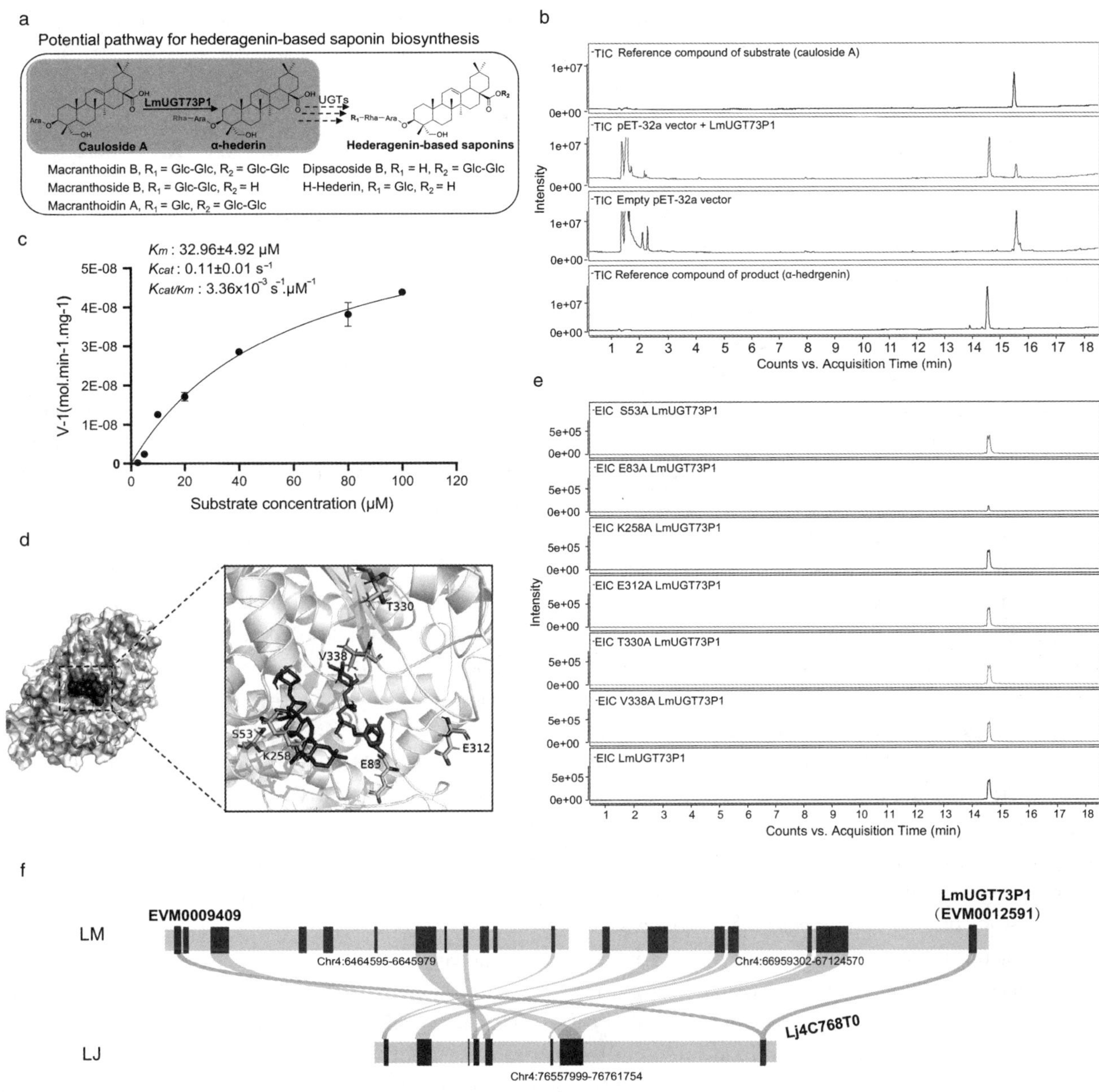


**Figure 5 Functional identification for LmUGT73P1**

(a) Potential glycosylation process of the hederagenin-based saponins. The step underlined in grey was confirmed in this study and other steps with dotted line remained to be explored. (b) *In vitro* assay of LmUGT73P1 in the catalysis of cauloside A to α-hederin. Total ion chromatogram (TIC) of the substrate, cauloside A ($m/z$ 603.39) and product compound, α-hederin ($m/z$ 749.45) was shown. (c) Determination of kinetic parameters for LmUGT73P1. The $K_m$ value was calculated using cauloside A as the substrate and UDP-Rha as the donor. (d) Overview of LmUGT73P1 model docked with the substrate cauloside A and the donor UDP-Rha. Cauloside A is shown in dark blue, UDP-Rha is shown in red, and the mutated amino acids around binding pocket marked with light blue. (e) Effect of amino acid mutation on LmUGT73P1 enzyme activity. Extracted ion chromatogram (EIC) of product compound, α-hederin ($m/z$ 749.45) was shown. (f) The colinearity relationship of *LmUGT73P1* between *Lonicera macranthoides* (LM) and *L. japonica* (LJ). The syntenic blocks are connected by grey lines. The syntenic target genes are connected by yellow lines. UDP-Rha, uridine 5-diphosphate rhamnose; *UGT*, *UDP-glycosyltransferase*.

generally serves as a chemical marker for the quality control of LM and its differentiation from LJ in the Chinese Pharmacopoeia. The hederagenin-based saponins have been demonstrated to possess strong antiviral functions. Particularly, intermediate α-hederin was reported to possess the therapeutic potential to combat COVID - 19 by *in silico* study. In addition, caffeoylquinic acids were also higher in LM than LJ. In contrast, iridoids and flavonoids were lower in LM than LJ. These findings will be useful to facilitate the quality control of LM and LJ.

Until now, only the genome of LJ had been reported among the ~100 *Lonicera* species. Thus, the high-quality genome of LM reported in this study, serves as an invaluable genome resource for evolutionary phylogenomic studies of the *Lonicera* genus. Similar to previous findings, we found a close relationship of LJ with the Asteraceae species, *C.*

*nankingense* and *L. sativa*. Furthermore, phylogenomic analysis demonstrated that the *Lonicera* genus (LM and LJ) was much closer to *D. carota* with an estimated divergence time of 71.2 MYA. It was reported that a specific WGD event occurred ~51 MYA in case of LJ. In close agreement, we have found that LM experienced a common WGD event dated approximately 53.9 - 55.2 MYA before the differentiation of the two *Lonicera* species. This minor difference in time of WGD event might be caused by different software and datasets. At the period of ~ 55 MYA called Palaeocene-Eocene Thermal Maximum, dramatic climate change happened on earth. It is possible that this linage-specific WGD event might enable the *Lonicera* genus to better cope with the drastic environmental changes experienced at that time.

Recent genomic studies have demonstrated that WGD event could affect metabolic diversification of secondary metabolites, such as triterpenes, wogonin, and triptolide. In accordance with these observations, results of our study indicated that the calculated WGD event impacted the duplications of genes involved in the biosynthesis of the hederagenin-based saponins in LM (Figure S21). Interestingly, these genes were arranged in several clusters on the chromosomes of LM (Figure S22). The divergence time of LM and LJ were estimated to 1.30 - 2.27 MYA. Intergenomic co-linearity analysis indicated that most genes were linearly arranged between the chromosomes of LM and LJ. It is important to note that chromosome inversions and translocations were partly found between them. Chromosome inversion and translocation usually mediate reduction of meiotic recombination and lead to genetic isolation and geographic differentiation. It is possible that this critical genetic architecture may provide evidence of the primordial force leading to speciation between LM and LJ. In addition, 3 854 genes were identified in the chromosome inversion-regions. Among them, 362 (9.39%) genes are highly and 209 (5.42%) are lowly expressed in LM compared to in LJ. Interestingly, 2 significantly changed hederagenin-based saponin biosynthetic genes (*EVM0008033* and *EVM0033113*) are located in this region (Figure S23), indicating chromosome inversions might affect saponin biosynthesis through regulating gene expression.

Genome-based transcriptome analysis indicated that the hederagenin-based saponin biosynthesis-related genes were more highly expressed in LM than in LJ. Specifically, at the transcript level, *LmOAS1* transcript was extremely high in LM but it was almost undetectable in LJ. LmOAS1 (EVM0008033), a type II cytochrome oxidase, belongs to the CYP716A family (Figure S24). CYP716A was reported to catalyse oxidation of β-Amyrin to yield oleanolic acid in plants, such as *Medicago truncatula* and *Glycyrrhiza uralensis*. In accordance with these reports, our results also demonstrated that LmOAS1 was expanded in LM and could catalyse the oxidation of β-Amyrin to produce oleanolic acid. The key amino acid sites for enzymatic activities of OAS family members are less studied. Using the single site mutation strategy, this work indicated that the amino acid residues K145, P146, A148, L149, and R150 were crucial in sustaining the catalytic activity of LmOAS1. Identification of these key amino acids would therefore provide a better understanding for the catalytic function of OAS. Additionally, we found that LmOAS1 lacking the 1 - 26 amino acid region also lost catalytic activity, suggesting an indispensable role for this transmembrane motif.

Many UGT genes were more highly expressed in LM than in LJ. *UGT*s encode enzymes that catalyse the formation of saponins with different backbones, including dammarane, cucurbitane, and oleanane. The UGT73 subfamily enzymes have been reported to catalyse the glycosylation of the oleanane saponins. In this work, *LmUGT73P1* was expanded in LM, and the results of *in vitro* and *in vivo* assays demonstrated that LmUGT73P1 is capable of effectively transferring a Rha residue on cauloside A to produce the intermediate α-hederin for macranthoidin B biosynthesis. Several studies have reported the substrate catalytic promiscuity of the UGTs. We showed substrate specificity of LmUGT73P1 for cauloside A but not for oleanolic acid and hederagenin. Importantly, site-directed mutagenesis indicated that the enzymatic activity of LmUGT73P1 was drastically reduced when the negatively charged E83 was mutated to the neutral A83, indicating that the charge of amino acids might be an important factor for the catalytic activity of the UGT73 subfamily members. Additionally, compared with its corresponding collinear genes in LJ, *LmOAS1* and *LmUGT73P1* had an interesting phenomenon of 'neighbourhood replication' in the LM genome. Both *LmOAS1* and *LmUGT73P1* had higher expression levels in LM compared with that of their collinear genes in LJ. The regulatory motifs in the 2 000-bp promoter regions (upstream of the translation start site) of *LmOAS1* and *LmUGT73P1* are different from those in the 2 000-bp promoter regions of their respective collinear genes (*Lj5A798G50* and *Lj4C768T0*, respectively) in LJ (Figure S25). The interesting 'neighbourhood replication' phenomenon and differences between the promoter regions of *OAS1* and *UGT73P1* genes of LM and LJ, in terms of regulatory motifs, might be an important reason leading to the differential production of these enzymes and related compounds in LM and LJ plants.

## 4 CONCLUSION

Remarkable differences between LM and LJ in terms of their metabolomes, genomes and transcriptomes were reported in this work. These findings provide insights into the genome evolution of *Lonicera* genus and the differential hederagenin-based saponin production in LM and LJ. The roles of LmOAS1 and LmUGT73P1 in the production of oleanolic acid and α-hederin, respectively, were identified using protein mutation and *in vitro* and *in vivo* enzyme activity assays. The challenge in genetic transformation of *Lonicera* plants should be solved to open the way to study the functions of genes encoding LmOAS1 and LmUGT73P1, as well as other genes encoding other enzymes involved in the hederagenin-based saponin production in *Lonicera* genus by a genetic means. In future studies, genes involved in the biosynthesis of the hederagenin-based saponins could be cloned and integrated into microbes, such as *E. coli* or yeast, to produce large quantities of the active compounds for therapeutic applications. Accordingly, the LM genome sequence can serve as a vital resource in studying the genetic foundation of secondary metabolite metabolism and in the design of molecular breeding strategies to produce high-quality honeysuckle cultivars.

## 5 MATERIALS AND METHODS

Plant material The LM cultivar collected from Longhui County, Hunan Province, China, was used for sequencing. Healthy fresh leaves were collected, and external contaminants were removed by washing with ultrapure water three times. The leaves were then frozen in liquid nitrogen and stored at −80 ℃ before DNA extraction. For metabolomic analyses, 22 batches of LJ were brought from Shandong Province, China, and 12 batches of LM were brought from Hunan Province, Hubei Province, and Chongqing city, China. For RNA-sequencing experiments, green bud flower samples were collected from the individuals and stored at −80 ℃. For genome survey, tender leaves were collected and used.

Metabolome profiling of LM and LJ Metabolites were extracted from LM and LJ using 50% methanol according to a previously published method with slight modification and analysed by LC‒QTOF‒MS. Details of this procedure are provided in methods section of the Supporting Information S1. The identification of metabolites was performed based on the mass spectra, retention times, and fragmentation patterns relative to reference compounds and literature. Reference standards for macranthoidin B, macranthoside A, dipsacoside B, asperosaponin VI, macranthoside, H-hederin, α-hederin, cauloside A, and hederagenin (Chengdu Alfa Biotechnology CO, LTD, Sichuan, China) were used to determine the concentrations of hederagenin-based saponins. The identified metabolites were then subjected to unsupervised principal component analysis and heatmap clustering using R v. 3. 5. 1 based on their peak areas.

Genome sequencing Genomic DNA of the LM leaves was obtained with the Plant DNA extraction Kit (TIANGEN) and fragmented randomly. DNA sequencing libraries were constructed in accordance with the standard Illumina library preparation protocols for the genome survey and contig polishing. Paired-end libraries, with an average insert size of around 220 bp, were then set up in accordance with the manufacturer's instructions (Illumina, San Diego, CA). A total of 56. 74 Gb high-quality data were produced for genome survey and contig polishing. Next, high-molecular-weight genomic DNA were screened by BluePippin electrophoresis. Libraries with an insert size of 15‒20 kb were constructed and analysed by the PacBio Sequel system with P6‒C4 chemistry. In total, nine single molecule real-time cells were sequenced, producing 107. 89 Gb of high-quality data for genome assembly. Hi-C libraries were constructed with reference to an earlier published method. A total of six Hi-C fragment libraries, comprising five *Dpn*II and one *Hin*dIII libraries with fragment sizes between 300 and 700 bp, were constructed and analysed by the Illumina HiSeqX Ten platform. In total, 121. 35 Gb of high-quality Hi-C data were generated.

Genome features estimation and assembly Genome size was evaluated using the k-mer frequency. Processing of the PacBio data involved the removal of sequencing adaptors, as well as low-quality reads using the PacBio SMRT Analysis package with stringent parameters (min Sub Read Length, 500). The high-quality PacBio subreads were qualified using Canu (version 1. 5) software with the parameter 'corrected error rate' set to 0. 045, and then subjected to contig assembly by wtdbg (https://github.com/ruanjue/wtdbg) and Canu software. The Quickmerge (version 0. 2) package was applied to merge both assembly results using the wtdbg contigs as reference input. The short reads (56. 74 Gb) from the secondary sequenced data were used to polish merged contigs using Pilon (version 1. 22) and BWA (version 0. 7. 10‒r789). Subsequently, the polished contigs were further scaffolded using Hi-C data.

In brief, a total of 121. 35 Gb of high-quality Hi-C data were generated after adaptor sequences were trimmed and low-quality (over 10% N base pairs or Q10 < 50%) paired-end reads were removed. BWA (version 0. 7. 10‒r789) was used to map Hi-C data based on the aln method. Scaffolding was performed using the uniquely mapped reads of quality > 20. HiC‒Pro (version 2. 8. 1) was used to perform duplicate removal, sorting, and quality checks. The Hi‒C links were combined in 50-kb bins and separately normalized for intra- and intercontig contacts. LACHESIS was used to order the contigs into scaffolds. A final genome size of 811. 06 Mb and scaffold N50 size of 82. 4 Mb were obtained.

Genome annotation The repeat sequences of the LM genome were identified and annotated with a combination of *de novo* and homologue search strategies. Prediction of gene structure was based on homology blast, *de novo* annotation, and transcriptome analysis. Gene function assignment of LM was performed with BLAST in public databases. The accuracy and completeness of the gene prediction were assessed with CEGMA pipeline search, expressed sequence tag (EST) alignment, and BUSCO datasets.

Genome comparison and evolution  The orthologous genes of the 13 representative plant genomes were identified through retrieval of their full genome sequences from websites. The phylogenetic tree was inferred with RAxML (version 8.2.12) using the GTRGAMMA model, 100 starting trees and 1 000 bootstrap replicates. Gene family expansions and contractions were identified by Café (version 4.2.1). Because the genome of *V. vinifera* did not undergo any other WGD event, and the genome of *D. carota* underwent another two WGD events (Dc-α, Dc-β) following the γ event, we selected these two species (*V. vinifera* and *D. carota*) as references to confirm the number of WGD events for the two honeysuckle species (LM and LJ). The WGD event times for LM and LJ were detected using wgd (version 3.0). The co-linearity analyses between the honeysuckle species and *V. vinifera* were performed using JCVI 1.0.5 (https://github.com/tanghaibao/jcvi). After that, the Ks distribution of LM was measured using the wgdi (version 0.51).

To compare the differences between the two honeysuckle species at the genome level, the shared and species-specific orthologous groups between LM and LJ were reanalyzed using OrthoFinder. KEGG enrichment analysis was performed for the species-specific orthologous groups in LM. The differences in chromosomal structure between LM and LJ were visualized by the co-linearity method using JCVI. The sequence similarities and Ks values between these gene pairs were calculated using EMBOSS Needle (version 6.6), and phylogenetic analysis was performed using maximum likelihood (PAML; version 4.9b).

Evolution of hederagenin-based saponin biosynthesis-related genes  To assess tandem duplications that might have taken place in every gene family in the biosynthetic pathway, we determined the positions of all genes identified in the assembly. Divergence time of gene duplication in the hederagenin-based saponins biosynthetic pathway was evaluated with reference to the phylogenetic tree of *Arabidopsis* genes. Selected paralogous gene pairs were subjected to Ks calculation using Nei and Gojobori in the PAML program (version 4.9b). The divergence time was subsequently calculated from the obtained Ks value based on the relation, $T = Ks/2r$, where '$r$' represents a substitution rate of $7.7 \times 10^{-9}$ mutations per site per year for eudicots.

Transcriptome profiling of LM and LJ  Total RNA was extracted from all samples for transcriptome analyses. The quality and concentrations of extracted RNA samples were determined, and cDNA library construction and sequencing were performed by the Biomarker Technologies Corporation (Beijing, China). After sequencing, clean data (clean reads) were obtained by removing reads containing adapter, reads containing poly-N, and low-quality reads from the raw data. Gene expression was calculated with Fragments Per Kilobase of exon model per Million mapped fragments (FPKM). The differential patterns of gene expression were analysed with count number by DESeq2 using a model based on the negative binomial distribution. The resulting *P* values were adjusted using the Benjamini and Hochberg's approach for controlling the false discovery rate. Genes with an adjusted $P$-value $< 0.05$ and fold change $>2$ or $<0.5$, were considered as DEGs.

Cloning and yeast transformation of LmOAS1  The full-length coding sequence (CDS) of *LmOAS1* was amplified from cDNA of LM using primers as described in the Table S18 following the protocol of Phanta Max Super-Fidelity DNA Polymerase (Vazyme, Nanjing, China). To obtain the EVM0008033 with 26 amino acids missing in the N-terminus of protein, primers pYES226cut0008033-F and pYES20008033-R listed in the Table S18 were used. The wild EVM0008033 and truncated EVM0008033 were cloned into yeast expression vector, respectively. Cytochrome P450 reductase ART1 obtained from *Arabidopsis thaliana* was also cloned into the yeast system.

The transformed yeasts were screened on synthetic dropout (SD)/-Leu/-Ura plates. The empty vector with pRS425-Leu-ART1 co-transformed strain was used as negative control. Each of the transformed yeast strains was verified according to the protocol of 2 × Rapid Taq Master Mix (TaKaRa, Kyoto, Japan) before cultivation. The yeast cells were harvested by centrifugation at 3 000 *g* for 10 min. Subsequent procedures were performed at 4 ℃ or on ice. Harvested cells were washed with 100 mM potassium phosphate buffer (pH 7.4) for three times and resuspended in the same buffer containing 1 mM EDTA. Glass beads were added to lyse the cells by vortexing 20 min. The lysed cells were centrifuged at 12 000 *g* for 10 min. The supernatant was collected and stored as crude yeast protein at −80 ℃ until use.

*In vitro* enzymatic activity assay of LmOAS1  The activity of LmOAS1 was tested in a 2 mL reaction mixture containing 20 mM Glc-6-phosphate, 2.5 units of Glc-6-phosphate dehydrogenase, 30 mg of β-Amyrin, 2 mmol/L NADPH and 1.8 mL of crude yeast proteins. After incubating the reaction mixture for 6 h at 28 ℃, the reaction was terminated and extracted with 2 mL of ethyl acetate. The extraction was evaporated and re-dissolved in 110 μL of 100% methanol and subjected to LC-QTOF-MS/MS analysis. Enzymatic metabolites were monitored by comparing both the retention time and mass spectra data with standard oleanolic acid (Yuanye Bio-Technology Co., Ltd Shanghai, China).

Molecular docking and site-directed mutagenesis of

LmOAS1 The three-dimensional LmOAS1 was constructed based on the X-ray structure of CYP120A (resolution: 2.10 Å) using Profiles-3D method. Substrate β-Amyrin was docked into the binding pocket of LmOAS1 model using the Autodock software. Amino acid residues surrounding the substrate at a distance less than 5 Å and facing the active site center were chosen as mutation candidates. Residues K145, P146, E147, A148, L149, and R150 were selected for subsequent site-directed mutagenesis to K145E, P146S, E147H, A148S, L149G, and R150N variants. The fragments of mutated LmOAS1 were amplified from the vector of pYES2-Ura-EVM0008033 using primers listed in the Table S1 following the protocol of Phanta Max Super-Fidelity DNA Polymerase (TaKaRa). Fragments of each Mutated LmOAS1 were ligated and cloned into the vector, pYES2-Ura according to the protocol of ClonExpress Ultra One Step Cloning Kit (Vazyme). The enzyme activities of mutated LmOAS1 versions were determined using *in vitro* enzymatic assay as described above.

Protein expression and purification of LmUGT73P1 The full length of the *LmUGT73P1* cDNA was amplified by polymerase chain reaction (PCR) using designed primers (Table S18) and inserted into the pET - 28a (+) vector (Invitrogen, Carlsbad, USA). The recombinant plasmid pET - 28a - LmGT73P1 was then introduced into *E. coli* BL21 (DE3; Transgen Biotech, Beijing, China) for heterologous expression. The target protein was induced and purified from the edited *E. coli* cells using Ni-NTA agarose (QIAGEN, Dusseldorf, Germany). The purified protein was then concentrated and desalted using the Amicon Centrifugal Filter (Millipore, Billerica, MA) and stored at −80 ℃ for *in vitro* assays. The activity of LmUGT73P1 was analysed by *in vitro* enzyme assay.

*In vitro* assays and kinetic measurements of LmUGT73P1 The function of LmUGT73P1 was characterized by co-incubating 20 μg purified protein, 0.1 mmol/L substrates (oleanolic acid, hederagenin, and cauloside A were separately used), and 0.5 mmol/L sugar donor (mixture of UDP - Rha, UDP - Ara, and UDP - Glu) in 100 μL of 50 mmol/L Tris-HCl buffer (pH 8.0, 37 ℃, 1 h). Reactions were quenched with ice cold methanol and centrifuged at 12 000 **g** for 10 min. The supernatants were dried and re-dissolved in methanol and subjected to LC - QTOF - MS/MS analysis.

Kinetic parameters of LmUGT73P1 were calculated using cauloside A as the substrate. Assays were performed in a final volume of 100 μL, consisting of 50 mM Tris-HCl (pH 7.5), 1 μg LmUGT73P1, 10 mmol/L of UDP-Rha, and different concentrations of the substrates (2.5, 5, 10, 20, 40, 80, 100 μmol/L). After incubating at 37 ℃ for 20 min, the reactions were quenched with ice cold methanol and centrifuged at 12 000 **g** for 10 min, and the supernatants were analysed by LC - QTOF - MS/MS. The value of *Km* was calculated with the Michaelis-Menten plotting method.

Molecular docking and site-directed mutagenesis of LmUGT73P1 The three-dimensional structures of the substrate and sugar donor were generated and optimized by Chem3D software (CambridgeSoft, Cambridge, MA, USA). The structure model of LmUGT73P1 was predicted by Robetta server (http://robetta.bakerlab.org/), and then the pocket and cavity were obtained by the web POCASA (https://g6altair.sci.hokudai.ac.jp/g6/service/pocasa/). Cauloside A and UDP - Rha were successfully docked into the substrate binding pocket using the AutoDock Vina with a grid box (30 Å × 30 Å × 40 Å) centered at (−1.1, 30.6, −35.5) Å. Amino acid residues surrounding binding pocket were chosen as candidates. Residues S53, E83, K258, E312, T330, and V338 were selected for subsequent site-directed mutagenesis to make S53A, E83A, K258A, E312A, T330A, and V338A variants. The fragments of mutated LmUGT73P1 were amplified from the vector of pET - 28a (+)- LmUGT73P1 using the primers listed in the Table S18 following the protocol of Phanta Max Super-Fidelity DNA Polymerase (TaKaRa). Fragments of each mutated LmUGT73P1 were ligated and cloned into the vector of pET - 28a (+) according to the protocol of ClonExpress Ultra One Step Cloning Kit (Vazyme). The enzyme activities of mutated LmUGT73P1 versions were analysed through *in vitro* enzymatic assay.

Expression of UDP-glycosyltransferase (LmUGT73P1) in *N. benthamiana* and product analysis The LmUGT73P1-encoding gene was amplified by PCR with gene-specific primers UGT73P1 - 3 × Flag-BamHI and UGT73P1 - 3 × Flag - SpeI and inserted into the pHB-3 × Flag vector. Upon PCR and DNA sequence verification, the pHB - UGT73P1 vector was transferred to the *Agrobacterium tumefaciens* GV3101 strain. The positive clones were cultured at 28 ℃ in LB liquid medium. After centrifugation at 4 000 **g** for 10 min, the *A. tumefaciens* cells were collected and resuspended in MMA buffer to obtain a final solution with an $OD_{600}$ of 0.8 for each transformant. After a 2 h culturing at room temperature, the solution prepared was injected into the leaves of *N. benthamiana*. *A. tumefaciens* solution without UGT73P1 (empty vector) was used as control. After growing in a glasshouse for 5 days, fresh leaves of infiltrated plants were harvested and dried at 40 ℃. Dried leaves were ground into a powder and metabolites were extracted by 50% methanol solution and analysed using the UPLC - QTOF - MS/MS method.

[尹小建,陆续,齐炼文,等. Plant Biotechnology Journal, 2023,21:1 - 15.]

# Structure-driven protein engineering for production of valuable natural products

## 1 THE ESSENCE OF ENZYMATIC ACTIVITY: PROTEIN STRUCTURE

In recent decades, advances in technology and techniques have facilitated great strides in protein structure analysis, which in turn have further promoted protein engineering as a powerful means of generating enzymes or proteins with desirable properties. As an effective toolbox, there have been many efforts to modulate metabolic pathways and improve biological networks by expanding libraries of reactive elements and enhancing, regulating, expanding, and innovating metabolic responses. In combination with traditional metabolic engineering strategies, protein engineering has shown promise in facilitating the production of many biobased products. In contrast to traditional metabolic engineering strategies, synthetic biology, chemoenzymatic approaches, and plant metabolic engineering, developed on the basis of protein engineering, have shown great promise in facilitating the production of valuable natural products.

The chemical essence of most enzymes is protein, and the complexity and diversity of structures lead to differences in function. Advances in structural biology have enabled investigators to reveal the relationship between structure and function. The core site of enzyme catalytic function is the active pocket, which is the surface or interior cavity of the functional protein with the ability to bind ligands. The amino acid residues surrounding the active pocket not only determine the physicochemical properties of the binding ligand and pocket but also affect the function through shape and size within the protein. These properties are used to assess the ability of the pocket to bind substrates and its promiscuity and specificity (Figure 1).

In the past two decades, developments in molecular biology, X-ray diffraction, NMR, and cryoelectron microscopy instrumentation, together with computational methods, have allowed nearly exponential growth of protein structure studies. A large number of proteins derived from animals, plants, and microbes have been identified, and their structures and mechanism have been defined. At the same time, based on statistical analysis of proteins with actual structures, multiple databases have been established to calculate virtual screening and molecular simulations for undisclosed proteins in 3D structures, and they use evolutionarily related sequences, multiple sequence alignments, and amino acid residue pair representations to improve the precision of protein structures. For example, SWISS-MODEL and Alphafold2, especially Alphafold2, were leveraged by Google's DeepMind team, which has achieved great advances in protein structure prediction. However, because the structure prediction database was developed on the basis of deep learning of proteins with existing actual structures, its accuracy is adequate for predicting proteins with structures/functions similar to known ones, whereas the prediction of completely new protein structures is not as good as expected. It can be seen that the future trend of structural biology is to use the continuous innovation and development of instrumentation to continuously optimize experimental conditions and then obtain higher-resolution structural information of biomolecules as close to nature as possible, which will provide a more reliable template for the subsequent development of artificial intelligence.

Recently, protein engineering has become a favored method to improve enzymatic activity, increase enzyme stability, and expand product spectra in natural product biosynthesis. Protein is one of the most important and resourceful biological macromolecules, and, given its relevance between structure and function, protein engineering has become a significant biotechnological intervention. Depending on the structural basis of the protein, protein engineering can be used to expand or narrow the substrate spectrum, change product types, and further improve catalytic efficiency while addressing product specialization. It provides an increasing number of catalytic elements for the production of valuable natural products.

## 2 PROTEIN ENGINEERING IN NATURAL PRODUCT SYNTHETIC BIOLOGY

Reshape enzyme performance  Synthetic biology offers opportunities to discover and optimize biosynthetic pathways by improving existing parts or engineering new circuits to produce novel molecules by applying the 'Design-Build-Test-Learn' principle. Protein engineering provides synthetic biology with new, more efficient components, especially enzymes.

Protein engineering can reshape enzyme performance through the following aspects: improving catalytic efficiency, broadening substrate spectrum, altering product promiscuity, improving protein stability, and broadening pH range

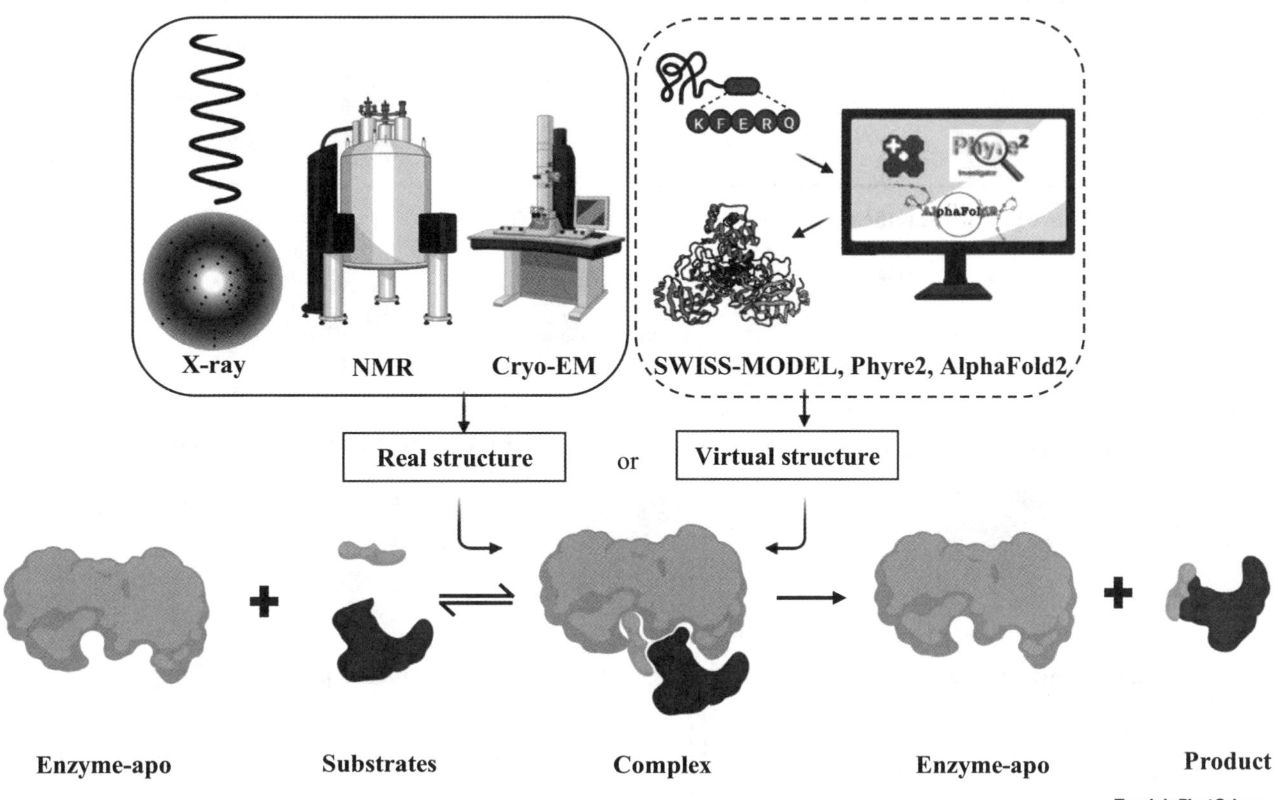


**Figure 1 Schematic representation of protein engineering based on structural biology**

The raw data of the protein samples were collected by using physical instruments [such as X-ray, scanning electron cryomicroscopy (Cryo-EM), and NMR], and the data were analyzed by using computational programs to obtain macromolecular structures or build protein homology models by using virtual software (such as SWISS-MODEL, Alphafold2, and Phyre2). Based on the structural biology, the mechanisms of enzyme catalysis were explained. Figure created with Biorender.com.

(Figure 2). In regard to protein engineering, enzymatic activity enhancement is the most common objective, among others. Ginsenoside Rh2 is a major bioactive ingredient isolated from ginseng. However, its low titer originating from a low catalytic capacity of uridine 5′-diphosphoglucuronosyltransferase (UGT) in microbial fermentation is a bottleneck for scaling up production. Owing to crystal structure-based rational design, the efficiency of glycosyltransferase UGT51 was boosted to ~1 800-fold in *Saccharomyces cerevisiae*, which laid a vital foundation for high-level production of ginsenoside Rh. As a high-value diterpenoid, forskolin is exclusively produced by *Coleus forskohlii*. Researchers have elucidated its complete biosynthetic pathway and found that the key rate-limiting enzyme is cryptic cytochrome P450. To enhance the enzymatic activity of P450, Victor *et al*. turned to protein engineering to study the substrate recognition sites (SRSs) of pathway-related P450s. The homology modelling results, together with functional experiments, indicated that a single point mutation in the SRS1 loop of CYP76AH15, a cytochrome P450 responsible for the first oxidative step in forskolin biosynthesis, could increase the catalytic efficiency greater than fivefold, yielding more 11-oxo-13R-mannoyl oxide in yeast cells. In certain circumstances, enzymes with undesired substrate selectivity and product promiscuity become bottlenecks in natural product biosynthesis. To fix this problem, protein engineering has been applied to create desired enzymes with either high specificity or diverse functions in metabolic pathways. In nature, the abundance of medium-chain (C6 - C12) fatty acids and lipids is significantly less than that of longer-chain compounds. Combining structure-inspired mutagenesis and optimized algorithms, *Escherichia coli*-derived ‘TesA mutants that exhibit distinct preferences towards medium-chain fatty acids were identified, contributing to the synthesis of value-added octanoic acid (C8) and dodecanoic acid (C12). Similar work was conducted on baker's yeast, where fatty acid synthase was reprogrammed according to its structural and functional data, mainly generating specific hexanoic acid (C6) and octanoic acid (C8) up to 464 mg/l altogether. Novel enzymes with new functions can also be redesigned through protein engineering to expand the biopart library for synthetic biology. Authentic structure-driven protein engineering

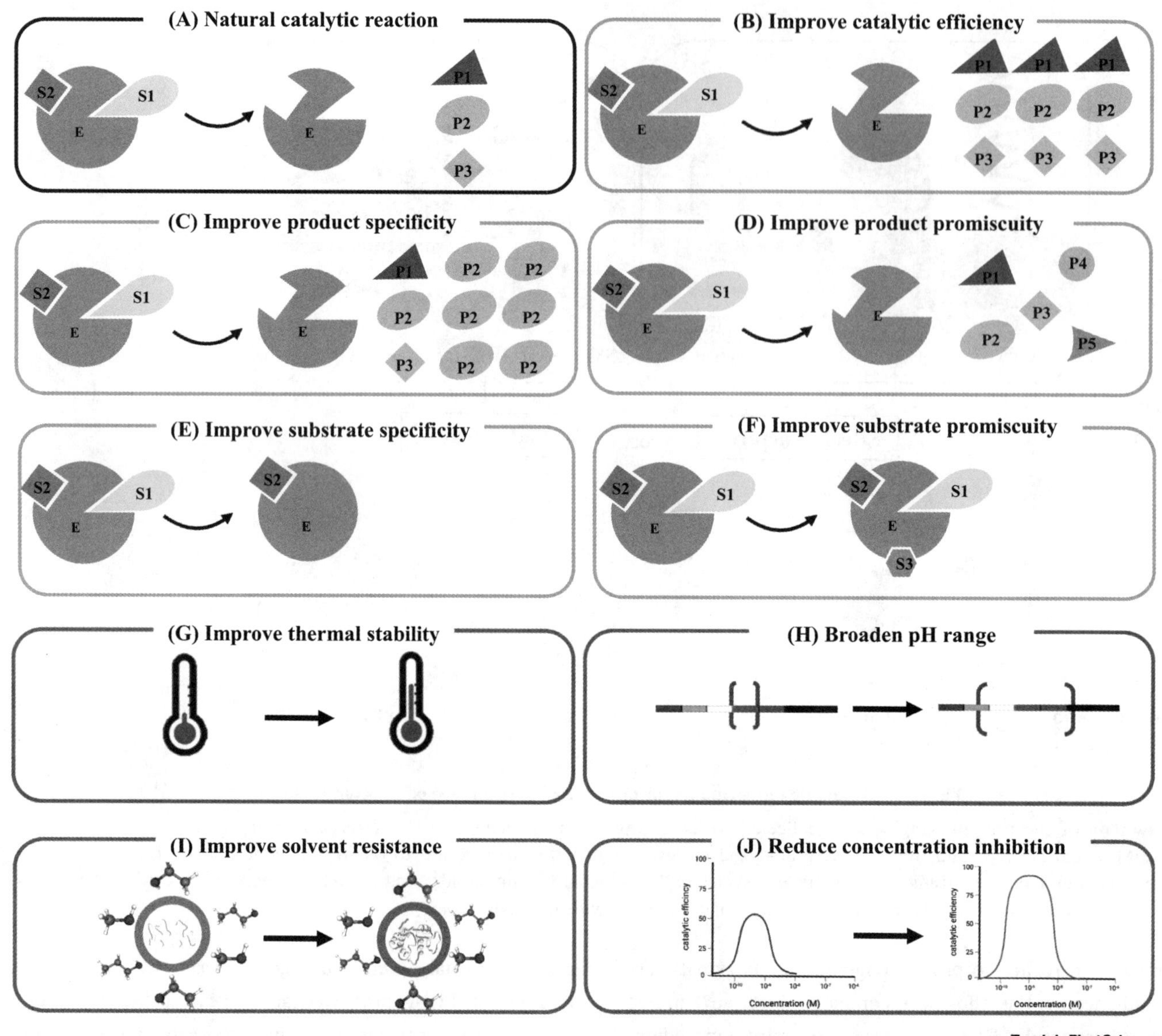


**Figure 2 Schematic representation of improved enzyme performance benefiting from protein engineering**

(A) The enzymatic reaction in the natural state, where enzyme (E) can catalyze substrates (S1 and S2) to form corresponding products (P1, P2, and P3). (B) The enzymatic reaction mediated by engineered protein, where the yield of products was obviously improved due to high catalytic efficiency. (C) The enzymatic reaction initiated by optimized protein, where the generation of a certain product (P2) was boosted, presenting product specificity. (D) The enzymatic reaction initiated by devised protein, where the types of products were enriched, exhibiting product promiscuity. (E) The enzymatic reaction catalyzed by rationally designed proteins, where the enzyme can only accept S2 as a substrate, indicating substrate specificity. (F) The enzymatic reaction catalyzed by the reformed protein, where the enzyme can additionally recognize S3 as a substrate, showing substrate promiscuity. (G－J) The inner properties of enzymes can be ameliorated through protein engineering in some aspects, such as thermal stability/pH tolerance range/solvent resistance/concentration inhibition. Figure created with Biorender. com.

of monoterpenoid synthase from *Salvia fruticosa*-SfCinS1 has been proved to be effective in shifting substrate bias from characteristic GPP (geranyl diphosphate) to atypical 2meGPP (2-methyl-GPP), harvesting promiscuous C11 terpenoid backbones.

Offer a favorable microenvironment　In addition to ameliorating target enzymes with desired properties, protein engineering can be applied to provide a better reactive environment for anabolism, accelerating the catalytic rate of the whole pathway. Protein scaffold engineering is a method that leverages structural information, such as peptide motifs and adaptor domains, to spatially organize enzymes participating in sequential reactions (Figure 3A). For instance, a pair of protein-peptide interaction domains (PSD95/Dlg1/zo-1) and their ligand (PDZ ligand) from metazoan cells were selected to optimize the biosynthesis route of flavonoids in *E. coli*,

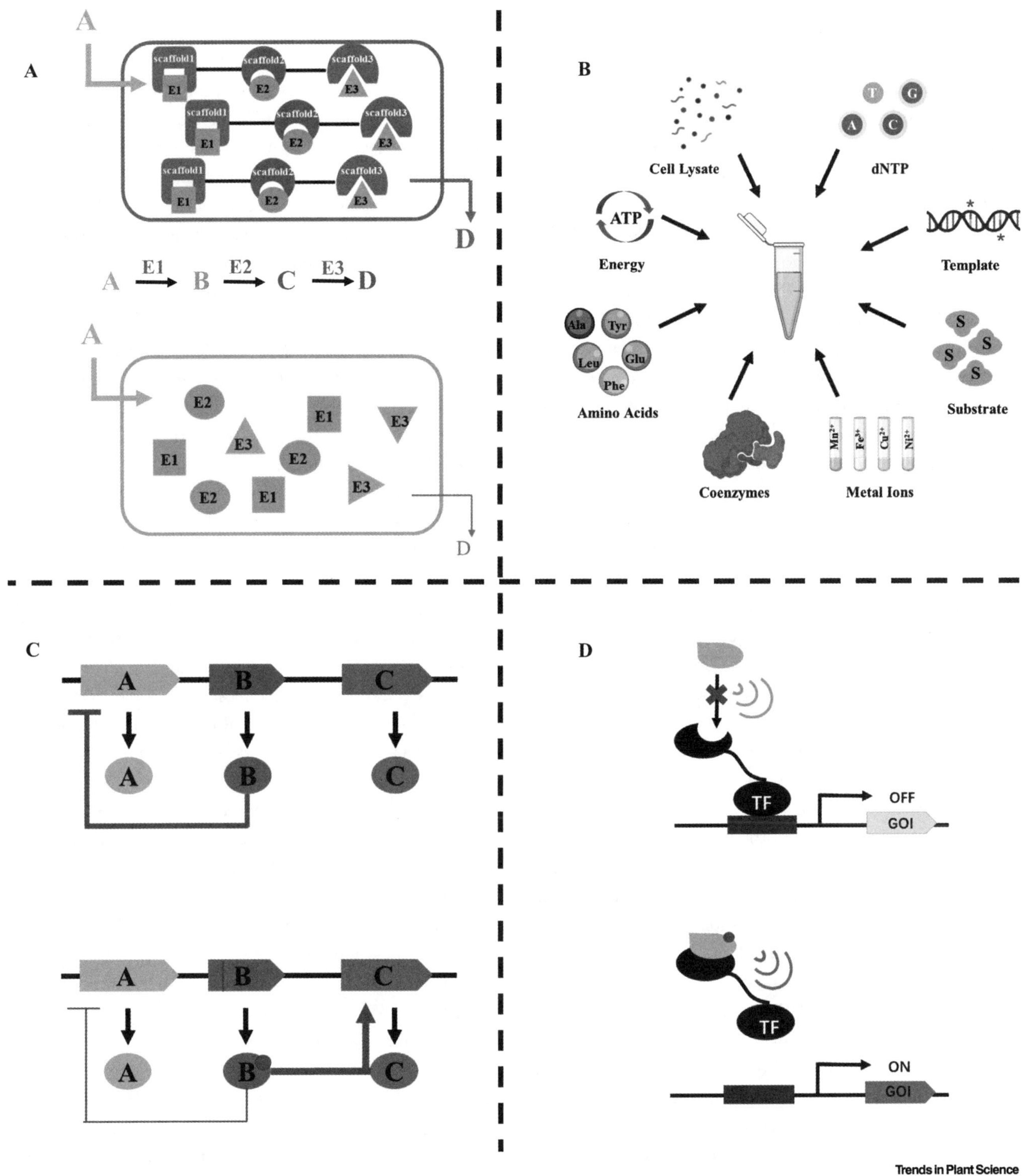


**Figure 3 Schematic representation of protein engineering applications in synthetic biology**

(A) On the basis of structural information of scaffold proteins, peptides or motifs with interactions can be modified to organize the enzymes involved in specific metabolic pathways in order, thus spatially organizing enzymes in the same pathway. (B) When the key catalytic site is validated, a cell-free system is worth trying to circumvent obstacles in traditional metabolic engineering, such as precursor shortage, intermediate toxicity, and membrane permeability. (C) Protein engineering (red dot) can be used in redirecting metabolic flux distribution, which in turn alleviates feedback inhibition in natural product biosynthesis, promoting highly efficient biosynthesis of target natural products. (D) As an important branch of synthetic biology, dynamic regulation can profit from directed protein engineering (red dot), maintaining balance between cell growth and target metabolite synthesis. Figure created with Biorender.com.

gaining 143.5 mg/l baicalein (6.6-fold improvement) and 120.4 mg/l scutellarein (1.4-fold improvement), respectively. Similarly, different protein scaffolds have been redesigned with a stoichiometric arrangement of enzymes engaged in 5-deoxy(iso)flavonoid biosynthesis, harvesting 97 mg/l total flavanone, which is a 1.4-fold increase. During the biosynthesis of complex compounds, tough problems, such as precursor supply, intermediate toxicity, and membrane permeability, are inevitable and can hardly be handled by usual metabolic engineering. An alternative way to circumvent these limitations is to com-bine protein engineering with cell-free systems, leveraging purified enzymes and cofactors to expedite the *in vitro* conversion of a substrate into a product (Figure 3B). Recently, for the sake of the high titer of cannabigerolic acid (CBGA), the rate-limiting enzyme prenyltransferase NphB was chosen for mutagenesis on the basis of *in silico* docking and Rosetta analysis. When the promising variant M32 was combined with a cell-free prenylating system, the final concentration of CBGA was 1.25 g/L over 24 h, a nearly 140-fold improvement compared with the nonoptimized pathway, highlighting the bright prospect of such a strategy.

Control of metabolic flux When a specific biosynthetic pathway is introduced into a heterologous system, flux imbalance caused by multiple enzyme assembly hinders the high-efficiency synthesis of final compounds. Therefore, it is necessary to redirect the flux distribution in cells by means of derived-protein engineering (Figure 3C). Homoserine acetyltransferase (MetX) is not only rigorously controlled by intermediates such as SAM and cysteine but also subjected to feedback inhibition by the end product. MetX was designed by evolutionary conservation analysis and structure-guided design to reduce its sensitivity towards *O*-acetylhomoserine (OAH). The replacement of the triple F147L - M182I - M240A mutant into *E. coli* resulted in a 57.14% increase in OAH production.

Apart from static regulation, protein engineering can also achieve dynamic control of a given metabolic pathway with the aid of regulatory-based biosensors (Figure 3D). To manage the trade-off between cell density and product synthesis, a previously developed engineering of uric acid-responsive HucR was focused on monitoring the concentration of substrate and product. To increase the accuracy of HucR, four crucial sites (W20, L44, D73, and R80) were selected within the effector binding pocket for several rounds of site-saturation mutagenesis, and a superior regulatory component responsive to both added ferulic acid and produced vanillin was finally obtained. The feedback activation, combined with cascade dynamic control, promised sufficient strain growth and vanillin output, showing the possibility for broad application in natural product synthetic biology.

## 3 STRUCTURE-BASED DESIGN FOR CHEMOENZYMATIC SYNTHESIS

Natural products represent a diversified family of chemicals with a broad variety of biological activities that have found multiple applications in the food, pharmaceutical, clothing, paper product, transportation fuel, and environmental industries. Due to the low bioavailability and structural complexity of active compounds from natural sources, as well as the fact that conventional chemical synthesis involves poor regioselectivity, stereoselectivity, and laborious protection-deprotection procedures for functional groups, meeting the growing demand remains a major challenge. Chemoenzymatic synthesis, which introduces biocatalysts into the chemical pathway, has been a promising alternative method with substantial benefits, such as better cost effectiveness, less synthetic steps, and environmental friendliness (Figure 4). Although multiple limitations towards enzyme stability, enzyme selectivity, substrate promiscuity, and reaction specificity have been met during chemoenzymatic procedures, protein engineering based on structures will be greatly helpful in guiding mutagenesis and modelling studies to over-come these obstacles for desired purposes.

The poor stability of biocatalysts when exposed to chemical conditions is one of the key reasons for their restricted practical applications. The thermostability is the most important factor; it is controlled by multiple factors and generally requires mutations to the peptide chain of amino acid residues composing the protein. To improve the thermostability of chitosanase-CsnTS, the potentially relevant serine residues were mutated through structure and sequence comparison with thermophilic homologous CelA from *Clostridium thermocellum*, and the engineered CsnTS can be applied in the industrial scale-up production of chitooligosaccharides. Optimizing reaction specificity is another goal for engineered proteins in chemoenzymatic synthesis. For example, homology modelling and bioinformatic analysis provided evidence for rational engineering of an iron- and α-ketoglutarate-dependent enzyme (GetI) to be 4-arginine hydroxylase by switching the substrate specificity. This novel enzyme was adapted in the concise chemoenzymatic synthesis of enduracidin analogues.

There is a set of complex enzymatic transformations involved in the biosynthetic pathways of natural products, whereas the limited substrate scope is always one of the chal-lenges to the effectiveness and scalability of these transfor-mations. AsqJ is an iron- and 2-oxoglutarate-dependent oxygenase that can be an alternative to chemical asymmetric epoxidation during viridicatin-type alkaloid production. Previous studies have elucidated the AsqJ-catalyzed mechanism on the basis of structural characterization. To explore substrate promiscuity, molecular dynamics (MD) simulations and *in*

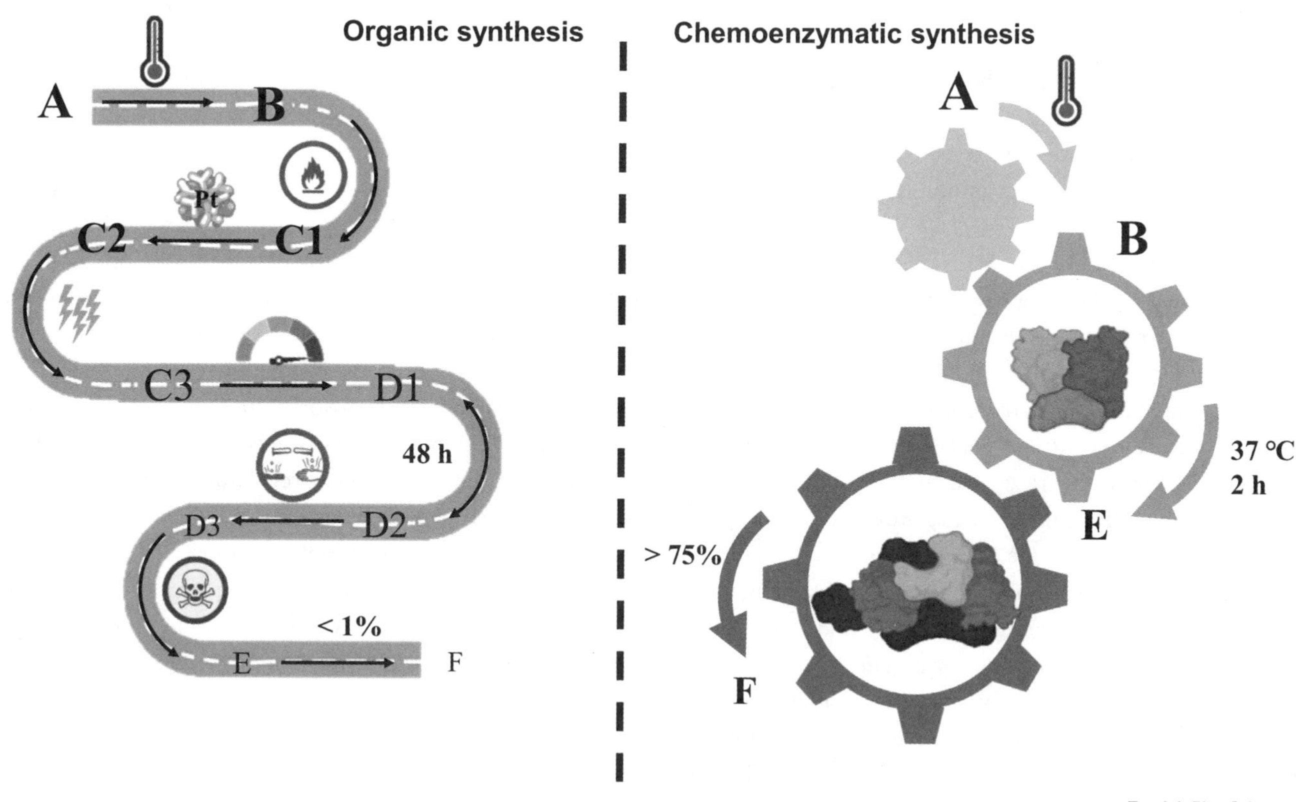


**Figure 4 Schematic comparison between organic synthesis and chemoenzymatic synthesis**

(A) A simple substrate. (B－E) Different intermediates. (F) The target product. In organic synthesis, the production of (F) is quite complicated, where the reaction requires high temperature and pressure, flammable and erosive agents, noble metal catalysts, and specific wavelengths, and the yield is far from satisfactory. In chemoenzymatic procedures, intermediate (B) derived from chemical synthesis can be efficiently converted to final product (F) using protein engineering under mild reaction conditions with higher yield. Figure created with Biorender.com.

*silico* analysis with crystallographic data were performed to effectively prepare suitable substrates. The reaction outcomes were consistent with the evaluated binding effects, which facilitated the chemoenzymatic synthesis of the quinolone alkaloid library. According to homology modelling and MD simulations, the versatile *C*-glycosyltransferases (AbCGT) from *Aloe barbadensis* showed the ability to catalyze glycosylate phenols lacking the acyl group. Following saturation mutagenesis on similar key amino acid residues (V183) in enzyme-binding sites, both the catalytic selectivity and the efficiency of AbCGT were improved, showing potential to generate more drug-candidate C-glycosides by chemoenzymatic routes. In light of structure-based protein engineering, the chemoenzymatic strategy has expanded the synthetic utility of valuable natural products, which contributes to future industrial production and opens the way to prospective new-to-nature derivatives.

## 4 RATIONAL DESIGN IN PLANT METABOLIC ENGINEERING

Metabolic engineering aims to modify the endogenous metabolic network of plants to obtain more useful functional characteristics, such as the production of a value-added compound and the improvement of plant resistance. Transforming the synthetic pathways in plants through genetic engineering techniques has become the most effective means of metabolic engineering. Unlike genetic engineering techniques, which obtain targets through mass disorderly screening, protein engineering methods and approaches have made it a reality quickly and easily, with better stability, higher catalytic activity, and, most important, a wider range of applicability of proteins.

Regarding the transformation of the substrate promiscuity of the protein complex, specific reshaping of the active sites of MOMT5 (T133L/E165I/F175I/F166WH169F) created enzymes that specifically methylate the condensed guaiacyl lignin precursor coniferyl alcohol, imposing an apparent steric hindrance that excludes bulkier lignin precursors. This provided an excellent target for modulating lignin composition and/or structure *in planta*. Replacing enzymes with a low catalytic rate and poor affinity and specificity with those with a higher catalytic rate in plants can achieve a better phenotype. A LysM receptor heteromer OsMYR1/OsLYK2 and OsCERK1 mediates the perception of arbuscular mycorrhizal fungi in rice. Replacing the ectodomains of OsMYR1 and OsCERK1 with those from the homologous Nod factor receptors MtNFP and MtLYK3 of *Medicago truncatula* increased calcium oscillations in response to Nod factors and significantly improved the recognition of nodulation factors in rice.

As seen above, there are relatively few cases of protein engineering-based regulation of secondary plant metabolism, but examples of using protein engineering to regulate plant immunity and energy conversion have been reported. By engineering the heavy metal-associated (HMA) structural domain of rice RGA5, it was confirmed that the modified RGA5 could specifically recognize and bind the pathogen effector protein AVR-PikD, which is not recognized by the original RGA5, extending the disease resistance of the crop. RbcS is a small subunit of Rubisco, and knocking out the OsRbcS (rice RbcS) multigene family and completely replacing OsRbcS with SbRbcS (sorghum RbcS) in rice Rubisco increased the photosynthetic $CO_2$ assimilation rate and photosynthetic efficiency, which can greatly improve plant growth and productivity. As with many life activities in plants, metabolic pathways involve the assembly of multiple enzymes; however, not all pathway enzymes are efficient and specific, often manifesting as imbalances in fluxes, redundant reactions, and the accumulation of unwanted intermediates. The transfer of metabolic fluxes from precursors to target metabolites can be enhanced, redirected, and truncated by modifying the properties of rate-limiting enzymes. One of the future trends in plant metabolic engineering is the reprogramming of plant metabolic pathways with greater fluxes and fewer steps. CRISPR/Cas9-assisted engineering now provides technical support for the replacement and removal of pathway enzymes, and protein engineering provides a basis for the creation of new enzymes that can build a rapid system for protein screening and modification *in vivo*, which offers the possibility of reshaping the secondary metabolic network in plants.

## 5 CONCLUDING REMARKS AND FUTURE PERSPECTIVES

Proteins are the most functional macromolecules and are key to the regulation of biological processes. Given their importance, protein engineering has become a significant biotechnological intervention. In the past few years, there has been tremendous progress in protein engineering with the development of techniques for the structural analysis of proteins. Protein engineering can permanently alter the catalytic and physical properties of enzymes and may significantly increase the potential for biocatalyst applications, facilitating the continued rapid development of biocatalysts and natural product biotransformation. Protein engineering has thus developed into a powerful tool that has made a prominent contribution to the development of metabolic engineering.

The main objective of metabolic engineering is to rationalize metabolic pathways based on knowledge of metabolic networks and to modify complex pathways and their regulation to efficiently synthesize target products. To date, it has evolved to construct new metabolic pathways by combining multiple enzyme molecules from different sources to achieve the coexpression of multiple genes. Due to the complexity of metabolic networks, it is much more difficult to find suitable modification targets from the thousands of metabolic reactions and their regulatory loops. However, the advent of structural biology has provided new ideas and methods to address these problems. Computational analysis can be used to design optimal synthetic pathways and identify suitable metabolic engineering modification strategies, and structural biology will contribute to constructing high-performance biological parts that act more precisely and perform more consistently with new functions, resulting in faster and better access to specific products. Synthetic biology optimizes artificially designed and constructed biological parts to synthesize new biological systems or modify biological systems and processes that exist in nature. Chemoenzymatic strategies have been developed in which chemical synthesis could be combined with enzyme-catalyzed reactions to reprogram existing non-natural active ingredients using modified enzymes. Plant metabolic engineering can combine structural biology with techniques such as the CRISPR/Cas9 system to enhance desired products by upregulating certain genes or downregulating others. Nonetheless, the relevant synthetic pathway could only be designed if the metabolite and the associated reaction are resolved, whereas a large number of unknown biochemical reactions are not included in these pathways. The rational design of enzymes with new catalytic activity will obtain new bioproducts, reconstruct biosynthetic pathways, or even synthesize new biomolecules that do not exist in nature. Moreover, the analytical or screening methods used in each study are often highly specific to a particular trait and therefore not always transferable to other situations. The applications of structure-driven protein engineering in metabolic engineering for the production of valuable natural products still have a number of bottlenecks that need to be addressed (see Outstanding questions). Rational protein engineering is therefore an important trend for the future of protein engineering. This relies on an in-depth understanding of protein structures/computational simulations and their catalytic mechanisms. With the new methods and avenues emerging rapidly in this area, protein engineering could very soon become an essential tool for synthetic biology, chemoenzymatic synthesis, and plant metabolic engineering, resulting in the efficient production of valuable natural products.

[王芸,张磊,等. Trends in Plant Science, 2023,28(4): 460-470.]

# Heterologous mogrosides biosynthesis in cucumber and tomato by genetic manipulation

The preference for food flavour pervades the entire evolutionary history of humans, and this preference has occasionally been higher than human nutritional requirements have been. Flavours have played a pivotal role in food preference, and tastiness afforded a sense of pleasure, which has important implications for improving appetite, digestion and increasing the use rate of nutrients. Moreover, humans have already begun improving vegetable and fruit flavours, which has ultimately led to the guidance of diet expenditure and improvement to human health. Over the past half century, the breeding goal of high crop productivity has indirectly caused a reduction in flavour and nutrients. Owing to genetic linkage, quality traits appear to be negatively related to yield, and desirable flavour, high yield and high quality are complex traits controlled by multiple genes. In general, therefore, plant breeding for flavour enhancement remains a major challenge on the basis of the high yield and good quality. Since 1983, major advances in transgenic biotechnology have allowed breeding for enhanced flavour and nutritional quality to be more simplified and feasible. As has been shown previously, there is an obvious absence of flavour-associated volatiles in modern commercial tomato cultivars. Consequently, scientists have modified tomato plants such that the fruits present a lemon flavour and a rose-like aroma via the expression of *Ocimum basilicum* geraniol synthase. Furthermore, *TomLoxC* has been widely acknowledged to affect tomato fruit flavour by catalysing lipid-derived C5 and C6 volatile biosynthesis. More-over, previous research has indicated the transformation of *VpVAN* gene regulating the vanillin biosynthesis has changed the unique flavour of pepper. Obviously, plant breeding involving homologous or heterologous transgenes associated with flavour has become a popular research topic likely to continue in the future.

Sweetness preference is a kind of human instinct, and sweet-ness has been described as a fundamental hedonic pleasure. Sweet foods with sugar as the essential ingredient have markedly increased obesity, diabetes and cardiovascular diseases in all age groups worldwide; thus, it is necessary to explore sugar-free sweeteners for use in daily diets. Equally, scientists transformed sweet-tasting proteins into cucumber, tomato, strawberry, pear, and lettuce for sweet-taste crops breeding. However, sweet proteins were commonly limited by high price, insufficient supply, poor taste and short shelf life and stability. In 1983, mogroside V, a non-sugar sweetener isolated from the unique *Siraitia grosvenorii* fruit (Cucurbitaceae; Luo-han-guo or monk fruit), was discovered in China, and were approved by FDA in 2010. Typically, mogrosides are divided into several sweet components, such as mogroside III, siamenoside I and mogroside V. The sweetness of mogrosides differ depending on the number of glycosylation and glycosylation sites. The great advantage of mogroside V is its superb flavour compared with that of stevio-sides, rubusoside and glycyrrhizin, which normally are slightly bitter tasting sweet. Interestingly, this natural sweetener with antiglycation effects has a high sweetness, has a low-calorie content and is nontoxic; its sweetness is approximately 300 times higher than that of sucrose; and its history of medicinal use is >300 years. Mogrosides have been approved and used by all kinds of recognised brands at home and abroad, and it has been applied in the >4, 300 products all over the world by the end of September 2019. In China, mogrosides is thought as a kind of safe, non-toxic and natural sweetener, which is widely used in the food, beverage and pharmaceutical industries and has great commercial potential worldwide. In 2011, our group investi-gated the mogroside V biosynthesis pathway, and 40 key enzyme-encoding genes were cloned for the first time, which provided donor genes for crop breeding for sweet flavour improvement. According to the literature, the precursor of mogroside V biosynthesis, 2,3-oxidosqualene, is extensively found in plants (Supplementary Fig. S1). Therefore, it is vitally important that various mogroside V synthase genes be transformed into candidate plants to develop sweet plants, and these transgenic plants can also be used as promising materials for mogroside V production.

During the past 30 years, many transgenic plants for which a single trait has been genetically improved have been applied to promote commercial cultivation in some countries and areas. With the development of metabolic engineering and synthetic biology, multigene transformation has been applied for regulating biosynthesis and improving multiple biological properties instead of single-gene transformation, which is an emerging trend in genetic breeding. To date, there have been numerous break-throughs in plants genetically engineered for the biofortification of micronutrients, phytonutrients and bioactive components, such as β-carotene-enriched Golden rice, potato, banana and canola, anthocyanin-, L-DOPA-, folate and flavonol-, betalain-biofortified tomato fruits, which were developed via multigene transformation involving targeted metabolite biosynthesis pathways. To achieve the de novo synthesis of mogroside V, the key problem is the integration of 6 mogrosides biosynthesis genes into candidate plants. We therefore developed a simple and efficient multigene expression system based on In-fusion technology and self-cleaving 2A peptides. Moreover, 6 mogroside V synthase genes have been successfully introduced into cucumber and tomato, and all genes had high transcript levels in the transgenic plants. Accordingly, we developed sweet cucumber transgenic plant with mogroside V and slightly sweet tomato with mogroside III (MIII) firstly. This study describes extensive prospective application in the field of vege-table and fruit flavour breeding and provides a valuable and captivating blueprint for elaborately developing exceptional plant germplasms with certain characteristic and multiple flavours.

## 1 RESULTS

Promoter activity assays  The AtUBQ10 and AtPD7 promoters were isolated from *Arabidopsis thaliana* and ligated into a pBI121 vector together with the GUS reporter gene (Fig. 1a). To assess the suitability of the promoters, transient expression was per-formed in the cotyledons of *Cucumis sativus* as described previously. Leaves of *Nicotiana benthamiana* and cotyledons of *Cucumis sativus* were infected with *Agrobacterium* harbouring pBI121 in which the GUS gene was driven by AtUBQ10, AtPD7 and CaMV 35S promoters under the same conditions. To char-acterize the function of these promoters, histochemical staining was performed as described previously. As expected, there was a high level of GUS activity under the control of the AtUBQ10 and AtPD7 promoters in *Cucumis sativus* and *Nicotiana benthamiana* (Fig. 1b, c), and the highest expression level was detected at 5 d after infiltration of *Cucumis sativus*. Therefore, the ability of the AtUBQ10 and AtPD7 promoters to drive gene transcription in *Cucumis sativus* and *Nicotiana benthamiana* was comparable to that of the CaMV 35S promoter, and there was no significant difference between these promoters (Fig. 1b and Fig. 1c). These promoters could therefore be used as strong constitutive promoters to drive gene expression in the multigene vector.

Design of multigene expression vector for mogrosides biosynthesis  It has been widely demonstrated that the precursor of mogrosides biosynthesis is 2, 3-oxidosqualene, which is syn-thesized through the mevalonate pathway and catalysed by a series of enzymes to synthesize mogroside V in *Siraitia grosvenorii* (Supplementary Fig. S1). Therefore, the binary plasmid pCAMBIA1300 harbouring the mogrosides synthesis-related enzyme-encoding genes *SgSQE1*, *SgCS*, *SgEPH2*, *SgP450*, *SgUGT269-1* and *SgUGT289-3* together with Hyg resistance gene (Hyg, selection marker) driven by AtPD7, AtUBQ10 and CaMV 35S promoters was constructed via In-fusion technology and self-cleaving 2A peptides (Supplementary Fig. S2a). First, all the target genes were ligated into pBI121 or pCAMBIA1300 to produce the first gene expression cassette. Second, the region harbouring the promoter, target gene and terminator was cloned and ligated into pCAMBIA1300 to produce a double-gene expression cassette. Then, combining the first gene expression cassette and the double-gene expression cassette, we constructed a triple-gene expression cassette. Finally, the triple-gene expression cassettes were ligated into the final vector by P2A peptides. (Supplemen-tary Fig. S2a). The corresponding U22p-SCE plasmid was iden-tified via PCR (Supplementary Fig. S2b). This multigene expression vector was large (the length from the left border to the right border was ~21.5 kb) and was used to synthesize mogro-sides. The U22p-SCE plasmid was introduced into *Agrobacterium tumefaciens* GV3101, and the transformants were further used for genetic transformation.

Transient expression assays  To further confirm the availability of the multigene vectors, a transient expression assay was performed in *Cucumis sativus*. All mogrosides biosynthesis-related genes were expressed in the cotyledons of *Cucumis sativus* via agroinfiltration. In accordance with the methods of our preliminary study, we sampled the cotyledons of *Cucumis sativus* at 5 d and the cotyledons of tobacco leaves at 48 h after infiltration for HPLC-ESI-MS/MS analysis. As indicated in the Supplementary Fig. S3a and S3b, MII-E and MIII accumulated slightly in the cotyledons of *Cucumis sativus* transformed with the U22p-SCE multigene expression vector, but MI-A1 was not detected. Unfortunately, no SI or MV was observed in the multiple transient expression assay. The lack of accumulation of SI and MV suggested at least two possibilities: ① the transient expression assay generally lasted for a short time, in this case, the accumulation of MIII substrate was inadequate for the production of SI and MV in the cotyledons of (*Cucumis sativus*). ② the multigene expression vector was too large to suppress the gene expression, which resulted in the reduction of MII-E and MIII. Nevertheless, the transient expression

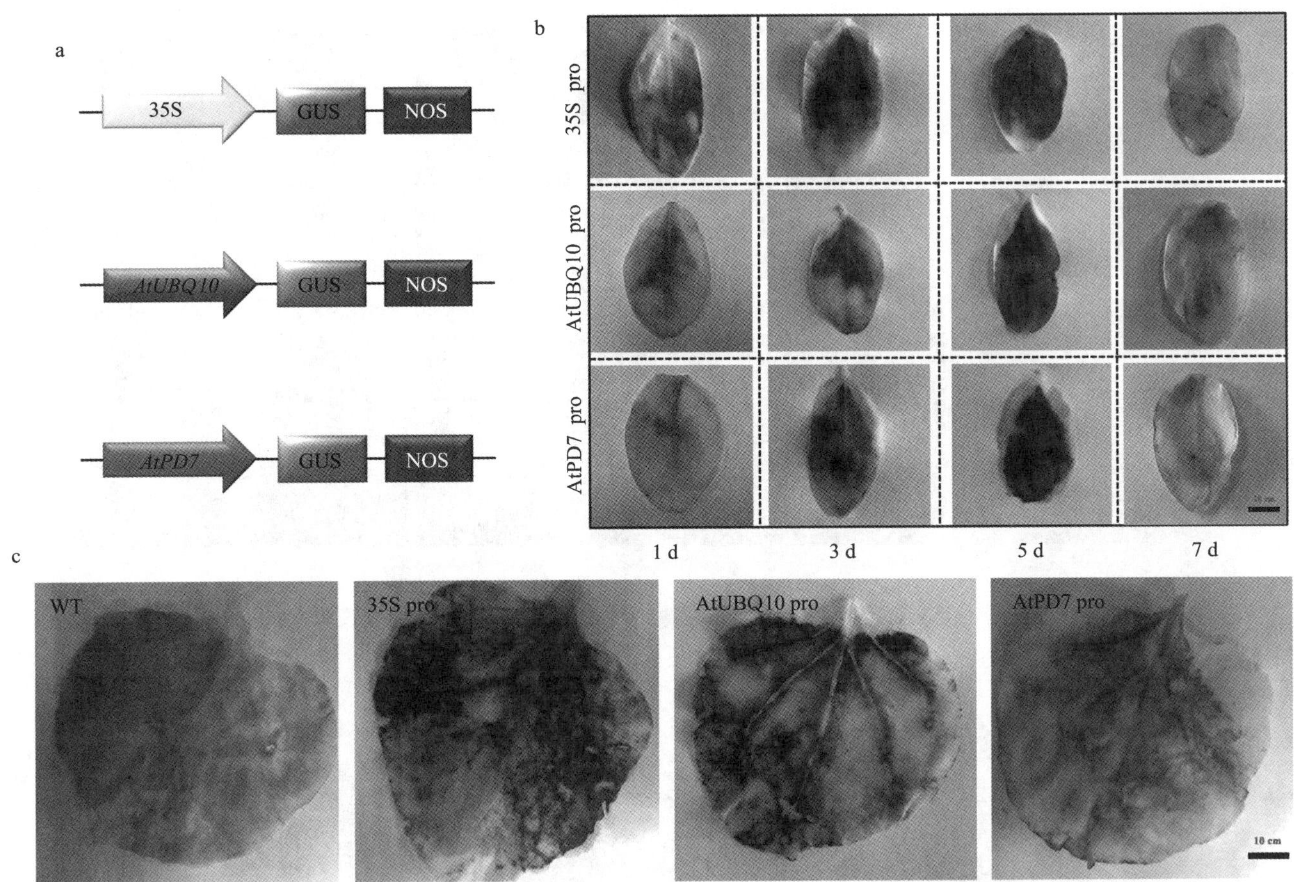


**Fig. 1 Cloning and analysis of candidate promoters in cucumber and tobacco**

(a) Recombinant plasmid with different promoters. (b) Histochemical GUS assay of transient expression in cucumber. (c) Histochemical GUS assay of transient expression was performed after 48 h of infiltration in tobacco. WT plants were used as negative controls. 35S pro: CaMV 35S promoter; AtUBQ10 pro: AtUBQ10 promoter; AtPD7 pro: AtPD7 promoter.

assay confirmed that multigene expression vector was available. Thus, the stable transformation of multigene expression vectors is required for their genetic transformation into *Cucumis sativus* and *Lyco-persicon esculentum*, which provides a new idea about mogrosides-accumulating vegetable breeding.

Generation of mogrosides-accumulating cucumber To enhance the nutritional characteristics of cucumber, the multigene expression vector U22p - SCE was introduced into *Agrobacterium tumefaciens* strain GV3101 and the mogrosides biosynthetic pathway was genetically engineered to produce mogrosides in cucumber plants. About 500 cucumber leaf ex-plants were subjected to *Agrobacterium*-mediated transfor-mation with the U22p - SCE vector. Among these, the total number of Hyg-resistant lines was about 15, but many Hyg-resistant lines were not able to root, survive and grow on seedling. Finally, only 5 transgenic plants were grown in the green house after domestication and trans-plantation. All transgenic plants and non-transformed plants were cultivated in the greenhouse with the consistent growth environment (Fig. 2a). To detect the integration of the transgenes into the genome of the cucumber plants (Fig. 2b), genomic DNA was extracted to determine the presence of target genes and Hyg genes using gene-specific primers by PCR (Supplementary Table S4). Fragments of the expected size were detected in all Hyg-resistant transgenic lines (Fig. 2c). A 1 587 bp fragment of *SgSQE1*, 2 280 bp fragment of *SgCS*, 951 bp fragment of *SgEPH2*, 1 421 bp fragment of *SgP450*, 1 253 bp fragment of *SgUGT269 - 1*, 1 026 bp fragment of *SgUGT289 - 3* and 392 bp fragment of the Hyg resistance gene were simultaneously detected in the one trans-genic plant (U1) but were not amplified from WT cucumber plants (Fig. 2c). Other plants almost never existed all six genes using PCR amplication. The data of the cucumber transformation experiment were listed in the Supplementary Table S1. In total, we obtained only one independent transgenic cucumber line after transformation with the U22p - SCE vector. Although the trans-formation frequency was relatively low in this study, this is the first study in which 6 genes were transformed simultaneously into the cucumber genome, and a large-vector transformation is unpredictable. Previous studies have suggested that the genetic transformation efficiency of cucumber is still highly variable and that the genotypes of explants that can be used are limited. To improve the

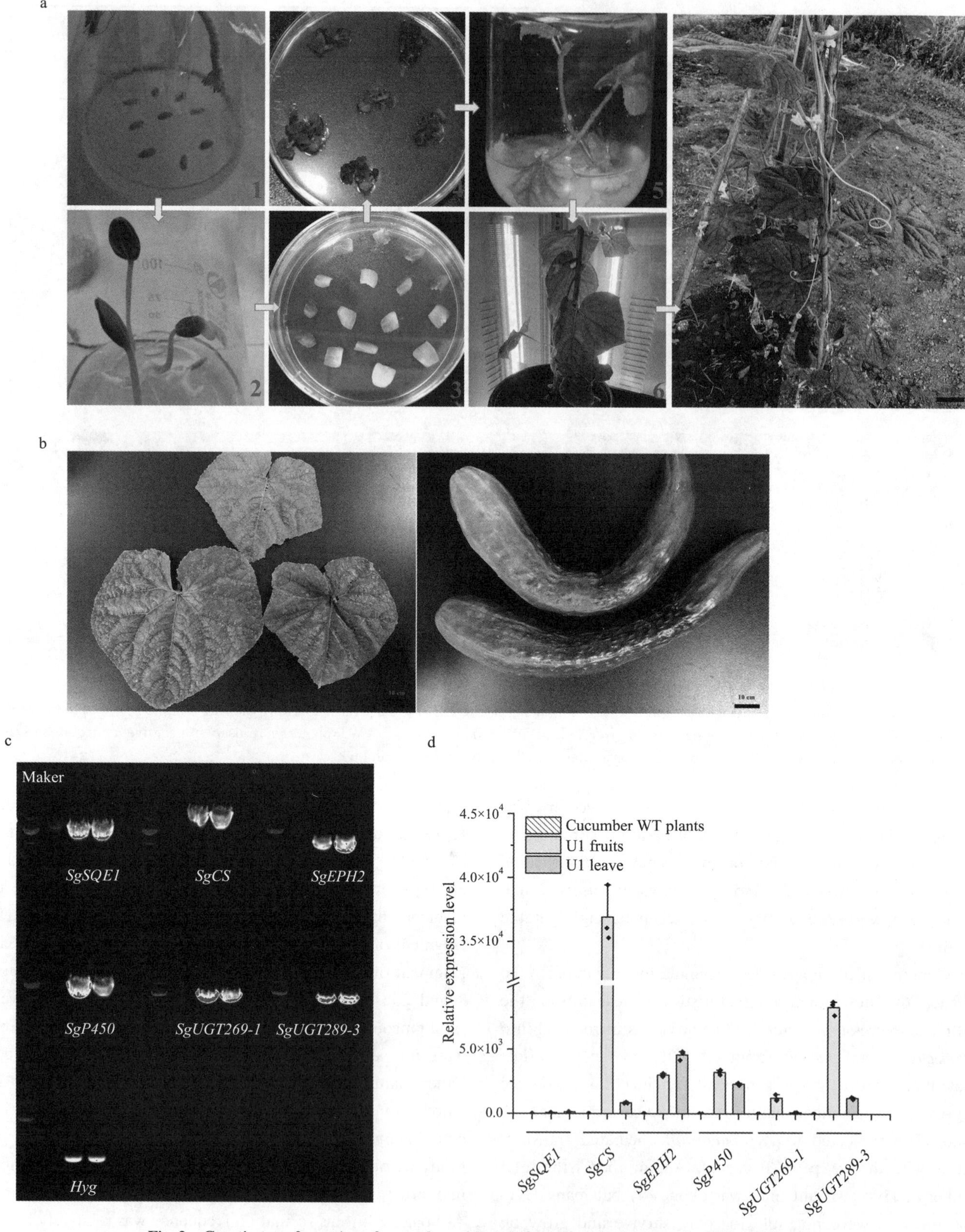


**Fig. 2　Genetic transformation of cucumber with *Agrobacterium* harbouring the U22p-SCE vector**

(a) Genetic transformation of cucumber with *Agrobacterium* harbouring the U22p-SCE vector. (1) Sterilized seeds. (2) 4-days-old seedlings. (3) The cotyledons were cut and used as explants. (4) The explants in the selected medium. (5) The regenerated plants in the rooting media. (6, 7) Regenerated plants. (b) Leaves and fruits of transgenic cucumber line U1. (c) PCR-based detection of U1. The lanes from left to right represent the Maker, WT, U1 fruits and U1 leaves. An image of the DNA marker (4. 5 kb) is in the bottom right-hand corner of the figure. (d) Transcript level analysis of transgenic cucumber line U1 according to qRT-PCR. The *Csactin* is used as an internal control. Expression of cucumber WT plants was set to 1. The data are presented as the mean values ±SDs, $n$ = 3 biologically independent samples.

transformation efficiency with multigene vector in an *Agrobacterium*-mediated system, the essential step in genetic transformation still need to optimized, which the key tasks and the targets for the next stage. We further measured the expression level of transgenes via qRT - PCR (Fig. 2d). Quantitative real-time PCR (qRT - PCR) analysis revealed that the *SgSQE1*, *SgCS*, *SgEPH2*, *SgP450*, *SgUGT269 - 1* and *SgUGT289 - 3* transcript levels were markedly higher in the WT plants. In this assay, the expression of 6 transgenes varied in the leaves and fruits. For example, in all six transgenes, the relatively lower *SgSQE* expression was detected in the both of leaves and fruits (Fig. 2d), which was located in the second gene position for 2A peptides construct driven by CaMV 35S promoter (Supplementary Fig. S2a). The gene expression level between the first and the second gene positions was commonly affected by the utilization of different 2A peptides. All in all, PCR and qRT - PCR detection indicated that the structural genes involved in mogrosides bio-synthesis were expressed in the transgenic lines of cucumber. Finally, only the U1 transgenic plant was acquired using *Agro-bacterium*-mediated transformation.

On the basis of a molecular analysis, the composition and content of mogrosides in the transgenic cucumber line were determined using HPLC - ESI - MS/MS. Mogrol, MI - A1, MII - E, MIII, SI and MV standards were detected at retention times of 4.01, 19.38, 13.88, 12.03, 10.14 and. 8.37 min, respectively (Fig. 3a and Supplementary Fig. S4a). As shown in Fig. 3b and Supplementary Fig. S4b, mogrol, MIA - 1, MII - E, MIII, and SI were detected in transgenic cucumber fruits and leaves, except for MV, which was found only in the fruits. MV accumulated to ~ 587 ng/g fresh weight (FW) in the fruits, and the contents of the other mogrosides is listed in Fig. 3b and Supplementary Fig. S4b. Mogrosides were not detected in the WT cucumber plants. Furthermore, the metabolites were further identified by UPLC - ESI - QTOF - MS/MS, and the total ion chromatographs in negative mode are shown in Fig. 4. According to the retention time, true molecular weight and mass spectrometry of standards, five mogrosides were observed in transgenic cucumber U1 fruits, including MI - A1, MII - E, MIII, SI and MV. And $[M+HCOO-H]^-$ and $[M-H]^-$ were commonly observed in the MS/MS spectrum at negative ion mode. The fracture mode of MV was as follows: the characteristic fragments easily obtained one molecule of formic acid, which resulted in product ions at $m/z$ 1 331.544 3 in MS spectrum. The deprotonated ions of $[M-H]^-$ ($m/z$ 1 285.550 7) was clearly observed in the MS/MS spectrum (Supplementary Fig. S5a). Moreover, SI obtained one molecule of formic acid to show $[M+HCOO-H]^-$ ($m/z$ 1 169.509 6) and generated a deprotonated ion $[M-H]^-$ at $m/z$ 1 123.533 0 (Supplementary Fig. S5b). Similarly, based on MS/MS spectra, compounds 3, 4 and 5 were identified as MIII, MII - E and MI - A1 (Supplementary Fig. S5c - e). Notably, the presence of mogrosides confirmed that the simultaneous expression of the 6 genes was successful in the transgenic cucumber line. Sweet cucumber was generated successfully by reconstructing mogrosides biosynthesis in trans-genic cucumber. Interesting, in the U1 leave, the presence of mogrosides was also proved to be a great potential for SI production using agricultural wastes. In our study, we developed a convenient and highly efficient multigene transformation strategy via In-fusion technology and 2A peptide linkers.

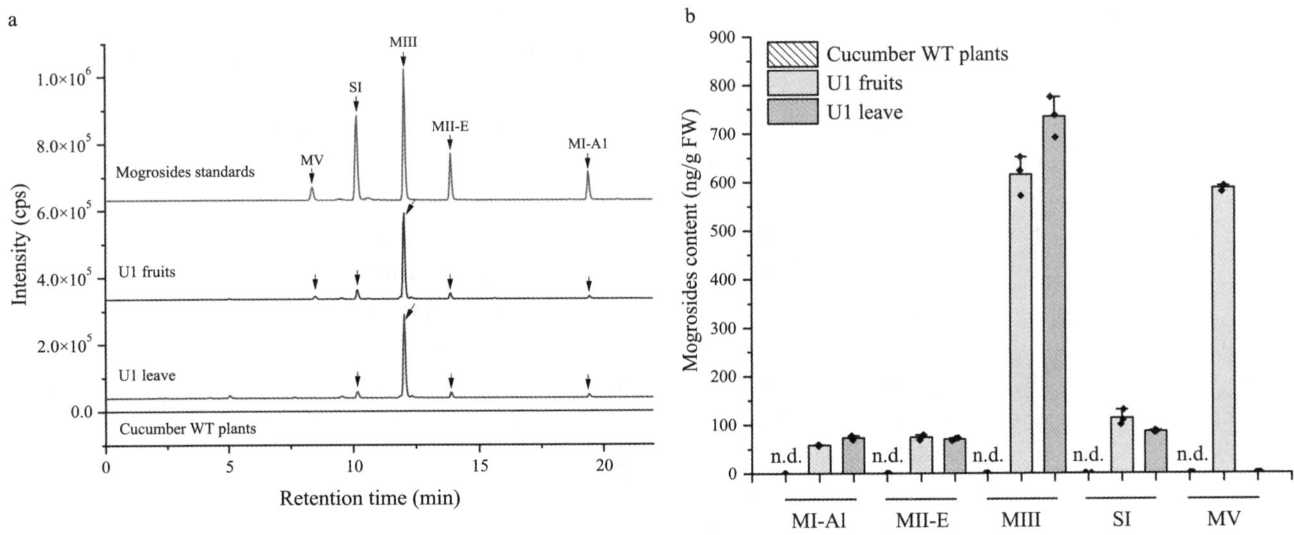


**Fig. 3 Production of mogrosides in transgenic cucumber line**

(a) HPLC - ESI - MS/MS analysis of mogrosides in transgenic cucumber line U1. The black arrows indicate the peak of mogrosides. (b) Accumulation of mogrosides in transgenic cucumber line U1. n.d., not detected. The data are presented as the mean values±SDs, $n=3$ biologically independent samples.

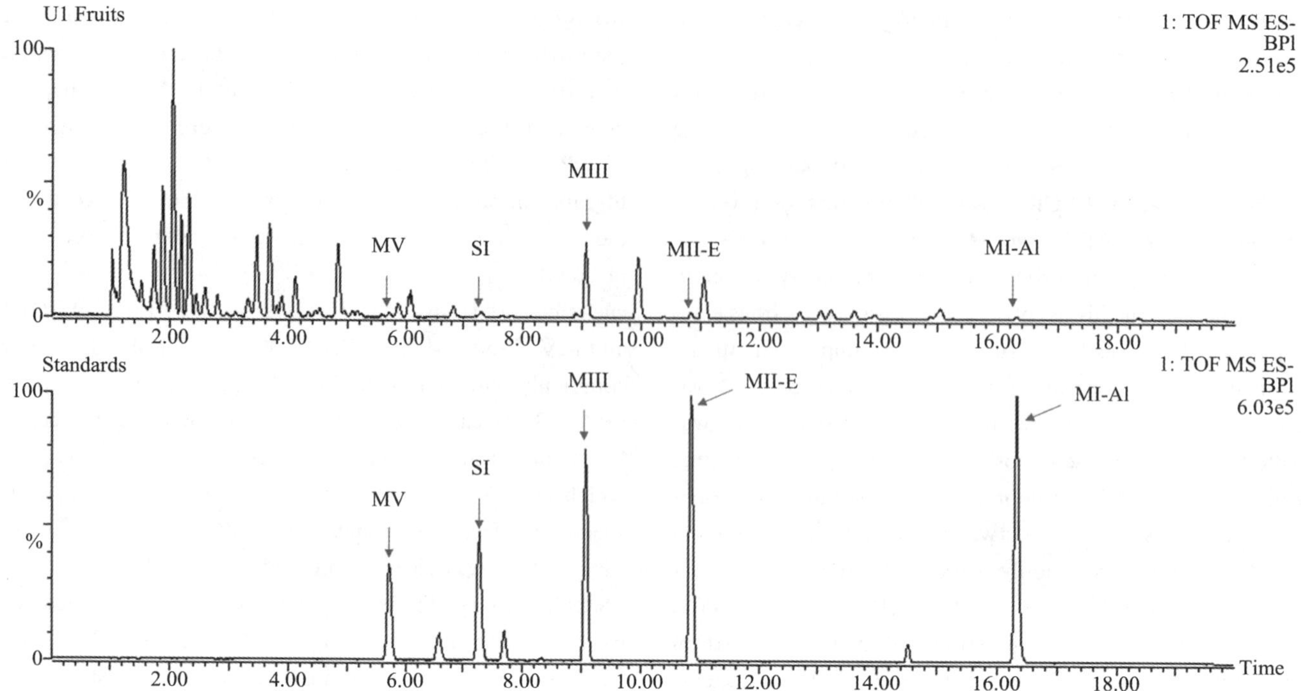


**Fig. 4 The total ion chromatogram of mogrosides in transgenic cucumber line U1 and standards**

MIA－1, MII－E, MIII, SI, and MV represented the mogroside I－A1, mogroside II－E, mogroside III, siamenoside I, and mogroside V, respectively.

These results indicate that this strategy could be applied in cucumber and have important implications for developing mogrosides-accumulating vegetables firstly.

Generation of MIII-accumulating tomato Similarly, the multigene vector was transformed into Micro-Tom tomato. About 500 explants were transformed in the assay, and twenty Hyg-resistant tomato transgenic lines were generated by multiple transformation methods. Among them, only four lines had mogrosides biosynthesis-related genes detected via PCR with specific primers for the *SgSQE1*, *SgCS*, *SgEPH2*, *SgP450*, *SgUGT269－1*, *SgUGT289－3* and Hyg genes. Fragments of the expected size were obtained from the genomic DNA of four candidate transgenic tomato lines. All the mogrosides biosynthesis-related genes were amplified from these four (S8, S10, S14 and S17) lines out of the twenty lines transformed with the U22p－SCE vector (Fig. 5a); none of the target genes were observed in the WT plants (Fig. 5b). That is, this multigene vector was successfully introduced in the tomato genome. To further confirm the transgenic lines, the expression level of the target genes was examined in the S8, S10, S14 and S17 lines via qPCR (Fig. 5c). All mogrosides biosynthesis-related genes were over-expressed, although there were relatively higher expression levels of all genes in the S10 line (Fig. 5c). No transcripts of the target genes were detected in the WT tomato plants, which indicated that 6 structural genes involved in mogrosides biosynthesis were expressed in transgenic tomato fruits. That is, the mogrosides pathway was successfully introduced into the transgenic tomato plants firstly.

The production of mogrosides in the four transgenic tomato fruits was measured by HPLC－ESI－MS/MS. The extracted ion chromatogram (EIC) of the HPLC suggested that a small amount of MIII accumulated in transgenic tomato line S10 (Fig. 6a), and the retention times were consistent with those of the mogrosides standards. No MIII was detected in the WT plants (Fig. 6a). The content of MIII was 25.92 ng/g FW (Fig. 6b), and we also found a small amount of MI－A1 (5.65 ng/g), MII－E (2.33 ng/g), SI and MV. However, the content of SI and MV is still below the limit of quantification (<LOQ) (Fig. 6a). The target compounds in tomato transgenic plants were further confirmed by UPLC－ESI－QTOF－MS/MS. The result has been shown in Supplementary Fig. S6a－f. In general, tomato transgenic plants also produced mogrosides, but the level was lower compared to mogrosides content in cucumber transgenic plants. As shown in Supple-mentary Fig. S4c and S4d, there were only minute amount of mogrol accumulation in the transgenic tomato lines S8 and S17. And the production of mogrol was absent in the Micro-Tom WT plants.

## 2 DISCUSSION

Cucumber is a commonly nutritious vegetable, yet it has a bland taste. Polyphenolic compounds and salivary proteins provide cucumbers with a subtle astringent taste, which causes some people to avoid eating cucumbers. To improve the flavour of cucumber, *Siraitia grosvenorii* mogrosides

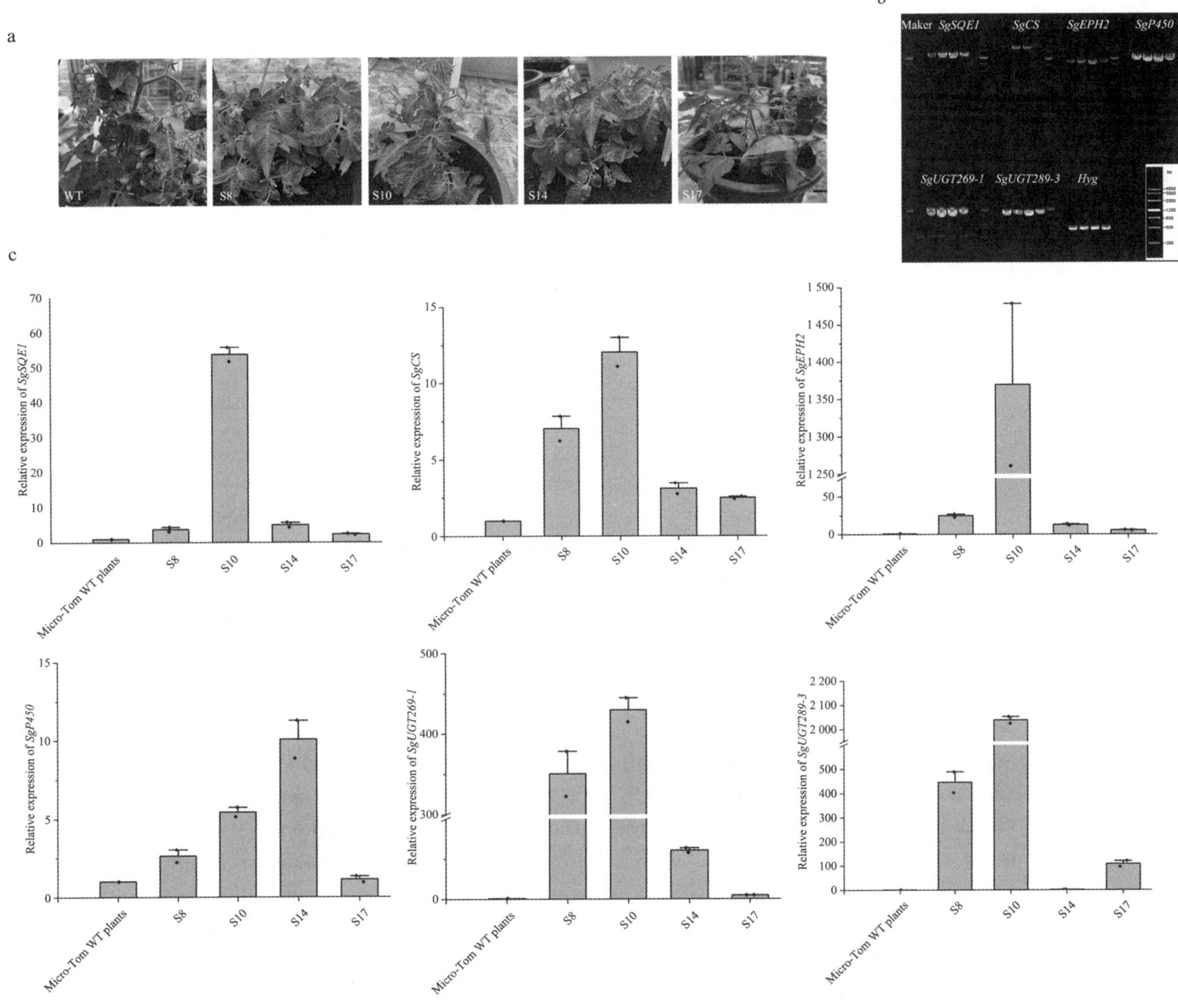


**Fig. 5 Molecular analysis and detection of mogrosides in transgenic tomato lines**

(a) Micro-Tom tomato wild-type plants (WT) and transgenic tomato plants. (b) PCR-based analysis of the transgenic tomato fruits. The lanes from left to right represent the Maker, WT, S8, S10, S14 and S17. An image of the DNA marker (4.5 kb) is in the bottom right-hand corner of the figure. (c) Relative expression level analysis of 6 mogrosides biosynthesis genes in transgenic tomato fruits. The *Leactin* is used as an internal control. Expression of tomato WT plants was set to 1. The data are presented as the mean values ±SDs, $n = 3$ biologically independent samples.

biosynthesis genes were transformed into cucumber plants, which produces a germplasm with mogroside V. And in the fruits of transgenic cucumber line U1, mogrol, MI - A, MII - E, MIII, and SI were found and the content were 36.88, 58, 74.3, 615, and 113 ng/g FW, respectively. Although it is well known that mogroside IA - 1, II - E are bitter-tasting glycosides, SI and MV are extremely sweet, MIII is tasteless or slightly sweet, which cultivate cucumbers to taste sweet, blend flavours, or totally new tastes to commonly known vegetables. And the content of MI - A and MII - E with bitter flavour were present at too low a level in the fruits of transgenic cucumber, and therefore the consequence for flavour of trans-genic cucumber is relatively small. Similarly, the transformation of tomato produced a small amount of mogroside III in tomato. The content of SI and MV is still below the limit of quantification (<LOQ) in the transgenic tomato lines. The taste description of MIII is weak or tasteless compared with mogroside V, and it is reported in literature that mogroside III is 195 times sweeter than sucrose, Previously its maltase inhibitory effect has been investigated previously, and MIII reduced pulmonary fibrosis and may have therapeutic potential for treating fibrosis. Combining with the natural flavour of tomato fruits, it is presumed that the taste of transgenic tomato fruits is slightly sweet, which allow vegetables to taste better. In general, tomato transgenic plants also produced mogrosides, but the level was lower com-pared to mogrosides content in cucumber transgenic plants. The reason for this phenomenon might be a lack of

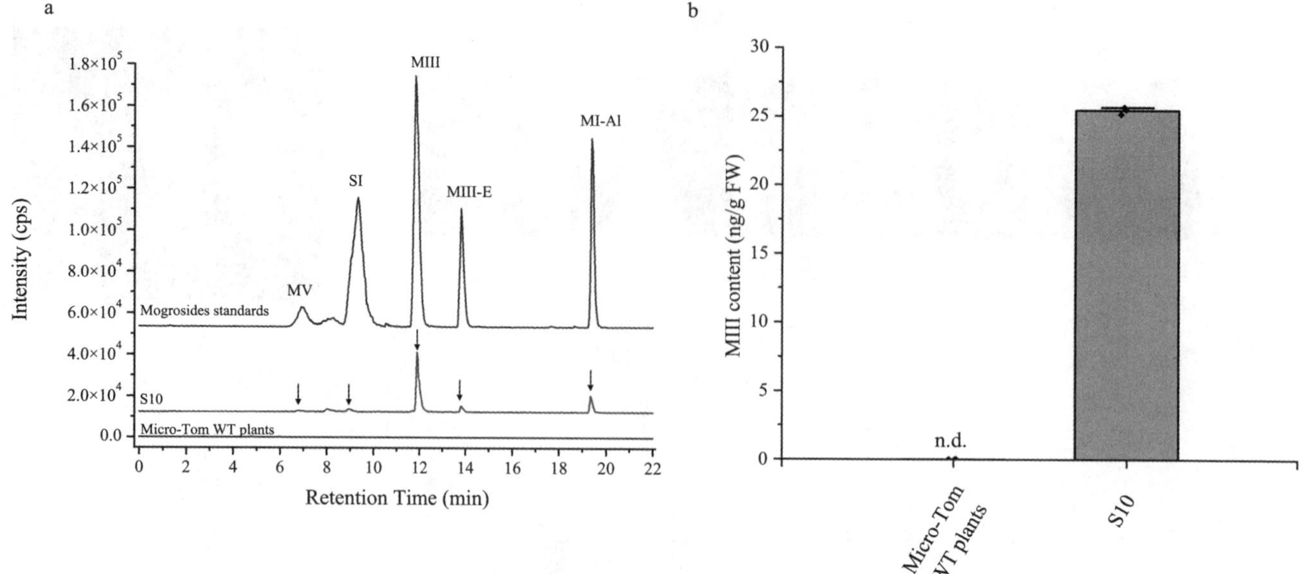


**Fig. 6 Production of mogrosides in tomato transgenic lines**

(a) HPLC-ESI-MS/MS analysis of mogrosides in transgenic tomato fruits. (b) Accumulation of MIII in transgenic tomato fruits. The black arrows indicate the peak of mogrosides. n. d., not detected. The data are presented as the mean values ±SDs, $n = 3$ biologically independent samples.

precursor accu-mulation, stepwise glycosylation strategy or T-DNA insertion position. To reduce the consumption of substrates, gene-editing technology such as clustered, regularly interspaced, short palin-dromic repeats (CRISPR)/CRISPR-associated 9 (Cas9), which have widely used for the functional verification of key enzymes and regulatory elements, can be applied to knock out genes involved in branch pathways. Overexpression of upstream genes encoding various rate-limiting enzymes, such as HMGR (encoding 3-hydroxy-3-methyl glutaryl coenzyme A reductase) and SQS (encoding squalene synthase), is beneficial to the accu-mulation of substrates. Despite this, 2, 3-Oxidosqualene is widely found in all kinds of plants, theoretically, it could be exploited to transfer mogrosides biosynthesis genes. Our study marks the success of the transformation of mogrosides bio-synthesis genes into heterologous plants, which offers a fresh perspective on breeding innovative tasty vegetables and producing plant materials that could serve as source of multiple mogrosides.

In our study, the morphological observation results of trans-genic tomato plants revealed that serious dwarfish was observed in the four independent tomato transgenic lines, but no obvious morphological changes were found in the transgenic cucumber plants. This result suggests that mogrosides can affect plant growth, which may produce metabolic toxic effects on transgenic tomato lines. The possible explanation for the absence of dwarfing in cucumber is that both cucumber and *Siraitia grosvenorii* are cucurbitaceae plants, and in cucumber itself there are many cucurbitane triterpene saponin such as cucurbitacin B and cucurbitacin C, and mogrosides are also triterpene saponin, in this case, there is no toxicity effect on the transgenic cucumber lines. Moreover, according to the previous researches, most studies have proven that transgenic engineering has caused a metabolic disturbance in gibberellin metabolism, which leads to the dwarfish in the transgenic tomato lines. And the insertion of transgenic genes often causes poor growth, serious dwarf in transgenic plants, for example, previous study showed that the integration of T-DNA into the genome will activate or inactivate other nonspecific genes expression, which has caused physiolo-gical disorders or plant resistance in transgenic plants. Therefore, we speculated that the dwarfish of transgenic tomato in this study may be correlated to the changes in gibberellin metabolism, but more information will be further introduced in several forthcoming experiments.

Multigene transformation can be used to introduce complete metabolic pathways into plants. Unlike the time-consuming and tedious steps of conventional cross breeding, re-transformation and co-transformation methods, emerging multigene vector transformation and polycistronic transgenes have excellent advantages. In particular, multiple vector transformation allows the assembly of multiple gene expression cassettes into a single T-DNA region and integration into the host chromosome genome. To date, there is no evidence to suggest that the maximum number of transgenes can be introduced into plants, and yet little research has been conducted on 6 or more transgene transformations in a single vector. Additionally, as the number of transgenes rises, unstable binary vectors can induce spontaneous gene loss in heterologous plants. Consequently, the schematic design of the multigene vector assembly in this research was important.

The Transgene Stacking II system (TGS II), Gateway Recombination system, Gibson Assembly and In-fusion technology have been widely used in multigene vector assembly. Among these, the Gateway recombination system remains a challenge with respect to the assembly of more than five genes due to operational difficulty. On this basis, TGS II was recently developed as a more convenient and efficient multigene vector system that can be used to transform 4-8 genes into het-erologous plants. Gibson assembly and In-fusion technology have been widely used to fuse multiple overlapping DNA frag-ments simultaneously in a single reaction. In addition, the max-imum vector size of In-fusion technology is 46 kb. Therefore, In-fusion technology allows the assembly of multiple gene expression cassettes. Considering repetitive sequences in a multigene vector, self-cleaving 2A peptides (16 to 20 amino acids) was introduced, which lead to relatively high levels of downstream protein expression compared to other strategies for multi-gene expression. However, the efficiency of protein expression mediated by different 2A sequences. In this study, *SgSQE1*, *SgCS*, *SgEPH2*, *SgP450*, *SgUGT269-1* and *SgUGT289-3* transcript levels were different in the transgenic cucumber leaves and fruits. One possible reason is that most of transgenes driven by a constitutive promoter, CaMV 35S promoter, which showed that marked variations in transcriptional activity depending on the tissue and organ type. CaMV 35S promoter drove β-glucuronidase (GUS) activity was higher in birch roots and axillary buds than in other birch organs. Green fluorescence protein (GFP) driven by CaMV 35S promoter had a higher activity in the tobacco leaf vascular tissues than other tissues. And physiological conditions and abiotic stress also affected the target transgenes expression. Therefore, to ensure high and stable transgene activity, con-siderable attention should be given to the multigene vector con-struction and growth condition further.

In summary, an In-fusion based gene stacking strategy for transgene stacking was developed, 6 mogrosides biosynthesis genes were transferred into cucumber and tomato, and transgenic sweet cucumber containing mogroside V and slightly sweet tomato containing mogroside III. This study displays the great potential in the genetic improvement of fresh-eating sweet plants. Our work fundamentally changes the traditional pattern of sweet-taste breeding, and offers a excellent mode for the transformation of non-sugar and non-protein sweet components instead of increasing sugar contents in fresh vegetables. Moreover, this study provides a possibility for mogrosides heterologous biosynthesis.

## 3 METHODS

Plant materials and strains *Cucumis sativus* (JinYan 4, ZY4) and *Lycopersicon esculentum* (Micro-Tom) were used for plant transformation. Transient expression experiments were carried out in *Cucumis sativus* ZY4 and tobacco. *Escherichia coli* strains DH5α and XL10-Gold (WeidiBio, Shanghai, China) were used in this experiment, and *Agrobacterium tumefaciens* strain GV3101 was used for transformation.

Promoter activity assays Appropriate promoters are crucial for driving the expression of target genes in multigene vectors. Ubiquitin 10 AtUBQ10 and serine carboxypeptidase-like *AtSCPL30* (AtPD7, 456 bp) promoters were cloned from *Arabidopsis thaliana* using KOD One PCR Master Mix (TOYOBO CO., LTD., Japan). The PCR conditions were as follows: initial activation at 98 ℃ for 5 min, followed by 35 cycles at 98 ℃ for 10 s, annealing temperature −5 ℃ for 5 s, and 68 ℃ for 10 s/kb, and a final extension at 68 ℃ for 7 min. To construct AtUBQ10: β-glucuronidase (GUS) and AtPD7: GUS vectors, each of these pro-moters was fused to a pBI121 plasmid at *Xba*I/*Bam*HI restriction sites (Fig. 1b). The primers were listed in the Supplementary Table S2. The resultant recombinant plasmids were confirmed by sequencing. pBI121 driven by the 35S cauliflower mosaic virus (CaMV 35S) promoter was used in this study as a positive control. All the plasmids were transformed into *Agrobacterium tumefaciens* strain GV3101 and used for transient assays in *Cucumis sativus* and *Nicotiana benthamiana*.

Multigene expression vector construction The cDNA of *Siraitia grosvenorii* fruits was used to amplify the coding se-quences of *SgSQE1* (squalene epoxidase), *SgCS* (cucurbitadi-enol synthase), *SgEPH2* (epoxide hydrolases), *SgP450* (cyto-chrome P450 monooxygenase), *SgUGT269-1* and *SgUGT289-3* (UDP-glucosyltransferases). To initiate the expression of all genes, the CaMV 35S promoter was isolated from the pBI121 plasmid, and the AtUBQ10 and AtPD7 promoters were amplified from *Arabidopsis thaliana* using KOD One PCR master Mix. In terms of transcriptional terminators, nopaline synthase (NOS) terminators were obtained from pBI121, and mannopine synthase (MAS) terminators and heat-shock protein (HSP) 18.2 terminators were chemically synthesized by GEN-EWIZ (Suzhou, China).

In the first round of gene assembly, each of these mogrosides biosynthesis-related genes was amplified via Phanta Max Super-Fidelity DNA Polymerase (Vazyme Biotech Co., Ltd., Nanjing, China), and then *SgCS*, *SgEPH2*, *SgP450* and *SgUGT289-3* were ligated into the *BamH*I and *Sac*I sites of the pBI121 vector using a ClonExpress II One Step Cloning Kit (Vazyme Biotech Co., Ltd., Nanjing, China). *SgSQE1* fused with AtPD7 promoter and HSP terminator, and *SgUgt269-1* together with the AtUBQ10 promoter and MAS terminator was inserted into pBI121 at the *Hin*dIII and *Eco*RI sites using a ClonExpress MultiS One Step Cloning Kit (Vazyme Biotech Co., Ltd., Nanjing, China), respectively. PD7: SgSQE1: Thsp, 35S:

SgCS: Tnos, 35S: SgEPH2: Tnos, 35S: SgP450: Tnos, 35S: SgUGT289 - 3: Tnos and UBQ10: SgUGT269 - 1: Tmas were generate. In the second round of gene assembly, each of the first gene expression cassettes containing the promoter, target gene and terminator was cloned via KOD One PCR Master Mix. PD7: SgSQE1: Thsp and 35S: SgCS: Tnos were inserted at the *Eco*RI/*Hin*dIII restriction sites of a pCAMBIA1300 binary plasmid via a ClonExpress MultiS One Step Cloning Kit. Similarly, UBQ: SgUGT269 - 1: Tmas and 35S:: SgUGT289 - 3: Tnos were ligated into the same restriction sites of the pCAMBIA1300 plasmid, yielding a double-gene expression cassette. In the third round of gene assembly, the regions of PD7: SgSQE1: Thsp:: 35S: SgCS: Tnos and 35S: SgEPH2: Tnos were amplified by PCR and subcloned into the UBQ10: SgUGT269 - 1: Tmas:: 35S: SgUGT289-3: Tnos *Eco*RI/*Hind*III sites of a pCAMBIA1300 plasmid. Then, the sequences of UBQ10: SgUGT269-1: Tmas:: 35S: SgUGT289 - 3: Tnos and 35S: SgP450: Tnos were isolated and inserted into the pCAMBIA1300 plasmid, and triple-gene expression cassettes were constructed. Subsequently, in the final round of gene assembly, the 6.1-kb sequence of UBQ10: SgUGT269 - 1: Tmas:: 35S: SgUGT289 - 3: Tnos:: 35S: SgP450 and SgSQE1: Thsp:: 35S: SgCS: Tnos:: 35S: SgEPH2: Tnos (6.5-kb) were isolated from the triple-gene expression cassettes. For the final multigene expression vector, above-mentioned fragments were ligated with a 2A peptide linker from porcine teschovirus (amino acid sequence is GSGATNFSLLKQAGDVEENPGP) (P2A) via a ClonExpress Ultra One Step Cloning Kit (Vazyme Biotech Co., Ltd., Nanjing, China). This final vector was referred to as the U22p - SCE vector in this study (Supplementary Fig. S2a). All primers used for multi-gene vector construction are listed in the Supplementary Table S3.

Transient expression To verify the multigene expression vectors and analyse the promoter activity, a transient expression assay was performed in *Cucumis sativus* ZY4 and tobacco. A multigene expression vector was transformed into *Agro-bacterium tumefaciens* strain GV3101 through the freeze-thaw method. The transformed *Agrobacterium* strains were cultured at 28 ℃ in LB media supple-mented with rifampicin and kanamycin until the $OD_{600}$ of the bacteria reached 0.6. All the cultures were centrifuged at 5 000 × g for 10 min, resuspended in buffer that included 10 mmol/L 2-(N-morpholino) ethanesulfonic acid (MES), 10 mmol/L MgSO4 and 200 μmol/L acetosyringone (AS), and then incubated for 2 - 4 h at room temperature. The suspension was infected via a needleless syringe into cotyledons of 8-day-old *Cucumis sativus* ZY4 plants and leaves of *Nicotiana benthamiana* (positive con-trol). To ensure accuracy, the transient expression procedures were repeated independently ten times.

GUS staining *Nicotiana benthamiana* was sampled at 48 h post-infiltration, and cotyledons of *Cucumis sativus* ZY4 were sampled at 1, 3, 5 and 7 d for GUS histochemical staining analyses according to a previous protocol. Images were taken using a Canon EOS 80D. The images were used to determine the intensity of blue staining. This experiment was repeated independently ten times.

Generation of engineered cucumber plants The seeds of *Cucumis sativus* line ZY4 were soaked in the 55 ℃ for 15 min, and then placed at room temperature for 2 h. The cucumber seeds were sterilized following Trulson et al. with minor modification. After soaking, seeds were sterilized with 75% alcohol for 30 s, followed by 3% NaClO for 15 min, then washed 5 times with sterile water, and inoculated on the Murashige and Skoog (MS) under darkness for 3 d. In order to obtain genetically engineered cucumber, we used the cotyledons of 4-day-old *Cucumis sativus* (cucumber) as explants. The cotyledons were cut from the seedlings and removed the growing point. The explants were placed on the pre-cultivation media, MS media containing 1 mg/L 6-benzylaminopurine (6 - BA), 0.5 mg/L abscisic acid (ABA) and 2 mg/L $AgNO_3$ for 1 day in the dark. Then, the explants were infected with *Agrobacterium* harbouring the multigene expression vector for 30 min. and co-cultivated on co-cultivation media (MS media with 1 mg/L 6 - BA, 0.5 mg/L ABA, 2 mg/L AgNO3 and 1.45 mg/L AS) for 2 day in the dark at 25 ℃. After co-cultivations, the explants were cultivated in selective medium (MS media with 1 mg/L 6 - BA, 0.5 mg/L ABA, 2 mg/L $AgNO_3$, 500 mg/L Cefotaxime sodium (Cef) and 5 or 8 mg/L hygromycin (Hyg) under 18 h light/6 h dark conditions). Hyg (5 mg/L) was used to select the transformed plants. Calli grew on MS media supplemented with Hyg (8 mg/L). Generally, the adventitious shoots that arose from calli reached were regenerated into green and healthy explants. Then, 2 - 3 cm segments of the regenerants were selected for cultivation in rooting media supplemented with 10 mg/L Hyg. After 1 month of cultivation, the regenerated cucumber seedlings were excised in vivo and then cultivated in a greenhouse (Fig. 2a). After that, the callus and regeneration plants were obtained by subculture continuously. To obtain transgenic lines, The regeneration plants were cultured on rooting media (MS media with 1 mg/L Gibberellin A3 (GA3), 400 mg/L Cef). The regenerated plants were cultured in a greenhouse at 28 ℃ under 18 h /6 h (light/dark).

Generation of transgenic Micro-Tom tomato plants The genetic transformation was performed following Sun et al. with modification. Seeds of Micro-Tom were sterilized in 70% ethanol for 30 s and in 10% NaClO for 10 min, rinsed four times with sterilized water and dried on sterilized filter paper. The seeds were germinated in the MS media. Using the leaves, cotyledons and hypocotyls of 10-day-old Micro-Tom plants as explants, leaves and cotyledons were cut into the pieces about 0.5 cm × 0.5 cm, the hypocotyls were cut into segments about 0.5 - 0.6 cm to allow them to adsorb the bacterial suspension. They were pre-cultured on the pre-cultivation media (MS media with 1 mg/L 6 - BA and 0.2 mg/L NAA) for 24 h. After pre-cultivation, explants were incubated for 30 min with *Agrobacterium* harbouring the multigene expression vector and then transferred to co-cultivation media (MS media containing 1 mg/L 6 - BA, 0.2 mg/L NAA, and 0.1 mmol/L AS) for 2 days. Then, the explants were transferred to selection media (2.0 mg/L zeatin (ZT), 0.2 mg/L indole-acetic acid (IAA), 10 mg/L Hyg and 500 mg/L carbenicillin). Afterwards, the buds were transferred to elongation media (1.0 mg/L ZT, 0.05 mg/L IAA, 500 mg/L Cef, 10 mg/L Hyg and 500 mg/L carbenicillin), and the regenerated shoots were allowed to grow to a length of 1 cm. The shoots were subsequently transferred to rooting culture media consisting of 1/2-strength MS media with 0.1 mg/L IAA, 2 mg/L Hyg, 500 mg/L Cef and 500 mg/L carbenicillin.

Molecular identification Genomic DNA was obtained from the transgenic lines using a Plant Genomic DNA Kit (Tiangen Biotech Co., Ltd., Beijing). Genomic PCR with KOD One PCR Master Mix was performed to verify the transgenic plants. In addition, genomic PCR was used to detect the transgenic lines obtained by Hyg resistance screening. Wild-type (WT) plant genomic DNA was used as a negative control. All the primers used for PCR detection are shown in Supple-mentary Table S4.

Total RNA was isolated from the leaves of the transgenic plants via a CWBIO RNA extraction kit (CWBIO. Co., Ltd., Beijing, China), and 1 μg of total RNA was used to reverse transcribe cDNA via *TransScript* ® One-Step gDNA Removal and cDNA Synthesis SuperMix (Transgen, Beijing, China). For quantitative real-time PCR (qRT-PCR), *PerfectStart*™ Green qPCR SuperMix (Transgen, Beijing, China) in conjunction with an ABI CFX96™ Real-Time System (USA) was used to quantify the expression levels according to the manufacturers' instructions. The thermal cycling was as follow: (1) 95℃ for 30 s; (2) 40 cycles of 3 s denaturation at 95 ℃, 10 s annealing at 55 ℃; (3) dissociation curve consisting of 15 s incubation at 95℃, 60 s incubation at 60℃, a ramp up to 95 ℃. The gene transcript levels were precisely quantified for target gene expression with the $2^{-\Delta\Delta CT}$ method, and *Csactin* and *Leactin* were used as internal control. This experiment was conducted for multiple technical replicates. All the primers used for qRT-PCR are listed in Supplementary Table S5.

Quantitative analysis of metabolites by HPLC-ESI-MS/MS All samples were ground in liquid nitrogen (cucumber, 10 g and tomato, 4 g), homogenized in 10 mL and 4 mL 80% methanol solution, respectively. And then an ultrasonic water-bath assisted extraction was performed at room temperature at 40 kHz for 1 h, and centrifuged at 5 000 × g for 20 min. Afterwards, the supernatant was collected and filtered using a 0.22 μmol/L Millipore filter.

For quantitative analysis of mogrosides and mogrol contents, an AB SCIEX QTRAP 4,500 LC-MS/MS (AB SCIEX, Toronto, Canada) system and an Agilent Technologies 1 260 Series LC system (Agilent, USA) equipped with an Agilent Poroshell 120 SB C18 column (100 mm × 2.1 mm, 2.7 μm) were used. The mobile phase consisted of (A) water (including 0.1% formic acid) and (B) acetonitrile (including 0.1% formic acid) with a gradient elution. The HPLC conditions for mogrosides were as follows: 0 min, 20% B; 3 - 5 min, 23% B; 18 min, 40% B; and 18.01 - 20.10 min, 20% B. The flow rate was 0.25 mL/min. For mogrol, the HPLC conditions were as follows: 0 min, 20% B; 0.5 min 30% B; 2 - 4 min, 88% B; and 5.50 - 8.00 min, 20% B. The HPLC-ESI-MS/MS parameters are listed in Table 1, and electrospray ionization (ESI) with multiple reaction monitoring (MRM) scanning was used in this study. Each experiment was performed three times. The above two methods have been developed for quantitative analysis in our previous work, and they are suitable for the accurate quantification of target components in this study. The quantitative analyses were performed by means of an external standard method.

All standards including mogroside I - A1 (MI - A1), mogroside II - E (MII - E), mogroside III (MIII), siamenoside I (SI), mogroside V (MV) and mogrol were purchased from Chengdu Must Bio-Technology Co., Ltd. (Sichuan, China) and solved into the methanol.

Qualitative analysis of metabolites using UPLC - ESI - QTOF - MS/MS To identify metabolites in transgenic plants were analyzed by a UPLC - ESI - QTOF - MS/MS system (Waters Corp.) with negative electrospray ionization (ESI). The MS con-ditions were in MSE continuum mode, with a scan range of $m/z$ 100 to 1 500. The collision voltage was 2.5 KV. The sampling cone voltage and extractor voltage were 40 KV and 4 KV, respectively. The source temperature and desolvation tempera-ture were 100 ℃ and 250 ℃, respectively. The cone gas flow was 50 L/hr, and desolvation gas flow was 600 L/hr; Collision energy was ramped from 15 to 45 eV for the collection of MS/MS data. Masslynx 4.1 software was used for data acquisition and processing.

Statistics and reproducibility The real-time quantitative analysis data are pre-sented as the means ±SEM of at least three independent experiments in the paper. Unless otherwise stated, all samples were obtained randomly and all independent samples or experiment were repeated more than three times. The average values and standard deviations were calculated using SPSS 16.0 statistics programme (IBM Co., Armonk,

Table 1 HPLC - ESI - MS/MS parameters

| Analytes | Molecular Formula | Retention time (min) | product ion ($m/z$) | DP (V) | CE (eV) |
|---|---|---|---|---|---|
| MV | $C_{60}H_{102}O_{29}$ | 7.38 | 1 285.8/1 123.7<br>1 285.8/961.7 | −220 | −90 |
| SI | $C_{54}H_{92}O_{24}$ | 9.62 | 1 123.6/961.6<br>1 123.6/799.2 | −220 | −75 |
| MIII | $C_{48}H_{82}O_{19}$ | 11.86 | 961.6/799.4<br>961.6/637.3 | −170 | −70 |
| MII - E | $C_{42}H_{72}O_{14}$ | 13.82 | 799.5/637.5<br>799.5/475.5 | −170 | −65 |
| MI - A | $C_{42}H_{72}O_{14}$ | 19.38 | 637.5/475.5<br>637.5/160.5 | −160 | −540 |
| Mogrol | $C_{30}H_{52}O_4$ | 4.01 | 459.3/441.2<br>459.3/423.3 | 80 | 20 |

| MS parameters | Mogrosides | Mogrol |
|---|---|---|
| Ion mode | Negative | Positive |
| Source temperature (℃) | 550 | 550 |
| Ionization voltage (V) | −4 500 | 5 500 |
| GS1 (psi) | 55 | 60 |
| GS2 (psi) | 55 | 50 |
| CUR (psi) | 20 | 20 |
| CAD | Medium | Medium |
| Dwell time (ms) | 100 | 200 |
| EP (V) | −10 | 10 |
| CXP (V) | −15 | 10 |

NewYork, USA). All plots were obtained using Origin 2019b (OriginLab Co., Northampton, MA, USA).

Reporting summary. Further information on research design is available in the Nature Portfolio Reporting Summary linked to this article.

[廖晶晶，马小军，等. Communications Biology, 2023, 6:191.]

# Simple phenylpropanoids: recent advances in biological activities, biosynthetic pathways, and microbial production

## 1 INTRODUCTION

Simple phenylpropanoids are a group of secondary metabolites comprising a phenyl ring linked with a three-carbon side chain (C6 - C3). In plants, they are primarily derived from the aromatic amino acid L-phenylalanine (L-Phe). These compounds can be classified into several subcategories associated with changes in the substituent on the benzene ring and the position of the propenyl double bond, such as phenylpropanoic acids (cinnamic and hydroxycinnamic acids), phenylpropanoic aldehydes, phenylpropanols, phenylpropene and simple coumarins. By serving as biogenetic precursors of various complex phenylpropanoids and other downstream metabolites, simple phenylpropanoids are essential for structural support, pigmentation, defence, and signalling throughout the plant kingdom. They also show a wide range of biological activities and are useful as raw materials applicable to high value-added chemical products, which have received considerable attention from agriculture, cosmetics, biofuel, biomaterials, and pharmaceutical industries.

Plants synthesize approximately 10 gigatons of phenylpropanoid molecules each year, which constitute approximately 20% of the total carbon in the terrestrial biosphere. Simple phenylpropanoids are mainly obtained from natural raw materials, particularly from millions of tons of agricultural wastes and forest litter produced per annum. Access to a sustainable supply of simple phenylpropanoids is restricted by a variety of factors, including sluggish growth and accumulation, variable synthesis fluctuations caused by climatic and environmental changes, challenging extraction and purification methods, as well as time-consuming and contaminating procedures. Development of more naturefriendly production methods has long been the subject of research owing to the intensifying contradiction between the increasing demand for simple phenylpropanoids and the urgent need for ecological conservation. Compared to plant extraction and chemical synthesis, microbial production is a promising alternative, not only for its much shorter production periods but also for being safer, low-cost, and environmentally friendly. Recent advances in the design-build-test-learn cycle associated with metabolic engineering, synthetic biology, systems biology, bioinformatics, and other advanced technologies have accelerated the development of microbial cell factories, resulting in the accumulation of simple phenylpropanoids from inexpensive and renewable sources. However, despite the tremendous progress made, several urgent challenges remain in advancing microbial engineering as a general approach for the biosynthesis of simple phenylpropanoids, including: ① non-specificity and inefficient cofactor supply of enzymes. ② unbalanced metabolic flux between glycolysis and pentose phosphate pathway (PPP). ③ low cell performance. ④ metabolic promiscuity in single cells.

In this review, we first summarize the extensive biological activities of simple phenylpropanoids, and emphasize the importance in food, cosmetic, nutraceutical, chemical, and, especially, the pharmaceutical industries. In addition, we outline biosynthetic pathways of simple phenylpropanoids in different species (plants, bacteria, and fungi), which provides inspiration for route design and optimization of microbial cell factories for heterologous synthesis. Next, we summarize effective engineering strategies for the microbial production of simple phenylpropanoids that are based on the reprogramming the metabolic flux toward aromatic amino acids (AAAs), and efficient microbial production of simple phenylpropanoids. Finally, we here discuss in detail the potential challenges for further improving titers of simple phenylpropanoids in microbial cell factories under the concept of the four-dimensional metabolic engineering. We also present some perspectives and constructive solutions to the current challenges.

## 2 BIOLOGICAL ACTIVITIES

Simple phenylpropanoids are widely found in fruits, vegetables, cereals, coffee, tea, and some traditional herbs. They possess various biological activities, including antioxidant, anti-inflammatory, antimicrobial, antidiabetic, neuroprotective, and anticancer properties. In addition to their pharmacological activities, simple phenylpropanoids are core precursors to many complex natural products, such as flavonoids, lignans, and polyphenols. Therefore, simple phenylpropanoids play a significant role in food, cosmetic, nutraceutical, chemical, and, especially, the pharmaceutical industries (Fig. 1).

### 2.1 Bioactivities of simple phenylpropanoids

**2.1.1 Ultraviolet protection** Due to their perfuming, antioxidant and ultraviolet (UV) protection properties, *trans*-cinnamic acid (*t*-CA) and its derivatives, such as cinnamyl aldehyde, cinnamyl alcohol, cinnamyl alcohol, have been widely used in cosmetics for decades. It is well known that UV irradiation of skin can lead to the increased expression of matrix metalloproteinase-1 (MMP-1) and tyrosinase, which are responsible for collagen breakdown and pigmentation, and reactive oxygen species (ROS) production. Caffeic acid (CaA) and sinapic acid can inhibit MMP-1 expression, ROS generation and collagen degradation *in vitro* through the inactivation of mitogen-activated protein kinases and nuclear factor κB (MAPKs/NFκB) signalling pathways. Therefore, these compounds are effective in the prevention and treatment of UV irradiation-induced skin photoaging. Tyrosinase is the ratelimiting step in melanogenesis in human skin. Because of their structural similarity to tyrosine, *t*-CA and cinnamyl aldehyde show antityrosinase activities and can be used to treat dermatological disorders by blocking the process of melanogenesis, such as occurs during pigmentation and melanoma. Cinnamic acid-derived *p*-coumaric acid (*p*-HCA) is a drug candidate that has been extensively tested *in vitro* and *in vivo* for the treatment of hyperpigmentation.

**2.1.2 Antimicrobial** Simple phenylpropanoids, such as *t*-CA, cinnamyl alcohol, have been utilized as functional ingredients for natural food preservatives because of their antimicrobial activities. Cinnamyl aldehyde is the most potent antimicrobial substance in cinnamon, and is active against multiple bacteria, such as *Staphylococcus aureus*, *Bacillus subtilis*, *Escherichia coli*, *Listeria monocytogenes*, and *Salmonella anatum*, as well as many fungi. *trans*-Cinnamyl aldehyde is identified as Generally Recognized as Safe by the United States Food and Drug Administration, and has not only served as a fungicide in agriculture, but is

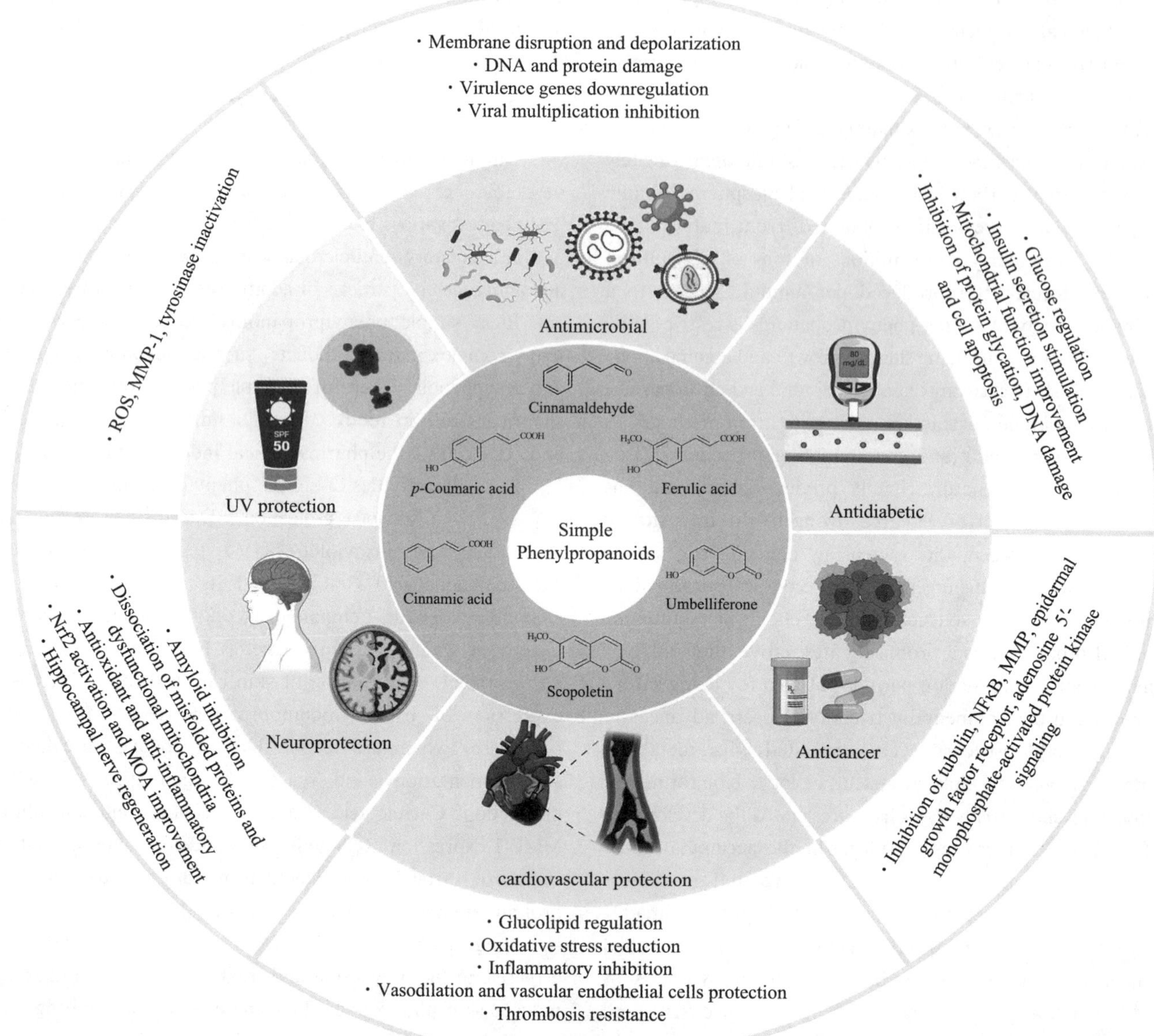


**Fig. 1 Biological activities and pharmacological functions of simple phenylpropanoids**

Abbreviations: NFκB, nuclear factor κB; MMP, matrix metalloproteinase; Nrf2, NF-E2-related factor 2; MOA, monoamine oxidase A; ROS, reactive oxygen species. Figure created with https://Biorender.com.

also added into edible antimicrobial films for inhibition of foodborne pathogens. There are many mechanisms involved in the antimicrobial activity of simple phenylpropanoids, which may differ for specific pathogens. CaA has been shown to relieve chronic infections induced by microorganisms (bacteria, fungi, and viruses), mainly through membrane disruption and depolarisation, by damaging DNA and protein structures, by downregulating virulence genes, and by inhibiting cellular proliferation. Interestingly, *t*-CA has been observed to generate multipletarget or synergistic effects in combination with classical antimalarial drugs. These results have inspired the exploration of the application of simple phenylpropanoids combined with other natural antimicrobials or medicinal antibiotics, which may revitalise conventional drugs and address antibiotic resistance issues. Recently, a mouse experiment evaluated the antiviral effects of *t*-CA against Zika virus. These plant-derived compounds have the potential to be used as a nutraceutical or drug candidate against pandemics.

2.1.3 Antidiabetic Diabetes, a metabolic disorder characterised by insulin resistance and hyperglycaemia, is associated with oxidative stress and increased inflammation. The inability to regulate blood glucose levels leads to multiple complications, including retinopathy and vascular lesions. *t*-CA and its derivatives have beneficial effects on diabetes and its complications. It regulates glucose metabolism by improving glucose tolerance and stimulating insulin secretion. Cinnamic aldehydes are effective in improving insulin sensitivity and mitochondrial function. Elevated plasma concentrations of methylglyoxal are associated with the onset and progression of diabetes, but ferulic acid (FA) can inhibit methyglyoxal-induced DNA damage, protein glycation, and cell apoptosis in pancreatic β-cells. Umbelliferone has antioxidant and anti-glycation activities in diabetic mice, and can delay diabetic nephropathy by attenuating ferroptosis *via* activation of the Nrf-2/HO-1 pathway.

2.1.4 Anticancer The ubiquitous presence of α, β-unsaturated acid groups in simple phenylpropanoids makes these derivatives potentially therapeutic in the treatment of cancer through different mechanisms. *t*-CA has anticancer effects by inhibiting a wide range of targets in cancer cells, including NFκB, tubulin, adenosine 5′-monophosphate-activated protein kinase signalling, epidermal growth factor receptor, and matrix metalloproteinase. *p*-HCA is known to display favourable inhibitory effects on lung cancer, breast cancer, liver cancer, colon adenocarcinoma and neuroblastoma, as it has apoptotic and antiproliferative effects. Treatment with CaA has been reported to selectively remove induced pluripotent stem cells (iPSCs) without affecting normal and iPSC-derived differentiated cells, indicating that it can be used as a safe and economical anti-teratoma agent in iPSCs-based therapy. Moreover, CaA can play multiple roles in different stages of chemotherapy. Pre-treatment can regulate chemoresistance, meaning that CaA and caffeic acid phenethyl ester enhance the sensitivity of cancer cells to chemotherapy. Co-administration with other antitumour drugs can display synergistic effects. CaA can also prevent cancer recurrence by directly targeting cancer stem cells. Through studies on network pharmacology and molecular docking, EGFR, BRAF, and AKT1 have been proven to be key targets of scopoletin against non-small cell lung cancer. Drug combination has been a popular strategy for the discovery and development of novel drugs. CaA and FA bound to resveratrol have shown stronger inhibitory effects on the proliferation of human colorectal cancer cells (HCT116). Accordingly, it is conceivable that simple phenylpropanoid-based hybrids can provide new ideas for discovering novel anticancer agents to improve therapeutic efficiency, reduce side effects, and overcome multidrug resistance.

2.1.5 Neuroprotection Cognitive impairment is an increasingly important public health issue in modern society. Aβ aggregation, mitochondrial dysfunction and oxidative stress are major factors associated with neurodegeneration in Alzheimer's disease (AD). Hydroxycinnamic acids can show neuroprotective and pro-cognitive effects by modulating oxidant machinery and inflammatory status. Hydroxyeinnamic acids can also activate autophagy and limit brain damage by breaking down misfolded proteins and dysfunctional mitochondria. Due to their activities as antioxidants, anti-inflammatories and for their ability to inhibit amyloid formation, FA has served as a scaffold to develop many potential analogues for AD therapy. As the α, β-unsaturated carbonyl group serving as an activator of NF-E2-related factor 2 (Nrf2), coniferaldehyde was screened from cinnamaldehyde analogues and was found to greatly attenuate AD-like pathology and preserve brain function in the APP/PS1 AD mouse model by activating Nrf2. By combining *t*-CA and a D-amino acid, a unique anti-neuroinflammatory compound was synthesised with some efficacy against AD, and was found to be able to bin d strongly the proinflammatory cytokine interleukin-1β (IL-1β). Recently, a number of non-clinical trials have supported antidepressant effects of phenylpropanoids. FA can achieve significant alleviation of depression in animal models by enhancing monoamine oxidase A (MOA) activity, promoting hippocampal nerve regeneration, anti-oxidative stress, and anti-inflammatory activity, and activating the protein kinase B/collapsin response mediator protein 2 (AKT/CRMP2) signalling pathway.

2.1.6 Cardiovascular protection Abnormal blood lipid levels are implicated in the pathogenesis of cardiovascular disease. The analysis of hyperlipidemic subjects revealed that FA could improve lipid profiles, and reduce levels of the oxidative stress biomarker and the inflammatory markers (hs-CRP). FA has antithrombotic activity and appears protective to vascular endothelial cells and is expected to be useful in preventing coronary heart disease and atherosclerosis. The mechanisms of *t*-CA and cinnamic aldehyde on ameliorating glucolipid metabolism are similar in mouse experiments and can improve mitochondrial function, reduce serotonin content and upregulate autophagy-mediated lipid clearance. Caffeic acid phenethyl ester, which is isolated from propolis, is the most studied CaA derivative. It has vasorelaxant, antihyper-tensive, anti-atherosclerotic and anti-angiogenic activities and is the most promising compound for clinical application. Because of their antioxidant and vasodilator effects, coumarins can be used as lipid-lowering agents. Umbelliferone has been shown to be an antidiabetic and antihyperlipidemic agent in hyperglycaemic rat models and exerts protective effects on the liver and kidney to reduce diabetic complications. A separate study on isoproterenol-induced myocardial injury showed that umbelliferone effectively protected normal cardiac function from oxidative and inflammatory responses and cell death by upregulating the Nrf2/HO-1 signalling pathway.

2.2 Bioactivities of complex phenylpropanoids In addition to serving as versatile phytochemicals, simple phenylpropanoids are key precursors of valuable complex natural products. The lignan compound podophyllotoxin has significant antitumor activity and is the raw material used in synthesis of etoposide, a clinically important chemotherapy drug. Silybin, a flavonolignan, exerts a therapeutic effect on hepatic disease. Icaritin is extracted from the Chinese *Herba Epimedii* and has been developed as a clinical drug for the treatment of liver cancer in China. Icaritin shows anti-inflammatory and immunomodulatory effects. Salvianolic acid B is the major bioactive water-soluble polyphenolic acid of *Salvia miltiorrhiza*, exhibits anti-inflammatory, anticancer, and cardioprotective activities, and has been clinically utilised to treat cardio- and cerebrovascular disorders.

Current efforts have developed novel forms such as nano-particles to enhance bioavailability, and many artificial derivatives based on simple phenylpropanoid scaffolds have been synthesised to further expand applications.

## 3 BIOSYNTHETIC PATHWAYS

The diversity and conservatism of simple phenylpropanoids are the result of efficient modification and amplification towards the fundamental "C6 - C3" structure through an orchestrated cascade of enzymes, including oxygenases, reductases, ligases and transferases. The biosynthesis of simple phenyl-propanoids are derived from the aromatic amino acids (AAAs) L-Phe and L-tyrosine (L-Tyr) in plants (Fig. 2). As nodes connecting primary and secondary metabolism, L-Phe and L-Tyr are synthesised from chorismate (CHA) *via* the AAA pathway. The condensation of two core precursors, phosphoenolpyruvate (PEP), derived from glycolysis, and erythrose 4-phosphate (E4P), derived from the pentose phosphate pathway (PPP), leads to a metabolic flux into the shikimate pathway for CHA synthesis. Therefore, the biosynthetic pathways of simple phenyl-propanoids can be divided into primary metabolism and plant-specific phenylpropanoid metabolism. Except for plant-specific $CO_2$ fixation (shown in green in Fig. 2), the AAA biosynthetic pathway is relatively conserved in plants and microorganisms (shown in red in Fig. 2). Biosynthetic pathways of simple phenylpropanoids and their derived complex phenylpropanoids usually exist in plants.

Plants absorb carbon dioxide to produce sugar, whereas glucose is the most direct carbon source for cellular biomass in bacteria and fungi. Central carbon metabolism converts glucose to PEP and E4P *via* glycolysis and nonoxidative steps in the PPP, respectively. Notably, PPP is related to the redox cofactor NADPH, which is critical for several downstream enzymes and the normal cellular energy metabolism. The pathway connecting central carbon metabolism and the AAA network is the shikimate pathway, which comprises seven enzymatic reactions and is ubiquitous in plants, fungi and bacteria. As the first committed step, studies have shown that the aldol condensation of PEP and E4P to produce 3-deoxy-D-arabino-heptulosonate 7-phosphate (DAHP) in a reaction catalysed by DAHP synthase is a rate limiting reaction.

The following steps to generate the final product of the

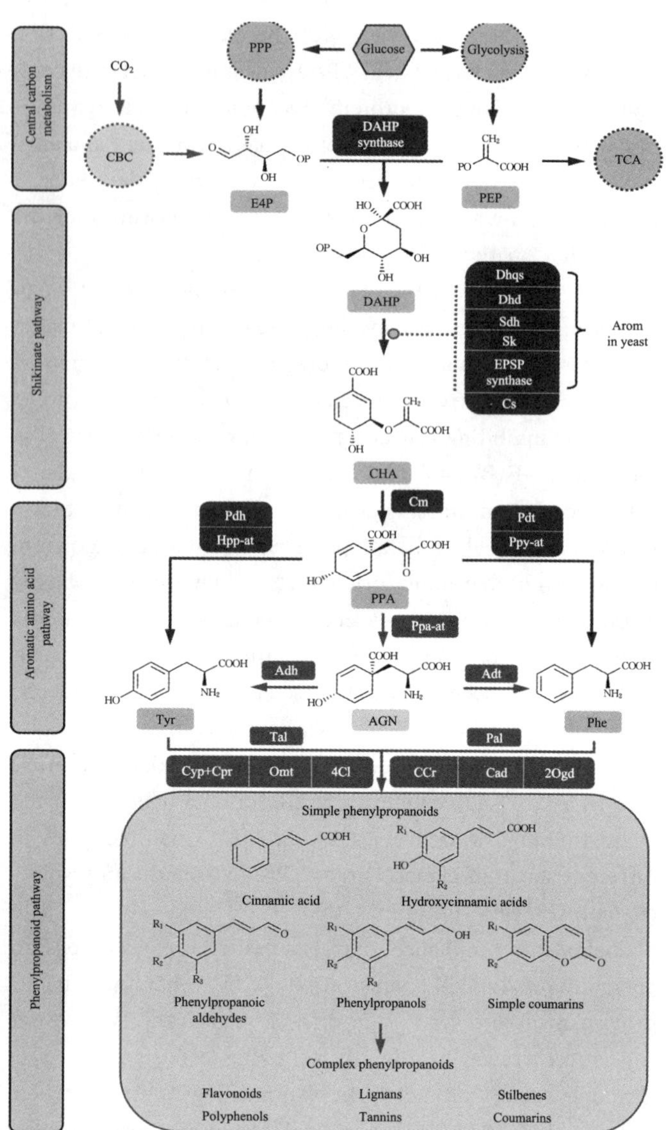


**Fig. 2 The schematic diagram of simple phenylpropanoids biosyn-thesis**

The conserved part of the pathway in plants and microorganisms (including glycolysis, pentose phosphate pathway (PPP), shikimate pathway, and aromatic amino acid pathway) and the specific part in plants (including $CO_2$ fixation and simple phenylpropanoid pathway) are shown in red and green, respectively. Abbreviations: $CO_2$, carbon dioxide; CBC, Calvin-Benson cycle, TCA, tricarboxylic acid cycle; PPP, pentose phosphate pathway; E4P, erythrose 4-phosphate; PEP, phosphoenolpyruvate; DAHP, 3-deoxy-D-arabino-heptulosonate 7-phosphate; CHA, chorismate; PPA, prephenate; AGN, L-arogenate. Enzymes: Dhqs, 3-dehydroquinate synthase; Dhd, 3-dehydroquinate dehydratase; Sdh, shikimate dehydrogenase; Sk, shikimate kinase; EPSP synthase, 5-enolpyruvate-shikimate-3-phosphate synthase; Cs. chorismate synthase; Cm, chorismate mutase; Pdh, prephenate dehydrogenase; Hpp-at, 4-hydroxyphenylpyruvate aminotransferase; Pdt, prephenate dehydratase; Ppy-at, Phenylpyruvate aminotrans-ferase; Ppa-at, prephenate aminotransferase; Adh, arogenate dehy-drogenase; Adt, arogenate dehydratase; Pal, phenylalanine ammonia-lyase; Tal, tyrosine ammonia-lyase; Cyp, cytochrome P450-depen-dent monooxygenase; Cpr, Cytochrome P450 reductase; Omt, *O*-methyltransferase; 4Cl, 4-coumarate-CoA ligase; Ccr, cinnamoyl-CoA reductase; Cad, cinnamyl alcohol dehydrogenase; 2Ogd, 2-oxoglutarate-dependent dioxygenase.

shikimate pathway, chorismate (CHA), are typically supported by individual monofunctional enzymes in plants and *E. coli*, including 3-dehydroquinate synthase (Dhps), 3-dehydroquinate dehydratase (Dqd), shikimate dehydrogenase (Sdh), shikimate kinase (Sk), 5-enolpyruvate-shikimate-3-phosphate synthase (Epsp synthase) and chorismate synthase (CS), whereas in *Saccharomyces cerevisiae*, a penta-functional protein (Arom) can directly catalyse the reaction of DAHP to 5-enolpyruvylshikimate-3-phosphate (EPSP). As a key branching point of the primary metabolic pathway to make aromatic amino acids, CHA firstly forms prephenate (PPA) in a reaction catalysed by chorismate mutase (Cm). The subsequent conversion to Phe and Tyr occurs *via* two routes in plants. One is conserved in both plants and microorganisms, where PPA catalyses the synthesis of L-Phe by prephenate dehydratase (Pdt) and phenylpyruvate amin-otrans-ferase (Ppy-at) or L-Tyr by prephenate dehydrogen-ase (Pdh) and 4-hydroxyphenylpyruvate aminotransferase (Hpp-at). PPA is converted to L-arogenate (AGN) by prephenate aminotransferase (Ppa-at), which is then converted in reactions catalysed by arogenate dehydratase (Adt) or arogenate dehydrogenase (Adh) to L-Phe or L-Tyr, respectively.

The biosynthetic pathway producing simple phenylpropanoids that occurs in plants has been heterologously established in microorganisms — the specific pathways involved are described in the following section. The conversion of L-Phe to *t*-CA is catalysed by phenylalanine ammonia-lyase (Pal). Studies have demonstrated that the broad substrate spectrum of Pal includes L-Phe and L-Tyr, and that the reverse reaction to i-Phe can also be catalysed by Pal in the presence of ammonia. *t*-CA is modified by the hydroxylation and methylation of the aromatic ring, giving rise to hydroxycinnamic acids. Among these, *p*-HCA can also be directly formed from the deamination of L-Tyr by the bifunctional Phe/Tyr ammonia-lyase (PTal) enzyme from monocot grasses of the Poaceae family, or from some bacterial and fungal species. The enzyme 4-coumarate-CoA ligase (4Cl) catalyses the conversion of phenylpropanoic acids to the coenzyme A (CoA) thioesters, which are then converted to the corresponding aldehydes by cinnamoyl-CoA reductase (Ccr), and subsequently to phenylpropanols by cinnamyl alcohol dehydrogenase (Cad), and simple coumarins by 2-oxoglutarate-dependent dioxygenase (2Ogd). Furthermore, simple phenylpropanoids are considered basic building blocks for downstream decorations to produce large quantities of secondary metabolites, such as flavonoids, stilbenes, lignans, polyphenols, and condensed tannins. These complex phenyl-propanoids and their derivatives have various biological and commercial values and are being intensively evaluated.

## 4 MICROBIAL PRODUCTION

As the compounds connecting the microbial innate pathway and the plant allogenic pathway, L-Phe and L-Tyr obtain carbon fluxes from the central carbon metabolic and shikimate pathways for the synthesis of simple phenylpropanoids (Fig. 2). Reprogramming the primary metabolic flux to AAAs (L-Phe and L-Tyr) is the basis for the high-level synthesis of simple phenylpropanoids. Therefore, the construction of a microbial cell factory for the efficient synthesis of simple phenylpropanoids requires two steps: construction of an AAA high-producing chassis (Fig. 3) and introduction and optimization of simple phenylpropanoid pathways (Fig. 4).

### 4.1 Efficient microbial production of AAAs

Multilevel metabolic engineering strategies have been studied to overproduce AAAs (L-Phe and L-Tyr), such as rewiring central carbon metabolism, relieving negative regulation, eliminating by-product formation, and engineering transport processes (Fig. 3). To rewire the central carbon flux towards the AAA pathway, an improved supply of PEP and E4P is required. The PPP is the exclusive pathway for glucose conversion to E4P, and its optimization is crucial for E4P supply. Since *S. cerevisiae* tends to quickly introduce metabolic flux into glycolysis for ethanol fermentation under anaerobic conditions and limits PPP, the deficiency of E4P is a major problem. In addition, E4P has been reported to be the primary limiting substrate for AAA biosynthesis in some bacteria, such as *E. coli*, *B. subtilis*, and *Corynebacterium glutamicum*. In *S. cerevisiae*, the optimization strategy for PPP depends on cell culture conditions because the upstream (Zwf and Gnd) and downstream (Tkl and Tal) enzymes of PPP are rate-limiting steps for E4P synthesis under high- and low-glucose concentrations, respectively. Therefore, different strategies should be used for PPP optimization to accommodate the use of high- and low-glucose-induced promoters. A novel PHK pathway consisting of phosphoketolase (Xfpk) can split xylose 5-phosphate (X5P) and/or fructose 6-phosphate (F6P) into acetyl-phosphate and glyceraldehyde-3-phosphate (G3P) /E4P, which is critical for rewiring the carbon metabolism of glycolysis into E4P. Therefore, simultaneous expression of Xfpk, Tal, and Tkl can significantly increase the metabolic flux towards E4P in *S. cerevisiae*. Although *S. cerevisiae* is not able to use xylose as a sole carbon source, it is clear that metabolic flux enters the PPP faster for E4P synthesis when xylose is used, which may be useful in further improving the E4P supply in yeast. In contrast with E4P, carbon flow towards PEP is usually sufficient because of its important position in glycolysis. Construction of a non-PTS route in *E. coli* has been proven to avoid PEP loss for glucose transport, ($>50\%$), thereby supporting the synthesis of downstream

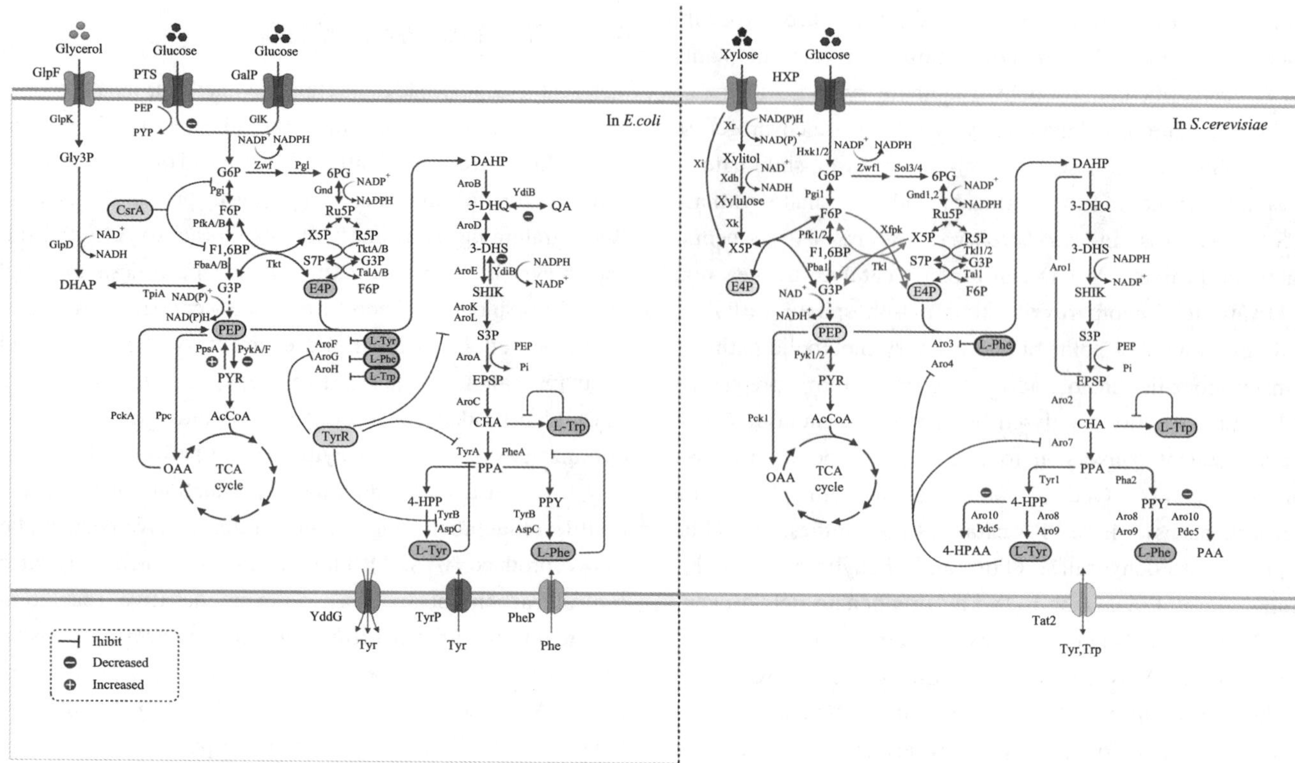


**Fig. 3 Overview of metabolic engineering strategies for efficient microbial production of AAAs in *E. coli* and *S. cerevisiae***

Endogenous AAA pathways are represented by the solid black arrows, the dashed arrows indicate multiple reactions, while the alternative pathway that have been evaluated are represented by yellow arrows. The blue arrows represent the increased fluxes by overexpressing genes, the red arrows represent the decreased fluxes by deletion of genes. The indicator arrows (red) show inhibitions by isoenzymes allosteric regulatory circuits and the transcriptional regulatory factors. Abbeviations: (a) in *E. coli*: GlpF, glycerol uptake facilitator; GlpK, glycerol kinase; Gly-3P, sn-glycerol-3-phosphate; GipD, glycerol 3-phosphate dehydrogenase; TpiA, triosephosphate isomerase; PTS, phosphoenolpyruvate phosphotransferase system; GalP, galactose permease; Glk, glucokinase; G6P, glucose 6-phosphate; Pgi, phosphoglucose isomerase; F6P, fructose 6-phosphate; PrkA/B, phosphofructokinase; F1, 6BP, fructose-1, 6-bisphosphate; FbaA/B, fructose 1, 6-bisphosphate aldolase; G3P, glyceraldehyde 3-phos-phate; Zwf, glucose-6-phosphate dehydrogenase; Pgl, 6-phosphogluconolactonase; 6PG, 6-phosphogluconate; Gnd, 6-phosphogluconate dehydrogenase; Ru5P, ribulose 5-phosphate; X5P, xylulose-5-phosphate; R5P, ribose 5-phosphate; S7P, sedoheptulose 7-phophate; F6P, fructose 6-phosphate; TalA/B, transaldolase; ThtA/B, transketolase; E4P, erythrose 4-phosphate; PEP, phosphoenolpyuvate; DAHP, 3-deoxy-D-arabino-heptulosonate 7-phosphate; PpsA, PEP synthase; PykA/F, pyruvate kinase; PckA, PEP carboxykinase; Ppc, PEP carboxylase; PYR, pyruvate; AcCoA, acetyl-CoA; OAA, oxaloccetate; TCA, tricarboxylic acid cycle; 3-DHQ, 3-dehydroquinate; 3-DHS, 3-dehydroshikimate; SHIK, shikimate; S3P, shikimate 3-phosphate; EPSP, 5-enolpyruvate-shikimate-3-phosphate; CHA, chorismate; PPA, prephenate; 4-HPP, 4-hydroxyphenytpyruvate; PPY, phenytpynvate. 4-HPAA. 4-hydroxyphenylacetaldehyde; PAA, phenylacetaldehyde; AroF/G/H, DAHP synthases; AroB, 3-dehydroquinate synthase; AroD, 3-dehydroquinate dehydratase; AroE, shikimate dehydrogenase; YdiB, quinate/shikimate dehydrogenase; AroK/L, shikimate kinase; AroA. Esp synthase; AroC, chorismate synthase, PheA/TyrA, chorismite mutase/prepherate dehydratase; TyrB, aromatic amino acid aminotransferase; AspC, aspartate aminotransferase; CsrA and TyrR, transcriptional repressors; YddG, TyrP, PheP, transporters of aromatic amino acids (b) in *S. cerevisiae*: Xr, xylose reductase; Xdh, xylitol dehydrogenase; Xi, xylose isomerase; Xk, xylulokinase; Mxk1/2, hexokinase; Pgil, phosphogluccose isomerase; Pfk1/2, phosphofructokinase; Fbal, fructose 1, 6-bisphosphate aldolase; Zwfi, glucose-6-phos-phate dehydrogenase; Sol3/4, 6-phosphogluconolactonase; Gndl/2, 6-phosphogluconate dehydrogenase; Tall, transaldolase; Tk11/2, trans-ketolase; Xfpk, phosphoketolase; Pyk1/2, pyruvate kinase; Pck1, PEP carboxykinase; Aro3/4; DAHP synthases; Arol, a penta-functional protein catalyzing DAHP to EPSP; Aro2, chorismate synthase; Aro7, chorismate mutase holoenzyme; Pha2, prephenate dehydratase: Tyr1, prephenate dehydrogenase. Aro8/9, aromatic amino transferases; Aro10, pheny lpyruvate decarboxylase; Pdc5, pyruvate decarboxylase; Tat2: tryptophan and tyrosine permease. Figure created with https://Biorender.com.

AAA. The availability of PEP and E4P can also be improved by adjusting the activity of precursor pathway enzymes, such as by deletion of pyruvate kinases (encoded by *PYKA* and *PYKF*), or by over-expression of PEP synthase (encoded by PPSA), transketolase (encoded by *TKTA*) and/or transaldolase (encoded by *TALB*). It is reasonable that the carbon flux between PEP and E4P is significantly different, thus it is essential to balance the availability of E4P and PEP (increase E4P and decrease PEP) to maintain high productivity. Promoter engineering by fine-tuning the strength of glycolysis and PEP alleviated this limitation in *S. cerevisiae*.

Since bypass inevitably diverts the flow of the target

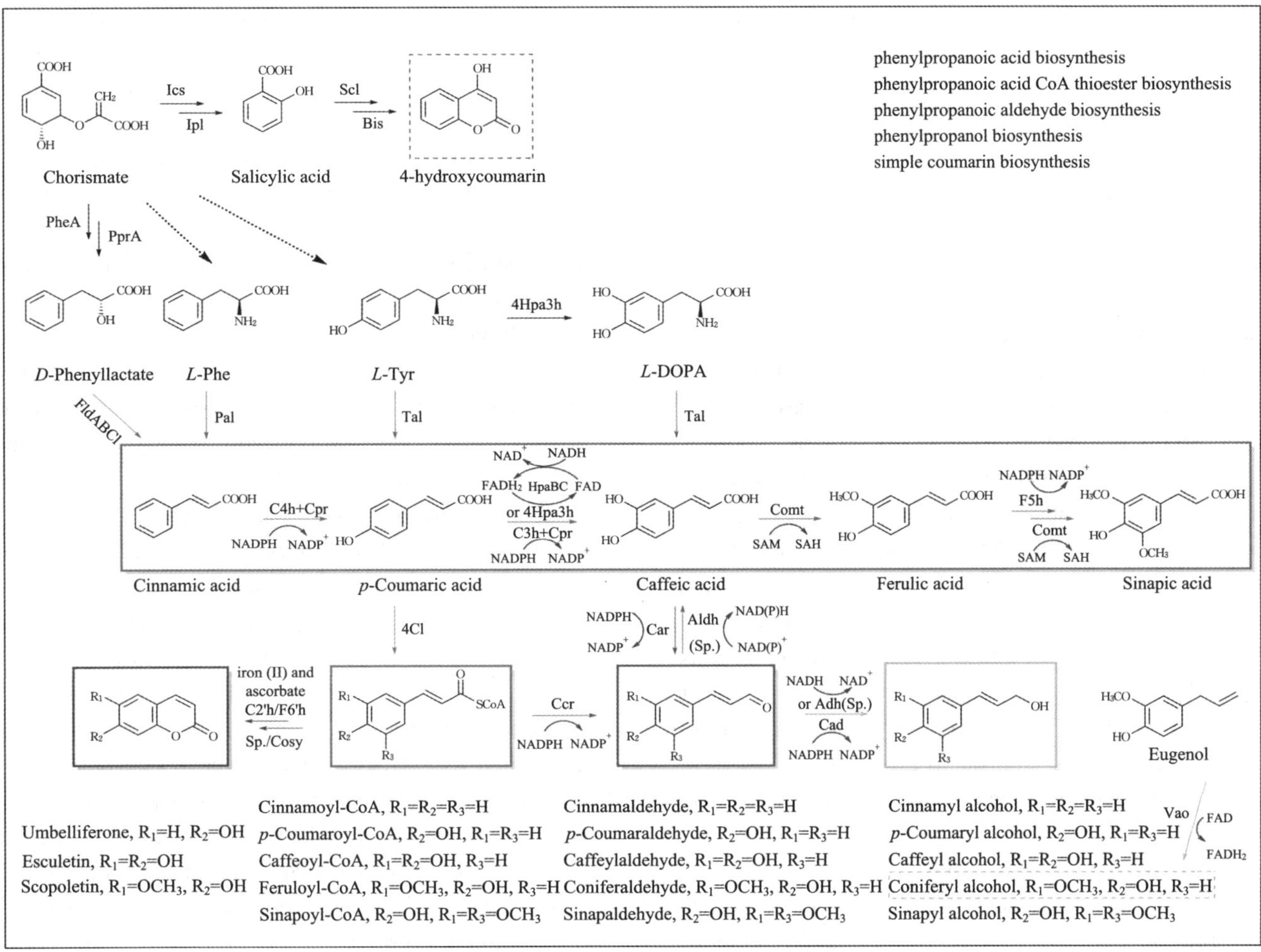


**Fig. 4 Biosynthesis of simple phenylpropanoids**

The multiple reactions are represented by the dashed arrow. Abbreviations: Ics, isochorismate synthase; lpl, isochorismate pyruvate lyase; Scl, salicylate-CoA ligase; Bis, biphenyl synthases; PheA, chorismate mutase; PprA, phenylpyruvate reductase; FldABCl phenyllactate dehydratase; Pal, pherylalanine ammonia-lyase; Tal, tyrosine armmonia-lyase; C4h/C3h, cytochrome P450-dependent monooxygenase; Cpr, Cytochrome P450 reductase; 4Hpa3h, 4-hydroxyphenylacetic acid 3-hydroxylase; HpaBC, *p*-hydroxyphenylacetate 3-hydroxylase; Comt, caffec acid/5-hydroxyferulic acid 3/5-*O*-methytransferase; F5h, ferutate 5-hydroxylase; 4Cl, 4-coumarate-CoA ligase; Ccr, cinnamoyl-CoA reductase; Cad, cinnamyl alcohol dehydrogenase; Car, carboylic acid reductase; Aldh/Adh, endogenous aldehyde/alcohol dehydrogenase; C2′h, coumaroyl-CoA 2′-hydroxylase; F6′h, feruloyi-CoA 6′-hydroxylase. Cosy, coumarin synthase; Sp., spontaneous reactions.

pathway, it is necessary to control the pathway by weakening its branches to facilitate product synthesis. In *E. coli*, the bifunctional enzyme (YdiB) was replaced by the monofunctional enzyme (AroE) to reduce the by-product formation of quinate in the shikimate pathway. In *S. cerevisiae*, increased flux in the AAA biosynthetic pathway results in the accumulation of undesired fusel alcohol/acids *via* the Ehrlich pathway, which can be relieved by a double knock-out of phenylpyruvate decarboxylase (Aro10) and pyruvate decarboxylase (Pdc5). interestingly, a recent report has found that the deletion of a novel gene HTZ1 significantly increased the tyrosine-producing capacity of yeast cells, although the underlying mechanism remains to be elaborated. Primary metabolism is strictly regulated by microorganisms, including yeasts. At the enzyme activity level, metabolic flux is controlled mainly by AAA-mediated feedback inhibition in the first and post-chorismate steps in the above-mentioned biosynthetic pathways. By protein structure analysis with site directed mutagenesis, the feedback-resistant (fbr) variants such as aro4$^{K229L}$ and aro7$^{G141S}$ have been widely utilized in *S. cerevisiae* to eliminate the allosteric regulation for the enhancement of the corresponding AAAs and derived metabolites. *CSRA*, encoding the carbon- storage regulator of *E. coli*, regulates enzymes in glycolysis, and over 2-fold increase in yield of v-Phe were achieved when CsrA was disrupted. TyrR is the tyrosine repressor that negatively regulate several genes transcription of Tyr-producing pathway in *E. coli*, and inactivation of TyrR led to an increase in the L-Tyr biosynthesis. Transport engineering contributes to strain development by addressing substrate uptake and product output, as well as loss of intermediates. The tyrosine-specific transporters TyrP and TyrR were mutated in *E. coli* overexpressing aroG$^{\Delta fbr}$, aroL and tyrC, leading to a maximum L-Tyr titre of 43.14 g/L by fed-batch fermentation.

Notably, the regulation of cell growth and highly tailored production should be carried out in an optimal and sustainable manner. A synthetic RNA (sRNA) strategy was employed in *E. coli* to fine-tune target gene expression, which could coordinate the flux balance between L-Tyr production and biomass accumulation. Adaptive laboratory evolution could also be useful as a way of enhancing the robustness of engineered strains. A *Pseudomonas putida* S12 mutant strain highly accumulating L-Phe was successfully screened by a combination of random mutagenesis and selection of toxic analogs. Recently, with the aid of biosensors as a high-throughput screening tool, recombinant strains with the desired properties for enhanced AAAs are likely to be identified in high efficiency. Researchers have explored the potential of non-conventional microbial chassis to generate AAAs, such as *Yarrowia lipolytica* and *C. glutamicum*, which have been an attractive platform optimized for aromatic compounds production.

4.2 Efficient microbial production of simple phenylpropanoids

4.2.1 Phenylpropanoic acids

4.2.1.1 Cinnamic acid Cinnamic acid belongs to a class of auxins that regulate cell growth and differentiation. Owing to its broad applicability, the microbial production of cinnamic acid, which is a relatively facile and green technology, has been actively explored over the last few decades. Cinnamic acid is the non-oxidative deamination product of L-Phe in a reaction catalysed by Pal and mostly occurs in the *trans* configuration (*t*-CA) (Fig. 4). Pal is the starting and limiting enzyme in the simple phenylpropanoids biosynthetic pathway, hence much effort has been made in identifying high-efficiency alternative enzymes for functional expression in heterologous microbes. The production titre of *t*-CA reached 6.9 g/L by heterologous expression of an efficient SmPal from *Streptomyces maritimus* in an engineered L-Phe-overproducing *E. coli*, together with cultivation optimization and casamino acid supplementation in a 2 litre bioreactor. In order to further optimize the catalytic function of *Sm*Pal, the combination of a *Sm*Pal-based whole-cell biocatalyst in *C. glutamicum* and a crossflow membrane-based cell recycling system was designed to produce *t*-CA from L-Phe with a yield of 75% (0.75 mol/mol). An alternative pathway harbouring a phenyllactate dehydratase encoded by FLDABCI genes from *Clostridium sporogenes* was developed for additional *t*-CA production from D-phenyllactate (Fig. 4), which exceeded the Pal-dependent pathway to achieve an 11-fold increase in *t*-CA yield. Most recently, a high-density culture system of the cyanobacterium *Synechocystis* sp. PCC 6 803 successfully synthesized approximately 0.8 g/L *t*-CA from $CO_2$ as the carbon source, which indicates that exploiting the primary metabolism of cyanobacteria has great potential for the green and sustainable production of phenylpropanoids. As the cytotoxicity of *t*-CA impairs cell proliferation, researchers have found that near-neutral culture pH and alcoholic carbon source might be useful to improve the cellular tolerance to *t*-CA inhibition.

4.2.1.2 Coumaric acid Coumaric acid, also known as hydroxycinnamic acid, naturally exists as three isomers (*ortho*-, *meta*-, and *para*-) with different substitution positions for the active hydroxyl group on the benzene ring. Among these, *para*-coumaric acid (*p*-HCA) occurs more often in nature. With advances in metabolic engineering, microbial production has become a promising alternative for obtaining large-scale yields of *p*-HCA. Starting with aromatic amino acids, L-Tyr can be directly converted to *p*-HCA by Tal, which is typically found in bacteria. Alternatively, the deamination product *t*-CA of L-Phe can be further hydroxylated to *p*-HCA by membrane bound cinnamate-4-hydroxylase (C4h) in plants. The Tal-dependent one-step biosynthesis is more convenient and economical; also, the Pal-C4h pathway requires plant-derived Cpr and cofactor NADPH to form the electron transport chain to complete the hydroxylation reaction (Fig. 4). Therefore, the onestep reaction catalysed by Tal is favoured for application in *p*-HCA production from microbial cell factories. However, this conversion is often limited by the poor activity of the heterologous Tal enzyme and the competitive inhibition of *p*-HCA on Tal and Pal. Therefore, it is necessary to identify novel enzymes with higher and more stable activities from different sources. The substrate specificity and activity of enzymes can be altered by rationally designing active amino acid residues. By the combination of directed evolution and high-throughput screening, a Tal variant from *Rhodotorula glutinis* with higher selectivity for L-Tyr and superior catalytic efficiency was screened, producing a *p*-HCA titre that was 2.2-fold higher than that of the control strain. Systematic bioinformatics analysis and enzyme characterization have been applied to identify Tals most suitable for *p*-HCA production in *E. coli* and yeast. Interestingly, when the *Fj*Tal protein was anchored to the yeast vacuole, *p*-HCA production was significantly enhanced. Although C4h as a membrane-bound Cyp is not amenable to expression in *E. coli*, a novel C4h from *Lycoris aurea* was identified and functionally expressed in *E. coli*, and when combined with the optimization of NADPH regeneration and Cpr expression enabled a *p*-HCA titre of 25.62 mg/L. In order to greatly enlarge the capacity of yeast in producing *p*-HCA, carbon metabolic allocation is optimized towards aromatic amino acid biosynthesis, which, together with the microbial Tal and introduction of a plant Pal-C4h, led to a high-level production of *p*-HCA (12.5 g/L) in fed-batch fermentation in *S. cerevisiae*. To eliminate the Crabtree effect, xylose as the carbon source for *p*-HCA production was investigated in *S. cerevisiae* and finally achieved a 45-fold increase in *p*-HCA production compared to the use of glucose as the carbon source under the same conditions. In recent years, the *de novo* synthesis of *p*-HCA in *Synechocystis* sp. PCC 6803 has been achieved. Using the fixation of $CO_2$ by solar energy as the carbon source, the highest total titre was up to 0.4 g/L in a high-density cultivation system. To eliminate the genetic and production instability of strains using episomal plasmid expression in the fermentation, a high *p*HCA-yielding *S. cerevisiae* was built through POT1-mediated delta integration, after which the titre and gene copy number remained stable for more than one hundred generations. Transporters are responsible for the efflux of small product molecules, and have showed significance in strain improvement. The deletion of a specific transporter (TAT1), which is responsible for transport of L-Tyr and L-Trp, led to a 50% increase in *p*-HCA titre. Upregulation of the aromatic acid transporter ESBP6 promoted increases in the *p*-HCA titre, as well as improvements in the yeast tolerance to toxicity. Although the microbial production of *p*-HCA has already achieved on a g/L scale, microbial cell factories still need to be further optimized for high-level synthesis, such as by targeting product degradation and inhibition, cofactor imbalance, and transcriptional regulation.

4.2.1.3 Caffeic acid CaA is a phytonutrient frequently found in plants, including vegetables. The biosynthesis of CaA involves the *ortho*-hydroxylation of *p*-HCA through the Cyp enzyme *p*-coumarate 3-hydroxylase (C3h) (Fig. 4), which is traditionally difficult to perform in bacteria. Therefore, identifying different C3h isozymes from other organisms is crucial for the synthesis of CaA in engineered cells. A microbial C3h encoded by SAM5 from *Saccharothrix espanaensis* and a site-directed mutant of CYP199A2 from *Rhodopseudomonas palustris* were shown to have activity when expressed in bacteria to synthesise CaA from *p*-HCA. The *de novo* biosynthesis of CaA in *E. coli* was also achieved by expressing endogenous 4-hydroxyphenylacetic acid 3-hydroxylase (4Hpa3h) that can hydroxylate both *p*-HCA and L-Tyr to generate CaA and L-3, 4-dihydroxyphenylalanine (L-DOPA), respectively, while L-Dopa was further converted to CaA by Tal from *Rhodobacter capsulatus*. An alternative pathway catalysed by bacteriacoupled enzymes HpaB (FAD-dependent 4-hydroxyphenylacetate-3-monooxygenase) and HpaC (NADH-flavin oxidoreductase) has been shown to be the most preferred strategy for CaA synthesis in both bacterial and fungal systems. In this pathway, the direct electron donor is $FADH_2$, rather than NADPH, and $FADH_2$-dependent enzymes are usually more adapted in microorganisms. The yield of CaA also depends on the compatibility of HpaB and HpaC in cell factories. Through orthogonal assays, the combination of HpaB from *Pseudomonas aeruginosa* and HpaC from *Salmonella enterica* was regarded as the best. By expressing this enzyme pair, combined with the cofactor optimization strategy, the yield of CaA in *S. cerevisiae* reached 5.5 g/L. This strategy using suitable cofactor engineering provides fundamental insights for future research in other natural product biosynthesis. Apart from enzyme screening and cofactor engineering, control of transport proteins has also been proven to be an effective strategy for reducing cytotoxicity and promoting CaA synthesis. By overexpressing the putative sugar ABC transporter permease (YcjP), which was identified through transcriptome data mining, the production of CaA was further enhanced to about 7.9 g/L in *E. coli* with the integration of other optimized factors. This is the highest known titre so far. Recently, the multi-copy integration expression strategies based on delta sites were applied to integrate the genes of the CaA pathway into yeast and resulted in an increase of CaA production by 50 times compared to that produced by the initial multi-copy-plasmid expression. Some other carbon sources and the whole-cell biocatalyst strategy have also been successfully used for CaA synthesis. By introducing the xylose assimilation pathway into *Candida glycerinogenes*, the advantage of using mixed sugars as carbon sources showed that the optimized strain eventually obtained 1.2-fold higher CaA than that using glucose. In addition, the generation of CaA can proceed in four steps, from L-Tyr through *p*-HCA, coumaroyl-CoA and caffeoyl-CoA, as CoA thioesterase can convert caffeoyl-CoA to CaA, although this pathway is inefficient.

4.2.1.4 Ferulic acid FA (*p*-hydroxy-3-methoxycinnamic acid), a phytomolecule crosslinked with lignin and hemicellulose in plant cell walls, is abundant in certain cereal raw materials and medicinal herbs. Caffeic acid/5-hydroxyferulic acid 3/5-*O*-methyltransferase (Comt) catalyses the methylation of the 3-hydroxyl group of CaA to generate FA, which can be further converted to sinapic acid (Fig. 4). SA has multiple pharmaceutical applications, but limited data are available on its microbial production. Most efforts have been devoted to constructing FA synthetic pathways in microbial hosts to produce FA using glucose or L-Tyr as substrates. For example, a recombinant *E. coli* harbouring plasmids with the pathway genes (TAL, C3H and COMT) produced 257.3 mg/L FA from L-Tyr. In another example, after the optimization of gene expression by changes to the promoter strength and copy number, coupled with enhanced NADPH levels to improve the conversion towards CaA, and overexpression of a methionine kinase, 212 mg/L of FA was produced in shake flash cultures. More recently, an engineered yeast achieved a yield of 3.8 g/L of FA in a fed-batch fermentation through cofactor engineering of that accelerated the methyl cycle and SAM regeneration. To address the insufficient supply of HpaBC-dependent cofactor $FADH_2$, a NAD(P)H-flavin reductase (Fre) was introduced to active $FADH_2$ regeneration, which promoted an 8.1-fold increase in efficiency of hydroxylation. Combined with the efforts on a L-Tyr overproducer and SAM reactivation, the total titre of FA reached 5.09 g/L in *E. coli* under the fed-batch condition. FA and SA can also be synthesized from the oxidation of coniferyl aldehyde and sinapoyl aldehyde, respectively, by the corresponding aldehyde dehydrogenase (Aldh), which indirectly detoxify the reactive aldehydes in cellular metabolic processes. Alternatively, the biotransformation of eugenol to FA was also established in a recombinant *S. cerevisiae* by expressing vanillyl-alcohol oxidase (*Ps*Vao) from *Penicillium simplicissimum*, and 16.9 g/L of FA was produced from eugenol feeding in a fermentor. Of special interest, the Vao family of enzymes involve many reactions with phenolic substrates and the FAD cofactor. Considering that eugenol is an inexpensive and readily available substrate, its bioconversion to FA is likely to expand to industrial levels. Notably, an alternative one-step production method based on microbial fermentation is of great interest, using feruloyl esterase to prepare FA from agro-industrial wastes (*e.g.*, wheat bran and brewery spent grain) with microbial fermentation. Feruloyl esterase is expected to be a catalyst for the production of biofuels from biomass.

4.2.2 Phenylpropanoic aldehydes Simple phenylpropanoic aldehydes include cinnamaldehyde, *p*-coumaraldehyde, caffeoylaldehyde, coniferaldehyde, and sinapaldehyde. Phenylpropanoic aldehydes are produced from phenylpropanoic acids by the actions of two enzymes, 4Cl and Ccr, in which the CoA thioester of the 4Cl products is converted to an aldehyde group using NADPH (Fig. 4). The co-expression of three plant enzymes Pal, 4Cl, and Ccr in *E. coli* achieved cinnamaldehyde production from L-Phe. The fusion of 4Cl1-Ccr was functionally overexpressed in *E. coli* to construct a metabolic channel for improved production of *p*-coumaraldehyde, caffealdehyde and coniferaldehyde from feedstocks consisting of the corresponding phenypropanoic acids. In addition, a novel microbial pathway consisting of an aryl carboxylic acid reductase (Car) and a phosphopantetheinyl transferase (EntD) were shown to synthesize cinnamaldehyde from *t*-CA without the presence of plant 4Cl. The *de novo* biosynthesis of cinnamaldehyde was carried out in L-Pheoverproducing *S. cerevisiae* using glucose as a substrate. Although the *de novo* biosynthesis of cinnamaldehyde was achieved in a strain of *S. cerevisiae* producing high levels of L-Phe, cell growth was affected by the concentration of cinnamaldehyde, and some unanticipated metabolites such as cinnamyl alcohol were detected in the fermentation broth. The toxicity of aldehyde chemicals is harmful to the growth and metabolism of microbes, which provides a reasonable explanation for the absence of natural accumulation of aldehydes in microorganisms. In contrast, the endogenous Aldh and alcohol dehydrogenase (Adh) in *S. cerevisiae* are thought to be spontaneously involved in the reversible conversion of aldehydes to alcohols and acids and are associated with sugar metabolism. Therefore, the spontaneous conversion from cinnamaldehyde to cinnamyl alcohols may be explained by a cellular Adh/Aldh-related detoxification mechanism, which could be an important target for further optimization to increase the production of aldehydes. By knocking out 10 endogenous Adh and Aldh enzymes and using some necessary engineering strategies, such as changes to cofactor supply, enzyme expression enhancement, auto-induction systems, and engineered *E. coli*, a maximum cinnamaldehyde titre of 3.8 g/L was achieved using glucose.

4.2.3 Phenylpropanoids Phenylpropanoids, also known as monolignols, are mainly synthesised through the monolignol pathway, in which cinnamyl alcohol dehydrogenase (Cad) catalyses the NADPH-mediated reversible conversion of aldehydes to their corresponding alcohols (Fig. 4).

The biotechnological production of natural phenylpropanols has been achieved by reconstructing the plant monolignol pathway in microbial hosts. Although the synthesis of cinnamyl alcohol and hydrocinnamyl alcohol has been achieved in *S. cerevisiae* and *E. coli* by expressing Cad or Ccr enzymes from different species, severe product inhibition is the key limiting factor in cinnamyl alcohol biosynthesis. Product inhibition was successfully removed using a dibutyl phthalate/water biphasic system, which constantly separated and concentrated cinnamyl alcohol synthesised by *E. coli* from *t*-CA into the organic phase. Coniferyl alcohol, a precursor of silybin and other natural pharmaceuticals, is the most abundant monolignol in plants. The co-expression of 4Cl, Ccr, and Cad from *Arabidopsis thaliana* in a FA producer achieved *de novo* synthesis of coniferyl alcohol with titres of 187.7 mg/L and 201.1 mg/L in *E. coli* and *S. cerevisiae* through fed-batch fermentation, respectively. Moreover, it is noteworthy that these enzymes responsible for the monolignol biosynthesis are known to be promiscuous on the substrate specificity, which is double-edged for the production of phenylpropanols. A study applied a co-culture strategy to the engineered *E. coli* hosts, which minimized the effect of promiscuous HpaBC catalysing the side reaction of L-Tyr to produce L-Dopa, reaching 534 mg/L caffeyl alcohol and 124.9 mg/L coniferyl alcohol. Additionally, a study used the *Ps*Vao to convert eugenol to coniferyl alcohol in *E. coli*, together with catalase (Ctal) from *S. cerevisiae* to avoid over-oxidation of coniferyl alcohol, which reached the final coniferyl alcohol titre of 53.9 g/L in a 5 L bioreactor with a conversion rate of 86.72%. In another study, *E. coli* was demonstrated to synthesize non-natural phenylpropanols through feeding of different precursors, such as 5-bromoconiferyl alcohol and 2-nitroconiferyl alcohol.

4.2.4 Simple coumarins Simple coumarins have a core skeleton of fused benzene and α-pyrone rings, and include compounds such as basic coumarin, umbelliferone (7-hydroxycoumarin), 4-hydroxycoumarin, esculetin (6, 7-dihydroxycoumarin), and scopoletin (7-hydroxy-6-methoxycoumarin). They are derived from the respective cinnamates by three consecutive reactions: an *ortho*-hydroxylation of the aromatic ring is catalysed by coumaroyl-CoA 2′-hydroxylase (C2′h) or feruloyl-CoA 6′-hydroxylase (F6′h) to form *o*-hydroxycin-namoyl-CoA thioesters, which is followed by spontaneous reactions (a *trans-cis*-isomerisation and a lactonisation) (Fig. 4). A new coumarin synthase (Cosy) was discovered recently with the capability to accomplish the final reactions and bypass the spontaneous steps, which may be helpful in enhancing coumarin production in the future. Multiple P450 enzymes are involved in the pathway and the *ortho*-hydroxylation step is considered to be a key stage for simple coumarin biosynthesis due to its irreversibility. The last two reactions take place partially spontaneously in the presence of the CoA group and *ortho*-hydroxyl group, catalysed by light at room temperature. By co-expressing Tal, 4Cl and C2′h, 2.43 mg/L umbelliferone was biosynthesized in *E. coli* without extra addition of 4-coumarate. Similarly, *de novo* synthesis of scopoletin was achieved in *E. coli* from glucose and glycerol by expressing a pathway containing Tal, HpaBC, 4Cl, Caffeoyl-CoA *O*-methyltransferase (CCoAomt) and F6′h. A recombinant *E. coli* strain harbouring F6′h and 4Cl genes was grown in culture supplemented with *p*-HCA, CaA, and FA, yielding 82.9 mg/L of umbelliferone, 79.5 mg/L of scopoletin, and 52.3 mg/L of esculetin.

To prevent the degradation of 4Cl-producing thioester intermediates, a predicted acyl-CoA thioesterase (YbgC) was deleted for higher production of esculetin and umbelliferone from glucose. A systematic study that overcame the limitation of 4Cl through protein engineering improved the supply of L-Tyr through metabolic flow remodelling and optimized fermentation conditions, obtaining 356.59 mg/L umbelliferone from L-Tyr. To overcome the inefficient spontaneous reactions, researchers established a novel artificial pathway condensing malonyl-CoA and salicylic acid by a biphenyl synthase (Bis) that was introduced into *E. coli* for the *de novo* synthesis of 4-hydroxycoumarin from glycerol. The resulting titre was 483.1 mg/L in 24 h. Furthermore, the production was enhanced to 935 mg/L in shake flasks by alleviating the thioesterase-mediated degradation of salicoyl-CoA. Nowadays, the use of lignin hydrolysate to produce valuable chemicals with benzene rings has attracted much interest in biotransformation technology. An engineered budding yeast expressing necessary enzymes to generate scopoletin from lignin hydrolysate was recently reported. The scopoletin production reached 4.79 mg/L, suggesting that this approach may offer new opportunities for improved biosynthesis of coumarins from renewable sources.

## 5 DISCUSSION AND FUTURE PERSPECTIVES

Driven by the important applications of simple phenylpropanoids, either because of their wide bioactivity or as precursors for the synthesis of complex natural product molecules, great progress has been achieved in the microbial production of simple phenylpropanoids (Table S1 provided as an attachment).[†] Although many simple phenylpropanoids have been synthesised at the g/L level in microorganisms with considerable engineering endeavours over the past 20 years, their titre, yield, and productivity (TYP) still require improvement to achieve industrial production. Some challenges that limit the high-level synthesis of simple phenylpropanoids must be addressed. Based on the three-dimensional metabolic engineering strategy proposed in the previous study, here we map these challenges to an upgraded four-dimensional metabolic engineering strategy (*i.e.*, "point-line-plane-system"), and suggest a potential technical proposal to meet these challenges (Fig. 5).

5.1 The "Point" level: the unsatisfied enzyme activity and cofactor utilization Enzymes are the most basic elements that fundamentally determine the synthetic efficiency in a cell factory through specific activities and cofactor supply. The catalytic promiscuity and low cofactor utilisation of enzymes in the simple phenylpropanoid pathway are key issues hindering synthetic efficiency. 4Cl is a rate-limiting enzyme with a broad substrate spectrum that generates CoA thioester intermediates from phenylpropanoic acids (Fig. 4), which may result in unexpected disruption of metabolic flux. For instance, when 4Cl is designed to react with FA, it preferentially reacts with upstream phenylpropanoic acids (*i.e.*, *t*-CA, *p*-HCA, and CaA), thereby blocking the metabolic flux towards FA. Given that several 4CL protein crystal structures have been resolved (UniProt Q42524, Q9SMT7, and Q94M3), and there have been some advances in changing the 4Cl substrate preference. It is expected that specific unnatural variants of 4Cl can be designed through classical structural biology-based protein rational modification. The continued evolution of machine-learning-assisted models will provide feasible clues for the virtual screening and

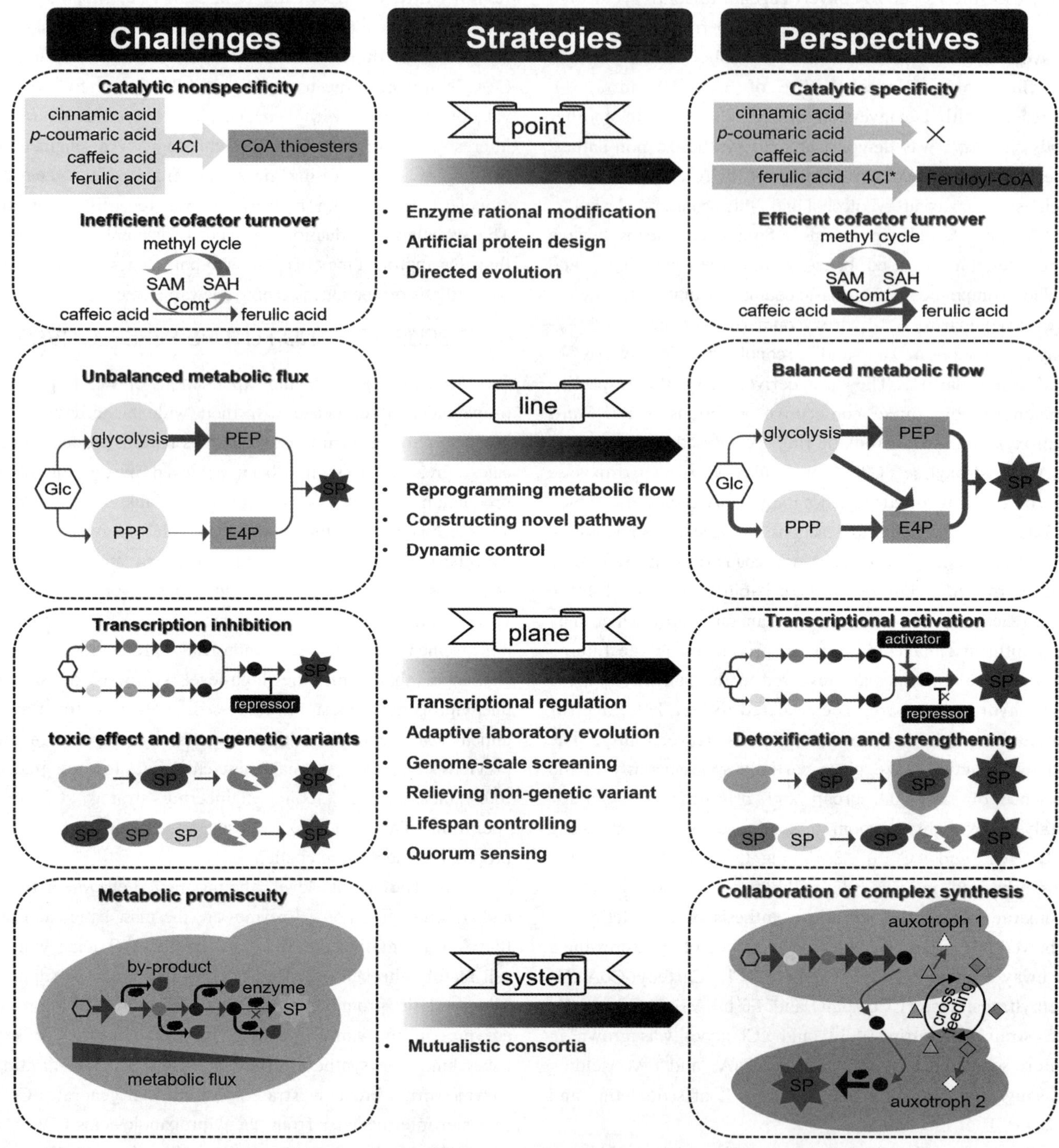


**Fig. 5 Challenges and perspectives of microbial synthesis of simple phenylpropanoids**

Potential challenges, corresponding strategies and expected results are mapped in the four-dimensional metabolic engineering strategy (*i. e.*, "point-line-plane-system"). Arrows represent multistep reactions and different colored circles represent metabolites in the pathway. 4Cl, 4-coumarate-CoA ligase; 4Cl*, mutated 4-coumarate-CoA ligase; Comt, caffeic acid *O*-methyltransferase; SAM, *S*-adenosyl-*l*-methion; SAH, *S*-adenosy-*l*-homocysteine; Glc, glucose; PPP, pentose phosphate pathway; PEP, phosphoenolpyruvate; E4P, erythrose-4-phosphate; SP, simple phenylpropanoids.

prediction of key enzymes. More importantly, the latest advances in deep learning-inspired language models may enable the *de novo* design of enzymes, which, in the case of ProGen, can be adapted to generate artificial protein sequences that are functionally identical to natural proteins.

Comt is the key enzyme in FA synthesis, and its low turnover of the methyl donor SAM results in low catalytic efficiency for CaA. Although the conversion rate of CaA to FA was increased from 28% to 64% through the metabolic engineering strategy of expressing an efficient form of Comt and by optimising the methyl cycle, more than 36% of CaA still failed to synthesise FA, and the catalytic problem of Comt itself has not been solved. Biosensors are an ideal strategy for high-throughput screening of enzymes based on intuitive phenotypic changes. A $FAR_{ON}$ switch system derived from a phenolic acid decarboxylase regulator (aPadR) was designed to respond to FA in mammalian cells. In addition, a sensitive synchronous fluorometric method based on the oxidation of FA with Ce(IV) in a sulfuric acid medium was used to detect FA *in vitro*. Therefore, optimization of the $FAR_{ON}$ biosensor and the Ce (IV)-dependent sensor to improve the cofactor turnover of Comt through directed evolution is expected to further increase FA production.

5.2 The "Line" level: the imbalance of multi-pathway metabolic fluxes Simple phenylpropanoids are derived from two AAAs (L-Phe and L-Tyr) condensed from two endogenous intermediates, *i.e.*, E4P from PPP and PEP from glycolysis. Therefore, an equal supply of E4P and PEP is advantageous for the synthesis of simple phenylpropanoids. Although glycolysis and PPP are the two fundamental routes for catabolizing glucose in most living cells, E4P has been reported to be the primary limiting substrate for simple phenylpropanoid biosynthesis in many microorganisms. To maintain the intracellular balance of $NADH/NAD^+$ and a fast growth rate, *S. cerevisiae* tends to introduce metabolic flux into glycolysis for ethanol fermentation and limits PPP when consuming sugars under anaerobic conditions. Some attempts to control heterologous expression under glucose-limited conditions, stretching PPP fluxes and weakening glycolysis have successfully increased the E4P supply and simple phenylpropanoid production in *S. cerevisiae*. Although yeast central metabolism has been extensively rewired to improve the supply of E4P, it is challenging to balance metabolic flux because of the metabolic competition between PPP and glycolysis. Considering that *S. cerevisiae* can be modified from an ethanol-producing to an oil-producing yeast, this strong metabolic plasticity implies the possibility of further improvement in the metabolic flux towards E4P through metabolic reprogramming. Furthermore, a novel PHK pathway consisting of phosphoketolase (Xfpk) and phosphotransacetylase (Pta) was introduced to channel more carbon flux towards E4P from F6P derived from glycolysis. Metabolic flux analysis indicated that the availability of E4P and the unbalanced supply of E4P and PEP remain key issues. To further alleviate this limitation, the introduction of an efficient xylose pathway may be a viable option to improve E4P supply. In addition, it may be possible to construct a self-adjusting system or optogenetic regulation to allow the dynamic control of metabolic flux towards glycolysis and PPP.

5.3 The "plane" level: the weakness of cell performance Even for well-studied microorganisms such as *E. coli* and *S. cerevisiae*, it is often not easy to accurately understand and correct the negative effects of metabolic engineering on whole cells. These negative effects may be caused by transcriptional regulation, accumulation of toxic products, and unknown mechanisms. Ric1 is a transcriptional repressor of multiple genes in the aromatic amino acid biosynthetic pathway in S. *cerevisiae*, and inhibition of Ric1 has been shown to increase the yield of shikimic acid, a precursor of simple phenylpropanoids. Although the identified targets can be used to optimize the synthesis levels, most targets for the global optimization of microbial synthesis performance are unknown. Aromatic compounds are generally toxic to microorganisms, which makes their high-level production in microbial hosts challenging. Adaptive laboratory evolution is a powerful tool used in the improvement of microbial cell factories at the entire cell level (the "plane" level), which emphasizes the importance of "collaboration" between scientists 'deliberate choices and microorganisms' initiative to achieve design goals, and compensates for the lack of comprehensive understanding of host strains. Coordination between adaptive laboratory evolution and whole-genome sequencing revealed that Esbp6 is an important transporter for the secretion of *p*-HCA and tolerance to aromatic acids, which can be used to optimize the production of simple phenylpropanoids. Inspired by this, we believe that evaluating the growth rate on a medium with high concentrations of aromatic acids in a genome-scale collection of *S. cerevisiae* gene-deletion strains will uncover novel strategies for improving aromatic acid tolerance.

During microbial fermentation, although the genetic information of all individual cells in a microbial population is identical, their contributions to compound synthesis and single-cell biosynthetic performance may vary greatly (up to a 10-fold difference) owing to nongenetic cell-to-cell variation, which could have a significant impact on group performance. Nongenetic cell-to-cell variations may be due to different epigenetic modifications and variation in the regulation of expression due to differences in developmental history (uneven cell division and different parent cells) or exposure to environmental factors (differences in the concentrations of various substances in the local medium). Understanding the key mechanisms affecting nongenetic variations requires longterm efforts that do not provide reliable short-term engineering strategies. In one study, a minority (15%) of the total cell population produced more than half of thc total free fatty acids, and the majority of cells performed very weakly in the fermentation of a fatty acid-producing *E. coli*. A quality control (PopQC) system was constructed to continuously select and kill low-performing nongenetic strains and maintain high-performing nongenetic variants for production. Since such genetic circuits for screening often rely on specific regulatory elements, biosensors that respond to simple phenylpropanoid concentrations should first be developed. Although this strategy alleviates the problems caused by nongenetic variants to some extent, it may inadvertently kill young cells with synthetic potential. Conversely, regulating cellular processes such as autophagy, apoptosis, and replication can extend the lifespan and the effective time available for product synthesis, thereby increasing the yield. Quorum sensing is a widespread bacterial mechanism for cell-to-cell communication that synchronises gene expression and has been successfully implemented to improve the synthetic performance of 4-hydroxycoumarin, flavonoids, and simple chemicals in bacteria. Although autoinducer-2 has been successfully used as a 'universal signal' for interspecies communication to improve CaA synthesis in *S. cerevisiae*, its mechanism and universality require further exploration. As an important mechanism of intercellular communication, an in-depth study of exosomes is expected to provide opportunities to improve the overall performance of cell factories.

5.4 The "system" level As multicellular organisms, plants often complete the oriented synthesis of natural products through the division of labour and metabolite transport of multiple cells, tissues, organs, and organelles. The synthesis of aromatic acids involves the cooperation of multiple organelles, which is important for ensuring an optimal catalytic environment and avoiding metabolic promiscuity. Although compartmentalisation strategies can significantly improve synthesis efficiency by the modularized expression of heterologous pathways in different organelles, it sometimes comes at the expense of an optimal reaction environment for catalytic enzymes. For example, to avoid side reactions and waste of metabolic flux caused by the catalytic promiscuity of 4Cl, 4Cl can be considered as a node to separate the upstream and downstream pathways for the synthesis of ferulate CoA, a key precursor of many phenylpropanoids. However, both the upstream and downstream pathways need to be expressed in the cytosol to ensure the necessary reaction environment, such as NADPH and SAM cofactors. Therefore, building a stable and mutualistic microbial consortium system that cooperates with plant cells could reasonably confer wider metabolic capabilities and achieve more complex synthesis, which is difficult to achieve in a single cell. In addition, mutualistic consortia also endow microorganisms with higher synthetic titres through unique abilities, such as balancing metabolic flow, relieving metabolic burden, optimising resource utilisation, enriching the cellular environment and cofactors, and adapting to fluctuating environments. Considering these advantages, microbial consortium strategies have been extended to construct bacterial, yeast, and yeast systems for the synthesis of terpenoids, phenylpropanoids, and polyketones, and alkaloids. However, most are simply mixed cultures formed by changing the initial inoculation ratio, which makes it difficult to form a stable community, and this instability is further amplified in largescale fermentation. Efforts to construct a mutualistic relationship for the members of microbial consortia to form stable mutualistic consortia is a viable approach to improve these strategies.

Overall, based on the current gram-scale synthesis of simple phenylpropanoids in microorganisms, the integration of multidisciplinary technologies and tools is expected to further break the bottlenecks and increase production levels. These strategies will provide a framework for the synthesis of complex phenylpropanoids and other types of natural products.

[朱展频，陈瑞兵，张磊，等. Natural Product Reports, 2024, 41: 6-24.]

# Biosynthetic pathway of prescription cucurbitacin Ⅱa and high-level production of key triterpenoid intermediates in engineered yeast and tobacco

## 1 INTRODUCTION

Cucurbitacins, a class of highly diverse and oxygenated triterpenoids primarily found in the Cucurbitaceae family, exhibit specific and potent bioactivities encompassing the treatment of cancer, inflammatory disease, and diabetes. Cucurbitacins are typically classified into 12 categories, cucurbitacins A-T, based on skeleton oxidation groups. The cucurbitacin F (CuF) class, which includes cucurbitacin IIa (CuIIa) and cucurbitacin IIb (CuIIb), is predominantly found in plants of the genus *Hemsleya*. Many of these plants are renowned traditional Chinese medicines with well-established pharmacological properties and therapeutic principles in China. Recently, Culla and Cullb were found to be novel anti-cancer agents; however, the biosynthetic pathway of CuFs is largely unknown.

Currently, cucurbitacin biosynthetic pathways are gradually being revealed in some cucurbitaceous plants. In *Cucurbita pepo*, the formation of 2, 3-oxidosqualene and 2, 3; 22, 23-diepoxysqualene is mediated by three squalene epoxidases (SEs). Cucurbitadienol (Cuol) is the first committed precursor of cucurbitacins synthesized from 2, 3-oxidosqualene by a specialized oxidosqualene cyclase (OSC) termed Cuol synthase (CBS). After initial construction of the triterpenoid skeleton by OSC, subsequent modifications, including oxidation and acylation, are facilitated by cytochrome P450 monooxygenases (CYPs) and BAHD-acetyltransferases (ATs).

In *Crocus sativus*, two CYP genes (CsCYP88L2 and CsCYP81Q58) were shown to be involved in cucurbitacin C (CuC) biosynthesis, catalyzing C19β-hydroxylation and C25 hydroxylation of the Cuol backbone (Shang et al., 2014). In *C. melo* and *C. lanatus*, Cm890 (CmCYP87D20) and Cl890 (ClCYP87D20) were identified as catalysts for C11 carboxylase and C20 hydroxylase, and Cm180 (CmCYP81Q59) and Cl180 (ClCYP81Q59) were found to catalyze C2 hydroxylation (Zhou et al., 2016b). CmACT and ClACT were found to catalyze the acetylation of cucurbitacin B (CuB) and cucurbitacin I from cucurbitacin D (CuD) and cucurbitacin E (CuE) in *C. melo* and *C. lanatus*, respectively (Zhou et al., 2016b). Three new CYP genes from *Momordica charantia* involved in cucurbitacin biosynthesis were recently reported: McCYP81AQ19 is responsible for Cuol C23 hydroxylation, McCYP88L7 catalyzes C19 hydroxylation and is involved in formation of C5 - C19 ether-bridged products, and McCYP88L8 functions as a C7 hydroxylase (Takase et al., 2019b). In *Iberis amara*, a member of the Brassicaceae family, two species-specific CYPs (CYP708A16 and CYP708A15) were identified that catalyze the unique C16 for C16β-hydroxyl and C22 hydroxylation of the Cuol backbone. Despite these advances, the precise pathway of CuF biosynthesis remains to be clarified, particularly with regard to C3α-hydroxyl, C16α-hydroxyl, and C22-carbonyl functionalities.

Cucurbitacins, valued for their diverse biological activities, face challenges in pharmaceutical applications due to low plant content and complex extraction procedures. Although synthetic biology shows potential for production of high-value natural drugs, heterologous biosynthesis of cucurbitacins has been limited to the precursor Cuol. Challenges include unknown enzymes for modification and scarce intermediate compounds for testing of enzyme activity. Heterologous synthesis and metabolic engineering have also emerged as effective strategies, providing ample substrates for validation and enabling high-throughput screening. Therefore, establishing a tobacco system and chassis for high-yield production of cucurbitacin intermediates is crucial for advancing metabolic engineering efforts.

A previous study reported the construction of two engineered yeast strains, EY10 and EGY48-CpCPQ (CBS in *C. pepo*), for production of Cuol (related output not reported). The construction strategy was to reuse the inducible pGAL promoter (GAL1 or GAL10), which has problems such as insufficient promoter strength, interference with galactose metabolism, and increased complexity of the *in vivo* expression system. Recently, strategies involving the use of constitutive promoters for production of triterpenoids have emerged; such strategies can maintain relatively stable transcript levels that are virtually unaffected by intracellular or extracellular stimuli. For instance, the yeast strain CS-021 achieved a promising titer of 63.00 mg/l through integration of the *SgCBS* gene and maintenance of a sufficient squalene precursor supply. Collectively, these findings suggest that metabolic engineering with constitutive promoters holds promise for enhancing cucurbitacin synthesis. For heterologous expression in a plant system, *Agrobacterium-mediated* transient expression in *Nicotiana benthamiana* is an efficient synthetic biological platform for triterpene production. A previous study reported that transient co-expression of CpSE2 and CpCPQ in *N. benthamiana* resulted in Cuol production of 0.02 ng/g dry weight (dw), and such low yields limit cucurbitacin production.

In this study, we functionally characterized key *SEs*, *OSCs*, *CYPs*, and *ATs* from *H. chinensis* (Figure 1). A Cuol-producing yeast chassis (Cuol01-1) was constructed by overexpressing and optimizing pathway genes, producing 133.21 mg/l and a maximum titer of 794.7 mg/l Cuol from glucose in shake flasks and fed-batch fermentation, respectively. A series of chassis cells based on Cuol01 - 1 were constructed by optimizing the oxidation efficiency of C11=O and C20 - OH. Efficient CYP87D20 catalytic elements from other species were screened to increase compatibility and elevate CYP87D20 expression levels. By combining all these engineering strategies, we constructed a yeast cell factory (DNCm87 - 03) that could produce 46.41 mg/L of 11-carbonyl-20β-hydroxy-Cuol and 126.47 mg/L of total cucurbitacin triterpenoids in shake flasks, the highest yields reported to date.

## 2 RESULTS

Culla accumulation in tubers of *H. chinensis* Culla and Cullb are widely distributed in *Hemsleya* plants, particularly in their tubers. We found that contents of Culla and Cullb were significantly higher in *H. chinensis* than in other species (Supplemental Table 1). Triterpenoid compounds, including Culla, Cullb, and oleanolic acid, accumulated specifically in the tubers, followed by the roots, and were

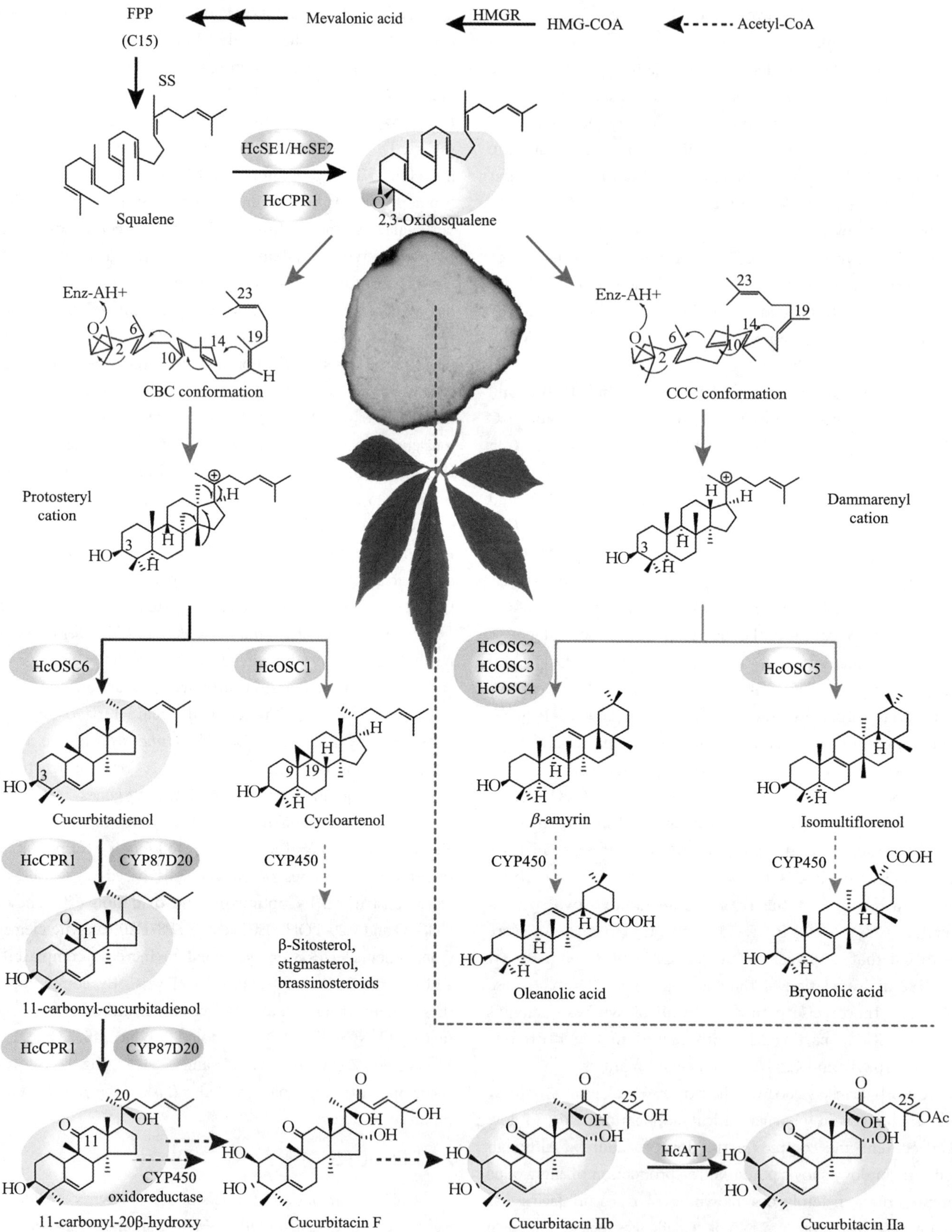


**Figure 1 Proposed biosynthetic pathway of cucurbitacin F in *Hemsleya chinensis***

The blue arrows indicate the proposed cucurbitacin F biosynthetic pathway, and the green arrows indicate proposed phytosterol and pentacyclic triterpene biosynthetic pathways. Dotted arrows indicate one or multiple proposed reactions steps; solid arrows indicate identified reactions. Enzymes identified in this study are in blue, and unidentified enzymes are in red. Enzyme abbreviations: SE, squalene epoxidase; OSC, oxidosqualene cyclase; CYP450, cytochrome P450 monooxygenase; AT, BAHD-acetyltransferase. Other abbreviations: CBC, chair-boat-chair; CCC, chair-chair-chair.

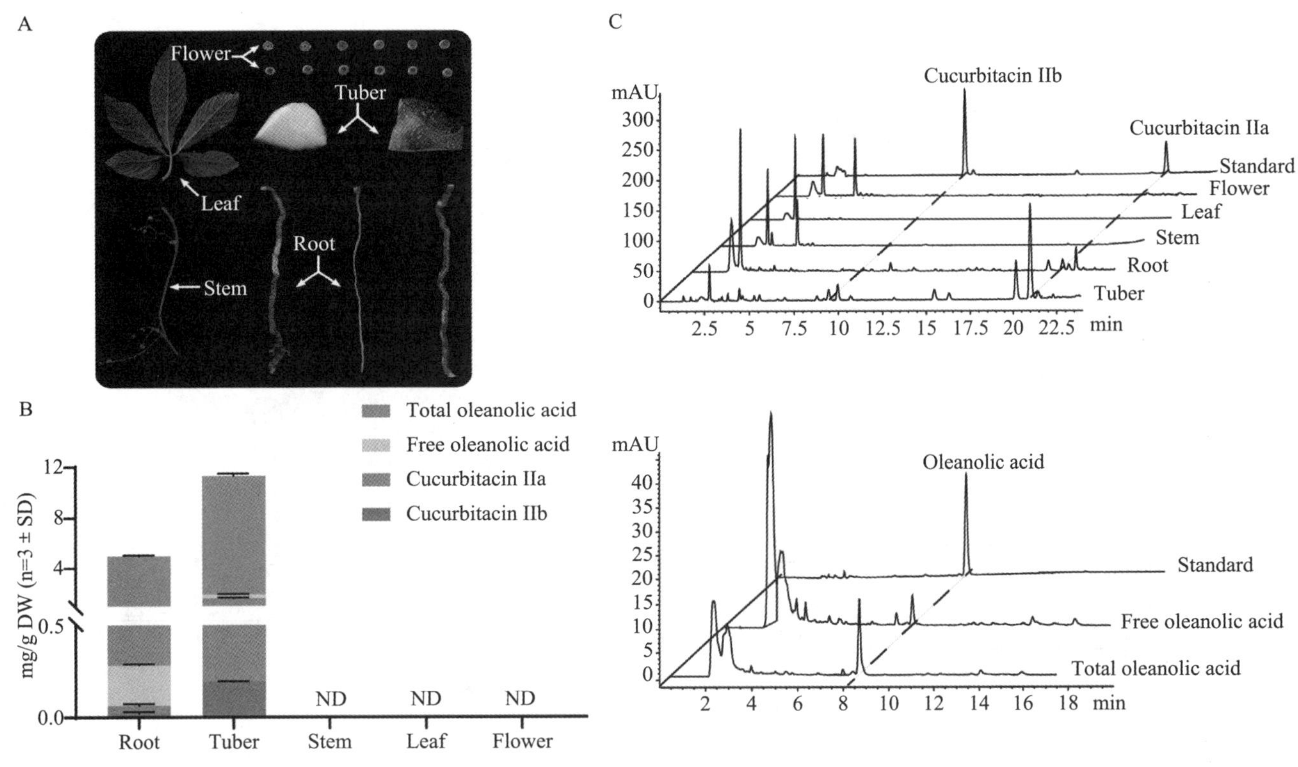


**Figure 2 Content of main triterpenoids in *Hemsleya chinensis***

(A) Images of different tissues of *H. chinensis* and RNA samples for RNA-seq analysis. (B) Quantification of cucurbitacin IIa, cucurbitacin IIb, and oleanolic acid in extracts from different *H. chinensis* tissues. Means of triplicates and standard deviations are shown (mg/g dw, $n=3\pm$SE). ND, not detected. (C) UHPLC analysis of cucurbitacin IIa, cucurbitacin IIb, and oleanolic acid contents in tissues of *H. chinensis*.

barely detectable in aboveground plant parts (Figure 2B – 2D). Biosynthetic pathway genes in plants are often co-regulated and co-expressed in a tissue-specific manner, forming co-expressed functional units that can be characterized by metabolomic and transcriptomic analysis. Several studies have shown that co-expression analysis is one of the most useful methods for screening candidate genes. To identify the genetic components involved in cucurbitacin biosynthesis, we obtained RNA sequencing (RNA-seq) data for multiple *H. chinensis* tissues and measured the distribution of CuIIa accumulation for subsequent identification of candidate genes (Figure 2A).

Functional characterization of *HcSE*, *HcOSC*, and *HcAT* genes A total of 50 061 733 *H. chinensis* RNA-seq reads were obtained and assembled into 52 923 contigs (Supplemental Table 2) (http://medicinalplants.ynau.edu.cn/transcriptomics/213); 32 742 of the contigs were annotated by BLAST searches of the National Center for Biotechnology Information (NCBI) non-redundant, Swiss-Prot, Kyoto Encyclopedia of Genes and Genomes, and Clusters of Orthologous Groups/Eukaryotic Orthologous Groups protein databases.

A BLAST search of the transcriptome data using previously reported sequences of SE, CPR, OSC, and AT proteins revealed three *SE* genes, two *CPR* (NADPH-cytochrome P450 reductase) genes, six *OSC* genes, and two *AT* genes (Supplemental Table 3). We used gene-specific primers (Supplemental Table 11) to clone the corresponding sequences from an *H. chinensis* cDNA library and performed additional bioinformatic and phylogenetic analyses of these candidate genes (Supplemental Figures 1 – 7). A prokaryotic system was used to express their proteins for enzyme activity (Supplemental Figure 8). Three SE candidate genes were ligated into a prokaryotic expression vector for enzyme production, and subsequent detection of the reaction products was performed by gas chromatography-mass spectrometry (GC – MS). The results revealed the emergence of a peak at 16.02 min, which was identified as 2, 3-oxidosqualene on the basis of characteristics exhibited by the primary ion peaks. However, no signal for 2, 3 : 22, 23-diepoxysqualene was detected in any of the experimental groups, indicating that CuF is likely derived directly from 2, 3-oxidosqualene rather than 2, 3 : 22, 23-diepoxysqualene in *H. chinensis* (Figure 3B). We failed to express HcSE3 protein in *Escherichia coli* (BL21 DE3), and no further enzyme activity tests were performed. These results indicate that the functions of the HcSEs differ from those of the CpSEs in *C. pepo*, and functional validation of SEs in other cucurbits have not been reported. 2, 3-oxidosqualene was not detected in the absence of HcCPR1 when squalene was supplemented as a control

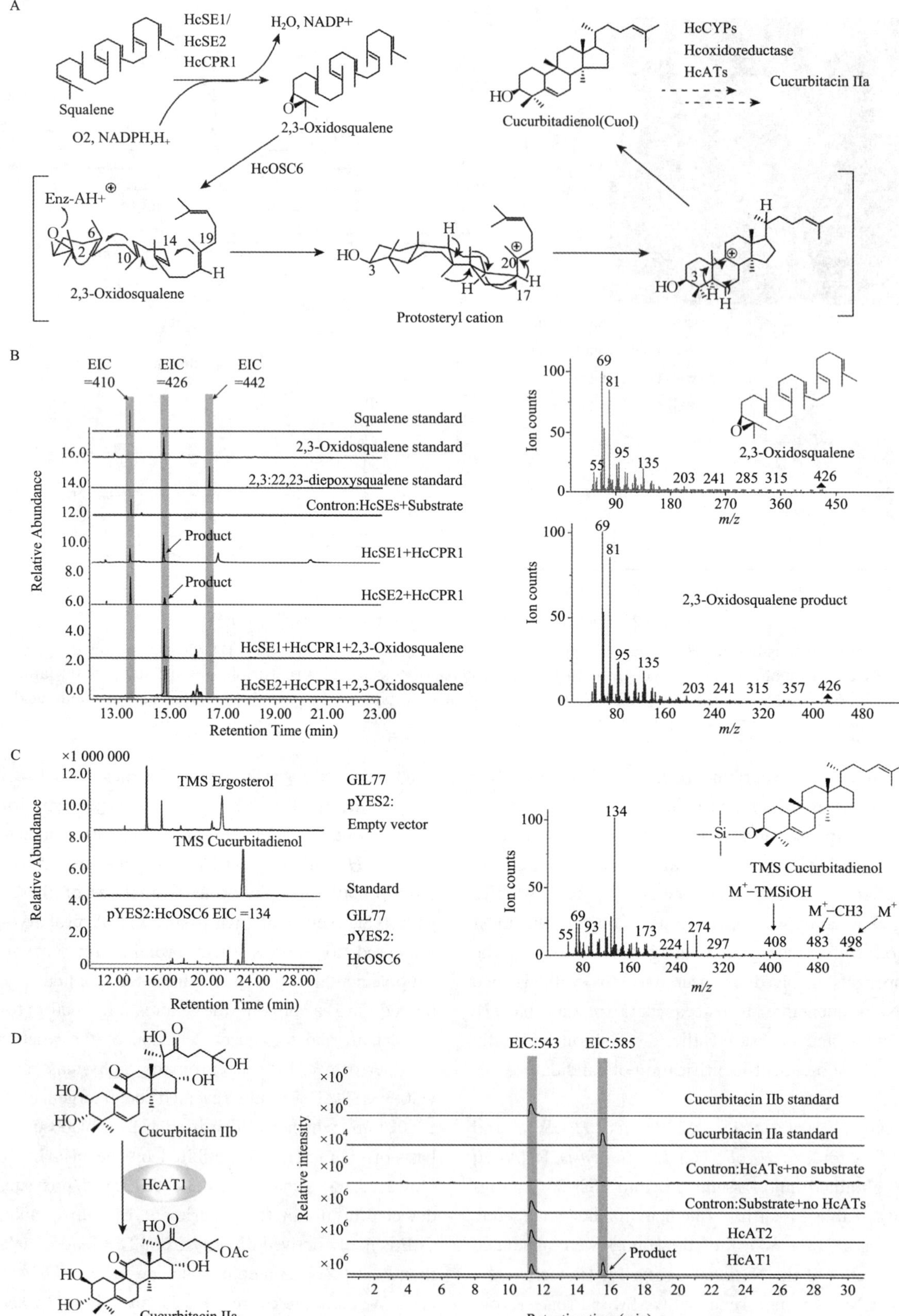


**Figure 3 SDS-PAGE of HcSEs, HcCPR1, and HcATs and enzyme activity of recombinant HcSE, HcCPR1, HcOSC6, and HcATs**

(A) Functional characterization of homologous genes in the biosynthetic pathway of cucurbitacin IIa. (B) GC-MS results of the HcSE1, HcSE2, and HcCPR1 enzymatic reactions and MS results revealed the primary ion peak of the 2, 3-oxidosqualene standard and the enzymatic product. (C) GC-MS analysis of the products in yeast strains containing the HcOSC6 expression plasmids and the empty vector. EIC 134, extracted ion chromatograms of the characteristic fragment ion of cucurbitadienol at a mass/charge ratio ($m/z$) of 134. (D) HcAT1 catalyzes the final step of cucurbitacin IIa synthesis and LC-MS results of the HcAT enzymatic reactions. The sample without HcAT1 protein or substrate served as the negative control.

(Figure 3B), as the epoxidation of squalene necessitates the involvement of an NADPH-dependent cytochrome P450 reductase. A previous study demonstrated that formation of 2, 3-oxidosqualene occurred exclusively when squalene and NADPH were incubated with the recombinant proteins DzSE and DzCPR derived from *Dioscorea zingiberensis*.

Multiple sequence alignments revealed that the deduced amino acid sequences of the six *HcOSCs* showed 42.71%-68.93% similarity (Supplemental Figure 2). All six *HcOSCs* contained the DCTAE motif, which is involved in substrate binding, and four QW motifs characteristic of the OSC superfamily (Supplemental Figure 3). The QW motifs may be involved in stabilizing carbocations during cyclization. *HcOSC2*, *HcOSC3*, and *HcOSC4* had the MWCYCR motif, which is predicted to be a highly conserved motif of β-amyrin synthase. To identify the cyclase that catalyzes the first step in formation of the cucurbitacin skeleton, we subcloned the complete open reading frames (ORFs) of six *HcOSCs* into the pYES2 vector and transformed the resulting constructs into lanosterol synthase-deficient yeast (GIL77). GC analysis revealed that extracts from GIL77 yeast expressing HcOSC1 exhibited a distinct peak at 22.10 min whose retention time and mass spectral characteristics were identical to those of the purified cycloartenol standard (Supplemental Figure 9A). Extracts from yeast harboring HcOSC2, HcOSC3, and HcOSC4 contained β-amyrin. The retention time of their product was consistently 24.80 min, and its mass spectral characteristics matched those of the authentic β-amyrin standard (Supplemental Figure 9B). The GIL77 strain expressing HcOSC5 produced a distinct product with a retention time of 24.20 min whose mass spectral characteristics were identical to those of the purified isomultiflorenol standard (Supplemental Figure 9C). Thin layer chromatography (TLC) showed that GIL77 strains expressing *HcOSC6* and *McCBS* (as a positive control) produced a product with the same $R_f$ value as the purified Cuol standard (Supplemental Figure 10A). This product exhibited a retention time and mass spectral characteristics identical to those of the purified Cuol standard, with an elution peak at 22.60 min in the GC-MS analysis (Figure 3C). The products of HcOSC1, HcOSC5, and HcOSC6 were also subjected to nuclear magnetic resonance (NMR) spectroscopy, and their NMR data were consistent with previous reports (Supplemental Figures 11 - 13 and Supplemental Table 4) (DavidáNes, 1991; Isaev, 1995; Yoshida et al., 1989). The results obtained from analysis of GC-MS and NMR spectra thus provide compelling evidence that HcOSC6 functions as a Cuol synthase.

CuIIb was used as the substrate for *in vitro* enzymatic reactions, and high-performance liquid chromatography (HPLC) revealed that HcAT1 effectively facilitated the acetylation of CuIIb to generate CuIIa (Supplemental Figure 14A). We also examined the enzymatic reaction of HcAT1 using cucurbitacin I as the substrate. The HPLC results demonstrated that HcAT1 also catalyzed acetylation of the C25 hydroxyl group on cucurbitacin I, leading to formation of cucurbitacin E (Supplemental Figure 14B). This finding was confirmed by liquid chromatography-mass spectrometry (LC-MS) using a commercial CuIIa standard. The product peak matched that of the CuIIa standard at 20.02 min, and their characteristic peaks were consistent; CuIIa was not detected in the reaction catalyzed by HcAT2 (Figure 3D). The parent mass of cucurbitacin IIa was determined to be 562.35, and the fragment feature exhibited a mass value of 585.35, indicating sodium adduct formation $[M+Na]^+$ (Supplemental Figure 14C). These results confirmed that HcAT1 catalyzes the final step in the CuIIa pathway.

**Identification of candidate genes involved in skeleton oxidation modification** To identify genes encoding oxidative-modification enzymes in CuIIa biosynthesis, we performed weighted gene co-expression network analysis (WGCNA) and gene co-expression correlation analysis. The transcriptome data from *H. chinensis* were divided into 17 modules based on their expression patterns, and *HcOSC6* and *HcAT1* with confirmed functions were used as bait genes to identify candidate genes. Thirty-six candidate genes were enriched in the terpenoid skeleton biosynthetic pathway (ko00900), sesquiterpene and triterpene biosynthesis pathway (ko00909), and steroid biosynthesis pathway (ko00100) (Supplemental Table 5) and were mainly assigned to the gray60, coral1, brow4, and other modules (Supplemental Figure 15). According to their correlation and connectivity values, the 36 candidate genes were displayed as three gene co-expression networks using Cytoscape software; genes involved in the oleanolic acid, saponin, and steroid pathways were found mainly in co-expression networks 1 and 2 (Figure 4B). One of the *CYP90B1*s was predicted to catalyze the hydroxylation of C22 and C16 on cholesterol. Eleven genes formed a strongly correlated co-expression network, network 3 (Figure 4B), which included the four *CYPs HcCYP87D20*, *HcCYP81Q58*, *HcCYP81Q59*, and *HcCYP87D19*. *HcCYP87D20* was predicted to be a homolog of *CmCYP87D20* and *ClCYP87D20*, which act as a C11 carboxylase and a C20 hydroxylase of Cuol; *HcCYP81Q58* was predicted to be the homolog of *CsCYP81Q58*, which acts as a C25 hydroxylase of Cuol; and *HcCYP81Q59* was predicted to act as a C2 hydroxylase, producing 11-carbonyl-20β-hydroxy-Cuol (Supplemental Table 5). A *CYP87D19* gene was also identified; its homolog *CsCYP87D19* was previously identified as a member of a gene cluster involved in CuC biosynthesis, but its function has not yet been determined. Phylogenetic analysis of the *CYP* sequences revealed that *HcCYP87D19* was located in

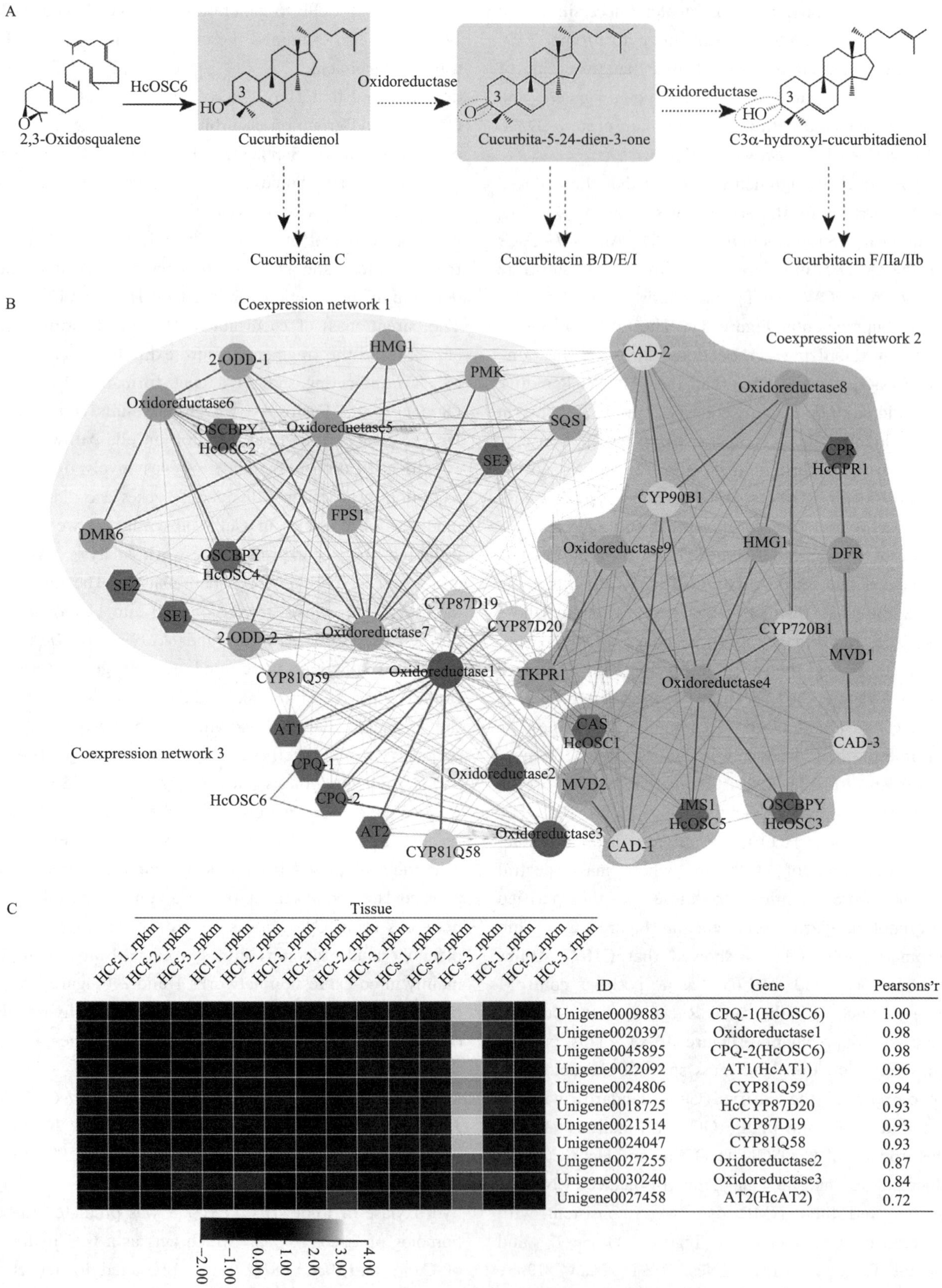

A

2,3-Oxidosqualene
HcOSC6
Cucurbitadienol
Oxidoreductase
Cucurbita-5-24-dien-3-one
Oxidoreductase
C3α-hydroxyl-cucurbitadienol
Cucurbitacin C
Cucurbitacin B/D/E/I
Cucurbitacin F/IIa/IIb

B

Coexpression network 1
Coexpression network 2
Coexpression network 3

C

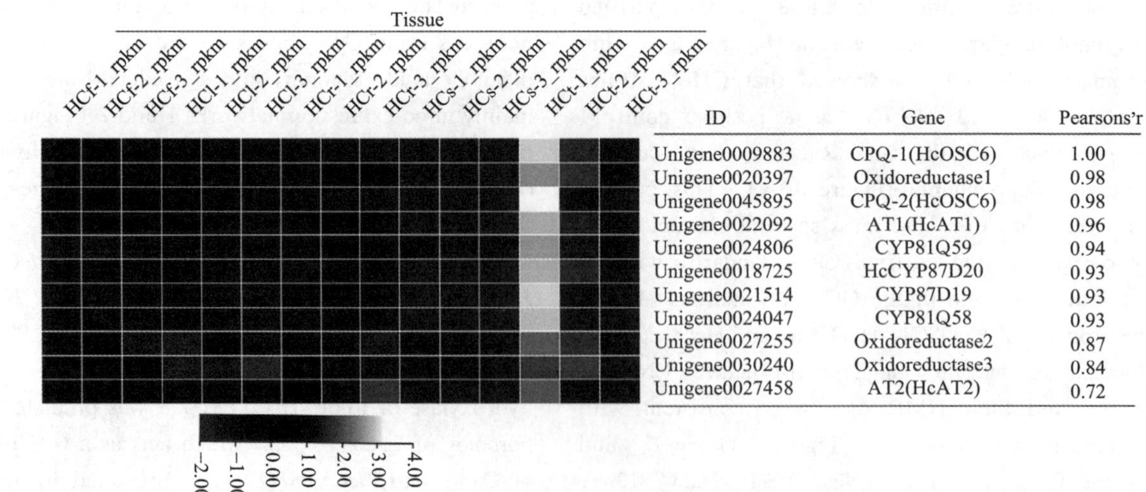


| ID | Gene | Pearsons'r |
|---|---|---|
| Unigene0009883 | CPQ-1(HcOSC6) | 1.00 |
| Unigene0020397 | Oxidoreductase1 | 0.98 |
| Unigene0045895 | CPQ-2(HcOSC6) | 0.98 |
| Unigene0022092 | AT1(HcAT1) | 0.96 |
| Unigene0024806 | CYP81Q59 | 0.94 |
| Unigene0018725 | HcCYP87D20 | 0.93 |
| Unigene0021514 | CYP87D19 | 0.93 |
| Unigene0024047 | CYP81Q58 | 0.93 |
| Unigene0027255 | Oxidoreductase2 | 0.87 |
| Unigene0030240 | Oxidoreductase3 | 0.84 |
| Unigene0027458 | AT2(HcAT2) | 0.72 |

**Figure 4 Identification of candidate genes involved in Culla biosynthesis by WGCNA and co-expression analysis and analysis of tissue expression of *HcSE*, *HcOSC*, and *HcAT* genes**

(A) Cuol undergoes epimerization mediated by an oxidoreductase enzyme to yield cucurbita-5-24-dien-3-one and C3α-hydroxyl cucurbitadienol. (B) Identification of 36 candidate genes involved in triterpene and steroid biosynthesis by WGCNA. (C) Identification of 11 candidate genes involved in Culla biosynthesis by co-expression analysis and Pearson's correlation coefficients of the *Oxidoreductase1* gene and *CYP87D19* with bait genes in the pathway.

a clade that contained *MICYP87D16*, whose encoded enzyme catalyzes the C - $16_{\alpha}$ oxidation of β-amyrin in *Maesa lanceolata* (Supplemental Figure 7) (Moses et al., 2015). *HcCYP87D19* was therefore predicted to be a hydroxylase for $C16_{\beta}$-hydroxylation of Cuol.

Three oxidoreductase family genes were also identified, with *oxidoreductase1* emerging as the central gene (Supplemental Table 6). This gene was predicted to encode zerumbone synthase (ZSD1), an alcohol dehydrogenase responsible for converting 8-hydroxy-a-humulene into zerumbone by reducing hydroxyl groups to carbonyl groups. in *Arabidopsis thaliana*, *At3g29250* (*THAR1*) and *At1g66800* (*THAR2*) encode a pair of promiscuous oxidoreductases; THAR1 was reported to convert the $C3_{\beta}$-hydroxys of thalianol and related compounds into C3 ketones, whereas THAR2 reduced C3-ketones to 3α alcohols. Notably, CuF possesses the distinctive molecular feature of a C3α-hydroxyl, which sets it apart from the C3β-hydroxyl of CuC and the C3-ketone of CuB. On the basis of this observation, we hypothesize that HcOSC6 catalyzes the formation of Cuol from 2, 3-oxidosqualene and that Cuol subsequently undergoes epimerization mediated by an oxidoreductase enzyme to yield cucurbita-5-24-dien-3-one and C3α-hydroxyl-cucurbitadienol (Figure 4A).

To further investigate the co-expression patterns and transcript expression profiles of these 11 genes, we performed hierarchical clustering and Pearson's correlation analysis (Figure 4C). We observed high expression levels of candidate genes involved in cucurbitacin biosynthesis in tubers (Supplemental Figure 16), consistent with the distribution patterns of CuIIa and CuIIb in *H. chinensis* (Figure 2). Pearson's correlation coefficients between the oxidoreductase1 gene and CYP87D19 and bait genes in the pathway were greater than 0.93 (Supplemental Table 6). Overall, our findings suggest that *oxidoreductase1* and *CYP87D19* are highly promising novel candidate genes implicated in oxidative modification of the cucurbitacin skeleton.

Construction of a yeast strain with high Cuol production

We next aimed to construct an engineered yeast platform for high-level Cuol production in order to characterize the functions of candidate genes encoding oxidation-modification enzymes (Figure 5A and 5B). Because 2, 3-oxidosqualene is a key precursor of Cuol, we used previously reported methods to overexpress truncated 3-hydroxy-3-methyl glutaryl coenzyme A reductase (*tHMG1*), farnesyl diphosphate synthase (*ERG20*), squalene synthase (*ERG9*), and 2, 3-oxidosqualene synthase (*ERG1*) genes in the engineered yeast strain EY10. HcOSC6 and HcCPR1 were also characterized and overexpressed to ensure sufficient Cuol production (Supplemental Figure 17A and 17B). We used a different constitutive promoter strategy to integrate seven expression-cassette DNA fragments into the delta DNA site of the yeast BY4742 genome via homologous recombination (Supplemental Figure 17A). Cuol in the engineered yeast was analyzed and identified using TLC and GC-MS (Figure 5C and Supplemental Figure 10B) and quantified using purified Cuol as an external standard. This analysis revealed a yield of 133.21 mg/L Cuol from glucose in shake flasks (Supplemental Table 7). We thus successfully developed an engineered yeast platform (Cuol01 - 1) for production of Cuol, the direct precursor of cucurbitacins (Figure 5E).

To further investigate the yield of our engineered yeast Cuol01 - 1, we performed a batch fermentation culture of Cuol01 - 1 with YPAD medium. When the initial medium was depleted of glucose, we started feeding to dynamically adjust the fermentation to maintain the pH at 5.8. Glucose was continuously fed throughout the fermentation process, ensuring that its content did not exceed 5 g/L (Supplemental Figure 17C) to avoid accumulation of ethanol and high osmotic pressure that would affect the growth of cells. After a 12 - h lag period, the dynamic fermentation entered the logarithmic growth phase until the dry cell weight of the engineered cells reached 81.6 g/L at 120 h. As the chassis cells entered the logarithmic growth phase, ethanol began to accumulate. The DO (dissolved oxygen) value was maintained at 40% by adjusting the speed and aeration to continuously ferment and accumulate products. The resulting yield of Cuol reached 794.7 mg/L at 120 h (Supplemental Figure 17C), the highest yield yet reported. The Cuol products were prepared by separation and purification (Supplemental Figure 17C). The yield of cucurbitacin could be further optimized by modulation of fermentation conditions in future work.

Functional characterization of candidate oxidation-modification genes The ORF sequences of five *CYPs* (*HcCYP87D20*, *HcCYP81Q58*, *HcCYP81Q59*, *HcCYP87D19*, and *HcCYP90B*) and three *oxidoreductases* were cloned and ligated into the expression vector YCplac33-PE (Y33). The transformed plasmid expressed each *CYP* and each *oxidoreductase* in Cuolproducing yeast Cuol01 - 1. An empty Y33 vector was also transformed into Cuol01 - 1 as a negative control (Supplemental Tables 8 - 9).

Initially, the expected trimethylsilylated cucurbitacin was not detected in the yeast extract through GC - MS analysis. In EI - MS fragmentation mode, the parent ion ($M^+$) of trimethylsilylated Cuol in the control group is 498 (426+TMSi); CYPs catalyze the hydroxylation modification of Cuol, resulting in a product with an $M^+$ of 586 (498+16+ TMSi). However, GC-MS analysis of the metabolites resulting from each CYP-catalyzed Cuol did not reveal the presence of a new peak with an $M^+$ value of 586. Similarly, in the control group, Cuol without trimethylsilylation treatment exhibited an $M^+$ value of 426. Oxidoreductase catalyzes the

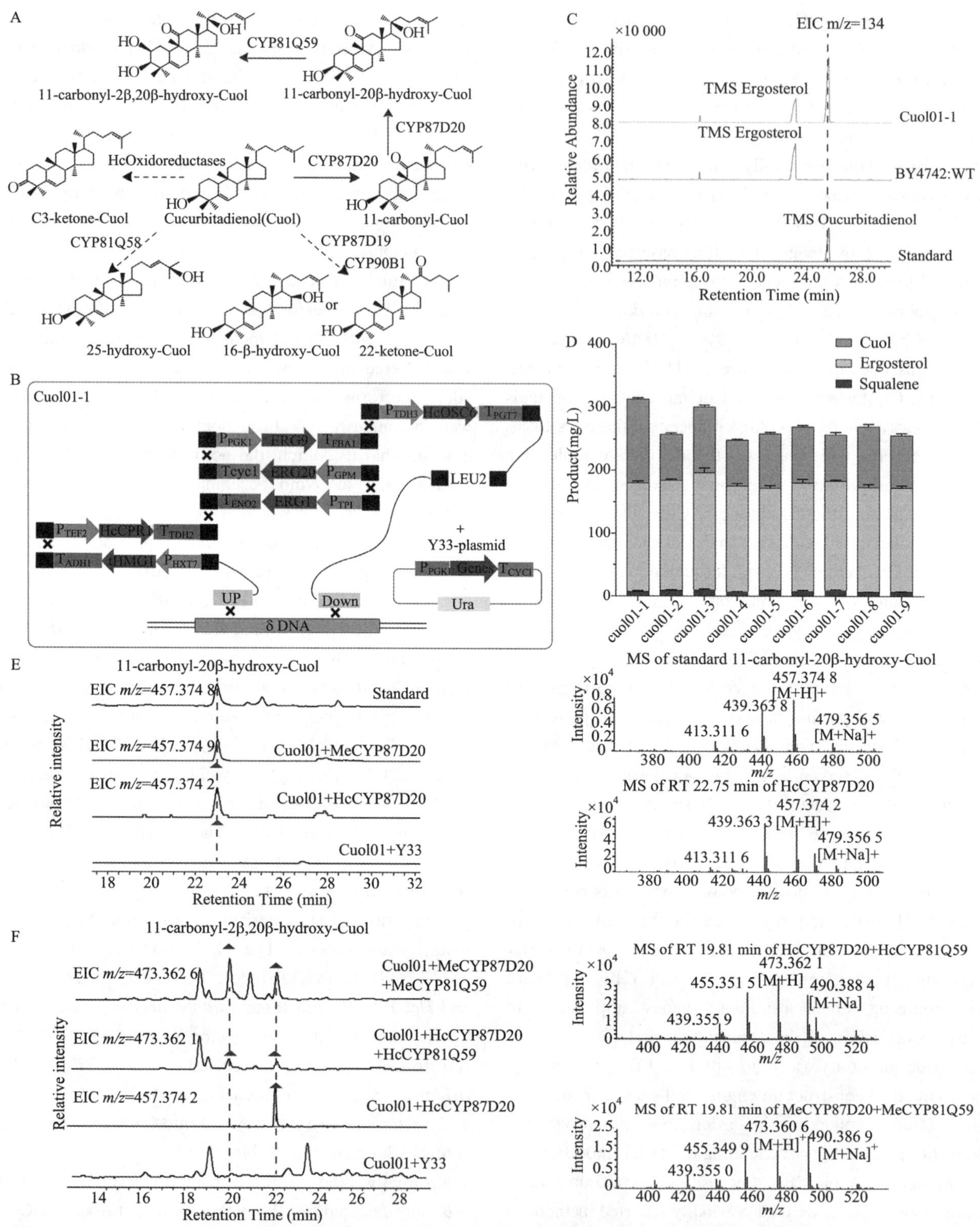

**Figure 5 Construction of an engineered yeast platform with high-level production of Cuol to characterize the functions of candidate oxidation-modification enzyme genes**

(A) Identified oxidative-modification enzyme genes related to Culla biosynthesis. (B) Design of the biosynthetic pathway in the engineered yeast platform (Cuo101 - 1); oxidative-modification enzyme genes were later verified by plasmid sequencing. (C) GC - MS detection of Cuol accumulation in the engineered yeast strain Cuol01 - 1. (D) Cuol production by different strains in shake flasks. (E) LC - MS reveals that HcCYP87D20 and MeCYP87D20 are functional in yeast. Overlaid ion chromatograms of extracts from strains expressing the target genes or the empty vector control (Cuol01 - Y33). Peaks potentially corresponding to saponins are labeled with the $m/z$ value of 11-carbonyl-20β-hydroxy-Cuol ($m/z$ 456). (F) LC - MS reveals that HcCYP81Q59 and MeCYP81Q59 are functional in yeast. Overlaid ion chromatograms of extracts from strains expressing the target genes or the empty vector control (Cuol01 - EV). Peaks potentially corresponding to saponins are labeled with the $m/z$ value of 11-carbonyl-2β, 20β-hydroxy-Cuol ($m/z$ 472). New peaks in the engineered strains are marked by green triangles, and the MS/MS spectra are shown.

C3β-hydroxylation of Cuol to form a C3-ketone, resulting in an $M^+$ value loss of two $H^+$, which corresponds to 424. GC-MS analysis of yeast extract subjected to the oxidoreductase-catalyzed Cuol reaction did not reveal any new peak with an $M^+$ value of 424 either. Furthermore, TLC analysis revealed that, compared with the negative control yeast extract, extracts derived from strain Cuol01 - 1 - PCm87 expressing *CmCYP87D20* and strain Cuol01 - 1 - PHc87 expressing *HcCYP87D20* both displayed two distinct bluish-purple spots; however, no additional blue-purple spots were observed in yeast extracts expressing *HcCYP81Q58*, *HcCYP81Q59*, or any oxidoreductase (Supplemental Figure 10C).

We next identified the two products by comparative TLC and LC - MS analysis using 11-carbonyl-Cuol and 11-carbonyl-20β-hydroxy-Cuol standards provided by Prof. Yi Shang (Figure 5E and Supplemental Figure 10C). After fermenting 10 l of yeast strain Cuol01 - 1 - PHc87, we separated and purified the extracted products to obtain the two target compounds, named 87D20 - 1 and 87D20 - 2. Subsequent NMR analysis revealed that both compounds exhibited two olefin signals in the low-field region, $^{\delta}$H 5.65 ($^{\delta}$C120.8, C-6) and $^{\delta}$H 5.08 ($^{\delta}$C124.3 - 125.1, C-24), and a carbonyl carbon signal, $^{\delta}$C214.7 - 216.5 (C11-carbonyl). The hydrogen atom on carbon-20 of 87D20 - 2 was substituted with a hydroxyl group, resulting in a down-field shift of the carbon-20 signal to 75.0 parts per million (ppm) ($^{\delta}$C 39.35), indicating that 87D20 - 1 corresponded to 11-carbonyl-Cuol and 87D20 - 2 corresponded to 11-carbonyl-20β-hydroxy-Cuol (Supplemental Figures 18 and 19 and Supplemental Table 4). The obtained NMR data were consistent with previous literature reports.

We fermented the Cuol01 - 1 - PHc87 strain in shake flasks and quantitatively analyzed the yeast extract using HPLC. The yields of Cuol, 11-carbonyl-Cuol, and 11-carbonyl-20β-hydroxy-Cuol were 123.56, 4.27, and 1.52 mg/l, respectively (Supplemental Table 7). However, the conversion efficiency of HcCYP87D20 in converting Cuol to 11-carbonyl-Cuol and 11-carbonyl-20β-hydroxy-Cuol was only 4.5% (calculated as [11-carbonyl-Cuol + 11-carbonyl-20β-hydroxy-Cuol]/[Cuol + 11-carbonyl-Cuol + 11-carbonyl-20β-hydroxy-Cuol]). Compared with other candidate oxidation-modification enzymes that lack the ability to catalyze synthesis of novel products from Cuol, HcCYP87D20 exhibits dominant catalytic activity by using Cuol as a substrate to generate downstream products. This finding is reminiscent of our previous study in which co-expression of *Cs890* (*CsCYP87D20*) and *Cs540* (*CsCYP88L2*) in Cuol-producing yeast resulted in detection of both 19-hydroxycucurbitadienol and 11-carbonyl-20-hydroxycucurbitadienol, highlighting the superior catalytic efficiency of CYP87D20 relative to CYP88L2. We therefore speculate that HcCYP87D20 may serve as the initial catalyst for oxidative modification subsequent to skeleton formation, whereas 11-carbonyl-20β-hydroxy-Cuol could potentially function as the primary intermediate in Culla biosynthesis.

We also explored the oxidative modification step after the formation of 11-carbonyl-20β-hydroxy-Cuol. A double-gene recombinant vector carrying *HcCYP87D20* and *HcCYP81Q59* was constructed by Gibson assembly, and a recombinant vector carrying *CmCYP87D20* and *CmCYP81Q59* (C2 hydroxylase) was constructed as a positive control. Transfer of the combined vectors into the Cuol-producing yeast strain Cuol01 - 1 produced the novel yeast strains Cuol01 - 1 - PHc87 + HcQ59 and Cuol01 - 1 - PCm87 + CmQ59 (Supplemental Tables 8 - 9). LC - MS analysis revealed the expected peak (mass/charge [$m/z$] 473.3620 [M+H]$^+$) in the yeast extract of Cuol01 - 1 - PHc87 + HcQ59, and an identical peak was also observed at 19.81 min in the positive control strain Cuol01 - 1 - PCm87 + CmQ59. We analyzed the fragment ion mass spectrum of this peak (positive ion mode, collision voltage 20 V) and found that it was consistent with the reported fragment ion mass spectrum of 11-carbonyl-2β, 20β-dihydroxy-Cuol (Figure 5F). Specifically, the fragment peaks at $m/z$ 455 and 437 are the quasi-molecular ion peaks of the compound, with 1 $H_2O$ and 2 $H_2O$ removed in sequence, and the important fragment ion at $m/z$ 179 produced by cleavage of its side chain with the loss of molecular weight of 126 ($C_8H_{14}O$) revealed additional oxygen on the side chain (Supplemental Figure 20). Unfortunately, despite performing shake flask fermentation and cultivating 20 l of yeast, we were unsuccessful in isolating the target compound owing to its exceptionally low yield. Only milligram-level 11-carbonyl-2β, 20β-dihydroxy-Cuol was obtained by culturing yeast harboring *CmBi* (*CBS* in *C. sativus*), *CPR*, *Cm890* (*CmCYP87D20*), and *Cm180* (*CmCYP81Q59*) in large-scale shake flasks in a previous study. These previous results led us to speculate that 11-carbonyl-20β-hydroxy-Cuol may not serve as a substrate for CYP81Q59, and further investigations of the mechanisms and genes underlying oxidative modification are warranted.

**High-level production of 11-carbonyl-20β-hydroxy-Cuol in engineered yeast** Currently, one of the more effective strategies for enhancing the expression level of *CYPs* involves optimizing the ratio of CYP oxidase and reductase, improving electron transport chain efficiency, and enhancing electron transfer efficiency. To optimize the expression of *CYP87D20* in yeast for increased cucurbitacin production (Figure 6A), we synthesized six codon-optimized CPR genes, including two from *H. chinensis* (*HcCPR1* and *HcCPR2*), one from *A. thaliana* (*ATR2*), one from *C. sativus* (*CsCPR1*), one from *Vitis vinifera* (*VvCPR1*), and one from *Panax ginseng* (*PgCPR1*) (Supplemental Figure

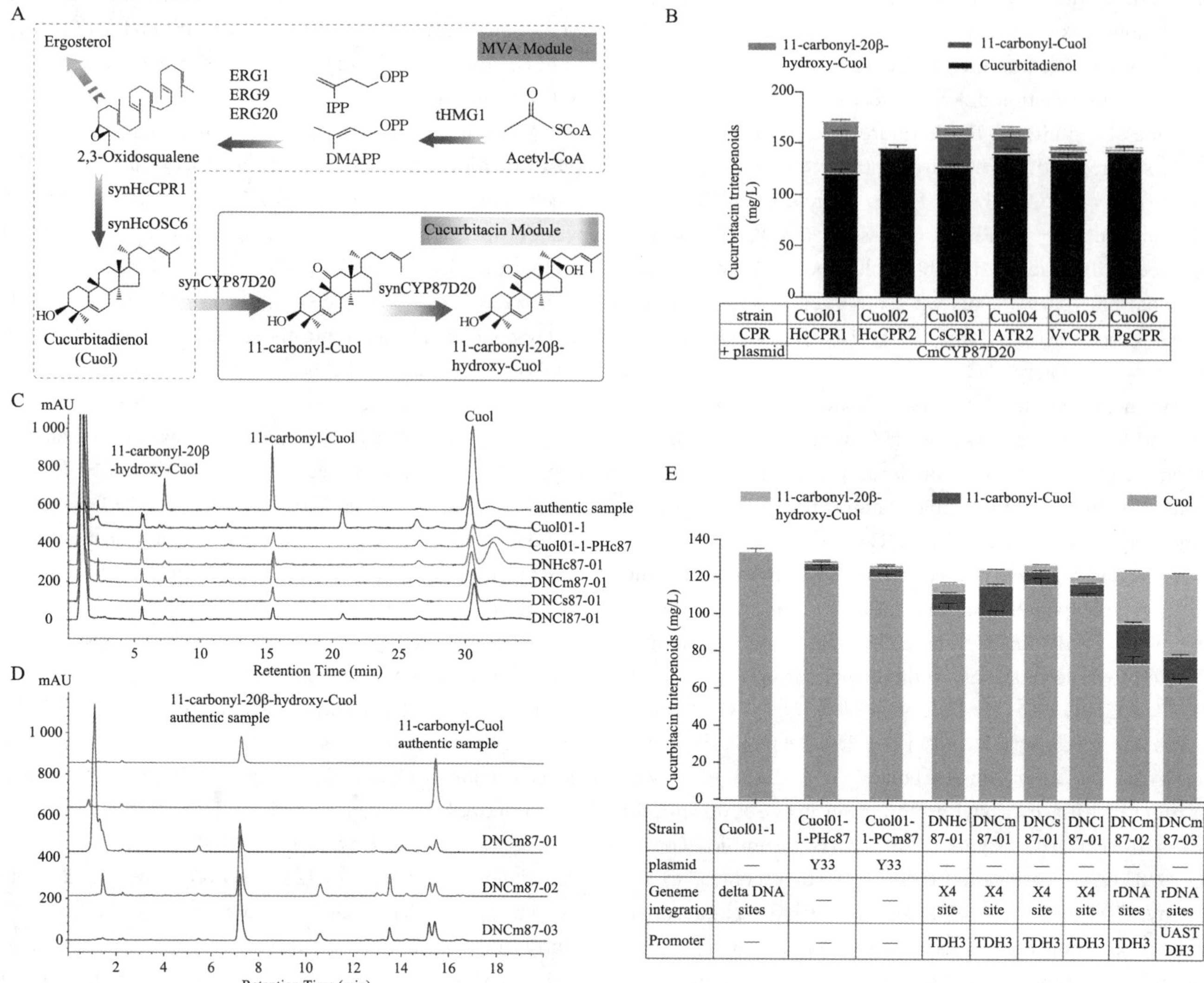


**Figure 6 Construction of a platform for production of 11-carbonyl-20β-hydroxy-Cuol in engineered yeast**

(A) Design of the biosynthetic pathway for production of 11-carbonyl-20β-hydroxy-Cuol in engineered yeast. (B) Quantification of triterpenoids in engineered strains harboring various CPRs. (C) HPLC analysis of cucurbitadienol (Cuol), 11-carbonyl-Cuol, and 11-carbonyl-20β-hydroxy-Cuol produced by Cuol01-1, Cuol01-1-PHc87, DNHc87-01, DNCm87-01, DNCs87-01, and DNCl87-01. (D) HPLC analysis of cucurbitadienol (Cuol), 11-carbonyl-Cuol, and 11-carbonyl-20β-hydroxy-Cuol produced by DNCm87-01, DNCm87-02, and DNCm87-03. (E) Quantification of Cuol, 11-carbonyl-Cuol, and 11-carbonyl-20β-hydroxy-Cuol produced by different strains. The error bars indicate the SEM of three biological replicates.

18A). We selected HcCPR1 (87.72%) and HcCPR2 (45.55%) on the basis of comparison with previously reported CsCPR homologs. To assess coupling efficiency between different *CPRs* and *CYPs*, we used a similar construction method in the engineered yeast strain Cuo01; specifically, candidate *CPRs* were used to replace the *HcCPR1* gene element in Cuo01, resulting in different engineered strains named Cuol02 (*HcCPR2*), Cuol03 (*CsCPR1*), Cuol04 (*ATR1*), Cuol05 (*VvCPR1*), and Cuol06 (*PgCPR1*). All engineered strains produced Cuol with yields that did not differ significantly from that of Cuol01 (*HcCPR1*).

Under the control of the PTDH3 promoter, *CmCYP87D20* was inserted into the single-copy X4 site of the engineered strains constructed above. The coupling efficiency was evaluated by monitoring the process of 11-carbonyl-Cuol and 11-carbonyl-20β-hydroxy-Cuol production. HPLC analysis showed that the engineered strain containing Cuol01 (*HcCPR1*) produced the highest titer of total triterpenes. No fermentation products were detected in the engineered yeast containing *HcCPR2*, but the other five CPRs were able to transfer electrons to the CYP. The relative amounts of fermentation products produced by engineered yeast with different CPRs were ranked *HcCPR1* > *CsCPR1* > *ATR2* > *VvCPR1* > *PgCPR1* > *HcCPR2* (Figure 6B). These results indicated that CPRs had varying degrees of influence on the catalytic activity of CYP87D20, which in turn affected the

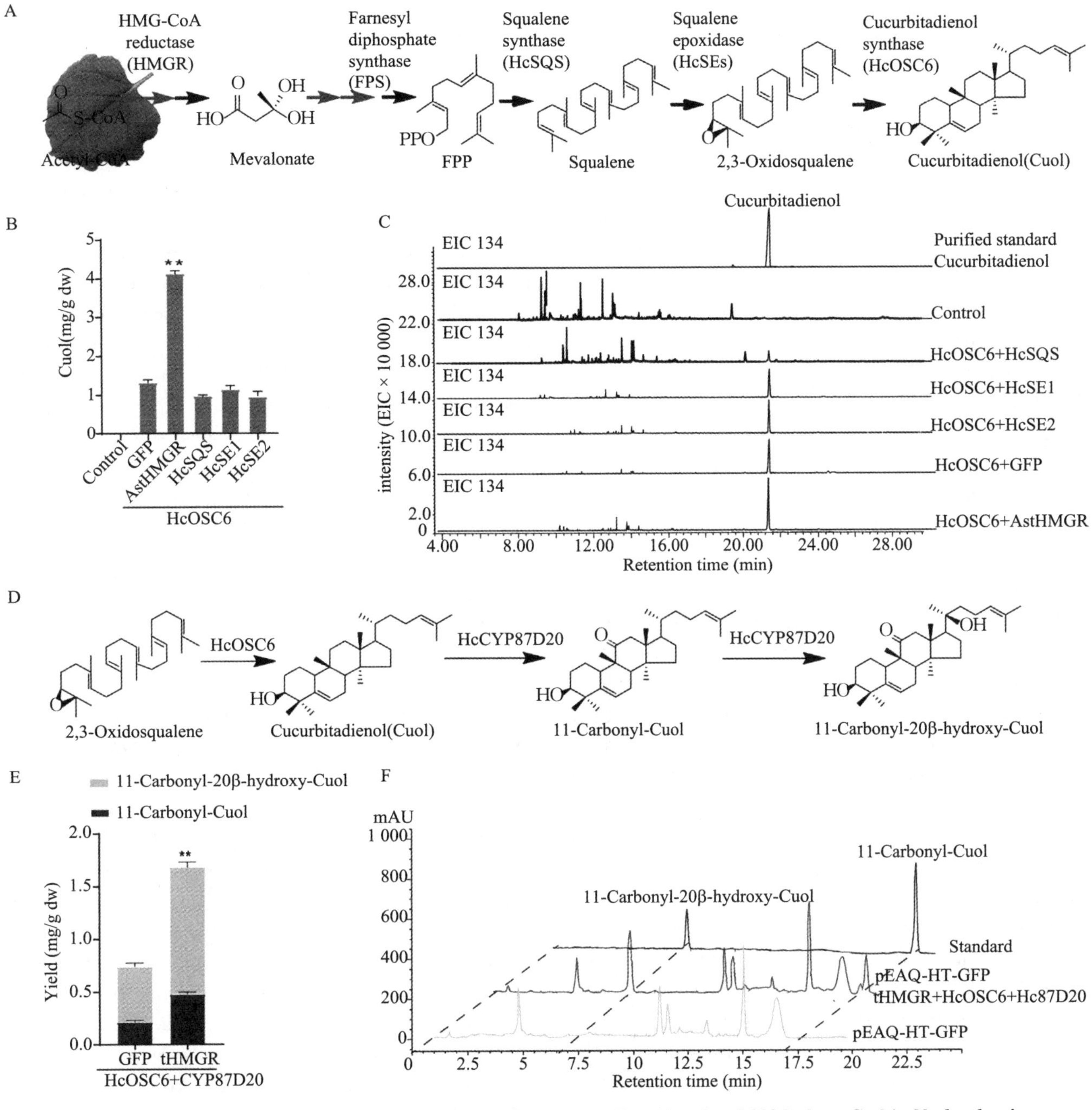


**Figure 7 Co-expression with AstHMGR enhances levels of the intermediate 11-carbonyl-20β-hydroxy-Cuol in *N. benthamiana***

(A) Biosynthesis of the triterpene cucurbitadienol (Cuol) occurs via the mevalonate pathway. (B) Cuol content of tobacco leaves co-expressing *HcOSC6* with *AstHMGR* (mean of three biological replicates±SE; control, empty vector [EV] or pEAQ-HT-DEST with *GFP* gene). * $P < 0.05$. (C) Total extracted ion chromatograms (EICs) of extracts from leaves expressing *HcOSC6* with *AstHMGR*. EIC 134, extracted ion chromatograms of the characteristic fragment ion of cucurbitadienol at a mass/charge ratio ($m/z$) of 134. (D) Oxygenation of the Cuol scaffold by HcCYP87D20 to produce 11-carbonyl-Cuol and 11-carbonyl-20β-hydroxy-Cuol. (E) 11-Carbonyl-Cuol and 11-carbonyl-20β-hydroxy-Cuol contents of leaves expressing *HcOSC6* and *HcCYP87D20* with *GFP* or *tHMGR* (mean of three biological replicates ± SE). * $P < 0.05$. (F) HPLC analysis of 11-carbonyl-Cuol and 11-carbonyl-20β-hydroxy-Cuol in tobacco leaf extract.

production of cucurbitacin triterpenes.

To enhance the yield of 11-carbonyl-Cuol and 11-carbonyl-20β-hydroxy-Cuol, we screened alternative CYP87D20 enzymes from four species to identify an efficient biosynthetic pathway for 11-carbonyl-20β-hydroxy-Cuol. Among the screened enzymes, only *Cs890*, *Cm890*, *Cl890A*, and *Cl890B* were found to participate in this catalytic reaction. Their amino acid sequences showed 83.01%-84.21% homology (Supplemental Figure 21C and Supplemental Table 3), which greatly limited the development of the current optimization strategy. To assess the biosynthetic efficiency of different CYP87D20s under the control of the strong structural promoter $P_{TDH3}$, four

CYP87D20 genes were synthesized by codon optimization (*synHcCYP87D20*, *synCmCYP87D20*, *synCsCYP87D20*, and *synClCYP87D20*) and introduced into the single-copy X4 site of Cuol01 - 1 (Figure 6E). The 11-carbonyl-Cuol and 11-carbonyl-20β-hydroxy-Cuol yields of the four resulting strains (DNHc87 - 01, DNCm87 - 01, DNCs87 - 01, and DNCl87 - 01) were higher than those of the plasmid-expressing strain Cuol01 - 1 - PHc87. The 11-carbonyl-Cuol and 11-carbonyl-20β-hydroxy-Cuol yields were 1.9- and 1.5-fold higher in DNCm87 - 01 than in the control strain DNHc87 - 01. We therefore speculated that the homolog CmCYP87D20 from *C. melo* has the highest catalysis activity for 11-carbonyl-20β-hydroxy-Cuol production (Figure 6C - 6E and Supplemental Table 7); even so, a large amount of Cuol (99.42 mg/l) still accumulated in DNCm87 - 01, indicating that only a small amount of Cuol was converted into 11-carbonyl-Cuol and 11-carbonyl-20β-hydroxy-Cuol. The oxidation conversion rate was only 20.2%, and the yield of the intermediate 11-carbonyl-Cuol was doubled compared with 11-carbonyl-20β-hydroxy-Cuol (Figure 6E and Supplemental Table 7).

We attempted to increase *CmCYP87D20* expression by introducing multiple copies of *CmCYP87D20* into the rDNA sites to obtain the strain DNCm87 - 02, which has hundreds of copies in the yeast chromosome (Supplemental Figure 21C). The 11-carbonyl-Cuol and 11-carbonyl-20β-hydroxy-Cuol yields of DNCm87 - 02 were increased to 21.7 and 28.45 mg/l, respectively, and the yield of 11-carbonyl-20β-hydroxy-Cuol was greater than that of 11-carbonyl-Cuol (Figure 6E and Supplemental Table 7). The strong artificial promoter $UAS_{TEF1}$ - $UAS_{CIT1}$ - $UAS_{CLB2}$ - $P_{TDH3}$ (hereafter referred to as *UAS - TDH3*) replaced the $P_{TDH3}$ promoter in the strain DNCm87 - 03 (Supplemental Figure 21C). As a result, production of 11-carbonyl-20β-hydroxy-Cuol increased to 46.41 mg/L, and production of 11-carbonyl-Cuol decreased to 15.85 mg/L (Figure 6E and Supplemental Table 7). The production of 11-carbonyl-20β-hydroxy-Cuol was three-fold higher than that of 11-carbonyl-Cuol. Cuol content was reduced to 64.21 mg/L, and the conversion rate of the oxidation product rose to 49.23%. Overall, production of 11-carbonyl-20β-hydroxy-Cuol was increased five-fold by increasing the expression level of *CmCYP87D20* in the Cuol chassis Cuol01-1 (Supplemental Figure 10E). These results suggest that increasing the expression of selected CYP genes can enhance the efficient conversion of Cuol into 11-carbonyl-20β-hydroxy-Cuol. The 11-carbonyl-20β-hydroxy-Cuol-accumulating strain DNCm87 - 03 can be used as a platform to further explore the functions of candidate enzymes and as a cell factory for production of cucurbitacin intermediates.

Reconstitution of 11-carbonyl-20β-hydroxy-Cuol biosynthesis in *N. benthamiana* leaves Plants offer several advantages as heterologous hosts for metabolic engineering, including their safety, cost-effectiveness, and potential for unlimited production of therapeutics in a rapid and flexible manner. Compared with yeast systems, plant systems may serve as better hosts for terpenoid production. To enhance the efficiency of leaf infiltration, we used a modified *Agrobacterium* infiltration process based on a previous report. In brief, *A. tumefaciens* strains containing each gene construct were cultured individually and mixed in equal volumes prior to co-infiltration into *N. benthamiana* leaves; six to eight plant leaves were vacuum infiltrated simultaneously to combine expressed genes. To establish a high-efficiency *Agrobacterium-mediated* transient expression system in tobacco leaves, the expression efficiency of *GFP* in different *Agrobacterium* strains was screened by $OD_{600}$ values and vacuum osmotic pressure. Three *Agrobacterium* strains (GV3101, EHA105, and LBA4404) carrying the *35Spro*: *GFP* gene vector were infiltrated into tobacco, and GFP expression reached the highest level at 4 days after infiltration. Under conditions of $OD_{600}$ = 0.8 and a vacuum pressure of 80 kPa, EHA105 exhibited the highest GFP fluorescence signal in transformed tobacco (Supplemental Figure 22A - 22D). EHA105 was therefore considered to be the optimal strain for construction of a transient expression system, consistent with previous findings.

Because precursor availability might be limited, we co-expressed *HcOSC6* with different upstream mevalonate pathway genes to determine their effects on Cuol production. GC - MS analysis of the *N. benthamiana* leaf extract revealed a single peak at 20.02 min that exhibited a mass fragment pattern and retention time consistent with the purified Cuol standard (Figure 7C). The product was quantified using Cuol as the external standard (Supplemental Table 10). The results demonstrated that expression of squalene synthase (*HcSQS*) and *HcSE* genes had little impact on Cuol content, whereas the AstHMG-CoA reductase (*tHMGR*) gene produced a significant, three-fold increase in Cuol yield (Figure 7B). The total Cuol content was 1.32 mg/g (dw) when *HcOSC6* was expressed ($35S_{pro}$: *HcOSC6* + $35S_{pro}$: *GFP*) and 4.18 mg/g (dw) when *HcOSC6* and *AstHMGR1* were co-infiltrated ($35S_{pro}$: *HcOSC6* + $35S_{pro}$: *AstHMGR*). Co-expression of *AstHMGR* can thus significantly increase triterpene production in a transient plant expression system (Figure 7B).

We also transiently co-expressed *HcCYP87D20* in combination with *HcOSC6* and *GFP* in tobacco (*35Spro*: *HcCYP87D20* + *35Spro*: *HcOSC6* + *35Spro*: *GFP*), and *HcCYP87D20* converted Cuol into the expected products, 0.32 mg/g of 11-carbonyl-Cuol and 0.58 mg/g of 11-carbonyl-20β-hydroxy-Cuol (Figure 7E). LC - MS analysis of co-infiltrated tobacco leaf extract revealed an ion peak with $m/z$ 457.3746 $[M+H]^+$ that showed the same retention time (6.75 min) as the 11-carbonyl-20β-hydroxyl-Cuol standard. No product was found in extract of tobacco infiltrated with the blank control pEAQ-HT-DEST1-GFP (Figure 7F). Transient expression of *HcCYP87D20*, *HcOSC6*, and *AstHMGR* (*35Spro*: *HcCYP87D20* + *35Spro*: *HcOSC6* + *35Spro*: *AstHMGR*) in tobacco yielded 0.63 mg/g of 11-carbonyl-Cuol and 1.28 mg/g of 11-carbonyl-20β-hydroxy-Cuol. Yields of both 11-carbonyl-Cuol and 11-carbonyl-20β-hydroxy-Cuol were thus increased two-fold when *AstHMGR was included* in the plant transient expression system (Figure 7E). 11-carbonyl-20β-hydroxy-Cuol may be easier to obtain in tobacco leaves than in the engineered yeast strain DNcm87 - 03. We also tried to transiently co-express *AstHMGR*, *HcOSC6*, *HcCYP87D20*, and *HcCYP81Q59* in tobacco and obtained a specific peak with fragment ions of *m/z* 473.362 5, *m/z* 455.349 8, and *m/z* 437.362 5, indicating the products of quasimolecular ion peaks that removed 1 $H_2O$ and 2 $H_2O$, similar to the reported 11-carbonyl-2β, 20β-dihydroxy-Cuol fragment mass spectra (Supplemental Figure 22E).

## 3 DISCUSSION

Cucurbitacins have been used extensively in recent decades owing to their diverse biological activities, with CuIIa and CuIIb being utilized as prescriptions. Identifying the enzymes involved in plant cucurbitacin metabolism would potentially enable the synthesis of cucurbitacins through a synthetic approach.

Here, through analysis of the *H. chinensis* transcriptome, we identified and functionally characterized two *SEs* (*HcSE1* and *HcSE2*), *HcOSC6*, *HcCYP87D20*, *HcCPR1*, and *HcAT1* involved in 11-carbonyl-20β-hydroxy-Cuol and CuIIa biosynthesis. WGCNA and co-expression cluster analysis were performed to identify additional genes potentially involved in CuIIa biosynthesis. *HcOSC6*, *HcCYP87D20*, *HcCYP81Q58*, *HcCYP81Q59*, *HcCYP87D19*, *HcOxidoreductase1*, and *HcAT1* emerged as the most significant candidate genes. It is presumed that *HcCYP87D19* catalyzes formation of the C16β-hydroxyl of Cuol and that HcOxidoreductase1 potentially converts the C3β-hydroxy of Cuol into C3 ketones, leading to formation of cucurbita-5-24-dien-3-one.

Functional characterization of six HcOSCs in a lanosterol-synthase-deficient yeast strain revealed their distinct substrate specificity. HcOSC2/3/4 exhibited monofunctional activity, catalyzing the cyclization of 2, 3-oxidosqualene to β-amyrin, which suggested their involvement in formation of the oleanolic acid skeleton. Surprisingly, HcOSC5 was identified as an isomultiflorenol synthase, converting 2, 3-oxidosqualene to isomultiflorenol, an intermediate in pentacyclic triterpene biosynthesis that is subsequently converted into bryonolic acid. Previous studies have demonstrated accumulation of bryosic acid in roots and cultured cells of diverse Cucurbitaceae species. Although bryonolic acid has not previously been reported in the *Hemsleya* genus, this study reports for the first time that HcOSC5 (isomultiflorenol synthase) functions as an OSC controlling the biosynthesis of the bryonolic acid skeleton in *H. chinensis*. This finding will contribute to future research on the biosynthetic pathways of bryonolic acid. Furthermore, our study highlights the essential role of multiple OSCs in generating triterpenoid diversity within the *Hemsleya* genus.

To identify the oxidative-modification enzymes involved in CuIIa biosynthesis, we focused specifically on CYPs and oxidoreductases, which have previously been documented to catalyze redox reactions of the triterpene skeleton. We functionally characterized the CYP and oxidoreductase candidate genes by expressing them in the Cuol-producing engineered yeast Cuol01-1. Expression of *HcCYP81Q58*, *HcCYP87D19*, and *HcOxidoreductase1 - 3* did not yield any new products, indicating that these enzymes were not suitable for catalyzing formation of Cuol. However, HcCYP87D20 and CmCYP87D20 were capable of continuously catalyzing production of 11-carbonyl-Cuol and 11-carbonyl-20β-hydroxy Cuol from Cuol, consistent with the observed catalytic functions of CsCYP87D20, CmCYP87D20, and ClCYP87D20. The catalysis of C-2 hydroxylation in 11-carbonyl-20β-hydroxy-Cuol to generate 11-carbonyl-2β, 20β-dihydroxy-Cuol resulted in an extremely low yield, suggesting that 11-carbonyl-20β-hydroxy-Cuol may not be a substrate for HcCYP81Q59. Consequently, it is plausible to consider HcCYP87D20 the initial enzyme involved in the oxidative modification of Cuol. Further investigations are necessary to explore different combinations of *CYP* and *Oxidoreductase* expression to identify the functional gene and its significance. Furthermore, a high-quality *H. chinensis* genome is necessary for mining candidate genes by gene cluster analysis.

The limited presence of cucurbitacins in Cucurbitaceae plants has hindered the exploration of their pharmaceutical activities and applications. There have also been few reports on the isolation of cucurbitacin intermediates, which exacerbates the challenge of speculating on the cucurbitacin pathway and screening enzyme gene activity. The present study presents a modular metabolic engineering approach in *Saccharomyces cerevisiae* that ensures sufficient precursor supply for the production of three cucurbitacin intermediate compounds. Under shake-flask conditions without process optimization, the chassis strain Cuol01 - 1 achieved a Cuol production of 133.21 mg/L. By optimizing fed-batch fermentation conditions, the dry cell weight of engineered cells reached 81.6 g/l, and the yield of Cuol approached gramscale levels at 794.7 mg/L. In addition, through optimization of *CYP* expression levels, high yields of *de novo*-synthesized 11-carbonyl-20β-hydroxy-Cuol (46.41 mg/l) and 11-carbonyl-Cuol (15.85 mg/L) were also obtained from glucose in shake flasks.

Nonetheless, the precursor concentration of Cuol in engineered yeast DNCm87 - 03 remained at 64.21 mg/L, perhaps because of the metabolic burden resulting from overexpression of multiple genes or the inhibitory effects of triterpenoids on cell growth. The strategy used here for construction of engineered yeast involved the use of various constitutive promoters, irrespective of their inducibility or repressibility, ensuring stable expression levels. This approach has been successfully implemented for production of numerous high-value compounds, including artemisinic acid, ginsenosides, breviscapine, and medicinal tropane alkaloids in yeast. High expression of recombinant *CYPs* in the host microorganism is essential for efficient, high-yield biosynthesis of natural products. To achieve high yield through enhanced expression and activity of *CYPs* in the future, we will explore additional metabolic strategies, including N-terminal modification, co-expression of chaperones, supplementation with prosthetic groups, and engineering of the endoplasmic reticulum. Recently, two multidrug and T-oxygen complex extrusion (MATE) proteins involved in the transport of cucurbitacin have been reported in plants. These proteins facilitate the directional extracellular transport of cucurbitacin, providing an alternative approach to enhancing yield by alleviating the effect of cucurbitacin on cell growth or toxicity, as well as simplifying the process of cucurbitacin purification from the medium.

In the tobacco transient expression system, we observed that co-expression with AstHMGR was sufficient to significantly enhance the synthesis of cucurbitacin intermediates. Co-expression of *AstHMGR1* and *HcOSC6* resulted in production of 4.18 mg/g (dw) of Cuol, which was 3.16-fold higher than that achieved by expressing *HcOSC6*, consistent with previous findings. Similarly, co-expression of *HcOSC6* and *HcCYP87D20* with *AstHMGR* resulted in a two-fold increase in production of 11-carbonyl-20β-hydroxy-Cuol compared with that observed in the absence of *AstHMGR*. Whereas the engineered yeast DNCm87 - 03 accumulated a substantial amount of the cucurbitacin intermediate 11-carbonyl-Cuol, conversion of the substrate Cuol to 11-carbonyl-20β-hydroxy-Cuol was enhanced in *N. benthamiana*, as plant-derived genes exhibit higher expression efficiency in tobacco than in microorganisms. This is attributed to the ability of tobacco plants to support accurate mRNA and protein processing, precise protein localization, and metabolic compartmentalization, as well as the fact that they possess a rich pool of essential metabolic precursors and co-enzymes.

Cucurbitacins are triterpenes that undergo extensive oxidative modifications, indicating their derivation from a complex and intricate biosynthetic pathway. Consequently, it is imperative to perform exhaustive screening of numerous genes encoding oxidative-modification enzymes in order to unravel the precise steps involved in the complete cucurbitacin pathway. Combinatorial expression of biosynthetic enzyme-encoding genes in *N. benthamiana* provides a robust platform for characterizing gene functions. For instance, this approach facilitated characterization of the biosynthetic pathway responsible for the distinctive 5, 6-spiroketal moiety in diosgenin through simultaneous expression of 29 full-length *Paris polyphylla* CYPs and 33 full-length *Trigonella foenumgraecum* CYPs. We reasoned that this approach would significantly enhance progress toward elucidating the complete cucurbitacin pathway and enable subsequent identification of specific *CYPs* and *oxidoreductases*. Co-expression of identified genes encoding pathway enzymes together with unknown *CYPs* and *oxidoreductases* in *N. benthamiana* can generate a plethora of cucurbitacin intermediates and monomers, thereby facilitating pathway analysis and heterologous synthesis of cucurbitacin.

## 4 MATERIALS AND METHODS

Plant materials and transcriptome sequencing  Mature (6-year-old) *H. chinensis* plant tissues were collected from Kunming City in Yunnan Province, China. Roots, tubers, stems, leaves, and flowers were harvested from three individuals, frozen with liquid nitrogen, and sent to Gene Denovo Biotechnology (Guangzhou, China) for library construction. Other *Hemsleya* plants were also used for analysis of Culla and Cullb content (Supplemental Table 1). Plant materials were identified by researcher Yunheng Ji (Kunming Institute of Botany), and the plant specimens are preserved in the herbarium of Kunming Institute of Botany, Chinese Academy of Sciences. Total RNA was extracted from 15 tissues of *H. chinensis* using the HiPure HP Plant Total RNA Kit (Magen, China). The isolated RNA was used for cDNA synthesis according to the manufacturer's instructions. The PrimeScript II 1st Strand cDNA Synthesis Kit (TaKaRa, Japan) was used for qPCR experiments, and the HiScript II 1st Strand cDNA Synthesis Kit (Vazyme Biotech) was used for gene cloning experiments. Sequencing was performed on an Illumina HiSeq 4000 platform by Gene Denovo Biotechnology. After purification of cDNA fragments, end repair and poly (A) tailing were performed before ligation to Illumina sequencing adapters. Pre-sequencing assessment of RNA quality was performed using an Agilent 2100 Bioanalyzer (Agilent Technologies, Palo Alto, CA).

UPLC analysis of Culla, Cullb, and oleanolic acid content in plant tissues  Samples of five tissues (tubers, roots, leaves, stems, and flowers) collected from *H. chinensis* and other species were vacuum freeze-dried (Christ ALPHA 1 - 2, Germany) and ground to a fine powder. Three replicate samples of each tissue (0.5 g) were collected.

The samples were accurately weighed and placed in stoppered conical flasks, and 25 mL of 70% methanol was added. After a second weighing, the samples were ultrasonicated (180 W power, 40 kHz frequency) for 40 min. They were allowed to cool and re-weighed before compensating for any weight loss using 70% methanol and thorough shaking. The resulting mixture was extracted three times with ethyl acetate, and the extracts were combined and concentrated. The concentrate was dissolved in methanol and diluted to a final volume of 10 mL. The supernatant was filtered through a 0.22 μm microporous membrane and subjected to ultra-HPLC (Agilent) to determine the content of CuIIa, CuIIb, and free oleanolic acid. An extract obtained using 70% methanol as described above was concentrated after centrifugation. Reflux was performed with 25 mL of 10% sulfuric acid in a water bath, maintaining slight boiling for 2 h. After cooling overnight, the mixture was filtered and the precipitate washed with water until neutral drying occurred. The dried precipitate was dissolved in methanol and transferred to a 10-ml volumetric flask for dilution up to the mark. An appropriate amount of solution was filtered through a 0.22 μm microporous membrane, and the resulting filtrate was used as the test solution for determining total oleanolic acid.

Content analysis was performed using an Agilent 1 290 Infinity II High Performance UHPLC System with a Phenomenex Kinetex C18 analytical column (4.6×100 mm, 2.6 μm) and a temperature maintained at 30℃. For detection of CuIIa and CuIIb, we used a gradient elution of 0.2% phosphoric acid aqueous solution (A) and acetonitrile (B): 0 - 15 min, 25%- 33% B; 15 - 20 min, 33%- 40% B; 20 - 24 min, 40%- 60% B; 24 - 28 min, 60% - 90% B; the detection wavelength was set to 212 nm. To determine oleanolic acid content, we used a gradient elution of 0.2% phosphoric acid aqueous solution (A) and acetonitrile (B): 0 - 10 min, 40%- 69% B; 10 - 15 min, 69% B; 15 - 20 min, 69%- 80% B; the detection wavelength was set to 201 nm. The flow rate was 0.8 ml/min, and the injection volume was 5 μl. CuIIa, CuIIb, cucurbitacin I, cucurbitacin E, and oleanolic acid standards (purchased from Desite Biotechnology, Chengdu, China) were used for quantification and qualitative analysis (Supplemental Table 10).

Cloning of *HcSE*, *HcOSC*, *HcCYP450*, *HcOxidoreductase*, and *HcAT* coding sequences *SE*, *OSC*, *CYP450*, *Oxidoreductase*, and *AT* candidate genes were identified from the *H. chinensis* transcriptome database. The protein-coding gene sequences of candidate genes were obtained from the transcriptome data of *H. chinensis*, and primers were designed for amplification of the *HcSE*, *HcOSC*, *HcCYP450*, *HcOxidoreductase*, and *HcAT* gene sequences (Supplemental Table 11). Coding sequences were amplified with the Phanta Max Super-Fidelity DNA Polymerase Kit (Vazyme Biotech), recovered from the gel, and ligated into expression vectors with the ClonExpress II One Step Cloning Kit (Vazyme Biotech). Finally, the gene sequences were cloned into the vector and transferred to *E. coli* DH5α by thermal excitation for sequencing and verification (Supplemental Table 12).

Sequence and phylogenetic analyses The online tool ORF Finder (http://www.ncbi.nlm.nih.gov/gorf) was used to acquire the ORFs and amino acid sequences of *HcSEs*, *HcOSCs*, *HcCYP450s*, and *HcATs*. Protein functional domains were identified through alignment. Multiple sequence alignment was performed using DNAMAN software, and Interpro (www.ebi.ac.uk/Tools/InterProScan) was used for domain identification. Amino acid sequences of OSCs from other species were obtained from the NCBI database and aligned using ClustalW. A phylogenetic tree was constructed in IQ-tree software using the maximum-likelihood method with 1 000 bootstrap replicates. To construct a phylogenetic tree of ATs, we downloaded reported ATs of different species from NCBI (Supplemental Table 13).

Tissue expression patterns and real-time qPCR The total RNA from five tissues of *H. chinensis* was reverse transcribed for real-time qPCR following the manufacturer's protocols and principles outlined in the HiScript III RT SuperMix for qPCR (+gDNAwiper) Kit (Vazyme Biotech). Specific primers for real-time qPCR (Supplemental Table 11) were designed using online software (http://www.primer3plus.com/), and gene expression was analyzed on the Applied Biosystems QuantStudio 5 real-time PCR system (Applied Biosystems, New York). The PCR conditions consisted of an initial incubation at 95℃ for 3 min, followed by 45 cycles of denaturation at 95℃ for 3 s and annealing/extension at 60℃ for 30 s, with subsequent melting curve analysis. The 18S rRNA gene was used as the reference for quantification of relative gene expression using the $2^{-\Delta\Delta Ct}$ method; triplicate measurements were obtained from three biological replicates.

Functional identification in *E. coli* The complete coding regions of HcSEs were cloned into the maltoprotein-tagged pMal-c2x vector through homologous recombination using the ClonExpress II One Step Cloning Kit (Vazyme Biotech). Following the instructions provided, the N-terminal transmembrane domain of HcCPR1 was truncated at 66 amino acid residues (M1 - V66) and ligated into the pET - 32a vector as described above. Protein purification and enzymatic detection of HcSE and HcCPR1 were performed following previously established protocols. HcSE was purified using an MBPTrap HP affinity column (Abbkine, China) and eluted with 10 mmol/L maltose, whereas HcCPR1 was purified using a Ni-NTA agarose affinity column and 80 mmol/L imidazole. All buffer systems used Tris-HCl. Recombinant proteins were quantified by 10% ( $W/V$ ) sodium dodecyl sulfate-polyacrylamide gel electrophoresis (SDS-PAGE) with BSA as the standard for determination of protein concentration. The enzymatic activity of the HcSEs was determined by adding HcCPR1 to the reaction system to provide hydrogen peroxide for oxygenation of the substrate squalene, resulting in production of either 2, 3-oxidosqualene or 2, 3:22, 23-diepoxysqualene. The 1 mL enzyme reaction mixture comprised the following components: 40 mmol/L squalene substrate (Sigma-Aldrich), 50 μg recombinant HcSE protein, 50 μg recombinant HcCPR1 protein, 1 mmol/L FAD, 1 mmol/L NADPH, Triton X-100 (1%), and 50 mmol/L Tris-HCl (pH 7.5). A negative control was included without the addition of 50 μg recombinant HcCPR1. After incubation overnight at 25℃, extracts from the enzyme reaction mixtures were subjected to GC-MS analysis.

HcAT protein expression, purification, and enzymatic activity detection were performed following previously established protocols. The HcATs were ligated into the pET32a vector. Positive colonies were cultured in LB medium, and cells were harvested after induction of protein expression with 0.1 mmol/L IPTG at 16℃ for 18 h. After cell disruption, recombinant His-tagged HcAT was purified by Ni affinity chromatography in a buffer system (50 mM sodium phosphate [pH 8.0], 500 mmol/L NaCl, 80 mM imidazole). Purified proteins were quantified by SDS-PAGE using BSA as a standard for quantification. The enzyme activity of the HcATs was determined by performing HPLC and LC-MS to analyze the presence of the Culla product in the enzyme reaction solution, which contained 40 μg purified HcATs, 400 μmol/L Cullb substrate, and a buffer consisting of 40 mmol/L acetyl-CoA and 50 mmol/L sodium phosphate (pH 7.5). A negative control without recombinant HcCPR1 was also used. Standards of the substrate Culla and the product Cullb were purchased from BioBioPha.

Immunoblotting Immunoblotting was used to detect purified HcCPR1 and HcAT proteins. The proteins were prepared in loading buffer containing SDS and loaded onto LK202 Omni-PAGE 10%-12% Bis-Tris gels (EpiZyme, China) for electrophoresis. A high-quality wet protein transfer machine (genscript, eBlot-L1, China) was used to transfer the proteins from the gel to the membrane, with parameters set to 17 min and a voltage of 50 V. The membranes were then blocked in PBST-buffered saline supplemented with 0.05% ( $V/V$ ) Tween 20 and incubated at room temperature with mouse monoclonal His-tag monoclonal antibody (GenStar, China) diluted in a solution containing 5% $W/V$ skimmed milk. After 1 h of incubation in PBST buffer and thorough washing steps, the membranes were incubated with IgG-HRP-conjugated secondary antibody (GenStar). The results were visualized using the StarSignal Plus Chemiluminescence Detection Kit (GenStar) (Tanon 5 200, China).

Functional identification in yeast and metabolite extraction *HcOSCs* obtained by cloning were ligated into the yeast expression vector pYES2 with the ClonExpress II One Step Cloning Kit. Plasmid extraction was performed following identification of positive colonies via sequencing (Vazyme Biotech). The plasmid was introduced into yeast cells via electroporation, and pYES2 without HcOSC was used as a negative control strain. The transformation procedure followed previously described methods. GIL77 yeast cells were cultured in YPD medium supplemented with ergosterol (20 μg/mL), heme (13 μg/mL), and Tween 80 (5 mg/mL) under shaking conditions. The yeast cells were harvested by centrifugation. After a washing treatment with water, 1 mol/L sorbitol, and 0.1 mol/L lithium acetate dissolved in 1 mol/L sorbitol, 100 μL of cells were transferred to a 0.2 cm electroporation cuvette and supplemented with 1 μg of plasmid DNA. Electroporation was performed using a GenePulser Electroporation System (Bio-Rad) with a voltage of 1.5 kV, resistance of 600 Ω, and capacitance of 25 μF. After the electroporated cells recovered in YPD medium for 1 h, the transformants were screened on solid medium without uracil (SC-Ura) for 2-3 days, and positive yeast strains were identified by sequencing. Culture of the positive transformants and detection of the HcOSC products were performed as described previously. The yeast cell culture was initially shaken in SC-Ura medium containing 2% glucose for 2 days, then switched to SC-Ura medium with 2% galactose for 1 day. The cells were then incubated ovemight at pH 7.0 with 2% glucose in a potassium phosphate buffer (0.1 mol/L). Finally, the extracted products from the yeast cells were analyzed by GC-MS. Products were extracted from the yeast cells either by ultrasonic extraction with methanol or by refluxing with 10 mL of 20% KOH and 50% EtOH for 5 min. The supernatant was then extracted three times with petroleum ether. Candidate genes responsible for oxidative modification were cloned into the YC-plac33 expression vector (Supplemental Table 9). The expression plasmid was transformed into yeast Cuol01-1 using the lithium acetate method, and the YCplac33 plasmid served as a negative control. For each candidate gene, three single colonies were used and inoculated into their respective screening SC medium for cultivation purposes. After 6 days of growth in a shaker, the products were analyzed by HPLC and LC-MS.

Purification and structural characterization of HcOSC1, HcOSC5, HcOSC6, 87D20-1, and 87D20-2 products The HcOSC-expressing GIL77 cells and Cuol01-1-PHc87 cells were cultured and harvested in 10 I each. HcOSCs and Cuol01-1-PHc87 were then obtained through saponification cleavage following previously established protocols. The extract was dissolved and separated by silica gel column chromatography (zcx. II, particle size 200 - 300; Haiyang, Qingdao, China) using a hexane:ethyl acetate solvent system (15 : 1 - 1 : 3, $V/V$). Compounds were eluted through a step gradient system, and the combined target products were analyzed via TLC. Further purification of the target products was performed using a reverse-phase HPLC semi-preparative column (Agilent Zorbax SB C18, 250×9.4 mm, 5 μm) for manual collection of the desired compounds. Cycloartenol (20 mg), isomultiflorenol (15 mg), and Cuol (55 mg), as well as 87D20 - 1 (48 mg) and 87D20 - 2 (16 mg) were purified from *S. cerevisiae* cultures expressing HcOSC1, HcOSC5, HcOSC6, and HcCYP87D20, respectively. The purified compounds were analyzed by NMR spectroscopy.

Recombinant yeast strains capable of producing Cuol and 11-carbonyl-20β-hydroxy-Cuol were constructed using the previously described method of yeast engineering through homologous recombination. The specific step involved PCR amplification to generate each gene expression cassette in the reconstituted pathway, with recombinant or fusion PCR using homologous sequences shared by these cassettes (Supplemental Figure 17A and 17B and Supplemental Table 11). Fusion fragments obtained through fusion PCR were then co-transformed into yeast strains using the lithium acetate method. Integration into chromosomes was achieved by sharing 40 - 75 bp of homologous sequences, followed by corresponding nutritional screening to generate yeast transformants.

Yeast cultivation and metabolite extraction  YPD medium was used for yeast growth culture following established protocols. Transformants were subsequently cultivated on SC solid medium supplemented with the corresponding auxotrophic marker to facilitate selection. The positive yeast transformants were shaken and cultured, after which seed liquid was acquired and inoculated in YPD medium for 96 h. The resulting fermentation broth was extracted using a 1 : 1 mixture of methanol and acetone to determine the titers of Cuol, 11-carbonyl-Cuol, and 11-carbonyl-20β-hydroxy-Cuol. Fed-batch fermentation, strain cultivation, batch fermentation cultivation, and feeding procedures were performed according to previously published protocols. After culturing the engineered yeast in 4 mL of YPD liquid for 24 h, seed medium was obtained and expanded to a volume of 100 ml. The seed medium was aseptically inoculated into a 1 L reactor medium to initiate fermentation. Throughout the fermentation process, culture media were collected at various time intervals for analysis of dry cell weight and cucurbitacin triterpene content.

Transient expression in *N. benthamiana* leaves  The genes sequences of *HcSE1 - 2*, *HcSQS*, *HcOSC6*, and *HcCYP87D20* from *H. chinensis* were cloned, along with the *GFP* gene from the pAN580 plasmid and a truncated 417-nucleotide portion of the HMGR gene from *Avena strigosa* (*AstHMGR*; GenBank accession number KY284573). These genes were subcloned into the pEAQ-HT-DEST1 binary vector using the ClonExpress II One Step Cloning Kit (Vazyme Biotech) and then transformed into an *A. tumefaciens* strain. The positive strains were confirmed by sequencing in EHA105 (Shanghai Weidi Biotechnology). *AstHMGR* has previously been reported to promote triterpenoid production. Following previously described methods, we co-expressed *HcOSC6* with *AstHMGR1* and introduced various strain combinations to evaluate gene interactions. In brief, the transformed *A. tumefaciens* were cultured in LB medium at 28℃ for 24 h, followed by cell harvesting using a solution containing 10 mmol/L MES [2-(N-morpholino)] ethanesulfonic acid), 10 mmol/L $MgCl_2$, and 100 mmol/L acetosyringone (4′-hydroxy-3′, 5′-dimethoxyacetophenone). The harvested cells were then suspended in the same solution to adjust the $OD_{600}$ to 0.8 and incubated in darkness with gentle shaking for 2 h. *A. tumefaciens* carrying *AstHMGR1* and *HcOSC6* genes were infiltrated into *N. benthamiana* leaves at week 5 using a modified vacuum infiltration method, and leaf samples were collected after 5 days for triterpenoid analysis.

Co-expression network analysis  Fifteen transcriptome datasets from *H. chinensis* were analyzed using the WGCNA package (v. 1.47) in R (v. 3.2.2). After filtering genes, 19 271 genes were used for WGCNA, and their expression values were imported to construct co-expression networks. The automatic network build function block with default settings was used to obtain modules, which were visualized using Cyto-scape_3.3.7 for analysis of gene co-expression relationships.

TLC and GC - MS analysis of extracts  For TLC analysis of target triterpenoids, yeast extract or tobacco extract was dissolved in 1 mL of ethyl acetate. The sample was loaded onto a TLC silica gel plate (Qingdao Haixiang, China) using a capillary tube. The developing solution consisted of n-hexane:ethyl acetate or petroleum ether:ethyl acetate at ratios ranging from 15 : 1 to 1 : 3. After development, the plate was dyed with a solution containing 10% sulfuric acid and ethanol, then heated to observe the color development of cucurbitadienol, ergosterol, 11-carbonyl-Cuol, and 11-carbonyl-20β-hydroxy-Cuol. Extracted samples were resuspended in 200 μL extraction solvent, and aliquots of 50 μL were dried under nitrogen gas. Dried aliquots were derivatized with 50 μL of trimethylsilyl (Sigma-Aldrich) and transferred to glass inserts within glass autosampler vials for GC - MS analysis using an Agilent 7890B GC system as described previously. In brief, a 1-μL sample (inlet temperature of 250℃) was injected in pulsed no-spigot mode (pulse pressure of 30 psi), using a program with an initial oven temperature of 170 ℃ for 2 min, followed by a ramp to 300 ℃ at a rate of 20 ℃/min and a hold at 300 ℃ for an additional 11.5 min. Detection was performed in scan mode (60 – 800 mass units) with a solvent delay set to 8 min and adjusted to precisely match the retention time. Data acquisition and analysis were performed using MassHunter Workstation software from Agilent Technologies. Quantitative and qualitative assessments were performed using squalene, 2, 3-squalene oxide, 2, 3:22, 23-dioxasqualene, and ergosterol standards purchased from Sigma-Aldrich for qualitative purposes, as well as Cuol standards obtained by purification (Supplemental Table 10).

HPLC and HPLC/ESIMS analysis of extracts The analytical method used to detect the target product in the HcAT reactions involved quantifying the contents of Culla and Cullb in the plant sample as described above, with 0.01% formic acid replacing 0.2% phosphoric acid. To detect 11-carbonyl-Cuol, 11-carbonyl-20β-hydroxy-Cuol, and 11-carbonyl-2β, 20β-dihydroxy-Cuol, we used a gradient elution of 0.01% formic acid aqueous solution (A) and acetonitrile (B): 0 – 12 min, 70%– 73% B; 12 – 16 min, 73%– 94% B; 16 – 26 min, 94% B. The detection wavelength was set to 210 nm. In addition, the extracts were analyzed using an Agilent 1290 UPLC/6540 Q-TOF system (Agilent Technologies) equipped with an Agilent Poroshell 120 EC C18 analytical column (4.6×100 mm, 2.7 μm). The ion source operated in positive ion mode with voltage settings as follows: 3 500 V voltage setting; 135 V fragmentation voltage; 60 V cone voltage; 750 V RF voltage. The scanning range spanned from 100 to 1 000 $m/z$. For quantification and qualitative purposes, we used a cucurbitadienol standard along with purified confirmed samples of 11-carbonyl-Cuol and 11-carbonyl-20β-hydroxy-Cuol (Supplemental Table 10).

NMR analysis The purified compounds were analyzed using $^{1}$H-NMR and $^{13}$C – NMR spectroscopy on Bruker AV – 600 MHz and 800 MHz spectrometers in $CDCl_3$ or $C_5D_5N$ solutions at the respective frequencies. Chemical shifts were recorded in ppm and referenced to the residual solvent peak. Multiplicities were denoted as follows: s, singlet; d, doublet; dd, doublet of doublets; dt, doublet of triplets; t, triplet; q, quartet; m, multiplet; br, broad; appt, apparent. Coupling constants are reported in Hertz.

[陈庚，张广辉，郝冰，等. Plant Communications, 2024, 5: 100835.]

# Discovering a mitochondrion-localized BAHD acyltransferase involved in calystegine biosynthesis and engineering the production of 3β-tigloyloxytropane

Plant secondary metabolites have been utilized as medicines by humans for thousands of years. Tropane alkaloids (TAs) are a class of secondary metabolites that are characterized by an 8-azabicyclo [3.2.1] octane core skeleton that contains a cycloheptane ring with a nitrogen bridge and are commonly referred to as a tropane moiety or tropane core. More than 300 TAs have been identified from the *Solanaceae*, *Convolvulaceae*, *Rhizophoraceae*, *Erythroxylaceae*, and other families. These compounds include the antricholinergic pharmaceuticals, hyoscyamine and scopolamine, which are synthesized by select genera of the *Solanaceae* family, and the narcotic cocaine, which is synthesized by the *Erythroxylaceae*.

Recent studies on *Atropa belladonna*, a species belonging to the *Solanaceae*, have comprehensively revealed the biosynthetic pathway of hyoscyamine and scopolamine. The tropane moiety of hyoscyamine and scopolamine is contributed by 3α-tropanol (also named tropine), which is biosynthesized by tropinone reductase I (TRI) using tropinone as a substrate. In addition, tropinone can be reduced to 3β-tropanol (also named pseudotropine) by tropinone reductase II (TRII) (Fig. 1). Calystegines, 3β-tropanol-derived TAs, are widely distributed in the plant kingdom and include several important vegetables in the *Solanaceae*, such as tomatoes, potatoes, eggplants, and hot peppers. Calystegines strongly inhibit glycosidase, might cause problems with nutrient absorption, and can be used in therapies for metabolic disorders. Despite being minor components in TA-producing plants, some 3β-tropanol esters are pharmaceutically important. For example, 3β-tigloyloxytropane, otherwise known as tigloidine or tropigline, is a substitute for atropine in the treatment of neurodegenerative disease; compared to atropine, 3β-tigloyloxytropane causes fewer side effects, including dry throat, mydriasis, and headache, than atropine. In addition, 3β-benzoyloxytropane, otherwise known as tropacocaine, is a potential ophthalmic and spinal anesthetic.

Comprehensive knowledge on the biosynthetic pathways of hyoscyamine, scopolamine, and cocaine has greatly facilitated their production in engineered plants and microbes. However, knowledge on the biosynthesis of 3β-tropanol derivatives is limited. Therefore, the efficient production of valuable 3β-tropanol esters, such as 3β-tigloyloxytropane and 3β-benzoyloxytropane, using metabolic engineering or synthetic biology approaches is also limited. Structurally, it was postulated that calystegines can be directly demethylated and hydroxylated from 3β-tropanol. Nevertheless, recent work challenges this long-standing speculation and propose the following roadmap: 3β-Tropanol is esterified into 3β-tigloyloxytropane (the key intermediate for the biosynthesis of calystegines), which undergoes demethylation and hydroxylation, followed by hydrolytic reactions, resulting in the production of calystegines. Although Robins and colleagues reported that catalytic activities associated with 3β-tropanol esterification occurred in *Datura stramonium* and *A. belladonna* in the 1990s, the genes that encode acyltransferases responsible for the formation of 3β-tropanol esters remain to be elucidated.

Esterification is among the most important chemical modifications of small molecules and involves the addition of an acyl moiety to produce esters and amides. Two enzyme families, serine carboxypeptidase-like acyltransferase (SCPL-AT) and BAHD acyltransferase (BAHD-AT), function as major acyltransferases that are involved in metabolite esterification in plants. SCPL-ATs usually employ 1-*O*-β-glucose as an acyl donors. For instance, in the biosynthesis of hyoscyamine and scopolamine, the SCPL-AT littorine synthase (LS), catalyzes the condensation of 3α-tropanol and phenyllactylglucose via esterification to generate littorine (Fig. 1). Interestingly, a recent study indicated that chicoric acid synthase (EpCAS), an SCPL-AT from *Echinacea purpurea*, uses chlorogenic acid as an acyl donor. However, BAHD-ATs normally use acyl-CoA thioesters. For instance, *Erythroxylum coca* cocaine synthase (EcCS), a member of the BAHD-AT family, is responsible for the biosynthesis of cocaine (a TA produced by the coca tree) through initiating esterification between methylecgonine (an intermediate with a tropane moiety) and benzoic acid.

SCPL-ATs and BAHD-ATs resulted from independent evolution. One of the fascinating aspects of metabolism is complex subcellular compartmentation. Many enzymes involved in secondary metabolite biosynthesis are located in the cytosol and multiple organelles. SCPL-ATs are usually localized in the vacuole, and this localization is essential for their function. Generally, BAHD-ATs do not possess a localization signal and occur freely in the cytosol. The enzymes involved in the biosynthesis of hyoscyamine and scopolamine are distributed throughout the cytosol, vacuole, and endoplasmic reticulum. Interestingly, although mitochondria are the center of nitrogen metabolism and TAs are nitrogenous secondary metabolites, no mitochondrial localization of enzymes involved in TA synthesis has been reported.

In this study, we functionally identified a mitochondrion-localized BAHD acyltransferase from *A. belladonna*, 3β-tigloyloxytropane synthase (TS). This enzyme catalyzes 3β-tropanol and tigloyl-CoA to produce 3β-tigloyloxytropane (Fig. 1). We also analyzed the tissue expression pattern of *TS*, observed its subcellular localization, studied its metabolic roles *in planta*, and analyzed its catalytic activities and mechanism. Finally, 3β-tigloyloxytropane was efficiently produced in engineered *E. coli*. This identification of TS enriches the knowledge on the biosynthesis of TAs and provides a biotechnological approach to produce 3β-tropanol-derived alkaloids through synthetic biology.

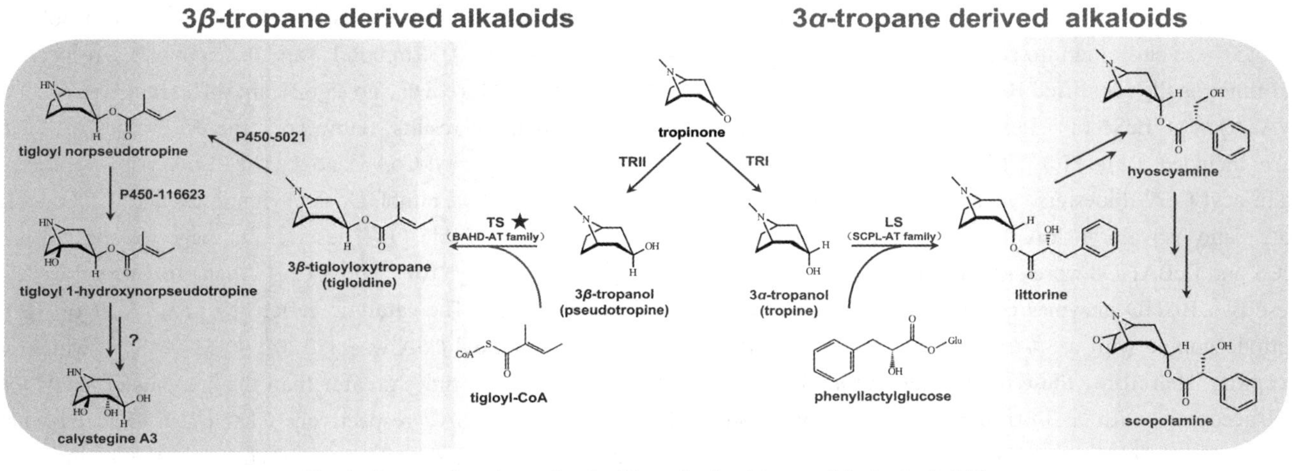

**Fig. 1 Proposed pathway for the biosynthesis of tropanol-derived alkaloids**

TRI tropine-forming reductase or tropinone reductase I, TRII pseudotropine-forming reductase or tropinone reductase II, LS littorine synthase, TS tigloidine synthase, the key finding of this study. The 3β-tropane alkaloid biosynthetic pathway is marked in blue, and the 3α-tropane alkaloid biosynthetic pathway is marked in green. P450-5021, 3β-tigloyloxytropane demethylase. P450-116623, tigloyl norpseudotropine hydroxylase.

## 1 RESULTS

The expression of *TS* is associated with the 3β-tigloyloxytropane distribution in *A. belladonna* To identify the genes responsible for 3β-tigloyloxytropane biosynthesis, we first analyzed the levels of 3β-tigloyloxytropane in different organs of *A. belladonna*. 3β-Tigloyloxytropane was detected in the primary and secondary roots, but not in any other tissues of *A. belladonna*, including mature seeds, ripe fruits, flowers, stems, green fruits, and leaves (Fig. 2A). With respect to 3β-tigloyloxytropane, 1.18 μg/g dry weight (DW) and 12.40 μg/g DW were detected in primary and secondary roots, respectively. The root-specific distribution of 3β-tigloyloxytropane suggested that the corresponding genes exhibited similar expression patterns, i.e., root-specific or root-preferring. Through HMMER search analysis, 46 BAHD-AT genes were identified from the *A. belladonna* transcriptome. Subsequently, metabolite and gene expression association analysis (MGAA) was used to screen out candidates that produce 3β-tigloyloxytropane. The MGAA results revealed that a putative BAHD gene (aba locus 5 896), named *TS*, was specifically expressed in primary and secondary roots and thus was tightly clustered with 3β-tigloyloxytropane (Fig. 2B). The expression pattern of *TS* was confirmed by qPCR after the full-length cDNA sequence was isolated (Fig. 2C).

Phylogenetic analysis of BAHD acyltransferases To determine the evolutionary relationship of TS, a phylogenetic tree of the BAHD-AT family was constructed, which included 46 BAHD-ATs of *A. belladonna* and 196 functionally identified BAHD-ATs from other plants (Fig. 2D and Supplementary Data 1-2). The phylogenetic tree was divided into clades 0-6, and these clades were the same as those in a previous report. Phylogenetic analysis revealed that TS were clustered into clade 3 (Fig. 2D). In clade 3, TS and functionally identified BAHD-ATs, such as PaASAT1-4, SlyASAT1-3, LeSAT1, LeAAT1, CaMAT and CaDAT, were included (Fig. 2E). These BAHDs recognize short-chain acyl-CoA thioesters, including acetyl-CoA, isobutyryl CoA, and isovaleryl-CoA, as acyl donors. Nonetheless, EcCS and EcBAHD8 were also included in clade 3 (Fig. 2E); these two BAHD enzymes catalyze cocaine formation using methylecgonine with a 3β-tropane ring skeleton as the acyl acceptor. Therefore, these results suggest that TS recognizes acyl acceptors with a 3β-tropane ring skeleton, and acyl donors of short-chain acyl-CoA thioesters.

TS catalyzes the esterification of 3β-tropanol To investigate the function of TS, we produced recombinant TS proteins in engineered *E. coli* and purified. First, we synthesized 3β-tropanol esters and tigloyl-CoA using chemical methods (Supplementary Figs. S1-S24 and Supplementary Data 3). In a reaction system with 3β-tropanol and tigloyl-CoA, TS produced a product with an $[M+H]^+$ $m/z$ of 224.1645, identical to that of the authentic 3β-tigloyloxytropane (Fig. 3A, B). Nonetheless, when TS was boiled, no products were detected (Fig. 3A). In a reaction system with 3α-tropanol and tigloyl-CoA, TS did not generate products (Fig. 3A). The above results indicated that TS catalyzes the condensation of 3β-tropanol with tigloyl-CoA to generate 3β-tigloyloxytropane via esterification reactions.

Furthermore, the optimum pH and temperature conditions for TS catalysis were investigated. The catalytic activities of TS treated with 3β-tropanol and tigloyl-CoA in the pH range of 6.0-10.6. The maximum activity of TS was detected at pH 8.6 (Supplementary Fig. S25A). The optimal pH conditions for the catalytic activity of most BAHD proteins are in a narrow alkaline range, approximately from 8 to 10. For example, the optimal pH conditions for EcCS, CiHCT2, and NtMAT1 are 9.4, 9.0, and 8.5, respectively. In addition, the catalytic activities of TS treated with 3β-tropanol and tigloyl-CoA between 20 ℃ and 50 ℃ were determined (Supplementary Fig. S25B). The maximum activity of TS was detected at 30 ℃. Next, the enzyme kinetic constants were measured under the optimal conditions (pH 8.6 and 30℃).

BAHD-AT family proteins generally exhibit substrate promiscuity. Therefore, we tested different acyl donors for TS. When 3β-tropanol and acetyl-CoA were used as substrates, TS produced 3β-acetoxytropane with a $[M+H]^+$ $m/z$ value of 184.1332 (Supplementary Fig. S26). When 3β-tropanol and benzoyl-CoA were used as substrates, TS produced 3β-benzoyloxytropane with a $[M+H]^+$ $m/z$ value of 246.1489 (Supplementary Fig. S27) in trace amounts. When tigloyl-CoA, acetyl-CoA, and benzoyl-CoA were used as acyl donors, the $K_m$ values of TS for 3β-tropanol were 0.36 mmol/L, 0.39 mmol/L, and 0.43 mmol/L, respectively (Table 1). Moreover, no significant difference was observed between these results. However, the $K_m$ values of TS for tigloyl-CoA, acetyl-CoA, and benzoyl-CoA were significantly different at 0.02 mmol/L, 0.09 mmol/L, and 0.92 mmol/L respectively (Table 1). These results suggested that TS has a greater affinity for tigloyl-CoA than for acetyl-CoA or benzoyl-CoA. The catalytic efficiency ($K_{cat}/K_m$) of TS for accessing tigloyl-CoA was 338 332.70 $M^{-1}$. $S^{-1}$, which was 743 and 26 473 times greater than the amounts of acetyl-CoA and benzoyl-CoA, respectively (Table 1). The enzymatic assays indicated that TS mainly catalyzes the formation of 3β-tigloyloxytropane.

Silencing of *TS* disrupts the biosynthesis of calystegine A3 *in planta* To determine the role of *TS* in the biosynthesis of 3β-tropanol esters *in planta*, *TS* was suppressed by virus-induced gene silencing (VIGS) in *A. belladonna* seedlings.

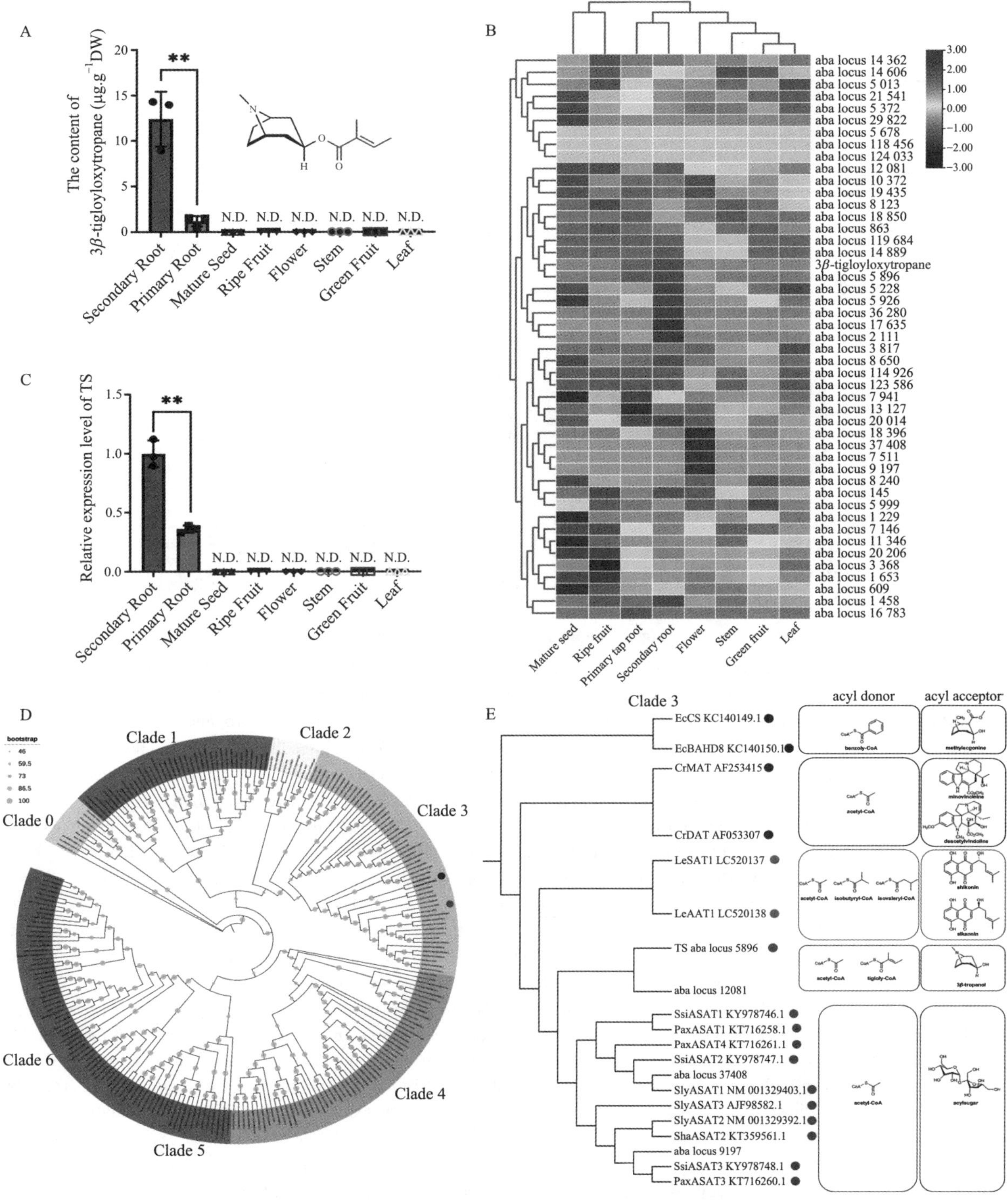


**Fig. 2 Metabolite, transcriptome, and phylogenetic association analysis**

(A) Tissue profile of 3$\beta$-tigloyloxytropane. Three independent plants were used in the tissue profile analysis of 3$\beta$-tigloyloxytropane. The data are presented as means values$\pm$s. d. ** $P=0.0032$. DW, dry weight. (B) Association analysis of the metabolites and BAHD gene family expression patterns. (C) Relative expression levels of TS in different organs, as indicated by qPCR. Three independent plants were used in the relative expression analysis of TS. The data are presented as means values $\pm$s. d. ** $P=0.0007$. (D) Phylogenetic analysis of the BAHD-AT gene family. The phylogenetic tree was divided into clades 0 - 6. (E) BAHD acyltransferases and their substrates in clade 3: TS, the BAHD acyltransferase identified in this study; EcCS, *Erythroxylum coca* cocaine synthase, a BAHD acyltransferase of the coca tree; EcBAHD8, the homolog of EcCS in *Erythroxylum coca*; PaxASAT1-4, an acylsugar acyltransferase in *Petunia axillaris*; SlyASAT1-3, an acylsugar acyltransferase in *Solanum lycopersicum*; SsiASAT1-3, an acylsugar acyltransferase in *Salpiglossis sinuata*; ShaASAT2, an acylsugar acyltransferase in *Solanum habrochaites*; LeSAT1, a shikonin *O*-acyl-transferase in *Lithospermum erythrorhizon*; LeAAT1, an alkannin *O*-acyltransferase in *Lithospermum erythrorhizon*; CrMAT, a minovincinine-19-hydroxy-*O*-acetyl-transferase in *Catharanthus roseus*; and CrDAT, a deacetylvindoline 4-*O*-acetyl-transferase in *Catharanthus roseus*. All functionally identified BAHD-ATs are labeled with their corresponding accession numbers. Statistical analysis was performed according to the two-sided independent sample *t*-test.

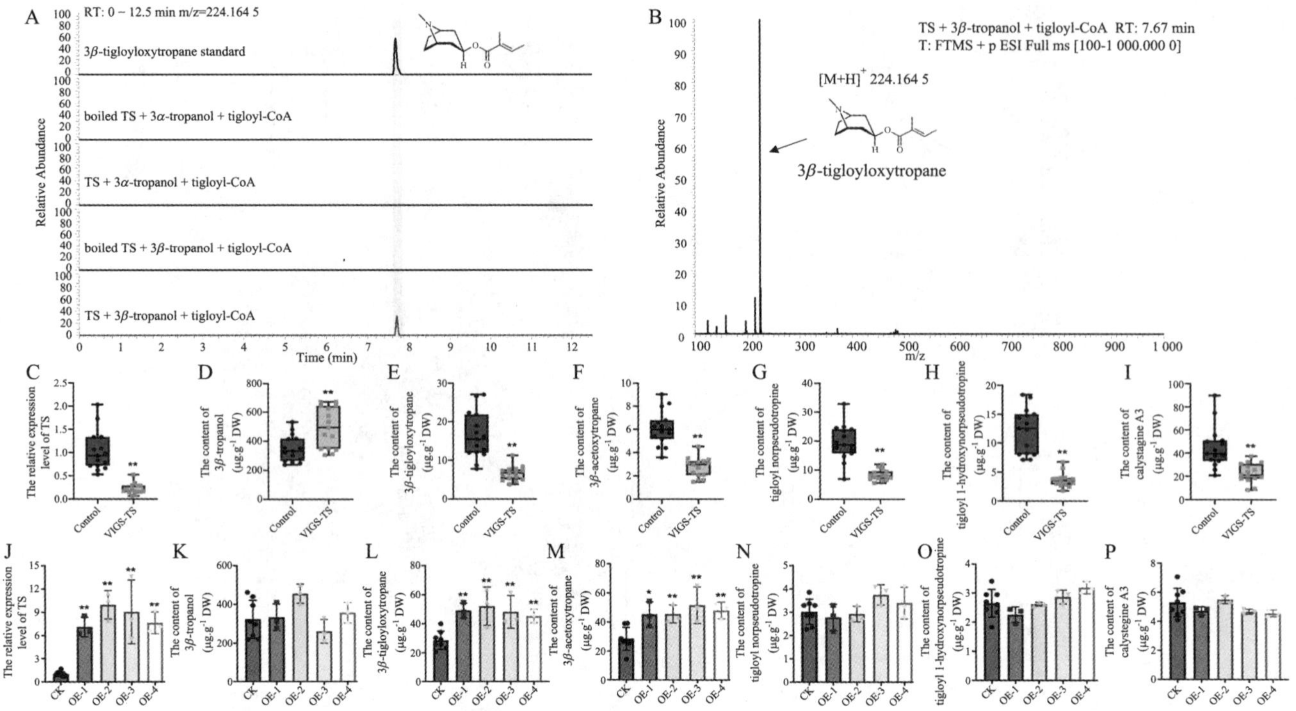

**Fig. 3 Functional characterization of TS**

(A) TS enzymatic assays with tigloyl-CoA as the acyl donor and 3$\beta$-tropanol as the acyl acceptor. (B) Mass spectrometry (MS) data of 3$\beta$-tigloyloxytropane. (C) Relative expression levels of *TS* in VIGS-*TS A. belladonna* seedlings. ** $P<0.0001$. (D) Contents of 3$\beta$-tropanol in VIGS-*TS A. belladonna* seedlings. ** $P=0.0024$. (E) Contents of 3$\beta$-tigloyloxytropane in VIGS-*TS A. belladonna* seedlings. ** $P<0.0001$. (F) Contents of 3$\beta$-acetoxytropane in VIGS-*TS A. belladonna* seedlings. ** $P<0.0001$. (G) Contents of tigloyl norpseudotropine in VIGS-*TS A. belladonna* seedlings. ** $P<0.0001$. (H) Contents of tigloyl 1-hydroxynorpseudotropine in VIGS-*TS A. belladonna* seedlings. ** $P<0.0001$. (I) Contents of calystegine A3 in VIGS-TS *A. belladonna* seedlings. ** $P=0.0002$. Control, control line obtained by empty plasmid transformation. VIGS-*TS*, TS-silenced line. Fifteen independent plants each from the control group and VIGS-*TS* group were used in the VIGS assays. Center line of box plot denotes the median value; lower and upper bounds denote first and third quartile; whiskers extend to the smallest and maximum values. (J) Relative expression levels of *TS* in *TS*-overexpressing *A. belladonna* hairy root cultures. ** $P<0.0001$ (OE-1), ** $P<0.0001$ (OE-2), ** $P<0.0001$ (OE-3), ** $P<0.0001$ (OE-4). (K) Contents of 3$\beta$-tropanol in *TS*-overexpressing *A. belladonna* hairy root cultures. (L) Contents of 3$\beta$-tigloyloxytropane in *TS*-overexpressing *A. belladonna* hairy root cultures. ** $P=0.0007$ (OE-1), ** $P=0.0024$ (OE-2), ** $P=0.0044$ (OE-3), ** $P=0.0025$ (OE-4). (M) Contents of 3$\beta$-acetoxytropane in *TS*-overexpressing *A. belladonna* hairy root cultures. * $P=0.0136$ (OE-1), ** $P=0.0087$ (OE-2), ** $P=0.0048$ (OE-3), ** $P=0.0039$ (OE-4). (N) Contents of tigloyl norpseudotropine in *TS*-overexpressing *A. belladonna* hairy root cultures. (O) Contents of tigloyl 1-hydroxynorpseudotropine in *TS*-over-expressing *A. belladonna* hairy root cultures. (P) Contents of calystegine A3 in *TS*-overexpressing *A. belladonna* hairy root cultures. CK, eight independently transformed root culture lines transformed with pBI121. OE denotes all independently transformed root culture lines overexpressing TS (three biological replicates for each line), including OE-1, OE-2, OE-3, and OE-4. The data are presented as means values ± s.d. Statistical analysis was performed according to the two-sided independent sample *t*-test. DW, dry weight.

As shown in Fig. 3C, *TS* was effectively suppressed in *A. belladonna* roots. In accordance with the decreased expression level of TS, the contents of 3$\beta$-tropanol, 3$\alpha$-tropanol, and tropanol hexosides in the TS-silenced lines were markedly greater than those in the control lines (Fig. 3D and Supplementary Fig. S28). The contents of 3$\beta$-tigloyloxytropane, 3$\beta$-acetoxytropane, tigloyl norpseudotropine, tigloyl 1-hydroxynorpseudotropine, and calystegine A3 in the TS-silenced lines were markedly lower than those in the control lines (Fig. 3E–I). However, the contents of the 3$\alpha$-tropanol derivatives littorine, hyoscyamine, and scopolamine, in *TS*-silenced plants did not significantly differ from those in the control plants (Supplementary Fig. S28). Both in-planta and in vitro assays showed that TS catalyzes the formation of 3$\beta$-tigloyloxytropane in the biosynthetic pathway of calystegine A3.

Overexpression of *TS* increases the content of 3$\beta$-tigloyloxytropane in hairy roots In addition, we overexpressed *TS* in hairy root cultures of *A. belladonna* to further investigate its role in the biosynthesis of 3$\beta$-tigloyloxytropane and explore its application in engineering. Genomic-PCR and qPCR analysis indicated that *TS* was integrated into the genome of *A. belladonna* and that its expression level was greatly increased in *TS*-over-expressing root lines (Fig. 3J, Supplementary Fig. S29). The contents of 3β-tigloyloxytropane and 3β-acetoxytropane were significantly greater in the *TS*-overexpressing lines than in the control lines (Fig. 3L, M), while no differences were observed in the production of 3β-tropanol, tigloyl norpseudotropine, tigloyl 1-hydroxynorpseudotropine and calystegine A3 (Fig. 3K, N-P). In addition, the contents of 3α-tropanol derivatives in the *TS*-overexpressing lines were not significantly different from those in the control lines (Supplementary Fig. S30). Overall, these results indicated that TS overexpression could increase the production of 3β-tigloyloxytropane in *A. belladonna* hairy roots.

TS is localized in the mitochondria  Previous studies reported that BAHD-ATs are localized in the cytosol. When analyzing the targeting signal sequence in the TS, we determined that the TS contains a potential mitochondrion-localizing signal sequence in its *N*-terminus (Supplementary Fig. S31). The subcellular localization of TS was subsequently investigated in tobacco protoplasts. TS fused with YFP (TS-YFP) and its mitochondrion-localizing signal peptide (the 32 amino acids at the N-terminus) fused with YFP (N32-YFP) were expressed in tobacco protoplasts. YFP signals in tobacco protoplasts overlapped with those derived from the mitochondrion-specific fluorescent dye Mito-Tracker Red (Fig. 4A). Furthermore, we performed a subcellular localization analysis of TS without the 32 amino acids at its N-terminus. Based on the results, TS without 32 amino acids ($TS^{Del\text{-}N32}$) still exhibited mitochondrial localization (Supplementary Fig. S32). Therefore, we speculate that the mitochondrial localization signal of TS is not only located at its N-terminus but also distributed at other regions. When $TS^{Del\text{-}N32}$ was expressed in *E. coli*, its catalytic activity decreased markedly (Supplementary Fig. S33A), suggesting that the 32-amino-acid sequence of TS plays a crucial role in enzymatic activity. Based on the 3D structure of TS generated by Alpha-Fold2, its 32-amino-acid sequence constitutes the core scaffold of TS (Supplementary Fig. S33B).

Next, we isolated mitochondria and supernatant from the secondary roots of *A. belladonna*. Voltage-dependent anion channel (VDAC) was used to detect mitochondria. The mitochondrion marker protein VDAC was detected in the mitochondrial fraction but not in the supernatant fraction (Fig. 4B). These results suggested that we successfully obtained mitochondria from *A. belladonna*. The catalytic activities of the crude protein from the mitochondria and supernatant were subsequently detected. The formation of 3β-tigloyloxytropane was catalyzed by the crude mitochondrial protein catalyzed but not the crude protein in the supernatant (Fig. 4C).

These results demonstrated that TS are localized mitochondria; this subcellular compartmentalization is different from that of previously reported BAHD-ATs, which are localized in the cytosol.

Catalytic mechanism of TS and improvements of TS inactivity  The catalytic mechanisms of BAHD-ATs with phenylpropanoids as acyl acceptors have been studied extensively; however, the mechanism through which BAHD-ATs recognize 3β-tropanol, a compound with very different structures from phenylpropanoids, as an acyl acceptor, has remained unknown. To explore the catalytic mechanism of TS and provide information for engineering, a complex model was constructed by molecular docking (Supplementary Fig. S34). We observed that His162 in the HXXXD motif forms a hydrogen bond with the oxygen of 3β-tropanol (3.0 Å), which is a universally conserved catalytic residue in BAHD-ATs, suggesting that His162 is the base catalyst in the catalytic pocket of TS (Fig. 5A). Consistent with our hypothesis, when His162 was mutated to alanine, $TS^{H162A}$ completely lost its catalytic activity (Fig. 5B). In addition, a binding pocket of 3β-tropanol formed by His162, Ile35, Gln39, Asn298, Leu300, Tyr280 and Trp340 was observed (Fig. 5C). To examine the roles of these residues in the binding pocket, site-directed mutants of TS were generated. Ile35, Gln39, Tyr280, Asn298, Leu300, and Trp340 were mutated to alanine, and the catalytic activities of the mutants were dramatically reduced (Fig. 5D). Together, our findings revealed that these residues in the binding pocket of 3β-tropanol play critical roles in governing TS activity.

The results of enzymatic kinetic analysis indicated that TS poorly utilizes benzoyl-CoA, suggesting that TS prefers short-chain acyl-CoA thioesters as acyl donors rather than benzoyl-CoA with an aromatic amino acid. The mechanism by which TS strictly govern acyl donor identification is interesting. We assumed that the greater steric hindrance of benzoyl-CoA relative to short-chain acyl-CoA thioesters, which is not suitable for the substrate pocket of TS, contributed to the low production of 3β-benzoyloxytropane. Through molecular docking, we compared the substrate pocket of TS with that of EcCS, which uses benzoyl-CoA as an acyl donor. A Phe46 residue was observed in TS that is 2.5 Å away from the benzene ring of benzoyl-CoA (Fig. 6A), whereas its corresponding residue in EcCS (Ile45) is 4.5 Å (Fig. 6C). When Phe46 in TS was mutated to isoleucine, the distance between the benzene ring of benzoyl-CoA and Ile46 was 4.1 Å (Fig. 6B). When the 46th amino acid of TS is phenylalanine, the distances to tigloyl-CoA and acetyl-CoA are 3.6 Å and 5.0 Å, respectively (Fig. 6D, E). However, when the 46th amino acid of TS is isoleucine, the distances increase to 4.9 Å and 6.3 Å, respectively (Fig. 6F, G). Subsequently, we conducted in vitro enzyme assays to verify the results of the molecular docking experiments. Consistent with our hypothesis, the F46I mutation significantly enhanced the activity of TS in the synthesis of 3βbenzoyloxytropane (Fig. 6H and Table 1) and significantly decreased the activity of TS in the synthesis of 3$\beta$-tigloyloxytropane (Table 1). The $K_{cat}/K_m$ value for benzoyl-CoA in $TS^{F461}$ was 99.32 $M^{-1}$. $S^{-1}$, which was 7.77 times greater than that of TS (Table 1). The $K_{cat}/K_m$ values for tigloyl-CoA and acetyl-CoA in $TS^{F461}$ were 3 588.34 $M^{-1}$ • $S^{-1}$ and 16.17 $M^{-1}$ • $S^{-1}$, which were 1.06% and 3.5%, respectively, of the TS (Table 1). The results above showed that Phe46 is the key amino acid residue that governs the use of short-chain acyl-CoA thioesters as acyl donors.

**Table 1 Kinetic parameters of TS**

| Product | Substrate | Enzyme | $K_m$(mM) | $K_{cat}$($s^{-1}$) | $K_{cat}/K_m$($M^{-1}$ • $s^{-1}$) |
|---|---|---|---|---|---|
| 3$\beta$-tigloyloxytropane | 3$\beta$-tropanol | TS | 0.36±0.05 | 6.84±0.30 | 19 045.07±1 658.79 |
| 3$\beta$-tigloyloxytropane | 3$\beta$-tropanol | $TS^{S40T}$ | 0.32±0.07 | 11.09±0.81 | 35 153.35±5 480.42 |
| 3$\beta$-tigloyloxytropane | 3$\beta$-tropanol | $TS^{F461}$ | 0.32±0.06 | 1.44±0.09 | 4 550.90±593.97 |
| 3$\beta$-tigloyloxytropane | 3$\beta$-tropanol | $TS^{S40T-F461}$ | 0.27±0.07 | 2.48±0.22 | 9 464.65±1 784.82 |
| 3$\beta$-tigloyloxytropane | tigloyl-CoA | TS | 0.02±0.004 | 7.38±0.25 | 338 332.70±49 061.33 |
| 3$\beta$-tigloyloxytropane | tigloyl-CoA | $TS^{S40T}$ | 0.02±0.003 | 11.42±0.34 | 572 303.6±72 285.97 |
| 3$\beta$-tigloyloxytropane | tigloyl-CoA | $TS^{F461}$ | 0.41±0.11 | 1.42±0.17 | 3 588.34±569.56 |
| 3$\beta$-tigloyloxytropane | tigloyl-CoA | $TS^{S40T-F461}$ | 0.15±0.02 | 2.27±0.10 | 14 809.27±1 370.76 |
| 3$\beta$-acetoxytropane | 3$\beta$-tropanol | TS | 0.39±0.11 | 0.048±0.005 | 126.03±23.98 |
| 3$\beta$-acetoxytropane | 3$\beta$-tropanol | $TS^{S40T}$ | 0.31±0.08 | 0.098±0.007 | 319.69±52.89 |
| 3$\beta$-acetoxytropane | 3$\beta$-tropanol | $TS^{F461}$ | 0.48±0.08 | 0.000 8±0.000 4 | 16.79±1.64 |
| 3$\beta$-acetoxytropane | 3$\beta$-tropanol | $TS^{S40T-F461}$ | 0.53±0.08 | 0.02±0.001 | 41.03±3.67 |
| 3$\beta$-acetoxytropane | acetyl-CoA | TS | 0.09±0.02 | 0.04±0.002 | 455.09±62.68 |
| 3$\beta$-acetoxytropane | acetyl-CoA | $TS^{S40T}$ | 0.07±0.01 | 0.09±0.004 | 1 191.44±155.40 |
| 3$\beta$-acetoxytropane | acetyl-CoA | $TS^{F461}$ | 0.35±0.12 | 0.005±0.000 8 | 16.17±3.42 |
| 3$\beta$-acetoxytropane | acetyl-CoA | $TS^{S40T-F461}$ | 0.27±0.03 | 0.02±0.000 9 | 73.93±5.33 |
| 3$\beta$-benzoyloxytropane | 3$\beta$-tropanol | TS | 0.43±0.05 | 0.006±0.000 3 | 14.55±1.18 |
| 3$\beta$-benzoyloxytropane | 3$\beta$-tropanol | $TS^{S40T}$ | 0.46±0.09 | 0.02±0.001 | 37.09±4.52 |
| 3$\beta$-benzoyloxytropane | 3$\beta$-tropanol | $TS^{F461}$ | 0.34±0.06 | 0.03±0.002 | 90.78±10.21 |
| 3$\beta$-benzoyloxytropane | 3$\beta$-tropanol | $TS^{S40T-F461}$ | 0.48±0.09 | 0.07±0.005 | 155.33±17.65 |
| 3$\beta$-benzoyloxytropane | benzoyl-CoA | TS | 0.92±0.58 | 0.01±0.004 | 12.78±3.57 |
| 3$\beta$-benzoyloxytropane | benzoyl-CoA | $TS^{S40T}$ | 0.84±0.38 | 0.03±0.006 | 32.73±6.77 |
| 3$\beta$-benzoyloxytropane | benzoyl-CoA | $TS^{F461}$ | 0.37±0.09 | 0.04±0.004 | 99.32±13.33 |
| 3$\beta$-benzoyloxytopane | benzoyl-CoA | $TS^{S40T-F461}$ | 0.26±0.08 | 0.08±0.008 | 304.94±54.07 |

To further improve the catalytic activity of TS, a consensus protein design was employed. Based on the conservative substitution analysis performed on residues within a 5 Å range of His162, we observed that only Ser40 did not fit the conservative replacement model TS (Supplementary Fig. S35A). Virtual mutation prediction revealed that substituting Ser40 with the conservative substitution threonine may change the hydrogen bonding network around the 3$\beta$-tropanol entry channel (Supplementary Fig. S35B, C). Thr40 established a new hydrogen bond with Asn135 in the adjacent coil (Supplementary Fig. S35B, C). Similarly, the Kcat values of $TS^{S40T}$ for synthesizing 3$\beta$-tropanol esters were significantly greater than those of the other samples, while the $K_m$ values were not significantly different (Table 1). The $K_{cat}/K_m$ values for 3$\beta$-tropanol and tigloyl-CoA in $TS^{S40T}$ were 35 153.35 $M^{-1}$ • $S^{-1}$ and 572 303.6 $M^{-1}$ • $S^{-1}$, which was 3.00 and 1.69 times greater than that of the wild-type TS (Table 1 and Supplementary Fig. S35D, E). The results above demonstrated that compared to wildtype TS, the $TS^{S40T}$ mutant could synthesize 3$\beta$-tropanol esters, including 3$\beta$-tigloyloxytropane, 3$\beta$-acetoxytropane and 3$\beta$-benzoyloxytropane, more efficiently.

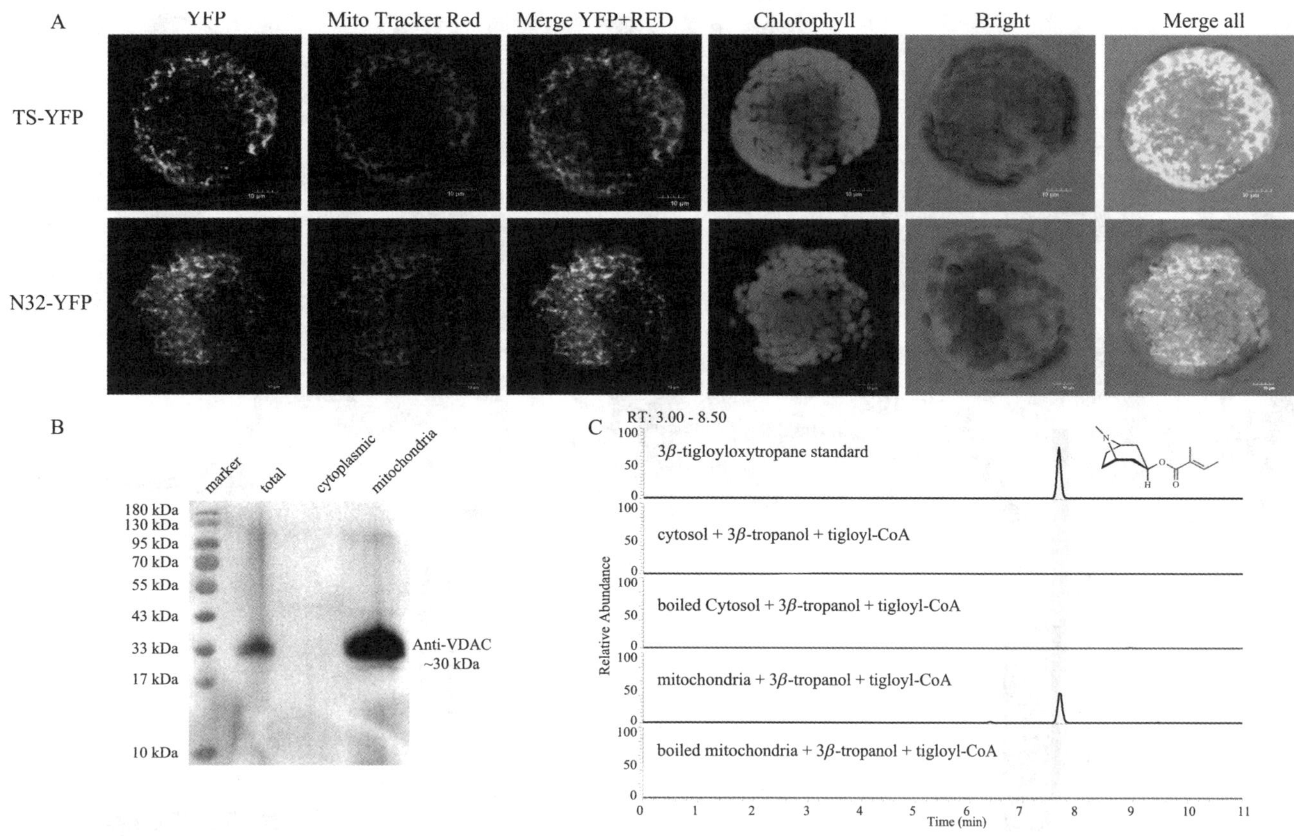


**Fig. 4 Subcellular localization analysis of TS**

(A) The localization of TS-YFP and N32-YFP in tobacco protoplasts was observed by confocal microscopy. YFP yellow fluorescence from YFP. MitoTracker Red, MitoTracker Red fluorescence-labeled mitochondria. Merge YFP+RED, the merged images for the yellow fluorescence and MitoTracker Red fluorescence. Chlorophyll, chlorophyll spontaneous fluorescence. Bright, bright field image. Overlapping images of all the channels mentioned above were merged. TS-YFP, TS fused with YFP. N32-YFP, mitochondrion-localizing signal peptide (the 32 amino acids at the N-terminus) of TS fused with YFP. All tobacco transformation and microscopic analyses were independently conducted three times with different plants. (B) Determination of *A. belladonna* mitochondria by Western blot analysis with an antibody against VDAC. Western blot analysis was independently conducted two times with different plants. (C) Crude protein from *A. belladonna* mitochondria-catalyzed tigloyl-CoA and 3β-tropanol to form 3β-tigloyloxytropane.

Biosynthesis of 3β-tigloyloxytropane in *N. benthamiana*

To further assess the function of TS and its application in 3β-tigloyloxytropane engineering in tobacco, we reconstructed the 3β-tropanol ester biosynthetic pathway in the leaves of *N. benthamiana*. Six upstream biosynthesis genes (*Erythroxylum novogranatense* ornithine decarboxylase, EnODC; *A. belladonna* putrescine *N*-methyltransferase, AbPMT; *A. belladonna* *N*-methylputrescine oxidase, AbMPO; *A. belladonna* type III polyketide synthase, AbPYKS; *A. belladonna* tropinone synthase, AbCYP82M3; and *Datura stramonium* tropinone reductase II, DsTRII), together with TS were transiently coexpressed in tobacco leaves (Fig. 7A). Control experiments were conducted in which yellow fluorescent protein (YFP) was expressed. Leaves that expressed these six enzymes and TS yielded tropinone, hygrine, 3β-tropanol, 3β-tigloyloxytropane and 3β-acetoxytropane (Fig. 7B – G). The control leaves did not yield any 3β-tigloyloxytropane or intermediates. To further promote the harvest of 3β-tigloyloxytropane from tobacco leaves, we substituted the wild-type TS with $TS^{S40T}$. $TS^{S40T}$ increased the levels of 3β-tigloyloxytropane and 3β-acetoxytropane by 1.33- and 5.02- fold respectively, compared with those in the wild-type TS. The highest contents of 3β-tigloyloxytropane and 3β-acetoxytropane were detected in tobacco leaves, which were 6.14 μg/g DW and 0.13 μg/g DW, respectively (Fig. 7F, G).

Although tobacco leaves coexpressed the seven biosynthetic genes involved in 3β-tigloyloxytropane biosynthesis, the production level was low. This low yield might result from the insufficient supply of tigloyl-CoA in plants. Increasing the synthesis of tigloyl-CoA may promote the accumulation of 3β-tigloyloxytropane. Tigloyl-CoA is a metabolite degraded from isoleucine in plants, but metabolic genes related to tigloyl-CoA formation have not been identified.

We hypothesized that CoA ligase catalyzes the formation of tigloyl-CoA using tiglic acid and CoA. In bacteria, *Pseudomonas chlororaphis* contains an isobutyryl CoA synthetase (PcICS) that catalyzes a reaction between isobutyric acid and CoA to

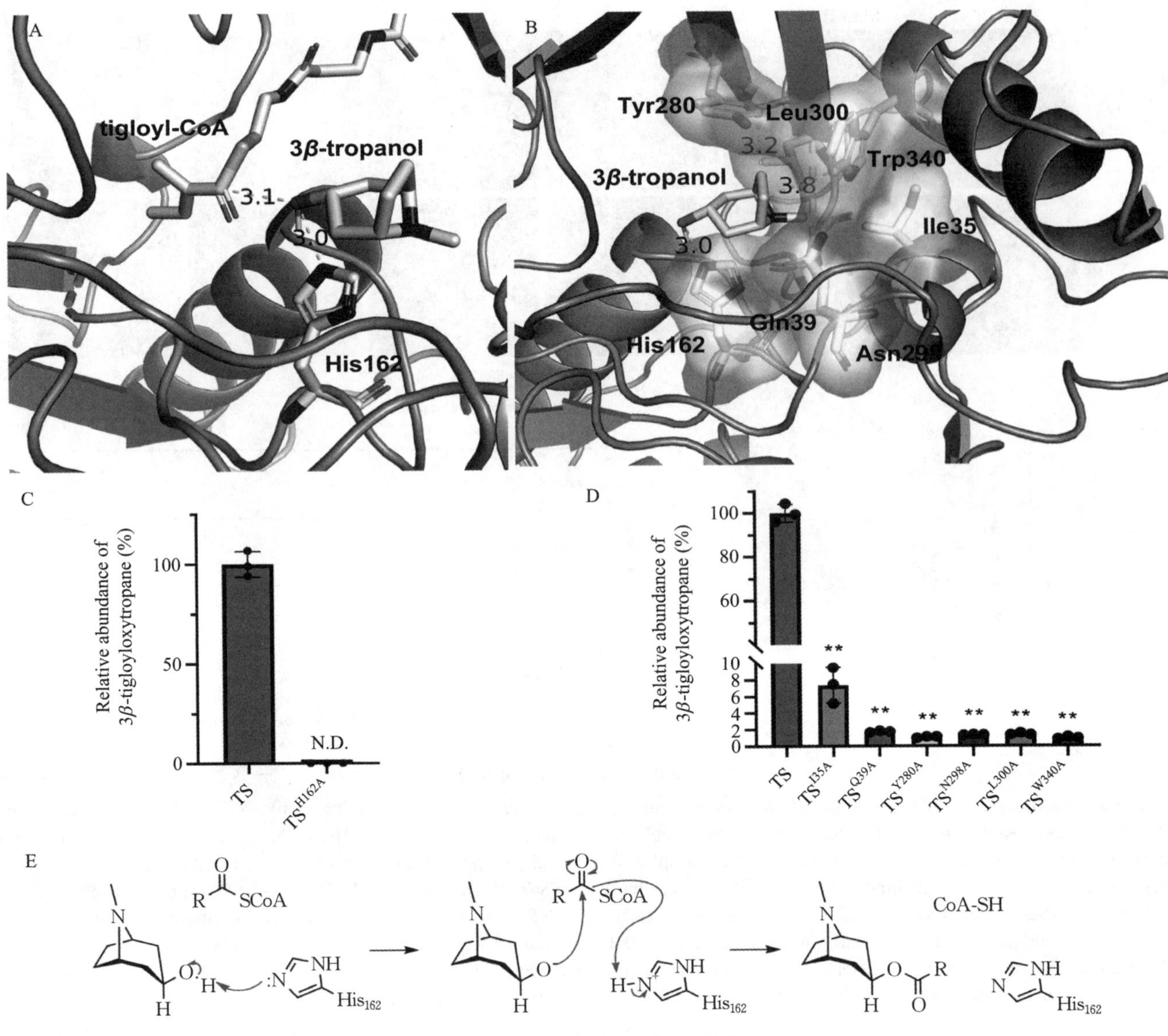


**Fig. 5 Catalytic mechanism of TS**

(A) Schematic model of the catalytic pocket that contains 3$\beta$-tropanol and tigloyl-CoA. (B) Comparison of the relative activities of TS and $TS^{H162A}$ using tigloyl-CoA as the acyl donor. (C) Key residues in the substrate pocket combined with 3$\beta$-tropanol. (D) Comparison of the relative activity of TS and TS mutants (3$\beta$-tropanol binding residues mutated to alanine) using tigloyl-CoA as the acyl donor. $^{**}P<0.0001$ ($TS^{I35A}$), $^{**}P<0.0001$ ($TS^{Q39A}$), $^{**}P<0.0001$ ($TS^{Y280A}$), $^{**}P<0.0001$ ($TS^{N298A}$), $^{**}P<0.0001$ ($TS^{L300A}$), $^{**}P<0.0001$ ($TS^{W340A}$). (E) 3$\beta$-Tropanol and acyl donors are converted to 3$\beta$-tropanol esters via the catalysis of TS. The data are presented as means values$\pm$s. d. Recombinant protein obtained from three independent transformants of TS and each mutant for activity test. Statistical analysis was performed according to the two-sided independent sample $t$-test.

produce isobutyryl CoA. We hypothesized that PcICS uses tiglic acid as a substrate because the structures of isobutyric acid and tiglic acid are similar. Consistent with this hypothesis, purified PcICS catalyzed the synthesis of tigloyl-CoA from CoA and tiglic acid (Fig. 8A, B). Unfortunately, when the six upstream biosynthesis genes, $TS^{S40T}$ and PcICS were coexpressed and tiglic acid was added to tobacco leaves, the level of 3$\beta$-tigloyloxytropane did not significantly increase (Supplementary Fig. S36), probably due to the insufficient supply of 3$\beta$-tropanol.

Then, we performed further experiments. When TS was expressed in tobacco leaves fed 3$\beta$-tropanol, 3$\beta$-tigloyloxytropane was produced at a much greater level than that produced during the de novo biosynthesis of 3$\beta$-tigloyloxytropane (Supplementary Fig. S37). When TS was expressed in tobacco leaves fed sufficient 3$\beta$-tropanol and tiglic acid, 3$\beta$-tigloyloxytropane was produced at a slightly increased level (Supplementary Fig. S37). When PcICS and $TS^{S40T}$ were coexpressed in tobacco leaves fed 3$\beta$-tropanol and tiglic acid, 3$\beta$-tigloyloxytropane was produced at markedly increased levels, reaching up to 293.86 μg/g DW (Supplementary Fig. S37). These results suggested that a sufficient supply of substrates through feeding facilitated the production of 3$\beta$-tigloyloxytropane in tobacco leaves.

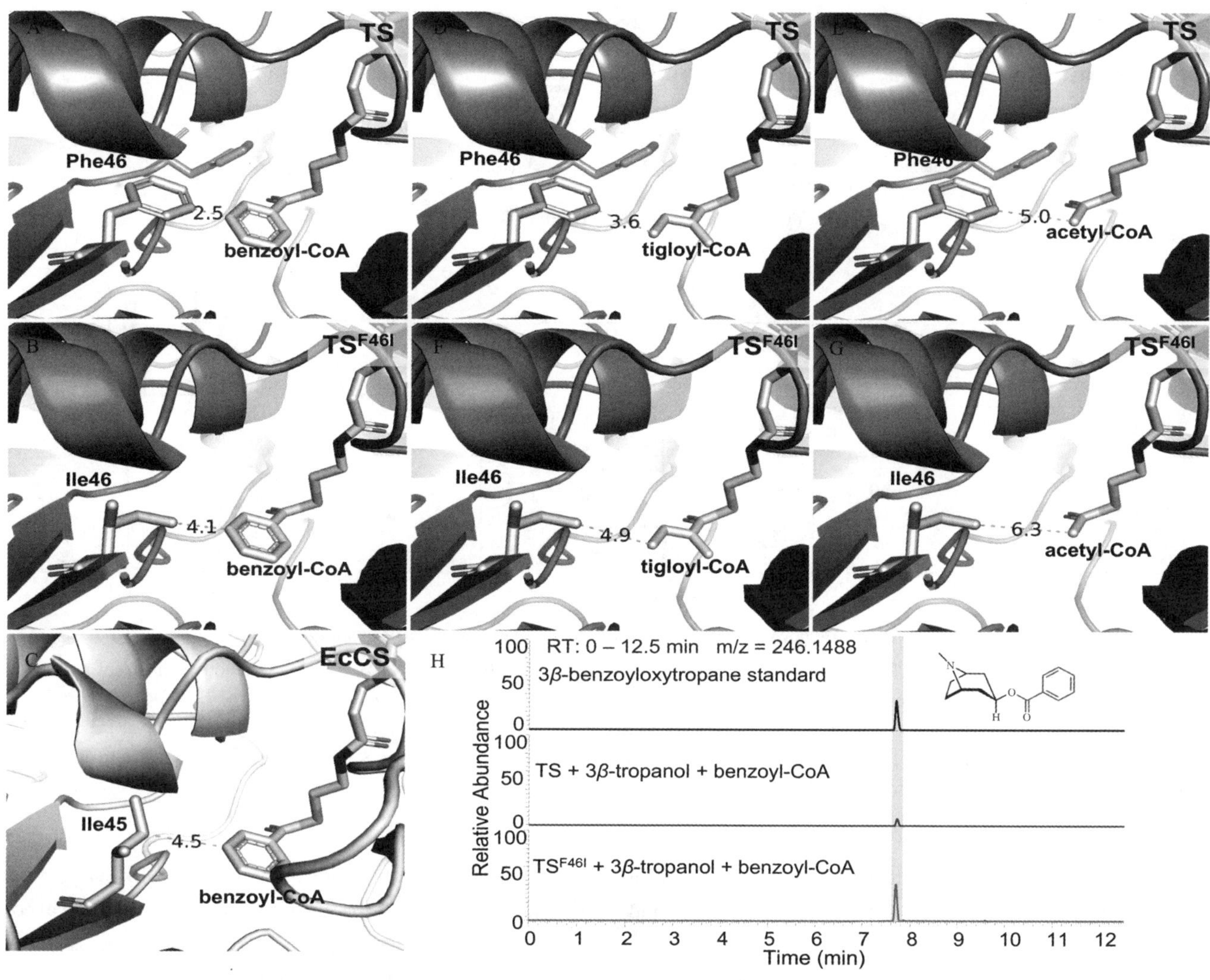


**Fig. 6 Improvement in the substrate promiscuity of TS**

(A) Catalytic pocket of TS that contains benzoyl-CoA. (B) Catalytic pocket of $TS^{F46I}$ that contains benzoyl-CoA. (C) Catalytic pocket of EcCS that contains benzoyl-CoA. (D) Catalytic pocket of TS that contains tigloyl-CoA. (E) Catalytic pocket of TS that contains acetyl-CoA. (F) Catalytic pocket of $TS^{F46I}$ that contains tigloyl-CoA. (G) Catalytic pocket of $TS^{F46I}$ that contains acetyl-CoA. (H) Enzymatic assays of TS and $TS^{F46I}$ with benzoyl-CoA as the acyl donor.

**Biosynthesis of 3β-tigloyloxytropane in *E. coli*** Due to the low production of 3β-tigloyloxytropane in plants, we constructed an efficient platform to produce this potential drug for treating neurodegenerative diseases. We therefore built an engineered *E. coli* bioreactor to produce 3β-tigloyloxytropane, by feeding the readily available substrates tiglic acid and 3β-tropanol (Fig. 8C).

To produce 3β-tigloyloxytropane, *E. coli* cells expressing TS were fermented in LB medium with 250 mg. $L^{-1}$ of 3β-tropanol. Although TS and $TS^{S40T}$ catalyzed the production of 3β-tropanol and tigloyl-CoA to 3β-tigloyloxytropane in plants and in vitro, we did not detect 3β-tigloyloxytropane in this fermentation system (Fig. 8D). This difference might be attributed to the absence of tigloyl-CoA in *E. coli*. Therefore, to produce 3β-tigloyloxytropane, a CoA ligase that catalyzes the synthesis of tigloyl-CoA from CoA and tiglic acid is necessary. Thus, PcICS was used to engineer *E. coli* to produce 3β-tigloyloxytropane together with TS or its mutants. The highest yield (357.40 mg/L with a conversion rate of 90.9%), was detected after 60 h of fermentation when $TS^{S40T}$ and PcICS were expressed (Fig. 8D).

## 2 DISCUSSION

Calystegines are potential anti-nutritional factors that have been found in various Solanaceous foods, such as potatoes and tomatoes. Recently, the discovery of two P450s involved in the biosynthesis of calystegines shed the light on the complete elucidation of the biosynthetic pathway of calystegines. However, the crucial esterification step leading to the formation of 3β-tigloyloxytropane remained elusive. In this study, we successfully identified 3β-tigloyloxytropane synthase (TS), a BAHD acyltransferase, that catalyzes the formation of 3β-tigloyloxytropane. Considering the glycosidase-inhibiting activities of calystegines and their putative applications

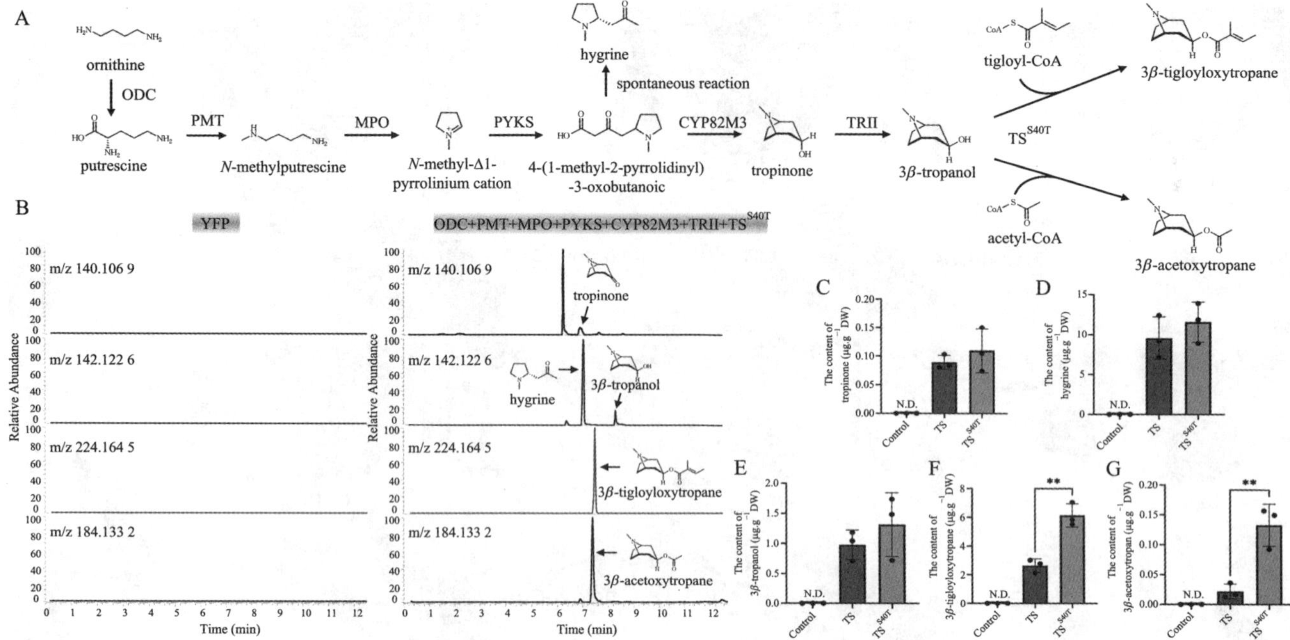

**Fig. 7 De novo synthesis of 3β-tigloyloxytropane in *N. benthamiana***

(A) Reconstruction of the 3β-tigloyloxytropane biosynthetic pathway in *N. benthamiana*. (B) LC-MS detection of target metabolites in tobacco leaves. (C) The contents of tropinone. (D) The contents of hygrine. (E) The contents of 3β-tropanol. (F) The contents of 3β-tigloyloxytropane. $^{**}P=0.003$. (G) The contents of 3β-acetoxytropane. $^{**}P=0.0068$. The control represents tobacco leaves expressing YFP. TS ($TS^{S40T}$) represents tobacco leaves coexpressing six TA genes and TS ($TS^{S40T}$). The data are presented as means values±s. d. Leaves from three independent plants of each line were used for metabolite analysis. Statistical analysis was performed according to the two-sided independent sample *t*-test.

in the therapy of metabolic disorders, our finding provides a target for breeding calystegines-free *Solanaceae* crops and synthesizing valuable calystegines in plants or microbes.

Proper subcellular localization is essential for enzyme activity. Although BAHD-ATs are generally localized in the cytosol, TS was localized in the mitochondria (Fig. 4). In particular, the 32 amino-acid in the N-terminal of TS plays an important role in TS activity, but it is sufficient but not essential for the mitochondrial localization of TS. The mitochondrial localization of TS was unexpected but reasonable. It is well established that tigloyl-CoA, a degradation product of isoleucine, is produced in mitochondria. The mitochondrial localization of TS suggests that this enzyme may utilize acyl donors in a rapid and economical manner. Earlier studies showed that mitochondria are a good organelle for the production of terpenes that require acetyl-CoA as a substrate. Thus, a more efficient metabolic engineering strategy for BAHD-AT-mediated esters biosynthesis may be achieved by this mitochondrial localization feature of TS.

Based on the ternary complex model (Fig. 5A), we found that the acyl acceptor binding pocket of TS, composed of Ile35, Gln39, His162, Tyr280, Asn298, Leu300, and Trp340, stabilized 3β-tropanol in a suitable catalytic conformation (Fig. 5B). Combined with the enzymatic activity assays of TS mutants, we proposed the catalytic mechanism of TS. The His162 in the conserved HXXXD domain of BAHD-ATs is a general base that deprotonates the 3-hydroxyl of 3β-tropanol, priming it for nucleophilic attack on the carbonyl carbon of the acyl donor (Fig. 5E). In this process, CoA is then, released from the tetrahedral intermediate as a leaving group to produce the 3β-tropanol ester (Fig. 5E).

Like reported BAHD-ATs, TS exhibits acyl donor promiscuity. TS mainly catalyzed the formation of 3β-tigloyloxytropane, because its affinity for tigloyl-CoA is much higher than that for acetyl-CoA and benzoyl-CoA (Table 1). This may be due to the aromatic ring of benzoyl-CoA exhibiting greater steric hindrance compared to shortchain acyl-CoA thioesters. For TS, Phe46 strictly controls the recognition of acyl donors through steric hindrance. When benzoyl-CoA was used as a substrate, the aromatic ring of Phe46 hinder the entry of benzoyl-CoA. Mutation of Phe46 to isoleucine decreased the steric hindrance significantly improved the utilization efficiency of benzoyl-CoA and greatly reduced the utilization efficiency of tigloyl-CoA (Fig. 6, Supplementary Fig. S35 and Table 1). Our findings on the catalytic mechanism of TS provided insights into the esterification mediated by BAHD-ATs and can be used to design diversity esters.

A highly efficient enzyme is key to the production of natural products by synthetic biology. A higher activity TS mutant, $TS^{S40T}$, was designed (Supplementary Fig. S35). Thr40 of $TS^{S40T}$ formed a novel hydrogen bond with Asn135,

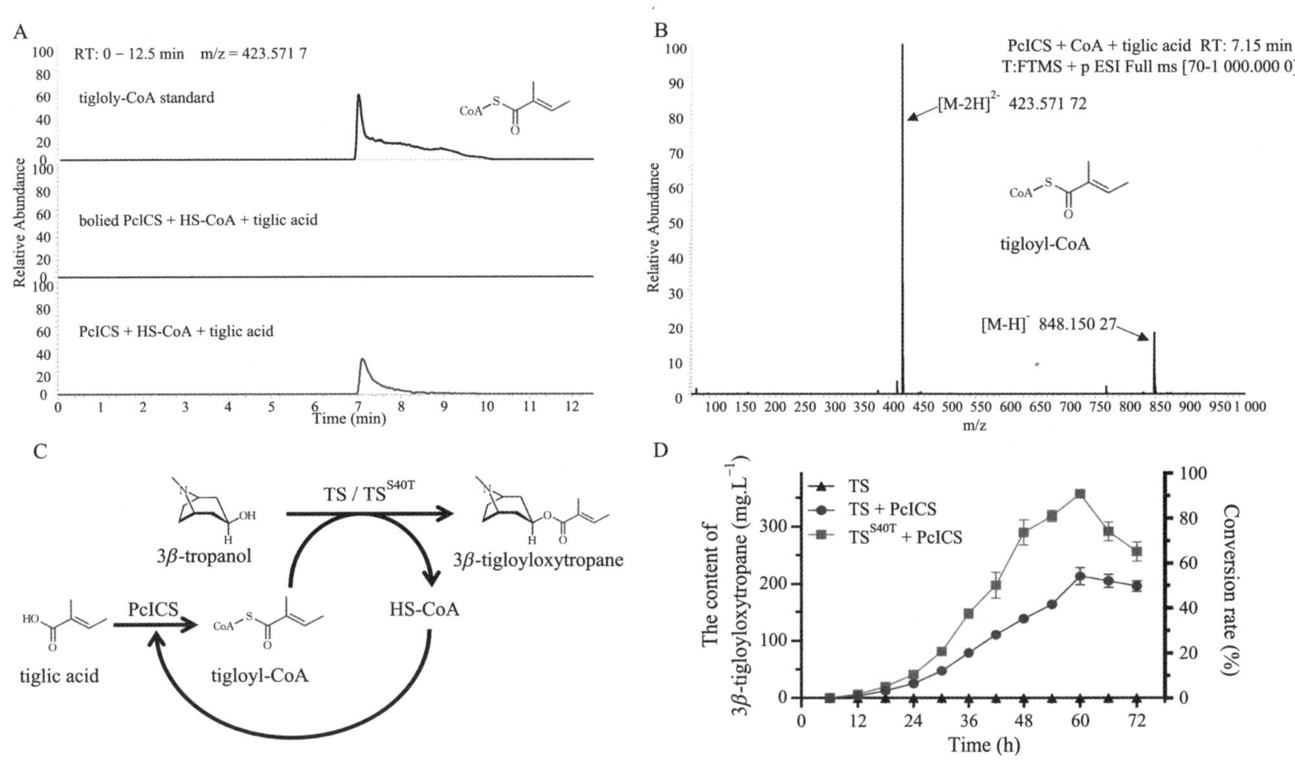


**Fig. 8 *E. coli* bioreactors for the biosynthesis of 3β-tropanol esters**

(A) PcICS enzymatic assays. (B) MS data of tigloyl-CoA. (C) Semi-biosynthetic route of 3β-tigloyloxytropane. (D) Production of 3β-tigloyloxytropane. Left Y-axis, the content of 3β-tigloyloxytropane. Right Y-axis, the conversion rate from 3β-tropanol to 3β-tigloyloxytropane. HS-CoA means coenzyme A (CoA). Three independent transformants of each engineered *E. coli* were used in the semi-biosynthesis of 3β-tigloyloxytropane. The data are presented as means values±s. d.

which was not present in TS. These intramolecular interactions play an important role in enzyme stability by rigidifying the active center. Thus, the hydrogen bond between Thr40 and Asn135 may contribute to the stability of the 3β-tropanol binding pocket, thereby improving the catalytic activity of the enzyme.

Consistent with the in vitro enzyme activity assays, the $TS^{S40T}$ also exhibited higher esterification activity than TS in engineered tobacco, in which a de novo biosynthetic pathway for 3β-tropanol esters was constructed (Fig. 7). Although our results demonstrated the feasibility of synthesizing 3β-tigloyloxytropane from tobacco, the very low levels of 3β-tigloyloxytropane prevented the use of tobacco as an ideal platform for 3β-tigloyloxytropane production. Most of the metabolic flux was directed toward hygrine rather than towards 3β-tigloyloxytropane, and an insufficient supply of intermediates might limit 3β-tigloyloxytropane production (Fig. 7). To produce 3β-tigloyloxytropane more efficiently, we designed engineered strains of *E. coli* for the semi-biosynthesis of 3β-tigloyloxytropane. To overcome the limitation of lack of tigloyl-CoA in *E. coli* and improve the efficiency, we employed PcICS from *Pseudomonas chlororaphis*. The advantages were obvious. On the one hand, using the substrate promiscuity of PcICS, synthesis of tigloyl-CoA from CoA and tiglic acid, increased the supply of tigloyl-CoA (Fig. 8C). On the other hand, CoA, the products of TS, can be used as substrates for PcICS (Fig. 8C). In this CoA recycling system, the expensive substrate, CoA, originated from *E. coli* itself and was continuously regenerated and utilized (Fig. 8C). Combined with the utilization of the highly efficient TS mutant, $TS^{S40T}$, we constructed a semi-biosynthesis 3β-tigloyloxytropane production system using only two readily available substrates, 3β-tropanol and tiglic acid and achieved 357.40 mg/L 3β-tigloyloxytropane production with 90.9% conversion rate (Fig. 8D).

To summarize, in this study, we identified the missing step in 3β-tigloyloxytropane formation by identifying the mitochondrion-localized BAHD acyltransferase 3β-tigloyloxytropane synthase (TS). We revealed the catalytic mechanism of TS and successfully improved its activity. Finally, we managed to reconstitute 3β-tigloyloxytropane biosynthesis in tobacco and *E. coli*. Our study helps characterize the enzymology and chemical diversity of TAs and provides an approach for producing 3β-tigloyloxytropane through synthetic biology.

## 3 METHODS

Chemical synthesis As commercial standards of 3β-tigloyloxytropane, 3β-acetoxytropane, 3β-benzoyloxytropane and tigloyl-CoA are not available, these three compounds were chemically synthesized in our laboratory. The synthetic methods used were described previously. The acids were converted to acyl chloride derivatives and then reacted with 3β-tropanol to prepare 3β-tropanol esters. Tigloyl-CoA thioesters were synthesized from CoA and free acid via the catalysis of PyBOP.

To generate tigloyl chloride/acetyl chloride/benzoyl chloride: Tiglic acid/acetic acid/benzoic acid (10 mmol, 1 equivalent) was added portion-wise to oxalyl chloride (20 mmol, 1.50 equivalent), followed by one drop of N, N-dimethylformamide. After 2.5 h, the excess oxalyl chloride was removed under reduced pressure to provide tigloyl chloride/acetyl chloride as a light-yellow liquid.

3β-Tigloyloxytropane/3β-acetoxytropane/3β-benzoyloxytropane: 3β-tropanol (0.79 mmol, 1 equivalent) was dissolved in 5 ml of anhydrous tetrahydrofuran in a round-bottomed flask with a molecular sieve (0.4 nm), after which 4-dimethylaminopyridine (DMAP; 0.04 mmol) and triethylamine (1.58 mmol, 2 equivalent) were added. An inert atmosphere was established and maintained by a continuous flow rate of nitrogen. The mixture was cooled in an ice bath, after which tigloyl chloride/acetyl chloride (2.37 mmol, 3 equivalents) was introduced dropwise. The reaction mixture was left at 25 ℃, under agitation, for 2 h, diluted with a saturated solution of $Na_2CO_3$ (10 mL) and distilled water (20 mL), and subsequently extracted with chloroform (3 × 30 mL). The organic portion was dried with anhydrous sodium salfate and concentrated under reduced pressure at 35 ℃. Then, the product was further purified by thin-layer chromatography and high-performance liquid chromatography (HPLC).

Tigloyi-CoA: Tiglic acid (50 μmol, 5.0 equivalent), PyBOP (16 μmol, 1.6 equivalent), and $K_2CO_3$ (40 μmol, 4.0 equivalent) were dissolved in 3 mL of freshly distilled tetrahydrofuran (THF) under argon. CoA (10 μmol, 1.0 equivalent) was dissolved in 1 mL of $H_2O$ ($O_2$ was removed by sonication) and added dropwise to the THF solution. After stirring at 25 ℃ for 3 h, the reaction mixture was directly subjected to a HPLC on C18 semi-preparative reversed-phase column.

The fragment ions were analyzed through high-resolution tandem mass spectrometry (MS/MS) analysis to preliminarily determine their structures (Supplementary Fig. S1 - S4). Nuclear magnetic resonance (NMR), specifically, $^1$H-NMR, $^{13}$C-NMR, and 2D-NMR, was used to further confirm the structures of the synthesized compounds (Supplementary Fig. S5 - S24 and Supplementary Data 1).

Bioinformatics analysis Hidden Markov Model (HMM) for BAHD-ATs (PF02458) was used to identify the BAHD genes through the hmmsearch program against *A. belladonna* transcriptomes from the Medicinal Plant Genomics Resource (http://mpgr.uga.edu/) in HMMER 3.3.2. Batch CD-Search (https://www.ncbi.nlm.nih.gov/Structure/bwrpsb/bwrpsb.cgi) was used to further confirm that the candidate genes belonged to the BAHD-AT family. TBtools-II v2.042 was used to construct a heatmap of the association analysis of the metabolites and BAHD gene family expression patterns. Amino acid sequence alignment was performed using the E-INS-I method in MAFFT v7.475. The phylogenetic tree was constructed using IQ-TREE v2.1.2 with the maximum likelihood model (LG+F+G4). The tree was rooted using the algal enzyme clade (clade 0) and classified according to the previous method. In addition, the tree was annotated and visualized with iTOL v6.

Expression analysis of *TS* Different organs, including the secondary roots, primary roots, mature seeds, ripe fruits, flowers, stems, green fruits, and leaves, were harvested from 4-month-old *A. belladonna* plants; these organs were used for RNA isolation and cDNA synthesis via kits from TIANGEN Biotech (Beijing, China). Real-time quantitative PCR was used to analyze the tissue profile of TS using an iQ5 system (Bio-Rad, USA), with *PGK* serving reference gene. Amplifications were carried out using SYBR Green PCR MasterMix (Novoprotein, Shanghai, China). The primers used for qPCR are listed in Supplementary Table S1.

Purification of MBP-tagged TS and enzymatic assay To obtain sufficient protein for biochemical characterization, the coding sequence of TS was synthesized according to the codon usage bias of *E. coli*, forming a codon-optimized version designated TSopt. The coding sequence of TSopt was amplified by a pair of primers with BamHI and PstI restriction sites and then inserted into pMAL-c5x to generate the prokaryotic expression plasmid, pMAL-c5x-TS. The primers used to construct the vectors are listed in Supplementary Table S1. The pMAL-c5x-TS plasmid was subsequently introduced into *E. coli* BL21 (DE3) for expression. Protein expression was induced overnight at 16℃ with 0.25 mmol/L IPTG in LB medium. The MBP-tagged TS protein was purified using amylose resin (Smart-Lifesciences). After desalting, fresh proteins were immediately subjected to enzymatic assays. 3β-Tropanol was combined with three different acyl donors (tigloyl-CoA, benzoyl-CoA, and acetyl-CoA) to form a substrate for three groups of enzymatic assays. The reaction mixture was 50 mmol/L glycine-NaOH buffer containing 20 μg of purified TS, 1 mmol/L 3β-tropanol and tigloyl-CoA (or benzoyl-CoA or acetyl-CoA).

To explore the optimal reaction conditions of TS, a pH range from 6 to 10.6 and a temperature range from 20 ℃ to 50 ℃ were tested with tigloyl-CoA and 3β-tropanol. Finally, the enzyme kinetics were measured at pH 8.6 and 30 ℃. Various concentrations of 3β-tropanol (0.01 - 2 mmol/L) and tigloyl-CoA (or benzoyl-CoA, acetyl-CoA) (0.01-1 mmol/L) were used for the analysis of enzyme kinetics.

Subcellular localization analysis Subcellular localization prediction of TS was performed using TargetP-2.0 (https://services.healthtech.dtu.dk/services/TargetP-2.0/). The coding sequence of TS, 32 amino acids at its N-terminus, and TS without 32 amino acids at its N-terminus were amplified by a pair of primers with *Bgl*II and *Hind*III restriction sites and then inserted into the plant expression vector pGD3G-YFP to generate pGD3G-TS-YFP, pGD3G-N32-YFP, and pGD3G-$TS^{Del\text{-}N32}$-YFP. The primers used for vector construction are listed in Supplementary Table S1. Subsequently, the constructs were subsequently transferred into the *A. tumefaciens* strain GV3101, which was subsequently cotransformed into *N. benthamiana* leaves. After 48 h of cultivation, the leaves were prepared into protoplasts and treated with MitoTracker Red (Beyotime, Shanghai, China). The Confocal microscopy (Olympus FV1200) was used to analyze the subcellular localization of TS. Red fluorescence was emitted from the MitoTracker Red. Yellow fluorescence was emitted from TS-YFP, N32-YFP, and $TS^{Del\text{-}N32}$-YFP.

To further determine the localization of TS in *A. belladonna*, mitochondria were extracted from the roots of 2-month-old *A. belladonna* plants. After differential centrifugation was performed to separate mitochondria, the following steps were performed: I. Ten grams of fresh roots were frozen in liquid nitrogen and ground thoroughly into a fine powder. II. Add Mitochondrial extraction buffer (70 mmol/L sucrose, 210 mmol/L mannitol, 10 mmol/L HEPES, 1 mmol/L EDTA, 1 mmol/L PMSF, pH 7.5) was added, and the samples were homogenized with a Dounce tissue grinder for 10 cycles. III. The homogenate obtained in the previous step was centrifuged at 600 × g for 10 min at 4 ℃, after which the supernatant was collected. IV. Centrifuge at 1 200 × g for 10 min at 4 ℃ and collect the supernatant. V. Centrifuge at 11,000 × g for 20 min at 4 ℃. The supernatant obtained at this stage was the cytosol, and the pellet was the mitochondria. Western blotting was also conducted to further determine the mitochondria and cytosol content. Western blotting was performed with an anti-VDAC1 antibody (rabbit, 1 : 2 000 dilution), which was used as a mitochondrial marker. The anti-VDAC1 antibody was purchased from Orizymes with Catalog Number PAB220312. Goat anti-rabbit IgG antibody (goat, 1 : 5 000 dilution) was used as the secondary antibody. The Goat anti-rabbit IgG antibody was purchased from Biosharp with Catalog Number BL003A. The chemiluminescent signals were detected using a Tanon 5 200 Fully Automatic Chemiluminescence Image Analysis System (TANON, Shanghai, China). Next, the cytosol and mitochondria were treated using ultrasound (20 kHz, ultrasound for 3 s, stop for 7 s, 50 cycles) and the protein concentration was measured using the BCA method. Then, the crude protein from the mitochondria/cytosol was incubated with the substrate for the enzymatic assay. The reaction mixture was 50 mmol/L glycine-NaOH buffer (pH 8.6) containing 50 μg of crude protein from mitochondria/cytosol, 1 mM 3β-tropanol, and tigloyl-CoA.

Virus-induced gene silencing (VIGS) A 538 bp TS fragment was inserted into the tobacco rattle virus (TRV) vector (pTRV2) using the restriction enzymes XhoI and KpnI to construct the plasmid pTRV2-TS. The primers used for vector construction are listed in Supplementary Table S1. Then, pTRV1 and pTRV2-TS were co-introduced into *Agrobacterium tumefaciens* GV3101, which was subsequently transiently transformed into 18-day-old *A. belladonna* cotyledons. The pTRV1 and pTRV2 plasmids were co-introduced as control groups. After 28 days, the roots were subjected to expression and metabolite analysis. The operation process of VIGS that was used in the present study was previously reported.

Overexpression of TS in hairy root cultures of *A. belladonna* The *TS* coding sequence was amplified by a pair of primers with *Bam*HI and *Sac*I restriction sites and then inserted into pBI121 to generate the plant expression vector, pBI121-TS. The primers used for vector construction are listed in Supplementary Table S1. To evaluate the effects of TS overexpression on the biosynthesis of TAs, we established root cultures of *A. belladonna* through *Agrobacterium*-mediated transformation. Root cultures of *A. belladonna* were established according to methods already described. The root cultures were grown in a flask containing 100 mL of Murashige and Skoog liquid media and harvested after they had been cultured for 28 days at 25 ℃ in darkness. Eight root lines, independently transformed with pBI121, were used as control root cultures (CK group). Four lines with significantly increased expression of target genes (OE-1, OE-2, OE-3, and OE-4), independently transformed by the corresponding engineered vectors, were randomly selected for metabolite analysis.

Metabolite analysis Freeze-dried root cultures, including those of the roots and hairy roots of *A. belladonna* and tobacco leaves, were ground into fine powder and used for alkaloid extraction. The extraction and detection of these TAs were based on a previously reported methodology. In brief, 250 mg of dry root powder was placed in 1 mL of extraction buffer (20% methanol, containing 0.1% formic acid) and shaken for 2 h at 200 r/min and 25 ℃. Each extract was passed through a 0.22 μm Nylon 66 filter (Jinteng, Tianjin, China), and the filtrate was subsequently diluted 100-fold for future analysis. The alkaloid content in the extract was analyzed by an Orbitrap Exploris 120 LC - MS (Thermo Scientific, Pittsburgh, PA, USA). Measurements were performed using electron spray ionization (ESI) in positive ion mode and full MS mode. The instrument parameters were set as follows: sheath gas flow rate of 35, aux gas flow rate of 10, spray voltage of 3.00 kV, capillary temperature of 350 ℃, S-lens RF level of 50, aux gas heater temperature of 350 ℃. The level of High Energy Collision Dissociation was 30 in MS/MS analysis.

3β-Acetoxytropane, hygrine, tropinone, 3α-tropanol, and 3β-tropanol were analyzed using a CORTECS UPLC HILIC column (2.1 mm × 100 mm, 1.6 μm) obtained from Thermo Scientific (Pittsburgh, PA, USA). The system's flow rate was 0.3 mL/min, and the temperature was 35 ℃. The sample solution per injection was 3 μL; the elution procedures are described in Supplementary Table S2.

3β-Tigloyloxytropane, 3β-benzoyloxytropane, littorine, hyoscyamine, anisodamine, scopolamine, tropanol hexosides, tigloyl norpseudotropine, tigloyl 1-hydroxynorpseudotropine and calystegines A3 were analyzed with a Hypersil GOLD C18 column (2.1 mm × 100 mm, 1.9 μm) obtained from Thermo Scientific (Pittsburgh, PA, USA), for which the sample solution per injection was 3 μL. The system's flow rate was 0.3 mL/min, and the temperature was 35 ℃. The corresponding elution procedures are detailed in Supplementary Table S3.

Molecular simulation  AlphaFold2 v2.3.0 was used for building the protein model of TS and predicting the substrate pocket. The ligands (3β-tropanol, acetyl-CoA, tigloyl-CoA and benzoyl-CoA) were downloaded from the Pub-Chem database (https://pubchem.ncbi.nlm.nih.gov/) and docked into the cofactor-binding site of TS using AutoDock Tools v1.5.6. Then, independent docking runs for different substrates with TS were generated and complex structures with lower binding energies and favorable orientations were selected. The interactions between the substrates and TS were analyzed using PLIP v2.3.0. PyMOL 2.1 (http://www.pymol.org) was used to view the molecular interactions and process the image.

Consensus protein design  Consensus protein design is based on the hypothesis that at a given position, compared with nonconserved amino acids, the respective consensus amino acid contributes more than average to the stability of the protein. Through BLASTP from NCBI server, genes with more than 50% identity to the TS amino acid sequence from the public database were obtained for consensus protein design. Conservative substitution analysis was performed on residues within the 5 Å range centered on His162 in TS. The seqlogo drawn by TBtools-II v2.042 displayed conservative substitutions.

Biosynthesis of 3β-tigloyloxytropane in *N. benthamiana*  For the de novo synthesis of 3β-tropanol esters in *N. benthamiana*, EnODC, AbPMT, AbMPO, AbPYKS, AbCYP82M3, DsTRII, and AbTS (or its mutants) were coexpressed in tobacco leaves. The coding sequences of these genes were amplified by a pair of primers with AgeI and XhoI restriction sites and then inserted into pEAQ-HT to generate a series of transient expression vectors. The primers used for vector construction are listed in Supplementary Table S1. These transient expression vectors were subsequently introduced into *Agrobacterium tumefaciens* GV3101 and transiently transformed into tobacco leaves. After 5 days of cultivation, the leaves were harvested and subjected to metabolite analysis.

In the semi-synthetic experiment of tobacco, PcICS optimized according to tobacco codons was constructed into pEAQ-HT. Then, AbTS (or its mutants) and PcICS were expressed in the tobacco leaves via a process mediated by GV3101. 2 Days later, tobacco leaves were fed 3β-tropanol and tiglic acid at a concentration of 1 mM. After 3 days of cultivation, the leaves were harvested and subjected to metabolite analysis.

Biosynthesis of 3β-tigloyloxytropane in *E. coli*  The coding sequences of TS (or its mutants) and PcICS were inserted into pETDuet-1 to generate a series of prokaryotic expression vectors. The primers used for vector construction are listed in Supplementary Table S1. Then, these prokaryotic expression vectors were introduced into *E. coli* (BL21). The engineered *E. coli* was cultured in 100 mL of LB liquid medium to an OD600 of 0.6. Next, IPTG was added to a final concentration of 0.25 mmol/L and substrate of 250 mg/L (tiglic acid and 3β-tropanol) of substrate was added to the culture medium. One milliliter of culture solution was added every 6 h for product content analysis.

Statistics and reproducibility  GraphPad Prism 8 software was used for regular statistical analysis and enzyme kinetic analysis. A two-tailed Student's *t*-test was used to calculate significant differences among samples or genotypes. Details of biological replicates used in various experiments are provided in the "Methods" section as well as in the main figures and Supplementary Figs. legends, wherever necessary. No statistical method was used to predetermine the sample size. No data were excluded from the analyses. Four lines with significantly increased expression of target genes (OE-1, OE-2, OE-3, and OE-4), independently transformed by the corresponding engineered vectors, were randomly selected for metabolite analysis.

[曾俊岗，廖志华，等. Nature Communications, 2024, 15: 3623.]

# A prenyltransferase participates in the biosynthesis of anthraquinones in *Rubia cordifolia*

## 1 INTRODUCTION

Natural anthraquinones (AQs) and their derivatives are the largest group of natural quinones, most of which are produced by plants, lichens, and fungi. Plant-derived AQs are mainly distributed in the families Polygonaceae, Rubiaceae, Leguminosae, Rhamnaceae, Scrophulariaceae, Liliaceae, Verbenaceae, and Valerianaceae. AQ-rich plants in these families, for instance, Chinese Rhubarb (*Rheum palmatum*), Heshouwu (*Polygoni multiflora*), Madder (*Rubia cordifolia*), Bajitian (*Morinda officinalis*), and Sicklepod (*Cassia obtusifolia*), have been used to treat various diseases for centuries in China. Modern pharmacological studies have proved that AQs had potent anticancer, antipathogenic microorganisms, antioxidation, antiosteoporosis, anti-inflammatory, anti-injury, antidepression, anticonstipation, and other pharmacological activities. In addition, due to the inclusion of numerous chromophore groups and auxochrome groups in the basic skeleton, natural AQs are dark in color and have been used as natural dyes since ancient times.

Plant-derived AQs have the most common structure of 9,10-AQ with three rings and can be classified as emodintype AQs or alizarin-type AQs based on the presence of two or one hydroxylated rings in the structure. Two main distinct biosynthetic pathways leading to AQs have been reported: the polyketide pathway for emodin-type AQs and the shikimate pathway for alizarin-type AQs. Tracer studies and phytochemical analyses support the view that alizarin-type AQs found in Rubiaceae, Bignoniaceae, and Verbenaceae are formed by the latter pathway. This pathway comprises three parts (Fig. 1): ① conversion of shikimate to the naphthoquinone (NQ) head-group precursor 1, 4-dihydroxy-2-naphthoic acid (DHNA), which gives rise to ring A and B of AQs. ② synthesis of 3, 3-dimethylallyl pyrophosphate (DMAPP), which is carried out via the MEP pathway in Rubiaceae. ③ attachment of DMAPP to the head group and ring closure to produce the ring C. The same biosynthetic logic also applies to NQs of plants, for example, shikonin and chimaphilin. In these compounds, ring A is derived from shikimate. The prenylation step and subsequent cyclization result in the formation of ring B (Fig. 1). Obviously, the DHNA-prenylation step is of key importance for the formation of the AQ structure in the shikimate pathway.

DHNA-prenylation reactions are generally catalyzed by membrane-bound prenyltransferases (PTs) belonging to the UbiA superfamily. DHNA PT, i. e. MenA, was identified in *Escherichia coli* as a DHNA-octaprenyltransferase involved in the biosynthesis of menaquinone. Then DHNA-phytyltransferases, homologs of MenA, were identified from cyanobacteria and land plants and confirmed to be involved in the synthesis of phylloquinone. In animals, UBIAD1, a homolog of MenA, is the PT for menaquinone-4 (MK4) biosynthesis and is associated with many physiological processes and diseases. However, the gene encoding the DHNA-dimethylallyltransferase (DHNA-DT) that leads to the formation of ring C in alizarin-type AQs is yet to be discovered. Whether it is also homologous to MenA remains unknown.

In this context, a cell suspension culture of *R. cordifolia*, a representative species of Rubiaceae, was used as material for analyzing the biosynthetic pathway of alizarin-type AQs. The microsomal fraction prepared from this material exhibited DHNA-DT activity. Then, the PT gene *Rubia cordifolia* dimethylallyltransferase 1 (*RcDT1*) was cloned from the cell suspension culture and proved to be responsible for the activity. RNA interference combined with expression profile and subcellular localization analyses confirmed the participation of RcDT1 in alizarin-type AQs biosynthesis. Biochemical studies and phylogenetic analyses highlighted the differences in reaction mechanism and evolution between RcDT1 and MenA. These results have deepened the understanding of AQ biosynthesis in the shikimate pathway and would have profound implications for elucidating the subsequent cyclization steps in AQ biosynthesis by the shikimate pathway.

## 2 RESULTS

Enzymatic activity of *R. cordifolia* microsomes Plant cell suspension cultures are fundamental research tools for elucidating the biosynthesis of plant specialized metabolites. In order to explore the DHNA-prenylation activity in alizarin-type AQ biosynthesis, *R. cordifolia*, a representative species of Rubiaceae, was chosen for research, and its cell suspension culture was established. As in a previous study, Munjistin (0.66% to 0.81% by dry weight) and purpurin (0.33% to 0.40% by dry weight) were identified as the major alizarin-type AQs produced by this plant material (Supplementary Fig. S1). The microsomal fraction was extracted and incubated with DHNA (**1**), the biosynthetic

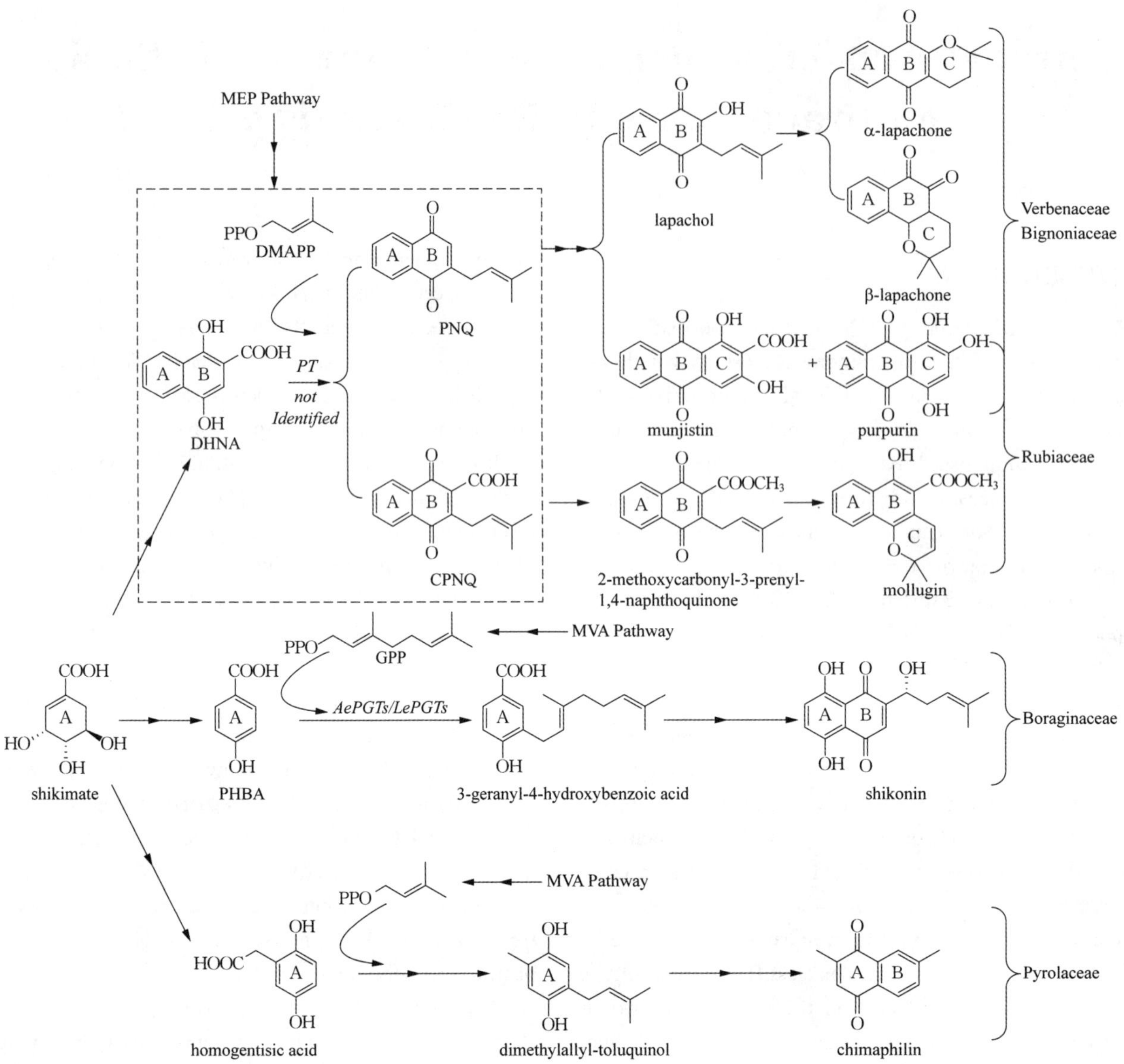

**Figure 1 Biosynthetic pathways of shikimate-derived naphthoquinones and AQs in land plants**

The problem addressed in this study is highlighted in the dotted box. MVA, mevalonate; MEP, methylerythritol 4-phosphate; DMAPP, dimethylallyl diphosphate; GPP, geranyl diphosphate; DHNA, 1, 4-dihydroxy-2-naphthoic acid; CPNQ, 2-carboxyl-3-prenyl-1, 4-naphthoquinone; PNQ, 3-prenyl-1, 4-naphthoquinone; PHBA, 4-hydroxybenzoic acid; PT, prenyltransferase.

intermediate of alizarin-type AQs, together with the prenyl donor DMAPP. Considering that UbiA PTs are strictly dependent on divalent metal ions, $Mg^{2+}$, the ion most commonly used by UbiA PTs, was also included in the reaction system. As a result, a major product **1a** and a minor product **1b** were detected simultaneously at retention times of 1.8 and 4.4 min (Fig. 2B). Product formation was strictly dependent on the presence of DHNA, DMAPP, $Mg^{2+}$, and the active microsomal protein. HPLC-UV/ESI MS analysis revealed that the molecular weight of the major product (**1a**) was 66 amu higher than DHNA (**1**), indicating that DHNA (**1**) was prenylated (68-amu increase in molecular weight) and oxidized to naphthoquinone (2-amu decrease in molecular weight) (Fig. 2D and E). Previously, tracer studies and phytochemical analyses have confirmed that prenylation during the biosynthesis of alizarin-type AQs in Rubiaceae occurred at the position C-3 of DHNA (**1**). Accordingly, the chemical structure of the major product **1a** was inferred to be 2-carbonyl-3-prenyl-1, 4-naphthoquinone (CPNQ), which was likely to be a branch point in the biosynthetic pathway leading to AQ and naphthohydroquinone (NHQ, e. g. mollugin) derivatives (Figs. 1 and 2A). Through comparing with an authentic standard using HPLC-UV/ESI MS analysis, the minor product **1b** was identified as 2-prenyl-1, 4-naphthoquinone (PNQ, i. e. deoxylapachol) (Fig. 2A, B, and F). Both the molecular weight of **1b** (44-amu less than **1a**) and the mass spectrometry fragmentation of **1a** and **1b** supported that decarboxylation of **1a** produced **1b** (Fig. 2E and F). Since $\beta$-keto acid decarboxylation was known in both organic chemistry and biocatalysis, PNQ (**1b**)

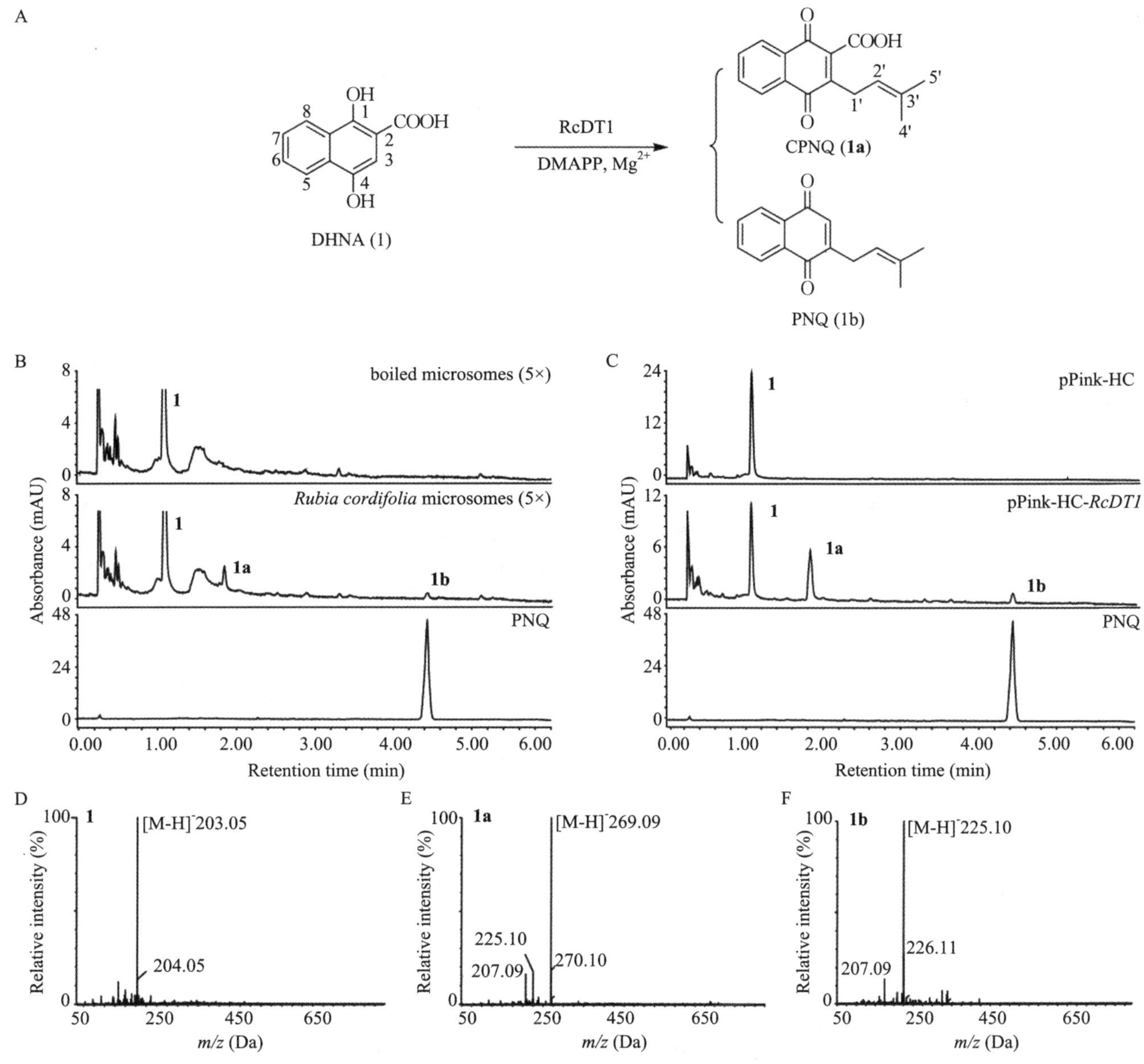


**Figure 2 Functional characterization of *R. cordifolia* microsomes and recombinant RcDT1**

The detection wavelength is set at 254 nm. PNQ is used as an authentic standard.
(A) Reaction mode diagram by *R. cordifolia* microsomes. The chemical structures of the compounds and corresponding peaks in UPLC chromatogram are marked as **1**, **1a**, and **1b**. (B) UPLC traces for the reactions containing DHNA (**1**) with active or boiled *R. cordifolia* microsomes. (C) UPLC traces for the reactions containing DHNA (**1**) with recombinant RcDT1 microsomes or microsomal extract from yeast transformed with empty vector. (D) ESI MS (negative mode) spectrum of DHNA (**1**). (E) ESI MS (negative mode) spectrum of the product **1a**. (F) ESI MS (negative mode) spectrum of the product **1b**. DHNA, 1, 4-dihydroxy-2-naphthoic acid; CPNQ, 2-carboxyl-3-prenyl-1, 4-naphthoquinone; PNQ, 3-prenyl-1, 4-naphthoquinone; $m/z$, mass to charge ratio.

was assumed to be formed through spontaneous decarboxylation of CPNQ (**1a**). This prenylation reaction mode was different from that observed in MenA, which catalyzed the C-2 prenylation of DHNA (**1**). Due to the instability of CPNQ (**1a**), the attempt to isolate **1a** in the solid state from the reaction system failed, and the decarboxylation of **1a** has not been further studied in vitro.

Cloning and characterization of *RcDTs* from the cell suspension culture of *R. cordifolia* To mine the DHNA (**1**) PT gene(s) responsible for the prenylati on catalyzed by cultured *R. cordifolia* cells, an RNA-seq library was prepared and then used for transcriptome analysis. Dark-maintained *R. cordifolia* cell suspension cultures in sucrose-containing MS medium were used for RNA-seq in culture day 10. An *ab*errant *c*hloroplast development relevant gene (*AtABC4*) homologous to MenA and involved in phylloquinone biosynthesis in Thale Cress (*Arabidopsis thaliana*), a *p*-hydroxybenzoate geranyltransferase (*LePGT1*) from Gromwell (*Lithospermum erythrorhizon*), a *p*-hydroxybenzoate geranyltransferase (*AePGT6*) from Ratanjot (*Arnebia* *euchroma*), and a naringenin *8-d*imethylallyltransferase (*SfN8DT-1*) from Kushen (*Sophora flavescens*) were employed as queries to search the transcriptome database independently. As a result, the search yielded six putative aromatic PT genes, *RcDT1* – *6*. No candidate gene with a certain similarity (*E*-value <1) to *AtABC4* was found. This is consistent with the finding that phylloquinone was not detected in the cell suspension culture of *R. cordifolia* (Supplementary Fig. S2), indicating that DHNA is mainly involved in the biosynthesis of AQs rather than phylloquinone. As described in a previous study, darkness cultivation and sucrose in the medium were thought to be responsible for the inhibition of phylloquinone biosynthesis.

The encoded polypeptides of *RcDT1* – *6* had 5 to 8 putative transmembrane α-helices as predicted by the DeepTMHMM program. A multiple alignment of the encoded polypeptides and query UbiA enzymes is shown in Supplementary Fig. S3. The polypeptides possessed two conserved aspartate-rich motifs N (Q/D) XXDXXXD and DXXDXXXD. The former motif is commonly thought to be involved in the binding of prenyl diphosphate. The latter motif exhibited a high degree of variability in the alignment. SignalP-6.0 predictions indicated that the polypeptides possess N-terminal signal peptides in the length range of 20 to 70. The above data matched the typical structural characteristics of plant aromatic PTs.

The methylotrophic yeast *Pichia pastoris* is now one of the standard tools used in molecular biology for the generation of recombinant protein, with the ability to produce foreign proteins at high levels and perform many eukaryotic posttranslational modifications. Previous studies had shown that N-terminal truncation usually increased the enzymatic activity of heterologously expressed UbiA enzymes. Consequently, *RcDT1* – *6* with an N-terminal truncation of 24 amino acids were expressed in *P. pastoris* to detect their prenylation activity against DHNA (**1**). As a result, incubation of DHNA (**1**) and DMAPP with the recombinant *RcDT1* microsomes in the presence of $Mg^{2+}$ led to the detection of CPNQ (**1a**) and PNQ (**1b**) (Fig. 2C). Product formation was strictly dependent on the presence of **1**, DMAPP and the active recombinant *RcDT1* microsomal protein. This was consistent with the results obtained with *R. cordifolia* microsome, and the transformation efficiency was increased substantially (Fig. 2B and C). We further compared the activities of truncated and untruncated *RcDT1*. As predicted by SignalP-6.0, *RcDT1* possesses an N-terminal signal peptide of 70 amino acids. Truncated *RcDT1* with a 24, 48, 72 amino acid deletion from the start codon were not substantially different in activity, which were 7.5 times more active than untruncated *RcDT1*. Since *RcDT1* shared high identities with *PGTs* (50.16% to 54.42% at the amino acid level) and *PGTs* possess no signal peptide, the signal peptide of *RcDT1* was finally determined through alignment with *PGTs* (Supplementary Fig. S3). In subsequent experiments, the truncated *RcDT1* with a 72 amino acid deletion at the N-terminal was selected to study the biochemical properties. Due to the lack of activity when using DHNA (**1**) as the substrate, the candidate genes *RcDT2* – *6* were not investigated further.

Biochemical properties of the recombinant RcDT1 Previous studies have shown that PT activity in plants was strongly affected by divalent cations, temperature and pH. Further investigations using DHNA (**1**) as the prenyl acceptor and DMAPP as the prenyl donor revealed that the optimum reaction temperature of recombinant RcDT1 was 30℃, and more than 60% of the activity was maintained at a temperature up to 50 ℃ (Fig. 3A). The analysis of the enzyme activity within the pH range of 6.5 to 10.5 revealed that the optimal pH value was about 8.5, and the activity decreased rapidly at pH above 9.0 (Fig. 3B). The activity of recombinant RcDT1 was observed to decrease in the order of $Mg^{2+} > Fe^{2+} > Mn^{2+} > Co^{2+} > Cu^{2+}$. $Ca^{2+}$, $Ni^{2+}$, and $Zn^{2+}$ did not lead to the production of CPNQ (**1a**) and PNQ (**1b**). No product was detected in the reaction buffer after the addition of EDTA (Fig. 3C).

Substrate specificities of the recombinant RcDT1 To investigate the prenyl acceptor specificities of recombinant RcDT1, we tested 23 potential acceptors, including various types of naphthoic acids and a naphthalene (**1** – **8**), benzoic acids (**9** – **18**), phenylacetic acids (**19**, **20**), and phenylpropanes (**21** – **23**) (Fig. 4B). The results showed that RcDT1 could accept both naphthoic acids **1** – **5** and benzoic acids **9** – **13** as prenyl acceptors (Fig. 4C). The enzymatic products of **2**, **3**, **9**, and **11** were prepared from larger scale assays and subjected to MS and NMR spectroscopic analyses (Fig. 4A and Supplementary Table S1). The chemical structure of the enzymatic product of **10** was confirmed by UPLC-UV/ESI MS analysis (Supplementary Fig. S10). The prenylated products of **4**, **5**, and **13** were not prepared successfully due to the relative low yields. For naphthoic acid substrates, one dimethylallyl moiety was introduced into the carboxyl-bearing ring at the position C-3 or C-4 (Fig. 4A). For benzoic acid substrates, one dimethylallyl moiety was regioselectively introduced into the *ortho* position of the 4-hydroxyl group (Fig. 4A).

The reactivities of RcDT1 toward different naphthoic acids and benzoic acids provided insight into the reaction mechanism and enzyme selectivity. First, the relative conversion rate of DHNA (**1**) was the highest among all the substrates, indicating that it was the natural substrate of RcDT1. Regarding the recognition of DHNA (**1**), the existence of unsubstituted 2-carboxyl was crucial because the

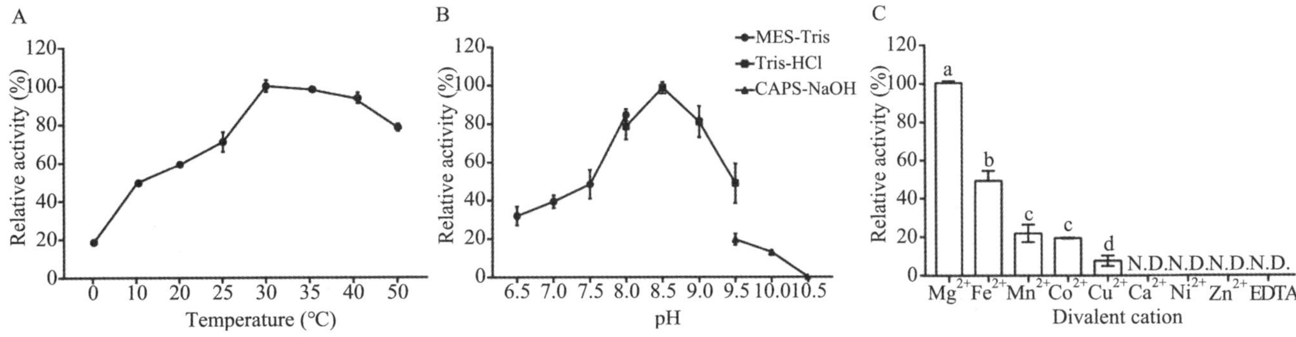


**Figure 3 Biochemical properties of the recombinant RcDT1**

(A) The effects of different temperatures on the activity of recombinant RcDT1. (B) pH dependences of recombinant RcDT1. (C) The effects of different divalent cations on the activity of recombinant RcDT1. One-way ANOVA was used to compare the relative activity. Different lowercase letters indicate significant differences ($P<0.05$). N. D., not detected. The maximum activity levels of RcDT1 were assumed to be 100%. All data represent the mean±SD of three biological replicates. MES, 2-morpholinoethanesulphonic acid; CAPS, N-cyclohexyl-3-aminopropanesulfonic acid; Tris, 2-amino-2- ( hydroxymethyl )-1, 3-propanediol; EDTA, ethylenediaminetetraacetic acid.

absence (**8**) or the methylation (**7**) of 2-carboxyl led to no enzymatic product generation. The prenylation could still take place in C-1/3/4 hydroxylated 2-naphthoic acid (**2**, **3**, and **5**) and 2-hydroxy-1-naphthoic acid (**4**). However, the loss of the hydroxyl groups in the carboxyl-bearing ring led to no prenylation (**6**). The unsubstituted ring in the recognized naphthoic acids (**1** - **5**) also played an important role in substrate recognition because the benzoic acid substructure fragments (**14** - **16**) of **1** - **5** could not be prenylated. To summarize, naphthoic acids with hydroxyl(s) in the carboxyl-bearing ring were putative substrates of RcDT1.

The prenylations are electrophilic substitution reactions, and the reaction mechanism includes a prenyl carbocation. As observed in the experiments, the prenyl substitution occurred at the position with sufficient electron density (e.g. C-4 of **3**). It is worth noting that decarboxylation is not observed for the other available naphthoic acids except DHNA (**1**). This result could be interpreted that β-keto in CPNQ (**1a**), which was generated by spontaneous oxidation, was a prerequisite for the decarboxylation. Therefore, the reaction mechanism of DHNA prenylation by RcDT1 could be summarized as follows: dimethylallyl moiety was firstly introduced into the C-3 of DHNA; then the naphthol structure was oxidized to NQ spontaneously to produce CPNQ (**1a**); at last, the decarboxylation of CPNQ (**1a**) led to the generation of PNQ (**1b**).

In addition to naphthoic acids, RcDT1 also exhibited relatively high catalytic activity toward benzoic acids (Fig. 4C). For the recognition of benzoic acid substrates, RcDT1 recognized only the benzoic acids with 4-hydroxyl group (**9** - **13**). And the prenylation occurred exclusively at an adjacent position of the 4-hydroxyl group (Fig. 4A). This prenylation reaction mode of RcDT1 for 4-hydroxyl benzoic acids resembled that of PHBA polyprenyltransferase (PPT) in ubiquinone biosynthesis and boraginaceous PGTs in shikonin biosynthesis.

In order to further understand the preference of recombinant RcDT1 to prenyl acceptors, the apparent *Km* values of all substances that can be catalyzed by recombinant RcDT1 were measured with the exception of 2-hydroxy-1-naphthoic acid (**4**), 3-hydroxy-2-naphthoic acid (**5**), and orsellinic acid (**13**), which were not measured due to the low conversion rate. The results showed that DHNA (**1**) was the most suitable substrate (*Km* 26.86±5.52 μmol/L). The apparent *Km* values of RcDT1 for **2**, **3**, **9**, **10**, **11**, and **12** were calculated as 59.23±11.20 μmol/L, 46.07±6.75 μmol/L, 54.43 ± 11.41 μmol/L, 78.46 ± 19.21 μmol/L, 76.50 ± 19.21 μmol/L, and 83.17 ± 11.59 μmol/L, respectively (Table 1).

DMAPP, geranyl diphosphate (GPP), and farnesyl pyrophosphate (FPP) were tested with DHNA (**1**) as the acceptor to explore the donor selectivity of RcDT1 (Fig. 4D). Consequently, only DMAPP could be recognized, which validated the strict prenyl donor specificity of RcDT1. The apparent *Km* value for DMAPP was calculated as 79.49± 5.93 μmol/L (Table 1).

Chemical inhibitor studies of the recombinant RcDT1

In order to obtain further information on the substrate recognition mechanism and confirm the role of *RcDT1* in the prenylation activity of *R. cordifolia* microsomes, various phenolic compounds were used for competitive analysis. The candidate inhibitors included **a** MenA inhibitor Ro 48 to 8071 (**24**), three phenol inhibitors for LePGT1 [homogentisic acid (**19**), catechol (**25**), and hydroquinone (**26**)], and simple naphthols (**8**, **27** - **30**) (Fig. 5A). Each of the candidate inhibitors was added to the reaction mixture at the same concentration of the substrate, and the effect on the activity of recombinant RcDT1 was examined. The competitive

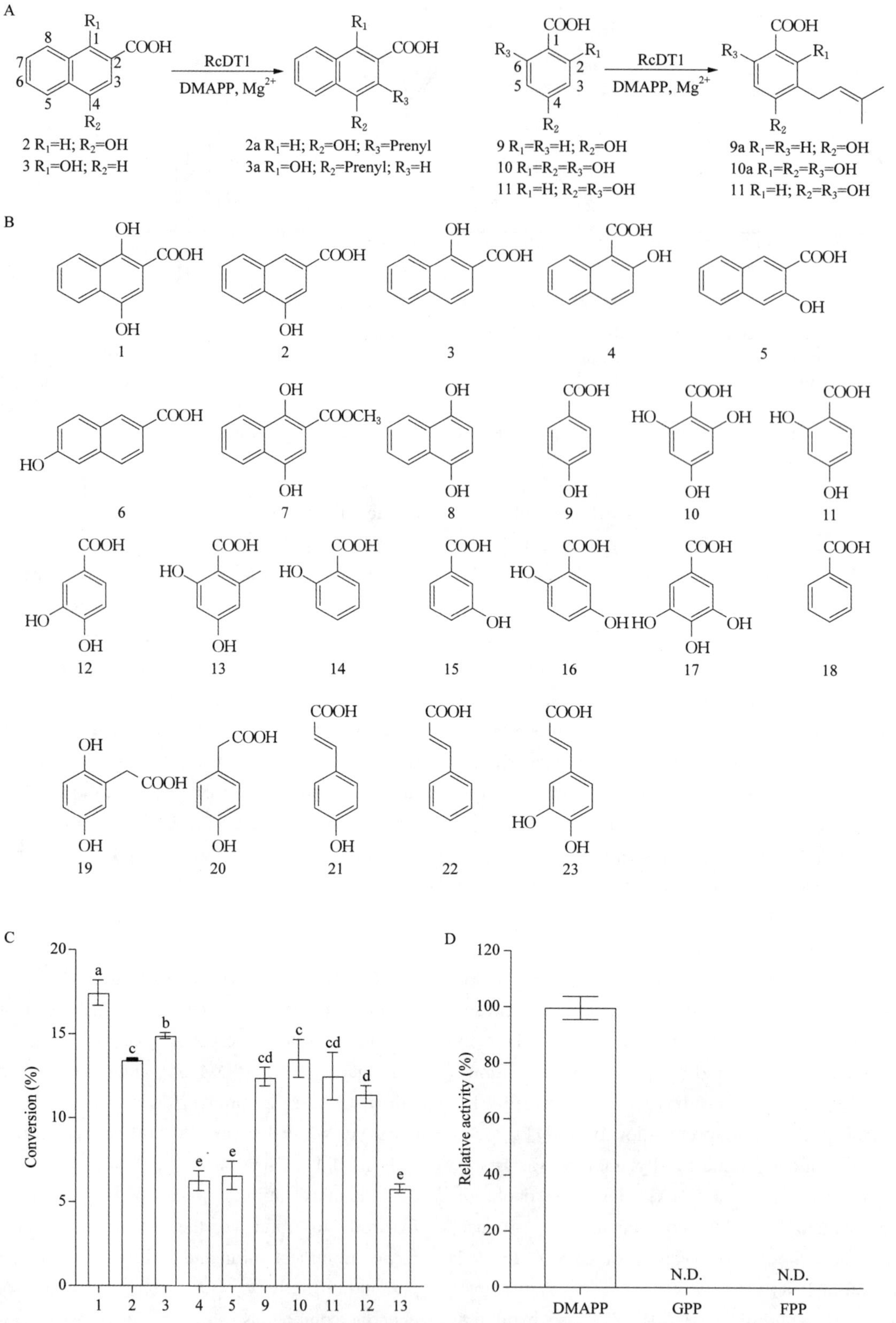

**Figure 4 Substrate specificities of the recombinant RcDT1**

(A) The reactions catalyzed by the recombinant RcDT1. (B) Chemical structures of the compounds for the substrate specificity analysis. (C) Enzymatic activities with the substrates in (B) as the prenyl acceptors and DMAPP as the prenyl donor. The reaction mixture (200 μL) for determining enzyme activity contained 50 mmol/L Tris-HCl (pH 8.5), 5 mmol/L $MgCl_2$, 200 μmol/L the prenyl acceptors, 400 μmol/L DMAPP, and 0.5 mg microsome protein. One-way ANOVA was used to compare the conversion. Different lowercase letters indicate significant differences ($P<0.05$). (D) Relative enzymatic activities with DMAPP, GPP, and FPP as the prenyl donors and DHNA (1) as the prenyl acceptor. The reaction mixture (200 μL) for determining enzyme activity contained 50 mM Tris-HCl (pH 8.5), 5 mmol/L $MgCl_2$, 200 μmol/L DHNA, 400 μmol/L prenyl donor, and 0.5 mg microsome protein. N. D., not detected. The maximum activity level of RcDT1 was assumed to be 100%. All data represent the mean±SD of three biological replicates. DMAPP, 3,3-dimethylallyl pyrophosphate; GPP, geranyl pyrophosphate; FPP, farnesyl pyrophosphate.

**Table 1 Kinetic parameters of RcDT1 with an N-terminal truncation of 72 amino acids**

| Substrate | *K*m (μM) | *Vmax* (pkat/μg protein) |
|---|---|---|
| DHNA (**1**) | 26.86±5.52 | 2.32±0.13 |
| 4-Hydroxy-2-naphthoic acid (**2**) | 59.23±11.20 | 1.44±0.11 |
| 1-Hydroxy-2-naphthoic acid (**3**) | 46.07±6.75 | 1.98±0.12 |
| 4-Hydroxybenzoic acid (**9**) | 54.43±11.41 | 1.45±0.11 |
| 2, 4, 6-Trihydroxybenzoic acid (**10**) | 78.46±19.21 | 1.38±0.09 |
| 2, 4-Dihydroxybenzoic acid (**11**) | 76.50±19.21 | 1.34±0.14 |
| 3, 4-Dihydroxybenzoic acid (**12**) | 83.17±11.59 | 1.24±0.11 |
| DMAPP | 79.49±5.93 | 0.85±0.02 |

analyses using DHNA (**1**) or PHBA (**9**) as the substrate produced nearly identical results; hence, only the results for DHNA (**1**) were shown. As seen in Fig. 5B, the MenA inhibitor Ro 48-8071 (**24**) exhibited no inhibition effect on the prenylation of DHNA (**1**) by RcDT1. Among the LePGT1 inhibitors, only catechol (**25**) showed a moderate inhibitory effect, which could reduce the activity of RcDT1 by 50.9%. These results highlighted the difference between MenA homologs, boraginaceous PGTs, and RcDT1 in the substrate recognition mechanism. Simple naphthols 1, 4-dihydroxynaphthalene (1, 4-DHN, **8**) and 1, 2-DHN (**27**) showed strong inhibition (5.7% and 0% activities of control reaction, respectively), and the prenylation of **8** or **27** was not detected. Considering that the prenylation of both DHNA (**1**) and PHBA (**9**) was strongly inhibited by simple naphthols but not phenols, it could be confirmed that RcDT1 primarily recognized naphthoic acids, and benzoic acids were prenylated through promiscuous recognition.

The best inhibitor of RcDT1, 1, 2-DHN (**27**), was then added to the reaction assay of *R. cordifolia* microsomes for competitive analysis. Like the recombinant RcDT1, 1, 2-DHN (**27**) completely inhibited the prenylation catalyzed by *R. cordifolia* microsomes (Fig. 5C). This result validated that RcDT1 was responsible for the prenylation catalyzed by *R. cordifolia* microsomes.

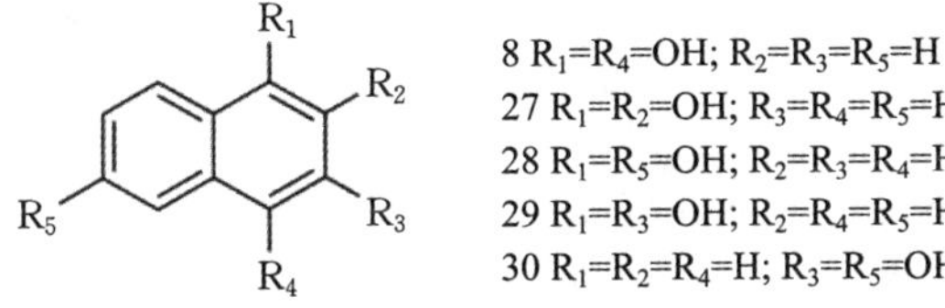


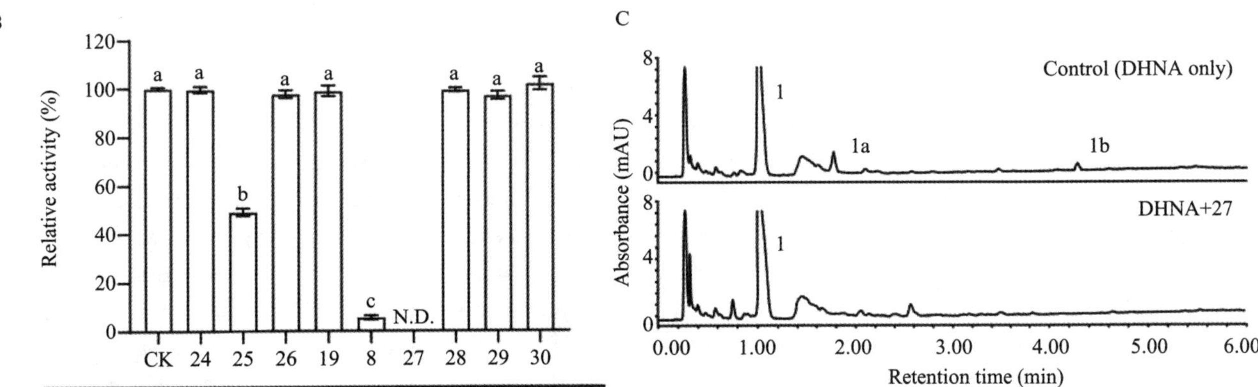


**Figure 5 Influence of aromatic compounds on the prenylation activities of recombinant RcDT1 and *R. cordifolia* microsomes**

(A) Structures of tested aromatic compounds in chemical inhibitor studies. (B) Relative prenylation activities for DHNA (**1**) by recombinant RcDT1 with different inhibitors. One-way ANOVA was used to compare the relative activity. Different lowercase letters indicate significant differences ($P<0.05$). CK, DHNA only. N.D., not detected. The enzyme activity level of the CK was assumed to be 100%. All data represent the mean±SD of three biological replicates. (C) UPLC traces for the reactions containing DHNA (**1**) with *R. cordifolia* microsomes in the presence or absence of 1, 2-dihydroxynaphthalene (**27**). DHNA, 1, 4-dihydroxy-2-naphthoic acid.

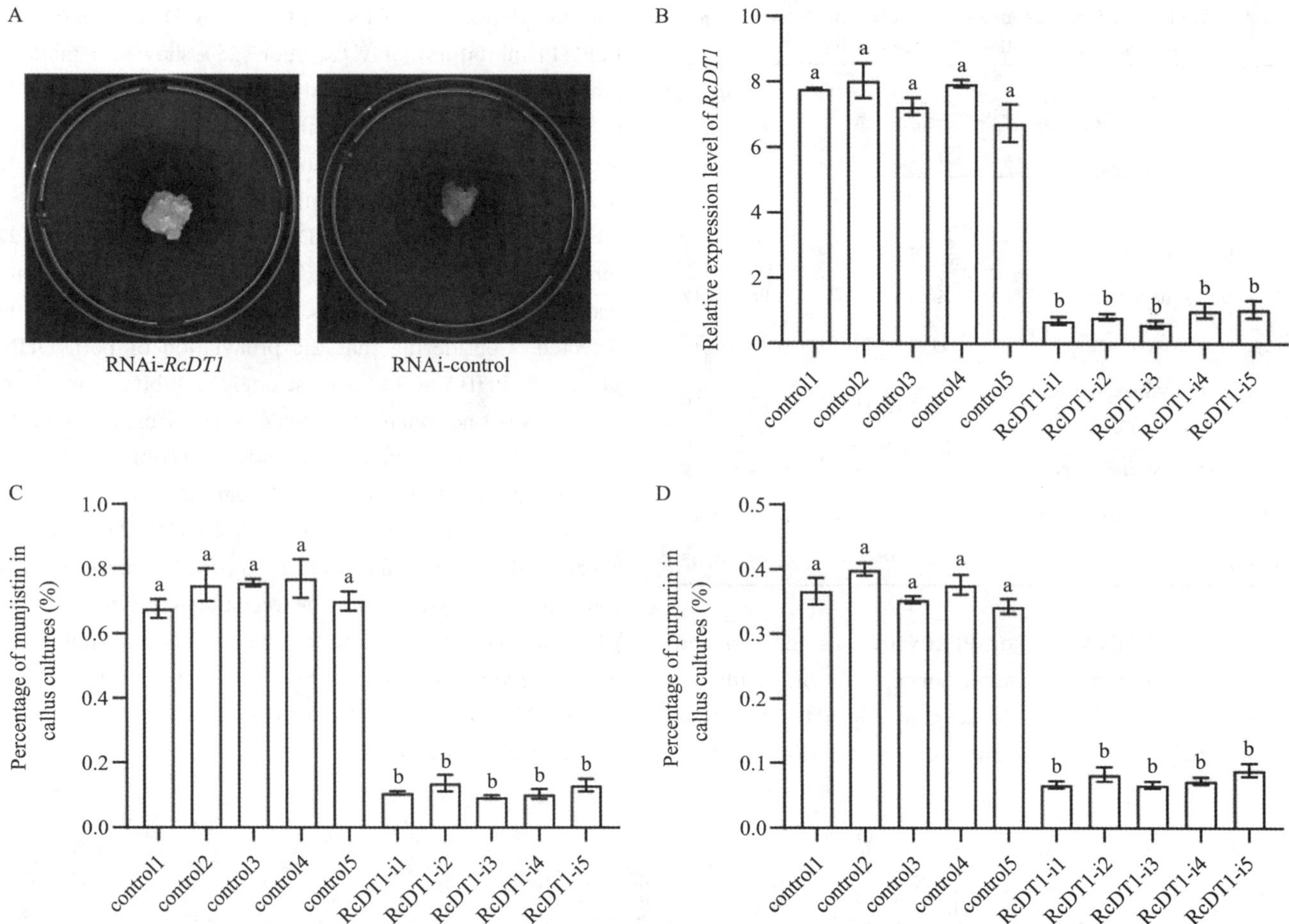


**Figure 6 Physiological function of *RcDT1* in vivo**

(A) Phenotypes of RNAi-*RcDT1* and control cell lines. (B) Expression levels of *RcDT1* in callus cultures of the five independent RNAi-*RcDT1* and control cell lines. (C) Percentage of munjistin in the dry weight of the five independent RNAi-*RcDT1* and control cell lines. (D) Percentage of purpurin in the dry weight of the five independent RNAi-*RcDT1* and control cell lines. In (B－D), one-way ANOVA was used to compare the *RcDT1* expression and anthraquinone content between callus cultures. Different lowercase letters indicate significant differences ($P<0.05$). All data represent the mean ±SD of three biological replicates.

Physiological function of *RcDT*1 *in vivo* To investigate the in vivo role of *RcDT1*, RNA interference (RNAi) was used to knock down its gene expression in *R. cordifolia* callus cells. A 300 bp specific fragment from *RcDT1* was cloned into the plant binary expression vector pK7GWIWG2D (II), which can generate self-complementary hairpin RNA fragments that induce specific gene silencing. The interfering vector pK7GWIWG2D (II)-*RcDT1* and the control vector were transferred to *R. cordifolia* explants via *Agrobacterium tumefaciens* to produce recombinant callus cells. Several indepemdent *RcDT1*-RNAi (*RcDT1*i) and control cell lines were generated, excised and transferred to MS medium. The callus cultures grew as friable tissues (Fig. 6A). The efficiency of *RcDT1* interference was evaluated using RT-qPCR. The results showed that the expression of *RcDT1* was suppressed efficiently in interfering callus cell lines (Fig. 6B).

As munjistin and purpurin represent 90% of the total AQs yield in callus cultures of *R. cordifolia* (Supplementary Fig. S1), their contents were measured to investigate the effects of *RcDT1* knockdown. Compared with the control lines, the contents of the major AQs in the *RcDT1*-RNAi cell lines significantly decreased (Fig. 6C and D). The contents of munjistin and purpurin in the *RcDT1*-RNAi cell lines were about 16% and 21% of the control lines, respectively. The expression of *RcDT1* is positively associated with the accumulation of AQs, indicating that *RcDT1* is involved in the biosynthesis of alizarin-type AQs in *R. cordifolia*.

Expression profile and subcellular localization of *RcDT1* Analysis of the organ-specific expression of *RcDT1* in intact *R. cordifolia* plants by RT-qPCR showed that the expression in roots was significantly higher than that in stems and leaves (Fig. 7A). This result is consistent with that the AQ content in the roots of *R. cordifolia* is much higher than that in other tissues.

To assess the subcellular localization of RcDT1 *in planta*, full-length RcDT1 or its first 72 amino acids representing the signal peptide were fused with the green fluorescent protein (GFP) and introduced into *A. thaliana*

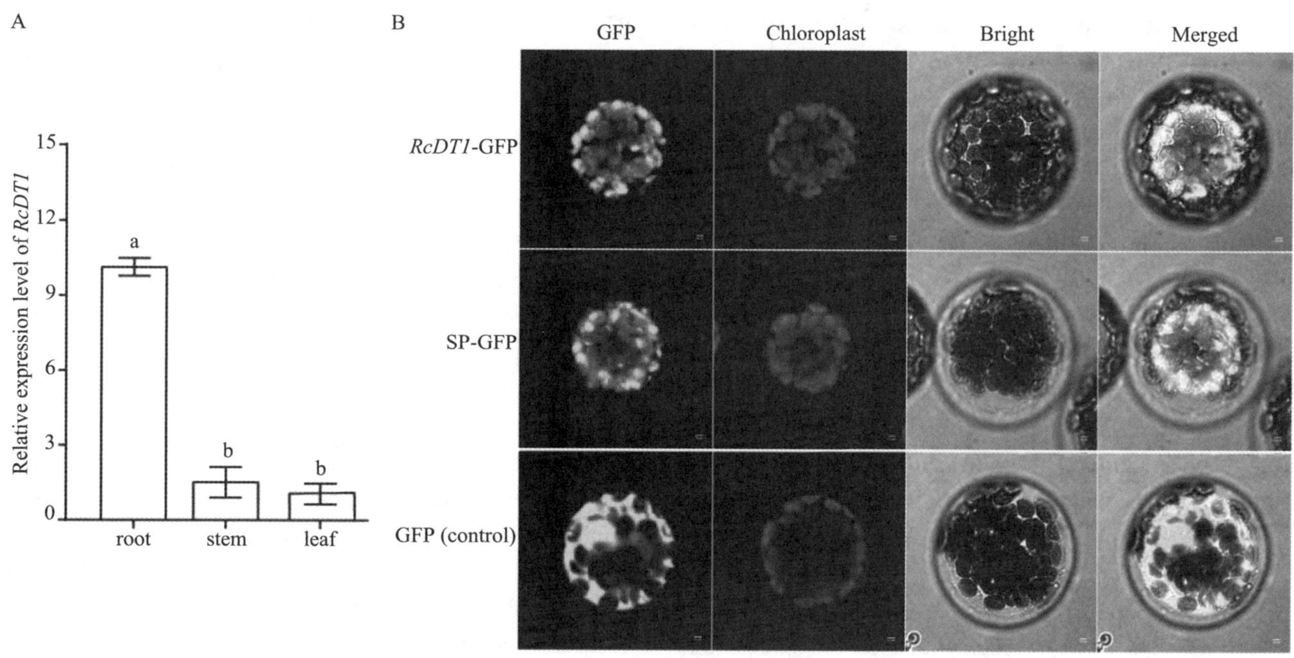


**Figure 7 Organ-specific gene expression and subcellular localization of *RcDT1***

(A) Expression of *RcDT1* in different organs of *R. cordifolia*. All experiments were performed in triplicate, each being repeated at least three times. The vertical bars represent the standard error of the means of independent replicates. One-way ANOVA was used to compare the expression difference between tissues. Different lowercase letters indicate significant differences ($P < 0.05$). (B) Subcellular localizations of full-length *RcDT1* and the signal peptide (the first 72 amino acids at the N terminus) of *RcDT1*. *RcDT1*-GFP, SP-GFP, and GFP (control) are introduced into *A. thaliana* protoplasts. Chloroplasts are revealed by red chlorophyll autofluorescence. SP, Signal peptide. Scale bars = 10 μm.

protoplasts. Confocal microscopy of the transformed protoplasts showed that the fluorescence pattern of chloroplast was similar to that of GFP co-localized with RcDT1 or its signal peptide, indicating chloroplast localization of both chimeric proteins (Fig. 7B). The results of subcellular localization suggest that RcDT1 functions in plastids of *R. cordifolia*, consistent with the plastid localization of the MEP pathway that provides DMAPP to constitute ring C of AQs in rubiaceous plants.

Functional validation of RcDT1 homologs in other Rubiaceous plants Considering that AQs found in Rubiaceae are all formed through the shikimate pathway, we attempt to verify whether homologs of RcDT1 in other rubiaceous plants have similar functions as in *R. cordifolia*. The polypeptide sequence of *RcDT1* was employed as a query to retrieve the genome databases of Arabian Coffee (*Coffea arabica*) and Eugenioides Coffee (*Coffea eugenioides*) (two classic examples of Rubiaceae) and the transcriptome database of *M. officinalis* (an AQ-rich medicinal plant widely cultivated in the Lingnan region of southern China) independently. Regarding *C. arabica* and *C. eugenioides*, the search for genes with identities greater than 60% to *RcDT1* yielded four and two homologs, respectively. After removing highly similar genes, three homologs termed *CaDT1*, *CaDT2*, and *CeDT1* were selected for following studies (Supplementary Table S2). As for *M. officinalis*, *MoDT1*, which is 73.79% identical with *RcDT1*, was investigated in follow-up experiments.

Truncated *CaDT1*, *CaDT2*, *CeDT1*, and *MoDT1* genes with a 72 amino acid deletion from the start codon were synthesized and expressed in *P. pastoris*. The investigation for the prenylation activity was carried out using DHNA (**1**) or PHBA (**9**) as the substrate with recombinant enzymes in the presence of DMAPP and $Mg^{2+}$. As a result, recombinant CaDT1 and MoDT1 could prenylate DHNA (**1**) and PHBA (**9**) in the same manner as recombinant RcDT1 (Supplementary Fig. S4). This suggests that the prenylation step of AQ biosynthesis in Rubiaceae is catalyzed by RcDT1 and its homologs. Recombinant CaDT2 did not exhibit any prenylation activity toward DHNA (**1**) and PHBA (**9**). Interestingly, recombinant CeDT1 could only accept PHBA (**9**) but not DHNA (**1**) as the prenyl acceptor (Supplementary Fig. S4). The promiscuous recognition of DHNA (**1**) and PHBA (**9**) by RcDT1 and its homologs support the view that DHNA PTs and PHBA PTs share a common evolutionary origin in Rubiaceae.

Phylogenetic analysis of *RcDT1* Although *Coffea* plants are not rich in AQs, the cognate genes of *RcDT1* identified from these plants still catalyze the prenylation of DHNA/PHBA. This leads us to infer that the emergence of *RcDT1* homologs is widespread in Rubiaceae, even in the plants that do not produce AQs. *RcDT1* was then used to query the NCBI Gene database (https://www.ncbi.nlm.nih.gov/gene) and OneKP database (https://db.cngb.org/onekp/search) to obtain homologous sequences from Rubiaceae. A maximum-likelihood tree was constructed to analyze the evolutionary relationships of *RcDT1* and its homologs with the other plant aromatic PTs (Fig. 8). *RcDT1* and its homologs turned out to form an independent branch neighboring the PGTs for shikonin formation in Boraginaceae and PPTs for ubiquinone formation. Correspondingly, *RcDT1* and its homologs in Rubiaceae could recognize PHBA (**9**) as the substrate. Therefore, it can be concluded that DHNA/PHBA DTs in Rubiaceae have evolved via recruitment from the ubiquinone biosynthetic pathway. On the other hand, the rubiaceous branch in the tree was clearly divergent from that of the MenA homologs for phylloquinone biosynthesis. This was verified by the result that recombinant RcDT1 and MenA were different in substrate recognition and prenylation mechanisms. These phylogenetic analyses suggested that DHNA-prenylation activities evolved convergently in distant clades of the UbiA superfamily.

## 3 DISCUSSION

The identification of RcDT1 clarifies a key step in alizarin-type AQ biosynthesis  Rubiaceous plants biosynthesize AQs through the combination of the shikimate pathway providing the DHNA moiety and the MEP pathway providing the prenyl (isoprenoid) chain. The key step in the coupling of the two pathways is catalyzed by a membrane-bound aromatic PT catalyzing the prenylation of DHNA. This PT has not previously been identified. The biosynthesis of phylloquinone in plants proceeds in a manner similar to that of AQs, where DHNA prenylation is catalyzed by homologs of MenA. Thus, the question arises whether the PT involved in the biosynthesis of AQs is also homologous to MenA. In this study, we started by establishing cell suspension cultures of *R. cordifolia* in which a DHNA-DT activity was detected. As previously observed in the cell suspension culture of *Morinda lucida* (a Rubiaceous plant rich in alizarintype AQs), darkness cultivation and the presence of sucrose-directed metabolic flux toward AQs rather than phylloquinone in suspension-cultured *R. cordifolia* cells. Then, a candidate PT gene belonging to the UbiA superfamily, *RcDT1*, was discovered to account for the prenylation activity. The involvement of *RcDT1* in the biosynthesis of alizarin-type AQs was demonstrated both in vitro and in vivo. Biochemical studies showed that recombinant RcDT1 and MenA differed in substrate recognition and prenylation mechanisms. Phylogenetic analyses confirmed that *RcDT1* evolved via recruitment from the ubiquinone but not the phylloquinone biosynthetic pathway. These results high-lighted the differences between *RcDT1* and MenA. For *RcDT1*, the key PT in alizarin-type AQ biosynthesis, its genetic information, enzymatic characteristics, reaction mechanism, resulting intermediates, and evolution have been elucidated.

The stepwise catalytic mechanism of RcDT1 leads to structurally diverse AQs/NQs  Compared with the identified DHNA PTs homologous to MenA, RcDT1 differed in the reaction mechanism. The tracer studies proved that the prenylation of DHNA by MenA occurred at the C-2 position and required the replacement of the carboxyl with the isoprenoid side chain. No intermediate or two separate reaction steps are observed for MenA-catalyzed prenylation. In contrast, the prenylation of DHNA by RcDT1 occurred at the C-3 position and was uncoupled from the decarboxylation. As in MenA-catalyzed prenylation, the introduction of dimethylallyl moiety by RcDT1 was accompanied by a spontaneous naphthol to naphthoquinone oxidation to produce CPNQ (**1a**). The formation of β-keto structure may facilitate the decarboxylation to generate PNQ (**1b**). A similar decarboxylation step was proposed in the laccase-catalyzed synthesis of 1, 4-naphthoquinone-2, 3-bis-sulfides from DHNA. The main biological importance of this stepwise mechanism is that it leads to the branch of the biosynthetic pathway toward AQs and NHQs in Rubiaceae (Fig. 1). Specifically, if **1a** was further methyl-esterified to form 2-methoxycarbonyl-3-prenyl-1, 4-naphthoquinone, its decarboxylation and subsequent cyclization to form AQs were prevented, and the metabolic flux was shifted to NHQs (Fig. 1). When incubated in the reaction buffer without proteins, 2-methoxycarbonyl-3-prenyl-1, 4-naphthoquinone was observed to spontaneously cyclize to form mollugin, a signature naphthoquinone of *R. cordifolia* (Supplementary Fig. S5). In contrast, the decarboxylation of **1a** to form **1b** triggered the subsequent cyclization and enabled entry into alizarin-type AQs (Fig. 1). In addition to Rubiaceae, alizarin-type AQs are also found in Bignoniaceae and Verbenaceae, where they are accompanied by the structure-related characteristic constituent lapachol. Therefore, it can be inferred that AQs and lapachol are both biosynthesized through the shikimate pathway, and PNQ (i. e. deoxy-lapachol, **1b**) is also the immediate precursor of lapachol and related quinones (Fig. 1).

Convergent and independent evolution of UbiA superfamily enzymes enable entry into quinones derived from the shikimate pathway  The above differences in reaction mechanism, together with the phylogenetic clustering, strongly suggest that the DHNA-prenylation activities evolved convergently from different ancestral UbiA progenitors in ubiquinone and phylloquinone biosynthesis, respectively. This evolutionary trajectory is in line with previous reports describing the convergent evolution of coumarin C-PTs in Apiaceae and Moraceae, coumarin O-PTs in Apiaceae and

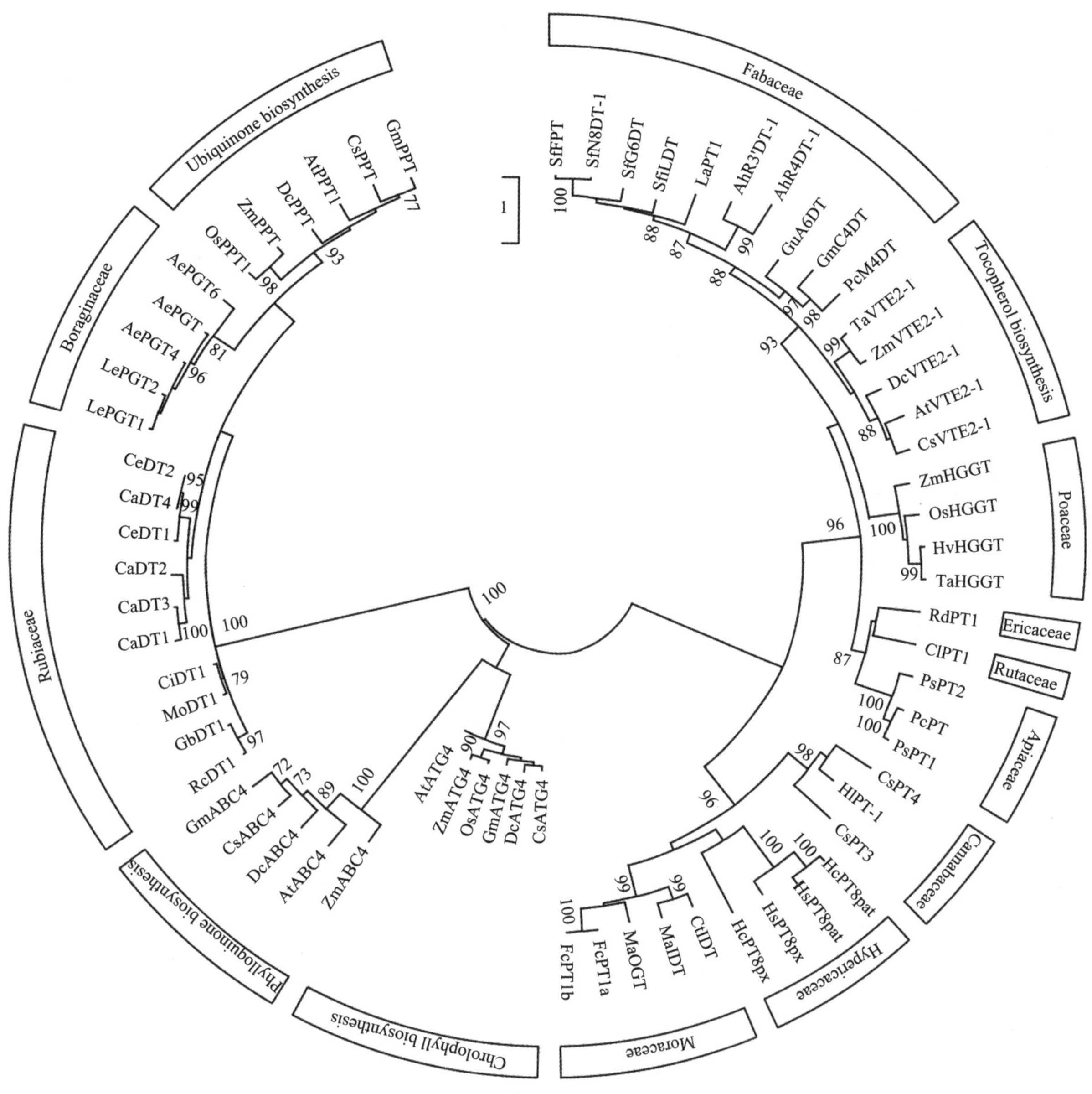


**Figure 8 Phylogenetic analysis of RcDT1**

The tree was constructed using the maximum-likelihood method applying 1,000 bootstrap replicates. Nodes with bootstrap values $>70$ are indicated by numbers on the branch. The scale bar represents 1 amino acid substitutions per site. SfFPT (*S. flavescens*; KC513505); SfN8DT-1 (*S. flavescens*; AB325579); LaPT1 (*Lupinus albus*; JN228254); SfG6DT (*S. flavescens*; AB604224); SfiLDT (*S. flavescens*; AB604223); GuA6DT (*Glycyrrhiza uralensis*; KJ123716); GmC4DT (*Glycine max*; LC140927); PcM4DT (*Psoralea corylifolia*; MH626730); AhR3′ DT-1 (*Arachis hypogaea*; KY565245); AhR4DT-1 (*A. hypogaea*; KY565244) TaVTE2-1 (*Triticum aestivum*; DQ231056); ZmVTE2-1 (*Zea mays*; EU973221); AtVTE2-1 (*A. thaliana*; DQ231056); CsVTE2-1 (*Citrus sinensis*; XM_006474143); DcVTE2-1 (*Daucus carota*; XM_017398463); HvHGGT (*Hordeum vulgare*; AY222860); TaHGGT (*T. aestivum*; AY222861); OsHGGT (*Oryza sativa*; AY222862); ZmHGGT (*Z. mays*; XM_008661550); ClPT1 (*Citrus limon*; AB813876); RdPT1 (*Rhododendron dauricum*; LC381857); PsPT2 (*Pastinaca sativa*; KM017084); PcpT (*Petroselinum crispum*; AB825956); PsPT1 (*P. sativa*; KM017083); CsPT3 (*Cannabis sativa*; BK010680); CsPT4 (*C. sativa*; BK010648); HlPT-1 (*Humulus lupulus*; AB543053); HcPT8pat (*Hypericum calycinum*; MH461103); HcPT8px (*Hy. calycinum*; MH461102); HsPT8px (*Hy. sampsonii*; MH461100); HsPT8pat (*Hy. sampsonii*; MH461101); CtIDT (*Cudrania tricuspidata*; KM262660); MaIDT (*Morus alba*; KM262659); FcPT1a (*Ficus carica*; LC369744); FcPT1b (*F. carica*; LC369745); OsATG4 (*O. sativa*; EF432576); ZmATG4 (*Z. mays*; NM_001148732); AtATG4 (*A. thaliana*; NM_115041); DcATG4 (*D. carota*; XM_017388300); CsATG4 (*C. sinensis*; XM_006481001); GmATG4 (*G. max*; NM_001252704); AtABC4 (*A. thaliana*; NM_001124046.2); CsABC4 (*C. sinensis*; XM_025093178); GmABC4 (*G. max*; XM_003532557); ZmABC4 (*Z. mays*; NM_001158698); DcABC4 (*D. carota*; AY222861); RcDT1 (*R. cordifolia*; OR493119); CaDT1 (*C. arabica*; XM_027266276); CaDT2 (*C. arabica*; XM_027266749); CaDT3 (*C. arabica*; XM_027269080); CaDT4 (*C. arabica*; XM_027124411); CeDT1 (*C. eugenioides*; XM_027313870); CeDT2 (*C. eugenioides*; XM_027313873); CiDT1 (*Carapichea ipecacuanha*; BQEQ_2057440); GbDT1 (*Galium boreale*; WQRD_2015494); AePGT (*A. euchroma*; DQ397513); AePGT4 (*A. euchroma*; KT991522); LePGT2 (*L. erythrorhizon*; AB055079); LePGT1 (*L. erythrorhizon*; AB055078); AePGT6 (*A. euchroma*; KT991524); DcPPT (*D. carota*; XM_017367441); AtPPT1 (*A. thaliana*; NM_118497); GmPPT (*G. max*; XM_006602661); CsPPT (*C. sinensis*; XM_015532016); OsPPT1 (*O. sativa*; AY222861); ZmPPT (*Z. mays*; NM_001155086). The sequence MoDT1 from *M. officinalis* can be found in Supplementary Table S4.

Rutaceae, as well as flavonoid and stilbene PTs in Moraceae and Fabaceae. These recurring neofunctionalization events could be due to a number of factors. Firstly, the UbiA superfamily is a large gene family, and its members are widely involved in the biosynthesis of both primary and specialized metabolites in microbes, plants, and animals. Diverse substrate specificities and expression profiles of UbiA PTs increase opportunities for neofunctionalization. Secondly, substrate promiscuity was repeatedly found in UbiA PTs of specialized metabolism, which served as the starting point for neofunctionalization. Finally, the end product of the pathway containing UbiA PTs may have abundant ecological functions in multiple niches, which forces the mutations to be preserved.

As the first pathway-specific enzyme of alizarin-type AQ biosynthesis, *RcDT1* independently evolved from the highly conserved PPT of ubiquinone biosynthesis. Both its promiscuous recognition of the benzoic acids with the 4-hydroxyl group and phylogenetic clustering support this conclusion. Interestingly, *CeDT1*, a homolog of *RcDT1* in *C. eugenioides*, lost the DHNA-prenylation activity but retained PHB-prenylation activity, confirming the evolutionary relevance of the two functions in Rubiaceae. A similar evolutionary event took place in Boraginaceae, wherein PGTs of shikonin biosynthesis evolved independently from PPTs. Both RcDT1 and boraginaceous PGTs function as the first pathway-specific enzyme of quinone biosynthesis. Similar cyclization. mechanisms were observed in the subsequent biosynthetic reactions of these two classes of quinones (Fig. 1). Taken together, it could be drawn that neofunctionalization events of PPTs in Rubiaceae and Boraginaceae may lead to taxon-specific metabolic pathways to form AQs and NQs. And homology might be predicted for subsequent steps in AQ and NQ biosynthesis. However, the remaining reaction steps in the shikimate pathway, especially the cyclization, remain to be fully elucidated.

Excluding AQs, shikonin and lapachone derivatives, the shikimate pathway has been found to form NQs such as chimaphilin in the distantly related plants from Pyroleae (Fig. 1). A deeper understanding is needed in terms of achieving analogous chemicals by convergent evolution of this pathway in different plants.

In conclusion, RcDT1, the first pathway-specific PT in the biosynthesis of alizarin-type AQs, was identified from *R. cordifolia*. The prenylation of DHNA by RcDT1 proceeds in a stepwise manner, yielding two products via direct prenylation and decarboxylation. Phylogenetic analysis further proved that RcDT1 and its rubiaceous homologs evolved convergently from ancestral UbiA progenitors in ubiquinone biosynthesis. As the branch point enzyme in the shikimate pathway, RcDT1 and its homologs opened the biosynthesis of alizarin-type AQs and NQs not only in Rubiaceae but possibly in other lamiids plants. Thus, the evolution of RcDT1 provides useful guidance for identifying additional and evolutionarily varied PTs that enable entry into quinones derived from the shikimate pathway. Moreover, the identification and characterization of RcDT1 will have profound implications for understanding the biosynthetic process of the AQ/NQ ring derived from the shikimate pathway.

## 4 MATERIALS AND METHODS

General experimental procedures $^{1}H$ and $^{13}C$ NMR spectra were recorded on Bruker DRX 500 spectrometer. The observed chemical shift values were reported in ppm. The UPLC and LC MS analyses of the enzymatic products were performed as previously described, with the exception that the solvent system comprised acetonitrile (containing 0.1% formic acid, A) and water (containing 0.1% formic acid, B) at 0.5 mL/min with the following gradient program: 0 min, 30% A; 6 min, 60% A; 6.5 min, 100% A; 8.5 min, 100% A. Concentrations are expressed using volume percent (% *V*/*V*). A Waters Acquity UPLC-I Class system (Waters Co., Milford, MA, USA) was equipped with a BEH Phenyl column (2.1×50 mm, 1.7 μm), and the absorbance at 254 nm was measured. For the isolation of the enzymatic product, the same approach as previously described was employed.

Plant materials and chemicals Young leaves of Madder (*R. cordifolia*) were collected on the campus of China Academy of Chinese Medical Sciences in August 2018 and used as explants to initiate calli. The initiation and maintenance of the calli were performed as previously described, except that MS medium supplemented with 1.0 mg/L naphthalene acetic acid and 0.5 mg/L 6-benzyla-minopurine was used. Approximately 5 g of cells was transferred to 250 mL Erlenmeyer flasks containing 60 mL of MS liquid medium mentioned above, maintained on a rotary shaker at 120 r/min, and grown at 25 ℃ in the dark. On culture day 10, suspension-cultured cells were collected for RNA and microsomal protein extraction.

Dimethylallyl diphosphate (DMAPP) was synthesized according to a previously described method, and other chemical reagents were purchased from Sigma-Aldrich (St. Louis, MO, USA) and Macklin (Shanghai, CHN).

RNA sequencing and bioinformatic processing The cDNA libraries of *R. cordifolia* cultured cells were sequenced on an Illumina HiSeq 2000 platform, and the raw sequencing data were deposited in the National Center for Biotechnology Information's Short Read Archive (SRA) under accession no. PRJNA1016061. The sequencing data were analyzed following the process described in a previous study. The raw sequencing data of *M. officinalis* (SRA accession no. SRP258544) were processed as above and used for homology search.

Total RNA extraction and RT-qPCR analysis  Total RNA from different tissues and cultured *R. cordifolia* cells were extracted using the E. Z. N. A. Plant RNA kit (Omega Bio-tek Inc., Doraville, GA, USA) following the manufacturer's instructions. First-strand cDNAs were synthesized with the PrimerScript First-strand cDNA Synthesis Kit at the same time [Takara Biomedical Technology (Beijing) Co., Ltd., Beijing, China]. RT-qPCR was performed using the TB Green *Premix Ex Taq*II [Takara Biomedical Technology (Beijing) Co., Ltd., Beijing, China] and an Applied Biosystems 7 500 realtime instrument. The primers used are listed in Supplementary Table S3. The *RcActin* was used as the endogenous control to normalize expression data. These PCRs were conducted using an amplification program consisting of initial denaturation at 95 ℃ for 2 min followed by 40 cycles of denaturation at 95 ℃ for 10 s, and elongation at 60 ℃ for 30 s. Amplification of the target sequences was confirmed by sequencing. The expression level of each gene was quantified using $2^{-\Delta\Delta Ct}$. At least three independent experiments were performed for each analysis.

cDNA cloning and heterologous expression in yeast  *AtABC4* (GenBank accession no. NP_001117518.1), *LePGT1* (GenBank accession no. BAB84122.1), *AePGT6* (GenBank accession no. ANC67959.1), and *SfN8DT-1* (GenBank accession no. BAG12671.1) were used as queries to retrieve the transcriptome database of *R. cordifolia* cell suspension cultures. As a result, six candidate genes numbered as *RcDT1-6* were selected for further analysis. Specific primers were designed to obtain the complete coding sequence of *RcDT1-6* from the cDNA of cultured *R. cordifolia* cells (Supplementary Table S3). Using the complete coding sequences as the templates, primers were designed to amplify truncated *RcDT1* (with a 24/48/72-amino acid deletion from the start codon) and truncated *RcDT2-6* (with a 24-amino acid deletion from the start codon). Complete and truncated PT sequences were subcloned into the *EcoR* I/*Kpn* I restriction sites of the pPink-HC plasmid, and the plasmid construction was verified by sequencing.

The expression vectors were introduced into the yeast PichiaPink Strain 2 using Frozen-EZ Yeast Transformation II (Zymo Research Co., Irvine, CA, USA). Recombinant strains were initially cultured in BMGY liquid medium at 30 ℃ for about 24 h. The cells were then harvested and resuspended into BMMY liquid medium to induce recombinant protein expression. The induction lasted 5 days at 30 ℃, and methanol was added to the final concentration of 0.5% on time every day.

In vitro enzyme activity assay  The prenylation activity was assayed for recombinant years and cultured *R. cordifolia* cells. The collected yeast cells were broken with an APV2000 continuous high-pressure crusher (AxFlow, Stockholm, Sweden). The cultured cells of *R. cordifolia* were ground in a mortar. The microsomal proteins were prepared by differential centrifugation as described previously. All these procedures were performed at 4 ℃. The total protein concentration was determined by the Bradford method.

The reaction mixture (200 μL) for determining enzyme activity contained 50 mmol/L Tris-HCl (pH 8.5), 5 mmol/L $MgCl_2$, 200 μmol/L the prenyl acceptors, 400 μmol/L DMAPP, and 0.5 mg microsome protein. The reaction mixtures were incubated at 30 ℃ for 30 min, and the reaction was terminated by the addition of 600 μL of acetonitrile. The protein was removed by centrifugation at 15 000 × *g* for 20 min, and the reaction was analyzed by UPLC-UV/ESI MS. Products detected by UPLC were used to calculate conversion with the following formula: conversion (%) = 100 × product content/(product content + substrate content).

Biochemical properties of the recombinant enzymes  The truncated *RcDT1* with a 72 amino acid deletion at the N-terminal was selected to study the biochemical properties. With DHNA as the prenyl acceptor and DMAPP as the prenyl donor, the biochemical characteristics of the recombinant enzyme were analyzed by calculating the yield of the main product. To investigate the optimal pH, the enzyme reactions were performed in reaction buffers with pH values in the range of MES-Tris (pH 6.5 to 8.0), Tris-HCl (pH 8.0 to 9.5), and CAPS-NaOH (pH 9.5 to 10.5) at 30 ℃ for 30 min. To investigate the optimal temperature, the reaction mixtures were incubated at eight different temperatures (0 ℃ to 50 ℃) in 50 mM Tris-HCl buffer (pH 8.5). To test the requirement of *RcDT1* activity for divalent cations, the reaction mixtures were incubated with 5 mM $MgCl_2$, $CaCl_2$, $FeCl_2$, $NiCl_2$, $MnCl_2$, $CuCl_2$, $ZnCl_2$, $CoCl_2$ and EDTA separately in 50 mM Tris-HCl buffer (pH 8.5) at 30 ℃ for 30 min. Relative activities of recombinant RcDT1 with prenyl diphosphate of different chain lengths were analyzed with DMAPP (C5), GPP (C10), and FPP (C15), respectively, at 30 ℃ for 30 min.

The apparent $K_m$ values for different prenyl acceptors were determined by incubating 200 μg of recombinant yeast microsomes with various concentrations of prenyl acceptors (12 to 400 μmol/L) and a fixed concentration of DMAPP (400 μmol/L) in 200 μL reaction mixtures at 30 ℃. The apparent $K_m$ values for DMAPP were determined using various concentrations of DMAPP (12 to 400 μmol/L) and a fixed concentration of DHNA (400 μmol/L) under the same conditions. For each prenyl acceptor or DMAPP, the incubation time was controlled separately so that the reaction was under 10% complete. Kinetic constants were calculated based on Michaelis-Menten kinetics using GraphPad Prism 8

(GraphPad Software Inc., San Diego, CA, USA). Three independent experiments were performed for each analysis.

Structure identification of enzymatic products The assays for the isolation of the enzymatic products (15 to 20 mL) contained 50 mmol/L Tris-HCl (pH 8.5), 5 mmol/L $MgCl_2$, 2 mmol/L the prenyl acceptors, 4 mmol/L DMAPP, and 30 mg of the recombinant RcDT1 microsome. The reaction mixtures were incubated at 30 ℃ for 12 h and subsequently extracted three times with ethyl acetate. After evaporation of the solvent under vacuum, the residues were dissolved in methanol and purified by reverse-phase semipreparative HPLC. The products were analyzed by MS, $^1$H NMR, and $^{13}$C NMR spectroscopy (Supplementary Figs. S6 - S10).

RNAi in callus cultures of *R. cordifolia* A 300 bp segment of *RcDT1* (nucleotides 366 to 665) was cloned into pENTR/SD/D-TOPO (Invitrogen; primers are shown in Supplementary Table S3) and subcloned into the binary vector pK7GWIWG2D (II) using Gateway LR Clonase Enzyme Mix (Invitrogen). The pK7GWIWG2D(II)-*RcDT1* and empty vector used as a negative control were then introduced into *A. tumefaciens* GV3101 via a freeze-thaw method. The sterile stem of *R. cordifolia* was soaked in the recombinant *A. tumefaciens* infection solution for 30 min to infect the stem explant. The stem explant was dried on sterile filter paper, placed on hormone-free MS medium, and cultivated in darkness at 25 ℃ for 2 days. Transfer the stem explants to MS agar medium supplemented with 50 mg/L kanamycin, 250 mg/L cefotaxime, 1.0 mg/L naphthalene acetic acid and 0.5 mg/L 6-benzylaminopurine. The explants were cultivated in darkness at 25 ℃ until callus cultures grew. Rapidly growing kanamycin-resistant lines were screened and transferred to MS medium supplemented with 1.0 mg/L naphthalene acetic acid and 0.5 mg/L 6-benzylaminopurine for cultivation in darkness at 25 ℃ for 30 days. The process of transgenic callus culture construction was shown in Supplementary Fig. S11. Part of the callus culture of *R. cordifolia* was subjected to RT-qPCR to determine the expression level of *RcDT1*, while the other part was freeze-dried to determine the content of alizarin-type AQs. Referring to the method previously described, 30 mg of dried callus powder impregnated with 0.15 mL 5 N HCl was extracted by ultrasonication in 1.5 mL of methanol. The filtered extract then underwent UPLC analysis. The solvent system comprised acetonitrile (containing 0.1% formic acid, A) and water (containing 0.1% formic acid, B) at 0.5 mL/min with the following gradient program: 0 min, 10% A; 5.5 min, 100% A; 7.5 min, 100% A. Concentrations are expressed using volume percent (% *V*/*V*). A Waters Acquity UPLC-I Class system (Waters Co., Milford, MA, USA) was equipped with a HSS T3 column (2.1×100 mm, 1.8 μm), and the absorbance at 254 nm was measured.

Subcellular localization of *RcDT1* The nucleotide sequence for full-length *RcDT1* or its N-terminal sequence (216 bp) was subcloned into the *BsaI*/*Eco31I* restriction sites of the pBWA (V) HS-ccdb-GLosgfp plasmid to give pBWA (V) HS-RcDT1, pBWA (V) HS-RcDT1-TP. Empty pBWA (V) HS-ccdb-GLosgfp plasmid was used as a negative control. *A. thaliana* protoplasts were isolated and transformed as described previously with modifications. The transformed protoplasts were examined with a light microscope and a laser confocal microscope (C2-ER; Nikon). For GFP detection, excitation at 488 nm and detection at 510 nm were used. For chloroplast detection, excitation at 640 nm and detection at 675 nm were used.

In silico sequence analysis The transmembrane regions and the transit peptides of RcDTs were predicted by Deep TMHMM (https://dtu.biolib.com/Deep TMHMM) and SignalP-6.0 (https://services.healthtech.dtu.dk/services/SignalP-6.0/), respectively. The protein sequences were aligned using Clustal W, and a phylogenetic tree was drawn by MEGA X. Phylogenetic relationships were reconstructed by the maximum-likelihood method based on the JTT/+G model (five categories) and a bootstrap of 1 000 replicates. Bootstrap values were indicated in percentages (only those > 70% were presented) on the nodes. The scale bar corresponded to 1.0 estimated amino acid changes per site.

Accession numbers The nucleotide sequences of *RcDT1* - *6* have been deposited in the GenBank database under the accession numbers OR493119 - OR493124, respectively.

[刘长征,黄璐琦,郭兰萍,等. Plant Physiology, 2024, DOI: 10.1093/plphys/kiae171.]

# Efficient heterologous biosynthesis of verazine, a metabolic precursor of the anti-cancer drug cyclopamine, in *Nicotiana benthamiana*

Among the large number of *Veratrum* steroid alkaloids, cyclopamine has been shown to have various inhibitory mechanisms against cancer, including inhibition of the hedgehog signaling pathway, improvement of tumor tissue microenvironment, inhibition of cell respiration, promotion of cell apoptosis, and reversal of tumor drug resistance. The biosynthetic pathway of verazine, a possible metabolic precursor of cyclopamine, has been discovered in *Veratrum californicum*. However, the content of *Veratrum* steroid alkaloids in plants is very low (Supplemental Figure 2), so reliance on direct extraction from plants for commercial production is not feasible. A more effective strategy is to synthesize rare plant secondary metabolites using synthetic biology technology.

About 1 mg verazine was extracted from dried *Veratrum nigrum* rhizome for qualitative and quantitative analyses of verazine, and the nuclear magnetic resonance results are shown in Supplemental Tables 1 and 2. To synthesize the precursor molecule cholesterol required for verazine metabolism, the genes involved in the cholesterol biosynthetic pathway of *Paris polyphylla* were expressed in *Nicotiana benthamiana*. Using a high-yielding cholesterol synthesis chassis in *N. benthamiana*, four enzymes involved in the synthesis of verazine in *V. californicum* were transiently co-expressed. *VcCYP90B27* (KJ869252) was confirmed to encode a cholesterol C-22 hydroxylase. However, the enzyme activity of VcCYP90B27 in *N. benthamiana* was not as high as expected, and the substrate utilization rate was less than 25% (Supplemental Figures 1A and 1B). Some key amino acid differences (Figure 1A) may have contributed to the low activity of VcCYP90B27 in *N. benthamiana*. As a result, the downstream enzymes VcCYP94N1 (KJ869255), VcGABAT (KJ869263), and VcCYP90G1 (KJ869260) may have had insufficient substrates for verazine synthesis.

Because of the low activity of VcCYP90B27 in *N. benthamiana*, it was necessary to find an alternative enzyme with high catalytic activity. We noted that *V. nigrum*, a traditional medicinal herb from China, also contains a wide variety of steroid alkaloids. We sequenced the full-length transcriptome of *V. nigrum* and obtained four candidate genes, *VnCYP90B27* (PP129547), *VnCYP94N2* (PP129548), *VnGABAT* (PP129549), and *VnCYP90G9* (PP129550), on the basis of their predicted amino acid sequence similarity to orthologs in *V. californicum*. These candidate genes had similar tissue expression specificities (Figure 1B) and the same accumulation patterns as verazine in *V. nigrum* (Figures 1I - 1M). Agrobacteria harboring these four genes were infiltrated into *N. benthamiana* leaves to test their functions. The substitution of VnCYP90B27 for VcCYP90B27 resulted in an approximately 20-fold increase in 22(*R*)-hydroxycho-lesterol content (Figure 1N). With the addition of VnCYP90B27, VcCYP94N1 was able to oxygenate the C-22 position of 22(*R*)-hydroxycholesterol, and the product 22, 26-dihydroxycholesterol was observed by gas chromatography-mass spectrometry. Liquid chromatography-tandem mass spectrometry revealed that VcGABAT replaces the C-22 aldehyde group of 22, 26-dihydroxycholesterol with an amino group, yielding 22-hydroxy-26-aminocholesterol. VcCYP90G1 then oxidizes the C-22 hydroxyl group of 22-hydroxy-26-aminocholesterol into a carbonyl group, which undergoes a ring formation reaction with the C-26 amino group to synthesize verazine (Figures 1E - 1H).

The yields of eight enzymes involved in the biosynthesis of verazine from *V. nigrum* and *V. californicum* were compared in different combinations (Figures 1N - 1Q). Because PpCYP90B27 has been confirmed to be a cholesterol C-22 hydroxylase, like VnCYP90B27 and VcCYP90B27, there were three candidate genes for CYP90B27 derived from *V. californicum*, *V. nigrum*, and *P. polyphylla*. VnCYP90B27 and PpCYP90B27 showed the same level of activity, and the production of VnCYP90B27 was slightly higher (Figure 1N). The second enzyme for comparison was CYP94N1, and the candidate enzymes were VnCYP94N2 and VcCYP94N1. The yield of VnCYP94N2 was slightly higher, about 1.4 times that of VcCYP94N1 (Figure 1O). The catalytic product yields of VcGABAT and VnGABAT were compared, and that of VnGABAT was significantly lower, approximately one-eighth that of VcGABAT (Figure 1P). Moreover, after addition of VnCYP90G9 on this basis, the amount of verazine synthesized was only 0.03 $\mu$g/g DW (Figure 1Q). On the basis of the aforementioned combinations, replacement of VnGABAT with VcGABAT significantly increased the downstream production of verazine. Overall, the combination of VnCYP90B27, VnCYP94N2, VcGABAT,

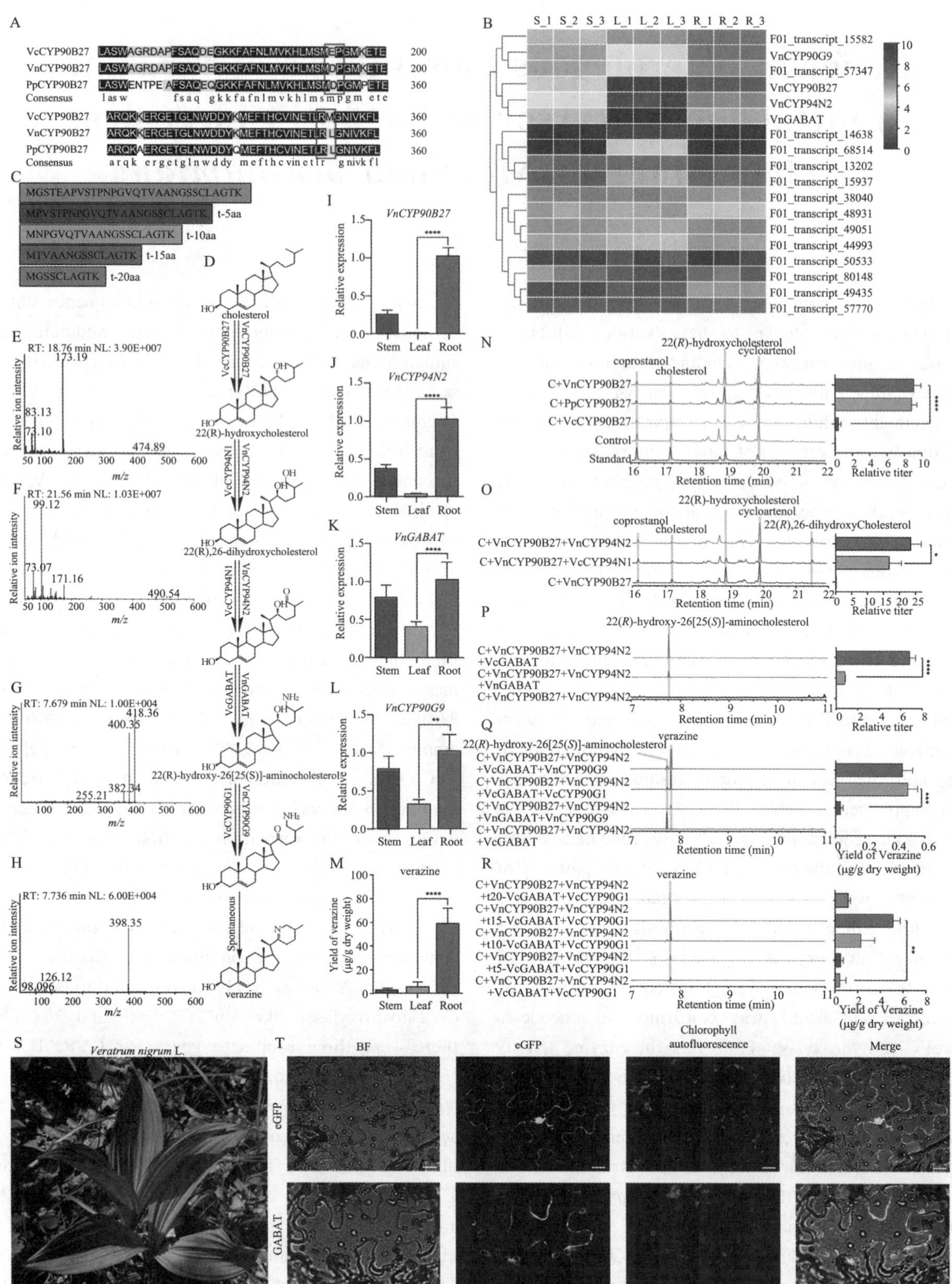

**Figure 1 Heterologous and efficient synthesis strategy of verazine from *N. benthamiana***

(A) Amino acid variations in CYP90B27 enzymes from different species. (B) Tissue-specific expression patterns of the VnCYP90 family, the VnCYP94 family, and VnGABAT. (C) Strategies for N-terminal signal peptide truncation of VcGABAT. (D) Strategies for the biosynthesis of verazine. (E–H) Mass spectra of verazine and its intermediates. (I–M) Expression levels of *VnCYP90B27*, *VnCYP94N2*, *VnCYP90G9*, and *VnGABAT* and verazine contents in different organs (* $P<0.05$, ** $P<0.01$, *** $P<0.001$, and **** $P<0.0001$). (N–Q) Yield comparison of genes with the same function from different species in *Nicotiana benthamiana* by gas chromatography-mass spectrometry (GC-MS) and liquid chromatography-tandem MS (LC-MS/MS) analysis. C, cholesterol heterologous synthesis chassis (* $P<0.05$, ** $P<0.01$, *** $P<0.001$, and **** $P<0.0001$). (R) Effects of different N-terminal truncations of GABAT on verazine yield. (S) *Veratrum nigrum* L (* $P<0.05$, ** $P<0.01$, *** $P<0.001$, and **** $P<0.0001$). (T) Subcellular localization of VcGABAT in *Nicotiana benthamiana* leaf cells observed by confocal laser scanning microscopy (Zeiss LSCM 800, Oberkochen, Germany). The sequence of EGFP is linked to the C terminus of *VcGABAT*. Bar=20 μm.

and VcCYP90G1 produced the highest verazine yield of 0.53 μg/g dry weight (DW) (Figure 1Q).

The three CYP450s involved in the metabolism of cholesterol to verazine are located on the endoplasmic reticulum (Supplemental Figure 1C). However, another key rate-limiting enzyme, GABAT, is localized in the chloroplast (Figure 1T). We speculated that differences in subcellular localization may affect the efficiency of GABAT in utilization of 22-dihydroxycholesterol-26-ol. Because GABAT is localized in chloroplasts and on the cytoplasmic membrane, we predicted that truncating its N-terminal signal peptide would increase its opportunity to bind with the substrate, thereby improving product yield. The strategy for truncating GABAT is shown in Figure 1C. Use of a truncated GABAT missing 15 amino acids, t15-VcGABAT, increased the verazine yield to 5.11 μg/g DW, about 10 times higher than that obtained with untruncated VcGABAT (Figure 1R). The metabolic pathway of verazine involves a metabolic branch: CYP94N1 catalyzes the formation of two isomers from 22(*R*)-hydroxycholesterol produced by CYP90B27, namely 22(*R*), 26[25(*R*)]-dihydroxycholesterol and 22(*R*), 26[25(*S*)]-dihydroxycholesterol. Only 22(*R*), 26[25(*S*)]-dihydroxycholesterol can be used to synthesize verazine. At the same time, CYP90G1 oxidizes the C-22 hydroxyl group of 22(*R*)-hydroxy-26[25(*S*)]-aminosterol, forming 22-ketohydroxycholesterol-26[25(*R*)]. This pathway not only leads to the loss of pathway intermediates but also wastes the catalytic activity of the enzyme. One potential strategy for further increasing the verazine yield is therefore to optimize the product specificity of VnCYP94N2 and the substrate selectivity of VcCYP90G1. Introduction of glutamate decarboxylase into the synthetic chassis to increase levels of γ-aminobutyric acid, the amino donor for GABAT, could be an alternative approach. In addition, the catalytic efficiency of enzymes is influenced by differences in amino acids in the active center. Further experiments have shown that saturation mutagenesis at key amino acid sites in the active center can produce highly efficient enzymes. Enzyme engineering through directed mutagenesis is based on this principle. Different species of *Veratrum* may have differences at multiple amino acid sites in these key enzymes (CYP90B27 and GABAT) that may lead to variations in their catalytic efficiency.

In summary, we completed the heterologous biosynthesis of verazine in *N. benthamiana*. We compared the activities of enzymes from different sources and identified the optimal enzyme combination. These genes make about 100 times as much verazine in *N. benthamiana* than in *Camelina sativa* seed. Heterologous biosynthesis of verazine provides new insight into the production mode of steroid alkaloids, as well as substrate support for the resolution of the verazine-to-cyclopamine metabolic pathway.

[寇呈熹，薛哲勇，麻鹏达，等. Plant Communications, 2024, 5: 100831.]

# A *Syringa pinnatifolia* genome assembly reveals the zerumbone biosynthesis machinery with a cytochrome P450-catalysed epoxidation reaction in eudicots

*Syringa pinnatifolia*, a shrub within the *Syringa* genus of the Oleaceae family (Figure S1), is valued in traditional Chinese medicine for its volatile chemical constituents. These principally include a suite of humulane-type monocyclic sesquiterpenoids with an 11-membered ring, notably zerumbone and its derivatives. Renowned for their cardioprotective, immunomodulatory and anti-carcinogenic properties, these compounds are found extensively in various monocot species yet are conspicuously present in the eudicot *S. pinnatifolia*. The biosynthesis pathway of zerumbone has been elucidated in the monocot *Zingiber zerumbet*, while it is still unclear in the eudicot *S. pinnatifolia*.

Seeking to characterize the biosynthetic pathway of zerumbone in *S. pinnatifolia*, we assembled a chromosome-level genome utilizing 105.17 Gb of Illumina sequencing data, 309.64 Gb of PacBio long reads and 123.54 Gb of Hi-C pairedend reads (Tables S1 – S3; Appendix S1). The PacBio data facilitated the construction of a contig-level genome assembly spanning 998.20 Mb (Table S4), and subsequent integration of Hi-C data that we anchored to the 23 pseudochromosomes (Figure S2; Tables S5 – S7). A *de novo* annotation predicted 43 197 genes, and a BUSCO analysis indicated gene coverage of 93.9% (Figure S3). An MCMCtree analysis suggested that *S. pinnatifolia* and *S.*

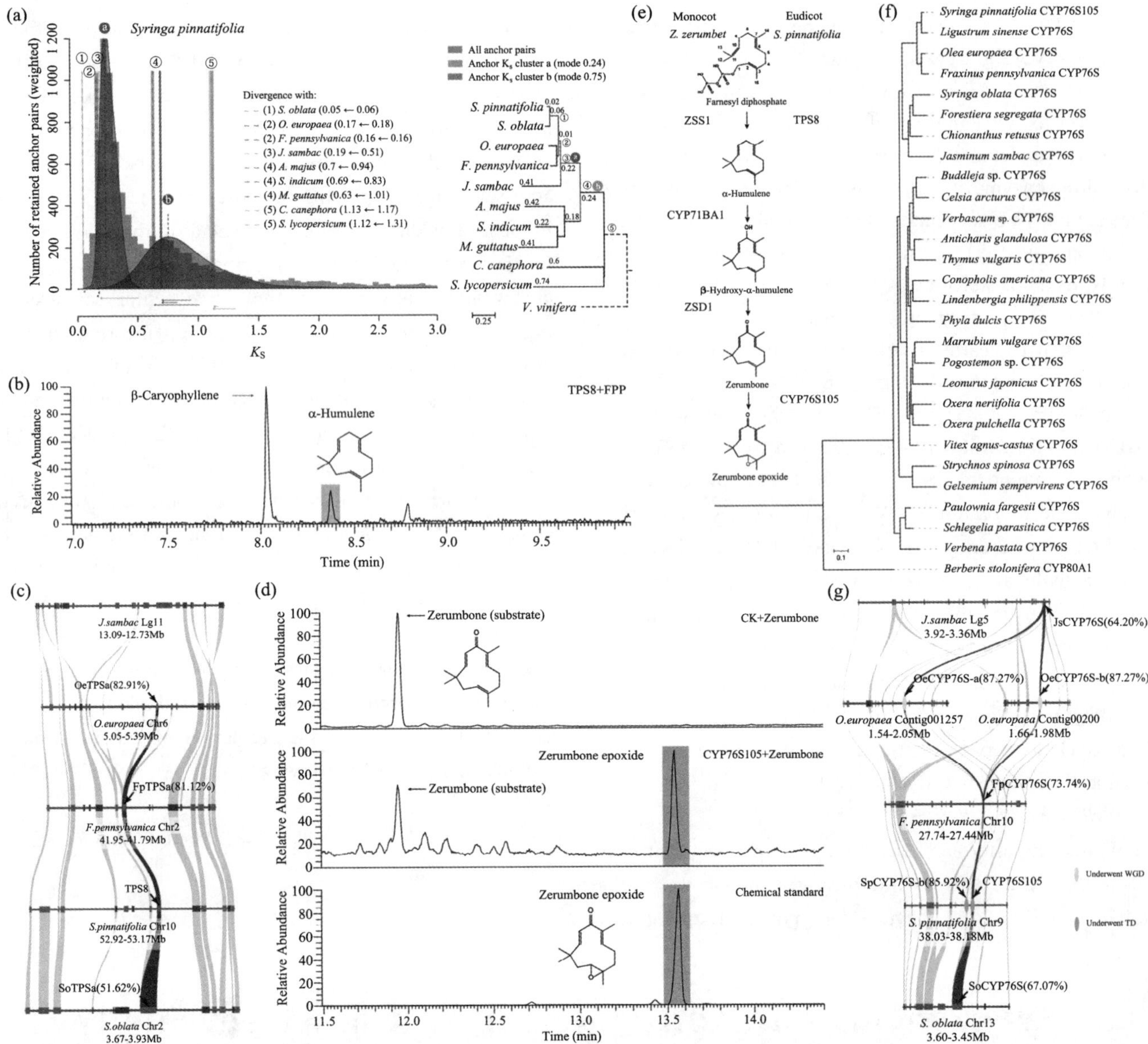


**Figure 1** (a) Substitution-rate-adjusted mixed paralog-ortholog synonymous substitutions per synonymous site (Ks) plot for *Syringa pinnatifolia* as produced by ksrates. The anchor-pair Ks distribution for *S. pinnatifolia* is shown in grey, with one putative whole-genome duplication (WGD) components inferred by lognormal mixture model clustering indicated in blue and red. Phylogram generated by ksrates from the input phylogenetic tree, with branch lengths set to the Ks distances estimated from ortholog Ks distributions. (b) The ion current chromatogram of the product from reaction mixture in which TPS8 catalysed the substrate FPP. (c) Microsyntenty analysis of TPS8 within family Oleaceae. The percentages behind the gene names are their values identical to TPS8. The blue line indicates the evolutionary trajectory of *TPS8* homologues. (d) The ion current chromatogram of the product from reaction mixtures in which **CYP76S105** catalysed the substrate zerumbone and the control group. (e) The zerumbone biosynthesis pathway in *S. pinnatifolia* and *Zingiber zerumbet*. (f) Maximum likelihood tree of the transcripts homologous to ***CYP76S105***. (g) Microsyntenty analysis of **CYP76S105** within family Oleaceae. The percentages behind the gene names are their values identical to **CYP76S105**. The red line indicates the evolutionary trajectory of ***CYP76S105*** homologues. The yellow and orange elliptical blocks represent the gene pair underwent WGD or tandem duplication events.

*oblata* diverged at the boundary of the Paleogene and Neogene periods (Figure S4). The *Ks* value distributions among anchored paralogs and orthologs indicated that at least two whole-genome duplication (WGD) events have occurred in *S. pinnatifolia* (Figure 1a), and an intragenomic synteny analysis revealed remnants of a WGD event common to Oleaceae species (Figure S5).

Comparative analysis of the volatile components of *S. pinnatifolia* and *Z. zerumbet* revealed identical compounds involved in the elucidated biosynthesis pathway of zerumbone, suggesting a conserved biosynthetic pathway in *S. pinnatifolia* (Figure S6). In the monocot *Z. zerumbet*, the biosynthesis pathway of zerumbone begins with the production of α-humulene by cyclization of farnesyl pyrophosphate (FPP) by ZSS1 (a terpene synthase). We identified 32 terpene synthase (TPS) genes divided into TPS-a, TPS-b, TPS-c, TPS-e/f and

TPS-g subfamilies of the TPS family in *S. pinnatifolia* (Figure S7). Subsequently, we employed the TPS belonging to TPS-a and TPS-g (Table S8), which are primarily responsible for sesquiterpenoid production in TPS family to seek the enzyme functioning to cyclization of FPP producing α-humulene. Using FPP as the substrate, we employed the *Escherichia coli* heterologous expression system to estimate the function of the TPS candidate genes (Figure S8; Appendix S1). It found that TPS8, which belongs to TPS-a subfamily in *S. pinnatifolia*, had the ability to facilitate the cyclization of FPP to generate α-humulene along with β-caryophyllene (Figures 1b and S9). Except for TPS8, we characterized six TPS functioning to generate 14 different sesquiterpenoids along with three TPS producing monoterpenoids (Figures S10 - S17).

The products of TPS8 is same as the α-humulene synthase in *Z. zerumbet* (ZSS1), and they both belong to TPS-a subfamily (Figure S18), although the identity of them was only 40.93%. In percentage, the ratio of the two products (α-humulene and β-caryophyllene) in ZSS1 is different from that in TPS8, we found that ZSS1 produced more α-humulene of the two products in *Z. zerumbet* (approximately 88%) and the number of TPS8 is about 23% (Figure S19a), which may be a factor resulting in higher zerumbone content in the monocot species as the zerumbone content comparison of the tissues where this component mainly accumulates in *S. pinnatifolia* (stem) and *Z. zerumbet* (rhizome) shown (Figure S19b). Analysing the homologous of *TPS8* within Oleaceae family, we identified three genes from the reported Oleaceae species genomes (Figure 1c). We estimated the their catalysing effects on FPP employing *E. coli* heterologous expression system and found that OeTPSa from *O. europaea* can produce α-humulene and β-caryophyllene as TPS8 did (Figure S20).

Cytochrome P450 (P450) enzymes perform various biooxidation reactions that collectively greatly expand the chemical diversity of terpenoids. Our annotation identified 217 putative CYP450 genes divided into eight clans (CYP51, CYP71, CYP72, CYP74, CYP710, CYP85, CYP86 and CYP97) in the *S. pinnatifolia* genome (Figure S21). CYP71, CYP72, CYP85 and CYP86 are multi-family clans with larger scales than the single-family clans, and CYP71 clan includes majority of the CYP450 families involved in sesquiterpenoid metabolism up to now. Focussing on CYP71 and the related clans, *in vitro* functional assays in which microsomes representing more than 100 P450s (from yeast cells) were fed zerumbone as the substrate revealed a new peak for the CYP76S105 reaction (Appendix S1). Comparison between the retention time (13.54 min) and mass spectrum ($m/z$ 234.22) with a chemical standard confirmed the product as zerumbone epoxide, apparently resulting from C2 to C3 epoxidation of zerumbone (Figures 1d and S22). In this way, we found a downstream P450-catalysed step of zerumbone biosynthesis pathway, which has not been revealed in the monocot *Z. zerumbet* (Figure 1e). Moreover, the epoxidation reaction that adds a single oxygen atom across a carbon-carbon double bond has not been reported in CYP76 family as far as we know.

To understand the evolutionary history of the *S. pinnatifolia CYP76S105*, we constructed a phylogenetic tree with the transcripts homologous to *CYP76S105* (one transcripts with highest identity each species) from the 1 000 Plant Transcriptome (1KP) database and the reported Oleaceae species genomes (Figure 1f; Table S9). Among the homologous transcripts, *Ligustrum sinense LsCYP76S* was the transcripts with the highest identity (92.86%) to *CYP76S105* from 1KP database; *O. europaea OeCYP76S* was the transcripts with the highest identity (87.27%) from the reported Oleaceae species genomes except for *S. pinnatifolia*. The microsynteny analysis illustrated the evolutionary trajectory of *CYP76S105* homologues within the Oleaceae family, and two homologous genes (*OeCYP76S-a/b*) with identical nucleotide sequences in different chromosomal locations (Figure 1g). Moreover, we found a *S. pinnatifolia SpCYP76S-b* with the highest identity (85.92%) to *CYP76S105* in this plant itself, and it located close to *CYP76S105* in chromosome 9. Employing zerumbone as substrate, we found that *L. sinense Ls*CYP76S (designated CYP76S110) and *O. europaea Oe*CYP76S (designated CYP76S63) can convert zerumbone to zerumbone epoxide (Figure S23), while the other candidates including the *S. pinnatifolia SpCYP76S-b* with a high identity to *CYP76S105* cannot. The two transcripts of *CYP76S63* emerged as duplicated gene from the WGD event, with catalysing effect on zerumbone; however, the gene pair (*CYP76S105/SpCYP76S-b*) formed from tandem duplication (TD) event did not encode the enzyme with same catalysing function on zerumbone, showing the complex evolutionary history about the loss and gain of the gene function in Oleaceae family (Figure 1g).

In summary, this study presents a chromosome-level assembly of *S. pinnatifolia* aimed at elucidating the zerumbone biosynthesis pathway in eudicots. We provided a TPS responsible for cyclization of FPP to facilitate the production of α-humulene, which is the sesquiterpene intermediate in the zerumbone biosynthesis pathway. The finding of the epoxidation reaction catalysed by CYP76 enzymes would broaden the insight of the functions in this family.

[高佳琪，刘娟，黄璐琦，等. Plant Biotechnology Journal，2024，DOI：10.1111/pbi.14376.]